PSYCHOPHARMACOLOGY
The Fourth Generation of Progress

An Official Publication of the
American College of Neuropsychopharmacology

PSYCHOPHARMACOLOGY
The Fourth Generation of Progress

An Official Publication of the
American College of Neuropsychopharmacology

Editors-in-Chief

Floyd E. Bloom, M.D.
Chairman
Department of Neuropharmacology
The Scripps Research Institute
La Jolla, California

David J. Kupfer, M.D.
Professor and Chairman
Department of Psychiatry
University of Pittsburgh School of Medicine
Western Psychiatric Institute and Clinic
Pittsburgh, Pennsylvania

Associate Editors

Benjamin S. Bunney, M.D.
Charles B. G. Murphy Professor and Chairman
Department of Psychiatry
Professor of Pharmacology
Yale University School of Medicine
New Haven, Connecticut

Roland D. Ciaranello, M.D.
Nancy Friend Pritzker Professor
Department of Psychiatry and Behavioral Sciences
Stanford University School of Medicine
Stanford, California

Kenneth L. Davis, M.D.
Professor and Chairman
Department of Psychiatry
Mount Sinai School of Medicine
New York, New York

George F. Koob, Ph.D.
Professor
Department of Neuropharmacology
The Scripps Research Institute
La Jolla, California

Herbert Y. Meltzer, M.D.
Douglas D. Bond Professor
Department of Psychiatry
Case Western Reserve University School of Medicine
University Hospitals of Cleveland
Cleveland, Ohio

Charles R. Schuster, Ph.D.
Intramural Research Program
National Institute on Drug Abuse
National Institutes of Health
Baltimore, Maryland

Richard I. Shader, M.D.
Professor
Department of Pharmacology and Experimental Therapeutics
Tufts University School of Medicine
Boston, Massachusetts

Stanley J. Watson, Jr., M.D., Ph.D.
Associate Director
Mental Health Research Institute
Associate Chair for Research
Department of Psychiatry
University of Michigan
Ann Arbor, Michigan

RAVEN PRESS ☙ NEW YORK

Raven Press, Ltd., 1185 Avenue of the Americas, New York, New York 10036

Made in the United States of America

Library of Congress Cataloging-in-Publication Data

Psychopharmacology: the fourth generation of progress/editors-in-
  chief, Floyd E. Bloom, David J. Kupfer; associate editors, Benjamin
  S. Bunney . . . [et al.]; in association with the American College of
  Neuropsychopharmacology.
      p. cm.
    Includes bibliographical references and index.
    ISBN 0-7817-0166-X
    1. Psychopharmacology. I. Bloom, Floyd E. II. Kupfer, David J.,
  1941–   . III. American College of Neuropsychopharmacology.
    [DNLM: 1. Central Nervous System—drug effects. 2. Psychotropic
  Drugs—pharmacology. 3. Mental Disorders—drug therapy. QV 77
  P9732 1994]
  RM315.P762 1994
  615'.78—dc20
  DNLM/DLC
  for Library of Congress   94-7409

9 8 7 6 5 4 3 2 1

In Memoriam

Daniel X. Freedman, M.D.

Daniel Freedman was known throughout the world as an early pioneer in neuropharmacology. He was among those few who understood that eventual, as-yet-unimagined developments in neuroscience would profoundly alter the future of psychiatry. Although Danny, as he liked to be called, was a talented clinician-scientist, he was first and foremost an educator. He was an inspiring mentor who had a lifelong commitment to advancing the careers and welfare of his students. Endowed with a powerful analytic intellect, a whimsical sense of humor, and seemingly unlimited energy, this man of small stature became a towering figure in academic medicine. Over nearly half a century, he played a unique role in the evolving science policy of the United States by becoming a trusted adviser to learned societies, leaders of Congress, and presidents. His untimely death is a tragic loss for our College and, indeed, for all of biomedical science in the United States.

Thomas Detre, M.D.
ACNP President, 1994

PSYCHOPHARMACOLOGY
The Fourth Generation of Progress
Section Contents

Part I: Preclinical

Overview

Critical Analysis of Methods

Transmitter Systems
   Amino Acids
   Amines
   Peptides
   New Transmitters

Integrative Concepts

Part II: Clinical

Overview

Critical Analysis of Methods

Psychiatric Disorders
   Mood Disorders
   Schizophrenia
   Anxiety Disorders
   Geriatric Disorders
   Neurologic Disorders
   Personality Disorders
   Eating Disorders
   Sleep Disorders
   Childhood Disorders
   Substance Abuse

Integrative Concepts

Part III: Special Topics

Subject Index

Contents

PART I. PRECLINICAL SECTION

Critical Analysis of Methods

Transmitter Systems
Amino Acids

Amines

Peptides

Psychiatric Disorders

Mood Disorders

Schizophrenia

Anxiety Disorders

Geriatric Disorders

Neurologic Disorders

Contributors

Elizabeth D. Abercrombie, Ph.D.
Assistant Professor of Neuroscience
Center for Molecular and Behavioral
* Neuroscience*
Rutgers University
197 University Avenue
Newark, New Jersey 07102

George K. Aghajanian, M.D.
Professor
Departments of Psychiatry and Pharmacology
Yale University School of Medicine
Connecticut Mental Health Center
34 Park Street
New Haven, Connecticut 06508

Huda A. Akil, Ph.D.
Professor of Psychiatry
Research Scientist
Mental Health Research Institute
University of Michigan
205 Zina Pitcher Place
Ann Arbor, Michigan 48109

George S. Alexopoulos, M.D.
Professor
Department of Psychiatry
Cornell University Medical College
Director, Division of Geriatric Services
Cornell Medical Center—Westchester
21 Bloomingdale Road
White Plains, New York 10605

Donna Ames, M.D.
Assistant Professor
Department of Psychiatry
University of California, Los Angeles
School of Medicine
760 Westwood Plaza
Los Angeles, California 90024

Stephen P. Arneric, Ph.D.
Project Leader
Cholinergic Channel
Project and Neuroscience Research D47W
Abbott Laboratories
One Abbott Park Road
Abbott Park, Illinois 60064-3500

Jean-Michel Arrang, Ph.D.
Unité de Neurobiologie et Pharmacologie
* (U.109) de l'INSERM*
Centre Paul Broca
2 ter rue d'Alésia
75014 Paris, France

Gary S. Aston-Jones, Ph.D.
Professor and Director
Division of Behavioral Neurobiology
Department of Mental Health Sciences
Hahnemann University Medical School
Broad and Vine Streets
Philadelphia, Pennsylvania 19102

Efrain C. Azmitia, Ph.D.
Professor
Department of Biology
New York University
100 Washington Square East
New York, New York 10003

Robert L. Balster, Ph.D.
Professor
Department of Pharmacology
Director, Center for Drug and Alcohol Studies
Virginia Commonwealth University
Medical College of Virginia
Richmond, Virginia 23298-0310

Heather A. Bannerman, B.S.P.H., M.P.A.
Department of Health Behavior and Health
* Education*
School of Public Health
University of North Carolina
Chapel Hill, North Carolina 27599

Michael J. Bannon, Ph.D.
Professor
Cellular and Clinical Neurobiology Program
Department of Psychiatry
Wayne State University School of Medicine
540 East Canfield
Detroit, Michigan 48201

Eric L. Barker, Ph.D.
Department of Anatomy and Cell Biology
Emory University School of Medicine
Atlanta, Georgia 30322-3030

Samuel H. Barondes, M.D.
Director, Center for Neurobiology and
*   Psychiatry*
Professor, Department of Psychiatry
University of California, San Francisco
401 Parnassus Avenue
San Francisco, California 94143-0984

Linda C. Barr, M.D.
Assistant Professor
Department of Psychiatry
Yale University School of Medicine
Connecticut Mental Health Center
34 Park Street
New Haven, Connecticut 06519

James E. Barrett, Ph.D.
Central Nervous System Research
Lederle Laboratories
American Cyanamid Company
Pearl River, New York 10965

Tamas Bartfai, Ph.D.
Professor
Department of Neurochemistry and
*   Neurotoxicology*
Stockholm University
Arrhenius Laboratories of Natural Sciences
Svante Arrhenius väg 21A
S-106 91 Stockholm, Sweden

Andrew Baum, Ph.D.
Professor of Psychology and Psychiatry
University of Pittsburgh
Director, Behavioral Medicine and Oncology
Pittsburgh Cancer Institute
3600 Forbes Avenue, Suite 405
Pittsburgh, Pennsylvania 15213

Lewis R. Baxter, Jr., M.D.
Professor
Department of Psychiatry and Biobehavioral
*   Sciences*
UCLA Neuropsychiatric Institute
760 Westwood Plaza
Los Angeles, California 90024

Andrew J. Bean, Ph.D.
Fellow
Department of Molecular and Cellular
*   Physiology*
Howard Hughes Medical Institute
Beckman Center B151
Stanford, California 94305

Margery C. Beinfeld, Ph.D.
Professor
Department of Pharmacological and
*   Physiological Science*
St. Louis University Medical Center
1402 South Grand Boulevard
St. Louis, Missouri 63104

George E. Bigelow, Ph.D.
Professor
Department of Psychiatry and Behavioral
*   Sciences*
Johns Hopkins University School of Medicine
BPRU, Behavioral Biology Research Center
5510 Nathan Shock Drive
Baltimore, Maryland 21224-6823

Boris Birmaher, M.D.
Associate Professor of Child Psychiatry
University of Pittsburgh School of Medicine
Western Psychiatric Institute and Clinic
3811 O'Hara Street
Pittsburgh, Pennsylvania 15213

Garth Bissette, Ph.D.
Associate Professor
Departments of Psychiatry and Pharmacology
Duke University Medical Center
Research Drive, 026 Carl Building
Durham, North Carolina 27710

Randy D. Blakely, Ph.D.
Assistant Professor and Woodruff Neuroscience
*   Investigator*
Department of Anatomy and Cell Biology
Emory University School of Medicine
Atlanta, Georgia 30322-3030

Barbara Blanchard
Research Associate
Finch University of Health Sciences
The Chicago Medical School
3333 Green Bay Road
North Chicago, Illinois 60064

Floyd E. Bloom, M.D.
Chairman
Department of Neuropharmacology
The Scripps Research Institute
10666 North Torrey Pines Road
La Jolla, California 92037

Charles Bowden, M.D.
Chief, Division of Biological Psychiatry
Nancy U. Karren Professor and Deputy
  Chairman
Department of Psychiatry
University of Texas Health Science Center
7703 Floyd Curl Drive
San Antonio, Texas 78284-7792

David L. Braff, M.D.
Professor
Department of Psychiatry
University of California, San Diego Medical
  Center
200 West Arbor Drive
San Diego, California 92093

George A. Bray, M.D.
Professor
Department of Medicine
Louisiana State University
Executive Director
Pennington Biomedical Research Center
6400 Perkins Road
Baton Rouge, Louisiana 70808-4124

J. Douglas Bremner, M.D.
Assistant Professor
Department of Psychiatry
Yale University School of Medicine and
West Haven VAMC
950 Campbell Avenue
New Haven, Connecticut 06516

David A. Brent, M.D.
Associate Professor of Child Psychiatry,
  Epidemiology and Pediatrics
University of Pittsburgh School of Medicine
Chief, Division of Child and Adolescent
  Psychiatry
Western Psychiatric Institute and Clinic
3811 O'Hara Street
Pittsburgh, Pennsylvania 15213

Richard J. Bridges, Ph.D.
Associate Professor of Pharmacology and
  Toxicology
Department of Pharmaceutical Science
University of Montana
Missoula, Montana 59812

Kelly J. Brown
Senior Graduate Fellow
Department of Medical and Clinical
  Psychology
Uniformed Services University of the Health
  Sciences
4301 Jones Bridge Road
Bethesda, Maryland 20814

Benjamin S. Bunney, M.D.
Charles B. G. Murphy Professor and
  Chairman
Department of Psychiatry
Professor of Pharmacology
Yale University School of Medicine
25 Park Street
New Haven, Connecticut 06519

Blynn Garland Bunney, Ph.D.
Director of Research Development and
  Education
Brain Imaging Center
Department of Psychiatry
University of California, Irvine
College of Medicine
Medical Science I
Irvine, California 92717

William E. Bunney, Jr., M.D.
Director of Research
Department of Psychiatry
University of California, Irvine
College of Medicine
Medical Science I
Irvine, California 92717

Michael J. Burke, M.D., Ph.D.
Professor, Department of Psychiatry
University of Kansas School of Medicine—
  Wichita
1010 N. Kansas
Wichita, Kansas 67214

Daniel J. Buysse, M.D.
Assistant Professor
Sleep and Chronobiology Center
Department of Psychiatry
University of Pittsburgh School of Medicine
Western Psychiatric Institute and Clinic
3811 O'Hara Street
Pittsburgh, Pennsylvania 15213

Joseph R. Calabrese, M.D.
Director, Mood Disorders Program
Associate Professor
Department of Psychiatry
Case Western Reserve University School of
  Medicine
University Hospitals of Cleveland
11400 Euclid Avenue, Suite #200
Cleveland, Ohio 44116

Hervé Canton, Ph.D.
Research Fellow
Department of Pharmacology
Vanderbilt University
School of Medicine
Nashville, Tennessee 37232-6600

Arvid Carlsson, M.D., Ph.D.
Department of Pharmacology
University of Göteborg
Medicinaregatan 7
S-413 90 Göteborg, Sweden

Daniel E. Casey, M.D.
Chief, Psychiatry, Research and
  Psychopharmacology
Veterans Administration Medical Center
  Psychiatry Service
3710 Southwest U.S. Veterans Hospital Road
Portland, Oregon 97207

Regina C. Casper, M.D.
Professor
Department of Psychiatry and Behavioral
  Sciences
Stanford University School of Medicine
Stanford, California 94305-5546

Marie-Noëlle Castel, Ph.D.
Department of Neuroscience
Karolinska Institute
S-171 77 Stockholm, Sweden

Dennis S. Charney, M.D.
Professor and Associate Chairman for
  Research
Department of Psychiatry
Yale University School of Medicine and
West Haven Veterans Affairs Medical Center
950 Campbell Avenue
West Haven, Connecticut 06516

Charles I. Chavkin, Ph.D.
Associate Professor
Department of Pharmacology
University of Washington
School of Medicine
Seattle, Washington 98195

Kevin J.-S. Chen, Ph.D.
Associate Research Professor
Department of Molecular Pharmacology
  and Toxicology
University of Southern California
School of Pharmacy
1985 Zonal Avenue
Los Angeles, California 90033

Louis A. Chiodo, Ph.D.
Professor and Chairman
Department of Pharmacology
Texas Tech University Health Sciences Center
School of Medicine
3601 4th Street
Lubbock, Texas 79430

Roland D. Ciaranello, M.D.
Nancy Friend Pritzker Professor
Department of Psychiatry and Behavioral
  Sciences
Stanford University School of Medicine
1201 Welch Road
Stanford, California 94305-5485

Olivier Civelli, Ph.D.
F. Hoffman-La Roche Ltd.
CH 4002 Basel, Switzerland

Emil F. Coccaro, M.D.
Director, Clinical Neuroscience Research Unit
Associate Professor
Department of Psychiatry
Medical College of Pennsylvania at
Eastern Pennsylvania Psychiatric Institute
3200 Henry Avenue
Philadelphia, Pennsylvania 19129

Donald J. Cohen, M.D.
Director, Child Study Center
Yale University
230 South Frontage Road
New Haven, Connecticut 06510-8009

Jonathan O. Cole, M.D.
Professor
Department of Psychiatry
Harvard Medical School
Boston, Massachusetts and
McLean Hospital
115 Mill Street
Belmont, Massachusetts 02178

T. J. Collier
Department of Neurological Sciences
Rush Medical School
Chicago, Illinois 60612

Jeremy D. Coplan, M.D.
Assistant Clinical Professor
Department of Psychiatry
Columbia University College of Physicians and
  Surgeons
New York State Psychiatric Institute
722 West 168th Street
New York, New York 10032

Carl W. Cotman, Ph.D.
Director, Irvine Research Unit in Brain
  Imaging
Professor
Department of Psychobiology and Neurology
University of California, Irvine
1305 Biological Sciences II
Irvine, California 92717-4550

John C. Crabbe, Jr., Ph.D.
*Professor, Medical Psychology and
    Pharmacology*
*Oregon Health Sciences University and
Research Career Scientist
Research Services (151W)
Veterans Affairs Medical Center
3710 SW U.S. Veteran's Hospital Road
Portland, Oregon 97201*

Karrie J. Craig
*Senior Research Associate
Uniformed Services University of the Health
    Sciences
4301 Jones Bridge Road
Bethesda, Maryland 20814*

Jacqueline N. Crawley, Ph.D.
*Chief, Section on Behavioral
    Neuropharmacology
Experimental Therapeutics Branch
National Institute of Mental Health
National Institutes of Health
Bethesda, Maryland 20892*

Raymond R. Crowe, M.D.
*Professor
Department of Psychiatry
University of Iowa College of Medicine
200 Hawkins Drive
Iowa City, Iowa 52242-1057*

John G. Csernansky, M.D.
*Gregory B. Couch Associate Professor
Departments of Psychiatry, Anatomy, and
    Neurobiology
Washington University School of Medicine
4940 Children's Place
St. Louis, Missouri 63110*

William E. Cullinan, Ph.D.
*Research Fellow
Mental Health Research Institute
University of Michigan
205 Zina Pitcher Place
Ann Arbor, Michigan 48109-0720*

Thomas E. Curran, Ph.D.
*Department of Molecular Oncology and
    Virology
Roche Institute of Molecular Biology
340 Kingsland Street
Nutley, New Jersey 07110*

Åke Dagerlind, Ph.D.
*Department of Neuroscience
Karolinska Institute
S-171 77 Stockholm, Sweden*

Ronald Dahl, M.D.
*Associate Professor of Child Psychiatry and
    Pediatrics
University of Pittsburgh School of Medicine
Western Psychiatric Institute and Clinic
3811 O'Hara Street
Pittsburgh, Pennsylvania 15213*

Svein G. Dahl, Ph.D.
*Professor
Department of Pharmacology
Institute of Medical Biology
University of Tromsö School of Medicine
N-9037 Tromsö, Norway*

Michael Davidson, M.D.
*Professor
Department of Psychiatry
Mount Sinai School of Medicine
New York, New York and
Veterans Affairs Medical Center
130 West Kingsbridge Road
Bronx, New York 10468*

Candace L. Davis, B.S.
*Chemist
Biological Psychiatry Branch
National Institute of Mental Health
National Institutes of Health
Bethesda, Maryland 20892*

Kenneth L. Davis, M.D.
*Professor and Chairman
Department of Psychiatry
Mount Sinai School of Medicine
1450 Madison Avenue
New York, New York 10029*

Michael E. Dawson, Ph.D.
*Professor
Department of Psychology
University of Southern California
5GM 501
Los Angeles, California 90089-1061*

Ted M. Dawson, M.D., Ph.D.
*Assistant Professor of Neurology and
    Neuroscience
Department of Neurology
Johns Hopkins University School of Medicine
600 North Wolfe Street
Baltimore, Maryland 21287*

Stephen J. DeArmond, M.D., Ph.D.
*Departments of Pathology and Neurology
University of California, San Francisco
Box 0506
San Francisco, California 94143-0506*

Errol B. DeSouza, Ph.D.
*Executive Vice President, Research and
    Development
Neuroendocrine Biosciences, Incorporated
3050 Science Park Road
San Diego, California 92121*

Ariel Y. Deutch, Ph.D.
*Associate Professor
Departments of Psychiatry and Pharmacology
Yale University School of Medicine
34 Park Street
New Haven, Connecticut 06508* and
*Psychiatry Service
Department of Veteran Affairs Medical Center
West Haven, Connecticut 06516*

D. P. Devanand, M.D.
*Associate Professor
Department of Biological Psychiatry
Columbia University College of Physicians and
    Surgeons
New York State Psychiatric Institute
722 West 168th Street
New York, New York 10032*

Michael J. Devlin, M.D.
*Assistant Professor of Clinical Psychiatry
Columbia University College of Physicians and
    Surgeons
Research Psychiatrist
New York State Psychiatric Institute
722 West 168th Street
New York, New York 10032*

Joseph A. DiMasi, Ph.D.
*Senior Research Fellow
Center for the Study of Drug Development
Tufts University
192 South Street
Boston, Massachusetts 02111*

Malgorzata Dukat, Ph.D.
*Research Assistant Professor
Department of Medicinal Chemistry
School of Pharmacy
Medical College of Virginia
Virginia Commonwealth University
Richmond, Virginia 23298*

Ronald S. Duman, Ph.D.
*Associate Professor of Psychiatry and
    Pharmacology
Department of Psychiatry
Yale University School of Medicine
Connecticut Mental Health Center
34 Park Street
New Haven, Connecticut 06508*

Adrian J. Dunn, Ph.D.
*Professor, and Department Head
Department of Pharmacology and Therapeutics
Louisiana State University Medical Center
1501 Kings Highway
Shreveport, Louisiana 71130*

Michael J. Eckardt, Ph.D.
*Laboratory of Clinical Studies
National Institute on Alcohol Abuse and
    Alcoholism
National Institutes of Health
Bethesda, Maryland 20892*

Frederick J. Ehlert, Ph.D.
*Associate Professor
Department of Pharmacology
University of California, Irvine
College of Medicine
Irvine, California 92717*

Thomas R. Elbert, Ph.D.
*Westfälische Wilhelms-Universität
Institut für Experimentelle Audiologie
Kardinal-von-Galen-Ring 10
DH 48129 Münster, Germany*

Gregory I. Elmer, Ph.D.
*Senior Staff Fellow
Preclinical Pharmacology Branch
Addiction Research Center
4940 Eastern Avenue
Baltimore, Maryland 21224*

John D. Elsworth, Ph.D.
*Research Scientist
Departments of Pharmacology and Psychiatry
Yale University School of Medicine
333 Cedar Street
New Haven, Connecticut 06520-8066*

Monique Ernst, M.D., Ph.D.
*Guest Researcher
Section on Clinical Brain Imaging
Laboratory of Cerebral Metabolism
National Institutes of Health
Bethesda, Maryland 20892*

Dwight L. Evans, M.D.
*Professor of Psychiatry, Medicine, and
    Neuroscience
Chairman, Department of Psychiatry
University of Florida College of Medicine
1600 Southwest Archer Road
Gainsville, Florida 32610-0256*

Barry J. Everitt, Ph.D.
Reader in Neuroscience
Department of Anatomy
University of Cambridge
Downing Street
Cambridge CB2 3EB, United Kingdom

H. Christian Fibiger, Ph.D.
Division of Neurological Sciences
Department of Psychiatry
University of British Columbia
2255 Wesbrook Mall
Vancouver, British Columbia, V6T 1Z3 Canada

Janet M. Finlay, Ph.D.
Research Assistant Professor
Department of Neuroscience
University of Pittsburgh
570 Crawford Hall
Pittsburgh, Pennsylvania 15260

Michael B. First, M.D.
Assistant Professor of Clinical Psychiatry
Columbia University College of Physicians and
  Surgeons
New York State Psychiatric Institute
722 West 168th Street
New York, New York 10032

Stephen L. Foote, Ph.D.
Professor
Department of Psychiatry
University of California, San Diego
School of Medicine
9500 Gilman Drive
La Jolla, California 92093

Judith M. Ford, Ph.D.
Senior Research Associate
Department of Psychiatry
Stanford University School of Medicine
Stanford, California
Palo Alto Veterans Affairs Medical Center
3801 Miranda Avenue
Palo Alto, California 94304

Casimir A. Fornal, Ph.D.
Research Psychologist
Department of Psychology
Princeton University
Green Hall
Princeton, New Jersey 08544

Allen Frances, M.D.
Professor and Chairman
Department of Psychiatry
Duke University Medical Center
Box 3950
Durham, North Carolina 27710

Ellen Frank, Ph.D.
Professor
Department of Psychiatry and Psychology
University of Pittsburgh School of Medicine
Western Psychiatric Institute and Clinic
3811 O'Hara Street
Pittsburgh, Pennsylvania 15213-2593

Arthur S. Freeman, Ph.D.
Associate Professor
Department of Pharmacology
Texas Tech University Health Sciences Center
3601 4th Street
Lubbock, Texas 79430

Arnold J. Friedhoff, M.D.
Professor
Department of Psychiatry
Director, Millhauser Laboratories
New York University Medical Center
550 First Avenue
New York, New York 10016

Timothy K. Gallaher, Ph.D.
Postdoctoral Fellow
Department of Molecular Pharmacology and
  Toxicology
University of Southern California
School of Pharmacy
1985 Zonal Avenue
Los Angeles, California 90033

Monique Garbarg, Ph.D.
Unité de Neurobiologie et Pharmacologie
  (U.109) de l'INSERM
Centre Paul Broca
2 ter rue d'Alésia
75014 Paris, France

James C. Garbutt, M.D.
Associate Professor of Psychiatry
University of North Carolina at Chapel Hill
Chapel Hill, North Carolina 27599-7600
Clinical Research Unit
Dorothea Dix Hospital
Raleigh, North Carolina 27603

George Gardos, M.D.
Associate Clinical Professor
Department of Psychiatry
Harvard Medical School
Boston, Massachusetts
McLean Hospital
115 Mill Street
Belmont, Massachusetts 02178

David S. Geldmacher, M.D.
Assistant Professor of Neurology
Case Western Reserve University
Assistant Director of Clinical Programs
Alzheimer Center
University Hospitals of Cleveland
11100 Euclid Avenue
Cleveland, Ohio 44106

Elizabeth Gettig, M.S.
Director of Genetic Counseling Program
Department of Human Genetics
University of Pittsburgh
130 DeSoto Street
Pittsburgh, Pennsylvania 15261

Mark A. Geyer, Ph.D.
Professor
Department of Psychiatry
University of California, San Diego
School of Medicine
9500 Gilman Drive
La Jolla, California 92093-0804

Richard A. Glennon, Ph.D.
Professor
Department of Medicinal Chemistry
School of Pharmacy
Medical College of Virginia
Virginia Commonwealth University
Richmond, Virginia 23298

Ira D. Glick, M.D.
Professor
Department of Psychiatry and Behavioral
  Sciences
Stanford University School of Medicine
101 Quarry Road
Stanford, California 94305-5546

Alison M. Goate, Ph.D.
Associate Professor of Genetics in Psychiatry
Department of Psychiatry
Washington University Medical School
4940 Children's Place
St. Louis, Missouri 63110

Andrew W. Goddard, M.D.
Assistant Professor
Department of Psychiatry
Yale University
Connecticut Mental Health Center
34 Park Street
New Haven, Connecticut 06519

James M. Gold, Ph.D.
Clinical Research Services Branch
NIMH Neurosciences Center at St. Elizabeths
2700 Martin Luther King, Jr. Avenue, SE
Washington, DC 20032

Terry E. Goldberg, Ph.D.
Chief, Unit on Neuropsychology
Clinical Brain Disorders Branch
NIMH Neuroscience Center at St. Elizabeths
2700 Martin Luther King, Jr. Avenue, SE
Washington, DC 20032

Menek Goldstein, Ph.D.
Professor of Neurochemistry
Department of Psychiatry
Neurochemistry Research Laboratory
New York University Medical Center
560 First Avenue
New York, New York 10016

Wayne K. Goodman, M.D.
Professor
Department of Psychiatry
University of Florida
College of Medicine
Gainesville, Florida 32610-0256

David A. Gorelick, M.D., Ph.D.
Adjunct Professor of Psychiatry
University of Maryland School of Medicine
Chief, Treatment Branch
National Institute on Drug Abuse
  Intramural Research Program
National Institutes of Health
P.O. Box 5180
Baltimore, Maryland 21224

Andrew J. Goudie, Ph.D.
Department of Psychology
University of Liverpool
Eleanor Rathbone Building
P.O. Box 147
Liverpool, L69 3BX, United Kingdom

Henry G. Grabowski, Ph.D.
Professor
Department of Economics
Duke University
Durham, North Carolina 27708-0097

Anthony A. Grace, Ph.D.
Associate Professor
Departments of Neuroscience and Psychiatry
University of Pittsburgh
458 Crawford Hall
Pittsburgh, Pennsylvania 15260

James G. Granneman, Ph.D.
Associate Professor
Cellular and Clinical Neurobiology Program
Department of Psychiatry
Wayne State University School of Medicine
540 East Canfield
Detroit, Michigan 48201

David J. Greenblatt, M.D.
Professor
Department of Pharmacology and
*   Experimental Therapeutics*
Tufts University School of Medicine
136 Harrison Avenue
Boston, Massachusetts 02111

Roland R. Griffiths, Ph.D.
Professor of Behavioral Biology
Departments of Psychiatry and Behavioral
*   Sciences and of Neuroscience*
Johns Hopkins University School of Medicine
Behavioral Biology Research Center
5510 Nathan Shock Drive
Baltimore, Maryland 21224-6823

Dimitri E. Grigoriadis, Ph.D.
Neurocrine Biosciences, Inc.
3050 Science Park Road
San Diego, California 92121

Raquel E. Gur, M.D., Ph.D.
Professor
Department of Psychiatry
University of Pennsylvania
University of Pennsylvania Hospital
3500 Spruce Street
Philadelphia, Pennsylvania 19104

Katherine A. Halmi, M.D.
Professor
Department of Psychiatry
Director, Eating Disorders Program
Cornell University Medical College
Cornell Medical Center—Westchester
21 Bloomingdale Road
White Plains, New York 10605

Jerold S. Harmatz
Department of Pharmacology and
*   Experimental Therapeutics*
Tufts University School of Medicine
136 Harrison Avenue
Boston, Massachusetts 02111

Vahram Haroutunian, Ph.D.
Associate Professor of Psychiatry and
*   Neurobiology*
Department of Psychiatry
Mount Sinai School of Medicine, and
Director, Psychopharmacology Laboratory
Veterans Affairs Medical Center
130 West Kingsbridge Road
Bronx, New York 10468

M. Jackuelyn Harris, M.D.
Assistant Professor
Department of Psychiatry
University of California, San Diego and
San Diego Veterans Affairs Medical Center
*   (116A)*
3350 La Jolla Village Drive
San Diego, California 92161

Markus Heilig, M.D., Ph.D.
Department of Psychiatry and Neurochemistry
University of Göteborg
Mölndals Sjukhus
S-431 80 Mölndal, Sweden

George R. Heninger, M.D.
Professor
Department of Psychiatry
Yale University School of Medicine
Connecticut Mental Health Center
34 Park Street
New Haven, Connecticut 06508

Jack E. Henningfield, Ph.D.
Chief, Clinical Pharmacology Branch
National Institute on Drug Abuse
Intramural Research Program
4940 Eastern Avenue
Baltimore, Maryland 21224

Mary M. Herman, M.D.
Special Expert in Neuropathology
Clinical Brain Disorders Branch
Intramural Research Programs
NIMH Neuroscience Center at St. Elizabeths
2900 Martin Luther King, Jr. Avenue, SE
Washington, DC 20032

Melvyn P. Heyes, Ph.D.
Visiting Scientist
Section on Analytical Biochemistry
Laboratory of Clinical Science
National Institute of Mental Health
National Institutes of Health
Bethesda, Maryland 20892

Stephen T. Higgins, Ph.D.
Associate Professor
Department of Psychiatry
University of Vermont
38 Fletcher Place
Burlington, Vermont 05401-1419

Robert M. A. Hirschfeld, M.D.
Professor and Chairman
Department of Psychiatry and Behavioral
*   Sciences*
University of Texas Medical Branch at
*   Galveston*
1014 Texas Avenue
Galveston, Texas 77555-0429

Tomas G. M. Hökfelt, M.D.
Professor of Histology and Cell Biology
Department of Neuroscience
Karolinska Institutet
S-17177 Stockholm, Sweden

Philip V. Holmes
Section on Behavioral Neuropharmacology
Experimental Therapeutics Branch
Department of Health and Human Services
National Institute of Mental Health
National Institutes of Health
Bethesda, Maryland 20892

Florian Holsboer, M.D., Ph.D.
Professor of Psychiatry
Clinical Institute
Max-Planck-Institute of Psychiatry
Kraepelinstrasse 10
80804 München, Germany

Thomas M. Hyde, M.D., Ph.D.
Clinical Brain Disorders Branch
Intramural Research Program
Neuroscience Center at St. Elizabeths
National Institute of Mental Health
2700 Martin Luther King, Jr. Avenue, SE
Washington, DC 20032

Robert B. Innis, M.D., Ph.D.
Associate Professor
Department of Psychiatry
Yale University School of Medicine
Veteran Affairs Medical Center
950 Campbell Avenue
West Haven, Connecticut 06516

Thomas R. Insel, M.D.
Director, Yerkes Regional Primate Research
* Center*
Professor, Department of Psychiatry
Emory University School of Medicine
954 Gatewood Road, N.E.
Atlanta, Georgia 30322

Michael Irwin, M.D.
Associate Professor
Department of Psychiatry
University of California, San Diego
9500 Gilman Drive
San Diego, California 92037

Barry L. Jacobs, Ph.D.
Program in Neuroscience
Princeton University
Green Hall
Princeton, New Jersey 08544

David S. Janowsky, M.D.
Professor of Psychiatry
Department of Psychiatry
University of North Carolina Medical School
Medical School Wing B
CB #7160
Chapel Hill, North Carolina 27599-7160

Murray E. Jarvik, M.D., Ph.D.
Professor Emeritus
Department of Psychiatry
University of California—Los Angeles School
* of Medicine*
Chief, Psychopharmacology Unit
Veterans Affairs Medical Center
Neuropsychiatric Institute
760 Westwood Plaza
Los Angeles, California 90024

Dilip V. Jeste, M.D.
Professor of Psychiatry and Neurosciences
Director, Geriatric Psychiatry Clinical
* Research Center*
University of California, San Diego
San Diego Veteran Affairs Medical Center
3350 La Jolla Village Drive
San Diego, California 92161

Chris-Ellyn Johanson, Ph.D.
Chief, Etiology Branch
National Institute on Drug Abuse
Intramural Research Program
National Institutes of Health
P.O. Box 5180
Baltimore, Maryland 21122

Jennifer S. Kahle, Ph.D.
Lecturer
Department of Psychobiology
Irvine Research Unit in Brain Aging
University of California, Irvine
Irvine, California 92717-4550

René S. Kahn, M.D., Ph.D.
Professor and Chairman
Department of Psychiatry
University Hospital Utrecht
Heidelberglaan 100
3584 CX Utrecht
Box 85500
3508 GA Utrecht, The Netherlands

John M. Kane, M.D.
Chairman, Department of Psychiatry
Hillside Hospital, A Division of Long Island
* Jewish Medical Center*
75-59 263rd Street
Glen Oaks, New York 11004

Gregory Kapatos, Ph.D.
Professor
Cellular and Clinical Neurobiology Program
Department of Psychiatry
Wayne State University School of Medicine
540 East Canfield
Detroit, Michigan 48201

Jordan Karp, B.A.
University of Pittsburgh
Western Psychiatric Institute and Clinic
3811 O'Hara Street
Pittsburgh, Pennsylvania 15213-2593

Jonathan L. Katz, Ph.D.
Chief
Psychobiology Section
National Institute on Drug Abuse
Intramural Research Program
National Institutes of Health
P.O. Box 5180
Baltimore, Maryland 21224

Donald F. Klein, M.D.
Director of Research
New York State Psychiatric Institute
722 West 168th Street
New York, New York 10032

Joel E. Kleinman, M.D., Ph.D.
Deputy Chief
Clinical Brain Disorders Branch
Intramural Research Programs
NIMH Neuroscience Center at St. Elizabeths
2900 Martin Luther King, Jr. Avenue, SE
Washington, DC 20032

James H. Kocsis, M.D.
Professor of Psychiatry
Cornell University Medical College and
The New York Hospital
525 East 68th Street
New York, New York 10021

George F. Koob, Ph.D.
Member
Department of Neuropharmacology
Scripps Research Institute
10666 North Torrey Pines Road
La Jolla, California 92037

Amos D. Korczyn, M.D., M.Sc.
Department of Physiology and Pharmacology
Sackler Faculty of Medicine
Tel Aviv University
Ramat Aviv 69978, Israel

Helena Chmura Kraemer, Ph.D.
Professor of Biostatistics in Psychiatry
Department of Psychiatry and Behavioral
  Sciences
Stanford University School of Medicine
101 Quarry Road
Stanford, California 94305

David J. Kupfer, M.D.
Professor and Chairman
Department of Psychiatry
University of Pittsburgh School of Medicine
Western Psychiatric Institute and Clinic
3811 O'Hara Street
Pittsburgh, Pennsylvania 15213

Michele C. LaBuda, Ph.D.
Assistant Professor
Department of Psychiatry and Behavioral
  Sciences
Johns Hopkins University School of Medicine
600 N. Wolfe Street
Baltimore, Maryland 21287-3325

Marc Laruelle, M.D.
Assistant Professor
Department of Psychiatry
Yale University School of Medicine, and
West Haven Veteran Affairs Medical Center
950 Campbell Avenue
West Haven, Connecticut 06516

Louis Lasagna, M.D., D.Sc.
Dean, Sackler School of Graduate Biomedical
  Sciences
Tufts University School of Medicine
136 Harrison Avenue
Boston, Massachusetts 02111

James F. Leckman, M.D.
Neison Harris Professor of Child Psychiatry
  and Pediatrics
Child Study Center
Yale University School of Medicine
230 South Frontage Road
New Haven, Connecticut 06520-7900

Michel Le Moal, M.D., Dr.Sci.
Professor of Neurosciences
INSERM, Psychobiology of Adaptive Behaviors
University of Bordeaux II
Domaine de Carreire Rue Camille Saint-Saëns
33077 Bordeaux Cedex, France

Corinne L. Lendon, Ph.D.
Research Instructor of Genetics in Psychiatry
Department of Psychiatry
Washington University School of Medicine
4940 Children's Place
St. Louis, Missouri 63110

Ting-Kai Li, M.D.
Distinguished Professor of Medicine and
 Biochemistry
Indiana University School of Medicine
545 Barnhill Drive
Indianapolis, Indiana 46202

Kelvin O. Lim, M.D.
Assistant Professor of Psychiatry
Department of Psychiatry and Behavioral
 Sciences
Stanford University School of Medicine
Palo Alto Veteran Affairs Medical Center and
 Psychiatry Service
3801 Miranda Avenue
Palo Alto, California 94304

Keh-Ming Lin, M.D., M.P.H.
Professor of Psychiatry
Director, Research Center on the
 Psychobiology of Ethnicity
Harbor-UCLA Research and Education
 Institute
Department of Psychiatry
Harbor-UCLA Medical Center
1124 West Carson Street
Torrance, California 90509

V. Markku I. Linnoila, M.D., Ph.D.
Scientific Director
National Institute on Alcohol Abuse and
 Alcoholism
National Institutes of Health
Bethesda, Maryland 20892

Keith J. Lookingland, Ph.D.
Associate Professor
Department of Pharmacology and Toxicology
Michigan State University
Life Sciences Building, B432
East Lansing, Michigan 48824

Linda J. Lotspeich, M.D., M.Ed.
Director, Pervasive Developmental Disorders
 Clinic
Division of Child Psychiatry and Child
 Development
Department of Psychiatry and Behavioral
 Sciences
Stanford University School of Medicine
101 Quarry Road
Stanford, California 94305

Avram H. Mack, A.B.
Research Associate
Department of Psychiatry
Duke University Medical Center
Box 3950
Durham, North Carolina 27710

Michael Maes, M.D., Ph.D.
Assistant Professor
Department of Psychiatry
Case Western Reserve University
School of Medicine
2040 Abingdon Road
Cleveland, Ohio 44106

Pierre J. Magistretti, M.D., Ph.D.
Institut de Physiologie
Faculté de Médecine
Université de Lausanne
7, rue du Bugnon
CH 1005 Lausanne, Switzerland

Robert T. Malison, M.D.
Assistant Professor
Department of Psychiatry
Yale University School of Medicine
Connecticut Mental Health Center
34 Park Street
New Haven, Connecticut 06508

J. John Mann, M.D.
Professor of Psychiatry
Department of Psychiatry and Behavioral
 Sciences
Laboratories of Neuropharmacology
University of Pittsburgh School of Medicine
Pittsburgh, Pennsylvania 15213
current address
Department of Neuroscience
New York State Psychiatric Institute
722 West 168th Street
New York, New York 10032

Alfred Mansour, Ph.D.
Research Investigator
Mental Health Research Institute
University of Michigan
205 Zina Pitcher Place
Ann Arbor, Michigan 48109

Stephen R. Marder, M.D.
Chief, Psychiatry Service
West Los Angeles Veterans Administration
 Medical Center
Department of Psychiatry
University of California, Los Angeles
School of Medicine
760 Westwood Plaza
Los Angeles, California 90024

Deborah B. Marin, M.D.
Assistant Professor
Department of Psychiatry
Mount Sinai School of Medicine
1 Gustave L. Levy Place
New York, New York 10029

Athina Markou, Ph.D.
Assistant Member
Department of Neuropharmacology
The Scripps Research Institute
10666 North Torrey Pines Road
La Jolla, California 92037

Jean-Luc Martin, Ph.D.
Institut de Physiologie
Faculté de Médecine
Université de Lausanne
7, rue du Bugnon
CH 1005 Lausanne, Switzerland

Billy R. Martin, Ph.D.
Louis and Ruth Harris Professor
Department of Pharmacology and Toxicology
Medical College of Virginia
Virginia Commonwealth University
Box 613 MCV Station
410 North 12th Street
Richmond, Virginia 23298-0613

George A. Mason, Ph.D.
Research Professor of Psychiatry
Department of Psychiatry
University of North Carolina School of
 Medicine
Chapel Hill, North Carolina 27599-7160

Josephine Mauskopf, M.A., M.H.A., Ph.D.
Section Head, Economics Research
Department of International Surveillance,
 Epidemiology, and Economics Research
Burroughs Wellcome Co.
3030 Cornwallis Road
Research Triangle Park, North Carolina 27709

Bruce S. McEwen, Ph.D.
Professor and Head
Laboratory of Neuroendocrinology
The Rockefeller University
1230 York Avenue
New York, New York 10021

Herbert Y. Meltzer, M.D.
Douglas Danford Bond Professor of Psychiatry
Department of Psychiatry
Case Western Reserve University School of
 Medicine
University Hospitals of Cleveland
2040 Abington Road
Cleveland, Ohio 44106-5000

Marek-Marsel Mesulam, M.D.
Professor of Neurology
Department of Neurology
Northwestern University Medical School
233 East Erie Street-Suite 614
Chicago, Illinois 60611

Klaus A. Miczek, Ph.D.
Moses Hunt Professor of Psychology and
 Psychiatry
Department of Psychology
Tufts University
490 Boston Avenue
Medford, Massachusetts 02155

Stephan E. Miller
Department of Psychobiology
Irvine Research Unit in Brain Imaging
University of California, Irvine
Irvine, California 92717-4550

Philip B. Mitchell, M.D., F.R.C. Psych.
Associate Professor
School of Psychiatry
University of New South Wales
Clinical Sciences Building
Prince Henry Hospital
Little Bay, NSW 2036, Australia

Richard C. Mohs, Ph.D.
Professor
Department of Psychiatry
Mount Sinai School of Medicine
Veteran Affairs Medical Center
130 West Kingsbridge Road
Bronx, New York 10468

Susan E. Molchan, M.D.
Section on Geriatric Psychiatry
National Institute of Mental Health
National Institutes of Health
Bethesda, Maryland 20892

Stuart A. Montgomery, M.D., F.R.C. Psych.
Professor
Department of Psychiatry
St. Mary's Hospital Medical School
Praed Street
London W2 1NY, United Kingdom

Kenneth E. Moore, Ph.D.
Professor and Chairperson
Department of Pharmacology and Toxicology
Michigan State University
Life Sciences Building
East Lansing, Michigan 48824-1317

M. Inés Morano, Ph.D.
Research Fellow
Mental Health Research Institute
University of Michigan
205 Zina Pitcher Place
Ann Arbor, Michigan 48109-0720

James I. Morgan, Ph.D.
Department of Neuroscience
Roche Institute of Molecular Biology
340 Kingsland Street
Nutley, New Jersey 07110

David A. Morilak, Ph.D.
Assistant Professor
Department of Pharmacology
University of Texas Health Sciences Center
7703 Floyd Curl Drive
San Antonio, Texas 78284-7764

Patrizia Morino, Ph.D.
Department of Neuroscience
Karolinska Institute
S-171 77 Stockholm, Sweden

Geoffrey K. Mumford, Ph.D.
Assistant Professor
Department of Psychiatry and Behavioral
* Sciences*
Johns Hopkins University School of Medicine
5510 Nathan Shock Drive
Baltimore, Maryland 21224-6823

Dennis L. Murphy, M.D.
Chief, Laboratory of Clinical Science
National Institute of Mental Health
National Institutes of Health
Bethesda, Maryland 20892

Charles B. Nemeroff, M.D., Ph.D.
Professor and Chairman
Department of Psychiatry and Behavioral
* Sciences*
Emory University School of Medicine
P.O. Drawer AF
Atlanta, Georgia 30322

Eric J. Nestler, M.D., Ph.D.
Elizabeth Mears and House Jameson Professor
* of Psychiatry and Pharmacology*
Laboratory of Molecular Psychiatry
Departments of Psychiatry and Pharmacology
Yale University School of Medicine
Connecticut Mental Health Center
34 Park Street
New Haven, Connecticut 06508

John G. Newcomer, M.D.
Assistant Professor
Department of Psychiatry
Washington University School of Medicine
Schizophrenia Research Program
Malcolm Bliss Mental Health Center
4940 Children's Place
St. Louis, Missouri 63110

Mitchell S. Nobler, M.D.
Assistant Professor of Clinical Psychiatry
Department of Biological Psychiatry
Columbia University College of Physicians and
* Surgeons*
New York State Psychiatric Institute
722 West 168th Street
New York, New York 10032

Keith H. Nuechterlein, Ph.D.
Professor of Medical Psychology
Department of Psychiatry and Behavioral
* Sciences*
University of California, Los Angeles
School of Medicine
300 UCLA Medical Plaza
Los Angeles, California 90024-6968

Charles P. O'Brien, M.D., Ph.D.
Professor and Vice-Chair
Department of Psychiatry
University of Pennsylvania
Veterans Affairs Medical Center
Treatment Research Center
3900 Chestnut Street
Philadelphia, Pennsylvania 19104-6178

David H. Overstreet, Ph.D.
Research Associate Professor
Department of Psychiatry
Center for Alcohol Studies
University of North Carolina at Chapel Hill
Chapel Hill, North Carolina 27599-7175

Michael J. Owens, Ph.D.
Assistant Professor
Department of Psychiatry and Behavioral
* Sciences*
Laboratory of Neuropsychopharmacology
Emory University School of Medicine
P.O. Drawer AF
Atlanta, Georgia 30322

Lisa S. Parker, Ph.D.
Assistant Professor
Department of Human Genetics
University of Pittsburgh
130 DeSoto Street
Philadelphia, Pennsylvania 15261

Barbara L. Parry, M.D.
Associate Professor
Department of Psychiatry
University of California, San Diego
9500 Gilman Drive
La Jolla, California 92093-0804

Paul H. Patterson, Ph.D.
Professor and Executive Officer of Biology
Division of Biology 216-76
California Institute of Technology
Pasadena, California 91125

Steven M. Paul, M.D.
Intramural Research Program
National Institute of Mental Health
National Institutes of Health
Bethesda, Maryland 20892
current address
Vice President
Lilly Research Laboratories
Eli Lilly and Company
Indianapolis, Indiana 46285

David L. Pauls, Ph.D.
Yale University School of Medicine
Child Study Center
230 South Frontage Road
New Haven, Connecticut 06520-7900

Jane S. Paulsen, Ph.D.
Assistant Professor
Department of Psychiatry
University of California, San Diego and
San Diego Veterans Affairs Medical Center
3350 La Jolla Village Drive
San Diego, California 92161

Godfrey D. Pearlson, M.D.
Professor
Department of Psychiatry and Behavioral
  Science
Johns Hopkins University School of Medicine
Director, Psychiatry Neuro-Imaging
Johns Hopkins Hospital
600 North Wolfe Street
Baltimore, Maryland 21287

Luc Pellerin
Institut de Physiologie
Faculté de Médecine
Université de Lausanne
7, rue du Bugnon
CH 1005 Lausanne, Switzerland

Diana O. Perkins, M.D., M.P.H.
Assistant Professor
Department of Psychiatry
University of North Carolina School of
  Medicine
Campus Box 7160
Chapel Hill, North Carolina 27599

James G. Pfaus, Ph.D.
Assistant Professor of Psychology
Center for Studies in Behavioural
  Neurobiology
Concordia University
1455 de Maisonneuve Boulevard West
Montreal, Quebec, H3G 1M8, Canada

Adolf Pfefferbaum, M.D.
Professor of Psychiatry
Department of Psychiatry and Behavioral
  Sciences
Stanford University School of Medicine and
Psychiatry Service 116A
Palo Alto Veteran Affairs Medical Center
3801 Miranda Avenue
Palo Alto, California 94304

Virginia M. Pickel, Ph.D.
Professor
Department of Neurology and Neuroscience
Cornell University Medical College
411 East 69th Street
New York, New York 10021

Roy W. Pickens, Ph.D.
Research Scientist
Molecular Neurobiology Branch
National Institute on Drug Abuse
Intramural Research Program
National Institutes of Health
P.O. Box 5180
Baltimore, Maryland 21224

Daniele Piomelli, Ph.D.
Directeur de Recherche
Unité Neurobiologie et Pharmacologie de
  l'INSERM
Centre Paul Broca
2 ter rue d'Alésia
75014 Paris, France

Andreas Plaitakis, M.D.
Professor of Neurology
Mount Sinai School of Medicine
One Gustave L. Levy Place
New York, New York 10029

Paul M. Plotsky, Ph.D.
Stress Neurobiology Laboratory
Department of Psychiatry and Behavioral
  Sciences
Emory University School of Medicine
1639 Pierce Drive
P.O. Drawer AF
Atlanta, Georgia 30322

Russell E. Poland, Ph.D.
Professor
Department of Psychiatry
Harbor-UCLA Medical Center
1000 West Carson Street
Torrance, California 90509

Matthew H. Porteus, M.D., Ph.D.
Children's Hospital
300 Longwood Avenue
Boston, Massachusetts 02115

Robert M. Post, M.D.
Chief, Biological Psychiatry Branch
National Institute of Mental Health
National Institutes of Health
Bethesda, Maryland 20892

William Z. Potter, M.D.
Chief, Section on Clinical Pharmacology
Experimental Therapeutics Branch
National Institute of Mental Health
National Institutes of Health
Bethesda, Maryland 20892

Arthur J. Prange, Jr., M.D.
Boshamer Professor of Psychiatry
Department of Psychiatry
University of North Carolina
School of Medicine
Chapel Hill, North Carolina 27599-7160

Sheldon H. Preskorn, M.D.
Professor and Vice Chairman
Department of Psychiatry
University of Kansas School of Medicine–
  Wichita
President and Medical Director
Psychiatric Research Institute
1100 N. St. Francis, Suite 200
Wichita, Kansas 67214

Kenzie L. Preston, Ph.D.
Associate Professor
Division of Behavioral Biology, Psychiatry and
  Behavioral Sciences
Johns Hopkins University School of Medicine
Chief, Clinical Trials Section
Treatment Branch
National Institute on Drug Abuse
Intramural Research Program
National Institutes of Health
P.O. Box 5180
Baltimore, Maryland 21224

Donald L. Price, M.D.
Professor
Departments of Pathology, Neurology, and
  Neuroscience
Johns Hopkins University School of Medicine
720 Rutland Avenue
Baltimore, Maryland 21205

Lawrence H. Price, M.D.
Associate Professor
Department of Psychiatry
Yale University School of Medicine
Connecticut Mental Health Center
34 Park Street
New Haven, Connecticut 06519

Robert F. Prien, Ph.D.
Chief, Clinical Treatment Research Branch
Division of Clinical and Treatment Research
National Institute of Mental Health
National Institutes of Health
5600 Fishers Lane
Rockville, Maryland 20857

Stanley B. Prusiner, M.D.
Department of Neurology, HSE-781
University of California, San Francisco
School of Medicine
San Francisco, California 94143-0518

Stanley I. Rapoport, M.D.
Chief, Laboratory of Neurosciences
National Institute on Aging
National Institutes of Health
Bethesda, Maryland 20892

Murray A. Raskind, M.D.
Professor
Department of Psychiatry and Behavioral
  Sciences—RP-10
University of Washington School of Medicine
1959 NE Pacific Street
Seattle, Washington 98195

D. Eugene Redmond, Jr., M.D.
Professor of Psychiatry
Neurobehavioral Lab, B422
Yale University School of Medicine
333 Cedar Street
New Haven, Connecticut 06520-8068

Peter B. Reiner, V.M.D., Ph.D.
Division of Neurological Sciences
Department of Psychiatry
University of British Columbia
2255 Wesbrook Mall
Vancouver, British Columbia, V6T 1Z3 Canada

Charles F. Reynolds III, M.D.
Professor of Psychiatry and Neurology
Department of Psychiatry
University of Pittsburgh School of Medicine
Western Psychiatric Institute and Clinic
3811 O'Hara Street
Pittsburgh, Pennsylvania 15213

Elliott Richelson, M.D.
Departments of Psychiatry and Psychology,
  and Pharmacology
Mayo Clinic Jacksonville
Birdsall Medical Research Building
4500 San Pablo Road
Jacksonville, Florida 32224

Karl Rickels, M.D.
Professor of Psychiatry and Pharmacology
University of Pennsylvania
University Science Center
3600 Market Street
Philadelphia, Pennsylvania 19104-2649

Linda Rinaman, Ph.D.
Postdoctoral Fellow
Department of Behavioral Neuroscience
University of Pittsburgh
446 Crawford Hall
Pittsburgh, Pennsylvania 15260

Trevor W. Robbins, Ph.D.
Reader
Department of Experimental Psychology
University of Cambridge
Downing Street
Cambridge CB2 3EB, United Kingdom

Donald S. Robinson, M.D.
Vice President, CNS Clinical Research
Bristol-Myers Squibb Company
1066 Spanish Wells Drive
Melbourne, Florida 32940

William R. Roeske, M.D.
Associate Chief, Section of Cardiology
Professor
Departments of Medicine and Pharmacology
University of Arizona
College of Medicine
1501 N. Campbell Avenue
Tucson, Arizona 85724

Margaret Rosenbloom
Psychiatry Service 116A
Palo Alto Veteran Affairs Medical Center
3801 Miranda Avenue
Palo Alto, California 94304

Ruth Ross, M.A.
Department of Psychiatry
Box 3950
Duke University Medical Center
Durham, North Carolina 27710

Bryan L. Roth, M.D., Ph.D.
Associate Professor of Psychiatry
Department of Psychiatry
Case Western Reserve University School of Medicine
2040 Abington Road
Cleveland, Ohio 44106

Robert H. Roth, Ph.D.
Professor
Departments of Psychiatry and Pharmacology
Yale University School of Medicine
333 Cedar Street
New Haven, Connecticut 06520-8066

Walton T. Roth, M.D.
Professor
Department of Psychiatry and Behavioral Sciences
Stanford University School of Medicine
Veterans Affairs Medical Center (116A3)
3801 Miranda Avenue
Palo Alto, California 94304

David R. Rubinow, M.D.
Clinical Director
National Institute of Mental Health
National Institutes of Health
Bethesda, Maryland 20892

A. John Rush, M.D.
Betty Jo Hay Distinguished Chair in Mental Health
Department of Psychiatry
University of Texas Southwestern Medical Center and
Mental Health Clinical Research Center at St. Paul
5953 Harry Hines Boulevard
Dallas, Texas 75235

Neal Ryan, M.D.
Associate Professor of Psychiatry
University of Pittsburgh School of Medicine
Western Psychiatric Institute and Clinic
3811 O'Hara Street
Pittsburgh, Pennsylvania 15213

Harold A. Sackeim, Ph.D.
Professor and Chief
Department of Biological Psychiatry
Columbia University College of Physicians and Surgeons
New York State Psychiatric Institute
722 West 168th Street
New York, New York 10032

Carl Salzman, M.D.
Professor of Psychiatry
Harvard Medical School
Massachusetts Mental Health Center
74 Fenwood Road
Boston, Massachusetts 02115

Elaine Sanders-Bush, Ph.D.
Professor
Department of Pharmacology
Vanderbilt University
School of Medicine
Nashville, Tennessee 37232

Alan F. Schatzberg, M.D.
Kenneth T. Norris, Jr. Professor and Chairman
Department of Psychiatry and Behavioral
  Sciences
Stanford University School of Medicine
101 Quarry Road, C-301
Stanford, California 94305-5548

Joseph J. Schildkraut, M.D.
Professor
Department of Psychiatry
Harvard Medical School
74 Fenwood Road
Boston, Massachusetts 02115

Thomas E. Schlaepfer, M.D.
Assistant Professor
Department of Psychiatry
Johns Hopkins University School of Medicine
Johns Hopkins Hospital
600 N. Wolfe Street
Baltimore, Maryland 21287

Lon S. Schneider, M.D.
Associate Professor of Psychiatry and
  Neurology
Department of Psychiatry
University of Southern California School of
  Medicine
2250 Alcazar Street
Los Angeles, California 90033

Leslie M. Schuh, Ph.D.
Clinical Pharmacology Branch
National Institute on Drug Abuse
Intramural Research Program
National Institutes of Health
P.O. Box 5180
Baltimore, Maryland 21224

Charles R. Schuster, Ph.D.
Senior Research Scientist
Treatment Research Branch
National Institute on Drug Abuse
National Institutes of Health
4940 Eastern Avenue
Baltimore, Maryland 21224

Jean-Charles Schwartz, Ph.D.
Professor
Unité de Neurobiologie et Pharmacologie
  (U.109) de l'INSERM
Centre Paul Broca
2ter rue d'Alésia
75014 Paris, France

Edward Schweizer, M.D.
Associate Professor of Psychiatry
University of Pennsylvania
University Science Center
3600 Market Street
Philadelphia, Pennsylvania 19104

Philip Seeman, M.D., Ph.D.
Department of Pharmacology and Psychiatry
Medical Sciences Building
University of Toronto
Toronto, Ontario M5S 1A8, Canada

Susan R. Sesack, Ph.D.
Assistant Professor
Department of Behavioral Neuroscience
University of Pittsburgh
446 Crawford Hall
Pittsburgh, Pennsylvania 15260

Richard I. Shader, M.D.
Professor
Department of Pharmacology and
  Experimental Therapeutics
Tufts University School of Medicine
136 Harrison Avenue
Boston, Massachusetts 02111

P. Shashidharan, Ph.D.
Instructor
Department of Neurology
Mount Sinai School of Medicine
One Gustave L. Levy Place
New York, New York 10029

Thomas G. Sherman, Ph.D.
Assistant Professor
Department of Behavioral Neuroscience
University of Pittsburgh
446 Crawford Hall
Pittsburgh, Pennsylvania 15260

Jean Chen Shih, Ph.D.
Boyd and Elsie Welin Professor
Department of Molecular Pharmacology and
  Toxicology
University of Southern California
School of Pharmacy
1985 Zonal Avenue
Los Angeles, California 90033

Larry J. Siever, M.D.
Professor of Psychiatry
Department of Psychiatry
Mount Sinai School of Medicine
One Gustave L. Levy Place
New York, New York 10029

George R. Siggins, Ph.D.
Department of Neuropharmacology
Scripps Clinic and Research Foundation
10666 N. Torrey Pines Road
La Jolla, California 92037

Raul R. Silva, M.D.
Assistant Professor
Department of Psychiatry
Millhauser Laboratories
New York University Medical Center
550 First Avenue
New York, New York 10016

Sangram S. Sisodia, Ph.D.
Assistant Professor
Department of Pathology
Neuropathology Laboratory
The Johns Hopkins University School of
  Medicine
720 Rutland Avenue
Baltimore, Maryland 21205

John R. Sladek, Jr., Ph.D.
Professor and Chairman
Department of Neuroscience
Finch University of Health Sciences
The Chicago Medical School
3333 Green Bay Road
North Chicago, Illinois 60064

Solomon H. Snyder, M.D.
Distinguished Service Professor of
  Neuroscience Pharmacology and Molecular
  Sciences, and of Psychiatry
Director, Department of Neuroscience
Johns Hopkins University School of Medicine
725 North Wolfe Street
Baltimore, Maryland 21205

Robert A. Stern, Ph.D.
Assistant Professor
Departments of Psychiatry and Human
  Behavior and Clinical Neurosciences
Brown University School of Medicine
Department of Psychiatry
Rhode Island Hospital
593 Eddy Street
Providence, Rhode Island 02903

Maxine L. Stitzer, Ph.D.
Professor of Behavioral Biology
Behavioral Biology Research Center
Johns Hopkins Bayview Medical Center
5510 Nathan Shock Drive
Baltimore, Maryland 21224

Edward M. Stricker, Ph.D.
Professor of Neuroscience and Psychiatry
Chairman
Department of Behavioral Neuroscience
University of Pittsburgh
479 Crawford Hall
Pittsburgh, Pennsylvania 15260

James P. Sullivan, Ph.D.
Group Leader
Molecular and Biochemical Pharmacology
Neuroscience Research D47W
Abbott Laboratories
One Abbott Park Road
Abbott Park, Illinois 60064

Trey Sunderland, M.D.
Chief, Section on Geriatric Psychiatry
National Institute of Mental Health
National Institutes of Health
Bethesda, Maryland 20892

John F. Tallman, Ph.D.
Scientific Director
Neurogen Corporation
35 Northeast Industrial Road
Branford, Connecticut 06405

Jane R. Taylor, Ph.D.
Research Scientist
Neurobehavior Laboratory
Department of Psychiatry
Yale University School of Medicine
333 Cedar Street
New Haven, Connecticut 06520-8066

Michael E. Thase, M.D.
Associate Professor of Psychiatry
Director, Division of Mood, Anxiety,
  Personality and Substance Abuse Disorders
Associate Director, Clinical Research Center
University of Pittsburgh School of Medicine
Western Psychiatric Institute and Clinic
3811 O'Hara Street
Pittsburgh, Pennsylvania 15213

Elisabeth Traiffort, Ph.D.
Unité de Neurobiologie and Pharmacologie
  (U.109) de l'INSERM
Centre Paul Broca
2ter rue d'Alésia
75014 Paris, France

George R. Uhl, M.D., Ph.D.
Associate Professor
Department of Neurology and Neuroscience
Johns Hopkins University School of Medicine
Chief, Molecular Neurobiology Branch
Acting Scientific Director
National Institute on Drug Abuse
Intramural Research Program
National Institutes of Health
P.O. Box 5180
Baltimore, Maryland 21224

Eberhard H. Uhlenhuth, M.D.
Professor of Psychiatry
Department of Psychiatry
University of New Mexico
2400 Tucker, NE
Albuquerque, New Mexico 87131

Jolanta Ułas, Ph.D.
Associate Researcher
Department of Psychobiology
Irvine Research Unit in Brain Imaging
University of California, Irvine
1305 Biological Sciences II
Irvine, California 92717

Rita J. Valentino, Ph.D.
Associate Professor
Department of Mental Health Sciences
Division of Behavioral Neurobiology
Hahnemann University Medical School
Broad and Vine Streets
Philadelphia, Pennsylvania 19102-1192

Theodore Van Putten, M.D. (deceased)
University of California, Los Angeles
  School of Medicine and
West Los Angeles Veterans Affairs Medical
  Center
11301 Wilshire Boulevard
Los Angeles, California 90073

Lisa L. von Moltke, M.D.
Research Assistant Professor
Department of Pharmacology and
  Experimental Therapeutics
Tufts University School of Medicine
136 Harrison Avenue
Boston, Massachusetts 02111

John J. Wagner, Ph.D.
Research Associate
Department of Physiology
University of Maryland at Baltimore
655 West Baltimore Street
Baltimore, Maryland 21201

Claus Wahlestedt, M.D., Ph.D.
Professor of Pharmacology
Astra Pain Research Unit
275, bis.boul. Armand Frappier
Laval, Quebec, H7V4A7 Canada

B. Timothy Walsh, M.D.
Professor of Clinical Psychiatry
Columbia University College of Physicians
  and Surgeons
Director, Eating Disorders Unit
New York State Psychiatric Institute
722 West 168th Street, Box 98
New York, New York 10032

Stanley J. Watson, Jr., M.D., Ph.D.
Associate Director
Mental Health Research Institute
Associate Chair Research
Department of Psychiatry
University of Michigan
205 Zina Pitcher Place
Ann Arbor, Michigan 48109-0720

Daniel R. Weinberger, M.D.
Chief, Clinical Brain Disorders Branch
Division of Intramural Research Programs
National Institute of Mental Health
National Institutes of Health
2700 Martin Luther King, Jr. Avenue, SE
Washington, DC 20032

Richard H. Weisler, M.D.
Adjunct Associate Professor
Department of Psychology
Duke University Medical Center
900 Ridgefield Drive
Raleigh, North Carolina 27609

Susan R. B. Weiss, Ph.D.
Research Psychologist
Biological Psychiatry Branch
National Institute of Mental Health
National Institutes of Health
Bethesda, Maryland 20892

Patricia M. Whitaker-Azmitia, Ph.D.
Associate Professor of Psychiatry
Department of Psychiatry and Behavioral
  Science
Health Science Center
State University of New York at Stony Brook
Stony Brook, New York 11794

Peter J. Whitehouse, M.D., Ph.D.
Director, Alzheimer Center
University Hospital of Cleveland
2074 Abington Road
Cleveland, Ohio 44106

Michael Williams, Ph.D., D.Sc.
Divisional Vice President
Neuroscience Research D-464
Pharmaceutical Products Division
Abbott Laboratories
One Abbott Park Road
Abbott, Illinois 60064

Paul Willner, M.A., D.Phil,
  C. Psychol., F.B.Ps.S.
Professor
Department of Psychology
University of Wales
University College of Swansea
Singleton Park
Swansea, SA2 8PP, United Kingdom

Gail Winger, Ph.D.
Associate Research Scientist
Department of Pharmacology
University of Michigan Medical School
301 E. Catherine
Ann Arbor, Michigan 48109-0626

William C. Wirshing, M.D.
University of California, Los Angeles
*   School of Medicine*
West Los Angeles Veterans Affairs Medical
*   Center*
11301 Wilshire Boulevard
Los Angeles, California 90073

Anna Wirz-Justice, Ph.D.
Professor of Biological Psychiatry
Psychiatrische Universitatsklinik
Wilhelm Klein Strasse 27
CH-4025 Basel, Switzerland

Susan I. Wolk, M.D.
Department of Psychiatry
Columbia University College of Physicians and
*   Surgeons*
New York State Psychiatric Institute
722 West 168th Street
New York, New York 10032

James H. Woods, Ph.D.
Professor
Department of Pharmacology
University of Michigan Medical School
1301 E. Catherine
Ann Arbor, Michigan 48109-0626

Mark J. Woyshville, M.D.
Director, Clinical Drug Trials Section
Mood Disorders Program
Assistant Professor
Department of Psychiatry
Case Western Reserve University School of
*   Medicine*
University Hospitals of Cleveland
11400 Euclid Avenue
Cleveland, Ohio 44106

Henry I. Yamamura, Ph.D.
Professor of Pharmacology, Biochemistry,
*   Neuroscience, and Psychiatry*
Department of Pharmacology
University of Arizona College of Medicine
1501 North Campbell Avenue
Tucson, Arizona 85724

Alice M. Young, Ph.D.
Professor
Department of Psychology
Wayne State University College of Science
71 W. Warren Avenue
Detroit, Michigan 48202

Alan Zametkin, M.D.
Section on Clinical Brain Imaging
Laboratory of Cerebral Metabolism
National Institute of Mental Health
National Institutes of Health
Bethesda, Maryland 20892-0001

Gary A. Zarkin, Ph.D.
Program Director, Health and Human
*   Resource Economics*
Center for Economics Research
Research Triangle Institute
3040 Cornwallis Road
Research Triangle Park, North Carolina 27709

Xu Zhang
Department of Neuroscience
Karolinska Institute
S-171 77 Stockholm, Sweden

Michael J. Zigmond, Ph.D.
Department of Behavioral Neuroscience
University of Pittsburgh
570 Crawford Hall
Pittsburgh, Pennsylvania 15260

George S. Zubenko, M.D., Ph.D.
Professor
Department of Psychiatry
Adjunct Professor of Biological Sciences
University of Pittsburgh
School of Medicine, and
Western Psychiatric Institute and Clinic
3811 O'Hara Street
Pittsburgh, Pennsylvania 15213

R. Suzanne Zukin, Ph.D.
Professor
Department of Neuroscience
Director of Neuropsychopharmacology Center
Albert Einstein College of Medicine
Rose F. Kennedy Center
1300 Morris Park Avenue
Bronx, New York 10461

Preface to the Third Edition

Psychopharmacology: The Third Generation of Progress is similar to the two preceding editions, in that it provides a definition of and treatise about the domain of psychopharmacology as understood by the American College of Neuropsychopharmacology (ACNP): to utilize drugs and other chemical agents to understand neural function, to prevent and treat mental illness, drug abuse, and alcoholism; and to understand how nontherapeutic psychoactive drugs and natural substances alter human mood, mentation, motor activity, endocrine, and other centrally mediated functions. A comparison of this edition with its predecessors reveals the remarkable developments in psychopharmacology, and why publication of a new volume is both desirable and timely. The explosion of information—a consequence of the huge increase in the number of neuroscientists and a more modest but nonetheless significant increase in the number of clinical investigators—has made some changes in format desirable. The book is divided into three major sections: Basic Neurobiology, Biological Psychiatry, and Clinical Psychopharmacology. The authors have, for the most part, eschewed textbook-type presentations in favor of critical evaluation of the most worthy research findings of the past nine years, often concluding with suggestions for future research.

This edition will help to educate scientists and clinicians who are encountering psychopharmacology for the first time, to broaden the knowledge of those already in the field, and to stimulate further research through an emphasis on the crucial areas of psychopharmacology where the opportunity for advancement is greatest.

Herbert Y. Meltzer

Preface

The accelerated pace of modern scientific research has inevitably reduced the length of a scientific generation to considerably less than the classic two decades. In fact, the history of this series has been one of progressively shorter and shorter intervals of assessment of the progress within our field. Like its predecessors, this volume seeks to redefine the scientific field of neuropsychopharmacology for its parent organization, The American College of Neuropsychopharmacology. In this iteration, the field's definition has been constructed from the two interrelated bodies of work that comprise the major working arms of the College: the *clinical* investigation of psychiatric and neurological disorders in terms of their biologically defined mechanisms of pathogenesis, treatment and prevention; and the *preclinical* foundations of neuropsychopharmacology in terms of the essential signaling mechanisms by which neurons interact to perform the behavioral level operations of the brain and mental activity. In these parallel tracks of effort, drugs are a tool to dissect the chemical signaling systems of the brain, as well as a means to restore functions disrupted by brain diseases. The better the characterization of the chemical signaling systems, the more insightful will be the analyses of the drugs in their therapeutic assessment.

A slight departure of this book from its predecessor volumes is the attempt to provide a more comprehensive overview of the clinical and preclinical arms of the field. Here the approach is designed first to provide new scholars with overviews of preclinical and clinical psychopharmacology, and then more detailed coverage to understand the methods by which data in each of these arms are assessed in research. The introductory sections provide a basis for the detailed coverage of the enormous amounts of progress that have been achieved since the previous volume. Finally, the coverage builds upon these foundations with assessments of the most recent cross-cutting issues. There is intentionally extensive cross-referencing between clinical and preclinical subjects. The text is designed to allow experts in both spheres to find the latest assessments of progress, while also permitting the less experienced readers to increase their appreciation of the work underway.

The cast of authorships is broad and international, by design going beyond the boundaries of the College's current membership. By providing a road map to the linkages between the major topics of today's research, the editors and authors hope to illuminate critically the most exciting discoveries, as well as to indicate the important gaps that need attention, while allowing room for the unexpected discoveries that will almost certainly emerge. We close this preface with our sincere appreciation to all those who worked with us on this effort.

Floyd E. Bloom
David J. Kupfer

PSYCHOPHARMACOLOGY
The Fourth Generation of Progress

An Official Publication of the
American College of Neuropsychopharmacology

Psychopharmacology: The Fourth Generation of Progress, edited by Floyd E. Bloom and David J. Kupfer. Raven Press, Ltd., New York © 1995.

CHAPTER 1

Introduction to Preclinical Neuropsychopharmacology

Floyd E. Bloom

Neuropsychopharmacology links the frontiers of basic neuroscience to the treatment of neurological and psychiatric diseases. On one level, this scientific field seeks to understand how drugs can affect the central nervous system (CNS) selectively to relieve pain, heighten attention, induce sleep, reduce fever or appetite, suppress disordered movement, or prevent seizures. Notably, this is the field that seeks to understand how drugs can treat anxiety, mania, depression, or schizophrenia without altering consciousness. On a more profound level, this field seeks to understand the biological basis for such complex mental states as the disordered cognition of the schizophrenic. On this level, the goal is not only to understand the nature of the alterations in biology which lead to altered emotions and thought processes, but also to develop specific therapeutic molecules to regulate their biological underpinnings—namely, the as yet unspecified sequences of multineuronal interactions by which these behaviors emerge.

Drugs can affect precise molecular targets in discrete cells within selected circuits to influence specific interconnected systems of neurons that mediate or generate behaviors. By illuminating this process, neuropsychopharmacologists stand at the threshold of a profound scientific challenge—namely, to understand the cellular and molecular basis for the enormously complex and varied functions of the human brain. Among the most profound research questions that now pose testable challenges for neuropsychopharmacologists are the detailed understanding of the brain operations that account for normal mental activity and the pathological mental states of emotion, cognition, and perception. In this effort, neuropsychopharmacologists employ drugs in two strategies: (i) to dissect the functional and structural systems that operate in the normal CNS, thereby defining the specificity of these drugs as well as the systems on which they act, and (ii) to provide the means to develop appropriate drugs to correct pathophysiological events in the abnormal CNS.

A BRIEF GUIDE TO THE PRECLINICAL NEUROPSYCHOPHARMACOLOGY CHAPTERS

Comprehending the sites and mechanisms of action of drugs and drug classes requires an understanding of (a) the molecular biology of the cell classes of the brain and (b) the means by which these properties define the anatomy, physiology, and chemistry of the nervous system. This chapter serves to introduce the preclinical portion of this *Generation of Progress* volume. For scholars with limited prior experience in the neurosciences, it will provide some fundamental principles and concepts for the comprehensive analysis of drug actions on the CNS. As an overview, this chapter provides (a) a summary of the principal methods by which preclinical data are obtained and analyzed (Chapters 2–6) and (b) a summary of the ensuing chapters (Chapters 7–57), which detail the recent progress on the basic elements of the pertinent brain systems and discuss the clinical implications of this progress. In addition, this chapter will survey some promising future developments that cut across diverse facets of the current research frontier (Chapters 58–69), many of which provide the thresholds to the next generation of progress.

Within these three preclinical sections, certain key goals were held as uniform targets: Section I, the Critical Analyses of Methods (Chapters 2–6) are intended to (a) provide new scholars of neuropsychopharmacology with a critical assessment of the primary research methods

F. E. Bloom: Department of Neuropharmacology, The Scripps Research Institute, La Jolla, California 92037.

being applied currently, (b) indicate their advantages and disadvantages, and (c) indicate what qualities of data they can or cannot now provide. Section II, The Transmitter Systems, focuses on the well-defined neurotransmitter systems which provide the molecular and cellular substrate by which drugs act to influence behavior and to treat neurological and psychiatric diseases. The transmitter systems are arbitrarily divided into three traditional chemical categories: (i) *amino acids* (Chapters 7 and 8); (ii) *aminergic neurons,* further subdivided into transmitters: acetylcholine (Chapters 9–13), dopamine (Chapters 14–26), noradrenaline (Chapters 27–34), histamine (Chapter 35), and serotonin (Chapters 36–42); and (iii) *neuropeptides* (Chapters 43–52). Within each of these transmitter systems, the authors have identified the essential starting premises from the previous *Generation of Progress* volume (5) and have focused their attention mainly on what are considered to be the most important elements of subsequent progress. Depending on the depth of neuropsychopharmacological relevance of these transmitter systems, each transmitter's coverage may include, to varying degrees, data from each of the principal levels of analysis, namely, molecular, cellular, systems, and behavioral (see below).

These chapters on the traditional transmitters are then followed by preliminary discussions on several signaling molecules that are likely to come into increased recognition as important members of the interneuronal signaling process: arachidonic acid (see Chapter 53, *this volume*), nitric oxide and related substances (see Chapter 54, *this volume*), purines (see Chapter 57, *this volume*), and the series of intercellular (see Chapter 55, *this volume*) and intracellular (see Chapter 56, *this volume*) growth and differentiation molecules which seem critical for normal nervous system development as well as for maintenance of function.

Section III examines integrative concepts which transcend individual transmitter systems, but which enlighten the means by which neuronal activity is normally coordinated to meet the demands of the internal and external environments faced by a given individual. These critical brief reviews examine brain energy metabolism (see Chapter 58, *this volume*), brain development (see Chapter 59, *this volume*), the development of behavior (see Chapter 60, *this volume*), intracellular mechanisms of adaptive plasticity (see Chapter 61, *this volume*), the interactions of the nervous system with the endocrine (see Chapters 62 and 67, *this volume*) and immune systems (see Chapter 63, *this volume*), the means by which animals become tolerant to the behavior altering effects of drugs (see Chapter 64, *this volume*), and the utility of genetic models (see Chapter 69, *this volume*), as well as more traditional animal models for abused drugs (see Chapter 66, *this volume*) and for psychiatric disorders (see Chapter 68, *this volume*) including dysfunctional sexual behavior (see Chapter 65, *this volume*).

These preclinical progress reports thus provide the basis for the specific therapeutic approaches to neurological and psychiatric disorders which are presented in the clinical chapters that follow (Sections IV–VI). The relationship is fruitfully bidirectional: Untreatable diseases and unexpected nontherapeutic side effects reveal ill-defined mechanisms of pathophysiology which can drive preclinical research to search for additional mechanisms of cellular regulation to link molecular processes to behavior.

HIERARCHICAL LEVELS OF RESEARCH IN NEUROSCIENCES

Four hierarchical levels of analysis epitomize the research strategies used to analyze the neuroscientific substrates of neuropsychological phenomena: molecular, cellular, multicellular (or systems), and behavioral. These terms constitute the minimal dissection of a complex hierarchical ensemble that we have previously noted to epitomize the principal methods of neuroscience research (see ref. 2). The main underlying concept of neuropsychopharmacology is that drugs which influence behavior and improve the functional status of patients with neurological or psychiatric diseases act by enhancing or blunting the effectiveness of chemical transmission at the sites of principal interneuronal communication, the specialized chemical junctions termed *synapses.*

The intensively exploited molecular level has been the traditional focus for characterizing drugs that alter behavior. Molecular discoveries provide biochemical probes for identifying the appropriate neuronal sites and their mediative mechanisms. Such mechanisms include the neurotransmitters' receptors as well as the auxiliary molecules that allow these receptors to influence the short-term biology of responsive neurons (through regulation of ion channels) and their longer-term regulation (through alterations in gene expression; see Chapters 2, 27, 31, 55, 56, and 61, *this volume*). Molecular level research also provides the pharmacologic tools to verify the working hypotheses of other molecular, cellular, and behavioral strategies and allows for a means to pursue their genetic basis (see Chapters 69, 153, and 155, *this volume*).

During the interval since the previous *Generation of Progress* volume (5), some of the most exciting and rigorous discoveries at the molecular level have been made, finally affording scientists a glimpse into the nature of the molecules that serve as ion channels, as neurotransmitter receptors, and as transporters for the reaccumulation of transmitter into some neurons after its release. At the level of the molecules that make up the transmitter storage and release sites (i.e., the small organelles termed *synaptic vesicles*), virtually every step of the physiological process of loading the transmitter into the vesicles, storing it, moving the vesicle close to the release sites, activating the Ca-dependent process of transmitter release, and then recycling the vesicle for re-use has now been identified (see ref. 4).

The most basic molecular phenomena of neurons are now becoming visualizable in terms of such discrete molecular entities. While it has been known for some time that the basic excitability of neurons was achieved through modifications of the ion channels that all neurons express in abundance in their plasma membranes, it is now possible to understand precisely how the three major cations—Na, K, and Ca—are regulated in their flow through highly discriminated ion channels, and it is also possible to determine how drugs, toxins, and imposed voltages can alter the excitability of a neuron, can allow it to become active spontaneously, or can lead to its death through prolonged opening of such channels. The scope of this work was deemed too detailed for this volume, but several recent compilations of such information may provide the interested reader with starting points (see refs. 1 and 3).

Research at the cellular level determines which specific neurons and which of their most proximate synaptic connections may mediate a behavior or the behavioral effects of a given drug. For example, research at the cellular level into the basis of emotion exploits both molecular and behavioral leads to determine the most likely brain sites at which behavioral changes pertinent to emotion can be analyzed, and it provides the preliminary clues as to the nature of the interactions in terms of interneuronal communication (i.e., excitation, inhibition, or more complex forms of synaptic interaction (see ref. 2; also see Chapter 5, *this volume,* for references).

At present, the most underilluminated phase of this multilevel strategic conceptualization is the multicellular, or systems, level—namely, the means by which events on the behavioral level can be linked to discrete cells and circuits, and obviously vice versa. Such an understanding of systems levels is obligatory, for example, in order to draw together the descriptive structural and functional properties of the central catecholamine neurons and their possible function at the behavioral level. For example, two decades ago brain catecholamines were implicated as "the" critical chemical mediators of a variety of physiological–behavioral outputs of the brain, ranging from feeding, drinking, thermoregulation, and sexual behavior to such abstract actions as pleasure, reinforcement, attention, motivation, memory, learning–cognition, and the major psychoses and their chemotherapy. While many such hypotheses were proposed, there was no conclusive proof that a monoamine "mediates" any behavior (see Chapter 32, *this volume*). Furthermore, a unifying hypothesis as to how any catecholamine cellular system could possibly be legitimately involved in so many global actions was difficult to conceive.

From a purely hypothetical view, one could argue that behavioral tests of a central catecholamine circuit do not require a database of molecular and cellular attributes. In contrast, a cellularly based neurobiologist would argue that until hypotheses of behavioral level functions integrate themselves with the known anatomy and cellular physiology of these transmitter systems, the behavioral interpretations cannot be validated at the cellular level. Thus, a behavioral event lacking intrinsically specified operations for particular cellular sequences is a relatively untestable hypothesis in terms of whether the cells and transmitter system are, in fact, essential for the behavior. For example, with the locus coeruleus system (see Chapters 29 and 33, *this volume*), the recent direct electrophysiological observations in the behaviorally responsive animal provide a far more detailed database on which to formulate specific testable hypotheses regarding a noradrenaline cellular role in specific types of behavior (also see Chapter 34, *this volume*). These cellular data indicate that the locus coeruleus system fires with the occurrence of novel external sensory events, rather than with learning or extinction per se, and that the neurons are under strong inhibitory influences during vegetative acts such as eating, grooming, or sleeping. If we were to take a "bottoms up" approach to analyzing noradrenergic relevant behavior based on these cellular analyses, the suggestion might be that tasks involving contingencies of sensory discrimination of novel objects or during significant environmental demand (stress) might be the most relevant conditions in which to demonstrate behavioral perturbations (see Chapter 32, *this volume*).

In regard to the dopaminergic systems (see Chapter 100, *this volume*), the cellular correlative approach to behavioral function has so far been less rewarding. Better clues to be followed in characterizing the dopaminergic neurons may, in contrast, be a "top down" approach, in which the optimal conditions for seeking cellular correlates would be based upon the results of the behavioral observations. The behavioral observations (see Chapter 25, *this volume*) suggest that a response initiation task would be most critically dependent upon dopaminergic function. If this view were valid, cellular correlates of neuronal firing should then become apparent in such tasks. Clearly, within the functional properties of dopamine neurons lies a robust capacity to maintain and restore their synaptic operations even under conditions in which they have been almost completely ablated (see Chapter 4, *this volume*).

Among the many profound problems awaiting future research is the riddle of how to evolve these tentative behavioral consequences in the normal brain to clarify the possible relevance of the central catecholamine neurons to the behavioral symptoms of the major psychopathologies. Although that extension currently seems unlikely to be realized in the near future, continued attention to a multidisciplinary, multilevel approach to central catecholamine neuron function (or any other specified cellular system) may eventually provide such answers.

Research at the behavioral level (see Chapters 6, 32,

64, 65, 66, and 68, *this volume*) centers on the integrative phenomena that link populations of neurons (often through operationally or empirically defined ways) into extended specialized circuits, ensembles, or more pervasively distributed "systems" that integrate the physiological expression of a learned, reflexive, or spontaneously generated behavioral response. The entire concept of "animal models" of human psychiatric diseases rests on the assumption that scientists can appropriately infer from observations of behavior and physiology (heart rate, respiration, locomotion, etc.) that the states experienced by animals are equivalent to the emotional states experienced by humans expressing these same sorts of physiological changes. Such hypotheses as the catecholamine hypothesis of depression or the dopamine hypothesis of schizophrenia are continuously tested by clinical observations on the neurochemical and neuropharmacological correlates of emotional diseases (e.g., major depression; see Chapter 16, *this volume*) and the anxiety disorders (see Chapter 34, *this volume*) as well as by the emotional consequences of the self-administration of drugs that are addictive in humans (see Chapter 66, *this volume*). Inferences as to the locus of the cells or cell systems central to experimental analysis of emotion have also been provided by lesions or stimulations of specific brain sites (see Chapter 6, *this volume*), and both approaches figure prominently into attempts to establish animals models for at least certain aspects of these complex human conditions (see Chapter 68, *this volume*).

HOW THE BRAIN IS ORGANIZED

The brain is an assembly of interrelated neural systems that regulate their own and each other's activity in a dynamic, complex fashion (2). The major visible regions of the brain can be linked superficially to coarse definitions of brain functions, and within and between these visible macroscopic regions lie interconnected cellular elements which provide their detailed and interdependent operations. Thus, the central nervous system can be subdivided into the forebrain (cerebral cortex, thalamus, and hypothalamus), the midbrain, the hindbrain (pons, medulla, and cerebellum), and the spinal cord. The largest mass consists of the cerebral hemispheres, comprised of the outer cellular zone or cortex, and a number of well-defined subcortical regions, named on the basis of their appearance or location, including several of immediate pertinence to neuropsychopharmacology: the hippocampal formation, the basal ganglia, the amygdaloid complex, the thalamus, and the hypothalamus.

Cerebral hemispheres, in turn, are typically classified into cortical regions on the basis of one of several characteristics such as the sensory modality subserved there (e.g., somatosensory, visual, auditory, or olfactory, while other regions are concerned with motor operations or are

termed "associational" to imply integrations between sensory modalities and motor performance) or the anatomical location (frontal, temporal, parietal, or occipital). An alternative scheme classifies the cortex microscopically in terms of the geometrical relationship between cell types—generally their size, shape, and packing density across the major cortical layers (so-called cytoarchitectonic classifications).

Within any given region of the cerebral cortex, the four or six layers of which it is composed will appear essentially uniform microscopically, and it is thought that ensembles of vertically connected neurons which span the layers comprise the elemental processing modules. The specialized functions of a cortical region arise from the interplay upon this basic module of connections to and from both other regions of the cortex (corticocortical systems) and noncortical areas of the brain (subcortical systems). Varying numbers of adjacent columnar modules may be functionally, but transiently, linked into larger information-processing ensembles. The pathology of Alzheimer's disease (see Chapter 115, *this volume*), for example, destroys the integrity of the columnar modules and the corticocortical connections.

CELLS OF THE BRAIN

At the most elemental level, the cell types found in the nervous system can be divided into neurons and non-neuronal cells. The non-neuronal cells are estimated to outnumber the neuronal cells by at least an order of magnitude. The non-neuronal cells of the central nervous system consist of the *macroglia*, the *microglia*, and the *cells of the vascular elements*, including the intracerebral vessels and the vasculature of the cerebrospinal fluid forming tissues found within the cerebral ventricles, the *choroid plexus*. The *macroglia*, like the neurons, arise from the neuroectoderm, but somewhat later during development (see Chapter 59, *this volume*). This cell class can be further divided into (a) the *astrocytes*, which are interposed between the vasculature and the neurons and which are regarded as serving supportive metabolic roles for the neurons especially within the gray matter of the brain and spinal cord (these metabolic and support functions are described in Chapter 58, *this volume*), and (b) the *oligodendroglia*, a class of cells that produce the myelin coating that allows some axons (the efferent process of neurons) to conduct bioelectric signals rapidly over long distances. The *microglia* are a second form of incompletely characterized central nervous system supportive cells; these cells are believed to be derived from mesodermal origin and are thought to be related to the macrophage monocyte cell lineage. This cell class has some members that are permanently resident in the brain, but the general class may be augmented from the peripheral circulation during injury or acute inflammatory responses (progress in the understanding of the interfaces between the neural and immune systems are described in Chapter 63, *this volume*).

Neurons are the class of cells whose physical interconnections constitute the circuitry of the brain, spinal cord, and the peripheral nervous system and give rise to the multicellular ensembles of neurons which carry out the functions of the nervous system. Neurons are thus regarded as the information-processing elements. Neurons differ widely in their size, shape, location, and other intrinsic properties. Neurons communicate chemically by releasing (or secreting) and responding to a wide range of chemical substances, referred to in the aggregate as *neurotransmitters*. The release of the neurotransmitters is tightly coupled temporally to neuronal activity according to rather stringent functional rules. The sets of chemical substances that neurons can secrete when they are active can also influence the non-neuronal cells. The functional activity of a neuron, measured either through changes in its excitability or by changes in its chemical operations, can also be modified by a different range of chemicals released from non-neuronal cells of the central or peripheral nervous system, and the latter substances are often referred to as *neuromodulators*. Products released by the non-neuronal cells of the immune system that may be present in the brain during acute infections form a major focus of attention in the considerations of neural-immune interactions (see Chapter 63, *this volume*).

Current research on neurotransmitters and neuromodulators is devoted to: (a) understanding the genes (see Chapter 2, *this volume*) that control the synthesis, storage, release, conservation (see Chapter 28, *this volume*), and metabolism of known neurotransmitters; (b) identifying new substances that meet the identifying criteria to be recognized as neurotransmitters; (c) understanding the molecular events by which neurons and other cells react to neurotransmitters (a process often termed *signal transduction,* which cells of the nervous system share with most other cells of the body) in the short-term (see Chapters 27 and 29, *this volume*) and long-term time frame (see Chapters 2 and 56, *this volume*); and (d) understanding the operations of neuronal communication in an integrative context of the circuits that release and respond to specific transmitters, and the way in which these neuronal circuits participate in defined types of behavior, either normal or abnormal.

CONCEPTS OF NEURONAL CIRCUITRY AND SIGNAL TRANSDUCTION IN THE NORMAL BRAIN

After two decades of increasingly precise examination, a very large part of the organization of the mammalian brain's circuitry has been resolved, at least in rodents (see Chapter 3, *this volume;* also see Chapter 23 for dopamin-ergic considerations, Chapter 12 for cholinergic considerations, and Chapter 39 for serotonergic considerations), and the major mechanisms and mediators of signal transduction have been determined (see Chapter 5, *this volume*). From this body of work, three sets of simplifying observations can be extracted for a modern, but hypothetically simplified, view of brain structure and function.

Brain Circuitry Patterns

Three main patterns of neuronal circuitry are recognized:

1. *long hierarchical circuits* (such as those characterizing the interconnected major pathways of the sensory, motor, and intracortical relay systems in which excitatory amino acids are generally the transmitter—see Chapter 7, *this volume*);
2. *local circuit neurons* (such as the short axon neurons, both excitatory and inhibitory, that regulate the extent to which afferent signals can spread, a role frequently subsumed by the inhibitory amino acid transmitters, GABA and GLY (see Chapter 8, *this volume*), and containing one or more neuropeptide co-transmitters (see Chapters 42–51); and
3. *single-source, divergent neurons* (such as those neurons of the brainstem's reticular core nuclei, whose axons diverge to target cells in many parts of the neuraxis, the format exhibited by virtually all of the aminergic neurons (see Chapter 12, *this volume*) and by some of the neuropeptide-containing neurons (see Chapters 46 and 47, *this volume*).

Neurotransmitter Organization

Against this simplified view of neuronal circuitry, the major chemical classes of neurotransmitters may be captured in a similar triadic fashion: *amino acid transmitters,* of which glutamate and aspartate (see Chapter 7, *this volume*) are recognized as the major excitatory transmitting signals, and gamma aminobutyrate (GABA) and glycine (see Chapter 8, *this volume*) as the major inhibitory transmitters; the *aminergic transmitters* (acetylcholine, epinephrine, norepinephrine, dopamine, serotonin, and histamine; each are described in a series of chapters in Section II); and the literally dozens of *peptides* (see Chapter 43, *this volume,* and related chapters that follow). A revolutionary finding has emerged here in concepts of brain system interactions: It would now seem that neuropeptides are almost certainly never the sole signal to be secreted by a central neuron that contains such a signaling molecule, but rather a companion signal to one or more potentially secreted signals. In the best-studied cases, neuropeptides are found with either an amino acid or an amine transmitter at intrasynaptic terminal concentrations a thousand- to a millionfold higher (see Chapter 18, *this volume*). The peptide-containing neurons may also contain a second or third peptide as well (see Chapter 43, *this volume*).

It is also likely, but not yet definitively established, that other kinds of molecules, from purines like adenosine triphosphate (see Chapter 57, *this volume*), lipids like arachidonic acid and prostaglandins (see Chapter 53, *this volume*), and steroids similar to those made and released by the adrenal cortex and the gonads (see Chapters 62, 63, 67, and 80, *this volume*), may also be made by neurons to play important auxiliary roles in intercellular transmission in the nervous system. A recent flurry of activity has revealed that under some conditions active neurons may synthesize gaseous signals (such as nitric oxide and carbon monoxide) that can carry rapidly evanescent signals over short distances (see Chapter 54, *this volume*). Some peptide growth factors can effect trophic actions on cells of the nervous system as well as on non-neuronal cells in many other tissues, while other polypeptide growth factors are selective in their trophic actions (see Chapter 55, *this volume*). Interestingly, some "neuropeptides" have considerable growth potential for non-neuronal cells outside of the central nervous system in addition to their effects in communication between neurons (see Chapter 51, *this volume*).

The bioelectric properties of neurons and their synaptic junctions in the CNS generally follow the general mechanisms of chemical transmission defined for the peripheral somatomotor and autonomic nervous systems (see Chapters 5 and 27, *this volume*). The series of defined steps in the transmission of chemical messages from neurons to their target cells each provide the potential for pharmacological intervention. Transmitters, or drugs that can either stimulate or antagonize them, act at specific molecular recognition sites, termed *receptors*. In molecular morphology, the known classes of receptors also conveniently break down into distinct categories.

In the simplest case, the "ionophore receptor," the receptor is oligomeric (i.e., formed as an assembly of four or five highly similar subunit molecules, which in this case are inferred from their chemical properties to exhibit four transmembrane domains, as well as intracytoplasmic loops that provide links to other transductive sequences). Such a macromolecule constitutes both the functional ion channel to be opened or closed by the action of the transmitter and also contains the sites for recognition and binding of the transmitter. Examples include receptors for GABA and glycine in the CNS (see Chapter 8, *this volume*), the excitatory amino acid glutamate (see Chapter 7, *this volume*), the nicotinic cholinergic receptor (see Chapter 9, *this volume*), and one of the several subtypes of serotonin receptors (see Chapter 38, *this volume*). Multiple forms of the mRNAs that encode one or more of the subunits of several ligand-regulated ion channels have been detected, and it is very likely that different forms

of these receptors are expressed in various types of neurons (see ref. 6).

The mechanism of action of the other major class of neurotransmitter receptors, termed *G-protein-coupled receptors* (see Chapter 61, *this volume*), is clearly more complex and involves the concerted function of a series of interacting macromolecules. These include: the plasma-membrane-bound receptor itself, with its extracellularly oriented ligand-binding domain; the membrane-associated "G proteins" [proteins that specifically bind guanosine triphosphate (GTP) and that hydrolyze it to guanosine monophosphate during this process], which act as transducers by coupling activation of the receptor to regulation of the activity of an effector protein; and the actual effector molecule of the transductive pathway, which may be either a membrane-bound enzyme (e.g., adenyl cyclase) or an ion channel. The genes encoding more than two dozen of these G-protein-coupled receptors have been sequenced, providing for further interesting generalizations. These include muscarinic cholinergic receptors (see Chapter 10, *this volume*), both α- and β-adrenergic receptors (see Chapter 27, *this volume*), all other types of tryptaminergic receptors (see Chapters 37 and 40, *this volume*), and the receptors for all known neuropeptides (see Chapter 43, *this volume*). All G-protein-coupled receptors consist of seven presumptive transmembrane spans, with intervening extracellular and cytoplasmic loops. The ligand-binding sites of these receptors are contributed by several amino acid residues that lie within the transmembrane-spanning segments. The cytoplasmic loops interact with the G protein. Depending on the receptor and the G protein involved, the ultimate result can be activation or inhibition of adenyl cyclase, activation of one or more phospholipases (see Chapter 11, *this volume*), or regulation of the activity of a variety of ion channels (e.g., for K^+ or Ca^{2+}; see Chapter 5, *this volume*).

DRUGS CAN SELECTIVELY MODIFY CNS FUNCTION

The structural and functional properties of neurons provide a means to specify the possible sites at which drugs could interact specifically or generally in the CNS. In this scheme, drugs that affect neuronal energy metabolism (see Chapter 58, *this volume*), membrane integrity, or transmembrane ionic equilibria would be generally acting compounds. Similarly general in action would be drugs that affect the two-way intracellular transport systems by which molecules are transported from the perinuclear cytoplasm of a neuron up the dendrites and down the axons and then back again (e.g., colchicine). These general effects can still exhibit different dose–response or time–response relationships among different neurons based, for example, on such neuronal properties as rate of firing, dependence of discharge on external stimuli or internal pacemakers, resting ionic fluxes, or axon length.

In contrast, when drug actions can be related to specific aspects of the metabolism, release, or function of a neurotransmitter, the site, specificity, and mechanism of action of a drug can be defined by systematic studies of dose–response and time–response relationships. From such data the most sensitive, rapid, or persistent neuronal event can be identified. Transmitter-dependent actions of drugs can be organized conveniently into *presynaptic* and *postsynaptic* categories. Each of these presynaptic or postsynaptic actions is potentially highly specific and can be envisioned as being restricted to a single, chemically defined subset of CNS cells.

The presynaptic category includes all of the events in the perikaryon and nerve terminal that regulate transmitter synthesis (including the acquisition of adequate substrates and cofactors), storage, release, reuptake, and catabolism. Transmitter concentrations can be lowered by blockade of synthesis, storage, or both. The amount of transmitter released per impulse is generally stable but can also be regulated. The effective concentration of transmitter may be increased by inhibition of reuptake or by blockade of catabolic enzymes. The transmitter that is released at a synapse can also exert actions upon the terminal from which it was released by interacting with receptors at these sites (termed *autoreceptors;* see Chapter 21, *this volume*). Activation of presynaptic autoreceptors can slow the rate of release of transmitter and thereby provide a feedback mechanism that controls the concentration of transmitter in the synaptic cleft. Coexisting peptides may also perform similar functions for other aminergic neurons (see Chapters 48 and 50, *this volume*).

The postsynaptic category includes all the events that follow release of the transmitter in the vicinity of the postsynaptic receptor—in particular, the molecular mechanisms by which occupation of the receptor by the transmitter produces changes in the properties of the membrane of the postsynaptic cell (shifts in membrane potential) as well as more enduring biochemical actions (changes in intracellular cyclic nucleotides, protein kinase activity, and related substrate proteins; see Chapters 12, 27, 38, 56, and 61, *this volume*).

FUTURE PERSPECTIVES

Current efforts in neuropsychopharmacology focus in part on the adaptive changes imposed on the nervous system by chronic treatment with drugs (see Chapter 61, *this volume*) and in part on the nature of the ongoing dynamic regulation of neuronal functions in proportion to the demands placed on the behaving organism. Clearly the metabolic and functional changes observed initially on acute treatments of normally behaved animals do not persist and are replaced at varying intervals by changes that may in fact be opposite to those seen acutely. With the ability to clone, sequence, and express the genes that encode receptor molecules for neurotransmitters, a new era in drug development is approaching. Such studies have permitted the identification of novel receptor subtypes that were undetected by traditional pharmacological approaches; the pace of such discovery will accelerate. It is now possible to create novel mouse transgenic mutants in which specific genes have been knocked out or amplified in a few or many cells (see Chapters 2 and 69, *this volume*). Likewise, in normal experimental animals it is possible to inject nucleic acid probes which can (a) hybridize to normal messenger RNAs (so-called antisense probes) for specific receptor proteins or their transductive intermediate proteins and (b) prevent the expression and hence the execution of a particular transductive pathway (see Chapter 48, *this volume*). Furthermore, the incredible number of subunit forms for every neurotransmitter receptor complex generates a molecular heterogeneity which provides an opportunity for still greater pharmacological selectivity. In situ hybridization with appropriate probes facilitates unambiguous cellular localization of individual forms of a receptor and expression of the receptor (see Chapter 19, *this volume*).

In the future, molecular modeling based on the primary amino acid sequence of a receptor should make it possible to define the precise structure of the ligand-binding site and should permit synthesis of novel compounds tailored to these sites (see Chapter 158, *this volume*). Future efforts to provide explanations for drug-induced neurological changes will undoubtedly continue to focus on synaptic transmitters and their mechanisms. If estimates of the complexity of brain-specific mRNA are any indication, many more transmitter-important molecules remain to be discovered (7).

REFERENCES

1. Adams M, Swanson G. Neurotoxins supplement. *Trends Neurosci* 1994;17(4)(Suppl):1–29.
2. Bloom FE. Neurohumoral transmission and the central nervous system. In: Gilman AG, Rall TW, Nies AS, Taylor P, eds. *Goodman and Gilman's: The pharmacological basis of therapeutics.* New York: Pergamon Press, 1990;244–268.
3. Hille B. *Ionic channels of excitable membranes,* 2nd ed. Sunderland, MA: Sinauer, 1992.
4. Jahn R, Südhof TC. Synaptic vesicles and exocytosis. *Annu Rev Neurosci* 1994;17:219–246.
5. Meltzer HY. *Psychopharmacology: The third generation of progress.* New York: Raven Press, 1987;1780.
6. Seeburg PH. The molecular biology of mammalian glutamate receptor channels. *Trends Neurosci* 1993;16(9):359–365.
7. Sutcliffe JG. mRNA in the mammalian nervous system. *Annu Rev Neurosci* 1988;11:157–198.

Psychopharmacology: The Fourth Generation of Progress, edited by Floyd E. Bloom and David J. Kupfer. Raven Press, Ltd., New York © 1995.

CHAPTER **2**

Basic Concepts and Techniques of Molecular Genetics

Samuel H. Barondes

Psychopharmacology has changed a great deal in the more than three decades since this series of books was initiated. Whereas the early emphasis was on direct studies of the effects of drugs on human and animal behavior, interest has progressively turned towards the examination of the brain proteins with which drugs react and of the molecular regulatory mechanisms that control the biosynthesis and cellular function of these proteins. This trend was already apparent in several contributions (including my own) to *Psychopharmacology: A Review of Progress, 1957–1967.* But at that time it was hard to imagine the power of molecular biology to address the structure and function of the myriad of proteins with which drugs interact, and it was also hard to imagine the enormous importance of this work for the development of drugs that influence behavior.

The practical impact of molecular biology, which would have seemed fanciful several decades ago, is now well known even to the general public. For example, the great popularity of the novel and motion picture *Jurassic Park* reflects public awareness of the wide applicability of the DNA revolution. I need not, then, pay much attention, in this chapter, to restating the case for the relevance of molecular genetics to psychopharmacology.

Instead, what I will do is review briefly some of the elementary facts that are assumed in the many applications of molecular genetics that appear throughout this book. I will also call attention to a few of the critical techniques that underlie work that will be considered by other contributors. These techniques are essential for the development of molecular psychopharmacology, a major theme of this volume. For readers who wish more detailed

descriptions of this information, several recent books may be consulted (1–3).

PROPERTIES OF DNA AND OF THE HUMAN GENOME

Genes are made up of deoxyribonucleic acid (DNA). DNA is a long polymer made up of four components, called *deoxyribonucleotides.* Each deoxyribonucleotide has one of the following constituents, called bases: adenine (A), guanine (G), thymine (T), and cytosine (C). A gene contains a few thousand to a few hundred thousand bases that are strung together in a particular sequence. The base sequence of a gene determines the structure of the gene's product, a protein. Other parts of the gene's base sequence determine the way that the gene is expressed during development of the individual and in response to various stimuli.

DNA's role in storing and transferring hereditary information depends on an inmate property of its four constituent bases. Each of these four bases has structural features which lead it to associate with one, and only one, of the other bases. Two bases that can associate with each other are said to be complementary. Guanine and cytosine are complementary to each other as are adenine and thymine.

Complementary base pairing plays an essential role in maintaining the stability of DNA and also in the transfer of its innate information. Stability is brought about because the DNA in our genes consists of two complementary strands which, by interacting with each other, shield the DNA from perturbations. Information is transferred by separating these two strands, which can then act as templates for the synthesis of new nucleic acid molecules.

DNA molecules may be used as templates in two critical ways. First the DNA is used as a template for replicat-

S. H. Barondes: Center for Neurobiology and Psychiatry, Department of Psychiatry, University of California—San Francisco, San Francisco, California 94143.

ing additional copies of DNA, which is essential for cell division. In this case, free deoxyribonucleotides bond with exposed complementary bases in each of the two template strands and are then linked together by an enzyme, DNA polymerase. The product is two new complementary chains which, together, reproduce the template. In DNA replication, complete DNA strands, made up of tens of millions of bases, are copied—so they can be transmitted to new cells. The other way that DNA is used as a template is more selective and has a different purpose. In this case, small bits of a strand are used as a template for the construction of molecules called *messenger RNAs* (mRNAs), each of which carries the message for the synthesis of a particular protein.

Messenger RNAs differ from DNA in a number of ways. First they are much shorter—generally on the order of a thousand to several thousand base pairs long. Second, they are made up of only a single strand (in contrast with double-stranded DNA) that contains all the requisite information to direct the synthesis of a particular protein. They also have a different sugar in their nucleic acid backbone—ribose rather than deoxyribose; and the thymine found in DNA is replaced with a similar base, uracil (U) in mRNA. Like thymine, uracil is complementary to adenine.

The entire human genome consists of about 100,000 genes distributed within a total DNA sequence of about 3 billion nucleotides. The DNA of the human genome is divided into 24 huge molecules, each the essential constituent of a particular chromosome (22 autosomes and two different sex chromosomes, X and Y). When we are conceived we receive 23 chromosomes from each parent, 22 autosomes and a sex chromosome.

As already indicated, a major function of a gene is to encode the structure of a specific protein. Translation of the information encoded in DNA (which is expressed in an alphabet of nucleotides) into a protein (which is expressed in an alphabet of amino acids) depends on a genetic code. In this code, sequences of three nucleotides, called a *codon*, represent one of the 20 amino acids that comprise the building blocks of all proteins. Because there are 64 possible codons that can be constructed from an alphabet consisting of four different bases, and only 20 different amino acids to be coded for, many amino acids are encoded by more than one particular codon. Three of the codons, called *stop codons*, are used to signal termination of translation.

Although all cells express certain genes that are required for their shared housekeeping functions, the distinctive differences between specialized cells (such as particular classes of neurons) are due to selective gene expression. For example, in the nervous system certain neurons use acetylcholine and others use dopamine as neurotransmitters. This results from selective expression of genes that encode specific proteins (in this case enzymes) that catalyze the biosynthesis of either acetylcho-

line or dopamine. Expression of these genes is ultimately under the control of specific regulatory proteins, called *transcription factors,* that bind to regions of the genes. These regulatory proteins control the transcription of mRNA from the genes they control. The regulatory proteins that control specific genes are, themselves, selectively expressed during the maturation of the particular classes of neurons.

Expression of enzymes that control biosynthesis of neurotransmitters is controlled not only by factors that operate during embryonic development, but also by factors that influence the adult organism. For example, the synthesis of certain of these enzymes depends, in part, on neuronal activation. When there is more neuronal activation, more of a critical enzyme is made and, as a result, the neuron makes more of the neurotransmitter. Complex regulation of genes involved in neurotransmitter biosynthesis (and of other genes for receptors and transporters that determine neurotransmitter function) may play important roles in the control of behavior. Regulation of genes also determines the response of the nervous system to drugs, the central concern of this volume.

The study of these genetic and cellular regulatory processes is one of the most active areas of contemporary biology. At present a great deal is being learned about the specific base sequences, called *regulatory sequences,* that surround the portions of the gene dedicated to encoding the sequence of a protein. These sequences are activated or inactivated by the specific transcription factors that bind to and control them. The complex interaction of regulatory sequences and transcription factors underlies adaptation of the brain to drugs. In the case of antidepressants and neuroleptics, these adaptive changes are essential for the therapeutic effect, which only develops after weeks of drug treatment. Because adaptive changes are essential, understanding them should lead to the design of new psychopharmacological agents.

MANIPULATING DNA

One of the ultimate goals of molecular genetics is to determine the exact base sequence of all 3 billion bases that comprise the human genome. This task is very challenging because DNA molecules are gigantic, which makes them extremely difficult to deal with.

A major step toward achieving this goal came from development of methods to isolate, and then examine, the bite-size pieces of DNA that had been transcribed into mRNAs. The information encoded into mRNAs can be isolated and amplified by a technique called cDNA cloning (Fig. 1). In this technique, a mixture, containing all the mRNAs from an organ, such as the brain, are first purified. The mixture of mRNAs are then treated with an enzyme, called *reverse transcriptase,* which transcribes the mRNAs into single complementary strands of DNA

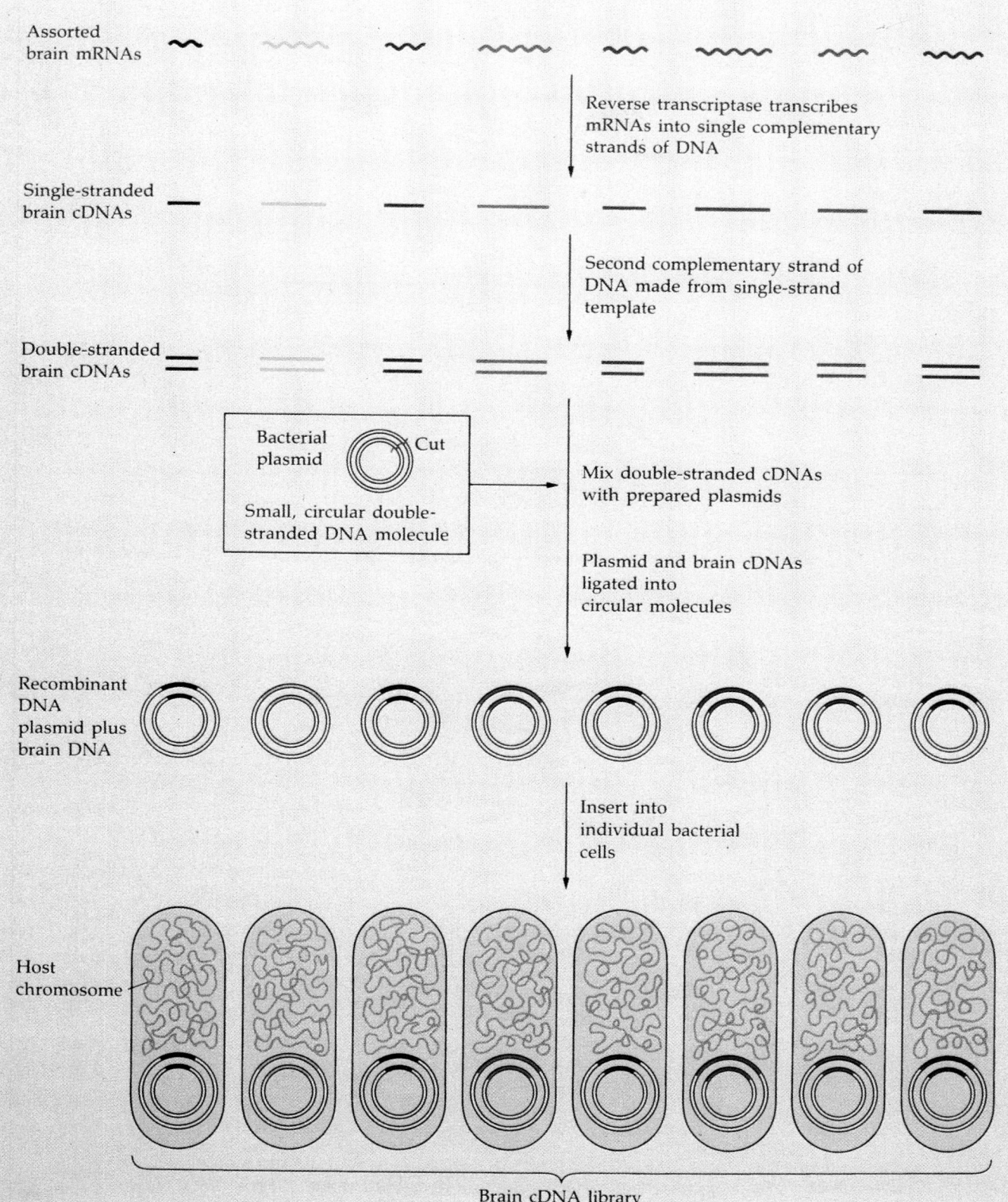

Assorted brain mRNAs

Reverse transcriptase transcribes mRNAs into single complementary strands of DNA

Single-stranded brain cDNAs

Second complementary strand of DNA made from single-strand template

Double-stranded brain cDNAs

Bacterial plasmid — Cut

Small, circular double-stranded DNA molecule

Mix double-stranded cDNAs with prepared plasmids

Plasmid and brain cDNAs ligated into circular molecules

Recombinant DNA plasmid plus brain DNA

Insert into individual bacterial cells

Host chromosome

Brain cDNA library

FIG. 1. Making a brain cDNA library. A mixture of brain mRNAs are transcribed to make cDNAs. Each cDNA is ligated into an opened plasmid, a circular piece of bacterial DNA engineered so it will accept cDNA. The plasmid is also engineered to contain regulatory elements so that the cDNA will be transcribed in appropriate cells (bacterial or human as required). The closed plasmids, each containing a cDNA, are then inserted into bacteria. When the bacteria grow and divide, they not only replicate their own DNA but also make copies of the plasmid with the cDNA. (From ref. 2.)

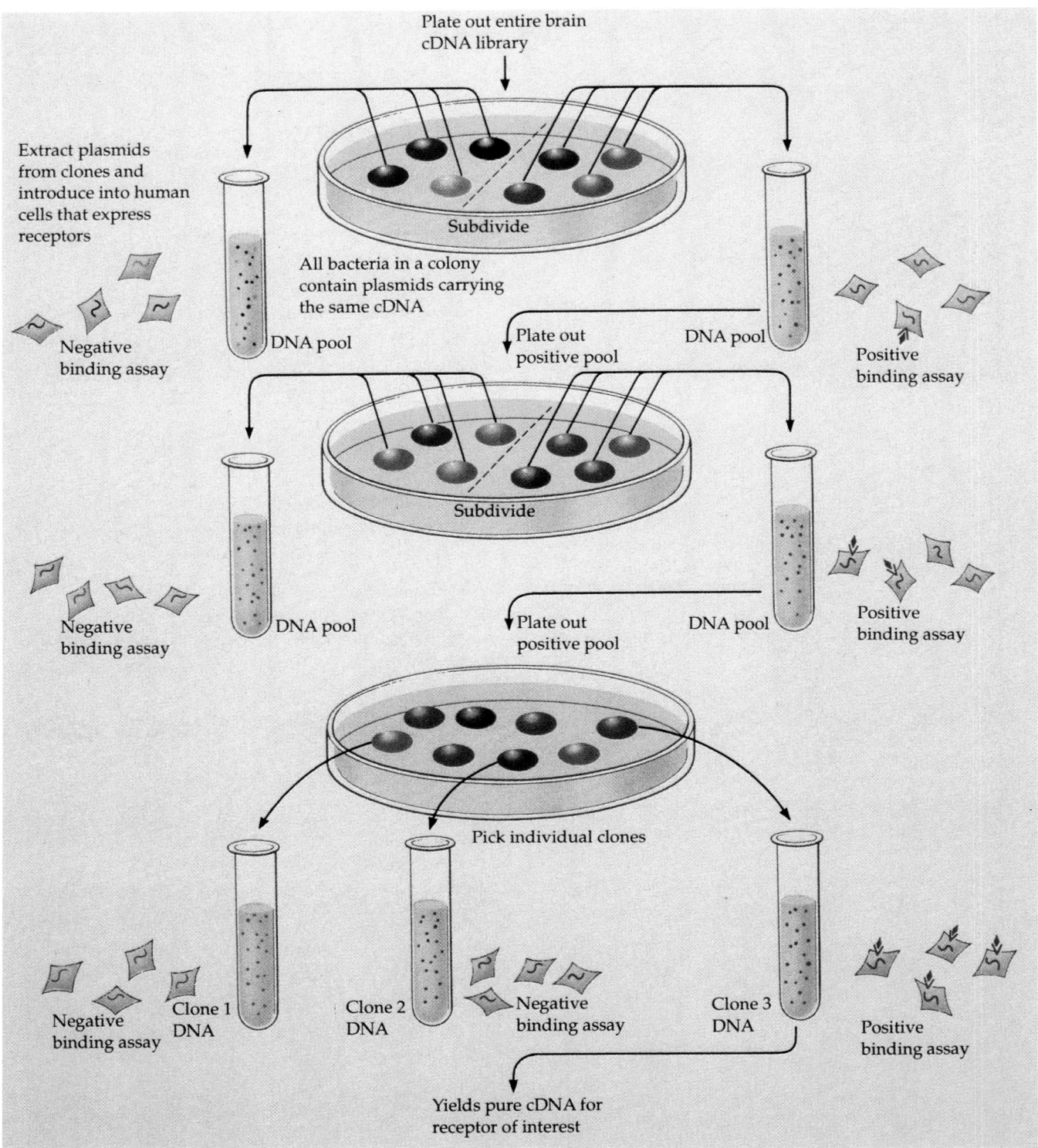

FIG. 2. Selecting a clone that contains the cDNA for a neurotransmitter receptor. A brain cDNA library is plated on a solid agar surface at a low density so that each bacterium in the library is widely separated from its neighbors. The agar contains nutrients enabling the bacteria to grow and divide. The descendants of each bacterium remain close to it and together are a clone, each member containing the same cDNA. To screen for the receptor of interest, the clones from each half of the plate are introduced into a population of human cells in tissue culture. If a clone encoding the receptor of interest is inserted into a human cell, the receptor is synthesized and inserted on the cell's surface. Cells containing this receptor are detected with a ligand-binding assay. The clones from the part of the plate that are found to be positive in this assay are then diluted (because each clone contains thousands of bacteria) and applied to a new plate. By repeating this process, most brain cDNAs are eliminated. It then becomes practical to sample and assay each remaining clone directly until the desired one is found. (From ref. 2.)

called *complementary DNA* (cDNA). Single-stranded cDNAs are then used as templates to make a second strand that is complementary to the first; and the double-stranded cDNAs are then inserted into bacterial plasmids to make products called *recombinant DNA plasmids*. The plasmids are then inserted into specially engineered bacteria in which they are replicated, along with the bacterial DNA, during the process of bacterial cell division. In this way many copies of the cDNAs are made. The bacterial population is comprised of many individual bacteria, each of which contains a particular plasmid with a particular cDNA derived from an mRNA from the original tissue sample. This mixed population is called a *cDNA library*.

To physically separate the individual members of the library, the bacteria are grown on a solid nutrient agar at low density. Each bacterium in the library is plated onto the agar at a large distance from the others. As each bacterium divides on the agar, it gives rise to a colony of descendants called a *clone*, which is physically separate from other clones derived from other bacteria that contain other cDNAs. Each member of a clone carries copies of the cDNA-containing plasmid that had been inserted into the clone's founder. Each clone may then be separately removed from the agar (without contamination with bacteria from other clones), and bacteria that all contain the particular cDNA may be grown up in large quantities. Then the cDNA within the plasmids can be excised, and its nucleotide sequence can be determined by chemical techniques. The cloned cDNA may also be used for many other purposes, a few of which are discussed later.

Of course the brain expresses many mRNAs that are also expressed by other tissues and that may have no special interest for neurobiological or pharmacological research. In most studies of brain cDNA the goal is to find the one that encodes the sequence of a particular protein of interest, such as a receptor protein for a particular neurotransmitter. There are many ways to go about searching for a specific cDNA (and its specific clone). One involves insertion of cDNA-containing plasmids (derived from bacterial clones) into cultured mammalian cells (such as fibroblasts) that can express the neurotransmitter receptor on their cell surface (in contrast with bacteria which do not process the cDNAs in the same way). The cDNA of interest is sought by reacting the mammalian cell population with a ligand (such as a neurotransmitter or a drug that binds the receptor that is being sought) and isolating the cells that bind the ligand, as shown schematically in Fig. 2.

Once a particular cDNA is isolated, it can be used to make limitless quantities of the protein whose sequence it encodes. For some proteins, this can be done in bacteria. In this case the plasmid can be induced to make mRNA that is translated by the bacterial protein-synthesizing machinery. However, in many cases the translation is done in mammalian cells, so that the protein product not only has the amino acids sequence encoded by the cDNA, but

also undergoes appropriate post-translational modifications, such as glycosylation, which do not occur with expression in bacterial cells. In the case of neurotransmitter receptors the desired product may not be a pure soluble receptor protein, but may instead be a mammalian population of cells that express the receptor as a protein integrated into the plasma membrane on the cell surface. Cells with a particular receptor on their surface can then be used to screen for drugs that bind this receptor.

Cloned cDNA can also be used as a reagent in a variety of biological and medical studies. These are generally based on the innate property of nucleic acids to undergo complementary base paring, so that a single-stranded cDNA will bind to complementary nucleic acid sequences in mixtures of human nucleic acid, or even in tissue sections, by a process called *hybridization*. If the cDNA probe has been prepared in a radioactive form, the amount of radioactive cDNA that hybridizes to an aliquot of a tissue extract provides a measure of the amount of the mRNA that is complementary to it in the tissue extract. The radioactive cDNA probe can also be applied to brain tissue sections to localize the mRNA in specific neuronal populations in the brain, by a process called *in situ* hybridization. In this way the distribution of a particular protein, such as a receptor, can be inferred by determining the distribution of the mRNA that codes for this protein. The distribution of a particular receptor may have important implications for the design of drugs that are targeted to a specific brain region.

MANIPULATING GENES

Once it became possible to isolate cDNAs that encode proteins of particular interest, a variety of techniques were developed to use the cDNAs to learn about the function of the proteins. The basic idea is to insert the cDNAs (modified by the addition of regulatory sequences that make possible their controlled expression; and, at times, also modified in other ways) into cells, then measure specific effects. Some of these studies are done in cells in tissue culture, whereas others are done by changing the genetic composition of intact organisms. This type of gene manipulation underlies very powerful approaches to the study of the function of given proteins, and it also provides cell types and animals with many applications in psychopharmacological research.

The simplest manipulation of this type is to introduce a new gene (or many additional copies of a particular gene) into a cultured cell line, a process called *transfection*. This is accomplished by engineering the cDNA into various vectors, such as appropriate plasmids, that will carry it into the cell and allow it to be expressed. In one form of transfection, called *stable transfection*, the cDNA (along with regulatory sequences) or other type of foreign DNA is stably integrated into the DNA of a chromosome.

When a cell of this type replicates its DNA for cell division, the integrated cDNA is also replicated and transmitted to the daughter cells. To obtain stably transfected cells it is necessary to select them from a population that consists largely of cells that have not integrated the cDNA of interest.

The desired cells may be selected from a mixed population that also consists of many cells that do not contain the desired cDNA by a trick of genetic engineering. The trick is to transfect the cDNA of interest along with other DNA that makes possible the survival of transfected cells under experimentally induced toxic conditions. For example, the transfected DNA may include a sequence for a protein that renders the recipient cell resistant to a toxic compound so that only cells containing the transfected DNA (including the cDNA of interest) will survive if this toxic compound is added to the culture medium. In this way, clones of cells that contain the cDNA of interest can be isolated and used for various purposes.

To make animals that express a particular segment of foreign DNA, it is possible to inject this particular DNA into one-celled embryos. The DNA is then integrated into the genome of the recipient embryo and into all its cells, including its germ cells, so that it will be transmitted to future generations. Most of these experiments are done with mice, and a single mouse with a segment of foreign DNA incorporated into its genome can give rise to a line of mice, each of which has the foreign DNA, which is called a *transgene*. Such mice are called *transgenic mice*. Regulatory sequences surrounding the coding sequence of the transgene may bring it under specific control. For example, certain regulatory sequences will direct expression of the transgene only in a particular cell type, such as muscle cells.

A particularly interesting variety of transgenic mice has a foreign gene inserted not in addition to, but in place of, a normal gene. This is accomplished by a technique in which a normal gene is removed from a chromosome in the same process in which the foreign gene is inserted. One common application of this approach is to replace a normal gene in the germ line with one that is inactive or defective, thereby giving rise to progeny that lack the normal gene and its function. By mating brothers and sisters each with one defective gene copy, progeny can be raised that have two defective genes (i.e., no normal copies of the gene). Such "*knockout experiments*" are one way of examining the normal biological role of the gene in question.

In some cases the results are not very informative because absence of the functional gene during early embryonic development results in the death of the embryo. In other cases, loss of a particular gene has no obvious effect, presumably because other genes take over for the one that was inactivated. In many cases, however, mice that lack a particular gene have proved useful for determining a particular gene's function. In the context of the present volume, mice lacking a particular receptor for a neurotransmitter may provide clues to this receptor's function in the cells that express it, and in the animal as a whole. Animals lacking a particular receptor may also prove useful for certain approaches to drug development.

IMPLICATIONS FOR PSYCHOPHARMACOLOGY

It should be apparent from this brief review that molecular genetics is already providing tools that will facilitate the design of new drugs that influence behavior. Just the simple availability of a specific cell line that expresses only one receptor for a neurotransmitter (in contrast with many, in usual neuronal cell lines) represents an important technical advance in drug screening procedures. The ability to screen brain sections by in situ hybridization with specific cDNAs allows for precise localization of neurotransmitter receptors and receptor subtypes (e.g., see Chapters 3 and 19, *this volume*) with an accuracy and detail not achievable by other approaches. There are also many potential applications of transgenic mice in drug design (see Chapters 69 and 158, *this volume*).

There may also come a time when genes themselves will be used as drugs (see Chapters 115, 132, 143, 153, and 159, *this volume*). Already attempts are being made to treat certain diseases, caused by the absence of a specific enzyme, by removing the patient's cells, transfecting them with the cDNA that directs the synthesis of the enzyme, and then injecting the cells back into the patient. In this way, sustained enzyme expression can be achieved. Applications of such cellular engineering to psychopharmacology are presently being considered. Molecular genetic techniques are also being used in human genome screening designed to search for genes that may be responsible for psychiatric disorders such as bipolar disorder and schizophrenia. Should such genes be found, their identity may point the way to specific psychopharmological treatment.

Given the increasing power of molecular genetics, it is safe to predict that its impact on psychopharmacology will become progressively more significant in the years to come. A decade from now, with the publication of the next volume in the series, there should be many new and interesting applications to consider.

REFERENCES

1. Alberts B, Bray D, Lewis J, Raff M, Roberts K, Watson JD. *Molecular biology of the cell,* 2nd ed. New York: Garland Publishing, 1989.
2. Barondes SH. *Molecules and mental illness.* New York: WH Freeman, 1993.
3. Watson JD, Gilman M, Witkowski J, Zoller M. *Recombinant DNA,* 2nd ed. New York: Scientific American Books, 1992.

Psychopharmacology: The Fourth Generation of Progress, edited by Floyd E. Bloom and David J. Kupfer. Raven Press, Ltd., New York © 1995.

CHAPTER 3

Cytology and Circuitry

Stanley J. Watson, Jr. and William E. Cullinan

This chapter is a discussion of the principles involved in the application of anatomical–biochemical methods to the study of the brain. It emphasizes the cell biological aspects of neuronal function, as well as neuronal operation in the context of multicellular circuits. The aim of this chapter, in conjunction with the preceding chapter on molecular biology and the following on neurochemistry, is that of (a) an appreciation of the larger principles governing genomic functioning at the cellular level and (b) a sense of the essentials of neurotransmission within neuronal circuits (see also Chapter 5, *this volume*).

The initial section is a brief review of molecular aspects of neurochemistry, enabling the reader to focus on key biochemical elements used to study cellular regulation. For example, it is important to appreciate the functions of different types of neuronal proteins in order to readily understand the techniques used to study them in cell and circuit contexts. Among such sets of proteins are the biosynthetic enzymes (e.g., tyrosine hydroxylase), receptors (e.g., D_2 dopamine receptor), and peptide precursors (e.g., pro-opiomelanocortin). Equally important is an understanding of the related actions of the gene encoding them, their transcription into messenger RNA (mRNA), and translation into protein. The body of the chapter focuses on the conceptual framework underlying the methods reviewed, rather than being a technical "cookbook." We will attempt to present a clear view of the rationale behind the method, followed by a brief analysis of particular advantages and limitations. Four main approaches will be emphasized: receptor autoradiography, immunocytochemistry, in situ hybridization histochemistry, and neuroanatomical tract-tracing. We hope to convey how the complementary nature of information gained through the application of these methods has helped move neuroscience research to a level of power and sophistication previously unattainable. The goal of this chapter is then really twofold: to briefly highlight key elements of neuronal cell biology, and to indicate the breadth of available tools for studying neuronal regulation in an anatomical context.

PRINCIPLES OF NEURONAL CELL BIOLOGY: RELEVANCE TO BIOCHEMICAL ANATOMY

Among the unique components of neurons are those focused on generating an action potential, producing neurotransmitters, and receiving transynaptic signals. Most of neurobiology and much of biological psychiatry thus depends in part on the analysis of these elements of brain functioning. At its core, the neuron is specialized in its ability to be "excited" by incoming signals and to pass that (modified) information on to other cells. As we look at a typical neuron (Fig. 1), some of the essential elements for this communication can be seen, including a host of specialized proteins. If we begin with a vesicle in a typical dopamine neuron in the substantia nigra, for example, we see that it contains a set of synthetic enzymes—in this case tyrosine hydroxylase and aromatic amino acid decarboxylase—which are responsible for the conversion of the amino acid tyrosine into dopamine. Furthermore, this dopamine vesicle might contain a peptide precursor (e.g., pro-neurotensin) and the enzymes necessary for its processing (as many as 3–6 different types of peptidases) into the final active peptide product, neurotensin. As this vesicle is moved from the cell body to the terminal by an elaborate transport system, these enzymes act to produce their final transmitter products. At the synapse, vesicles are accumulated so that at the appropriate electrochemical signal (involving another major class of proteins) their products are released into the synaptic cleft. The postsynaptic cell "senses" the released dopamine and neurotensin by their action on specific dopamine and neurotensin receptors, which had been previously

S. J. Watson, Jr. and W. E. Cullinan: Mental Health Research Institute, University of Michigan, Ann Arbor, Michigan 48109.

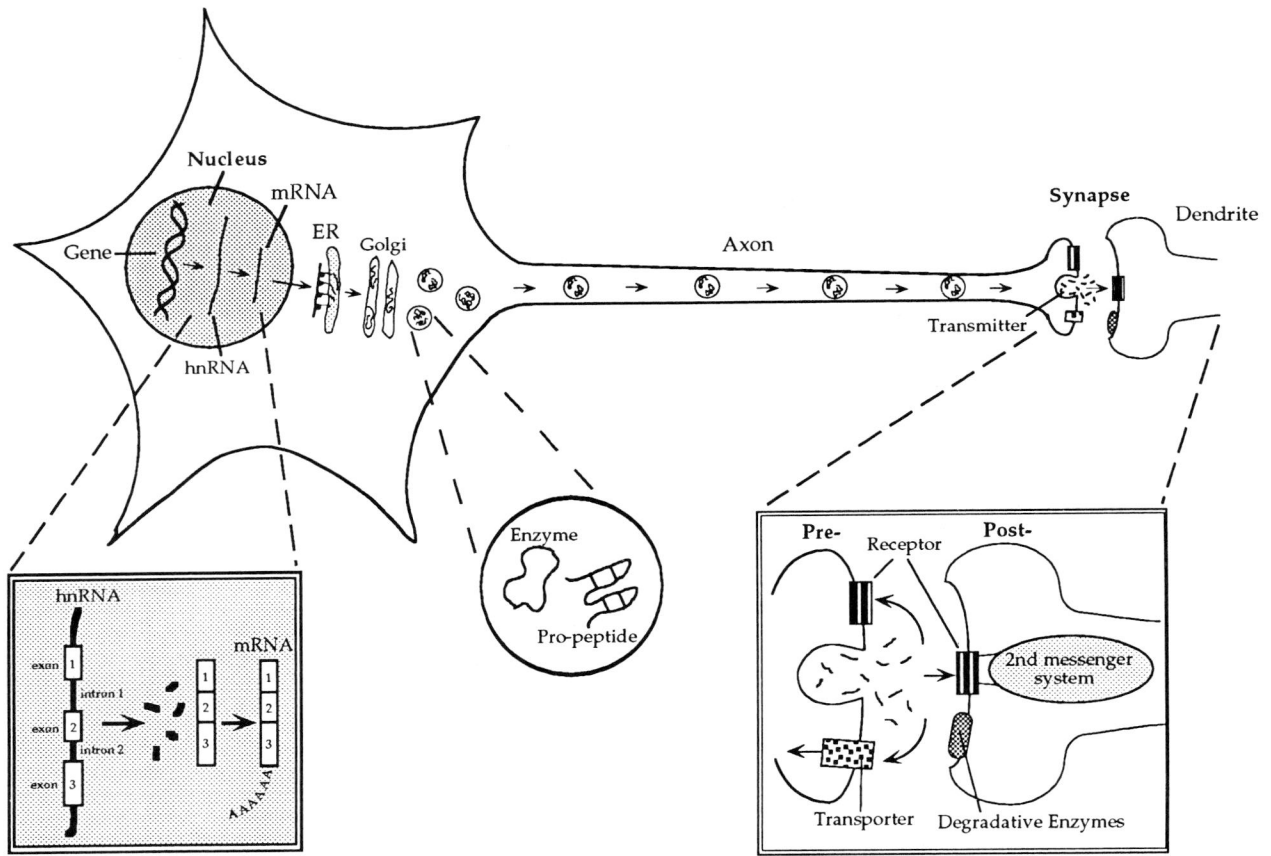

FIG. 1. Diagram illustrating the biosynthesis and transport of neurotransmitters, their synthesizing enzymes, and neuropeptides, as well as neurotransmitter release.

synthesized and inserted into the membrane. It is clear that many other types of proteins are active in this signaling process. For example, transduction from the receptor to a series of second- and third-order messenger proteins involves a host of molecules, among them channels, G proteins, cyclases, kinases, and transacting factors (see Chapters 11, 27, and 38, *this volume*). Beyond this array of postsynaptic activity are a series of residual actions on the presynaptic side. For example, monoamines are usually removed from the synapse into the cytosol by a transmitter-specific transporter (see Chapters 11 and 28, *this volume*); there the transmitter (dopamine) can be moved into the vesicle for re-use (an event accomplished by yet another specific protein), or it can be metabolized by degradative enzymes (e.g., monoamine oxidase). Dopamine remaining in the synapse can also activate another dopamine receptor subtype on the dopamine-producing cell. This dopamine "autoreceptor" inhibits further dopamine release into the synapse (see Chapter 10, *this volume*).

The foregoing discussion was presented in order to highlight the diversity of proteins needed for effective neurotransmission. It is indeed these very proteins which can be used to study neuronal regulation in brain. The reader may notice that this discussion began with a complement of mature proteins in neurons. Neurobiology texts often begin there in part because this was basically the extent of our knowledge regarding them 10–15 years ago. As the fields of cell biology and molecular biology have grown, it has become clear that all cells use the same fundamental genetic and protein synthetic machinery. The proteins critical to neuronal functioning are thus the products of standard transcriptional and translational processes. We now turn to a brief description of some of these early events, before describing the aforementioned histochemical and anatomical methods.

GENE TRANSCRIPTION AND RNA TRANSLATION INTO PROTEIN

As seen in Fig. 1, the double-stranded DNA of the gene is transcribed into a long, single-stranded RNA molecule. This primary RNA transcript [itself a member of a family of RNAs known as *heteronuclear RNA* (hnRNA)] is a full copy of the gene containing introns and exons alike. Introns are parts of the gene which are not represented in the final mature mRNA; exons are the parts of the gene which comprise the mRNA. After production of this primary transcript, it is then acted upon by a series of splicing enzymes which remove all introns, so all that remains is a series of connected exons. Prior to moving out of the nucleus, this RNA is capped at its 5′ end with a special nucleotide, and a 3′ tail of adenines is attached (often 100–200 A's in length). It is now a mature mRNA and passes into the cytoplasm for translation into protein. Free mRNA forms a complex with ribosomal and transfer RNA machinery, ultimately leading to the formation of the peptide chain. Thus, regardless of whether the focus of study is a protein in the form of an enzyme, peptide precursor, or receptor, it is possible to examine the process of its synthesis in the cell body by quantitating hnRNA (to estimate rates of gene transcription) or, much more commonly, mRNA (to infer the ability of the cell to rapidly synthesize protein).

RECEPTOR AUTORADIOGRAPHY

The study of a receptor protein could be carried out in a number of ways. The protein could be localized by the use of antibodies (immunocytochemistry), its mRNA

could be detected (in situ hybridization), or, as described below, it could be localized by virtue of its binding by a radiolabeled ligand (receptor autoradiography). Each of these methods provides a distinct class of information. While immunocytochemistry reflects protein localization, and in situ hybridization can give information about the cell bodies of origin and amount of a specific mRNA, receptor autoradiography reflects the location and amount of binding activity of the receptor protein itself. The central issue in the use of this method is that the *binding activity* of the protein must be expressed in the tissue preparation under study. It is generally assumed that the receptor protein is intact, is properly inserted in the membrane (if that is its natural location), and is in a chemically proper environment (or at least a workable one). For example, inappropriate salts, fixatives, or protein degradative agents can alter binding. Below we discuss this method in more detail and emphasize some advantages and limitations.

Method

The original work on receptor autoradiography actually began with the infusion of radiolabeled ligands into living

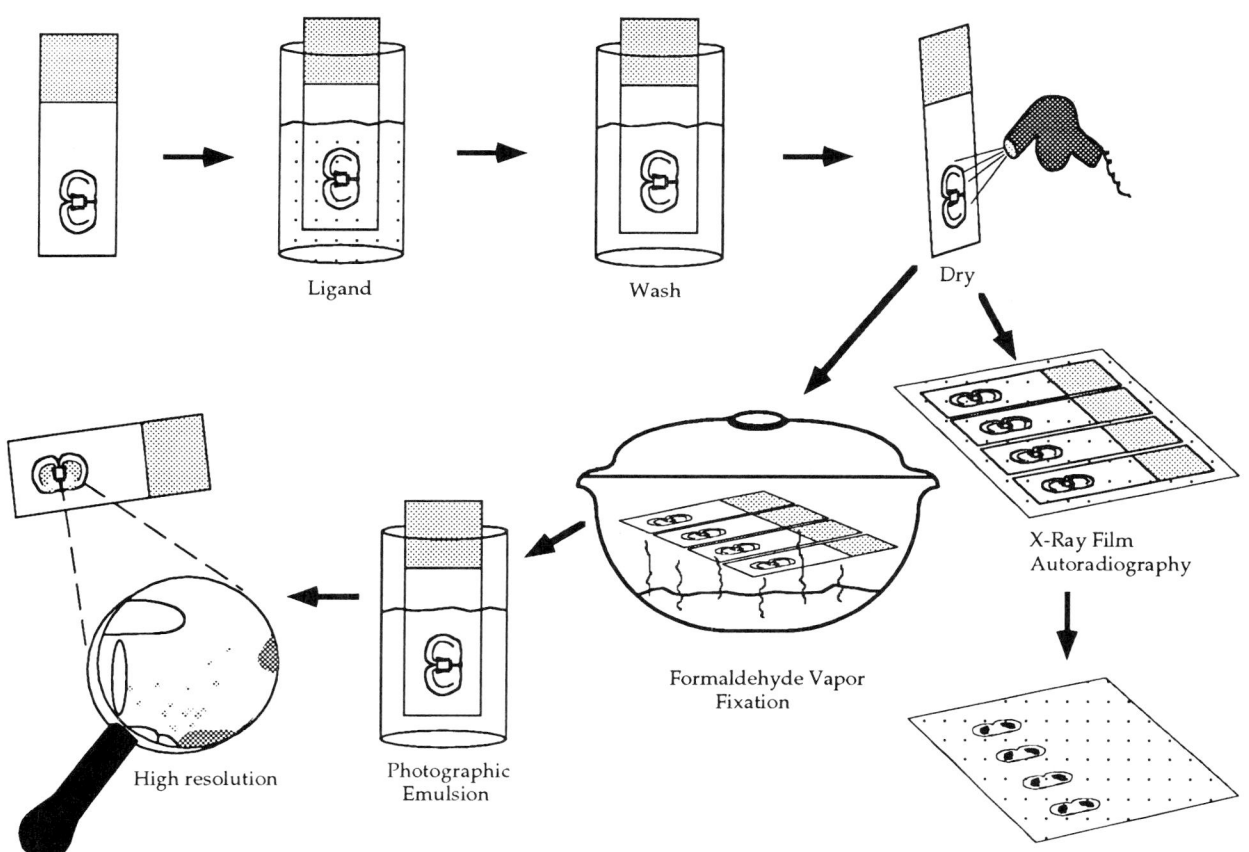

FIG. 2. Summary diagram of steps involved in the receptor autoradiographic method.

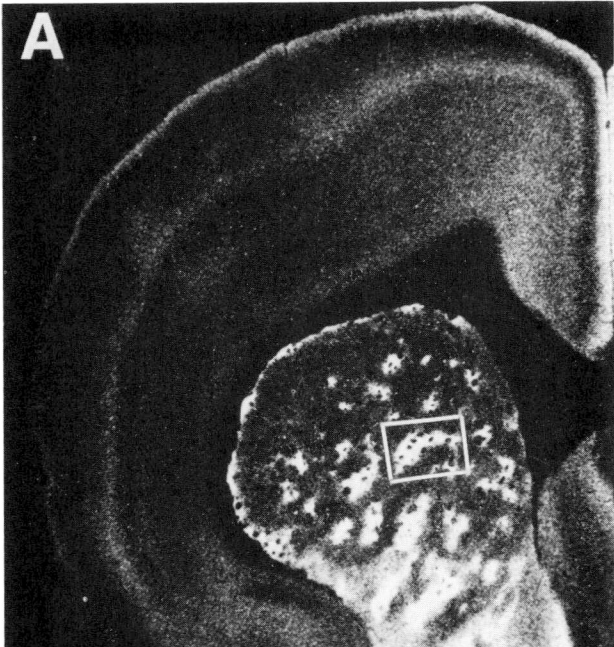

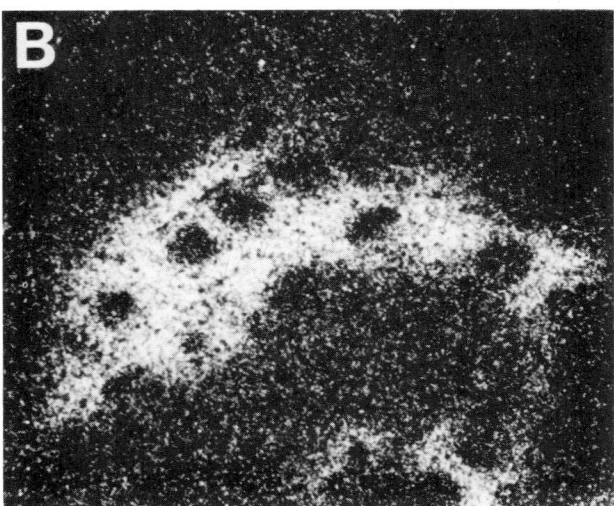

FIG. 3. **A:** Dark-field photomicrograph illustrating distribution of mu opioid receptor binding sites in a coronal hemisection of rat forebrain labeled by [³H]-DAGO. Note the patchy appearance of binding within the striatum. **B:** Boxed area in **A** is shown at higher magnification. (Courtesy of Dr. Alfred Mansour.)

animals (21). Under the proper conditions, the ligand passed into the central nervous system (CNS) and was bound, and this ligand–receptor complex could be visualized autoradiographically. This early method was very expensive, time-consuming, and complex. A real revolu-

tion in ease, flexibility, and efficiency occurred with the introduction of the tissue slice method (see Fig. 2) (17,27,28,44). In brief, whole frozen rat brain was sectioned on a freezing microtome (or cryostat) and slide-mounted. These tissue sections (10–30 μm) contained relatively undamaged membranes, including most of the receptor proteins in them. The slides were briefly washed in an appropriate buffer and subsequently immersed in a vial of buffered radiolabeled ligand, during which the receptor–ligand complex forms. (Often the investigator must invest considerable initial effort in establishing the proper binding parameters and conditions, including the buffer composition and concentration, time and temperature of incubation, and, of course, the appropriate ligand and its concentration. It can take many carefully planned runs to optimize these conditions.) Following binding, the slides are usually washed in a cooled buffer to remove unbound ligand (nonspecific binding), thereby leaving specific binding on the tissue section. Again, time, temperature, and the composition of buffer involved in this step are often carefully studied to establish optimal conditions. Finally the slides are removed from the wash and rapidly dried (in a stream of air). The goal here is to remove water quickly to prevent diffusion of the ligand away from the binding site, thus preserving the anatomical precision of the binding.

The binding step itself is often modified for a variety of technical purposes. For example, adding excess unlabeled ligand (or a pharmacological analog) during the binding step is a method for addressing pharmacological specificity and pharmacokinetic issues (K_d, B_{max}, etc.). It is often at this step that receptor subtypes and ligand "cross-reactivity" issues can be clarified, in that different ligands and conditions can be compared between serial or sequential sections containing the same anatomical structures and receptor composition.

After drying, the slides can be placed next to x-ray film in a light-tight cassette for a period of time ranging from a few hours to months (see Fig. 2). The range of exposure time of the tissue sections against the x-ray film is determined by the specific activity of the ligand, the number of bound receptors in the section, and the nature of the radioactive marker attached to the ligand. In order to produce higher-resolution information, slides can be fixed and subsequently dipped in photographic emulsion and later developed (Fig. 2). This thin coating of radiation-sensitive particles is capable of providing 1- to 2-μm resolution (in the case of a low-energy ³H emitter). Thus, even intracellular resolution is possible.

Both methods (x-ray film and liquid emulsion) require that the investigator determine the appropriate exposure period. Emulsions, either liquid or film, have a range 10- to 15-fold from threshold detection to complete saturation. For example, if one had a signal 50-fold that of the threshold after 2 days of exposure, the autoradiogram would exceed saturation and be overexposed. For the investigator to attempt reasonable quantitation, it is essential to keep the exposure time within the linear range of the film (roughly the middle 10-fold from threshold to saturation).

Thus, in the example above (50-fold signal at 2 days), one would need to decrease the exposure intensity (from 50-fold to about 5-fold), which could be done by reducing the exposure time by a factor of 10 (to 4.8 hours). Of course, the labeled tissue may be re-exposed to different x-ray films until a correct exposure is obtained. For emulsion-dipped slides, several series of test slides are developed after different time periods to establish optimal exposure time for the body of the experiment. The photomicrograph in Fig. 3 illustrates the results of such an autoradiographic study, in this case involving the localization of a class of opiate receptors.

Having established a set of binding conditions for a particular ligand and also having produced autoradiograms within the dynamic range of the emulsion, it is now possible to quantitate the binding. Such quantitation is usually undertaken to compare specific binding across anatomical regions, to evaluate receptor subtypes within a tissue region, or to study changes in receptor levels within regions after various treatments. The methods commonly used in quantitation of autoradiographic data involve digitization of the x-ray (or emulsion dipped) signal, and passage of data to a common personal computer. Along with the digitized value of the autoradiographic signal, separate values for the background area, and area containing only nonspecific binding are usually taken. Through subtraction of background and nonspecific binding, an estimate value for specific binding is obtained. By comparing the signal density (per square micron) with densities produced by a series of known radioactive standards, and knowing the specific activity of the ligand, it is possible to calculate the number of moles of labeled ligand per gram of tissue.

Advantages

The advantages of receptor autoradiography have become increasingly clear over the last decade, making it a standard technique in a large part of biology. The validity of the method has been supported by data using alternative methods for localization of receptors (or their mRNAs) such as immunocytochemistry and in situ hybridization (see below and Chapter 19, *this volume*). Advantages include:

1. Pharmacological relevance in an anatomical context.
2. Medium to high level of anatomical resolution.
3. Ability to quantitate receptor binding, and thereby estimate number and affinity of receptor binding sites, allowing the study of regulation of receptor systems in a large number of tissues, systems, and conditions.

Limitations

1. Because receptor proteins are largely transported along axonal or dendritic processes, much ambiguity can arise in the distinction between neuronal perikarya and other cellular processes.
2. The slice autoradiographic method is limited with respect to complex biochemical techniques. For example, the best binding conditions for the natural ligand may be different than those for a pharmacological analogue, and might be difficult to process on a tissue slice. Moreover, the second messenger system coupling actions of the receptor may differentially affect the affinity of the natural ligand or analogue for the site.
3. Finally, even with our best pharmacological efforts, it is clear that we do not have ligands capable of selectively binding to many of the receptors that have been cloned, and thus it is probable that in some instances more than one receptor type is bound. While this issue is slowly being resolved as new clones and ligands come to the fore, it is important not to lose sight of the fact that one is detecting ''binding activity'' only, rather than a specific gene product or protein itself.

IMMUNOCYTOCHEMISTRY

Immunocytochemistry is a method for studying proteins in an anatomical context through the use of specific antibodies directed to detect a particular antigen in tissue (see ref. 34). Briefly, the tissue to be studied is fixed so that the antigen (protein) is kept in place (and not degraded). An antibody directed against that target protein binds it in a thinly sectioned piece of tissue. After washing to remove excess antibody, a second series of antibodies or other marker protein is used to visualize the original (or primary) antibody, thereby indirectly marking the location of the protein in question. As applied to neuroanatomy, this protein might be a neurotransmitter molecule, neurotransmitter-synthesizing enzyme, receptor, or other protein. In addition to neuronal localization, the technique is also widely used to provide valuable information on glia and other non-neuronal cells.

Prior to addressing the method itself, it is valuable to review some basic aspects of the structure of immunoglobulins (IgG in particular) and the antibody–antigen interaction. Antibodies are divided into five classes, with immunoglobulin G (IgG) type being the most commonly used in immunochemical methods. IgGs are 160-kD proteins comprised of two heavy chains and two light chains connected by disulfide bonds (Fig. 4A). The structure of the IgG molecule is divided into three domains: hypervariable, variable, and constant. The hypervariable region is the primary source of antigen-binding specificity. Most of the flexibility of IgG binding is genomically deter-

A

IgG

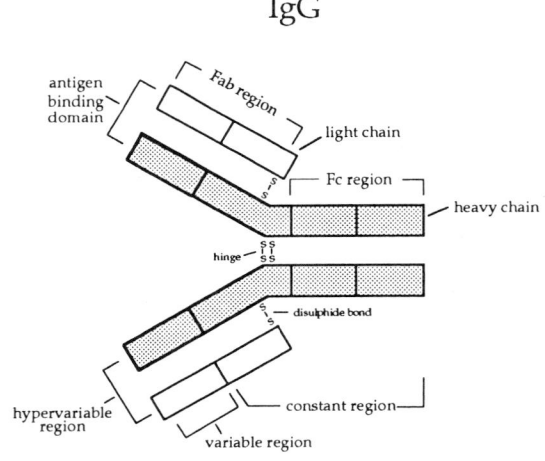

B

FIG. 4. A: Diagram illustrating structure of the IgG molecule. B: Schematic diagram depicting multiple epitopes within a typical protein.

mined in this region. The variable region contributes additional sources of protein variation in the unique binding qualities of any particular IgG clone. Finally, the constant region is a nonvariable "structural" component of IgG. This region is common to all IgGs in a particular species. It is known that the hypervariable and variable part of the molecule are the receptor portions of the IgG molecule. Fragments of IgG which contain these regions continue to exhibit active binding. In contrast, the constant region of the IgG molecule can itself serve as an antigen. Thus, in an immunocytochemical reaction the very same IgG may bind antigen (at its hypervariable segment) while its constant region acts an antigen for a second antibody (Figs. 4A and 5). Hence, a series of antibodies can be layered, and this amplification can be used to enhance signal strength (35).

An additional set of concepts, that regarding *antigen* and *epitope*, warrant discussion. By definition, an antigen is a protein (usually) which can be bound by a specific IgG. An epitope is the few amino acids in the antigen

protein to which a specific IgG binds. Figure 4B illustrates the protein sequence with several epitopes (they are often "bends" in the protein. One epitope sequence is highlighted (ABCDE) to indicate the small size of the average epitope (about 4–6 amino acids). Any one IgG molecule (from a single B lymphocyte which itself has been grown in a clonal fashion) binds to only one epitope. In the case of a monoclonal antibody, a single species of specific IgG molecules is used that is specific for a single epitope. A polyclonal antiserum contains multiple IgG species which may bind to any of a number of available epitopes. Interestingly, a monoclonal antibody may be very precise, but because the average epitope is small compared to the total size of the protein (e.g., 4–6 out of 400), one must be concerned about the potential for "cross-reactivity" with an identical sequence in another protein. A polyclonal antiserum reacts with any of several epitopes on the target protein, but the diversity of IgG types may cause cross-reactivity with similar epitopes on other molecules. Overcoming the problem of cross-reactivity often requires fairly thoughtful strategies: multiple antisera, biochemical extraction and characterization of antigen, affinity purification of antibody, and so on.

While the production of antisera and preparation of pure proteins are beyond the scope of this chapter, a few points are worth mentioning. The use of an impure protein preparation (containing multiple proteins) to stimulate antibody production will most likely generate an antiserum with IgGs directed against the protein of interest as well as against protein contaminants. Such a serum may bind some, many, or most of the proteins in an antigen mix. Furthermore, if a large excess of this same antigen mixture is incubated with the antiserum (before it is used on the tissue section), as is commonly performed as a control, the specific signal will probably be blocked and the remaining staining inferred to be specific! Thus, use of a dirty antigen for antibody production can be a source of a mixed antiserum and improper controls.

Assuming that one has a clean antigen and a good antiserum, some considerable effort is then put into establishing optimal conditions for the procedure. Probably the most troublesome is the need to establish fixation chemistry conditions. There is a complex list of fixative reagents, buffers, mixtures, and times which can be tested. Generally, most investigators begin with a neutral buffered 4% paraformaldehyde solution, and then vary mixtures of additional reagents (glutaraldehyde, acroline, picric acid, alcohols, etc.). It is possible to use carbohydrate or lipid fixatives, or even nucleic acid fixatives. The goal is to preserve the antigen in its original cellular context and prevent degradation, while still rendering it ''visible'' to the antiserum. It is worth noting that cross-linking proteins with fixatives may hide epitopes normally available in the native state; thus, excessive fixation is also a consideration. Once a fixation condition is established, a ''working titer'' of the antibody is determined. Generally this refers to the dilution of the original antiserum that produces optimal signal while minimizing nonspecific background. Most good antisera can be used in the dilution range of 1:500 to 1:50,000 or more! Other variables include antibody buffer conditions, tissue thickness, and length of incubation. Finally, a detection system (peroxidase histochemistry, fluorescence, etc.) is chosen based on individual needs and level of analysis. This step may also require some fine-tuning.

Method

In the preceding section we have focused on a variety of concepts and issues related to immunocytochemical methods. Here we attempt to present some more detailed considerations concerning application of the technique. The example chosen involves peroxidase histochemistry for visualization, although many of the principles apply to other detection methods as well.

Prior to sectioning, the tissue of interest is usually treated with a protein fixative (e.g., paraformaldehyde). As noted above, the fixation and associated parameters are usually determined empirically. The next step is to dilute the primary antiserum and apply it to the section for 16–48 hours. For the purposes of demonstration, let us begin with a rabbit anti-enkephalin IgG applied to a slice of rat caudate. After incubation with this primary antiserum, the tissue sections are thoroughly washed and a second antiserum is applied for a period of few hours, up to 24 hours. This secondary IgG was produced in goat and raised against rabbit IgG (remember, the primary IgG protein acts as antibody when binding enkephalin, but it acts as antigen when bound by the goat anti-rabbit IgG). We thus have a section with enkephalin bound by a rabbit IgG, which itself is bound by goat IgG directed against rabbit IgG. Following another wash, the next step is the addition of another rabbit IgG for 1–2 hours. This antibody is directed against the enzyme horseradish peroxidase (HRP), but is bound at its constant domain by the remaining binding site of the secondary IgG (goat anti-rabbit). [Note: All IgGs have two binding sites and can thus capture two molecules of antigen.] Following another wash, the tissue is incubated for 1–2 hours in a solution containing the enzyme HRP. [Note: the latter two steps can be replaced with the peroxidase–antiperoxidase (PAP) complex—see ref. 35]. Finally, the tissue is reacted with the HRP substrate hydrogen peroxide in the presence of a chromagen (e.g., diaminobenzidine), resulting in a colored precipitate at the site of this whole antigen–antibody complex. After washing and dehydrating, this precipitate is visible as a brown stain within the antigen-containing structures. The general method can be used at a very high level of resolution (including ultrastructural analysis) and across a large number of proteins (and nonproteins as well). This immunocytochemical sequence, as well as a related strategy (18) involving biotinylated IgGs and the avidin–biotin peroxidase complex (ABC), is outlined in Fig. 5, and an example of its application is shown in Fig. 6.

Technical controls are a very central part of this method. At a basic level it is important to know that the staining seen after the reaction sequence is specific to a particular protein. Criteria that need to be satisfied include the following: (a) absence of staining when the protocol is run with deletion of the primary antibody, (b) absence of staining when antisera is applied that was preincubated in the presence of a large excess of antigen, and (c) lack of staining with application of the enzyme or substrate alone. (Interestingly, some tissues have endogenous peroxidase activity that can be confused with specific staining following immunocytochemical protocols involving this enzyme; this problem can usually be avoided by pretreatment with hydrogen peroxide.) In addition, some non-antigen-related signals are considered to be false-positives. It is important to realize that a ''nonimmune''

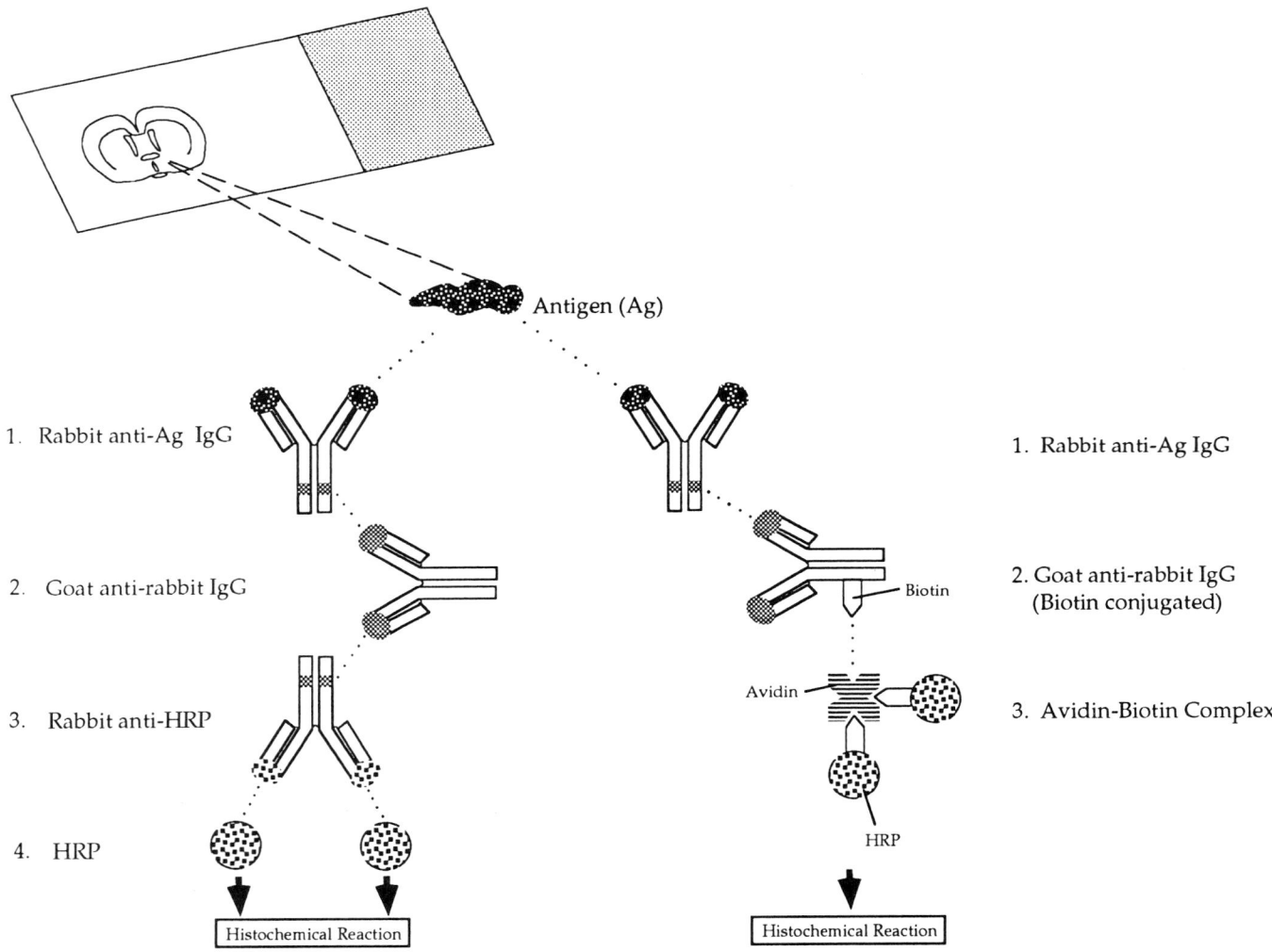

FIG. 5. Schematic diagram illustrating two variations of an immunocytochemical protocol utilizing peroxidase histochemistry.

rabbit serum (often used to block nonspecific IgG sites in tissues) is actually loaded with IgGs produced by the rabbit over time, and can therefore be the source of non-specific labeling. This potential pitfall can be overcome through the use of blocking agents not derived from normal serum (e.g., addition to the incubation mix of carrageenan, a gum that is effective at blocking nonspecific IgG binding sites in tissues). Perhaps the most elaborate control for specificity is the extraction of antigen from tissue, followed by biochemical characterization and quantitation. Other approaches to specificity and precision may be seen in the use of multiple antisera against the same antigen, or even antisera directed against different epitopes on the same antigen.

Advantages

1. Immunocytochemistry is a broad-based and powerful method for analyzing specific biochemical structures and sequences at the cellular level.

2. Multiple cellular compartments may be amenable to study, including the cell body, axons, and dendrites.
3. Minute levels of protein can be visualized in cellular compartments and membranes.

Limitations

1. Perhaps the greatest concern in immunocytochemistry is the question of specificity. It can be quite difficult to prove antigen specificity, particularly in view of the potential for cross-reactivity.
2. Immunocytochemistry is generally not quantitative. There are a number of reasons for this, including multiple epitopes, different affinities for different sizes and sequences of various protein versions, variable fixation, and variable tissue penetration by antisera.

There are several other considerations that can make immunocytochemistry a complex, expensive, and often

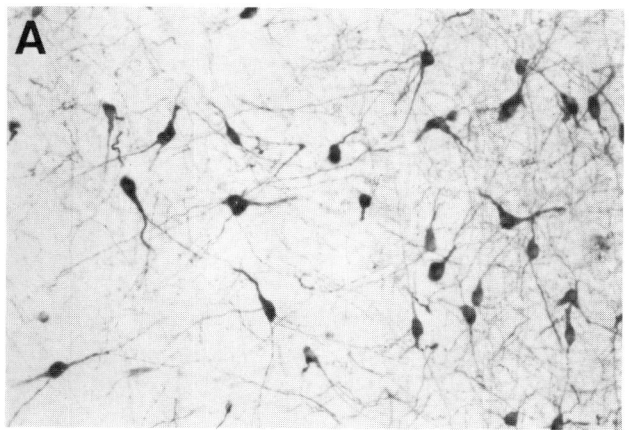

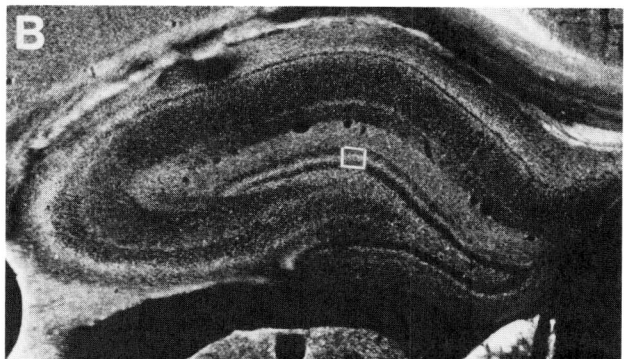

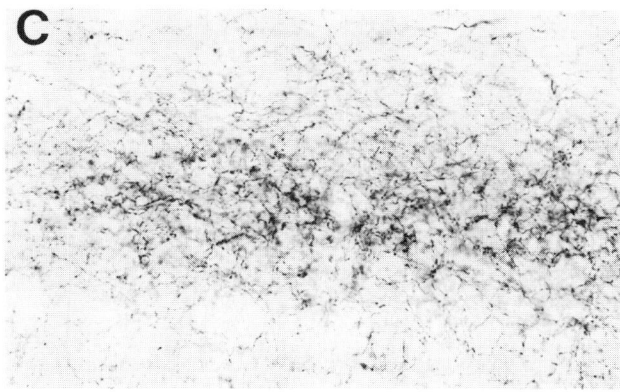

FIG. 6. Immunocytochemical detection of choline acetyltransferase, the acetylcholine-synthesizing enzyme, using a protocol outlined in Fig. 5. Cholinergic cell bodies and dendrites located within the medial septal nucleus are seen in **A**. These neurons are part of the origin of the cholinergic septohippocampal pathway. The low-magnification darkfield photomicrograph in **B** illustrates the distribution pattern of cholinergic fibers and terminals within the dentate gyrus. The boxed area in **B** is seen in **C** under brightfield illumination. (Courtesy of Dr. László Záborszky.)

technically demanding procedure. Adequate amounts of antigen for blocking studies are often hard to produce, particularly when the antigen is a protein. Even the vaunted specificity of monoclonal antibodies might be defeated by the occurrence of a common epitope in several different antigens. For example, the first four amino

acids of all of the opioid peptides are tyrosine-glycine-glycine-phenylalanine. This sequence is found once in the β-endorphin/adrenocorticotropic hormone (ACTH) precursor, three times in the pro-dynorphin precursor, and seven times in the pro-enkephalin precursor! A monoclonal antibody directed against this epitope could potentially find 11 targets in any of three propeptides (see ref. 23). The use of polyclonal antisera can also be somewhat problematic, because they are produced in limited amounts. Moreover, polyclonal antisera can react with different epitopes over different bleeds from the same source.

IN SITU HYBRIDIZATION

In situ hybridization is a method which allows for the detection of mRNA molecules, usually within their cells of origin (10,11,19,30,32,37,38,43). In a sense the method is similar to receptor autoradiography and immunocytochemistry, in that all three techniques rely on some form of binding to form stable complexes. Receptor autoradiography involves binding of receptor by radiolabeled ligand, and immunocytochemistry involves binding of antigen by antibodies. In in situ hybridization, binding occurs between mRNA in the cytosol and an externally produced radiolabeled RNA or DNA probe capable of forming a hybrid with it. Detection of the radiolabeled probe is then performed by methods similar to those used in receptor autoradiography (x-ray film or photographic emulsion).

The most important concept for understanding this technique is that of "hybridization." Two strands of RNA, two strands of DNA, or one RNA and one DNA can bind (or hybridize) through specific hydrogen bonding between chains. In Fig. 7, two strands of RNA are depicted (see inset box). One (AUGCCUCAU) represents a short strand of mRNA; the strand below it (UACGGA-GUA) is complementary to it (called cRNA). Inspection of the figure shows that A always binds U and that G always binds C. In fact, A shares two hydrogen bonds with U (or T in a DNA strand), and G shares three hydrogen bonds with C. While any single hydrogen bond is weak, a series of them can form a quite stable complex. In the example shown in Fig. 7 there are 5 A-U pairs (10 hydrogen bonds) and 4 G-C pairs (12 hydrogen bonds), resulting in a fairly stable hybrid of 22 hydrogen bonds. A stable combination of RNA–RNA strands is easily obtainable by as few as 25–30 bases (50–75 hydrogen bonds). This simple piece of chemistry forms the basis for a large number of molecular biological methods (in situ hybridization, Northern analysis, Southern analysis, cDNA library screening, etc.), not to mention its central role in stabilization of the double-stranded DNA of the genome itself!

The in situ hybridization method is described below. It is not very different from many aspects of receptor

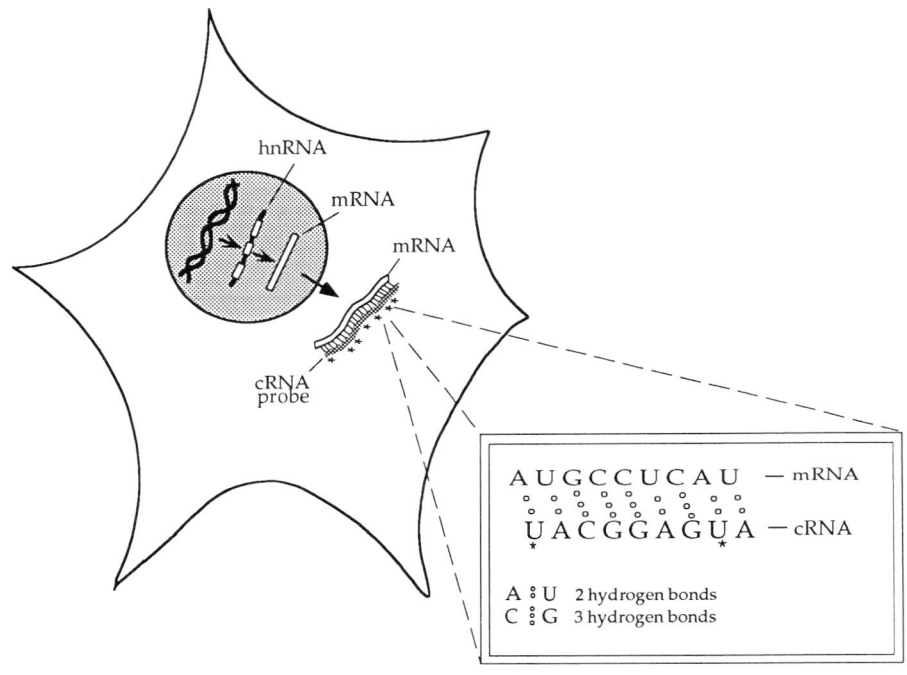

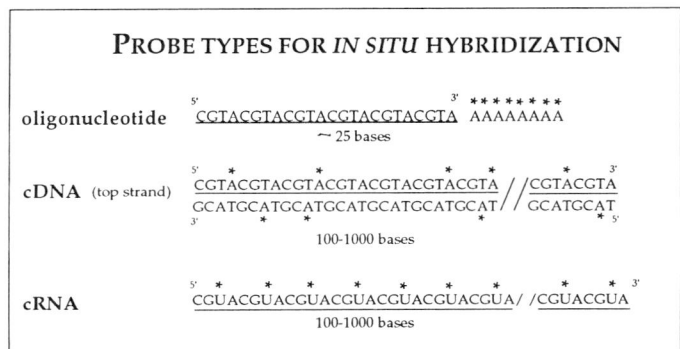

FIG. 7. Schematic diagram illustrating bonding principles and probe types involved in in situ hybridization histochemistry.

autoradiography and immunocytochemistry. In fact, some aspects of its early development were borrowed directly from these methods. We will center our discussion largely to the application of longer cRNA probes (see Fig. 7), although it should be noted that the method can be applied with some variation for cDNA and oligonucleotide probes as well.

Method

In situ hybridization is usually carried out on brain tissue that has been previously sectioned and immersed in a formaldehyde fixative. It may also be performed on tissue that has been fixed by perfusion and subsequently sectioned, although this is usually at the expense of some sensitivity. It is important to realize that mRNA molecules are not themselves fixed by a protein fixative such as formaldehyde,

but are essentially immobilized by the fixed proteins. Without protein fixation, mRNA can be subjected to the ubiquitous degradative enzyme RNase and/or diffuse away from the tissue section into the buffer. After washing and drying, the tissue is exposed to reagents designed to make it porous to radiolabeled probe. The most common permeabilizer is proteinase K, an enzyme which hydrolyzes many proteins. The tissue is then treated to reduce its net charge (acetylation), which reduces the tendency of the probe to stick to tissues nonspecifically. After another wash step, the sections are incubated with radiolabeled cRNA probe for 12–48 hours. During this period, the cRNA probe (which is applied in great excess) can form stable hybrids with endogenous mRNA. It is this RNA–RNA hybrid which provides the basis for signal localization, as well as a series of specificity controls. Following hybridization the tissue is incubated in the enzyme RNase, which digests all single-stranded RNA and thus digests nonhybridized probe, thereby dramatically

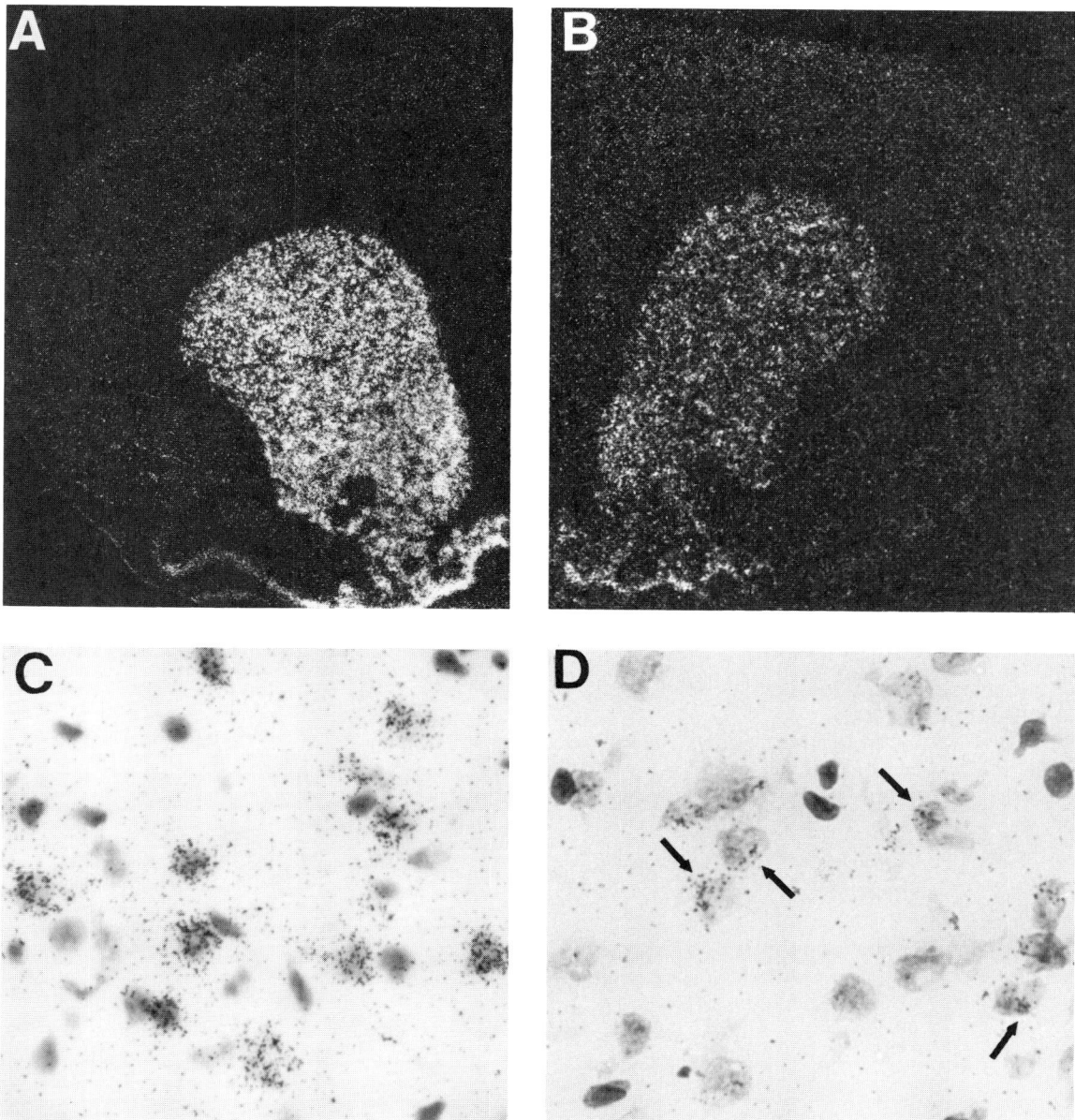

FIG. 8. Dark-field photomicrographs in **A** and **B** illustrate distribution pattern of neurons expressing mRNA transcripts encoding the D_2 dopamine receptor in the rat forebrain as revealed by in situ hybridization. The riboprobe used in the experiment shown in **A** was directed against an exonic portion of the D_2 mRNA, whereas the probe applied in the experiment in **B** was specific for an intronic segment of the D_2 hnRNA. Cellular labeling from the two cases is seen at higher magnification in the bright-field photomicrographs in **C** and **D**, which were from sections that were dipped in emulsion and Nissl-counterstained. Note the cytoplasmic distribution of grains from the experiment involving the exonic probe **C**, in contrast to the largely nuclear distribution of grains following application of the intronic probe **D**. (Courtesy of Dr. Charles A. Fox and Dr. Alfred Mansour.)

reducing a prominent source of background. After the RNase step, the sections are washed in low salt buffers at 45–65°C. This important step removes nonspecifically adherent probe, as well as probe that is only weakly hybridized. The tissue section is then dried, and subsequently it is exposed to x-ray film or is dipped in photographic emulsion. Quantitation is performed almost identically to receptor au-

toradiography (see previous section). An example of the results of a typical in situ hybridization experiment is illustrated in Fig. 8.

Technical Issues

A number of technical issues are important in understanding in situ hybridization technology. The preceding description was centered around the use of longer cRNA probes (approximately 200–1000 bases) or riboprobes, in which labeled nucleotides are incorporated into the RNA strand. An alternative method is to use short cDNA probes (generally 20+ bases) to hybridize to mRNA. These *oligonucleotide* probes have some advantages, particularly concerning tissue penetration, which is facilitated as a result of their small size. They are also easier to use than cRNA probes, but cannot be labeled to an equivalent high specific activity. This loss of sensitivity can be overcome through the use of multiple nonoverlapping oligonucleotide probes. It is also notable that in addition to an isotope of sulfur (^{35}S) as label, other isotopes are available for use, such as ^{32}P and ^{33}P. ^{32}P is a very-high-energy label with wide scatter, and it generally produces a less desirable signal compared to ^{35}S, which is only half the specific activity of ^{32}P but offers 30–50 times higher resolution. ^{33}P offers a resolution and specific activity that is intermediate, though closer to that of ^{35}S than ^{32}P. The shorter half-life of ^{33}P makes it attractive relative to ^{35}S in terms of safety and disposal, although it presently is more expensive than either ^{35}S or ^{32}P. It should be noted that nonradioactive markers are being increasingly used to produce a high-resolution signal for in situ hybridization (reviewed in refs. 30 and 43). These materials are usually simple molecules which are coupled to a nucleotide and which, once incorporated into probe and applied to tissue, can be detected with methods involving or resembling immunocytochemistry. While presenting an obvious appeal in terms of rapid detection, ease, and safety of use, these methods are typically not as sensitive as their radiolabeled counterparts (30,43). However, in some cases, immunocytochemical detection of the nucleotide-coupled molecule can provide further signal amplification (22). Also, a number of protocols have recently been advanced for the simultaneous detection of two mRNA species in brain by combining radioactive and nonradioactive detection methods (see Fig. 9F) (25,26,42). The in situ hybridization technique may also be adapted for studies at the ultrastructural level, particularly those methods involving histochemical detection of nonisotopic probes (40).

Another important issue concerns specificity controls. Probes are capable of ''cross-hybridization'' in a fashion analogous to the cross-reactivity of antibodies. In the event that an investigator suspects cross-reactivity, the first and conceptually simplest control for this phenomenon is degradation (using RNase) of all RNA in the section prior to hybridization, which should remove the signal. A second control is the use of a ''sense'' strand RNA probe, which can be created by transcribing the opposite strand of the gene (opposite to that used to create the usual cRNA or ''antisense'' probe). This radiolabeled sense probe should not yield a signal, because it is actually identical to a part of the mRNA sequence. Assuming that the RNase and sense strand controls are negative, the

investigator may then want to establish a very stringent set of temperature and salt conditions for the wash step of the mRNA–cRNA hybrid. Mismatched strands giving rise to a false signal can be melted apart with increasing temperature and decreasing salt conditions. Finally, of course, mRNA localization should be compared to known data concerning protein expression or localization.

Advantages

1. In situ hybridization is a major step forward in the ability to understand neuronal cell biology in an anatomical context at the level of gene product regulation. The technique can allow for detection and quantitation of mRNA in the cytosol, or even hnRNA within the nucleus (a reflection of the transcription rate of a single gene in individual cells).
2. The technique allows for identification of cell bodies of origin of specific molecules which may not be stored to a detectable degree in the soma.
3. The method is very specific with a wide degree of control afforded to the investigator in terms of probe design.
4. Current in situ hybridization technology is very sensitive in that it can differentiate mRNAs varying by a few percent, and can do so down to tens of copies of mRNA per cell.

Limitations

The method, in its most sensitive form (use of riboprobes), is complex, expensive, and requires skills in molecular biology.

NEUROANATOMICAL TRACT-TRACING

The methods presented above (receptor autoradiography, immunocytochemistry, and in situ hybridization) involve the study of biochemical processes and structures. In contrast, neuroanatomical tract-tracing is performed to answer fundamental questions concerning neuronal projections and connectivity. The past two decades have seen great advances in the development of new and highly sensitive methods for tracing neuronal connections, and even a superficial survey of all of these techniques is well beyond the scope of the present chapter. In general, many modern neuroanatomical tracing methods involve the injection of various types of compounds or dyes that are subsequently transported in an anterograde or retrograde fashion (or both) in relation to neuronal cell bodies. These compounds may be visible through fluorescence microscopy or may be detected using standard histochemical or immunocytochemical techniques. Through the placement of discrete injections within a given brain region, it is

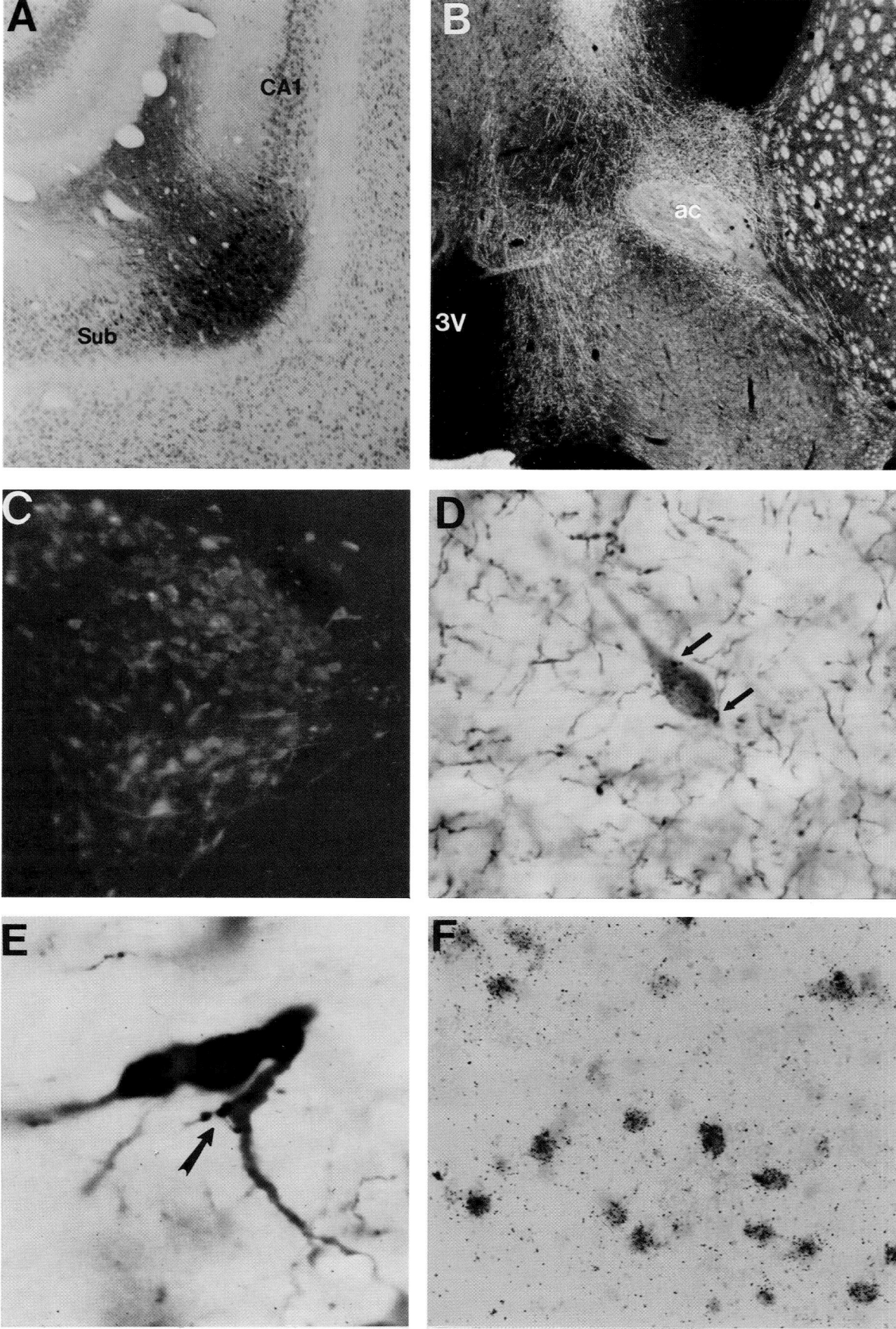

thus possible to confirm the inputs and outputs of an area. Multiple compounds can be injected in the same animal to address issues such as axonal collateralization (e.g., two or more retrograde compounds) (1,29,41) or to establish neuronal chains (through the use of multiple tracers) (7,8). The capacity to visualize many of these compounds at the ultrastructural level has added a new level of power in defining synaptic connectivity (3,13,14,24,45). Moreover, many of these methods are compatible with immunocytochemistry (29,33) or with in situ hybridization (6,39), making it possible to reveal not only the presence of a given projection, but also its biochemical composition (e.g., neurotransmitter content) in the same experiment. A sampling of some of these applications is illustrated in Fig. 9A–E.

At the technical level, a number of issues require consideration (for discussion, see refs. 2, 15, 16, and 24). For example, it is obviously desirable to limit the extent of tracer diffusion to the specific anatomical structure under study, because spread outside the target area confounds interpretation. In many cases this can be accomplished by iontophoretic delivery or, alternatively, by limiting injection volumes. Individual characteristics of the tracer compound must also be considered, such as tendency to label fibers-of-passage, toxicity, diffusibility, and tendency for transport in the direction opposite to that desired. Fixation parameters are also of importance, particularly for experiments requiring immunocytochemical detection or those that will ultimately rely on electron microscopic evaluation.

Let us briefly return to our example of the dopamine neurons in the substantia nigra presented in the early part of this chapter. As part of the classic nigrostriatal pathway, this projection (as well as nonstriatal projections of these neurons) could be demonstrated using an anterograde tracer (e.g., PHA-L, biocytin, Fluoro-Ruby). These

cells also could be retrogradely labeled from the striatum with any of a number of compounds (e.g., Fluoro-gold, true blue, rhodamine beads, WGA-HRP, or a cholera toxin B-HRP conjugate) and in a combined immunocytochemical experiment shown to contain dopamine (or one of its synthesizing enzymes, such as tyrosine hydroxylase). Such retrogradely labeled cells could also be shown to express a neuropeptide transmitter or a specific dopamine receptor subtype (or their respective mRNA transcripts) in an experiment combining retrograde tracing with immunocytochemistry (or in situ hybridization). Of course, as with any combination of methods, a set of technical issues and limitations concerning compatibility must be considered in the design of the experiment. Nevertheless, recent advances in such combined applications have made it possible to characterize brain regions in substantial detail with a high degree of flexibility (3,4,6–9,14,20,29,33,39,45). For illustrative purposes, brief descriptions of an anterograde tracing method (PHA-L) and a retrograde tracing technique (Fluoro-gold) presently in common use are included below.

Anterograde tract-tracing using the lectin *Phaseolus vulgaris*-leucoagglutinin (PHA-L) was first introduced in 1984 by C. Gerfen and P. Sawchenko (12). This protein is delivered by iontophoresis, incorporated largely by dendrites at the site of injection, and is subsequently transported along the axon (at a relatively slow rate of approximately 4–6 mm/day). Thus, it is possible to label all neurons giving rise to a projection (including substantial portions of their dendritic arbors, in many cases resembling preparations using the Golgi method), as well as produce a rather complete picture of axonal trajectories and terminal arborizations. Importantly, when delivered under the appropriate conditions (iontophoresis of a 2.5% solution), this tracer is apparently neither incorporated by passing fibers, nor transported retrogradely by terminals

FIG. 9. A: An injection site of the anterograde neuronal tracer PHA-L within the ventral hippocampus. The tracer was detected immunocytochemically, resulting in a brown precipitate in neurons that have incorporated PHA-L. The section has been Nissl-counterstained. **B:** Dark-field photomicrograph illustrating the distribution of PHA-L-labeled fibers (gold) within the rat forebrain from the injection in **A**. **C:** Dual immunofluorescence combined with retrograde tracing. Triple exposure reveals distribution of neurons within the hypothalamic paraventricular nucleus which contain vasopressin (fluorescein-immunolabeled, green) or CRH (rhodamine-immunolabeled, red), as well as those retrogradely labeled from the spinal cord using the tracer true blue. (Figure kindly provided by Drs. Larry W. Swanson and Paul E. Sawchenko. From ref. 36, with permission.) **D:** Retrograde neuronal tracing in combination with anterograde tracing. A neuron located within the bed nucleus of the stria terminalis is retrogradely labeled with the tracer Fluoro-gold, which was injected into the hypothalamic paraventricular nucleus and detected immunocytochemically. This neuron is approached by axon terminals (*arrows*) labeled with PHA-L, following an injection of this anterograde tracer in the ventral subiculum. **E:** Anterograde neuronal tract-tracing combined with ChAT immunocytochemistry. PHA-L-labeled terminal boutons are seen in apposition to a cholinergic neuron located in the basal forebrain following delivery of the tracer to the lateral hypothalamus. **F:** Dual in situ hybridization. Striatal neurons expressing enkephalin mRNA (purple) have been detected with a nonradioactive in situ hybridization technique using a digoxigenin-labeled cRNA probe. Grains located over these cells represent labeling from a radioactive cRNA probe specific for D_2 dopamine receptor mRNA. (Courtesy of Dr. Eileen J. Curran.)

in the vicinity of the injection site (12). Following survival periods, perfusion fixation (usually with a buffered formaldehyde or paraformaldehyde solution) is performed and brains removed and subsequently sectioned. The lectin is then detected in tissue sections using standard immunocytochemical methods (typically involving the avidin–biotin method as outlined in Fig. 6), rendering the technique compatible with a wide array of immunocytochemical procedures. For example, neurochemical identification of PHA-L labeled axons may be performed with double-immunofluorescence methods, and biochemical characterization of the targets of PHA-L-labeled afferents may be accomplished in combination with immunocytochemical techniques (see Fig. 9E). The method may also be extended to analyses at the electron microscopic level, in which synaptic interconnections can be unequivocally demonstrated (13,14,45). A disadvantage of the method is the somewhat limited penetration of the anti-PHA-L antibody. This can be particularly troublesome for analysis of synaptic connectivity in electron microscopic studies that require the omission of the membrane-solubilizing detergents in order to preserve ultrastructure.

Perhaps one of the most versatile fluorescent compounds available for retrograde tract-tracing is Fluorogold. Fluoro-gold is a stilbene derivative first introduced in the mid-1980s by L. Schmued and J. Fallon (31). Although the mechanism of incorporation is unknown, Fluoro-gold is transported relatively rapidly in the retrograde direction and produces visible labeling within neurons within 24–48 hours. Longer survival times (10–14 days) typically produce a stronger fluorescence signal, including extensive visualization of dendrites. The tracer is compatible with many standard fixation protocols and is amenable to numerous combinations, including those involving multiple fluorescent markers, in situ hybridization histochemistry, and immunocytochemical methods. Additionally, the recent development of an antibody directed against Fluoro-gold (5) has made it possible to detect the tracer immunocytochemically (see Fig. 9D), allowing important advantages in terms of increased sensitivity, enhanced resolution (particularly of dendritic processes), and compatibility with ultrastructural analyses. A limitation of the technique is its apparent ability to be taken up by fibers-of-passage.

In summary, the advent of a new generation of sensitive and versatile tract-tracing methods has helped make it possible to define neuronal circuits with a new level of sophistication and precision. We have highlighted only two of these tools in an effort to illustrate their suitability for combined studies; these obviously represent only a small fraction of the tracing compounds currently available for neuroanatomical investigation. A number of excellent texts are available for detailed descriptions of modern neuroanatomical methods, particularly with respect combined applications (see refs. 2, 15, 16, and 24).

SUMMARY

The study of brain in cellular and circuit contexts has relied heavily on the methods overviewed in the present chapter. Each of these techniques (receptor autoradiography, immunocytochemistry, in situ hybridization histochemistry, and neuroanatomical tract-tracing) can be used to provide fundamentally different classes of information concerning specific neuronal elements. We have attempted to highlight some of the basic principles underlying these techniques. While each method presents its own set of advantages and limitations, both individually and in concert with other techniques, new and creative combinations continue to emerge that have enabled characterization of neuronal microcircuitry in ever-increasing detail. The ultimate power of these approaches lies in the ability to provide functional insights by the coupling of information gained from them. Such circuit analyses are contributing substantially to our understanding of fundamental mechanisms underlying brain function in health and disease states.

ACKNOWLEDGMENTS

We wish to thank Dr. Derek T. Chalmers and Dr. Charles A. Fox for helpful comments regarding the manuscript. We would also like to thank the following for photomicrograph contributions: Drs. Eileen J. Curran, Charles A. Fox, Alfred Mansour, Paul E. Sawchenko, Larry W. Swanson, and László. Záborszky.

REFERENCES

1. Bentivoglio M, Molinari M. Fluorescent retrograde triple labeling of brainstem reticular neurons. *Neurosci Lett* 1984;46:121–126.
2. Björklund A, Hökfelt T, Wouterlood FG van den Pol AN, eds. *Handbook of chemical neuroanatomy, vol 8. Analysis of neuronal microcircuits and synaptic interaction.* Amsterdam: Elsevier, 1990.
3. Bolam JP, Ingham CA. Combined morphological and histochemical techniques for the study of neuronal microcircuits. In: Björklund A, Hökfelt T, Wouterlood FG, van den Pol AN, eds. *Handbook of chemical neuroanatomy, vol 8. Analysis of neuronal microcircuits and synaptic interactions.* Amsterdam: Elsevier, 1990;125–198.
4. Buhl EH, Schwerdtfeger WK, Germroth P. Intracellular injection of neurons in fixed brain tissue combined with other neuroanatomical techniques at the light and electron microscopic level. In: Björklund A, Hökfelt T, Wouterlood FG, van den Pol AN, eds. *Handbook of chemical neuroanatomy, vol 8. Analysis of neuronal microcircuits and synaptic interactions,* Amsterdam: Elsevier, 1990;273–304.
5. Chang HT, Kuo H, Whittaker JA, Cooper NG. Light and electron microscopic analysis of projection neurons retrogradely labeled with Fluoro-gold: notes on the application of antibodies to Fluoro-gold. *J Neurosci Methods* 1990;1:31–37.
6. Chronwall BM, Lewis ME, Schwaber JS, O'Donohue TL. In situ hybridization combined with retrograde fluorescent tract tracing. In: Heimer L, Zaborszky L, eds. *Neuroanatomical tract-tracing methods 2. Recent progress.* New York: Plenum, 1989;265–295.
7. Cliffer KD, Giesler GJ Jr. Postsynaptic dorsal column pathway of the rat. III. Distribution of ascending afferent fibers. *J Neurosci* 1989;9:3146–3168.
8. Cullinan WE, Herman JP, Watson SJ. Ventral subicular interaction with the hypothalamic paraventricular nucleus: evidence for a relay

in the bed nucleus of the stria terminalis. *J Comp Neurol* 1993;332:1–20.

9. Freund TF, Somogyi P. Synaptic relationships of Golgi-impregnated neurons as identified by electrophysiological or immunocytochemical techniques. In: Heimer L, Zaborszky L, eds. *Neuroanatomical tract-tracing methods 2. Recent progress.* New York: Plenum, 1989;201–238.

10. Gall JG, Pardue ML. Formation and detection of RNA–DNA hybrid molecules in cytological preparations. *Proc Natl Acad Sci* 1969;63:378–383.

11. Gee CE, Roberts JL. In situ hybridization histochemistry: a technique for the study of gene expression in single cells. *DNA* 1983;2:157–163.

12. Gerfen CR, Sawchenko PE. An anterograde neuroanatomical tracing method that shows the detailed morphology of neurons, their axons and terminals: immunohistochemical localization of an axonally transported plant lectin, *Phaseolus vulgaris* leucoagglutinin (PHA-L). *Brain Res* 1984;290:219–238.

13. Gerfen CF, Sawchenko PE, Carlsen J. The PHA-L anterograde axonal tracing method. In: Heimer L, Zaborszky L, eds. *Neuroanatomical tract-tracing methods 2. Recent progress.* New York: Plenum, 1989;19–47.

14. Groenewegen HJ, Wouterlood FG. Light and electron microscopic tracing of neuronal connections with Phaseolus vulgaris-leucoagglutinin (PHA-L), and combinations with other neuroanatomical techniques. In: Björklund A, Hökfelt T, Wouterlood FG, van den Pol AN, eds. *Handbook of chemical neuroanatomy, vol 8. Analysis of neuronal microcircuits and synaptic interactions.* Amsterdam: Elsevier, 1990;47–124.

15. Heimer L, Robards MJ, eds. *Neuroanatomical tract-tracing methods.* New York: Plenum, 1981.

16. Heimer L, Záborszky L, eds. *Neuroanatomical tract-tracing methods 2. Recent progress.* New York: Plenum, 1989.

17. Herkenham M, Pert CB. Light microscopic localization of brain opiate receptors: a general autoradiographic method which preserves tissue quality. *J Neurosci* 1982;2:1129–1149.

18. Hsu S, Raine L, Fanger H. Use of avidin-biotin-peroxidase complex (ABC) in immunoperoxidase techniques: a comparison between ABC and unlabeled antibody (PAP) procedures. *J Histochem Cytochem* 1981;29:577–580.

19. John HA, Birnstiel ML, Jones KW. RNA-DNA hybrids at the cytological level. *Nature* 1969;223:582–587.

20. Kitai ST, Penney GR, Chang HT. Intracellular labeling and immunocytochemistry. In: Heimer L, Zaborszky L eds. *Neuroanatomical tract-tracing methods 2. Recent progress.* New York: Plenum, 1989;173–199.

21. Kuhar MJ, Yamamura HI. Light autoradiographic localization of cholinergic muscarinic receptors in rat brain by specific binding of a potent antagonist. *Nature* 1975;253:560–561.

22. McQuaid S, Allan GM. Detection protocols for biotinylated probes: optimization using multistep techniques. *J Histochem Cytochem* 1992;40:569–574.

23. Meo T, Gramsch C, Inan R, Hollt V, Weber E, Herz A, Riethmuller G. Monoclonal antibody to the message sequence Tyr-Gly-Gly-Phe of opioid peptides exhibits the specificity requirements of mammalian opioid receptors. *Proc Natl Acad Sci* 1983;80:4084–4088.

24. Mesulam M-M, ed. *Tracing neural connections with horseradish peroxidase.* New York: John Wiley & Sons, 1982.

25. Normand E, Bloch B. Simultaneous detection of two mRNAs in the central nervous system: a simple two-step in situ hybridization procedure using a combination of radioactive and non-radioactive probes. *J Histochem Cytochem* 1991;39:1575–1578.

26. Marks DL, Wiemann JN, Burton KA, Lent KL, Clifton DK, Steiner RA. Simultaneous visualization of two cellular mRNA species in individual neurons by use of a new double in situ hybridization method. *Mol Cell Neurosci* 1992;3:395–405.

27. Rogers AW, ed. *Techniques of autoradiography,* 2nd ed. New York: Elsevier, 1979.

28. Roth LJ, Diab IM, Watanabe M, Dinerstein RJ. A correlative radioautographic, fluorescent, and histochemical technique for cytopharmacology. *Mol Pharmacol* 1974;10:986–988.

29. Sawchenko PE, Swanson LW. A method for tracing biochemically defined and immunohistochemical techniques. *Brain Res* 1982;210:31–52.

30. Schäfer MK-H, Herman JP, Watson SJ. In situ hybridization. In: London ED, ed. *Imaging drug action in the brain.* Boca Raton, FL: CRC Press, 1993;337–378.

31. Schmued LC, Fallon JH. Fluoro-gold: a new fluorescent retrograde axonal tracer with numerous unique properties. *Brain Res* 1986;377:147–154.

32. Simmons DM, Arriza JL, Swanson LW. A complete protocol for in situ hybridization of messenger RNAs in brain and other tissues with radio-labeled single-stranded RNA probes. *J Histotechnol* 1989;12:169–181.

33. Skirboll LR, Thor K, Helke C, Hökfelt T, Robertson B, Long R. Use of retrograde fluorescent tracers in combination with immunohistochemical methods. In: Heimer L, Zaborszky L, eds. *Neuroanatomical tract-tracing methods 2. Recent progress.* New York: Plenum, 1989.

34. Sternberger LA. *Immunocytochemistry,* 3rd ed. New York: John Wiley & Sons, 1986.

35. Sternberger LA, Hardy PH, Cuculis JJ, Meyer HG. The unlabeled-enzyme method of immunocytochemistry. Preparation and properties of soluble antigen–antibody complex (horseradish peroxidase-anti-horseradish peroxidase) and its use in identification of spirochetes. *J Histochem Cytochem* 1970;18:315–333.

36. Swanson LW, Sawchenko PE, Lind RW. Regulation of multiple peptides in CRF parvocellular neurosecretory neurons: implications for the stress response. In: Hökfelt T, Fuxe K, Pernow B, eds. *Progress in brain research, vol 68,* Amsterdam: Elsevier Science Publishers, 1986;169–190.

37. Uhl GR, ed. In situ *hybridization in brain.* New York: Plenum, 1986.

38. Valentino KL, Eberwine JH, Barchas JD, eds. In situ *hybridization. Applications to neurobiology.* New York: Oxford University Press, 1987.

39. Watts AG, Swanson LW. The combination of in situ hybridization with immunocytochemistry and retrograde tract-tracing. In: Conn PM, ed. *Methods in neurosciences, vol 1. Genetic probes.* New York: Academic Press, 1989;127–136.

40. Webster HF, Lamperth L, Favilla JT, Lemke G, Tesin D, Manuelidis L. Use of biotinylated probe and in situ hybridization for light and electron microscopic localization of Po mRNA in myelin-forming Schwann cells. *Histochemistry* 1987;86:441–444.

41. Wessendorf MW. Characterization and use of multi-color fluorescence microscopic techniques. In: Björklund, A, Hökfelt T, Wouterlood FG, van den Pol AN, eds. *Handbook of chemical neuroanatomy, vol 8. Analysis of neuronal microcircuits and synaptic interactions.* Amsterdam: Elsevier, 1990;1–45.

42. Young WS III. Simultaneous use of digoxigenin- and radiolabeled oligodeoxyribonucleotide probes for hybridization histochemistry. *Neuropeptides* 1989;13:271–274.

43. Young WS III. In situ hybridization histochemistry. In: Björklund A, Hökfelt T, Wouterlood FG, van den Pol AN, eds. *Handbook of chemical neuroanatomy, vol 8. Analysis of neuronal microcircuits and synaptic interactions.* Amsterdam: Elsevier, 1990;481–512.

44. Young WS III, Kuhar MJ. A new method for receptor autoradiography: [³H] opioid receptors in rat brain. *Brain Res* 1979;179:255–270.

45. Zaborszky L, Heimer L. Combinations of tracer techniques, especially HRP and PHA-L, with transmitter identification for correlated light and electron microscopic studies. In: Heimer L, Zaborszky L, eds. *Neuroanatomical tract-tracing methods 2. Recent progress.* New York: Plenum, 1989.

Psychopharmacology: The Fourth Generation of Progress, edited by Floyd E. Bloom and David J. Kupfer. Raven Press, Ltd., New York © 1995.

CHAPTER 4

A Critical Analysis of Neurochemical Methods for Monitoring Transmitter Dynamics in the Brain

Janet M. Finlay and Michael J. Zigmond

Chemical techniques were first applied to the study of the nervous system in a systematic way in the late 19th Century. At that time, "neurochemistry" meant describing the inorganic and organic constituents of neuronal tissue, an endeavor referred to as "chemical statics" by the parent of neurochemistry, J. W. L. Thudichum. There was some appreciation for the fact that the major task of the brain, the processing of information, was dynamic rather than static in nature. Yet for many decades the study of communication between neurons was mainly within the domain of electrophysiology, a tool which seemed to offer what neurochemistry could not: anatomical specificity and high temporal resolution. However, by the middle of the 20th century it had become clear that the great majority of the information transfer between neurons involved chemical signals, even in the brain, and neurochemical approaches began to be developed to monitor this process. Moving from bioassays to the use of high-performance liquid chromatography, from whole-brain analyses to microdissection, and from assays of postmortem tissue to assays of extracellular fluid sampled in vivo, continuing improvements in technology have made neurochemistry an evermore important partner in our efforts to understand the activity of the nervous system.

In this chapter we explore the neurochemical methods available to monitor the activity of specific neuronal systems in the central nervous system (CNS). We comment briefly on older methods, because some papers utilizing such methods remain an important part of the literature. However, our focus is on approaches that have undergone major development over the past decade (e.g., in vivo

microdialysis and voltammetry) and on certain more established methods that are still in frequent use (e.g., release from tissue slices) (for additional reviews on these and related subjects see refs. 30, 47, 60, 64, 70). In considering these approaches we will critically evaluate them, noting where appropriate the distinction between the neurobiological variables of interest and what is actually measured in the laboratory. Often the examples chosen involve the catecholamines, norepinephrine (NE) and dopamine (DA), or the indoleamine, serotonin [5-hydroxytryptamine (5-HT)]. This is both because these biogenic amines are the transmitters with which the authors are most familiar and because at present a disproportionate amount of information is available regarding them. However, our focus on these examples should not detract from the generality of the themes that we wish to emphasize in this review: First, for any neurotransmitter there are many variables that one could hope to assess; each of these is presumably of biological significance, yet only a few are directly related to the two processes that are usually of greatest interest: transmitter release and the resulting postsynaptic response. Second, the plethora of feedback loops that participate in the synthesis, release, and degradation of a neurotransmitter or in its transduction to a postsynaptic event can be expected to complicate the task of monitoring transmitter dynamics because methods that influence these homeostatic processes can alter the variables under investigation, often making the proper interpretation of observations difficult.

POSTMORTEM ANALYSES

Steady-State Conditions

A major concern in postmortem studies is the impact of death and postmortem delay on the variables under

J. M. Finlay and M. J. Zigmond: Department of Neuroscience, University of Pittsburgh, Pittsburgh, Pennsylvania 15260.

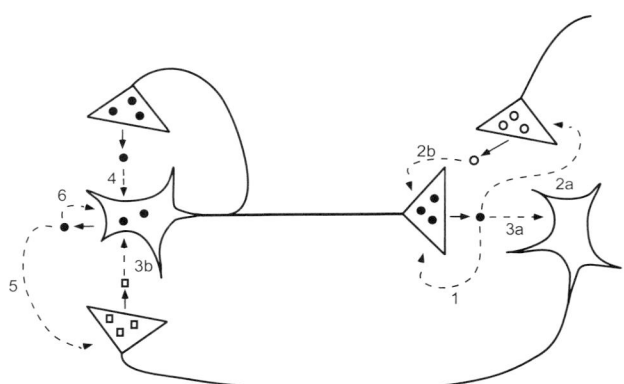

FIG. 1. Regulatory pathways influencing neurotransmitter dynamics. Shown are some of the feedback loops that act to keep the output of a neuron relatively constant. These may include: (1) terminal autoreceptor regulation; (2a + 2b) terminal–terminal heteroreceptor regulation; (3a + 3b) multisynaptic feedback loops; (4) axon collaterals; (5 + 3b) dendritic–terminal heteroreceptor regulation; and (6) dendritic autoreceptor regulation. Not shown are even longer feedback systems that may involve physiological or even behavioral components.

study (see Chapters 75, 84, 100, 118, 123, 128, 141, and 142, *this volume*). We will focus on another critical issue: the biological significance of measurements in postmortem tissue. In most such experiments animals are killed, either by decapitation or anesthesia, tissues are dissected, and the samples are homogenized in strong acid to break down cellular compartments and liberate the compounds of interest. These, in turn, are isolated and measured using one of many possible methods for quantification.

Transmitter Content

The analysis of the amount of neurotransmitter present in tissue represented the earliest attempt to investigate the activity of chemically identified neuronal systems. At first, large regions of the CNS were examined; subsequently, improvements in dissection and in analysis permitted the measurement of increasingly smaller subdivisions of brain. Yet the assumption that changes in transmitter content would tell us much about the dynamics of cell-to-cell communication has proven incorrect, at least in most instances. Instead, a key aspect of transmitter dynamics appears to be "synthesis–secretion coupling," with the maintenance of constant transmitter stores in the face of changing rates of utilization (Fig. 1) (78).

There are exceptions. For example, because the biosynthesis of neuropeptides occurs primarily in the cell body and preterminal axon, there is little capacity for rapid adjustments to changing rates of release (13). In addition, whereas acetylcholine (ACh) is synthesized in the nerve terminal at a rate that usually matches the rate of ACh utilization, ACh content in the neostriatum is inversely

correlated with release (32,62). In general, however, the concentration of a given transmitter has no value as a measure of transmitter dynamics. Indeed, transmitter content is such a stable property of a given class of neurons that it has been used as an index of the number of neuronal elements present in the tissue.

Transmitter Metabolites

Whereas the level of transmitter in neuronal tissue has not generally proven to be very useful, in the case of the monoamines considerable insight has been provided by measurement of transmitter metabolites in postmortem samples (see also Chapter 103, *this volume*). For example, although stimulation of DA neurons within a physiological range does not deplete tissue of its transmitter stores, it does increase the level of the deaminated metabolite, dihydroxyphenylacetic acid (DOPAC). As a result, numerous studies have been performed in which changes in tissue levels of DOPAC are used to examine the impact of a drug or an alteration in the environment on the release of DA (41,61). This approach has led to numerous insights. However, in interpreting changes in tissue levels of metabolites formed from neurotransmitters, several issues should be taken into consideration. For example, metabolites often can be formed in intracellular compartments and need not reflect changes in transmitter release. DOPAC can be formed from newly synthesized DA that has not been released, as well as from DA that has been released and taken back up into the terminal. Moreover, there often exist more than one catabolic pathway with different pathways associated with different cellular compartments. To make matters more complicated, the metabolites that are formed, as well as their biological significance, can change with brain region as well as with the experimental animal (71).

Another possible difficulty in interpreting metabolite data is that synthesis, release, and metabolism need not always co-vary. This is particularly true when drugs are used as part of the experimental protocol. For example, by blocking high-affinity catecholamine uptake as well as monoamine oxidase activity, amphetamine can greatly *reduce* the rate of formation of deaminated metabolites of catecholamines while presumably *increasing* catecholamine release. And even when drugs are not involved, one can expect dissociations among these variables. For example, a transmitter that is released can be taken back up and reutilized without being subject to metabolism; a change in transmitter metabolism can occur without any change in release; and the rate of clearance of a metabolite might change, altering the amount that is recovered without any modification in its rate of formation.

A third problem can arise under conditions in which there is a high background level of metabolite already present. For example, changes in the concentrations of choline and acetic acid that occur during the release and degradation of ACh may not be readily detected against the high background of preexisting choline and acetic acid present in tissue and extracellular fluid. The same may be true of glutamine formed from glutamate, succinic semialdehyde formed from gamma-aminobutyric acid (GABA), and many of the presumptive degradation products of peptides.

Finally, a problem may arise when metabolic data are presented as *ratios* of the concentration of a given metabolite to that of its parent transmitter levels. Because the transmitter content of a particular neuron usually is relatively constant (see above), such ratios can be useful in helping to correct for changes in the density of innervation of the tissue sample being analyzed. Yet such an interpretation is valid only if the transmitter content of the tissue is unaffected by the treatment, and this cannot be determined by the reader unless both the concentration of transmitter and of metabolite are provided separately.

In summary, a large body of useful information has been obtained by measurement of transmitter metabolites in postmortem tissue, particularly in the case of the biogenic amines, and at present these approaches represent the only commonly available approach to the study of human postmortem tissue. In interpreting such data, however, it is important to remember that the variable being measured is quite removed from release per se, and that the significance of particular metabolite routes may differ for different transmitters, different species, and different experimental conditions.

Conversion of Radiolabeled Precursors to a Transmitter

Because transmitter release usually is coupled with transmitter synthesis, investigators often turn to monitoring synthesis in an attempt to evaluate changes in the rate at which a transmitter is being released. A classical way in which to examine the rate of a biochemical reaction in such cases is to introduce a radiolabeled precursor and measure the accumulation of a labeled product. A variant of the approach is to introduce a radiolabeled form of the product and follow its rate of disappearance. The use of radiolabeled tracers has been utilized widely in studies of neurotransmitter dynamics in brain since the 1960s (33,55). To determine the rate of synthesis of a compound from such an experiment, one must know two quantities: the specific activity of the precursor and the amount of labeled product formed. In practice, neither of these quantities can be known with certainty. First, in general it is not possible to measure the specific activity of the pool of precursor that is utilized in the biosynthetic reaction, but only to obtain some indirect estimate, such as the specific activity in plasma or in the entire tissue under investigation. Second, once formed, the transmitter not

only *accumulates*, but also is *utilized*. As a result, synthesis rate can only be estimated from a determination of the accumulation of radiolabeled product during the earliest stages of an experiment, or through the use of multiple data points and complex equations (16,79).

A central assumption of any such study is that the radiolabeled tracer is handled precisely as is the natural precursor. However, each of the known transmitters is synthesized from a precursor that itself can be formed at least in part from endogenous sources and that can participate in more than one reaction. For example, the tyrosine used in the synthesis of catecholamines can be taken up from plasma, synthesized from phenylalanine, or formed through the degradation of protein. Moreover, the percentage of available tyrosine that is utilized to form catecholamines is very small, with the majority of tyrosine being incorporated into protein or transaminated into *p*-hydroxyphenylpyruvic acid. Thus the rates of many biochemical pathways that involve tyrosine (which could be influenced by the condition under investigation) can have a significant influence on its availability for conversion to catecholamines. As a result, it is never possible to use radiolabeled tyrosine to obtain an exact calculation of the rate of DA synthesis, because the precise specific activity of the precursor pool can never be determined. Moreover, one must be wary of the possibility that an experimental condition under investigation will alter that specific activity.

Transmitter-Synthesizing Enzymes

In some cases, changes in transmitter release are accompanied by changes in the activity of one or more transmitter-synthesizing enzymes. An example of this is the increase in tyrosine hydroxylase (TH) activity that often occurs in catecholaminergic neurons during conditions of increased impulse flow (see Chapter 17, *this volume*). These changes in enzyme activity can occur rapidly as a result of modification of existing TH molecules, or they can occur more slowly due to a change in the rate of formation, degradation, and/or delivery of TH molecules. Such changes can be identified by the appropriate measurement of the kinetics of the reaction and the amount of enzyme protein, and they can sometimes be used to monitor changes in neuronal activity. There are, however, ways in which transmitter biosynthesis might be altered that are less readily monitored; for example, the delivery of some constituent of the reaction could change as could the availability of an inhibitor or an activator of the biosynthetic process. Thus, the *absence* of a change in the isolated form of a biosynthetic enzyme itself need not indicate that transmitter synthesis is unchanged. A particularly interesting example of this phenomenon involves the synthesis of ACh. In this case, the synthesizing enzyme choline acetyltransferase does not appear to be subject to short-term covalent modulation. On the other hand, the high-affinity transporter that provides choline, a precursor for ACh, often is responsive to the rate at which the axon terminal is depolarized, and choline transport can sometimes be used to monitor ACh turnover (63; although also see ref. 62).

If the concentration of biosynthetic enzymes can be altered during changes in transmitter synthesis, the concentration of the relevant mRNAs might be expected to be altered as well, and can sometimes be of value in detecting longer-term changes in transmitter synthesis. Moreover, because specific mRNAs usually can be monitored by in situ hybridization, histochemical techniques can be used to provide a neuroanatomical precision that is not otherwise available in neurochemical studies. As in the case of changes in transmitter synthesizing enzymes, however, the presence or absence of changes in mRNAs must be interpreted with caution.

Non-Steady-State Conditions

In studies involving experimental animals, one approach to overcoming the impact of synthesis–secretion coupling on postmortem analyses has been to couple the measurement of transmitter level with a pharmacological intervention. For example, synthesis might be blocked and the rate of disappearance of transmitter determined. Alternatively, catabolism might be inhibited and transmitter accumulation monitored. Of course, whenever steady-state conditions are disrupted, one must be concerned about the physiological significance of the resulting observation. One reason for this derives from the existence of numerous homeostatic feedback loops, which can cause a treatment that modifies one step in neurotransmission (e.g., release) to induce changes in other steps as well (e.g., synthesis). Because this problem often cannot be avoided, it is important to use more than one method to estimate the variable of interest, determining whether approaches that disturb the system in different ways nonetheless yield similar results. Another consequence of this problem of disrupting feedback loops is that measurements of changes in transmitter dynamics are usually more useful for rough, qualitative estimates than for more precise quantitative conclusions. A second potential source of problems results from the fact that newly synthesized transmitter often appears to be released preferentially.

The first attempts to overcome the problems imposed by synthesis–secretion coupling by pharmacological means involved the biogenic amines. Several approaches were taken, including (a) inhibiting transmitter metabolism and monitoring the accumulation of the amine under study (53), (b) inhibiting biogenic amine synthesis at the initial, rate-limiting step and determining the rate of transmitter disappearance (12), and (c) inhibiting amine syn-

thesis at the second step, decarboxylation of DOPA or 5-HT, and measuring the accumulation of precursor (15). Despite the problems with non-steady-state techniques, these approaches proved to be an important advance. For example, using α-methyl-p-tyrosine, an inhibitor of tyrosine hydroxylase, it was soon shown that certain stressors altered the rate of disappearance of NE, although stress-induced changes in NE content had not been detected without drug pretreatment. Several of these pharmacological approaches remain in use today.

IN VITRO PREPARATIONS

An alternative to postmortem analysis is to use an in vitro preparation in which the processes of synthesis and release are ongoing and can be monitored. One of the first such preparations was the tissue slice, introduced in the 1930s as a method for studying the respiration of central neural tissue. Over the years, other in vitro preparations have been developed, including explants, isolated nerve ending fractions or synaptosomes, and cultured cells. In this section we will focus on the use of brain slices, but many of our comments are relevant to these other preparations as well.

The basic methods for preparing and incubating brain slices have been reviewed elsewhere (22,43,58). In most cases, the slices are prepared using a mechanical device, such as a tissue chopper or "vibratome," although in earlier experiments the slices were prepared freehand or with a simple guide. Slices are generally between 300 μm and 500 μm in thickness in order to allow for adequate diffusion of gases, and they are incubated in a buffered iso-osmotic salt solution. Typically, slices are then depolarized and the incubation medium collected for analysis of transmitter content.

Initial studies involved monitoring the efflux of radiolabeled tracers, and these approaches are still in use. As in the case of studies in which tracers are administered in vivo (see above), care must be taken in interpreting such results. In some cases, analytical techniques have advanced to the point where one can measure the endogenous, non-radiolabeled transmitter directly. In some cases these analytical methods are combined with the use of drugs that inhibit the inactivation of the transmitter in question. For example, acetylcholinesterase inhibitors might be used to block the degradation of ACh, or an inhibitor of the DA transporter might be employed to inhibit the reuptake of DA. Whereas the objective in such cases is to increase the sensitivity of the method, the danger is that which is inherent in any study involving a disturbance of the usual life cycle of a transmitter: the possibility of interfering with a normal homeostatic process. Thus, inhibitors of ACh hydrolysis or DA reuptake will increase extracellular concentration of the respective transmitter and may thereby influence synthesis and/or release modulating autoreceptors.

A variety of stimuli can be used to examine the response to depolarization of the neuronal membranes. One of the most common depolarizing stimuli is elevated K^+; others include veratridine and ouabain. Although each of these conditions causes depolarization by a different mechanism, they share a common drawback. Whereas a piece of neuronal membrane is normally in a depolarized state for less than 10% of the time (assuming a 1-msec action potential and a frequency of less than 100 Hz), each of these approaches causes a continuous state of depolarization. Although it is never possible to mimic the physiological state with regard to the characteristics of the stimulus or the number of neurons affected, a major advance in this direction is provided by the use of electrical field depolarization, an approach which permits the use of a wide variety of frequencies, pulse durations, and patterns. On the other hand, any procedure that involves exposing an entire slice to depolarizing conditions will produce a highly unphysiological mix of transmitters in the extracellular compartments, thereby producing interactions that bear little resemblance to the normal state. There have been a few attempts to deal with this problem by selectively stimulating certain fiber tracts (7,18), but although such approaches are the rule for electrophysiology they are still in their infancy in neurochemistry. Despite these problems, the use of in vitro preparations such as the tissue slice has provided many important insights that were not available from biochemical analyses of tissue. For the first time it was possible to measure the transmitter content of an *extracellular* compartment. Moreover, serial measurements could be made on the same tissue sample, increasing both the power and the efficiency of experiments.

IN VIVO PREPARATIONS

Although in vitro preparations can provide insights not readily available from analysis of postmortem samples, they utilize tissue that has had both neural and vascular connections transected and is incubated in a fluid that is at best only a rough approximation of extracellular fluid. For a more accurate index of transmitter dynamics under physiological conditions, one must move to an in vivo preparation. In this section we will focus on several approaches that have been used to monitor extracellular levels in intact animals (Fig. 2). Particular attention will be paid to two methods whose use has grown dramatically over the past several years: microdialysis and voltammetry.

Cortical Cup

The first in vivo preparation developed for sampling the extracellular environment was the cortical cup (Fig. 2a). As early as 1953, the cortical cup was used to demon-

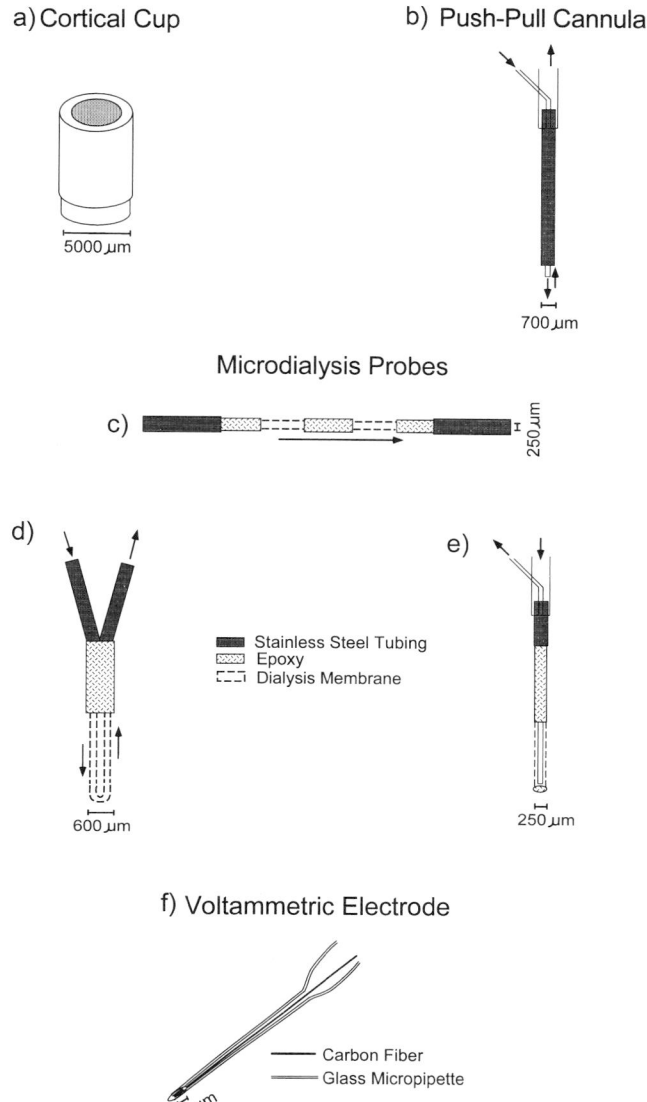

FIG. 2. Methods for measuring neurotransmitter release in vivo. Shown schematically are (**a**) cortical cup, (**b**) push–pull cannula, (**c**) transverse microdialysis probe, (**d**) U-shaped microdialysis probe, (**e**) vertical concentric microdialysis probe, and (**f**) carbon fiber voltammetric electrode. Scale bars represent the approximate size of these devices as used to study neurochemical events in the extracellular fluid of rat.

strate that ACh release was related to the spontaneous electrical activity of the cortex (45). With this method the skull overlaying the cortical area of interest is removed and a cylinder is placed in tight contact with the cortical surface (for details of the method see ref. 51). The cylinder is then filled with a buffered solution comparable to that used with in vitro preparations. The fluid is collected (either by continuous flow or by sequential washes), and it is analyzed for the compounds of interest. This method has been used to study factors regulating

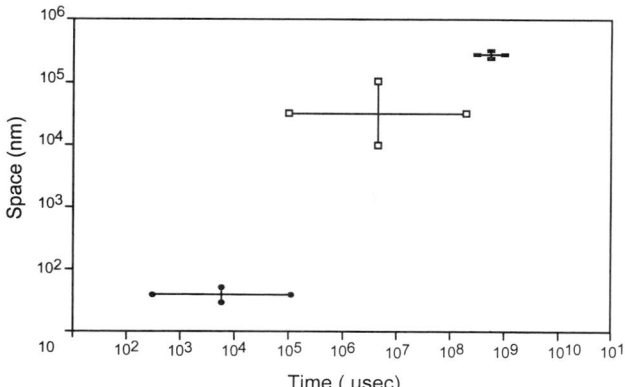

FIG. 3. A representation of the relation between the dynamics of transmitter release at the synaptic cleft (●) and the in vivo sampling methods of voltammetry (□) and microdialysis (■) with respect to the temporal and spatial domains. Calculations are based on a synaptic cleft of 30–50 nm with a synaptic delay of 0.3–100 msec, voltammetric electrodes of 10- to 100-μm diameter with a sampling interval of 100 msec to 3 min, and microdialysis probes of 250- to 300-μm diameter and a sampling interval of 5–15 min.

neurotransmitter efflux from cortex of both anesthetized and unanesthetized preparations (52). In many ways the procedure is analogous to the in vitro slice preparation except that the superfusion is performed in the intact living organism. However, the method has limited applications because it can only be applied to the cortical surface.

Push–Pull Cannula

Development of the push–pull cannula method in the early 1960s provided the first opportunity to evaluate neurochemical events in discrete structures deep within the intact CNS (28,29). Present forms of the method developed from the merging of two independent push–pull cannula techniques; one was designed to monitor cerebrospinal fluid (8,9,25), and the other was designed to sample the chemical environment of subcutaneous tissue (26).

Over the years, many refinements of this method have appeared (54,59). In general, however, the push–pull cannula consists either of two concentric tubes, as originally designed (28; Fig. 2b), or of two parallel tubes (19). The cannula is implanted into the brain so that the tip is located in the brain structure of interest. A perfusion solution is forced down one of the tubes and pulled up the other tube using two pumps working in synchrony as pushing and pulling devices. The push–pull method can be performed in an acute anesthetized preparation or in freely moving animals, either by implantation of the push–pull cannula directly or by implantation of the guide cannula and subsequent implantation of the push–pull cannula. Although the method is conceptually straightforward, its proper use requires very close attention to details associated with the perfusion itself (30,57). For example, the distance be-

tween the tips of the inner and outer tubes of the concentric cannula generates a siphon and must be accurately adjusted in order to obtain a constant flow rate and avoid having tissue being pulled into the perfusion medium. In addition, the rate of push and pull of the perfusion solution must be carefully adjusted in order to reach a constant flow. The perfusion solution, once collected, can be analyzed by any suitable analytical method, providing a way of continuously sampling the microenvironment of the brain under in vivo conditions.

One major disadvantage of the push–pull method is the tissue perturbation produced by directly infusing a perfusion solution into the area from which neurotransmitter efflux is being determined (30). A related problem is the damage produced by the cannula itself, disrupting as it does a large region of brain in the very center of the area of measurement. Nonetheless, the method has been of great value in the study of transmitter dynamics and continues to be used by a number of research groups to examine the release of endogenous ACh, catecholamines, amino acids, and peptides, as well as efflux of radiolabeled transmitters following administration of labeled precursors (57).

Microdialysis

Several years after the introduction of the push–pull cannula technique, it was proposed that the principles of dialysis could be applied to a method for sampling the extracellular fluid of brain, thereby circumventing the problems associated with having a perfusion solution coming into direct contact with brain tissue. This method involves introducing a dialysis membrane between the perfusion solution and the extracellular fluid. Molecules that are sufficiently small to pass through the dialysis membrane will then diffuse across the membrane from an area of high concentration to an area of low concentration. In a first attempt to dialyze the extracellular fluid, Bito et al. (10) implanted *dialysis sacs* into the cerebral hemispheres of dogs; after several days, these sacs were removed and the amino acid levels of the dialysate determined. A few years later, Delgado and collaborators (20,21) developed the *dialytrode*, a push–pull cannula with a small permeable bag attached to the end. Relative to the dialysis sac, this method offered the advantage of providing an opportunity for continuous sampling of the extracellular environment. These early attempts to dialyze the extracellular fluid of brain laid the foundation for subsequent work in this area. However, popularization of this method can be attributed to the seminal work of Ungerstedt and colleagues (66,67).

Ungerstedt began by inserting dialysis tubing transversely through brain tissue and measuring radiolabeled DA efflux (67). Subsequently, endogenous DA also was measured (68,76), primarily due to the parallel development of an analytical method with sufficient sensitivity for detection of endogenous catecholamines, high pressure liquid chromatography with electrochemical detection developed by Adams and colleagues (2,40). When first introduced, the microdialysis probe consisted of a hollow tube of dialysis membrane inserted transversely through a region of brain (Fig. 2c) (66). Such transverse probes are simple to make, but they cause severe damage to muscle and skull as well as to an extensive area of CNS through which they pass. The development of the loop probe provided a means of reducing the extent of surgically induced injury. This probe consists of a loop of dialysis membrane which is implanted vertically into the brain via a single hole in the skull (Fig. 2d). Still less damage is produced by a vertical concentric-style dialysis probe (Fig. 2e). This probe consists of a single piece of dialysis tubing blocked off at one end with glue; the inlet and/or outlet portions of the probe pass down into the dialysis tubing. Whereas these probes are technically more difficult to make, their smaller overall diameter (typically about 200 μm) and subsequent reduction in tissue damage has resulted in their widespread use (4).

The advantages of microdialysis over earlier in vivo methods have been summarized (65,74). Most of these advantages are directly related to the presence of the dialysis membrane at the tip of the microdialysis probe. Because the membrane prevents the perfusion solution from directly contacting the tissue, this provides a barrier to turbulence and infection. As with any invasive technique, mechanical injury to CNS tissue occurs during implantation of a microdialysis probe, and this can elicit neurotransmitter release that is not physiological. However, several hours after implantation of a microdialysis probe, transmitter efflux generally appears to be almost entirely due to physiological processes as demonstrated by its sensitivity to manipulation of extracellular Ca^{2+} and blockade of voltage-sensitive Na^+ channels (73). In contrast, this has not been established for the use of push–pull cannulae. Indeed, the blockade of Na^+ channels only partly inhibits the release of DA from striatum as measured by push–pull cannula and furthermore stimulates DA release from the substantia nigra (56). This may suggest that mechanical disruption of the tissue, such as that produced by turbulence, plays a continuing role in producing the transmitter efflux measured by the push–pull method.

The dialysis membrane also acts as a filter to prevent the diffusion of large molecules from extracellular fluid into the perfusion medium. This provides certain advantages for the analysis of transmitter content in the dialysate. First, the membrane can prevent large molecules such as enzymes from entering the perfusion solution and thereby halt the continuous enzymatic degradation of neurotransmitters once they have entered the perfusion solution. Also, by virtue of its ability to exclude molecules from the perfusion solution, the membrane partially puri-

fies samples prior to their analysis. The presence of the dialysis membrane also provides certain technical advantages. For example, the size of the perfused area can be controlled by limiting the active surface of the membrane. In addition, the perfusion is greatly simplified because it is not necessary to adjust inflow and outflow accurately in order to prevent build-up of pressure or clogging of the cannula as with the push–pull technique.

Of course, implantation of the dialysis probe results in several reactions within the CNS tissue. Knowledge of the time course of these events is critical in determining the interval during which microdialysis experiments can be performed with minimal interference from tissue reactions (3,4,60). In general, it is thought that dialysis experiments should not be performed either very soon (≤ 10 hr) or very long (several days to weeks) after probe implantation and that the optimal interval for performing microdialysis experiments is approximately 16–48 hr after implantation of the dialysis probe. Efforts have been made to develop methods whereby sampling can be carried out over many days in a single subject using either chronic implantation of a dialysis probe or implantation of a guide cannula followed by multiple insertions of a probe over days. However, these have generally been unsuccessful (60). In addition to the postoperative time at which samples are collected, other important variables include (a) the ionic composition of the dialysate and (b) the rate of perfusion. It is clear that the composition of the dialysate should mimic the ionic constituents of extracellular fluid in brain as closely as possible (5,50,57,72), and that the flow rate of the dialysate should be as low as possible (usually approximately 0.1–5.0 μl/min) (4).

In vivo microdialysis undoubtedly provides information about *qualitative* changes in the extracellular concentration of a neurochemical. In addition, methods for establishing *quantitative* information regarding extracellular concentrations have recently been developed. Originally, extracellular concentrations of molecules were estimated based on the in vitro recovery of the dialysis probe— that is, the concentration of a compound that appeared in dialysate as a percentage of the concentration present in a beaker into which the probe had been placed (68,77). However, because the mass transport of substances in brain tissue is very different from that in an aqueous solution, this led to errors (6). Subsequently, many approaches have been developed to generate quantitative data using the microdialysis technique. These approaches can be divided into those based primarily on a theoretical approach and those employing an empirical approach (38). Recently, empirical approaches to estimating in vivo concentrations have been developed that involve extrapolation to zero flow (35) or calculation of the equilibration concentration, also referred to as the method of no net flux (44); these approaches have been applied extensively to the study of extracellular DA levels in CNS (36).

In vivo microdialysis is itself only a sampling technique. The ability to measure compounds within dialysate is entirely dependent upon the sensitivity of an appropriate analytical method. As in the case of in vitro preparations, under conditions when the analytical method is not sufficiently sensitive to detect dialysate levels of a particular compound, several approaches have been taken. Pharmacological tools have been used to compensate for inadequate sensitivity by increasing the level of substance to be analyzed. For example, acetylcholinesterase inhibitors have been used to enable detection of ACh in dialysate (17). Another approach has been to prelabel neurons by infusing isotopes of the transmitter or precursors and assaying the radiolabeled compounds (42). The problems with these approaches have been previously discussed. In some instances, such as the study of endogenous DA in extracellular fluid of certain brain regions, it has become fairly routine to detect dialysate levels of neurotransmitter using high-pressure liquid chromatography coupled with electrochemical detection. However, even under these conditions, microdialysis requires the collection of dialysate over several minutes, and therefore it cannot be used to answer questions about rapid changes in extracellular fluid concentrations of a compound. Finally, in cases of compounds such as glutamate, where both neurotransmitter and nontransmitter functions are being subserved, one must interpret results with particular caution.

Despite the several concerns that have been noted, use of microdialysis in neuroscience has increased rapidly since its development. Its popularity can be attributed to the fact that, relative to earlier methods, microdialysis does offer several distinct advantages, including (a) an opportunity to examine changes in the concentration of compounds in extracellular fluid derived from anatomically discrete brain regions with minimal disruption of the tissue and the blood–brain barrier and (b) the ability to sample extracellular fluid on a continuous basis. Microdialysis is now used extensively for the study of several transmitters in the CNS. In addition to its widespread use for assay of endogenous biogenic amines, there are laboratories that are using the approach to monitor amino acids (4), ACh (17), and peptides (46). The method also has been used to examine the efflux of cyclic adenosine monophosphate in extracellular fluid to provide a measure of in vivo receptor function (24). In addition to its extensive use in experimental animals, the method has been used to a limited extent in clinical neuroscience to monitor extracellular fluid in human patients during focal brain ischemia (34) and seizures (23).

Voltammetry

Adams and his colleagues (1,39) published the first report of an in vivo electrochemical method which allows the direct monitoring of a specific subset of molecules within extracellular fluid of brain. Voltammetry makes use of the fact that certain compounds are readily oxidizable. The method typically employs a working electrode, a reference electrode, and an auxiliary electrode. These electrodes are positioned in electrical continuity with one another, the working electrode being positioned in the brain structure of interest. A controlled potential is then applied between the working and reference electrode, and the resultant current that flows from the working electrode provides a measure of the amount of electroactive material in the solution (2).

In most in vivo voltammetric experiments, the applied voltage is not held at a constant value but instead consists of a waveform generated by pulsing a voltage (chronoamperometry), applying a voltage sweep (cyclic voltammetry), or a combination of the two (differential pulse voltammetry). Those methods which alter the applied potential during the detection interval (i.e., cyclic voltammetry) provide information about the chemical identity of the compound being oxidized, whereas those that employ a single voltage pulse during the detection interval do not (i.e., chronoamperometry) (37,48). In addition, the various voltammetric methods differ in terms of their sensitivity and time resolution (see Fig. 1).

The design of voltammetric electrodes has changed considerably since the first use of this method leading to reduction in size and improvements in selectivity. A major technical advance has been the development of electrodes that range in size from 1 to 30 μm in diameter and that provide the best available spatial resolution of any method for studying neurochemical events in vivo. In contrast, improving the selectivity of voltammetric electrodes has been a much more difficult and less successful objective. Voltammetry makes use of the fact that several neurotransmitters, including DA, NE, and 5-HT, are readily oxidizable at potentials at which most other compounds in the extracellular fluid do not oxidize. However, even within this range of potentials there are other molecules that will oxidize and thereby complicate the detection of these neurotransmitters. For example, oxidation of DOPAC and ascorbate occur within the same voltage range as the catecholamines, and under basal conditions both DOPAC and ascorbate are present in extracellular fluid at much higher concentrations than the catecholamines. In methods involving the collection of extracellular fluid prior to analysis, it is possible to separate molecules with similar oxidation potentials from one another by high-pressure liquid chromatography before they reach the working electrode. However, separation of this sort cannot be achieved with voltammetry alone, and therefore the molecular specificity of a particular in vivo voltammetric technique must be demonstrated convincingly in order to validate the method (75).

At present, the best methods for improving the selectivity of in vivo voltammetry involve modification of the electrode surface itself (49). For example, coating electrodes with the negatively charged polymer Nafion increases the selectivity of the electrode for cations (such as DA and NE) relative to anions (such as ascorbate and DOPAC) by reducing the likelihood that the latter compounds will gain access to the surface of the working electrode (31). Improved selectivity of voltammetric methods has also been achieved by other means. First, because the neurochemical content of different regions of the brain vary considerably, a certain amount of selectivity can be achieved by selection of an appropriate target site for the voltammetric electrode. For example, by placing an electrode in the striatum, which has a high DA content but very little NE, one can usually be confident that most of the current generated is not due to oxidation of NE. Second, pharmacological manipulations of compounds in the extracellular environment have also been used to enhance selectivity. For example, pargyline pretreatment has been used to prevent formation of DOPAC. This permits the detection of DA without interference from its principal metabolite, although it creates the problems inherent in pharmacological pretreatments that have already been discussed. Improved selectivity may also be attained by restricting the in vivo voltammetric determination of a compound to an interval during which the axons of the neurons of interest are directly stimulated. Under these conditions, the immediate increase in current should be due to release of the parent neurotransmitter. However, the approach is limited by the fact that transmitter release can only be determined under conditions of electrical stimulation of axons or cell bodies, requires the presence of a discrete site for the selective stimulation of a specific set of neurons, and may not reflect the type of response elicited by more physiological increases in neuronal firing.

Comparison of Dialysis and Voltammetry

Microdialysis and voltammetry each makes a unique contribution to this field of study as a result of differing temporal and spatial resolution (Fig. 3), chemical resolution, and sensitivity (74). For example, voltammetric measurements of compounds in the extracellular fluid have been made at intervals as short as 100 msec, whereas dialysis measurements represent an integration of changes that have occurred over a 5- to 20-min interval. As a result, voltammetry and microdialysis are best suited to examination of momentary versus long-lasting changes in the content of extracellular fluid, respectively. Voltammetric electrodes sample from a very small area because their size ranges from 1 to 30 μm in diameter. In fact, it has been demonstrated that a 10-μm carbon fiber electrode can be used to sample DA from a distance of less than 10 μm from the electrode surface (37). In contrast, dialysis probes are 200–300 μm in diameter or larger. Moreover, due to continuous removal of the substances from the extracellular fluid as a result of perfusion

through the probe, concentrations gradients are set up that may extend several millimeters into the tissue (14). As indicated previously, the chemical resolution of voltammetric electrodes has improved greatly in recent years such that a number of compounds can be detected with confidence. However, to date, the use of voltammetry has been limited to the detection of readily oxidizable species. In contrast, the range of chemicals that can be examined using in vivo microdialysis is limited only by the ability of a given compound to pass through the dialysis membrane and the availability of an appropriate analytical technique. As a result, in vivo microdialysis has seen a wider range of applications than in vivo voltammetry. The sensitivity of in vivo voltammetry varies depending upon the electrode and the voltammetric method. However, in general, this method is not sufficiently sensitive to measure basal extracellular levels of neurotransmitters and thus, as a result, cannot be used to examine the impact of treatments thought to *decrease* extracellular neurotransmitter levels. In contrast, basal levels of catecholamines are readily detectable using in vivo microdialysis. In summary, it is clear that these methods are capable of providing complementary rather than redundant information about the behavior of molecules in the extracellular fluid.

CONCLUDING COMMENTS

In this chapter we have tried to focus on interpretational issues: What do the results mean in biological terms, what are the pitfalls, and what are the relative advantages? We have focused on some of the major methods in use today, along with some others that are important for historical reasons. However, we have not exhausted the available approaches to measuring transmitter dynamics. Among the others deserving of attention that we are not able to discuss in this brief review are (a) the use of antibody microprobes and electrodes treated with immobilized enzymes and (b) the monitoring of use-dependent changes in such variables as receptor number, specific gene products (including those of immediate early genes), second messengers, and deoxyglucose utilization (e.g., see ref. 64).

We wish to close by dealing briefly with a question that often is overlooked in studies such as those we have outlined here, yet is perhaps the most important: In measurements of transmitter "release," what is the true relation between the quantity measured and release itself? This is not an issue for all chemical signals, because some hormones, such as adrenaline or corticosterone from the adrenal gland, can be readily collected and assayed. But most, if not all, neurotransmitters released from neurons do not remain in extracellular fluid for long. Instead they are either inactivated enzymatically or taken up into local cells by a specific transporter. Thus, what can actually be collected is generally a small fraction of the amount of material that was originally released. Attempts often are made to circumvent this problem by blocking transmitter inactivation. For example, in the case of the biogenic amines and the amino acids one can block the high-affinity transporter, whereas in the case of ACh one can inhibit acetylcholinesterase. In each of these instances there occurs a dramatic increase in the amount of material that can be collected. However, the drawback of such pharmacological manipulations has already been discussed: Altering the concentration of transmitter in extracellular fluid interferes with the normal feedback processes and alters the response to subsequent depolarization.

Thus it would seem that at present one is generally forced to choose between two imperfect states: measuring *overflow* (the small amount of transmitter that manages to escape from the synapse) or using a drug to promote that escape. Yet, is it possible that in some cases "overflow" is not a result of an imperfect system of private synaptic transmission but actually a means of cell-to-cell communication? Might the extracellular pool of transmitter that is sampled in studies of in vitro slices, microdialysis, and voltammetry actually be a *physiological* pool of transmitter, allowing some neurons to communicate over a wide field very much in the manner of a hormone?

Much has been written on this subject. For example, it has been noted that paracrine-like communication appears to occur in the invertebrate, in the mammalian autonomic nervous system, and even in the mammalian CNS (e.g., see refs. 27 and 69). Moreover, some authors have commented on (a) the relative absence of synaptic contacts made by certain types of neurons, (b) the presence of high-affinity receptors capable of responding to the low concentration of transmitter that often are detected in extracellular fluid, and (c) the apparent mismatch of receptors and the terminals containing an appropriate transmitter. On the other hand, it also has been argued that in none of these cases is there incontrovertible evidence for nonsynaptic transmission in the mammalian CNS (for references, see ref. 27).

Until such evidence is provided, those of us who aspire to measure the release of neurotransmitters must remember that synaptic transmission is at best being monitored indirectly and that nonsynaptic transmission may not exist at all. And yet, how far we have come from the earliest days in which all that could be measured were concentrations of a small number of transmitters in large regions of the brain. Surely, this progress will continue into the next generation of methods.

ACKNOWLEDGMENTS

We wish to thank Adrian Michael and Alan F. Sved for helpful comments on this chapter. This work was supported, in part, by U.S. Public Health Service grants NS19608, MH29670, MH45156, and MH00058 and by grants from the Tourette Syndrome Association, the Schizophrenia Research Program of the Scottish Rite, and the National Alliance of Research in Schizophrenia and Affective Disorders.

REFERENCES

1. Adams RN. Probing brain chemistry with electroanalytical techniques. *Anal Chem* 1976;48:1128A–1138A.
2. Adams RN, Marsden CA. Electrochemical detection methods for monoamine measurements in vitro and in vivo. In: Iversen LL, Iversen SD, Snyder SH, eds. *Handbook in psychopharmacology.* New York: Plenum Press, 1982;1–74.
3. Benveniste H, Hansen AJ. Practical aspects of using microdialysis for determination of brain interstitial concentrations. In: Robinson TE, Justice JB Jr. *Microdialysis in the neurosciences, Techniques in the behaviorial and neural sciences.* New York: Elsevier Science Publishers, 1991;7:81–96.
4. Benveniste H, Hüttemeier PC. Microdialysis—theory and application. *Prog Neurobiol* 1990;35:195–215.
5. Benveniste H, Hansen AJ, Ottosen NS. Determination of brain interstitial concentrations by microdialysis. *J Neurochem* 1990;52:1741–1750.
6. Benveniste H. Brain microdialysis. *J Neurochem* 1989;52:1667–1679.
7. Bernath S, Berger TW, Zigmond MJ. Glutamate release in the striatum promoted by stimulation of the corticostriatal pathway in a complex slice preparation. *Soc Neurosci Abstr* 1993;19:920.
8. Bhattacharya BK, Feldberg W. Perfusion of cerebral ventricles: assay of pharmacologically active substances in the effluent from the cisterna and the aqueduct. *Br J Pharmacol* 1958;13:163–174.
9. Bhattacharya BK, Feldberg W. Perfusion of cerebral ventricles: effects of drugs on outflow from the cisterna and the aqueduct. *Br J Pharmacol* 1958;13:156–162.
10. Bito R, Davson H, Levin EM, Murray M, Snider N. The concentration of free amino acids and other electrolytes in cerebrospinal fluid, in vivo dialysate of brain and blood plasma of the dog. *J Neurochem* 1966;13:1057–1067.
11. Boulton AA, Baker GB, eds. *Neuromethods, series I: Neurochemistry, vol 1. General neurochemical techniques.* Clifton, NJ: Humana Press, 1985.
12. Brodie BB, Costa E, Dlabac A, Neff NH, Smookler HH. Application of steady-state kinetics to the estimation of synthesis rate and turnover time of tissue catecholamines. *J Pharmacol Exp Ther* 1966;154:493–498.
13. Brownstein MJ. Neuropeptides. In: Siegel GJ, Agranoff BW, Albers RW, Molinoff PB, eds. *Basic neurochemistry,* 5th ed. New York: Raven Press, 1994;341–365.
14. Bungay RL, Morrison PF, Dedrick RL. Steady-state theory for quantitative microdialysis application to in vivo sampling of tritiated water. *Life Sci* 1990;46:105–119.
15. Carlsson A, Davis JN, Kehr W, Lindqvist M, Atack CV. Simultaneous measurement of tyrosine and tryptophan hydrozylase activities in brain in vivo using an inhibitor of the aromatic amino acid decarboxylase. *Naunyn Schmiedebergs Arch Pharmacol* 1972;275:153–168.
16. Costa E, Neff NH. Estimation of turnover rates to study the metabolic regulation of the steady-state level of neuronal monoamines. In: Lajtha A, ed. *Handbook of neurochemistry,* vol 4. New York: Plenum Press, 1970;45–90.
17. Damsma G, Westerink HC. A microdialysis and automated on-line analysis approach to study central cholinergic transmission in vivo. In: Robinson TE, Justice JB Jr, eds. *Microdialysis in the neurosciences. Techniques in the behavioral and neural sciences.* New York: Elsevier Science Publishers, 1991;7:237–249.
18. Davis MD, Gerhardt GA. Stimulus frequency-dependent dopamine autoreceptor activity investigated in vitro using rat nigrostriatal "core" explants and microelectrode electrochemistry. *Soc Neurosci Abstr* 1989;15:1002.
19. Delgado JMR. Pharmacological modifications of social behavior.

In: Paton WDM, ed. *Pharmacological analysis of central nervous action.* Oxford: Pergamon Press, 1962;265–292.

20. Delgado JMR. Telecommunication in brain research. *Proc IV Int Congr Pharmacol* 1970;5:270–278.
21. Delgado JMR, De Feudis FV, Roth RH, Ryugo DK, Mitruka BM. Dialytrode for long term intracerebral perfusion in awake monkeys. *Arch Int Pharmacodyn* 1972;198:9–21.
22. Dingledine R, ed. *Brain slices.* New York, Plenum Press, 1984.
23. During M. In vivo neurochemistry of the conscious human brain: intrahippocampal microdialysis in epilepsy. In: Robinson TE, Justice JB Jr, eds. *Microdialysis in the neurosciences. Techniques in the behavioral and neural sciences.* New York: Elsevier Science Publishers, 1991;425–441.
24. Egawa M, Hoebel BG, Stone EA. Use of microdialysis to measure brain noradrenergic receptor function in vivo. *Brain Res* 1988; 458:303–308.
25. Feldberg W, Sherwook SL. A permanent cannula for intraventricular injections in cats. *J Physiol (Lond)* 1953;120:3P–5P.
26. Fox RH, Hilton SM. Bradykinin formation in human skin as a factor in heat vasodilation. *J Physiol (Lond)* 1953;142:219–232.
27. Fuxe K, Agnati LF, eds. *Advances in neuroscience, vol 1: Transmission in the brain: novel mechanisms for neural transmission.* New York: Raven Press, 1991.
28. Gaddum JH. Push–pull cannulae. *J Physiol (Lond)* 1961;155:1P.
29. Gaddum JH. Substances released in nervous activity. In: Paton WD, Lindgren P eds. *Pharmacological analysis of central nervous action.* London: Pergamon Press, 1962;1–6.
30. Gardner EL, Chen J, Paredes W. Overview of chemical sampling techniques. *J Neurosci Methods* 1993;48:173–197.
31. Gerhardt GA, Oke AF, Nagy G, Moghaddam B, Adams RN. Nafion-coated electrodes with high selectivity of CNS electrochemistry. *Brain Res* 1984;290:390–395.
32. Glick SD, Szilagyi PIA, Crane LA, Green JP. Haloperidol-induced decrease in striatal acetylcholine content in rats killed by either decapitation or microwave radiation. *Brain Res* 1976;118:550–602.
33. Glowinski J, Iversen LL. Regional studies of catecholamines in the rat brain: the disposition of 3H-norepinephrine, 3H-dopamine, 3H-dopa in various regions of the brain. *J Neurochem* 1966;13:665–669.
34. Hillered L, Persson L. Microdialysis for metabolic monitoring in cerebral ischemia and trauma: experimental and clinical studies. In: Robinson TE, Justice JB Jr, eds. *Microdialysis in the neurosciences. Techniques in the behavioral and neural sciences.* New York: Elsevier Science Publishers, 1991;7:389–403.
35. Jacobson I, Sandbergh M, Hamberger A. Mass transfer in brain dialysis devices—a new method for the estimation of extracellular amino acid concentration. *J Neurosci Methods* 1985;15:263–268.
36. Justice JB Jr. Quantitative microdialysis of neurotransmitters. *J Neurosci Methods* 1993;48:263–276.
37. Kawagoe KT, Zimmerman JB, Wightman RM. Principles of voltammetry and microelectrode surface states. *J Neurosci Methods* 1993;48:225–240.
38. Kehr J. A survey on quantitative microdialysis: theoretical models and practical implications. *J Neurosci* 1993;48:251–261.
39. Kissinger PT, Hart JB, Adams RN. Voltammetry in brain tissue—a new neurophysiological measurement. *Brain Res* 1973;55:209–213.
40. Kissinger PT, Refshauge CJ, Dreiling R, Blank L, Freeman R, Adams RN. An electrochemical detector for liquid chromatography with picogram sensitivity. *Anal Lett* 1973;6:465–477.
41. Korf J, Grasdijk L, Westerink BHC. Effects of electrical stimulation of the nigrostriatal pathway of the rat on dopamine metabolism. *J Neurochem* 1976;26:579–584.
42. Lehmann A, Sandberg M, Huxtable RJ. In vivo release of neuroactive amines and amino acids from the hippocampus of seizure-resistant and seizure-susceptible rats. *Neurochem Int* 1986;8:513–520.
43. Lipton P. Brain slices: Uses and abuses. In: Boulton AA, Baker GB, eds. *Neuromethods, series I: Neurochemistry, vol 1. General neurochemical techniques.* Clifton, NJ: Humana Press, 1985.
44. Lonnroth P, Jannson P-A, Smith U. A microdialysis method allowing characterization of intercellular water space in humans. *Am J Physiol* 1987;253:E228–E231.

45. MacIntosh FC, Oborin PE. Release of acetylcholine from intact cerebral cortex. *Abstr XIX Int Physiol Congr* 1953;580–581.
46. Maidment NT, Evans CJ. Measurement of extracellular neuropeptides in the brain: microdialysis linked to solid-phase radioimmunoassays with sub-femtomole limits of detection. In: Robinson TE, Justice JB Jr. *Microdialysis in the neurosciences. Techniques in the behavioral and neural sciences* vol 7. New York: Elsevier Science Publishers, 1991;275–301.
47. Marsden CA, ed. *Measurement of neurotransmitter release* in vivo. New York: John Wiley & Sons, 1984;127–148.
48. Marsden CA, Braxell MP, Maidment NT. An introduction to in vivo electrochemistry. In: Marsden CA, ed. *Measurement of neurotransmitter release* in vivo. New York: John Wiley & Sons, 1984;127–148.
49. Marsden CA, Joseph MH, Kruk ZL, Maidment NT, O'Neill RD, Schenk JO, Stamford JA. In vivo voltammetry—present electrodes and methods. *Neuroscience* 1988;25(2):389–400.
50. Moghaddam B, Bunney BS. Ionic composition of microdialysis perfusing solution alters the pharmacological responsiveness and basal outflow of striatal dopamine. *J Neurochem* 1989;53:652–654.
51. Moroni F, Pepeu G. The cortical cup technique. In: Marsden CA, ed. *Measurement of neurotransmitter release* in vivo. *IBRO handbook series: Methods in the neurosciences* vol 6. New York: John Wiley & Sons, 1984;63–76.
52. Myers RD. Development of push–pull systems for perfusion of anatomically distinct regions of the brain of the awake animal. *Ann NY Acad Sci* 1986;473:21–41.
53. Neff NM, Tozer TN. In vivo measurement of brain serotonin turnover. *Adv Pharmacol* 1968;6a:97–109.
54. Nieoullon A, Cheramy A, Glowinski J. Release of dopamine in vivo from cat substantia nigra. *Nature* 1977;266:375–377.
55. Nyback H, Sevall G. Effect of chlorpromazine on accumulation and disappearance of catecholamines formed from tryosine-14C in brain. *J Pharmacol Exp Ther* 1968;162:294–301.
56. Osborne PG, O'Connor WT, Ungerstedt U. Effect of varying the ionic concentration of a microdialysis perfusate on basal striatal dopamine levels in awake rats. *J Neurochem* 1990;56:452–456.
57. Philippu A. Use of push–pull cannulae to determine the release of endogenous neurotransmitters in distinct brain areas of anaesthetized and freely moving animals. In: Marsden CA, ed. *Measurement of neurotransmitter release* in vivo. *IBRO handbook series: Methods in the neurosciences,* vol 6, New York: John Wiley & Sons, 1984;3–30.
58. Reid KH, Edmonds HL Jr, Schurr A, Tseng MT, West CA. Pitfalls in the use of brain slices. *Prog Neurobiol* 1988;31:1–18.
59. Robinson TE, Camp DM. The feasibility of repeated microdialysis for within-subjects design experiments: studies on the mesostriatal dopamine system. In: Robinson TE, Justice JB Jr, eds. *Microdialysis in the neurosciences. Techniques in the behavioral and neural sciences,* vol 7, New York: Elsevier Science Publishers, 1991;189–218.
60. Robinson TE, Justice JB Jr, eds. *Microdialysis in the neurosciences. Techniques in the behavioral and neural sciences.* New York: Elsevier Science Publishers, 1991;7:81–96.
61. Roffler-Tarlov S, Sharman DF, Tegerdine P. 3,4-Dihydroxyphenylacetic acid and 4-hydroxy-3-methoxyphenylacetic acid in the mouse striatum: a reflection of intra- and extraneuronal metabolism of dopamine? *Br J Pharmacol* 1971;42:343–351.
62. Sherman KA, Hanin I, Zigmond MJ. The effect of neuroleptics on acetylcholine concentration and choline uptake in striatum: implications for regulation of acetylcholine metabolism. *J Pharmacol Exp Ther* 1978;621:677–686.
63. Simon JR, Atweh S, Kuhar MJ. Sodium-dependent high affinity choline uptake: a regulatory step in the synthesis of acetylcholine. *J Neurochem* 1976;26:909–922.
64. Stamford JA, ed. Monitoring neuronal activity: a practical approach. Oxford: IRL Press, 1992.
65. Ungerstedt U. Introduction to intracerebral microdialysis. In: Robinson TE, Justice JB Jr, eds. *Microdialysis in the neurosciences. Techniques in the behavioral and neural sciences,* vol 7, New York: Elsevier Science Publishers, 1991;3–18.
66. Ungerstedt U. Measurement of neurotransmitter release by intracranial dialysis. In: Marsden CA, ed. *Measurement of neurotrans-*

mitter release in vivo. *IBRO handbook series: methods in the neurosciences,* vol 6, New York: John Wiley & Sons, 1984;81–105.

67. Ungerstedt U, Pycock C. Functional correlates of dopamine neurotransmission. *Bull Schweiz Akad Med Wiss* 1974;30:44–55.

68. Ungerstedt U, Herrera-Marshcitz M, Jungnelius U, Ståhle L, Tossman U, Zetterstöm T. Dopamine synaptic mechanisms reflected in studies combining behavioral recordings and brain dialysis. In: Kotisaka M, Shomori T, Tsukada Y, Woodruff GM. *Advances in dopamine research.* New York: Pergamon Press, 1982;219–231.

69. Vizi ES. *Non-synaptic interactions between neurons: modulation of neurochemical transmission.* New York: Wiley & Sons, 1984.

70. Weiner N. A critical assessment of methods for determination of monoamine synthesis and turnover rate in vivo. In: Usdin E, ed. *Neuropsychopharmacology of the monoamines and their regulatory enzymes.* New York: Raven Press, 1974:143.

71. Westerink BHC. Sequence and significance of dopamine metabolism in the rat brain. *Neurochem Int* 1985;7:221–227.

72. Westerink BHC, Hofsteede HM, Damsma G, de Vries JB. The significance of extracellular calcium for the release of dopamine, acetylcholine and amino acids in conscious rats, evaluated by brain microdialysis. *Naunyn Schmiedebergs Arch Pharmacol* 1988;337:373–378.

73. Westerink BHC, De Vries JB. Characterization of the in vivo dopamine release as determined by brain microdialysis after acute and subacute implantations; methodological aspects. *J Neurochem* 1988;51:683–687.

74. Westerink BHC, Justice JB. Microdialysis compared with other in vivo release models. In: Robinson TE, Justice JB Jr, eds. *Microdialysis in the neurosciences. Techniques in the behavioral and neural sciences,* vol 7 New York: Elsevier Science Publishers, 1991;23–40.

75. Wightman RM, Brown DS, Huhr WG, Wilson RL. Molecular specificity of in vivo electrochemical measurements. In: Justice JB, ed. *Voltammetry in the neurosciences.* 1987;103–108.

76. Zetterström T, Sharp T, Marsden CA, Ungerstedt U. In vivo measurement of dopamine and its metabolites by intracerebral dialysis: changes after *d*-amphetamine. *J Neurochem* 1983;41:1769–1773.

77. Zetterström T, Vernet L, Ungerstedt U, Tossman U, Jonzon B. Purine levels in the intact rat brain. Studies with an implanted perfused hollow fibre. *Neurosci Lett* 1982;29:111–115.

78. Zigmond MJ, Stricker EM. Adaptive properties of monoaminergic neurons. In: Lajtha A, ed. *Handbook of neurochemistry,* vol 9 New York: Plenum Press, 1985;87–102.

79. Zilversmit DB. The design and analysis of isotope experiments. *Am J Med* 1960;2:832–848.

Psychopharmacology: The Fourth Generation of Progress, edited by Floyd E. Bloom and David J. Kupfer. Raven Press, Ltd., New York © 1995.

CHAPTER 5

Electrophysiology

Gary S. Aston-Jones and George R. Siggins

Neurons are cells specialized for the integration and propagation of electrical events. It is through such electrical activity that neurons communicate with each other as well as with muscles and other end organs. Therefore, an understanding of basic electrophysiology is fundamental to appreciating the function and dysfunctions of neurons, neural systems, and the brain.

The purpose of this chapter is to describe, for the non-electrophysiologist, the methods used in animal studies to understand the electrical functioning of neurons in the central nervous system (CNS), particularly as related to drug actions and mental function and dysfunction. This chapter is divided into sections devoted to different methods, models, preparations, and concepts used in electrophysiology. These methods differ fundamentally in the level of analysis, and our survey will review them from subcellular (patch-clamping single-ion channels) to behavioral approaches (neuronal recordings in awake primates). Noninvasive electrophysiological techniques, such as electroencephalography (EEG) and event-related potential recordings, are discussed in Chapters 77 and 78 (*this volume*). Methods of metabolic imaging to measure neuronal activity are discussed in Chapters 76, 87, 99, 109, and 119 (*this volume*).

Within each section we describe techniques, give specific examples of their application, and point out their strengths and limitations. Each section will also discuss how a method's particular procedures and level of analysis relate to neuropsychopharmacology. Substantial technical development in electrophysiology has arisen from studies in nonmammalian species (e.g., aplysia, squid). However, to remain most directly relevant to neuropsychopharmacology in the space available, we will consider only techniques used in mammalian preparations. Unfor-

tunately, because of space constraints we are compelled to neglect several very important but lesser-used methods and models, such as noise analysis of ion channel activity (1), and various forms of electrophysiological analyses in intraocular grafts (2), brain "chunks," or in vitro perfused explants (see, e.g., ref. 3). The reader should refer to the cited references and the excellent "methods" book by Kettenmann and Grantyn (4) for details on these and other novel approaches.

The introductory descriptions of neurons (see Chapter 1, *this volume*) provide a background for the following sections on specific electrophysiological techniques. Throughout this chapter, we will draw upon knowledge reviewed by Barondes (Chapter 2), Watson and Cullinan (Chapter 3), Zigmond (Chapter 4), and Roth and colleagues (Chapter 78, *this volume*). Readers are referred to those chapters for details.[1]

TECHNIQUES AND MODELS TO STUDY MEMBRANE CHANNEL FUNCTION

At the cellular level, electrical activity of neurons consists of the movement of charges (ions) through neuronal surface membranes. The major charge carrying ions are sodium (Na^+), potassium (K^+), chloride (Cl^-) and calcium (Ca^{2+}). The surface membranes of neurons are primarily composed of lipids (resistive elements, in electrical terms) which do not allow ionic flow. Instead, these semi-permeable membranes are spanned by large specialized protein aggregates that form pores or channels through the lipid membrane. There are specific channel protein assemblies (usually more than one) for each of the ionic charge carriers, as well as those for certain cations in

G. S. Aston-Jones: Division of Behavioral Neurobiology, Department of Mental Health Sciences, Hahnemann University Medical School, Philadelphia, Pennsylvania 19102.

G. R. Siggins: Department of Neuropharmacology, Scripps Clinic and Research Foundation, La Jolla, California 92037.

[1] To comply with editorial limitations on length, references cited were purposely curtailed to include only detailed descriptions of specific methods, reviews of these techniques, or recent reports in which application of such methods have yielded important neuropsychopharmacological insights.

general, that confer a semipermeable nature to the membrane. The ability of these channels to permit ion flow is determined by several factors, most prominently the electrical potential that exists across the membrane, the gradient of ions set up by membrane pumps, and the semipermeable nature of the channels, as well as by responses of receptors, guanosine triphosphate (GTP)-binding proteins (termed G proteins), and second messengers to neurotransmitters and hormones. For more detail on these aspects of neuronal membrane and channel properties, (see Chapters 11, 27, and 38, *this volume*); also see larger works by Siggins and Gruol (5), Hille (6) and Shepherd (7).

Artificial Membrane-Channel Preparations

Description

There is a long history of electrophysiological studies on artificial lipid bilayer membranes that were designed in large part to determine whether bioelectric events result from membrane ion pores (channels) or transmembrane ion carriers (active transport). The results of these studies were important for substantiating the view cited above of cellular-level events involved in bioelectric activity. Studies on pore-forming antibiotic models by Mueller and Rudin (reviewed in ref. 6) laid a strong biophysical foundation (such as the involvement of water molecules) for subsequent understanding of natural ion channels, and they were largely predictive of subsequent single-channel recordings of biological channels (see below). Later refinements of this method included insertion of natural ion channels prepared from a variety of cell types or organelles. In brief, the artificial bilayer membranes are usually made by forming a sheet of lipid (such as phosphatidylserine) across a partition with a small hole separating two aqueous compartments. A vesicle preparation (e.g., "liposomes") containing either the antibiotic protein (e.g., gramacidin), a fractionated membrane containing ion channels, or (in later studies) reconstituted vesicles with purified channels is added to one of the compartments (see ref. 8 for review); under the right conditions, the vesicles fuse with the lipid bilayer membrane and insert channels. Standard voltage-clamp recordings (see below) are then performed between the two compartments, and drugs and ion changes can be applied to either side of the artificial membrane.

Studies using natural membranes with artificially inserted foreign but natural receptor-channel complexes have given even more validity to the pore theory and provided another powerful model for testing pharmacological agents. The procedure here typically involves injection of a channel preparation directly into a large living cell (tolerant to insertion of large injection and recording pipettes) such as the *Xenopus laevis* oocyte or several types of cell lines. The channel source is usually either (a) vesicles prepared from fractionated channel-bearing membrane, (b) vesicles with reconstituted, purified channel (glyco)protein, or (c) channels newly synthesized by foreign DNA or RNA injected into the oocyte via large pipettes (Fig. 1). Of course, the more purified the protein or DNA/RNA, the more homogenous will be the channel population eventually inserted.

Example Studies

In terms of their great potential for dissection of the molecular mechanisms of pharmacological action, studies using these artificial, reconstituted or "cloned" channels are still in their infancy. However, there have already been too many fine examples of the use of the methods to adequately recount here. Notwithstanding, we would be remiss not to mention the elegant molecular and pharmacological studies of the gamma-aminobutyric acid (GABA) receptor–ionophore complex by Eric Barnard, Robert MacDonald, and co-workers (9), as well as of the various glutamate receptor-channel subtypes by the Dingledine and Heinemann groups (10,11) (see also Chapters 7 and 8, *this volume*). Moreover, recent studies of ethanol effects on brain GABA and glutamate receptor channels expressed in *Xenopus* oocytes (12) and cell lines (13) have provided considerable insight into these two major sites of alcohol action (14) and provide prime examples of the potential uses of these methods for the study of the molecular mechanisms of action of psychopharmacological agents. Future studies of this type, in combination with site-directed mutagenesis, will help delineate the molecular site(s) of drug actions on a wide range of neuronal receptors.

Single-Channel Patch Clamp

Description

The discovery and development, by Sakmann and Neher (15), of the "patch-clamp" method for recording from single-ion channels provided decisive proof of the aqueous pore theory for the origin of neuronal excitability and led to a long string of seminal studies culminating in their Nobel prize. This method originally required fabricating and fire-polishing of specific types of glass micropipettes (with large tip diameters relative to the "sharp" pipettes used in traditional intracellular recording), so that the tips could form a high-resistance (gigohm) seal when pushed onto a cultured or acutely isolated cell. The gigohm seal (and new electronic breakthroughs) essentially allowed the high current gain, low noise amplification necessary for recording the small, brief currents (under voltage-clamp conditions) passing through single ionic channels. Imagine the excitement when Sakmann and Neher saw the now familiar "box-like" currents suggesting the abrupt opening and closing of channels (Fig. 2; see ref. 15). There were other surprises not predicted

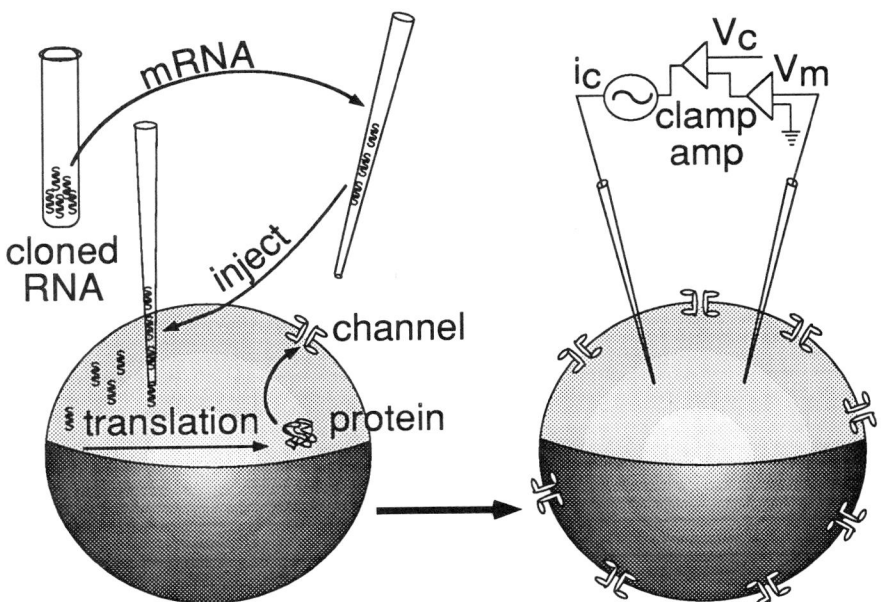

FIG. 1. Schematic of oocyte expression system and voltage-clamp recording method. **Left:** RNA (or DNA, not shown) prepared from a cloned gene for a membrane channel is injected from a micropipette into a frog oocyte. The oocyte contains the necessary processing systems to translate this RNA (or DNA) into the specific protein, which is then incorporated into the outer membrane of the oocyte as a functional channel. **Right:** Voltage-clamp recording is used to examine the properties of this newly expressed channel. The large size of the oocyte allows two-electrode voltage clamp. The recording pipette transmits the membrane potential (V_m) to the clamp amplifier, which also receives a voltage command (V_c). The comparative difference between V_m and V_c is used to generate a clamping current (I_c) which is injected into the cell to bring V_m to equal V_c. In this way, V_m is "clamped" to the value of V_c; the I_c needed to maintain this V_m is equal to currents flowing across the membrane at any time-point and can be examined as a function of drug application or changes in V_c, or small changes in the composition of cloned RNA/DNA (and therefore the channel protein). These manipulations can help isolate the parts of the inserted channel responsible for each unique property of that channel (e.g., sites for antagonist or G-protein binding).

by the biophysical models, such as the rapid open-and-closed "flickering" and burst-like openings of the channels in many cases.

The patch-clamp method can be applied in at least four configurations (Fig. 2), giving the technique formidable adaptability for testing the molecular mechanisms of receptors and their associated ion channels and second messengers. Three of these configurations (cell-attached patch, inside-out patch, and outside-out patch) allow study of individual ion channels under different conditions. In the *cell-attached* configuration, after formation of the gigohm seal, recording of single channels is made without disruption of the cell membrane. In the other two single-channel preparations, the membrane patch is detached from the neuron after a gigohm seal is formed, and single-channel activity is recorded in isolation from the cell. In the *inside-out* configuration, the patch of membrane is gently pulled away from the cell, and the patch remains attached to the pipette with its cytoplasmic surface now exposed to the bathing solution. Preparation of the *outside-out* patch begins by making a whole-cell configuration (see below) whereby, after forming the gigohm

seal, the membrane patch under the pipette is ruptured by applying a strong vacuum through the recording pipette. Then the pipette is gently pulled away from the cell, carrying a piece of membrane with it. The detached membrane seals over the pipette tip during this maneuver, in favorable cases forming a membrane patch in which the extracellular membrane surface is exposed to the bathing solution. The *whole-cell* configuration will be described below.

Example Studies

Once again, examples of the use of single-channel patch-clamp methods are far too numerous to itemize here. However, psychopharmacologists interested in the use of these methods in elucidating the pharmacology of NMDA, GABA, and opiate receptors may wish to consult the work of Barker and colleagues (16), MacDonald and colleagues (17), and North and co-workers (18). These papers contain abundant detail on the elegant methods used to record single channels and test the action of various psychopharmacological agents.

Patch Configurations

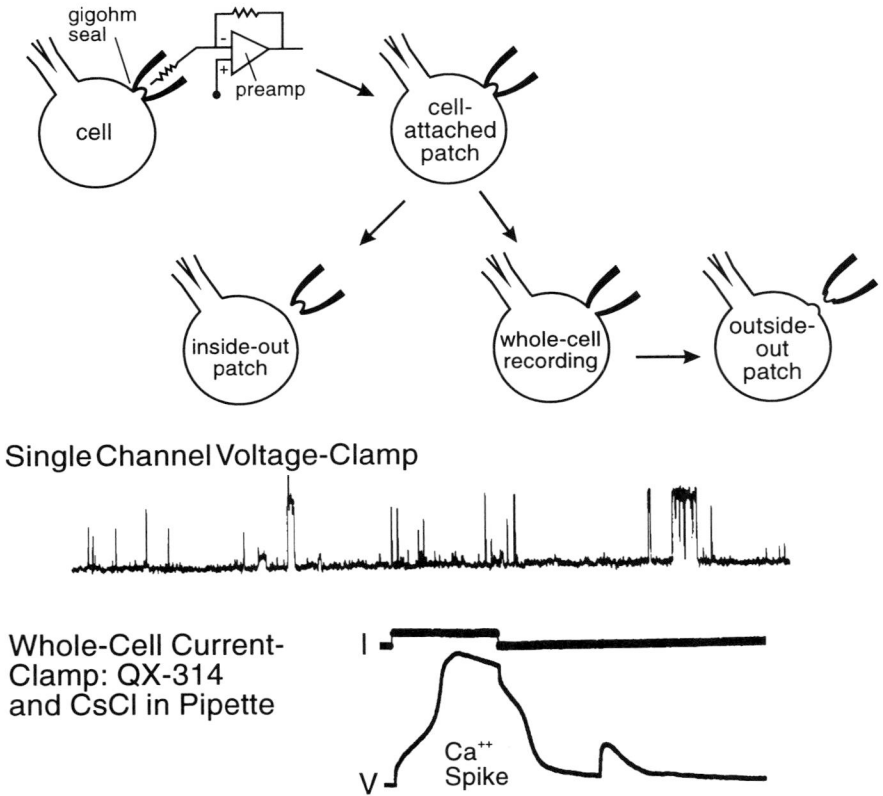

Single Channel Voltage-Clamp

Whole-Cell Current-Clamp: QX-314 and CsCl in Pipette

I

V

Ca^{++} Spike

FIG. 2. Schematic of patch-clamp configurations and representative single-channel and whole-cell records. **Upper panel:** The same patch pipette and voltage-clamp amplifier setup can be used to record in four different configurations (see text for details). Single-channel recordings can be taken from three of the four configurations: cell-attached, inside-out and outside-out patches. Breaking the patch under the pipette (by suction) allows whole-cell voltage or current recording. **Middle panel:** A representative cell-attached patch recording (voltage-clamp mode) from a cultured CNS neuron, showing currents flowing through single ion channels. Single-channel activity appears as box-like upward events. At least two channels are present in this patch, as indicated by the different event amplitudes. Brief upward events are channel openings not fully resolved due to recording limitations (D. L. Gruol, *unpublished observations*). **Lower panel:** Representative whole-cell current-clamp recording of a hippocampal neuron in a slice preparation, recorded with a pipette containing QX-314 to block Na^+ channels (fast spikes) and 140 mM CsCl to block K^+ channels (G. R. Siggins, *unpublished observations*). This record was taken about 5 min after patching on and breaking into the cell; the Ca^{2+}-dependent action potential (a broad depolarizing plateau without a fast Na^+ component or afterhyperpolarizing potential) evoked by depolarizing current injection indicates the rapid equilibration allowed by this configuration, between the contents of the pipette and the cellular constituents. I = current, V = voltage. (Modified from Fig. 10 of ref. 5.)

Whole-Cell Clamp

The whole-cell clamp, illustrated in Fig. 2, is a form of the cell-attached configuration that uses the same pipette type and gigohm seal method described above but that, by rupturing the membrane under the tip, allows recording of the "macroscopic" or summed currents flowing through all channels in the entire cellular membrane, rather than through a single channel. In this configuration, after the pipette is sealed to the membrane, another slightly stronger vacuum is applied to the pipette tip (via the tube attached to the pipette holder) to rupture the membrane under the tip with-

out disrupting the gigohm seal or cell viability. During current-clamp recording, successful "break-in" is signaled by a negative shift in the recorded potential (to the cell resting membrane potential) and a large reduction in the input resistance of the system (now due only to the series resistance of the pipette and the input resistance of the total cell). In this configuration, the diffusable contents of the pipette then exchange over time with those of the cell.

Example Studies

Again, there are numerous examples in the literature over the last 10 years of whole-cell patch recording of neurons in isolated systems and an ever-increasing number of whole-cell patch-clamp studies of neurons in slice preparations (see below). From a pharmacological viewpoint, the whole-cell patch studies of the MacDonald (17) and North groups (18) on second messenger and G-protein mediation or regulation of GABA, opiate, catecholamine, and somatostatin effects deserve special reference. See the chapter by Foote and Aston-Jones (*this volume*) for details on such studies in rat locus coeruleus neurons.

Voltage and Ion-Sensitive Dyes and Resins

Description

Over the last 30 years, a variety of nonelectrophysiological (and sometimes even noninvasive) methods have been explored to measure the membrane properties and ionic constituents of excitable cells. Purely optical recording methods (without dyes) were originally applied to isolated axons (e.g., from squid or crab) and revealed changes in both light scattering and membrane birefringence during stimulus-evoked action potentials. Later studies infused a potentiometric merocyanine dye intracellularly and used signal averaging methods to show that optical absorption or fluorescence changes closely followed the time course of the action potential (19), indicating that these were useful methods for studying membrane potential by relatively noninvasive methods. The development of newer, more effective voltage-sensitive dyes offer pharmacologists the opportunity to follow membrane potential changes optically, without penetration or other disruption of the neuronal membrane other than extracellular treatment with the dye. The reader is referred to recent reviews (e.g., refs. 20 and 21) for details on the types and mechanisms of these membrane potential indicators.

Dyes can also be used to measure the intracellular and extracellular concentrations of certain free ions (or better, their activities). While there are now a variety of indicator dyes relatively selective for several different ions (including H^+, Na^+, and Cl^-), by far the most research has been done with Ca^{2+}-sensitive dyes (see ref. 21). Metallochromatic indicator dyes like arsenazo III were found useful for the measurement of cytosolic free Ca^{2+}, as first tested in squid giant axons. The luminescent photoprotein aequorin also had its heyday as an indicator of intracellular free Ca^{2+}. However, most of these methods involved the injection of the indicator into the cell, therefore requiring the study of larger neurons. The newer fluorescent probes (quin-2, fura-2, indo-1, and fluo-3) based on the Ca^{2+}-chelator ethyleneglycol bis(aminoethyl ether)tetraacetate (EGTA) model (see ref. 21) also generally requires the use of fluorescent (ultraviolet or near-ultraviolet) illumination on relatively isolated neurons (e.g., neuronal cultures, very thin slices, or acutely isolated neurons) or

isolated axon bundles. However, these newer indicators can now be loaded into neurons without injection or penetration by using their hydrolyzable esters such as acetoxymethyl (MA) ester. These esterified indicators can merely be applied extracellularly; the ester confers hydrophobicity, allowing the indicator to pass through the membrane into the cytoplasm, where the ester is removed by endogenous esterases, trapping the indicator inside. Furthermore, the recent development of scanning confocal microscopy (which can optically section a neuron without contamination by out-of-focus objects), in combination with these Ca^{2+} indicators, has made it possible to observe spatial or compartmental changes in intracellular free Ca^{2+} even in neurons within relatively thick preparations (21,22).

However, as implied above, unless a confocal microscope is available (still a rather large expense), all of these methods require a certain degree of isolation of the neurons under study. Therefore, if the chosen model is an in vivo or thick-slice preparation, the use of ion-sensitive electrodes containing ion-exchange resins, although difficult to implement (see ref. 23 for details on electrode fabrication), can be of considerable advantage. These electrodes can be inserted blindly into thick brain slices, or even into brain regions in vivo, to record absolute values or changes in ion activities. These electrodes achieve their ionic selectivity by virtue of the resin which generates a current flow in the electrode in proportion to the concentration of a specific ionic species. K^+ and Ca^{2+} ion activities are the most often measured. Whereas the ion-exchange resin method is best at measuring extracellular ionic activities (because the high resistance of the resin usually requires the use of rather large-tipped micropipettes), under the right conditions intracellular measures can also be obtained with this method (23).

Examples

Considerable information about neuronal and synaptic mechanisms and the effects of drugs on these mechanisms has been obtained with either the extracellular or intracellular application of ion-sensitive microelectrodes. For example, Lux, Heinemann, and colleagues (see ref. 23) have used these microelectrodes in various preparations to follow the extracellular K^+ and Ca^{2+} levels with epileptiform activity or synaptic action via stimulation of afferent pathways.

As for the ion-sensitive fluorescent probes, fura-2 has been used to measure intracellular Ca^{2+} in innumerable studies. However, the ability of this indicator to measure compartmentally (spatially) distinct and time-dependent changes of intracellular calcium levels in several neuron types, with alteration of these changes by neurotransmitters, drugs (e.g., caffeine), and ion changes, is an especially exciting use of this method (21). This method also has great applicability for non-neuronal cells: Holliday and Gruol (24) recently used fura-2 imaging to show that the cytokine interleukin-1β dramatically increases intracellular Ca^{2+} levels in cortical astrocyte cultures and also enhances the increased Ca^{2+} evoked by the glutamate receptor agonist quisqualate.

Advantages and Disadvantages—Isolated Preparations and Patch-Clamp Analyses

The artificial membrane, reconstituted receptor/channel, and patch-clamp methods have allowed the use of isolated membrane components, isolated mRNA, foreign (non-neural) cells, and acutely isolated (enzymatically dissociated) or cultured neurons. As a result, there are several global advantages for these methods. First, these isolated preparations represent greatly simplified systems whose electrophysiological responses are not confounded by uncontrolled synaptic or hormonal inputs. Indeed, the total external and internal milieu of the cells and channels can be controlled by the experimenter, thus providing unprecedented capabilities for testing the influence of countless influences and variables. For example, the researcher can adjust the ionic compositions on either side of the membrane or channel so that the voltage differential is exactly opposite (i.e., positive on the inside surface) to that in normal cells; this facilitates greater isolation of membrane conductances involved in certain membrane and synaptic functions.

Another advantage of these isolated membranes and systems is their suitability for use of molecular and genetic techniques (described by Baronds, *this volume*). Thus, as implied above, one can easily test the effects of minute modifications of the molecular structure of receptors and their associated channels, as well as the individual components (subunits) of G proteins and second messenger systems (described by Zigmond, *this volume*). As a result, researchers can now answer many physiological questions at the molecular level. For example, one can determine exactly where [i.e., at what codon(s) in the RNA or amino acid(s) in the protein] in the channel molecule or subunit that an antagonist or drug acts, or at what point protein phosphorylation (e.g., via protein kinases) can modulate receptor function. Thus, using combined electrophysiology and molecular biology, for the first time we can begin to make a definitive connection between structure and function at the molecular level.

The several disadvantages of these models are principally derived from the isolation process itself. Hence, these isolated preparations, because they lack normal synaptic connections with other neurons, may be functioning under conditions greatly different than normally seen in the living organism, and thus may provide answers not relevant to the "real world." In addition, one is never certain that the "extracellular" and "intracellular" media used do not constitute a totally artificial environment that would not be relevant to a living neuron in vivo. The lack

of normally circulating agents such as steroids, hormones, plasma proteins, and other colloidal substances could lead to drastic changes in the function of the molecules and channels under study. Finally, this inability to examine receptor and channel function in the context of an intact functioning system may cloud the application of findings derived from these models to the behavior of living organisms.

The patch-clamp method is nearly ideal for the study of the mechanisms of drug action at the single-channel level. Some of the advantages of this method include the following: (a) Ions, toxins, neurochemicals, and other pharmacological agents can be applied easily (either in the bath or in the pipette), in defined concentrations, to both the external and internal surfaces of the membrane; (b) several chemicals or ions can be tested on one patch (or channel) either together or in sequence; and (c) several different drug or ion concentrations can be tested on the same membrane patch, thus facilitating generation of dose–response curves. In addition, the gating mechanism(s) behind the opening of channels can be pharmacologically tested more easily in a patch configuration.

The single-channel, cell-attached, and inside-out patch-clamp methods are particularly well-suited for the study of second messenger systems, and particularly for those systems (such as G-protein-mediated events) that are "membrane-delimited" (see, e.g., ref. 25). Thus, in the cell-attached configuration, if a transmitter or other receptor regulator (first messenger) applied externally in the bathing solution—but not when applied from within the pipette—alters single-channel function (e.g., opening or closing of the channel recorded), the receptor must be remote from the recorded channel and mediation of the event by a diffusible second messenger is suspected. If the transmitter or regulator alters channel function even when applied via the recording pipette to an inside-out patch (where a soluble second messenger would diffuse away from the system), a membrane-delimited system is a likely candidate (see ref. 18) for an elegant example of this approach in opiate responses of locus coeruleus neurons.

A major disadvantage of the single-channel patch-clamp method is the necessity to use cultured or acutely isolated cells; such models seem to allow formation of better gigohm seals, probably because the relative lack of overlying glia or other supporting cells facilitates close apposition and seal of the pipette to the neuronal membrane. In addition, compared to cells lying within a slice preparation, the thin or nonexistent level of tissue and/or fluid overlying the recorded neuron reduces the capacitance in the recording system and allows better recording characteristics for the small-current signals generated by single channels. Therefore, most single-channel studies to date have been limited to cultured or isolated neurons. However, new refinements have allowed whole-cell patch (and some single-channel) recording in brain slices, and even in vivo (see below).

In part because of the free exchange of contents between the cell and the pipette, the whole-cell method has several additional advantages and disadvantages. First, unlike the single-channel methods, the whole-cell method can be used routinely in brain-slice preparations (see below and refs. 26 and 29) as well as in vivo. Also, with this method one can adjust the ionic balance and contents of the cell merely by placing the appropriate buffers and salts in the pipette solution. Furthermore, second messengers and drugs affecting them can be placed directly in the pipette solution for diffusion into the cell. For selective blockade of certain channel types (e.g., K^+-selective channels), toxins (e.g., tetraethylammonium) or appropriate ions (e.g., Cs^+) can also be placed in the pipette. And finally, dyes such as lucifer yellow or biocytin can be placed in the pipettes for quicker and more complete filling of the neurons than with the standard intracellular ''sharp'' pipettes.

The major disadvantages of the whole-cell method usually stem from the same properties that confer the advantages. Thus, because it is usually not possible to know the exact ionic or second messenger composition of the normal resting cell, there is always the risk that essential cell constituents (e.g., cyclic AMP) will diffuse out of the cell into the pipette (which usually constitutes a much larger volume than that of the cell). It is thought that such diffusion accounts for the slow ''run-down'' in some cells of certain currents such as the L-type Ca^{2+} current. Attempting to replace such lost constituents (e.g., cyclic AMP, ATP, GTP) by adding them to the pipette solution can help alleviate some of these problems. The use of a nystatin ''barrier'' in the pipette tip (see ref. 27), which allows passage of small monovalent ions (e.g., for current injection) but prevents the diffusion of most divalent and large nonionic constituents (e.g., proteinaceous buffers and components of phosphorylation systems) from the cell, is another procedure for reducing these problems.

As alluded to above, there are many advantages of the various imaging approaches, the most important being the ability to measure ionic or potential changes via relatively noninvasive methods. However, it should be remembered that most of these methods require dyes and/or light exposure of some sort that can distinctly alter cell function over time. In addition, most of these methods require relatively isolated or thin preparations, so that microscopic observation can be performed.

Relevance to Neuropsychopharmacology

Implicit in these studies of ion channels and their related receptors is the idea that a substantial molecular and electrophysiological understanding of the function of each structural element or subelement will allow the rational development of more effective and selective pharmacological agents and, ultimately, better therapeutic drugs. For example, understanding what part (amino acid residues, phosphorylated region, etc.) of the *N*-methyl-D-

aspartate (NMDA) receptor-channel complex is affected by alcohol could lead to the development of a drug to blunt the alcohol antagonism of NMDA receptor function. Because the anti-NMDA effect of ethanol is thought to account for many aspects of alcohol intoxication (14), this drug could be the ''silver bullet,'' sought by alcohol researchers for years, for rapidly reversing ethanol-induced intoxication. In addition, all of the single-channel methods have the capability of being applied to human samples (e.g., slices or cultures from biopsies), both from normal tissue and from diseased brains. The single-channel (and molecular) data from these two sources could then be compared for indications of the structural source of the abnormalities or malfunction; with this sort of knowledge base, more rational drug development or intervention procedures would lead to new, more effective treatments for the disease.

TECHNIQUES TO STUDY CELLULAR ELECTRICAL FUNCTION

The above discussion concerns parts of cells or individual channels. However, there are many motives for electrophysiological study of intact neurons in isolation or semi-isolation. Activity in a single channel typically has little influence on the overall electrical activity of a postsynaptic cell. A neuron usually receives synapses from thousands of other neurons, and many of those inputs may be active at approximately the same time (synchrony). The way in which this postsynaptic cell integrates these numerous inputs and alters its own electrical activity is the fundamental basis of neuronal integration and information processing in the brain. The researcher may need to understand the integration between different parts of the neuron, or how an action at one locus (e.g., an ion channel) can lead to transmission of information to another locus (e.g., by a second messenger), without interference from outside events. To accomplish this understanding, the electrophysiologist uses the numerous tools and models that have been developed to study intact neurons.

Isolated Neurons and Neuronal Cultures

The most completely isolated yet relatively intact cellular preparation is the *acutely isolated neuron* model. Such isolated neurons are prepared by mild enzymatic digestion and gentle agitation and trituration of brain slices (28). Neurons can be isolated from most brain regions; when prepared correctly, they have most of the properties of neurons in culture and slice preparations, but are free of the glial investments and debris that prevent formation of gigohm seals in patch-clamp studies. Although the distal dendrites can be truncated by this procedure (with possible loss of important channels or receptors), the reduced dendritic length greatly reduces space-clamp difficulties in voltage-clamp recordings (see below).

Chronically cultured neurons and cell lines (such as those also used for single-channel studies) have been a major cellular source for electrophysiological studies (see, e.g., refs. 9 and 16), as have single neurons within *brain slices* (see below for methods of preparation). Acutely isolated or cultured neurons have the advantage of direct microscopic visualization and manipulation; however, neurons in brain slices (described later) also can be visualized now using new optical methods such as Nomarski microscopy combined with sensitive video imaging (29,30). Another relatively new model, the *slice culture,* has been developed by the Gähwiler group (31). Slice cultures are prepared by long-term incubation of brain slices in a rotating drum (''roller tubes''), where the slices develop into a monolayer of neurons that retain their local cytoarchitectonic relationships and that can be individually manipulated under microscopic visualization.

Although there are usually synaptic connections among neurons of all these models except acutely isolated neurons and some cell lines, for purely cellular studies the neurons can be chemically isolated by blocking synaptic transmission with Na^+ or Ca^{2+} channel antagonists such as tetrodotoxin or low concentrations of Ca^{2+} with high concentrations (8–12 mM) of Mg^{2+}. The researcher can then study the neurons individually with little influence from remote synaptic effects. Another method of electrical isolation is to bathe the slice in isotonic sucrose (without salts) and then apply a small amount of (conductive) Ringer's solution via a small-bore pipette to the neuronal region under study; this is a cellular application of the old ''sucrose gap'' method. Methods such as these should always be used as controls in any study testing the effects of exogenously applied drugs or transmitters: if the isolation procedure blocks the drug effects, then indirect (remote) effects are suspected.

Examples

For details on the preparation and use of these and other cellular models, we direct the reader to two excellent books on methods, edited by Shahar et al. (32) and by Kettenmann and Grantyn (4).

Current and Voltage-Clamp Recording in Vitro

Both of these methods involve recording membrane potential with an electrode inserted into, or in contact

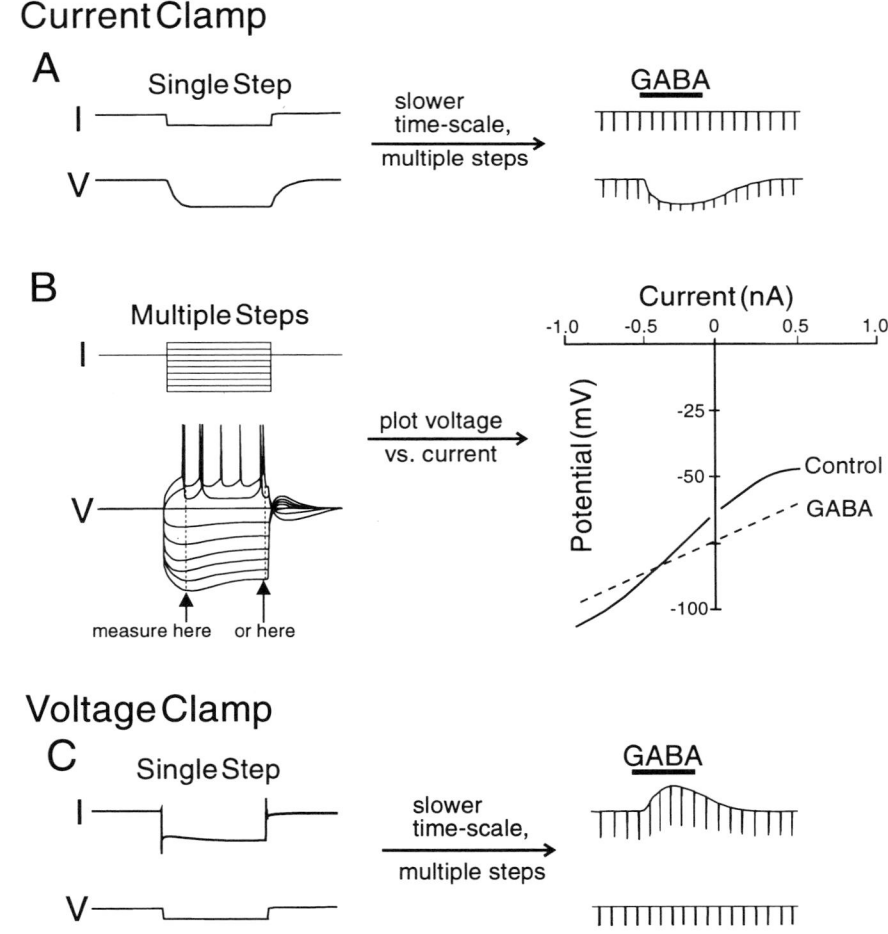

with, the intracellular compartment. Such *intracellular recordings* are required for several types of analyses—including, for example, observation of pacemaker activity or subthreshold synaptic effects.

Current-clamp is a method of intracellular recording involving measurement of the voltage difference across the cellular membrane while injecting constant positive or negative current (as "square" d.c. pulses) into the cell. Voltage recording without current injection or other perturbation will usually tell the researcher only what the membrane potential is (usually around -60 to -80 mV in resting neurons). However, by injecting repetitive constant current pulses (or steps) into the cell and using appropriate "bridge" methods to balance out the resistive influence of the recording micropipette, the electrophysiologist can obtain from the voltage response a relative measure of the resistance (or, inversely, of conductance: g) of the membrane. Ohm's law ($E = IR$) can be applied here to obtain a simple relationship between the current injected (I), the voltage recorded (E), and the "input resistance" (R) of the membrane. If a drug or transmitter is then applied to the cell, a change in the size of the voltage response to the current pulse indicates a change in ionic conductance ($g = 1/R$). By incrementally varying the amplitudes of the current steps over a wide range (typically from 0.1 to 1 nA in mammalian CNS neurons), a family of voltage responses can be obtained for construction of a voltage–current ($V–I$) curve (where voltage is typically plotted as a function of injected current; see Fig. 3). This curve reveals much about the "macroscopic" currents (that is, the aggregate currents flowing through many ionic channels) passing through the neuronal membrane at different membrane potentials. Any drug treatment that alters ionic conductance will also alter the slope and shape of the $V–I$ curve. Thus, a reduction in the slope of the $V–I$ curve indicates increased ionic conductance, whereas a steeper slope indicates decreased conductance.

In practice, current-clamp recording is usually performed by inserting a single sharp micropipette into a neuron while recording voltage and injecting current through the same pipette. Penetration of the cell is sig-

---

FIG. 3. Schematic of typical protocols for current- and voltage-clamp recording. **A:** Current-clamp. *Left panel:* Membrane potential is recorded with a brief injection (20–500 msec) of a rectangular negative (hyperpolarizing) current (*I*) pulse through the recording barrel; a hyperpolarizing voltage (*V*) response (deflection) is recorded that reflects the impedance (resistive) properties of the membrane (effects of electrode resistance are subtracted). The slowness of the onset and offset of the voltage response represents the effect of membrane capacitance and resistance. The amplitude of the voltage response is proportional to membrane resistance; this value times the current injected allow the calculation of "input resistance" (by Ohm's law). *Right panel:* During injection of multiple current pulses at regular intervals (2–10 sec) and recording at a slower time-base, voltage responses appear as brief downward deflections. Application of a conventional inhibitory transmitter such as GABA reveals the expected hyperpolarization associated with a reduction of the size of the downward deflections, indicating reduced input resistance. **B:** To allow better analysis of voltage-dependent drug effects (see Fig. 4) and to determine their reversal or equilibrium potentials, construction of voltage–current curves are required. Here, multiple pulses or steps of current of both polarities and various intensities (e.g., 0.05–2 nA) are injected at regular intervals and resultant voltage responses displayed superimposed at high oscilloscope speed, as shown at left. The "sag" in the voltage responses often seen at more hyperpolarized potentials results from a time-dependent current [e.g., the M-current (see Fig. 4) or the *Q* or *h* current, a hyperpolarization-dependent inward rectifying current involved in pacemaker potentials]. Plotting the size of these potentials (at either the peak or the steady state: *dotted lines*) against the current (the independent variable) yields a $V–I$ curve (*right panel*) with properties characteristic for each cell. Repeating this procedure during drug application may then reveal changes in the position and slope of the $V–I$ curve. For example, GABA lowers the curve and reduces the slope, indicating hyperpolarization with reduced input or slope resistance (or increased conductance). The intersection of the control and GABA curves at around -80 mV denotes the reversal potential of the GABA effect, as would be expected of increased Cl^- conductance and recording with a pipette filled with an anion that does not alter the intracellular Cl^- concentration. **C:** A simple voltage-clamp protocol, in which the membrane current is the measured, dependent variable. Voltage is the independent variable: Using a single hyperpolarizing voltage command (V_c), with the membrane potential clamped (at holding potential: V_h, often around resting potential), one can obtain a relative estimate of the "macroscopic" current (*left panel*) flowing through multiple ion channels (see text). The slow time-dependent inward "relaxation" in the current trace during the command potential represents the so-called Q or h current. When multiple voltage commands of the same size are applied repetitively at slow chart speed (*right panel*), one can determine whether a drug increases or decreases ionic conductance (directly proportional to the size of each current response); thus, in this case, GABA increases ionic conductance. *Not shown:* Delivery of multiple depolarizing and/or hyperpolarizing voltage commands of different intensities can be used to generate current–voltage curves similar (although with axis rotated 90 degrees and the curve inverted) to the $V–I$ curves of current-clamp recordings (see part **B**, *right panel*). Such $I–V$ curves give an estimate of "slope conductance" of the macroscopic currents over a large membrane potential range. Here, increased slope would indicate increased conductance (decreased resistance). (Modified from Fig. 7 of ref. 5.)

naled by an abrupt transition to a large negative voltage (about −70 mV), accompanied by an increase in input resistance (as typically reflected in the voltage deflection produced by a current pulse). After successful settling ("sealing") of the pipette into the membrane, control V–I curves and synaptic activations can be generated (usually nowadays by sophisticated computer methods); drug administration by superfusion or pipette application (see below) is then followed by repeated V–I and synaptic measures for statistical comparison to the control measures. Reversal of any drug effects by washout with the vehicle (artificial cerebrospinal fluid) alone assures the researcher that any changes are not merely the result of a rundown (e.g., slow death) of the cell or a slowly improving penetration "seal." The usual measures taken in current clamp include: resting membrane potential, input resistance, I–V curves, and voltage responses (excitatory postsynaptic potentials or inhibitory postsynaptic potentials) to activation of inhibitory or excitatory synaptic afferents. In addition, much information about membrane and drug properties can be obtained from the rebound voltage responses (so-called "anodal break" depolarizations, due to activation of several possible currents) immediately following strong hyperpolarizing current steps, or from the prolonged hyperpolarizations [afterhyperpolarizations (AHPs) due to Ca^{2+}-dependent K^+ conductances] following the burst of spikes evoked by strong depolarizing current steps. Many neurotransmitters have been shown to potently alter the latter measure (see ref. 5).

In *voltage-clamp* recording, the investigator measures the current required to hold a neuron at a constant voltage; voltage "commands" are typically applied as steps or as a steady voltage (termed "holding potential"; see Fig. 3). A major advantage of this method over current-clamp recording is that the investigator can directly measure ionic currents, and not just the reflection of currents passing through channels (i.e., voltage response, which may vary with other changes). In addition, by using abrupt voltage-command jumps, one can measure the changes (and their kinetics) in the currents flowing at the original potential as the channels slowly adjust (open or close) to the new potential. Thus, with this method, voltage-dependent and time-dependent ionic conductances, and the effects of drugs on these conductances, can be directly monitored.

In practice, voltage-clamp recording of mammalian CNS neurons in vitro involves the same sorts of micropipettes and other methods as those used in current-clamp recording (most high-performance commercial headstage amplifiers allow switching between the two modes). In fact, one usually penetrates a neuron with the micropipette under current-clamp mode. Then after the cell stabilizes, a series of adjustments of the recording characteristics can allow stable switching to voltage clamp.

Until recently, most research on brain-slice preparations (described below) has applied either extracellular recording or standard intracellular recording with "sharp" pipettes. Because these pipettes usually have the

unfortunate feature of high electrical resistance (because of the need for fine tips to penetrate small cells with little injury), recording properties were not optimal. Because early voltage-clamp methods generally required insertion of two pipettes into large (invertebrate) cells, early studies of brain-slice neurons typically employed "current-clamp" methods (described above). Later, a novel "switch-clamp" method was developed whereby a single pipette is used to switch rapidly (at about 2–7 kHz) back and forth between current injection and voltage measurement modes (see ref. 33). As with the two-electrode voltage-clamp method, the measured voltage is compared to a desired voltage (the "holding" or "command" potential) and the difference is used during the next brief current-injection cycle to inject the appropriate current to bring the membrane to the desired voltage. However, the switch-clamp method has several disadvantages, including the need to keep pipette resistance and capacitance to a minimum (usually 50–70 MΩ or less) so that the cell and not the pipette potential is clamped. Another disadvantage is the difficulty in clamping remote membrane areas (e.g., in the dendrites and other processes), which can lead to "space-clamp" artifacts.

Some of these disadvantages can be minimized with new methods recently devised to perform whole-cell patch-clamping in slice preparations (so-called "patch-slice" methods; see above for whole-cell recording techniques). Prior to about 1988 this feat was considered impossible because of the postulated "fouling" of the pipette tip with cellular debris arising from the tissue in the slice overlying the neuron to be recorded. One method (29) got around this problem by observing the slice under Nomarski optics and "cleaning away" the cells and debris overlying the target neuron with puffs of saline applied from a large-bore pipette. However, a more straightforward method (26) entailed the slow, "blind" penetration of the slice with a non-fire-polished patch pipette until the telltale small increase in resistance occurred. Then a gigohm seal was formed exactly as in the patch-clamp methods described above. With the single-pipette, whole-cell method, the pipette tip resistance is low (3–8 MΩ) and continuous-mode clamping or a faster (5–10 kHz) form of switch-clamping can be performed, with consequent reduction in artifactual clamping of the pipette tip potential. In addition, with whole-cell clamp it is much easier to inject ions and toxins into the cell to eliminate major sources of large conductances, thus helping to reduce the remote or space-clamp problem.

Examples

An example of the use of voltage clamp is provided by analysis of the M-current. The M-current is a voltage-dependent conductance that is only active (but persistently so) at membrane potentials slightly depolarized from resting potential (−60 to −10 mV); if one holds the membrane potential at about −40 mV (where the M-current is permanently "on") and then applies a hyperpolarizing step towards −60 mV or so, a slowly changing inward current develops (actually, a reduction of an outward K^+ current; the M-current "relaxation") that signals the slow closing of M-channels caused by bringing the membrane potential out of the range of M-current activation. Figure 4 shows the enhancing effects of the opioid peptide dynorphin A on this current in hippocampus (34). Without voltage-clamp methods, this unusual but important con-

ductance (or channel type), and its alteration by transmitters, probably would not have been discovered (reviewed in ref. 5).

Advantages and Disadvantages

These cellular methods have added powerful tools to the armamentarium of the neuropsychopharmacologist. First, because they use isolated preparations or relatively

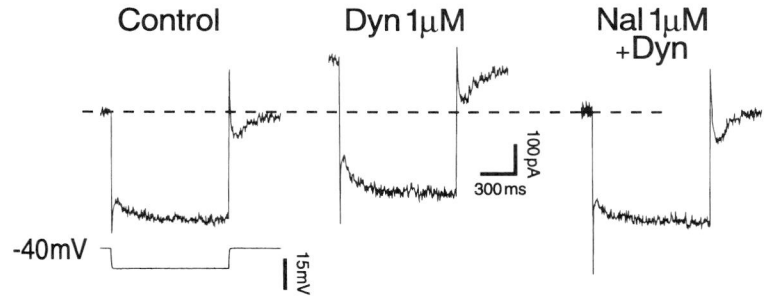

FIG. 4. Schematic of a simple voltage-clamp protocol for recording the M-current, and representative M-current records showing opioid effects. **A:** The M-current was one of the first voltage-dependent conductances shown to be altered by neurotransmitters. The *left panels* show the expected current response to a small (5−10 mV) hyperpolarizing voltage command if there were no open M-channels in the membrane (for example, at holding potentials of −65 or more hyperpolarized). Here, only an abrupt, non-voltage-dependent "ohmic" drop (due to the so-called leak current) is evoked, giving rise to a rectangularly shaped current response. However, if the membrane is depolarized by clamping it at around −50 mV or more depolarized, and the same-sized voltage command is delivered (*right panel*), the abrupt ohmic drop is followed by an inward current relaxation that is actually due to the slow (time- and voltage-dependent) closing of many M-channels that were persistently open at the more depolarized potential (i.e., a reduction of an outward K^+ current). A measure of the M conductance at the holding potential can be obtained by measuring the current difference between the end of the ohmic drop and the "steady-state" current toward the end of the hyperpolarizing command. Duration of voltage command: about 1 sec. **B:** Typical M-current recordings from a CA1 hippocampal pyramidal neuron using a single-electrode voltage clamp and a holding potential of −40 mV. Note the dynorphin-evoked increase in the size of the M-current, as manifested by the increased slope of the inward relaxation during the 15-mV hyperpolarizing voltage command (protocol at *lower left*) and the overall size of the current response (a conductance increase). The large outward shift in the baseline (holding) current is also consistent with an increase in the M-current evoked by dynorphin at depolarized membrane potentials. All these effects of dynorphin are reversed by naloxone (*right panel*), indicating involvement of an opiate receptor. *Dotted line:* Original control holding current. (from ref. 34.)

simple systems, they allow study of neuronal properties and cellular integrative mechanisms without the confounds of outside influence (e.g., from other neurons or hormones, etc.). Second, the ability to use known concentrations of drugs (with application by perfusion) allows the researcher to attempt to (i) mimic the concentrations of neurotransmitters released synaptically, (ii) adjust applied drug concentrations to those known to exist in blood or brains of humans with systemically administered drugs, or (iii) use drug concentrations within the known range for selective action at target receptors. For example, opiates or alcohol can be perfused onto neurons over a range of concentrations known to cause intoxication in humans. In addition, unlike single-channel studies where a large sample of channels must be studied one at a time, these cellular methods allow a more rapid survey of the effects of drugs on many types of conductances. Finally, synaptic events are also available for study with these methods (provided chemical isolation is not used); even in the acutely isolated neuron, intact synaptic boutons can remain attached and exhibit spontaneous transmitter release (35).

Obviously, some of the same advantageous features of the isolated preparations also confer disadvantages. Thus, the lack of normal connections between sets of functioning neurons lessens the utility of these models for the study of hodology, neuronal networks, or the normal interactions between brain regions. Still, some of these confounds can be overcome to a degree by the proper preparation of brain slices or brain "chunks": cutting large slices of tissue in the proper orientation (e.g., nucleus accumbens with attached A10 area or cortex). Still, the fact that the cells are always maintained in a somewhat artificial environment—or, in the case of cultures, may have abnormal developmental properties—are problems not so easily circumvented in these preparations.

Relevance to Neuropsychopharmacology

These cellular-level approaches are crucial to drug development. As our knowledge of the structure, function, and enormous specificity of receptor proteins increases, we are better able to design drugs that have specific targeted effects at the cellular level on identified neurons; for example, the design of neuroleptics that interfere with a particular subset of dopamine receptors on cortical neurons is one currently feasible goal. Such specific drug design demands neuropharmacological testing at the cellular level using the techniques described above.

A considerable advantage of these methods for clinical work is that in many cases human samples can be directly explored. For example, it is feasible to extract mRNA of a receptor protein from diseased human brain, express it in a test cellular system (e.g., oocyte), and determine its functional status (Fig. 1).

Overall, these cellular level methods have enormous potential for the future of neuropsychopharmacology by virtue of the fact that they interface extremely well with molecular biological manipulations. Thus, new developments in the genetics or molecular biology of mental disease can find direct application using these cellular electrophysiological techniques.

BRAIN SLICES TO STUDY NEURAL CIRCUIT FUNCTION

McIlwain first discovered that if a brain is rapidly removed from the skull and rapidly cooled, a "slice" or slab of brain tissue could be cut that would survive for many hours in the proper organ culture environment in vitro. Whereas originally developed for studies of metabolism, neurochemistry, and neurotransmitter release from the cerebral cortex (see Chapter 4, *this volume*), this technique has now been widely applied to many brain regions for the study of electrophysiology of neurons and local brain circuits.

Description

With minor variations for different brain areas, the method for removal and incubation of a brain slice is straightforward. The techniques for slices of various types from various brain areas are described in detail elsewhere (reviewed in ref. 4). The brain is rapidly removed from the skull and placed in ice-cold saline or artificial cerebrospinal fluid (ACSF) saturated with carbogen (95% O_2, 5% CO_2) gas. Using either a vibrating microtome or a tissue chopper, a thin (usually 100–400 μM) slice of fresh brain is cut through the area of interest. This slice is rapidly placed in cold carbongenated ACSF and (perhaps later) transferred to a slice recording chamber containing ACSF. Recording is usually performed after 1–2 hr of incubation to allow recovery from the insult of the surgery. Although recording chambers vary somewhat in their design, they all have the ability to continuously perfuse the slice with fresh ACSF and to add drugs to the ACSF perfusate at known concentrations (as well as by the pipette methods described in the section on in vivo studies). The two most common slice techniques are (i) submerged slices, in which the tissue is fully submerged in the bath with continuous superfusion, or (ii) "interface" slices, in which the bath fluid extends just to the upper surface of the tissue (to interface with a layer of warm, moist carbogen gas). While in the recording chamber, the temperature is best maintained in the physiological range so that normal processes may be studied. With practice, the brain-slice preparation in most cases will remain viable and yield excellent electrophysiological recordings as well as neurochemical measurements for 12 hr or more.

Finally, we would be remiss to omit the isolated brain in vitro (36). Seeming like science fiction, in this method the entire brain (or brainstem plus cerebellum) is removed and kept alive in an incubation environment where various electrophysiological experiments can be performed. This exciting preparation has many advantages of the slice in terms of recording stability and ease of intracellular recordings, yet is nearly fully intact like the in vivo brain. While technically difficult and not yet used extensively for pharmacology questions, this approach holds great promise for future neuropharmacology studies. A related but technically more feasible preparation is the isolated brainstem–spinal cord, which has been used to great advantage in studies of the physiology of respiration (37).

Example Studies

The brain-slice technique has been widely used over the last two decades, so that slices of most brain areas have been studied. One of the first, and by far the most widely studied, of these preparations has been the hippocampal slice. This preparation has been a key factor in working out mechanisms underlying long-term potentiation, postsynaptic effects of various transmitters at the membrane level, and actions of a variety of drugs. Although far too numerous to list in full, the reader is referred to work by Madison and Nicoll (38) and by Siggins and colleagues (34,39) for specific examples of the utility of this preparation.

Another preparation that has been used to great advantage in understanding the cellular effects of opiates is the locus coeruleus (LC) slice. The extensive studies of opiates in LC slices by Aghajanian and colleagues and by North, Williams, and co-worker are described in more detail in Foote and Aston-Jones (*this volume*).

Advantages and Disadvantages

The brain-slice method allows the repeatable application of known concentrations of drugs to the cells being studied, an important advantage in drawing conclusions concerning receptor identity and postsynaptic mechanisms. A second important advantage compared to most in vivo methods is the relative ease of obtaining long-term, stable intracellular recordings without anesthetics or immobilizing agents, so that the effects of drugs on membrane properties of identified neurons can be directly ascertained. An equally important advantage of the brain slice for electrophysiological studies is that the local circuits and cytoarchitecture of the tissue are relatively intact. This allows straightforward identification of the neuron being studied by visualization of its position with respect to known landmarks and other characteristics (e.g., the LC is clearly evident in the slice as a translucent group of cells adjacent to the fourth ventricle). This contrasts with studies in cultured neurons, where the neurochemical or nuclear identity of the neuron under study may be difficult or impossible to determine. Finally, the

relatively intact local anatomy of the slice preparation also allows one to study synaptic responses of brain neurons as in some culture preparations (see above). Finally, the physiology and pharmacology of neurons can be studied in semi-isolation from the confounds of the ongoing behaviors of a freely moving animal.

Perhaps the most significant disadvantage here again is that the slice is a relatively isolated preparation, and neurons in the slice lack many normal afferent inputs and efferent targets. Of course, neurons in the slice are also isolated from any circulating influences such as hormones or steroids. Thus, properties observed in slice studies must always be considered with the caveat that results may reflect the artificial nature of the preparation and may differ from those obtained in the intact organism. Similarly, the slice is, of necessity, situated in an artificial environment rather than the natural and more complex milieu of the brain. The properties of neurons observed vary widely with minor changes in the slice environment, so that results may be heavily biased by the particular experimental conditions employed in an individual lab (for example, depending upon whether interface or submersion slice chambers are used). Also, by being isolated from the behaving organism, neurons within the slice are not amenable to study in the intact, functioning circuits in which they normally reside. Responses of neurons to transmitters are often best revealed when the neuron is challenged by other afferents, which may be lacking in the slice. Similarly, one cannot use this preparation to test the role of a set of neurons in a particular circuit function or behavior. Thus, slice studies are, of necessity, limited to the cellular level of analysis. However, when used in combination with studies in the intact organisms (reviewed next), experiments in the brain slice provide a powerful adjunctive analysis of an important range of phenomena.

Relevance to Neuropsychopharmacology

The same advantages for neuropsychopharmacology listed above for cellular techniques apply to approaches using brain slices, because these techniques also allow a cellular-level examination of function. However, slices have the additional advantage that neuronal structure is better preserved than in isolated or culture situations, so that drug development can be carried out more easily at identified neurons and synapses.

Slices can also take advantage of animal models of disease to examine underlying cellular changes in identified neurons and synapses. One example here are models of drug abuse (using chronic drug administration) where slice studies have provided important insights into underlying neuronal changes (e.g., see Chapters 15, 20, and 25, *this volume*). Other animal models (e.g., transgenic mice) could also be profitably explored using slice methods.

IN VIVO SINGLE-CELL ELECTROPHYSIOLOGY TO STUDY NEURAL CIRCUIT FUNCTION

Description

The intact, functioning brain is readily explored with microelectrodes in anesthetized animals. In this approach, the animal is anesthetized, most commonly with a barbiturate, urethane, chloralose, or halothane. The animal is then placed in a stereotaxic instrument which positions the skull in an exact position and orientation with respect to submillimeter scales in three dimensions on the instrument. By positioning the microelectrode tip at a desired coordinate along these scales, determined by reference to a stereotaxic atlas of the brain of that species, any site within the brain can be found and cellular activity recorded. X-ray or magnetic resonance imaging methods may also be used for this purpose in human studies.

In these experiments, impulse activity of neurons is typically recorded extracellularly, in contrast to the intracellular recordings discussed above. In extracellular recordings, the tip of a microelectrode (typically $1-10$ μm in diameter) is positioned immediately adjacent to, but outside of, a neuron. When in close proximity to the neuron, current fields generated by action potentials in that cell are detected by the microelectrode as small voltage deflections (typically $0.1-1$ mV).

There are many experimental applications of in vivo single-cell electrophysiology. Below we briefly describe three: iontophoresis and local drug application, stimulation recording, and antidromic activation.

Iontophoresis and Local Drug Application

In neuropharmacology experiments it is often useful to study the direct effects of neurotransmitter agents or drugs on neurons in the intact brain to mimic or alter responses to synaptically released transmitters. The ability of an exogenously applied agent to mimic the actions of the endogenously released transmitter is one of the cardinal criteria for establishing the identity of a neurotransmitter at a particular synapse (5). Also, such direct application of drugs obviates interpretive problems of systemic drug application, where direct effects might be confounded with indirect effects mediated by the drug acting at multiple sites in the CNS or periphery.

Curtis first used the iontophoretic technique, showing that charged drug molecules in a solution would be carried out of the tip of a micropipette by electrical current flow of the same polarity as the charge on the drug ion. Thus, by passing current through a glass micropipette, one can apply drug into the local area of the neuron being simultaneously recorded by another, adjacent pipette. This technique, denoted initially as microelectrophoresis but later as iontophoresis, was further developed in the CNS by

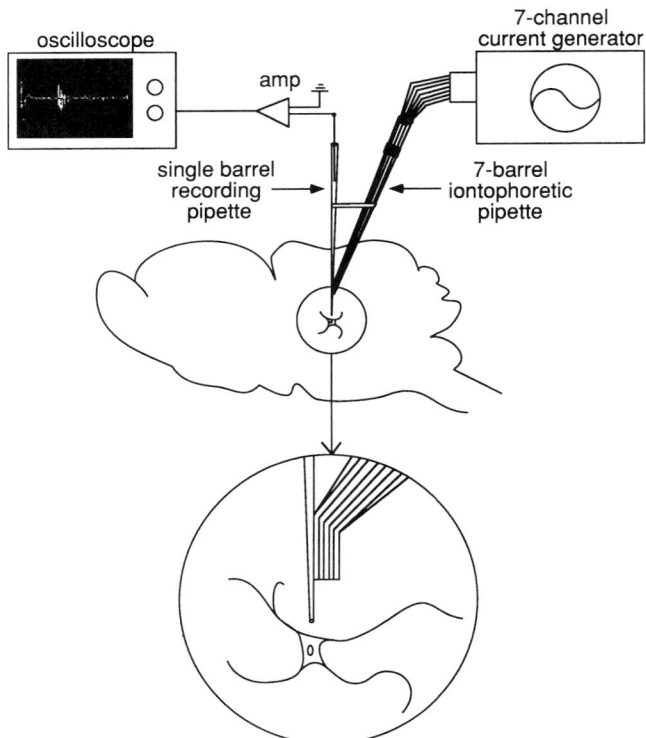

FIG. 5. Schematic of one type of multibarrel micropipette used for local application of drugs by iontophoresis or micropressure while recording neuronal activity. In the method shown, a 7-barrel drug pipette is glued adjacent to a single-barrel recording micropipette. The recording pipette tip extends $10-20$ μm beyond the drug pipette tip, yielding recordings with large spikes and minimizing artifacts due to iontophoretic current or pressure from the drug tips.

Krnjevic and Salmoiraghi and colleagues (see ref. 5 for review). In brief, a multibarrel glass micropipette is manufactured so that $5-7$ tips are adjacent to one another. A single micropipette is used for recording neural impulses extracellularly; this may be one barrel of the multibarrel pipette assembly, or (better) it may be an adjacent pipette affixed (glued) to the iontophoretic multibarrel electrode so as to protrude $10-20$ μm, as illustrated in Fig. 5. The iontophoretic barrels are filled with drug or salt solutions. It is important that one barrel be filled with NaCl, so that current of opposite polarity to that being passed through a drug barrel can be applied at the same time as the drug ion, to neutralize stray currents and minimize artifacts. Once stable impulse activity from a neuron is recorded, current (usually $5-200$ nA) of appropriate polarity is then applied to the barrel containing the drug of interest and the resulting effect on neural activity is monitored, usually using a ratemeter-type recording of firing rate (Fig. 6). When the drug is not being applied (during control conditions), a "backing" or "holding" current of appropriate intensity (usually $5-20$ nA) and polarity to attract the drug ion is applied to prevent unwanted leakage of drug from the tip. It is most advantageous to use an iontophoretic device designed to apply the drugs at precise intervals and automate the control procedures.

An important variant of iontophoresis is local application of drugs from micropipettes by pressure (denoted micropressure application). In this method, a multibarrel micropipette similar to the iontophoretic assembly is employed, but controlled automated pneumatic pressure instead of electrical current is used to eject drug from the tip. This method is often necessary to apply large or uncharged molecules (e.g., large peptides) that do not readily move with iontophoresis. It is possible to configure the pipette so that both iontophoresis and micropressure techniques can be used from the same barrel. If similar results are obtained with both methods of local drug delivery, it is less likely that the results are due to artifacts associated with either technique alone. See ref. 40 and Chapter 33, (this volume) for recent examples of this combined method.

Local micropressure application has several advantages over iontophoresis. One of the major drawbacks of iontophoresis is that one does not know the concentration of drug applied. This is because the drug is carried by current, and for most drug solutions the physiochemical properties determining the relative transport of drug molecules in an electrical field in the micropipette glass are not known. It is possible that very high concentrations are ejected even with low currents (for easily ionized drugs), while even high currents may eject very little of another, poorly ionizable drug. There is also considerable release variability across micropipettes. In contrast, with local pressure application the solution ejected is the same concentration as that in the pipette. While the absolute concentration at the recorded cell is uncertain due to diffusion and dilution in the extracellular milieu, at least the highest possible concentration is known. This is important, because the receptor specificity of drugs are dependent upon their use within a certain concentration range. By increasing the volume of solution ejected, pressure application may also allow a larger area of tissue to be infused than with iontophoresis. For this reason, pressure is typically the method of choice when trying to locally antagonize synaptically mediated events that may reflect inputs onto distal or remote dendrites of the neuron being recorded. However, there are caveats with this method, such as artifacts due to pressure (movement), pH, or osmolarity changes; iontophoresis usually allows a greater range of drugs to be applied to the same neurons, and it is often associated with more stable and successful recording.

It is important for both microiontophoresis and micropressure application of drugs that the proper controls for current, pH, and volume effects be conducted, and that drug application follows a regularly timed protocol to minimize "warm-up" effects and possible experimenter bias (see ref. 5 for review).

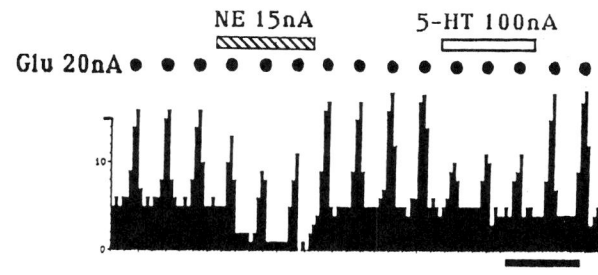

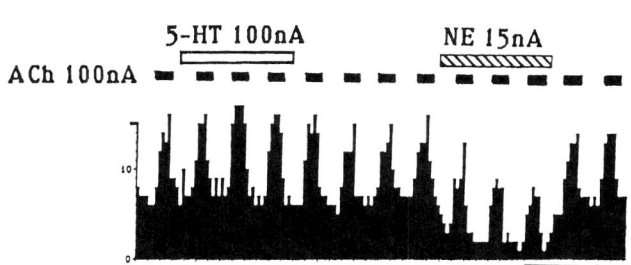

FIG. 6. Comparison of norepinephrine (NE) and 5-hydroxytryptamine (5-HT) effects on responses to glutamate (Glu) and acetylcholine (ACh) for the same LC neuron. NE applied iontophoretically (at hatched bars) inhibits basal activity but leaves responses evoked by Glu (applied at solid circles, **upper trace**) or ACh (applied at solid bars, **lower trace**) intact. In contrast, 5-HT (iontophoresed at open bars) does not affect basal discharge rate but attenuates responses to Glu (**upper trace**). Note, however, that in the same neuron 5-HT does not attenuate responses to ACh (**lower trace**). Calibrations: abscissae, number of spikes per 5 sec; ordinates, 2 min. For more details see ref. 40.

Stimulation Recording

This is the simple but requisite procedure for discerning the functional effect of an afferent input to a neuron. There are two methods available for this purpose: (i) the classical approach of electrically stimulating the afferents while recording the target neuron and (ii) a more recent method (especially important for studies in such complex tissues as brain) using local chemical (instead of electrical) stimulation to activate the input source.

With the former method, pulses of electrical stimulation are applied to a stimulating electrode to activate neurons that project to the area where a target cell is recorded. Extracellular recordings are typically used to measure the functional effect of the input. Most commonly, responses are measured in displays called peri-stimulus time histograms (PSTHs), where neural activity recorded for many successive stimulus trials is accumulated, synchronized with the stimulus presentation (Fig. 7). By accumulating activity in such a histogram, even relatively weak responses can be revealed due to the summation over many trials. This type of analysis allows quantitation of response magnitude, onset latency, and duration. These parameters can then be compared before and after drug

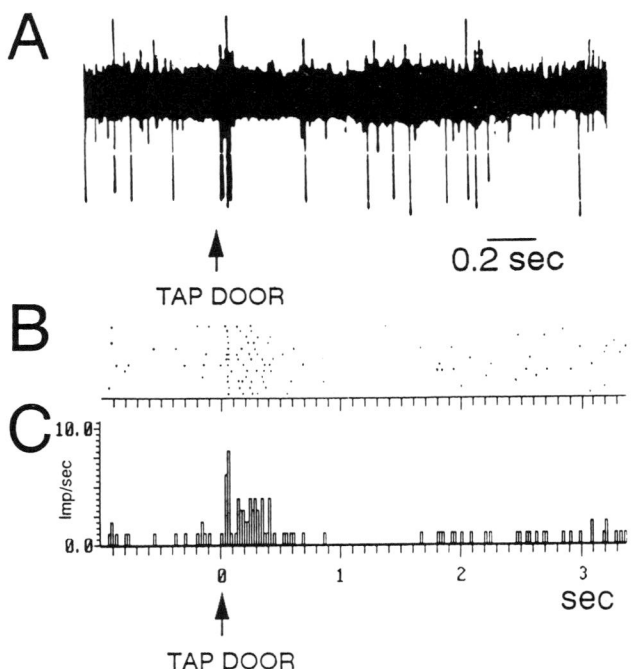

FIG. 7. A: Slow-speed recording from an LC neuron in a waking, chair-restrained monkey in response to a single tap on the door of the experimental chamber (at arrow). Note the stable spike size, and the phasic activation followed by post-activation inhibition, typical of LC (and other) neurons. **B:** Raster display of activity of this same LC neuron in response to a series of door taps (at arrow below panel **C**). Each dot represents an impulse from this neuron, and activity for 13 trials is arranged in rows from top to bottom. Note the consistent activation followed by postactivation inhibition for these stimuli. **C:** A cumulative peri-stimulus time histogram (PSTH) of activity seen in panel **B**, but summated in one display for all 13 trials. Time base in panel **C** applies also to panel **B**. For more details on properties of monkey LC neurons see Foote and Aston-Jones (*this volume*) and ref. 43.

administration to determine, for example, the effect of a particular receptor antagonist on the response to activation of an input and thereby help determine the likely transmitter candidate in that afferent. The reader is referred to the review by Ranck (41) for a detailed treatment of factors determining types of neural elements activated with different parameters of electrical stimulation.

A major drawback of electrical stimulation is that both cell bodies in the area of the stimulating electrode, and fibers of passage derived from cells located in other areas, will be activated by the stimuli applied. Therefore, the origin of the responses obtained is uncertain. This problem is surmounted by using local chemical stimulation, which activates the input neurons by infusion of a neural activator such as glutamate or one of its analogues into the area of the cell bodies or dendrites. Because stimulation by this method relies on receptor activation, and receptors are thought to reside only on somata and dendrites of neurons, this approach does not activate passing axons that originate from neurons elsewhere. However,

while the origin of responses are better identified with this method, the temporally imprecise activation by chemical microinfusion does not allow accurate determination of response latencies. A second important limitation of chemical stimulation is that neurons can be *inactivated* by stimulating chemicals such as glutamate, if too high a concentration is applied. That is, too much of a chemical activator (e.g., glutamate) can depolarize neurons into a state of *depolarization block*, where the neuron is maintained in a depolarized state and thus cannot generate action potentials due to persistent inactivation of Na^+ channels. Thus, what is thought to be stimulation can actually inhibit neurons of interest. A procedure that minimizes such concerns is to apply a range of concentrations of the chemical activator and examine the corresponding dose–response curve in the target cell. This should reveal the minimum dose for obtaining an effect, which with glutamate is presumably due to excitation of neurons near the site of infusion. Another way around this potential problem is to record the response of neurons in the infusion site during application of the chemical stimulant. This not only allows direct confirmation of the effect of the infused agent on those cells, but also gives the time that activity in the local neurons is affected; this can greatly improve the temporal accuracy of such stimulation–response studies. Without such procedures, results obtained with local chemical stimulation are difficult to interpret.

Local Synaptic Decoupling

A similar method is used in combination with stimulation-recording experiments to test the involvement of a particular brain region as a circuit element mediating an evoked response. Instead of infusing an excitatory neurochemical, however, the solution microinfused is one that inactivates or synaptically decouples local neurons. As illustrated in Fig. 8, a composite recording/infusion pipette can be used so that neuronal recordings help localize the area desired for infusion as well as verify the effect of the infusion on neurons at the infusion site. One approach is to locally infuse a local anesthetic (e.g., lidocaine) to block local activity while conducting the stimulation-recording experiment (42). However, anesthetics block impulse conduction in passing fibers as well as in local somata, so that this approach does not test the role of local neurons as a possible relay in the circuit response being examined. Alternatively, the infusion solution contains either (i) a strongly inhibitory neurotransmitter agent (e.g., GABA, or a GABA agonist such as muscimol) or (ii) a synaptic decoupling agent (e.g., divalent ions such as low Ca^{2+}/high Mg^{2+}, Cd^{2+}/Mn^{2+}, or Co^{2+}). By inhibiting neurons in the infusion area, the first approach prevents them from responding to synaptic inputs, while in the latter approach interference with Ca^{2+}-dependent neurotransmitter release "synaptically decouples'' the local area infused. Because passing fibers are not thought to be sensitive to these agents, in either case the result is that local neurons but not passing fibers are functionally removed from circuit activity, and their role in the circuit response being examined can be directly tested. See Fig. 8 and (43) for an example of the use of these methods to investigate the role of the ventral medulla in sensory responses of locus coeruleus neurons.

Antidromic Activation

Antidromic activation has at least two major uses: (i) to confirm a projection to an area and (ii) to determine the time required for conduction of an impulse along a projection pathway. In this procedure, an electrical stimulation electrode is placed in the projection area of a neuron while a microelectrode in the soma region records neurons that are ''backfired'' from the target area. This technique

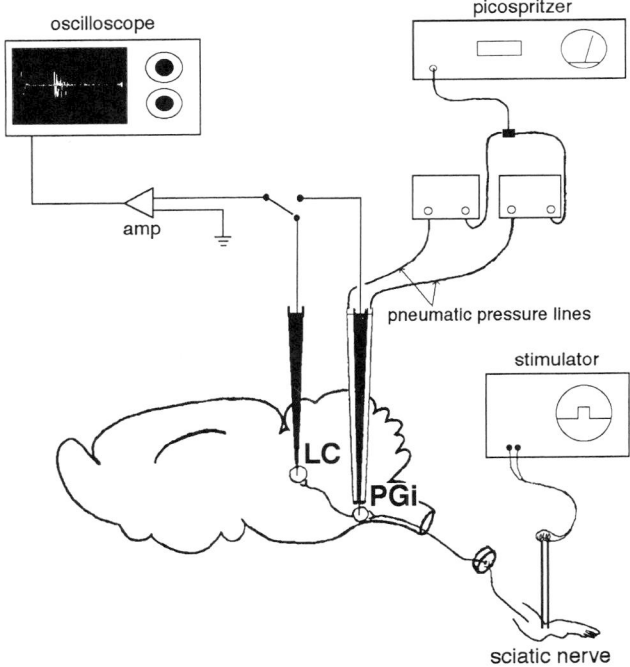

FIG. 8. Schematic of the use of local drug microinfusion combined with stimulation recording in vivo to trace functional circuitry. In this case, the sciatic nerve was stimulated electrically and impulse activity of LC neurons was recorded extracellularly with a glass micropipette. A composite recording/injection pipette was placed in a major afferent to the LC, the nucleus paragigantocellularis (PGi). The smaller central barrel (*dark shading*) was used to record neuronal activity to aid in the proper placement of the injection assembly. In this case, two drug barrels (*unshaded area*) are glued adjacent to the recording pipette. Drug solutions were injected there using pneumatic pressure. Inactivation of the PGi via local microinfusions of lidocaine, GABA, or a synaptic decoupling solution blocked or attenuated responses of LC neurons to sciatic stimulation, indicating that the PGi is a synaptic relay for sciatic influences on LC neurons (43).

is based upon the fact that axons will conduct impulses in both directions. Although under most conditions impulses are generated at the source of the axon (soma) and only travel orthodromically, antidromic (''backwards'') conduction is a powerful and convenient property. By stimulating the target area and recording an antidromically driven response elsewhere, one can conclude that the neuron recorded sends an axon to the region being stimulated (Fig. 9). This is often done to confirm anatomical evidence of a projection. Note, however, that because this employs electrical stimulation a positive response does not indicate that the recorded neuron *terminates* at the site of stimulation, only that the neuron sends a fiber (possibly en route elsewhere) to that region; additional (orthodromic) tests must be performed to indicate a synaptic input (e.g., as described under *Stimulation Recording,* above). In addition, such activation yields the time required for the impulse to travel the length of the axon (conduction velocity is the same in both directions along the axon). This latency of impulse conduction is useful in interpreting stimulation-recording experiments, because synaptic (orthodromic) responses at a similar latency may be due to a direct monosynaptic (versus indirect, polysynaptic) projection from the input neuron stimulated.

There are three tests that should be performed to confirm that a driven impulse is antidromic: (i) It should have a very constant latency of activation (synaptically driven responses usually exhibit a few milliseconds of ''jitter''); exceptions to this constant latency rule can occur for very-small-diameter unmyelinated fibers (e.g., see ref. 44); (ii) the driven response should faithfully follow high-frequency activation above 100 Hz (e.g., two stimuli at a 5-msec interpulse interval should drive two spikes); and (iii) orthodromic (spontaneously occurring) spikes should collide with and eliminate the driven spike (collision test).

Example Studies

Because these methods have been in wide use for several decades, there are literally hundreds of specific examples that could be described. The reader is referred to the text by Shepherd (7) for additional references and descriptions of applications of these methods in sensory and motor systems of the brain. These methods have been used to determine the origin of the hyperactivity of locus coeruleus neurons during opiate withdrawal (45) and to demonstrate that systemic nicotine potently activates the LC indirectly (46) (see also Chapter 33, *this volume*). These results could not be realized in cultured LC neurons, or in LC slice preparations.

Advantages and Disadvantages

The advantages of in vivo electrophysiology compared to the in vitro methods described previously are obviously

A

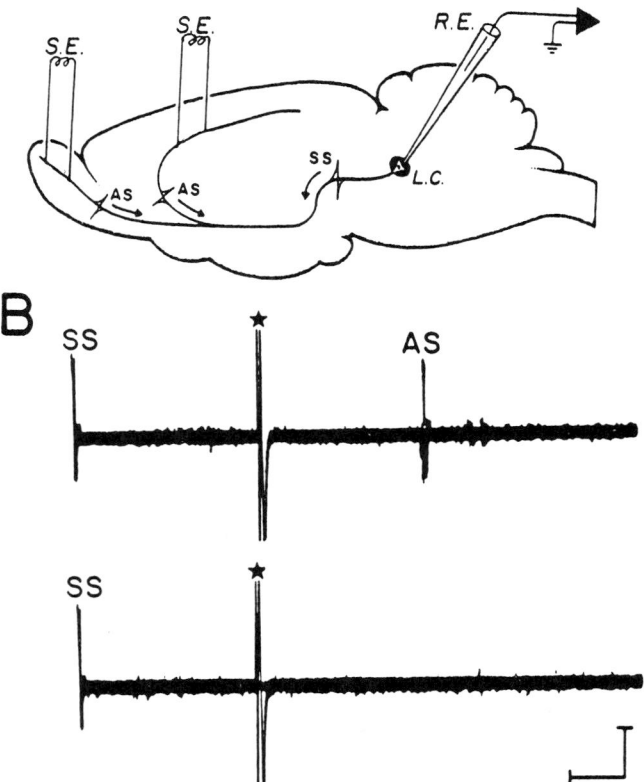

B

FIG. 9. Schematic of antidromic stimulation procedure. **A:** Micropipette recording electrode (R.E.) is used to record impulse activity extracellularly from a neuron in the LC. Stimulating electrodes (S.E.) in the cingulate cortex and olfactory bulb are used to evoke antidromic spikes (AS; traveling towards the soma) along LC axons. Note a spontaneously occurring spike (SS) which travels orthodromically (away from the soma) along the LC axon. **B:** Collision technique. Spontaneously occurring spikes (SS) are used to trigger stimulation of the cingulate cortex after a precise delay. In the upper trace, stimuli presented 65 msec after SS evoked constant latency spikes (denoted AS) 60 msec later. As seen in the lower trace, when the stimulation followed SS by 63 msec (sum of conduction time plus absolute refractory period), no driven spikes are observed, demonstrating collision between SS and AS along the same axon and also demonstrating that AS are antidromic. (Modified from ref. 44.)

due to the more intact preparation in vivo. With these in vivo methods, one can study brain regions or neurons in their intact state with its normal complement of inputs and targets, and in their natural milieu of circulating hormones and factors. The cells being studied usually have not been severed or damaged, as is almost always the case with slice studies, and have developed normally in the intact organism, in contrast to the culture preparation. These considerations lend additional credibility and

fewer caveats to results concerning neuronal activity in vivo.

There are several experimental questions that require an intact organism, and they cannot be pursued in vitro. For example, to mimic the clinical situation it is important to determine the effect of a *systemically* administered drug (e.g., abused drugs like ethanol or opiates) upon activity in a particular brain region. In this way even if the drug has several sites of action in the brain, one sees the "net effect" of human-like drug exposure on the neurons of interest. The intact in vivo preparation is also necessary for determining the effect of certain organismic physiological manipulations on particular neurons (e.g., effects of changes in cardiovascular activity or steroid levels). Similarly, the effects of functionally defined inputs typically must be examined in the intact organism (e.g., sensory or painful stimuli). Finally, a significant advantage of the in vivo preparation for electrophysiology is that it is more readily correlated with anatomical studies than in in vitro models. Antidromic activation can more directly confirm projections found in anatomical experiments, and stimulation-recording studies can establish the functional effect and neurotransmitter of a pathway, again confirming results seen with anatomical tract-tracing and immunohistochemical experiments (for anatomical approaches to these issues see Chapter 3, *this volume*).

However, there are also several disadvantages of in vivo preparations. In addition to the relative difficulty in performing many of the intracellular and whole-cell studies described above (and therefore in obtaining data on membrane mechanisms of drug action), the researcher does not have as much knowledge as in the in vitro preparations of actual drug concentrations at the cell under study. Therefore, drug and transmitter responses are less confidently identified with a specific receptor or channel. In addition, there may be other confounds, such as the presence of anesthetics (or in awake animals, immobilization stress) that could alter the normal electrophysiological responses to drugs and transmitters.

Relevance to Neuropsychopharmacology

Several applications of in vivo electrophysiological methods lend themselves particularly well to clinically relevant questions of special interest to neuropsychopharmacology. In addition to the points above, the in vivo preparation allows the study of neural activity and drug responses in animal models of human disorders. Studies of locus coeruleus activity in opiate withdrawal (see Chapters 33, 61, and 148, *this volume*) are obvious examples of this application, but others abound. There are animal models of other abused drugs (e.g., alcohol and cocaine) and several disorders, including schizophrenia, depression, and anxiety, all of which promise to make (or already have made) significant contributions to neuropsychopharmacology, and which require electrophysiological testing in the intact organism (for descriptions of animal models see Chapters 6, 32, 41, 64, 68, and 69, *this volume*). In addition, because these techniques are needed for study of effects of systemically administered drugs, they can be an important step in new drug development.

TECHNIQUES TO STUDY NEURAL–BEHAVIORAL LINKAGES

Behavioral Electrophysiology: Researching the Spark of Cognition

In addition to interactions between individual neurons, there are other, more complex organizations in the nervous system. Neurons are typically associated in functionally related groups and circuits. Function at the behavioral level is a product of these neuronal networks rather than simply the product of properties of individual neurons. There are networks and circuits specialized for sensory and motor functions, and others specialized for associative activities. It seems highly likely that the elements of such neuronal networks have evolved within the context of network function(s) to have specific and perhaps unique properties tailored for that network.

As has been stated above for in vivo techniques, many questions concerning neuropsychopharmacology require experiments in the intact animal. This is perhaps most true for questions regarding cognition. While molecular and cellular experiments are important for understanding details of processes involved in mental dysfunction or drug responses, they are unable to integrate such results to ultimately and completely explain cognitive functions such as attention, perception, emotion, or memory. An analogous relationship exists between physics and chemistry: While the principles of physics are critical to our understanding of chemistry, they are not sufficient to fully understand or predict the properties of chemical reactions. It is fundamentally necessary to conduct experiments in chemistry per se or, as is the case at hand, in cognitive neuroscience.

Hence, most studies in the electrophysiology of cognitive processes involve recording single neurons in behaving animals. These methods will be briefly described below, followed by a description of methods used to locally manipulate neurons in behaving animals to test hypotheses generated by correlations found with recording experiments.

Single-Cell Recording in Behaving Animals

These methods rely on the same principles as described above with some modifications for behaving animals. Most such studies employ extracellular recordings from a metal microelectrode held in a miniature microposi-

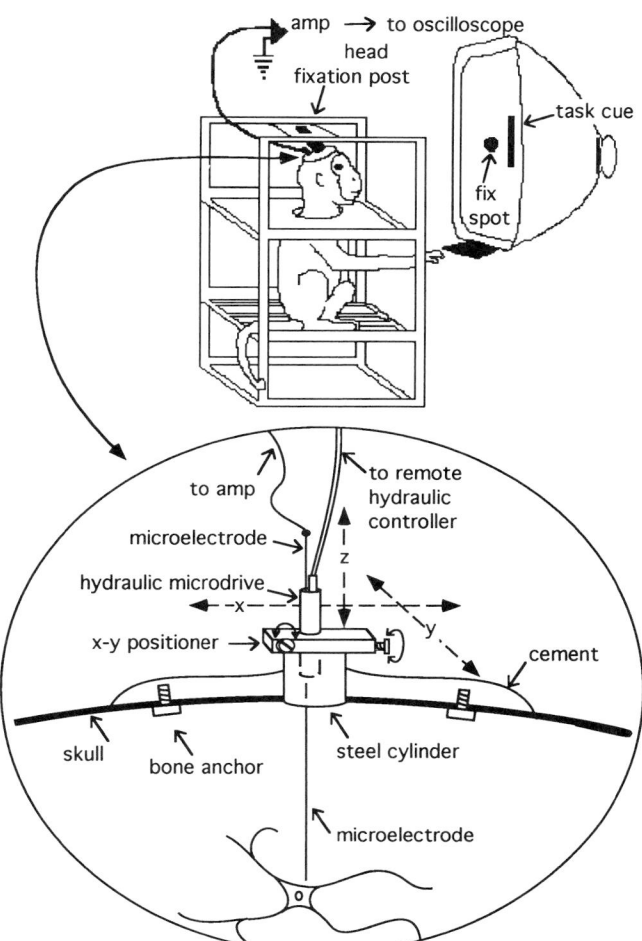

FIG. 10. Schematic of one type of recording technique used in behaving monkey. At top is shown a monkey in a restraining chair with head fixation. The monitor in front of the monkey displays a spot which the animal must visually fixate to initiate each trial; this ensures that the animal is attending to the task when cues are presented. The animal presses the nearby lever after target cues for juice reward. The head-mounted assembly for recording impulse activity of brain neurons is shown in more detail below. A steel cylinder is cemented to the animal's skull and bone anchors. This cylinder is fitted with an X–Y positioner and a remotely controlled hydraulic microdrive. The X–Y positioner allows lateral repositioning of the electrode between penetrations in the brain, while the hydraulic microdrive lowers the electrode along each penetration. Electrical activity recorded on the electrode is relayed to amplifiers and other electronics for analysis.

tioner on the animal's head. As illustrated in Fig. 10, the micropositioner is typically attached to a chronically implanted steel chamber or cylinder that is stereotaxically positioned and permanently cemented to the skull in a prior surgery. These chambers often allow lateral repositioning of the recording microelectrode for multiple penetrations, while the micropositioner allows the electrode to be lowered into the brain to the desired target along a particular track. Additional details on such methods can be found in refs. 47–49.

The most common types of microelectrodes used for recording from neurons in behaving animals are (a) etched tungsten or platinum–iridium wires, insulated with either glass or lacquer except for ~20 μm from the tip, or (b) thin microwires that are typically 25–62 μm in diameter and lacquer-insulated except for the bluntly cut tip. Neurons of different brain areas are recorded more easily with one or another type of electrode; for example, locus coeruleus neurons in awake rats and monkeys (43) are more easily recorded using the more flexible microwires. In general, microwires are advantageous for experiments entailing long-term recordings from neurons in deep structures in behaving animals, whereas etched, stiff microelectrodes are advantageous for studies where penetration of the dura mater is needed or where numerous penetrations in a small area are desired.

Two general approaches are used with microwire electrodes. Perhaps most commonly the microwires are simply implanted and glued in place with no further movement of the wires possible after surgery. In this method, a large number of wires (often more than 40) are implanted and each wire is monitored daily over the course of months for unit activity. Activity occurs on enough wires over time that many long-term and very stable recordings can often be obtained (e.g., see refs. 50 and 51). The second method is to attach a small number of microwires (two to six) to a movable microdrive which allows the wires to be repositioned vertically, and sometimes laterally as well, for new penetrations after surgery (e.g., see ref. 43). This approach has the advantage of obtaining many more recordings from a single subject than the fixed wire approach, an important consideration when subjects are in limited supply (e.g., monkeys) or when extensive training is required for each animal recorded.

High-gain amplification of signals from the head of a moving animal often yields considerable movement-related electrical artifacts; these are the bane of a behavioral electrophysiologist. These problems are typically overcome by including a miniature first-stage amplifier in the fixed implant on the animal's head, so that recordings from the microelectrode can be amplified and converted to low-impedance signals before traveling over long distances of flexing cables.

As with all extracellular recordings, it is important to know whether activity seen on an individual electrode is generated from one neuron only, or from several nearby neurons simultaneously recorded. Results of the latter, termed *multiple-cell recording* or *multi-unit recording,* are more difficult to interpret because neurons in the multiple cell population may be physiologically heterogeneous. In that case, opposite changes in different cells recorded may appear as no change in the multiple-cell data. In addition, it is more difficult to ensure the stability of the recorded signal over time with multiple-cell activity.

In recordings in awake monkeys, the animal's head is usually fixed in place by a post that is cemented to the skull and anchoring screws, so that such movement artifacts are minimized (Fig. 10). This technique also allows precise measurement of the direction of gaze by monitoring eye position, an especially valuable aspect in studies where monitoring and controlling attention is important. However, this approach does not allow free movement of the animal and may produce uncontrolled effects of immobilization stress.

A key element in behavioral electrophysiology is the computer system that is used to acquire and analyze the data. Because so many events are typically recorded simultaneously (e.g., two or more cells, EEG, EMG, markers for different sensory stimuli and behavioral events, video time markers, X and Y eye positions), it is necessary to have a system that can rapidly record large amounts of data on-line with millisecond temporal resolution. In the last few years, affordable microcomputers with sufficient speed and disk storage have become available to accomplish this data storage task. In addition, sophisticated software is required so that neuronal activity or other data can be tabulated (typically in PSTHs) with respect to an arbitrarily chosen type of event out of the many recorded. For example, it may be desired to construct PSTHs of neuronal activity synchronized with a particular type of sensory stimulus out of the many presented, or synchronized with a particular type of sensory stimulus that elicits a specific behavioral response (e.g., to examine neuronal activity associated with non-target conditioned cues for trials in which the animal mistakenly elicited a behavioral response). The most challenging (but important) aspect of developing such software is to make it easy to use and easy to abstract results from very large data files, but also make it sufficiently flexible so that new subroutines can be written and integrated to analyze electrophysiological data. The latter is an ever-present need, so that typically the behavioral physiologist must be quite computer-literate!

Example Studies

Recordings of neuronal activity in animals performing structured behavioral tasks have proven invaluable in understanding the neural bases of various types of cognitive activity. Of the many studies using this approach, one example for activity of locus coeruleus neurons in a monkey performing an attention task is found in ref. 47 (see also Chapters 29, 33, 34, and 41, *this volume*). Similarly, recent studies by Schultz and colleagues recording putative dopamine neurons in waking monkeys (52) hold great promise for further understanding this system and its importance in neuropsychopharmacology. For other examples of the use of behavioral electrophysiology to decipher the neurobiology of cognition, the reader is referred to work by Goldman-Rakic and colleagues (47) and by Wise, Desimone, and colleagues (48,49).

Acute Manipulation of Specific Neurons and Neural Groups in Behaving Animals

Description

Studies of the causal role of a brain area in a specific behavior or cognitive process commonly employ lesions of one type or another. The simplest approach is to remove or destroy the area of brain by excision or electrolytic lesion and tissue coagulation. However, these approaches have serious drawbacks that limit the interpretability of results obtained, most prominently (i) passing fibers originating from neurons located elsewhere are lesioned and (ii) recovery of function may occur (via adaptive changes in remaining brain structures) during the weeks needed for the animal to recuperate from such a gross insult. This effect may lead to false-negative results concerning the role of the lesioned brain structure. The reader is referred to the elegant studies of Newsome and colleagues (53) for an example of recovery of function following chronic lesion manipulations.

A better approach to such causal behavioral studies is to (a) acutely manipulate (e.g., activate or inactivate) the neurons in question using local infusions of selective chemical agents and (b) examine the effect on behavior during the acute effect. This approach avoids the two concerns listed above. These studies employ techniques similar to those described under *Stimulation Recording* (above) to locally infuse drugs into a target group of neurons. Optimally, the investigator employs a combination recording/infusion electrode that allows neuronal recording from cells in the immediate area during infusions of chemical agents (e.g., see Fig. 8). This permits several advantages: (i) The desired infusion site can be precisely localized by recording characteristic neuronal activity prior to infusion, (ii) the time of onset and offset of altered activity in the target neurons can be monitored and compared to the timing of behavioral changes, and (iii) individual infusion trials can be directly confirmed as to their effectiveness in altering neuronal activity at the infusion site in the desired fashion.

Examples

One example of this approach is found in recent studies by Foote, Valentino, and colleagues in studies of the impact of activity in locus coeruleus neurons on EEG in rats. As described in more detail in Chapter 29, *this volume*, local intra-coeruclear infusions of the cholinergic drug pilocarpine to activate locus coeruleus neurons also activated the EEG, whereas local infusions of clonidine (that powerfully and selectively attenuated locus coeruleus activity) led to EEG synchronization. Recordings from locus coeruleus neurons during the infusions confirmed the effectiveness of the manipulations and revealed

that the EEG changes were closely time-locked to the changes induced in LC activity.

A second example of the power of this approach to test hypotheses generated by electrophysiology in behaving animals is found in the work of Goldman-Rakic and colleagues. Recording experiments suggested that the dorsolateral prefrontal cortex may be involved in spatial working memory (47). To test the role of dopamine in this proposed function, Sawaguchi and Goldman-Rakic (54) infused selective D1 antagonists into this area and found that animals apparently could not remember a specific location for objects; the same objects in surrounding locations were not affected. Hence, this method can also be used to test the role of transmitter influences in a particular brain area on behavioral functions.

Advantages and Disadvantages

The advantages of behavioral electrophysiological methods for neuropsychopharmacology are numerous. These are the only methods whereby one can directly correlate neural activity with behavior. This can be especially powerful when the behavior being measured is itself a measure or reflection of a cognitive process. In addition, there is no confounding effect of anesthesia on neuronal activity recorded. Finally, because these studies take place in the intact animal, one can relate results to anatomical and neurochemical properties of the relevant circuits.

Extending electrophysiology with acute chemical manipulations of specific brain neurons can directly test the causality of hypotheses generated from the correlative results of behavioral electrophysiology experiments. This approach obviates problems of nonspecificity and recovery of function encountered with more conventional lesion manipulations. By using local infusions of neurotransmitters or related drugs, this method also provides results that can be directly related to anatomical and neurochemical results on the same system. Together, these techniques provide a powerful means of investigating the neural basis of cognitive function.

Disadvantages of this approach are also considerable. First, because these experiments take place in the behaving animal, it is difficult (if not impossible) to control all of the possible relevant variables that may affect the activity being recorded (e.g., behavioral state, stress, training differences, individual differences in task ability, etc.). Second, the behavioral measures obtained may not be temporally precise, or may only indirectly reflect the process of interest (e.g., attentional studies). Third, these studies are slow, technically difficult, and require tedious and long (often months-long) training of the animals before recording experiments can even begin. Finally, elegant though they are, these behavioral-recording studies yield only correlative data. It is necessary to extend such experiments with manipulations of the systems of interest using activation or inactivation of select groups of neurons (employing methods described below) to test causal hypotheses of their roles in specific behaviors.

Relevance to Neuropsychopharmacology

The importance of these approaches to neuropsychopharmacology lies in the fact that many mental disorders are problems of complex cognitive function; the neural bases of these normal cognitive functions are only partly understood (if at all). Substantial progress in understanding and developing new treatments for disorders of memory, attention, drug craving, and the like require a more complete understanding of the underlying biological processes. As stated above, such an understanding will require experiments combining neurobiology and cognitive testing, particularly electrophysiology and local acute manipulations in animals performing sophisticated cognitive tasks. In addition, studies by Georgopoulous et al. (55) and by Houk et al. (56), among others (50), are revealing the power of analyzing activity in networks of neurons to understand the neural bases of cognition and behavior. If combined with drug administration and testing, such experiments analyzing neuronal populations in behaving animals could prove to be very valuable for future neuropsychopharmacological analyses. Such models of normal function can be used not only to understand the neural processes involved and to develop new drug treatments of related disorders, but also to test putative drug treatments in animals in a clinically relevant manner before their application to the human patient.

FUTURE STUDIES

In this review we have only briefly surveyed the myriad electrophysiological methods available to study nervous system function. Advances in these methods have been very rapid, and it is expected that this pace will continue. The direction of future studies will be determined to a great extent by technical advances. One example: The recent rapid advances in speed and storage capabilities of microcomputer systems have greatly aided (and in some cases enabled) the above experimental procedures. Moreover, the reduced cost of these systems and commercial availability of experimentally oriented software packages has markedly increased access to sophisticated electrophysiological analyses.

It is increasingly clear that any one method or level of analysis is insufficient to provide a detailed and yet complete understanding of neural function as needed to drive rapid progress in neuropsychopharmacology. Integration among these methods and levels of analysis will prove to be very important in increasing not only our understanding of neuropsychological function, but also our ability to pharmacologically manipulate it and treat its disorders.

ACKNOWLEDGMENTS

We thank S. Aston-Jones and C. Chiang for artwork. This work was supported by PHS grants NS24698, DA06241, DA03665, MH44346, AA06420, and MH47680 and by the Air Force Office of Scientific Research, Air Force Systems Command, USAF, under grant numbers AFOSR-90-0147 and F49620-93-1-0099.

REFERENCES

1. Dionne VE. Noise analysis. *Tech Cell Physiol* 1982;II:1–19.
2. Hoffer B, Seiger A, Freedman R, Olson L, Taylor D. Electrophysiology and cytology of hippocampal formation transplants in the anterior chamber of the eye. II. Cholinergic mechanism. *Brain Res* 1977;119:107–132.
3. Jarvis CR, Bourque CW, Renaud LP. Depolarizing action of cholecystokinin on rat supraoptic neurones in vitro. *J Physiol (Lond)* 1992;458:621–632.
4. Kettenmann H, Grantyn R, eds. *Practical electrophysiological methods. A guide for in vitro studies in vertebrate neurobiology.* New York: Wiley–Liss, 1992;322.
5. Siggins GR, Gruol DL. Mechanisms of transmitter action in the vertebrate central nervous system. In: Bloom FE, eds. *Handbook of physiology. The nervous system IV.* Bethesda, MD: The American Physiological Society, 1986;1–114.
6. Hille B. *Ionic channels of excitable membranes,* 2nd ed. Sunderland, MA: Sinauer Associates, 1992;607.
7. Shepherd GM. *Neurobiology,* 2nd ed. New York: Oxford University Press, 1988;689.
8. Miller C. *Ion channel reconstitution.* New York: Plenum, 1986;577.
9. Moss SJ, Smart TG, Porter NM, et al. Cloned GABA receptors are maintained in a stable cell line: allosteric and channel properties. *Eur J Pharmacol* 1990;189:77–88.
10. Hollmann M, Oshea GA, Rogers SW, Heinemann S. Cloning by functional expression of a member of the glutamate receptor family. *Nature* 1989;342:643–648.
11. Dingledine R. New wave of non-NMDA excitatory amino acid receptors. *Trends Pharmacol Sci* 1991;12(10):360–362.
12. Harris AR, Allan AM. Alcohol intoxication: ion channels and genetics. *FASEB J* 1989;3:1689–1695.
13. Lovinger DM. High ethanol sensitivity of recombinant AMPA-type glutamate receptors expressed in mammalian cells. *Neurosci Lett* 1993;159:83–87.
14. Lovinger DM, White G, Weight FF. NMDA receptor-mediated synaptic excitation selectively inhibited by ethanol in hippocampal slices from adult rat. *J Neurosci* 1990;10:1372–1379.
15. Sakmann B, Neher E, eds. *Single channel recording.* New York: Plenum, 1983;503.
16. Mathers DA, Barker JL. Chemically induced ion channels in nerve cell membranes. *Int Rev Neurobiol* 1982;23:1–34.
17. Twyman RE, MacDonald RL. Neurosteroid regulation of GABAA receptor single-channel kinetic properties of mouse spinal cord neurons in culture. *J Physiol (Lond)* 1992;456:215–245.
18. Miyake M, Christie M, North R. Single potassium channels opened by opioids in rat locus ceruleus neurons. *Proc Natl Acad Sci USA* 1989;86:3419–3422.
19. Cohen L, Landowne D, Loew L, Salzberg B. Optical signals: changes in membrane structure, recording of membrane potential, and measurement of calcium. *Curr Top Membr Transp* 1985;22:423–443.
20. Loew LM, ed. *Spectroscopic membrane probes.* Boca Raton, FL: CRC Press, 1988;297.
21. Tsien RY. Fluorescent probes of cell signaling. *Am Rev Neurosci* 1989;12:227–253.
22. Holliday J, Adams RJ, Sejnowski TJ, Spitzer NC. Calcium-Induced release of calcium regulates differentiation of cultured spinal neurons. *Neuron* 1991;7:787–796.
23. Heinemann U, Arens J. Production and calibration of ion-sensitive microelectrodes. In: Kettenmann H, Grantyn R, eds. *Practical elec-*

trophysiological methods. A guide for in vitro studies in vertebrate neurobiology. New York: Wiley–Liss, 1992;206–212.

24. Holliday J, Gruol D. Cytokine stimulation increases intracellular calcium and alters the response to quisqualate in cultured cortical astrocytes. *Brain Res* 1993;621(2):233–241.

25. Armstrong DL, White RE. An enzymatic mechanism for potassium channel stimulation through pertussis-toxin-sensitive G proteins. *Trends Neurol Sci* 1992;15(10):403–408.

26. Blanton MG, Lo Turco JJ, Kriegstein AR. Whole cell recording from neurons in slices of reptilian and mammalian cerebral cortex. *J Neurosci Meth* 1989;30:203–210.

27. Grantyn R, Kraszewski K, Richthof S, Kettenmann H. The nystatin method of whole-cell patch clamp recording. In: Kettenmann H, Grantyn R, eds. *Practical electrophysiological methods. A guide for in vitro studies in vertebrate neurobiology.* New York: Wiley–Liss, 1992;274–278.

28. Kay AR. A procedure for isolating neurons from the mature mammalian brain. In: Shahar A, de Vellis J, Vernadakis A, Haber B, eds. *A dissection and tissue culture manual of the nervous system.* New York: Alan R Liss, 1989;54–59.

29. Edwards FA, Konnerth A, Sakmann B, Takahashi T. A thin slice preparation for patch clamp recordings from neurones of the mammalian central nervous system. *Pflugers Arch* 1989;414:600–612.

30. Dodt H-U. Infrared videomicroscopy of living brain slices. In: Kettenmann H, Grantyn R, eds. *Practical electrophysiological methods. A guide for in vitro studies in vertebrate neurobiology.* New York: Wiley–Liss, 1992;6–10.

31. Gahwiler B. Slice cultures of nervous tissue. In: Shahar A, de Vellis J, Vernadakis A, Haber B, eds. *A dissection and tissue culture manual of the nervous system.* New York: Alan R Liss, 1989;65–68.

32. Shahar A, de Vellis J, Vernadakis A, Haber B, eds. *A dissection and tissue culture manual of the nervous system.* New York: Alan R Liss, 1989;371.

33. Finkel AS, Redman SJ. Optimal voltage clamping with single microelectrodes. In: Smith TG, Lecar H, Redman SJ, Gage PW, eds. *Voltage and patch clamping with microelectrodes.* In: Baltimore: Williams & Wilkins, 1985;95–120.

34. Moore SD, Madamba SM, Schweitzer P, Siggins GR. Voltage-dependent effects of opioid peptides on hippocampal CA3 pyramidal neurons in vitro. *J Neurosci* 1994;14:809–820.

35. Drewe J, Childs G, Kunze D. Synaptic transmission between dissociated adult mammalian neurons and attached synaptic boutons. *Science* 1988;241:1810–1813.

36. Llinas R, Muhlethaler M. An electrophysiological study of the in vitro perfused brainstem-cerebellum of adult guinea-pig. *J Physiol (Lond)* 1988;404:215–240.

37. Feldman JL. Neurophysiology of breathing in mammals. In: Bloom FE, ed. *Handbook of physiology, section 1. The nervous system, vol IV: Intrinsic regulatory systems of the brain.* Bethesda, MD: American Physiological Society, 1986;463–524.

38. Madison DV, Nicoll RA. Control of the repetitive discharge of rat CA1 pyramidal neurons in vitro. *J Physiol* 1987;354:319–331.

39. Schweitzer P, Madamba S, Siggins GR. Arachidonic acid metabolites as mediators of somatostatin-induced increase of neuronal M-current. *Nature* 1990;346:464–467.

40. Aston-Jones G, Akaoka H, Charlety P, Chouvet G. Serotonin selectively attenuates glutamate-evoked activation of locus coeruleus neurons in vivo. *J Neurosci* 1991;11:760–769.

41. Ranck JBJ. Which elements are excited in electrical stimulation of mammalian central nervous system: a review. *Brain Res* 1975;(98):417–440.

42. Sandkühler J, Maisch B, Zimmerman M. The use of local anaesthetic microinjections to identify central pathways: a quantitative evaluation of the time course and extent of the neuronal block. *Exp Brain Res* 1987;(68):168–178.

43. Aston-Jones G, Chiang C, Alexinsky T. Discharge of noradrenergic locus coeruleus neurons in behaving rats and monkeys suggests a role in vigilance. *Prog Brain Res* 1991;88:501–520.

44. Aston-Jones G, Segal M, Bloom FE. Brain aminergic axons exhibit marked variability in conduction velocity. *Brain Res* 1980;195(1):215–222.

45. Aston-Jones G, Shiekhattar R, Rajkowski J, Kubiak P, Akaoka H. Opiates influence noradrenergic locus coeruleus neurons by potent indirect as well as direct effects. In: Hammer R, ed. *The neurobiology of opiates.* New York: CRC Press, 1993;175–202.

46. Chen Z, Engberg G. The rat nucleus paragigantocellularis as a relay station to mediate peripherally induced central effects of nicotine. *Neurosci Lett* 1989;101(1):67–71.

47. Funahashi S, Bruce CJ, Goldman-Rakic PS. Mnemonic coding of visual space in the monkey's dorsolateral prefrontal cortex. *J Neurophysiol* 1989;61(2):331–349.

48. Spitzer H, Desimone R, Moran J. Increased attention enhances both behavioral and neuronal performance. *Science* 1988;240:338–340.

49. Wise SP, Desimone R. Behavioral neurophysiology: insights into seeing and grasping. *Science* 1988;242:736–741.

50. Nicolelis MA, Lin RC, Woodward DJ, Chapin JK. Dynamic and distributed properties of many-neuron ensembles in the ventral posterior medial thalamus of awake rats. *Proc Natl Acad Sci* 1993;90(6):2212–2216.

51. Callaway CW, Henriksen SJ. Neuronal firing in the nucleus accumbens is associated with the level of cortical arousal. *Neuroscience* 1992;51(3):547–553.

52. Schultz W, Romo R. Dopamine neurons of the monkey midbrain: contingencies of responses to stimuli eliciting immediate behavioral reactions. *J Neurophysiol* 1990;63(3):607–624.

53. Newsome WT, Wurtz RH. Probing visual cortical function with discrete chemical lesions. *Trends Neurol Sci* 1988;11:394–400.

54. Sawaguchi T, Goldman-Rakic P. D1 dopamine receptors in prefrontal cortex: involvement in working memory. *Science* 1991;25:947–950.

55. Georgopoulos AP, Taira M, Lukashin A. Cognitive neurophysiology of the motor cortex. *Science* 1993;260(5104):47–52.

56. Houk JC, Keifer J, Barto AG. Distributed motor commands in the limb premotor network. *Trends Neurol Sci* 1993;16(1):27–33.

Psychopharmacology: The Fourth Generation of Progress, edited by Floyd E. Bloom and David J. Kupfer. Raven Press, Ltd., New York © 1995.

CHAPTER **6**

Behavioral Techniques in Preclinical Neuropsychopharmacology Research

James E. Barrett and Klaus A. Miczek

Behavioral measurements of the effects of drugs have been a central component of the field of neuropsychopharmacology since its inception some 40 years ago. The discovery of chlorpromazine and the subsequent demonstration that this drug produced differential effects on avoidance and escape behavior provided a strong impetus for the development of assays for evaluating the behavioral effects of potential antipsychotic drugs (9,12). The early growth of neuropsychopharmacology coincided also with the development and spread of the field of operant conditioning. Indeed, many of the techniques and procedures used to control and monitor operant behavior were adopted and enthusiastically endorsed by behavioral pharmacologists emphasizing the importance of behavior in determining the effects of drugs (15,29,44). Early researchers understood quickly the utility and the power of behavioral techniques in demonstrating specific and systematic effects in the integrated organism, and the field of behavioral pharmacology emerged as a discipline within the larger context of neuropsychopharmacology.

In a general sense, behavioral research in this context can be viewed as having two major objectives. In the first case, behavior is used to answer questions where the primary interest is in pharmacology, and a behavioral measure is studied to evaluate drug effects in much the same way as any other experimental preparation. For example, a behavior such as locomotor activity or lever pressing maintained by food permits a comparison of dose–response relationships and pharmacological antagonism, and it can also be developed as a method for "screening" new clinical compounds provided that it meets certain other criteria that are described in more detail below. In the second case, the study of behavior has been the primary interest, and drugs have been used to dissect and elucidate certain behavioral phenomena. For example, several studies have shown that existing environmental conditions or prior behavioral experiences can modify profoundly the qualitative and quantitative effects of a drug (4,35,37). The sensitivity of behavior to these influences has implications for understanding the significance of environmental conditions on the neuropharmacological substrates at which drug effects occur and unify behavioral and neuropharmacological analyses of drug action. Whether pharmacological or behavioral endpoints are of primary interest, both research areas have contributed substantially to (a) our understanding of drugs affecting the central nervous system and (b) our appreciation of how those effects can be determined by preexisting and current environmental conditions.

Research using behavioral techniques has continued to evolve over the several decades since the emergence of neuropsychopharmacology as a scientific discipline. As the field of neuropsychopharmacology continues its seemingly inevitable progression towards more molecular analyses, it will be of continued importance to maintain the experimental and conceptual rigor that has characterized the study of behavior as it has developed within the broader context of this field. It will also be critical for behavioral pharmacologists to adapt and address the information stemming from this progress. Although the actions of drugs affecting the central nervous system are studied at many different levels, it is inevitable that a thorough analysis will eventually address issues of a behavioral nature. Experiments involving the study of the actions of molecular signaling systems at the cellular level take on added significance when those processes can be

J. E. Barrett: Central Nervous System Research, Lederle Laboratories, American Cyanamid Company, Pearl River, New York 10965.

K. A. Miczek: Department of Psychology, Tufts University, Medford, Massachusetts 02155.

related meaningfully to the integrated activities of the behaving organism. As our understanding of molecular mechanisms and targets of drug action increases, it will be of increasing importance to understand the functional relationships of those processes to the expression of various behaviors.

There is a particular irony in the current situation in which it appears that as the understanding of molecular events underlying synaptic transmission and neuroregulation has assumed increasing complexity and sophistication, the procedures used to evaluate the relationship of those events to behavior are, in many cases, often rather simple. The fact that some of the current efforts to integrate molecular biology with behavioral pharmacology appear to have regressed to the use of simpler procedures should not be interpreted as a disregard for the sophisticated advances that have occurred in behavioral pharmacology over the past several decades. In some sense, this situation is similar to that which existed early in the field of neuropsychopharmacology where relatively simple procedures were used initially to assess the actions of drugs such as chlorpromazine, chlordiazepoxide, and imipramine. These drugs were brought into the experimental behavior laboratory after unequivocal evidence of clinical efficacy. The establishment of clinical activity could then be used to develop more complex procedures that would differentiate among the compounds possessing different clinical utility and different neuropharmacological actions. Indeed, behavioral procedures such as conditioned avoidance and ''conflict'' or punishment have been extraordinarily successful in predicting clinical efficacy and activity for the antipsychotic and anxiolytic drugs, respectively. Newer procedures have also been introduced for the evaluation of antidepressant activity, providing a reasonably broad array of behavioral procedures with relatively good predictive value for numerous clinical disorders (46,49). Despite these significant advances, there is a continuing need for new procedures that address emerging disciplines, and there is also a necessity for continued analysis and refinement of existing techniques. Until newer research directions involving, for example, ''knockout'' studies, transgenic animals, or other techniques become firmly established (see Chapters 2 and 69, *this volume*), it is perhaps best to rely on relatively simple and straightforward procedures. Some of these directions are discussed at the end of this chapter.

The main objective of this chapter is to provide a foundation for, and an overview of, the use and assessment of behavioral techniques in the study of drug action. The scope will necessarily be somewhat limited because several excellent monographs are available that provide detailed information on both behavioral principles and procedures in behavioral pharmacology (e.g., see refs. 26 and 59). This chapter will also attempt to address the means by which more recent techniques can be meaning-fully and productively incorporated into the field of behavioral neuropsychopharmacology.

PRINCIPLES OF BEHAVIOR

A detailed review of guiding principles underlying the study of behavior is beyond the scope of this chapter. However, it is of critical importance to appreciate the complex processes involved when neuropsychopharmacological research is escalated to include behavioral questions. One of the more striking aspects of many who evaluate behavioral research often has been the lack of appreciation for seemingly simple principles that, upon intensive scrutiny and experimental analysis, are of overwhelming importance. Often, for example, great care is taken in the preparation of solutions, mixtures of brain homogenates, and other experimental details, while considerably less attention is given to matters surrounding the acclimation of animals to the experimental testing conditions, handling, and so on despite the fact that these variables also can be of critical significance. Some of these concerns can, of course, be overcome by studying variables that are strong enough to override the influence of such intrusions, but, in many cases, this is not possible because the variables controlling behavior exert subtle but disruptive influences.

Substantial progress has been made in the development of techniques that permit the objective and quantitative study of behavior that is stable over time, manipulable over a range of controlling parameter values, reproducible within and across species, and sensitive to a number of pharmacological and environmental interventions. In the field of neuropsychopharmacology, the adoption and widespread use of these procedures has had the multiple benefit of broadening our understanding of behavior, elucidating the principles and mechanisms of drug action, and demonstrating the dynamic interactions between behavior and the neurochemical substrates influencing both behavior and drug action.

Reflexive Behavior and Conditioned Reflexes

One basic type of behavior that has been utilized in research on the behavioral effects of drugs is *respondent* or *reflexive* behavior. This type of behavior is elicited by specific stimuli and usually involves no specific training or conditioning in that the responses are typically part of the behavioral repertoire of the species and are expressed under suitable environmental conditions. Although factors responsible for the occurrence of these behaviors presumably lie in the organism's distant evolutionary past, certain unconditioned responses, called *reflexes,* can be brought under more direct and immediate experimental control through the use of procedures first discovered and systematically explored by Pavlov. Such procedures consist of expanding the range of stimuli capable of producing or eliciting a response. For instance, considerable use has been made of a procedure for the study of anxiolytic drugs in which a stimulus paired with the delivery of electric shock enhances the response to a loud auditory stimulus that elicits a startle response (13). When the startle reflex is reduced by the presentation of a brief stimulus presented immediately before the eliciting startle stimulus, "prepulse inhibition" results; this phenomenon has been useful in the evaluation of neuroleptic drugs (52). For the study of drugs that impair or enhance memory, conditioned reflexes such as those by the nictitating membrane of the rabbit eye have proven informative (24). These behaviors depend primarily on antecedent events that elicit specific responses. Typically, these responses do not undergo progressive differentiation in that the responses to either a conditioned or unconditioned stimulus are generally quite similar. Such procedures do not establish new responses, but the range of stimuli to which that response occurs is expanded. Protocols for eliciting conditioned and unconditioned reflexes have been automated, and the measurement techniques for reflexes in response to startle, eyeblink, or nociceptive stimuli result in precise and accurate data.

In some cases the elicited behavior is elicited by the administration of a drug, and then the particular behavior is used to define or assess pharmacological activity. For example, the administration of high doses of amphetamine can elicit stereotyped behavior; 5-HT$_{1A}$ agonists, such as 8-hydroxy-di-n-propylamino tetralin (8-OH-DPAT) can elicit the "serotonin syndrome" consisting of head weaving, reciprocal forepaw treading, and hindlimb abduction. When there is a particular behavior elicited by a drug, this often suggests that the behavior is mediated by a specific neurotransmitter receptor. Drug-induced behavior has been quite useful for studying the pharmacology of various neurotransmitter systems. Technically, drug-induced behavior is assessed by trained observers who employ rating scales. Video-tracking systems have been developed to automate the detection of stereotyped behavior.

In contrast to respondent behavior, *operant behavior* is controlled by consequent events in that it is established, maintained, and further modified by its consequences. Operant behavior occurs for reasons that are not always specifiable. Such responses may have some low probability of occurrence, or they may never have occurred previously. Novel or new responses are typically established by the technique of "shaping," in which a behavior resembling or approximating some final desired form or characteristic is selected, increased in frequency, and then further differentiated by the provision of a suitable consequence such as food presentation to a food-deprived organism. This technique has been used widely to develop operant responses such as (a) lever pressing by rodents, humans, and nonhuman primates or (b) key pecking by

pigeons. Behavior that has evolved under such contingencies may bear little or no resemblance to its original form and can perhaps only be understood by careful examination of the organism's history. Although some behaviors often appear unique or novel, it is likely that the final product emerged as a continuous process directly and sequentially related to earlier conditions. The manner in which operant responses have been developed and maintained, as well as further modified, has been the subject of extensive study and has had a tremendous impact on the development of behavioral neuropsychopharmacology. Many of the potent variables that influence the occurrence of behavior, such as reinforcement, punishment, and precise schedules under which these events occur, also are of critical import in determining how a drug will affect behavior.

Ethological Analysis of Behavior Patterns

Experimental procedures that engender more complex species-specific behavior patterns in animals have been the focus of the ethological approach. These types of behaviors have evolved in situations of survival. Selection pressure has resulted in the development of sensory and motor functions, sexual behavior, care of the young, social cohesion and dispersion, and interactions with other species in the ecological niche. These elaborate behavior patterns are the result of phylogenetic and ontogenetic processes; they are typical for the species and require no explicit conditioning for their expression, although they can be modified by experience. It is possible to reproduce under controlled conditions the essential features of situations promoting the display of those elements of the behavioral repertoire that are characteristic of exploration, foraging and appetite, reproduction, maternal care, attachment to and separation from the group, as well as aggression and defense (8,32,36).

Particularly relevant to neuropsychopharmacology are the ethological approaches to the study of drug action on emotional behavior that derive their rationale from Darwin's argument of emotions having evolved just as did an organism's morphology. Ethological analyses of emotional behavior attempt to delineate its distal and proximate causation in the phylogeny and ontogeny of the organism and to determine its function. When experimental techniques succeed in engendering emotional behavior with an adaptive function such as distress calls by an individual who is separated from the group, then selective drug action on this behavior points to modulation of functionally significant biological mechanisms. Adequate measurements of the behavioral expressions of affect require detailed familiarity with the species-typical displays in order to avoid impressionistic and anthropomorphic accounts, colored by the bias of the observer. Quantitative ethological methods have proven most informative when comprehensive analyses, usually on the basis of audio and video records, incorporate the traditional behavioral measurements of latency, frequency, and duration parameters, as well as a quantification of the temporal and sequential pattern (39). Increasingly more sophisticated levels of analysis assess not just the presence or absence of these behaviors, but also whether or not the species-typical acts, postures, displays, and gestures are fully developed in intensity, latency, and patterning. Precise analyses of the salient elements in an animal's repertoire detect behaviorally selective drug action; that is, they assess the "behavioral cost" for a desired drug effect. As the availability of agents to treat various neurological and psychiatric disorders increases, and the selectivity of the drugs available to treat those disorders improves, it will be possible to use this information to design even more sensitive and selective procedures for the evaluation of pharmacological activity.

Schedules of Reinforcement

One of the more important techniques to emerge from the field of behavioral research is the study of behavior using schedules of reinforcement. Many features of operant conditioning, including its frequency of occurrence, idiosyncratic form, and susceptibility to further modification and intervention, depend on the schedule of reinforcement. A schedule of reinforcement is, by definition, a prescription for the initiation and termination of reinforcing or discriminative stimuli in time and in relation to an organism's responses (42). Most schedules are variations on conditions that arrange for a consequent event to follow a response either after a specified number of responses (*ratio* schedules) or after a specified period of time (*interval* schedules). Under both ratio and interval schedules, reinforcement can be arranged to follow either a fixed or a variable number of responses or a fixed or a variable period of time. Under most laboratory conditions, and indeed under most environmental conditions, behaviorally relevant consequences occur intermittently. Properties of behavior that have useful analytical dimensions, such as the rate and patterning of responses, often can be seen only under conditions where consequent events are intermittently scheduled. Although it may seem paradoxical, behavior is actually strengthened and intensified by carefully scheduled intermittent rather than continuous reinforcement. Schedules of reinforcement have allowed and encouraged the creation of reliable quantitative, reproducible features of behavior and have permitted the study of behavioral processes that are of general importance.

In addition to their ability to establish and maintain durable behavior that occurs with reliability and orderliness, schedules of reinforcement offer other practical advantages. When food presentation is arranged intermit-

tently under a schedule to engender and maintain behavior, it is possible to sustain behavior over long periods of time with less concern about satiation, thereby permitting adequate evaluation of the time course of pharmacological activity. If the maintaining event is the self-administration of a drug, it is possible to capture the essence of the dynamic aspects of drug abuse because stimuli can be paired with the drug injection and the behavior can be brought under the control of those stimuli as well as the drug (28). There has been a progressive evolution of newer approaches and procedures to address new developments or issues in the field of drug abuse such as "craving" and withdrawal. The behavioral techniques used in this field have served as the foundation not only for the evaluation of drugs of abuse but also of the principles (such as reinforcement) that initiate, perpetuate, and maintain the process of addiction and dependence (see Chapter 66, *this volume*).

BEHAVIORAL METHODOLOGY AND DRUG EVALUATION

The number of methods employed to evaluate various behavioral processes and to examine the behavioral effects of drugs has increased dramatically in recent years. One main reason for this increase has been the growing availability of a number of drugs that, on the basis of either neurochemical or traditional receptor binding studies, would be expected to possess certain types of activity, thereby warranting study using sensitive and selective in vivo techniques. There is also heightened interest in newer procedures because many of the new chemical entities are based on molecular techniques that involve the use of cloned receptors; these developments, while offering tremendous potential, also remain to be validated using behavioral techniques. Finally, in recent years a number of drugs have appeared to be clinically effective yet their activity in traditional animal "models" has been inconsistent or absent, thus prompting the need to reevaluate existing procedures and/or develop new ones. The field of behavioral pharmacology is far from static; these developments, coupled with the results obtained in clinical studies, promise to result in newer techniques that provide better sensitivity and selectivity for studying the behavioral effects of drugs.

Punishment Procedures

Among the more compelling principles in the study of operant behavior are those of *reinforcement* and *punishment*. Though commonly used terms, these principles refer precisely to processes that, respectively, increase and decrease specific responses following the presentation or termination of some event. Reinforcement and punishment are descriptive, empirical processes that refer to relationships between behavior and its consequences. The use of punishment procedures, as will be discussed below, has provided one of the dominant methods for evaluating drugs effective in the treatment of anxiety. Recent work on the neurobiology of anxiety and the development of anxiolytic drugs with novel mechanisms of action also illustrates some of the successes and challenges of preclinical behavioral research. Procedures such as those developed in the early period of modern experimental psychopharmacology by Geller and Seifter (20) that began to characterize the behavioral actions of anxiolytic drugs have been refined further (10,45,47) and have added to the utility of these procedures. The use of punished behavior (sometimes referred to as a *conflict procedure*), in which the food-maintained responding of an animal is suppressed by a stimulus such as electric shock, has provided a sensitive and systematic procedure for the study of dose-dependent effects of benzodiazepine-type anxiolytics that could be prevented or reversed by benzodiazepine receptor antagonists (5). A hallmark of these procedures is that they enabled the monitoring of graded drug effects over time and on repeated occasions on behavioral parameters predictive of clinically relevant anxiolytic actions as compared to those indicative of sedative or suppressive effects. These features satisfy fundamental pharmacological and behavioral criteria and are obtained in various animal species, including humans. Moreover, these procedures have continued to play an integral role in the analysis of drug activity with the more recent development of partial benzodiazepine agonists that have lower positive intrinsic efficacy but retain significant therapeutic advantages (23,34). Undoubtedly, these procedures will continue to play an important role in the development of anxiolytic drugs that are devoid of unwanted side effects.

Newer Developments in Behavioral Methods to Study Anxiolytic Drugs

Some of the impetus for other recent developments in the field of anxiolytic behavioral pharmacology appears to have been the discovery of drugs acting through novel mechanisms where conventional punishment procedures appeared less effective. This was the case, for example, with 5-HT$_{1A}$-type drugs such as buspirone which, though clinically active, were not easily detected using typical rodent models of anxiety such as the Geller–Seifter procedure, and there was a need for different or more sensitive methods to detect the actions of these drugs (6). In this case, punishment procedures using the pigeon provided a useful means of evaluating the novel 5-HT$_{1A}$ anxiolytics and antidepressants. This area of research and the use of animal models for other clinical disorders is discussed in Chapter 68 (*this volume*).

A result of these expanded efforts, however, has been the heightened interest in different methods for evaluating anxiolytic drug activity, including methods using ethologically based approaches (30). An intriguing ethological approach to the study of anxiolytics has focused on vocal responses in mammals in situations where they appear to communicate an affective state. The range of vocalizations includes the following: (a) monotonous ultrasounds emitted by rat pups that are separated from their littermates, (b) modulated calls by juvenile rhesus monkeys, and (c) the more extensive vocal repertoire emitted by adults exposed to environmental and social demands (18,27,41,60). Vocal responses have been effectively modulated in a systematic, dose-dependent, antagonist reversible fashion by prototypic anxiolytics as well as by several classes of substances with potentially anxiolytic effects such as those with actions on serotonergic, N-methyl-D-aspartate (NMDA), and peptidergic receptor subtypes. The behavioral specificity of these drug effects can be assessed by comparing effects on vocalizations with those on laryngeal, respiratory, and thermoregulatory changes.

Drugs as Discriminative Stimuli

One of the more popular methods to emerge in behavioral pharmacology has been the use of drugs as discriminative stimuli. In essence, this procedure consists of establishing a drug as a stimulus in the presence of which a particular response is reinforced. The use of a drug to gain discriminative control over behavior is very different from that mentioned earlier in which a drug *elicits* a reflexive-like behavior. When a drug is developed as a discriminative stimulus, it is often said to "set the occasion" for a response, indicating that it does not by its administration merely produce the response but makes the response more likely to occur because of past consequences in the presence of that stimulus. Typically, when a drug is established as a discriminative stimulus, a single dose of a drug is selected and, following its administration, one of two responses are reinforced (usually, with rodents or nonhuman primates this consists of pressing one of two simultaneously available levers, with reinforcement scheduled intermittently after a fixed number of correct responses). Alternatively, when saline is administered, responses on the other device are reinforced. Over a number of experimental sessions, a discrimination develops between the administration of the drug and saline, with the interoceptive stimuli produced by the drug seen as "guiding" or controlling behavior in much the same manner as any external stimulus such as a visual or auditory stimulus. Once established, it is possible to perform several additional studies to investigate aspects of the drug stimulus in the same way as one might investigate other physical stimuli. Thus, it is possible to determine "intensity" gradients or dose–effect functions as well as generalization functions that are directed towards determining how similar the training drug dose is to a different dose or to another drug that is substituted for the training stimulus. It has also been possible to use drug discrimination techniques as a means for exploring changes in neurotransmitter function following exposure to neurotoxins or other types of interventions that may alter receptors in the central nervous system (7,11).

One of the more striking aspects of this technique is the finding of a strong relationship between the generalization profile and the receptor binding characteristics of various drugs. For instance, animals trained to discriminate a benzodiazepine anxiolytic (such as chlordiazepoxide) from saline respond similarly to other drugs that also interact with the receptor site(s) for benzodiazepine ligands (5,48). However, anxiolytic drugs that produce their effects through other mechanisms, such as the 5-HT_{1A} compounds, do not engender responding similar to that occasioned by benzodiazepines, suggesting that it is actually receptor-mediated activity that is established using this technique and not the action of the drug on a hypothetical psychological construct (3,33,43).

While the utility of receptor-selective drug discrimination procedures have become increasingly apparent to pharmacologists and medicinal chemists, the behavioral significance of stimuli correlated with drug administration has only recently been of experimental interest. Recently, the discriminative stimulus properties of "anxiogenic" drugs such as pentylenetetrazol (PTZ) or benzodiazepine inverse agonists, as well as other compounds such as barbiturates and psychomotor stimulants, have been of interest as a means of assessing subjective states (31). For example, rats trained to discriminate PTZ from saline responded on the lever appropriate for PTZ administration when threatened by an aggressive opponent or when exposed to the odor of a cat (19,55,56). In addition, the fear-like state of the threatened animal, as assessed by PTZ-appropriate responding, was antagonized by benzodiazepine anxiolytics. Such observations suggest that the drug-induced "anxiogenic" stimulus overlaps considerably with a behavioral fear-like state that is engendered by specific environmental events. Thus, it may be possible to mimic certain behavioral "states" by the administration of a drug, and the drug-related state then can be used to assess certain environmental conditions that may engender the same set of stimuli as those encountered in the environment. This technique has also received attention in attempting to determine whether withdrawal from a drug also produces an anxiogenic response similar to that engendered by PTZ (16; see also Chapter 66, *this volume*). These studies warrant further exploration and evaluation but provide a possibly useful means for assessing potential "emotional" states induced by specific environmental conditions.

Related Areas of Behavioral Research—Challenges and Problems

The area of drug abuse research has relied heavily on behavioral methodology and has broadened considerably in scope over the past several years. Drugs of abuse have been analyzed using the same conditioning principles outlined above and have relied heavily on behavioral procedures to analyze the processes of tolerance, dependence, withdrawal, and addiction (see Chapter 66, *this volume*). An area of continuing development, and perhaps the most complex and as yet unresolved, is that pertaining to the field of learning and memory ("cognition"). As yet, there are no prototypical drugs available and, as a result, no validated tests or procedures that engender experimental confidence. Despite a plethora of models and procedures, as well as a pressing need to evaluate potential drugs for the treatment of age-related dementia such as Alzheimer's disease, it is difficult to evaluate these drugs because such models appear to lack predictive value and also because there is, as yet, little understanding of the mechanisms involved in the disease process. Many of these behaviors—that is, those in which behavior is in "transition," such as during sensitization, tolerance, and habituation, as well as in complex forms of learning and maturation—require special research strategies and techniques because exposure of the individual animal to these conditions may produce long-lasting or even irreversible effects.

Another formidable challenge to preclinical research is the development of experimental and analytic procedures that adequately capture behavioral events that are episodic, infrequent, or cyclic in nature. Many affective disorders are characterized by explosive and intense behavior such as psychotic outbursts or depressive phases that may intrude into the behavioral repertoire only once or twice a year. In preclinical research, productive experimental protocols have only begun to emerge that engender intense aggressive behavior (40) or that encompass the assessment of behavioral and biological rhythms (53). While the significance of these phasic and infrequent events for neuropsychopharmacology is apparent, they too require novel experimental and analytical methodologies.

One of the main problems in each of these areas of research—anxiety, drug abuse, learning and memory, and aggression—is that the proliferation of procedures frequently has surpassed their careful experimental evaluation and validation. For example, in the study of anxiolytic drug effects, there are at least 30 different procedures ranging from the traditional Geller–Seifter conflict procedure to procedures utilizing ultrasonic vocalization, conditioned startle responses, or open field activity. During the last decade a range of procedures were introduced that attempted to avoid elaborate conditioning protocols and used exploratory and social behavior suppressed by aversive consequences such as bright light or an unfamiliar environment (17,30,54). While these procedures offer the convenience of being rapid and simple, and also have the appeal of increased face validity, these advantages have to be contrasted with the problems surrounding extensive involvement of the experimenter (e.g., more subjective measurements, time to perform evaluations and analyze results), single use of each subject due to rapid habituation, and the apparent variability depending on a host of uncontrolled variables. Furthermore, another potential difficulty is that the uncritical selection of a procedure for the evaluation of a drug may yield information that is of limited utility. The problem is complex because of the acknowledged difficulty of any type of in vitro or in vivo drug evaluation that may be quite good for the discovery of a drug that functions through the particular mechanism for which the test was designed, but which may not detect comparable potential clinical activity of a drug that functions through a different biochemical mechanism to which the screens are not sensitive. This dilemma can only be resolved by a close and detailed understanding of the behavioral, biochemical, and clinical issues as progress in each of these areas continues to unfold.

FUTURE DIRECTIONS

As mentioned earlier in this chapter, there have been a number of recent developments in the field of molecular neurobiology that, in conjunction with behavioral techniques, provide powerful experimental tools for examining the relationship between receptors and behavior. Two techniques that will undoubtedly receive more widespread use in neuropsychopharmacology involve antisense oligonucleotides and the generation of animals with specific gene mutations.

Antisense Oligonucleotide Approaches in Neuropsychopharmacology

Significant advances have occurred in the molecular biology of receptor subtypes for several neurotransmitter systems, including dopamine and serotonin. Although in some cases the functional significance of the different receptor subtypes is reasonably well understood [e.g., the 5-HT_{1A} receptor appears to be involved in 5-HT synthesis and release that is related to anxiety and depression (62)], for the most part the functional relevance of numerous receptors remains unclear. The use of antisense oligonucleotides to target and inhibit the information flow from gene to protein allows for the development of selective pharmacological tools for better understanding receptor-mediated activity in the central nervous system and also permits the development of therapeutics targeted towards specific genes (57). Recently, an antisense oligodeoxynucleotide of the rat neuropeptide Y1 (NPY-Y1) receptor was used to evaluate the role of this receptor for which there is as yet no specific receptor antagonist (58) (see Chapters 2 and 48, *this volume*). The addition of this antisense oligodeoxynucleotide to rat cortical neuron cultures reduced the density of Y1 receptors while having

no effect on Y2; in addition, there was a concomitant reduction in the decrease in cAMP that typically occurs after Y1 receptor activation. Injection of the oligodeoxynucleotide directly into the lateral cerebral ventricle of rats also resulted in a reduction of cortical Y1 receptors, but produced little effect on Y2 receptors. These animals also were tested in an elevated plus maze used frequently to measure exploratory behavior and to study the effects of anxiolytic and anxiogenic drugs. The maze, which consists of two open and two closed arms, assesses the tendency of rodents to explore the two compartments; normally, less time is spent in the open arms, a result believed to reflect the fear of open spaces by rodents. Anxiolytic drugs increase the proportion of time spent in the open compartments, whereas anxiogenic drugs reduce this time. In the antisense-treated animals there was a decrease in the number of entries and amount of time spent in the open portion of the elevated maze, reflecting an anxiogenic-like effect. Thus, these results support (a) the hypothesis that NPY is involved in anxiety and (b) prompt additional studies using other types of behavioral procedures to extend these findings and to also evaluate NPY involvement in other areas (such as feeding) where it also has been implicated.

A similar approach using antisense was adopted to study the function of the dopamine D2 receptor (61). Intracerebroventricular administration of an oligodeoxynucleotide antisense to the D2 dopamine receptor messenger RNA in mice resulted in a reduction in the levels of D2 receptors and D2 receptor mRNA but had little effect on D1 receptors or D1 mRNA. In antisense-treated mice that also received 6-hydroxydopamine lesions of the corpus striatum, the customary contralateral rotations produced by the D2 dopamine receptor agonists quinpirole and N-propyl-N-2-thienylethylamine-5-hydroxytetralin were significantly inhibited. Importantly, effects of the dopamine D1 receptor agonist 1-phenyl-2,3,4,5-tetrahydro-1H-3 benzazepine-7,8-diol HCl or the muscarinic cholinergic receptor agonist oxotremorine were not affected.

These studies with NPY and dopamine receptors suggest that it is possible to use antisense techniques to selectively block specific receptors in the central nervous system, and they indicate that this approach may be a valuable alternative to the use of traditional receptor antagonists to probe the behavioral significance of those receptors. The further use and extension of these powerful technologies to include increasingly more complex behaviors promises to yield (a) a better understanding of the roles of specific receptors in neuropharmacology and (b) more selective tools and therapeutics.

Gene Inactivation Techniques: Mutant Mice and "Knockout" Studies

With the development of technology for targeting and manipulating specific genes, it is possible to produce animals with specific mutations in any gene that has been cloned. The methodology for this approach involves the introduction of a desired gene mutation into embryonic stem cells and the eventual development of a line of mutant animals (22). A number of studies have now shown that inactivation or "knockout" of certain protein kinases produce animals deficient in performing certain tasks. For instance, studies of mice with mutations of α-Ca^{2+}-calmodulin-dependent kinase II (α-CaMKII), a synaptic protein that is enriched in the hippocampus, have been shown to be deficient in learning a spatial navigational task and are also deficient in demonstrating long-term potentiation (LTP), believed to be a synaptic marker of learning and memory (50,51). Behavioral experiments with the mutant and wild-type mice were conducted using the Morris water maze task, a procedure in which mice are placed in a pool of water and must swim to a platform that is located below the water level. In some cases the platform is indicated by a marker, whereas in other cases it is not; both tasks are believed to assess the learning involving spatial stimuli. The α-CaMKII-deficient mice took longer than the wild-type control subjects to learn the location of both the marked and hidden platform, suggesting an impairment in spatial learning ability. Other test procedures were also used to characterize possible differences between the mutant and wild-type animals. For example, animals with hippocampal lesions not only show deficits similar to those of the mutant mice in these studies in the water maze task, but also demonstrate characteristic increases in locomotor or exploratory behavior, effects shown also by the α-CaMKII mutant animals. Other studies have now also demonstrated impaired learning of spatial tasks involving the water maze, as well as impaired LTP induction in mice with mutations of *fyn*, a tyrosine kinase gene, and in mice lacking the γ subtype of protein kinase (PKC), an enzyme involved in signal transduction in a number of physiological systems (1,2,21). Due, in part, to the fact that this research is in its nascent phases, there are still several questions that remain, and certain concerns have already been raised about the nature and specificity of the deficits and about the view that something as complex as learning can be reduced to a single gene (14). However, these developments remain one of the most promising directions for the integration of behavior, pharmacology, and cell biology that may provide insight into an area of research that has been rather stagnant for a lengthy time period.

Finally, knockout studies have also been conducted with specific neurotransmitter receptors and provide additional compelling evidence of the potential utility of this technique in neuropsychopharmacology (25). The 5-HT_{1B} receptor, which is the rodent homologue of the 5-$HT_{1D\beta}$ (see Chapters 36–38, *this volume*), has been demonstrated in several studies to play an important role in feeding, aggression, and locomotor activity (62). Mutant mice, generated by homologous recombination, lacking the 5-HT_{1B} receptor show diminished locomotor activity compared to wild-type animals and do not respond to the typical locomotor-enhancing effects of the 5-$HT_{1A/1B}$ agonist RU 24969. Additionally, the mutant mice are also hyperaggressive, suggesting that the pharmacological analyses of the role of this receptor as subserving a role in locomotor activity and aggression are due to activity of this receptor subtype.

These developments in molecular biology and genetics provide a new set of tools with which to explore the complex interrelationships between neuropharmacological systems and behavior and promise a fertile means for generating insight into processes that previously could only be speculative. At present, the behavioral techniques have been rather basic when compared to some of those outlined in this chapter, but, as was suggested earlier, it is necessary to use uncomplicated procedures initially and then move to more complex techniques. Undoubtedly, this will occur as the field of molecular neuropsychopharmacology continues to grow and as more individuals embrace the combined approaches of behavior and molecular neurobiology.

SUMMARY AND CONCLUSIONS

The techniques and principles of behavioral analysis and drug action summarized in this chapter point to the richness and potential benefits derived from combining the careful study of behavior with the analysis of drug effects. A drug is not simply a molecule with static, unitary effects but can exert an array of behavioral effects depending on several well-characterized features of the previous and immediate environment. The study of drugs within the context of neuropsychopharmacology contributes both to an understanding of behavior and to the systems that subserve drug action and behavior. There are an overwhelming number of procedures that have been developed to study the behavioral effects of drugs over the period of time since the discipline of neuropsychopharmacology was initially established. Many have been used repeatedly and have served the science well, helping to establish a prominent place in the field for characterizing the behavioral effects of drugs and for understanding neuropharmacological mechanisms underlying behavioral processes. With the advent and incorporation of new molecular techniques into the field of neuropsychopharmacology, it will be a challenging time to adapt and extend existing procedures to provide the type of synergy possible when different fields merge.

ACKNOWLEDGMENTS

We wish to thank Kathleen O'Sullivan for her assistance in the preparation of the manuscript.

REFERENCES

1. Abeliovich A, Chen C, Goda Y, Silva AJ, Stevens CF, Tonegawa S. *Cell* 1993;75:1253–1262.
2. Abeliovich A, Paylor R, Chen C, Kim JJ, Wehner JM, Tonegawa S. *Cell* 1993;75:1263–1271.
3. Andrews JS, Stephens DN. *Pharmacol Ther* 1992;47:267–280.
4. Barrett JE. In: Meltzer HY, ed. *Psychopharmacology: the third generation of progress.* New York: Raven Press, 1987;1493–1501.
5. Barrett JE, Gleeson S. In: Rodgers RJ, Cooper SJ, eds. *5-HT_{1A} agonists, 5-HT_3 antagonists and benzodiazepines: their comparative behavioural pharmacology.* New York: Wiley, 1991;59–105.
6. Barrett JE, Vanover KE. *Psychopharmacology* 1993;112:1–12.
7. Barrett JE, Monaghan MM, Rosenzweig-Lipson S. Vanover KE. *Drug Dev Res* 1994;[in press].
8. Blundell JE. In: Eversen LL, Iversen SD, Snyder SH, eds. *Handbook of psychopharmacology, new directions in behavioral pharmacology,* vol 19. New York: Plenum Press, 1987;123–182.
9. Cook L, Weidley E. *Ann NY Acad Sci* 1957;66:740–752.
10. Cook L, Sepinwall J. *Fed Proc* 1975;34:1889–1897.
11. Cory-Schlechta DA, Widzowski DV, Polora MJ. *Neurotoxicology* 1993;14:105–114.
12. Courvoisier S, Fournel J, Ducrot R, Kolsky M, Koetschet P. *Arch Int Pharmacodyn* 1953;92:305–361.
13. Davis M. *Pharmacol Ther* 1990;24:147–165.
14. Deutsch JA. *Science* 1993;262:760–763.
15. Dews PB. *J Pharmacol Exp Ther* 1955;113:393–401.
16. Emmett-Oglesby MW, Mathis DA, Moon RTY, Lal H. *Psychopharmacology* 1990;101:292–309.
17. File SE. *Neuropsychobiology* 1985;13:55–62.
18. Gardner CR. *J Pharmacol Methods* 1985;14:181–187.
19. Gauvin DV, Holloway FA. *Pharmacol Biochem Behav* 1991;39:521–523.
20. Geller I, Seifter J. *Psychopharmacologia* 1962;1:482–492.
21. Grant AGN, O'Dell TJ, Karl KA, Stein PL, Soriano P, Kandel ER. *Science* 1992;258:1903–1910.
22. Grant SGN, Silva AJ. *Trends Pharmacol Sci* 1994;17:71–75.
23. Haefely W, Martin JR, Schoch P. *Trends Pharmacol Sci* 1990;11:452–456.
24. Harvey JA. In: Meltzer HY, ed. *Psychopharmacology: the third generation of progress.* New York: Raven Press, 1987;1485–1490.
25. Hen R, Boschert U, Lemeur M, Dierich A, Dit Amara D, Buhot MC, Segu L, Missin R, Saudou F. *Soc Neurosci Abstr* 1993;19:632.
26. Iversen IH, Lattal KA. *Experimental analysis of behavior,* parts 1 and 2. New York: Elsevier, 1991.
27. Kalin NH. *Science* 1989;243:1718–1721.
28. Katz JL, Goldberg SR. In: Bozarth MA, ed. *Methods of assessing the reinforcing properties of abused drugs.* New York: Springer-Verlag, 1987;105–115.
29. Kelleher RT, Morse WH. *Ergeb Physiol Chem Exp Pharmakol* 1968;60:1–56.
30. Lister RG. *Pharmacol Ther* 1990;46:321–340.
31. Lubinski D, Thompson T. *Brain Behav Sci* 1993;16:627–642.
32. Mackintosh JH, Chance MRA, Silverman AP. In: Iversen LL, Iversen SD, Snyder SH., eds. *Handbook of psychopharmacology-principles of behavioral pharmacology,* vol 7. New York: Plenum Press, 1977;3–35.
33. Mansbach RS, Barrett JE. *J Pharmacol Exp Ther* 1987;240:364–369.
34. Martin JR, Schoch P, Jenck F, Moreau J-L, Haefely WE. *Psychopharmacology* 1993;111:415–422.
35. McKearney JW, Barrett JE. In: Blackman DE, Sanger DJ, eds. *Contemporary research in behavioral pharmacology.* New York: Plenum Press, 1978;1–68.
36. Miczek KA. In: Spiegelstein MY, Levy A., eds. *Behavioral models and the analysis of drug action.* Amsterdam: Elsevier, 1982;225–239.
37. Miczek KA, Thompson ML, Shuster L. *Science* 1982;215:1520–1522.
38. Miczek KA, Tornatzky W, Vivian JA. In: Olivier B, Mos J, Slangen JL, eds. *Animal models in psychopharmacology,* Basel: Birkhauser Verlag, 1991;409–427.
39. Miczek KA, Weerts EM, DeBold JF, Vatne T. *Psychopharmacology* 1992;107:551–563.
40. Miczek KA, Weerts EM, Haney M, Tidey J. *Neurosci Biobehav Rev* 1994;18:97–110.
41. Miczek KA, Weerts EM, Vivian JA, Barros H. *Psychopharmacology* 1994;in press.
42. Morse WH. In: Honig WK, ed. *Operant behavior.* New York: Appleton–Century–Crofts, 1966;52–108.
43. Nader MA, Hoffmann S, Gleeson S, Barrett JE. *Behav Pharmacol* 1989;1:57–67.
44. Pickens R. In: Thompson T, Dews PB, eds. *Advances in behavioral pharmacology,* vol 1, New York: Academic Press, 1977;229–257.
45. Pollard GT, Howard JL. *Pharmacol Ther* 1990;45:403–424.
46. Porsolt RD, Lenègre A, McArthur, RA. In: Olivier B, Slangen J, Mos J, eds. *Animal models in psychopharmacology.* Basel: Birkhauser Verlag, 1991;137–159.
47. Sanger DJ. In: Boulton A, Baker G, Martin-Iverson M., eds. *Neuromethods, animal models in psychiatry II,* vol 19. Clifton, NJ: Humana Press, 1991:147–198.
48. Sanger DJ, Benavides J. *Psychopharmacology* 1993;111:315–322.
49. Seiden LS, O'Donnell JM. In: Seiden LS, Balster RL, eds. *Neurology and neurobiology,* vol 13. *Behavioral pharmacology: the current status.* New York: Alan R. Liss. 1985;323–338.
50. Silva AJ, Paylor R, Wehner JM, Tonegawa S. *Science* 1992;257:206–211.
51. Silva AJ, Stevens CF, Tonegawa S, Wang Y. *Science* 1992;257:201–206.
52. Swerdlow NR, Braff DL, Taaid N, Geyer MA. *Arch Gen Psychiatry* 1994;51:139–154.
53. Teicher MH, Barber NI, Lawrence JM, Balderssarini RJ. In: Koob GF, Ehlers CL, Kupfer DJ, eds. *Animal models of depression.* Basel: Birkhauser, 1989;135–161.
54. Treit D. *Neurosci Biobehav Rev* 1985;9:203–222.
55. Vellucci SV, Martin PJ, Everitt BJ. *J Psychopharmacol* 1988;2:80–93.
56. Vivian JA, Weerts EM, Miczek KA. *Psychopharmacology* 1994; [in press].
57. Wahlestedt C. *Trends Pharmacol Sci* 1994;15:42–46.
58. Wahlestedt C, Pich EM, Koob GF, Yee F, Heilig M. *Science* 1993;259:528–531.
59. Willner P. *Behavioural models in psychopharmacology.* New York: Cambridge University Press, 1991.
60. Winslow JT, Insel TR. *Trends Pharmacol Sci* 1991;12:402–404.
61. Zhou L-W, Zhang S-P, Qin, Z-H, Weiss, B. *J Pharmacol Exp Ther* 1994;268:1015–1023.
62. Zifa E, Fillion G. *Pharmacol Rev* 1992;44:401–457.

Psychopharmacology: The Fourth Generation of Progress, edited by Floyd E. Bloom and David J. Kupfer. Raven Press, Ltd., New York © 1995.

CHAPTER 7

Excitatory Amino Acid Neurotransmission

Carl W. Cotman, Jennifer S. Kahle, Stephan E. Miller, Jolanta Ułas, and Richard J. Bridges

The amino acid L-glutamate is now recognized as the major excitatory neurotransmitter in the central nervous system (CNS). Accumulating evidence suggests that the glutamate system is involved not just in fast synaptic transmission, but also in plasticity and higher cognitive functions. It is becoming clear that the glutamate transmitter system is organized at a high level of sophistication. This is evident in the organization of the glutamate receptor subtypes, which include both ionotropic and metabotropic receptor families. Ionotropic glutamate receptors (see Chapters 1 and 5, *this volume*) can be distinguished pharmacologically by specific binding of the agonists N-methyl-D-aspartate (NMDA), kainic acid (KA), and α-amino-3-hydroxy-5-methyl-4-isoxazole propionic acid (AMPA) (Table 1) and include receptors that gate both voltage-dependent and voltage-independent currents carried by Na^+, K^+, and, in some cases, Ca^{2+}. Because Ca^{2+} can act as a second messenger, it can initiate a wide range of intracellular responses. Metabotropic glutamate receptors (mGluRs) provide for another level of response complexity through their links with the phosphoinositide (PI) and cyclic nucleotide (cAMP) second messenger systems. Thus, different combinations of receptor subtypes can influence the specific functional capability of individual synapses and neurons. In contrast to a relatively simpler system, such as the neuromuscular junction, this complexity provides the infrastructure necessary of a system involved in higher cognitive function (see Chapters 101, 118, 132, and 134, *this volume*).

This organization, however, appears to come at a cost. The processes of information integration, association, and storage utilize cellular mechanisms for which there is a narrow range of normal function. An imbalance at any one of many key points of the processes can lead to the destruction of the neurons involved and the disruption of circuitries and associated functions. This is most clearly illustrated by the process of excitotoxic-mediated neuronal injury, which may contribute to CNS pathology in a variety of neurodegenerative conditions.

The concept of the pervasiveness and homogeneity of glutamate as the principal transmitter is yielding to an understanding of the highly sophisticated specialized combinations of receptors discretely organized to carry out specific functions. The goal of this chapter is to provide an updated overview of the excitatory amino acid (EAA) transmitter system, in particular, focusing on the glutamate receptors and transport proteins. We have chosen to emphasize two areas that are rapidly developing: (i) the pharmacology of the ligand binding sites on the receptors and transporters (Table 1) and (ii) the molecular biology of the receptors (Tables 2–4). Progress in molecular techniques has led to the cloning and expression of many of the components of the glutamate receptor system. This provides a valuable strategy to examine the independent function of the subunits in defined combinations from reconstitution experiments. In parallel, advances in pharmacology have been directed toward the characterization of binding-site pharmacophores and the design of conformationally restrained glutamate analogues. As an acyclic molecule, glutamate can assume a staggered conformer as a result of rotation about its $\alpha\beta$ and $\beta\gamma$ sp^3 carbon bonds. Conformationally restricted analogues, which mimic stable conformations of glutamate, allow the exploration of the specific stereochemistry of the subunit pharmacology. The integration of molecular biology and pharmacology and the organization of the specific receptors in the CNS holds great promise for the characterization of the complex structure–function relationships within this transmitter system in health and disease.

C. W. Cotman, J. S. Kahle, S. E. Miller, and J. Ułas: Irvine Research Unit in Brain Aging, University of California, Irvine, Irvine, California 92717-4550.

R. J. Bridges: Department of Pharmaceutical Science, University of Montana, Missoula, Montana 59814.

TABLE 1. *Glutamate receptor pharmacology*[a]

	NMDA		AMPA		Kainate	Metabotropic
	Competitive	Modulatory	Competitive	Modulatory[b]		
Agonists	NMDA L-CCG-IV ACBD	Glycine	AMPA ATPA 5-Fluorowillardiine Br-HIBO	Aniracetam 1-BCP Cyclothiazide	Kainate Domoate	trans-ACPD L-CCG-I L-AP4 3,5-Dihydroxy- phenylglycine trans-2,4-ADA

Antagonists	D-AP5
	
	CGS19755
	
	CGP37849
	D-CPP
	D-CPPene
		7-Chloro-
		  kynurenate
		5,7-Dichloro-
		  kynurenate
		MNQX
		L689,560
		HA966
			NBQX	GYKI 52466		L-AP3
						
						(+)-MCPG
						
						(S)-4CPG

Channel blockers	MK801 PCP					

[a] This table provides a partial list of agonists and antagonists of each receptor type with emphasis on the more selective agents. Abbreviations: L-CCG-IV, (2S,3R,4S)-α(carboxycyclopropyl)glycine; D-AP5, D-2-amino-5-phosphonopentanoic acid; ACBD, 1-amincyclobutane-1,3-dicarboxylate; CGS19755, cis-4-(phosphonomethyl)piperidine-2-carboxylic acid; CGP37849, D,L-(E)-2-amino-4-methyl-5-phosphono-3-pentenoic acid; CPP, 3-(2-carboxypiperazin-4-yl)propyl-1-phosphonic acid; CPPene, (E)-4-(3-phosphono-2-propenyl)piperaziiine-2-carboxylic acid; MK801, dizocilpine; PCP, phencyclidine; MNQX, 5,7-dinitroquinoxaline-2,3-dione; L689,560, (±)-4-trans-2-carboxy-5,7-dichloro-4-phenylaminocarbonylamino-1,2,3,4-tetrahydroquinoline; ATPA, α-amino-3-hydroxy-5-tertbutyl-4-isoxazole-propionate; HA966, 3-amino-1-hydroxypyrrolidin-2-one; Br-HIBO, (S)-4-bromohomoibotenate; NBQX, 2,3-dihydro-6-nitro-7-sulfamoyl-benzo(F)-quinoxaline; aniracetam, 1-(4-methoxybenzoyl)-2-pyrrolidinone; 1-BCP, 1-(1,3-benzodioxol-5-ylcarbonyl)-piperidine; GYKI 52466,1-(4-aminophenyl)-4-methyl-7,8-methylenedioxy-5H-2,3-benzodiazepine; trans-ACPD, 1-aminocyclopentane-trans-1,3-dicarboxylic acid; L-CCG-I, (2S,3S,4S)-α-(carboxycyclopropyl)glycine; L-AP-4, L-2-amino-4-phosphonobutyric acid; trans-2,4-ADA, trans-azetidine-2,4-dicarboxylic acid; L-AP-3, L-2-amino-3-phosphonopropionic acid; (+)-MCPG, (+)-α-methyl-4-carboxyphenylglycine; (S)-4CPG, (S)-4-carboxyphenylglycine.
[b] The sites of action of the non-competitive modulators of AMPA receptors have not been well-characterized.

IONOTROPIC GLUTAMATE RECEPTORS

NMDA Receptors

Receptor/Channel Properties

NMDA receptors were initially identified and separated pharmacologically from other EAA receptors by selective activation by the agonist NMDA. The recent explosion of research on this receptor subtype has revealed that its activity is highly regulated via several allosteric regulatory binding sites on the receptor/channel complex. Activation of the receptor and concurrent depolarization results in the development of a relatively slow-rising, long-lasting current mediated primarily by the influx of Ca^{2+}. Calcium entering the cell can also mediate longer-lasting cellular responses. NMDA receptors appear to have a pivotal role in long-term potentiation (LTP), long-term depression (LTD), and developmental plasticity. Overactivation of NMDA receptors, however, appears to cause damage via excitotoxicity.

At a single CNS synapse, NMDA receptors usually coexist with either AMPA or KA receptors and are thought to be involved in amplification of the glutamate signal, although examples of primarily NMDA-mediated synaptic responses have been reported (70). At resting potentials, NMDA channels are normally blocked by Mg^{2+} and there must be sufficient concurrent depolarization of the postsynaptic neuronal membrane (to about -30 mV) before the Mg^{2+} block is relieved and the NMDA channel can contribute to the electrical response of the cell. The level of concurrent depolarization depends on AMPA/KA activation and/or other modulatory postsynaptic signals controlling depolarization.

Precise modulation of NMDA channel activity is required for normal neuronal function, and, as expected, there are several regulatory sites on the NMDA receptor/channel complex which control NMDA-mediated activity further. The binding of glycine to the receptor/channel complex increases the frequency of agonist-induced channel opening. Glycine binding appears to be an absolute requirement for NMDA channel activation. Studies of the NMDA receptor/channel complex at the molecular level indicate that binding of two glycines and two glutamate molecules is required for channel activation (23). The receptor/channel complex also includes a polyamine binding site which, when activated, potentiates the NMDA current by increasing channel open probability. This is due, in part, to an increase in glycine binding. At higher concentrations, the polyamine spermine binds to a second site which results in a reduction of the NMDA current potentiation and a decrease in the channel conductance

TABLE 2. *Ionotropic glutamate receptors: NMDA[a]*

Subunit	Channel assembly	Characteristics
NMDAR1	Homomeric or heteromeric	Seven splice variants NMDAR1A-G
NMDAR2	Heteromeric only	Four splice variants NMDAR2A-D increases current when assembled with NMDAR1

[a] NMDA receptors are characterized by high Ca^{2+} permeability and voltage-sensitive Mg^{2+} blockade which are mediated by an asparagine residue in the second transmembrane domain in a homologous location to the Q/R site in AMPA/KA receptors. NMDAR1 corresponds to NR1 or $\zeta 1$ in mouse; NMDAR2 corresponds to NR2 or $\epsilon 1-\epsilon 4$.

and/or mean open time. The NMDA receptor/channel complex can also be inhibited via a Zn^{2+} binding site. In addition, there is a distinct site within the channel that binds MK-801 and PCP inhibiting channel opening (for review see ref. 34). Thus, there is capacity for several different mechanisms for both positive and negative control of NMDA channel function.

NMDA-Mediated Plasticity

The voltage-dependent properties of NMDA-mediated Ca^{2+} current provides the capacity for Hebbian-type plasticity at synapses where NMDA receptors are located (see ref. 13 for discussion). Repetitive or concurrent activation can depolarize the postsynaptic cell to the level at which Mg^{2+} block of NMDA-mediated current is relieved and where these channels begin to contribute additional currents to the postsynaptic response. Furthermore, the influx of calcium through this channel initiates long-term synaptic and cellular modification. Thus, NMDA receptor/channels have a key role in plastic events at the synaptic, cellular, and behavioral level.

On the other hand, increasing evidence indicates that the complex mechanisms controlling synaptic plasticity in the brain also introduce points of vulnerability to pathology. In this case, too much intracellular free calcium can be toxic to neurons, and overstimulation can result in excitotoxic cell death. A breakdown of any one of the points of modulation of NMDA channel activity can lead to excitotoxicity. This type of cell death appears to contribute to brain pathology in several conditions, including epilepsy and ischemia, and, possibly, Alzheimer's disease and Huntington's disease (12).

Molecular Characterization

The NMDA receptor subtype has recently been cloned and appears to include two families of subunits (Table 2). NMDAR1 (also called NR1 or $\zeta 1$ in mouse) exhibits the major electrophysiological and pharmacological char-

acteristics of the NMDA receptor/channel complex when expressed in isolation in *Xenopus* oocytes. However, the current carried by the channel is much smaller than that observed in native receptor/channel complexes (36). Presently, seven splice variants have been described and called NMDAR1A–NMDAR1G (NR1a–NR1g). The basic pharmacological and electrophysiological characteristics of channels formed from these splice variants are reminiscent of native NMDA receptors, with slight shifts in specific characteristics (e.g., binding affinities) (56). However, there are several marked differences that have been described. For example, it appears that the NMDA-induced current through NMDAR1B channels are not potentiated by exposure to the polyamine spermine (15).

NMDAR2A–NMDAR2D (also called NR2A–NR2D or $\epsilon 1-\epsilon 4$ in mouse), the second family of subunits to be cloned, are considered to be modulatory subunits and do not form channels by themselves (homomeric channels), but form heteromeric channels (channels consisting of more than one type of subunit). Thus, when NMDAR2 subunits are expressed with NMDAR1A, heteromeric channels are formed that exhibit much greater currents than those of homomeric NMDAR1 channels. Different combinations of specific NMDAR2 subunits and NMDAR1A subunits appear to produce NMDA receptor/channel complexes with subtly different electrophysiological properties. For example, NMDAR1 and NMDAR2C heteromers exhibit an increased current relative to those of NMDAR1 and NMDAR2A (20).

Distribution

The distribution of different NMDA receptor subunit expression is distinct throughout the brain. In general, the patterns of mRNA expression appear to be consistent with heteromeric receptors made up of a common subunit (NMDAR1) with various NMDAR2 subunit combinations. Thus NMDAR1 is expressed at high levels in most neurons (36), while NMDAR2 mRNAs show distinct temporal and spatial patterns in the developing and adult brain. Previous autoradiographic studies have suggested that NMDA receptors are a heterogeneous population including agonist-preferring and antagonist-preferring receptors (35). Agonist-preferring sites are observed, for example, in the medial striatum, while antagonist-preferring sites are found in the lateral thalamus. These two populations of NMDA receptors may be related to different combinations of NMDA subunits from the two families. The NMDAR2A subunit, for example, has a distribution very similar to that of the antagonist-preferring NMDA subtype (labeled by the antagonist ^{3}H-CPP). Furthermore, when reconstituted in oocytes, NMDAR1/NMDAR2A receptors have a higher affinity for antagonists whereas NMDAR1/NMDAR2B receptors have a higher affinity for agonists (9). Such studies are providing a direct link between subunit composition and receptor physiology.

Pharmacology

Agonists

Besides NMDA, several other dicarboxylic amino acids are also agonists at the NMDA binding site. These include L-glutamate, S-sulfo-L-cysteine, L-homocysteate, L-aspartate, homoquinolinate, L-homo-cysteinesulfinate, L-cysteinesulfinate, L-serine-O-sulfate, L-cysteate, and quinolinate, in order of potency from greatest to least (31). Several conformationally restricted agonists have been identified, some of which are more potent than NMDA. For example, one of the most potent rigid agonists is *trans*-1-aminocyclobutane 1,3 dicarboxylate (*trans*-ACBD), a natural product of a seed (genus *Atelia*). The fact that this analogue is selective and potent is consistent with the suggestion that decreasing conformational flexibility increases selectivity. Modeling studies based on a variety of conformers have led to a proposed stereochemical arrangement of functional groups for the NMDA receptor (10,42).

Competitive and Non-competitive Antagonists

The pharmacology of the NMDA receptor/channel complex indicates three major possible mechanisms of antagonism. Several well-characterized competitive antagonists include: D-AP5, D-AP7, D-α-amino adipate, CPP, and CPPene. Antagonists in which the intervening carbons have been rigidified (such as in a cyclic conformation) have led to the synthesis of compounds more potent than AP5 or AP7 (e.g., CGP37849). Several non-competitive antagonists have been identified that bind to a site within the channel itself (e.g., MK-801 and PCP) (34). There are also non-competitive antagonists that bind to the glycine binding site: kynurenate, 5,7-dichloro-kynurenate, MNQX, and L689,560 (29). The study of cyclic derivatives which are conformationally constrained will allow for a rigorous analysis of the structure–activity relationship of the distinct subunits.

Non-NMDA Receptors

Characteristics of Ligand-Gated Responses

Both KA and AMPA receptors mediate fast excitatory synaptic transmission and are associated primarily with voltage-independent channels that gate a depolarizing current primarily carried by an influx of Na^+ ions (see ref. 34 for review). The natural plant product KA (isolated from *Digenea simplex*) and a synthetic analogue of quisqualic acid, AMPA, have had a pivotal role in the characterization of the non-NMDA glutamate receptor subclass. Early electrophysiological studies with these potent excitants (often in combination with EAA antagonists) demonstrated the presence of EAA receptor subtypes that were easily distinguishable from NMDA receptors. Thus, the classification of these receptors as "non-NMDA" evolved as a result of being able to use NMDA antagonists (e.g., D-AP5, MK-801) to easily differentiate KA and AMPA receptor-mediated responses from NMDA receptor-mediated responses, but not from each other. Glutamate activation of AMPA receptors initiates a current comprised of a fast desensitizing component and a steady-state component. Importantly, specific combinations of subunits regulate the differing desensitization kinetics. This desensitization, in turn, appears to be controlled by an allosteric site that binds compounds in the aniracetam family (68). In the presence of these modulators, desensitization of the receptor is delayed and the synaptic current is correspondingly enhanced. The site is important because aniracetam analogues appear to enhance synaptic activity and improve learning in animal models (63). Receptors relatively specific for KA have been identified with ligand binding (34); however, KA and AMPA can show overlapping patterns and ligand cross-reactivity.

Molecular Characterization

Molecular biology studies on the non-NMDA receptors have not only confirmed the existence of the KA and AMPA classes, but indicate that the potential heterogeneity within these receptor families reveals a remarkable degree of complexity. AMPA receptor channels can be formed by reconstituting one or any two of four subunits (GluR1–GluR4, also called GluRA–GluRD), while the KA subclass of receptors includes GluR5–GluR7 and KA-1–KA-2 (Table 3).

AMPA receptors are approximately 900 amino acids in length and occur in two forms distinguished by the presence or absence of an alternatively spliced exonic sequence of 38 residues preceding the last transmembrane domain (TM IV) (62) (for explanation see Chapter 2, *this volume*). This alternative splicing of GluR1–GluR4 results in the so-called "flip" or "flop" variants. The "flip" forms give rise to a larger sustained current (slower to desensitize) than do the "flop" forms. Any one or two of the four subunits assemble into ion channels and are activated by AMPA and, to a lesser degree, KA. The ionic specificity of the assembled channels (e.g., Na^+ or K^+ versus Ca^{2+}) has been shown to be dependent upon the combination of subunits expressed. GluR1, GluR3, and GluR4 are Ca^{2+}-permeable, while GluR2 appears to possess an optional Ca^{2+}-permeability that is dependent upon the amino acid composition at a single residue. The amino acid composition of this site is controlled by RNA editing. That is, a CAG codon (glutamine) in transmembrane domain II is edited to CIG (arginine) via the enzyme adenosine deaminase. Thus, brain cells can regulate the extent of Ca^{2+}-permeability by controlling the level of GluR2 expression and by RNA editing.

Calcium influx through glutamate receptor channels is

TABLE 3. *Ionotropic glutamate receptors: AMPA/kainate[a]*

Subunit	Channel assembly	Characteristics	Agonist selectivity
AMPA-preferring			
GluR1 GluR2 GluR3 GluR4	Homomeric or heteromeric	RNA splicing generates alternate "flip" or "flop" variants In heteromeric channels, GluR2 limits Ca^{2+} permeability[b]	AMPA > KA
Kainate-preferring			
GluR5 GluR6	Homomeric or heteromeric	Low-affinity KA binding	KA ≫ AMPA
GluR7	Heteromeric only	Low-affinity KA binding	KA ≫ AMPA
KA1 KA2	Heteromeric only	High-affinity KA binding	KA ≫ AMPA

[a] Adapted from ref. 29.
[b] The low Ca^{2+} permeability of GluR2 appears to be conferred by RNA editing to change a single residue in the second transmembrane domain from a glutamine to an arginine. Similar RNA editing of this "Q/R site" in GluR5 and GluR6 generates two alternate forms of these subunits with different Ca^{2+} permeabilities. GluR1–GluR4 are also known as GluRA–GluRD.

thought to play a causal role in glutamate-mediated excitotoxicity. Following transient global ischemia, expression of GluR2, which limits calcium permeability in heteromeric channels, is suppressed in CA1, a region susceptible to ischemic injury, but not in CA3 or the dentate gyrus, regions which are resistant to ischemic injury (45). Such differential regulation suggests that the ratios of expression of the individual receptor subunits is an important determinant in maintaining or disrupting cell viability.

The KA subclass of receptors includes GluR5–GluR7, which correspond to the previously described low-affinity site, and KA1–KA2, which correspond to the high-affinity site. Homomeric expression of GluR5 or GluR6 (but not GluR7) yields a binding pharmacology consistent with a high-affinity site and the formation of ion channels that are activated by KA but not AMPA. In contrast, homomeric expression of KA1 or KA2 subunits does not generate functional ion channels, though binding studies are consistent with a high-affinity KA site. Functional channels are produced, however, if KA1 or KA2 is heteromerically expressed with GluR5 or GluR6. Both GluR5 and GluR6 (not GluR7 or KA1-2) occur in two forms with respect to the Q/R site controlling Ca^{2+} permeability in the transmembrane II domain that can be modified by RNA editing. These two forms occur at different frequencies in the CNS.

Distribution

Autoradiographic studies with radioligands clearly demonstrate that while both KA and AMPA sites are principally localized in telencephalic regions, each exhibits a distinctive distribution. The combined patterns of the five-subunit mRNAs of KA approximate the patterns observed for high-affinity ³H-KA sites in the rat brain. KA binding sites are relatively enriched in the hippocampal CA3 stratum lucidum, striatum, deep cortical layers, reticular nucleus of the thalamus, and granule cell layer of the thalamus (14). At present, *in situ* hybridization studies of the AMPA subunits are difficult to interpret and match with autoradiographic studies. Distribution studies with ³H-AMPA demonstrate that the binding sites are concentrated in CA1 stratum radiatum, outer cortical layers, lateral septum, and molecular layer of the cerebellum (14). This distribution is similar to that exhibited by the NMDA receptors and is consistent with their common action as a functional pair.

Pharmacology

The respective pharmacologies of KA and AMPA receptors are similar enough that they are more often distinguished by the relative rank order of potencies of a series of agonists rather than by the action of a single selective compound. Electrophysiological studies demonstrate that the relative potencies of non-NMDA agonists (e.g., KA, domoate, QA, AMPA) vary according to the brain area examined. These studies, however, have been carried out in physiological preparations where the precise receptor subunit compositions of the recorded neurons has yet to be determined. It is clear that the development of more selective agonists and antagonists will play an important role in correlating the receptor structure and function. Considerable progress, however, has been made in identifying agonists that exhibit preferential activity at KA or AMPA receptors (Table 1).

Agonists

KA, a di-substituted proline derivative, contains an embedded L-glutamate moiety that is conformationally restricted about the α,β bond which is probably responsible for the reduced affinity of KA for NMDA receptors, metabotropic receptors, and the high-affinity Na^+-dependent glutamate transporter (10). KA can, however, assume several envelope conformers, mimic a number of glutamate conformations, and therefore interact with several types of GluRs (10). The KA derivatives, acromelic acid and domoic acid, have been shown to be more potent than KA as specific KA receptor agonists. Domoic acid is of particular interest because consumption of this neurotoxin by humans has been shown to produce pathological damage to the hippocampus as well as dementia (64). AMPA shows good specificity for AMPA receptors and itself has limited conformational flexibility. Several conformationally constrained analogues of AMPA have been shown to be more potent and selective agonists at the AMPA receptor (27). Other competitive-site AMPA agonists include ATPA, 5-fluorowillardiine, Br-HIBO, and β-L-ODAP, the EAA agonist identified as the causative agent in neurolathyrisms (8). A separate set of agonists exhibit non-competitive modulatory effects on AMPA receptors via action at an allosteric site(s) involved in attenuating receptor desensitization, thereby enhancing synaptic current. Agonists with such allosteric action include aniracetam (68), related analogues [e.g., 1-BCP (63)], and a series of benzothiadiazides [e.g., cyclothiazide (72)].

Antagonists

At present, the most potent and selective of the non-NMDA antagonists are a series of dihydroxyquinoxaline derivatives, CNQX, DNQX, and NBQX. Although these antagonists will competitively block both of the non-NMDA receptors, NBQX may provide insight into the design of more specific antagonists, because it appears to exhibit the greatest selectivity for AMPA receptors. Few KA-selective compounds have been developed, but recently NS-102 has been reported to competitively antagonize low-affinity kainate binding with some selectivity (21). A promising new class of 2,3-benzodiazepines (particularly GYKI 52466) has been demonstrated to noncompetitively block both AMPA- and KA-induced responses (50). Importantly, many of the newly developed competitive and non-competitive antagonists have been shown to potently attenuate ischemic neuronal injury in animal models, highlighting the potential role of non-NMDA receptors in CNS pathology. Structural comparisons and molecular modeling with these antagonists and agonists is beginning to shed some light on the respective pharmacophores of the KA and AMPA receptors (10,27). Progress will no doubt accelerate as analogues are examined in detail on homomeric and heteromeric subunits.

METABOTROPIC GLUTAMATE RECEPTORS

Unlike the ionotropic glutamate receptors which are directly coupled to cation-specific ion channels and mediate fast excitatory synaptic responses, the more recently characterized mGluRs are coupled to a variety of signal transduction pathways via guanine-nucleotide-binding proteins (G proteins) (see Chapters 1 and 27, *this volume*), producing alterations in intracellular second messengers and generating slower synaptic responses. The prevalence of glutamate as a neurotransmitter in combination with the widespread distribution of metabotropic receptors points to this system as a major modulator of second messengers in the mammalian CNS.

Characteristics of Ligand-Gated Second Messenger Responses

Different subtypes of mGluRs are linked to at least two major signal transduction cascades: PI hydrolysis and the adenylate cyclase/cyclic AMP system. The ability of glutamate to stimulate PI hydrolysis has been extensively characterized in a variety of preparations, including tissue slices, cultured neurons, cultured astrocytes, and transfected cell lines (see ref. 54 for review). Stimulation of PI hydrolysis results from activation of a receptor coupled to a G protein that activates phospholipase C, initiating a signaling cascade by cleaving phosphatidylinositol-4,5-bisphosphate into two second messengers: diacylglycerol which activates protein kinase C and inositol 1,4,5-trisphosphate (IP_3) which elicits the release of Ca^{2+} from intracellular stores.

Metabotropic glutamate receptors can also regulate cAMP levels. Synthesis of cAMP by adenylate cyclase can be altered by activation of either stimulatory G_s proteins or inhibitory G_i proteins which produce opposing effects on adenylate cyclase. In contrast to the excitatory actions of glutamate on ionotropic receptors and PI hydrolysis, glutamate produces an inhibitory effect on cAMP accumulation, an action that has now been characterized in a number of preparations. Some studies have also demonstrated a stimulation of cAMP accumulation with mGluR activation, and evidence exists for coupling of mGluRs to other transduction pathways, including phospholipase D, arachidonic acid, and direct G-protein coupling to cation channels (54).

In addition to biochemical studies, electrophysiological consequences of mGluR activation have also been extensively studied. These studies have been greatly facilitated by the identification of a selective agonist 1-aminocyclopentane-*trans*-1,3-dicarboxylic acid (*trans*-ACPD), a conformationally restricted analogue of glutamate which activates metabotropic, but not ionotropic, glutamate receptors (44). Electrophysiologically, activation of mGluRs results in both excitatory and inhibitory actions (54). For example in the hippocampus, *trans*-ACPD can

TABLE 4. *Metabotropic glutamate receptors*[a]

Subgroup	Gene	Effector system	Agonist selectivity
I	mGluR1 mGluR5	Stimulates phospholipase C	QA > Glu ≥ Ibo > t-ACPD ≫ AP4
II	mGluR2 mGluR3	Inhibits adenylate cyclase	Glu ≥ t-ACPD > Ibo ≫ QA ≫ AP4
III	mGluR4 mGluR6	Inhibits adenylate cyclase	Ap4 > Glu > SOP > ACPD > QA > Ibo AP4 > SOP > Glu ≫ ACPD > QA/Ibo

[a] The six metabotropic glutamate receptor subtypes have been classified into three subgroups based upon similarities in their sequence homology, effector coupling in artificial expression systems, and agonist selectivity. In addition to those shown above, other coupling mechanisms have been characterized, including stimulation of cyclic AMP accumulation, stimulation of arachadonic acid metabolism, inhibition of cation channels, and stimulation of phospholipase D. Adapted from refs. 29 and 67.

produce depolarization and reduction of the after-hyperpolarization via a blockade of a Ca^{2+}-activated potassium current. It has also been shown to block accommodation of cell firing, increase the amplitude of population spikes, induce generation of multiple spikes, decrease paired-pulse inhibition, and decrease evoked inhibitory postsynaptic potentials. Inhibitory actions of *trans*-ACPD in the hippocampus include reduction of the field excitatory postsynaptic potential via a presynaptic action.

Molecular Characterization

To date, six different cDNA clones of mGluRs (mGluR1–mGluR6), all with highly conserved amino acid sequences, have been isolated from rat cDNA libraries (38) (Table 4). It has been shown that the family of mGluRs does not share overall sequence similarities with other G-protein-coupled receptors (66). In contrast to ionotropic glutamate receptors, mGluRs contain three structural domains: a large extracellular hydrophilic NH_2-terminal sequence, seven membrane-spanning domains characteristic of G-protein-linked receptors, and a hydrophilic intracellular COOH-terminal sequence. Members of the mGluR family can be divided into three subgroups according to their sequence similarities, signal transduction properties, and pharmacological profile (i.e., relative potencies of QA, glutamate, ACPD, and AP4) when expressed in cell lines (67).

The members of the first group, mGluR1 (2) and mGluR5 (1), are coupled to PI hydrolysis when expressed in Chinese hamster ovary (CHO) cells. In addition, mGluR1 stimulates cAMP formation and arachidonic acid release with the same order of agonist selectivity (2). Two splice variants of mGluR1 with truncated carboxy terminals have also been isolated (46,66). The second subgroup, comprised of mGluR2 and mGluR3, are negatively coupled to adenylate cyclase in CHO cells (66,67). The members of the third group, mGluR4 and mGluR6, also inhibit cAMP accumulation but have a different agonist selectivity (37,67,69).

Distribution

As a group, the mGluRs are widely expressed throughout the brain. The individual subtypes are differentially distributed although sometimes overlap. Considering first the receptors coupled to PI hydrolysis, *in situ* hybridization (46,58) and immunocytochemistry (30) have shown a wide distribution of mGluR1 in rat brain, with particularly prominent expression in hippocampal dentate gyrus granule cells, CA4 cells, CA2–CA3 pyramidal cells, cerebellar Purkinje cells, mitral and tufted cells of the olfactory bulb, and neurons of the thalamus and lateral septum. The receptor appears to be localized postsynaptically, and no glial staining has been demonstrated (30). Expression of mGluR5, the other PI-coupled subtype, is prominent in the cerebral cortex, dentate gyrus granule cells, pyramidal cells in CA1–CA4, subiculum, lateral septum, internal granule layer of the olfactory bulb, anterior olfactory nucleus, striatum, and nucleus accumbens (1).

Of the adenylate-cyclase-inhibiting receptors, the distribution of mGluR2 is more restricted than that of the PI-coupled receptors. *In situ* hybridization showed the most prominent expression in Golgi cells of the cerebellum, mitral cells of the accessory olfactory bulbs, and pyramidal neurons of the entorhinal cortex and parasubicular cortex, as well as in the dentate gyrus (40). It has been suggested that mGluR2 may serve as a presynaptic receptor in the cortico-striatal glutamate projection (40). mGluR3, the subtype with the greatest homology to mGluR2, is more widely distributed. Prominent expression of mGluR3 mRNA was found in neurons of the cerebral cortex, thalamic reticular nucleus, caudate-putamen, supraoptic nucleus, and granule cells in the dentate gyrus (67). In addition to the neuronal localization, mGluR3 mRNA was found in glial cells in the corpus callosum, anterior commissure, and throughout the brain (67).

The final subgroup of receptors is comprised of mGluR4 and mGluR6 which also have distinct patterns of expression. mGluR4 is most prominently expressed in cerebellar granule cells, neurons of the internal granule layer of the main olfactory bulb, thalamus, lateral septum, pontine nucleus, and entorhinal cortex, with weaker expression in dentate gyrus and CA3 of the hippocampus (26,67). The selectivity of mGluR4 for L-AP4 and its expression in the entorhinal cortex suggest that mGluR4 corresponds to the AP4 receptor, a presynaptic autoreceptor initially described in physiological studies (24,69). The distribution of the final receptor subtype, mGluR6, is the most restricted of all the mGluRs. Appreciable expression was observed only in the inner nuclear layer of the retina (37), the area of the ON-bipolar cells, known to be hyperpolarized by glutamate or L-AP4.

It is interesting to note the degree of differential expression not only between regions but also within a region. In the cerebellum, for example, there is prominent expression of three separate subtypes: mGluR1 in the Purkinje cells, mGluR2 in the Golgi cells, and mGluR4 in granule cells. Such precise segregation of receptors implies an important role for the subtypes in functional specialization.

Pharmacology

Agonists

Glutamate, QA, and IBO were extensively used in the initial studies of mGluRs. These agonists, however, do not differentiate between ionotropic and metabotropic receptors: Glutamate, of course, activates all receptor subtypes, QA also activates AMPA receptors and IBO cross-reacts with NMDA receptors. To further examine the functional roles of mGluR activation required the development of pharmacological tools specific for the mGluRs such as trans-ACPD (44) and (2S,3S,4S)-α-(carboxycyclopropyl) glycine [L-CCG-I (59); see Table 1)]. However, recent discoveries of the molecular heterogeneity of mGluRs and the coupling of mGluRs to multiple signal transduction pathways have necessitated identification of even more selective agonists to pharmacologically differentiate between mGluR subtypes. The original pharmacological studies of metabotropic responses were conducted primarily with brain slices or primary cultures, which are complex systems with multiple receptor subtypes present. More recently, individual subtypes have been expressed in CHO or baby hamster kidney (BHK) cells allowing examination of the agonist profiles of individual receptors as described above. Among other findings, these studies have demonstrated that L-AP4 is the most potent agonist of mGluR4 and mGluR6 but has little effect on the other receptor subtypes (26,37,67). Similarly, L-CCG-I was shown to activate mGluR2 at concentrations that have little effect on mGluR1 and mGluR4 (19). Two promising agonists which have recently been developed and may have some selectivity for specific receptor subtypes are (2S,1'R,2'R,3'R)-2-(2,3-dicarboxycylopropyl)glycine [DCG-IV (59)] and (−)-trans-azetidine-2,4-dicarboxylic acid [t-ADA (16)].

Antagonists

Studies of the physiological roles of metabotropic receptors have long been hampered by a lack of effective antagonists. Unlike the overlap with ionotropic receptors in agonist specificity, the mGluRs do not appear to share antagonists with any other glutamate receptor. L-2-Amino-3-phosphonopropionic acid (L-AP3), which has been used most extensively, typically displays a pharmacological action characteristic of a weak partial agonist, but its efficacy varies widely between preparations (54). Recently, a promising series of phenylglycine derivatives, e.g., α-methyl-4-carboxyphenylglycine (MCPG) have been developed which have been shown to competitively inhibit ACPD-stimulated PI hydrolysis and antagonize ACPD-induced depolarization (4) (Table 1). Although they have yet to be fully characterized, it appears that some of these analogues may differentially antagonize individual receptor subtypes.

Roles in Plasticity and Pathology

A substantial body of evidence now exists indicating that mGluRs have important roles in development and plasticity. For example, the developmental peak of EAA-stimulated PI hydrolysis occurs between 6 and 12 days of age in neonatal rats and exhibits a high correlation with periods of intense synaptogenesis (39). More direct evidence for a role of mGluRs in plasticity is provided by studies of LTP. Bath application of trans-ACPD can produce LTP in the absence of concomitant tetanic stimulation (5) or can potentiate LTP when applied in conjunction with tetanic stimulation (33). Most recently it has been shown that the newly characterized metabotropic antagonist MCPG can block the induction of LTP without affecting baseline synaptic transmission or previously established LTP (3).

Evidence indicates that activation of mGluRs can have both neuroprotective and neurotoxic effects. Koh et al. (25) demonstrated that trans-ACPD can attenuate NMDA-induced excitotoxicity using a murine cortical culture system. Although other neuroprotective actions of trans-ACPD have been subsequently demonstrated both in vitro and in vivo (11,41,48,61), some recent studies have indicated neuropathological effects of mGluR agonists (28,32,53). Whether the net effect of an mGluR agonist is neuroprotective or neuropathological may depend upon the relative expression of specific metabotropic receptor subtypes coupled to either excitatory or inhibitory transduction mechanisms. Expression of the subtypes is differentially regulated according to region, cell type, and developmental state, and the ratios of receptors expressed may represent homeostatic mechanisms that have roles in determining the balance between plasticity and pathology.

EXCITATORY AMINO ACID TRANSPORT

While most of the attention and effort aimed at the study of the EAA system has focused specifically on the neurotransmitter receptors, an integrated model of the synapse should include the other steps in synaptic transmission, such as transmitter inactivation. The rapid removal of glutamate, and related transmitters, from the synaptic cleft by high-affinity uptake is thought to contribute to (a) the termination of the excitatory signal, (b) the maintenance of extracellular glutamate levels below those that could induce excitotoxic damage, and (c) the recycling of the transmitter via the glutamine cycle (18,51, 55,57).

The uptake process, as well as the potential consequences of decreases in transport capacity, is particularly significant in view of the excitotoxic properties of L-glutamate. This inverse relationship between transport capacity and excitotoxic sensitivity is supported by both in vivo and in vitro studies in which a reduction of transport capacity is associated with a concomitant increase in the damage produced by EAA agonists (51). Interestingly, decreases in the binding density of the transport substrate ^{3}H-D-aspartate have been reported in Alzheimer's disease (43), while the maximum uptake velocity (V_{max}) of glutamate is reduced in synaptosomes prepared from the spinal cords of patients with amyotrophic lateral sclerosis (ALS) (52). Such deficits may ultimately contribute to the excitotoxic vulnerability of neurons in these diseases.

Analogous to the heterogeneity found within the receptor systems, accumulating evidence indicates that there are a number of distinct EAA transporters. Currently, these uptake systems can be distinguished on the basis of: (a) their ionic dependency, Na$^+$ versus Cl$^-$ versus Ca^{2+}; (b) cell type, neuronal versus glial; (c) anatomical location, forebrain versus cerebellar; (d) substrate, glutamate versus homocysteate; and (e) cell organelle, synaptosome versus synaptic vesicle. Among these various systems, the Na$^+$-dependent high-affinity transporter appears to be the dominant species and is the most thoroughly characterized in regard to pharmacology, distribution, mechanism, and molecular biology (10,22,47,49,65).

Molecular Characterization

Three glutamate transport genes (22,47,65) have been identified, each of which share the common features of: (a) being expressed in brain, (b) lacking apparent signal sequences, (c) containing carbohydrate moieties, and (d) having molecular weights of about 57–64 kD. Importantly, when the proteins are pharmacologically characterized in expression systems, they demonstrate a strong Na$^+$-dependency, are appropriately enantioselective (i.e., D-aspartate, L-aspartate and L-glutamate are substrates, whereas D-glutamate is not), and are inhibited by well-characterized uptake blockers, such as dihydrokainate, β-

threo-hydroxy-aspartate, and L-trans-2,4-pyrrolidine dicarboxylate (L-trans-2,4-PDC). Two of these proteins appear to be of glial origin, while the third is reported to be found in neurons, although each exhibits a specific distribution in the CNS.

Sequence analysis demonstrates that while the three transporters share about 50% homology among themselves, they exhibit little homology with any other eukaryotic protein, including the superfamily of neurotransmitter transporters that mediate the uptake of GABA, noradrenaline, serotonin, dopamine, glycine, and choline (for review see ref. 71). Examination of the sequences of each of the three proteins has led to the identification of both glycosylation sites and potential phosphorylation sites, as well as the prediction that each contains a distinct number of membrane-spanning regions (i.e., six, eight, and ten).

Pharmacology

Early studies of the pharmacology of the Na$^+$-dependent high-affinity glutamate uptake system identified the basic specificity of the system by quantifying the ability of a large number of glutamate analogues to inhibit the uptake of radiolabeled substrates (e.g., ^{3}H-L-glutamate and ^{3}H-D-aspartate) in a variety of preparations (e.g., synaptosomes, cultured astrocytes, tissue slices). In this manner, it was demonstrated that uptake inhibitors generally share the common features of being α-amino acids with a second acidic group separated from the α-COOH by 2–4 methylene groups. Structure–activity studies indicate that the distal COOH group can be derivatized to a hydroxamate (e.g., L-aspartate-β-hydroxamate) or replaced by a sulfonate group (e.g., cysteic acid). Some modification of the carbon backbone is also tolerated, because β-THA and DHK are well-known competitive inhibitors. The system also exhibits enantioselectivity, because D-glutamate is a very weak inhibitor, although L- and D-asparate are excellent substrates.

A major advance in the pharmacological characterization of this system came with the identification of transport inhibitors that are conformationally restricted analogues of L-glutamate, such as L-trans-2,4-PDC (7), L-CCG-III (60), and cis-1-aminocyclobutane-1,3-dicarboxylate (CACB) (17). In contrast to the conformational flexibility of the acyclic molecules, these more rigid analogues are considerably more useful in defining the pharmacophore of the transporter binding site and, in the long term, developing selective transport inhibitors that do not cross-react with the other EAA receptors. Toward this goal, L-trans-2,4-PDC has been shown to be one of the most potent uptake blockers identified, yet it exhibits little or no activity at the NMDA, KA, or AMPA receptors (7).

With the aid of molecular modeling, comparisons have been made between energetically stable envelope conformations of L-trans-2,4-PDC and preferred staggered conformers of L-glutamate. Using this approach, a folded conformation of L-glutamate has been identified that exhibits a high degree of functional group overlap with L-*trans*-2,4-PDC (6,10). The specific L-*trans*-2,4-PDC conformer is one in which the distal carboxyl group occupies an axial-like position at the flap of the pyrrolidine envelope. The L-glutamate conformer, in turn, corresponds to the relatively abundant folded conformation found in solution. Additional modeling studies with CCG-III and CACB further supported this arrangement of functional groups, because significant overlap was also observed with these conformationally restricted uptake blockers (6). These results support the hypothesis that a partially folded conformer of glutamate represents the active conformation at the Na$^+$-dependent transporter and provides a firm basis for further modeling of the binding site pharmacophore and the design of new inhibitors.

SUMMARY AND CONCLUSIONS

As discussed in this chapter, the EAA receptors are a complex class with heterogeneous ligand specificity and subtle differences in the time course and magnitude of current flow even within each subtype. This specificity is created by various combinations of subunits, alternative splicing, and RNA editing. In the case of the ionotropic receptors there are at least 16 cDNAs identified, whereas in the metabotropic class there are over six subtypes, with the number still growing. Their varied distributions suggest that different combinations of EAA receptor and transporter subtypes are essential for functional specialization of individual cell types and at individual synapses. Recent advances in approaches to pharmacological examination of the EAA transmitter system will continue to allow a progressively more detailed understanding of these functions and how they can be modified during dysfunction.

REFERENCES

1. Abe T, Sugihara H, Nawa H, Shigemoto R, Mizuno N, Nakanishi S. Molecular characterization of a novel metabotropic glutamate receptor mGluR5 coupled to inositol phosphate/Ca^{2+} signal transduction. *J Biol Chem* 1992;267:13361–13368.
2. Aramori I, Nakanishi S. Signal transduction and pharmacological characteristics of a metabotropic glutamate receptor, mGluR1, in transfected CHO cells. *Neuron* 1992;8:757–765.
3. Bashir ZI, et al. Induction of LTP in the hippocampus needs synaptic activation of glutamate metabotropic receptors. *Nature* 1993;363: 347–350.
4. Birse EF, et al. Phenylglycine derivatives as new pharmacological tools for investigating the role of metabotropic glutamate receptors in the central nervous system. *Neuroscience* 1993;52:481–488.
5. Bortolotto ZA, Collingridge GL. Activation of glutamate metabotropic receptors induces long-term potentiation. *Eur J Pharmacol* 1992;214:297–298.
6. Bridges RJ, Lovering FE, Humphrey JM, Stanley, MS, et al. Conformationally restricted inhibitors of the high affinity L-glutamate transporter. *Bioorg Med Clem Lett* 1993;3:115–121.
7. Bridges RJ, Stanley MS, Anderson MW, Cotman CW, Chamberlin AR. Conformationally defined neurotransmitter analogues.

8. Selective inhibition of glutamate uptake by one pyrrolidine-2,4-dicarboxylate diastereomer. *J Med Chem* 1991;34:717–725.
8. Bridges RJ, Stevens DR, Kahle JS, Nunn PB, Kadri M, Cotman CW. Structure–function studies on *N*-oxalyl-diamino-dicarboxylic acids and excitatory amino acid receptors: evidence that beta-L-ODAP is a selective non-NMDA agonist. *J Neurosci* 1989;9:2073–2079.
9. Buller AL, Morrisett RA, Monaghan DT. The NR2 subunit contributes to the pharmacological diversity of native NMDA receptors. *Soc Neurosci Abstr* 1993;19:1356.
10. Chamberlin AR, Bridges RJ. Conformationally constrained acid amino acids as probes of glutamate receptors and transporters. In: Kozikowski AP, ed. *Drug design for neuroscience.* New York: Raven Press, 1993;231–259.
11. Chiamulera C, Albertini P, Valerio E, Reggiani A. Activation of metabotropic receptors has a neuroprotective effect in a rodent model of focal ischaemia. *Eur J Pharmacol* 1992;216:335–336.
12. Choi DW. Excitotoxic cell death. *J Neurobiol* 1992;23:1261–1276.
13. Cotman CW, Monaghan DT, Ganong AH. Excitatory amino acid neurotransmission: NMDA receptors and Hebb-type synaptic plasticity. *Annu Rev Neurosci* 1988;11:61–80.
14. Cotman CW, Monaghan DT, Offersen OP, Storm-Mathisen J. Anatomical organization of EAA receptors and their pathways. *Trends Neurosci* 1987;10:273–280.
15. Durand GM, Gregor P, Zheng X, Bennett MV, Uhl GR, Zukin RS. Cloning of an apparent splice variant of the rat *N*-methyl-D-aspartate receptor NMDAR1 with altered sensitivity to polyamines and activators of protein kinase C. *Proc Natl Acad Sci USA* 1992;89:9359–9363.
16. Favaron M, Manev RM, Canedo P, Arban R, et al. *Trans*-azetidine-2,4-dicarboxylic acid activates neuronal metabotropic receptors. *Neuroreport* 1993;4:967–970.
17. Fletcher EJ, Mewett KN, Drew CA, Allan RD, Johnston GAR. Inhibition of high affinity L-glutamic acid uptake into rat cortical synaptosomes by the conformationally restricted analogue of glutamic acid: *cis*-1-aminocyclobutane-1,3-dicarboxylic acid. *Neurosci Lett* 1991;121:133–135.
18. Hamberger AC, Chiang GH, Nylen ES, Scheff SW, Cotman CW. Evaluation of glucose and glutamine as precursors for the synthesis of preferentially released glutamate. *Brain Res* 1979;168:513–530.
19. Hayashi Y, Tanabe Y, Aramori I, Masu M, et al. Agonist analysis of 2-(carboxycyclopropyl)glycine isomers for cloned metabotropic glutamate receptor subtypes expressed in Chinese hamster ovary cells. *Br J Pharmacol* 1992;107:539–43.
20. Ishii T, Moriyoshi K, Sugihara H, Sakurada K, et al. Molecular characterization of the family of the *N*-methyl-D-aspartate receptor subunits. *J Biol Chem* 1993;268:2836–2843.
21. Johansen TH, Drejer J, Watjen F, Nielsen EO. A novel non-NMDA receptor antagonist shows selective displacement of low-affinity [^{3}H]kainate binding. *Eur J Pharmacol* 1993;246:195–204.
22. Kanai Y, Hediger MA. Primary structure and functional characterization of a high-affinity glutamate transporter. *Nature* 1992;360:467–471.
23. Kemp JA, Leeson PD. The glycine site of the NMDA receptor—five years on. *Trends Pharmacol Sci* 1993;14:20–25.
24. Koerner JF, Cotman CW. Micromolar L-2-amino-4-phosphonobutyric acid selectively inhibits perforant path synapses from lateral entorhinal cortex. *Brain Res* 1981;216:192–198.
25. Koh JY, Palmer E, Cotman CW. Activation of the metabotropic glutamate receptor attenuates *N*-methyl-D-aspartate neurotoxicity in cortical cultures. *Proc Natl Acad Sci USA* 1991;88:9431–9435.
26. Kristensen P, Suzdak PD, Thomsen C. Expression pattern and pharmacology of the rat type IV metabotropic glutamate receptor. *Neurosci Lett* 1993;155:159–162.
27. Krogsgaard-Larsen P, Nielsen EO, Engfesgaard A, Lauridsen J, Brehm L, Hansen JJ. *Amanita muscaria* in medicinal chemistry. II. Ibotenic acid analogues as specific agonists at central glutamate receptors. *Natural Prod Drug Dev: Alfred Benzen Symp* 1984;20:525–545.
28. Lipartiti M, Fadda E, Savoini G, Siliprandi R, et al. In rats, the metabotropic glutamate receptor-triggered hippocampal neuronal damage is strain-dependent. *Life Sci* 1993;52:PL85–PL90.
29. Lodge D, Schoepp D. Excitatory amino acids. *Trends in Pharmacological Science Receptor Nomenclature Supplement* 1993; 4th ed: insert.
30. Martin LJ, Blackstone CD, Huganir RL, Price DL. Cellular localiza-

tion of a metabotropic glutamate receptor in rat brain. *Neuron* 1992;9:259–270.

31. Mayer ML, Benveniste M, Patneau DK, Vyklicky LJ. Pharmacologic properties of NMDA receptors. *Ann NY Acad Sci* 1992;648:194–204.

32. McDonald JW, Fix AS, Tizzano JP, Schoepp DD. Seizures and brain injury in neonatal rats induced by 1*S*,3*R*-ACPD, a metabotropic glutamate receptor agonist. *J Neurosci* 1993;13:4445–4455.

33. McGuinness N, Anwyl R, Rowan M. The effects of *trans*-ACPD on long-term potentiation in the rat hippocampal slice. *NeuroReport* 1991;2:688–690.

34. Monaghan DT, Bridges RJ, Cotman CW. The excitatory amino acid receptors: their classes, pharmacology, and distinct properties in the function of the central nervous system. *Annu Rev Pharmacol Toxicol* 1989;29:365–402.

35. Monaghan DT, Olverman HJ, Nguyen L, Watkins JC, Cotman CW. Two classes of *N*-methyl-D-aspartate recognition sites: differential distribution and differential regulation by glycine. *Proc Natl Acad Sci USA* 1988;85:9836–9840.

36. Moriyoshi K, Masu M, Ishii T, Shigemoto R, Mizuno N, Nakanishi S. Molecular cloning and characterization of the rat NMDA receptor. *Nature* 1991;354:31–37.

37. Nakajima Y, Iwakabe H, Akazawa C, Nawa H, et al. Molecular characterization of a novel retinal metabotropic glutamate receptor mGluR6 with a high agonist selectivity for L-2-amino-4-phosphonobutyrate. *J Biol Chem* 1993;268:11868–11873.

38. Nakanishi S. Molecular diversity of glutamate receptors and implications for brain functions. *Science* 1992;258:597–603.

39. Nicoletti F, Iadarola MJ, Wroblewski JT, Costa E. Excitatory amino acid recognition sites coupled with inositol phospholipid metabolism: developmental changes and interaction with α_1-adrenoreceptors. *Proc Natl Acad Sci USA* 1986;83:1931–1935.

40. Ohishi H, Shigemoto R, Nakanishi S, Mizuno N. Distribution of the messenger RNA for a metabotropic glutamate receptor, mGluR2, in the central nervous system of the rat. *Neuroscience* 1993;53:1009–1018.

41. Opitz T, Reymann KG. (1*S*,3*R*)-ACPD protects synaptic transmission from hypoxia in hippocampal slices. *Neuropharmacology* 1993;32:103–104.

42. Ortwine DF, Malone TC, Bigge CF, Drummond JT, et al. Generation of *N*-methyl-D-aspartate agonist and competitive antagonist pharmacophore models. Design and synthesis of phosphonoalkyl-substituted tetrahydroisoquinolines as novel antagonists. *J Med Chem* 1992;35:1345–1370.

43. Palmer AM, Proctor AW, Stratman GC, Bowen DM. Excitatory amino acid-releasing and cholinergic neurones in Alzheimer's disease. *Neurosci Lett* 1986;60:199–204.

44. Palmer E, Monaghan DT, Cotman CW. Trans-ACPD, a selective agonist of the phosphoinositide-coupled excitatory amino acid receptor. *Eur J Pharmacol* 1989;166:585–587.

45. Pellegrini-Giampietro DE, Zukin RS, Bennett MV, Cho S, Pulsinelli WA. Switch in glutamate receptor subunit gene expression in CA1 subfield of hippocampus following global ischemia in rats. *Proc Natl Acad Sci USA* 1992;89:10499–10503.

46. Pin J-P, Waeber C, Prezeau L, Bockaert J, Heineman SF. Alternative splicing generates metabotropic glutamate receptors inducing different patterns of calcium release in *Xenopus* oocytes. *Proc Natl Acad Sci USA* 1992;89:10331–10335.

47. Pines G, Danbolt NC, Bjoras M, Bendahan A, et al. Cloning and expression of a rat brain L-glutamate transporter. *Nature* 1992;360:464–467.

48. Pizzi M, Fallacara C, Arrighi V, Memo M, Spano PF. Attenuation of excitatory amino acid toxicity by metabotropic glutamate receptor agonists and aniracetam in primary cultures of cerebellar granule cells. *J Neurochem* 1993;61:683–689.

49. Robinson MB, Sinor JD, Dowd LA, Kerwin JF. Subtypes of sodium-dependent high-affinity L-[³H]glutamate transport activity: pharmacologic specificity and regulation by sodium and potassium. *J Neurochem* 1993;60:167–179.

50. Rogawski MA. Therapeutic potential of excitatory amino acid antagonists: channel blockers and 2,3-benzodiazepines. *Trends Pharmacol Sci* 1993;14:325–331.

51. Rosenberg PA, Amin S, Leitner M. Glutamate uptake disguises neurotoxic potency of glutamate agonists in cerebral cortex in dissociated cell culture. *J Neurosci* 1992;12:56–61.

52. Rothstein JD, Martin LJ, Kuncl RW. Decreased glutamate transport by the rat brain and spinal cord in amyotrophic lateral sclerosis. *N Engl J Med* 1992;326:1464–1468.

53. Sacaan AI, Schoepp DD. Activation of hippocampal metabotropic excitatory amino acid receptors leads to seizures and neuronal damage. *Neurosci Lett* 1992;139:77–82.

54. Schoepp DD, Conn PJ. Metabotropic glutamate receptors in brain function and pathology. *Trends Pharmacol Sci* 1993;14:13–20.

55. Schousboe A, Larsson P, Krogsgaard-Larsen P, Drejer J, Hertz L. Uptake and release processes for neurotransmitter amino acids in astrocytes. In: Norenberg MD, Hertz L, Schousboe A, eds. *The Biochemical Pathology of Astrocytes*. New York: Alan R Liss, 1988;381–394.

56. Seeburg PH. The molecular biology of mammalian glutamate receptor channels. *Trends Pharmacol Sci* 1993;14:297–303.

57. Shank RP, Aprison MH. Present status and significance of the glutamine cycle in CNS tissue. *Life Sci* 1981;28:837–842.

58. Shigemoto R, Nakanishi S, Mizuno N. Distribution of the mRNA for a metabotropic glutamate receptor (mGluR1) in the central nervous system: an in situ hybridization study in adult and developing rat. *J Comp Neurol* 1992;322:121–135.

59. Shinozaki H, Ishida M. Excitatory amino acids: physiological and pharmacological probes for neuroscience research. *Acta Neurobiol Exp (Warsz)* 1993;53:43–51.

60. Shinozaki H, Ishida M, Shimamoto K, Ohfune Y. Potent NMDA-like actions and potentiation of glutamate responses by conformational variants of glutamate analogue in rat spinal cord. *Br J Pharmacol* 1989;98:1213–1224.

61. Siliprandi R, Lipartiti M, Fadda E, Sautter J, Manev H. Activation of the glutamate metabotropic receptor protects retina against *N*-methyl-D-aspartate toxicity. *Eur J Pharmacol* 1992;219:173–174.

62. Sommer B, Keinanen K, Verdoorn TA, Wisdem W, et al. Flip and flop: a cell-specific functional switch in glutamate-operated channels of the CNS. *Science* 1990;249:1580–1585.

63. Staubli U, Rogers G, Lynch G. Facilitation of glutamate receptors enhances memory. *Proc Natl Acad Sci USA* 1994;91:777–781.

64. Stewart GR, Zorumski CF, Price MT, Olney JT. Domoic acid: a dementia-inducing excitotoxic food poison with kainic acid receptor specificity. *Exp Neurol* 1990;110:127–138.

65. Storck T, Schulte S, Hofmann K, Stoffel W. Structure, expression, and functional analysis of a Na⁺-dependent glutamate/aspartate transporter from rat brain. *Proc Natl Acad Sci USA* 1992;89:10955–10959.

66. Tanabe Y, Masu M, Ishii T, Shigemoto R, Nakanishi S. A family of metabotropic glutamate receptors. *Neuron* 1992;8:169–179.

67. Tanabe Y, Nomura A, Masu M, Shigemoto R, Mizuno N, Nakanishi S. Signal transduction, pharmacological properties, and expression patterns of two rat metabotropic receptors, mGluR3 and mGluR4. *J Neurosci* 1993;13:1372–1378.

68. Tang C-M, Shi Q-Y, Katchman A, Lynch G. Modulation of the time course of fast EPSCs and glutamate channel kinetics by aniracetam. *Science* 1991;254:288–290.

69. Thomsen C, Kristensen P, Mulvihill E, Haldeman B, Suzdak PD. L-2-Amino-4-phosphonobutyrate (L-AP4) is an agonist at the IV metabotropic glutamate receptor which is negatively coupled to adenylate cyclase. *Eur J Pharmacol Mol Pharmacol Section* 1992;227:362–362.

70. Thomson AM. A magnesium-sensitive post-synaptic potential in rat cerebral cortex resembles neuronal responses to *N*-methylaspartate. *J Physiol* 1986;370:531–549.

71. Uhl GR. Neurotransmitter transporters: a promising new gene family. *Trends Neurosci* 1992;15:265–268.

72. Yamada KA, Tang C. Benzothiadiazides inhibit rapid glutamate receptor desensitization and enhance glutamatergic synaptic currents. *J Neurosci* 1993;13:3904–3915.

*Psychopharmacology: The Fourth
Generation of Progress,* edited by
Floyd E. Bloom and David J. Kupfer.
Raven Press, Ltd., New York © 1995.

CHAPTER 8

GABA and Glycine[1]

Steven M. Paul

Amino acids are among the most abundant of all neurotransmitters present within the central nervous system (CNS). Studies which have characterized the high-affinity uptake of amino acids, in either brain slices or subcellular fractions, support current dogma that the majority of neurons in the mammalian brain utilize either glutamate or γ-aminobutyric acid (GABA) as their primary neurotransmitters. In effect, GABA and glutamate serve to regulate the excitability of virtually all neurons in brain and, not surprisingly, therefore have been implicated as important mediators of many critical physiological as well as pathophysiological events that underlie brain function and/or dysfunction. Pharmacological studies utilizing drugs which selectively block or augment the actions of GABA or glutamate support the notion that these two neurotransmitters, by virtue of their often opposing excitatory and inhibitory actions, control, to a large degree, the overall excitability of the CNS. Thus, drugs which enhance inhibitory synaptic events mediated by GABA often decrease opposing excitatory events mediated by glutamate and vice versa (see Chapters 7, 101, 132, 134, and 152 *this volume*). The behavioral consequences of such pharmacologically induced changes in the "balance" between inhibition and excitation are often profound (e.g., following administration of convulsant or anesthetic drugs which are known to alter GABAergic or glutamatergic neurotransmission).

GABA and glycine are arguably the most important inhibitory neurotransmitters in the brain and brainstem/spinal cord, respectively. These inhibitory amino acids are of particular interest to the neuropsychopharmacologist, because many commonly studied (and therapeutically useful) drugs work by selectively affecting these two neurotransmitter systems. What follows is a review of these two inhibitory amino acid neurotransmitters, with an em-

phasis on the important role they play in mediating the actions of a variety of neuropsychopharmacologic agents.

GABA: AN ABUNDANT AND UBIQUITOUS INHIBITORY NEUROTRANSMITTER

In 1950, GABA was independently identified and reported to be present in the vertebrate brain by Roberts and Frankel (40) and by Awapara et al. (2). These investigators also demonstrated the presence of glutamic acid decarboxylase (GAD) in mouse brain and showed that active enzyme, capable of decarboxylating glutamate to GABA, required pyridoxal 5'-phosphate (PLP) as cofactor (18). Early electrophysiological work carried out primarily in crustaceans firmly established GABA as an inhibitory neurotransmitter in invertebrates (34). Although GABA was originally shown to be present in very high (up to millimolar) concentrations in the vertebrate CNS, it proved considerably more difficult to unequivocally establish its role as a neurotransmitter in the mammalian brain. By the early 1970s, however, GABA had been shown to satisfy all of the classical criteria of a neurotransmitter (25,39).

Part of the difficulty in establishing GABA's role as a neurotransmitter stemmed from the very widespread distribution of GABAergic neurons throughout the CNS (in contrast to more discretely localized and less abundant neurotransmitters such as the biogenic amines) and the lack of suitable reagents to positively identify GABAergic neurons. Following the purification of GAD and the generation of GAD antisera, immunohistochemical studies revealed that many (if not most) GABAergic neurons in brain are interneurons and are therefore uniquely able to alter the excitability of local circuits within a given brain region (39). From these (and other) studies it has been

S. M. Paul: CNS Discovery Research, Lilly Research Laboratories, Eli Lilly and Company, Indianapolis IN 46285.

[1] Dedicated to the memory of Daniel X. Freedman—friend, colleague, and mentor.

estimated that 30–40% of all CNS neurons utilize GABA as their primary neurotransmitter!

GABA: SYNTHESIS, UPTAKE, AND METABOLISM

GABA is formed in vivo via a metabolic pathway called the *GABA shunt*. The initial step in this pathway utilizes α-ketoglutarate formed from glucose metabolism via the Krebs cycle. α-Ketoglutarate is then transaminated by α-oxoglutarate transaminase (GABA-T) to form glutamate, the immediate precursor of GABA. Finally, glutamate is decarboxylated to form GABA by the enzyme(s) glutamic acid decarboxylase (GAD) (18,39). GAD is expressed only in GABAergic neurons and in certain peripheral tissues which are also known to synthesize GABA (see below). Like most neurotransmitters, GABA is stored in synaptic vesicles and is released in a Ca^{2+}-dependent manner upon depolarization of the presynaptic membrane. Following release into synaptic cleft, GABA's actions are terminated principally by reuptake into presynaptic terminals and/or surrounding glia. GABA is also metabolized by GABA-T to form succinic semialdehyde. This transamination will regenerate glutamate when it occurs in the presence of α-ketoglutarate. Succinic semialdehyde is oxidized by succinic semialdehyde dehydrogenase (SSADH) to succinic acid which then reenters the Krebs cycle.

The reuptake of GABA occurs via highly specific transmembrane transporters which have recently been shown to be members of a large family of Na^+-dependent neurotransmitter transporters. GABA uptake is temperature- and ion-dependent (both Na^+ and Cl^- ions are required for optimal uptake). Affinity purification of the GABA transporter protein has recently led to its molecular cloning (20). The principal neuronal GABA transporter appears to be a 70- to 80-kDa glycoprotein which, based on its deduced amino acid sequence, is predicted to contain 12 hydrophobic membrane-spanning domains. To date, at least two other GABA transporter cDNAs have been cloned (9). However, the physiological and pharmacological significance of this heterogeneity is unknown. Nonetheless, specific inhibitors of GABA uptake which directly bind to the transporter itself have been synthesized, and several have been shown to have anticonvulsant and/or antinociceptive properties in laboratory animals.

GLUTAMIC ACID DECARBOXYLASE: TWO FORMS ENCODED BY SEPARATE GENES

Unlike the other enzymes involved in GABA synthesis, GAD is expressed only in neurons and certain peripheral tissues which make or utilize GABA for signaling and/or endocrine functions (18). Early work strongly suggested the existence of at least two GAD enzymes which differed in their interaction(s) with PLP as well as in their subcellular distributions (18). Native GAD appears to exist as a dimer—probably a homodimer of two subunits of approximately 60 kDa each. GAD activity is quite high in brain, and it is now clear that approximately 50% of the enzyme(s) exists as apo-GAD (not bound to PLP) whereas the rest is bound to PLP (holo-GAD). Interestingly, there is also evidence that increased neuronal activity (e.g., that induced by depolarizing conditions) results in an increase in local GABA synthesis by promoting the association of PLP with apo-GAD to form active enzyme (18). Although the presence of two GAD isoforms was strongly supported by both biochemical and immunochemical data, their similarities and differences were not fully appreciated until both forms were cloned in an elegant series of studies by Tobin and colleagues (17,18).

GAD is also expressed outside the CNS. For example, both GAD isozymes are present in β cells of the pancreatic islets where GABA is suspected to play a role in pancreatic endocrine function. (Immunohistochemical and lesion studies with β-cell toxins such as streptozotocin have shown that GAD and insulin coexist in the β cell.) In this regard, Baekkeskov et al. (3) have shown that antibodies to the 64-kDa form of GAD (which appears to be related to GAD_{65}) occur in most, if not all, patients with insulin-dependent diabetes, and their presence appears to precede the clinical onset of disease. Autoantibodies to GAD may therefore underlie the development of insulin-dependent (type I) diabetes as well as that of the relatively rare neurological disorder known as *stiff-man syndrome*.

GABA_A RECEPTORS: PHYSIOLOGY TO PHARMACOLOGY

Receptors for both inhibitory and excitatory amino acid neurotransmitters are either ionotropic (i.e., their activation results in enhanced membrane ion conductance) or metabotropic (i.e., their activation results in increased intracellular levels of second messenger) in nature. GABA_A receptors are ionotropic receptors leading to increased Cl^- ion conductance, whereas GABA_B receptors are metabotropic receptors which are coupled to G proteins and thereby *indirectly* alter membrane ion permeability and neuronal excitability (see below). Electrophysiological studies using voltage-clamp and single-channel recording techniques have yielded a rather detailed description and understanding of the operation of the GABA_A receptor-gated Cl^- ion channel (10,28). Activation of the GABA_A receptor by agonist results in an increase in Cl^- ion conductance via the receptor-gated ion channel or pore. This increase in Cl^- ion conductance, which requires the binding and cooperative interaction of two molecules of GABA, is actually due to an increase in the mean open

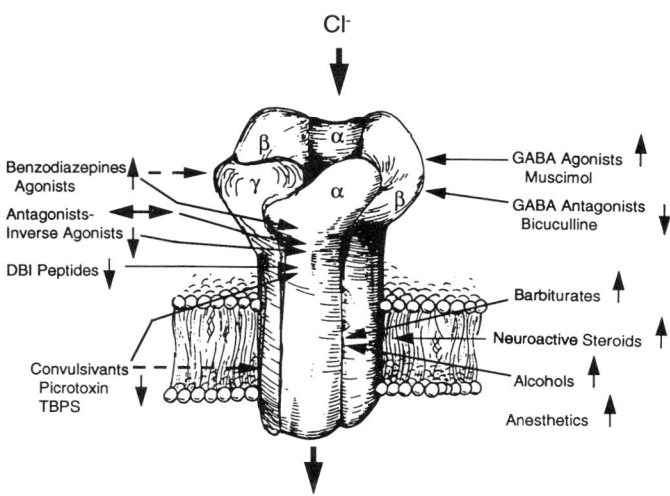

Fig. 1. Hypothetical pentameric structure of a GABA$_A$ receptor containing two α and β subunits and a single γ subunit to form an intrinsic Cl⁻ ion channel. Also shown are many of the drugs and putative ligands known to interact at one or more sites associated with GABA$_A$ receptors to either positively (↑) or negatively (↓) modulate GABA-gated Cl⁻ ion conductance. Although many of these compounds have been shown to augment GABA-mediated Cl⁻ ion conductance rather selectively (e.g., benzodiazepines picrotoxin/cage convulsants) several (e.g., barbiturates, alcohols, and anesthetics) have been shown to bind to and affect other receptors and channels as well.

time of the Cl⁻ ion channel itself (28). (GABA activates the GABA$_A$ receptor at low micromolar concentrations, suggesting that it must be highly compartmentalized within nervous tissue.) The increase in Cl⁻ ion conductance observed following activation of GABA$_A$ receptors results in a localized hyperpolarization of the neuronal membrane and therefore leads to an increase in the "threshold" required for excitatory neurotransmitters to depolarize the membrane in order to generate an action potential. This decrease in neuronal membrane "excitability" results in the inhibitory actions of GABA.

GABA$_A$ Receptor Agonists and Antagonists

GABA$_A$ receptors, like most receptors, can be defined by the drugs (and other ligands) which selectively bind to, and either stimulate or block, receptor activity (Fig. 1). A variety of GABA receptor agonists have been discovered and have been shown to selectively activate GABA$_A$ receptors. Muscimol, a rigid GABA analogue isolated from the hallucinogenic mushroom *Amanita muscaria*, is one of the most selective and potent GABA agonists known. Muscimol is also not a substrate for the GABA transporter, which makes it useful for electrophysiological and biochemical studies. Both competitive and noncompetitive GABA$_A$ receptor antagonists have also

been described (16). Bicuculline is the prototypical competitive antagonist and directly competes with GABA for binding to the receptor complex. Bicuculline reduces both the frequency and mean open time of the GABA-gated Cl⁻ ion channel. Picrotoxin and other extremely potent cage convulsants such as *t*-butylbicyclophosphorothionate (TBPS) are noncompetitive GABA receptor antagonists which do not compete directly with GABA for its recognition site(s) but, instead, bind to a separate and distinct recognition site(s) associated with the receptor complex (44). Not surprisingly, both classes of GABA$_A$ receptor antagonists produce seizures when administered to laboratory animals. The affinity of cage convulsants such as TBPS for GABA$_A$ receptors is so high that they have proven to be useful radioligands for measuring GABA$_A$ receptors in vitro and for their subsequent biochemical and pharmacological characterization (44). These studies have revealed that GABA$_A$ receptors have multiple allosteric binding sites for drugs which, when occupied, modulate (positively or negatively) the inhibitory actions of GABA.

Benzodiazepines and Barbiturates Act at GABA$_A$ Receptors

The observation that sedative–hypnotic drugs, which are classified behaviorally as CNS depressants, can augment the inhibitory properties of GABA was first established in 1975 for both benzodiazepines and barbiturates using electrophysiological techniques (23,32). Benzodiazepines were discovered and developed in large measure to circumvent the potential lethal effects of barbiturates. It is most curious that benzodiazepines and barbiturates, which are structurally dissimilar and which were discovered with no knowledge of their underlying mechanisms of action, actually share the same molecular target(s).

In 1977, specific high-affinity receptors for benzodiazepines were discovered in the brains of many species, including man (30,43). The excellent correlations between receptor affinity measured in vitro and the in vivo pharmacological potencies of a series of benzodiazepines strongly indicated that these receptors mediate most, if not all, of the pharmacological actions of benzodiazepines (30,43). In the ensuing 17 years, the pharmacological significance of these receptors has been amply confirmed by many laboratories. It is now clear that *all* of the major centrally mediated actions of benzodiazepines—that is, their anxiolytic, anticonvulsant, muscle-relaxant, and sedative–anesthetic properties—are mediated by benzodiazepine receptors. Moreover, it has also been shown that the benzodiazepine receptor first demonstrated in 1977 is really a subtype of GABA$_A$ receptor (see below) (48,49).

While both benzodiazepines and barbiturates bind to GABA$_A$ receptors to augment GABA-mediated responses, they do so in different ways. Barbiturates have dual actions to enhance GABA_A receptor-mediated Cl⁻ ion conductance (42,45). At low (subanesthetic) concentrations, barbiturates augment the affinity of the GABA_A receptor for GABA and increase the mean channel opening time induced by GABA. At higher (anesthetic) concentrations, barbiturates directly increase channel openings, even in the absence of GABA. Benzodiazepines, on the other hand, have no direct effects on channel opening but only increase the affinity of the receptor for GABA as well as the frequency of GABA-activated channel openings (28,45). This is an important distinction because it means that benzodiazepines will markedly augment GABA's actions at low intrasynaptic GABA concentrations, but will have little to no effect at saturating concentrations of GABA (i.e., benzodiazepines "shift" the concentration–response curve for GABA slightly to the left) (54). These differences undoubtedly contribute to the relatively low toxicity of benzodiazepines compared to barbiturates.

There is now considerable evidence that a number of other sedative-hypnotic-anesthetic drugs also interact with GABA_A receptors and at pharmacologically-relevant concentrations. Parenthetically, these studies (cited below) were among the first to suggest that the behavioral effects of alcohols and anesthetics were due, at least in part, to their "specific" actions at critical membrane protein targets, notably ligand-gated ion channels. (It had been widely assumed for over 100 years that the behavioral effects of alcohols and anesthetics were due to their "nonspecific" effects on membrane lipids.)

Ethanol, one of the most commonly used (and abused) sedative-hypnotic agents, has been shown by several investigatiors to augment GABA-activated Cl⁻ ion conductance in a variety of intact and isolated neuronal membrane preparations (46). To date, however, electro-physiological studies of ethanol's actions in augmenting GABA-activated Cl⁻ ion conductance have yielded somewhat mixed results (see ref. 31 for review). More recent studies have generally confirmed that pharmacologically-relevant concentrations of ethanol (10–100 mM) weakly (but significantly) augment GABA-activated Cl⁻ ion conductance (31) as do longer chain-length alcohols and general anesthetics (31,51). Moreover, several imidazobenzodiazepine inverse agonists of the benzodiazepine receptor (see below) have been reported to "antagonize" the sedative/ataxic effects of ethanol (47)—further implicating the GABA_A receptor as one of the key central sites mediating at least some of ethanol's neuropharmacological effects. The effects of ethanol on GABA_A receptors, coupled with its more recently described actions in inhibiting glutamate (NMDA) receptor-mediated depolarizing events (51), likely contribute to the anxiolytic and sedative effects of alcohols.

Agonists, Antagonists, and Inverse Agonists

Since the discovery of the benzodiazepine receptor (recognition site), a large number of benzodiazepine and nonbenzodiazepine drugs have been found to interact with these receptors—and in unexpected ways. In addition to those receptor ligands which augment GABA responses (now called *agonists*), two other broad classes of ligands have now been characterized. Selective antagonists such as the imidazobenzodiazepine Ro15-1788 (flumazenil) bind with high affinity to GABA_A receptors but are devoid of intrinsic activity of their own (22). However, these antagonists completely block the actions of benzodiazepine receptor agonists in augmenting GABA-mediated responses. Selective antagonists like flumazenil also block (or reverse) the actions of *inverse agonists*. The latter are benzodiazepine receptor ligands which *decrease* GABA-activated Cl⁻ ion conductance (by decreasing the frequency of channel openings). The GABA_A receptor can thus be *positively* or *negatively* modulated by compounds which range in activity from full agonists to full inverse agonists (22). Along this continuum lie compounds with different degrees of intrinsic efficacy—that is, compounds with only partial agonist or inverse agonist actions. Behaviorally, full agonists have sedative–anesthetic properties, whereas full inverse agonists are convulsants (14). Partial benzodiazepine receptor agonists (now in development by several pharmaceutical companies) may prove to be effective anxiolytics, devoid of the sedative effects generally observed with full agonists (22). The fact that benzodiazepine receptor agonists reduce anxiety and that inverse agonists are profoundly anxiogenic, coupled with recent observations that the "sensitivity" of animals to inverse agonists can be altered (in some cases increased) by pharmacological or environmental factors, has prompted considerable speculation that GABA_A receptors are involved in at least some forms of human anxiety (see refs. 24 and 54 for reviews).

The large number of drug recognition sites associated with GABA_A receptors (which are clearly distinct from those which recognize GABA itself) have led several investigators to propose the existence of endogenous receptor ligands. Several such "candidate" ligands have been identified; however, with the possible exception of two, there is little compelling evidence at present that any interact with GABA_A receptors in vivo. One of these ligands is an endogenous peptide called *diazepam-binding inhibitor* (DBI), which was initially isolated by Guidotti et al. (21) and was shown to interact with GABA_A receptors and to have anxiogenic properties (similar to inverse agonists). The other postulated endogenous ligand(s) include two natural reduced steroid metabolites of progesterone and deoxycorticosterone (allopregnanalone and allotetrahydro-DOC) (29). These neuroactive steroids bind with high affinity to GABA_A receptors and have "barbiturate-like" actions in augmenting GABA-mediated responses (for review see ref. 35). The plasma and brain levels of these neuroactive steroids increase dramatically following exposure of rats to various stressors. Plasma allopregnanolone levels are also quite high during the third trimester of pregnancy, and they decrease dramatically following parturition (35). None of these putative natural ligands, however, have yet been unequivocally demonstrated to subserve any physiological function.

GABA$_A$ RECEPTORS: MOLECULAR HETEROGENEITY UNDERLIES DIVERSITY OF FUNCTION

In 1987, Barnard, Seeburg, and colleagues (4,41), using partial amino acid sequences from purified bovine brain GABA$_A$ receptors succeeded in cloning several of the subunits which comprise the GABA$_A$ receptor(s). The deduced amino acid sequences of the α- and β-subunit cDNAs isolated by these investigators indicated that each subunit was approximately 50–60 kDa in size and had four α-helical hydrophobic membrane-spanning sequences of approximately 20–30 amino acids. The predicted structure of the receptor was based on strong evidence that the GABA$_A$ receptor is a member of a large superfamily of ligand-gated ion channels which includes the nicotinic-cholinergic, ionotropic glutamate, and glycine receptors (there is approximately 10–20% sequence identity between members of this superfamily) (4,33).

Currently, it is believed that, like the nicotinic-cholinergic receptor, the GABA$_A$ receptor is a heteropentameric glycoprotein of approximately 275 kDa (33) (Fig. 1). To date, five distinct classes of polypeptide subunits (α, β, γ, δ, and ρ) have been cloned and multiple isoforms of each have been shown to exist (e.g., there have been six α-subunit cDNAs isolated so far!) (15). There is approximately 70% sequence identity between the polypeptide subunits within a given class, but only approximately 30% between classes.

Although the exact subunit composition of most GABA$_A$ receptor(s) is unknown, it appears that their composition varies from brain region to region—and even between neurons within a given region. In situ hybridization studies (now complemented by immunocytochemical studies) have revealed, for example, that some α subunits (e.g., α_1) are widely expressed throughout the brain whereas others are only expressed in discrete populations of neurons. Remarkably, a recently cloned α-subunit isoform (α_6), which also confers unique pharmacology to recombinantly expressed GABA$_A$ receptors, is *only* expressed in a single neuron subtype—the cerebellar granule neuron (26).

What is the pharmacological and physiological significance of the surprising heterogeneity of GABA$_A$ receptor subunit isoforms expressed in brain? A few examples serve to illustrate the critical importance of subunit composition with respect to the pharmacological actions of drugs which, as previously discussed, work by interacting with GABA$_A$ receptors. Following the initial report describing the cloning and expression of α and β subunits, it was soon realized that coexpression of these subunits

in various combinations reproduced many, but not all, of the properties of native GABA$_A$ receptors. The notable exception was the lack of a reproducible response to benzodiazepines when only α and/or β subunits were expressed. It is now clear that coexpression of an additional subunit, called γ, is necessary to observe the potentiation of GABA responses by benzodiazepines that is characteristic of most native receptors (38). Moreover, coexpression of individual γ-subunit variants (γ_1, γ_2, γ_3), which have now been identified (with α and β subunits), results in varying degrees of modulation by benzodiazepine receptor ligands (agonists, antagonists, inverse agonists). Photaffinity labelling studies suggest that the GABA binding site itself resides on the β subunit, while the benzodiazepine binding site resides on the α subunit (Fig 1) (33). Although these experiments have clearly delineated an important role for individual subunits (such as α and γ) in determining the ligand-gating and pharmacological properties of GABA$_A$ receptors, it is still not entirely clear where each of the ligand binding sites resides on native GABA$_A$ receptors.

Although expression of the γ subunit is essential for conferring the modulatory actions of benzodiazepines on recombinant GABA$_A$ receptors, it appears that α-subunit heterogeneity determines the diversity of physiological and pharmacological responses characteristic of native GABA$_A$ receptors (36,37). When coexpressed with β_1 subunits, for example, the α_1 subunit yields a receptor with a relatively high affinity for GABA. (Recall that the α_1 subunit is the most widely and abundantly expressed α subunit in brain.) By contrast, coexpression of the α_2 or α_3 subunits (with the β_1 subunit) results in GABA$_A$ receptors with far lower affinities for GABA. Thus, the subunit composition of a given receptor may determine the local "response" to synaptically released GABA (27). There are also multiple forms of the β subunit expressed in brain (15,27). Although their exact role in GABA$_A$ receptor function has yet to be determined, each contains a consensus sequence for phosphorylation by protein kinase A. There is some evidence that phosphorylation of the β subunit may result in receptor desensitization seen with continuous exposure to GABA.

Subunit heterogeneity seems also to be relevant to the pharmacological differences observed between drugs, such as the benzodiazepines, which interact with GABA$_A$ receptors. Receptors which are composed of α_3 subunits (together with β_1 and α_2 subunits) yield much greater responses to benzodiazepines than do receptors which contain α_1 or α_2 subunits (27). Early work by Lippa and colleagues delineated pharmacologically distinct subtypes of GABA$_A$ receptors (type I versus type II) based on their affinity for CL 218,872 and their regional distribution in brain (see refs. 36 and 54 for discussion of those subtypes). Type I receptors had high affinity for CL 218,872 and were predominantly expressed in cerebellum, whereas type II had relatively low affinity for CL 218,872 and were enriched in the hippocampus. A combination of α_1, β_1, and γ_2 subunits results in type I receptors with high affinity for CL 218,872 (type I receptors are enriched in the cerebellum where α_1 subunit mRNA is highly expressed) (36). Type I receptors seem to have a high affinity for sedative–hypnotic benzodiazepines as well as for the nonbenzodiazepine hypnotic zolpidem. Type II receptor pharmacology can be reproduced with receptors containing α_2 or α_3 subunits, and the transcripts for these subunits are expressed in the hippocampus (36). In retrospect, it is not surprising, given the structural simplicity of GABA, that the complexity and diversity of its many functions would require the evolution of a large and heterogeneous number of GABA receptors now known to be expressed in both neurons and glia throughout the brain.

GABA_B RECEPTORS

While attempting to identify functional GABA receptors on peripheral nerve terminals, Bowery and Hudson (13) (see ref. 12 for review) described a bicuculline-insensitive action of GABA in reducing the release of [^{3}H]norepinephrine. Subsequently, these investigators extended their findings to the CNS, where it became clear that GABA could also potently inhibit the depolarization-induced release of [^{3}H]norepinephrine from brain slices. Early on, it also became apparent that many GABA_A receptor (bicuculline-sensitive) agonists were unable to mimic the actions of GABA in inhibiting neurotransmitter release—leading to the proposal to divide GABA receptors into two subtypes, GABA_A and GABA_B. Moreover, one compound, β-p-chlorophenyl-GABA (baclofen), which was designed to be a centrally active GABA analogue (and which is still marketed as an antispastic agent), was found to be inactive at GABA_A receptors but quite active at GABA_B receptors (12). Therefore, baclofen proved to be the first selective GABA_B receptor agonist and is still used extensively for characterizing GABA_B receptors. Phaclofen, the phosphonic derivative of baclofen, is a selective, albeit weak, GABA_B receptor antagonist. Several newer, more potent GABA_B antagonists have been discovered; however, the published data on these compounds are rather limited (12). Nonetheless, administration of GABA_B antagonists to laboratory animals does not result in the profound behavioral sequelae observed following administration of GABA_A receptor antagonists (e.g., seizures). This suggests that GABA_A receptors are tonically (and continuously) activated, whereas GABA_B receptors may only be activated under certain physiological conditions.

Activation of GABA_B receptors in many brain regions results in an increase in K^+ channel conductance with a resultant hyperpolarization of the neuronal membrane (10,12). This increase in K^+ conductance is often blocked by pretreatment with pertussis toxin, indicating that many postsynaptic GABA_B receptors are indirectly coupled to K^+ channels through an intervening G protein (1). There is considerable evidence that a large proportion of GABA_B receptors are coupled to G proteins, but there is also evidence that some presynaptic GABA_B receptors may be directly linked to K^+ channels. The fact that GABA_B receptors are coupled to G proteins may also explain, in part, the reported effects of GABA_B receptor agonists on Ca^{2+} conductance and secondarily neurotransmitter release (12). Very little data is available on the structure of the GABA_B receptor. To date, attempts to clone the GABA_B receptor by microsequencing a portion of the purified protein or by expression cloning in oocytes have proven to be unsuccessful.

GLYCINE: SYNTHESIS AND UPTAKE

Glycine is the major inhibitory neurotransmitter in the brainstem and spinal cord, where it participates in a variety of motor and sensory functions. Glycine is also present in the forebrain, where it has recently been shown to function as a coagonist at the N-methyl-D-aspartate (NMDA) subtype of glutamate receptor. In the latter, context glycine promotes the actions of glutamate, the major excitatory neurotransmitter (for a discussion of glycine's role as a coagonist of the NMDA receptor, see Chapter 7, *this volume*). Thus, glycine subserves both inhibitory and excitatory functions within the CNS.

Glycine is formed from serine by the enzyme serine hydroxymethyltransferase (SHMT). Glycine, like GABA, is released from nerve endings in a Ca^{2+}-dependent fashion. The actions of glycine are terminated primarily by reuptake via Na^+/Cl^--dependent, high-affinity glycine transporters. The specific uptake of glycine has been demonstrated in the brainstem and spinal cord in regions where there are also high densities of inhibitory glycine receptors.

Recently, two glycine transporters have been cloned and shown to be expressed in the CNS as well as in various peripheral tissues (11,19). These glycine transporters are members of the large family of Na^+/Cl^--dependent neurotransmitter transporters, and both share approximately 50% sequence identity with the GABA transporters discussed above. The deduced amino acid sequence of both cDNAs predicts the typical 12 transmembrane domains characteristic of these transporters. The two glycine cloned transporters have been named GLYT-1 and GLYT-2 in the order that they were reported (11). These transporter cDNAs are transcribed from the same gene and are quite similar in their 3' nucleotide sequences. They differ in their 5' noncoding regions as well as in the first 44 nucleotides of their coding sequence. Expression of GLYT-1 and GLYT-2 yield transporters with similar kinetic and pharmacological properties. Interestingly, however, the distribution of GLYT-1 and

GLYT-2 transcripts measured by in situ hybridization are different. GLYT-1 mRNA also closely parallels the distribution of the glycine receptor. These data suggest that GLYT-1 is primarily a glial glycine transporter whereas GLYT-2 is primarily a neuronal transporter. The mapping of both glycine transporter mRNAs, as well as the glycine receptor subunit mRNAs, confirm the importance of this neurotransmitter in the brainstem and spinal cord, but support a more widespread distribution in supraspinal brain regions than was previously suspected.

GLYCINE RECEPTORS

Inhibitory glycine receptors are blocked by the plant alkaloid strychnine, which was also first used to label glycine receptors in spinal cord membranes (52,53). Strychnine poisoning results in muscular contractions and tetany as a result of glycinergic disinhibition and overexcitation. Electrophysiological studies primarily carried out in rodent spinal cord neurons have demonstrated that glycine activates Cl^- ion conductance (8). Like GABA, this increase in Cl^- ion conductance results in a hyperpolarization of the neuronal membrane and an antagonism of other depolarizing stimuli. Other α- and β-amino acids, including β-alanine and taurine, also activate glycine receptors, but with lower potency (6,8).

The glycine receptor was first successfully solubilized and purified by Betz and colleagues using affinity purification over an affinity matrix derivatized with aminostrychnine (8). The affinity-purified glycine receptor was shown to consist of two polypeptide subunits of approximately 48 kD (α) and 58 kD (β), respectively. Reconstitution of these polypeptide subunits into lipid vesicles resulted in functional receptors, and intramolecular cross-linking experiments suggested that the native glycine receptor is a pentameric structure. Photoaffinity labeling of the glycine receptor with [^{3}H]strychnine revealed that both the strychnine and glycine binding sites are located on the 48-kD α subunit. Purification of the α- and β-receptor subunits was followed closely by their molecular cloning (7).

The deduced amino acid sequences of the α- and β-glycine-receptor subunits predict structures quite homologous to the subunits of other ligand-gated ion channels, including the $GABA_A$ receptor (7). Each subunit has four hydrophobic membrane-spanning sequences, and each shares considerable sequence identity with the other. Several glycine-receptor α-subunit variants have now been identified (α_{1-4}), and, not surprisingly, they differ in their pharmacological properties and level of expression. As mentioned, both the agonist and antagonist binding sites are located on the α subunit, but at different amino acids (50). Interestingly, glycine receptors comprised of α_1 subunits are efficiently gated by taurine and β-alanine, whereas α_2-containing receptors are not (8). The α_1 and α_2 genes are expressed in the adult and neonatal brain, respectively. Interestingly, the β-subunit transcript is expressed at relatively high levels in the cerebral cortex and cerebellum, where no α transcripts or specific [^{3}H]-strychnine binding sites have been observed. Coexpression of β subunits with α subunits (as opposed to homo-oligomeric α-subunit glycine receptors) results in glycine receptors with pharmacological properties quite similar to native glycine receptors. Nonetheless, the widespread distribution of β-subunit mRNA in brain suggests that other, perhaps strychnine-insensitive glycine receptor isoforms will be found.

Recently, the expression of α_1 and α_2 subunits has been shown to be developmentally regulated with a switch from the neonatal α_2 subunit (strychnine-insensitive) to the adult α_1 form (strychnine-sensitive) at about 2 weeks postnatally in the mouse (8). The timing of this "switch" corresponds with the development of spasticity in the mutant *spastic* mouse (5), prompting speculation that insufficient expression of the adult isoform may underlie some forms of spasticity.

CONCLUSIONS

A convergence of scientific effort—involving molecular pharmacologists, molecular biologists, and medicinal chemists—has revealed a remarkable and, for the most part, unsuspected degree of complexity and heterogeneity in the biosynthetic enzymes, transporters, and receptors for GABA and glycine. For the neuropsychopharmacologist, GABA and glycine-containing and receptive neurons are of particular significance because they are among the best-characterized of all drug targets. Many psychoactive drugs which alter (increase or decrease) CNS excitability do so by effecting GABAergic or glycinergic neurotransmission. Some of these drugs (e.g., benzodiazepine and nonbenzodiazepine anxiolytic–hypnotics) are commonly prescribed for a variety of disorders. It is likely that the wealth of new information on GABA and glycine will result in an even better understanding of their potential role(s) in various neuropsychiatric disorders and in the discovery even more of effective therapeutic agents.

REFERENCES

1. Andrade R, Malenka RC, Nicoll RA. A G-protein couples serotonin and GABA_B receptors to the same channels in hippocampus. *Science* 1986;234:1261–1265.
2. Awapara J, Landua A, Fuerst R, Seale B. Free gamma-aminobutyric acid in brain. *J Biol Chem* 1950;187:35–39.
3. Baekkeskov S, Landin M, Kristensen J, et al. Antibodies to a 64,000 M_r human islet cell antigen precede the clinical onset of insulin-dependent diabetes. *J Clin Invest* 1987;79:926–934.
4. Barnard EA, Darlison MG, Seeburg P. Molecular biology of the GABA_A receptor: the receptor channel superfamily. *Trends Neurosci* 1987;10:502–509.
5. Becker C-M. Disorders of the inhibitory glycine receptor: the *spastic* mouse. *FASEB J* 1990;4:2767–2774.

6. Betz H, Becker C-M. The mammalian glycine receptor: biology and structure of a neuronal chloride channel protein. *Neurochem Int* 1988;13:137–146.

7. Betz H. Ligand-gated ion channels in the brain: the amino acid receptor superfamily. *Neuron* 1990;5:383–392.

8. Betz H. Structure and function of inhibitory glycine receptors. *Q Rev Biophys* 1992;25:381–394.

9. Borden LA, Smith KE, Hartig PR, Branchek TA, Weinshank RL. Molecular heterogeneity of the gamma-aminobutyric acid (GABA) transport system. *J Biol Chem* 1992;267:21098–21104.

10. Bormann J. Electrophysiology of GABA$_A$ and GABA$_B$ receptor subtypes. *Trends Neurosci* 1988;11:112–116.

11. Borowsky B, Mezey E, Hoffman BJ. Two glycine transporter variants with distinct localization in the CNS and peripheral tissues are encoded by a common gene. *Neuron* 1993;10:851–863.

12. Bowery NG. GABA$_B$ receptor pharmacology. *Annu Rev Pharmacol Toxicol* 1993;33:109–117.

13. Bowery NG, Hudson AI. Gamma-aminobutyric acid reduces the evoked release of ^{3}H-noradrenaline from sympathetic nerve terminals. *Br J Pharmacol* 1979;66:108P.

14. Breier A, Paul SM. Anxiety and the benzodiazepine–GABA receptor complex. In: Roth M, Noyes R, Burrows GC, eds. *Handbook of anxiety.* Amsterdam: Elsevier, 1988;1.

15. Burt DR, Kamatchi GL. GABA$_A$ receptor subtypes: from pharmacology to molecular biology. *FASEB J* 1991;5:2916–2923.

16. Curtis DR, Duggan AW, Felix D, Johnston GAR. GABA, bicuculline and central inhibition. *Nature* 1970;226:1222–1224.

17. Erlander MG, Tillakaratne NJK, Feldblum S, Patel N, Tobin AJ. Two genes encode distinct glutamate decarboxylases. *Neuron* 1991;7:91–100.

18. Erlander MG, Tobin AJ. The structural and functional heterogeneity of glutamic acid decarboxylase: a review. *Neurochem Res* 1991;16:215–226.

19. Guastella J, Brecha N, Weigmann C, Lester H, Davidson N. Cloning, expression, and localization of a rat brain high-affinity glycine transporter. *Proc Natl Acad Sci USA* 1992;89:7189–7193.

20. Guastella J, Nelson N, Nelson H, et al. Cloning and expression of a rat brain GABA transporter. *Science* 1990;249:1303–1306.

21. Guidotti A, Forchetti C, Corda M, Kondel D, Bennett C, Costa E. Isolation, characterization and purification to homogeneity of an endogenous polypeptide with agonistic action on benzodiazepine receptors. *Proc Natl Acad Sci USA* 1983;80:3531–3535.

22. Haefely W. The GABA–benzodiazepine interaction fifteen years later. *Neurochem Res* 1990;15:169–174.

23. Haefely W, Kulcsar A, Mohler H, Pieri L, Polc P, Schaffner R. Possible involvement of GABA in the central actions of benzodiazepines. In: Costa E, Greengard P, eds. *Mechanism of action of benzodiazepines.* New York: Raven Press, 1975;131–151.

24. Hommer DW, Skolnick P, Paul SM. The benzodiazepine GABA receptor complex and anxiety. In: Meltzer HY, ed. *Psychopharmacology: the third generation of progress.* New York: Raven Press, 1987;977–983.

25. Krnjevic K. Chemical nature of synaptic transmission in vertebrates. *Physiol Rev* 1974;54:418–540.

26. Lüddens H, Pritchett DB, Köhler M, et al. Cerebellar GABA$_A$ receptor selective for a behavioral alcohol antagonist. *Nature* 1990;346:648–651.

27. Lüddens H, Wisden W. Function and pharmacology of multiple GABA$_A$ receptor subunits. *Trends Pharmacol Sci* 1991;12:49–51.

28. Macdonald RL, Twyman RE. Biophysical properties and regulation of GABA$_A$ receptor channels. *Semin Neurosci* 1991;3:219–230.

29. Majewska MD, Harrison NL, Schwartz RD, Barker JL, Paul SM. Steroid hormone metabolites are barbiturate-like modulators of the GABA receptor. *Science* 1986;232:1004–1007.

30. Möhler H, Okada T. Benzodiazepine receptor: demonstration in the central nervous system. *Science* 1977;198:849–851.

31. Narahashi T, Arakawa O, Brunner EA, et al. Modulation of GABA receptor-channel complex by alcohols and general anesthetics. In: Biggio G, Concas A, Costa E, eds. *GABAergic synaptic transmission.* New York: Raven Press, 1992;325–334.

32. Nicoll R, Eccles J, Oshima T. Prolongation of hippocampal inhibitory postsynaptic potentials by barbiturates. *Nature* 1975;258:625–627.

33. Olsen RW, Tobin AJ. Molecular biology of GABA$_A$ receptors. *FASEB J* 1990;4:1469–1480.

34. Otsuka J, Iversen LL, Hall ZW, Kravitz EA. Release of gamma-aminobutyric acid from inhibitory nerves of lobster. *Proc Natl Acad Sci USA* 1966;56:1110–1115.

35. Paul SM, Purdy RH. Neuroactive steroids. *FASEB J* 1992;6:2311–2322.

36. Pritchett DB, Lüddens H, Seeburg P. Type I and type II GABA$_A$ benzodiazepine receptors produced in transfected cells. *Science* 1989;245:1389–1392.

37. Pritchett DB, Sontheimer H, Borman CM, et al. Transient expression shows ligand gating and allosteric potentiation of GABA$_A$ receptor subunits. *Science* 1988;242:1306–1308.

38. Pritchett D, Sontheimer H, Shivers BD, et al. Importance of a novel GABA$_A$ receptor subunit for benzodiazepine pharmacology. *Nature* 1989;338:582–585.

39. Roberts E. GABA: the road to neurotransmitter status. In: Olsen RW, Venter CJ, eds. *Benzodiazepine/GABA receptors and chloride channels: structural and functional properties.* New York: Alan R Liss, 1986;1–39.

40. Roberts E, Frankel S. Gamma-aminobutyric acid in brain: its formation from glutamic acid. *J Biol Chem* 1950;187:55–63.

41. Schofield PR, Darlison MG, Fujita N, et al. Sequence and functional expression of the GABA$_A$ receptor shows a ligand gated receptor superfamily. *Nature* 1987;328:221–227.

42. Skolnick P, Moncada V, Barker J, Paul S. Pentobarbital has dual actions to increase brain benzodiazepine receptor affinity. *Science* 1981;211:1448–1450.

43. Squires RF, Braestrup C. Benzodiazepine receptors in rat brain. *Nature* 1977;266:732–734.

44. Squires RF, Casida JE, Richardson M, Saederup E. [^{35}S]*t*-Butylbicyclophosphorothionate binds with high affinity to brain specific sites coupled to γ-aminobutyric acid-A and ion recognition sites. *Mol Pharmacol* 1983;23:326–336.

45. Study RE, Barker JL. Diazepam and (−)-pentobarbital: fluctuation analysis reveals different mechanisms for potentiation of γ-aminobutyric acid responses in cultured central neurons. *Proc Natl Acad Sci USA* 1981;78:7180–7184.

46. Suzdak PD, Schwartz RD, Skolnick P, Paul SM. Ethanol stimulates γ-aminobutyric acid receptor-mediated chloride transport in rat brain synaptoneurosomes. *Proc Natl Acad Sci USA* 1986;83:4071–4075.

47. Suzdak PD, Paul SM, Crawley JN. Effects of Ro15-4513 and other benzodiazepine receptor inverse agonists on alcohol-induced intoxication in the rat. *J Pharmacol Exp Ther* 1988;245(3):880–886.

48. Tallman J, Thomas J, Gallager D. GABAergic modulation of benzodiazepine binding site sensitivity. *Nature* 1978;274:383–385.

49. Tallman JF, Paul SM, Skolnick P, et al. Receptors for the age of anxiety: pharmacology of the benzodiazepines. *Science* 1980;207:274–281.

50. Vandenberg RJ, Handford CA, Schofield PR. Distinct agonist- and antagonist-binding sites on the glycine receptor. *Neuron* 1992;491–496.

51. Weight FF, Aguayo LG, White G, et al. GABA- and glutamate-gated ion channels as molecular sites of alcohol and anesthetic action. In: Biggio G, Concas A, Costa E, eds. *GABAergic synaptic transmission.* New York: Raven Press, 1992;335–347.

52. Young AB, Snyder SH. Strychnine binding in rat spinal cord membranes associated with the synaptic glycine receptor: cooperativity of glycine interactions. *Mol Pharmacol* 1974;10:790–809.

53. Young AB, Snyder SH. The glycine synaptic receptor: evidence that strychnine binding is associated with the ionic conductance mechanism. *Proc Natl Acad Sci USA* 1974;71:4002–4005.

54. Zorumski CF, Isenberg KE. Insights into the structure and function of GABA-benzodiazepine receptors: ion channels and psychiatry. *Am J Psychiatry* 1991;148:162–173.

Psychopharmacology: The Fourth Generation of Progress, edited by Floyd E. Bloom and David J. Kupfer. Raven Press, Ltd., New York © 1995.

CHAPTER 9

Neuronal Nicotinic Acetylcholine Receptors

Novel Targets for Central Nervous System Therapeutics

Stephen P. Arneric, James P. Sullivan, and Michael Williams

Acetylcholine (ACh) receptors in the mammalian central nervous system (CNS) can be divided into muscarinic (mAChR) (see Chapters 10, 11, and 12, *this volume*) and nicotinic (nAChR) subtypes based on the ability of the natural alkaloids, muscarine and nicotine, to mimic the effects of ACh as a neurotransmitter (59). Until recently, the neuropsychopharmacological effects of ACh have focused studies on mAChRs (7,66), whereas nAChRs have been evaluated primarily for their role in mediating neuromuscular and ganglionic transmission in the parasympathetic and sympathetic nervous systems (59).

Over the past 30 years, chemical efforts directed towards therapeutic agents acting at ACh receptors have almost exclusively focused on ligands acting at the mAChR subtype with very limited clinical success. The negative connotations associated with the use of nicotine in tobacco products and the deleterious effects of the latter on health diminished interest in developing ligands for the neuronal nAChR subtype. However, this trend has changed following recent preclinical and clinical studies indicating that neuronal nAChRs may have a substantial role in mediating cognitive performance, in modulating affect, and in enhancing critical brain functions and the release of transmitters involved in the facilitation of cognitive performance (6).

In the past decade, workers at the Salk Institute and at the Institut Pasteur have established that the muscle nAChR is a ligand-gated ion channel (LGIC) receptor composed of α, β, γ, δ, and ε subunits that are developmentally regulated (10). Like other members of the LGIC

receptor superfamily, nAChR subunit genes encode for peptides that have a relatively hydrophilic amino-terminal portion, constituting a major extracellular domain of the receptor protein where ACh is thought to bind, followed by three hydrophobic transmembrane domains (M1–M3), a large intracellular loop, and a fourth hydrophobic transmembrane domain (M4) (10). More recently, 10 nAChR subunit genes have been identified in rat and chick brain, providing for a multitude of potential combinations suggesting that many functional subtypes of neuronal nAChR are possible (16,51).

The wide distribution of the α2, α3, α4, and β2 transcripts in mammalian brain indicates that neuronal nAChRs represent a major neurotransmitter receptor superfamily related to other LGICs including gamma-aminobutyric acid (GABA$_A$ subtype) (see Chapter 8, *this volume*), *N*-methyl-D-aspartate (NMDA) (see Chapter 7, *this volume*), and glycine. However, in contrast to these other LGICs where established pharmacology rapidly segued into the molecular biology, the pharmacology of neuronal nAChRs is only beginning to emerge as a result of the rapid advances in the molecular biology of the nAChR family.

The majority of evidence defining potential therapeutic targets involving nAChRs in nervous tissue has resulted from studies on the effects of (−)-nicotine in a variety of preclinical and, to a lesser extent, clinical models. And, while a significant number of neuronal nAChR receptor subtypes have been potentially identified based on subunit structure at the molecular level, little is known regarding the physiological role of most of these receptor subtypes beyond what can be deduced from their discrete localization within brain tissue. The development of receptor-subtype-selective ligands, especially antagonists, may be

S. P. Arneric, J. P. Sullivan, and M. Williams: Neuroscience Discovery, Pharmaceutical Products Division, Abbott Laboratories, Abbott Park, Illinois 60064.

anticipated to facilitate the definition of receptor subtype function. In this chapter the molecular biology of neuronal nAChRs is discussed within the context of the pharmacology of agonists, antagonists, and allosteric modulators. In addition, the potential CNS therapeutic targets for nAChRs are reviewed.

NICOTINIC RECEPTORS: CLASSIFICATION, TRANSITION STATES, AND SITES OF INTERACTION

Receptor nomenclature in the nAChR area has been derived from classical pharmacology approaches, including receptor sensitivity to snake toxins and by the characterization of the subunit structure of the receptor. Following from Dale's conceptualization of ACh receptor subtypes nearly 80 years ago, Barlow and Ing and Paton and Zaimis showed that the antagonist decamethonium (C10) was more effective than hexamethonium (C6) in blocking muscle nAChRs, whereas C6 was effective in autonomic ganglia (59). This led to the description of "C10" (muscle) and "C6" (neuronal) receptors. More

recently, an "N" nomenclature has evolved. N_1 muscle receptors are selectively activated by phenyltrimethylammonium, elicit membrane depolarization in the presence of bis quaternary agents such as C10, are preferentially blocked by the competitive antagonist d-tubocurarine, and are pseudo-irreversibly blocked by α-bungarotoxin (α-BgT). N_2 receptors found in ganglia are (a) preferentially activated by 1,1-dimethyl-4-phenylpiperazinium (DMPP), (b) competitively blocked by trimethaphan (Fig. 1), (c) blocked by bis-quaternary agents, with C6 being the most potent, and (d) resistant to snake α-toxins, yet sensitive to neuronal bungarotoxin (n-BgT; also known as κ-BgT, α-BgT 3.1, or toxin F). Structure–activity studies based on C6 and C10 led to the development of the first effective antihypertensive agents that included pentolinium, trimethaphan, and mecamylamine (Fig. 1), compounds that show selectivity between the ganglion and neuromuscular nAChRs, albeit with significant side-effect liabilities.

In mammalian brain, two major neuronal nAChR subclasses can be delineated (12,57) using radioligand binding: those recognizing α-BgT and n-BgT with high affinity (BgTnAChRs; $K_d \sim 0.5$ nM using $[^{125}I]\alpha$- or n-BgT)

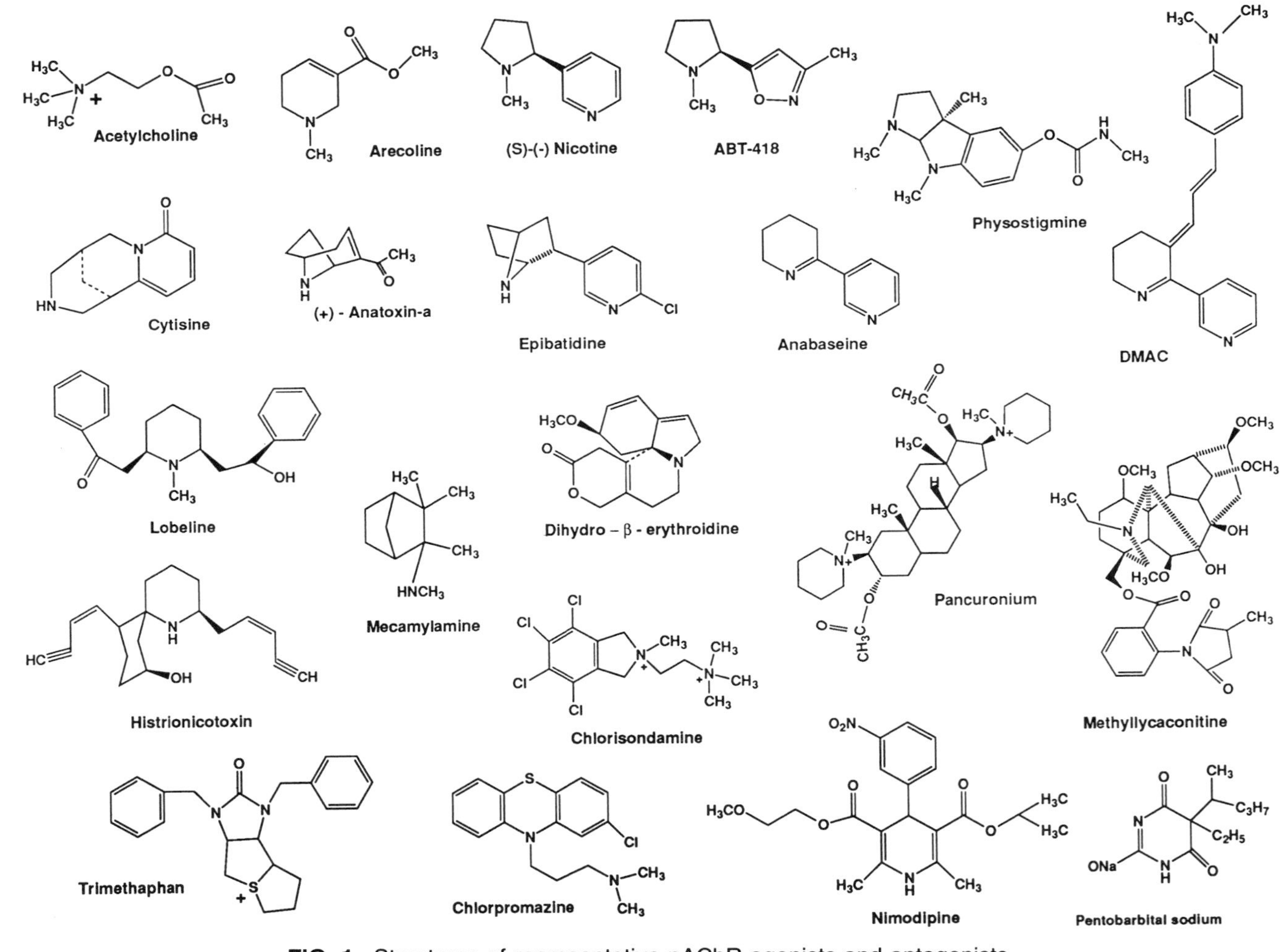

FIG. 1. Structures of representative nAChR agonists and antagonists.

and those that do not (nAChRs). BgTnAChRs have low affinity for (−)-nicotine, whereas nAChRs have high affinity ($K_d = 0.5-5$ nM using [3H](−)-nicotine, [3H]ACh, [3H]methylcarbamylcholine, and [3H]cytisine) for (−)-nicotine (see Fig. 1) (41). All four of these [3H]agonist ligands are thought to interact with the same ACh binding sites on the nAChR. The competitive antagonist, dihydro-β-erythroidine (DHβE) (Fig. 1), an alkaloid isolated from *erythina* seeds, also appears to bind directly to the neuronal nAChR in brain in a manner comparable to that of nAChR agonists (41). Although each of these nAChR ligands gives comparable results in terms of binding parameters and pharmacology in given brain regions, [3H]-cytisine is by far the best radioligand to use with respect to reproducibility and ease of use (e.g., radiochemical stability, high specific binding, binding kinetics). Greater than 90% of the high-affinity [3H](−)-nicotine binding sites in rat can be precipitated by antibodies raised against the α4 and β2 subunits (18).

Although less well studied, at least two additional sites on the nAChR have been identified that appear distinct from those sites revealed by [3H](−)-nicotine or snake toxins. The noncompetitive antagonist, mecamylamine, does not bind to the same site on the neuronal nAChR as does (−)-nicotine (34). However, (−)-nicotine, some of its analogues, and selected calcium channel antagonists compete for the [3H]mecamylamine site (34). Most recently, the presence of a novel site located on the α subunit of nAChRs and α-BgTnAChRs has been identified using [3H]1-methyl-physostigmine (45; see below), which can be competitively displaced by physostigmine (Fig. 1), benzoquinonium, galanthamine, and FK1, a nAChR-specific antibody raised against rat muscle nAChR α subunits, but not by competitive neuronal nAChR antagonists.

Transition States

In addition to structurally distinct subtypes of nAChRs, there are functionally distinct transition states for an individual nAChR. Current evidence regarding the states of activation and desensitization of nAChRs derives primarily from work on the muscle nAChR, a protein oligomer with defined properties of symmetry that can undergo transitions that adopt distinct binding characteristics and states of ion channel opening (25). Distinct ligand binding sites, some sensitive to ACh and (−)-nicotine and others involving distinct classes of allosteric modulator on, and between, the various receptor subunits, can cooperatively modify, either positively or negatively, the equilibrium between the receptor states affecting the proportion of receptors existing in each state but not significantly altering the intrinsic binding and physiological properties of the states themselves. Thus, the nAChR functions within the context of the classical allosteric "concerted scheme"

(10,25) for oligomeric proteins that incorporates the multiple state concept originally proposed by Katz and Thesleff for the nAChR.

The allosteric transition state model considers a minimum of four interconvertible states with differing rates of interconversion: a resting state (R); an activated state (A) with the channel opening in the microsecond to millisecond timescale and having low affinity (10 μM to 1 mM) for agonists; and two "desensitized" closed channel states (I or D) that are refractory to activation on a millisecond (I) to minute (D) timescale but exhibit a high affinity (1−1000 nM) for nAChR agonists and some antagonists. nAChR ligands may therefore be considered to differentially stabilize the conformational states to which they preferentially bind.

A more persistent modulation of nAChR function can occur by phosphorylation of the receptor protein (25). While little is known regarding phosphorylation of neuronal nAChRs, the sites of phosphorylation and the associated protein kinases have been well characterized in the *Torpedo* receptor. At least four kinases differentially phosphorylate muscle and *Torpedo* nAChR subunits: cAMP-dependent kinase (PKA); protein kinase C (PKC), which also phosphorylates the neuronal receptor; a tyrosine kinase; and a Ca^{2+}-calmodulin kinase. Phosphorylation can enhance the rate of nAChR desensitization and increase the frequency of spontaneous channel openings. Interestingly, a large pool of silent receptors may be converted into activatable receptors through a cAMP-dependent process presumably linked to phosphorylation, a finding consistent with the supposition that cAMP causes a shift of the allosteric equilibrium from the desensitized state to the activatable resting state. Furthermore, substance P, which is present in ganglionic cells, can activate a PKC pathway in ganglia, indicating a potential indirect modulation of the equilibrium transition states of the nAChR by neuropeptides as neuromodulatory agents.

Sites of nAChR−Ligand Interaction

Evidence is rapidly emerging to indicate that the nAChR channel may be activated through sites distinct from the classical ACh binding sites and suggests that "cholinergic channel activators" (ChCAs) may be a more appropriate, and all encompassing, classification for those compounds that activate nAChRs. In addition, there are a number of presumably separate sites involving one or more subunits where ligands can bind to noncompetitively inhibit activator-gating of nAChR channel mediated ion conductance.

The ACh Binding Site

Binding sites for cholinergic ligands on the nAChR were initially thought to reside solely on the α subunit.

More recently, site-directed mutagenesis studies have shown that binding sites for cholinergic ligands on the muscle nAChR are located at the interfaces between the α and β subunits and the α and δ subunits (10). Ligand binding sites on neuronal nAChRs may be formed in a similar manner because both α and β subunits are involved in determining the pharmacological properties of these receptors (31). For example, neuronal nAChRs formed by $\alpha2$ or $\alpha3$ subunits differ dramatically in their sensitivity to nicotinic agonists and antagonists. Analysis of chimeric subunits consisting of portions of these two α subunits have indicated that: (a) the region from the amino terminus to position 84 is important in determining sensitivity to the agonists, ACh and $(-)$-nicotine; (b) positions 84 to 121 and from position 121 to 181 contain amino acid residues important in determining n-BgT-sensitivity; and (c) the sequence segment from position 195 to 215 is important for both agonist and antagonist sensitivity. In particular, the amino acid residue at position 198 (glutamine in $\alpha3$ and proline in $\alpha2$) is believed to be important in determining the sensitivity of neuronal nAChRs. A similar approach has been used to identify amino acid residues responsible for the contribution of the β subunits.

Alternative Channel "Activator" Sites

Neuronal nAChR function may also be enhanced via ligand binding sites distinct from those at which ACh or $(-)$-nicotine interact (45). These sites are thought to be present at the level of the α subunit and are not subject to the same desensitization mechanisms described for $(-)$-nicotine. Compounds that interact with this novel site to increase neuronal nAChR-mediated ion conductance have been termed "channel activators" (45). The cholinesterase inhibitors physostigmine (Fig. 1) and galanthamine are examples of compounds that act as channel activators at this site, which is distinct from the $(-)$-nicotine site, via a mechanism that occurs independent of cholinesterase inhibition. However, physostigmine which has a variety of pharmacological actions including open channel blockade, and cholinesterase inhibition may actually interfere with the channel activation process. Thus, nonselective effects of compounds such as physostigmine detract from their potential utility as CNS therapeutics.

$(+)$-2-Methylpiperidine is a putative positive allosteric modulator of neuronal nAChRs that stereoselectively "unmasks" the number of available nAChRs without affecting the affinity of agonists for the high-affinity nAChR binding site (6). The compound can thus enhance the receptor interaction with which the endogenous ligand, ACh, binds to the nAChR, thus enhancing only ongoing or evoked cholinergic neurotransmission and reducing the potential for side-effect liability (6). This type of compound is similar in conceptual effect to glycine

antagonists acting at NMDA receptors or the various allosteric modulators of the GABA/benzodiazepine receptor complex.

Alternative Ligand Binding Sites That Antagonize nAChR Function

Based primarily on work from the muscle nAChR, and supported by preliminary work from the neuronal nAChR, there is evidence to indicate that there are a number of other ligand binding sites that can antagonize neuronal nAChR function.

Noncompetitive (Negative Allosteric Modulators) Blockers

A number of chemically diverse molecules, including histrionicotoxin (Fig. 1), chlorpromazine (Fig. 1), phencyclidine (PCP), MK 801, local anesthetics, lipophilic agents (such as detergents), fatty acids, barbiturates, volatile anesthetics, and n-alcohols, can modify the properties of the nAChR without interacting with the ACh binding site, or directly affecting the binding of ACh (25,70). These noncompetitive blockers (NCBs) interact with at least two distinct sites that differ from those of the competitive blockers. The first site binds ligands in the low micromolar range, is found within the pore, and is composed of amino acids in the M2 segments of the five subunits. Binding of NCBs is facilitated by agonist binding, is sensitive to inhibition by histrionicotoxin, and has a stoichiometry of one site per receptor. Single-channel experiments suggest that interaction at this site causes either a rapid reversible channel blockade or simply shortens channel opening times in a voltage-sensitive manner (25). Blockade of this high-affinity site blocks ion conductance by simple steric hindrance and can increase the affinity of the receptor for other nicotinic ligands. Thus, NCBs acting at this site appear to stabilize the desensitized (D) state of the nAChR. A second low-affinity site has a distinct pharmacology in that NCBs accelerate desensitization of the nAChR by shifting the equilibrium towards the desensitized state (25). Such sites are numerous (10–20 per molecule of nAChR in $Torpedo$ membrane), are of relatively low affinity ($K_i > 100\ \mu M$), and are insensitive to histrionicotoxin. Because the ligands to these sites are generally lipophilic and the number of sites calculated per receptor in reconstitution experiments depends on the lipid-to-protein ratio, it has been suggested that these sites lie at the interface between the nAChR protein and membrane lipids. Thus, function of nAChRs may well be modulated by the lipid environment. Fatty acids, phospholipases, detergents, general anesthetics, and several local anesthetics enhance the rate of desensitization and increase the affinity of the receptor for nAChR ligands. Thus, lipids and lipid-perturbing agents block the electrogenic action of ACh (25).

More recent data (70) suggest that the binding sites for NCBs may provide an additional mechanism by which sedative hypnotic barbiturates such as pentobarbital (Fig. 1) can decrease neuronal excitability mediated through the increased open channel times of GABA$_A$ receptors and associated chloride conductances.

Steroid Binding Sites

Steroids can inhibit neuronal nAChRs expressed in oocytes, chromaffin cells, and brain. This is not surprising considering the clinical effect of the steroid-like, neuromuscular blocking agent, pancuronium (Fig. 1). Steroids are thought to desensitize the nAChR at an allosteric site distinct from both the ACh binding site and the ion channel. Progesterone and testosterone coupled to bovine serum albumin, but not cholesterol or pregnenolone, inhibit the chick neuronal $\alpha 4\beta 2$ nAChR in a voltage-insensitive manner (25). In chromaffin cells, it has been reported that dexamethasone, hydrocortisone, and prednisolone behave as noncompetitive inhibitors of the nAChRs, and in vivo there is an intriguing association between circulating corticosteroids, [^{125}I]α-BgT binding proteins, and behavioral sensitivity to (−)-nicotine (44). Adrenalectomy results in corticosterone-reversible increases in the sensitivity to (−)-nicotine in a variety of behavioral and physiological tests in mice, and chronic corticosterone selectively reduces the density of [^{125}I]α-BgTnAChRs. In vitro corticosterone (high micromolar concentrations) inhibited binding of [^{125}I]α-BgT to rat brain membranes and reduced the affinity of (−)-nicotine for this binding site, which is consistent with a negative allosteric interaction. Physiologically, this site of modulation would work in concert with the effects of neurosteroids such as alfaxalone and the 5α-reduced metabolites of progesterone, which enhance GABA$_A$-receptor-mediated Cl$^-$ conductance in rat brain by prolonging the Cl$^-$ channel open time (25).

Dihydropyridine Binding Site

The neuronal nAChR may also be a target at clinically relevant (low micromolar) concentrations of dihydropyridines (29) such as nimodipine (Fig. 1). This may, in part, contribute to the overall antihypertensive effects of dihydropyridines by limiting the vasoconstricting effects of excess circulating catecholamines elicited by increased central sympathetic outflow. Both the L-type Ca^{2+} channel (see Chapter 5, *this volume*) activator, Bay K 8644, and the antagonists nimodipine, nifedipine, nitrendipine, and furnidipine inhibit the uptake of [^{45}Ca^{2+}] into bovine chromaffin cells elicited by DMPP depolarization due to Na$^+$ entry, but do not diminish the effects of K$^+$ depolarization. These findings suggest that neuronal nAChRs

present on chromaffin cells contain a dihydropyridine site whose occupation blocks ligand-gated Na$^+$ entry through the ionophore, which limits the ensuing membrane depolarization, firing of action potentials, recruitment of Ca^{2+} channels, and entry of Ca^{2+} in the cells. In the medial habenula, physiological concentrations of Ca^{2+} increase the opening frequency of single nAChR channels without changing the duration of channel opening (25,43). Ca^{2+} may in these circumstances act to reverse desensitization or enhance the opening rate of the nAChR. Thus, compounds that affect the dynamics of Ca^{2+} flux may also indirectly affect nAChR function.

NEURONAL NICOTINIC RECEPTOR PHARMACOLOGY

The multiplicity of CNS actions of (−)-nicotine to interact with nAChRs may be related to: (a) the subunit combination on the nAChR (i.e., receptor-subtype-activated); (b) the neuronal system affected (e.g., dopaminergic versus noradrenergic) in a brain region mediating a specific behavior; and (c) the intrinsic channel properties of the subtype activated (i.e., ion selectivities and channel conductance properties).

Functional and Behavioral Effects of (−)-Nicotine

(−)-Nicotine is a potent modulator of CNS function because of its enhancement of ion flux and neurotransmitter release, augmentation or gating of a number of neuronal systems, and elicitation of a variety of behavioral states. These effects are generally assumed to be mediated in a manner similar to the fast excitation observed in autonomic ganglia. Although definitive evidence that central synaptic transmission is mediated by nAChRs only exists at the motor neuron–Renshaw cell synapse in the spinal cord (51), (−)-nicotine responses can also be observed in retina, spinal cord, hippocampus, respiratory nuclei of the brainstem, cerebral cortex, cerebellar cortex, thalamus, hypothalamus, interpeduncular nucleus, septal nucleus, substantia nigra, striatum, and locus coeruleus (43).

(−)-Nicotine interacts with presynaptic nAChRs to facilitate the release of a variety of neurotransmitters, including ACh, dopamine, norepinephrine, serotonin, GABA and glutamate (69), many of which have been implicated in mediating/modulating a number of behavioral tasks (15).

The basal forebrain (BF) cholinergic system coordinates/regulates a number of CNS functions including aspects of attention, cognitive performance, cerebral blood flow (CBF), cerebral glucose utilization (CGU), and neocortical electrical activity as assessed by the electroencephalogram (EEG). Each of these aspects of brain function can be augmented by (−)-nicotine and other centrally acting nicotinic agonists, diminished by the centrally acting nAChR channel blocker mecamylamine, attenuated by age-related decrements of the BF cholinergic system, or abolished by excitotoxin-elicited destruction of this enabling system (2,6,9,23,26,27,36,38,39,50).

(−)-Nicotine also can improve learning and memory performance in a variety of preclinical paradigms (9,23,26). A reported lack of effect has been related to genetic factors that modulate the ability of (−)-nicotine to enhance cognitive performance (26). Administration of (−)-nicotine over days or weeks has also been found to improve memory performance, a persistent effect. Thus, acute injections of (−)-nicotine can improve delayed matching-to-sample accuracy in monkeys not only 10 minutes after injection but also 24 hours later (9). Even more remarkable is the persistent enhanced performance shown in a radial-arm maze choice accuracy task 2 weeks after withdrawal from a 3-week chronic administration of (−)-nicotine (26). The mechanisms for the persistent effects of (−)-nicotine are currently unknown, but may involve up-regulation of nAChRs in various brain regions including those involved with learning and memory such as the cerebral cortex and hippocampus (67). Alternatively, the effect may be related to the longer-acting effects of (−)-nicotine on other neurotransmitter systems. Acute injection of (−)-nicotine can increase tyrosine hydroxylase (TH) activity and norepinephrine release in the hippocampus for up to 28 days (23). The ability to elicit long-term effects is likely to involve nAChR-dependent modulation of neuronal transcription and translation processes (24).

(−)-Nicotine can also reverse deficits in several models of impaired cognitive performance (26). Improvements were seen in (a) impairment of Morris water maze performance following septal lesions, (b) deficits in radial-arm maze performance elicited by either basal forebrain lesions with ibotenic acid or chronic treatment with alcohol, and (c) impairments in radial-arm maze performance caused by lesions of the fimbria-fornix.

(−)-Nicotine is known to cause desynchronization of the cortical EEG (55). This is thought to occur through augmentation of the BF cholinergic system-mediated suppression of cortical slow-wave and thalamic rhythmic oscillatory activity (36). Loss of the BF system may be responsible for the loss of attentional acuity in Alzheimer's disease (AD) patients (50,65), while the ability of (−)-nicotine to enhance performance of attentionally driven tasks in AD patients suggests that (−)-nicotine therapy may be useful in normalizing this disorder-related deficit.

Cholinergic neurons arising from the BF participate in the neurogenic control of cortical CBF. Electrical or chemical microstimulation of the BF elicits remarkable increases in cortical CBF (up to 250% of control) that are uncoupled to changes in metabolism. This response is selectively decreased by the noncompetitive nAChR antagonist, mecamylamine, demonstrates age-related impairments, and can be enhanced by (−)-nicotine (27).

nAChR Diversity

All subunit genes encode for a protein with two cysteines separated by 13 residues that align with cysteines 128 and 142 of the muscle α subunit. Of the neuronal genes, seven ($\alpha2-\alpha8$) code for α subunits (see refs. 16 and 51 for reviews) based on the presence of adjacent cysteine residues in the predicted protein sequences, in a region homologous to the putative agonist binding site of the muscle α subunit ($\alpha1$) (10). A conserved lysine in the N-terminal extracellular domain of these subunits is believed to be important in the binding of channel activators (16; also see below). Three neuronal non-α subunits have been identified in rat ($\beta2-\beta4$) and chick ($n\alpha1-n\alpha3$) (16,51). Human $\alpha2-\alpha5$, $\beta2$, and $\beta4$ subunits (51,58) and the human $\alpha7$ gene (17) have been cloned. Rat, human, and chick nAChR genes of the same name are highly homologous (>70% amino acid identity). As a group, however, β subunits are as different from each other as they are from α subunits (16,51). Comparison of the rat $\alpha7$-subunit sequence with that of other rat sequences suggests that this subunit is distinct (52), a finding that may in part explain the unique pharmacological properties of the functional $\alpha7$ homopentamer (see below). Surprisingly, the human $\alpha7$ gene does not show this divergence from the other available nAChR sequences (17). Whether this difference in the evolution of the rat and human nAChR subunit gene superfamilies translates into differences in expression, regulation, and pharmacological characteristics has yet to be elucidated.

CNS Expression of Neuronal nAChRs

Both nAChRs and α-BgTnAChRs have been extensively mapped in rodent brain and, to some extent, in human brain. Using radioligand binding and in situ hybridization, the topographical distribution of nAChRs corresponds well with the effects elicited by (−)-nicotine and the known functions associated with each brain region.

Those high-affinity nAChR sites revealed by [^{3}H](−)-nicotine are abundant in selective areas of the cerebral cortex (predominantly layers III and IV), thalamus, interpeduncular nucleus, and the superior colliculus but are of low to moderate abundance in the hippocampus and hypothalamus (12) (Table 1). The second class of sites, labeled by [^{125}I]α-BgT, is enriched in the hippocampus, hypothalamus, and layers I and IV of the cerebral cortex (12). The distribution of nAChR subunit mRNAs in rodents correlates reasonably well with the distribution of high-affinity nicotine/ACh and α-BgT binding sites (Table 1). In situ hybridization assays have demonstrated that at least one nAChR gene is expressed in numerous areas

TABLE 1. *Autoradiographic and in situ hybridization analysis of the distribution of nicotinic receptor binding sites and mRNA in rat brain[a,b]*

Region	Ligand binding		Subunit distribution								
	Nicotine	BgT	α_2	α_3	α_4	α_5	α_6	α_7	β_2	β_3	β_4
Forebrain											
Cortex	+++	++	(+)	++	+++	+	−	+	+	−	+
Hippocampus	+	+++	(+)	+	++	++	−	+++	++	−	++
Thalamus	+++	(+)	−	++	+++	−	++	+	+++	++	++
Hypothalamus	+	+++	−	(+)	+	−	+	++	+	−	+
Amygdala	++	(+)	−	(+)	++	−	+	−	+	−	(+)
Septum	++		(+)	−	++	−	−	+	+	−	(+)
Brainstem											
Motor nuclei	++	−	−	+++	+	−	−	−	++	+	++
LC	++	++	−	+++	(+)	−	+	−	++	−	+
IPN	+++	+++	+++	+	+	++	−	−	++	−	++
Cerebellum	(+)	(+)	−	−	++	(+)	−	+	++	−	(+)
Cortex	+	++	−	+	+	−	−	++	++	−	+

[a] Data for autoradiographic studies were derived from ref. 12; *in situ* hybridization data were derived from refs. 16, 51 and 64. Note that the relative abundance within a given subunit is internally consistent; but may not translate across subunits.

[b] Key: −, not detectable; (+), very weak signal; +, weak signal; ++, moderate signal; +++, strong signal; IPN, interpeduncular nucleus; LC, locus coeruleus.

within rat brain and that each gene is expressed in a distinct pattern (51,52,63) (Table 1). For example, the α_4 subunit is expressed strongly in a number of areas, including the ventral tegmental area, the medial habenula, and the substantia nigra pars compacta, whereas the α_2 subunit is expressed at high levels only in parts of the interpeduncular nucleus (51). Among the β subunits, β_2 and β_4 are expressed in almost all areas of the brain whereas the expression of β_3 is more restricted (51) (Table 1). The distribution of the $\alpha_4\beta_2$ subunit combination coincides with the distribution of high-affinity nicotine binding sites in rat brain (Table 1) and supports studies demonstrating that greater than 90% of the high-affinity nicotine binding sites in rat can be precipitated by antibodies raised against the α_4 and β_2 subunits (51). A reasonably good correlation has also been noted between the distribution of the α_7 gene and that of the high-affinity binding sites for α-BgT in rodent brain (52).

Much less is known about the expression of nAChR subunit genes in human brain. However, it is likely that differences do exist in the regional distribution of these subunits across species in light of autoradiography studies

showing differences in the distribution of α-BgT and nicotine in rat, monkey, and human brain (Table 2). For example, [^{125}I] α-BgT binding is high in rat hippocampus (12) but is not detectable in monkey hippocampus (11), while [^{3}H]($-$)-nicotine binding in cortex is low in human (1) but high in rat. Whether these differences translate into differences in pharmacological properties across species will require further investigation.

Identification of Potential nAChR Subtypes with Differing Channel Functions

Oocyte expression studies have provided considerable information on the properties of different subunit combinations. The ion conductance of a channel is determined by the conformation and amino acid sequence composition of the ion channel itself (10,43). Thus, subunits which have different sequences in their transmembrane domains will have different single-channel conductances. Indeed, the Ca^{2+}/Na^+ permeability ratios of several neuronal nAChRs are significantly higher than that of the muscle

TABLE 2. *Species differences exist in the distribution of nicotinic and α-bungarotoxin binding sites in brain[a,b]*

Region	Rat (12)		Monkey (11)		Human (1)	
	Nicotine	BgT	Nicotine	BgT	Nicotine	BgT
Cortex	+++	++	−	+	+	++
Hippocampus	+	+++	−	−	(+)	++
Thalamus	+++	(+)	++	+++	+++	++
Basal ganglia	++	(+)	−	−	+	(+)

[a] References where the data are derived from are indicated for each species.

[b] Key: −, not detectable; (+), very weak signal; +, weak signal; ++, moderate signal; +++, strong signal.

nAChR in various preparations (52,62). The potential for long-term modulation through second messenger cascades elicited by the influx of Ca^{2+} clearly exists as is well documented for the NMDA receptor. Thus, it is plausible that subtype-selective activators of nAChRs will be able to cause cell-selective and regionally selective modulation of synaptic function.

Functional responses occur in oocytes transfected with pairwise combinations of α and β subunits, confirming biochemical findings which suggest that native nAChRs consist of α/β heteromers (16). $\alpha7$ and $\alpha8$ gene products differ from other members of the nAChR superfamily in that they can form functional receptors in oocytes when expressed as homo-oligomers (52; J. Lindstrom, *personal communication*). However, not all subunit combinations form functional nAChRs. The rat $\beta3$ gene, for example, in combination with $\alpha2$, $\alpha3$, or $\alpha4$ genes does not form a functional nAChR (16). Similarly, rat $\alpha5$ and $\alpha6$ genes do not participate in the formation of functional nAChR channels when coexpressed with various β subunits. Nonetheless, the channel conductance properties of the $\alpha4\beta2$ subunit combination can be altered in the presence of $\alpha5$ subunits (L. Role, *personal communication*), thus adding to the complexity of potential neuronal nAChR subunit combinations and providing a possible explanation for some of the discrepancies in channel properties between the oocyte expression studies and the receptors expressed in vivo (see Table 3 and discussion below).

Studies of the single-channel properties of neuronal nAChRs expressed in oocytes indicate considerable diversity among heterologously expressed subunit combinations (43). For example, two distinct populations of open-channel conductances can be observed after injection of either $\alpha2\beta2$ or $\alpha3\beta2$ subunits into oocytes. In contrast, the $\alpha4\beta2$ subunit combination generates only a single type of channel. Of the $\beta2$-containing receptors, the current of the $\alpha3\beta2$ receptor is the most sustained whereas the $\alpha2\beta2$ combination gives the greatest peak current. nAChRs containing the $\beta2$ subunit are thus likely to generate brief synaptic currents in vivo, creating the potential for rapid signal processing. In contrast, currents for the $\alpha3\beta4$ subunit combination are of a smaller conductance but do not desensitize as rapidly. Accordingly, if $\alpha3\beta4$ receptors predominate at synapses, responses may be prolonged, providing more time to organize a cellular response. Recent electrophysiological studies in cultured hippocampal cells are consistent with these suppositions (3).

Validation of the Emerging Pharmacological Diversity of Neuronal nAChRs

The rank order of potency for four nAChR activators—ACh, (−)-cytisine, DMPP, and tetramethylammonium—on receptors formed from rat $\beta2$ or $\beta4$ subunits in combination with $\alpha2$, $\alpha3$, or $\alpha4$ subunits (30) has established the importance of both α and β subunits in defining the pharmacological properties of the nAChR with these distinct subunit combinations. Receptors including the $\beta4$ subunit were most sensitive to (−)-cytisine (Fig. 1), whereas those containing the $\beta2$ subunit were (−)-cytisine-insensitive. Interestingly, (−)-cytisine competitively inhibited the ACh response of $\beta2$-containing subunits (30,43), suggesting that the tertiary structure of the complete nAChR defines whether a molecule will have agonist or antagonist properties. However, these findings are in contrast to studies in a cell line stably transfected with the $\alpha4\beta2$ combination where (−)-cytisine was found to be as efficacious as (−)-nicotine in stimulating cation efflux (S. Wonnacott, *personal communication*).

TABLE 3. *In vitro model systems used to evaluate the antagonist pharmacology of neuronal nAChR subtypes[a]*

Antagonist	$\alpha_2\beta_2$	$\alpha_4\beta_2$	Thalamic synaptosome [$^{86}Rb^+$] flux ($\alpha_4\beta_2$)	$\alpha_3\beta_2$	PC$_{12}$ cells/ sympathetic ganglia "ganglionic-like" ($\alpha_3\alpha_z\beta_4\beta_z$)	Striatal DA release ($\alpha_3\beta_x$)	Types of response for cultured hippocampal cells[b] IA	II	III	$\alpha7$	$\alpha_1\beta_1\delta\gamma$
α-BgT	0	0	0	0	0	0	+++	0	0	+++	+++
n-BgT	0	+	+	+++	+++	+	+++	++	0	0	0
MLA	NT	++	0	NT	+	+	+++	++	0	+++	0
DHβE	NT	++	++	NT	0	++	0	+++	0	+	+
NSTX	+++	+++	NT	+++	+++	+++	NT	NT	NT	NT	+
MEC	++	++	++	++	++	++	0	+	++	+	+
(−)-Cytisine	NT	++	(+)	++	NT	0	NT	NT	NT	(+)	NT
(−)-Lobeline	NT	NT	(+)	NT	(+)	++	NT	NT	NT	NT	NT
α-Conotoxins	0	0	NT	0	NT	NT	NT	NT	NT	NT	+++

[a] Key: 0, no antagonism; (+), partial agonist with some blocking effect; +, moderately potent (0.1–10 μM) partial antagonist effects; ++, moderately potent (0.1–10 μM), full antagonist; +++, potent (<100 nM), full antagonist; NT, not tested.

[b] Data derived from recent work in cultured hippocampal cells (3). Data for the specific subunit combinations are derived from *Xenopus* oocyte expression work (32). The subunit combinations for the other assay systems are the possible subunit combinations that may exist based on the known mRNA transcripts present in the preparation (22,28,33).

Rat and chick $\alpha7$ and chick $\alpha8$ subunits expressed as homo-oligomers in oocytes also form functional cation channels gated by nicotinic agonists with differing pharmacological properties (4; J. Lindstrom, *personal communication*). The agonist sensitivities of chick $\alpha7$ and $\alpha8$ expressed in oocytes showed that the $\alpha8$ homomers exhibited higher affinity for nicotinic agonists as compared to $\alpha7$ homomers. The order of potency for $\alpha8$ was $(-)$-nicotine $= (-)$-cytisine (EC$_{50} = 1\ \mu M$) $\sim$ ACh $>$ DMPP $>$ tetramethylammonium. In contrast, DMPP was a very weak partial agonist for $\alpha7$ and tetramethylammonium had no effect. Importantly, these pharmacological differences between $\alpha7$ and $\alpha8$ were also observed with native $\alpha7$ and $\alpha8$ subunits immunoisolated from chick retina. The finding that the rank order of potency for agonists was similar for both native $\alpha7$ and the homo-oligomeric subunit expressed in oocytes is in contrast to studies demonstrating differences in electrophysiological properties of this subunit in these two systems (4). These differences were attributed to the presence of an as yet unidentified structural subunit in the native subunits, which is consistent with the neuromuscular junction receptor complex where the absence of the ε subunit during development alters the channel conductance properties but not the agonist sensitivity of the receptor.

Information from heterologous expression studies combined with in situ hybridization studies has identified intact in vitro model systems in which the pharmacology of compounds acting at putative subtypes of neuronal nAChRs can be evaluated using electrophysiological (3) and biochemical (22,33) techniques (see Table 3). For example, greater than 90% of the binding of the nAChR agonist, [^{3}H]$(-)$-cytisine, occurs at nAChRs that contain the $\alpha4\beta2$ subunit isoform (18). Correspondingly, this receptor subtype appears to modulate the flux of monovalent ions as measured by efflux of [^{86}Rb$^+$] from thalamic synaptosomes (33) and is believed to play a role in the release of ACh from rat hippocampus. The $\alpha3$ subunit combined with other structural subunits has been implicated in mediating neurotransmitter release from mouse striatal slices based on the finding that n-BgT is a potent inhibitor of nicotine-induced dopamine release in this tissue (22) (Table 3).

The most striking pharmacological characteristic of the α-BgT-sensitive $\alpha7$ homo-oligomeric receptor is its marked permeability to calcium ions both in heterologous expression systems (52) and in tissue preparations (62). This finding, coupled with the unique distribution pattern of this receptor in brain (12,62), has led to heightened interest in the $\alpha7$ subtype as a potential therapeutic target. It is noteworthy that most of the structures with the highest abundance of $\alpha7$ transcript in rodents are major components of the limbic system (62). A role for this receptor subtype in the regulation of neurite outgrowth and survival has also been suggested (19; also see below).

While studies in oocytes have yielded some clues as

to the physiological/pharmacological roles of the different nAChR subunits in vivo, caution is required in interpreting these findings because of the atypical nature of the oocyte environment. The phenotype of the oocyte may modulate receptor expression in a manner different to that occurring in mammalian cells. Similarly, different subunit combinations may alter the relative expression levels of the component subunits leading to pentamers that are atypical in nature. Thus, it is not surprising that in a number of cases, attempts to match native nAChRs with heterologously expressed nAChRs of defined composition have failed. The expression of multiple nicotinic receptor genes in central and peripheral tissues suggests that some nAChR subtypes in these areas may contain more than two types of subunit (61), a finding that would explain why some of the pharmacological properties of receptors formed by injection of a single subunit ($\alpha7$) or by the pairwise combination of α/β subunits do not correlate well with the properties of receptors found in neurons (4). For example, in cultured chick sympathetic neurons which express $\alpha3$, $\alpha4$, $\alpha5$, $\alpha7$, $\beta2$, and $\beta4$ subunit mRNAs, α-BgT binds with high affinity to the cell surface but does not block nAChR function (28). However, n-BgT does block sympathetic ganglia responses and, remarkably, shows a preference to block $\alpha3\beta2$ instead of $\alpha7$ responses (32; refer to Table 3). Nonetheless, antisense oligonucleotide experiments suggest that $\alpha7$ subunits contribute to functional nAChRs in these cells (28). The pharmacological properties of $\alpha7$ isolated from embryonic chick brain differed from those of the chick $\alpha7$ gene expressed in oocytes (4). Thus, it appears that $\alpha7$-containing nAChRs are not homo-oligomers in some tissue preparations; rather, they can combine with certain other α and/or β subunits.

Antagonists

Neurotoxins can be used to distinguish between neuronal nAChR receptor subunit combinations (32,34). Lophotoxins are a family of related neurotoxins isolated from marine soft coral that nondiscriminantly inhibit both neuronal and muscle subtypes of nAChRs (32). Neosugurotoxin (NSTX), isolated from the Japanese ivory mollusc (*Babyloni japonica*), exerts potent blocking action in autonomic ganglia, antagonizes $(-)$-nicotine-induced antinociception in mice, inhibits $(-)$-nicotine-evoked release of [^{3}H] dopamine from rat striatal synaptosomes, and blocks ACh-elicited currents in oocytes containing $\alpha2\beta2$, $\alpha4\beta2$, and $\alpha3\beta2$ (but not $\alpha7$ and $\alpha1\beta1\delta\gamma$) nAChR subtypes (34; see Table 3). The rat and chick $\alpha7$ gene expressed as a homo-oligomer in oocytes is highly sensitive to α-BgT (51), and ACh-gated currents can be completely blocked by nanomolar concentrations of this toxin (Table 3). Neuronal bungarotoxin (n-BgT) completely blocks ACh-induced currents in oocytes injected with $\alpha3\beta2$ but is ineffective at blocking $\alpha2\beta2$ and $\alpha4\beta2$ function (32). Both the $\alpha3$ and $\beta2$ genes are also expressed in the peripheral nervous system. Thus, this combination of subunits may compose all or part of the α-BgT-insensitive, n-BgT-sensitive receptor subtype detected in peripheral ganglia. As discussed below for the agonist sensitivities of nAChR ligands, the nature of the β subunit influences the effects of antagonists on expressed nAChRs as illustrated by the insensitivity of $\alpha3\beta4$ nAChR currents to n-BgT. These distinct agonist/antagonist sensitivities observed in oocytes suggest that it may be possible to develop novel agents that distinguish different nAChR subtypes in vivo.

Methyllycoconitine (MLA) (Fig. 1), isolated from the plant *Delphinium brownii*, is a very potent ($K_i = 1$ nM) inhibitor of [^{125}I]α-BgT binding in rat forebrain preparations, produces a potent reversible blockade of $\alpha7$ (but not $\alpha3\beta2$ or $\alpha4\beta2$) responses in oocytes, and is inactive at the muscle nAChR (68). Thus, MLA is the only available antagonist that clearly differentiates between BgT-sensitive sites on neuronal and muscle nAChRs (see Table 3). Initial studies with the immunomodulatory peptide thymopoietin suggested that it too interacted with α-BgT-sensitive nAChRs. However, subsequent work has established that this putative activity of thymopoietin is due to the presence of snake venom toxins in the preparations of the peptide (M. Quik, *personal communication*).

Agonists

Currently no agonist ligands are available that are known to specifically label the major subtype of nAChR, $\alpha4\beta2$. Moreover, in contrast to the availability of antagonists that discriminate between nAChR subunit combinations, most of the available agonist ligands do not demonstrate absolute selectivity. For example, the ability of a classical agonist like (−)-cytisine to act as a channel activator or an antagonist is remarkably affected by the structural β subunits present (see Table 3 and discussion below). Conceptually, this is an important issue to consider when interpreting receptor binding data using [^{3}H]cytisine as a nAChR probe, or in examining the whole-animal response to ligands with a similar profile. This pharmacologic dilemma is probably not unique to (−)-cytisine.

(−)-Lobeline (Fig. 1) is another nicotinic agonist with high affinity for the neuronal nAChR ($K_i = 1.5$ nM) with a nonclassical pharmacology. In particular, (−)-lobeline is a full antagonist at preventing (−)-nicotine-elicited [^{3}H]dopamine release from striatal slices in vitro (J. Sullivan, *unpublished observation*) and is a full agonist in enhancing cognitive performance in rats (14), but it does not elicit a "nicotine cue" and does not cross-discriminate with (−)-nicotine (56). Much less is known about this atypical nAChR ligand at other putative subtypes of nAChRs.

(+)-Anatoxin-a (AnTx) (Fig. 1), an alkaloid produced by the freshwater cyanobacterium *Anabaena flos aqua*, is eightfold more potent than ACh at the vertebrate muscle endplate, and in a variety of in vitro brain preparations it is between 3 and 50 times more potent than (−)-nicotine and 20 times more potent than ACh (60). Less than 10-fold separation exists for AnTx to activate $\alpha7$ homo-oligomers reconstituted in *Xenopus* oocytes (EC$_{50}$ = 580 nM), and the $\alpha4\beta2$ nAChR transfected into M10 cells (EC$_{50}$ = 48 nM) (60).

Epibatidine (Fig. 1), a chloropyridine natural product isolated from the venom of the "poison arrow" frog (*Epipedobates tricolor*), is the most potent nicotinic ligand yet reported (47): $K_i = 40$ pM at [^{3}H]cytisine sites, and $K_i = 300$ nM at sites in brain labeled by [^{125}I]α-BgT. Functionally, it is more than 1000-fold more potent than (−)-nicotine in eliciting nAChR-mediated channel currents in PC12 cells (J. Daly, *personal communication*), a cell line rich in $\alpha3$ subunits.

2,4-Dimethylcinnamylidene anabaseine (DMAC) (Fig. 1) and 2,4-dimethoxybenzylidene anabaseine (DMXB) act as agonists at $\alpha7$ nAChRs (37). These analogues and anabaseine (Fig. 1) interact with both the $\alpha7$ and $\alpha4\beta2$ binding sites. In particular, DMXB is equipotent at both subtypes, while DMAC is the only reported nAChR agonist that demonstrates preferential affinity for sites in brain labeled by [^{125}I]α-BgT ($K_i = 48$ nM) as compared to those sites labeled by [^{3}H]cytisine, ($K_i = 176$ nM) (37). Functionally, DMXB appears to act as potent partial agonist at the $\alpha7$ subtype, but is a very weak partial agonist at the $\alpha4\beta2$ subtype blocking the effects of ACh in a noncompetitive manner. DMAC has an EC$_{50}$ of 2 μM for the $\alpha7$ subunit. DMXB facilitated hippocampal LTP in a mecamylamine-sensitive manner consistent with the memory-enhancing effects of this agent in a number of behavioral models. When DMXB was applied to hippocampal slices at concentrations greater than 10 μM, there was a decrease in LTP suggesting two modes of action in this in vitro model for learning and memory. However, it is not clear whether it is the agonist or antagonist effects of DMXB that are responsible for the effects of this agent on LTP.

ABT-418 (5) (Fig. 1), an isoxazole isostere of (−)-nicotine, is a potent, stereoselective, cholinergic ligand with selectivity for the neuronal [^{3}H]cytisine binding site ($K_i = 3$ nM), but not the [^{125}I]α-BgT binding sites on rat brain membranes or *Torpedo* electroplax tissue ($K_i > 10,000$ nM). Ligand binding studies with [^{3}H]ABT-418 indicate that it has a distribution in rat brain that differs from [^{3}H]cytisine and that chronic administration of ABT-418 does not elicit the same up-regulation of nAChR binding sites following chronic administration as does (−)-nicotine (J. Sullivan, *unpublished observation*). ABT-418 is fourfold less potent than (−)-nicotine in activating channel currents in PC12 cells, an effect that is prevented by the noncompetitive nAChR channel blocker, mecamylamine, and it stimulates the release of [³H]dopamine from striatal slices with an EC$_{50}$ value of 380 nM, showing 10-fold lower potency than (−)-nicotine (EC$_{50}$ = 40 nM), suggestive of lower affinity for the $\alpha 3$ subunit (5). Changes in rubidium flux in the mouse thalamus are thought to result from activation of the $\alpha 4\beta 2$ form of the nAChR (22) and in this assay, ABT-418 and (−)-nicotine had equivalent activity (EC$_{50}$ values, 500 and 700 nM, respectively). It is noteworthy that no other "classical" nAChR agonists that have been evaluated in this assay were both as potent and as efficacious as (−)-nicotine (22). For example, (−)-cytisine, while twice as potent as (−)-nicotine, elicited a significantly lower maximum efflux. In contrast, ACh, MCC, and DMPP behaved as full agonists but were less potent than (−)-nicotine. Thus, the in vitro pharmacodynamic effects of ABT-418 indicate that it has an activity profile that is substantially different than (−)-nicotine. When compared directly with (−)-nicotine in a variety of test systems, it appears to be the most selective compound available to activate nAChRs of the $\alpha 4\beta 2$ subtype.

THERAPEUTIC TARGETS

Preclinical and clinical research (26,49,53,65) in the area of neuronal nicotinic agonists has, to date, been limited primarily to the pharmacological evaluation of (−)-nicotine and other related, naturally occurring alkaloids, because, as already noted, pharmacologically selective ligands for neuronal nAChRs are limited in number. The identification of multiple ligand sites on nAChRs has focused attention on the concept that site- and/or subtype-selective modulation of nAChRs is possible. These findings parallel findings in the area of NMDA and BDZ receptor complexes where compounds have been identified that allosterically modulate these ligand-gated ion channel receptors in a manner distinct from directly acting ligands that consequently have the potential for reduced side effects. Those agonists termed "cholinergic channel activators" (ChCAs) define a broad group of ligands that directly or allosterically activate one or more subtypes of the nAChR. The therapeutic outcome of a selective ChCA would be twofold: (i) focused efficacy at a subtype of neuronal nAChR that has a defined role in mediating a CNS function and (ii) potentially diminished side-effect liability as a result of restricted activity at other nAChRs (6). (+)-2-Methylpiperidine and ABT-418 (Fig. 1) represent the first reported ChCAs that selectively activate neuronal nAChRs without eliciting the dose-limiting side effects typically observed with (−)-nicotine (6,14).

Cognition Enhancement/Alzheimer's Disease

(−)-Nicotine, by increasing vigilance and resistance to extinction, also improves learning and memory in various

preclinical models. At the molecular level, the various cognitive effects of nicotine are mediated by different neurotransmitter systems: resistance to extinction involves ascending noradrenergic pathways and an increase in tyrosine hydroxylase expression, while increased vigilance involves a direct effect on ascending cholinergic pathways (23). Nicotine can also enhance glutamate-evoked responses in the rat prefrontal cortex, providing an additional mechanism for the cognition enhancing activities of this nAChR agonist (63).

In AD brain tissue, cortical nAChRs are markedly reduced (57), reflecting the cholinergic deficits associated with AD as well as the characteristic cortical perfusion abnormality seen in AD (6,20). The nAChR antagonist, mecamylamine, but not the mAChR antagonist, scopolamine, reduces resting cortical perfusion in the parieto-temporal cortex of humans, the area most consistently implicated in functional brain imaging of AD patients (20) (see Chapters 118 and 120, *this volume*). Two pilot clinical studies (39,50), using systemically administered (−)-nicotine, have shown an enhancement of cognitive performance in AD patients. In contrast, mecamylamine can impair performance in normal subjects (37). Pharmacoepidemiological studies have shown a reduced incidence of AD in populations of individuals who have previously smoked (54), an effect that when carefully adjusted for all major risk factors suggests a dose-related protection that has been attributed to nicotine. More well documented is a reduced incidence of Parkinson's disease (PD) in smokers (54), again attributed to chronic (−)-nicotine consumption.

While controlled delivery of (−)-nicotine represents a feasible approach to the treatment of smoking cessation (42), the potential use of this compound in the treatment of AD is problematic especially as related to chronic usage in an aged patient population. (−)-Nicotine activates the sympathetic nervous system directly via central activation of sympathetic outflow and indirectly through the enhanced release of circulating catecholamines—resulting in elevated blood pressure, an increased workload to the heart (6,42) that may evoke acute myocardial infarction, and sudden death—and elevates plasma lipids, an action that would potentially predispose an individual to atherosclerosis. An additional concern in aged patients who generally exhibit significant sleep disturbances and abnormal EEG patterns is the additional sleep disruption resulting from elevated levels of (−)-nicotine (55) which, with chronic usage, may lead to a further exacerbation of the cognitive and affective decline associated with AD. The gastrointestinal and addiction liabilities associated with (−)-nicotine are of lesser concern but nonetheless would preclude the use of (−)-nicotine in AD patients.

In nonsmokers, (−)-nicotine patch usage is frequently associated with nausea and gastrointestinal distress (42). The dose-related side-effect liabilities of (−)-nicotine, relative to the benefits, will be: (a) a major issue for the further development of this compound and (b) a major milestone for any related ChCAs.

In animal models of the cholinergic deficits associated with AD involving loss of cholinergic afferents from the nucleus basalis, nicotine, the selective ChCA, ABT-418 (M. Decker, *personal communication*), and the anabaseine analogue, DMXB (Fig. 1), reversed the performance deficits elicited by acute lesions (E. Meyer, *personal communication*) or age-related loss of this input (D. Woodruff-Pak, *personal communication*). In a single-, rising dose study in young, normal, healthy male subjects, ABT-418 administered in a transdermal patch formulation was well-tolerated in smokers and nonsmokers over a range of doses which elevated plasma level to 200 ng/ml (J. Grebb, *personal communication*). This is quite remarkable considering that (−)-nicotine patches given acutely to a nonsmoking adults frequently cause nausea and emesis when plasma levels > 25 ng/ml are achieved (42). The increased safety of ABT-418 as compared to the reported effects of (−)-nicotine patches is consistent with the preclinical safety and efficacy profile. In mice, ABT-418 is 3–10 more potent in memory enhancement and anxiolytic test paradigms via a mecamylamine-sensitive mechanism when compared to (−)-nicotine, and it is less potent in eliciting hypothermia, seizures, locomotor activity reduction, and death (14). In rats, ABT-418 maintains behavioral efficacy in both the memory enhancement and anxiolytic test paradigms following 14 days of continuous subcutaneous infusion and normalized the hyperactivity response elicited by lesions of the medial septum (M. Decker, *personal communication*). Similar levels of ABT-418 are rapidly achieved in brain (5–50 ng/g) and plasma (5–55 ng/ml) following doses that enhance behavioral performance (J. Brioni, *personal communication*). In monkeys, ABT-418 enhances performance of a delayed matching-to-sample task to a greater degree and over a broader dose range than (−)-nicotine (J. Buccafusco, *personal communication*). In dogs, ABT-418 has significantly lower pressor activity than (−)-nicotine when given intravenously, and it has less emetic liability (14). Although not the most potent nAChR ligand reported, ABT-418 is one of the more selective activators of neuronal nAChRs that may potentially provide safe and effective palliative treatment of AD.

Neuroprotection

In addition to its palliative actions in reversing cognitive deficits, (−)-nicotine may have neuroprotective actions, preventing the presynaptic loss of function following hemitransection or MPTP lesions of the nigrostriatal system as well as the transneuronal degeneration observed following neurotoxic destruction of the basal forebrain system (40). Other nicotinic agonists such as DMXB can also prevent neurite and cell loss following removal of

nerve growth factor (NGF) from NGF-differentiated PC12 cells, an effect prevented by the nAChR blocker, mecamylamine (35).

The mechanistic basis of the neuroprotective actions of (−)-nicotine is unknown but, like the long-term effects of the agonist on cognitive performance, may involve receptor-mediated activation of transcriptional factors (24) involved in neurotrophin production. (−)-Nicotine has been reported to elicit NGF induction, while α-BgT increases NGF and BDNF (brain derived neurotrophic factor) mRNA levels (19). Thus, nAChR subtypes may be differentially involved in the expression of a variety of neurotrophins. It is tempting to speculate that the reported neuroprotective effects of (−)-nicotine in PD may be the result of induction of BDNF formation, which has substantial neurorestorative effects in dopaminergic neuronal populations, while the neuroprotective effects reported in AD may involve NGF production.

Smoking Cessation

Tobacco smoke contains a large variety of substances; however, the addictive nature of smoking is attributable to the reinforcing actions of nicotine (56) which appear to involve the mesolimbic dopaminergic systems. Nicotine reinforcement is a complex phenomenon involving receptor cognition enhancement, stress adaptation, subjective euphoria, a paradoxical receptor up-regulation (67), and relief from the withdrawal syndrome (see Chapter 147, *this volume*).

The severe health liabilities and high mortality rates associated with tobacco usage have resulted in major efforts to identify therapeutic treatments, most notably that of nicotine replacement therapy. Nicotine gum and nicotine patches have been developed as aids in smoking cessation. Patch formulations are an accepted method for delivering (−)-nicotine for periods of up to 24 hours to maintain constant plasma levels (42), potentially reducing abuse potential, and diminishing the potential gastrointestinal liabilities seen with oral administration of (−)-nicotine gum.

The initial optimism of a "cure" for smoking via nicotine replacement therapy in the form of gum and patches has been dampened by patient disillusionment due to the inability of either nicotine formulation to replace the nicotine provided in cigarettes as well as overcome the psychological cues associated with smoking (e.g., smoke inhalation and oral and hand cues). This has been compounded by anecdotal reports of heart attacks associated with patch usage and concurrent cigarette smoking. Nonetheless, second-generation nicotine replacement therapy is focused on increasing the amount of (−)-nicotine being delivered by gum or patch in the hopes that the psychological and behavioral aspects of smoking may be overcome.

Alternative therapies under development are the "non-nicotine," nicotinic agonists and partial agonists with reduced side-effect liability, as well as combined agonist/antagonist treatment. (−)-Lobeline (Fig. 1), an nAChR ligand with full agonist, partial agonist, and full antagonist properties depending on the test paradigm examined, is entering Phase III clinical trials as a once-a-week, subcutaneous, controlled release formulation, inpatient treatment for smoking cessation. However, (−)-lobeline is a compound that also selectively inhibits the CYP2D6 isoform of the drug metabolism enzyme P_{450}, and its utility for other CNS indications may be limited due to interference with medications such as the tricyclic antidepressants (D. Rodrigues, *personal communication*). The ChCA, ABT-418, which has minimal cardiovascular liabilities as compared to (−)-nicotine, may be another approach, because this compound can also prevent the anxiogenic response of rats to abrupt withdrawal from (−)-nicotine (J. Brioni, *personal communication*). The use of partial agonists in drug dependence therapy combines both substitution (agonist) and blockade of reinforcement (antagonist) in a single molecule, a concept that has been argued (49) to 'insulate' the addicted individual from reinforcement while preventing withdrawal symptoms. This combined agonist/antagonist concept has been validated in a recent randomized, double-blind, placebo-controlled trial that evaluated concurrent orally administered mecamylamine with (−)-nicotine skin patch treatment for smoking cessation (48). The improved effects of adding mecamylamine were to increase abstinence by reducing craving for cigarettes, negative affect, and appetite.

From an addiction viewpoint, however, it is probable that no single replacement approach will result in complete abstinence, and it has been argued (48) that nicotine maintenance via patch or gum may be safer than smoking for both the smoker and those subject to side smoke, although the cardiovascular toxicity of (−)-nicotine may confound this approach.

Anxiety Disorders

(−)-Nicotine has anxiolytic actions in humans (46) and preclinical models of anxiety (14). In the latter, these anxiolytic-like effects can be blocked by both mecamylamine and the benzodiazepine "inverse agonist," flumazenil (J. Brioni, *personal communication*). The latter finding suggests that (−)-nicotine may indirectly produce its anxiolytic actions by enhancing the release of endogenous benzodiazepine-like substances which, in turn, interact with the central benzodiazepine–GABA$_A$ receptor complex. However, unlike diazepam, (−)-nicotine enhanced cognitive performance and is nonsedating. The ChCA, ABT-418 has antianxiety effects similar to those seen with (−)-nicotine and has no sedating or alcohol

potentiating actions (6,14) (see also Chapters 113 and 114, *this volume*).

Schizophrenia

An increased sensitivity to auditory stimuli in schizophrenics and their immediate relatives involves a diminished gating of a brain wave designated as P_{50} in humans and N_{40} in rats (2) (see Chapter 104, *this volume*). The N_{40} originates in the hippocampal CA3 region and involves a nicotinic component which is blocked by α-BgT, but not by mecamylamine. Interestingly, hippocampal tissue from schizophrenics is deficient in α-BgT binding sites and in $\alpha7$ mRNA. Among psychiatric patients, those with schizophrenia are more likely to be smokers (88%) than those with other psychiatric diagnoses. Administration of (−)-nicotine gum to nonsmoking relatives of schizophrenics can restore the deficient P_{50} sensory gating, although this is a short-lived effect possibly due to nAChR desensitization (2). In an animal model of sensory gating, (−)-nicotine, but not (−)-lobeline, enhanced sensory gating (M. Decker, *personal communication*). The possibility that nicotinic agonists that do not show diminished responsiveness with repeated administration may have potential use in schizophrenia remains to be examined.

Attention-deficit disorder (ADD), with or without hyperactivity, is a behavioral disorder characterized by distractibility and impulsiveness that has been treated with stimulants like pemoline. Because (−)-nicotine, but not (−)-lobeline (M. Sarter, *personal communication*), can improve concentration and task performance, it (or compounds such as DMXB or ABT-418) may be a useful acute treatment for the deficits in attention seen in ADD.

Tourette's Syndrome

Classical neuroleptics are used to treat Tourette's syndrome but are limited in their usefulness due to sedation, exacerbation of learning difficulties, and potentially tardive dyskinesia liability. (−)-Nicotine can potentiate the behavioral effects of neuroleptics such as haloperidol in a number of preclinical models of behavior, and thus it may be useful in potentiating the beneficial actions of neuroleptics while diminishing their side-effect profile. Pilot clinical trials have indicated that both (−)-nicotine gum and (−)-nicotine patches are effective in ameliorating the symptoms of Tourette's syndrome (i.e., complex motor and verbal tics) in nonsmoking adolescents who are not satisfactorily controlled with neuroleptics (53). This remains a promising and largely unexplored area of opportunity for examining the role of ChCA therapy (see Chapter 143, *this volume*).

Analgesia

(−)-Nicotine has antinociceptive actions that may involve L-type calcium channels or, alternatively, dihydropyridine-sensitive binding sites on the neuronal nAChR (13). The modulatory effects of the dihydropyridines are manifest in their potent blockade of (−)-nicotine-mediated analgesia. Nifedipine and nimodipine block (−)-nicotine-induced analgesia in mice, whereas the calcium channel activator Bay K 8644 actually potentiates the analgesic action of (−)-nicotine. Conversely, intrathecal injection of mecamylamine blocks the antinociception produced by intrathecal administration of Ca^{2+}, Bay K 8644, the ionophore A23187, and thapsigargin, suggesting that nAChRs may affect independent intracellular Ca^{2+} signaling dynamics (13). The observation that mecamylamine and (−)-nicotine do not compete for [^{3}H]-nitrendipine binding ($K_i > 10 \ \mu M$) is consistent with a distinct, noncompetitive, negative allosteric modulation by the dihydropyridines. Epibatidine (Fig. 1), which is 200-fold more potent than morphine as an analgesic, is also the most potent competitive ligand at neuronal nAChRs described to date. The analgesic action of epibatidine is blocked by mecamylamine but not by the opiate antagonist, naloxone (47). (±)-Epibatidine is also an exceptionally toxic nAChR agonist and is greater than 100-fold more potent than (−)-nicotine in causing death in mice (M. Decker, *unpublished observation*). Separation of the side-effect liabilities of this novel neuronal nAChR agonist from its efficacy at nAChR subtypes mediating analgesia would represent a major breakthrough in the field of analgesic therapy, potentially replacing the opiates.

Depression

Both retrospective (21) and prospective (8) clinical studies have demonstrated a relationship between smoking and major depression. This is apparently not a causal relationship but results from shared predispositions involving genetic or environmental factors (8). Depression increases the probability of smoking, as well as nicotine and other dependencies (21). The potential role of nicotinic agonists in the treatment of major depression remains to be determined (see also Chapters 96 and 147, *this volume*).

FUTURE ASPECTS

It is evident that considerable progress has been made in defining the molecular properties of nAChRs and in focusing efforts, both chemical and pharmacological, on their therapeutic potential over the past 6 years, since the previous edition of this monograph was published (66).

The pentameric structure of the neuronal nAChR and the considerable molecular diversity in subunits offers the possibility of a large number of nAChR subtypes, which, based on pharmacological precedent, may be anticipated to subserve a variety of discrete functions within the CNS and thus represent novel targets for therapeutic agents. To capitalize on this opportunity, given the paucity and conflicting nature of therapeutic data to date, will require characterization of functionally relevant subunit combinations with respect to their localization within the CNS together with the identification of selective ligands that modulate receptor function as both direct and allosteric agonists and antagonists. The variety of pharmacophores active at nAChRs (Fig. 1), especially antagonists, provides a wealth of interesting tools to complement the molecular diversity of the receptor.

In the next decade, the potential for developing nAChR ligands for use in AD, smoking cessation, anxiety, depression, and schizophrenia as well as novel analgesics appears high, providing a challenge and a emerging therapeutic opportunity that is comparable in many ways to the identification and development of selective ligands with demonstrated therapeutic utility for the ever-expanding serotonin receptor superfamily.

ACKNOWLEDGMENTS

The authors would like to acknowledge the contributions of Neal Benowitz, Jerry Buccafusco, Clark Briggs, Al Collins, Mike Decker, Bob Freedman, Barry Hoffer, Mark Holladay, John Long, Michael Marks, Paul Newhouse, Jim Pauly, Clement Stone, Peter Whitehouse, and Sue Wonnacott. Because of space constraints, the authors were limited in citing original article and abstracts and have relied extensively on review articles and personal communications.

REFERENCES

1. Adem A, Gillberg PG, Jossan SS, Sara V, Nordberg A. Distribution of nicotinic acetylcholine receptors in the human brain: quantitative autoradiography using [^{3}H] nicotine. In: Clementi F, Gotti C, Sher E, eds. *Nicotinic acetylcholine receptors in the nervous system.* NATO ASI Series. Berlin: Springer, 1988:331–350.
2. Adler LE, Hoffer LJ, Griffith J, Waldo MC, Freedman R. Normalization by nicotine of deficient auditory sensory gating in the relatives of schizophrenics. *Biol Psychiatry* 1992;32:607–616.
3. Alkondon M, Albuquerque EX. Diversity of nicotinic acetylcholine receptors in rat hippocampal neurons. I. Pharmacological and functional evidence for distinct structural subtypes. *J Pharmacol Exp Ther* 1993;265:1455–1473.
4. Anand R, Peng X, Lindstrom J. Homomeric and native α7 acetylcholine receptors exhibit remarkably similar but non-identical pharmacological properties, suggesting that the native receptor is a heteromeric protein complex. *FEBS Lett* 1993;327:241–246.
5. Arneric SP, Sullivan JP, Briggs C, et al. ABT-418: a novel cholinergic ligand with cognition enhancing and anxiolytic activity. I. *In vitro* activity. *J Pharmacol Exp Ther* 1994;[*in press*].
6. Arneric SP, Williams M. Nicotinic agonists in Alzheimer's disease: Does the molecular diversity of nicotine receptors offer the opportunity for developing CNS selective cholinergic channel activators?

In: *Recent advances in the treatment of neurodegenerative disorders and cognitive function. Int Acad Biomed Drug Res* 1993;7:30.

7. Bartus RT, Dean RL, Flicker C. Cholinergic psychopharmacology: an integration of human and animal research on memory. In: Meltzer H, ed. *Psychopharmacology: the third generation of progress,* New York: Raven Press, 1987;219–232.

8. Breslau N, Kilbey MM, Andreski P. Nicotine dependence and major depression. New evidence from a prospective investigation. *Arch Gen Psychiatry* 1993;50:31–35.

9. Buccafusco JJ, Jackson WJ. Beneficial effects of nicotine administered prior to a delayed matching-to-sample task in the young and aged monkeys. *Neurobiol Aging* 1991;12:233–238.

10. Changeux J-P, Galzi J-L, Devillers-Thiery A, Betrand D. The functional architecture of the acetylcholine nicotinic receptor explored by affinity labeling and site-directed mutatgenesis. *Q Rev Biophys* 1992;25:395–432.

11. Cimino M, Marini P, Fornasari D, Cattabeni F, Clementi F. Distribution of nicotinic receptors in cynomolgus monkey brain and ganglia: localization of α3 subunit mRNA, α-bungarotoxin and nicotine binding sites. *Neuroscience* 1992;51:77–86.

12. Clarke PBS, Schwartz RD, Paul SM, Pert CD, Pert A. Nicotinic binding in rat brain autoradiographic comparison of [^{3}H]-acetylcholine, [^{3}H]nicotine, and [^{125}I]-L-Bungarotoxin. *J Neurosci* 1985;5:1307–1315.

13. Damaj MI, Welch SP, Martin BR. Involvement of calcium and L-type channels in nicotine-induced antinociception. *J Pharmacol Exp Ther* 1993;266:1330–1338.

14. Decker MW, Brioni J, Sullivan JP, et al. ABT-418: a novel cholinergic ligand with cognition enhancing and anxiolytic activity. II. *In vivo* activity. *J Pharmacol Exp Ther* 1994;[in press].

15. Decker MW, McGaugh JL. The role of interactions between the cholinergic system and other neuromodulatory systems in learning and memory. *Synapse* 1991;7:151–168.

16. Deneris ES, Connolly J, Rogers SW, Duvoisin R. Pharmacological and functional diversity of neuronal nicotinic acetylcholine receptors. *Trends Pharmacol Sci* 1991;12:34–40.

17. Doucette-Stamm L, Monteggia L, Donnelly-Roberts D, Wang WT, Tian JL, Giordano T. Cloning and sequence of the human α7 nicotinic acetylcholine receptor. *Drug Dev Res* 1993;30:252–256.

18. Flores CM, Rogers SW, Pabreza LA, Wolfe B, Kellar KJ. A subtype of nicotinic cholinergic receptor is composed of α4 and β2 subunits and is upregulated by chronic nicotine treatment. *Mol Pharmacol* 1992;41:31–37.

19. Freedman R, Weltmore C, Stromberg I, Leonard S, Olson L. α-Bungarotoxin binding to hippocampal interneurons: immunocytochemical characterization and effects on growth factor expression. *J Neurosci* 1993;13:1965–1975.

20. Gitelman DR, Prohovnik I. Muscarinic and nicotinic contributions to cognitive function and cortical blood flow. *Neurobiol Aging* 1992;13:313–318.

21. Glassman AH, Stetner F, Walsh BT, et al. Heavy smokers, smoking cessation and clonidine. Results of a double-blind, randomized trial. *J Am Med Assoc* 1988;259:2863–2866.

22. Grady S, Marks MJ, Wonnacott S, Collins AC. Characterization of nicotinic receptor mediated [^{3}H]dopamine release from synaptosomes prepared from mouse striatum. *J Neurochem* 1992;59:848–856.

23. Gray JA, Mitchell SN, Joseph MH, Grigoryan G, Dawe S, Hodges H. Neurochemical mechanisms mediating the behavioral and cognitive effects of nicotine. *Drug Dev Res* 1994;31:3–17.

24. Greenberg ME, Ziff EB, Greene LA. Stimulation of neuronal acetylcholine receptors induces rapid gene transcription. *Science* 1986;234:80–83.

25. Léna C, Changeux, J-P. Allosteric modulations of the nicotinic acetylcholine receptor. *Trends Neurosci* 1993;16:181–186.

26. Levin E. Nicotinic systems and cognitive function. *Psychopharmacol* 1992;108:417–421.

27. Linville, DG, Williams S, Raskiewicz, JL and Arneric SP. Nicotinic agonists modulate basal forebrain (BF) control of cortical cerebral blood flow in anesthetized rats. *J Pharmacol Exp Ther* 1993;267:440–461.

28. Listerud M, Brussard AB, Devay P, Colman DR, Role LW. Functional contribution of neuronal AChR subunits revealed by antisense oligonucleotides. *Science* 1991;254:1518–1521.

29. Lopez MG, Fonteriz RI, Gandia L, et al. The nicotinic acetylcholine receptor of the bovine chromaffin cell, a new target for dihydropyridines. *Eur J Pharmacol Mol Pharmacol Section* 1993;247:199–207.

30. Luetje CW, Patrick J. Both α- and β-subunits contribute to the agonist sensitivity of neuronal nicotinic acetylcholine receptors. *J Neurosci* 1991;11:837–845.

31. Luetje CW, Piattoni M, Patrick J. Mapping of ligand binding sites of neuronal nicotinic acetylcholine receptors using chimeric α subunits. *Mol Pharmacol* 1993;44:657–666.

32. Luetje CW, Wada K, Rogers S, et al. Neurotoxins distinguish between different neuronal nicotinic acetylcholine receptor subunit combinations. *J Neurochem* 1990;55:632–640.

33. Marks MJ, Garnham DA, Grady SR, Collins AC. Nicotinic receptor function determined by stimulation of rubidium efflux from mouse brain synaptosomes. *J Pharmacol Exp Ther* 1993;264:542–552.

34. Martin BR, Martin TJ, Fan F, Damaj MI. Central actions of nicotine antagonists. *Med Chem Res* 1993;2:564–577.

35. Martin EJ, Panickar KS, King MA, Deyrup M, Hunter BE, Meyer EM. Cytoprotective actions of 2,4-dimethoxybenzylidene anabaseine in differentiated PC12 cells and septal cholinergic neurons. *Drug Dev Res* 1994;135–141.

36. McCormick DA. Cellular mechanism of cholinergic control of neocortical and thalamic neuronal excitability. In: Steriade M, Biesold D, eds. *Brain cholinergic systems,* New York: Oxford University Press, 1990;pp 236–264.

37. Meyer EM, de Fiebre CM, Hunter BE, Simpkins CE, Frauworth N, de Fiebre NEC. Effects of anabaseine-related analogs on rat brain nicotinic receptor binding and on avoidance behaviors. *Drug Dev Res* 1994;31:127–134.

38. Newhouse PA, Potter A, Corwin J, Lenox R. Modeling the nicotinic receptor loss in dementia using the nicotinic antagonist mecamylamine: effects on human cognitive functioning. *Drug Dev Res* 1994;31:71–79.

39. Newhouse P, Sunderland T, Tariot P, et al. Intravenous nicotine in Alzheimer's disease: a pilot study. *Psychopharmacology* 1988;95:171–175.

40. Owman C, Fuxe K, Jason AM, Kahrstrom J. Studies of protective actions of nicotine on neuronal and vascular functions in the brain of rats: comparison between sympathetic noradrenergic and mesostriatal dopaminergic fiber system, and the effect of a dopamine agonist. *Prog Brain Res* 1989;79:267–276.

41. Pabreza LA, Dhawan S, Kellar KJ. [^{3}H] Cytisine binding to nicotinic cholinergic receptors in brain. *Mol Pharmacol* 1991;39:9–12.

42. Palmer KJ, Buckley MM, Faulds D. Transdermal nicotine: a review of its pharmacodynamic and pharmacokinetic properties, and therapeutic efficacy as an aid to smoking cessation. *Drugs* 1992;44:498–529.

43. Papke RI. The kinetic properties of neuronal nicotinic acetylcholine receptors: Genetic basis of functional diversity. *Prog Neurobiol* 1993;41:509–531.

44. Pauly JR, Grun EU, Collins AC. Glucocorticoid regulation of sensitivity to nicotine. In: Lippiello PM, Collins AC, Gray JA, Robinson JH, eds. *The biology of nicotine: current research issues.* 1992;121–139. New York: Raven Press.

45. Pereira EFR, Reinhardt-Maelicke S, Schrattenholz A, Maelicke A, Albuquerque EX. Identification and functional characterization of a new agonist site on nicotinic acetylcholine receptors of cultured hippocampal neurons. *J Pharmacol Exp Therap* 1993;265:1474–1491.

46. Pomerleau OF. Nicotine as a psychoactive drug: Anxiety and pain reduction. *Psychopharmacol Bull* 1986;22:865–869.

47. Qian C, Li T, Shen TY, Libertine-Garahan L, Eckman J, Biftu T, Ip S. Epibatidine is a nicotinic analgesic. *Eur J Pharmacol* 1993;250:R13–R14.

48. Rose JE, Behm FM, Westman EC, Levin ED, Stein RM, Ripka GV. Mecamylamine combined with nicotine skin patch facilitates smoking cessation beyond nicotine patch treatment alone. *Clin Pharmacol Therap.* 1994;55:[in press].

49. Rose JE, Levin ED. Concurrent agonist-antagonist administration for the analysis and treatment of drug dependence. *Pharm Biochem Behav* 1991;41:219–226.

50. Sahakian B, Jones G, Levy R, Gray J, Warburton D. The effects of nicotine on attention, information processing, and short term

memory in patients with dementia of the Alzheimer type. *Br J Psychiatry* 1989;154:797–800.

51. Sargent PB. The diversity of neuronal nicotinic acetylcholine receptors. *Ann Rev Neurosci* 1993;16:403–443.

52. Seguela P, Wadiche J, Dineley-Miller K, Dani JA, Patrick JW. Molecular cloning functional properties, and distribution of rat brain $\alpha 7$: A nicotinic cation channel highly permeable to calcium. *J Neurosci* 1993;13:596–604.

53. Silver AA, Sanberg PR. Transdermal nicotine patch and potentiation of haloperidol in Tourette's syndrome. *Lancet* 1993;342:182.

54. Smith CJ, Giacobini E. Nicotine, Parkinson's and Alzheimer's disease. *Rev Neurosci* 1992;3:25–42.

55. Soldatos CR, Kales JD, Scharf MB, Bixler EO, Kales A. Cigarette smoking associated with sleep difficulty. *Science* 1980;207:551–553.

56. Stolerman IP, Shoaib M. The neurobiology of nicotine addiction. *Trends Pharmacol Sci* 1991;12:467–473.

57. Sugaya K, Giacobini, Chiappinelli VA. Nicotinic acetylcholine receptor subtypes in human frontal cortex: changes in Alzheimer's disease. *J Neurosci Res* 1990;27:349–359.

58. Tarroni P, Rubboli F, Chini B, et al. Neuronal-type nicotinic receptors in human neuroblastoma and small-cell lung carcinoma cell lines. *FEBS Lett* 1992;312:66–70.

59. Taylor P. Agents acting at the neuromuscular junction and autonomic ganglia. *Goodman and Gilman's, The pharmacological basis of therapeutics,* 8th ed. New York: Pergamon Press, 1990;166–186.

60. Thomas P, Stephens M, Wilkie G, etc. (+)-Anatoxin-a is a potent agonist at neuronal nicotinic acetylcholine receptors. *J Neurochem* 1993;39, 2308–2311.

61. Vernallis AB, Conroy WG, Berg DK. Neurons assemble acetylcholine receptors with as many as three kinds of subunits while maintaining subunit segregation among receptor subtypes. *Neuron* 1993;10:451–464.

62. Vernino S, Amador M, Luetje CW, Patrick J, Dani JA. Calcium modulation and high calcium permeability of neuronal nicotinic acetylcholine receptors. *Neuron* 1992;8:127–134.

63. Vidal C. Nicotinic potentiation of glutamatergic synapses in the prefrontal cortex: new insight into the analysis of the role of nicotinic receptors in cognitive functions. *Drug Dev Res* 1994;31:120–126.

64. Wada E, Wada K, Boulter J, Deneris E, Heinemann S, et al. Distribution of $\alpha 2$, $\alpha 3$, $\alpha 4$ and $\beta 2$ neuronal nicotinic receptor subunit mRNAs in the central nervous system: a hybridization histochemical study in rat. *J Comp Neurol* 1989;284:314–335.

65. Warburton DM. Nicotine as a cognitive enhancer. *Prog Neuropsychopharmacol Biol Psychiatry* 1992;16:181–191.

66. Watson M, Roeske WR, Yamamura HI. Cholinergic receptor heterogeneity. In: Meltzer HY, ed. *Psychopharmacology: the third generation of progress.* New York: Raven Press, 1987;241–248.

67. Wonnacott S. The paradox of nicotinic acetylcholine receptor upregulation by nicotine. *Trends Pharmacol Sci* 1990;11:216–219.

68. Wonnacott S, Albuquerque EX, Bertrand D. Methyllycaconitine: a new probe that discriminates between nicotinic acetylcholine receptor subclasses. *Methods Neurosci* 1993;12:263–275.

69. Wonnacott S, Irons J, Rapier C, Thorne B, Lunt GG. Presynaptic modulation of transmitter release by nicotinic receptors. In: Norderg A, Fuxe K, Holmstedt B, Sundwall A, eds. *Progress in Brain Research.* Amsterdam: Elsevier, 1990;157–163.

70. Yost SC, Dodson BA. Inhibition of nicotinic acetylcholine receptor by barbiturates and by procain: Do they act at different sites? *Cell Mol Neurobiol* 1993;13:159–172.

Psychopharmacology: The Fourth Generation of Progress, edited by Floyd E. Bloom and David J. Kupfer. Raven Press, Ltd., New York © 1995.

CHAPTER 10

Molecular Biology, Pharmacology, and Brain Distribution of Subtypes of the Muscarinic Receptor

Frederick J. Ehlert, William R. Roeske, and Henry I. Yamamura

It has been 80 years since Dale (13) divided the actions of acetylcholine into nicotinic and muscarinic. These effects are now known to be mediated by two quite distinct classes of receptors which show little in common except their ability to bind acetylcholine. The muscarinic class of acetylcholine receptors are widely distributed throughout the body and subserve numerous vital functions in both the brain and autonomic nervous system (50). Activation of muscarinic receptors in the periphery causes a decrease in heart rate, a relaxation of blood vessels, a constriction in the airways of the lung, an increase in the secretions and motility of the various organs of the gastrointestinal tract, an increase in the secretions of the lacrimal and sweat glands, and a constriction in the iris sphincter and ciliary muscles of the eye. In the brain, muscarinic receptors participate in many important functions such as learning, memory, and the control of posture.

Until the early 1980s, muscarinic receptors seemed to represent a fairly homogeneous class of receptors, although pharmacological evidence to the contrary had actually existed since the early 1950s. Unequivocal evidence for muscarinic receptor heterogeneity came in the late 1980s when five different subtypes of the muscarinic receptor were identified using molecular biological techniques (6,42,43,54,60,62). This result was somewhat of a surprise because, up to that time, only three subtypes of the muscarinic receptor could be reasonably identified using selective muscarinic antagonists.

The aims of this chapter are to review the pharmacology and molecular biology of the muscarinic class of acetylcholine receptors and to describe their distribution in the brain and the methods that are currently in use to study these receptors. In addition, the implications for the treatment of neuropsychiatric disease will be mentioned.

EARLY PHARMACOLOGICAL EVIDENCE FOR SUBTYPES OF THE MUSCARINIC RECEPTOR

The first evidence for subtypes of the muscarinic receptor came soon after the introduction of gallamine as an adjunct in general anesthesia when it was noted that this neuromuscular blocking agent caused sinus tachycardia as a side effect (74). The results of experiments on isolated tissues showed that, while gallamine opposed the negative inotropic and chronotropic effects of acetylcholine on the heart, it was much less effective at antagonizing the actions of muscarinic agonists on intestinal smooth muscle (12,64). Other neuromuscular blocking agents were identified which shared the cardioselective antimuscarinic effects of gallamine (64). Thus, muscarinic receptors in the heart appeared to be different from those located at other sites in smooth muscle and exocrine glands. In an elegant series of experiments, Clark and Mitchelson (12) and Stockton et al. (67) demonstrated that the blocking action of gallamine on the heart differed from competitive inhibition, but could be rationalized by an allosteric mechanism. Thus, the pharmacological specificity of muscarinic receptors is determined not only by the primary recognition site where acetylcholine binds but also by the secondary allosteric site where gallamine binds.

F. J. Ehlert: Department of Pharmacology, College of Medicine, University of California, Irvine, California 92717.

W. R. Roeske: Department of Medicine, College of Medicine, University of Arizona, Tucson, Arizona 85724.

H. I. Yamamura: Department of Pharmacology, College of Medicine, University of Arizona, Tucson, Arizona 85724.

TABLE 1. *Subtypes of the muscarinic receptor*

Nomenclature					
Molecular:	m1	m2	m3	m4	m5
Pharmacological:	M1	M2	M3		
Selective antagonists:	Pirenzepine	AF-DX 116	HHSiD	—	—
	Telenzepine	Gallamine	p-F-HHSiD		
Tissue distribution:	Brain	Heart	Exocrine glands	Lung	
	Autonomic ganglia	Smooth muscle	Smooth muscle	Striatum	
				Olfactory tubercle	

Evidence for additional complexity in muscarinic receptor heterogeneity came in the early 1960s when Rowskowski (65) described the properties of the novel compound, McN-A-343, which had properties of a muscarinic ganglionic stimulant. When injected into cats, McN-A-343 caused an increase in blood pressure which was antagonized by atropine but not by hexamethonium. This effect was shown to be caused by an action on sympathetic ganglia. Remarkably, McN-A-343 was almost completely inactive at other muscarinic sites, including heart and smooth muscle. Thus, as early as 1961, pharmacological evidence for three subtypes of the muscarinic receptor existed: (i) muscarinic receptors in sympathetic ganglia triggering a rise in blood pressure, (ii) muscarinic receptors on pacemaker cells mediating a slowing in heart rate, and (iii) muscarinic receptors eliciting contraction in smooth muscle. For the most part, the subsequent development of selective pharmacological agents has served to reinforce the designation of these three subtypes of the muscarinic receptor, although additional subtypes have been identified through gene cloning (see below).

Perhaps the first time that strong pharmacological evidence for the existence of subtypes of the muscarinic receptor appeared was in the early 1980s when the novel binding properties of the selective muscarinic antagonist pirenzepine were first described. This compound had been in use in Europe as an antiulcer drug. Unlike other muscarinic antagonists, it blocked gastric acid and pepsinogen secretion at doses which had little or no influence on intestinal motility, salivary secretions, and heart rate (56). It was shown subsequently that pirenzepine bound with high affinity to a subclass of the muscarinic receptor that was abundant in the cerebrum and in peripheral ganglia, whereas it displayed intermediate binding affinity for receptors in exocrine glands and low affinity for receptors

in the heart (34,35). Pirenzepine was shown to block the pressor response to McN-A-343 with high potency, whereas it only weakly antagonized the bradycardia caused by vagal stimulation (35). In contrast, more conventional muscarinic antagonists, such as N-methylscopolamine (NMS), are approximately equipotent at blocking these two effects. A variety of subsequent pharmacological experiments have demonstrated that pirenzepine can be used to divide muscarinic receptors into the same three classes mentioned above, namely, a major subtype in brain and peripheral ganglia (high affinity for pirenzepine), a cardiac subtype (low affinity for pirenzepine), and a subtype mediating responses in exocrine glands and smooth muscle (intermediate affinity for pirenzepine). These three subtypes of the muscarinic receptor are known as M1, M2, and M3, respectively. A complete definition of muscarinic receptor subtypes is given below (also see Table 1).

In addition to the agents mentioned above, several other muscarinic antagonists have been useful in the classification of muscarinic receptor subtypes. Some compounds, such as 4-diphenylacetoxy-N-methylpiperidine methiodide (4-DAMP) and hexahydrosiladifenidol (HHSiD), were shown to antagonize M3-mediated contractions of intestinal smooth muscle more potently than M2-mediated cardiac responses, which led to their designation as M3-selective antagonists (2,47). However, these compounds actually exhibit high affinity for all subtypes of the muscarinic receptor except the M2, indicating that they are more appropriately defined as non-M2 antagonists. Another group of compounds, including gallamine and AF-DX 116 (11-[2-[(diethylamino)-methyl]-1-piperidinyl]acetyl-5,11-dihydro-6H-pyrido-[2,3b][1,4]benzodiazepine-6-one), exhibit the converse selectivity—that is, high affinity for M2 muscarinic receptors and low affinity for the other subtypes (59). It is important to note that, whereas gallamine has high affinity for the secondary allosteric site on M2 muscarinic receptors, AF-DX 116 exhibits high affinity for the primary recognition site where acetylcholine, atropine, and other competitive agents bind.

In general, none of the currently available muscarinic antagonists is highly selective. Typically, most of the compounds only exhibit about a 10-fold difference in affinity between the subtype for which they are selective and the other subtypes (see Tables 2 and 3). Conse-

TABLE 2. *Dissociation constants of subtype selective muscarinic antagonists in transfected murine fibroblasts[a]*

Antagonists	−Log (K_D)				
	M1	M2	M3	M4	M5
Atropine	9.29	9.00	9.28	9.66	9.43
Pirenzepine	7.89	6.38	6.72	7.07	7.06
AF-DX 116	6.27	7.04	5.95	6.54	5.66
HHSiD	7.85	6.71	7.99	7.69	7.37
4-DAMP	8.92	8.21	9.19	9.15	8.92

[a] Data were taken from Kashihara et al. (41).

TABLE 3. *Dissociation constants of subtype selective antagonists for native muscarinic receptors*[a]

	$-\text{Log}\ (K_D)$					
	M1		M2		M3	
Antagonists	Binding	Function	Binding	Function	Binding	Function
Atropine	9.4	9.3	9.1	9.0	9.5	9.1
Pirenzepine	8.0	8.0	6.1	6.5	6.6	6.9
AF-DX 116	6.5	6.9	7.3	7.2	6.0	6.2
HHSiD	7.8	7.7	6.7	6.4	8.1	7.9
4-DAMP	9.1	9.1	8.2	7.8	8.9	8.8

[a] The binding data were taken from Pedder et al. (59), except for the values for 4-DAMP which were taken from Delmendo et al. (14). The functional estimates are the means of values taken from Barlow et al. (2), Eltze (22), Giachetti et al. (30), and Lambrecht et al. (47). Other details are given in the text.

quently, it is necessary to employ a group of antagonists to characterize a particular pharmacological response before it can be concluded what receptor subtype is involved. Unfortunately, there are no agonists available which have strong subtype-selectivity. The agonist, McN-A-343, is moderately M1-selective (37) and is very useful as a tool to activate M1 receptors in a few pharmacological assays; however, its selectivity is insufficient for widespread application as a standard M1 agonist. The problem in the use of agonists is that a high degree of selectivity is required to overcome the variation in receptor reserve (i.e., the differences in receptor density and the efficiency of coupling of a receptor to a particular response) that exists in different tissues. This variation in signal amplification can lead to large variations in agonist potency which are unrelated to differences in the ability of the agonist to discriminate among receptor subtypes.

CLONING OF MUSCARINIC RECEPTOR GENES

In 1986, Numa and his colleagues (42,43) cloned the m1 and m2 subtypes of the muscarinic receptor by screening cDNA libraries prepared from porcine cerebrum and heart, respectively. These libraries were screened with degenerate oligonucleotide probes that were synthesized to correspond with sequence information obtained from partial tryptic digests of the muscarinic receptor purified from porcine cerebrum and heart using the affinity chromatography procedure developed by Haga and Haga (33). In the next year, three more receptor subtypes (m3–m5) were cloned by screening both cDNA and genomic libraries under low-stringency conditions using oligonucleotide probes corresponding to regions of high homology between the m1 and m2 sequences (6,54,62). On the basis of the pharmacological properties of the expressed recombinant receptors and the distribution of their mRNA (55), it appears that the m1, m2, and m3 cloned subtypes correspond to the M1, M2, and M3 subtypes identified using pharmacological procedures (see below). The current convention is to use an uppercase "M" or a lowercase "m" to designate subtypes depending upon whether pharmaco-

logical (M) or molecular biological (m) criteria are used to identify the subtype. However, because there is correspondence between the two classification schemes with regard to the first three subtypes, we will use a single "uppercase" scheme throughout the rest of this chapter to avoid confusion.

The relationship between the pharmacological and molecular biological classification schemes for subtypes of the muscarinic receptor is summarized in Table 1. The M1 subtype exhibits high affinity for pirenzepine and is abundant in forebrain and sympathetic ganglia (21,32, 35,41,82). The M2 subtype has high affinity for AF-DX 116 and gallamine and is expressed in the mammalian myocardium, where it accounts for essentially the total muscarinic receptor population (41,70). The M2 receptor is also expressed at a relatively low, uniform density throughout the brain (21,82), and, surprisingly, it represents the major muscarinic receptor in smooth muscle (11). It does not participate directly in the contraction of smooth muscle, but it does modulate contraction by preventing the effects of smooth muscle relaxants, such as isoproterenol and forskolin (69). The M3 muscarinic receptor has high affinity for the non-M2 antagonists, HHSiD and 4-DAMP, and represents the major muscarinic receptor in exocrine glands (41,59). It also triggers direct contractions of smooth muscle; however, it only represents a minor fraction of total muscarinic receptor population in most smooth muscles (11). Finally, it is expressed in relatively low density throughout the brain (82). The M4 muscarinic receptor also has high affinity for 4-DAMP and HHSiD in addition to himbacine (41). It represents the major muscarinic receptor in the peripheral lung of rabbits (48), but not humans (5) and rats (27). It is also expressed abundantly in various regions of the forebrain, particularly the corpus striatum and olfactory tubercle (82). The M5 muscarinic receptor also has high affinity for the non-M2 antagonists 4-DAMP and HHSiD and is typified by its low affinity for AF-DX 116 (41). It does not appear to be expressed to any significant extent in peripheral tissues, and it represents less than 2% of the total density of muscarinic receptors in various regions of the brain (82).

STRUCTURAL IMPLICATIONS OF THE PRIMARY SEQUENCE

Analysis of the primary sequences of the muscarinic subtypes shows that these receptors are members of a superfamily of genes including the opsins and numerous receptors which signal through G proteins (6,42). A more complete description of G proteins is given in Chapters 11, 27, and 38, in the section entitled "Signal Transduction and GTP-Binding Proteins." This family of receptors is typified by the presence of seven hydrophobic regions in their sequence which are thought to form alpha helixes which span the membrane (see Fig. 1). The transmembrane (TM) segments of the muscarinic receptor represent the regions of highest homology among the different subtypes and across other members of this large family of G-protein-linked receptors. If the sequences of the five subtypes of the muscarinic receptor are aligned to achieve maximum identity, it can be seen that differences in the lengths of the sequences arise from differences in the

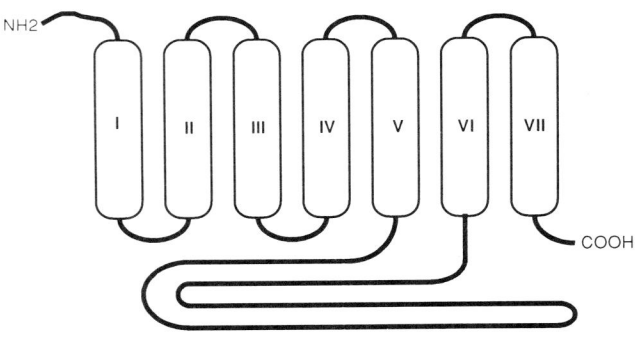

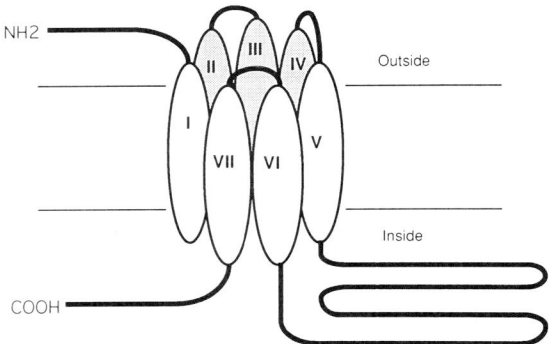

FIG. 1. Structure of the muscarinic receptor. **Top:** The sequence of the muscarinic receptor is illustrated schematically. The sequence contains seven transmembrane-spanning (TM) domains that are labeled with Roman numerals. The seven TM segments are connected together via three extracellular loops and three intracellular loops. The protein has an extracellular amino terminis and an intracellular carboxy terminis. **Bottom:** The hypothetical arrangement of the seven TM segments within the plane of the membrane.

extracellular amino terminis, the cytoplasmic carboxy terminis, and the third intracellular (i3) loop. The remaining portions of the protein—namely, the seven TM segments, the three extracellular loops, and the first two cytoplasmic loops—are all the same length. There is 63% identity among the amino acids of seven TM segments of the human M1–M5 subtypes, and most of the remaining residues in these segments are conservative replacements. The greatest divergence arises from the third cytoplasmic (i3) loop. This loop varies in length from 156 (M1) to 239 (M3) residues in the five human sequences, and it accounts for 34–45% of the total number of amino acids. A comparison of the sequences shows that the M1, M3, and M5 subtypes show maximum homology with each other, whereas the M2 and M4 subtypes constitute a separate homologous group.

The overall structure of the muscarinic receptor and other G-protein-linked receptors has not been determined, but it seems likely that it might be analogous to that of bacteriorhodopsin, the only member of this family whose structure has been determined (25). Accordingly, the seven TM segments are thought to form the staves of a barrel-like structure having a central pore (see Fig. 1). Using a "helical wheel" model of the muscarinic receptor, Hulme et al. (38) have predicted that most of the conserved residues in the TM segments form the inner lining of the central pore, whereas the few nonconserved residues are on the outside. Acetylcholine and other muscarinic ligands are thought to bind at a site within this pore, and Hulme et al. (38) have pointed to the highly conserved nature of the central pore as the explanation for the present lack of highly selective muscarinic agonist and antagonists. As described below, large molecules [i.e., antibodies and toxins (63)] showing a high degree of discrimination among the subtypes have been developed; however, these agents interact with more nonconserved regions of the receptor.

LIGAND BINDING SITE

It has long been known that muscarinic agonists require a positive charge to be active (10,36). This cationic requirement is also shared by many muscarinic antagonists, and it suggests the existence of a complementary anionic site on the muscarinic receptor (4,18). On the basis of the pH dependence of the binding of the muscarinic agonist [^{3}H]cis-dioxolane to cerebral muscarinic receptors, it was speculated that a carboxylic acid group forms the anionic site on the muscarinic receptor (20). There is now convincing evidence that the carboxyl group from a highly conserved aspartic acid residue in the third TM segment of the muscarinic receptor (aspartic acid 105, human M1 sequence) provides the negative charge for ligand binding. This evidence includes the results of peptide mapping and sequencing studies indicating that [^{3}H]propylbenzilylcholine mustard ([^{3}H]PrBCM) covalently attaches itself to cognate aspartic acids 105 and 111 in the M1 and M4 sequences, respectively (39). The site of covalent attachment of [^{3}H]PrBCM to the muscarinic receptor is likely to be the anionic site involved in ligand binding because the chemically reactive aziridinium group of [^{3}H]PrBCM is structurally similar to the quaternary ammonium head group of many muscarinic ligands including benzilylcholine itself. Moreover, mutation of aspartate 105 to an asparaginine in the M1 sequence abolished ligand binding and the phosphoinositide response, whereas point mutations in the other conserved aspartic acids at positions 71, 99, and 122 in the M1 sequence had little or no effect on ligand binding (26).

Site-directed mutagenesis studies have also shown that conserved threonine and tyrosine residues are essential for agonist, but not antagonist, affinity. Point mutations in threonine 234 and tyrosine 506 in the M3 sequence caused 40- and 60-fold reductions, respectively, in the binding affinity of acetylcholine for M3 muscarinic receptors without affecting the binding of the antagonist, [^{3}H]*N*-methylscopolamine ([^{3}H]NMS) (78,79). Interestingly, although these residues are on TM segments V (threonine 234) and VI (tyrosine 506), the molecular modeling studies of Brann et al. (7) suggest that both residues are adjacent to the conserved aspartic acid 105 (M1) in TM segment III. Collectively, these results provide an internally consistent picture of the residues involved with the binding of acetylcholine.

SIGNALING MECHANISMS OF MUSCARINIC RECEPTOR SUBTYPES

It appears that the structural properties of the individual subtypes of the muscarinic receptor determine, in part, their signaling mechanism (see Chapter 11, *this volume*, for a more complete description of muscarinic receptor signaling mechanisms). Presumably, this specificity arises as a result of the selective coupling of the receptor subtypes to G proteins. The results of studies in which the individual receptor genes were transfected into cells previously lacking muscarinic receptors have demonstrated that the M1, M3, and M5 subtypes stimulate phosphoinositide hydrolysis, whereas activation of the M2 and M4 subtypes causes a pertussis-toxin-sensitive inhibition of adenylate cyclase (1,44,46,53,61). In most instances, the muscarinic phosphoinositide response is insensitive to pertussis toxin. However, in a few cells a pertussis-toxin-sensitive phosphoinositide response has been observed for M1 receptors (57). These observations imply that at least two types of G proteins are involved in the muscarinic phosphoinositide response. It can be seen from the foregoing observations that, at least in general terms, muscarinic receptors can be divided into two categories depending upon whether they inhibit adenylate cyclase activity (M2 and M4) or cause a robust stimulation of phosphoinositide hydrolysis (M1, M3, and M5). Interest-

ingly, muscarinic receptor subtypes can be divided into the same two groups on the basis of sequence homology (see above).

The pattern of selective receptor coupling seen in transfected cells is also apparent in various tissues expressing a mixture of receptor subtypes. For example, the phosphoinositide response in the rat cerebral cortex is potently antagonized by the M1-selective antagonist pirenzepine (31). In smooth muscle, the phosphoinositide response is potently antagonized by HHSiD, but not by pirenzepine, which indicates the involvement of M3 receptors (11). In contrast, inhibition of adenylate cyclase in mammalian heart and intestinal smooth muscle is potently antagonized by the M2-selective antagonist AF-DX 116 (11). Interestingly, muscarinic agonists inhibit adenylate cyclase in the corpus striatum, yet the pharmacological profile of this response does not agree with the M1, M2, or M3 subclasses (19). Consequently, it is likely that the M4 receptor mediates this response in the corpus striatum, a conclusion that is supported by the great abundance of M4 receptors in this region (see below).

The division of the receptor subtypes into two categories based on coupling mechanisms seems inherently accurate even though several empirical observations would appear unadaptable to this scheme. For example, M2 and M4 muscarinic receptors have been shown to stimulate phosphoinositide hydrolysis; however, the magnitude of the response is weak, and it only occurs in cells expressing high densities of these receptors (61). Moreover, it is sensitive to pertussis toxin (1,46), unlike the phosphoinositide response to M1, M3, and M5 receptors which is usually, but not always, pertussis-toxin-insensitive. It has also been noted that M1, M3, and M5 receptors stimulate cyclic AMP accumulation in intact cells (45,61). However, this response may be downstream from the phosphoinositide response, resulting from calcium or protein kinase C activation of adenylate cyclase. The discovery that the $\beta\gamma$ subunits of heterotrimeric G proteins activate the type II and IV adenylate cyclases (28,68) provides another mechanism for muscarinic enhancement of adenylate cyclase activity that could be demonstrable in a broken cell preparation. This mechanism is dependent upon simultaneous activation by the α subunit of G$_S$ (stimulatory guanine-nucleotide-binding protein) and may represent the mechanism by which M4 muscarinic receptors stimulate adenylate cyclase activity in homogenates of the olfactory tubercle (58). In addition to the second messenger pathways mentioned above, muscarinic receptors can affect inwardly rectifying potassium channels by direct G-protein coupling [see Jones (40)].

An interesting difference between the two signaling groups of muscarinic receptors mentioned above is that M2- and M4-mediated inhibition of adenylate cyclase activity is practically always much more sensitive than M1, M3, and M5-stimulated phosphoinositide hydrolysis (3,11). That is, the potency of agonists (such as carbachol and oxotremorine) for inhibiting adenylate cyclase activity is usually much greater than their respective potencies for stimulating phosphoinositide hydrolysis. This difference in sensitivity cannot be rationalized by assuming that these agonists are M2-selective, because the binding affinities of carbachol and oxotremorine for M2 and M3 receptors are practically the same when measured under physiological conditions [i.e., in the presence of GTP and physiological concentrations of salt; see Ehlert (16)]. Also, these agonists are not M2-selective on the basis of efficacy in the sense that each agonist has the same relative efficacy at M2- and M3-mediated responses, although the intrinsic efficacy of carbachol is greater than that of oxotremorine (16). There is evidence that the difference in sensitivity is related to G-protein activation. Lazareno et al. (49) have noted that nonselective muscarinic agonists are at least 10-fold more potent at stimulating $[^{35}S]$-GTPγS binding and GTPase activity at M2 and M4 muscarinic receptors as compared to M1 and M3 receptors. Also, several investigators have noted that guanine nucleotides cause a greater reduction in agonist affinity at M2 and M4 receptors as compared to M1 and M3 receptors [e.g., see Baumgold and Drobnick (3)]. Thus, the M2 and M4 receptors can cause a greater activation of G proteins as compared to the M1 and M3 receptors, which might explain the difference in sensitivity between the two second messenger responses. This difference could be caused by either (a) structural differences in the receptors and their complementary G proteins or (b) differences in the size of the G-protein pool with which the receptors interact. For example, a greater expression of G_i relative to G_q might cause a more sensitive M2-mediated inhibition of adenylate cyclase as compared to M3-stimulated phosphoinositide hydrolysis.

Although the mechanism for this coupling difference is unclear, it is tempting to speculate that it maintains the sensitivity of the M2 and M4 signaling pathways in the body. Many receptor signaling pathways have a series or cascade of events between the initial receptor activation and the final cellular response. This cascade provides many opportunities for amplification in the signaling process so that a relatively low level of receptor activation can elicit a near maximal response. This situation appears to reflect M3-mediated contractions of smooth muscle, where a low level of receptor occupancy by an efficacious agonist can lead to a maximum contractile response [see Candell et al. (11)]. In other words, the final response can be highly amplified without having a very sensitive initial transduction mechanism (i.e., phosphoinositide hydrolysis). In contrast, M2 and M4 signaling pathways do not typically exhibit many steps in the signaling cascade. The M2-mediated increase in potassium conductance in pacemaker cells of the heart is the result of direct G-protein coupling to potassium channels. In other words, there is only one step in the signaling pathway between G-protein activation and an increase in potassium conductance. If this hyperpolarizing response is to be as sensitive as M3-mediated contractions of smooth muscle, then the M2

activation of G proteins must be highly amplified. It is also possible that M2 and M4 activation of G_i must be highly amplified in order to achieve a sensitive and effective physiological antagonism of responses elicited by an increase in cyclic AMP by G_s-linked receptors.

STRUCTURAL DETERMINANTS OF G-PROTEIN COUPLING

A variety of evidence indicates that the i3 loop of the muscarinic receptor is important for G-protein coupling. Perhaps the most spectacular evidence of this sort comes from a study on a chimeric receptor in which the entire i3 loop of the D_2 dopamine receptor was replaced with the analogous portion from the M1 muscarinic receptor (24). The chimeric receptor bound dopaminergic ligands with affinities similar to those of native D_2 dopamine receptors. However, unlike the native receptor, which typically inhibits adenylate cyclase and has little influence on Ca^{2+}, the chimeric receptor increased intracellular Ca^{2+} levels in response to dopamine. These data indicate that the i3 loop of the M1 muscarinic receptor is involved in coupling the receptor to G proteins which ultimately trigger calcium mobilization, presumably through phosphoinositide hydrolysis. Conversely, the M1 muscarinic receptor can be persuaded to stimulate adenylate cyclase activity via G_s if its i3 loop is replaced with that of the β-adrenergic receptor (80).

Studies on chimeric receptors constructed from different subtypes of the muscarinic receptor provide further evidence that the i3 loop plays a major role in determining whether the receptor couples to stimulation of phosphoinositide hydrolysis or to inhibition of adenylate cyclase. Replacement of the i3 loop of the M2 receptor with the corresponding portion of the M3 receptor resulted in an M2/M3-i3 chimer which, like the native M3 receptor, stimulated phosphoinositide hydrolysis in a pertussis-toxin-insensitive manner but did not inhibit adenylate cyclase (77). In contrast, when the i3 loop of the M3 receptor is replaced with the corresponding M2 sequence, the resulting M3/M2-i3 chimer has the coupling properties of a native M2 receptor; that is, it inhibits adenylate cyclase and causes a weak, pertussis-toxin-sensitive stimulation of phosphoinositide hydrolysis (77). Similar results have been obtained with M1/M2 chimeric receptors. Lai et al. (45) have constructed three chimeric M1/M2 receptors having splices between M1 and M2 sequence in TM segments IV and VI and have also found that the i3 loop has a major role in determining functional coupling. In these studies, the coupling behavior of the chimeric receptors could be predicted from the source of the i3 loop. The two chimeric receptors having M2 sequence in the i3 loop had no effect on phosphoinositide hydrolysis but inhibited adenylate cyclase activity, whereas the chimeric receptor having M1 sequence in the i3 loop stimulated phosphoinositide hydrolysis and increased, rather than decreased, cyclic AMP accumulation. The increase in cyclic AMP accumulation caused by this chimeric M2/M1 receptor was actually fourfold greater than that caused by the native M1 receptor, yet the maximum phosphoinositide response of the same chimeric receptor was only 30% that of the M1 response. These observations suggest that the increase in cyclic AMP is triggered by a mechanism distinct from phosphoinositide hydrolysis.

An interesting property of the i3 loop of the muscarinic receptors is that it contains an abundance of charged residues, particularly in the regions adjacent to TM segments V and VI. These residues make up approximately 30% of the total number of residues in the i3 loop of the various subtypes. Moreover, there is an excess (35–127%) of positive charge relative to negative in the i3 loop. This excess of positive charge also applies to the two other cytoplasmic loops and the cytoplasmic carboxy terminis. The positively charged nature of the i3 loop is striking when one considers that some highly negatively charged compounds have been shown to uncouple M2 muscarinic receptors as well as other G-protein-linked receptors. These compounds, including heparin, dextran sulfate, and trypan blue, have been shown to prevent M2-receptor-mediated inhibition of adenylate cyclase activity (29). These compounds also reduce high-affinity agonist binding to M2 muscarinic receptors in the heart without influencing antagonist binding (29). The high-affinity agonist receptor complex is thought to represent the receptor–G-protein complex (16). Collectively, these results are consistent with the postulate that heparin, dextran sulfate, and trypan blue uncouple M2 muscarinic receptors from G_i. Perhaps these highly negatively charged compounds bind to the abundant, positively charged residues on the i3 loop and sterically hinder the association of the receptor and G protein.

PHARMACOLOGICAL PROPERTIES OF THE SUBTYPES OF THE MUSCARINIC RECEPTOR

Defining the pharmacological properties of the subtypes of the muscarinic receptor is an important goal because it provides a means of establishing the function of these receptors in the body and fosters the development of useful drugs for medicine and basic research. At the present time, none of the currently available muscarinic antagonists is selective enough to block a response mediated by one subtype completely without also dampening responses mediated by the other subtypes. Consequently, when assessing the ability of an antagonist to interfere with a muscarinic response, it is essential to apply the principles of competitive antagonism (or, if appropriate, allosterism; see ref. 17) to estimate the dissociation constant (K_D) of the antagonist. This functional estimate of K_D can then be compared with that measured in competitive radioligand binding experiments on cells transfected with subtypes of the muscarinic receptor. A match between

the functional values and the binding affinity profile of a receptor subtype provides strong evidence that the subtype mediates the response. Although the discriminatory power of hybridization and immunoprecipitation techniques greatly exceeds that of competitive muscarinic antagonists, the former methods are used primarily to identify which receptors are present in a tissue. The identification of the major receptor subtype in a given tissue does not constitute proof that this is the subtype which mediates the response of the tissue. For example, the techniques of ligand binding (11), immunoprecipitation (52), and Northern analysis (55) all demonstrate that the major muscarinic receptor in intestinal smooth muscle is the M2. However, the pharmacology of the contractile response is inconsistent with the idea that M2 receptors mediate contraction. Rather, the functional K_D values of muscarinic antagonists in the intestine are in close agreement with the binding properties of recombinant m3 muscarinic receptors and a minor population of binding sites in the intestine (11). Thus, using several different techniques it is possible to conclude with certainty that M3 muscarinic receptors mediate contraction of intestinal smooth muscle.

Antagonist Binding Properties of Recombinant Subtypes of the Muscarinic Receptor

The binding affinities of selective muscarinic antagonists for subtypes of the muscarinic receptor have been estimated in competitive binding assays on cells transfected with the M1 through M5 genes. Table 2 shows a compilation of results from studies in which the competitive inhibition of [^{3}H]N-methylQNB binding by various antagonists was measured in murine fibroblasts transfected with recombinant rat muscarinic receptors (41,57). An important feature of these particular studies is that the binding assay was carried out at 37°C in tissue culture media so that the ionic composition of the assay buffer resembles physiological conditions. It can be seen that none of the compounds shows greater than a sixfold difference in affinity between the receptor for which it has highest affinity and the other subtypes. Pirenzepine has highest affinity for M1 receptors ($pK_i = 7.9$), intermediate affinity for M3, M4, and M5 receptors ($pK_i \approx 7.0$), and low affinity for m2 receptors ($pK_i = 6.4$). AF-DX 116 has highest affinity for M2 receptors ($pK_i = 7.0$), intermediate affinity for M4 receptors ($pK_i = 6.5$), and low affinity for M1, M3, and M5 ($pK_i \approx 6.0$). Both HHSiD and 4-DAMP have high affinities for all the subtypes except the M2. The data shown in Table 2 are generally consistent with the results of similar studies by Buckley et al. (9) and Dörje et al. (15) which were carried out in 25 mM phosphate buffer containing 5 mM $MgCl_2$. The biggest discrepancy is in the affinity values of AF-DX 116. This difference can probably be attributed to differences in the assay buffer, because Pedder et al. (59) have demonstrated that the affinity of AF-DX 116 is markedly influenced by ionic strength.

Antagonist Binding Properties of Native Muscarinic Receptor Subtypes in Various Tissues of the Rat

The binding affinities of selective muscarinic antagonists have also been measured in tissues of the rat expressing predominantly one receptor subtype. A convenient means of measuring the binding properties of M1 muscarinic receptors is to run competition experiments in the rat cerebral cortex using a low concentration of [^{3}H]-pirenzepine to label M1 receptors selectively (76). The binding properties of M2 receptors can be easily measured by running competitive binding experiments on the mammalian heart which expresses M2 receptors exclusively (70). M3 receptors can be assessed by running experiments on various exocrine glands. Table 3 gives the dissociation constant of various muscarinic antagonist for M1, M2, and M3 muscarinic receptors measured in binding studies on the rat using the strategy described above (14,59). The binding assays were carried out at 30–32°C, in a buffer having an ionic strength similar to physiological conditions. It can be seen that the results in Table 3 are in excellent agreement with those shown in Table 2, indicating that the murine fibroblast transfection system provides an accurate pharmacological picture of native muscarinic receptor subtypes. None of the values in the two tables differ by more than 1.9-fold (0.28 log units; see pirenzepine, M2, and 4-DAMP, M3). The average of the absolute values of the differences between the estimates in the two tables is only 0.14 log units (i.e., 1.4-fold), and the standard deviation of this estimate is 0.09 log units.

It is informative to compare the estimates of affinity made in binding assays with those obtained from the results of antagonism studies on tissues whose functional responses are thought to be mediated by the M1, M2, and M3 subtypes of the muscarinic receptor. The functional assay system that is commonly used to screen for M1 antagonism is the rabbit vas deferens, where the M1 agonist, McN-A-343, causes an inhibition of the twitch response elicited by transmural stimulation (22,23,47). The standard assay for the M2 receptor is the electrically paced or spontaneously beating guinea-pig atria which exhibits a decrease in contractile force or in beating rate, respectively, when stimulated by muscarinic agonists (2,22,30,47). Finally, the M3 system that is commonly used is the isolated guinea-pig ileum which contracts to muscarinic agonists (2,30,47). The K_D values that have been measured for subtype-selective muscarinic antagonists in the functional assays described above are listed in Table 3 together with the estimates of K_D from binding studies on tissues of the rat. It can be seen that there is general agreement between the two estimates, which validates the use of the biological assay system.

DISTRIBUTION OF MUSCARINIC RECEPTOR SUBTYPES IN THE BRAIN

The distribution of subtypes of the muscarinic receptor in the brain has been mapped out using a variety of methods. Radioligand binding techniques provided the first direct demonstration of the distribution of muscarinic receptors in the brain and also provided a reasonable picture of the distribution of the major subtypes. More recently, the development of subtype-selective antibodies for the M1–M5 subtypes has provided an unequivocal demonstration of the regional distribution of the subtypes in the brain. In general, there is striking agreement between the results of the two methods. Finally the results of in situ hybridization studies have demonstrated that the distribution of mRNA for the subtypes generally parallels the distribution of their protein. Convergence of the results of several types of methodologies to the same conclusion is gratifying and provides a strong validation of the results. In the remainder of this section, the distribution of muscarinic receptors in the brain will be described by reviewing the results of studies using the variety of techniques mentioned above.

Radioligand Binding Studies

Early studies on the binding properties of the muscarinic antagonist [^{3}H](−)QNB established the distribution of muscarinic receptors in the brain (81). These studies showed that the density of muscarinic receptors was highest in various regions of the forebrain but declined in more caudal regions of the brain. In general, the distribution of ligand binding paralleled the distribution of other cholinergic markers such as acetylcholinesterase, cholineacetyltransferase, and high-affinity choline uptake. These results provided convincing evidence for the distribution of the total density of muscarinic receptors in the brain because [^{3}H](−)QNB was highly specific for muscarinic receptors, and it labeled all subtypes of the muscarinic receptor uniformly.

By measuring the ability of subtype-selective muscarinic antagonists to inhibit the binding of a nonselective radioligand competitively, it was possible to identify subtypes of the muscarinic receptor in brain and to establish their regional distribution. The results of studies in brain where the specific binding of [^{3}H]NMS was competitively inhibited by the M1-selective antagonist pirenzepine demonstrated that the resulting pirenzepine/[^{3}H]NMS competition curves were inconsistent with a simple one-site model but could be rationalized by a model incorporating two sites with differential affinity for pirenzepine (21,32). The proportion of high-affinity pirenzepine sites was highest in the forebrain and lowest in more caudal regions of the brain. When similar studies were carried out with the M2-selective antagonist AF-DX 116, analogous results were obtained except that the proportion of high-affinity AF-DX 116 sites showed exactly the converse distribution as that of the high-affinity pirenzepine sites (21,32). That is, sites with high affinity for AF-DX 116 represented the majority of the muscarinic receptors in the cerebellum and a minor fraction of the receptors in more rostral regions of the brain. These results were also verified by direct binding studies with [³H]pirenzepine (76) and [³H]AF-DX 116 (75). Collectively, these results demonstrated that M1 receptors represented the majority of the muscarinic sites in the forebrain, whereas the M2 receptor was the most abundant site in more caudal regions of the brain.

Although the nature of the pirenzepine/[³H]NMS and AF-DX 116/[³H]NMS competition curves mentioned above were both consistent with two-site models, it was impossible to rationalize the competition data in terms of only two types of binding sites. The inadequacy of the two-site model was particularly apparent in the corpus

striatum, where the sum of the densities of the high-affinity binding sites for pirenzepine (M1, 31%) and AF-DX 116 (M2, 7%) only amounted to 38% of the total density of muscarinic receptors in this brain region (19). Clearly there must be a large population of sites lacking high affinity for both AF-DX 116 and pirenzepine. The simplest hypothesis to account for the data is a three-site model incorporating a high-affinity pirenzepine site (M1), a high-affinity AF-DX 116 site (M2), and third site (non-M1, non-M2) lacking high affinity for both AF-DX 116 and pirenzepine. This model predicts that AF-DX 116 has similar, but perhaps not identical, affinities for the M1 and the non-M1, non-M2 site and that pirenzepine has about the same affinities for the M2 site and the non-M1, non-M2 site.

The question then arises, What is the relationship between these three binding sites and the five cloned subtypes (M1–M5) of the muscarinic receptor? It seems clear

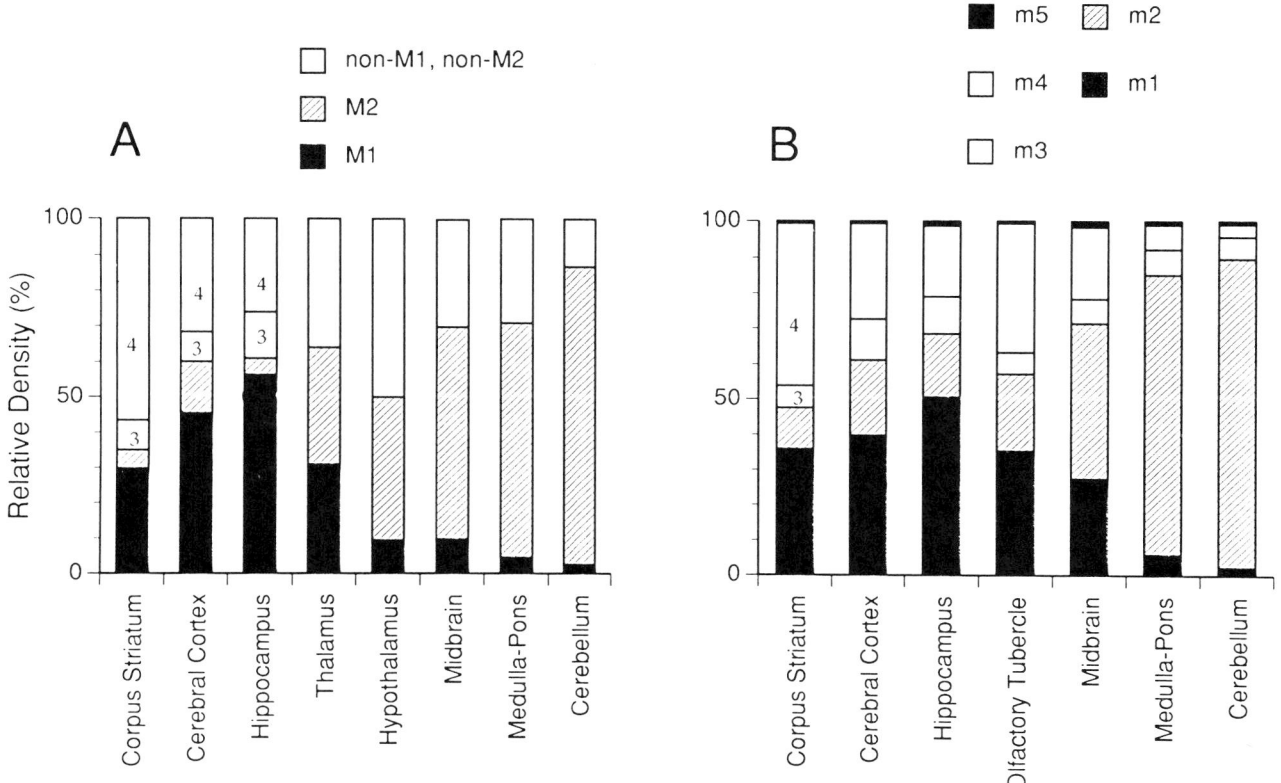

FIG. 2. Relative distribution of subtypes of the muscarinic receptor in brain. **A:** The percentage of M1, M2, and non-M1, non-M2 binding sites in the rat brain are the average of values given by Ehlert and Tran (21), Giraldo et al. (32) and Waelbroeck et al. (70). The non-M1, non-M2 class of binding sites has been further subdivided into the M3 and M4 subtypes in the cerebral cortex, corpus striatum, and hippocampus according to the estimates given by Waelbroeck et al. (71). **B:** The relative distribution of the M1 through M5 subtypes of the muscarinic receptor determined by immunoprecipitation with subtype selective antibodies. The data have been normalized with respect to the total amount of muscarinic receptors immunoprecipitated, and they have been estimated from Fig. 8 of Yasuda et al. (82). The M3 and M4 subtypes are both designated by open bars to allow easy comparison with the data in **A,** and they are designated with the numbers "3" and "4," respectively, in the corpus striatum. In all cases, the relative densities of the subtypes are shown sequentially, starting with M1 at the bottom of each bar and M5 at the top.

that the high-affinity pirenzepine and AF-DX 116 sites represent the M1 and M2 subtypes, respectively, because of the reasons described above (see Table 2). It follows that the non-M1, non-M2 site represents the remainder of the subtypes (i.e., M3, M4, and M5). However, because the results of immunoprecipitation studies with M5-selective antibodies indicate very little M5 subtype in brain (less than 2% of the total, see below), it seems appropriate to designate the non-M1, non-M2 binding site as the sum of the densities of the M3 and M4 subtypes. The consequences of this hypothesis indicate that, whereas the high-affinity component of the pirenzepine/[^{3}H]NMS competition curve in brain represents the M1 receptor, the low-affinity component is composed of the M2, M3, and M4 receptors. A comparison of the negative log of the K_D of the high-affinity pirenzepine site in rat brain (pK_H = 7.82; see ref. 21) shows good agreement with that (7.89) determined for recombinant rat M1 receptors (see Table 2). Moreover, the estimate of pK_H was essentially the same in various regions of the brain, indicating that the high-affinity component of pirenzepine binding represented a single type of site (21). In contrast, the low-affinity K_D (pK_L) of pirenzepine varied from a low value of 6.15 in the cerebellum to a high value of 6.65 in the corpus striatum. This variation is consistent with the postulate that the low-affinity component actually represents a mixture of sites whose affinities are similar, but not identical, and that the measured pK_L of pirenzepine in a given brain region represents the weighted average of pK_D values for the M2, M3, and M4 receptors (6.38, 6.72, 7.07, respectively; see Table 2). Accordingly, the low pK_L value of pirenzepine in the cerebellum (6.15) is consistent with the great abundance of M2 receptors in this tissue which have the lowest affinity for pirenzepine (pK_D = 6.38; see Table 2). Also, the high pK_L value in the corpus striatum (6.65) is consistent with the great abundance of M4 receptors in this tissue which have relatively high affinity (i.e., compared to M2 and M3) for pirenzepine (pK_D = 7.07; see Table 2). An analogous type of argument can be made for the behavior of the AF-DX 116/[^{3}H]NMS competition curves in various regions of the brain. Thus, it can be seen that the method of fitting the pirenzepine/[^{3}H]NMS and AF-DX 116/[^{3}H]-NMS competition curves to a two-site model is an approximation; nevertheless, the error associated with this technique is low as indicated by the good agreement between this method and the immunoprecipitation method described below.

The results of the studies described above on the regional binding properties of muscarinic receptors in the brain are summarized in Fig. 2. It can be seen in Fig. 2A that the proportion of M1 and non-M1, non-M2 sites (M3 + M4) was greatest in various telencephalic structures and decreased proportionately the more caudal the brain region. In contrast, the proportion of M2 sites was greatest in the cerebellum and decreased proportionately the more rostral the brain region. The actual densities of

the M1, M2, and non-M1, non-M2 sites (M3 + M4) can be calculated by multiplying their respective proportions by the total density of muscarinic receptors in various regions of the brain. Figure 3 shows the distribution of the M1, M2, and non-M1, non-M2 sites (M3 + M4) in various regions of the brain. It can be seen that in terms of absolute density, the M2 site has a relatively low uniform density throughout the brain, whereas the M1 and non-M1, non-M2 sites (M3 + M4) are most abundant in the forebrain and decrease in more caudal regions of the brain.

By taking advantage of the slow rate at which [^{3}H]NMS dissociates from M3 and M4 receptors relative to the M1 and M2 receptors, Waelbroeck et al. (71) have actually

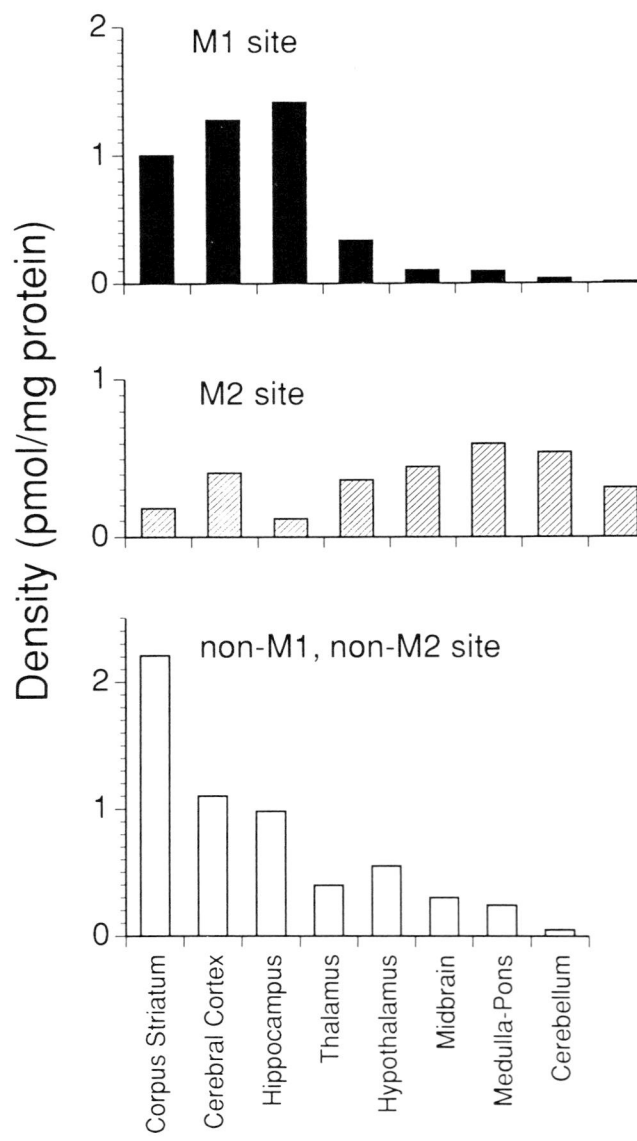

FIG. 3. Absolute densities of the M1, M2, and non-M1, non-M2 classes of muscarinic binding sites in the brain. The binding values have been calculated from the data in Fig. 2A and the total density of [^{3}H]NMS binding sites in various regions as determined by Ehlert and Tran (21).

estimated the proportion of the M3 and M4 receptors in some regions of the brain. These investigators have obtained himbacine/[³H]NMS and methoctramine/[³H]NMS competition curves after [³H]NMS has been washed off the M1 and M2 sites. Because himbacine and methoctramine have much higher affinity for M4 receptors relative to M3, it was possible to divide the non-M1, non-M2 class of sites into M3 and M4 receptors. The estimates of the proportion of M3 and M4 receptors made by Waelbroek et al. (71) in the cerebral cortex, hippocampus, and corpus striatum are also given in Fig. 2A.

Quantitative Autoradiography

Quantitative autoradiography has been used to map out the distribution of M1, M2, and non-M1, non-M2 receptors in the brain. The distributions of the M1 and M2 sites have been determined by directly labeling these receptors with [³H]pirenzepine and [³H]AF-DX 116, respectively (66). The distribution of the non-M1, non-M2 site was determined by labeling these sites with [³H]NMS in the presence of pirenzepine and AF-DX 116 so that radioligand binding to the M1 and M2 sites was blocked (66). Table 4 shows the results of a quantitative autoradiographic analysis by Smith et al. (66) in which the strategy described above was used to map out the distribution of the M1, M2, and non-M1, non-M2 subtypes in the brain. It can be seen that the M1 and the non-M1, non-M2 sites represent the most abundant receptor classes in the brain, with high densities occurring in various regions of the forebrain. In contrast, the M2 receptor has a very low, uniform distribution throughout the brain. These results are in general agreement with those shown in Figs. 2 and 3. The highest densities of M1 receptors occur in the hippocampus, various subcortical telencephalic nuclei, and various layers of the cerebral cortex. The highest densities of the non-M1, non-M2 site occur in the islands of Calleja, olfactory tubercle, caudate putamen, and nucleus accumbens. High densities also occur in other subcortical telencephalic structures, the hippocampus, and various layers of the cerebral cortex (see also Chapter 18, *this volume*).

Immunoprecipitation

The development of subtype-selective antibodies has provided a powerful means of measuring the distribution of subtypes of the muscarinic receptor in different regions of the brain. Two groups of investigators (51,82) have raised antisera to fusion proteins containing the i3 loop of the different subtypes of the muscarinic receptor. The high selectivity of these antibodies rests on the divergent nature of the i3 loop of the different subtypes of the muscarinic receptor. Wolfe and co-workers (52,72,73,82) were able to immunoprecipitate all five subtypes of the muscarinic receptor from brain. Moreover, the total

amount of receptors immunoprecipitated in various regions of the brain varied from 86% to 99% of the total amount of [³H](−)QNB binding sites. These data indicate the highly quantitative recovery of protein that is achievable using the antibodies. These data also indicate that it is unlikely that there are significant amounts of additional subtypes of the muscarinic receptor in brain because the total amount of receptors that can be immunoprecipitated

TABLE 4. *Autoradiographic analysis of the distribution of M1, M2, and non-M1, non-M2 subtypes of the muscarinic receptor in various regions of the rat brain*[a]

Brain region	Regional binding (fmol/mg tissue wet wt)		
	M1	M2	Non-M1, non-M2
Cerebral cortex			
Frontoparietal cortex, somatosensory area			
Layers I–II	244	24	292
Layers III–IV	162	9	219
Layer V	132	15	238
Layer VI	166	9	179
Primary olfactory cotex	252	9	239
Subcortical telencephalon			
Olfactory bulb, external plexiform layer	149	57	340
Anterior olfactory nucleus	254	12	270
Olfactory tubercle	193	18	413
Lateral septum	52	25	191
Medial septum	26	22	76
Vertical limb, diagonal band	41	9	86
Islands of Calleja	243	24	417
Caudate putamen	263	27	389
Nucleus accumbens	228	15	371
Basolateral amygdala	204	16	156
Lateral amygdala	181	21	177
Hippocampal subfields			
CA1, oriens	259	9	254
CA1, pyramidale	259	9	232
CA1, radiatum	259	9	279
CA3	143	6	154
Dentate gyrus	270	6	195
Diencephalon			
Ventrolateral thalamic nucleus	30	6	58
Anteroventral thalamic nucleus	39	34	166
Medial geniculate nucleus	50	6	95
Anterior hypothalamic nucleus	25	13	60
Ventromedial hypothalamic nucleus	27	12	58
Mesencephalon			
Superior colliculus	29	54	147
Inferior colliculus	22	18	61
Central gray	20	15	84
Rhombencephalon			
Motor trigeminal nucleus	—	36	57
Cerebellum lobules	—	21	—

[a] Data are from Smith et al. (66). The binding values do not represent absolute receptor densities, but rather the magnitude of radioligand binding measured under the conditions of the experiment.

from CHO cells transfected with the M1–M5 subtypes ranges from 83% to 95%.

The data in Fig. 2B show the relative distribution of the M1–M5 subtypes of the muscarinic receptor in various regions of the rat brain. The data have been estimated from Fig. 8 in the publication by Yasuda et al. (82) and have been normalized with respect to the total amount of receptors immunoprecipitated. It can be seen that there is very little M5 muscarinic receptor expressed in the brain, and that it accounts for less than 2% of the total receptor population. The M1 and M4 muscarinic receptors represent the most abundant receptors in various forebrain regions, and their relative proportion declines in more caudal regions of the brain. In contrast, the relative abundance of the M2 receptor is low in various forebrain regions; however, it represents the major receptor in more caudal regions of the brain. When the absolute densities of the subtypes of the muscarinic receptor are considered, it can be seen that the M1 and M4 subtypes are most abundant in the forebrain, and their density declines in more caudal regions of the brain. In contrast, the M2 receptor has a low, relatively uniform distribution throughout the brain. The M3 receptor is not expressed to a great extent in the brain; however, its density is greatest in the forebrain, and it decreases in more caudal regions of the brain. It can be seen by comparison of the binding data in Fig. 2A with the immunoprecipitation data in Fig. 2B that there is a striking agreement between the two sets of data.

In Situ Hybridization Histochemistry

The results of a study (8) using in situ hybridization histochemistry has demonstrated that the relative abundances of mRNA for the M1 and M4 subtypes of the muscarinic receptor are greatest in various forebrain structures such as the cerebral cortex, hippocampus, and caudate putamen and that the message for these receptors declines in more caudal regions of the brain. The abundance of M3 mRNA was greatest in the cerebral cortex and hippocampus, but low in the caudate putamen and in caudal regions of the brain. In contrast, M2 mRNA had a relatively low, uniform distribution throughout the brain. In summary, it can be seen that the distribution of mRNA for subtypes of the muscarinic receptor generally agrees with the distribution of these proteins as determined by radioligand binding and immunoprecipitation (see Fig. 2A and 2B).

CONCLUSIONS

A variety of different techniques can be used to study the pharmacology, signaling mechanisms, regional distribution, and molecular biology of subtypes of the muscarinic receptor. Molecular biological and immunological techniques have provided the most powerful methods for

the identification of subtypes of the muscarinic receptor. Moderately selective muscarinic antagonists have been developed which discriminate among the different subtypes of the muscarinic receptor. By using a panel of antagonists including pirenzepine, AF-DX 116, and HHSiD, it is possible to determine whether a given response is mediated by an M1, M2, or M3 subtype of the muscarinic receptor. If methoctramine or himbacine is used in combination with the other antagonists, it should be possible to discriminate among the M1–M4 subtypes. To date, few agonists have been developed which exhibit high selectivity for the different subtypes of the muscarinic receptor. The great abundance of M1 receptors in the cortex and hippocampus suggests that perhaps M1-selective agonists which penetrate the brain might be efficacious in the treatment of neurological conditions associated with hypocholinergic function in the forebrain (e.g., Alzheimer's disease). Moreover, the existence of a secondary allosteric site on the muscarinic receptor suggests that it might be possible to develop novel allosteric muscarinic agonists that potentiate the effects of endogenous acetylcholine much in the same way that benzodiazepines potentiate GABA. Presumably, allosteric muscarinic agonists would only activate muscarinic receptors that are occupied by acetylcholine. Consequently, they offer an advantage to muscarinic agonists which act at the primary recognition site in that they should preserve the temporal pattern of receptor activation. Moreover, overdose from an allosteric muscarinic agonist should have less disastrous consequences than a directly acting agonist, because the effect of an allosteric agonist would have a ceiling depending upon how much it potentiated endogenous acetylcholine. Although no such allosteric muscarinic agonists have been identified to date, they could be very efficacious in the treatment of Alzheimer's disease. Finally, the great abundance of M4 receptors in the caudate putamen suggests that centrally active M4-selective muscarinic antagonists might be useful in the treatment of parkinsonism. Such agents would lack the peripheral side effects of classic muscarinic antagonists which block M2- and M3-mediated responses throughout the parasympathetic nervous system. Centrally active M4-selective muscarinic antagonists might be useful in parkinsonism by themselves or as adjuncts to levodopa.

ACKNOWLEDGMENTS

Portions of the authors' work cited in this chapter were supported by National Institutes of Health grants NS-26511, NS-30882, HL-20984, and MH-45051 and by the American Heart Association. Frederick J. Ehlert is a recipient of a United States Public Health Service, Research Career Development Award from the National Institute of Neurological Disorders and Stroke.

REFERENCES

1. Ashkenazi A, Winslow JW, Peralta EG, Peterson GL, Schimerlik MI, Capon DJ, Ramachandran J. An M2 muscarinic receptor subtype coupled to both adenylyl cyclase and phosphoinositide turnover. *Science* 1987;238:672–675.
2. Barlow RB, Berry KJ, Glenton PAM, Nikolaou NM, Soh KS. A comparison of affinity constants for muscarine-sensitive acetylcholine receptors in guinea-pig atrial pacemaker cells at 29°C and in ileum at 29°C and 37°C. *Br J Pharmacol* 1976;58:613–620.
3. Baumgold J, Drobnick A. An agonist that is selective for adenylate cyclase-coupled muscarinic receptors. *Mol Pharmacol* 1989;36:465–470.
4. Birdsall NJM, Chan S-C, Eveleigh P, Hulme EC, Miller KW. The modes of binding of ligands to cardiac muscarinic receptors. *Trends Pharmacol Sci* 1990; (suppl):31–34.
5. Bloom JW, Halonen M, Yamamura HI. Characterization of muscarinic cholinergic receptor subtypes in human peripheral lung. *Mol Pharmacol* 1988;244:625–632.
6. Bonner TI, Buckley NJ, Young AC, Brann MR. Identification of a family of muscarinic acetylcholine receptor genes. *Science* 1987;237:527–532.
7. Brann MR, Klimkowski VJ, Ellis J. Structure/function relationships of muscarinic acetylcholine receptors. *Life Sci* 1993;52:405–412.
8. Buckley NJ, Bonner TI, Brann MR. Localization of a family of muscarinic receptor mRNAs in rat brain. *J Neurosci* 1988;8(12):4646–4652.
9. Buckley NJ, Bonner TI, Buckley CM, Brann MR. Antagonist binding properties of five cloned muscarinic receptors expressed in CHO-K1 cells. *Mol Pharmacol* 1989;35:469–476.
10. Burgen ASV. The role of ionic interactions at the muscarinic receptor. *Br J Pharmacol* 1965;25:4–7.
11. Candell LM, Yun SH, Tran LLP, Ehlert FJ. Differential coupling of subtypes of the muscarinic receptor to adenylate cyclase and phosphoinositide hydrolysis in the longitudinal muscle of the rat ileum. *Mol Pharmacol* 1990;38:689–697.
12. Clark AL, Mitchelson F. The inhibitory effect of gallamine on muscarinic receptors. *Br J Pharmacol* 1976;58:323–331.
13. Dale HH. The action of certain esters and ethers of choline, and their relation to muscarine. *J Pharmacol Exp Ther* 1914;6:147–190.
14. Delmendo RE, Michel AD, Whiting RL. Affinity of muscarinic receptor antagonists for three putative muscarinic receptor binding sites. *Br J Pharmacol* 1989;96:457–464.
15. Dörje F, Wess J, Lambrecht G, Tacke R, Mutschler E, Brann MR. Antagonist binding profiles of five cloned human muscarinic receptor subtypes. *J Pharmacol Exp Ther* 1991;256:727–733.
16. Ehlert FJ. The relationship between muscarinic receptor occupancy and adenylate cyclase inhibition in the rabbit myocardium. *Mol Pharmacol* 1985;28:410–421.
17. Ehlert FJ. Estimation of the affinities of allosteric ligands using radioligand binding and pharmacological null methods. *Mol Pharmacol* 1988;33:187–194.
18. Ehlert FJ, Delen FM. Influence of pH on the binding of scopolamine and *N*-methylscopolamine to muscarinic receptors in the corpus striatum and heart of rats. *Mol Pharmacol* 1990;38:143–147.
19. Ehlert FJ, Delen FM, Yun SH, Friedman DJ, Self DW. Coupling of subtypes of the muscarinic receptor to adenylate cyclase in the corpus striatum and heart. *J Pharmacol Exp Ther* 1989;251:660–671.
20. Ehlert FJ, Roeske WR, Yamamura HI. Regulation of muscarinic receptor binding by guanine nucleotides and *N*-ethylmaleimide. *J Supramol Struct* 1980;14:149–162.
21. Ehlert FJ, Tran LLP. Regional distribution of M1, M2 and non-M1, non-M2 subtypes of muscarinic binding sites in rat brain. *J Pharmacol Exp Ther* 1990;255:1148–1157.
22. Eltze M. Muscarinic M$_1$- and M$_2$-receptors mediating opposite effects on neuromuscular transmission in rabbit vas deferens. *Eur J Pharmacol* 1988;151:205–221.
23. Eltze M, Gmelin G, Wess J, Strohmann C, Tacke R, Mutschler E, Lambrecht G. Presynaptic muscarinic receptors mediating inhibition of neurogenic contractions in rabbit vas deferens are of the ganglionic M$_1$-type. *Eur J Pharmacol* 1988;158:233–242.
24. England BP, Ackerman MS, Barrett RW. A chimeric D$_2$ dopamine/m1 muscarinic receptor with D$_2$ binding specificity mobilizes intracellular calcium in response to dopamine. *FEBS Lett* 1991;279:87–90.
25. Findlay JBC, Pappin DJC. The opsin family of proteins. *Biochem J* 1986;238:625–642.
26. Fraser CM, Wang C-D, Robinson DA, Gocayne JD, Venter JC. Site-directed mutagenesis of m$_1$ muscarinic acetylcholine receptors: conserved aspartic acids play important roles in receptor function. *Mol Pharmacol* 1989;36:840–847.
27. Fryer AD, El-Fakahany EE. Identification of three muscarinic receptor subtypes in rat lung using binding studies with selective antagonists. *Life Sci* 1990;47:611–618.
28. Gao B, Gilman AG. Cloning and expression of a widely distributed (type IV) adenylyl cyclase. *Proc Natl Acad Sci USA* 1991;88:10178–10182.
29. Gerstin EH, Luong T, Ehlert FJ. Heparin, dextran and trypan blue allosterically modulate M$_2$ muscarinic receptor binding properties and interfere with receptor-mediated inhibition of adenylate cyclase. *J Pharmacol Exp Ther* 1992;263:910–917.
30. Giachetti A, Micheletti R, Montagna E. Cardioselective profile of AF-DX 116, a muscarine M$_2$ receptor antagonist. *Life Sci* 1986;38:1663–1672.
31. Gil DW, Wolfe BB. Pirenzepine distinguishes between muscarinic receptor-mediated phosphoinositide breakdown and inhibition of adenylate cyclase. *Mol Pharmacol* 1985;232:608–616.
32. Giraldo E, Hammer R, Ladinsky H. Distribution of muscarinic receptor subtypes in rat brain as determined in binding studies with AF-DX 116 and pirenzepine. *Life Sci* 40:833–840.
33. Haga K, Haga T. Purification of the muscarinic acetylcholine receptor from porcine brain. *J Biol Chem* 1985;260:7927–7935.
34. Hammer R, Berrie CP, Birdsall NJM, Burgen ASV, Hulme EC. Pirenzepine distinguishes between different subclasses of muscarinic receptors. *Nature* 1980;283:90–92.
35. Hammer R, Giachetti A. Muscarinic receptor subtypes: M1 and M2 biochemical and functional characterization. *Life Sci* 1982;31:2991–2998.
36. Hanin I, Jenden DJ, Cho AK. The influence of pH on the muscarinic action of oxotremorine, arecoline, pilocarpine, and their quaternary ammonium analogues. *Mol Pharmacol* 1966;2:352–359.
37. Hu J, El-Fakahany EE. Selectivity of McN-A-343 in stimulating phosphoinositide hydrolysis mediated by M1 muscarinic receptors. *Mol Pharmacol* 1990;38:895–903.
38. Hulme EC, Birdsall NJM, Buckley NJ. Muscarinic receptor subtypes. *Annu Rev Pharmacol Toxicol* 1990;30:633–673.
39. Hulme EC, Curtis CAM, Wheatley M, Aitken A, Harris AC. Localization and structure of the muscarinic receptor ligand binding site. *Trends Pharmacol Sci* 1990; (Suppl):22–25.
40. Jones SVP. Muscarinic receptor subtypes: modulation of ion channels. *Life Sci* 1993;52:457–464.
41. Kashihara K, Varga EV, Waite SL, Roeske WR, Yamamura HI. Cloning of the rat M3, M4 and M5 muscarinic acetylcholine receptor genes by the polymerase chain reaction (PCT) and the pharmacological characterization of the expressed genes. *Life Sci* 1992;51:955–971.
42. Kubo T, Fukuda K, Mikami A, Maeda A, Takahashi H, Mishina M, Haga T, Haga K, Ichiyama A, Kangawa K, Kojima M, Matsuo H, Hirose T, Numa S. Cloning, sequencing and expression of complementary DNA encoding the muscarinic acetylcholine receptor. *Nature* 1986;323:411–416.
43. Kubo T, Maeda A, Sugimoto K, et al. Primary structure of porcine cardiac muscarinic acetylcholine receptor deduced from the cDNA sequence. *FEBS Lett* 1986;209:367–372.
44. Lai J, Mei L, Roeske WR, Chung F-Z, Yamamura HI, Venter JC. The cloned murine M$_1$ muscarinic receptor is associated with the hydrolysis of phosphatidylinositols in transfected murine B82 cells. *Life Sci* 1988;42:2489–2502.
45. Lai J, Nunan L, Waite SL, Ma S-W, Bloom JW, Roeske WR, Yamamura HI. Chimeric M$_1$/M$_2$ Muscarinic receptors: correlation of ligand selectivity and functional coupling with structural modifications. *J Pharmacol Exp Ther* 1992;262:173–180.
46. Lai J, Waite SL, Bloom JW, Yamamura HI, Roeske WR. The m$_2$ muscarinic acetylcholine receptors are coupled to multiple signaling pathways via pertussis toxin-sensitive guanine nucleotide regulatory proteins. *J Pharmacol Exp Ther* 1991;258:938–944.
47. Lambrecht G, Feifel R, Wagner-Röder M, Strohmann C, Zilch H, Tacke R, Waelbroeck M, Christophe J, Boddeke H, Mutschler E.

Affinity profiles of hexahydro-sila-difenidol analogues at muscarinic receptor subtypes. *Eur J Pharmacol* 1989;168:71–80.

48. Lazareno S, Buckley NJ, Roberts FF. Characterization of muscarinic M_4 binding sites in rabbit lung, chicken heart, and NG108-15 cells. *Mol Pharmacol* 1990;38:805–815.

49. Lazareno S, Farries T, Birdsall NJM. Pharmacological characterization of guanine nucleotide exchange reactions in membranes from CHO cells stably transfected with human muscarinic receptors M1-M4. *Life Sci* 1993;52:449–456.

50. Lefkowitz RJ, Hoffman BB, Taylor P. Neurohumoral transmission: the autonomic and somatic motor nervous systems. In: Gilman AG, Rall TW, Nies AS, Taylor P, eds. *The pharmacological basis of therapeutics.* New York: Pergamon Press, 1990;84–121.

51. Levey AI, Kitt CA, Simonds WF, Price DL, Brann MR. Identification and localization of muscarinic acetylcholine receptor proteins in brain with subtype-specific antibodies. *J Neurosci* 1991;11:3218–3226.

52. Li M, Yasuda RP, Wall SJ, Wellstein A, Wolfe BB. Distribution of m2 muscarinic receptors in rat brain using antisera selective for m2 receptors. *Mol Pharmacol* 1991;40:28–35.

53. Liao C-F, Schilling WP, Birnbaumer M, Birnbaumer L. Cellular responses to stimulation of the M5 muscarinic acetylcholine receptor as seen in murine L cells. *J Biol Chem* 1990;265:11273–11284.

54. Liao C-F, Themmen APN, Joho R, Barberis C, Birnbaumer M, Birnbaumer L. Molecular cloning and expression of a fifth muscarinic acetylcholine receptor. *J Biol Chem* 1989;264:7328–7337.

55. Maeda A, Kubo T, Mishina M, Numa S. Tissue distribution of mRNAs encoding muscarinic acetylcholine receptor subtypes. *FEBS Lett* 1988;239:339–342.

56. Matsuo Y, Seki A. Actions of pirenzepine dihydrochloride (LS-519 Cl) on gastric juice secretion, gastric motility and experimental gastric ulcer. *Arzneimittelforsch* 1979;29:1028–1035.

57. Mei L, Lai J, Roeske WR, Fraser CM, Venter JC, Yamamura HI. Pharmacological characterization of the M_1 muscarinic receptors expressed in murine fibroblast B82 cells. *J Pharmacol Exp Ther* 1989;248:661–670.

58. Olianas MC, Onali P. Muscarinic stimulation of adenylate cyclase activity of rat olfactory bulb. II Characterization of the antagonist sensitivity and comparison with muscarinic inhibitions of the enzyme in striatum and heart. *J Pharmacol Exp Ther* 1991;259:680–686.

59. Pedder EK, Eveleigh P, Poyner D, Hulme EC, Birdsall NJM. Modulation of the structure-binding relationships of antagonists for muscarinic acetylcholine receptor subtypes. *Br J Pharmacol* 1991;103:1561–1567.

60. Peralta EG, Ashkenazi A, Winslow JW, Smith DH, Ramachandran J, Capon DJ. Distinct primary structures, ligand-binding properties and tissue-specific expression of four human muscarinic acetylcholine receptors. *EMBO J* 1987;6:3923–3929.

61. Peralta EG, Ashkenazi A, Winslow JW, Ramachandran J, Capon DJ. Differential regulation of PI hydrolysis and adenylyl cyclase by muscarinic receptor subtypes. *Nature* 1988;334:434–437.

62. Peralta EG, Winslow JW, Peterson GL, Smith DH, Ashkenazi A, Ramachandran J, Schimerlik MI, Capon DJ. Primary structure and biochemical properties of an M_2 muscarinic receptor. *Science* 1987;236:600–605.

63. Potter LT, Hanchett-Valentine H, Liang J-S, Max SI, Purkerson SL, Silberberg HA, Strauss WL. m1-Toxin. *Life Sci* 1993;52:433–440.

64. Riker WF, Wescoe WC. The pharmacology of flaxedil with observations on certain analogs. *Ann NY Acad Sci* 1951;54:373–394.

65. Roskowski AP. An unusual type of sympathetic ganglionic stimulant. *J Pharmacol Exp Ther* 1961;132:156–170.

66. Smith TD, Annis SJ, Ehlert FJ, Leslie FM. N-[^{3}H]-Methylscopolamine labeling of non-M_1, non-M_2 muscarinic receptor binding sites in rat brain. *J Pharmacol Exp Ther* 1990;256:1173–1181.

67. Stockton JM, Birdsall NJM, Burgen ASV, Hulme EC. Modification of the binding properties of muscarinic receptors by gallamine. *Mol Pharmacol* 1982;23:551–557.

68. Tang W-J, Gilman AG. Type-specific regulation of adenylyl cyclase by G protein bg subunits. *Science* 1991;254:1500–1503.

69. Thomas EA, Baker SA, Ehlert FJ. Functional role for the M_2 muscarinic receptor in smooth muscle of guinea pig ileum. *Mol Pharmacol* 1993;44:102–110.

70. Waelbroeck M, Gillard M, Robberecht P, Christophe J. Kinetic studies of [^{3}H]N-methylscopolamine binding to muscarinic receptors in rat central nervous system: evidence for the existence of three classes of binding sites. *Mol Pharmacol* 1986;30:305–314.

71. Waelbroeck M, Tastenoy M, Camus J, Christophe J. Binding of selective antagonists to four muscarinic receptors (M_1 to M_4) in rat forebrain. *Mol Pharmacol* 1990;38:267–273.

72. Wall SJ, Yasuda RP, Hory F, Flagg S, Martin BM, Ginns EI, Wolfe BB. Production of antisera selective for m1 muscarinic receptors using fusion proteins: distribution of m1 receptors in rat brain. *Mol Pharmacol* 1991;39:643–649.

73. Wall SJ, Yasuda RP, Li M, Wolfe BB. Development of an antiserum against m3 muscarinic receptors: distribution of m3 receptors in rat tissues and clonal cell lines. *Mol Pharmacol* 1991;40:783–789.

74. Walton FA. Flaxedil: a new curarizing agent. *Can Med Assoc J* 1950;63:123–129.

75. Wang JX, Roeske WR, Gulya K, Yamamura HI. [^{3}H]AF-DX 116 labels subsets of muscarinic cholinergic receptors in rat cerebral cortical and cardiac membranes. *Life Sci* 1987;41:1751–1760.

76. Watson M, Yamamura HI, Roeske WR. A unique regulatory profile and regional distribution of [^{3}H]pirenzepine binding in the rat provide evidence for distinct M1 and M2 muscarinic receptor subtypes. *Life Sci* 1983;32:3001–3011.

77. Wess J, Bonner TI, Dörje F, Brann MR. Delineation of muscarinic receptor domains conferring selectivity of coupling to guanine nucleotide-binding proteins and second messengers. *Mol Pharmacol* 1990;38:517–523.

78. Wess J, Gdula D, Brann MR. Site-directed mutagenesis of the m3 muscarinic receptor: identification of a series of threonine and tyrosine residues involved in agonist but not antagonist binding. *EMBO J* 1991;10:3729–3734.

79. Wess J, Maggio R, Palmer JR, Vogel Z. Role of conserved threonine and tyrosine residues in acetylcholine binding and muscarinic receptor activation. *J Biol Chem* 1992;267:19313–19319.

80. Wong SK-F, Parker EM, Ross EM. Chimeric muscarinic cholinergic β-adrenergic receptors that activate G_s in response to muscarinic agonists. *J Biol Chem* 1990;265:6219–6224.

81. Yamamura HI, Kuhar MJ, Greenberg D, Snyder SH. Muscarinic cholinergic receptor binding: regional distribution in monkey brain. *Brain Res* 1974;66:541–546.

82. Yasuda RP, Ciesla W, Flores LR, Wall SJ, Li M, Satkus SA, Weisstein JS, Spagnola BV, Wolfe BB. Development of antisera selective for m4 and m5 muscarinic cholinergic receptors: distribution of m4 and m5 receptors in rat brain. *Mol Pharmacol* 1992;43:149–157.

Psychopharmacology: The Fourth Generation of Progress, edited by Floyd E. Bloom and David J. Kupfer. Raven Press, Ltd., New York © 1995.

CHAPTER 11

Cholinergic Transduction

Elliott Richelson

There are two classes of acetylcholine receptors, muscarinic and nicotinic (see Chapter 10, *this volume*). These receptors play major roles in the function of the body. In brain, evidence suggests a role for muscarinic receptors in memory function (28,71) and in the pathophysiology of affective illness (46,47,79) and schizophrenia (24,50,85,86). Because of their putative role in cognitive function, muscarinic receptors have been a focus of research in Alzheimer's disease (see Chapter 120, *this volume*).

Researchers defined the two classes of cholinergic receptors early in this century on the basis of tissue responses to certain agonists and antagonists (22). A response caused by muscarine, an alkaloid derived from a poisonous mushroom (*Amanita muscaria*), and antagonism of a response caused by atropine, an alkaloid from the deadly nightshade (*Atropa belladonna*—a favorite of poisoners in past centuries), defined muscarinic receptors in a tissue. On the other hand, response to nicotine and blockade by *d*-tubocurarine (one of the alkaloids from the South American arrow poisons) defined nicotinic receptors. These definitions for the two types of cholinergic receptors are still used today.

Muscarinic receptors are widely distributed throughout the body. They mediate various types of responses in many different tissues—such as cardiac tissue, smooth muscle, and exocrine glands—and in cells throughout the peripheral and central nervous system. Within the nervous system, muscarinic receptors are present on some axon endings (heteroreceptors and autoreceptors), regulating neurotransmitter release (1,67,68,90). These receptors are also on the soma and dendrites of many types of neurons, including cholinergic and noncholinergic neurons (67,95).

In the past several years, discoveries by molecular biologists have made the field of muscarinic receptors immensely interesting and complex. At a time when pharmacologists could identify at most three subtypes of muscarinic receptors, molecular biologists showed that at least five different muscarinic receptors exist on the basis of molecular cloning experiments (15,16,54,55,63). Much knowledge about these receptors has come from the use of transfected cell lines that have incorporated into their genome and express the gene encoding the specific muscarinic receptor.

This chapter will focus mainly on the biochemical events associated with activation of muscarinic receptors. The concepts of receptors, their effectors, and second messengers will be presented along with a general discussion of the types of membrane-bound receptors. Specific aspects of transduction at cholinergic receptors will be presented along with a brief discussion of the neuropsychopharmacology of muscarinic receptors.

RECEPTORS

The concept of a receptor was put forth in the latter part of the nineteenth century and the early part of this century by Professors J. N. Langley and Paul Ehrlich. Professor Ehrlich has stated "the toxin must unite . . . with 'receptors' in order for the toxin to have its effects" (30). Professor Langley used the term "receptive substance" (56).

A receptor is a highly specialized protein, which, in most cases, is a transmembrane spanning protein on the cellular surface (receptors for steroid hormones are intracellular). This receptor protein has the unique ability to recognize (bind) specific molecules. All neurotransmitters, neuromodulators, and hormones have specific receptors. Many neurotransmitters are known to have more than one type of receptor to which they bind.

Currently, receptors may be classified into four groups based upon their signal transduction mechanisms: (i) receptors that are ligand-gated ion channels [e.g., the nico-

E. Richelson: Department of Psychiatry and Psychology and Department of Pharmacology, Mayo Foundation, and Mayo Clinic Jacksonville, Jacksonville, Florida 32224.

tinic acetylcholine (21,65) and gamma-aminobutyric acid (GABA) receptors (13,75)]; (ii) receptors that are enzymes [e.g., the insulin receptor, which is a tyrosine kinase (42); and the atrial natriuretic peptide receptor, which is a particulate form of guanylate cyclase (78)]; (iii) receptors that couple to guanosine triphosphate (GTP)-binding proteins [e.g., muscarinic acetylcholine receptors and a multitude of others (44,81)]; and (iv) receptors with unknown signal transduction mechanisms (e.g., the sigma receptor).

SIGNAL TRANSDUCTION AND GTP-BINDING PROTEINS

The term *signal transduction* refers to the mechanism used by the first messenger (the neurotransmitter, neuromodulator, or hormone) of the transmitting cell to convert its information into a second messenger within the receiving cell. Signal transduction will involve a receptor for the first messenger and may involve both *transducers* and *effectors*. In the field of receptors, a *transducer* may be defined as a molecule that translates one form of "energy" (e.g., the neurotransmitter) into another form, the second messenger. *Effector* is a molecule that mediates a specific effect (e.g., an ion channel).

The classical example of a transducer is a GTP-binding protein or G protein (70), of which there are many (36,58,81). Even light and olfaction make use of G proteins in the transduction mechanisms for these sensations. G proteins consist of three different proteins (a heterotrimer) labeled as G_α, G_β, and G_γ, in the order of decreasing molecular weight. Biochemical studies as well as molecular cloning experiments have identified a multitude (nearly 20) of G_α subtypes and several (at least four each) G_β and G_γ subtypes. Among the G_α subtypes are those involved with stimulating adenylate cyclase ($G_{\alpha s}$) and those involved with inhibiting ($G_{\alpha i}$) this enzyme. Recent evidence suggests that the $\beta\gamma$ subunits may also be involved in activation or inhibition of adenylate cyclase, depending on the type of adenylate cyclase (87).

G proteins can be broadly classified into four groups, according to their sensitivity to two different bacterial toxins—cholera toxin and pertussis toxin. Both toxins, which are enzymes, adenosine triphosphate (ADP)-ribosylate specific sites on the G proteins. The four classes are as follows: (i) cholera-toxin-sensitive; (ii) pertussis-toxin-sensitive; (iii) pertussis- and cholera-toxin-sensitive; and (iv) pertussis- and cholera-toxin-insensitive (58,81). The pertussis-toxin-sensitive $G_{\alpha o}$ is the most abundant in brain, comprising about 1–2% of brain membrane protein.

The neurotransmitter (or hormone, etc.), its receptor, and a G protein, to which is bound guanosine diphosphate (GDP), form a ternary complex. This complex binds the neurotransmitter with high affinity. When GTP displaces GDP, the complex dissociates into its components, in-

cluding a form of the receptor that binds neurotransmitter with low affinity. Support for this mechanism comes from radioligand binding studies showing that GTP (or an analogue) added to the binding reaction shifts the equilibrium dissociation constant for the agonist to a lower affinity. This lower-affinity binding results kinetically from GTP, causing an acceleration of the dissociation of the agonist from its binding site. Compounds with lower affinity dissociate more rapidly from their binding sites than do compounds with higher affinity.

The prime example of an effector is adenylate cyclase, the enzyme that synthesizes the second messenger cyclic adenosine $3',5'$-monophosphate (cyclic AMP) from adenosine triphosphate (ATP) (84). For example, norepinephrine causes the second messenger cyclic AMP to form within the cell by the following mechanism, involving the binding to a β-adrenoceptor. First, norepinephrine binds to its receptor. The G protein in the ternary complex (norepinephrine–receptor–G protein) is then released when GDP is exchanged for GTP. The G protein dissociates to $G_{\alpha s}$-GTP and the $\beta\gamma$ dimer. $G_{\alpha s}$-GTP is then available to activate adenylate cyclase and increase intracellular levels of cyclic AMP.

There are several subtypes of the muscarinic receptor, and there are many different types of cellular responses which depend upon the subtype of muscarinic receptor and the cells in which the receptor resides. Most, if not all, of these responses are dependent on G proteins. On the other hand, signal transduction is relatively simple at nicotinic acetylcholine receptors. The nicotinic receptor, consisting of five subunits surrounding an internal channel, is its own ligand-gated ion channel (21,65). After binding two molecules of acetylcholine, the nicotinic receptor channel opens to allow the flow of sodium ions. As such, these sodium ions are the second messengers for nicotinic cholinergic neurotransmission.

PHARMACOLOGICAL, BIOCHEMICAL, AND MOLECULAR BIOLOGICAL EVIDENCE FOR MUSCARINIC RECEPTOR DIVERSITY

In general, pharmacologists define receptors in an experimental system (for example, measurement of agonist-mediated second messenger synthesis by cultured cells) on the basis of selectivity of agonists and antagonists. However, antagonists are more selective for receptor subtypes than are agonists (51). For the muscarinic cholinergic receptor, the agonist muscarine and antagonist atropine have defined this receptor for most of this century.

More recently, pharmacologists had divided muscarinic receptors into two major groups, M_1 and M_2, with an agonist labeled McN-A-343 being selective for the M_1 subtype (38).* However, only when the muscarinic antag-

---

* The nomenclature for muscarinic receptors is as follows: Capital letters and subscripts are used to denote pharmacological subtypes, and lowercase letters with numbers are used to denote genetic subtypes (12).

TABLE 1. *Muscarinic receptor subtypes[a]*

Pharmacologic subtype:	M$_1$	M$_2$	M$_3$	M$_4$	—
Molecular subtype:	m1	m2	m3	m4	m5
Some relatively selective antagonists:	Pirenzepine	—	—	—	—
Principal regions of expression:	Brain Exocrine glands	Heart Smooth muscle Brain	Exocrine glands Brain Smooth muscle	Brain	Brain
Major biochemical response:	Inositol phosphate release	Inhibit cyclic AMP	Inositol phosphate release	Inhibit cyclic AMP	Inositol phosphate release

[a] Adapted from ref. 12.

onist and antiulcer drug pirenzepine (29) became available did researchers have a convincing pharmacologic tool to prove the existence of more than one type of muscarinic receptor. Unlike the classical muscarinic antagonist atropine, pirenzepine blocked different muscarinic receptor effects with different potencies (41). Blockade by pirenzepine at low concentrations (high potency) defined the muscarinic M$_1$ receptor.

Even more recently, pharmacologists suggested that they could subdivide muscarinic receptors into four groupings (M$_1$, M$_2$, M$_3$, and M$_4$) based upon selective antagonists (91). On the other hand, molecular biologists have so far identified five subtypes of the muscarinic receptor (m1–m5)[1] (Table 1).

The "brain" (m1) (55) and "heart" (m2) (54,63) receptors were molecularly cloned from the partial amino acid sequences of the purified proteins. The remaining receptors (m3, m4, m5) were cloned by screening for homologous DNA sequences in DNA libraries (15,16). All five receptors from humans and rats have been molecularly cloned. Studies with these cloned receptors expressed in transfected cell lines have added to our understanding of the selectivity of drugs for these subtypes and the transduction mechanisms associated with these subtypes.

With the use of oligonucleotide probes selective for each of the five subtypes of muscarinic receptors, researchers can show the locations of the cell bodies that synthesize the various receptor subtypes in brain. In particular, messenger RNA (mRNA) for the m1, m3, and m4 subtypes are abundantly and broadly detected in rat brain, including the cerebral cortex, striatum, and hippocampus (18; see also Chapter 10, *this volume*). Next in abundance is mRNA for the m2 receptor. The m5 receptor message is least abundant in brain (57,89). Heart is a rich source for the m2 receptor, and exocrine glands and smooth muscle are rich in the m3 subtype (Table 1).

MUSCARINIC RECEPTORS BELONG TO A SUPERFAMILY OF G-PROTEIN-COUPLED RECEPTORS

All five muscarinic receptors are homologous proteins consisting of between 460 and 590 amino acids for the

human receptors (15,62). There is a very high degree of homology at the amino acid level for each receptor across species (for example, human m1 has 98.9% identity with porcine m1) (62). Homology between the muscarinic receptor, other receptors (specifically, the β-adrenoceptor), and opsin (55) led to the conclusion that the muscarinic receptors are in the family of seven-transmembrane-spanning receptors that link to G proteins. The number of proteins in this family numbers greater than 100 at this time. Included among these proteins are receptors for many biogenic amine neurotransmitters (e.g., norepinephrine, dopamine, serotonin) and for many neuropeptides (e.g., substance P, neurotensin).

The fact that all five muscarinic receptors are in this superfamily of G-protein-coupled receptors is important for understanding cholinergic transduction at these receptors. Thus, muscarinic cholinergic transduction at all five muscarinic receptor subtypes depends mostly on the coupling of each receptor to G proteins. This coupling is thought to involve the third intracellular loop of the protein (Fig. 1) (see Chapters 10 and 27, *this volume*).

CAN MUSCARINIC RECEPTORS BE CLASSIFIED PHARMACOLOGICALLY?

To discuss cholinergic transduction at specific muscarinic receptor subtypes and to interpret studies with animal tissues, one must first have knowledge of the pharmacological identification of these receptors. The corollary question of that posed above is: are there drugs that specifically or selectively block or stimulate muscarinic receptor subtypes?

A compound that is specific for a receptor binds to only one receptor. A compound that is selective for a receptor binds to one receptor with a higher affinity than that for its binding to another receptor. It is generally considered that a compound shows selectivity for a receptor when its affinity for one receptor is at least 10-fold greater than that for another receptor.

The definitive answer to the question posed above has come from studies with different transfected cell lines, each expressing a different subtype (m1–m5) of the muscarinic receptor. Currently, there is no selective or specific

Muscarinic m1, m3, or m5 receptor

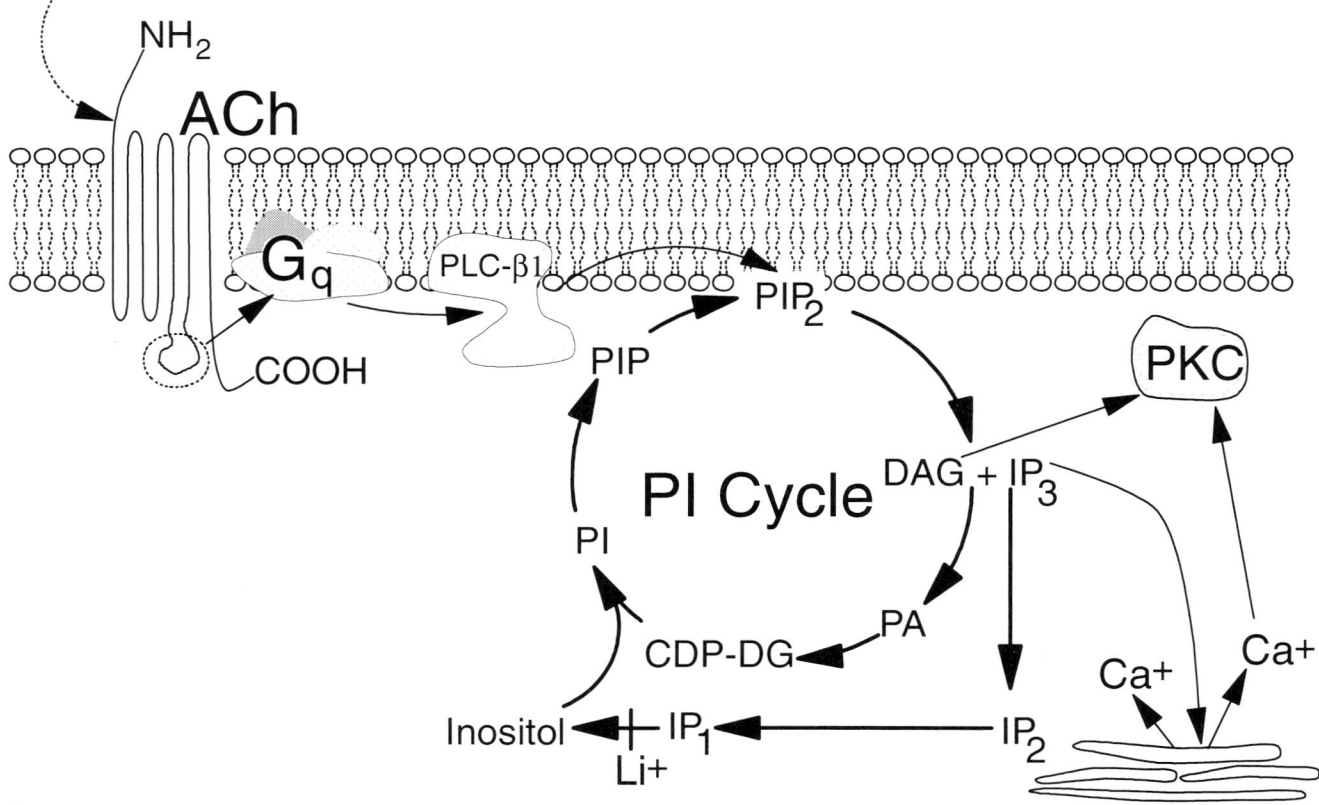

FIG. 1. Muscarinic Receptors and the Phosphatidylinositol (PI) Cycle. Abbreviations: ACh, acetylcholine; G_q, GTP-binding protein; PLC-β1, phospholipase C, β1 isozyme; PI, phosphatidylinositol; PIP_2, phosphatidylinositol 4,5-bisphosphate; DAG, 1,2-diacyl-sn-glycerol; IP_3, D-myo-inositol 1,4,5-trisphosphate; IP_2, D-myo-inositol 1,4-trisphosphate; IP_1, D-myo-inositol 1-trisphosphate; PA, phosphatidic acid; CDP-DG, cytidine diphosphodiacylglycerol; PIP, phosphatidylinositol 4-phosphate; PKC, protein kinase C.

antagonist or agonist of the five muscarinic receptors (14,27,96). Thus, pirenzepine, the "M₁-selective" antagonist, is not sufficiently selective to distinguish m1 from m4 receptors, although it will distinguish m1 from m2, m3, and m5 receptors (14,27) (Table 2). The "M₁-selective" agonist McN-A-343 has effects on all five receptors, with perhaps its best effects on m1 and m4 receptors (96). Until the chemistry and pharmacology catches up with the molecular biology, a combination of pharmacology and molecular biology must be used to classify a particular muscarinic response with a specific receptor subtype (see Chapter 10, *this volume*). Therefore, this review will emphasize results with the molecularly cloned muscarinic receptors expressed in host cells.

There are caveats to consider when generalizing results with experiments involving cloned receptors to what occurs with receptors in their natural setting. In these experiments the host cell provides the machinery necessary for the signal transduction to occur. In this case the host cell may not have the necessary apparatus (as discussed below for muscarinic-receptor-mediated cyclic GMP synthesis) or may have components that are not present in those

cells in vivo expressing these receptors. In addition, expression of these receptors (measured as B_{max} in a radioligand binding assay) can be orders of magnitude greater than that found in the natural state. As a result, these receptors can couple to transduction mechanisms that would not occur if the receptors were expressed at lower levels. High levels of receptors can also increase the efficacy of agonists for these receptors (51).

BIOCHEMICAL ASPECTS OF MUSCARINIC CHOLINERGIC TRANSDUCTION

Muscarinic Receptors Stimulate Membranal Phospholipid Turnover

Coupling to Phospholipase C (PLC)

About 40 years ago, Hokin and Hokin (43) first reported the "phospholipid labeling effect" for acetylcholine at muscarinic receptors. More specifically, these researchers showed that acetylcholine and the cholinergic agonist car-

TABLE 2. *Binding of antidepressants, antimuscarinics, and neuroleptics to human muscarinic receptor subtypes*

Drug	Human muscarinic receptor subtype				
	m1	m2	m3	m4	m5
	Geometric mean of K_d (nM)				
Antidepressants[a]					
Amitriptyline	14.7	11.8	12.8	7.2	15.7
Bupropion	>35,000	>35,000	>35,000	>35,000	>35,000
Etoperidone	>35,000	>35,000	>35,000	>35,000	>35,000
Femoxetine	92	150	220	470	400
Fluoxetine	1030	2700	1000	2900	2700
Lofepramine	67	330	130	340	460
Paroxetine	300	340	80	320	650
Sertraline	1300	2100	1300	1400	1900
Venlafaxine	>35,000	>35,000	>35,000	>35,000	>35,000
Antimuscarinics[b]					
Benztropine	0.231	1.4	1.1	1.1	2.8
Biperiden	0.48	6.3	3.9	2.4	6.3
Pirenzepine	8	270	150	28	170
Procyclidine	4.6	25	12.4	7	24
Scopolamine	1.1	2.0	0.4	0.8	2.1
Trihexyphenidyl	1.6	7.0	6.4	2.6	15.9
Neuroleptics[b,c]					
Chlorpromazine	25	150	67	40	42
Chlorprothixene	11	28	22	18	25
Clozapine	3.1	48	20	11	11
Fluperlapine	8.8	71	41	14	17
Melperone	15,000	2400	15,000	4400	15,000
Mesoridazine	10	15	90	19	60
Rilapine	190	470	1400	1000	1100
Risperidone	11,000	3700	13,000	2900	15,000
Thioridazine	2.7	14	15	9	13
Zotepine	18	140	73	77	260

[a] Data from ref. 82.
[b] Data from ref. 14.
[c] All but chlorpromazine, chlorprothixene, mesoridazine, and thioridaze are considered atypical neuroleptics.

bamylcholine, which cause enzyme secretion in the pancreas, markedly increase the incorporation of ^{32}P into phospholipids in tissue slices of pigeon pancreas. The effects of these agonists were blocked by the muscarinic antagonist atropine, establishing the muscarinic nature of this effect.

This phospholipid labeling effect of muscarinic agonists is the result of the breakdown of a membranal phospholipid, phosphatidylinositol 4,5-bisphosphate (PIP$_2$), caused by muscarinic receptor (m1, m3, or m5) activation of the enzyme phospholipase C (PLC-β1 isozyme) through a G protein called G$_q$ (Fig. 1). This activation of PLC leads to a cascade of events. As illustrated in Fig. 1, these events, with a time course measured in seconds, begin with the breakdown of PIP$_2$ into 1,2-diacyl-*sn*-glycerol (diacylglycerol, DAG) and D-*myo*-inositol 1,4,5-trisphosphate (IP$_3$) (10,33).

DAG is recycled, in a series of reactions, back to PIP$_2$ (Fig. 1). Additionally, DAG becomes available to activate the enzyme protein kinase C (PKC), of which there are several subtypes (34). In its activated form, PKC can then phosphorylate proteins, thereby regulating their functions.

For example, activation of PKC by phorbol esters can inhibit muscarinic-receptor-mediated release of inositol phosphates in cultured murine neuroblastoma cells (49). These results suggest a feedback role for DAG in signal transduction through PKC. DAG can also be degraded by diglyceride lipase to form arachidonic acid, the pivotal substrate for the synthesis of prostaglandins, leukotrienes, epoxides, and related compounds.

Lithium ion inhibits the enzyme inositol 1-monophosphatase, which hydrolyzes IP$_1$ into inositol (40). Thus, in vitro lithium ion is used to amplify the signal resulting from receptor-mediated release of inositol phosphates (9). It is uncertain whether this action of lithium ion plays a role in its therapeutic effects in treating affective disorders. However, it may play a role in some of its adverse effects (11).

IP$_3$ has receptors on smooth endoplasmic reticulum (23), which release stored calcium ions after the IP$_3$ receptor is activated (8) (Fig. 1). Increased intracellular levels of calcium ions then cause a myriad of events to occur within the cell, including the potentiation of the effects of PKC.

Receptor-mediated activation of PLC is by no means exclusive to muscarinic subtypes m1, m3, and m5, or to muscarinic receptors in general. The odd-numbered muscarinic receptors are most efficiently coupled to this response and give the most robust responses, compared to those of the even-numbered receptors (3,64). In addition, the odd-numbered muscarinic receptors activate PKC (β1 isozyme) by a pertussis-toxin-insensitive G protein (G_q). The other two receptors mediate this activation by a pertussis-toxin-sensitive G protein, likely $G_{\alpha i}$ (25). There is an extensive list of receptors that mediate the release of inositol phosphates. A few examples of these are the α_1-adrenergic, histamine H_1, serotonin 5-HT_2, and neurotensin receptors. Finally, there are receptors (e.g., dopamine D_1) that inhibit receptor-mediated inositol phosphate release, including that at muscarinic receptors (94).

Coupling to Phospholipase D (PLD)

Phospholipases of the D type are enzymes that cleave choline from the membranal phospholipid, phosphatidylcholine (lecithin), yielding phosphatidic acid and choline, an acetylcholine precursor (19,31). A phosphatidate-phosphohydrolase acting on phosphatidic acid yields DAG. Thus, PLD acting on phosphatidylcholine provides another source of DAG to activate PKC, which is known to activate PLD (39). In fact, phosphatidylcholine, being much more abundant, provides a greater and more sustained source of DAG than does PIP_2.

All receptors that stimulate the breakdown of PIP_2 may also stimulate the breakdown of phosphatidylcholine. Muscarinic receptors activate PLD by a mechanism that appears to involve G proteins (66,72,74). As with the coupling to PLC, the odd-numbered muscarinic receptors are more efficiently and robustly coupled to PLD (73). This type of signal transduction has been much less well-characterized than that involving the phosphatidyl-inositol-specific PLC. However, this coupling of muscarinic receptors to PLD may be of importance to cholinergic transmission in general, by providing the precursor of acetylcholine and by providing other compounds that may affect other signal transduction mechanisms.

Coupling to Phospholipase A_2 (PLA$_2$)

Arachidonic acid is a bioactive compound that serves as a precursor of many compounds derived from the action of lipoxygenases, epoxygenases, and cyclooxygenases. Additionally, arachidonic acid is involved with the activation of PKC (see Chapter 53, *this volume*).

Several different receptors, including the odd-numbered muscarinic receptors (20,32,80,83), can mediate the release of arachidonic acid. Thus, by itself or through a metabolite, arachidonic acid is a second messenger.

The principal effector involved in this receptor-mediated arachidonic acid release is PLA_2 (7). This enzyme acting on a variety of phospholipids at the 2-position releases arachidonic acid with the formation of lysophospholipids. Another enzyme that can release arachidonic acid is diglyceride lipase, which releases this compound from DAG, produced by the action of PLC on phosphatidylinositol 4,5-bisphosphate (26). There is good evidence to suggest a role for G proteins in receptor-mediated PLA_2 activation (7,53), although other mechanisms have been suggested (17,32). The exact subtype of G protein involved with PLA_2 activation is unknown.

Muscarinic Receptor Activation Changes Intracellular Levels of Cyclic Nucleotides

Increase in Intracellular Levels of Cyclic GMP

Cyclic guanosine 3′,5′-monophosphate (cyclic GMP) and the enzymes (soluble and particulate) that synthesize this cyclic nucleotide are widely distributed in brain and elsewhere in the body (37,93). Cyclic GMP formation mediated by acetylcholine was first reported over two decades ago with rat heart (35). Shortly thereafter, muscarinic responses in other tissues were reported. The dependence of the response on calcium ions was established early (77). All the major target organs of parasympathetic cholinergic fibers contain muscarinic receptors that mediate an increase in cyclic GMP (37). Muscarinic receptors in sympathetic ganglia and in brain also mediate cyclic GMP synthesis.

Many different established cell lines of nervous system origin have muscarinic receptors that mediate cyclic GMP synthesis. A widely studied example is murine neuroblastoma clone N1E-115 cells (2,59,69). In this model system, the muscarinic receptor and six others that increase intracellular levels of the second messenger cyclic GMP in a calcium-dependent manner mediate the release of inositol phosphates (69). Calcium-dependent, receptor-mediated cyclic GMP synthesis occurs only with intact cells. Calcium ions and nitric oxide (NO) (60,61) are very likely involved in this receptor-mediated stimulation of soluble guanylate cyclase. NO, which is synthesized from L-arginine by the enzyme NO synthase in a calcium/calmodulin-dependent manner (61), directly stimulates soluble guanylate cyclase.

NO, a free radical, is a novel second messenger of muscarinic and other receptors. It may be involved with both intracellular and intercellular communication of neurons (see Chapter 54, *this volume*).

The role of G proteins in muscarinic receptor-mediated cyclic GMP synthesis has not been defined. However, it may be that synthesis of NO and, subsequently, cyclic GMP following receptor activation is secondary to the increase in intracellular calcium ions, resulting from the release of IP_3 from PIP_2 by the action of PLC.

The human muscarinic receptors expressed in Chinese

hamster ovary cells, despite robust release of inositol phosphates, do not mediate cyclic GMP synthesis. These cells lack NO synthase and guanylate cyclase. These facts likely explain the absence of muscarinic-receptor-mediated cyclic GMP synthesis in Chinese hamster ovary cells.

With clone N1E-115 cells, there is a very close association between the activation of muscarinic M_1 (and other) receptors and the formation of inositol phosphates and cyclic GMP. These results suggest that the two events are linked to one another and that one (cyclic GMP response) could be dependent on the other (inositol phosphate release). However, with rat brain tissue, there is evidence to suggest that different subtypes of the muscarinic receptor mediate these responses independently (52,88). Although more research needs to be done on this topic, these data could be explained in part by the absence of NO synthase in certain cells that have muscarinic receptors (see Chapter 54, *this volume*).

Decrease in Intracellular Levels of Cyclic AMP

Another biochemical property established early for muscarinic receptors is their "negative coupling" to adenylate cyclase (37), the enzyme that synthesizes cyclic AMP from ATP. Negative coupling means the inhibition by the muscarinic receptor of adenylate cyclase activation mediated by a second receptor. Other types of receptors negatively couple to adenylate cyclase (e.g., α_2-adrenoceptors, delta-opioid receptors). It is mediated by the $G_{\alpha i}$ subunit of the G protein, although the $\beta\gamma$ subunits may also be involved (87). The even-numbered muscarinic receptors, m2 and m4, are the ones that use this type of signal transduction mechanism.

Muscarinic receptor activation can reduce cyclic AMP levels by another mechanism (45), involving the activation of cyclic AMP phosphodiesterase, the enzyme that degrades cyclic AMP. This effect appears to be secondary to mobilization of intracellular calcium ions by the action of PLC and the subsequent activation of a calcium/calmodulin-dependent phosphodiesterase. So far, this muscarinic response has been shown to occur only with a human astrocytoma cell line. This cell line has the adenosine receptor that inhibits adenylate cyclase activity by a pertussis-toxin-sensitive mechanism, indicating a requirement for $G_{\alpha i}$. These results suggest that, unlike the molecularly cloned muscarinic receptors, the muscarinic receptor in these tumor cells is incapable of coupling to this type of G protein.

ELECTRICAL ASPECTS OF MUSCARINIC CHOLINERGIC TRANSDUCTION

Activation of muscarinic receptors leads to a diverse array of electrical responses within cells. The type of response depends upon the subtype of muscarinic receptor and the type of cell involved. Some examples of these responses are inhibition and stimulation of inward rectifier currents (see Chapter 5, *this volume*). As might be expected from the preceding, studies with the molecularly cloned receptors appear to show that the odd-numbered muscarinic receptors evoke similar electrical responses and that these responses are different from those of the even-numbered receptors. All these electrical responses appear to require coupling to G proteins. The reader is referred to a recent publication (48) for an in-depth review of this topic.

ALTERATIONS OF MUSCARINIC CHOLINERGIC TRANSDUCTION IN NEUROPSYCHIATRIC DISEASE

Researchers have published hypotheses and supporting data implicating the muscarinic cholinergic system in affective disorders (46,47,79) and in schizophrenia (24,50, 85,86). Only one study, involving manic patients, has looked at muscarinic receptor transduction (76). Other studies in the literature involving muscarinic transduction used brain material from patients who died from Alzheimer's disease. One group suggests that muscarinic receptor coupling to G proteins is altered in brains of Alzheimer's patients (97; see also Chapter 120, *this volume*).

Animal studies suggest that lithium ion inhibits the coupling of muscarinic and β-adrenergic receptors to G proteins (5). More specifically, these studies showed that agonist-induced increases in the binding of [^{3}H]GTP to pertussis-toxin-sensitive (muscarinic receptor) and cholera-toxin-sensitive (β-adrenergic receptor) G proteins in cerebral cortex was blocked by treatment of rats for 12–21 days with lithium carbonate. This effect is reversed in vitro by magnesium ions (4). Consistent with these data, this treatment abolished the GTP shift of the agonist to a lower-affinity state as measured in binding assays with a nonselective muscarinic radioligand. The pertussis toxin-sensitivity of this effect suggests that G_i or G_o is involved and not G_q.

Evidence was presented to suggest that the muscarinic receptor involved is the M_1 subtype (6). More work needs to be done to prove this point (for example, obtaining equilibrium dissociation constants for a series of antagonists and not IC_{50} values) because this conclusion does not fit with the molecular biology and molecular pharmacology. It is more likely that the m4 receptor is involved (see Chapter 10, *this volume*).

These animal studies suggested that receptor coupling at muscarinic and β-adrenergic receptors is awry in bipolar disorder, the illness effectively treated with lithium salts. Therefore, the same researchers sought clinical data to test this idea (76). The source of receptors was mononuclear leukocytes. These were obtained from untreated bipolar patients in the manic phase of their illness, from euthymic patients treated with lithium salts, and from healthy volunteers. Similar to the results found in the cerebral cortex of rat, agonists of the two receptors stimulated the binding of an analogue of GTP to membranes from the leukocytes. In addition, this stimulation was abolished at muscarinic and β-adrenergic receptors by pertussis toxin and cholera toxin, respectively.

Interestingly, there was a much more robust stimulation of the binding at both receptors for leukocytes from untreated manic patients compared to that for controls. In addition, the effects of agonists with the membranes of cells from the treated, euthymic bipolar patients were no different from those of controls. Although these studies need to be replicated, it does suggest that a defect exists in certain types of G proteins in bipolar patients.

THE NEUROPSYCHOPHARMACOLOGY OF MUSCARINIC RECEPTORS

Antidepressants, neuroleptics, and antiparkinsonism drugs antagonize muscarinic receptors with varying degrees of potency and selectivity. Interruption of muscarinic cholinergic transduction is effectively achieved by this muscarinic receptor blockade.

We have studied many compounds within these three classes of drugs at the five cloned human muscarinic receptors expressed in Chinese hamster ovary cells (14,82) (Table 2). No drug is specific or selective (as defined above) for the five receptors. However, some compounds are relatively potent and relatively selective. For example, the classical tricyclic compound amitriptyline is the most potent antidepressant at all five muscarinic subtypes. The neuroleptic clozapine is very potent and relatively selective for the m1 subtype. This selectivity may explain clozapine's unusual efficacy in refractory schizophrenic patients and its low incidence of extrapyramidal side effects. However, because most other atypical neuroleptics studied lacked high affinity and selectivity at muscarinic receptor subtypes, it is likely that other mechanisms are involved as well. Potent blockade of muscarinic receptors can also cause a number of adverse effects such as memory dysfunction (possibly m1), sinus tachycardia (m2), and dry mouth (possibly m3).

CONCLUSIONS

The existence of muscarinic receptors has been known for most of this century. We enter the next century with the knowledge that there are at least five different muscarinic receptors that can play a whole host of "instruments" to control many aspects of the functioning of the organism. In the total picture, however, muscarinic receptors are several among the perhaps hundreds of receptors for neurotransmitters, neurohormones, and neuromodulators. There are many interactions that are known between muscarinic and other receptors. Many more are yet to be found.

There are suspicions based upon experimental data that a few more muscarinic receptors are waiting to be found. In the future, these other muscarinic receptor subtypes may be molecularly cloned. If this were the case, muscarinic receptor pharmacology would become even more complex. As it is we must await breakthroughs from the chemists, collaborating with molecular biologists and pharmacologists to obtain the truly specific or truly selective muscarinic receptor ligands. However, these receptors are so highly homologous, especially in regions where they are thought to bind agonists and antagonists, that some think we may never obtain the desired compounds.

How else will we be able to assign function to these receptors in the brain as we await the specific and selective compounds? One approach to consider is antisense technology. This technique can selectively inhibit the expression of a gene of interest. By observing function or behavior and after knocking out the gene (92), we may be able to assign function to each of the five muscarinic subtypes. Whether antisense technology will provide new muscarinic receptor "antagonists" is the subject for some exciting future research.

ACKNOWLEDGMENTS

The writing of this chapter was supported in part by the Mayo Foundation and U.S.P.H.S. Grant MH27692.

REFERENCES

1. Akaike A, Sasa M, Takaori S. Muscarinic inhibition as a dominant role in cholinergic regulation of transmission in the caudate nucleus. *J Pharmacol Exp Ther* 1988;246:1129–1136.
2. Amano T, Richelson E, Nirenberg M. Neurotransmitter synthesis by neuroblastoma clones. *Proc Natl Acad Sci USA* 1972;69:258–263.
3. Ashkenazi A, Peralta EG, Winslow JW, Ramachandran J, Capon DJ. Functionally distinct G proteins selectively couple different receptors to PI hydrolysis in the same cell. *Cell* 1989;56:487–493.
4. Avissar S, Murphy DL, Schreiber G: Magnesium reverses lithium inhibition of beta adrenergic and muscarinic receptor coupling to G-proteins. *Biochem Pharmacol* 1991;41:171–175.
5. Avissar S, Schreiber G, Danon A, Belmaker RH. Lithium inhibits adrenergic and cholinergic increases in GTP binding in rat cortex. *Nature* 1988;331:440–442.
6. Avissar S, Schreiber G. Muscarinic receptor subclassification and G-proteins: significance for lithium action in affective disorders and for the treatment of the extrapyramidal side effects of neuroleptics. *Biol Psychiatry* 1989;26:113–130.
7. Axelrod J, Burch RM, Jelsema CL. Receptor-mediated activation of phospholipase A_2 via GTP-binding proteins: arachidonic acid and its metabolites as second messengers. *Trends Neurosci* 1988;11:117–123.
8. Berridge MJ, Irvine RF. Inositol trisphosphate, a novel second messenger in cellular signal transduction. *Nature* 1984;312:315–321.
9. Berridge MJ, Downes CP, Hanley MR. Lithium amplifies agonist-dependent phosphatidylinositol responses in brain and salivary glands. *Biochem J* 1982;206:587–595.
10. Berridge MJ. Rapid accumulation of inositol trisphosphate reveals that agonists hydrolyse polyphosphoinositides instead of phosphatidylinositol. *Biochem J* 1983;212:849–858.
11. Bersudsky Y, Vinnitsky I, Grisaru N, et al. The effect of inositol

on lithium-induced polyuria-polydipsia in rats and humans. *Hum Psychopharmacol Clin Exp* 1992;7:403–407.

12. Birdsall N, Buckley N, Doods H, et al. Nomenclature for muscarinic receptor subtypes recommended by symposium. *Trends Pharmacol Sci* 1989;Dec(Suppl):VII.
13. Blair LAC, Levitan ES, Marshall J, Dionne VE, Barnard E. Single subunits of GABA_A receptor form ion channels with properties of the native receptor. *Science* 1988;242:577–579.
14. Bolden C, Cusack B, Richelson E. Antagonism by antimuscarinic and neuroleptic compounds at the five cloned human muscarinic cholinergic receptors expressed in Chinese hamster ovary cells. *J Pharmacol Exp Ther* 1992;260:576–580.
15. Bonner TI, Young AC, Brann MR, Buckley NJ. Cloning and expression of the human and rat m5 muscarinic acetylcholine receptor genes. *Neuron* 1988;1:403–410.
16. Bonner TI, Buckley NJ, Young AC, Brann MR. Identification of a family of muscarinic acetylcholine receptor genes. *Science* 1987;237:527–532.
17. Brooks RC, McCarthy KD, Lapetina EG, Morell P. Receptor-stimulated phospholipase A_2 activation is coupled to influx of external calcium and not to mobilization of intracellular calcium in C62B glioma cells. *J Biol Chem* 1989;264:20147–20153.
18. Buckley NJ, Bonner TI, Brann MR. Localization of a family of muscarinic receptor mRNAs in rat brain. *J Neurosci* 1988;8:4646–4652.
19. Chalifour RJ, Kanfer JN. Microsomal phospholipase D of rat brain and lung tissues. *Biochem Biophys Res Commun* 1980;96:742–747.
20. Conklin BR, Brann MR, Buckley NJ, Ma AL, Bonner TI, Axelrod J. Stimulation of arachidonic acid release and inhibition of mitogenesis by cloned genes for muscarinic receptor subtypes stably expressed in A9 L cells. *Proc Natl Acad Sci USA* 1988;85:8698–8702.
21. Conti-Tronconi BM, Hunkapiller MW, Lindstrom JM, Raftery A. Subunit structure of the acetylcholine receptor from electrophorus electricus. *Proc Natl Acad Sci USA* 1982;79:6489–6493.
22. Dale HH. The action of certain esters and ethers of choline, and their relation to muscarine. *J Pharmacol Exp Ther* 1914;6:147–190.
23. Danoff SK, Ferris CD, Donath C, et al. Inositol 1,4,5-trisphosphate receptors: distinct neuronal and nonneuronal forms derived by alternative splicing differ in phosphorylation. *Proc Natl Acad Sci* 1991;88:2951–2955.
24. Davis KL, Hollister LE, Berger PA, Barchas JD. Cholinergic imbalance hypotheses of psychoses and movement disorders: strategies for evaluation. *Psychopharmacol Commun* 1975;1:533–543.
25. Dell'Acqua ML, Carroll RC, Peralta EG. Transfected m2 muscarinic acetylcholine receptors couple to G_{αi2} and G_{αi3} in Chinese hamster ovary cells—activation and desensitization of the phospholipase-C signaling pathway. *J Biol Chem* 1993;268:5676–5685.
26. Diaz-Meco MT, Larrodera P, Lopez-Barahona M, Cornet ME, Barreno PG, Moscat J. Phospholipase C-mediated hydrolysis of phosphatidylcholine is activated by muscarinic agonists. *Biochem J* 1989;263:115–120.
27. Dorje F, Wess J, Lambrecht G, Tacke R, Mutschler E, Brann MR. Antagonist binding profiles of five cloned human muscarinic receptor subtypes. *J Pharmacol Exp Ther* 1990;256:727–733.
28. Drachman DA, Leavitt J. Human memory and the cholinergic system. A relationship to aging? *Arch Neurol* 1974;30:113–121.
29. Eberlein VW, Schmidt G, Reuter A, Kutter E. Anti-ulcer agent pirenzepine (L-S 519)—a tricyclic compound with particular physico-chemical properties. *Arzneimittelforschung/Drug Res* 1977;27:356–359.
30. Ehrlich P. Veber den jetzigen Stand der Chemotherapie. *Ber Dtsch Chem Ges* 1909;42:17–47.
31. Exton JH. Signaling through phosphatidylcholine breakdown. *J Biol Chem* 1990;265:1–4.
32. Felder CC, Dieter P, Kinsella J, et al. A transfected m5 muscarinic acetylcholine receptor stimulates phospholipase A_2 by inducing both calcium influx and activation of protein kinase C. *J Pharmacol Exp Ther* 1990;255:1140–1147.
33. Fisher SK, Agranoff BW. Receptor activation and inositol lipid hydrolysis in neural tissues. *J Neurochem* 1987;48:999–1017.
34. Fukami Y, Nishizuka Y. The protein kinase c family in signal transduction and cellular regulation. In: Papa S, Azzi A, Tager J, eds. *Adenine nucleotides in cellular energy transfer and signal transduction.* Basel: Birkhäser Verlag, 1992;201–205.

35. George WJ, Polson JB, O'Toole AG, Goldberg ND. Elevation of guanosine 3',5'-cyclic phosphate in rat heart after perfusion with acetylcholine. *Proc Natl Acad Sci USA* 1970;66:398–403.
36. Gilman AG. G proteins: transducers of receptor-generated signals. *Annu Rev Biochem* 1987;56:615–649.
37. Goldberg N:R, Haddox MT. Cyclic GMP. *Adv Cyclic Nucleotide Res* 1973;3:155–223.
38. Goyal RK, Rattan S. Neurohumoral, hormonal and drug receptors for the lower esophageal sphincter. *Gastroenterol* 1978;74:598–619.
39. Gustavsson L, Hansson E. Stimulation of phospholipase D activity by phorbol esters in cultured astrocytes. *J Neurochem* 1990;54:737–742.
40. Hallcher LM, Sherman WR. The effects of lithium ion and other agents on the activity of myoinositol-1-phosphatase from bovine brain. *J Biol Chem* 1980;255:10896–10901.
41. Hammer R, Berrie CP, Birdsall NJM, Burgen ASV, Hulme EC. Pirenzepine distinguishes between different subclasses of muscarinic receptors. *Nature* 1980;283:90–92.
42. Herrera R, Rosen OM. Regulation of the protein kinase activity of the human insulin receptor. *J Recept Res* 1987;7:405–415.
43. Hokin MR, Hokin LE. Enzyme secretion and the incorporation of P^{32} into phospholipides of pancrease slices. *J Biol Chem* 1953;203:967–977.
44. Houslay MD. Review: G-protein linked receptors—a family probed by molecular cloning and mutagenesis procedures. *Clin Endocrinol* 1992;36:525–534.
45. Hughes AR, Harden TK. Adenosine and muscarinic cholinergic receptors attenuate cyclic AMP accumulation by different mechanisms in 1321N1 astrocytoma cells. *J Pharmacol Exp Ther* 1986;237:173–178.
46. Janowsky DS, El-Yousef MK, Davis JM, Sekerke HJ. Parasympathetic suppression of manic symptoms by physostigmine. *Arch Gen Psychiatry* 1973;28:542–545.
47. Janowsky DS, El-Yousef MK, Davis JM, Sekerke HJ. A cholinergic–adrenergic hypothesis of mania and depression. *Lancet* 1972;1:632–635.
48. Jones SVP. Muscarinic receptor subtypes—modulation of ion channels. *Life Sci* 1993;52:457–464.
49. Kanba S, Kanba KS, Richelson E. The protein kinase C activator, 12-O-tetradecanoylphorbol-13-acetate (TPA), inhibits muscarinic (M_1) receptor-mediated inositol phosphate release and cyclic GMP formation in murine neuroblastoma clone (N1E-115). *Eur J Pharmacol* 1986;125:155–156.
50. Karson CN, Garcia-Rill E, Biedermann J, et al. The brain stem reticular formation in schizophrenia. *Psychiatry Res Neuroimaging* 1991;40:31–48.
51. Kenakin TP. The classification of drugs and drug receptors in isolated tissues. *Pharmacol Rev* 1984;36:165–222.
52. Kendall DA. Cyclic GMP formation and inositol phosphate accumulation do not share common origins in rat brain slices. *J Neurochem* 1986;47:1483–1489.
53. Kim D, Lewis DL, Graziadai L, Neer EJ, Gar-Sagi D, Clapham DE. G-protein βγ-subunits activate the cardiac muscarinic K^+-channel via phospholipase A_2. *Nature* 1989;337:557–560.
54. Kubo T, Maeda A, Sugimoto K, et al. Primary structure of porcine cardiac muscarinic acetylcholine receptor deduced from the cDNA sequence. *FEBS Lett* 1986;209:367–372.
55. Kubo T, Fukuda K, Mikami A, et al. Cloning, sequencing and expression of complementary DNA encoding the muscarinic acetylcholine receptor. *Nature* 1986;323:411–416.
56. Langley JN. On the reaction of cells and of nerve-endings to certain poisons, chiefly as regards the reaction of striated muscle to nicotine and to curare. *J Physiol (Lond)* 1905;374–413.
57. Liao CF, Themmen APN, Joho R, Barberis C, Birnbaumer M, Birnbaumer L. Molecular cloning and expression of a fifth muscarinic acetylcholine receptor. *J Biol Chem* 1989;264:7328–7337.
58. Manji HK. G-proteins—implications for psychiatry. *Am J Psychiatry* 1992;149:746–760.
59. Matsuzawa H, Nirenberg M. Receptor-mediated shifts in cGMP and cAMP levels in neuroblastoma cells. *Proc Natl Acad Sci USA* 1975;72:3472–3476.
60. Mckinney M, Bolden C, Smith C, Johnson A, Richelson E. Selective blockade of receptor-mediated cyclic GMP formation in N1E-115 neuroblastoma cells by an inhibitor of nitric oxide synthesis. *Eur J Pharmacol* 1990;178:139–140.

61. Moncada S, Palmer RMJ, Higgs EA. Nitric oxide—physiology, pathophysiology, and pharmacology. *Pharmacol Rev* 1991;43:109–142.

62. Peralta EG, Ashkenazi A, Winslow JW, Smith DH, et al. Distinct primary structures, ligand-binding properties and tissue-specific expression of four human muscarinic acetylcholine receptors. *EMBO J* 1987;6:3923–3929.

63. Peralta EG, Winslow JW, Peterson GL, et al. Primary structure and biochemical properties of an M2 muscarinic receptor. *Science* 1987;236:600–605.

64. Peralta EG, Ashkenazi A, Winslow JW, Ramachandran J, Capon DJ. Differential regulation of PI hydrolysis and adenylyl cyclase by muscarinic receptor subtypes. *Nature* 1988;334:434–437.

65. Popot JL, Sugiyame H, Changeux JP. Studies on the electrogenic action of acetylcholine with torpedo marmorata electric organ II. The permeability response of the receptor-rich membrane fragments to cholinergic agonists in vitro. *J Mol Biol* 1976;106:469–483.

66. Qian Z, Drewes LR. Muscarinic acetylcholine receptor regulates phosphatidylcholine phospholipase D in canine brain. *J Biol Chem* 1989;264:21720–21724.

67. Raiteri M, Marchi M, Paudice P, Pittaluga A. Muscarinic receptors mediating inhibition of γ-aminobutyric acid release in rat corpus striatum and their pharmacological characterization. *J Pharmacol Exp Ther* 1990;254:496–501.

68. Raiteri M, Leardi R, Marchi M. Heterogeneity of presynaptic muscarinic receptors regulating neurotransmitter release in the rat brain. *J Pharmacol Exp Ther* 1984;228:209–214.

69. Richelson E, Kanba S, Kanba KS, Pfenning M. Phosphoinositides and cyclic GMP in neural cells. In: Tucek S, ed. *Synaptic transmitters and receptors.* Chichester: John Wiley & Sons, 1987;315–318.

70. Rodbell M, Birnbaumer L, Pohl SL, Krans MJ. The glucagon-sensitive adenyl cyclase system in plasma membranes of rat liver. V. An obligatory role of guanyl nucleotides in glucagon action. *J Biol Chem* 1971;246:1877–1882.

71. Safer DJ, Allen RP. The central effects of scopolamine in man. *Biol Psychiatry* 1971;3:347–355.

72. Sandmann J, Peralta EG, Wurtman RJ. Coupling of transfected muscarinic acetylcholine receptor subtypes to phospholipase-D. *J Biol Chem* 1991;266:6031–6034.

73. Sandmann J, Peralta EG, Wurtman RJ. Coupling of transfected muscarinic acetylcholine receptor subtypes to phospholipase-D. *J Biol Chem* 1991;266:6031–6034.

74. Sandmann J, Wurtman RJ. Phospholipase D and phospholipase C in human cholinergic neuroblastoma (LA-N-2) cells: modulation by muscarinic agonists and protein kinase C. In: Nishizuka Y, Endo M, Tanaka C, eds. *The biology and medicine of signal transduction.* New York: Raven Press, 1990;176–181.

75. Schofield PR, Darlison MG, Fujita N, et al. Sequence and functional expression of the GABA receptor shows a ligand-gated receptor super-family. *Nature* 1987;328:221–227.

76. Schreiber G, Avissar S, Danon A, Belmaker RH: Hyperfunctional G proteins in mononuclear leukocytes of patients with mania. *Biol Psychiatry* 1991;29:273–280.

77. Schultz G, Hardman JG, Schultz K, Baird CE, Sutherland W. The importance of calcium ions for the regulation of guanosine 3',5'-monophosphate levels. *Proc Natl Acad Sci USA* 1973;70:3889–3893.

78. Singh S, Lowe DG, Thorpe DS, Rodriguez H, et al. Membrane guanylate cyclase is a cell-surface receptor with homology to protein kinases. *Nature* 1988;334:708–712.

79. Sitaram N, Nurnberger JI, Gershon ES, Gillin JC. Faster cholinergic REM sleep induction in euthymic patients with primary affective illness. *Science* 1980;208:200–202.

80. Snider RM, McKinney M, Forray C, Richelson E. Neurotransmitter receptors mediate cyclic GMP formation by involvement of phospholipase A_2 and arachidonic acid metabolites. *Proc Natl Acad Sci USA* 1984;81:3905–3909.

81. Spiegel AM, Shenker A, Weinstein LS. Receptor–effector coupling by g-proteins—implications for normal and abnormal signal transduction. *Endocr Rev* 1992;13:536–565.

82. Stanton TT, Bolden-Watson C, Cusack B, Richelson E. Antagonism of the five cloned human muscarinic cholinergic receptors expressed in CHO-K1 cells by antidepressants and antihistaminics. *Biochem Pharmacol* 1993;45:2352–2354.

83. Strosznajder J, Samochocki M. Ca^{2+}-independent, Ca^{2+}-dependent, and carbachol-mediated arachidonic acid release from rat brain cortex membrane. *J Neurochem* 1991;57:1198–1206.

84. Sutherland E. Studies on the mechanism of hormone action. *Science* 1972;177:401–408.

85. Tandon R, Dequardo JR, Goodson J, Mann NA, Greden JF. Effect of anticholinergics on positive and negative symptoms in schizophrenia. *Psychopharmacol Bull* 1992;28:297–302.

86. Tandon R, Shipley JE, Greden JF, Mann NA, Eisner WH, Goodson J. Muscarinic cholinergic hyperactivity in schizophrenia—relationship to positive and negative symptoms. *Schizophrenia Res* 1991;4:23–30.

87. Tang WJ, Gilman AG. Type-specific regulation of adenylyl cyclase by G-protein $\beta\gamma$-subunits. *Science* 1991;254:1500–1503.

88. Tonnaer JADM, Cheung CL, De Boer T. cGMP formation and phosphoinositide turnover in rat brain slices are mediated by pharmacologically distinct muscarinic acetylcholine receptors. *Eur J Pharmacol Mol Pharmacol Sect* 1991;207:183–188.

89. Vilaro MT, Palacios JM, Mengod G. Localization of m5 muscarinic receptor mRNA in rat brain examined by in situ hybridization histochemistry. *Neurosci Lett* 1990;114:154–159.

90. Vizi ES, Kobayashi O, Torocsik A, et al. Heterogeneity of presynaptic muscarinic receptors involved in modulation of transmitter release. *Neuroscience* 1989;31:259–267.

91. Waelbroeck M, Tastenoy M, Camus J, Christophe J. Binding of selective antagonists to four muscarinic receptors (M_1 to M_4) in rat forebrain. *Mol Pharmacol* 1990;38:267–273.

92. Wahlestedt C, Pich EM, Koob GF, Yee F, Heilig M. Modulation of anxiety and neuropeptide Y-Y1 receptors by antisense oligodeoxynucleotides. *Science* 1993;259:528–531.

93. Waldman SA, Murad F. Cyclic GMP synthesis and function. *Pharmacol Rev* 1987;39:163–196.

94. Wallace MA, Claro E. A novel role for dopamine: inhibition of muscarinic cholinergic-stimulated phosphoinositide hydrolysis in rat brain cortical membranes. *Neurosci Lett* 1990;110:155–161.

95. Wamsley JK, Zarbin MA, Kuhar MJ. Distribution of muscarinic cholinergic high and low affinity agonist binding sites: a light microscopic autoradiographic study. *Brain Res Bull* 1984;12:233–243.

96. Wang S-Z, El-Fakahany EE. Application of transfected cell lines in studies of functional receptor subtype selectivity of muscarinic agonists. *J Pharmacol Exp Ther* 1993;266(1):237–243.

97. Warpman U, Alafuzoff I, Nordberg A. Coupling of muscarinic receptors to GTP proteins in postmortem human brain—alterations in Alzheimer's disease. *Neurosci Lett* 1993;150:39–43.

Psychopharmacology: The Fourth Generation of Progress, edited by Floyd E. Bloom and David J. Kupfer. Raven Press, Ltd., New York © 1995.

CHAPTER 12

Structure and Function of Cholinergic Pathways in the Cerebral Cortex, Limbic System, Basal Ganglia, and Thalamus of the Human Brain

Marek-Marsel Mesulam

The cerebral cortex, thalamus, and basal ganglia of the human brain provide neural templates for the transformation of simple movements and sensations into exceedingly complex psychological acts and experiences. These transformations occur through the orderly transfer of information along parallel and serial pathways that lead to the formation of large-scale distributed networks. The thousands of neural pathways that contribute to the formation of these networks can be divided into two major groups. One group contains *point-to-point* (discrete) projections such as those that interconnect individual thalamic nuclei with their cortical targets. The second group contains equally important *regulatory* (diffuse) neural projections which (a) innervate the entire cerebral cortex, (b) arise from relatively small nuclei, and (c) employ small amines such as dopamine, histamine, norepinephrine, serotonin, and acetylcholine as the transmitter substances. These regulatory pathways are less involved in determining the specific contents of experience than in modulating its general flavor and impact on the individual. Each of these regulatory pathways has been implicated in the modulation of global behavioral states such as emotion, motivation, and arousal (39; see also Chapter 1, *this volume*).

Every complex psychological phenomenon represents an intermingling of contributions from discrete and regulatory pathways. The content of a memory, for example, is probably dependent on the specific information transported along discrete point-to-point pathways that interconnect association cortex with limbic structures. The

emotional tone of the recollection and perhaps the speed and efficiency of recall, on the other hand, may be determined by the activity of regulatory pathways that innervate the same parts of the brain. Among the various components of complex behavior, those that represent the contributions of the regulatory pathways are the most amenable to psychopharmacological treatment. In fact, the vast majority of modern neuropharmacology is based on drugs that alter the activity along one or more of these transmitter-specific regulatory pathways. This is one reason why regulatory pathways have attracted such a great deal of interest. This chapter will deal with one of these regulatory pathways, namely, the one that employs acetylcholine as its transmitter substance.

Cholinergic pathways are phylogenetically ancient and anatomically ubiquitous. Their presence is identified by markers such as acetylcholinesterase (AChE), muscarinic and nicotinic receptors (see Chapters 9–11, *this volume*), and choline acetyltransferase (ChAT). Of these markers, ChAT is confined to presynaptic cholinergic elements whereas the other two are found in both presynaptic cholinergic neurons and also in the postsynaptic cholinoceptive neurons. All peripheral motor nerves (cranial and spinal) and a substantial portion of the autonomic nervous system are cholinergic. In this chapter, however, the emphasis will be on cholinergic pathways that are exclusively distributed within the central nervous system.

There are eight major cholinergic cell groups that project to other central nervous system structures. Most of these cholinergic cell groups do not respect traditional nuclear boundaries, and their constituent cholinergic cells are intermixed with other noncholinergic neurons. We

M-M Mesulam: Department of Neurology, Northwestern University Medical School, Chicago, Illinois 60611.

have therefore introduced the Ch1–Ch8 nomenclature in order to classify the cholinergic neurons within these eight cell groups (38).

According to this nomenclature, Ch1 designates the cholinergic cells associated with the medial septal nucleus, Ch2 those associated with the vertical nucleus of the diagonal band, Ch3 those associated with the horizontal limb of the diagonal band nucleus, Ch4 those associated with the nucleus basalis of Meynert, Ch5 those associated with the pedunculopontine nucleus of the rostral brainstem, Ch6 those associated with the laterodorsal tegmental nucleus also in the rostral brainstem, Ch7 those in the medial habenula, and Ch8 those in the parabigeminal nucleus.

Tracer experiments in a number of animal species have shown that Ch1 and Ch2 provide the major cholinergic innervation for the hippocampal complex, Ch3 for the olfactory bulb, Ch4 for the cerebral cortex and amygdala, Ch5 and Ch6 for the thalamus, Ch7 for interpeduncular nucleus, and Ch8 for the superior colliculus. There are also lesser connections from Ch1–Ch4 and Ch8 to the thalamus and from Ch5–Ch6 to the cerebral cortex (38,72).

All basal ganglia display widespread cholinergic innervation. The cholinergic innervation of the striatum is mostly intrinsic, arising from cholinergic interneurons. The striatum also receives a lesser cholinergic innervation from Ch4 and from Ch5–Ch6. The cholinergic innervation of other basal ganglia such as the globus pallidus, the subthalamic nucleus, and the pars compacta of the substantia nigra is exclusively extrinsic, probably originating mostly from Ch5–Ch6.

In the rodent brain, there are intrinsic cholinergic interneurons which may provide up to 30% of the cholinergic innervation in the cerebral cortex. No such cholinergic interneurons have been reported in the adult primate cerebral cortex or in the thalamus of any species studied this far. Therefore, the cholinergic innervation of the adult primate cerebral cortex and thalamus is exclusively extrinsic.

THE CHOLINERGIC NEURONS OF THE BASAL FOREBRAIN

The basal forebrain of the primate brain contains four overlapping constellations of cholinergic projection neurons. Studies in the monkey brain show that approximately 10% of perikarya within the boundaries of the medial septal nucleus are cholinergic and belong to the Ch1 cell group, approximately 70% of neurons in the vertical limbic nucleus of the diagonal band are cholinergic and belong to the Ch2 cell group, approximately 1% of neurons in the horizontal nucleus of the diagonal band are cholinergic and belong to the Ch3 cell group, and approximately 90% of the large neurons in the nucleus basalis of the substantia innominata are cholinergic and

belong to the Ch4 cell group. Of these four cholinergic cell groups, the Ch4 group is by far the largest and the one that has been most extensively studied in the human brain (41,47).

Because nearly 90% of the nucleus basalis (NB) neurons in the human brain express choline acetyltransferase (and therefore belong to Ch4), this cell group can also be designated as the NB–Ch4 complex. The more general "NB" term can be used to designate all of the components in this nucleus (large and small cells, cholinergic and noncholinergic), whereas the more restrictive Ch4 designation is reserved for the contingent of cholinergic NB neurons as revealed by ChAT immunohistochemistry.

The human NB–Ch4 extends from the level of the olfactory tubercle to that of the anterior hippocampus, spanning a distance of 13–14 mm in the sagittal plane. It attains its greatest mediolateral width of 18 mm within the substantia innominata (subcommissural gray) (Fig. 1). Arendt et al. (1) have estimated that the human NB–Ch4 complex contains 200,000 neurons in each hemisphere. Thus, the NB–Ch4 contains at least ten times as many

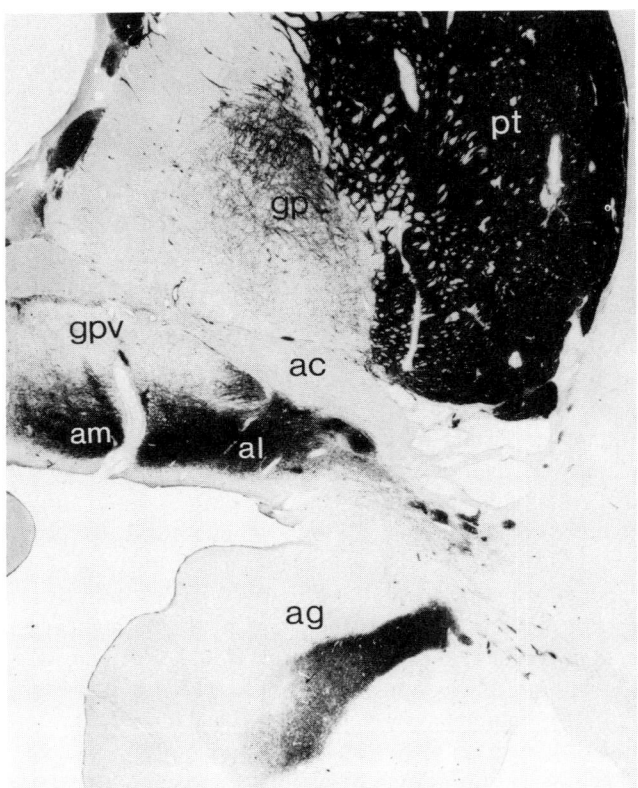

FIG. 1. AChE histochemistry of a coronal section through the anterior sector of NB–Ch4 showing its anteromedial (am) and anterolateral (al) subsector. Medial is to the left, dorsal is to the top. At this level, the NB–Ch4 complex is surrounded by the anterior commissure (ac), the amygdala (ag), and the ventral globus pallidus (gpv). This section also passes through the putamen (pt) and the more dorsal part of the globus pallidus (gp). From the brain of a 91-year-old subject. Magnification ×5. (From ref. 41.)

neurons as the nucleus locus coeruleus, which has approximately 15,000 neurons in the adult human brain (69). On topographical grounds, the constituent neurons of the human NB–Ch4 complex can be subdivided into six sectors that occupy its anteromedial (Ch4am), anterolateral (NB–Ch4al) anterointermediate (NB–Ch4ai), intermediodorsal (NB–Ch4id) intermedioventral (NB–Ch4iv), and posterior (NB–Ch4p) regions.

Gorry (16) has pointed that the NB displays a progressive evolutionary trend, becoming more and more extensive and differentiated in more highly evolved species, especially in primates and cetacea. Our observations are consistent with this general view and show that the human NB–Ch4 is a highly differentiated and relatively large structure. Although many morphological features of the human NB–Ch4 are similar to those described for the rhesus monkey, there is also a sense of increased complexity and differentiation. For example, a prominent Ch4ai sector is easily identified in the human brain but not in the rhesus monkey. In addition to these ''compact'' neuronal sectors, the Ch4 complex also contains ''interstitial'' elements which are embedded within the internal capsule, the diagonal band of Broca, the anterior commissure, the ansa peduncularis, the inferior thalamic peduncle, and the ansa lenticularis. The physiological implications of this intimate association with fiber bundles are unknown. Conceivably, the NB–Ch4 complex, and especially its interstitial components, could monitor and perhaps influence the physiological activity along these fiber tracts. The presence of these interstitial components outside the traditional boundaries of the nucleus basalis is another reason why Ch4 and NB are not synonymous terms.

There is no strict delineation between the boundaries of NB–Ch4 and adjacent cell groups such as those of the olfactory tubercle, preoptic area, hypothalamic nuclei, striatal structures, nuclei of the diagonal band, amygdaloid nuclei, and globus pallidus. In addition to this ''open'' nuclear structure, the neurons of NB–Ch4 are heteromorphic in shape and have an isodendritic morphology with overlapping dendritic fields, many of which extend into fiber tracts traversing the basal forebrain. These characteristics are also present in the nuclei of the brainstem reticular formation and have led to the suggestion that the NB–Ch4 complex could be conceptualized as a telencephalic extension of the brainstem reticular core (58).

All neurons of the Ch1–Ch4 cell groups contain AChE and ChAT in the perikarya, dendrites, and axons. Approximately 90% of Ch1–Ch4 neurons express the p75 low-affinity nerve growth factor receptor (NGFr) (44,53). Nearly all Ch1–Ch4 cholinergic neurons of the human brain also express calbindin D28K (14). There are considerable interspecies differences in the cytochemical signature of basal forebrain cholinergic neurons (14). For example, 20–30% of cholinergic neurons in the basal forebrain of the rat contain reduced nicotinamide-

adenine-dinucleotide-phosphate-diaphorase (NADPHd) activity [which is now known to overlap with nitric oxide synthase activity (70)], whereas none of the basal forebrain cholinergic neurons in the monkey or human brain do so. Furthermore, the basal forebrain cholinergic neurons of the rat do not express calbindin D28K, whereas almost all Ch1–Ch4 neurons of the monkey and human do. There are differences even within primates. For example, Ch1–Ch4 neurons of the monkey express galanin, whereas this does not occur in the human brain (30). Such cytochemical differences need to be taken into account when developing animal models for human diseases that effect the basal forebrain cholinergic cell groups.

The Ch1–Ch4 groups are the only neurons which regularly express large amounts of NGFr in the adult human central nervous system. The NGFr is expressed in the perikaryon and is transported intraaxonally to the cerebral cortex, where it binds cortically produced NGF (23). The NGF–NGFr complex is then transported retrogradely to the Ch1–Ch4 cell body, which is dependent on this retrogradely transported NGF for its survival. Because all Ch1–Ch8 cholinergic neurons express ChAT, the presence of this enzyme in an axon designates it as cholinergic but does not help to identify its origin. Because only Ch1–Ch4 neurons express NGFr, axonal NGFr helps to identify the axon not only as cholinergic but also as originating in the basal forebrain. However, because not all Ch1–Ch4 neurons are NGFr-positive, the absence of NGFr in a cholinergic axon does not rule out the possibility that the axon originates in the basal forebrain.

CHOLINERGIC INNERVATION OF THE CEREBRAL CORTEX

Axonal transport experiments combined with AChE histochemistry or ChAT immunocytochemistry in the monkey have shown that Ch1 and Ch2 provide the major source of cholinergic innervation for the hippocampal complex, that Ch3 provides the major source of cholinergic innervation for the olfactory bulb, and that Ch4 is the major source of cholinergic projections for the entire cerebral cortex and the amygdala. This type of experimental evidence is not available for the human brain. However, there is indirect support for the existence of a similar organization. For example, in patients with Alzheimer's disease, cell loss in the NB–Ch4 complex is almost always significantly correlated with the magnitude of ChAT depletion in the cerebral cortex (11).

Experimental neuroanatomical methods in the monkey brain have shown that different cortical areas receive their major cholinergic input from individual sectors of the NB–Ch4 complex. Thus, Ch4am provides the major source of cholinergic input to medial cortical areas including the cingulate gyrus; Ch4al to frontoparietal and opercular regions and the amygdaloid nuclei; Ch4id–Ch4iv to laterodorsal frontoparietal, peristriate and midtemporal regions; and Ch4p to the superior temporal and temporopolar areas (47). The experimental methods that are needed to reveal this topographic arrangement cannot be used in the human brain. However, indirect evidence for the existence of a similar topographical arrangement can be gathered from patients with Alzheimer's disease. We described two patients in whom extensive loss of cholinergic fibers in temporopolar but not frontal opercular cortex was associated with marked cell loss in the posterior (Ch4p) but not the anterior (Ch4am + Ch4al) sectors of Ch4 (41). This relationship is consistent with the topography of the projections in the monkey brain.

The distribution of cholinergic innervation in the human cerebral cortex has been studied in detail with the help of AChE histochemistry, ChAT immunocytochemistry, and NGFr immunocytochemistry (13,43,45). All cytoarchitectonic regions and layers of the cerebral cortex display a dense cholinergic innervation (Fig. 2). These fibers have numerous varicosities and, on occasion, complex preterminal profiles arranged in the form of dense

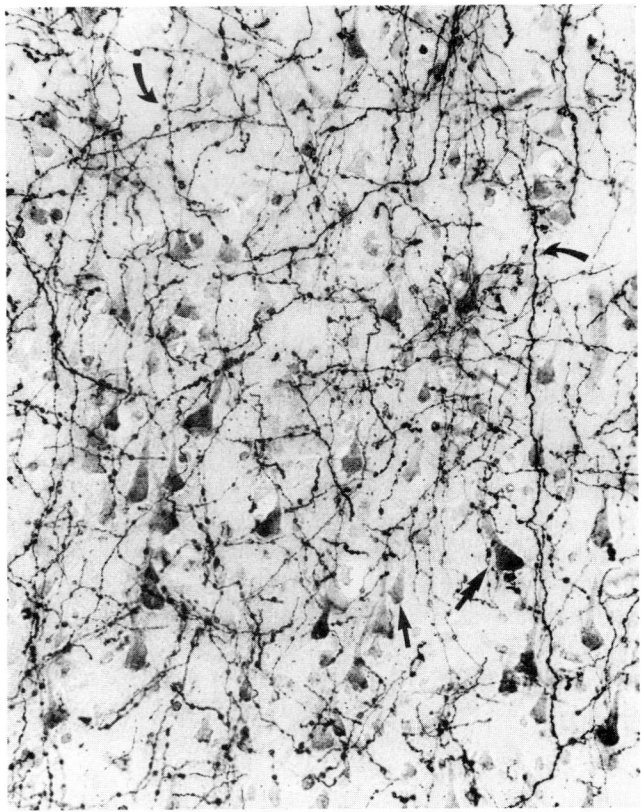

FIG. 2. AChE histochemistry in layer III of inferotemporal visual association cortex of 22-year-old subject. Dorsal is to the top. The AChE-rich axons (which are also ChAT-positive) form a dense plexus. The axons (*curved arrows*) display numerous swellings which may constitute sites of axonal varicosities and synaptic contact. The axons come in close association with cortical neurons that are AChE-rich (*double arrow*) as well as with those that are not (*single arrow*). Magnification ×415. (From ref. 41.)

clusters. The density of cholinergic axons is higher in the more superficial layers (layers I and II and the upper parts of layer III) of the cerebral cortex. Distinct patterns of lamination exist in individual cytoarchitectonic regions.

There are also major and statistically significant differences in the overall density of cholinergic axons among the various cytoarchitectonic areas (Fig. 3). The cholinergic innervation of primary sensory, unimodal and heteromodal association areas is lighter than that of paralimbic and limbic areas. Within unimodal association areas, the density of cholinergic axons and varicosities is lower in the upstream (parasensory) sectors than in the downstream sectors. Within paralimbic regions, the nonisocortical sectors have a higher density of cholinergic innervation than the isocortical sectors. The highest density of cholinergic axons occurs in core limbic structures such as the hippocampus and the amygdala.

Within the hippocampal complex, the highest density of AChE-rich cholinergic fibers is seen in a thin band along the inner edge of the molecular layer of the dentate gyrus and within parts of the CA2, CA3, and CA4 sectors. The subiculum has a cholinergic innervation that is lighter than that of the other hippocampal sectors (17). In the amygdala, each nucleus has a slightly different profile of cholinergic innervation (10). The density is highest in the central and basal lateral nuclei and lightest in the lateral nucleus. The medial nucleus is the only region of the amygdala that has virtually no cholinergic innervation.

In all cortical and hippocampal fields, NGFr axonal staining is of approximately equivalent density as that of axonal ChAT, providing further evidence that the majority of cholinergic innervation to these regions arises from the Ch1–Ch4 cell groups (46). The one exception occurs in the amygdala, especially in the basolateral nucleus, which contains very light NGFr staining, raising the possibility that the cholinergic innervation to this nucleus and perhaps to other parts of the amygdala arises from NGFr negative Ch1–Ch4 neurons or from cholinergic neurons in the brainstem.

POSTSYNAPTIC COMPONENTS OF CORTICAL CHOLINERGIC PATHWAYS

Electronmicroscopic studies in rodents indicate that most cortical cholinergic axons are unmyelinated and that they make symmetrical and asymmetrical synaptic contacts with large numbers of cortical neurons (12,71). It is also thought that some acetylcholine may be re-leased outside of traditional synaptic contacts and that it may exert its effect by diffusion into receptor-containing sites (68).

The acetylcholine released from presynaptic cholinergic axons of the cerebral cortex exerts its neurotransmitter effects through the mediation of nicotinic and muscarinic receptors. Muscarinic receptors predominate in the mammalian cerebral cortex. Five subtypes of muscarinic cholinergic receptors (m1–m5) have been recognized, each

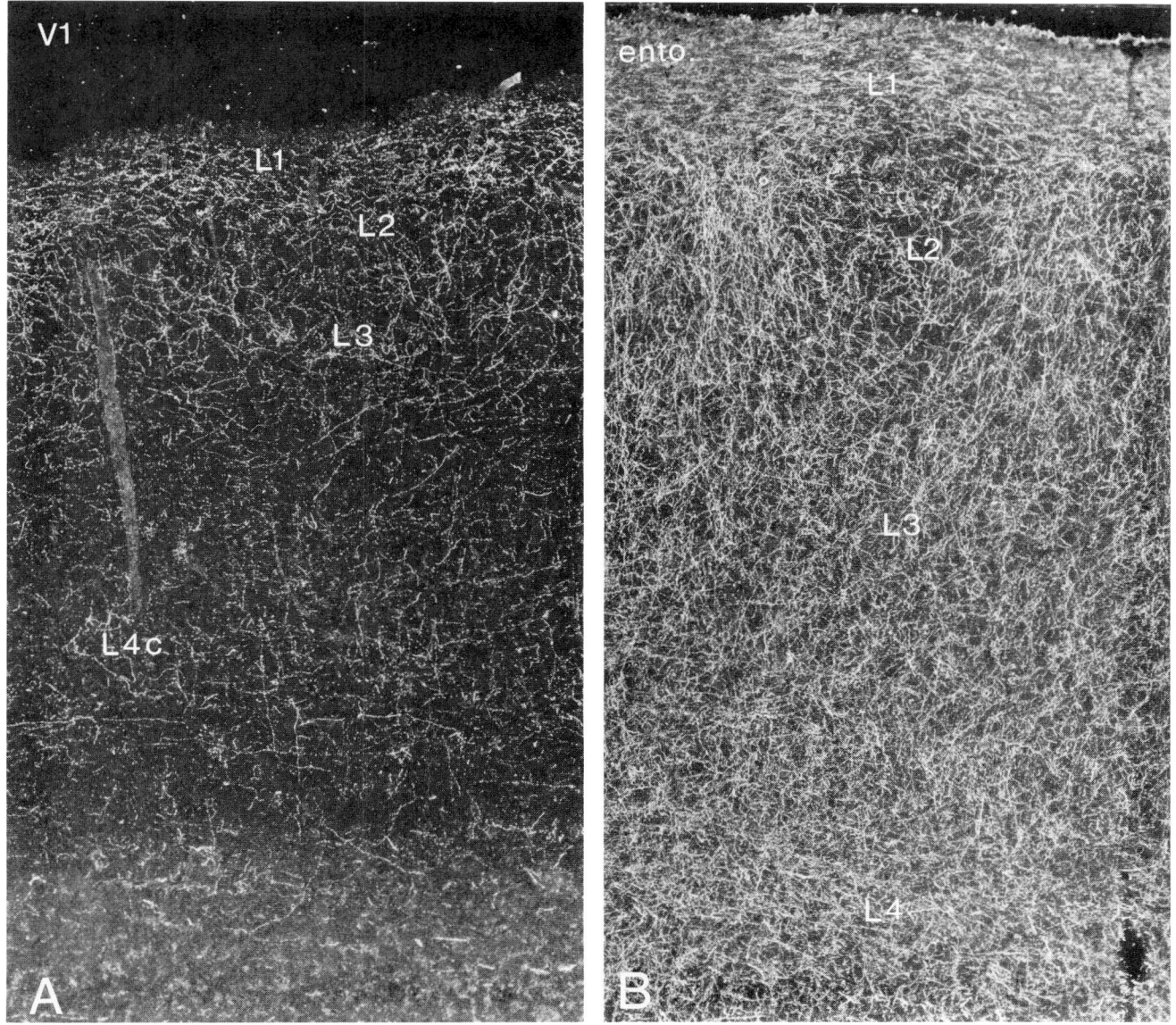

FIG. 3. Dark-field photomicrograph showing the differential density and lamination of cholinergic axons in primary visual cortex (V1) (**A**) and in enterorhinal cortex (**B**). Note the very substantial difference in overall density. Magnification ×62. (From ref. 45.)

the product of a different gene (3,26). Three muscarinic receptor subtypes have been characterized pharmacologically (M1–M3), and of these the M1 and M2 subtypes have received the greatest attention. Autoradiographic experiments in the rhesus monkey showed that the pirenzepine-sensitive M1 receptors were far more numerous than M2 receptors. The M1 receptor density reaches the highest levels in components of limbic and association cortex. In contrast, the M2 receptors reach their highest densities in primary sensory and motor areas of the cortex (34).

Immunocytochemical studies in the human brain have identified cortical neurons which express nicotinic and muscarinic receptors. Such neurons are localized predom-

inantly in the pyramidal neurons of layers III and V. Approximately 30% of immunopositive pyramidal neurons were found to display immunoreactivity for both muscarinic and nicotinic receptors (62).

It is thought that all cholinoceptive neurons express AChE in order to hydrolyze acetylcholine. However, only a subset of cholinoceptive neurons give an AChE-rich histochemical reaction (21,40,42). Some of these AChE-rich neurons are polymorphic in shape and are distributed preferentially in the deeper cortical layers and the subjacent white matter. Others are pyramidal in shape and are located in layers III and V, especially in association cortex. It is interesting to note that such AChE-rich neurons have a low density in limbic and paralimbic areas, although these parts of the cerebral cortex contain the highest presynaptic cholinergic innervation.

In addition to postsynaptic receptors, cholinergic axons are also thought to contain presynaptic autoreceptors. These presynaptic autoreceptors may be involved in the autoregulation of acetylcholine release.

THE CHOLINERGIC PROJECTION CELLS OF THE UPPER BRAINSTEM

Nearly all of the hyperchromic neurons in the pedunculopontine nucleus (pars compacta) of the human brain are intensely ChAT-positive and constitute the compact sector of the Ch5 cell group (Ch5c). The Ch5c component is surrounded by a diffuse-interstitial component (Ch5d) containing slightly smaller ChAT-positive neurons embedded within passing fiber systems such as the superior cerebellar peduncle and especially the central tegmental tract. Isolated Ch5 neurons are also seen in the traditional boundaries of the cuneiform nucleus, the parabrachial nuclei, the subcoeruleus zone, and the lateral lemniscus. The interstitial Ch5 neurons are at least as numerous as those within the compact pedunculopontine region (44).

Approximately 10% of neurons within the compact sector of the pedunculopontine nucleus fail to give a detectable ChAT reaction, even though they have an identical appearance in Nissl preparations. The frequency of noncholinergic neurons can be as high as 75% in regions containing the interstitial components of Ch5. Some of the noncholinergic neurons intermingled with Ch5 are catecholaminergic (tyrosine hydroxylase-positive), but the transmitter identity of most of these neurons remains unknown.

The Ch6 complex has its center of gravity within the laterodorsal tegmental nucleus, but its neurons spread into the adjacent parts of the central gray, into the medial longitudinal fasciculus, and even into the regions of the nucleus locus coeruleus. The Ch6 complex reaches peak density at a level somewhat more caudal than the region of peak density for Ch5. The Ch6 neurons are slightly smaller than those of Ch5c. The laterodorsal tegmental nucleus contains a relatively pure population of cholinergic neurons. However, the surrounding zones of the central gray which contain interstitial Ch6 neurons also contain many tyrosine hydroxylase-positive catecholaminergic neurons.

There is no precise delineation between Ch5 and Ch6. The two groups are related to each other in the form of partially overlapping constellations rather than discrete nuclei with firm boundaries. Here as in the basal forebrain, the lack of correspondence with traditional cytoarchitectonic boundaries and the intermingling of cholinergic with noncholinergic neurons justifies the use of the Ch designation.

Experiments in a number of animal species indicate that Ch5–Ch6 neurons provide the vast majority of cholinergic innervation for the thalamus and that this thalamic projection constitutes the major output for Ch5–Ch6 (18,47). The Ch5–Ch6 cell groups may also provide a relatively sparse projection to parts of the cerebral cortex, the basal forebrain, and a number of extrapyramidal structures such as the striatum, globus pallidus, subthalamic nucleus, and substantia nigra (see refs. 44 and 46 for review).

Animal experiments indicate that the connectivity of Ch5 is not identical to that of Ch6. The Ch5 neurons appear to be more closely interconnected with extrapyramidal structures than the Ch6 neurons (75). Furthermore, the Ch6 group sends relatively few projections to sensory relay nuclei of the thalamus, but it figures prominently in projections to its limbic nuclei (18,75). In keeping with the limbic affiliations of Ch6, projections have been described from the laterodorsal tegmental nucleus of the baboon to such extrathalamic limbic structures as the cingulate and subicular cortices but not to parietal neocortex (49). Furthermore, the cholinergic neurons of the laterodorsal tegmental nucleus (Ch6) have more extensive projections than those of Ch5 to the lateral septum and medial prefrontal cortex (60). Therefore, it appears that Ch6 is more closely associated with the limbic system, whereas Ch5 participates more extensively in the neural systems subserving sensory processing and extrapyramidal motor control. This distinction further justifies the delineation of Ch5 from Ch6 despite the absence of strict cytoarchitectonic demarcations.

THE CHOLINERGIC INNERVATION OF THE THALAMUS

Choline acetyltransferase-positive axonal staining shows that the human thalamus receives substantial and widespread cholinergic innervation (22). The highest levels of ChAT axonal staining are found in intralaminar nuclei (except for the parafascicular nucleus), the reuniens nucleus, the anterodorsal nucleus, medially situated patches in the mediodorsal nucleus, the lateral geniculate nucleus, and the reticular nucleus. The lowest levels are found in the pulvinar and the medial geniculate nucleus. The remaining nuclei display an intermediate density of ChAT-positive cholinergic staining. The cholinergic axons in these nuclei display multiple varicosities and other complex preterminal profiles.

Based on animal experiments, we assume that the majority of these thalamic projections originate in the Ch5–Ch6 cell groups. The existence of NGFr-immunoreactive axonal profiles suggested that some thalamic nuclei of the human brain also receive a second cholinergic innervation from the basal forebrain. Nuclei with the most extensive NGFr immunoreactivity included the mediodorsal nucleus (especially the medially situated patches) as well as the intralaminar and reticular nuclei. The other thalamic nuclei contained only rare NGFr-positive axonal profiles. In each of these areas, the density of ChAT-immunoreactive axonal profiles was always higher, and in most instances much higher, than the density of NGFr-immunoreactive profiles, suggesting that even in the nuclei with a prominent dual cholinergic innervation, the preponderant cholinergic input arises from the brainstem. These observations show that some thalamic nuclei—especially the mediodorsal, intralaminar, and reticular—are under complex dual cholinergic influence, one arising from the basal forebrain and the other arising from the brainstem. In contrast to the cerebral cortex, the thalamus contains more M2 than M1 receptors (6) and also a high level of nicotinic binding (76).

CHOLINERGIC INNERVATION OF THE BASAL GANGLIA

The distribution of ChAT-positive varicose axons indicated that the human striatum, globus pallidus, subthalamic nucleus, red nucleus, and substantia nigra receive substantial cholinergic innervation (46). The density of cholinergic innervation is very high in the striatum, high in the subthalamic nucleus and red nucleus, moderate in the globus pallidus and ventral tegmental area, and low in the pars compacta of the substantia nigra. This cholinergic innervation displays a very orderly but also complex organization within each of these subcortical structures.

The overall cholinergic innervation of the four striatal components (caudate, putamen, olfactory tubercle, and nucleus accumbens) is of comparable intensity, but each component shows a complex mosaic of ChAT-positive varicosities organized in the form of light and dark patches. Numerous ChAT-positive perikarya are distributed throughout the striatal components (Fig. 4).

Animal experiments indicate that the vast majority of striatal cholinergic innervation arises from these cholinergic interneurons. However, we also found that the striatum, especially the putamen, contains NGFr-immunoreactive axons, suggesting that there is a second but lesser cholinergic input from the Ch1–Ch4 neuronal groups. Observations in monkeys show that the striatum may also receive cholinergic projections from the Ch5–Ch6 cell groups of the brainstem (63).

The density of ChAT-positive axons and varicosities in the globus pallidus was modest in comparison to that of the striatum. The rarity of ChAT-positive axonal staining within the striatopallidal bundles eliminates the striatum as the major source of this input. The presence of some NGFr-positive varicosities shows that part of this cholinergic input (especially in the anterior and external pallidal segments) is likely to arise from the Ch1–Ch4 cell groups of the basal forebrain. The majority of the cholinergic innervation for the globus pallidus, especially for its internal sector (which corresponds to the entopeduncular nucleus of nonprimates), however, appears to arise from cholinergic cells outside of the forebrain or from NGFr-

negative neurons of the Ch1–Ch4 cell groups. Most of this projection is likely to come from the Ch5–Ch6 cell groups.

The perikarya of the subthalamic nucleus and red nucleus were embedded within a dense matrix of ChAT-positive varicosities. The paucity of NGFr-like immunoreactivity in these two structures suggested that almost all of this cholinergic innervation arises from sources outside of the basal forebrain. A substantial component of this input probably originates from the Ch5 and Ch6 cell groups. There has been considerable controversy, however, concerning the magnitude of the Ch5–Ch6 projection to the subthalamic nucleus (see ref. 46 for review). Conceivably, the subthalamic nucleus and the red nucleus could receive cholinergic input from brainstem sources other than Ch5–Ch6. It has been suggested (but not yet confirmed), for example, that the red nucleus may receive the bulk of its cholinergic input from ChAT-positive neurons of the cerebellum (27).

The melanin-containing (presumably dopaminergic) neurons of the human substantia nigra also receive ChAT-positive axonal innervation. Axonal NGFr is nearly absent in the substantia nigra. Some experiments in rats have suggested that the Ch5–Ch6 cell groups provide the major source of nigral cholinergic input while other reports provide conflicting evidence. Within the substantia nigra, we found that the medially situated pigmented neurons of the ventral tegmental area received a more intense cholinergic innervation than the more laterally situated neurons of the pars compacts. Such neurochemical differences may underlie the different behavioral affiliations displayed by these two major groups of dopaminergic neurons. The pars compacta of the substantia nigra plays a major role in extrapyramidal motor control, whereas the ventral tegmental area seems to be more closely affiliated with the modulation of motivation and related functions of the limbic system.

Electron microscopic investigations in the striatum of the rat show that the dominant mode of cholinergic neurotransmission occurs through symmetrical synapses upon the medium-sized and noncholinergic (presumably GABAergic) projection neurons (55,57). Assuming that symmetrical synapses are mostly inhibitory, such an input on inhibitory GABAergic projection neurons would have a net excitatory effect upon the targets of striatofugal GABAergic pathways such as the substantia nigra and the globus pallidus. Only 2–3% of cholinergic terminals in the striatum were found to make synaptic contact with cholinergic interneurons (57). It is not known if the extrinsic cholinergic terminals that arise from the basal forebrain have a synaptic organization that sets them apart from the far more numerous intrinsic terminals. In the monkey, muscarinic receptor autoradiography shows that the striatum contains considerably more M1 than M2 receptors (34). Physiological experiments in tissue slices show that muscarinic agonists have complex excitatory and inhibitory effects on striatal neurons (9).

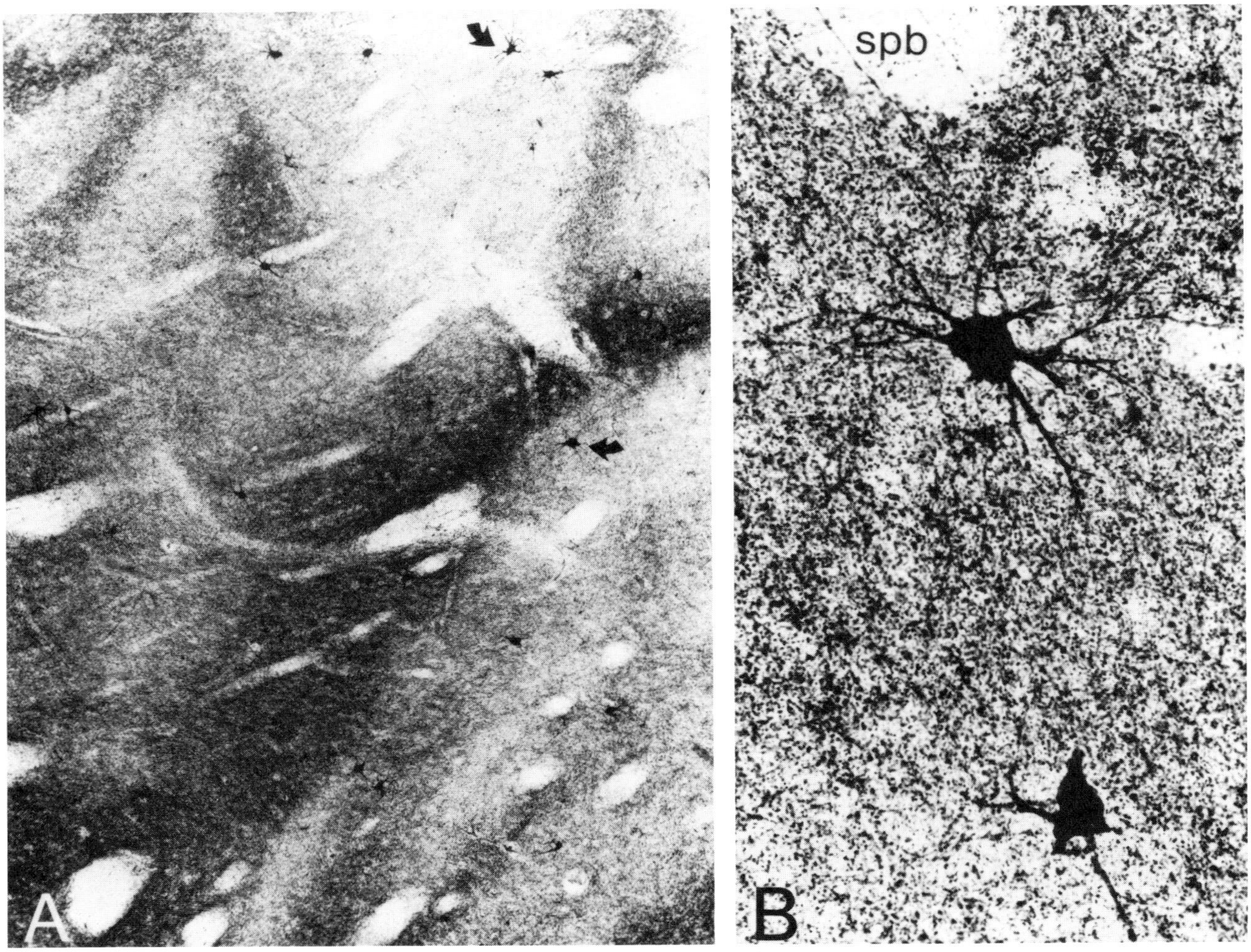

FIG. 4. Choline acetyltransferase (ChAT) immunocytochemistry in the putamen. **A:** Multipolar cholinergic neurons (*curved arrows*) are interspersed throughout the putamen. The ChAT-positive varicosities display intricate variations of density. The lightest areas correspond to the striatal patches (or striasomes), and the more intensely stained areas correspond to the matrix. There is no obvious relationship between the density of ChAT-positive neurons and the density of neuropil staining. Dorsal towards the top, lateral towards the left. Magnification ×64. **B:** Detail of putaminal ChAT immunopositivity. Two ChAT-positive multipolar neurons are embedded in a dense bed of ChAT-positive preterminal profiles (or varicosities). From the brain of a 55-year-old subject. Magnification ×343. (From ref. 46.)

In contrast to the predominance of symmetrical contact within the striatum, the predominant type of cholinergic contact in the subthalamic nucleus and substantia nigra is of the asymmetrical and presumably excitatory type (33,66). In the pars compacta of the substantia nigra and in the ventral tegmental area, cholinergic neurotransmission is mediated predominantly by M1-like receptors and tends to increase the rate of spontaneous action potential of the dopaminergic neurons (31).

Clinical evidence shows that cholinergic agents tend to produce tremor, whereas anticholinergic agents are quite effective for treating the rigidity and bradykinesia of Parkinsonism (54). The influence of cholinoactive substances upon motor activity has traditionally been attributed to the well-established cholinergic innervation of the striatum. Our observations show that the globus pallidus, red nucleus, substantia, and subthalamic nucleus may also participate in mediating the effects of cholinergic agents upon extrapyramidal function.

PHYSIOLOGICAL AND BEHAVIORAL IMPLICATIONS

The physiological effect of acetylcholine on cholinoceptive cortical neurons is exceedingly complex. The major effect of acetylcholine is to cause a relatively prolonged reduction of potassium conductance so as to make cortical cholinoceptive neurons more susceptible to other excitatory inputs (36,64; see also Chapter 5, *this volume*). However, the effect of acetylcholine on cortical neurons can also be inhibitory, either directly or through the mediation of GABAergic interneurons.

Because all regions of the cerebral cortex receive intense cholinergic innervation, it is not surprising that all aspects of cortical function are influenced by cholinergic neurotransmission. In primary visual cortex, for example, cholinergic stimulation does not alter the orientation specificity of a given neuron but increases the likelihood that the neuron will fire in response to its preferred stimulus (61). An analogous effect has been described in somatosensory cortex (48).

The Ch1–Ch4 cell groups of the basal forebrain can be considered as a telencephalic extension of the brainstem reticular formation and also as a direct extension of basomedial limbic cortex. This dual identity helps to understand why arousal and memory are the two major behavioral affiliations of the Ch1–Ch4 cell groups. Thus, experiments in rats have shown that the cortical cholinergic projections from the basal forebrain play a major role in sustaining at least one component of the hippocampal theta rhythm and also the arousal-related low-voltage fast activity of the cortical electroencephalogram (EEG) (5,65). In a number of animal species, lesions of the Ch4 cell group can cause severe impairments of memory that can be reversed by the systemic administration of agonists (28,59). We are beginning to understand the cellular bases for these two behavioral affiliations.

Single-unit studies in monkeys have shown that the neurons of the nucleus basalis (Ch4) are particularly sensitive to stimulus novelty and to the motivational relevance of sensory cues (73,74). The novelty and behavioral significance of a sensory event can therefore influence the cortical release of acetylcholine, which, in turn, modulates the cortical response to the sensory event. Cortical cholinergic pathways are thus in a position to alter the neural impact of sensory experiences according to their behavioral significance. It is easy to see how such a circuitry would have a major influence on cortical arousal. In keeping with this interpretation, the muscarinic blocking agent scopolamine attenuates the cortical P-300 arousal response that is normally elicited by novel or surprising stimuli (19).

The relationship of the Ch1–Ch4 cell groups and of cortical cholinergic innervation to memory function is quite complex. Limbic and paralimbic regions of the cerebral cortex are known to play a critical role in memory and learning. The preferential concentration of cholinergic innervation in these parts of cortex may explain why cholinergic antagonists and cholinoactive drugs seem to have a preferential effect on memory, learning, and other limbic functions such as mood, reward, and aggressive behaviors (15,77,78). The role of acetylcholine in hippocampal long-term potentiation (67) may provide another mechanism that underlies the relationship of cholinergic pathways to memory. Recent brain-slice experiments in piriform cortex of the rat have shown that acetylcholine can selectively suppress excitatory intrinsic synaptic transmission through a presynaptic mechanism, while leaving excitatory afferent input unaffected. In a computa-

tion model, this selective suppression can prevent interference from previously stored patterns during the learning of new patterns. Hasselmo et al. (20) have argued that this could provide a novel mechanism through which cortical cholinergic innervation could participate in new learning. Buzsaki (4) has proposed a different model according to which the cholinergic innervation, especially of the hippocampal complex, plays a major role in switching from on-line attentive processing, characterized by the hippocampal theta rhythm, to an off-line period of consolidation, characterized by sharp wave activity (see ref. 7 for review). Cholinergic innervation may even participate in cortical plasticity and axonal sprouting (2,32). We have speculated, for example, that the exceedingly complex presynaptic "dense cluster" profiles displayed by cholinergic axons of the cerebral cortex may reflect events of local plasticity and reorganization in response to individual experience (45).

Another mechanism that links cholinergic axons to memory and learning may be related to the differential regional density of cortical cholinergic innervation. Experimental evidence leads to the conclusion that sensory–limbic pathways play pivotal roles in a wide range of behaviors related to emotion, motivation, and especially memory (37,50). The primary sensory areas of the cerebral cortex which provide a portal for the entry of sensory information into cortical circuitry. These primary areas project predominantly to upstream (parasensory) unimodal sensory association areas, which, in turn, project to downstream unimodal areas and heteromodal cortex. The heteromodal and downstream unimodal areas collectively provide the major source of sensory information into paralimbic and limbic areas of the brain. Our observations show that the density of cholinergic innervation is lower within unimodal and heteromodal association areas than in paralimbic areas of the brain. Moreover, in the unimodal areas the downstream sectors had a higher density of cholinergic innervation than the upstream sectors. Within all major paralimbic areas, we found that the non-isocortical subsectors, known to have the more extensive interconnections with limbic structures, also had a higher density of cholinergic innervation. Core limbic areas such as the amygdala and hippocampus had the highest densities of cholinergic innervation.

This pattern of differential distribution led us to suggest that sensory information is likely to come under progressively greater cholinergic influence as it is conveyed along the multisynaptic pathways leading to the limbic system. As a consequence of this arrangement, cortical cholinergic innervation may help to channel (or gate) sensory information into and out of the limbic system in a way that is sensitive to the behavioral relevance of the associated experience. The memory disturbances that arise after damage to the Ch1–Ch4 cell groups or after the systemic administration of cholinergic antagonists may therefore reflect a disruption of sensory–limbic interactions which are crucial for effective memory and learning.

In addition to Ch1–Ch4, the cholinergic neurons of the upper brainstem are also intimately involved in the modulation of arousal. Moruzzi and Magoun (52) had introduced the concept of an ascending reticular activating system (ARAS) that acted to desynchronize the cortical electroencephalogram via a relay in the thalamus. Subsequent work revealed that a most important component in this system consists of a cholinergic reticulothalamic pathway that facilitates the activation of corticopetal relay neurons in the thalamus (8,24,25,35,56). The physiological relevance of this pathway to the reticular activating system was demonstrated by Kayama et al. (29). They identified the Ch5–Ch6 neurons with NDPHd histochemistry and showed that electrical stimulation of these neurons causes a scopolamine-sensitive activation of lateral geniculate neurons and even an occasional enhancement of their response to photic stimulation. Thus, the Ch5–Ch6 neurons can facilitate the transthalamic (and ultimately corticopetal) processing of sensory information in ways that could modulate arousal and attention.

Electrical stimulation of Ch5 causes a hyperpolarization of GABAergic neurons in the reticular nucleus of the thalamus. Because the neurons of the reticular nucleus have an inhibitory effect on thalamic relay neurons, the net effect of Ch5 stimulation is to facilitate transthalamic processing by the excitation of relay nuclei and also through a process of disinhibition (64). The reticular nucleus, which plays a pivotal role in the regulation of many processes related to arousal, attention, and sleep, receives a dual cholinergic innervation, one from Ch5–Ch6 and a second from Ch4.

Acetylcholine appears to be the neurotransmitter responsible for switching the burst firing mode of thalamic neurons during EEG-synchronized sleep toward a tonic firing mode associated with waking and rapid eye movement (REM) sleep (64). The Ch5–Ch6 cell groups are also directly involved in brainstem mechanisms which trigger REM sleep (51).

TOWARDS AN EXPANDED ARAS

These observations show that the original concept of the ARAS needs to be expanded to include at least two sources of ascending cholinergic projections, a traditional one in the upper brainstem (Ch5–Ch6) and a second one in the basal forebrain (Ch1–Ch4). Noncholinergic regulatory pathways which arise from the hypothalamus (histaminergic; see Chapter 35), ventral tegmental area (dopaminergic; see Chapters 15, 22, and 25), nucleus locus coeruleus (noradrenergic; see Chapters 29 and 32), and brainstem raphe (serotonergic; see Chapters 39 and 41, *this volume*) and which send widespread projections to the cerebral cortex and thalamus probably also need to be included into this expanded ARAS. Each of these cholinergic and noncholinergic projections can exert a powerful influence on the information-processing state of the thalamus and cerebral cortex in ways that influence attentional, motivational, and arousal states. These ascending regulatory pathways provide the physiological matrix (or state) within which the discrete point-to-point projections that interconnect the cortex, thalamus, and basal ganglia set the vectors of complex behaviors.

ACKNOWLEDGMENTS

I want to thank Leah Christie for expert secretarial assistance. This work was supported in part by a Javits Neuroscience Investigator Award (NS20285).

REFERENCES

1. Arendt T, Bigl V, Tennstedt A, Arendt A. Neuronal loss in different parts of the nucleus basalis is related to neuritic plaque formation in cortical target areas in Alzheimer's disease. *J Neurosci* 1985; 14:1–14.
2. Bear MF, Singer W. Modulation of visual cortical plasticity by acetylcholine and noradrenaline. *Nature* 1986;320:172–176.
3. Bonner TI. The molecular basis of muscarinic receptor diversity. *Trends Neurol Sci* 1989;12:148–151.
4. Buzsaki G. Commentary: Two-stage model of memory trace formation: a role for "noisy" brain states. *Neuroscience* 1989;31:551–570.
5. Buzsaki G, Bickford RG, Ponomareff G, Thal LJ, Mandel R, Gage FH. Nucleus basalis and thalamic control of neocortical activity in the freely moving rat. *J Neurosci* 1988;8:4007–4026.
6. Cortes R, Probst A, Palacios JM. Quantitative light microscopic autoradiographic localization of cholinergic muscarinic receptors in the human brain: forebrain. *Neuroscience* 1987;20:65–107.
7. Churchland PS, Sejnowski TJ. The computational brain. In: *Plasticity: cells, circuits, brains and behavior*. Cambridge, MA: MIT Press, 1992;239–329.
8. Dingledine R, Kelly JS. The brainstem stimulation and the acetylcholine-invoked inhibition of neurons in the feline nucleus reticularis thalami. *J Physiol* 1977;271:135–154.
9. Dodt HU, Misgeld U. Muscarinic slow excitation and muscarinic inhibition of synaptic transmission in the rat neostriatum. *J Physiol (Lond)* 1986;380:593–608.
10. Emre M, Heckers S, Mash DC, Geula C, Mesulam M-M. Cholinergic innervation of the amygdaloid complex in the human brain and its alterations in old age and Alzheimer's disease. *J Comp Neurol* 1993;336(1):117–134.
11. Etienne P, Robitaille Y, Wood P, Gauthier S, Nair NPV, Quirion R. Nucleus basalis neuronal loss, neuritic plaques and choline acetyltransferase activity in advanced Alzheimer's disease. *J Neurosci* 1986;19:279–1291.
12. Frotscher M, Leranth C. Cholinergic innervation of the rat hippocampus as revealed by choline acetyltransferase immunocytochemistry: A combined light and electron microscopic study. *J Comp Neurol* 1985;239:237–246.
13. Geula C, Mesulam M-M. Cortical cholinergic fibers in aging and Alzheimer's disease: a morphometric study. *Neuroscience* 1989;33:469–481.
14. Geula C, Schatz CR, Mesulam M-M. Differential localization of NADPH-Diaphorase and calbindin-D 28K within the cholinergic neurons of the basal forebrain, striatum and brainstem in the rat, monkey, baboon and human. *Neuroscience* 1993;54(2):461–476.
15. Gillin JC, Sutton L, Ruiz C, Kelsoe J, Dupont RM, Dovko D, Risch SC, Golshan S, Janowsky D. The cholinergic rapid eye movement induction test with arecholine in depression. *Arch Gen Psychiatry* 1991;48:264–270.
16. Gorry JD. Studies on the comparative anatomy of the ganglion basale of Meynert. *Acta Anat (Basel)* 1963;55:51–104.
17. Green RC, Mesulam M-M. Acetylcholinesterase fiber staining in the human hippocampus and parahippocampal gyrus. *J Comp Neurol* 1988;273:488–499.

18. Hallanger AE, Levey AI, Lee HJ, Rye DB, Wainer BH. The origins of cholinergic and other subcortical afferents to the thalamus in the rat. *J Comp Neurol* 1987;262:105–124.
19. Hammond EJ, Meador KJ, Aunq-Din R, Wilder BJ. Cholinergic modulation of human P3 event-related potentials. *Neurology* 1987;37:346–350.
20. Hasselmo ME, Anderson BP, Bower JM. Cholinergic modulation of cortical associative memory function. *J Neurophysiol* 1992;67:1230–1246.
21. Heckers S, Geula C, Mesulam M-M. Acetylcholinesterase-rich pyramidal neurons in Alzheimer's disease. *Neurobiol Aging* 1992;13:455–460.
22. Heckers S, Geula C, Mesulam M-M. Cholinergic innervation of the human thalamus: dual origin and differential nuclear distribution. *J Comp Neurol* 1992;325:68–82.
23. Hefti F, Hartikka J, Salvaterra A, Weiner WJ, Mash D. Localization of nerve growth factor receptors in cholinergic neurons of the human basal forebrain. *Neurosci Lett* 1986;69:37–41.
24. Hoover DB, Baisden RH. Localization of putative cholinergic neurons innervation the anteroventral thalamus. *Brain Res Bull* 1980;5:519–524.
25. Hoover DB, Jacobowitz DM. Neurochemical and histochemical studies of the effect of a lesion of the nucleus cuneiformis on the cholinergic innervation of discrete areas of the rat brain. *Brain Res* 1979;70:113–122.
26. Hosey MM. Diversity of structure, signaling and regulation within the family of muscarinic cholinergic receptors. *FASEB J* 1992;6:845–852.
27. Ikeda M, Houtani T, Ueyama T, Sugimoto T. Choline acetyltransferase immunoreactivity in the cat cerebellum. *Neuroscience* 1991;45:671–690.
28. Irle E, Markowitsch HJ. Basal forebrain-lesioned monkeys are severely impaired in tasks of association and recognition memory. *Ann Neurol* 1987;22:735–743.
29. Kayama J, Takagi M, Ogawa T. Cholinergic influence of the laterodorsal tegmental nucleus on neuronal activity in the rat lateral geniculate nucleus. *J Neurophysiol* 1986;56:1297–1309.
30. Kordower JH, Mufson EJ. Galanin-like immunoreactivity within the primate basal forebrain: differential staining patterns between humans and monkeys. *J Comp Neurol* 1990;294:281–292.
31. Lacey MG, Calabresi P, North RA. Muscarine depolarizes rat substantia nigra zona compacta and ventral tegmental neurons in vitro through M1-like receptors. *J Pharmacol Exp Ther* 1990;253:395–400.
32. Layer PG, Sporns O. Spatiotemporal relationship of embryonic cholinesterases with cell proliferation in chicken brain and eye. *Proc Natl Acad Sci USA* 1987;84:284–288.
33. Martinez-Murillo R, Villalba RM, Rodrigo J. Electron microscopic localization of cholinergic terminals in the rat substantia nigra: an immunocytochemical study. *Neurosci Lett* 1989;96:121–126.
34. Mash DC, White WF, Mesulam M-M. Distribution of muscarinic receptor subtypes within architectonic subregions of the primate cerebral cortex. *J Comp Neurol* 1988;278:265–274.
35. McCance I, Phillis JW, Westerman RA. Acetylcholine-sensitivity of thalamic neurons: its relationship to synaptic transmission. *Br J Pharmacol* 1986;32:635–651.
36. McCormick DA. Cellular mechanisms of cholinergic control of neocortical and thalamic neuronal excitability. In: Steriade M, Biesold D, eds. *Brain cholinergic systems.* New York: Oxford University Press, 1990;236–264.
37. Mesulam M-M. Patterns in behavioral neuroanatomy. In: Mesulam M-M, ed. *Principles of behavioral neurology.* Contemporary Neurology Series. Philadelphia: FA Davis, 1985;1–70.
38. Mesulam M-M. Central cholinergic pathways: neuroanatomy and some behavioral implications. In: Avoli M, Reader TA, Dykes RW, Gloor P, eds. *Neurotransmitters and cortical function.* New York: Plenum Press, 1988;237–260.
39. Mesulam M-M. Large scale neurocognitive networks and distributed processing for attention, language and memory. *Ann Neurol* 1990;28:597–613.
40. Mesulam M-M, Geula C. Acetylcholinesterase-rich pyramidal neurons in the human neocortex and hippocampus: absence at birth, development during the life span, and dissolution in Alzheimer's disease. *Ann Neurol* 1988;24:765–773.
41. Mesulam M-M, Geula C. Nucleus basalis (Ch4) and cortical cholinergic innervation of the human brain: observations based on the distribution of acetylcholinesterase and choline acetyltransferase. *J Comp Neurol* 1988;275:216–240.
42. Mesulam M-M, Geula C. Acetylcholinesterase-rich neurons of human cerebral cortex: cytoarchitectonic and ontogenetic patterns of distribution. *J Comp Neurol* 1991;306:193–220.
43. Mesulam M-M, Geula C. Overlap between acetylcholinesterase-rich and choline acetyltransferase-positive (cholinergic) axons in human cerebral cortex. *Brain Res* 1992;577:112–120.
44. Mesulam M-M, Geula C, Bothwell MA, Hersh LB. Human reticular formation: cholinergic neurons of the pedunculopontine and laterodorsal tegmental nuclei and some cytochemical comparisons to the forebrain cholinergic neurons. *J Comp Neurol* 1989;281:611–633.
45. Mesulam M-M, Hersh LB, Mash DC, Geula C. Differential cholinergic innervation within functional subdivisions of the human cerebral cortex: a choline acetyltransferase study. *J Comp Neurol* 1992;318:316–328.
46. Mesulam M-M, Mash D, Hersh L, Bothwell M, Geula C. Cholinergic innervation of the human striatum, globus pallidus, subthalamic nucleus, substantia nigra and red nucleus. *J Comp Neurol* 1992;323:252–268.
47. Mesulam M-M, Mufson EJ, Levey AI, Wainer BH. Cholinergic innervation of cortex by the basal forebrain: cytochemistry and cortical connections of the septal area, diagonal band nuclei, nucleus basalis (substantia innominata) and hypothalamus in the rhesus monkey. *J Comp Neurol* 1983;214:170–197.
48. Metherate R, Tremblay N, Dykes RW. The effects of acetylcholine on response properties of cat somatosensory cortical neurons. *J Neurophysiol* 1988;59:1231–1252.
49. Mikol J, Menini M, Brion S, Guicharnaud L. Connections of the laterodorsal nucleus of the thalamus in the monkey. Study of efferents. *Rev Neurol (Paris)* 1984;140:615–624.
50. Mishkin M. A memory system in the monkey. *Philos Trans R Soc Lond [Biol]* 1982;298:85–92.
51. Mitani A, Ito K, Hallanger AE, Wainer BH, Kataoka K, McCarley RW. Cholinergic projections from the laterodorsal and pedunculopontine tegmental nuclei to the pontine gigantocellular tegmental field in the cat. *Brain Res* 1988;451:397–402.
52. Moruzzi G, Magoun HW. Brain stem reticular formation and activation of the EEG. *Electroencephalogr Clin Neurophysiol* 1949;1:459–473.
53. Mufson EJ, Bothwell M, Hersh LB, Kordower JH. Nerve growth factor receptor immunoreactive profiles in the normal, aged human basal forebrain: colocalization with cholinergic neurons. *J Comp Neurol* 1989;285:196–217.
54. Penney JB, Young AB. Speculations on the functional anatomy of basal ganglia disorders. *Annu Rev Neurosci* 1983;6:73–94.
55. Phelps PE, Houser CR, Vaughn JE. Immunocytochemical localization of choline acetyltransferase within the rat striatum: a correlated light and electron microscopic study of cholinergic neurons and synapses. *J Comp Neurol* 1985;238:286–307.
56. Phillis JW, Tebecis AK, York DH. A study of cholinoceptive cells in the lateral geniculate nucleus. *J Physiol* 1967;192:695–713.
57. Pickel VM, Chan J. Spiny neurons lacking choline acetyltransferase immunoreactivity are major targets of cholinergic and catecholaminergic terminals in rat striatum. *J Neurosci Res* 1990;25:263–280.
58. Ramon-Moliner E, Nauta WJH. The isodendritic core of the brain. *J Comp Neurol* 1966;126:311–336.
59. Ridley RM, Murray TK, Johnson JA, Baker HF. Learning impairment following lesion of the basal nucleus of Meynert in the marmoset: modification by cholinergic drugs. *Brain Res* 1986;376:108–116.
60. Satoh K, Fibiger HC. Cholinergic neurons of the laterodorsal tegmental nucleus: efferent and afferent conditions. *J Comp Neurol* 1986;253:277–302.
61. Sato H, Hata V, Hagihara K, Tsumoto T. Effects of cholinergic depletion on neuron activities in the cat visual cortex. *J Neurophysiol* 1987;58:781–794.
62. Schröder H, Giacobini E, Struble RG, et al. Muscarinic cholinoceptive neurons in the frontal cortex in Alzheimer's disease. *Brain Res Bull* 1991;227:631–636.
63. Smith Y, Parent A. Differential connections of caudate and putamen in the squirrel monkey (*Saimiri sciureus*). *Neuroscience* 1986;18:347–371.
64. Steriade M, Gloor P, Llinas RR, Lopes da Silva FH, Mesulam

M-M. Basic mechanisms of cerebral rhythmic activities. *Electroencephalogr Clin Neurophysiol* 1990;76:481–508.

65. Steward DF, Macfabe DF, Vanderwolf CH. Cholinergic activation of the electrocorticogram: role of the substantia innominata and effects of atropine and quinuclidinyl benzilate. *Brain Res* 1984; 322:219–232.

66. Sugimoto T, Hattori T. Organization and efferent projections of nucleus tegmenti pedunculopontinus pars compacta with special reference to its cholinergic aspects. *Neuroscience* 1984;11:931–946.

67. Tanaka Y, Sakurai M, Hayashi S. Effect of scopolamine and HP029, a cholinesterase inhibitor, on long-term potentiation in hippocampal slices of guinea pig. *Neurosci Lett* 1989;98:179–183.

68. Umbriaco D, Watkins KF, Descarries L, Cozzari C, Hartman B. Ultrastructural features of acetylcholine axon terminals in adult rat cerebral cortex. *Soc Neurosci Abstr* 1990;16:1057.

69. Vijayashankar N, Brody H. A quantitative study of the pigmented neurons in the nuclei locus coeruleus and sub coeruleus in man as related to aging. *J Neuropathol Exp Neurol* 1979;38:490–497.

70. Vincent SR, Hope BT. Neurons that say no. *Trends Neurol Sci* 1992;15:108–113.

71. Wainer BH, Bolam JP, Freund TF, Henderson Z, Totterdell S, Smith AD. Cholinergic synapses in the rat brain: a correlated light and electron microscopic immunohistochemical study employing a monoclonal antibody against choline acetyltransferase. *Brain Res* 1984;308:69–76.

72. Wainer BH, Mesulam M-M. Ascending cholinergic pathways in the rat brain. In: Steriade M, Biesold D, eds. *Brain cholinergic systems.* New York: Oxford University Press, 1990;65–119.

73. Wilson FAW, Rolls ET. Neuronal responses related to reinforcement in the primate basal forebrain. *Brain Res* 1990;509:213–231.

74. Wilson FAW, Rolls ET. Neuronal responses related to novelty and familiarity of visual stimuli in the substantia innominata, diagonal band of Broca and periventricular region of the primate basal forebrain. *Exp Brain Res* 1990;80:104–120.

75. Woolf NJ, Butcher LL. Cholinergic systems in the rat brain. III. Projections from the pontomesencephalic tegmentum to the thalamus, tectum, basal ganglia, and basal forebrain. *Brain Res Bull* 1986;16:603–637.

76. Xuereb JH, Perry EK, Candy JM, Bonham JR, Perry RH, Marshall E. Parameters of cholinergic neurotransmission in the thalamus in Parkinson's disease and Alzheimer's disease. *J Neurol Sci* 1990;99:185–197.

77. Yeomans JS, Kofman O, McFarlane V. Cholinergic involvement in lateral hypothalamic rewarding brain stimulation. *Brain Res* 1984;329:19–26.

78. Yoshimura H, Ueki S. Biochemical correlates in mouse-killing behavior of the rat: prolonged isolation and brain cholinergic function. *Pharmacol Biochem Behav* 1977;6:193–196.

Psychopharmacology: The Fourth Generation of Progress, edited by Floyd E. Bloom and David J. Kupfer. Raven Press, Ltd., New York © 1995.

CHAPTER 13

Functional Heterogeneity of Central Cholinergic Systems

Peter B. Reiner and H. Christian Fibiger

Cholinergic neurons are widely distributed throughout the mammalian central nervous system, and they exist as both projection neurons and interneurons. Amongst the projection neurons, two prominent cell groups have received the lion's share of attention in recent years: basal forebrain cholinergic neurons (located in the medial septum, vertical and horizontal limbs of the diagonal band of Broca, and the nucleus basalis) and brainstem cholinergic neurons (found in the laterodorsal and pedunculopontine tegmental nuclei). Basal forebrain cholinergic neurons innervate the cerebral cortex, while brainstem cholinergic neurons primarily innervate the thalamus (see Chapter 12, *this volume*). Within the basal forebrain cholinergic system, subdivisions exist: Cholinergic neurons in the medial septum/vertical limb project primarily to the hippocampus, while the axon terminals of cholinergic neurons found in the horizontal limb and nucleus basalis are directed primarily towards the neocortex. As will be argued below, it is beginning to appear that these anatomical distinctions may have considerable functional relevance. In particular, there is growing evidence that anatomically distinct cholinergic neurons subserve distinct functions.

Based upon the continuous distribution of the "cholinergic basal nucleus complex" (56) and a continuous caudal-to-rostral gradient of development (57), earlier formulations suggested that basal forebrain cholinergic neurons might reasonably be viewed as a single functional unit. Histochemical data now argue against such a view. While most, if not all, basal forebrain cholinergic neurons express nerve growth factor (NGF) receptors (4; see also Chapter 55, *this volume*), substance P receptors (23), and

P. B. Reiner and H. C. Fibiger: Division of Neurological Sciences, Department of Psychiatry, University of British Columbia, Vancouver, B.C. V6T 1Z3, Canada.

estrogen receptors (67; see also Chapter 65, *this volume*), there appears to be considerable heterogeneity with respect to colocalized neuroactive agents. In the rat, for example, only those basal forebrain cholinergic neurons localized within the medial septum and vertical limb of the diagonal band (which project to the hippocampus) express the enzyme nitric oxide synthase (25,44) and the neuropeptide galanin (37). Thus, it is clear that not all basal forebrain cholinergic neurons exhibit the same phenotype and that cotransmitter status is correlated with terminal fields. The functional significance of this phenomenon is not yet clear, there are marked species differences in expression of several of these phenotypic markers (25,35,71). Nonetheless, these data demonstrate that, at least in the rat, there are chemical differences between subpopulations of basal forebrain cholinergic neurons. To date, brainstem cholinergic neurons appear relatively uniform, but this question has not been examined in sufficient detail. These observations have important implications for pharmacological manipulation of central cholinergic neurons, for therapies based upon transplantation of cholinergic neurons, and for behavioral formulations of central cholinergic function.

ELECTROPHYSIOLOGY OF CENTRAL CHOLINERGIC SYSTEMS

One way of understanding the functional role of central cholinergic neurons is to study the activity of *identified* cholinergic neurons in behaving animals during the execution of complex behaviors. To date, such studies have not been technically feasible. Rather, recordings have been obtained from neurons in regions that contain dense but not pure populations of cholinergic neurons, with or without the additional criterion of antidromic invasion from known postsynaptic targets. While data obtained with this approach are interesting, because it has not been possible to be certain that recordings were indeed obtained from cholinergic neurons, their precise relationship to central cholinergic function remains uncertain.

Several studies have examined state-related changes in firing rate of basal forebrain neurons in rats and cats. The results have been as diverse as the neurons from which the recordings were obtained: Some neurons increase their firing during waking, whereas others exhibit increased activity during slow-wave sleep (13,65). In the primate, nucleus basalis neurons consistently increase their firing rate in response to reinforcing stimuli, but this cannot be construed as a "signature" of cholinergic neurons because cells in noncholinergic regions of the forebrain respond similarly (48,53). Nonetheless, the increase in firing rate in the region of the nucleus basalis can be dissociated from both the sensory and motoric aspects of the task (50,73). At present, it remains unclear to what extent such responses reflect a change in arousal or other complex contingencies associated with the rewarding task (49,74).

An enduring problem, of course, is the absence of definitive phenotypic identification of these neurons as cholinergic, an issue of critical import. This obstacle has been overcome in studies of basal forebrain cholinergic neurons in brain slices, where the combination of intracellular labelling and choline acetyltransferase (ChAT) immunohistochemistry has permitted unambiguous identification of the intrinsic properties of cholinergic neurons. In nucleus basalis, identified basal forebrain cholinergic neurons have intrinsic ionic conductances which endow them with the capability of generating bursts of action potentials (32). Surprisingly, such bursting behavior is much more difficult to evoke in identified cholinergic neurons in the medial septum (Gorelova and Reiner, *unpublished observations*), where bursts of action potentials are commonly found "pacing" the theta rhythm (63). At present, it is difficult to place these in vitro studies into a behavioral context. However, it is of considerable interest that similar regional differences exist in both physiological and anatomical phenotypes (see above), further supporting the notion that functional subdivisions exist within the cholinergic basal forebrain.

Mesopontine cholinergic neurons have also been intensively studied in recent years. As with basal forebrain neurons, the state-related discharge of brainstem neurons in regions containing dense accumulations of cholinergic neurons is heterogeneous; at least some neurons exhibit discharge properties consistent with a role in electroencephalographic (EEG) desynchrony (see below) as well as in synchrony with ponto-geniculo-occipital (PGO) waves during rapid eye movement (REM) sleep (61). Once again, the heterogeneous nature of the nuclei in question and the absence of definitive identification of the cholinergic phenotype in such neurons has hindered the generation of strong hypotheses of brainstem cholinergic function. However, studies of identified brainstem cholinergic neurons in brain slices have produced results with clear behavioral implications. At least in the rat, it is the cholinergic neurons of the brainstem that are capable of generating bursts of action potentials (31), and this provides a plausible cellular mechanism for the generation of PGO waves (34).

ROLE OF CENTRAL CHOLINERGIC NEURONS IN EEG DESYNCHRONIZATION

During the waking state, the neocortical electroencephalogram (EEG) is dominated by a low-voltage, high-frequency pattern known as *EEG desynchrony*. It is well established that systemic administration of muscarinic antagonists blocks neocortical EEG desynchrony during most waking behaviors (33,68,70). The implication is that central cholinergic mechanisms are involved in control of the EEG, in particular in the generation of EEG desynchrony. A key question relates to the locus of the antimuscarinic effect upon the cortical EEG. The two most likely candidate cholinergic systems are those arising in the brainstem mesopontine tegmentum and the basal forebrain. The notion that brainstem cholinergic systems are involved in EEG desynchrony has a rich history. The most effective sites for electrically evoked EEG desynchrony in the cat brain (39) coincide with regions containing dense accumulations of cholinergic neurons (29,47). Retrograde tracing studies have confirmed the early conjecture of Shute and Lewis (58) that there exists a prominent cholinergic pathway from the mesopontine tegmentum to the thalamus (28,55). This is an important point, because it has been argued that the membrane potential of thalamic neurons is central to neuronal control of the cortical EEG, with depolarization associated with desynchrony and hyperpolarization associated with synchrony of the EEG (60). Consistent with this notion, acetylcholine depolarizes thalamic relay neurons in brain slices (36), as does stimulation of the mesopontine tegmentum in vivo (43). In unanesthetized animals, at least some mesopontine neurons fire at higher rates during EEG desynchronized states than during slow-wave sleep (20,59). Taken together, it is plausible that activation of brainstem cholinergic neurons may be involved in EEG desynchrony.

However, not all data are congruent with this hypothesis, and in recent years an ever-increasing body of evidence has accumulated suggesting that at least some aspects of EEG desynchrony are due to release of acetylcholine from the axon terminals of basal forebrain cholinergic neurons. Acetylcholine release from the cerebral cortex is highly correlated with EEG desynchrony (8), and this finding has been supported by recent studies using in vivo microdialysis (see below). Because the predominant cholinergic innervation of the cerebral cortex derives from the basal forebrain, these observations alone suggest that basal forebrain cholinergic neurons may be central to the phenomenon. A key observation derives from studies using excitotoxic lesions. While extensive damage of the mesopontine tegmentum has only minimal effects upon the cortical EEG (72), similar lesions of the basal forebrain essentially abolish atropine-sensitive EEG desynchrony (62). When such excitotoxic lesions are confined to one side of the brain, the contralateral EEG behaves normally while the ipsilateral EEG exhibits a marked increase in slow delta waves (7), and normal EEG desynchrony can be largely restored by cholinergic agonists (69). Taken together, these data argue that atropine-sensitive EEG desynchrony is due to an increase in the release of acetylcholine in the cerebral cortex from the axon terminals of basal forebrain cholinergic neurons.

BEHAVIORAL PHARMACOLOGY OF MUSCARINIC RECEPTORS

There is substantial pharmacological evidence that central cholinergic neurons are important in the acquisition and post-acquisition performance of a variety of learned behaviors (see refs. 21 and 27 for reviews). Many studies have demonstrated that antimuscarinic agents such as scopolamine and atropine have deleterious affects on such behaviors. Similarly, compounds (such as physostigmine) that enhance central cholinergic tone by inhibiting the catabolic enzyme acetylcholinesterase (AChE) can, under certain circumstances, enhance performance in learning and memory tasks. In addition, at appropriate doses a variety of muscarinic receptor agonists can enhance performance on tests of learning and memory. This body of pharmacological research has provided strong evidence that unspecified cholinergic systems in the brain play important roles in the acquisition and performance of learned tasks.

At present, there is no consensus about the psychological mechanisms underlying antimuscarinic-induced deficits. Disruptions of behavioral inhibition, working (short term) memory, retrieval from reference (long term) memory, attention, decisional processes, movement and strategy selection, and altered sensory processing are among the variables that have been proposed as mediating the disruptive effects of muscarinic receptor blockade (21). As has been indicated previously (22), hypotheses concerning the nature of the psychological mechanism that underlies antimuscarinic-induced deficits in the acquisition and performance of learned behaviors are flawed because they have occurred in the absence of neuroanatomical realities. We now know, for example, that cholinergic neurons innervate virtually the entire neuraxis and that muscarinic receptors are distributed throughout the central nervous system. This being the case, it is virtually

certain that cholinergic mechanisms are involved in a disparate variety of central nervous system functions and that antimuscarinic-induced deficits are multifactorally determined. Viewed in this light, it is quite conceivable that systemically administered scopolamine disrupts the acquisition and performance of a learned behavior via simultaneous actions on, for example, attention (e.g., cerebral cortex?), working memory (e.g., hippocampus?), and sensory gating (e.g., thalamus?). In addition, given that scopolamine is a competitive antagonist, the net level of functional blockade in each structure will be determined in part by the level of ACh release in that structure, which can in turn be influenced by a variety of factors. As a result, the extent to which each of the above-mentioned mechanisms contributes to the impaired performance may be determined by variables such as level of training, motoric demands, drug dose, genetics, state of arousal, and so on (see ref. 22).

Questions regarding the behavioral and psychological correlates of cholinergic activity in discrete regions of the central nervous system are of considerable importance. Unfortunately, for the reasons outlined above, these questions cannot be addressed in experiments using systemically administered cholinergic agents. However, local intracerebral administration of such compounds are proving to be a useful alternative in this regard (5,6). In a particularly interesting application of this strategy, Dunnett et al. (17) found that intrahippocampal injections of scopolamine produced delay-dependent impairments in the performance of a "delayed, non-matching to position" task in rats. Such delay-dependent effects are consistent with the hypothesis that the drug produces deficits in short-term memory when injected into the hippocampus, and they agree with data from many other sources that implicate the hippocampus in short-term memory functions (38,42). In contrast to its hippocampal effects, when Dunnett et al. (17) injected scopolamine into the prefrontal cortex it produced dose-dependent but delay-independent deficits in performance, suggesting a non-mnemonic, possibly attentional, basis to this disturbance.

CHOLINERGIC BASAL NUCLEAR COMPLEX: LESION STUDIES

Although various aspects had been considered earlier (14,15), the formal presentation of the "cholinergic hypothesis of geriatric memory dysfunction" was proposed by Bartus et al. in 1982 (3). The two central notions of the hypothesis were that (a) forebrain cholinergic systems provide an essential substrate for a variety of cognitive processes, particularly those involved in learning and memory, and (b) the learning and memory deficits of aging are attributable, at least in part, to a decline in the functional integrity of those forebrain cholinergic systems. In its original formulation, this hypothesis was considered in the context of normal aging. However, several lines of evidence, including the loss of cortical cholinergic markers in Alzheimer's disease (AD), the discovery of a correlation between these biochemical measures and mental test scores in AD patients, and the loss/atrophy of the basal forebrain neurons themselves, led Coyle et al. (9) to extend the cholinergic hypothesis to Alzheimer's dementia—that is, to suggest that the more profound memory deficits of AD may also be attributable to extensive degeneration of the same forebrain cholinergic systems. However, many other neuroanatomical and neurochemical systems also degenerate in AD, so that it is extremely difficult to establish a causal relationship with the cholinergic decline specifically. With this issue in mind, the formulation of the cholinergic hypothesis in 1982 stimulated a large number of studies in the subsequent decade which sought to investigate whether the explicit destruction of magnocellular cholinergic neurons in the basal forebrain by axon-sparing excitotoxins would produce a profile of deficits in experimental animals similar to the changes observed in the aged animal or comparable to more profound changes in learning and memory capacity that is such a distinctive feature of human dementia. The expectation was that reproduction of comparable deficits by an explicit and selective experimental intervention would provide direct evidence in favor of the cholinergic systems having a truly causal role in their genesis. Unfortunately, the early enthusiasm that accompanied the introduction of this strategy has been tempered by subsequent findings that have identified a number of its shortcomings. These issues have been discussed extensively elsewhere and are therefore not reviewed in detail here (18,19,22). Suffice it to say that the most serious limitation of the lesion strategy derives from the fact that wherever they occur in the basal forebrain, cholinergic neurons are intermingled with populations of noncholinergic cells. This being the case, it is uncertain that the deficits in behavior that are produced by excitotoxin lesions of the basal forebrain are due specifically to the loss of cholinergic neurons. What is needed for lesion-based strategies to contribute definitive information concerning the functions of central cholinergic systems is a toxin that is selective for cholinergic neurons. Unfortunately, at present no such compound exists. Despite the above-mentioned limitation of excitotoxin-lesion-based strategies, it is increasingly clear that animals with extensive lesions of the cholinergic neurons that form the nucleus basalis magnocellularis (nBM) (see Chapter 12, *this volume*) can perform normally in a variety of learning and memory tests (18,22). This is particularly evident in studies that have used quisqualic acid or α-amino-3-hydroxy-5-methyl-4-isoxazole propionic acid (AMPA) to lesion the basal forebrain in the region of the nBM. On the basis of such evidence, Dunnett et al. (18) have proposed that the mnemonic deficits described in the earlier studies that utilized ibotenic acid lesions of the basal forebrain are not attributable

to destruction of cholinergic neurons but occur as a result of damage to corticostriatal output systems that course through the globus pallidus. If this is correct, what then are the functional consequences of damage to the telencephalic projections of the nBM? Recent data suggest that impaired attentional function may be one important consequence. One of the first studies to demonstrate this was conducted by Robbins et al. (52), who used a 5-choice serial reaction time task to show that quisqualic acid lesions in the region of the nBM produced deficits in visual attentional function in rats. Subsequently this group of investigators has demonstrated that AMPA-induced lesions of the nBM produce similar impairments in this test of visual attention and that these deficits can be ameliorated by low doses of the AChE inhibitor physostigmine (40). While reversibility by procholinergic drugs does not prove that a lesion-induced deficit is due to a damaged cholinergic system (22), this is clearly the most straightforward explanation for such a finding. In addition, and as will be seen below, data from a variety of other sources are compatible with the hypothesis that cortical projections of the cholinergic basal nuclear complex are neural substrates for some attentional functions.

FUNCTIONAL CORRELATES OF CORTICAL ACETYLCHOLINE RELEASE

It has been known for nearly 30 years that acetylcholine (ACh) release in the cortex increases markedly during EEG desynchronization (8,30). This is consistent with data from other approaches showing that the activity of neurons in the region of the nBM is increased during EEG desynchrony (7,13) and that lesions of the nBM produce EEG slowing (7,51). Day et al. (10) have shown that behavioral measures of arousal such as locomotor activity also correlate positively with cortical ACh release. In the context of the attentional hypothesis of cortical cholinergic function, recent data obtained with brain microdialysis have provided significant support. Specifically, Day and Fibiger (11) have shown that *d*-amphetamine potently increases ACh release in the cortex of awake, behaving animals. Methylphenidate has similar actions (Day and Fibiger, *unpublished observations*). Inasmuch as these compounds are known to improve attention in humans (41,64) and are the treatment of choice in attention deficit disorder, their positive actions on cortical ACh release are entirely consistent with this hypothesis. Subsequent pharmacological analysis has shown that stimulation of D_1 dopamine receptors is the primary mechanism through which *d*-amphetamine produces these effects and raises the possibility that D_1 receptor agonists may have therapeutic applications in the treatment attention deficit disorders (11,12). The fact that scopolamine impairs performance on some attentional tasks in humans, particularly those that require active allocation of attentional capacity, is also consistent with the attentional hypothesis (16,46). Similarly, Sahakian et al. (54) recently demonstrated that tetrahydroaminoacridine (THA), which among other actions is an AChE inhibitor, improves performance on certain tests of attentional function in patients with mild to moderate Alzheimer's disease. It is noteworthy that this occurred in the absence of significant effects on tests of mnemonic function. While these results suggest that central cholinergic mechanisms are involved in the regulation of attentional processes, they do not of course provide any information about the anatomical locus of such effects. At present, the only data pointing to a role for the nBM-cortical projection are the above-mentioned excitotoxin lesion studies in rodents, and as indicated earlier the interpretation of these results is far from straightforward. In summary, while existing evidence is compatible with a role for this cholinergic projection in attention, definitive evidence regarding the validity of this hypothesis awaits the results of future research.

CLINICAL SIGNIFICANCE OF CHOLINERGIC DEGENERATION IN ALZHEIMER'S DISEASE: IMPLICATIONS FOR CHOLINERGIC-BASED PHARMACOTHERAPIES

As indicated above, the functions of the telencephalic projections of the cholinergic basal nuclear complex are not yet firmly established in animals. Similarly, the behavioral consequences of the degeneration of this complex in Alzheimer's disease remain unknown (see also Chapters 118, 120, and 123, *this volume*). Despite this, over the past decade many drug discovery programs have been based on the assumption that the cholinergic hypothesis of Alzheimer's dementia will eventually be validated and that pharmacological restoration of central cholinergic tone will therefore be of significant therapeutic value in the treatment of this condition. There are, however, a number of reasons to be skeptical about this line of reasoning. Perhaps the most important is that this strategy assumes that postsynaptic targets of degenerating cholinergic terminals remain relatively intact in Alzheimer's disease. While postsynaptic muscarinic receptors are generally considered to be unaffected in the hippocampus and cortex of Alzheimer's patients (1), there is abundant evidence that these structures undergo marked degeneration during the course of the disease (2,45,66). Indeed, it is possible that the primary pathological processes in Alzheimer's disease occur in these telencephalic structures and that the damage to the cholinergic neurons in the basal forebrain is secondary and represents retrograde degeneration (24). Given this, the question arises as to whether pharmacological enhancement of cholinergic transmission in these cytoarchitecturally damaged target structures would be expected to reduce the cognitive

deficits in Alzheimer's disease. Unless the loss of basal forebrain neurons in Alzheimer's disease is the earliest degenerative event and unless there is a significant period during which the hippocampus and cortex remain relatively intact, hopes for successful cholinomimetic replacement therapies are poorly founded. In addition, the fact that the neuropathology of Alzheimer's disease is increasingly being understood to involve many noncholinergic, chemically defined systems (26) adds to the concern that procholinergic drugs may not benefit Alzheimer's patients. In this context, it is perhaps understandable that this pharmacological strategy has not yet produced clinically significant improvements in these patients. This is not to say that the development of procholinergic drugs may not eventually find important applications in other patient populations. As discussed above, there is evidence that central cholinergic systems may be important neural substrates for attention, an important component of the larger process termed *cognition*. This being the case, cholinomimetic drugs may prove to be useful in the treatment of attention deficit disorder. In addition, they may also find applications in the treatment of more mildly impaired, more neurologically intact geriatric individuals such as those suffering from age-related memory loss. A better understanding of the normal functions of central cholinergic systems will be a key step in exploring these possibilities.

ACKNOWLEDGMENTS

This work was supported by grants from the Medical Research Council of Canada, the Alzheimer's Society of British Columbia (PBR), and an unrestricted grant from Bristol-Myers Squibb (HCF).

REFERENCES

1. Araujo DM, Lapchak PA, Robitaille Y, Gauthier S, Quirion R. Differential alteration of various cholinergic markers in cortical and subcortical regions of human brain in Alzheimer's disease. *J Neurochem* 1988;50:1914–1923.
2. Ball MJ, Hachinski V, Fox A, et al. A new definition of Alzheimer's disease: a hippocampal dementia. *Lancet* 1985;8419:14–16.
3. Bartus RT, Dean RL, Beer B, Lippa AS. The cholinergic hypothesis of geriatric memory dysfunction. *Science* 1982;217:408–417.
4. Batchelor PE, Armstrong DM, Blaker SN, Gage FH. Nerve growth factor receptor and choline acetyltransferase colocalization in neurons within the rat forebrain: response to fimbria–fornix transection. *J Comp Neurol* 1989;284:187–204.
5. Blokland A, Honig W, Raaijmakers WGM. Effects of intra-hippocampal scopolamine injections in a repeated spatial acquisition task in the rat. *Psychopharmacology* 1992;109:373–376.
6. Brito GNO, Davis BJ, Stopp LC, Stanton ME. Memory and the septohippocampal cholinergic system in the rat. *Psychopharmacology* 1983;82:315–320.
7. Buzsaki G, Bickford RG, Ponomareff G, Thal LJ, Mandel R, Gage FH. Nucleus basalis and thalamic control of neocortical activity in the freely moving rat. *J Neurosci* 1988;8:4007–4026.
8. Celesia GG, Jasper HH. Acetylcholine released from cerebral cortex in relation to state of activation. *Neurology* 1966;16:1053–1063.

9. Coyle JT, Price DL, DeLong MR. Alzheimer's disease: a disorder of cortical cholinergic innervation. *Science* 1983;219:1184–1190.
10. Day J, Damsma G, Fibiger HC. Cholinergic activity in the rat hippocampus, cortex and striatum correlates with locomotor activity: an in vivo microdialysis study. *Pharmacol Biochem Behav* 1991;38:723–729.
11. Day J, Fibiger HC. Dopaminergic regulation of cortical acetylcholine release. *Synapse* 1992;12:281–286.
12. Day J, Fibiger HC. Dopaminergic regulation of cortical acetylcholine release: effects of dopamine receptor agonist. *Neuroscience* 1993;54:643–648.
13. Detari L, Vanderwolf CH. Activity of identified cortically projecting and other basal forebrain neurones during large slow waves and cortical activation in anaesthetized rats. *Brain Res* 1987;437:1–8.
14. Deutch JA. The cholinergic synapse and the site of memory. *Science* 1971;174:788–794.
15. Drachman DA, Sahakian BJ. Memory, aging and pharmacosystems. In: Stein D, ed. *The psychobiology of aging: problems and perspectives*. Amsterdam: Elsevier/North-Holland, 1980;347–368.
16. Dunne MP, Hartley LR. Scopolamine and the control of attention in humans. *Psychopharmacology* 1986;89:94–97.
17. Dunnett SB, Wareham AT, Torres EM. Cholinergic blockade in prefrontal cortex and hippocampus disrupts short-term memory in rats. *NeuroReport* 1990;1:61–64.
18. Dunnett SB, Everitt BJ, Robbins TW. The basal forebrain–cortical cholinergic system: interpreting the functional consequences of excitotoxic lesions. *Trends Neurosci* 1991;14:494–501.
19. Dunnett SB, Fibiger HC. Role of forebrain cholinergic systems in learning and memory: relevance to the cognitive deficits of aging and Alzheimer's dementia. *Prog Brain Res* 1993;98:413–420.
20. El-Mansari M, Sakai K, Jouvet M. Unitary characteristics of presumptive cholinergic tegmental neurons during the sleep–waking cycle in freely moving cats. *Exp Brain Res* 1989;76:509–529.
21. Fibiger HC. Central cholinergic systems and memory. In: Squire LR, Lindenlaub E, eds. *The biology of memory*, Symposia Medica Hoechst 23. New York: Springer-Verlag, 1990;381–398.
22. Fibiger HC. Cholinergic mechanisms in learning, memory and dementia: a review of recent evidence. *Trends Neurosci* 1991;14:220–223.
23. Gerfen CR. Substance P (neurokinin-1) receptor mRNA is selectively expressed in cholinergic neurons in the striatum and basal forebrain. *Brain Res* 1991;556:165–170.
24. German DC, White III CL, Sparkman DR. Alzheimer's disease: neurofibrillary tangles in nuclei that project to the cerebral cortex. *Neuroscience* 1987;21:305–312.
25. Geula C, Schatz CR, Mesulam M-M. Differential localization of NADPH-diaphorase and calbindin-D_{28k} within the cholinergic neurons of the basal forebrain, striatum and brainstem in the rat, monkey, baboon and human. *Neuroscience* 1993;54:461–476.
26. Gottfries CG. Neurochemical aspects of dementia disorders [Review]. *Dementia* 1990;1:56–64.
27. Hagan JJ, Morris RGM. The cholinergic hypothesis of memory: a review of animal experiments. In: Iversen LL, Iversen SD, Snyder SH, eds. *Handbook of psychopharmacology*, vol 20. New York: Plenum Press, 1988;217–323.
28. Hallanger AE, Levey AI, Lee HJ, Rye DB, Wainer BH. The origins of the cholinergic and other subcortical afferents to the thalamus in the rat. *J Comp Neurol* 1987;262:105–124.
29. Jones BE, Beaudet A. Distribution of acetylcholine and catecholamine neurons in the cat brain stem: a choline acetyltransferase and tyrosine hydroxylase immunohistochemical study. *J Comp Neurol* 1987;261:15–32.
30. Kainai T, Szerb JC. Mesencephalic reticular activating system and cortical acetylcholine output. *Nature* 1965;205:80–82.
31. Kamondi A, Williams JA, Hutcheon B, Reiner PB. Membrane properties of mesopontine cholinergic neurons studied with the whole-cell patch-clamp technique: implications for behavioral state control. *J Neurophysiol* 1992;68:1359–1372.
32. Khateb A, Muhlethaler M, Alonso A, Serafin M, Mainville L, Jones BE. Cholinergic nucleus basalis neurons display the capacity for rhythmic bursting activity mediated by low-threshold calcium spikes. *Neuroscience* 1992;51:489–494.
33. Longo VG. Behavioral and electroencephalographic effects of atropine and related compounds. *Pharmacol Rev* 1966;18:965–996.
34. Luebke JI, Greene RW, Semba K, Kamondi A, McCarley RW, Reiner PB. Serotonin hyperpolarizes cholinergic low threshold burst neurons in the rat laterodorsal tegmental nucleus in vitro. *Proc Natl Acad Sci USA* 1992;89:743–747.
35. Martin LJ, Blackstone CD, Levey AI, Huganir RL, Price DL. Cellular localizations of AMPH glutamate receptors within the basal forebrain magnocellular complex of rat and monkey. *J Neurosci* 1993;13:2249–2263.
36. McCormick DA. Cholinergic and noradrenergic modulation of thalamocortical processing. *Trends Neurosci* 1989;12:215–221.
37. Melander T, Staines WA, Hökfelt T, et al. Galanin-like immunoreactivity in cholinergic neurons of the septum–basal forebrain complex projecting to the hippocampus of the rat. *Brain Res* 1985;360:130–138.
38. Mishkin M. A memory system in the monkey. *Philos Trans R Soc Lond [Biol]* 1982;298:83–95.
39. Moruzzi G, Magoun HW. Brainstem reticular formation and activation of the EEG. *Electroencephalogr Clin Neurophysiol* 1949;1:455–473.
40. Muir JL, Everitt BJ, Robbins TW. AMPA-induced excitotoxic lesions of the basal forebrain: a significant role for the cortical cholinergic system in attentional function. *J Neurosci* 1994;14:2313–2326.
41. Newhouse PA, Belenky G, Thomas M, Thorne D, Sing HC, Fertig J. The effects of *d*-amphetamine on arousal, cognition, and mood after prolonged total sleep deprivation. *Neuropsychopharmacology* 1989;2:153–164.
42. Olton DS, Becker JT, Handelmann GE. Hippocampus, space, and memory. *Behav Brain Sci* 1979;2:313–365.
43. Pare D, Steriade M, Deschenes M, Bouhassira D. Prolonged enhancement of anterior thalamic synaptic responsiveness by stimulation of a brain-stem cholinergic group. *J Neurosci* 1990;10:20–33.
44. Pasqualotto BA, Vincent SR. Galanin and NADPH-diaphorase coexistence in cholinergic neurons of the rat basal forebrain. *Brain Res* 1991;551:78–86.
45. Pearson RCA, Esiri MM, Hiorns RW, Wilcock GK, Powell TPS. Anatomical correlates of the distribution of the pathological changes in the neocortex. *Proc Natl Acad Sci USA* 1985;82:4531–4534.
46. Preda L, Alberoni M, Bressi S, et al. Effects of acute doses of oxiracetam in the scopolamine model of human amnesia. *Psychopharmacology* 1993;110:421–426.
47. Reiner PB, Vincent SR. Topographic relations of cholinergic and noradrenergic neurons in the feline pontomesencephalic tegmentum: an immunohistochemical study. *Brain Res Bull* 1987;19:705–714.
48. Richardson RT, DeLong MR. Nucleus basalis of Meynert neuronal activity during a delayed response task in monkey. *Brain Res* 1986;399:364–368.
49. Richardson RT, DeLong MR. A reappraisal of the functions of the nucleus basalis of Meynert. *Trends Neurosci* 1988;11:264–267.
50. Richardson RT, DeLong MR. Context-dependent responses of primate nucleus basalis neurons in a go/no-go task. *J Neurosci* 1990;10:2528–2540.
51. Riekkinnen Jr. P, Sirvio J, Hannila T, Miettinen R, Riekkinen P. Effects of quisqualic acid nucleus basalis lesioning on cortical EEG, passive avoidance and water maze performance. *Brain Res Bull* 1990;24:839–842.
52. Robbins TW, Everitt BJ, Marston HM, Wilkinson J, Jones GH, Page KJ. Comparative effects of ibotenic acid- and quisqualic acid-induced lesions of the substantia innominata on attentional function in the rat: further implications for the role of the cholinergic neurons of the nucleus basalis in cognitive processes. *Behav Brain Res* 1989;35:221–240.
53. Rolls ET, Sanghera MK, Roper-Hall A. The latency of activation of neurones in the lateral hypothalamus and substantia innominata during feeding in the monkey. *Brain Res* 1979;164:121–135.
54. Sahakian BJ, Owen AM, Morant NJ, et al. Further analysis of the cognitive effects of tetrahydroaminoacridine (THA) in Alzheimer's disease: assessment of attentional and mnemonic function using CANTAB. *Psychopharmacology* 1993;110:395–401.
55. Satoh K, Fibiger HC. Cholinergic neurons of the laterodorsal tegmental nucleus: efferent and afferent connections. *J Comp Neurol* 1986;253:277–302.
56. Schwaber JS, Rogers WT, Satoh K, Fibiger HC. Distribution and organization of cholinergic neurons in the rat forebrain demon-

strated by computer-aided data acquisition and three-dimensional reconstruction. *J Comp Neurol* 1987;263:309–325.

57. Semba K, Fibiger HC. Time of origin of cholinergic neurons in the rat basal forebrain. *J Comp Neurol* 1988;269:87–95.

58. Shute CCD, Lewis PR. The ascending cholinergic reticular system: neocortical, olfactory and subcortical projections. *Brain* 1967; 90:497–520.

59. Steriade M, Datta S, Pare D, Oakson G, Dossi RC. Neuronal activities in brain-stem cholinergic nuclei related to tonic activation processes in thalamocortical systems. *J Neurosci* 1990;10:1541–1559.

60. Steriade M, Jones EG, Llinas RR. *Thalamic oscillations and signalling.* New York: John Wiley & Sons, 1990.

61. Steriade M, McCarley RW. *Brainstem control of wakefulness and sleep.* New York: Plenum Press, 1990.

62. Stewart DJ, MacFabe DF, Vanderwolf CH. Cholinergic activation of the electrocorticogram: role of substantia innominata and effects of atropine and quinuclidinyl benzylate. *Brain Res* 1984;322:219–232.

63. Stewart M, Fox SE. Do septal neurons pace the hippocampal theta rhythm? *Trends Neurosci* 1990;13:163–168.

64. Sykes DH, Douglas VI, Morgenstern G. The effect of methylphenidate (Ritalin) on sustained attention in hyperactive children. *Psychopharmacologia* 1972;25:262–274.

65. Szymusiak R, McGinty D. Sleep–waking discharge of basal forebrain projection neurons in cats. *Brain Res Bull* 1989;22:423–430.

66. Terry RD, Katzman R. Senile dementia of the Alzheimer's type. *Ann Neurol* 1983;14:497–506.

67. Toran-Allerand CD, Miranda RC, Bentham WDL, et al. Estrogen receptors colocalize with low-affinity nerve growth factor receptors in cholinergic neurons of the basal forebrain. *Proc Natl Acad Sci USA* 1992;89:4668–4672.

68. Vanderwolf CH. Cerebral activity and behavior: control by central cholinergic and serotonergic systems. *Int Rev Neurobiol* 1988; 30:225–340.

69. Vanderwolf CH, Raithby A, Snider M, Cristi C, Tanner C. Effects of some cholinergic agonists on neocortical slow wave activity in rats with basal forebrain lesions. *Brain Res Bull* 1993;31:515–521.

70. Vanderwolf CH, Robinson TH. Reticulocortical activity and behavior: a critique of the arousal theory and a new synthesis. *Behav Brain Sci* 1981;4:459–514.

71. Walker LC, Rance NE, Price DL, Young WS. Galanin mRNA in the nucleus basalis of Meynert complex of baboons and humans. *J Comp Neurol* 1991;303:113–120.

72. Webster HH, Jones BE. Neurotoxic lesions of the dorsolateral pontomesencephalic tegmentum–cholinergic cell area in the cat. II. Effects upon sleep–waking states. *Brain Res* 1988;458:285–302.

73. Wilson FAW, Rolls ET. Neuronal responses related to reinforcement in the primate basal forebrain. *Brain Res* 1990;509:213–231.

74. Wilson FAW, Rolls ET. Learning and memory is reflected in the responses of reinforcement-related neurons in the primate basal forebrain. *J Neurosci* 1990;10:1254–1267.

Psychopharmacology: The Fourth Generation of Progress, edited by Floyd E. Bloom and David J. Kupfer. Raven Press, Ltd., New York © 1995.

CHAPTER 14

Molecular Biology of the Dopamine Receptor Subtypes

Olivier Civelli

Until recently, our understanding of the dopaminergic system has been based on the interactions of one neurotransmitter, dopamine, with two receptors, the D1 and D2 receptors. In the last few years, the application of molecular biological techniques has led to the identification of three new dopamine receptors (for review see ref. 11; see also Chapters 19, 26, and 27, *this volume*). The discovery of these "unexpected" dopamine receptor subtypes has had a revolutionary impact on the study of the dopaminergic system and their implications in human disorders.

THE CLASSICAL VIEW OF THE DOPAMINERGIC SYSTEM

Dopamine is present in most parts of the central nervous system (CNS) but in particular in the nigrostriatal pathway comprising the neurons of the substantia nigra (A9) and projecting to neurons of the neostriatum and the mesocorticolimbic pathway composed of neurons of the ventral tegmental area (A10) connecting with those of the limbic cortex and other limbic structures (5).

The involvement of the dopaminergic nigrostriatal pathway in extrapyramidal dysfunctions was shown by the discovery that degeneration of this pathway occurs in the brains of patients afflicted with Parkinson's disease (18,49). The depletion of dopamine resulting from the degeneration of the nigrostriatal pathway led to the development of dopamine-replacement therapies which are successful in alleviating Parkinson's disease (4,29). The hypothesis that dopamine is involved in the pathogenesis of psychosis, in particular schizophrenia, rests on the finding that most antipsychotic drugs are dopamine recep-

tor antagonists and that agents which cause excessive release of dopamine mimic schizophrenia-like states (7,8,12,50). The mesocorticolimbic pathway has been implicated as the principal dopaminergic pathway involved in the etiology of psychoses. These data explain the dilemma associated with dopamine-related drug therapies: The blockade of the dopaminergic system, desired for reducing psychoses, induces extrapyramidal dysfunctions and vice versa.

In 1979, Kebabian and Calne found that dopamine exerts its effects by binding to two receptors, known as the D1 and D2 receptors (30). These receptors could be differentiated pharmacologically, biologically, physiologically, and by their anatomical distribution (for review see ref. 13). Pharmacologically, the hallmark of the D1 receptor is to bind the benzazepine antagonist SCH 23390, while that of the D2 receptor is to recognize with high affinity the butyrophenones: spiperone and haloperidol. These two receptors exert their biological actions by coupling to and activating different G protein complexes. The D1 receptor interacts with the G_s complex to activate adenylyl cyclase, whereas the D2 interacts with G_i to inhibit cAMP production. The anatomical distributions of these two receptors overlap in the CNS, yet their quantitative ratios differ significantly in particular anatomical areas. With respect to mental disorders, it is noteworthy that both D1 and D2 receptors are present in the nigrostriatal and mesocorticolimbic pathways.

For 10 years, this two-subtype classification has accounted for most of the activities attributed to the dopaminergic system. The existence of other dopamine receptors has been proposed but had been refuted when the "new" receptors were recognized to represent different affinity states of the canonical D1 and D2 receptor (2,31). However, this classification was dramatically changed

O. Civelli: F. Hoffmann–La Roche Ltd., CH-4002 Basel, Switzerland.

with the application of recombinant DNA technology to the molecular characterization of the dopamine receptors.

MOLECULAR CHARACTERIZATION OF THE DOPAMINE RECEPTORS

Cloning of the D2 Receptor

The cloning of the D2 dopamine receptor resulted from the recognition that, on the basis of its inhibitory activity on adenylyl cyclase, it would belong to the supergene family of the G-protein-coupled receptors (17,27; see also Chapter 27, *this volume*). Consequently, the use of a cloning strategy based on the sequence homology known to exist among G-protein-coupled receptors could lead to the molecular characterization of the D2 receptor. The D2 dopamine receptor was cloned using the hamster β2-adrenergic receptor coding sequence as hybridization probe under conditions which would detect sequentially related DNA fragments (6). Via genomic and cDNA screenings, a rat brain cDNA was identified and shown to encode a protein featuring the characteristics expected for a G-protein-coupled receptor. The receptor encoded by this cDNA had the pharmacological profile and biological activity of the dopamine D2 receptor found in the brain and pituitary, demonstrating that this cloned receptor is the same D2 receptor as the one described in 1979 (1,6,45).

Application of the Homology Screening Approach: Discovery of the Dopamine Receptor Heterogeneity

The success of the homology approach in the cloning of the D2 receptor opened the door for the cloning of other dopamine receptors. Successful cloning of the D1 receptor was reported by several groups (15,41,56,63). The sequences derived from these clones share the characteristics expected of G-protein-coupled receptors in general and of the catecholamine receptors in particular (63). These putative receptors were expressed by DNA transfection and were shown to bind D1 receptor ligands and to stimulate adenylyl cyclase activity, the two hallmarks of the D1 receptor. Molecular characterization of the D1 receptor had been achieved.

The generality of the homology approach allowed for the search of other unexpected dopamine receptors. Using a D2-receptor-specific DNA fragment as probe under low-stringency hybridization conditions, Sokoloff et al. (54) identified another dopamine receptor, the D3 receptor. When expressed in eukaryotic cells, this receptor was shown to bind D2 but not D1 ligands. Its structure and binding characteristics thus permitted its classification as a new dopamine receptor called the D3 receptor. Noteworthy is its ability to affect second messenger systems, which has thus far not been demonstrated.

Furthermore, by analyzing the mRNAs of human neuroepithelioma SK-N-MC cells with D2 receptor cDNA probes under conditions of low stringency, another D2-related mRNA was detected (58). The corresponding cDNA and gene analyses led to the characterization of the D4 receptor. The D4 receptor, when expressed in COS-7 cells, binds D2 antagonists with a pharmacological profile that is distinct but reminiscent of that of the D2 receptor. The D4 receptor was shown to couple to G proteins, although its potential at inducing second messenger systems is still being determined.

Finally, the D1 receptor clone was used as a hybridization probe to identify D1-related genes. A human D5 and a rat D1b receptor have been characterized (26,55,57). They display the same pharmacological profile, reminiscent of that of the D1 receptor, and are able to stimulate adenylyl cyclase activity. On the basis of their sequences, the D5 and D1b receptors are human and rat equivalents of the same receptor, respectively.

Thus the application of homology screening techniques not only led to the deciphering of the molecular structures of the D1 and D2 receptors, but also led to the characterization of three new dopamine receptors: D3, D4, and D5. These discoveries have, of course, medical implications. For example, most of what is known about dopamine agonists' and antagonists' actions has to be reevaluated in view of the existence of the different dopamine receptors. Our renewed knowledge of the dopaminergic system begins with the study of the dopaminergic receptor family.

COMMON FEATURES OF THE DOPAMINE RECEPTORS

Primary Sequences

In their putative transmembrane domains, the D1 and D5 receptors are 79% identical but are only 40–45% identical to the D2, D3, and D4 receptors. Conversely, the D2, D3, and D4 receptors are between 75% and 51% identical to each other, the first indication that the five receptors can be divided into the D1-like and D2-like receptor subfamilies. The topologies of the five dopamine receptors are predicted to be the same as all the other G-protein-coupled receptors. They should contain seven putative membrane-spanning helices which would form a narrow dihedral hydrophobic cleft surrounded by three extracellular and three intracellular loops. The receptor polypeptides are probably further anchored to the membranes through palmitoylation of a conserved Cys residue found in their C-tails (347 in D1, the C-terminus in D2-like receptors) (46). The dopamine receptors are probably glycosylated in their N-terminal domains; in addition, the D1-like subtypes have potential glycosylation sites in their first extracytoplasmic loop.

Genomic Organization

The genomic organization of the dopamine receptors also supports the notion that they derive from the divergence of two gene subfamilies, the D1-like and D2-like receptor genes. The D1 and D5 receptor genes do not contain introns in their protein coding regions, whereas the D2, D3, and D4 genes do. Furthermore, most of the introns in the D2-like receptor genes are located in similar positions (25,54,56,58,63).

Ligand Binding and Second Messenger Inductions

The cloned dopamine receptors, when expressed by transfection, exhibit binding profiles which can also differentiate them into the D1-like and D2-like subfamilies. The D1-like receptors bind with high-affinity D1 and not D2 antagonists. A prototypic ligand for the D1-like receptors is the benzazepine SCH23390 ($K_{is} < 1$ nM); on the other hand, they bind the butyrophenone spiperone with low affinity (K_{is} in the micromolar range). In contrast, the D2-like receptors efficiently bind spiperone ($K_{is} < 1$ nM) and not SCH23390 (K_{is} for D2 in the micromolar range); they also recognize most of the neuroleptics. Because there are 21 amino acid residues which differentiate D1-like from D2-like receptors in the transmembrane domains, these might participate in the selective recognition process. While there presently exists no ligand to differentiate the D1 from the D5 receptor, several D2 antagonists can distinguish the different D2-like receptors. The compound 7-OH-DPAT is selective for the D3 receptor (33), whereas clozapine has the highest affinity for the D4 receptor. It is noteworthy that dopamine binds to the D3, D4, and D5 receptors with nanomolar or submicromolar affinity constants, while its corresponding constants for the D1 and D2 receptors are in the micromolar ranges.

The predominant biological activities associated with D1 and D2 receptor stimulation are the activation and inhibition of adenylyl cyclase activity, respectively. Stimulation of the D1 and D5 receptors in transfected cells has been shown to result in activation of adenylyl cyclase, indicating similar pathways of second messenger induction for the D1-like receptors. On the other hand, the D3 and D4 receptors have, thus far, not been shown to induce second messenger systems, thus preventing their subfamily classification based on biological activity. However, because receptors' interactions with G proteins involve the cytoplasmic loops (16,32) and because D2-like receptors have a large third cytoplasmic loop and a short C-terminal tail representative of the catecholamine receptors coupled to Gi proteins, the D2-like relative homology suggests that they might couple to the same set of G proteins.

Thus, on the basis of their primary sequences, of their genomic organization, and of their pharmacological and, at least partly, biological activities, the different dopamine receptors can be classified into the D1-like and D2-like subtypes. This, and the fact that the D3, D4, and D5 receptors are present in significantly lower amounts than are the D1 and D2 receptors, suggest that the existence of the former ones could not be found by pharmacological analyses.

PARTICULARITIES OF THE DIFFERENT DOPAMINE RECEPTORS

Pharmacological Profiles

As mentioned above, no selective ligand has been described which is able to differentiate the D1 from the D5 receptor. On the other hand, the pharmacological profiles of the D3 or D4 receptors show distinct striking differences when compared to that of the D2 receptor.

Most neuroleptics were developed as D2 receptor antagonists and thus are expected to bind to the D2 receptor with higher affinity than to the D3 and D4 receptors. This is true for the majority of the neuroleptics, which implies that those neuroleptics are acting predominantly at D2 receptors in the human brain. However, a few neuroleptics have been found to show selectivity for the D3 or D4 receptors; through these, some aspects of the functions of the D3 and D4 receptors may be revealed.

Two antagonists, UH232 and AJ76, bind to the D3 receptor with a higher affinity than they do to the D2 receptor (54). These compounds are classified as selective for presynaptic receptors or for autoreceptors. In addition, it was found that dopamine binds the D3 receptor with a 20-fold higher affinity than the D2 receptor, a characteristic expected for autoreceptors. Furthermore, the presence of D3 receptor mRNA in the substantia nigra, a center of dopamine production, supports the hypothesis that the D3 receptor may be a presynaptic receptor. Noteworthy is that the D2 receptor mRNA is the predominant dopamine receptor mRNA in the substantia nigra (38) and that, as for the D3 receptor, 6-OHDA lesions show its presence in the dopamine-secreting neurons (9,21,34,35,54). Therefore both the D2 and the D3 receptors are autoreceptors. Interestingly, the recent involvement of the D3 receptor in modulating cocaine self-administration has also been associated with its autoreceptor properties.

Clozapine, an "atypical" neuroleptic (i.e., a neuroleptic whose actions are not accompanied by adverse motor control side effects), shows a higher selectivity for the D4 receptor than for any other D2-like receptors. In schizophrenia therapy, clozapine is administered at a concentration 10-fold lower than its affinity constant for the D2 receptor, indicating that clozapine may not be primarily acting at the D2 receptor. The D4 receptor binds clozapine with a 10-fold higher affinity than does the D2 receptor (58). Therefore the D4 receptor may be the specific target of clozapine. A corollary of this is that antagonism of dopamine binding to the D4 receptor could be an important step in prevention of psychoses, a hypothesis reinforced by the low abundance of D4 mRNA in the striatum (58). Thus the lack of extrapyramidal side effects observed with clozapine treatment may be a reflection of D4 receptor localization in the CNS. These observations point to the D4 receptor as an important molecule in the etiology of psychoses (see also Chapters 100 and 108, *this volume*).

Tissue Distribution

Because there are no current antibodies against all the different dopamine receptors, our knowledge of their tissue distribution comes primarily from in situ hybridization experiments. In the CNS, the five dopamine receptors exhibit overlapping but also distinct localizations. In the periphery, the different receptors are mostly expressed in a tissue-specific fashion.

The tissue distribution of the D1 and D2 mRNAs in the CNS supports their participation in the different aspects of dopaminergic neurotransmission which have been described on the basis of ligand binding and receptor autoradiography experiments. The D1 and D2 receptor mRNAs are present in all dopaminoceptive regions of the rat brain (20,34,36,38,39,44,62). High levels of D1 and D2 mRNAs are present in the caudate-putamen, nucleus accumbens, and olfactory tubercule, and lower levels are present in the septum, hypothalamus, and cortex. Regions where D2 but no D1 mRNAs were detected are the substantia nigra and ventral tegmental area, where the D2 mRNA is expressed at a high level, and the hippocampus. Conversely, the amygdala contains D1 mRNA but little, if any, D2 mRNA.

The D3, D4, and D5 receptor mRNAs are mostly present in tissues where the D1 and/or the D2 mRNAs are also expressed. However, their relative abundances are one to two orders of magnitude lower than that of the D1 or D2 mRNAs (54,58). It has been shown that, relative to the D1 or D2 receptors, the D3 and D4 receptors are more selectively associated with the ''limbic'' brain, a region which receives its dopamine input from the ventral tegmental area and is known to be associated with cognitive, emotional, and endocrine functions. The location of the D5 receptor mRNA, on the other hand, is highly specific. The D5 mRNA is found only in the hippocampus, the hypothalamus, and the parafascicular nucleus of the thalamus and thus might be involved in affective, neuroendocrine, or pain-related aspects of dopaminergic functions (37). Finally, using in situ hybridization experiments, it has also been possible to demonstrate that D1 and D2 mRNA are colocalized in 26–40% of all caudate-putamen cells and in about 50% of all dopamine receptor mRNA-positive cells (38).

Dopamine receptor reactivities have also been described in several peripheral organs. mRNA detection by Northern blot analyses have shown that neither D1 nor D3 receptor mRNA are detectable outside the CNS (54,63). On the other hand, the D2 receptor mRNA is expressed at high levels in the pituitary (6) and in the adrenal gland and also in the retina. Of particular interest are the kidney and the heart in which both D1- and D2-like activities have been described (2,19). The D5 receptor mRNA is expressed, albeit at low levels, in the kidney (J. H. Meador-Woodruff and D. K. Grandy, *unpublished data,* 1992). Whether it is the expected D1-like receptor has yet to be demonstrated. None of the cloned D2-like receptor mRNAs is present in the kidney. On the other hand, the D4 mRNA is expressed in the heart (47) and might account for the expected D2-like reactivity reported for this tissue. None of the D1-like receptor mRNAs exists in significant amount in the heart. These data open the possibility that the D4 and D5 receptors carry the dopamine receptor reactivities detected in the kidney and the heart.

In conclusion, one can foresee that an advantage for the organism of having heterogeneous population of receptors is that it permits tissue-specific expression. mRNA detection experiments show that the different dopamine receptors exhibit specificity in their tissue distribution in the periphery, while in the CNS they often share tissue locations and, possibly, individual neurons as in the case of the D1 and D2 receptors. Although selectivity in cellular distributions has also been found in the CNS, it does not seem to be the rule for the different receptor subtypes. Another factor to consider in our understanding of the importance of the receptor diversity is the comparison of the relative abundance of the subtypes. Variable levels of distinct receptors, added to the fact that interactions between different dopamine receptor subtypes exist (3,51,60,61), generate a high degree of diversity in responses that reflect the broad spectrum of the physiological activities known to be regulated by dopamine.

Alternative Splicing and Gene Polymorphism

Although the human genome contains five dopamine receptor genes, the number of dopamine receptor mRNA species that it encodes is higher. This results from the fact that polymorphism and alternative splicing events play a role in dopamine receptor gene expression and leads to the existence of more than five different receptor binding sites.

First was the discovery that there exist two forms of D2 dopamine receptors (10,14,23,25,40,42,48,52). These two forms differ in 29 amino acid residues located in the putative third cytoplasmic loop of the receptor. They are generated by an alternative splicing event which occurs during the maturation of the D2 receptor pre-mRNA

(14,25,48). The two D2 receptor forms are neither species- nor tissue-specific; they coexist in all tissues analyzed but at a highly variable ratio. Because of its location in the third cytoplasmic loop, the 29-residue addition was expected to affect G protein coupling and consequently second messenger systems. It has been shown that both forms can inhibit cAMP accumulation (14) and that their efficiencies are somewhat variable (28,43). Alternative splicing events have also been shown to occur during the maturation of the D3 dopamine receptor pre-mRNA (22,53).

The existence of different variants of the human D4 receptor has also been demonstrated, although their generation is not by alternative splicing. These variants differ in the number of 48 base-pair repeats contained in their putative third cytoplasmic loop (59) and they have been detected in the genomes of different individuals, showing that a genetic polymorphism is responsible for the generation of the D4 receptor variants. These repeats are not present in the rat gene, making the polymorphism specific to humans. When expressed by DNA transfection, the variants containing 2, 4, and 7 repeats bind clozapine with equal affinities in the presence of sodium chloride. In the absence of sodium ions, however, the variants containing 2 and 4 repeats had a six- to eightfold lower dissociation constant for clozapine, while the affinity of the variant containing seven repeats was practically unaffected (59). Although it is not understood what effects the sodium ions have on receptors, these data indicate that the variants can behave differently with respect to the mechanism of ligand recognition.

Finally, the D5 receptor gene is peculiar among the G-protein-coupled receptors because it is associated with two pseudogenes in the human genome (26). The three D5-related genes are found on different chromosomes (24). Only one gene (DRD5, chromosome 4 q15.1-q15.3) codes for the active receptor; the two others contain an 8-base-pair insertion which leads to a frame shift and are genuine pseudogenes. Interestingly, these pseudogenes appear to be specific to humans, suggesting that the evolution of the D5 pseudogenes is a very recent event which may be restricted to primates.

DISCUSSION

The discovery of the "unexpected" dopamine receptors has and will continue to impact our understanding of the dopaminergic system. Of immediate interest is whether agonists or antagonists to the new dopamine receptors can be of therapeutic value like the D2 receptor antagonists are. The D3 and D4 receptors have two similar particularities. They bind most of the neuroleptics with less affinity than the D2 receptor, which indicates that, as commonly carried out, neuroleptic treatments may have not affected their activities. Furthermore, the D3 and

D4 receptors are found predominantly in the limbic system and are relatively absent in the nigrostriatal system, and thus are associated preferentially with the etiology of psychoses instead of locomotion dysfunctions. The D4 receptor carries the further characteristic of binding clozapine with an affinity corresponding to its therapeutic concentration. Although clozapine can also bind to other receptors, its affinity to the D4 receptor might begin to explain its activity in the dopaminergic system. Consequently, the atypical effect of clozapine may be derived from the relative absence of D4 receptor in the basal ganglia. Whether this hypothesis proves valid will require the synthesis of specific antagonists. Finally, the D5 receptor may also be of therapeutic interest. It is present in very low amounts and is restricted only to a few tissues in the CNS. Its interest may stem from its presence in the kidney, whose function is improved by dopamine in cases of shock and low cardiac input. Thus a D5 agonist with low affinity for other catecholamine receptors could be valuable.

In conclusion, the discovery of the new dopamine receptors is too new to be conclusively evaluated with regard to potential therapies. Yet the few data that have already been obtained show promising characteristics and will hopefully lead to the development of tools which, in turn, will help further our understanding of the dopaminergic system and of its physiological implications.

REFERENCES

1. Albert PR, Neve KA, Bunzow JR, Civelli O. Coupling of a cloned rat dopamine D2 receptor to inhibition of adenylyl cyclase and prolactin secretion. *J Biol Chem* 1990;265:2098–2104.
2. Andersen PH, Gingrich JA, Bates MD, et al. Dopamine receptor subtypes: beyond the D_1/D_2 classification. *Trends Pharmacol Sci* 1990;11:231–236.
3. Bertorello AM, Hopfield JF, Aperia A, Greengard P. Inhibition by dopamine of $(Na^+ + K^+)$ ATPase activity in neostriatal neurons through D_1 and D_2 dopamine receptor synergism. *Nature* 1990;347:386–388.
4. Birkmayer W, Hornykiewicz O. Der L-Dioxyphenylalanin (=L-DOPA)-Effekt beim Parkinson-Syndrom des Menschen: Zur Pathogenese and Behandlung der Parkinson-Akinese. *Arch Psychiatr Nervenkr* 1962;203:560–574.
5. Bjorklund A, Lindvall O. Dopamine-containing systems in the CNS. In: Bjorklund A, Hokfelt T, eds. *Classical transmitters in the CNS. Handbook of chemical neuroanatomy.* Amsterdam: Elsevier, 1964;55–122.
6. Bunzow JR, Van Tol HHM, Grandy DK, et al. Cloning and expression of a rat D_2 dopamine receptor cDNA. *Nature* 1988;336:783–787.
7. Carlsson A. The current status of the dopamine hypothesis of schizophrenia. *Neuropsychopharmacology* 1988;1:179–186.
8. Carlsson A, Lindqvist M. Effect of chlorpromazine and haloperidol on the formation of 3-methoxytyramine in mouse brain. *Acta Pharmacol* 1963;20:140–144.
9. Chen JF, Qin ZH, Szele F, Bai G, Weiss B. Neuronal localization and modulation of the D_2 dopamine receptor mRNA in brain of normal mice and mice lesioned with 6-hydroxydopamine. *Neuropharmacology* 1991;30:927–941.
10. Chio CL, Hess GF, Graham RS, Hugg RM. A second molecular form of D_2 dopamine receptor in rat and bovine caudate nucleus. *Nature* 1990;343:266–269.

11. Civelli O, Bunzow JR, Grandy DK. Molecular diversity of the dopamine receptors. *Annu Rev Pharmacol Toxicol* 1992;32:281–307.

12. Creese I, Burt DR, Snyder SH. Dopamine receptor binding predicts clinical and pharmacological potencies of antischizophrenic drugs. *Science* 1976;192:481–483.

13. Creese I, Fraser CM. *Dopamine receptors.* New York: Alan R Liss, 1987.

14. Dal Toso R, Sommer B, Ewert M, et al. The dopamine D2 receptor: two molecular forms generated by alternative splicing. *EMBO J* 1989;8:4025–4034.

15. Dearry A, Gingrich JA, Falardeau P, Fremeau RT, Bates MD, Caron MG. Molecular cloning and expression of the gene for a human D_1 dopamine receptor. *Nature* 1990;347:72–76.

16. Dixon RAF, Sigal IS, Strader CD. Structure-function analysis of the β-adrenergic receptor. *Cold Spring Harbor Symp* 1988;53:487–498.

17. Dohlman HG, Caron MG, Lefkowitz RJ. A family of receptors coupled to guanine nucleotide regulatory proteins. *Biochemistry* 1987;26:2657–2664.

18. Ehringer H, Hornykiewicz O. Verteilung von Noradrenalin and Dopamin (3-Hydroxytyramin) im Gehirn des Menschen und ihr Verhalten bei Erkrankungen des Extrapyramidalen Systems. *Klin Wochenschr* 1960;38:1236–1239.

19. Felder RA, Felder CA, Eisner GM, Jose PA. The dopamine receptor in adult and maturing kidney. *Am J Physiol* 1989;257:F315–F327.

20. Fremeau RT Jr, Duncan GE, Fornaretto MG, et al. Localization of D_1 dopamine receptor mRNA in brain supports a role in cognitive, affective, and neuroendocrine aspects of dopaminergic neurotransmission. *Proc Natl Acad Sci USA* 1991;88:3772–3776.

21. Gerfen CR, Engber TM, Mahan LC, et al. D_1 and D_2 dopamine receptor-regulated gene expression of striatonigral and striatopallidal neurons. *Science* 1990;250:1429–1430.

22. Giros B, Martres MP, Pilon C, Sokoloff P, Schwartz JC. Shorter variants of the D_3 dopamine receptor produced through various patterns of alternative splicing. *Biochem Biophys Res Commun* 1991;176:1584–1592.

23. Giros B, Sokoloff P, Martres MP, Rious JF, Emorine LJ, Schwartz JC. Alternative splicing directs the expression of two D_2 dopamine receptor isoforms. *Nature* 1989;342:923–926.

24. Grandy DK, Allen LJ, Zhang Y, Zhou QY, Magenis RE, Civelli O. Chromosomal localization of the three human D_5 dopamine receptor genes. *Genomics* 1992;13:968–973.

25. Grandy DK, Marchionni MA, Makam H, et al. Cloning of the cDNA and gene for a human D_2 dopamine receptor. *Proc Natl Acad Sci USA* 1989;86:9762–9766.

26. Grandy DK, Zhang Y, Bouvier C, et al. Multiple D_5 dopamine receptor genes: a functional receptor and two pseudogenes. *Proc Natl Acad Sci USA* 1991;88:9175–9179.

27. Hall ZA. Three of a kind: the β-adrenergic receptor, the muscarinic acetylcholine receptor, and rhodopsin. *Trends Neuro Sci* 1987;10:99–100.

28. Hayes G, Biden TJ, Selbie LA. Structural subtypes of the dopamine D_2 receptor are functionally distinct: expression of the cloned D_{2A} and D_{2B} subtypes in a heterologous cell line. *Mol Endocrinol* 1992;6:920–926.

29. Hornykiewicz O. Dopamine and brain function. *Pharmacol Res* 1966;18:925–964.

30. Kebabian JW, Calne DB. Multiple receptors for dopamine. *Nature* 1979;277:93–96.

31. Leff SE, Creese I. Interactions of dopaminergic agonists and antagonists with dopaminergic D3 binding sites in rat striatum: evidence the [^{3}H]dopamine can label a high affinity agonist-binding state of the D_1 dopamine receptor. *Mol Pharmacol* 1985;27:184–192.

32. Lefkowitz RJ, Kobilka BK, Benovic JL, et al. Molecular biology of adrenergic receptors. *Cold Spring Harbor Symp* 1988;53:507–514.

33. Levesque D, Diaz J, Pilon C, et al. Identification, characterization and localization of the dopamine D_3 receptor in the brain using 7-[^{3}H]hydroxy-*N'N*-di-*n*-propyl-2-amino tetralin. *Proc Natl Acad Sci USA* 1992;89:8155–8159.

34. Mansour A, Meador-Woodruff J, Bunzow J, Civelli O, Akil H, Watson S. Localization of dopamine D_2 receptor mRNA and D_1 and D_2 receptor binding in the rat brain and pituitary: an in situ hybridization-receptor audoradiographic analysis. *J Neurosci* 1990;10:2587–2600.

35. Mansour A, Meador-Woodruff JH, Camp DM, et al. *The effects of nigrostriatal 6-hydroxydopamine lesions on dopamine D2 receptor mRNA and opioid systems.* Alan R. Liss, Inc., 1989.

36. Meador-Woodruff JH, Mansour A, Bunzow JR, Van Tol HHM, Watson S, Civelli O. Distribution of D_2 dopamine receptor mRNA in rat brain. *Proc Natl Acad Sci USA* 1989;86:7625–7628.

37. Meador-Woodruff JH, Mansour A, Grandy DK, Damask SP, Civelli O, Watson SJ. Distribution of D_5 dopamine receptor mRNA in rat brain. *Neurosci Lett* 1992;145:209–212.

38. Meador-Woodruff JH, Mansour A, Healty DJ, et al. Comparison of the distributions of D_1 and D_2 dopamine receptor mRNAs in rat brain. *Neuropsychopharmacology* 1991;5:231–242.

39. Mengod G, Martinez-Mir MI, Vilaro MT, Palacios JM. Localization of the mRNA for the dopamine D_2 receptor in the rat brain by in situ hybridization histochemistry. *Proc Natl Acad Sci USA* 1989;86:8560–8564.

40. Miller JC, Wang Y, Filer D. Identification by sequence analysis of a second rat brain cDNA encoding the dopamine D_2 receptor. *Biochem Biophys Res Commun* 1990;166:109–112.

41. Monsma FJ Jr, Mahan LC, McVittie LD, Gerfen CR, Sibley DR. Molecular cloning and expression of a D_1 dopamine receptor linked to adenylyl cyclase activation. *Proc Natl Acad Sci USA* 1990;87:6723–6727.

42. Monsma FJ Jr, McVittie LD, Gerfen CR, Mahan LC, Sibley DR. Multiple D2 dopamine receptors produced by alternative RNA splicing. *Nature* 1989;342:926–929.

43. Montmayeur JP, Borrelli E. Transcription mediated by a cAMP-responsive promoter element is reduced upon activation of dopamine D2 receptors. *Proc Natl Acad Sci USA* 1991;88:3135–3139.

44. Najlerahim A, Barton AJL, Harrison PJ, Heffernan J, Pearson RCA. Messenger RNA encoding the D_2 dopaminergic receptor detected by in situ hybridization histochemistry in rat brain. *FEBS Lett* 1989;255:335–339.

45. Neve KA, Henningsten RA, Bunzow JR, Civelli O. Functional characterization of a rat dopamine D_2 receptor cDNA expressed in mammalian cell lines. *Mol Pharmacol* 1989;36(3):446–451.

46. O'Dowd BF, Hnatowich M, Caron MG, Lefkowitz RJ, Bouvier M. Palmitoylation of the human β_2-adrenergic receptor. *J Biol Chem* 1989;264:7564–7569.

47. O'Malley KL, Harmon S, Tang L, Todd RD. The rat dopamine D_4 receptor: sequence, gene, structure, and demonstration of expression in the cardiovascular system. *New Biol* 1992;4:137–146.

48. O'Malley KL, Mack KJ, Gandelman KY, Todd RD. Organization and expression of the rat D_{2A} receptor gene: identification of alternative transcripts and a variant donor splice site. *Biochemistry* 1990;29:1367–1371.

49. Poirier LJ, Sourkes TL. Influence of the substantia nigra on the catecholamine content of the striatum. *Brain* 1965;88:181–192.

50. Seeman P, Lee T, Chan-Wong M, Wong K. Antipsychotic drug doses and neuroleptic/dopamine receptors. *Nature* 1976;261:717–719.

51. Seeman P, Niznik HB, Guan H-C, Booth G, Ulpian C. Link between D_1 and D_2 dopamine receptors is reduced in schizophrenia and Huntington diseased brain. *Proc Natl Acad Sci USA* 1989;86:10156–10160.

52. Selbie LA, Hayes G, Shine J. The major dopamine D_2 receptors: molecular analysis of the human D_{2A} subtype. *DNA* 1989;8:683–689.

53. Snyder LA, Roberts JL, Sealfon SC. Alternative transcripts of the rat and human dopamine D_3 receptor. *Biochem Biophys Res Commun* 1991;180:1031–1035.

54. Sokoloff P, Giros B, Martres MP, Bouthenet ML, Schwartz JC. Molecular cloning and characterization of a novel dopamine receptor (D_3) as a target for neuroleptics. *Nature* 1990;347:146–151.

55. Sunahara RK, Guan HC, O'Dowd BF, et al. Cloning of the gene for a human dopamine D_5 receptor with higher affinity for dopamine than D_1. *Nature* 1991;350:614–619.

56. Sunahara RK, Niznik HB, Weiner DM, et al. Human dopamine D_1 receptor encoded by an intronless gene on chromosome 5. *Nature* 1990;347:80–83.

57. Tiberi M, Jarvie KR, Silvia C, et al. Cloning, molecular characterization and chromosomal assignment of a gene encoding a second

D_1 dopamine receptor subtype: differential expression pattern in rat brain compared with the D_1 receptor. *Proc Natl Acad Sci USA* 1991;88:7491–7495.

58. Van Tol HHM, Bunzow JR, Guan HC, et al. Cloning of a human dopamine D_4 receptor gene with high affinity for the antipsychotic clozapine. *Nature* 1991;350:610–614.

59. Van Tol HMM, Wu CM, Guan HC, et al. Multiple dopamine D_4 receptor variants in the human population. *Nature* 1992;358:149–152.

60. Waddington JL. Functional interactions between D_1 and D_2 dopamine receptor systems: their role in the regulation of psychomoter behavior, putative mechanisms, and clinical relevance. *J Psychopharmacol* 1989;3:54–63.

61. Walters JR, Bergstrom DA, Carlson JH, Chase TN, Braun AR. D_1 dopamine receptor activation required for postsynaptic expression of D_2 agonist effects. *Science* 1987;269:719–722.

62. Weiner DM, Brann MR. The distribution of a dopamine D_2 receptor mRNA in rat brain. *FEBS Lett* 1989;253:207–213.

63. Zhou QY, Grandy D, Thambi L, et al. Cloning and expression of human and rat D_1 dopamine receptors. *Nature* 1990;347:76–80.

*Psychopharmacology: The Fourth
Generation of Progress,* edited by
Floyd E. Bloom and David J. Kupfer.
Raven Press, Ltd., New York © 1995.

CHAPTER 15

Electrophysiological Properties of Midbrain Dopamine Neurons

Anthony A. Grace and Benjamin S. Bunney

The neurotransmitter, dopamine (DA), has had a comparatively short but momentous history (cf. ref. 20). The discovery of DA as an independent neurotransmitter occurred in 1958 by Dr. Arvid Carlsson. Five years after its discovery, this neurotransmitter was implicated in the mode of action of antipsychotic drugs, and the degeneration of DA neurons was discovered to be the etiological basis of Parkinson's disease. As a consequence, the DA system itself has been subjected to extensive analysis by investigators utilizing a variety of approaches to better understand this important but complex neurochemical system.

The electrophysiological analysis of DA-containing neurons began with a paper published in 1973 (4), in which combined physiological, neurochemical, and histochemical techniques were brought to bear in defining this system. As a result of this effort, substantial progress has been made in the past two decades in which the physiology of this system has been dissected in preparations ranging from in vitro recordings of isolated neurons to recording their activity in freely behaving primates. Therefore, although the physiology of the DA neuron has been reviewed in every volume of this series, including the last one published only 7 years ago, sufficient data have accumulated to devote two chapters to the analysis of this system: This chapter deals with the basic physiological properties of the DA neuron, and in Chapter 21 the pharmacological responses of the DA neuron are examined in detail. In the present chapter, primary emphasis will be placed on the more recent in vitro recordings,

with comparisons drawn to in vivo data reviewed in the last volume (see also Chapters 22 and 25 for differential functional emphases, and Chapter 29 for noradrenergic neurons, *this volume*).

IDENTIFICATION

The electrophysiological analysis of neurons is capable of providing substantial insight into the function of these neuronal elements, and comparisons between their discharge properties and biochemical measures of neurotransmitter regulation can provide the basis for novel ideas regarding the multifaceted modes of regulation present in the nervous system. Indeed, such a coordinated biochemical and electrophysiological analysis of defined systems has led the way to substantial advances in our knowledge of the catecholamine systems. However, when the electrophysiological study involves neurochemically defined neurons, the physiologist has the burden of providing a level of proof that can be taken for granted in most biochemical investigations: that the neurons one is studying are indeed the cells that release the neurotransmitter of interest. Although identification of neurons on the basis of location or morphology may suffice when the investigator is studying the postsynaptic actions of these neurohumors, meaningful data cannot be collected from the cells that synthesize and release a given neurotransmitter unless this identification is definitive.

DA-containing neurons in the midbrain of rats have undergone a series of identification techniques ranging from indirect to direct, depending on the capabilities of the techniques employed. The first identification was accomplished in vivo, and it relied on the ability to cause DA in tissue slices to fluoresce when treated with substances that combine with DA to form a fluorescent prod-

A. A. Grace: Departments of Neuroscience and Psychiatry, Center for Neuroscience, University of Pittsburgh, Pittsburgh, Pennsylvania 15260.

B. S. Bunney: Department of Psychiatry, Yale University School of Medicine, New Haven, Connecticut 06519.

uct, such as formaldehyde vapor or glyoxylic acid. Thus, utilizing extracellular recording techniques, the DA precursor L-DOPA was locally applied by iontophoresis to midbrain neurons in the substantia nigra that exhibited a unique action potential waveform. The result was the recovery of a group of highly fluorescent, presumably dopaminergic neurons that had taken up the L-DOPA, converted it to DA, and as a result showed higher levels of fluorescence than observed in DA neurons located only a few hundred microns from the ejection site (4). This identification was later verified using in vivo intracellular recording techniques to inject the L-DOPA directly into a single DA-containing neuron, thereby providing precise identification of the single cell impaled as being of the dopaminergic cell type (22). This was further confirmed using other techniques to augment the DA content (i.e., intracellular injection of the tyrosine hydroxylase cofactor or intracellular injection of colchicine to cause somatic buildup of DA), and hence histochemical fluorescent intensity, of single DA neurons (23). Adjunct techniques including DA-specific lesions and antidromic activation provided further support for the accuracy of this identification (23,31). As a result of these investigations, a unique action potential waveform and firing pattern could be accurately associated with identified DA-containing neurons, thereby enabling accurate studies of the physiology and pharmacology of this important neurochemical system.

Unfortunately, the criteria used to identify this class of neurons in the in vivo preparation proved to be insufficient to be utilized in most in vitro recording studies. This was due to three factors: (i) The neurons recorded in the substantia nigra in the in vitro midbrain slice did not fire with the same discharge pattern as that linked with identified DA neurons recorded in vivo, (ii) identification based on antidromic activation from DA axon target sites was not possible in a 400-μm-thick slice, and (iii) because most in vitro studies involved intracellular recordings, the unique extracellular action potential waveform of the DA cell was not an appropriate identification criterion. Indeed, one of the most unusual features of the spike discharge of the DA neuron in vivo was the highly variable nature of the spike waveform generated from a single neuron; however, because this variability was apparently derived from the interaction with afferent fibers, this characteristic was not observed in the in vitro preparation. Furthermore, because studies have shown the presence of nondopaminergic neurons within the zona compacta region (32), localization of the recorded neuron was not sufficient to identify these neurons. Indeed, reliance on location within the zona compacta has led several investigators to ascribe characteristics to DA neurons, such as rebound burst firing and prominent low-threshold calcium events, even though these properties have never been observed in any of the studies that have used reliable identification techniques. In fact, studies that relied on histochemical identi-

fication of neurons have universally ascribed these properties to the nondopaminergic neurons within the substantia nigra (29,69). As a result, a different set of criteria based on new identification procedures were required.

Because of the high variability in the intraneuronal concentrations of DA present within neurons located at different depths within the midbrain slice recorded in vitro, it was difficult to identify DA neurons using the techniques previously utilized in vivo. Instead, the first direct identification of DA neurons in vitro relied on immunocytochemistry. Thus, because only catecholamine-synthesizing neurons contain the enzyme tyrosine hydroxylase, and given the absence of the enzyme DA-β-hydroxylase (a norepinephrine- and epinephrine-specific enzyme) within neurons in this brain region, DA cell identification was accomplished using combined intracellular staining with immunocytochemical localization of tyrosine hydroxylase. In order to reliably separate the fluorescence of the intracellular stain from that of the tyrosine hydroxylase immunolocalization within the same brain section, the putative DA neuron was injected intracellularly with the highly fluorescent dye Lucifer yellow, which could be readily separated from the rhodamine-labeled secondary antibody employed in the immunocytochemical localization of tyrosine hydroxylase. Using this method, DA-containing neurons within the midbrain ventral tegmental area and substantia nigra were accurately identified during in vitro recordings in the midbrain slice (29,69). Unlike that reported in vivo, in both cases the DA-containing cells were identified as the non-burst-firing cell class, with the cells showing prominent rebound burst firing shown to be the nondopaminergic zona reticulata neurons. Furthermore, this study provided the basis for another distinct criterion that could be used for the electrophysiological identification of DA-containing neurons during intracellular recordings in brain slices: the presence of a large-amplitude, slow depolarization that was responsible for driving spike activity in these cells (18,29). More recently, DA-containing neurons have been identified using direct histochemical detection of catecholamine fluorescence or immunocytochemistry in dissociated substantia nigra tissue (33,64) as well as in primary neuron cultures (8,54).

MORPHOLOGY

Intracellular injection of Lucifer yellow was also used for examining the morphology of DA neurons in thick slices. In general, DA neurons of the substantia nigra could be divided into two classes: The DA neurons located in the more dorsal regions of the zona compacta of the substantia nigra were typically fusiform in appearance, with somata averaging 15–25 μm in diameter and with 2–5 dendrites emanating from the poles of the neuron. The dendrites branched sparsely within the substantia nigra, but remained confined to the zona compacta region of this nucleus. In contrast, the more ventrally located DA neurons were multipolar in shape, having somata that were approximately 20–35 μm in diameter. The dendrites also emanated from the poles of the soma and extended laterally within the zona compacta region. However, unlike the dorsal neurons, DA cells in the ventral region also had a long dendritic process that entered into and branched within the zona reticulata. The DA neurons stained within the ventral tegmental region ranged from large fusiform to multipolar in appearance. They also had 3–5 dendrites emanating from the soma that extended in a radial array from the soma, probably owing to the comparative lack of spatial constraints within the ventral tegmentum. Analysis of neurons using an image analysis system revealed that the neuron and its dendritic field typically extended over a mediolateral and dorsoventral region of approximately 400–2500 μm; however, the neurons were comparatively constrained in the anteroposterior direction, typically extending only 100–200 μm in this dimension (Fig. 1). Similar morphological properties of zona compacta neurons have been described using intracellular injection of horseradish peroxidase (41,67).

DA neurons in both the ventral tegmentum and the substantia nigra have several atypical morphological characteristics that may contribute to their distinctive physiological properties. One of these unusual properties is that DA neurons appear to be capable of storing and releasing DA within the substantia nigra and ventral tegmentum in a calcium-dependent, tetrodotoxin (TTX)-sensitive manner (6). However, this release does not appear to be derived from local axonal collaterals. The axon of the DA neuron in almost all cases is not derived from the soma of the neuron, but instead emanates from a major dendrite or from a somatic appendage. The thin, unmyelinated axon projects out of the somatodendritic field before turning in an anterior direction and exiting the plane of the slice. Local axonal branching or collaterals have not been observed. On the other hand, the long, sparsely branched dendrites of the DA neuron appear in all cases examined to end in a forked process. The forks of this process are thin and highly recursive, giving the appearance of an axonal branch encircling a postsynaptic element. Although speculative, the axon-like morphology of the dendrite and the absence of recurrent axonal terminals suggest that these distally located, specialized dendritic arborizations may represent the dendritic DA release sites associated with these neurons.

The dendrites of the DA neurons are mostly smooth in morphology. However, the dendrites are also observed to

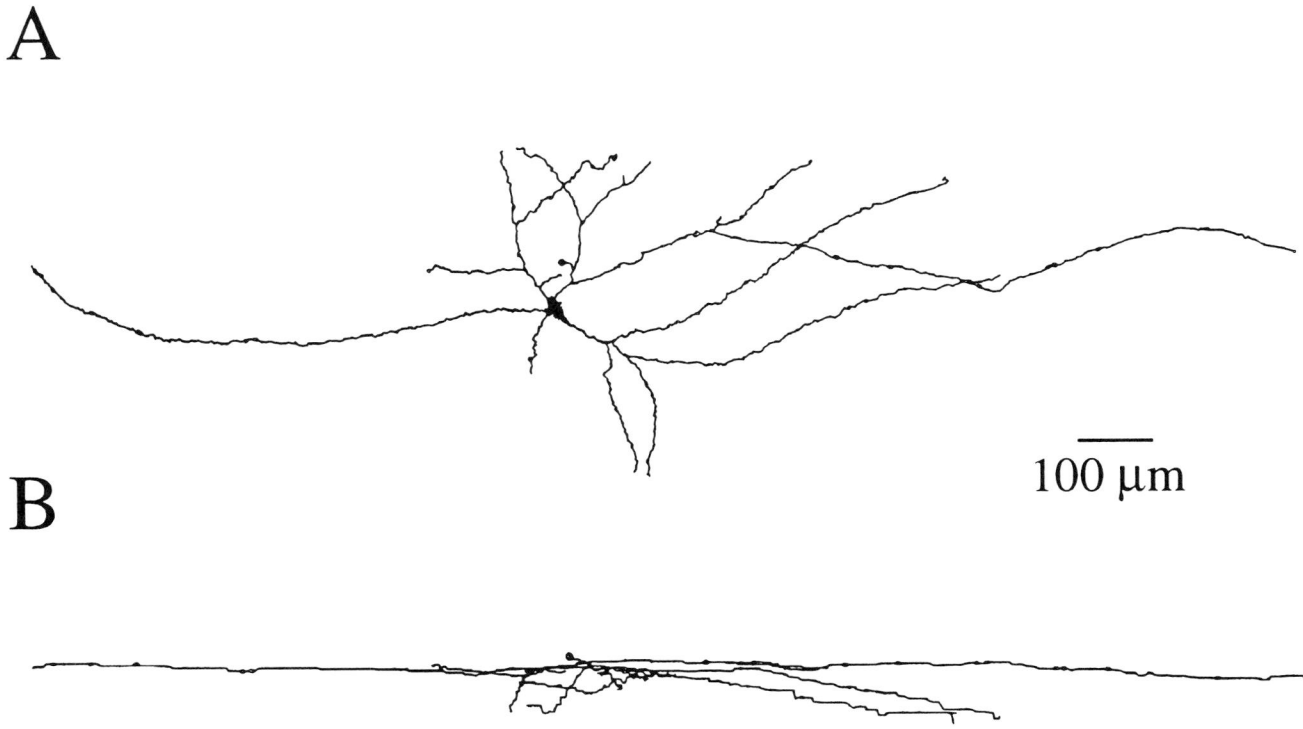

FIG. 1. Computer reconstruction of a substantia nigra DA neuron stained by Lucifer yellow. **A:** Examined in a frontal plane, the DA neuron dendrites are observed to extend for hundreds of microns in the dorsal/ventral plane (*top/bottom of figure*) and in the medial/lateral plane (*left/right of figure*). **B:** However, examined from a dorsal viewpoint, the anterior/posterior extent of the neuron (*top/bottom of figure*) is highly compressed. (Pucak and Grace, *unpublished observations.*)

possess short cytoplasmic extensions that occur infrequently along the length of the process. These branchlets are approximately 0.5–2.0 μm in diameter and extend from 5 to 50 μm from the dendrite without branching. These branchlets are not unlike those associated with axon terminal attachment sites in other brain regions (see also Chapter 23, *this volume,* for ultrastructural progress).

BASIC ELECTROPHYSIOLOGICAL PROPERTIES

Passive Membrane Properties

The membrane properties of DA neurons appear to depend, to some extent, on the preparation used. Stable intracellular recordings from DA neurons in vivo have shown them to have a moderate input resistance, averaging 31 ± 7 megohms (range: 18–45 megohms) (23). In contrast, identified DA neurons recorded in vitro exhibit input resistances approximately three- to fivefold greater, with input resistances averaging 168 ± 61 megohms (range: 80–320 megohms) (16,29,45). Nonetheless, in both cases the membranes are characterized by a prominent anomalous rectification when hyperpolarized (Fig. 2) (16,18,23,41,43,45). This anomalous rectification is

comprised of two components: an instantaneous component and a time-dependent component that showed maximal activation at membrane potentials of −63 mV and −78 mV, respectively (18). In addition, at the termination of a brief membrane hyperpolarization the DA cell exhibits a pronounced voltage-dependent delayed repolarization (13,16,18,29,64). Both in terms of its voltage dependency and its effects on membrane repolarization, this conductance resembles that described in other preparations as the I_A current. However, unlike the I_A described in other regions, this conductance is not affected by application of the potassium blocker 4-aminopyridine (Fig. 2).

Pacemaker Potential

One of the unusual properties of DA neurons noted during extracellular recording is the prominent negative phase of the spike and the highly variable shape of their spike waveform, even when recording a series of spikes from a single, well-isolated neuron. Intracellular recordings performed from DA neurons both in vivo (23,25) and in vitro (17,18,29) have provided a potential explanation for this observation. First, in both preparations the

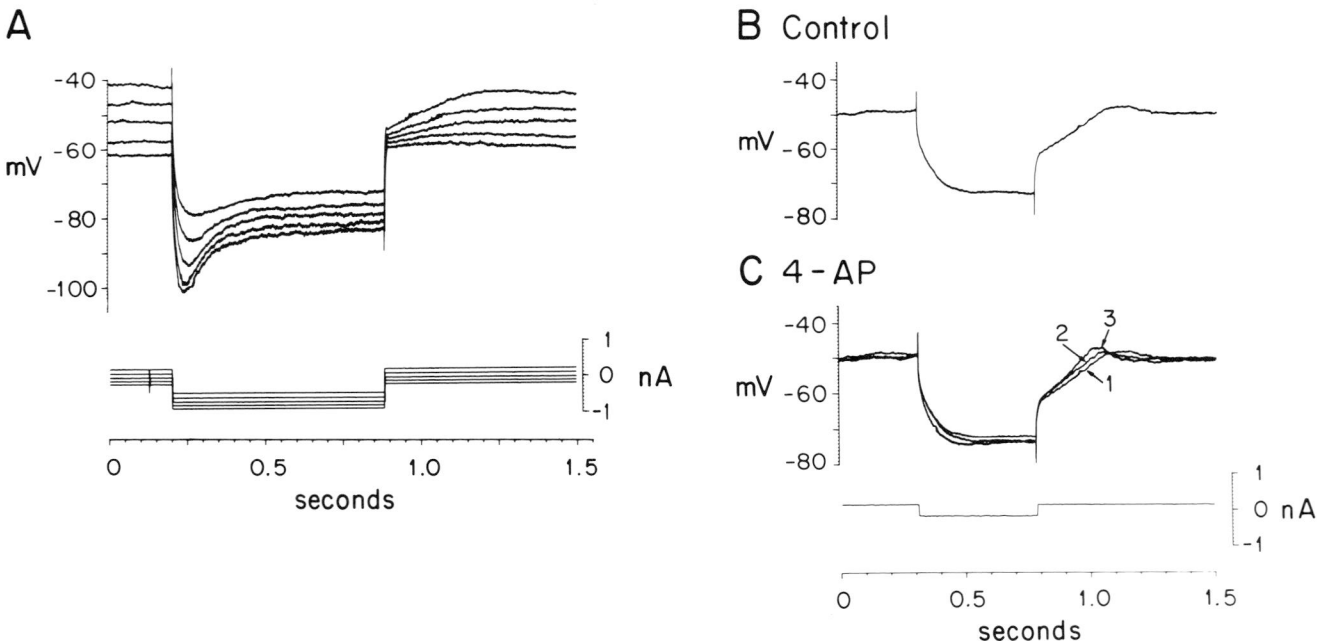

FIG. 2. The anomalous rectification and the I_A-like delayed repolarization observed during a brief membrane hyperpolarization exhibit voltage-dependent properties. **A:** In a nondischarging DA neuron, progressive steady-state hyperpolarization of the membrane by current injection (*bottom trace*) increased the amplitude of the anomalous rectification observed at the initiation of the hyperpolarizing pulse and caused a decrease in the I_A-like delayed repolarization observed at the offset of the pulse. **B, C:** Injection of a hyperpolarizing current pulse into this tetrodotoxin (TTX)- and tetraethylammonium (TEA)-treated DA neuron reveals the delayed repolarization at the offset of the pulse. Although the form of the delayed repolarization is similar to that described for the I_A conductance described elsewhere, it does not exhibit the characteristic sensitivity to administration of 4-aminopyridine (4-AP). Concentrations of 4-AP: 1 = control; 2 = 5 mM; 3 = 20 mM. (From ref. 29, with permission.)

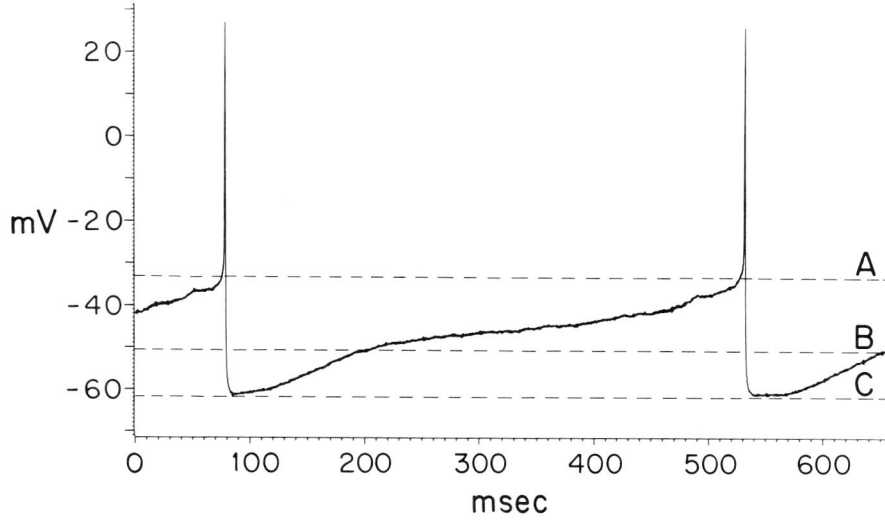

FIG. 3. DA neurons recorded intracellularly in vivo and in vitro exhibit characteristic pacemaker-like slow depolarizations and high spike thresholds. In this recording from a spontaneously discharging DA neuron recorded in vitro from a rat midbrain slice, a slow membrane depolarizing conductance depolarizes this neuron from its resting potential (**B**) to the atypically high membrane potential threshold for spike generation that is characteristic for these neurons, which in this case is −33 mV (**A**). The action potential is followed by a calcium-dependent afterhyperpolarization (**C**), which then decays prior to the initiation of a subsequent slow depolarization. (From ref. 29, with permission.)

DA neuron action potential is triggered from a comparatively depolarized membrane potential, averaging −41 mV in vivo and −36 mV in vitro. Thus, the DA neuron membrane must be depolarized approximately 15–25 mV in order to depolarize the membrane from its resting potential (average RMP = −57 ± 4 mV) to this high threshold for spiking. In fact, it is these depolarized spike thresholds that likely prevent antidromic activation of DA neurons from eliciting a full-amplitude action potential, since even the initial segment (IS) spike is not of sufficient amplitude to provide this level of depolarization (17,23). The spontaneous discharge of the DA neuron is therefore highly dependent on the presence of a slow, large-amplitude pacemaker depolarization (Fig. 3). This pacemaker conductance is a voltage-dependent depolarization that drives spontaneous spike generation in DA neurons as shown in both in vivo (23,25) and in vitro (14, 16,18,29,41) preparations. It is the alternation of this pacemaker with the spike and its associated afterhyperpolarization that underlies the highly regular firing pattern observed in DA neurons in the in vitro brain-slice preparation (29) as well as in dissociated dopaminergic neurons (33). Although DA neurons recorded in vivo rarely fire

in a pacemaker-like pattern, intracellular injection of the calcium chelator ethyleneglycol bis(aminoethyl ether)tetraacetate (EGTA) has been shown to change an irregularly discharging or a burst-firing neuron in vivo to one firing in a highly regular pacemaker pattern identical to that found in vitro. This pacemaker conductance appears to be comprised of both sodium- and calcium-dependent conductances, because administration of either TTX or cobalt will block spontaneous spike generation of DA neurons in vitro.

Calcium-Mediated Spikes

Blockade of sodium conductances in DA neurons by administration of TTX readily blocks spontaneous spike activity and reveals the presence of two cobalt-sensitive (and hence presumably calcium-mediated) active membrane events. Following TTX treatment, a low-amplitude, brief hyperpolarization of the membrane will evoke a rebound depolarizing all-or-none wave (16,29,41,52) that in many ways resembles the low-threshold calcium spike (LTS) reported in other brain regions. The presence of

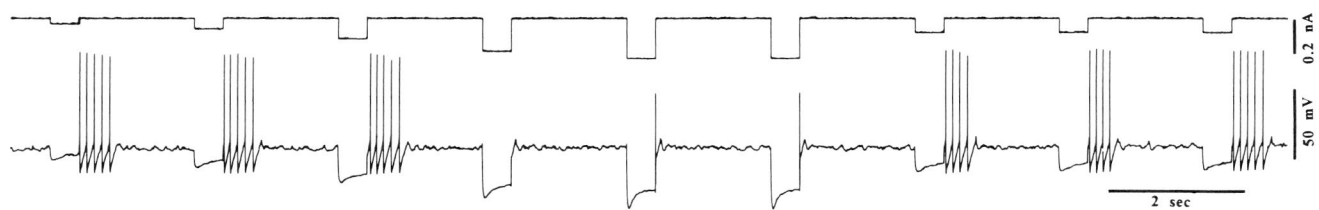

FIG. 4. Injection of low-amplitude, brief hyperpolarizing pulses (*top trace*) into a nonfiring DA neuron will often evoke rebound action potential discharge (*bottom trace;* first three events). On the other hand, increases in the amplitude of the hyperpolarizing pulse will eventually trigger the I_A-like delayed repolarization of the membrane, effectively blocking the rebound depolarization and spike discharge (third through sixth events). As a consequence, large-amplitude rebound bursts of spikes are not observed in this class of neurons. (From ref. 18, with permission.)

---

this rebound event is highly dependent on the membrane potential: It cannot be evoked by brief hyperpolarizing pulses injected into a hyperpolarized neuron, whereas depolarizing the neuron will typically reveal this rebound event. However, if the amplitude of the hyperpolarizing pulse is increased, the rebound event is obscured by the I_A-like delayed repolarization (Fig. 2). Indeed, the constraints placed on the amplitude of the LTS by its voltage-dependency and that of the putative I_A most likely underlie the inability to evoke large-amplitude rebound depolariza-

tions or bursts, but appear to be sufficient to enable small-amplitude hyperpolarizing events to elicit sustained rebound spike firing (Fig. 4). Because this LTS can be evoked by injecting very-small-amplitude depolarizing pulses into the soma, is highly dependent on the membrane potential of the soma, and has an activation threshold that is not altered by potassium blockers, this event is most likely generated proximal to the soma (17,44).

In TTX-treated neurons, injection of large-amplitude depolarizing current pulses fails to evoke any additional

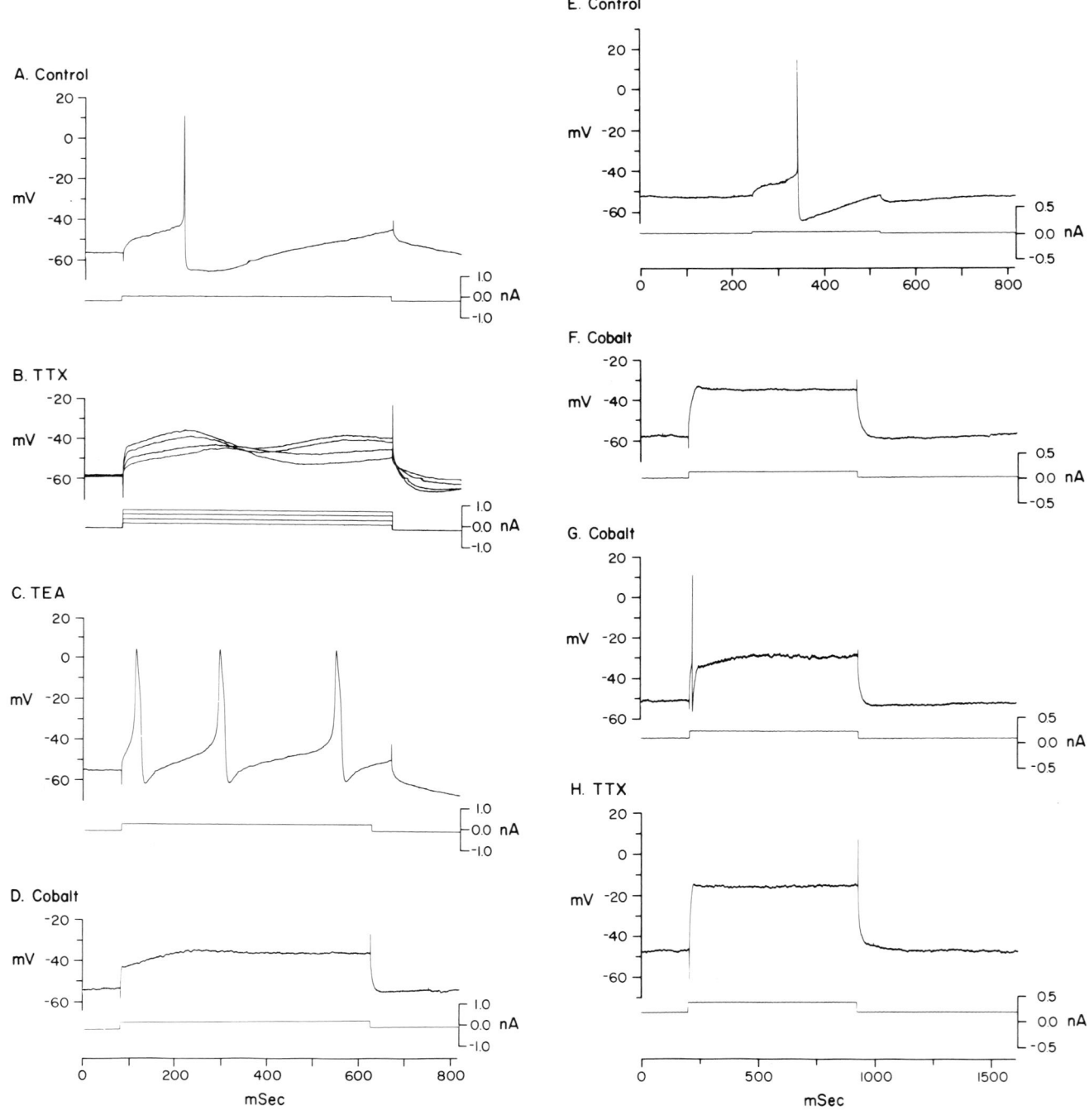

active membrane events. However, after administration of the potassium blocker tetraethylammonium (TEA) to the bath, comparatively small-amplitude depolarizations of the membrane will evoke large-amplitude (i.e., 60–85 mV), long-duration (i.e., 7–20 msec), cobalt-sensitive spikes with prominent afterhyperpolarizations (Fig. 5) (16,17,29,41) that resemble the high-threshold calcium spikes (HTSs) observed in other preparations. TEA is known to block the delayed rectifier of neurons, allowing current to spread more effectively into the distal dendrites and making them more isopotential with the soma. The fact that these events cannot be evoked by direct somatic depolarization without the presence of TEA suggests that they are generated distally to the soma, possibly at the distal dendritic regions (44). Indeed, the calcium-dependent nature of these spikes and their generation at distal dendritic sites suggest that these spikes may at least contribute to the dendritic release of DA from these neurons (29,44). These HTSs apparently give rise to the prolonged afterhyperpolarizations associated with the slow firing frequency of these neurons. The afterhyperpolarization itself appears to be composed of two components: (i) a fast component that inactivated near −63 mV independent of the membrane potential and (ii) a slower, larger-amplitude component that increased in amplitude with hyperpolarization of the membrane (18). A long-latency afterhyperpolarization that exhibited summation with subsequent spikes in a train similar to that observed in vivo (25) was not observed in the in vitro preparation (18).

The pharmacology of these calcium-dependent events has recently been investigated in detail (53). It appears that the oscillatory calcium conductance that underlies the TTX-insensitive portion of the oscillatory pacemaker potential can be abolished by treatment with nifedipine, whereas the HTS is little affected by this blocker. Furthermore, both nifedipine and apamin also attenuated the slow component of the spike afterhyperpolarization (53,63). In contrast, the HTS can be partially blocked by administration of ω-conotoxin.

Sodium-Mediated Spikes

As found with blockade of sodium conductances with TTX, administration of the calcium blocker cobalt to DA neurons recorded in vitro causes a cessation of spontaneous spike activity. However, strong depolarizations of the membrane will trigger a rapid burst of fast, small-amplitude spikes (Fig. 5). These spikes have little or no afterhyperpolarizations and can be blocked by TTX. Although administration of TEA does not affect these events, application of 4-aminopyridine (4-AP) causes a substantial lowering of their threshold, enabling these spikes to be evoked by moderate depolarization of the membrane. In terms of their amplitude, duration, and absence of an afterhyperpolarization, these spikes resemble the IS spikes triggered during antidromic activation of DA-containing neurons in vivo.

Properties of DA Neuron Action Potentials

Perhaps the most distinctive feature of DA cells is the irregular but unique spike waveform they produce. These action potentials are unusual in having an atypically depolarized spike threshold (i.e., −41 mV in vivo and −36 mV in vitro at RMP) that varies with the membrane potential; indeed, the threshold decreases by approximately 5 mV with a 7-mV hyperpolarization of the membrane. Studies have shown that, as with most other neurons, the action potential is comprised of a short-duration (0.8–1.5 msec) initial segment (IS) spike followed by a longer-duration (1.5–3 msec) somatodendritic (SD) spike; however, in DA cells the IS spike is only approximately one-fourth to one-third the size of the SD spike. The IS is the lowest-threshold region of the neuron, and therefore it determines

FIG. 5. Action potentials recorded in vitro in DA neurons can be differentiated pharmacologically into two components. **A:** Injection of a depolarizing pulse (*bottom trace*) evokes a membrane depolarization and action potential discharge (*top trace*) in an identified DA neuron. **B:** After the administration of 1 μm of the sodium channel blocker tetrodotoxin (TTX) into the superfusion fluid, the depolarization-evoked spike discharge is blocked even when the amplitude of the membrane depolarization is increased severalfold. **C:** Administration of the selective potassium channel blocker tetraethylammonium (TEA; 2 mM) enables moderate amplitudes of membrane depolarization to elicit a series of large-amplitude, long-duration spikes with prominent spike afterhyperpolarizations. **D:** Subsequent application of the calcium blocker cobalt (2 mM) prevents the occurrence of these depolarization-elicited high-threshold spikes (HTSs). Other experiments show that this HTS underlies the somatodendritic component of the action potential. **E:** Depolarization of the membrane of a DA neuron in control conditions evokes action potential discharge. **F:** Administration of the calcium blocker cobalt to the superfusion fluid blocks spike activity in this neuron. **G:** However, if sufficient amplitudes of membrane depolarization are delivered, the cell discharges a moderate-amplitude, fast spike. This spike is brief in duration and is associated with very little spike afterhyperpolarization. **H:** Subsequent administration of the sodium channel blocker TTX blocks this depolarization-elicited spike discharge. Other experiments show that this TTX-sensitive spike underlies the initial segment spike of the action potential. (From ref. 17, with permission.)

the action potential threshold. The IS spike in DA neurons is likely to be generated at a site that is comparatively distal and not isopotential with respect to the soma, because (a) the morphological studies reviewed earlier showed that in DA neurons, the axon does not arise from the soma but instead arises at a more distal location on a primary dendrite, (b) the IS spike is smaller in amplitude than the SD spike, (c) its threshold varies with the membrane potential, and (d) administration of 4-AP lowers the action potential threshold as well as the threshold of the IS spike, without affecting the SD spike. TEA, on the other hand, lowers the threshold of the calcium-mediated HTS spike and increases the duration of the SD spike without affecting the IS spike. Furthermore, as shown during antidromic activation of DA neurons in vivo, activation of the IS spike is not sufficient to trigger the SD spike unless the membrane is depolarized by the pacemaker potential.

Spike Generation in DA Neurons

Based on the data presented in this section, a model of spike generation in DA neurons may be derived (18): The action potential sequence is initiated when the membrane is depolarized by the pacemaker potential. The IS segment is depolarized fastest because of its smaller volume and proximity to the pacemaker potential source. The depolarization at the soma lags behind the IS potential due to a 4-AP sensitive conductance. Indeed, a 4-AP-sensitive I_A located between the IS and the soma could contribute to this lag by shunting the slow depolarization. Such a 4-AP-sensitive I_A conductance has been identified in the more electrotonically compact, higher input resistance dissociated DA neuron preparation (64), in which normally electrotonically distal events may be more easily assessed by a whole-cell clamp at the soma. As a consequence, the apparent threshold of the IS as measured at the soma would be substantially higher than at the IS, and would vary depending on the voltage-dependent activation of the putative 4-AP-sensitive I_A. The IS would then spread across the somatodendritic region already depolarized by the slow depolarization, and thereby cause a sufficient level of depolarization in the distal dendritic regions (possibly the site of the recursive dendritic arbors and putative DA release sites) to trigger the HTS/SD spike component. The Ca-mediated HTS then hyperpolarizes the cell by activating a $I_{K(Ca)}$, which upon decay activates the LTS and the next slow depolarization. Another potential function of the HTS would be to trigger calcium-dependent dendritic DA release. Note that this is only one of several possible ways to fit the data into a sequential model. Nevertheless, it can serve as a basis for analyzing the functional compartmentalization of the DA neuron until more substantial data can be derived.

ACTIVITY STATES AND PATTERNS OF ACTIVITY IN MIDBRAIN DA NEURONS

Studies have shown that the pharmacological or physiological activation of DA neurons occurs across three dimensions (3,16,35): (i) firing rate, (ii) spike discharge pattern (25,26), and (iii) the proportion of neurons that are spontaneously active. Thus, systemic administration of DA antagonists (3,4), iontophoretic application of glutamate (26), or large depletions of striatal DA (35) will increase the firing rate of active neurons, increase the number of spontaneously active neurons recorded per electrode track in the substantia nigra, cause the DA neurons to fire in bursts, and cause them to change from a single-spiking to a burst-firing pattern of discharge.

Burst Firing

One activity state that has received increased attention recently is that of firing pattern. DA cells show a comparatively limited range of activity, with spontaneous firing rates averaging approximately 4.5 Hz in the anesthetized rat, but are only capable of firing at a maximum of approximately 10 Hz. However, an increase in DA cell activity is typically accompanied by a shift from an irregular single-spiking pattern to one of burst firing (25,26). Burst firing found to occur in DA cells is distinct from that observed in areas more typically associated with burst discharge, such as the hippocampus or thalamus, in that the DA cells have an exceptionally long interspike interval between spikes in the burst, the bursts can consist of 15 spikes or more, and the bursts are associated with depolarization of the DA neuron membrane (26). Stimulation studies have shown that activation of the DA neuron axon in patterns resembling burst discharge will release two to three times more DA than is released by an equivalent number of evenly spaced stimuli (15). Therefore, an alteration in firing pattern is likely to cause a more substantial alteration in synaptic DA release than that produced by an increase in discharge rate alone. For this reason, the regulation of DA cell discharge pattern has been the focus of considerable attention in recent years.

DA neurons recorded in vivo will fire in bursts upon depolarization of their membrane. One of the most potent activators of burst firing in these neurons is the direct application of glutamate to the neurons (26), or by activating glutamatergic afferents that innervate DA neurons (65). Furthermore, glutamatergic stimulation appears to be a prerequisite for inducing burst firing in vivo. Thus, inactivation of glutamatergic afferents to DA neurons (65,66) or administration of a glutamate antagonist such as kynurenic acid (5) or an N-methyl-D-aspartate (NMDA) blocker (7,55) will cause DA neurons to enter a single-spiking mode. Nonetheless, glutamatergic stimulation alone does not appear to be sufficient to cause burst firing. Several studies have now shown that positively identified DA neurons do not fire in bursts when recorded in vitro in midbrain slices, nor can they be induced to fire by depolarization or hyperpolarization of the membrane (18,29,69). Furthermore, application of glutamate or NMDA agonists alone will not cause DA neurons recorded in vitro to fire in bursts (62). Indeed, the only instances in which activity partially resembling burst firing has been induced in the in vitro preparations are cases in which one or more potassium channel blockers have been applied to the neuron (39,63).

Therefore, the current data are insufficient to adequately account for the mechanisms underlying burst firing in DA neurons. However, one thing that is apparent about the mechanism responsible is that, although burst firing is typically associated with increased firing rate, studies have shown that these characteristics appear to be regulated by different systems. Thus, the correlation between firing rate and burst firing is reported to be substantially different when nicotine instead of glutamate is used to stimulate these neurons (30). This can also be illustrated in studies in which the subthalamic nucleus is activated. Stimulation of the subthalamic nucleus appears to activate direct glutamatergic afferents to DA neurons as well as afferents to GABAergic neurons in the substantia nigra that inhibit DA cell firing. Thus, activation of the subthalamus nucleus will inhibit the firing rate of DA neurons. However, upon cessation of the stimulation, the DA cell shows a significant activation of burst firing as it recovers toward its basal rate of firing (65). Thus, burst firing appears to be regulated by a system that has a different time course from that controlling firing rate.

Homeostatic Regulatory Influences on DA Cell Activity States

Each of the activity states reviewed above appears to be under a homeostatic regulatory influence. Thus, when DA demand is increased by administering a DA blocker, such as haloperidol, each of these dimensions of DA cell activity are increased (3,28). Another method that has been used to place a demand on the DA system is the production of 6-OHDA-induced partial lesions of the nigrostriatal DA system. Studies using this technique provide a substantial example of the enormous recovery potential present in this system. Thus, rats depleted of 95% or more of their striatal DA will, after approximately 1 month, exhibit spontaneous recovery of function (70). This recovery is mediated by several homeostatic changes within the nigrostriatal DA system, including decreased DA uptake sites, increased DA synthesis, DA receptor supersensitivity, and so on (cf. refs. 19 and 70). However, the electrophysiological activity of the remaining DA neurons is at its basal level; indeed, even the proportion of neurons active remains constant after correcting for cell loss (35). On the other hand, all of these parameters of DA cell activity are increased if the lesion size exceeds approximately 97%, at which point the rat fails to recover. Furthermore, in lesion-recovered rats, introduction of additional demand on the DA system, such as a low dose of haloperidol, causes a rapid depolarization blockade of DA cell firing and a return of profound motor deficits (37). Therefore, it appears that DA neurons are required to be at their basal level of activity in order to maintain a normal behavioral condition. On this basis, it appears that the homeostatic changes take place over time at the biochemical and receptor level in order to maintain a maximal dynamic range of electrophysiological response, thereby enabling a maximal, rapid increase in DA cell firing and DA release in response to an immediate behavioral demand (35).

An additional state of DA cell activity is depolarization block of spike generation (3,28). In depolarization block, DA cells are in a state of overexcitation, resulting in the inactivation of spike firing. However, unlike the other states of activity, depolarization block appears to only occur in association with pharmacological manipulation of the nigrostriatal system. Thus, repeated administration of DA blockers (3,28), or acute administration of a DA blocker in DA-lesioned and recovered rats (37), will induce this state in DA neurons. Interestingly, decreased DA receptor stimulation by repeated haloperidol administration will readily induce depolarization block, whereas the diminished DA receptor stimulation occurring after a partial DA lesion fails to induce block. One potential explanation for this difference could be that haloperidol administration also pharmacologically circumvents a major homeostatic influence on DA neurons—that is, somatodendritic autoreceptor-mediated inhibition. Thus, with 6-OHDA-induced depletion of only 50% or more of striatal DA, the DA cells in the substantia nigra show evidence of autoreceptor supersensitivity (56). Furthermore, the subsequent pharmacological blockade of these autoreceptors by acute administration of a DA blocker immediately induces a state of depolarization block (37). Therefore, the DA system appears to be capable of compensating for physiological deficits; however, pharmacological interference with its autoreceptor-mediated feedback regulatory system causes the system to lose stability and inactivate due to overdepolarization.

DA NEURON REGULATION BY DENDRODENDRITIC INTERACTION WITH NEIGHBORING DA CELLS

In the previous section, recent advances into the membrane mechanisms that influence the discharge properties of individual DA neurons were reviewed. In this section, evidence for DA neuron regulation via interaction with neighboring dopaminergic neurons is summarized. This interaction has been shown to occur via two distinct and independent mechanisms: (i) electrical interactions and (ii) dendritic release of DA.

Electrical Interactions

This topic has been reviewed in detail in prior publications of this volume, and it will only be mentioned briefly here. Autoreceptor-mediated inhibition via dendritic interactions between DA neurons have been known for some time. However, this type of inhibitory interaction cannot account for data showing that neighboring DA neurons often fire simultaneously with very short interspike intervals (24). Studies using in vivo intracellular recording and injection of the dye Lucifer yellow provided evidence that subsets of DA neurons appear to be interconnected by gap junctions (24). This hypothesis has received support by the recent demonstration of the presence of connexin immunoreactivity within the zona compacta region of the substantia nigra (51), because connexin has been shown to be a monomeric component of the gap junction structure.

Somatodendritic Autoreceptors

The high degree of sensitivity of DA neurons to their own transmitter (4) and the release of DA from dendritic stores (6) have been known for some time; however, clear evidence of a functional role for this system has been lacking. Thus, several investigators cast doubt about whether tonic autoreceptor stimulation is present on DA neurons, because iontophoretic application of DA antagonists (1) or the systemic administration of DA blockers in rats following kainic acid-induced lesions of the striatum (42) have been reported to cause an activation of DA neuron firing similar to that observed after systemic DA antagonist administration to intact rats (4). This observation suggested that systemically administered DA antagonists activated DA cells via the blockade of this neurotransmitter at postsynaptic sites. However, more recent data suggested that this was not the case. Thus, infusion of large amounts of DA blockers directly onto DA neurons using pressure ejection was found to activate DA cell firing (68). Furthermore, acute transection of the striatonigral feedback pathway 1 hour prior to testing did not alter the ability of DA antagonists to activate DA cell firing (57). In addition, recent evidence obtained during in vitro intracellular recordings from DA neurons demonstrated that L-DOPA administration inhibited DA cell firing in control media but was ineffective when the decarboxylation of L-DOPA to DA is blocked by carbidopa administration (46). Furthermore, DA antagonists are capable of activating DA neuron firing when administered to the in vitro slice (58). Therefore, this evidence provided substantial support for the tonic inhibition of DA neuron

activity via autoreceptor stimulation by locally released DA within the confines of the substantia nigra. One question that remained, however, was whether the dopaminergic inhibition occurred through autoinhibition of the cell releasing the DA, or whether the DA released by individual cells formed a "pool" of neurotransmitter that inhibited neighboring DA neurons as well. Although not conclusive, studies showing the development of DA cell autoreceptor supersensitivity following partial 6-OHDA-induced lesions (56) suggests that lesion-induced loss of neighboring DA neurons will decrease the biophase concentration of DA within the substantia nigra, leading to supersensitivity of the residual neurons. The pharmacology and biophysics of this mode of regulation is covered in detail in the next chapter in this volume (Chiodo and Bunney).

STRIATONIGRAL FEEDBACK REGULATION OF DA NEURON ACTIVITY

DA neurons receive afferent inputs from a number of brain regions. However, the majority of the inputs to the substantia nigra arise either directly or indirectly from the striatum. DeLong and co-workers (2) have described two efferent projection systems from the striatum: a direct pathway and an indirect pathway. Recent studies show that these afferent systems may form a parallel feedback regulatory input to the substantia nigra DA-containing neurons as well.

Striatonigral GABAergic Projection

As reviewed in detail previously, stimulation of the striatum will evoke a short-latency inhibitory postsynaptic potential (IPSP) in zona compacta dopaminergic neurons and in zona reticulata neurons (27). However, stimulation of the striatum in trains will actually cause an activation of DA neuron firing. This DA cell activation occurs in concert with an inhibition of zona reticulata GABAergic neurons that normally inhibit DA neuron activity (21,27). These GABAergic inhibitory neurons may represent collaterals of nigrothalamic neurons (9) or a short-axon interneuron located near the zona compacta (10). Therefore, striatal stimulation appears to exert two actions on DA neuron electrophysiology: a direct GABAergic inhibition and an indirect disinhibition. A similar dichotomy between interneurons and dopaminergic cells has been proposed to exist within the ventral tegmentum as well (38).

Striatal Regulation of Subthalamonigral Glutamate Projection

The striatum is known to send a large number of GABAergic inhibitory projections to the globus pallidus, which, in turn, sends GABAergic fibers to the subthalamic nucleus (36,40,59). Recent physiological and metabolic studies have shown that extensive lesions of the nigrostriatal DA system activate the striatopallidal pathway, thereby disinhibiting the subthalamus (49,50). Single-pulse stimulation of the subthalamus has been shown to produce short-latency excitation of both dopaminergic and nondopaminergic neurons within the substantia nigra (34,52,65), and glutamatergic excitatory postsynaptic potentials (EPSPS) have been evoked in DA neurons recorded in vitro (38,47). However, maintained stimulation of the subthalamic nucleus has been shown to exert substantially different effects. During early periods of sub-

thalamus activation, there is an excitation of zona reticulata neuron firing and a concomitant inhibition of DA cell activity. However, as the activation diminishes, the DA neuron regains its baseline firing rate. Moreover, this is accompanied by a significant activation of burst firing (65). In contrast, lesions of the subthalamus were found to produce a regularization of firing pattern primarily in the DA cells located in more lateral regions of the substantia nigra (Fig. 6) (65). The activation of this feedback system in rats with large DA depletions (49,50) may therefore underlie the increase in burst firing without a similar activation of firing rate that occurs in the residual DA neurons recorded after such lesions (35).

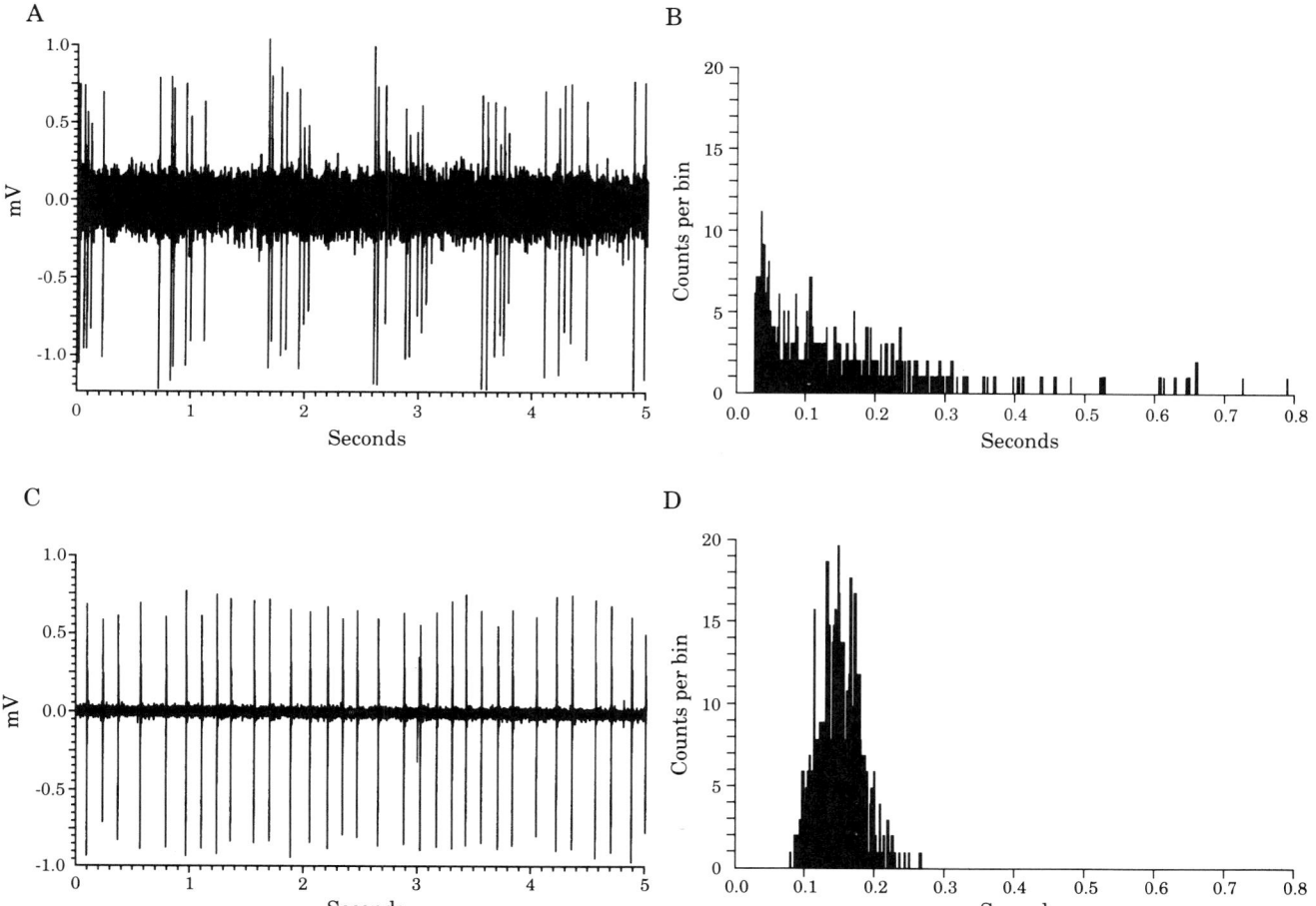

FIG. 6. Rapidly firing DA neurons typically exhibit burst firing activity. A: In this DA neuron recorded in vivo in the substantia nigra of a rat, the spike activity is showing the characteristic pattern of burst firing in DA neurons: bursts of 3–10 spikes with comparatively brief interspike intervals (e.g., 80–160 msec) separated by extended periods of post-burst inactivity. The DA neuron in this example is discharging at 7.2 Hz. B: Plotting the spike discharge pattern in the form of an interspike interval histogram reveals the multimodal form of this activity. The initial peak at 40 to 60-msec intervals represents the interspike intervals within the burst events, whereas the long intervals illustrate the intervals between the termination of one burst and the onset of the subsequent event. C: In rats in which an electrolytic lesion of the subthalamic nucleus had been performed, DA cells located in the lateral portions of the substantia nigra often exhibited pacemaker-like discharge patterns. This DA cell is discharging at a rate (i.e., 7.0 Hz) comparable to that observed in A. D: As revealed in the interspike interval histogram for this neuron, the intervals between spikes in this neuron show a much narrower distribution. (From ref. 65, with permission.)

Synthesis

The above evidence suggests that the striatonigral feedback system has at least two major modes of regulation over the DA neuron, with each of these modes apparently having opposing actions on DA cell activity. However, it should be noted that in each case, stimulation of the striatum or the subthalamus was done in such a manner as to activate a large number of neurons projecting to the nigra. Instead of causing opposing influences, a more likely scenario is that the system is capable of independently activating feedback inhibitory or feedback excitatory influences in order to rapidly and potently alter DA neuron activity. For example, during periods of DA demand the striatal system that activates the direct subthalamic excitatory input to the DA neuron may be co-activated with the striatonigral GABAergic projection that preferentially inhibits GABAergic interneurons, thereby disinhibiting the DA neuron. Conversely, during periods of decreased DA demand, the striatum may activate the excitatory projections from the subthalamus to the GABAergic interneurons while also activating inhibitory GABAergic afferents to the DA neurons (65). Whether the anatomy of the system coincides with this model remains to be examined using highly specific tract tracing techniques.

As shown by the data reviewed above, the striatum can potentially exert substantial feedback inhibitory control over the substantia nigra dopaminergic neurons. On the other hand, transection of striatonigral interconnections has been reported to cause little or no change in DA neuron activity (56,57). In contrast, transection of striatonigral connections appears to exert prominent effects on nigral cell activity in a rat in which a demand has been placed upon the DA system, such as during chronic haloperidol administration (3). Therefore, it appears that the striatonigral feedback system exerts little exogenous regulation on DA neuron activity except in cases in which a pharmacological perturbation has caused an increased DA demand on the system.

BEHAVIORAL RELEVANCE OF DA NEURON DISCHARGE: RECORDINGS FROM DA NEURONS IN FREELY BEHAVING PRIMATES

For some time, studies of the activities of DA neurons in awake animals and its correlation with behavior have involved studies of the rodent or in several cases the cat. In these studies, DA cells have been shown to behave similar in some respects to those recorded in the anesthetized animal, showing a somewhat similar proportion of neurons spontaneously discharging action potentials and firing in both single-spiking and burst-discharge modes (11,12). However, one property that was somewhat unusual is the report that DA neurons in awake rats are capable of rapid switching from a single-spiking to a burst firing pattern of activity (12), as contrasted to their comparatively stable firing patterns recorded in the anesthetized animal (25,26). Furthermore, several studies have correlated this burst-driven activation with the presentation of behaviorally relevant stimuli—that is, stimuli requiring a behavioral response (48).

Recent advances in the behavioral relevance of DA neuron discharge have been made in studies of DA cells recorded in the primate. By using an organism that is capable of acquiring and performing complex tasks, specific questions regarding the precise role of the DA system in behavioral processes may be elucidated. In general, studies have shown that, as in the rat, DA neurons are activated when the primate is presented with a behaviorally relevant stimulus requiring a response. However, the DA system appears to be primarily involved during the acquisition phase of this event, with little or no activation present when the animal is overtrained on the task (61). Therefore, as suggested by studies of the DA system in reward behavior (60), DA neuron discharge appears to be necessary during the phase in which the behavioral relevance of the stimulus is being defined.

SUMMARY

The DA neuron exhibits at least three electrophysiological dimensions along which it is capable of activating postsynaptic transmitter release: a change from inactive to spontaneously discharging state, an increase in the rate of spontaneous spike discharge, and an alteration from single-spiking to a burst-discharge mode of activity. A fourth state, one of depolarization block, occurs when an abnormally large demand, typically mediated by an exogenous pharmacological agent, causes the system to be overdriven to the state of inactivity. DA neurons have been shown to be under a number of complex regulatory influences. These factors range from characteristics related to their membranes and their morphology to properties derived from the influences of their afferents. Thus, the membrane properties that drive spike activity in the DA neuron enable it to fire spontaneously in the absence of afferent activation, and to accommodate rapidly to maintained excitatory influences and regain its basal level of activity. Dendrodendritic interactions appear to underlie synchronization of activity as well as provide autoreceptor-mediated local feedback modulation of the activity of the neuron, with drug administration or lesions causing alteration in the sensitivity of the autoreceptor, resulting in the restoration of basal activity states within this system. The influences of afferent and feedback processes further define the responsivity of this system: They apparently play a minor role when the system is in a basal state, but provide a substantial impact on the discharge pattern and level of activity when the system is challenged pharmacologically or physiologically.

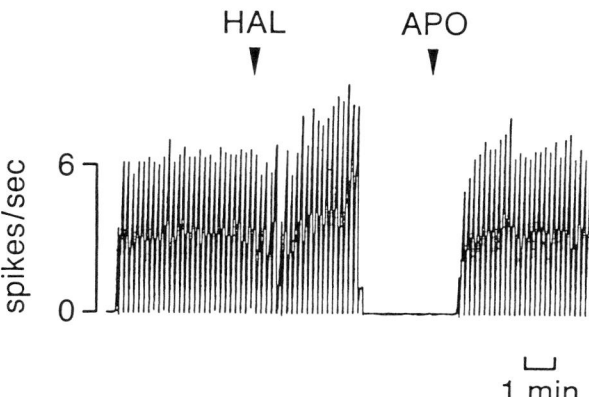

FIG. 7. A ratemeter recording of a DA neuron recorded in a rat 4–6 weeks following a partial depletion of striatal DA by 6-hydroxydopamine administration (∼79–90% DA depletion). In control rats, systemic administration of the DA antagonist haloperidol typically causes an increase in DA cell discharge rate. However, following partial depletions of striatal DA, a comparatively low dose of haloperidol (HAL; 0.1 mg/kg, i.v.) caused a large increase in the firing rate of this substantia nigra DA neuron, followed by a decrease in spike amplitude, increase in spike duration, and finally cessation of spontaneous spike discharge. Subsequent administration of the DA agonist apomorphine (0.1 mg/kg, i.v.) caused a reinstatement of spontaneous spike discharge in this DA neuron. Administration of additional doses of apomorphine caused an inhibition of DA cell discharge (not shown).

In each case, these multiple homeostatic factors appear to act in concert to enable the DA neuron to maintain a basal level of activity. This would be consistent with experimental evidence showing that the DA system is under extensive homeostatic regulation and can readily compensate for maintained changes in afferent drive or residual capacity. Therefore, it would appear that the discharge of DA neurons is not involved in the maintenance of long-term changes in the nigrostriatal system, but instead only alters their activity states phasically in response to short-term demand (35). Therefore, by preserving basal levels of electrophysiological activity, the DA neuron conserves the dynamic range of electrophysiological response that can be rapidly drawn upon when required by the system. Indeed, the property of the DA system to maintain basal activity levels when faced with a tonic demand but respond rapidly with a massive phasic increase when required is consistent with the behavioral studies showing that DA neuron discharge is only altered when the system is changing state, as occurs with the learning of a novel stimulus paradigm. On the other hand, when the DA system is driven in a manner such that the biochemical compensations are inadequate to respond to the demand [resulting in a tonic activation of DA cell firing (e.g., with chronic neuroleptic treatment or near maximal DA depletions)] or if one of the primary regulatory responses is thwarted (e.g., administering a DA blocker to a system recovered from a lesion), the ultimate

consequence appears to be depolarization block of DA cell discharge and a reinstatement of the deficit state (Fig. 7) (37). However, under conditions in which the DA system appears to be showing an abnormal increased responsivity, such as schizophrenia (19), the induction of depolarization block may be the most effective way to circumvent behaviorally mediated activation of this system (19,20,37).

REFERENCES

1. Aghajanian GK, Bunney BS. Central dopaminergic neurons: Neurophysiological identification and responses to drugs. In: Snyder SH, Usdin E, eds. *Frontiers in catecholamine research.* New York: Pergamon Press, 1973;643–648.
2. Alexander GE, DeLong MR, Strick PL. Parallel organization of functionally segregated circuits linking basal ganglia and cortex. *Annu Rev Neurosci* 1986;9:357–381.
3. Bunney BS, Grace AA. Acute and chronic haloperidol treatment: comparison of effects on nigral dopaminergic cell activity. *Life Sci* 1978;23:1715–1728.
4. Bunney BS, Walters JR, Roth RH, Aghajanian GK. Dopaminergic neurons: Effect of antipsychotic drugs and amphetamine on single cell activity. *J Pharmacol Exp Ther* 1973;185:560–571.
5. Charléty PJ, Grenhoff J, Chergui K, de la Chapelle B, Buda M, Svensson TH, Chouvet G. Burst firing of mesencephalic dopamine neurons is inhibited by somatodendritic application of kynurenate. *Acta Physiol Scand* 1991;142:105–112.
6. Chéramy A, Leviel V, Glowinski J. Dendritic release of dopamine in the substantia nigra. *Nature* 1981;289:537–542.
7. Cherugi K, Charléty PJ, Akaoka H, Saunier CF, Brunet J-L, Buda M, Svensson TH, Chouvet G. Tonic activation of NMDA receptors causes spontaneous burst discharge of rat midbrain dopamine neurons in vivo. *Eur J Neurosci* 1993;5:137–144.
8. Chiodo LA, Kapatos G. Mesencephalic neurons in primary culture: Immunohistochemistry and membrane physiology. In: Chiodo LA, Freeman AS, eds. *The neurophysiology of dopamine systems.* Detroit: Lake Shore Publications, 1987;67–91.
9. Deniau JM, Féger J, LeGuyader C. Striatal evoked inhibition of identified nigrothalamic neurons. *Brain Res* 1976;104:245–256.
10. Francois C, Percheron G, Yelnick J, Heyner S. Demonstration of the existence of small local circuit neurons in the Golgi-stained primate substantia nigra. *Brain Res* 1979;172:160–164.
11. Freeman AS, Bunney BS. Activity of A9 and A10 dopaminergic neurons in unrestrained rats: further characterization and effects of apomorphine and cholecystokinin. *Brain Res* 1987;405:46–55.
12. Freeman AS, Meltzer LT, Bunney BS. Firing properties of substantia nigra dopaminergic neurons in freely moving rats. *Life Sci* 1985;36:1983–1994.
13. Fujimura K, Matsuda Y. Responses to ramp current stimulation of the neurons in substantia nigra pars compacta in vitro. *Brain Res* 1988;475:177–181.
14. Fujimura K, Matsuda Y. Autogenous oscillatory potentials in neurons of the guinea pig substantia nigra pars compacta in vitro. *Neurosci Lett* 1989;104:53–57.
15. Gonon FG. Nonlinear relationship between impulse flow and dopamine released by rat midbrain dopaminergic neurons as studied by in vivo electrochemistry. *Neuroscience* 1988;24:19–28.
16. Grace AA. The regulation of dopamine neuron activity as determined by in vivo and in vitro intracellular recordings. In: Chiodo LA, Freeman AS, eds. *The neurophysiology of dopamine systems.* Detroit: Lake Shore Publications, 1987;1–66.
17. Grace AA. Evidence for the functional compartmentalization of spike generating regions of rat midbrain dopamine neurons recorded in vitro. *Brain Res* 1990;524:31–41.
18. Grace AA. Regulation of spontaneous activity and oscillatory spike firing in rat midbrain dopamine neurons recorded in vitro. *Synapse* 1991;7:221–234.
19. Grace AA. Phasic versus tonic dopamine release and the modulation

of dopamine system responsivity: a hypothesis for the etiology of schizophrenia. *Neuroscience* 1991;41:1–24.

20. Grace AA. Cortical regulation of subcortical dopamine systems and its possible relevance to schizophrenia. *J Neural Transm* 1993;91:111–134.

21. Grace AA, Bunney BS. Paradoxical GABA excitation of nigral dopaminergic cells: indirect mediation through reticulata inhibitory interneurons. *Eur J Pharmacol* 1979;59:211–218.

22. Grace AA, Bunney BS. Nigral dopamine neurons: intracellular recording and identification with L-DOPA injection and histofluorescence. *Science* 1980;210:654–656.

23. Grace AA, Bunney BS. Intracellular and extracellular electrophysiology of nigral dopaminergic neurons. I. Identification and characterization. *Neuroscience* 1983;10:301–315.

24. Grace AA, Bunney BS. Intracellular and extracellular electrophysiology of nigral dopaminergic neurons. III. Evidence for electrical coupling. *Neuroscience* 1983;10:333–348.

25. Grace AA, Bunney BS. The control of firing pattern in nigral dopamine neurons: single spike firing. *J. Neurosci* 1984;4:2866–2876.

26. Grace AA, Bunney BS. The control of firing pattern in nigral dopamine neurons: burst firing. *J Neurosci* 1984;4:2877–2890.

27. Grace AA, Bunney BS. Opposing effects of striatonigral feedback pathways on midbrain dopamine cell activity. *Brain Res* 1985;333:271–284.

28. Grace AA, Bunney BS. Induction of depolarization block in midbrain dopamine neurons by repeated administration of haloperidol: analysis using in vivo intracellular recording. *J Pharmacol Exp Ther* 1986;238:1092–1100.

29. Grace AA, Onn S-P. Morphology and electrophysiological properties of immunocytochemically identified rat dopamine neurons recorded in vitro. *J Neurosci* 1989;9:3463–3481.

30. Grenhoff J, Aston-Jones G, Svensson TH. Nicotinic effects on the firing pattern of midbrain dopamine neurons. *Acta Physiol Scand* 1986;128:351–358.

31. Guyenet PG, Aghajanian GK. Antidromic identification of dopaminergic and other output neurons of the rat substantia nigra. *Brain Res* 1978;150:69–84.

32. Guyenet PG, Crane JK. Non-dopaminergic nigrostriatal pathway. *Brain Res* 1981;213:291–305.

33. Hainsworth AH, Roper J, Kappor R, Ashcroft FM. Identification and electrophysiology of isolated pars compacta neurons from guinea-pig substantia nigra. *Neuroscience* 1991;43:81–93.

34. Hammond C, Deniau JM, Rizk A, Feger J. Electrophysiological demonstration of an excitatory subthalamonigral pathway in the rat. *Brain Res* 1978;151:235–244.

35. Hollerman JR, Grace AA. The effects of dopamine-depleting brain lesions on the electrophysiological activity of rat substantia nigra dopamine neurons. *Brain Res* 1990;533:203–212.

36. Hollerman JR, Grace AA. Subthalamic nucleus cell activity in the 6-OHDA-treated rat: basal activity and response to haloperidol. *Brain Res* 1992;590:291–299.

37. Hollerman JR, Abercrombie ED, Grace AA. Electrophysiological, biochemical, and behavioral studies of acute haloperidol-induced depolarization block of nigral dopamine neurons. *Neuroscience* 1992;47:589–601.

38. Johnson SW, North RA. Two types of neurone in the rat ventral tegmental area and their synaptic inputs. *J Physiol* 1992;450:455–468.

39. Johnson SW, Seutin V, North R. Burst firing in dopamine neurons induced by N-methyl-D-aspartate: role of electrogenic sodium pump. *Science* 1992;258:665–667.

40. Kita T, Chang HT, Kitai ST. Pallidal inputs to subthalamus: intracellular analysis. *Brain Res* 1983;264:255–265.

41. Kita T, Kita H, Kitai ST. Electrical membrane properties of rat substantia nigra compacta neurons in an in vitro slice preparation. *Brain Res* 1986;372:21–30.

42. Kondo Y, Iwatsubo K. Diminished responses of nigral dopaminergic neurons to haloperidol and morphine following lesions in the striatum. *Brain Res* 1980;181:237–240.

43. Lacey MG, Mercuri NB, North RA. Two cell types in rat substantia nigra zona compacta distinguished by membrane properties and the actions of dopamine and opioids. *J Neurosci* 1989;9:1233–1241.

44. Llinás R, Greenfield SA, Jahnsen H. Electrophysiology of pars compacta cells in the in vitro substantia nigra—a possible mechanism for dendritic release. *Brain Res* 1984;294:127–132.

45. Mercuri NB, Calabresi P, Bernardi G. Effects of glycine on neurons in the rat substantia nigra zona compacta: in vitro electrophysiological study. *Synapse* 1990;5:190–200.

46. Mercuri NB, Calabresi P, Bernardi G. Responses of rat substantia nigra compacta neurones to L-DOPA. *Br J Pharmacol* 1990;100:257–260.

47. Mereu G, Costa E, Armstrong DM, Vicini S. Glutamate receptor subtypes mediate excitatory synaptic currents of dopamine neurons in midbrain slices. *J Neurosci* 1991;11:1359–1366.

48. Miller JD, Sanghera MK, German DC. Mesencephalic dopaminergic activity in the behaviorally conditioned rat. *Life Sci* 1981;29:1255–1265.

49. Miller WC, DeLong MR. Altered tonic activity of neurons in the globus pallidus and subthalamic nucleus in the primate MPTP model of parkinsonism. In: Carpenter MB, Jayaraman A, eds. *The basal ganglia II—structure and function: current concepts.* New York: Plenum, 1987;415–427.

50. Mitchell IJ, Clarke CE, Boyce S, Robertson RF, Peggs D, Sambrook MA, Crossman AR. Neural mechanisms underlying parkinsonian symptoms based upon regional uptake of 2-deoxyglucose in monkeys exposed to 1-methyl-4-phenyl-1,2,3,6-tetrahydropyridine. *Neuroscience* 1989;32:213–226.

51. Nagy JI, Yamamoto T, Shiosaka S, Dewar KM, Whittaker ME, Hertzberg EL. Immunohistochemical localization of gap junction protein in rat CNS: a preliminary account. In: Hertzberg EL, Johnson R, eds. *Modern cell biology.* Alan R Liss, 1988;375–389.

52. Nakanishi H, Kita H, Kitai ST. Intracellular study of rat substantia nigra pars reticulata neurons in an in vitro slice preparation: electrical membrane properties and response characteristics to subthalamic stimulation. *Brain Res* 1987;437:45–55.

53. Nedergaard S, Flatman JA, Engberg I. Nifedipine- and ω-conotoxin-sensitive Ca²⁺ conductances in guinea-pig substantia nigra pars compacta neurons. *J Physiol (Lond)* 1993;466:727–747.

54. Ort CA, Futamachi KJ, Peacock JH. Morphology and electrophysiology of ventral mesencephalon nerve cell cultures. *Dev Brain Res* 1988;39:205–215.

55. Overton P, Clark D. Iontophoretically administered drugs acting at the N-methyl-D-aspartate receptor modulate burst firing in A9 dopamine neurons in the rat. *Synapse* 1992;10:131–140.

56. Pucak ML, Grace AA. Partial dopamine depletions result in an enhanced sensitivity of residual dopamine neurons to apomorphine. *Synapse* 1991;9:144–155.

57. Pucak ML, Grace AA. Blockade of somatodendritic autoreceptors on nigral dopamine neurons contributes to the firing rate-increasing effects of dopamine antagonists. *Soc Neurosci Abstr* 1991;17:1352.

58. Pucak ML, Grace AA. Effects of dopamine antagonist administration on the activity of midbrain dopamine neurons recorded in vitro. *Soc Neurosci Abstr* 1992;18:277.

59. Rouzaire-Dubois B, Hammond C, Hamon B, Féger J. Pharmacological blockade of the globus pallidus-induced inhibitory response of subthalamic cells in the rat. *Brain Res* 1980;200:321–329.

60. Schultz W. Activity of dopamine neurons in the behaving primate. *Semin Neurosci* 1992;4:129–138.

61. Schultz W, Apicella P, Ljungberg T. Responses of monkey dopamine neurons to reward and conditioned stimuli during successive steps of learning a delayed response task. *J Neurosci* 1993;13:900–913.

62. Seutin V, Verbanck P, Massotee L, Dresse A. Evidence for the presence of N-methyl-D-aspartate receptors in the ventral tegmental area of the rat: an electrophysiological in vitro study. *Brain Res* 1990;514:147–150.

63. Shepard PD, Bunney BS. Effects of apamin on the discharge properties of putative dopamine-containing neurons in vitro. *Brain Res* 1988;463:380–384.

64. Silva NL, Pechuar CM, Barker JL. Postnatal rat nigrostriatal dopaminergic neurons exhibit five types of potassium conductances. *J Neurophysiol* 1990;64:262–272.

65. Smith ID, Grace AA. The regulation of nigral dopamine neuron firing by afferents from the subthalamic nucleus. *Synapse* 1992;12:287–303.

66. Svensson TH, Tung C-S. Local cooling of pre-frontal cortex induces

pacemaker-like firing of dopamine neurons in rat ventral tegmental area in vivo. *Acta Physiol Scand* 1989;136:135–136.

67. Tepper JM, Sawyer SF, Groves PM. Electrophysiologically identified nigral dopaminergic neurons intracellularly labeled with HRP: light-microscopic analysis. *J Neurosci* 1987;7:2794–2806.

68. Wuerthele SM, Freed WJ, Olson L, Morihisa J, Spoor L, Wyatt RJ, Hoffer BJ. Effect of dopamine agonists and antagonists on the electrical activity of substantia nigra neurons transplanted into the lateral ventricle of the rat. *Exp Brain Res* 1981;44:1–10.

69. Yung WH, Hausser MA, Jack JB. Electrophysiology of dopaminergic and non-dopaminergic neurones of the guinea-pig substantia nigra pars compacta in vitro. *J Physiol (Lond)* 1991;436:643–667.

70. Zigmond MJ, Berger TW, Grace AA, Stricker EM. Compensatory responses to nigrostriatal bundle injury: studies with 6-hydroxydopamine in an animal model of parkinsonism. *Mol Chem Neuropathol* 1989;10:185–200.

Psychopharmacology: The Fourth Generation of Progress, edited by Floyd E. Bloom and David J. Kupfer. Raven Press, Ltd., New York © 1995.

CHAPTER 16

The Dopamine Transporter

Potential Involvement in Neuropsychiatric Disorders

Michael J. Bannon, James G. Granneman, and Gregory Kapatos

Although dopamine (DA)-containing neurons constitute less than 1 in every 10^5–10^6 neurons in the mammalian brain, DA cells have been studied intensively, in large part due to their established role in the pathophysiology of Parkinson's disease and drug abuse and their purported role in other neuropsychiatric disorders. DA neurotransmission is combinatorially controlled by postsynaptic DA receptor/signal transduction mechanisms (Civelli; Chiodo and Bunney, *this volume*) and by presynaptic regulation of synaptic DA concentrations. Presynaptic control of synaptic DA, in turn, involves the regulation of DA synthesis and release (see Chapters 17 and 20, *this volume*) and the activity of the DA transporter (DAT). The DAT is a member of a family of substrate-specific, high-affinity, Na^+-dependent membrane transporters (2,87; Blakely, *this volume*). DAT-mediated recapture of released DA is generally thought to be the primary mechanism for limiting the extent, duration, and area of DA receptor activation. The DAT is also an important means of *releasing* DA under some pharmacological (and perhaps physiological) conditions. Finally, the DAT is an important target for a variety of psychostimulants and for catecholamine-selective neurotoxins. In this chapter we will review briefly the recent explosion of information about the DAT within the context of DAT studies conducted over the last 25 years.

DISCOVERY OF THE DA TRANSPORTER

By the mid-1960s, an uptake mechanism for norepinephrine (NE) had been described and many of its proper-

ties elucidated (see Chapter 28, *this volume*). At about this same time, the existence of distinct DA-containing nigrostriatal neurons had been demonstrated (see ref. 11). The substantial accumulation of radiolabeled NE seen in the striatum following intraventricular ^{3}H-NE injection was correctly attributed to the ability of nigrostriatal DA cells to accumulate ^{3}H-NE (28). Subsequently, Snyder and Coyle (15,84) directly compared DA and NE uptake in various brain regions. These investigators reported that ^{3}H-DA accumulated more readily than ^{3}H-NE in all brain regions studied, consistent with the finding that DA is actually the preferred substrate for the NE transporter (see Chapter 28, *this volume*). Within the striatum, a distinct uptake process was identified with higher affinity (submicromolar K_t) for DA but lesser affinity and a different isomeric selectivity for NE compared to the typical nonstriatal NE transporter. Thus the study of the DAT had begun. During the following two decades, many biochemical and pharmacological properties of the rat and human DAT were elucidated (5,35,36,48,53).

The advent of radiolabeled DAT ligands, including cocaine and analogues [e.g., WIN 35,065-2, WIN 35,428, and RTI-55 (10,48,58,72), mazindol (41), methylphenidate (39), GBR-12935 (3,7), and nomifensine (19)], has greatly facilitated the characterization of the DAT. Advantages of DAT radioligand binding compared to DA uptake include the ability to conduct analyses in the absence of metabolically competent nerve terminals (thus allowing the anatomical resolution of tissue slices as well as human postmortem analyses) and the ability to image the DAT in vivo by positron emission tomography (PET) and single photon emission computerized tomography (SPECT) analyses (22,37,80). The potencies of compounds to inhibit DA uptake by striatal synaptosomes and DAT antagonist binding to striatal membranes are

M. J. Bannon, J. G. Granneman, and G. Kapatos: Cellular and Clinical Neurobiology Program, Department of Psychiatry, Wayne State University School of Medicine, Detroit, Michigan 48201.

essentially identical (12), consistent with the idea that the one receptor mediates both uptake and binding (but see the discussion of DAT mutagenesis data below). In the same vein, the developmental appearance of striatal DA uptake and DAT ligand binding exhibit identical postnatal time courses (9).

FUNCTIONAL PROPERTIES AND ACUTE MODULATION OF DAT

Characterization of the kinetic properties of the DAT (36,53) and of the highly homologous NE transporter (86; Blakely, *this volume*), as well as the extensive analysis of the native and cloned gamma-aminobutyric acid (GABA) transporter (47,59), illuminates DAT function and its potential for modulation. Based on these data, a simplified scheme of DAT function would predict that 1 or 2 Na^+, 1 Cl^-, and 1 DA molecule bind sequentially to the DAT and are transported, making DA transport an electrogenic process. The initial binding of Na^+ may orient the DAT until DA binding and DAT translocation. Given the transmembrane Na^+ gradient, most DATs would therefore be expected to be outwardly oriented. The voltage dependency of Na^+ binding to the DAT is probably the primary determinant of the voltage dependency of DAT function, which results in greater inward DA transport with increasing hyperpolarization and an inhibition of transport during periods of depolarization. Such a mechanism would serve to sharpen DA-mediated neurotransmission by allowing maximal synaptic DA concentrations during depolarization-induced release and a rapid recapture of DA as the DA cell membrane repolarizes. As discussed below, indirectly acting amines such as amphetamine are thought to reverse DA transport by increasing the effective DA concentration at the inner membrane surface of the DAT. Conditions that inhibit Na^+ extrusion (ouabain treatment, hypoxia, or glucose deprivation) or increase Na^+ influx (veratridine, excitatory amino acid receptor agonists) also cause substantial Ca^{2+}-independent transporter-mediated release of neurotransmitters (33,70). The potential reversal of transport by neurotransmitter-mediated local changes in Na^+ gradient adds another level of complexity to transporter control of synaptic transmitter levels. Given the slow rate of transporter cycling (<10/sec), the contribution of DA transport in regulating DA transmission will be dependent upon net inward (versus outward) DA transport, local DAT density, and the affinity of the various DA receptors for synaptic DA.

Numerous manipulations (e.g., depolarization and changes in Ca^{2+} or phospholipase A_2-mediated release of arachidonic acid) have been shown to alter choline and glutamate transport (see ref. 2; Blakely, *this volume*). In the case of the DAT, DA uptake is reportedly rapidly increased in mesolimbic/mesocortical (but not nigrostriatal) DA nerve terminals in animal subjected to stressors known to activate mesolimbic/mesocortical DA neurons

(32). Moreover, DAT activity in cultured hypothalamic cells is rapidly stimulated in response to cell-permeant cAMP analogues (44). Inhibitors of arachidonic acid metabolism potently inhibit DA uptake in striatal slices (13). The recent identification of putative consensus sequences for several protein kinases within the DAT and related transporter sequences (see below) suggests a means by which various signal transduction pathways might acutely regulate DAT function. Nevertheless, there is no evidence that the DAT is in fact a phosphoprotein or that the effects on DAT function are direct effects (versus effects secondary to altered ion channel function or electrochemical gradients). The development of molecular probes (discussed below) will help to elucidate potential post-translational regulation.

DAT STRUCTURE AND MOLECULAR BIOLOGY

DAT Protein Characterization

Despite characterization of the DAT as a functional entity, sequence information about the DAT protein and its gene are clearly necessary for a more complete understanding of the regulation of DAT biosynthesis and function. One experimental approach has utilized radiolabeled photoaffinity ligands with relative selectivity for the DAT. Such studies have identified a labeled polypeptide of approximately 80 kD (although earlier estimates of molecular weights varied substantially) with the anticipated regional distribution and whose labeling is prevented by preincubation with DAT-specific ligands (8,29,55,74). Studies with various exo- and endonucleases indicate that the DAT is an N-linked glycoprotein containing *N*-acetylglucosamine and terminal sialic acid residues (8,29,55,74). While differences in glycosylation apparently account for slight differences in the molecular weight of the DAT in different brain regions (56), the role for these carbohydrates in DAT substrate recognition/transport is unclear (56,94).

DAT cDNA Cloning

The first neurotransmitter transporter cloned, a GABA transporter clone (GAT-1), was obtained by protein purification and partial sequencing and standard plaque hybridization methods, whereas the NE transporter was cloned shortly thereafter using a mammalian expression system (see Chapter 28, *this volume*). For the cloning of the DAT, regions of high sequence homology between the NE and GAT-1 GABA transporters were used to design degenerate oligonucleotides as probes or as primers for polymerase chain reaction-derived probes. Within a short period of time, DAT cDNA clones were obtained from rat (26,49,81), bovine (88), and human (4,27,89) tissues.

As expected, the deduced primary (619- or 620-amino-

TABLE 1. *Comparison of the K_i values of drugs at cloned and native dopamine transporters[a]*

Drug	Cloned human dopamine transporter[b]	Cloned rat dopamine transporter[b]	Rat striatal synaptosomes[c]
Dopamine	1220	890, 885,[d] 1190[e]	105, 300
Mazindol	11	23, 70,[d] 30[e]	85, 280
GBR12783	13	22	2
GBR12209	17	17	51
Nomifensine	17	60, 150[d]	50, 100, 220, 780, 48, 85
Benztropine	55	109	170, 100
Cocaine	58	330, 2000,[d] 1000[e]	310, 670, 1400
Amfebutamone	330	521	600
D-Amphetamine	2260	2160	240, 980, 640
Desipramine	13,000	12,000	20,000
L-Amphetamine	22,000	22,600	2900
MPP$^+$	23,000	23,000	400

[a] From ref. 25, with permission. Note the lower affinity of the heterologously expressed transporters for various substrates.
[b] Data taken from ref. 27.
[c] Data taken from ref. 36.
[d] Data taken from ref. 49.
[e] Data taken from ref. 81.

acid) sequences and predicted secondary structure of the cloned DATs are highly homologous with other members of this gene family (and especially with other monoamine transporters) (for comprehensive reviews, see refs. 2,25, and 87; also see Chapter 28, *this volume*). The most highly conserved sequences are thought to encompass the 12 hydrophobic (membrane spanning) domains and flanking amino acids, with the predicted intracellular amino and carboxyl termini and extracellular loops exhibiting less sequence similarity. The presence of three or four potential glycosylation sites in the large second extracellular loop is consistent with the identification of a photoaffinity-labeled DAT glycoprotein (see above). As mentioned above, putative consensus sequences for various protein kinases could be involved in post-transcriptional DAT regulation by phosphorylation, although little direct evidence for this possibility exists at present.

Reasoning by analogy from studies of catecholamine receptors, aspartate and serine residues conserved within certain transmembrane domains of the DAT and other monoamine transporters have been examined for their possible role in DA binding and transport (51). Replacement of an aspartate in transmembrane domain 1 resulted in a dramatically reduced uptake of DA and reduced affinity for the cocaine analogue CFT. Mutations of several serines in transmembrane domain 7 (but not 8) also substantially altered these parameters. It has been hypothesized (51) that the conserved aspartate interacts with the amine group of DA while the serines interact with its catechol group. The presence of leucine zipper motifs and other conserved features of neurotransmitter transporters (including the DAT) conjectured to be involved in intra- or intermolecular interactions, protein positioning, or substrate binding and/or translocation have been reviewed in detail elsewhere (2).

To date, little information has been reported on the

kinetic properties (e.g., ionic and voltage dependence, stoichiometry of transport, turnover rate) of the cloned DATs, in contrast to the detailed analyses of the cloned GABA transporter GAT-1 (47,59). Interestingly, DAT clones exhibit 3- to 200-fold lower affinity for DA and other DAT substrates than that obtained in rat striatal synaptosomal preparations (26,27,49,81,88; see Table 1). It has been pointed out (92) that this discrepancy does not exist in the case of cloned versus native GABA transporters, possibly due to either (a) the lower substrate affinity of the native GABA transporter or (b) a lesser dependence of GABA transport upon some accessory tissue factor(s) missing in heterologous expression systems. It is also conceivable that the apparent decrease in substrate affinity for the DAT in heterologous expression systems is due to the absence of vesicular transport and sequestration which, in nerve terminals, serves to limit cytoplasmic concentrations of DA and other DAT substrates and minimize reverse transport. The other pharmacological properties of the cloned, heterologously expressed DATs (e.g., affinities for DAT antagonists) are in reasonable agreement with the native DATs. Interestingly, the cloned human DAT exhibits a higher affinity for cocaine than either the cloned or native rat DATs (25; see Table 1).

DAT mRNA and Gene Analyses

The distribution of mRNA determined by either in situ hybridization (26,49,81,82,88) or sensitive solution hybridization analysis (4,91) is consistent with its exclusive expression in DA cell dendrites and soma. The highest DAT mRNA levels are seen in the substantia nigra, with somewhat lower levels within the nuclei of the ventral tegmental area and very low levels of expression within the olfactory bulb and hypothalamus. DAT mRNA is not detected in DA terminal fields or other brain regions examined (e.g., caudate, putamen, nucleus accumbens, cerebral cortex, or cerebellum). A single rat DAT RNA band of 3.6–3.7 kb has been identified by Northern blot analysis (81). Solution hybridization experiments to date (4,91) are also consistent with a single mRNA species encoding the DAT, although the possibility of RNA splice variants cannot be ruled out at the present time. Interestingly, a series of unique 40-bp repetitive elements are located in the 3′ untranslated region of the human (but not rat) DAT cDNA (89). It is conceivable that these elements might alter some property (e.g., half-life or translation) of DAT mRNA and in this manner regulate DAT gene expression. To date, little characterization of the DAT gene has been published. A single human DAT gene has been localized to the distal end of chromosome 5 (5p15.3) (27). It appears that the rat and human genes are both interrupted (intron-containing) genes (27,89) and that the human gene is highly polymorphic (25,89).

THE DAT AS A PHENOTYPIC MARKER FOR DA NEURONS

Almost since its discovery, high-affinity DA uptake has served as a neurochemical index of the density and structural integrity of nigrostriatal DA nerve terminals. Numerous studies have shown that lesions of the nigrostriatal DA pathway produce parallel losses of DA levels and the DAT (measured by DA uptake and ligand binding) (1,3,39,40,48), supporting the use of the DAT as a marker for DA nerve terminals. DA uptake has also been used to identify embryonic DA neurons maintained in culture (6) [although pharmacological characterization of DA accumulation in these cells suggests that an immature form of the DAT, characterized by inhibition by desipramine but not benztropine, is present early in development (20,69)]. Changes in DA uptake within cultures of midbrain DA neurons have been used as a measure of survival and/or terminal arborization in response to co-culture with appropriate or inappropriate neural targets (69), trophic factors (54), or neurotoxins (75,76).

Overall, these in vivo and in vitro observations (pertaining primarily to nigrostriatal neurons) suggest that the DAT could be considered a better phenotypic marker for DA neurons and their nerve terminals than tyrosine hydroxylase, which is expressed in all catecholaminergic neurons and is highly regulated (87). Nevertheless, it is clear that the level of DAT expression varies significantly among DA cell groups and that embryonic midbrain DA neurons express tyrosine hydroxylase and DA well before the expression of the DAT (4,18,61,82). Furthermore, even within a given DA cell population, the level of DAT expression may be subject to regulation (see discussions above and below). These observations indicate that the DAT is a very good, but not invariant, phenotypic marker for DA neurons. As is the case for tyrosine hydroxylase

and peptide co-transmitter content, the level of DAT expression seemingly can be modified to meet the particular requirements of different DA neurons.

DAT AS A RECEPTOR FOR PSYCHOSTIMULANTS AND NEUROTOXINS

As outlined above, the DAT plays a critical role in the physiological control of synaptic DA levels. DA neurons (especially mesolimbic DA cells) are implicated in the reinforcing properties of a variety of drugs of abuse (52). In the case of psychostimulants such as cocaine and amphetamines, this effect is mediated primarily through interaction with the DAT (73). Cocaine and related drugs bind to the DAT and prevent DA transport, although the nature of the interaction at a kinetic level of analysis is disputed (for a discussion, see ref. 12). Amphetamines serve as substrates for the DAT, thereby inhibiting DA uptake while themselves being accumulated in DA terminals. Once in the terminal, amphetamines release DA from vesicular stores (perhaps by altering vesicular pH), thereby increasing free intracellular DA concentrations and evoking a reverse transport of DA. The net acute effect of the psychostimulants is to increase synaptic DA levels. Blockade of the somatodendritic DAT may be critical for the initiation of stimulant-induced behavioral sensitization, a progressive increase in responsiveness with repeated drug administration that may have a clinical counterpart in humans (21,45). In contrast, nerve terminal DATs may play a role in the altered DA transmission apparently underlying the continued expression of this sensitization (45; see also Chapters 66 and 145, *this volume*).

The literature pertaining to the effects of psychostimulants on DAT expression is inconsistent, presumably due to critical differences in drug treatment regimes and the measures of DAT function employed (38,63,67,79,91,93). Understanding the regulation of the DAT is an important step towards elucidation of the molecular bases of stimulant drug abuse. The development of new reagents (e.g., cDNA clones and DAT-directed antisera) should further this line of investigation. Understanding stimulant modulation of DAT expression may also help to illuminate the therapeutic actions of amphetamine and the related drug methylphenidate (Ritalin) used in the treatment of children with attention deficit disorder.

The DAT also has assumed importance in the study of toxin-induced and idiopathic Parkinson's disease. The selectivity of DA neurotoxins [e.g., 6-hydroxydopamine and, to an even greater extent, 1-methyl-4-phenylpyridine (MPP^+)] is largely based on their high affinity for the DAT. Once transported, these toxins destroy DA neurons and ultimately produce parkinsonism in both animal models and humans (42). Expression of the cloned DAT in COS cells confers sensitivity to MPP^+ toxicity (51). MPP^+ resistance may also be related to sequestration of cytosolic toxin by vesicular amine transporters (71) inasmuch as expression of a vesicular transporter clone confers toxin resistance in sensitive CHO cells (57). Thus it is conceivable that the levels of DAT and vesicular transporter expression combinatorially dictate the response to exogenously or endogenously generated neurotoxins. In this regard, it is of interest to note that regional differences in the levels of DAT expression (see above) correlate well with the extent of DA cell loss in Parkinson's disease or after MPP$^+$ treatment (23,24,34).

THE DAT AND CLINICAL STUDIES

Parkinson's Disease

One of the primary pathological features of Parkinson's disease is the substantial loss of ventral mesencephalic DA cell bodies and a corresponding decrease of DA within the caudate and putamen (50,62). Numerous studies have quantitated changes in DAT content within the caudate and putamen using radiolabeled DAT ligands. Surprisingly, only a 20–60% decrease in DAT binding has routinely been reported in homogenates of Parkinson's disease specimens exhibiting >90% DA depletion (40,60,66,77,78). Most (but not all) of these studies were conducted using the ligand GBR-12935. It should be noted that experimental destruction of nigrostriatal DA neurons in the rat results in a profound loss of striatal DAT, as determined using the same ligands (see above).

More recent analyses (64,78) suggest that GBR binding to an additional, non-DAT site in human tissue may have resulted in significant underestimates of the extent of DAT loss in Parkinson's disease. Recent quantitative autoradiographic studies with the cocaine analogue WIN 35,428 and mazindol (14,46) demonstrate a profound loss of DAT binding in Parkinson's disease which parallels the regional decline in DA levels (Fig. 1). Thus, DAT ligand binding may provide a sensitive marker for the density of human DA nerve terminals, but special attention must be paid to experimental parameters such as the choice and concentration of probe and tissue handling (46; see also Chapter 126, *this volume*).

Normal Aging

Gradual age-related decreases in DAT ligand binding in human caudate and putamen have been reported (17,95). Strikingly, DAT mRNA in human substantia nigra decreases precipitously with age (4), as evidenced by in situ hybridization (Fig. 2) and solution hybridization (Fig. 3A). In an effort to rule out potentially confounding variables (such as differing tissue sources, causes of death, and postmortem intervals), levels of caudate DAT ligand binding have been determined (in collaboration with Drs. M. J. Kuhar and J. Boja) in the caudates of the same individuals for whom DAT mRNA values were previously reported. Consistent with previous reports, Fig. 3B shows a gradual but significant age-related decrease in specific WIN 35,428 binding in the same subjects who exhibited profound decreases in DAT mRNA (Fig. 3A). (Note that all data are presented on a log scale). Thus, a dramatic increase in the DAT ligand binding/DAT mRNA ratio occurs with age (Fig. 3C).

While this dissociation of DAT mRNA and protein is initially surprising, striking dissociations of TH mRNA and TH protein within DA neurons have also been observed. For example, the linear age-related decline in TH mRNA in human substantia nigra (4) roughly parallels earlier estimates of the rate of DA cell loss (62), but stands in contrast to the stable TH protein content and relative number of TH-positive nerve terminals in human caudate with age (90). A provocative model for these changes is seen after partial neurotoxin-induced lesions of DA cells (65), in which TH mRNA concentrations within surviving DA neurons continue to decline many months after lesioning, at a time when the levels of TH protein, TH activity, and DA have returned to control values within the striatum. (Importantly, the decreased TH mRNA is not indicative of a generalized metabolic change in DA cells inasmuch as the β-tubulin mRNA concentration within these same cells is unaltered.) In each case, the maintenance of normal or near-normal levels of DAT or TH protein following a substantial decrease in the number of DA cells strongly suggests that the remaining DA neurons each contain significantly more of

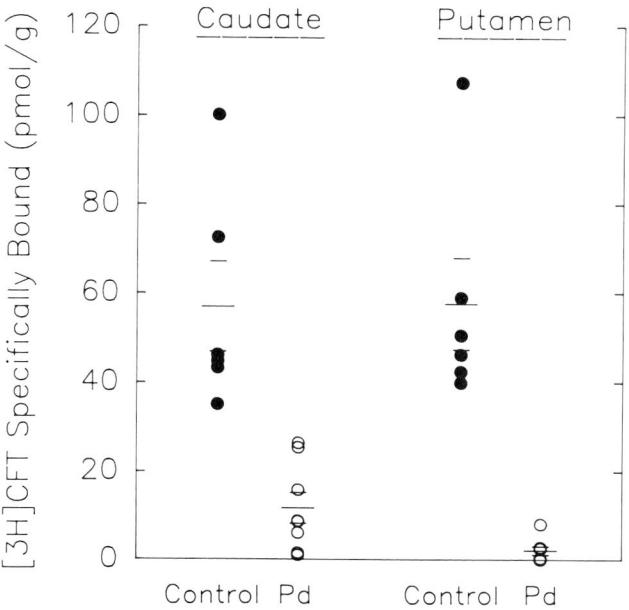

FIG. 1. Comparison of specific [^{3}H]CFT (cocaine analogue) binding in postmortem caudate and putamen from control and Parkinson's disease (Pd) subjects. Bars indicate means and SEMs. Note the profound loss of transporter binding sites in Parkinson's disease. (From ref. 46, with permission.)

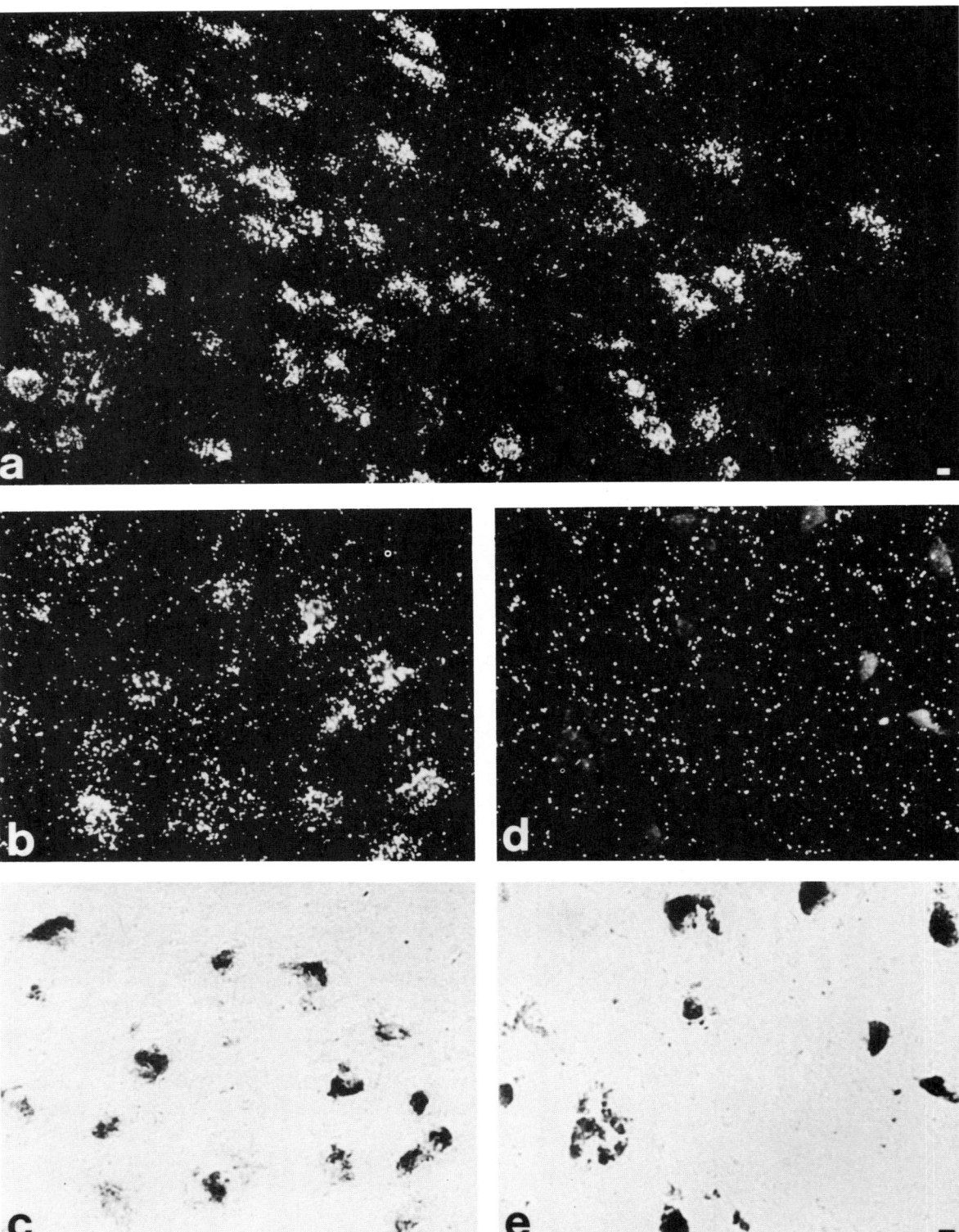

FIG. 2. Localization by in situ hybridization of dopamine transporter mRNA in human substantia nigra. **a:** Dark-field photomicrograph of a tissue section from the 42-year-old subject showing intense labeling for dopamine transporter mRNA. **b, c:** Dark-field and bright-field views, respectively, of a field in a tissue section from this subject. Note that all transporter-positive cells (**b**) are also melanin-positive (**c**). **d, e:** Dark-field and bright-field views, respectively, of a field from a tissue section of a 60-year-old subject. Note the presence of numerous melanin-positive but transporter mRNA-negative neurons. Bars represent 10 μm. (From ref. 4, with permission.)

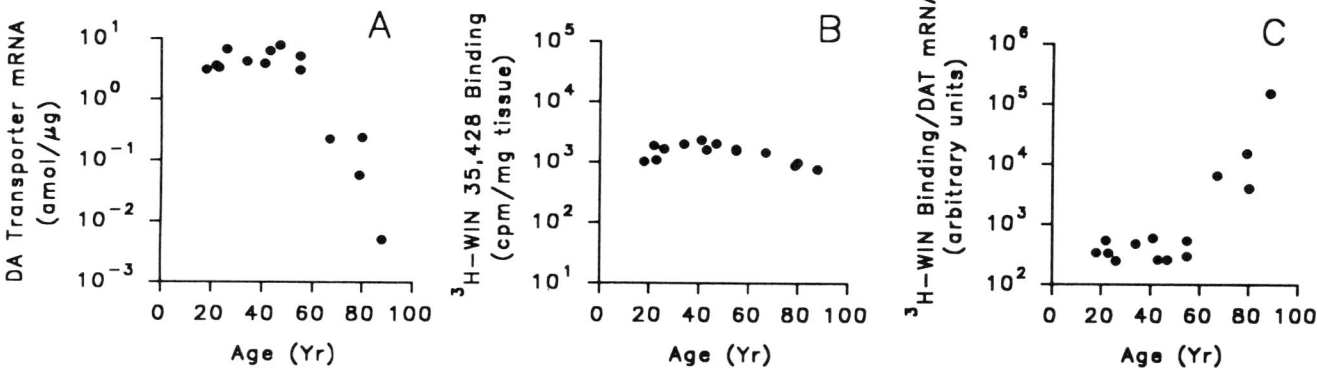

FIG. 3. Age-dependent changes in dopamine transporter mRNA versus binding sites. **A:** Precipitous decrease in substantia nigra dopamine transporter mRNA with age. (From ref. 4, with permission.) **B:** Gradual, modest age-related decrease in WIN binding in caudates from the same subjects. (Note that all data are presented on a log scale.) (Unpublished data of MJB, JGG, GK, and Drs. John Boja and Michael Kuhar.) **C:** A dramatic increase in the amount of transporter ligand binding per unit transporter mRNA occurs with age.

these DA phenotypic proteins within their terminal arbor. The mechanism underlying this phenomenon is presently unknown; sprouting of remaining DA terminals within the striatum, changes in DAT and TH protein stability, or altered DAT and TH mRNA translational efficiency have been discussed (65,90) as possible explanations for the observed changes. The use of animal models for age- or disease-related DA cell loss may shed some light on the molecular adaptations elicited in compromised DA neurons and may reveal how these adaptations contribute to functional compensation and perhaps further decompensation.

Schizophrenia and Tourette's Syndrome

The possible involvement of DA systems in the etiology of schizophrenia has led to a number of studies investigating the status of the DAT in this disorder. Predicated on the observation that viable nerve terminals

expressing high-affinity DA uptake can be prepared from frozen human brain under certain conditions (30,31,85), DA uptake has been measured in postmortem caudate and nucleus accumbens of schizophrenics and age-matched controls. The V_{max} and K_m for DA uptake into nerve terminals isolated from the brains of schizophrenic subjects were reportedly increased two- to threefold relative to age- and sex-matched subjects (30,31). In contrast to these functional studies of the DAT, a number of investigators have been unable to detect any change in DAT ligand binding associated with schizophrenia (16,66,68). These studies are, however, presumably prone to the same difficulties in interpretation as the Parkinson's disease analyses (discussed above) using the same ligands. A quantitative autoradiographic analysis of mazindol binding (which *has* detected changes in Parkinson's disease; see ref. 14) was also unable to detect a significant difference between normal and schizophrenic subjects (43). The basis for the discrepancy between the uptake and binding studies is unclear.

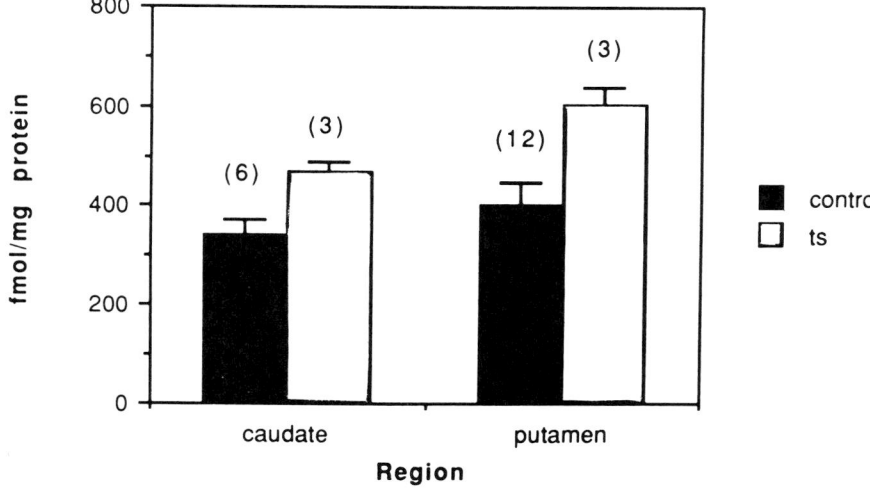

FIG. 4. [³H]Mazindol binding to dopamine transporter in the caudate and putamen of control and Tourette's subjects. Means and SEM are indicated; n values are given in parentheses. The increased ligand binding in Tourette's subjects (ts) is statistically significant in both tissues. (From ref. 83, with permission.)

Interestingly, a significant increase in membrane mazindol binding has been reported in a small number of Tourette's syndrome subjects (83) (Fig. 4). This observation warrants replication with a larger number of subjects and a different DAT ligand and/or functional DA uptake analyses (see also Chapters 26, 100, and 103, *this volume*).

FUTURE DEVELOPMENTS RELATED TO THE DAT

Insights into the molecular nature of the DAT are already resulting in a greater understanding of the function of the DAT in controlling dopaminergic neurotransmission. The potential role of the DAT in various pathophysiological states can now be explored in greater depth. DAT expression in heterologous systems should aid in the development of new, more selective DAT antagonists. Preliminary mutagenesis data suggest that it may be possible to develop agents that can prevent cocaine binding to the DAT while allowing normal DA transport, supporting the feasibility of developing cocaine antagonists for the treatment of cocaine addiction, withdrawal, or overdose. Exploring the subtleties of the DAT may also lead to new drugs useful in the treatment of depression or Parkinson's disease.

If membrane components of dying DA cells find their way into the cerebrospinal fluid, it may be possible to use anti-DAT antibodies to screen presymptomatic or very-early-stage patients for evidence of the DA cell death which precedes the symptomatology of Parkinson's disease. In this case, therapeutic strategies (e.g., deprenyl) aimed at slowing or halting the progression of the disease could be more effective. Likewise, DAT ligands used for in vivo imaging might be more routinely employed for diagnosis, for following the progression of disease and response to treatment, and for purifying human embryonic DA cells and monitoring their viability and outgrowth once transplanted into parkinsonian recipients. In short, it is likely that our newly found knowledge of the DAT will rapidly be translated into therapeutic advances in the treatment of brain diseases.

ACKNOWLEDGMENTS

This work was supported by NIH grants DA06470, MH43026, and NS26081.

REFERENCES

1. Altar CA, Jakeman LB, Acworth IN, Soriano R, Dugich-Djordjevic M. Regionally restricted loss and partial recovery of nigrostriatal dopamine input following intrastriatal 6-hydroxydopamine. *Neurodegeneration* 1992;1:123–133.
2. Amara SG, Kuhar MJ. Neurotransmitter Transporters. *Annu Rev Neurosci* 1993;16:73–93.
3. Andersen PH. Biochemical and pharmacological characterization of [³H]GBR 12935 binding in vitro to rat striatal membranes: labeling of the dopamine uptake complex. *J Neurochem* 1987;48:1887–1896.
4. Bannon MJ, Poosch MS, Xia Y, Goebel DJ, Cassin B, Kapatos G. Dopamine transporter mRNA content in human substantia nigra decreases precipitously with age. *Proc Natl Acad Sci USA* 1992;89:7095–7099.
5. Bannon MJ, Xue C-H, Shibata K, Dragovic LJ, Kapatos G. Expression of a human cocaine-sensitive dopamine transporter in *Xenopus laevis* oocytes. *J Neurochem* 1990;54:706–708.
6. Berger B, Di Porzio U, Daquet MC, Gay M, Vigny A, Glowinski J, Prochiantz A. Long-term development of mesencephalic dopaminergic neurons of mouse embryos in dissociated primary cultures: morphological and histochemical characteristics. *Neuroscience* 1982;7:193–205.
7. Berger P, Janowsky A, Vocci F, Skolnick P, Schweri MM, Paul SM. [³H]GBR-12935: a specific high affinity ligand for labeling the dopamine transport complex. *Eur J Pharmacol* 1985;107:289–290.
8. Berger P, Martenson RE, Laing P, Thurkauf A, Decosta B, Rice KC, Paul SM. Photoaffinity labeling of the dopamine reuptake carrier protein with 3-azido [³H]GBR-12935. *Mol Pharmacol* 1991;39:429–435.
9. Bonnet J-J, Costentin J. Correlation between (³H)dopamine specific uptake and (³H)GBR 12783 specific binding during the maturation of rat striatum. *Life Sci* 1989;44:1759–1765.
10. Calligaro DO, Eldefrawi ME. Central and peripheral cocaine receptors. *J Pharmacol Exp Ther* 1987;243:61–67.
11. Carlsson A. Monoamines of the central nervous system: a historical perspective. In: Meltzer HY, ed. *Psychopharmacology: the third generation of progress*. New York: Raven Press, 1987;39–48.
12. Carroll FI, Lewin AH, Boja JW, Kuhar MJ. Cocaine receptor: biochemical characterization and structure–activity relationships of cocaine analogues at the dopamine transporter. *J Med Chem* 1992;35:969–981.
13. Cass WA, Larson G, Fitzpatrick FA, Zahniser NR. Inhibitors of arachidonic acid metabolism: effects on rat striatal dopamine release and uptake. *J Pharmacol Exp Ther* 1991;257:990–996.
14. Chinaglia G, Alvarez FJ, Probst A, Palacios JM. Mesostriatal and mesolimbic dopamine uptake binding sites are reduced in Parkinson's disease and progressive supranuclear palsy: a quantitative autoradiographic study using [³H]mazindol. *Neuroscience* 1992;49:317–327.
15. Coyle JT, Snyder SH. Catecholamine uptake by synaptosomes in homogenates of rat brain: stereospecificity in different areas. *J Pharmacol Exp Ther* 1969;170:221–231.
16. Czudek C, Reynolds GP. [³H]GBR 12935 binding to the dopamine uptake site in postmortem brain tissue in schizophrenia. *J Neural Transm* 1989;77:227–230.
17. De Keyser J, Ebinger G, Vauquelin G. Age-related changes in the human nigrostriatal dopaminergic system. *Ann Neurol* 1990;27:157–161.
18. Demerest KY, Moore KE. Lack of a high affinity transport system for dopamine in the median eminence and posterior pituitary. *Brain Res* 1979;171:545–551.
19. Dubocovich ML, Zahniser NR. Binding characteristics of the dopamine uptake inhibitor [³H]nomifensine to striatal membranes. *Biochem Pharmacol* 1985;34:1137–1144.
20. Engele J, Pilgrim C, Kirsch M, Reisert I. Different developmental potentials of diencephalic and mesencephalic dopaminergic neurons in vitro. *Brain Res* 1989;483:98–109.
21. Fischman MW. Cocaine and the amphetamines. In: Meltzer HY, ed. *Psychopharmacology: the third generation of progress*. New York: Raven Press, 1987;1543–1554.
22. Fowler JS, Volkow ND, Wolf AP, Dewey SL, Schlyer DJ, MacGregor RR, Hitzemann R, Logan J, Bendriem B, Gatley SJ, Christman D. Mapping cocaine binding sites in human and baboon brain in vivo. *Synapse* 1989;4:371–377.
23. German DC, Dubach M, Askari S, Speciale SG, Bowden DM. 1-Methyl-4-phenyl-1,2,3,6-tetrahydropyridine-induced parkinsonian syndrome in macaca fascicularis: which midbrain dopaminergic neurons are lost? *Neuroscience* 1988;24:161–174.
24. German DC, Manaye K, Smith WK, Woodward DJ, Saper CB. Midbrain dopaminergic cell loss in Parkinson's disease: computer visualization. *Ann Neurol* 1989;26:507–514.
25. Giros B, Caron MG. Molecular characterization of the dopamine transporter. *Trends Pharmacol Sci* 1993;14:43–49.

26. Giros B, El Mestikawy S, Bertrand L, Caron MG. Cloning and functional characterization of a cocaine-sensitive dopamine transporter. *FEBS Lett* 1991;295:149–154.

27. Giros B, El Mestikawy S, Godinot N, Zheng K, Han H, Yang-Feng T, Caron MG. Cloning, pharmacological characterization, and chromosome assignment of the human dopamine transporter. *Mol Pharmacol* 1992;42:383–390.

28. Glowinski J, Iversen LL. Regional disposition of catecholamines in the rat brain-I: the disposition of [³H]norepinephrine, [³H]-dopamine and [³H]dopa in various regions of the brain. *J Neurochem* 1966;13:655–669.

29. Grigoriadis DE, Wilson AA, Lew R, Sharkey JS, Kuhar MJ. Dopamine transport sites selectively labeled by a novel photoaffinity probe: ¹²⁵I-DEEP. *J Neurosci* 1989;9:2664–2670.

30. Haberland N, Hetey L. Studies in postmortem dopamine uptake. I. Kinetic characterization of the synaptosomal dopamine uptake in rat and human brain after postmortem storage and cryopreservation. Comparison with noradrenaline and serotonin uptake. *J Neural Transm* 1987;68:289–301.

31. Haberland N, Hetey L. Studies in postmortem dopamine uptake. II. Alterations of the synaptosomal catecholamine uptake in postmortem brain regions in schizophrenia. *J Neural Transm* 1987;68:303–313.

32. Hadfield MG. Mesocortical vs nigrostriatal dopamine uptake in isolated fighting mice. *Brain Res* 1981;222:172–176.

33. Haycock JW, Levy WB, Denner LA, Cotman CW. Effects of elevated (K⁺)ₒ on the release of neurotransmitters from cortical synaptosomes: efflux or secretion? *J Neurochem* 1978;30:1113–1123.

34. Hirsch E, Graybiel AM, Agid YA. Melanized dopaminergic neurons are differentially susceptible to degeneration in Parkinson's disease. *Nature* 1988;334:345–348.

35. Holtz RW, Coyle JT. The effects of various salts, temperature and the alkaloids veratridine and batrachotoxin on the uptake of [³H]-dopamine into synaptosomes from rat striatum. *Mol Pharmacol* 1974;10:746–758.

36. Horn AS. Dopamine uptake: a review of progress in the last decade. *Prog Neurobiol* 1990;34:387–400.

37. Innis R, Baldwin R, Sybirska E, Zea Y, Laruelle M, Al-Tikriti M, Charney D, Zoghbi S, Wisniewski G, Hoffer P, Wang S, Millius R, Neumeyer J. Single photon emission computer tomography imaging of monoamine reuptake sites in primate brain with [¹²³I]CIT. *Eur J Pharmacol* 1991;200:369–370.

38. Izenwasser S, Cox BM. Daily cocaine treatment produces a persistent reduction of [³H]dopamine uptake in vitro in rat nucleus accumbens but not in striatum. *Brain Res* 1990;531:338–341.

39. Janowsky A, Schweri MM, Berger P, Long R, Skolnick P, Paul SM. The effects of surgical and chemical lesions on striatal [³H]-threo-(±)-methylphenidate binding: correlation with [³H]dopamine uptake. *Eur J Pharmacol* 1985;108:187–191.

40. Janowsky A, Vocci F, Berger P, Angel I, Zelnik N, Kleinman JE, Skolnick P, Paul SM. [³H]GBR 12935 binding to the dopamine transporter is decreased in the caudate nucleus in Parkinson's disease. *J Neurochem* 1987;49:617–621.

41. Javitch JA, Blaustein RO, Snyder SH. [³H]Mazindol binding associated with neuronal dopamine uptake sites in corpus striatum membranes. *Eur J Pharmacol* 1983;90:461–462.

42. Javitch JA, D'Amato RJ, Strittmatter SM, Snyder SH. Parkinsonism-inducing neurotoxin, *N*-methyl-4-phenyl-1,2,3,6-tetrahydropyridine: uptake of the metabolite *N*-methyl-4-phenylpyridine by dopamine neurons explains toxicity. *Proc Natl Acad Sci USA* 1985; 82:2173–2177.

43. Joyce JM, Lexow N, Bird E, Winokur A. Organization of dopamine D1 and D2 receptors in human striatum: receptor autoradiographic studies in Huntington's disease and schizophrenia. *Synapse* 1988;2:546–557.

44. Kadowaki K, Hirota K, Koike K, Ohmiche M, Kiyama H, Miyake A, Tanizawa O. Adenosine 3′,5′-cyclic monophosphate enhances dopamine accumulation in rat hypothalamic cell culture containing dopaminergic neurons. *Neuroendocrinology* 1990;52:256–261.

45. Kalivas PW, Stewart J. Dopamine transmission in the initiation and expression of drug- and stress-induced sensitization of motor activity. *Brain Res Rev* 1991;16:223–244.

46. Kaufman MJ, Madras BK. Severe depletion of cocaine recognition sites associated with the dopamine transporter in Parkinson's disease striatum. *Synapse* 1991;9:43–49.

47. Kavanaugh MP, Arriza JL, North RA, Amara SG. Electrogenic uptake of γ-aminobutyric acid by a cloned transporter expressed in *Xenopus* oocytes. *J Biol Chem* 1992;267:22007–22009.

48. Kennedy LT, Hanbauer I. Sodium-dependent cocaine binding to rat striatal membrane: possible relationship to dopamine uptake sites. *J Neurochem* 1983;41:172–178.

49. Kilty JE, Lorang D, Amara SG. Cloning and expression of a cocaine-sensitive rat dopamine transporter. *Science* 1991;254: 578–579.

50. Kish SJ, Shannak K, Hornykiewicz O. Uneven pattern of dopamine loss in the striatum of patients with idiopathic Parkinson's disease. *N Engl J Med* 1988;318:876–880.

51. Kitayama S, Shimada S, Xu H, Markham L, Donovan DM, Uhl GR. Dopamine transporter site-directed mutations differentially alter substrate transport and cocaine binding. *Proc Natl Acad Sci USA* 1992;89:7782–7785.

52. Koob GF, Bloom FE. Cellular and molecular mechanisms of drug dependence. *Science* 1988;242:715–723.

53. Kruger BK. Kinetics and block of dopamine uptake in synaptosomes from rat caudate nucleus. *J Neurochem* 1990;55:260–267.

54. Leon A, Dal Toso R, Presti D, Benvegnu D, Facci L, Kirschner G, Tettamanti G, Toffano G. Development and survival of serum-free cell cultures. II. Modulatory effects of gangliosides. *J Neurosci* 1988;8:746–753.

55. Lew R, Grigoriadis DE, Wilson A, Boja JW, Simantov R, Kuhar MJ. Dopamine transporter: deglycosylation with exo- and endoglycosylases. *Brain Res* 1991;539:239–246.

56. Lew R, Patel A, Vaughan RA, Wilson A, Kuhar MJ. Microheterogeneity of dopamine transporters in rat striatum and nucleus accumbens. *Brain Res* 1992;584:266–271.

57. Liu Y, Peter D, Roghani A, Schuldiner S, Prive G, Eisenberg D, Brecha N, Edwards RH. A cDNA that suppresses MPP⁺ toxicity encodes a vesicular amine transporter. *Cell* 1992;70:539–551.

58. Madras BK, Spealman RD, Fahey MA, Neumeyer JL, Saha JK, Milius RA. Cocaine receptors labeled by [³H]2β-carbomethoxy-3β-94-fluorophenyltropane. *Mol Pharmacol* 1989;36:518–524.

59. Mager S, Naeve J, Quick M, Labarca C, Davidson N, Lester HA. Steady states, charge movements, and rates for a cloned GABA transporter expressed in *Xenopus* oocytes. *Neuron* 1993;10:177–188.

60. Maloteaux J-M, Vanisberg M-A, Laterre C, Javoy-Agid F, Agig Y, Laduron PM. [³H]GBR 12935 binding to dopamine uptake sites: subcellular localization and reduction in Parkinson's disease and progressive supranuclear palsy. *Eur J Pharmacol* 1988;156:331–340.

61. Marshall JF, O'Dell SJ, Navarrete R, Rosenstein AJ. Dopamine high-affinity transport site topography in rat brain: major differences between dorsal and ventral striatum. *Neuroscience* 1990;37:11–21.

62. McGeer PL, McGeer EG, Sukuki JS. Aging and extrapyramidal function. *Arch Neurol* 1977;34:33–35.

63. Missale C, Castelletti L, Govoni S, Spano PF, Trabucchi M, Hanbauer I. Dopamine uptake is differentially regulated in rat striatum and nucleus accumbens. *J Neurochem* 1985;45:51–56.

64. Niznik HB, Fogel EF, Fassos FF, Seeman P. The dopamine transporter is absent in parkinsonian putamen and reduced in the caudate nucleus. *J Neurochem* 1991;56:192–198.

65. Pasinetti GM, Osterburg HH, Kelly AB, Kohama S, Morgan DG, Reinhard JF Jr, Stellwagen RH, Finch CE. Slow changes of tyrosine hydroxylase gene expression in dopaminergic brain neurons after neurotoxin lesioning: a model for neuron aging. *Mol Brain Res* 1992;13:63–73.

66. Pearce RKB, Seeman P, Jellinger K, Tourtellotte WW. Dopamine uptake sites and dopamine receptors in Parkinson's disease and schizophrenia. *Eur Neurol* 1989;30:9–14.

67. Peris J, Boyson SJ, Cass WA, Curella P, Dwoskin LP, Larson G, Lin L-H, Yasuda RP, Zahniser NR. Persistence of neurochemical changes in dopamine systems after repeated cocaine administration. *J Pharmacol Exp Therap* 1990;253:38–44.

68. Pimoule C, Schoemaker H, Reynolds GP, Langer SZ. [³H]SCH 23390 labeled D₁ receptors are unchanged in schizophrenia and Parkinson's disease. *Eur J Pharmacol* 1985;114:235–237.

69. Prochiantz A, di Porzio U, Kato A, Berger B, Glowinski J. *In vitro* maturation of mesencephalic dopaminergic neurons from mouse embryos is enhanced in the presence of their striatal target cells. *Proc Natl Acad Sci USA* 1979;76:5387–5391.

70. Raiteri M, Cerrito F, Cervoni AM, Levi G. Dopamine can be released by two mechanisms differentially affected by the dopamine

transport inhibitor nomifensine. *J Pharmacol Exp Ther* 1979; 208:195–202.

71. Reinhard JF Jr, Diliberto EJ Jr., Viveros OH, Daniels AJ. Subcellular compartmentalization of 1-methyl-4-phenylpyridinium with catecholamines in adrenal medullary chromaffin vesicles may explain the lack of toxicity to adrenal chromaffin cells. *Proc Natl Acad Sci USA* 1987; 84:8160–8164.

72. Ritz MC, Boja JW, Grigoriadis D, Zaczek R, Carroll FI, Lewis AH, Kuhar MJ. [³H]WIN 35,065-2: a ligand for cocaine receptors in striatum. *J Neurochem* 1990; 55:1556–1562.

73. Ritz MC, Lamb RJ, Goldberg SR, Kuhar MJ. Cocaine receptors on dopamine transporters are related to self-administration of cocaine. *Science* 1987; 237:1219–1223.

74. Sallee FR, Fogel EL, Schwartz E, Choi SM, Curran DP, Niznik HB. Photoaffinity labeling of the mammalian dopamine transporter. *FEBS Lett* 1989; 256:219–224.

75. Sanchez-Ramos JR, Michel P, Weiner WJ, Hefti F. Selective destruction of cultured dopaminergic neurons from fetal rat mesencephalon by 1-methyl-4-phenylpyridinium: cytochemical and morphological evidence. *J Neurochem* 1988; 50:1934–1944.

76. Schnelli S, Zuddas A, Kopin IJ, Barker JL, Di Porzio U. 1-Methyl-4-phenyl-1,2,3,6-tetrahydropyridine metabolism and 1-methyl-4-phenylpyridinium uptake in dissociated cell cultures from the embryonic mesencephalon. *J Neurochem* 1988; 50:1900–1907.

77. Schoemaker H, Pimoule C, Arbilla S, Scatton B, Javoy-Agid F, Langer SZ. Sodium dependent [³H]cocaine binding associated with dopamine uptake sites in the rat striatum and human putamen decrease after dopaminergic denervation and in Parkinson's disease. *Naunyn Schmiedebergs Arch Pharmacol* 1985; 329:227–235.

78. Seeman P, Niznik HB. Dopamine receptors and transporters in Parkinson's disease and schizophrenia. *FASEB J* 1990; 4:2737–2744.

79. Sharpe LG, Pilotte NS, Mitchell WM, DeSouza EB. Withdrawal of repeated cocaine decreases autoradiographic [³H]mazindol-labelling of dopamine transporter in rat nucleus accumbens. *Eur J Pharmacol* 1991; 203:141–144.

80. Shaya EK, Scheffel U, Dannals RF, Ricaurte GA, Carroll FI, Wagner HN Jr, Kuhar MJ, Wong DF. In vivo imaging of dopamine reuptake sites in the primate brain using single photon emission computed tomography (SPECT) and iodine-123 labeled RTI-55. *Synapse* 1992; 10:169–172.

81. Shimada S, Kitayama S, Lin C-L, Patel A, Nanthakumar E, Gregor P, Kuhar M, Uhl G. Cloning and expression of a cocaine-sensitive dopamine transporter complementary DNA. *Science* 1991; 254:576–578.

82. Shimada S, Kitayama S, Walther D, Uhl G. Dopamine transporter mRNA: dense expression in ventral midbrain neurons. *Mol Brain Res* 1992; 13:359–362.

83. Singer HS, Hahn I-H, Moran TH. Abnormal dopamine uptake sites in postmortem striatum from patients with Tourette's syndrome. *Ann Neurol* 1991; 30:558–562.

84. Snyder SH, Coyle JT. Regional differences in H³-norepinephrine and H³-dopamine uptake into rat brain homogenates. *J Pharmacol Exp Ther* 1969; 165:78–86.

85. Stenstrom A, Oreland L, Hardy J, Wester P, Winblad B. The uptake of serotonin and dopamine by homogenates of frozen rat and human brain tissue. *Neurochem Res* 1985; 10:591–599.

86. Trendelenburg U. Functional aspects of the neuronal uptake of noradrenaline. *Trends Pharmacol Sci* 1991; 12:334–337.

87. Uhl GR. Neurotransmitter transporters (plus): a promising new gene family. *Trends Neurol Sci* 1992; 15:265–268.

88. Usdin TB, Mezey E, Chen C, Brownstein MJ, Hoffman BJ. Cloning of the cocaine-sensitive bovine dopamine transporter. *Proc Natl Acad Sci USA* 1991; 88:11168–11171.

89. Vandenbergh DJ, Persico AM, Uhl GR. A human dopamine transporter cDNA predicts reduced glycosylation, displays a repetitive element and provides racially-dimorphic Taq I RFLPs. *Mol Brain Res* 1992; 15:161–166.

90. Wolf ME, LeWitt PA, Bannon MJ, Dragovic LJ, Kapatos G. Effect of aging on tyrosine hydroxylase protein content and the relative number of dopamine nerve terminals in human caudate. *J Neurochem* 1991; 56:1191–1200.

91. Xia Y, Goebel DJ, Kapatos G, Bannon MJ. Quantitation of rat dopamine transporter mRNA: effects of cocaine treatment and withdrawal. *J Neurochem* 1992; 59:1179–1182.

92. Xia Y, Poosch MS, Whitty CJ, Kapatos G, Bannon MJ. GABA transporter mRNA: in vitro expression and quantitation in neonatal rat and postmortem human brain. *Neurochem Int* 1993; 22:263–270.

93. Yi S-J, Johnson KM. Effects of acute and chronic administration of cocaine on striatal uptake, compartmentalization and release of [³H]dopamine. *Neuropharmacol* 1990; 29:475–486.

94. Zaleska MM, Ericinska M. Involvement of sialic acid in high-affinity uptake of dopamine by synaptosomes from rat brain. *Neurosci Lett* 1987; 107:–112.

95. Zelnick N, Angel I, Paul SM, Kleinman JE. Decreased density of human striatal dopamine uptake sites with age. *Eur J Pharmacol* 1986; 126:175–176.

Psychopharmacology: The Fourth Generation of Progress, edited by Floyd E. Bloom and David J. Kupfer. Raven Press, Ltd., New York © 1995.

CHAPTER 17

Long- and Short-Term Regulation of Tyrosine Hydroxylase

Menek Goldstein

Tyrosine hydroxylase (TH) (EC 1.14.16.2) catalyzes the enzymatic conversion of L-tyrosine to L-3,4-dihydroxyphenylalanine (L-dopa), the first step in the biosynthesis of dopamine (DA), norepinephrine (NE), and epinephrine (E). TH is subject to short- and long-term regulation; the latter occurs at transcriptional as well as at translational levels, and the former occurs at post-translational levels. The findings that dibutyryl cyclic AMP (dB-cAMP) stimulates L-dopa biosynthesis from L-tyrosine in striatal slices (4), and that phosphorylation of TH mediated by cAMP-dependent protein kinase A (PKA) phosphorylates and activates TH in vitro, have provided the first evidence that protein kinase-mediated phosphorylation plays a role in regulation of the enzyme activity and catecholamine biosynthesis. Subsequently it was shown that various protein kinases catalyze phosphorylation of TH at multiple serine sites of the enzyme (10,45). The findings that long- and short-term regulation of TH activity at transcriptional, translational, and post-translational levels, respectively, involve similar second messenger signals raises the possibility that these pathways are interdependent.

Many advances in the mechanisms involving regulation of TH gene and enzyme activity have been made in the last few years, and we will review only some of them. We will focus on areas that have recently made rapid progress and discuss strategies to be pursued in future research.

LONG-TERM REGULATION OF TYROSINE HYDROXYLASE

The long-term regulation of TH occurs at transcriptional and translational levels. Several studies have shown

M. Goldstein: Department of Psychiatry, New York University Medical Center, New York, New York 10016.

that cAMP and glucocorticoids regulate TH mRNA levels primarily by stimulating the transcription rate of TH gene. Both elevate TH protein as well as mRNA and gene transcription rate in cultured PC12 cells and in adrenal glands (38,39,56,57). The 5′ flanking region of the TH gene possesses the same response elements which mediate the regulation of several other genes by cAMP and glucocorticoids (39). The absence of the cAMP response element in the TH gene promoter region results in a loss of response to elevated cAMP (39,56). The transcription rate of the TH gene as estimated from the run-off assays was found to be stimulated 5- to 20-fold by treatment of PC18 cells (a variant of PC12 cells) with cAMP analogues or dexamethasone (14). The pulse-labeling experiments with 4-thiouridine have shown that treatment with a cAMP analogue or dexamethasone increases the rate of TH mRNA synthesis. However, the enhanced stability may also, in part, contribute to the increased steady-state TH mRNA levels elicited by cAMP (14). Because protein kinase C (PKC) seems to mediate both short- and long-term Ca^{2+}-dependent cellular functions, its involvement in the regulation of TH at transcriptional and post-transcriptional levels was investigated (10). Activation of PKC by the phorbol ester, TPA, leads to an increase of TH gene transcription, as well as to the post-translational modulation of TH gene expression in PC12 cells (61). Thus, PKA and PKC are involved in transcriptional regulation of TH, and both pathways may converge to amplify TH expression and activity in some physiological and/or pathological states.

Regulation of TH in Dopaminergic and Noradrenergic Neurons

The TH gene regulation in dopaminergic (DA) and noradrenergic (NE) neurons has been the subject of numerous studies. It became apparent that regulation of TH activity and TH enzyme protein in NE neurons differs from that in DA neurons. In the central nervous system (CNS) the reserpine effect on TH activity is restricted to NE neurons, and it does not have an effect on TH activity in the DA neurons of the substantia nigra (51). Nevertheless, one study reports that reserpine slightly increased TH protein levels without affecting the enzymatic activity in the DA neurons of substantia nigra (35). The time course of the induction of TH by reserpine was analyzed in adrenals, locus coeruleus, and substantia nigra (13). Reserpine caused in locus coeruleus and adrenals a significant increase in TH mRNA and in TH activity, while no effect was observed in the substantia nigra (13). The exposure of rats to chronic stress increases the levels of TH mRNA and TH protein in the locus coeruleus (44,52), but it does not alter TH in the substantia nigra or ventral tegmentum (44). It is noteworthy that a single study reports that isolation stress results in a small transient increase in TH mRNA in both the substantia nigra and ventral tegmental area (VTA); the magnitude of increase is much smaller than in locus coeruleus (5). Repeated administration of morphine increases TH mRNA levels in the locus coeruleus but not in the substantia nigra (22), while chronic treatment with antidepressants decreases the firing rate of NE neurons as well as the steady-state TH mRNA levels and TH protein in locus coeruleus but not in the midbrain DA neurons (44,52). Because stress activates the hypothalamic–pituitary–adrenal axis, which results in increased levels of adrenocorticotropic hormone (ACTH) and corticotropin-releasing factor (CRF), it was suggested that these neuropeptides might be involved in the regulation of TH. Indeed, CRF seems to mediate the induction of TH in response to chronic footshock and noise stress (43).

Several lines of evidence suggest that the cAMP second messenger system contributes to adaptive responses of NE neurons in locus coeruleus (3). Thus, the cAMP system mediates the long-term effects of stress, catecholamine depletion, and various drug and hormone treatments in NE neurons but not in DA neurons (44). It is of considerable interest that TH phosphorylated at Ser40 position by PKA was localized immunohistochemically in E and NE neurons of the brainstem, and in only a small population of DA neurons in substantia nigra and VTA (36,37). The findings that E and NE neurons in the steady state are phosphorylated by PKA at TH Ser40, and that most DA neurons are not, imply that a large capacity for phosphorylation of TH above basal levels exists in some midbrain DA neurons.

SHORT-TERM REGULATION OF TYROSINE HYDROXYLASE

Feedback Inhibition and Autoreceptor Regulation

The question of whether the feedback inhibition of TH activity in vitro by the enzymatic end products L-dopa

and DA and by other catecholamines (47,55) is of physiological significance was extensively studied. The intracellular concentration of free catecholamines might be too low for regulating TH activity, and feedback inhibition of the enzyme by the enzymatic end products might play a role only when intracellular levels are elevated under physiological or pathological conditions. Our findings that site-directed mutagenesis of TH at serine 40 (Ser was substituted with Leu or Tyr) produces an activated form of the enzyme which is less sensitive to feedback inhibition and increases L-dopa synthesis in situ (18,63) illustrates the effects of reduced inhibition on L-dopa biosynthesis. It was also reported that feedback inhibition involves competition between the catecholamines and the pteridine cofactor for the oxidized form of the enzyme, and catecholamines bind to TH by a direct coordination to Fe^{3+} at the active enzyme site (24).

The autoreceptor regulation of TH activity was also extensively studied (17,62), and it was shown that stimulation of autoreceptors by DA or other DA D_2/D_3 agonists inhibits striatal TH activity and release of DA from nerve terminals, as well as decreases the phosphorylation of TH (17,62). The question of whether DA autoreceptors which regulate synthesis and release of the transmitter represent the same or different receptor proteins requires further investigation. The findings that DA autoreceptors regulating synthesis of the transmitter are linked to pertussis-toxin-sensitive G proteins, whereas those regulating release are not (6,8,25), indicate that these receptors are not coupled to the same effector systems. In light of the available data that DA D_2 receptors are coupled to G proteins whereas DA D_3 receptors are not, one can postulate that DA autoreceptors regulating DA biosynthesis are DA D_2 receptors whereas those regulating release of DA are DA D_3 receptors (see also Chapters 14 and 20, *this volume*).

Activation of TH

In vitro incubation of the enzyme with polyanions, phospholipids, mucopolysaccharides such as heparin, and ribonucleic acid results in increased TH activity (34,48). The activation of TH by macromolecules seems to be an electrostatic phenomenon rather than a result of a specific chemical interaction, and the physiological relevance is questionable. The activation of TH by protein-kinase-mediated phosphorylation leads to a covalent modification of the enzyme, and phosphorylation/dephosphorylation of TH represents an important mechanism in the short-term regulation of the enzymatic activity. It is now well established that the amino-terminal segment of the enzyme contains several potential phosphorylation sites and that each Ser site is phosphorylated by a distinct protein kinase (Fig. 1).

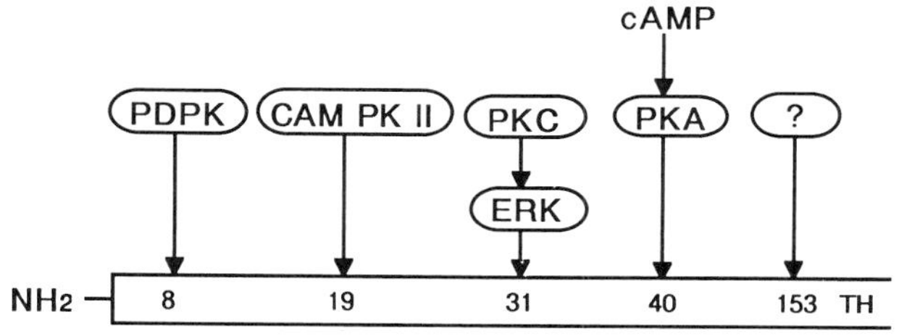

FIG. 1. Schematic presentation of TH phosphorylation at multiple serine sites of the enzyme (Ser19, Ser31, and Ser40) by distinct protein kinases.

PKA

TH is a substrate for phosphorylation by PKA, and phosphorylation correlates with increased catalytic activity (42,46). In purified TH preparations from cultured PC12 cells, PKA increased [^{32}P] incorporation from [γ-^{32}P]ATP, and the radioactivity is associated with the 62-kD subunit of the enzyme (42). The enzyme phosphorylated by PKA has a higher affinity for the pteridine cofactor and a lower inhibitory affinity for catechols (40,42,59). The activity of the nonphosphorylated enzyme has a pH optimum at 6.0, whereas that of the phosphorylated has a broad optimum in the physiological pH range (42). The kinetic parameters and the activity optimum at physiological pH values of the phosphorylated enzyme suggest that phosphorylation of TH by PKA is of importance in regulation of TH activity and catecholamine biosynthesis. The phosphorylated and activated TH is dephosphorylated by phosphatase 2A, suggesting a role of specific phosphatases in the regulation of TH activity by dephosphorylation (23,58).

PKC

TH is phosphorylated by the Ca^{2+}-phospholipid-dependent PKC (see Fig. 1), and the kinetic properties of the enzyme phosphorylated by this kinase are similar to those phosphorylated by PKA (2). A comparison of phosphopeptides generated by tryptic digestion of TH phosphorylated by PKA and those by PKC revealed that both kinases phosphorylate the enzyme at a similar site (2). However, it was reported that phosphorylation by PKA and not by PKC results in activation of the enzymatic activity (15). As a possible explanation it was suggested that PKC phosphorylates only two out of the four subunits of the enzyme without affecting the enzyme activity, whereas PKA phosphorylates all four subunits, resulting in an increase in the enzymatic activity. The availability of TH antibodies which recognize specifically TH phosphorylated at Ser40 site, anti-TH Ser40p, makes it possible to further investigate the stoichiometry of phosphorylation by PKA and PKC (36,37). The findings that TH at Ser31 is indirectly phosphorylated by PKC and directly

by ERK1 and ERK2 kinases (31) will provide new insights on the regulation of TH by these protein kinases.

Ca^{2+}/Calmodulin-Dependent Protein Kinase II (Ca^{2+}/CaMpKII)

Ca^{2+} CaMpKII phosphorylates TH, but its phosphorylation is not associated with an increase in enzymatic activity (64). Some studies suggest that an "activator protein" is required for increased catalytic activity, and the cloning of cDNA coding for the protein kinase-dependent activator has been reported (32). Other explanations for the lack of enhanced catalytic activity following phosphorylation by Ca^{2+}/CaMpKII—such as the enzyme is phosphorylated at multiple sites, and these sites modulate the activity in a way that the activation is nullified (20)—were also suggested. The idea that Ca^{2+}/CaMpKII, like PKC, phosphorylates only two of the four subunits of the enzyme, which is not sufficient for activation of the enzyme, has also been proposed (20).

Growth Factor-Stimulated Protein Kinases

A number of serine/threonine kinases which are stimulated in response of cells to growth factors were described. Some of these involve enzymes which are regulated by second messengers, whereas others seem to be independent of them. The second-messenger-independent serine/threonine protein kinases which are activated by growth factors include ribosomal protein S6 kinase (1,12) and MAP kinase (ERK 1 and ERK 2) (1,9,12,19,31,53,54). Treatment of intact PC12 cells with bradykinin or nerve growth factor (NGF) increased the phosphorylation of TH in situ and the catalytic activity of ERKs (31). TH phosphorylation at the Ser31 site is regulated by multiple signaling pathways which converge at or prior to activation of ERKs (31). The presence in PC12 cells of an NGF-activated protein kinase, designated as N-kinase, was described (53). N-kinase is rapidly activated in PC12 cells by treatment with NGF, epidermal growth factor (EGF), basic fibroblast growth factor (bFGF), phorbol ester or dB-cAMP. Thus, N-kinase can be activated via multiple second messenger pathways, and it might play a role in mediating shared intracellular responses to various extracellular signals (54).

Site-Specific Phosphorylation (see Fig. 1)

TH is phosphorylated by distinct protein kinases at five phosphorylation sites: Ser8, Ser19, Ser31, Ser40 and Ser153 in the N-terminal region of the enzyme (10,31). TH is phosphorylated at Ser19 by CaMpKII, at Ser40 by PKA and PKC (and to a small extent by CaMpKII), and at Ser31 by ERK1 and ERK2 kinases and indirectly by

PKC. Electrical stimulation of the medial forebrain bundle increases phosphorylation at Ser19, Ser31, and Ser40 of the enzyme (26). Although Ser153 is a substrate for phosphorylation by PKA, no evidence for in situ phosphorylation at this enzymatic site was obtained.

Cellular Mechanisms Regulating TH Activity

Ser8 Phosphorylation

The proline-directed protein kinase (PDPK) isolated from PC12 cells was shown to phosphorylate Ser8 in vitro (60). The levels of this kinase are very low in brain and adrenal glands, but relatively high in PC12 cells. PDPK activity is increased in response to NGF, and this effect seems to be mediated by the high-affinity NGF receptors (59). Inhibition of phosphatase-2A by treatment of synaptosomes with okadaic acid increases by severalfold the [^{32}P] incorporation into Ser8, suggesting a high turnover rate of phosphate on Ser8 (29).

Ser19 Phosphorylation

CaM-protein kinase is the only protein kinase known to phosphorylate TH at Ser19, and this kinase is activated in nerve terminals by depolarization (50). The activation of CaMpKII seems to be linked to depolarization-dependent Ca^{2+} influx, and phosphorylation of TH by this kinase is of physiological significance. The temporal changes following depolarization of striatal terminals on phosphorylation of TH were investigated (29). At relatively short treatment durations the effects of K^+ and veratradine were restricted to Ser19 phosphorylation. At longer treatment durations (up to 4 min), an increase in Ser31 phosphorylation and a smaller increase in Ser19 phosphorylation was observed (29). A biphasic increase in Ser19, but not in Ser31, was also observed in chromaffin cells following prolonged exposure to acetylcholine (27,30). The increased activity and phosphorylation by nicotine and muscarine is primarily associated with phosphorylation of the enzyme at Ser19 site (30).

Ser31 Phosphorylation

TH Ser31 was found to be a substrate for ERK1 and ERK2 (31), and a number of receptor systems in PC12 cells stimulate ERKs activity and Ser31 phosphorylation. Thus, muscarinic, bradykinin, ATP, and NGF receptor activation increases Ser31 phosphorylation. Two intracellular signaling pathways, an NGF and a PKC activation pathway, seem to be linked with the ERKs-mediated Ser31 phosphorylation of TH. Muscarine, bradykinin, and ATP activate G-protein-linked receptors, resulting in an increase of phosphatidyloinositol phosphate turnover and

activation of PKC. However, the pathways associated with NGF-stimulated increases in Ser31 phosphorylation are not yet established. The high-affinity NGF receptor has been identified as trk-B (the proto-oncogene product), and NGF increases its tyrosine phosphorylation in PC12 cells (33). Although phosphorylation of Ser31 increases TH activity by 20–40% (31), its physiological significance might not be relevant in view of much greater increases associated with phosphorylation of TH at Ser40 by PKA. The interactions between Ser31 phosphorylation and that of Ser40 and/or Ser19 are under investigation.

Ser40 Phosphorylation

The enzyme is phosphorylated at Ser40 in vitro by several protein kinases including PKA, PKC, CaMpKII, PKN, and S6 kinase, but the phosphorylation by PKA plays the predominant role in vivo (26). The adenylyl cyclase/cAMP-dependent protein kinase system stimulates TH activity in intact striatal synaptosomes and slices, as well as in vivo by increased phosphorylation of Ser40. Vasoactive intestinal polypeptide and related peptides stimulate TH activity in various catecholaminergic tissues by PKA-mediated increased phosphorylation of Ser40. In intact PC12 cells the substrate specificity of Ser40 seems to be restricted to PKA (27). The involvement of CaMp-KII in phosphorylation of Ser40 seems unlikely, because in synaptosomes maximal increases in Ser19 phosphorylation produced by elevated K^+ failed to increase Ser40 phosphorylation. On the other hand, the possible involvement of PKC in phosphorylation of Ser40 cannot be excluded because treatment of synaptosomes for a longer time period (15 min) with phorbol dibutyrate increased the phosphorylation of Ser31 and, to a smaller extent, Ser40 (29,30).

Modification of TH by Site-Directed Mutagenesis

In order to determine the degree to which phosphorylation at serine sites 19, 31, and 40 contributes to an increase in TH activity, we individually substituted the corresponding serine with leucine or tyrosine and transfected AtT-20 cells with TH cDNA constructs (63). The specific enzymatic activity of transiently expressed TH mutant Ser40m was higher as compared with the wild-type enzyme or the mutants Ser19 and Ser31 (63). Kinetic studies with stably expressed recombinant TH revealed that Ser40m has a lower K_M for the cofactor 6-methyltetrahydropteridine and a higher K_i for the end product DA than the wild-type enzyme (63). These findings suggest that Ser40 exerts an inhibitory influence on the enzymatic activity; and its replacement with another amino acid (AA) by site-directed mutagenesis, or its modification by phosphorylation, leads to a change in confirmation with an increase in enzymatic activity. The phosphorylation of

TH mediated by PKA increases the enzymatic activity of the wild type but has no effect on Ser40m activity, indicating the essential role of Ser40 in the activation of TH by PKA (63).

Multiple Forms of Human TH

TH is the product of a single gene, and in most species a single TH mRNA is translated to produce a single form of the protein. However, three additional forms of human TH mRNA which were formed by alternative splicing were detected. The three additional mRNA forms have 12, 81, or 12 + 81 additional nucleotides (21,49). Antibodies to each of the four forms of TH protein identified all four isoforms of TH in human adrenal glands, in human pheochromocytoma, and in several neuroblastoma cell lines (27). The physiological and pathological significance of the four TH isoforms in the regulation of TH activity is not yet known. It is of interest that the addition of 12 nucleotides transforms the sequence surrounding Ser35 in hTH-2 and -4 (Arg-Gly-Gln-Ser) in such a way that it represents a putative site for phosphorylation by a Ca/CaMpKII.

DISCUSSION AND FUTURE PERSPECTIVES

Considerable progress was made in elucidating the mechanisms involving short- and long-term regulation of TH. Phosphorylation by distinct protein kinases at specific Ser phosphorylation sites of the enzyme were characterized, but their individual contribution to the regulation of TH and catecholamine biosynthesis has to be further investigated. A large body of experimental evidence suggests that phosphorylation at Ser40 by the cAMP-dependent protein kinases increases enzymatic activity. However, Ser40 can be phosphorylated in vitro by a number of other protein kinases such as PKC, Ca/CaMpKII, PKN, and so on, and the role of each of these kinases in the stimulation of enzymatic activity has not yet been established. A Ca^{2+}-dependent activation of TH by depolarization in peripheral and central nervous system has been demonstrated, and this activation is linked to Ca/CaMpKII phosphorylation of TH at the Ser19 site of the enzyme. Studies with mutant enzymes in which single and multiple phosphorylation sites are systematically eliminated will further elucidate the relationships between different sites and their effects on TH activity. With this in mind, we investigated the phosphorylation and activation of TH mutants in which Ser40, Ser31, or Ser19 was substituted with another AA. Our studies indicate that removal of the phosphorylation site at Ser40 affects the magnitude of phosphorylation at other sites (18). The findings that in situ L-dopa biosynthesis in AtT-20 cells catalyzed by TH Ser40m is higher than that by TH WT (18) infer that a single AA mutation might be associated

with the overproduction of catecholamines in some specific disorders. It is noteworthy that PKC exhibits both negative and positive cross-talk with multifunctional Ca^{2+}/CaM protein kinase in PC12 cells (41), and multiple signaling pathways might be involved in the regulation of TH activity.

The resistance of TH to regulation by various exogenous and endogenous stimuli in DA, but not in NE/E neurons, suggests that different intracellular transduction pathways converge upon TH in these neuronal populations. cAMP-dependent systems play an essential role in the regulation of neuronal noradrenergic activity, but the intracellular pathways in the DA neurons were not yet fully elucidated. Most studies on phosphorylation of TH mediated by trophic factors [e.g., NGF, acidic fibroblast growth factor (aFGF) or bFGF] were carried out in PC12 cells. However, the importance of these signaling systems in nervous tissues remains to be determined. The presence of neurotrophic factors such as aFGF or bFGF in mesencephalic DA neurons (7,11) indicates that these factors might modulate TH activity in these neurons. The findings that NGF induction of TH in PC12 cells is regulated by the c-fos gene family (16) raises the possibility that the expression of early genes is associated with regulation and dysregulation of TH neuronal activity. The generation of phospho/dephospho-specific antibodies against a segment of TH (36,37) will be a useful tool in investigations of the basic regulatory features of TH in catecholamine neurons and their dysregulation in disease state.

ACKNOWLEDGMENTS

The author gratefully acknowledges the support of NIMH, Career Scientist Award MH 14918, and MH 02717.

REFERENCES

1. Ahn NG, Waiel JE, Chan CP, Krebs EG. Identification of multiple epidermal growth factor-stimulated protein serine/threonine kinase from Swiss 3T3 cells. *J Biol Chem* 1990;266:11495–11501.
2. Albert KA, Helmer-Matyjek E, Nairn AC, et al. Calcium/phospholipid-dependent protein kinase (protein kinase C) phosphorylates and activates tyrosine hydroxylase. *Proc Natl Acad Sci USA* 1984;81:7713–7717.
3. Alreja M, Aghajanian GK. Pacemaker activity of locus coeruleus neurons: whole cell recordings in brain slices show dependence on cAMP and protein kinase A. *Brain Res* 1991;556:339–343.
4. Anagnoste B, Shirron C, Friedman E, Goldstein M. Effect of dibutyryl cyclic AMP on ^{14}C-dopamine biosynthesis in rat brain striatal slices. *J Pharmacol Exp Ther* 1974;191:370–376.
5. Angulo JA, Printz D, Ledoux M, McEwen BS. Isolation stress increases tyrosine hydroxylase mRNA in the locus coeruleus and midbrain and decreases proenkephalin mRNA in the striatum and nucleus accumbens. *Mol Brain Res* 1991;11:301–308.
6. Bean AJ, Shepard PD, Bunney BS, Nestler EJ, Roth RH. The effects of pertussis toxin on autoreceptor-mediated inhibition of dopamine synthesis in the rat striatum. *Mol Pharmacol* 1988;34:715–718.
7. Bean AJ, Elde R, Cao Y, et al. Expression of acidic and basic

fibroblast growth factors in the substantia nigra of rat, monkey and human. *Proc Natl Acad Sci USA* 1991;88:10237–10241.

8. Bowyer JF, Weiner N. K$^+$ channel and adenylate cyclase involvement in regulation of Ca^{2+}-evoked release of [^{3}H]dopamine from synaptosomes. *J Pharmacol Exp Ther* 1989;248:514–520.

9. Boulton TG, Nye SH, Robbins DJ, et al. ERKs: A family of protein-serine/threonine kinases that are activated and tyrosine phosphorylated in response to insulin and NGF. *Cell* 1991;65:663–675.

10. Campbell DG, Hardie DG, Vulliet PR. Identification of four phosphorylation sites in the N-terminal region of tyrosine hydroxylase. *J Biol Chem* 1986;261:10489–10492.

11. Cintra A, Cao Y, Oellig C, et al. Basic FGF is present in dopaminergic neurons of the ventral midbrain of the rat. *NeuroReport* 1991;2:597–600.

12. Erikson E, Maller JL. In vivo phosphorylation and activation of ribosomal protein S6 kinases during *Xenopus* oocyte maturation. *J Biol Chem* 1989;264:13711–13717.

13. Faucon Biguet N, Buda M, Lamouroux A, Samolyk D, Mallet J. Time course of the changes of TH mRNA in rat brain and adrenal medulla after a single injection of reserpine. *EMBO J* 1986;5:287–291.

14. Fossom LH, Sterling CR, Tank AW. Regulation of tyrosine hydroxylase gene transcription rate and tyrosine hydroxylase mRNA stability by cyclic AMP and glucocorticoid. *Mol Pharmacol* 1992;42:989–908.

15. Funakoshi H, Okuno S, Fujisawa H. Different effects on activity caused by phosphorylation of tyrosine hydroxylase at serine 40 by three multifunctional protein kinases. *J Biol Chem* 1991;266:15614–15620.

16. Gizang-Ginsberg E, Ziff EB. Nerve growth factor regulates tyrosine hydroxylase gene transcription through a nucleoprotein complex that contains c-Fos. *Genes Dev* 1990;4:447–491.

17. Goldstein M, Harada K, Meller E, Schalling M, Hokfelt T. Dopamine autoreceptors: biochemical, pharmacological and morphological studies. In: Kalsner S, Westfall TC, eds. *Presynaptic receptors and the question of autoregulation of neurotransmitter release*, vol 604. New York: NY Academy of Sciences, 1990;69–75.

18. Goldstein M, Wu J, Tang D, Haycock J. L-Dopa formation and phosphorylation of tyrosine hydroxylase (TH) in AtT-20 cells expressing wild type or a serine 40 mutant of TH. *Soc Neurosci* 1993;19:6958.

19. Gomez N, Tonks NK, Morrison C, Harmar T, Cohen P. Evidence for communication between nerve growth factor and protein tyrosine phosphorylation. *FEBS Lett* 1990;271:119–122.

20. Griffith LC, Schulman H. The multifunctional Ca^{2+}/calmodulin-dependent protein kinase mediates Ca^{2+}-dependent phosphorylation of tyrosine hydroxylase. *J Biol Chem* 1988;263:9542–9549.

21. Grima B, Lamouroux A, Boni C, Julien JF, Javoy-Agid F, Mallet J. A single human gene encoding multiple tyrosine hydroxylases with different predicted functional characteristics. *Nature* 1987;326:707–711.

22. Guitart X, Hayward M, Nisenbaum LK, Beitner-Johnson DB, Haycock JW, Nestler EJ. Identification of MARPP-58, a morphine- and cyclic AMP-regulated phosphoprotein of 58 kDa, as tyrosine hydroxylase: evidence for regulation of its expression by chronic morphine in the rat locus coeruleus. *J Neurosci* 1990;10:2649–2659.

23. Haavik J, Schelling D, Campbell DG, Andersson KK, Flatmark T, Cohen P. Identification of protein phosphatase 2A as the major tyrosine hydroxylase phosphatase in adrenal medulla and corpus striatum: evidence from the effects of okadaic acid. *FEBS Lett* 1989;251:36–42.

24. Haavik J, Le Bourdelles B, Martinez A, Flatmark T, Mallet J. Recombinant human tyrosine hydroxylase isozymes: reconstitution with iron and inhibitory effect of other metal ions. *Eur J Biochem* 1991;199:371–378.

25. Harada K, Meller E, Goldstein M. Effects of pertussis toxin on inhibition of synaptosomal tyrosine hydroxylase activity by apomorphine. *Eur J Pharmacol Mol Pharmacol Section* 1990;188:123–128.

26. Haycock JW. Phosphorylation of tyrosine hydroxylase *in situ* at serine 8, 19, 31 and 40. *J Biol Chem* 1990;265:11682–11691.

27. Haycock JW. Multiple signaling pathways in bovine chromaffin cells regulate tyrosine hydroxylase phosphorylation at Ser19, Ser31, and Ser40. *Neurochem Res* 1993;18:15–26.

28. Haycock JW. Multiple forms of tyrosine hydroxylase in human neuroblastoma cells: quantitation with isoform-specific antibodies. *J Neurochem* 1993;60:493–502.

29. Haycock J, Haycock DA. Tyrosine hydroxylase in rat brain dopaminergic nerve terminals: multiple phosphorylation *in vivo* and in synaptosomes. *J Biol Chem* 1991;266:5650–5657.

30. Haycock JW, Wakade AR. Activation and multiple-site phosphorylation of tyrosine hydroxylase in perfused rat adrenal glands. *J Neurochem* 1992;58:57–64.

31. Haycock JW, Ahn NG, Cobb MH, Krebs EG. ERK1 and ERK2, two microtubule-associated protein 2 kinases, mediate the phosphorylation of tyrosine hydroxylase at serine-31 *in situ*. *Proc Natl Acad Sci USA* 1992;89:2365–2369.

32. Ichimura T, Isobe T, Okuyama T, et al. Molecular cloning of cDNA coding for brain-specific 14-3-3 protein, a protein kinase-dependent activator of tyrosine and tryptophan hydroxylases. *Proc Natl Acad Sci USA* 1984;85:7084–7088.

33. Kaplan DR, Hempstead BL, Martin-Zanca D, Chao MV, Parada LF. The trk proto-oncogene product: a signal transducing receptor for nerve growth factor. *Science* 1991;252:554–558.

34. Katz IR, Tamauchi T, Kaufman S. Activation of tyrosine hydroxylase by polyanions and salts: an electrostatic effect. *Biochem Biophys Acta* 1976;429:84–95.

35. Labatut R, Buda M, Berod A. Long-term changes in rat brain tyrosine hydroxylase following reserpine treatment: a quantitative immunochemical analysis. *J Neurochem* 1988;50:1375–1380.

36. Lee KY, Lew JY, Wu J, Tang D, Goldstein M. The recognition of phosphatase and site-specific tyrosinse hydroxylase (TH) by anti-pTH-16. *Proc Soc Neurosci* 1993;19:303.2.

37. Lew JY, Lee KY, Goldstein M, Deutch A. Generation of state-specific antibodies to a segment of tyrosine hydroxylase (TH). *Proc Soc Neurosci* 1992;18:578.13.

38. Lewis EJ, Tank AW, Weiner, Chikaraishi DM. Regulation of tyrosine hydroxylase mRNA by glucocorticoids and cyclic AMP in a rat pheochromocytoma cell line: isolation of cDNA clone for tyrosine hydroxylase mRNA. *J Biol Chem* 1983;258:14632–14637.

39. Lewis EJ, Harrington CA, Chikaraishi DM. Transcriptional regulation of the tyrosine hydroxylase gene by glucocorticoid and cyclic AMP. *Proc Natl Acad Sci USA* 1987;84:3550–3554.

40. Lovenberg WE, Bruckwick EA, Hanbauer I. ATP, cyclic AMP, and magnesium increase the affinity of rat striatal tyrosine hydroxylase for its cofactor. *Proc Natl Acad Sci USA* 1975;72:2955–2958.

41. MacNico M, Schulman H. Cross-talk between protein kinase C and multifunctional Ca^{2+}/calmodulin protein kinase. *J Biol Chem* 1992;267:12197–12201.

42. Markey KA, Kondo S, Shenkman L, Goldstein M. Purification and characterization of tyrosine hydroxylase from a clonal pheochromocytoma cell line. *Mol Pharmacol* 1980;17:79–85.

43. Melia KR, Duman RS. Involvement of corticotropin releasing factor in chronic stress regulation of the brain noradrenergic system. *Proc Natl Acad Sci USA* 1991;88:8382–8386.

44. Melia KR, Rasmussen K, Terwilliger RZ, Haycock JW, Nestler EJ, Duman RS. Coordinate regulation of the cyclic AMP system with firing rate and expression of tyrosine hydroxylase in the rat locus coeruleus: effects of chronic stress and drug treatments. *J Neurochem* 1992;58:494–502.

45. Mitchell JP, Hardie DG, Vulliet PR. Site-specific phosphorylation of tyrosine hydroxylase after KCl depolarization and nerve growth factor treatment of PC12 cells. *J Biol Chem* 1990;265:22358–22364.

46. Morgenroth VI III, Hegstrand LR, Roth RH, Greengard P. Evidence for involvement of protein kinase in the activation by adenosine 3'5'-monophosphate of brain tyrosine 3-monooxygenase. *J Biol Chem* 1975;250:1946–1948.

47. Nagatsu T, Levitt BG, Udenfriend S. Tyrosine hydroxylase: the initial step in norepinephrine biosynthesis. *J Biol Chem* 1964;238:2910–2917.

48. Nelson TJ, Kaufman S. Interaction of tyrosine hydroxylase with ribonucleic acid and purification with DNA-cellulose or poly(A)-sepharose affinity chromatography. *Arch Biochem Biophys* 1987;257:69–84.

49. O'Malley KL, Anhalt MJ, Martin BM, Kelsoe JR, Winfield SL,

Ginns EI. Isolation and characterization of the human tyrosine hydroxylase gene: identification of 5' alternative splice sites responsible for multiple mRNAs. *Biochemistry* 1987;26:6910–6914.

50. Ouimet CC, McGuinness TL, Greengard P. Immunocytochemical localization of calcium/calmodulin-dependent protein kinase II in rat brain. *Proc Natl Acad Sci USA* 1984;81:5604–5608.

51. Reis DJ, Joh TG, Ross RA, Pickel VM. Reserpine selectively increases tyrosine hydroxylase and dopamine-β-hydroxylase enzyme protein in central noradrenergic neurons. *Brain Res* 1974;81:380–386.

52. Richard F, Faucon-Biguet M, Labatut R, Rollet D, Mallet J, Buda M. Modulation of tyrosine hydroxylase gene expression in rat brain and adrenals by exposure to cold. *J Neurosci Res* 1988;20:32–37.

53. Rowland E, Muller TH, Goldstein M, Greene LA. Cell-free detection and characterization of a novel nerve growth factor-activated protein kinase in PC12 cells. *J Biol Chem* 1987;262:7504–7513.

54. Rowland-Gagne E, Greene LA. Multiple pathways of N-kinase activation in PC12 cells. *J Neurochem* 1990;54:424–433.

55. Spector S, Gordon R, Sjoerdsma A, Udenfriend S. Endproduct inhibition of tyrosine hydroxylase as a possible mechanism for regulation of norepinephrine synthesis. *Mol Pharmacol* 1967;3:549–555.

56. Tank AW, Curella P, Ham L. Induction of tyrosine hydroxylase by cyclic AMP and glucocorticoids in a rat pheochromocytoma cell line: evidence for the regulation of tyrosine hydroxylase synthesis by multiple mechanisms in cells exposed to elevated levels of both inducing agents. *Mol Pharmacol* 1986;30:497–503.

57. Tank AW, Ham L, Curella P. Induction of tyrosine hydroxylase by cyclic AMP and glucocorticoids in a rat pheochromocytoma cell line: effect of the inducing agents alone or in combination on the enzyme levels and rate of synthesis of tyrosine hydroxylase. *Mol Pharmacol* 1986;30:486–496.

58. Vrana KE, Roskoski R Jr. Tyrosine hydroxylase inactivation following cAMP-dependent phosphorylation activation. *J Neurochem* 1983;40:1692–1700.

59. Vulliet PR, Langan TA, Weiner N. Tyrosine hydroxylase: a substrate of cyclic AMP-dependent protein kinase. *Proc Natl Acad Sci USA* 1980;77:92–96.

60. Vulliet PR, Hall FL, Mitchell JP, Hardie DG. Identification of a novel proline-directed serine/threonine protein kinase in rat pheochromocytoma. *J Biol Chem* 1989;264:16292–16298.

61. Vyas S, Faucon Biguet N, Mallet J. Transcriptional and post-transcriptional regulation of tyrosine hydroxylase gene by protein kinase C. *EMBO J* 1990;9:3707–3712.

62. Wolf ME, Roth RH. Autoreceptor regulation of dopamine synthesis. In: Kalsner S, Westfall TC, eds. *Presynaptic receptors and the question of autoregulation of neurotransmitter release,* vol 604. New York: NY Academy of Sciences, 1990;323–343.

63. Wu J, Filer D, Friedhoff AJ, Goldstein M. Site-directed mutagenesis of tyrosine hydroxylase: role of serine-40 in catalysis. *J Biol Chem* 1992;267:17373–17378.

64. Yamauchi T, Nakata H, Fujisawa H. Tyrosine 3-monooxygenase is phosphorylated by Ca^{2+}-calmodulin-dependent protein kinase followed by activation by activator protein. *Biochem Biophys Res Commun* 1981;100:807–813.

Psychopharmacology: The Fourth Generation of Progress, edited by Floyd E. Bloom and David J. Kupfer. Raven Press, Ltd., New York © 1995.

CHAPTER 18

Colocalization in Dopamine Neurons

Ariel Y. Deutch and Andrew J. Bean

It has been a generation since the discovery that multiple chemical messengers can be present in a single neuron. The definition of generation in this case is the conventional temporal one of 20 years. In contrast, the generation in the title of the series *Psychopharmacology: Generation of Progress* is an intellectual one, which seems to occur about every 5 years. Both definitions apply to colocalization in central neurons, because in the 20-odd years since colocalization has been documented there have been marked advances in our understanding of the varieties of colocalization and the mechanisms that are operative in neurons with multiple messengers.

The presence of multiple transmitters or proteins in single cells also presents other problems in terminology. The term *coexistence* may be inappropriate because it implies the presence of two or more transmitters in the same vesicle. Moreover, the adjective *peaceful* is frequently used to modify coexistence, yet there are hints that multiple transmitters may have antagonistic effects, both pre- and postsynaptically. We suggest that colocalization may offer a slight advantage, although it is clearly not ideal.

Colocalization of neuroactive substances occurs in virtually all types of neurons. In this chapter, we review briefly the status of colocalization in central dopamine (DA) neurons. Several recent reviews cover the general field of colocalization from different perspectives and emphasize different aspects (2,31,33). By necessity, our review is selective. We have attempted to convey the richness and complexity of colocalization in DA neurons, and to relate in certain cases the significance of colocalization

to neuropsychiatric disorders (see also Chapter 43, *this volume*).

GENERAL CONSIDERATIONS

Dale's Principle

Almost concurrent with the discovery (if not acceptance) of chemical neurotransmission, Dale (13) hypothesized that a neuron extends its metabolic activity from the soma to all of its processes. In its most basic form, this principle posits only that metabolic processes that occur in the soma can reach or influence events occurring in distal parts of the neurons. Dale's principle was restated and expanded by Eccles (17) to suggest that a neuron releases the same transmitter at all of its processes. Both of these formulations can accommodate multiple messengers in a single neuron, requiring only that the molecules be distributed in all processes. However, recent data indicate that multiple peptide transmitters are targeted to different processes within a single *Aplysia* neuron (57); the degree to which such compartmentation is present in mammals is not clear (however, see ref. 30). The presence of the same peptide in different processes indicates that there are exceptions to Dale's principle, and it suggests that single neurons containing multiple transmitters may have the ability to spatially direct different types of output.

Physiological Mechanisms of Differential Release of Colocalized Messengers

The functional significance of colocalization within a single neuron remains unclear. Spatially directed output of different transmitters has been described only in certain simple systems. The difficulties in defining the functional role(s) of colocalization stem from the lack of much basic information concerning both pre- and postsynaptic as-

A. Y. Deutch: Departments of Psychiatry and Pharmacology, Yale University School of Medicine, and Psychiatry Service, New Haven, Connecticut; and Department of Veteran Affairs Medical Center, West Haven, Connecticut 06508.

A. J. Bean: Howard Hughes Medical Institute, Department of Molecular and Cellular Physiology, Stanford University, Stanford, California 94305.

pects of neurotransmission, particularly those processes that package and prepare for release chemical messengers. We briefly review these processes below.

Despite the gaps in our knowledge, we are beginning to catch glimpses of the functions of multiple chemical messengers. Using simple systems in which peptide effects are well-defined, peptides have been shown to act at sites distant to the immediate postsynaptic membrane (37). Differences in presynaptic release mechanisms (44,63) have also provided a clue to the physiological role of colocalized messengers. Evidence gathered from experiments in simple defined systems has suggested that peptide and nonpeptide messengers may provide both temporally and spatially resolved signals (37,44).

Two pathways are used by neurons to secrete proteins. The constitutive pathway, which is not triggered by extracellular stimulation, is used to secrete membrane components, viral proteins, growth factors, and extracellular matrix molecules; this pathway acts by continuous fusion of Golgi-derived vesicles with the plasma membrane. In contrast, the release of chemical messengers is controlled by extracellular signals and uses the so-called regulated pathway (39). The usual route followed by peptide proteins secreted via the regulated pathway involves synthesis of precursors containing an N-terminal signal sequence, which are targeted to the endoplasmic reticulum (ER) and subsequently translocated into the ER lumen. The complex is then transported from the *cis-* to the *trans-*Golgi compartment and to the *trans-*Golgi network where peptides are packaged into large (~100 nm) dense-core vesicles (DCVs), which are moved to the terminal (39).

Another population of vesicles, the synaptic vesicles (SVs), can be distinguished from DCVs on the basis of size, content, and membrane composition. These small (~50 nm) vesicles are electron-lucent and contain classical transmitters such as DA. SVs are formed from the ER and transported to the terminal, or directly recycled at the terminal, and transmitters are accumulated by specific transporters that are driven by proton pumps of the vesicular membrane (39). Thus, peptide and nonpeptide transmitters are for the most part segregated in their formation and localization in the cell. Recent evidence points to distinct but related molecular mechanisms responsible for the release of DCV and SV contents (7).

The release of multiple messengers, and the molar ratios of release of the colocalized substances, depends upon cellular activity (2,9,36,60). Both firing frequency and the pattern of cell firing govern the relative release of colocalized messengers. Increases in firing frequency promote increases in the ratio of peptide/nonpeptide release (2,44,60), while short bursts of high-frequency stimulation may preferentially activate processes responsible for peptide release (44).

Thus, there are two sets of processes that synthesize and package transmitters and that govern the activity-dependent release of these compounds. What brings these two sets of processes together may be differences in the temporal and spatial characteristics of intraterminal calcium levels (56).

Methodological Issues

The ability to define colocalization requires the unambiguous definition of a uniform population of cells. This has led to immunohistochemical methods being the main approach to defining colocalization, although biochemical techniques have been useful adjunct methods. In contrast, biochemical and electrophysiological methods have in general been more useful for elucidating the functional significance of colocalization.

The problems inherent in immunohistochemical approaches to colocalization have been discussed in several recent reviews (see refs. 31 and 33). Nonetheless, several methodological issues may be worth discussing. Most studies of colocalization focus on the cell body of neurons, because the soma generally contains more of the protein and because of the difficulty in unambiguously defining preterminal axons under light-microscopic conditions. This can be problematic, because different parts of the same neuron do not invariably express a given protein (30,57). The use of confocal microscopy may lead to a greater emphasis on defining colocalization in axons.

The use of *in situ* hybridization histochemistry to define specific mRNAs has opened new doors to the study of colocalization, particularly in primates. The underlying assumption is that the mRNA is appropriately translated and post-translationally modified to yield a functional protein. Unfortunately, it is difficult to verify this assumption. Still more problematic is the possibility that certain mRNAs are not expressed under basal conditions, but are expressed only under certain challenge conditions (see refs. 5 and 14).

A factor not often discussed is the nature of the colocalized substances. In cases of colocalization between two presumptive transmitters, we generally assume that the compounds are indeed neurotransmitters. Those criteria that are commonly used to define a transmitter are based on data derived from studies of classical (autonomic) transmitters, perhaps biasing the designation of other categories, such as peptidergic transmitters. Nonetheless, as the numbers of colocalized ''transmitters'' grow in parallel with the numbers of journal issues, it is appropriate to consider whether a designated molecule functions as a transmitter or has another role.

FORMS OF COLOCALIZATION

A large number of studies have addressed the anatomical and physiological aspects of colocalization between DA and transmitters. Much less frequently considered is the colocalization between DA and nontransmitter proteins and peptides, despite the fact that these forms of colocalization may be more prevalent. We have previously suggested an organizational framework in which to place different forms of colocalization (26).

Perhaps the simplest form of colocalization is the presence of DA and a protein or peptide that does not subserve a role as a transmitter, receptor, or transporter. Obviously, among such examples could be enzymes that are ubiquitously present in cells (hexose-6-phosphate) or neurons (neuron-specific enolase) of the mature central nervous system (CNS). The uniform presence of these enzymes suggests that the inclusion of this form of colocalization is not very helpful in attempts to arrive at an organizing scheme. However, a number of proteins and peptides are heterogeneously distributed in the CNS and are found in certain DA neurons. An example is the vitamin D_{28} calcium-binding protein calbindin (24).

Transporter proteins serve an important role as a means of terminating transmitter action, and therefore are generally (although not invariably) associated with neurons from which their substrate is released. Thus, the dopamine transporter mRNA is present in most (if not all) DA neurons, although the extent to which the actual transporter protein is expressed and functional is not clear (see below). Similarly, neurons can express proteins that serve as autoreceptors or heteroceptors. Among the former are the release-modulating autoreceptor of DA neurons (which biochemical studies suggest is present on all DA neurons) and the synthesis-modulating autoreceptor of DA neurons (expressed in most, but not all, DA neurons). DA neurons also contain a large number of heteroceptors, including ligand-gated ion channel receptors (e.g., nicotinic acetylcholine receptor) and G-protein-coupled receptors (e.g., neurotensin receptor), emphasizing the importance of afferent regulation for DA neurons.

Colocalization of classical transmitters is still another category. For example, several groups of DA neurons also contain γ-aminobutyric acid (GABA). Colocalization of classical and nonclassical transmitters represent the form of colocalization most frequently discussed. Peptidergic transmitters are found in a number of different DA cell groups, ranging from the presence of cholecystokinin (CCK) in midbrain DA neurons to growth-hormone-releasing factor (GH-RF) in dopaminergic cells of the arcuate nucleus.

Finally, there are a number of cells that express higher-order combinations of the above-described categories. For example, some midbrain DA neurons contain DA, a peptide (neurotensin or CCK, or both), and a nontransmitter protein (calbindin; see ref. 24).

COLOCALIZATION OF DA AND NONTRANSMITTER NEUROACTIVE PEPTIDES AND PROTEINS

There are a large number of nontransmitter proteins and peptides that are present in central DA neurons. These range from receptors to proteins involved in calcium se-

questration. Although in many cases the functional significance of these forms of colocalization remains to be determined, the functional characteristics of the colocalized molecule in other parts of the nervous system or in non-neural tissues have led to speculations that can be empirically examined.

There are several examples in which transcripts for various transmitters or receptors have been identified in brain, but for which conclusive evidence of colocalization, such as dual staining procedures, is not available. In most brain areas the DA neurons represent but one ingredient in a stew of neurons. However, in the pars compacta of the substantia nigra (SN) the DA neurons are tightly packed, such that ≥90% of pars compacta cells are dopaminergic. Given the characteristic gross structure of the pars compacta, we have included several examples of *presumptive* colocalization based on presence in this midbrain structure. However, it is important to recognize that these examples are presumptive and that they require confirmatory studies. An excellent illustration of this problem is the fact that although 5-HT$_{2c}$ transcripts are present in cells of the pars compacta, these receptors are expressed uniformly on GABAergic, but not dopaminergic, neurons (19).

Classical Transmitter Receptors

There are almost no definitive dual-staining anatomic studies indicating the presence of receptors for classical transmitters on DA neurons. However, anatomical studies of the distribution of receptor mRNAs or proteins, electrophysiological data, and the presence of transmitter-specific terminals all strongly suggest that DA neurons express receptors for certain classical transmitters.

Dopamine Receptors

DA receptors serve as autoreceptors to regulate release and synthesis of DA and the activity of DA neurons. Thus, there are release-modulating, synthesis-modulating, and impulse-modulating autoreceptors on DA neurons (see Chapters 20 and 21, *this volume*). In situ hybridization studies have detected the presence of the D_2 DA receptor mRNA in many DA cell-body regions (see Chapter 19, *this volume*); this is consistent with pharmacological data indicating that autoreceptors in the adult exhibit a D2-like pharmacological profile. The best current data suggest that the D_2 receptors, but not the D_3 or D_4 receptors, are present on DA cells in the rodent and primate (see Chapter 19, *this volume*). If the different functional DA autoreceptors are D_2 receptors, this suggests that the type of autoreceptor role manifested is a function of transduction mechanisms rather than a function of the receptor differences.

Although it is clear that there are D_2 DA receptor transcripts in midbrain cells, there are no published studies documenting the invariant association of D2 mRNA and DA in neurons using dual-label procedures (see Chapters 14 and 19, *this volume*). While the distribution of D_2 mRNA-containing cells in the rat suggests an excellent correspondence, preliminary data in the primate suggests that midline DA cells may not express the D_2 receptor (J. Meador-Woodruff, *personal communication*).

Nicotinic Acetylcholine Receptors

Immunohistochemical studies of the nicotinic cholinergic receptor (see Chapter 9, *this volume*) have revealed dense immunoreactivity of cells in the pars compacta of the SN and ventral tegmental area (VTA) (15). Studies of the distribution of mRNAs encoding different subunits of the nicotinic acetylcholine receptor also suggest the presence of α_1, α_3, α_4, α_5, and β_2 subunits on A9 and A10 DA neurons (62). While most of the subunits that form heteromeric channels are present in the midbrain DA neurons, it appears that some are not (e.g., α_2 and α_7). The precise assembly of the subunits may confer different receptor properties on different DA neurons.

GABA$_A$ Receptors

The GABA$_A$ receptor complex is a multimeric ion channel assembly with several associated allosteric modulatory sites. There are over 10 subunits, which are differentially expressed; different subunit compositions of the receptor confer different functional properties (59). The α_3, α_4, β_3, and β_4 are present in the pars compacta, suggesting that these subunits may be expressed in A9 DA cells (64). The use of subunit specific antibodies has led to the conclusion that DA cells of the pars compacta express a GABA$_A$ receptor that consists of subunits α_3 and γ_2 (22). A large body of data indicates the presence of GABA$_A$ receptors on both DA and non-DA neurons in the SN and VTA.

Excitatory Amino Acid Receptors

Receptors for excitatory amino acids, including glutamate and aspartate, are present on most neurons in the CNS, including DA cells (see Chapter 7, *this volume*). Both N-methyl-D-aspartate (NMDA) and non-NMDA excitatory amino acid receptors are thought to be present in certain DA neurons. For example, the GluR1 AMPA family receptor is expressed in VTA and pars compacta neurons, and both flip and flop forms of the GluR1 mRNA are seen in the SN and VTA (46). Other AMPA family receptors (GluR2/3 and GluR4) are also present in the SN and VTA. Pharmacological studies also indicate that these excitatory amino acid receptors are present on DA neurons, but more conclusive dual-staining procedures are required to confirm this (see Chapter 7, *this volume*).

Serotonin Receptors

There is a paucity of information on the direct electrophysiological effects of serotonin on central DA neurons, and there is a similar lack of anatomical data suggesting the presence of serotonin receptors on DA neurons. There are over a dozen serotonin receptors (the rate at which new ones are cloned suggests that it is prudent not to specify an exact number), some of which are present only in certain species (see Chapter 37, *this volume*). 5-HT$_{2c}$ (previously designated 5-HT$_{1c}$) receptor transcripts are present in cells of the pars compacta, suggestive of colocalization in the A9 DA neurons. However, Chesselet and colleagues (19) have found that those pars compacta cells that express 5-HT$_{2c}$ mRNA are exclusively nondopaminergic.

Peptide Receptors

Electrophysiological and biochemical pharmacology as well as autoradiographic studies suggest the presence of a number of peptidergic receptors on DA neurons. In many cases, *in situ* hybridization and immunohistochemistry, or studies using lesion methods, have confirmed the presence of peptidergic receptors on DA neurons (see Chapter 43, *this volume*).

Tachykinin Receptors

Three tachykinin receptors (NK1, NK2, and NK3) respond to central tachykinins, including substance P, neurokinin A, and neurokinin B (41). A high density of NK1 receptor sites has been demonstrated by autoradiographic studies, and *in situ* hybridization suggests that these receptors are present on DA neurons of the pars compacta. There are substantial species differences in expression of tachykinin receptors, both across different rodents as well as between rodents and primates. The presence of a few scattered tachykinin-containing neurons in the VTA of the rat suggests the possibility that these cells exhibit tachykinin autoreceptors; further studies will be required to determine if these tachykinin-containing cells are also dopaminergic.

Neurotensin Receptors

Neurotensin (NT) is colocalized with certain midbrain DA neurons and DA neurons in the arcuate nucleus (20), as are NT-containing axon terminals. Autoradiographic studies have indicated a high density of NT receptors in the SN that are associated with DA neurons, as have recent in situ hybridization data (18,65). It is not clear if the coexistent DA–NT cells express NT receptors. Surprisingly, although several lines of evidence indicate that NT receptors are expressed on nigral DA neurons, the

NT innervation of the SN is directed to the non-DA neurons (65), suggesting a ligand–receptor mismatch (see also Chapter 51, *this volume*).

Cholecystokinin Receptors

There are two forms of CCK receptors, CCK-A and CCK-B, both showing considerable species variability in distribution. The regulation of the mesotelencephalic DA neurons through CCK receptors has been extensively examined using pharmacological approaches. Many of these data suggest that CCK modulates DA function primarily through CCK-A receptors. However, a recent in situ hybridization study indicates that CCK-B, but not CCK-A, transcripts are present in the pars compacta and VTA (35), suggesting colocalization; dual staining procedures have not yet been performed.

Because CCK is found in most nigral DA neurons in the rat (see below), the presence of the CCK-B receptor in many neurons of the pars compacta raises the possibility that the CCK-B site functions as an autoreceptor on these neurons (see also Chapter 52, *this volume*).

Opioid Receptors

A large body of data indicates that opioid peptides regulate DA neurons in the hypothalamus and midbrain. Autoradiographic data indicate a moderate density of κ receptors throughout the hypothalamus, including the arcuate nucleus. In the pars compacta and VTA, there is a high density of μ-opioid receptors but a low density of κ sites (45). However, the μ receptors revealed by autoradiography in the pars compacta appear to be primarily associated with afferents, because μ transcripts are present only in scattered neurons in the SN and VTA (58). In contrast, an mRNA encoding for the κ receptor is abundant in the pars compacta (48). Thus, the present data suggest that κ receptors are expressed in many DA neurons of the SN; this interpretation requires confirmation using dual-labeling procedures (see also Chapter 46, *this volume*).

Glucocorticoid Receptor

Autoradiographic studies and the availability of antisera to the glucocorticoid receptor led to the finding that although glucocorticoid receptors are distributed almost homogeneously across the CNS if one considered very low levels, certain neurons stand out sharply by expressing large amounts of the protein. The monoaminergic cells of the brain are among the sites in which the glucocorticoid receptor is present in high amounts. All DA neurons in the hypothalamic arcuate nucleus (A12 cell group), the majority of cells in the A13 cell group (zona incerta), and all of the A14 cells (periventricular hypothal-

amus) expressed the glucocorticoid receptor (29). In the midbrain, 40–70% of the DA cells expressed the glucocorticoid receptor, with A10 DA cells in the VTA having strong immunoreactivity. Although there has been a wide appreciation of the role of glucocorticoids in the hypothalamo-hypophyseal axis, less is known about how glucocorticoids impact on the dopaminergic function in the mesotelencephalic system. Recent data suggest that glucocorticoids may play an important permissive role in the development of sensitization of DA neurons to drugs of abuse (see also Chapters 62 and 67, *this volume*).

Other Receptors

There are several receptors for which pharmacological data indicate a role in regulating central DA neurons, particularly in the hypothalamus; indeed, there are data to support virtually every peptide as a regulator in this region. In virtually all of these studies, it is impossible to parcel out direct and indirect effects. Because conclusive data concerning colocalization with these receptors are lacking, we will not review these data.

Colocalization of Transporters and DA

A large number of transport molecules have recently been cloned. These do not appear to share a single-membrane topography, but they all function in the reuptake of released transmitter.

Membrane DA Transporter

Dopamine neurons express a membrane reuptake process that is the major means of terminating dopaminergic transmission. The DA transporter (DAT) has recently been cloned, and the DAT mRNA is expressed at detectable levels in most, but not all, DA neurons (1,47). Pharmacological data suggest that a functional DAT is not present on tuberoinfundibular DA neurons; DAT transcripts are either absent or below detection threshold in DA neurons of the ventrolateral arcuate nucleus (47). There have been suggestions that distinct DATs may arise from regionally specific differences in post-translational processes, particularly glycosylation; there are no current data to indicate the presence of more than one DAT mRNA. Interestingly, the DA transporter has reasonable affinities for norepinephrine, serotonin, and epinephrine as well as for DA (see Chapter 16, *this volume*).

Vesicular Monoamine Transporter

In addition to the membrane DA transporter, a vesicular monoamine transporter has recently been cloned (43). This transporter is present in DA neurons, and it is thought to be of importance in packaging DA into the vesicle for subsequent release. In addition, the sequestering of DA by the vesicular monoamine transporter may be of importance in preventing DA from attack by free radicals.

Other Transporters

There are suggestive data concerning the presence of several other transporters in nigral DA neurons. These include the GAT-3 (previously termed GAT-B) GABA transporter (12), one form of the alternatively spliced glycine transporter (10), and SV2, a synaptic vesicle transporter of unknown function (8).

DA and Non-receptor, Non-transporter Proteins

There are several examples of proteins which are heterogeneously distributed in the CNS but which are not transmitters, receptors, or transporters and which are present in DA neurons. We briefly discuss a few well-documented cases.

Acetylcholinesterase

Probably the best known of these is acetylcholinesterase (AChE), which conventional histochemical methods showed to be present in high concentrations in catecholaminergic neurons, prominently including the A9 DA cells of the SN (see ref. 27). AChE in nigral DA neurons does not appear to function (at least predominantly) as a metabolic enzyme for acetylcholine, although there is a sparse cholinergic input to this region. AChE has been documented to be released from dendrites of these DA neurons in response to certain stimuli (27). The specific functions subserved by AChE in DA neurons remain unclear (27).

Vitamin D$_{28}$ Calcium-Binding Protein

Calbindin is present in distinct subsets of midbrain DA neurons (23,24). Neurons in the dorsal tier of the pars compacta, which project to the islandic (patch) compartment of the striatum, contain calbindin, as do certain DA neurons in the VTA (23). The functional role of calbindin (other than regulation of intracellular calcium stores) in these neurons remains obscure, although there have been speculations that the enzyme may play a neuroprotective role (see below).

NADPH Cytochrome P450 Reductase

Microsomal mixed function oxidases that are of importance in xenobiotic metabolism are found in high concentration in the liver. Antibodies generated against the purified hepatic enzyme NADPH cytochrome P450 reductase stain monoaminergic cells of the brainstem, including the midbrain DA neurons and the A11, A12, and A13 cells of the hypothalamus (28). Although most DA neurons in these regions are immunoreactive for the enzyme, there are also non-DA cells that express NADPH cytochrome P450 reductase. The functional significance of this colocalized protein is not known, although its hepatic function suggests that it may play a role in metabolism of, and hence protection from, certain toxins.

DT Diaphorase

NAD(P)H:quinone oxidoreductase (DT diaphorase) is a dicoumarol-sensitive enzyme that catalyzes the reduction of NADH and NADPH in the presence of quinones. DT diaphorase is present in a subset of midbrain DA neurons, as well as in glial cells (52). The function of this enzyme in DA neurons is not known, but because it reduces catecholamine quinones to hydroquinones it may be of importance in protecting DA neurons from toxic free radicals.

Growth Factors

One of the most interesting groups of proteins that are colocalized with DA neurons are neurotrophic factors. Several neurotrophic factors, including acidic and basic fibroblast growth factors (6), brain-derived neurotrophic factor (53), and neurotropin-3 (53), are expressed in midbrain DA neurons. In contrast, other trophic factors, including nerve growth factor and NT-4, are not present in detectable amounts, and still others (ciliary neurotrophic factor, transforming growth factor α) have not been examined (53). Glial-derived growth factor is presumably not present in DA neurons, but this remains to be determined.

Although the proposed function of growth factors is obvious, the presence of growth factors in DA neurons leads to several questions. Growth factors are thought to provide trophic support for afferent neurons. Because several of the growth factors appear to be of benefit in preventing DA cell death or enhancing cell survival in various paradigms, it is not clear if the function of the growth factors present in DA cells is to support afferents (e.g., striatonigral neurons) or to support the same DA neurons that elaborate the growth factors. Alternatively, the growth factors could provide trophic support for adjacent DA cells or intramesencephalic DA afferents.

COLOCALIZATION OF DA AND CLASSICAL TRANSMITTERS

There are perhaps fewer examples of coexistence of DA and classical transmitters than any other category. This may simply be due to there being fewer so-called "classical" transmitters than "modern" (and even "post-modern," e.g., nitric oxide) transmitters.

GABA-DA Colocalization

The only well-documented classical transmitter that is present in central DA neurons is GABA. Colocalized DA–GABA neurons are found in the arcuate nucleus of the hypothalamus and in the periglomerular cells of the olfactory bulb (20,21). Despite the fact that there are few cases of colocalization of classical transmitters and DA, DA–GABA colocalization in the olfactory bulb is seen across several species, being present in insects and reptiles as well as in mammals (16,40).

Glutamate–DA Colocalization

In addition to GABA, there is some evidence that glutamate may be colocalized with DA neurons in the midbrain. Midbrain DA neurons are strongly immunoreactive for phosphate-activated glutaminase (38), which is thought to be the biosynthetic enzyme for the transmitter pool of glutamate. The colocalization of DA and glutamate awaits verification using other approaches.

COLOCALIZATION OF DA AND PEPTIDE TRANSMITTERS

Probably the best-known form of colocalization is that of the DA and a neuropeptide transmitter. There are a large number of peptidergic transmitters that are found in DA neurons; in many cases two peptides are present with DA in single cells. Despite the fact that peptidergic neurons in the arcuate nucleus of the hypothalamus are so frequent as to resemble a pointilistic construction, perhaps the best-characterized colocalized populations of DA–peptide cells are those in the ventral mesencephalon.

Neurotensin–DA Colocalization

NT–DA-containing neurons are found in the mesencephalon and hypothalamus of the rat. There is a colocalized population of neurons in the arcuate nucleus (20), and NT cells are present in the A10 DA neurons of the VTA (32). NT is also found in CCK-containing DA neurons in the VTA (55). NT-containing neurons of the VTA are clearly seen in the rat using immunohistochemical methods, but in contrast are not apparent in primate species (15). A recent in situ hybridization paper has revealed that the NT/neuromedin N (NMN) transcript is present in a small population of cells in the ventral mesencephalon of primates, including that of humans (4). It is not known if the NT/NMN mRNA is translated to the mature peptide species in primates.

NT–DA colocalized cells in the VTA project to a num-

ber of forebrain targets, including the prefrontal cortex (PFC). In fact, all NT axons in the PFC have been suggested to contain DA (see ref. 14). The presence of a colocalized population of NT-containing axons in the PFC, a region that does not receive NT-containing innervations from regions other than the ventral midbrain, has allowed the in vivo investigation of features governing the release of colocalized neurons (2).

One other aspect of NT–DA colocalization in midbrain DA cells suggests a novel function of colocalization. Under certain conditions, NT injected directly into the striatum is taken up by nigrostriatal DA terminals and retrogradely transported to the SN (11) via a rapid transport process. The mechanism through which NT is taken up by the DA terminals is not clear, but may represent internalization of a ligand–receptor complex. The number of pars compacta cells expressing TH mRNA after intrastriatal injection of either NT or its active fragment NT_{8-13} has been reported to be increased by ~40% (11). This is clearly an unusual role for a colocalized peptide, particularly in light of the suggestion that the retrogradely transported peptide increases the number of neurons expressing TH mRNA rather than increasing the abundance of the transcript per cell (see ref. 14). In any event, this represents a novel form of colocalization and if verified may suggest a trophic role for NT (see Chapter 51, *this volume*).

CCK–DA Cells

CCK-containing DA neurons are present in the A8, A9, and A10 cell groups of the midbrain (34). As noted above, many of these cells also contain NT and thus innervate the same forebrain targets. Also similar to NT, there are species differences in the localization of CCK (see below). Initially, CCK was thought to represent a relatively small subpopulation of A9 cells. However, the use of fixatives that preserve the antigen better and the availability of several different antibodies to CCK have revealed that most nigral DA neurons of the rat express CCK. There are considerable species differences in the degree to which CCK is expressed in DA neurons (50) (see Chapter 52, *this volume*).

Other Peptides

Several other peptides have been demonstrated to coexist in central DA neurons, particularly in the arcuate nucleus. Among these are galanin, GH-RF, and the opioid peptides dynorphin, met-enkephalin, and leu-enkephalin (20). In addition, somatostatin-containing DA cells are present in the A13 cell group of the zona incerta (20), as are some DA cells that contain calcitonin-gene related peptide (49). There are several cases of A12 DA neurons containing more than one peptide (20).

DA cells are scattered through the supramammillary

nucleus at the mes-diencephalic border. Several peptides have been found in these DA neurons, including peptide histidine isoleucine/vasoactive intestinal peptide (PHI/VIP), substance P, and CCK (54); a few of these cells contain DA, CCK, and PHI/VIP.

COLOCALIZATION AND NEUROPSYCHIATRIC DISORDERS

It is easy to understand the significance of colocalization for neuropsychiatric disorders if one simply thinks of receptor changes in various disorders. For example, there are changes in D_2 DA receptors that are seen in Parkinson's disease, including the loss of D_2 receptors related to the late-stage atrophy of dendritic spines on dopaminoceptive neurons; this results in patients who are refractory to DA replacement therapy. Less well characterized but even better known is the proposed increase in the density of striatal D_2 receptors in schizophrenic subjects. In addition to changes in receptor systems, several recent postmortem studies have led to findings that graphically illustrate the potential significance of colocalization in DA neurons. We have chosen examples from schizophrenia and Parkinson's disease (PD).

Schizophrenia

The presence of both CCK and NT in certain midbrain DA neurons has long fueled speculation that there may be alterations in both peptidergic and dopaminergic function in schizophrenia. An initial report concerning the distribution of CCK mRNA in the human brain noted that nonhuman primates do not express discernible amounts of the transcript in the SN (50); this finding fits well with reports NT-like immunoreactive neurons could not be demonstrated in the several monkey species (14). Subsequent careful studies in the human midbrain by Hökfelt and colleagues (51) fortuitously used tissue from schizophrenic subjects and found moderate expression of the CCK in the nigra, but in contrast noted that CCK mRNA is present in low abundance or below the threshold for detection in control subjects. Animal studies suggest that this difference is not due to the effects of chronic neuroleptic treatment; moreover, age, sex, and postmortem interval do not appear to contribute (51).

As mentioned above, there are species differences in NT–DA colocalization in the midbrain: NT-like immunoreactive neurons are not seen in the ventral mesencephalon of nonhuman primates (14). Again, the use of probes to the human neurotensin/neuromedin N (NT/M) gene led to the finding that there is a small population of human midbrain DA neurons that express NT/M (4). However, in contrast to CCK, there is no significant difference in the number of cells expressing NT/N and DA (or melanin) in the SN of schizophrenics (4).

While these studies illustrate the potential significance

of colocalization for clinical conditions, they paradoxically alert us to the difficulties in attempting to define the extent and role of neuronal colocalization. There are clear species differences present that unfortunately limit the ability to extrapolate from nonhuman subjects, particularly rodents. Another problem is that although the gene for a particular colocalized transmitter may be expressed, it remains unclear if the corresponding protein product is translated. Even more difficult to assess are the factors that promote transcription. For example, the degree to which CCK mRNA is expressed in the midbrain of humans appears to be quite low under normal conditions, yet given the appropriate state or trait, the CCK gene appears to be induced. It is not clear to what degree this reflects a state problem (i.e., the contribution of antipsychotic drugs) or a trait problem (schizophrenia). Thus, the study of one issue that on the surface appears relatively simple—namely, the degree to which CCK is expressed in the midbrain DA neurons of humans—opens up issues of (a) species dependency, state, and trait characteristics of the subject from whom the tissue is obtained, (b) mRNA stability and translation, and (c) factors that regulate gene expression.

Parkinson's Disease

In contrast to the coexistence of CCK or NT and DA, calbindin in midbrain DA neurons does not appear to play a direct transmitter role. Instead, calbindin appears to be of significance in sequestration of intracellular calcium stores and thus appears to be of potential importance as a neuroprotective agent. Several studies have documented that calbindin-containing DA neurons in the SN of nonhuman subjects are preferentially spared following systemic administration of the neurotoxin MPTP (42). Studies of the midbrain from PD patients have led to the same finding: There is a preferential sparing of those neurons that contain calbindin (25,61). Although there is scant evidence for direct calcium-mediated excitotoxicity in PD, these observations that calbindin-containing DA cells are resistant to the neuropathological process in PD may lead to new ideas concerning the pathophysiology of the disorder.

ACKNOWLEDGMENTS

We are indebted to Tomas Hökfelt for frequent and illuminating discussions and encouragement. We also thank Richard Scheller for his support and encouragement. This work was supported by grant MH-45124 and by the Howard Hughes Medical Institute, the National Parkinson Foundation Center of Excellence at Yale University, and the Veterans Administration National Centers for Schizophrenia Research and for Post-Traumatic Stress Disorder, West Haven VA Medical Center.

REFERENCES

1. Augood SJ, Westmore K, McKenna PJ, Emson PC. Co-expression of dopamine transporter mRNA and tyrosine hydroxylase mRNA in ventral mesencephalic neurons. *Mol Brain Res* 1993;20:328–334.
2. Bartfai T, Iverfeldt K, Fisone G, Serfozo P. Regulation of the release of coexisting neurotransmitters. *Annu Rev Pharmacol Toxicol* 1988;28:285–310.
3. Bean AJ, Roth RH. Extracellular dopamine and neurotensin in rat prefrontal cortex in vivo: effects of median forebrain bundle stimulation frequency, pattern, and dopamine autoreceptors. *J Neurosci* 1991;11:2694–2702.
4. Bean AJ, Dagerlind A, Hökfelt T, Dobner PR. Cloning of human neurotensin/neuromedin N genomic sequences and expression in the ventral mesencephalon of schizophrenics and age/sex matched controls. *Neuroscience* 1992;50:259–268.
5. Bean AJ, During MJ, Deutch AY, Roth RH. The effects of dopamine depletion on striatal neurotensin: biochemical and immunohistochemical studies. *J Neurosci* 1989;9:4430–4438.
6. Bean AJ, Elde R, Cao YH, et al. Expression of fibroblast growth factors in the substantia nigra of rat, monkey, and human. *Proc Natl Acad Sci USA* 1991;88:10237–10241.
7. Bean AJ, Zhang X, Hökfelt T. Peptide secretion: what do we know? 8:630–638.
8. Bennett M, Scheller RH. A molecular description of synaptic vesicle membrane trafficking. *Annu Rev Neurosci* 1994;63:63–100.
9. Bloom SR, Edwards AV, Garrett JR. Effects of stimulating the sympathetic innervation in bursts on submandibular vascular and secretory function in cats. *J Physiol* 1987;393:91–106.
10. Borowsky B, Mezey E, Hoffman BJ. Two glycine transporter variants with distinct localization in the CNS and peripheral tissues are encoded by a common gene. *Neuron* 1993;10:851–863.
11. Burgevin M-C, Castel M-N, Quarteronet D, Chevet T, Laduron PM. Neurotensin increases tyrosine hydroxylase messenger RNA-positive neurons in substantia nigra after retrograde axonal transport. *Neuroscience* 1992;49:627–633.
12. Clark J, Deutch AY, Gallipoli PZ, Amara S. Functional expression and CNS distribution of a β-alanine-sensitive neuronal GABA transporter. *Neuron* 1992;9:337–348.
13. Dale H. Pharmacology and nerve endings. *Proc R Soc Med* 1935;28:319–332.
14. Deutch AY, Zahm DS. The current status of neurotensin–dopamine interactions: issues and speculations. *Ann NY Acad Sci* 1992;668:232–252.
15. Deutch AY, Holliday J, Roth RH, Chun LLY, Hawrot E. Immunohistochemical localization of a neuronal nicotinic acetylcholine receptor in mammalian brain. *Proc Natl Acad Sci USA* 1987;84:8697–8701.
16. Distler P. Synaptic connections of dopamine immunoreactive neurons in the antennal lobes of *Periplaneta americana*. Colocalization with GABA-like immunoreactivity. *Histochem* 1990;93:401–408.
17. Eccles JC. Chemical transmission and Dale's principle. *Prog Brain Res* 1986;68:3–13.
18. Elde R, Schalling M, Ceccatelli S, Nakanishi S, Hökfelt T. Localization of neuropeptide receptor mRNA in rat brain: initial observations using probes for neurotensin and substance P receptors. *Neurosci Lett* 1990;120:134–138.
19. Eberle-Wang K, Mikeladze Z, Chesselet M-F. Expression of 5-HT1c receptor mRNA in the basal ganglia of rats. *Soc Neurosci Abstr* 1993;19:132.
20. Everitt BJ, Meister B, Hökfelt T, et al. The hypothalamic arcuate nucleus–median eminence complex: immunohistochemistry of transmitters, peptides and DARPP-32 with special reference to coexistence in dopamine neurons. *Brain Res Rev* 1986;11:97–155.
21. Gall CM, Hendry SHC, Seroogy KB, Jones EG, Haycock JW. Evidence for coexistence of GABA and dopamine in neurons of the rat olfactory bulb. *J Comp Neurol* 1987;266:307–318.
22. Fritschy J-M, Benke D, Mertens S, Oertel WH, Bach T, Mohler H. Five subtypes of type A gamma-aminobutyric acid receptors identified in neurons by double and triple immunofluorescence staining with subunit-specific antibodies. *Proc Natl Acad Sci USA* 1992;89:6726–6730.
23. Gerfen CR, Herkenham M, Thibault J. The neostriatal mosaic. III.

Biochemical and developmental dissociation of patch-matrix mesostriatal systems. *J Neurosci* 1987;7:3915.
24. German DC, Liang C-L. Neuroactive peptides in the midbrain dopaminergic neurons that contain calbindin-D_{28k}. *Neuroreport* 1993;4:491–494.
25. Gibb WR. Melanin, tyrosine hydroxylase, calbindin, and substance P in the human midbrain and substantia nigra in relation to nigrostriatal projections and differential neuronal susceptibility in Parkinson's disease. *Brain Res* 1992;581:283–291.
26. Goldstein M, Deutch AY. The inhibitory action of neuropeptide Y and galanin on ^{3}H-norepinephrine release in the central nervous system: Relation to a proposed hierarchy of neuronal molecular coexistence. In: Mutt V, Fuxe K, Hökfelt T, Lundberg JM, eds. *Neuropeptide Y*. New York: Raven Press, 1989;153–162.
27. Greenfield SA. A noncholinergic action of acetylcholinesterase (AChE) in the brain: from neuronal secretion to the generation of movement. *Cell Mol Neurobiol* 1991;11:55–77.
28. Haglund L, Kohler C, Haaparanta T, Goldstein M, Gustafsson J-A. Presence of NADPH-cytochrome P450 reductase in central catecholamine neurons. *Nature* 1984;307:259–262.
29. Harfstrand A, Fuxe K, Cintra A, et al. Glucocorticoid receptor immunoreactivity in monoaminergic neurons of rat brain. *Proc Natl Acad Sci USA* 1986;83:9779–9783.
30. Hattori T, Takada M, Moriizumi, van der Kooy D. Single dopaminergic nigrostriatal neurons form two chemically distinct synaptic types: possible transmitter segregation within neurons. *J Comp Neurol* 1991;309:391–401.
31. Hökfelt T. Neuropeptides in perspective: the last ten years. *Neuron* 1991;7:867–879.
32. Hökfelt T, Everitt BJ, Theodorsson-Norheim E, Goldstein M. Occurrence of neurotensinlike immunoreactivity in subpopulations of hypothalamic, mesencephalic, and medullary catecholamine neurons. *J Comp Neurol* 1984;222:543–559.
33. Hökfelt T, Johansson O, Holets V, Meister B, Melander T. Distribution of neuropeptides with special reference to their coexistence with classical transmitters. In: Meltzer HY, ed. *Psychopharmacology: the third generation of progress*. New York: Raven Press, 1987;401–416.
34. Hökfelt T, Skirboll L, Rehfeld JF, Goldstein M, Markey K, Dann O. A subpopulation of mesencephalic dopamine neurons projecting to limbic areas contains a cholecystokinin-like peptide: evidence from immunohistochemistry combined with retrograde tracing. *Neuroscience* 1980;5:2093–2124.
35. Honda T, Wada E, Dattey JF, Tank SA. Differential gene expression of CCK$_A$ and CCK$_B$ receptors in the rat brain. *Mol Cell Neurosci* 1993;4:143–154.
36. Iverfelt K, Serfozo P, Diaz AL, Bartfai T. Differential release of coexisting neurotransmitters: frequency dependence of the efflux of substance P, thyrotrophin releasing hormone, and [^{3}H]-serotonin from tissue slices of rat ventral spinal cord. *Acta Physiol Scand* 1989;137:63–71.
37. Jan YN, Jan LY. Some features of peptidergic transmission. *Prog Brain Res* 1983;58:49–59.
38. Kaneko T, Akiyama H, Nagatsu I, Mizuno N. Immunohistochemical demonstration of glutaminase in catecholaminergic and serotonergic neurons of rat brain. *Brain Res* 1990;507:151–154.
39. Kelley RB. Storage and release of neurotransmitters. *Cell* 1993;72:43–53.
40. Kosaka T, Kosaka K, Nagatsu I. Tyrosine hydroxylase-like immunoreactive neurons in the olfactory bulb of the snake, *Elaophe quadrivirgata*, with special reference to the colocalization of tyrosine hydroxylase- and GABA-like immunoreactivities. *Exp Brain Res* 1991;87:353–362.
41. Krause JE, Bu JY, Takeda Y, et al. Structure, expression and second messenger-mediated regulation of the human and rat substance P receptors and their genes. *Regul Pept* 1993;46:59–66.
42. Levoie B, Parent A. Dopaminergic neurons expressing calbindin in normal and parkinsonian monkeys. *Neuroreport* 1991;2:601–604.
43. Liu Y, Peter D, Roghani A, et al. A cDNA that suppresses MPP + toxicity encodes a vesicular amine transporter. *Cell* 1992;70:539–551.
44. Lundberg JM. Peptide and classical transmitter mechanisms in the autonomic nervous system. *Arch Int Pharmacodyn Ther* 1990;303:9–19.
45. Mansour A, Watson SJ. In: Herz A, ed. *Opioids I. Handbook of*

experimental pharmacology, vol 104. Berlin: Springer-Verlag, 1993;79–106.

46. Martin LJ, Blackstone CD, Levey AI, Huganir RL, Price DL. AMPA glutamate receptor subunits are differentially distributed in rat brain. *Neuroscience* 1993;53:327–358.

47. Meister B, Elde R. Dopamine transporter mRNA in neurons of the rat hypothalamus. *Neuroendocrinology* 1993;58:388–395.

48. Meng F, Xie GX, Thompson RC, et al. Cloning and pharmacological characterization of a rat kappa opioid receptor. *Proc Natl Acad Sci USA* 1993;90:9954–9998.

49. Orazzo C, Pierebone VA, Ceccatelli S, Ternenius L, Hökfelt T. CGRP-like immunoreactivity in A11 dopamine neurons projecting to the spinal cord and a note on CGRP-CCK cross-reactivity. *Brain Res* 1993;600:39–48.

50. Savasta M, Palacios JM, Mengod G. Regional distribution of the messenger RNA coding for the neuropeptide cholecystokinin in the human brain examined by in situ hybridization. *Mol Brain Res* 1990;7:91–104.

51. Schalling M, Friberg K, Seroogy K, et al. Analysis of expression of cholecystokinin in dopamine cells in the ventral mesencephalon of several species and in humans with schizophrenia. *Proc Natl Acad Sci USA* 1990;87:8427–8431.

52. Schultzberg M, Segura-Aguilar J, Lind C. Distribution of DT diaphorase in the rat brain: biochemical and immunohistochemical studies. *Neuroscience* 1988;27:763–776.

53. Seroogy KB, Gall CM. Expression of neurotrophins by midbrain dopaminergic neurons. *Exp Neurol* 1993;124:119–128.

54. Seroogy K, Tsuruo Y, Hökfelt T, et al. Further analysis of presence of peptides in dopamine neurons. *Exp Brain Res* 1988;72:523–534.

55. Seroogy KB, Ceccatelli S, Schalling M. A subpopulation of dopaminergic neurons in rat ventral mesencephalon contains both neurotensin and cholecystokinin. *Brain Res* 1988;455:88–98.

56. Smith S, Augustine GJ. Calcium ions, active zones, and synaptic transmitter release. *Trends Neursci* 1988;11:458–465.

57. Sossin WS, Sweet-Cordero A, Scheller RH. Dale's hypothesis revisited: different neuropeptides derived from a common prohormone are targeted to different processes. *Proc Natl Acad Sci USA* 1990;87:4845–4848.

58. Thompson RC, Mansour A, Akil H, Watson SJ. Cloning and pharmacological characterization of a rat mu opioid receptor. *Neuron* 1993;11:903–913.

59. Verdoorn TA, Draguhn A, Ymer S, Seeburg PH, Sakmann B. Functional properties of recombinant rat GABA$_A$ receptors depend upon subunit composition. *Neuron* 1990;4:919–928.

60. Verhage M, McMahon HT, Ghijsen WE. Differential release of amino acids, neuropeptides, and catecholamines from isolated nerve terminals. *Neuron* 1991;6:517–524.

61. Yamada T, McGeer PL, Baimbridge KG, McGeer EG. Relative sparing in Parkinson's disease of substantia nigra dopamine neurons containing calbindin-D28K. *Brain Res* 1990;526:303.

62. Wada E, Wada K, Boulter J, et al. Distribution of alpha 2, alpha 3, alpha 4, and beta 2 neuronal nicotinic receptor subunit mRNAs in the central nervous system: a hybridization histochemistry study in the rat. *J Comp Neurol* 1989;284:314–335.

63. Whim MD, Lloyd PE. Frequency dependent release of peptide cotransmitters from identified cholinergic motor neurons in *Aplysia. Proc Natl Acad Sci USA* 1989;86:9034–9038.

64. Wisden W, Laurie DJ, Monyer H, Seeburg PH. The distribution of 13 GABA$_A$ receptor subunit mRNAs in the rat brain. I. Telencephalon, diencephalon, mesencephalon. *J Neurosci* 1992;12:1040–1062.

65. Wolfe J, Beaudet A. Neurotensin terminals form synapses primarily with neurons lacking detectable tyrosine hydroxylase immunoreactivity in the rat substantia nigra and ventral tegmental area. *J Comp Neurol* 1992;321:163–176.

*Psychopharmacology: The Fourth
Generation of Progress,* edited by
Floyd E. Bloom and David J. Kupfer.
Raven Press, Ltd., New York © 1995.

CHAPTER 19

Dopamine Receptor Expression in the Central Nervous System

Alfred Mansour and Stanley J. Watson, Jr.

The cloning of the D_2 dopamine receptor (6) in 1988 and the subsequent identification of multiple dopamine receptors referred to as D_1, D_3, D_4, and D_5 (10,35, 46,48,49,52,54,59) has profoundly changed our understanding of dopamine receptor anatomy and pharmacology. Prior to the isolation of these dopamine receptor subtypes, the dopamine field distinguished two subtypes of dopamine receptors (referred to as D_1 and D_2) that differed in their coupling to G-proteins, their distribution in the central nervous system (CNS), and their pharmacology (5,47,56). The cloning of these receptors and their genes has given us a better appreciation of a larger number of dopamine receptors present in the nervous system and how they may be organized in specific neuronal circuits. Given the multiple introns present in the D_2, D_3, and D_4 receptor genes, alternative splicing can yield several forms of these receptors, adding further to this complexity, and may be the basis for more subtle pharmacological differences.

This chapter will focus on the anatomical distribution of the dopamine receptors and will primarily examine the mRNA expression of the D_1, D_2, D_3, and D_5 receptors in the rat CNS. The D_4 receptor, despite its clinical importance as the site where clozapine and other atypical antipsychotics are thought to mediate their therapeutic effects (43,54), will not be discussed because its level is so low in the rat CNS that it has thus far been difficult to reliably detect. We have chosen to concentrate our efforts on the rat brain, because with the exception of a few publications in the human and primate brain (20,21,31), the vast majority of anatomical information concerning the localization and circuitry of the dopamine receptor messenger ribonucleic acids (mRNAs) has been derived from the rat

CNS. The chapter begins with a description of the receptor mRNA distributions in the brain, followed by a comparative analysis of dopamine receptor binding sites defined by selective ligands and receptor autoradiographic techniques. Next we focus on the basal ganglia, where on the basis of lesion and colocalization studies, the dopamine receptors have been suggested to be localized in different circuits and perhaps mediate distinct physiological effects. The chapter concludes with a discussion of the possible directions anatomical studies will take in the future to elucidate the role of the multiple dopamine receptors in the CNS. For further information concerning the molecular biology of the dopamine receptor subtypes, readers should refer to Chapters 14, 20, and 27, (*this volume*).

ANATOMICAL LOCALIZATION OF DOPAMINE RECEPTOR mRNAs

The cloned dopamine receptors (D_1–D_5) can be divided into two groups of receptors that correspond to the D_1 and D_2 receptor classification that had been previously identified pharmacologically. The D_1 and D_5 receptors have a D_1-like pharmacology, whereas the D_2, D_3, and D_4 receptors have a D_2-like pharmacological profile. In general, the D_1 and D_2 receptor mRNAs have a wider distribution and are more abundant in the CNS as compared to their pharmacologically related counterparts. The D_5 receptor mRNA, for example, is restricted to specific thalamic and hypothalamic nuclei and to the cells of the hippocampus, whereas the D_1 receptor mRNA is detected in numerous regions of the CNS. Similarly, cells expressing D_3 receptor mRNA are detected in far fewer nuclei than those expressing D_2 receptor mRNA. The wider distributions of cells expressing D_1 and D_2 receptor mRNA may be reflective of the broader number of functions mediated by these receptors in the CNS, including the modu-

A. Mansour and S. J. Watson, Jr.: Mental Health Research Institute and Department of Psychiatry, University of Michigan, Ann Arbor, Michigan 48109.

lation of cognitive, sensorimotor, and neuroendocrine effects, as compared to more limited functions that may be mediated by the other dopamine receptor types.

Several laboratories have described the mRNA distributions of the dopamine receptors in the CNS (4,14,34, 57,58), and while in large part there is agreement, differences do exist. These differences may be methodological or in some cases reflect technical differences such as the use of radiolabeled oligonucleotides in some studies and cRNA probes in others. The anatomical description that follows is based on findings largely generated from this laboratory (26–30,32).

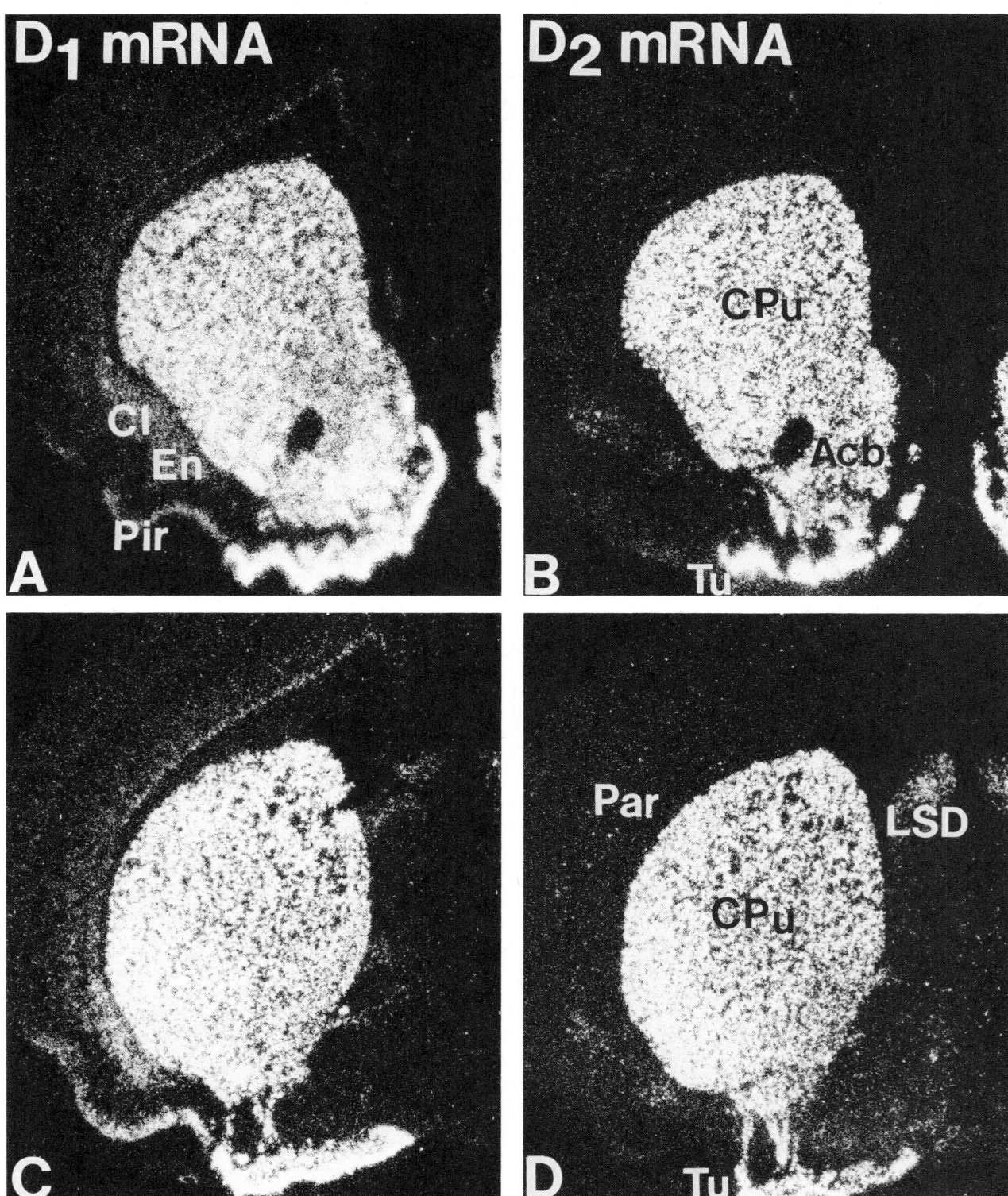

FIG. 1. *Continues on opposite page.*

TELENCEPHALON

The dopamine receptor mRNAs vary in their cortical distributions. Cells expressing D_1 are widely distributed in both neocortical and palleocortical areas, with the highest levels of expression in the anterior cingulate, orbital, insular, piriform, and entorhinal cortex (Figs. 1 and 2). Neocortical areas, such as the frontal, parietal, temporal, and occipital cortex, also express D_1 receptor mRNA, with cells localized predominantly in layers V and VI. In contrast, cells expressing high levels of D_2 receptor mRNA are observed only in the entorhinal cortex, with moderate levels of expression in the anterior cingulate, orbital, and insular cortex. Scattered cells in layers IV–VI of the frontal, parietal, temporal, and occipital cortex also express D_2 mRNA (Figs. 1 and 2). Cells expressing D_3 and D_5 receptor mRNAs are not detected in either neocortical or palleocortical areas.

The olfactory nuclei similarly demonstrate a heterogeneity of dopamine receptor mRNA expression. Cells expressing D_1 receptor mRNA are localized in all the divisions of the anterior olfactory nuclei, including the dorsal, lateral, ventral, and medial divisions, whereas cells expressing D_2 receptor mRNA are primarily in the dorsal and lateral divisions. Cellular expression of D_2 in the dorsal and lateral olfactory nuclei is comparatively low. In contrast, no cells expressing D_3 receptor mRNA are detected in any division of the anterior olfactory nucleus.

More caudally, D_1, D_2, and D_3 receptor mRNA expression is high within the rat striatum (Figs. 1 and 3A,C). Cells expressing high levels of D_1 and D_2 receptor mRNA are found in all levels of the caudate-putamen and extend ventrally into the nucleus accumbens. Medial–lateral differences are observed with higher levels of cellular expression of both D_1 and D_2 in the lateral caudate-putamen (Fig. 1). In contrast, cells expressing D_3 receptor mRNA are predominantly in the nucleus accumbens, with fewer scattered cells expressing comparatively lower levels of D_3 mRNA in the medial caudate-putamen (Fig. 3A,C). The cellular expression within the nucleus accumbens is also heterogeneous with high levels of expression and more cells expressing D_3 mRNA in the accumbens shell and septal pole. Cellular expression of D_1 and D_2 receptor mRNAs is also higher in the accumbens shell and septal pole, but the precise distribution of cells expressing the three mRNAs differ (Figs. 1A,B and 3C). In addition,

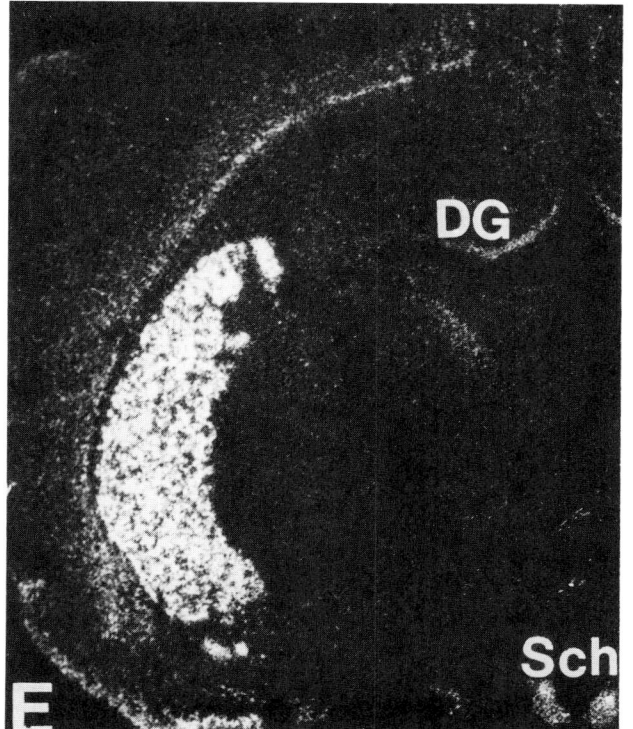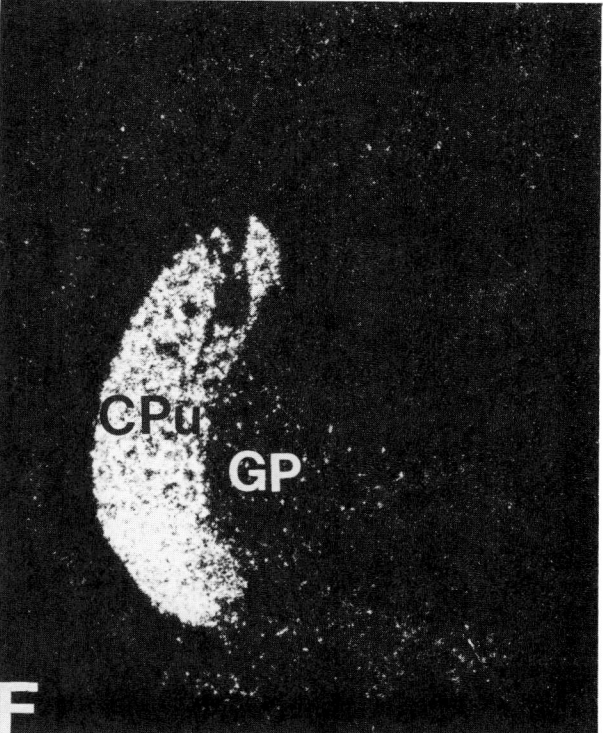

FIG. 1. Dark-field autoradiograms comparing the distributions of D_1 (**A, C, E**) and D_2 (**B, D, F**) receptor mRNAs in the rostral forebrain of the rat. D_1 and D_2 receptor mRNA expression is high in the caudate-putamen (CPu), nucleus accumbens (Acb), and olfactory tubercle (Tu). D_1 expressing cells are extensively distributed in neo- and palleocortical areas with particularly high levels in the piriform cortex (Pir). Other cells expressing D_1 receptor mRNA are localized in the dentate gyrus (DG), claustrum (Cl), endopiriform nucleus (En), and the suprachiasmatic nucleus of the hypothalamus (Sch). Cells expressing D_2 receptor mRNA demonstrate a different distribution, with cells localized in the lateral dorsal septum (LSD), in the globus pallidus (GP), and in scattered cells of the parietal (Par) and frontal cortex.

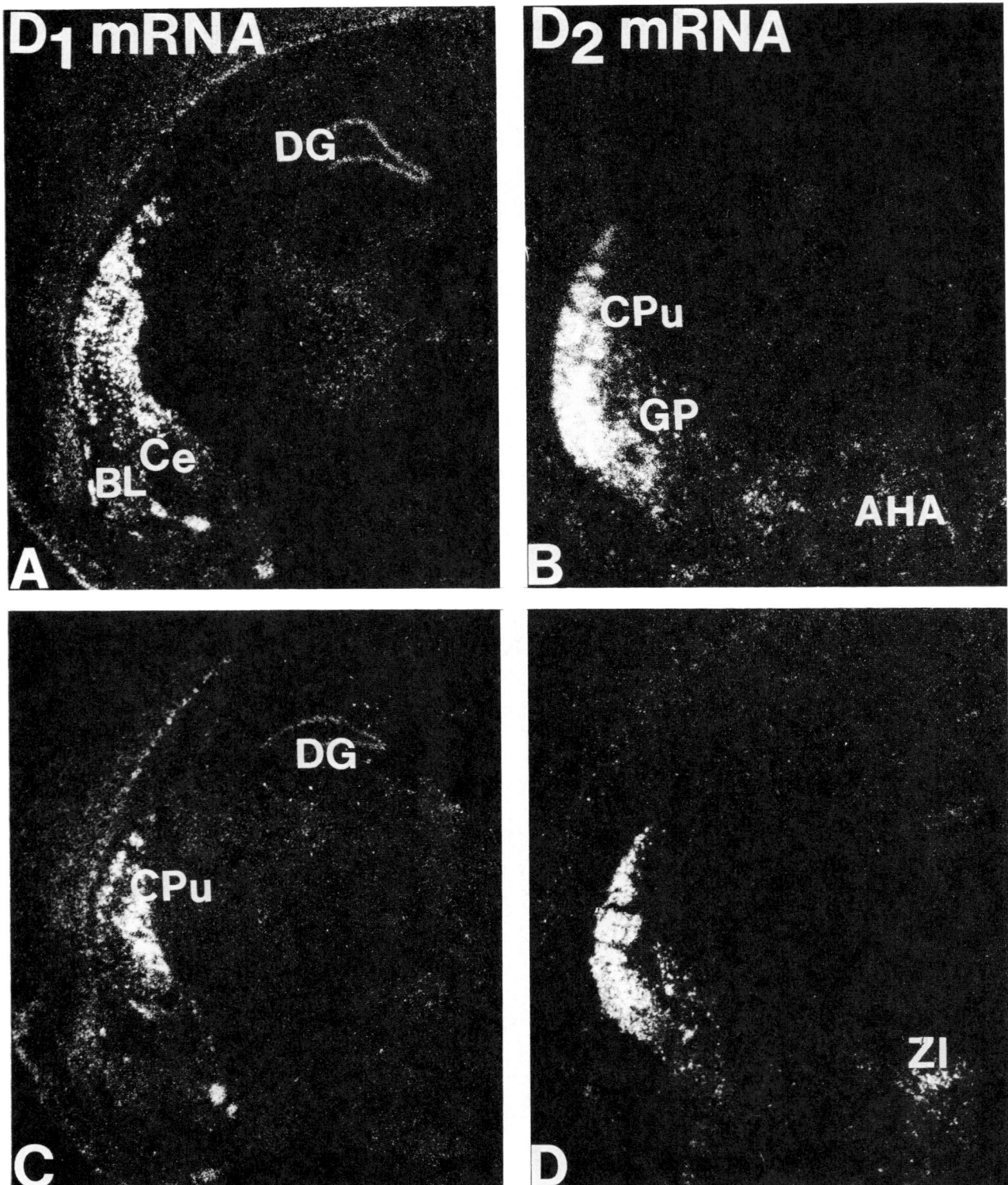

FIG. 2. *Continues on opposite page.*

there are higher levels of expression of D_1 and D_2 mRNA in the accumbens core relative to accumbens shell than observed with D_3. More ventrally, cells in the islands of Calleja express high levels of D_3 mRNA and no D_1 and D_2 receptor mRNA, whereas the cells of the olfactory tubercle express high levels of D_1 and D_2 receptor mRNA

and no D_3 receptor mRNA (Figs. 1A,B and 3A,C). The expression of D_3 receptor mRNA in the islands of Calleja is the highest observed in the CNS and appears to be selective for D_3.

The globus pallidus, a major efferent pathway of the striatum, shows a heterogeneity in dopamine receptor

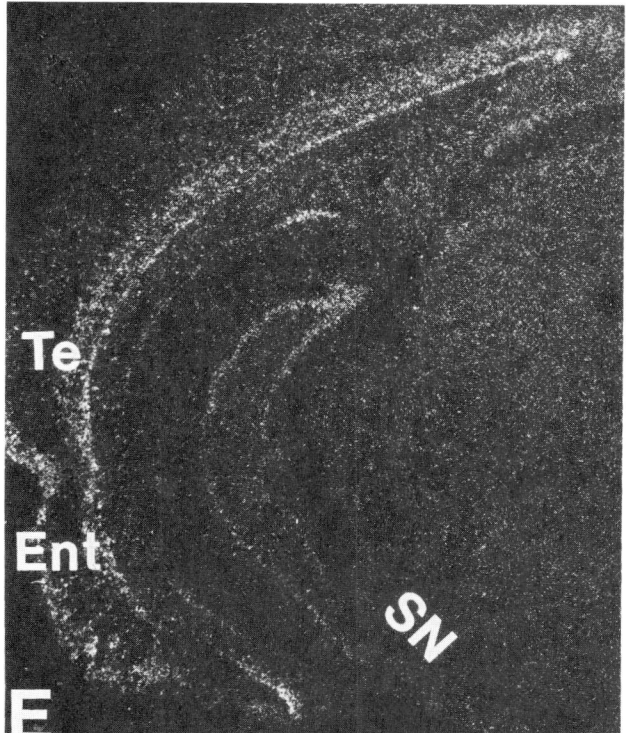
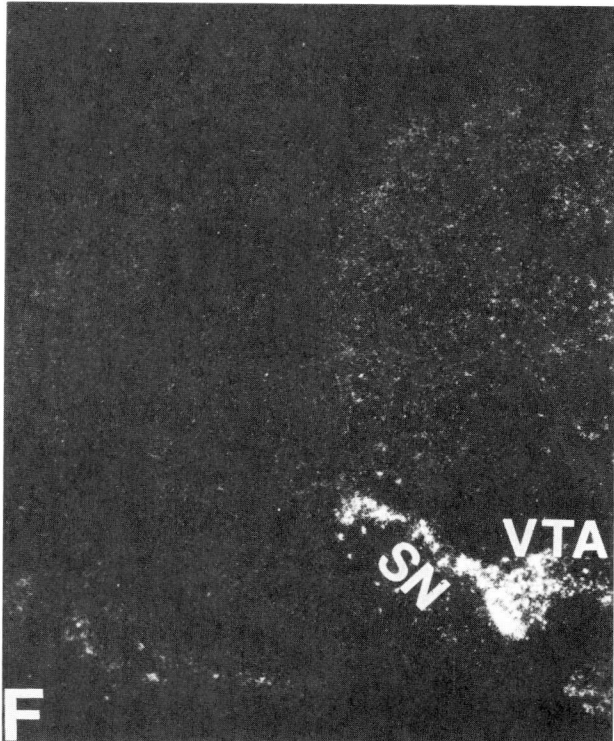

FIG. 2. Dark-field autoradiograms comparing the distribution of D₁ (**A, C, E**) and D₂ (**B, D, E**) receptor mRNAs in the rat di- and mesencephalon. Cells expressing D₁ and D₂ receptor mRNAs are differentially distributed, with cells expressing D₁ in the caudate-putamen (CPu), dentate gyrus (DG), basolateral (BL) amygdala and in the temporal (Te) and entorhinal (Ent) cortex. In contrast, cells expressing D₂ receptor mRNA are localized in the caudate-putamen (CPu), globus pallidus (GP), scattered cells of the anterior hypothalamic area (AHA), zona incerta (ZI), central amygdala (Ce), substantia nigra (SN), and ventral tegmental area (VTA).

mRNA expression. Of the dopamine receptor mRNAs examined, only D₂ is present in the large cells of the globus pallidus (Figs. 1F and 2B). Levels of D₂ receptor mRNA expression are lower compared to the striatum, with cells scattered throughout the globus pallidus and extending into the ventral pallidum. The number of cells expressing D₂ receptor mRNA are comparatively lower in the ventral pallidum. Interestingly, in the ventral pallidum, which receives direct projections from the shell portion of the nucleus accumbens, few scattered D₃ receptor expressing cells are detected.

In the septal nuclei, cells expressing D₁ receptor mRNA are primarily localized in the dorsal division of the lateral septum, whereas those cells expressing D₂ mRNA extend more medially and ventrally from the dorsal lateral septum to the intermediate lateral septum (Fig. 1C,D). Scattered cells expressing D₂ receptor mRNA are also observed in the medial septum and extend into the diagonal band of Broca, where D₂ receptor expression is prominent in the horizontal limb. Cells expressing D₃ receptor mRNA are localized in the medial portion of the lateral septum, with scattered cells in the medial septum and diagonal band of Broca.

Rostral–caudal differences are observed in the dopa-

mine receptor expression in the hippocampal formation. While few, if any, D₁ expressing cells can be detected in the dorsal hippocampus, in the ventral hippocampus numerous cells express D₁ in the CA1–CA3 fields (Fig. 1E versus Fig. 2E). D₁ mRNA expression levels in these cells are low compared to the high levels of expression observed in the cells of the dentate gyrus (Figs. 1E and 2A,C). Scattered cells expressing low levels of D₂ and D₅ receptor mRNA are found in the dorsal and ventral hippocampus, and as can be seen in Fig. 3B, D₃ expressing cells are detected in the hippocampus and dentate gyrus.

Cells expressing D₁ mRNA are extensively distributed throughout the amygdaloid complex. Highest levels of D₁ receptor mRNA expression are found in the intercalated nuclei of the basolateral amygdala (Fig. 2A). D₁ expressing cells are also localized in the basolateral, medial, central, and cortical amygdala. In contrast, D₂ expressing cells are primarily localized in the lateral division of the central nucleus, with scattered cells in the basomedial amygdala. Only a few scattered cells expressing D₃ mRNA are detected in the medial amygdala.

Other regions in the telencephalon, where distribution of the dopamine receptors differ, include the endopiriform nucleus and claustrum. Cells in these areas express D₁

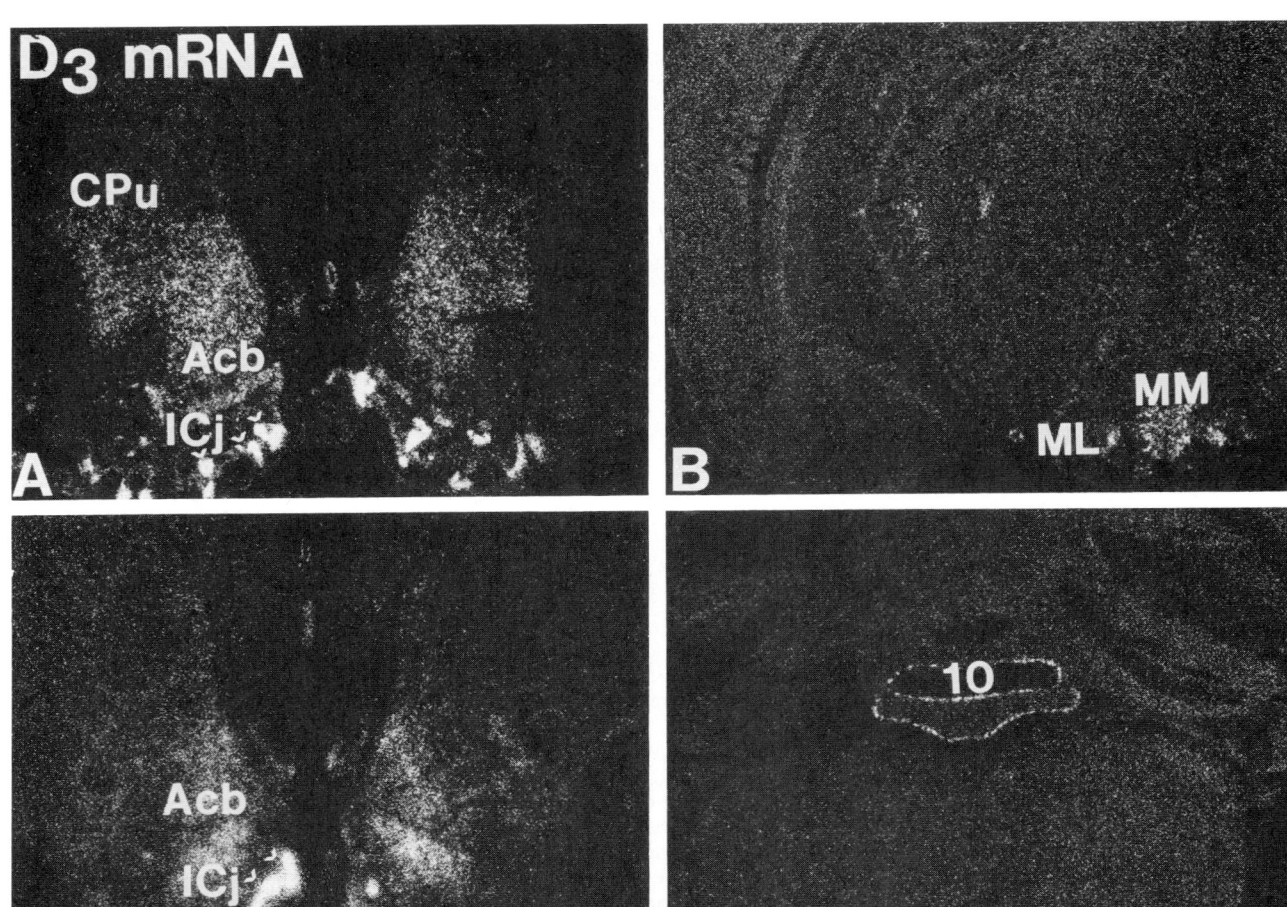

FIG. 3. Dark-field autoradiograms showing the distribution of D₃ receptor mRNA at two levels of the nucleus accumbens (**A** = rostral, **C** = caudal), caudal hypothalamus (**B**), and cerebellum (**D**). Cells expressing D₃ receptor mRNA are localized in the islands of Calleja (ICj), nucleus accumbens (Acb), medial caudate-putamen (CPu), medial (MM) and mediolateral (ML) mammillary nuclei of the hypothalamus, and lobule 10 of the cerebellum (10).

receptor mRNA (Fig. 1A) and no detectable D₃ or D₅ mRNA. Cells in the bed nucleus of the stria terminalis similarly express D₂ receptor mRNA, with no detectable D₁, D₃, or D₅.

DIENCEPHALON

The level of dopamine receptor mRNA expression in the thalamus is low compared to other regions of the CNS. Of the dopamine receptor mRNAs, D₁ is expressed most widely in the thalamus, with D₁ expressing cells in the anterior dorsal, anterior ventral, centromedial, paracentral, ventromedial, ventrolateral, and posterior nuclei, as well as the lateral habenula and dorsolateral geniculate body. The distribution of cells expressing D₂ receptor mRNA is more restricted, with high levels of expression in the cells of the zona incerta (Fig. 2D). Cells expressing D₃ mRNA are prominent in the paraventricular nucleus,

with scattered cells in the centromedial, gelatinosus, ventromedial, ventrolateral nuclei, as well as the zona incerta and lateral and medial geniculate bodies. D₅ receptor mRNA expression is limited to the cells of the parafascicular nucleus.

In the hypothalamus, cells expressing D₁ receptor mRNA have a more limited distribution and are localized in the supraoptic, suprachiasmatic (Fig. 1E), paraventricular, and rostral arcuate nuclei. In contrast, cells expressing the D₂ receptor mRNA are more widely scattered in the hypothalamus and are found in the large cells of the lateral preoptic area, anterior hypothalamic area (Fig. 2B), and lateral hypothalamus. More caudally, cells in the posterior division of the arcuate nucleus and the ventral and dorsal premammillary nuclei express D₂ receptor mRNA. The distribution of cells expressing D₂ and D₃ mRNAs are clearly differentiated in the mammillary nuclei, where high levels of D₂ receptor mRNA are expressed in the cells of the lateral mammillary nuclei, whereas D₃ expressing cells are localized in the medial and mediolateral mammillary nuclei (Fig. 3B). In the posterior medial mammillary nucleus, however, both D_2 and D_3 receptor mRNAs are expressed. Tiberi et al. (52) suggest that cells expressing D_5 receptor mRNA are also localized in the lateral mammillary nuclei. Large scattered cells of the lateral hypothalamus also express D_3 receptor mRNA, suggesting that the D_3 receptors may also play a role in hypothalamic regulation.

MESENCEPHALON

Of the cloned dopamine receptors, cells expressing D_2 receptor mRNA are more widely distributed in the midbrain and hindbrain, and may be involved in a host of autonomic functions and in the regulation of dopamine release. Cells expressing D_2 receptor mRNA are prominent, for example, in the dopaminergic cells of the substantia nigra and ventral tegmental area, where their expression levels are high (Fig. 2F). Within the substantia nigra, cells expressing D_2 receptor mRNA are primarily in the pars compacta, with a few cells in the pars reticulata (Fig. 2F). Higher numbers of cells expressing D_2 receptor mRNA are observed in the caudal portion of the pars reticulata. In addition to the dopaminergic cells of the substantia nigra and ventral tegmental area, D_2 receptor mRNA is also localized in the magnocellular cells of the red nucleus that are part of the rubrospinal pathway. In contrast, while there are high levels of D_1 receptor binding in the substantia nigra, pars reticulata, no cells expressing D_1 receptor mRNA could be detected in the substantia nigra or ventral tegmental area. Similarly, while some reports suggest the localization of D_3 receptor mRNA in the cells of the substantia nigra (4,46), research from our laboratory has failed to replicate these findings.

More dorsally in the superior colliculus, cells expressing D_2 receptor mRNA are localized in the intermediate and deep layers, with no cells detected in the superficial layer of the superior colliculus, where D_2 receptor binding is localized. Cells in both the central and external cortex of the inferior colliculus express moderate levels of D_2 receptor mRNA. In contrast, cells expressing D_1, D_3, or D_5 are not detected in either the superior or inferior colliculus.

Cells expressing D_2 receptor mRNA are also localized in the periaqueductal gray. D_2 expressing cells are visualized in both the dorsal and ventral central gray; however, there are higher numbers of D_2 cells in the ventral division, where they may be important in modulating analgesic responses. Large scattered cells in the midbrain reticular nuclei and more caudally in the pontine reticular and gigantocellular reticular nuclei of the hindbrain express moderate to high levels of D_2 receptor mRNA. These cells have been implicated in morphine-induced analgesia, and these findings are consistent with the role of D_2 receptors in the modulation of analgesic responses.

Cells in the rostral division of the interpeduncular nucleus express low levels of D_3 receptor mRNA. This represents a relatively selective dopamine receptor expression as D_1, D_2, and D_5 receptor mRNA is not detected in the interpeduncular nucleus.

MET- AND MYLENCEPHALON

D_2 receptor mRNA expression is high in a number of raphe nuclei, where they may serve to regulate serotonin release. Cells expressing the D_2 receptor mRNA are visualized in the dorsal and caudal linear raphe, as well as the large cells of the raphe magnus. Cells expressing D_1 receptor mRNA are also observed in the raphe nuclei, where their primary localization is in the dorsal raphe. D_2 receptor mRNA is moderate to high in a number of brainstem nuclei (including the dorsal tegmental, lateral lemniscus, locus coeruleus, parabrachial, and trigeminal) and the rostral nucleus of the solitary tract. Within the trigeminal nuclei, it is primarily the cells of the sensory and spinal trigeminal that express D_2 receptor mRNA. Scattered cells, comparatively few in number, also express D_2 receptor mRNA in the medial vestibular, hypoglossal, cuneate, and gracilis nuclei. D_1 receptor mRNA expression is more limited in the hindbrain, with D_1 expressing cells detected in the locus coeruleus, lateral parabrachial, and facial nuclei.

While D_3 receptor mRNA expression is not easily measured in most hindbrain nuclei, low levels of D_3 mRNA are observed in the inferior olivary nucleus. Low levels of D_2 receptor mRNA expression are also seen in the inferior olive.

In the cerebellum, there is a heterogeneity of dopamine receptor mRNA expression. High levels of D_1 mRNA expression are observed in the granular cells of the cerebellum. D_3 receptor mRNA expression, on the other hand, is limited to lobules 9 and 10 and in the parafluculus, where it is localized in large Purkinje cells (Fig. 3D). In contrast, no cells expressing either D_2 or D_5 receptor mRNA can be detected in the lobules of the cerebellum, but D_2 expressing cells are observed in the lateral cervical nucleus of the cerebellum.

MULTIPLE DOPAMINE RECEPTOR mRNA FORMS

Given the intronic organization of the D_2, D_3, and D_4 genes, multiple mRNA transcripts may be generated by each gene by alternative splicing. While variant and truncated forms of the D_3 and D_4 receptors have been reported (13,16,41,55), two forms of the D_2 receptor that differ by a 29-amino-acid insertion in the third cytosolic loop have been studied most extensively (3,17,18,36,37,39,45,53). In situ hybridization studies in pituitary and brain suggest that both mRNAs are expressed in the same cells, with the longer D_2 form (444 amino acids) being the more abundant species (29,45,53). The relative ratios of $D_{2(444)}$ and $D_{2(415)}$, however, do vary with brain area, and some studies have suggested that the D_2 receptor forms may be differentially regulated with antipsychotics or denervation (3,39,45). This is of both clinical and physiological relevance, because it suggests that there may be cellular mechanisms regulating the rate of splicing and the final ratios of receptor products that are inserted into the cell membrane. Several studies, for example, have demonstrated that the shorter form of D_2 [$D_{2(415)}$] is more efficiently coupled to G-proteins (18,36,37), suggesting that a change in receptor ratios of $D_{2(415)}/D_{2(444)}$ may result in an enhanced cellular response. A similar observation has been noted with the D_4 receptor, where the least number of insertions in the third cytosolic loop showed the highest affinity for dopamine receptor ligands and coupled more effectively to G-proteins (55).

In localization and regulatory studies, it is imperative, therefore, that multiple forms of the dopamine receptors are considered in interpreting the results. Multiple probes spanning different domains of the dopamine receptors need to be examined in order to evaluate distribution and regulatory effects on several dopamine receptor variants. This is more easily accomplished using cRNA protection assays, but can also be accomplished with in situ hybridization using oligomers that bridge divergent regions of two receptor forms. The importance of examining the dopamine receptor variants has recently been highlighted by Schmauss et al. (41), who report a differential loss of D_3 receptor mRNA forms in the parietal and motor cortex of schizophrenics (see also Chapter 100, *this volume*).

COMPARISON OF THE DISTRIBUTION OF DOPAMINE RECEPTOR mRNAs AND BINDING SITES

The cloning of the dopamine receptors has allowed the direct comparison of the cells synthesizing the mRNA encoding these receptors to the sites of ligand binding as defined by receptor autoradiographic techniques. While such comparisons are never perfect because binding sites are localized in both cell bodies and terminals, and the mRNAs are predominantly in cell bodies, they do provide several kinds of valuable information concerning the anatomical organization of the receptor systems. First, receptors and other proteins are often cloned from cell lines that express a receptor at high levels. Localization of the mRNA encoding this receptor by in situ hybridization and the subsequent comparison to receptor autoradiographic distributions is important in determining whether the receptor is expressed in the CNS and has any physiological relevance. Second, by examining the anatomical connections in areas of the brain where there is an apparent mismatch between the expression of the mRNA and the binding, one may glean insights into the possible transport of receptors and the cellular origins of a receptor protein

(26,28). Third, a mismatch between mRNA expression and receptor binding may be indicative of the labeling of additional receptors that have not been pharmacologically characterized or identified with molecular biological techniques. Examples of how comparisons of receptor binding and receptor mRNA have been useful in understanding dopamine receptor anatomy follow.

In general, studies examining the distributions of cells expressing the dopamine receptor mRNAs and dopamine receptor binding sites have shown a good agreement between distributions (24,26,28). For example, D_2 receptor binding sites and the cells expressing D_2 receptor mRNA are similarly distributed in the caudate-putamen, nucleus accumbens, olfactory tubercle, globus pallidus, substantia nigra, ventral tegmental area, locus coeruleus, lateral parabrachial nucleus, and the nucleus of the solitary tract. Clear differences are seen in the zona incerta, where there are high levels of receptor mRNA but little, if any, receptor binding, which may be indicative of receptor transport. The converse is observed in the superior colliculus, where high levels of D_2 receptor binding are detected in the superficial layer, with no D_2 receptor mRNA expression. Because the superficial layer receives direct projections from retinal ganglia cells, the cell bodies and, therefore, the mRNA encoding these D_2 receptor sites is likely localized in the retina. This has been confirmed by in situ hybridization studies (58).

Clearly, not all mismatches observed in receptor binding and receptor mRNA distributions are due to receptor transport. The choice of receptor ligand and binding conditions are critical to ensure the labeling of a single receptor population. A particularly relevant example of this problem can be demonstrated with the "selective" D_2 ligand sulpiride. Many of the differences noted in the distribution of cells expressing D_2 mRNA and D_2 receptor binding when sulpiride was used as the labeling ligand may have been due to the binding of sulpiride to D_3 receptor sites. For example, the labeling of the islands of Calleja, medial mammillary nuclei, and lobule 9 and 10 of the cerebellum by sulpiride (56) suggest the labeling of D_3 binding sites and would have been interpreted as a mismatch when compared to the mRNA distribution visualized by D_2-selective cRNA probes.

Similar comparisons of the cells expressing D_1 receptor mRNA and D_1 receptor binding defined by [³H]SCH 23390 in the presence of ketanserin show a good correspondence in regions such as the neocortex, caudate-putamen, nucleus accumbens, amygdala, and the suprachiasmatic nucleus, whereas other regions show a lack of correspondence (28). For example, high levels of D_1 receptor binding are observed in the entopeduncular nucleus and the substantia nigra, pars reticulata (Fig. 4), whereas no D_1 mRNA can be detected in these areas. This lack of correspondence is suggestive that D_1 receptors are synthesized in the striatum and transported to efferent projections in the entopeduncular nucleus and substantia nigra, with some portion of D_1 binding sites remaining

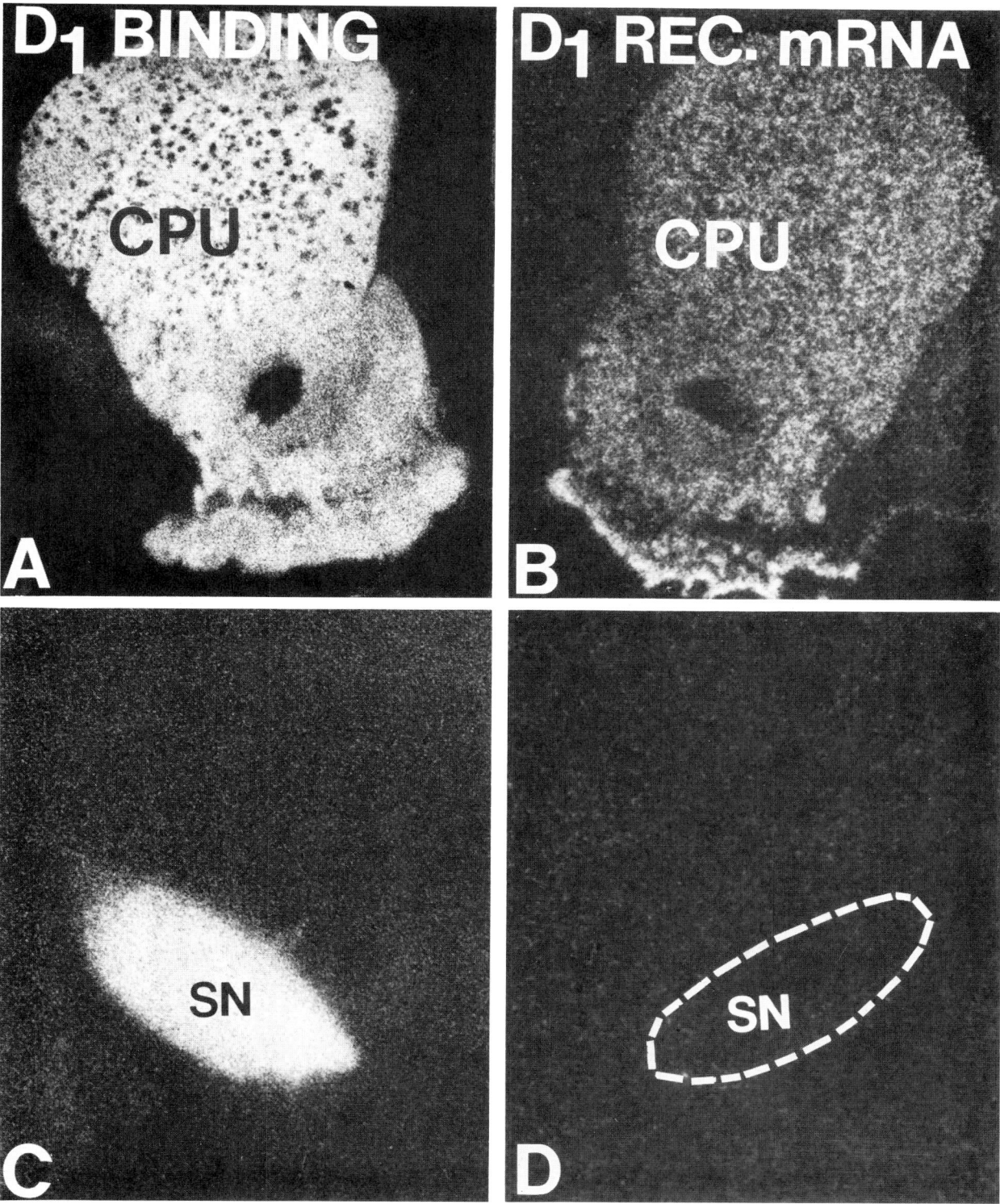

FIG. 4. Dark-field autoradiograms comparing the distribution of D_1 receptor binding (**A, C**) defined by [^{3}H]SCH 23390 in the presence of 1 μM ketanserin to D_1 receptor mRNA (**B, D**) in the rat striatum and substantia nigra. While there is a good correspondence between D_1 receptor mRNA expression and D_1 receptor binding in the caudate-putamen (CPU), nucleus accumbens, and olfactory tubercle, there is a lack of correspondence in the substantia nigra (SN), where high levels of D_1 receptor binding are observed and no D_1 receptor mRNA.

in striatal cell bodies. Ibotenic acid lesions in the striatum are consistent with this conclusion, and they demonstrate a coordinate loss of D_1 receptor mRNA and binding in the caudate-putamen that is accompanied by a degeneration of fibers projecting to the entopeduncular nucleus and substantia nigra (28). Differences in the laminar distribution of D_1 binding and D_1 receptor mRNA in the dentate gyrus and the cerebellum may also be due to receptor transport. Cells expressing D_1 receptor mRNA are localized in the granular cell layer of the dentate gyrus and cerebellum, while D_1 receptor binding is detected in the molecular layer of these brain areas. It is likely, then, that the granular cells in the dentate gyrus and the cerebellum synthesize D_1 receptors that are subsequently transported to either their dendritic or axonal fields, respectively, in the molecular layer.

A good correspondence between the distribution of cells expressing D_3 receptor mRNA and D_3 receptor binding defined by 7-OH-DPAT (24) and 7-*trans*-OH-PIPAT (33) has also been reported. High levels of D_3 receptor mRNA expression and D_3 binding are observed in the islands of Calleja, the rostral portion of the nucleus accumbens and in lobules 9 and 10 of the cerebellum. Lower densities of 7-*trans*-OH-PIPAT binding were also observed in medial caudate-putamen, substantia nigra, inferior olive, interpeduncular nucleus, and selected nuclei of the hypothalamus and thalamus. Interestingly, the D_3 binding observed in the substantia nigra was restricted to the pars reticulata (33), and not the dopaminergic cells of the pars compacta, as would be expected if D_3 receptors were autoreceptors. Given the lack of D_3 receptor mRNA expression detected by this laboratory in the rat substantia nigra, these findings suggest that the D_3 binding observed in the pars reticulata may be on extrinsic fibers projecting to the substantia nigra. Similarly, the localization of D_3 receptor mRNA in the Purkinje cells of lobules 9 and 10 of the cerebellum, along with the presence of D_3 receptor binding in the molecular layer of lobules 9 and 10, again suggests D_3 receptor transport.

The presence of relatively high levels of both D_1 and D_3 receptor binding and mRNA expression in the cells of the cerebellum is somewhat surprising, given the lack of a known dopaminergic projection to this region. This receptor–neurotransmitter mismatch has been observed in several other neurotransmitter systems and is suggestive that perhaps not all receptors are in direct synaptic contact with their transmitter. In some cases—such as in the hippocampus and dentate gyrus, where a dopamine receptor–neurotransmitter mismatch has been suggested—a small dopaminergic projection has been reported by some investigators (51). Whether this projection to the hippocampus and dentate gyrus from the ventral tegmental area and medial tip of the substantia nigra (51) is functional and results in the formation of specific synaptic contacts with cells expressing dopamine receptors remains to be determined.

LESION AND COLOCALIZATION STUDIES

Selective lesion and dual mRNA localization studies have been very useful in differentiating the neuronal circuits in which the dopamine receptors may be localized. Because of the relative abundance of the D_1, D_2, and D_3 receptors in the basal ganglia and their clinical importance in schizophrenia, Parkinson's disease, and Huntington's chorea, most studies have focused on these brain regions. Both lesion and colocalization studies in the striatum suggest that the dopamine receptors are differentially distributed and organized into distinct neuronal systems.

With regard to the dopamine binding sites found within the caudate-putamen, lesions designed to selectively destroy cell bodies suggest that the vast majority of D_1 binding sites are postsynaptic and localized in intrinsic striatonigral cells (2,11). In contrast, D_2 binding sites in the striatum are largely on presynaptic terminals originating most likely from cells in the cortex and midbrain (12,38,42). Only a small proportion of D_2 binding sites found within the striatum are postsynaptic and localized in striatal neurons. Of the intrinsic striatal neurons expressing D2 receptor mRNA, colocalization and tract-tracing studies suggest that a small proportion are localized in cholinergic neurons (9,23), whereas the vast majority of cells examined in the dorsal striatum are colocalized with proenkephalin and project to the globus pallidus (15,23). The vast majority of cells expressing D_1 receptor mRNA, on the other hand, coexpress prodynorphin and substance P mRNAs (15,22) and project to the substantia nigra and entopeduncular nucleus, with a small proportion (10–20%) of cholinergic cells intrinsic to the striatum also expressing D_1 receptor mRNA (22). Cells expressing D_1 receptors are therefore localized in the dynorphin striatonigral pathway, whereas cells expressing D_2 receptors are part of the enkephalinergic striatopallidal pathway.

As indicated earlier, comparison of D_3 mRNA and D_3 binding distributions suggests that D_3 binding sites are largely synthesized by cells intrinsic to the striatum. Given the presence of D_3 binding and no D_3 receptor mRNA in the substantia nigra, pars reticulata, the D_3 binding sites are likely synthesized in the striatum, with a portion transported to the substantia nigra. This organization is very similar to the D_1 receptor, but lesion and tract-tracing studies need to be performed to confirm this conclusion. Given the lack of D_3 receptor binding reported in the entopeduncular nucleus, D_3 receptors may be localized only in a subpopulation of striatonigral neurons. A complete colocalization of D_3 and D_1 receptors is unlikely because D_3 expressing cells have a more restricted distribution, being localized in the ventral striatum and medial portion of the dorsal striatum, whereas D_1 expressing cells are seen throughout the dorsal and ventral striatum.

While colocalization and lesion experiments suggest that D_1 and D_2 receptors are present in distinct populations of striatal cells and in different neuroanatomical circuits, electrophysiological studies suggest a high degree of D_1 and D_2 receptor colocalization (for review, see ref. 8). A possible explanation of these discrepant findings is that early electrophysiological studies may have used ligands that did not discriminate between D_2 and D_3 receptors, resulting in an apparent colocalization of D_1 and D_2. More recently, however, using a polymerase chain reaction (PCR) strategy, it has been suggested that D_1, D_2 and D_3 receptors may be colocalized in the same striatonigral neurons. Surmeier et al. (50) demonstrated that they could amplify D_1, D_2, and D_3 mRNAs from individual dissociated striatonigral neurons, and the vast majority of neurons tested showed a coexpression of all three dopaminergic receptors. It is presently unclear whether these mRNAs may have been induced in the process of tissue culturing, or are representative of a high incidence of colocalization of the dopamine receptors. It is certainly possible that striatal neurons may express all three dopamine receptor mRNAs to different extents, so that when a PCR strategy is used, each mRNA would be amplified, but when a colocalization approach is used, mRNAs expressed at low levels would go undetected. Further research is needed to resolve the extent of dopamine receptor colocalization.

DOPAMINE AUTORECEPTORS

Since the pioneering research of Carlsson (7), it has been clear that the activity of dopaminergic neurons in the midbrain can be modulated by the release or the exogenous application of dopamine. These receptors were termed ''autoreceptors'' and are thought to be important in maintaining dopaminergic activity in the nigrostriatal and mesolimbic dopamine systems (1,44). With the cloning of the multiple dopamine receptors, the question arose as to which member of this family could serve as an autoreceptor. The available evidence suggests that the cloned D_2 receptor is the most likely candidate for a dopaminergic autoreceptor. Several lines of evidence support this conclusion: (i) D_2 receptor mRNA and binding is localized in the substantia nigra and the ventral tegmental area (30,34,57); (ii) colocalization studies demonstrate that D_2 receptor mRNA and tyrosine hydroxylase are expressed in the same dopaminergic neurons of the substantia nigra and the ventral tegmental area (29); and (iii) 6-hydroxydopamine lesions in the medial forebrain bundle result in simultaneous loss of tyrosine hydroxylase and D_2 receptor mRNA in the substantia nigra and the ventral tegmental area (27,29).

It has been suggested by others that the D_3 may also function as an autoreceptor, but the evidence is not compelling. In situ hybridization studies performed in this laboratory in the rat suggest that the cells of the substantia nigra and ventral tegmental area do not express D_3 receptor mRNA and that D_3 receptor binding is localized in the pars reticulata of the substantia nigra and not the pars

compacta, as would be expected for an autoreceptor. High levels of D_3 receptor mRNA have been reported in the lateral division of the substantia nigra pars compacta (4), but we have been unable to replicate these results. We can detect cells expressing D_3 receptor mRNA in the peripeduncular nucleus, which is in close proximity to the lateral substantia nigra. The expressed D_3 receptor has a somewhat higher affinity for dopamine than does the D_2 receptor (46), but the anatomical evidence suggests it may not function as an autoreceptor in terms of modulating mesencephalic dopaminergic release. Similarly, the lack of a D_1 and D_5 receptor mRNA localization in the substantia nigra and ventral tegmental argues against these receptors serving as autoreceptors.

FUTURE DIRECTIONS

Future anatomical studies are likely to focus on several questions. In situ hybridization procedures need to be developed to specifically label the D_4 dopamine receptor. One report has suggested that the D_4 receptor mRNA is more abundant in the periphery (40), but this finding has not been confirmed by other laboratories. Northern blot analysis suggests that the D_4 receptor mRNA is expressed in the cortex and striatum of primates (54) at one-tenth the levels observed for the D_2 receptor. It is presently unclear whether the difficulty in detecting the D_4 receptor mRNA in the rat reflects a species difference in the level of expression or the lack of D_4 receptor mRNA expression in the rat CNS.

Further colocalization studies are also needed to more specifically define subpopulations of cells expressing dopamine receptors. Thus far, most colocalization studies have concentrated on the striatum, with relatively few neurotransmitters and receptors being explored. Colocalization studies need to be extended to a wider number of neurotransmitters and to other regions of the CNS. In conjunction with tract-tracing studies, such investigations will provide a better appreciation of dopamine receptor anatomy and circuitry, which is imperative in understanding of how dopaminergic drugs may function in the brain. These basic anatomical findings provide the framework for posing more precise questions concerning the regulation of the dopamine receptors and in addressing the neural systems that may be dysfunctional in psychiatric disorders such as schizophrenia (see Chapters 26, 106, and 107, *this volume*), as well as in neurological diseases such as Huntington's and Parkinson's disease (Chapter 126, *this volume*). Dysregulation of the dopamine systems has also been implicated with the development of movement disorders or tardive dyskinesia, with chronic neuroleptic treatment (Chapter 107, *this volume*) and in opiate and cocaine addiction (Chapters 145 and 148, *this volume*).

The recent development of specific antibodies for D_1 and D_2 receptors (19,25) has provided a means for examining the cellular distributions of these proteins with immunohistochemical techniques. These antibodies have provided a new means for examining dopamine receptor pathways in the CNS, and will be invaluable in examining the subcellular organization of the dopamine receptors. The development of these antibodies will also allow the study of receptor regulation at a third level, that of protein translation. This complements the ongoing studies examining receptor regulation at the gene transcription and ligand binding levels. Similar efforts are needed to develop selective antibodies for the D_3, D_4, and D_5 dopamine receptors.

ACKNOWLEDGMENTS

We are grateful to Stephanie McWethy for expert secretarial assistance in the preparation of this manuscript, and to Charles Fox and Eileen Curran for their thoughtful participation in the writing of this manuscript. This work was supported by grants from The Markey Charitable Trust, Theophile Raphael, NIDA (DA 02265), NIMH (MH 42251), and The Gastrointestinal Hormone Research Center (P30 AM34933).

REFERENCES

1. Aghajanian GK, Bunney BS. Pharmacological characterization of dopamine "autoreceptors" by microiontophoretic single cell recording studies. *Adv Biochem Psychopharmacol* 1977;16:433–438.
2. Altar CA, Marien MR. Picomolar affinity of ^{125}I-SCH 23982 for D_1 receptors in brain demonstrated with digital subtraction autoradiography. *J Neurosci* 1987;7:213–222.
3. Arnauld E, Arsaut J, Demotes-Mainard J. Differential plasticity of the dopaminergic D_2 receptor mRNA isoforms under haloperidol treatment, as evidenced by *in situ* hybridization in rat anterior pituitary. *Neurosci Lett* 1991;130:12–16.
4. Bouthenet M-L, Souil E, Martres M-P, Sokoloff P, Giros B, Schwartz J-C. Localization of dopamine D_3 receptor mRNA in the rat brain using *in situ* hybridization histochemistry: comparison with dopamine D_2 receptor mRNA. *Brain Res* 1991;564:203–219.
5. Boyson SJ, McGonigle P, Molinoff PB. Quantitative autoradiographic localization of the D_1 and D_2 subtypes of dopamine receptors in rat brain. *J Neurosci* 1986;6:3177–3188.
6. Bunzow JR, Van Tol HHM, Grandy DK, et al. Cloning and expression of a rat D_2 dopamine receptor cDNA. *Nature* 1988;336:783–787.
7. Carlsson A. Receptor-mediated control of dopamine metabolism. In: Usdin E, Bunney WE, eds. *Pre- and postsynaptic receptors*. New York: Marcel Dekker, 1975;49–65.
8. Clark D, White FJ. D_1 dopamine receptor—the search for a function: a critical evaluation of the D_1/D_2 dopamine receptor classification and its functional implications. *Synapse* 1987;1:347–388.
9. Dawson VL, Dawson TM, Filloux FM, Wamsley JK. Evidence for dopamine D-2 receptors on cholinergic interneurons in the rat caudate-putamen. *Life Sci* 1988;42:1933–1939.
10. Dearry A, Gingrich JA, Falardeau P, Fremeau RT Jr, Bates MD, Caron MG. Molecular cloning and expression of the gene for a human D_1 dopamine receptor. *Nature* 1990;347:72–76.
11. Filloux F, Dawson TM, Wamsley JK. Localization of nigrostriatal dopamine receptor subtypes and adenylate cyclase. *Brain Res Bull* 1988;20:447–459.
12. Filloux F, Liu TH, Hsu CY, Hunt MA, Wamsley JK. Selective cortical infarction reduces [^{3}H]sulpiride binding in rat caudate-putamen: autoradiographic evidence for presynaptic D2 receptors on corticostriate terminals. *Synapse* 1988;2:521–531.
13. Fishburn CS, Belleli D, David C, Carmon S, Fuchs S. A novel short isoform of the D_3 dopamine receptor generated by alternative

14. Fremeau RT Jr, Duncan GE, Fornaretto M-G, et al. Localization of D_1 dopamine receptor mRNA in brain supports a role in cognitive, affective, and neuroendocrine aspects of dopaminergic neurotransmission. *Proc Natl Acad Sci USA* 1991;88:3772–3776.
15. Gerfen CR, Engber TM, Mahan LC, et al. D_1 and D_2 dopamine receptor-regulated gene expression of striatonigral and striatopallidal neurons. *Science* 1990;250:1429–1432.
16. Giros B, Martres M-P, Pilon C, Sokoloff P, Schwartz J-C. Shorter variants of the D_3 dopamine receptor produced through various patterns of alternative splicing. *Biochem Biophys Res Commun* 1991;176:1584–1592.
17. Giros B, Sokoloff P, Martres M-P, Riou J-F, Emorine LJ, Schwartz J-C. Alternative splicing directs the expression of two D_2 dopamine receptor isoforms. *Nature* 1989;342:923–926.
18. Hayes G, Biden TJ, Selbie LA, Shine J. Structural subtypes of the dopamine D2 receptor are functionally distinct: expression of the cloned D2$_A$ and D2$_B$ subtypes in a heterologous cell line. *Mol Endocrinol* 1992;6:920–926.
19. Huang Q, Zhou D, Chase K, Gusella JF, Aronin N, DiFiglia M. Immunohistochemical localization of the D_1 dopamine receptor in rat brain reveals its axonal transport, pre- and postsynaptic localization, and prevalence in the basal ganglia, limbic system, and thalamic reticular nucleus. *Proc Natl Acad Sci USA* 1992;89:11988–11992.
20. Huntley GW, Morrison JH, Prikhozhan A, Sealfon SC. Localization of multiple dopamine receptor subtype mRNAs in human and monkey motor cortex and striatum. *Mol Brain Res* 1992;15:181–188.
21. Landwehrmeyer B, Mengod G, Palacios JM. Dopamine D_3 receptor mRNA and binding sites in human brain. *Mol Brain Res* 1993;18:187–192.
22. Le Moine C, Normand E, Bloch B. Phenotypical characterization of the rat striatal neurons expressing the D_1 dopamine receptor gene. *Proc Natl Acad Sci USA* 1991;88:4205–4209.
23. Le Moine C, Normand E, Guitteny AF, Fouque B, Teoule R, Bloch B. Dopamine receptor gene expression by enkephalin neurons in rat forebrain. *Proc Natl Acad Sci USA* 1990;87:230–234.
24. Lévesque D, Diaz J, Pilon C, et al. Identification, characterization, and localization of the dopamine D_3 receptor in rat brain using 7-[^{3}H]hydroxy-*N,N*-di-*n*-propyl-2-aminotetralin. *Proc Natl Acad Sci USA* 1992;89:8155–8159.
25. Levey AI, Hersch SM, Rye DB, et al. Localization of D_1 and D_2 dopamine receptors in brain with subtype-specific antibodies. *Proc Natl Acad Sci USA* 1993;90:8861–8865.
26. Mansour A, Meador-Woodruff JH, Bunzow JR, Civelli O, Akil H, Watson SJ. Localization of dopamine D_2 receptor mRNA and D_1 and D_2 receptor binding in the rat brain and pituitary: an *in situ* hybridization-receptor autoradiographic analysis. *J Neurosci* 1990;10:2587–2600.
27. Mansour A, Meador-Woodruff JH, Camp DM, et al. The effects of nigrostriatal 6-hydroxydopamine lesions on dopamine D_2 receptor mRNA and opioid systems. *The international narcotics research conference (INRC) '89*. New York: Alan R Liss, 1990;227–230.
28. Mansour A, Meador-Woodruff JH, Zhou Q-Y, Civelli O, Akil H, Watson SJ. A comparison of D_1 receptor binding and mRNA in rat brain using receptor autoradiographic and *in situ* hybridization techniques. *Neuroscience* 1991;45:359–371.
29. Meador-Woodruff JH, Mansour A. Expression of the dopamine D_2 receptor gene in brain. *Biol Psych* 1991;30:985–1007.
30. Meador-Woodruff JH, Mansour A, Bunzow JR, Van Tol HHM, Watson SJ, Civelli O. Distribution of D_2 receptor mRNA in rat brain. *Proc Natl Acad Sci USA* 1989;86:7625–7628.
31. Meador-Woodruff JH, Mansour A, Civelli O, Watson SJ. Distribution of D_2 dopamine receptor mRNA in the primate brain. *Prog Neuropsychopharmacol Biol Psychiatry* 1991;15:885–893.
32. Meador-Woodruff JH, Mansour A, Grandy DK, Damask SP, Civelli O, Watson SJ Jr. Distribution of D_5 dopamine receptor mRNA in rat brain. *Neurosci Lett* 1992;145:209–212.
33. McGonigle P, Artvmvshvn RP, McElligott S, Kung MP, Kung H. Determination of dopamine D_3 receptor distribution in rat brain using [^{125}I]7-Trans-OH-PIPAT. *Soc Neurosci Abstr* 1993;2:1369.
34. Mengod G, Martinez-Mir MI, Vilaró, Palacios JM. Localization of the mRNA for the dopamine D_2 receptor in the rat brain by *in situ* hybridization histochemistry. *Proc Natl Acad Sci USA* 1989;86:8560–8564.

splicing in the third cytoplasmic loop. *J Biol Chem* 1993;268:5872–5878.

35. Monsma FJ Jr, Mahan LC, McVittie LD, Gerfen CR, Sibley DR. Molecular cloning and expression of a D_1 dopamine receptor linked to adenylyl cyclase activation. *Proc Natl Acad Sci USA* 1990;87:6723–6727.

36. Montmayeur J-P, Borrelli E. Transcription mediated by a cAMP-responsive promoter element is reduced upon activation of dopamine D_2 receptors. *Proc Natl Acad Sci USA* 1991;88:3135–3139.

37. Montmayeur J-P, Guiramand J, Borrelli E. Preferential coupling between dopamine D2 receptors and G-proteins. *Mol Endocrinol* 1993;7:161–170.

38. Nagy JI, Lee T, Seeman P, Fibiger HC. Direct evidence for presynaptic and postsynaptic dopamine receptors in brain. *Nature* 1978;274:278–281.

39. Neve KA, Neve RL, Fidel S, Janowsky A, Higgins GA. Increased abundance of alternatively spliced forms of D2 dopamine receptor mRNA after denervation. *Proc Natl Acad Sci USA* 1991;88:2802–2806.

40. O'Malley KL, Harmon S, Tang L, Todd RD. The rat dopamine D_4 receptor: sequence, gene structure, and demonstration of expression in the cardiovascular system. *New Biol* 1992;4:137–146.

41. Schmauss C, Haroutunian V, Davis KL, Davidson M. Selective loss of dopamine D_3-type receptor mRNA expression in parietal and motor cortices of patients with chronic schizophrenia. *Proc Natl Acad Sci USA* 1993;90:8942–8946.

42. Schwarcz R, Creese I, Coyle JT, Snyder SH. Dopamine receptors localised on cerebral cortical afferents to rat corpus striatum. *Nature* 1978;271:766–768.

43. Seeman P. Dopamine receptor sequences—therapeutic levels of neuroleptics occupy D_2 receptors, clozapine occupies D_4. *Neuropsychopharmacology* 1992;7:261–284.

44. Skirboll LR, Grace AA, Bunney BS. Dopamine auto- and postsynaptic receptors: electrophysiological evidence for differential sensitivity to dopamine agonists. *Science* 1979;206:80–82.

45. Snyder LA, Roberts JL, Sealfon SC. Distribution of dopamine D_2 receptor mRNA splice variants in the rat by solution hybridization/protection assay. *Neurosci Lett* 1991;122:37–40.

46. Sokoloff P, Giros B, Martres M-P, Bouthenet M-L, Schwartz J-C. Molecular cloning and characterization of a novel dopamine receptor (D_3) as a target for neuroleptics. *Nature* 1990;347:146–151.

47. Stoof JC, Kebabian JW. Two dopamine receptors: biochemistry, physiology and pharmacology. *Life Sci* 1984;35:2281–2296.

48. Sunahara RK, Guan H-C, O'Dowd BF, et al. Cloning of the gene for a human dopamine D_5 receptor with higher affinity for dopamine than D_1. *Nature* 1991;350:614–619.

49. Sunahara RK, Niznik HB, Weiner DM, et al. Human dopamine D_1 receptor encoded by an intronless gene on chromosome 5. *Nature* 1990;347:80–83.

50. Surmeier DJ, Eberwine J, Wilson CJ, Cao Y, Stefani A, Kitai ST. Dopamine receptor subtypes colocalize in rat striatonigral neurons. *Proc Natl Acad Sci USA* 1992;89:10178–10182.

51. Swansom LW. The projections of the ventral tegmental area and adjacent regions: a combined fluorescent retrograde tracer and immunofluorescence study in the rat. *Brain Res Bull* 1982;9:321–353.

52. Tiberi M, Jarvie KR, Silvia C, et al. Cloning, molecular characterization, and chromosomal assignment of a gene encoding a second D_1 dopamine receptor subtype: differential expression pattern in rat brain compared with the D_{1A} receptor. *Proc Natl Acad Sci USA* 1991;88:7491–7495.

53. Toso RD, Sommer B, Ewert M, et al. The dopamine D_2 receptor: two molecular forms generated by alternative splicing. *EMBO J* 1989;8:4025–4034.

54. Van Tol HHM, Bunzow JR, Guan H-C, et al. Cloning of the gene for a human dopamine D_4 receptor with high affinity for the antipsychotic clozapine. *Nature* 1991;350:610–614.

55. Van Tol HHM, Wu CM, Guan H-C, et al. Multiple dopamine D4 receptor variants in the human population. *Nature* 1992;358:149–152.

56. Wamsley JK, Gehlert DR, Filloux FM, Dawson TM. Comparison of the distribution of D-1 and D-2 dopamine receptors in the rat brain. *J Chem Neuroanatomy* 1989;2:119–137.

57. Weiner DM, Levey AI, Brann MR. Expression of muscarinic acetylcholine and dopamine receptor mRNAs in rat basal ganglia. *Proc Natl Acad Sci USA* 1990;87:7050–7054.

58. Weiner DM, Levey AI, Sunahara RK, et al. D_1 and D_2 dopamine receptor mRNA in rat brain. *Proc Natl Acad Sci USA* 1991;88:1859–1863.

59. Zhou Q-Y, Grandy DK, Thambi L, et al. Cloning and expression of human and rat D_1 dopamine receptors. *Nature* 1990;347:76–80.

Psychopharmacology: The Fourth
Generation of Progress, edited by
Floyd E. Bloom and David J. Kupfer.
Raven Press, Ltd., New York © 1995.

CHAPTER 20

Dopamine Autoreceptor Signal Transduction and Regulation

Louis A. Chiodo, Arthur S. Freeman, and Benjamin S. Bunney

The electrophysiological investigation of dopamine (DA) neurons within the mammalian brain has spanned some 24 years. This area of investigation, when coupled with the dramatic advances in our knowledge of the biochemistry, molecular biology, anatomy, and behavior of these neuronal systems, has yielded many insights into the regulation of these cells and their role in normal and perhaps aberrant behavior. Several guiding principles have emerged in our conceptualization of the membrane physiology of these clinically important cells. One such principle is that these cells possess presynaptic dopamine receptors that serve as autoreceptors [a term coined by Arvid Carlsson (9)]. That is, DA neurons have receptors that are sensitive to the neurotransmitter released by these cells—DA itself. The analysis of the precise role that autoreceptors play in regulating the physiological activity of these neurons has received extensive study (13; see also Chapter 15, *this volume*), in part, because changes in these regulatory mechanisms may be involved in clinical disorders in which dopaminergic neuronal systems have been implicated. We now know that most mesencephalic DA neurons possess DA autoreceptors that modulate membrane excitability (thereby controlling the level of spontaneous action potential generation), DA synthesis, and DA release (see Chapter 21, *this volume*). In contrast to most midbrain DA cells, those that project to certain frontal cortical regions possess only release-modulating nerve terminal autoreceptors (12,24). Given the current conceptual understanding that DA autoreceptors play a critical self-regulatory (self-inhibitory) role in these cells, why do subpopulations of mesencephalic DA neurons

lack certain functional autoreceptor mechanisms? Moreover, how is the expression of these autoreceptor-modulated functions determined, and how might they be altered? Although the answers to these questions are yet to be found, an understanding has been gained as to the coupling of DA autoreceptors, located on the somal and dendritic membranes of these cells (called somatodendritic DA autoreceptors), to transmembrane ionic currents that underlie the ability of these receptors to alter DA cell excitability. We will review the current understanding of the regulation of both potassium- and calcium-dependent currents in DA neurons and discuss our present knowledge of the signal transduction mechanisms that are involved.

In recent years, it has become apparent that we need to revise our concept of autoreceptors with respect to DA neurons. It has been demonstrated that the peptides cholecystokinin (CCK) and neurotensin are differentially colocalized with DA in subpopulations of midbrain DA neurons. These peptides can be released from the DA neuron and stimulate their specific receptors also located on the DA cell membrane. Thus, we now need to conceptualize DA neurons as possessing not only DA autoreceptors, but also CCK and neurotensin autoreceptors. Moreover, these peptides have the ability to modulate DA autoreceptor function. Recent studies of the effects of these peptides on impulse-regulating DA autoreceptors will be discussed.

IMPULSE-MODULATING DOPAMINE AUTORECEPTORS

In the early 1970s, it was observed that the local microiontophoretic application of either DA or the mixed D_1/D_2 receptor agonist apomorphine inhibited the spontaneous electrical activity of mesencephalic DA neurons when

L. A. Chiodo and A. S. Freeman: Department of Pharmacology, Texas Tech University Health Sciences Center, Lubbock, Texas 79430.
B. S. Bunney: Department of Psychiatry, Yale University School of Medicine, New Haven, Connecticut 06519.

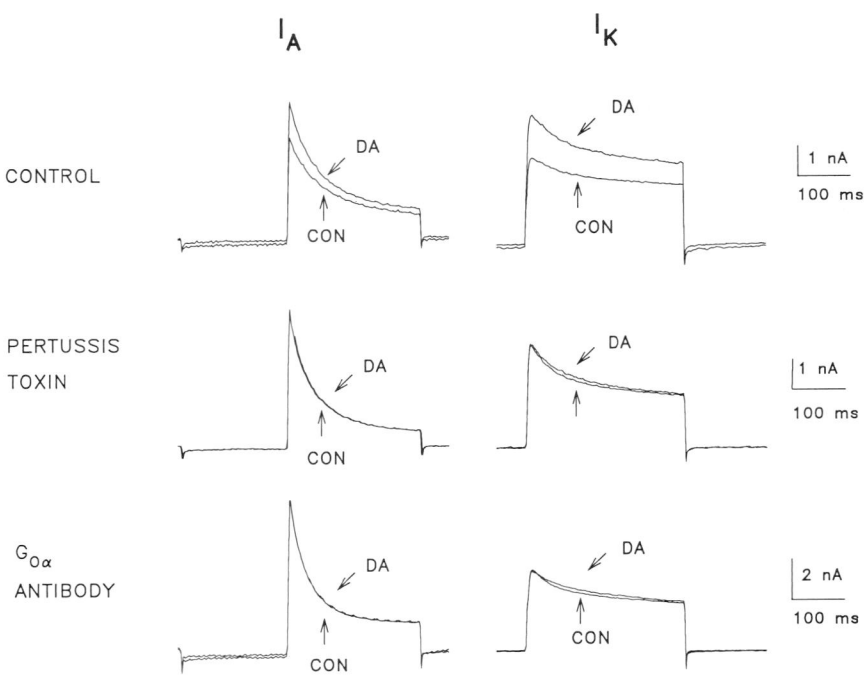

FIG. 1. Illustration of the effects of the local application of DA on both I_A and I_K observed in DA neurons maintained in primary culture. The whole-cell current traces were obtained from cells under control conditions (CONTROL), after the pretreatment with pertussis toxin (PERTUSSIS TOXIN), and after the intracellular application of a polyclonal antibody selective for the α subunit of G_o ($G_{o\alpha}$ ANTIBODY). It can be seen that under control conditions the application of DA (100 μM in the pressure ejection pipette) readily increased the magnitude of I_A and I_K. In contrast, the other two treatments completely blocked these responses to DA autoreceptor stimulation. Both currents were measured under whole-cell patch recording conditions. To measure I_A, the membrane was held at -40 mV and then stepped to -90 mV for 200 msec before jumping to the test membrane potential of 30 mV. To measure I_K, the membrane was held at -60 mV and jumped to a test potential of 30 mV. (See ref. 42 for complete discussion.)

applied onto the soma and dendrites of these cells (1,2). Since then, this effect has been demonstrated numerous times (for review, see ref. 13), and it is now taken as a hallmark attribute of this neurochemical class of cells (i.e., these cells possess somatodendritic DA autoreceptors that regulate impulse flow as part of their normal electrophysiological behavior). These receptors are of the D_2 receptor subtype that is part of the superfamily of G-protein-coupled receptors (59; see also Chapters 14 and 27, *this volume*). In support of this classification, pretreatment with pertussis toxin, which inactivates both G_i and G_o, blocks the inhibitory effects of somatodendritic autoreceptors (34).

IMPULSE-REGULATING DOPAMINE AUTORECEPTORS AND POTASSIUM CURRENTS

Several lines of evidence have shown that D_2 DA receptor activation increases potassium conductances in a variety of tissues, including the MMQ clonal pituitary cell line (43), dissociated striatal neurons (23), and lactotrophs (11). Similarly, it has been observed that DA autoreceptor stimulation increases potassium conductances in mesencephalic DA neurons in both (a) the in vitro slice (38) and (b) primary dissociated cell culture preparations (14,17). The whole-cell potassium conductance of these cells is mediated by several distinct potassium currents (15,17,51,61). Indeed, it is now known that mesencephalic DA neurons possess an anomalous rectifier current functioning at hyperpolarized membrane potentials (I_{ANOM}), two different calcium-dependent outward currents (one that is apamin-sensitive, termed I_{AHP}) that are im-

portant in the afterhyperpolarization that follows the action potential, the delayed rectifier (I_K), a transient A current (I_A), and apparently an ATP-sensitive current (I_{ATP}).

The regulation of distinct potassium currents has recently been studied in some detail. It is now known that direct stimulation of the DA somatodendritic autoreceptor increases at least three different potassium currents: I_K, I_{ANOM}, and I_A (18,42). It was shown recently that the coupling of D_2 receptors to both I_A and I_K utilize a common signal transduction pathway that involves G_o (18,42). Thus, the increase in the magnitude of both these currents is pertussis-toxin-sensitive, blocked by intracellular application of GDPβS, mimicked by GTPγS, and abolished by the intracellular application of an antibody directed against the $G_{o\alpha}$ subunit (see Fig. 1). At this time, it is not clear whether the activated α subunit of G_o directly influences both I_A and I_K channels or influences the observed whole-cell current via some additional intracellular mechanism. Although direct α-subunit modulation of potassium channels has been shown in other tissues (6,37,44,65,67), the activated subunit could influence other cellular transduction systems. It would appear, however, that changes in intracellular levels of cAMP are probably not involved (58).

IMPULSE-REGULATING DOPAMINE AUTORECEPTORS AND CALCIUM CURRENTS

It has been known for some time that DA neurons possess both high- and low-threshold calcium conductances (14,27,28). These conductances are generally thought to be critically involved in the regulation of DA cell excitability. It has been shown that DA cells possess

A

B

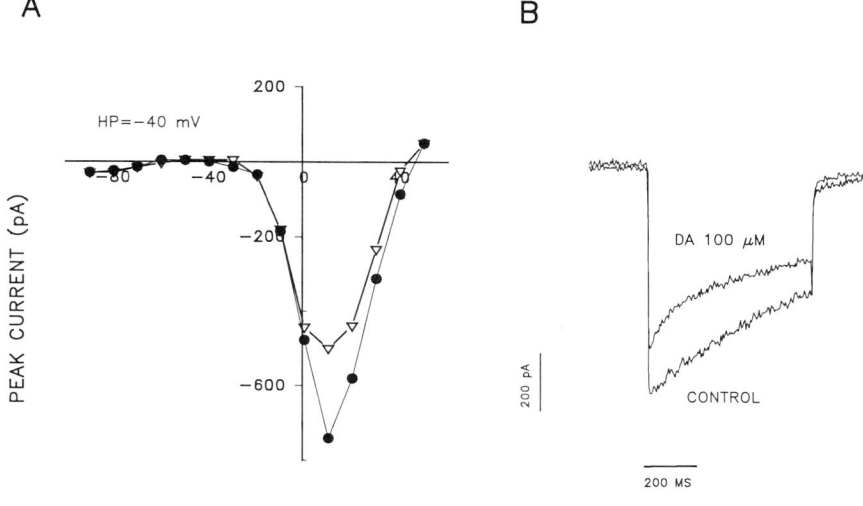

HP=−40 mV

PEAK CURRENT (pA)

MEMBRANE POTENTIAL (mV)

DA 100 μM

CONTROL

200 pA

200 MS

FIG. 2. Illustration of DA-induced inhibition of I_L in cultured mesencephalic DA neurons. **A:** Whole-cell current traces showing I_L before (●, Control) and after the local application of DA (△, DA 100 μM). The membrane was held at −40 mV and stepped to a potential of 10 mV. **B:** The current−voltage relationship for the cell shown in **A**.

three different calcium currents: I_N, I_T, and I_L (39,40). I_T is a low-voltage-activated current (activated at −50 mV) that displays a rapid inactivation and is blocked partially by amiloride or nickel. I_L may be activated by depolarizing voltage steps from a holding potential of −40 mV. This current slowly and incompletely inactivates, and is blocked completely by nifedipine. I_N is also observed in DA neurons, and it activates at the same thresholds as I_L, but it requires prior hyperpolarization of the membrane (to −90 mV) and is ω-conotoxin-sensitive. Both I_L and I_N, but not I_T, are reduced by stimulation of the DA autoreceptor (Fig. 2). The coupling of the DA autoreceptor to these currents involves a pertussis-toxin-sensitive G protein because pertussis toxin pretreatment blocks the coupling of the somatodendritic autoreceptor to both I_N and I_L (Fig. 3). Additional studies are required to determine which G proteins are utilized and whether the different currents are coupled to the DA autoreceptor by similar or different transduction pathways.

EXPRESSED D₂ RECEPTORS IN TRANSFECTED CELLS

Analysis of the D₂ receptor gene has shown that at least two molecular forms of this receptor are produced via alternative splicing of mRNA (8,44,45,59). These two distinct isoforms are termed D₂-short (D₂S) and D₂-long (D₂L) and differ by a 29-amino-acid sequence contained within the third cytoplasmic loop. Given that this cytoplasmic loop is critically important for receptor interactions with G proteins, it has been hypothesized that these receptor isoforms may couple to effector systems within cells via different signal transduction pathways. Because the mRNA for these receptors are colocalized within the same neurons (including DA neurons; see refs. 25, 47–49, and 64) and selective pharmacological agents are not available (20,26), individual expression of these isoforms

in a single cell line has been used by several groups to begin to examine this issue. When expressed in NG108-15 neuroblastoma × glioma hybrid cells, the D₂ selectivity of these receptors is maintained and these receptors couple to potassium channels in the cell membrane. In this expression system, it has been shown that the D₂S isoform couples to potassium currents via a pertussis-toxin-insensitive mechanism (10), whereas D₂L receptors couple to the same currents via a pertussis-toxin-sensitive process (41). These observations raise the possibility that the D₂ receptor isoforms, when expressed in the same cells (as is the case with the DA neurons), can influence transmembrane currents in similar ways but via independent transduction pathways. The precise nature of D₂ isoform modulation of a variety of physiological events in the DA neuron will surely be studied extensively over the next few years. The information obtained will likely change our understanding of the molecular diversity of DA autoreceptor regulation in these cells. The use of expression systems such as the NG108 cell line should prove to be of great value in these investigations.

OTHER DA AUTORECEPTORS?

Recent work by several groups has demonstrated that DA neurons in the midbrain possess not only mRNA for both isoforms of the D₂ receptors, but also a message for the closely related D₃ receptor (5,63). This has raised the intriguing possibility that DA neurons possess a variety of functionally distinct DA autoreceptors. To date, it has been hard to ascertain the role of D₃ receptors in vivo because the available drugs that are relatively selective for these receptors also exert strong actions at D₂ receptors. Thus, initial studies have begun to examine these D₃ receptors following their stable expression in NG108-15 cells (19). This work has shown that the D₃ receptor couples to outward potassium currents in these cells in a

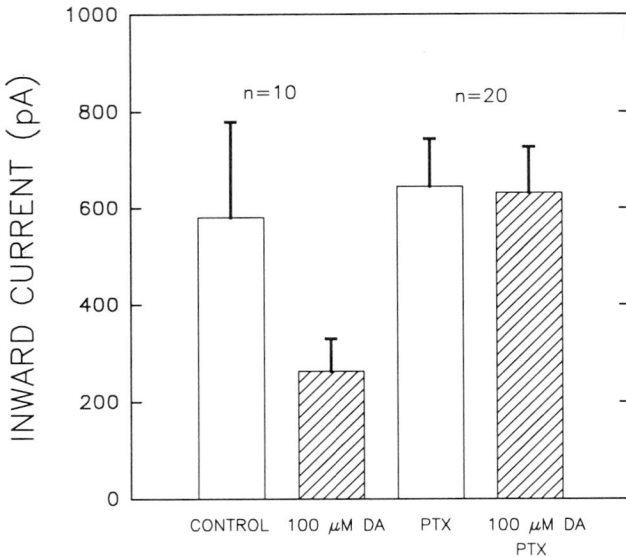

FIG. 3. Bars graphs demonstrating the effects of pertussis toxin pretreatment on the calcium current, I_L, observed in cultured mesencephalic DA neurons. It can be seen that the normal reduction in I_L, which is produced by stimulating the DA autoreceptors with DA (100 μM), is completely abolished by pertussis toxin pretreatment.

manner similar to that observed for D_{2S} and D_{2L}. The coupling of this receptor to potassium currents is pertussis-toxin-sensitive, and the intracellular application of an antibody directed against the $G_{o\alpha}$ subunit completely blocked D_3-mediated inhibition of these currents.

PEPTIDES COLOCALIZED WITH DA MAY INFLUENCE AUTORECEPTOR MECHANISMS

Many DA neurons in the rat ventral tegmental area and medial substantia nigra pars compacta contain the peptide cotransmitter CCK (30,53,54), which is present in the brain mainly in its sulfated octapeptide form (4,21,22,50). A subpopulation of these DA/CCK neurons contains a second peptide cotransmitter, neurotensin (52). In addition to the acknowledged autoregulatory role of nonsynaptic somatodendritically released DA, the similar release of these peptides may result in additional phasic autoregulatory influences on the transmembrane currents and impulse activity of DA neurons. The midbrain also receives a sparse input from CCK-containing axon terminals (52) and receives a more dense input from neurotensin-containing terminals (see below and Chapter 18, *this volume*).

Exogenously administered CCK and neurotensin influence the sensitivity of impulse-regulating DA autoreceptors to DA agonist-induced inhibition of firing rate. To date, these studies have been limited to extracellular electrophysiological experiments. After intravenous (i.v.) administration to rats, CCK potentiates the inhibitory effects of i.v. administration of the mixed DA agonist apo-

morphine (32,33), and of the D2 agonist quinpirole (36), on DA cell firing rate. Microiontophoresis of CCK into the vicinity of the somatodendritic region of DA cells also potentiates the inhibitory effects of similarly applied DA (16). Bath-applied CCK potentiates the inhibitory effects of DA and quinpirole in midbrain brain slices in vitro (7,66). Although not proof, these studies suggest that the effect of CCK on DA autoreceptor-mediated inhibition of impulse flow is due to a direct interaction with the DA cell membrane. Similarly, a substantial portion of the excitatory effects of i.v. CCK on DA cell firing rate was concluded to be due to direct effects on DA cells (31). Intracellular studies are required to elucidate the nature of the specific ionic conductances involved in the interaction of CCK with autoreceptor mechanisms.

CCK binds to both CCK-A and CCK-B receptors (46). Unsulfated CCK and CCK tetrapeptide are selective CCK-B agonists, and they have been used to explore the question of which receptor subtype is associated with the modulatory effects of CCK on DA autoreceptor function. There are reports of involvement of CCK-A receptors (36) and CCK-B receptors (33) in these effects.

In contrast to CCK, the tridecapeptide neurotensin attenuates the inhibitory effects of DA autoreceptor stimulation on DA neuronal firing rate. Intracerebroventricular administration of neurotensin antagonizes the inhibitory effects of i.v. quinpirole on DA cell activity (56). In in vitro midbrain slices, neurotensin also attenuates the inhibitory effects of DA (57) and the DA agonist BHT 920 (55) on DA cell firing rate. Neurotensin exerts this effect through a cAMP-dependent mechanism: This effect is mimicked by 8-Br-cAMP, by forskolin, by inhibition of phosphodiesterase, and by inhibition of protein kinase A (58).

In the ventral tegmental area, it appears that all neurotensin-immunoreactive perikarya also contain DA (3,29,52). Some of these perikarya are in direct apposition to another DA neuron (3), which provides the anatomical basis for intercellular effects of somatodendritic neurotensin and DA on DA cells. In addition, neurotensin-containing axon terminals exist in the midbrain (3,29,35,52,68). About one-third of the targets of these terminals are DA cells (3). As with CCK, detailed analysis of the effects of neurotensin on transmembrane ionic currents should enhance our understanding of the mechanism of action of this peptide in the modulation of impulse-regulating DA autoreceptors. The opposing effects of CCK and neurotensin on DA autoreceptor function may represent a fine-tuning mechanism for the control of DA autoreceptor sensitivity.

FUTURE PERSPECTIVES

As reviewed above, our understanding of the nature of somatodendritic autoreceptor modulation of DA cell activity has changed over the last few years. We now know that a variety of specific potassium and calcium currents in these cells are modulated by DA autoreceptor stimulation. The increase in the magnitudes of I_A and I_K, when coupled with the decrease in magnitudes of I_L and I_N, serves as a direct and effective means of decreasing DA cell membrane excitability. It remains to be determined which G proteins are involved in the coupling of DA autoreceptors with inward calcium currents. An understanding of the transduction mechanisms that influence these inward currents is critical to determining which individual currents are affected by autoreceptor stimulation. For example, it is now clear that, because I_A and I_K share a common transduction pathway, they are modulated simultaneously by agonist stimulation of the autoreceptor. If I_L and I_N are shown to be associated with G proteins different from those associated with I_A and I_K, it would suggest that the autoreceptor-mediated increase in outward and decrease in inward currents could be affected differentially.

REFERENCES

1. Aghajanian GK, Bunney BS. Central dopaminergic neurons: neurophysiological identification and response to drugs. In: Usdin E, Snyder SH, eds. *Frontiers of catecholamine research.* New York: Pergamon Press, 1973;643–648.
2. Aghajanian GK, Bunney BS. Pre- and postsynaptic feedback mechanisms in central dopaminergic neurons. In: Seeman P, Brown GM, eds. *Frontiers of neurology and neuroscience research.* Toronto: University of Toronto Press, 1974;4–11.
3. Bayer VE, Towle AC, Pickel VM. Ultrastructural localization of neurotensin-like immunoreactivity within dense core vesicles in perikarya, but not terminals, colocalizing tyrosine hydroxylase in the rat ventral tegmental area. *J Comp Neurol* 1991;311:179–196.
4. Beinfeld MC, Meyer DK, Eskay RL, Jensen RT, Brownstein MJ. The distribution of cholecystokinin immunoreactivity in the central nervous system of the rat as determined by radioimmunoassay. *Brain Res* 1981;212:51–57.
5. Bouthenet ML, Souil E, Matres MP, Sokoloff P, Giros B, Schwartz JC. Localisation of dopamine D3 receptor mRNA in the rat brain using in situ hybridisation histochemistry: comparison with dopamine D2 receptor mRNA. *Brain Res* 1991;564:203–219.
6. Breitwieser GE. G protein-mediated ion channel activation. *Hypertension* 1991;17:684–692.
7. Brodie MS, Dunwiddie TV. Cholecystokinin potentiates dopamine inhibition of mesencephalic dopamine neurons in vitro. *Brain Res* 1987;425:106–113.
8. Bunzow JR, VanTol HHM, Grandy DK, Albert P, Salon J, Christie M, Machida CA, Neve KA, Civelli O. Cloning and expression of a rat D_2 dopamine receptor cDNA. *Nature* 1988;336:783–787.
9. Carlsson A. Dopaminergic autoreceptors. In: Almgren O, Carlsson A, Engel J, eds. *Chemical tools in catecholamine research,* vol 11. Amsterdam: North-Holland, 1975;219–224.
10. Castellano MA, Liu L-X, Monsma FJ Jr, Sibley DR, Kapatos G, Chiodo LA. Transfected D_2 short dopamine receptors inhibit voltage-dependent potassium current in neuroblastoma × glioma hybrid (NG108-15) cells. *Mol Pharmacol* 1993;44:649–656.
11. Castelletti L, Memo M, Missale C, Spano PF, Valerio A. Potassium channels involved in the transduction mechanism of dopamine D-2 receptor in rat lactotrophs. *J Physiol (Lond)* 1989;410:251–265.
12. Chiodo LA, Bannon MJ, Grace AA, Roth RH, Bunney BS. Evidence for the absence of impulse-regulating somatodendritic and synthesis-modulating nerve terminal autoreceptors on subpopulations of midbrain dopamine neurons. *Neuroscience* 1984;12:1–16.
13. Chiodo LA. Dopamine-containing neurons in the mammalian central nervous system: electrophysiology and pharmacology. *Neurosci Biobehav Rev* 1988;12:49–90.
14. Chiodo LA, Kapatos G. Mesencephalic dopamine-containing neurons in culture: morphological and electrophysiological characterization. In: Chiodo LA, Freeman AS, eds. *Neurophysiology of dopamine neuronal systems—current status and clinical perspectives.* Grosse Pointe, MI: Lakeshore Publishing Co., 1987;67–91.
15. Chiodo LA. Dopamine autoreceptor signal transduction in the DA cell body: a "current" view. *Neurochem Int* 1992;20:18S–84S.
16. Chiodo LA, Freeman AS, Bunney BS. Electrophysiological studies on the specificity of the cholecystokinin antagonist proglumide. *Brain Res* 1987;410:205–211.
17. Chiodo LA, Kapatos G. Membrane properties of identified mesencephalic dopamine neurons in primary dissociated cell culture. *Synapse* 1992;11:294–309.
18. Chiodo LA, Liu L-X, Kapatos G. $G_{o\alpha}$ mediates transduction of DA autoreceptor modulation of three different K^+ currents. *Soc Neurosci Abstr* 1992;18:1516.
19. Chiodo LA, Liu L-X, Monsma FJ Jr, Sibley DR. Transfected D3 dopamine receptors inhibit voltage-dependent potassium current in neuroblastoma × glioma hybrid (NG108-15) cells. *Soc Neurosci Abstr* 1993;19:79.
20. Dal Toso R, Sommer B, Ewert M, Herb A, Pritchett DB, Bach A, Shiver BD, Seeburg PH. The dopamine D_2 receptor: two molecular forms generated by alternative splicing. *EMBO J* 1989;8:4025–4034.
21. Dockray GJ. Cholecystokinin in rat cerebral cortex: identification, purification and characterization by immunochemical methods. *Brain Res* 1980;188:155–165.
22. Freeman AS, Chiodo LA, Lentz S, Wade K, Bannon MJ. Release of CCK from midbrain slices and modulatory influence of D2 DA receptor stimulation. *Brain Res* 1991;555:281–287.
23. Freedman JE, Weight FF. Quinine potently blocks single K^+ channels activated by dopamine D-2 receptors in rat corpus striatum. *Eur J Pharmacol* 1989;164:341–346.
24. Galloway MP, Wolf ME, Roth RH. Regulation of dopamine synthesis in the medial prefrontal cortex is mediated by release modulating autoreceptors: studies in vivo. *J Pharmacol Exp Ther* 1986;236:689–698.
25. Gandelman KY, Harmon S, Todd RD, O'Malley KL. Analysis of the structure and expression of human dopamine D2A receptor gene. *J Neurochem* 1991;56:1024–1029.
26. Giros B, Sokoloff P, Matres MP, Riou JF, Emorine LJ, Schwartz JC. Alternative splicing directs the expression of two D_2 dopamine receptor isoforms. *Nature* 1989;343:923–926.
27. Grace AA. The regulation of dopamine neurons as determined by in vivo and in vitro intracellular recordings. In: Chiodo LA, Freeman AS, eds. *Neurophysiology of dopamine neuronal systems—current status and clinical perspectives.* Grosse Pointe, MI: Lakeshore Publishing Co., 1987;1–66.
28. Grace AA, Onn S-P. Morphology and electrophysiological properties of immunocytochemically identified rat dopamine neurons recorded in vitro. *J Neurosci* 1989;9:3463–3481.
29. Hökfelt T, Everitt BJ, Theodorsson-Norheim E, Goldstein M. Occurrence of neurotenson-like immunoreactivity in subpopulations of hypothalamic, mesencephalic and medullary catecholamine neurons. *J Comp Neurol* 1984;222:543–559.
30. Hökfelt T, Skirboll L, Rehfeld JF, Goldstein M, Markey K, Dann O. A subpopulation of mesencephalic dopamine neurons projecting to limbic areas contains a cholecystokinin-like peptide: evidence from immunohistochemistry combined with retrograde tracing. *Neuroscience* 1980;5:2093–2124.
31. Hommer DW, Palkovits M, Crawley JN, Paul SM, Skirboll LR. Cholecystokinin-induced excitation in the substantia nigra: evidence for peripheral and central components. *J Neurosci* 1985;6:1387–1392.
32. Hommer DW, Skirboll LR. Cholecystokinin-like peptides potentiate apomorphine-induced inhibition of dopamine neurons. *Eur J Pharmacol* 1983;91:151–152.
33. Hommer DW, Stoner G, Crawley JN, Paul SM, Skirboll LR. Cholecystokinin-dopamine coexistence: electrophysiological actions corresponding to cholecystokinin receptor subtype. *J Neurosci* 1986;6:3039–3043.
34. Innis RB, Aghajanian GK. Pertussis toxin blocks autoreceptor-mediated inhibition of dopaminergic neurons in rat substantia nigra. *Brain Res* 1987;411:139–143.
35. Jennes L, Stumpf WE, Kalivas PW. Neurotensin: topographical

distribution in rat brain by immunocytochemistry. *J Comp Neurol* 1982;210:211–224.

36. Kelland MD, Chiodo LA, Freeman AS. Receptor selectivity of cholecystokinin effects on mesoaccumbens dopamine neurons. *Synapse* 1991;8:137–143.

37. Kurachi Y, Tung RT, Ito H, Nakajima T. G protein activation of cardiac muscarinic K^+ channels. *Prog Neurobiol* 1992;39:229–246.

38. Lacey MG, Mercuri NB, North RA. Dopamine acts on D2 receptors to increase potassium conductances in neurones of the rat substantia nigra zona compacta. *J Physiol* 1987;392:397–416.

39. Liu L-X, Kapatos G, Chiodo LA. Voltage-clamp analysis of calcium-dependent inward currents in cultured mesencephalic dopamine neurons. *Soc Neurosci Abstr* 1991;17:1350.

40. Liu L-X, Kapatos G, Chiodo LA. DA autoreceptor modulation of different calcium currents in DA neurons. *Soc Neurosci Abstr* 1992;18:1516.

41. Liu L-X, Monsma FJ Jr, Sibley DR, Chiodo LA. Coupling of D_2-long receptor isoform to K+ currents in neuroblastoma × glioma (NG108-15) cells. *Soc Neurosci Abstr* 1993;19:79.

42. Liu L-X, Shen R-Y, Kapatos G, Chiodo LA. Dopamine neuron membrane physiology: characterization of the transient outward current (I_A) and demonstration of a common signal transduction pathway for I_A and I_K. *Synapse* 1994;[*in press*].

43. Login IS, Pancrazio JJ, Kim YI. Dopamine enhances a voltage-dependent transient K^+ current in the MMQ cell, a clonal pituitary line expressing functional D_2 dopamine receptors. *Brain Res* 1990;506:331–334.

44. Man-Son-Hing H, Codina J, Abramowitz J, Haydon PG. Microinjection of the α-subunit of the G protein G_{o2}, but not G_{o1}, reduces a voltage-sensitive calcium current. *Cell Signaling* 1992;4:429–441.

45. Monsma FJ, McVittie LD, Gerfen CR, Mahan LC, Sibley DR. Multiple D_2 dopamine receptors produced by alternative RNA splicing. *Nature* 1989;342:926–929.

46. Moran TH, Robinson PH, Goldrich MS, McHugh PR. Two brain cholecystokinin receptors: implications for behavioral actions. *Brain Res* 986;62:175–179.

47. Neve KA, Henningsen RA, Bunzow JR, Civelli O. Functional characterization of a rat dopamine D-2 receptor cDNA expressed in a mammalian cell line. *Mol Pharmacol* 1989;36:446–451.

48. Neve KA, Neve RL, Fidel S, Janowsky A, Higgins GA. Increased abundance of alternatively spliced forms of D_2 dopamine receptor mRNA after denervation. *Proc Natl Acad Sci USA* 1991;88:2802–2806.

49. O'Malley KL, Mack KJ, Gandelman KY, Todd RD. Organization and expression of the rat $D2_A$ receptor gene: identification of alternative transcripts and a variant donor splice site. *Biochemistry* 1990;29:1367–1371.

50. Rehfeld JF. Immunochemical studies on cholecystokinin. II. Distribution and molecular heterogeneity in the central nervous system and small intestine of man and hog. *J Biol Chem* 1978;253:4022–4030.

51. Roeper J, Hainsworth AH, Ashcroft FM. Tolbutamide reverses membrane hyperpolarization induced by activation of D2 receptors and GABAB receptors in isolated substantia nigra neurones. *Eur J Pharmacol* 1990;416:473–475.

52. Seroogy KB, Ceccatelli S, Schalling M, Hökfelt T, Frey P, Dockray G, Buchan A, Goldstein M. A subpopulation of dopaminergic neurons in the rat ventral mesencephalon contain both neurotensin and cholecystokinin. *Brain Res* 1988;455:88–98.

53. Seroogy KB, Dangaran K, Lim S, Haycock JW, Fallon JH. Ventral mesencephalic neurons containing cholecystokinin- and tyrosine hydroxylase-like immunoreactivities project to forebrain regions. *J Comp Neurol* 1989;279:397–414.

54. Seroogy K, Schalling M, Brene S, Dagerlind A, Chai SY, Hökfelt T, Persson H, Brownstein M, Huan R, Dixon J, Filer D, Schlessinger D, Goldstein M. Cholecystokinin and tyrosine hydroxylase messenger RNAs in neurons of rat mesencephalon: peptide/monoamine coexistence studies using in situ hybridization combined with immunocytochemistry. *Exp Brain Res* 1989;74:149–162.

55. Seutin V, Massotte L, Dresse A. Electrophysiological effects of neurotensin on dopaminergic neurones of the ventral tegmental area of the rat in vitro. *Neuropharmacology* 1989;28:949–954.

56. Shi W-X, Bunney BS. Neurotensin attenuates dopamine D2 agonist quinpirole-induced inhibition of midbrain dopamine neurons. *Neuropharmacology* 1990;29:1095–1097.

57. Shi W-X, Bunney BS. Neurotensin modulates autoreceptor mediated dopamine effects on midbrain dopamine cell activity. *Brain Res* 1991;543:315–321.

58. Shi W-X, Bunney BS. Roles of intracellular cAMP and protein kinase A in the actions of dopamine and neurotensin on midbrain dopamine neurons. *J Neuroscience* 1992;12:2433–2438.

59. Sibley DR, Monsma FJ Jr. Molecular biology of dopamine receptors. *Trends Pharmacol Sci* 1992;13:61–69.

60. Sibley DR. Cloning of a D_3 receptor subtype expands dopamine receptor family. *Trends Pharmacol Sci* 1991;12:7–9.

61. Silva NL, Bunney BS. Intracellular studies of dopamine neurons in vitro: pacemakers modulated by dopamine. *Eur J Pharmacol* 1988;149:307–315.

62. Silva NL, Barker JL. Calcium currents recorded from nigrostriatal dopamine neurons acutely dissociated from the postnatal rat. *Soc Neurosci Abstr* 1989;15:1001.

63. Sokoloff P, Giros B, Martres MP, Bouthenet ML, Schwartz JC. Molecular cloning and characterization of a novel dopamine receptor (D3) as a target for neuroleptics. *Nature* 1990;347:146–151.

64. Snyder LA, Roberts JL, Sealfon SC. Distribution of D_2 receptor mRNA splice variants in the rat by solution hybridization/protection assay. *Neurosci Lett* 1991;122:37–40.

65. Sternweis PC, Pang IH. The G protein-channel connection. *Trends Neurosci* 1990;13:122–126.

66. Stittsworth JD, Mueller AL. Cholecystokinin octapeptide potentiates the inhibitory response mediated by D_2 dopamine receptors in slices of the ventral tegmental area of the brain of the rat. *Neuropharmacology* 1990;29:119–127.

67. Szabo G, Otero AS. G protein mediated regulation of K^+ channel in heart. *Annu Rev Physiol* 1990;52:293–305.

68. Woulfe J, Beaudet A. Neurotensin terminals form synapses primarily with neurons lacking tyrosine hydroxylase immunoreactivity in the rat substantia nigra and ventral tegmental area. *J Comp Neurol* 1992;321:163–176.

*Psychopharmacology: The Fourth
Generation of Progress,* edited by
Floyd E. Bloom and David J. Kupfer.
Raven Press, Ltd., New York © 1995.

CHAPTER 21

Biochemical Pharmacology of Midbrain Dopamine Neurons

Robert H. Roth and John D. Elsworth

ANATOMICAL AND FUNCTIONAL CONSIDERATIONS

Over the past quarter century, the dopamine cells of the ventral mesencephalon have been among the most intensively studied of the chemically defined neuronal groups. At first believed to be two rather homogeneous groups of tyrosine-hydroxylase-positive cells localized to the substantia nigra and ventral tegmental area, midbrain dopamine neurons have turned out to be heterogeneous populations consisting of dopamine neurons projecting to a variety of overlapping areas in the telencephalon. Since the original histochemical description of the monoaminergic neurons in brain during the mid-1960s, anatomical studies have focused on the delineation of the telencephalic projections of the midbrain dopamine neurons. Over the past 30 years, advances in neuroanatomical methodologies have led to an appreciation of the striking heterogeneity of the mesencephalic dopamine neurons both in terms of their connectivity and in reference to the transmitters and proteins localized to these neurons.

Neurochemical, pharmacological, and electrophysiological investigations have revealed corresponding heterogeneities in midbrain dopamine neurons and have led to an appreciation of the diversity of both intrinsic and extrinsic control mechanisms that regulate these systems. A conceptual approach that utilizes these anatomical and neurochemical heterogeneities to define functional subpopulations of dopamine cells seems most likely to yield information that may enable the rational pharmacological manipulation of dopaminergic function. The dopamine neurons of the ventral mesencephalon have been desig-

nated the A8, A9, and A10 cell groups. There are no clear anatomical boundaries between the neurons of the different cell groups (16,25) and the dopamine neurons forming these populations appear at the same time during development (see Chapter 24, *this volume*). These facts, coupled with the overlap in projection fields of the A8, A9, and A10 cell groups, have led to the suggestion that these neurons be collectively designated the *mesotelencephalic dopamine system* (16,25). Such anatomical overlap in the innervation pattern of dopamine neurons on to terminal field targets suggest that there may exist a considerable degree of heterogeneity not only between but also within a given terminal field. Such heterogeneities are apparent in the striatum in which there are two distinct nerve terminal dopamine systems termed the *islandic* and *diffuse* systems. These two types of dopamine innervations originate from different populations of neurons within the midbrain dopamine cell groups and exhibit both different basal dopamine turnover rates and different responsiveness to dopamine agonists and antagonists (27,30). Recent anatomical data suggest that the nucleus accumbens can also be divided into two compartments: (i) a core region related to the caudate-putamen and (ii) a shell region associated with the limbic system, receiving enriched innervation from A9 and A10 dopamine cell groups, respectively (33,72). These two accumbal segments can be further distinguished on the basis of their response to both environmental and pharmacological challenges (15). Such heterogeneities in dopamine innervation, coupled with histochemically distinct compartments in the dorsal and ventral striatum with which the different dopamine systems are in register, suggest that there may be multiple levels of input/output organization that may be reflected in the functional characteristics of these pathways.

Midbrain dopamine neurons also project extensively to

R. H. Roth and J. D. Elsworth: Departments of Pharmacology and Psychiatry, Yale University School of Medicine, New Haven, Connecticut 06520.

cortical sites, including the prefrontal cortices, cingulate cortex, and certain allocortical sites. Recent data indicate that dopaminergic fibers innervate neocortical sites that were previously thought to be devoid of dopamine input such as the visual and association cortices. Although it is not clear to what degree dopaminergic innervation patterns differ between species, the neocortical dopamine system appears to be considerably more extensive in primates than in rodents. There appear to be extensive connections among the dopamine terminal regions and also efferents from the terminal field regions on to the midbrain cell body areas forming feedback loops. Such pathways are currently the focus of considerable attention because these interconnections are believed to function in the integration of dopaminergic activity within the telencephalon.

GENERAL NEUROCHEMICAL CHARACTERISTICS OF MIDBRAIN DOPAMINE NEURONS

While it is apparent that midbrain dopamine neurons exhibit anatomical, biochemical, and pharmacological heterogeneity, their functional organization generally reflects features of transmitter dynamics that are shared by all dopamine neurons. These features have been most thoroughly studied in the nigrostriatal pathway (52) and are summarized below (see Fig. 1).

Dopamine Synthesis

Dopamine synthesis, like that of all catecholamines in the nervous system, originates from the amino acid precursor tyrosine, which must be transported across the blood–brain barrier into the dopamine neuron. A number of conditions can affect tyrosine transport, diminishing its availability and thus altering dopamine formation. The rate-limiting step in dopamine synthesis once tyrosine gains entry into the neuron is the conversion of L-tyrosine to L-dihydroxyphenylalanine (L-DOPA) by the enzyme tyrosine hydroxylase. DOPA is subsequently converted to dopamine by L-aromatic amino acid decarboxylase. This latter enzyme turns over so rapidly that DOPA levels in the brain are negligible under normal conditions. Because of the high activity of this enzyme and the low endogenous levels of DOPA normally present in the brain, it is possible to dramatically enhance the formation of dopamine by providing this enzyme with increased amounts of this substrate. Because the levels of tyrosine in the brain are relatively high and are above the K_m for tyrosine hydroxylase, it is not feasible, under most circumstances, to significantly augment dopamine synthesis by increasing brain levels of this amino acid. However, as noted below, there are some exceptions to this generality. Because tyrosine hydroxylase is the rate-limiting en-

zyme in the biosynthesis of dopamine, this enzyme sets the pace for the formation of dopamine and is particularly susceptible to physiological regulation and pharmacological manipulation. Endogenous mechanisms for regulating the rate of dopamine synthesis in dopamine neurons primarily involve modulation of the activity of this key enzyme.

Dopamine Release

Calcium-dependent release of dopamine from the nerve terminal is thought to occur in response to invasion of the terminal by an action potential. The extent of dopamine release appears to be a function of the rate and pattern of firing (8,29). The burst-firing mode leads to an enhanced release of dopamine. Dopamine release is also modulated by presynaptic release-modulating autoreceptors. In general, dopamine agonists inhibit, whereas dopamine antagonists enhance, the evoked release of dopamine. Much evidence gathered over the last 20 years has indicated that dopamine can be released not only from nerve terminals but also from dendrites of dopamine neurons that originate in the mesencephalon. The enzymes necessary for synthesis of the dopamine are located in perikarya and dendrites of the neurons, and dopamine release has been shown to be calcium-dependent and tetrodotoxin-sensitive. A variety of drugs (e.g., haloperidol, amphetamine) have been found to produce qualitatively similar effects on dopamine synthesis, release, or metabolism in terminal and cell body regions, although the magnitude of the response has tended to be greater in the terminals. Based on the effects of apomorphine or haloperidol on the rate of disappearance of dopamine in the substantia nigra after alpha-methylparatyrosine, it has been suggested that dopamine release in the substantia nigra is not regulated by local dopamine autoreceptors (44). More recently, however, it has been shown that intra-nigral administration of either a D2 dopamine receptor agonist or antagonist is capable of eliciting a synchronous decrease or increase in dopamine release, respectively, in both the substantia nigra and the striatum (68).

Several distinct differences in dopamine biochemistry have been noted between the terminal and dendrites of nigrostriatal dopamine neurons. For instance, the substantia nigra possesses a pool of dopamine that has a much faster turnover than the terminals in the striatum. In addition, in contrast to the striatum, it appears that a considerable proportion of released dopamine in the substantia nigra is taken up into nondopaminergic cells. Another important difference is that nigral dopamine release is partially reserpine-insensitive, and it appears that dopamine in the dendrites of nigrostriatal dopamine neurons is stored both in classical storage vesicles and in smooth endoplasmic reticulum.

Dopamine is released from proximal dendrites in the

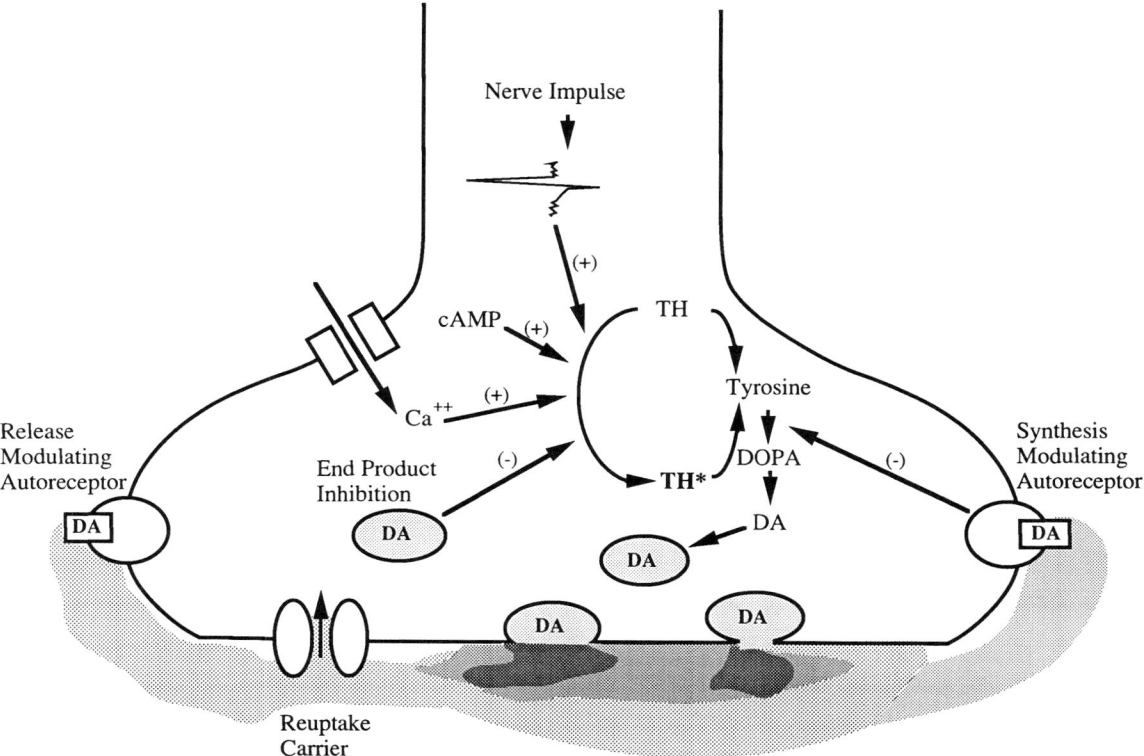

FIG. 1. Schematic model of a prototypic dopaminergic nerve terminal illustrating the life cycle of dopamine and depicting mechanisms which modulate dopamine release and synthesis. Invasion of the terminal by a nerve impulse results in the Ca^{2+}-dependent release of dopamine. This release process is attenuated by release of modulating autoreceptors. Increased impulse flow also stimulates tyrosine hydroxylation. This appears to involve the phosphorylation of tyrosine hydroxylase (TH), resulting in the conversion to an activated form with greater affinity for tetrahydrobiopterin cofactor. The rate of tyrosine hydroxylation can be attenuated by (a) activation of synthesis-modulating autoreceptors, which may function by reversing the kinetic activation of TH, and (b) end-product inhibition by intraneuronal dopamine which competes with cofactor for a binding site on TH. Release- and synthesis-modulating autoreceptors may represent distinct sites. Alternatively, one site may regulate both functions through distinct transduction mechanisms. The dopamine transporter is a unique component of the dopamine terminal, which serves an important physiological role in the inactivation and recycling of dopamine release into the synaptic cleft.

substantia nigra para compacta of nigrostriatal neurons and from distal dendrites that arborize in the substantia nigra para reticulata. Dopamine released in the pars compacta can act at D2-like autoreceptors located on soma and dendrites of nigrostriatal neurons to reduce their firing rate. Dopamine released in the pars reticulata may act in a paracrine fashion on D1-like receptors to increase release of gamma-aminobutyric acid (GABA) from GABAergic striatal efferents that innervate the substantia nigra pars reticulata. Increased GABA release in the pars reticulata in turn is inhibitory to neurons that project to other regions (e.g., nigrothalamic neurons). A behavioral effect of dopamine-induced GABA release in the pars reticulata appears to be facilitated locomotion. In fact, evidence has accumulated recently to suggest that part of the antiparkinsonian effects of L-DOPA treatment may involve activation of D1 receptors in the substantia pars reticulata (50).

Dopamine Uptake and the Dopamine Transporter

Dopamine nerve terminals possess high-affinity dopamine uptake sites which are important in terminating transmitter action and in maintaining transmitter homeostasis. Uptake is accomplished by a membrane carrier which is capable of transporting dopamine in either direction, depending on the existing concentration gradient. The dopamine transporter is a unique component of the functioning dopamine nerve terminal, which plays an important physiological role in the inactivation and recycling of dopamine released into the synaptic cleft by actively pumping extracellular dopamine back into the nerve terminal. The action of dopamine at synapses is terminated by a high-affinity reuptake into presynaptic nerve terminals via the action of Na^+- and Cl^--dependent transporter protein. There is no evidence to date to suggest that different midbrain dopamine neurons have unique dopamine transporters. Although some heterogeneity in dopamine transporter proteins have been detected, this heterogeneity may be the result of differential glycosylation of the same protein (46; see also Chapter 16, *this volume*).

Dopamine Autoreceptors

Autoreceptors can exist on most portions of dopamine cells, including the soma, dendrites, and nerve terminals (53). Stimulation of dopamine autoreceptors in the somatodendritic region slows the firing rate of dopamine neurons, whereas stimulation of autoreceptors located on dopamine nerve terminals results in an inhibition of dopamine synthesis and release (70). Somatodendritic autoreceptors may also regulate dopamine release and synthesis by changing impulse flow. Thus, somatodendritic and nerve terminal autoreceptors work in concert to exert feedback regulatory effects on dopaminergic transmission. Three types of autoreceptors can be defined according to their functional effects: impulse modulating autoreceptors, release modulating autoreceptors, and synthesis modulating autoreceptors. In general, all dopamine autoreceptors can be classified as D2 dopamine receptors (see also Chapters 14 and 26, *this volume*).

Available data suggest that nerve terminal and somatodendritic autoreceptors have similar pharmacological properties. Both are relatively more sensitive to dopamine agonists than postsynaptic dopamine receptors and exhibit similar pharmacological profiles. It is conceivable that a single receptor protein might be responsible for modulating such diverse functions as transmitter release, tyrosine hydroxylation, and action potential generation. For example, all of these functions may share a common sensitivity to the initiating signal (hyperpolarization) triggered by autoreceptor occupation. However, it is more likely that different second messenger systems are ultimately responsible for transducing the signal of autoreceptor occupation into changes in dopamine release, synthesis, and impulse generation.

A number of differences also exist between D2 dopamine receptors in different brain regions. For example, D2 dopamine receptors in the nucleus accumbens do not inhibit adenylate cyclase, whereas the striatum appears to contain both D2 dopamine receptors that inhibit adenyalte cyclase and D2 dopamine receptors that act independently of adenylate cyclase. The striatal D2 dopamine receptors which are not coupled to adenylate cyclase appear to be located on nerve terminals, whereas those D2 dopamine receptors that inhibit adenylate cyclase are located on intrinsic neurons. The D2 dopamine receptors not coupled to adenylate cyclase activity are likely those that mediate inhibition of dopamine and acetylcholine release in the striatum and nucleus accumbens. These release-modulating D2 dopamine receptors may work by increasing potassium conductance. Indeed, if any signal transduction proves universal to all D2 dopamine receptors, it may be the ability to open potassium channels and thereby hyperpolarize target cells. This has been observed for postsynaptic D2 dopamine receptors on striatal neurons, for somatodendritic dopamine autoreceptors, and for pituitary lactotrophs (70). Terminal excitability studies also suggest that stimulation of nerve terminal autoreceptors may exert a hyperpolarizing effect (63). However, there are exceptions to this generalization. For example, stimulation of D2 dopamine receptors on the terminals of hippocampal accumbens neurons increases their terminal excitability, suggesting that D2 dopamine receptors at this site exert a depolarizing action (71). Thus, it appears that there is no consistent feature of D2 dopamine receptor function.

Autoreceptors also differ from postsynaptic D2 dopamine receptors with respect to their interaction with D1 dopamine receptors. It is now well-established that D1 and D2 dopamine receptors act synergistically in many behavioral and electrophysiological models (13). Stimulation of D1 receptors appears to play an enabling role; that is, D1 receptor occupancy is necessary for the full expression of the functional effects of postsynaptic D2 dopamine receptor stimulation. Interestingly, this does not appear to be the case for either synthesis-modulating or impulse-modulating autoreceptors (64), where synergy with D1 receptors is not observed.

SITES OF DRUG ACTION ON DOPAMINERGIC NEURONS

There are many potential sites at which drugs can influence the function of midbrain dopamine neurons (69). The potential sites for modulation of dopamine function are illustrated in Fig. 2. For the purpose of discussion, drug effects can be divided into three broad categories: (i) non-receptor-mediated effects exerted on presynaptic function; (b) dopamine-receptor-mediated effects; and (iii) effects mediated indirectly as a result of drug interactions with other chemically defined transmitter systems that modulate the function of dopamine neurons. The relative importance of the latter two potential sites of drug action will vary among different dopamine systems dependent upon factors such as the presence or absence of autoreceptors, the efficiency of postsynaptic-receptor-mediated neuronal feedback loops, and the nature of the afferent inputs impinging upon the dopamine neurons in question or upon their terminal fields.

Nonreceptor-Mediated Effects

There are several stages in the life cycle of dopamine where drugs can influence transmitter dynamics (see Fig. 1). Many useful pharmacological tools are available for

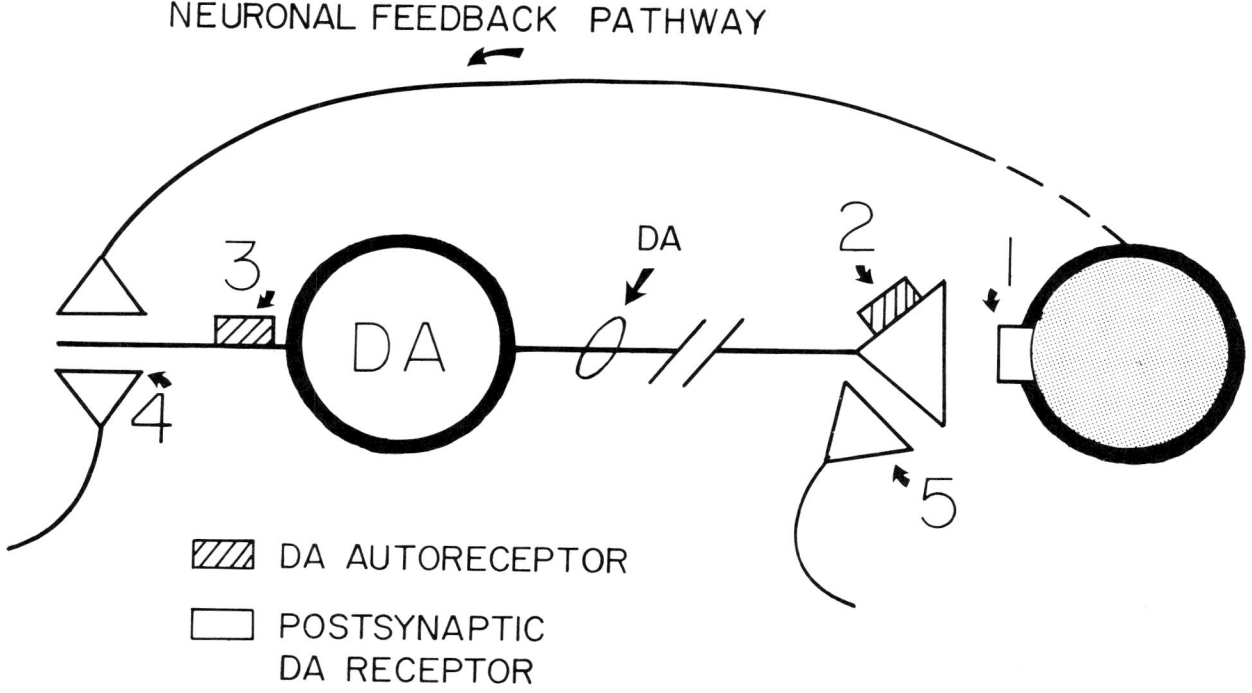

NEURONAL FEEDBACK PATHWAY

Site		Consequences
	Modulatory Effects at DA Receptors	
1. Stimulate postsynaptic DA receptors	A. B.	Enhance dopaminergic transmission Enhance function of neuronal feedback loops
Block postsynaptic DA receptors	A. B.	Block dopaminergic transmission Interfere with function of neuronal feedback loops
2. Stimulate presynaptic DA autoreceptors	A.	Decrease DA synthesis and release
Block presynaptic DA autoreceptors	A.	Increase DA synthesis and release
3. Stimulate somatodendritic DA autoreceptors	A. B.	Decrease firing rate and diminish DA output from nerve terminal Decrease somatodendritic DA turnover (?)
Block somatodendritic DA autoreceptors	A. B.	Interfere with feedback regulation of firing rate and DA output from terminal Interfere with feedback regulation of somatodendritic DA turnover
	Modulatory Effects at Non-DA Receptors on DA neurons	
4. Modify afferent input to cell body (i.e., block or mimic effects of transmitter released by afferent terminal)	A. B.	Alter firing rate of DA cell and thus alter DA output from nerve terminal Alter somatodendritic turnover of DA (and co-localized peptides?)
5. Modify afferent input to nerve terminal	A.	Alter release from nerve terminal of DA (and co-localized peptides?)

FIG. 2. Potential sites for modulation of dopaminergic function.

modifying dopaminergic activity and manipulating dopaminergic function. However, most of these agents are not very selective for dopaminergic synapses and will interact with other catecholamines (norepinephrine and epinephrine) systems and in some cases with other monoamine (5-hydroxytryptamine) systems as well. The major exception to this generality is that there are drugs which target the specific monoamine transporters. Recently, uptake blockers in the GBR series have been characterized which appear to be highly selective for the dopamine transport complex and should prove to be valuable experimental tools perhaps leading to the development of therapeutic agents which can selectively augment dopamine function or be useful as diagnostic aids for visualization of the integrity of dopamine systems in vivo. In fact, striking results have been obtained with several new cocaine derivatives such as 3β-(4-fluorophenyl)tropane-2β-carboxylate (CFT) and 3β-(4-iodophenyl)tropane-2β-carboxylate (β-CIT), which exhibit high affinity for the dopamine transporter. These agents have been used in autoradiographic experiments and employed in PET and SPECT studies to image the striatal dopamine transporter in both normal and parkinsonian monkeys and humans (21,26,36,40,42). These studies have demonstrated (a) loss of striatal dopamine transporters in both experimental and idiopathic Parkinson's disease and (b) the restoration of dopamine transporter density associated with the presence of nigral grafts in the caudate of transplanted MPTP monkeys with improved behavioral functions.

Dopamine-Receptor-Mediated Effects

Drugs that affect dopamine receptors can be subdivided into two groups: (i) receptors on nondopamine-containing cell types, which are usually referred to as *postsynaptic receptors* because they are postsynaptic to a dopamine-releasing cell (site 1), and (ii) receptors on dopamine cells or their processes, which are termed *autoreceptors* to indicate their sensitivity to the neurons own transmitter (sites 2 and 3). Dopamine agonists and antagonists may act on both types of dopamine receptors to elicit biochemical changes in the metabolism of dopamine and alter the functional output of dopaminergic systems (Fig. 2). The overall effect of a drug on dopaminergic activity will depend on both its pre- and postsynaptic effects. This can be illustrated by considering the interaction of a reversible dopamine antagonist with various types of dopamine receptors. Blockade of postsynaptic dopamine receptors is usually considered to be the primary effect of neuroleptic administration; at a given synapse, this will result in a decrease in dopaminergic transmission. However, for some dopamine neurons (e.g., nigrostriatal cells) this immediate effect is opposed by compensatory feedback mechanisms. For example, blockade of presynaptic autoreceptors by neuroleptics will result in increased synthesis

and release of dopamine from the dopaminergic terminal. The resulting increase in synaptic dopamine may act to competitively overcome the blockade of dopamine receptors produced by the antagonist. In addition to this local feedback mechanism, long-loop neuronal feedback pathways can also come into play. As noted above, striatal neurons communicate with dopamine cell bodies in the substantia nigra by way of striatonigral feedback loops. During periods of enhanced postsynaptic dopamine receptor stimulation, these loops exert negative feedback effects on dopamine cell firing. Conversely, then, blockade of postsynaptic receptors by antagonists will produce a compensatory increase in dopamine cell firing. Because dopamine synthesis, release, and turnover in dopamine neurons are coupled to firing rate and firing pattern under most conditions, this results in increased dopamine release. Similar to the effects elicited by autoreceptor blockade, the resulting changes in synaptic dopamine will ultimately contribute to lessening the effectiveness of the antagonist at blocking both pre- and postsynaptic dopamine receptors.

Even though the consequences of receptor blockade by an antagonist differ at autoreceptors and postsynaptic receptors, if the dopamine antagonist in question is equipotent in blocking receptors at both sites, the functional output of the dopamine system should be diminished. If the antagonist has a more potent effect on postsynaptic receptors, the blockade of dopaminergic function should be prolonged and more effective, because it will not be overwhelmed or competitively reversed by synaptic dopamine. On the other hand, if autoreceptor blockade predominates, the resultant increase in transmitter outflow will competitively antagonize the blockade at postsynaptic receptors and compromise the drug-induced blockade of dopaminergic function. These considerations suggest that neuroleptics can exert a multiplicity of effects on dopamine neurons and that the net outcome of these effects will depend, in part, on the relative importance of pre- and postsynaptic dopamine receptors in regulating the activity of a particular group of dopamine neurons. Unfortunately, less is known about the neuronal feedback pathways from mesolimbic and mesocortical target sites back to dopamine cell bodies in the A9 and A10 regions. Indirect biochemical and electrophysiological evidence suggests that feedback pathways are less important for mesocortical and mesolimbic dopamine neurons than for nigrostriatal dopamine cells. These considerations, as well as the lack of (or diminished number of) synthesis and impulse-modulating autoreceptors on subpopulations of dopamine neurons, are important to keep in mind when attempting to predict the biochemical responsiveness of particular dopamine systems to dopamine receptor blockade.

Non-Dopamine-Receptor (Heteroreceptor)-Mediated Effects

Dopaminergic function can be influenced by modulating afferent input to the dopamine cell soma or dendrites by blocking or mimicking the effects of transmitter release by the afferent terminals (site 4). Function can also be modulated by modifying afferent input to the dopamine nerve terminal (site 5), which can lead to alterations in the release of dopamine and colocalized peptides from the dopamine nerve terminals. Pharmacological modulation at sites 4 and 5 will depend upon the chemical nature of the afferent inputs to the dopamine neurons in question.

CHARACTERISTICS OF MESOTELENCEPHALIC DOPAMINE NEURONS

The previous section indicated that the functional output of a given dopamine neuron depends on both (a) intrinsic regulatory properties such as the presence of autoreceptors and (b) extrinsic regulatory properties such as the nature of afferent inputs to cell body regions. In the following section, consideration will be given to differences exhibited by subpopulations of mesotelencephalic dopamine neurons with respect to these parameters and how these heterogeneities might explain differences in the responsiveness of various dopamine systems to both pharmacological and environmental manipulations.

Presence or Absence of Autoreceptors

Many of the differences in responsiveness among various midbrain dopamine neurons can be explained in part by differences in their autoreceptor function. The terminals of all midbrain dopamine neurons examined to date—nigrostriatal, mesoaccumbens, mesoprefrontal, mesocingulate, mesoentorhinal, and mesoamygdaloid—have been found to possess release modulating autoreceptors (53,70). This is not the case for synthesis- and impulse-modulating autoreceptors. For example, whereas most nigral and many ventral tegmental dopamine neurons possess somatodendritic-impulse-modulating and nerve-terminal-synthesis-modulating autoreceptors, the dopamine neurons which project to the prefrontal and cingulate cortices as well as those projecting to the amygdaloid nucleus appeared either to have a greatly diminished number of these receptors or to lack them entirely (5,41,53). Of interest is recent evidence which suggests that dopamine-synthesis-modulating autoreceptors appear transiently during development in the prefrontal cortex and that they may belong to the D1 class of receptors (62). The functional significance of the transient expression of the D1 autoreceptor in the prefrontal cortex is unknown. However, in adult rats the absence or diminished numbers of these important modulatory receptors on mesoprefrontal and mesocingulate dopamine neurons, and perhaps also on mesoamygdaloid neurons, appears in part to be responsible for some of the unique characteristics of these neurons when compared to other mesotelencephalic dopamine neurons which possess autoreceptors (nigrostriatal,

mesolimbic, and mesopiriform systems) (51). For example, electrophysiological studies have revealed that midbrain dopamine neurons lacking somatodendritic autoreceptors possess a higher basal rate of physiological activity and exhibit a different pattern of activity characterized by a greater degree of burst firing (5,6). These electrophysiological studies complement biochemical studies which demonstrate that the turnover rate of dopamine in the cingulate and prefrontal cortices is greater than that observed in the piriform cortex or in the projection fields of other midbrain dopamine neurons which possess autoreceptors (51).

Autoreceptors also appear to play a prominent role in controlling the response of various dopamine projections to acute and chronic treatment with dopamine antagonists such as haloperidol, as well as in controlling their response to dopamine agonists (6,51). While dopamine neurons possessing autoreceptors exhibit dramatic alterations in parameters such as firing rate, dopamine synthesis, and dopamine metabolism in response to acute administration of dopamine antagonists and agonists, mesoprefrontal and mesocingulate dopamine cells are relatively unresponsive both biochemically and electrophysiologically to these agents. For example, administration of haloperidol produces large increases in dopamine synthesis and the accumulation of dopamine metabolites in nigrostriatal and mesoaccumbens and mesopiriform dopamine terminals but has only a modest effect on mesoprefrontal, mesocingulate, and mesoamygdaloid dopamine neurons. Dopamine cell bodies in A8, A9, and A10 areas also exhibit significant differences in their biochemical responsiveness to neuroleptics which may be related to autoreceptor distribution (52).

Acute treatment with haloperidol significantly increases dopamine synthesis in the medial and central substantia nigra, whereas the lateral substantia nigra is unaffected. Within the ventral tegmental area, the lateral area (primary source of the mesolimbic efferents) exhibits a significant increase in synthesis in response to haloperidol, whereas no increase is observed in the medial sector of the ventral tegmental area (primary source of the mesocortical innervation). This biochemical finding is most likely related to the fact that mesoprefrontal and mesocingulate dopamine neurons lack both synthesis-modulating and somatodendritic autoreceptors. No haloperidol-induced increase in dopamine synthesis is observed in either the medial or lateral sectors of the retrorubral field (A8 region), suggesting that A8 dopamine neurons may also lack synthesis-modulating autoreceptors. Failure of the lateral sector of the substantia nigra to respond to haloperidol may similarly reflect an absence or diminished number of somatodendritic autoreceptors in this region.

Although most studies have dealt with the acute effects of neuroleptics on dopamine neurons, chronic studies may be of considerably greater clinical relevance because both the therapeutic effects and extrapyramidal side effects produced by repeated administration of antipsychotic drugs in patients appear only after a latency of several weeks. Interestingly, dopamine neurons which lack autoreceptors respond very differently to chronic treatment with dopamine antagonists such as haloperidol (51). Following chronic treatment with haloperidol, tolerance develops to the elevation of dopamine metabolites levels elicited by a challenge dose of the dopamine agonist in nigrostriatal, mesolimbic, and mesopiriform dopamine neurons. Furthermore, the time course for the development of tolerance closely parallels the development of autoreceptor supersensitivity. In contrast, dopamine neurons projecting to the prefrontal and cingulate cortices appear to be relatively resistant to the development of biochemical tolerance. These studies in rodents have been extended to nonhuman primates, where tolerance development is observed in caudate, putamen, and olfactory tubercles but not in the dopamine systems projecting to the frontal and cingulate cortices (4). Thus, it seems likely that autoreceptors may be involved in the development of biochemical tolerance to antipsychotic drugs after long-term administration. The lack of biochemical tolerance observed in mesoprefrontal and mesocingulate dopamine neurons parallels the lack of tolerance to the therapeutic effects of antipsychotic drugs observed in patients and suggests that sustained biochemical alterations in mesocortical dopamine neurons may be related to the persistent therapeutic actions of these agents.

It is noteworthy that electrophysiological studies have also revealed differences in the responsiveness of dopamine cells to chronic antipsychotic drug administration (11). After repeated administration of antipsychotic drugs to rats, the number of actively firing dopamine cells in both A9 and A10 cell groups is decreased. This state of quiescence, which is thought to reflect depolarization block, appears to result from tonic depolarization of these neurons and can be reversed by hyperpolarizing current or neurotransmitters which hyperpolarize dopamine cells. These treatments help to repolarize the cell and thus restore its ability to fire. Certain dopamine cells appear to be resistant to depolarization block following repeated administration of antipsychotic drugs (11). These are the dopamine cells projecting to the prefrontal or cingulate cortices. Although this observation makes it tempting to speculate that autoreceptors play some role in depolarization block, numerous other mechanisms are likely operative. Dopamine metabolites or ratios of parent amine to metabolite have not proven to be useful biochemical markers of depolarization block. However, monitoring of in vivo tyrosine hydroxylation by following the short-term accumulation of DOPA after inhibition of DOPA decarboxylase has provided a useful biochemical correlate of depolarization block in dopamine projections following chronic administration of typical and atypical neuroleptics (18).

The enhanced susceptibility of mesoprefrontal and mesocingulate dopamine neurons to precursor control of transmitter synthesis may also be related to the absence of dopamine autoreceptors. These dopamine neurons selectively increase their synthesis rate following administration of physiologically relevant doses of precursor tyrosine (51). Precursor dependency has been suggested to be closely related to the physiological firing rate of catecholamine neurons. The mesoprefrontal and mesocingulate dopamine neurons exhibit the highest firing frequency and the most bursting of the mesotelencephalic dopamine cells, possibly because they lack impulse modulating somatodendritic autoreceptors (5). Thus, it is not surprising that this subset of dopamine neurons is most susceptible to precursor regulation of transmitter synthesis.

The findings outlined above have focused primarily on differences between mesocortical, mesolimbic, and nigrostriatal dopamine neurons. Recent findings, however, suggest that dopamine neurons terminating in the striatum must also be considered a heterogeneous population. Dopamine nerve terminals in the striatum can be divided into two distinct groups referred to as the *islandic* and *diffuse* systems (30). These two systems exhibit different basal rates of transmitter turnover and respond in a fashion quantitatively different from that of dopamine agonists and antagonists (27). Furthermore, because these two distinct dopamine systems appear to be in register with distinct histochemical compartments, it is likely that the two dopamine systems differentially regulate output characteristics of the striatum.

The striatum also exhibits other types of regional variations in pharmacological responsiveness. For example, the magnitude of the increase in dopamine metabolite accumulation and dopamine synthesis elicited by dopamine antagonists exhibits a twofold regional variability in the striatum: Areas in the striatum which exhibit the greatest increase in both parameters receive their dopamine innervation from the medial and central regions of the A9 dopamine cell group. Areas exhibiting low responsiveness are predominantly innervated by A10 and A8 neurons. Those areas intermediate in responsiveness receive mixed A9 and A10 inputs. Because differences in biochemical responsiveness of different dopamine cell body regions correlates with striatal heterogeneity, it appears likely that certain dopamine neurons which innervate the striatum may lack, or have a different density of, synthesis-modulating autoreceptors. This distinction is readily lost when the entire striatum is examined as a homogeneous structure. As indicated earlier, anatomical data suggest that the nucleus accumbens can also be parceled into two compartments, namely, a core and a shell region (33). These two compartments can be distinguished on the basis of anatomical markers, such as differences in the density of a number of transmitters and receptors and differences in their efferent projections. Recent anatomical findings suggest that the dopamine innervations of core and shell can also be distinguished on the basis of vulnerability to neurotoxic challenges (7). Using biochemical methods, dopamine innervations of the nucleus accumbens core and shell regions have been further characterized and shown to exhibit significant differences indicating that they can be distinguished on the basis of their response to both environmental and pharmacological challenges (15). The biochemical data are consistent with the anatomical data indicating that the dopamine innervation of the nucleus accumbens core is associated with the nigrostriatal system, whereas that of the nucleus accumbens shell is more closely related to the mesolimbic system.

Modulation by Afferent Inputs

Dopamine neurons also differ in the nature of their interaction with other neurotransmitter systems in the brain. A prototypic example of such interactions is that which occurs between dopamine and acetylcholine in the striatum. Axonal release of dopamine in the striatum inhibits acetylcholine release from cholinergic interneurons; conversely, acetylcholine appears to facilitate dopamine release within the striatum. While such presynaptic regulation of dopamine release is of great importance in the striatum, it appears that this type of interaction is regionally specific; although cholinergic interneurons are present in the nucleus accumbens, the olfactory tubercle, and the medial prefrontal cortex, there does not appear to be a functional dopamine/acetylcholine link in these mesoaccumbens or mesocortical areas. Thus, transmitter interactions such as those occurring at the presynaptic (i.e., independent of dopaminergic impulse flow) level can differ across various brain regions by virtue of the presence or absence of a particular neuron and receptors for its transmitter or physiological factors of local importance.

The ventral tegmental area receives a large number of afferents from telencephalic, diencephalic, and hindbrain regions (47). Moreover, afferents to the ventral tegmental area do not innervate the region diffusely but rather innervate specific nuclei within the ventral tegmental area (47), although dopamine neurons are distributed throughout the region. For example, the nucleus interfascicularis, situated in the most medial aspect of the ventral mesencephalic tegmentum, receives afferents from the medial habenulae and raphe, but does not appear to receive prominent projections from telencephalic dopamine-rich areas (47). Projections to the ventral tegmental area from the nucleus accumbens are relatively sparse, and GABAergic projections from the nucleus accumbens to the ventral tegmental area are predominantly restricted to the anteromedial ventral tegmental area (66). the relatively distinct termination pattern of afferents to the ventral tegmental area, coupled with the topographic organization of the A10 dopamine neurons onto the telencephalon (25), suggests that specific afferents to the ventral tegmental area may regulate sub-

sets of midbrain dopamine neurons, such as those innervating the prefrontal cortex.

A number of recent studies have focused on the chemical nature and differences of afferent input to the somatodendritic region of subpopulations of A10 dopamine neurons in the ventral tegmental area (38). Many of these studies have suggested that subpopulations of A10 dopamine cells can be differentially modulated by afferent inputs. For example, experimental evidence suggests that substance P terminals in A10 may play an important role in modulating the activity of mesocortical dopamine neurons, whereas substance K, a related member of the tachykinin family of peptides, appears to be more important in modulating mesoaccumbens dopamine neurons (17). Thus, it is tempting to speculate that selective substance P or substance K antagonists might be useful in the differential modulation of mesoprefrontal and mesoaccumbens dopamine activity. Other endogenous peptide-containing afferents which innervate the ventral tegmental area also appear to selectively modulate distinct subsets of dopamine neurons. Thus, calcitonin gene-related peptide appears to selectively activate mesoprefrontal but not other mesocortical, mesolimbic, or nigrostriatal dopamine neurons (19).

The presence of GABAergic neurons in the substantia nigra and ventral tegmental area has been shown using immunocytochemical detection of both GABA and the GABA synthetic enzyme glutamic acid decarboxylase. In situ hybridization for glutamic acid decarboxylase mRNA also reveals a moderate density of GABAergic cells within the ventral tegmental area and substantia nigra. Whereas greater than 60% of the neurons in the substantia nigra pars reticulata are GABAergic, only 20% of the neurons in the ventral tegmental area express mRNA for glutamic acid decarboxylase. The intrinsic GABA neurons in the ventral tegmental area synapse on dopaminergic cells as well as project outside the ventral mesencephalon to influence other limbic and motor structures. GABAergic neurons projecting to the ventral tegmental area originate primarily in the nucleus accumbens and ventral pallidum. The GABAergic projection is topographically organized with the shell of the nucleus accumbens and ventromedial ventral pallidum projecting to the ventral tegmental area and the accumbal core and dorsolateral ventral pallidum projecting to the substantia nigra (33). GABAergic efferents to the substantia nigra and ventral tegmental area synapse on both dopaminergic and nondopaminergic neurons, which may explain the paradoxical electrophysiological observation that low doses of GABA$_A$ agonists increase the firing frequency of dopamine cells. This increase in dopamine cell firing is associated with a decrease in the firing frequency of nondopamine cells, and it is speculated that the inhibition of GABAergic interneurons results in the disinhibition of dopamine cells and their enhanced firing frequency. GABA does not appear to alter D2 receptor function.

However, because GABA$_B$-receptor-mediated membrane polarizations arise from the same potassium conductance as D2 receptors, an increase in GABA$_B$ receptor stimulation could compensate for D2 receptor desensitization. This modulatory effect might become most prevalent when D2 receptor desensitization arises from excessive somatodendritic release of dopamine, such as that observed during cocaine sensitization. Elevated synaptic dopamine would stimulate D1 receptors located presynaptically on GABAergic afferents to dopamine cells, thus augmenting GABA release.

Midbrain dopamine cells are also modulated by excitatory amino acids (EAAs). Glutamatergic innervation of the ventral tegmental area arises from three potential sources: EAA projections from the medial prefrontal cortex; the pedunculopontine region; and the subthalamic nucleus. Numerous data demonstrate that EAA input to the ventral tegmental area is at least partially responsible for converting pacemaker-like firing in dopamine cells into burst firing patterns. Prefrontocortical afferents appear to play a major role in regulating N-methyl-D-aspartate (NMDA)-dependent burst firing of ventral tegmental area dopamine cells. Electrical stimulation or direct application of glutamate in the prefrontal cortex converts dopamine neuronal activity in the ventral tegmental area into bursting patterns, and cooling the prefrontal cortex converts spontaneous burst firing dopamine cells back to pacemaker-like firing. Thus afferent EAA tone appears to be an important determinant of whether the firing pattern of dopamine cells will be pacemaker-like or bursting (12). This in vivo activity contrasts strikingly with the pacemaker activity of the same dopamine neurons recorded in vitro when the afferent inputs are disrupted. Burst firing of dopamine neurons in vitro can be induced by application of NMDA (37). Pharmacological studies also indicate that the burst firing of midbrain dopamine neurons in vivo result from tonic activation of NMDA receptors by endogenous EAAs (12). It has been suggested that the EAA inputs to midbrain dopamine neurons may constitute a major physiological mechanism in the control of synaptic dopamine levels in target projection areas. In fact, the neuronal discharge pattern, independent of the mean discharge rate, has been shown to exert a potent control over the release of dopamine and colocalized peptides (such as neurotensin) from terminal fields (8,29). The observation that bursting activity elicits more terminal dopamine release per action potential than pacemaker activity and that bursting elicits release of co-peptide transmitters more readily than nonbursting patterns has focused attention on the functional significance of bursting activity in midbrain dopamine neurons (see also Chapter 100, *this volume*).

Pharmacological Heterogeneity

Some of the differences in pharmacological responsiveness between subpopulations of dopamine neurons appear to be due to differences in the responsivity of these cells to afferent inputs. For example, recent neurochemical studies have directly demonstrated that EAA receptors may be involved in the selective metabolic activation of subsets of dopamine neurons within the ventral tegmental area which project to the prefrontal cortex (38,39). Stimulation of NMDA receptors more selectively activates the dopamine projection to the prefrontal cortex, whereas stimulation of non-NMDA receptors activates mesoaccumbens and nigrostriatal neurons. The NMDA receptor complex is an EAA-ligand-gated ion channel which is selectively activated by NMDA and regulated at several pharmacologically distinct sites including a high-affinity, strychnine-insensitive glycine binding site. Competitive antagonists of the strychnine-insensitive glycine site which cross the blood–brain barrier have become available, making possible in vivo pharmacological manipulation of the NMDA receptor through this regulatory site. One such high-affinity selective antagonist at the NMDA receptor glycine site, (+)-HA-966, is the recently resolved enantiomer of the drug (±)-3-amino-1-hydroxy-2-pyrolidinone (59). Systemic administration of this agent to the rat has been shown to normalize dopamine neuron firing patterns (57). The neurochemical and behavioral effects of (+)-HA-966 have been studied in several paradigms (restraint stress and conditioned fear) that are known to cause a metabolic activation of mesoprefrontal and mesoaccumbens dopamine neurons. (+)-HA-966 given systemically or injected into the ventral tegmental area prevents the stress-induced increase in dopamine metabolism in the prefrontal cortex without altering the response in the nucleus accumbens (43). Similarly, systemic administration of the noncompetitive antagonist of the NMDA receptor, MK-801, blocked the stress-induced rise in dopamine metabolism in the prefrontal cortex but not the nucleus accumbens. The negative enantiomer of HA-966 did not produce a selective antagonism of the stress-induced dopamine metabolism in the prefrontal cortex. The role of the NMDA receptor and its glycine modulatory site in the rat conditioned-fear paradigm has also been investigated (28). Aversive conditioning results in selective dopamine and serotonergic metabolic activation in the medial and lateral prefrontal cortex, elevation in serum corticosterone, ultrasonic vocalization, and freezing behavior. Pretreatment with (+)-HA-966 abolished the dopamine metabolic activation in the medial and lateral prefrontal cortex. Serotonergic metabolic activation in the medial prefrontal cortex and dopamine metabolic activity in nucleus accumbens were not affected by (+)-HA-966 pretreatment, indicating neurochemical and regional specificity of the (+)-HA-966 blocking effect. Pretreatment with (+)-HA-966 did not effect serum corticosterone elevation, but facilitated extinction of the freezing response. These data indicate that the NMDA receptor complex and associated glycine modulatory site may play an important role in the afferent control of the mesoprefrontal cortical dopamine system during restraint or conditioned fear, suggesting a potential target for pharmacological modulation of this dopamine projection. These results also support previous data, which suggest that the mesocortical and mesoaccumbens dopamine neurons respond to excitatory input through different glutamate receptor mechanisms. Recent studies have demonstrated that microinjection of NMDA antagonists into the ventral tegmental area can prevent the initiation of behavioral sensitization to systemic cocaine (39), which poses the interesting possibility that the NMDA-dependent induction of burst firing in ventral tegmental area dopamine cells may be a critical factor in establishing sensitized motor behavior. In view of the observation that EAA afferents from the prefrontal cortex play an important role in burst firing, these data argue that EAA afferents from the prefrontal cortex may have a permissive function in initiating behavioral sensitization. Midbrain dopamine neurons also differ in the types of neurotransmitter systems which influence dopamine turnover at the level of the nerve terminals (see Fig. 2), although comparatively little is known about this type of interaction in mesolimbic and mesocortical projection fields compared to the striatum.

It is now well-documented that the mesoprefrontal cortical dopamine system is activated by certain stress conditions (mild footshock stress and conditioned fear) which do not produce an appreciable metabolic activation of other mesotelencephalic dopamine systems (nigrostriatal mesolimbic or other mesocortical) or central noradrenergic systems. The stress-induced activation of mesoprefrontal dopamine neurons is antagonized by anxiolytic agents such as lorazepam or diazepam, which target the benzodiazepine site of the GABA$_A$ receptor. Furthermore, the anxiolytic properties of these agents as well as their ability to block the stress-induced activation of mesoprefrontal dopamine neurons are reversed by benzodiazepine antagonists, implicating the involvement of benzodiazepine GABA receptors in the stress-induced alterations in mesoprefrontal dopamine function (20). The observation that mesoprefrontal dopamine neurons differ from nigrostriatal and mesolimbic dopamine neurons in that they lack impulse modulating and synthesis modulating autoreceptors prompted the speculation that the lack of autoreceptors might account in part for the unique responsiveness of this system to mild stress. However, the experimental evidence to date is not entirely consistent with the correlation between lack of autoreceptors and enhanced responsiveness to stress. For example, dopamine neurons that innervate the cingulate cortex also lack synthesis- and impulse-modulating autoreceptors but are not activated by mild stress. Thus, extrinsic influences over midbrain dopamine neurons such as peptidergic, EAA, serotonergic, and noradrenergic inputs are thought to play an instrumental role in the production of this phenomena (20,38). Consistent with this speculation, it

has been demonstrated that infusion into the ventral tegmental area of monoclonal antibodies directed against substance P effectively prevents the footshock-induced increase in prefrontal cortical DOPAC. It therefore seems likely that distinct afferents to different areas within the mesencephalon may, in part, account for the selective response of various dopamine systems to stress rather than solely the presence or absence of somatodendritic and synthesis-modulating nerve terminal autoreceptors. Also, more recently, it has also been shown, as alluded to above, that administration of the glycine site antagonist of the NMDA receptor, HA966, can block the metabolic activation of the mesoprefrontal dopamine neurons induced by restraint stress and aversive conditioning without altering the metabolic activation which occurs in the mesoaccumbens, suggesting a differential regulation of mesocortical and mesoaccumbens dopamine neurons by NMDA receptors (28; see also Chapters 7, 61, and 67, *this volume*).

In addition to being selectively activated by mild stress, mesoprefrontal dopamine neurons also exhibit increased dopamine turnover in response to administration of anxiogenic beta carbolines. These agents are believed to act as inverse agonists at the benzodiazepine recognition site on the GABA$_A$ benzodiazepine receptor complex and are known to antagonize the various central effects of benzodiazepines. One of the anxiogenic beta carbolines, FG7142 (*N*-methyl-β-carboline-3-carboxamide), produces a dose-dependent increase in dopamine metabolism in the prefrontal cortex and ventral tegmental area of rats without causing any significant increase in dopamine metabolism in other mesocortical, mesolimbic, or nigrostriatal sites (51). The metabolic activation observed in the prefrontal cortex is blocked by anxiolytic benzodiazepines and by benzodiazepine antagonists, implicating the involvement of benzodiazepine/GABA receptors in this response (51). Because all midbrain dopamine cells examined to date have been shown to be inhibited by GABA, the selective effects of this beta carboline on mesoprefrontal dopamine neurons suggests that cell bodies of mesoprefrontal dopamine neurons may be wired in a unique manner to the GABA-benzodiazepine-dependent mechanisms in the ventral tegmental area or be enriched in a particular subtype of GABA$_A$ receptor. The fact that mesoprefrontal dopamine neurons are uninfluenced or less responsive to autoreceptor-mediated regulation of firing rate may explain why these cells might be more sensitive to the inhibitory effects of GABAergic inputs.

Other evidence suggests that dopamine systems may also be differentially modulated by serotonin and noradrenergic neurons. For example, dopamine utilization is selectively enhanced in the nucleus accumbens but decreased in the prefrontal cortex in a temporally specific fashion following electrolytic lesions of the median raphe. Lesions of the dorsal raphe increase dopamine utilization in the nucleus accumbens but do not alter dopamine turnover in the prefrontal cortex (34). Systemic administration of 8-hydroxy-dipropylaminotetralin (8-OH-DPAT), a 5-HT$_{1a}$ agonist, increases the firing rate and bursting of A10 dopamine neurons (2) and also increases the in vivo release of dopamine from the prefrontal cortex (1). A postmortem increase in dopamine turnover as assessed by measures of the DOPAC/dopamine ratio is also observed in the prefrontal cortex (Rasmusson, Goldstein, and Roth, *unpublished observations*). Furthermore, dopamine utilization is decreased in the prefrontal cortex but remains unaltered in the nucleus accumbens following 6-OHDA-induced degeneration of the norepinephrine fibers projecting to the ventral tegmental area. Although the ventral tegmental area is known to receive both serotonergic and noradrenergic afferents from brainstem monoamine neurons, it is not clear whether the regulatory interaction described above occurs at the level of the cell bodies of origin of the various dopaminergic projections; interactions at the level of the terminal field are equally possible.

Colocalization with Neuropeptides

The possibility of an additional type of interaction between dopamine and neuropeptides is suggested by recent findings which indicate that dopamine, like other classical neurotransmitters, is often colocalized in single neurons with neuropeptides and nontransmitter proteins. For example, certain midbrain dopamine neurons contain the peptide cholecystokinin (CCK) (14), whereas other subpopulations of mesencephalic dopamine neurons contain the peptide neurotensin and a third group of dopamine neurons in the ventral tegmental area contains CCK, neurotensin, and dopamine (56). Similarly, dopamine is colocalized in certain mesencephalic neurons with nontransmitter proteins, including acetylcholinesterase, protein-*O*-carboxymethyltransferase, cytochrome P-450 reductase, and a vitamin-D-dependent calcium-binding protein (see Chapter 18, *this volume*).

The functional significance of such colocalization is not clear. However, because receptors for certain colocalized peptides such as neurotensin are present on dopamine neurons in the midbrain, activity of these dopamine neurons may be regulated by peptide autoreceptors in a fashion analogous to somatodendritic dopamine autoreceptor modulation of impulse flow and dopamine synthesis. Furthermore, because it appears that release mechanisms for dopamine and colocalized peptides may be dissociated under certain conditions (e.g., dependent on the firing pattern and firing frequency of the neuron (8), colocalized peptides may serve as part of a hierarchical array of neuronal regulatory features. In this regard, it is of interest that nerve terminal autoreceptors in the prefrontal cortex have been shown to exert reciprocal effects on dopamine and neurotensin release. Stimulation of dopamine autore-

ceptors diminishes dopamine release and enhances neurotensin release, whereas blockade of dopamine receptors augments dopamine release and diminishes neurotensin release. The functional implications of these findings for the activity of follower cells in the prefrontal cortex is presently uncertain, but it could allow the prefrontal cortex dopamine neurons to differentially modulate the physiological activity of cortical postsynaptic follower cells.

Although the functional correlates of peptide-amine colocalization in mesencephalic dopamine neurons remains to be clearly established, it appears likely that colocalization of peptides or nontransmitter proteins and dopamine will prove to reliably define certain subpopulations of dopamine neurons. Thus, CCK-dopamine colocalized neurons of the ventral tegmental area project to the caudal, but not rostral, nucleus accumbens. Such distinctions may have important implications for regionally specific function of dopamine in psychiatric and neurological disorders, as well as for the response of specific dopamine systems in these pathological conditions or to pharmacological treatment. The coexistence with neurotensin in particular mesencephalic dopamine neurons has not been observed in primates (9). However, this might not be a permanent phenotype. The possibility of a transient coexpression either in pathological states like schizophrenia or during ontogeny similar to the transient multicolocalization of tyrosine hydroxylase with peptides observed in the rodent amygdala (somatostatin and substance P) seems plausible. In fact, Hökfelt and collaborators (55) have recently found that the CCK gene is expressed in the midbrain of humans and specifically in the substantia nigra of schizophrenic patients, whereas CCK mRNA is low or nondetectable in the mesencephalon of normal subjects. Although neurotensin and CCK appear to modulate the function of mesotelencephalic dopamine neurons (14,58), their role in normal brain function or their possible dysregulation in neurological or psychiatric disorders or in stress- or drug-induced sensitization is still unclear. However, the availability of potent, bioavailable antagonists should lead to new insight concerning their importance and help to elucidate the role played by these neuropeptides in both normal and abnormal brain function (14,32).

Much of the latter part of this chapter has been concerned with the heterogeneity of central dopamine neurons and the implications of these differences in the pharmacology and pathology of dopamine neurons. A summary is presented in Table 1.

Sensitivity to MPTP

A number of neurotoxins have been reported to damage certain mesotelencephalic dopamine neurons. Among these toxins are (a) heavy metals such as manganese and lead and (b) a variety of organic compounds such as

TABLE 1. *Biochemical pharmacology of central dopamine neurons*[a,b]

	N-STR	M-ACC	M-PFR	M-PIR	M-AMY	TINF	THYP	IHYP	OLF-B	RETN
Perikarya location:	A9 > A8 > A10	A10 > A8 > A9	A10	A9 > A8	A8, A9, A10	A12	A12	A11, A13, A14	A16	A17
Efferent fiber length:	Long	Long	Long	Long	Long	Interm.	Interm.	Interm. and long	Short	Short
Possible functions:	Motor	Reward, emotion	Cognition	Cognition	Integration of sensory stimuli	Pituitary hormone release	Pituitary hormone release	Pituitary hormone release	Olfaction	Light/dark adaptation
High-affinity DA uptake:	Yes	Yes	Yes	Yes	No?	No	No	Yes	No	Yes
6-OHDA sensitivity:	Yes	Yes	Yes	Yes	Low	No	No	Yes	?	Yes
Synthesis-modulating autoreceptor:	Yes	Yes	No	Yes	No	No	Yes/no (mixed)c	Yes	?	Yes
Tyrosine dependency—basal:	No	No	Yes	?	?	?	?	?	?	No
Tyrosine dependency—activated:	Yes	Yes	Yes	?	Yes	?	?	?	?	Yes
Response to agonist (decrease in DA synthesis, catabolism, turnover):	Yes	Yes	Yes (small)	Yes	Yes	Yes (delayed)	Yes	Yes	?	Yes
Response to antagonist (increase DA synthesis, catabolism, turnover):	Yes	Yes	Yes (small)	Yes	Yes	Yes (delayed)	Yes	Yes	?	Yes
Tolerance to chronic typical neuroleptic:	Marked	Yes	Less	?	Yes/no (mixed)c	No	No	?	?	Less
Response to mild stress (BZ-sensitive, increase in synthesis and metabolism):	No	Yes (shell)	Yes	No	Yes/no (mixed)c	No	No	?	?	?
Response to beta cabolines (increase in DA catabolism):	No	No (core) Yes (shell)	Yes	No	No	?	?	?	?	?
Psychostimulant sensitization (augmentation of DA release):	Moderate	High	Low	?	?	?	?	?	?	?
Cocaine withdrawal (decrease in B_{max} for transporter):	No	?	Yes	?	?	?	?	?	?	?

[a] For references, see citations in text; also see refs. 10 and 35.

[b] Abbreviations: N-STR, nigrostriatal; M-ACC, mesoaccumbens; M-PRF, mesoprefrontal; M-PIR, mesopiriform; M-AMY, mesoamygdaloid; TINF, tuberoinfundibular; THYP, tuberohypophyseal; IHYP, incertohypothalamic; OLF-B, olfactory bulb; RETN, retina; interm., intermediate.

[c] *Mixed* indicates that the response differs within the category, depending on the neuronal subset examined.

TABLE 2. *Known biochemical and pharmacological differences between primate and rodent catecholamine neurons*[a,b]

Characteristic	Rodent	Primate	References
Tyrosine hydroxylase (mRNA transcripts)	Single	Multiple	32
Monoamine oxidase (relative abundance in striatum)	Type A > Type B	Type B > Type A	45
Dopamine metabolism (major end metabolites)	DOPAC + HVA	HVA	3
Norepinephrine metabolism (major end metabolites)	DHPG + MHPG sulfates	MHPG	24
Phenolsulfotransferase (affinity for DA and NE)	Low	High	54
Phenolsultotransferase (affinity for deaminated and O-methylated DA and NE metabolites)	High	Low	54
Adenylate cyclase (efficacy of partial D1 agonist to stimulate)	High	Low	48 (but see ref. 67)
Neurotensin colocalization (in DA neurons)	Present	Low	7,9,56
CCK colocalization (in mesocortical DA neurons)	Present	Low	55,56
Susceptibility to MPTP (nigrostriatal DA toxicity)	Low	High	23
D1/D2 receptor interaction	Established	Uncertain	65

[a] Some differences in the biochemical pharmacology of central catecholamine neurons between the rodent and primate. In addition, the amino acid sequence of transporter proteins and some of the metabolic enzymes are different between the species, although these have not been related to functional differences.

[b] Abbreviations: DA, dopamine; NE, norepinephrine; HVA, homovanillic acid; DOPAC, dihydroxyphenylacetic acid; MHPG, 3-methoxy-4-hydroxyphenylglycol; DHPG, 3,4-dihydroxyphenylglycol.

3-acetylpyridine. The toxic effects of such compounds, however, are relatively nonspecific and result in the loss of nondopaminergic as well as dopaminergic neuronal elements throughout the brain. 1-Methyl-4-phenyl-1,2,3,6-tetrahydropyridine (MPTP) is a neurotoxin which appears to exert its effects in a relatively selective manner to effect a depletion of striatal dopamine stores, and thus result in a parkinsonian syndrome in primates (see Chapter 126, *this volume*).

Rats are relatively resistant to the neurotoxic effects of systemic MPTP administration. The susceptibility of primate species to MPTP is a striking example of the differences that exist in the biochemistry or pharmacology of rodent and primate central dopamine neurons (Table 2). In fact, due to the relative paucity of research on primates, there are doubtless other discrepancies that are not yet known. In areas where distinct differences occur, caution is needed when relating the significance of observations obtained in rodents to human or nonhuman primates.

Initial reports of MPTP-induced neuropathology indicated that the toxin resulted in a selective loss of the nigrostriatal dopaminergic system of primate species, whereas mesolimbic and mesocortical dopamine systems were spared. However, more recent data (22,23) indicate that certain mesolimbic/cortical dopamine neurons are also damaged by MPTP. In contrast to idiopathic Parkinson's disease, in which other monoamine systems are impacted, the susceptibility of serotonergic and noradrenergic neurons to the toxic effects of MPTP appear to be minimal.

The primary toxicity of MPTP appears to be manifested at the terminal field level, because most of the midbrain dopamine cell bodies of origin of the striatal dopamine innervation do not disappear until well after the striatal dopamine depletion is maximal. It has been possible to exploit the temporal disparity between terminal and somatodendritic degeneration to examine the possible preferential vulnerability of different populations of midbrain dopamine neurons. Several studies indicate that the lateral A8 and central dorsal A9 dopamine neurons are preferentially vulnerable to MPTP, and that only later do medial A9 neurons of the substantia nigra show degenerative changes. The dorsomedial A10 dopamine neurons of the ventral tegmental area are also lost following MPTP treatment, consistent with the partial loss of the septal dopamine innervation seen following exposure to the neurotoxin. In addition, there is heterogeneity of dopamine loss in striatal regions after MPTP (22).

The key question generated by the studies of MPTP has been to determine the mechanisms whereby MPTP exerts such selective effects on central dopamine neurons. Not only is there remarkable specificity in the neuronal damage induced by MPTP, but, furthermore, MPTP toxicity is manifested in its complete form only in primate species. Administration of MPTP to infraprimate species, including mice, cats, and dogs, can result in striatal dopamine depletion; however, the loss of striatal dopamine in these species is not of the magnitude observed in primates treated with far lower doses of MPTP. These data suggest that some feature restricted to specific subpopulations of dopamine neurons of primates may render these dopamine neurons more vulnerable to the toxic effects of MPTP. In fact, recent data are consistent with the possibility that the calcium-binding protein, calbindin, might exert a neuroprotective effect on dopamine neurons. The dopamine neurons which do not express calbindin are preferentially vulnerable to Parkinson's disease and to the neurotoxic effects of MPTP. Identification of the corresponding biochemical heterogeneity may allow the development of specific strategies aimed at the prevention of Parkinson's disease. In the interim, the MPTP-treated parkinsonian primate has provided a very useful model in which to examine therapeutic strategies for the treatment of Parkinson's disease. In fact, this model has already been successfully exploited to design, refine, and evaluate neuronal transplantation techniques (23,49,60) and to test new pharmacological strategies for the therapeutic management of Parkinson's disease (61).

CONCLUSION

On the basis of biochemical, anatomical, and electrophysiological studies, there is now compelling evidence that the organization of ascending dopamine neurons arising from the substantia nigra, ventral tegmental area, and retrorubral field is much more complex than originally suspected. The initial classification scheme indicating the existence of three major systems, namely the nigrostriatal, mesolimbic, and mesocortical systems, no longer seems fully appropriate. It is now recognized that distinct dopamine subsystems are responsible for the dopamine innervations of well-defined cortical areas as well as mesolimbic structures. It is also clear that the substantia nigra contains dopamine cells that project not only to the striatum, but to certain cortical and mesolimbic sites as well; furthermore, certain ventral tegmental area neurons contribute to the striatal dopaminergic innervation. These interdigitating dopamine subsystems can be distinguished not only on the basis of their origin with the midbrain dopamine cell groups, but also by virtue of the type of dopamine neurons they comprise (e.g., shape of the cell body and nature of the dendritic arborization, characteristic axonal morphology, presence of axon collaterals, coexistence of identified peptides or enzymes, existence of autoreceptors), by their physiological profile (e.g., firing rate, degree of bursting, transmitter turnover), by their respective specific afferents, and by their specific reactivity to pharmacological treatments or environmental stimuli. In mesocortical dopamine systems, such distinctions have been examined extensively in relation to the medial prefrontal cortical dopaminergic innervation of the rat. Much remains to be done to characterize in a similar way the properties of dopamine neurons innervating other cortical regions as well as to extend these studies in rodents to primates.

The findings discussed above suggest that it may be plausible to design drugs which would selectively target specific dopamine cells through interaction with distinct regulatory features of these neurons. For example, certain subsets of dopamine neurons exhibit striking differences in intrinsic regulatory properties such as the presence of autoreceptors or coexistence with neuropeptides. They also possess distinct differences in extrinsic regulatory properties such as the nature of afferent inputs to their cell body regions or terminal fields. It is conceivable that drugs might be targeted to exploit these differences. It may be possible to take advantage of interactions between specific dopamine systems and other neurotransmitters in order to selectively alter the activity of subpopulations of midbrain dopamine neurons. For example, it appears that substance K and substance P preferentially modulate mesolimbic and mesocortical dopamine neurons, respectively. Thus, if stable, bioavailable specific substance P agonists or antagonists were developed, it might prove possible to selectively manipulate mesocortical dopamine function. Mesoprefrontal and mesolimbic dopamine neurons may also be differentially modulated by serotonergic and noradrenergic afferents originating from brainstem sites as well as by enkephalinergic and other peptidergic afferents. Some midbrain dopamine neurons in the ventral tegmental area appear to be differentially sensitive to excitatory glutamatergic input, thereby allowing their activity to be differentially modulated by NMDA receptors. Differences in afferent input or the responsivity of heteroreceptors on dopamine neurons could provide the rationale for the design of novel agents which would interact selectively with subpopulations of dopamine neurons, or they suggest conditions in which traditional antipsychotic agents might be more effective if used in combination with drugs which affect other transmitter systems or target selective dopamine systems.

In conclusion, there have been considerable advances in the last decade in the understanding of the diversity of central nervous system dopamine neurons and the chemical basis of this diversity. The next challenge is to apply this knowledge to the development of useful diagnostic agents and more selective therapeutic agents for both the evaluation and treatment of neurological and psychiatric disorders which involve dopamine dysfunction.

REFERENCES

1. Aborelius L, Nomikos GG, Hacksell U, Svensson TH. (R)-8-OH-DPAT preferentially increases dopamine release in rat medial prefrontal cortex. *Acta Physiol Scand* 1993;148:465–466.
2. Arborelius L, Chergui K, Murase S, Nomikos GG, Höök BB, Chouvet G, Hacksell U, Svensson TH. The 5-HT$_{1a}$ receptor selective ligands, (R)-8-OH-DPAT and (S)-UH-301, differentially affect the activity of midbrain dopamine neurons. *Naunyn Schmiedebergs Arch Pharmacol* 1993;347:353–362.
3. Bacopoulos NG, Mass JW, Hattox SE, Roth RH. Regional distribution of dopamine metabolites in human and primate brain. *Commun Psychopharmacol* 1978;2:281–286.
4. Bacopoulos NG, Spokes EG, Bird ED, Roth RH. Antipsychotic drug action in schizophrenic patients: selective effect on cortical dopamine metabolism after chronic treatment. *Science* 1979;205:1405–1407.
5. Bannon MJ, Freeman AS, Chiodo LA, Bunney BS, Roth RH. The pharmacology and electrophysiology of mesolimbic dopamine neurons. In: Iversen LL, ed. *Handbook of psychopharmacology,* vol 19. New York: Plenum Press, 1987;329–374.
6. Bannon MJ, Roth RH. Pharmacology of mesocortical dopamine neurons. *Pharmacol Rev* 1983;35(1):53–68.
7. Bean AJ, Dagerlind A, Hokfelt T, Dobner PR. Cloning of human neurotensin/neuromedin N genomic sequences and expression in

the ventral mesencephalon of schizophrenics and age/sex matched controls. *Neuroscience* 1992;50(2):259–268.

8. Bean AJ, Roth RH. Extracellular dopamine and neurotensin in rat prefrontal cortex in vivo: effects of median forebrain bundle stimulation frequency, stimulation pattern and dopamine autoreceptors. *J Neurosci* 1991;11:2694–2702.

9. Berger B, Gaspar P, Verney C. Dopaminergic innervation of the cerebral cortex: unexpected differences between rodents and primates. *TINS* 1991;14:24–27.

10. Bodis-Wollner I, Piccolini M, eds. *Dopaminergic mechanisms in vision.* New York: Alan R Liss, 1988;1–276.

11. Bunney BS. Antipsychotic drug effects on the electrical activity of dopaminergic neurons. *TINS* 1984;7:212–215.

12. Chergui K, Charléty PJ, Akaoka H, Saunier CF, Brunet J-L, Buda M, Svensson TH, Chouvet G. Tonic activation of NMDA receptors causes spontaneous burst discharge of rat midbrain dopamine neurons in vivo. *Eur J Neurosc* 1993;5:137–144.

13. Clark D, White FJ. Review: D1 dopamine receptor—the search for a function: a critical evaluation of the D1/D2 dopamine receptor classification and its functional implications. *Synapse* 1987;1:347–388.

14. Crawley JN. Cholecystokinin–dopamine interactions. *Trends Pharmacol Sci* 1991;12:232–236.

15. Deutch AY, Cameron DS. Pharmacological characterization of dopamine systems in the nucleus accumbens core and shell. *Neuroscience* 1992;46:49–56.

16. Deutch AY, Goldstein M, Baldino F Jr, Roth RH. Telencephalic projections of the A8 dopamine cells group. *Ann NY Acad Sci* 1988;537:27–50.

17. Deutch AY, Maggio JE, Bannon MJ, Kalivas PW, Tam S-Y, Goldstein M, Roth RH. Substance K and substance P differentially modulate mesolimbic and mesocortical systems. *Peptides* 1985;6:113–122.

18. Deutch AY, Roth RH. Alterations in dopamine synthesis induced by chronic neuroleptic administration: a possible biochemical correlate of depolarization inactivation. *Soc Neurosci Abstr* 1988;14:27.

19. Deutch AY, Roth RH. Calcitonin gene-related peptide in the ventral tegmental area: selective modulation of prefrontal cortical dopamine metabolism. *Neurosci Lett* 1987;74:169–174.

20. Deutch AY, Roth RH. The determinants of stress-induced activation of the prefrontal cortical dopamine system. In: Uylings HBM, Van Eden CG, DeBruin JPC, Corner MA, Feenstra MGP, eds. *Progress in brain research,* vol 85. Amsterdam: Elsevier Science Publishers BV, 1990;367–403.

21. Elsworth JD, Al-Tikriti M, Sladek JR Jr, Taylor JR, Innis RB, Redmond DE Jr, Roth RH. A novel radioligand for the dopamine transporter demonstrates presence of nigral grafts in caudate nucleus of MPTP monkey with improved behavioral function. *Exp Neurol* 1994;[in press].

22. Elsworth JD, Deutch AY, Redmond DE Jr, Taylor JR, Sladek JR Jr, Roth RH. Symptomatic and asymptomatic 1-methyl-4-phenyl-1,2,3,6-tetrahydropyridine (MPTP)-treated primates: biochemical changes in striatal regions. *Neuroscience* 1989;33:323–331.

23. Elsworth JD, Redmond DE Jr, Sladek JR Jr, Deutch AY, Collier TJ, Roth RH. Reversal of MPTP-induced Parkinsonism in primates by fetal dopamine cell transplants. In: Franks AJ, Ironside JW, Mindham RHS, eds. *Function and dysfunction of the basal ganglia.* Manchester: Manchester University Press, 1989;161–180.

24. Elsworth JD, Roth RH, Redmond DE Jr. The relative importance of 3-methoxy-4-hydroxyphenylglycol (MHPG) and 3,4-dihydroxyphenylglycol (DHPG) as norepinephrine metabolites in rat, monkey and human tissue. *J Neurochem* 1983;41(3):786–793.

25. Fallon JH. Topographic organization of ascending dopaminergic projections. *Ann NY Acad Sci* 1988;537:1–9.

26. Frost JJ, Rosier AJ, Reich SG, Smith JS, Ehlers MD, Snyder SH, Ravert HT, Dannals RF. Positron emission tomographic imaging of the dopamine transporter with 11C-WIN 35,428 reveals marked declines in mild Parkinson's disease. *Ann Neurol* 1993;34:423–431.

27. Fuxe K, Agnati LF, Ogren S-O, Kohler C, Calzu L, Benfenati F, Goldstein M, Anderson K, Neroth P. The heterogeneity of the dopamine systems in relation to the actions of dopamine agonists. *Acta Pharm Suec [Suppl]* 1983;1:60–79.

28. Goldstein LE, Rasmusson AM, Bunney BS, Roth RH. The NMDA glycine site antagonist (+)-HA-966 selectively regulates psychological stress-induced metabolic activation of the mesoprefrontal cortical dopamine but not serotonin systems: a behavioral, neuroendocrine, and neurochemical study in the rat. *J Neurosci* 1994;in press.

29. Gonon FG. Nonlinear relationship between impulse flow and dopamine released by rat midbrain dopaminergic neurons as studied by in vivo electrochemistry. *Neuroscience* 1988;24:19–28.

30. Graybiel AM. Correspondence between the dopamine islands and striosomes of the mammalian striatum. *Neuroscience* 1984;13:1157.

31. Gully D, Canton M, Boigegrain R, Jeanjean R, Molimard F, Pancelet J-C, Gueudét C, Heaulme M, Leyris R, Brouard A, Pelaprat D, Labbé-Jullié, Mazella J, Soubrié P, LeFur G. Biochemical and pharmacological profile of a potent and selective nonpeptide antagonist of the neurotensin receptor. *Proc Natl Acad Sci USA* 1993;90:65–69.

32. Haycock JW. Four forms of tyrosine hydroxylase are present in human adrenal medulla. *J Neurochem* 1991;56:2139–2142.

33. Heimer L, Zahm DS, Churchill L, Kalivas PW, Wohltmann C. Specificity in the projection patterns of accumbal core and shell. *Neuroscience* 1991;41:89–126.

34. Herve D, Simon H, Blanc G, LeMoal M, Glowinski J, Tassin JP. Opposite changes in dopamine utilization in the nucleus accumbens and the frontal cortex after electrolytic lesion of the median raphe in the rat. *Brain Res* 1981;261:422–428.

35. Hitri A, Wyatt J. Regional differences in rat brain dopamine transporter binding: function of time after chronic cocaine. *Clin Neuropharmacol* 1993;16:525–539.

36. Innis R, Seibly J, Wallace E, Scanley E, Laruele M, Abi-Dargham A, Zea-Ponce Y, Zoghbi S, Charney D, Wang S, Gao Y, Neumeyer J, Baldwin R, Marek R, Hoffer P. SPECT imaging demonstrates loss of striatal dopamine transporters in Parkinson's disease. *Proc Natl Acad Sci USA* 1994;90:11965–11969.

37. Johnson SW, Seutin V, North RA. Burst firing in dopamine neurons induced by *N*-Methyl-D-aspartate: role of electrogenic sodium pump. *Science* 1992;258:665–667.

38. Kalivas PJ. Neurotransmitter regulation of dopamine neurons in the ventral tegmental area. *Brain Res Rev* 1993;18:75–113.

39. Kalivas PW, Alesdattger JE. Involvement of *N*-methyl-D-aspartate receptor stimulation in the ventral tegmental area and amygdala in behavioral sensitization to cocaine. *J Pharmacol Exp Ther* 1993;267:486–495.

40. Kaufman M, Madras B. Severe depletion of cocaine recognition sites associated with the dopamine transporter in Parkinson's diseased striatum. *Synapse* 1991;49:43–49.

41. Kilts CD, Anderson CM, Ely TD, Nishita JK. Absence of synthesis-modulating nerve terminal autoreceptors on mesoamygdaloid and other mesolimbic dopamine neuronal populations. *J Neurosci* 1987;7:3961–3975.

42. Laruelle M, Baldwin RM, Malison RT, Zea-Ponce Y, Zoghbi SS, Al-Tikriti MS, Sybirska EH, Zimmerman RC, Wisniewski G, Neumeyer JL, Milius RA, Want S, Charney D, Roth RH, Hoffer PB, Innis RB. SPECT imaging of dopamine and serotonin transporters with [123I]-b-CIT: pharmacological characterization of brain uptake in nonhuman primates. *Synapse* 1993;13:295–309.

43. Morrow BA, Clark WA, Roth RH. Stress activation of mesocorticolimbic dopamine neurons: effects of a glycine/NMDA receptor antagonist. *Eur J Pharmacol* 1993;238:255–262.

44. Nissbrant H, Sundström E, Jonsson G, Hjorth S, Carlsson A. Synthesis and release of dopamine in rat brain: comparison between substantia nigra pars compacta, pars reticulata, and striatum. *J Neurochem* 1989;52:1170–1182.

45. Oreland L. Monoamine oxidase, dopamine and Parkinson's disease. *Acta Neurol Scand* 1991;84:60–65.

46. Papel A, Uhl G, Kuhar MJ. Species differences in dopamine transporters: postmortem changes and glycosylation differences. *J Neurochem* 1993;61:496–500.

47. Phillipson OT. Afferent projections to the ventral tegmental area of Tsai and interfascicular nucleus: a horseradish peroxidase study in the rat. *J Comp Neurol* 1979;187:117–143.

48. Pifl C, Reither H, Hornykiewicz O. Lower efficacy of the dopamine D1 agonist, SKF 38393, to stimulate adenylyl cyclase activity in primate than in rodent striatum. *Eur J Pharmacol* 1991;202:273–276.

49. Redmond DE Jr, Roth RH, Spencer DD, Naftolin F, Leranth C,

Robbins RJ, Marek KL, Elsworth JD, Taylor JR, Sass KJ, Sladek JR Jr. Neural transplantation for neurodegenerative disease: past, present, and future. In: Nitsch RM, Crowdon JH, Corkin S, eds. *Disease: amyloid precursors and proteins, signal transductions, and neuronal transplantation.* Cambridge, MA: Center for Brain Sciences and Metabolism Charitable Trust, 1993;51–60.

50. Robertson HA. Dopamine receptor interactions: some implications for the treatment of Parkinson's disease. *Trends Neurol Sci* 1992;15:201–205.

51. Roth RH, Tam S-Y. Regulatory control of midbrain dopamine neurons. In: Kaufman S, ed. *Amino acids in health and disease: new perspectives. UCLA Symposia on Molecular and Cellular Biology, New Series, Volume 55.* Alan R Liss, New York, 1987;159–178.

52. Roth RH, Wolf ME, Deutch AY. Neurochemistry of midbrain dopamine systems. In: Meltzer HY, ed. *Psychopharmacology: the third generation of progress.* New York: Raven Press, 1987;81–94.

53. Roth RH. CNS dopamine autoreceptors: distribution, pharmacology and function. *Ann NY Acad Sci* 1984;430:27–53.

54. Sandler M, Usdin E, eds. *Phenolsulfo-transferase in mental health research.* New York: Macmillan, 1981.

55. Schalling M, Friberg K, Seroogy K, Riederer P, Bird E, Schiffman SN, Mailleux P, Vansderhaeghen J-J, Kuga S, Goldstein M, Kitahama K, Lumm PH, Jouvet M, Hökfelt T. Analysis of expression of cholecystokinin in dopamine cells in the ventral mesencephalon of several species and in humans with schizophrenia. *Proc Natl Acad Sci USA* 1990;87:8427–8431.

56. Seroogy KB, Mehta A, Fallon JH. Neurotensin and cholecystokinin coexist within neurons of the ventral mesencephalon: projections to the forebrain. *Exp Brain Res* 1987;68:277–289.

57. Shepard PD, Lehmann H. (±)-1-Hydroxy-3-aminopyrrolidone-2 (HA-966) inhibits the activity of substantia nigra dopamine neurons through a non-*N*-methyl-D-aspartate receptor-mediated mechanism. *J Pharmacol Exp Ther* 1992;261(2):387–394.

58. Shi WX, Bunney BS. Actions of neurotensin: a review of the electrophysiological studies. *Ann NY Acad Sci* 1992;669:129–145.

59. Singh L, Donald AE, Foster AC, Hutson PH, Iversen LL, Iversen SD, Kemp JA, Leeson PD, Marshall GR, Oles RJ, Priestley T, Thorn L, Tricklebank MD, Vass CA, Williams BJ. Enantiomers of HA-966 (3-amino-1-hydroxypyrrolid-2-one) exhibit distinct central nervous system effects: (+)-HA-966 is a selective glycine/*N*-methyl-D-aspartate receptor antagonist, but (−)-HA-966 is a potent gamma-butyrolactone-like sedative. *Proc Natl Acad Sci USA* 1990;87:347.

60. Sladek JR Jr, Elsworth JD, Roth RH, Evans LE, Collier TJ, Cooper SJ, Taylor JR, Redmond DE Jr. Fetal dopamine cell survival after transplantation is dramatically improved at a critical donor gestational age in nonhuman primates. *Exp Neurol* 1993;122:16–27.

61. Taylor JR, Lawrence MS, Redmond DE Jr, Elsworth JD, Roth RH, Nichols DE, Mailman RB. Dihydrexidine, a full dopamine D_1 agonist, reduces MPTP-induced parkinsonism in African green monkeys. *Eur J Pharmacol* 1991;199:389–391.

62. Teicher MH, Gallitano AL, Gelbard HA, Evans HK, Marsh ER, Booth RG, Baldessarini RJ. Dopamine D1 autoreceptor function: possible expression in developing rat prefrontal cortex and striatum. *Dev Brain Res* 1991;63:229–235.

63. Tepper JM, Groves PM, Young SJ. The neuropharmacology of the autoinhibition of monoamine release. *Trends Pharmacol Sci* 1985;6:251.

64. Wachtel SR, Hu XT, Galloway MP, White FJ. D1 dopamine receptor stimulation enables the postsynaptic, but not autoreceptor, effects of D2 dopamine agonists in nigrostriatal and mesoaccumbens dopamine systems. *Synapse* 1989;4(4):327–346.

65. Waddington JL, O'Boyle KM. Drugs acting on brain dopamine receptors: a conceptual reevaluation five years after the first selective D1 antagonist. *Pharm Ther* 1989;43:1–52.

66. Walaas I, Fonnum F. Biochemical evidence for γ-aminobutyrate containing fibres from the nucleus accumbens to the substantia nigra and ventral tegmental area in the rat. *Neuroscience* 1980;5:63–72.

67. Watts VJ, Lawler CP, Gilmore JH, Southerland SB, Nichols DE, Mailman RB. Dopamine D1 receptors: efficacy of full (dihydrexidine) vs. partial (SKF38393) agonists in primates vs. rodents. *Eur J Pharmacol* 1993;242:165–172.

68. Westerink BHC, Santiago M, DeVries JB. In vivo evidence for a concordant response of terminal and dendritic dopamine release during intranigral infusions of drugs. *Naunyn Schmiedebergs Arch Pharmacol* 1992;346:637–643.

69. Wolf ME, Roth RH. Heterogeneity of midbrain dopamine neurons: Implications for psychiatry. *Psychiatry Lett* 1988;VI(1-6);24–32.

70. Wolf ME, Roth RH. Autoreceptor regulation of dopamine synthesis. *Ann NY Acad Sci* 1990;604:323–343.

71. Yang CR, Mogenson GJ. Dopamine enhances terminal excitability of hippocampal-accumbens neurones via D-2 receptor: role of dopamine in presynaptic inhibition. *J Neurosci* 1986;6:2470–2478.

72. Zahm DS, Brog JS. On the significance of subterritories in the "accumbens" part of the rat ventral striatum. *Neuroscience* 1992;751–767.

Psychopharmacology: The Fourth Generation of Progress, edited by Floyd E. Bloom and David J. Kupfer. Raven Press, Ltd., New York © 1995.

CHAPTER **22**

Dopaminergic Neuronal Systems in the Hypothalamus

Kenneth E. Moore and Keith J. Lookingland

In a previous review published in 1987 (51) it was pointed out that there are differences in the characteristics of neurons that comprise the various anatomically differentiated dopaminergic (DA) neuronal systems in the mammalian brain. Evidence available at that time revealed that neurochemical properties and responses to pharmacological and endocrinological manipulations of the major ascending mesotelencephalic DA neurons are often quite different from those DA neurons that originate in the diencephalon [i.e., those DA neurons identified as the A_{11}, A_{12}, A_{13}, and A_{14} cell groups by the alphanumeric system of Dählström and Fuxe (8)]. This chapter provides an updated review of these hypothalamic DA neurons.

ANATOMICAL OVERVIEW

Details of the anatomy of DA perikarya in the rat diencephalon are provided by Björklund et al. (6), and the location of their perikarya are depicted schematically in Fig. 1. There are more DA perikarya in the rat diencephalon (A_{11}, A_{12}, A_{13}, and A_{14} consist of approximately 8000 cells) than in the substantia nigra (A_8 and A_9 consist of approximately 7000 cells), which is generally considered to be the major locus of DA neurons in the brain (69). The most familiar hypothalamic DA neurons are those that comprise the tuberoinfundibular dopaminergic (TIDA) system; perikarya of these neurons (A_{12}), which are located in the mediobasal hypothalamus (dorsomedial region of the arcuate nucleus and the adjacent region of the periventricular nucleus), project to the external layer of the median eminence (Fig. 2). Although TIDA neurons have been studied more extensively than other DA neu-

rons in the diencephalon, they actually represent a minority ($\sim$2800 cells; see ref. 55) of these DA neurons. The majority of diencephalic DA neurons are located in dorsal regions of the hypothalamus and ventral thalamus, as well as in regions adjacent to the third ventricle. A small number of relatively large DA perikarya (A_{11}) are located in the posterior regions of the dorsal hypothalamus and the periventricular gray of the central thalamus; axons from some of these neurons project to the spinal cord. These diencephalospinal DA neurons will not be discussed in this chapter.

Approximately 900 small DA perikarya, identified as the A_{13} cell group, are clustered in the rostral regions of the medial zona incerta (MZI). These perikarya, along with the A_{14} DA neurons located in the rostral periventricular nucleus, comprise the incertohypothalamic dopaminergic (IHDA) system. These neurons were believed to give rise to axons that project short distances to various regions within the hypothalamus, but results of recent neurochemical and anatomical studies suggest that some A_{13} DA neurons project out of the hypothalamus to such regions as the diagonal band of Broca, septum, and central nucleus of the amygdala (Wagner, Eaton, Moore, and Lookingland, *unpublished data*).

DA neurons projecting to the posterior pituitary were reported initially to originate from rostral A_{12} cells in the arcuate and periventricular nuclei; accordingly, they were referred to as *tuberohypophysial DA neurons.* More recent studies (16,29) have revealed that DA neurons projecting to the intermediate lobe of the pituitary originate from a subpopulation of A_{14} DA cells in the periventricular nucleus (Fig. 2). In this review, DA neurons projecting to the intermediate lobe of the pituitary will be identified as the *periventricular–hypophysial dopaminergic (PHDA) neurons,* although in the majority of earlier references these neurons are referred to as *tuberohypophysial DA neurons.* The remaining A_{14} periventricular DA neu-

K. E. Moore and K. J. Lookingland: Department of Pharmacology and Toxicology, Michigan State University, East Lansing, Michigan 48824.

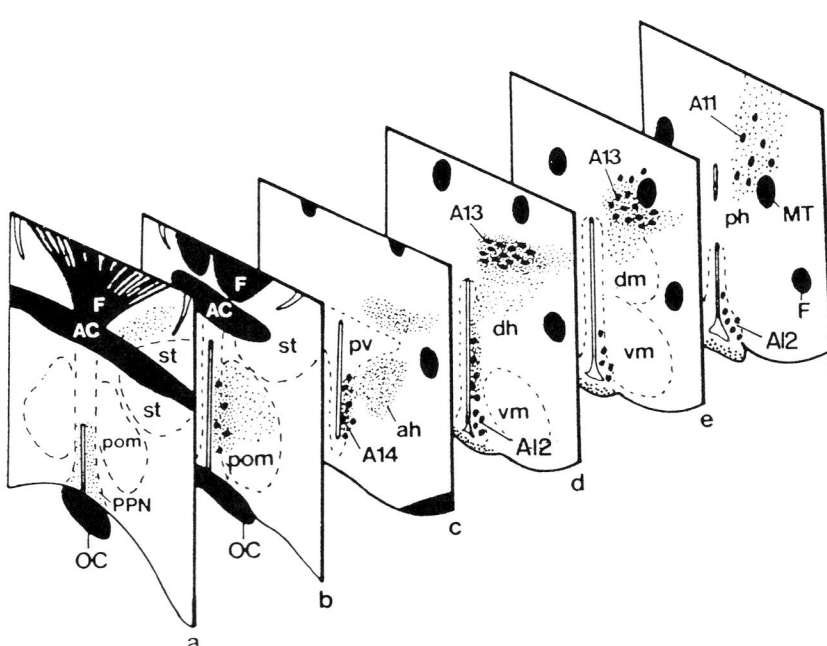

FIG. 1. Location of dopaminergic perikarya ($A_{11}-A_{14}$) are depicted schematically on frontal sections through the diencephalon of the rat. AC, anterior commissure; ah, anterior hypothalamic area; $A_{11,12,13,14}$, DA cell groups; dh, dorsal hypothalamic area; dm, dorsomedial nucleus; F, fornix; MT, mammillothalamic tract; OC, optic chiasm; ph, posterior hypothalamus; pom, medial preoptic area; PPN, preoptic periventricular nucleus; pv, paraventricular nucleus; st, bed nucleus of the stria terminalis. (Modified from ref. 6.)

rons are believed to project laterally into adjacent regions (e.g., medial preoptic area, anterior hypothalamic area). Additional details of the distribution of TIDA, PHDA, IHDA, and periventricular DA neurons can be found in the following sections dealing with each of these neuronal systems.

ESTIMATION OF THE ACTIVITY OF HYPOTHALAMIC DA NEURONS

Only a few investigators have attempted to measure the activity (or impulse flow) of hypothalamic DA neurons. For example, Sanghera (57) and Eaton and Moss (10) recorded electrical activity from neurons in the MZI in response to a variety of pharmacological manipulations using both in situ and in vitro slice preparations. Loose et al. (38) and Lin et al. (30) recorded electrical activity in slices of the mediobasal hypothalamus, particularly from DA neurons in the arcuate nucleus. Only Loose et

al. (38) determined unequivocally that recordings were made from DA neurons.

Alternatively, investigators have employed a variety of neurochemical techniques to estimate impulse flow in hypothalamic DA neurons. The basis of these biochemical techniques is that the release of dopamine (DA) is coupled to the rates of synthesis and metabolism of DA in terminals and dendrites of DA neurons. Procedures that increase or decrease activity of DA neurons generally do not alter steady-state concentrations of DA but produce corresponding increases or decreases, respectively, in rates of synthesis, turnover, and metabolism of this amine. The utility of various neurochemical procedures for estimating activity of hypothalamic DA neurons has been discussed previously (51), and it is only reviewed briefly and updated in this section.

A number of investigators have employed in vitro techniques to characterize neurochemical properties of TIDA and PHDA neurons, but because this chapter will focus

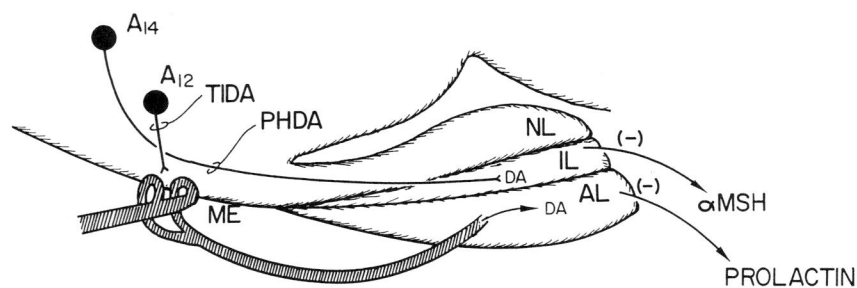

FIG. 2. Parasagittal section through the mediobasal hypothalamus and pituitary of the rat illustrating schematically the location of axonal projections of A_{12} and A_{14} DA neurons. The roles of these neurons in the regulation of prolactin and αMSH secretion are also illustrated. AL, anterior lobe; IL, intermediate lobe; ME, median eminence; NL, neural lobe; PHDA, periventricular–hypophysial DA neurons; TIDA, tuberoinfundibular DA neurons. (From ref. 15.)

on the responses of hypothalamic DA neuronal systems to physiological and pharmacological manipulations, discussions will be limited to results obtained using in vivo techniques. Early in vivo attempts to estimate the activity of central catecholaminergic neurons involved studies that employed α-methyltyrosine, an inhibitor of tyrosine hydroxylase. Following administration of α-methyltyrosine the concentrations of catecholamines are reduced in an exponential manner at a rate that is proportional to the activity of the neurons that contain these amines. The advantage of this technique is that it permits concurrent estimation of DA and norepinephrine (NE) turnover in the same hypothalamic brain region. There are, however, several disadvantages to this procedure: (a) measurement of catecholamines must be made in groups of animals killed immediately before, and at least two different times after, α-methyltyrosine administration in order to ensure that an exponential rate of decline has occurred; (b) rapid measurements cannot be made which prohibits its use for short-term experimental manipulations; and (c) by virtue of its ability to block synthesis, α-methyltyrosine reduces catecholamine release, which compromises neuronal function. This is a problem when studying TIDA neurons in that blockade of DA synthesis in TIDA neurons reduces DA release into the hypophysial portal blood and thereby causes an increased secretion of prolactin from the anterior pituitary. Prolactin feeds back to increase activity of TIDA neurons.

The rate of catecholamine synthesis is regulated at the step catalyzed by tyrosine hydroxylase so estimates of catecholaminergic activity can be obtained from measurements of the activity of this enzyme. This can be accomplished in vivo by administering 3-hydroxybenzylhydrazine (NSD 1015), an inhibitor of aromatic amino acid decarboxylase. The concentration of 3,4-dihydroxyphenylalanine (DOPA) in brain tissue is essentially zero because once it is synthesized from tyrosine, it is immediately decarboxylated to DA. Following the administration of NSD 1015, DOPA accumulates in catecholaminergic nerve terminals at a rate that is proportional to the activity of these neurons. The advantages of this procedure over the α-methyltyrosine technique are that fewer measurements are needed (DOPA concentrations are so low that "zero-time" values are unnecessary), and they can be made over a shorter time frame (i.e., 15 min after intravenous NSD 1015). As with α-methyltyrosine, NSD 1015 disrupts catecholamine synthesis and thereby alters the properties of the catecholaminergic neurons (e.g., NSD 1015, like α-methyltyrosine, increases plasma levels of prolactin). Finally, DOPA accumulates in both DA and noradrenergic (NE) neurons after the administration of NSD 1015. This has little consequence when DOPA accumulation is measured in terminals of TIDA and PHDA neurons in the median eminence or intermediate lobe of the pituitary, because the concentrations and turnover of DA greatly exceed that of NE. In most hypothalamic regions the concentrations of NE greatly exceed that of

DA, so this procedure cannot be employed to estimate IHDA or periventricular DA neuronal activity.

In brain regions containing a preponderance of DA over NE nerve terminals the concentrations of 3,4-dihydroxyphenylacetic acid (DOPAC), a major metabolite of DA, reflect the activity of DA neurons. It has been shown empirically that increases and decreases in TIDA and PHDA neuronal activities are accompanied by concurrent increases and decreases in DOPAC concentrations in the median eminence and intermediate lobe of the pituitary, respectively (32,35). In contrast to techniques that require administration of α-methyltyrosine or NSD 1015, no drug pretreatments are required prior to the measurement of DOPAC concentrations; accordingly, measurements can be made within minutes after initiating a manipulation.

In the following discussions, alterations in hypothalamic DA neuronal activity (i.e., increases or decreases in impulse flow) were estimated using one or more of the neurochemical methods described above.

TUBEROINFUNDIBULAR DOPAMINERGIC NEURONS

Anatomy

Perikarya of TIDA (A_{12}) neurons are located in the arcuate and periventricular nuclei of the rat mediobasal hypothalamus (8). Within the arcuate nucleus, two populations of tyrosine hydroxylase-containing neurons have been identified on the basis of their size and location in either the dorsomedial or ventrolateral regions of this nucleus (13). In the dorsomedial arcuate nucleus and adjacent periventricular nucleus, relatively small DA perikarya have dendrites oriented in the dorsoventral plane (69) and axons which project ventrally to terminate in the external layer of the median eminence (7). DA released from terminals of these neurons in the median eminence diffuses through fenestrated capillaries and is transported in the hypophysial portal blood to the anterior pituitary where it activates D_2 receptors on lactotrophs and tonically inhibits the secretion of prolactin from these cells. Tyrosine hydroxylase-containing perikarya in the ventrolateral arcuate nucleus are larger in size (13), with dendrites oriented in the mediolateral plane (69) and axons that terminate in the lateral portion of the median eminence (7). These neurons lack L-aromatic amino acid decarboxylase (13,48), and they do not express DA transporter protein mRNA as do the DA-containing neurons in the dorsomedial portion of the arcuate nucleus (49). "DOPAergic" neurons have also been identified in the ventrolateral arcuate nucleus of the human brain, and although their functional significance is not known, it has been suggested that DOPA released from these neurons may be decarboxylated to DA in the hypothalamic–pituitary vasculature (48).

TIDA neurons in the dorsomedial arcuate nucleus also

synthesize a number of substances reported to have either inhibitory [gamma-aminobutyric acid (GABA), galanin, enkephalin] or stimulatory (neurotensin) effects on DA release from these neurons (13). It has been postulated that these colocalized neurotransmitters may be selectively synthesized and released under different physiological conditions, thereby modulating (a) TIDA neuronal regulation of prolactin secretion and (b) the responsiveness of these neurons to hormonal and neuronal feedback (47).

Neurochemistry

Each of the neurochemical techniques described above in the Introduction has been used effectively to estimate TIDA neuronal activity and have provided consistent results. The terminal region of these neurons, the median eminence, is well-defined and relatively easy to dissect, and the concentration and rate of turnover of DA are much higher than those of NE, so there is no difficulty in relating changes in DOPA accumulation or DOPAC concentrations to TIDA activity (23,35). The activity of these neurons has also been estimated from measurements of the amount of DA released into hypophysial portal blood, but because this technique involves use of anesthetized animals following radical surgery, there has been little use of this technique in recent years. Neurochemical estimates of TIDA neuronal activity have been correlated with reciprocal changes in circulating levels of prolactin. One should be cognizant, however, that while the primary control of prolactin secretion is exerted by the inhibitory actions of TIDA neurons, the secretion of prolactin under some circumstances is influenced by prolactin-releasing factors.

Regulation of Activity

The properties and responses of TIDA neurons differ in many respects from those of other DA neuronal systems in the mammalian brain. Some of these differences were discussed in previous reviews (51); additions to, and updates of, these differences are described below.

Gender Differences

There are marked differences in the activities of TIDA neurons of male and female rats. Although there is no gender difference in the density of TIDA nerve terminals (as reflected in the concentration of DA in the median eminence) the rates of turnover, synthesis, and metabolism of DA in this region, and the concentration of DA in hypophysial portal blood is two to three times higher in female than in male rats. TIDA neuronal activity is increased in the male and decreased in the female after castration, and these effects are reversed by replacement

with testosterone (66) or with estrogen (68), respectively. The ability of estrogen to increase TIDA neuronal activity in ovariectomized rats is secondary to the ability of this hormone to increase circulating levels of prolactin.

There are also major gender differences in the responses of TIDA neurons to a variety of pharmacological and physiological manipulations. TIDA neurons in females are more responsive to the stimulating actions of prolactin, to the inhibitory effects of stress (36), and to the administration of kappa opioid agonists (44) and the N-methyl-D-aspartate receptor antagonist MK801 (71). On the other hand, activation of TIDA neurons after administration of bombesin (67) and a kappa opioid antagonist (44) is more pronounced in the male. Additional details of the responses of TIDA neurons in male and female rats is provided in the following sections which describe the actions of individual drugs.

There are obvious changes in the properties and activity of TIDA neurons that occur exclusively in female rats—for example, those that occur during pregnancy, lactation, and suckling. These topics will not be discussed here but have been reviewed elsewhere (51; see also Chapters 62, 65, and 67, *this volume*).

Effects of Prolactin

Under most physiological situations the activity of TIDA neurons is regulated, to a large extent, by circulating levels of prolactin; other DA neurons are unresponsive to this hormone. TIDA neuronal activity is reduced during periods of hypoprolactinemia, such as that induced by hypophysectomy or by the administration of DA agonists or prolactin antibody. The reduction of TIDA neuronal activity is more pronounced in the female; indeed, following several hours of low circulating levels of prolactin the activity of these neurons in the female rat is equivalent to that seen in a male with normal prolactin levels. On the other hand, TIDA neuronal activity is increased during periods of hyperprolactinemia—for example, following implantation of prolactin-secreting tumors, administration of DA antagonists or estrogen, and the central or systemic administration of prolactin. TIDA neurons in the female rat are more sensitive and responsive to prolactin than they are in the male. The mechanism by which prolactin activates TIDA neurons has not been elucidated.

Putative Afferent Neurotransmitters

To date, the majority of studies on TIDA neurons has focused on responses of these neurons to changes in the hormonal milieu (e.g., prolactin, gonadal steroids; see ref. 51). It is apparent, however, that TIDA neurons are also acutely responsive to afferent neuronal influences as evidenced by the rapid responses of these neurons in female rats to stressful manipulations and suckling, both of which promptly inhibit TIDA neuronal activity and thereby increase plasma concentrations of prolactin (51). The neuronal circuits responsible for stress- or suckling-induced inhibition of TIDA neurons have not been well-defined, but because the responses can be attenuated by antagonists of recognized neurotransmitters [e.g., 5-hydroxytryptamine (5-HT), acetylcholine], it is reasonable to assume that neurons utilizing these transmitters are located somewhere in neuronal circuits activated by stressful or suckling stimuli. A number of attempts have been made to employ pharmacological techniques to uncover roles played by putative aminergic and peptidergic neurotransmitters in regulating TIDA neuronal activity. The following sections review some of the effects of putative neurotransmitters, and of their agonists and antagonists, on TIDA neuronal activity and secretion of prolactin.

Drugs which act as selective agonists or antagonists at mu, kappa, or delta opioid receptors produce characteristic patterns of responses of different DA neurons. Morphine and a variety of mu opioid agonists increase the activity of the major mesotelencephalic DA neurons terminating in the striatum and limbic forebrain regions (51) and of IHDA neurons (65); on the other hand, these compounds inhibit PHDA and TIDA neurons. Inhibition of TIDA neurons is responsible, at least in part, for increased circulating levels of prolactin produced by mu opioid agonists. The inhibitory action of mu opioids on TIDA neurons appears due to the ability of these compounds to hyperpolarize these neurons by increasing potassium conductance (38).

Endogenous mu opioids may play a role in the physiological regulation of TIDA neurons. For example, in lactating rats but not in male or estrous female rats, TIDA neurons synthesize enkephalin (50). In lactating animals, enkephalin may be released from TIDA neurons, act on autoreceptors to inhibit DA release, and thereby maintain high circulating levels of prolactin and milk production.

Drugs that act at kappa opioid receptors also influence the activity of DA neurons, but unlike mu opioid agonists, which, depending on the system, can increase or decrease the activity of DA neurons, kappa agonists exert only inhibitory actions; the degree of inhibition is generally dependent upon the level of activity of the DA neurons at the time the kappa agonist is administered. U50,488, a selective kappa agonist, inhibits PHDA neurons but appears to exert minimal inhibitory actions on nigrostriatal, mesolimbic, or TIDA neurons unless these neurons are activated (42). Thus, U50,488 reduces the high level of activity of TIDA neurons in female rats but is without effect in males unless the latter animals are injected with prolactin or are orchidectomized in order to activate their TIDA neurons (44). On the other hand, the selective kappa opioid receptor antagonist, norbinaltorphimine, increases TIDA neuronal activity in male but not in female rats, suggesting that TIDA neurons in the male are tonically inhibited by an endogenous kappa opioid, such as dynorphin. Consistent with this suggestion, intracerebroventricular (i.c.v.) administration of dynorphin antibodies

to male rats increases the activity of TIDA and PHDA neurons, but has no effect on nigrostriatal or mesolimbic DA neurons, prompting the suggestion that the former hypothalamic DA neurons are under tonic inhibitory tone of endogenous dynorphin (45).

There have been few studies on the responses of hypothalamic DA neurons to drugs that act at delta opioid receptors, but results of a recent study (46) reveal that these drugs exert a pattern of effects that is different from that of drugs acting on mu or kappa opioid receptors. In male rats, i.c.v. injection of [D-Pen^2, D-Pen^5]enkephalin, a delta opioid receptor agonist, has no effect on nigrostriatal or PHDA neurons, but increases the activity of TIDA and mesolimbic DA neurons terminating in nucleus accumbens. These effects are blocked by naltrindole, a selective delta opioid receptor antagonist, but this antagonist has no effect per se on DA neuronal systems.

Several neuroactive peptides stimulate TIDA neurons; the most potent of these is bombesin. Intracerebroventricular injection of this peptide into male rats at doses as low as 1 ng causes a marked but relatively short-lasting increase in TIDA neuronal activity and a concomitant decrease in plasma concentrations of prolactin (43). At higher doses this peptide also activates PHDA neurons terminating in the intermediate lobe of the pituitary, but is without effect on activities of nigrostriatal or mesolimbic DA neurons. These stimulatory effects of bombesin are mimicked by equimolar concentrations of gastrin-releasing peptide (GRP), a bombesin-like peptide found in mammalian brain. The activation of TIDA and PHDA neurons by bombesin and GRP are blocked by a bombesin antagonist (MDL 101,562), but because this antagonist has no effect per se it appears that under basal conditions these hypothalamic DA neurons are not under tonic excitatory control of a bombesin-like peptide (Manzanares, Edwards, Lookingland, and Moore, *unpublished data*). The stimulatory effect of bombesin on TIDA neurons does not involve prolactin, but because the response is pronounced in ovariectomized but not in gonadally intact rats it would appear that the stimulatory actions of bombesin in the female are reduced by estrogen (67).

Two other peptides have been reported to activate TIDA neurons, namely, alpha-melanocyte-stimulating hormone (α-MSH) and neurotensin. α-MSH, when administered i.c.v., increases TIDA neuronal activity, and thereby reduces circulating concentrations of prolactin (33). In the same experiment, α-MSH did not alter the activity of PHDA, nigrostriatal, or mesolimbic DA neurons. Neurotensin is a peptide colocalized with DA in TIDA neurons (24). Following i.c.v. administration of this peptide, TIDA neurons are activated; it also activates mesolimbic DA neurons (19). The neurotensin-induced activation of TIDA is related temporally with a decrease in plasma concentrations of prolactin (53).

Galanin is a peptide reported to inhibit the activity of TIDA neurons in both female and male rats (15; see also Chapter 50, *this volume*). The effects of this peptide on TIDA neurons is activity-dependent in that galanin only inhibits the activity of TIDA neurons under stimulated conditions and has no effect on the basal activity of these neurons in either gender. This may represent an autoregulatory feedback mechanism by which galanin colocalized and released from TIDA neurons regulates DA release.

A number of amino acid-derived neurotransmitters presumably released from hypothalamic interneurons are reported to have either stimulatory (e.g., excitatory amino acids) or inhibitory (e.g., GABA) effects on the activity of TIDA neurons. Glutamate acting at N-methyl-D-aspartate (NMDA) receptors tonically stimulates the basal activity of TIDA neurons in female, but not male, rats (71). This gender difference in NMDA-receptor-mediated regulation of TIDA neuronal activity is likely due to estrogen-induced stimulation of glutamate release by a prolactin-independent mechanism (71). In both genders, endogenous excitatory amino acids acting at non-NMDA, α-amino-3-hydroxy-5-methylisoxazole-4-propionic acid (AMPA) receptors tonically inhibit the basal activity of TIDA neurons (72) by a mechanism involving $GABA_A$ receptors (Wagner, Moore, and Lookingland, *unpublished data*). Activation of $GABA_B$ receptors also decreases the basal activity of TIDA neurons, but these neurons are not tonically inhibited by endogenous GABA acting at $GABA_B$ receptors (Wagner, Goudreau, Moore, and Lookingland, *unpublished data*).

Psychoactive Drugs

Antipsychotics

Acute administration of "classical" antipsychotics with D_2 DA-receptor antagonistic properties (e.g., haloperidol) activates DA neurons that comprise the mesolimbic, nigrostriatal, periventricular–hypophysial, and incertohypothalamic systems, but has no direct action on TIDA neurons. On the other hand, TIDA neurons are activated indirectly several hours after administration of haloperidol and other D_2 antagonists as a result of their ability to increase circulating concentrations of prolactin (51). By contrast, some atypical neuroleptics, exemplified by clozapine, increase acutely TIDA neuronal activity (20). Although it has been proposed that the ability of clozapine to activate TIDA neurons involves interactions with D_1 DA receptors and/or neurotensin, the mechanism by which clozapine increases the activity of these neurons remains to be elucidated. This action of clozapine may, however, be responsible for the drug's brief elevation of plasma prolactin levels compared to the long duration of its other effects. That is, the clozapine-enhanced release of DA from TIDA neurons may counteract the antagonistic actions it has on release of prolactin from lactotrophs in the anterior pituitary (see Chapter 106, *this volume*).

DA Agonists

By activating autoreceptors and/or DA receptor-mediated neuronal feedback loops, nonselective DA agonists (e.g., apomorphine, bromocriptine) reduce the activities of those DA neurons that comprise the periventricular–hypophysial, incertohypothalamic, mesolimbic, and nigrostriatal systems. On the other hand, TIDA neurons are unresponsive to the acute administration of these drugs (51). Therefore, it was unexpected that recently developed, more selective D_1 and D_2 DA agonists have pronounced and opposite actions on TIDA neurons; D_1 agonists (e.g., SKF 38393, CY 208-243) exert inhibitory effects, whereas ergoline-derived D_2 agonists (e.g., quinpirole, quinelorane) stimulate TIDA neurons.

Although D_1 DA agonists have little effect on the basal activity of TIDA neurons in male rats, they reduce the increased activity of these neurons following activation by neurotensin or the haloperidol-induced elevation of circulating levels of prolactin (4). Selective D_1 antagonists (SCH 23390, loxapine), while having no effect per se, block the inhibitory actions of the D_1 agonists on TIDA neurons. Quinpirole and quinelorane, like other DA agonists, reduce the activity of periventricular–hypophysial, mesolimbic and nigrostriatal DA neurons; in contrast, these drugs increase TIDA neuronal activity (5,12). This latter effect is blocked by haloperidol and raclopride, but not by the selective D_1 antagonist SCH 23390, indicating that TIDA neuronal activation by these ergoline-derived DA agonists is mediated by D_2 receptors. Results of earlier studies showing a lack of effect on TIDA neurons by "classical" DA agonists may have resulted from opposing actions on D_1 and D_2 receptors, although there is no direct evidence in support of this suggestion.

PERIVENTRICULAR-HYPOPHYSIAL DOPAMINERGIC NEURONS

Anatomy

DA axons terminating in the posterior pituitary were postulated initially to constitute a distinct tuberohypophysial DA neuronal system originating from A_{12} perikarya located in the most rostral extent of the arcuate nucleus (7). More recent anatomical (29) and neurochemical studies (16) have revealed that DA neurons terminating in the intermediate lobe of the posterior pituitary originate from a subpopulation of A_{14} DA neurons located in the periventricular nucleus dorsal to the retrochiasmatic area of the anterior hypothalamus. These PHDA neurons have dendrites oriented in the dorsoventral plane (69) and axons that project ventrally through the internal layer of the median eminence and pituitary stalk to terminate in close proximity to intermediate lobe melanotrophs. DA released from PHDA neurons tonically inhibits the secretion of the pro-opiomelanocortin-derived peptide hormones

α-MSH (16) and β-endorphin from melanotrophs in the intermediate lobe. In addition, DA neurons terminating in the intermediate lobe have been implicated in the regulation of prolactin secretion (2).

PHDA neurons colocalize substances known to have both stimulatory (neurotensin; see ref. 26) and inhibitory (GABA; see ref. 70) effects on the release of DA in the intermediate lobe. In addition, terminals of PHDA neurons take up and store 5-HT (56), but the role of this amine and other colocalized neurotransmitters in the regulation of PHDA neurons and melanotroph hormone secretion is unknown.

Neurochemistry

Concentrations and rates of turnover of DA greatly exceed those of NE in the intermediate lobe of the pituitary, the terminal region of PHDA neurons, so increases and decreases in PHDA neuronal activity are reflected in concurrent changes in (a) rates of DA turnover and DOPA accumulation (23) and (b) concentrations of DOPAC in this region (32). Changes in neurochemical estimations of the activity of these neurons are reflected in changes in their function. That is, increases and decreases of PHDA neuronal activity are associated with decreases and increases, respectively, in circulating concentrations of α-MSH (31).

Regulation of Neuronal Activity

PHDA neurons terminating in the intermediate lobe of the pituitary, unlike the anatomically related TIDA neurons, do not exhibit pronounced gender differences and are not responsive to changes in circulating levels of gonadal steroids (21). On the other hand, PHDA neurons resemble the major ascending mesotelencephalic DA neurons in that they are regulated by DA receptor-mediated mechanisms. Acute administration of DA agonists and antagonists cause prompt decreases and increases, respectively, of PHDA neuronal activity (51).

Putative Afferent Neurotransmitters

Agonists and antagonists of mu (51) or delta (46) opioid receptors do not alter PHDA neuronal activity. On the other hand, agonists and antagonists of kappa opioid receptors decrease and increase, respectively, the activity of PHDA neurons and cause reciprocal changes in circulating concentrations of αMSH (40,41). The ability of dynorphin antibodies to mimic the stimulatory effects of kappa opioid antagonists on PHDA neurons suggests that these neurons are inhibited tonically by an endogenous dynorphin-containing neuronal system (45). Other peptides have stimulatory actions on PHDA neurons; i.c.v. administration of bombesin, GRP (43), and neurotensin

(53) increase PHDA neuronal activity and cause concomittant decreases in concentration of α-MSH in plasma.

Neither increasing activity at histaminergic receptors by i.c.v. administration of histamine nor facilitating release of endogenous histamine influences basal PHDA activity; neither do drugs that inhibit histamine synthesis or block histaminergic receptors (14). Thus, while histaminergic neuronal systems do not influence basal activity of PHDA neurons, they do play a role in stress-induced inhibition of these neurons (see below). Similarly, disruption of 5-HT transmission processes fails to alter basal PHDA neuronal activity, but pharmacological activation of 5-HT_2 receptors does reduce PHDA neuronal activity and increase α-MSH secretion (17). Furthermore, 5-HT neurons are involved in stress-induced inhibition of PHDA neurons (18).

GABA, a dominant inhibitory neurotransmitter in the hypothalamus, is colocalized with DA in neurons innervating the posterior pituitary, and $GABA_A$ and $GABA_B$ receptors are widely distributed in the hypothalamus. The activity of PHDA neurons is unaltered by pharmacological manipulations of $GABA_A$ receptors, but the $GABA_B$-receptor agonist baclofen reduces PHDA neuronal activity and increases circulating concentrations of α-MSH (Goudreau, Wagner, Lookingland, and Moore, *unpublished data*). Selective $GABA_B$ antagonists block these effects of baclofen but have no effect on PHDA neurons per se. This suggests that under basal conditions GABA neurons are quiescent so that $GABA_A$ and $GABA_B$ receptors are unoccupied and therefore unresponsive to the administration of GABA receptor antagonists. GABA neurons, however, are involved in the stress-induced inhibition of PHDA neurons (see below).

Stress

While stressful manipulations activate mesolimbic and mesocortical DA neurons, they inhibit PHDA neurons and consequently increase secretion of α-MSH from the intermediate lobe of the pituitary (37). Results of pharmacological studies suggest that neurons that transmit information by histamine, 5-HT, and GABA all play a role in the response of PHDA neurons to stress (see also Chapter 67, *this volume*).

Histaminergic neurons are activated during stress and are involved in the stress-induced inhibition of PHDA neurons; drugs that inhibit histamine synthesis or block H_1 receptors attenuate the reduction of PHDA neuronal activity during stress (Fleckenstein, Lookingland, and Moore, *unpublished data*). 5-HT neurons also appear to be involved with stress-induced inhibition of PHDA neurons because this response is blocked or attenuated in rats pretreated with 5,7-dihydroxytryptamine to destroy 5-HT neurons, with 8-hydroxy-2-(di-*n*-propylamino)-tetralin to inhibit 5-HT neuronal activity, and with 5-HT_2-receptor antagonists (17). Because these pretreatments do not alter basal activity of PHDA neurons, it would appear that during nonstressful conditions 5-HT neurons are quiescent, but become activated by stressful manipulations. Because activation of 5-HT$_2$ receptors depolarizes and excites postsynaptic membranes, it is unlikely that 5-HT neurons inhibit PHDA neurons directly, but during stress act indirectly by activating inhibitory interneurons. Current evidence supports a role for GABA inhibitory interneurons. Administration of 2-hydroxysaclofen, a GABA$_B$ antagonist, blocks the inhibition of PHDA neurons and the secretion of α-MSH resulting from both the administration of a 5-HT$_2$ agonist and restraint stress (Goudreau, Wagner, Lookingland, and Moore, *unpublished data*).

In summary, stressful manipulations activate a chain of neuronal events that are translated into a hormonal response, namely, the release of α-MSH from melanotrophs in the intermediate lobe of the pituitary. This response is the result of two concurrent events: (i) the release from the adrenal medulla of epinephrine, which, in turn, releases α-MSH by activating β_2 receptors on melanotrophs, and (ii) the removal of inhibitory tone on the melanotroph exerted by PHDA neurons. Stress-induced inhibition of these neurons appears to be mediated by histaminergic, 5-HTergic, and GABAergic neurons; the latter two may be arranged in series. Thus, it appears that PHDA neurons receive a convergence of inhibitory inputs which are important for removing the tonic inhibition of melanotroph secretion during stress.

INCERTOHYPOTHALAMIC DOPAMINERGIC NEURONS

Anatomy

IHDA (A$_{13}$) neurons are located in the most rostral portion of the MZI (6,7). Perikarya of these densely packed DA neurons have short dendrites oriented in the ventral plane which overlap ventromedially with dendrites of A$_{14}$ DA neurons in the adjacent periventricular nucleus (69). Although little is known about the efferent projections of A$_{13}$ DA neurons, early reports using glyoxylic acid histochemical fluorescence techniques suggested that these DA neurons project to the surrounding anterior, dorsomedial, and posterior regions of the hypothalamus (6,7). The results of more recent studies suggest that A$_{13}$ DA neurons project to a number of extrahypothalamic brain regions, including the horizontal limb of the diagonal band of Broca and central nucleus of the amygdala (Wagner, Eaton, Moore, and Lookingland, *unpublished data*).

Neurochemistry

There are two major problems using neurochemical techniques to estimate IHDA neuronal activity. The first of these relates to a lack of knowledge of the anatomical distribution of the A$_{13}$ DA neurons and to the possibility that IHDA neurons project to regions that are also innervated by mesolimbic DA neurons. Accordingly, changes in DA neurochemistry within these regions cannot be attributed exclusively to changes in IHDA neuronal activity. Because a "pure" IHDA projection region has yet to be identified, investigators have relied on neurochemical evaluation of changes in (a) the MZI, which contains soma, dendrites, and possibly terminals of IHDA neurons, and (b) the dorsomedial nucleus (DMN), which is reported to contain dendrites and some terminals of A$_{13}$ DA neurons.

A second problem associated with biochemical estimation of DA neuronal activity in the MZI and DMN is that these regions are densely innervated by NE neurons. Using the tedious α-methyltyrosine technique, DA and NE turnover rates have been quantified (51), but DA turnover rates are not useful for determining rapid and/or short-lasting changes in IHDA neuronal activity. Following NSD 1015 administration, DOPA accumulates in both DA and NE neurons within the MZI and DMN, so this technique is not useful for estimating IHDA neuronal activity unless NE innervation to these regions has been eliminated.

With some precautions, changes in concentrations of DOPAC and DA in the MZI and DMN can be used to estimate changes in IHDA neuronal activity (64). DA is a precursor of NE, and as such is present in low concentrations in NE neurons. When impulse flow in NE neurons increases, tyrosine hydroxylase is activated and the synthesis of DA within NE neurons increases. Because of limitations imposed by transport of DA into synaptic vesicles and/or the activity of dopamine-β-hydroxylase, which is located within these vesicles, the concentration of DA within NE neurons increases, and some of the amine is metabolized to DOPAC. Thus, a concurrent increase in both DOPAC and DA concentrations within a region without a significant change in the DOPAC/DA ratio is usually indicative of an increase in the activity of NE neurons in this region. If this is the case, the increase in DA and DOPAC will be accompanied by an increase in the concentrations of 3-methoxy-4-hydroxyphenylethylene glycol (MHPG), a major metabolite of NE. An increase in DOPAC without a change in DA concentrations (increase in DOPAC/DA ratio) usually signifies an increase in DA neuronal activity within a region. In order to substantiate this conclusion, it is advisable to determine that concentrations of MHPG do not change and to measure DOPAC/DA ratios in brains in which NE neurons have been destroyed by intracerebral injections of 6-hydroxydopamine (64).

Regulation of Neuronal Activity

IHDA neurons are regulated by DA receptor mediated mechanisms (51,64) and in this respect resemble neurons comprising the major ascending mesotelencephalic DA systems. DA-receptor agonists such as apomorphine decrease, whereas DA-receptor antagonists such as haloperidol increase the activity of IHDA neurons (51,64). In addition, local application of DA inhibits the firing rate of neurons in the MZI, possibly by activating autoreceptors on A_{13} DA perikarya or dendrites (10,57). These effects are likely mediated by D_3 (or possibly a subtype of D_2) DA receptors because IHDA neurons are responsive to the mixed D_2/D_3 antagonist raclopride, but not the selective D_2 antagonist remoxipride (11).

IHDA neurons are activated following acute administration of morphine by a mechanism involving mu opioid receptors (51,64). Activation of kappa opioid receptors has no effect on the activity of IHDA neurons (64). The stimulatory effects of mu opioid receptor activation on IHDA neurons are not dependent upon the presence of 5-HT neurons because neurotoxin-induced disruption of 5-HT innervation to the hypothalamus has no effect on the ability of morphine to stimulate the activity of IHDA neurons (64). In this respect, IHDA neurons resemble extrahypothalamic mesotelencephalic DA neurons rather than hypothalamic TIDA neurons.

Another difference between IHDA and TIDA neurons is that IHDA neurons are not responsive to experimentally induced changes in circulating levels of gonadal steroids or prolactin. There is no gender difference in the basal activity of IHDA neurons, and neither castration nor steroid hormone treatment alters the activity of IHDA neurons (22) or tyrosine hydroxylase gene expression in the MZI of either gender (52,59). Furthermore, IHDA neurons in the MZI are not responsive to chronic elevations in prolactin concentrations (1,51,59), suggesting that these neurons are not involved in the regulation of basal prolactin secretion and do not mediate the effects of hyperprolactinemia on reproductive function.

Although IHDA neurons are unresponsive to hormonal feedback regulation, they have been reported to stimulate the preovulatory surge of luteinizing hormone and ovulation (39,58). Direct injection of DA or its agonists into the MZI increases luteinizing hormone secretion and causes ovulation by a mechanism involving D_1 receptors (27,39). Conversely, lesions of the MZI block the proestrous surge of luteinizing hormone (58) and disrupt estrous cyclicity (39). The role of efferent projections of IHDA neurons to the horizontal diagonal band of Broca, a region containing gonadotropin-releasing hormone perikarya, in regulating preovulatory surges of luteinizing hormone remains to be elucidated.

PERIVENTRICULAR DOPAMINERGIC NEURONS

Anatomy

Perikarya of A_{14} DA neurons are distributed in the periventricular nucleus throughout the entire rostrocaudal extent of the third ventricle (69). Dendrites of these neurons are oriented in the dorsoventral plane and overlap extensively with dendrites from adjacent DA neurons. A_{14} DA perikarya are also distributed laterally along the ventral surface of the brain near the supraoptic and suprachiasmatic nuclei (69), and dorsally in the parvocellular region of the paraventricular nucleus (34). In the paraventricular nucleus, DA neurons receive axosomatic synapses from corticotropin-releasing hormone neurons, suggesting that these neurons may mediate stress-induced changes in pituitary hormone secretion (63). In the rostroventral region of the periventricular nucleus, the distribution of DA neurons is sexually dimorphic in that the number of tyrosine hydroxylase-immunoreactive cells and fibers is two- to threefold higher in females as compared with males (61). Although little information is available regarding the efferent projections of A_{14} DA neurons, fibers of these neurons in the rostral periventricular nucleus extend laterally into the adjacent medial preoptic nucleus and anterior hypothalamic area (7).

A number of neuropeptides including neurotensin (26), cholecystokinin, and vasoactive intestinal polypeptide (60) are colocalized with DA in periventricular DA neurons, but little information is available regarding the effects of these neurotransmitters on the activity or function of periventricular DA neurons.

Neurochemistry

Comments on neurochemical estimation of the activity of IHDA neurons (see above) are also pertinent for periventricular DA neurons.

Regulation of Neuronal Activity

Periventricular DA neurons are regulated by DA receptor mediated mechanisms and in this respect resemble IHDA neurons in the MZI (51). Acute administration of DA-receptor antagonists and agonists increase and decrease, respectively, the activity of DA neurons in the periventricular nucleus and adjacent medial preoptic nucleus and anterior hypothalamic area. Furthermore, inhibition of neuronal activity following administration of gamma-hydroxybutyrolactone results in an apomorphine-reversible increase in DA concentrations in these regions, suggesting that periventricular DA neurons are regulated, at least in part, by DA autoreceptors located on dendrites, perikarya, and/or axon terminals of these neurons (51).

DA neurons in the rostral periventricular nucleus and medial preoptic nucleus are activated following acute administration of morphine by a mechanism involving mu opioid receptors (51). No information is available regarding the effects of kappa or delta opioid receptor activation or blockade on the activity of these neurons.

In contrast to IHDA neurons, periventricular DA neurons in the rostral hypothalamus are responsive to experimentally induced changes in circulating levels of gonadal steroids and prolactin. There is a gender difference in the basal activity of DA neurons in the rostral periventricular, and medial preoptic nuclei, with the activity in females being 20–30% higher than that in males (22). This gender difference in the activity of DA neurons in the medial preoptic nucleus could be due, in part, to the inhibitory effects of testosterone in males (62) and/or the stimulatory effects of estrogen in females (51). Testosterone treatment of orchidectomized males has also been reported to have a stimulatory effect on the activity of DA neurons in the medial preoptic area (22). Experimental manipulations which produce elevations in circulating prolactin decrease the activity of DA neurons in the medial preoptic area of gonadally intact males (51), and they counteract the inhibitory effects of testosterone on these neurons in orchidectomized males (28).

Although the function of periventricular DA neurons is currently unknown, compelling evidence suggests that those neurons terminating in the medial preoptic area are important in regulating male sexual behavior. Indeed, neurotoxin-induced lesions of DA neurons in the medial preoptic nucleus (3) or direct injection of a DA antagonist into this region (54) decreases male copulatory behavior by a mechanism involving D_2 DA receptor regulation of reflexive and motivational factors, rather than locomotion (73). This is supported by the recent observation that DA neuronal activity is increased in the medial preoptic area in males during copulation (25). In females, DA neurons in the medial preoptic area have been implicated in the regulation of estrogen-induced sexual receptivity (74) and in the desensitization of the negative feedback effects of estrogen on luteinizing hormone secretion that occurs during puberty (9).

HYPOTHALAMIC DOPAMINERGIC NEURONS IN THE HUMAN

Information on hypothalamic DA neurons provided above has been obtained primarily from studies conducted in the rat. There have been relatively few studies on DA neurons in the human brain, and the majority of these, as in the rat, have focused on those DA neurons that comprise the nigrostriatal, mesolimbic, and mesocortical systems. Functional studies in humans have revealed that administration of drugs that disrupt DA synthesis or block D_2 DA receptors increases circulating concentrations of prolactin. This suggests that, as in the rat, the secretion of prolactin is tonically inhibited by DA released from neurons terminating near the primary capillary loops of the hypophysial portal system.

There is no evidence to support the existence in humans of a DA neuronal system comparable to PHDA neurons in the rat. A distinct intermediate lobe is present in human fetal and neonatal pituitaries, but the size of this lobe diminishes with age so that in the adult there is no well-defined intermediate lobe. Although melanotrophs are dispersed throughout the human anterior pituitary, it is not known if these cells are innervated by DA neurons or if they respond to the administration of DA agonists and antagonists. As noted above, little is known about the functions and precise anatomical projections of A_{13} and rostral A_{14} DA cell bodies in the rat, and there have been no studies on comparable neurons in the human brain.

SUMMARY AND CONCLUSIONS

A review of hypothalamic DA neurons published in the last volume of *Psychopharmacology: The Third Generation of Progress* (51) focused primarily on TIDA neurons that tonically inhibit the secretion of prolactin from the anterior pituitary. It was noted that many properties of these DA neurons are distinctly different from those of the major ascending nigrostriatal and mesolimbic DA neuronal systems. Although the importance of the hormonal regulation of TIDA neurons was emphasized, it was also recognized that these neurons respond acutely to sensory stimuli, but the chemical characteristics of afferent neurons that influence TIDA neurons was largely unknown at that time. Since 1987 the characteristic responses of TIDA neurons to putative neurotransmitters, and to compounds that mimic the actions of these transmitters, have been documented and reviewed here.

Over the past few years much has been learned about the hypothalamic DA neurons that innervate the intermediate lobe of the pituitary. These PHDA neurons, unlike TIDA neurons, are not responsive to changes in hormonal milieu, but are inhibited by stress and are activated or inhibited by a variety of compounds that interfere with or mimic the actions of aminergic or peptidergic neurotransmitters.

Studies on the mechanisms by which TIDA and PHDA neurons are regulated have been assisted greatly by knowledge of the anatomical distribution and functions of these neurons. This is not the case with two other hypothalamic DA neuronal systems, the IHDA and periventricular DA neurons. Studies of these neurons have been hampered by a lack of information of their anatomical projections and functions. The endocrinological consequences of psychoactive drugs that mimic, facilitate, or block DA neurotransmission of TIDA and PHDA neurons are well-recognized. The challenge now is to characterize further the anatomy and functions of the IHDA and periventricular DA neurons. Only then will it be possible to evaluate potential therapeutic or adverse effects of pharmacological manipulations that modify these two, as yet poorly understood, hypothalamic DA systems.

ACKNOWLEDGMENTS

The authors' studies cited in this review were supported by NIH grants NS 15911 and MH42802.

REFERENCES

1. Arbogast LA, Voogt JL. Hyperprolactinemia increases and hypoprolactinemia decreases tyrosine hydroxylase messenger ribonucleic acid levels in the arcuate nuclei, but not the substantia nigra or zona incerta. *Endocrinology* 1991;128:997–1005.
2. Ben-Jonathan N, Laudon M, Garris PA. Novel aspects of posterior pituitary function: regulation of prolactin secretion. *Front Neuroendocrinol* 1991;12:231–277.
3. Bitran D, Hull EM, Holmes GM, Lookingland KJ. Regulation of male copulatory behavior by preoptic incertohypothalamic dopamine neurons. *Brain Res Bull* 1988;20:323–331.
4. Berry SA, Gudelsky GA. D$_1$ receptors function to inhibit the activation of tuberoinfundibular dopamine neurons. *J Pharmacol Exp Ther* 1990;254:677–682.
5. Berry SA, Gudelsky GA. Effect of D$_2$ dopamine agonists on tuberoinfundibular dopamine neurons. *Neuropharmacology* 1991;30:961–965.
6. Björklund A, Lindvall O, Nobin A. Evidence of an incertohypothalamic dopamine neuronal system in the rat. *Brain Res* 1975;89:29–42.
7. Björklund A, Lindvall O. Dopamine-containing systems in the CNS. In: Björklund A, Hökfelt T, eds. *Handbook of chemical neuroanatomy. Classical transmitters in the CNS, part I.* Amsterdam: Elsevier, 1984;2:55–122.
8. Dåhlström A, Fuxe K. Evidence of the existence of monoamine containing neurons in the central nervous system. I. Demonstration of monoamines in cell bodies of brain stem neurons. *Acta Physiol Scand* 1964;62(Suppl 232):1–55.
9. Döcke F, Rohde W, Oelssner W, Schleussner E, Gutenschwager I, Dörner G. Influence of the medial preoptic dopaminergic activity on the efficiency of the negative estrogen feedback in prepubertal and cyclic female rats. *Neuroendocrinology* 1987;46:445–452.
10. Eaton MJ, Moss RL. Electrophysiology and pharmacology of neurons of the medial zona incerta: an in vitro slice study. *Brain Res* 1989;502:117–126.
11. Eaton MJ, Tian Y, Lookingland KJ, Moore KE. Remoxipride and raclopride differentially alter the activity of incertohypothalamic dopaminergic neurons. *Neuropharmacology* 1992;31:1121–1126.
12. Eaton MJ, Gopalan C, Kim E, Lookingland KJ, Moore KE. Comparison of the effects of the D$_2$ agonist quinelorane on tuberoinfundibular dopaminergic neuronal activity in male and female rats. *Brain Res* 1993;629:53–58.
13. Everitt BJ, Meister B, Hökfelt T, et al. The hypothalamic arcuate nucleus-median eminence complex: immunohistochemistry of transmitters, peptides and DARPP-32 with special reference to coexistence in dopamine neurons. *Brain Res Rev* 1986;11:97–155.
14. Fleckenstein AE, Lookingland KJ, Moore KE. Differential effects on the activity of hypothalamic dopaminergic neurons in the rat. *J Pharmacol Exp Ther* 1994;268:270–276.
15. Gopalan C, Tian Y, Moore KE, Lookingland KJ. Neurochemical evidence that the inhibitory effect of galanin on tuberoinfundibular dopamine neurons is activity dependent. *Neuroendocrinology* 1993;58:287–293.
16. Goudreau JL, Lindley SE, Lookingland KJ, Moore KE. Evidence that hypothalamic periventricular dopamine neurons innervate the intermediate lobe of the rat pituitary. *Neuroendocrinology* 1992;56:100–105.
17. Goudreau JL, Manzanares J, Lookingland KJ, Moore KE. 5HT$_2$ receptors mediate the effects of stress on the activity of periventricular–hypophysial dopaminergic neurons and the secretion of α-melanocyte-stimulating hormone. *J Pharmacol Exp Ther* 1993;265:303–307.
18. Goudreau JL, Lookingland KJ, Moore KE. 5-Hydroxytryptamine$_2$ receptor-mediated regulation of periventricular-hypophysial dopaminergic neuronal activity and the secretion of α-melanocyte-stimulating hormone. *J Pharmacol Exp Ther* 1994;268:270–276.
19. Gudelsky GA, Berry SA, Meltzer HY. Neurotensin activates tuberoinfundibular dopamine neurons and increases serum corticosterone concentrations in the rat. *Neuroendocrinology* 1989;49:604–609.
20. Gudelsky GA, Meltzer HY. Activation of tuberoinfundibular dopamine neurons following the acute administration of atypical antipsychotics. *Neuropsychopharmacology* 1989;2:45–51.
21. Gunnet JW, Lookingland KJ, Moore KE. Effects of gonadal steroids on tuberoinfundibular and tuberohypophysial dopaminergic neuronal activity in male and female rats. *Proc Soc Exp Biol Med* 1986;183:48–53.
22. Gunnet JW, Lookingland KJ, Moore KE. Comparison of the effects of castration and steroid replacement on incertohypothalamic dopaminergic neurons in male and female rats. *Neuroendocrinology* 1986;44:269–275.
23. Gunnet JW, Lookingland KJ, Lindley SE, Moore KE. Effects of electrical stimulation of the arcuate nucleus on neurochemical estimates of tuberoinfundibular and tuberohypophysial dopaminergic neuronal activities. *Brain Res* 1987;424:371–378.
24. Hökfelt T, Everitt B, Theodorsson-Norheim E, Goldstein M. Occurrence of neurotensin-like immunoreactivity in subpopulations of hypothalamic, mesoencephalic and medullary catecholamines. *J Comp Neurol* 1984;222:543–559.
25. Hull EM, Eaton RC, Moses J, Lorrain D. Copulation increases dopamine activity in the medial preoptic area. *Life Sci* 1993;52:935–940.
26. Ibata Y, Kawakami F, Fukui K, et al. Morphological survey of neurotensin-like immunoreactive neurons in the hypothalamus. *Peptides* 1984;5:109–120.
27. James MD, MacKenzie FJ, Tuohy-Jones PA, Wilson CA. Dopaminergic neurones in the zona incerta exert a stimulatory control on gonadotropin release via D$_1$ dopamine receptors. *Neuroendocrinology* 1987;43:348–355.
28. Kalra PS, Simpkins JW, Kalra SP. Hyperprolactinemia counteracts the testosterone-induced inhibition of the preoptic area dopamine turnover. *Neuroendocrinology* 1981;33:118–122.
29. Kawano H, Daikoku S. Functional topography of the rat hypothalamic dopamine neuron systems: retrograde tracing and immunohistochemical study. *J Comp Neurol* 1987;265:242–253.
30. Lin JY, Li CS, Pan JT. Effects of various neuroactive substances on single-unit activities of hypothalamic arcuate neurons in brain slices. *Brain Res Bull* 1993;31:587–594.
31. Lindley SE, Gunnet JW, Lookingland KJ, Moore KE. Effects of alterations in the activity of tuberohypophysial dopaminergic neurons on the secretion of α-melanocyte stimulating hormone. *Proc Soc Exp Biol Med* 1988;188:282–286.
32. Lindley SE, Gunnet JW, Lookingland KJ, Moore KE. 3,4-Dihydroxyphenylacetic acid concentrations in the intermediate lobe and neural lobe of the posterior pituitary gland as an index of tuberohypophysial dopaminergic neuronal activity. *Brain Res* 1990;506:133–138.
33. Lindley SE, Lookingland KJ, Moore KE. Activation of tuberoinfundibular but not tuberohypophysial dopaminergic neurons following intracerebroventricular administration of alpha-melanocyte-stimulating hormone. *Neuroendocrinology* 1990;51:394–399.
34. Liposits Zs, Phelix C, Paull WK. Electron microscopic analysis of tyrosine hydroxylase, dopamine-β-hydroxylase and phenylethanolamine-N-methyl-transferase immunoreactive innervation of the hypothalamic paraventricular nucleus in the rat. *Histochemistry* 1986;84:105–120.
35. Lookingland KJ, Gunnet JW, Moore KE. Electrical stimulation of the arcuate nucleus increases the metabolism of dopamine in terminals of tuberoinfundibular neurons in the median eminence. *Brain Res* 1987;436:161–164.
36. Lookingland KJ, Gunnet JW, Toney TW, Moore KE. Comparison of the effects of ether and restraint stress on the activity of tuberoinfundibular dopaminergic neurons in female and male rats. *Neuroendocrinology* 1990;52:99–105.
37. Lookingland KJ, Gunnet JW, Moore KE. Stress-induced secretions of alpha-melanocyte stimulating hormone is accompanied by a decrease in the activity of tuberohypophysial dopaminergic neurons. *Neuroendocrinology* 1991;53:91–96.
38. Loose MD, Ronnekleiv OK, Kelly MJ. Membrane properties and responses to opioids of identified dopamine neurons in the guinea-pig hypothalamus. *J Neurosci* 1990;10:3627–3634.
39. MacKenzie FJ, Hunter AJ, Daly C, Wilson CA. Evidence that the dopaminergic incerto-hypothalamic tract has a stimulatory effect on ovulation and gonadotropin release. *Neuroendocrinology* 1984;39:289–295.
40. Manzanares J, Lookingland KJ, Moore KE. Kappa opioid receptor-mediated regulation of α-melanocyte-stimulating hormone secretion and tuberohypophysial dopaminergic neuronal activity. *Neuroendocrinology* 1990;52:200–205.
41. Manzanares J, Lookingland KJ, LaVigne SD, Moore KE. Activation

of tuberohypophysial dopamine neurons following intracerebroventricular administration of the selective kappa opioid receptor antagonist nor-binaltorphimine. *Life Sci* 1991;48:1143–1149.

42. Manzanares J, Lookingland KJ, Moore KE. Kappa opioid receptor-mediated regulation of dopaminergic neurons in the rat brain. *J Pharmacol Exp Ther* 1991;256:500–505.

43. Manzanares J, Toney TW, Lookingland KJ, Moore KE. Activation of tuberoinfundibular and tuberohypophysial dopamine neurons following intracerebroventricular administration of bombesin. *Brain Res* 1991;565:142–147.

44. Manzanares J, Wagner EJ, LaVigne SD, Lookingland KJ, Moore KE. Sexual differences in kappa opioid receptor-mediated regulation of tuberoinfundibular dopaminergic neurons. *Neuroendocrinology* 1992;55:301–307.

45. Manzanares J, Wagner EJ, Lookingland KJ, Moore KE. Effects of immunoneutralization of dynorphin$_{1-17}$ and dynorphin$_{1-8}$ on the activity of central dopaminergic neurons in the male rat. *Brain Res* 1992;587:301–305.

46. Manzanares J, Durham RA, Lookingland KJ, Moore KE. δ-Opioid receptor-mediated regulation of central dopaminergic neurons in the rat. *Eur J Pharmacol* 1993;249:107–112.

47. Meister B, Hökfelt T. Peptide- and transmitter-containing neurons in the mediobasal hypothalamus and their relation to GABAergic systems: possible roles in control of prolactin and growth hormone secretion. *Synapse* 1988;2:585–605.

48. Meister B, Hökfelt T, Steinbusch HWM, et al. Do tyrosine hydroxylase-immunoreactive neurons in the ventrolateral arcuate nucleus produce dopamine or only L-DOPA? *J Chem Neuroanat* 1988;1:59–64.

49. Meister B, Elde R. Dopamine transporter mRNA in neurons of the rat hypothalamus. *Neuroendocrinology* 1993;58:388–395.

50. Merchenthaler I. Induction of enkephalin in tuberoinfundibular dopaminergic neurons during lactation. *Endocrinology* 1993;133:2645–2651.

51. Moore KE. Hypothalamic dopaminergic neuronal systems. In: Meltzer HY, ed. *Psychopharmacology: the third generation of progress.* New York: Raven Press, 1987;127–139.

52. Morrell JI, Rosenthal MF, McCabe JT, Harrington CA, Chikaraishi DM, Pfaff DW. Tyrosine hydroxylase mRNA in the neurons of the tuberoinfundibular region and zona incerta examined after gonadal steroid hormone treatment. *Mol Endocrinol* 1989;3:1426–1433.

53. Pan J-T, Tian Y, Lookingland KJ, Moore KE. Neurotensin-induced activation of hypothalamic dopaminergic neurons is accompanied by a decrease in pituitary secretion of prolactin and α-melanocyte-stimulating hormone. *Life Sci* 1992;50:2011–2017.

54. Pehek EA, Warner RK, Bazzett TJ, Bitran D, Band LC, Eaton RC, Hull EM. Microinjection of *cis*-flupenthixol, a dopamine antagonist, into the medial preoptic area impairs sexual behavior of male rats. *Brain Res* 1988;443:70–76.

55. Reymond MJ, Arita J, Dudley CA, Moss RL, Porter JC. Dopaminergic neurons in the mediobasal hypothalamus of old rats: evidence for a decreased affinity of tyrosine hydroxylase for substrate and cofactor. *Brain Res* 1984;304:215–223.

56. Saland LC, Wallace JA, Samora A, Gutierrez L. Co-localization of tyrosine hydroxylase (TH)- and serotonin (5-HT)-immunoreactive innervation in the rat pituitary gland. *Neurosci Letts* 1988;94:39–45.

57. Sanghera MK. Electrophysiological and pharmacological properties of putative A$_{13}$ incertohypothalamic dopamine neurons in the rat. *Brain Res* 1989;483:361–366.

58. Sanghera MK, Anselmo-France J, McCann SM. Effect of medial

59. Selmanoff MK, Shu C, Hartman RD, Barraclough CA, Petersen SL. Tyrosine hydroxylase and POMC mRNA in the arcuate region are increased by castration and hyperprolactinemia. *Mol Brain Res* 1991;10:277–281.

60. Seroogy K, Tsuruo Y, Hökfelt T, et al. Further analysis of presence of peptides in dopamine neurons: cholecystokinin, peptide histidine-isoleucine/vasoactive intestinal polypeptide and substance P in rat supramammillary region and mesencephalon. *Exp Brain Res* 1988;72:523–534.

61. Simerly RB, Swanson LW, Gorski RA. The distribution of monoaminergic cells and fibers in a periventricular preoptic nucleus involved in the control of gonadotropin release: immunohistochemical evidence for a dopaminergic sexual dimorphism. *Brain Res* 1985;330:55–64.

62. Simpkins JW, Kalra PS, Kalra SP. Inhibitory effects of androgens on preoptic area dopaminergic neurons in castrate rats. *Neuroendocrinology* 1980;31:177–181.

63. Thind KK, Goldsmith PC. Corticotropin-releasing factor neurons innervate dopamine neurons in the periventricular hypothalamus of juvenile macaques: synaptic evidence for a possible companion neurotransmitter. *Neuroendocrinology* 1989;50:351–358.

64. Tian Y, Lookingland KJ, Moore KE. Contribution of noradrenergic neurons to 3,4-dihydroxyphenylacetic acid concentrations in regions of the rat brain containing incertohypothalamic dopaminergic neurons. *Brain Res* 1991;555:135–140.

65. Tian Y, Eaton MJ, Manzanares J, Lookingland KJ, Moore KE. Characterization of opioid receptor-mediated regulation of incertohypothalamic dopamine neurons: lack of evidence for a role of 5-hydroxytryptaminergic neurons in mediating the stimulatory effects of morphine. *Brain Res* 1992;591:116–121.

66. Toney TW, Lookingland KJ, Moore KE. Role of testosterone in the regulation of tuberoinfundibular dopaminergic neurons in the male rat. *Neuroendocrinology* 1991;54:23–29.

67. Toney TW, Manzanares J, Moore KE, Lookingland KJ. Sexual differences in the stimulatory effects of bombesin on tuberoinfundibular dopaminergic neurons. *Brain Res* 1992;598:279–285.

68. Toney TW, Pawsat DE, Fleckenstein AE, Lookingland KJ, Moore KE. Evidence that prolactin mediates the stimulatory effects of estrogen on tuberoinfundibular dopamine neurons in female rats. *Neuroendocrinology* 1992;55:282–289.

69. van den Pol AN, Herbst RS, Powell JF. Tyrosine hydroxylase-immunoreactive neurons of the hypothalamus: a light and electron microscopic study. *Neuroscience* 1984;13:1117–1156.

70. Vuillez P, Carbajo Perez S, Stoeckel ME. Colocalization of GABA and tyrosine hydroxylase immunoreactivities in the axons innervating the neurointermediate lobe of the rat pituitary: an ultrastructural immunogold study. *Neurosci Lett* 1987;79:53–58.

71. Wagner EJ, Moore KE, Lookingland KJ. Sexual differences in N-methyl-D-aspartate receptor-mediated regulation of tuberoinfundibular dopaminergic neurons in the rat. *Brain Res* 1993;611:139–146.

72. Wagner EJ, Moore KE, Lookingland KJ. Non-NMDA receptor-mediated regulation of hypothalamic dopaminergic neurons in the rat. *Eur J Pharmacol* 1994;254:105–112.

73. Warner RK, Thompson JT, Markowski VP, et al. Microinjection of the dopamine antagonist *cis*-flupenthixol into the MPOA impairs copulation, penile reflexes and sexual motivation in male rats. *Brain Res* 1991;540:177–182.

74. Wilson CA, Thody AJ, Hole DR, Grierson JP, Celis ME. Interaction of estradiol, alpha-melanocyte-stimulating hormone, and dopamine in the regulation of sexual receptivity in the female rat. *Neuroendocrinology* 1991;54:14–22.

Psychopharmacology: The Fourth Generation of Progress, edited by Floyd E. Bloom and David J. Kupfer. Raven Press, Ltd., New York © 1995.

CHAPTER 23

Electron Microscopy of Central Dopamine Systems

Virginia M. Pickel and Susan R. Sesack

Availability of antisera and development of improved labeling methods have permitted considerable recent advancement in our knowledge of the ultrastructure and synaptic circuitry of dopamine neurons. These advances are crucial for understanding the cellular basis for electrophysiological properties of dopamine neurons and their functional interactions with other transmitter systems (see also Chapters 15, 20, 21, 22, and 25, *this volume*). We review the methodological advances and their contribution to the known ultrastructural features of the nigrostriatal and mesocorticolimbic dopamine neurons. These two major dopamine systems are then compared to dopamine neurons in other brain regions including the diencephalon, olfactory bulb, retina, and brainstem. In the final portion of this review, we briefly discuss the structural correlates of altered function in plasticity and neurodegenerative disorders, focusing in particular on the nigrostriatal dopamine neurons. The descriptions are based exclusively on the most recent literature. For earlier studies, see Pickel and Milner in the previous volume of *Psychopharmacology* and also see reference lists referred to in other specified publications.

METHODOLOGICAL ADVANCES

The advances in methodology that have been the most influential in improving current understanding of the ultrastructure of dopamine neurons include: (i) the production and characterization of highly specific antibodies against dopamine and its receptors and (ii) the use of these antibodies in combination with tract-tracing methods or

V. M. Pickel: Department of Neurology and Neuroscience, Cornell University Medical College, New York, New York 10021.
S. R. Sesack: Department of Behavioral Neuroscience, University of Pittsburgh, Pittsburgh, Pennsylvania 15260.

immunocytochemical labeling of other antigens. These technologies have permitted significant advances in determining the cellular substrates for transmitter synthesis and release, interaction of dopamine with specific receptor subtypes, and synaptic as well as nonsynaptic associations between dopamine neurons and neurons containing other identifiable transmitters.

Dopamine-Specific Antibodies

The production of antibodies against glutaraldehyde conjugates of monoamines has been an important recent advance for morphological studies of central dopamine neurons. [See review by Steinbusch and Tilders (70)]. The specificity of dopamine antibodies was established partly on the basis of light microscopic immunocytochemical distribution. This labeling was abundantly distributed in dopamine-enriched brain regions such as the substantia nigra and caudate-putamen nuclei. These same regions also contain tyrosine hydroxylase (TH), an enzyme necessary for the first step in catecholamine biosynthesis, but are largely devoid of dopamine beta-hydroxylase (DBH), the enzyme converting dopamine to noradrenaline. These findings support the utility of anti-TH antibodies as markers for dopamine neurons in brain regions such as the substantia nigra and ventral tegmental area containing no other known catecholamine perikarya. Antibodies raised against TH have been used extensively in studies of dopamine neurons, because this enzyme is mainly soluble and highly abundant in these cells. TH also is usually more easily detected in dopamine versus noradrenaline terminals (46). However, except in regions such as the caudate-putamen nuclei where the levels of catecholamines other than dopamine are low, TH is not an exclusive marker for dopamine terminals. Thus, antibodies against dopamine have proven most useful in ultrastructural studies of regions containing dopamine axons or perikarya extensively intermixed with other catecholamines (40,57). However, because dopamine antibodies were produced against glutaraldehyde conjugates, relatively high concentrations of glutaraldehyde are required for electron microscopic immunocytochemistry, limiting the numbers of compatible antisera available for dual labeling studies.

Dual Labeling

Recent ultrastructural studies of dopamine neurons have relied on refinements in dual labeling electron microscopic immunocytochemical or combined immunocyto-

chemical and tract-tracing methods. [For detailed methods and references see Leranth and Pickel (38), Pickel and Chan (50), and Smith and Bolam (66).] The electron-dense secondary markers primarily include: autoradiographic silver grains, gold particles with or without silver intensification, and osmium-darkened peroxidase reaction product. These methods provide a means to examine whether observed pharmacological and physiological associations attributed to selective interactions of dopamine and other transmitter systems involve (i) direct or multisynaptic connections, (ii) presynaptic modulation, (iii) coexistence of transmitters, or (iv) convergence of afferents on common targets. Additionally, the symmetry or asymmetry of synaptic junctions provides information relative to potential sites for inhibition or excitation of the dopa-

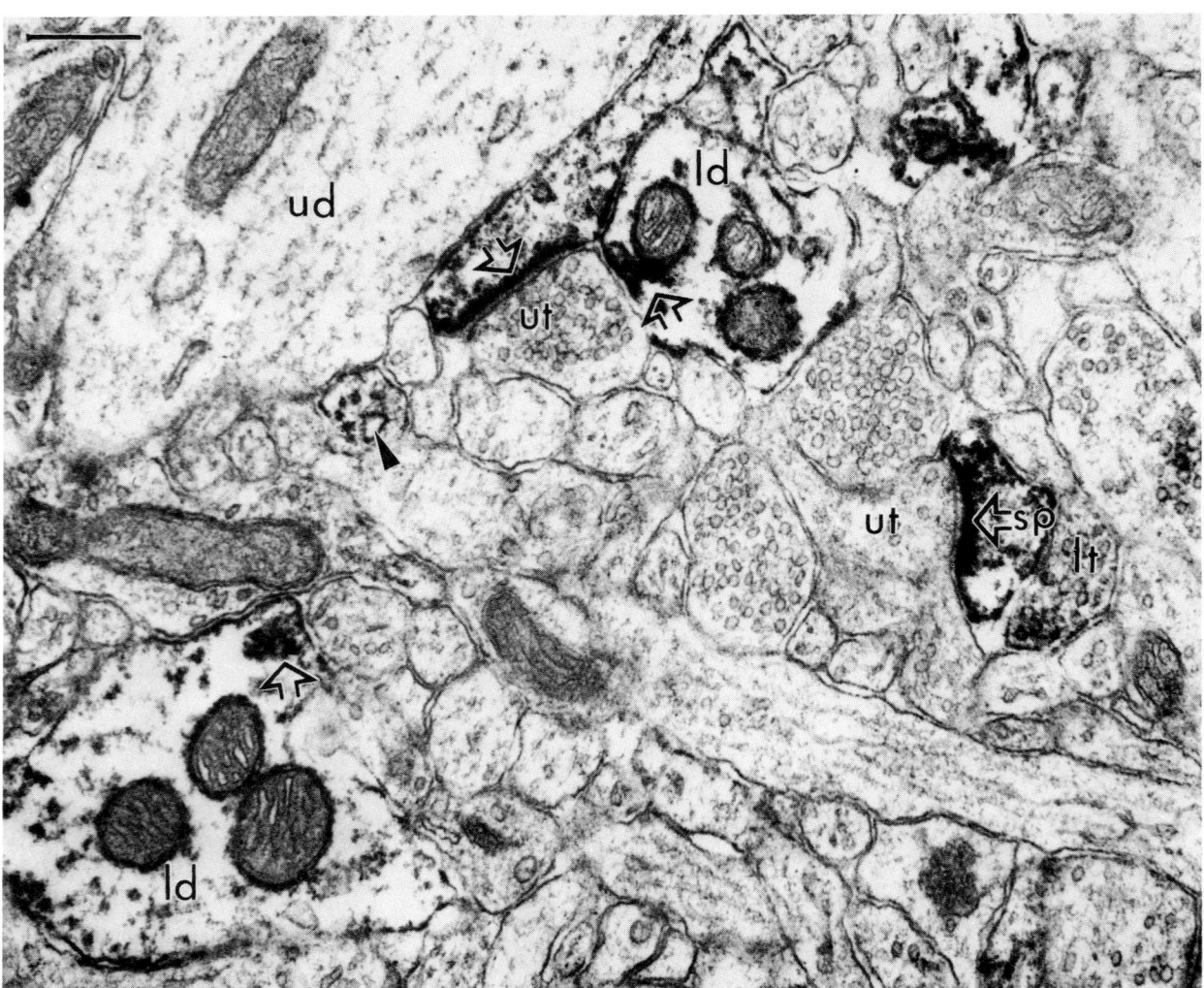

FIG. 1. Immunoperoxidase labeling for site-directed antiserum against a cytoplasmic peptide sequence found within the D_2 receptor protein. Dense peroxidase reaction product is seen in aggregates (*open arrows*) in labeled dendrites (ld) and spines (sp). The labeled spines are postsynaptic to unlabeled terminals (ut) containing marked differences in their content of synaptic vesicles. A densely labeled saccule (*arrowhead*) of smooth endoplasmic reticulum is seen in a small unmyelinated axon. Peroxidase reaction product also is detectable in a small, vesicle-filled axon terminal (lt) that is apposed to the immunoreactive spine in the right portion of the micrograph. An unlabeled dendrite (ud) is seen in the neuropil along with numerous other unlabeled terminals. Bar represents 0.2 μm.

mine neurons. This is based on biochemical analysis of postsynaptic proteins and morphological evidence that inhibitory amino acids are found in terminals that form symmetric junctions, whereas excitatory amino acids are found in terminals forming asymmetric junctions (13,36). Location of terminals on soma and proximal dendrites as opposed to distal dendrites also provides information relative to the synaptic potency of afferents to the dopamine neurons (78).

Dopamine Receptor Localization

An understanding of the sites and mechanisms whereby dopamine elicits modulatory effects on target cells can perhaps best be appreciated through morphological studies of the cellular and subcellular localization of dopamine receptor subtypes (for a review of dopamine receptors see Chapters 14, 19, and 26, *this volume*). Autoradiography of binding sites has been useful for light microscopic examination of receptor distributions, but requires extensive quantification for cellular and subcellular localization (45). Recent cloning of dopamine receptor subtypes has permitted the production of site-directed antibodies for use in light and electron microscopic localization of the putative receptors (5,61,85). Most extensive morphological analyses thus far have examined the localization of peptides within the D_1 and D_2 dopamine receptors. D_1 dopamine receptor antibodies were regionally localized to dopamine-enriched portions of the basal ganglia (27). Electron microscopic studies further showed that D_1-receptor-like immunoreactivity was found in dendrites and dendritic spines, as well as axon terminals in the caudate-putamen nuclei (85). D_2-receptor-like immunoreactivity also was seen in both spiny dendrites and axons in this region (Fig. 1). (See ref. 61 for detailed description and review of the literature.) By combining immunogold silver labeling of TH with immunoperoxidase labeling of a peptide fragment from the D_2 receptor, we have shown colocalization of the enzyme and receptor in the same axon terminals in the caudate-putamen nuclei (61). However, the majority of the terminals containing D_2-receptor-like immunoreactivity did not contain detectable immunolabeling for TH. These results provide the first ultrastructural evidence that a D_2-receptor-like protein is strategically positioned to subserve autoreceptor functions in axon terminals and also may act presynaptically of other afferents in the caudate nuclei. The demonstration of D_2-receptor-like immunoreactivity in TH-labeled dendrites in the midbrain tegmentum further supports a favorable location for autoreceptor function (61).

DOPAMINE SOMATA AND DENDRITES

Substantia Nigra and Ventral Tegmental Area

Dopamine somata and dendrites in the substantia nigra and ventral tegmental area are relatively large (10–20

μm) and multipolar. In both regions, spines are occasionally seen on the soma as well as on dendrites. Other distinguishing features of these neurons include: content of organelles, dendritic appositions, and synaptic input. [For a more detailed description and pertinent references see Bayer and Pickel (7) and Pickel et al. (52).]

Subcellular Organelles

Midbrain dopamine neurons contain Golgi lamellae, large dense-core vesicles, rough and smooth endoplasmic reticulum, lysosomes, and other usual organelles (48). The elaborate perinuclear array of Golgi lamellae are responsible (i) for the ordered processing and sorting of biosynthetic products from the rough endoplasmic reticulum and (ii) for packaging this product into secretory-type large dense-core vesicles (42). Consistent with this function, dopamine neurons in the substantia nigra have large (100–150 nm) dense-core vesicles occasionally located in close proximity to the lateral saccules of the Golgi lamellae (Fig. 2A). Following intraventricular injections of colchicine, there is a pronounced increase in these large dense-core vesicles in many of the dopamine neurons within the ventral tegmental area. This microtubule toxin reduces interneuronal transport of secretory material from the endoplasmic reticulum to the Golgi apparatus and also reduces vesicular transport in axons (1). The large dense-core vesicles within dopamine neurons in the ventral tegmental area contain neurotensin (9) and/or cholecystokinin (30). These vesicles are often located along nonsynaptic portions of the plasmalemma of both perikarya and dendrites. This suggests sites for exocytotic release of the peptides to activate receptive sites identified on midbrain dopamine neurons. The large dense-core vesicles seen in conventionally stained electron micrographs are clearly distinct from smaller vesicles containing dense central cores only following treatment with permanganate or loading with 5-hydroxydopamine. (See ref. 9 and Pickel and Milner in the previous edition of *Psychopharmacology.*)

Saccules of rough endoplasmic reticulum and clusters of polyribosome are distributed in the cytoplasm between the Golgi lamellae and the plasmalemma. In this portion of the cytoplasm of dopamine neurons in the substantia nigra, immunogold silver labeling shows an enrichment of TH immunoreactivity (Fig. 2A). In contrast to the rough endoplasmic reticulum, smooth-surfaced endoplasmic reticulum is seen near the nuclear envelope and Golgi lamellae and immediately beneath the plasma membrane. The smooth endoplasmic reticulum near the surface of the neuron sometimes is arranged in lamellar folds called *subsurface cisternae*. [See additional references in Bayer and Pickel (7).] Less organized individual saccules of smooth endoplasmic reticulum also are seen near the plasmalemma. We have postulated that transport within the smooth reticulum to or from the cell surface may account

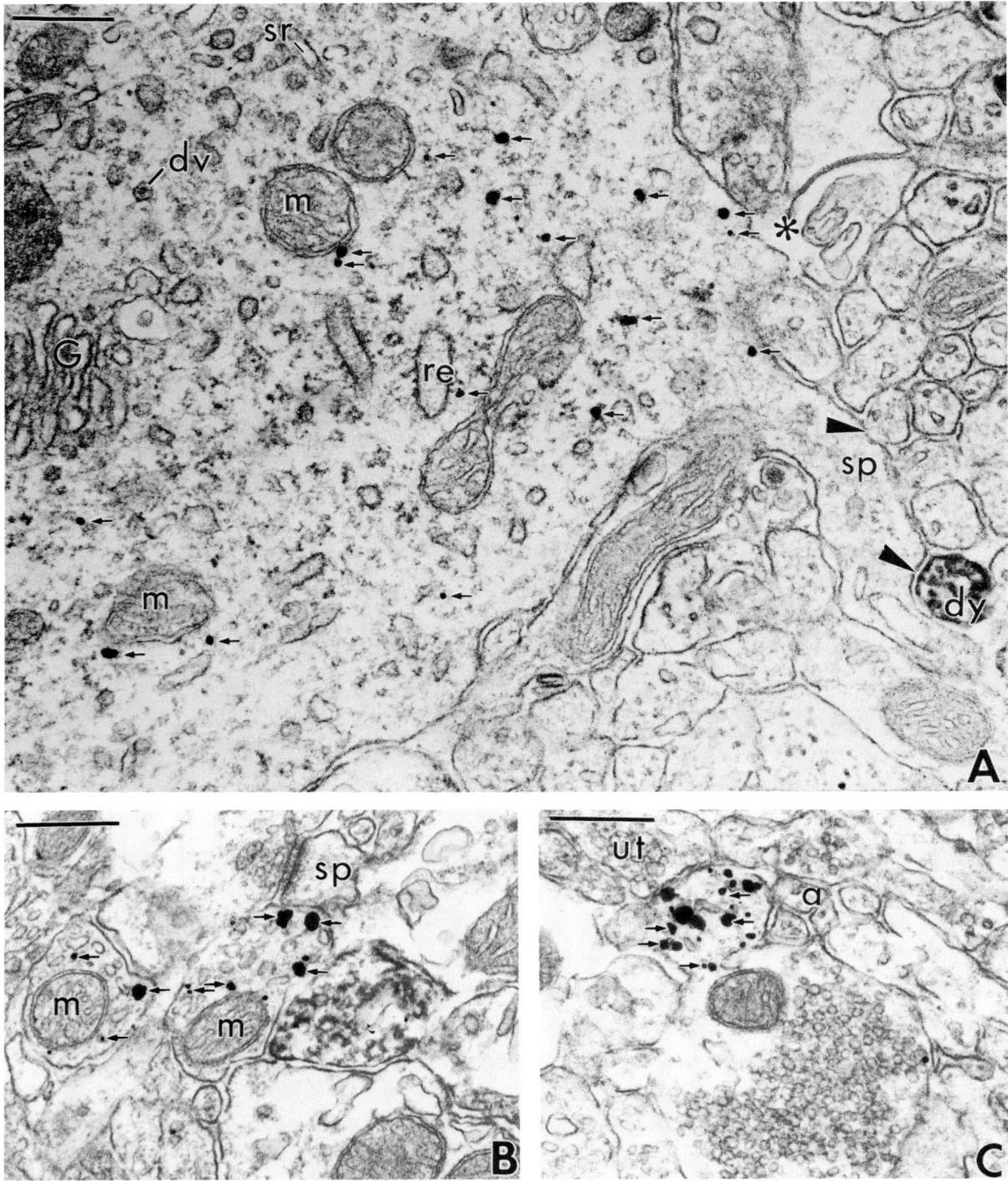

FIG. 2. Ultrastructural immunogold silver localization of tyrosine hydroxylase. **A:** Perikaryon in the substantia nigra shows gold–silver labeling (*small arrows*) in portions of the cytoplasm between the Golgi lamellae (G) and the plasmalemma. The labeled cytoplasmic region contains abundant rough endoplasmic reticulum (re) and numerous mitochondria (m). A dense-core vesicle (dv) and saccules of smooth endoplasmic reticulum (sr) are seen near the upper left of the micrograph near the nucleus (out of field to left of micrograph). A somatic spine (sp) emerges from the labeled cell and is apposed (*arrowheads*) to unlabeled and dynorphin (dy)-immunoperoxidase labeled axons. The perikaryon is directly contacted by glial processes (*asterisk*). **B** and **C:** TH-immunolabeled terminals in the caudate-putamen nuclei contain numerous gold–silver particles (*small arrows*). In **B,** one heavily labeled TH terminal is apposed to an unlabeled dendritic spine (sp) and an electron-dense terminal showing peroxidase immunolabeling for enkephalin. Both gold–silver TH-labeled terminals contain mitochondria (m). In **C,** the immunogold TH-labeled terminal is apposed to an unlabeled axon (a) and to an unlabeled terminal (ut). Bar represents 0.2 μm.

for the frequent detection of D_2-receptor-like immunoreactivity in association with this organelle (61). However, other functions, including the binding of intracellular calcium, also have been proposed for the smooth endoplasmic reticulum (72).

Multivesicular bodies and lysosomes both contain acid phosphatase, but have differential ultrastructural features in midbrain dopamine neurons. The multivesicular bodies range from 0.3 to 0.6 μm in diameter and contain numerous electron-lucent vesicles surrounded by a unit membrane (48). These organelles are major sites for endocytosis and membrane recycling. [See Castel et al. (14) for other related references.] Lysosomes contain an abundance of other degradative enzymes packaged in the Golgi apparatus. These enzymes contribute to their content of finely dense granular material as seen by electron microscopy (48). A variety of structures having ultrastructural features similar, but not identical, to either the conventional multivesicular body or lysosome can be seen in dopamine soma. These probably represent intermediate organelles formed by the fusion of lysosomes with multivesicular bodies and the ongoing process of membrane degradation (48).

Dendritic Appositions

Dendrites of dopamine neurons in the ventral tegmental area and substantia nigra are often closely apposed to each other and to other dendrites lacking TH immunoreactivity. The apposed dendrites show equally spaced plasma membranes. Occasionally, the dopamine dendrites contain a few small (30–40 nm) or large (80–100 nm) vesicles. In conventionally stained materials the smaller vesicles are usually lucent whereas larger vesicles have a dense central core. The location of vesicles in apposed dendrites supports the concept that dopamine or neuropeptides may be released from the dendrites in the midbrain. Moreover, our recent localization of D_2-receptor-like immunoreactivity in TH-labeled and unlabeled midbrain dendrites may reflect receptive sites for dopamine released from dendrites, because relatively few TH-immunoreactive terminals were identified (61). [See Le Boulch et al. (37) for more references on dendritic release of dopamine.]

Electronic coupling offers another viable option for functional interactions between apposed dopamine dendrites (see also Chapters 15, 20, 21, 22, and 25, *this volume*). This type of interaction is thought to occur through gap junctions, the known cellular substrates for electrical coupling. Such junctions have not been identified between apposed dopamine and nondopamine neurons in the midbrain by electron microscopy using conventional staining methods. However, subsurface cisternae found near dendritic appositions exhibit immunoreactivity against gap junction proteins (80). Moreover, as mentioned above, the subsurface cisternae may be stores for calcium, a known modulator of gap junction perme-

ability. Finally, the localization of D_2-receptor-like immunoreactivity along apposed plasmalemmas of dendrites in the substantia nigra and ventral tegmental area is consistent with autoreceptor regulation of electrical coupling [see also Chapter 15, *this volume,* and discussion by Sesack et al. (61).]

Afferent Input

Afferents to dopamine neurons in midbrain derive extensively from the striatum, caudate-putamen nuclei, and nucleus accumbens (20). In addition, neocortical afferents [presumably utilizing glutamate as a transmitter (64)] and cholinergic terminals (12) also form direct synapses with midbrain dopamine neurons. In contrast to the more motor connections of dopamine neurons in the substantia nigra, the dopamine neurons in the ventral tegmental area receive more prominent input from limbic regions, including the nucleus accumbens, prefrontal cortex, and amygdaloid nuclei. (See refs. 12 and 64 for additional references.) However, in both substantia nigra and ventral tegmental area, dopamine neurons receive synaptic input from terminals containing gamma-aminobutyric acid (GABA), substance P, and opioid peptides.

GABA terminals provide one of the more prominent inputs to dopamine neurons in the substantia nigra and ventral tegmental area. [For a detailed description and citation of earlier literature see Bayer and Pickel (8) and Bolam and Smith (13).] The GABA afferents originate mainly from perikarya in the striatum, but also from neurons in the globus pallidus (65) and most likely from local GABAergic neurons (43). The GABA terminals usually synapse on soma and large proximal dendrites, thus exerting a potentially powerful modulation of the dopamine target neurons. Moreover, the density of cytoplasmic TH immunoreactivity in individual cells and dendrites directly corresponds to the relative abundance of their GABA innervation. For example, lightly TH-immunoreactive dendrites receive proportionally greater numbers of GABA-labeled terminals (8). This suggests that the greater inhibitory input from GABA, or alternatively the proportionally less excitatory input, may regulate the synthesis of dopamine by modulation of the levels of the rate-limiting TH enzyme in these neurons.

Substance P terminals with and without detectable GABA immunoreactivity form synapses with dopamine neurons in the substantia nigra and are derived from the striatum (13). The substance-P-immunoreactive terminals also form synapses with GABA neurons within the substantia nigra (43) and with dopamine dendrites in the ventral tegmental area (73). The substance P immunoreactivity within axon terminals is prominently associated with large dense-core vesicles. Most of the substance-P-labeled terminals in the midbrain form symmetric synapses. This is consistent with their colocalization of GABA or inhibitory actions on the target neurons.

However, substance P terminals also form asymmetric, excitatory-type contacts with dendrites of dopamine as well as nondopamine neurons in the substantia nigra and ventral tegmental area. These junctions could reflect the known excitatory actions of substance P or possibly co-release of other excitatory transmitters.

Opioid peptides, enkephalin, dynorphin, and their respective receptor subtypes are differentially distributed in the ventral tegmental area and substantia nigra. [See German et al. (21) and Speciale et al. (68) for additional references.] The enkephalin and dynorphin terminals form primarily symmetric synapses with TH-immunoreactive dendrites, but they also form asymmetric ones (39,63). These terminals usually contain one or more large dense-core vesicles intensely labeled for the opioid peptides and also contain more abundant small clear vesicles that are less notably immunoreactive in their central lumen. However, many terminals also lacked detectable large dense-core vesicles within the sections that were examined (52). The heterogeneous morphological features may suggest co-storage of opiate peptides with GABA or other transmitters as seen for substance P. The opioid containing large dense-core vesicles in terminals forming synapses with dopamine dendrites were often located along non-synaptic portions of the plasmalemma. This is consistent with nonsynaptic release to activate not only the dopamine target, but also neighboring axons and glia. (See ref. 52 for further discussion and references.)

Astrocytic Associations

Exclusive of sites of synaptic contact or dendritic appositions, the plasma membranes of dopamine neurons in the substantia nigra and ventral tegmental area are closely ensheathed in astrocytic processes (Fig. 2A) (7,52). These have irregular contours and contain microfilaments as well as a few vesicles having electron-dense granular matrix thought to be associated with iron storage (41,48). The extension or retraction of the glial processes between pairs of dendrites or between dendrites and their afferent terminals is thought to play a major role in neuroglia plasticity in several brain regions. [See review by Raisman (56).] Further studies are needed to determine whether such mechanisms are also relevant to modulation of dopamine neurons.

Comparative Morphology in Other Regions

Diencephalon

Dopamine neurons of the hypothalamus have been examined by both light and electron microscopy. [For description and citations of earlier studies see Van den Pol et al. (77).] Many of these cells are located in the arcuate nucleus and send axons to the median eminence. These soma are smaller (averaging 10 μm in cross-sectional diameter) and more ovoid than the dopamine neurons in the mesencephalon. Hypothalamic dopamine neurons also usually have a thinner rim of cytoplasm, but contain most of the same organelles as described above for midbrain dopamine neurons.

Appositions are seen between dopamine dendrites and other soma as well as dendrites in the hypothalamus. In the arcuate nucleus, the TH-labeled soma are in apposition only to other TH-labeled dendrites, whereas the TH-labeled dendrites directly appose both TH-labeled and unlabeled dendrites. Dendritic appositions usually do not show aggregates of vesicles. The morphological features suggest that hypothalamic dopamine neurons may interact through nonvesicular signals, and possibly through electronic coupling as described above for midbrain dopamine neurons.

Coexistence of dopamine with other transmitters occurs within hypothalamic neurons in the arcuate nucleus of the hypothalamus. Some of these cells colocalize GABA, whereas others colocalize acetylcholine. [See Tinner et al. (75) for additional references.] The hypothalamic dopamine neurons are similar to those in the ventral tegmental area in that they also (i) contain neurotensin (33) and (ii) receive afferent input from terminals containing GABA and/or neuropeptides. They specifically receive input from terminals containing corticotropin-releasing factor (CRF) (74). The CRF-containing terminals form primarily asymmetric synapses with dopamine dendrites, thus suggesting a substrate for activation of the dopamine neurons in response to stress. (See ref. 74 and their references.) Except for points of contact with the afferent terminals, the hypothalamic dopamine neurons are ensheathed by glial processes containing abundant dense iron-storing granules (83).

Olfactory Bulb and Retina

Other groups of dopamine neurons that have been characterized ultrastructurally include those in the periglomerular portion of the olfactory bulb, some of which also colocalize GABA. [See Gall et al. (18) for colocalization and references.] These dopamine cells include the superficial tufted cells and small periglomerular neurons. The soma are small (about 10 μm in mean diameter) and have a thin rim of cytoplasm containing typical organelles. The periglomerular dopamine neurons have somatic spines and receive relatively few somatic or dendritic synapses. Dendrodendritic appositions are commonly seen between TH-labeled and unlabeled periglomerular neurons.

Dopamine cells in the retina (amacrine and/or interplexiform neurons) are distributed fairly evenly in the inner nuclear and inner plexiform layers. [See ref. 79 for review and references.] These cells are 10–15 μm in diameter and have a thin rim of cytoplasm, again with typical organelles (34). Plasmalemmal appositions without recognized synaptic densities are often seen between dopamine dendrites and other dopamine and nondopamine dendrites (81). The synaptic input to TH-immunoreactive dendrites in the retina are from unlabeled bipolar cells and from TH-labeled and unlabeled amacrine terminals many of which contain GABA (81).

Brainstem

Dopamine neurons have been detected immunocytochemically in the ventrolateral and dorsomedial medulla, including the area postrema, nucleus tractus solitarii (NTS), and dorsal motor nuclei of the vagus (40). Their ultrastructural features have not been described.

DOPAMINE TERMINALS

Caudate-Putamen Nuclei and Nucleus Accumbens

Ultrastructure

The ultrastructure and circuitry of dopamine terminals in the caudate-putamen nuclei and nucleus accumbens have been extensively examined. [See Gerfen (20) and Pickel and Milner in the previous edition of *Psychopharmacology*.] In both regions the findings are similar, possibly reflecting the fact that until recently most studies have focused on core regions of the nucleus accumbens (84). The core of the nucleus accumbens has considerable structural and functional homologies with the caudate-putamen nuclei [see Heimer et al. (23)].

In the caudate-putamen nuclei and core of the nucleus accumbens, dopamine terminals have a cross-sectional diameter of 0.15–1.00 μm and contain primarily small clear vesicles (Fig. 2B and 2C). The small vesicles are usually distributed throughout the terminal without notable aggregation at sites of contact with other neurons. Most dopamine (TH-immunoreactive) terminals contact the necks of dendritic spines. The apposed membranes of the dopamine terminal and dendritic spine are equally spaced and electron-dense when observed in optimal planes of sections. These features of symmetric synapses are less commonly seen when the dopamine terminals contact proximal dendrites or soma and are never seen in appositions between the dopamine terminal and other axon terminals.

In contrast with the core subregion, TH-immunoreactive terminals in the shell region of the nucleus accumbens have a smaller cross-sectional diameter and more frequently contact dendritic shafts. Their other morphological features are similar to those in the core of the nucleus accumbens. [See Zahm (84) and references on core and shell.]

Target Neurons

Dopamine terminals in the striatum form synapses with spiny neurons projecting to the substantia nigra, many of which contain GABA (4). Spiny GABAergic neurons in the ventral striatum (mainly core subregion of the nucleus accumbens) also are major targets of dopamine terminals. [See Pickel et al. (55) for dual labeling and earlier references.] Certain GABA-containing spiny striatal neurons colocalize enkephalin, a peptide also demonstrated immunocytochemically in targets of dopamine terminals in the caudate nuclei. (See ref. 51 and relevant citations of earlier studies.) In contrast to the GABA- and enkephalin-containing neurons, we were unable to demonstrate a direct synaptic input to cholinergic neurons in either the caudate nucleus or nucleus accumbens (49). However, others have used dual labeling methods to support a postsynaptic action of dopamine on cholinergic neurons in the caudate nucleus. [See discussion and references reviewed by Pickel and Chan (49) and by Chang (15).] Moreover, choline acetyltransferase and D_2-receptor mRNA are found in the same striatal neurons (6). This localization of the D_2-receptor does not, however, necessarily indicate a postsynaptic action of dopamine on the cholinergic neurons and is consistent with other presynaptic types of interactions (see below).

Dendritic and Axonal Appositions

As indicated above, dopamine terminals in contact with larger dendrites, soma, or other axons rarely show well-defined synaptic specializations. In most cases, these have not been extensively examined in serial sections; but if present, random samples would be expected to reveal the densities with frequencies similar to those on dendritic spines. Appositions without recognized densities have been most commonly reported between dopamine terminals and aspiny neurons containing GABA, acetylcholine, and neuropeptide Y. (See the results and references in refs. 2,49, and 55.) This might indicate that in these neurons dopamine acts through different receptor subtypes or second messengers. [See Landis (36) for cytoplasmic structure of synaptic junctions.]

Direct appositions also have been described between dopamine terminals and other axons in the caudate-putamen nuclei (49) and in the nucleus accumbens (62,64). These are characterized by closely apposed axonal membranes that are not separated by glial processes. Examples of appositions between dopamine terminals and other axons and terminals are shown in Fig. 2B and 2C. Dopamine terminals confined to the small space around the head of dendritic spines are likely to be in apposition to other converging afferents, especially those forming asymmetric synapses on the same spines (62,64). Such an arrangement may partially account for the frequent detection of appositions between TH-immunoreactive terminals and cortical afferents, both of which preferentially contact dendritic spines (64). Additionally, TH-immunoreactive terminals have been shown in direct apposition to terminals containing several other transmitters, including GABA (55), substance P (53), enkephalin (51), and acetylcholine (49). In most of these contacts, there was no obvious clustering of synaptic vesicles to suggest presynaptic release sites in either the dopamine or nondopamine terminal. More rarely, one of the pairs of axons was filled with vesicles and directly apposed a presynaptic small-diameter axon containing relatively few vesicles (51). Except in serial section analysis, this type of contact is only detectable in favorable planes of section revealing the small axon in continuity with its terminal varicosity. Thus, the frequency of such contacts are likely to be underestimated, and many small unmyelinated axons may be mistakenly identified as the necks of spines. Studies localizing a D_2-receptor-like protein to small axons support the contention that axonal appositions may reflect sites where dopamine acts to release other transmitters (61). However, appositions between TH-labeled and unlabeled axons also may reflect morphological substrates for presynaptic modulation of dopamine release by acetylcholine and a variety of other transmitters in the striatum. (See ref. 19 for discussion and references pertinent to presynaptic regulation of dopamine release.)

Convergence

Use of dual-labeling electron microscopic techniques has established the cellular substrates for physiological interactions involving convergence of dopamine and other afferents on striatal spiny neurons (Fig. 3). Convergence of dopamine terminals with extrinsic excitatory afferents has been shown using anterograde degeneration and immunocytochemistry. Prefrontal cortical terminals identified ultrastructurally with anterograde markers [lesion-induced degeneration or transport of *Phaseolus vulgaris* leucoagglutinin (PHA-L)] form synapses with spines receiving input from dopamine terminals in the nucleus accumbens. [See Sesack and Pickel (64) and their references to related studies in the caudate nuclei.] Convergence between dopamine terminals and hippocampal afferents also has been demonstrated using similar methods in the nucleus accumbens (62). The junctions of dopamine terminals and cortical or hippocampal afferents on spines may provide a cellular basis for modulation of the overall excitability of target neurons through changes in spine responses to excitatory afferents.

Convergence between dopamine terminals and collaterals of known inhibitory projection neurons also has been shown using dual labeling for TH combined with either GABA (55) or enkephalin (51). (See Schematic in Fig. 3.) However, the incidence of detected conversion was significantly greater for GABA than for enkephalin (55). This may indicate either more frequent conversion between dopamine and GABA terminals, or, more likely, a greater abundance of GABA terminals. The convergence of dopamine terminals with both GABA and enkephalin on cells having morphological characteristics of spiny

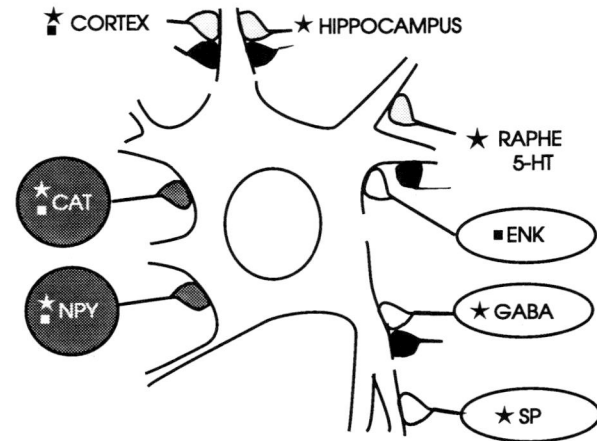

FIG. 3. Summary diagram showing convergence between dopamine terminals and terminals identified using either anterograde tracing from cortex and hippocampus or immunocytochemistry in caudate-putamen nuclei (*box*) and/or nucleus accumbens (*star*). Instances of most noted convergences are shown by contact of dopamine and nondopamine terminals on an uninterrupted segment of the neuronal surface (*continuous black lines*). These include: (i) extrinsic afferents from cortex (prefrontal or somatosensory) and hippocampus and (ii) terminals from GABA and enkephalin (ENK) containing spiny projection neurons. Terminals in contact with morphologically similar striatal neurons, but rarely showing detectable convergence with dopamine terminals in single sections, are illustrated on segments of the neuronal surface separated by a broken line. These include: (i) serotonin (5-HT) terminals presumably from the raphe nuclei, (ii) terminals of interneurons containing choline acetyl transferase (CAT) and neuropeptide Y (NPY), and (iii) terminals of spiny projection neurons containing substance P (SP).

neurons provides a substrate for their dual modulation of the outflow from the striatum.

In contrast with cortical afferents and GABA and enkephalin terminals, axons containing certain other immunocytochemically identified transmitters rarely, if ever, show morphological evidence of convergence with dopamine terminals. For example, striatal afferents from the raphe containing serotonin [5-hydroxytryptamine (5-HT)] infrequently contact the same target as TH-immunoreactive terminals in either subregion of the nucleus accumbens (76). These 5-HT terminals form primarily asymmetric synapses in the core subregion of the nucleus accumbens, but in the shell the terminals are larger, contain more numerous large dense-core vesicles, and preferentially form symmetric junctions with dendrites (76). The 5-HT terminals in the caudate nucleus are morphologically similar to those in the core of the nucleus accumbens (67). However, their relative incidence of convergence with dopamine terminals has not been examined in this region.

Terminals containing substance P, a known coexisting

peptide in serotonin terminals and the major tachykinin in collaterals of striatal projection neurons, also rarely show evidence of convergence with TH-immunoreactive terminals in the nucleus accumbens (53). Similarly, terminals derived from striatal interneurons containing choline acetyltransferase (49) or neuropeptide Y (3) rarely contact dendrites receiving afferent input from dopamine terminals as seen in single or small series of serial sections. However, these terminals do form synapses on spiny neurons morphologically similar to those receiving dopamine synapses. Thus failure to detect convergence may reflect preferential distributions of the dopamine terminals on more distal spinous dendrites and more proximal inputs from the other terminals. Alternatively, separate sets of spiny neurons may be selectively targeted by dopamine and certain extrinsic or intrinsic terminals in the striatum. Studies identifying the afferent inputs to single neurons identified though intracellular filling with biocytin or other dyes are needed to resolve this issue.

Comparative Morphology of Dopamine Terminals in Other Target Regions

Forebrain

In the central nucleus of the amygdala and the neocortex, dopamine afferent terminals form primarily symmetric junctions with dendrites. These terminals contain many small round vesicles and a few large dense-core vesicles. (See description and references in refs. 10 and 59.) In the central nucleus of the amygdala, a population of large dense-core vesicles has been shown to contain neurotensin and most likely originate from neurons in the ventral tegmental area (10). Targets of the TH- and/or neurotensin-immunoreactive terminals in the amygdala contain neurotensin as well as other transmitters.

In cortical regions, dopamine terminals form synapses with spines, dendritic shafts, and soma of pyramidal neurons (22,59). The synaptic incidence, proximal versus distal location of synapses, and symmetry or asymmetry of the synaptic specialization vary depending on the cortical region examined. Spines postsynaptic to dopamine terminals in cortex are usually also postsynaptic to unlabeled terminals forming asymmetric junctions (22,59). This arrangement is similar to that seen for dopamine terminals described above in the dorsal caudate-putamen nuclei and suggests common modulatory interactions involving dopamine and excitatory afferents to pyramidal neurons in the cerebral cortex.

In the lateral septum, dopamine afferents are round to ovoid, have a diameter of $0.2-1.0$ μm, and contain mostly small clear and, rarely, large dense-core vesicles. (See ref. 28 and their references.) These terminals form asymmetric as well as symmetric contacts on cholinergic neurons in the septal nuclei (44). A recent study demonstrated the dual origin of this septal dopamine innervation. One of

these originated from the periventricular and basolateral hypothalamus and colocalized somatostatin, whereas the second derived from the ventral tegmental area and coexpressed neurotensin (29). Multiple lines of evidence suggest that these inputs mediate opposing inhibitory and excitatory functional influences in the septum.

Diencephalon and Pituitary

Dopamine neurons in the rostral parvocellular arcuate nucleus and more dorsal periventricular regions of the hypothalamus send efferents to the median eminence and the neurointermediate lobe of the pituitary (58,71). Because D_2 receptors are also located in the anterior lobe of the pituitary, which is devoid of dopamine axons, dopamine is thought to be released nonsynaptically in the neurointermediate lobe and then diffuse to its receptive sites (71).

Projections of dopamine neurons between hypothalamic nuclei have also been described in ultrastructural studies. (See ref. 26 for detailed localization and reference listing.) More specifically, TH-containing afferents most likely derived from the anterior periventricular area of the hypothalamus form synapses on dendrites in the medial preoptic area. These dendrites contain immunoreactivity for either luteinizing-hormone-releasing hormone (LHRH) or glutamic acid decarboxylase, an enzymatic marker for GABA.

Olfactory Bulb and Retina

Terminals of periglomerular and certain other types of interneurons in the olfactory bulb are immunoreactive for TH and/or GABA. (See description and references in ref. 18.) These terminals form primarily symmetric junctions with dendrites. Additionally, these terminals are apposed to, and sometimes show synaptic specializations with, other nondopamine axon terminals.

In the retina, the dopamine amacrine cells are distinguished largely by their highly collateralized and varicose axons extending widely beyond the dendritic tree (16,34). The axon varicosities have similar size and content of vesicles as seen in the caudate-putamen nuclei. The dendritic junctions formed by these terminals are characterized by thin symmetric synaptic specializations (25). Anatomical and physiological studies support their role in movement of rods in the outer retina (17) and regulation of gap junctional permeability between amacrine cells (47).

Brainstem and Spinal Cord

Dopamine varicosities are seen by light microscopy in several brainstem regions, including the NTS, dorsal motor nuclei of the vagus, inferior olive, and the spinal trigeminal, hypoglossal, cuneate, gracile, and raphe nuclei (40). Pharmacological studies of dopamine D_1 receptors indicate that dopamine terminals in the NTS may provide direct synaptic input to tachykinin-containing neurons (69). Ultrastructural studies of dopamine terminals in the brainstem are lacking. However, in the spinal cord, dopamine terminals form mainly symmetric, axodendritic junctions in the ventral horn and intermediolateral cell column and are largely nonsynaptic in the cervical dorsal horn (57). This may reflect regional differences in function or differences in methods of analysis.

STRUCTURAL CORRELATES OF ALTERED FUNCTION

Plasticity

Compensatory changes to retain function are well documented for central dopamine neurons (35). Recently, we have characterized the ultrastructure of TH-labeled terminals in the caudate-putamen nuclei of adult animals that received intranigral injections of the dopamine neurotoxin 6-hydroxydopamine (6-OHDA) while neonates (54). As expected, there were significantly fewer TH-labeled terminals in the caudate-putamen nucleus ipsilateral to the lesions. However, we also observed that the remaining terminals were significantly larger than those in the contralateral unlesioned hemisphere or in either hemisphere of unlesioned animals. Larger terminals associated with a concomitant increase in the number of synaptic vesicles and mitochondria are potentially capable of greater dopamine release. (See ref. 54 for discussion and references on dopamine release.)

Neurodegeneration

A comprehensive coverage of neurodegenerative ultrastructure of dopamine neurons is beyond the scope of this chapter. However, recent studies showing a critical role for iron and iron chelators in the neurodegeneration of dopamine neurons (60) are of particular interest relative to this review. Postmortem human studies have shown evidence for ongoing toxic processes involving lipid peroxidation, altered iron metabolism, and impaired mitochondrial function thought to increase cell death in neurodegenerative disorders such as Parkinson's disease (31). Iron serves as a catalyst of free radical formation (11,32) and is elevated in the substantia nigra in Parkinson's disease (24). Moreover, disturbances of metal-containing glia, particularly in the olfactory bulb, have been postulated as a potential cause underlying memory dysfunctions in Alzheimer's disease (82). As reviewed above, many dopamine neurons are closely contacted by astrocytic processes containing deposits of iron. Further ultrastructural and molecular analysis of these astrocytes in relation to dopamine neurons may be important for understanding the mechanisms of several major neurodegenerative disorders.

CONCLUSIONS

Ultrastructural studies of central dopamine neurons provide interesting parallels in all systems thus far examined. Many, if not all, dopamine neurons (i) are extensively synaptically linked with GABA neurons, (ii) show potential sites for nonsynaptic transmitter release and/or electrical coupling between dendrites, (iii) have elaborate terminal arborizations extending beyond the confines of soma and dendrites, and (iv) have terminals that form thin symmetric junctions or lack recognized membrane specializations. These features provide numerous structural substrates for dopamine's role in diverse physiological functions in normal brains and possibly form the basis for abnormalities in neurodegenerative disorders involving dopamine systems.

ACKNOWLEDGMENT

We wish to thank Dr. Teresa A. Milner for comments on the manuscript, and we also thank June Chan for her input on the immunogold labeling. This work was supported by grants from NIMH (MH40342, MH48776, and MH00078) and from NIDA (DA04600).

REFERENCES

1. Alonso G. Effects of colchicine on the intraneuronal transport of secretory material prior to the axon: a morphofunctional study in hypothalamic neurosecretory neurons of the rat. *Brain Res* 1988;453:191–203.
2. Aoki C, Pickel VM. Neuropeptide Y-containing neurons in the rat striatum: ultrastructure and cellular relations with tyrosine hydroxylase containing terminals and astrocytes. *Brain Res* 1988;459:205–225.
3. Aoki C, Pickel VM. Neuropeptide Y in cortex and striatum. Ultrastructural distribution and coexistence with classical neurotransmitters and neuropeptides. *Ann NY Acad Sci* 1990;611:186–205.
4. Arai R, Kojima Y, Geffard M, Kitahama K, Maeda T. Combined use of silver staining of the retrograde tracer WGAapoHRP-Au and pre-embedding immunocytochemistry for electron microscopy: demonstration of dopaminergic terminals in synaptic contact with striatal neurons projecting to the substantia nigra in the rat. *J Histochem Cytochem* 1992;40:889–892.
5. Ariano MA, Fisher RS, Smyk-Randall W, Sibley DR, Levine MS. D2 dopamine receptor distribution in the rodent CNS using antipeptide antisera. *Brain Res* 1993;609:71–80.
6. Aubry J-M, Schulz M-F, Pagliusi S, Schulz P, Kiss JZ. Coexpression of dopamine D_2 and substance P (neurokinin-1) receptor messenger RNAs by a subpopulation of cholinergic neurons in the rat striatum. *Neuroscience* 1993;53:417–424.
7. Bayer VE, Pickel VM. Ultrastructural localization of tyrosine hydroxylase in the rat ventral tegmental area: relationship between immunolabeling density and neuronal associations. *J Neurosci* 1990;10:2996–3013.
8. Bayer VE, Pickel VM. GABA-labeled terminals form proportionally more synapses with dopaminergic neurons containing low densities of tyrosine hydroxylase-immunoreactivity in rat ventral tegmental area. *Brain Res* 1991;559:44–55.
9. Bayer VE, Towle AC, Pickel VM. Ultrastructural localization of

neurotensin-like immunoreactivity within dense core vesicles in perikarya, but not terminals, colocalizing tyrosine hydroxylase in the rat ventral tegmental area. *J Comp Neurol* 1991;311:179–196.

10. Bayer VE, Towle AC, Pickel VM. Vesicular and cytoplasmic localization of neurotensin-like immunoreactivity (NTLI) in neurons postsynaptic to terminals containing NTLI and/or tyrosine hydroxylase in the rat central nucleus of the amygdala. *J Neurosci Res* 1991;30:398–413.

11. Ben-Shachar D, Eshel G, Riederer P, Youdim MBH. Role of iron and iron chelation in dopaminergic-induced neurodegeneration: implication for Parkinson's disease. *Ann Neurol* 1992;32(Suppl): S105–S110.

12. Bolam JP, Francis CM, Henderson Z. Cholinergic input to dopaminergic neurons in the substantia nigra: a double immunocytochemical study. *Neuroscience* 1991;41:483–494.

13. Bolam JP, Smith Y. The GABA and substance P input to dopaminergic neurones in the substantia nigra of the rat. *Brain Res* 1990;529:57–78.

14. Castel M-N, Woulfe J, Wang X, Laduron PM, Beaudet A. Light and electron microscopic localization of retrogradely transported neurotensin in rat nigrostriatal dopaminergic neurons. *Neuroscience* 1992;50:269–282.

15. Chang HT. Dopamine–acetylcholine interaction in the rat striatum: a dual-labeling immunocytochemical study. *Brain Res Bull* 1988;21:295–304.

16. Dacey DM. The dopaminergic amacrine cell. *J Comp Neurol* 1990;301:461–489.

17. Gabriel R, Zhu BS, Straznicky C. Tyrosine hydroxylase-immunoreactive elements in the distal retina of *Bufo marinus*: a light and electron microscopic study. *Brain Res* 1991;559:225–232.

18. Gall CM, Hendry SH, Seroogy KB, Jones EG, Haycock JW. Evidence for coexistence of GABA and dopamine in neurons of the rat olfactory bulb. *J Comp Neurol* 1987;266:307–318.

19. Gauchy C, Desban M, Krebs MO, Glowinski J, Kemel ML. Role of dynorphin-containing neurons in the presynaptic inhibitory control of the acetylcholine-evoked release of dopamine in the striosomes and the matrix of the cat caudate nucleus. *Neuroscience* 1991;41:449–458.

20. Gerfen CR. Synaptic organization of the striatum. *J Electron Microsc Tech* 1988;10:265–281.

21. German DC, Speciale SG, Manaye KF, Sadeq M. Opioid receptors in midbrain dopaminergic regions of the rat. I. Mu receptor autoradiography. *J Neural Transm* 1993;91:39–52.

22. Goldman Rakic PS, Leranth C, Williams SM, Mons N, Geffard M. Dopamine synaptic complex with pyramidal neurons in primate cerebral cortex. *Proc Natl Acad Sci USA* 1989;86:9015–9019.

23. Heimer L, Zahm DS, Churchill L, Kalivas PW, Wohltmann C. Specificity in the projection patterns of accumbal core and shell in the rat. *Neuroscience* 1991;41:89–125.

24. Hirsch EC. Why are nigral catecholaminergic neurons more vulnerable than other cells in Parkinson's disease. *Ann Neurol* 1992;32(Suppl):S88–S93.

25. Hokoc JN, Mariani AP. Tyrosine hydroxylase immunoreactivity in the rhesus monkey retina reveals synapses from bipolar cells to dopaminergic amacrine cells. *J Neurosci* 1987;7:2785–2793.

26. Horvath TL, Naftolin F, Leranth C. Luteinizing hormone-releasing hormone and gamma-aminobutyric acid neurons in the medial preoptic area are synaptic targets of dopamine axons originating in anterior periventricular areas. *J Neuroendocrinol* 1993;5:71–79.

27. Huang Q, Zhou D, Chase K, Gusella JF, Aronin N, DiFiglia M. Immunohistochemical localization of the D_1 dopamine receptor in rat brain reveals its axonal transport, pre- and postsynaptic localization, and prevalence in the basal ganglia, limbic system, and thalamic reticular nucleus. *Proc Natl Acad Sci USA* 1992;89:11988–11992.

28. Jakab RL, Leranth C. Catecholaminergic, GABAergic, and hippocamposeptal innervation of GABAergic "somatospiny" neurons in the rat lateral septal area. *J Comp Neurol* 1990;302:305–321.

29. Jakab RL, Leranth C. Presence of somatostatin or neurotensin in lateral septal dopaminergic axon terminals of distinct hypothalamic and midbrain origins: convergence on the somatospiny neurons. *Exp Brain Res* 1993;92:420–430.

30. Jayaraman A, Nishimori T, Dobner P, Uhl GR. Cholecystokinin and neurotensin mRNAs are differentially expressed in subnuclei of the ventral tegmental area. *J Comp Neurol* 1990;296:291–302.

31. Jenner P. Oxidative stress as a cause of Parkinson's disease. *Acta Neurol Scand* [*Suppl*] 1991;136:6–15.

32. Jenner P. Parkinson's disease: pathological mechanisms and actions of piribedil. *J Neurol* 1992;239(Suppl 1):S2–S8.

33. Kasckow J, Nemeroff CB. The neurobiology of neurotensin: focus on neurotensin-dopamine interactions. *Regul Pept* 1991;36:153–164.

34. Kolb H, Cuenca N, Wang HH, Dekorver L. The synaptic organization of the dopaminergic amacrine cell in the cat retina. *J Neurocytol* 1990;19:343–366.

35. Kuchel GA, Zigmond RE. Functional recovery and collateral neuronal sprouting examined in young and aged rats following a partial neural lesion. *Brain Res* 1991;540:195–203.

36. Landis DM. Membrane and cytoplasmic structure at synaptic junctions in the mammalian central nervous system. *J Electron Microsc Tech* 1988;10:129–151.

37. Le Boulch NL, Truong-Ngoc NA, Gauchy C. Role of dendritic dopamine of the substantia nigra in the modulation of nigrocollicular gamma-aminobutyric acid release: *in vivo* studies in the rat. *J Neurochem* 1991;57:1080–1083.

38. Leranth C, Pickel VM. Electron microscopic pre-embedding double immunostaining methods. In: Heimer L, Zaborszky L, eds. *Neuroanatomical Tract Tracing Methods 2*, New York: Plenum Press, 1989:129–172.

39. Liang C-L, Kozlowski GP, German DC. Leucine⁵-enkephalin afferents to midbrain dopaminergic neurons: light and electron microscopic examination. *J Comp Neurol* 1993;332:269–281.

40. Maqbool A, Batten TFC, Berry PA, McWilliam PN. Distribution of dopamine-containing neurons and fibers in the feline medulla oblongata: a comparative study using catecholamine-synthesizing enzyme and dopamine immunohistochemistry. *Neuroscience* 1993; 53:717–733.

41. McLaren J, Brawer JR, Schipper HM. Iron content correlates with peroxidase activity in cysteamine-induced astroglial organelles. *J Histochem Cytochem* 1992;40:1887–1897.

42. Meller ST, Dennis BJ. A multiple Golgi analysis of the periaqueductal gray in the rabbit. *J Comp Neurol* 1990;302:66–86.

43. Mendez I, Elisevich K, Flumerfelt B. Substance P synaptic interactions with GABAergic and dopaminergic neurons in rat substantia nigra: an ultrastructural double-labeling immunocytochemical study. *Brain Res Bull* 1992;28:557–563.

44. Milner TA. Cholinergic neurons in the rat septal complex: ultrastructural characterization and synaptic relations with catecholaminergic terminals. *J Comp Neurol* 1991;314:37–54.

45. Morelli M, Mennini T, Di Chiara G. Nigral dopamine autoreceptors are exclusively of the D_2 type: quantitative autoradiography of [¹²⁵I]iodosulpride and [¹²⁵I]SCH 23982 in adjacent brain sections. *Neuroscience* 1988;27:865–870.

46. Noack HJ, Lewis DA. Antibodies directed against tyrosine hydroxylase differentially recognize noradrenergic axons in monkey neocortex. *Brain Res* 1989;500:313–324.

47. Pereda A, Triller A, Korn H, Faber DS. Dopamine enhances both electronic coupling and chemical excitatory postsynaptic potentials at mixed synapses. *Proc Natl Acad Sci USA* 1992;89:12088–12092.

48. Peters A, Palay SL, Webster HdeF. *The fine structure of the nervous system*, 3rd ed. New York: Oxford University Press, 1991;1–494.

49. Pickel VM, Chan J. Spiny neurons lacking choline acetyltransferase immunoreactivity are major targets of cholinergic and catecholaminergic terminals in rat striatum. *J Neurosci Res* 1990;25:263–280.

50. Pickel VM, Chan J. Electron microscopic immunocytochemical labelling of endogenous and/or transported antigens in rat brain using silver-intensified one-nanometer colloidal gold. In: Cuello AC, ed. *Immunohistochemistry II.* New York: John Wiley & Sons, 1993;265–280.

51. Pickel VM, Chan J, Sesack SR. Cellular basis for interactions between catecholaminergic afferents and neurons containing Leu-enkephalin-like immunoreactivity in rat caudate-putamen nuclei. *J Neurosci Res* 1992;31:212–230.

52. Pickel VM, Chan J, Sesack SR. Cellular substrates for interactions between dynorphin terminals and dopamine dendrites in rat ventral tegmental area and substantia nigra. *Brain Res* 1993;602:275–289.

53. Pickel VM, Joh TH, Chan J. Substance P in the rat nucleus accumbens: ultrastructural localization in axon terminals and their relation to dopaminergic afferents. *Brain Res* 1988;444:247–264.

54. Pickel VM, Johnson E, Carson M, Chan J. Ultrastructure of spared

dopamine terminals in caudate-putamen nuclei of adult rats neonatally treated with intranigral 6-hydroxydopamine. *Dev Brain Res* 1992;70:75–86.

55. Pickel VM, Towle AC, Joh TH, Chan J. Gamma-aminobutric acid in the medial rat nucleus accumbens: ultrastructural localization in neurons receiving monosynaptic input from catecholaminergic afferents. *J Comp Neurol* 1988;272:1–14.

56. Raisman G. Glia, neurons, and plasticity. *Ann NY Acad Sci* 1991;633:209–213.

57. Ridet J-L, Sandillon F, Rajaofetra N, Geffard M, Privat A. Spinal dopaminergic system of the rat: light and electron microscopic study using an antiserum against dopamine, with particular emphasis on synaptic incidence. *Brain Res* 1992;598:233–241.

58. Schimchowitsch S, Vuillez P, Tappaz ML, Klein MJ, Stoeckel ME. Systematic presence of GABA-immunoreactivity in the tubero-infundibular and tubero-hypophyseal dopaminergic axonal systems: an ultrastructural immunogold study on several mammals. *Exp Brain Res* 1991;83:575–586.

59. Seguela P, Watkins KC, Descarries L. Ultrastructural features of dopamine axon terminals in the anteromedial and the suprahinal cortex of adult rat. *Brain Res* 1988;442:11–22.

60. Sengstock GJ, Olanow CW, Menzies RA, Dunn AJ, Arendash GW. Infusion of iron into the rat substantia nigra: nigral pathology and dose-dependent loss of striatal dopaminergic markers. *J Neurosci Res* 1993;35:67–82.

61. Sesack SR, Aoki C, Pickel VM. Ultrastructural localization of D2 receptor-like immunoreactivity in midbrain dopamine neurons and their striatal targets. *J Neurosci* 1994;14(1):88–106.

62. Sesack SR, Pickel VM. In the rat medial nucleus accumbens, hippocampal and catecholaminergic terminals converge on spiny neurons and are in apposition to each other. *Brain Res* 1990;527:266–279.

63. Sesack SR, Pickel VM. Dual ultrastructural localization of enkephalin and tyrosine hydroxylase immunoreactivity in the rat ventral tegmental area: multiple substrates for opiate–dopamine interactions. *J Neurosci* 1992;12:1335–1350.

64. Sesack SR, Pickel VM. Prefrontal cortical efferents in the rat synapse on unlabeled neuronal targets of catecholamine terminals in the nucleus accumbens septi and on dopamine neurons in the ventral tegmental area. *J Comp Neurol* 1992;320:145–160.

65. Smith Y, Bolam JP. The output neurones and the dopaminergic neurones of the substantia nigra receive a GABA-containing input from the globus pallidus in the rat. *J Comp Neurol* 1990;296:47–64.

66. Smith Y, Bolam JP. Combined approaches to experimental neuroanatomy: combined tracing and immunocytochemical techniques for the study of neuronal microcircuits. In: Bolam JP, ed. *Experimental neuroanatomy, a practical approach.* Oxford: IRL Press, 1992;239–266.

67. Soghomonian JJ, Descarries L, Watkins KC. Serotonin innervation in adult rat neostriatum. II. Ultrastructural features: a radioautographic and immunocytochemical study. *Brain Res* 1989;481:67–86.

68. Speciale SG, Manaye KF, Sadeq M, German DC. Opioid receptors in midbrain dopaminergic regions of the rat. II. Kappa and delta receptor autoradiography. *J Neural Transm* 1993;91:53–66.

69. Srinivasan M, Yamamoto Y, Brodin E, Persson H. Chronic treatment with SCH-23390, a selective dopamine D₁ receptor blocker decreases preprotachykinin-A mRNA levels in nucleus tractus soli-

tarii of the rabbit: role in respiratory control. *Mol Brain Res* 1991;9:233–238.

70. Steinbusch HWM, Tilders FJH. Immunohistochemical techniques for light microscopical localization of dopamine, noradrenaline, adrenaline, serotonin and histamine in the central nervous system. In: Steinbusch HWM, ed. *Monoaminergic neurons: light microscopy and ultrastructure.* New York: John Wiley & Sons, 1993:125–166.

71. Stoof JC. Localization and pharmacology of some dopamine receptor complexes in the striatum and the pituitary gland: synaptic and non-synaptic communication. *Acta Morphol Neerl Scand* 1988;26:115–130.

72. Takei K, Stukenbrok H, Metcalf A, Mignery GA, Südhof TC, Volpe P, De Camilli P. Ca²⁺ stores in Purkinje neurons: endoplasmic reticulum subcompartments demonstrated by the heterogeneous distribution of the InsP₃ receptor, Ca²⁺-ATPase, and calsequestrin. *J Neurosci* 1992;12:489–505.

73. Tamiya R, Hanada M, Kawai Y, Inagaki S, Takagi H. Substance P afferents have synaptic contacts with dopaminergic neurons in the ventral tegmental area of the rat. *Neurosci Lett* 1990;110:11–15.

74. Thind KK, Goldsmith PC. Corticotropin-releasing factor neurons innervate dopamine neurons in the periventricular hypothalamus of juvenile macaques. Synaptic evidence for a possible companion neurotransmitter. *Neuroendocrinology* 1989;50:351–358.

75. Tinner B, Fuxe K, Kohler C, Hersh L, Andersson K, Jansson A, Goldstein M, Agnati LF. Evidence for the existence of a population of arcuate neurons costoring choline acetyltransferase and tyrosine hydroxylase immunoreactivities in the male rat. *Neurosci Lett* 1989;99:44–49.

76. Van Bockstaele EJ, Pickel VM. Ultrastructure of serotonin-immunoreactive terminals in the core and shell of the rat nucleus accumbens: cellular substrates for interactions with catecholamine afferents. *J Comp Neurol* 1993;334:603–617.

77. Van den Pol AN, Herbst RS, Powell JF. Tyrosine hydroxylase-immunoreactive neurons of the hypothalamus: a light and electron microscopic study. *Neuroscience* 1993;13:1117–1156.

78. Wilson CJ. Cellular mechanisms controlling the strength of synapses. *J Electron Microsc Tech* 1988;10:293–313.

79. Witkovsky P, Schutte M. The organization of dopaminergic neurons in vertebrate retinas. *Vis Neurosci* 1991;7:113–124.

80. Yamamoto T, Hertzberg EL, Nagy JI. Epitopes of gap junctional proteins localized to neuronal subsurface cisterns. *Brain Res* 1990;527:135–139.

81. Yazulla S, Zucker CL. Synaptic organization of dopaminergic interplexiform cells in the goldfish retina. *Vis Neurosci* 1988;1:13–29.

82. Young JK. Alzheimer's disease and metal-containing glia. *Med Hypotheses* 1992;38:1–4.

83. Young JK, McKenzie JC, Baker JH. Association of iron-containing astrocytes with dopaminergic neurons of the arcuate nucleus. *J Neurosci Res* 1990;25:204–213.

84. Zahm DS. An electron microscopic morphometric comparison of tyrosine hydroxylase immunoreactive innervation in the neostriatum and the nucleus accumbens core and shell. *Brain Res* 1992;575:341–346.

85. Zhou D, Huang Q, Gusella JF, Aronin N, DiFiglia M. Subcellular localization of D1-dopamine receptors in rat basal ganglia. *J Neurosci* 1994 [*in press*].

*Psychopharmacology: The Fourth
Generation of Progress,* edited by
Floyd E. Bloom and David J. Kupfer.
Raven Press, Ltd., New York © 1995.

CHAPTER 24

Development of Mesencephalic Dopamine Neurons in the Nonhuman Primate

Relationship to Survival and Growth Following Neural Transplantation

John R. Sladek, Jr., Barbara Blanchard, T. J. Collier, John D. Elsworth,
Jane R. Taylor, Robert H. Roth, and D. Eugene Redmond, Jr.

DEVELOPMENT OF MESENCEPHALIC DOPAMINE NEURONS IN MAMMALS

Independent studies have characterized the appearance of dopamine (DA) biochemically and histochemically in mesencephalic neurons in the mouse and rat during early ontogenesis (4,9,11,12,13,18,20,26,27,33,34,40). Similar studies have not been performed in comparable detail in nonhuman primates, but considerable data do exist for human brain (5,19,21,23,24,29). Our understanding of the temporal events in the development of the mesencephalic DA neurons consequently is based primarily on analysis of rodents. While this information is useful, it may prove difficult to apply to experimental designs involving primates because of major differences in the timing of neurogenesis and the expression of transmitters. For example, DA histofluorescence was first noted during the latter half of gestation in the rat at approximately embryonic day 12.5 (i.e., E 12.5), which corresponds to a surge in the number of labeled cells seen during neurogenesis of the

ventral mesencephalic neuron population (10). The presence of tyrosine hydroxylase was first detected in these neurons also at E 12.5, which suggests a temporal relationship that is consistent with the production of dopamine soon after the onset of neurogenesis. DA exists in neurons as they migrate through the deeper layers of the mesencephalon after division in the germinal zone. In fact, dopamine has been reported in neurons while still in the germinal zone, which reflects biosynthesis immediately after mitosis. Thus, dopamine is present during the latter half of gestation in the rat, whereas it is seen during the first trimester of primate development as described in more detail below. The early presence of dopamine in the primate brain may reflect a role for this neurotransmitter in neurogenesis. For example, interruption of the biosynthesis of a monoamine transmitter, serotonin, by prenatal administration of parachlorphenylalanine (PCPA) results in the delay of differentiation of target neurons of the serotonin system, particularly in the hippocampus (12). If similar mechanisms exist in primate brain, then the relatively early appearance of DA could be influential in the differentiation of critical targets such as the striatum and frontal cortex (see also Chapters 59, 60, and 98, *this volume*).

DOPAMINE IN THE DEVELOPING PRIMATE BRAIN

The timing of the expression of DA in mesencephalic neurons in monkeys is understood incompletely and can-

J. R. Sladek, Jr. and B. Blanchard: Department of Neuroscience, The Chicago Medical School, North Chicago, Illinois 60064.
T. J. Collier: Department of Neurological Sciences, Rush Medical School, Chicago, Illinois 60612.
J. D. Elsworth, J. R. Taylor, R. H. Roth, and D. E. Redmond: Departments of Psychiatry and Pharmacology, Yale University School of Medicine, New Haven, Connecticut 06510.

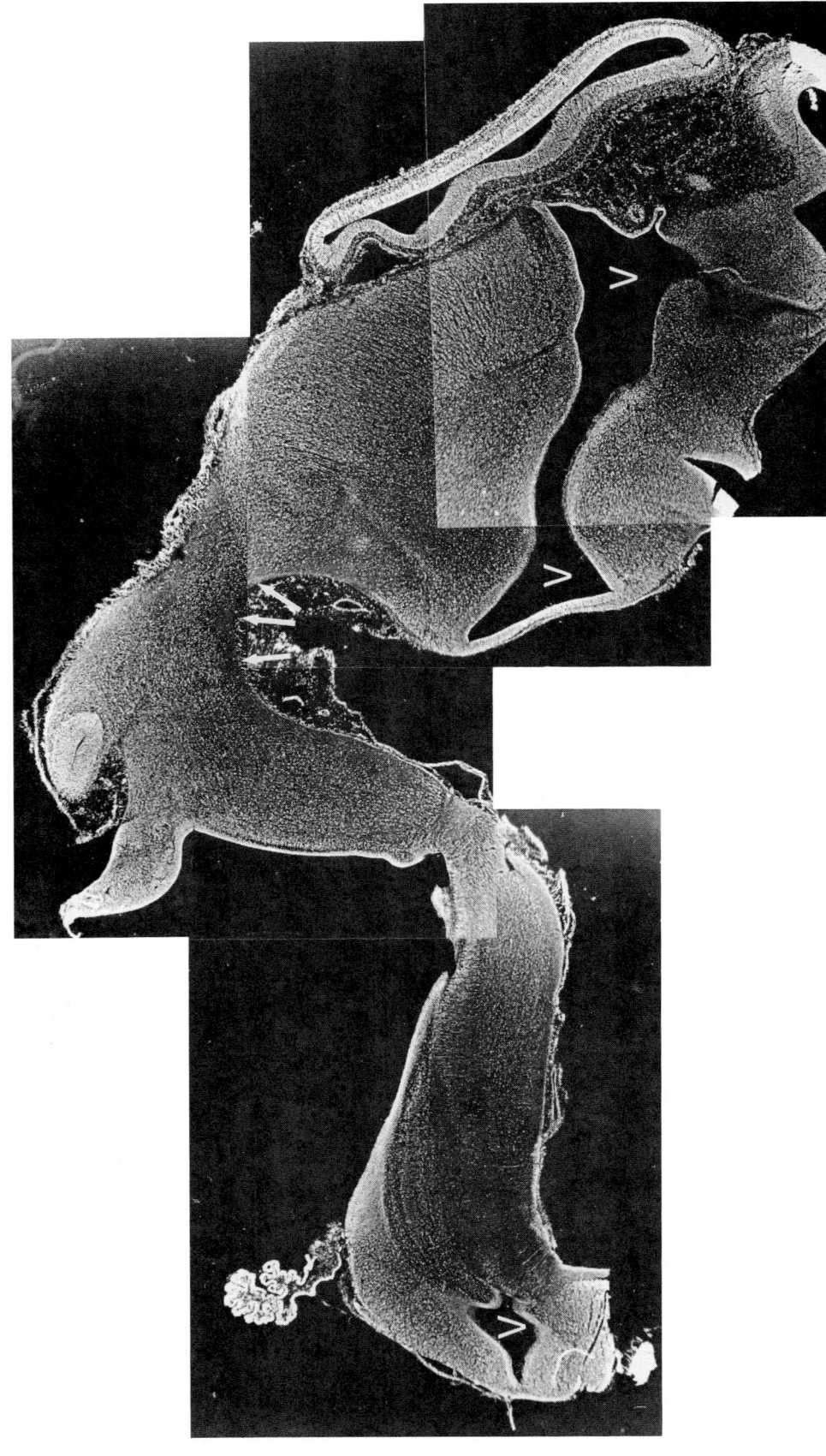

FIG. 1. This dark-field photomontage of an E 40–41 African green monkey shows the full extent of brain development from the forebrain (**right**) to the hindbrain (**left**). The ventricular system (V) forms a prominent cavity which can serve as a useful neuroanatomical landmark. The mesencephalic flexure (*arrows*) demarcates the developing ventral mesencephalon. This region is illustrated in greater detail in Fig. 2.

not be extrapolated from data generated from either the rat or human brain. DA is seen in mesencephalic neurons early in human gestation, but relatively later in the rat. Our examination of this question, although preliminary at present, is described below as a framework for comparison to other mammalian species, including human. A number of studies have been conducted on aborted human material as described below, but the utility of such information with respect to the design of experiments to test developmental hypotheses in primates is far too limited. Thus, knowledge of similar phenomena in nonhuman primates provides an important database for experimental manipulation of the developing DA systems in order to test theories on transmitter expression or differentiation (for example) which could not be examined in developing human brain.

The Mesencephalic Groups at E 40 in Nonhuman Primate

According to Levitt and Rakic (14), neurogenesis of the substantia nigra occurs in the rhesus monkey between E 36 and E 43. The expression of the DA phenotype in nigral neurons in a closely related Old World macaque, the African green monkey, occurs at a similar time as demonstrated by the presence of the synthetic enzyme tyrosine hydroxylase and shown at day E 40 in Figs. 1–4. This is consistent with a generalized "mammalian plan" which results in the biosynthesis of monoamine transmitters early in development, shortly after the initial wave of neurogenesis. The newly formed DA neurons are small and generally rounded, with an average perikaryal length of 9.2 μm (range: 7.4–12.2 μm). Many possess short, dorsally projecting neurites that are about the same length as the perikarya of the mesencephalic neurons (Fig. 2). Others have dorsal neurites that can be traced for distances of 4–5 times (29.6–55.0 μm) the length of the DA perikarya in a single histological section through the mesencephalon. These neurites, at this point in ontogeny, are not recognizable as a rostrally projecting pathway into or toward the striatum or basal forebrain. These migratory neurons occur throughout the depth of the embryonic mesencephalon (Fig. 2) with a high concentration dorsally at the germinal zone, as well as ventrally within the developing mesencephalic tegmentum. The density of neurons is exceptionally high, which provides a predominant appearance of cellularity in the E 40 mesencephalon.

The Mesencephalic Groups at E 55 and E 61

The picture of dopamine neurons changes substantially by E 55 in the African green monkey. At this time, the DA neurons form a recognizable cluster in the ventral mesencephalon, although the separation into three distinct groups is not complete. Distinct groups are recognizable

at E 61 based on size, shape, and staining density. Also, neurite extension is more extensive at this later stage. At E 55, the individual neurons have increased in size to an average diameter of 14.3 μm (range: 9.8–24.6 μm) and the extension of axons rostrally has proceeded to the level of the striatum (Fig. 5), approximately 2 mm rostral to the ventral mesencephalon. The density of tyrosine-hydroxylase-stained fibers is modest as seen in the ascending DA pathway associated with the medial forebrain bundle (Fig. 5) and in the vicinity of the internal capsule where it separates the caudate nucleus from the putamen. However, the ascending monoamine pathways collectively form a prominent bundle at this age, and it is difficult to determine what component is attributable to nigrostriatal axons in the absence of tracer studies or the use of more specific antisera.

The DA perikarya at this age stain with a higher intensity than at E 40 (Fig. 3). DA neurons are not present in the germinal zone, and migration through the tegmentum appears complete. Some tyrosine-hydroxylase-stained neurons are present in the mesencephalic periaqueductal gray and within the region of nucleus raphe dorsalis and could be misinterpreted as components of the germinal zone. It is likely that they represent the small number of catecholaminergic neurons that are present in the adult macaque in the dorsal raphe and periaqueductal gray of the mesencephalon (8).

The Mesencephalic Groups at E 90

By E 90 the mesencephalic DA neurons have attained an adult-like appearance with respect to shape, size, neurite outgrowth, and position (Figs. 7–9). Perikaryal diameters have enlarged to approximately 17.4 μm (range: 11.7–24.3 μm), and individual neurons resemble those seen in adults in all three mesencephalic cell groups (Fig. 9). Neurite extension has progressed over 3.7 mm to reach the striatum where the initial innervation is seen in the form of early patch matrix, or tyrosine-hydroxylase-fiber-rich "islands" (Fig. 6) similar to those first described by Tennyson et al. (37,38) in rabbit neostriatum and by Olson and Seiger (20) in the rat. A prominent bundle of tyrosine-hydroxylase-positive fibers is present rostral to the mesencephalon and appears as a continuous pathway into the striatum (Figs. 6 and 7). Dendrite bundles, another feature of the adult substantia nigra, also exist from the zona compacta to the zona reticulata of the substantia nigra (Figs. 8 and 9D). The neuropil of the ventral mesencephalon reflects highly developed DA systems with considerable interwoven fibers in the local environment (Fig. 9).

Although preliminary at this time (one or two determinations at each time point), we have performed biochemical determinations of DA content in dissected striatum and ventral mesencephalon of fetal African green monkey brains at stages of development comparable to stages re-

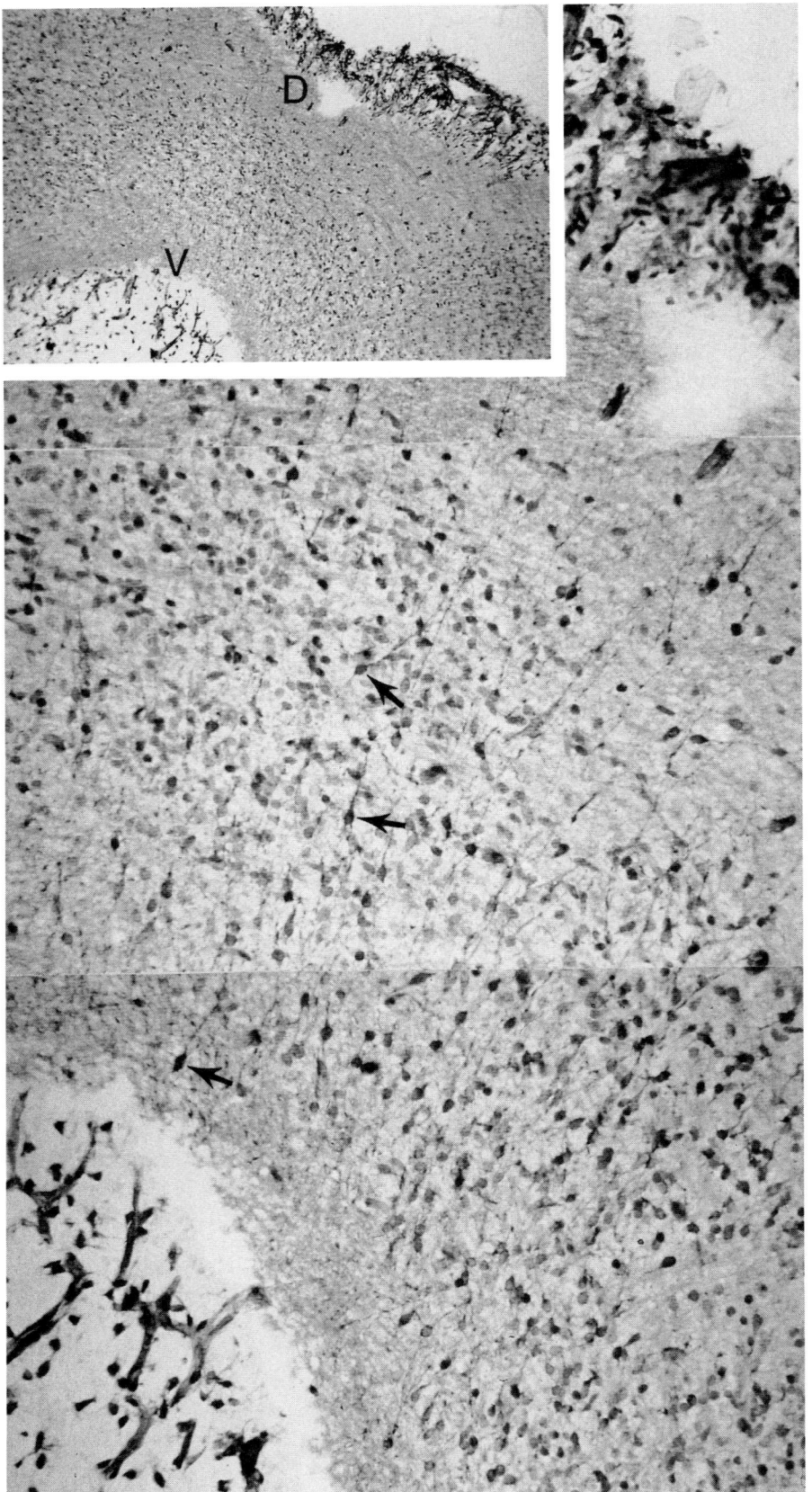

FIG. 2. The low-power insert illustrates the region of the mesencephalic flexure through its full dorsal (D) to ventral (V) extent. This section is adjacent to the midline; therefore the aqueduct of the mesencephalon is not visible. Nevertheless, newly born DA neuroblasts migrate from the germinal epithelium ventrally, and in so doing they provide the appearance seen in the high-power photomontage of small, bipolar neurons with elongated neurites that extend in a dorsoventral plane. The migrating neurons (*arrows*) are stained for tyrosine hydroxylase and demonstrate the early onset of transmitter enzyme in these neurons as depicted at E 40–41.

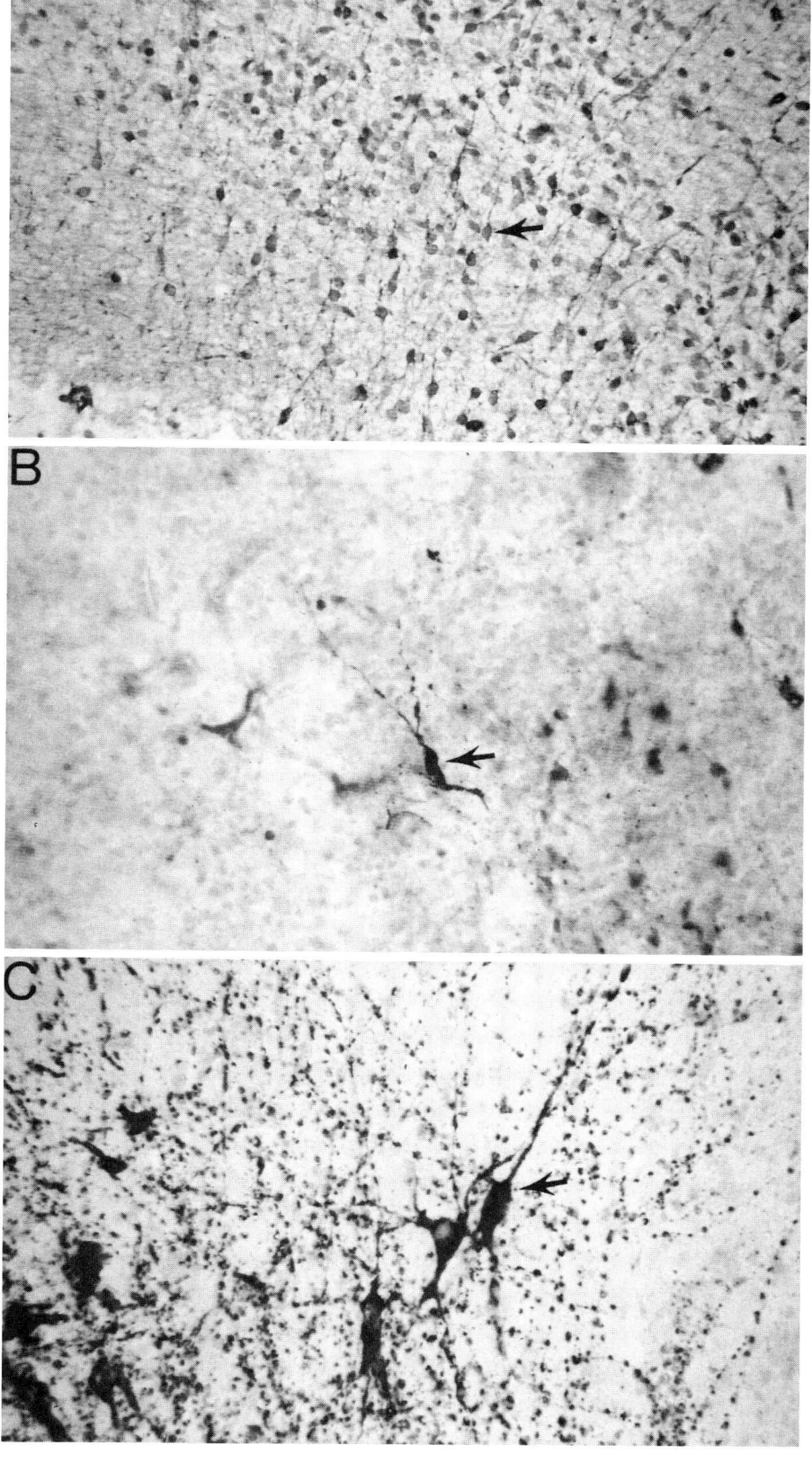

FIG. 3. The three panels illustrate the growth of DA neurons (*arrows*) of the ventral mesencephalon at three developmental ages: (**A**) E 40–41, (**B**) E 55, (**C**) E 90. The dramatic perikaryal growth and neuritic complexity is particularly evident because these three micrographs were taken at identical magnifications.

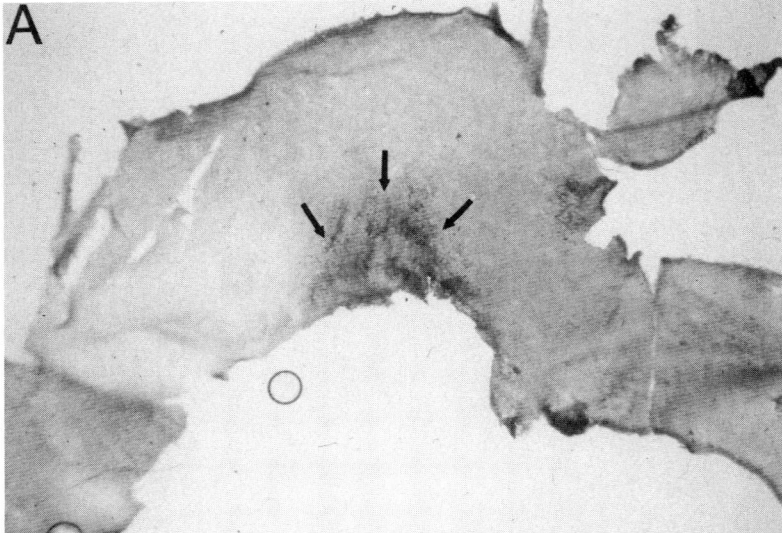

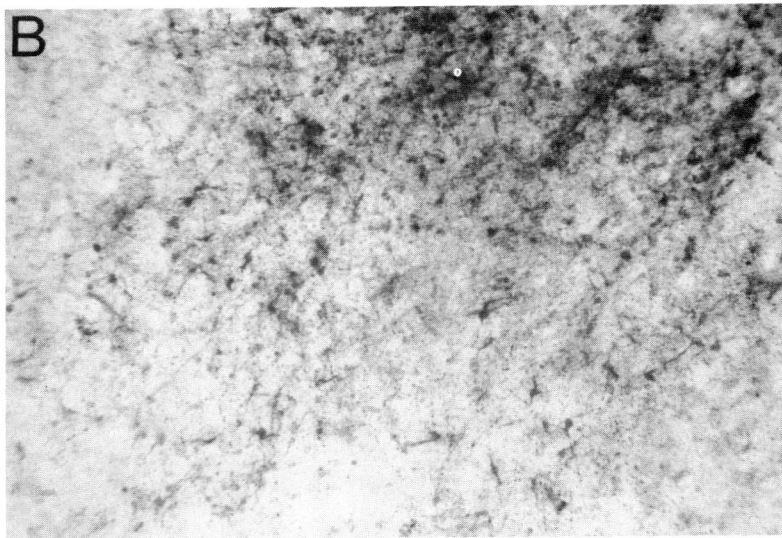

FIG. 4. The brainstem and basal forebrain are illustrated at E 55 following staining for tyrosine hydroxylase; rostral is to the left. In **A**, it is apparent that the ventral mesencephalon is filled with DA neurons (*arrows*) that have completed their migration from the germinal epithelium. In **B**, they appear densely packed and have minimal neuritic arborization at this level.

ported above. The concentration of homovanillic acid, the main end metabolite of DA in this species, parallels that of DA. At E 47, DA concentration, although relatively low, is higher in the ventral mesencephalon than in the striatum. Later, at about 70–90 days, DA levels in the striatum rise sharply, consistent with synaptogenesis in the striatum. At this time, striatal DA concentration is 53.5 ng/mg protein; by comparison this value is 5.05 at E 70 and 0.415 at E 47.

APPLICATION TO TRANSPLANTATION STUDIES IN PRIMATES

Transplantation of neurons into the central nervous system has been studied for over 100 years (39). This technique provides a useful tool for the analysis of neuronal development and can be used to test the specificity of connections between transmitter-defined neural systems.

For the past decade, neural grafts have been tested as a therapeutic intervention in neurodegenerative disorders, particularly Parkinson's disease (7,15,31; see also Chapter 126, *this volume*). Considerable work in nonhuman primates (1,25,32) and with xenografting of human neurons (2,3,22,36) has demonstrated the feasibility of neural transplants in highly ordered primate brain to produce functional, DA-producing grafts that are capable of reversing motor deficits in animal models of Parkinson's disease. Recent reports from several centers suggest that the implantation of embryonic DA neuroblasts can result in some degree of improvement in advanced parkinson patients (6,16,17,35), particularly if the symptoms were caused by the (unknowing) intake of a DA-specific neurotoxin (41). Approximately 300 parkinson patients worldwide have received neural grafts of embryonic mesencephalic neurons, and the recent lifting of a federal restriction on the use of federal support for this experimental surgery will prompt additional attempts at this

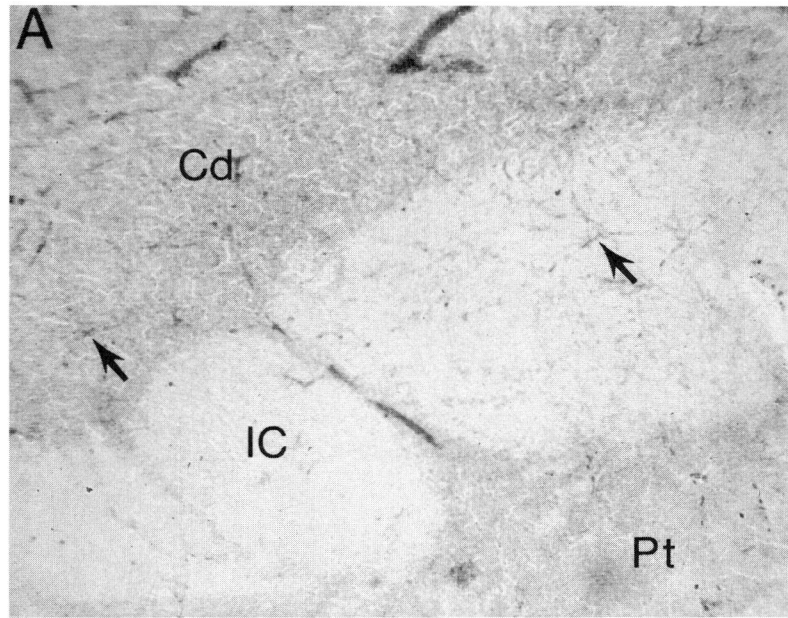

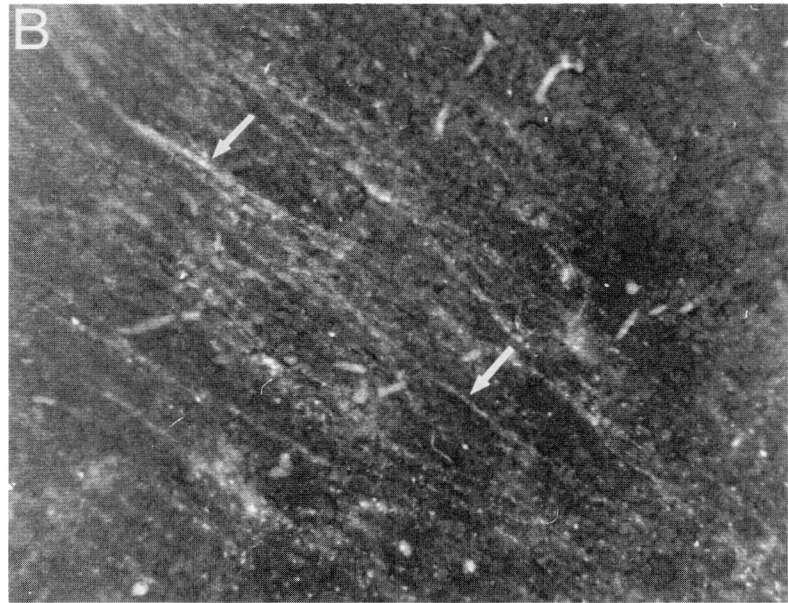

FIG. 5. A: Some axons (*arrows*) of the ventral mesencephalon at E 55 appear to course through the internal capsule (IC) as they ascend through the putamen (PT) and caudate nucleus (CD). **B:** Components of the ascending monoaminergic systems are seen as they pass through the region of the medial forebrain bundle at a diencephalic level. Although identifiable, the fiber density is minimal in comparison to stage E 90 as illustrated in Fig. 6.

experimental clinical approach. Yet a number of critical characteristics of the developing DA neurons are incompletely understood such as the optimal embryonic age for survival of grafted neurons in primates, including human.

Knowledge gained from basic developmental studies can be applied to questions of neuronal survival following transplantation. For example, if the outgrowth of neurites is considered as a potential determinant of viability following the extirpation of DA neurons from embryonic brain, then the observation of neurite extension from the region of the developing substantia nigra to the striatum in the E 55 monkey described above suggests that neurons from this age are too well developed to survive the obligatory axotomy that accompanies the extirpation. In fact,

we have observed between one-tenth and one-twentieth as many DA neurons following grafting of mesencephalon from later-stage embryos such as E 55 in monkey in comparison to younger donor grafts (Fig. 10). Moreover, the "window" for the best survival probably is quite narrow. Ten times as many DA neurons were seen following grafting of E 44 tissue in comparison to E 49 in African green monkey (30), and our recent observations suggest that maximal DA neuron survival is achieved from donor tissue during a 48-hr period, at E 41–42. If we consider that gestation in the monkey is approximately 6 months, as compared to 9 months for the human, then the window for human tissue might be 50% longer and perhaps span a 3-day period at a critical point in neurogen-

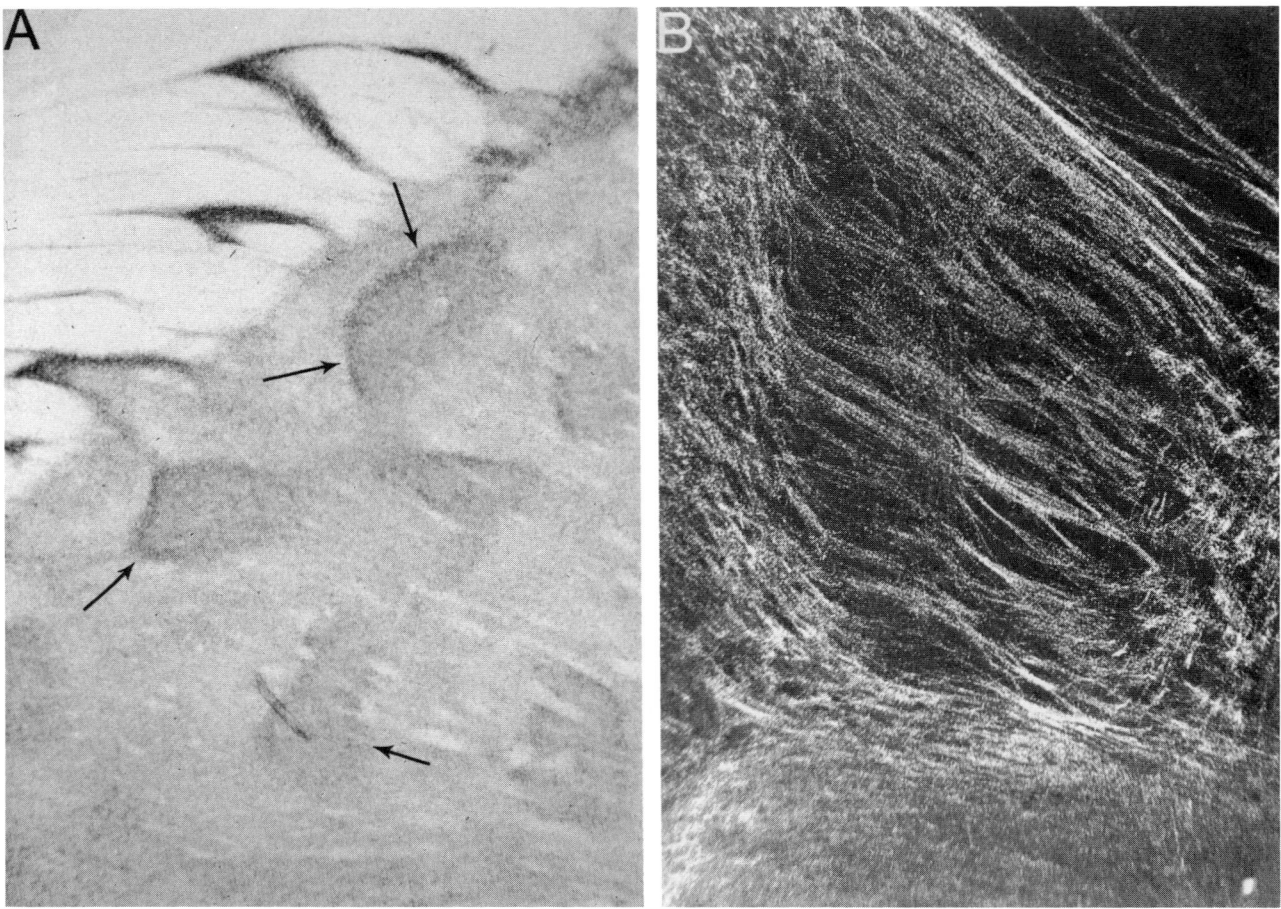

FIG. 6. The ascending DA axons are highly developed at E 90 and are seen as a dense parallel array of fibers (**B**) as they approach the neostriatum. Their terminal fields in the caudate nucleus are seen in **A,** where the presence of numerous "patches" of DA fibers (*arrows*) begins to be manifested. This is also seen in the overview in Fig. 7.

esis or neuronal differentiation. The determination of that critical point is an essential next step for neural grafting experiments in humans. This is particularly crucial because a relatively wide range of embryonic ages has been used in the extant human experiments in parkinson patients (6,16,17,35). The predictive nature of developmental studies in human material is underscored by the observations described below that attempt to characterize transmitter expression, neurite extension, and the growth

of terminal plexuses of DA neurons as a template for transplantation. Thus, the presumption is that survival is influenced by the degree to which axons have extended from the perikarya; that is, extension past a specific distance renders neurons incapable of surviving grafting if axons are severed during the dissection. In this case, only those neurons or neuroblasts that appear as rounded cells with no or short processes will survive grafting. This pool would include that percentage of neuroblasts that

FIG. 7. This photomontage illustrates the position of developing catecholamine systems in the brainstem, the ascending axons caudal to the putamen, and the dense patch-matrix appearance of the developing striatum. Three large clusters of perikarya are identified ventrally in the brainstem (**right**); these correspond to the ventral noradrenergic neuronal groups (A1, A2, A5, A7) that give rise to the ventral noradrenergic pathway, seen here immediately caudal to the second group, the locus coeruleus (A6). The third, and most prominent, cluster represents the DA neurons of the ventral mesencephalon which form an exceptionally dense cluster of intensely stained neurons (A8, A9). Ascending nigrostriatal axons (*arrows*) and the dense patch-matrix appearance of the caudate (CD) and putamen (PT) are prominent features. AC, anterior commissure; IC, internal capsule; IOC, inferior olivary complex; SC, superior colliculus.

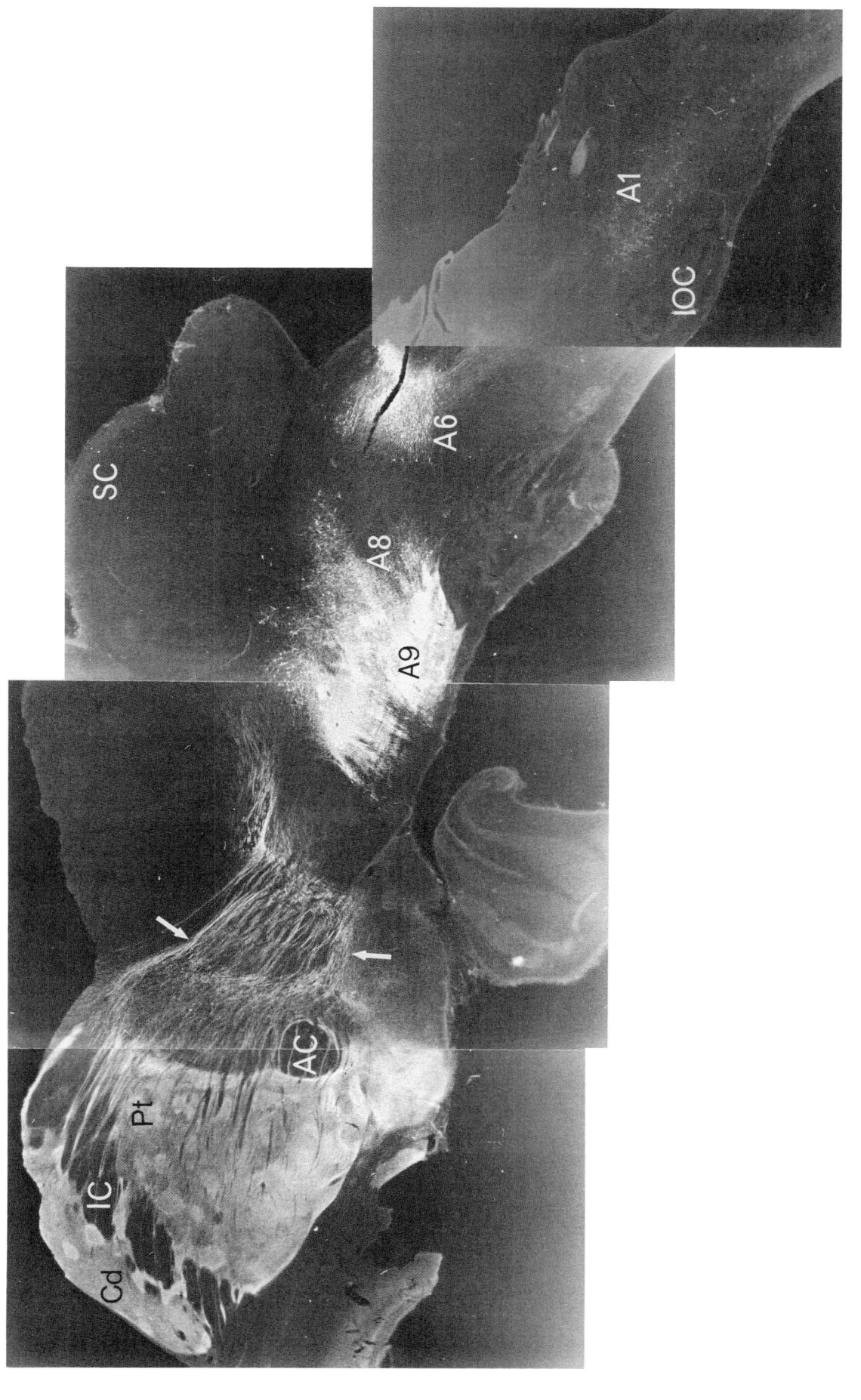

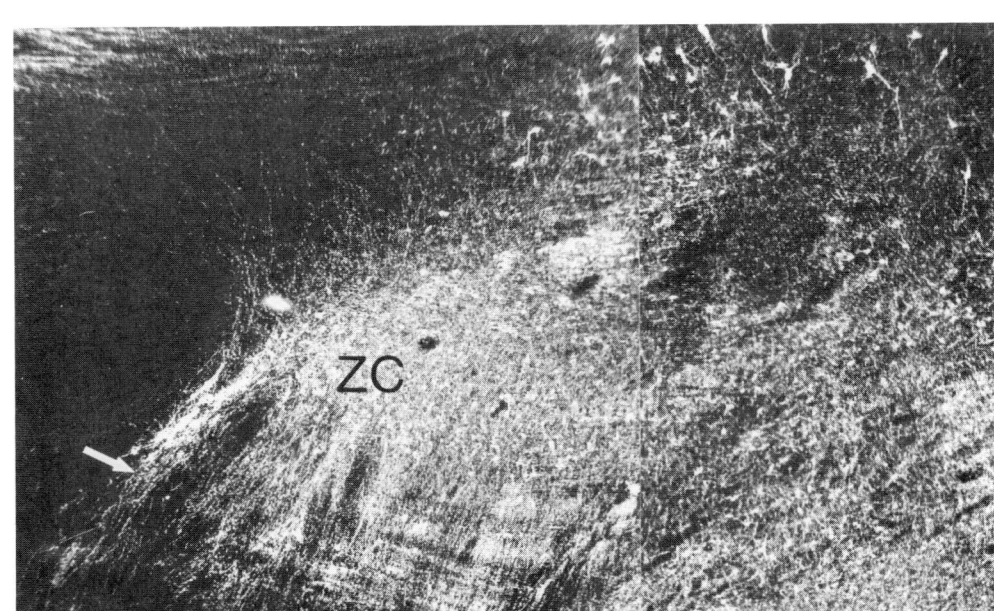

FIG. 8. This higher-power view of the ventral mesencephalon at age E 90 illustrates the dense packing of DA neurons as well as the highly developed dendritic bundles (*arrows*) that course from the substantia nigra zona compacta (ZC) into the zona reticulata (ZR). Ascending axons en route to the striatum are seen in the upper left corner of this photograph.

are "born" immediately prior to grafting. Neurogenesis takes place over at least 1 week in monkeys, and Freeman et al. (5) reported that tyrosine-hydroxylase-positive neuroblasts were present in the germinal zone in humans as late as 10 weeks, which is 3.5 weeks after they were first seen in this region. This suggests that neurogenesis of the human substantia nigra may occur over a considerably longer period than that in monkeys and that a certain percentage of neurons are capable of surviving grafting at any point during this 3.5-week period. This has been verified in our studies in monkeys where survival of DA neurons was observed in late-stage tissue (27,32), and predictably the number of grafted tyrosine-hydroxylase-positive neurons was exceptionally low (i.e., often fewer than 100/animal).

Factors other than axon elongation may play a critical role in determining cell survival following transplantation. The development of intracellular messengers, DA autoreceptors, transporter mechanisms, availability of trophic factors, and gene regulation of transmitters and associated enzymes all could influence the ability of embryonic neuroblasts to survive neural transplantation. Systematic

analysis of these, as well as other, potential variables is needed to provide a clear understanding of this question in human as well as nonhuman primate brain.

COMPARISON TO HUMAN DEVELOPMENT

A number of investigators have examined events in the development of human monoaminergic neuron systems, particularly with histofluorescence and immunohistochemical techniques as indices of transmitter expression. The first description by Olson et al. (21) noted (a) the relatively early appearance of monoamines in human neuroblasts of the mesencephalon and (b) the gradual growth of fluorescent ascending axons and striatal patches of catecholamine histofluorescence. At 7 weeks, fluorescence attributed to serotonin and catecholamines was seen within small, round neuroblasts that generally possessed few processes (0–2/cell). By 10 weeks of gestation the neurons were situated in the ventral mesencephalon in groups, but were not subdivided into the A8–A10 subgroups. Some fluorescent axons were present in the stria-

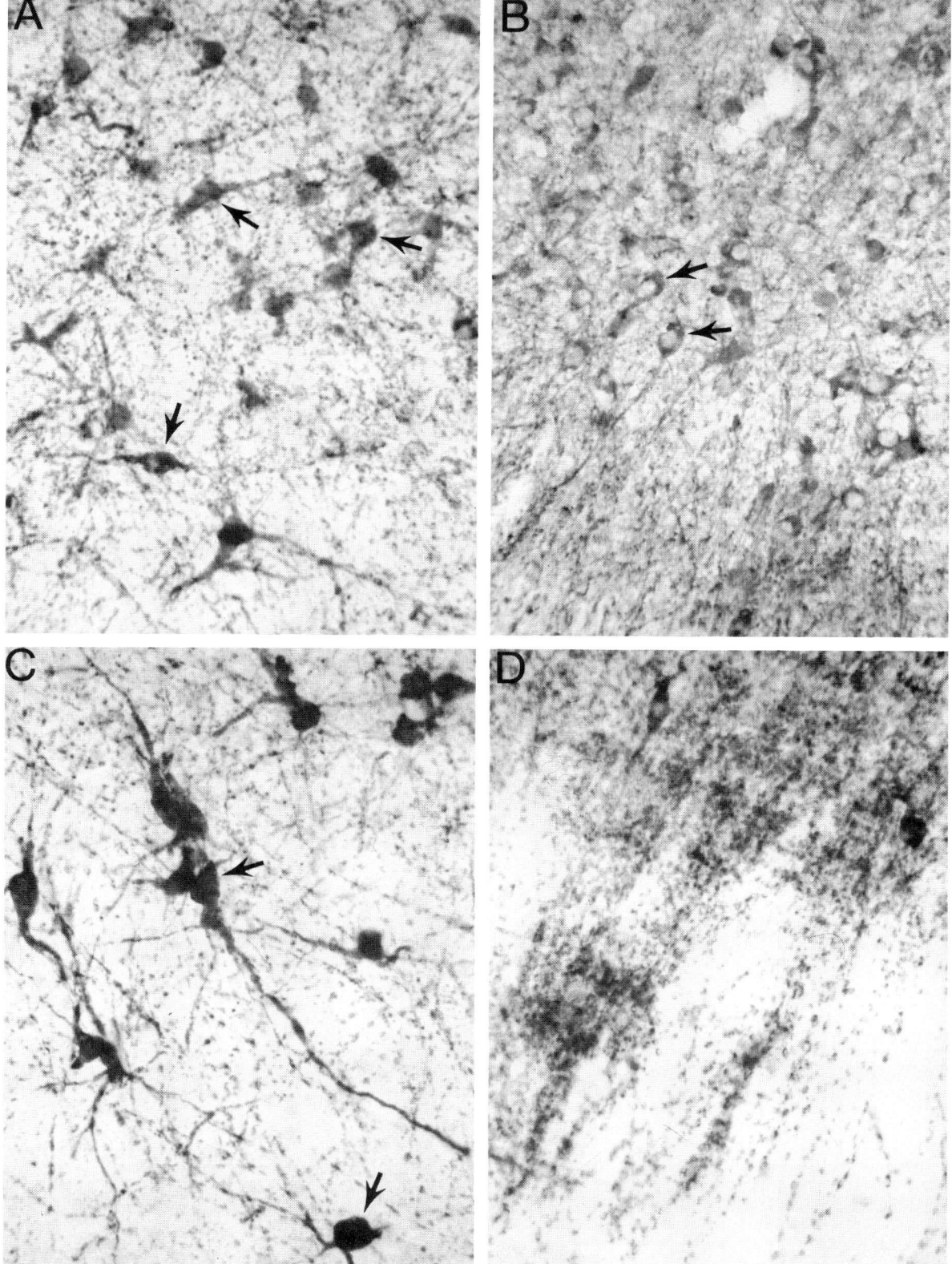

FIG. 9. These four panels illustrate various cell types (*arrows*) seen within the developing mesencephalon at age E 90. In **A,** densely packed neurons reminiscent of zona compacta are seen, whereas in **B** the smaller, more oval neurons of the ventral tegmental area (A10) are illustrated. Panel **C** represents the more dorsally and caudally placed neurons of the retrorubal group (A8), while panel **D** illustrates dendritic bundles ventral to the zona compacta.

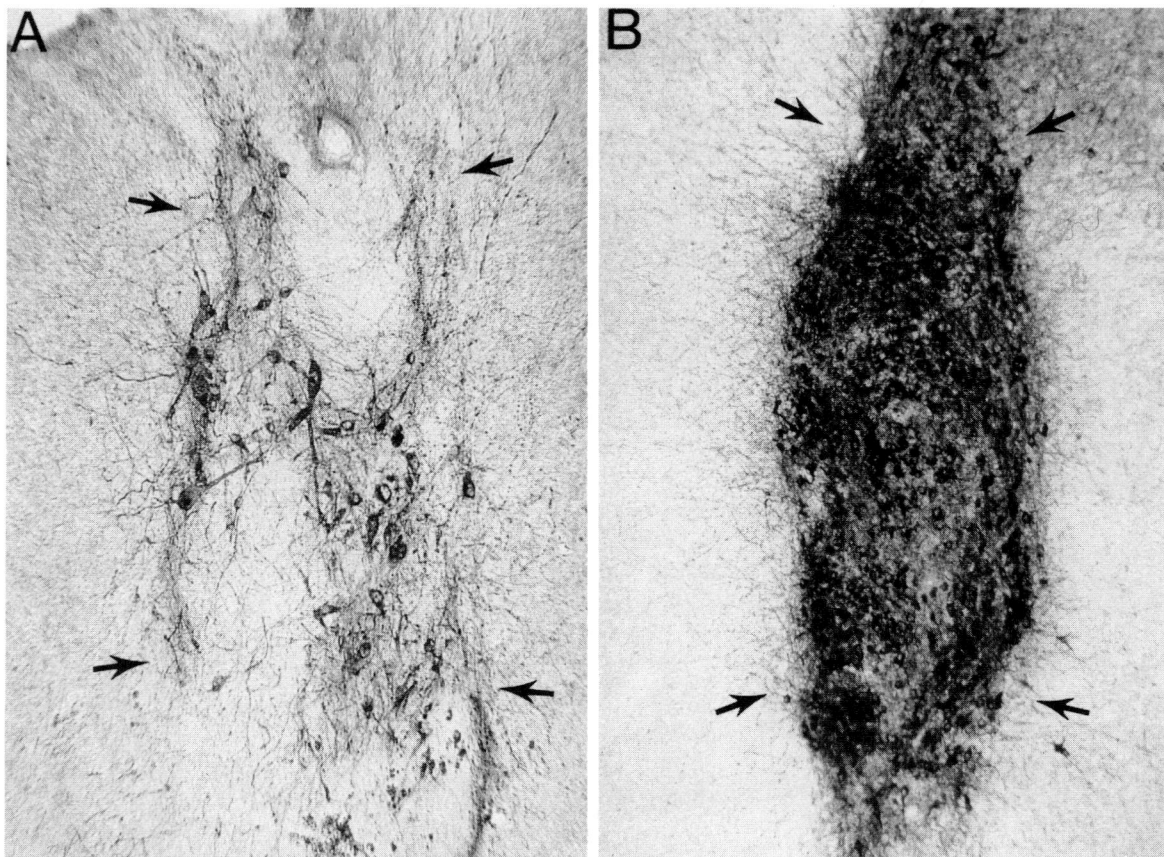

FIG. 10. Representative transplants (*arrows*) of embryonic DA neurons are seen in two adult African green monkeys at the same magnification. This comparison of grafted neurons collected from an optimally aged donor (**B**) versus those of an older donor (**A**) illustrates the dramatic increase in viability seen following grafting of the younger tissue. These illustrations are representative of grafts that contain approximately 500 (older donor) and 5000 (younger donor) tyrosine-hydroxylase-positive neurons as reflected by the density of perikarya. This enhanced survival undoubtedly relates to the immature stage of neuritic development at the earlier time, but may be attributed to other factors as well.

tum, although the development of islands was not seen until 12.5 weeks. The more caudally placed putamen received a DA innervation prior to that of the caudate, which is consistent with the directional course of the ascending DA fiber bundle which approaches the striatal complex in a caudal-to-rostral direction. The mesencephalic complex of DA neurons was "heavily subdivided" by 15.5 weeks, and the striatum was more heavily supplied with a dense patchy pattern of terminals of nigrostriatal origin. Thus, over the relatively short period of 10 weeks the mesencephalic DA neurons are born, grow into the host striatum, and develop a terminal pattern reminiscent of adults. By comparison, the mesocortical pathways were reported by these investigators to follow a somewhat later time course with respect to terminal innervation, although the histofluorescence technique was less capable of demonstrating cortical monoamine fibers than were later versions of the method as described below. A parallel study by Nobin and Björklund (19) basically confirmed these findings and noted that the overall stage of develop-

ment of the monoamine systems in the human fetus was comparable to that of the rat during the second week after birth, which raises questions about the potential role of the relatively early appearing DA in the human brain.

More recent investigations of human gestation by Freeman et al. (5) using immunohistochemistry noted the presence of tyrosine hydroxylase in mesencephalic neuroblasts at 6.5 weeks and neurite extension at 8 weeks. Tyrosine hydroxylase fibers were reported first in the putamen at 9 weeks, and, remarkably, putative DA neurons were seen adjacent to the ventricle, presumably in the germinal zone, at 10 weeks of gestation. A similar study by Silani et al. (28) reported a few tyrosine hydroxylase cells in the germinal zone of the mesencephalon as early as 5.5 weeks in human material. Thus, the systems apparently begin to produce synthetic enzyme in advance of the first reported demonstration of DA fluorescence, and the presence of DA is an early event that begins during and shortly after neurogenesis. The role of DA at these early stages has been the subject of investigation as described earlier and will undoubtedly continue to be examined carefully, for example, with molecular techniques as interest on the development of monoamine neurons, particularly those that utilize DA, continues to focus on neurologic and psychiatric disorders that may in part be due to abnormal development.

ACKNOWLEDGMENTS

This research was made possible by the contributions of the staff of St. Kitt's Biomedical Research Institute. This study was funded by NIH grants PO1 NS 24032 and RSA MH 00643 (D.E.R.) and by the Axion Research Foundation.

REFERENCES

1. Bakay RAE, Fiandaca MS, Barrow DL, Schiff A, Collins DC. Preliminary report on the use of fetal tissue transplantation to correct MPTP-induced Parkinson-like syndrome in primates. *Appl Neurophysiol* 1985;48:358–361.
2. Brundin P, Nilsson OG, Strecker RE, Lindvall O, Astedt B, Björklund A. Behavioral effects of human fetal dopamine neurons grafted in a rat model of Parkinson's disease. *Exp Brain Res* 1986;65:235–240.
3. Brundin P, Strecker RE, Widner H, Clarke DJ, Nilsson OG, Astedt B, Lindvall O, Björklund A. Human fetal dopamine neurons grafted in a rat model of Parkinson's disease: immunological aspects, spontaneous and drug-induced behavior, and dopamine release. *Exp Brain Res* 1988;70:192–208.
4. Coyle JT. The development of catecholaminergic neurons of the central nervous system. *Neurosci Res* 1973;5:35–52.
5. Freeman TB, Spence MS, Boss BD, Spector DH, Strecker RE, Olanow CW, Kordower JH. Development of dopaminerig neurons in the human substantia nigra. *Exp Neurol* 1991;113:344–353.
6. Freed CR, Breeze RE, Rosenberg NL, Schneck SA, Kriek E, Qi J-X, et al. Survival of implanted fetal dopamine cells and neurologic improvement 12 to 46 months after transplantation for parkinson's disease. *N Engl J Med* 1992;327(2):10–16.
7. Freed WJ. Substantia nigra grafts and Parkinson's disease: from animal experiments to human therapeutic trials. *Res Neurol Neurosci* 1991;3:109–134.
8. Garver DL, Sladek JR Jr. Monoamine distribution in primate brain. I. Catecholamine-containing perikarya in the brain stem of *Macaca speciosa*. *J Comp Neurol* 1975;159:289–304.
9. Golden GS. Prenatal development of the biogenic amine systems of the mouse brain. *Dev Biol* 1973;33:300–311.
10. Hanaway J, McConnell JA, Netsky MG. Histogenesis of the substantia nigra, ventral tegmental area of Tsai and interpeduncular nucleus: an autoradiographic study of the mesencephalon in the rat. *J Comp Neurol* 1971;142:59–73.
11. Lauder JM, Bloom FL. Ontogeny of monoamine neurons in the locus coeruleus, raphe nuclei and substantia nigra of the rat. *J Comp Neurol* 1974;155:469–482.
12. Lauder JM, Krebs H. Effects of *p*-chlorophenylalanine on time of neuronal origin during embryogenesis in the rat. *Brain Res* 1976;107:638–644.
13. Levitt P, Moore RY. Development of the noradrenergic innervation of neocortex. *Brain Res* 1979;162:243–259.
14. Levitt P, Rakic P. The time of genesis, embryonic origin and differentiation of the brain stem monoamine neurons in the rhesus monkey. *Dev Brain Res* 1982;4:35–57.
15. Lindvall O. Transplantation into the human brain: present status and future possibilities. *J Neurol Neurosurg Psychiatry* 1989:39–54.
16. Lindvall O, Rehncrona S, Brundin P, et al. Human fetal dopamine neurons grafted into the striatum in two patients with severe Parkinson's disease. *Arch Neurol* 1989;46:615–631.
17. Lindvall O, Brundin P, Widner H, et al. Grafts of fetal dopamine neurons survive and improve motor function in Parkinson's disease. *Science* 1990;247:574–577.
18. Loizou LA. The postnatal ontogeny of monamine-containing neurones in the central nervous system of the albino rat. *Brain Res* 1972;40:395–418.
19. Nobin A, Björklund. Topography of the monoamine neuron systems in the human brain as revealed in fetuses. *Acta Physiol Scand Suppl* 1973;388:1–40.
20. Olson L, Seiger Å. Early prenatal ontogeny of central monoamine neurons in the rat: fluorescence histochemical observations. *Z Anat Entwicklungsgesch* 1972;137:301–316.
21. Olson L, Boreus LO, Seiger Å. Histochemical demonstration and mapping of 5-hydroxytryptamine- and catacholamine-containing neuron systems in the human fetal brain. *Z Anat Entwicklungsgesch* 1973;139:259–282.
22. Olson L, Strömberg I, Bygdeman M, Granholm A-Ch, Hoffer B, Freedman R, Seiger Å. Human fetal tissues grafted to rodent hosts: structural and functional observations of brain, adrenal and heart tissues in oculo. *Exp Brain Res* 1987;67:163–178.
23. Pearson J, Brandeis L, Goldstein M. Appearance of tyrosine hydroxylase immunoreactivity in the human embryo. *Dev Neurosci* 1980;3:140–150.
24. Pickel VM, Spect LA, Krushdev KS, Joh TH, Reis DJ, Hervonen A. Immunocytochemical localization of tyrosine hydroxylase in the human fetal nervous system. *J Comp Neurol* 1980;194:465–474.
25. Redmond DE Jr, Roth RH, Elsworth JD, Sladek JR Jr, Collier TJ, Deutch AY, Haber SN. Fetal neuronal grafts in monkeys given methylphenyltetrahydropyridine. *Lancet* 1986;1125.
26. Schlumpf M, Shoemaker WJ, Bloom FE. Innervation of embryonic rat cerebral cortex by catecholamine-containing fibers. *J Comp Neurol* 1980;192:361–376.
27. Seiger Å, Olson L. Late prenatal ontogeny of central monoamine neurons in the rat: fluorescence histochemical observations. *Z Anat Entwicklungsgesch* 1973;140:281–318.
28. Silani V, Mariani D, Donato FM, Ghezzi C, Mazzucchelli F, Buscaglia M, et al. Development of dopaminergic neurons in the human mesencephalon and in vitro effects of basic fibroblast growth factor treatment. *Exp Neurol* 1994;[in press].
29. Sladek JR Jr, Collier TJ, Haber SN, Roth RH, Redmond DE Jr. Survival and growth of fetal catecholamine neurons transplanted into primate brain. *Brain Res Bull* 1986;17:809–818.
30. Sladek JR Jr, Elsworth JD, Roth RH, Evans LE, Collier TJ, Cooper SJ, Taylor JR, Redmond DE Jr. Fetal dopamine cell survival after transplantation is dramatically improved at a critical donor gestational age in nonhuman primates. *Exp Neurol* 1993;122:16–27.
31. Sladek JR Jr, Gash DM. Nerve-cell grafting in Parkinson's disease. *J Neurosurg* 1988;68:337–351.
32. Sladek JR Jr, Redmond DE Jr, Collier TJ, Haber SN, Elsworth JD, Duetch AY, Roth RH. Transplantation of fetal dopamine neurons in primate brain reverses MPTP induced parkinsonism. *Prog Brain Res* 1987;71:309–323.
33. Specht LA, Pickel VM, Joh TH, Reis DJ. Light-microscopic immunocytochemical localization of tyrosine hydroxylase in prenatal rat brain. I. Early ontogeny. *J Comp Neurol* 1981;199:233–253.
34. Specht LA, Pickel VM, Joh TH, Reis DJ. Light-microscopic immunocytochemical localization of tyrosine hydroxylase in prenatal rat brain. II. Late ontogeny. *J Comp Neurol* 1981;199:255–276.
35. Spencer DD, Robbins RJ, Naftolin F, Phil D, Marek KL, Vollmer T, Leranth C, Roth RH, Price LH, Gjedde A, Bunney BS, Sass KJ, Elsworth JD, Kier EL, Makuch R, Hoffer PB, Redmond DE Jr. Unilateral transplantation of human fetal mesencephalic tissue into the caudate nucleus of patients with Parkinson's disease. *N Eng J Med* 1992;327(22):1541–1548.
36. Strömberg I, Bygdeman M, Goldstein M, Seiger Å, Olson L. Human fetal substantia nigra grafted to the dopamine-denervated striatum if immunosuppressed rats: evidence for functional reinnervation. *Neurosci Lett* 1986;71:271–276.
37. Tennyson VM, Barrett RE, Cohen G, Cote L, Heikkila R, Mytilineou C. The developing neostriatum of the rabbit: correlation of

fluorescence histochemistry, electron microscopy, endogenous dopamine levels and H3-dopamine uptake. *Brain Res* 1972;46:251–255.

38. Tennyson VM, Mytilineou C, Barrett RE. Fluorescence and electron microscopic studies of the early development of the substantia nigra and area ventralis tegmenti in the fetal rabbit. *J Comp Neurol* 1973;149:233–258.

39. Thompson WG. Successful brain grafting. *NY Med J* 1890;51:701.

40. Voorn P, Kalsbeek A, Jorritsma-Byham, Groenewegen HJ. The pre- and postnatal development of the dopaminergic cell groups in the ventral mesencephalon and the dopaminergic innervation of the striatum of the rat. *Neuroscience* 1988;25:857–887.

41. Widner H, Tetrud J, Rehngrona S, Snow B, Brundin P, Gustavii B, et al. Bilateral fetal mesencephalic grafting in two patients with parkinsonism induced by 1-methyl-4-phenyl-1,2,3,6-tetrahydropyridine (MPTP). *N Eng J Med* 1992;327(22):1556–1563.

Psychopharmacology: The Fourth Generation of Progress, edited by Floyd E. Bloom and David J. Kupfer. Raven Press, Ltd., New York © 1995.

CHAPTER 25

Mesocorticolimbic Dopaminergic Neurons

Functional and Regulatory Roles

Michel Le Moal

DOPAMINE: CHALLENGES WITH A FUNCTIONAL APPROACH

In 1978, Moore and Bloom (26) observed that progress had been slow in elucidating the role of the dopaminergic (DA) neurons and, in particular, their fundamental functional property. While still valid, few neuronal systems have provoked as much investigative efforts as the DA neurons, as noted in other chapters in this volume. DA neurons are the source of hypotheses concerning sensorimotor and psychotic defects, the pathophysiology of drug abuse, and favored targets for drug development and grafting replacement therapy (see Chapters 66, 100, 126, 145, and 147, *this volume*).

The nonstriatal projections, generally referred to as a separate set often labeled "mesolimbic" or A10, have received somewhat less attention than the "nigrostriatal" A9 DA neurons. The mesolimbic neurons—later the "mesocorticolimbic" group—have subsequently been divided into numerous subsets denoted in the terms of the region of the projection, of which about 20 have been noted. The cellular subgroups are intermingled within the ventral mesencephalon while some limbic projections have their origin in the substantia nigra and vice versa such that selective inactivation of each system is not only difficult, but has caused confusion in interpreting pharmacological manipulations. Consequently the list of the "functions" attributed to the "mesolimbic" neurons is as varied as the behavioral paradigms used to study them. Furthermore, no disease or clinical syndrome with ana-

tomical or biochemical abnormalities primarily involving these structures has yet been demonstrated. In this chapter, I extend a working hypothesis formulated in 1984 and extended recently (21). The conclusions can be summarized briefly as follows: (i) DA neurons do not have specific functions; (ii) they regulate and enable integrative functions in the neuronal systems onto which they project; (iii) lesion of their terminals induces neuropsychological deficits that are characteristic of the functions of the neuronal systems they regulate; and (iv) the deficits observed depend on the behavioral situations or the tasks used to explore them.

FUNCTIONAL CHARACTERIZATION OF THE DA PROJECTIONS: ANALYTICAL APPROACH

Mesencephalic Cell Bodies: Functional Studies

The Medial Ventral Mesencephalon as an Anatomicofunctional Entity

The DA cells are embedded within dense tracts of ascending and descending fibers (among them the medial forebrain bundle) through which they communicate with large regions, such as the limbic–forebrain and the limbic–midbrain structures, defined by Nauta (27). The ventral mesencephalon, which encompasses the ventral tegmental area (VTA), is an anterior part of the reticular formation. The DA cells receive signals of all sorts, and numerous peptides and transmitters have been found in this area (15).

Destruction of the VTA with radio-frequency (RF) lesions produces a behavioral syndrome [see (21) for refer-

M. Le Moal: Psychobiologie des Comportements Adaptatifs, INSERM—Université de Bordeaux II, Bordeaux 33077, France.

ences] characterized by: (i) a high level of locomotor activity and hypoexploration; (ii) profound deficits in behavioral suppression capacity (10); (iii) disappearance of the behavioral patterns essential to the survival of the individual or the species [e.g., social, maternal (9), and hoarding behaviors (44)]; (iv) deficits defined operationally in terms of (a) the facilitation of active (one way) avoidance learning, (b) deficits in approach behaviors with continuous or fixed-interval schedules of reinforcement due to a lack of behavioral suppression ability, and (c) deficits in intracranial self-stimulation and in self-administration of psychostimulant drugs; and (v) profound deficits in attentional and representational cognitive processes as measured by delayed alternation tasks without deficits in a visual discrimination (10). The hypokinetic–hypoattentional deficits are correlated with a decrease in dopamine in the anteromedian frontal cortex and to a lesser extent in the nucleus accumbens, whereas no correlation was observed with the dopamine levels in the nucleus caudatus or the serotonin and noradrenaline levels in the forebrain.

Effects of Neurochemically Selective Lesions of the Mesolimbic and Mesocortical DA Cell Bodies

Local injections of 6-hydroxydopamine (6-OHDA) confirmed some of the results obtained after RF lesions: hyperactivity and disruption of behavioral capacities (18,21,31,32), but without the aphagia, adipsia, or motor disorders. Moreover, these deficits were unlike those resulting from local destruction of DA terminals within the nucleus accumbens or within the frontal cortex (see ref. 21). Extended investigations have led to a clarification of five deficits.

Locomotor Activity

Extensive studies (19,20) using RF techniques and different doses of 6-OHDA in the cell bodies and accumbens regions as well as in combined lesions led to the following conclusions: (i) large 6-OHDA lesions of the VTA or of the nucleus accumbens produce hypoactivity, a complete blockade of the locomotor stimulating effects of amphetamine, and a profound supersensitive response to apomorphine; (ii) smaller VTA lesions produce significant increases in spontaneous daytime and nocturnal locomotor activity, with the largest effect occurring at the lowest dose; (iii) the hyperactivity produced by RF lesions to the VTA is unresponsive to amphetamine, but it decreases after apomorphine and is blocked by the addition of a 6-OHDA lesion to the nucleus accumbens; and (iv) these combined lesions produce a blockade of the stimulating effects of amphetamine and a potentiated response to apomorphine which was identical to that observed with a nucleus accumbens lesion alone. These results suggest

that dopamine may play an essential role in the expression of both spontaneous and stimulant-induced activity (28). Furthermore, the much larger increase in spontaneous activity observed in the VTA-RF group than in the VTA-6-OHDA groups suggests that an as yet unidentified powerful inhibitory influence is exerted on the DA neurons within the mesencephalon or at the level of the terminal fields.

Aphagia and Adipsia

Aphagia and adipsia result from lesions of the nigrostriatal neurons or from added damage of mesocorticolimbic neurons and of a trigeminal sensory component. Extensive studies (see ref. 21) allow us to conclude the following: (i) the most effective site for producing aphagia and adipsia after RF lesion to the mesencephalon is an intermediate zone between the substantia nigra and the VTA; (ii) 6-OHDA in this intermediate zone led to a less severe feeding deficit than that observed with RF lesions, suggesting that both DA and non-DA neurons are involved in the mesencephalic aphagic syndrome; (iii) rats with RF lesions of the sensory trigeminal nucleus are aphagic; but when they recover, their deficit is less severe than after RF lesion; and (iv) a 6-OHDA lesion of the mesencephalic intermediate zone combined with a RF lesion of the trigeminal sensory nucleus led to the more severe deficits observed. These results demonstrate that the DA neurons projecting to the cortical and limbic regions contribute to the aphagic syndrome but are not essential for it.

Initiation of Responding, Incentive, and Active Avoidance

After 6-OHDA infusion in various terminal areas and combined lesions of these terminal areas, only rats with combined 90% total depletion of dopamine showed a severe deficit in initiation and incentive to respond in an active avoidance task (19). These rats showed no response to a low or high dose of amphetamine, and they remained cataleptic as if receiving high doses of neuroleptics for the duration of the experiment but rapidly recovered from transient aphagia and adipsia (less than 10 days post lesion). These findings show that major psychomotor deficits are prevalent after the total lesion of the DA fibers in the whole forebrain and that the existence of interactions between DA projections is a prerequisite for the initiation and development of a fully adaptive response. This cooperation supports the hypothesis that interrelationships exist between the various terminal fields of the DA network.

Sensorimotor Integration and Motivation

Dozens of studies, mainly using DA receptor blockade, suggest a role for dopamine in sensorimotor integration as well as in goal-directed response and motivational arousal. It is generally assumed that the cortical and limbic projections—that is, the neurons from the VTA—do not modulate sensorimotor integration. However, limbic and frontal neglect syndromes have been described when at least one-third of the system is destroyed. The extent of the resulting neglect was correlated (see ref. 21) with the overall damage to the substantia nigra and VTA, rather than to any individual region within this DA continuum. Damage to the corticolimbic projections potentiates the severity of the neglect produced by nigrostriatal lesions. Thus, the involvement of the individual subclasses of mesotelencephalic DA neurons in the neglect syndrome is more widespread than was previously thought to be the case. Do these changes result from deficits in motivation, impaired stimulus perception, or inadequate sequence of motor responses? Numerous tests under various levels of motivation have shown (32) that rats are insensitive to motivational stimuli only when DA lesions are placed in the medial ventral mesencephalon.

Learning Processes

The disruption of instrumental conditioning after blockade of central DA neurotransmission with drugs or lesions has been explained as an inability to initiate movements rather than as a disruption of learning mechanisms per se. However, an attentional impairment following disruption of mesofrontal or mesoseptal DA systems has been inferred (30) from performance on an alternation hole board learning task (conditioned blocking). Here increases in behaviors collateral to task performance were observed after dopamine-depleting lesions of the frontal cortex, septum, and medial ventral mesencephalon. The level of DA activity (or the balance between the DA and noradrenaline projections) in frontal and limbic regions can contribute to both efficient associative conditioning and the normal ability of rats not to ignore a redundant stimulus (see ref. 21).

Mesoaccumbens DA Transmission and Ventral Striatum System

Studies on the ventral striatum have led to the hypothesis that this region mediates communications between neural systems involved in motivation, emotion, and movement or ongoing behavior (4,25). Several behavioral investigations (see ref. 21) led to the conclusion that DA terminal lesions induce hypoexploration, failure to inhibit response strategies, and, more generally, a perseveration syndrome with reduced distraction caused by irrelevant information and decreased behavioral switching and flexibility and paradoxical locomotor disinhibition in an emotional context. In addition, these lesioned animals exhibited an enhanced latency in the initiation of motor

responses, disturbances in the acquisition of spatial discrimination, and great difficulty in reversing previously learned habits. However, after acquisition has taken place, subsequent lesions do not impair retention.

The behavioral changes caused by these lesions appear to result partly from an inability to switch from one behavioral activity to another and to organize complex behaviors, such as hoarding activities (see ref. 21). Such lesions also disrupt the acquisition of a displacement activity, such as schedule-induced polydipsia. DA neurons in the ventral striatum have been implicated in psychostimulant self-administration; both acquisition and retention are suppressed after lesion of these neurons. Also, a direct relationship has been found to exist between dopamine utilization in the ventral striatum and the intensity of physical, environmental or social stimuli: The more stressful the signal, the more altered the DA activity (see ref. 21).

However, it is difficult to destroy the mesoaccumbens DA projections without affecting the other DA forebrain projections that course through this area. Vigorous sprouting of remaining axons associated with increased rates of transmitter synthesis and an enhancement of postsynaptic dopamine receptor plasticity occur in this region (see Chapter 4, *this volume*). In addition, anatomical and functional considerations suggest that the prefrontal cortex exerts descending influences upon subcortical regions, nucleus accumbens, septum, and the ventral mesencephalon itself. For instance, both dopamine receptors and turnover increase in accumbens after selective lesion in the prefrontal cortex.

Mesocortical DA Transmission

Increased Reactivity of Cortical DA Neurons During Arousal, Environmental Challenges, and Stressful Situations

Data from many groups suggest that the corticofrontal region is important for the representation and the evaluation of situations as being potential stress. In a conditioned fear situation (i.e., after exposure to an environment previously paired with footshocks), increased dopamine utilization is a general phenomenon related to various types of anxiety, adaptive situations, and representations (see ref. 21). A 3-min electric footshock session more effectively enhanced dopamine utilization in the frontal cortex of isolated rats when compared to those living in groups. However, long-term isolation in the rat greatly reduces dopamine utilization in the mesofrontal DA transmission (12 weeks of isolation), but it increases utilization in the mesoaccumbens or mesostriatal projections. After rats that had been isolated for 8 weeks were kept in groups for 4 weeks, a relative increase in the DA metabolites occurred, with values between those of the controls and those of rats isolated for 12 weeks (2). These results also suggested the existence of interneuronal regulations between the various DA projections, because an increase in dopamine utilization in a given projection field was accompanied by a decrease in another field and suggested that the meso-prefrontal DA neurons may exert inhibitory effects on the activity of DA neurons innervating subcortical structures (21). Further support for this hypothesis comes from studies of electrolytic lesions of the ventral tegmentum (see ref. 21) where the correlation between the increase in locomotor activity and the decrease in dopamine content in the frontal cortex and nucleus accumbens suggests that DA neurons play a prominent and inhibitory role in prefrontal cortex functioning.

DA mesoaccumbens activation may indirectly reflect the functioning of the prefrontal cortex in adaptive, representational, or stressful situations and may explain why in some situations the mesoaccumbens DA projection is also activated. A mild, 8-min tail pressure causes a large and sustained (longer than 2 hr) increase in dopamine utilization in the nucleus accumbens but not in the prefrontal cortex, as measured by extracellular DOPAC using in vivo voltammetry (22). A specific increase in DOPAC levels was also observed in the nucleus accumbens 1 hr after stress in postmortem biochemical assays (6). Moreover, the increase in DA metabolites was antagonized by pretreatment with benzodiazepine or other anxiolytic drugs. It is interesting to note that restraint associated with cold increases DOPAC levels in the frontal cortex but not in the nucleus accumbens (21), whereas electric footshock stress increases DOPAC in both brain regions (21,47), and immobilization stress increases dopamine utilization selectively in the nucleus accumbens (48). Carlson et al. (5) showed that 24 hr of food deprivation in rats produced an increase in DOPAC levels in the medial prefrontal cortex but not in the ventral or dorsal striatum. Explanations for these differences may include the anatomical relationships of the frontal cortex. The frontal cortex may be considered as a visceral cortex involved in the recognition of autonomic signals and reciprocally connected with the hypothalamus. Stimulation of the medial frontal cortex decreases gastric motility, and the prefrontal cortex seems to have an inhibitory pathway to the medial hypothalamus, which has also been implicated in the regulation of feeding.

The Mesocortical DA Projections and Cognitive Processes

It is now generally agreed that the prefrontal neuronal system mainly includes the prefrontal cortex and the anteromedial part of the striatum which receives afferents not only from the mediodorsal thalamic nucleus but also from the prefrontal cortex. The prefrontal cortex in the rat is defined anatomicofunctionally as the region to which ef-

ferent fibers project from the mediodorsal thalamic nucleus. However, some VTA DA neurons project to the anteromedial part of the caudate nucleus (see ref. 26).

Delayed-response tasks are generally considered to be particularly susceptible to cognitive deficits after lesions of the prefrontal system in all species of mammals. The mesoprefrontal DA projections are also involved in cognitive processes, especially those required for performing delayed alternation tasks. 6-OHDA lesion of the terminals in the prefrontal cortex or in the anterior and medial parts of the striatum induced a deterioration of the preoperative performance of lesioned rats (see Table 1). During the postoperative learning period, treated rats exhibited collateral behaviors (suggestive of enhanced distractability such as rearing, stopping, and returning) before entering the chosen arm of the T maze, but these same rats were able to learn normally a visual discrimination task for food reward. Similar deficits were observed after prefrontal cortex and anteromedial striatum lesions, resembling the effects of a large lesion of the frontal cortex. Thus, the deficits observed characterized a kind of DA disconnection syndrome for the region to which the DA neurons projected. However, the exact nature of the impaired function is more difficult to explain.

In support of this hypothesis, 6-OHDA lesions of DA terminals in monkey prefrontal association cortex impaired performance of delayed alternation spatial tasks (3,12). This impairment was nearly as severe as that caused by surgical ablation of the same area, but could be temporarily reversed by systemic injections of either L-dopa or apomorphine. Dopamine augments the activity of prefrontal neurons involved in temporal integration of external cues and motor performance, including spatial short-term memory and predictive processes (42). Moreover, an activation of D1-type dopamine receptors appears to be responsible for the increased activity in prefrontal neurons related to the performance of the task. In this respect, it is interesting that the frontal syndrome has also been interpreted in terms of impaired selective attention. The increased locomotor activity that occurs after 6-OHDA-selective or RF lesion of the medial prefrontal cortex or of the DA cells in the ventral mesencephalon may be related to attentional deficits, and the hyperactivity–hypoexploration syndrome caused by RF lesion of the mesencephalic cell bodies is at least partly due to a complex imbalance within the DA cortical system (see ref. 21).

Conclusion

Taken as a whole, data from frontal cortex, nucleus accumbens, and septal and amygdala regions (for details, see ref. 21) demonstrate that the functional effects of DA terminal lesions are as varied as the number of projections investigated. However, lesions of the cell bodies induce

TABLE 1. *Acquisition and retention of a delayed alternation task.*
Effect of different DA terminal regions in corticolimbic systems

Group	Errors in the 60 first trials (mean ± SEM)		Trials for learning criterion	
	Preoperative	Postoperative	Preoperative	Postoperative
Control	17.6 ± 0.9	6.9 ± 8.4	190.0 ± 8.4	86.7 ± 11.4
Anterior striatum	17.2 ± 0.7	18.2 ± 3.0**,a	183.3 ± 46.4	2132.3 ± 46.4*,a
Prefrontal cortex	17.6 ± 0.9	17.3 ± 2.7**,a	193.3 ± 16.1	153.3 ± 27.7*,a
Nucleus accumbens	17.3 ± 1.2	14.2 ± 1.2**,a	160.0 ± 12.7	192 ± 42.7*,a

[a] Nonsignificantly different from preoperative measures.
Student's *t*-test: * $p < 0.01$; ** $p < 0.001$.

profound adaptive disability, presumably reflecting deficits in all the projection areas. Selective lesions of the different DA projections provoke different behavioral syndromes which characterize the deafferentated neuronal system. The various projections function in an interdependent manner and are stimulated either from the bottom (i.e., the reticular formation) or from the top (i.e., the various integrative regions where they project). This integrated set defines the network (Fig. 1).

These considerations confirm a nonspecific activational role of the DA transmission, necessary but not sufficient for organization of adaptive behaviors. DA neurons are necessary because if they are not present—and only minute amounts may be necessary—the neurophysiological functions and integrative processes do not operate. They are not sufficient because if the other systems are pushed

or if the external or internal environments have urgent needs, the systems in imbalance can temporarily recover. DA neurons do not appear to regulate specific function or behavior, and the patterns of activity of these neurons do not support such an integrative capability.

DA NETWORK AND BRAIN FUNCTIONING: A HOLISTIC APPROACH

Behavioral Correlates of the Activation of DA Neurons

When DA neurons are stimulated—for instance, by high doses of psychostimulant drugs—the behavioral response rate also increases but, in parallel, the responses show less variation or adaptability, leading to stereotypy (repetition of invariant sequences of behavior). This drug response phenomenon yields an inverted "U-shaped" dose–response curve to increasing doses of psychostimulant. As described elegantly by Lyon and Robbins (23), a shift occurs from a progressive facilitation of response sequencing to a progressively disorganized and fragmented behavior, from complex patterns to simple ones, and from a sensorimotor facilitation and environment exploration, flexibility, and adaptation to a channeling of sensorimotor integration and eventually to a massive activation of the motor output system which closes the organism to the environment and binds the subject to stereotypy and routines (23) (see Fig. 2). It can be inferred that the more these executive systems are stimulated, the greater the number of routines that are selected and the fewer the number of environmental controls that are possible—that is the greater the number of extrapyramidal output systems that are involved, repeating motor schemes over and again (39).

Based on local infusion of agonists and lesion studies, psychostimulant-induced locomotion may result from a facilitation of the DA transmission in the nucleus accumbens and not of dorsal striatum (21,23). For example, DA transmission blockade or 6-OHDA lesion of the dorsal striatum blocks amphetamine-induced stereotypy, while lesion of the ventral striatum has no such effect, but

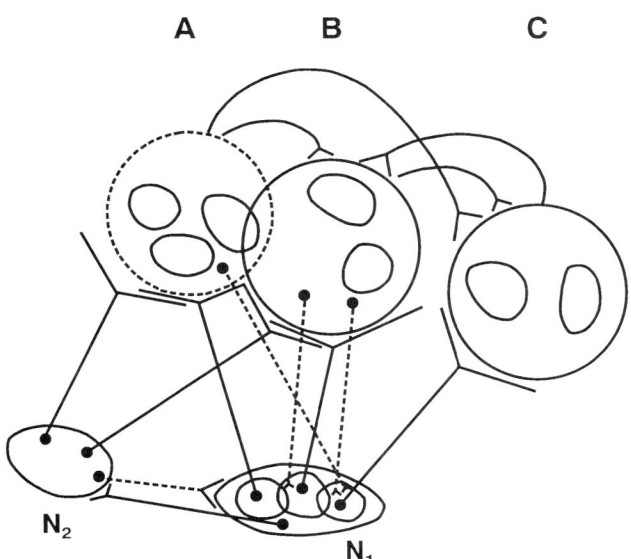

FIG. 1. Symbolic representation of the DA neuroregulation. Selective groups of DA neurons (N1) project onto different forebrain regions (A, B, and C) that are assumed to have integrative and executive functions. Feedback does exist between these regions and DA neurons; moreover, the integrative regions communicate. The DA neurons are themselves modulated by other neurotransmitters N2 (such as serotonin) and by steroids.

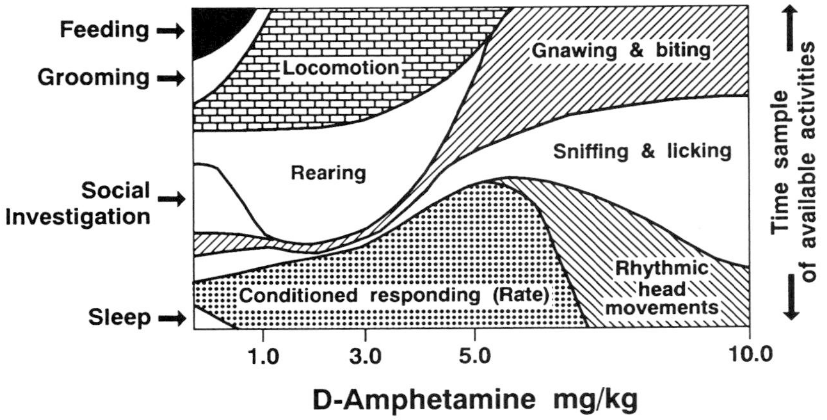

FIG. 2. Schematic drawing depicting the relative distribution of various behavioral activities within a given time sample relative to increasing doses of dextroamphetamine. Note that as the dose increases, the number of activities decreases but the rate of behavior within a given behavioral activity increases. (Redrawn from ref. 23, with permission.)

blocks the locomotor activation produced by amphetamines. However, this anatomical functional dichotomy—that is, dorsal striatum stereotypy versus ventral striatum locomotion—has probably been oversimplified. DA activation of the dorsal striatum might be a necessary but certainly not sufficient condition for amphetamine-induced stereotypy. Intra-accumbens injection of psychostimulants dose-dependently increases locomotion as well as stereotypy, so the ventral striatum may have a more important role than the dorsal striatum in the initiation of the locomotor and stereotyped effects of the psychostimulants than was previously thought (see ref. 21).

The whole striatum operates under the control of the neuronal systems involved in motivation, arousal, and cognitive processes. These processes modulate investigative behaviors initiated by motivation and trigger activity in the striatal DA system essential for appropriate sensorimotor coordination (14). At lower psychostimulant drug doses, stimulation of the DA mesoaccumbens pathway appears first, modifying the ventral striatum–ventral pallidum output system. Then the ventral striatum promotes further activity in the DA projection to the anteromedial and anteroventral striatum and lastly then enhances the activation of the mesostriatal (dorsolateral caudatus) pathway. These successive instructions are translated into behavioral sequences: locomotion, head and oral movements, then stereotyped features. As the dose of stimulant increases, the behavioral responses are occluded, arising from the occurrence of intense head and oral movements, sniffing, and the disappearance of locomotor hyperactivity. Of course, this succession of actions also involves non-DA output pathways and a diffuse set of regions and subsystems (see ref. 21). Various chemical stimulations and lesions have been found to replicate or reduce the psychostimulant-induced locomotor or stereotyped responses: sniffing and biting are induced via the substantia nigra reticulata, oral stereotypies are obtained via the superior colliculus, the thalamus is involved in posture, the reticular formation is involved in head turns, and the ventral pallidum and the mesencephalic locomotor regions mediate some aspects of the locomotor response.

In conclusion, the DA projections of the ventral and dorsal striatum may serve as filtering and gating mechanisms for signals from the limbic regions (i.e., for basic biological drives and motivational variables) and from the neocortex (i.e., for signals of a cognitive nature), which have to be synchronized and eventually translated into motor acts through the pallidal and pontine motor nuclei (9,25). This synchronization of sensorimotor integration (dorsal striatum) and motivational and energizing processes (ventral striatum) allows the initiation of specific responses appropriate to the moment-to-moment changes in the environment as the behavioral sequence progresses. Multiple motor subsystems exist (Fig. 3) which function normally at a low dose of psychostimulant in a coordinated manner, and dopamine regulates the entity which dissolves into dysfunctional parts when the neuroregulator fails to act in a coordinated fashion.

Adaptive Responses and Involvement of the DA Neurons

Any change in the functioning of the DA neurons will have repercussions on adaptive capacities and their brain–body indexes. For example, schedule-induced behaviors have frequently been used as behavioral models of adaptation. Dopamine depletion in the ventral striatum blocks the acquisition of water intake response during a scheduled food delivery test. Lesion of the DA mesoseptal projection leads to the reverse effect—that is, to an increase in the acquisition rate with the same type of behavioral response (21). Thus, animals placed under scheduled food delivery conditions have significantly increased plasma corticosterone, brain endorphin levels, and analgesia compared to rats given nonscheduled food. Conversely, rats which were free to engage in excessive drinking or other displacement activities showed a significant reduction in these hormonal responses (45,46). Interestingly, a DA terminal lesion in the ventral striatum abolished the increase in corticosterone levels in rats subjected to a schedule of food delivery. This suggests that the DA

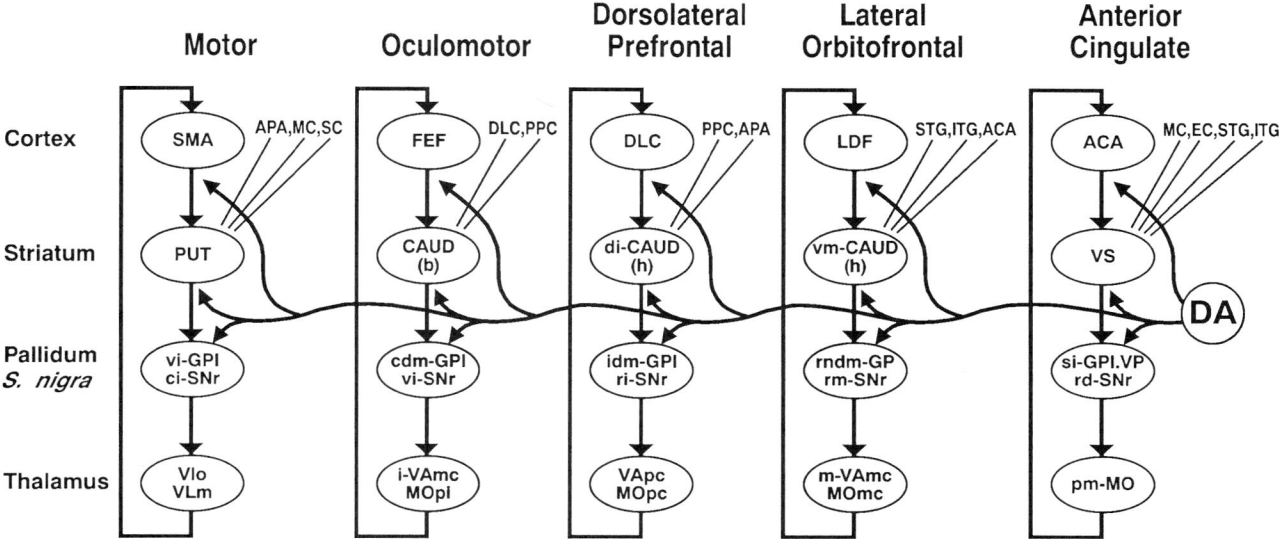

FIG. 3. Parallel organization of the five ganglia-thalamocortical circuits. Note that each circuit engages specific regions at four levels of integration of the forebrain and that the DA network regulates and coordinates the functioning of each circuit from a set of cells and allows each element to function in relation to the others. ACA, anterior cingulate area; APA, arcuate premotor area; CAUD, caudate; b, body; h, head; DLC, dorsolateral prefrontal cortex; EC, entorhinal cortex; FEF, frontal eye fields; GPi, internal segment of globus pallidus; HC, hippocampal cortex; ITG, inferior temporal gyrus; LOF, lateral orbitofrontal cortex; MC, motor cortex; MDpl, medialis dorsalis pars paralamellaris; MDmc, medialis dorsalis pars magnocellularis; MDpc, medialis dorsalis pars parvocellularis; PPC, posterior parietal cortex; PUT, putamen; SC, somatosensory cortex; SMA, supplementary motor area; SNr, substantia nigra pars reticulata; STG, superior temporal gyrus; VAmc, ventralis anterior pars magnocellularis; Vaps, ventralis anterior pars parvocellularis; VLm, ventralis lateralis pars medialis; VLo, ventralis lateralis pars oralis; VP, ventral pallidum; VS, ventral striatum; cl, caudolateral; cdm, caudal dorsomedial; dl, dorsolateral; l, lateral; ldm, lateral dorsomedial; m, medial; mdm, medial dorsomedial; pm, posteromedial; rd, rostrodorsal; rl, rostrolateral; rm, rostromedial; vm, ventromedial; vl, ventrolateral. (Redrawn from ref. 1, with permission.)

pathways are involved at a more general level in this kind of adaptive response.

Recent data have indicated that the DA neurons possess receptors to corticosterone (13) which might make them receptive to arousing or stressful situations. Glucocorticoids may potentiate the activation of biogenic amine response to stress and then help the neuronal system to oppose the neural action of this potentially deleterious stress and restore the homeostatic balance. Repeated intermittent treatment with the psychostimulant or stress and induced increases in plasma corticosterone produced enduring changes in the response of DA neurons and that of the pituitary to subsequent stress. Stress clearly changes the dopamine metabolism in the ventral striatum as well as in the frontal cortex (21,47).

The linking of DA functioning, adaptive capacities, and coping is particularly evident with stress that cannot be controlled. For example, rats receiving an identical amount of stress from electric footshock, but allowed to control its duration, displayed much less stereotypy than did stressed rats (21). These data are integrated between several well-established findings: (i) the inducing and precipitating role of psychostimulants in psychopathological

states; (ii) the role of stress in the relapse and precipitation of these psychopathological states; (iii) the sensitizing effects of either psychostimulants or stress—both of which are interchangeable—on the DA neurons; and (iv) the importance of individual differences as regards the vulnerability and the sensitivity to the drug or stress precipitating effects.

These findings have led to the hypothesis that the effects of stress or sensitization to psychostimulants may depend on these individual coping mechanisms. As described above, displacement activity such as schedule-induced polydipsia stabilizes an organism that is disrupted by conflicts or by being prevented from reaching a goal and is adaptive roles through its de-arousing effects as shown by the decrease of costicosterone level and blockade of endogenous pain inhibitory systems (45,46). Moreover, repeated administrations of psychostimulants and DA neuron manipulation facilitate the development of displacement activities, and coping with conflicting situations is related to enhanced activity in the dopaminergic neurons. Stress-reducing properties of adjunctive behavior reduces responsiveness to psychostimulants. Some rats learn the task and drink whereas others never learn, even after repeated sessions. Only the polydipsic rats displayed a lower behavioral activation in response to a low dose of amphetamine, whereas the nonpolydipsic rats and the rats without access to water and which were not able to engage in a displacement activity did not; that is, a reduced activation and desensitization of the DA neurons were revealed by the lower response to amphetamine. These results support the hypothesis that the effects of stress are determined by an individual's self-perceived ability to cope with stressors.

Individual Differences for Dopamine Utilization and for Brain Lateralization

Two other sources of individual differences involve brain asymmetry and sex hormones. Rotational or turning preferences or asymmetrical orienting responses and other lateralized activities in normal animals may be related to differences in DA activity between the left and right basal ganglia, the left and right frontal cortex, and hippocampus (8,21).

Inheritable or epigenetic determinants and sexual hormones such as testosterone also have been shown to contribute to lateralization as well as to sex-related differences in responses to drugs acting on the DA neurons which seem sexually dimorphic. The in vivo presence or absence of gonadal steroids modulate the release of dopamine measured in vitro from striatal tissue fragments obtained from female, but not male, rats (21). Similar differences have been reported in dopamine turnover and fluctuation across the estrous cycle (see ref. 21 for references). The effects of gonadal steroids on the behavioral responses modulated by the DA neurons have been extensively documented, and estrous cycle has been found to influence DA mechanisms in the frontal cortex and possibly in the tuberoinfundibular system (16). Female rats are more sensitive to amphetamine, and they have higher dopamine levels after drug administration in the striatum contralateral to the dominant direction of rotation. Thus, the general reaction of the organism under stress is partly dependent on individual differences to which DA sex-related neuronal asymmetry may contribute, although these individual differences are not yet frequently taken into account.

Plasticity at the Level of the DA Transmission

Behavioral Sensitization After Drug Administration

Chronic administration of indirect DA agonists induces reverse tolerance, or behavioral sensitization (37), to many of the effects on these drugs such as hypothermia, hyperactivity, stereotypy, and even seizures at the higher doses. When the same dose of stimulant is repeated, a progressive increase in locomotor activity occurs. This phenomenon has several characteristics: (i) it reflects a long-lasting change in responsivity which persists weeks and months after withdrawal of the drug; (ii) it involves changes in both the magnitude and the triggering of hyperactivity and stereotypy; (iii) females seem to be more sensitive than males; and (iv) it has been observed in a great variety of animals. Some studies have shown the environmental context and conditioning to play an important role in the process of sensitization and to be crucial for the ultimate degree of expression of drug-induced behavior. However, besides this obviously associative form of sensitization, a more subtle and complex form of long-lasting, time-dependent sensitization has been demonstrated (38). This kind of sensitization is a ubiquitous phenomenon, is demonstrable with a broad spectrum of agents, does not require daily treatment, can be obtained after a simple exposure to a low-to-moderate dose of various psychopharmacologically active drugs or to a stressful situation, is subject to cross-sensitization, and becomes more visible with the passage of time. Dopamine receptor antagonists have been found to block the development of sensitization but not to block it once it has developed (i.e., when given on the test day), suggesting that dopamine transmission is necessary to the occurrence and development of, but not to the expression of, stimulant-induced sensitization (40).

Controversies exist about the respective role of drug–environment conditioning and nonassociative sensitization in the development of behavioral sensitization (40). However, both drug–environment conditioning and sensitization, whether they be considered independently or together, involve long-lasting changes in the neural systems that mediate the behavioral responses measured.

Numerous data show enhanced dopamine metabolism in animals to which a subsequent challenge injection of amphetamine has been administered (for reviews, see refs. (40 and 49), and these changes may be at least partly responsible for behavioral sensitization. These results suggest that repeated exposure to the abnormally high concentration of transmitter released after repeated drug administration causes autoreceptors situated on presynaptic terminals, cell body, and/or dendrites of neurons to become subsensitive. Because these receptors are thought to control dopamine synthesis and release and the discharge rate (see Chapters 15 and 20, *this volume*), any subsensitivity of these receptors would trigger enhanced dopamine release by reducing the negative feedback. However, electrophysiological data here are somewhat contradictory (40). The electrophysiological effects dissipate quickly, unlike the behavioral and biochemical effects; they do not appear after a single drum administration and are often opposite to those predicted by the hypothesis. Also, in vitro, release of dopamine elicited by amphetamine is not modulated by presynaptic autoreceptors. More research is needed to explore the cascade of cellular events underlying the observed behavioral and neurochemical consequences of sensitization.

Involvement of the DA Networks in Electrical and Drug Reinforcement

Electrical stimulation of specific restricted regions of the brain, particularly the medial forebrain bundle and its connections, can initiate and maintain operant behaviors and has provided a powerful means of studying of the neural mechanisms involved in reinforcement and appetitively or aversively motivated learning. Given that DA neurons modulate the activity of most of these regions through the medial forebrain bundle, it is not surprising that considerable modifications of brain stimulation effects have been observed after manipulating the DA transmissions.

Two hypotheses were developed for the role of dopamine in neuronal mechanisms. The first argued for a unitary system, and the DA neurons were said to be a critical link and were misleadingly said to form the ''pleasure centers,'' leading to the ''DA theory of reward'' (50). The second strategy (multiple brain substrates for reward) was based on the fact that self-stimulation has been observed from a large diversity of structures, from all regions of the brain. The highest rates of self-stimulation obtained in the brain are in the VTA and even more in the mesencephalic and pontine raphe nuclei (21), regions through which the dense ascending and descending fibers linking the limbic forebrain–midbrain areas pass.

Furthermore, self-stimulation of many regions of the brain persists after lesion of the DA neurons or of their terminals. The existence of numerous areas from which such self-stimulation can be obtained without any DA influence is incompatible with the concept of a unitary substrate for brain stimulation reward. DA neurons were neither sufficient nor necessary (see ref. 21 for references) for self-stimulation, but may appear to be involved only because they modulate regions which are the authentic neural substrates for reinforcement or for performance (33).

Finally, the use of a quantitative technique for measuring changes in glucose utilization showed that self-stimulation of the medial forebrain bundle including DA fibers activates large neuronal systems including the dorsomedial thalamus, septum, ventral striatum, prefrontal cortex, amygdala, and hippocampus (36), implying that integration across any neuronal brain region plays a more important role than any specific neurotransmitter.

Less artificial than the self-stimulation phenomenon, intravenous drug self-administration (21, 50, and 51) has been studied routinely for the last two decades. Research in this field has direct important strategic implications for the study of drug-seeking addiction and dependence. In one view, a given drug may have a limited neurobiologi-

cal specificity but can activate neuronal circuitries linked to one of the brain's reinforcement systems. Another view promotes the existence of a unique brain mechanism for the reward processes, of which the DA neurons are taken to be the most important component. Alternatively, the various classes of drugs may each have their own impact on specific receptors and synaptic transmissions, in which addiction results from a complex interplay between these separate networks (17). In this view, the DA pathways would be viewed as a more specific substrate for psychostimulant drugs.

In support of this hypothesis, nearly 20 years ago low doses of a dopamine receptor antagonist were reported to increase the response rate for amphetamine and cocaine self-administration in rats (52). These paradoxical results were interpreted as a reduction of the reinforcing effects of the self-administered drug. The partial blockade of the dopamine receptors by low doses of antagonist led the animal to respond more strongly, because higher doses of the drug were now required to maintain the same level of drug reward. The increase in self-administration rate, observed after the dopamine receptor blockade, was qualitatively similar to the effects of decreasing the dose of drug per injection. Higher doses of antagonist induced a complete blockade of the transmission and caused complete extinction of self-administration (52). Large 6-OHDA lesions of the mesocorticolimbic DA system can also produce extinction of already established self-administration (21).

However, in contrast to studies in rats trained for drug self-administration, in drug-naive rats RF or 6-OHDA lesions of the mesocortical or mesolimbic DA cell bodies produce an increase in the rate of acquisition of amphetamine intravenous self-administration (21). This result indicated that the lesioned animals were more sensitive to the effects of the psychostimulant. These studies had three important characteristics which provide some unique insights into the role of the mesocorticolimbic DA system in psychostimulant reinforcement: (i) The dose of amphetamine available per lever-press or nose-poke was very small (7.5 μg/kg was generally used as compared to the usually available dose of at least 100 μg/kg); such low doses make it difficult, if not impossible, for a normal rat to acquire drug self-administration; (ii) most of the other studies (see ref. 21 for references) used an experimental paradigm in which the animals were experimentally manipulated (lesion or receptor blockade) after acquisition and stabilization of the self-administration response rate; and (iii) a two-nose-poke procedure was used during acquisition of drug self-administration, so that it is possible to study the rat's capacity to discriminate between the drug and the vehicle. These results suggest that partial lesions of the DA system may increase vulnerability to acquire self-administration of psychostimulants, perhaps via release of dopamine from remaining terminals

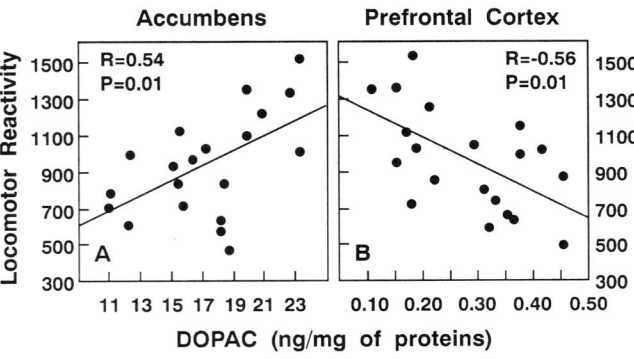

FIG. 4. Dopaminergic activity reduced in the prefrontal cortex and increased in the nucleus accumbens of rats predisposed to develop amphetamine self-administration. **Top:** DOPAC/dopamine ratio of HR and LR animals in basal condition (Basal) and after 30 min [Novelty (30')] and 120 min [Novelty (120')] exposure to novelty (Postmortem measures). HR animals had a lower ratio in the prefrontal cortex ($F_{1,42}$ = 2.89, $p < 0.05$) and a higher one in the nucleus accumbens ($F_{1,42}$ = 13,40, $p < 0.001$) and dorsal striatum ($F_{1,42}$ = 8.41, $p < 0.01$). *$p < 0.05$; **$p < 0.01$. **Bottom:** Correlation between DOPAC content in basal condition and the locomotor reactivity to a mild stress (novelty) in the two regions (nucleus accumbens positively and frontal cortex negatively). (From ref. 34, with permission.)

acting on supersensitive postsynaptic receptors (see Chapter 4, *this volume*).

Lesions of neurons containing the transmitter, serotonin, can also facilitate the acquisition of amphetamine self-administration. The role of serotonin can be explained through changes in dopamine turnover in other regions. After lesion of the raphe, dopamine utilization is enhanced in the nucleus accumbens but decreases in the prefrontal cortex (see ref. 21). Chronic rearing isolation and DA lesion in the amygdala induced the same biochemical pattern and also induced an increased sensitivity to the self-administered drug (7,43). For example,

rats housed in groups reliably fail to self-administer cocaine, whereas weanling rats housed under isolated conditions readily acquired an operant conditioning task to receive infusions of cocaine. Stress or food deprivation also induced changes in stimulant self-administration (20). These data suggest that environmental factors which induce changes in dopamine utilization in some parts of the DA network determine individual differences in the propensity to self-administer the drug. Conversely, a near total lesion of the noradrenergic dorsal bundle leads to the reverse pattern: a decrease in dopamine turnover at the cortical level without any changes in the nucleus accumbens level (see review in ref. 21).

During the last few years, research has focused on individual differences in vulnerability to drug intake and dependence, a fact largely emphasized by clinicians (29), and on factors which may predict such vulnerability. For instance, vulnerability and locomotor reactivity to stressful situations differentiate individuals, and such parameters predict individual vulnerability to drug self-administration (34). Such sensitive animals present a specific pattern of DA activity: The transmitter is reduced in the prefrontal cortex and increased in the nucleus accumbens (35) (Fig. 4); moreover, these vulnerable animals present a higher and longer stress-induced increase in dopamine concentrations in the nucleus accumbens (41).

CONCLUSION

DA neurons have homeostatic and regulatory roles in that they allow the forebrain and cortical neuronal systems to function normally. The DA neurons are closely interrelated and controlled by so many feedbacks that it may be incorrect to conclude that the symptoms observed after restricted manipulations are directly and solely due to a unique set of neurons. A local lesion can bring about increases or decreases in dopamine utilization in the other regions and provokes a new pattern of regulation within the network. A lesion of the DA neurons disturbs many of the brain integrative functions not directly related to the sensory and motor processes (i.e., learning and memory, cognitive functions, and reinforcement processes). These deficits explain why organisms cannot normally survive without dopamine and why DA regulation is essential for the adaptive psychobiological capacities. After lesion these capacities are paradoxically virtually present but latent (i.e., not overtly expressed). They can be restored by L-dopa or various pharmacological treatments or by changes in the external (more than internal) environment (e.g., stress, strong emotional stimulation, arousing situations or stimuli, and cues previously paired with a reinforcer).

Manipulations of the DA neurons may help us to better understand the neurobiological function of the regions to which they project. Dopamine, besides the signal it translates, has a general role in activation; more dopamine, within the physiological limits, increases the adaptative capabilities and the vigor and probability of responses. Thus, a functional concept of the dopamine signal is to activate the final common pathway of several integrative processes.

REFERENCES

1. Alexander GE, De Long MR, Strick PL. Parallel organization of functionally segregated circuits linking basal ganglia and cortex. *Annu Rev Neurosci* 1986;9:357–381.
2. Blanc G, Herve D, Simon H, Lisoprawski A, Glowinski J, Tassin JP. Response to stress of mesocortico-frontal dopaminergic neurones in rats after long-term isolation. *Nature* 1980;284:265–267.
3. Brozoski TJ, Brown RM, Rosvold HE, Goldman PS. Cognitive deficit caused by regional depletion of DA in prefrontal cortex of rhesus monkey. *Science* 1979;205:929–931.
4. Cador M, Robbins JW, Everitt BJ, Simon H, Le Moal M, Stinus L. Limbic–striatal interactions in reward-related processes: modulation by the dopaminergic system. In: Willner P, Sheel-Krüger J, eds. *The mesolimbic dopamine system: from motivation to action.* John Wiley & Sons, 1991;225–250.
5. Carlson JN, Herrick KF, Baird JL, Glick SD. Selective enhancement of dopamine utilization in the rat prefrontal cortex by food deprivation. *Brain Res* 1987;400:200–203.
6. D'Angio M, Serrano A, Rivy JP, Scatton B. Tail-pinch stress increases extracellular DOPAC levels (as measured by in vivo voltammetry) in the rat nucleus accumbens but not frontal cortex: antagonism by diazepam and zolpidem. *Brain Res* 1987;409:169–174.
7. Deminiere JM, Taghzouti K, Tassin JP, Le Moal M, Simon H. Increased sensitivity to amphetamine and facilitation of amphetamine self-administration after 6-hydroxydopamine lesions of the amygdala. *Psychopharmacology* 1988;94:232–236.
8. Diaz-Palarea MD, Gonzalez MC, Rodriguez M. Behavioral lateralization in the T-maze and monoaminergic brain asymmetries. *Physiol Behav* 1987;40:785–789.
9. Gaffori O, Le Moal M. Disruption of maternal behavior and appearance of cannibalism after ventral mesencephalic tegmentum lesions. *Physiol Behav* 1979;23:317–323.
10. Galey D, Jaffard R, Le Moal M. Alternation behavior, spatial discrimination and reversal after electrocoagulation of the ventral mesencephalic tegmentum in the rat. *Behav Neural Biol* 1979;26:81–88.
11. Glick SD, Hinds PA, Carlson JN. Food deprivation and stimulant self-administration in rats: difference between cocaine and *d*-amphetamine. *Psychopharmacology* 1987;91:372–374.
12. Goldman-Rakic PS. Dopamine-mediated mechanisms of the prefrontal cortex. *Semin Neurosci* 1992;4:149–159.
13. Gustafsson JA, Carlstedt-Duke J, Poellinger L, et al. Biochemistry, molecular biology and physiology of the glucocorticoid receptor. *Endocr Rev* 1987;8:185–234.
14. Iversen SD. Brain dopamine system and behavior. In: Iversen LL, Iversen SD, Snyder SH, eds. *Handbook of psychopharmacology,* vol 8. New York: Plenum Press, 1977;334–384.
15. Kalivas PW. Neurotransmitter regulation of dopaminergic neurons in the ventral tegmental area. *Brain Res Rev* 1993;18:75–113.
16. Kazandjian A, Spyraki C, Papadopoulou Z, Sfikakis A, Varonos DD. Behavioral and biochemical effects of haloperidol during the oestrous cycle of the rat. *Neuropharmacology* 1988;27:73–78.
17. Koob GF, Goeders N. Neuroanatomical substrates of drug self-administration. In: Liebman JM, Cooper SJ, eds. *Neuropharmacological basis of reward,* vol 6. New York: Oxford University Press, 1989;214–264.
18. Koob GF, Riley SJ, Smith SC, Robbins TW. Effects of 6-hydroxydopamine lesions of the nucleus accumbens septi and olfactory tubercle on feeding, locomotor activity, and amphetamine anorexia in the rat. *J Comp Physiol Psychol* 1978;92:917–927.
19. Koob GF, Simon H, Herman JP, Le Moal M. Neuroleptic-like

20. Koob GF, Stinus L, Le Moal M. Hyperactivity and hypoactivity produced by lesions to the mesolimbic DA system. *Behav Brain Res* 1981;3:341–359.
21. Le Moal M, Simon H. Mesocorticolimbic dopaminergic network: functional and regulatory roles. *Physiol Rev* 1991;71:155–234.
22. Louilot A, Le Moal M, Simon H. Opposite influences of dopaminergic pathways to the prefrontal cortex or the septum on the dopaminergic transmission in the nucleus accumbens. An in vivo voltammetric study. *Neuroscience* 1989;29:45–56.
23. Lyon M, Robbins TW. The action of central nervous system stimulant drugs: a general theory concerning amphetamine effects. In: Essman W, Valzelli L, eds. *Current developments in psychopharmacology, vol 2.* New York: Spectrum Publications, 1975;79–163.
24. Mittleman GM, Castaneda E, Robinson TE, Valenstein ES. The propensity for nonregulatory ingestive behaviour is related to differences in dopamine systems: behavioural and biochemical evidence. *Behav Neurosci* 1986;100:213–220.
25. Mogenson GJ. Limbic-motor integration. In: Sprague J, Epstein AN, eds. *Progress in psychobiology and physiological psychology, vol. 12.* New York: Academic Press, 1987;117–170.
26. Moore RY, Bloom FE. Central catecholamine neuron system: anatomy and physiology of the dopamine systems. *Annu Rev Neurosci* 1978;1:129–169.
27. Nauta WJH. Hippocampal projections and related neural pathways to the midbrain in the cat. *Brain* 1958;81:319–340.
28. Nisenbaum ES, Stricker EM, zigmond MJ, Berger TW. Long-term effects of dopamine-depleting brain lesions on spontaneous activity of type II striatal neurons: relation to behavioral recovery. *Brain Res* 1986;398:221–230.
29. O'Brien CP, Ehrman RN, Terns JM. Classical conditioning in human opioid dependence. In: Goldberg SR, Stolerman IP, eds. *Behavioral analysis of drug dependence.* London: Academic Press, 1986;329.
30. Oades RD, Rivet JM, Taghzouti K, Kharouby M, Simon H, Le Moal M. Catecholamines and conditioned blocking: effects of ventral tegmental, septal and frontal 6-hydroxydopamine lesions in rats. *Brain Res* 1987;406:136–146.
31. Oades RD, Taghzouti K, Rivet JM, Simon H, Le Moal M. Locomotor activity in relation to dopamine and noradrenaline in the nucleus accumbens, septal and frontal areas: a 6-hydroxydopamine study. *Neuropsychobiology* 1986;16:37–42.
32. Papp M, Bal A. Separation of the motivational and motor consequences of 6-hydroxydopamine lesions of the mesolimbic or nigrostriatal system in rats. *Behav Brain Res* 1987;23:221–229.
33. Phillips AG, Jakubovic A, Fibiger HC. Increased in vivo tyrosine hydroxylase activity in rat telencephalon produced by self-stimulation of the ventral tegmental area. *Brain Res* 1987;402:109–116.
34. Piazza PV, Deminiere J-M, Le Moal M, Simon H. Factors that predict individual vulnerability to amphetamine self-administration. *Science* 1989;245:1511–1513.
35. Piazza PV, Rouge-Pont F, Deminiere JM, Kharouby M, Le Moal M, Simon H. Dopamine activity is reduced in the prefrontal cortex and increased in the nucleus accumbens of rats predisposed to develop amphetamine self-administration. *Brain Res* 1991;567:169–174.
36. Porrino LJ, Esposito RU, Seeger TF, Crane AM, Pert A, Sokoloff L. Metabolic mapping of the brain during rewarding self-stimulation. *Science* 1984;224:306–309.
37. Post RM, Contel NR. Human and animal studies of cocaine: implications for development of behavioral pathology. In: Creese I, ed. *Stimulants: neurochemical, behavioral and clinical perspectives.* New York: Raven Press, 1983;169–203.
38. Post RM, Weiss SRB, Pert A. The role of context and conditioning in behavioral sensitization to cocaine. *Psychopharmacol Bull* 1987;23:425–429.
39. Robbins TW, Everitt BJ. Functional studies of the central catecholamines. *Int Rev Neurobiol* 1982;23:303–365.
40. Robinson TE, Becker JB. Enduring changes in brain and behavior produced by chronic amphetamine administration: a review and evaluation of animal models of amphetamine psychosis. *Brain Res Rev* 1986;11:157–198.

41. Rouge-Pont F, Piazza PV, Kharouby M, Le Moal M, Simon H. Higher and longer stress-induced increase in dopamine concentrations in the nucleus accumbens of animals predisposed to amphetamine self-administration. A microdialysis study. *Brain Res* 1993;602:169–174.

42. Sawaguchi T, Matsumuea M, Kubota K. Catecholaminergic effects on neuronal activity related to a delayed response task in monkey prefrontal cortex. *J Neurophysiol* 1990;63:1385–1400.

43. Simon H, Taghzouti K, Gozlan H, et al. Lesion of dopaminergic terminals in the amygdala produces enhanced locomotor response to *d*-amphetamine and opposite changes in dopaminergic activity in prefrontal cortex and nucleus accumbens. *Brain Res* 1988;447:335–340.

44. Stinus L, Gaffori O, Simon H, Le Moal M. Disappearance of hoarding and disorganization of eating behavior after ventral mesencephalic tegmentum lesion in rats. *J Comp Physiol Psychol* 1978;92:288–296.

45. Tazi A, Dantzer R, Le Moal M. Schedule-induced polydipsia experience decreases locomotor response to amphetamine. *Brain Res* 1988;445:211–215.

46. Tazi A, Dantzer R, Mormede P, Le Moal M. Pituitary–adrenal correlates of schedule-induced polydipsia and wheel running in rats. *Behav Brain Res* 1986;19:249–256.

47. Thierry AM, Tassin JP, Blanc G, Glowinski J. Selective activation of the mesocortical dopaminergic system by stress. *Nature* 1976;263:242–244.

48. Watanabe H. Activation of dopamine synthesis in mesolimbic dopamine neurons by immobilization stress in the rat. *Neuropharmacology* 1984;23:1335–1338.

49. Willner P, Sanger M, Emmett-Oglesby M. Behavioural sensitization. *Behav Pharmacol* 1993;4:298–463.

50. Wise RA. The dopamine synapse and the notion of "pleasure centers" in the brain. *Trends Neurosci* 1980;3:91–94.

51. Wise RA, Bozarth MA. A psychomotor stimulant theory of addiction. *Psychol Rev* 1987;94:469–492.

52. Yokel RA, Wise RA. Attenuation of intravenous amphetamine reinforcement by central dopamine blockade in rats. *Psychopharmacology* 1976;48:311–318.

Psychopharmacology: The Fourth Generation of Progress, edited by Floyd E. Bloom and David J. Kupfer. Raven Press, Ltd., New York © 1995.

CHAPTER **26**

Dopamine Receptors

Clinical Correlates

Philip Seeman

DOPAMINE RECEPTORS, SCHIZOPHRENIA, PARKINSON'S DISEASE, AND HUNTINGTON'S CHOREA

Brain dopamine receptors are the primary targets in the treatment of schizophrenia, Parkinson's disease, and Huntington's chorea. Dopamine receptor antagonists, or neuroleptics, are often effective in blocking hallucinations and delusions which occur in these diseases, whereas dopamine receptor agonists such as bromocriptine are effective in alleviating the signs of Parkinson's disease.

The discovery and direct detection of dopamine receptors originally depended on the existence of stereoselective antipsychotic drugs (50). While the antipsychotic drugs then permitted the discovery of dopamine receptors, the cloned dopamine receptors are now in turn facilitating the search and discovery of more selective antipsychotic drugs and antiparkinsonian drugs. A current hope is that more selective therapy can be achieved by developing drugs which are more selective for a particular subtype of the dopamine receptors (49) (see also Chapters 14, 19, 20, 100, 106, and 109, *this volume*).

DOPAMINE D1-LIKE AND D2-LIKE RECEPTORS

The original classification of two main groups of dopamine receptors—namely, D1-like and D2-like dopamine receptors—still stands (61). The currently known and cloned dopamine receptors fall into these two classes.

The dopamine D1-like receptors include D1 and D5

P. Seeman: Departments of Pharmacology and Psychiatry, University of Toronto, Toronto, Ontario M5S 1A8, Canada.

(63,64), with two pseudogenes related to D5 (37). The pseudogenes are so named because they code for incomplete forms of the dopamine D5 receptor, wherein the protein stops at 154 amino acids instead of an expected full-length dopamine D5 receptor of 477 amino acids. These 154-amino-acid proteins (37) are not expected to have the usual receptor functions.

There are three main types of dopamine D2-like receptors: D2, D3, and D4. The dopamine D2 receptor has two variants, D2(short) and D2(long), the difference being a 29-amino-acid peptide coded by an exon which is missing (i.e., spliced out) in D2short (40). The dopamine D3 receptor (25,59) also has two variants: D3(long) (25) and D3(short) (23).

The dopamine D4 receptor (41,66,67), the gene for which is at the end of the short arm of chromosome 11, has at least eight polymorphic variants in the human. Each variant has a different number of repeat units (located in the third cytoplasmic loop of the receptor protein). Each repeat consists of 16 amino acids. Most humans (50–70%, depending on the ethnic composition) have four repeats, and this receptor is named the dopamine D4.4 receptor. No humans have yet been found to have dopamine D4.0, D4.1, or D4.9 receptors (33), as indicated in Table 1.

In addition to the number of repeats varying in the human dopamine D4 receptor, there are at least 21 different types of repeat units (33), each repeat type identified as α, β, θ, η, ε, ζ, γ, κ, ν, σ, ρ, μ, ψ, δ, ι, λ, o, π, or ξ. For example, one person may have a dopamine D4.4 receptor with repeat types α, β, θ, and ζ, such that his/her D4.4 receptor may be named D4.4$\alpha\beta\theta\zeta$. The first and last repeat types (repeat types α and ζ) are the same in all individuals (33). Table 1 lists examples of these different dopamine D4 receptors.

TABLE 1. *Examples of human variants of dopamine D4 receptors*

D4.0	Not found
D4.1	Not found
D4.2	D4.2 $\alpha\zeta$
D4.3	D4.3 $\alpha\beta\zeta$
D4.4	D4.4 $\alpha\beta\alpha\zeta$
	D4.4 $\alpha\beta\beta\zeta$
	D4.4 $\alpha\beta\theta\zeta$
	D4.4 $\alpha\beta\delta\zeta$
	D4.4 $\alpha\beta\lambda\zeta$
	etc.
D4.5	D4.5 $\alpha\beta$ooζ
	D4.5 $\alpha\beta$ooζ
	etc.
D4.6	D4.6 $\alpha\beta$oooζ
	D4.6 $\alpha\beta$oooζ
	etc.
D4.7	D4.7 $\alpha\beta$ooooζ
	etc.
D4.8	D4.8 $\alpha\beta$oooooζ
	etc.
D4.9	Not found
D4.10	D4.10 $\alpha\beta$oooooooooζ
	etc.

Where o indicates any repeat unit of the 21 types: α, β, γ, δ, ϵ, θ, . . . , ζ.

The different phenotypes and genotypes of the human dopamine D4 receptor preclude a simple nomenclature for the D2-like receptors, such as D2A for D2, D2B for D3, or D2C for D4, as has been suggested by others (17,58). Otherwise, the D4.4 receptor would be D2C.4 or D2C.4$\alpha\beta\theta\zeta$, both excessively complex to remember or to use verbally. Moreover, at present there is considerable confusion on the use of D2A and D2B. For example, D2B has been used to refer to D2(short) (15), to D3 (58), and to D4 (17).

PHARMACOLOGY OF DOPAMINE RECEPTORS

The drug sensitivities of the cloned D1 and D5 dopamine receptors are generally the same as those for D1 receptors in native tissues, as summarized in Tables 2 and 3. This is readily apparent for the antagonists (Table 3), including a higher stereoselective potency for R-(+)-sulpiride compared to S-(−)-sulpiride.

For dopamine agonists, however, it has been difficult to obtain accurate comparisons of the agonist sensitivities of the cloned receptors with those in native tissues. This is because dopamine receptors in native tissues can adopt

TABLE 2. *Agonist dissociation constants for dopamine receptors*

		D1-like group			D2-like group			
Agonist	State*	D1 native[a] (nM)	D1 clones (nM)	D5 clones (nM)	D2 native[b] (nM)	D2 clones (nM)	D3 clones (nM)	D4 clones (nM)
Apomorphine-(−)	High[c]	0.7			0.7	39		
	Low[d]	206	417	252	127	86	32	
Bromocriptine	[e]	439	672	454	4.8	12	4.8	285
Dopamine	High	0.9	~250	~18	7.5	~33	~4	~30
	Low	383	~2,000	228	4,300	924	31	50−150
Fenoldopam-R	High	0.8		~0.6	2.8			
	Low	45	~33	~18	1,000			
Pergolide	High	0.8	0.8		~0.8			
	Low	322	1,363	918	60	~20	~1.5	
(+)PHNO	High	80			0.5	~81		
	Low	5,000			645	147		
Quinpirole	High	1,200	1,900		4.8	~4.8		
	Low	42,000	42,000	50,000	3,680	~800	~17	
SKF 38393	High	1.1		~0.5	157			
	Low	381	~128	~80	8,800	~9,560	5,000	

[a] Native: Calf brain striatum and/or calf parathyroid used for native D1 receptors.
[b] Native: Pig anterior pituitary and/or canine brain striatum used for native D2 receptors.
[c] High = high-affinity state of receptor.
[d] Low = low-affinity state of receptor, or dissociation constant from IC50%.
[e] High- and low-affinity states for bromocriptine are identical.

D1 references: 16,48,63−65.
D2 references: 10,14,24,31,36,42,59,60,62.
D3 references: 42,45,59,60.
D4 references: 66,67.
D5 references: 29,48,64,65,69.

TABLE 3. *Antagonist dissociation constants for dopamine receptors*

Antagonist	D1-like group			D2-like group			
	D1 native[a] nM	D1 clones nM	D5 clones nM	D2 native[b] nM	D2 clones nM	D3 clones nM	D4 clones nM
Chlorpromazine	94	73	133	3	1.4	4.4	35
Clozapine (no Na)				86			6
Clozapine (with Na)	172	141	331	229	216	174	21
Emonapride				0.06	0.06	0.3	0.09
Haloperidol	55–102	26	98	1.2	1	~4–10	2.3
Melperone				240	182		~460
Olanzapine				45			27
Raclopride	18,000			1.8	1.8	3.5	1500
Remoxipride				~300	178	2,300	~2,000
Risperidone				5.6			7
SCH 23390	0.17	0.37	0.3	1,690	634	780	~3,000
Spiperone	212	~350	~3,500	0.06	0.07	0.6	0.08
Sulpiride-S-(−)	57,000	34,500	77,270	15	18	~13	1,005
Sulpiride-R-(+)	12,000	25,800	28,636	868	347	422	965

[a] Native: Calf brain striatum and/or calf parathyroid used for native D1 receptors.
[b] Native: Pig anterior pituitary and/or brain striatum (human or canine) for native D2.

D1 references: 16,29,63–65,69.
D2 references: 10,12,22,24,28,45,59,60,62.
D3 references: 2,32,45,59,60.
D4 references: 66,67.
D5 references: 63–65,69.

either a high-affinity state or a low-affinity state for an agonist, whereas tissue culture cells vary in their ability to reveal the high-affinity state. For example, African green monkey kidney tissue culture cells, which are often used to express the cloned dopamine receptors, do not have sufficient or appropriate G-protein subunits to allow the high-affinity state of the receptor to exist. Thus, the high-affinity data for agonists in Table 2 are incomplete at present. However, an important consistent difference between the D1 and D5 receptors is that dopamine itself is about 10 times more potent at the D5 receptor.

Accurate values for many of the agonist potencies on the dopamine D2, D3, and D4 receptors are not currently available, for the same reason as just mentioned above for D1 receptors. Nevertheless, some important selectivities are clearly emerging. For example, bromocriptine is about two orders of magnitude more potent at D2 and D3, compared to D4, as indicated in Table 2. Moreover, 7-hydroxy-dipropylaminotetralin (or 7-DPAT) is approximately 10-fold more potent at D3, compared to D2 (see D3 references of Tables 2 and 3).

In the case of antagonists, clozapine is approximately one order of magnitude more potent at D4 than at D2 or D3, as shown in Table 3. Chlorpromazine, however, is about one order weaker at D4, while raclopride is about two orders weaker at D4, compared to D2 or D3. Sulpiride is not stereoselective at D4.

SCHIZOPHRENIA, CLOZAPINE AND DOPAMINE RECEPTORS

The dopamine hypothesis of schizophrenia proposes that brain dopamine synapses are overactive in schizo-phrenia (see references in ref. 47). This overactivity may stem from either an excess release of dopamine or an overactive response by the dopamine receptors. Most evidence for the hypothesis of dopamine overactivity in schizophrenia relies on the fact that neuroleptics block dopamine D2 receptors in direct relation to their clinical antipsychotic potencies (47,50) (see also Chapters 100, 106, and 107, *this volume*).

Up to now, however, clozapine had been an exception to this rule, because clozapine blocks dopamine D2 receptors at concentrations which are 20 times higher than the concentration range of 10–20 nM found in the spinal fluid of clozapine-treated patients (data of J. Lieberman et al., 1991, as analyzed in ref. 47).

Hence, the cloning of the dopamine D4 receptor now provides new insight on the dopamine hypothesis, because this receptor is blocked at precisely the clozapine concentrations (10–20 nM) found in the spinal fluid of clozapine-medicated patients. As indicated in Fig. 1, the affinities of the various neuroleptics for the dopamine D2 and D4 receptors indicate that therapeutic concentrations of antipsychotic drugs act at dopamine D2 receptors—except for clozapine, which acts at dopamine D4 receptors.

Although it may also be argued that the atypical neuroleptic action of clozapine stems from its ability to block serotonin or muscarinic receptors, the minimum view would be that the D4 receptor is the primary target for clozapine, thus being compatible with the general rule that all presently used neuroleptics are antidopaminergic. In more detail, while clozapine can also block muscarinic

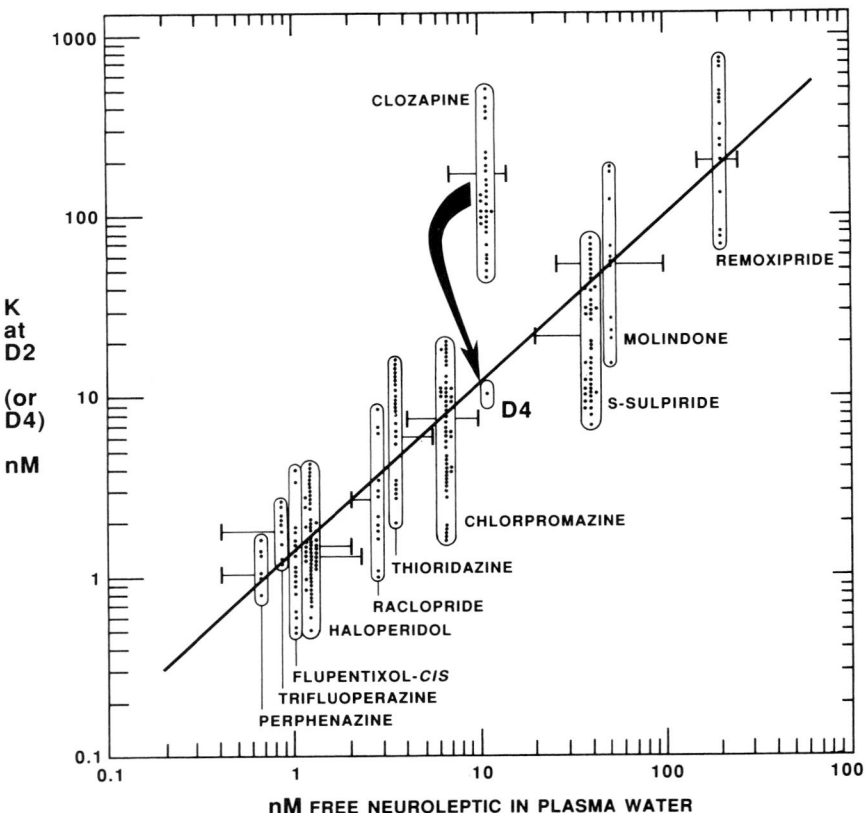

FIG. 1. The neuroleptic dissociation constants (K) at the dopamine D2 receptor closely match the free neuroleptic concentrations in the patients' plasma water or spinal fluid. Each point indicates a K value published from a different laboratory. Clozapine is the only drug that does not fit the D2 correlate, but its affinity at D4 (*arrow*) does. The plasma molarities for *cis*-flupentixol and for S-sulpiride are half those published for the racemates (which are used clinically). (From ref. 47, with permission.)

receptors, serotonin S2 receptors, and dopamine D1 receptors, the blockade of these sites does not adequately explain the lack of parkinsonian side effects by clozapine. For example, clozapine is known to be clinically superior (that is, clozapine provides better antipsychotic action in treatment-resistant patients and causes fewer parkinsonian side effects) than a combination of haloperidol (for dopamine D2 receptor block) and benztropine (for muscarinic receptor block) (30). As for serotonin S2 receptors, the possible blockade of serotonin S2 receptors by clozapine is unlikely to explain the atypical action of clozapine, based on the following considerations. First, Wadenberg (68) found that ritanserin, a serotonin S2 antagonist, did not antagonize catalepsy in rats caused by the blockade of dopamine D2 receptors with raclopride. Second, Casey (11) found that ritanserin did not block the haloperidol-induced dystonia in monkeys, while clozapine is known to do so in this animal model of neuroleptic-induced parkinsonism. Third, Chouinard et al. (13) found that risperidone (which blocks both dopamine D2 and serotonin S2 receptors) produced parkinsonian signs in only about 30% of patients, when given at 6 mg/day, but elicited parkinsonian signs in about 50% of patients when given at 16 mg/day. In other words, if serotonin S2 receptor blockade by risperidone alleviated the parkinsonian side effects of dopamine D2 receptor blockade, the protective "window" (or dose range) of serotonin S2 receptor blockade was small (between 6 and 16 mg/day).

DOPAMINE D2 AND D4 RECEPTOR DENSITIES IN SCHIZOPHRENIA

The density of dopamine D2-like receptors is elevated in postmortem schizophrenia brain tissues (47,52), compatible with the idea of dopamine overactivity in schizophrenia. This elevation, however, is only found in vivo using [^{11}C]methylspiperone (70) but not [^{11}C]raclopride (20), the discrepancy partly attributable to endogenous dopamine reducing the binding of radioactive raclopride but not methylspiperone (53). This discrepancy is further resolved by the following findings that the density of dopamine D4 receptors is markedly elevated in postmortem schizophrenia tissues, while the combined density for D2 and D3 receptors is only raised by 15%.

In control human striata the average density of [^{3}H]-spiperone sites is 12.9 pmol/g (Fig. 2). In striata from schizophrenic patients, the density of [^{3}H]spiperone sites is elevated by 56% to a value of 20.2 pmol/g, as previously reported (52). It is not possible, however, to compare such [^{3}H]spiperone data with [^{3}H]raclopride data, because the cloned dopamine receptor binds approximately two [^{3}H]raclopride molecules (or two [^{3}H]-emonapride molecules) for each [^{3}H]spiperone molecule (56). This indicates that [^{3}H]raclopride binds to the monomer of the D2 receptor while [^{3}H]spiperone binds to a dimer of the D2 dopamine receptors (56).

Although there is no drug currently available which is

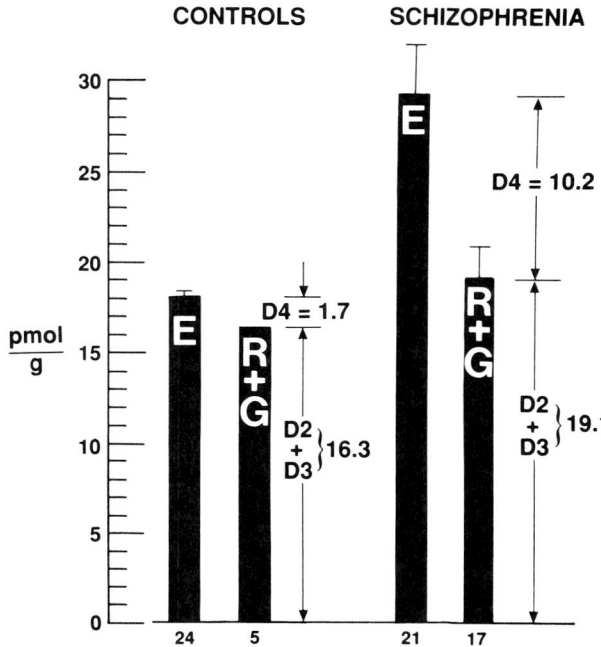

FIG. 2. Summary (52,57) indicating that the density of dopamine D4 receptors is elevated by sixfold in schizophrenia. The density of [³H]emonapride (**E**) sites (which includes dopamine D2, D3, and D4 receptors) averaged 18.0 ± 1.3 pmol/g in control brains and 29.3 ± 2.8 pmol/g in schizophrenia (57). In the presence of guanine nucleotide (**G**) (used to remove the inhibiting effect of endogenous dopamine on [³H]racopride binding), the density of [³H]raclopride sites (which only includes dopamine D2 and D3 receptors, because raclopride has a low affinity for D4) was 16.3 ± 5 pmol/g in control striata and 19.1 ± 1.8 pmol/g in schizophrenia, an increase of approximately 15%. The density of dopamine D4 receptors, however, measured as the difference between the [³H]emonapride and [³H]raclopride (with nucleotide) densities, increased sixfold in schizophrenia.

highly selective for D4, Table 3 indicates how dopamine D4 receptors can be measured indirectly in brain tissue, using [³H]emonapride and [³H]raclopride. Emonapride (or YM-09151-2) binds to dopamine D2, D3, and D4 receptors with dissociation constants of between 0.06 nM and 0.3 nM. Raclopride, however, binds to dopamine D2 and D3 receptors with dissociation constants of between 1.8 nM and 3.5 nM, but has a very low affinity for dopamine D4 receptors.

Thus, [³H]emonapride readily labels dopamine D2, D3, and D4 receptors, while [³H]raclopride readily labels dopamine D2 and D3 receptors. Any difference in the binding densities of these two ligands, therefore, may be attributed to dopamine D4 receptors. Hence, using this approach, the density of dopamine D4 receptors in the human striatum is between 1 and 2 pmols/g. (This compares to a density of 12 pmols/g for dopamine D2 receptors.)

As shown in Fig. 2, the difference between the [³H]-emonapride and [³H]raclopride densities reveals the dopamine D4 density to be 1.7 pmol/g in control striata and

10.2 pmol/g in schizophrenia, a sixfold elevation. It is important to emphasize here that when the D4 density is determined by this subtraction method, it is essential that the density of [³H]raclopride sites be measured in the presence of guanine nucleotide to remove the interfering effect of endogenous dopamine on the binding of [³H]-raclopride.

As also shown in Fig. 2, the combined density of dopamine D2 and D3 receptors, as labeled by [³H]raclopride in the presence of guanine nucleotide, rises only 15% in schizophrenia, in agreement with the in vivo data reported by Farde et al. (20), using [¹¹C]raclopride.

This analysis resolves the apparent discrepancy, mentioned above, wherein the density of [¹¹C]methylspiperone-

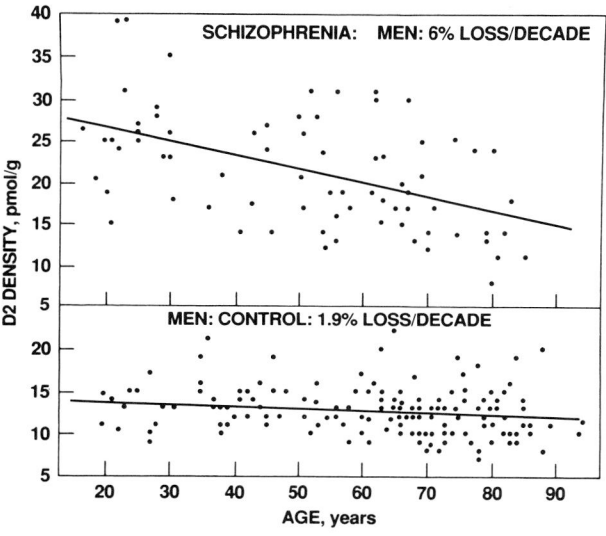

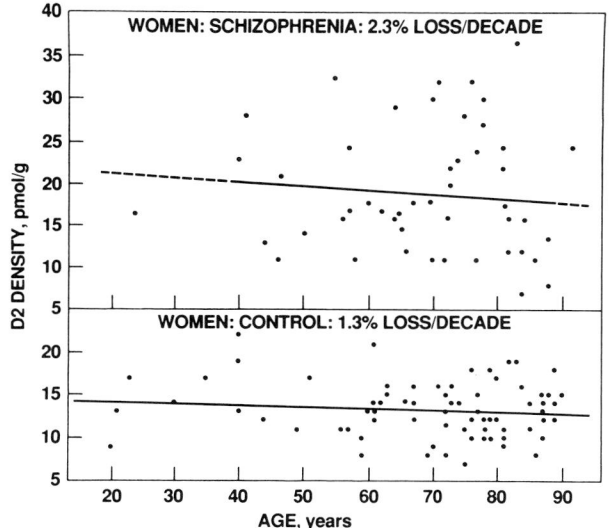

FIG. 3. The density of D2-like receptors (i.e., D2, D3, and D4) in postmortem human striatal tissues, as measured by [³H]spiperone, falls by 6% per 10-year period in schizophrenic men but only by 2.3% per decade in schizophrenic women.

labeled sites (70) (i.e., D2, D3, and D4), but not that for [^{11}C]raclopride-labeled sites (20) (i.e., D2 and D3), was found elevated in the striata of schizophrenics.

DOPAMINE D2-LIKE RECEPTORS IN BRAIN STRIATA FROM MALE AND FEMALE SCHIZOPHRENIC PATIENTS

Figure 3 illustrates that the elevated density of the D2-like receptors in striata from schizophrenics falls as the patients age (51,52). The rate of fall for the schizophrenic men is about three times faster than that for the schizophrenic women. Clinically, these data may be related to the slow, but steady, clinical improvement found in schizophrenic men as they get older (46).

DOPAMINE D2-LIKE RECEPTORS ARE ELEVATED ON THE RIGHT SIDE OF SCHIZOPHRENIC BRAINS, COMPATIBLE WITH LEFTWARD TURNING OF SCHIZOPHRENIC PATIENTS

Patients with schizophrenia turn more often toward their left side, in contrast to normal individuals who turn to their left or right equally often (3,4,34). The same is true for a small subgroup of nonschizophrenic, but severely psychotic, patients (35). Such rotational preference is not related to handedness in normal controls (5) and not related to handedness or medication in the psychotic patients (3,34,35). There is, however, a correlation between the severity of delusions and the extent of left-turning (8).

On a neurochemical basis, it has been found that rotation of the body is commonly toward the brain side containing less dopaminergic activity. This holds for both animals (27) and humans (6,7,26).

In order to study why patients with schizophrenia turn more often toward their left side, we examined whether there was an asymmetry in the densities of dopamine D2-like receptors in the left and right postmortem schizophrenia brain striata. Using [^{3}H]emonapride to label dopamine D2-like receptors (38), the density of receptors on the right side was higher than that of the left side in 13 of 16 pairs (81%) of the striata from schizophrenics (Fig. 4). This right-side finding with [^{3}H]emonapride is identical to that which we found previously with [^{3}H]spiperone (44). However, using [^{3}H]raclopride, only 6 of the 16 pairs (38%) revealed higher densities of [^{3}H]raclopride sites on the right side. The absolute densities for [^{3}H]raclopride were always about 25–30% lower than those for [^{3}H]-emonapride. Because the binding of [^{3}H]raclopride to these receptors is reduced by the presence of endogenous dopamine (55), while the binding of [^{3}H]emonapride is less affected, the data with [^{3}H]emonapride more appropriately reflect the true densities of the dopamine D2-like

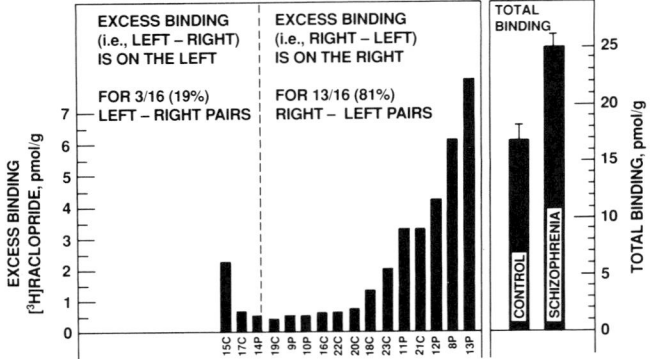

FIG. 4. Of the 16 pairs of left and right sides of striata (from schizophrenics) measured for dopamine D2-like receptors with [^{3}H]emonapride, 13 pairs (81%) had more receptors on the right side. "Excess binding" was the difference between the receptor densities on the left and the right. "Total binding" refers to total specific binding. Compared to control values, the density of dopamine receptors in schizophrenia was elevated by 8.2 pmol/g for [^{3}H]emonapride (*right*).

receptors. Thus, if the extra dopamine D2-like receptors on the right are functional and active, then the individual would turn toward the left, in keeping with the general principle that both animals and humans rotate toward the side where the brain hemisphere is relatively hypodopaminergic.

LINK BETWEEN D1 AND D2 RECEPTORS REDUCED IN PSYCHOSIS

There are many psychomotor activities where the dopamine D1 and D2 receptors are cooperative or synergistic (see references in ref. 54). One molecular basis for this synergism may be through the $\beta\gamma$ subunits of the G proteins which are associated with both of these dopamine receptors (54). Most interesting is the observation that the D1–D2 link is reduced or absent in approximately two-thirds of postmortem striatal tissues from schizophrenic patients and from late-stage Huntington patients (54). Normally, the D1 receptor appears to keep D2 in its low-affinity state. Any reduction in the D1 influence on D2 would therefore be expected to result in D2 retaining its high-affinity (or functional) state. Hence, clinically, a reduced influence of D1 on D2 would be expected to result in a more active set of psychotic symptoms.

RELATION BETWEEN CLINICAL SIGNS AND D2 BLOCKADE

As a result of many studies using positron emission tomography to measure the occupancy of D2 receptors in neuroleptic-treated patients (1,9,18,19,21,39,43), there is a clear relation between clinical signs and D2 block.

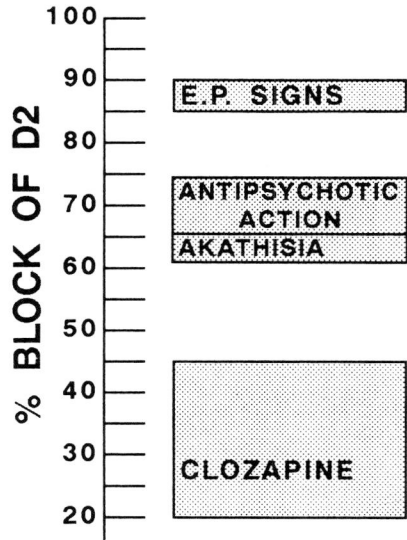

FIG. 5. Relation between clinical signs and dopamine D2 receptor block, as obtained by studies using positron emission tomography to measure the occupancy of D2 receptors in neuroleptic-treated patients (1,9,18,19,21,39,43).

Akathisia occurs at around 60–65% D2 blockade, antipsychotic action occurs at about 65–75% D2 block, and extrapyramidal parkinsonian signs occur at approximately 90% block of D2 receptors, as summarized in Fig. 5.

CONCLUSION

Practical benefits are emerging from the dopamine hypothesis and from the cloning strategies. As just noted above, there is a clear relation between clinical signs and D2 receptor blockade. Hence, the art of psychiatry is rapidly becoming the quantitative science of psychiatry. In addition, with the discoveries that clozapine targets to the dopamine D4 receptor and that dopamine D4 receptors are markedly elevated in schizophrenia, the development of new clozapine-like neuroleptics (which do not cause parkinsonism and do not cause tardive dyskinesia) is desirable and possible. A new generation of selective neuropsychopharmacology is on the horizon.

REFERENCES

1. Baron JC, Martinot JL, Cambon H, et al. Striatal dopamine receptor occupancy during and following withdrawal from neuroleptic treatment: correlative evaluation by positron emission tomography and plasma prolactin levels. *Psychopharmacology* 1989;99:463–472.
2. Boundy VA, Luedtke RR, Gallitano AL, et al. Expression and characterization of the rat D3 dopamine receptor: pharmacologic properties and development of antibodies. *J Pharmacol Exp Ther* 1993;264:1002–1011.
3. Bracha HS. Asymmetric rotational (circling) behavior, a dopamine-related asymmetry: preliminary findings in unmedicated and never-medicated schizophrenic patients. *Biol Psychiatry* 1987;22:995–1003.
4. Bracha HS. Is there a right hemi-hyper-dopaminergic psychosis? *Schizophrenia Res* 1989;2:317–324.
5. Bracha HS, Seitz DJ, Otemaa J, Glick SD. Rotational movement (circling) in normal humans: sex difference and relationship to hand, foot and eye preference. *Brain Res* 1987;411:231–235.
6. Bracha HS, Shults C, Glick SD, Kleinman JE. Spontaneous asymmetric circling behavior in hemi-parkinsonism: a human equivalent of the lesion-circling rodent behavior. *Life Sci* 1987;40:1127–1130.
7. Bracha HS, Lyden PD, Khansarinia S. Delayed emergence of striatal dopaminergic hyperactivity after anterolateral ischemic cortical lesions in humans; evidence from turning behavior. *Biol Psychiatry* 1989;25:265–274.
8. Bracha HS, Livingston RL, Clothier J, Linington BB, Karson CN. Correlation of severity of psychiatric patients' delusions with right hemispatial inattention (left-turning behavior). *Am J Psychiatry* 1993;150:330–332.
9. Brücke T, Roth J, Podreka I, Strobl R, Wenger S, Asenbaum S. Striatal dopamine D2-receptor blockade by typical and atypical neuroleptics. *Lancet* 1992;339:497.
10. Bunzow JR, Van Tol HHM, Grandy DK, et al. Cloning and expression of a rat D2 dopamine receptor cDNA. *Nature* 1988;336:783–787.
11. Casey DE. The effect of a serotonin S2 antagonist, ritanserine, and an anticholinergic benztropine on haloperidol-induced dystonia in nonhuman primates [Abstract]. *Am College Neuropsychopharmacol* 1991;30:127.
12. Castro SW, Strange PG. Differences in the ligand binding properties of the short and long versions of the D2 dopamine receptor. *J Neurochem* 1993;60:372–375.
13. Chouinard G, Jones B, Remington G, et al. A Canadian multicenter placebo-controlled study of fixed doses of risperidone and haloperidol in the treatment of chronic schizophrenic patients. *J Clin Psychopharmacol* 1993;13:25–40.
14. Cox BA, Henningsen RA, Spanoyannis A, Neve KA. Contributions of conserved serine residues to the interactions of ligands with dopamine D2 receptors. *J Neurochem* 1992;59:627–635.
15. Dal Toso R, Sommer B, Ewert M, et al. The dopamine D2 receptor: two molecular forms generated by alternative splicing. *EMBO J* 1989;8:4025–4034.
16. Dearry A, Gingrich JA, Falardeau P, Fremeau Jr RT, Bates MD, Caron MG. Molecular cloning and expression of the gene for a human D1 dopamine receptor. *Nature* 1990;347:72–76.
17. De Keyser J. Subtypes and localization of dopamine receptors in human brain. *Neurochem Int* 1993;22:83–93.
18. Farde L. Selective D₁- and D₂-dopamine receptor blockade both induces akathisia in humans—a PET study with [¹¹C]SCH 23390 and [¹¹C]raclopride. *Psychopharmacology* 1992;107:23–29.
19. Farde L, Wiesel F-A, Halldin C, Sedvall G. Central D2-dopamine receptor occupancy in schizophrenic patients treated with antipsychotic drugs. *Arch Gen Psychiatry* 1988;45:71–76.
20. Farde L, Wiesel, F-A, Stone-Elander S, et al. D₂ dopamine receptors in neuroleptic-naive schizophrenic patients: a positron emission tomography study with [¹¹C]raclopride. *Arch Gen Psychiatry* 1990;47:213–219.
21. Farde L, Nordström A-L, Wiesel F-A, Pauli S, Halldin C, Sedvall G. Positron emission tomographic analysis of central D₁ and D₂ dopamine receptor occupancy in patients treated with classical neuroleptics and clozapine. *Arch Gen Psychiatry* 1992;49:538–544.
22. Figur LM, Evans DL, Stratman NC, Lahti RA. The dopamine D4 and D2 receptors: comparison of neuroleptic binding affinities. *Soc Neurosci Abstr* 1992;18:Abstr 158.3.
23. Fishburn CS, Belleli D, David C, Carmon S, Fuchs S. A novel short isoform of the D₃ dopamine receptor generated by alternative splicing in the third cytoplasmic loop. *J Biol Chem* 1993;268:5872–5878.
24. Giros B, Sokoloff P, Martres M-P, Riou J-F, Emorine LJ, Schwartz J-C. Alternative splicing directs the expression of two D2 dopamine receptor isoforms. *Nature* 1989;342:923–926.
25. Giros B, Martres M-P, Sokoloff P, Schwartz J-C. Clonage de gène du récepteur dopaminergique D3 humain et identification de son chromosome. *C R Acad Sci (Paris)* 1990;311:501–508.
26. Glick SD, Ross DA. Lateralization of function the rat brain mecha-

nisms may be operative in humans. *Trends Neurosci* 1981;4:196–199.

27. Glick SD, Jerussi TP, Fleisher LN. Turning in circles: the neuropharmacology of rotation. *Life Sci* 1976;18:889–896.

28. Grandy DK, Marchionni MA, Makam H, et al. Cloning of the cDNA and gene for a human D2 dopamine receptor. *Proc Natl Acad Sci USA* 1989;86:9762–9766.

29. Grandy DK, Zhang Y, Bouvier C, et al. Multiple human D5 dopamine receptor genes: a functional receptor and two pseudogenes. *Proc Natl Acad Sci USA* 1991;88:9175–9179.

30. Kane J, Honigfeld G, Singer J, Meltzer H, and the Clozaril collaborative study group. Clozapine for the treatment-resistant schizophrenic. *Arch Gen Psychiatry* 1988;45:789–796.

31. Lahti RA, Figur LM, Piercey MF, Ruppel PL, Evans DL. Intrinsic activity determinations at the dopamine D2 guanine nucleotide-binding protein-coupled receptor: utilization of receptor state binding affinities. *Mol Pharmacol* 1992;42:432–438.

32. Lévesque D, Diaz J, Pilon C, et al. Identification, characterization, and localization of the dopamine D3 receptor in rat brain ssing 7-[³H]hydroxy-*N,N*-di-*n*-propyl-2-aminotetralin. *Proc Natl Acad Sci USA* 1992;89:8155–8159.

33. Lichter JB, Barr CL, Kennedy JL, Van Tol HHM, Kidd KK, Livak KJ. A hypervariable segment in the human dopamine receptor D_4 (*DRD4*) gene. *Hum Mol Gen* 1993;2:767–773.

34. Lyon N, Satz P. Left turning (swivel) in medicated chronic schizophrenic patients. *Schizophrenia Res* 1991;4:53–58.

35. Lyon N, Satz P, Fleming K, Green MF, Bracha HS. Left turning (swivel) in manic patients. *Schizophrenia Res* 1992;7:71–76.

36. Neve KA, Cox BA, Henningsen RA, Spanoyannis A, Neve RL. Pivotal role for aspartate-80 in the regulation of dopamine D2 receptor affinity for drugs and inhibition of adenyl cyclase. *Mol Pharmacol* 1991;39:733–739.

37. Nguyen T, Sunahara R, Van Tol HHM, Seeman P, O'Dowd BF. Transcription of a human dopamine D5 pseudogene. *Biochem Biophys Res Commun* 1991;181:16–21.

38. Niznik HB, Grigoriadis DE, Pri-Bar I, Buchman O, Seeman P. Dopamine D_2 receptors selectively labeled by a benzamide neuroleptic: [³H]-YM-09151-2. *Naunyn Schmiedebergs Arch Pharmacol* 1985;329:333–343.

39. Nordstöm A-L, Farde L, Wiesel F-A, et al. Central D2-dopamine receptor occupancy in relation to antipsychotic drug effects: a double-blind PET study of schizophrenic patients. *Biol Psychiatry* 1993;33:227–235.

40. O'Dowd BF, Nguyen T, Tirpak A, et al. Cloning of two additional catecholamine receptors from rat brain. *FEBS Lett* 1990;262:8–12.

41. O'Malley KL, Harmon S, Tang L, Todd RD. The rat dopamine D4 receptor: sequence, gene structure, and demonstration of expression in the cardiovascular system. *New Biol* 1992;4:137–146.

42. Patel S, Marwood R, Emms FA, Knowles MR, Mcallister G, Freedman SB. Pharmacological studies on the human dopamine D3 receptor expressed in stable cell lines. *Br J Pharmacol* 1992;107:297P.

43. Pilowsky LS, Costa DC, Ell PJ, Murray RM, Verhoeff NPLG, Kerwin RW. Clozapine, single photon emission tomography, and the D2 dopamine receptor blockade hypothesis of schizophrenia. *Lancet* 1992;340:199–202.

44. Reynolds GP, Czudek C, Bzowej N, Seeman P. Dopamine receptor asymmetry in schizophrenia. *Lancet* 1987;i:979.

45. Seabrook GR, Patel S, Marwood R, et al. Stable expression of human D3 dopamine receptors in GH4C1 pituitary cells. *FEBS Lett* 1992;312:123–126.

46. Seeman, MV, ed. *Gender and psychopathology.* Washington, DC: American Psychiatric Association, 1994;[*in press*].

47. Seeman P. Dopamine receptor sequences. Therapeutic levels of neuroleptics occupy D2 receptors, clozapine occupies D4. *Neuropsychopharmacology* 1992;7:261–284.

48. Seeman P, Niznik HB. Dopamine D1 receptor pharmacology. *ISI Atlas Sci Pharmacol* 1988;2:161–170.

49. Seeman P, Van Tol HHM. Dopamine receptor pharmacology. *Curr Opin Neurol Neurosurg* 1993;6:602–608.

50. Seeman P, Chau-Wong M, Tedesco J, Wong K. Brain receptors for antipsychotic drugs and dopamine: direct binding assays. *Proc Natl Acad Sci USA* 1975;72:4376–4380.

51. Seeman P, Bzowej NH, Guan H-C, et al. Human brain dopamine receptors in children and aging adults. *Synapse* 1987;1:399–404.

52. Seeman P, Bzowej NH, Guan H-C, et al. Human brain D_1 and D_2 dopamine receptors in schizophrenia, Alzheimer's, Parkinson's and Huntington's diseases. *Neuropsychopharmacology* 1987;1:5–15.

53. Seeman P, Guan H-C, Niznik HB. Endogenous dopamine lowers the dopamine D2 receptor density as measured by [³H]raclopride: implications for positron emission tomography of the human brain. *Synapse* 1989;3:96–97.

54. Seeman P, Niznik HB, Guan H-C, Booth G, Ulpian C. Link between D1 and D2 dopamine receptors is reduced in schizophrenia and Huntington diseased brain. *Proc Natl Acad Sci USA* 1989;86:10156–10160.

55. Seeman P, Niznik HB, Guan H-C. Elevation of D2 dopamine receptors in schizophrenia is underestimated by radioactive raclopride. *Arch Gen Psychiatry* 1990;47:1170–1172.

56. Seeman P, Guan H-C, Civelli O, Van Tol HHM, Sunahara RK, Niznik HB. The cloned dopamine D_2 receptor reveals different densities for dopamine antagonist ligands. Implications for human brain positron emission tomography. *Eur J Pharmacol Mol Pharmacol Sect* 1992;227:139–146.

57. Seeman P, Guan H-C, Van Tol HHM. Dopamine D4 receptors elevated in schizophrenia. *Nature* 1993;365:441–445.

58. Sibley DR, Monsma Jr FJ. Molecular biology of dopamine receptors. *Trends Pharmacol Sci* 1992;13:61–69.

59. Sokoloff P, Giros B, Martres M-P, Bouthenet M-L, Schwartz J-C. Molecular cloning and characterization of a novel dopamine receptor (D3) as a target for neuroleptics. *Nature* 1990;347:146–151.

60. Sokoloff P, Andrieux M, Besançon R, et al. Pharmacology of human dopamine D3 receptor expressed in a mammalian cell line: comparison with D2 receptor. *Eur J Pharmacol Mol Pharmacol Sect* 1992;225:331–337.

61. Spano PF, Govoni S, Trabucchi M. Studies on the pharmacological properties of dopamine receptors in various areas of the central nervous system. *Adv Biochem Psychopharmacol* 1978;19:155–165.

62. Stormann TM, Gdula DC, Weiner DM, Brann MR. Molecular cloning and expression of a dopamine D2 receptor from human retina. *Mol Pharmacol* 1990;37:1–6.

63. Sunahara RK, Niznik HB, Weiner DM, et al. Human dopamine D1 receptor encoded by an intronless gene on chromosome 5. *Nature* 1990;347:80–83.

64. Sunahara RK, Guan H-C, O'Dowd BF, et al. Cloning of the gene for a human dopamine D5 receptor with higher affinity for dopamine than D1. *Nature* 1991;350:614–619.

65. Tiberi M, Jarvie KR, Silvia C, et al. Cloning, molecular characterization, and chromosomal assignment of a gene encoding a second D1 dopamine receptor subtype: differential expression pattern in rat brain compared with the D1A receptor. *Proc Natl Acad Sci USA* 1991;88:7491–7495.

66. Van Tol HHM, Bunzow JR, Guan H-C, et al. Cloning of a human dopamine D4 receptor gene with high affinity for the antipsychotic clozapine. *Nature* 1991;350:614–619.

67. Van Tol HHM, Wu CM, Guan H-C, et al. Multiple dopamine D4 receptor variants in the human population. *Nature* 1992;358:149–152.

68. Wadenberg M-L. Antagonism by 8-OH-DPAT, but not ritanserin, of catalepsy induced by SCH 23390 in the rat. *J Neural Transm* 1992;89:49–59.

69. Weinshank RL, Adham N, Macchi M, Olsen MA, Branchek TA, Hartig PR. Molecular cloning and characterization of a high affinity dopamine receptor (D1β) and its pseudogene. *J Biol Chem* 1991;266:22427–22435.

70. Wong DF, Wagner HN Jr, Tune LE, et al. Positron emission tomography reveals elevated D2 dopamine receptors in drug-naive schizophrenics. *Science* 1986;234:1558–1563.

Psychopharmacology: The Fourth Generation of Progress, edited by Floyd E. Bloom and David J. Kupfer. Raven Press, Ltd., New York © 1995.

CHAPTER 27

Signal Transduction Pathways for Catecholamine Receptors

Ronald S. Duman and Eric J. Nestler

Until relatively recently, synaptic transmission was conceptualized as a set of processes by which neurotransmitters, acting through their receptors, caused changes in the conductances of specific ion channels to produce excitatory or inhibitory postsynaptic potentials. According to this view, the human brain could be viewed as a very complex digital computer with its complexity derived largely from its wiring diagram. Over the past 20 years, however, it has become evident that neurotransmitters elicit diverse and complicated effects in target neurons. This has led to a much more complete view of synaptic transmission (20). Thus, in addition to the rapid elicitation of postsynaptic potentials, neurotransmitter–receptor interactions influence virtually every aspect of a target neuron's functioning through a complex network of intracellular messenger systems (Fig. 1). The purpose of this chapter is to present a brief overview of these intracellular messenger systems in the brain and to describe how these systems mediate the many effects of catecholamines and their numerous receptors on target neuron functioning (see also Chapters 11, 14, 21, 29, and 37, *this volume*).

OVERVIEW OF INTRACELLULAR MESSENGER SYSTEMS IN BRAIN

Extracellular signals, generated by neurotransmitter activation of catecholamine receptors and most other types of receptors, are transmitted to intracellular sites via G-protein coupling factors (Fig. 1). G proteins then "couple" receptors to various effector proteins. These effectors include ion channels and numerous intracellular

second messenger pathways. Generation of second messengers leads to diverse physiological effects via cascades of intracellular messengers. In most cases, these intracellular cascades ultimately involve changes in protein phosphorylation—the addition (via protein kinases) or removal (via protein phosphatases) of phosphate groups from target phosphoproteins. Altered phosphorylation of phosphoproteins, which can be considered "third messengers," alters their physiological activity.

As with all neurotransmitters, catecholamine regulation of second messenger and protein phosphorylation pathways influences virtually all aspects of neuronal function through the phosphorylation of diverse types of neural proteins (Fig. 1). Such intracellular processes produce some of the rapid responses to the neurotransmitter, such as regulation of ion channels and neuronal firing rate. In addition, these processes produce short-term modulatory effects on neuronal function, such as regulation of the responsiveness of the neuron to the same or different neurotransmitters (e.g., via altered receptor sensitivity). Finally, these processes produce more long-term modulatory effects on neuronal function, including changes that are achieved through the regulation of gene expression. Such changes can include altered synthesis of receptors, ion channels, and other cellular proteins and can ultimately involve forms of learning and memory. Individual steps in these intracellular cascades are given below in greater detail.

G Proteins in Brain Signal Transduction

With the exception of synaptic transmission mediated via receptors that contain intrinsic ion channels, the family of G proteins may be involved in all other transmembrane signaling in the nervous system (Fig. 1; see refs. 27 and 38). G proteins are so-named because of their

R. S. Duman and E. J. Nestler: Laboratory of Molecular Psychiatry, Departments of Psychiatry and Pharmacology, Yale University School of Medicine, Connecticut Mental Health Center, New Haven, Connecticut 06508.

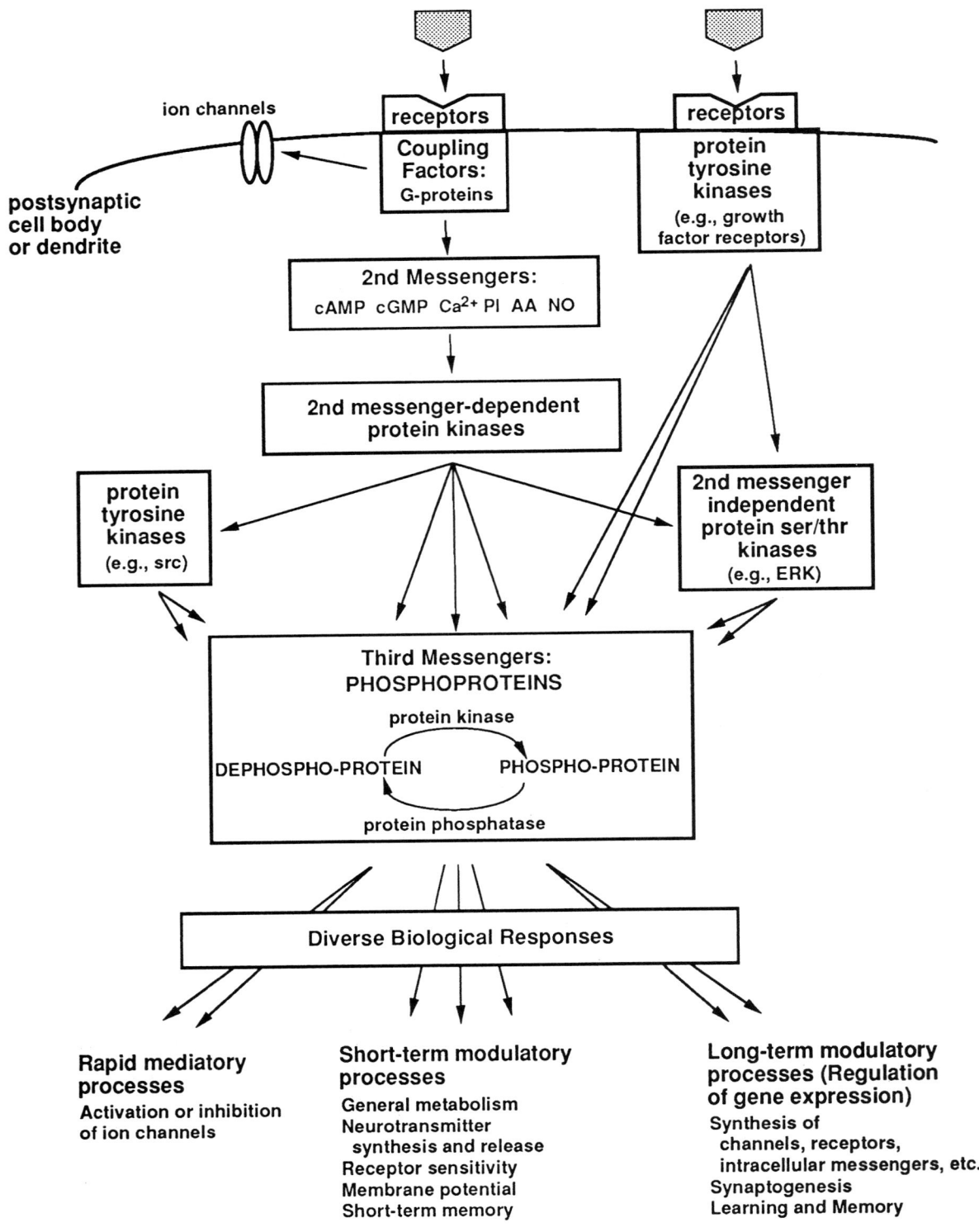

ability to bind the guanine nucleotides, guanosine triphosphate (GTP) and guanosine diphosphate (GDP). As stated above, G proteins serve to couple receptors to specific intracellular effector systems (Fig. 2). Four major types of G proteins (Gs, Gi, Go, and Gq) are involved in transduction of signals produced by neurotransmitter binding, and multiple subtypes exist for each. Rhodopsin, the light-sensitive molecule of photoreceptor cells in the retina, can also be viewed as a G-protein-linked receptor: light activates rhodopsin, which then, through a fifth type of G protein called *transducin* (Gt), regulates the electrical properties of photoreceptor cells. Each type of G protein is a heterotrimer composed of single α, β, and γ subunits. Distinct α subunits confer specific functional activity on the different types of G proteins, which appear to share some common subtypes of $\beta\gamma$ subunits. Regulation of the functional activity of G proteins is shown schematically in Fig. 2.

G-Protein Regulation of Ion Channels

G proteins have been shown to couple neurotransmitter receptors to multiple types of intracellular effector proteins. In some cases, G proteins couple neurotransmitter receptors directly to certain types of ion channels (e.g., Fig. 3) (31). In this case, it appears that the α subunit released from the G-protein–receptor interaction directly gates (i.e., opens or closes) the channel. The best established example of this type of mechanism in brain is the coupling of many types of receptors, via subtypes of Go and Gi in many types of neurons, to the activation of an inward rectifying K^+ channel and to the inhibition of a voltage-dependent Ca^{2+} channel, actions that hyperpolarize cells. There are also reports that $\beta\gamma$ subunits may regulate ion channel function in some cases.

G-Protein Regulation of Intracellular Second Messengers

In addition to direct regulation of ion channels, G proteins transduce the activation of neurotransmitter receptors into alterations in intracellular levels of second messengers in target neurons. Prominent second messengers in brain include cyclic AMP (cAMP), cyclic GMP (cGMP), calcium, the major metabolites of phosphatidylinositol (PI) [inositol triphosphate (IP$_3$) and diacylglycerol] and of arachidonic acid, and nitric oxide (NO). As discussed above, altered levels of second messengers me-

FIG. 1. Schematic illustration of the role played by intracellular messenger systems in synaptic transmission in the brain. Recent studies in neuroscience have provided a complex view of synaptic transmission. These studies have focused on the involvement of intracellular messenger systems, involving coupling factors (termed G proteins), second messengers [e.g., cAMP, cGMP, Ca^{2+}, nitric oxide (NO), and the metabolites of phosphatidylinositol (PI) and arachidonic acid (AA)], and protein phosphorylation (involving the phosphorylation of phosphoproteins by protein kinases and their dephosphorylation by protein phosphatases), in mediating multiple actions of neurotransmitters on their target neurons. Prominent in brain are numerous protein serine/threonine kinases that are activated directly by various second messengers, and they are referred to as second messenger-dependent protein kinases. Brain also contains numerous protein serine/threonine kinases that are not regulated directly by second messengers (see Table 1). In addition, the brain contains numerous types of protein tyrosine kinases; some reside in the receptors for most growth factors, whereas others are not associated with growth factor receptors (see Table 1). These various protein kinases are all highly regulated by extracellular stimuli. The second-messenger-dependent protein kinases are regulated by receptor–second-messenger pathways as shown in Fig. 3. The receptor-associated protein tyrosine kinases are activated upon growth factor binding to the receptor. The second-messenger-independent protein serine/threonine kinases and the protein tyrosine kinases that are not receptor-associated seem to be regulated indirectly by second messengers and second-messenger-dependent protein kinases and by protein tyrosine kinases, although the precise mechanisms are not yet known in most cases. The brain also contains numerous types of protein serine/threonine and protein tyrosine phosphatases, which are also subject to regulation by extracellular stimuli. The figure illustrates three major roles subserved by these intracellular messenger pathways. In some cases, intracellular messengers mediate the actions of some neurotransmitters in opening or inhibiting particular ion channels. However, intracellular messengers mediate most of the many other actions of neurotransmitters on their target neurons. Some are relatively short-lived and involve modulation of the general metabolic state of the neurons, their ability to synthesize or release neurotransmitter, and the functional sensitivity of their various receptors and ion channels to various synaptic inputs. Others are relatively long-lived and are achieved through the regulation of gene expression in the target neurons. Thus, neurotransmitters, through the regulation of intracellular messenger pathways and alterations in gene transcription and protein synthesis, alter the numbers and types of receptors and ion channels in target neurons, the functional activity of the intracellular messenger systems in those neurons, and even the shape and numbers of synapses the neurons form. The figure is drawn to illustrate the amplification that intracellular messenger systems can give to neurotransmitter action. Thus, a single event of a neurotransmitter binding to its receptor (the first messenger level) can act through the second, third, fourth, and so on, messenger levels to produce an increasingly wider array of physiological effects.

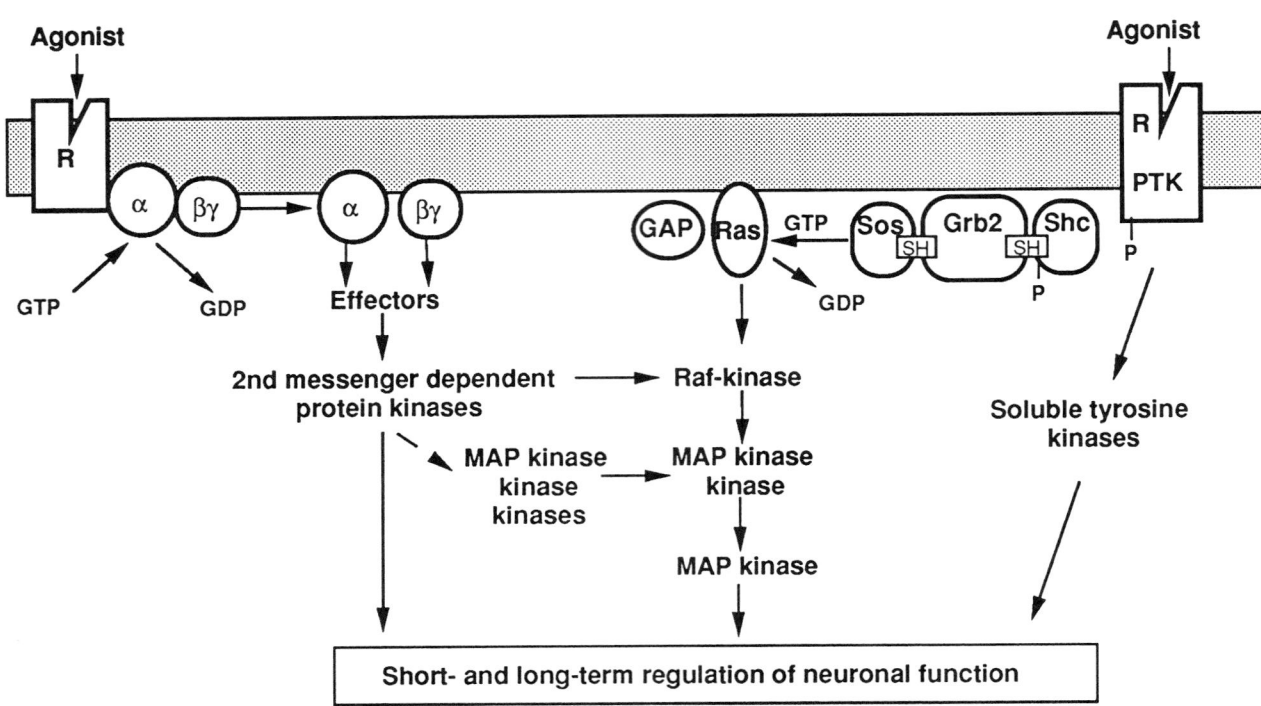

FIG. 2. Schematic illustration of the mechanisms by which G-protein-coupled receptors and receptor-associated protein tyrosine kinases function in the brain. G-protein-coupled receptors and receptor-associated protein tyrosine kinases employ distinct mechanisms for activation of intracellular signal transduction pathways. **A:** Activation of G-protein-coupled receptors (R) leads to association of the receptor with a heterotrimeric G protein comprised of single α, β, and γ subunits. This leads to the binding of GTP to the α subunit and the displacement of GDP from the subunit. GTP binding induces the generation of free α subunit by causing the dissociation of the α subunit from its $\beta\gamma$ subunits and the receptor. Free α subunit, bound to GTP, is functionally active and directly regulates a number of effector proteins, which, depending on the type of α subunit and cell involved, can include ion channels, adenylyl cyclase, phospholipase C, and phosphodiesterases. Free $\beta\gamma$ subunits also appear to directly regulate the same effector proteins. GTPase activity intrinsic to the α subunit hydrolyzes GTP to GDP. This leads to the reassociation of the α and $\beta\gamma$ subunits, which, along with the dissociation of ligand from the receptor, leads to restoration of the basal state. **B:** Activation of growth factor (e.g., neurotrophin) receptors (R-PTK) stimulates protein tyrosine kinase activity intrinsic to the receptor. This leads to phosphorylation of the receptor itself and adaptor proteins with Src homology (SH) domains, such as Shc. The SH proteins, or phosphorylated receptor in some cases, then associate with Grb2. Grb2 then complexes with Sos (and related Ras effector proteins) via SH domains to promote GTP binding to Ras. The function of Ras is also negatively regulated by GAP (GTPase activating protein), which stimulates Ras GTPase activity and the hydrolysis of GTP to GDP. Ras, bound to GTP, is functionally active and directly stimulates Raf by an unknown mechanism. Raf, a protein serine/threonine kinase, phosphorylates and activates MAP-kinase kinase, which then activates MAP-kinase by phosphorylating it on threonine and tyrosine residues. Raf and possibly other MAP-kinase kinase kinases can also be regulated by second-messenger-dependent protein kinases. This provides a pathway by which G-protein-coupled receptors can influence this major growth factor–Ras cascade. In addition to the MAP-kinase pathway, receptor-protein tyrosine kinases can also influence cellular responses by phosphorylation and activation of soluble protein tyrosine kinases (tyrosine kinases which lack a receptor domain).

diate the actions of neurotransmitter–receptor activation on some types of ion channels, as well as on numerous other physiological responses as outlined in Fig. 1.

Second Messengers in Brain Signal Transduction

cAMP

The molecular mechanism by which neurotransmitters regulate cAMP levels is well established (Fig. 3). Gs couples certain receptors to adenylyl cyclase, the enzyme responsible for the synthesis of cAMP, such that the enzyme is stimulated by receptor activation. In contrast, Gi (and possibly Go) couples other receptors to adenylyl cyclase such that the enzyme is inhibited by receptor activation (38,40). A variant form of Gi, termed Gz, may also mediate receptor inhibition of adenylyl cyclase in some cell types. Six forms of adenylyl cyclase have been cloned (9–11,27). These enzymes show different regional distributions in brain, as well as distinct regulatory properties. The enzymes differ in their ability to be activated or inhibited upon binding free $\beta\gamma$ complexes or Ca^{2+}-calmodulin complexes (see Fig. 3) (27).

cGMP and Nitric Oxide

Neurotransmitters regulate cellular cGMP levels via several different mechanisms (Fig. 3) (27,42). In some cases, nitric oxide (NO) appears to act as an intracellular second messenger in mediating the ability of certain receptors to activate guanylyl cyclase, the enzyme that catalyzes the synthesis of cGMP. It is thought that these receptors elicit an increase in intracellular Ca^{2+} levels (as described below), which activates NO synthetase, the enzyme responsible for the synthesis of NO (4). NO then directly activates cytoplasmic forms of guanylyl cyclase. In other cases, as with the atrial natriuretic peptide receptor and related systems, the enzyme guanylyl cyclase resides within the receptor protein. In still other cases, it is conceivable, though not proven, that some neurotransmitter receptors are coupled via specific G proteins to guanylyl cyclase (see also Chapter 54, *this volume*).

In addition to activating guanylyl cyclase, NO has been shown to regulate ADP-ribosylation, a process whereby ADP-ribose groups are transferred from NAD (nicotinamide adenine dinucleotide) to specific substrate proteins. The addition of ADP-ribose then alters the physiological activity of the protein. Brain contains high levels of ADP-ribosyltransferases which catalyze this reaction, and some forms of the enzyme are activated by NO (8,41). Although most of the physiological substrates for these NO-sensitive and -insensitive enzymes remain unknown, recent studies demonstrate that growth-associated protein of 43 kD (GAP-43) and glyceraldehyde-3-phosphate dehydrogenase are substrates in vitro, although more work is needed to define how the function of these proteins is

altered by ADP-ribosylation. (Cholera and pertussis toxins can also be considered ADP-ribosyltransferases in that they catalyze the ADP-ribosylation of specific G-protein subunits, but their activity is not affected by NO.) Further research is needed to determine which of the second messenger roles of NO in the brain are mediated via regulation of ADP-ribosylation. In any case, it is notable that recent studies to identify a retrograde messenger involved in long-term potentiation have implicated NO and ADP-ribosylation: Inhibition of NO synthesis or ADP-ribosylation has been reported to block the formation of long-term potentiation. However, this remains controversial, because not all laboratories have been able to replicate these findings (see 27).

Phosphodiesterases

Cyclic nucleotide levels in neurons are highly regulated by the metabolism, as well as the synthesis, of these second messengers. This is accomplished by phosphodiesterases (PDEs), a family of enzymes which catalyze the conversion of cAMP and cGMP into 5'-AMP and 5'-GMP, respectively (1,27). The different forms of PDE display different affinities for cyclic nucleotides and are differentially regulated and distributed in brain. PDE I isozymes account for more than 90% of enzyme activity in brain and can hydrolyze either cAMP or cGMP. These PDEs are stimulated by Ca^{2+}/calmodulin and are thereby regulated by extracellular stimuli that regulate Ca^{2+} levels. PDE II enzymes are regulated by binding cGMP and also hydrolyze both cAMP and cGMP. PDE IV is specific for cAMP, and there are reports that the enzyme is regulated by guanine nucleotides, suggesting a possible role for G proteins. Other forms of PDE, namely PDE III and PDE V, are expressed in peripheral tissues and rod outer segments but to date have not been found in brain.

Calcium and the Phosphatidylinositol System

The ways in which neurotransmitters alter intracellular Ca^{2+} levels are more complex compared to those for cyclic nucleotides and involve two types of mechanisms that operate to different extents in different cell types (Fig. 3). Neurotransmitter receptor activation can alter the flux of extracellular Ca^{2+} into neurons or can regulate release of Ca^{2+} from intracellular stores. Once released, Ca^{2+} can exert multiple actions on neuronal function via intracellular regulatory proteins (Fig. 3). Receptors can directly regulate the conductance of specific voltage-gated Ca^{2+} channels via coupling with G proteins, as mentioned above. In addition, activation of other second messenger systems can alter Ca^{2+} channel conductance; for example, cAMP, and neurotransmitters that act through cAMP, can increase the conductance of some voltage-gated Ca^{2+} channels (see below). Depolarization of a neuron by any means will activate voltage-gated Ca^{2+} channels, which

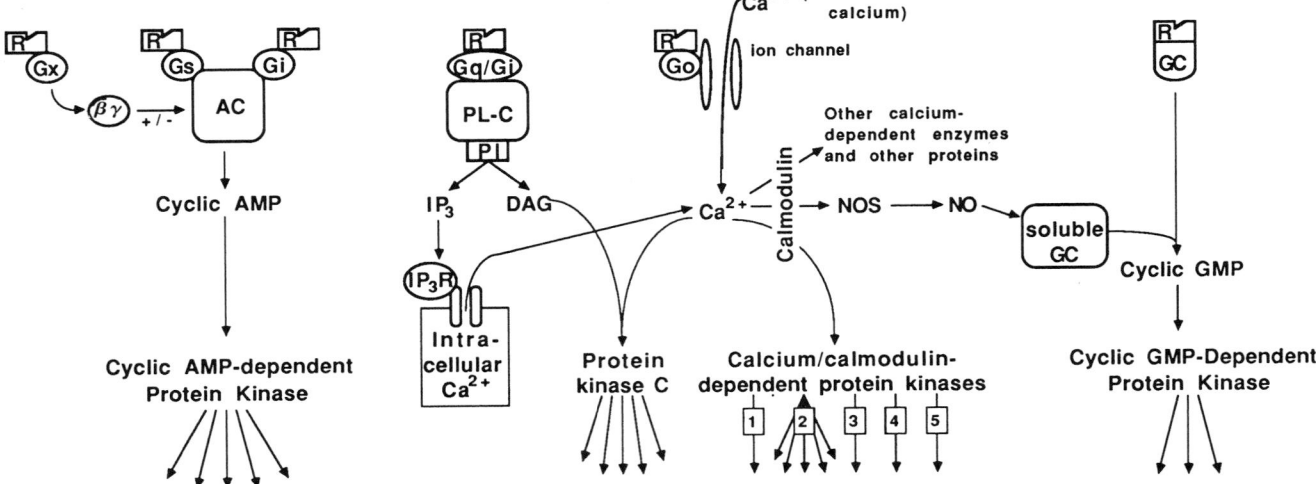

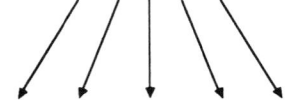

FIG. 3. Schematic illustration of major second messenger pathways in the brain. Gs and Gi/o, respectively, mediate the ability of neurotransmitter receptors (R) to activate or inhibit adenylyl cyclase, the enzyme that catalyzes the synthesis of cAMP. Also shown in the figure is the ability of G-protein $\beta\gamma$ subunits, released potentially by any type of G protein, to stimulate or inhibit different forms of adenylyl cyclase. Gi/o and Gq mediate the ability of neurotransmitter receptors to regulate phospholipase C (PLC), which metabolizes phosphatidylinositol (PI) into the second messengers inositol triphosphate (IP_3) and diacylglycerol (DAG). IP_3 then acts on specific IP_3 receptors (IP_3R) to increase intracellular levels of free Ca^{2+} (also a second messenger in brain) by releasing Ca^{2+} from internal stores. Increased levels of intracellular Ca^{2+} also result from the flux of Ca^{2+} across the plasma membrane through Ca^{2+} and other ion channels, a flux stimulated by nerve impulses and certain neurotransmitters. As discussed in the text, G proteins mediate many of the actions of neurotransmitters on such channels. Increased levels of Ca^{2+} activate nitric oxide synthetase (NOS), leading to increased levels of nitric oxide and the activation of cytoplasmic guanylyl cyclase (the enzyme that catalyzes the synthesis of cGMP) and of ADP-ribosyltransferases (not shown). Other forms of guanylyl cyclase reside in specific plasma membrane receptors. These second messengers, in turn, activate specific types of protein kinases. Brain contains one major type of cAMP-dependent protein kinase and of cGMP-dependent protein kinase, although subtypes of these enzymes are differentially expressed throughout the brain. These enzymes phosphorylate a specific array of substrate proteins, which can be considered third messengers. cAMP-dependent protein kinase has a broad substrate specificity; that is, it phosphorylates many substrate proteins and mediates most of the numerous second messenger actions of cAMP in the nervous system. The substrate specificity of cGMP-dependent protein kinase appears to be less broad, although by analogy with the cAMP system, it is likely that it mediates many of the second messenger functions of cGMP. Brain contains two major classes of Ca^{2+}-dependent protein kinase. One is activated by Ca^{2+} and calmodulin and is referred to as Ca^{2+}/calmodulin-dependent protein kinase. Brain contains at least five distinct types of this enzyme: Ca^{2+}/calmodulin-dependent protein kinases I, II (several subtypes of this enzyme are known), and III; phosphorylase kinase; and myosin light-chain kinase. The other major class is activated by Ca^{2+} in conjunction with DAG and various phospholipids and is referred to as Ca^{2+}/DAG-dependent protein kinase or protein kinase C; there are at least seven closely related variants of this enzyme present in the brain. Protein kinase C and Ca^{2+}/calmodulin-dependent protein kinase II have broad substrate specificities (as indicated by the multiple arrows in the figure), and each probably mediates many of the numerous second messenger actions of Ca^{2+} in the nervous system. (The figure also illustrates that some of the second messenger actions of Ca^{2+} in brain are mediated through proteins other than protein kinases.) Not shown in the figure is the fact that some protein phosphatases are also subject to regulation by second messengers. For example, protein phosphatase 2B, or calcineurin, is activated upon binding Ca^{2+}/calmodulin. Phosphorylation of substrate proteins by these various second-messenger-dependent protein kinases alters their physiological activity in such a way as to lead to the biological responses of the extracellular messengers either directly or indirectly through intervening fourth, fifth, sixth, and so on, messengers. (Modified from ref. 20.)

will lead to the flux of Ca^{2+} into the cells. Finally, extracellular Ca^{2+} can pass through some ligand-gated channels, such as the nicotinic cholinergic and N-methyl-D-aspartate (NMDA)-glutamate receptors.

Receptors can increase intracellular levels of free Ca^{2+} through regulation of the phosphatidylinositol system and subsequent actions on intracellular Ca^{2+} stores (Fig. 3) (2). Thus, many types of neurotransmitter receptors are coupled through G proteins to an enzyme called phospholipase C (PLC) (also referred to as phosphoinositidase C). Depending on the cell type, subtypes of Gq, Gi, and Go have been implicated in coupling receptors to PLC (38). Multiple forms of PLC which show different anatomical and regulatory properties have been identified in brain: PLC-β1 is stimulated by G-protein α subunits, PLC-β2 is stimulated by $\beta\gamma$ subunits, and PLC-γ is activated upon phosphorylation by protein tyrosine kinases (see below). PLC catalyzes the breakdown of PI, resulting in the generation of IP_3, which, through binding to a specific IP_3 receptor located on intracellular organelles (e.g., endoplasmic reticulum), releases Ca^{2+} from intracellular stores. The IP_3 receptor, like the related ryanodine receptor, forms a Ca^{2+} channel that responds to IP_3 by releasing Ca^{2+} stores. In addition, Ca^{2+} itself can exert a stimulatory effect on IP_3 and ryanodine receptors, which may underlie "oscillations and waves" in Ca^{2+} levels in some neurons and other cell types (2); this effect of Ca^{2+} represents a type of positive feedback which promotes the spread of the Ca^{2+} signal throughout the cell.

Arachidonic Acid Metabolites

The prostaglandins and leukotrienes represent another family of intracellular messengers (see Piomelli, *this volume,* for detailed discussion). Briefly, this family of messengers is generated by activation of an enzyme called phospholipase A_2, which cleaves membrane phospholipids to yield free arachidonic acid. The activity of phospholipase A_2 may be regulated by certain neurotransmitter–receptor interactions via G proteins, although this remains speculative. Next, arachidonic acid is cleaved by cyclooxygenase (an enzyme inhibited by aspirin and other nonsteroidal anti-inflammatory drugs) to yield, after numerous additional enzymatic steps, several types of prostaglandins and other cyclic endoperoxides (e.g., prostacyclins and thromboxanes), or it is cleaved by lipoxygenase to yield the leukotrienes. These endoperoxides and leukotrienes exert many effects on cell function by influencing directly the activity of adenylyl cyclase, guanylyl cyclase, ion channels, protein kinases, and other cellular proteins (35; also see Chapter 53, *this volume,* for detailed discussion).

Protein Phosphorylation as a Final Common Pathway in the Regulation of Neuronal Function

Despite the large number of second messengers that can be activated within neurons, there is a relatively uni-

form way in which these signaling pathways work. While second messenger molecules may occasionally have direct actions as effectors (e.g., cAMP can bind to and directly gate ion channels in neurons of the olfactory epithelium, and Ca^{2+} can bind to and directly regulate the activity of several enzymes), most of the known effects of intracellular second messengers are mediated, as stated earlier, by protein phosphorylation—that is, by stimulating the addition or removal of phosphate groups from specific amino acid residues in target proteins. Phosphate groups alter the conformation and charge of proteins and thereby alter their function (28,29).

The regulation of protein function by phosphorylation plays a paramount role in signal transduction within the brain, a view originally proposed by Greengard and co-workers over 25 years ago. In most cases, neurotransmitters regulate protein phosphorylation through second messenger-mediated activation of enzymes called *protein kinases*. Protein kinases transfer phosphate groups from ATP to serine, threonine, or tyrosine residues in specific substrate proteins. Neurotransmitters can also regulate protein phosphorylation through second-messenger-mediated regulation of protein phosphatases, enzymes that remove phosphate groups from proteins through hydrolysis. Each protein kinase and protein phosphatase acts on a specific array of substrate proteins.

Protein Kinases

The best-studied protein kinases in brain are those activated by the second messengers cAMP, cGMP, Ca^{2+}, and diacylglycerol (Table 1) (19,28,29). These protein kinases are named for the second messengers that activate them. Brain contains one major class of cAMP-dependent protein kinase and one major class of cGMP-dependent protein kinase (Fig. 3), although isoforms of these enzymes are now known. In contrast, two major classes of Ca^{2+}-dependent protein kinases have been described (Fig. 3). One is activated by Ca^{2+} in conjunction with the Ca^{2+}-binding protein calmodulin and is referred to as Ca^{2+}/calmodulin-dependent protein kinase. The other is activated by Ca^{2+} in conjunction with diacylglycerol and other lipids and is referred to as protein kinase C (32). The brain contains several subtypes of each of these Ca^{2+}-dependent enzymes, which exhibit different regulatory properties and are expressed differentially in neuronal cell types throughout the nervous system.

The brain contains numerous additional types of protein serine/threonine kinases, which are not directly activated by second messengers, and numerous types of protein tyrosine kinases, which phosphorylate substrate proteins specifically on tyrosine residues (see Fig. 1). It is likely that many of these protein kinases also play critically important roles in brain signal transduction, although the mechanisms involved are not as clearly established as for the second messenger-dependent enzymes.

TABLE 1. *Protein kinases in the brain*

Protein serine-threonine kinases
Second messenger-dependent protein kinases
    cAMP-dependent protein kinase
    cGMP-dependent protein kinase
    Ca^{2+}/calmodulin-dependent protein kinases
    Protein kinase C
Second-messenger-independent protein kinases
    MAP kinases (or ERKs)
    cdc kinases
    Casein kinases
    raf kinase
    rsk (ribosomal S6 kinase)
    mos kinase
    ste kinase
    Many others

Protein tyrosine kinases
Receptor-associated kinases
    Insulin receptor
    Epidermal growth factor receptor
    Neurotrophin receptors (trk)
    Many others
Not receptor-associated
    src
    yes
    fes
    Many others

An example of a second-messenger-independent protein serine/threonine kinase is the MAP-kinases [also referred to as *e*xtracellular signal-*r*egulated *k*inases (ERKs)], first identified on the basis of their association with, and phosphorylation of, microtubule-associated proteins (MAPs) (3,6). MAP-kinases have since been shown to phosphorylate a number of other proteins in brain and elsewhere, including tyrosine hydroxylase and numerous DNA-binding proteins. The activity of MAP-kinases are regulated by many extracellular signals, apparently through cAMP-dependent and Ca^{2+}-dependent protein kinases and protein tyrosine kinases. Thus, those neurotransmitters, including catecholamines (see below), that initially influence the cAMP and Ca^{2+} pathways would be expected to ultimately regulate (and produce certain physiological effects via) the MAP-kinase system.

The activity of MAP-kinases themselves is controlled through complex cascades involving protein phosphorylation. MAP-kinases are activated via their phosphorylation on threonine and tyrosine residues by another protein kinase, termed MAP-kinase kinase (also referred to as MEK or *MAP*-kinase/*ERK* kinase), which in turn can be phosphorylated and activated by several MAP-kinase kinase kinases (also referred to as MEK-kinases or ERK-kinase kinases), such as Raf-kinase. The mechanisms by which these enzymes are influenced by second messenger-dependent protein kinases and by protein tyrosine kinases is becoming increasingly well known and are summarized in Fig. 2. This system highlights the complex interrelationships among intracellular messenger pathways and their regulation of cell function.

The best-studied protein tyrosine kinases are those that are associated with plasma membrane receptors for many types of growth factors (see ref. 19). Receptors for most growth factors, including insulin, epidermal growth factor, nerve growth factor, and various neurotrophins, possess protein tyrosine kinase enzyme activity within the receptor complex. Many forms of these receptor-kinases are known. The neurotrophins activate a class of receptor-kinases, called *trk* proteins. Recent studies (see refs. 3 and 6) have revealed some of the mechanisms by which activation of these receptors lead to biological responses (see Fig. 2). Binding of growth factor to its receptor leads to activation of the receptor-associated protein tyrosine kinase and to phosphorylation of the receptor itself as well as other proteins with Src homology (SH) adaptor domains. The phosphorylated receptor and other proteins then interact with a series of other proteins, leading eventually to activation of the MAP-kinase pathway. This probably represents a common mechanism for activation of intracellular signal transduction pathways by most receptor-kinases.

The other major class of protein tyrosine kinase (e.g., src) lacks a receptor domain. The mechanism underlying their regulation has remained elusive, although early evidence indicates that some of these enzymes might transiently become associated with specific receptors or other membrane proteins via SH domains and thereby transduce extracellular signals into changes in intraneuronal function. In addition, these protein tyrosine kinases may be phosphorylated and activated by receptor-protein tyrosine kinases.

Protein Phosphatases

Protein phosphatases can be divided into two major classes based on the types of amino acids they dephosphorylate: serine/threonine phosphatases and tyrosine phosphatases (19,37). There are two known mechanisms by which neurotransmitters can influence protein phosphorylation through the regulation of protein serine/threonine phosphatases. One phosphatase, referred to as *calcineurin* or *phosphatase type 2B*, can be activated directly by binding Ca^{2+}/calmodulin. Presumably, neurotransmitters that alter cellular Ca^{2+} levels influence the phosphorylation of cellular proteins through alterations in calcineurin activity. The other mechanism is indirect and involves a class of protein referred to as *protein phosphatase inhibitors*. The best-known protein phosphatase inhibitors are phosphatase inhibitors-1 and -2 and DARPP-32, the latter an inhibitor protein expressed in specific neuronal cell types in the brain (see below). These proteins are potent inhibitors of protein phosphatase type 1, and their phosphorylation by cAMP-dependent or other protein kinases alters their inhibitory activity. Presumably, in neurons that contain these phosphatase inhibitors, neurotransmitters that alter cellular cAMP levels influence the phosphorylation of cellular proteins through alterations in type 1 protein phosphatase activity. Less is known about the physiological regulation of protein tyrosine phosphatases in the brain.

Regulation of Proteins by Phosphorylation

Following the regulation of protein kinase or protein phosphatase activity, the next step in intracellular signal transduction involves regulation of the phosphorylation state of specific neuronal phosphoproteins. These phosphoproteins are referred to as *third messengers*. Virtually every type of neural protein is now known to be regulated by phosphorylation (Table 2), indicating the widespread role of protein phosphorylation in the regulation of diverse aspects of neuronal function. This includes the regulation of ion channel conductance, activity of various transporters, neurotransmitter receptor sensitivity, neurotransmitter synthesis and release, axoplasmic transport, elaboration of dendritic and axonal processes, development and maintenance of differentiated characteristics of neurons, and gene expression. (See Chapter 61, *this volume*, for further discussion of gene expression and neuronal plasticity.)

The above discussion of signal transduction pathways portrays protein phosphorylation as the major molecular currency with which protein function is regulated in response to extracellular stimuli, a view supported by over a generation of research. Thus, although proteins are known to be covalently modified in many other ways (e.g., by ADP-ribosylation, carboxymethylation, acetylation, myristoylation, palmitoylation, tyrosine sulfation, isoprenylation, and glycosylation), none of these mechanisms is as widespread and readily subject to regulation by synaptic stimuli as phosphorylation.

Heterogeneity in Brain Signal Transduction Pathways

As with receptors and ion channels, molecular biological studies have demonstrated extraordinary heterogeneity

TABLE 2. *Types of phosphoproteins in the brain regulated by catecholamines*

Signal transduction proteins
  Neurotransmitter receptors
  G proteins
  Second messenger enzymes (e.g., cyclases, phospholipases, phosphodiesterases
  Protein kinases
  Protein phosphatases
Ion channels and pumps
Neurotransmitter synthetic enzymes
Cytoskeletal proteins
Synaptic-vesicle-associated proteins
Proteins involved in protein synthesis
Proteins involved in gene expression
General metabolic enzymes

in intracellular messenger pathways, a degree of heterogeneity not suspected by classical biochemical, pharmacological, or physiological studies. For example, whereas biochemical and pharmacological studies indicated the existence of five major types of G proteins (i.e., Gs, Gi, Go, Gq, and Gt), two types of cAMP-dependent protein kinase, and just one type of protein kinase C, molecular cloning studies now indicate the existence of over 20 distinct G-protein subunits, six distinct subunits of cAMP-dependent protein kinase, and seven subtypes of protein kinase C. Such heterogeneity is due to a combination of the existence of numerous distinct genes for each of the proteins plus alternative splicing of some common genes. Comparison of the individual subtypes of these proteins has indicated that they possess different regulatory properties and exhibit varying levels of expression in different neuronal cell types. This high degree of heterogeneity indicates still greater potential for functional specificity within and between neuronal cell types in the brain. Such heterogeneity also raises the possibility of developing drugs targeted for specific subtypes of intracellular messengers, drugs that would represent novel approaches in the treatment of neuropsychiatric disorders.

INTRACELLULAR SYSTEMS COUPLED TO CATECHOLAMINE RECEPTORS: PROXIMAL EFFECTS

All known receptors for catecholamine neurotransmitters belong to the family of G-protein-coupled receptors, which possess seven transmembrane domains and produce all of their physiological effects via interactions with G proteins. Known catecholamine receptors are listed in Table 3 and discussed elsewhere in this text. These receptors, and the intracellular messenger pathways through which they produce their physiological effects, can be categorized based on the species of G protein with which they interact initially. In this section, we focus on the mechanisms by which catecholamine receptors, via their interactions with G proteins and intracellular messengers, produce rapid electrophysiological effects. In the next section, we illustrate how the same recruitment of intracellular messengers also results in the regulation of many additional neural processes.

Before discussing signal transduction pathways for specific catecholamine receptors, it is important to emphasize the technical difficulties in delineating these pathways experimentally. For example, to support a second messenger role of cAMP in the electrophysiological actions of a catecholamine receptor, it is necessary to show that agents that directly activate the cAMP pathway mimic receptor activation. This is not straightforward, because cAMP analogues applied extracellularly cannot elevate intracellular cAMP levels as rapidly and to the same extent as receptor activation. As a result, numerous reports of the inability of cAMP or other second messengers to mimic receptor activation must be viewed with extreme caution. Similar technical problems exist for demonstrating that agents that directly inhibit cAMP, or other second messenger pathways, block the consequences of receptor activation. Ultimately, the signal transduction cascades for individual receptors must be studied by patch-clamp and related techniques, which permit direct access to the intracellular milieu.

Receptors Coupled to Gs

β_1- and β_2-adrenergic and D_1- and D_5-dopamine receptors are believed to produce their physiological actions via interactions with Gs (Table 3) and the subsequent stimulation of adenylyl cyclase and cAMP-dependent protein kinase (see ref. 39). This cascade mediates the electrophysiological actions of these receptors through the phosphorylation of ion channels and pumps. Most, and possibly all, types of channels and pumps are acutely regulated via their phosphorylation by many types of protein kinases. The electrophysiological actions of β-adrenergic and $D_{1/5}$-dopamine receptors therefore depend on the types of channels and pumps expressed in a particular type of target cell that can be phosphorylated by cAMP-dependent protein kinase. For example, β-adrenergic receptor stimulation depolarizes cardiac myocytes via the phosphorylation and activation of voltage-dependent Ca^{2+} channels. β-Adrenergic receptor stimulation also promotes depolarization of hippocampal pyramidal and many other neurons, although in this case the effect is mediated via phosphorylation and inhibition Ca^{2+}-activated K^+ channels (31), as well as via the phosphorylation and facilitation of glutamate receptor function (12). It should be noted that this latter mechanism may mediate the ability of β-adrenergic receptors to influence long-term potentiation in the hippocampus. In contrast, β-adrenergic receptor stimulation promotes gamma-aminobutyric acid (GABA)-induced hyperpolarization of cerebellar Purkinje cells (36), possibly via the phosphorylation and facilitation of $GABA_A$ receptor-chloride channel function (23). Most known effects of $D_{1/5}$ receptor stimulation are hyperpolarizing, although the specific ion channels involved have not yet been identified in most cases.

Other signal transduction pathways for these receptors have been reported in the literature (39), although the extent to which they mediate physiological actions of the receptors in brain remains most uncertain. In the heart, free $Gs\alpha$ generated via activation of β-adrenergic receptors may activate voltage-dependent Ca^{2+} channels in two ways: (i) via stimulation of adenylyl cyclase, leading eventually to channel phosphorylation (as outlined above), and (ii) by directly binding to and activating the channels. In certain tissues, activation of D_1-dopamine receptors is claimed to activate PI hydrolysis, leading to the speculation that some of the effects of D_1 receptors are

TABLE 3. *Signal transduction pathways for catecholamine receptors*

Receptor	G protein[a]	Effectors[b]
Adrenergic		
β_1, β_2	Gs	Adenylyl cyclase (↑)
α_{1A}[c]	Gi/o	Ca^{2+} (↑)
α_{1B}[c]	Gq	Inositol triphosphate (↑)
α_{1C}[c]	Gq	Inositol triphosphate (↑)
α_{1D}[c]	Gq	Inositol triphosphate (↑)
$\alpha_{2A/D}$[d]	Gi	Adenylyl cyclase (↓), K^+ (↑), Ca^{2+} (↓)
α_{2B}	$Gi_{2,3}$[e]	Adenylyl cyclase (↓)
α_{2C}	Go[e]	Adenylyl cyclase (↓)
Dopaminergic		
D_1, D_5	Gs	Adenylyl cyclase (↑)
D_2, D_3, D_4	Gi/o	Adenylyl cyclase (↓), K^+ (↑), Ca^{2+} (↓)

[a] G protein utilized by each receptor could vary depending on the brain region and effector systems present. Pertussis toxin has been useful in determining the type of G protein utilized by different receptors: Gq and Gz are insensitive, whereas Gi and Go are inactivated by toxin treatment. Gz is not included in the table; it is reported to mediate inhibition of adenylyl cyclase in cultured cells, but a role in mediating catecholamine receptor regulation of adenylyl cyclase has not been demonstrated.

[b] The table lists the primary action(s) mediated by G-protein α subunits. Different, and sometimes opposing, effects may be produced by G-protein $\beta\gamma$ subunits.

[c] There are several cases of α-adrenergic stimulation of cGMP levels, presumably mediated via Ca^{2+} stimulation of nitric oxide synthetase and subsequent nitric oxide stimulation of guanylyl cyclase.

[d] α_{2A} and α_{2D} receptors appear to be human and rat homologues, respectively, with slightly different pharmacological profiles.

[e] α_{2B} and α_{2C} prefer these G-protein subtypes when expressed in cultured cells, but may utilize other G-protein subtypes in vivo.

mediated via the IP_3, Ca^{2+}, and protein kinase C cascade. However, these studies have not ruled out the alternative explanation that D_1-induced activation of PI hydrolysis may be mediated via the cAMP pathway.

Receptors Coupled to Gi/Go

Catecholamine receptors coupled to the Gi/Go family of G proteins are listed in Table 3, and they include several subtypes of the α_2-adrenergic receptor and the D_2-, D_3-, and D_4-dopamine receptors (39). In addition, there are reports that the α_{1A}-adrenergic receptor subtype also utilizes these G proteins. The role of Gi and Go in mediating the actions of these receptors is based on the ability of pertussis toxin, which ADP-ribosylates and inactivates these G proteins, to block various physiological actions of receptor activation. However, it remains unanswered in most cases as to which subtype of Gi and/or

Go mediates the various effects of a certain receptor in a given cell type.

The α_2-adrenergic and D_{2-4}-dopamine receptors, and probably all other types of receptors that are coupled to Gi and Go, produce their rapid physiological actions via two major mechanisms, which can occur in the same target neurons (31,39). In one mechanism, receptor stimulation leads to the activation of an inward rectifying K^+ channel and/or to the inhibition of a voltage-dependent Ca^{2+} channel. In smooth muscle, α_{1A}-adrenergic receptors are reported to stimulate dihydropyridine-sensitive Ca^{2+} channels; whether a similar mechanism operates in brain remains to be determined. These various actions are thought to be mediated via direct G-protein coupling: Free $G\alpha i/o$ (or $\beta\gamma$) subunit binds to and gates the channel. In the other mechanism, receptor stimulation leads to inhibition of adenylyl cyclase. This action is thought to be mediated primarily via receptor–G-protein interaction and the generation of free $G\alpha i/o$ subunit, which then binds to and inhibits adenylyl cyclase. Inhibition of adenylyl cyclase would then lead to some of the electrophysiological effects of receptor stimulation via inhibition of cAMP-dependent phosphorylation of various types of channels and pumps, depending on the neuronal cell type involved, as described above.

Free $\beta\gamma$ subunits generated by receptor–G-protein interactions may also contribute to adenylyl cyclase inhibition, at least for some forms of the enzyme (e.g., the type I, calmodulin-sensitive enzyme) expressed in some cell types (27). Other forms of adenylyl cyclase (e.g., the type II, calmodulin-insensitive enzyme) have been shown to be stimulated by free $\beta\gamma$ subunits in vitro. This leads to the theoretical possibility that receptors coupled to Gi and Go might even stimulate adenylyl cyclase in some cell types. Although this has not been directly demonstrated for the α_2-adrenergic or D_{2-4}-dopamine receptors, such a mechanism could explain reports of α_2-adrenergic receptor enhancement of cAMP responses in brain.

There are isolated reports that some of these same catecholamine receptors may activate the PI system in vitro (39). These actions are reported to occur via coupling with Gi/o through mechanisms analogous to those described below for Gq.

Receptors Coupled to Gq

Of the large number of neurotransmitter receptors known to activate phosphatidylinositol hydrolysis, only one class of catecholamine receptor, the α_1-adrenergic receptor, is known to produce its physiological actions primarily via this second messenger pathway (see Table 3) (39). In most cell types, neurotransmitter-receptor-induced activation of the phosphatidylinositol pathway is mediated via pertussis-toxin-insensitive G proteins (Gq), although in some cases toxin-sensitive G proteins (Gi and/or Go) are involved (38). Despite the fact that activa-

tion of several subtypes of the α_1-adrenergic receptor has been shown to lead to PI hydrolysis in numerous tissues, the specific type of G protein involved in various neuronal cell types remains unknown in most cases.

Activation of the PI pathway could theoretically lead to regulation of ion channels via several mechanisms, although the specific mechanisms pertinent to the α_1-receptor are not known. Activation of the PI pathway would lead, via the generation of diacylglycerol and IP_3-mediated release of Ca^{2+} from internal stores, to the activation of protein kinase C and to the phosphorylation and regulation of many types of channels and pumps, depending on the cell type. Release of Ca^{2+} from internal stores would also lead to activation of Ca^{2+}/calmodulin-dependent protein kinases and the subsequent phosphorylation and regulation of other channels and pumps. In addition, release of Ca^{2+} from internal stores would influence directly Ca^{2+}-activated K^+ channels.

α_1-Adrenergic receptors also indirectly activate the cAMP system in brain (7). While activation of α_1-adrenergic receptors alone has little or no effect, α_1-adrenergic receptor activation enhances the cAMP response to receptors that couple to Gs, including the β-adrenergic and vasoactive intestinal peptide receptors. This may occur via formation of IP_3, elevated Ca^{2+} levels, and activation of protein kinase C. Alternatively, it could involve activation of adenylyl cyclase by free G-protein $\beta\gamma$ subunits released upon receptor–G-protein coupling to Gq.

Activation of α_1-adrenergic receptors is also known to increase cellular levels of cGMP in nervous tissue (39). The most likely mechanism is via Ca^{2+}-induced activation of NO synthetase and the subsequent activation of guanylyl cyclase by nitric oxide. The physiological consequences of α_1-adrenergic receptor stimulated increases in the cGMP and NO pathways remain to be determined. However, it should be mentioned that certain ion channels are known to be phosphorylated and regulated by cGMP-dependent protein kinase (28,29).

INTRACELLULAR SYSTEMS COUPLED TO CATECHOLAMINE RECEPTORS: DISTAL EFFECTS

This section discusses the diverse effects that catecholamine receptors exert on target cells through the regulation of intracellular messenger pathways. As discussed in the preceding section and in other chapters of this volume (see Chapters 15, 20, 21, 25, 29, and 33, *this volume*), catecholamine regulation of the electrical properties of target neurons are important for mediating the most rapid effects of catecholamines in the brain. However, in addition to these rapid effects, catecholamines exert many other actions on their target neurons that produce short- and long-term modulatory effects on neuronal function (see Fig. 1). These modulatory effects, which are mediated predominantly (if not solely) via intracellular messenger pathways, include regulation of the activity of receptors, ion channels, second messenger effector enzymes, and neurotransmitter synthetic enzymes, as well as regulation of the synthesis and degradation of these and other neuronal proteins. In fact, these modulatory effects can be viewed as catecholamine-mediated neural plasticity, some examples of which are discussed below. Given that the formation of mental symptoms is gradual, as is their reversal in response to psychotropic drug treatment and other therapies, it is possible that these modulatory effects of catecholamines are more relevant for psychiatric phenomena than the regulation of ion channels or pumps per se. The physiological relevance of these modulatory processes to specific psychiatric phenomena is the subject of a later chapter (Chapter 61, *this volume*).

Short-Term Modulatory Processes

Activation of catecholamine receptors exerts short-term modulatory effects on several cellular systems. In most cases, these actions are mediated through the regulation of specific protein kinases and protein phosphatases. A few examples of such short-term modulatory effects are discussed below. The reader is referred elsewhere for a more detailed discussion (20).

Regulation of Receptor Function

Activation of catecholamine receptors can trigger numerous processes that influence the functional state of that receptor system. Agonist treatment has been shown to alter receptor affinity for its ligand, receptor coupling to G proteins, receptor accessibility to the extracellular space (e.g., sequestration and internalization), receptor degradation, and receptor synthesis. Receptor phosphorylation by multiple protein kinases appears to mediate many of these phenomena (18,22). These processes are best established for the β-adrenergic receptor and are presented in greater detail below.

Regulation of Neurotransmitter Metabolism

Activation of catecholamine receptors can influence the ability of target neurons to synthesize their own neurotransmitter. One mechanism by which this is achieved is through the phosphorylation of neurotransmitter synthetic enzymes. This is best established for tyrosine hydroxylase, the rate-limiting enzyme in the synthesis of the catecholamines, which is phosphorylated and activated by cAMP-dependent protein kinase, Ca^{2+}/calmodulin-dependent protein kinase II, and protein kinase C, as well as by MAP-kinase and probably other second-messenger-independent protein kinases (29,44). In most cases, phosphorylation increases the V_{max} of tyrosine hydroxylase

(i.e., increases the maximal catalytic activity of a single enzyme molecule) or the affinity of the enzyme for its pterin cofactor (which would make the enzyme more active at subsaturating concentrations of cofactor). Dephosphorylation of the enzyme (achieved via inhibition of the cAMP or Ca^{2+} pathways as discussed above) could mediate the ability of α_2-adrenergic or D_2-dopamine autoreceptors to reduce catecholamine synthesis. Phosphorylation of tyrosine hydroxylase also mediates the ability of many other types of neurotransmitter receptor, which act through the cAMP or Ca^{2+} systems, to rapidly regulate tyrosine hydroxylase activity and, as a result, the capacity of catecholaminergic neurons to synthesize their neurotransmitter. This provides a critical homeostatic control mechanism that enables catecholaminergic neurons to alter their functional activity in response to a variety of synaptic inputs.

Activation of catecholamine receptors can also influence the synthesis of other neurotransmitters by regulating the expression of peptide neurotransmitters in target neurons, as discussed below.

Regulation of Neurotransmitter Release

Activation of catecholamine receptors located on presynaptic nerve terminals can regulate the release of neurotransmitter from those terminals. One mechanism probably involves regulation of the phosphorylation of nerve terminal ion channels or pumps and the subsequent regulation of Ca^{2+} entry into the terminals and the release of neurotransmitter. For example, by hyperpolarizing nerve terminals, α_2-adrenergic and D_{2-4}-dopamine receptors would be expected to reduce neurotransmitter release via activation of K^+ channels or inhibition of Ca^{2+} channels.

Another critical mechanism appears to involve the phosphorylation of a family of synaptic-vesicle-associated proteins, the best-studied of which are the synapsins (13). The synapsins comprise a family of phosphoproteins present in virtually all nerve terminals in brain that are phosphorylated by cAMP-dependent and Ca^{2+}/calmodulin-dependent protein kinases. Synapsin phosphorylation increases the amount of neurotransmitter released from nerve terminals in response to physiological stimuli. Phosphorylation of synapsins appears to augment neurotransmitter release by altering their binding affinity for synaptic vesicles and other cytoskeletal proteins. Such changes in synapsin binding affinities are thought to regulate synaptic vesicle traffic within nerve terminals and, possibly, the process of exocytosis. Phosphorylation of the synapsins is regulated by a number of neurotransmitters, which influence cAMP or Ca^{2+} levels in nerve terminals, and appears to mediate the ability of these neurotransmitters to produce relatively long-lasting changes in the functional activity of those terminals. For example, stimulation of β-adrenergic or D_1-dopamine receptors, via activation of the cAMP pathway, has been shown to stimulate synapsin phosphorylation in a variety of neural preparations, and this probably contributes to the ability of these receptors to increase neurotransmitter release. In contrast, α_2-adrenergic and D_{2-4}-dopamine receptor inhibition of the cAMP and Ca^{2+} pathways and of synapsin phosphorylation would be expected to contribute to receptor inhibition of neurotransmitter release.

Long-Term Modulatory Processes

Activation of catecholamine receptors can also result in more long-term regulation of neuronal function. A brief overview of these processes is given below. More detailed information of these mechanisms, and their role in mediating the chronic actions of psychotropic drug treatments on the brain, is presented later (see Chapter 61, *this volume*).

Regulation of Protein Levels

A prominent mechanism by which catecholamines exert long-term effects on the brain involves regulation of the types and amounts of proteins present in target neurons. Thus, in addition to regulation by covalent modifications, the functional activity of a given protein in a neuron can be influenced by the amount of protein that is expressed. Catecholamine-induced alterations in protein levels can thereby exert profound and persistent changes in target neurons. As some examples, altered levels of a neurotransmitter receptor would produce long-lasting changes in the neuron's responsiveness to that neurotransmitter, altered levels of an ion channel would produce long-lasting changes in the neuron's electrical excitability, and altered levels of a neurotransmitter synthetic enzyme would produce long-lasting changes in the neuron's capacity to transmit its signals to subsequent neurons.

Catecholamine regulation of protein levels appears to be achieved by the regulation of every conceivable step involved, including alterations in gene transcription, the processing of mRNA and its transport into the cytoplasm, the stability and translatability of mRNA, the posttranslational processing of proteins and their localization to specific subcellular compartments, and their enzymatic degradation. Once again, protein phosphorylation appears to be the most important mechanism by which each of these processes is influenced by extracellular signals. This occurs through the phosphorylation, and consequent regulation of the physiological activity, of specific regulatory proteins involved in transcription, translation, and posttranslational processing.

Through these various mechanisms it is becoming increasingly apparent that catecholamines influence the expression of diverse types of neuronal proteins. One prominent example is regulation of the expression of peptide neurotransmitters and growth factors. For example, based on the actions of haloperidol (as a D_2 receptor antagonist)

and stimulants (as indirect dopamine agonists), it is clear that dopamine can regulate the expression of proenkephalin and other neuropeptides in specific brain regions in vivo (see ref. 20).

One aspect of gene expression which has received a great deal of attention is regulation of nuclear transcription factors. Transcription factors are proteins that bind to specific sequences of DNA present in certain genes and thereby increase or decrease the rate of transcription of those genes (20,26). One class of transcription factor (e.g., Fos and Jun), encoded by immediate early genes, would appear to have an important role in long-term modulatory processes, because they are induced rapidly in brain in response to a variety of extracellular stimuli, including activation of adrenergic and dopaminergic receptors (26). Another class of transcription factor, an example of which is the *cyclic AMP response element binding* protein (CREB), is also rapidly regulated in brain, but in this case by protein phosphorylation by cAMP-dependent (and probably Ca^{2+}-dependent) protein kinases. Catecholamine receptors that result in alterations in the cAMP (or Ca^{2+}) pathway would be expected to result in altered CREB phosphorylation and altered transcriptional activity (20). Regulation of these transcription factors, and other pathways for regulation of gene expression in the brain, are discussed in further detail elsewhere in this volume (see Chapter 61, *this volume*).

Regulation of Neuronal Growth and Differentiation

It is likely that catecholamines influence cell growth, differentiation, and movement (including axoplasmic transport and sprouting of dendrites and axons) in their target cells, although the details of the mechanisms involved remain obscure. This view is based on the ability of catecholamines to regulate, as discussed above, the critical intracellular messenger pathways known to control these cellular processes. Moreover, recent studies have demonstrated that activation of adrenergic and dopaminergic receptors increases the expression of neurotrophins in primary neuronal cultures and in brain (25,33,43). These findings, while preliminary, support trophic-like consequences of catecholamine receptor activation and suggest that regulation of neurotropins may be one of the mechanisms involved.

Regulation of Learning and Memory

Every instance in which a protein is phosphorylated, or the amount of a protein changes, can be viewed as molecular memory. This is because a change in a protein's phosphorylation or amount leads to a change in that protein's, and hence its neuron's, function—a molecular record of that neuron's prior experience. These individual examples of molecular memory then accumulate to lead successively to changes in the physiological properties of individual neurons, to changes in the physiological properties of larger neural networks, and ultimately to changes in the behavior of the organism. It is well known that catecholamines can influence processes of learning and memory at the behavioral level (see Chapters 32 and 33, *this volume*). Identification of the myriad molecular steps underlying such phenomena is a major challenge for the future (see Chapter 61, *this volume*).

Regulation of Intracellular Messenger Pathways

The ability of catecholamine receptors to initiate specific intracellular cascades means that these receptors also influence, albeit less directly, numerous other intracellular messenger pathways in their target cells. This is based on the now extensive evidence that most of the protein components of intracellular messenger systems are themselves regulated by phosphorylation. This permits extraordinarily complex cross-talk between signaling pathways, which permits cells to coordinate their responses to environmental stimuli (20,28,29).

Several types of G proteins have been reported to undergo phosphorylation by a variety of protein kinases. Proteins that control the synthesis of the cyclic nucleotide second messengers (adenylyl cyclase and guanylyl cyclase), as well as the degradation of cyclic nucleotides (phosphodiesterases), are regulated by phosphorylation. Similarly, proteins that control intracellular Ca^{2+} levels or the PI system (e.g., PLC, Ca^{2+} channels, the Ca^{2+}/ Mg^{2+}-ATPase pump, the IP_3 receptor) are regulated by phosphorylation. Moreover, phospholipase A_2, which generates arachidonic acid metabolites (e.g., prostaglandins) that modulate cyclic nucleotide and Ca^{2+} levels, is also subject to phosphorylation. Many protein kinases are themselves phosphorylated and regulated by other protein kinases, and protein phosphatase type 1 is regulated by protein phosphatase inhibitor proteins, which themselves are regulated by phosphorylation. In addition, most, and possibly all, protein kinases undergo autophosphorylation whereby they phosphorylate themselves.

It is clear from the above discussion that each second messenger system in the brain influences all the others. This means that although the systems are drawn as distinct pathways in Fig. 3, they do not operate as distinct pathways, but operate instead as a complex web of interacting pathways (see Fig. 1). Thus, any time a catecholamine or other neurotransmitter produces its primary effect on one second messenger system, many other systems will also be influenced eventually, with such interactions mediated for the most part through protein phosphorylation. For example, β-adrenergic and $D_{1/5}$-dopamine receptors, which produce their primary effects through the activation of the cAMP pathway, could potentially influence the Ca^{2+} and PI systems via cAMP-dependent phosphorylation of G proteins, phospholipases, Ca^{2+} and K^+ channels, electrogenic pumps, Ca^{2+}-dependent protein kinases, and

the IP_3 receptor, as well as the many proteins that can be phosphorylated by both cAMP-dependent and Ca^{2+}-dependent protein kinases.

In addition, there is also potential for interactions between these catecholamine-receptor-activated pathways and the second-messenger-independent protein kinase pathways, including those regulated by the receptor-associated protein tyrosine kinases (see Figs. 1 and 2). Thus, second messenger kinases can phosphorylate and activate Raf-kinase and possibly other MAP-kinase kinase kinases. These enzymes are the first step in the MAP-kinase pathway, and they function (as stated earlier in this chapter) by phosphorylating and activating MAP-kinase kinases, which, in turn, function by phosphorylating and activating MAP-kinases. This provides a mechanism whereby catecholamine-receptor-activated second messenger pathways may interact with and regulate, in either a stimulatory or inhibitory manner, the same pathways regulated by neurotrophins and other growth factor receptors.

Examples of Distal Actions of Catecholamine Receptor Activation

β-Adrenergic Receptor

Activation of the β-adrenergic receptor (βAR) results, via Gs, in activation of the cAMP second messenger system and thereby initiates a cascade of intracellular events regulated by this pathway. Some of these events, which have been studied in detail, include receptor desensitization and down-regulation, activation and translocation of cAMP-dependent protein kinase, regulation of transcription factors, and expression of specific target genes (see Fig. 4) (21,22,24).

Desensitization of the βAR has been studied extensively and involves alterations of practically every point of the βAR-coupled cAMP system, including regulation of receptor and effector protein expression (Fig. 4). Agonist binding to the βAR leads to formation of cAMP and activation of cAMP-dependent protein kinase which, in turn, phosphorylates the receptor and functionally uncouples it from Gs. This involves phosphorylation of specific serine residues in the third cytoplasmic and carboxy-terminus domains of the receptor and results in a reduced sensitivity to agonist, as measured by a rightward shift in dose response. Continued exposure to high concentrations of agonist results in phosphorylation of the receptor by a second protein kinase, termed βAR kinase (βARK), which only phosphorylates the agonist-activated form of the receptor at serine residues in the carboxy-terminus domain. Once these sites are phosphorylated, another protein, β-arrestin, binds to this domain of the receptor and competes with Gs; this reduces the maximal response to agonist stimulation. More recent studies indicate that various forms of βAR kinase and β-arrestin are not spe-

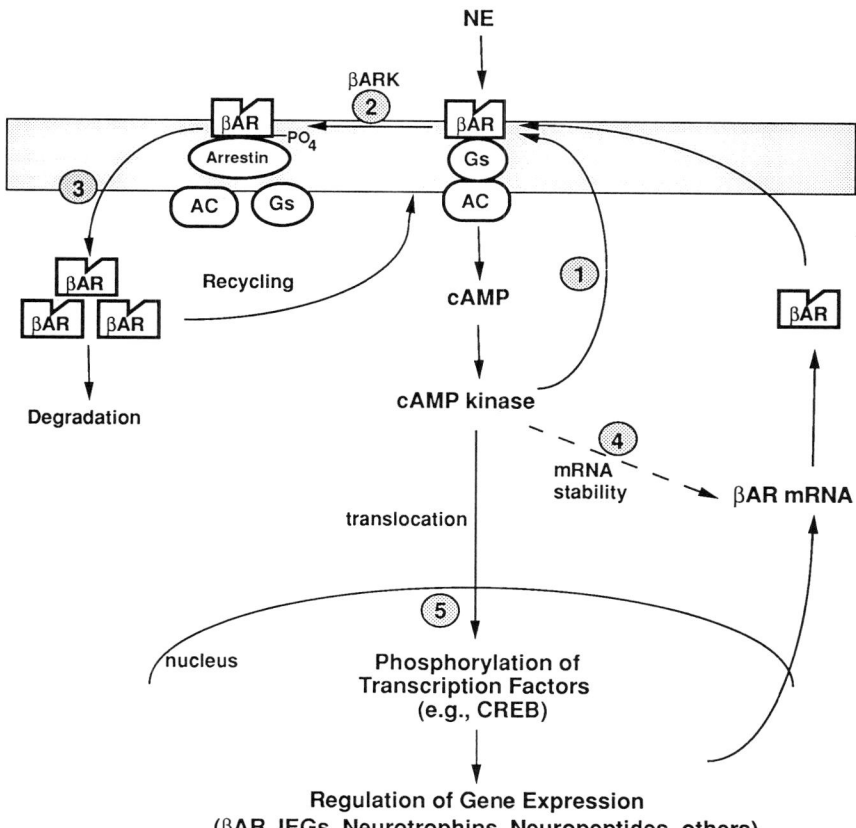

FIG. 4. Schematic illustration of multiple mechanisms underlying regulation of the βAR. One of the best-characterized actions of βAR activation is regulation of the receptor itself, which involves several points controlling receptor function and expression. (1) βAR stimulation of the cAMP system results in phosphorylation of the receptor by cAMP-dependent protein kinase, which leads to uncoupling of the receptor from Gs. The activated protein kinase would also phosphorylate many other proteins, not shown in the figure, which would then mediate many of the actions of βAR activation. (2) Prolonged activation of the receptor leads to phosphorylation by another kinase, βAR kinase (βARK), which only phosphorylates the agonist-activated form of the receptor. This results in binding of the receptor to β-arrestin, which competes with Gs and thereby inhibits βAR-stimulation of adenylyl cyclase (AC). (3) Loss of βARs from the membrane occurs when receptors are internalized and sequestered into intracellular vesicles. This pool of receptors is then available for either recycling back to the membrane or degradation. Such sequestration, internalization, degradation, and membrane re-insertion may be mediated via receptor phosphorylation and dephosphorylation involving the cAMP and/or βARK pathways. Another mechanism by which receptor activation leads to down-regulation of the βAR is via regulation of receptor mRNA levels, which may occur by two primary mechanisms. (4) The level of receptor mRNA is regulated by the stability or half-life of the mRNA. Although the mechanisms responsible for regulation of mRNA stability have not been identified, they may also involve cAMP-dependent protein kinase. (5) The level of receptor mRNA is also regulated via changes in βAR gene transcription. This effect is mediated by the cAMP pathway and appears to involve the translocation of cAMP-dependent protein kinase catalytic subunit into the nucleus and the phosphorylation of constitutively expressed transcription factors (e.g., CREB). It might also depend upon the subsequent induction of other transcription factors [e.g., immediate early gene (IEG) products such as c-Fos]. In addition to regulation of receptor gene transcription, such regulation of transcription factors would mediate the effects of βAR activation on the expression of many other genes—for example, those for G proteins, cAMP-dependent protein kinase, neurotrophins, and neuropeptides. This, in turn, would mediate many of the more long-term effects of βAR activation on brain function.

cific for the βAR and probably mediate agonist-induced desensitization of many other G-protein-coupled receptors, including other catecholamine receptors.

Loss of βAR binding sites from the cell membrane involves at least two mechanisms, receptor sequestration and degradation (down-regulation). In the presence of high concentrations of agonist, receptors are internalized and are then sequestered into intracellular vesicles; these receptors are accessible to hydrophobic ligands, which penetrate the vesicle membrane, but not to hydrophilic ligands. This pool of receptors is available for recycling back to the plasma membrane, apparently upon receptor dephosphorylation. Alternatively, internalized receptors may be transported to lysosomes where they are degraded rapidly.

Down-regulation of the βAR in response to agonist exposure also occurs via regulation of receptor expression, an action apparently mediated through the cAMP-dependent protein phosphorylation pathway. The amount of receptor protein expressed appears to be regulated by changes in βAR mRNA stability as well as in the rate of βAR gene transcription, depending on the cell type or tissue being examined. Agonist treatment is reported to regulate both β_2AR mRNA stability and gene expression in a smooth muscle cell line (5,14,15), whereas agonist treatment regulates β_1AR gene expression, with no change in mRNA stability, in a glioma cell line (16,17). In either case, decreased expression of βAR mRNA and protein would contribute to the down-regulation of receptor in response to agonist treatment. These mechanisms of receptor regulation may have particular relevance to the actions of psychotropic drugs, such as antidepressants, which require several weeks of treatment (see Nestler and Duman, *this volume*).

In some systems, prolonged activation of the βAR has been shown to result in altered levels of proteins, in addition to the receptor itself, in the βAR signal transduction pathway. This would contribute further to agonist-induced down-regulation of βAR function. Such βAR-induced down-regulation has been observed for G proteins and cAMP-dependent protein kinase (see refs. 14 and 28).

The physiological actions of βAR activation are presumably mediated by many target proteins. βAR-stimulation of the cAMP pathway would be expected to lead to the phosphorylation and regulation of numerous cellular proteins and consequently to the regulation of numerous cellular processes, as discussed in previous sections of this chapter. This would include changes in gene expression via regulation of transcription factors (e.g., Fos, CREB). One mechanism by which βAR activation may lead to transcription factor regulation is by inducing the nuclear translocation of cAMP-dependent protein kinase (see ref. 30). While regulation of these transcription factors can be used as a marker for studying the brain regions influenced by βAR activation, at this time there is little known about the specific target genes for these transcription factors in specific neuronal cell types in the brain. Potential target genes of the βAR, as mentioned above, are those for neuropeptides and neurotrophins, which possess DNA response elements sensitive to these transcription factors and show regulation by βAR ligands in cultured cells and brain.

The D_1-Dopamine Receptor and DARPP-32

Activation of the D_1-dopamine receptor would be expected to result in many of the same types of effects in target neurons as outlined above for the βAR, because the actions of both receptors are mediated via the cAMP pathway. However, an additional type of signal transduction mechanism has been elaborated for the D_1 receptor. This mechanism involves DARPP-32 (*d*opamine and cAMP *r*egulated *p*hospho*p*rotein of 32 kD) and highlights the complex interactions, mediated via intracellular messenger pathways, that occur among neurotransmitter actions in the brain.

DARPP-32 was discovered during a study of the regional distribution of neuronal phosphoproteins in rat brain (34). It is one of several substrates for cAMP-dependent protein kinase that are highly concentrated in the basal ganglia. DARPP-32 is phosphorylated in vitro on a single threonine residue by cAMP-dependent or by cGMP-dependent protein kinase. Phospho-DARPP-32, but not the dephospho form of the protein, is a highly potent and specific inhibitor of protein phosphatase 1. DARPP-32 is also phosphorylated on serine residues by casein kinases I and II; casein kinases are second-messenger-independent serine/threonine protein kinases (Table 1). Such phosphorylation influences the ability of the threonine residue to be phosphorylated by cAMP-dependent protein kinase.

DARPP-32 is highly enriched in neurons in the brain that possess D_1-dopamine receptors, and it appears to be present in all such neurons. It is also present in renal tubular epithelial cells, parathyroid-hormone-producing cells in the parathyroid gland, and tanocytes, all of which are known to express the D_1 receptor. However, DARPP-32 has been found in one cell type that does not possess D_1-dopamine receptors, namely, choroid epithelial cells.

The state of phosphorylation of DARPP-32 can be regulated in many cell types by various hormones and neurotransmitters that activate the cAMP or cGMP pathway; one notable example is stimulation of DARPP-32 phosphorylation in striatal neurons via activation of D_1-dopamine receptors. Changes in the phosphorylation state and phosphatase inhibitory activity of DARPP-32 indirectly influence the phosphorylation state of other proteins, and thereby mediate some of the effects of dopamine and other first messengers on cell function. The full spectrum of proteins regulated by DARPP-32 phosphorylation in this way have not yet been identified, although the Na^+/K^+-ATPase represents one target protein. Regulation of this protein by DARPP-32 provides one mechanism by which alterations in DARPP-32 phosphorylation can lead to changes in the electrical excitability of neurons and in ion transport properties of nonexcitable peripheral tissues.

Several types of physiological actions for DARPP-32 can be envisioned. First, DARPP-32 phosphorylated and activated in response to dopamine (or another first messenger) and cAMP (or cGMP) can act as a positive feedback signal for these messengers by reducing the dephosphorylation of other substrates for the same protein kinase. Second, DARPP-32 can reduce the dephosphorylation of substrate proteins for other protein kinases and, in so doing, can mediate the effects of first- and second-messenger systems on one another. Third, DARPP-32, through its phosphorylation by cAMP (or cGMP)-dependent protein kinase and its dephosphorylation by Ca^{2+}/calmodulin-dependent protein phosphatase (calcineurin), can integrate certain physiological effects of first messengers that influence the cAMP and Ca^{2+} systems.

An example of this latter mechanism is illustrated in Fig. 5. In this scheme, extracellular signals that activate

the cAMP pathway would phosphorylate and activate DARPP-32, whereas extracellular signals that activate the Ca^{2+} pathway would dephosphorylate and inactivate DARPP-32. Changes in DARPP-32 activity would then lead to altered activity of protein phosphatase 1 and, as a result, to altered dephosphorylation of Na^+/K^+-ATPase, a prominent substrate for this enzyme. Changes in the phosphorylation state of the Na^+/K^+-ATPase would result in altered sodium transport across the cell membrane and, in excitable cells, to altered membrane potential. Considerable evidence has been obtained to support this scheme in several cell types. Moreover, the scheme can account for some of the antagonist actions of dopamine (acting through cAMP) and glutamate (acting through Ca^{2+}) on neuronal excitability in striatal neurons (34).

REFERENCES

1. Beavo JA. Multiple isozymes of cyclic nucleotide phosphodiesterase. *Adv Sec Mess Phosphoprotein Res* 1988;22:1–37.
2. Berridge MJ. Inositol triphosphate and calcium signaling. *Nature* 1993;361:315–325.
3. Blenis J. Signal transduction via the MAP kinases: proceed at your own RSK. *Proc Natl Acad Sci USA* 1993;90:5889–5892.
4. Bredt DS, Snyder SH. Nitric oxide, a novel neuronal messenger. *Neuron* 1992;8:3–11.
5. Collins S, Bouvier M, Bolanowski MA, Caron MG, Lefkowitz RJ. cAMP stimulates transcription of the β_2-adrenergic receptor gene in response to short-term agonist exposure. *Proc Natl Acad Sci USA* 1989;86:4853–4857.
6. Davis RJ. The mitogen-activated protein kinase signal transduction pathway. *J Biol Chem* 1993;268:14553–14556.
7. Duman RS, Karbon EW, Harrington C, Enna SJ. An examination of the involvement of phospholipases A2 and C in the α-adrenergic and γ-aminobutyric acid receptor modulation of cyclic AMP accumulation in rat brain slices. *J Neurochem* 1986;47:800–810.
8. Duman RS, Terwilliger RZ, Nestler EJ. Endogenous ADP-ribosylation in brain: initial characterization of substrate proteins. *J Neurochem* 1991;57:2124–2132.
9. Feinstein P, Schrader K, Bakalyar H, et al. Molecular cloning and characterization of a Ca^{2+}/calmodulin-insensitive adenylyl cyclase from rat brain. *Proc Natl Acad Sci USA* 1991;88:10173–10177.
10. Gao B, Gilman AG. Cloning and expression of a widely distributed (type IV) adenylyl cyclase. *Proc Natl Acad Sci USA* 1991;88:10178–10182.
11. Glatt CE, Snyder SH. Cloning and expression of an adenylyl cyclase localized to the corpus striatum. *Nature* 1993;361:536–538.
12. Greengard P, Jen J, Nairn AC, Stevens CF. Enhancement of the glutamate response by cAM-dependent protein kinase in hippocampal neurons. *Science* 1991;253:1132–1335.
13. Greengard P, Valtorta F, Czernik AJ, Benfenati F. Synaptic vesicle phosphoproteins and regulation of synaptic function. *Science* 1993;259:780–785.
14. Hadcock JR, Malbon CC. Agonist regulation of gene expression of adrenergic receptors and G proteins. *J Neurochem* 1993;60:1–9.
15. Hadcock JR, Wang H-Y, Malbon CC. Agonist-induced destabilization of β-adrenergic receptor mRNA. *J Biol Chem* 1989;264:19928–19933.
16. Hosoda K, Feussner G, Fishman PH, Duman RS. Agonist and cyclic AMP mediated regulation of β_1-adrenergic receptor mRNA and gene transcription in rat C6 glioma cells. *J Neurochem* 1994;[in press].
17. Hough C, Chuang D-M. Differential down-regulation of β_1- and β_2-adrenergic receptor mRNA in C6 glioma cells. *Biochem Biophys Res Commun* 1990;170:46–52.
18. Huganir RL, Greengard P. Regulation of neurotransmitter receptor desensitization by protein phosphorylation. *Neuron* 1990;5:555–567.
19. Hunter T, Sefton BM, eds. Protein phosphorylation. Parts A and B.

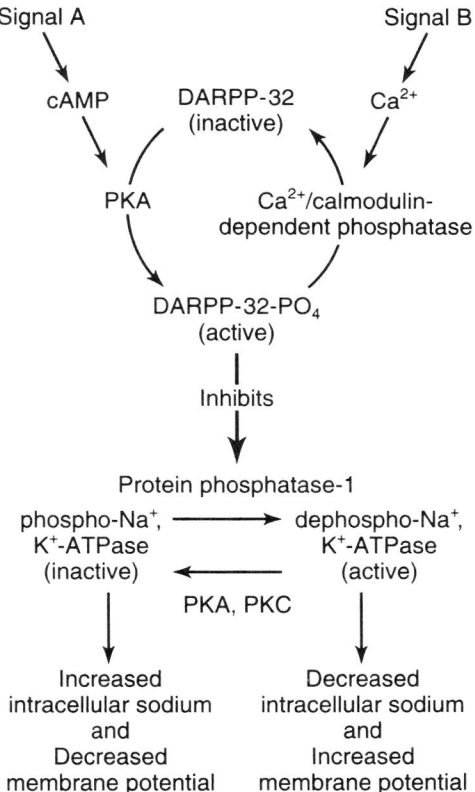

FIG. 5. Scheme illustrating the hypothetical role of DARPP-32 in mediating the effects of first messengers with opposing physiological actions and in the regulation of Na^+/K^+-ATPase activity. This scheme, involving bidirectional control of Na^+/K^+-ATPase activity, may be applicable to various tissues, including brain and kidney. cAMP-PK, cAMP-dependent protein kinase; PKC, protein kinase C. (From ref. 34.)

Methods in enzymology, vols 200 and 201. New York: Academic Press, 1991.

20. Hyman SE, Nestler EJ. *The molecular foundations of psychiatry.* Washington, DC: American Psychiatric Press, 1993.

21. Kobilka B. Adrenergic receptors as models for G protein-coupled receptors. *Annu Rev Neurosci* 1992;15:87–114.

22. Lefkowitz RJ. G protein coupled receptor kinases. *Cell* 1993; 74:409–412.

23. Leidenheimer NJ, Browning MD, Harris RA. GABA$_A$ receptor phosphorylation: multiple sites, actions, and artifacts. *Trends Pharmacol Sci* 1991;12:84–87.

24. Liggett SB, Ostrowski J, Chesnut LC, Kurose H, Raymond JR, Caron MG, Lefkowitz RJ. Sites in the third intracellular loop of the α_{2A}-adrenergic receptor confer short term agonist-promoted desensitization. *J Biol Chem* 1992;267:4740–4746.

25. Mocchetti I, De Bernardi MA, Szekely AM, Alho H, Brooker G, Costa E. Regulation of nerve growth factor biosynthesis by β-adrenergic receptor activation in astrocytoma cells: a potential role of c-Fos protein. *Proc Natl Acad Sci USA* 1989;86:3891–3895.

26. Morgan JI, Curran T. Stimulus-transcription coupling in the nervous system. *Annu Rev Neurosci* 1991;14:421–452.

27. Nestler EJ, Duman RS. G-proteins and cyclic nucleotides in the nervous system. In: Siegel G, Agranoff B, Albers RW, Molinoff P, eds. *Basic neurochemistry,* 5th ed. New York: Raven Press, 1994;429–448.

28. Nestler EJ, Greengard P. *Protein phosphorylation in the nervous system.* New York: John Wiley & Sons, 1984.

29. Nestler EJ, Greengard P. Protein phosphorylation and the regulation of neuronal function. In: Siegel G, Agranoff B, Albers RW, Molinoff P, eds. *Basic neurochemistry,* 5th ed. New York: Raven Press, 1994;449–474.

30. Nestler EJ, Terwilliger RZ, Duman RS. Chronic antidepressant administration alters the subcellular distribution of cyclic AMP-dependent protein kinase in rat frontal cortex. *J Neurochem* 1989;53:1644–1647.

31. Nicoll RA. The coupling of neurotransmitter receptors to ion channels in the brain. *Science* 1988;241:545–551.

32. Nishizuka Y. Intracellular signaling by hydrolysis of phospholipids and activation of protein kinase C. *Science* 1992;258:607–614.

33. Okazawa H, Murata M, Watanabe M, Kamei M, Kanazawa I. Dopaminergic stimulation up-regulates the in vivo expression of brain-derived neurotrophic factor (BDNF) in the striatum. *FEBS Lett* 1992;313:138–142.

34. Pessin MS, Snyder GL, Halpain S, Girault J-A, Aperia A, Greengard P. DARPP-32/protein phosphatase-1/Na$^+$/K$^+$ATPase system: a mechanism for bidirectional control of cell function. In: *Proceedings of the 1992 Wenner Gren International Symposium,* Stockholm. 1994;in press.

35. Piomelli D, Greengard P. Lipoxygenase metabolites of arachidonic acid in neuronal transmembrane signalling. *Trends Pharmacol Sci* 1990;11:367–373.

36. Sessker FN, Mouradian RD, Cheng J-T, Yeh HH, Liu W, Waterhouse BD. Noradrenergic potentiation of cerebellar Purkinje cell responses to GABA: evidence for mediation through the β-adrenoceptor-coupled cyclic AMP system. *Brain Res* 1989;499:27–38.

37. Shenolikar S, Nairn AC. Protein phosphatases: recent progress. *Adv Second Messenger Phosphoprotein Res* 1991;23:1–121.

38. Simon MI, Strathman MP, Gautam N. Diversity of G proteins in signal transduction. *Science* 1991;252:802–808.

39. Summers RJ, McMartin LR. Adrenoceptors and their second messenger systems. *J Neurochem* 1993;60:10–23.

40. Taussig R, Iniguez-Lluhi JA, Gilman AG. Inhibition of adenylyl cyclase by Giα. *Science* 1993;261:218–221.

41. Williams MB, Li X, Gu X, Jope RS. Modulation of endogenous ADP-ribosylation in rat brain. *Brain Res* 1992;592:49–56.

42. Yuen PST, Garbers DL. Guanylyl cyclase-linked receptors. *Annu Rev Neurosci* 1992;15:193–225.

43. Zafra F, Lindholm D, Castren E, Hartikka J, Thoenen H. Regulation of brain-derived neurotrophic factor and nerve growth factor mRNA in primary cultures of hippocampal neurons and astrocytes. *J Neurosci* 1992;12:4793–4799.

44. Zigmond RE, Schwarzschild MA, Rittenhouse AR. Acute regulation of tyrosine hydroxylase by nerve activity and by neurotransmitters via phosphorylation. *Annu Rev Neurosci* 1989;12:415–461.

Psychopharmacology: The Fourth Generation of Progress, edited by Floyd E. Bloom and David J. Kupfer. Raven Press, Ltd., New York © 1995.

CHAPTER 28

Norepinephrine and Serotonin Transporters

Molecular Targets of Antidepressant Drugs

Eric L. Barker and Randy D. Blakely

The monoamine neurotransmitters norepinephrine (NE) and serotonin (5-hydroxytryptamine, 5HT) play important roles in an array of behaviors including sleep, appetite, memory, and mood. At a molecular level, monoamine signaling is dynamically regulated by a diverse set of macromolecules including biosynthetic enzymes, secretory proteins, ion channels, pre- and postsynaptic receptors, and transporters (Fig. 1). NE and 5HT are synthesized from simple amino acid precursors, packaged into synaptic vesicles, and released into the synapse in response to depolarizing stimuli, eliciting pre- and postsynaptic responses through receptor activation. Subsequently, transmitter is efficiently cleared from the extracellular space by transporter proteins localized in the plasma membranes of presynaptic terminals (Fig. 1). Transmitter reuptake is believed to have three important consequences. First, levels of transmitter in the synapse are reduced faster than can be achieved by simple diffusion, allowing for improved temporal discrimination of consecutive release events. Second, the effects of released transmitter are constrained to a smaller area, permitting dense packing of chemically identical but functionally distinct synapses. Finally, transmitter can be recycled for another round of release once it is transported back across the presynaptic membrane and into synaptic vesicles. The neurotransmitter transporter proteins that carry out NE and 5HT clearance are of much interest because they are molecular targets for many antidepressants, such as the tricyclics, fluoxetine, and sertraline as well as substances

of abuse such as cocaine and amphetamines (1,22,30). Antidepressants and cocaine share the ability to alter neuronal signaling by blocking NE and 5HT transport. Unlike the antidepressants, cocaine also impedes dopamine (DA) clearance and thereby leads to a distinct spectrum of behavioral alterations (see Chapter 16, *this volume*). With transporter-mediated clearance pharmacologically inhibited, extracellular levels of transmitter remain elevated longer and can activate receptors at greater distances away from the synapse. Chronic alterations in transporter-mediated clearance may seriously compromise the ability of brain synapses to function properly. Changes in 5HT uptake sites, for example, have long been associated with major affective disorders, particularly depression (49). Thus, neurons may carefully set the level of NE and 5HT transporter expression to match synaptic demands for clearance, with a disruption in transporter expression or regulation providing a molecular liability to mental illness (see Chapter 16 for the dopamine transporter, *this volume*).

Although the involvement of transporters in NE and 5HT clearance has been clear for several decades (30), progress in understanding transporter structure and regulation has been limited, largely due to difficulties associated with transporter protein purification. Recently, expression and homology-based cloning efforts have (5,28,50,52) revealed that NE transporters (NETs) and 5HT transporters (SERTs) are members of a large gene family comprised of carriers for other neurotransmitters, osmolytes, and nutrients (1). Expression of NETs and SERTs in non-neuronal cells has been achieved (5,28,50), establishing model systems for analysis of the structural basis of transporter specificity for neurotransmitters and

---

E. L. Barker and R. D. Blakely: Department of Anatomy and Cell Biology, Emory University School of Medicine, Atlanta, Georgia 30322.

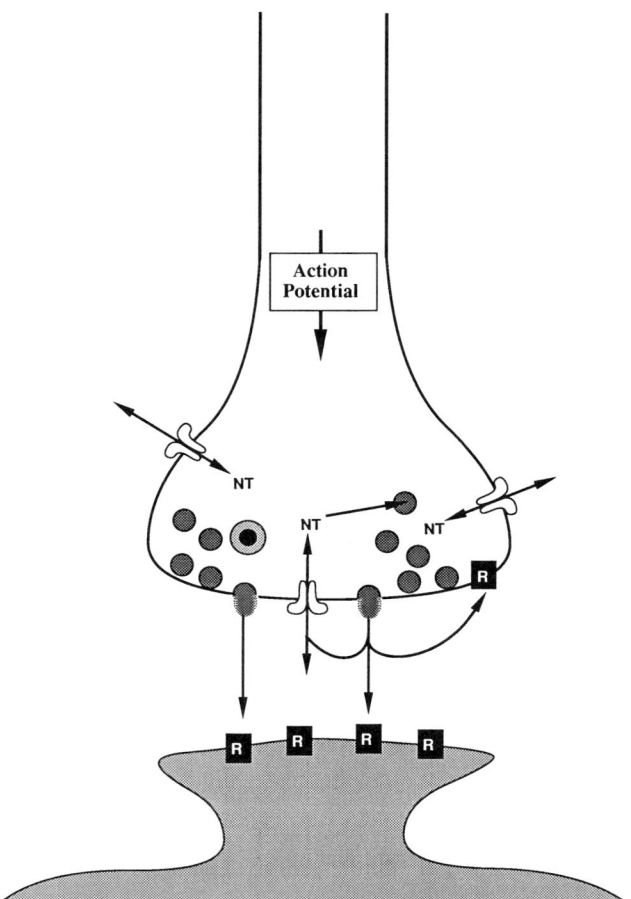

FIG. 1. Schematic representation of a synapse showing vesicular release of biogenic amines and transmitter reuptake by presynaptic transporters. Transmitter movements by transporters are given bidirectional arrows to indicate a capacity for both influx and efflux. Transmitter vesicles within the presynaptic cytoplasm are shown colocalized with large dense-core secretory granules containing neuropeptides. NT, neurotransmitter undergoing uptake and being packaged into synaptic vesicles for subsequent release; R, receptors on presynaptic and postsynaptic membranes.

antagonists. Indeed, it now appears that, unlike previous suggestions, most (if not all) antagonists block uptake by binding directly to the transporter protein. Mechanistic models for how transport is achieved are now more readily testable with overexpression in transfected cells providing opportunities for electrophysiological measurements of transporter turnover as a function of membrane potential, ion gradients, and cytosolic regulators. Furthermore, the availability of transporter-specific antibodies and nucleic acid probes has renewed interest in the endogenous control mechanisms acutely regulating NE and 5HT transport in vivo and whether chronic alterations in NET and SERT genes underlie neuropsychiatric disorders. Below we review our present understanding of NE and 5HT transport and the new insights achieved from molecular cloning and regulation studies.

GENERAL CHARACTERISTICS OF NOREPINEPHRINE AND 5HT TRANSPORTERS (NETs AND SERTs)

Ionic Requirements of NE and 5HT Transport

It is important to understand the ionic and voltage sensitivities for transporters because these properties may dictate uptake rates, thereby controlling the speed by which transporters can clear NE or 5HT from synapses and ultimately the duration of postsynaptic responses. Although the speed of NE and 5HT clearance from central nervous system (CNS) synapses by NETs and SERTs has not been determined, elegant work on a voltage-dependent 5HT uptake process in leech serotonergic synapses (10) provides convincing support for the ability of neurotransmitter transporters to dictate the duration and magnitude of postsynaptic responses. One of the first common properties recognized for NE and 5HT transport was an absolute dependence on extracellular Na^+ (Fig. 2), a feature now known to be characteristic of Na^+/cotransport processes where energy for inward solute transfer is coupled to the energetically favorable influx of Na^+ down its concentration gradient (for a comprehensive review of ion dependence of monoamine transporters, see ref. 58). In addition, extracellular Cl^- is absolutely necessary for NE and 5HT transport (58), although the halide specificity appears less rigid than the Na^+ requirement: Other anions such as NO_2^- and Br^- are capable of substituting, at least partially, for Cl^-. For SERT, a model for this multisubstrate uptake process has been proposed in which Na^+, Cl^-, and a protonated 5HT molecule binds to the transporter, forming a quaternary complex which then undergoes a conformational change to release the neurotransmitter and the ions into the cytoplasm (58). Subsequently, intracellular K^+ has been proposed to associate with SERT and promote the reorientation of the unloaded carrier for another transport cycle. Thus, intracellular K^+ accelerates 5HT influx, presumably by facilitating a conformational change required for external exposure of unoccupied 5HT binding sites on the unloaded transporter (58). Surprisingly, SERT and NET appear to differ in the role of intracellular K^+ in transport (Fig. 2); NE influx also is sensitive to intracellular K^+, but available data are more consistent with K^+ stimulation at a modulatory site rather than direct K^+ efflux as observed with SERT. If such a difference exists, the net charge movement per cycle for NETs and SERTs would be distinct and might lead to differences in the voltage sensitivity of transport. Among other transporters in this gene family, sensitivity to intracellular ions such as K^+ seems to be far more variant than extracellular ion requirements; the homologous GABA transporter (GAT), for example, appears to lack sensitivity for intracellular K^+ altogether (32), suggesting that

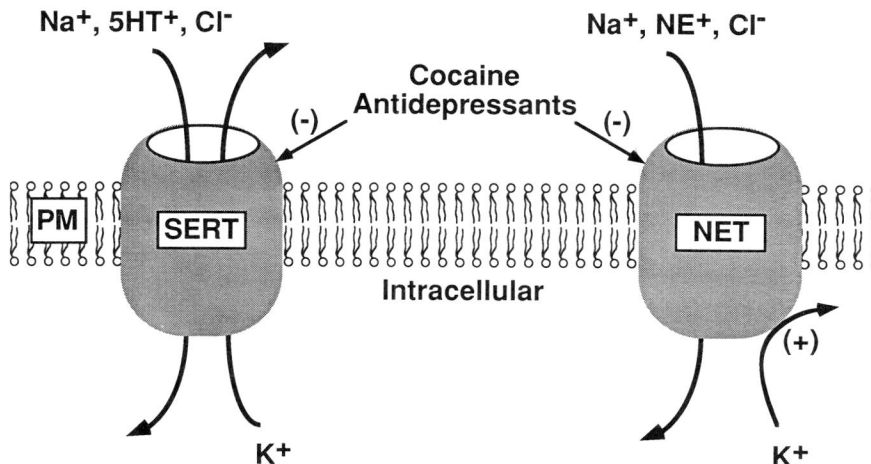

FIG. 2. General model of ion-coupled NE and 5HT uptake. **Left:** Proposed mechanism for the 5HT transporter (SERT) whereby uptake of 5HT is dependent upon cotransport of Na^+ and Cl^- and countertransport of K^+. **Right:** Norepinephrine transporter (NET) model showing Na^+ and Cl^--dependent NE uptake with intracellular K^+ stimulation of NE uptake, but no associated K^+ efflux. Both transporters are inhibited by antidepressants and cocaine. PM, plasma membrane.

structural similarities among transporter family members may mask important mechanistic distinctions acquired in the evolutionary divergence from a common ancestral transporter. Recent progress in recording NET and SERT transporter currents by whole-cell patch-clamp techniques (L. DeFelice and R. Blakely, *unpublished results*) suggests that both carriers move net charge per transport cycle in a voltage-sensitive manner.

Another consequence of neurotransmitter uptake driven by transmembrane ion gradients is transporter-mediated *efflux* of substrate, as well as influx, if ion gradients are reversed and/or membranes are depolarized (43). For example, reversed NE transport from sympathetic nerves accompanies moderate periods of cardiac ischemia when internal Na^+ concentrations rise and the plasma membrane becomes depolarized, possibly contributing to fatal cardiac arrhythmias (43). By analogy, adrenergic receptors might be bathed inappropriately with NE during CNS ischemia accompanying stroke. As transporter-mediated efflux is antagonized by transporter inhibitors, these antagonists may find new uses in the prevention of inappropriate transmitter efflux until normal ion gradients and resting potentials can be restored.

Pharmacological Profiles of NETs and SERTs

As mentioned previously, SERTs and NETs are the pharmacological targets for a variety of therapeutic antidepressants and abused substances (Table 1). Tricyclic antidepressant sensitivity is shared by NETs and SERTs, but not by DA transporters (DATs; see Chapter 16, *this volume*) (5,28,37,50). Tertiary amine tricyclics (imipramine, amitriptyline) are more potent at SERTs as compared to the NET-preferring secondary amine tricyclics desipramine and nortriptyline. The steric interactions by which the addition of a single methyl group increases potency of the tertiary amines for SERT are not known;

however, mutagenesis of the SERT protein should prove useful in identifying residues important in this effect and allow predictions concerning binding of ligands to the transporter (see below). Other potent NET antagonists include nomifensine, mazindol, and nisoxetine. Highly selective antagonists for SERTs such as paroxetine and fluoxetine have been developed whose chemical structures differ from the tricyclic nucleus, but which are effective antidepressants supporting alterations in serotonin neurons as targets in affective disorders (22). Cocaine is a nonselective, competitive antagonist of NE, 5HT, and DA transport. The addictive potential of cocaine is though to be a consequence of actions on CNS DATs, whereas the life-threatening cardiovascular effects of cocaine may involve blockade of NETs at sympathetic and CNS autonomic synapses. In addition to cocaine, other drugs of

TABLE 1. *Inhibitor Profiles for NET and SERT*

Inhibitor	K_i or K_m (nM)[a]	
	hNET	hSERT
Fluoxetine	—	3.1
Sertraline	—	0.8
Paroxetine	310	0.25
Citalopram	>1000	5.0
Imipramine	65	2.1
Desipramine	4.0	40
Clomipramine	—	0.3
Amitriptyline	100	15
Nortriptyline	16.5	130
D-Amphetamine	55	>10,000
Cocaine	140	4200
Nomifensine	8.0	840
Mazindol	1.4	100
5HT	>10,000	460
Norepinephrine	460	>10,000
Dopamine	140	>10,000

[a] The K_i or K_m values were obtained from assays using cells transfected with cDNAs for indicated transporter as reported in refs. 50 and 52, and in unpublished results.

abuse including *p*-chloroamphetamine, fenfluramine, and (3,4-methylenedioxy)methamphetamine (MDMA, "ecstasy") also are inhibitors of 5HT uptake. Interestingly, MDMA and the other amphetamines are neurotoxic substrates for SERTs and additionally cause efflux of 5HT by a transported-mediated exchange process (59).

Like the binding of substrates, antagonist binding to NETs and SERTs also is dependent on extracellular Na^+, although ion dependency appears to be complex and varies for different antagonists. For example, the binding of [^{3}H]desipramine (39) and [^{3}H]mazindol (31) to NETs is Na^+- and Cl^--dependent, suggesting that these antagonists bind to the carrier in the conformation by which NET recognizes substrates. For SERT, the binding of [^{3}H]imipramine appears to require the presence of 2 Na^+ ions per imipramine molecule (30), whereas the Na^+ dependence of other 5HT transport antagonists varies depending upon the compound (29). Perhaps all ligands share a single Na^+-modulated binding site, with additional Na^+-linked sites recruited in an antagonist-specific manner. The cocaine analogue 3β-[4-[^{125}I]iodophenyl]tropan-2β-carboxylic acid methyl ester ([^{125}I]RTI-55) labels SERTs and NETs in platelet membranes in a largely Na^+-dependent manner (66); however, in contrast to other ligands, RTI-55 binding is independent of Cl^-. Unlike imipramine binding, RTI-55 binding to SERTs is markedly pH-sensitive, perhaps indicating the influence of titratable amino acid side chains near the cocaine binding pocket. These data suggest that cocaine and its congeners interact with SERT and NET in a manner distinct from substrates and antidepressants, possibly reflecting contact sites outside of the substrate binding pocket. Given the structural differences between the simple phenylethylamine and tryptamine substrates and the heterocyclic antagonists such as cocaine and antidepressants, it seems naive to assume complete correspondence between substrate and antagonist transporter contact points.

While antidepressants and cocaine are thought to be competitive antagonists of NETs, other ligands which antagonize NE transport and [^{3}H]desipramine binding, such as phencyclidine (PCP) and the sigma opiate ligands, may do so through allosteric mechanisms. At present, it is not clear whether this antagonism is mediated directly by recognition sites on NET or through the aegis of a distinct protein. For example, sites labeled by [^{3}H]desipramine in adrenal medulla are reported to be displaced noncompetitively by the sigma ligands haloperidol and (+)-3-PPP as well as by the PCP$_1$-selective ligand MK-801 (56). The size of PCP/sigma receptor targets (21–33 kD) from photoaffinity-labeling and purification studies (65) appears to be different from that expected for NET (45,50); however, the rank order of potency for antagonism of [^{3}H]-desipramine binding by sigma ligands does not match any characterized sigma or PCP receptor subclass (56). Clarification of the commonality and divergence of these

sites using cloned proteins could reveal novel strategies for the therapeutic blockade of NETs, particularly if allosteric modulation of transport is involved. Thus, antagonists which block the actions of cocaine yet permit substrate translocation might be powerful tools in the fight against drug abuse.

Distribution of NETs and SERTs in the CNS and Periphery

High-affinity neuronal NE transport was first described in postganglionic neuronal terminals of sympathetically innervated peripheral tissues including the heart, spleen, and vas deferens (then termed "Uptake 1"; see ref. 30) before being identified in CNS nerve terminal preparations. Neuronal lesions in periphery and brain support a localization of NETs to innervating terminals rather than targets. Kinetically indistinguishable NE transport activities also are present in adrenal chromaffin cells, lung, and placental brush-border membranes. However, NE accumulation alone is not a definitive measure of the noradrenergic character of the preparation under study because NE also is a substrate for the DAT (1). In fact, DA is actually a better substrate (lower K_m) than NE for both the NET and DAT, presenting a problem. How do we determine which transporter is responsible for the uptake activity present in a particular tissue? Exploitation of the pharmacological selectivity of transporter antagonists has, until recently, been the principal means of addressing this question. Catecholamine transport into terminals of peripheral sympathetic and CNS noradrenergic neurons is abolished by nanomolar concentrations of the tricyclic antidepressant desipramine; catecholamine uptake in striatal synaptosomes, where DA is the primary neurotransmitter, is largely insensitive to antidepressants yet sensitive to a number of cocaine derivatives (e.g., GBR12909 and GBR12935) which lack potency for NETs (1,50). These pharmacological distinctions, among others, originally helped establish brain NETs and DATs as separate activities, likely to be the products of distinct transporter molecules, and identified NETs as the most prevalent catecholamine transporter in the periphery (30).

Whereas transport measurements provide a sensitive measure of the capacity for catecholamine accumulation, more direct approaches are required to identify and quantitate the distribution of NETs in situ. Historically, the most informative strategies have relied upon the binding of selective radiolabeled antagonists to brain sections and the subsequent anatomic localization of bound ligand by autoradiographic techniques. Initially, [^{3}H]desipramine and [^{3}H]mazindol were exploited as ligands to identify sites of NETs in rodent brain membranes and slices (37); however, [^{3}H]desipramine exhibits high nonspecific binding and [^{3}H]mazindol labels both NE and DA uptake sites.

More recently, [³H]nisoxetine has been introduced as a potent and selective agent for labeling NE transport sites (61). Studies by Tejani-Butt (61) demonstrate (a) a high density of [³H]nisoxetine binding sites in rat brain regions containing a high density of noradrenergic soma or terminals, including the locus coeruleus and hypothalamic nuclei, and (b) a low density in regions receiving sparse noradrenergic innervation, such as the striatum (61). A marked loss of [³H]nisoxetine labeled sites occurs following chemical brain lesions with the neurotoxins 6-hydroxydopamine (6-OHDA) and DSP-4, indicating that forebrain labeling is most likely associated with noradrenergic terminals rather than targets or surrounding glia, although a small perisynaptic contribution which disappears with loss of innervation cannot be excluded.

Sites of 5HT uptake have been similarly characterized through the binding of [³H]imipramine, which bears moderately higher affinity for SERTs than for NETs (Table 1). However, because of the high nonspecific binding of [³H]imipramine in brain preparations, more recent investigations have utilized more selective ligands such as [³H]paroxetine, [³H]citalopram, and [³H]nitroquipazine. Autoradiographic studies using [³H]citalopram and [³H]-imipramine (16) identify the amygdala, thalamus, hypothalamus, CA3 region of the hippocampus, substantia nigra, locus coeruleus, and the raphe nuclei of the midbrain as the rat and human brain regions with the highest level of 5HT uptake sites. As with NET localization, toxin-induced lesions of serotonergic neurons in rat brain reduce antidepressant binding sites in raphe projection areas consistent with a presynaptic origin of SERTs in vivo (16). Whereas SERT expression appears to be confined to neurons in the adult CNS, antidepressant-sensitive 5HT uptake has been reported for primary cultures of astrocytes (33). However, until SERT expression in glia can be directly established in vivo, reports of glial 5HT uptake may represent an altered or embryonic phenotype of cells in primary culture.

In addition to neuronal expression, 5HT uptake has been identified in platelets, placenta, pulmonary endothelium, and mast cells (21). In the lung, 5HT transporters efficiently clear plasma-borne 5HT and, with the help of platelets, keep blood levels of free 5HT low. Placental SERTs may protect the heavily vascularized tissue from premature constriction arising from circulating maternal 5HT. Platelet SERTs have become a widely used peripheral index of central serotonergic neuronal systems (for review, see refs. 37 and 49). Although not a universal finding, many studies have found decreased activity and density of platelet SERTs in depressed patients (37,49). The validity in extrapolating platelet SERT data to disturbances in CNS SERT levels or function assumes identical SERTs in the CNS and periphery with a parallel responsiveness to alterations induced by psychiatric disease. Recent advances in the molecular biology of SERTs has

begun to clarify this clinically important issue (see below). Because of the absence of a facile peripheral measure of the NET similar to the SERT-expressing platelet, NET alterations in depression or other affective disorders has received far less attention. Because NET-selective antagonists also have antidepressant activities, further studies are warranted to quantitate potential alterations in NETs accompanying mental illness (see Chapters 89 and 90, *this volume*).

MOLECULAR BIOLOGY OF NOREPINEPHRINE TRANSPORTERS (NETs) AND SEROTONIN TRANSPORTERS (SERTs)

Cloning of Transporter cDNAs

Protein purification strategies have achieved only limited success in the elucidation of neurotransmitter transporter structure; therefore, to clone transporter cDNAs in the absence of protein-derived sequence information, Pacholczyk et al. (50) turned to expression cloning in COS cells where transport activity induced by cDNA clones could be efficiently screened. These efforts led to the cloning of the first monoamine transporter, the human NET, from the SK-N-SH neuroblastoma cell line. The primary sequence of the human NET cDNA predicts a highly hydrophobic 617-amino-acid polypeptide of ~67 kD with 12 potential transmembrane domains (TMDs) (Fig. 3). Although there is little amino acid sequence homology between NET and the facilitated or Na⁺-coupled glucose transporters, the 12 TMD structure appears as a common motif for transporter proteins. Indeed, this multiple transmembrane domain motif is common to membrane-associated proteins, particularly those responsible for ion and solute transport. Comparison of the predicted primary amino acid sequence for the human NET with that of a previously cloned GABA transporter (GAT) revealed 46% absolute identity, establishing the existence of an Na⁺/Cl⁻-dependent neurotransmitter transporter gene family. The sequence similarity evident between NET and GAT cDNAs provided a route to clone SERTs from rat brain (5) and a rat basophilic leukemia (RBL) cell line by homology screening (28). Despite sequence differences in the original reports, both brain- and RBL-cell-derived rat SERT cDNAs now are known to encode a GAT/NET homologue of 630 amino acids (6,52) with a predicted size of ~68 kD and 50% identity to human NET. Furthermore, the cloning of the identical SERTs from rat brain and a rat mast cell line provides strong support for identical peripheral and CNS SERTs, particularly important in light of the frequent use of human platelet SERTs as a diagnostic tool for psychiatric disease (37,49). Recently, Ramamoorthy et al. (52) have identified a functional human SERT, which bears 92% se-

Serotonin Transporter (SERT)　　　Norepinephrine Transporter (NET)

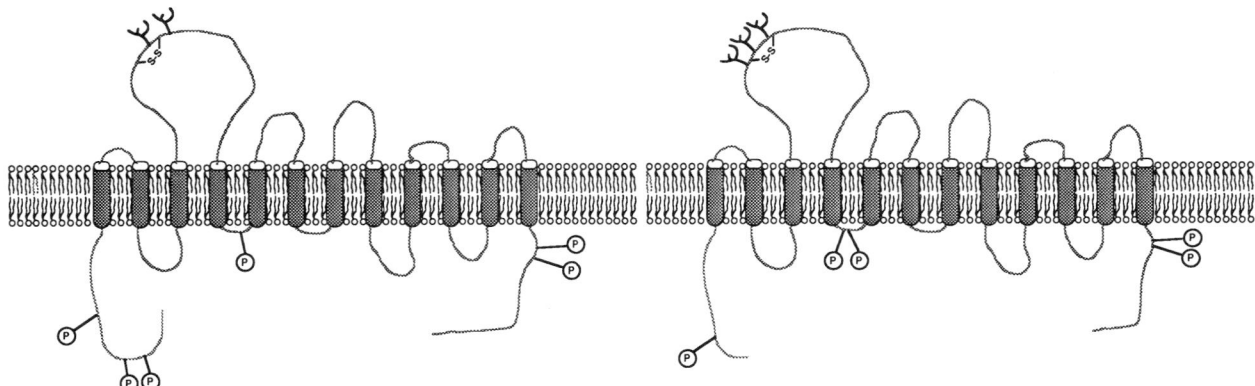

γ N-Linked Glycosylation Sites
S-S Potential Intramolecular Disulfide Bridge
Ⓟ Potential Ser/Thr Phosphorylation Sites

FIG. 3. Proposed transmembrane topology and structural features of SERT and NET subunits. Note the 12 proposed transmembrane domains (TMDs), the large extracellular loop between TMD3 and TMD4 bearing multiple N-linked glycosylation sites, cytoplasmic -NH₂ and -COOH tails, and sites for potential intramolecular or intermolecular disulfide bridge formation and phosphorylation.

quence homology with the rat SERT, and have verified its functional properties in transfected cells. A murine SERT also has recently been cloned and characterized (13).

The cloning of NET and SERT cDNAs has provided important new tools to define the tissue and cellular distribution of transporter gene expression. Thus, in situ hybridization studies on rat brain sections hybridized with specific NET oligonucleotide (20) and cRNA (44) probes confirm the synthesis of NETs in brainstem nuclei, thereby corroborating radioligand binding data observed using [³H]antidepressants. However, autoradiography of [³H]ligand binding does not possess sufficient spatial resolution to resolve actual membrane sites of NET expression. Thus, the high density of NETs reported in noradrenergic nuclei may arise from carriers expressed on the cell soma, dendrites, or axons, and it also could reflect intracellular access of ligands. Antibodies that specifically recognize NETs have been developed (45) and are currently being used to discern whether these transporters are tightly localized near neurotransmitter release sites on presynaptic membranes or whether they are distributed uniformly across axonal and dendritic membranes. Presumably, for clearance of NE to affect spatial and temporal aspects of synaptic signaling, NETs should be present at or near sites of release and response. A more diffuse membrane distribution on axons or surrounding glia might indicate a cooperative role among NETs on adjacent terminals to provide a more compartmental reduction of extracellular NE levels.

Examination of SERT distribution by Northern blot hybridization of rat and mouse RNAs reveals single SERT

mRNA species in brainstem, midbrain, lung, spleen, gut, and adrenal gland (5,13,28). In situ localization of SERT mRNA in both rodent and human brain demonstrates prominent expression in the serotonergic neurons of the median and dorsal raphe nuclei (3,5,13,28). Interestingly, Lesch et al. (41), using sensitive polymerase chain reaction techniques, have obtained evidence for low levels of SERT mRNA in forebrain regions lacking serotonergic soma, although the cellular sites for this expression remain unknown. Anti-SERT antibodies, which detect the transporter in vivo (46), provide a means to assess the legitimacy of proposed nonneuronal SERT expression in the CNS. As expected, antibody staining of rat brain sections reveals abundant SERT expression in the raphe neurons and within serotonergic axons and varicosities, consistent with autoradiographic data; however, no SERT immunoreactivity is detected in surrounding glia (R. D. Blakely, *unpublished results*).

What Are the Common Structural Features of NET and SERT?

Comparisons of the predicted sequences of the cloned NET and SERTs reveal multiple topological similarities, many of which are shared by other GAT/NET gene family members as well. The NH₂ termini of NETs and SERTs lack hydrophobicity characteristics of a signal sequence for membrane insertion and bear no asparagine-linked glycosylation sites; thus, as for many other transport proteins, the NH₂ termini are predicted to reside in the cytoplasm. An even number of TMDs following the NH₂ terminus places the COOH terminus also in the cytoplasm (Fig. 3). Following TMD3, both SERT and NET contain a large extracellular loop with multiple canonical asparagine-linked glycosylation sites, suggesting an extracellular localization of this domain. Glycosylation of membrane proteins can contribute to their folding, stability, trafficking, or ligand recognition. Human NETs undergo sequential glycosylation in transfected cells, modifications that appear critical for transporter stability and/or trafficking (45), similar to observations for β-adrenergic receptors (36). Analogous studies with recently developed anti-SERT antibodies confirm that both native and transfected SERTs exist as glycoproteins with asparagine-linked sugars. Furthermore, preliminary studies with these antibodies suggest that brain and platelet SERTs may undergo differential post-translational modifications. Thus, while the primary amino acid sequences of CNS and peripheral SERTs appear identical, tissue-specific structural modifications are apparent, suggesting caution in absolute extrapolation of platelet SERT studies to CNS SERTs in psychiatric disease. Additionally, conserved cysteine residues are located within the large extracellular loop between TMDs 3 and 4 and may serve, via potential disulfide bridge formation, to maintain a functional conformation of the protein as has been shown for the nicotinic acetylcholine receptor (7). Protein phosphorylation at serine, threonine, and tyrosine residues is involved in the acute regulation of many proteins. The putative cytoplasmic domains of NETs and SERTs contain multiple, canonical sites for serine/threonine phosphorylation (Fig. 3), and acute regulation of transporter activity by exogenous hormones has been reported (see below); however, validation of the phosphorylation of any of these sites has not been achieved, limited largely by an absence of purification methods suitable for phosphoprotein analysis. Progress on NET and SERT phosphorylation as well as other post-translational modifications (e.g., acylation) should be accelerated by the recent development of antibodies capable of immunoprecipitating NET and SERT proteins (45,46).

Because the transport activities conferred by cloned transporter cDNAs is inhibited by tricyclic antidepressants, amphetamine, and cocaine, over appropriate concentration ranges, the cloning of NET and SERT defined each transporter's primary structure and established a single protein subunit as competent for drug recognition as well as transport activity; however, still lacking is a knowledge of the native stoichiometry of transporter monomers and whether accessory proteins are organized with the transporters in an active complex. Site-directed mutagenesis of the transporter proteins leading to altered or abolished ligand binding supports the cloned transporters as direct targets for antagonists (35; R. D. Blakely, *unpublished results*). In support of a larger functional entity, native placental SERTs sized by gel filtration are

much larger than the size of a single SERT monomer (54); however, the contributions of detergent and lipid to these estimates cannot be completely discounted. Expression of NETs and SERTs in non-neuronal hosts, yet bearing drug sensitivities similar to those of transporters found in native membranes, suggests that if any additional subunits exist, such accessory proteins are likely to be modulatory rather than essential to function.

The shared structural features visible in a comparison of NET and SERT sequences subsequently has been observed in a large number of related transporter homologues. These include carriers for DA, glycine, taurine, proline, creatine, and betaine transporters (1), among others (Fig. 4). Estimates from genomic hybridization studies suggest as many as 30 members within the GAT/NET gene family; indeed, additional GAT/NET homologues have been cloned by several laboratories that, at present, lack defined substrates. The Na^+/L-glutamate and $Na^+/$ glucose cotransporters reside in distinct gene families unrelated to the GAT/NET group (1). Interestingly, these latter transporters do not exhibit a requirement for extracellular Cl^-, providing one mechanistic feature likely to help in the categorization of as yet uncloned transport activities. Approximately 40% identity is detected in 2×2 comparisons of human NET with other GAT/NET homologues; DA, NE, and 5HT transporters are most closely related to each other, defining a small subdivision

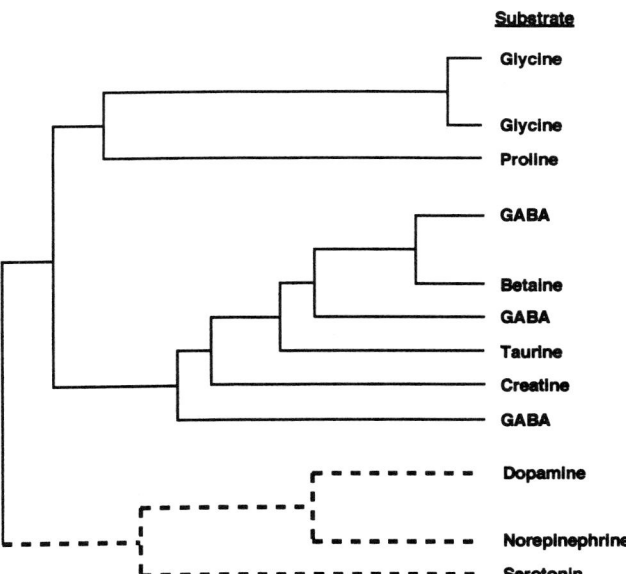

FIG. 4. GAT/NET gene family tree. Transporters are identified by their most likely endogenous substrate. Multiple species variants of the transporters presented are not included, nor are additional gene products with yet unidentified substrates. The monoamine transporter subdivision is highlighted with dashed lines. The length of horizontal lines is inversely proportional to relatedness of homologues connected by branch points.

united by both sequence and pharmacology (Fig. 4). At the primary amino acid level, approximately 20% of NET and SERT residues are absolutely conserved across all GAT/NET family members. Interestingly, this sequence identity is distributed nonuniformly, with particularly high conservation evident in TMDs 1–2 and 5–8 (1,5). These shared residues most likely represent sites involved in common properties such as Na^+ and Cl^- binding; alternatively, they may dictate the global architecture required for substrate translocation across the plasma membrane.

One feature which separates the NE, 5HT, and DA transporters from other GAT/NET homologues is high-affinity recognition of the psychoactive agents cocaine and amphetamine, and, for NET and SERT, the tricyclic antidepressants. Although the sites of antagonist recognition have yet to be directly established, the expression of cloned and mutant NETs, SERTs, and DATs in transfected cells is rapidly illuminating functional properties of shared structural features. Sequence comparisons show the NH_2 and COOH termini to be poorly conserved and, thus, potentially involved in unique attributes of each carrier. However, chimera studies wherein these domains are swapped between NETs and SERTs reveal no alteration in substrate or antagonist selectivity (6); furthermore, removal by mutagenesis of GAT tails fails to alter transport properties (4), suggesting NH_2 and COOH termini to be inconsequential for ligand recognition. The NH_2 and COOH tails, which contain multiple sites for protein phosphorylation, may comprise regulatory domains specific for each transporter, whereas the regions comprised of transmembrane domains between these tails are likely to contribute to the formation of the translocation pore and antagonist binding sites.

The simple structure of the neurotransmitters NE and 5HT invites comparisons between modes of monoamine recognition by receptors and transporters. In adrenergic receptors, the protonated NH_2 group on NE is believed to ion pair with an intramembrane aspartate residue, while catechol OH groups form hydrogen bonds with serine residues on a nearby TMD (36). Likewise, structural features of catecholamines required for high-affinity recognition by NETs and SERTs confirm the importance of ring hydroxyl groups and a protonated, unsubstituted NH_2 group (30). Furthermore, TMD aspartate and serine residues are among the handful of residues specific to the NET, SERT, DAT wing of the GAT/NET gene family, raising possibilities of similar strategies for the recognition of neurotransmitters by transporters and receptors (35). Site-directed mutagenesis of the TMD1 aspartate residue in NET, SERT (R. D. Blakely, *unpublished results*), and DAT (35) markedly alters substrate and antagonist recognition. For DAT, retention of low-affinity cocaine binding and substrate recognition suggests a selective alteration in the ligand binding pocket by the aspartate mutation rather than a gross destabilization of

transporter protein. Antibody studies reveal no difference between wild-type and TMD1 aspartate-mutant NET and SERT proteins, similarly consistent with a direct alteration at the binding site rather a global modification of protein stability. Nonetheless, the idea that the TMD1 aspartate residue directly coordinates the catecholamine NH_2 group via salt-bridge formation is problematic in light of the fact that other GAT/NET proteins have an uncharged glycine residue in the position occupied by the NET, DAT, and SERT aspartate, and yet they bind substrates with protonated NH_2 groups. Moreover, what is unique about NE, DA, and 5HT as GAT/NET substrates is not the presence of a protonated NH_2 group to possibly bind the TMD1 aspartate, but rather the absence of an acidic side chain linked to the substrates' α-carbon. One or more of the residues shared by NET, SERT, and DAT but not by other GAT/NET homologues, such as the TMD1 aspartate, may represent a binding site for the decarboxylated catecholamine and indoleamine substrates. Finally, the differential drug sensitivities observed between species variants of the same transporter may assist in the search for molecular determinants of antagonist binding. For example, the recent identification of a *Drosophila* SERT that transports 5HT selectively but recognizes NET antagonists like mazindol with high affinity (15) may provide important clues to how antagonists bind and block transport.

Are There Multiple Subtypes of SERT and NET?

Are all endogenous NETs and SERTs identical to the transporters identified by recent cloning, or do multiple subtypes of the transporters exist as has been found for other membrane proteins such as ion channels and receptors? Virtually identical transport activities can arise from more than one gene product, suggesting caution in extrapolating beyond available data. For example, distinct genes are known to encode two functionally similar vesicle transporters responsible for intracellular NE packaging in adrenal gland and neural tissues (17). Multiple genes also encode several pharmacologically distinct GABA transporter isoforms (8) (Fig. 4). Tissue-specific differences in ligand recognition by NETs have been reported (30), although these discrepancies may reflect assay differences more than the properties of NET structural variants. A single human genomic locus for NETs has been identified, spanning a locus of at least 10 kB on chromosome 16q12.2 (11) with multiple introns evident. Multiple mRNA species are revealed by human NET cDNA probes in SK-N-SH and PC-12 cells as well as by rat and human primary tissues (44,50,55). It is possible that these multiple RNA species reflect differential use of noncoding elements in the NET mRNAs synthesized and have little or no impact on the structure of the expressed protein. Coding region variants also could be derived from the single human NET gene. For example, alternative splicing of RNAs derived from a single glycine transporter gene (represented in Fig. 4) results in two transporters with different NH$_2$ termini, but indistinguishable transport activities (9). Further studies on NETs cloned from different sources should aid in the evaluation of NET variants.

The identification of α- and β-adrenergic receptor subtypes which show pharmacological selectivity for NE and epinephrine, respectively, raises questions of whether epinephrine-selective transporters exist within the GAT/NET gene family. Epinephrine can be accumulated by sympathetic terminals through NETs, although its affinity as a substrate is lower than that of NE. To date, no data support a unique epinephrine carrier in the mammalian peripheral nervous system. Indeed, the hormonal nature of epinephrine in the peripheral nervous system would not appear to require a specialized transport system because epinephrine's actions are not spatially constrained to the same degree as catecholamine release at synapses. However, studies with antibodies to phenylethanolamine N-methyl transferase (PNMT), the enzyme that converts NE to epinephrine, reveal the presence of putative epinephrine-synthesizing neurons and terminals within the rodent and human brainstem. Unlike other brainstem neurons that secrete NE, these PNMT-positive neurons do not express NET mRNAs (44). Perhaps PNMT-positive neurons synthesize a unique NET homologue specialized to retrieve epinephrine at synaptic sites. Such a transporter has actually been reported at amphibian sympathetic synapses. Sympathetic terminals in the frog release epinephrine rather than NE and express a desipramine-sensitive catecholamine uptake activity (37). The frog transporter, unlike the mammalian NET, prefers epinephrine over NE as a substrate, and can be detected with [^{3}H]desipramine in radioligand binding assays. Could some of the nonspecific effects of antidepressants be due to antagonism of epinephrine transporters on epinephrine terminals innervating brainstem autonomic control centers? Because the physiological relevance of PNMT expression in brainstem neurons is controversial, cloning and characterization of mammalian epinephrine transporters, if indeed these proteins exist, could provide new tools to investigate the role of epinephrine as a transmitter in the mammalian brain.

The search for multiple subtypes of SERTs commands special attention due to the frequent use of platelet SERTs as a peripheral marker of CNS 5HT neurons. Using the polymerase chain reaction, Lesch et al. (42) have amplified identical SERT cDNAs from human platelet and brain mRNAs consistent with the aforementioned single identity of peripheral and CNS rodent SERTs, at least at the amino acid level. While tissue-specific posttranslational modifications of SERT may occur, these data support the derivation of human peripheral and CNS

SERTs from a common gene. Whether platelet and brain SERTs are regulated equivalently in psychiatric disease, however, remains to be determined, an issue that must be resolved if the diagnostic use of platelet SERTs is to continue as a window into CNS serotonergic function. In the rat, a single RNA species hybridizes to SERT cDNA probes on Northern blots of various tissues, whereas at least three SERT mRNAs are detected on blots of human tissues and cell lines (3,52). The significance of these multiple human SERT RNAs is presently unknown, but, like the human NET gene, the human SERT gene (located on chromosome 17q11.1–17q12) possesses multiple exons (52). To date, no subtypes of SERT have been identified, but future progress into potential SERT structural variants should be accelerated by the recent cloning of the human SERT genomic locus (R. D. Blakely, *unpublished results*).

REGULATORY PROCESSES INFLUENCING NETs AND SERTs

Regulation of NETs

Many aspects of noradrenergic neurotransmission, including biosynthesis and release of transmitter, are tightly regulated. Given that transporters control the temporal aspects of transmitter actions after release, it would not be surprising that NETs also are subject to acute regulation by membrane and cytoplasmic factors. Because transport activity is a function of neurotransmitter concentration, synaptic NET activity is expected to increase as the concentration of extracellular NE increases until NETs reach maximal velocity at saturating NE concentrations. The kinetic properties of NETs in native and transfected cells demonstrate a K_m of ~0.5 μM, indicating transporter saturation at low micromolar concentrations. Synaptic concentrations of NE at peripheral synapses, which generally have wide synaptic spaces, may reach high micromolar levels; even higher concentrations may be reached transiently in the more confined synaptic spaces in the CNS. At saturation, NETs must either be converted to a more active state or be joined by other NETs previously held in intracellular compartments; otherwise, synaptic recovery will not keep pace with release, NE may spillover to extrasynaptic sites, and less NE will be recovered for repackaging. Alternatively, an alteration in the activity or number of NETs at noradrenergic synapses could be utilized to alter the level and lifetime of synaptic NE independent of control mechanisms regulating release. Gillis first demonstrated a rapid increase in the retention of NE by cat atrium after stimulation of the heart's sympathetic innervation (25). Rorie et al. (57), utilizing electrical stimulation of adrenergic fibers in the dog saphenous vein and measurement of both NE overflow and metabolite production, detected enhanced NE transport paralleling the increase in impulse flow. Similar findings have been reported by Eisenhofer et al. (18) using pharmacological manipulation of peripheral sympathetic neurons in unanesthetized rabbits in vivo. These studies indicate that NE uptake increases in parallel with increased firing rate and release. Whether the increased NET activity simply reflects an increased turnover of a fixed number of NETs as substrate levels rise or involves an alteration in NET density remains to be determined. Sustained elevation of intracellular Ca^{2+} following repetitive terminal depolarization could provide an intrinsic signal to move transporters from subcellular sites to the terminal membrane.

NE release is altered by a number of endogenous agents which act on presynaptic terminals; likewise, acute hormonal regulation of NET activity has been reported. Multiple groups (e.g., see refs. 60 and 63) have found NETs in central and peripheral nervous systems to be sensitive to angiotensin peptides. Angiotensin II or III typically reduces transport and increases release, although acute stimulation of transport has been reported for rat brainstem neuronal cultures (60). Atrial natriuretic peptide has been reported to acutely elevate NET activity and reverse the inhibitory effects of angiotensin II and III at dosages subthreshold for its own response (62,64). Insulin, in rat brain synaptosomes and PC12 cells, produces a rapid (within 1 min), dose-dependent reduction in NE uptake (19,51). In synaptosomes, insulin reduces NET V_{max} with no effect on K_m, consistent with either a reduction in surface pools of NETs or an alteration in capacity of a fixed number of transporters (51). Insulin's effects are observed in PC12 cells despite reserpine depletion of vesicular catecholamine stores and thus are not likely to arise from alterations in DA or NE release (19). Although the intracellular effectors of these peptide responses are not known, direct treatment of bovine adrenal chromaffin cells in vitro with agents that elevate or mimic intracellular cAMP is reported to reduce NE uptake (12). Clearly, the presence of serine/threonine phosphorylation sites on human NETs raises questions as to whether any of these effects are mediated by protein phosphorylation. Unfortunately, only a few studies report a kinetic basis for hormone-altered transport, and the presence of an NE release pathway (often modulated in parallel) confounds analysis. Use of purified NET proteins and stably transfected cell systems should help clarify these effects and permit a direct evaluation of NET protein phosphorylation.

Hormones may also modulate NE uptake capacity by altering NET gene expression. For example, Figlewicz et al. (20) have shown that chronic intraventricular administration of insulin to rats in vivo significantly reduces steady-state levels of NET mRNA in the locus coeruleus. In vitro, chronic insulin treatment reduces NE uptake and

levels of desipramine-labeled NETs in PC12 cells (19). Pertussis toxin treatment of chromaffin cells also appears to modulate NET expression in a delayed fashion most compatible with reduced gene expression or mRNA stability (12). Regardless, these studies indicate that expression levels of NETs can be modulated by external hormonal influences; these findings are of potential clinical relevance particularly where endocrine dysfunction is suspected. Indeed, sympathetic NETs have been reported to be up-regulated in human diabetic cardiomyopathy (24) as well as in rodents where insulin-secreting β cells have been destroyed with streptozotocin (23). NETs also can be regulated in parallel with tissue NE concentrations: Depletion of brain NE with reserpine causes a decrease in uptake sites, whereas increased synaptic NE availability due to monoamine-oxidase inhibitors results in an increase in sites as labeled by [³H]desipramine (40). An inability of the NET gene to respond to hormonal cues in CNS neurons could result in inappropriate levels of synaptic NE clearance and improper receptor stimulation, precipitating behavioral disturbances. Although this idea is clearly speculative, DNA and antibody probes are now available to examine human NET protein and gene regulation in the context of human neuropsychiatric disorders.

Regulation of SERTs

Analysis of the amino acid sequences of the cloned human SERT reveals six potential sites of phosphorylation by protein kinase A and protein kinase C (52); five of these recognition sites also are conserved in rat SERT (5,28). Acute and chronic regulation of SERT by protein kinase C and cAMP have been reported, possibly involving one or more of these potential phosphorylation sites. Activation of protein kinase C with phorbol esters causes a dose-dependent inhibition of SERT activity in bovine pulmonary endothelial cells, platelets, and RBL cells that is blocked by protein kinase C inhibitors (2,47,48). However, in the RBL cell line, activation of adenosine receptors coupled to the phosphoinositide hydrolysis signaling pathway also should activate protein kinase C and, in contrast, increase SERT activity, suggesting differential regulation by protein kinase C and/or additional pathways engaged in these cells (47). After cholera toxin and forskolin treatment, human placental choriocarcinoma (JAR) cells display enhanced SERT activity and increased cell-surface transporter density; however, the delayed nature of this effect compared to the rapid rise in intracellular cAMP levels suggests an effect on mRNA stability or gene transcription (14). Indeed, the levels of SERT mRNA are markedly elevated by cholera toxin treatment (53). The effects of cAMP on SERT expression may reflect a cell or species-specific sensitivity of the human SERT gene to second messengers in that increases in cAMP levels have been reported to induce down-regulation of SERT activity in rat PC12 cells and C33-14-B1 mouse fibroblasts (34). Regardless, SERTs and NETs, like other molecules involved in neurotransmitter signalling, appear to be sensitive to chronic changes in intracellular regulatory cascades and could be inappropriately regulated in mental illness.

Blockade of 5HT uptake is an immediate effect of the antidepressant 5HT uptake inhibitors, whereas the therapeutic effects of these drugs are observed only after 2–3 weeks of treatment. Compensatory responses at pre- and/or postsynaptic receptors resulting from prolonged transporter blockade are generally thought to be involved in the therapeutic actions of the antidepressants; thus, potential adaptive responses in SERT expression associated with chronic antidepressant treatment also are of much interest. For example, chronic treatment with the tricyclic antidepressant clomipramine decreases [³H]-imipramine binding in platelets from healthy human volunteers. Conversely, amitriptyline treatment reportedly increases SERT sites, whereas imipramine has no effect on platelet [³H]imipramine binding (37). At the molecular level, long-term treatment with selective SERT antagonists, but not monoamine-oxidase inhibitors, decreases the steady-state levels of SERT mRNA in rat brains (41), consistent with differential effects of these agents on rat brain SERT sites measured with radioligand binding (26). Because these studies were performed in animals and healthy subjects, a more pertinent clinical question becomes, How are SERTs regulated in depressed patients? Several postmortem brain studies as well as the previously mentioned platelet SERT data report that [³H]imipramine binding is reduced in patients with affective disorders (37,49) (Alterations in platelet and brain SERTs observed in depression also are reviewed in Nemeroff et al., *this volume*). In some (but not all) studies, a delayed increase in platelet [³H]imipramine binding has been observed in depressed patients following clinical improvement resulting from antidepressant treatments, lending some credence to the use of platelet SERTs as a diagnostic marker for depression (37). However, an absolute correlation between platelet SERT levels and severity of clinical depression remains to be established (see Chapters 89 and 90, *this volume*).

In addition to depression, SERT inhibitors have found clinical usefulness in the treatment of obsessive–compulsive disorder, panic disorder, eating disorders, alcoholism, and premenstrual syndrome (22), although none of these disorders has as yet been directly linked to altered SERT gene expression. The identification of the human genetic locus for SERT and the isolation of human SERT genomic clones will assist in evaluating possible hereditary SERT variations that might underlie a predisposition to psychiatric disease. In addition, greater inspection of SERT expression in humans in vivo should be feasible due to the combination of advanced brain imaging techniques with potent and selective SERT ligands (38). Modeling of SERT-related disorders in rodents may be facilitated by the cloning of the murine SERT, now known to be localized to mouse chromosome 11 (13,27), and its use in the generation of targeting vectors for transgenic ablation of the SERT locus.

STUDIES FOR THE NEXT GENERATION

Although uptake of the monoamine neurotransmitters has been studied for almost three decades, our basic knowledge of NET and SERT structure and regulation is rudimentary. The cloning of NET and SERT cDNAs has provided (a) information regarding primary transporter sequence and (b) the necessary tools to more directly examine the many biophysical and pharmacological properties associated with their activities. Although significant progress has been achieved in defining ionic and substrate specificity of native and cloned transporters, we know little about how substrates bind to the transporters and are thereby shuttled across the plasma membrane, or how antagonists bind. The role of protein phosphorylation or other post-translational modifications in regulating transporter function is only beginning to be evaluated, but it promises to be a fertile area for future studies now that NET and SERT proteins can be visualized. Hints of altered NET and SERT gene regulation after hormonal stimulation suggest significant gains to be acquired from systematic analysis of genomic regulatory elements that control transporter expression. For many, the focus has shifted from establishment of the primary structures of NETs and SERTs to exploiting new DNA and antibody tools for an understanding of how these molecules bind and transport substrates and antagonists, how they become localized to synaptic sites, the degree to which they respond to regulatory cues, and whether hereditary genetic variations contribute to neuropsychiatric disorders.

REFERENCES

1. Amara SG, Kuhar MJ. Neurotransmitter transporters: recent progress. *Ann Rev Neurosci* 1993;16:73–93.
2. Anderson GM, Horne WC. Activators of protein kinase C decrease serotonin transport in human platelets. *Biochim Biophys Acta* 1992;1137:331–337.
3. Austin MC, Bradley CC, Mann JJ, Blakely RD. Expression of serotonin transporter mRNA in the human brain. *J Neurochem* 1994;62:2362–2367.
4. Bendahan A, Kanner BI. Identification of domains of a cloned rat brain GABA transporter which are not required for its functional expression. *FEBS Lett* 1993;318:41–44.
5. Blakely RD, Berson HE, Fremeau RTJ, et al. Cloning and expression of a functional serotonin transporter from rat brain. *Nature* 1991;354:66–70.
6. Blakely RD, Moore KR, Qian Y. Tails of serotonin and norepinephrine transporters: deletions and chimeras retain function. In: Reuss L, Russell JM, Jennings ML, eds. *Molecular biology and function*

of carrier proteins, vol 48. New York: Rockefeller University Press, 1993;283–300.

7. Blount P, Merlie JP. Mutational analysis of muscle nicotinic acetylcholine receptor subunit assembly. *J Cell Biol* 1990;111:2613–2622.

8. Borden LA, Smith KE, Hartig PR, Branchek TA, Weinshank RL. Molecular heterogeneity of the γ-aminobutyric acid (GABA) transport system. *J Biol Chem* 1992;267:21098–21104.

9. Borowsky B, Mezey E, Hoffman BJ. Two glycine transporter variants with distinct localization in the CNS and peripheral tissues are encoded by a common gene. *Neuron* 1993;10:851–863.

10. Bruns D, Engert F, Lux HD. A fast activating presynaptic reuptake current during serotonergic transmission in identified neurons of hirudo. *Neuron* 1993;10:559–572.

11. Brüss M, Kunz J, Lingen B, et al. Chromosomal mapping of the human gene for the tricyclic antidepressant-sensitive noradrenaline transporter. *Hum Genet* 1993;91:278–280.

12. Bunn SJ, O'Brien KJ, Boyd TL, Powis DA. Pertussis toxin inhibits noradrenaline accumulation by bovine adrenal medullary chromaffin cells. *Naunyn Schmiedebergs Arch Pharmacol* 1992;346:649–656.

13. Chang AS, Chang SM, Starnes DM, Blakely RD. Cloning and expression of the mouse brain serotonin transporter. *Neurosci Abstr* 1993;19:206.10.

14. Cool DR, Leibach FH, Bhalla VK, Mahesh VB, Ganapathy V. Expression and cyclic AMP-dependent regulation of a high affinity serotonin transporter in the human placental choriocarcinoma cell line (JAR). *J Biol Chem* 1991;266:15750–15757.

15. Demchyshyn LL, Pristupa ZB, Sugamori KS, et al. Cloning, expression and localization of a chloride-facilitated, cocaine-sensitive serotonin transporter from *Drosophila melanogaster. Proc Natl Acad Sci USA* 1994;91:5158–5162.

16. Duncan GE, Little KY, Kirkman JA, Kaldas RS, Stumpf WE, Breese GR. Autoradiographic characterization of imipramine and citalopram binding in rat and human brain: species differences and relationships to serotonin innervation patterns. *Brain Res* 1992;591:181–197.

17. Edwards RH. The transport of neurotransmitters into synaptic vesicles. *Curr Op Neurobiol* 1992;2:594–596.

18. Eisenhofer G, Cox HS, Esler MD. Parallel increases in noradrenaline reuptake and release into plasma during activation. *Naunyn Schmiedebergs Arch Pharmacol* 1990;341:192–199.

19. Figlewicz DP, Bentson K, Ocrant I. The effect of insulin on norepinephrine uptake by PC12 cells. *Brain Res Bull* 1993;32:425–431.

20. Figlewicz DP, Szot P, Israel PA, et al. Insulin reduces norepinephrine transporter mRNA in vivo in rat locus ceruleus. *Brain Res* 1993;602:161–164.

21. Fozard J, ed. *Peripheral actions of 5-hydroxytryptamine.* New York: Oxford University Press, 1989.

22. Fuller RW, Wong DT. Serotonin uptake and serotonin uptake inhibition. *Ann NY Acad Sci* 1990;600:68–78.

23. Fushimi H, Inoue T, Kishino B, et al. Abnormalities in plasma catecholamine response and tissue catecholamine accumulation in streptozotocin diabetic rats: a possible role for diabetic autonomic neuropathy. *Life Sci* 1984;35:1077–1081.

24. Ganguly PK, Dhalla KS, Innes IR, Beamish RE, Dhalla NS. Altered norepinephrine turnover and metabolism in diabetic cardiomyopathy. *Circ Res* 1986;59:684–693.

25. Gillis CN. Increased retention of exogenous norepinephrine by cat atria after electrical stimulation of the cardioaccelerator nerves. *Biochem Pharmacol* 1963;12:593–595.

26. Graham D, Tahraoui L, Langer SZ. Effect of chronic treatment with selective monoamine oxidase inhibitors and specific 5-hydroxytryptamine uptake inhibitors on [^{3}H]paroxetine binding to cerebral cortical membranes of the rat. *Neuropharmacology* 1987;26:1087–1092.

27. Gregor P, Patel A, Shimada S, et al. Murine serotonin transporter: sequence and localization to chromosome 11. *Mamm Genome* 1993;4:283–284.

28. Hoffman BJ, Mezey E, Brownstein MJ. Cloning of a serotonin transporter affected by antidepressants. *Science* 1991;254:579–580.

29. Humphreys CJ, Levin J, Rudnick G. Antidepressant binding to the

porcine and human platelet serotonin transporters. *Mol Pharmacol* 1988;33:657–663.

30. Iversen LL. Uptake processes for biogenic amines. In: Iversen LL, Iversen SD, Snyder SH, eds. *Handbook of psychopharmacology* New York: Plenum Press, 1975;3:381–442.

31. Javitch JA, Blaustein RO, Snyder SH. [^{3}H]Mazindol binding associated with neuronal dopamine and norepinephrine uptake sites. *Mol Pharmacol* 1984;26:35–44.

32. Kanner BI, Schuldiner S. Mechanism of transport and storage of neurotransmitters. *CRC Crit Rev Biochem* 1987;22:1–38.

33. Kimelberg HK, Katz DM. Regional differences in 5-hydroxytryptamine and catecholamine uptake in primary astrocyte cultures. *J Neurochem* 1986;47:1647–1652.

34. King SC, Tiller AA, Chang AS, Lam DM. Differential regulation of the imipramine-sensitive serotonin transporter by cAMP in human JAr choriocarcinoma cells, rat PC12 pheochromocytoma cells, and C33-14-B1 transgenic mouse fibroblast cells. *Biochem Biophys Res Commun* 1992;183:487–491.

35. Kitayama S, Shimada S, Xu H, Markham L, Donovan DM, Uhl GR. Dopamine transporter site-directed mutations differentially alter substrate transport and cocaine binding. *Proc Natl Acad Sci USA* 1992;89:7782–7785.

36. Kobilka B. Adrenergic receptors as models for G protein-coupled receptors. *Annu Rev Neurosci* 1993;15:87–114.

37. Langer SZ, Schoemaker H. Effects of antidepressants on monoamine transporters. *Prog Neuropsychopharmacol Biol Psychiatry* 1988;12:193–216.

38. Laruelle M, Baldwin RM, Malison RT, et al. SPECT imaging of dopamine and serotonin transporters with β-CIT: pharmacological characterization of brain uptake in nonhuman primates. *Synapse* 1993;13:295–309.

39. Lee CM, Javitch JA, Snyder SH. Characterization of [^{3}H]-desipramine binding associated with neuronal norepinephrine uptake sites in rat brain membranes. *J Neurosci* 1982;2:1515–1525.

40. Lee CM, Javitch JA, Snyder SH. Recognition sites for neurotransmitter uptake: regulation by neurotransmitter. *Science* 1983;220:626–629.

41. Lesch KP, Aulakh CS, Wolozin BL, Tolliver TJ, Hill JL, Murphy DL. Regional brain expression of serotonin transporter mRNA and its regulation by reuptake inhibiting antidepressants. *Mol Brain Res* 1993;17:31–35.

42. Lesch KP, Wolozin BL, Murphy DL, Reiderer P. Primary structure of the human platelet serotonin uptake site: identity with the brain serotonin transporter. *J Neurochem* 1993;60:2319–2322.

43. Levi G, Raiteri M. Carrier-mediated release of neurotransmitter. *Trends Neurosci* 1993;16:415–419.

44. Lorang D, Amara SG, Simerly RB. Cell-type specific expression of catecholamine transporters in the rat brain. *J Neurosci* 1994;[in press.]

45. Melikian HE, MacDonald JK, Gu H, Rudnick G, Moore KR, Blakely RD. Human norepinephrine transporter: biosynthetic studies using a site-directed polyclonal antibody. *J Biol Chem* 1994;269:12290–12297.

46. Melikian HE, Moore KR, Qian Y, et al. Structure and function of plasma membrane serotonin transporters. *Neurosci Abstr* 1993;19:206.1.

47. Miller KJ, Hoffman BJ. Regulation of the serotonin transporter by PKC and adenosine receptor activation. *Neurosci Abstr* 1993;19:95.9.

48. Myers CL, Lazo JS, Pitt BR. Translocation of protein kinase C is associated with inhibition of 5-HT uptake by cultured endothelial cells. *Am J Physiol* 1989;257:L253–L258.

49. Owens MJ, Nemeroff CB. The role of serotonin in the pathophysiology of depression: focus on the serotonin transporter. *Clin Chem* 1994;40:288–295.

50. Pacholczyk T, Blakely RD, Amara SG. Expression cloning of a cocaine and antidepressant-sensitive human noradrenaline transporter. *Nature* 1991;350:350–354.

51. Raizada MK, Shemer J, Judkins JH, Clarke DW, Masters BA, LeRoith D. Insulin receptors in the brain: Structural and physiological characterization. *Neurochem Res* 1988;13:297–303.

52. Ramamoorthy S, Bauman AL, Moore KR, et al. Antidepressant- and cocaine-sensitive human serotonin transporter: molecular cloning,

expression, and chromosomal localization. *Proc Natl Acad Sci USA* 1993;90:2542–2546.

53. Ramamoorthy S, Cool DR, Mahesh VB, et al. Regulation of the human serotonin transporter: cholera toxin-induced stimulation of serotonin uptake in human placental choriocarcinoma cells is accompanied by increased serotonin transporter mRNA levels and serotonin transporter-specific ligand binding. *J Biol Chem* 1993; 268:21626–21631.

54. Ramamoorthy S, Leibach FH, Mahesh VB, Ganapathy V. Partial purification and characterization of the human placental serotonin transporter. *Placenta* 1993;14:449–461.

55. Ramamoorthy S, Prasad PD, Kulanthaivel P, Leibach FH, Blakely RD, Ganapathy V. Expression of a cocaine-sensitive norepinephrine transporter in the human placental syncytiotrophoblast. *Biochemistry* 1993;32:1346–1353.

56. Rogers C, Lemaire S. Characterization of [³H]desmethylimipramine binding in bovine adrenal medulla: interactions with σ- and (or) phencyclidine-receptor ligands. *Can J Physiol Pharmacol* 1992; 70:1508–1514.

57. Rorie DK, Hunter LW, Tyce GM. Dihydroxyphenylglycol as an index of neuronal uptake in dog saphenous vein. *Am J Physiol* 1989;257:H1945–H1951.

58. Rudnick G, Clark J. From synapse to vesicle: the reuptake and storage of biogenic amine neurotransmitters. *Biochim Biophys Acta Bio-Energetics* 1993;1144:249–263.

59. Rudnick G, Wall SC. The platelet plasma membrane serotonin

60. Sumners C, Raizada MK. Angiotensin II stimulates norepinephrine uptake in hypothalamus-brain stem neuronal cultures. *Am J Physiol* 1986;250:C236–244.

61. Tejani-Butt SM. [³H]Nisoxetine: a radioligand for quantitation of norepinephrine uptake sites by autoradiography or by homogenate binding. *J Pharmacol Exp Ther* 1992;260:427–436.

62. Vatta MS, Bianciotti LG, Fernandez BE. Influence of atrial natriuretic factor on uptake, intracellular distribution, and release of norepinephrine in rat adrenal medulla. *Can J Physiol Pharmacol* 1993;71:195–200.

63. Vatta MS, Bianciotti LG, Locatelli AS, Papouchada ML, Fernandez BE. Monophasic and biphasic effects of angiotensin II and III on norepinephrine uptake and release in rat adrenal medulla. *Can J Physiol Pharmacol* 1992;70:821–825.

64. Vatta MS, Bianciotti LG, Papouchada ML, Locatelli AS, Fernandez BE. Effects of atrial natriuretic peptide and angiotensin III on the uptake and intracellular distribution of norepinephrine in medulla oblongata of the rat. *Comp Biochem Physiol* 1991;99C:293–297.

65. Walker JM, Bowen WD, Walker FO, Matsumoto RR, De Costa B, Rice KC. Sigma receptors: biology and function. *Pharmacol Rev* 1990;42:355–402.

66. Wall SC, Innis RB, Rudnick G. Binding of the cocaine analog 2β-carbomethoxy-3 β-(4-[¹²⁵I]iodophenyl)tropane to serotonin and dopamine transporters: different ionic requirements for substrate and 2β-carbomethoxy-3β-(4-[¹²⁵I]iodophenyl)tropane binding. *Mol Pharmacol* 1993;43:264–270.

transporter catalyzes exchange between neurotoxic amphetamines and serotonin. *Ann NY Acad Sci* 1992;648:345–347.

Psychopharmacology: The Fourth Generation of Progress, edited by Floyd E. Bloom and David J. Kupfer. Raven Press, Ltd., New York © 1995.

CHAPTER **29**

Pharmacology and Physiology of Central Noradrenergic Systems

Stephen L. Foote and Gary S. Aston-Jones

The purpose of this chapter is to summarize and critically evaluate selected major recent developments in our understanding of the cellular physiology and pharmacology of brain noradrenergic neurons. There has been substantial progress in these areas since the previous edition of this volume. We have chosen to focus on particular subsets of data that form "critical masses" of information relevant to prominent functional issues. These include data obtained using both in vitro and in vivo preparations to accomplish detailed studies of the noradrenergic neurons of the locus coeruleus (LC) as well as their target cells. Those findings having clear implications for understanding systems-level physiology and pharmacology, as well as those findings with readily apparent behavioral implications, have been emphasized.

IN VITRO STUDIES OF NORADRENERGIC NEURONS

Pharmacology of LC Neurons: The In Vitro Slice Preparation

Recordings obtained from LC neurons in brain slices have proved enormously valuable in characterizing the pharmacologic properties of these cells. Such in vitro preparations have numerous advantages for pharmacological studies of CNS neurons (reviewed in Chapter 5, *this volume*).

The LC slice has been used to greatest advantage in the study of two prominent receptors on this cell popula-

tion, the alpha-2 adrenoceptor and the mu opiate receptor. Because of space constraints, the present summary of recent data concerning LC pharmacology as studied in the slice preparation is focused on these receptors. The reader is also referred to numerous reports in the literature (11–13,45,48–51,55,64) for descriptions of other pharmacologic properties of LC neurons in the slice.

Alpha-2 Adrenoceptor Mechanisms in LC Neurons

Early in vivo studies by Aghajanian and colleagues provided evidence for potent inhibition of LC neurons by alpha-2 adrenergic agonists, such as clonidine (reviewed in ref. 25). In vivo studies indicated that one possible role of these receptors is autoinhibition of LC neurons via recurrent collaterals (12,25). While these extracellular studies indicated that norepinephrine (NE) and epinephrine strongly suppressed LC impulse activity, and that alpha-2 receptors were the most prominent adrenoceptor on LC cells, they revealed little about the underlying membrane effects of these agents on LC neurons.

Intracellular studies in LC slices revealed important aspects of the cellular events triggered by alpha-2 adrenoceptor activation. Egan et al. (23) found that electrical field stimulation of the slice yielded potent hyperpolarizing synaptic potentials in LC neurons that were mediated by alpha-2 receptors, consistent with the proposed alpha-2 mediation of collateral inhibition. Other studies (5) questioned the role of alpha-2 receptors in autoinhibition; however, this conflict with results of previous in vivo studies from the same laboratory may reflect the limiting effects of severed axonal or dendritic collaterals in the slice preparation.

Williams et al. (60) used voltage-clamp analysis in slices to show that alpha-2-mediated hyperpolarization of

S. L. Foote: Department of Psychiatry, School of Medicine, University of California, San Diego, La Jolla, California 92093.

G. S. Aston-Jones: Division of Behavioral Neurobiology, Department of Mental Health Sciences, Hahnemann University Medical School, Philadelphia, Pennsylvania 19102.

LC neurons resulted from opening an inwardly rectifying potassium channel. Williams and North (62) also found that NE acting at alpha-2 receptors on LC neurons reduced calcium influx into these cells, which contributed to the inhibition of discharge. Subsequent studies (2,44) showed that the alpha-2-induced increase in potassium conductance was mediated through a G-protein intermediary and caused a decrease in adenylate cyclase activity and intracellular cAMP levels (reviewed in Chapters 27 and 61, *this volume*). Interestingly, however, the alpha-2-evoked opening of K channels and subsequent hyperpolarization was not mimicked by forskolin (an activator of adenylate cyclase) or blocked by inhibitors of the cAMP-protein kinase A pathway (43). These observations indicate that the potassium channel is linked to the alpha-2 receptor directly by a G protein without an intermediary diffusible second messenger, such as cAMP. The role of cAMP, and its regulation by alpha-2 adrenoceptor activity, remains uncertain and controversial (6,44).

Together, the above studies yield a clear picture of the action of adrenergic agonists on LC neurons. Acting almost entirely through alpha-2 receptors (at least in adults; see refs. 41 and 61, for differences in LC pharmacologic properties in young rats), NE or epinephrine increases an inwardly rectifying potassium conductance. It appears that the alpha-2 receptor is linked to a G-protein mechanism (perhaps within the membrane) and that the G protein is directly linked to the K channel which it opens without the assistance of a diffusible second messenger. The details of alpha-2 adrenoceptor action are probably better understood for LC neurons than any other class of central neuron. However, other brain areas that have been examined with intracellular recordings in slice preparations have exhibited similar membrane responses, indicating that the LC slice may serve as a generalizable model system for alpha-2 receptor actions.

Mu Opiate Receptor Actions in LC Neurons

LC neurons in rat are densely invested with opiate receptors, particularly of the mu subtype (25). This nucleus is also prominently innervated by endogenous opioid fibers (13). Early studies using extracellular recordings in vivo demonstrated that systemic or iontophoretic opiates strongly inhibited LC discharge activity (reviewed in ref. 25). These findings, and the proposed role of the LC system in opiate abuse (see Chapters 27, 33, and 61, *this volume*), motivated a series of elegant studies of the effects of opiates on membrane properties of LC neurons.

Intracellular studies in slice preparations by Williams, North, and colleagues first showed that enkephalin acted at mu receptors on LC neurons to increase a K conductance and hyperpolarize the membrane (reviewed in ref. 11). Later studies (42) showed that this action of enkephalin also inhibited calcium action potentials in LC neurons,

a second mechanism (besides hyperpolarization) by which opioids may inhibit LC discharge activity. Additional experiments determined that the potassium conductance activated by opioids in LC neurons was inwardly rectifying and operated through a G-protein mechanism (2,44). Biochemical studies revealed that acute opiate treatment decreased adenylate cyclase activity and cAMP levels in LC neurons (see Chapters 27 and 61, *this volume*). Some studies indicated that the hyperpolarization induced by opiates in LC cells was linked to the reduction of cAMP, as it could be attenuated by administration of certain cAMP analogues to the slice bath (6). However, patch-clamp experiments by Miyake et al. (39) showed that opioids potently activate a potassium conductance in LC neurons in the absence of any intermediary diffusible second messenger such as cAMP. The role of cAMP in responses of LC neurons to opioids remains unclear. However, recent studies have demonstrated that increases in cAMP in LC neurons (e.g., as brought about by other transmitter inputs) markedly increase the hyperpolarization evoked in LC neurons by opiates (reviewed in ref. 11).

Examination of the properties listed above for alpha-2 adrenoceptor- and mu opiate receptor-mediated actions in LC neurons reveals striking similarities: Both open an inwardly rectifying potassium channel through a G-protein mechanism, both inhibit calcium influx into LC neurons, and both decrease cAMP levels in these cells. Many of these common features were shown to reflect the fact that alpha-2 and mu receptors are linked to the same potassium channel (2,44). The main evidence for this intriguing finding is that during a maximal electrophysiological response to an agonist at one receptor, application of an agonist at the other receptor does not further increase K conductance. This and other evidence indicate that the two receptors share the same K channels. This is one of the first and best characterized examples of shared channels among different receptors in central nervous system (CNS) neurons, but other examples also exist.

The LC has also been used as a model system to study potential cellular mechanisms underlying opioid tolerance and dependence. It has been known from early in vivo studies that LC neurons become tolerant to the inhibitory effects of opiates with chronic administration, and that opiate withdrawal potently activates LC neurons (reviewed in ref. 11). Detailed examination of changes in LC response to opiates using intracellular recordings in vitro revealed that tolerance may be due primarily to a decrease in the coupling of the mu receptor to the G protein, which, in turn, activates the K channel (17). The mechanism of withdrawal hyperactivity revealed some interesting and unexpected twists. First, it was found that although LC neurons in slices of morphine-treated rats exhibited tolerance, they exhibited little dependence; that is, the withdrawal-induced hyperactivity typical of LC neurons in vivo was relatively lacking when examined in the in vitro slice (reviewed in Chapter 33, *this volume,* as well as in ref. 11). This indicated that most of the opiate dependence of LC neurons was due to a change in afferent drive to these cells rather than a change in the

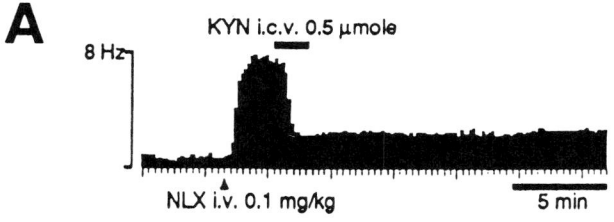

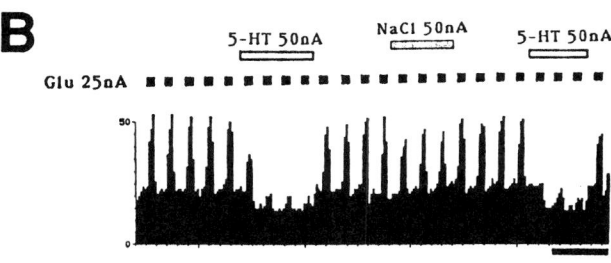

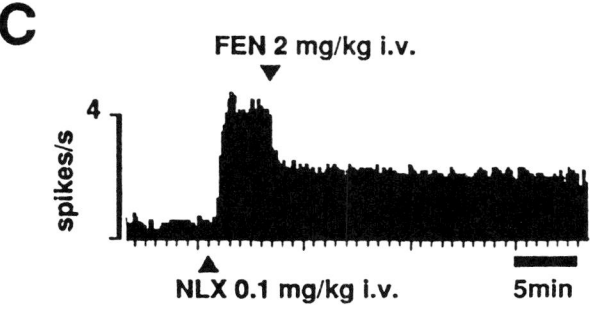

FIG. 1. A: Intracerebroventricular injection of the excitatory amino acid antagonist kynurenate (KYN) (0.5 μmol in 5 μl) strongly attenuated the withdrawal hyperactivity of LC neurons precipitated by intravenous naloxone (NLX: 0.1 mg/kg). (From ref. 3.) **B:** Computer-generated integrated activity–time histograms, revealing interactive effects of 5-HT and Glu on LC discharge. Pulses of Glu (applied at *solid bars*) activate a typical LC neuron. Co-iontophoresis of 5-HT (applied at *open bars*), but not of saline (applied at *stippled bar*), attenuates Glu response but has little effect on basal discharge. (From ref. 7.) **C:** Effects of intravenous administration of the indirect 5-HT agonist d-fenfluramine (FEN) on the activity of LC neurons during opiate withdrawal. Ratemeter record illustrating the attenuation of withdrawal-induced activation of LC neurons by d-fenfluramine. d-Fenfluoramine (2 mg/kg i.v.) strongly but incompletely reversed the activation of this typical LC neuron following morphine withdrawal precipitated by i.v. naloxone (0.1 mg/kg). (From ref. 4.)

membrane properties of the cells themselves. This was supported by several findings. First, intracellular studies showed little, if any, change in intrinsic membrane properties of LC neurons in slices taken from chronically morphine-treated rats (17). Second, excitatory amino acid antagonists, administered either intracerebroventricularly or locally into the LC in vivo, substantially attenuated the hyperactivity elicited by morphine withdrawal in intact, morphine-pretreated rats (Fig. 1). Finally, lesions of the nucleus paragigantocellularis, a prominent afferent to the LC that utilizes an excitatory amino acid transmitter to activate LC neurons, also attenuated withdrawal-induced hyperactivity of these cells. Together, these results strongly indicate that the bulk of opiate withdrawal response in the LC is mediated via augmented amino acid drive to the LC from the nucleus paragigantocellularis.

These findings, in view of previous results showing that serotonin decreases LC response to excitatory amino acids (Fig. 1) (7), suggested the clinically interesting possibility that serotonergic drugs may attenuate LC hyperactivity during opiate withdrawal. Indeed, Akaoka and Aston-Jones (4) have recently reported that fenfluramine, fluoxetine, or sertraline have this effect, suggesting that they may be useful clinically in treating withdrawal (Fig. 1) (see Chapter 33, *this volume*).

It should also be noted that while most of the withdrawal response can be accounted for by extrinsic afferent drive, recent studies reveal that a small amount of the withdrawal response (~20%) may reflect local intracoerulear changes that may involve alterations in adenylate cyclase activity (see Chapters 27 and 61, *this volume*).

IN VIVO STUDIES OF NORADRENERGIC NEURONS

Spontaneous LC Discharge and the Sleep–Waking Cycle

It has long been hypothesized that a principal function of the LC is participation in the control of various stages of the sleep–waking cycle (reviewed in ref. 9). In rat, spontaneous LC discharge covaries consistently with stages of the sleep–waking cycle: These neurons fire fastest during waking, more slowly during slow-wave sleep, and become virtually silent during paradoxical sleep (PS) (8). These observations support previous proposals that a similar subpopulation of neurons within the neurochemically heterogeneous cat LC are noradrenergic (8). However, other activity profiles of purported noradrenergic neurons have been reported in cat LC (18). Similar fluctuations in LC discharge with levels of alertness are also seen in the monkey (8). Although these animals do not exhibit normal sleep and waking under our experimental conditions of chair restraint, LC activity has been observed during alertness and drowsiness as measured by electroencephalography (EEG). As described above for rat LC, monkey LC neurons vary their activity closely with the state of arousal, even during unambiguous waking. Thus, periods of drowsiness are accompanied by decreased LC discharge, whereas alertness is consistently associated with elevated LC activity. Also as in rat, such changes in LC activity preceded the corresponding changes in EEG state by a few hundred to several hundred milliseconds.

Spontaneous LC Discharge and Waking Behavior

It has further been observed that LC discharge is altered during certain spontaneous waking behaviors. During both grooming and consumption of a glucose solution, rat LC discharge decreases compared to that in other behavioral episodes characterized by approximately the same degree of EEG arousal (8). Similar results have been obtained for LC activity in behaving primates. These results indicate that LC discharge is reduced not only for periods of low arousal (drowsiness or sleep), but also during certain behaviors (grooming and consumption) during which animals are in an active waking state but are inattentive to most environmental stimuli.

LC discharge rates also covary reliably with orienting behavior. In both rats and monkeys, the highest discharge rates observed for LC neurons were consistently associated with spontaneous or evoked behavioral orienting responses (8). LC discharge associated with orienting behavior is phasically most intense when automatic, tonic behaviors (sleep, grooming, or consumption) are suddenly disrupted and the animal orients toward the external environment.

LC Sensory Responsiveness

In addition to the above fluctuations in LC spontaneous discharge, it has also been observed that these neurons in unanesthetized rats and monkeys are responsive to non-noxious environmental stimuli (8). In waking rats, LC activity is markedly phasic, yielding short-latency (15–50 msec) responses to simple stimuli in every modality tested (auditory, visual, somatosensory, and olfactory). Responses were most consistently evoked by intense, conspicuous stimuli, though sporadic responses were also observed for nonconspicuous stimuli as well. These responses were similar for the different sensory modalities, and they consisted of a brief excitation followed by diminished activity lasting a few hundred milliseconds.

While sensory responsiveness was qualitatively similar for LC neurons in rats and monkeys, there were important differences as well. In rats, any of a variety of intense stimuli evoked LC responses in a majority of sensory trials. In contrast, monkey LC was less strongly influenced by such stimuli, with responses fading after the first few trials. However, more complex stimuli, such as a new face or a meaningful but unpredictable stimulus (see below), were consistently capable of eliciting LC responses in monkeys (8). In both species, stimuli that interrupted behavior and elicited orienting responses were those that most reliably evoked LC responses.

LC Responsiveness to Complex Stimuli During an "Oddball" Discrimination/Vigilance Task

The results described above indicated that LC neurons are robustly activated by intense stimuli because their intensity elicited behavioral orienting responses. However, it was hypothesized that nonintense stimuli that demand a behavioral response may also elicit responses in LC neurons. To explicitly test this possibility, Aston-Jones et al. (8,10) have recorded LC activity in unanesthetized monkeys trained in an "oddball" visual discrimination task. This task involves discriminating different colored lights, or vertical versus horizontal line segments, on a video monitor. Target cues (CS+) are presented on 10–20% of trials, intermixed in a semirandom fashion with non-target cues (CS−). Neurons in the LC area were recorded along with cortical surface slow waves [averaged event-related potentials (AERPs)] and behavioral responses (hits, misses, false alarms, and correct rejections). LC neurons exhibited phasic as well as tonic activity during this task, an observation that links this system to attentional processing.

In terms of phasic responses, LC neurons consistently and uniformly were activated by CS+ stimuli but not by other task events. In addition, these phasic responses to CS+ stimuli occurred with a short latency (mean 108 msec). This is far in advance of behavioral responses which occur at 250–300 msec, indicating that LC responses may participate in (e.g., facilitate) the behavioral response to CS+ cues. Recordings during reversal training revealed that these responses were specifically related to the imperative nature of stimuli, not to their physical attributes. As illustrated in Fig. 2, when the stimulus meaning was reversed, LC neurons quickly reversed their stimulus responsiveness, so that responses were soon selectively elicited for the new CS+ (previous CS−) while responses for the old CS+ (new CS−) rapidly faded. It is noteworthy that these changes varied closely with behavioral performance, so that responses to the new CS+ increased (and responses to the new CS− decreased) in parallel with the increasing percentage of correct behavioral responses to the new contingency.

In addition, cortical activity exhibited a similar set of properties. AERPs recorded from the frontal and parietal cortices at latencies of 200–300 msec post-stimulation were selectively augmented by CS+ cues (8), as reported by others in both humans (31) and monkeys (46). There is evidence that these potentials in nonhuman primates

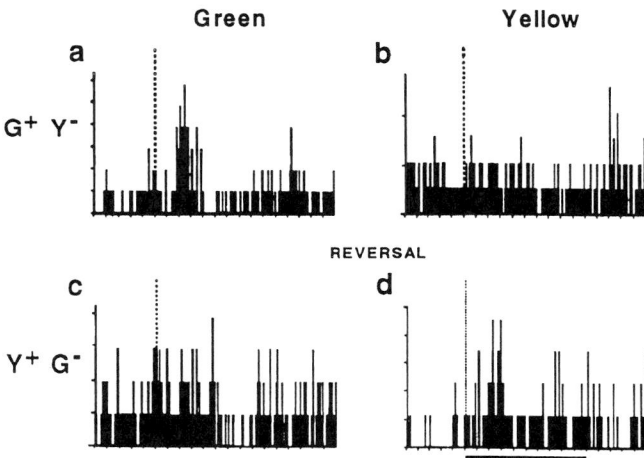

Green **Yellow**

REVERSAL

FIG. 2. A reversal procedure in a visual discrimination task in monkeys reveals responses for LC neurons specific to meaningful stimuli. Target stimuli occur on 10% of trials, and non-target stimuli occur on 90%; stimuli are presented at *vertical dashed lines* in each histogram. The animal receives a drop of juice when it responds after a target stimulus. **a** and **b**: Post-stimulus-time histograms (PSTHs) for response of an LC neuron to green (target), but not to yellow (non-target) stimuli. **c** and **d**: Similar PSTHs for the same LC neuron after reversal training such that target stimuli are now yellow and non-target stimuli green. Note that green stimuli (**c**) no longer elicit responses, whereas yellow stimuli (**d**) now elicit a small response. Thus, the response is selectively elicited by meaningful stimuli. Calibration bar represents 1 sec. (From ref. 8.)

are similar to the P3 or P300 potentials in humans (46). During reversal training, the AERPs altered their selectivity in a manner similar to that of neurons in the LC area to become selectively responsive to the new CS+ and no longer responsive to the previous CS+ (new CS−) (8). As with the brainstem neurons, these changes in cortical evoked activity followed a time course that closely paralleled behavioral discrimination performance during reversal. Pineda et al. (46) have shown that such AERP responses in monkeys are attenuated by lesions of the LC. The present results support their suggestion that the LC may contribute to these cortical slow-wave events.

Tonic activity of monkey LC neurons also changed in an intriguing manner during this task (47). In one version of the task, the animal must visually fixate a spot on the video monitor for a few hundred milliseconds to initiate each trial. Such foveation is effortful and reflects focused attentiveness to the task. As noted above, during drowsiness LC activity is very low (<0.5 spike/sec) and there is typically no task performance. It was observed that during continuous alertness and task performance the frequencies of both LC discharge and successful foveation fluctuated over short (10–30 sec) and long time intervals (10–30 min). Periods of high foveation frequency were associated with (a) stable gaze directed at the center of the monitor and (b) good overall task performance. Epochs of

low foveation frequency, in contrast, were associated with frequent eye movements and poor overall performance. Changes in fixation frequency and task performance were consistently inversely correlated with LC discharge rate, such that slightly elevated LC activity (by about 1–2 spikes/sec) was accompanied by decreased foveation frequency and poorer task performance. Correlation analyses revealed that this relationship was highly significant (typically $r = -0.4$, $p < 0.001$). Thus, a strong relationship exists among tonic LC discharge rate, sensory responsiveness of LC neurons, and vigilance performance. Very low LC activity is associated with drowsiness and inattentiveness, whereas high tonic LC discharge corresponds with labile scanning attention; optimal focusing of attention occurs with intermediate levels of tonic LC activity (47; see also Chapters 32 and 33, *this volume*).

The Role of the LC in Stress

The substantial involvement of the LC, along with enhanced NE release, in stress responses has been further documented and elaborated in recent years (see Valentino and Aston-Jones, *this volume*).

POSTSYNAPTIC EFFECTS OF NOREPINEPHRINE AND LOCUS COERULEUS STIMULATION

Three techniques have commonly been used to assess the impact of LC on the electrophysiological activity of its target neurons: (i) in vivo microiontophoretic or pressure application of NE (and/or agonists or antagonists), (ii) in vivo LC activation (or inactivation), and (iii) in vitro application of NE and related agents (see Chapter 5, *this volume*).

NE and LC Stimulation Effects on Sensory-Elicited Activity of Individual Neocortical Neurons

There have been numerous studies focused on the issue of how NE and/or LC stimulation alter the spontaneous and sensory-evoked discharge patterns of neocortical neurons (see refs. 25,26, and 63 for reviews). These studies have yielded generally consistent findings indicating that these manipulations are capable of enhancing the responsiveness of these neurons to sensory stimulation while at the same time reducing or not altering spontaneous activity. In recent years, Waterhouse and colleagues (e.g., see refs. 40,58, and 59) have extended and refined this body of data, examining the ability of NE application and/or LC stimulation to "gate" inputs to target neurons so that previously subthreshold synaptic input becomes suprathreshold for eliciting discharge activity. As in their previous work, these investigators find evidence for NE enhancement of both excitatory and inhibitory inputs to neocortical target cells. For example, the effects of iontophoretically applied NE on visually elicited responses of neurons in area 17 of anesthetized rat have been examined (58,59). For the majority of cells tested, NE application was found to enhance both the vigor and the precision of visually evoked responses.

NE and LC Stimulation Effects on Evoked Activity in Hippocampus

Within the last decade, there have been numerous demonstrations obtained from both in vitro and in vivo preparations that exogenous NE and/or LC stimulation can substantially enhance various measures of synaptically driven neuronal responses in the hippocampus. The early demonstrations of such phenomena followed the pioneering studies of Madison and Nicoll (33) demonstrating that NE reduces spike frequency adaptation, elicited by current injection, via actions on specific conductances in individual hippocampal neurons. These earlier studies, not summarized here, demonstrated facilitatory NE effects on various types of synaptically elicited activity in hippocampus (reviewed in ref. 27). Recent studies have confirmed and extended these previous observations. For example, both exogenous NE and LC stimulation have been shown to increase the amplitude of the population spike elicited in the dentate gyrus by perforant path stimulation, and it has been demonstrated that this enhancement can be blocked by beta-receptor antagonists and reduced by NE depletion (e.g., see refs. 20,28,29,52, and 57; see ref. 29 for limitations on the effects of beta blockers). It has also been recently shown that this beta-dependent potentiation can be elicited by stimulation of a major LC afferent, the nucleus paragigantocellularis (14). A long-lasting, beta-mediated enhancement of the population spike evoked in CA1 by Schaffer collateral stimulation has also been documented (22,30). In addition to these effects, which can be elicited without previous high-frequency stimulation of the non-NE afferent, there have also been numerous demonstrations of NE enhancement of long-term potentiation in CA3 and the dentate gyrus (28,32,52).

Thus, the literature demonstrating LC/NE enhancement of synaptically driven activity in hippocampus is impressive in several regards: Compatible observations have been made in vivo and in vitro; NE application and LC stimulation produce similar effects; several laboratories have replicated the basic findings, indicating that they are robust and consistent; and similar effects have been demonstrated for various hippocampal synapses.

Characterization of NE Effects on State-Related Activity of Individual Neurons in Thalamus and Neocortex

One of the most significant advances in understanding the possible mechanisms underlying the functional impact of the LC–NE system on behavioral state has been the delineation of the profound effects of exogenous NE on patterns of neuronal discharge activity in thalamus and neocortex in in vitro brain-slice preparations. A cohesive set of findings has been generated by McCormick and his colleagues (e.g., see refs. 34–38, and 56), who have obtained intracellular recordings from neurons in numerous thalamic and cortical areas in such preparations. These experiments show that NE activates these cells and changes their discharge patterns from one that in the in vivo preparation is generally observed during slow-wave sleep to one that is characteristic of the EEG state that indexes alertness and arousal. In addition, these investigators have been able to specify the membrane events underlying these pattern changes. For example, in studies of neurons from several thalamic nuclei, NE induced a slow depolarization that was apparently due to a decrease in potassium conductance (35,37,38). This slow depolarization suppressed burst firing and enhanced single-spike activity, changes in discharge pattern that mimic those that occur in these neurons in vivo during the transition from slow-wave sleep to waking and are presumed to underlie the parallel changes observed in corticothalamic EEG indices. Thus, these in vitro studies have provided evidence that a cellular substrate exists that could well serve to mediate profound LC effects on behavioral state as measured by thalamocortical EEG measures.

Effects of LC Activation on Forebrain EEG Measures

Recently, in vivo experiments have been conducted in which LC activity has been manipulated via local drug infusions while being simultaneously monitored with microelectrode recordings. This method achieves selective, acute, potent, and verifiable activation of LC, using a combined recording/infusion probe, as previously described (1,24). The electrophysiological recordings facilitate the accurate placement of peri-coerulear infusions of drugs that alter LC neuronal discharge rates. The close proximity of the infusion site to the LC allows the use of small volumes, reducing the spread of the infusion into other brainstem structures while at the same time not damaging the LC itself. The microelectrode recordings obtained before and after the infusion provide quantitative verification of the LC manipulation and permit analyses of temporal relationships between the onset and offset of LC activation/inactivation and any observed physiological effects.

Recently, this technique has been used to determine whether peri-LC bethanechol infusions produce reliable forebrain EEG activation, whether this EEG activation is dependent on enhancement of LC neuronal discharge rates, and whether this effect can be blocked by antagonizing noradrenergic neurotransmission. In a total of 39 halothane-anesthetized animals, the findings were as follows

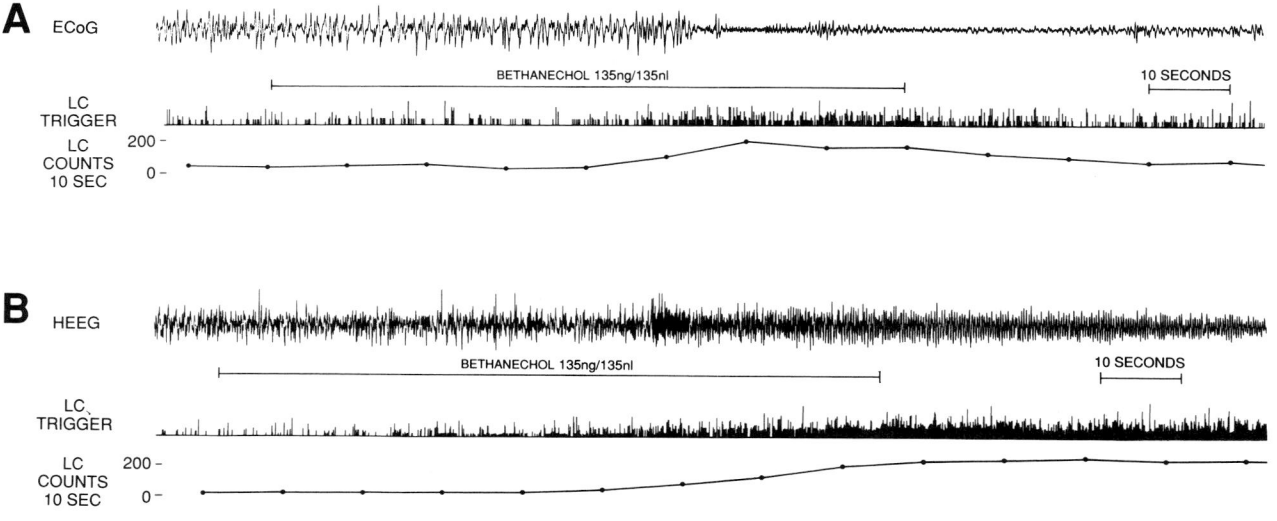

FIG. 3. Relationship of LC activity to cortical (ECoG; **A**) and hippocampal EEG (HEEG; **B**) before, during, and after peri-LC bethanechol infusions. **A** and **B** represent data from separate experiments. In each experiment, bethanechol-induced changes in EEG activity were observed simultaneously in both the ECoG and HEEG recordings. Bethanechol was infused at a constant rate throughout the interval indicated. EEG activity is shown in the *top trace* of each panel, the raw trigger output from LC activity is shown in the *middle trace,* and the integrated trigger output (10-sec intervals) is shown in the *bottom trace.* In **A,** LC activity is seen to increase during the latter part of the infusion; several seconds later, reduced amplitude and increased frequency become evident in the ECoG trace. As LC activity begins to decrease following the infusion, ECoG amplitude begins to increase and its frequency decreases. In **B,** enhanced LC activity becomes evident in the latter part of the infusion period; several seconds later, theta rhythm begins to dominate the HEEG trace. For the remainder of the trace, LC activity remains elevated and theta rhythm predominates. (From ref. 15.)

(15; examples are shown in Fig. 3): (a) LC activation was consistently followed, within 5–30 sec, by a shift from low-frequency, high-amplitude to high-frequency, low-amplitude activity in the neocortical EEG; (b) these EEG responses followed LC activation with similar latencies whether infusions were made lateral or medial to the LC; (c) infusions placed at a distance of more than 500–600 μm from the LC were not followed by these EEG responses; (d) following infusion-induced activation, EEG returned to preinfusion patterns with about the same time course as the recovery of LC activity; and (e) the infusion-induced changes in EEG were blocked or severely attenuated by pretreatment with the alpha-2 agonist clonidine (50 μg/kg, iv) or the beta-antagonist propranolol (200 μg, icv). These observations indicate that enhanced LC discharge activity is the crucial mediating event for the infusion-induced changes in forebrain EEG activity observed under these conditions. This demonstration that LC activation is followed by cortical EEG desynchronization is especially interesting because it indicates that LC activity levels are not only correlated with, but can be causally related to, EEG measures of forebrain activation.

Effects of LC Inactivation on Neocortical EEG Activity

It is well known that systemic administration of alpha-2 adrenergic agonists produces behavioral and EEG mea-

sures of sedation. Because these drugs act to inhibit LC neuronal discharge activity and NE release (see preceding discussion), these observations are consistent with an action of the LC–NE system in the maintenance of an activated forebrain. The possibility that inhibition of LC activity might be a major mediating mechanism for these actions has been enhanced by the observation that intrabrainstem administration of alpha-2 agonists into the region of the LC has similar sedative effects (19,21). However, interpretation of these results is complicated by a variety of factors, such as the small size of the LC and its close proximity to other nuclei known to affect behavioral and EEG states (53,54). These factors, together with the absence of electrophysiological measures documenting the relationship between changes in LC neuronal activity and EEG state following such infusions, preclude specific conclusions regarding the site(s) of action for the sedative effects of intrabrainstem administered alpha-2 agonists.

In recent studies (16), small clonidine infusions (35 nl or 150 nl; 1 ng/nl) were made either immediately adjacent to, or at a distance of approximately 1000 μm from, LC in halothane-anesthetized rats using a recording/infusion probe, as described above. These infusions were made under conditions in which high-frequency, low-voltage activity predominated in the neocortical EEG. The following results were obtained (see Fig. 4 for examples): (a)

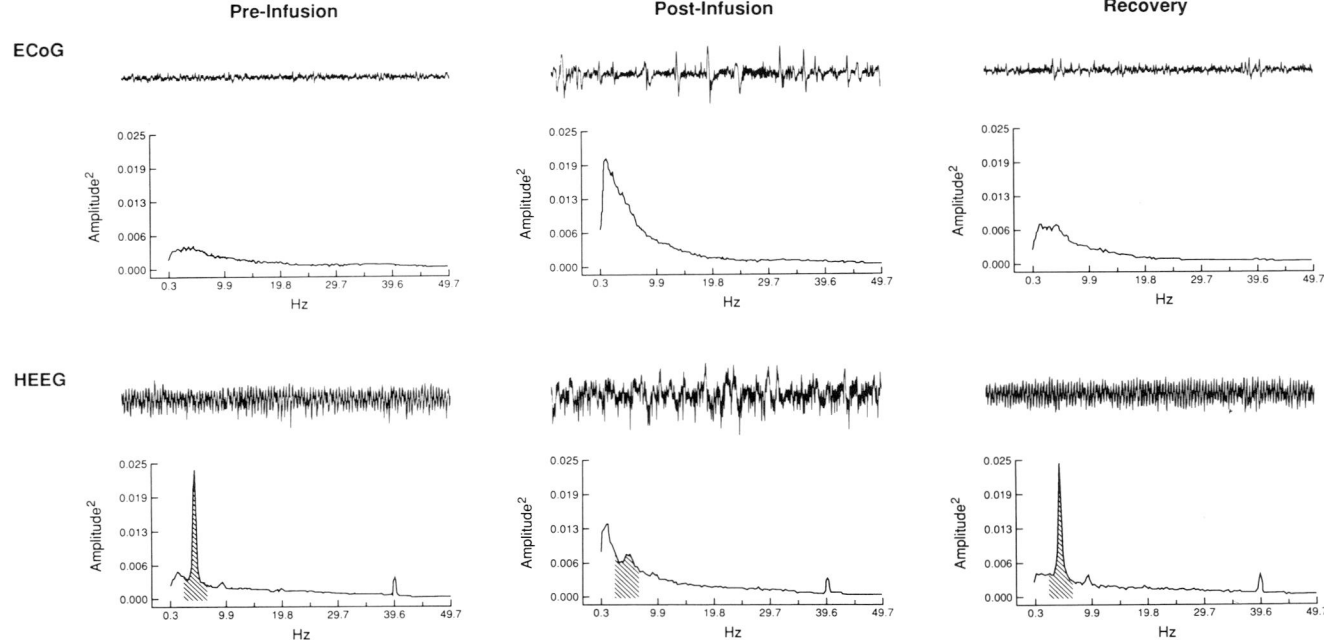

FIG. 4. Effects of bilateral, peri-LC clonidine infusions on EEG measures in halothane-anesthetized rat. The infusions completely suppressed LC discharge activity. Power-spectrum analyses are shown for ECoG and HEEG samples from preinfusion, postinfusion, and recovery periods. A 25-sec raw EEG trace representative of the entire 8-min period from which the PSA was computed is shown above each power spectrum. The most striking postinfusion changes in the ECoG are the increase in power of the slowest frequencies, and those in the HEEG are the appearance of mixed-frequency activity. Shading indicates the theta frequency band (2.3–6.9 Hz) in the HEEG power spectra. (From ref. 16.)

cortical EEG activity was not substantially affected following unilateral clonidine-induced LC inactivation; (b) bilateral clonidine infusions that completely suppressed LC neuronal discharge activity in both hemispheres induced a shift in neocortical EEG to low-frequency, large-amplitude activity; (c) 35-nl infusions placed 800–1200 μm from the LC did not induce a complete suppression of LC activity and did not alter forebrain EEG; (d) 150-nl infusions placed 800–1200 μm from LC were either ineffective at completely suppressing LC neuronal discharge activity or did so with a longer latency to complete LC inhibition and a shorter duration of inhibition; (e) in all cases, the onsets of EEG responses coincided with the complete bilateral inhibition of LC discharge activity, and these EEG effects persisted throughout the period during which bilateral LC neuronal discharge activity was completely suppressed (60–240 min); and (f) the resumption of preinfusion EEG activity patterns closely followed the recovery of LC neuronal activity or could be induced with systemic administration of the alpha-2 noradrenergic antagonist, idazoxan. These results suggest that the clonidine-induced EEG changes were dependent on the complete bilateral suppression of LC discharge activity and that, under the present experimental conditions, the LC–NA system exerts a potent and tonic activating influence on forebrain EEG state such that activity within

this system is necessary for the maintenance of an activated forebrain EEG state.

In these studies of neocortical EEG and manipulation of LC activity by drug infusion, hippocampal EEG activity was also recorded. It was consistently observed that LC activation was followed by intense hippocampal theta activity, whereas LC inactivation diminished the occurrence of EEG activity in this frequency range.

CONCLUSION

In summary, there have been a large number of observations from both in vivo and in vitro preparations indicating that changes in LC activity accompany, and participate in producing, changes in behavioral state. There is substantial evidence that this occurs in terms of the sleep–wake cycle, where elevated LC discharge activity precedes spontaneous waking and its associated EEG alerting. Moreover, activating LC with local drug infusions induces neocortical and hippocampal EEG activation, and NE produces discharge patterns characteristic of activated EEG states in individual thalamic and neocortical neurons.

There is also evidence from LC recordings obtained from waking rats, cats, and monkeys that LC activity is modulated within the waking state to produce a more fine-grained control of vigilance. In a parallel set of observations, the application of exogenous NE or LC activation has been found to enhance the robustness and precision of neocortical neuronal responses to defined sensory input while reducing or not altering "background" or "spontaneous" activity. Additionally, NE and/or LC activation enhance several indices of hippocampal synaptic responsiveness, both at the level of individual neurons and at the level of cell populations. Recent evidence indicates that moderate LC activation accompanies optimal information processing, whereas high discharge rates accompany, and perhaps produce, a hyperarousal that may lead to poor performance in circumstances requiring focused, sustained attention.

These latter results suggest that focused attentiveness varies with tonic LC discharge in an inverted U relationship (Aston-Jones, Rajkowski, and Kubiak, *in preparation*). This relationship between LC activity and performance resembles the Yerkes–Dodson law, suggesting that LC activity changes may in part underlie this classical relationship between "arousal" and performance. It is worthwhile to compare these results for LC activity with those for lesions of the LC system. Lesions of the ascending projections from the LC have led investigators to posit that no or low LC activity may promote attention to contextual, distant cues in the environment, whereas high LC activity (as presumably occurs during stress) may facilitate more focused attention, centered on conditioned or proximal cues (reviewed in Chapter 32, *this volume*). While these lesion results lead to a similar functional dimension for the LC as the cellular recordings (indicating a role in attentional focussing), the specific prediction is the opposite: Recordings predict less focused attention with high LC activity, whereas lesion studies predict more focused attention with high LC activity. These different results may reflect the different species or behavioral paradigms employed. Alternatively, this difference may reveal limitations of the lesion techniques commonly employed in behavioral studies, where weeks are allowed for recovery from surgery before testing and where substantial functional recovery may occur in the lesioned or other systems. More readily interpretable results may be found using acute reversible inactivations of the LC system, where possible recovery of function could not occur (discussed in Chapter 32, *this volume*). Future studies are necessary to test this and other possibilities for the intriguing differences predicted for LC functions from cell recordings as compared to lesion studies.

MAJOR ISSUES TO BE ADDRESSED IN THE NEXT GENERATION

Despite the continuing progress that characterizes studies of the LC–NE system, some major limitations of the currently available database are readily evident. Four areas ripe for exploitation are the following:

More precise determination of the behavioral correlates of LC discharge. While progress has been made in determining how LC discharge activity is correlated with certain aspects of behavior in well-defined paradigms, much remains to be done. The variety of paradigms in which LC activity has been assessed needs to be expanded, and the number of behavioral, autonomic, and electrographic correlates that are simultaneously indexed and correlated with measures of LC activity must be enlarged.

Moving toward unanesthetized, in vivo preparations in experiments manipulating LC activity. The goal of manipulating LC activity in some specific way and then determining the behavioral consequences of such treatment has remained elusive throughout the history of this field. The experiments described above involving local drug infusions and simultaneous electrophysiological monitoring offer promise in this regard, but they are currently limited to anesthetized preparations. Convincing demonstrations of LC function will depend both on detailed correlative experiments as indicated in the preceding paragraph and on corresponding manipulative experiments that can demonstrate causal relationships between changes in LC discharge activity and indices of behavioral or state variables.

Specifying relationships between LC–NE and other alerting systems. It is almost certain that the LC–NE system performs its functions in such a way that its actions are coordinated with those of other ascending modulatory systems. Systematic study of these interactions will be imperative for understanding the control of forebrain levels of alertness and/or vigilance.

Determining the afferent inputs and efferent targets of LC neurons. The current status of knowledge on this topic is reviewed elsewhere in this volume (see Chapter 33, *this volume*). Understanding the functional status of the LC in brain and behavioral activities requires a thorough comprehension of its input–output relationships, as has proved to be so critical in understanding the functions of other brain areas (e.g., sensory, motor). This analysis will reveal the functional correlates of the LC system in brain circuitry, providing important knowledge about the function of the LC system itself.

REFERENCES

1. Adams LM, Foote SL, Neville HJ. Effects of locally infused pharmacological agents on spontaneous and sensory-evoked activity of locus coeruleus neurons. *Brain Res* 1988;21:395–400.
2. Aghajanian GK, Wang YY. Common alpha-2 and opiate effector mechanisms in the locus coeruleus: intracellular studies in brain slices. *Neuropharmacology* 1987;26:789–800.
3. Akaoka H, Aston-Jones G. Opiate withdrawal-induced hyperactivity of locus coeruleus neurons is substantially mediated by augmented excitatory amino acid input. *J Neurosci* 1991;11:3830–3839.

4. Akaoka H, Aston-Jones G. Indirect serotonergic agonists attenuate neuronal opiate withdrawal. *Neuroscience* 1993;54:561–565.

5. Andrade R, Aghajanian GK. Locus coeruleus activity in vitro: intrinsic regulation by a calcium-dependent potassium conductance but not alpha 2-adrenoceptors. *J Neurosci* 1984;4(1):161–170.

6. Andrade R, Aghajanian GK. Opiate- and α2-adrenoceptor-induced hyperpolarizations of locus ceruleus neurons in brain slices: reversal by cyclic adenosine 3':5'-monophosphate analogues. *J Neurosci* 1985;5(9):2359–2364.

7. Aston-Jones G, Akaoka H, Charlety P, Chouvet G. Serotonin selectively attenuates glutamate-evoked activation of locus coeruleus neurons in vivo. *J Neurosci* 1991;11:760–769.

8. Aston-Jones G, Chiang C, Alexinsky T. Discharge of noradrenergic locus coeruleus neurons in behaving rats and monkeys suggests a role in vigilance. *Prog Brain Res* 1991;88:501–520.

9. Aston-Jones G, Foote SL, Bloom FE. Anatomy and physiology of locus coeruleus neurons: functional implications. In: Ziegler M, Lake CR, eds. *Norepinephrine. Frontiers of clinical neuroscience, vol 2.* Baltimore: Williams & Wilkins, 1984;92–116.

10. Aston-Jones G, Rajkowski J, Kubiak P, Alexinsky T. Locus coeruleus neurons in the monkey are selectively activated by attended stimuli in a vigilance task. *J Neurosci* 1994;in press.

11. Aston-Jones G, Shiekhattar R, Rajkowski J, Kubiak P, Akaoka H. Opiates influence noradrenergic locus coeruleus neurons by potent indirect as well as direct effects. In: Hammer R, ed. *The neurobiology of opiates.* New York: CRC Press, 1993;175–202.

12. Aston-Jones G, Shipley MT, Ennis M, Williams JT, Pieribone VA. Restricted afferent control of locus coeruleus neurons revealed by anatomic, physiologic and pharmacologic studies. In: Marsden CA, Heal DJ, eds. *The pharmacology of noradrenaline in the central nervous system.* Oxford: Oxford University Press, 1990;187–247.

13. Aston-Jones G, Shipley MT, Chouvet G, et al. Afferent regulation of locus coeruleus neurons: anatomy, physiology and pharmacology. *Prog Brain Res* 1991;88:47–75.

14. Babstock DM, Harley W. Paragigantocellularis stimulation induces β-adrenergic hippocampal potentiation. *Brain Res Bull* 1992;28:709–714.

15. Berridge CW, Foote SL. Effects of locus coeruleus activation on electroencephalographic activity in neocortex and hippocampus. *J Neurosci* 1991;11:3135–3145.

16. Berridge CW, Page ME, Valentino RJ, Foote SL. Effects of locus coeruleus inactivation on electroencephalographic activity in neocortex and hippocampus. *Neuroscience* 1993;55:381–393.

17. Christie MJ, Williams JT, North RA. Cellular mechanisms of opioid tolerance: studies in single brain neurons. *Mol Pharmacol* 1987;32(5):633–638.

18. Chu NS, Bloom FE. Activity patterns of catecholamine-containing potine neurons in the dorsolateral tegmentum of unrestrained cats. *J Neurobiol* 1974;5:527–544.

19. Correa-Sales C, Rabin BC, Maze M. A hypnotic response to dexmedetomidine, and α2-agonist, is mediated in the locus coeruleus in rats. *Anesthesiology* 1992;76:948–952.

20. Dahl D, Sarvey JM. Norepinephrine induces pathway-specific long-lasting potentiation and depression in the hippocampal dentate gyrus. *Proc Natl Acad Sci USA* 1989;86:4776–4780.

21. De Sarro GB, Ascioti C, Froio F, Libri V, Nistico G. Evidence that locus coeruleus is the site where clonidine and drugs acting at alpha-1- and alpha-2-adrenoceptors affect sleep and arousal mechanisms. *Br J Pharmacol* 1987;90:675–685.

22. Dunwiddie TV, Taylor M, Heginbotham LR, Proctor WR. Long-term increases in excitability in the CA1 region of rat hippocampus induced by β-adrenergic stimulation: possible mediation by cAMP. *J Neurosci* 1992;12(2):506–517.

23. Egan TM, Henderson G, North RA, Williams JT. Noadrenaline-mediated synaptic inhibition in rat locus coeruleus neurones. *J Physiol* 1983;345:477–488.

24. Foote SL, Berridge CW, Adams LM, Pineda JA. Electrophysiological evidence for the involvement of the locus coeruleus in alerting, orienting, and attending. *Prog Brain Res* 1991;88:521–532.

25. Foote SL, Bloom FE, Aston-Jones G. The nucleus locus coeruleus: new evidence of anatomical and physiological specificity. *Physiol Rev* 1983;63:844–914.

26. Foote SL, Morrison JH. Extrathalamic modulation of neocortical function. *Annu Rev Neurosci* 1987;10:67–95.

27. Harley CW. A role for norepinephrine in arousal, emotion and learning: limbic modulation by norepinephrine and the Kety hypothesis. *Prog Neuropsychopharmacol Biol Psychiatry* 1987;11:419–458.

28. Harley C. Noradrenergic and locus coeruleus modulation of the performant path-evoked potential in rat dentate gyrus supports a role for the locus coeruleus in attentional and memorial processes. In: Barnes CD, Pompeiano O, eds. *Progress in brain research.* Amsterdam: Elsevier Science Publishers, 1991;307–321.

29. Harley C, Milway JS, LaCaille J-C. Locus coeruleus potentiation of dentate gurus responses: evidence for two systems. *Brain Res Bull* 1989;22:643–650.

30. Heginbotham LR, Dunwiddie TV. Long-term increase in the evoked population spike in the CA1 region of rat hippocampus induced by β-adrenergic receptor activation. *J Neurosci* 1991;11:2519–2527.

31. Hillyard SA. Electrophysiology of human selective attention. *Trends Neurosci* 1985;8:400–405.

32. Hopkins WF, Johnston D. Noradrenergic enhancement of long-term potentiation at mossy fiber synapses in the hippocampus. *J Neurophysio* 1988;59(2):667–687.

33. Madison DV, Nicoll RA. Noradrenaline blocks accommodation of pyramidal cell discharge in the hippocampus. *Nature* 1982;299:636–638.

34. McCormick DA. Cellular mechanisms underlying cholinergic and noradrenergic modulation of neuronal firing mode in the cat and guinea pig dorsal lateral geniculate nucleus. *J Neurosci* 1992;12(1):278–289.

35. McCormick DA. Neurotransmitter actions in the thalamus and cerebral cortex and their role in neuromodulation of thalamocortical activity. *Prog Neurobiol* 1992;39:337–388.

36. McCormick DA. Cholinergic and noradrenergic modulation of thalamocortical processing. *Trends Neurosci* 1989;12(6):215–221.

37. McCormick DA, Prince DA. Noradrenergic modulation of firing pattern in guinea pig and cat thalamic neurons, in vitro. *J Neurophysiol* 1988;59(3):978–996.

38. McCormick DA, Wang Z. Serotonin and noradrenaline excite GABAergic neurones of the guinea-pig and cat nucleus reticularis thalami. *J Physiol* 1991;442:235–255.

39. Miyake M, Christie M, North R. Single potassium channels opened by opioids in rat locus ceruleus neurons. *Proc Natl Acad Sci USA* 1989;86:3419–3422.

40. Mouradian RD, Sessler FM, Waterhouse BD. Noradrenergic potentiation of excitatory transmitter action in cerebrocortical slices: evidence for mediation by an α1 receptor-linked second messenger pathway. *Brain Res* 1991;546:83–95.

41. Nakamura S, Sakaguchi T. Development and plasticity of the locus coeruleus: a review of recent physiological and pharmacological experimentation. *Prog Neurobiol* 1990;34(6):505–526.

42. North RA, Williams JT. Opiate activation of potassium conductance inhibits calcium action potentials in rat locus coeruleus neurones. *Br J Pharmacol* 1983;80(2):225–228.

43. North RA, Williams JT. On the potassium conductance increased by opioids in rat locus coeruleus neurones. *J Physiol* 1985;364:265–280.

44. North RA, Williams JT, Surprenant A, Christie MJ. Mu and delta receptors belong to a family of receptors that are coupled to potassium channels. *Proc Natl Acad Sci USA* 1987;84:5487–5491.

45. Osmanovic SS, Shefner SA. Gamma-aminobutyric acid responses in rat locus coeruleus neurones in vitro: a current-clamp and voltage-clamp study. *J Physiol* 1990;421:151–170.

46. Pineda JA, Foote SL, Neville HJ, Holmes T. Endogenous event-related potential in squirrel monkeys: the role of task relevance, stimulus probability, and behavioral response. *Electroencephalogr Clin Neurophysiol* 1988;70:155–171.

47. Rajkowski J, Kubiak P, Aston-Jones G. Activity of locus coeruleus neurons in behaving monkeys varies with focussed attention: short- and long-term changes. *Soc Neurosci Abstr* 1992;18:538.

48. Regenold JT, Illes P. Inhibitory adenosine α1-receptors on rat locus coeruleus neurones. An intracellular electrophysiological study. *Naunyn Schmiedebergs Arch Pharmacol* 1990;341(3):225–231.

49. Shen KZ, North RA. Muscarine increases cation conductance and decreases potassium conductance in rat locus coeruleus neurones. *J Physiol* 1992;455:471–485.

50. Shen KZ, North RA. Substance P opens cation channels and closes

potassium channels in rat locus coeruleus neurons. *Neuroscience* 1992;50(2):345–353.

51. Shen KZ, North RA. Excitation of rat locus coeruleus neurons by adenosine 5′-triphosphate: ionic mechanism and receptor characterization. *J Neurosci* 1993;13(3):894–899.

52. Stanton PK, Sarvey JM. Norepinephrine regulates long-term potentiation of both the population spike and dendritic EPSP in hippocampal dentate gyrus. *Brain Res Bull* 1987;18:115–119.

53. Steriade M, Datta S, Pare D, Oakson G, Dossi RC. Neuronal activities in brain-stem cholinergic nuclei related to tonic activation processes in thalamocortical systems. *J Neurosci* 1990;10:2541–2559.

54. Vanderwolf CH. Cerebral activity and behavior: control by central cholinergic and serotonergic systems. *Int Rev Neurobiol* 1988;30:225–341.

55. Wang YY, Aghajanian GK. Excitation of locus coeruleus neurons by vasoactive intestinal peptide: role of a cAMP and protein kinase A. *J Neurosci* 1990;10(10):3335–3343.

56. Wang Z, McCormick DA. Control of firing mode of corticotectal and corticopontine layer V burst-generating neurons by norepinephrine, acetylcholine, and 1S,3R-ACPD. *J Neurosci* 1993;13:2199–2216.

57. Washburn M, Moises HC. Electrophysiological correlates of presynaptic α2-receptor-mediated inhibition of norepinephrine release at locus coeruleus synapses in dentate gyrus. *J Neurosci* 1989;9:2131–2140.

58. Waterhouse BD, Azizi A, Burne RA, Woodward DJ. Modulation of rat cortical area 17 neuronal responses to moving visual stimuli during norepinephrine and serotonin microiontophoresis. *Brain Res* 1990;546:276–292.

59. Waterhouse BD, Sessler FM, Cheng J, Woodward DJ, Azizi A, Moises HC. New evidence for a gating action of norepinephrine in central neuronal circuits of mammalian brain. *Brain Res Bull* 1988;21:425–432.

60. Williams JT, Henderson G, North RA. Characterization of alpha 2-adrenoceptors in rat locus coeruleus neurones. *Neurosci* 1985;14(1):95–101.

61. Williams JT, Marshall KC. Membrane properties and adrenergic responses in locus coeruleus neurons of young rats. *J Neurosci* 1987;7(11):3687–3694.

62. Williams JT, North RA. Catecholamine inhibition of calcium actin potentials in rat locus coeruleus neurones. *Neuroscience* 1985;14(1):103–109.

63. Woodward DJ, Moises HC, Waterhouse BD, Hoffer BJ, Freedman R. Modulatory actions of norepinephrine in the central nervous system. *Fed Proc* 1979;38:2109–2116.

64. Xiong HG, Marshall KC. Angiotensin II modulation of glutamate excitation of locus coeruleus neurons. *Neurosci Lett* 1990;118(2):261–264.

Psychopharmacology: The Fourth Generation of Progress, edited by Floyd E. Bloom and David J. Kupfer. Raven Press, Ltd., New York 1995.

CHAPTER **30**

Coexisting Neurotransmitters in Central Noradrenergic Neurons

Philip V. Holmes and Jacqueline N. Crawley

The noradrenergic neurons in the mammalian central nervous system (CNS) are localized in the nucleus locus coeruleus (LC), or A6 cell group, and in medullary nuclei designated A1, A2, A5, and A7. As diagrammed in Fig. 1, reviewed in ref. 14, and described further in chapters by Valentino and Aston-Jones and by Robbins and Everitt in this volume, the LC is a bilateral nucleus in the dorsal tegmentum, just ventral and lateral to the fourth ventricle. Each LC contains approximately 1500 densely packed neurons, with extensively branching axons forming five major noradrenergic tracts. The ascending projections of the LC comprise the dorsal noradrenergic bundle, the central gray dorsal longitudinal facsiculus, and the ventral tegmental–medial forebrain bundle, which project to the hypothalamus, thalamus, and telencephalon. Additional projections innervate the cerebellar cortex and the ventrolateral spinal cord. The A7 noradrenergic cell group is located in the lateral tegmental area ventral to the LC. The A1, A2, and A5 cell groups are situated more caudally in the medulla. The ascending projections of the A1, A2, A5, and A7 cell groups comprise the ventral noradrenergic bundle, innervating forebrain areas including the septum and hypothalamus. The LC and the A1 and A2 cell groups are the most extensively studied of the noradrenergic cell groups with respect to coexistence of transmitters and will therefore be the focus of the present review.

The noradrenergic neurons of the LC contain two neuropeptides, galanin (GAL) and neuropeptide Y (NPY) (26,34). Neuropeptides are short sequences of amino acids, localized in high concentrations in neurons. The majority of neuropeptides were discovered in the brain during the 1970s, with the advent of radioimmunoassay

and immunohistochemical techniques developed for applications to the nervous system (25). At least 50 neuropeptides have been conclusively identified in the mammalian CNS (25; also see Chapter 43, *this volume*). Functional studies are in progress for many peptides, to determine whether the criteria (i.e., neuronal synthesis, vesicular storage, release, specific receptors, effectors, and physiological actions) for a neurotransmitter are satisfied for a candidate neuropeptide (14). Following closely upon the discovery of the many putative peptide transmitters was the discovery of coexistence, the phenomenon of two or more neurotransmitters synthesized within the same neuron (25). Histochemical techniques, including double-labeling, tract-tracing, and lesion studies, demonstrate that neuropeptides are often localized within the same neuron as a well-known "classical" neurotransmitter (25; also see Chapter 43, *this volume*). The coexistence of GAL and NPY with norepinephrine in neurons of the LC provides an excellent model for investigating the functional interactions of a triple coexistence (see also Chapters 18 and 43, *this volume*).

ANATOMY

GAL and NPY in the Locus Coeruleus

Current histochemical evidence suggests that GAL is the predominant neuropeptide coexisting with norepinephrine (NE) in LC neurons in the rat brain (26,37; see also Chapter 50, *this volume*). GAL is a 29-amino-acid peptide that is regionally distributed throughout the mammalian CNS (37,51). GAL apparently belongs to a distinct family of peptides, because it contains no significant sequence homologies with other known peptides (27,58). The cDNA encoding this putative neurotransmitter has

P. V. Holmes and J. N. Crawley: Section on Behavioral Neuropharmacology, Experimental Therapeutics Branch, National Institute of Mental Health, Bethesda, Maryland 20892.

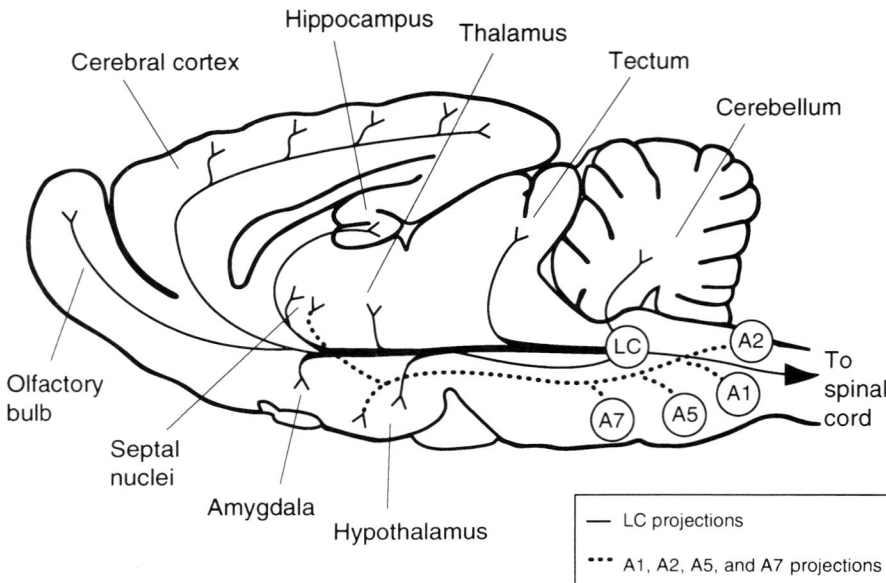

FIG. 1. Summary of the noradrenergic nuclei and their projections in the rat brain. *Solid lines* indicate the major projections of the LC, including the dorsal noradrenergic bundle and central gray longitudinal fasciculus (*thick line*) and ventral tegmental bundle (*thin line*). *Dotted lines* indicate the projections of the A1, A2, A5, and A7 cell groups comprising the ventral noradrenergic bundle. (Adapted from ref. 14.)

been cloned and sequenced (27,58). GAL-like-immunoreactive (GAL-LI) and GAL mRNA-containing cell bodies are densely clustered in the hypothalamic paraventricular, arcuate, and dorsomedial nuclei, the bed nuclei of the stria terminalis, and the nucleus tractus solitarius in addition to the LC (37,51). GAL coexists with other neurotransmitters, including cholinergic neurons of the basal forebrain and serotonergic neurons of the dorsal raphe (25,26).

GAL-LI is present in approximately 80% of noradrenergic LC neurons in the rat (26). The coexistence of GAL with NE was demonstrated by immunocytochemical double-staining techniques using the synthetic enzymes tyrosine hydroxylase (26) and dopamine-β-hydroxylase (34) as markers for noradrenergic neurons. GAL-LI is not typically observed in the absence of dopamine-β-hydroxylase or tyrosine hydroxylase, suggesting that GAL is present only within NE-containing neurons of the LC (26,34). GAL-LI is present throughout the LC, with a slightly higher density in the dorsal aspect of the LC (26,34). The distribution of GAL mRNA detected by in situ hybridization matches well with the immunocytochemical distribution. GAL mRNA is present throughout the LC, showing highest levels in the dorsal LC (3,15).

NPY coexists with NE in LC neurons of the rat, to a lesser extent than GAL. NPY is a 36-amino-acid peptide that is widely distributed throughout the mammalian CNS (19,32; see Chapter 48, *this volume*). NPY-LI neurons are present in high concentrations in the rat cerebral cortex, hippocampus, and arcuate nucleus of the hypothalamus (19,32), with densely clustered NPY-LI cell bodies in the brainstem catecholaminergic neurons (19,47). NPY-like immunoreactivity is present in moderate concentrations in the LC (26,47,55), where double-labeling studies indicate that approximately 20–40% of noradrenergic neurons in the LC contain NPY-LI (19,26). NPY, like GAL, appears

to be present in the LC only in tyrosine hydroxylase (TH)-immunoreactive neurons (47).

Efferents of GAL- and NPY-Containing Locus Coeruleus Neurons

Figure 2 diagrams the major noradrenergic pathways containing GAL and NPY in the rat brain. Combined immunocytochemistry and axonal transport studies have demonstrated that approximately 30% of GAL-LI LC neurons project to the hypothalamus, primarily terminating in the parvocellular subdivision of the paraventricular nucleus (PVN) of the hypothalamus (26,34), corresponding closely with the location of preganglionic autonomic neurons (34). Electron microscopic analysis indicates that GAL-LI terminals in the PVN, containing dense-core vesicles characteristic of peptide storage, synapse predominantly on those parvocellular cells lacking in well-developed Golgi cisternae and secretory granules (34). Noradrenergic LC neurons containing GAL-LI also project to the medial thalamus, terminating on thalamic neurons that process and relay ascending nociceptive input from the spinothalamic tract (8,33). LC neurons containing GAL-LI and dopamine-β-hydroxylase-LI project to the cerebral cortex, hippocampus, and spinal cord (26,37). Holets et al. (26) estimated that approximately 14% of GAL-LI noradrenergic neurons in the LC project to ipsilateral cerebral cortex and 3% project to either ipsilateral or contralateral spinal cord.

Few NPY-LI neurons project to the hypothalamus, and these projections do not terminate in the PVN (76), indicating that NPY in the hypothalamus arises from sources other than the LC (46,47). NPY projections to thalamus appear to terminate exclusively in the medial division

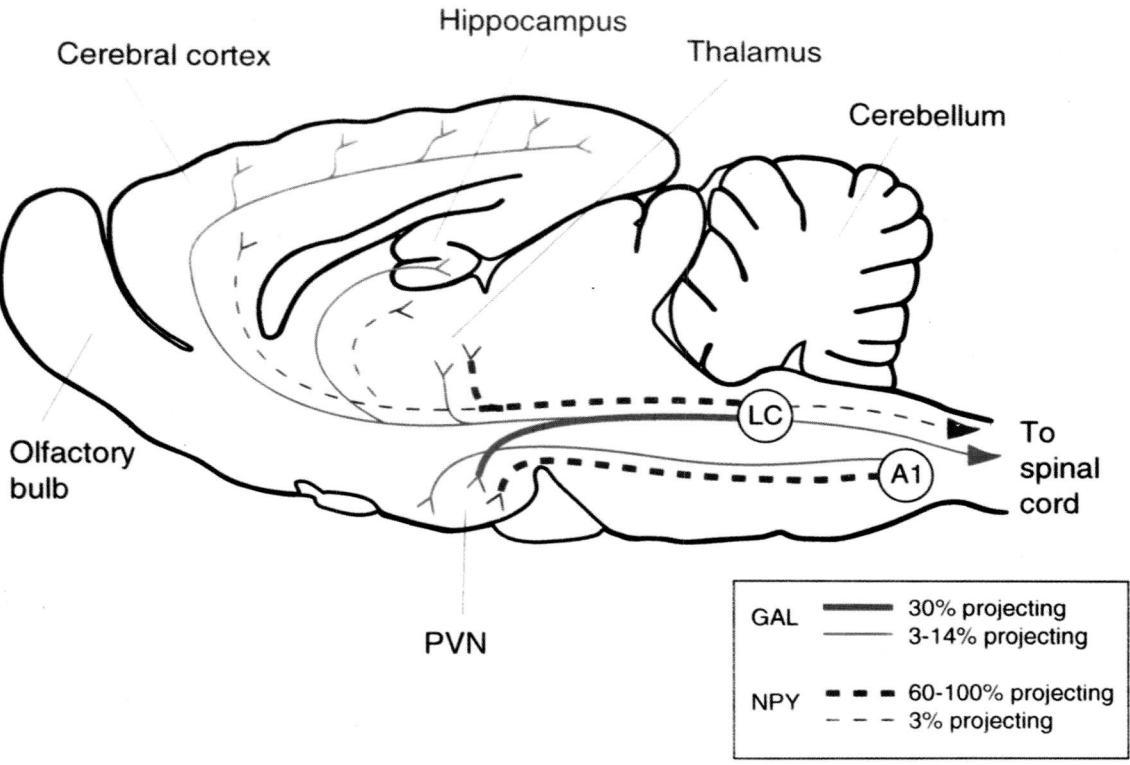

Cerebral cortex

Hippocampus

Thalamus

Cerebellum

Olfactory
bulb

LC

A1

To
spinal
cord

PVN

GAL	———	30% projecting
	———	3-14% projecting
NPY	– – –	60-100% projecting
	– – –	3% projecting

FIG. 2. Peptides coexisting with norepinephrine (NE): projections in the rat CNS. Schematic drawing of a parasagittal view of the rat brain depicting the coexistence of galanin (GAL), neuropeptide Y (NPY), and NE in the locus coeruleus and A1 cell groups and their ascending and descending projections. *Solid green lines* indicate GAL projections. *Dashed red lines* indicate NPY projections. Line thickness indicates the percentage of peptidergic neurons projecting to terminal regions. (Adapted from refs. 26, 34, and 47.)

(33). The coexistence of NE and NPY in this coeruleo-thalamic projection has not been established by double-labeling techniques, but the extent of NPY-LI found in this pathway is almost 100% (33). NPY-LI fibers comprise a small percentage of the ipsilateral projection from LC to the entorhinal, medial, and lateral cortical areas and to the ventral hippocampus (26,62). Approximately 3% of NPY-LI LC neurons project either ipsilaterally or contralaterally to the spinal cord (26).

GAL and NPY in the A1 and A2 Cell Groups

GAL coexists with NE in neurons of the A1 cell group, but to a much lesser degree than in the LC, with approximately 15% of A1 neurons immunoreactive for both dopamine-β-hydroxylase and GAL (34). A high density of GAL-LI neurons are located in the A2 noradrenergic region of the caudal nucleus tractus solitarius (24,34,37, 51). However, double-labeling studies reveal that GAL does not coexist with NE in this cell group (34). GAL-immunoreactive fibers from the A1 group are widely scattered throughout the PVN, projecting to the parvocellular and magnocellular subdivisions of the PVN (34).

NPY-LI coexists with NE in a high proportion of neurons in the rostral and ventral portion of the A1 cell group. Estimates of the degree of coexistence range from 50% to 90% (19,47). A1 cells expressing immunoreactivity for NPY without dopamine-β-hydroxylase are rare, suggesting that NPY is present only as a coexisting transmitter in the A1 cell group. Retrograde tracing and double-labeling studies indicate that about 60% of A1 noradrenergic neurons sending axons to the PVN contain NPY-LI, densest in the parvocellular division, which contains high levels of hypophyseal hormones (47). In the A2 cell group, approximately 10–30% of noradrenergic neurons contain NPY-LI (19,47).

Other Peptides in Central Noradrenergic Systems

Neurons immunoreactive for atrial natriuretic factor, bombesin, calcitonin gene-related peptide, enkephalin, neurotensin, substance P, and vasoactive intestinal peptide have been observed in the LC (33,55). However, there is no evidence to date that these peptides coexist with NE in LC neurons. Basic fibroblast growth factor (BDNF), a 24-amino-acid peptide, was recently discovered to coexist with NE in LC, A1, A5, and A7 perikarya of the rat, which will be of interest in light of the trophic actions of BDNF at other brain sites (10).

FUNCTIONAL INTERACTIONS

A neuropeptide coexisting with a "classical" neurotransmitter may act as a primary transmitter producing independent actions, may interact with the "classical" transmitter as a facilitatory or inhibitory modulator, or may serve a minor function only under specialized physiological conditions or during discrete developmental stages. Investigations of the role of a coexisting neuropeptide include: (a) studies of synthesis, using in situ hybridization and Northern blot analysis of messenger RNA (mRNA) levels; (b) studies of storage in synaptic vesicles, using electron microscopy combined with immunocytochemistry; (c) studies of release, using tissue slice preparations and in vivo microdialysis; (d) studies of receptors, using high-affinity binding assays and quantitative autoradiography; (e) studies of effector mechanisms, using biochemical assays for adenylate cyclase, phosphoinositide hydrolysis, potassium and chloride channels; (f) studies of neurophysiology, using tissue slice and in vivo recording techniques; and (g) studies of behavior, using animal behavior paradigms and central microinjections. Functional interactions of GAL and NPY with NE in the LC have not been extensively characterized, despite the fact that the percentage of LC neurons containing GAL is higher than any other reported coexistence (26,37). Preliminary findings published to date are described below.

Synthesis

Coexisting neurotransmitters may be synthesized at the same rate, or their synthesis may be regulated differentially. Quantitative analysis of neuropeptide synthesis has been limited by the unavailability of selective agents that uniquely stimulate or inhibit synthesis of a specific peptide. Unlike NE, for example, in which synthesis can be inhibited through the rate-limiting synthetic enzyme TH, both GAL and NPY appear to be cleaved from larger, pre-pro peptides by relatively nonselective enzymes (27,58). The methods in current use to quantitate peptide synthesis are Northern blot and in situ hybridization histochemistry for the mRNA specific to the peptide (see Fig. 3). Employing quantitative in situ hybridization, GAL mRNA was found to increase concomitantly with TH mRNA in the LC, after treatment with the catecholamine-depleting agent reserpine (3). Treatments that did not increase TH mRNA in the LC (e.g., cold water swim stress) did not increase GAL mRNA in the LC (3). Desmethylimipramine blocked the reserpine-induced increase in TH mRNA, but only partially attenuated the increase in GAL mRNA, suggesting a selective interaction of the antidepressant desmethylimipramine with reserpine on the regulation of TH, but not GAL, gene expression (48).

Release

Similarly, coexisting neurotransmitters may be released simultaneously or differentially, depending on neuronal ac-

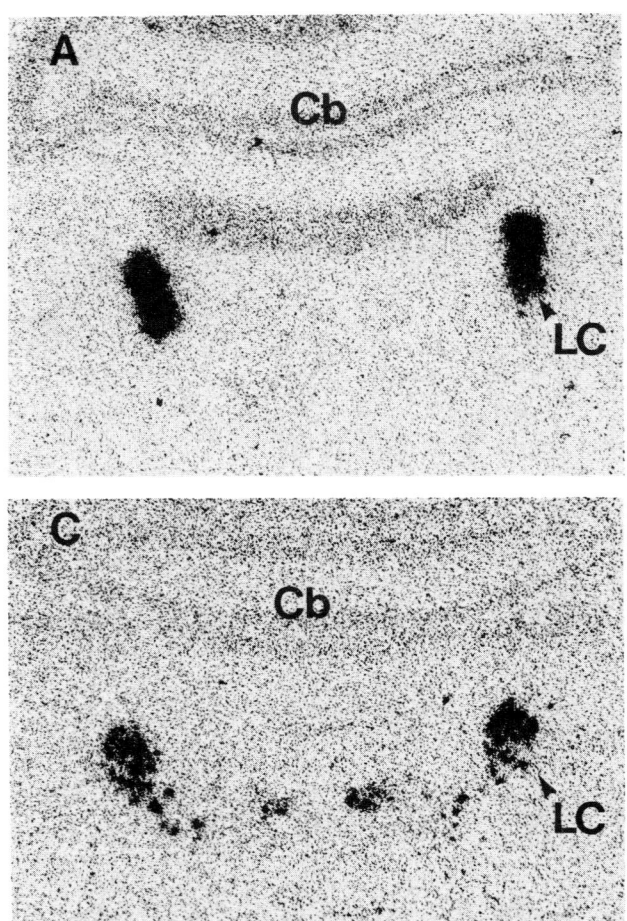

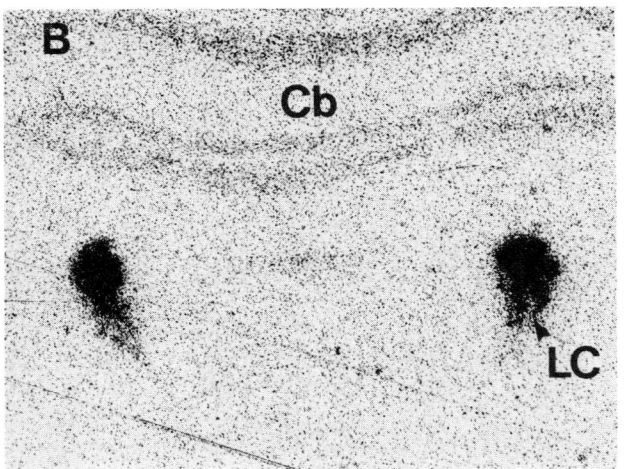

FIG. 3. Expression of mRNA for (**a**) tyrosine hydroxylase (TH), (**b**) galanin (GAL), and (**c**) neuropeptide Y (NPY) in the locus coeruleus. ^{35}S-oligodeoxynucleotide probes were used for hybridization of TH, GAL, and NPY mRNAs in 12-μm sections through the rat locus coeruleus (LC) as previously described (3). Slides were exposed to autoradiography film for 3–5 days (Holmes and Crawley, *unpublished autoradiographs*). Cb, cerebellum.

tivity. Analysis of the release of endogenous GAL and NPY in vivo has been limited by the sensitivity of existing radioimmunoassays. Investigations have begun on the ability of GAL and NPY to modulate NE release. GAL and NPY both inhibited ^{3}H-NE release in tissue slices from rat hypothalamus, a terminal field region of the LC (22,57). However, in vivo microdialysis studies in the paraventricular nucleus of the hypothalamus of freely moving rats reported that GAL microinjected into the paraventricular nucleus significantly increased NE levels in the microdialysate in either the presence or the absence of food (30). NPY increased NE release in this paradigm when food was present, but decreased NE release when food was absent (30). These contradictory data suggest that GAL has opposite actions on NE release in vitro versus in vivo.

Receptors and Second Messengers

Distinct receptors for NE, GAL, and NPY are well established (see Chapters 27 and 43, *this volume*). GAL binds to a pertussis-toxin-sensitive, ADP-ribosylated G_i/G_o protein-coupled high-affinity receptor (4,31). GAL receptor activation may involve opening of an ATP-

sensitive or -insensitive potassium channel, reduction in intracellular calcium, stimulation of phosphatidyl inositol hydrolysis, or inhibition of adenylate cyclase activity (4,12,41). Specific, high-affinity binding sites for ^{125}I-GAL are regionally distributed in the locus coeruleus, hypothalamus, thalamus, amygdala, hippocampus, septum, striatum, and cerebral cortex, demonstrating a relatively good match between the distribution of GAL-LI terminals and GAL receptors (31,38,52). Two subtypes of high-affinity NPY receptors have been identified: (i) NPY-Y1, linked to intracellular calcium mobilization, and (ii) NPY-Y2, with high affinity for the C-terminal NPY 13–36 sequence (59). Both receptor subtypes are associated with inhibition of adenylate cyclase, and they may interact functionally with alpha-2-adrenergic receptors (59). Specific, high-affinity binding sites for ^{125}I-NPY are regionally distributed in the cerebral cortex, hippocampus, thalamus, hypothalamus, septum, striatum, and brainstem, sites which receive NPY innervation (59).

Neurophysiology

GAL (10^{-9} to 10^{-7} M) inhibits the firing rate of locus coeruleus neurons in tissue slices from the rat hindbrain

(49,50). This inhibition is similar to that induced by alpha-adrenergic and μ-opiate receptor agonists such as NE and [Met^5]enkephalin, respectively. The mechanism for the inhibitory action of GAL on LC firing rate may involve an indirect interaction between GAL receptors and μ-opiate receptors, but not between GAL receptors and alpha-adrenergic receptors. GAL-induced hyperpolarization was unaffected by the alpha-adrenergic antagonist, idazoxan, but was potentiated by the μ-opiate receptor antagonist, naloxone (50). NPY depressed noradrenergic inhibitory postsynaptic potentials of LC neurons in rat pontine slices (20). In vivo studies of the neurophysiological actions of GAL and NPY in the LC have not been performed to date.

Behavior

GAL and NPY both stimulate feeding (16,17,29,54). Microinjected into the PVN, both GAL and NPY increase food consumption in satiated rats (17,29,54). GAL also increased food consumption when microinjected into the amygdala (16). These effects of GAL may be mediated through interactions with NE in terminal fields of LC projections. The ability of GAL to preferentially increase consumption of a high-fat diet was blocked by treatment with alpha-2-adrenergic receptor antagonists and by depletion of endogenous norepinephrine with alpha-methyl-para-tyrosine, whereas NPY-induced feeding was independent of noradrenergic antagonists (29). GAL has been implicated in pain transmission. Intrathecally administered GAL potentiated the analgesic effects of morphine in unanesthetized rats (61). GAL directly antagonized the spinal reflex in decerebrate rats (63), suggesting that the mechanism of action of GAL is via primary sensory neurons, not through descending spinal projections from the LC. GAL administered into the lateral ventricle or into the ventral hippocampus has an inhibitory effect on spatial memory tasks in rats, including T-maze delayed alternation, delayed non-matching to sample, the sunburst maze, and the Morris water maze (35,36,42,44). However, it is not known whether these performance deficits induced by GAL are mediated through cholinergic pathways, noradrenergic pathways, and/or other mechanisms (18). NPY has been reported to improve retention of a step-down passive avoidance task and a T-maze active avoidance task when administered intraventricularly to mice (21). The projections of NPY-containing neurons of the LC are one possible set of sites for this NPY action on a memory paradigm. NPY administered into the lateral ventricle of rats produced an anxiolytic-like action on punished conflict responding (23). Intraventricular administration of an NPY antisense oligodeoxynucleotide to rats produced an anxiolytic-like action on the elevated plus maze (60), suggesting a function for endogenous NPY, arising from the LC and/or from other sources, in the reduction of anxiety-

related behaviors. GAL administered intraventricularly produced inhibitory effects on sexual behaviors in male rats (43), whereas GAL microinjected into the preoptic nucleus facilitated copulatory behavior in male rats (9). NPY administered into the third ventricle stimulated the release of luteinizing-hormone-releasing hormone (an NE-like effect), thereby initating ovulation (45). Hypothalamic receptors innervated by GAL- and NPY-containing LC projections to the hypothalamus (26) could be mediating these sexual and reproductive behaviors.

CLINICAL IMPLICATIONS

Clinical investigations of GAL and NPY levels in cerebrospinal fluid and in postmortem brain tissue, including terminal fields for LC projections, have been conducted for several disease states. In cerebrospinal fluid of patients with anorexia and bulimia, NPY levels were elevated whereas GAL levels were normal (7). GAL levels were normal in cerebrospinal fluid from Alzheimer's disease patients, as compared to age-matched controls (7). In postmortem brain tissue from Alzheimer's patients, GAL-like immunoreactivity was found in the senile plaques (28). Tissue assays from Alzheimer's disease detected normal levels of GAL in cerebral cortex and hippocampal regions, in the same samples in which choline acetyltransferase levels were significantly reduced (5). Conversely, increased concentrations of GAL were found in the cholinergic cell body regions of the nucleus basalis of Meynert in Alzheimer's brains as compared to age-matched controls, whereas in the same samples NPY levels were normal and choline acetyltransferase was reduced (6). Histological analysis revealed that small, GAL-immunoreactive interneurons, which innervate the large cholinergic nucleus basalis of Meynert neurons in the human brain, and additional extrinsic GAL-LI axons, possibly from the LC, hyperinnervate the nucleus basalis of Meynert neurons in Alzheimer's brains (11,39). This finding of greatly increased numbers of GAL-LI terminals on cholinergic basal forebrain neurons does not appear to be a nonspecific, or space-filling, artifact resulting from the progressive loss of cholinergic neurons, because GAL hyperinnervation did not occur in Down's syndrome, in which cholinergic neurons also degenerate (39).

The coexistence of GAL and NPY with NE in the LC, along with the inhibitory actions of both peptides to reduce the firing rate of LC neurons in vitro, suggests that these two coexisting neuropeptides may be inhibitory modulators, serving as inhibitory feedback to noradrenergic actions mediated by the LC. Noradrenergic pathways of the LC are thought to mediate aspects of depression, anxiety, withdrawal from drug addiction, arousal, attention, response to novelty, learning, memory, and feeding (1,2,13,23,40,53,60; also see Chapters 27, 29, 32, 33, and 61, *this volume*). The few functional studies performed to date and described above, which investigate the actions of GAL and NPY in relevant animal behavior models and clinical conditions, indicate that GAL has inhibitory effects on memory (35,36,42,44) and hyperinnervates the cholinergic neurons remaining after degeneration in Alzheimer's disease (6,11,39). NPY may be elevated in a human feeding disorder (7), and it acts as an anxiolytic in an animal model (23). Both peptides stimulate feeding (16,17,29,54). The recent availability of GAL antagonists (4), NPY antagonists (56), and NPY receptor antisense (60) will enable direct studies of the contributions of endogenous GAL and NPY to LC functions in animal behavior models. Future experiments will determine whether endogenous GAL and/or NPY are functionally important in these animal paradigms and whether GAL and/or NPY are implicated in the etiology of neuropsychiatric disorders. It is interesting to speculate that GAL and NPY agonists may be useful as treatments for anxiety, or withdrawal from drug addiction, and that GAL and NPY antagonists, alone or together with NE agonists and cholinergic therapies, may be useful as treatments for feeding disorders, depression, and Alzheimer's disease (see also Chapters 118, 136, and 138, *this volume*).

REFERENCES

1. Akaoka H, Aston-Jones G. Opiate withdrawal-induced hyperactivity of locus coeruleus neurons is substantially mediated by augmented excitatory amino acid input. *J Neurosci* 1991;11:3830–3839.
2. Angulo JA, Printz D, Ledoux M, McEwen BS. Isolation stress increases tyrosine hydroxylase mRNA in the locus coeruleus and midbrain and decreases proenkephalin mRNA in the striatum and nucleus accumbens. *Mol Brain Res* 1991;11:301–308.
3. Austin MC, Cottingham SL, Paul SM, Crawley JN. Tyrosine hydroxylase and galanin mRNA levels in locus coeruleus neurons are increased following reserpine administration. *Synapse* 1990;6:351–357.
4. Bartfai T, Fisone G, Langel Ü. Galanin and galanin antagonists: molecular and biochemical perspectives. *Trends Pharmacol Sci* 1992;6:351–357.
5. Beal MF, Clevens RA, Chattha GK, MacGarvey UM, Mazurek MF, Gabriel SM. Galanin-like immunoreactivity is unchanged in Alzheimer's disease and Parkinson's disease dementia in cerebral cortex. *J Neurochem* 1988;51:1935–1941.
6. Beal MF, MacGarvey U, Swartz KJ. Galanin immunoreactivity is increased in the nucleus basalis of Meynert in Alzheimer's disease. *Ann Neurol* 1990;28:157–161.
7. Berrettini WH, Kaye WH, Sunderland T, May C, Gwirtsman HE, Mellow A, Albright A. Galanin immunoreactivity in human CSF: studies in eating disorders and Alzheimer's disease. *Neuropsychobiology* 1988;19:64–68.
8. Blasco I, Alvarez FJ, Villalba RM, Solana ML, Martinez-Murillo R, Rodrigo J. Light and electron microscopic study of galanin-immunoreactive nerve fibers in the rat posterior thalamus. *J Comp Neurol* 1989;283:1–12.
9. Bloch GJ, Butler PC, Kohler JG, Bloch DA. Microinjection of galanin into the medial preoptic nucleus facilitiates copulatory behavior in the male rat. *Physiol Behav* 1993;54:615–624.
10. Chadi G, Tinner B, Agnati LF, Fuxe K. Basic fibroblast growth factor (bFGF, FGF-2) immunoreactivity exists in the noradrenaline, adrenaline and 5-HT nerve cells of the rat brain. *Neurosci Lett* 1993;160:171–176.
11. Chan-Palay V. Galanin hyperinnervates surviving neurons of the human basal nucleus of Meynert in dementias of Alzheimer's and Parkinson's disease: a hypothesis for the role of galanin in accentu-

ating cholinergic dysfunction in dementia. *J Comp Neurol* 1988;273:543–557.
12. Chen Y, Laburthe M, Amiranoff B. Galanin inhibits adenylate cyclase of rat brain membranes. *Peptides* 1992;13:339–341.
13. Cole BJ, Robbins TW, Everitt BJ. Lesions of the dorsal noradrenergic bundle simultaneously enhance and reduce responsivity to novelty in a food preference test. *Brain Res Rev* 1988;13:325–349.
14. Cooper JR, Bloom FE, Roth RH. *The biochemical basis of neuropharmacology,* 6th ed. New York: Oxford University Press, 1991.
15. Cortes R, Ceccatell S, Schalling M, Hökfelt T. Differential effects of intracerebroventricular colchicine administration on the expression of mRNAs for neuropeptides and neurotransmitter enzymes, with special emphasis on galanin: an in situ hybridization study. *Synapse* 1990;6:369–391.
16. Corwin RL, Robinson JK, Crawley JN. Galanin antagonists block galanin-induced feeding in the hypothalamus and amygdala of the rat. *Eur J Neurosci* 1993;5:1528–1533.
17. Crawley JN, Austin MC, Fiske SM, Martin B, Consolo S, Berthold M, Langel U, Fisone G, Bartfai T. Activity of centrally administered galanin fragments on stimulation of feeding behavior and on galanin receptor binding in the rat hypothalamus. *J Neurosci* 1990; 10:3695–3700.
18. Crawley JN, Wenk GL. Coexistence of galanin and acetylcholine: is galanin involved in memory processes and dementia? *Trends Neurosci* 1989;12:278–282.
19. Everitt BJ, Hökfelt T. The coexistence of neuropeptide-Y with other peptides and amines in the central nervous system. In: Mutt V, Fuxe K, Hökfelt T, Lundberg JM, eds. *Neuropeptide Y.* New York: Raven Press, 1989;61–71.
20. Finta EP, Regenold JT, Illes P. Depression by neuropeptide Y of noradrenergic inhibitory postsynaptic potentials of locus coeruleus neurons. *Naunyn Schmiedebergs Arch Pharmacol* 1992;346:472–474.
21. Flood JF, Hernandez EN, Morley JE. Modulation of memory processing by neuropeptide Y. *Brain Res* 1987;421:280–290.
22. Goldstein M, Deutch AY. The inhibitory actions of NPY and galanin on ³H-norepinephrine release in the central nervous system: Relation to a proposed hierarchy of neuronal coexistence. In: Mutt V, Fuxe K, Hökfelt T, Lundberg JM, eds. *Neuropeptide Y.* Karolinska Institute Nobel Conference Series. New York: Raven Press, 1989;153–162.
23. Heilig M, McLeod S, Brot M, Heinrichs S, Menzaghi F, Koob GF, Britton KT. Anxiolytic-like action of neuropeptide Y (NPY), but not other peptides in an operant conflict test. *Neuropsychopharmacology* 1993;8:357–363.
24. Herbert H, Saper CB. Cholecystokinin-, galanin-, and corticotropin-releasing factor-like immunoreactive projections from the nucleus of the solitary tract to the parabrachial nucleus in the rat. *J Comp Neurol* 1990;293:581–598.
25. Hökfelt T, Millhorn D, Seroogy K, Tsuruo Y, Ceccatelli S, Lindh B, Meister B, Melander T, Schalling M, Bartfai T, Terenius L. Coexistence of peptides with classical neurotransmitters. *Experientia* 1987;43:768–780.
26. Holets VR, Hökfelt T, Rökaeus Å, Terenius L, Goldstein M. Locus coeruleus neurons in the rat containing neuropeptide Y, tyrosine hydroxylase or galanin and their efferent projections to the spinal cord, cerebral cortex and hypothalamus. *Neuroscience* 1988; 24:893–906.
27. Kaplan LM, Spindel ER, Isselbacher KJ, Chin WW. Tissue-specific expression of the rat galanin gene. *Proc Natl Acad Sci USA* 1988;85:1065–1069.
28. Kowall NW, Beal MF. Galanin-like immunoreactivity is present in human substantia innominata and in senile plaques in Alzheimer's disease. *Neurosci Lett* 1989;98:118–123.
29. Kyrkouli SE, Stanley BG, Hutchinson R, Seirafi RD, Leibowitz SF. Peptide–amine interactions in the hypothalamic paraventricular nucleus: analysis of galanin and neuropeptide Y in relation to feeding. *Brain Res* 1990;521:185–191.
30. Kyrkouli SE, Stanley BG, Leibowitz SF. Differential effects of galanin and neuropeptide Y on extracellular norepinephrine levels in the paraventricular hypothalamic nucleus of the rat: a microdialysis study. *Life Sci* 1992;51:203–210.
31. Lagny-Pourmir I, Epelbaum J. Regional stimulatory and inhibitory effects of guanine nucleotides on [¹²⁵I]galanin binding in rat brain:

relationship with the rate of occupancy of galanin receptors by endogenous galanin. *Neuroscience* 1992;49:829–847.

32. Larhammar D, Ericsson A, Persson H. Structure and expression of the rat neuropeptide Y gene. *Proc Natl Acad Sci USA* 1987;84:2068–2072.

33. Lechner J, Leah JD, Zimmermann M. Brainstem peptidergic neurons projecting to the medial and lateral thalamus and zona incerta in the rat. *Brain Res* 1993;603:47–56.

34. Levin MC, Sawchenko PE, Howe PRC, Bloom SR, Polak JM. Organization of galanin-immunoreactive inputs to the paraventricular nucleus with special reference to their relationship to catecholaminergic afferents. *J Comp Neurol* 1987;261:562–582.

35. Malin DH, Novy BJ, Lett-Brown AE, Plotner RE, May BT, Radulescu SJ, Crothers MK, Osgood LD, Lake JR. Galanin attenuates retention of one-trial reward learning. *Life Sci* 1992;50:939–944.

36. Mastropaolo J, Nadi N, Ostrowski NL, Crawley JN. Galanin antagonizes acetylcholine on a memory task in basal forebrain-lesioned rats. *Proc Natl Acad Sci USA* 1988;85:9841–9845.

37. Melander T, Hökfelt T, Rokaeus A. Distribution of galaninlike immunoreactivity in the rat central nervous system. *J Comp Neurol* 1986;248:475–517.

38. Melander T, Kohler C, Nilsson S, Hökfelt T, Brodin E, Theodorsson E, Bartfai T. Autoradiographic quantitation and anatomical mapping of ^{125}I-galanin binding sites in the rat central nervous system. *J Chem Neuroanat* 1988;1:213–233.

39. Mufson EJ, Cochran E, Benzing W, Kordower JH. Galaninergic innervation of the cholinergic vertical limb of the diagonal band (Ch2) and bed nucleus of the stria terminalis in aging, Alzheimer's disease and Down's syndrome. *Dementia* 1993;4:237–250.

40. Nestler EJ. Molecular mechanisms of drug addiction. *J Neurosci* 1992;12:2439–2450.

41. Nishibori M, Oishi R, Itoh Y, Saeki K. Galanin inhibits noradrenaline-induced accumulation of cyclic AMP in the rat cerebral cortex. *J Neurochem* 1988;51:1953–1955.

42. Ögren SO, Hökfelt T, Kask K, Langel Ü, Bartfai T. Evidence for a role of the neuropeptide galanin in spatial learning. *Neuroscience* 1992;51:1–5.

43. Poggioli R, Rasori E, Bertolini A. Galanin inhibits sexual behavior in male rats. *Eur J Pharmacol* 1992;213:87–90.

44. Robinson JK, Crawley JN. Intraventricular galanin impairs delayed non-matching to sample performance in rats. *Behav Neurosci* 1993;107:458–467.

45. Sabatino FD, Collins P, McDonald JK. Neuropeptide Y stimulation of luteinizing hormone-releasing hormone secretion from median eminence in vitro by estrogen dependent and Ca^{+2} independent mechanisms. *Endocrinology* 1989;124:2089–2098.

46. Sawchenko PE, Pfeiffer SW. Ultrastructural localization of neuropeptide Y and galanin immunoreactivity in the paraventricular nucleus of the hypothalamus in the rat. *Brain Res* 1988;474:231–245.

47. Sawchenko PE, Swanson LW, Grzanna R, Howe PRC, Bloom SR, Polak JM. Colocalization of neuropeptide Y immunoreactivity in brainstem catecholaminergic neurons that project to the paraventricular nucleus of the hypothalamus. *J Comp Neurol* 1985;241:138–153.

48. Schultzberg M, Austin MC, Crawley JN, Paul SM. Repeated administration of desmethylimipramine blocks the reserpine-induced increase in tyrosine hydroxylase mRNA in locus coeruleus neurons of the rat. *Mol Brain Res* 1991;10:307–314.

49. Seutin V, Verbanck P, Massotte L, Dresse A. Galanin decreases the activity of the locus coeruleus neurons in vitro. *Eur J Pharmacol* 1989;164:373–376.

50. Sevcik J, Finta EP, Illes P. Galanin receptors inhibit the spontaneous firing of locus coeruleus neurones and interact with μ-opiate receptors. *Eur J Pharmacol* 1993;230:223–230.

51. Skofitsch G, Jacobowitz DM. Quantitative distribution of galanin-like immunoreactivity in the rat central nervous system. *Peptides* 1985;7:609–613.

52. Skofitsch G, Sills MA, Jacobowitz DM. Autoradiographic distribution of ^{125}I-galanin binding sites in the rat central nervous system. *Peptides* 1986;7:1029–1042.

53. Smith MA, Brady LS, Glowa J, Gold PW, Herkenham M. Effects of stress and adrenalectomy on tyrosine hydroxylase mRNA levels in the locus coeruleus by in situ hybridization. *Brain Res* 1991;544:26–32.

54. Stanley BG, Leibowitz SF. Neuropeptide Y injected in the paraventricular hypothalamus: a powerful stimulant of feeding behavior. *Proc Natl Acad Sci USA* 1985;82:3940–3943.

55. Sutin EL, Jacobowitz DM. Immunocytochemical localization of peptides and other neurochemicals in the rat laterodorsal tegmental nucleus and adjacent area. *J Comp Neurol* 1988;270:243–270.

56. Tatemoto K. Neuropeptide Y and its receptor antagonists. In: Allen JM, Koenig JI, eds. *Central and peripheral significance of neuropeptide Y and its related peptides.* New York: New York Academy of Sciences, 1990;1–6.

57. Tsuda K, Tsuda S, Goldstein M, Masuyama Y. Effects of neuropeptide Y on norepinephrine release in hypothalamic slices of spontaneously hypertensive rats. *Eur J Pharmacol* 1990;182:175–179.

58. Vrontakis ME, Peden LM, Duckworth ML, Friesen HG. Isolation and characterization of a complementary DNA (galanin) clone from estrogen-induced pituitary tumor messenger RNA. *J Biol Chem* 1987;262:16755–16758.

59. Wahlestedt C, Grundemar L, Hakanson R, Heilig M, Shen GH, Zukowska-Grojec Z, Reis DJ. Neuropeptide Y receptor subtypes, Y1 and Y2. In: *Central and peripheral significance of neuropeptide Y and its related peptides.* Allen JM, Koenig JI, eds. New York: New York Academy of Sciences, 1990;7–26.

60. Wahlestedt C, Pich EM, Koob GF, Yee F, Heilig M. Modulation of anxiety and neuropeptide Y-Y1 receptors by antisense oligodeoxynucleotides. *Science* 1993;259:528–531.

61. Wiesenfeld-Hallin Z, Xu XJ, Hakanson R, Feng DM, Folkers K. Low-dose intrathecal morphine facilitates the spinal flexor reflex by releasing different neuropeptides in rats with intact and sectioned peripheral nerves. *Brain Res* 1990;551:157–162.

62. Wilcox BJ, Unnerstall JR. Identification of a subpopulation of neuropeptide Y-containing locus coeruleus neurons that project to the entorhinal cortex. *Synapse* 1990;6:284–291.

63. Xu XJ, Wiesenfeld-Hallin Z, Villar MJ, Fahrenkrug J, Hökfelt T. On the role of galanin, substance P and other neuropeptides in primary sensory neurons of the rat: studies on spinal reflex excitability and peripheral axotomy. *Eur J Neurosci* 1990;2:733–743.

*Psychopharmacology: The Fourth
Generation of Progress,* edited by
Floyd E. Bloom and David J. Kupfer.
Raven Press, Ltd., New York © 1995.

CHAPTER 31

Modification of Central Catecholaminergic Systems by Stress and Injury

Functional Significance and Clinical Implications

Elizabeth D. Abercrombie and Michael J. Zigmond

Central neuronal systems utilizing the catecholamines norepinephrine (NE) and dopamine (DA) play an important role in hypotheses concerning the biological bases of many neurological and psychiatric disorders, as well as the mechanisms of action of drugs used in their treatment. This has helped to stimulate much of the basic research focused on better understanding the roles of these transmitters and to promote the development of specific pharmacological tools for the manipulation of catecholaminergic function. Because the details of recent advances in our understanding of the physiological, pharmacological, and behavioral characteristics of the major central catecholaminergic systems are presented in other chapters of this volume, only brief comments on these topics are included here. The primary goal of this chapter is to review the nature of cellular responses brought about in central catecholaminergic neurons in response to conditions of chronically increased demand and to consider the functional significance of such changes.

HYPOTHESES OF CATECHOLAMINERGIC FUNCTION

It is not surprising that catecholamines have been implicated in many cellular and behavioral phenomena (see Chapters 25, 29, 32, and 33, *this volume*). In the mammal, the neuronal systems that utilize NE or DA as their trans-

mitter comprise widespread networks, usually innervating multiple target structures. Consistent with this diffuse anatomy are the relations between the activity of several catecholamine systems and arousal. Most prominent is the relation between the firing rate of NE neurons of the locus coeruleus (LC) and the sleep–wake cycle, with LC active during the waking state and relatively inactive or even silent during stages of sleep. Furthermore, LC neurons emit a burst of activity when the organism is presented with a novel environmental stimulus and show further tonic elevations in firing rate during exposure of the organism to an environmental stressor (1–4). The tonic level of activity of the DA cells in the substantia nigra (SN) also varies between wakefulness and sleep, although far less than does activity in LC (5). Evoked responses are obtained from DA cells in response to phasic sensory stimuli, and, similar to the case for LC neurons, these responses lessen in magnitude with decreasing arousal level and increase in magnitude if the stimulus has acquired behavioral significance (6–8). Postmortem biochemical determinations as well as measurements of extracellular levels of NE and DA obtained using in vivo microdialysis are consistent with the electrophysiological data in demonstrating arousal-related alterations in catecholamine efflux at a number of forebrain sites (9–13).

Postsynaptically, NE and DA appear to play key roles in modulating cellular excitability at their diverse targets, usually via relatively slow second-messenger-mediated mechanisms. In the case of NE, this modulation typically is manifest as an increase in evoked responding of the target neuron relative to the spontaneous level of activity, whereas postsynaptic modulation by DA apparently can be either facilitatory or inhibitory depending on the mo-

E. D. Abercrombie: Center for Molecular and Behavioral Neuroscience, Rutgers University, Newark, New Jersey 07102.
M. J. Zigmond: Department of Behavioral Neuroscience, University of Pittsburgh, Pittsburgh, Pennsylvania 15260.

mentary state of the target cell membrane (14–17). Specificity of signaling in such systems can be achieved by the simultaneous activation of the diffuse, relatively slow catecholaminergic inputs along with the pathways that rapidly transmit primary information (18).

Based on the general attributes described above, it would seem that the central catecholaminergic systems are best viewed as important in determining the overall state of arousal of the organism, the concomitant efficiency of ongoing sensorimotor processing, and, ultimately, the ability of the organism to react flexibly and appropriately to continuously changing environmental demands. In this regard they play a role in the broad task of maintaining homeostasis, as do the catecholaminergic cells in the periphery. This view should be contrasted with the types of explanatory models that emerged during the 1960s and the 1970s, positing a primary role for one or another catecholamine system in subserving specific behavioral processes.

The concept of homeostasis is relevant not only to what catecholamines do but also to how they do it. Catecholamine neurons themselves exhibit a wide range of homeostatic properties. For example, when these neurons are exposed to conditions of increased demand, cellular changes occur that enhance their capacity to synthesize and release transmitter (19). Two examples are given in this chapter to illustrate this phenomenon: (i) the alterations in the NE-containing neurons of the LC that take place in response to conditions of chronic stress and (ii) the alterations in the DA-containing neurons of the SN that occur following partial injury to that system.

NORADRENERGIC NEURONS AND CHRONIC STRESS: RESPONSE TO A SUBSEQUENT STRESSOR

A wide variety of acutely presented stressful stimuli, including footshock, cold environment, and immobilization, have been shown to affect indices of activity in NE-containing neurons originating in the LC (20,21). Among the changes that occur as a result of acute stress are increases in the tonic firing rate of NE neurons in LC (1), decreases in brain NE content (22,23), increases in NE turnover (24,25), and increases in the extracellular level of NE (9,26). Following chronic exposure to stress, the reductions in brain NE levels that occur after acute stress no longer are observed (27,28). Indeed, brain NE levels may actually be increased in response to chronic stress exposure (23,25,29–31). Based on such results, it has been hypothesized that chronic stress leads to a compensatory increase in the biosynthesis of NE which then permits a sustained increase in NE release such that NE content does not decline and may even increase.

It is well established that the activity of tyrosine hydroxylase (TH) is regulated in response to the demand for catecholamines. Electrical stimulation of both central and peripheral catecholamine neurons results in an apparent activation of TH which persists following the termination of the stimulation period (32,33). Furthermore, an activation of TH occurs in response to other stimuli known to increase the activity of central NE neurons, including administration of catecholamine-depleting drugs, partial injury to the LC system, and various forms of stress (33–36). In addition to these increases in TH activity, which represent immediate adaptation to increased transmitter utilization, a second process may come into play after prolonged increases in the activity of NE neurons. This latter mechanism is reflected by an apparent increase in the maximal velocity of TH, which appears to be due to an actual increase in the number of active enzyme molecules (34,37–39). Presumably, the increase in TH protein permits a further increase in the capacity for catecholamine biosynthesis and release, although direct support for this hypothesis currently is lacking.

Recent experiments have examined the impact of stress-induced alterations in LC neurons on their response to a subsequent stressor (40,41). Extracellular NE in the dorsal hippocampus was measured under resting conditions and in response to 30 min of intermittent tail-shock using in vivo microdialysis methods. Two groups of rats were studied, a naive control group and a group that previously had been housed for 3–4 weeks at 4°C, a condition known to produce an increase in maximal TH activity within the cell bodies of the LC (39,42,43). The basal extracellular concentration of NE in hippocampus was found to be the same in the naive and chronically cold-stressed rats. However, 30 min of exposure to an

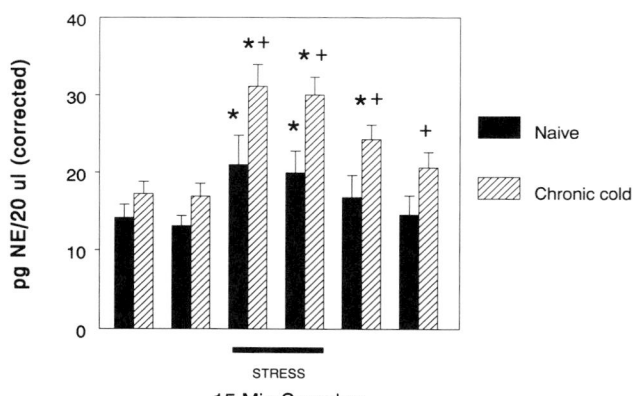

FIG. 1. The effect of acute tail shock on extracellular NE in hippocampus of naive and chronically cold-stressed rats. Thirty minutes of intermittent tail shock (*line*) was administered after obtaining at least four stable baseline samples. Basal NE levels did not differ between the two groups. In naive rats (*solid bars*), tail shock produced a 54% increase in extracellular NE ($n = 9$), whereas in chronically cold-stressed rats (*hatched bars*) an 82% increase above baseline occurred ($n = 9$). Results are expressed as mean ± SEM; *, $p < 0.05$ versus respective baseline; †, $p < 0.05$ chronically cold-stressed versus naive rats. (From ref. 41).

intermittent tail-shock paradigm produced a 52% greater elevation of extracellular NE in the cold-stressed animals compared to the naive control animals (Fig. 1).

To examine changes in NE biosynthesis after chronic stress, subsequent experiments employed a method in

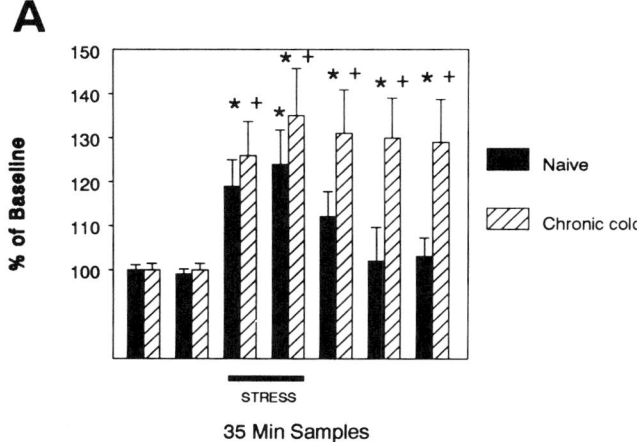

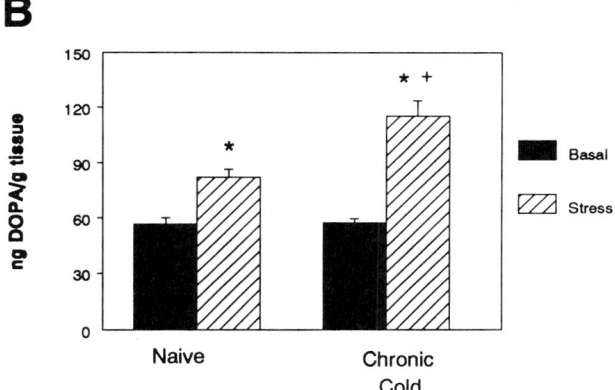

FIG. 2. The effect of acute tail shock on two indices of hippocampal NE synthesis in naive and chronically cold-stressed rats. A: Extracellular DOPA accumulation during local infusion of NSD-1015 via the dialysis probe. Basal DOPA levels did not differ significantly between the two groups. In naive rats (*solid bars*), 30 min of intermittent tail shock (*line*) resulted in a 24% increase in extracellular DOPA (*n* = 6), whereas in chronically stressed rats (*hatched bars*) a 35% increase above baseline was recorded (*n* = 6). (From ref. 40.) B: Tissue DOPA accumulation after systemic administration of NSD-1015. Rats were injected with NSD-1015 (100 mg/kg, i.p.) and either placed back in their home cages for 30 min or exposed to 30 min of intermittent tail shock. All rats were then immediately decapitated, and hippocampus dissected out. Basal accumulation of DOPA (*solid bars*) did not differ between naive and chronically cold-stressed rats. Following 30 min of intermittent tail shock (*hatched bars*), DOPA accumulation was increased 45% over basal level in naive rats (*n* = 10) and 101% over basal level in chronically stressed rats (*n* = 12). (From ref. 41.) All results are expressed as mean ± SEM; *, $p < 0.05$ versus respective baseline; †, $p < 0.05$ chronically cold-stressed versus naive rats.

which an inhibitor of aromatic amino acid decarboxylase (AADC), NSD-1015, is administered via the dialysis probe and the resulting accumulation of DOPA in the extracellular fluid is measured (44). In rats previously exposed to chronic cold, NE synthesis in hippocampus did not differ from that observed in naive controls. However, acute tail shock produced a significantly greater and more prolonged increase in hippocampal NE synthesis in chronically stressed rats than in control animals (Fig. 2A). This issue also was examined by utilizing the more traditional method of measuring the postmortem accumulation of DOPA in tissue after inhibition of AADC (45). In agreement with the in vivo microdialysis data, these results revealed that NE synthesis was elevated to a greater extent in hippocampus of chronically stressed rats exposed to acute tail shock than in naive controls (Fig. 2B).

Taken together, these data suggest that under basal conditions NE release and ongoing tyrosine hydroxylation are not altered by prior exposure to chronic stress. However, the increases in release and synthesis of NE evoked by a novel stressor are larger in magnitude in hippocampus of chronically cold-stressed rats than in that of controls. These changes, then, represent alterations in LC–NE neurons in response to conditions of increased demand.

There is reason to believe that the phenomenon described above is not limited to LC neurons or to the particular combination of stimuli used in the experiments outlined. For example, similar effects of long-term stress on subsequent responsiveness are also observed in the mesolimbic DA system (46) and with chronic injection of saline instead of exposure to cold (Abercrombie and Zigmond, *unpublished data*). Moreover, these observations may be related to a larger group of findings in which exposure to a stimulus (often a drug) leads to an enhanced responsiveness to a subsequent exposure to the same stimulus (''sensitization'') or to another stimulus (''cross-sensitization'') (reviewed in refs. 47 and 48).

DOPAMINERGIC NEURONS AND PARTIAL INJURY

Injury to the nigrostriatal DA system does not lead to gross neurological deficits unless the extent of the injury is very great. In the adult rat, for example, few permanent behavioral deficits are observed in the resting state unless the loss of tissue DA content in striatum exceeds 95%. There is a considerable body of evidence to suggest that this phenomenon reflects compensatory changes occurring in the remaining DA neurons—including elevated rates of transmitter synthesis and release (49–52), as well as decreased reuptake of released transmitter (52–54). These events seem adequate to maintain a normal level of dopaminergic function in the resting state despite extensive neuronal degeneration (55). Up to a certain point, compensatory modifications in DA neurons may even

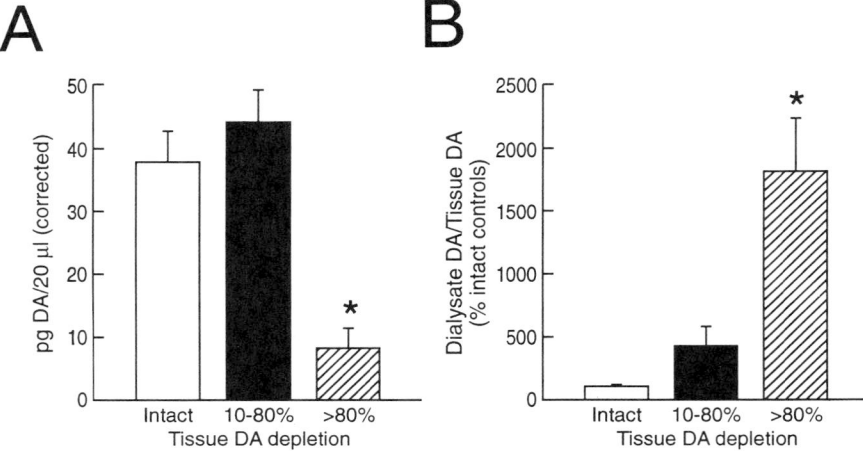

FIG. 3. Effects of 6-OHDA-induced depletion of tissue DA in striatum on extracellular DA. The data were organized a posteriori into the following groups: intact (*open bars; n* = 13), 10–80% tissue DA depletion (*solid bars; n* = 7), and >80% tissue DA depletion (*hatched bars; n* = 12). **A:** The absolute amount of DA obtained in striatal dialysates was not significantly affected unless tissue DA level in striatum was decreased by more than 80%. **B:** Because dialysate DA level was decreased by a lesser amount than was tissue DA level, the ratio of these two measures increased with increasing lesion size. This ratio is an estimate of the contribution of each surviving DA terminal to the pool of extracellular DA. Results are expressed as mean ± SEM; *, $p < 0.05$ versus intact. (From ref. 56.)

permit continued responding under conditions where stimulus-evoked increases in DA release are brought about, such as stress (13).

Recently, the relation between the loss of striatal DA terminals and extracellular DA level in striatum has been directly determined by using in vivo microdialysis to monitor extracellular DA in intact rats and in rats sustaining depletions of DA in striatal tissue (56; see also refs. 57 and 58). The depletions were produced by central administration of the catecholaminergic neurotoxin 6-hydroxydopamine (6-OHDA). The concentration of DA measured in the extracellular fluid of striatum was not significantly reduced by prior 6-OHDA treatment unless the depletion of DA in striatal tissue exceeded 80% (Fig. 3A). Importantly, this also is the approximate level of DA loss required for behavioral deficits to be observed (59,60).

Because the concentration of DA in extracellular fluid was decreased by a lesser amount than was the concentration of DA in tissue, the ratio of these two measures increased with increasing lesion size (Fig. 3B). These and other results (see above) suggest that after the partial degeneration of central dopaminergic terminals, those terminals that remain compensate to maintain the extracellular concentration of DA at a normal level. When functional impairments eventually do occur, it is assumed that it is because these compensatory processes are limited. Data compatible with this conceptual framework also have been obtained in studies of central serotonergic and noradrenergic systems and in the peripheral sympathoadrenal system (34,61–65).

MODIFICATION OF CATECHOLAMINERGIC FUNCTION

General Principles

It appears that alterations in the demands placed on a catecholaminergic neuron can significantly alter the subsequent characteristics of that neuron. We have illustrated this with two different examples. In the instance of NE and chronic stress, the number of neuronal elements was held constant and the environment was altered by exposure to the chronic stressor. The result was enhanced responsivity of the neurons to a subsequent novel stressor. In the example of DA and partial injury, we illustrated how biochemical adaptations in catecholamine neurons can occur when the environment is constant and the number of neuronal elements is reduced. These two cases involve apparent increases in function, but downward regulation also is possible. For example, compensatory down-regulation of a number of cellular parameters has been noted to occur in NE neurons of the LC after chronic treatment with antidepressant drugs (66,67).

It is proposed that a fundamental property of catecholaminergic neurons is the capacity to adjust levels of transmitter synthesis and release as a function of past history of activity or of ongoing changes in activity requirements. This capacity for cellular homeostasis in catecholaminergic neurons can account for the phenomena described in this chapter as well as similar phenomena described for responses to other stimuli or for other catecholaminergic systems (see above).

Clinical Implications

The functional significance of stimulus-induced modifications in the responsiveness of catecholaminergic neurons is not yet clear. It seems likely that the underlying mechanisms evolved to serve some adaptive function. For example, enhanced catecholamine synthesis during chronic stress may protect against the depletion of stores, permitting an organism to react more effectively to a novel challenge. However, it also may be that under certain conditions overresponsiveness may result in maladaptive behavior, as occurs during clinical anxiety or in post-traumatic stress disorder. Might genetic or acquired differences in the regulation of transmitter dynamics during conditions of altered use underlie the normal range of individual differences in the ability to successfully respond to environmental challenge? Furthermore, might certain disease states represent "neuroregulatory disorders" of compensatory responding in these neurons, leading to behavioral disorders of arousal and mood such as schizophrenia and affective illness?

A consideration of the properties of biochemical adaptation inherent to catecholaminergic neurons may also be relevant to an understanding of the dissociation between neuropathology and symptomatology that appears to occur in many disorders, including Parkinson's disease. Parkinson's disease is a progressive neurological disorder caused by the degeneration of DA neurons in the nigrostriatal system. As in the case of 6-OHDA-lesioned animals, patients with Parkinson's disease show marked clinical deficits only after the near-total loss of the dopaminergic innervation of the striatum (50). Presumably, the increase in DA synthesis and release that has been documented in the animal model (see above) also develops in parkinsonism and underlies the extensive preclinical phase of the disease. In support of this hypothesis is the observation that the concentrations of DA metabolites are less dramatically affected by the disease than is DA itself, leading to a ratio of DA metabolites to DA whose value sometimes reached more than 10 times that observed in control tissue (50,68). A related hypothesis deriving from such data is that perhaps age-related deficits in the homeostatic capacities of catecholaminergic neurons results in the accelerated rates of behavioral decline seen in senescence (69–72) (see Chapters 118, 123, and 126, this volume).

In summary, exposure to chronic environmental stress or partial injury to the neurons in a particular cell group can alter the functional characteristics of catecholaminergic neurons, leading to changes in transmitter synthesis and release. These changes may be maladaptive, as may occur under certain conditions of chronic stress, or they may be adaptive, as appears to be the case in Parkinson's disease. Further examination of these phenomena and their functional implications may provide some insights into a variety of neurological and psychiatric conditions as well as their treatment.

ACKNOWLEDGMENTS

This work was supported by United States Public Health Service grants MH-43947, MH-00058, and NS-19608, the American Parkinson's Disease Association, and the National Alliance for Research on Schizophrenia and Depression. We are indebted to the many colleagues and students who importantly contributed to these efforts and whose work is cited in this review.

REFERENCES

1. Abercrombie ED, Jacobs BL. Single-unit response of noradrenergic neurons in the locus coeruleus of freely moving cats. I. Acutely presented stressful and nonstressful stimuli. *J Neurosci* 1987;7:2837–2843.
2. Aston-Jones G, Bloom FE. Activity of norepinephrine-containing locus coeruleus neurons in behaving rats anticipates fluctuations in the sleep–waking cycle. *J Neurosci* 1981;1:876–886.
3. Foote SL, Aston-Jones G, Bloom FE. Impulse activity of locus coeruleus neurons in awake rats and monkeys is a function of sensory stimulation and arousal. *Proc Natl Acad Sci USA* 1980;77:3033–3037.
4. Rasmussen K, Morilak DA, Jacobs BL. Single unit activity of locus coeruleus neurons in the freely moving cat. I. During naturalistic behaviors and in response to simple and complex stimuli. *Brain Res* 1986;371:324–334.
5. Steinfels GF, Heym J, Strecker RE, Jacobs BL. Behavioral correlates of dopaminergic unit activity in freely moving cats. *Brain Res* 1983;258:217–228.
6. Ljungberg T, Apicella P, Schultz W. Responses of monkey dopamine neurons to external stimuli: changes with learning. In: Bernardi G, Carpenter MB, DiChiara G, eds. *Basal ganglia III.* New York: Plenum Press, 1991;469–476.
7. Steinfels GF, Heym J, Strecker RE, Jacobs BL. Response of dopaminergic neurons in cat to auditory stimuli presented across the sleep–waking cycle. *Brain Res* 1983;277:150–154.
8. Strecker RE, Jacobs BL. Substantia nigra dopaminergic unit activity in behaving cats: effect of arousal on spontaneous discharge and sensory evoked activity. *Brain Res* 1985;361:339–350.
9. Abercrombie ED, Keller RW, Zigmond MJ. Characterization of hippocampal norepinephrine release as measured by microdialysis perfusion: pharmacological and behavioral studies. *Neuroscience* 1988;27:897–904.
10. Abercrombie ED, Keefe KA, DiFrischia DS, Zigmond MJ. Differential effect of stress on in vivo dopamine release in striatum, nucleus accumbens, and medial frontal cortex. *J Neurochem* 1989;52:1655–1658.
11. Church WH, Justice JB, Neill DB. Detecting behaviorally relevant changes in extracellular dopamine with microdialysis. *Brain Res* 1987;412:397–399.
12. Dunn AJ, File SE. Cold restraint alters dopamine metabolism in frontal cortex, nucleus accumbens, and neostriatum. *Physiol Behav* 1983;31:511–513.
13. Keefe KA, Stricker EM, Zigmond MJ, Abercrombie ED. Environmental stress increases extracellular dopamine in striatum of 6-hydroxydopamine-treated rats: in vivo microdialysis studies. *Brain Res* 1990;527:350–353.
14. Hu X-T, Wachtel SR, Galloway MP, White FJ. Lesions of the nigrostriatal dopamine projection increase the inhibitory effects of D1 and D2 dopamine agonists on caudate-putamen neurons and relieve D2 receptors from the necessity of D1 receptor stimulation. *J Neurosci* 1990;10:2318–2329.
15. Surmeier DJ, Eberwine J, Wilson CJ, Cao Y, Stefani A, Kitai ST. Dopamine receptor subtypes colocalize in rat striatonigral neurons. *Proc Natl Acad Sci USA* 1992;89:10178–10182.
16. Waterhouse BD, Sessler FM, Cheng J-T, Woodward DJ, Azizi SA, Moises HC. New evidence for a gating action of norepinephrine in central neuronal circuits of mammalian brain. *Brain Res Bull* 1988;21:425–432.
17. Woodward DJ, Waterhouse BD, Hoffer BJ, Freedman R. Modula-

tory actions of norepinephrine in the central nervous system. *Fed Proc* 1979;38:2109–2116.

18. Foote SL, Bloom FE, Aston-Jones G. Nucleus locus ceruleus: new evidence of anatomical and physiological specificity. *Physiol Rev* 1983;63:844–914.

19. Zigmond MJ, Stricker EM. Adaptive properties of monoaminergic neurons. In: Lajtha A, ed. *Handbook of neurochemistry. Alterations of metabolites in the nervous system.* New York: Plenum Press, 1985;87–102.

20. Anisman H, Zacharko RM. Multiple neurochemical and behavioral consequences of stressors: implications for depression. *Pharmacol Ther* 1990;46:119–136.

21. Stone EA. Stress and catecholamines. In: Friedhoff AJ, ed. *Catecholamines and behavior, vol 2.* New York: Plenum Press, 1975;31–72.

22. Bliss E, Ailion J, Zwanziger J. Metabolism of norepinephrine, serotonin and dopamine in rat brain with stress. *J Pharmacol Exp Ther* 1968;164:122–134.

23. Kvetnansky R, Palkovits M, Mitro A, Torda T, Mikulaj L. Catecholamines in individual hypothalamic nuclei of acutely and repeatedly stressed rats. *Neuroendocrinology* 1977;23:257–267.

24. Korf J, Aghajanian GK, Roth RH. Increased turnover of norepinephrine in the rat cerebral cortex during stress: role of the locus coeruleus. *Neuropharmacology* 1973;12:933–938.

25. Thierry AM, Javoy J, Glowinski J, Kety SS. Effects of stress on the metabolism of norepinephrine, dopamine and serotonin in the central nervous system of the rat. I. Modifications of norepinephrine turnover. *J Pharmacol Exp Ther* 1968;163:163–171.

26. Kalen P, Rosegren E, Lindvall O, Bjorklund A. Hippocampal noradrenaline and serotonin release over 24 hours as measured by the dialysis technique in freely moving rats: correlation to behavioural activity state, effect of handling and tail-pinch. *Eur J Neurosci* 1989;1:181–188.

27. Ritter S, Ritter RC. Protection against stress-induced brain norepinephrine depletion after repeated 2-deoxy-D-glucose administration. *Brain Res* 1977;127:179–184.

28. Zigmond MJ, Harvey JA. Resistance to central norepinephrine depletion and decreased mortality in rats chronically exposed to electric foot shock. *J Neuro-Visc Rel* 1970;31:373–381.

29. Adell A, Garcia-Marquez C, Armario A, Gelpi E. Chronic stress increases serotonin and noradrenaline in rat brain and sensitizes their responses to a further acute stress. *J Neurochem* 1988;50:1678–1681.

30. Irwin J, Ahluwalia P, Zacharko RM, Anisman H. Central norepinephrine and plasma corticosterone following acute and chronic stressors: influence of social isolation and handling. *Pharmacol Biochem Behav* 1986;24:1151–1154.

31. Roth KA, Mefford IM, Barchas JD. Epinephrine, norepinephrine, dopamine and serotonin: differential effects of acute and chronic stress on regional brain amines. *Brain Res* 1982;239:417–424.

32. Morgenroth VH III, Boadle-Biber MC, Roth RH. Tyrosine hydroxylase: activation by nerve stimulation. *Proc Natl Acad Sci USA* 1974;71:4283–4287.

33. Salzman PM, Roth RH. Poststimulation catecholamine synthesis and tyrosine hydroxylase activation in central noradrenergic neurons. I. In vivo stimulation of the locus coeruleus. *J Pharmacol Exp Ther* 1980;212:64–73.

34. Acheson AL, Zigmond MJ. Short and long term changes in tyrosine hydroxylase activity in rat brain after subtotal destruction of central noradrenergic neurons. *J Neurosci* 1981;1:493–504.

35. Iuvone PM, Dunn AJ. Tyrosine hydroxylase activation in mesocortical 3,4-dihydroxyphenylethylamine neurons following footshock. *J Neurochem* 1986;47:837–844.

36. Stone EA, Freedman LS, Morgano LE. Brain and adrenal tyrosine hydroxylase activity after chronic footshock stress. *Pharmacol Biochem Behav* 1978;9:551–553.

37. Chuang D, Costa E. Biosynthesis of tyrosine hydroxylase in rat adrenal medulla after exposure to cold. *Proc Natl Acad Sci USA* 1974;71:4570–4574.

38. Fluharty SJ, Snyder GL, Stricker EM, Zigmond MJ. Tyrosine hydroxylase activity and catecholamine biosynthesis in the adrenal medulla of rats during stress. *J Pharmacol Exp Ther* 1985;233:32–38.

39. Thoenen H. Induction of tyrosine hydroxylase in peripheral and central adrenergic neurones by cold-exposure of rats. *Nature* 1970;228:861–862.

40. Nisenbaum LK, Abercrombie ED. Enhanced tyrosine hydroxylation in hippocampus of chronically stressed rats upon exposure to a novel stressor. *J Neurochem* 1992;58:276–281.

41. Nisenbaum LK, Zigmond MJ, Sved AF, Abercrombie ED. Prior exposure to chronic stress results in enhanced synthesis and release of hippocampal norepinephrine in response to a novel stressor. *J Neurosci* 1991;11:1478–1484.

42. Richard F, Faucon-Biguet N, Labautu R, Rollet D, Mallet J, Buda M. Modulation of tyrosine hydroxylase gene expression in rat brain and adrenals by exposure to cold. *J Neurosci Res* 1988;20:32–37.

43. Zigmond RE, Schon F, Iversen LL. Increased tyrosine hydroxylase activity in the locus coeruleus of rat brain stem after reserpine treatment and cold stress. *Brain Res* 1974;70:547–552.

44. Westerink BHC, DeVries JB, Duran R. The use of microdialysis for monitoring tyrosine hydroxylase activity in the brain of conscious rats. *J Neurochem* 1990;54:381–387.

45. Carlsson A, Davis JN, Kehr W, Lindqvist M, Atack CV. Simultaneous measurement of tyrosine and tryptophan activities in brain in vivo using an inhibitor of the aromatic amino acid decarboxylase. *Naunyn Schmiedebergs Arch Pharmacol* 1972;275:153–168.

46. Kalivas PW, Duffy P. Similar effects of daily cocaine and stress on mesocorticolimbic dopamine neurotransmission in the rat. *Biol Psychiatry* 1989;25:913–928.

47. Kalivas PW, Stewart J. Dopamine transmission in the initiation and expression of drug- and stress-induced sensitization of motor activity. *Brain Res Rev* 1991;16:223–244.

48. Robinson TE, Becker JB. Enduring changes in brain and behavior produced by chronic amphetamine administration: a review and evaluation of animal models of amphetamine psychosis. *Brain Res Rev* 1986;11:157–198.

49. Agid Y, Javoy F, Glowinski J. Hyperactivity of remaining dopaminergic neurons after partial destruction of the nigro-striatal dopaminergic system in the rat. *Nature* 1973;245:150–151.

50. Bernheimer H, Birkmayer W, Hornykiewicz O, Jellinger K, Seitelberger F. Brain dopamine and the syndromes of Parkinson and Huntington: clinical, morphological and neurochemical correlations. *J Neurol Sci* 1973;20:415–455.

51. Hefti F, Melamed E, Wurtman RJ. Partial lesions of the nigrostriatal system in rat brain: biochemical characterization. *Brain Res* 1980;195:123–137.

52. Zigmond MJ, Acheson AL, Stachowiak MK, Stricker EM. Neurochemical compensation after nigrostriatal bundle injury in an animal model of preclinical parkinsonism. *Arch Neurol* 1984;41:856–861.

53. Altar CA, Marien MR, Marshall JF. Time course of adaptations in dopamine biosynthesis, metabolism, and release following nigrostriatal lesions: implications for behavioral recovery from brain injury. *J Neurochem* 1987;48:390–399.

54. Stachowiak MK, Keller RW, Stricker EM, Zigmond MJ. Increased dopamine efflux from striatal slices during development and after nigrostriatal bundle damage. *J Neurosci* 1987;7:1648–1654.

55. Zigmond MJ, Abercrombie ED, Berger TW, Grace AA, Stricker EM. Compensations after nigrostriatal bundle injury: some clinical and basic implications. *Trends Neurosci* 1990;13:290–296.

56. Abercrombie ED, Bonatz AE, Zigmond MJ. Effects of L-DOPA on extracellular dopamine in striatum of normal and 6-hydroxydopamine-treated rats. *Brain Res* 1990;525:36–44.

57. Altar CA, Marien MR. Preservation of dopamine release in the denervated striatum. *Neurosci Lett* 1989;96:329–334.

58. Robinson TE, Whishaw IQ. Normalization of extracellular dopamine in striatum following recovery from a partial unilateral 6-OHDA lesion of the substantia nigra: a microdialysis study in freely moving rats. *Brain Res* 1988;450:209–224.

59. Marshall JF, Berrios N, Sawyer S. Neostriatal dopamine and sensory inattention. *J Comp Physiol Psychol* 1980;94:833–846.

60. Ungerstedt U. 6-Hydroxydopamine induced degeneration of central monoamine neurons. *Eur J Pharmacol* 1968;5:107–110.

61. Abercrombie ED, Zigmond MJ. Partial injury to central noradrenergic neurons: reduction of tissue norepinephrine content is greater than reduction of extracellular norepinephrine measured by microdialysis. *J Neurosci* 1989;9:4062–4067.

62. Bjorklund A, Wiklund L. Mechanisms of regrowth of the bulbospinal serotonin system following 5,6-dihydroxytryptamine induced axotomy. I. Biochemical correlates. *Brain Res* 1980;191:109–127.

63. Fluharty SJ, Rabow LE, Zigmond MJ, Stricker EM. Tyrosine hydroxylase activity in the sympathoadrenal system under basal and stressful conditions: effect of 6-hydroxydopamine. *J Pharmacol Exp Ther* 1985;235:354–360.

64. Mueller RA, Thoenen H, Axelrod J. Adrenal tyrosine hydroxylase: compensatory increase after chemical sympathectomy. *Science* 1969;163:468–469.
65. Stachowiak MK, Stricker EM, Jacoby JH, Zigmond MJ. Increased tryptophan hydroxylase activity in serotonergic nerve terminals spared by 5,7-dihydroxytryptamine. *Biochem Pharmacol* 1986; 35:1241–1248.
66. Melia KR, Rasmussen K, Terwilliger RZ, Haycock JW, Nestler EJ, Duman RS. Coordinate regulation of the cyclic AMP system with firing rate and expression of tyrosine hydroxylase in the rat locus coeruleus: effects of chronic stress and drug treatments. *J Neurochem* 1992;58:494–502.
67. Nestler EJ, McMahon A, Sabban EL, Tallman JF, Duman RS. Chronic antidepressant administration decreases the expression of tyrosine hydroxylase in the rat locus coeruleus. *Proc Natl Acad Sci USA* 1990;87:7522–7526.
68. Hornykiewicz O, Kish SJ. Biochemical pathophysiology of Parkinson's disease. *Adv Neurol* 1987;45:19–34.
69. Date I, Felten DL, Felten SY. Long-term effect of MPTP in the mouse brain in relation to aging: neurochemical and immunocytochemical analysis. *Brain Res* 1990;519:266–276.
70. Finch CE, Randall PK, Marshall JF. Aging and basal ganglia function. In: Eisdorfer C, ed. *Annual review of gerontology and geriatrics.* New York: Springer, 1981;49–87.
71. Marshall JF, Rosenstein AJ. Age-related decline in rat striatal dopamine metabolism is regionally homogeneous. *Neurobiol Aging* 1990;11:131–137.
72. Nishi K, Kondo T, Narabayashi H. Difference in recovery patterns of striatal dopamine content, tyrosine hydroxylase activity and total biopterin content after 1-methyl-4-phenyl-1,2,3,6-tetrahydropyridine (MPTP) administration: a comparison of young and older mice. *Brain Res* 1989;489:157–162.

Psychopharmacology: The Fourth Generation of Progress, edited by Floyd E. Bloom and David J. Kupfer. Raven Press, Ltd., New York © 1995.

CHAPTER 32

Central Norepinephrine Neurons and Behavior

Trevor W. Robbins and Barry J. Everitt

The neurobiological data reviewed in past and present articles in the Generation of Progress series (35; see Chapters 29 and 33, *this volume*) and summarized in Table 1 provide several clues to the functions of the locus coeruleus (LC) in the behaving animal. However, extrapolations from such data to psychological processes must be made with care. Clearly, the widespread nature of the coeruleo-cortical projection indicates that activation of this noradrenergic cell group will have pervasive effects in diverse terminal regions such as the neocortex, the hippocampus, and the amygdala. It is perhaps no surprise that the LC has been implicated in such distinct processes as learning, memory, attention, and anxiety, which clearly depend to different degrees on these discrete regions of the forebrain. Two critical questions are: (i) what effect, if any, does such activation have on cognitive and behavioral processes? and (ii) under what circumstances does such activation normally occur? The first question can only be answered by studying the behaving animal and inferring changes in psychological function. Thus it is predicted that manipulations of coeruleo-cortical function will affect various psychological processes including associative learning, different forms of memory, and attention depending, in large part, on which terminal domains of the noradrenergic projection are especially engaged during the task under study. Presumably, the distributed nature of these effects represents an integrated, adaptive response to the environmental and behavioral setting. The electrophysiological data and also neurochemical indices show that LC neurons are especially active during relatively high states of arousal, including exposure to stressful environments and salient, phasic stimuli (see Chapter 29, *this volume*). Thus, in stressful circumstances it may

TABLE 1. *Neurobiological clues to LC function*

- Widely ramifying projections
- Diffuse innervation of cortex
- Laminar complementarity
- Regional selectivity of innervation
- Restricted nature of LC afferents
- Monotonic relationship between unit firing and arousal stages
- Phasic responses to novel/intense stimuli
- Neurochemical evidence of increased NE turnover in stress
- Enhanced signal-to-noise ratios in terminal regions

[a] See ref. 35; also see Chapters 29 and 33, *this volume*.

be useful not only to consolidate memories more efficiently, but also to focus attention on salient features of the environment; the coeruleo-cortical noradrenergic system is clearly suited to such a function.

BEHAVIORAL FUNCTIONS OF THE LOCUS COERULEUS (LC)

Electrophysiological Studies in the Behaving Animal

Measuring LC activity concomitantly with behavior provides useful information on the functions of the LC–norepinephrine (NE) neurons, although it must be borne in mind that any correlative study of this sort does not establish the overall significance of the LC in particular behavioral processes. The mere presence of neuronal activity, even if highly correlated with environmental events, does not necessarily identify causal factors in behavior, which are best assessed by interventions which affect noradrenergic function more directly.

The observation that LC-noradrenergic neurons are active during stressful circumstances is clearly consistent with suggestions that they may be involved in the learning

T. W. Robbins and *B. J. Everitt: Departments of Experimental Psychology and *Anatomy, University of Cambridge, Cambridge CB2 3EB, United Kingdom.

of aversively motivated tasks (see below). It is noteworthy, therefore, that Jacobs (35) has demonstrated marked increases in NE neuron unit activity during presentation of a conditioned stimulus (CS) previously paired with an aversive air puff to the face of a cat. The selectivity of this response of LC neurons was emphasized by the observation that the same CS previously paired with a rewarding stimulus did not evoke increases in NE neuronal firing. While these data strongly suggest LC involvement in learning associated with stressful stimuli, for which there is considerable support from behavioral studies (see below), they do not account for the observation that learning of some appetitively motivated tasks is significantly retarded following lesions of the coeruleo-cortical noradrenergic projection (26).

Indeed, recent data suggest that LC neurons are active during appetitive learning. In rats, there was an immediate response of LC cells to any change in stimulus-reinforcer contingencies in appetitive and aversive conditioning, often prior to the behavioral expression of conditioning (57). The changes were even more reliable than the responses to novelty and were unrelated to movements, disappearing when the behavioral response was well established. In primates, LC neurons are active during the performance of a vigilance or ''oddball'' visual discrimination task that is appetitively motivated. Monkeys were trained to release a lever after a target cue light that occurred randomly in 10% of trials and to withhold responding during non-target cues. LC neurons responded selectively to the target cues on this task, and they reversed this salience if the non-target stimuli became relevant instead. High levels of LC discharge were related to decreased foveation, restlessness, and impaired task performance (7). Importantly, cortical, event-related potentials were elicited in this task selectively by the same stimuli that evoked

LC responses, suggesting that the LC activation was associated with cortical processing mechanisms.

At the cortical level, P-300-like potentials have been recorded in squirrel monkeys in other ''oddball'' paradigms where the animal responds to low probability auditory stimuli (48). The generation and modulation of the P-300-like auditory potential was shown to be impaired by electrolytic lesions of the LC, although more specific destruction of ascending NE fibers failed to have the same effects (see also Chapter 29, *this volume*).

In general, these electrophysiological studies are consistent with a role for LC-NE neurons in processes related to the processing of novelty, including new contingencies that require learning.

Effects of Neurotoxic Lesions of the Dorsal Bundle on Behavioral Function

Another approach to investigating the functions of the LC-NE system has been to define (a) the behavioral effects of selectively removing the rostral, noradrenergic projections of the LC and (b) the environmental circumstances under which such effects occur. Profound levels of forebrain NE depletion can be achieved by injecting the selective catecholamine neurotoxin 6-hydroxydopamine (6-OHDA) into the trajectory of the LC axons in the midbrain—namely, into the dorsal noradrenergic bundle (DB). The rationale underlying this neurochemically highly specific approach to studying LC function has been discussed extensively elsewhere (46,53) and will not be labored here. With optimal parameters (Fig. 1) it is feasible to deplete the telencephalic projection zones of NE to less than 10% of control values without any effect on any other known neurotransmitter system. Indeed, such

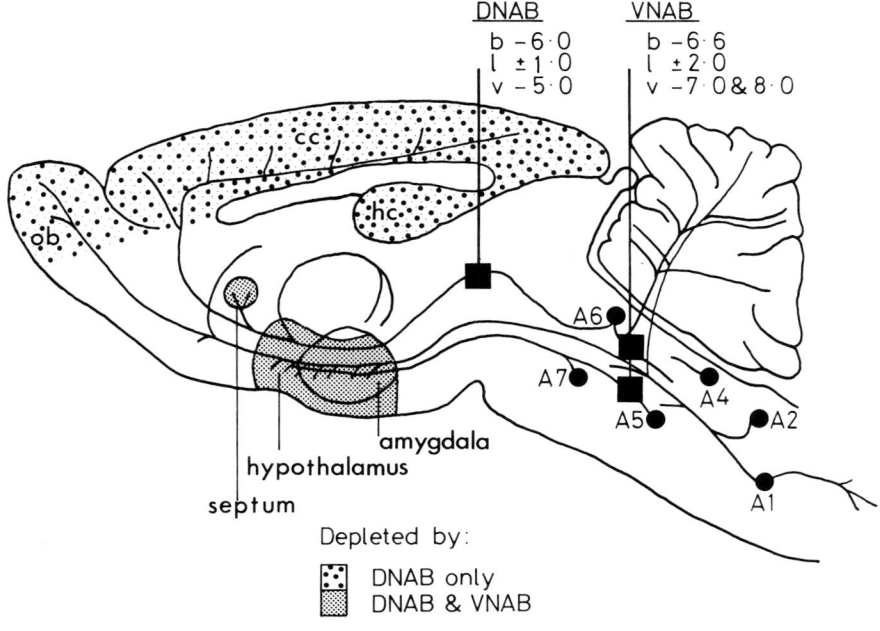

FIG. 1. Sagittal section of the rat brain showing the origin and course of the dorsal and ventral noradrenergic bundles from the locus coeruleus (cell group A6) (DNAB) and cell groups (A1–5,7) in the rostral medulla oblongata (VNAB). Also shown are the optimal parameters for making lesions of these projections using intracerebral administration of the catecholamine neurotoxin 6-hydroxydopamine. Terminal areas sustaining depletion are shaded. Typically greater than 90% depletion of neocortical and hippocampal NE is obtained following lesions of the DNAB (e.g., see refs. 14, 46, and 59) and about 70% of hypothalamic NE following depletion of the VNAB (e.g., see refs. 55 and 62). Abbreviations: ob, olfactory bulb; cc, cerebral cortex; hc, hippocampus. (Figure provided by B. J. Cole.)

potent degrees of depletion, as assessed by tissue levels of NE, are essential if comparable reductions of extracellular NE are to be achieved (1). Smaller degrees of depletion clearly enhance possible plastic and recuperative responses of noradrenergic neurons to 6-OHDA lesions, including up-regulation of adrenoceptor populations (2,22). Such problems may also make difficult the interpretation of the effects of the alternative noradrenergic neurotoxin DSP-4, which can lead to cortical NE loss of less than 70% (e.g., see ref. 72). Conclusions concerning the lack of involvement of central NE in particular psychological processes such as memory and learning are clearly unsafe if depletions are substantially less than 90%. On the other hand, several groups have consistently demonstrated robust and long-lasting behavioral deficits associated with depletion over 90% of telencephalic NE, which would seem hard to explain in terms of changes leading to overcompensation of the damaged system (see ref. 53). However, there are two major problems specifically related to the effects of DB lesions: (i) assessing the possible contaminating effects of hypothalamic NE depletion caused unavoidably by diffusion of the neurotoxin to fibers projecting from the cell bodies of the medulla oblongata contributing to the so-called ventral noradrenergic bundle (VB); this can be addressed by making control lesions of this structure (e.g., see Fig. 1) which, of course, also contribute to our understanding of the role of hypothalamic NE; and (ii) isolating the critical terminal region for a particular effect; this problem will be addressed in the section entitled "Interactions of LC with Specific Terminal Regions." While there are undoubtedly problems associated with the use of neurotoxic lesions of the DB or VB to understand the behavioral functions of the central NE systems, these have to be weighed against the difficulties of interpreting effects of systemic treatments with adrenergic receptor agents—for example, because of lack of pharmacological specificity and peripheral factors. However, such experiments can be helpful in providing converging sources of evidence and will be mentioned as appropriate.

Effects on Unconditioned Behavior

DB lesions have no obvious effect on gross behavior in the rat, such as eating, drinking, or spontaneous locomotor activity. This contrasts markedly with the changes produced in these forms of behavior by central dopamine depletion, as well as the increases in body weight and feeding often observed following hypothalamic NE depletion (33,55). This lack of effect of DB lesions on gross ingestive and locomotor responses simplifies the interpretation of many of the other effects of the lesion. However, it is evident that DB lesions do affect some forms of unconditioned behavior (e.g., behavioral responses to novelty), as might be expected from the single-unit studies that show stimulus novelty to be an effective trigger

for LC neurons. As will become obvious for many of the effects of these lesions, however, the sequelae appear to depend on subtle features of the testing situation (for a review see ref. 16). For example, DB lesions can reduce feeding overall in the threatening situation of a highly illuminated open field, and yet attenuate the suppression of eating normally shown to a novel food. Steketee et al. (67) have recently replicated the attenuation of this food neophobia in novel situations following DB lesions and have found that it can be attenuated by icv treatment with the beta receptor agonist isoproterenol (68).

Effects on Conditioning and Conditioned Behavior

One of the most important generalizations to have emerged about the effects of DB lesions is that they tend to impair the acquisition of new behavior to a greater extent than previously established performance. The concept that the DB is implicated in learning is by now quite venerable, but some of the original experiments were not convincing and there are many forms of learning that are not reliably affected by DB lesions. However, there is some evidence that under well-defined conditions, DB lesions reliably retard the gradual learning of an appetitive, conditional discrimination task, in which the rat is required to learn a rule (press right or left lever) to guide its response to one of two discriminative stimuli (e.g., lights flashing at one of two different frequencies). On the other hand, such lesions do not impair its performance if the lesion is made following the establishment of the discrimination by preoperative training (26). This clearly rules out many explanations of the effects of DB lesions based on simple performance factors such as changes in sensory capacity or motivation.

The dichotomy between acquisition and performance has also been observed for aversive conditioning; thus, conditioned suppression of food-maintained operant responding in the presence of a light acting as an aversive CS is attenuated in acquisition following surgery, but is unaffected if established prior to surgery (14). This dissociation argues against a simple explanation of the acquisition deficit in terms of an intervening variable such as "anxiety," and this is supported by demonstrations of a lack of effect of DB lesions on response suppression in the Geller–Seifter conflict paradigm (39). Furthermore, the acquisition of a possible oral coping response (e.g., gnawing, eating) to an unconditioned aversive event, tail-pinch, is impaired following DB lesions, but not if the response is established by experience prior to surgery (55). However, we should emphasize that associative processes are not always impaired by such lesions. For example, simultaneous visual discriminations, where the rat simply has to approach the rewarded stimulus, and the effects of reversing the contingencies so that the animal has to approach the formerly nonreinforced cue, are not affected by DB lesions (25). Conditioned taste aversion has also proved particularly resistant to disruption following DB lesions (23). Moreover, the effects on other forms of aversive learning and performance are complex and may depend on such factors as the nature and intensity of the aversive reinforcer, time elapsed between the DB lesion and testing, and the precise conditioning contingencies and test situation used (for a review see ref. 62). In general, VB lesions do not affect acquisition of appetitive or aversive conditioning, although they have been found to increase resistance to extinction of the latter, both for conditioned suppression and conditioned taste aversion (14,23). It seems plausible that these effects of VB lesions on extinction represent possible interactions with neuroendocrine mechanisms in the hypothalamic–pituitary axis, and that at least some of the earlier reports of extinction deficits following DB lesions (46) might be attributable to effects on neurons of the VB.

Contextual aversive conditioning (that is, conditioning to the background cues rather than to an explicit CS) is also spared by DB lesions; in fact, such conditioning may be *enhanced* by coeruleo-cortical NE loss, either when an explicit CS is also present (59) or when it is not (62). The difference between aversive conditioning to discrete, explicit cues and to the wider contexts in which they occur has obvious applicability to various forms of clinical anxiety. Plasma corticosterone is also affected by such lesions, but only in a manner predicted by the conditioned behavioral response (59). However, the complementary pattern of impaired CS conditioning and enhanced contextual conditioning seen in rats with DB lesions is another piece of evidence against a simple anxiolytic view of their effects, and it may instead argue for effects on attentional function (see below).

A possibly related effect of DB lesions on contextual conditioning is seen in spatial learning in the Morris swim maze, where the rat is required to learn to use distal cues around the room to locate a safe, but invisible, platform. DB lesions again may actually enhance acquisition of the task (40), especially if the rat is swimming in cold water (60). In this situation the DB lesion appears to protect the rat against the deleterious effects on learning in water sufficiently cold to lead to hypothermia, while having no effect by itself on body temperature in the swim maze or on plasma corticosterone levels (60). In contrast, VB lesions have no effects on spatial (60) or contextual (62,63) conditioning, although they do affect plasma corticosteroid levels to the shock (63), thereby showing a dissociation between effects on conditioning (by DB lesions) and endocrine status (by VB lesions) which probably corresponds to the relative roles of these systems in cognitive and vegetative functions, respectively.

In attempting to resolve the initially bewildering pattern of effects of coeruleo-cortical NE depletion on these different forms of learning, strong unifying themes can in fact be found. One such theme is the difficulty or sensitivity of the learning procedure, while another is the task-associated level of arousal; either factor might explain

the relatively greater sensitivity of aversive paradigms to learning deficits following DB lesions. Thus, the conditional appetitive discrimination task which has repeatedly shown (26,53) deficits in DB-lesioned rats typically takes many sessions to learn, even for a normal rat. Another factor is the attentional requirements of the tasks; it is possible that some of the DB lesion effects result not from deficits in associative processes, but from deficits in the input to the associative mechanisms. Thus, the dissociation between CS and contextual learning may suggest that DB rats are utilizing more distal cues than the normal rat, which in some situations may produce a paradoxical enhancement of acquisition. This prediction was tested directly in the water-maze task with a discrimination between two *local* sets of cues (platforms with vertical or horizontal stripes). The DB lesion *impaired* acquisition, despite facilitating acquisition of the spatial variant of the task (60), thus again showing a dissociation of effects on local versus distal cues, which possibly results from shifts in attention.

Effects on Attention

Since the original Segal and Bloom (58) findings of enhanced signal-to-noise ratios following iontophoretically applied NE in hippocampus, there has been a rash of hypotheses concerning the role of the LC in selective attention (46,53). An earlier review (53) made it clear that direct tests of this hypothesis employing paradigms including latent inhibition, blocking, and nonreversal shift have not generally confirmed earlier positive findings (47). However, there have been some interesting findings that probably require further investigation (e.g., see refs. 42 and 71), and a recent paper by Devauges and Sara (21) has suggested that activation of central NE mechanisms by the alpha-2 receptor antagonist, idazoxan, can lead to apparent improvements in shifting of attention between different types of cues, although it will be necessary in subsequent studies to control for the cue properties of the drug and possible state-dependency.

In assessing the role of the LC in attentional mechanisms, it is notable that there are several different forms of attention, including selective (focused) attention, divided attention, and sustained attention, including vigilance. Deficits can be observed following DB lesions in a continuous performance task which requires some of these attentional capacities, under certain conditions (10,18). As might be predicted, these deficits only occurred under very specific test conditions, namely when bursts of loud white noise were interpolated immediately prior to expected visual targets, when the rats were treated with amphetamine, or when the stimuli were temporally unpredictable, a manipulation that increases arousal. There were no such deficits in attention when the task was merely made more difficult by, for example, reducing the brightness of the discriminanda or by increasing the frequency of their presentation. The effect of white noise is manifestly consistent with the demonstration that LC neurons fire in response to such phasic stimuli (35; also see Foote and Aston-Jones, *this volume*) and also with demonstrations of enhanced distractibility in the maze situation (54), and possibly the enhanced reactivity of DB lesioned rats in the open field setting (9), as described above. The effect of temporal unpredictability is important in that it suggests that the LC can be activated in quite complex ways—namely, not only in response to the initial occurrence of a novel stimulus, but also to the omission of an expected event. One of the concomitant effects of white noise is to produce behavioral activation, which can be manifested as quicker reaction times and a propensity to impulsive responding (10). Such behavioral activation is also produced by the dopaminergic agonist, D-amphetamine, especially when infused into the region of the nucleus accumbens septi (15,17). Thus, it would be expected that discriminative accuracy in the visual vigilance task would also be impaired in rats with DB lesions following intra-accumbens infusions of amphetamine, and this result has been found (15). The degree of behavioral activation produced by amphetamine was unaffected by the DB lesion (15). Thus, under conditions of *equivalent* behavioral activation resulting from the endogenous cue of dopamine release, DB-lesioned rats became less efficient at detecting brief visual signals. The parallel with the effects of white noise is enhanced by evidence that dopamine depletion within the ventral striatum attenuates the activating effects of this stimulus as well as those of D-amphetamine (17).

Interactions of LC with Specific Terminal Regions

It is clear that DB lesions can affect a variety of behavioral processes in carefully defined conditions, but it is less clear how readily these may be attributed to the different projection fields of the LC. There are several strategies available for addressing this problem; one is to attempt to mimic the effects of a DB lesion with a manipulation of a discrete terminal zone, including local NE depletion or the acute modulation of NE function via intracerebral administration of specific adrenoceptor agonists or antagonists. In the former case, there are problems posed by the considerable plasticity following damage to terminal regions, which is undoubtedly greater than following damage at the level of the cell body or fiber bundle. In the latter instance, the problems of interpretation resulting from diffusion and local concentration are equally challenging, but they leave open the possibility of boosting local NE function and predicting an effect opposite to that of DB lesions. Not surprisingly, progress in this area has been limited.

In considering the effects of DB lesions on conditioning, it is of interest that recent neuropsychological analyses are helping to delineate the critical foci for the effects.

For example, acquisition of the rule-learning conditional discrimination task is surprisingly not affected by cell body lesions of the hippocampus or amygdala, but is disrupted by manipulations of the prefrontal and cingulate cortex (45; Burns et al., *unpublished findings*). In fact, 6-OHDA-induced lesions of these regions can mimic the effects of DB lesions described above (Ryan, Robbins, and Everitt, *unpublished findings*). Another recent study has shown an important role for NE fibers ascending to the cingulate cortex and anterior ventral thalamus of rabbits during discriminative instrumental avoidance training, following local NE depletion (66).

When interpreting the effects of DB lesions on aversive conditioning, there is considerable evidence of an involvement of the amygdala in learning about aversive CSs (20,30,43), whereas recent evidence has suggested a role for the hippocampus in aversive conditioning to context (61). Local depletion of NE from the region of the amygdala impairs conditioning to aversive CSs in the same way as does DB lesions (59), although local depletion of hippocampal NE on contextual conditioning has not been studied. The behavioral consequences of NE depletion from both regions following DB lesions may depend, therefore, on the relative degree of engagement of hippocampal versus amygdaloid mechanisms in any particular task or situation.

This principle may also apply to the case of choosing between familiar and novel food in a novel environment, especially because both amygdala and hippocampal lesions probably affect the responses to different aspects of novelty. There has been relatively little investigation of the effects of terminal NE manipulations on the response to novelty. However, Borsini and Rolls (8) found that 6-OHDA lesions of, and also NE infusions into, the amygdala affected the response to novel foods, although these two manipulations did not have the expected opposite pattern of effects. In assessing a locomotor response to a novel environment, Flicker and Geyer (28) found that chronic infusions of NE into the dentate gyrus retarded the habituation of spatial exploration. These two sets of results are intriguing in that they suggest that terminal NE manipulations can affect different aspects of the response to novelty at distinct neural sites, a conclusion fully consistent with findings of the different effects of DB lesions on response to different aspects of novelty (see above).

With respect to the neocortex, there has similarly been little direct investigation of the role of NE in behavioral paradigms. Performance of the 5-choice attentional task described above is known to depend on the rat neocortex, especially medial prefrontal cortex (Muir, Everitt, and Robbins, *unpublished data*). Other evidence has shown the involvement of NE mechanisms in processes of working memory in the primate prefrontal cortex, using the delayed response paradigm. The decline in working memory in aged rhesus monkeys is significantly ameliorated by systemic treatment with the alpha-2 adrenergic agonist, clonidine (5). Arnsten and Goldman-Rakic (5) further showed that prefrontal cortical ablation (around the *sulcus principalis*), or local noradrenergic denervation of this area induced by 6-OHDA, disrupt performance on the task—confirming its dependence on this area of neocortex. Clonidine was able to reduce the NE lesion-induced deficit, but not the cortical ablation-induced deficit, emphasizing the interpretation that not only does delayed response performance depend on the prefrontal cortex, but that NE interacting with postsynaptic alpha-2 receptors in this site appears to be an important component of the processes occurring there (5). Guanfacine, a more specific alpha-2 agonist with less sedative and cardiovascular effects, was even more potent than clonidine in improving memory in this spatial delayed response paradigm (6).

While beneficial effects of clonidine have also been observed in a delayed matching-to-sample task in monkeys (34), other investigators have failed to observe effects of systemic clonidine on delayed response performance in aged monkeys (19); this discrepancy might depend on subtle differences in test setting and procedure. For example, the delayed response task in these two studies was implemented in different ways; notably the latter investigation (19) employed an automated procedure, whereas the studies by Arnsten and colleagues (4–6) utilize a manual procedure in an environment susceptible to distraction. The possible importance of the attentional requirements of the task is provided by the recent study of Arnsten and Contant (4) showing that alpha-2 receptor agonists have strong protective effects against extraneous distraction in the aged animals during performance of the delayed response task, and that these effects can be blocked by treatment with an alpha-2 receptor antagonist acting predominantly at postsynaptic receptors. These findings are compatible with evidence reviewed above suggesting that DB lesions enhance distractibility in certain settings in the rat.

Overall, these results provide evidence that the effects of noradrenergic transmission through the coeruleo-cortical system are mediated through quite specific areas of its termination, whether neocortical, archaecortical (hippocampus), or involving subcortical structures of the limbic forebrain such as the amygdala (although the basolateral component of this nuclear complex may, in fact, be more cortical than subcortical in terms of both structure and connections).

Role of Coeruleo-cortical NE in Memory and Other Forms of Plasticity

Early theories of LC function emphasized its possible role in memory consolidation, which may contribute to some of the selective effects of DB lesions on acquisition (see ref. 52). This can be contrasted with the considerable evidence, in the rat, of spared short-term memory function following DB lesions, for example, in delayed matching

to position (37) and delayed alternation (49) tasks. It appears that, as well as having a role in the acute effects on attentional mechanisms, the DB may also be implicated in rather longer-term plastic changes in synaptic function that contribute to learning, perhaps particularly in tasks requiring lengthy training (see above). Experiments utilizing post-trial noradrenergic manipulations on the retention of one-trial aversive conditioning tasks have examined possible direct or modulatory roles of NE in the consolidation of memory traces (30,41,43). In general, the data suggest that low doses of NE infused into the amygdala facilitate retention (41), but higher doses are either without effect (41) or are amnesic (24). Furthermore, intra-amygdala beta-blockers are also amnesic in their effects (30). Evidence suggests that central NE mechanisms, probably within the amygdala, are a final common pathway for a variety of amnestic and promnestic treatments—for example, adrenaline infusions (43) and treatment with corticotropin-releasing factor (11), respectively.

A further locus of plastic change is the hippocampus, a structure typically associated with aspects of learning and memory, and there is evidence that depletion of NE can reduce long-term potentiation in the dentate gyrus, a finding supported by demonstrations of an initiation of short- and long-term potentiation of the dentate gyrus response to perforant path input by the exogenous or endogenous application of NE (for a review see ref. 32).

In parallel with the early theorizing on memory consolidation were suggestions that manipulation of cortical NE could affect visual development (36). However, these effects are controversial and are in the process of reevaluation (50). Destruction of central NE systems in neonatal rats does influence the degree of recovery from frontal cortex lesions when assessed behaviorally during adulthood (38). Perhaps most surprisingly, destruction of the DB prevents the adaptive changes resulting from damage to the mesolimbicocortical dopamine system, leading to an abolition of both neurochemical changes (in D1 dopamine receptors) and behavioral deficits (hyperactivity, impaired delayed alternation performance) normally associated with such depletion (69). In this context, it is of considerable interest that the disruption by fornix lesions of performance of an 8-arm radial maze task, which is correlated with reductions in cholinergic hippocampal markers, is completely ameliorated by central NE depletion induced by DSP-4 (56). Thus, again central NE depletion actually benefits behavioral recovery, and this emphasizes the importance of considering interactions and balances with activity in other neurotransmitter systems.

THEORETICAL SYNTHESES

There have been several dominant ideas in theories of LC–NE function, based largely on experiments in animals, ranging from notions of reinforcement and arousal (see ref. 52) to the mediation of anxiety (31,51) and the control of selective attention (46,52). Each theory commands its own set of supporting behavioral phenomena, but it is probably fair to say that no single construct can adequately explain the functions of the LC. While it is natural (though sometimes insightful) to ignore evidence that does not fit into a particular theory (and we are aware that a brief chapter such as this is unlikely to be free of this tendency), it is desirable that the theory be as precise but as all-embracing as possible. It seems likely, in fact, that the LC has rather general functions which bear on aspects of attention, learning, and anxiety. These functions are based on two very clear points. First, activity in LC neurons is monotonically related to increased arousal. Second, this activity probably improves the processing of salient external events evoking neuronal activity in diverse forebrain sites, whether these events are novel, salient because of conditioning, or even internalized, as representations of stimulus events receiving further processing in memory consolidation and retrieval.

An early theoretical suggestion (3) was that the LC functioned rather like the cognitive arm of a central sympathetic ganglion, and this notion has recently been extended by others (7). "Thus activation of the peripheral sympathetic system prepares the animal physically for adaptive phasic responses to urgent stimuli, while parallel activation of LC increases attention and vigilance, preparing the animal cognitively for adaptive responses to such stimuli" (ref. 7, p. 516). The notion of adaptive preparation or coping with the consequences of sympathetic arousal is also to be found in the earlier review (3), and it has also been stated by us (52,53) previously in terms such as the DB functions to preserve attentional selectivity especially under elevated levels of arousal (52). This is related to psychological theories such as that of Easterbrook (see ref. 27), who argues that high levels of arousal cause attentional focusing. Another probably related formulation is that the LC is implicated in "controlled" or "effortful," as distinct from "automatic," processing (18); that is, the system modulates attentional capacity. Presumably, LC activity would be part of that mechanism that effectively focuses attention onto salient events in threatening or demanding situations. This theory explains why the LC is more implicated in the acquisition of learning tasks than in the performance of these tasks, why aversive situations are more sensitive to manipulations of the LC, why attentional function is disrupted under certain conditions in DB-lesioned rats, and why the LC is active during orienting responses to novel stimuli. According to this view, the LC does not mediate anxiety or stress per se, but rather a state of arousal that is correlated with anxiety or stress, leading to attentional and cognitive change. This state of arousal can be self-regulated to a point, and there is evidence to implicate LC neurons in some of the phenomena of "learned helplessness." Specifically, central NE activity is affected by environmental

contingencies such as the availability of effective avoidance or "coping" responses; in situations where the animal is exposed to inescapable, uncontrollable stress, NE function is depressed (64; for a review see Chapter 33, *this volume*), but can be restored by treatment with adrenoceptor agents infused in the vicinity of the LC, leading to attenuation of those responses characteristic of "behavioral despair" (64). From a consideration of the cognitive sequelae of manipulations of central NE reviewed in this chapter, it is obvious that some of the major cognitive features not only of learned helplessness, but also of depression, including problems in attention and learning, could result from LC dysfunction.

Several of the effects of DB lesions (e.g., reduced food neophobia and conditioned suppression) would be expected if such depletion had anxiolytic effects, and the role for NE mechanisms of the LC in mediating certain elements of the opiate withdrawal syndrome (70) is also suggestive of a role in aversive motivation. However, the limited nature of the conditioned suppression deficits—in particular the apparent enhancement of contextual conditioning, the lack of effect on punished responding, and the different effects of chlordiazepoxide and DB lesions (16) in the food neophobia setting—is inconsistent with a simple form of the anxiety hypothesis. On the other hand, it is clear from studies with humans that anxiety often leads to enhanced distractibility rather than enhanced focusing, and that there is evidence from several sources (7,56,60) that elevated LC activity, far from improving performance, may actually impair it. A parsimonious account would then invoke the inverted U-shaped function relating arousal level to efficiency of performance (for review see ref. 27). The decrements in performance at high levels of arousal have been often been attributed to the attention the subject begins to pay to visceral cues arising from sympathetic arousal, such as palpitation, which may become correlated with subjective feelings of anxiety (27).

IMPLICATIONS FOR HUMAN COGNITIVE FUNCTION AND PSYCHOPATHOLOGY

Some of the experimental work on behavioral functions of the LC in animals fits surprisingly well with human psychopharmacological experiments on cognitive effects of adrenoceptor agonists and antagonists. Thus, Clark et al. (12) found that the mixed alpha1, alpha2 agonist clonidine impaired performance in a set of dichotic listening tasks (both divided and focused attention), presumably via its presynaptic actions to reduce LC firing. They suggested that the drug reduced alertness or arousal, and thereby increased the demands of the tasks on the volunteers. In contrast, a dopamine receptor blocker, while also impairing performance, reduced the activational state of the subjects or their readiness for action. Clark et al. (12), following a similar suggestion (52), make the useful distinction between the dual roles of the LC–NE system and central dopamine pathways: the former is concerned with regulating the capacity for conscious registration of external stimuli, whereas the latter regulates the capacity to respond to them.

Other effects of clonidine are fully compatible with the evidence concerning effects of DB lesions in animals. First, clonidine has been shown to impair the learning of difficult paired associates (29). Second, the drug reduces the cost (in reaction time) of shifting attention to a spatial cue (13); this is perhaps analogous to the changes in attentional distribution produced by DB lesions. It is of interest that a recent study of the alpha-2 antagonist, idazoxan, actually produced what appears to be the complementary effect of increased attention to the location of the previous cue (65).

Such results certainly have clinical potential. One of the more remarkable examples of "cognitive enhancement" by psychotropic drugs has been the improvements in cognitive performance in Korsakoff patients by clonidine (44). While this result is not readily predicted by the effects reviewed here on normal volunteers, it is possible that the presynaptic degeneration of NE neurons may enhance the contribution of postsynaptic effects of the drug, in a way possibly reminiscent of the effects of clonidine in aged monkeys reviewed above. These results hold some promise for the treatment of other neurodegenerative disorders associated with coeruleo-cortical NE loss, including Parkinson's and Alzheimer's diseases. The former is associated with significant cognitive deficits, often resembling effects of frontal lobe damage, but the possible role of the LC and therapeutic possibilities of treatment with adrenoceptor agents remain largely unexplored. While the cognitive syndrome in Alzheimer's disease is probably multifactorial, it is possible that a malfunctioning coeruleo-cortical system may make patients more susceptible to the abrupt decline in cognitive status often associated with transfer to a new environment such as a nursing institution. A major problem for further work in this area is to decide on the optimal method for enhancing noradrenergic function using drugs such as clonidine or idazoxan, which exert a balance of effects at both pre- and postsynaptic receptors.

In a more general sense, it is likely that possible malfunctioning of the LC is important in those human disorders in which there is an important interface between cognition and emotion, including depression, post-traumatic stress disorder, anxiety, and drug-withdrawal states. In some of these conditions, it is possible that the LC is overactive, and, as we have seen, this may also result in cognitive problems, which may exacerbate the emotional state. For example, it is plausible in panic disorder that noradrenergic overactivity helps to concentrate attention on dominant events or pathological cognitive schemas, promoting their consolidation and thus slowing the extinction of their influence over the subject's behavior. Many of these hypotheses will be tested in the clinical setting in the next generation of research, when their heuristic value is expected to become apparent.

ACKNOWLEDGMENTS

Our research is supported by the Wellcome Trust and the Medical Research Council. We thank our colleagues for their efforts and thank Dr. B. J. Cole for kindly providing Fig. 1.

REFERENCES

1. Abercrombie ED, Keller RW, Zigmond MJ. Characterization of hippocampal norepinephrine release as measured by microdialysis perfusion: pharmacological and behavioral studies. *Neuroscience* 1988;27:897–904.
2. Acheson A, Zigmond MJ, Stricker EM. Compensatory increases in tyrosine hydroxylase activity in the rat brain after intraventricular injection of 6-hydroxydopamine. *Science* 1980;207:537–540.
3. Amaral DG, Sinnamon HM. The locus coeruleus: neurobiology of a central noradrenergic nucleus. *Prog. Neurobiol* 1977;9:147–196.
4. Arnsten AFT, Contant TA. Alpha-2 adrenergic agonists decrease distractibility in aged monkeys performing the delayed response task. *Psychopharmacology* 1992;108:159–169.
5. Arnsten AFT, Goldman-Rakic PS. Alpha 2-adrenergic mechanisms in prefrontal cortex associated with cognitive decline in aged nonhuman primates. *Science* 1985;230:1273–1276.
6. Arnsten AFT, Cai JX, Goldman-Rakic PS. The alpha-2 adrenergic agonist guanfacine improves memory in aged monkeys without sedative or hypotensive side effects: evidence for alpha-2 receptor subtypes. *J Neurosci* 1988;8:4287–4298.
7. Aston-Jones G, Chiang C, Alexinsky T. Discharge of noradrenergic locus coeruleus neurons in behaving rats and monkeys suggests a role in vigilance. *Prog Brain Res* 1991;88:501–520.
8. Borsini F, Rolls ET. Role of noradrenaline and serotonin in the basolateral regions of the amygdala in food preference and learned taste aversion in the rat. *Physiol Behav* 1984;33:37–43.
9. Britton DR, Ksir C, Thatcher-Britton K, Young D, Koob GF. Brain-norepinephrine-depleting lesions selectively enhance behavioral responses to novelty. *Physiol Behav* 1984;33:473–478.
10. Carli M, Robbins TW, Evenden JL, Everitt BJ. Effects of lesions to ascending noradrenergic neurons on performance of a 5-choice serial reaction task in rats: implications for theories of dorsal noradrenergic bundle function based on selective attention and arousal. *Behav Brain Res* 1983;9:361–380.
11. Chen MF, Chiu TH, Lee EH. Noradrenergic mediation of the memory enhancing effect of corticotrophin releasing factor in the locs coeruleus of rats. *Psychoendocrinology* 1992;17:113–124.
12. Clark CR, Geffen GM, Geffen LB. Catecholamines and attention. II. Pharmacological studies in normal humans. *Neurosci Biobehav Rev* 1987;11:353–364.
13. Clark CR, Geffen GM, Geffen LB. Catecholamines and the covert orienting of attention. *Neuropsychologia* 1986;27:131–140.
14. Cole BJ, Robbins TW. Dissociable effects of lesions to the dorsal or ventral noradrenergic bundle on the acquisition, performance and extinction of aversive conditioning. *Behav Neurosci* 1987;101:476–488.
15. Cole BJ, Robbins TW. Amphetamine impairs the discrimination performance of rats with dorsal noradrenergic bundle lesions on a 5-choice serial reaction time task: new evidence for central dopaminergic-noradrenergic interactions. *Psychopharmacology* 1987;91:458–466.
16. Cole BJ, Robbins TW, Everitt BJ. Lesions of the dorsal noradrenergic bundle simultaneously enhance and reduce responsivity to novelty in a food preference test. *Brain Res Rev* 1988;13:325–349.
17. Cole BJ, Robbins TW. Effects of 6-hydroxydopamine lesions of the nucleus accumbens septi on performance of a 5 choice serial reaction time task in rats; implications for theories of selective attention and arousal. *Behav Brain Res* 1989;33:165–179.
18. Cole BJ, Robbins TW. Forebrain norepinephrine: role in controlled

information processing in the rat. *Neuropsychopharmacology* 1992;7:129–141.

19. Davis HP, Callahan MJ, Downs DA. Clonidine disrupts aged monkey delayed response performance. *Drug Dev Res* 1988;12:279–286.

20. Davis M, Hitchock JM, Rosen JB. Anxiety and the amygdala: pharmacological and anatomical analysis of the fear-potentiated startle paradigm. In: Bower G, ed. *The psychology of learning and motivation.* New York: Academic Press, 1987;263–305.

21. Devauges V, Sara SJ. Activation of the noradrenergic system facilitates an attentional shift in the rat. *Behav Brain Res* 1990;39:19–28.

22. Dooley DJ, Jones, GH, Robbins TW. Noradrenaline- and time-dependent changes in neocortical $\alpha 2$- and $\beta 1$-adrenoceptor binding in dorsal noradrenergic bundle-lesioned rats. *Brain Res* 1987;420:152–156.

23. Dunn LT, Everitt BJ. The effects of lesions to the noradrenergic projections from the locus ceruleus and lateral tegmental cell groups on conditioned taste aversion in the rat. *Behav Neurosci* 1987;101:409–422.

24. Ellis ME, Kesner RP. The noradrenergic system of the amygdala and aversive information processing. *Behav Neurosci* 1983;97:399–415.

25. Evenden JL, Marston HM, Jones GH, Giardini V, Lenard L, Everitt BJ, Robbins TW. Effects of excitotoxic lesions of the substantia innominata, ventral and dorsal globus pallidus on visual discrimination acquisition, performance and reversal in the rat. *Behav Brain Res* 1989;32:129–149.

26. Everitt BJ, Robbins TW, Gaskin M, Fray PJ. The effects of lesions to noradrenergic neurons on discrimination learning and performance in the rat. *Neuroscience* 1983;10:397–410.

27. Eysenck MW. *Attention and arousal.* Berlin: Springer-Verlag, 1982.

28. Flicker C, Geyer M. Behavior during hippocampal microinfusions. I. Norepinephrine and diverse exploration. *Brain Res Rev* 1982;4:79–103.

29. Frith CD, Dowdy J, Ferrier N, Crow TJ. Selective impairment of paired associate learning after administration of a centrally-acting adrenergic agonist (clonidine). *Psychopharmacology* 1985;87:490–493.

30. Gallagher M, Kapp BS, Musty RE, Driscoll, PA. Memory formation: evidence for a specific neurochemical system in the amygdala. *Science* 1977;198:423–425.

31. Gray JA. *The neuropsychology of anxiety.* Oxford: Clarendon Press, 1982.

32. Harley C. Noradrenergic and locus coeruleus modulation of the performant path-evoked potential in the rat dentate gyrus supports a role for the locus coeruleus in attentional and memorial processes. *Prog Brain Res* 1991;88:307–321.

33. Hernandez L, Hoebel BG. Overeating after midbrain 6-hydroxydopamine: prevention by central injection of selective catecholamine re-uptake blockers. *Brain Res* 1982;245:333–343.

34. Jackson WJ, Buccafusco JJ. Clonidine enhances delayed matching-to-sample performance by young and aged monkeys. *Pharmacol Biochem Behav* 1991;39:79–84.

35. Jacobs BL. Central monoaminergic neurons: single unit studies in behaving animals. In: Meltzer HY, ed. *Psychopharmacology: the third generation of progress.* New York: Raven Press, 1987;159–169.

36. Kasamatsu T. Neuronal plasticity maintained by the central norepinephrine system in the cat visual cortex. In: Sprague JM, Epstein AN, eds. *Progress in psychobiology and physiological psychology,* vol 10. New York: Academic Press, 1983;1–112.

37. Koger SM, Mair RG. Depletion of cortical norepinephrine in rats by 6-hydroxydopamine does not impair performance of a delayed matching to sample task. *Behav Neurosci* 1992;106:718–721.

38. Kolb B, Sutherland RJ. Noradrenaline depletion blocks behavioral sparing and alters cortical morphogenesis after neonatal frontal cortex damage in rats. *J Neurosci* 1992;12:2321–2330.

39. Koob GF, Thatcher-Britton K, Britton DR, Roberts DCS. Destruction of the locus coeruleus or the dorsal NE bundle does not alter the release of punished responding by ethanol and chlordiazepoxide. *Physiol Behav* 1984;33:479–485.

40. Langlais PJ, Connor DJ, Thal L. Comparison of the effects of single and combined lesions of the nucleus basalis magnocellularis and the dorsal noradrenergic bundle on learning and memory in the rat. *Behav Brain Res* 1993;54:81–90.

41. Liang KC, McGaugh JL, Yao H-Y. Involvement of amygdala pathways in the influence of post-training amygdala norepinephrine and peripheral epinephrine on memory storage. *Brain Res* 1990;508:225–233.

42. Lorden JF, Rickert EJ, Dawson RJ Jr, Pelleymounter M. Forebrain norepinephrine and the selective processing of information. *Brain Res* 1980;190:569–573.

43. McGaugh JL, Liang KC, Bennett C, Sternberg DB. Adrenergic influences on memory storage: interaction of peripheral and central systems. In: Lynch G, McGaugh JL, Weinberger NM, eds. *Neurobiology of learning and memory.* New York: The Guilford Press, 1984;313–332.

44. Mair RG, McEntee WJ. Cognitive enhancement in Korsakoff's psychosis by clonidine: a comparison with L-DOPA and ephedrine. *Psychopharmacology* 1986;88:374–380.

45. Marston HM, Everitt BJ, Robbins TW. Comparative effects of excitotoxic lesions of the hippocampus and septum/diagonal band on conditional visual discrimination and spatial learning. *Neuropsychologia* 1993;31:1099–1118.

46. Mason ST, Iversen SD. Theories of the dorsal bundle extinction effect. *Brain Res Rev* 1979;1:107–137.

47. Mason ST, Lin D. Dorsal noradrenergic bundle and selective attention. *J Comp Physiol Psychol* 1980;94:819–832.

48. Pineda JA, Foote SL, Neville HJ. Effects of locus coeruleus lesions on auditory, long-latency, event-related potentials in monkey. *J Neurosci* 1989;9:81–93.

49. Pisa M, Fibiger HC. Evidence against a role of the rat's dorsal noradrenergic bundle in selective attention and place memory. *Brain Res* 1983;272:319–329.

50. Rauschecker JP. Mechanisms of visual plasticity: Hebb synapses, NMDA receptors and beyond. *Physiol Rev* 1991;71:587–615.

51. Redmond DE. New and old evidence for the involvement of a brain norepinephrine system in anxiety, In: Fann WG, Karacan I, Pokorny D, Williams RL, eds. *Phenomenology and treatment of anxiety.* New York: Spectrum, 1979;153–203.

52. Robbins TW. Cortical noradrenaline, attention and arousal. *Psychol Med* 1984;14:13–21.

53. Robbins TW, Everitt BJ, Cole BJ, Archer T, Mohammed A. Functional hypotheses of the coeruleo-cortical noradrenergic projection: a review of recent experimentation and theory. *Physiol Psychol* 1985;13:127–150.

54. Roberts DCS, Price MTC, Fibiger HC. The dorsal tegmental noradrenergic projection: an analysis of its role in maze learning. *J Comp Physiol Psychol* 1976;90:363–372.

55. Sahakian BJ, Winn P, Robbins TW, Dooley RJ, Everitt BJ, Dunn LT, Wallace M, James WPT. Changes in body weight and food-related behaviour induced by destruction of the ventral or dorsal noradrenergic bundle. *Neuroscience* 1983;10:1405–1420.

56. Sara SJ, Dyon-Laurent G, Gilbert B, Leviel V. Noradrenergic hyperactivity after partial fornix section; role in cholinergic dependent memory performance. *Exp Brain Res* 1992;89:125–132.

57. Sara SJ, Segal M. Plasticity of sensory responses of locus coeruleus neurons in the behaving rat; behavioral implications. *Prog Brain Res* 1991;88:571–585.

58. Segal M, Bloom FE. The action of norepinephrine in the rat hippocampus. IV. The effects of locus coeruleus stimulation on evoked hippocampal activity. *Brain Res* 1976;107:513–525.

59. Selden NRW, Robbins TW, Everitt BJ. Enhanced behavioral conditioning to context and impaired behavioral and neuroendocrine responses to conditioning stimuli following ceruleo-cortical noradrenergic lesions: support for an attentional hypothesis of central noradrenergic function. *J Neurosci* 1990;10:531–539.

60. Selden NRW, Cole BJ, Everitt BJ, Robbins TW. Damage to ceruleo-cortical noradrenergic projections impairs locally cued but enhances spatially cued water maze acquisition. *Behav Brain Res* 1990;39:29–52.

61. Selden NRW, Everitt BJ, Jarrard LE, Robbins TW. Complementary roles for the amygdala and hippocampus in aversive conditioning to explicit and contextual cues. *Neuroscience* 1991;2:335–350.

62. Selden NRW, Everitt BJ, Robbins TW. Telencephalic but not diencephalic noradrenaline depletion enhances behavioral but not endocrine measures of fear conditioning to contextual stimuli. *Behav Brain Res* 1992;43:139–154.

63. Selden NRW, Robbins TW, Everitt BJ. Diencephalic noradrenaline depletion impairs the corticosterone response to footshock but does not affect conditioned fear. *J Neuroendocrinol* 1993;4:773–779.

64. Simson PG, Weiss JM, Hoffman LJ, Ambrose MJ. Reversal of behavioral depression by infusion of an alpha-2 adrenergic agonist into the locus ceruleus. *Neuropharmacology* 1986;25:385–389.

65. Smith AP, Wilson SJ, Glue P, Nutt DJ. The effects and after-effects of the alpha-2-adrenoceptor antagonist idazoxan on mood, memory and attention in normal volunteers. *J Psychopharmacol* 1992; 6:385–389.

66. Sparenborg S, Gabriel M. Local norepinephrine depletion and learning-related neuronal activity in cingulate cortex and anterior thalamus of rabbits. *Exp Brain Res* 1992;92:267–285.

67. Steketee JD, Silverman PB, Swann AC. Forebrain norepinephrine involvement in selective attention and neophobia. *Physiol Behav* 1989;46:577–583.

68. Steketee JD, Silverman PB, Swann AC. Noradrenergic mechanisms in neophobia. *Psychopharmacology* 1992;106:136–142.

69. Tassin J-P, Herve D, Vezina P, Trovero F, Blanc G, Glowinski J. Relationships between mesocortical and mesolimbic dopamine neurons: functional correlates of D1 receptor heteroregulation. In: Willner P, Scheel-Kruger J, eds. *The mesolimbic dopamine system: from motivation to action.* Chichester: Wiley, 1991;175–196.

70. Taylor JR, Elsworth JD, Garcia EJ, Grant SJ, Roth RH, Redmond DE Jr. Clonidine infusions into the locus coeruleus attenuate behavioral and neurochemical changes associated with naloxone-precipitated withdrawal. *Psychopharmacology* 1988;96:121–134.

71. Tsaltas E, Preston GC, Gray JA. The effects of dorsal bundle lesions on serial and trace conditioning. *Behav Brain Res* 1983;10:361–374.

72. Wenk G, Hughey D, Boundy V, Kim A, Walker L, Olton D. Neurotransmitters and memory; role of cholinergic, serotonergic and noradrenergic systems. *Behav Neurosci* 1987;101:325–332.

Psychopharmacology: The Fourth Generation of Progress, edited by Floyd E. Bloom and David J. Kupfer. Raven Press, Ltd., New York © 1995.

CHAPTER 33

Physiological and Anatomical Determinants of Locus Coeruleus Discharge

Behavioral and Clinical Implications

Rita J. Valentino and Gary S. Aston-Jones

The locus coeruleus (LC) noradrenergic system has been viewed as a broadly projecting system with nonspecific functions. This view of the LC was based in part on early anatomic findings which indicated that LC efferent projections were widespread, that single LC neurons send divergent projections to target cells of very different function, and that the nucleus was not topographically organized in a manner that could confer specificity. Similarly, early studies of LC afferents suggested a diversity nearly as great as its efferent projections, implying a lack of specificity in the types of stimuli that could affect LC activity and function. This concept of the LC as a "nonspecific" system was further supported by initial electrophysiological studies demonstrating that the effect of norepinephrine (NE) application or LC stimulation on postsynaptic targets was generally inhibition, regardless of the postsynaptic site studied. The last decade has brought advances in anatomic, physiological, and behavioral technology that has allowed for a more sophisticated analysis of the input and output relations of the LC–NE system. This chapter reviews recent studies that are refining our view of the LC–NE system as one that shows specifity in its response to various stimuli and in its effects on different target neurons (see Chapters 29 and 32 for other aspects, *this volume*).

ANATOMY

The anatomical and physiological characteristics of the LC have been most studied in the rat, cat, and primate.

The most obvious species difference is that LC neurons are homogeneously noradrenergic in rat and primate LC, although other neurotransmitters may be colocalized with norepinephrine in these neurons (see Chapter 30, *this volume*). In contrast, NE-containing neurons are interspersed with non-noradrenergic neurons in the LC of other species including cat. In order to limit discussion here to LC-noradrenergic neurons, most of the data reviewed will represent rat or primate studies, except where noted.

LC Afferents

Localization

The LC was originally thought to receive neurochemically and regionally diverse inputs. This was based on the numerous different neurochemically identified fibers in the LC area. The localization of binding sites for many of these neurotransmitters in the LC and their reported physiological effects on LC activity supported the notion that the LC received diverse afferent input. Table 1 summarizes the putative neurotransmitters that have been identified immunohistochemically in fibers in the LC region, neurotransmitter binding sites in the LC, and neurochemicals that directly affect LC neurons. However, these findings can be misleading and do not by themselves establish a particular neurotransmitter role for a substance in the LC. For example, the localization of neurotransmitter receptors does not necessarily match localization of nerve terminals containing the neurotransmitter. Additionally, the finding that a particular neurochemical affects LC discharge does not confirm that this is a physiologically relevant phenomena as opposed to a phar-

R. J. Valentino and G. S. Aston-Jones: Division of Behavioral Neurobiology, Department of Mental Health Sciences, Hahnemann University Medical School, Philadelphia, Pennsylvania 19102.

TABLE 1. *Evidence for neurotransmitter candidates in the LC locus coeruleus[a]*

Neurotransmitter[b]	Immunoreactive fibers	Binding sites	Effects
Acetylcholine	57	56	27
ACTH	70		47
Angiotensin II	21	43	72
CRF	66	12	66
Enkephalin	6, 37	7	Foote chapter, *this volume*
Epinephrine	44	73	6
Excitatory amino acids	18		5
GABA	46		69
Galanin	62		
Neuropeptide Y	60		
Neurotensin	64		47
Serotonin	50	71	5
Somatostatin	34	22	47
Substance P	51	52	27, 47
Vasopressin	13		47
VIP	14	42	67

[a] The numbers in columns 2–4 are reference numbers.
[b] ACTH, adrenocorticotropic hormone; CRF, corticotropin-releasing hormone; GABA, gamma-aminobutyric acid; VIP, vasoactive intestinal peptide.

macologic phenomena. Finally, the presence of neurotransmitter immunoreactivity in fibers in the LC region without ultrastructural confirmation of synapses is not convincing evidence for neurotransmission (e.g., fibers may be passing through to terminate elsewhere). Thus far, the most convincing evidence of functionally relevant input to the LC has come from a combination of (a) studies using tract tracers and immunohistochemistry to neurochemically identify and confirm afferents to the LC and (b) studies involving stimulation of putative afferents with simultaneous LC recording to physiologically confirm these inputs (see also Chapters 3 and 23, *this volume*).

Early retrograde tract-tracing studies of afferent input to LC which utilized the horseradish peroxidase (HRP)–diaminobenzidine (DAB) technique reported that more than 30 nuclei were labeled after injection of the tracer into the LC (6). Such findings suggested that the LC could be influenced by many structures and supported prevailing views that this was a general nonspecific system. The development in the last decade of tract tracers that could produce more focal injections has refined the number of nuclei projecting to the LC. These tracers include wheat germ agglutinin (WGA)-conjugated HRP, WGA-apoHRP coupled to colloidal gold (WGA-apoHRP-Au), the beta subunit of cholera toxin (CTb), and the fluorescent tracer, Fluoro-Gold. Using these tracers it has been demonstrated that the LC receives a far more restricted set of inputs than was originally believed (6). Two medullary nuclei, the nucleus paragigantocellularis (PGi) and nucleus prepositus hypoglossi (PrH), are prominent afferents to LC based on recent retrograde tract-tracing studies and electrophysiological evidence demonstrating that these nuclei directly impact on LC (see below). The PGi, localized in the rostral ventrolateral medulla, is of interest as an LC afferent because of its role in somatic, autonomic, and

visceral functions. Less is known about the function of cells in the PrH. However, oculomotor function has been attributed to the PrH, suggesting that this input to LC may integrate visual shifts in attention with cognitive shifts. Other areas that appear to send projections into the LC include the dorsal cap of the paraventricular nucleus of the hypothalamus, the intermediate zone of the spinal cord, the Kolliker-Fuse, periaqueductal gray, the lateral hypothalamus, and the preoptic area. However, it should be noted that fewer projections to the LC are found from these areas compared to PGi or PrH (6), and that these areas require further study to confirm direct projections to the LC proper. The involvement of some of these nuclei in stress and autonomic activity suggest possible routes whereby this information may reach the LC.

Anterograde tracing studies have confirmed that the PGi, the PrH, the ventrolateral periaqueductal gray, the Kolliker-Fuse, and the medial preoptic area project to the LC (6). However, dendrites of non-LC neurons extend into the LC nucleus, so that ultrastructural and electrophysiological studies are needed to confirm inputs to noradrenergic LC neurons; such electrophysiologic studies have confirmed functional inputs from the PGi and PrH (see below). In contrast, anterograde labeling from injections into areas previously thought to innervate the LC—including the VTA, the dorsal horn of the spinal cord, the rostral solitary nucleus, and the prefrontal cortex—was not apparent in the LC but was observed in structures surrounding LC (6). These findings indicate that these structures may innervate distal dendrites of LC neurons that extend into pericoerulear areas or that they may communicate with the LC only indirectly, perhaps by innervating pericoerulear regions. Anterograde labeling from amygdala, which was initially reported as a prominent LC afferent, was meager and was confined to the extreme rostral pole of the LC where NE neurons are interdigitated with non-NE neurons (6). Interestingly, the projections from the periaqueductal gray and from the preoptic nucleus terminate, for the most part, in pericoerulear regions that contain LC dendrites. Ultrastructural analysis of this region is necessary to evaluate the functional innervation of these dendrites. It is also possible that neurons in close proximity to the LC (i.e., Barrington's nucleus, lateral dorsal tegmentum) provide afferent input to the LC. However, it is difficult to determine whether these nuclei project to the LC using the available tracers because the close proximity of these nuclei to the LC prohibits any distinction between spread of tracer and actual retrograde labeling.

Neurochemical Identity

Many of the neurotransmitters reported to innervate the LC based on immunohistochemical localization of fibers in the LC are found in neurons of two major LC afferents, the PGi and PrH. These include PMNT (a marker for adrenaline) (31), excitatory amino acids (18), enkephalin (6,37), corticotropin-releasing factor (CRF) (66), substance P (38), serotonin (5-HT) (50), and gamma-aminobutyric acid (GABA) (46). Double labeling studies combining retrograde tract tracing and immunohistochemistry for glutaminase reveal putative glutaminergic neurons in PGi that project to the LC (6). This input has been confirmed physiologically and has been shown to mediate the well-characterized activation of LC neurons by footshock, as well as LC activation associated with opiate withdrawal (see below). Adrenergic innervation of the LC derives primarily from the PGi, where more than 20% of LC afferent neurons are PMNT-immunoreactive, although a small percentage of adrenergic LC innervation may also derive from PrH (6). Ultrastructural studies revealed numerous PNMT-immunoreactive varicosities making conventional symmetric and asymmetric synapses onto LC dendrites, further supporting a neurotransmitter role for adrenaline in the LC (44). Indeed, adrenaline may mediate a part of the postactivation inhibition associated with LC responses to footshock (see below). The PrH contains a large percentage (>40%) of LC projecting neurons that are GAD- or GABA-immunoreactive (6). Other nuclei, including the PGi, contain GAD- and GABA-immunoreactive neurons that project to the LC (46). The LC receives a rich enkephalinergic innervation (6), and ultrastructural studies indicate that enkephalin-immunoreactive terminals synapse on LC neurons (51), suggesting that the LC is an important target for opioid neurotransmission in the brain. This is consistent with the potent effects of opiates on LC neurons (see Chapters 27, 29, 46, 61, and 148, *this volume*). Recent double labeling studies revealed that a surprisingly large percentage of the LC projecting neurons in both PGi and PrH are immunoreactive for enkephalin (6).

The CRF innervation of the LC is noteworthy because the LC–NE system is sensitive to different stressors (see below). CRF was initially characterized as the hypothalamic hormone responsible for releasing adrenocorticotropin in response to stress and, therefore, as the initiator of the endocrine cascade of the stress response (65). Shortly after its characterization, numerous anatomic and behavioral studies suggested that CRF also acted as a neurotransmitter outside of the hypothalamic–pituitary axis to initiate other aspects of stress (66). The criteria for a neurotransmitter role for CRF have been most rigorously tested in the LC, and the results of these studies indicate that CRF acts as a neurotransmitter to activate the LC during hypotensive stress (see below). CRF input to LC appears to originate predominantly from the PGi (66). Interestingly, hypotensive stress also activates PGi neurons. Additionally, some CRF-immunoreactive neurons in the dorsal cap of the paraventricular nucleus are retrogradely labeled from the LC, and there are numerous pericoerulear CRF-containing neurons along the lateral border of the LC and rostromedial to the LC in Barrington's nucleus that may be a source of CRF fibers in LC (66).

Ultrastructural studies indicate that afferent terminations in the LC synapse on dendrites ranging between 0.5 and 2.5 μm in diameter and onto spine-like appendages on dendrites and cell bodies (26). Most of these synapses fall into four categories: (i) synapses with small round, densely packed vesicles (41%); (ii) those with large rounded vesicles (20%); (iii) synapses with large flattened vesicles (23%); and (iv) those with numerous small flattened vesicles (11%). The remaining 5% had mixtures of these and/or contained dense-core vesicles. Interestingly, there was no apparent segregation of symmetric and asymmetric junctions. If these different morphologic characteristics represent different afferents, this could suggest that different inputs converge in a common spatial distribution and that the net effect of inputs to an LC neuron will be an integration of these converging inputs.

Thus, afferent input to LC appears to be more restricted than previously believed, although it is neurochemically diverse. The physiological relevance of the LC afferents proposed from anatomic studies is described below. Their identity has been useful in understanding how various stimuli communicate with the LC.

LC Efferents

Localization

Numerous immunohistochemical studies have described NE innervation of the central nervous system (CNS); and in combination with LC lesions or tract tracing, the distribution of the massive divergent LC projection system has been described (see ref. 17 for review). An important finding revealed by these studies is that the

LC is the sole source of norepinephrine in the forebrain, as well as a major contributor to other regions. The detailed distribution will not be described here except where it is applicable to the functional correlates of the LC described below.

That the LC is important in sensory processing is suggested by its innervation of the spinal cord and sensory nuclei in brainstem and pons. The target of spinally projecting LC neurons has been the subject of controversy, because earlier studies suggested that this was the ventral horn, implicating the LC in motor function (17). However, several more recent studies convincingly demonstrate a bilateral innervation from the LC to the dorsal horn, terminating particularly in superficial layers such as the substantia gelatinosa (20). There has been general agreement that the LC does not innervate intermediolateral column of the thoracic cord (20). This pattern of innervation supports a role for the LC in analgesia and sensory information processing, as opposed to motor or autonomic function. The pattern of LC innervation of brainstem and pontine nuclei are also consistent with a role in sensory information processing rather than autonomic function. Most LC innervation of the pons is to sensory and association nuclei, whereas autonomic nuclei receive norepinephrine innervation from other noradrenergic nuclei (19). It is noteworthy, for example, that the LC densely innervates the trigeminal nucleus—particularly pars caudalis, which is involved in sensory information from the face (19).

The LC is the sole source of NE in the cerebellum (17). Ultrastructural studies of this innervation reveal NE synapses onto Purkinje cell dendrites (17). These findings led to numerous electrophysiological and pharmacological studies of the effects of NE and LC stimulation on Purkinje cell activity which have served as a model for studying the postsynaptic impact of this system (see below).

In contrast to many brain areas, the hypothalamus receives only a minor noradrenergic innervation from LC that is localized in the medial part of the parvocellular paraventricular nucleus of the hypothalamus, a region containing neurons that project to the median eminence (17). This innervation suggests that the LC may modulate neuroendocrine function. Interestingly, although the LC receives a minor input from the paraventricular nucleus of the hypothalamus, cells that project to the LC are localized more dorsally, arguing against the possibility of reciprocal communications (66). The LC also projects to the preoptic nucleus and bed nucleus stria terminalis. Interestingly, the preoptic nucleus is a minor source of afferents to the LC, suggesting the possibility of reciprocal communications between the LC and this nucleus. The LC innervates thalamic sensory relay nuclei for the visual and somatosensory cortex, the lateral geniculate nucleus, and ventrobasal complex, respectively, and there is a dense NE innervation from the LC to the thalamic reticular nucleus which coordinates thalamocortical activity

(17). The effects of LC stimulation or NE application on thalamic neuronal activity have been one of the more well-characterized postsynaptic effects of this system. These effects suggest a model whereby LC activation can produce a shift from drowsiness to the alert state, perhaps underlying the importance of the LC in arousal (see Chapter 29, *this volume*).

The LC is the sole source of NE in the hippocampus and neocortex, and the projection is predominantly (90%) unilateral (17). The pattern of LC innervation of cortex shows a distinct laminar distribution with little variation between different areas of cortex. The patterns of innervation of these structures and specific projection pathways from LC have been described in detail elsewhere (17).

Another LC target of interest is the olfactory bulb, which receives all NE innervation from the LC (58). The termination patterns suggest that the major target cell in this structure is the granule cell, a GABA interneuron that provides inhibitory feedback to the major output cells of the olfactory bulb, namely, the mitral and tufted cells.

An interesting characteristic of LC projections is their divergence, suggesting that changes in LC activity can influence neurons of diverse functions. This has been studied using multiple injections of retrograde tracers into the same structure but in different hemispheres or into different structures (17). The results of these studies indicate that a single LC neuron can project to different cortical hemispheres: to hippocampus and cortex, to thalamus and cortex, to thalamus and hippocampus, and to forebrain and spinal cord. This divergence supports the idea that changes in LC discharge can simultaneously impact on functionally diverse targets, and this could be one way in which the LC could coordinate the activity of multiple systems into a symptom complex as has been hypothesized to occur in opiate withdrawal or stress (see Chapters 27 and 148, *this volume*).

Topography

In spite of the clear evidence for the divergence of LC projections, it is becoming recognized that there is some topographical organization of LC efferents, which implies a greater specificity in the effects of this system than was originally believed. Recent studies indicate that topographically organized LC neurons with specific projections may also be distinguished morphologically (17). This is perhaps most apparent for projections to spinal cord which appear to originate from large multipolar neurons in the ventral third of the LC (17). These neurons may also project to the cerebellum. Although this population overlaps spatially with LC cortically projecting neurons, it appears to be distinct. Anterior large multipolar neurons are thought to project primarily to the hypothalamus and perhaps the septum (17). Additionally, small round neurons in the ventral LC project to the hypothalamus. In the core, medium multipolar neurons project to multiple targets, including the neocortex, the hippocampus, the hypothalamus, the cerebellum, and the spinal cord. However, there appears to be a modest topographic organization within the core as well: Core cells in the dorsal two-thirds of the LC project to the neocortex, the hippocampus, the hypothalamus, and the cerebellum, but not to the spinal cord, and core cells in the ventral third project primarily to the spinal cord and the cerebellum, but not to the hippocampus (17). Fusiform cells on the dorsal edge of the LC are thought to project to the hippocampus (17). Waterhouse et al. (68) detailed the topography of cortically projecting LC neurons. In this study, cortically projecting LC neurons were localized in the caudal three-fifths of the dorsal ipsilateral LC nucleus. Within this region, groups of cells identified as projecting to occipital, sensorimotor, or frontal cortex were observed to form a dorsal-to-ventral gradient, whereas occipital-projecting neurons tended to be more caudal. The frontal cortex received innervation from LC neurons in both dorsal and ventral subdivisions of the nucleus. These findings differ with earlier studies concluding that cortically projecting LC neurons are randomly distributed in the nucleus with the exception of the ventral division. It is possible that LC neurons sharing similar morphology and topography within the nucleus may also share other characteristics (such as afferents or colocalization of other neurotransmitters) with NE. While further studies are needed to explore such possibilities, this would be one mechanism whereby specialization of LC function could be conferred.

Ultrastructural Studies

Early reports using electron microscopic (EM) autoradiographic examination of NE terminals in the cerebral cortex concluded that most NE terminals did not make synaptic contacts, but rather existed as nonsynaptically arranged terminals to provide NE in a paracrine fashion to a local cortical area (11). In contrast, quantitative studies in hippocampus demonstrated that NE terminals formed specialized synaptic junctions with other neurons as frequently as did non-NE terminals (17). In addition, more recent studies using serial EM reconstruction of NE synapses in cerebral cortex identified with dopamine-β-hydroxylase (DBH) immunohistochemistry found that a great majority of NE terminals form conventional synaptic contact onto neuronal profiles (49). These studies are consistent with those of Olschowka et al. (48), who found that most DBH-immunoreactive terminals in areas of the diencephalon, cerebellum, and limbic cortex form axodendritic synapses characterized by specialized junctional appositions. Thus, considerable evidence exists to indicate that this system does use conventional synaptic transmission at many, if not all, of its terminations. It is also possible that both synaptic and paracrine modes of neurotransmission exist at the same or different NE terminals.

Other ultrastructural studies reveal tyrosine hydroxlyase terminals in apposition to astrocytic processes that stain for β-receptor antibody, suggesting that one mode of communication of LC with its targets may be via alterations in glial function (4). Future ultrastructural studies are necessary to confirm the mechanism by which the LC communicates with its numerous targets.

PHYSIOLOGY

Afferents

Antidromic Studies

The anatomic demonstration of specific inputs to the LC is not sufficient to verify function; this requires physiological confirmation. Thus, electrical stimulation of sources of LC afferents should alter activity of LC neurons, and LC stimulation should antidromically activate neurons that project to the LC. These techniques have been used to confirm afferents from the PGi and PrH proposed by anatomic studies. Electrical stimulation of the LC was found to antidromically activate >20% of neurons recorded in the PGi and PrH, but few or no neurons in the nucleus tractus solitarius, contralateral LC, or lateral reticular nucleus (6). Interestingly, these studies suggested at least two physiologically distinct populations of LC afferents in PGi, based on differential latencies to antidromic stimulation of the LC.

Orthodromic Activation

Electrical stimulation of PGi produces two effects on LC neurons. An excitation of short latency which is sensitive to non-N-methyl-D-aspartate (non-NMDA) excitatory amino acid receptor antagonists is most often observed (6). This putative excitatory amino acid afferent appears to be important in LC activation by a number of stimuli. For example, the characteristic response of LC neurons to footshock or pressure is also prevented by excitatory amino acid antagonists that are selective for non-NMDA receptors and by reversible inactivation of the PGi with local lidocaine or GABA injections (6) (also see below). An inhibitory response to PGi stimulation has also been reported and is thought to be due to activation of adrenaline-containing C1 neurons because it is prevented by the α2 antagonist, idazoxan (6). These findings confirm the anatomic studies which indicate that the LC receives a major adrenergic input from the PGi.

In contrast to PGi stimulation, electrical stimulation of PrH primarily inhibited LC neurons (6). This inhibition was eliminated by GABA antagonists, but not by opiate or α2 receptor antagonists, implicating GABA in this response. This is consistent with immunohistochemical observations of GABA-containing neurons in the PrH.

Similar physiological evidence for a functionally substantive projection to LC from other proposed afferents has not been obtained to date. Electrical stimulation of the central nucleus of the amygdala, nucleus of the solitary tract, or medial prefrontal cortex does not consistently alter LC activity, although earlier anatomic studies implicated these regions as LC afferents (6). Stimulation of these regions more often resulted in synaptic activation of areas adjacent to the LC such as the parabrachial nucleus or Barrington's nucleus. These results confirm the more recent anatomic studies revealing projections to these pericoerulear regions but not to the LC nucleus proper.

Thus, electrophysiological and pharmacologic studies are beginning to confirm anatomic studies suggesting a relatively restricted input to LC. An important aspect of these studies is the neurochemical diversity of afferents to LC from a common region. These results suggest that specificity of LC responses to various stimuli may be conferred by different neurotransmitter inputs. This appears to be the case for different stressors, as discussed below.

Efferents

Electrophysiological Studies

The postsynaptic effects of NE application or LC stimulation on targets of this system are described elsewhere in this volume (see Foote and Aston-Jones, *this volume*) and will only be reviewed briefly here. Of interest to this chapter it is important to note that just as the LC–NE system initally appeared to be "nonselective" because of its anatomic characteristics, the initial physiological studies of the system supported this general view. Thus, early investigations into the postsynaptic effects of the LC–NE system demonstrated a generalized inhibition of target cells. This effect was initially characterized in detail on cerebellar Purkinje neurons and subsequently noted in hippocampus, cortex, thalamus, and hypothalamus, suggesting that a global effect of the LC–NE system was inhibition (see ref. 17 for review). However, later studies revealed more complex effects of NE application that were concentration-dependent, whereby low doses selectively enhanced the effects of afferent inputs (evoked activity) relative to basal or spontaneous discharge, while higher doses resulted in inhibition. These effects were observed in the cerebellum, the cortex, and the hypothalamus and led to the idea that LC activation increases the "signal-to-noise" ratio of activity in postsynaptic neurons (17). More support for this idea came from studies demonstrating that NE and LC stimulation potentiated the effects of both excitatory and inhibitory neurotransmitters on the same neuron (17). Taken together, these effects suggested that the LC–NE system functioned to increase processing of information about incoming sensory stimuli, as opposed to solely altering basal discharge rate.

Although comparable effects of LC activation are observed on different postsynaptic targets, the net effect on a particular neuron may depend on properties of the circuit in which the neuron functions. For example, one effect attributed to NE is gating of postsynaptic activity, whereby a cell which was previously unresponsive to a stimulus becomes responsive in the presence of NE. This effect was demonstrated for visually evoked responses of cerebellar Purkinje neurons in the parafloccular lobe (69). Another related effect of NE, observed in the visual cortex of the cat, is to refine receptive fields. NE application onto visual cortical neurons resulted in more sharply defined transitions between stimulus-induced inhibition and excitation; that is, it sharpened the receptive field (69). This effect would be predicted to enhance the ability to detect stimulus movement across receptive field boundaries. Another effect of NE and LC stimulation may be to alter patterns of neuronal firing. For example, in the thalamus NE can shift the pattern of neuronal activity from a "bursting" mode, which is associated with slow-wave sleep and drowsiness, to a single-spike firing mode, which is associated with (a) transmission of sensory stimuli to the cerebral cortex and (b) waking and attention. This pattern shift may, in part, underlie LC effects on arousal (see Chapter 29, *this volume*).

Neurochemical Studies

Although it is generally assumed that LC discharge rate is proportional to NE release in target areas, this relationship has yet to be systematically characterized. This is important because some hypothesized functions of the LC–NE system have been generated by integrating (a) studies that quantify LC discharge rate under different conditions and (b) studies characterizing the effects of NE on target cell activity. The assumption that increases in LC discharge produce sufficient NE release in targets to mimic the effects reported in postsynaptic studies underlies the integration of these two types of studies into a hypothesis of LC function. Unfortunately, this assumption can only be tested in studies that combine recordings of activity in both LC and target regions simultaneously during manipulation, and these studies are few (however, see Chapter 29, *this volume*). The link between LC discharge and target cell effect (i.e., NE release) has recently been examined in voltammetry and microdialysis studies. These studies have demonstrated that stimuli that are known to increase LC rate also increase NE levels in extracellular fluid or increase the NE signal as measured by voltammetry in postsynaptic targets (cortex, hippocampus, and thalamus) of the LC–NE system. These stimuli include footshock, restraint stress, electrical and chemical stimulation of the LC or dorsal noradrenergic bundle, and administration of α_2 receptor antagonists (1,8,29). Interestingly, some studies demonstrate that NE release increases in a nonlinear manner with increasing frequencies of dorsal bundle stimulation, suggesting that during bursts of high-frequency activity, such as when LC discharge is evoked by phasic sensory stimuli, NE release per action potential is greater than when LC discharge is tonically elevated (8). Unfortunately, in the above neurochemical studies, LC discharge was not recorded simultaneously, so that the relationship between LC discharge and NE release still remains to be established. For example, it is not known to what extent, and for how long a duration, LC discharge must be elevated to produce increases in NE release in targets, and whether the amount of release is target-specific. An interesting finding of the neurochemical studies is that NE release in a particular region may be dependent on the mode of sensory stimulus that activates the LC. This was recently demonstrated in a study of the effects of visual stimulation on NE release (measured by voltammetry) in different cortical regions (41). This study demonstrated that NE release in monkey striate cortex exhibits an ocular dominance paralleling the ocular dominance for cortical neuron activation. Moreover, in the cat, visual stimuli that elicited NE release in visual cortex failed to do so in somatosensory cortex. A possible explanation for the local specificity of NE release is that it may be regulated presynaptically by cortical afferents activated by specific stimuli. This type of presynaptic heteroregulation of NE release could be a mechanism for conferring specificity on the LC–NE system within terminal areas.

FUNCTIONS

The proposed functions attributed to the LC–NE system have been based on lesion studies, pharmacologic studies, and electrophysiological recordings from LC neurons under different conditions (see Chapters 29 and 32, *this volume*). The putative roles of the LC in arousal, vigilance, attention, and learning are discussed in detail in other chapters in this volume and will not be reviewed here. This chapter focuses on putative functions derived from new knowledge of the input–output relations of the LC.

Pain and Analgesia

One characteristic of LC neurons that has implicated this nucleus in pain is that they are conspicuously activated by noxious stimuli. In waking animals, LC cells are activated by low-level stimuli of many modalities (described in ref. 17). However, these neurons are most reliably activated by either noxious or stressful stimuli. This fact is best illustrated by comparing LC sensory responsiveness in anesthetized versus unanesthetized animals.

The sensory sensitivity of LC neurons is markedly reduced under anesthesia. Indeed, reduced LC activity and responsiveness may be one of the hallmark actions of

anesthetic treatments. For example, LC neurons are potently activated by a variety of stimuli in waking animals, including auditory, visual, and non-noxious somatosensory events. In contrast, these cells recorded under anesthesia do not respond to any of these stimuli, but are activated exclusively by noxious stimuli such as foot or tail pinch or sciatic nerve activation (17). As another example, the magnitude of LC activation by hypotensive stress is more than 10 times greater in unanesthetized rats than in anesthetized ones (66). Similarly, the effects of pharmacological agents on LC discharge are dependent on the state of anesthesia. Thus, the stress neurohormone, corticotropin-releasing factor (CRF), increases LC spontaneous discharge rate and is more potent and efficacious in unanesthetized rats than in anesthetized ones (66). In contrast, morphine, which inhibits LC spontaneous discharge rate, is much less potent and less efficacious in unanesthetized rats than in anesthetized rats (66).

As noted above, under anesthesia LC neurons lose their responsiveness to nearly all low-level stimuli and become selectively sensitive to strongly noxious or stressful events. A particularly well-studied noxious stimulus that potently activates LC neurons is sciatic nerve or subcutaneous electrical footshock stimulation; similar results are seen with tail or paw pinch. Short-lasting stimuli of this type elicit a brisk, phasic activation of LC neurons consistently over many presentations. This is seen under a variety of anesthetics when LC neurons are insensitive to non-noxious auditory, tactile, or visual stimuli. These findings indicate that LC neurons are particularly responsive to noxious sensory stimuli. Recent studies by our group reveal that activation of peripheral C fibers (thought to mediate painful stimuli) by high-intensity stimuli yields a specific, long-latency response of LC neurons not observed with stimuli that activate only rapidly conducting peripheral nerves. This C-fiber-mediated response summates with the response to lower-threshold fast-conducting fibers to produce a substantially greater response in the LC for nociceptive versus non-nociceptive stimuli. This indicates that the LC system may play a role in processing of painful stimuli, a result consistent with antinociceptive effects of LC activity (discussed below).

Another important aspect of these responses is that all LC neurons are similarly activated, so that a noxious stimulus elicits concerted activation from the entire LC nucleus. This homogeneity of LC activity is true for all other physiological properties examined as well. Recent evidence reveals that LC activation by footshock and tail or paw pinch is due to an excitatory amino acid (EAA; i.e., glutamate or aspartate) transmitter input (6); this suggests avenues for pharmacologic manipulation of LC responses to painful stimuli. Because of the problems of maintaining recordings during abrupt, severe movements, the effects of painful stimuli on LC activity have not been well-studied in unanesthetized animals.

LC activation is associated with antinociception via projections to the spinal cord. Recent neurophysiological work by a number of groups indicates that LC activation can produce potent antinociception. For example, Jones and Gebhart (35,36) have shown that electrical or chemical activation of the LC area in lightly anesthetized rats can substantially increase the threshold for nociception, measured as increased latency for tail-flick to avoid a heat stimulus. Using a variety of receptor antagonists, these workers also found that this antinociceptive action of LC stimulation was mediated by spinal α_2-type adrenoceptors. Consistent with this, pharmacological studies have shown that intrathecal administration of α-adrenergic agonists produces dose-dependent analgesia (55). The mechanism for the antinociceptive effect associated with LC stimulation is indicated by studies of activity of neurons in the spinal dorsal horn in response to LC stimulation. Results indicate that LC activation significantly decreases the response of these cells that are early in the pain pathway to noxious stimuli (30). Furthermore, the effect of LC activation appeared to be somewhat selective because responses of dorsal horn neurons to noxious stimuli and input mediated by C and Aδ fibers were inhibited to a greater extent by LC activation than were responses of the same neurons to non-noxious stimuli or inputs mediated by faster-conducting fibers (45). These results have given rise to the idea of a descending noradrenergic antinociceptive system from the LC to the spinal dorsal horn and trigeminal system. These findings fit well with the above results for potent activation of LC neurons by noxious stimuli, and they suggest that antinociception may be part of a global influence of the activated LC system to facilitate rapid and adaptive responses to urgent stimuli (discussed below).

Drug Dependence and Withdrawal

Virtually all classes of abused drugs affect LC discharge characteristics at doses that are in the range of those abused by humans. These include hallucinogens, stimulants, opiates, alcohol, nicotine, and benzodiazepines. Much of the work on the LC in substance abuse has focused on physical dependence and withdrawal symptoms. This interest has, in part, been generated by the usefulness of α_2-adrenergic agonists such as clonidine, which suppresses LC activity, in the alleviation of withdrawal symptoms for several dependence-producing substances. However, pharmacological investigations into the acute effects of some of these agents on LC discharge suggest that the LC may also play a role in other central effects of these drugs, and they are revealing the importance of particular LC afferents in these effects.

Nicotine

Nicotine produces a potent activation of LC neurons when administered systemically (16). Surprisingly, recent evidence indicates that this effect of nicotine is not mediated in the LC, or even initiated in the brain, but results from nicotinic activation of primary sensory C-fiber afferents (28). For example, in contrast to intravenous (i.v.) administration, local iontophoretic application of nicotine is ineffective on LC activity (16). Systemic administration of quaternary nicotinic agonists, which would not be expected to cross the blood–brain barrier, mimic the effects of nicotine, and systemic administration of quaternary nicotinic antagonists prevent the effect of i.v. nicotine, consistent with the idea that nicotine is acting at peripheral receptors. Several findings indicate that LC activation by systemic nicotine is mediated by primary sensory C-fiber afferents and subsequent activation of excitatory amino acid LC afferents from PGi. Thus, nicotine effects on LC are prevented by capsaicin lesion of primary sensory C-fiber afferents (28), by excitatory amino acid antagonists, and by chemical inactivation of the PGi (16). In addition to increasing LC discharge, nicotine also alters discharge pattern such that burst activity is more frequent. Assuming that NE release from LC neurons is greater during burst modes, the net effect of nicotine may be to elicit more effective NE release in targets and, via effects on thalamocortical activity, produce short-lasting periods of enhanced arousal (see also Chapter 147, *this volume*).

Cocaine

Like nicotine, cocaine and amphetamine-like drugs produce arousal and heightened vigilance at certain doses. However, in contrast to nicotine, the action of these CNS stimulants on LC activity is primarily inhibitory, presumably through activation of presynaptic α_2 receptors by increased levels of synaptic NE. Because synaptic levels of NE are also elevated in postsynaptic targets by these stimulants, the net effect of a dose of cocaine or amphetamine will be an integration of these two opposing effects. In this regard, doses of cocaine that inhibit LC discharge rate enhanced cerebellar responsiveness to synaptic activation and iontophoretically applied neurotransmitters in a manner similar to the effects of iontophoretically applied NE (33). These studies suggest that cocaine effects on NE release in terminal regions predominate over inhibitory effects on LC cell bodies. It is likely that there is an optimal dose of cocaine at which the function of the LC–NE system is enhanced. Consistent with this, in unanesthetized rats, doses of cocaine that are in the intermediate range of the dose response for LC inhibition (0.3–3.0 mg/kg, i.v.) (10) are similar to those that have been shown to improve performance by rats in tasks requiring sustained attention (2.5 mg/kg) (25). Doses higher than this did not improve performance (see also Chapter 147, *this volume*).

Opiates

The prominent enkephalinergic input to LC, taken together with the high density of opiate receptors in this nucleus and the potent effects of opioid peptides and synthetic opiates on LC discharge, has implicated the LC as integral to endogenous opioid function as well as to the pharmacologic effects of opiates. Unfortunately, the role of LC in endogenous opioid function has been difficult to determine because opiate antagonists have little effect on LC discharge, indicating that this input is not tonically active. The LC is not unique in this regard because opiate antagonists have also been reported to have little effect in other brain regions that contain opioid peptidergic terminals (e.g., hippocampus). Future studies aimed at determining conditions under which the opioid input to LC is active will be necessary to determine the function of the LC in endogenous opioid effects.

In contrast to their lack of effect in naive animals, opiate antagonists produce a dramatic, potent, long-lasting excitation of LC neurons of rats that have chronically received opiates (see Chapters 5 and 29, *this volume*). This effect has been the basis for rationalizing the use of clonidine, which inhibits LC discharge, in the treatment of opiate withdrawal (23). Only a fraction of this excitation occurs in vitro, suggesting that a critical site of action of opiate antagonists is on cell bodies of LC afferents rather than on LC neurons or presynaptic terminals of LC afferents (9).

An excitatory amino acid input from PGi has been implicated in the bulk of LC activation associated with opiate withdrawal. Excitatory amino acid antagonists administered into the LC prior to opiate antagonists attenuate LC withdrawal excitation, and the same drugs significantly reverse this response when given after withdrawal is precipitated (2). Excitatory amino acid antagonists selective for non-NMDA receptors are more effective than selective NMDA antagonists, although both produce a significant attenuation of the activation. PGi lesions also attenuate increases in LC discharge associated with opiate withdrawal (53). The finding that excitatory amino acid antagonists do not completely reverse withdrawal-induced LC activation suggests that although a major component of this activation is mediated by opiate antagonist actions on cell bodies of excitatory amino acid LC afferents, a minor component is mediated by nonexcitatory amino acid mechanisms.

The elucidation of the circuitry underlying LC activation during opiate withdrawal has led to novel approaches of manipulating this activation. Initial studies focused on directly inhibiting LC discharge using α_2-adrenergic agonists, such as clonidine. More recent studies suggest that serotonergic agents may attenuate LC activation without affecting basal LC discharge. Iontophoresis of serotonin onto LC neurons markedly attenuated activation of LC neurons by the EAA glutamate, but had no consistent effect on either basal activity or acetylcholine-evoked activity of LC neurons (5; see also Chapters 5 and 29, *this volume*). Because EAAs mediate hyperactivity of LC neurons during opiate withdrawal, these results led to the prediction that augmentation of serotonergic neurotrans-

mission within the LC may attenuate withdrawal-induced hyperactivity. Indeed, our group has recently found that intravenous administration of indirect serotonin agonists, including the uptake blockers fluoxetine or sertraline or the serotonin releaser/uptake blocker fenfluramine, substantially attenuates the hyperactivity of LC neurons associated with morphine withdrawal (3). A similar effect was also seen in preliminary studies using local administration of fenfluramine, indicating that a possible site of action was within the LC. Furthermore, this attenuation of withdrawal hyperactivity was prevented by depletion of serotonin with PCPA, indicating that the effect was mediated through endogenous serotonin systems. Because hyperactivity of LC neurons has been implicated in a number of symptoms of opiate withdrawal, these results suggest a new pharmacotherapy for treating withdrawal which may be without the side effects of presently used agents.

The translation of LC activation to behavioral or physiological withdrawal symptoms remains controversial. The LC area was found to be the most sensitive site for the elicitation of motor aspects of opiate withdrawal by intracerebrally injected quaternary opiate antagonists (40). Moreover, electrolytic lesion of the LC attenuated wet dog shakes, mastication, rearing, piloerection, hyperactivity, ptosis, and eye twitch associated with precipitated opiate withdrawal, although these elicited signs were not completely abolished (39). Interestingly, attenuation of LC activation by administration of excitatory amino acid antagonists does not consistently alter the withdrawal syndrome as determined by scoring elicited behaviors in rats (54). However, as mentioned above, these agents do not completely abolish LC activation associated with precipitated withdrawal (see Chapters 27, 29, 61, and 148, *this volume*).

Stress and Physiological Challenges

LC and LC Afferents

Neurochemical and electrophysiological studies over the past 15 years support a strong link between stress and activation of the LC–NE system. The earliest studies implicating the LC in stress demonstrated that stress was associated with increased NE turnover in brain regions known to receive their sole NE input from the LC (i.e., hippocampus, cortex), suggesting that stress increases NE release (see ref. 66 for review). More recently, this has been substantiated by microdialysis studies, which provide a better indication of NE release (1). A likely cause of enhanced NE release during stress is increased discharge of LC neurons, and this is supported by findings that stress increases tyrosine hydroxylase expression in LC cell bodies (see Chapters 27 and 61, *this volume*). Electrophysiological studies in which LC activity is recorded during stress have provided more direct evidence that the increases in NE function in postsynaptic targets is due to increased LC activity. In unanesthetized cats, both environmental and physiological challenges including hypoglycemia, hyperthermia, hemorrhage, hypotension, restraint, and aversive auditory stimuli increase LC discharge, and this is usually accompanied by autonomic activation (32,66). Similarly, in anesthetized rats, physiological challenges such as hypotension and hypercarbia increase LC discharge rate and activate sympathetic nerve discharge (63,66). The frequent coactivation of sympathetic activity and LC discharge may be functionally significant and may reflect the fact that the PGi prominently innervates both the LC and the preganglionic sympathetic nucleus in spinal lateral horn. However, it should be noted that coactivation of sympathetic and LC activity does not always occur and the two effects are not always temporally correlated, suggesting that sympathetic activation is neither the initial stimulus for, or a consequence of, LC activation (15,63). In spite of this distinction, the finding that both LC and the autonomic nervous system are often activated in parallel is consistent with the possibility that a common brain site (e.g., nucleus PGi) relays stress-related information to both the LC and autonomic nervous system.

Although stressors and physiological challenges have long been associated with activation of the LC–NE system, only recently has the circuitry underlying this activation been investigated. Particularly, it was not clear whether stressors of different modalities activated the LC via a common "stress" pathway or by different afferents, specific for the type of stressors. Recent studies have addressed this by pharmacologically characterizing LC activation by two physiological challenges, namely, hypotension and bladder distention. These studies suggest that LC activation by different stressors is mediated by different neurotransmitter inputs. Several findings indicate that LC activation by hypotension is mediated by CRF afferents to LC. For example, hypotensive stress elicited by i.v. nitroprusside infusion mimics the effects of intracerebroventricularly administered CRF on LC discharge; that is, it increases spontaneous discharge rate and disrupts LC responses to phasic sensory stimuli. Intracerebroventricular (i.c.v.) administration or intracoerulear microinfusion of CRF antagonists prevents LC activation by hypotensive stress, but not LC activation by footshock (66). This is in contrast to excitatory amino acid antagonists which prevent LC activation by footshock, but not by hypotensive stress (66). Taken together, these findings suggest that hypotensive stress is associated with neuronal CRF release within the LC which then activates LC neurons.

Similar pharmacologic experiments have elucidated the neurotransmitter involved in LC activation by bladder distention (66). In contrast to LC activation by hypotension, LC activation by bladder distention is largely prevented by i.c.v. or local administration of excitatory amino acid antagonists, but not by i.c.v. administration of the CRF antagonist, α-helical CRF$_{9-41}$. Antagonists

that are more selective for non-NMDA receptors are much more effective than NMDA-type receptor antagonists. Thus, the pharmacology for LC activation by bladder distention is similar to that for LC activation by footshock and opiate withdrawal and may involve similar LC afferents.

The studies cited above indicate that LC activation by stressors of different modalities is mediated by different neurotransmitter inputs to LC. Figure 1 illustrates the potential pathways and neurotransmitters thought to be involved in LC activation by different challenges. Thus, LC activation by footshock, bladder distention, nicotine, and opiate withdrawal require excitatory amino acid neurotransmission in LC which may originate (at least in part) from the nucleus PGi. In contrast, LC activation by hypotensive stimuli require CRF afferents to the LC. This argues against the idea of a common neural substrate for LC activation by stressors and suggests a certain degree of specificity with regard to responses of LC neurons to stress. Because the LC is activated by a variety of stressors, the elucidation of the neurotransmitters and pathways involved in the effects of specific stressors will likely be a focus of future investigations.

LC Efferents

Recent studies combining LC unit recording with cortical electroencephalographic (EEG) activity have begun to address the functional consequences of elevated LC discharge during stress. These studies demonstrated that LC activation produced by hypotension is accompanied by, and necessary for, forebrain EEG activation (66). Bilateral LC inactivation produced by intracoerulear clonidine injection prevented EEG activation associated with hypotension (66). Likewise, bilateral injection of CRF antagonists into the LC prevented both LC and EEG activation by hypotensive challenge (66). These studies suggest that CRF serves as a neurotransmitter to activate the LC during hypotensive stress and that one function of this is to maintain or increase EEG arousal. Interestingly, LC activation during hypotensive stress does not appear to impact on autonomic function because when this is prevented by CRF antagonists, the magnitude and duration of the hypotensive response is unaltered (66). This is consistent with anatomic findings that the LC does not substantially project to autonomic nuclei.

Other findings are consistent with the view that cortical arousal may be a common consequence of LC activation by multiple stimuli. Bladder distention, like hypotensive stress, increases LC discharge and activates the electroencephalogram, and both of these effects are prevented by pretreatment with excitatory amino acid antagonists (66). Recently, selective pharmacologic manipulation of LC discharge has been shown to have profound effects on forebrain electrophysiology recorded as electroencephalogram (see Chapters 5 and 29, *this volume*). Taken to-

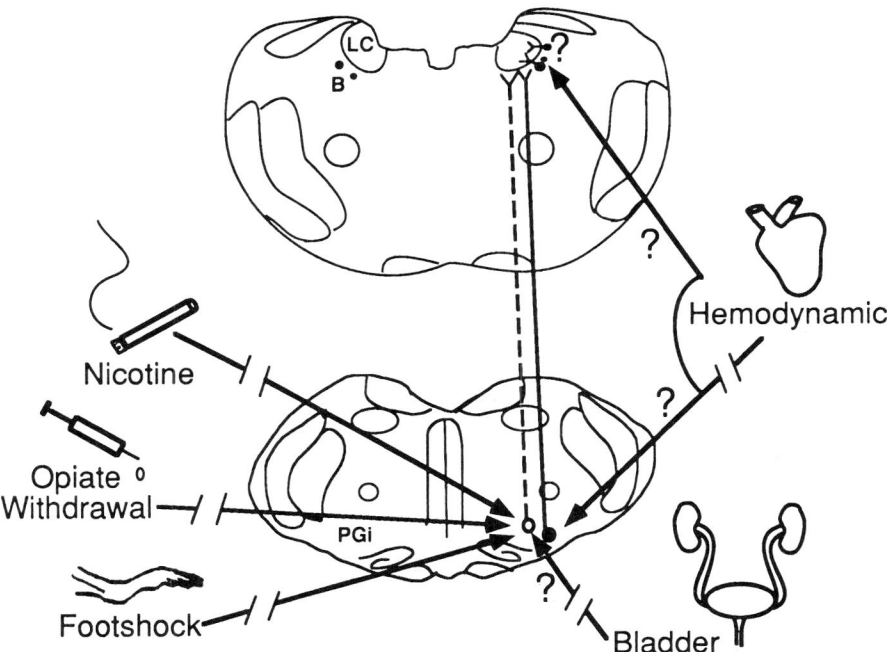

FIG. 1. Schematic illustrating possible pathways involved in LC activation by different stimuli. The top coronal section is at the level of LC. The bottom coronal section is at the level of the PGi. Substantial evidence suggests that LC activation produced by nicotine, opiate withdrawal, and footshock is mediated by excitatory amino acid afferents (*open circle, dotted line*) from PGi. Although LC activation by bladder distention requires excitatory amino acid afferents to the LC, the source of these afferents have not been determined (indicated by "?"). LC activation by hemodynamic stress requires CRF input to the LC (*solid circles, solid line*), although the source of these afferents has not been established (indicated by "?"). Potential sources of CRF input to LC that may mediate this activation include the PGi, pericoerulear CRF neurons such as Barrington's nucleus (B), or the dorsal cap of the paraventricular nucleus of the hypothalamus (not shown). Breaks in the lines leading from the stimulus to the brainstem indicate that the circuitry underlying the activation of LC afferents by the different stimuli is unknown.

gether, these results argue for at least one common consequence of LC activation regardless of the input (i.e., EEG arousal).

Psychiatric Disorders

Because of the limitations of animal models of psychiatric disease, it has been more difficult to ascertain a role of the LC or its afferents in specific psychiatric disorders. Of the clinical phenomena that have implicated the LC–NE system, depression has been the most thoroughly studied, perhaps because of the neurochemical and pharmacological evidence that strongly supported the original biogenic amine hypothesis of depression. This hypothesis has been much revised since its original formulation such that it is now thought that dysfunctions, rather than decreased functions, of serotonin or norepinephrine systems are important (59). In addition to biogenic amine function, hypothalamic–pituitary–adrenal function is also abnormal in depression (61). However, the relationship between dysfunctions in these two systems was relatively understudied. The integration of findings from basic and clinical studies in the last few years has suggested that CRF

may be an important link between neuroendocrine and biogenic amine dysfunctions in depression. This has been partly based on the dual role of CRF as a hypothalamic neurohormone that initiates endocrine components of the stress response and as a neurotransmitter serving to activate the LC–NE system in stress. Substantial clinical neuroendocrine findings implicate enhanced hypothalamic CRF activity in the endocrine dysfunctions that characterize depression (24). A parallel increase in CRF neurotransmitter activity in the LC would be predicted to cause persistent activation of this nucleus, with disrupted responses to brief sensory stimuli. The consequences of this may be hyperarousal and inability to concentrate, two symptoms that are characteristic of depression. Nonetheless, these predictions are dependent on the assumption that hypothalamic and extrahypothalamic CRF are hypersecreted in parallel in depression, and this has yet to be demonstrated (see Chapters 45 and 84, *this volume*).

There are numerous other conditions in which the LC–NE system has clearly been implicated and which deserve mention. Dysfunction of the LC–NE system may be involved in attention deficit disorder based on the role of the LC in attention which is reviewed in more detail elsewhere in this volume (see Chapters 29 and 32). Indeed, drugs that are effective in this disorder profoundly affect LC activity and NE in postsynaptic targets. Future treatments of attention deficit disorder may focus on more controlled pharmacological manipulation of this system.

Marked parallels between the symptoms of post-traumatic stress disorder (PTSD) and LC hyperactivity suggest that LC dysfunction may be involved in this phenomenon. For example, PTSD is precipitated by stressful events, and stressors activate the LC. Certain symptoms of PTSD, including hypervigilance and sleep abnormalities, are also predictable signs of LC hyperactivity. Other symptoms of PTSD are characterized by autonomic hyperactivity (tachycardia, hypertension, pallor, flushing, and sweating), and there appear to be mechanisms by which peripheral sympathetic and central noradrenergic function can be activated in parallel (see above). These similarities between PTSD and LC function suggest that this may be a key nucleus whose dysregulation leads to perhaps some of the symptoms of PTSD (see also Chapter 34, *this volume*).

CONCLUSIONS

In the last four years, detailed analyses of the anatomy and physiology of the LC–NE system have provided substantial evidence that this system is more specifically organized than previously thought. Future questions will be directed at the level of specificity of this system and the mechanisms by which specificity is conferred. The studies necessary to answer these questions must focus on a better understanding of the topography of LC afferents and efferents, identification of the circuitry and neuromediators underlying LC responses to stimuli, more detailed analysis of the cellular effects of norepinephrine and/or LC stimulation on different postsynaptic targets, and quantification of the translation of LC discharge to postsynaptic effect. These future studies will help reveal the function of the LC–NE system in normal and pathologic conditions and how this system can be pharmacologically or behaviorally manipulated to treat psychiatric disorders.

REFERENCES

1. Abercrombie ED, Keller RW, Zigmond MJ. Characterization of hippocampal norepinephrine release as measured by microdialysis perfusion: pharmacological and behavioral studies. *Neuroscience* 1988;27:897–904.
2. Akaoka H, Aston-Jones G. Opiate withdrawal-induced hyperactivity of locus coeruleus neurons is substantially mediated by augmented excitatory amino acid input. *J Neurosci* 1991;11:3830–3839.
3. Akaoka H, Aston-Jones G. Indirect serotonergic agonists attenuate neuronal opiate withdrawal. *Neuroscience* 1993;54:561–565.
4. Aoki C. Beta-adrenergic receptors: astrocytic localization in the adult visual cortex and their relation to catecholamine axon terminals as revealed by electron microscope immunohistochemistry. *J Neurosci* 1992;12:781–792.
5. Aston-Jones G, Akaoka H, Charlety P, Chouvet G. Serotonin selectively attenuates glutamate-evoked activation of noradrenergic locus coeruleus neurons. *J Neurosci* 1991;11:760–769.
6. Aston-Jones G, Shipley MT, Chouvet G, Ennis M, Van Bockstaele, EJ, Pieribone V, Shiekhattar R, Akaoka H, Drolet G, Astier B, Charlety P, Valentino R, and Williams JT. Afferent regulation of locus coeruleus neurons: anatomy, physiology and pharmacology. *Prog Brain Res* 1991;85:47–75.
7. Bird SJ, Kuhar MJ. Iontophoretic application of opiates to the LC. *Brain Res* 1977;122:523–533.
8. Brun P, Suaud-Chagny MF, Lachuer J, Gonon F, Buda M. Catecholamine metabolism in locus coeruleus neurons: a study of its activation by sciatic nerve stimulation in the rat. *Eur J Neurosci* 1991;3:397–406.
9. Christie MJ, Williams JT, North RA. Cellular mechanisms of opioid tolerance: studies in single brain neurons. *Mol Pharmacol* 1987;32:633–638.
10. Curtis AL, Conti E, Valentino RJ. Cocaine effects on brain noradrenergic neurons of anesthetized and unanesthetized rats. *Neuropharmacology* 1993;32:419–428.
11. Descarries L, Watkins KC, and Lapierre Y. Noradrenergic axon terminals in the cerebral cortex of rat. III. Topometric ultrastructural analysis. *Brain Res* 1977;133:197–222.
12. De Souza EB. Corticotropin-releasing factor receptors in the rat central nervous system: characterization and regional distribution. *J Neurosci* 1987;7:88–100.
13. De Vries GJ, Buijs RM, Van Leeuwen FW, Caffe AR, Swaab DF. The vasopressinergic innervation of the brain in normal and castrated rats. *J Comp Neurol* 1985;233:236–254.
14. Eiden LE, Nilaver G, Palkovits M. Distribution of vasoactive intestinal polypeptide (VIP) in the rat brain stem nuclei. *Brain Res* 1982;231:472–477.
15. Elam M, Svensson TH, Thoren P. Differentiated cardiovascular afferent regulation of locus coeruleus neurons and sympathetic nerves. *Brain Res* 1985;358:77–84.
16. Engberg G. Nicotine induced excitation of locus coeruleus neurons is mediated via release of excitatory amino acids. *Life Sci* 1989;44:1535–1540.
17. Foote SL, Bloom FE, Aston-Jones G. Nucleus locus coeruleus: new evidence of anatomical and physiological specificity. *Physiol Rev* 1983;63:844–914.
18. Forloni G, Grzanna R, Blakely RD, Coyle JT. Co-localization of *N*-acetyl-aspartyl-glutamate in central cholinergic, noradrenergic, and serotonergic neurons. *Synapse* 1987;1:455–460.
19. Fritschy J-M, Grzanna R. Distribution of locus coeruleus axons within the rat brainstem demonstrated by PHA-L anterograde tracing in combination with dopamine-β-hydroxylase immunofluorescence. *J Comp Neurol* 1990;293:616–631.
20. Fritschy J-M, Lyons WE, Mullen CA, Kosofsky BE, Molliver ME, Grzanna R. Distribution of locus coeruleus axons in the rat spinal cord: a combined anterograde transport and immunohistochemical study. *Brain Res* 1987;437:176–180.
21. Fuxe K, Ganten D, Hokfelt T, Bolme P. Immunohistochemical evidence for the existence of angiotensin II-containing nerve terminals in the brain and spinal cord in the rat. *Neurosci Lett* 1976;2:229–234.
22. Gagne C, Moyse E, Kocher L, Bour H, Pujol JF. Light microscopic localization of somatostatin binding sites in the locus coeruleus of the rat. *Brain Res* 1990;530:196–204.
23. Gold MS, Pottash AC. The neurobiological implications of clonidine HCl. *Ann NY Acad Sci* 1981;362:191–202.
24. Gold PW, Goodwin FK, Chrousos GP. Clinical and biochemical manifestations of depression. *N Engl J Med* 1988;319:413–420.
25. Grilly DM, Grogan TW. Cocaine and levels of arousal: effects on vigilance task performance of rats. *Pharmacol Biochem Behav* 1990;35:269–271.
26. Groves PM, Wilson CJ. Monoaminergic presynaptic axons and dendrites in rat locus coeruleus seen in reconstructions of serial sections. *J Comp Neurol* 1980;193:853–862.
27. Guyenet PG, Aghajanian GK. Acetylcholine Substance P and met-enkephalin in the LC: pharmacological evidence for independent sites of action. *Eur J Pharmacol* 1979;53:319–328.
28. Hajos M, Engberg G. Role of primary sensory neurons in the central effects of nicotine. *Psychopharmacology* 1988;94:468–470.
29. Heureux RL, Dennis T, Curet O, Scatton B. Measurement of endogenous noradrenaline release in the rat cerebral cortex in vivo by transcortical dialysis: effects of drugs affecting noradrenergic transmission. *J Neurochem* 1986;46:1794–1801.
30. Hodge CJ, Apkarian AV, Stevens RT, Vogelsang GD, Wisnicki

HJ. Locus coeruleus modulation of dorsal horn unit responses to cutaneous stimulation. *Brain Res* 1981;240:415–420.

31. Hokfelt T, Fuxe K, Goldstein M, Johansson O. Immunohistochemical evidence for the existence of adrenaline neurons in the rat brain. *Brain Res* 1974;66:235–251.
32. Jacobs BL. Central monoaminergic neurons: single-unit studies in behaving animals. In: Meltzer HY, ed. *Psychopharmacology: the third generation of progress*. New York: Raven Press, 1987;159–170.
33. Jimenez-Rivera CA, Waterhouse BD. Effects of systemically and locally applied cocaine on cerebrocortical neuron responsiveness to afferent synaptic inputs and glutamate. *Brain Res* 1991;546:287–296.
34. Johansson O, Hokfelt T, Elde RP. Immunohistochemical distribution of somatostatin-like immunoreactivity in the central nervous system of the adult rat. *Neuroscience* 1984;13:265–339.
35. Jones SL, Gebhart GF. Characterization of coeruleospinal inhibition of the nociceptive tail-flick reflex in the rat: mediation by spinal alpha 2-adrenoceptors. *Brain Res* 1986;364:315–330.
36. Jones SL, Gebhart GF. Inhibition of spinal nociceptive transmission from the midbrain, pons and medulla in the rat: activation of descending inhibition by morphine, glutamate and electrical stimulation. *Brain Res* 1988;460:281–296.
37. Khachaturian H, Lewis M, Watson SJ. Enkephalin systems in the diencephalon and brainstem of the rat. *J Comp Neurol* 1983;220:310–320.
38. Ljungdahl A, Hokfelt T, Nilsson G. Distribution of substance P-like immunoreactivity in the central nervous system of the rat. I. Cell bodies and nerve terminals. *Neuroscience* 1978;3:63–80.
39. Maldonado R, Koob GF. Destruction of the locus coeruleus decreases physical signs of opiate withdrawal. *Brain Res* 1993;605:128–138.
40. Maldonado R, Stinus L, Gold LH, Koob GF. Role of different brain structures in the expression of the physical morphine-withdrawal syndrome. *J Pharmacol Exp Ther* 1992;261:669–677.
41. Marrocco RT, Lane RF, McClurkin JW, Blaha CD, Alkire MF. Release of cortical catecholamines by visual stimulation requires activity in thalmocortical afferents of monkey and cat. *J Neurosci* 1987;7:2756–2767.
42. Martin JL, Dietl MM, Hof PR, Palacios JM, Magistretti PJ. Autoradiographic mapping of [mono[^{125}I]iodo-Tyr10, MetO17] vasoactive intestinal peptide binding sites in the rat brain. *Neuroscience* 1987;23:539–565.
43. Mendelsohn FAO, Quirion R, Saavedra JM, Aguilera G, Catt KJ. Autoradiographic localization of angiotensin II receptors in rat brain. *Proc Natl Acad Sci USA* 1984;81:1575–1579.
44. Milner TA, Abate C, Reis DJ, Pickel VM. Ultrastructural localization of phenylethanolamine *N*-methyltransferase-like immunoreactivity in the rat locus coeruleus. *Brain Res* 1989;478:1–15.
45. Mokha SS, McMillan JA, Iggo A. Descending influences on spinal nociceptive neurones from locus coeruleus: actions, pathway, neurotransmitters and mechanisms. In: Bonica JJ, Lindblom U, Iggo A, eds. *Advances in pain research and therapy*, vol 5. New York: Raven Press, 1983;387–392.
46. Mugnaini E, Oertel WH. An atlas of the distribution of GABAergic neurons and terminals in the rat CNS as revealed by GAD immunohistochemistry. In: Bjorklund A, Hokfelt T, eds. *Handbook of chemical neuroanatomy, vol 4. GABA and neuropeptides in the CNS.* Amsterdam: Elsevier Science Publishers, 1985;436–608.
47. Olpe HR, Steinmann MW, Pozza MF, Haas HL. Comparative investigation into the actions of ACTH$_{1-24}$, somatostatin, neurotensin, substance P and vasopressin on LC neuronal activity *in vitro*. *Naunyn Schmiedebergs Arch Pharmacol* 1987;336:434–437.
48. Olschowka JA, Molliver ME, Grzanna R, Rice FL, Coyle JT. Ultrastructural demonstration of noradrenergic synapses in the rat central nervous system by dopamine-beta-hydroxylase immunocytochemistry. *J Histochem Cytochem* 1981;29:271–280.
49. Papadopoulos GC, Parnavelas JG, Buijs RM. Monoaminergic fibers form conventional synapses in the cerebral cortex. *Neurosci Lett* 1990;76:275–279.
50. Pickel VM, Joh TH, Reis DJ. A serotonergic innervation of noradrenergic neurons in the nucleus locus coeruleus: demonstration by immunocytochemical localization of the transmitter specific enzymes tyrosine hydroxylase and tryptophan hydroxylase. *Brain Res* 1977;131:197–214.
51. Pickel VM, Joh TH, Reis DJ, Leeman SE, Miller RJ. Electron

microscopic localization of substance P and enkephalin in axon terminals related to dendrites of catecholaminergic neurons. *Brain Res* 1979;160:387–400.
52. Quirion R, Shults CW, Moody TW, Pert CB, Chase TN, O'Donahue TL. Autoradiographic distribution of substance P receptors in rat central nervous system. *Nature* 1983;303:714–716.
53. Rasmussen K, Aghajanian GK. Withdrawal-induced activation of locus coeruleus neurons in opiate-dependent rats: attenuation by lesion of the nucleus paragigantocellularis. *Brain Res* 1989;505:346–350.
54. Rasmussen K, Beitner-Johnson DB, Krystal JH, Aghajanian GK, Nestler EJ. Opiate withdrawal and rat locus coeruleus: behavioral, electrophysiological, and biochemical correlates. *J Neurosci* 1990;10:2308–2317.
55. Reddy SV, Maderdrut JL, Yaksh TL. Spinal cord pharmacology of adrenergic agonist-mediated antinociception. *J Pharmacol Exp Ther* 1980;213:525–533.
56. Rooter A, Birdsall NJM, Field PM, Raisman G. Muscarinic receptors in the central nervous system of the rat. II. Distribution and binding of [^{3}H] propylbenzilylcholine mustard in the midbrain and hindbrain. *Brain Res Rev* 1979;1:167–183.
57. Ruggiero DA, Giuliano R, Anwar M, Stornetta R, Reis DJ. Anatomical substrates of cholinergic-autonomic regulation in the rat. *J Comp Neurol* 1990;292:1–53.
58. Shipley MT, Halloran FJ, De La Torre J. Surprisingly rich projection from locus coeruleus to the olfactory bulb in rat. *Brain Res* 1985;329:294–299.
59. Siever LJ. Role of noradrenergic mechanisms in the etiology of the affective disorders. In: Meltzer HY, ed. *Psychopharmacology: the third generation of progress*. New York: Raven Press, 1987;493–504.
60. Smith Y, Parent A, Kerkerian L, Pelletier G. Distribution of neuropeptide Y immunoreactivity in the basal forebrain and upper brainstem of the squirrel monkey (*Saimiri sciurens*). *J Comp Neurol* 1985;236:71–89.
61. Stokes PE, Sikes CR. Hypothalamic-pituitary-adrenal axis in affective disorders. In: Meltzer HY, ed. *Psychopharmacology: the third generation of progress*. New York: Raven Press, 1987;589–608.
62. Sutin EL, Jacobowitz DM. Immunocytochemical localization of peptides and other neurochemicals in the rat laterodorsal tegmental nucleus and adjacent area. *J Comp Neurol* 1988;270:243–270.
63. Svensson TH. Peripheral, autonomic regulation of locus coeruleus noradrenergic neurons in brain: putative implications for psychiatry and psychopharmacology. *Psychopharmacology* 1987;92:1–7.
64. Uhl GR, Goodman RR, Snyder SH. Neurotensin-containing cell bodies, fibers and nerve terminals in brainstem of the rat: immunohistochemical mapping. *Brain Res* 1979;167:77–91.
65. Vale W, Spiess J, Rivier C, Rivier J. Characterization of a 41-residue ovine hypothalamic peptide that stimulates secretion of corticotropin and beta-endorphin. *Science* 1981;213:1394–1397.
66. Valentino RJ, Foote SL, Page ME. The locus coeruleus as a site for integrating corticotropin-releasing factor and noradrenergic mediation of stress responses. *Ann NY Acad Sci* 1993;697:171–187.
67. Wang YY, Aghajanian GK. Excitation of locus coeruleus neurons by vasoactive intestinal peptide: evidence for a G-protein-mediated inward current. *Brain Res* 1989;500:107–118.
68. Waterhouse BD, Lin CS, Burne RA, Woodward DJ. The distribution of neocortical projection neurons in the locus coeruleus. *J Comp Neurol* 1983;217:418–431.
69. Waterhouse BD, Sessler FM, Liu W, Lin C-S. Second messenger-mediated actions of norepinephrine on target neurons in central circuits: a new perspective on intracellular mechanisms and functional consequences. *Prog Brain Res* 1991;88:351–362.
70. Watson SJ, Richard CW, Barchas JD. Adrenocorticotropin in rat brain: immunohistochemical localization in cells and axons. *Science* 1978;200:1180–1182.
71. Weissmann-Nanupoulos D, Mach E, Magre J, Demassey Y, Pujol JF. Evidence for the localization of 5HT$_{1A}$ binding sites on serotonin containing neurons in the raphe dorsalis and raphe centralis nucleus of the rat brain. *Neurochem Int* 1985;7:1061–1072.
72. Xiong H, Marshall KC. Angiotensin II modulation of glutamate excitation of LC neurons. *Neurosci Lett* 1990;118:261–264.
73. Young WS III, Kuhar MJ. Noradrenergic α1 and α2 receptors: autoradiographic visualization. *Eur J Pharmacol* 1979;59:317–319.

Psychopharmacology: The Fourth Generation of Progress, edited by Floyd E. Bloom and David J. Kupfer. Raven Press, Ltd., New York © 1995.

CHAPTER 34

Noradrenergic Neural Substrates for Anxiety and Fear

Clinical Associations Based on Preclinical Research

Dennis S. Charney, J. Douglas Bremner, and D. Eugene Redmond, Jr.

Preclinical studies investigating the physiological mechanisms of fear and anxiety states have strongly suggested that multiple brain neurochemical and neuropeptide systems, including noradrenergic, benzodiazepine, serotonergic, and corticotropin-releasing hormone, are involved in the pathophysiology of human anxiety. In addition, the evidence implicates specific brain structures such as the amygdala, thalamus, hypothalamus, central gray, hippocampus, locus coeruleus, and prefrontal cortex as mediators of the broad range of behaviors and physiological responses associated with anxiety and fear.

The focus of this review is the role of brain noradrenergic neural systems in the development of human anxiety disorders—clinical associations based on preclinical research. Neuroanatomical, neurochemical, neurophysiological, and behavioral studies of the noradrenergic system provide a basis for relating increased activity of this system to the expression of anxiety and fear and the somatic symptoms and cardiovascular changes that accompany severe anxiety states (Table 1). We will first review some of the main preclinical findings and then describe the status of clinical studies largely based on these preclinical data (see also Chapters 29, 32, and 33, *this volume*).

PRECLINICAL STUDIES

Neuroanatomy of the Locus Coeruleus

The neuroanatomy of the largest central noradrenergic nucleus, the locus coeruleus (LC), is characterized by an extensive efferent projection system and a more restricted afferent input (5,20,40). A retrograde labeling study of afferent input to the LC using iontophoretic horseradish peroxidase (HRP) injections found that forebrain structures, such as the neocortex, amygdala, and hypothalamus, project to the LC. The hypothalamic innervation is noteworthy because it provides a potential regulatory role for the LC with regard to autonomic function. Brainstem monoaminergic neurons, such as the raphe nuclei and a variety of sensory relay areas, also project to the LC. The existence of these sensory afferents from the spinal cord and the nucleus of the solitary tract provide insight into the mechanisms by which the LC is responsive to noxious stimuli and alterations in cardiovascular function (10). Consistent with these observations, a recent neuroanatomical investigation involving anterograde labeling with PHA-L in the cat and monkey found terminal fibers in the LC following injections in lamina I of the spinal or medullary dorsal horn (20). These observations are supported by an electrophysiological mapping study which revealed that spinal cord lamina I cells terminated in the LC (40). There are reports, in contradiction to the above, that direct afferents to the LC almost exclusively come from the paragigantocellularis (PGi) and the prepositus hypoglossi (PrH) (4). These studies used very small injections of wheat germ agglutinin conjugated to HRP (WGA-HRP) that were restricted to the LC in the rat. The discrepant observations may be due to the fact that WGA-HRP is not an efficient retrograde marker for lamina I neurons (21). The finding of additional afferents to the LC using choleratoxin B subunit as a retrograde tracer instead of WGA-HRP is consistent with this assertion (38). The hypothesis that PGi and PrH are the predominant afferents

D. S. Charney, J. D. Bremner, and D. E. Redmond, Jr.: Department of Psychiatry, Yale University School of Medicine; West Haven and Veterans Affairs Medical Center, West Haven, Connecticut 06516.

TABLE 1. *The role of noradrenergic neuronal systems in anxiety and fear: the locus coeruleus*

Neuroanatomy		Neurochemistry
Afferent pathways	Efferent pathways	
Cortex	Cortex	Major norepinephrine containing nucleus in brain
Amygdala	Thalamus	Highly regulated by benzodiazepine, opiate,
Hippocampus	Amygdala	serotonin, CRH, NMDA, and ACH systems
Nucleus	Hypothalamus	
Paragigantocellularis	Hippocampus	
Nucleus	Cerebellum	
Prepositus hypoglossi	Spinal Cord	

Behavior			Clinical Implications
Stimulation	Lesions	Neuronal Activity	
Fear Induced Behaviors	Reduced fearful Behavior	↑With Threat ↑Fear Conditioning ↑Chronic Stress ↑With reduced blood pressure ↑With elevated CO_2 ↑With blood loss ↑With Distention of bladder, colon, rectum ↑With hypoglycemia	The LC-norepinephrine system may help determine whether, under threat, an individual directs attention toward external, sensory stimuli or to internal vegatative events. The system may be important in facilitating the planning and execution of behaviors important for survival. The LC is a key component in the efferent arm of the neural circuitry of anxiety. Abnormalities in noradrenergic function hypothesized to be involved with pathophysiology of Panic Disorder and PTSD

to the LC is also not supported by the demonstration that destruction of these nuclei fail to block LC responses to somatosensory stimuli (51).

If not the primary LC afferent, the PGi remains an important afferent to the LC and is a key sympathoexcitatory region in brain (5). There are widespread afferents to the PGi from diverse brain areas (81). The PGi may be an integrative pathway for activating the LC by a variety of mechanisms. The PGi is involved in control of arterial blood pressure, cardiopulmonary reflexes, and parasympathetic function. It has been suggested that the peripheral sympathetic nervous system is activated in parallel with the LC by projections to both areas from the PGi (5). The LC also appears to be activated by projections responsive to corticotropin-releasing factor (CRF), and considerable evidence suggests that CRF has anxiogenic properties. Intracerebroventricular infusion of CRF increases norepinephrine (NE) turnover in several forebrain areas (24). In a dose-dependent fashion, CRF increases the firing rate of LC–NE neurons (80). Stress, which activates NE neurons, markedly increases CRF concentrations in the LC (11). Moreover, it has recently been demonstrated that infusion of CRF into the LC produces anxiogenic activity and significant increases in the NE metabolite 3,4-dihydroxyphenylglycol in forebrain areas such as the amygdala and hypothalamus (6).

The LC has diffuse projections to the entire cortical mantle, as well as thalamus, hypothalamus, amygdala, hippocampus, cerebellum, and spinal cord. Through this broad efferent network the LC can mediate a range of cognitive, neuroendocrine, cardiovascular, and skeletal motor responses that accompany anxiety and fear.

The LC is the primary source of NE fibers in a number of neocortical regions in the primate. Consistent with postsynaptic inhibitory effects of NE, activation of the LC neurons produce inhibition of neuronal activity in brain regions receiving projections from the LC, including the cochlear nucleus, cerebral and cerebellar cortices, spinal trigeminal nucleus, hippocampus, caudate, and superior colliculus. Similarly, LC stimulation reduces cerebral metabolism and blood flow in these areas (31,58). Because NE has greater inhibitory effects on spontaneous than on evoked neuronal activity, it has been suggested that a function of the LC–NE system is to enhance neuronal responses to inputs of behavioral significance or, put another way, to increase the signal-to-noise ratio (3); (also see Chapters 29 and 32, *this volume*).

Behavioral Effects of Locus Coeruleus Stimulation

Electrical stimulation of the LC produces a series of behavioral responses similar to those observed in naturally occurring or experimentally induced fear (55). These behaviors are also elicited by administration of drugs, such as yohimbine and piperoxone, which activate the LC by blocking alpha-2-adrenergic autoreceptors. Drugs which decrease the function of the LC by interacting with inhibitory opiate (morphine), benzodiazepine (diazepam), and alpha-2 (clonidine) receptors on the LC decrease fearful behavior and partially antagonize the effects of electrical stimulation of the LC in the monkey (53). These studies suggest that abnormally high levels of LC activity producing increased release of NE at postsynaptic projec-

TABLE 2. *Major preclinical evidence supporting noradrenergic contributions to anxiety and fear*

	References
Stress and fear inducing stimuli increase firing rate.	37,47,52,64
Stress induces increase in norepinephrine (NE) turnover in Limbic Brain Regions.	29,70,71
Stress and LC activation increase tyrosine hydroxylase and C-fos expression in the LC.	42,66
Conditioned fear is associated with increased LC neuronal activity and increased NE turnover in LC projection sites.	52,74
Electrical and Pharmacological activation of LC results in anxiety and fear behavior.	53,54,55
Drugs, which have anxiolytic activity, decrease stress induced increases in NE turnover and LC firing rate.	29,54,62,67,69

tion sites throughout the brain may act to augment some forms of fear or pathological anxiety, depending on the environmental conditions (19).

A single report of electrical stimulation of the region of the LC in humans reported that the subjects experienced feelings of fear and imminent death. In a subject with chronically implanted stimulation electrodes in the vicinity of the LC, electrical stimulation during sleep was associated with marked insomnia (32) (Table 2).

Behavioral Effects of Locus Coeruleus Lesions

Bilateral lesions of the LC in the monkey decrease the natural occurrence of these behavioral responses in a social group situation and in response to threatening confrontations with humans (53). Agents which decrease the function of the LC also decrease fearful behavior and partially antagonize the effects of electrical stimulation of the LC in the monkey. Lesions of the dorsal bundle which originates in the LC and projects mostly to the neocortex, hippocampus, and cerebellar cortex produce anxiolytic-type responses in anxiogenic behavioral test situations (82).

Many studies in rodents using the neurotoxin 6-hydroxydopamine (6-OHDA) have shown effects on a variety of behavioral tests which have been interpreted as inconsistent with the hypothesis that noradrenergic systems are critically involved in anxiety and fear (41). The validity of these behavioral paradigms to reflect anxiety and fear has been the subject of much debate (34,53,54).

Locus Coeruleus Activity and Behavioral States Associated with Stress and Fear

In laboratory rats, chronic stress results in an increased firing of the LC (47,64). Animals exposed to chronic inescapable shock, which is associated with learned helplessness, have an increase in responsiveness of the LC to an excitatory stimulus in comparison to animals exposed to escapable shock (64).

The effect of stressful and fear-inducing stimuli on LC activity has been assessed in freely moving cats (37,52). Conditions which are behaviorally activating, but not stressful, such as exposure to inaccessible rats or food, do not increase LC firing in cats as they do in rats (see Chapter 29, *this volume*). In contrast, stressful and fear-inducing stimuli, such as loud white noise, air puff, restraint, and confrontation with a dog, produce a rapid, robust, and sustained increase in LC activity (37). Of interest, these increases in LC function are accompanied by sympathetic activation. Generally, the greater the sympathetic activation in response to the stressor, as indicated by heart rate, the greater the correlation observed. Thus, a stimulus intensity threshold for coactivation of central and peripheral NE systems may exist.

A parallel activation of LC neurons and splanchnic sympathetic nerves is produced by noxious stimuli. The LC, like sympathetic, splanchnic activity, is highly responsive to various peripheral cardiovascular events, such as alterations in blood volume or blood pressure. Internal events that must be responded to for survival, such as thermoregulatory disturbance, hypoglycemia, blood loss, an increase in pCO_2, or a marked reduction in blood pressure, cause robust and long-lasting increases in LC activity (67).

There are also peripheral visceral influences on LC activity. In rats, distention of the urinary bladder, distal colon, or rectum activates LC neurons. These findings suggest that changes in autonomic or visceral function may result in specific behavioral responses via the brain LC–NE system. The LC–NE network may help determine whether, under threat, an individual turns attention toward external, sensory stimuli or to internal vegetative events. The system, when functioning normally, may be important in facilitating the planning and execution of behaviors important for survival (67) (Table 2).

Effects of Stressful and Fear-Inducing Stimuli on Biochemical Indices of Noradrenergic Function

Stressful stimuli of many types produce marked increases in brain noradrenergic function. Stress produces regionally selective increases in NE turnover in the LC, limbic regions, and cerebral cortex. It has recently been demonstrated that immobilization stress, footshock stress, and tail-pinch stress increase noradrenergic metabolism in the hypothalamus and amygdala (29,70,71). Stress also increases tyrosine hydroxylase levels in the LC (42). Anxiolytic agents reverse the effects of stress on noradrenergic metabolism (29,62,69). Consistent with these findings, acute cold restraint stress results in decreased density of alpha-2-adrenergic receptors in the hippocampus and amygdala (73). The stress-induced increase in NE turnover is also associated with a decrease in postsynaptic beta receptor density (79) (Table 2).

Noradrenergic Effects of Conditioning and Sensitization

Fear Conditioning

Several behavioral paradigms indicate an important role for noradrenergic neuronal systems in the processes involved in fear conditioning. Neutral stimuli paired with shock produce increases in brain NE metabolism and behavioral deficits similar to those elicited by the shock (88). In the freely moving cat, the firing rate of cells in the LC can be increased by presenting a neutral acoustic stimulus previously paired with an air puff to the whiskers, which also increases firing and is aversive to the cat (52). There is also a body of evidence indicating that an intact noradrenergic system may be necessary for the acquisition of fear conditioned responses (74).

Behavioral Sensitization

Sensitization generally refers to the increase in behavioral or physiological responsiveness that occurs following repeated exposure to a stimulus. Behavioral sensitization can be generally context-dependent or conditioned, such that animals will not demonstrate sensitization if the stimulis is presented in a different environment (50). However, if the intensity of the stimulis or drug dose is high enough, behavioral sensitization will occur even if the environment is changed. It has been suggested that different mechanisms are called into play with environment-independent sensitization (84).

Behavioral sensitization to stress involves alterations in noradrenergic function. Limited shock exposure that does not increase NE utilization in control rats does increase NE release in animals previously exposed to the stressor. Moreover, changes in noradrenergic function in animals subjected to long-term shock require lower shock currents (decreased stressor intensity) than required under acute conditions (30). An in vivo study observed augmented extracellular NE concentrations in the hippocampus, whereas ex vivo measurements of noradrenergic metabolites in response to chronic stress indicated a sensitized response in the hypothalamus but not in the hippocampus (45). It is not clear to what degree this reflects differences in metabolic disposition of NE in the two regions, as opposed to actual differences in sensitization processes. Nonetheless, regional specificity in bio-

chemical indices of the expression of sensitization may be important. A recent in vivo dialysis investigation demonstrated stress-induced sensitization of NE release in the medial prefrontal cortex (26).

Noradrenergic Function and Gene Expression

Stress and learning alter gene expression by modifying the binding of transcriptional activator proteins to each other and to the regulatory regions of genes (8). It has been suggested that immediate early genes, such as C-fos, whose proteins, acting in the nucleus as "third messengers," produce stable modifications in the transcriptions of late genes to long-term memory (1). Immediate early genes may serve a variety of functions in mediating genomic responses to extracellular stimuli (66).

Recently, it has been demonstrated that C-fos and other immediate early genes in the brain are activated by increases in brain noradrenergic neurotransmission. For example, yohimbine, an alpha-2-receptor antagonist, increases c-fos expression in rat cerebral cortex (66).

In support of studies that demonstrated that acute and chronic stress activate brain NE systems, stress increases expression of c-fos immunoreactivity in the LC (9). Furthermore, activation of the LC with glutamate produces marked and widespread increases in c-fos protein in brain regions receiving projections from the LC. If c-fos induction is a component of the noradrenergic signal transduction pathways, then basal levels of c-fos mRNA in brain could represent a summation of activity of noradrenergic neurons (see also Chapters 29, 32, and 33, this volume).

CLINICAL STUDIES

Clinical Investigation of Noradrenergic Function in Healthy Subjects and Anxiety Disorder Patients (Table 3)

Healthy Human Subjects

Accumulated evidence suggests that brain noradrenergic systems play a role in mediating normal state anxiety and the response to stress in healthy human subjects. States of anxiety or fear appear to be associated with an increase in NE release in healthy subjects (83).

Levels of the NE metabolite, MHPG, have also been found to increase in healthy subjects during emotional stress (36). Plasma MHPG was correlated with state anxiety in healthy subjects exposed to the anticipatory stress of receiving an electric shock, while there was no such correlation in the absence of the electric shock threat (75,78). Significant within-individual correlations between changes in urinary MHPG and changes in state anxiety have been found in healthy human subjects (68).

TABLE 3. *Major clinical evidence supporting noradrenergic contribution to the pathophysiology of Panic Disorder and PTSD*

	Disorder	References
Potentiated cerebral blood flow, cerebral metabolic, anxiogenic, biochemical, and cardiovascular responses to yohimbine	Panic Disorder PTSD	15,16,18,65,75,86
Potentiated blood pressure and MHPG responses to clonidine	Panic Disorder	18,19,46,77
Blunted growth hormone response to clonidine	Panic Disorder	18,19,46,77
Increased basal urinary epinephrine and norepinephrine	PTSD	12,35,87
Decreased platelet alpha-2 adrenergic receptor binding	PTSD	12
Sympathetic system activation during traumatic reminders	PTSD	12

Studies of Noradrenergic Function in Panic Disorder and PTSD Patients

In comparison to other anxiety disorders, the evidence for an abnormality in noradrenergic function is most compelling for panic disorder and Post-traumatic stress disorder (PTSD). Panic disorder and PTSD patients frequently report cardiovascular, gastrointestinal, and respiratory symptoms. Because the LC is responsive to peripheral alterations in the function of these systems, minor physiological changes in these patients may result in abnormal activation of LC neurons and, consequently, panic attacks and flashbacks. These functional interactions may explain the association of anxiety symptoms with tachycardia, tachypnea, hypoglycemia, and visceral and organ distention, as well as the marked sensitivity of panic disorder and PTSD patients to interoceptive simuli. The important role of the noradrenergic system in fear conditioning may account for the development of phobic symptoms in these patients. Finally, the involvement of noradrenergic neurons in learning and memory may relate to the persistence of traumatic memories in PTSD.

Peripheral Catecholamine Levels

Generally, measurement of peripheral NE and its metabolites have revealed concentrations in panic disorder patients similar to those in controls. Several studies have not found elevated plasma catecholamines following spontaneous or situationally provoked panic attacks (7,85). Moreover, plasma and urinary catecholamine levels (43,44), as well as cerebrospinal fluid (CSF) MHPG levels, in panic disorder patients are generally not different from those in healthy controls (25,76; B Lydiard, *personal communication,* April 1992).

Two studies have found significantly elevated 24-h urine NE excretion in combat veterans with PTSD compared to healthy subjects or patients with schizophrenia or major depression (35,87). A wide variety of investigations have been conducted to evaluate sympathetic nervous system (SNS) function in panic disorder. These studies have produced markedly divergent findings yielding no firm

consensus on whether an SNS dysfunction exists in panic disorder (57).

Regulation of Noradrenergic Function in Panic Disorder and PTSD

Yohimbine

The regulation of noradrenergic neuronal function has been examined by determining the behavioral, biochemical, and cardiovascular effects of oral and intravenous yohimbine, an alpha-2-adrenergic receptor antagonist, in a spectrum of psychiatric disorders, including schizophrenia, major depression, obsessive–compulsive disorder, generalized anxiety disorder, panic disorder, and PTSD (19). Specific abnormalities have been identified in panic disorder and PTSD. Approximately 60–70% of panic disorder patients experience yohimbine-induced panic attacks, and these patients have larger yohimbine-induced increases in plasma MHPG, blood pressure, and heart rate than do healthy subjects and those with other panic psychiatric disorders (15,16,18).

Similar to the panic disorder patients, approximately two-thirds of PTSD patients experience yohimbine-induced panic attacks, and, in addition, 40% report flashbacks after yohimbine. As a group, PTSD patients also have greater yohimbine-induced increases in plasma MHPG, sitting systolic blood pressure, and heart rate than do healthy subjects. A striking effect of yohimbine is its ability to increase the severity of the core symptoms associated with PTSD, such as intrusive traumatic thoughts, emotional numbing, and grief (65). This may be due to the involvement of noradrenergic systems in the mechanisms by which memories of traumatic experiences remain indelible for decades and are easily reawakened by a variety of stimuli and stressors.

Recently, the effects of yohimbine on regional cerebral blood flow (rCBF) and metabolism have been evaluated in panic disorder and PTSD patients. In panic disorder patients, yohimbine significantly reduced frontal rCBF rates in patients compared to healthy subjects (86). Similar to these observations, administration of yohimbine decreased regional glucose metabolic rates in several cortical regions in PTSD patients, but not in healthy subjects. Because cortical rCBF, metabolism, and spontaneous neuronal activity all generally decrease with noradrenergic stimulation, these data are consistent with a role for excessive stimulation of noradrenergic projections to the cortex in the pathophysiology of panic disorder and PTSD.

Clonidine

A consistent finding in the literature is that the growth hormone rise induced by clonidine is blunted in panic disorder patients (77). In a recent investigation, clonidine-growth hormone response was found primarily in the patients who experienced yohimbine-induced panic attacks (18). This suggests that the diminished postsynaptic alpha-2-adrenergic receptor function reflected by the blunted clonidine–growth-hormone response may relate to presynaptic noradrenergic neuronal hyperactivity.

Several previous investigations observed that clonidine produced greater decreases in plasma MHPG and blood pressure in panic disorder patients compared to healthy subjects (18,46; J. D. Coplan and colleagues, *personal communication,* December 1993). The clonidine-induced decreases in plasma MHPG may be greatest in the panic disorder patients who experienced yohimbine-induced panic attacks (18), suggesting that there is a distinct subgroup of panic disorder patients who manifest noradrenergic neuronal dysfunction. The effects of clonidine on these parameters have not been investigated in PTSD patients.

Beta-Adrenergic Receptor Function

Infusion of isoproterenol, a peripherally acting compound that is selective for the beta adrenoceptor, has been reported to trigger anxiety responses in panic patients compared with controls (49). Successful treatment of panic patients with tricyclic antidepressants blunted isoproterenol-induced anxiety and systolic blood pressure responses (48). These studies are consistent with the hypothesis of increased beta-1-adrenoceptor sensitivity in panic disorder, which is normalized by effective pharmacotherapy (48).

Noradrenergic Function and Treatment for Panic Disorder

Evidence is emerging that the efficacy of some tricyclic and monoamine oxidase inhibitor drugs against panic may be related to their regulatory effects on noradrenergic activity (14). The effects of chronic treatment with these agents on the regulation of noradrenergic activity are complex. Some of these effects, such as reduced tyrosine

hydroxylase activity, LC firing rate, NE turnover, and postsynaptic beta-adrenergic receptor sensitivity, diminish noradrenergic function. It is interesting that the only antidepressant drugs that do not exhibit antipanic efficacy—bupropion and trazodone—have effects on noradrenergic function different from those of the tricyclic and monoamine inhibitors (60). In the rat brain, bupropion does not down-regulate beta-adrenergic receptors or decrease NE turnover. While trazodone does down-regulate the beta-adrenergic receptors, it does not decrease the LC firing rate or the spontaneous activity of cortical neurons receiving noradrenergic innervation.

Benzodiazepines are highly effective treatments for panic disorder, generally at higher doses than those needed for generalized anxiety disorder. Clearly, the anxiolytic effects of benzodiazepines are related to their agonist actions at benzodiazepine receptors at a variety of brain sites. However, it has been hypothesized that the antipanic properties of benzodiazepines may also relate to inhibitory effects on noradrenergic function, because these drugs reduce LC neuronal activity (13).

The antipanic efficacy of the potent serotonin reuptake inhibitors (SRIs) such as clomipramine, fluvoxamine, zimelidine and fluoxetine is well-documented. The mechanism of action of SRIs in panic disorder has not been established. However, $5-HT_2$, $5-HT_{1C}$, and $5-HT_{1A}$ receptors are unlikely to be directly involved because ritanserin, a $5-HT_2$ and $5-HT_{1C}$ antagonist, and buspirone, a $5-HT_{1A}$ agonist, lack antipanic efficacy (23,61).

It is possible that interactions between the serotonin (5-HT) and noradrenergic systems may be related to the antipanic properties of SRIs. Preclinical studies suggest that 5-HT–NE interactions occur between the LC and the dorsal raphe. Direct application of 5-HT to LC neurons results in a tonic inhibition of electrical activity. Phasic 5-HT inhibition of LC function may be mediated by an excitatory amino acid (EAA) pathway from the nucleus paragigantocellularis, possibly via a $5-HT_{1A}$ receptor (2). In this context it is notable that fluvoxamine has been found to alter EAA receptor mRNA expression throughout the brain (28). The interactions between the noradrenergic and serotonin systems are supported by the finding that fluvoxamine, but not placebo treatment, reduced yohimbine-induced anxiety in panic disorder patients (27).

If the noradrenergic system is dysregulated in panic disorder, the mechanism of action of antipanic therapy may be its ability to decrease the wide and unpredictable fluctuations in noradrenergic activity and improve efficiency by reducing basal activity (decreasing noise) while effecting a more specific responsiveness to specific stimuli (increasing signal-to-noise ratio).

The treatment implications of the reported abnormalities in noradrenergic function in PTSD patients remain to be established. Specific PTSD symptoms (anxiety, flashbacks, and autonomic arousal) may be particularly responsive to drugs that reduce noradrenergic function

(33). It should be noted, however, that patients with panic disorder and those with PTSD have different therapeutic responses to tricyclic, SRI, and benzodiazepine compounds. Patients with panic disorder derive great benefit from these drugs, whereas those with PTSD have more modest responses. This may be related to the large number of neural systems that are affected by stress and likely to be involved in the pathophysiology of PTSD (12).

Noradrenergic Contributions to Anxiety in Other Psychiatric Disorders

Generalized Anxiety Disorder (GAD)

There is little clinical evidence supporting a primary role for the noradrenergic system in the pathophysiology of GAD. Plasma MHPG levels have been shown to be both increased (59) and not different (17) compared to normal controls. Similarly, increases in resting plasma NE in GAD patients have been reported in some studies (59) but not others (39). Growth hormone response to clonidine has been found to be blunted in GAD patients (22). Patients with GAD have been found to have normal responses to the alpha-2 antagonist, yohimbine (17).

Obsessive–Compulsive Disorder and Phobic Disorder

Very limited evidence supports any important role for noradrenergic systems in the pathophysiology of obsessive–compulsive disorder or phobic disorder, but full review of the literature is beyond the scope of this chapter (63,72).

Depression

Some studies have shown evidence for a relationship between CSF MHPG and anxiety (but not depression) in patients with major depressive disorders. Successful antidepressant treatment also seemed to begin with improvements in anxiety during the first week of treatment. These and other interactions with noradrenergic function in depression are consistent with a noradrenergic role in the emotion of anxiety or fear (56). Some data also exist showing increased noradrenergic function during mania, but like many of the correlative measurements they are confounded by physical activity and other extraneous factors.

CONCLUDING COMMENTS

While preclinical and clinical studies suggest that dysfunction of brain noradrenergic neurons may be involved in the development of specific human anxiety disorders, clinical anxiety is unlikely to be due entirely to abnormalities in a single neurotransmitter system. First, it is gener-

ally agreed that models which postulate too little or too much of a single neurotransmitter are not consistent with the complex regulation of neurotransmitter systems which involve multiple neurotransmitter receptor subtypes. Second, there are major functional interactions among different neurotransmitter and neuropeptide systems which make single neurotransmitter theories simplistic.

Similar arguments can be made against hypotheses that overemphasize a single brain structure to account for the spectrum of symptoms associated with human anxiety disorders. Brain structures, such as the amygdala, hypothalamus, hippocampus, and LC, are neuroanatomically and functionally interrelated and are probably responsible for different components of anxiety disorder syndromes.

Clinical research findings in panic disorder support these assertions. Drugs that produce descriptively similar panic anxiety states, such as yohimbine, MCPP, FG-7142, caffeine, lactate, and CCK-4, have many actions on neurotransmitter function, neuropeptide secretion, and cardiovascular and respiratory function. A task for future investigations of the pathophysiology of anxiety disorders is to develop clinically applicable biological tests that can assess the functional interactions among different neurotransmitter and neuropeptide systems and specific brain structures. Successful development of such paradigms could result in improved diagnostic classification and prediction of treatment response of human anxiety disorders.

ACKNOWLEDGMENTS

This work was supported by the National Center for Post Traumatic Stress Disorder, West Haven (Connecticut) Veterans Affairs Medical Center, by grants RO1-MH40140 and MH30929 from the National Institute of Mental Health, Bethesda, Maryland (Dr. Charney), and by Research Scientist Award MH00643 (Dr. Redmond). The authors thank Evelyn Testa and Karen Tyler for excellent manuscript preparation.

REFERENCES

1. Anokhin KV, Mileusnic R, Shamakina IY, Rose SPR. Effects of early experience on c-fos gene expression in the chick forebrain. *Brain Res* 1991;544:101–107.
2. Aston-Jones G, Akaoka H, Charlety P, Chouvet G. Serotonin selectively attenuates glutamate-evoked activation of noradrenergic locus coeruleus neurons. *J Neurosci* 1991;11:760–769.
3. Aston-Jones G, Chiang C, Alexinsky T. Discharge of noradrenergic locus coeruleus neurons in behaving rats and monkeys suggests a role in vigilance. In: Barnes CD, Pomeiano O, eds. *Progress in brain research.* Amsterdam: Elsevier, 1991;501–519.
4. Aston-Jones G, Ennis M, Pieribone J, Nickel WT, Shipley MT. The brain nucleus locus coeruleus: restricted afferent control over a broad efferent network. *Science* 1986;234:734–737.
5. Aston-Jones G, Valentino RJ, Van Bockstaele EJ, Meyerson AT. Locus coeruleus, stress and post traumatic stress disorder: neurobiological and clinical parallels. In: Murburg M, ed. *Catecholamine function in post traumatic stress disorder: emerging concepts.* Washington, DC: American Psychiatric Press, 1994;in press.
6. Butler PD, Weiss JM, Stout JC, Nemeroff CB. Corticotropin-

releasing factor produces fear-enhancing and behavioral activating effects following infusion into the locus coeruleus. *J Neurosci* 1990;10:(1):176–183.

7. Cameron OG, Lee MA, Curtis GC, McCann DS. Endocrine and physiological changes during spontaneous panic attacks. *Psychoneuroendocrinology* 1987;12:321–331.

8. Campean S, Hayward MD, Hope BT, Rosen JB, Nestler EJ, Davis M. Induction of the c-FOS proto-oncogene in rat amygdala during unconditioned and conditioned fear. *Brain Res* 1991;565:349–352.

9. Ceccatelli S, Villar MJ, Goldstein M, Hokfelt T. Expression of c-fos immunoreactivity in transmitter-characterized neurons after stress. *Proc Natl Acad Sci USA* 1989;86:9569–9573.

10. Cedarbaum JM, Aghajanian GK. Afferent projections to the rat locus coeruleus as determined by a retrograde tracing technique. *J Comp Neurol* 1978;178:1–16.

11. Chappell PB, Smith MA, Kilts CD, Bissette G, Ritchie J, Anderson C, Nemeroff CB. Alterations in corticotropin-releasing factor-like immunoreactivity in discrete rat brain regions after acute and chronic stress. *J Neurosci* 1990;6:2908–2914.

12. Charney DS, Deutch AY, Krystal JH, Southwick SM, Davis M. Psychobiologic mechanisms of posttraumatic stress disorder. *Arch Gen Psychiatry* 1993;50:294–305.

13. Charney DS, Heninger GR. Noradrenergic function and the mechanism of action of antianxiety treatment. I. The effect of long-term alprazolam treatment. *Arch Gen Psychiatry,* 1985;42:458–467.

14. Charney DS, Heninger GR. Noradrenergic function and the mechanism of action of antianxiety treatment. II. The effect of long-term imipramine treatment. *Arch Gen Psychiatry* 1985;41:473–481.

15. Charney DS, Heninger GR, Breier A. Noradrenergic function in panic anxiety: effects of yohimbine in healthy subjects and patients with agoraphobia and panic disorder. *Arch Gen Psychiatry* 1984;41:751–763.

16. Charney DS, Woods SW, Goodman WK, Heninger GR. Neurobiological mechanisms of panic anxiety: biochemical and behavioral correlates of yohimbine-induced panic attacks. *Am J Psychiatry* 1987;144:1030–1036.

17. Charney DS, Woods SW, Heninger GR. Noradrenergic function in generalized anxiety disorder. Effects of yohimbine in healthy subjects and patients with generalized anxiety disorder. *Psychiatry Res* 1987;27:173–182.

18. Charney DS, Woods SW, Krystal JH, Nagy LM, Heninger GR. Noradrenergic neuronal dysregulation in panic disorder: the effects of intravenous yohimbine and clonidine in panic disorder patients. *Acta Psychiatr Scand* 1992;86:273–282.

19. Charney DS, Woods SW, Price LH, Goodman WK, Glazer WM, Heninger, GR. Noradrenergic dysregulation in panic disorder. In: Ballenger JC, ed. *Neurobiology of panic disorders.* New York: Alan R Liss, 1990;91–105.

20. Craig AD. Spinal and trigeminal lamina 1 input to the locus coeruleus anterogradely labeled with *Phaseolus vulgaris* leucoagglutinin (PHA-L) in the cat and monkey. *Brain Res* 1992;584:325–328.

21. Craig AD, Linington AJ, Kniftki K-D. Significant differences in retrograde labeling of spinothalamic tract cells by horseradish peroxidase and fluorescent tracers fast blue and diamidino yellow. *Exp Brain Res* 1989;74:431–436.

22. Curtis G, Lee MA, Glitz DA, Cameron OG, Abelson J, Bronzo M. Growth hormone response to clonidine in anxiety disorders. *Biol Psychiatry* 1989;25:6A.

23. denBoer JA, Westenberg HGM. Serotonin function in panic disorder. A double blind placebo controlled study with fluvoxamine and ritanserin. *Psychopharmacology* 1990;102:85–94.

24. Dunn AJ, Berridge CW. Corticotropin-releasing factor administration elicits a stress like activation of cerebral catecholaminergic systems. *Pharmacol Biochem Behav* 1987;27:27(4):685–691.

25. Edlund. MJ, Swann AC, Davis CM. Plasma MHPG in untreated panic disorder. *Biol Psychiatry* 1987;22:1491–1495.

26. Finaly JM, Abercrombie ED. Stress induced sensitization of norepinephrine release in the medial prefrontal cortex. *Soc Neurosci Abstr* 1991;17:151.

27. Goddard AW, Woods SW, Sholomskas DE, Goodman WK, Charney DS, Heninger GR. Effects of the serotonin reuptake inhibitor fluvoxamine on noradrenergic function in panic disorder. *Psychiatry Res* 1993;48:119–133.

28. Havard HL, Buckland PR, O'Donovan MC, McGuffin P. The effect of antidepressant drugs on kainate receptor mRNA levels. *Neuropharmacology* 1991;30(6):675–677.

29. Ida Y, Tanaka M, Tsuda A, Tsujimaru S, Nagasaki N. Attenuating effect of diazepam on stress-induced increases in noradrenaline turnover in specific brain regions of rats: antagonism by Ro 15-1788. *Life Sci* 1985;37:2491–2498.

30. Irwin J, Ahluwalia P, Anisman H. Sensitization of norepinephrine activity following acute and chronic footshock. *Brain Res* 1986;379:98–103.

31. Justice A, Feldman SM, Brown LL. The nucleus locus coeruleus modulates local cerebral glucose utilization during noise stress in rats. *Brain Res* 1989;490:73–84.

32. Kaitin KI, Bliwise DL, Gleason C, Nino-Murcia G, Dement WC, Libet B. Sleep disturbance produced by electrical stimulation of the locus coeruleus in a human subject. *Biol Psychiatry* 1986;21:710–716.

33. Kinzie JD, Leung P. Clonidine in Cambodian patients with post traumatic stress disorder. *J Nerv Ment Dis* 1989;177:546–550.

34. Koob GF, Thatcher-Britton K, Britton Dr, Roberts DCS, Bloom FE. Destruction of the locus coeruleus or the dorsal NE bundle does not alter the release of punished responding by ethanol or chlordiazepoxide. *Physiol Behav* 1984;33:479–485.

35. Kosten TR, Mason JW, Giller EL, Ostroff RB, Harkness L. Sustained urinary norepinephrine and epinephrine elevation in posttraumatic stress disorder. *Psychoneuroendocrinology* 1987;12:13–20.

36. Lader M. The peripheral and central role of the catecholamines in the mechanisms of anxiety. *Int Pharmacopsychiatry* 1974;9:125–137.

37. Levine ES, Litto WJ, Jacobs BL. Activity of cat locus coeruleus noradrenergic neurons during the defense reaction. *Brain Res* 1990;531:189–195.

38. Luppi PH, Aston-Jones G, Akaoka H, Charlety P, Kovelowski C, Shipley MT, Zhu Y, Ennis M, Fort P, Chouvet G, Touvet M. Afferents to the rat locus coeruleus using choleteratoxin B subunit as a retrograde tracer. *Neurosci Abstr* 17:1991;1540.

39. Mathew RJ, Ho BT, Francis DJ, Taylor DL, Weinman ML. Catecholamines and anxiety. *Acta Psychiatr Scand* 1982;65(2):142–147.

40. McMahon SB, Wall PD. Electrophysiological mapping of brain stem projections of spinal cord lamina 1 cells in the rat. *Brain Res* 1985;333:19–26.

41. McNaughton N, Mason ST. The neuropsychology and neuropharmacology of the dorsal ascending noradrenergic bundle—a review. *Prog Neurobiol* 1980;14:157–219.

42. Melia KR, Nestler EJ, Duman RS. Chronic imipramine treatment normalized levels of tyrosine hydroxylase in the locus coeruleus of chronically stressed rats. *Psychopharmacology* 1992;108:23–26.

43. Nesse RM, Cameron OG, Buda AJ, McCann DS, Curtis CG, Huber-Smith MJ. Urinary catecholamines and mitral valve prolapse in panic anxiety patients. *Psychiatry Res* 1985;14:67–75.

44. Nesse RM, Cameron OG, Curtis GC, McCann DS, Huber-Smith MJ. Adrenergic function in patients with panic anxiety. *Arch Gen Psychiatry* 1984;41:771.

45. Nisenbaum LK, Zigmund MJ, Sved AF, Abercrombie ED. Prior exposure to chronic stress results in enhanced synthesis and release of hippocampal norepinephrine in response to a novel stressor. *J Neurosci* 1991;11:1478–1484.

46. Nutt DJ. Altered alpha2-adrenoceptor sensitivity in panic disorder. *Arch Gen Psychiatry* 1989;46:165–169.

47. Pavcovich LA, Cancela LM, Volosin M, Molina VA, Ramirez OA. Chronic stress-induced changes in locus coeruleus neuronal activity. *Brain Res Bull* 1990;24:293–296.

48. Pohl R, Yeragani VK, Balon R. Effects of isoproterenol in panic disorder patients after antidepressant treatment. *Biol Psychiatry* 1990;28:203–214.

49. Pohl R, Yeragani VK, Balon R, Rainey JM, Lycaki H, Ortiz R, Berchou R, Weinberg P. Isoproterenol induced panic attacks. *Biol Psychiatry* 1988;24:891–902.

50. Post RM. Transduction of psychosocial stress into the neurobiology of recurrent affective disorders. *Am J Psychiatry* 1992;149:999–1010.

51. Rasmussen K, Aghajanian GK. Failure to block responses to locus coeruleus neurons to somatosensory stimuli by destruction of two major afferent nucli. *Synapse* 1989;4:162–164.

52. Rasmussen K, Morilak DA, Jacobs BL. Single unit activity of locus coeruleus neurons in the freely moving cat. I. During naturalistic behaviors and in response to simple and complex stimuli. *Brain Res* 1986;371(2):324–334.

53. Redmond DE Jr. Studies of the nucleus locus coeruleus in monkeys and hypotheses for neuropsychopharmacology. In: Meltzer HY, ed. *Psychopharmacology: the third generation of progress*. New York: Raven Press, 1987;467–974.

54. Redmond DE, Huang YH. New evidence for a locus coeruleus norepinephrine connection with anxiety. *Life Sci* 1979;25:2149–2162.

55. Redmond DE Jr, Huang YH, Snyder DR, Maas JW. Behavioral effects of stimulation of the locus coeruleus in the stumptail monkey (*Macaca arctoides*). *Brain Res* 1976;116:502–507.

56. Redmond DE Jr, Katz MM, Maas JW, Swann A, Casper R. Cerebrospinal fluid biogenic amine metabolite relationships with behavioral measurements in unipolar and bipolar depressed manic and healthy control subjects. *Arch Gen Psychiatry* 1986;43:938–947.

57. Roth WT, Margraf J, Ehlers A, Taylor CB, Maddock RJ, Davies S, Agras WS. Stress reactivity in panic disorder. *Arch Gen Psychiatry* 1992;49:301–310.

58. Savaki HE, Kadekaro M, McCulloch J, Sokoloff L. The central noradrenergic system in the rat: metabolic mapping with alpha adrenergic blocking agents. *Brain Res* 1982;234:65–79.

59. Sevy S, Papadimitriou GN, Surmont DW, Goldman S, Mendlewicz J. Noradrenergic function in generalized anxiety disorder, major depressive disorder, and healthy subjects. *Biol Psychiatry* 1989;25:141–152.

60. Sheehan DV, Davidson J, Manschrek T. Lack of efficacy of a new antidepressant (bupropion) in the treatment of panic disorder with phobias. *J Clin Psychopharmacol* 1983;3:28–31.

61. Sheehan DV, Raj AB, Sheehan KH, Soto S. The relative efficacy of buspirone, imipramine, and placebo in panic disorder. A preliminary report. *Pharmacol Biochem Behav* 1988;29:815–817.

62. Shirao I, Tsuda A, Yoshisshige I, Tsujimaru S, Satoh H, Oguchi M, Tanaka M, Inanaga K. Effect of acute ethanol administration on noradrenaline metabolism in brain regions of stressed and nonstressed rats. *Pharmacol Biochem Behav* 1988;30:769–773.

63. Siever LJ, Insel TR, Jimerson DC, Lake CR, Uhde TW, Aloi J, Murphy DL. Growth hormone response to clonidine in obsessive–compulsive patients. *Br J Psychiatry* 1983;142:184–187.

64. Simson PE, Weiss JM. Altered activity of the locus coeruleus in an animal model of depression. *Neuropsychopharmacology* 1988;1:287–295.

65. Southwick SM, Krystal JH, Morgan CA, Johnson D, Nagy LM, Nicolau A, Heninger GR, Charney DS. Abnormal noradrenergic function in post-traumatic stress disorder. *Arch Gen Psychiatry* 1993;181:31–37.

66. Stone EA, Zhang Y, John S, Filer D, Bing G. Effect of locus coeruleus lesion on c-fos expression in the cerebral cortex caused by yohimbine injection or stress. *Brain Res* 1993;603:181–185.

67. Svensson TH. Peripheral, autonomic regulation of locus coeruleus noradrenergic neurons in brain. Putative implications for psychiatry and psychopharmacology. *Psychopharmacology* 1987;92:1–10.

68. Sweeney DR, Maas JW, Heninger GR. State anxiety, physical activity, and urinary 3-methoxy-4-hydroxyphenethylene glycol excretion. *Arch Gen Psychiatry* 1978;35:1418–1423.

69. Tanaka M, Kohno V, Tsuda A, Nakagawa R, Ida Y, Limori K, Nagasaki N. Differential effects of morphine on noradrenaline release in brain regions of stressed and nonstressed rats. *Brain Res* 1983;275:105–115.

70. Tanaka T, Yokoo H, Mizoguchi K, Yoshida M, Tsuda A, Tanaka M. Noradrenaline release in rat amygdala is increased by stress: studies with intracerebral microdialysis. *Brain Res* 1991;544:174–181.

71. Tanaka T, Yokoo H, Tsuda A, Tanaka M. Stress increased hypothalamic noradrenaline release studied by intracerebral dialysis method. *Neuroscience* 1990;16:293–300.

72. Tancer ME, Uhde TW. Neuroendocrine, physiologic, and behavioral responses to clonidine in patients with social phobia. *Biol Psychiatry* 1989;25:189–190.

73. Torda T, Kvetnansky R, Petrikova M. Effect of repeated immobilization stress on rat central and peripheral adrenoceptors. In: Usdin E, Kvetnansky R, Axelrod J, eds. *Stress: the role of catecholamines and other neurotransmitters*. New York: Gordon & Breach, 1984;691–701.

74. Tsaltas E, Gray JA, Fillenz M. Alleviation of response suppression to conditioned aversive stimuli by lesions of the dorsal noradrenergic bundle. *Behav Brain Res* 1987;13:115–127.

75. Uhde TW, Boulenger J-P, Post RM, Siever LJ, Vittone BJ, Jimerson DC, Roy-Byrne PP. Fear and anxiety: relationship to noradrenergic function. *Psychopathology* 1984;17(suppl 3):8–23.

76. Uhde TW, Joffe RT, Jimerson DC, Post RM. Normal urinary free cortisol and plasma MHPG in panic disorder: clinical and theoretical implications. *Biol Psychiatry* 1988;23:575–585.

77. Uhde TW, Murray MB, Vittone BJ, Siever LJ, Bouelenger JP, Klein E, Mellman TA. Behavioral and physiological effects of short-term and long-term administration of clonidine in panic disorder. *Arch Gen Psychiatry* 1989;46:170–177.

78. Uhde TW, Siever IJ, Post RM, Jimerson DC, Boulenger J-P, Buchsbaum MS. The relationship of plasma-free MHPG to anxiety and psychophysical pain in normal volunteers. *Psychopharmacol Bull* 1982;18:129–132.

79. U'Prichard DC, Kvethansky R. Central and peripheral adrenergic receptors in acute and repeated immobilization stress. In: Usdin E, Kvetnansky R, Kopin IJ, eds. *Catecholamines and stress: recent advances*. Amsterdam: Elsevier, 1980;299–308.

80. Valentino RJ, Foote SL. Corticotropin-releasing hormone increases tonic but not sensory-evoked activity of noradrenergic locus coeruleus neurons in unanesthetized rats. *J Neurosci* 1988;8:1016–1025.

81. Van Bockstaele EJ, Pieribone VA, Aston-Jones G. Diverse afferents converge on the nucleus paragigantocellularis in the rat ventrolateral medulla: retrograde and anterograde tracing studies. *J Comp Neurol* 1989;290:561–584.

82. Verleye M, Bernet F. Behavioral effects of lesions of the central noradrenergic bundles in the rat. *Pharmacol Biochem Behav* 1983;19:407–414.

83. Weiner H. The psychobiology of anxiety and fear. In: *Diagnosis and treatment of anxiety disorders*. Washington, DC: American Psychiatric Press, 1984;33–62.

84. Weiss SRB, Post RM, Pert A, Woodward R, Murman D. Context-dependent cocaine sensitization: differential effect of haloperidol on development versus expression. *Pharmacol Biochem Behav* 1989;34:655–661.

85. Woods SW, Charney DS, McPherson CA, Gradman AH, Heninger GR. Situational panic attacks: behavioral, physiological, and biochemical characterization. *Arch Gen Psychiatry* 1987;44:365–375.

86. Woods SW, Hoffer PB, McDougle CJ, Seibyl JP, Krystal JH, Heninger GR, Charney DS. Cerebral noradrenergic function in panic disorder. *Submitted for publication*.

87. Yehuda R, Southwick SM, Giller EL. Urinary catecholamine excretion and severity of post-traumatic stress disorder in Vietnam combat veterans. *J Nerv Ment Dis* 1992;180:321–325.

88. Yokoo H, Tanaka M, Yoshida M, Tsuda A, Tanaka T, Mizoguchi K. Direct evidence of conditioned fear-elicited enhancement of noradrenaline release in the rat hypothalamus assessed by intracranial microdialysis. *Brain Res* 1990;536:305–308.

Psychopharmacology: The Fourth Generation of Progress, edited by Floyd E. Bloom and David J. Kupfer. Raven Press, Ltd., New York © 1995.

CHAPTER 35

Histamine

Jean-Charles Schwartz, Jean-Michel Arrang, Monique Garbarg, and Elisabeth Traiffort

In a certain way, histaminergic systems have had a great, although indirect, historical importance in the development of neuropsychopharmacology. Indeed the discovery of both the neuroleptic and tricyclic antidepressant drugs in the 1950s was derived from the clinical study of behavioral actions of "antihistamines," a class of antiallergic drugs now designated H_1-receptor antagonists.

Nevertheless, the histaminergic neuronal system in brain, although already unraveled by the mid-1970s, has remained largely unexploited in drug design. Thus, only the traditional brain-penetrating H_1-receptor antagonists, used as over-the-counter sleeping pills, are known to interfere with histaminergic transmissions in the central nervous system (CNS). This contrasts with emergence, during the last decade, of a detailed knowledge of the system revealing that it shares many biological and functional properties with other aminergic systems overexploited in CNS drug design.

Histamine and its receptors in the brain have recently been the subject of two comprehensive reviews (22,62). Therefore, in order to limit the length of the present chapter we have deliberately selected to summarize the detailed information that can be found in these reviews, adding only more recent information and major references.

ORGANIZATION OF THE HISTAMINERGIC NEURONAL SYSTEM

One decade after the first evidence by Garbarg et al. of an ascending histaminergic pathway obtained by lesions of the medial forebrain bundle, the exact localiza-

tion of corresponding perikarya in the posterior hypothalamus was revealed immunohistochemically. Since then, the distribution, morphology, and connections of histaminergic neurons have been determined. Data were recently reviewed (49,66,68,73) and will only be summarized briefly here.

All known histaminergic perikarya constitute a continuous group of mainly magnocellular neurons (about 2000 in the rat), located in the posterior hypothalamus and collectively named the *tuberomammillary nucleus.* It can be subdivided into medial, ventral, and diffuse subgroups extending longitudinally from the caudal end of the hypothalamus to the midportion of the third ventricle. A similar organization was described in humans, except that histaminergic neurons are more numerous ($\sim$64,000) and occupy a larger proportion of the hypothalamus (2). Besides their large size (25–35 μm), tuberomammillary neurons are characterized by few thick primary dendrites, with overlapping trees, displaying few axodendritic synaptic contacts. Another characteristic feature is the close contact of dendrites with glial elements in a way suggesting that they penetrate into the ependyma and come in close contact with the cerebrospinal fluid, perhaps to secrete or receive still unidentified messengers.

The histaminergic neurons are characterized by the presence of an unusually large variety of markers for other neurotransmitter systems: glutamic acid decarboxylase, the gamma-aminobutyric acid (GABA)-synthesizing enzyme; adenosine deaminase, a cytoplasmic enzyme possibly involved in adenosine inactivation; galanin, a peptide colocalized with all other monoamines; (Met[5]) enkephalyl-Arg[6]Phe[7], a product of the proenkephalin A gene; and other neuropeptides, such as substance P, thyroliberin, or brain natriuretic peptide. Tuberomammillary neurons also contain monoamine oxidase B, an enzyme responsible for deamination of tele-methylhistamine, a major histamine metabolite in brain. Finally, a subpopula-

J.-C. Schwartz, J.-M. Arrang, M. Garbarg, and E. Traiffort: Unité de Neurobiologie et Pharmacologie (U. 109) de l'INSERM, Centre Paul Broca, 75014 Paris, France.

tion of histaminergic neurons is able to uptake and decarboxylate exogenous 5-hydroxytryptophan, a compound that they do not synthesize, however (66). Unraveling the functions of such a high number of putative co-transmitters in the same neurons remains an exciting challenge.

In analogy with other monoaminergic neurons, histaminergic neurons constitute long and highly divergent systems projecting in a diffuse manner to many cerebral areas. Immunoreactive, mostly unmyelinated, varicose or nonvaricose fibers are detected in almost all cerebral regions, particularly limbic structures. It was confirmed that individual neurons project to widely divergent areas (36). Ultrastructural studies suggest that these fibers make few typical synaptic contacts.

Fibers arising from the tuberomammillary nucleus constitute two ascending pathways: one laterally, via the medial forebrain bundle, and the other periventricularly. These two pathways combine in the diagonal band of Broca to project, mainly in an ipsilateral fashion, to many telencephalic areas—for example, in all areas and layers of the cerebral cortex, the most abundant projections being to the external layers. Other major areas of termination of these long ascending connections are the olfactory bulb, the hippocampus, the caudate putamen, the nucleus accumbens, the globus pallidus, and the amygdaloid complex. Many hypothalamic nuclei exhibit a very dense innervation—for example, the suprachiasmatic, supraoptic, arcuate, or ventromedial nuclei.

Finally, a long descending histaminergic subsystem arises also from the tuberomammillary nucleus to project to a variety of mesencephalic and brainstem structures such as the cranial nerve nuclei (e.g., the trigeminal nerve nucleus), the central gray, the colliculi, the substantia nigra, the locus coeruleus, the dorsal raphe nucleus, the cerebellum (sparse innervation), and the spinal cord.

Several anterograde tracing studies by Wouterloud and colleagues (73) established the existence of afferent connections to the histaminergic perikarya—namely, from the infralimbic division of the prefrontal cortex, the septum–diagonal band complex, the medial preoptic area, and the hippocampal area (subiculum).

MOLECULAR PHARMACOLOGY AND LOCALIZATION OF HISTAMINE RECEPTOR SUBTYPES

Three histamine receptor subtypes (H_1, H_2, and H_3) have been defined by means of functional assays and, subsequently, design of selective agonists and antagonists (22,63). All three seem to belong to the superfamily of receptors with seven transmembrane domains and coupled to guanylnucleotide-sensitive G proteins (Table 1) (see also Chapter 27, *this volume*).

The Histamine H_1 Receptor

The H_1 receptor was initially defined in functional assays (e.g., smooth muscle contraction) and the design of potent antagonists, the so-called "antihistamines" (e.g., mepyramine), most of which display prominent sedative properties.

Biochemical and localization studies of the H_1 receptor were made feasible with the design of reversible and irreversible radiolabeled probes such as [³H]mepyramine, [¹²⁵I]iodobolpyramine, and [¹²⁵I]iodoazidophenpyramine (20,50,56).

Initial biochemical studies indicated that the cerebral guinea-pig H_1 receptor was a glycoprotein of apparent molecular size of 56 kD with critical disulfide bonds and that agonist binding was regulated by guanyl nucleotides, implying that the receptor belongs to the superfamily of receptors coupled to G proteins. In addition, various intracellular responses were found to be associated with H_1-

TABLE 1. *Properties of three histamine receptor subtypes*

Property	H_1	H_2	H_3
Coding sequence	491 a.a. (bovine)	358 a.a. (rat)	?
	488 a.a. (guinea pig)	359 a.a. (dog, human)	
	486 a.a. (rat)		
Chromosome localization	Chromosome 3	?	?
Highest brain densities	Thalamus	Striatum	Striatum
	Cerebellum	Cerebral cortex	Frontal cortex
	Hippocampus	Amydgala	Substantia nigra
Autoreceptor	No	No	Yes
Affinity for histamine	Micromolar	Micromolar	Nanomolar
Characteristic agonists	2(*m*-chlorophenyl)histamine	Impromidine	(R)α-methylhistamine
		Sopromidine	Imetit
Characteristic antagonists	Mepyramine (pyrilamine)	Cimetidine	Thioperamide
Radioligands	[³H]Mepyramine	[³H]Tiotidine	[³H](R)α-methylhistamine
	[¹²⁵I]Iodobolpyramine	[¹²⁵I]Iodoaminopotentidine	[¹²⁵I]Iodophenpropit
Second messengers	Inositol phosphates (+)	cAMP (+)	Inositol phosphates (−)
	Arachidonic acid (+)	Arachidonic acid (−)	
	cAMP (potentiation)	Ca^{2+} (+)	

receptor stimulation: inositol phosphate release, increase in Ca^{2+} fluxes, cyclic AMP or cyclic GMP accumulation in whole cells, and arachidonic acid release (22). It was not known, however, whether such a variety of responses corresponds to a single receptor or to distinct isoreceptors. Indeed, several photoaffinity-labeled proteins of slightly different sizes, but similar H_1 pharmacology, were detected in some tissues (56).

In spite of preliminary attempts using affinity columns with a mepyramine derivative, the H_1 receptor was never purified to homogeneity. Nevertheless, the deduced amino acid sequence of a bovine H_1 receptor was recently disclosed after expression cloning of a corresponding cDNA. The latter was based upon the detection of a Ca^{2+}-dependent Cl^- influx into microinjected *Xenopus* oocytes. Following the transient expression of the cloned cDNA into COS-7 cells, the identity of the protein as an H_1 receptor was confirmed by binding studies (75).

Starting from the bovine sequence, the H_1-receptor DNA was also cloned in the guinea pig (23,69), a species in which the pharmacology of the receptor is better established. Although marked species differences in H_1-receptor pharmacology had been reported (62), the sequence homology between the putative transmembrane domains (TMs) of the two proteins is rather high (90%).

In both species, characteristic amino acid residues thought to bind the histamine molecule at the level of the ammonium and imidazole groups are found: an aspartate (Asp^{116} in the guinea pig) in TM3, and a threonine (Thr^{203}) and an asparagine (Asn^{207}) in TM5, respectively. Also the "anatomy" of the H_1 receptor, with a long i_3 (third intracellular domain) and a short C-terminal tail, is similar to that of other receptors positively coupled to phospholipases A_2 and C. Amino acid sequence homology between the TMs of the H_1 and of the muscarinic receptors ($\sim$45%) is higher than between those of H_1 and H_2 receptors ($\sim$40%). H_1-receptor antagonists often display significant antimuscarinic activity but only limited H_2-receptor antagonist properties.

A single intronless gene seems to encode the guinea-pig H_1 receptor, and mRNAs of similar size were detected in brain areas and peripheral tissues (69). Thus the two pharmacologically indiscernible isoforms of the H_1 receptor of 56 and 68 kD, detected after photolabeling and sodium dodecyl sulfate–polyacrylamide gel electrophoresis (SDS-PAGE) in some tissues (56), may correspond either to the same protein with different degrees of glycosylation or to the product of another similar gene revealed by Southern blot analysis (23).

When stably expressed in transfected fibroblasts, the guinea-pig H_1 receptor was found to trigger a large variety of intracellular signals involving or not coupling to pertussis-toxin-sensitive G proteins (Gi or Go)—namely, Ca^{2+} transients, inositol phosphates, or arachidonate release (33). H_1-receptor stimulation potentiates cAMP accumulation induced by forskolin in the same transfected fibro-

blasts, a response which resembles the H_1 potentiation of histamine H_2- or adenosine A_2-receptor-induced accumulation of cAMP in brain slices. All these responses mediated by a single H_1 receptor were known to occur in distinct cell lines or brain slices but could have been due to stimulation of isoreceptors.

The H_1 receptor mediates various excitatory responses in brain (21). In addition, in lateral geniculate relay neurons, it was recently shown to be responsible for a slow depolarization due to decrease in a K^+ current (39).

H_1-receptor distribution in the guinea-pig brain was established autoradiographically using [^{3}H]mepyramine or the more sensitive probe [^{125}I]iodobolpyramine (50) and the information complemented by in situ hybridization of the mRNA (23,69). For instance, the high density of H_1 receptors in the molecular layers of cerebellum and hippocampus seems to correspond to dendrites of Purkinje and pyramidal cells, respectively, in which the mRNA is highly expressed. H_1 receptors are also abundant in guinea-pig thalamus, hypothalamic nuclei (e.g., ventromedial nuclei), nucleus accumbens, amygdaloid nuclei, and frontal cortex but not in neostriatum (50), whereas they are more abundant in the human neostriatum (37).

The H_1 receptor was visualized in the primate and human brain by positron emission tomography using [^{11}C]-mepyramine (76).

The widespread distribution of the H_1 receptor in cerebral areas involved in wakefulness and cognition presumably accounts for the sedative properties of "antihistamines" of the first generation.

The Histamine H_2 Receptor

Molecular properties of the H_2 receptor have remained largely unknown for a long time. For instance, reversible labeling of the H_2 receptor was achieved only recently using [^{3}H]tiotidine or, more reliably, [^{125}I]-iodoaminopotentidine (62). Irreversible labeling, using a photoaffinity probe, followed by SDS-PAGE led to the identification of H_2-receptor peptides from the guinea pig (56).

By screening cDNA or genomic libraries with homologous probes, the gene encoding the H_2 receptor was first identified in dogs (18) and, subsequently, in rats (55) and humans (17). The H_2 receptor is organized like other receptors positively coupled to adenylyl cyclase; that is, it displays a short third intracellular loop and a long C-terminal cytoplasmic tail.

Initially, binding of the histamine molecule in the H_2 receptor seemed to involve (a) the carboxylate of Asp^{98} in TM3 as a counterion for the ammonium and (b) Asp^{186} and Thr^{190} for proton transfer and hydrogen bonding with the imidazole ring, but this idea found only partial support from site-directed mutagenesis (16).

Using transfected cell lines, not only the well-established positive linkage of the H_2 receptor with adenylyl cyclase (28) was confirmed, but also the unexpected inhibition of arachidonate release (71) and stimulation of Ca^{2+} transients (13). Hence H_2-receptor stimulation can trigger intracellular signals either opposite or similar to those evoked by H_1-receptor stimulation. Parallel observations were made for a variety of biological responses mediated by the two receptors in peripheral tissues.

Helmut Haas and colleagues showed that, in hippocampal pyramidal neurons, H_2-receptor stimulation potentiates excitatory signals by decreasing a Ca^{2+}-activated K^+ conductance, presumably via cAMP production (21). H_2-receptor activation depolarizes thalamic relay neurons slightly, increasing markedly apparent membrane conductance, a response due to enhancement of the hyperpolarization-activated cation current I_h (39).

The sole selective H_2-receptor antagonist known to enter the brain is zolantidine, a compound used sometimes in animal behavioral studies but never introduced in therapeutics (15). However, a number of tricyclic antidepressants are known to block H_2-receptor-linked adenylylcyclase quite potently and interact with $[^{125}I]$-iodoaminopotentidine binding in a complex manner (72).

Autoradiographic localization of H_2 receptors in guinea pig performed using $[^{125}I]$iodoaminopotentidine shows them distributed heterogeneously in a manner suggesting their major association with neurons (50). H_2 receptors are found in most areas of the cerebral cortex, with the highest density in the superficial layers, the piriform and occipital cortices, which contain low H_1-receptor density. The caudate putamen, ventral striatal complex, and amygdaloid nuclei (bed nucleus of the stria terminalis) are among the richest brain areas. In the hippocampal formation, H_2 receptors display a laminated pattern with labeling of lacunosum moleculare, radiatum, and oriens layers; the partial overlap with H_1 receptors may account for their synergistic interaction in cAMP accumulation. H_2 receptors in human brain were characterized and localized using $[^{125}I]$iodoaminopotendine (70).

The Histamine H_3 Receptor

The H_3 receptor was initially detected as an autoreceptor controlling histamine synthesis and release in brain. Thereafter it was shown to inhibit presynaptically the release of other monoamines in brain and peripheral tissues as well as of neuropeptides from unmyelinated C fibers (3).

The molecular structure of the H_3 receptor remains to be established. Reversible labeling of this receptor was first achieved using the highly selective agonist $[^3H](R)\alpha$-methylhistamine (62); then $[^3H]N\alpha$-methylhistamine, a less selective agonist, was also proposed (20) as well as, more recently, $[^{125}I]$iodophenpropit, an antagonist (27). The binding of $[^3H](R)\alpha$-methylhistamine is regulated by

guanyl nucleotides, strongly suggesting that the H_3 receptor, like the other histamine receptors, belongs to the superfamily of receptors coupled to G proteins (62). Constitutive H_3 receptors in a gastric cell line appear to be negatively coupled to phospholipase C via a mechanism sensitive to both pertussis and cholera toxins (6). In contrast, H_3 receptors in vascular smooth muscle mediate voltage-dependent Ca^{2+}-channel stimulation via a pertussis-insensitive G protein (44).

Recently, two highly potent and selective H_3-receptor agonists—$(R)\alpha,(S)\beta$-dimethylhistamine (35) and imetit (19)—were designed. Like $(R)\alpha$-methylhistamine, they are able to decrease brain histamine synthesis and release after systemic administration in low dosage (3,19,62). Thioperamide, a systemically active H_3 antagonist, markedly increases histamine turnover in brain (3) and, because no other class of drug is available for this purpose, is widely used in behavioral studies.

Functional studies have evidenced inhibitory H_3 receptors on nerve terminals not only of histaminergic (3,62) but also noradrenergic (58), serotoninergic (14), dopaminergic (59), cholinergic (7), and peptidergic neurons (38).

Autoradiography of H_3 receptors in rat (12,51) and monkey brain (37) shows them highly concentrated in neostriatum, nucleus accumbens, cingulate and infralimbic cortices, bed nucleus of stria terminalis, and substantia nigra pars lateralis. In contrast, their density is relatively low in the hypothalamus (including the tuberomammillary nucleus), which contains the highest density of histaminergic axons (and perikarya), indicating that the majority of H_3 receptors are not autoreceptors. In agreement, intrastriatal kainate strongly decreases H_3 binding sites in forebrain (as well as in substantia nigra, consistent with their presence in striatonigral neurons) (12,51).

HISTAMINERGIC NEURON ACTIVITY AND THEIR CONTROL

Electrophysiological Properties

Cortically projecting histaminergic neurons share with other aminergic neurons a number of electrophysiological properties evidenced by extracellular recording. They fire spontaneously slowly and regularly, and their action potentials are of long duration (21). In addition, they exhibit inward rectification attributed to an I_h current that may increase whole-cell conductance and decrease the efficacy of synaptic inputs during periods of prolonged hyperpolarization (see Chapter 5, *this volume*)—that is, when histaminergic neurons fall silent (29).

Modulation of Histamine Synthesis and Release In Vitro

The autoreceptor-regulated modulation of histamine synthesis in, and release from, brain neurons is now well-documented (62). It was initially evidenced in brain slices or synaptosomes after labeling the endogenous pool of histamine using the ^{3}H precursor. Exogenous histamine decreases the release and formation of [^{3}H]histamine induced by depolarization, and analysis of these responses led to the pharmacological definition of H_3 receptors. The autoregulation was found in various brain regions known to contain histamine nerve endings, suggesting that all terminals are endowed with H_3 autoreceptors. A regulation of histamine synthesis was also observed in the posterior hypothalamus, possibly indicating the existence of autoreceptors at the level of histaminergic perikarya or dendrites (3).

Galanin, a putative co-transmitter of a subpopulation of histaminergic neurons, regulates histamine release only in regions known to contain efferents of this subpopulation—that is, in hypothalamus and hippocampus but not in cerebral cortex or striatum (4). In brain slices, galanin also hyperpolarizes and decreases the firing rate of tuberomammillary neurons (60). It is not known, however, whether these galanin "autoreceptors" modulate galanin release from histaminergic nerve terminals. Other putative co-transmitters of histaminergic neurons failed to affect [^{3}H]histamine release from slices of rat cerebral cortex (61).

[^{3}H]Histamine synthesis and release are inhibited in various brain regions by stimulation of not only autoreceptors but also α_2-adrenergic receptors, M_1-muscarinic receptors, and κ-opioid receptors (62). Muscarinic receptors also inhibit endogenous histamine release in hypothalamus (48). Since these regulations are also observed with synaptosomes (61), all these receptors presumably represent true presynaptic heteroreceptors. In contrast, histamine release is enhanced by stimulation of nicotinic receptors in rat hypothalamus (48) and by μ-opioid receptors in mouse cerebral cortex (62).

Changes in Histaminergic Neuron Activity In Vivo

Both neurochemical and electrophysiological studies indicate that the activity of histaminergic neurons is high during arousal. In rat hypothalamus, histamine levels are low whereas synthesis is high during the dark period, suggesting that neuronal activity is enhanced during the active phase (62). Histamine release from the anterior hypothalamus of freely moving rats, evaluated by in vivo microdialysis, gradually increases in the second half of the light period and is maintained at a maximal level during the active phase (40). Such state-related changes are also found in single-unit extracellular recordings performed in the ventrolateral posterior hypothalamus of freely moving cats. Neurons with properties consistent with those of histaminergic neurons exhibited a circadian rhythm of their firing rate, falling silent during deep slowwave or paradoxical sleep (62).

A feeding-induced increase in the activity of histaminergic neurons has also been shown by microdialysis performed in the hypothalamus of conscious rats (26). Changes in the metabolism and release of histamine observed in vivo after occlusion of the middle cerebral artery in rats suggest that the histaminergic activity is also enhanced by cerebral ischemia (1).

Whereas H_1 and H_2 receptors are apparently not involved, inhibition mediated by H_3 autoreceptors constitutes a major regulatory mechanism for histaminergic neuron activity under physiological conditions. Administration of selective H_3-receptor agonists reduces histamine turnover (62) and release, as shown by microdialysis (24). In contrast, H_3-receptor antagonists enhance histamine turnover (62) and release in vivo (25,41), suggesting that autoreceptors are under tonic stimulation by endogenous histamine.

Agents inhibiting histamine release in vitro via stimulation of presynaptic α_2-adrenergic or muscarinic heteroreceptors reduce histamine release and turnover in vivo, but systemic administration of antagonists of these receptors does not generally enhance histamine turnover, suggesting that heteroreceptors are not tonically activated under basal conditions (9,45,52,61).

Activation of central nicotinic (45), 5-HT$_{1A}$ serotonergic (46), and dopaminergic receptors (53) inhibits histamine turnover, but the presynaptic location of these receptors remains to be demonstrated. Histamine turnover in the brain is also rapidly reduced after administration of various sedative drugs such as ethanol, Δ^9-tetrahydrocannabinol, barbiturates, and benzodiazepines (62). The effect of the latter compounds may result from their interaction in vivo with GABA receptors present on nerve endings of a subpopulation of histaminergic neurons containing GABA (66).

In contrast, stimulation of μ-opioid (62) and N-methyl-D-aspartate (NMDA) receptors (47) enhances histamine release and turnover in brain. Morphine increases histamine release in the periaqueductal gray (5).

The effect of reserpine on brain histamine turnover appears to be controversial: Both enhancement (62) and inhibition (42) were reported.

PHYSIOLOGICAL ROLES OF HISTAMINERGIC NEURONS

In spite of many different suggestions mainly derived from the observations of responses to locally applied histamine, only few physiological roles of histaminergic neurons appear relatively well-documented.

Arousal

Following our initial proposal in 1977, a large body of experimental evidence has accumulated to indicate that histaminergic neurons play a critical role in cortical activation and arousal mechanisms (62).

Intracerebral injection of histamine, particularly in the cat ventrolateral hypothalamus, where the density of histaminergic axons is high, increases wakefulness via stimulation of postsynaptic H_1 receptors. Endogenous histamine presumably plays a similar role because inhibition of its synthesis by an L-histidine decarboxylase inhibitor, inhibition of its release by an H_3-receptor agonist, and inhibition of its action by an H_1-receptor antagonist all increase deep slow-wave sleep and decrease wakefulness in several animal species; conversely, inhibitors of histamine methylation or H_3-receptor antagonists, which facilitate the amine release, both increase arousal (34,62). The role of histaminergic neurons in arousal is also shown by the decreased wakefulness following lesions of the posterior hypothalamus, particularly those aimed at destruction of the tuberomammillary nucleus.

Finally, histaminergic neurons share with other cortically projecting aminergic neurons which control behavioral states a number of electrophysiological properties, including increased activity during wakefulness (see preceding section).

Cellular modes of action of histamine mediated by H_1 and H_2 receptors may well account for its "arousing effect." On thalamic relay neurons, histamine, acting through these receptors, exerts a double depolarizing action and thereby facilitates a change of neuronal activity from one of endogenous oscillation and poor responsiveness to sensory inputs which predominates during sleep, to one dominated by single-spike activity and a more accurate and faithful relay of sensory information which characterizes arousal (67). In addition, histamine will facilitate further processing of sensory information in the neocortex through the reduction of spike frequency adaptation resulting from a block of a Ca^{2+}-activated K^+ current mediated by the H_2 receptor (21). These various actions seem shared by other neurotransmitters (including acetylcholine, noradrenaline, serotonin, and glutamate) which collectively innervate the forebrain and, possibly via shifts in oscillatory states of thalamocortical networks, promote the characteristic changes in firing occurring between sleep and arousal (67).

All these cellular modes of action of histamine, taken together with observations indicating that its release from activated tuberomammillary neurons is maximal during wakefulness, suggest that the histaminergic systems make an important contribution to the ascending control of arousal, attention, sensory information processing, and cognition.

Accordingly, in humans, many H_1-receptor antagonists induce drowsiness, impair performances requiring attention, increase the tendency to sleep, and are ingredients of over-the-counter sleeping pills. These sedative effects are stereoselective (43). Conversely, a new generation of "antihistamines," unable to block cerebral H_1 receptors,

are devoid of sedative properties. A rather large number of antidepressant (e.g., mianserin or doxepin) and antipsychotic agents (e.g., clozapine) display high H_1-receptor antagonist potency which presumably accounts for their sedative side effects (54).

Control of Pituitary Hormone Secretion

Exogenous and, in some cases, endogenous histamine were shown to affect the secretion of both posterior and anterior pituitary hormones (32,62).

Supraoptic nucleus neurons are typically excited by application of histamine, their firing rate being increased during secretory bursts of activity and the depolarizing afterpotential being enhanced (65). This effect is mediated by H_1 receptors and causes circulating vasopressin levels to rise. Histaminergic neurons may participate in the physiological control of vasopressin secretion because inhibition of histamine synthesis impairs the vasopressin response to adrenalectomy and stimulation of the tuberomammillary nucleus causes phasic supraoptic nucleus neurons to become more excitable (77). This control, however, may not be a tonic one because H_1-receptor antagonists do not appear to modify vasopressin secretion. It is not known whether the increase in water consumption elicited by an H_3-receptor agonist is related to an effect on supraoptic nucleus neurons (8).

Endogenous histamine may be involved in stress-, estrogen- or morphine-induced release of prolactin because the response is prevented by blockade of histamine synthesis or of postsynaptic H_1 or H_2 receptors or activation of presynaptic H_3 autoreceptors (32). Being also prevented by antibodies to vasopressin, the action of histamine may involve this neuropeptide. Endogenous histamine, acting primarily at H_1 receptors, may also be involved in the secretory responses of adrenocorticotropic hormone and β-endorphin induced by restraint or insulin hypoglycemia.

Although exogenous histamine predominantly inhibits the release of growth hormone and thyroid-stimulating hormone, the role of histaminergic neurons in the control of these hormones secretion is not established.

Control of Appetite

Weight gain is often experienced by patients receiving H_1 antihistamines or tricyclic antidepressants displaying potent H_1-receptor antagonist properties. It is likely that this reflects an inhibitory role of histamine neurons projecting to the ventromedial and paraventricular hypothalamic nuclei on feeding as shown by the effects of histamine synthesis inhibitors or H_3-receptor ligands (57). In addition, the extracellular concentration of the amine in rat hypothalamus increases during feeding (26).

Regulation of Seizure Susceptibility

The action of drugs affecting histamine synthesis or methylation, as well as of H_1- and H_3-receptor antagonists, suggests that endogenous histamine may restrict the manifestations of electrically and pentetrazole-induced seizures in rodents (78,79).

Regulation of Vestibular Reactivity

Some H_1 antagonists are the most commonly used anti-motion-sickness drugs, but it is not clear whether this is related to blockade of H_1 receptors. Histamine depolarizes neurons in vestibular nuclei and modulates quite effectively static vestibular reflexes through interaction with both H_2 and H_3 receptors (64,74). A beneficial effect of H_3-receptor antagonists in vertigo or motion sickness was suggested by these data.

DO HISTAMINERGIC NEURONS HAVE A ROLE IN NEUROPSYCHIATRIC DISEASES?

Among the various approaches that tend to establish the implication of other aminergic neuronal systems in neuropsychiatric diseases, so far only a few were (or could be) applied to histamine.

Postmortem studies in basal ganglia of patients with Parkinson's disease (62) or in a rodent model of this disease (10) show no change in the activity of the histamine-synthesizing enzyme.

In the hypothalamus of Alzheimer's disease patients, numerous neurofibrillary tangles and typical senile plaques were detected in the tuberomammillary area; it was not clear, however, whether the number of histamine-immunoreactive neurons was decreased (2). Because reports on histamine levels in such patients have been conflicting, a role of histamine in the etiopathology of Alzheimer's disease remains doubtful. In addition, it may be of significance that 9-amino-1,2,3,4-tetrahydroacridine (THA), an anticholinesterase drug which was found useful in Alzheimer's disease, is also a rather potent inhibitor of histamine methylation (11).

The effects of antipsychotics at dopamine receptors strongly suggested the role of dopamine in schizophrenia. In contrast, the interaction of psychotropic drugs with histamine receptors are of limited help to deduce a role of histaminergic neurons in psychiatry. Over a decade ago, the cerebral H_2 receptor was proposed by J. P. Green, P. Greengard, and colleagues to represent an important target for most tricyclic and other antidepressant drugs that interact with relatively high affinity with the receptor coupled to the cyclase (54). The strong dependence of the apparent affinity of these compounds for the H_2 receptor upon the experimental conditions of the assay leaves some doubt, however, about the therapeutic significance

of this observation (72). It remains that a number of side effects of several antidepressant drugs as well as some neuroleptics (e.g., sedation or weight gain) are attributable to the blockade of cerebral H_1 receptors (54).

Unfortunately, the effects of drugs able to stimulate the three cerebral histamine receptor subtypes or to block H_2 or H_3 receptors in neuropsychiatric diseases are not known. Therefore, these receptors remain important potential targets for novel classes of psychotropic agents, particularly "cognition/arousal enhancers" acting via facilitation of histaminergic neurotransmission in brain.

REFERENCES

1. Adachi N, Itoh Y, Oishi R, Saeki K. Direct evidence for increased continuous histamine release in the striatum of conscious freely moving rats produced by middle cerebral artery occlusion. *J Cereb Blood Flow Metab* 1992;12:477–483.
2. Airaksinen MS, Paetau A, Paliärui L, Reinikainen K, Riekkinen P, Suomalainen R, Panula P. Histamine neurons in human hypothalamus: anatomy in normal and Alzheimer diseased brains. *Neurosci* 1991;44:465–481.
3. Arrang JM, Garbarg M, Schwartz JC. H_3-receptor and control of histamine release. In: Schwartz JC, Haas HL, eds. *The histamine receptor.* New York: Wiley–Liss, 1992;145–159.
4. Arrang JM, Gulat-Marnay C, Defontaine N, Schwartz JC. Regulation of histamine release in rat hypothalamus and hippocampus by presynaptic galanin receptors. *Peptides* 1991;12:1113–1117.
5. Barke KE, Hough LB. Morphine-induced increases of extracellular histamine levels in the periaqueductal grey in vivo: a microdialysis study. *Brain Res* 1992;572:146–153.
6. Cherifi Y, Pigeon C, Le Romancier M, Bado A, Reyl-Desmars F, Lewin MJM. Purification of a histamine H_3 receptor negatively coupled to phosphoinositide turnover in the human gastric cell line HGT1. *J Biol Chem* 1992;267:25315–25320.
7. Clapham J, Kilpatrick GJ. Histamine H_3 receptor modulate the release of [³H]acetylcholine from slices of rat entorhinal cortex: evidence for the possible existence of H_3 receptor subtypes. *Br J Pharmacol* 1992;107:919–923.
8. Clapham J, Kilpatrick GJ. Histamine H_3-receptor mediated modulation of water consumption in the rat. *Eur J Pharmacol* 1993;232:99–103.
9. Cumming P, Damsma G, Fibiger HC, Vincent SR. Characterization of extracellular histamine in the striatum and bed nucleus of the stria terminalis of the rat: an in vivo microdialysis study. *J Neurochem* 1991;56:1797–1803.
10. Cumming P, Jakubovic A, Vincent SR. Cerebral histamine levels are unaffected by MPTP administration in the mouse. *Eur J Pharmacol* 1989;166:299–301.
11. Cumming P, Reiner PB, Vincent SR. Inhibition of rat brain histamine-N-methyltransferase by 9 amino 1,2,3,4tetrahydroacridine-(THA). *Biochem Pharmacol* 1990;40:1345–1350.
12. Cumming P, Shaw C, Vincent SR. High affinity histamine binding site is the H_3 receptor: characterization and autoradiographic localization in rat brain. *Synapse* 1991;8:144–151.
13. Delvalle J, Wang L, Gantz I, Yamada T. Characterization of H_2 histamine receptor: linkage to both adenylate cyclase and [Ca²⁺]ᵢ signaling systems. *Am J Physiol* 1992;263:G967–G972.
14. Fink K, Schlicker E, Neise A, Göthert M. Involvement of presynaptic H_3 receptors in the inhibitory effect of histamine on serotonin release in the rat brain cortex. *Naunyn Schmiedebergs Arch Pharmacol* 1990;342:513–519.
15. Ganellin CR. Pharmacochemistry of H_1 and H_2 receptors. In: Schwartz JC, Haas HL, eds. *The histamine receptor.* New York: Wiley–Liss, 1992;1–56.
16. Gantz I, Delvalle J, Wang LD, Tashiro T, Munzert G, Guo YJ, Konda Y, Yamada T. Molecular basis for the interaction of histamine with the histamine H_2 receptor. *J Biol Chem* 1992;267:20840–20843.

17. Gantz I, Munzert G, Tashiro T, Schaffer M, Wang L, Delvalle J, Yamada T. Molecular cloning of the human histamine H_2 receptor. *Biochem Biophys Res Commun* 1991;178:1386–1392.

18. Gantz I, Schaffer M, Delvalle J, Logsdon C, Campbell V, Uhler M, Yamada T. Molecular cloning of a gene encoding the histamine H_2 receptor. *Proc Natl Acad Sci USA* 1991;88:429–433.

19. Garbarg M, Arrang JM, Rouleau A, Ligneau X, Dam Trung Tuong M, Schwartz JC, Ganellin CR. S-[2-(4-Imidazolyl)ethyl]isothiourea, a highly specific and potent histamine H_3-receptor agonist. *J Pharmacol Exp Ther* 1992;263:304–310.

20. Garbarg M, Traiffort E, Ruat M, Arrang JM, Schwartz JC. Reversible labelling of H_1, H_2 and H_3 receptors. In: Schwartz JC, Haas HL, eds. *The histamine receptor*. New York: Wiley–Liss, 1992;73–95.

21. Haas HL. Electrophysiology of histamine receptors. In: Schwartz JC, Haas HL, eds. *The histamine receptor*. New York: Wiley–Liss, 1992;161–177.

22. Hill SJ. Distribution, properties and functional characteristics of three classes of histamine receptor. *Pharmacol Rev* 1990;42:45–83.

23. Horio Y, Mori Y, Higuchi I, Fujimoto K, Ito S, Fukui H. Molecular cloning of the guinea pig histamine H_1 receptor gene. *J Biochem* 1993;114:408–414.

24. Itoh Y, Oishi R, Adachi N, Saeki K. A highly sensitive assay for histamine using ion-pair HPLC coupled with postcolumn fluorescent derivatization: its application to biological specimens. *J Neurochem* 1992;58:884–889.

25. Itoh Y, Oishi R, Nishibori M, Saeki K. Characterization of histamine release from the rat hypothalamus as measured by in vivo microdialysis. *J Neurochem* 1991;56:769–774.

26. Itoh Y, Oishi R, Saeki K. Feeding-induced increase in the extracellular concentration of histamine in rat hypothalamus as measured by in vivo microdialysis. *Neurosci Lett* 1991;125:235–237.

27. Jansen FP, Rademaker B, Bast A, Timmerman H. The first radiolabelled histamine H_3 receptor antagonist, [^{125}I]iodophenpropit: saturable and reversible binding to rat cortex membranes. *Eur J Pharmacol* 1992;217:203–205.

28. Johnson CL. Histamine receptors and cyclic nucleotides. In: Schwartz JC, Haas HL, eds. *The histamine receptor*. New York: Wiley–Liss, 1992;129–143.

29. Kamondi A, Reiner PB. Hyperpolarization-activated inward current in histaminergic tuberomammillary neurons of the rat hypothalamus. *J Neurophysiol* 1991;66:1902–1911.

30. Kjaer A, Knigge U, Vilhardt H, Bach FW, Warberg J. Involvement of vasopressin V_1 and V_2 receptors in histamine and stress induced secretion of ACTH and β-endorphin. *Neuroendocrinology* 1993;57:503–509.

31. Kjaer A, Knigge U, Vilhardt H, Warberg J. Involvement of vasopressin in histamine and stress-induced prolactin release: permissive, mediating or potentiating role? *Neuroendocrinology* 1993;57:314–321.

32. Knigge U, Warberg J. Minireview: the role of histamine in the neuroendocrine regulation of pituitary hormone secretion. *Acta Endocrinol* 1991;124:609–619.

33. Leurs R, Traiffort E, Arrang JM, Tardivel-Lacombe J, Ruat M, Schwartz JC. Guinea pig histamine H_1 receptor. II. Stable expression in Chinese hamster ovary cells reveals the interaction with three major signal transduction pathways. *J Neurochem* 1994;62:519–527.

34. Lin JS, Sakai K, Vanni-Mercier G, Arrang JM, Garbarg M, Schwartz JC, Jouvet M. Involvement of histaminergic neurons in arousal mechanisms demonstrated with H_3-receptor ligands in the cat. *Brain Res* 1990;523:325–330.

35. Lipp R, Arrang JM, Garbarg M, Luger P, Schwartz JC, Schunack W. Synthesis, absolute configuration, stereoselectivity, and receptor selectivity of $(\alpha R, \beta S)$-α, β-dimethylhistamine, a novel highly potent histamine H_3-receptor agonist. *J Med Chem* 1992;35:4434–4441.

36. Losier B, Semba K. Dual projections of single cholinergic and aminergic brainstem neurons to the thalamus and basal forebrain in the rat. *Brain Res* 1993;604:41–52.

37. Martinez Mir MI, Pollard H, Moreau J, Arrang JM, Ruat M, Traiffort E, Schwartz JC, Palacios JM. Three histamine receptors (H_1, H_2 and H_3) visualized in the brain of human and non-human primates. *Brain Res* 1990;526:322–327.

38. Matsubara T, Moskowitz MA, Huang Z. UK-14, 304, R($-$)-α-methylhistamine and SMS 201-995 block plasma protein leakage within dura mater by prejunctional mechanisms. *Eur J Pharmacol* 1992;224:145–150.

39. McCormick DA, Williamson A. Modulation of neuronal firing mode in cat and guinea pig LGNd by histamine: possible cellular mechanisms of histaminergic control of arousal. *J Neurosci* 1991;11:3188–3199.

40. Mochizuki T, Yamatodani A, Okakura K, Horii A, Inagaki N, Wada H. Circadian rhythm of histamine release from the hypothalamus of freely moving rats. *Physiol Behav* 1992;51:391–394.

41. Mochizuki T, Yamatodani A, Okakura K, Takemura M, Inagaki N, Wada H. In vivo release of neuronal histamine in the hypothalamus of rats measured by microdialysis. *Naunyn Schmiedebergs Arch Pharmacol* 1991;343:190–195.

42. Muroi N, Oishi R, Saeki K. Effect of reserpine on histamine metabolism in the mouse brain. *J Pharmacol Exp Ther* 1991;256:967–972.

43. Nicholson AN, Pascoe PA, Turner C, Ganellin CR, Greengrass PM, Casy AF, Mercer AD. Sedation and histamine H_1 receptor antagonist studies in man with the enantiomers of chlorpheniramine and dimethindene. *Br J Pharmacol* 1991;104:270–276.

44. Oike M, Kitamura K, Kuriyama H. Histamine H_3-receptor activation augments voltage-dependent Ca^{2+} current via GTP hydrolysis in rabbit saphenous artery. *J Physiol* 1992;448:133–152.

45. Oishi R, Adachi N, Okada K, Muroi N, Saeki K. Regulation of histamine turnover via muscarinic and nicotinic receptors in the brain. *J Neurochem* 1990;55:1899–1904.

46. Oishi R, Itoh Y, Saeki K. Inhibition of histamine turnover by 8-OH-DPAT, buspirone and 5-hydroxytryptophan in the mouse and rat brain. *Naunyn Schmiedebergs Arch Pharmacol* 1992;345:495–499.

47. Okakura K, Yamatodani A, Mochizuki T, Horii A, Wada H. Glutamatergic regulation of histamine release from rat hypothalamus. *Eur J Pharmacol* 1992;213:189–192.

48. Ono J, Yamatodani A, Kishino J, Okada S, Wada H. Cholinergic influence of K^+-evoked release of endogenous histamine from rat hypothalamic slices in vitro. *Methods Find Exp Clin Pharmacol* 1992;14:35–40.

49. Panula P, Airaksinen MS. The histaminergic neuronal system as revealed with antisera against histamine. In: Watanabe T, Wada H, eds. *Histaminergic neurons: morphology and function*. Boca Raton, FL: CRC Press, 1991;127–144.

50. Pollard H, Bouthenet ML. Autoradiographic visualization of the three histamine receptor subtypes in the brain. In: Schwartz JC, Haas HL, eds. *The histamine receptor*. New York: Wiley–Liss, 1992;179–192.

51. Pollard H, Moreau J, Arrang JM, Schwartz JC. A detailed autoradiographic mapping of histamine H_3-receptors in rat brain areas. *Neuroscience* 1993;52:169–189.

52. Prast H, Heistracher M, Philippu A. In vivo modulation of the histamine release in the hypothalamus by adrenoreceptor agonists and antagonists. *Naunyn Schmiedebergs Arch Pharmacol* 1991; 344:183–186.

53. Prast H, Heistracher M, Philippu A. Modulation by dopamine receptors of the histamine release in the rat hypothalamus. *Naunyn Schmiedebergs Arch Pharmacol* 1993;347:301–305.

54. Richelson E. Histamine receptors in the central nervous system. In: Schwartz JC, Haas HL, eds. *The histamine receptor*. New York: Wiley–Liss, 1992;271–295.

55. Ruat M, Traiffort E, Arrang JM, Leurs R, Schwartz JC. Cloning and tissue expression of a rat histamine H_2-receptor gene. *Biochem Biophys Res Commun* 1991;179:1470–1478.

56. Ruat M, Traiffort E, Schwartz JC. Biochemical properties of histamine receptors. In: Schwartz JC, Haas HL, eds. *The histamine receptor*. New York: Wiley–Liss, 1992;97–107.

57. Sakata T, Fukagawa K, Ookuma K, Fujimoto K, Yoshimatsu H, Yamatodani A, Wada H. Hypothalamic neuronal histamine modulates ad libitum feeding by rats. *Brain Res* 1990;537:303–306.

58. Schlicker E, Behling A, Lümmen G, Göthert M. Histamine H_{3A} receptor-mediated inhibition of noradrenaline release in the mouse brain cortex. *Naunyn Schmiedebergs Arch Pharmacol* 1992; 345:489–493.

59. Schlicker E, Fink K, Detzner M, Göthert M. Histamine inhibits

dopamine release in the mouse striatum via presynaptic H_3 receptors. *J Neural Transm* 1993;93:1–10.

60. Schönrock B, Büsselberg D, Haas HL. Properties of tuberomammillary histamine neurons and their response to galanin. *Agents Actions* 1991;33:135–137.

61. Schwartz JC, Arrang JM, Garbarg M, Gulat-Marnay C, Pollard H. Modulation of histamine synthesis and release in brain via presynaptic autoreceptors and heteroreceptors. *Ann NY Acad Sci* 1990;604:40–54.

62. Schwartz JC, Arrang JM, Garbarg M, Pollard H, Ruat M. Histaminergic transmission in the mammalian brain. *Physiol Rev* 1991;71:1–51.

63. Schwartz JC, Haas HL, eds. *The histamine receptor.* New York: Wiley–Liss, 1992.

64. Serafin M, Khateb A, Vibert N, Vidal PP, Mühlethaler M. Medial vestibular nucleus in the guinea pig: histaminergic receptors. I. An in vitro study. *Exp Brain Res* 1992;93:242–248.

65. Smith BN, Armstrong WE. Histamine enhances the depolarizing afterpotential of immunohistochemically identified vasopressin neurons in the rat supraoptic nucleus via H_1 receptor activation. *Neuroscience* 1993;53:855–864.

66. Staines WA, Nagy JI. Neurotransmitter coexistence in the tuberomammillary nucleus. In: Watanabe T, Wada H, eds. *Histaminergic neurons: morphology and function.* Boca Raton, FL: CRC Press, 1991;163–176.

67. Steriade M, McCormick DA, Sejnowski TJ. Thalamocortical oscillations in the sleeping and aroused brain. *Science* 1993;262:679–685.

68. Tohyama M, Tamiya R, Inagaki N, Takagi H. Morphology of histaminergic neurons with histidine decarboxylase as a marker. In: Watanabe T, Wada H, eds. *Histaminergic neurons: morphology and function.* Boca Raton, FL: CRC Press, 1991;107–126.

69. Traiffort E, Leurs R, Arrang JM, Tardivel-Lacombe J, Diaz J, Schwartz JC, Ruat M. Guinea pig histamine H_1 receptor. I. Gene cloning, characterization and tissue expression revealed by in situ hybridization. *J Neurochem* 1994;62:507–518 .

70. Traiffort E, Pollard H, Moreau J, Ruat M, Schwartz JC, Martinez Mir MI, Palacios JM. Pharmacological characterization and autoradiographic localization of histamine H_2 receptors in human brain identified with [^{125}I]iodoaminopotentidine. *J Neurochem* 1992;59:290–299.

71. Traiffort E, Ruat M, Arrang JM, Leurs R, Piomelli D, Schwartz JC. Expression of a cloned rat histamine H_2 receptor mediating inhibition of arachidonate release and activation of cAMP accumulation. *Proc Natl Acad Sci USA* 1992;89:2649–2653.

72. Traiffort E, Ruat M, Schwartz JC. Interaction of mianserin, amitriptyline and haloperidol with guinea pig cerebral histamine H_2 receptors studied with [^{125}I]iodoaminopotentidine. *Eur J Pharmacol* 1991;207:143–148.

73. Wouterlood FG, Steinbusch HWM. Afferent and efferent fiber connections of histaminergic neurons in the rat brain: comparison with dopaminergic, noradrenergic and serotonergic systems. In: Watanabe T, Wada H, eds. *Histaminergic neurons: morphology and function.* Boca Raton, FL: CRC Press, 1991;145–162.

74. Yabe T, de Waele C, Serafin M, Vibert N, Arrang JM, Mühlethaler M, Vidal PP. Medial vestibular nucleus in the guinea pig: histaminergic neurons. II. An in vivo study. *Exp Brain Res* 1993;93:249–258.

75. Yamashita M, Fukui H, Sugawa K, Horio Y, Ito S, Mizuguchi H, Wada H. Expression cloning of a cDNA encoding the bovine histamine H_1 receptor. *Proc Natl Acad Sci USA* 1991;88:11515–11519.

76. Yanai K, Watanabe T, Yokoyama H, Hatazawa J, Iwata R, Ishiwata K, Meguro K, Itoh M, Takahashi T, Ido T, Matsuzawa T. Mapping of histamine H_1 receptors in the human brain using [^{11}C]pyrilamine and positron emission tomography. *J Neurochem* 1992;59:128–136.

77. Yang QZ, Hatton GI. Histamine and histaminergic inputs: responses of rat supraoptic nucleus neurons recorded intracellularly in hypothalamic slices. *Biomed Res* 1989;10:135–144.

78. Yokoyama H, Onodera K, Linuma K, Watanabe T. Effect of thioperamide, a histamine H_3 receptor antagonist on electrically induced convulsions in mice. *Eur J Pharmacol* 1993;234:129–133.

79. Yokoyama H, Onodera K, Maeyama K, Yanai K, Linuma K, Tuomisto L, Watanabe T. Histamine levels and clonic convulsions of electrically induced seizure in mice: the effects of α-fluoromethylhistidine and metoprine. *Naunyn Schmiedebergs Arch Pharmacol* 1992;346:40–46.

Psychopharmacology: The Fourth Generation of Progress, edited by Floyd E. Bloom and David J. Kupfer. Raven Press, Ltd., New York © 1995.

CHAPTER 36

Molecular Biology of Serotonin Receptors

A Basis for Understanding and Addressing Brain Function

Jean Chen Shih, Kevin J.-S. Chen, and Timothy K. Gallaher

For decades it has been suggested that the factors involved in mediating mental states, including mental illness, are neurochemical. Successful drug therapies for mental illnesses have been developed which reinforce the causative nature of the neurochemical environment and the role it plays in mental states. Such empirical knowledge has preceded the physiological basis for the actions of both therapeutic drugs and injurious drugs of abuse. Recently, data have been emerging from the field of molecular biology to provide a molecular basis for the neurochemical workings of the brain. Specifically, the receptors for numerous neurotransmitters and drugs have been cloned and their molecular structures have been determined. The number of different receptors identified by molecular cloning has provided insight into the complexity of the nervous system and allows us to begin devising novel methods for studying the brain and nervous system.

This chapter will discuss key concepts of our knowledge base concerning serotonin [5-hydroxytryptamine (5-HT)] receptors and present new approaches to study the brain and nervous system. The approaches discussed here for 5-HT receptors are also applicable to other neurotransmitter systems, and, indeed, an integrative approach encompassing all neurotransmitter systems will be necessary to further our understanding of the brain and nervous system (see also Chapters 11, 14, 19, 27, and 35, *this volume*).

Molecular cloning has provided solid molecular evidence concerning the structures of receptors and has provided cDNA which is of use in many ways for studying the brain. Many receptors have been cloned, and the data conclusively confirm the identification of multiple 5-HT receptors. The knowledge of the primary structures of the receptors is of great use for studying the function and architecture of the brain and how it may relate to mental states (see also Chapters 37 and 38, *this volume*).

A MOLECULAR BASIS FOR 5-HT RECEPTOR CLASSIFICATION

Classification schemes for 5-HT receptors have been used for more than 30 years. Initially, Gaddum and Picarelli (13) described D- and M-type receptors. Later pharmacological studies defined 5-HT1a, 1b, 1c, 1d, and 1e receptors and a 5-HT2 receptor. A 5-HT3 classification was later added. Each of these nomenclature schemes was based upon the ligand specificities of the individual receptors. Such approaches have proven to be valuable in our gaining knowledge of the 5-HT receptors, but also have inherent limitations. A new basis for their classification has arisen with the advent of molecular cloning techniques which make possible the determination of primary structures and gene structures. These structures provide a solid foundation on which to base 5-HT receptor classification. Using the molecular information presents the best approach to this task in that the data provided for the basis of the classification is the most unequivocal available. The goal of an objective and unambiguous classification scheme can hopefully be met using this data.

J. C. Shih, K. J.-S. Chen, and T. K. Gallaher: Department of Molecular Pharmacology and Toxicology, School of Pharmacy, University of Southern California, Los Angeles, California 90033.

Eventually the limitations of this molecular-based scheme may become apparent, but currently the classifications as will be described here may be the best we can do. Refinements to the classification nomenclature presented here might be in order, but the general basis and classification should hold, at least for awhile, until our understanding and knowledge increases to a point where this system also becomes too tenuous. It may be time for receptorologists to devise a nomenclature along the lines of enzyme nomenclature where the receptors can be classified as objectively as possible. Granted that the nature of the numerous receptor families makes this task more difficult than with enzymes, nonetheless we should approach the task wholeheartedly.

Two types of 5-HT receptors have been determined by molecular cloning: G-protein-coupled 5-HT receptors (42) and ligand-gated ion channels (18). Both types of 5-HT receptors fall into distinct supergene families of receptors which are related to each other and which are defined by their structure and function.

THE LIGAND-GATED 5-HT3 RECEPTOR

5-HT3 receptors are members of the ion-gated family of receptors (27). The model protein for this family is the nicotinic acetylcholine receptor, and this family includes cation channels (the nAchR, 5-HT3 receptor) and anion channels (GABAa receptor, glutamate receptor). The 5-HT3 receptor primary sequence indicates that it contains four transmembrane domains as determined by hydrophobicity analysis of its primary structure. It also contains the putative ligand binding domain which is found in the extracellular region of the protein, and it is characteristically seen in the primary structure of a receptor of this class in a disulfide loop region near the amino terminal of the protein. Also, the M4 helix is seen to contain numerous serine residues which may form an aqueous channel for the ion transport. The 5-HT3 receptor is clearly of this class, yet only one subunit has been cloned. Most members of this family are pentameric and consist of heterologous subunits. The 5-HT3 receptor subunit which has been cloned is able to form a 5-HT-gated ion channel, so it is possible that the 5-HT3 receptor is a homomeric pentamer, but given the diversity of the different subunits found in this family (e.g., the GABA receptor has upwards of 10 different subunits determined by molecular cloning) it is likely that more 5-HT3 subunits will be found by molecular cloning. The 5-HT3 receptor was designated 5-HT3 to keep in accord with the nomenclature scheme of designating the 5-HT receptor class with a number. The 5-HT1 and 5-HT2 classes had been defined pharmacologically, so the clearly unique 5-HT ligand-gated ion channel receptor was deemed the 5-HT3 receptor. Molecular cloning confirmed this assignment.

G-PROTEIN-COUPLED 5-HT RECEPTORS

All known 5-HT receptors except for 5-HT3 receptors are members of the G-protein-coupled (GPR) family of signal transducing receptors. Four different classes of 5-HT GPR receptors have been cloned: 5-HT1, 5-HT2, 5-HT5, and 5-HT6. Another class, the 5-HT4, has been identified but has yet to have had a member cloned. Multiple subtypes of 5-HT GPR receptors in each class have been observed as well. The nomenclature used to describe the receptors is based upon the pharmacological classification of Peroutka and Snyder (36), but is taken a step further to consistently integrate the classification of receptors based upon the data obtained from cloning with the pre-cloning pharmacologically based classification scheme; that is, new subclasses are numbered sequentially. Originally, two types of 5-HT receptors (designated 5-HT1 and 5-HT2) were defined (36) based upon their differing affinities for 5-HT and the neuroleptic antagonist spiperone. Currently, classification is based upon primary sequence homologies (and, to a lesser degree, second messenger responses). The strength of the pharmacological assignments has been demonstrated by the cloning data in that receptors classified as members of the 5-HT1 family (1a, 1b, 1c, 1d, 1e, and 1f) share greater sequence similarity with each other, with 30–50% sequence identity among the 5-HT1 receptors compared to the 5-HT2 receptors, which share less than 30% identity with the 5-HT1 receptors but greater than 30% with other 5-HT2 class receptors. The one exception here is the 5-HT1c receptor, which is clearly a member of the 5-HT2 receptor class (20,38) but was originally classified in the 5-HT1 class due to its high affinity for 5-HT compared to the 5-HT2 receptor. Consequently, a revised nomenclature has been presented to more appropriately reflect the relationships between the receptors determined by molecular cloning.

Another subclass has been defined and called the 5-HT4 receptor (4,8). These receptors demonstrated distinct pharmacological profiles and were positively linked to cyclic AMP production. The uniqueness of these observations merited the definition of the new 5-HT4 class of 5-HT receptors. This 5-HT4 class is the only defined subclass not to have a member cloned, so the primary sequences of any of this class are not known, and consequently the validity of the designation at a molecular level cannot be assessed. Because pharmacological and physiological definitions have been accurate, it is likely that the 5-HT4 receptors will stand as a class once the molecular data have been determined. Newer receptor clones (5-HT5 and 5-HT6 subtypes) have been obtained which do not fit the criteria for any pharmacologically defined 5-HT receptor subtype in either their pharmacological profile or, more importantly, their primary sequences. To continue using the nomenclature for the 5-HT receptors, the newest receptor was deemed the 5-

TABLE 1. *G-protein-coupled serotonin receptors*

Receptor subtype	Number of amino acids	Number of introns	Second messenger	Species and references
5-HT1a	421 (human) 421 (rat)	0	cAMP↓, K$^+$ channel, IP$_3$	Human (9), rat (3)
5-HT1b	390 (human) 386 (mouse)	0	cAMP↓	Human (1), mouse (28) rat (48)
5-HT1d	377	0	cAMP↓	Human (16)
5-HT1e	365	0	cAMP↓	Human (24,30)
5-HT1f	366	0	cAMP↓	Human (2)
5-HT2a (5-HT2)[a]	471	3	IP$_3$	Human (5,41), rat (20,38) mouse (52), hamster (47)
5-HT2b (5-HT2f)	479	≥2	IP$_3$	Rat (10,23)
5-HT2c (5-HT1c)	460 (rat, human) 459 (mouse)	3	IP$_3$	Human (5), rat (19) mouse (53)
5-HT5a	357	1	Unknown	Mouse (29,37)
5-HT5b	370	1	Unknown	Mouse (29)
5-HT6	437	≥1	cAMP↑	Rat (32)
dro-1	564	0	cAMP↑	Drosophila (51)
dro-2a	834	0	cAMP↓, IP$_3$	Drosophila (40)
dro-2b	645	4	cAMP↓, IP$_3$	Drosophila (40)

[a] Subtypes in parentheses indicate the original name of the receptor.

HT5 receptor (37). Since this initial 5-HT5 receptor was cloned, another 5-HT5 receptor was cloned and so these two receptors are designated 5-HT5a and 5-HT5b (29). Another GPR 5-HT receptor has been cloned which is unique in primary sequence, pharmacological profile, and physiological response and has been deemed the 5-HT6 receptor (32). This receptor activates adenylate cyclase, but its pharmacological profile indicates that it is not a 5-HT4 receptor, and its primary sequence cannot place it in the 5-HT1, 5-HT2, or 5-HT5 class of receptors. Whether or not a 5-HT6b receptor or 5-HT7 subtype will be found is not known, but chances are likely that newer subtypes will continue to be cloned. It is also possible that 5-HT6 receptors may turn out to be 5-HT4 receptors based upon sequence similarities because the pharmacological profiles can be misleading in indicating primary structure.

The classifications of the 5-HT receptors that have so far been cloned are presented in Table 1. These include four classes of mammalian GPR 5-HT receptors, including 11 individual receptors. Also included in Table 1 are the three 5-HT receptors which have been cloned in drosophila, namely, the cloned 5-HT4 subtype and the ligand-gated ion channel 5-HT3 receptor. With this inundation of molecular data, and likely more coming, it is time to examine what these data tell us and how we can use these data to determine how the brains works.

STRUCTURE AND FUNCTION OF 5-HT RECEPTORS

Now that we have such a wealth of primary sequence data, can we use these data to determine the molecular workings of the receptors? The answer is yes, and these types of studies have just begun. The comparisons of the primary structures have provided clues as to which amino acid residues are necessary for the functioning of the specific receptors. Also, experiments on other receptor and GPR proteins have contributed greatly to the understanding of 5-HT receptors. The initial cloning of the β-adrenergic receptor (βAR) (6) and the discovery that it is homologous to rhodopsin provided the first key in understanding the potential ligand binding sites for the GPR receptors. Deletion analysis of the βAR provided the initial evidence that the ligand binding site resides in the intramembrane regions of the GPR receptor (7). This observation established an analogy for receptor agonist-induced allosteric activation with the light-induced allosteric activation of rhodopsin that is mediated by the retinal chromophore known to be located in the intramembrane domains of the protein. Perusal of catecholamine receptor primary sequences pointed to potential sites on the protein for ligand interactions. Conserved aspartic acid residues in the second and third transmembrane domains of the receptors for biogenic amine agonists were obvious candidates as ligand binding residues. Site-directed mutagenesis served to support these ideas and indicate that aspartic acid in the third transmembrane acts as a counterion for the agonist amine group (44,49). The 5-HT GPR receptors all contain the analogous TMD3 aspartic acid, and mutagenesis of this residue in the 5-HT2 receptor (Asp155) to asparagine results in profound losses of affinity of the ligand (agonists and agonists) to the receptor (50).

Thus data from the amino acid sequences derived from molecular cloning pointed to potential residues important for ligand recognition. This sort of comparative examination takes into account evolutionary considerations in that it is considered that the receptors have arisen from divergent evolution from a common ancestral structure. The unique properties of the myriad receptors stems from the accumulated differences in primary sequences. The more similar the binding properties, the more similar may be the primary sequences. Or at least certain functionally important residues may be present at analogous sites in the various primary sequences.

Support for the role of the TMD3 aspartic acid in ligand binding is found in the examination of primary sequences of all the known GPR. Only in GPR where there is an aliphatic amine in the agonist structure is this TMD3 aspartic acid found. In receptors for ligands which do not contain aliphatic amine groups, such as the adenosine receptor (43) and cAMP receptor (39), no Asp appears in the third TMD. Conversely, an aspartic acid in the second transmembrane domain is conserved in all GPR receptors without respect to ligand structure. The results of mutagenesis studies of this residue in catecholamine (44,49), muscarinic (12), and 5-HT (50) receptors indicates that it is not as necessary for agonist binding as the TMD3 aspartic acid and that it is necessary for the activation of the second messenger response. The second messenger response is allosterically mediated, and the Asp in TMD 2 does play a role in allosterism (17), but its absolute necessity for second messenger response in all GPR receptors is unclear (46). These observations are indicative of how comparison of the primary sequences of these structurally related receptors in an evolutionary perspective can provide clues to their molecular workings.

An asparagine residue at the interface of the third extracellular loop and the seventh transmembrane domain has been shown to be necessary for the binding of aryloxyalkylamine antagonists (e.g., pindolol, propanolol, and alprenolol) to 5-HT1a receptors and rat 5-HT1b receptors. When this asparagine (Asn385 in 5-HT1a) is mutated to valine, the binding of aryloxyalkyamines to the 5-HT1a receptor is decreased 40- to 150-fold, but other agonists and antagonists demonstrate only minor changes in binding affinity (15). Also, the rat 5-HT1b receptor binds aryloxyalkylamine antagonists, but the human 5-HT1b receptor (also known as 5-HT1Dβ) has almost a thousandfold lower affinity for the aryloxyalkylamines. Rat 5-HT1b receptors contain asparagine at the cognate position, whereas the human receptor contains threonine. When the threonine of the human receptor (THR355) is mutated to asparagine, high-affinity binding of the aryloxyalkylamine antagonists is conferred (31,33,34). These experiments are excellent examples of how comparison of primary structures and ligand binding profiles can indicate functionally important amino acid residues.

Another example of this approach for exploring the structure of 5-HT receptor binding sites is seen in the 5-HT2 receptor and the differences in the human and rat primary structures. The primary sequences of human, rat, and mouse (Fig. 1) share great homology, especially in the transmembrane regions where only three amino acid

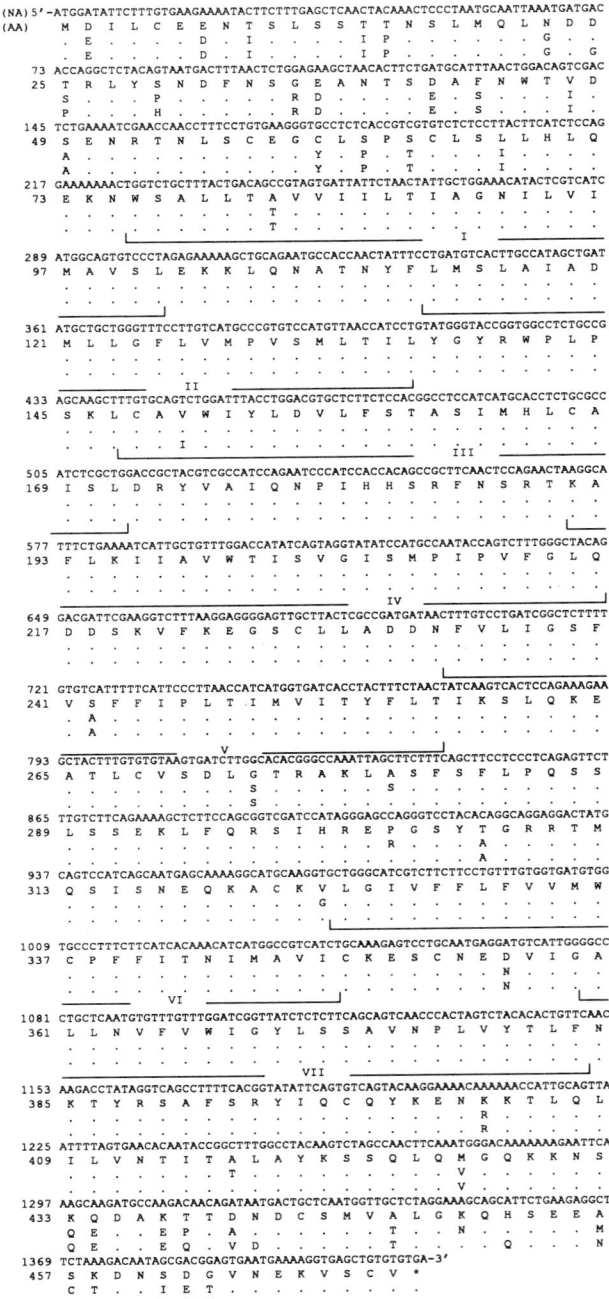

FIG. 1. DNA sequence of human 5-HT2 receptor cDNA and deduced amino acid sequence of the human (H), rat (R), and mouse (M) 5-HT2 receptors. The seven proposed transmembrane domains are bracketed. Intron−exon junctions are indicated by *arrows*, and exons are labeled E1, E2, and E3. Amino acids in rat or mouse receptors that are different than those in the human are shown—as opposed to identical residues, which are designated with *dots*.

differences are observed. One of the differences is at position 242 in the primary sequence that is found in the putative fifth transmembrane domain. In rat and mouse this residue is an alanine, but in the human 5-HT2 receptor a serine is found in this position (5,52). An analysis of position 242 and its proximity or contribution to the binding site of 5-HT2 receptors has been carried out using tryptamine agonists (14). Two naturally occurring compounds, bufotenin (5-hydroxy-N,N-dimethyltryptamine, 5-OH-DMT) and psilocin (4-hydroxy-N,N-dimethyltryptamine, 4-OH-DMT), were examined for their binding to human and rat 5-HT2 receptors. These two compounds differ only in their hydroxy substituent at the indole ring. Psilocin is at the four position and bufotenin is at the five position, which is the analogous position to the endogenous agonist 5-HT. It was observed that bufotenin binds with near equal affinity to both human and rat 5-HT2 receptors, whereas psilocin exhibited 15-fold higher affinity for the human receptor than for the rat receptor and that the binding of psilocin to the human receptor was comparable in affinity to the binding of bufotenin to either the rat or human 5-HT2 receptor. These results indicate that a determinant for psilocin binding is present in the human receptor but not in the rat receptor. Our knowledge of the binding mechanism of GPR agonists suggests that Ser242 of the human 5-HT2 receptor is the psilocin-specific determinant.

The results of βAR mutagenesis studies provide a strong analogy with which to analyze the psilocin binding to rat and human receptors (45). βAR agonists have two hydroxyl groups on their aromatic rings. βAR receptors also have serines at positions in their primary structure analogous to positions 239 and 242 in the 5-HT2 receptors. Site-directed mutagenesis has shown that these two serines serve as agonist binding residues. The evolutionary consideration that GPR receptors will conserve their basic functional mechanisms suggests that the 5-HT receptor agonists will bind analogously. The examination of numerous TMD5 sequences support the notion that residues of particular importance for specific ligand binding have been conserved. All receptors with dihydroxy-substituted aromatic rings contain the Ser-X-X-Ser sequence motif, whereas 5-HT receptors, which contain only one hydroxy substituent on the aromatic indole ring, contain only one serine or threonine in the fifth TMD that corresponds to the first serine of the S-X-X-S motif (Ser239 in the 5-HT2 receptor). Only the human 5-HT2 receptor contains the full S-X-X-S motif. Furthermore, the receptors for muscarinic receptors do not contain any analogous serines in the fifth TMD. The loss of these serines in the muscarinic receptors during evolution (or, conversely, the gain of the serines in the receptors for hydroxy-substituted agonists) is consistent with the evolutionary analysis of these GPR receptors. In the human 5-HT2 receptors the presence of the serine at position 242 provides a binding site for the 4-hydroxy group of psilo-

cin. The geometries of the two tryptamine agonists and the helical fifth transmembrane domain peptide structure indicate that if 4-OH-DMT and 5-OH-DMT bind analogously, then 242 can serve as a hydrogen bond site for psilocin and 239 can serve as the site for the 5-hydroxy-substituted bufotenin. Based on a normal α-helical structure the 239 and 242 serines would be 60° apart and 4.5Å would separate them in the membrane. Correspondingly, 4- and 5-substituted indoles differ by 60° with respect to the planar aromatic ring. The pharmacological properties of psilocin binding to rat and human 5-HT2 receptors support a binding site structure where the 4- or 5-hydroxy groups of the indole ring can interact with either Ser242 or Ser239, respectively. Such a prediction is in accord with the proposed binding site of the βAR receptor (26).

Another study has demonstrated the importance of position 242 in the 5-HT receptor in ligand binding. It has long been recognized that human and porcine 5-HT2 receptors differed in pharmacological profile with respect to one antagonist, mesulergine (35), which is seen to have a much lower affinity for the human and pig receptors than for the rat receptors. Site-directed mutagenesis of the human receptor where Ser242 was mutated to alanine indicated that this residue is the determinant for the difference in mesulergine affinity in rat and human receptors. Substitution of serine with alanine caused the mutant receptor to exhibit much greater affinity for mesulergine than the wild type, and the K_i value for this binding was nearly identical to that of the wild-type rat 5-HT2 receptor (21). The results are interesting because, while they do not indicate a binding site epitope, they do indicate that position 242 is in the binding site region.

Suggestions for ligand binding sites in 5-HT receptors based upon primary structure data in combination with pharmacological data serve to provide solid bases on which to build an accurate model of 5-HT receptor structure and function. These data must be applied to any computer modeling of the receptors as valuable constraints. The modeling, in turn, can reflect back on the feasibility of the proposed interactions of the ligands with the receptors. The data from the psilocin experiments, when examined in molecular model building, indicate the existence of a binding site where the 4 or 5 hydroxy can hydrogen bond with serine 242 or 239, respectively (unpublished observations). Furthermore, when the agonist is placed in this position, such a binding geometry of the indole nucleus reflects the basis for the differing affinities of mesulergine for the rat and human receptor. Serine 242 of human receptor is in a position to interact with the nonpolar saturated carbon of the mesulergine, which would cause a destabilization in its binding site. On the other hand, the nonpolar alanine does not present the same electrostatic destabilization for the saturated carbon of mesulergine that is in the vicinity of position 242. Such hypothetical model building will serve us until more precise physical methods such as x-ray crystallography

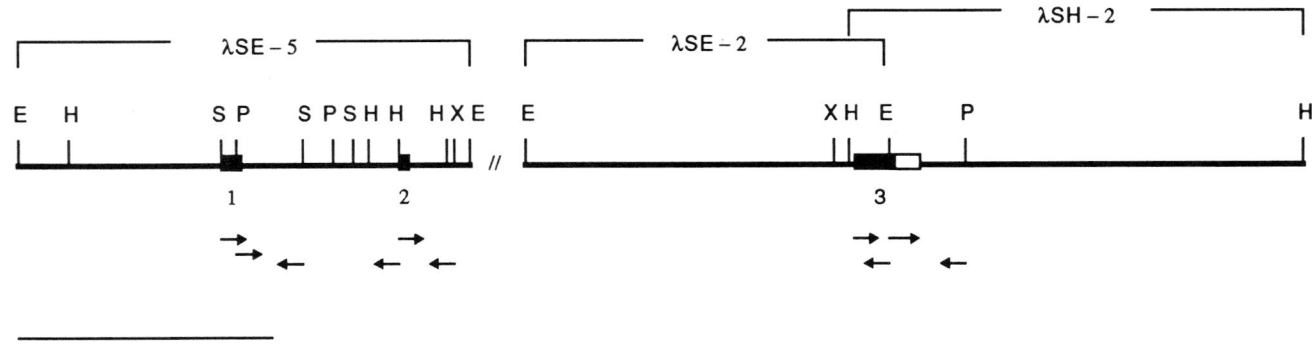

FIG. 2. Partial structural map of the human 5-HT2 receptor gene. λSE, λSE-2, and λSH-2 are restriction fragments isolated from genomic DNA libraries. *Filled boxes* represent the coding regions, and the *open box* is the untranslated region. The intron gap between genomic clones is represented by //. *Arrows* indicate the start site and direction of sequencing.

or nuclear magnetic resonance are made possible with the availability of sufficient amounts of purified receptor.

GENES FOR 5-HT RECEPTORS

The study of the genes for 5-HT receptors has also provided insights into their relationships with each other and with other GPR family members. 5-HT receptors fall into one of two categories with respect to their gene structures: either intronless genes or intron-containing genes. The 5-HT1a receptor was the first 5-HT receptor gene to be isolated due to its sequence similarity to the βAR and was seen to be intronless (9,22). Numerous 5-HT1 receptor subtypes (5-HT1a, 1b, 1d, 1e, 1f) are coded for by intronless genes. This is an important finding because it provides one more basis to categorize these receptors as a distinct subclass. To the classification of these receptors into the 5-HT1 class based upon pharmacological, physiological, and molecular structures is added their intronless nature.

5-HT2 receptor subclass members contain introns. The 5-HT2 receptor was the first 5-HT receptor to be shown to contain introns (5,52). The gene consists of three exons separated by two introns (Fig. 2). The other members of the 5-HT2 family, the 5-HT1c (also known as 5-HT2c) and the 5-HT2F (also known as 5-HT2b), now have also been shown to be intron-containing genes (11). Their evolutionary closeness is indicated by a partial conservation of intron−exon structure in all three of these 5-HT2 receptor subtypes. Two intron−exon junction structures are shared in each of the three 5-HT2 receptors and indicate that, as for the 5-HT1 subclass, the pharmacologically, physiologically, and molecularly defined class of 5-HT2 receptors is also defined by gene structure.

These findings reflect the divergent and convergent nature of the evolutionary processes that have resulted in the 5-HT subclass of GPR family receptors. Presumably all GPR family members have a common ancestral source, and divergent evolution has resulted in the receptors that bind the different ligands. As for the 5-HT receptors, we can see how receptors converged during evolution to use the same ligand as their activator. This is seen in the close relationship between the 5-HT1 receptors and the βAR class of receptors. Despite the fact that the 5-HT1 and 5-HT2 receptors share the same activating ligand, the 5-HT1 receptors are more closely evolutionarily related to the βAR receptors as determined by their primary sequence homologies. 5-HT1 receptors all share 50−60% sequence identity with each other but only approximately 30% identity with 5-HT2 receptors. The genetic data where the 5-HT1 receptor genes are all intronless whereas the 5-HT2 receptor genes contain a shared intronic structure further supports this assessment.

The most recently found members of the 5-HT receptor subgroup of GPR receptors contain introns. The 5-HT5a and 5-HT5b receptors each have one intron found in the region of the protein that constitutes the third intracellular loop (29). Furthermore, a cDNA for the 5-HT6 receptor was isolated that contained an unspliced intron (32), indicating that the 5-HT6 receptor has at least one intron. The presence of introns in the gene structures of these two 5-HT receptors, along with the 30−40% sequence identity shared with both 5-HT1 and 5-HT2 receptors, supports the conclusion that they reflect new 5-HT receptor subclasses and are not members of the 5-HT1 subclass.

FUTURE

The data garnered from, and the techniques made available by, molecular biological methods for studying 5-HT receptors provide new avenues to approach fundamental questions in neurobiology. One clear benefit is the ability to pharmacologically assess a pure receptor population. Pharmacological assays using brain tissue preparations have proven to be of great benefit in characterizing receptors and in developing specific ligands for receptors but have built-in limitations. Tissue preparations always contain multiple receptors and receptor subtypes. The ability to separate the individual receptors is overcome by the availability of cDNA for individual receptors and the ability to express the receptor in a mammalian cell. Such a "clean" environment can be used to screen newly synthesized drugs and can identify receptors in the brain that are being affected by a particular drug. This approach can also be of use in determining the basis of actions for therapeutic treatments. For example, tricyclic antidepressants used therapeutically are successful in treating certain mental disorders. The newly cloned 5-HT6 receptor is seen to have high affinity for this class of compounds and may indicate at least one of the sites in the brain where the tricyclic antidepressants exert their effects.

This same ability to express receptors in mammalian cell lines can also be of use in physiological studies where second messenger responses generated by a receptor, and the basis of the receptor-mediated response, will be examined. For example, the 5-HT1a receptor initiates different responses due to 5-HT stimulation depending on the cell line in which the cDNA is expressed (25). One can envision future "mixing and matching" experiments where receptors are transfected into cell lines that have known a G protein being expressed to do an inventory of, and obtain rank orders of potency for, the interactions of the receptors and the various G proteins.

The availability of the cDNA also makes it possible to express the receptors in a high yield expression system where large amounts of receptor can be produced. Such a technique can provide protein sufficient for reconstitution studies where the receptors can be reconstituted with various G proteins. Such a method would not only provide information concerning interactions between specific receptors and specific G proteins, but would also provide an environment where kinetic analysis of the GTP hydrolysis reaction which takes place in GPR-mediated signal transduction could be examined. A rigorous biochemical analysis of the signal transduction event will be of great use for computer-based simulations of neural function in providing accurate constants upon which to base the simulation's algorithms.

We also can foresee that the above-mentioned approaches can be seen as part of a comprehensive whole where a multidisciplinary examination of brain function is done based upon a neuromolecular anatomical mapping of the brain. The brain and nervous system are made up of billions of cells providing a myriad of neural connections between cells. Each cellular connection serves to communicate with and regulate its connected neighbor. The patterns of these connections and the effect of the neural networks on brain activity are believed to account for all behavioral and psychological activity of the organism. Drugs work by binding to a specific receptor and altering

the endogenous regulation of the neurotransmitter-regulated brain activity. Until recently it was impossible to try to identify the components of these systems at more than an unrefined basic level. With the availability of specific genes that code for 5-HT receptors, the distribution of individual 5-HT receptors can be examined in nervous tissue. This method makes use of already existing techniques for mapping anatomical structure using the method of thin brain slicing and in situ hybridization. Using the computer-assisted technique to store and analyze this topographical information, a map of all known 5-HT-receptor-containing neurons in terms of their anatomical location can be achieved. Computer-aided visualization of brain based upon these data would provide an amazing anatomical insight at a higher level than mere structural topology. The methods of anatomy, combined with the molecular biological methods of identifying nucleic acids by hybridization, provide a greater analysis of the organization of the brain than ever before.

REFERENCES

1. Adham N, Romanienko P, Hartig P, Weinshank RL, Branchek T. The rat 5-hydroxytryptamine$_{1B}$ receptor is the species homolog of the human 5-HT$_{1D\beta}$ receptor. *Mol Pharmacol* 1992;41:1–7.
2. Adham N, et al. Cloning of another human serotonin receptor (5-HT1F): a 5-HT1 receptor subtype coupled to the inhibition of adenylate cyclase. *Proc Natl Acad Sci USA* 1993;90:408–412.
3. Albert PR, Zhou Q-Y, Van To, HHM, Bunzow JR, Civelli O. Cloning, functional expression, and mRNA tissue distribution of the rat 5-hydroxytryptamine$_{1A}$ receptor gene. *J Biol Chem* 1990;265:5825–5832.
4. Becker BN, Gettys TW, Middleton JP, Olsen CL, Albers FJ, Lee S-L, Fanburg BL, Raymond JR. 8-Hydroxy-2-(di-*n*-propylamino) tetralin-responsive 5-hydroxytryptamine$_4$-like receptor expressed in bovine pulmonary artery smooth muscle cells. *Mol Pharmacol* 1992;42:817–825.
5. Chen K, Yang W, Grimsby J, Shih JC. The human 5-HT$_2$ receptor is encoded by a multiple intron–exon gene. *Mol Brain Res* 1992;14:20–26.
6. Dixon RAF, et al. Cloning of the gene and cDNA for mammalian β-adrenergic receptor and homology with rhodopsin. *Nature* 1986;321:75–79.
7. Dixon RAF, Sigal IS, Rands E, Register RB, Candelore MR, Blake AD, Skades CD. Ligand binding to the β-adrenergic receptor involves its rhodopsin-like core. *Nature* 1987;326:73–77.
8. Dumuis A, Bouhelal R, Sebben M, Cory R, Bockaert J. A nonclassical 5-hydroxytryptamine receptor positively coupled with adenylate cyclase in the central nervous system. *Mol Pharmacol* 1988;34:880–887.
9. Fargin A, Raymond JR, Lohse MJ, Kobilka BK, Caron MG, Lefkowitz RJ. The genomic clone of G-21 which resembles a β-adrenergic receptor sequence encodes the 5-HT1A receptor. *Nature* 1988;335:358–360.
10. Foguet M, Hoyer D, Pardo LA, Parekh A, Kluxen FW, Kalkman HO, Stuhmer W, Lubbert H. Cloning and characterization of the rat stomach fundus serotonin receptor. *EMBO J* 1992;11:4381–3487.
11. Foguet M, Nguyen H, Le H, Lubbert H. Structure of the mouse 5-HT$_{1C}$, 5-HT$_2$ and stomach fundus serotonin receptor genes. *Neuroreport* 1992;3:345–348.
12. Fraser CM, Wang C-D, Robinson DA, Gocayne JD, Venter JC. Site-directed mutagenesis of m$_1$ muscarinic receptors: conserved aspartic acids play important roles in receptor function. *Mol Pharmacol* 1989;36:840–847.

13. Gaddum JH, Picarelli ZP. Two kinds of tryptamine receptors. *Br J Pharmacol* 1957;12:323–328.
14. Gallaher TK, Chen K, Shih JC. Higher affinity of psilocin for human than rat 5-HT2 receptor indicates binding site structure. *Med Chem Res* 1993;3:52–66.
15. Guan X-M, Peroutka SJ, Kobilka BK. Identification of a single amino acid residue responsible for the binding of a class of β-adrenergic receptor antagonists to 5-hydroxytryptamine$_{1a}$ receptors. *Mol Pharmacol* 1992;41:695–698.
16. Hamblin MW, Metcalf MA. Primary structure and functional characterization of a human 5-HT$_{1D}$-type serotonin receptor. *Mol Pharmacol* 1991;40:143–148.
17. Horstman DA, Brandon S, Wilson AL, Guyer CA, Cragoe EJ, Limbird LE. An asparatate conserved among G-protein receptors confers allosteric regulation of α2-adrenergic receptors by sodium. *J Biol Chem* 1990;265:21590–21595.
18. Julius D. Molecular biology of serotonin receptors. *Annu Rev Neurosci* 1991;14:335–360.
19. Julius D, MacDermot AB, Axel R, Jessell TM. Molecular characterization of a functional cDNA encoding the serotonin 1c receptor. *Science* 1988;241:558–564.
20. Julius D, Huang KN, Livelli TJ, Axel R, Jessell TM. The 5-HT2 receptor defines a family of structurally distinct but functionally conserved serotonin receptors. *Proc Natl Acad Sci USA* 1990;87:928–932.
21. Kao H-T, Adham N, Olsen MA, Weinshank RL, Branchek TA, Hartig PR. Site-directed mutagenesis of a single residue changes the binding properties of the serotonin 5-HT$_2$ receptor from a human to a rat pharmacology. *FEBS Lett* 1992;307:324–328.
22. Kobilka BK, Frielle T, Collins S, Yang-Feng T, Kobilka TS, Francke U, Lefkowitz RJ, Caron MG. An intronless gene encoding a potential member of the family of receptors coupled to guanine nucleotide regulatory proteins. *Nature* 1987;329:75–79.
23. Kursar JD, Nelson DL, Wainscott DB, Cohen ML, Baez M. Molecular cloning, functional expression, and pharmacological characterization of a novel serotonin receptor (5-hydroxytryptamine$_{2F}$) from rat stomach fundus. *Mol Pharmacol* 1992;42:549–557.
24. Levy FO, Gudermann T, Birnbauer M, Kaumann AJ, Birnbauer L. Molecular cloning of a human gene (S31) encoding a novel serotonin receptor mediating inhibition of adenylyl cyclase. *FEBS Lett* 1992;296:201–206.
25. Liu YF, Albert PR. Cell-specific signalling of the 5-HT1A receptor. *J Biol Chem* 1991;266:23689–23697.
26. Maloney-Huss K, Lybrand TP. Three-dimensional structure for the β2 adrenergic receptor protein based on computer modeling studies. *J Mol Biol* 1992;225:859–871.
27. Maricq AV, Peterson AS, Brake AJ, Myers RM, Julius D. Primary structure and functional expression of the 5-HT3 receptor, a serotonin-gated ion channel. *Science* 1991;254:432–437.
28. Maroteaux L, Sadou F, Amlaiky N, Boschert U, Plassat JL, Hen R. Mouse 5HT1B serotonin receptor: cloning, functional expression, and localization in motor control centers. *Proc Natl Acad Sci USA* 1992;89:3020–3024.
29. Matthes H, Boschert U, Amlaiky N, Grailhe R, Plassat J-L, Muscatelli F, Mattei M-G, Hen R. Mouse 5-hydroxytryptamine5A and 5-hydroxytryptamine 5B receptors define a new family of serotonin receptors: cloning, functional expression, and chromosomal localization. *Mol Pharmacol* 1993;43:313–319.
30. McAllister G, Charlesworth A, Snodin C, Beer MS, Noble AJ, Middlemis DN, Iversen LL, Whiting P. Molecular cloning of a serotonin receptor from human brain (5HT1E): a fifth 5-HT1-like subtype. *Proc Natl Acad Sci USA* 1992;89:5517–5521.
31. Metcalf MA, McGuffin RW, Hamblin, MW. Conversion of the human 5-HT$_{1Dβ}$ serotonin receptor to the rat 5-HT$_{1B}$ ligand-binding phenotype by THR^{355}ASN site directed mutagenesis. *Biochem Pharmacol* 1992;44:1917–1920.
32. Monsma FJ, Shen Y, Ward RP, Hamblin MW, Sibley DM. Cloning and expression of a novel serotonin receptor with high affinity for tricyclic psychotropic drugs. *Mol Pharmacol* 1993;43:320–327.
33. Oskenberg D, Marsters SA, O'Dowd BF, Jin H, Havlik S, Peroutka SJ, Ashkenazi A. A single amino-acid difference confers major pharmacological variation between human and rodent 5-HT$_{1B}$ receptors. *Nature* 1992;360:161–163.
34. Parker EM, Griesel DA, Iben LG, Shapiro RA. A single amino acid difference accounts for the pharmacological distinctions between the rat and human 5-hydroxytryptamine$_{1B}$ receptors. *J Neurochem* 1993;60:380–383.
35. Pazos A, Hoyer D, Palacios JM. Mesulergine, a selective serotonin-2 ligand in the rat cortex, does not label these receptors in porcine and human cortex: evidence for species differences in brain serotonin-2 receptors. *Eur J Pharmacol* 1984;106:531–538.
36. Peroutka SJ, Snyder SH. Differential binding of [^{3}H]5-hydroxytryptamine, [^{3}H]lysergic acid diethylamide and [^{3}H]spiroperidol. *Mol Pharmacol* 1979;16:687–699.
37. Plassat J-L, Boschert U, Amlaiky N, Hen R. The mouse 5HT5 receptor reveals a remarkable heterogeneity within the 5HT1D receptor family. *EMBO J* 1992;11:4779–4786.
38. Pritchett DB, Bach AWJ, Wozny M, Taleb O, Dal Toso R, Shih JC, Seeberg PH. Structure and functional expression of cloned rat serotonin 5-HT2 receptor. *EMBO J* 1988;7:4135–4140.
39. Pupillo M, Klein P, Vaughn R, Pitt G, Lilly P, Sun T, Devreotes P, Kumagai A, Firtel R. cAMP receptor and G-protein interactions control development in *Dictyostelium*. *Cold Spring Harbor Symp Quant Biol* 1988;53:657–665.
40. Saudou F, Boschert U, Amlaiky N, Plassat J-L, Hen R. A family of *Drosophila* serotonin receptors with distinct intracellular signalling properties and expression patterns. *EMBO J* 1992;11:7–17.
41. Saltzman AG, Morse B, Whitman MM, Ivanschenko Y, Jaye M, Felder S. Cloning of the human serotonin 5-HT2 and 5-HT1C receptor subtypes. *Biochem Biophys Res Commun* 1991;181:1469–1478.
42. Shih JC, Yang W, Chen K, Gallaher T. Molecular biology of serotonin (5-HT) receptors. *Pharmacol Biochem Behav* 1990;40:1053–1058.
43. Stiles GL. Adenosine receptors. *J Biol Chem* 1992;267:6451–6454.
44. Strader CD, Sigal IS, Candelore MR, Rands E, Hill W, Dixon RAF. Conserved aspartic acids 79 and 113 of the β-adrenergic receptor have different roles in receptor function. *J Biol Chem* 1988;263:10267–10271.
45. Strader CD, Candelore MR, Hill WS, Sigal IS, Dixon RAF. Identification of two serine residues involved in agonist activation of the adrenergic receptor. *J Biol Chem* 1989;264:13572–13578.
46. Supranant A, Horstman DA, Akbarali H, Limbird LE. A point mutation of the α2-adrenoceptor that blocks coupling to potassium but not calcium currents. *Science* 1992;257:977–980.
47. Van Obberghen-Schilling E, Vouret-Craviari V, Haslam RJ, Chambard J-C. Cloning, functional expression and role in cell growth of a hamster 5-HT2 receptor subtype. *Mol Endocrinol* 1991;5:881–889.
48. Voight MM, Laurie DJ, Seeberg PH, Bach A. Molecular cloning of a rat brain cDNA encoding a 5-hydroxytryptamine$_{1B}$ receptor. *EMBO J* 1991;10:4017–4023.
49. Wang C-D, Buck MA, Fraser CM. Site-directed mutagenesis of α$_{2A}$-adrenergic receptors: identification of amino acids involved in ligand binding and receptor activation by agonists. *Mol Pharmacol* 1991;40:168–179.
50. Wang C-D, Gallaher TK, Shih JC. Site-directed mutagenesis of serotonin 5-HT2 receptors: identification of amino acids necessary for ligand binding and receptor activation. *Mol Pharmacol* 1993;43:931–940.
51. Witz P, Amlaiky N, Plassat J-L, Maroteaux L, Borreli E, Hen R. Cloning and characterization of a *Drosophila* serotonin receptor that activates adenylate cyclase. *Proc Natl Acad Sci USA* 1990;87:8940–8944.
52. Yang W, Chen K, Lan NC, Gallaher TK, Shih JC. Gene structure and expression of the mouse 5-HT2 receptor. *J Neurosci Res* 1992;33:196–204.
53. Yu L, Nguyen H, Le H, Bloem LJ, Kozak CA, Hoffman BJ, Snutch TP, Lester HA, Davidson N, Lubbert H. The mouse 5-HT$_{1C}$ receptor contains eight hydrophobic domains and is X-linked. *Mol Brain Res* 1991;11:143–149.

Psychopharmacology: The Fourth Generation of Progress, edited by Floyd E. Bloom and David J. Kupfer. Raven Press, Ltd., New York © 1995.

CHAPTER 37

Serotonin Receptor Subtypes

Richard A. Glennon and Malgorzata Dukat

Serotonin (5-hydroxytryptamine, 5-HT) mediates a wide range of physiological functions by activating multiple receptors. Likewise, 5-HT has been implicated as playing important roles in certain pathological and psychopathological conditions. In the past decade, no fewer than four major families of 5-HT receptors have been identified (5-HT1, 5-HT2, 5-HT3, 5-HT4); recently, three new receptor types (5-HT5, 5-HT6, 5-HT7) have been described. Of these, at least 15 subpopulations have now been cloned. Serotonin has become one of the most exciting and fastest-paced areas in neurochemistry. In fact, a recent literature (MEDLINE) search reveals nearly 10,000 entries on 5-HT in just the past 3 years. This plethora of 5-HT receptors should allow us to better understand the different and complex processes in which 5-HT is involved. On the other hand, this ever-expanding list of 5-HT receptors has become a nightmare for those involved in identifying or developing site-selective agonists and antagonists. So-called "selective" agents must be continually reevaluated so as to ensure their selectivity as new populations of 5-HT receptors are discovered (see also Chapters 36 and 38, *this volume*).

SEROTONIN RECEPTORS

Serotonin was discovered in the late 1940s, and within a decade there was evidence that it existed in the central nervous system of animals and that it might function as a neurotransmitter (see the previous edition of *Psychopharmacology* (48) for a detailed discussion of the early history of 5-HT). By 1957, there was evidence for 5-HT receptor heterogeneity in the periphery, and in 1979 two distinct populations of 5-HT receptor/binding sites were identified in rat brain. These two sites were termed 5-

R. A. Glennon and M. Dukat: Department of Medicinal Chemistry, School of Pharmacy, Medical College of Virginia, Virginia Commonwealth University, Richmond, Virginia 23298.

HT1 and 5-HT2. Soon thereafter, it became apparent that 5-HT1 sites were heterogeneous. An additional population of sites, distinct from 5-HT1 and 5-HT2 receptors, was also identified; these were termed 5-HT$_3$ receptors. In an attempt to organize the rapidly proliferating nomenclature of 5-HT receptors, specific definitions and criteria were suggested. The different populations of sites were classified as 5-HT1-like, 5-HT2, and 5-HT3. The 5-HT2 receptors and 5-HT3 receptors seemed to correspond to the peripheral 5-HT-D and 5-HT-M receptors, respectively, identified by Gaddum and Picarelli in the late 1950s. Although many of the classification criteria are still applied today, advances in molecular biology and the discovery of additional populations of sites that seemingly fail to meet the above criteria and definitions have resulted in some modifications in nomenclature. For example, 5-HT1-like sites were originally defined, at least in part, as those possessing a high affinity for 5-HT and a structurally related agent 5-carboxamidotryptamine. Certain newly identified 5-HT1 sites are now recognized to bind 5-carboxamidotryptamine only with low affinity (e.g., 5-HT1E sites), and some non-5-HT1 sites (e.g., 5-HT7) bind both 5-HT and 5-carboxamidotryptamine with sub-nanomolar affinity. 5-HT$_2$ sites were originally defined by their low affinity for 5-HT (i.e., $K_i > 500$ nM); but it has now been demonstrated, using appropriate ligands (e.g., [^{125}I]DOI, [^{3}H]DOB), that 5-HT binds at 5-HT$_2$ sites with high (i.e., $K_i < 10$ nM) affinity. More recently, it has been shown that most 5-HT1-like receptors share an amino acid sequence homology of at least 50%, display high affinity for 5-HT, and couple to the inhibition of adenylate cyclase activity as a primary coupling pathway (25). However, 5-HT1C receptors possess a 78% sequence homology with 5-HT2 receptors and, like 5-HT2 receptors, are coupled to a phosphoinositol second messenger system. 5-HT1C receptors are now considered members of the 5-HT2 family and have been variously termed 5-HT2B, 5-HT2β, and 5-HT2C receptors, relative to the originally defined 5-HT2 receptors which have been

TABLE 1. *Populations of 5-HT receptors*

Populations and subpopulations	Newer names	Comments (see text for clarification)
5-HT1		
5-HT1A	5-HT1A	Cloned and pharmacological 5-HT1A sites.
5-HT1B	5-HT1B	Rat homologue of human 5-HT1Dβ receptors.
	5-HT1Bβ	Mouse homologue of human 5-HT1Dβ receptors.
5-HT1D	5-HT1D	Sites identified by binding studies.
5-HT1Dα	5-HT1Dα	A cloned human 5-HT1D population.
5-HT1Dβ	5-HT1Dβ	A second cloned human 5-HT1D population.
5-HT1E	5-HT1E	5-HT1E sites identified by binding.
	5-HT1Eα	Alternate name for human 5-HT1E receptors.
	5-HT1Eβ	A cloned mouse homologue of 5-HT1F.
5-HT1F	5-HT1F	A cloned human 5-HT1-like receptor.
5-HT1P		A peripheral 5-HT1-like receptor.
5-HT1R		Rabbit 5-HT1D-like receptor.
5-HT1S		5-HT1-like receptor in spinal cord.
5-HT2		
5-HT2	5-HT2A	Original 5-HT2 (5-HT2α) receptors.
5-HT2F	5-HT2B	5-HT2-like receptors in rat fundus.
5-HT1C	5-HT2C	Original 5-HT1C (5-HT2β) receptors.
5-HT3		
5-HT3	5-HT3	An ion channel receptor.
5-HT4		
5-HT4	5-HT4	Not yet cloned.
5-HT5		
5-HT5A	5-HT5A	Cloned mouse 5-HT receptor.
5-HT5B	5-HT5B	Cloned mouse 5-HT5A-like receptor.
5-HT6		
5-HT6	5-HT6	Cloned rat 5-HT receptor.
5-HT7		
5-HT7	5-HT7	Two cloned receptors have been given this name.

referred to as 5-HT2A, 5-HT2α, or, simply, 5-HT2 receptors. In the remainder of this chapter, the newly proposed 5-HT nomenclature (Serotonin Nomenclature Committee, Houston, 1992) will be employed. That is, the original 5-HT2 receptors will be referred to as 5-HT2A receptors and the 5-HT1C receptors will be referred to as 5-HT2C receptors (Table 1). The different terminology often makes it quite difficult to comprehend and appreciate 5-HT receptor classification. Even more bewildering is the selectivity of various 5-HT agonists and antagonists; many agents considered selective for a particular population of sites only a few years ago are now realized to be considerably less selective and, in a few instances, even nonselective. This has led to the concept of semiselective agents—agents with selectivity for only two or three populations of 5-HT receptors. Judicious selection of several semiselective agents can often aid in classification of a particular functional activity or response as possibly being mediated by a given population of 5-HT receptors by a process of elimination. Indeed, binding profiles of a series of agents are commonly used to characterize newly identified 5-HT receptors. Nevertheless, there are very few serotonergic agents that are selective for one population of 5-HT receptors versus another (19).

The first two families of 5-HT receptors to be described,

5-HT1 and 5-HT2 (now 5-HT2A) receptors, were the result of radioligand binding studies and were an extension of the discovery that the dopaminergic label [^{3}H]-spiperone is capable of labeling what appeared to be a population of 5-HT receptors. Since then, several different techniques have been used to initially characterize and define the various populations of 5-HT receptors. Although discussed in greater detail below, for purpose of introduction it is sufficient to say that radioligand binding (5-HT1A, 5-HT1B, 5-HT1D, 5-HT1E, 5-HT1R, 5-HT1S, 5-HT2A), autoradiography and binding (5-HT2C), molecular biology (5-HT1Dα, 5-HT1Dβ, 5-HT1Eβ, 5-HT1F, 5-HT2B, 5-HT5A, 5-HT5B, 5-HT6, 5-HT7), and various functional assays (5-HT1P, 5-HT3, 5-HT4) accounted for the discovery of the different populations of sites. Some of the originally described 5-HT receptors already have been the subject of extensive review. Consequently, for these receptors, more references will be made to review articles than to the original literature.

SEROTONERGIC AGENTS

Numerous agents have been used to investigate 5-HT receptors. Serotonin itself binds at most populations of

5-HT receptors with low nanomolar affinity. No agent displays an absolute specificity for one population of 5-HT receptors versus the others, and very few agents possess significant selectivity for a particular population of 5-HT receptors. Agents that have been useful in identifying and investigating the different populations of 5-HT receptors will be mentioned under the appropriate headings. However, a few general comments regarding serotonergic agents and their classification will be made here.

Subpopulation specificity, and indeed agonist versus antagonist activity, is not so much a matter of chemical class as it is a matter of substituent type. Table 2 lists some classes of agents that bind at 5-HT receptors (also see Fig. 1). Within most of these different classes can be found examples of agents that bind at various populations of 5-HT receptors; that is, a particular chemical class of agents is not typically associated with only one receptor population (18). Small structural changes can result in agents with greater selectivity (i.e., in more selective or in semiselective agents). A case in point is 5-HT. 5-HT is an indolealkylamine; it binds in a rather nonselective manner at all populations of 5-HT receptors. The simple quaternization of 5-HT to the N,N,N-trimethyl derivative 5-HTQ enhances its affinity for 5-HT3 receptors by an order of magnitude. Furthermore, 5-HTQ binds with low affinity at most other populations of 5-HT receptors. An appropriate example of substituent groups modifying agonist versus antagonist activity is seen with the aminotet-

TABLE 2. *Classes of chemical agents that bind at 5-HT receptors[a]*

---

1. Indolealkylamines
   a. Tryptamines
   b. Partial ergolines
   c. Ergolines
2. Aminotetralins
3. Arylpiperazines
   a. Simple arylpiperazines
   b. Long-chain arylpiperazines
4. Alkyl- and arylpiperidines
5. Aryloxyalkylamines
6. Arylbiguanides
7. Keto compounds
   a. Benzoic acid derivatives
      i. Benzoate esters
      ii. Benzamides
   b. Ketoindoles
      i. Indolecarboxylic esters
      ii. Indolecarboxylic amides
      iii. Benzimidazoles
      iv. γ-Carolines
      v. Carbazoles
   c. Other heteroaryl esters and amides
   d. Ureas and carbamates
8. Miscellaneous agents

---

[a] Classification encompasses most classes of serotonergic agonists and antagonists. Many bioisoteres are not listed separately but are considered as members of an already mentioned class of agents. General structures are shown in Fig. 1.

ralin derivative 8-hydroxy-2-(di-*n*-propylamino)tetralin (8-OH DPAT). The R(−)-isomer of 8-OH DPAT is a full 5-HT1A agonist, whereas its S(+)-enantiomer is a partial agonist. Furthermore, introduction of a 5-fluoro group results in an antagonist. Thus, small structural changes can influence agonist versus antagonist character as well as selectivity (17).

The classification of serotonergic agents is complicated by the existence of bioisosteres. For example, using the above-mentioned 8-OH DPAT, replacement of the 4-position methylene group by an oxygen atom affords a chroman derivative. The chroman analogue of 8-OH DPAT retains 5-HT1A character. Thus, in order to simplify the chemical classification scheme shown in Table 2, certain bioisosteres, such as the chromans, are not specifically mentioned. In contrast, replacement of the 3-position carbon atom of the indole nucleus with a nitrogen atom affords the bioisosteric benzimidazoles; because these are a relatively widely used and recognized class of agents, they have been specifically mentioned in the classification scheme. Also mentioned are ureas and carbamates. Benzoic acid esters and amides, indolecarboxylic acid esters and amides, and other miscellaneous heteroaryl carboxylic acid esters and amides bind at 5-HT3 (and certain other populations of 5-HT) receptors. Their reverse esters and amides (i.e., esters and amides where the ester oxygen or amide nitrogen has been moved from one side of the carbonyl group to the other) also bind. Thus, it would not be unlikely for structurally related compounds with a nitrogen atom on both sides of the carbonyl group (i.e., ureas) or an oxygen on one side and a nitrogen on the other (i.e., carbamates) to bind also. Indeed, there are numerous examples of such agents (18). Thus, although ureas and carbamates may be considered bioisosteric with their corresponding esters and amides, they too are listed separately in Table 2 for purposes of clarity.

Indolealkylamines are notoriously nonselective agents. But, as mentioned above, small structural changes can result in enhanced selectivity. Typically, however, tryptamines and ergolines are quite nonselective. Ergolines, for example, bind at all populations of 5-HT receptors except for 5-HT3 and 5-HT4. Nevertheless, ergolines constitute an important class of agents in that various examples bind with very high affinity at many populations of 5-HT receptors. Consequently, due to their large size and shape and their stereochemically defined nature, they can reveal useful information about 5-HT receptors. In addition, tritiated and radioiodinated forms of various ergot derivatives (e.g., [³H]mesulergine, [¹²⁵I]iodo-LSD) are frequently used to label the different populations of 5-HT binding sites. Arylpiperazines lacking a piperazine N4 substituent (i.e., simple arylpiperazines) are usually nonselective; however, depending upon the presence and nature of an N4 substituent, arylpiperazines (i.e., long-chain arylpiperazines) bind with high affinity and/or selectivity at, in particular, 5-HT1A and 5-HT2A receptors. The nature of this N4 substituent also influences intrinsic

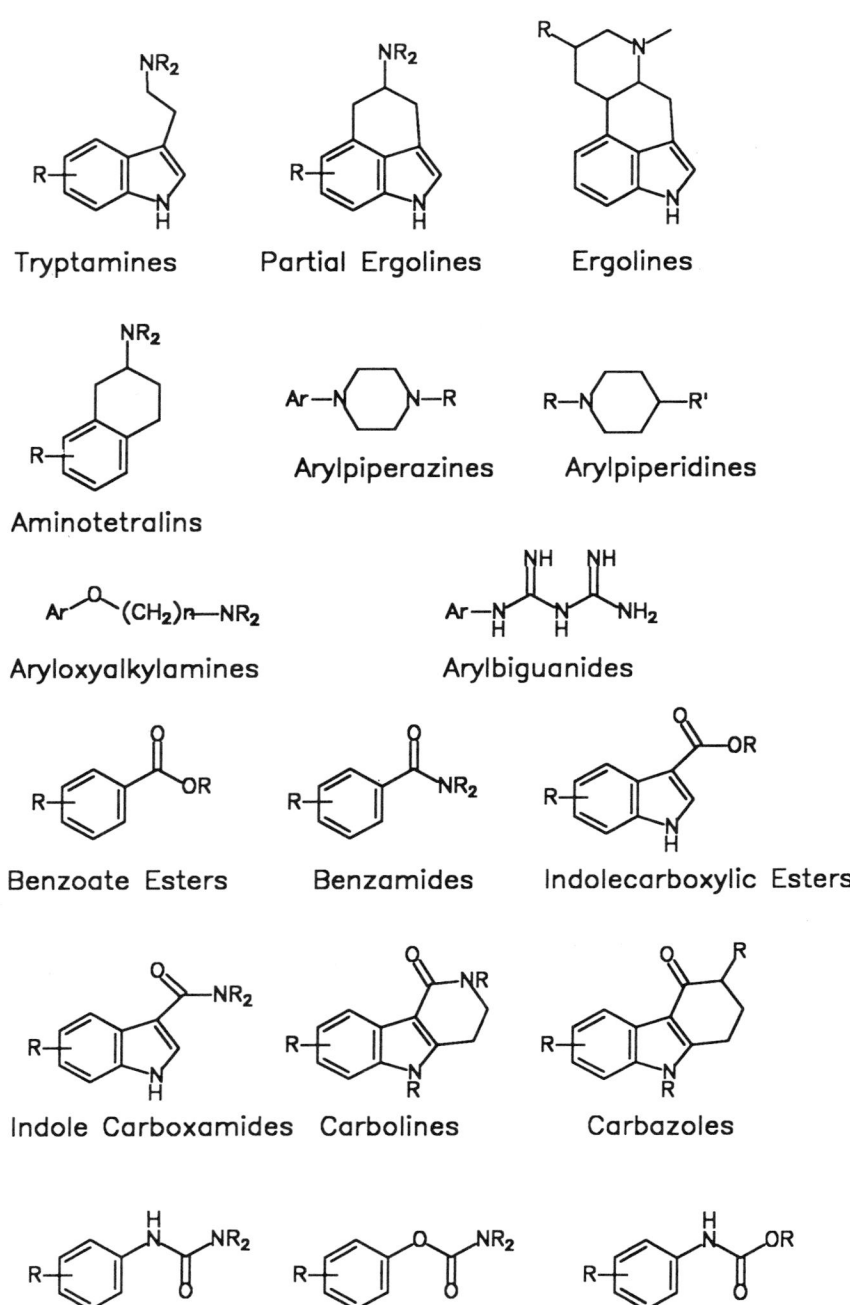

Tryptamines Partial Ergolines Ergolines

Aminotetralins Arylpiperazines Arylpiperidines

Aryloxyalkylamines Arylbiguanides

Benzoate Esters Benzamides Indolecarboxylic Esters

Indole Carboxamides Carbolines Carbazoles

Ureas Carbamates Carbamates

FIG. 1. General chemical structures of serotonergic agents described in Table 2.

activity. The alkyl- and arylpiperidines include agents such as the 5-HT1A/5-HT2A antagonist spiperone (which also binds at 5-HT7 receptors) and the 5-HT2A/5-HT2C antagonist ketanserin (which, incidentally, binds with low affinity at 5-HT2B sites). Most of these agents were developed primarily as 5-HT2A antagonists, but few show any selectivity for 5-HT2A versus 5-HT2C receptors. Aryloxyalkylamines, such as the β-adrenergic antagonists propranolol and pindolol, bind at 5-HT1A and 5-HT1B receptors; with the appropriate structural modifications, aryloxyalkylamines can be made selective for 5-HT1A

receptors. Arylbiguanides constitute a very poorly investigated class of agents; to date, the few arylbiguanides that have been studied appear to be selective for 5-HT3 receptors. The keto compounds constitute one of the largest chemical categories of serotonergic agents. Most of these compounds were developed as 5-HT3 ligands (primarily antagonists); however, a number of these agents have been demonstrated in recent years to act as 5-HT1P or 5-HT4 agonists or antagonists. Small structural modifications have resulted in newer agents that appear selective for 5-HT4 versus 5-HT3 receptors.

With the recent discovery of some of the newer populations of 5-HT receptors, the selectivity of the few "selective" agents comes into question. It also remains to be seen how examples of the different classes of agents bind at some of these newly identified sites.

SEROTONIN RECEPTOR SUBTYPES AND THEIR CHARACTERISTICS

Space constraints do not allow here a comprehensive review of the 5-HT literature. The present account will focus primarily on the more recent literature, with mention of the neuropharmacological or neuropsychiatric implications of 5-HT receptors. Several general overviews of 5-HT receptors have been recently published (27,70). Descriptions of some of the newer 5-HT ligands, as well as the medicinal chemistry and structure–activity relationships of serotonergic agents, are also available (18,20,27) (see also Chapters 36 and 38, *this volume*).

5-HT1A Receptors

5-HT1A receptors were originally defined as those 5-HT1 sites labeled in rat brain homogenates by [³H]5-HT that display high affinity for spiperone; 5-HT1 sites with low affinity for spiperone were termed 5-HT1B receptors. Nearly coincidental with the discovery of these sites was the development of a novel serotonergic agent: 8-hydroxy-2-(di-*n*-propylamino)tetralin (8-OH DPAT). Although it required several years, two French groups subsequently and independently identified 8-OH DPAT as a 5-HT1A-selective (relative to 5-HT1B and 5-HT2A) agent and [³H]8-OH DPAT was introduced as a radioligand for labeling 5-HT1A sites. To date, this remains one of the most selective serotonergic agents available, and although a number of other radioligands have been explored over the years, [³H]8-OH DPAT still remains the radioligand of choice for labeling 5-HT1A sites.

The regional distribution of 5-HT1A receptors in brain of various animal species has been examined, and the highest density appears to be in the hippocampus, the septum, the amygdala, and the cortical limbic area. 5-HT1A receptors located in the raphe nuclei correspond to somatodendritic autoreceptors. 5-HT1A receptors are, for the most part, negatively coupled to an adenylate cyclase second messenger system. There is also evidence that 5-HT1A receptors are positively coupled to adenylate cyclase; this may be accounted for either by the existence of different types of 5-HT1A receptors or by the coupling of 5-HT1A receptors to different G proteins (70).

Rat, mouse, and human 5-HT1A receptors were among the first 5-HT receptors to be cloned (3,11,14,25,47). Like other G-protein-coupled receptors, and like all other cloned 5-HT receptors with the exception of 5-HT3 receptors, the 5-HT1A receptors consist of seven transmembrane (TM) helices connected by intra- and extracellular loops. 5-HT1A receptors differ significantly from most other 5-HT receptors and exhibit a substantial similarity to adrenergic receptors; this may explain why a number of adrenergic agents, including propranolol, pindolol, oxymetazoline, and WB-4101, bind at 5-HT1A receptors with high affinity. (For additional discussion of cloned 5-HT1A receptors, see refs. 29 and 70.)

The membrane-spanning portions of rat and human 5-HT1A receptors exhibit a high (99%) degree of homology (25). The results of various receptor cloning experiments have led to several generalizations regarding receptor similarity (25). Any two receptors whose amino acid sequences are about 70–80% identical in their membrane-spanning segments may have highly similar, to nearly indistinguishable, pharmacological profiles and/or second messenger systems. Such closely related receptors (i.e., an *intermediate-homology group*) can be considered members of the same subfamily. In addition, there is a *low-homology group* (~35–55% TM homology) that consists of distantly related receptor subtypes from the same neurotransmitter family, and there is also a *high-homology group* (95–99% TM homology) that consists of species homologues from the same gene in different species (25). Furthermore, species homologues of the same gene reveal high sequence conservation in regions outside the transmembrane domains, whereas intra species receptor subtypes are usually quite divergent (25). Because ligand binding likely occurs in the membrane-spanning regions, similarities in these regions may account for the nonselectivity of various ligands. For example, human 5-HT1A receptors exhibit 50–55% TM homology with 5-HT1D receptors, and one of the problems in identifying 5-HT1D-selective agents is their high affinity for 5-HT1A receptors. On the other hand, even a high sequence homology between two receptors does not preclude the identification of "selective agents." For example, spiperone binds at 5-HT2A sites versus 5-HT2C sites with about 1000-fold selectivity even though the two receptors share 78% sequence homology.

5-HT1A Receptor Ligands

The prototypic 5-HT1A receptor agonist ligand is the aminotetralin derivative 8-OH DPAT. Long-chain arylpiperazines bind with modest to high affinity at 5-HT1A receptors. Some of the more widely used arylpiperazine (partial) agonists include buspirone, gepirone, and ipsapirone. Structurally related piperazine derivatives such as BMY 7378 and NAN-190 possess 5-HT1A antagonist character (17). Hundreds of arylpiperazine derivatives have been synthesized in order to explore their therapeutic potential (18). The alkylpiperidine spiperone is a 5-HT1A antagonist but, as already mentioned, lacks selectivity.

Clinical Significance

Buspirone is clinically available as an anxiolytic agent. Indeed, a number of structurally related agents hold the promise of being novel nonbenzodiazepine anxiolytics (49). 5-HT1A agents might also be useful in the treatment of depression (61), and there may be a relationship between serotonin metabolism, depression, and violent behavior. Certain 5-HT1A agents display antiaggressive behavior, and measurement of the density of 5-HT1A receptors in frontal cortex of suicide victims reveals that nonviolent suicide victims had a significantly higher B_{max} than did controls and violent suicide victims (42). The presence of alcohol is also associated with a decreased density of 5-HT1A receptors in certain brain regions (9). In the first clinical trial of its kind, gepirone was found to produce marked improvement in several depressed patients (51). Buspirone was effective in the treatment of mixed anxious–depressive patients (62). 5-HT1 (5-HT1A?) receptors may be involved in obsessive–compulsive disorders. 5-HT1A receptors also appear to be involved in sexual behavior, appetite control, thermoregulation, and cardiovascular function (reviewed in refs. 15 and 61). To date, most investigations have employed agents that are either 5-HT1A agonists or partial agonists. Although compounds such as BMY 7378 and NAN-190 possess 5-HT1A antagonist character, they appear to be postsynaptic antagonists but presynaptic agonists (reviewed in ref. 17). Recently, WAY 100135, a structural relative of BMY 7378 and NAN-190, has been demonstrated to be both a pre- and postsynaptic 5-HT1A antagonist (53). Human evaluation of silent and selective 5-HT1A antagonists should prove interesting and could open new vistas in 5-HT1A research.

5-HT1B/1D Receptors

5-HT1B Receptors

5-HT1B receptors were one of the first 5-HT1-like receptors to be described (reviewed in refs. 21 and 70). It was later shown that the distribution and second messenger coupling of 5-HT1B receptors in rodent brain was similar to that of 5-HT1D receptors in mammalian brain, leading to speculation that 5-HT1B and 5-HT1D receptors might constitute species variants of the same receptor (70). 5-HT1B receptors were initially identified in rodent brain using radioligand binding techniques and were defined as sites labeled by [³H]5-HT with low affinity for spiperone. The highest density of 5-HT1B receptors in rat and mouse brain is found in the substantia nigra, globus pallidus, dorsal subiculum, and superior colliculi. 5-HT1B receptors are located both postsynaptically and presynaptically and constitute terminal autoreceptors regulating the release of 5-HT (70). 5-HT1B receptors are negatively coupled to adenylate cyclase. Rat (1,64) and mouse (41) 5-HT1B receptor genes have been cloned. The cloned mouse 5-HT1B receptor (termed 5-HT1Bβ) (41) exhibits 100% identity to the rat 5-HT1B receptor (64) in the transmembrane region and differs overall by a total of

only five amino acids. This will be further discussed below.

5-HT1B Receptor Ligands

Early studies on ligand selectivity for 5-HT1B receptors can be rather confusing; much of the early work was done at a time when only two populations of 5-HT1 sites were recognized: 5-HT1A and 5-HT1B. Because it was possible to mask binding at 5-HT1A sites, residual binding was presumed to be attributable to 5-HT1B receptors. Most agents originally found to be 5-HT1B-selective are now realized to be fairly nonselective. For example, the simple arylpiperazine TFMPP was long used as a 5-HT1B-selective agonist, but it is now realized that TFMPP binds at multiple populations of 5-HT receptors with less than 10-fold selectivity. Further adding to their nonselective nature, TFMPP and RU 24969 (another agent long used as a "selective" 5-HT1B agonist) have been shown to enhance release of 5-HT.

To date, no 5-HT1B-selective ligands have been identified. Two of the more selective agents are the RU 24969 analogue CP-93,129 (and related derivatives) and serotonin O-carboxymethylglycyltyrosinamide. A radioiodinated version of the latter compound has been used in autoradiographic and radioligand binding studies. Both of these agents also bind at 5-HT1D receptors. Aryloxyalkylamines such as propranolol and pindolol bind at 5-HT1B receptors, and, under the appropriate masking conditions, tritiated iodocyanopindolol has been used to label 5-HT1B sites. The aryloxyalkylamine isomoltane binds at 5-HT1B receptors and appears to be an antagonist; in contrast, propranolol and pindolol are partial agonists. (For further discussion of these and related agents, see refs. 21 and 70. For comparisons of binding profiles and intrinsic activities, see ref. 59.)

5-HT1B Receptors: Clinical Significance

Rodent 5-HT1B receptors have been implicated as playing a role in thermoregulation, respiration, appetite control, sexual behavior, aggression, and anxiety (reviewed in ref. 21). Past studies, however, utilized agents that are now recognized as lacking selectivity for 5-HT1B receptors. In addition, the recent identification of multiple populations of 5-HT1B receptors and the discovery of the relationship between 5-HT1B and 5-HT1D receptors have raised new questions. The functional significance of 5-HT1B receptors begs reexamination, but such studies must await the development of agents with greater selectivity. At one time it was thought that 5-HT1B-type actions in rodents might be extrapolated to 5-HT1D-like actions in humans. Because of differences in receptor structure, rat 5-HT1B receptors may be poor models for the development of human drugs (25).

5-HT1D Receptors

5-HT1D receptors were first identified in bovine caudate by radioligand binding techniques and have been demonstrated to be widely distributed throughout the central nervous system (reviewed in refs. 21 and 70). They are G-protein-linked and are coupled to inhibition of adenylate cyclase. A 5-HT1D-like receptor, termed 5-HT1R, has been identified in rabbit brain.

Because of the manner in which binding studies were conducted (i.e., by masking other 5-HT1-like receptors known at that time), there was early speculation about the possible existence of additional 5-HT1-like receptors or of 5-HT1D receptor heterogeneity (e.g., ref. 33). Indeed, further investigation eventually led to the discovery of 5-HT1E receptors (33). The controversy surrounding the possible existence of 5-HT1D receptors in rat brain further confounded 5-HT1D research. This situation was subsequently remedied by molecular biology. A canine 5-HT1D receptor (RDC4) (37) and a human 5-HT1D receptor (24) were cloned and found to display about 90% amino acid sequence homology in their transmembrane domains. Hartig et al. (25) have suggested that the genes encoding these receptors are species homologues and have termed the cloned human 5-HT1D receptor 5-HT1Dα. A human gene encoding a second 5-HT1D receptor has also been cloned, and this second receptor has been termed 5-HT1Dβ (8,28,35,36,66). The human 5-HT1Dα and 5-HT1Dβ receptors display about 77% sequence homology; however, their pharmacological properties are nearly indistinguishable (25). The gene encoding 5-HT1Dα has been localized to chromosome 1, whereas that encoding 5-HT1Dβ is located on chromosome 6 (8,28). Cloning and characterization of rat (24,64) and mouse (41) 5-HT1B receptors reveals a high degree of similarity with human 5-HT1Dβ receptors. A mouse 5-HT1B receptor (5-HT1Bβ), identical to rat 5-HT1B receptors in the TM region, exhibits greater than 90% homology with human 5-HT1Dβ receptors, only 59% homology with human 5-HT1Dα receptors, and is distinct from a second mouse receptor (5-HT1Bα?) that possesses 89% homology with human 5-HT1Dα receptors (41). It appears, then, that human brain expresses two closely related intraspecies 5-HT1D receptors (5-HT1Dα and 5-HT1Dβ), whereas in rat and mouse the equivalent genes encode receptors whose pharmacological properties are associated with two separate pharmacological sites (5-HT1D and 5-HT1B) (25). That is, human 5-HT1Dα receptors appear to have species equivalents in dog (RDC4), rat (5-HT1D), and mouse (5-HT1Bα), as do human 5-HT1Dβ receptors in rat (5-HT1B) and mouse (5-HT1Bβ).

5-HT1D Ligands

Most investigations of 5-HT1D receptors were conducted prior to the discovery of 5-HT1Dα and 5-HT1Dβ receptors. Thus, binding data for most agents necessarily reflect "overall 5-HT1D" character. To date, there are no 5-HT1D-selective ligands. The one agent commonly referred to as a 5-HT1D agonist is sumatriptan (5-HT1D; $K_i = 20$–30 nM). However, sumatriptan binds at 5-HT1D receptors with only 2- to 20-fold selectivity over 5-HT1A and 5-HT1B receptors, and it also binds at 5-HT1Eβ and 5-HT1F sites. Its affinities for 5-HT1Dα sites ($K_i = 5.8$ nM) and for 5-HT1Dβ sites ($K_i = 7.7$ nM) are nearly identical (66). A newer ligand for 5-HT1D receptors is L-694,247, which reportedly binds at 5-HT1D receptors with 50-fold selectivity over 5-HT1A receptors (45). Structure–activity relationships for the binding of various agents at 5-HT1D receptors have been reported (see ref. 21 and references therein). Many indolealkylamines bind with high affinity but with little selectivity. Arylpiperazines have been shown to bind, and 1-[2-(4-amino)-phenylethyl]-4-(3-trifluoromethylphenyl)piperazine (PAPP), a fairly common 5-HT1A ligand, binds with no selectivity for 5-HT1A versus 5-HT1D receptors. Interestingly, however, the aryloxyalkylamine (−)pindolol, which binds at 5-HT1A and 5-HT1B receptors, displays little affinity for 5-HT1D receptors (58). Yohimbine and rauwolscine bind with 50- and 250-fold selectivity at 5-HT1D versus 5-HT1B receptors (58). Relatively few agents have been examined at 5-HT1Dα versus 5-HT1Dβ receptors; however, to date, no agent displays significant selectivity for one 5-HT1D subpopulation versus the other. For a diverse series of 19 agents, 5-HT1Dα binding was highly correlated ($r = 0.96$) with 5-HT1Dβ binding; interestingly, however, nearly all agents seemed to bind with slightly higher affinity for the 5-HT1Dα receptor (66).

5-HT1D Receptors: Clinical Significance

The clinical significance of 5-HT1D receptors is largely unknown. There has been speculation that these receptors might be involved in anxiety, depression, and other neuropsychiatric disorders, but this remains, for the most part, to be substantiated. Sumatriptan has been shown to be effective in the treatment of migraine, and logical extrapolation implies a role for 5-HT1D receptors in this disorder. However, there is considerable controversy regarding the nature of the actual 5-HT receptors involved in migraine (see ref. 21 for further discussion and key references). The finding that sumatriptan binds nearly equally well at 5-HT1Dα and 5-HT1Dβ receptors (66), and that it also binds at 5-HT1F sites (2), only adds further fuel to this controversy.

5-HT1E Receptors

Using [^{3}H]5-HT as radioligand, initial reports of 5-HT1E receptors in human cortical homogenates were based on binding studies where the masking of 5-HT1A, 5-HT1B, and 5-HT1C receptors led to biphasic competition curves for certain ligands (33). One component of these curves was associated with 5-HT1D binding, whereas the other was attributed to a new population of sites: 5-HT1E receptors. The low affinity of 5-carboxamidotryptamine and ergotamine for 5-HT1E receptors allowed their differentiation from 5-HT1D receptors. High-affinity [³H]5-HT binding was sensitive to guanine nucleotides, but functional coupling to a second messenger system was not reported. Preliminary studies also indicated the presence of 5-HT1E receptors in bovine and rat brain (33).

The cloning of human 5-HT1E receptors was independently reported by three laboratories (23,44,69). The sequence was identical to that reported by Levy et al. (35) earlier in 1992 for a novel 5-HT receptor which, at the time, was not identified as a 5-HT1E receptor. Consistent with the results of the initial radioligand binding study (33), the cloned 5-HT1E receptors are rather unique in that they display low affinity for most serotonergic agents. Even simple O-methylation of 5-HT reduces affinity by about 100- to 300-fold (23,69). Other than for 5-HT, the only agents shown to bind at 5-HT1E receptors with K_i values of less than 100 nM are lysergol, ergonovine, and methylergonovine (69). Functional studies, in cells stably expressing 5-HT1E receptors, indicate that the receptor is negatively coupled to adenylate cyclase. Methiothepin, which only binds at 5-HT1E receptors with modest affinity ($K_i \approx 200$ nM) (44,69), proved to be a weak competitive antagonist (44,69). On the basis of its sequence homology (64%) to 5-HT1Dα and 5-HT1Dβ receptors, 5-HT1E receptors may be viewed as a distantly related member of the 5-HT1D family (44,69).

A mouse 5-HT1E receptor has also been cloned; originally referred to as a "5-HT6" receptor, it has now been renamed 5-HT1Eβ because of its significant TM sequence homology (62%) with human 5-HT1E receptors. Accordingly, it has been suggested that human 5-HT1E receptors be termed 5-HT1Eα (43). Mouse 5-HT1Eβ receptors also display similarity to human 5-HT1Dα (56%) and mouse 5-HT1Bβ (54%) receptors (43). In addition, it appears that the mouse 5-HT1Eβ receptor is a species homologue of human 5-HT1F receptors (see next section).

5-HT1F Receptors

The newest 5-HT1 receptor to be cloned is the human 5-HT1F receptor. The 5-HT1F receptor exhibits intermediate transmembrane homology with several other 5-HT1 receptors: 5-HT1E (70%), 5-HT1Dα (63%), 5-HT1Dβ (60%), and 5-HT1A (53%) (2). Despite its similarity to 5-HT1E receptors, 5-HT1F receptors bind 5-methoxytryptamine and certain ergot derivatives with high affinity ($K_i < 100$ nM). The 5-HT1D agonist sumatriptan also binds at 5-HT1F sites; in contrast, 5-carboxamidotryptamine ($K_i = 717$ nM) binds only with modest affinity.

The cloned human 5-HT1F receptor couples to inhibi-tion of adenylate cyclase. Agonist effects of 5-HT were completely, and apparently competitively, antagonized by the nonselective 5-HT antagonist methiothepin (2). Detection of 5-HT1F receptors in the uterus and mesentery suggests a possible role in vascular contraction. Although distribution in the brain appears limited, there are distributional similarities with 5-HT1Dβ receptors. This, together with the high affinity of sumatriptan, suggests that 5-HT1F receptors may be involved in migraine (2).

There is a high degree of homology between human 5-HT1F receptors and mouse 5-HT1Eβ receptors. In fact, their TM regions differ only by two amino acid residues, one in TM helix 4 and one in TM helix 5. Thus, it is likely that these two receptor types are interspecies homologues.

5-HT1P Receptors

5-HT1P sites are labeled by [³H]5-HT and display a pharmacology distinct from that of other 5-HT receptors. 5-HT1P receptors are found in the gut; but because they have not been identified in the central nervous system, they will not be discussed here.

5-HT1S Receptors

Early studies suggested that 50% of sites labeled by [³H]5-HT in rat spinal cord were either 5-HT1A or 5-HT1B receptors. Subsequent investigations afforded similar results but additionally identified the remaining 5-HT receptors as a novel population that lacked characteristics of other 5-HT sites. These were termed 5-HT1S sites (68). 5-HT1S sites display high affinity for 5-HT ($K_i = 6.3$ nM) and tryptamine ($K_i = 6.9$ nM), modest affinity ($K_i = 200–300$ nM) for methiothepin, cyproheptadine, and metergoline, and micromolar affinity for 8-OH DPAT, TFMPP, RU 24969, propranolol, quipazine, methysergide, mianserin, ketanserin, and tropisetron (ICS 205-930). Saturation studies performed in the presence of guanine nucleotides showed that GTP and Gpp(NH)p significantly reduced the number of 5-HT1S receptors labeled by [³H]5-HT with a corresponding increase in apparent K_d values. In contrast, ATP had no effect on kinetic parameters. Although 5-HT1S receptors appear to be the predominant 5-HT1 receptor population in spinal cord, no significant density of 5-HT1S receptors was found in brainstem or frontal cortex. 5-HT1S receptors may be involved with modulation of pain input to the spinal cord (68).

5-HT2A Receptors

5-HT2A (also referred to as 5-HT2 and 5-HT2α) receptors were among the first populations of 5-HT receptors to be identified and, consequently, have been extensively reviewed (e.g., see refs. 27 and 70). 5-HT2A receptors are widely distributed, although at varying densities, throughout the brain; the highest density occurs in the neocortex. 5-HT2A receptors are directly coupled to a phosphoinositol second messenger system. In certain brain regions, 5-HT stimulates phospholipase A_2 via a 5-HT2 mechanism.

Early on, many actions—both central and peripheral—of serotonergic agents were attributed to a 5-HT2A as opposed to a 5-HT1 mechanism. This was due, in large part, to the availability of what was then considered a very selective 5-HT2A (versus 5-HT1) antagonist: ketanserin. [^{3}H]Ketanserin is still the radioligand of choice for binding studies. With the subsequent discovery of 5-HT2C (i.e., 5-HT1C, 5-HT2β) receptors, and the finding that many 5-HT2A ligands bind nearly equally well at both types of receptors, came the realization that some of the roles attributed to 5-HT2A receptors may in fact be mediated by 5-HT2C receptors. For example, ketanserin, the most widely used 5-HT2A antagonist, has been reported to bind with as little as 2-fold to as much as 140-fold selectivity for 5-HT2A versus 5-HT2C receptors. Most findings, however, are closer to the lower end of this range. Agents such as DOI and DOB act as 5-HT2 agonists, or partial agonists, but display less than 10-fold selectivity for 5-HT2A versus 5-HT2C receptors. Another confounding factor in 5-HT2 research was the initial finding that 5-HT, as well as other agents with 5-HT2A agonist activity, displays low affinity for [^{3}H]ketanserin-labeled 5-HT2A sites. Evidence was subsequently provided suggesting that 5-HT2A receptors exist in a high-affinity state (5-HT2H) and a low-affinity state (5-HT2L). This equilibrium appears to lie heavily in favor of the 5-HT2L state, and the tritiated antagonist ketanserin binds at both states with comparable affinity. In contrast, radiolabeled agonists such as [^{3}H]DOB and [^{125}I]DOI appear to label the 5-HT2H state (e.g., see ref. 27). Although this concept is not without controversy (see ref. 70 for further discussion), 5-HT and the more selective 5-HT2A agonists bind with 50- to 100-fold higher affinity at agonist-labeled sites than at [^{3}H]ketanserin-labeled sites.

Rat (30), mouse (13,38), hamster (6), and human (56) 5-HT2A receptors have been cloned, and they exhibit a high degree (>90%) of homology. In addition, there is significant (78%) homology in the TM portions of 5-HT2A receptors and cloned 5-HT2C receptors (39). This may, to some extent, explain the observed similarities in the binding of various ligands at the two receptor populations.

5-HT2A Ligands

The structure–activity relationships of 5-HT2A ligands have been reviewed (18,20). Indolealkylamines, which typically bind with higher affinity at [^{3}H]DOB- or [^{125}I]DOI-labeled sites than at [^{3}H]ketanserin-labeled sites, are nonselective 5-HT2A ligands. Various phenyl-alkylamines (such as DOB and DOI) act as 5-HT2A agonists or partial agonists, are significantly more selective than the indolealkylamines, and also bind with higher affinity at agonist-labeled versus antagonists-labeled 5-HT2A sites.

One of the largest, and more selective, classes of 5-HT2A ligands is the N-alkylpiperidines. The best known example is ketanserin. Another widely used 5-HT2A antagonist is ritanserin; but ritanserin also binds at 5-HT2B, 5-HT6, and 5-HT7 sites. Although numerous ketanserin-related derivatives have been reported, their structure–activity relationships have not been well-documented. Unlike ketanserin, which binds at 5-HT2C sites, spiperone displays about a 1000-fold selectivity for 5-HT2A versus 5-HT2C sites. Spiperone has been employed as a 5-HT2A antagonist; however, spiperone is also a dopamine antagonist, a 5-HT1A antagonist, and a 5-HT7 ligand. Various structurally related agents, such as the piperazine derivative irindalone, also act as 5-HT2A antagonists. Many 5-HT2A antagonists, although fairly selective for 5-HT2A and 5-HT2C receptors versus most other populations of 5-HT receptors, bind with modest to high affinity at other (particularly dopaminergic, histaminergic, and/or adrenergic) neurotransmitter receptors. Various tricyclic agents (e.g., tricyclic neuroleptics and tricyclic antidepressants) also bind at 5-HT2A receptors. In general, although ketanserin and spiperone are among the more widely used antagonists, and DOB and DOI are useful agonists, there do not seem to be any truly selective 5-HT2A agents (19).

Clinical Implications

It should be realized that many of the clinical implications of 5-HT2A receptors may actually involve 5-HT2C receptors, or a combination of 5-HT2A and 5-HT2C receptors. The potential therapeutic roles of 5-HT2A ligands, and the possible involvement of 5-HT2A receptors, in modulating normal physiological functions and various pathological and psychopathological conditions have been extensively reviewed (15,61,70). 5-HT2A receptors appear to play a role in appetite control, thermoregulation, and sleep. They are also involved, along with various other 5-HT receptor populations, in cardiovascular function and muscle contraction. They have also received considerable attention from a neuropsychiatric standpoint. Various neuroleptic agents and antidepressants bind with relatively high affinity at 5-HT2A receptors. Although there is no direct correlation between their receptor affinities and clinically effective doses, there is strong evidence that these disorders involve, at least to some extent, 5-HT2A (or perhaps 5-HT2C) receptors. For example, chronic administration of 5-HT2A antagonists results in a paradoxical down-regulation of 5-HT2A receptors; such a down-regulation would be of benefit in the treatment of depression. Several 5-HT2A antagonist are currently in clinical trials as potential neuroleptic agents. Many 5-

HT2A antagonists additionally bind at dopamine receptors. Although this may cloud the role of 5-HT2A antagonism versus dopamine antagonism as being the more important for neuroleptic activity, it has been suggested that certain types of schizophrenia may actually be more responsive to this combined effect. From animal studies there are indications that 5-HT2A antagonists possess anxiolytic properties; one 5-HT2A antagonist, ritanserin, appears to produce an antianxiety effect in humans. The role of 5-HT receptors in anxiety has been reviewed (49). It has been proposed that 5-HT2A (and/or 5-HT2C) receptors may be involved in the actions of the classical hallucinogens (reviewed in ref. 16). Although indolealkylamine (e.g., 5-methoxy-N,N-dimethyltryptamine) and ergot-related (e.g., LSD) classical hallucinogens are fairly nonselective agents that bind at multiple populations of 5-HT receptors, the phenylalkylamine hallucinogens (e.g., DOB, DOI) are much more 5-HT2-selective. However, to date, there have been no attempts to block the effect of classical hallucinogens in humans with 5-HT2A antagonists.

5-HT2B Receptors

The rat stomach fundus preparation has been used as a functional assay for serotonergic action for over 35 years. Questions concerning the pharmacological similarily of fundus receptors to the 5-HT2 family of receptors led to its recent cloning (see ref. 65 and references therein). 5-HT2B receptors (originally termed 5-HT2F receptors, and not to be confused with 5-HT2B terminology occasionally used to describe what were once called 5-HT1C receptors) exhibit about 70% homology to 5-HT2A and 5-HT2C (5-HT1C) receptors and, like 5-HT2A receptors, appear to couple functionally to phophoinositol hydrolysis. Using [^{3}H]5-HT as radioligand, 5-HT binds with high (K_i = 9 nM) affinity. The standard 5-HT2A antagonist ketanserin binds with low affinity (K_i = 3559 nM), whereas the 5-HT2A antagonist ritanserin retains high affinity (K_i = 5.18 nM) for 5-HT2B receptors (65). The 5-HT$_{2A/2C}$ agonist DOI also binds with high affinity (K_i = 27.5 nM). Agonists generally showed higher affinity for 5-HT2B receptors when binding assays were conducted at 0°C than at 37°C, whereas antagonists showed no difference in affinity; thus, binding at the two temperatures was found to be predictive for agonist versus antagonist activity (65). Rat fundus 5-HT2B receptors exhibit 96% homology to 5-HT receptors cloned from mouse stomach fundus (13).

5-HT2C Receptors

5-HT2C receptors, previously referred to as 5-HT1C or 5-HT2β receptors, were originally identified using autoradiographic and radioligand binding techniques (reviewed in refs. 26 and 70). Initially characterized in porcine choroid plexus, low densities of 5-HT2C sites have

now been found in various brain regions of a number of different animal species. Mouse (13,67), rat (29,39), and human (56) 5-HT2C receptors have been cloned and display a high homology with 5-HT2A receptors. Like 5-HT2A receptors, 5-HT2C receptors are coupled to phosphoinositol hydrolysis. There is some new evidence that 5-HT2C receptors may also be linked to stimulation of cGMP production (26). Many agents initially thought to be selective for 5-HT2A receptors were subsequently found to bind with high affinity at 5-HT2C receptors; in fact, the 5-HT2A affinities of various agents typically parallel their 5-HT2C affinities, and there are presently no 5-HT2C-selective agents. Consequently, many pharmacological functions once attributed to 5-HT2A receptors, on the basis of their being produced by DOB or DOI and/or their being antagonized by ketanserin and related agents, may actually involve a 5-HT2C mechanism. For example, the hyperthermic activity of a series of phenylisopropylamines is significantly correlated with their 5-HT2A affinity; later studies have shown a similar correlation between hyperthermic activity and 5-HT2C receptor affinity (16). Numerous atypical antipsychotic agents bind at 5-HT2A and 5-HT2C receptors; however, there is no correlation between their atypical nature and binding (52). 5-HT2C receptors may play a greater role than 5-HT2A receptors in migraine. Recent attempts have been made to sort out what behaviors might be 5-HT2A-mediated relative to those that are 5-HT2C-mediated (reviewed in ref. 32). But, in the absence of selective agents, this has been a difficult task. Spiperone, a 5-HT1A and dopamine antagonist, displays about a 1000-fold selectivity for 5-HT2A versus 5-HT2C sites; amperozide and pimozide also bind with comparable selectivity (52). Theoretically, such agents might be useful in defining the potential involvement of 5-HT2A versus 5-HT2C receptors as being important in a given functional effect. One interesting potential difference between 5-HT2A and 5-HT2C receptors is that the former may undergo allosteric regulation whereas the latter may not (see ref. 55 and references therein). Clearly, however, more selective agents are required.

5-HT3 Receptors

5-HT3 receptors constitute one of the first three families of 5-HT receptors to be studied. Unlike most of the other 5-HT receptors where functional assays were slow to be identified (and, in some cases, have yet to be identified), early 5-HT3 pharmacology involved only the use of functional assays. Because of the pharmacological similarity between 5-HT3 receptors and 5-HT-M receptors, it might be said that 5-HT3 research actually began in 1957; however, the first radioligand binding studies were not reported until 30 years later. 5-HT3 receptors are unique amongst the families of 5-HT receptors in that they are nonselective Na$^+$/K$^+$ ion channel receptors. They are found in the periphery and also in central nervous system, particularly in the area postrema, entorhinal cortex, frontal cortex, and hippocampus (31,70). The pharmacological and electrophysiological characteristics of the cloned 5-HT3 receptor are largely consistent with the properties of the native receptors (40).

5-HT3 Ligands

As might be expected, indolealkylamines typically bind at 5-HT3 receptors in a nonselective manner. Ergolines do not bind or bind only with very low affinity. 5-HT is a nonselective 5-HT3 agonist that binds only with modest affinity ($K_i \approx 500$ nM). 2-Methyl 5-HT is a somewhat more selective agent that binds with slightly lower affinity than 5-HT; although it may be only a partial agonist, it has found widespread application in 5-HT3 research. The quaternary amine derivative 5-HTQ binds with about 10 times the affinity of 5-HT, is much more selective than 5-HT or 2-methyl 5-HT, and, because of its quaternary nature, will likely not penetrate the blood–brain barrier. Phenylbiguanide is another example of a low-affinity ($K_i \approx 1000$ nM) 5-HT3 agonist. Its 3-chloro derivative, meta-chlorophenylbiguanide (mCPBG), binds in the low nanomolar range and retains agonist character.

MDL 72222 was the first selective 5-HT3 antagonist. Its development resulted from the structural modification of cocaine, an agent that had been previously shown to be a weak 5-HT-M receptor antagonist. Since then, numerous 5-HT3 antagonists have been identified. Almost all of these agents belong to the structural class of compounds referred to as *keto compounds* (Table 2). Some of the more widely used agents include ondansetron, tropisetron (ICS 205-930), zacopride, granisetron, and renzapride. It might be noted that many keto compounds also bind at 5-HT1P and/or 5-HT4 receptors. Simple arylpiperazine (e.g., meta-chlorophenylpiperazine, quipazine) bind with high affinity and are typically nonselective; it is not clear whether these agents are 5-HT3 agonists or antagonists. Long-chain arylpiperazines and alkylpiperidine derivatives lack affinity, or bind with very low affinity, at 5-HT3 receptors. The structure–activity relationships of 5-HT3 ligands have been reviewed in detail (18–20,31).

Clinical Implications

5-HT3 antagonists have proven quite effective for the treatment of chemotherapy induced or radiation-induced nausea and vomiting (31). There are also indications that they may be effective in the treatment of migraine (31). Animal studies suggest that 5-HT3 antagonists enhance memory, possess anxiolytic activity, and act as atypical neuroleptics (31); however, clinical trials are required to substantiate these claims. 5-HT3 receptors can control dopamine release and may also be involved acetylcholine release and control of the GABAergic system (70). This

intimate relationship could explain some of the pharmacological properties of 5-HT3 ligands. Interestingly, however, phenylbiguanide induces carrier-mediated release of [³H]dopamine independent of a 5-HT3 mechanism (57). Finally, there is evidence that 5-HT3 antagonists may suppress the behavioral consequences of withdrawing chronic treatment for drugs of abuse, including alcohol, nicotine, cocaine, and amphetamine (31) (see Chapters 145, and 147–149, *this volume*).

5-HT4 Receptors

A novel population of 5-HT receptors, originally identified in primary cell cultures of mouse embryo colliculi, was later called 5-HT4 receptors (reviewed in refs. 4 and 70). 5-HT4 receptors enjoy a broad tissue distribution and are positively coupled to adenylate cyclase. In the brain, 5-HT4 receptors appear to be localized on neurons and may mediate slow excitatory responses to 5-HT (70). In collicular and hippocampal neurons, 5-HT4 receptors stimulate adenylate cyclase; the mechanism by which these receptors inhibit K^+ channels in collicular neurons has been demonstrated to involve cAMP production and consequent activation of cAMP-dependent protein kinase A (4). Peripherally, 5-HT4 receptors facilitate acetylcholine release in guinea-pig ileum and may play a role in peristalsis.

5-HT4 receptors have not yet been cloned, and radioligand binding studies have not been widely used to investigate this population of receptors. Indeed, until most recently, selective agents had not been identified. Most of the work done with 5-HT4 receptors has involved various functional (isolated tissue) assays, and certain inconsistencies have raised the possibility of the existence of 5-HT4 receptor subpopulations (4). The previous lack of selective agents has hampered investigations of clinical significance; however, it has been speculated that because of its association with the cholinergic system there may be some relevance of 5-HT4 receptors to the acetylcholine-deficit concept of cognitive disorders (4).

Initially, no agents demonstrated selectivity for 5-HT4 receptors, and functional characterization relied heavily on a weak antagonist (the 5-HT3 antagonist tropisetron) and several other structurally related 5-HT3 antagonists which display 5-HT4 agonist properties. Within the past year, however, a number of new compounds have been identified. The potent 5-HT3 antagonists BIMU1 and BIMU8 (10) act as 5-HT4 agonists, whereas SC-49518 (a mixture of 1S,8R and 1R,8S isomers) and its optical isomer SC-53116 (12) are 5-HT4 agonists with relatively low affinity ($K_i > 150$ nM) for 5-HT3 receptors. Newly identified 5-HT4 antagonists include DAU 6285 (10), SDZ 205-557 (5), RS-23597-190 (34), and SC-53606 (12). The tritiated version of another new antagonist, GR113808, has recently been used to label 5-HT4 receptors in guinea-pig brain employing radioligand binding techniques (22). Some representative results using this assay are as follows: 5-HT (pK_i = 7.3), 5-methoxytryptamine (pK_i = 6.5), α-methyl 5-HT (pK_i = 5.8), 5-carboxamidotryptamine (pK_i = 5.3), tropisetron (pK_i = 7.2), SDZ 205-557 (pK_i = 8.2), GR113808 (pK_i = 9.5) (22).

5-HT5 Receptors

A functional mouse 5-HT receptor that is expressed primarily in the central nervous system has recently been identified (50). The 5-HT5 amino acid sequence is not closely related to other 5-HT receptors, but the pharmacological properties of this receptor resemble those of 5-HT1D receptors. A closely related receptor, 5-HT5B, has also been cloned, leading to the renaming of the original 5-HT5 receptor as 5-HT5A (43). The two 5-HT5 receptors exhibit 77% amino acid sequence homology, but less than 50% homology with other cloned 5-HT receptors (43). The 5-HT5A gene is on mouse chromosome 5, whereas the 5-HT5B gene is on chromosome 1.

5-HT5A and 5-HT5B receptors are both labeled with [^{125}I]I-LSD. 5-HT binds with modest affinity (K_i = 250 nM), whereas 5-carboxamidotryptamine binds with about 10-fold higher affinity at both receptors. It is the low affinity of 5-HT that has excluded the classification of these receptors as 5-HT1-like. Furthermore, preliminary studies suggest that neither receptor efficiently couples to G protein, leading to speculation that they may be coupled to ion channels (43).

The pharmacological profile of 5-HT5 receptors bears some similarity to 5-HT1D receptors, prompting conjecture that 5-HT5A receptors may correspond to pharmacologically defined rat 5-HT1D receptors or to a fraction of these sites (50). It might be noted, however, that there exists only a 35% sequence homology between mouse 5-HT5A and human 5-HT1Dα receptors. Nevertheless, potential 5-HT1D-like roles have been proposed for 5-HT5 receptors, including involvement in motor control, feeding, anxiety, and depression (43,50). 5-HT5A receptors may also play a role in brain development (43).

5-HT6 Receptors

A cDNA encoding a novel G-protein-coupled 5-HT receptor, which appears to be localized exclusively in the central nervous system and predominantly in the corpus striatum and in various limbic and cortical regions, has been cloned from rat brain (46). This receptor, termed 5-HT6, exhibits only 36–41% TM homology with 5-HT1A, 5-HT1B, 5-HT1D, 5-HT1E, 5-HT2A, and 5-HT2C receptors. Both [^{125}I]I-LSD and [^{3}H]5-HT label 5-HT6 sites, and 5-HT displays an affinity of 151 and 56 nM, respectively. With [^{125}I]I-LSD, certain ergots bind with high affinity (e.g., lisuride), whereas others (e.g., mesulergine) bind only with micromolar affinity. 5-Carboxamidotryp-

tamine binds only with modest affinity. Of interest is that a number of typical and atypical neuroleptic agents and tricyclic antidepressants bind with K_i values of less than 100 nM. In HEK-293 cells stably transfected with this receptor, 5-HT was shown to produce a potent dose-dependent increase in cAMP levels. As such, this is the first cloned 5-HT receptor that is coupled to activation of adenylate cyclase. 5-Methoxytryptamine and 5-carboxamidotryptamine behaved in a similar manner, lisuride acted as a partial agonist, and amoxipine, clozapine, and methiothepin acted as antagonists. It has been suggested that 5-HT6 receptors may be involved in neuropsychiatric disorders (46).

5-HT7 Receptors

Two new populations of 5-HT receptors have been termed 5-HT7 receptors (54,60). Although they are not identical, they are rather similar. Both, unlike 5-HT6 receptors, bind [^{3}H]5-HT with high affinity ($K_D \approx$ 1 nM). One, shown to be positively coupled to adenylate cyclase, possesses transmembrane homologies of less than 55% with most other 5-HT receptors: 5-HT1A (51%), 5-HT1B (55%), 5-HT1D (52%), 5-HT1E (53%), 5-HT1F (52%), 5-HT2A (43%), 5-HT2B (40%), 5-HT2C (42%), 5-HT5 (48%), 5-HT6 (45%) (54). The "5-HT1" ligand 5-carboxamidotryptamine binds at these sites with very high affinity (K_i = 0.12 nM). Certain ergots (e.g., LSD, lisuride), neuroleptic agents and antidepressants (e.g., spiperone, chlorpromazine, mianserin, cyproheptadine), and the nonclassical neuroleptic agent clozapine bind with K_i values of about 5–70 nM (54). It has been speculated that these receptors might be involved in mood and learning, as well as in neuroendocrine and vegetative behaviors. The second 5-HT7 receptor also displays about 50% homology with other 5-HT receptors: 5-HT1A (45%), 5-HT1B (50%), 5-HT1D (47%), 5-HT1E (45%), 5-HT1F (48%), 5-HT2A (39%), 5-HT2B (37%), 5-HT2C (40%), 5-HT5A/B (46%), 5-HT6 (44%) (60). Here, too, 5-carboxamidotryptamine (K_i = 0.16 nM) binds with high affinity; the 5-HT2 ligand ritanserin (K_i = 15 nM), certain ergots (LSD, lisuride, mesulergine), tricyclic antidepressants (e.g., amitriptyline), and nonclassical neuroleptic agents (e.g., clozapine, loxapine) bind with K_i values of less than 100 nM (60). On this basis, it has been speculated that this 5-HT7 receptor may play a role in psychotic disorders (60).

SUMMARY

The last edition of *Psychopharmacology* (48), published just 6 years ago, described only four populations of 5-HT receptors: 5-HT1A, 5-HT1B, 5-HT1C (now 5-HT2C), and 5-HT2 (now 5-HT2A) receptors. Many of the claims made for these populations of receptors at that

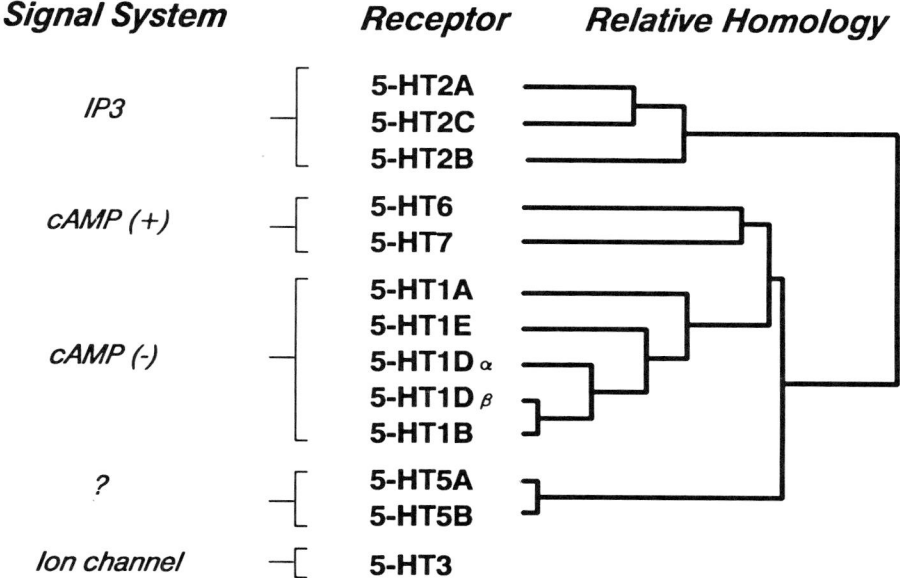

Signal System **Receptor** **Relative Homology**

IP3 — 5-HT2A, 5-HT2C, 5-HT2B

cAMP (+) — 5-HT6, 5-HT7

cAMP (-) — 5-HT1A, 5-HT1E, 5-HT1D α, 5-HT1D β, 5-HT1B

? — 5-HT5A, 5-HT5B

Ion channel — 5-HT3

FIG. 2. Structural relationships (approximate transmembrane sequence homology) and second messenger systems identified for some recently cloned 5-HT receptors. The data were adapted from refs. 43, 50, and 60.

time are still valid. The number of populations has simply increased. Figure 2 provides a brief summary of some of the cloned 5-HT receptors, their structural relationships, and their second messenger systems. Although the existence of the newer 5-HT receptor/binding sites should eventually aid our understanding of neuropsychiatric disorders, they are presently creating some short-term problems. For example, more than ever before there exists a shortage of site-selective agents. Certain fairly selective agents are now being shown to bind at some of the more recently identified sites; many other agents have yet to be examined.

There has been a shift in the focus of techniques used to identify new populations of 5-HT receptors. Whereas radioligand binding was responsible for many of the early discoveries, molecular biology has now assumed a commanding role; almost all new 5-HT receptor populations are being identified via cloning techniques. Such investigations allow a better understanding of 5-HT receptors at a molecular level. Site-directed mutagenesis and the synthesis of chimeric receptors (e.g., see ref. 7) can aid this process. Furthermore, knowledge of amino acid sequence data has allowed the construction of hypothetical three-dimensional graphics models of various populations of 5-HT receptors (e.g., see refs. 21 and 63). Once appropriate models have been identified, it should be possible to design novel and highly selective serotonergic agents.

Enormous strides have been made in the identification of new 5-HT receptor populations and in the development of novel serotonergic agents. Likewise, evidence continues to mount in support of important roles for 5-HT recep-

tors in various neuropsychiatric disorders. Anxiety, depression, schizophrenia, migraine, and drug abuse are at the top of the list. 5-HT receptors may also play important roles in appetite control, aggression, sexual behavior, and cardiovascular disorders.

REFERENCES

1. Adham N, Romanienko P, Hartig P, Weinshank R, Branchek T. The rat 5-hydroxytryptamine-1B receptor is the species homologue of the human 5-hydroxytryptamine-1Dβ receptor. *Mol Pharmacol* 1992;41:1–7.
2. Adham N, Kao HT, Schechter LE, Bard J, Olsen M, Urquhart D, Durkin M, Hartig PR, Weinshank RL, Branchek TA. Cloning of another human serotonin receptor (5-HT1F): a fifth 5-HT₁ receptor subtype coupled to the inhibition of adenylate cyclase. *Proc Natl Acad Sci USA* 1993;90:408–412.
3. Albert PR, Zhou QY, Van Tol HHM, Bunzou JR, Cirelli O. Cloning, functional expression and mRNA tissue distribution of the rat 5-hydroxytryptamine 1A receptor gene. *J Biol Chem* 1990;265:5825–5832.
4. Bockert J, Fozard JR, Dumuis A, Clarke DE. The 5-HT4 receptor: a place in the sun. *Trends Pharmacol Sci* 1992;13:141–145.
5. Buchheit K-H, Gamse R, Pfannkuche H-J. SDZ 205-557, a selective, surmountable antagonist for 5-HT4 receptors in the isolated guinea pig ileum. *Naunyn Schmiedebergs Arch Pharmacol* 1992;345:387–393.
6. Chambard JC, Obberghen-Schilling EV, Haslam RJ, Vouret V, Pouyssegur J. Chinese hamster serotonin (5-HT) type 2 receptor cDNA sequence. *Nucleic Acids Res* 1990;18:5282.
7. Choudhary MS, Craigo S, Roth BL. Identification of receptor domains that modify ligand binding to 5-hydroxytryptamine2 and 5-hydroxytryptamine1C serotonin receptors. *Mol Pharmacol* 1992;42:627–633.
8. Demchyshyn L, Sunahara RK, Miller K, Teitler M, Hoffman BJ, Kennedy JL, Seeman P, Van Tol HHM, Niznik HB. A human serotonin 1D receptor variant (5-HT1Dβ) encoded by an intronless

gene on chromosome 6. *Proc Natl Acad Sci USA* 1992;89:5522–5526.

9. Dillon KA, Gross-Isseroff R, Israeli M, Biegon A. Autoradiographic analysis of 5-HT1A receptor binding in the human brain postmortem: effect of age and alcohol. *Brain Res* 1991;554:56–64.

10. Dumuis A, Gozlan H, Sebben M, Ansanay H, Rizzi CA, Turconi M, Monferini E, Giraldo E, Schiantarelli P, Ladinsky H, Bockaert J. Characterization of a novel 5-HT4 receptor antagonist of the azabicycloalkyl benzimidazolone class: DAU 6285. *Naunyn Schmiedebergs Arch Pharmacol* 1992;345:264–269.

11. Fargin A, Raymond JR, Lohse MJ, Kobilka BK, Caron MJ, Lefkowitz RJ. The genomic clone G-21 which resembles a β-adrenergic receptor sequence encodes the 5-HT1A receptor. *Nature* 1988;335:358–360.

12. Flynn DL, Zabrowski DL, Becker DP, Nosal R, Villamil CI, Gullikson GW, Moummi C, Yang D-C. SC-53116: the first selective agonist at the newly identified serotonin 5-HT4 receptor subtype. *J Med Chem* 1992;35:1486–1489.

13. Foguet M, Nguyen H, Le H, Lubbert H. Structure of the mouse 5-HT1C, 5-HT2 and stomach fundus receptor genes. *Neuroreport* 1992;3:345–348.

14. Fujiwara Y, Nelson DL, Kashihara K, Varga E, Roeske WR, Yamamura HI. The cloning and sequence analysis of the rat serotonin-1A receptor gene. *Life Sci* 1990;47:PL-127–PL-132.

15. Glennon RA. Serotonin receptors: clinical implications. *Neurosci Biobehav Rev* 1990;14:35–47.

16. Glennon RA. Do hallucinogens act as 5-HT2 agonists or antagonists? *Neuropsychopharmacology* 1990;56:509–517.

17. Glennon RA. Concepts for the design of 5-HT1A serotonin agonists and antagonists. *Drug Dev Res* 1992;26:251–274.

18. Glennon RA, Dukat M. 5-HT receptor ligands—update 1992. *Current Drugs: Serotonin* 1993;1:1–45.

19. Glennon RA, Dukat M. Serotonin receptors and their ligands: a lack of selective agents. *Pharmacol Biochem Behav* 1991;40:1009–1017.

20. Glennon RA, Westkaemper RB, Bartyzel P. Medicinal chemistry of serotonergic agents. In: Peroutka SJ, ed. *Serotonin receptor subtypes.* New York: Wiley–Liss, 1991;19–64.

21. Glennon RA, Westkaemper RB. 5-HT1D receptors: A serotonin receptor population for the 1990's. *Drug News Perspect* 1993;3:317–334.

22. Grossman CJ, Kilpatrick GJ, Bunce KT, Oxford AW, Gale JD, Whitehead JF, Humphrey PPA. Development of a radioligand binding assay for the 5-HT4 receptor: use of a novel antagonist. In: *Second international symposium on serotonin*, Houston, TX, September 15–18, 1992. Abstract, p. 31.

23. Gudermann T, Levy FO, Birnbaumer M, Birnbaumer L, Kaumann AJ. Human S31 serotonin receptor clone encodes a 5-hydroxytryptamine$_{1E}$-like serotonin receptor. *Mol Pharmacol* 1993;43:412–418.

24. Hamblin MW, Metcalf MA. Primary structure and functional characterization of a human 5-HT1D-type serotonin receptor. *Mol Pharmacol* 1991;40:143–148.

25. Hartig PR, Branchek TA, Weinshank RL. A subfamily of 5-HT1D receptor genes. *Trends Pharmacol Sci* 1992;13:152–159.

26. Hartig PR, Hoffman BJ, Kaufman MJ, Hirata F. The 5-HT1C receptor. *Ann NY Acad Sci* 1990;600:149–167.

27. Herndon JL, Glennon RA. Serotonin receptors, agents, and actions. In: Kozikowsky A, ed. *Drug design, molecular modeling, and the neurosciences.* New York: Raven Press, 1993;167–212.

28. Jin H, Oksenberg D, Ashkenazi A, Peroutka SJ, Duncan AMV, Rozmahel R, Yang Y, Mengod G, Palacios JM, O'Dowd BF. Characterization of the human 5-hydroxytryptamine-1B receptor. *J Biol Chem* 1992;267:5835–5838.

29. Julius D. Molecular biology of serotonin receptors. *Annu Rev Neurosci* 1991;14:335–360.

30. Julius D, Huang KN, Lirelli TJ, Axel R, Jessel TM. The 5-HT2 receptor defines a family of structurally distinct but functionally conserved serotonin receptors. *Proc Natl Acad Sci USA* 1990;87:928–932.

31. Kilpatrick GJ, Bunce KT, Tyers MB. 5-HT3 receptors. *Med Res Rev* 1990;10:441–475.

32. Koek W, Jackson A, Colpaert FC. Behavioral pharmacology of antagonists at 5-HT2/5-HT1C receptors. *Neurosci Biobehav Rev* 1992;16:95–105.

33. Leonhardt S, Herrick-Davis K, Titeler M. Detection of a novel serotonin receptor subtype (5-HT$_{1E}$) in human brain: interaction with a GTP-binding protein. *J Neurochem* 1989;53:465–471.

34. Leung E, Perkins LA, Bonhaus DW, Loury DN, Clark R, Eglen RM. RS-23597-190: a selective high-affinity antagonist for 5-HT4 receptors. In: *Second international symposium on serotonin*, Houston, TX. September 15–18, 1992. Abstract p. 49.

35. Levy FO, Gudermann T, Birnbaumer M, Kaumann AJ, Birnbaumer L. Molecular cloning of a human gene (S31) encoding a novel serotonin receptor mediating inhibition of adenylate cyclase. *FEBS Lett* 1992;296:201–206.

36. Levy FO, Gudermann T, Perez-Reyes E, Birnbaumer M, Kaumann AJ, Birnbaumer L. Molecular cloning of a human serotonin receptor (S12) with a pharmacological profile resembling that of the 5-HT1D subtype. *J Biol Chem* 1992;267:7553–7562.

37. Libert F, Parmentier M, Lefort A, Dinsart C, Van Sande J, Maenhaut C, Simons MJ, Dumont JE, Vassart G. Selective amplification and cloning of four new members of the G protein-coupled receptor family. *Science* 1989;244:569–572.

38. Liu J, Chien Y, Kozak CA, Yu L. The 5-HT2 serotonin receptor gene Htr-2 is tightly linked to Es-10 on mouse chromosome 14. *Genomics* 1991;11:231–234.

39. Lubbert H, Hoffman BJ, Snutch TP, Van Duke T, Levine AJ, Hartig PR, Lester H, Davidson N. cDNA cloning of a serotonin 5-HT1C receptor by electrophysiological assays of mRNA-injected *Xenopus* oocytes. *Proc Natl Acad Sci USA* 1987;84:4332–4336.

40. Maricq AV, Peterson AS, Brake AJ, Myers RM, Julius D. Primary structure and functional expression of the 5-HT3 receptor, a serotonin gated ion channel. *Science* 1991;254:432–437.

41. Maroteaux L, Saudou F, Amlaiky N, Boschert V, Plassat JL, Hen R. Mouse 5-HT1B serotonin receptor: cloning, functional expression, and localization in motor control centers. *Proc Natl Acad Sci USA* 1992;89:3020–3024.

42. Matsubara S, Arora RC, Meltzer HY. Serotonergic measures in suicide brain: 5-HT1A binding sites in frontal cortex of suicide victims. *J Neural Trans* 1991;85:181–194.

43. Matthes H, Boschert V, Amlaiky N, Grailhe R, Plassat JL, Muscatelli F, Mattei MG, Hen R. Mouse 5-hydroxytryptamine-5A and 5-hydroxytryptamine-5B receptors define a new family of serotonin receptors: cloning, functional expression, and chromosomal localization. *Mol Pharmacol* 1993;43:313–319.

44. McAllister G, Charlesworth A, Snodin C, Beer MS, Noble AJ, Middlemiss DN, Iversen LL, Whiting P. Molecular cloning of a serotonin receptor from human brain (5-HT1E): a fifth 5-HT1-like subtype. *Proc Natl Acad Sci USA* 1992;89:5517–5521.

45. Middlemiss DN, Wilkinson LO, Hawkins LM, Beer MS, Noble AJ, Stanton JA, McAllister G. Functional correlates of 5-HT1-like receptors. In: *Second international symposium on serotonin*, Houston, TX, September 15–18, 1992. Abstract, p. 3.

46. Monsma FJ, Shey Y, Ward RP, Hamblin MW, Sibley DR. Cloning and expression of a novel serotonin receptor with high affinity for tricyclic psychotropic drugs. *Mol Pharmacol* 1993;43:320–327.

47. Oakey RJ, Caron MG, Lefkowitz RJ, Seldin MF. Genomic organization of adrenergic and serotonin receptors in the mouse: linkage mapping of sequence-related genes provides a method for examing mammalian chromosome evolution. *Genomics* 1991;10:338–344.

48. Peroutka SJ. Serotonin receptors. In: Meltzer HY, ed. *Psychopharmacology: the third generation of progress.* New York: Raven Press, 1987;303–311.

49. Perregaard J, Sanchez C, Arnt J. Recent developments in anxiolytics. *Curr Opin Ther Pat* 1993;3:101–126.

50. Plassat JL, Boschert U, Amlaiky N, Hen R. The mouse 5-HT5 receptor reveals a remarkable heterogeneity within the 5-HT1D receptor family. *EMBO J* 1992;11:4779–4786.

51. Rausch JL, Ruegg R, Moeller FG. Gepirone as a 5-HT1A agonist in the treatment of major depression. *Psychopharmacol Bull* 1990;26:169–171.

52. Roth BL, Ciaranello RD, Meltzer HY. Binding of typical and atypical antipsychotic agents to transiently expressed 5-HT1C receptors. *J Pharmacol Exp Ther* 1992;260:1361–1365.

53. Routledge C, Gurling J, Wright I, Dourish CT. Stereospecific effects of WAY100135, a selective and silent 5-HT1A receptor antagonist, on hippocampal 5-hydroxytryptamine release *in vivo. Second international symposium on serotonin*, Houston, TX. September 15–18, 1992. Abstract, p. 29.

54. Ruat M, Traiffort E, Leurs R, Tardivel-Lacombe J, Diaz J, Arrang

J-M, Schwartz J-C. Molecular cloning, characterization, and localization of a high-affinity serotonin receptor (5-HT$_7$) activating cAMP formation. *Proc Natl Acad Sci USA* 1993;90:8547–8551.

55. Sahin-Erdemli I, Schoeffter P, Hoyer D. Competitive antagonism by recognized 5-HT2 receptor antagonists at 5-HT1C receptors in pig choroid plexus. *Naunyn Schmiedebergs Arch Pharmacol* 1991; 344:137–144.

56. Saltzman AG, Morse B, Whitman MM, Ivanshchenko Y, Jaye M, Felder S. Cloning of the human serotonin 5-HT2 and 5-HT1C receptor subtypes. *Biochem Biophys Res Commun* 1991;181:1469–1478.

57. Schmidt CJ, Black CK. The putative 5-HT3 agonist phenylbiguanide induces carrier-mediated release of [^{3}H]dopamine. *Eur J Pharmacol* 1989;167:309–310.

58. Schoeffter P, Hoyer D. 5-Hydroxytryptamine (5-HT)-induced endothelium-dependent relaxation of pig coronary arteries is mediated by 5-HT receptors similar to the 5-HT1D receptor subtype. *J Pharmacol Exp Ther* 1991;252:387–395.

59. Schoeffter P, Hoyer D. Interaction of arylpiperazines with 5-HT1A, 5-HT1B, 5-HT1C, and 5-HT1D receptors. Do discriminatory 5-HT1B receptor ligands exist? *Naunyn Schmiedebergs Arch Pharmacol* 1989;339:675–683.

60. Shen Y, Monsma FJ Jr, Metcalf MA, Hamblin MW, Sibley DR. Molecular cloning and expression of a 5-hydroxytryptamine$_7$ serotonin receptor subtype. *J Biol Chem* 1993;268:18200–18204.

61. Sleight AJ, Pierce PA, Schmidt AW, Hekmatpanah CR, Peroutka SJ. The clinical utility of serotonin receptor active agents in neuropsychiatric disease. In: Peroutka SJ, ed. *Serotonin receptor subtypes.* New York: Wiley–Liss, 1991;211–227.

62. Tollefson GD, Lancaster SP, Montague-Clouse J. The association of buspirone and its metabolite 1-pyrimidinylpiperazine in the remission of comorbid anxiety with depressive features and alcohol dependency. *Psychopharmacol Bull* 1991;27:163–170.

63. Trumpp-Kallmeyer S, Bruinvels A, Hoflack J, Hibert M. Recognition site mapping and receptor modeling: application to 5-HT receptors. *Neurochem Int* 1991;19:397–406.

64. Voigt MM, Laurie DJ, Seeburg PH, Bach A. Molecular cloning and characterization of a rat brain cDNA encoding a 5-hydroxytryptamine-1B receptor. *EMBO J* 1991;10:4017–4023.

65. Wainscott DB, Cohen ML, Schenck KW, Audia JE, Nissen JS, Baez M, Kursar JD, Lucaites VL, Nelson DL. Pharmacological characteristics of the newly cloned 5-hydroxytryptamine-2F receptor. *Mol Pharmacol* 1993;43:419–426.

66. Weinshank RL, Zgombick JM, Macchi MJ, Branchek TA, Hartig PR. Human serotonin 1D receptor is encoded by a subfamily of two distinct genes: 5-HT1Dα and 5-HT1Dβ. *Proc Natl Acad Sci USA* 1992;89:3630–3634.

67. Yu L, Nguyen H, Le H, Bloem LJ, Kozak CA, Hoffman BJ, Snutch TP, Lester HA, Davidson N, Lubbert H. The mouse 5-HT1C receptor contains eight hydrophobic domains and is X-linked. *Mol Brain Res* 1991;11:143–149.

68. Zemlan FP, Schwab EF. Characterization of a novel serotonin receptor subtype (5-HT$_{1S}$) in rat CNS: interaction with a GTP binding protein. *J Neurochem* 1991;57:2092–2099.

69. Zgombick JM, Schechter LE, Macchi M, Hartig PR, Branchek TA, Weinshank RL. Human gene S31 encodes the pharmacologically definded serotonin 5-hydroxytryptamine-1E receptor. *Mol Pharmacol* 1992;42:180–185.

70. Zifa E, Fillion G. 5-Hydroxytryptamine receptors. *Pharmacol Rev* 1992;44:401–458.

Psychopharmacology: The Fourth Generation of Progress, edited by Floyd E. Bloom and David J. Kupfer. Raven Press, Ltd., New York © 1995.

CHAPTER 38

Serotonin Receptors

Signal Transduction Pathways

Elaine Sanders-Bush and Hervé Canton

Two major receptor-linked signal transduction pathways exist: a multistep enzyme mediated pathway and a direct regulation of ion channels. Both require a guanine nucleotide triphosphate (GTP)-binding protein (G protein) to link the receptor to the effector molecule. The sequence of steps involved in enzyme-dependent biochemical signaling is: cell-surface receptor → G protein → effector enzyme → second messenger → protein kinase → phosphoprotein. This multistep scheme applies to receptors linked to activation and inhibition of adenylate cyclase and to activation of phospholipase C. These enzyme-dependent pathways lead to amplification of cellular signals. Each step involves proteins that exist in multiple forms. For example, G proteins are composed of α, β, and γ subunits, each of which exists in multiple isoforms. More than 15 α subunits and at least three β and γ subunits have been identified, leading to a tremendous diversity in G proteins. Multiple isozymes of both adenylate cyclase and phospholipase C have been found, and more than one isoform is involved in signal transduction. In addition, protein kinase A, protein kinase C, and calcium/calmodulin-dependent kinase exist as multiple isoforms. A final level of complexity, which may serve to integrate various signals, is protein phosphorylation. The protein substrates are numerous, and it is impossible to list them. Key proteins regulated by phosphorylation include neurotransmitter and growth factor receptors, G proteins, protein kinases, protein phosphatases, ion channels, neurotransmitter synthetic and metabolic enzymes, transport molecules, and DNA transcription factors. This brief discussion serves to illustrate the multitude of cellular responses that may result when neurotransmitters such as 5-hydroxytryptamine (5-HT) activate receptors that couple to the adenylate cyclase and phospholipase C pathways. 5-HT receptors are numerous, and at least one receptor subtype is linked to each of the major signal transduction pathways (Table 1) (see also Chapters 36 and 37, *this volume*).

RECEPTORS LINKED TO ACTIVATION OF ADENYLATE CYCLASE

Stimulation of adenylate cyclase was the first signal transduction pathway to be linked to 5-HT—in invertebrates as well as in immature rat brain. However, the specific receptor mediating activation of adenylate cyclase has only recently been identified. This receptor, named 5-HT$_4$, was first characterized in mouse collicular neurons (21). It is also found in hippocampus and in peripheral tissues such as guinea-pig ileum, rat esophagus, and human atrium (12). In the past 2 years, a second receptor (5-HT$_6$) has been conclusively shown to couple positively to adenylate cyclase by cloning and functional expression in cell lines (51). Abstracts of recent or upcoming meetings suggest that still other 5-HT receptor subtypes will be linked to activation of adenylate cyclase.

Proximal cellular events that result from an increase in cyclic 3',5'-adenosine monophosphate (cAMP) include activation of protein kinase A, which, in turn, regulates the activity of cellular proteins by phosphorylation (Fig. 1). Electrophysiological studies in collicular and hippocampal neurons suggest that one consequence of activation of 5-HT$_4$ receptors is an inhibition of a voltage-

E. Sanders-Bush and H. Canton: Department of Pharmacology, Vanderbilt University School of Medicine, Nashville, Tennessee 37232.

TABLE 1. *Major signal transduction pathways for serotonin receptors*

Receptor subtype	G protein	Effector pathway
5-HT$_{1A}$	G$_i$	Inhibition of adenylate cyclase
	G$_i$	Opening of K$^+$ channel
	G$_o$	Closing of Ca^{2+} channel
5-HT$_{1B}$	G$_i$	Inhibition of adenylate cyclase
5-HT$_{1D\alpha}$		
5-HT$_{1D\beta}$	↓	↓
5-HT$_{1E}$		
5-HT$_{2A}$[a]	G$_q$[d]	Phosphoinositide hydrolysis
5-HT$_{2B}$[b]		
5-HT$_{2C}$[c]	↓	↓
5-HT$_3$	No G protein	Ligand-gated ion channel
5-HT$_4$	G$_s$	Activation of adenylate cyclase
5-HT$_6$	↓	↓

[a] New nomenclature [Humphrey et al. (36)]; formerly 5-HT$_2$.

[b] New nomenclature [Humphrey et al. (36)]; formerly 5-HT$_{2F}$.

[c] New nomenclature [Humphrey et al. (36)]; formerly 5-HT$_{1C}$.

[d] The specific G-protein subtype has not been identified. It is assumed that a member of the G$_q$ family links to PLC. However, in some tissues, 5-HT$_{2A}$-receptor-mediated phosphoinositide hydrolysis is pertussis-toxin-sensitive.

dependent K$^+$ current (6). cAMP was proposed as the mediator based on the following evidence: A cell-permeated analogue of cAMP and forskolin, a direct activator of adenylate cyclase, mimic the effects of 5-HT; a specific protein kinase A inhibitor blocks the effect of 5-HT; and, lastly, a phosphatase inhibitor, okadaic acid, potentiates 5-HT. In Fig. 1, the K$^+$ channel is depicted as the phosphorylation substrate; however, it is not clear whether this is the case or whether another protein is phosphorylated and, in turn, depresses K$^+$ channel activity. Depression of K$^+$ current may lead to depolarization, calcium influx, and subsequent enhancement of neurotransmitter release. Such events are known to be important in 5-HT-induced changes in synaptic plasticity in *Aplysia*. It is intriguing to consider that similar mechanisms may play a role in synaptic plasticity in vertebrates.

RECEPTORS LINKED TO INHIBITION OF ADENYLATE CYCLASE

5-HT$_1$ receptors are a large family of receptors that are negatively coupled to adenylate cyclase via the G$_i$ family of G proteins (Fig. 2). Additional subtypes in addition to those listed in Table 1 are suggested based on functional assays. The 5-HT$_{1A}$ receptor is the most well-characterized member of this family. In addition to adenylate cyclase coupling, 5-HT$_{1A}$ receptors are linked directly to voltage-sensitive K$^+$ channels via a G$_i$-like protein (7), with no intervening second messenger signaling (Fig. 2). Dual coupling with both adenylate cyclase and K$^+$ channels is now recognized as a hallmark of G$_i$-linked receptors and is likely to occur with other members of the 5-HT$_1$ receptor family. In addition, direct coupling to L-type Ca^{2+} channels has been described as a third signal transduction pathway for the G$_i$-linked family of receptors (Fig. 2). Activation of G$_i$-linked receptors leads to enhancement of K$^+$ channel activity and, conversely, blunting of Ca^{2+} channel activity. One important question is whether these different signal transduction pathways, which are mediated by G$_i$-like proteins, reflect multiple signaling mechanisms for a single receptor or multiple receptor subtypes that cannot be differentiated with the available drugs. There is good evidence that a single G$_i$-linked receptor can in fact couple to all three pathways: The cloned α2-adrenergic receptor, expressed in pituitary GH3 cells, couples to inhibition of adenylate cyclase, activation of K$^+$ conductance, and inhibition of a calcium current (67). It is, however, possible that not every receptor couples to all three signals in the native state. Considering the diversity of pertussis-toxin-sensitive G$_i$-like proteins, it is also possible that different members of the G$_i$ family are involved in the coupling to each of these signaling pathways. Furthermore, evidence suggests that different G proteins may couple different receptors to the same effector. In elegant experiments using antisense strategies, different G$_o$ subtypes were found to couple muscarinic and somatostatin receptors to inhibition of calcium currents (43). This diversity at several key points in the signal

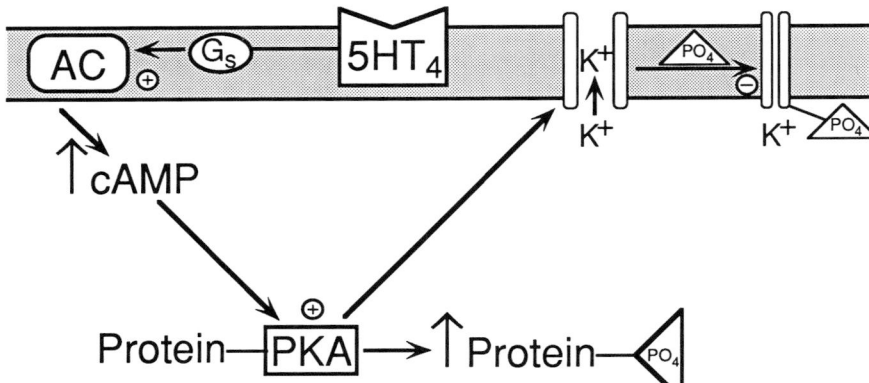

FIG. 1. Schematic representation of the 5-HT$_4$ receptor linked to adenylate cyclase (AC) activation. Receptor–effector coupling is via a G protein, G$_s$. One possible pathway of activation of a K$^+$ current is illustrated. PKA, protein kinase A.

Coupling to Adenylate Cyclase

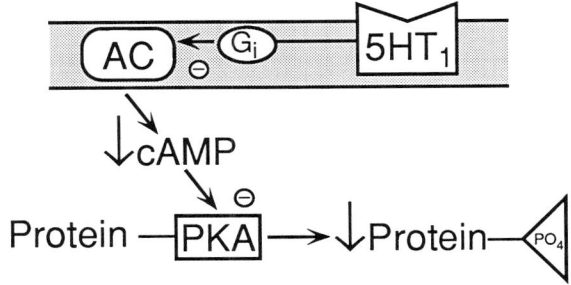

Coupling to Ion Channels

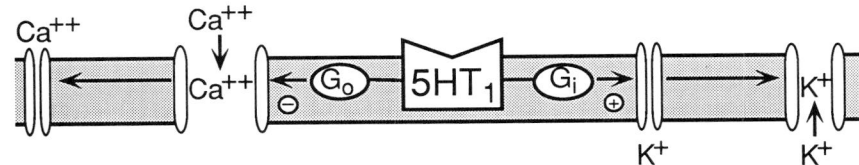

FIG. 2. Schematic representation of the dual coupling of G_i-linked 5-HT_1 receptor family. In this case, the coupling to K^+ and Ca^{2+} channels is direct via a G protein and not mediated by a second messenger. Note that receptor activation opens K^+ channels and closes Ca^{2+} channels.

transduction pathway portends tremendous complexity in G_i-linked responses.

5-HT_{1A} receptors on raphe cells function as somatodendritic autoreceptors, depressing neuronal firing rate when activated (for review see ref. 31). The mechanism involves membrane hyperpolarization elicited by increased K^+ conductance; 5-HT_{1A} receptors have also been characterized at postsynaptic sites, such as hippocampus (74) and cortex (9). At these sites, 5-HT_{1A} receptor activation elicits hyperpolarization by enhancing K^+ channel activity. Rodent 5-HT_{1B} receptors and the human homologue, 5-$HT_{1D\beta}$, function as axon terminal autoreceptors (31), where inactivation of Ca^{2+} channels may mediate the inhibition of 5-HT release. A significant portion of 5-HT_{1B} receptors are localized on postsynaptic structures where their function is unknown. Interestingly, although 5-HT_{1B} receptor-mediated inhibition of adenylate cyclase is pertussis-toxin-sensitive (52), studies in brain slices suggest that the terminal 5-HT_{1B} receptors in hippocampus regulating neurotransmitter release are not blocked by pertussis toxin (11). These results suggest that axon terminal 5-HT_{1B} autoreceptors may not be coupled to a G_i-like protein.

The functional correlates of inhibition of adenylate cyclase are not well-defined. Inhibition of protein kinase A with a subsequent reduction in the phosphorylation of its substrates would presumably alter cellular activity because many crucial proteins are regulated by changes in their phosphorylation state. To explore the consequences of 5-HT_{1A}-receptor-mediated inhibition of adenylate cyclase, Andrade (5) recently looked at the functional interaction of 5-HT_{1A} receptors and β-adrenergic receptors

linked to activation of adenylate cyclase in single pyramidal cells in the CA1 region of the hippocampus. Because these two receptors have opposing effects on adenylate cyclase activity, 5-HT_{1A} receptor activation was expected to inhibit β-adrenergic-receptor-induced reduction in afterhyperpolarization, which is mediated by activation of adenylate cyclase. Surprisingly, the opposite was found: 5-HT_{1A} receptor activation enhanced the β-adrenergic-receptor-mediated response. An explanation for this paradoxical effect may be related to the recent evidence that G-protein $\beta\gamma$ subunits can regulate adenylate cyclase activity (68). Interestingly, although $G\beta\gamma$ activates type II and type IV adenylate cyclase, it inhibits type I adenylate cyclase. Several other adenylate cyclase isoforms are insensitive to $G\beta\gamma$. This isoform-specific regulation of adenylate cyclase suggests remarkable flexibility. Thus, G_i-linked receptor activation by increasing free $G\beta\gamma$ could activate or inhibit adenylate cyclase depending on the isoform of adenylate cyclase present in the particular cell. In hippocampal pyramidal cells, where 5-HT_{1A} receptors potentiate a β-adrenergic-receptor/adenylate-cyclase-mediated response (5), the mechanism may be release of $G\beta\gamma$, which, in turn, activates type II adenylate cyclase. In other cell types, where type I adenylate cyclase predominates, activation of 5-HT_{1A} and other G_i-linked receptors may inhibit adenylate-cyclase-mediated responses. Such heterogeneity may explain the conflicting reports that appeared in the early literature of 5-HT_{1A}-receptor-mediated inhibition and activation of adenylate cyclase in different preparations.

Recombinant 5-HT_{1A} receptors expressed in transfected cells have been found to enhance phosphate uptake (61)

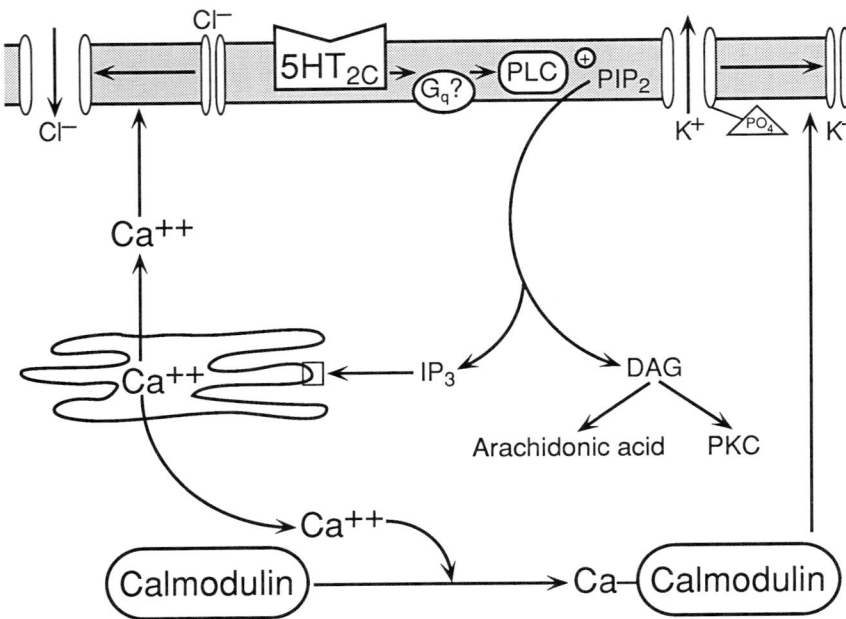

FIG. 3. Schematic representation of the coupling of 5-HT$_2$ receptor family to phospholipase C (PLC). The G protein involved has not been identified; it is assumed to be a member of the G$_q$ family. Examples of the physiological consequences of the two bifurcating pathways are given. These have been characterized in *Xenopus* oocytes expressing the cloned 5-HT$_{2C}$ receptor.

and to activate Na$^+$/K$^+$-ATPase (50). Although adenylate cyclase inhibition occurs in these cells, this signal transduction pathway apparently does not mediate these effects. Rather, a previously unrecognized, alternative signal transduction pathway, activation of phospholipase C appears to be involved. The biological significance of this alternative signaling will be discussed later.

One consequence of 5-HT$_{1B}$-receptor-linked inhibition of adenylate cyclase may be a mitogenic response. In fibroblasts, 5-HT acts via a pertussis-toxin-sensitive G protein to increase DNA synthesis in synergy with fibroblast growth factor (65). Although pertussis-toxin-sensitive inhibition of adenylate cyclase occurred in these cells, evidence suggests that the mitogenic effect of 5-HT in smooth muscle cells is independent of this response (42). One possible mechanism may be pertussis-toxin-sensitive coupling to phospholipase C, which, for the 5-HT$_{1A}$ receptor, predisposes fibroblasts to enhanced proliferation by serum-derived factors (1).

RECEPTORS LINKED TO ACTIVATION OF PHOSPHOLIPASE C

Phospholipase C (PLC), a membrane-bound enzyme, catalyzes the degradation of the inositol lipid, phosphatidylinositol 4,5-bisphosphate (PIP$_2$), with the production of inositol 1,4,5-triphosphate (IP$_3$) and diacylglycerol (DAG) (Fig. 3). IP$_3$ mobilizes Ca^{2+} from an intracellular storage site by interacting with specific receptors. Ca^{2+} induces multiple responses in the cell, including activation of calcium/calmodulin-dependent protein kinases, enzymes which phosphorylate/dephosphorylate key protein substrates in the cell. DAG activates another kinase

family, protein kinase C (PKC). PKC regulates numerous processes of cell function. DAG is also hydrolyzed by a specific lipase to release arachidonic acid with the subsequent formation of prostaglandins and prostacyclins. Thus, PLC activation induces diverse changes in the cell, leading to the regulation of many cellular processes.

The newly named 5-HT$_2$ receptor family is comprised of previously characterized receptors that are all coupled primarily to PLC (Table 1). The first evidence of a putative coupling of 5-HT receptors to phosphoinositide breakdown came from studies of insect salivary gland. Subsequently, it was shown that 5-HT is able to stimulate PLC activity in slices of rat cerebral cortex. Extensive pharmacological characterization of this response demonstrated the involvement of the 5-HT$_{2A}$ binding sites (64). Interestingly, in newborn rats, 5-HT induced a higher level of phosphoinositide hydrolysis than in adult rats (18). The mechanism of this supersensitivity is still unknown. Also, the exact identity of the G protein involved in 5-HT$_{2A}$-receptor-mediated activation of PLC remains to be determined. The G$_q$ family of G proteins activates PLC in a pertussis-toxin-insensitive manner. Some investigators have found the stimulation of phosphoinositide hydrolysis by the 5-HT$_{2A}$ receptors to be insensitive to pertussis toxin, supporting the conclusion that a G$_q$-type protein is involved (8,38). In contrast, pretreatment with pertussis toxin reduces 5-HT-induced formation of inositol phosphates in cerebellar granule cells (4), suggesting that a pertussis-toxin-sensitive protein of the G$_i$ family couples 5-HT$_{2A}$ receptors to PLC in the immature cerebellum. Thus the 5-HT$_{2A}$ receptor does not agree with the precept that a specific receptor couples with a single G protein. As discussed later, it is becoming increasingly evident that the nature of receptor–G-protein coupling is subject to variation, dependent not only on the structure of the receptor, but also on the particular cell type. In addition, multiple isozymes of PLC exist in the brain. Each one could be activated by different subunits of the G protein: Signals that activate the G_q family could result in the activation of PLC-β1 and PLC-β3 by the corresponding G_α subunits, while the $\beta\gamma$ subunits of G_i or G_o could activate PLC-β and PLC-δ1 isozymes (63).

Stimulation of phosphoinositide hydrolysis in rat choroid plexus is not mediated by the 5-HT$_{2A}$ receptor. In this structure the 5-HT-induced increase in PLC activity results from the activation of the 5-HT$_{2C}$ receptors (see ref. 64 for review). The only other area of the brain in which 5-HT$_{2C}$-receptor-mediated phosphoinositide hydrolysis has been definitively characterized is the immature rat hippocampus (19). Recently a new receptor belonging to the 5-HT$_2$ family was cloned: 5-HT$_{2B}$ receptors (29,44). Present in the stomach fundus, this receptor, when expressed in AV-12 cells, increases the production of IP$_3$. Another 5-HT receptor family, the 5-HT$_3$ receptor, has also been linked to the phosphoinositide hydrolysis cascade as discussed in detail later.

The functional correlates of activation of PLC by 5-HT$_2$ receptors are multiple. An increase in the intracellular concentration of calcium induces a rapid Cl$^-$ current through a Ca^{2+}-dependent chloride channel when receptors are expressed in *Xenopus* oocytes (Fig. 3). This response has been characterized for the three members of the 5-HT$_2$ receptor family and seems to be mediated through the PLC–IP$_3$ pathway (29,47,59). 5-HT$_{2C}$-receptor-mediated activation of chloride current in oocytes involves a pertussis-toxin-sensitive G protein (20) and an upstream calcium/calmodulin-dependent protein kinase (70). 5-HT$_{2A}$ receptor activation also induces the closing of a K$^+$ channel, leading to a depolarization of the cell. This effect (3) is mediated by a G protein. It will be interesting to identify the G protein involved and determine if a direct action inhibits the K$^+$ conductance as suggested by Aghajanian (3) or if a PLC-generated product is involved. More is known about putative mechanisms mediating the closing of K$^+$ channels via activation of the 5-HT$_{2C}$ receptor. In *Xenopus* oocytes coexpressing 5-HT$_{2C}$ receptors and a K$^+$ channel cloned from the brain, the suppression of K$^+$ conductance by 5-HT involves a calcium/calmodulin-activated phosphatase (34). It was postulated that the activated phosphatase dephosphorylates the K$^+$ channel, leading to its closing as illustrated in Fig. 3. Recovery from suppression seems to be due to the action of a protein kinase, because the protein kinase inhibitor H-7 blocked recovery (34). Cloned 5-HT$_{2C}$ receptors have been expressed in A9 cells as well as *Xenopus* oocytes and have been found to regulate Cl$^-$ and K$^+$ conductance. The exact pathways involved are not completely elucidated and may vary with the model used. For example, both calcium-dependent and calcium-

independent mechanisms have been found to regulate K$^+$ currents (34,55). These results illustrate that a cloned receptor expressed heterologously may couple to multiple signal transduction pathways (see later discussion). Recent patch-clamp studies of choroid plexus (37) demonstrated that 5-HT activates Cl$^-$ currents and inhibits K$^+$ currents in choroid plexus. It will be interesting to determine if the intracellular pathways in the choroid plexus epithelium are comparable to those described for oocytes.

One of the cellular events controlled by activation of the 5-HT$_{2C}$ receptor may be ion exchange between the central nervous system and the cerebrospinal fluid. 5-HT$_{2C}$ receptors are expressed at high density in the choroid plexus and are concentrated on the apical surface of the epithelial cells (37) in direct contact with the cerebrospinal fluid. Thus, 5-HT$_{2C}$ receptors are located suitably to regulate the composition of the cerebrospinal fluid. In choroid plexus epithelial cells in primary culture, 5-HT regulates the level of transferrin by activation of 5-HT$_{2C}$ receptors (24). Transferrin is an iron carrier protein and also has growth-factor-like actions. The choroid plexus may be an important source of transferrin and iron for brain cells, suggesting a role for the 5-HT$_{2C}$ receptor in brain development and homeostasis. 5-HT$_{2A}$ and 5-HT$_{2C}$ receptors expressed heterologously in fibroblasts activate Na$^+$/K$^+$/2Cl$^-$ co-transport (49), but this function could not be reproduced in native choroid plexus epithelial cells. Another important property of the 5-HT$_{2C}$ receptor is its ability to function as a proto-oncogene when expressed in non-neuronal cells such as NIH-3T3 fibroblasts (39). The 5-HT$_{2A}$ receptor similarly acts as a proto-oncogene in NIH-3T3 fibroblasts (40). Introduction of functional 5-HT$_{2A}$ or 5-HT$_{2C}$ receptors into these cells results in the generation of transformed foci. Moreover, generation and maintenance of the transformed foci requires continued activation of the receptor by 5-HT. Nevertheless, when expressed in other types of fibroblast cell lines (41) or in choroid plexus epithelial cells (24), the 5-HT$_{2C}$ receptor does not induce a transformed phenotype, thus distinguishing this protein from strong dominantly acting oncogene products (41).

5-HT$_3$ RECEPTORS: LIGAND-GATED ION CHANNELS

The 5-HT$_3$ receptor differs from the other 5-HT receptors. The receptor itself forms an ion channel that regulates ion flux in a G-protein-independent manner. The 5-HT$_3$ receptor is a member of the large family of ligand-gated ion channels of which the nicotinic cholinergic receptor is the prototype. 5-HT$_3$ receptors are unique among ligand-gated ion channels because only a single subunit has been found (48), although an alternative splice variant with a six-amino-acid deletion in the cytoplasmic loop has been recently described (35). Many drugs exist that interact specifically with the 5-HT$_3$ receptor, thus facilitating studies of its function. Results obtained in vivo suggest multiple 5-HT$_3$-like receptors, and the search goes on for other subunit proteins that might explain this pharmacological heterogeneity.

5-HT$_3$ receptors were first found on peripheral autonomic, sensory, and enteric neurons, where they mediate excitation. 5-HT$_3$ receptors in brain are primarily localized on nerve terminals (58), where they function in the regulation of the release of neurotransmitters, including 5-HT (30). The cloned 5-HT$_3$ receptor protein forms a homomeric multisubunit protein that regulates the gating of cations (48), and it presumably mediates the rapid, transient depolarization that occurs on 5-HT$_3$ receptor activation (56).

5-HT$_3$ receptors have been shown to activate phosphoinositide hydrolysis in the medial prefrontal cortex and entorhinal cortices (22), suggesting another family of 5-HT$_3$ receptors linked to G proteins. Thus, 5-HT$_3$ receptors may be analogous to the glutamate receptors, which were first characterized as ionotropic receptors and later shown to also exist as G-protein-linked (metabotropic) receptors. It is difficult, however, to rule out that 5-HT$_3$-receptor-mediated phosphoinositide hydrolysis is secondary to an influx of Ca^{2+} via the ligand-gated receptor, rather than being an independent signal transduction pathway. Furthermore, there is no convincing evidence of a role for a G protein in the phosphoinositide hydrolysis response. On the other hand, the agonists' and antagonists' profiles for the phosphoinositide-hydrolysis-linked receptor (22) differ somewhat from the profiles for the 5-HT$_3$ ionotropic receptors. Moreover, electrophysiological studies have shown that 5-HT$_3$-like receptors in the medial prefrontal cortex produce a slow depression of cell firing (72), rather than the fast activation of firing that has been described for the ligand-gated 5-HT$_3$ receptor. Thus, both biochemical and electrophysiological results suggest that 5-HT$_3$ receptors are heterogeneous, with respect to subtypes and intracellular signal transduction mechanisms. However, more studies are needed to determine conclusively whether the multiple 5-HT$_3$ receptors include members in both the ionotropic and metabotropic receptor superfamilies. For example, studies in cell-free systems are required in order to demonstrate direct coupling of the 5-HT$_3$ receptor to PLC.

OTHER SIGNAL TRANSDUCTION PATHWAYS

In the early literature, it was found that 5-HT stimulates the activity of phospholipase A2 in membranes of guinea-pig cerebral cortex. Phospholipase A2 releases arachidonic acid, resulting in the production of arachidonic acid metabolites by lipoxygenase and cycloxygenase pathways with the formation of eicosanoids. More recently, it has been found that 5-HT stimulates the production of arachidonic acid in a number of brain tissues—including hippocampal neurons, where its action is mediated by the 5-HT$_{2A}$ receptor subtype (28). Evidence was presented that this effect involves a direct activation of phospholipase A2 and is independent of the release of arachidonic acid induced by hydrolysis of DAG, which occurs when a receptor is coupled to phosphoinositide hydrolysis (28). The mechanism of this apparently direct activation of phospholipase A2 by 5-HT and/or its mediation by a specific G protein is still unknown.

Recently, it has been shown that the 5-HT$_{2C}$ receptor is linked not only to activation of PLC, but also to an elevation of cyclic-3',5'-guanosine monophosphate (cGMP) in the choroid plexus (33). The mechanism presumably involves the activation of phospholipase A2 and the release of arachidonic acid, a potent activator of guanylate cyclase. Other pathways might also contribute to elevation of arachidonic acid, such as activation of PLC by the 5-HT$_{2C}$ receptor and subsequent liberation of arachidonate by hydrolysis of DAG. 5-HT also has been shown to stimulate the formation of cGMP in a clonal cell line of glial origin (54) by a mechanism which could involve the 5-HT$_{2A}$ receptor and an increase of intracellular calcium mediated by PLC. A rise in the level of cGMP apparently mediated by the 5-HT$_3$ receptor was described in neuronal cell lines (62), the mechanism of which may involve the production of arachidonic acid and/or formation of nitric oxide. Because the elevation of cGMP by 5-HT does not seem to involve a direct activation of guanylate cyclase but rather is the consequence of interacting pathways, this may be an example of cross-talk between the various signal transduction mechanisms after activation of 5-HT receptors (see later section for a further discussion of cross-talk).

SIGNAL TRANSDUCTION IN HETEROLOGOUS CELL LINES EXPRESSING CLONED 5-HT RECEPTORS

Cloned receptors expressed in heterologous cell lines (cells that have been genetically engineered to express receptors that are not naturally present) have many advantages, including a pure population of receptors that can be studied without problems associated with receptor interactions or drug nonspecificity. These scientific factors combined with practical considerations, such as improved sensitivity and convenience, are responsible for the surging popularity of transfected cell lines. However, artifacts such as aberrant G-protein coupling or receptor cross-talk may be a consequence of overexpression of receptors in cells that do not normally synthesize those receptors (see next section). The pharmacological properties of the receptor are generally thought to be independent of other cellular constituents, so studies of receptor pharmacology in transfected cells should be valid. For example, the intrinsic activity of a drug (full agonist versus partial agonist versus pure antagonist) can be accurately accessed in transfected cells that give a strong biochemical signal. However, intrinsic activity varies with receptor density (71), and transfected cells with high receptor levels may not reproduce the endogenous system. For example, the partial agonist properties of pindolol at the 5-HT$_{1B}$ receptor were masked in high-expressing transfected cells, where this partial agonist behaved as a full agonist (2). The opposite may also occur—a partial agonist converts to an antagonist—as has been illustrated for 5-HT$_{1A}$ receptors expressed in HeLa cells (13). In these instances, receptor density appears to be the key variable, although it is also conceivable that the properties of a drug may change depending on the G protein involved or the cellular response. All of these considerations suggest that caution should be used when interpreting pharmacological studies in transfected cell lines. In vivo studies of 5-HT$_1$ receptors illustrate that drug properties at a given receptor may also be site-specific. For example, the degree of 5-HT$_{1A}$ receptor reserve varies markedly in different brain

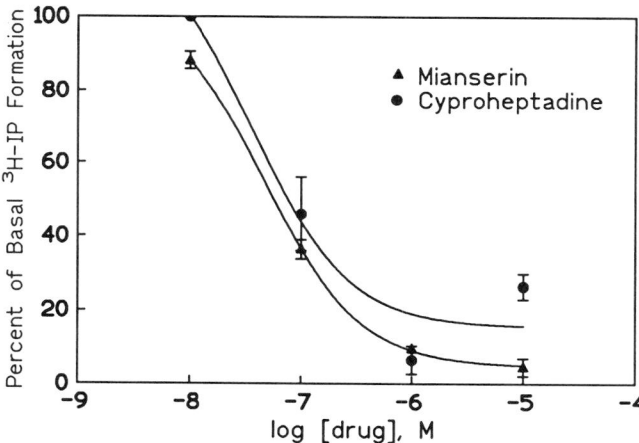

FIG. 4. Serotonin antagonists have negative intrinsic activity in cells transfected with the 5-HT$_{2C}$ receptor. NIH-3T3 fibroblasts were transfected with 5-HT$_{1C}$ receptor cDNA (obtained from Dr. David Julius, University of California, San Francisco), and a clonal line expressing a receptor density of about 600 fmol/mg protein was isolated. Cells were labeled overnight with [^{3}H]inositol in medium without serum. Phosphoinositide hydrolysis was evaluated by quantitating the formation of [^{3}H]inositol monophosphate (^{3}H-IP) in the presence of lithium as described previously (15). The values plotted are means ± SEM of triplicate determinations. Basal refers to ^{3}H-IP formation in the absence of agonist—that is, constitutive activity (basal values were about 1000 cpm in a typical experiment). The putative antagonists mianserin and cyproheptadine produced a dose-dependent reduction in basal activity. In other experiments, a maximum concentration of 5-HT produced a four- to fivefold increase in ^{3}H-IP formation. In nontransfected fibroblasts, basal activity was much lower than that found in transfected cells and was resistant to the negative effects of mianserin and cyproheptadine. These studies were done in collaboration with a graduate student, Eric Barker (9a).

sites. 5-HT$_{1A}$ somatodendritic autoreceptors in raphe possess a large receptor reserve, whereas postsynaptic 5-HT$_{1A}$ receptors in hippocampus lack receptor reserve (73). Partial agonists at postsynaptic 5-HT$_{1A}$ receptors became full agonists at raphe 5-HT$_{1A}$ receptors.

An example of the utility of heterologous expression systems is the resolution of a recent controversy concerning the existence of multiple, distinct 5-HT$_{2A}$ receptors versus multiple affinity states. Pierce and Peroutka (57) proposed the existence of two different 5-HT$_{2A}$ receptors, based on agonist radioligand binding studies in membranes from rat and human cerebral cortex. One subtype was characterized as having high affinity for agonists; the other, low affinity for agonists. Antagonists possessed equally high affinities for both of the putative receptor subtypes. In contrast, other investigators proposed the existence of two different affinity states for agonists at a single 5-HT$_{2A}$ receptor. Using cloned rat 5-HT$_{2A}$ receptors expressed in heterologous cell lines, Teitler et al. (69) and Branchek et al. (14) showed that a single 5-HT$_{2A}$ receptor protein binds agonists with two different affinity states, ruling out the postulated two-receptor theory. Thus, in this example, unambiguous data were obtained using a pure population of receptors expressed in cells that do not normally express the protein.

An intriguing result, obtained in a fibroblast cell line expressing the human 5-HT$_{1A}$ receptor, suggests that some 5-HT antagonists distinguish between G-protein-coupled and -uncoupled receptors (66). This study showed that the binding of 5-HT$_{1A}$ receptor agonists decreases in the presence of guanine nucleotides, a common property of G-protein receptor systems. Unexpectedly, the binding of the antagonist spiperone actually increases. Because guanine nucleotides destabilize the receptor–G-protein coupled form, these data suggest that spiperone has a higher affinity for the uncoupled receptor. Other antagonists were equipotent at binding to both the coupled and uncoupled state. If confirmed, studies such as these may lead to a reclassification of drugs that act at the 5-HT$_{1A}$ receptor. We have found evidence for a novel classification of 5-HT$_{2C}$ receptor antagonists using fibroblast cell lines expressing the cloned 5-HT$_{2C}$ receptor (9a). One cell line had a high basal level of phosphoinositide hydrolysis, indicating that the receptor was constitutively active in these cells. Common 5-HT antagonists reduced basal activity in the absence of agonist (Fig. 4), suggesting that these drugs have negative intrinsic activity at the receptor. This represents a novel property because drugs such as these are generally thought to function as silent antagonists, occupying the receptor and blocking an agonist, but having no effect in the absence of agonist. We are currently exploring the significance of negative intrinsic activity in the mechanism of the atypical down-regulation of 5-HT$_{2C}$ receptors by these antagonists and also in behavioral paradigms that may be sensitive to negative intrinsic activity.

PROMISCUOUS COUPLING VERSUS CROSS-TALK BETWEEN SIGNAL TRANSDUCTION PATHWAYS

A given receptor may couple to more than one signal transduction pathway. The example of 5-HT$_{1A}$ receptor coupling to inhibition of adenylate cyclase as well as directly activating a K$^+$ channel has already been discussed. When a receptor couples to a previously unrecognized signal cascade, especially if the cloned receptor is overexpressed in cell lines, this multiple signaling is referred to as *promiscuous coupling*. An example is G$_i$-linked receptors that couple to *activation* of adenylate cyclase in transfected cell lines. It is entirely possible that many, if not all, of the incidences of promiscuous coupling can be explained by cross-talk between the various signal transduction pathways. The numerous and diverse possibilities of cross-talk are just beginning to be worked out. Recent evidence suggest that G-protein $\beta\gamma$ subunits may play a central role in cross-talk between signaling pathways (10). Both adenylate cyclase and phospholipase Cβ are activated by G$\beta\gamma$ in an isoform-specific manner. G$\beta\gamma$ stimulation of PLC and adenylate cyclase requires high receptor occupancy and high expression levels. Thus the functional consequences of receptor–G-protein activation may vary from cell to cell, depending on both (a) the receptor and its level of expression and (b) the component of effector molecules within a given cell. Such complexities make results obtained in transfected cell lines difficult to relate back to the in vivo situation.

Emerging evidence suggests that, in addition to coupling to inhibition of adenylate cyclase and to the regulation of K$^+$ and Ca^{2+} channels, the 5-HT$_{1A}$ receptor also couples to PLC. These studies were done in transfected cell lines expressing a high density of the cloned human 5-HT$_{1A}$ receptor. In COS and HeLa cells, 5-HT is 100 times more potent at inhibiting adenylate cyclase than activating PLC (26). In other cell lines, the difference in potency for activating the two signals is smaller or nonexistent (46). Still another signal pathway is activated in transfected CHO cells, a 5-HT$_{1A}$-receptor-mediated augmentation of the release of arachidonic acid by substances such as ATP and thrombin (60). All three responses—inhibition of adenylate cyclase, activation of PLC, and augmentation of arachidonic acid release—are mediated by a G$_i$ protein(s) with equal sensitivity to inactivation by pertussis toxin. Arachidonic acid release has only been demonstrated in intact cells. This, combined with the finding that down-regulation of PKC abolishes 5-HT augmentation of arachidonic acid release (60), is consistent with an indirect mechanism for this response. On the other hand, an indirect mechanism for the activation of PLC in cell membranes is less likely. As discussed earlier, some isoforms of PLC are activated by $\beta\gamma$ subunits of G proteins. Coupling of the 5-HT$_{1A}$ receptor to G$_i$ protein and inhibition of adenylate cyclase would lead

to release of G$\beta\gamma$, which in turn could regulate PLC (Fig. 5). Based on the antibody blocking profile, G$_i$3 appears to mediate both inhibition adenylate cyclase and stimulation of PLC (25), which is consistent with interacting mechanisms. Alternatively, it is possible that the same receptor, coupled to the same G protein, can independently regulate distinct transmembrane effector pathways (Fig. 5). Definitive studies of coupling to multiple G proteins require antisense strategies or blocking antibodies directed against specific G proteins. Regardless of the mechanism, it is not at all clear that multiple signaling occurs with the native 5-HT$_{1A}$ receptor. It is possible that expression of high levels of 5-HT$_{1A}$ receptors in cells that do not normally express the protein creates artifacts, such as aberrant coupling to alternative G proteins or effector pathways. Consistent with this interpretation is the finding of cell-specific signaling of the 5-HT$_{1A}$ receptor—that is, different patterns of coupling of the cloned transfected receptor in different cell types (26,46). Also, the physiological consequences of alternative coupling of the 5-HT$_{1A}$ receptor to PLC varies as a function of cell type. In HeLa cells, an epithelial cell line, activation of 5-HT$_{1A}$ receptors enhances phosphate uptake, but this effect is not evident in transfected CHO cells, a fibroblast line

Dual Coupling

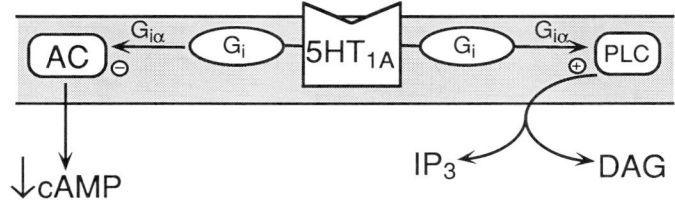

Crosstalk

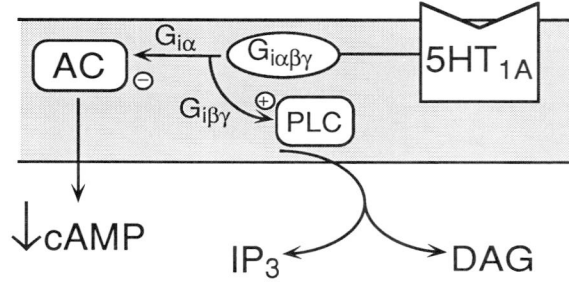

FIG. 5. Dual coupling versus cross-talk between G$_i$-linked receptors and the phospholipase C pathway. 5-HT$_{1A}$ receptor activation of phosphoinositide hydrolysis has been demonstrated in transfected cell lines. Two possible explanations are illustrated.

(61). These examples of cell-type-specific coupling to G proteins, effector enzymes, and downstream regulatory events highlight the limitations of studying receptor function in transfected cell lines.

Surprisingly, functional coupling of the 5-HT$_{1A}$ receptor to activation of adenylate cyclase via G$_s$ has not been demonstrated in transfected cells even though 5-HT$_{1A}$-receptor-mediated activation of adenylate cyclase has been described in vivo. The α2-adrenergic receptor, initially described in vivo as a G$_i$-linked receptor coupled to inhibition of adenylate cyclase, has been found to activate adenylate cyclase via G$_s$ in transfected cells. The coupling to G$_s$ requires high receptor expression and high agonist concentration and may be mediated by G protein $\beta\gamma$ subunits liberated by activation of the G$_i$-mediated pathway (27).

Examples of cross-talk between receptor/signal transduction pathways have been described in native expression systems. The enhancement of β-adrenergic-receptor-mediated hyperpolarization by 5-HT$_{1A}$ receptor activation may be an in vivo physiological correlate of G$\beta\gamma$ activation of type II adenylate cyclase (5). In astroglial cells in primary culture, 5-HT augments β-adrenergic receptor stimulation of cAMP formation (32). This effect is mediated by the 5-HT$_{2A}$ receptor, which activates phosphoinositide hydrolysis in these cells. This may be a version of the mechanism of cross-talk described many years ago (23) in which PKC activation potentiates cAMP formation by β-adrenergic agonists, perhaps by PKC-mediated phosphorylation of the catalytic subunit of adenylate cyclase. Also, in cultured astrocytes, the alpha$_2$ agonist clonidine potentiates 5-HT$_{2A}$-receptor-mediated phosphoinositide hydrolysis (32), perhaps reflecting G$\beta\gamma$ activation of phospholipase Cβ. Astrocyte cultures appear to be especially suitable for studying cross-talk between intracellular signaling cascades, although subpopulations of astrocytes that respond differently to 5-HT may compromise interpretation of results in these cells (53). An example of cross-talk between G$_i$-linked 5-HT$_{1A}$ receptors and muscarinic receptors linked to phosphoinositide hydrolysis was described, where 5-HT attenuates carbachol-stimulated phosphoinositide hydrolysis (16). This was initially interpreted as evidence for negative coupling of the 5-HT$_{1A}$ receptor to PLC. More recently, a mechanism involving activation of phospholipase A2 has been proposed in which phospholipase-A2-dependent release of arachidonic acid activates PKC, which then down-regulates either the muscarinic receptor or PLC (17). Interested readers are referred to a recent review in which many other possible mechanisms of cross-talk among the various signal-activated phospholipases are discussed (45).

CONCLUDING REMARKS

This chapter has attempted to bring the reader up-to-date about the signal transduction pathways for 5-HT receptors. Additional 5-HT receptors will undoubtedly be discovered, and it is possible that the signaling of these new receptors will follow one of the pathways described in this review. However, the recent description of novel mediators of signal transduction, such as nitric oxide and carbon monoxide, suggests that we should keep an open mind about the future possibilities.

ACKNOWLEDGMENTS

Dr. Sanders-Bush's research is supported by USPHS grants MH 34007 and DA 05181 and by an unrestricted research grant from Bristol Myers Squibb Corporation. Hervé Canton is partially supported by a fellowship from Groupe De Recherche Servier. The authors thank Ms. Edna Kunkel for preparing the illustrations.

REFERENCES

1. Abdel-Baset H, Bozovic V, Szyf M, Albert PR. Conditional transformation mediated via a pertussis toxin-sensitive receptor signalling pathway. *Mol Endocrinol* 1992;6:730–740.
2. Adham N, Ellerbrock B, Hartig P, Weinshank RL, Branchek T. Receptor reserve masks partial agonist activity of drugs in a cloned rat 5-hydroxytryptamine$_{1B}$ receptor expression system. *Mol Pharmacol* 1993;43:427–433.
3. Aghajanian GK. Serotonin-induced inward current in rat facial motoneurons: evidence for mediation by G proteins but not protein kinase C. *Brain Res* 1990;524:171–174.
4. Akiyoshi J, Hough C, Chuang D-M. Paradoxical increase of 5-hydroxytryptamine$_2$ receptors and 5-hydroxytryptamine$_2$ receptor mRNA in cerebellar granule cells after persistent 5-hydroxytryptamine$_2$ receptor stimulation. *Mol Pharmacol* 1993;43:349–355.
5. Andrade R. Enhancement of β-adrenergic responses by G$_i$-linked receptors in rat hippocampus. *Neuron* 1993;10:83–88.
6. Andrade R, Chaput Y. 5-Hydroxytryptamine 4-like receptors mediate the slow excitatory response to serotonin in rat hippocampus. *J Pharmacol Exp Ther* 1991;257:930–937.
7. Andrade R, Malenka RC, Nicoll RA. A G protein couples serotonin and GABA B receptors to the same channels in hippocampus. *Science* 1986;234:1261–1265.
8. Apud JA, Grayson DR, De Erausquin E, Costa E. Pharmacological characterization of regulation of phosphoinositide metabolism by recombinant 5-HT$_2$ receptors of the rat. *Neuropharmacology* 1992;31:1–8.
9. Araneda R, Andrade R. 5-Hydroxytryptamine$_2$ and 5-hydroxytryptamine$_{1A}$ receptors mediate opposing responses on membrane excitability in rat association cortex. *Neuroscience* 1991;40:399–412.
9a.Barker E, Westphal RS, Schmidt D, Sanders-Bush E. Constitutively active 5-hydroxytryptamine$_{2C}$ receptors reveal novel inverse agonist activity of receptor ligands. *J Biol Chem* 1994; 269: 11687–11690.
10. Birnbaumer L. Receptor-to-effector signaling through G proteins: roles for $\beta\gamma$ dimers as well as α subunits. *Cell* 1992;71:1069–1072.
11. Blier P. Terminal serotonin autoreceptor function in the rat hippocampus is not modified by pertussis and cholera toxins. *Naunyn Schmiedebergs Arch Pharmacol* 1991;344:160–166.
12. Bockaert J, Fozard JR, Dumuis A, Clarke DE. The 5-HT$_4$ receptor: a place in the sun. *Trends Pharmacol Sci* 1992;13:141–145.
13. Boddeke HWGM, Fargin A, Raymond JR, Schoeffter P, Hoyer D. Agonist/antagonist interactions with cloned human 5-HT$_{1A}$ receptors: variations in intrinsic activity studied in transfected HeLa cells. *Naunyn Schmiedebergs Arch Pharmacol* 1992;345:257–263.
14. Branchek T, Adham N, Macchi M, Kao H-T, Hartig PR. [³H]-DOB(4-bromo-2,5-dimethoxyphenylisopropylamine) and [³H]-

ketanserin label two affinity states of the cloned human 5-hydroxy-tryptamine$_2$ receptor. *Mol Pharmacol* 1990;38:604–609.

15. Burris KD, Breeding M, Sanders-Bush E. (+)Lysergic acid diethyl-amide, but not its nonhallucinogenic congeners, is a potent serotonin 5HT$_{1C}$ receptor agonist. *J Pharmacol Exp Ther* 1991;258:891–896.

16. Claustre Y, Bénavidès J, Scatton B. 5-HT$_{1A}$ receptor agonists inhibit carbachol-induced stimulation of phosphoinositide turnover in the rat hippocampus. *Eur J Pharmacol* 1988;149:149–153.

17. Claustre Y, Bénavidès J, Scatton B. Potential mechanisms involved in the negative coupling between serotonin 5-HT$_{1A}$ receptors and carbachol-stimulated phosphoinositide turnover in the rat hippo-campus. *J Neurochem* 1991;56:1276–1285.

18. Claustre Y, Rouquier L, Scatton B. Pharmacological characteriza-tion of serotonin-stimulated phosphoinositide turnover in brain re-gions of the immature rat. *J Pharmacol Exp Ther* 1988;244:1051–1056.

19. Claustre Y, Eudeline B, Bénavidès J, Scatton B. 5-HT1C receptors mediate phosphoinositide turnover activation in the immature rat hippocampus. *Eur J Pharmacol* 1992;225:37–41.

20. Dascal N, Ifune C, Hopkins R, et al. Involvement of a GTP-binding protein in mediation of serotonin and acetylcholine responses in *Xenopus* oocytes injected with rat brain messenger RNA. *Mol Brain Res* 1986;1:201–209.

21. Dumuis A, Bouhelal R, Sebben M, Cory R, Bockaert J. A nonclassi-cal 5-hydroxytryptamine receptor positively coupled with adenylate cyclase in the central nervous system. *Mol Pharmacol* 1988;34:880–887.

22. Edwards E, Harkins K, Ashby CR Jr, Wang RY. Effect of 5-hy-droxytryptamine$_3$ receptor agonists on phosphoinositide hydrolysis in the rat fronto-cingulate and entorhinal cortices. *J Pharmacol Exp Ther* 1991;256:1025–1032.

23. Enna SJ, Karbon EW. Receptor regulation: evidence for a relation-ship between phospholipid metabolism and neurotransmitter recep-tor-mediated cAMP formation in brain. *Trends Pharmacol Sci* 1987;8:21–24.

24. Esterle TM, Sanders-Bush E. Serotonin agonists increase transferrin levels via activation of 5-HT$_{1C}$ receptors in choroid plexus epithe-lium. *J Neurosci* 1992;12:4775–4782.

25. Fargin A, Yamamoto K, Cotecchia S, et al. Dual coupling of the cloned 5-HT$_{1A}$ receptor to both adenylyl cyclase and phospholipase C is mediated via the same G$_i$ protein. *Cell Signal* 1991;3:547–557.

26. Fargin A, Raymond JR, Regan JW, Cotecchia S, Lefkowitz RJ, Caron MG. Effector coupling mechanisms of the cloned 5-HT1A receptor. *J Biol Chem* 1989;264:14848–14852.

27. Federman AD, Conklin BR, Schrader KA, Reed RR, Bourne HR. Hormonal stimulation of adenyl cyclase through G$_i$-protein $\beta\gamma$ sub-units. *Nature* 1992;356:159–161.

28. Felder CC, Kanterman RY, Ma AL, Axelrod J. Serotonin stimulates phospholipase A$_2$ and the release of arachidonic acid in hippocampal neurons by a type 2 serotonin receptor that is independent of inosi-tolphospholipid hydrolysis. *Proc Natl Acad Sci USA* 1990;87:2187–2191.

29. Foguet M, Hoyer D, Pardo LA, et al. Cloning and functional charac-terization of the rat stomach fundus serotonin receptor. *EMBO J* 1992;11:3481–3487.

30. Galzin AM, Langer SZ. Modulation of 5-HT release by presynaptic inhibitory and facilitatory 5-HT receptors in brain slices. In: Langer SZ, Galzin AM, Costentin J, eds. *Presynaptic receptors and neu-ronal transporters.* Oxford: Pergamon Press, 1991;82:59–62.

31. Hamon M, Lanfumey L, El Mestikawy S, et al. The main features of central 5-HT$_1$ receptors. *Neuropsychopharmacology* 1990;3:349–360.

32. Hansson E, Simonsson P, Alling C. Interactions between cyclic AMP and inositol phosphate transduction systems in astrocytes in primary culture. *Neuropharmacology* 1990;29:591–598.

33. Hartig PR, Hoffman BJ, Kaufman MJ, Hirata F. The 5-HT$_{1C}$ recep-tor. In: Whitaker-Azmitia PM, Peroutka SJ, eds. *The neuropharma-cology of serotonin.* New York: The New York Academy of Sci-ences, 1990;149–167.

34. Hoger JH, Walter AE, Vance D, Yu L, Lester HA, Davidson N. Modulation of a cloned mouse brain potassium channel. *Neuron* 1991;6:227–236.

35. Hope AG, Downie DL, Sutherland L, Lambert JJ, Peters JA, Bur-chell B. Cloning and functional expression of an apparent splice variant of the murine 5-HT$_3$ receptor A subunit. *Eur J Pharmacol* 1993;245:187–192.

36. Humphrey PPA, Hartig P, Hoyer D. A proposed new nomenclature for 5-HT receptors. *Trends Pharmacol Sci* 1993;14:233–236.

37. Hung BCP, Loo DDF, Wright EM. Regulation of mouse choroid plexus apical Cl$^-$ and K$^+$ channels by serotonin. *Brain Res* 1993;617:285–295.

38. Ivins KJ, Molinoff PB. Serotonin-2 receptors coupled to phospho-inositide hydrolysis in a clonal cell line. *Mol Pharmacol* 1990;37:622–630.

39. Julius D, Livelli TJ, Jessell TM, Axel R. Ectopic expression of the serotonin 1c receptor and the triggering of malignant transformation. *Science* 1989;244:1057–1062.

40. Julius D, Huang KN, Livelli TJ, Axel R, Jessell TM. The 5HT2 receptor defines a family of structurally distinct but functionally conserved serotonin receptors. *Proc Natl Acad Sci USA* 1990;87:928–932.

41. Kahan C, Julius D, Pouysségur J, Seuwen K. Effects of 5-HT$_{1C}$-receptor expression on cell proliferation control in hamster fibro-blasts: serotonin fails to induce a transformed phenotype. *Exp Cell Res* 1992;200:523–527.

42. Kavanaugh WM, Williams LT, Ives HE, Coughlin SR. Serotonin-induced deoxyribonucleic acid synthesis in vascular smooth muscle cells involves a novel, pertussis toxin-sensitive pathway. *Mol Endo-crinol* 1988;2:599–605.

43. Kleuss C, Hescheler J, Ewel C, Rosenthal W, Schultz G, Wittig B. Assignment of G-protein subtypes to specific receptors inducing inhibition of calcium currents. *Nature* 1991;353:43–48.

44. Kursar JD, Nelson DL, Wainscott DB, Cohen ML, Baez M. Molec-ular cloning, functional expression, and pharmacological character-ization of a novel serotonin receptor (5-hydroxytryptamine$_{2F}$) from rat stomach fundus. *Mol Pharmacol* 1992;42:549–557.

45. Liscovitch M. Crosstalk among multiple signal-activated phospholi-pases. *Trends Biochem Sci* 1992;17:393–399.

46. Liu YF, Albert PR. Cell-specific signaling of the 5-HT$_{1A}$ receptor. *J Biol Chem* 1991;266:23689–23697.

47. Lübbert H, Snutch TP, Dascal N, Lester HA, Davidson N. Rat brain 5-HT$_{1C}$ receptors are encoded by a 5–6 kbase mRNA size class and are functionally expressed in injected *Xenopus* oocytes. *J Neurosci* 1987;7:1159–1165.

48. Maricq AV, Peterson AS, Brake AJ, Myers RM, Julius D. Primary structure and functional expression of the 5HT3 receptor, a seroto-nin-gated ion channel. *Science* 1991;254:432–437.

49. Mayer, SE, and Sanders-Bush, E. 5HT$_{2A}$ and 5HT$_{2C}$ receptors linked to Na$^+$, K$^+$ and Cl$^-$ co-transport. *Mol Pharmacol* 1994;[*in press*].

50. Middleton JP, Raymond JR, Whorton AR, Dennis VW. Short-term regulation of Na$^+$/K$^+$ adenosine triphosphatase by recombinant hu-man serotonin 5-HT$_{1A}$ receptor expressed in HeLa cells. *J Clin Invest* 1990;86:1799–1805.

51. Monsma FJ Jr, Shen Y, Ward RP, Hamblin MW, Sibley DR. Clon-ing and expression of a novel serotonin receptor with high affinity for tricyclic psychotropic drugs. *Mol Pharmacol* 1993;43:320–327.

52. Murphy TJ, Bylund DB. Characterization of serotonin-1B receptors negatively coupled to adenylate cyclase in OK cells, a renal epithe-lial cell line from the opossum. *J Pharmacol Exp Ther* 1989;249:535–543.

53. Nilsson M, Hansson E, Rönnbäck L. Heterogeneity among astroglial cells with respect to 5HT-evoked cytosolic Ca^{2+} responses. A mi-crospectrofluorimetric study on single cells in primary culture. *Life Sciences* 1991;49:1339–1350.

54. Ogura A, Ozaki K, Kudo Y, Amano T. Cytosolic calcium elevation and cGMP production induced by serotonin in a clonal cell of glial origin. *J Neurosci* 1986;6:2489–2494.

55. Panicker MM, Parker I, Miledi R. Receptors of the serotonin 1C subtype expressed from cloned DNA mediate the closing of K$^+$ membrane channels encoded by brain mRNA. *Proc Natl Acad Sci USA* 1991;88:2560–2562.

56. Peters JA, Malone HM, Lambert JJ. Recent advances in the electro-physiological characterization of 5HT$_3$ receptors. *Trends Pharmacol Sci* 1992;13:391–397.

57. Pierce PA, Peroutka SJ. Evidence for distinct 5-hydroxytryptamine$_2$ binding site subtypes in cortical membrane preparations. *J Neuro-chem* 1989;52:656–658.

58. Pratt GD, Bowery NG. The 5-HT$_3$ receptor ligand, [^{3}H]BRL 43694, binds to presynaptic sites in the nucleus tractus solitarius of the rat. *Neuropharmacology* 1989;28:1367–1376.

59. Pritchett DB, Bach AWJ, Wozny M, Taleb O, Dal Toso R, Shih JC, Seeburg PH. Structure and functional expression of cloned rat serotonin 5-HT-2 receptor. *EMBO J* 1988;7:4135–4140.

60. Raymond JR, Albers FJ, Middleton JP. Functional expression of human 5-HT$_{1A}$ receptors and differential coupling to second messengers in CHO cells. *Naunyn Schmiedebergs Arch Pharmacol* 1992;346:127–137.

61. Raymond JR, Fargin A, Middleton JP, et al. The human 5-HT$_{1A}$ receptor expressed in HeLa cells stimulates sodium-dependent phosphate uptake via protein kinase C. *J Biol Chem* 1989;264:21943–21950.

62. Reiser G. Mechanism of stimulation of cyclic-GMP level in a neuronal cell line mediated by serotonin (5-HT$_3$) receptors. *Eur J Biochem* 1990;189:547–552.

63. Rhee SG, Choi KD. Regulation of inositol phospholipid-specific phospholipase C isozymes. *J Biol Chem* 1992;267:12393–12396.

64. Sanders-Bush E. 5-HT receptors coupled to phosphoinositide hydrolysis. In: Sanders-Bush E, ed. *The serotonin receptors.* Clifton, NJ: Humana Press, 1988;181–198.

65. Seuwen K, Magnaldo I, Pouysségur J. Serotonin stimulates DNA synthesis in fibroblasts acting through 5-HT$_{1B}$ receptors coupled to a G$_i$-protein. *Nature* 1988;335:254–256.

66. Sundaram H, Newman-Tancredi A, Strange PG. Characterization of recombinant human serotonin 5HT$_{1A}$ receptors expressed in chinese hamster ovary cells. *Biochem Pharmacol* 1993;45:1003–1009.

67. Surprenant A, Horstman DA, Akbarali H, Limbird LL. A point mutation of the α_2-adrenoceptor that blocks coupling to potassium but not calcium currents. *Science* 1992;257:977–980.

68. Tang W-J, Gilman A. Type-specific regulation of adenylyl cyclase by G protein $\beta\gamma$ subunits. *Science* 1991;254:1500–1503.

69. Teitler M, Leonhardt S, Weisberg EL, Hoffman BJ. 4-[^{125}I]Iodo-(2,5-dimethoxy)phenylisopropylamine and [^{3}H]ketanserin labeling of 5-hydroxytryptamine$_2$ (5-HT$_2$) receptors in mammalian cells transfected with a rat 5-HT$_2$ receptor subtypes. *Mol Pharmacol* 1990;38:594–598.

70. Tohda M, Nakamura J, Hidaka H, Nomura Y. Inhibitory effects of KN-62, a specific inhibitor of Ca/calmodulin-dependent protein kinase II, or serotonin-evoked Cl$^-$ current and ^{36}Cl$^-$ efflux in *Xenopus* oocytes. *Neurosci Lett* 1991;129:47–50.

71. Varrault A, Journot L, Audigier Y, Bockaert J. Transfection of human 5-hydroxytryptamine$_{1A}$ receptors in NIH-3T$_3$ fibroblasts: effects of increasing receptor density on the coupling of 5-hydroxytryptamine$_{1A}$ receptors to adenylyl cyclase. *Mol Pharmacol* 1992;41:1007–1007.

72. Wang RY, Ashby CR Jr, Zhang JY. Functional roles of 5-HT$_3$-like receptors in the medial prefrontal cortex. *Adv Biosci* 1992;85:81–96.

73. Yocca FD, Iben L, Meller E. Lack of apparent receptor reserve at postsynaptic 5-hydroxytryptamine$_{1A}$ receptors negatively coupled to adenylyl cyclase activity in rat hippocampal membranes. *Mol Pharmacol* 1992;41:1066–1072.

74. Zgombick JM, Beck SG, Mahle CD, Craddock-Royal B, Maayani S. Pertussis toxin-sensitive guanine nucleotide-binding protein(s) couple adenosine A$_1$ and 5-hydroxytryptamine$_{1A}$ receptors to the same effector systems in rat hippocampus: biochemical and electrophysiological studies. *Mol Pharmacol* 1989;35:484–494.

Psychopharmacology: The Fourth Generation of Progress, edited by Floyd E. Bloom and David J. Kupfer. Raven Press, Ltd., New York © 1995.

CHAPTER 39

Anatomy, Cell Biology, and Plasticity of the Serotonergic System

Neuropsychopharmacological Implications for the Actions of Psychotrophic Drugs

Efrain C. Azmitia and Patricia M. Whitaker-Azmitia

The serotonin-producing neurons in the brainstem raphe nuclei form the largest and most complex efferent system in the human brain. This system surpasses that described for the brainstem catecholamine-producing neurons or the descending cortical projecting system. The amino acid transmitters are greater in absolute abundance throughout the brain, but they lack the strict anatomical boundaries characteristic of serotonin-producing neurons. Ramon y Cajal (36) described these giant neurons in the brainstem midline but was unable to follow their extensive projections. Dahlstrom and Fuxe's work with histochemical fluorescence provided details concerning the anatomical architecture (21). It was immediately clear that these ancient neurons, located near the ventricular canals of the brain, innervated the entire neuroaxis. Our work with [^{3}H]proline injections and radioautography mapped the numerous and sometimes redundant projection pathways (4). The application of immunocytochemistry developed by Steinbusch revealed the precise cellular details of the massive axonal branches flowing both up and down the brain (38).

Serotonin (5-hydroxytryptamine, 5-HT) was isolated by a chemist from the blood as a *ser*um factor that increased smooth muscle *tone* (34). Professor D. W. Woolley, a chemist at The Rockefeller Institute, described the comparable actions of LSD and serotonin in the cortex of the cat. This finding so intrigued him that he wrote a prophetic book in 1962 entitled *The Biochemical Basis of Psychosis: The Serotonin Hypothesis About Mental Disease* (47). Brodie and Shore (18) proposed that serotonin and the catecholamines function as the autonomic nervous system of the brain by providing counteracting influences on affective states. Today, the list of eminent psychiatrists that have recognized the importance of serotonin in psychiatric disorders is impressive (see clinical chapters).

The explosion of 5-HT pharmacology has provided clinicians with an array of drugs to manipulate the 5-HT system by interacting with individual 5-HT receptor subtypes. The 5-HT$_{1A}$ is the cell body autoreceptor localized on raphe neurons and also found in target neurons, astrocytes, and ependymal cells (10). It occurs in high amounts in the hippocampus, amygdala, and cortex and is thus sometimes referred to as the *limbic serotonin receptor* (35). The 5-HT$_{1A}$ receptor is the target of drugs used to treat anxiety and depression. The 5-HT$_2$ receptor is postsynaptic and is associated with the fine serotonergic fibers in the middle layers of cortex, especially motor areas (see Chapters 40 and 41, *this volume*). It may underlie many of the motor effects of 5-HT, and it is involved in the action of the major hallucinogenic drugs. The 5-HT$_3$ receptor is seen in limbic areas, where it may serve a role in anxiety and psychosis and in the area postrema, where it plays a role in chemically induced emesis. Functions for the other 5-HT receptors, totaling over 15, await additional research (see Chapters 36–38, *this volume*).

E. C. Azmitia: Department of Biology, New York University, New York, New York 10003.
P. M. Whitaker-Azmitia: Department of Psychiatry, Health Sciences Center, State University of New York, Stony Brook, New York 11791.

Drugs acting on particular receptors have proven useful at correcting chemical imbalances. In many instances, pharmacological treatment must be sustained indefinitely with the added burden of increasing dosage due to decreasing efficacy of the drug. Furthermore, morphological deficits may be responsible for the chemical imbalance. For example, if serotonin fibers are physically damaged in the rodent brain, the animal's behavior is altered. It may become more aggressive or sexually receptive. Hormonal secretion and daily rhythms may be disrupted. Body temperature, eating, and sleeping can become abnormal. However, given time, usually several weeks to months, the remaining 5-HT fibers can sense an increase in available growth factors and begin to recolonize the vacant 5-HT tissue (7). The resetting of the trophic signal appears to be triggered when these receptors are unoccupied.

In addition to the role of endogenous levels of serotonin or of serotonin agonists, steroids can influence the ability of the serotonergic system to undergo regrowth. Glucocorticoids have a normal diurnal rhythm with peak levels in the early morning during sleep. Cortisol is also secreted in high amounts during stress. These hormones function to increase the differentiation of the brain. Treatment with glucocorticoids early in development results in a brain containing a fewer number of cells (17). These same steroids increase 5-HT synthesis and turnover (11). Thus, 5-HT has a diurnal rhythm and is increased during stress in parallel with circulating adrenal steroids. In fact, when the glucocorticoid system is suppressed, the sprouting of 5-HT neurons is also suppressed (48). Thus, in adrenalectomized animals the hippocampal serotonergic fibers do not regrow after a partial lesion, whereas in the animals with an intact adrenal system, regrowth is evident. This growth retardation has also been demonstrated in young pups (39). Therefore, in seeking to promote recuperative sprouting, both neural and endocrine factors are important.

The following sections outline the anatomy and cellular biology of the ascending 5-HT neurons. In addition, the conditions for activation of neuronal growth factors in promoting fiber sprouting are presented. The purpose of this chapter is to emphasize the two roles of serotonin in the mammalian brain: neurotransmitter and neuronotrophic factor. It is important for the reader to appreciate that 5-HT plays both roles throughout the life of the brain. Moreover, both these roles should be kept in mind in order to understand serotonergic disorders and the actions of psychotrophic drugs. The following section, therefore, highlights not only the anatomy and cell biology, but also the development and plasticity, of central nervous system (CNS) serotonergic neurons and the cells they innervate.

THE ASCENDING 5-HT SYSTEM

Superior Raphe Nuclei

The description of the anatomy and development of the brainstem raphe nuclei that have projections to the forebrain has been reviewed previously (6,40). The following is a brief summary of the main nuclear groupings for the interested reader.

According to Wallace and Lauder (42), during early prenatal development two groups of serotonergic neurons are visible: (i) a superior group at the boundary between the midbrain and pons and (ii) a separate inferior group that stretches from the caudal pons to the cervical spinal cord (not discussed in this chapter). The developing 5-HT superior neurons express 5-HT as they migrate and immediately begin to send fine processes. Within hours, 5-HT-IR fibers are seen crossing the midline (29,42). The *superior group* of 5-HT neurons has been described as having two collections of neurons: rostral and caudal. The *rostral collection* gives rise to the caudal linear nucleus and most of the dorsal raphe nucleus (Fig. 1). The *caudal collection* descends from the ependymal zone in two streams of cells that meet in the midline to form the superior central nucleus (median raphe nucleus and the interfascicular portion of the dorsal raphe nucleus). In humans, the dorsal raphe nucleus is the largest of the ascending nuclei and has 235,000 5-HT-immunoreactive neurons (12).

1. *Caudal Linear Nucleus (CLN).* The most rostral group is the CLN, which starts at the level of the red nucleus. The 5-HT neurons are located between the rootlets of the oculomotor nuclei and extend dorsally from the anterior edge of the interpeduncular nucleus to blend with the rostral dorsal raphe nucleus. The projections from these regions extend to the thalamus and cortex.

2. *Dorsal Raphe Nucleus (DRN).* The DRN is divided into medial, lateral (the wings), and caudal components. The medial component can be further divided into a medial [ventral subdivision of Baker et al. 1990 (12)] and an interfascicular component (Fig. 1). The superior component is in the central gray just below the cerebral aqueduct. The interfascicular component surrounds the medial longitudinal fibers (MLFs) and is especially prominent between the fasciculi. These neurons blend with the caudal median raphe nucleus.

The lateral component (the wings) forms the larger division of the DRN and extends as far rostrally as the oculomotor nuclei. In the human, the lateral wings can be divided into a dorsal and ventrolateral subdivision (40).

3. *Median Raphe Nucleus (MRN).* The MRN is a paramedian and median cluster of cells, lying below and caudal to the superior cerebellar decussation (SCD) (Fig. 2). Scattered 5-HT cells of the MRN are seen ventrolateral to the MLF. These laterally situated cells lie in the nucleus pontis centralis oralis (33) and form a ring around the central tegmental tract, one of the most primitive ascending pathways carrying reticulothalamic axons. According to Olsewski and Baxter's human brain atlas (33), the MRN is but one part of the larger superior central nucleus (SCN) which includes the interfascicular aspect of the DRN. Although there is substantial anatomical,

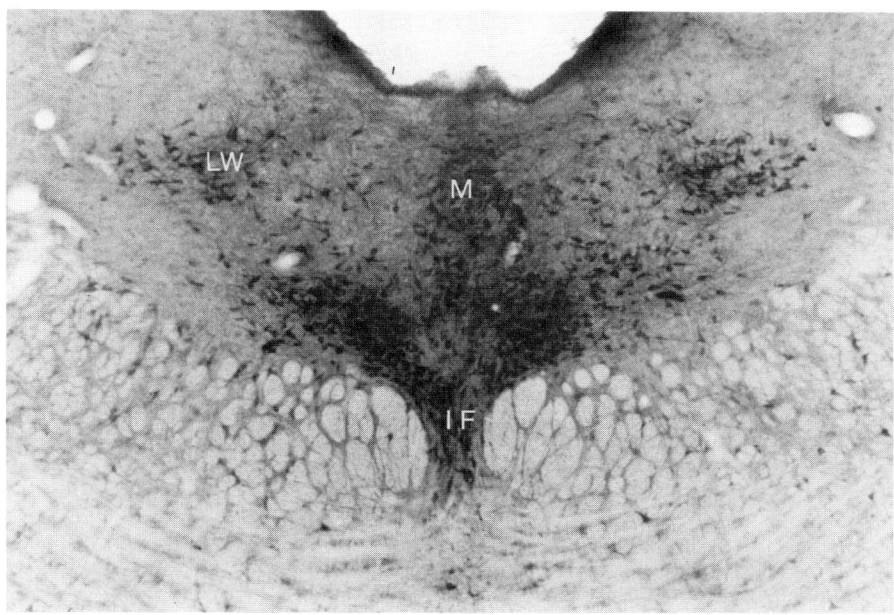

FIG. 1. A photograph of the dorsal raphe nucleus of the rat stained with a specific antipeptide antibody raised against amino acids 66–84 of the tryptophan hydroxylase molecule. IF, interfasciculus; LW, lateral wings; M, medial.

developmental, and functional evidence to support the inclusion of the DRN interfascicular neurons in the SCN, current usage prescribes keeping the original classification of DRN and MRN proposed by Dahlstrom and Fuxe (21).

4. *Supralemniscal Nucleus (SLN)*. This group is located along the superior surface of the medial lemniscus from the rostral border of the inferior olive to the level of the red nucleus. These cells are occasionally continuous with the cells of the MRN and form the ventral border of the ring of scattered cells that surrounds the central tegmental tract in the pontine reticular formation.

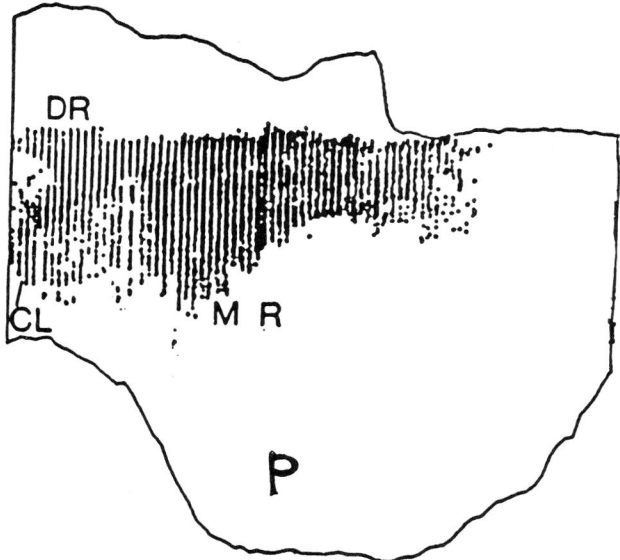

FIG. 2. The rostral serotonergic cell groups of the raphe nuclei of the human brainstem on a computer-generated sagittal section. Rostral is to the left. CL, caudal linear nucleus; DR, dorsal raphe nucleus; MR, medial raphe nucleus. (Adapted from ref. 40.)

Innervation of the Forebrain

The serotonergic fibers projecting to the forebrain originate mainly in the superior group of raphe nuclei (6). Several pathways have been described in rats and primates (Fig. 3). In the rat the largest pathway is the medial forebrain bundle which carries fibers from the MRN and the DRN to a wide range of target areas in the forebrain. In primates, a significant number of these fibers (~25%) are heavily myelinated. Furthermore, in primates the largest pathway appears to be the dorsal raphe cortical tract which enters the cortex through the internal capsule network. Virtually every cell in the brain is in close proximity to a 5-HT fiber. In the adult forebrain, a dense 5-HT innervation is seen in the suprachiasmatic nucleus (rhythm center), the substantia nigra (source of dopamine neurons), the Papez circuit and related limbic centers, and around and in the ventricles. Serotonergic fibers in the cortex are abundant in limbic areas, and the primary sensory and association areas. The lowest levels are found in the motor regions in the frontal lobe. The serotonergic fibers have been described as making classical synaptic contacts with specific target neurons or secreting 5-HT into the neurophil without forming specialized contacts (6). The morphological variation may contribute to the two roles played by 5-HT in the brain: transmitter and trophic factor.

In the cortex, the 5-HT fibers are the first afferent system to arrive and the last to establish its innervation pattern (29). The 5-HT fibers stream across the superficial and deep layers of the primordial cortex to innervate all cortical layers diffusely. More extensive branching proceeds in the granular cell layers (layer IV of cortex). The close association between 5-HT fibers and granule neurons is seen in all cortical areas—even the hippocampus, where the granule neurons are confined to the dentate

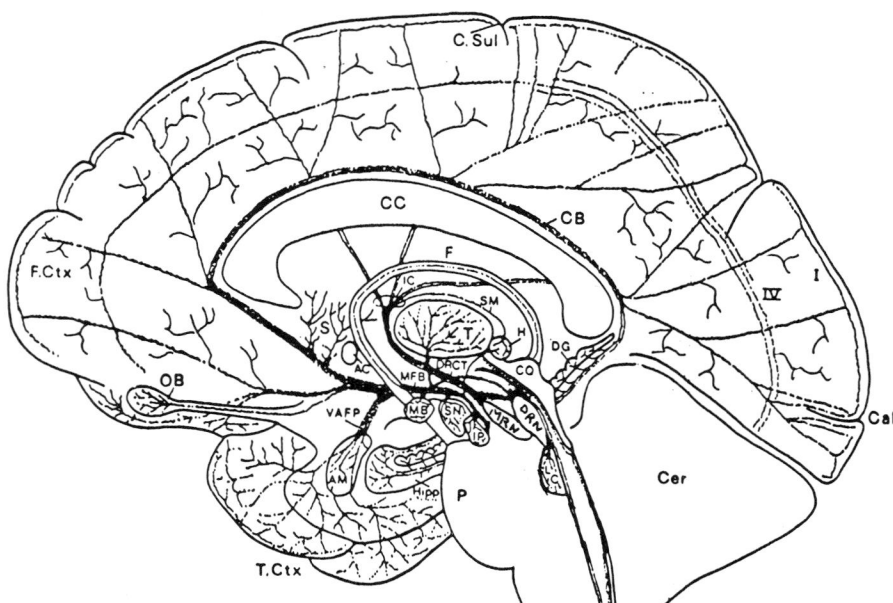

FIG. 3. Summary diagram of the ascending primate serotonergic system. The DRN and MRN nuclei are shown. The fiber pathways are shown as *broken lines.* AC, anterior commissure; Am, amygdaloid nuclei; CC, corpus callosum; CQ, corpus quadrigimini; Csul, central sulcus; DG, dentate gyrus; DRCT, dorsal raphe cortical tract; DRN, dorsal raphe nucleus; F, fornix; F.Ctx, FCII, frontal cortex; Hipp, hippocampus; IC, internal capsule; IP, interpeduncular nucleus; LC, locus coeruleus; MB, mammillary body; MFB, medial forebrain bundle; MRN, median raphe nucleus; OB, olfactory bulb; P, pons; S, septum; SM, stria medullaris; SN, substantia nigra; STC, superior temporal cortex; T, thalamus; T.Ctx, temporal cortex; VAFP, ventroamygdalofugal pathway. (From ref. 13, with modification.)

gyrus. These granule cells complete their final mitosis in the adult brain long after the pyramidal neuron (3). Granule neurons receive direct thalamocortical connections, so 5-HT would be positioned to modulate the electrical entry into the cortex and influence cognitive functioning.

The 5-HT projections from a single neuron or group of neurons can innervate several synaptically interconnected target regions. For example, the MRN innervates the cingulate cortex, septal nuclei, and the hippocampus, whereas the DRN innervates the substantia nigra, the corpus striatum, the amygdala, and the nucleus accumbens. Individual neurons in the DRN and MRN of rat may project to sensorimotor portions of both cerebral and cerebellar cortex, or to visual portions of both (43). The connections made by synaptically linked neurons could be matured by the collaterals of a single serotonergic neuron. When serotonergic neurons are active (e.g., during motor activity or arousal; see Chapter 41, *this volume*), the con-

nections would become stabilized, but when the 5-HT neurons are silent (e.g., during sleep), the target neurons would be exposed to a de-differentiating influence. As mentioned above, 5-HT fibers are the last extrinsic afferents to complete their innervation of the cortex and hippocampus. It was proposed that the serotonin innervation signals the completion of various neuronal circuits and is involved in verification and consolidation of interneuronal contacts (29). However, we propose that neuronal circuits are never complete (finished, stabilized), but we advance the idea that neuronal circuits are normally capable of continual modification and correction to accommodate a changing environment.

CELLULAR RELEASE OF 5-HT

Once the fibers have reached their targets, 5-HT must be released to exert both its electrical and neuronotrophic

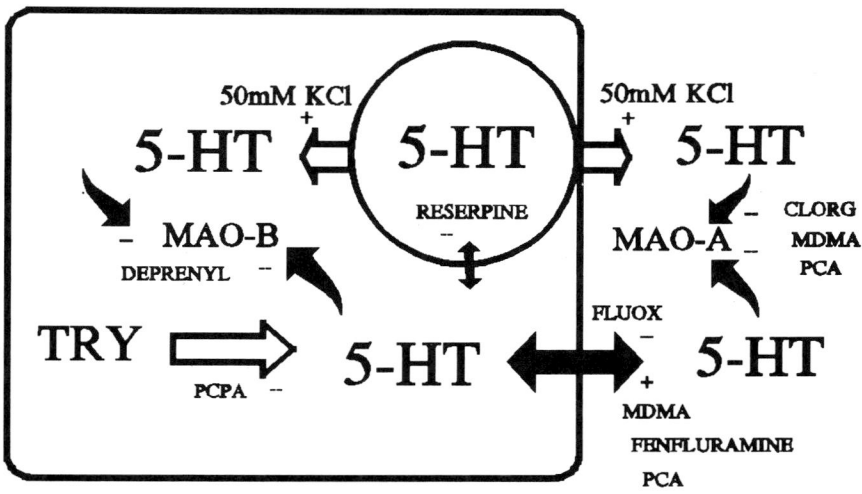

FIG. 4. A schematic drawing of a 5-HT terminal showing two forms of 5-HT release: Vesicular release induced by depolarization is Ca^{2+}-dependent, and cytoplasmic release occurs through the transporter protein by exchange diffusion and is driven by the Na^+ gradient. Monoamine oxidase A (MAO A) metabolizes intracellular 5-HT, and MAO B metabolizes extracellular 5-HT. Note that the vesicular 5-HT is available for release from the cytoplasm by the transporter mechanism. CLORG, clorgyline; FLUOX, fluoxetine; PCA, para-chloroamphetamine; PCPA, para-chlorophenylalanine; TRY, tryptophan.

functions, but depolarization is not the only means to release 5-HT. A schematic drawing of a 5-HT terminal is shown in Fig. 4.

5-HT is synthesized from tryptophan, an essential amino acid that is preferentially taken up by serotonergic neurons. The synthesis of 5-HT, blocked by parachlorophenylalanine, is increased by a Ca^{2+}-dependent stimulation in the presence of adrenal glucocorticoids (24). The newly synthesized 5-HT is stored in vesicular pools and can be released when the neuron fires. Extracellular 5-HT is destroyed by monoamine oxidase (MAO) A (inhibited by clorgyline), which is present in a wide variety of neurons (e.g., dopaminergic, pyramidal neurons) and non-neuronal cells (endothelial, astrocytes) (30).

Extracellular 5-HT that escapes metabolism is quickly taken back (reuptake) into the cytoplasm of the 5-HT neuron (Fig. 4) (see Chapter 28, *this volume*). This process is mediated by transporter protein driven by an Na^+ gradient (16). The 5-HT in the cytoplasm can be stored, transported to vesicles, or degraded by MAO B (inhibited by deprenyl). The 5-HT is transported into the synaptic vesicles by a reserpine sensitive transporter protein (37). The 5-HT is degraded by MAO B only when its levels reach approximately 10^{-3} M, because this form of MAO has a lower affinity for 5-HT than does MAO A. The 5-HT remaining in the cytoplasm is available for an alternate form of release, that mediated by the serotonin transporter. This release by exchange diffusion can be initiated by a variety of drugs, including fenfluramine, para-chloramphetamine (PCA), and 3,4-dioxymethylene-methamphetamine (MDMA) (14). Interestingly, these same drugs at low doses can inhibit the reuptake of 5-HT. Cocaine and fluoxetine are mainly 5-HT reuptake blockers and can inhibit the release of 5-HT by fenfluramine, MDMA, and PCA (14).

The 5-HT stored in cytoplasmic and vesicular pools are in a steady-state relationship (41). When 5-HT is released from one pool, 5-HT can be taken from the other pool (23). For example, neurons stimulated by MDMA release 5-HT through the 5-HT transporter (Fig. 4). However, a component of the 5-HT released actually originates from the vesicular stores. Reserpine, an inhibitor of 5-HT uptake into vesicles, depletes the vesicular stores of 5-HT and also reduces the amount of 5-HT that exits the cell after MDMA exposure. Also, if MAO B is inhibited by deprenyl, the depolarization-induced release of 5-HT is augmented. When depolarization and MDMA are combined, a greater-than-additive release is seen.

Finally, stored 5-HT may actually be received in the cell body from a distant target cell after retrograde transport through 5-HT axons (5).

5-HT$_{1A}$ RECEPTOR: A 5-HT–GLIAL LINK IN DEVELOPMENT AND PLASTICITY

We can propose a neurotrophic role for 5-HT by focusing on a single receptor subtype. The 5-HT$_{1A}$ receptors,

the first 5-HT receptors expressed in forebrain, actually appear before the 5-HT fibers reach the cortex and are modified before birth (44). 5-HT$_{1A}$ receptors can be seen on astrocytes and radial glial cells that contain high amounts of the neuronotrophic factor S-100β (8,46). The expression of these glial receptors can be down-regulated by 5-HT$_{1A}$ receptor agonists or up-regulated by dexamethasone and PCPA (28,45).

S-100β is an important factor in regulating the development of cortical neurons and astrocytes (8,9). Therefore, any factor which influences the release of S-100β from the astrocytes where it is produced will also regulate development. Most of the cortical release of this factor appears to be through the stimulation of 5-HT$_{1A}$ receptors on the astrocyte, and thus any change in the level of serotonin may have profound effects on cortical development. For example, depletion of serotonin by prenatal injections of para-chlorophenylalanine (PCPA, a specific 5-HT synthesis inhibitor) during early development of the rat retards the maturation of target neurons (27). In the somatosensory cortex, neonatal injections of 5,7-dihydroxytryptamine (5,7-DHT, a specific 5-HT neurotoxin) block the formation of barrel fields (15) and result in cortical pyramidal neurons with fewer and stunted primary dendrites (22). In addition, prenatal injection of cocaine to pregnant rats reduces the 5-HT density in cortex at birth and produces a severely stunted cortical mantle (1). Interestingly, if the cocaine-treated pups at birth are given daily injections of a 5-HT$_{1A}$ receptor agonist, the cortex expands to reach normal levels within 1 week (2). Giving the right drug at the right time can be successful.

In humans, 5-HT$_{1A}$ receptors are highest early in gestation (13) and decrease with aging (20,32). The potential for plasticity shows a corresponding fall as the brain matures. The fall in astrocytic 5-HT$_{1A}$ receptors might indicate that the neurotrophic actions of the 5-HT system, mediated by neuronal–glial interactions, is dormant in the adult brain (8) (see also Chapter 58, *this volume*).

Developmental disorders, such as Down's syndrome, are associated with changes in the levels of 5-HT$_{1A}$ receptors. Given the recent interest in schizophrenia as a developmental disorder, it may be pertinent that 5-HT$_{1A}$ receptors have been reported to be increased dramatically in the schizophrenic brain (26).

STRESS STEROIDS AND SPROUTING

Endocrine factors outside of the brain can have profound effects on the 5-HT system. A relationship exists between circulating adrenal steroids and brain 5-HT synthesis, turnover, and tryptophan hydroxylase levels (10). Stress has significant effects on brain 5-HT metabolism which are blocked by adrenalectomy (ADX) and restored by corticosterone or dexamethasone replacement.

The increase in synthesis and turnover of 5-HT is asso-

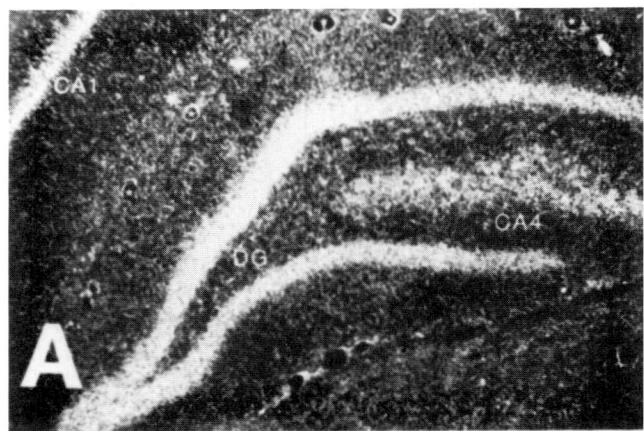

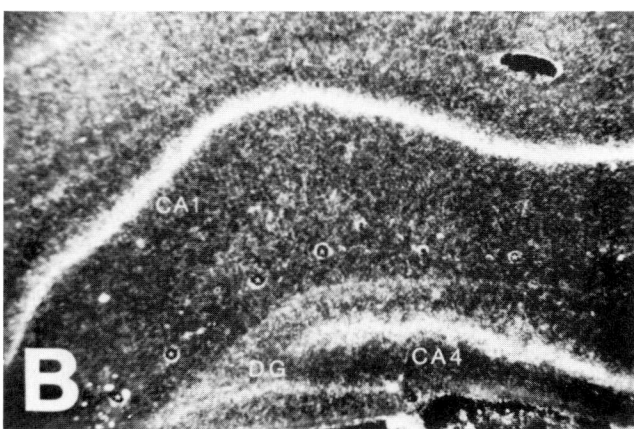

FIG. 5. Bright-field photomicrographs of dorsal hippocampus in coronal section counterstained with methyl green. **A:** Sham ADX. **B:** Two months after ADX. DG, dentate gyrus; g, granular cell layer; s, superior blade of granular cell; i, inferior blade of granular cell layer; CA1 and CA3, CA1 and CA3 regions of Ammon's horn; p, pyramidal cell layer. Bar represents 200 μm.

ciated with changes in the 5-HT$_{1A}$ receptor (Fig. 5). Short-term adrenalectomy increases the binding of 8-OH-DPAT to hippocampal membranes (31). In situ hybridization studies indicate an increased expression of 5-HT$_{1A}$ receptor mRNA in the cornu Ammonis of the hippocampus that appears to be mediated by the type 1, mineralocoid receptor (MR) (19). In contrast, long-term adrenalectomy results in a decreased expression of 5-HT$_{1A}$ mRNA in the dentate gyrus (28). This decrease is reversed by dexamethasone, an agonist at the type 2, glucocorticoid receptor (GR). It is possible that these changes may reflect a neuronal versus a glial localization of the 5-HT$_{1A}$ receptor, with the glial 5-HT$_{1A}$ receptor regulated by GR and the neuronal by MR. This would be consistent with the block of the 5-HT$_{1A}$-receptor-mediated change in a Ca^{2+}-independent K$^+$ channel on neurons by mineralcorticoids (25) (see also Chaptes 62, 65, and 67, *this volume*).

CONCLUSION

In the last few years, it has become increasingly evident that communication between neurons and their supporting glial cells is crucial for normal functioning of the mammalian brain. The functions thus regulated include not only the normal homeostatic mechanisms for providing energy and removing wastes, but also more vital functions—the development and aging of the entire brain. One result of signaling between serotonergic neuron and astrocyte is the release of S-100β. This soluble protein is a potent neurite extension factor for serotonergic neurons, cortical neurons, and spinal motoneurons (9). 5-HT neurons can thus regulate their own growth (autotropic) and induce the maturation of a variety of target cells through this glial protein.

Trauma-, drug-, or stress-induced 5-HT imbalances can alter the architecture of the brain during development and result in mental disorders that can be treated by using drugs to encourage glial activation and neuronal sprouting. This neuroglial link may be an important insight to neuropsychopharmacologists interested in the permanent redesigning of the defective brain in order to correct mental disorders.

ACKNOWLEDGMENTS

We would like to thank Efethemia Kokotos, Bao Liao, and Xi Gu for their critical reading of the chapter, and we are grateful to Oscar Pulido for the preparation of the manuscript. This work was supported by grants from the NIDA and NIA.

REFERENCES

1. Akbari HM, Kramer HK, Whitaker-Azmitia PM, Spear LK, Azmitia EC. Prenatal cocaine exposure disrupts the development of the serotonergic system. *Brain Res* 1992;572:57–63.
2. Akbari HM, Whitaker-Azmitia PM, Azmitia EC. Prenatal cocaine decreases the trophic factor S-100β and induced microcephaly: reversal by postnatal 5-HT$_{1A}$ receptor agonist *Neurosci Lett* 1994;170:141–144.
3. Altman J, Bayer SA. Mosaic organization of the hippocampal neuroepithelium and the multiple germinal sources of dentate granule cells. *J Comp Neurol* 1990;301:325–342.
4. Azmitia EC, Segal M. An autoradiographic analysis of the differential ascending projections of the dorsal and median raphe nuclei in the rat. *J Comp Neurol* 1978;179:641–659.
5. Azmitia EC. Bilateral serotonergic projections to the dorsal hippocampus of the rat: simultaneous localization of ³H-5HT and HRP after retrograde transport. *J Comp Neurol* 1981;203:737–743.
6. Azmitia EC. The primate serotonergic system: progression towards a collaborative organization. In: Meltzer H, ed. *Psychopharmacology: the third generation of progress.* New York: Raven Press, 1987;61–74.
7. Azmitia EC, Davila M, Frankfurt M, Whitaker-Azmitia PM, Zhou FC. Plasticity of fetal and adult CNS serotonergic neurons: role of growth-regulatory factors. *Neuropharmacol Serotonin* 1990;16:343–365.
8. Azmitia EC, Whitaker-Azmitia PM. Awakening the sleeping giant: anatomy and plasticity of the brain serotonergic system. *J Clin Psychopharmacol* 1991;52:4–16.

9. Azmitia EC, Griffin WST, Marshak DR, Van Eldik LJ, Whitaker-Azmitia PM. S100β and serotonin: a possible astrocytic–neuronal link to neuropathology of Alzheimer's disease. *Prog Brain Res* 1992;94:459–473.

10. Azmitia EC, Yu I, Akbari HM, Kheck N, Whitaker-Azmitia PM, Marshak DR. Antipeptide antibodies against the 5-HT$_{1A}$ receptor. *J Chem Neuroanat* 1992;5:289–298.

11. Azmitia EC, Liao B, Chen YS. Increase of tryptophan hydroxylase enzyme protein by dexamethasone in adrenalectomized rat midbrain. *J Neurosci* 1993;13:5041–5055.

12. Baker KG, Halliday GM, Törk I. Cytoarchitecture of the human dorsal raphe nucleus. *J Comp Neurol* 1990;301:147–161.

13. Bar-Peled O, Growss-Isseroff R, Ben-Hur M, et al. Fetal human brain exhibits a prenatal peak in the density of serotonin 5-HT$_{1A}$ receptors. *Neurosci Lett* 1991;127:173–176.

14. Berger UV, Gu XF, Azmitia EC. The substituted amphetamines methylenedioxymethamphetamine, methamphetamine, *p*-chloroamphetamine and fenfluramine induce 5-HT release via a common mechanism which is blocked by fluoxetine and cocaine. *Eur J Pharmacol* 1992;215:153–160.

15. Blue ME, Molliver ME. Serotonin influences barrel formation in developing somatosensory cortex of the rat. *Soc Neurosci Abstr* 1989;15:419.

16. Bogdanski DF, Brodie BB. Role of sodium and potassium ions in storage of norepinephrine by sympathetic nerve endings. *Life Sci* 1966;5:1563.

17. Bohn MC, Lauder JM. Cerebellar granule cell genesis in the hydrocortisone-treated rat. *Dev Neurosci* 1980;3:81–89.

18. Brodie BB, Shore PA. On a role for serotonin and norepinephrine as chemical mediators in the central autonomic nervous system. In: Hoagland H, ed. *Hormones, brain, function and behavior*. New York: Academic Press, 1957.

19. Chalmers DT, Kwak SP, Mansour A, Akil H, Watson SJ. Corticosteroids regulate brain hippocampal 5-HT$_{1A}$ receptor mRNA expression. *J Neurosci* 1993;13(3):914–923.

20. Cross AJ. Serotonin in Alzheimer's-type dementia. *Ann NY Acad Sci* 1990;600:405–415.

21. Dahlstrom A, Fuxe K. Evidence for the existence of monoamine-containing neurons in the central nervous system. I: demonstrations of monoamines in the cell bodies of brainstem neurons. *Acta Physiol Scand* 1964;62(Suppl 232):1–55.

22. Daugherty JA, Haring JH. Effects of neonatal serotonin depletion upon development of rat somatosensory cortex. *Soc Neurosci Abstr* 1989;15:1050.

23. Gu XF, Azmitia EC. MDMA and PCA increases 5-HT levels extracellularly in cultured raphe cells grown in serum free media: potentiation by deprenyl and depolarization and attenuation by reserpine and nimodipine. *Eur J Pharmacol, Mol Sect* 1993;235:51–57.

24. Hamon M, Bourgoin S, Henry F, Simmonet G. Activation of tryptophan hydroxylase by adenosine triphosphate, magnesium and calcium. *Mol Pharmacol* 1987;14:99–110.

25. Joëls M, Hesen W, deKloet ER. Mineralocorticoid hormones suppress serotonin-induced hyperpolarization of rat hippocampal CA1 neurons. *J Neurosci* 1991;11(8):2288–2294.

26. Joyce JN, Shane A, Lexow N, Winokur A, Casanova MF, Kleinman JE. Serotonin uptake sites and serotonin receptors are altered in the limbic system of schizophrenics. *Neuropsychopharmacology* 1993;8(4):315.

27. Lauder JM, Krebs H. Serotonin as a differentiation signal in early neurogenesis. *Dev Neurosci* 1978;1:15–30.

28. Liao B, Miesak BH, Azmitia EC. Loss of 5-HT$_{1A}$ receptor mRNA in the dentate gyrus of the longterm adrenalectomized rat and rapid reversal by dexamethasone. *Mol Brain Res* 19:328–332.

29. Lidov HGW, Molliver ME. An immunohistochemical study of serotonin neuron development in the rat: ascending pathways and terminal fields. *Brain Res Bull* 1982;8:389–430.

30. Levitt P, Pintar JE, Breakefield XO. Immunocytochemical demonstration of monoamine oxidase B in brain astrocytes and serotonergic neurons. *Proc Natl Acad Sci USA* 1982;79:6385–6389.

31. Mendelson SD, McEwen BS. Adrenalectomy increases the density of 5-HT$_{1A}$ receptors in rat hippocampus. *Neuroendocrinol Lett* 1990;12:353.

32. Middlemiss DN, Palmer AM, Edel N, et al. Binding of the novel serotonin agonist 8-hydroxy-2-(di-*n*-propylamino) tetralin in normal and Alzheimer brain. *J Neurochem* 1986;9:743–758.

33. Olszewski J, Baxter D. *Cytoarchitecture of the human brainstem.* Philadelphia: JB Lippincott, 1954.

34. Page IH. The vascular action of natural serotonin, 5- and 7-hydroxytryramine and tryptamine. *J Pharmacol Exp Ther* 1952;105:58.

35. Palacios JM, Dietl MM. Autodiographic studies of serotonin receptors. In: Sanders-Bush E, ed. *The serotonin receptors.* Clifton, NJ: Humana Press, 1988;89–138.

36. Ramon y Cajal S. *Histologie du système nerveux de l'homme et des vertèbres.* France: A Malone, 1911.

37. Slotkin AT. Reserpine, in neuropoisons. In: Simpson LL, Curtin DR, eds. *Their pathophysiological actin.* New York: Plenum Press, 1974;1–69.

38. Steinbusch HWM, Mulder AH. Immunoreactivity in the central nervous system of the rat-cell bodies and terminals. *Neuroscience* 1981;4:557–618.

39. Sze PY. Glucocorticoids as a regulatory factor for brain tryptophan hydroxylase during development. *Dev Neurosci* 1980;3:217–223.

40. Törk I. Anatomy of the serotonergic system. In: Whitaker-Azmitia PM, Perouka SJ, eds. *The neuropharmacology of serotonin.* New York: The New York Academy of Sciences, 1990;9–35.

41. Tracqui P, Morot-Gaudry Y, Staub JF, Brezillon P, Perault-Staub AM, Bourgoin C, Hamon M. Model of brain serotonin metabolism, I. Structure determination-parameter estimation. II—physiological interpretation. *Am J Physiol* 1983;244:R193–R206.

42. Wallace JA, Lauder JM. Development of the serotonergic system in the rat embryo: an immunocytochemical study. *Brain Res Bull* 1983;10:459–479.

43. Waterhouse BD, Mihailoff GA, Baack JC, Woodward DJ. Topographical distribution of dorsal and median raphe neurons projecting to motor, sensorimotor and visual cortical areas in the rat. *J Comp Neurol* 1986;249:460–476.

44. Whitaker-Azmitia PM, Lauder JM, Shemer A, et al. Postnatal changes in 5-HT$_1$ receptors following prenatal alterations in serotonin levels: further evidence for functional fetal 5-HT$_1$ receptors. *Dev Brain Res* 1987;33:285–295.

45. Whitaker-Azmitia PM, Murphy R, Azmitia EC. Stimulation of astroglial 5-HT$_{1A}$ receptors releases the serotonin growth factor, protein S-100, and alters glial morphology. *Brain Res* 1990;528:155–158.

46. Whitaker-Azmitia PM, Clarke C, Azmitia EC. 5-HT$_{1A}$ immunoreactivity in brain astrocytes colocalized with GFAP. *Synapse* 1993;14:201–205.

47. Woolley DW. *The biochemical basis of psychosis: the serotonin hypothesis about mental diseases.* New York: John Wiley & Sons, 1962.

48. Zhou FC, Azmitia EC. Effect of adrenalectomy and corticosterone on the sprouting of serotonergic fibers in hippocampus. *Neurosci Lett* 1985;54:111–116.

Psychopharmacology: The Fourth Generation of Progress, edited by Floyd E. Bloom and David J. Kupfer. Raven Press, Ltd., New York © 1995.

CHAPTER **40**

Electrophysiology of Serotonin Receptor Subtypes and Signal Transduction Pathways

George K. Aghajanian

More than a decade ago a multiplicity of serotonin (5-hydroxytryptamine, 5-HT) receptors in brain were defined pharmacologically by radioligand binding and other methods. Within the past 5 years, molecular cloning techniques have confirmed that 5-HT receptor subtypes (e.g., 5-HT$_1$, 5-HT$_2$, 5-HT$_3$), as predicted from radioligand binding, represent separate and distinct gene products (see Chapters 36–38, *this volume*). This knowledge has revolutionized electrophysiological approaches to the 5-HT system. For example, electrophysiological studies can now be directed toward neurons that express specific 5-HT receptor subtypes based on in situ hybridization maps of receptor mRNA expression. Within each neuron, 5-HT receptor subtypes interact with their own set of G proteins, second messengers, and ion channels, accounting for the wide range of electrophysiological actions produced by 5-HT throughout the brain and spinal cord.

In this rapidly developing field, emphasis must be placed upon more recent contributions to 5-HT electrophysiology, particularly those that have emerged since the publication in 1987 of *Psychopharmacology: The Third Generation of Progress* (see ref. 2 for a more detailed review of earlier studies).

5-HT$_1$ RECEPTORS

Physiology

Many electrophysiological studies on the 5-HT$_1$ receptor subtype have been conducted in areas with a dense

concentration of 5-HT$_{1A}$ binding sites and a high level of 5-HT$_{1A}$ mRNA expression such as the dorsal raphe nucleus and the hippocampal pyramidal cell layer (18,42,51). Studies in these and other regions will be reviewed in the following sections.

Dorsal Raphe Nucleus

Serotonergic neurons of the dorsal raphe nucleus can be inhibited by their own transmitter, 5-HT. Because it is located in the vicinity of the soma, the receptor mediating this effect has been termed a *somatodendritic autoreceptor* (as opposed to the prejunctional autoreceptor). Early studies showed that lysergic acid diethylamide (LSD) and other indoleamine hallucinogens are powerful agonists at the somatodendritic 5-HT autoreceptor (see ref. 2). Functionally, the somatodendritic 5-HT autoreceptor has been shown to mediate collateral inhibition within the raphe nuclei (see ref. 2). Studies in the brain-slice preparation have revealed that the ionic basis for the autoreceptor-mediated inhibition, by either 5-HT or LSD, is an opening of K$^+$ channels (see ref. 2); these channels are characterized by their inwardly rectifying properties (68).

The somatodendritic autoreceptor of dorsal raphe neurons appears to be predominantly of the 5-HT$_{1A}$ subtype as indicated by the fact that a variety of drugs with 5-HT$_{1A}$ selectivity (e.g., 8-OH-DPAT and the anxiolytic drugs buspirone and ipsapirone) share the ability to potently inhibit raphe cell firing in a dose-dependent manner (see ref. 2). Furthermore, intracellular recordings from dorsal raphe neurons in brain slices show that 5-HT$_{1A}$ agonists fully mimic 5-HT in hyperpolarizing the cell membrane and decreasing input resistance. While the classical 5-HT antagonists have proven ineffective in

G. K. Aghajanian: Departments of Psychiatry and Pharmacology, Yale School of Medicine and the Abraham Ribicoff Research Facilities, Connecticut Mental Health Center, New Haven, Connecticut 06508.

blocking the electrophysiological effects of 5-HT at the autoreceptor, acute intravenous administration of the drug spiperone, which has moderate affinity for the 5-HT$_1$ receptor binding site, rapidly blocks the effects of the 5-HT$_{1A}$ agonist 8-OH-DPAT in the dorsal raphe (10,36). Spiperone also rapidly blocks the inhibitory effects of locally applied 5-HT in the dorsal raphe (see ref. 2). In contrast, spiperone is relatively ineffective in blocking the inhibitory effect of 5-HT on postsynaptic CA3 neurons of the hippocampus, suggesting that pre- and postsynaptic 5-HT$_{1A}$ receptors may not be identical (11). However, the basis for this difference is unclear because only one 5-HT$_{1A}$ clone has been reported to date.

Receptor binding and behavioral studies have suggested that the β-adrenoceptor antagonists such as (−)-propranolol may also possess 5-HT$_{1A}$ antagonistic properties (see Chapter 37, *this volume*). Furthermore, electrophysiological studies have shown that low microiontophoretic currents of the β-blocker (−)-propranolol effectively block the suppressant effects of the 5-HT$_{1A}$ agonists (e.g., ipsapirone and 8-OH-DPAT) on raphe cell firing (see ref. 2). These results fit with cloning data which reveal a remarkable degree of sequence homology between the β_2-adrenoceptor and the 5-HT$_{1A}$ receptor (especially in the membrane-spanning segments), providing a molecular basis for the interaction between β-adrenoceptor antagonists and 5-HT$_{1A}$ agonists (see Chapter 38, *this volume*).

In addition to an opening of K$^+$ channels, whole-cell recordings from acutely dissociated raphe neurons have shown that 5-HT decreases high-threshold calcium currents, probably via 5-HT$_{1A}$ receptors because this effect is mimicked by 8-OH-DPAT (49). This calcium current is virtually insensitive to L-type calcium channel blockers but is partially sensitive to ω-conotoxin, an N-type channel blocker (50).

Other Subcortical Regions

Inhibitory or hyperpolarizing responses to 5-HT have been reported in a wide variety of neurons in the spinal cord, brainstem, and diencephalon. In general, such responses have been attributed to an action on 5-HT$_1$ receptors. In sensory neurons of dorsal root ganglia a 5-HT$_1$-like receptor has been reported to reduce the calcium component of action potentials and to produce hyperpolarizations which can be mimicked by 5-HT$_{1A}$ agonists such as 8-OH-DPAT (57,66). In cerebellar Purkinje cells, 5-HT-induced inhibition but not excitation is mediated through 5-HT$_{1A}$ receptors (23). In brain slices of the nucleus prepositus hypoglossi, focal electrical stimulation evokes inhibitory postsynaptic potentials which have been shown to be mediated by endogenous 5-HT acting on 5-HT$_{1A}$ receptors to activate a K$^+$ conductance (15). In the ventromedial hypothalamus (45) and lateral septum (30), 5-HT produces inhibitory effects through 5-HT$_{1A}$ recep-

tors and also by activating a potassium conductance. In the locus coeruleus, 5-HT suppresses depolarizing synaptic potentials, apparently through both 5-HT$_{1A}$ and 5-HT$_{1B}$ receptors (13). In addition, 5-HT appears to selectively suppress the excitatory response of locus coeruleus neurons to locally applied glutamate through a 5-HT$_{1A}$ receptor (20). In the rat laterodorsal tegmental nucleus (LDT), bursting cholinergic neurons are hyperpolarized by 5-HT via 5-HT$_1$ receptors (35). It has been suggested that the removal of a tonic inhibitory 5-HT influence from these cholinergic neurons may be responsible for the emergence of PGO spikes during rapid eye movement (REM) sleep.

Hippocampus

In CA1 pyramidal cells 5-HT produces a membrane hyperpolarization and reduction in input resistance due to an opening of potassium channels (see ref. 2). The receptors mediating these events appear to be of the 5-HT$_{1A}$ subtype because 8-OH-DPAT and other 5-HT$_{1A}$ (but not 5-HT$_{1B}$) agonists elicit similar, although weaker, changes in membrane potential and input resistance (5,55,59). However, two other postsynaptic responses to 5-HT—a reduction in the amplitude of the slow after hyperpolarization and a late depolarization—do not appear to be mediated by any of the 5-HT$_1$ receptor subtypes (5,9). In addition to direct postsynaptic effects on pyramidal cells, 5-HT has also been reported to depress spontaneous synaptic potentials (both IPSPs and EPSPs) in CA1 cells; a 5-HT$_{1A}$ receptor may be involved because 8-OH-DPAT produces similar effects (56). Furthermore, there is a subpopulation of interneurons in the hippocampus even more sensitive than pyramidal cells to the hyperpolarizing effect mediated by 5-HT$_{1A}$ receptors (58). Thus, 5-HT may attenuate slow inhibitory postsynaptic potentials in CA1 pyramidal cells by inhibiting a population of feedforward interneurons that are highly sensitive to 5-HT$_{1A}$ receptor stimulation.

Cerebral Cortex

Hyperpolarizing 5-HT$_{1A}$ responses in the cerebral cortex have been described in a number of studies (6,24,60). However, cortical neurons typically show mixed inhibitory and excitatory responses to 5-HT which involve dual actions at 5-HT$_{2/1C}$ and at 5-HT$_{1A}$ receptors expressed by the same neuron. These mixed responses are described below (see *5-HT$_2$ Receptors: Physiology*).

Signal Transduction Mechanisms

There is evidence that the opening of K$^+$ channels via 5-HT$_{1A}$ receptors in dorsal raphe neurons is mediated by a pertussis-toxin-sensitive G protein. Pertussis toxin cata-

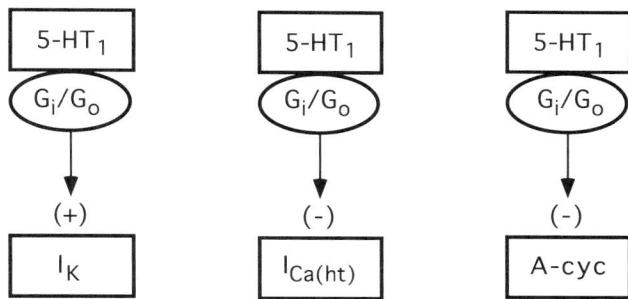

FIG. 1. Schematic representation of the three known transduction pathways for 5-HT₁ receptors: an increase in an inwardly rectifying K$^+$ current (I_K); a decrease in a high threshold Ca^{2+} current ($I_{Ca(ht)}$); and inhibition of adenylyl cyclase (A-cyc). All of these actions are mediated through the pertussis-toxin-sensitive G proteins G$_i$ and/or G$_o$. Although G$_i$ has traditionally been regarded as the G protein that couples to adenylyl cyclase, recent evidence indicates that the form of G$_o$ which is found in the brain also couples negatively to adenylyl cyclase (17).

lyzes the ADP ribosylation of the alpha subunit of certain G proteins (e.g., G$_i$ and G$_o$), causing an irreversible uncoupling of the G protein from its receptor. Extracellular and intracellular experiments in the dorsal raphe nucleus have shown that a 48-hr preinjection with pertussis toxin (local or intracerebroventricular) causes an almost total blockade of the inhibitory and hyperpolarizing effect of 5-HT (29,68). Consistent with their 5-HT$_{1A}$ binding properties, the inhibitory effects of ipsapirone and LSD in the dorsal raphe are also blocked by pertussis toxin (29). G-protein coupling to 5-HT$_1$ receptors in the dorsal raphe is also shown by the fact that intracellular injection of GTPγS, a nonhydrolyzable analogue of GTP which induces an irreversible activation of G proteins, mimics and is nonadditive with the hyperpolarizing action of 5-HT (29). Intracellular GTPγS also renders irreversible the suppression of high-threshold calcium currents in dorsal raphe neurons (50).

As in the dorsal raphe, the hyperpolarizing effects of 5-HT are blocked by pertussis toxin pretreatment in the hippocampus (see ref. 2). Pertussis toxin also blocks GABA$_B$ (see ref. 2) and adenosine (72) responses in the hippocampus. Because the hyperpolarizing effects of 5-HT are nonadditive with GABA$_B$ and adenosine agonists, this suggests a common G-protein-mediated transduction mechanism. Although 5-HT is negatively coupled to adenylate cyclase via a pertussis-toxin-sensitive G protein, the hyperpolarizing effect of 5-HT on membrane potential does not appear to involve cAMP because neither bath application of the membrane-soluble analogue of cAMP, 8-Br-cAMP, nor intracellular injection of cAMP reduces the response (see ref. 2). On this basis, it appears that the 5-HT$_{1A}$-induced hyperpolarizing response is mediated by a membrane-delimited coupling of G proteins to K$^+$ channels rather than through a diffusible second messenger system.

Other areas where pertussis toxin blockade of inhibitory responses to 5-HT has been demonstrated include dorsal root ganglion cells (22) and neurons of the ventromedial hypothalamus (46).

Signal transduction pathways for 5-HT$_1$ receptors are depicted schematically in Fig. 1.

5-HT₂ RECEPTORS

Physiology

Quantitative autoradiographic studies show high concentrations of 5-HT$_2$ binding sites and mRNA expression in certain regions of the forebrain such as the neocortex (layers IV/V), piriform cortex, claustrum, and olfactory tubercle (41). With few exceptions (e.g., facial nucleus and the nucleus tractus solitarius), relatively low concentrations of 5-HT$_2$ receptors or mRNA expression are found in the brainstem. Studies aimed at examining the physiological role of 5-HT$_2$ receptors in several of these regions are discussed in the following sections.

Facial Nucleus and Spinal Cord

Facial motoneurons have a high density of 5-HT$_2$ receptor binding sites, and in situ hybridization shows a high level of 5-HT$_2$ receptor mRNA in these neurons (41). Early studies in vivo showed that 5-HT applied microiontophoretically does not by itself induce firing in the normally quiescent facial motoneurons but does facilitate the subthreshold and threshold excitatory effects of glutamate (see ref. 2). Intracellular recordings from facial motoneurons in vivo or in brain slices in vitro (3,32) show that 5-HT induces a slow, subthreshold depolarization associated with an increase in input resistance, suggesting a decrease in a resting K$^+$ conductance. Similar effects of 5-HT also have been described in spinal motoneurons (67,71). Recently, it has been shown that 5-HT also increases the excitability of facial motoneurons by enhancing a hyperpolarization-activated cationic current I_h (26,31). In contrast, the depolarizing effect of norepinephrine on facial motoneurons appears to involve only a closure of K$^+$ channels (31).

The 5-HT$_2$ antagonist ritanserin is able to selectively block the excitatory effects of 5-HT in facial motoneurons (54). On the other hand, the selective 5-HT$_{1A}$ agonist 8-OH-DPAT, although it increases facial motoneuron excitability when given in vivo by systemic injection, fails to produce excitation when applied locally either by microiontophoresis or by bath application in brain slices. Thus, this selective 5-HT$_{1A}$ ligand does not appear to have any *direct* excitatory effect on facial motoneurons. However, 5-carboxamidotryptamine (5-CT), a broad-spectrum 5-HT$_1$ agonist, acts directly to enhance facial motoneuron excitability. Surprisingly, ritanserin is able to block the effects of 5-CT as well as those of 5-HT. Because ritanserin has extremely low affinity for all 5-HT$_1$ receptors except 5-HT$_{1C}$, it is possible that it is the 5-HT$_{1C}$ component of 5-CT's receptor profile that is responsible for its effect on facial motoneurons. The 5-HT$_{1C}$ receptor has a high degree of homology with the 5-HT$_2$ receptor, accounting for the difficulty in distinguishing the two sites pharmacologically. Indeed, it has been proposed that the 5-HT$_{1C}$ now be reclassified as the 5-HT$_{2C}$ receptor and that the original 5-HT$_2$ receptor now be termed 5-HT$_{2A}$ (see Chapter 37, *this volume*).

A large number of studies, using behavioral, ligand-binding, and electrophysiological techniques, have shown that indoleamine (e.g., LSD and psilocin) and phenethylamine (e.g., mescaline and DOI) hallucinogens share the property of interacting with 5-HT$_2$ receptors (see Glennon, *this volume*). The iontophoretic administration of LSD, mescaline, or psilocin, although having relatively little effect by themselves, produce a prolonged facilitation of facial motoneuron excitability (see ref. 2). Intracellular studies in brain slices show that the enhancement is due in part to a small but persistent depolarizing effect of the hallucinogens (26,54). In addition, LSD and the phenethylamine hallucinogen DOI enhance the cationic current I_h even to a greater degree than does 5-HT itself, suggesting that this action may be more important quantitatively than the closure of K$^+$ channels in explaining the increase motoneuronal excitability produced by these drugs (26). All of these effects of the hallucinogens are reversed by spiperone and ritanserin, consistent with mediation by 5-HT$_2$ receptors.

Locus Coeruleus

Systemically administered mescaline or LSD induces a simultaneous decrease in spontaneous activity and increase in sensory responsivity of noradrenergic cells in the locus coeruleus (LC) (see ref. 2). That the effects of LSD and mescaline (and other phenethylamine hallucinogens) on LC neurons are mediated by 5-HT$_2$ receptors is suggested by the fact that they can be reversed by low doses of 5-HT$_2$ antagonists such as ritanserin and LY-53857. In addition to reversing the effects of hallucinogens, the 5-HT$_2$ antagonists induce a small but significant increase in basal LC firing rates, suggesting the existence of a tonic 5-HT$_2$ inhibitory influence (see ref. 2). The latter electrophysiological findings are paralleled by voltammetric studies which show an increase in the catechol metabolite DOPAC in the LC following systemic injections of the 5-HT$_2$ antagonist ritanserin (21). Antipsychotics with affinity for 5-HT$_2$ binding sites are also able to reverse the actions of hallucinogens in the LC independently of their actions at dopamine and other types of receptors (53). The relative potencies of hallucinogens in their action on LC neurons correlates with their affinity

for 5-HT$_2$ receptors (see ref. 2). However, the effects of hallucinogens in the LC are not direct because they are not mimicked by the local, iontophoretic application onto LC cell bodies. Thus, the hallucinogens are likely to be acting indirectly on LC neurons via afferents to this nucleus.

Other Subcortical Regions

In brain slices of the medial pontine reticular formation, 5-HT induces a hyperpolarization in some cells (34%) and a depolarization in other cells (56%) (63). The hyperpolarizing responses are associated with an increase in membrane conductance and have a 5-HT$_1$ pharmacological profile. The depolarizing responses have a 5-HT$_2$ pharmacology and are associated with a decrease in membrane conductance resulting from a decrease in an outward K$^+$ current. These two actions of 5-HT do not appear to coexist in the same neurons, because none of the cells display dual responses to selective agonists. In the nucleus accumbens the great majority of neurons are depolarized by 5-HT, inducing them to fire (47). The depolarization is associated with an increase in input resistance due to a reduction in an inward rectifier K$^+$ conductance. Pharmacological analysis shows that the depolarization is mediated by a 5-HT$_2$ rather than a 5-HT$_1$ or 5-HT$_3$ receptor.

Marked depolarizing responses to 5-HT, associated with a decrease in a resting or "leak" K$^+$ conductance, have been reported in GABAergic neurons of the nucleus reticularis thalami; these excitatory responses to 5-HT are blocked by the 5-HT$_{2/1C}$ antagonists ketanserin and ritanserin (38). The 5-HT-induced slow depolarization potently inhibits burst firing in these cells and promotes single-spike activity. It has been suggested that this 5-HT-induced switch in firing mode from rhythmic oscillation to single-spike activity, which occurs during states of arousal and attentiveness, contributes to the enhancement of information transfer during these states.

Cerebral Cortex

The electrophysiological effects of 5-HT have been studied in several cortical regions. In vivo, 5-HT$_2$ agonists applied by microiontophoresis have been reported to have primarily inhibitory effects on the firing of unidentified neurons in prefrontal cortex (8); these inhibitions are blocked by 5-HT$_2$ antagonists. (Note that the inhibitions produced by 5-HT itself are not blocked by 5-HT$_2$ antagonists but are blocked by 5-HT$_3$ antagonists; see below.) In brain slices, pyramidal cells in various regions of the cerebral cortex have been found to respond to 5-HT by either a small hyperpolarization, depolarization, or no change in potential (6,24,39,60). Based on pharmacological evidence, the depolarizations appear to be mediated by 5-HT$_2$ or 5-HT$_{1C}$ receptors. In rat association cortex it has been shown that there can be a coexistence of 5-HT_{1A} and 5-HT_2 receptors on a single neuron (6). Thus, in the presence of the 5-$HT_{2/1C}$ antagonist ketanserin, 5-HT_{1A}-mediated hyperpolarizing responses can be elicited in cells which originally exhibit only a depolarizing response. Excitatory responses to 5-HT in pyramidal cells are due to a reduction in K^+ conductances (38,61). Three different types of conductances appear to be involved: a resting K^+ conductance, a depolarization-activated K^+ conductance (M current), and a Ca^{2+}-activated K^+ conductance. There is pharmacological evidence that the excitatory effects of 5-HT on pyramidal cells in piriform cortex are mediated by 5-HT_{1C} rather than 5-HT_2 receptors (61).

Recently, we have observed a novel effect of 5-HT in piriform cortex, namely, an induction of IPSPs (60) in pyramidal cells. The IPSPs are blocked by the GABA antagonist bicuculline, suggesting that the IPSPs arise from GABAergic interneurons that are excited by 5-HT. Accordingly, a subpopulation of interneurons (at the border of layers II and III) has been found that is excited by 5-HT. Somewhat less frequently, neurons within this same subpopulation of interneurons also tend to be excited by dopamine and norepinephrine (27). Excitation by 5-HT of these interneurons (as well as associated IPSPs in pyramidal cells) is blocked by 5-HT_2 antagonists. The hallucinogens LSD and DOM behave as partial agonists in this system, producing a modest activation by themselves but occluding the full effect of 5-HT. We have found a similar partial agonist effect of hallucinogens in the medial septal nucleus, where 5-HT also has an excitatory effect on GABAergic neurons (Alreja and Aghajanian, *unpublished data*).

In piriform cortex, the 5-HT_2 antagonist ritanserin blocks the activation of interneurons more readily than it blocks the depolarization of pyramidal cells (60). Ritanserin has a nearly 10-fold higher affinity for the 5-HT_2 receptor than for the 5-HT_{1C} receptor, suggesting that the action of 5-HT on these interneurons might be through 5-HT_2 receptors whereas the action of 5-HT on the pyramidal cells might be through 5-HT_{1C} receptors. This hypothesis is consistent with recent findings that mRNA for the 5-HT_2 receptor is located in cortical interneurons while mRNA for the 5-HT_{1C} receptor is found in pyramidal cells (40,41). Recent studies in the piriform cortex employing a new, highly selective antagonist (MDL 100,907) with a 300-fold greater affinity for the 5-HT_2 than for 5-HT_{1C} receptors also suggest that 5-HT_2 rather than 5-HT_{1C} receptors are responsible for the 5-HT excitation of interneurons (Marek and Aghajanian, *unpublished data*).

Signal Transduction Mechanisms

The role of G proteins in mediating the 5-HT_2-induced slow inward current has been evaluated in facial motoneu-

rons by using the hydrolysis-resistant guanine nucleotide analogues $GTP\gamma S$ and $GTP\beta S$ (1). The 5-HT-induced inward current becomes largely irreversible in the presence of intracellular $GTP\gamma S$. Mediation by G proteins is also suggested by the fact that the inward current is reduced by intracellular $GTP\beta S$ which prevents G-protein activation. The identity of the G protein(s) mediating the electrophysiological responses remains to be determined.

In addition to the electrophysiological effects mediated by 5-HT_2 and 5-HT_{1C} receptors, there is an activation phospholipase C which hydrolyzes phosphatidylinositol (PI) to yield two major intracellular messengers, diacylglycerol (DAG) and inositol trisphosphate (IP_3) (see Chapter 38, *this volume*). LSD and DOM act as partial agonists of this effect. An increase in IP_3 resulting from the activation of 5-HT_2 receptors would be expected to release intracellular stores of Ca^{2+} from its intracellular stores. Recently, 5-HT-induced increase in cytoplasmic Ca^{2+} levels has been directly demonstrated in cultured local interneurons of mouse olfactory bulb by Ca^{2+} imaging techniques using the fluorescent indicator fura-2 (65). This effect of 5-HT was blocked by ritanserin, indicating the involvement of 5-HT_2 receptors.

DAG, by activating protein kinase C (PKC), would be expected to affect many long-term cellular responses through protein phosphorylation. The effect of protein kinase inhibitors on the response of facial motoneurons to 5-HT has been tested (1). Two protein kinase inhibitors with different mechanisms of action, 1-(5-isoquinolylsulfonyl)-2-methylpiperazine (H7), a nonselective protein kinase inhibitor, and sphingosine, a selective PKC inhibitor, in concentrations that have no effect of their own (100 and 10 μM, respectively), both markedly enhance and prolong the excitation of facial motoneurons induced by 5-HT. Conversely, phorbol esters that are known to activate PKC reduce the excitatory effect of serotonin. These results suggest that activation of PI turnover, perhaps through receptor phosphorylation, has a negative feedback effect on 5-HT-induced excitations in the facial nucleus. Similar findings have also been obtained in the cerebral cortex using the grease-gap method for assessing the 5-HT enhancement of N-methyl-D-aspartate (NMDA)-induced depolarizations (52). In the latter studies, phorbol esters and DAG rather than mimicking the ability of 5-HT to enhance NMDA depolarizations, promoted 5-HT desensitization. An interesting implication of the negative feedback model is the possibility that the partial agonist properties of hallucinogens with respect to 5-HT-stimulated PI hydrolysis may contribute to, rather than interfere with, their electrophysiological actions (see Chapter 38, *this volume*).

The activation of 5-HT_2 receptors can have long-term effects through an alteration in immediate early gene expression. Within 30 min following systemic injections of the 5-HT_2 agonist 1-(2,5-dimethoxy-4-iodophenyl)-2-aminopropane (DOI), a dramatic increase in Fos protein

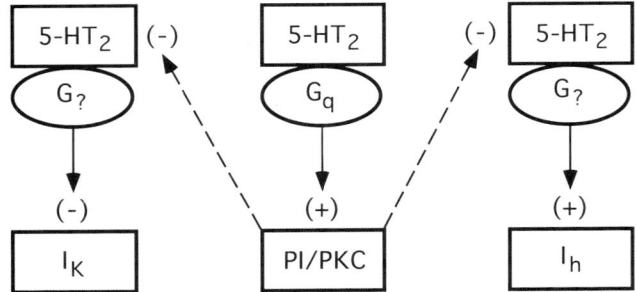

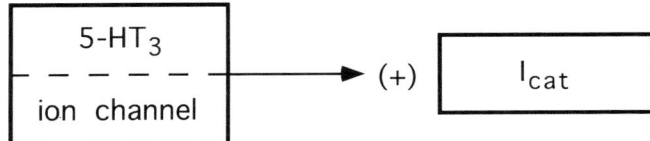

FIG. 2. Schematic representation of the three known transduction pathways for 5-HT$_2$ receptors: a decrease in certain resting and voltage-activated K$^+$ currents (I_K); positive coupling to the phosphoinositide (PI) second messenger pathway; and an increase in the hyperpolarization-activated cationic current I_h. The *dashed lines* indicate a proposed negative feedback between the activation of protein kinase C (PKC) and 5-HT$_2$ receptors, presumably through phosphorylation of the receptor. Activation of the PI pathway is presumably mediated by a member of the Gq subfamily (62); ion channel coupling may also be through Gq, but there are no data as yet on this point. This scheme is intended to apply to both the 5-HT$_{2A}$ and 5-HT$_{2C}$ receptors (formerly known as 5-HT$_2$ and 5-HT$_{1C}$, respectively).

FIG. 3. Schematic representation of the 5-HT$_3$ receptor as a ligand-gated ion channel where activation of the receptor produces a cationic current without the involvement of a G protein or a second messenger.

(the product of the immediate early gene c-fos) can be detected in neurons in middle layers of cerebral cortex, including piriform cortex (33). It is not known as yet whether this effect on immediate early gene expression is mediated through an activation of PKC.

Signal transduction pathways for 5-HT$_2$ receptors are summarized in Fig. 2.

5-HT$_3$ RECEPTORS

There are rapidly desensitizing depolarizing responses to 5-HT in the periphery that are mediated by 5-HT$_3$ receptors (formerly known as M receptors). In brain, excitatory responses to 5-HT have been found in cultured mouse hippocampal and striatal neurons which have many of the characteristics of peripheral 5-HT$_3$ responses: rapid onset and rapid desensitization, features that are typical of ligand-gated ion channels rather than G-protein-coupled receptor responses (69,70). In cultured NG108-15 cells the permeation properties of the 5-HT$_3$ channel are indicative of a cation channel with relatively high permeability to Na$^+$ and K$^+$ and low permeability to Ca^{2+} (70). Recently, a 5-HT-gated ion channel has been cloned which has physiological and pharmacological properties appropriate for a 5-HT$_3$ receptor (37). In the oocyte expression system, this receptor shows rapid desensitization and is blocked by 5-HT$_3$ antagonists (e.g., ICS 205-930 and MDL 72222). Because of its sequence homology with the nicotinic acetylcholine receptor (27%), the β_1 subunit of the GABA$_A$ receptor (22%), and the 48K subunit of the glycine receptor (22%), it is likely that this 5-HT$_3$ receptor clone is a member of the ligand-gated ion channel superfamily.

Rapidly desensitizing 5-HT$_3$ responses have also been reported in brain slices. In slices containing the lateral nucleus of the amygdala, 5-HT$_3$-mediated fast excitatory synaptic responses to focal electrical stimulation can be demonstrated when glutamate receptors are blocked; these synaptic responses show rapid cross-desensitization with bath-applied 5-HT (64). In hippocampal slices, 5-HT has been reported to increase GABAergic IPSPs, most likely through a 5-HT$_3$-receptor-mediated excitation of inhibitory interneurons; these responses also show fading with time (55).

While fast, rapidly inactivating excitation has generally become accepted as characteristic of 5-HT$_3$ receptors, nondesensitizing responses have also been reported. In dorsal root ganglion cells a relatively rapid but *noninactivating* depolarizing response has been described which has a 5-HT$_3$ pharmacological profile (66). In neurons of the nucleus tractus solitarius in a brain-slice preparation, there is a postsynaptic depolarizing response to 5-HT$_3$ agonists which does not appear to be rapidly desensitizing (28). In the latter preparation there are also enhancements of presynaptic responses (both IPSPs and EPSPs). In medial prefrontal cortex a slow *inhibitory* response to micro-iontophoretic applied 5-HT has been described which also has a 5-HT$_3$-like pharmacology (7). This effect is mimicked by the 5-HT$_3$ agonist 2-methylserotonin and blocked by the 5-HT$_3$ antagonists BRL 43693 and ICS205930. At this juncture, it is not clear whether there is more than just a superficial pharmacological relationship among these various so-called 5-HT$_3$ responses.

Figure 3 depicts the 5-HT$_3$ receptor as a ligand-gated cationic channel.

5-HT$_4$ RECEPTORS

The existence of the 5-HT$_4$ receptor in the central nervous system was first suspected on the basis of biochemical data showing positive coupling of 5-HT responses to adenylyl cyclase (16). Thus, this receptor differs from the 5-HT$_1$ subfamily, which is negatively coupled to adenylyl cyclase. Very recently, two novel 5-HT receptors positively coupled to adenylyl cyclase have been cloned; however, because their pharmacology differs from that of the previously described 5-HT₄ site, they have been tentatively designated as 5-HT₆ and 5-HT₇ receptors (34,43). The original 5-HT₄ receptor has not as yet been cloned and is characterized primarily by its pharmacological properties. The latter is generally unaffected by 5-HT₁, 5-HT₂, and 5-HT₃ agonists or antagonists, but certain benzamides (e.g., BRL 24923, zacopride, and metoclopramide) can act as agonists while ICS 205-930 (in contrast to other 5-HT₃ antagonists) shows antagonism, but with low potency and poor selectivity (16).

Up to this point there have been few electrophysiological studies performed on putative 5-HT₄ responses in the brain. In hippocampal CA1 pyramidal cells, 5-HT induces a slow depolarization (unmasked after blockade of 5-HT₁ₐ hyperpolarizing responses) and a reduction in the amplitude of the calcium-activated potassium conductance (afterhyperpolarization). These responses are not sensitive to the usual 5-HT₁, 5-HT₂, and 5-HT₃ agents, whereas they are blocked by BRL 24924 and certain other substituted benzamides and ICS 205-930 (4,19), suggesting a 5-HT₄-like pharmacology. However, these responses do not appear to be mediated through the cAMP signal transduction pathway (4). Another electrophysiological action of 5-HT with a 5-HT₄ profile has been reported in cultured mouse collicular neurons (25). In these cells, 5-HT reduces slowly inactivating voltage-activated potassium currents; this effect is generally insensitive to 5-HT₁, 5-HT₂, and 5-HT₃ drugs but is responsive to a variety of 5-HT₄-active agents including the substituted benzamides. However, in contrast to CA1 pyramidal cells, the effects of 5-HT in collicular neurons do appear to be mediated through the cAMP transduction pathway because they are mimicked by cAMP analogues and are blocked by intracellular application of PKI, a specific inhibitor of cAMP-dependent protein kinase.

In a number of regions, cAMP has been shown to mimic the ability of 5-HT to enhance the hyperpolarization activated cationic current (I_h). For example, in neurons of the nucleus prepositus hypoglossi the augmentation of I_h can be mimicked by cAMP-active agents (e.g., 8-bromo-cAMP and forskolin) (14). However, since this effect is also mimicked by 5-HT₁ agonists, the precise identification of the 5-HT receptor subtype is unclear because 5-HT₁ receptors are generally coupled negatively to adenylate cyclase. The newly cloned 5-HT₇ receptor, which has relatively high affinity for certain 5-HT₁ₐ ligands (34), must now be considered as a possible mediator of the increase in I_h in these cells. An augmentation of I_h by 5-HT (and norepinephrine) has also been reported for several thalamic nuclei such as the dorsal lateral and medial geniculate nuclei of the thalamus (48). The increase in I_h results in a reduced ability of thalamic neurons to generate rhythmic burst firing. It has been suggested that this reduction in burst firing (which is associated with sleep spindles) increases the efficacy of transfer of

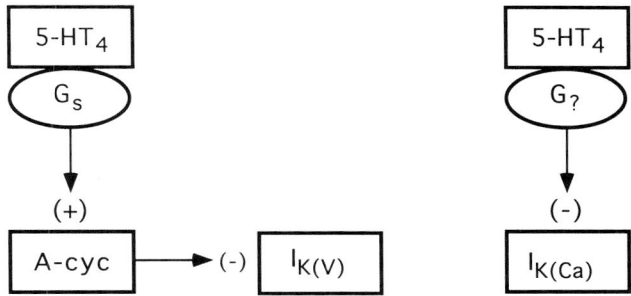

FIG. 4. Schematic representation of two proposed 5-HT₄ transduction pathways. The positive coupling to adenylyl cyclase is presumably through Gₛ, leading to a reduction in certain voltage-dependent K⁺ currents ($I_{K(V)}$) through the protein kinase A phosphorylation pathway. The coupling of 5-HT₄ receptors to the calcium-activated potassium current ($I_{K(Ca)}$) does not appear to involve cAMP.

information through the thalamus during periods of increased arousal and attentiveness. The increase in I_h in the thalamus is not blocked by 5-HT₁ or 5-HT₂ antagonists but is mimicked by membrane-permeable cAMP analogues or the adenylate cyclase activator forskolin. However, it has not been determined as yet whether this response is mediated by 5-HT₄ receptors. In brain slices, a non-5-HT₁, 5-HT₂-mediated increase in I_h has also been reported for dopaminergic neurons of the substantia nigra pars compacta (44). However, as yet there have been no reports on the role of cAMP or 5-HT₄ receptors in this effect.

Possible signal transduction pathways for 5-HT₄ receptors are depicted in Fig. 4.

SUMMARY AND OVERVIEW

5-HT Receptor Subtypes, Ion Channels, and Second Messenger Systems

The extraordinarily diverse electrophysiological actions of 5-HT in the central nervous system can now be categorized according to receptor subtypes and their respective effector mechanisms. The following generalizations are emerging: (a) Inhibitory effects of 5-HT are mediated by 5-HT₁ receptors linked to the opening of K⁺ channels or the closing of Ca²⁺ channels, both via pertussis-toxin-sensitive G proteins; (b) there are facilitatory effects of 5-HT that involve the closing of K⁺ channels which are mediated by 5-HT₂ receptors, with the PI second messenger system and PKC acting as a negative feedback loop; (c) other facilitatory effects of 5-HT are mediated by 5-HT₄ receptors through a reduction in $I_{K(Ca^{2+})}$ or voltage-dependent K⁺ current, apparently in some cases through the cAMP pathway and in other cases not; and (d) fast excitations are mediated by 5-HT₃ receptors through a ligand-gated cationic ion channel which does not require coupling with a G protein or a second messenger. Thus, the electrophysiological actions of 5-HT encompass the two major neurotransmitter superfamilies: the G-protein-coupled receptors (i.e., 5-HT$_1$, 5-HT$_2$, 5-HT$_4$) and the ligand-gated channels (5-HT$_3$).

Relevance to Clinical Disorders and Drug Actions

The diversity of receptors and transduction pathways that underlie the varied electrophysiological actions of 5-HT, together with the differential expression of these receptors in different neuronal populations, helps to explain how it is possible for one transmitter to be linked to such a large array of behaviors, clinical conditions, and drug actions. For example, alterations in 5-HT function have been implicated in affective disorders, anxiety states, schizophrenia, obsessive compulsive disorder, eating disorders, migraine, and sleep disorders (see Chapter 42, *this volume*). There is an equally wide range of drugs that interact with 5-HT neurotransmission, including antidepressants (e.g., selective 5-HT uptake blockers), atypical antipsychotics (e.g., clozapine), anxiolytics (e.g., buspirone), antiemetics (e.g., ondansetron), hallucinogens (e.g., LSD), antimigraine drugs (e.g., sumatriptan), and appetite suppressants (e.g., fenfluramine).

Role of 5-HT in Neuronal Networks

The direct actions of 5-HT at a cellular level, as detailed in this review, do not have a simple relationship to the overall input–output relations. For example, while 5-HT$_{1A}$ agonists are directly inhibitory upon serotonergic neurons in the raphe nuclei (possibly at doses insufficient to affect postsynaptic 5-HT$_{1A}$ receptors), the net effect of this inhibition may be disinhibitory for postsynaptic neurons that express 5-HT$_{1A}$ receptors and simultaneously disfacilitatory for postsynaptic neurons that express 5-HT$_2$, 5-HT$_3$, and 5-HT$_4$ receptors. Similarly, while 5-HT$_2$ agonists may be directly excitatory at a subpopulation of GABAergic interneurons in the cerebral cortex that express 5-HT$_2$ receptors, the net effect of this excitation may be inhibitory for those pyramidal cells that receive inputs from these interneurons. In general, to understand the functional consequences of the discrete cellular actions of 5-HT, these must be viewed within the context of the neuronal networks where they occur.

Integrative Action of 5-HT

This review has described the individual cellular actions of 5-HT in many different regions of the brain and spinal cord. Do these discrete and disparate effects of 5-HT have an integrated function greater than the sum of the parts? Suggestive of this possibility is the fact that (a) serotonergic neurons are clustered in a relatively small number nuclei within the brainstem (i.e., the raphe nuclei), projecting diffusely to almost every other region of the neuraxis (see Chapter 39, *this volume*), and (b) in unanesthetized animals, the tonic firing of serotonergic neurons *as a group* varies according to behavioral state, such that activity is greatest during behavioral arousal, diminished during slow-wave sleep, and virtually absent during REM sleep (see Chapter 41, *this volume*).

Do the individual cellular actions of 5-HT in different regions of the central nervous system serve to coordinate overall behavioral states? The possibility of an integrative action of 5-HT can be illustrated for three disparate sets of neurons as follows. During the waking state, when serotonergic neurons are in a tonic firing mode, the following conditions would prevail: (a) Motoneurons would be in a relatively depolarized, excitable state (via 5-HT$_2$ receptors) and thus would be receptive to the initiation of movement; (b) neurons of the nucleus reticularis thalami would be in a depolarized, single-spike mode (via 5-HT$_2$ receptors) and thus would be conducive to thalamocortical sensory information transfer (38,48); and (c) neurons of the laterodorsal tegmental nucleus would be hyperpolarized (via 5-HT$_1$ receptors) and therefore not able to generate the bursting activity of REM sleep (35). With a reduction in serotonergic activity during various stages of sleep, the above conditions would reverse such that motoneurons would become less excitable, thalamocortical sensory information transfer would be diminished, and sleep spindles and PGO waves would emerge. Thus, serotonergic neurons can be seen as functioning as part of a complex, coordinated modulation of motor, sensory, and other systems to promote a given behavioral state. It remains to be seen whether *all* the diverse cellular actions of 5-HT can be incorporated into this kind of holistic scheme or whether there are subsets of serotonergic neurons that operate different groups of postsynaptic neurons in an independent fashion.

ACKNOWLEDGMENTS

This work was supported by USPHS grants MH 17871 and MH 15642 and by the State of Connecticut.

REFERENCES

1. Aghajanian GK. Serotonin-induced inward current in rat facial motoneurons: evidence for mediation by G proteins but not protein kinase C. *Brain Res* 1990;524:171–174.
2. Aghajanian GK, Sprouse JS, Rasmussen K. Physiology of the midbrain serotonin system. In: Meltzer HY, ed. *Psychopharmacology: The third generation of progress.* New York: Raven Press, 1987; 141–149.
3. Aghajanian GK, Rasmussen K. Intracellular studies in the facial nucleus illustrating a simple new method for obtaining viable motoneurons in adult rat brain slices. *Synapse* 1989;3:331–338.
4. Andrade R, Chaput Y. 5-HT$_4$-like receptors mediate the slow excitatory response to serotonin in the rat hippocampus. *J Pharmacol Exp Ther* 1991;257:930–937.

5. Andrade R, Nicoll RA. Pharmacologically distinct actions of serotonin on single pyramidal neurones of the rat hippocampus recorded in vitro. *J Physiol (Lond)* 1987;394:99–124.

6. Araneda R, Andrade R. 5-Hydroxytryptamine$_2$ and 5-hydroxytryptamine$_{1A}$ receptors mediate opposing responses on membrane excitability in rat association cortex. *Neuroscience* 1991;40:399–412.

7. Ashby CR Jr, Edwards E, Harkins K, Wang RY. Characterization of 5-hydroxytryptamine-3 receptors in the medial prefrontal cortex: a microiontophoretic study. *Eur J Pharmacol* 1989;173:193–196.

8. Ashby CR Jr, Jiang LH, Kasser RJ, Wang RY. Electrophysiological characterization of 5-hydroxytryptamine-2 receptors in rat medial prefrontal cortex. *J Pharmacol Exp Ther* 1989;252:171–178.

9. Beck SG. 5-Carboxyamidotryptamine mimics only the 5-HT elicited hyperpolarization of hippocampal pyramidal cells via 5-HT$_{1A}$ receptor. *Neurosci Lett* 1989;99:101–106.

10. Blier P, Lista A, deMontigny C. Differential properties of pre- and postsynaptic 5-hydroxytryptamine$_{1A}$ receptors in the dorsal raphe and hippocampus. I. Effect of spiperone. *J Pharmacol Exp Ther* 1992;265:7–15.

11. Blier P, Steinberg S, Chaput Y, deMontigny C. Electrophysiological assessment of putative antagonists of 5-hydroxytryptamine receptors: a single-cell study in the dorsal raphe nucleus. *Can J Physiol Pharmacol* 1989;67:98–105.

13. Bobker DH, Williams JT. Serotonin agonists inhibit synaptic potentials in the rat locus ceruleus in vitro via 5-hydroxytryptamine$_{1A}$ and 5-hydroxytryptamine$_{1B}$ receptors. *J Pharmacol Exp Ther* 1989;250:37–43.

14. Bobker DH, Williams JT. Serotonin augments the cationic current I_h in central neurons. *Neuron* 1989;2:1535–1540.

15. Bobker DH, Williams JT. Serotonin-mediated inhibitory postsynaptic potential in guinea-pig prepositus hypoglossi and feedback inhibition by serotonin. *J Physiol (Lond)* 1990;422:447–462.

16. Bockaert J, Fozard JR, Dumuis A, Clarke DE. The 5-HT$_4$ receptor: a place in the sun. *Trends Pharmacol Sci* 1992;13:141–145.

17. Carter BD, Medzihradsky F. G$_o$ mediates the coupling of the μ opioid receptor to adenylyl cyclase in cloned neural cells and brain. *Proc Natl Acad Sci USA* 1993;90:4062–4066.

18. Chalmers DT, Watson SJ. Comparative anatomical distribution of 5-HT$_{1A}$ receptor mRNA and 5-HT$_{1A}$ binding in rat brain—a combined in situ hybridisation/in vitro receptor autoradiographic study. *Brain Res* 1991;561:51–60.

19. Chaput Y, Araneda RC, Andrade R. Pharmacological and functional analysis of a novel serotonin receptor in the rat hippocampus. *Eur J Pharmacol* 1990;182:441–456.

20. Charlety PJ, Aston-Jones G, Akaoka H, Buda M, Chouvet G. 5-HT decreases glutamate-evoked activation of locus coeruleus neurons through 5-HT 1A receptors. *Neurophysiology* 1991;421–426.

21. Clement HW, Gemsa D, Wesemann W. Serotonin-norepinephrine interactions: a voltammetric study on the effect of serotonin receptor stimulation followed in the N. raphe dorsalis and the locus coeruleus of the rat. *J Neural Trans* 1992;88:11–23.

22. Crain SM, Crain B, Makman MH. Pertussis toxin blocks depressant effects of opioid, monoaminergic and muscarinic agonists on dorsal-horn network responses in spinal cord-ganglion cultures. *Brain Res* 1987;400:185–190.

23. Darrow EJ, Strahlendorf HK, Strahlendorf JC. Response of cerebellar Purkinje cells to serotonin and the 5-HT$_{1A}$ agonists 8-OH-DPAT and ipsapirone in vitro. *Eur J Pharmacol* 1990;175:145–153.

24. Davies MF, Deisz RA, Prince DA, Peroutka SJ. Two distinct effects of 5-hydroxytryptamine on single cortical neurons. *Brain Res* 1987;423:347–352.

25. Fagni L, Dumuis A, Sebben M, Bockaert J. The 5-HT$_4$ receptor subtype inhibits K$^+$ current in colliculi neurones via activation of a cyclic AMP-dependent protein kinase. *Br J Pharmacol* 1992;105:973–979.

26. Garratt JC, Alreja M, Aghajanian GK. LSD has high efficacy relative to serotonin in enhancing the cationic current I_h: intracellular studies in rat facial motoneurons. *Synapse* 1993;13:123–134.

27. Gellman RL, Aghajanian GK. Pyramidal cells in piriform cortex receive a convergence of inputs from monoamine activated GABAergic interneurons. *Brain Res* 1993;600:63–73.

28. Glaum SR, Brooks PA, Spyer KM, Miller RJ. 5-Hydroxytryptamine-3 receptors modulate synaptic activity in the rat nucleus tractus solitarius in vitro. *Brain Res* 1992;589:62–68.

29. Innis RB, Nestler EJ, Aghajanian GK. Evidence for G protein mediation of serotonin- and GABA$_B$-induced hyperpolarization of rat dorsal raphe neurons. *Brain Res* 1988;459:27–36.

30. Joels M, Shinnick-Gallagher P, Gallagher JP. Effect of serotonin and serotonin analogues on passive membrane properties of lateral septal neurons in vitro. *Brain Res* 1987;417:99–107.

31. Larkman PM, Kelly JS. Ionic mechanisms mediating 5-hydroxytryptamine- and noradrenaline-evoked depolarization of adult rat facial motoneurones. *J Physiol (Lond)* 1992;456:473–490.

32. Larkman PM, Penington NJ, Kelly JS. Electrophysiology of adult rat facial motoneurones: the effect of serotonin (5-HT) in a novel in vitro brainstem slice. *J Neurosci Methods* 1989;28:133–146.

33. Leslie RA, Moorman JM, Coulson A, Grahame-Smith DG. Serotonin$_{2/1C}$ receptor activation causes a localized expression of the immediate-early gene c-fos in rat brain: evidence for involvement of dorsal raphe nucleus projection fibres. *Neuroscience* 1993;53:457–463.

34. Lovenberg TW, Baron BM, de Lecea L, Miller JD, Prosser RA, Rea MA, Foye PE, Racke M, Slone AL, Siegel BW, Danielson PE, Sutcliffe JG, Erlander MG. A novel adenylyl cyclase-activating serotonin receptor (5-HT$_7$) implicated in the regulation of mammalian circadian rhythms. *Neuron* 1993;11:449–458.

35. Luebke JI, Greene RW, Semba K, Kamond A, McCarley RW, Reiner PB. Serotonin hyperpolarizes cholinergic low-threshold burst neurons in the rat laterodorsal tegmental nucleus in vitro. *Proc Natl Acad Sci USA* 1992;89:743–747.

36. Lum JT, Piercey MF. Electrophysiological evidence that spiperone is an antagonist of 5-HT$_{1A}$ receptors in the dorsal raphe nucleus. *Eur J Pharmacol* 1987;149:9–15.

37. Maricq AV, Peterson AS, Brake AJ, Myers RM, Julius D. Primary source and functional expression of the 5-HT$_3$ receptor, a serotonin-gated ion channel. *Science* 1991;254:432–437.

38. McCormick DA, Wang Z. Serotonin and noradrenaline excite GABAergic neurones of the guinea-pig and cat nucleus reticularis thalami. *J Physiol (Lond)* 1991;442:235–255.

39. McCormick DA, Williamson A. Convergence and divergence of neurotransmitter action in human cerebral cortex. *Proc Natl Acad Sci USA* 1989;86:8098–8102.

40. Mengod G, Nguyen H, Lee H, Waeber C, Lubbert H, Palacios JM. The distribution and cellular localization of 5-HT$_{1C}$ receptor mRNA in the rodent brain examined by in situ hybridization histochemistry. Comparison with receptor binding distribution. *Neuroscience* 1990;35:577–592.

41. Mengod G, Pompeiano M, Martinez-Mir MI, Palacios JM. Localization of the mRNA for the 5-HT$_2$ receptor by in situ hybridization histochemistry. Correlation with the distribution of receptor sites. *Brain Res* 1990;524:139–143.

42. Miquel MC, Doucet E, Boni C, El Mestikawy S, Matthiessen L, Daval G, Verge D, Hamon M. Central serotonin$_{1A}$ receptors: respective distributions of encoding mRNA, receptor protein and binding sites by in situ hybridization histochemistry, radioimmunohistochemistry and autoradiographic mapping in the rat brain. *Neurochem Int* 1991;19:453–465.

43. Monsma FJ Jr, Shen Y, Ward RP, Hamblin MW, Sibley DR. Cloning and expression of a novel serotonin receptor with high affinity for tricyclic psychotropic drugs. *Mol Pharmacol* 1993;43:320–327.

44. Nedergaard S, Flatman JA, Engberg I. Excitation of substantia nigra pars compacta neurones by 5-hydroxytryptamine in vitro. *NeuroReport* 1991;2:329–332.

45. Newberry NR. 5-HT$_{1A}$ receptors activate a potassium conductance in rat ventromedial hypothalamic neurones. *Eur J Pharmacol* 1992;210:209–212.

46. Newberry NR, Priestley T. A 5-HT$_1$-like receptor mediates a pertussis toxin-sensitive inhibition of rat ventromedial hypothalamic neurons in vitro. *Br J Pharmacol* 1988;95:6–8.

47. North RA, Uchimura N. 5-Hydroxytryptamine acts at 5-HT$_2$ receptors to decrease potassium conductance in rat nucleus accumbens neurones. *J Physiol (Lond)* 1989;417:1–12.

48. Pape HC, McCormick DA. Noradrenaline and serotonin selectively modulate thalamic burst firing by enhancing a hyperpolarization-activated cation current. *Nature* 1989;340:715–718.

49. Penington NJ, Kelly JS. Serotonin receptor activation reduces calcium current in an acutely dissociated adult central neuron. *Neuron* 1990;4:751–758.

50. Pennington NJ, Kelly JS, Fox AP. A study of the mechanism of Ca^{2+} current inhibition produced by serotonin in rat dorsal raphe neurons. *J Neurosci* 1991;11:3594–3609.

51. Pompeiano M, Palacios JM, Mengod G. Distribution and cellular localization of mRNA coding for 5-HT$_{1A}$ receptor in the rat: correlation with receptor binding. *J Neurosci* 1992;12:440–453.

52. Rahman S, Neuman RS. Activation of 5-HT$_2$ receptors facilitates depolarization of neocortical neurons by *N*-methyl-D-aspartate. *Eur J Pharmacol* 1993;231:347–354.

53. Rasmussen K, Aghajanian GK. Potency of antipsychotics in reversing the effects of a hallucinogenic drug on locus coeruleus neurons correlates with 5-HT$_2$ binding affinity. *Neuropsychopharmacology* 1988;1:101–107.

54. Rasmussen K, Aghajanian GK. Serotonin excitation of facial motoneurons: receptor subtype characterization. *Synapse* 1990;5:324–332.

55. Ropert N. Inhibitory action of serotonin in CA1 hippocampal neurons in vitro. *Neuroscience* 1988;26:69–81.

56. Ropert N, Guy N. Serotonin facilitates GABAergic transmission in the CA1 region of rat hippocampus in vitro. *J Physiol (Lond)* 1991;441:121–136.

57. Scroggs RS, Anderson EG. 5-HT$_1$ receptor agonists reduce the Ca^{++} component of sensory neuron action potentials. *Eur J Pharmacol* 1990;178:229–232.

58. Segal M. Serotonin attenuates a slow inhibitory postsynaptic potential in rat hippocampal neurons. *Neuroscience* 1990;36:631–641.

59. Segal M, Azmitia EC, Whitaker-Azmitia PM. Physiological effects of selective 5-HT$_{1A}$ and 5-HT$_{1B}$ ligands in rat hippocampus: comparison to 5-HT. *Brain Res* 1989;502:67–74.

60. Sheldon PW, Aghajanian GK. Serotonin (5-HT) induces IPSPs in pyramidal layer cells of rat piriform cortex: evidence for the involvement of a 5-HT$_2$-activated interneuron. *Brain Res* 1990;506:62–69.

61. Sheldon PW, Aghajanian GK. Excitatory responses to serotonin (5-HT) in neurons of the rat piriform cortex: evidence for mediation by 5-HT$_{1C}$ receptors in pyramidal cells and 5-HT$_2$ receptors in interneurons. *Synapse* 1991;9:208–218.

62. Smrcka AV, Hepler JR, Brown KO, Sternweis PC. Regulation of polyphosphoinositide-specific phospholipase C activity by purified G_q. *Science* 1991;251:804–808.

63. Stevens DR, McCarley RW, Greene RW. Serotonin$_1$ and serotonin$_2$ receptors hyperpolarize and depolarize separate populations of medial pontine reticular formation neurons in vitro. *Neuroscience* 1992;47:545–553.

64. Sugita S, Shen KZ, North RA. 5-Hydroxytryptamine is a fast excitatory transmitter at 5-HT$_3$ receptors in rat amygdala. *Neuron* 1992;8:199–203.

65. Tani A, Yoshihara Y, Mori K. Increase in cytoplasmic free Ca^{2+} elicited by noradrenalin and serotonin in cultured local interneurons of mouse olfactory bulb. *Neuroscience* 1992;49:193–199.

66. Todorovic S, Anderson EG. 5-HT$_2$ and 5-HT$_3$ receptors mediate two distinct depolarizing responses in rat dorsal root ganglion neurons. *Brain Res* 1990;511:71–79.

67. White SR, Fung SJ. Serotonin depolarizes cat spinal motoneurons in situ and decreases motoneuron afterhyperpolarizing potentials. *Brain Res* 1989;502:205–213.

68. Williams JT, Colmers WF, Pan ZZ. Voltage- and ligand-activated inwardly rectifying currents in dorsal raphe neurons in vitro. *J Neurosci* 1988;8:3499–3506.

69. Yakel JL, Jackson MB. 5-HT$_3$ receptors mediate rapid responses in cultured hippocampus and a clonal cell line. *Neuron* 1988;1:615–621.

70. Yakel JL, Shao XM, Jackson MB. The selectivity of the channel coupled to the 5-HT$_3$ receptor. *Brain Res* 1990;533:46–52.

71. Yamazaki J, Fukuda H, Nagao T, Ono H. 5-HT$_2$/5-HT$_{1C}$ receptor-mediated facilitatory action on unit activity of ventral horn cells in rat spinal cord slices. *Eur J Pharmacol* 1992;220:237–242.

72. Zgombick JM, Beck SG, Mahle CD, Craddock-Royal B, Maayani S. Pertussis toxin-sensitive guanine nucleotide-binding protein(s) couple adenosine A1 and 5-hydroxytryptamine$_{1A}$ receptors to the same effector system in rat hippocampus: biochemical and electrophysiological studies. *Mol Pharmacol* 1989;35:484–494.

Psychopharmacology: The Fourth Generation of Progress, edited by Floyd E. Bloom and David J. Kupfer. Raven Press, Ltd., New York © 1995.

CHAPTER 41

Serotonin and Behavior

A General Hypothesis

Barry L. Jacobs and Casimir A. Fornal

Serotonin is an enigma. It is at once implicated in virtually everything, but responsible for nothing. Its name also adds to this mystery. Unlike other neurotransmitters, such as glutamate, acetylcholine, and gamma-aminobutyric acid (GABA), whose names evoke images of test tubes and tiled laboratories, serotonin (5-hydroxytryptamine; 5-HT) conjures up visions of the esoteric and the exotic. This characterization was fostered by early theories and research which linked it to hallucinogenic drug action, schizophrenia, and depression. Modern neuroscience has added to the mystique surrounding 5-HT: Axon terminals containing 5-HT are found in even the remotest reaches of the central nervous system (CNS); the release of 5-HT may not be subject to classical synaptic physiology; and 5-HT acts at a bewildering diversity of pre- and postsynaptic receptor subtypes.

Research over the past several decades has led to the development of specific theories regarding the function of the related brainstem-originating neurotransmitter systems, dopamine and norepinephrine. Thus, as detailed in other chapters in this volume, dopamine appears to be involved primarily in response initiation and reward, whereas norepinephrine is believed to be concerned primarily with vigilance. By contrast, hypotheses regarding 5-HT's role in the CNS remain wide-ranging and include regulation of processes as diverse as cardiovascular and respiratory activity, sleep, aggression and sexual behavior, nutrient intake, anxiety, mood, motor output, neuroendocrine secretion, and nociception and analgesia (67).

This chapter sets forth a general theory of 5-HT func-

B. L. Jacobs and C. A. Fornal: Program in Neuroscience, Princeton University, Princeton, New Jersey 08544.

tion within the CNS. It is based largely upon our own single-unit studies of 5-HT neuronal activity in behaving cats. We believe that the primary function of 5-HT neurons is to facilitate gross motor output in both the tonic and repetitive modes. Concurrently, the system acts to inhibit sensory information processing and to coordinate autonomic and neuroendocrine function with the demands of ongoing motor output. Under certain conditions, when the 5-HT system is inactivated, these relationships are reversed: Tonic motor output is disfacilitated and sensory information processing is disinhibited.

We propose that the diversity of behavioral and physiological processes in which 5-HT has been implicated can be subsumed within this integrative perspective. Additionally, we believe that the elucidation of 5-HT's role in human psychopathology is embedded within its basic biology. Accordingly, this chapter focuses upon the motor aspects of the 5-HT system, with some attention also given to its role in sensory and physiological processes (see also Chapters 39 and 40, *this volume*).

ANATOMY

From the time of its initial description with fluorescence histochemistry, the anatomy of the CNS 5-HT system was known to be extremely widespread (see Chapter 39, *this volume*). Of all the neurotransmitter systems within the vertebrate CNS, the 5-HT system is the most expansive. Nonetheless, this innervation pattern is neither ubiquitous nor nonspecific. Even within a particular target site some portions may receive a very dense 5-HT input, whereas neighboring regions may be only sparsely innervated. Additionally, some brain regions are almost devoid of 5-HT innervation.

Of special note regarding the distribution of 5-HT axon terminals is a preferential targeting of primary and secondary motor areas in the CNS (56). For example, in the rat there is a very dense innervation of the ventral horn, the motor nucleus of the trigeminal (MoV), the facial motor nucleus (MoVII), the substantia nigra, and the globus pallidus. As many as 13% of all the synaptic contacts in MoV of the rat are 5-HT-immunoreactive (54). Another interesting feature of the input to motor areas is its lack of homogeneity. In the ventral horn of the spinal cord, for example, the 5-HT input preferentially innervates motoneurons projecting to axial rather than distal musculature (56). In the brainstem of a variety of species there is dense innervation of motoneurons projecting to the large muscles of the jaw, face, and neck, but the extraocular muscles receive only sparse 5-HT input (56,60). Also noteworthy is the fact that the input to the cerebellum is relatively sparse. This pattern of differential innervation of motor structures reveals something about the function of the 5-HT system. It implies that 5-HT should be more strongly associated with movements employing gross skeletal muscles rather than those utilizing fine or discrete muscles. Thus, as we have seen, there is a denser input to the medial portion of the ventral horn, where axial motoneurons serving the trunk and limbs are found, as compared to the lateral portions, where distal motoneurons serving paws and digits are found. Similarly, in the brainstem, there is a much denser 5-HT input to MoV and MoVII, controlling jaw and facial muscles, respectively, as compared to the nuclei controlling eye movements. Consistent with this is the relatively weak 5-HT projection to the cerebellum, a structure associated more with the smoothing or adjustment of movements rather than with their direct execution.

If 5-HT neurons in the CNS projected exclusively to motor nuclei, this fact alone would constitute a strong case for the primacy of motor function for this system. There are, however, a multitude of other projections, some quite dense, to non-motor targets such as the hippocampus, the dorsal horn, dorsal column nuclei (DCN), and so on. This anatomical pattern is part of a larger picture that interrelates motor outflow to sensory information processing and to autonomic and neuroendocrine regulation. A couple of examples may help to clarify this point. It is known that 5-HT plays an important role in the regulation of the theta rhythm in the hippocampus and that this rhythm is often related to different types of motor patterns (35,62). Although the DCN are primary sensory nuclei, the dense 5-HT input to these sites in cats and monkeys selectively innervates those portions of the nuclei involved in motor function (i.e., projections to cerebellum, pretectum, inferior olive, etc.) rather than those

portions involved in fine somatosensory discrimination (i.e., projections to VPL of the thalamus) (6).

Finally, it is worth noting that the basic plan of 5-HT cell bodies and axon terminals is a primitive one, found in the simplest vertebrate brains, and one that remains remarkably conserved across phylogeny (45).

5-HT AND BEHAVIOR

One of the earliest findings regarding 5-HT and behavior came from studies employing its biosynthetic precursors L-5-hydroxytryptophan (5-HTP) and L-tryptophan. When these compounds are administered to any of a variety of mammals, a distinctive and complex syndrome, comprised of tonic and repetitive motor outputs, is produced. Its most conspicuous signs are tremor, rigidity, hindlimb abduction, Straub tail, head shakes or "wet dog" shakes, lateral head weaving, and reciprocal treading of the forepaws (20). (Similar effects are also seen in infra-mammalian vertebrates.) It is also clear that most of these motor signs can be elicited by drug treatment very early in ontogeny (e.g., in 3- to 4-day-old rat pups), thus implying that the system is at least partially functional at or near birth (50).

Equally relevant for the present discussion is the less-well-known fact that this "serotonin syndrome" is also seen in human patients administered 5-HT drugs (58). Most important is the fact that the effects observed are restricted almost exclusively to motor signs (myoclonus, tremor, shivering), with few, if any, indications of significant sensory alterations. Consistent with this, various drugs influencing 5-HT neurotransmission have also been reported to produce repetitive chewing or bruxism (tooth grinding) in rats and humans (46,59).

The actions of 5-HT drugs on more discrete aspects of behavior, such as treadmill-induced locomotion in spinal cats, have also been examined (3). The most prominent action of 5-HT here is to increase the flexor and extensor burst amplitude (a smaller increase is seen in burst duration) during locomotion. In this preparation 5-HT cannot by itself trigger locomotion and is assumed to act by increasing motoneuron excitability (4). In paralyzed rabbits, 5-HTP can enhance or even evoke reciprocal flexor and extensor hindlimb nerve activity, with the dominant effect seen in the flexors (64). We have examined the effects of injecting 5-HT directly into MoV in awake cats, and we have observed increases in both the amplitude of the tonic electromyogram (EMG) of the masseter muscle and the amplitude of an externally elicited jaw-closure (masseteric) reflex (49). Finally, 5-HT agonists or precursors evoke repetitive swallowing in anesthetized rats (5). These latter effects continued to be seen in decerebrate preparations, demonstrating that brainstem neural mechanisms were sufficient for their manifestation.

The varied species in which similar motor effects of 5-HT are seen supports the position that this 5-HT system subserves a common functional role across the vertebrates (20).

EFFECTS ON TARGET CELLS

The effects of 5-HT on motoneurons has been examined in the rat spinal cord and brainstem (36,68). By itself, 5-HT produces little or no change in neuronal activity (however, it is important to bear in mind that such studies are typically carried out on animals with reduced excitatory drive to these neurons—that is, either those under anesthesia or in reduced preparations). However, when 5-HT is combined with direct application of excitatory amino acids or with electrical stimulation of dorsal roots or motor cortex, it produces a strong facilitation of neuronal activity. This effect has been characterized as a bistability with a 5-HT-induced shift from a stable hyperpolarized state, with little or no neuronal activity, to a new stable depolarized "plateau" state, with tonic neuronal activity (19).

Similar analyses have also been carried out in a more complex situation, where cortical stimulation is used to elicit rhythmic masticatory-like activity in anesthetized guinea pigs (27). The activity of digastric (jaw opener) motoneurons is directly facilitated by the iontophoretic application of 5-HT, but, as above, only in the presence of glutamate or electrical excitation of these neurons. Additionally, iontophoretic application of 5-HT can facilitate and bring to threshold rhythmic digastric motoneuronal discharges during subthreshold repetitive cortical stimulation. A similar picture is seen when one examines the influence of 5-HT upon the neuronal mechanisms mediating fictive locomotion (swimming) in the isolated spinal cord of the lamprey (15). When applied to the spinal cord or to reticulospinal neurons, 5-HT elicits a depression of the afterhyperpolarization (AHP) that normally follows the action potential. Because the AHP is the primary factor in determining discharge frequency, this depression produces an increase in motoneuron discharge. If 5-HT is applied to the solution bathing the isolated spinal cord during fictive locomotion, motoneuronal bursts become more intense and longer, and the burst rate increases. 5-HT also modulates the intersegmental phase delay in the lamprey spinal cord, an integral component of coordinated swimming (18).

Although the literature is not as extensive and the data perhaps not as clearcut as its effects on motoneurons, 5-HT consistently is reported to inhibit primary sensory neurons in the forebrain. Once again, these studies are conducted primarily in anesthetized rats (see ref. 38 for a review). Iontophoretic application of 5-HT to relay neurons in the rat dorsal lateral geniculate nucleus (LGN)

suppressed spontaneous activity as well as that evoked by light flashes or electrical stimulation of the optic chiasm (51). In related experiments, high-frequency stimulation of 5-HT cell bodies produced an inhibition of LGN activity lasting for periods as long as several tens of seconds (28).

Comparable effects of 5-HT are seen in neocortex of anesthetized rats. When neurons are activated by somatosensory stimuli, iontophoretically applied 5-HT consistently suppresses this evoked activity to a greater degree than background or basal activity, resulting in a decrease in signal/noise ratio (66). Similar effects are seen when 5-HT's actions are examined on primary visual cortex neurons. The responses evoked by stimuli moving across the visual field were suppressed by 5-HT to a greater extent than was the basal activity of these cells (65). Of particular interest is the fact that norepinephrine consistently produces a complementary effect to that of 5-HT in both the LGN and neocortex—that is, an increase in signal/noise ratio (see ref. 38 for a review).

In summary, 5-HT's effect on alpha motoneurons is one of excitation, whereas its effect on primary sensory neurons is that of inhibition.

BASIC PROPERTIES OF 5-HT NEURONS

Over the past 20 years, much of the basic neurophysiology of 5-HT neurons in the various brainstem raphe nuclei—dorsalis (DRN), medianus (NRM), magnus (MRN), and pallidus (NRPa)—has been worked out (22). The neurons are autoactive, discharging in a stereotyped, almost clock-like manner, with an intrinsic frequency of 1–5 spikes/sec. The membrane properties that accompany this slow regular activity have been described, as have the ionic currents and channels mediating it (see Chapter 40, *this volume*). Additionally, at least in the rat, these basic neuronal properties are manifested early in development (3–4 days prenatal). Finally, there is a negative feedback mechanism which limits 5-HT neuronal activity. As activity increases and 5-HT is released locally from dendrites or axon collaterals, it acts upon somatodendritic 5-HT "autoreceptors" to inhibit neuronal activity. The mechanism functions only under physiological conditions in the sense that it is inoperative with low levels of neuronal activity, but becomes increasingly engaged as neuronal activity increases (see below) (23). Dysfunction of this regulatory mechanism may be implicated in some forms of human pathology, and therefore drugs targeted at these autoreceptors provide a potentially important site of therapeutic intervention.

One of the first significant discoveries about brain 5-HT neurons was that their activity was dramatically altered across the sleep–wake–arousal cycle (23,39). From a stable, slow, and regular discharge pattern of, for example, 3 spikes/sec during quiet waking, neuronal activity displays a gradual decline as the animal becomes drowsy and enters slow-wave sleep. A decrease in the regularity of firing accompanies this overall slowing of activity during sleep. During rapid eye movement (REM) sleep, 5-HT neuronal activity falls silent, but in anticipation of awakening, neuronal activity returns to its basal level, or above, several seconds prior to the end of the REM sleep epoch. During an aroused or active waking state, discharge rate may increase to 4 or 5 spikes/sec.

RESPONSE OF 5-HT NEURONS TO CHALLENGES

Because brain 5-HT has been implicated in such a variety of physiological processes (thermoregulation, cardiovascular control, respiration, etc.) and behaviors (aggression, nutrient intake, sleep, etc.), it was deemed imperative to examine 5-HT neuronal activity under a wide diversity of conditions. Accordingly, while recording the activity of 5-HT neurons in the DRN, MRN, or NRM, we exposed cats to the following conditions: loud noise, physical restraint, a natural enemy (dog), a variety of mildly painful stimuli, a heated environment or systemic administration of a pyrogen, drug-induced increases or decreases in blood pressure, or insulin-induced glucoprivation.

Exposing a cat to 100 dB of white noise for 15 min elicits strong sympathetic activation, as indicated by significant increases in tonic heart rate and plasma norepinephrine levels. It also evokes a stereotyped behavioral response of crouching, with ears flattened. Despite this, during the presentation of this stimulus, the activity of DRN 5-HT neurons was not significantly different from that observed during an undisturbed active waking baseline (70).

Similarly, when cats were physically restrained for 15 min, this also evoked a strong sympathetic activation. Struggling and vocalizations during the restraint provided additional behavioral evidence for the stressful nature of the stimulus. Once again, despite the behavioral and physiological activation produced by restraint, the activity of DRN neurons was not significantly different from that observed during the pre-stress baseline condition (70).

In the final experiment in this series, a dog was brought into proximity of the cat for 5 min. This evoked the typical stereotyped feline defense reaction of arched back, facing broadside, piloerection, often growling and hissing, and physiologic indices of sympathetic activation. However, despite this behavioral and physiological activation evoked by the dog, the discharge rate of DRN neurons was once again unchanged from that observed during an undisturbed active waking baseline (70).

A related series of studies examined the response of 5-HT neurons in the NRM to a variety of phasic or tonic painful stimuli. There was no change in neuronal activity in response to any of these stimuli, when compared to an active waking baseline (2). There was also no change in activity in response to the systemic administration of morphine in a dose that produced analgesia (2). These results are consistent with a recent study reporting that identified NRM 5-HT neurons in the rat are not activated by painful stimuli eliciting the withdrawal reflex (47).

Thus, as a whole, these data indicate that the activity of 5-HT neurons cannot easily be driven above the level observed during an undisturbed active waking baseline. This is in spite of the fact that the stimuli employed in these studies evoked a variety of different forms of behavioral arousal and strong sympathetic activation. Finally, contrary to the present results with 5-HT neurons, the same stimuli were effective in strongly activating a neighboring brainstem neurochemical system, the noradrenergic neurons of the locus coeruleus (LC) (reviewed in ref. 21).

Paralleling these studies of behavioral/environmental challenges, we also examined the response of DRN 5-HT neurons during perturbation of several physiological regulatory systems.

The activity of DRN neurons was examined in response to both increased ambient temperature and pyrogen-induced fever, stimuli eliciting opposite thermoregulatory responses (11). For environmental heating, the temperature in the experimental chamber was raised to 43°C. The activity of DRN neurons remained unaffected during the interval when ambient temperature was increased from 25°C to 43°C. During this initial phase of heating, no appreciable behavioral or physiologic responses were seen. However, following prolonged heat exposure, cats displayed intense continuous panting, relaxation of posture, and a progressive rise in body/brain temperature (range: 0.5°C to 2.0°C). Once again, however, no change in DRN single-unit activity was observed. DRN neuronal activity was also examined during the febrile response elicited by systemic administration of a synthetic pyrogen (muramyl dipeptide). Following drug administration, body/brain temperature began to increase within 30 min, reached a peak at 1–2 hr, and returned to predrug level by 6 hr. The peak elevation of body temperature that was attained was typically 1.5°C to 2.5°C. Once again, no change in DRN single-unit activity was observed during any phase of the pyrogen-induced febrile response.

The response of DRN neurons was also studied in relation to changes in blood pressure induced by peripherally acting drugs: Phenylephrine induces increases in blood pressure, sodium nitroprusside phasically decreases blood pressure, and hydralazine produces prolonged hypotension (13). Over a range of 20- to 70-mmHg increases and 10- to 50-mmHg decreases in mean arterial pressure, there was no change in the discharge rate of DRN 5-HT neurons. This is despite the fact that these blood pressure changes were of sufficient magnitude to produce significant reflexive changes in heart rate and plasma catecholamines.

The final study in this series manipulated blood glucose levels in both directions. The activity of DRN 5-HT neurons in behaving cats was not significantly altered by bolus injection of glucose (500 mg/kg, i.v.) that elevated blood glucose levels threefold (12). Likewise, the activity of these neurons was not significantly affected by the administration of a dose of insulin (2–4 IU/kg, i.v.), which lowered blood glucose by 50% or more, or following the rapid reversal of this hypoglycemia by subsequent glucose administration.

As we have seen with environmental stressors, physiologic challenges to the animal also fail to significantly activate brain 5-HT neurons above the level seen during an undisturbed active waking state. Once again, this is in spite of the fact that these manipulations produce behavioral arousal as well as activate the organism's sympathetic nervous system. And as with environmental stressors, these same physiologic challenges do significantly activate noradrenergic neurons in the cat LC (reviewed in ref. 21).

5-HT NEURONAL ACTIVITY AND MOTOR FUNCTION

A fundamental feature of REM sleep is a paralysis mediated by inhibition of motoneurons controlling antigravity muscle tone. Because the activity of 5-HT neurons is totally suppressed during REM sleep, we examined the possibility that there might be a relationship between these two phenomena. Lesions of the dorsomedial pons produces a condition which permits investigation of this issue. Cats with this lesion enter a stage of sleep which by all criteria appears to be REM sleep except antigravity muscle tone is present and the animals are thus capable of movement and even coordinated locomotion (26) [this condition has also been observed in humans (34)].

During both waking and slow-wave sleep, the activity of DRN 5-HT neurons in these pontine-lesioned cats was similar to that in normal animals (61). However, when these animals entered REM sleep, neuronal activity increased instead of displaying the decrease typical of this state. Those animals displaying the greatest amount of muscle tone and overt behavior during REM sleep showed the highest levels of neuronal activity, with some of their 5-HT neurons discharging at a level approximating that of the waking state.

If the cholinomimetic agent carbachol is microinjected into this same pontine area, a condition somewhat reciprocal to non-atonia REM sleep can be produced. These animals were awake, as demonstrated by their ability to track stimuli visually, but were otherwise paralyzed. However, the activity of their DRN 5-HT neurons was silent (57). In the same study, we found that peripheral paralysis, induced by blocking transmission at the neuromuscular junction, had no effect on 5-HT neuronal activity, but that a centrally acting muscle relaxant also completely suppressed 5-HT neuronal activity.

These data suggest that a strong relationship exists between tonic motor activity and 5-HT neuronal discharge. More recently, we observed a relationship between 5-HT neuronal activity and another general type of motor output. When cats engage in a variety of types of central pattern generator (CPG)-mediated oral–buccal activities, such as chewing/biting, licking, or grooming the body surface with the tongue, approximately one-fourth of DRN and MRN 5-HT neurons increase their activity by as much as two- to fivefold (22,48). (The remaining 5-HT neurons simply maintain their state-related or tonic-motor-related clock-like activity.) The increased neuronal activity often precedes the onset of movement by several seconds, but typically terminates coincident with the offset of the behavior. It is also occasionally phase-locked to the repetitive responses. Some of these neurons are also activated by somatosensory and proprioceptive stimulation of the head and neck area. During a variety of other purposive episodic or phasic movements, even those involving the oral–buccal area, no increase in neuronal activity is observed; in fact a slight decrease is often seen. Under some conditions involving gross behavior, a dramatic decrease in neuronal activity is observed. For example, if an arousing stimulus elicits an orienting response (evidenced by suppression of overt behavior and foveation toward the source of the stimulus), 5-HT neuronal activity in the DRN or MRN may fall silent for several seconds and then resume its normal activity (25).

A somewhat complementary picture emerges when one examines the activity of NRP 5-HT neurons, the primary source of 5-HT innervation of ventral horn motoneurons. These 5-HT neurons are activated (two- to threefold) in association with repetitive behaviors mediated by spinal cord CPGs, such as treadmill locomotion or hyperpnea (induced by exposure to CO_2) (63). In some cases there is a strong positive correlation between neuronal activity and speed of locomotion or rate/depth of respiration. Neuronal activity may also increase in association with tonic motor changes such as postural shifts. As with DRN neurons, the activity of NRP 5-HT neurons is occasionally phase-locked to the repetitive responses.

These cellular data from behaving animals have led us to the following conclusions. There is a general relationship between level of tonic motor activity and 5-HT neuronal activity. Superimposed upon this in some neurons is an additional relationship in which a further, often dramatic, neuronal activation is seen in association with repetitive CPG-mediated behaviors. Reciprocally, during the active inhibition of gross behavior (e.g., during orientation), 5-HT neuronal activity is suppressed. We hypothesize that the processing of sensory information is inhibited during the activation of tonic or repetitive motor activity but is disinhibited during the suppression of gross motor outflow.

RELATIONSHIP BETWEEN MOTOR AND SENSORY PROCESSES

The study of motor and sensory systems is typically carried out separately. However, there is abundant information that these two systems often interact to influence each other. For example, in both animals and humans, there is evidence that sensory transmission is suppressed during gross bodily movements (8,9). This is illustrated by the fact that just prior to and during arm movements in the monkey, somatosensory evoked potentials elicited by an irrelevant peripheral stimulus are depressed by as much as 60–70% at the lemniscal, thalamic, and cortical levels (9). Additionally, the single-unit response of thalamic and cortical neurons to somatosensory stimuli is suppressed during locomotion in the rat (55). Relevant to these physiological results, the anatomy of 5-HT inputs to sensory neurons indicates that they exert a direct influence at an early stage of processing. For example, in the primate visual cortex, 5-HT preferentially innervates layer IV, suggesting an effect on those cortical neurons that are the direct recipients of the inputs deriving from the LGN (10).

We believe that a similar motor–sensory interaction mechanism may explain 5-HT's well-established involvement in analgesia. As noted above, 5-HT neurons in NRM are neither activated by a variety of painful stimuli nor activated by an analgesic dose of morphine (2,47). Thus, the NRM 5-HT system does not constitute a pure primary antinociception or analgesic system per se. However, under physiological conditions, the suppression of nociception by 5-HT, at both forebrain and spinal levels, may occur as a concomitant of tonic or repetitive motor outflow. Reciprocally, as discussed above, sensory transmission may be enhanced during periods when the activity of 5-HT neurons is suppressed—for example, during orientation. Consistent with this, it is well known that ponto-geniculate-occipital cortex (PGO) waves are held under tonic 5-HT inhibition (53) and that these potentials can be evoked by exposing the behaving animal to strong phasic stimuli which elicit orienting responses (7). Additionally, under pharmacologic conditions, when 5-HT neurotransmission is compromised, this disinhibition of sensory processing is manifested as increased responsiveness or enhanced excitability or sensitivity in a variety of paradigms, including nociception (31,69) (see further discussion of this issue in the final section of this chapter).

In a similar manner, we hypothesize that 5-HT neurons facilitate the well-known sympathetic activation that accompanies, and even anticipates, motor activity (16). For a recent review of the sympathoexcitatory effects of 5-HT in the intermediolateral column of the spinal cord, see ref. 37. 5-HT has also been shown to facilitate the activity of respiratory (phrenic nerve) motor neurons in the rat spinal cord (e.g., see ref. 42). In this context, recall, as described above, that 5-HT neuronal activation often precedes increases in motor activity or muscle tone. Thus, an important ancillary role of 5-HT neurons may be the activation of physiological regulatory systems, such as those controlling cardiovascular activity and respiration, in the service of increasing motor demands.

GENERALITY ACROSS PHYLOGENY

5-HT function in invertebrates provides striking parallels to many aspects of the data from vertebrates described in this chapter. This is impressive, in view of the enormous differences in their gross bodily morphology, ecological niche (terrestrial versus aquatic for the invertebrates in these studies), and general organizational pattern of their nervous systems (brain versus ganglionic). Several examples will help to make this point. First, direct injection of 5-HT into the systemic circulation of several arthropods results in a general motor change (29,33). Second, when it has been examined, for example in lobsters, 5-HT neurons are found to be endogenously active (33). In both lobsters and aplysia, 5-HT neurons discharge with a slow and regular pattern (0.5–1.0 Hz) that can increase to 2–5 Hz during feeding or with postural changes (30,33). Furthermore, in Aplysia the 5-HT metacerebral cell alters its somewhat regular firing pattern to become phase-locked to oral–buccal movements during feeding (30). Third, in several molluscs, arthropods, and annelids, 5-HT modulates, rather than mediates, motor outflow, often by acting on CPGs (17). The involvement in motor control appears to be with both tonic (e.g., posture) (29) and repetitive (e.g., swimming, biting, etc.) outputs (17,43). Finally, in Aplysia and leeches, 5-HT exerts its effects on behavior at multiple levels (e.g., directly on muscles, on CPGs, on the cardiovascular system, etc.) (30,32).

CLINICAL IMPLICATIONS

As detailed in other chapters in this volume, 5-HT has been implicated strongly in the etiology and/or treatment of several forms of psychopathology, most notably depression and obsessive–compulsive disorders (OCDs). Do these results from basic research on brain 5-HT provide any insights into these clinical disorders? Recall that the activity of the brain 5-HT neurons is at an elevated level during increased tonic motor output and that for a subgroup of neurons it achieves an even higher level of activity during repetitive motor acts. Thus, if there is a deficit in 5-HT neurotransmission in at least some forms of depression, then it might be beneficial for such patients to increase their tonic motor activity or to engage in some form of simple repetitive motor task, such as riding a bicycle or jogging. Consistent with this, there are scattered reports of the salutary effects of jogging or other forms of exercise for depressed patients (e.g., see refs. 14,41, and 44) and, more generally, reports of exercise exerting mood-altering effects in nondepressed subjects (e.g., see refs. 40 and 52).

On the basis of our research we have also arrived at a novel way of viewing OCDs. Because repetitive or compulsive motor acts increase 5-HT neuronal activity, we believe that patients with OCD may be engaging in such behaviors as a means of self-treatment. In other words, they are activating their brain 5-HT system in a physiological manner in order to derive some (as yet unknown) benefit or rewarding effect. Treating them with drugs that block the reuptake of 5-HT into the presynaptic neuron accomplishes the same neurochemical endpoint and thus allows them to disengage from time-consuming, socially unacceptable, and often physically harmful behaviors. (The same case could also be made for repetitive obsessional thoughts, but this, obviously, is difficult to examine in the laboratory.)

Finally, because 5-HT neuronal activity, and therefore neurotransmitter release, is under negative feedback control, this provides a potentially productive avenue for drug intervention in the clinic. Administration of precursors of 5-HT, such as tryptophan or 5-HTP, are of limited value for elevating synaptic levels of brain 5-HT because they produce a compensatory decrease in neuronal activity through this negative feedback mechanism (1). However, if these treatments were combined with a low dose of an autoreceptor (5-HT$_{1A}$) antagonist drug, they might be of therapeutic value and thus capitalize on the advantage of employing natural biological precursors rather than synthetic drugs. Additionally, because of the rate-dependency of the feedback mechanism, our data suggest that autoreceptor antagonist drugs might be ineffective in quiescent, lethargic, or somnolent patients, but quite effective in spontaneously active patients or perhaps those activated by artificial means.

SUMMARY AND OVERVIEW

During an undisturbed waking state, brain 5-HT neurons discharge in a slow and rhythmic manner that is a manifestation of their endogenous pacemaker activity. This regular firing during waking creates a steady synaptic release of 5-HT which provides a tonic excitatory drive

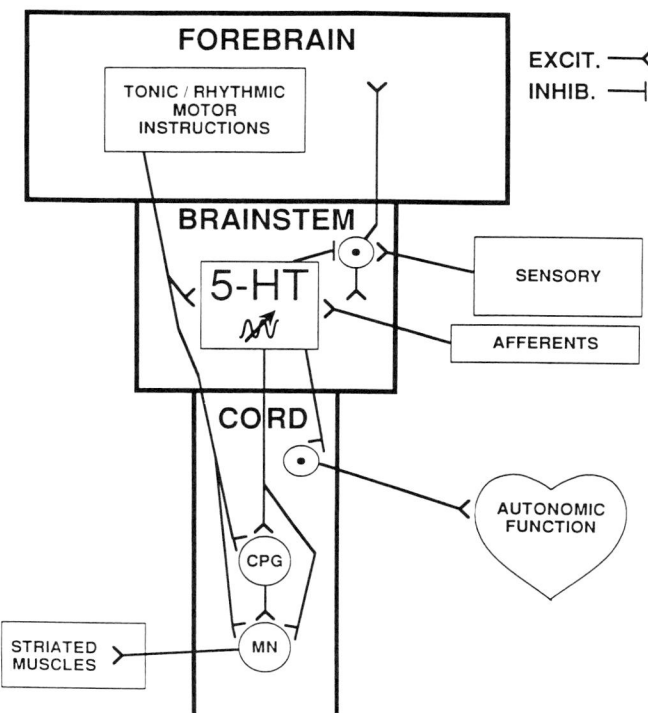

FIG. 1. Schematic representation of the major components of the motor hypothesis of 5-HT function. When voluntary tonic or rhythmic motor outflow is initiated, forebrain motor commands are simultaneously sent to alpha motoneurons (MN) and/or brainstem or spinal cord central pattern generators (CPG) and to brainstem 5-HT neurons. The output of 5-HT neurons serves several functions simultaneously: It facilitates CPG and α motoneuron activity, orchestrates autonomic and neuroendocrine (not shown) output with motor outflow, and inhibits sensory information processing. 5-HT neurons are shown to be driven by an endogenous oscillator (*sine wave with arrow*) and to be phasically activated by various afferents. Not shown is the possibility that different groups of 5-HT neurons may facilitate different motor functions (e.g., NRPa and respiration, DRN and oral–buccal movements, etc.). (Adapted from ref. 24.)

that modulates motor system neuronal activity. During gross repetitive motor behaviors that are mediated by brainstem and spinal cord CPGs, subpopulations of 5-HT neurons are activated (Fig. 1), attaining discharge levels several times greater than that observed during undisturbed waking. This activation, seen in association with chewing, grooming, running, and so on, is sometimes phase-locked to the cycling motor output. The distribution of 5-HT axon terminals in the spinal cord and brainstem is consistent with 5-HT's involvement in patterned movement employing gross skeletal muscles rather than those movements utilizing fine or more discrete muscles.

Several important functions may be served by these 5-HT inputs to motor structures. They may smooth motor outputs and may also obviate the need for continuous repetitive excitatory inputs to maintain a continuous output in motor systems. By augmenting weak or polysynaptic inputs, 5-HT may also bring motoneurons to threshold. The anticipation of motor activity by 5-HT neurons suggests that they may serve a priming function for motor output. 5-HT may also serve a timing or integrative function. The simultaneous inhibition of ''irrelevant'' sensory information processing acts to suppress inputs that might disrupt motor output (Fig. 1). Reciprocally, when 5-HT neuronal activity is phasically decreased, for example, during orientation, this serves to sharpen sensory function while disfacilitating tonic or repetitive motor output and thereby preventing it from disrupting sensory processing. Furthermore, motoneurons are now poised to respond phasically to discrete excitatory inputs. Finally, 5-HT's involvement in autonomic and neuroendocrine regulation serves a support function for the demands of changes in the level of motor output (Fig. 1), such as (a) increased oxygenation of the blood and increased blood flow to skeletal muscles or (b) increased carbohydrate consumption for maintaining a stable glucose supply to the brain.

It is parsimonious to hypothesize that 5-HT serves an integrative and overarching function in the CNS, rather than to assume that it is discretely and separately involved in a diversity of behavioral and physiological processes. The apparent involvement of 5-HT in this variety of functions is attributable to the fact that it is a widely projecting system that exerts a biasing influence over its target structures. In most experimental studies in this field the level of 5-HT synaptic transmission is perturbed far beyond the physiological range achieved under environmental or biological conditions, such as those described above. This comes about because, typically, the manipulations grossly influence 5-HT either by destroying 5-HT neurons, inhibiting its synthesis, blocking its receptors, preventing its reuptake into the presynaptic terminal, or by precursor loading. This, in turn, either by causing a general increase in motor activity or skeletal muscle tone, or by making the organism generally overreactive to environmental stimuli, biases whatever behavioral or physiological output is under examination (Also see Chapters 25 and 32 for behavioral overviews of other monoamine systems.)

ACKNOWLEDGMENTS

The authors' research described in this chapter was supported by grants from the AFOSR (90-0294) and the NIMH (MH 23433). Special thanks to Ms. Arlene Kronewitter for preparing this manuscript.

REFERENCES

1. Aghajanian GK. Feedback regulation of central monoaminergic neurons: evidence from single cell recording studies. In: Youdim MBH, Lovenberg W, Sharman DR, Lagnado JR, eds. *Essays in neurochemistry and neuropharmacology.* New York: John Wiley & Sons, 1978;1–32.
2. Auerbach S, Fornal C, Jacobs BL. Response of serotonin-containing neurons in nucleus raphe magnus to morphine, noxious stimuli, and periaqueductal gray stimulation in freely moving cats. *Exp Neurol* 1985;88:609–628.
3. Barbeau H, Rossignol S. The effects of serotonergic drugs on the locomotor pattern and on cutaneous reflexes of the adult chronic spinal cat. *Brain Res* 1990;514:55–67.
4. Barbeau H, Rossignol S. Initiation and modulation of the locomotor pattern in the adult chronic spinal cat by noradrenergic, serotonergic and dopaminergic drugs. *Brain Res* 1991;546:250–260.
5. Bieger D. Role of bulbar serotonergic neurotransmission in the initiation of swallowing in the rat. *Neuropharmacology* 1981; 20:1073–1083.
6. Blomqvist A, Broman J. Serotonergic innervation of the dorsal column nuclei and its relation to cytoarchitectonic subdivisions: an immunohistochemical study in cats and monkeys (*Aotus trivirgatus*). *J Comp Neurol* 1993;327:584–596.
7. Bowker RM, Morrison AR. The startle reflex and PGO spikes. *Brain Res* 1976;102:185–190.
8. Chapin JK. Modulation of cutaneous sensory transmission during movement: possible mechanisms and biological significance. In: Wise SP, ed. *Higher brain functions: recent explorations of the brain's emergent properties.* New York: John Wiley & Sons, 1987;181–209.
9. Chapman CE, Jiang W, Lamarre Y. Modulation of lemniscal input during conditioned arm movements in the monkey. *Exp Brain Res* 1989;72:316–334.
10. Foote SL, Morrison JH. Extrathalamic modulation of cortical function. *Annu Rev Neurosci* 1987;10:67–95.
11. Fornal CA, Litto WJ, Morilak DA, et al. Single-unit responses of serotonergic dorsal raphe nucleus neurons to environmental heating and pyrogen administration in freely moving cats. *Exp Neurol* 1987;98:388–403.
12. Fornal CA, Litto WJ, Morilak DA, et al. Single-unit responses of serotonergic neurons to glucose and insulin administration in behaving cats. *Am J Physiol* 1989;257:R1345–R1353.
13. Fornal CA, Litto WJ, Morilak DA, et al. Single-unit responses of serotonergic dorsal raphe neurons to vasoactive drug administration in freely moving cats. *Am J Physiol* 1990;259:R963–R972.
14. Greist JH, Klein MH, Eischens RR, Faris J, Gurman AS, Morgan WP. Running as treatment for depression. *Compr Psychiatry* 1979;20:41–54.
15. Grillner S, Wallen P, Brodin L, Lansner A. Neuronal network generating locomotor behavior in lamprey: circuitry, transmitters, membrane properties, and simulation. *Annu Rev Neurosci* 1991;14:169–199.
16. Guyton AC. *Textbook of medical physiology,* 6th ed. Philadelphia: WB Saunders, 1981;344–346.
17. Harris-Warrick RM. Chemical modulation of central pattern generators. In: Cohen AH, ed. *Neural control of rhythmic movements in vertebrates.* New York: John Wiley & Sons, 1988;285–331.
18. Harris-Warrick RM, Cohen AH. Serotonin modulates the central pattern generator for locomotion in the isolated lamprey spinal cord. *J Exp Biol* 1985;116:27–46.
19. Hounsgaard J, Hultborn H, Jesperson B, Kiehn O. Bistability of α-motoneurons in the decerebrate cat and in the acute spinal cat after intravenous 5-hydroxytryptophan. *J Physiol* 1988;405:345–367.
20. Jacobs BL. An animal behavior model for studying central serotonergic synapses. *Life Sci* 1976;19:777–785.
21. Jacobs BL. Locus coeruleus neuronal activity in behaving animals. In: Heal DJ, Marsden CA, eds. *The pharmacology of noradrenaline in the central nervous system.* New York: Oxford University Press, 1990;248–265.
22. Jacobs BL, Azmitia EC. Structure and function of the brain serotonin system. *Physiol Rev* 1992;72:165–229.
23. Jacobs BL, Fornal CA. Activity of brain serotonergic neurons in the behaving animal. *Pharmacol Rev* 1991;43:563–578.
24. Jacobs BL, Fornal CA. 5-HT and motor control: a hypothesis. *Trends Neurosci* 1993;16:346–352.
25. Jacobs BL, Metzler CW, Fornal CA. Suppression of 5-HT neuronal

activity during orientation in awake cats. *Soc Neurosci Abstr* 1993;19:743.

26. Jouvet M, Delorme F. Locus coeruleus et sommeil paradoxal. *C R Soc Biol* 1965;159:895–899.

27. Katakura N, Chandler SH. An iontophoretic analysis of the pharmacologic mechanisms responsible for trigeminal motoneuronal discharge during masticatory-like activity in the guinea pig. *J Neurophysiol* 1990;63:356–369.

28. Kayama Y, Shimada S, Hishikawa Y, Ogawa T. Effects of stimulating the dorsal raphe nucleus of the rat on neuronal activity in the dorsal lateral geniculate nucleus. *Brain Res* 1989;489:1–11.

29. Kravitz EA. Hormonal control of behavior: amines and the biasing of behavioral output in lobsters. *Science* 1989;241:1775–1781.

30. Kupfermann I, Weiss KR. The role of serotonin in arousal and feeding behavior of *Aplysia*. In: Jacobs BL, Gelperin A, eds. *Serotonin neurotransmission and behavior*. Cambridge, MA: MIT Press, 1981;255–287.

31. LeBars D. Serotonin and pain. In: Osborne NN, Hamon M, eds. *Neuronal serotonin*. New York: John Wiley & Sons, 1988;171–229.

32. Lent CM. Serotonergic modulation of the feeding behavior of the medicinal leech. *Brain Res Bull* 1985;14:643–655.

33. Ma PM, Beltz BS, Kravitz EA. Serotonin-containing neurons in lobsters: their role as gain-setters in postural control mechanisms. *J Neurophysiol* 1992;68:36–54.

34. Mahowald MH, Schenck CH. REM sleep behavior disorder. In: Kryger MH, Roth T, Dement WC, eds. *Principles and practice of sleep medicine*. Philadelphia: WB Saunders, 1989;389–401.

35. Marrosu F, Fornal CA, Tada K, Metzler CW, Jacobs BL. 5-HT$_{1A}$ autoreceptor agonists induce hippocampal rhythmic slow activity (RSA) in freely moving cats. *Soc Neurosci Abstr* 1991;17:1437.

36. McCall RB, Aghajanian GK. Serotonergic facilitation of facial motoneuron excitation. *Brain Res* 1979;169:11–27.

37. McCall RB, Clement ME. Identification of serotonergic and sympathetic neurons in medullary raphe nuclei. *Brain Res* 1989;477:172–182.

38. McCormick DA. Neurotransmitter actions in the thalamus and cerebral cortex and their role in neuromodulation of thalamocortical activity. *Prog Neurobiol* 1992;39:337–388.

39. McGinty DJ, Harper RM. Dorsal raphe neurons: depression of firing during sleep in cats. *Brain Res* 1976;101:569–575.

40. McGowan RW, Pierce EF, Jordan D. Mood alterations with a single bout of physical activity. *Percep Mot Skills* 1991;72:1203–1209.

41. McNeil JK, LeBlanc EM, Joyner M. The effect of exercise on depressive symptoms in the moderately depressed elderly. *Psychol Aging* 1991;6(3):487–488.

42. Mitchell GS, Sloan HE, Jiang C, Miletic V, Hayashi F, Lipski J. 5-Hydroxytryptophan (5-HTP) augments spontaneous and evoked phrenic nerve discharge in spinalized rats. *Neurosci Lett* 1992;141:75–78.

43. Nusbaum MP, Kristan WB. Swim initiation in the leech by serotonin-containing interneurons, cells 21 and 61. *J Exp Biol* 1986;122:277–302.

44. Pappas GP, Golin S, Meyer DL. Reducing symptoms of depression with exercise. *Psychosomatics* 1990;31:112–113.

45. Parent A. The anatomy of serotonin-containing neurons across phylogeny. In: Jacobs BL, Gelperin A, eds. *Serotonin neurotransmission and behavior*. Cambridge, MA: MIT Press, 1981;3–34.

46. Paulus MP, Geyer MA. The effects of MDMA and other methylene-dioxy-substituted phenylalkylamines on the structure of rat locomotor activity. *Neuropsychopharmacology* 1992;7:15–31.

47. Potrebic S, Fields HL, Mason P. Serotonin immunocytochemistry of physiologically identified neurons in the rat rostral ventromedial medulla. *Soc Neurosci Abstr* 1992;18:683.

48. Ribeiro-do-Valle LE, Fornal CA, Litto WJ, et al. Serotonergic dorsal raphe unit activity related to feeding/grooming behaviors in cats. *Soc Neurosci Abstr* 1989;15:1283.

49. Ribeiro-do-Valle LE, Metzler CW, Jacobs BL. Facilitation of mas-

50. Ristine LA, Spear LP. Is there a "serotonergic syndrome" in neonatal rat pups? *Pharmacol Biochem Behav* 1985;22:265–269.

51. Rogawski MA, Aghajanian GK. Norepinephrine and serotonin: opposite effects on the activity of lateral geniculate neurons evoked by optic pathway stimulation. *Exp Neurol* 1980;69:678–694.

52. Roth DL, Holmes DS. Influence of aerobic exercise training and relaxation training on physical and psychologic health following stressful life events. *Psychosom Med* 1987;49:355–365.

53. Ruch-Monachon MA, Jalfre M, Haefely W. Drugs and PGO waves in the lateral geniculate body of the curarized cat. II. PGO wave activity and brain 5-hydroxytryptamine. *Arch Int Pharmacodyn Ther* 1976;219:269–286.

54. Saha S, Appenteng K, Batten TFC. Light and electron microscopical localization of 5-HT-immunoreactive boutons in the rat trigeminal motor nucleus. *Brain Res* 1991;559:145–148.

55. Shin HC, Chapin JK. Movement induced modulation of afferent transmission to single neurons in the ventroposterior thalamus and somatosensory cortex in rat. *Exp Brain Res* 1990;81:515–522.

56. Steinbusch HWM. Distribution of serotonin-immunoreactivity in the central nervous system of the rat—cell bodies and terminals. *Neuroscience* 1981;4:557–618.

57. Steinfels GF, Heym J, Strecker RE, Jacobs BL. Raphe unit activity in freely moving cats is altered by manipulations of central but not peripheral motor systems. *Brain Res* 1983;279:77–84.

58. Sternbach H. The serotonin syndrome. *Am J Psychiatry* 1991;148:705–713.

59. Stewart BR, Jenner P, Marsden CD. Induction of purposeless chewing behaviour in rats by 5-HT agonist drugs. *Eur J Pharmacol* 1989;162:101–107.

60. Takeuchi Y, Kojima M, Matsuura T, Sano Y. Serotonergic innervation on the motoneurons in the mammalian brainstem. *Anat Embryol* 1983;167:321–333.

61. Trulson ME, Jacobs BL, Morrison AR. Raphe unit activity during REM sleep in normal cats and in pontine lesioned cats displaying REM sleep without atonia. *Brain Res* 1981;226:75–91.

62. Vanderwolf CH, Baker GB, Dickson C. Serotonergic control of cerebral activity and behavior: models of dementia. In: Whitaker-Azmitia PM, Peroutka SJ, eds. *The neuropharmacology of serotonin*. New York: New York Academy of Sciences, 1990;366–382.

63. Veasey SC, Fornal CA, Metzler CW, Milman W, Jacobs BL. Firing rates of subpopulations of medullary serotonergic neurons in cats are increased with respiratory and locomotor challenges. *Soc Neurosci Abstr* 1993;19:743.

64. Viala D, Buser P. The effects of DOPA and 5-HTP on rhythmic efferent discharges in hind limb nerves in the rabbit. *Brain Res* 1969;12:437–443.

65. Waterhouse BD, Azizi SA, Burne RA, Woodward DJ. Modulation of rat cortical area 17 neuronal responses to moving visual stimuli during norepinephrine and serotonin microiontophoresis. *Brain Res* 1990;514:276–292.

66. Waterhouse BD, Moises HC, Woodward DJ. Interaction of serotonin with somatosensory cortical neuronal responses to afferent synaptic inputs and putative neurotransmitters. *Brain Res Bull* 1986;17:507–518.

67. Whitaker-Azmitia PM, Peroutka SJ, eds. *The neuropharmacology of serotonin*. New York: New York Academy of Sciences, 1990.

68. White SR, Neuman RS. Facilitation of spinal motoneurone excitability by 5-hydroxytryptamine and noradrenaline. *Brain Res* 1980;188:119–127.

69. Wilkinson LO, Dourish CT. Serotonin and animal behavior. In: Peroutka SJ, ed. *Serotonin receptor subtypes: basic and clinical aspects*. Wiley–Liss, 1991;147–210.

70. Wilkinson LO, Jacobs BL. Lack of response of serotonergic neurons in the dorsal raphe nucleus of freely moving cats to stressful stimuli. *Exp Neurol* 1988;101:445–457.

seter EMG and masseteric (jaw closure) reflex by serotonin in behaving cats. *Brain Res* 1991;550:197–204.

Psychopharmacology: The Fourth Generation of Progress, edited by Floyd E. Bloom and David J. Kupfer. Raven Press, Ltd., New York © 1995.

CHAPTER 42

Indoleamines

The Role of Serotonin in Clinical Disorders

George R. Heninger

Since 1948 when serotonin (5-hydroxytryptamine, 5-HT) was first isolated, identified, and synthesized, there has been exponential growth in the information available on its biochemical, physiologic, and behavioral effects. 5-HT is involved in many physiologic and behavioral systems, and this is reflected by the use of numerous 5-HT-based drugs applied as treatments across a wide variety of very different clinical conditions. Even though alterations in 5-HT system function have been observed in many of these clinical conditions, definitive evidence of a ''serotonin disease'' (aside from carcinoid tumors) that demonstrates clear abnormalities at the genetic, anatomic, and biochemical levels remains to be demonstrated. Thus, at the present time, even though there are extensive therapeutics directed at increasing or decreasing 5-HT function at selected sites, considerable additional research will be necessary to clarify the causative pathogenic role of the many 5-HT-dependent mechanisms involved in the widely different clinical conditions where 5-HT-based treatments are used (see also Chapters 28, 29, and 102, *this volume*).

Initial research focused on defining the pathways for synthesis and degradation of 5-HT and the discovery of drugs interacting with these processes. One of the first applications of this new understanding was the use of the 5-HT synthesis inhibitor, parachorophenylalanine (PCPA), as a treatment to reduce the excessive 5-HT secretion from carcinoid tumors (58). The development of monoamine oxidase inhibitors and their effectiveness in the treatment of depression provided the initial evidence of the importance of 5-HT in these disorders, and the psychometimetic effects of lysergic acid diethylmide (LSD) pointed to the involvement of 5-HT in psychosis and schizophrenia (58). Early studies attempting to demonstrate the efficacy of 5-HT precursors as treatments provided some additional evidence of 5-HT involvement in affective disorders and in the control of myoclonus (58,68). In more recent times, the development and widespread clinical use of selective 5-HT reuptake inhibitors (SSRIs), along with the preclinical delineation of the multiple 5-HT receptor subtypes and their coupling to intracellular messenger systems and the development of drugs selectively acting on these systems, have catalyzed an explosion of new research information in this field. At present there is a great deal of new information on the molecular biology, physiology, and pharmacology of the 5-HT receptor subtypes (see preceding chapters). The role of the 5-HT system in the normal regulation of physiologic and behavioral processes is increasingly better understood, so that it is now clear that the 5-HT systems are extremely diverse and that they are involved in a multitude of physiologic and behavioral processes (see Chapters 40 and 41, *this volume*).

The major evidence for 5-HT alterations in clinical disease states derives from the symptomatic change following treatments that alter the 5-HT system. The utilization of 5-HT precursors and 5-HT receptor agonists and antagonists has provided some evidence that 5-HT function may be altered in some clinical conditions. However, the direct assessment of the anatomic integrity of the 5-HT systems and 5-HT synthesis and turnover in brain has been difficult to achieve. When cerebrospinal fluid 5-hydroxy indolacetic acid (5-HIAA) has been used as a measure of 5-HT turnover, it has provided much less

G. R. Heninger: Department of Psychiatry, Yale University School of Medicine, Connecticut Mental Health Center and the Abraham Ribicoff Research Facilities, New Haven, Connecticut 06508.

TABLE 1. *Clinical areas influenced by altered 5-HT function*

Affective disorders	Substance abuse
Anxiety disorders	Pain sensitivity
Obsessive–compulsive disorder	Emesis
	Mycoclonis
Schizophrenia	Neuroendocrine regulation
Eating disorders	Circadian rhythm regulation
Sleep disorders	Stress disorders
Sexual disorders	Carcinoid syndrome
Impulse disorders	
Developmental disorders	
Aging and neurodegenerative disorders	

evidence of abnormally in the clinical conditions where it has been studied (21).

The information reviewed in the six preceding chapters covering the molecular, biochemical, anatomical, physiological, pharmacologic, and behavioral dimensions of the 5-HT system clearly document the diversity of this predominantly modulatory system. Table 1 lists the number of the clinical areas where the involvement of the 5-HT system has been demonstrated. Because of the difficulties of isolating the function of such a diverse modulatory

system in humans, in none of these conditions has it been possible to definitively prove that there is a primary abnormality in 5-HT function. Certainly many alterations in 5-HT function have been demonstrated, but because of the complicated interdependency of the 5-HT system with other neurotransmitter and biochemical systems, these changes may easily be secondary to more primary abnormalities in other systems. In many instances, active treatments that alter 5-HT function are known to produce beneficial therapeutic effects even though abnormalities in the 5-HT system have not been clearly demonstrated for that clinical condition (e.g., diabetic neuropathy) (41,57).

Figure 1 is a schematic diagram illustrating several of the steps involved in 5-HT neurotransmission. It can be seen that there are a large number of cellular processes involved in 5-HT metabolism which could be altered in clinical conditions or altered by pharmacologic treatment. Over the history of research in the field, initial understanding was obtained regarding the overall 5-HT metabolic pathways such as synthesis and degradation and reuptake inhibition. Only more recently have the details of 5-HT receptor pharmacology, receptor effector coupling, and short- and long-term effects of 5-HT receptor stimulation on intracellular processes begun to be understood. In addi-

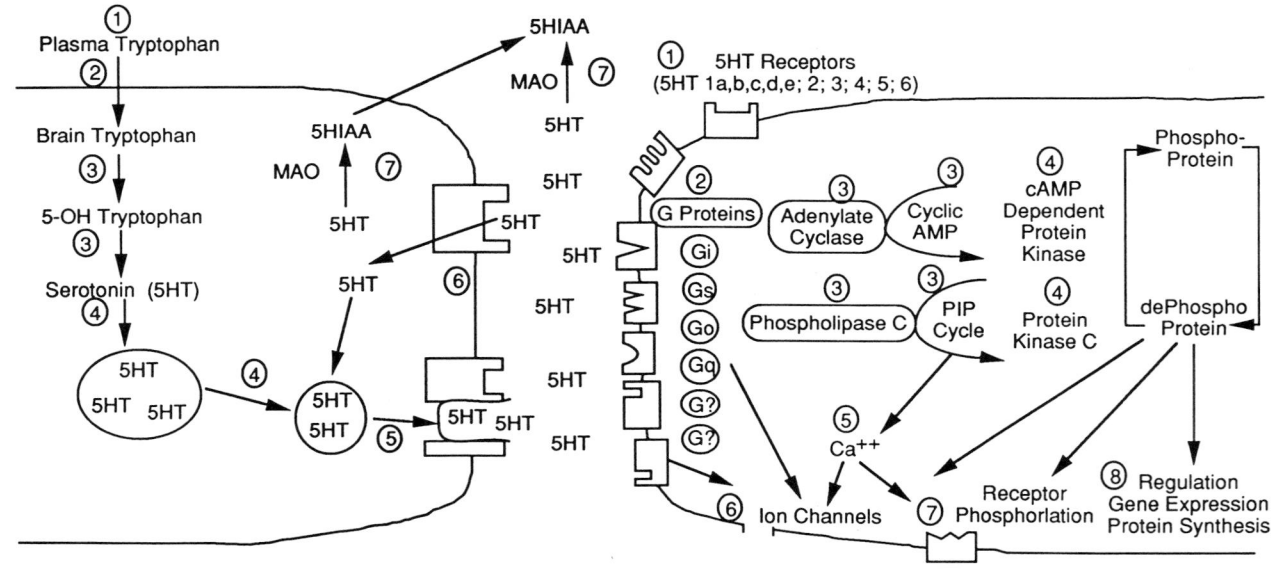

PRESYNAPTIC FACTORS

1. Plasma Level Tryptophan
2. Transport into CNS
3. Synthesis of 5HT
4. Storage
5. Release
6. Reuptake
7. 5HT Degradation

POSTSYNAPTIC FACTORS

1. 5HT binding to Receptor Subtypes
2. Receptor G Protein Coupling
3. 2nd Messenger Generating Systems
4. Protein Phosphorylation Systems
5. Calcium Release
6. Regulation Ion Channels
7. Regulation Receptor Function
8. Regulation Gene and Protein Expression

FIG. 1. A schematic diagram of aspects of serotonergic neurotransmission that could be modified by pharmacologic treatments or that may be altered in disease states.

tion to the biochemical diversity of the different 5-HT cellular systems, the numerous 5-HT receptor subtypes, the anatomic location of the different receptors (e.g., pre- versus postsynaptic, etc.), the different neural circuits involved, and the interaction with other neurotransmitter systems add additional layers of complexity. At present, even though a great deal is known regarding postsynaptic cellular mechanisms, their investigation at the clinical level is very difficult and their elucidation in a variety of clinical states and the effect of modification of 5-HT neurotransmission on them are only now beginning to be understood.

DIVERSITY OF 5-HT INVOLVEMENT AT THE CLINICAL LEVEL

The diverse nature of 5-HT involvement in different clinical conditions can be illustrated by reviewing four examples where the complexity of different aspects of the 5-HT systems may contribute to the variable clinical response to 5-HT-based treatments:

1. Differential sensitivity to 5-HT precursor levels.
2. Influence of 5-HT receptor subtype and location.
3. Interactions with other neurotransmitter systems.
4. Treatment-responsive dimensions to SSRIs across diverse clinical conditions.

The more specific details on the biochemical abnormalities, the response to 5-HT agonist or antagonist challenge, and the details of the response to 5-HT-based treatments can be found in subsequent chapters dealing with the specific clinical conditions such as depression, schizophrenia, eating disorders, and so on.

Differential Sensitivity of Depression and Obsessive Compulsive Disorder to Plasma Tryptophan Depletion Following SSRI-Induced Remission

One of the more compelling lines of evidence for the involvement of 5-HT in affective disorders was reported in the mid-1970s when Shopsin et al. (54,55) administered the tryptophan hydroxylase inhibitor, parachlorophenylalanine (PCPA) to patients who, while being treated with imipramine or tranylcypromine, had recently recovered from depression. In Table 2, the results of those experiments are summarized. It can be seen that in the two patients who recovered following imipramine treatment and in the four patients who recovered following tranylcypromine treatment, there was always a rapid and very robust return of depressive symptoms within 1 to 4 days after starting the PCPA. All patients recovered from the increase in symptoms 2–7 days after the PCPA was stopped. However, when PCPA was given to patients with carcinoid tumors, a clear and consistent production of depressive symptoms was not seen (58). Unfortunately,

no other experiments utilizing PCPA to study affective disorders have been reported.

Another method for producing a short-term alteration in 5-HT synthesis has been utilized by Young and colleagues (59,73). Because synthesis of 5-HT is dependent on brain levels of tryptophan and depletion of plasma tryptophan results in reduction in brain tryptophan, a method was developed to reduce plasma tryptophan levels and consequently produce a reduction in brain 5-HT turnover. The ingestion of a high amino acid load stimulates protein synthesis. Following the ingestion of a high amino acid load that does not include tryptophan, there is a marked drop in plasma-free and total tryptophan levels. The lowered tryptophan levels in conjunction with the higher neutral amino acid levels which compete with tryptophan for uptake into brain has been shown to lower brain tryptophan, serotonin, and 5-HIAA in nonhuman primates (72). This method has been utilized by Delgado et al. (10) to extend the prior studies on the role of 5-HT in depression. The method was modified by utilizing a low tryptophan diet preceding the ingestion of the large amino acid load without tryptophan. A control test was accomplished utilizing a large amino acid load with tryptophan present. Utilizing this methodology there is approximately a mean drop of 80% in free or total plasma tryptophan levels 5 hr following the amino acid ingestion. When this method has been applied to the study of previously depressed patients who had recently recovered on a variety of antidepressant treatments, it was found that 60% of them had a symptomatic relapse equal to or greater than a 50% increase in their Hamilton depression rating scale scores at 5 or 7 hr following the amino acid drink. In contrast, when this same procedure was utilized in highly symptomatic depressed patients not on medication, there was no consistent increase in depressive symptoms following the amino acid drink (13,14). These results are illustrated in Fig. 2, where it can be seen that the patients recently improved on antidepressant treatment had a mean increase of almost 12 points in the Hamilton rating scale. In contrast, the much more symptomatic patients who were off medication only had a mean change of 3 points, which was not statistically significant. Thus, the consistency of the results across the PCPA study and the tryptophan depletion study indicate that short-term maintenance of the clinical response to antidepressants is dependent adequate 5-HT function. However, the lack of effect of the tryptophan depletion in symptomatic drug-free patients remains unexplained. It is of interest also that PCPA does not produce depression in patients who are treated for carcinoid tumors (58).

The initial tryptophan depletion study suggested that patients on SSRIs and monoamine oxidase inhibitors were more vulnerable to the tryptophan depletion effects (10). However, patients had not been randomly assigned to the treatments, and this could have confounded the differences between treatments. In order to more objectively

TABLE 2. *Summary of previously reported effects of PCPA, a serotonin synthesis inhibitor, on depressive symptoms in six patients who had improved on imipramine or tranylcypromine treatment[a]*

Reference number of original report/ number of patient	Ongoing treatment	Age	Sex	Diagnosis	Days until relapse	Cumulative grams of PCPA taken until relapse	Rating scale	Magnitude of induced symptom change at relapse (sum change from prior rating/ number of rating items reported)	Days to recover after PCPA stopped
55/4	I	a	F	U	1	0.75	H	31/21	3
55/5	I	a	M	B	3	2.50	—	"Precipitous depression"	2
54/1	T	32	F	U	4	<7.50	H	21/10	7
54/2	T	47	M	B	1.5	1.25	BPRS	15/5	3
54/3	T	58	F	U	2	1.5	H	30/21	2
54/4	T	55	F	B	1	0.75	H	30/21	3

[a] Adapted from refs. 54 and 55.
—, data not reported; a, age between 28 and 52; I, imipramine; T, tranylcypromine; U, unipolar; B, bipolar; H, Hamilton rating scale; BPRS, brief psychiatric rating scale.

evaluate this possibility, a subsequent study was conducted where patients were randomly assigned to the SSRI fluoxetine or to the selective norepinephrine (NE) uptake inhibitor desipramine (12). On the left side of Fig. 3, the interaction of drug treatment with the tryptophan depletion effect is illustrated, and it can be seen that recently recovered patients on fluoxetine are significantly more vulnerable to relapse than similar recently recovered patients on desipramine. In order to assess the specificity of this effect relative to 5-HT depletion versus catecholamine depletion, a second study was conducted utilizing alpha methylparatyrosine to deplete catecholamine levels (11). The right half of Fig. 3 illustrates the findings from this study. It can be seen that all five recently recovered patients receiving the selective catecholamine uptake inhibitors desipramine or mazindol had a relapse but that

only one of 12 recently recovered patients receiving an SSRI did. Thus, not only do these data indicate that maintaining an antidepressant response is dependent on adequate 5-HT function, there is also specificity as to the drug treatment utilized, because patients recovering on SSRIs are more vulnerable to tryptophan depletion than patients on desipramine. This finding in conjunction with the specificity of the catecholamine depletion to produce relapse predominantly in patients treated with catecholamine-uptake-inhibiting drugs points to a specific role for the 5-HT system in affecting the antidepressant response to 5-HT-based treatments in depression.

Another clinical area where 5-HT has been implicated is in the treatment response in obsessive–compulsive disorder (OCD). Patients with the severe forms of OCD had previously proven refractory to many drug treatments.

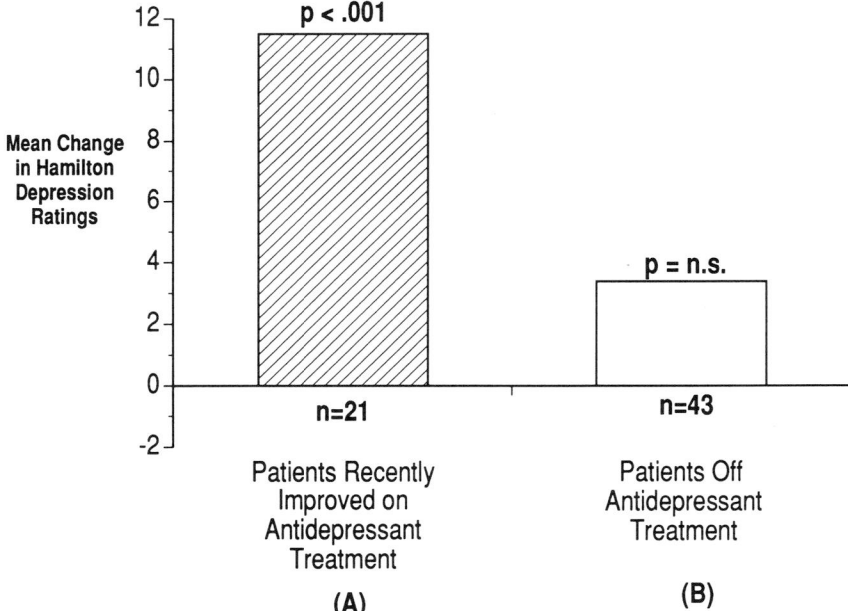

FIG. 2. A: Patients recently improved on at least 4 weeks of antidepressant treatment had an amino acid drink with tryptophan (control nondepletion) and an amino acid drink without tryptophan (active depletion) administered an average of 6 days apart. The ratings before the drink were subtracted from the ratings 7 hr after the drink in order to obtain the effect for each of the control and active drinks. The change plotted above is the active drink effect minus the control drink effect. (Adapted from ref. 10.) B: Patients off medication for at least 21 days had the amino acid drinks administered and the Hamilton rating scale scores calculated as described above. (Adapted from refs. 13 and 14.)

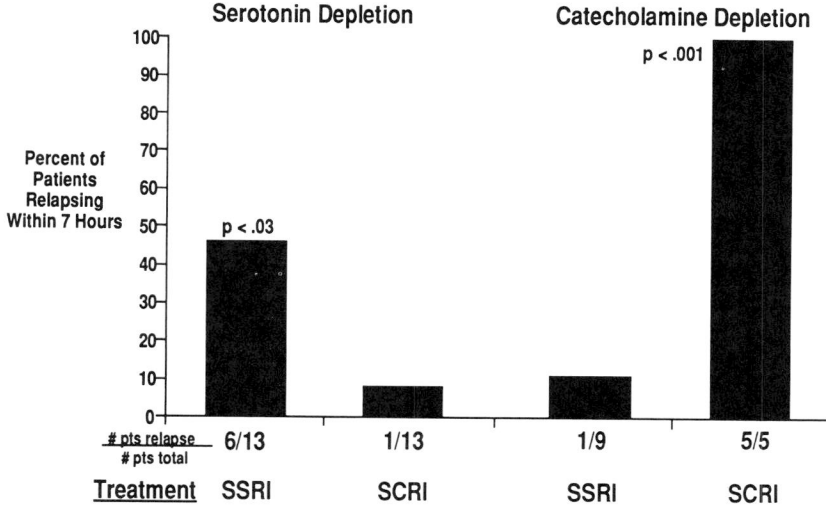

FIG. 3. Serotonin depletion was produced utilizing the amino acid drink without trypto-phan. Catecholamine depletion was produced utilizing 5 g of alpha-methyl paratyrosine given over 30 hr prior to Hamilton depression ratings. Relapse was defined as a greater than 50% increase in Hamilton depression ratings and a score greater or equal to 18. (Adapted from refs. 11 and 12.)

Subsequently, it has been clearly demonstrated that SSRIs are an effective treatment for this disorder (7,20). In Fig. 4 it can be seen that in comparison to placebo, clomipramine, which has strong 5-HT reuptake inhibitor properties, produces a decrease of 35% in OCD ratings over an 8-week treatment period and fluvoxamine, a more specific SSRI, produces a comparable decrease of 29%. It is of interest that the specific NE uptake inhibitor desipramine did not produce any change in OCD symptoms during the 8-week treatment trial. This is consistent with

several other studies comparing cloipramine and desipramine in OCD and other behavioral disorders such as trichotillomania (61), onychlphagia (36), and autistic disorder (22), where cloripramine was found to be more clearly effective than desipramine. These treatment response data suggest that OCD symptoms and certain stereotyped repetitive behaviors are specifically responsive to SSRI treatment.

Given the specificity of the response of OCD symptoms to SSRI treatment, it would have been reasonable to as-

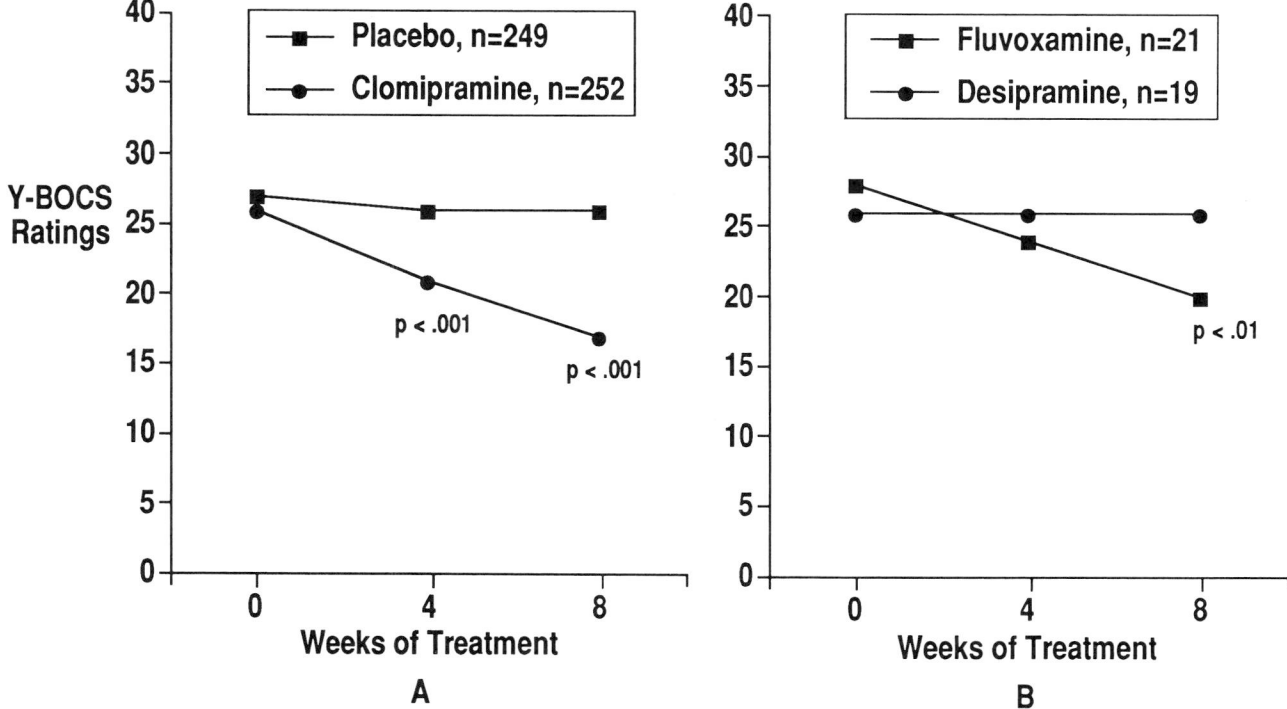

FIG. 4. Comparison of symptom reduction between cloimipramine and placebo treatment (**A**) and between fluvoxamine and desipramine treatment (**B**) in patients with obsessive compulsive disorder. [Adapted from refs. 7 (clomipramine versus placebo) and 20 (fluvoxamine versus desipramine).]

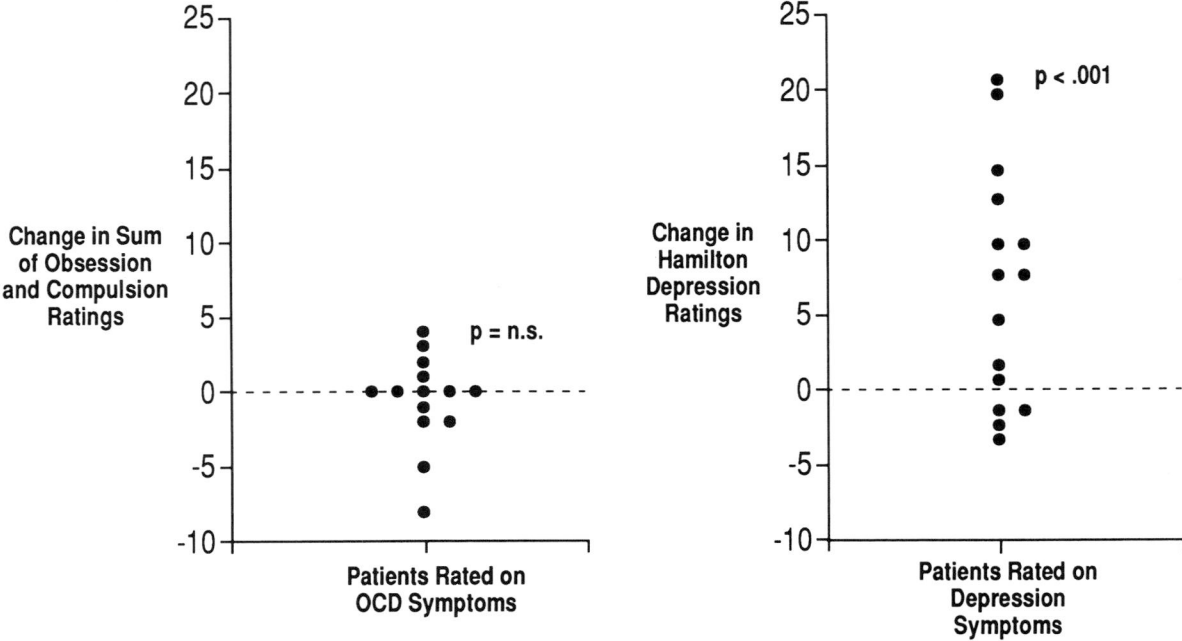

FIG. 5. Following at least 5 weeks of successful treatment with serotonin reuptake inhibitors, 15 patients diagnosed with obsessive–compulsive disorder received two tests 7–10 days apart, a trypto-phan-containing amino acid drink (control nondepletion) and an amino acid drink without tryptophan (active depletion). Ratings before the drink were subtracted from ratings 7 hr after the drink to obtain the drink effect for each of the control and active drinks. The change plotted above is the active drink effect minus the control drink effect. (Adapted from ref. 3.)

sume that OCD symptoms would worsen with the trypto-phan depletion procedure. However, when patients with OCD who had responded to SSRI treatment were studied with tryptophan depletion procedure, it was found that only depressive symptoms worsened and that there was no change in ratings of OCD symptoms (3). These data are illustrated in Fig. 5, where it can be seen that the tryptophan depletion in the SSRI-responding OCD pa-tients produced a significant increase in depressive symp-toms but no change in OCD symptoms. Thus it would appear that the 5-HT-dependent systems responsible for improvement of OCD symptoms following SSRI treat-ment are different in their biochemical pharmacology than the 5-HT systems related to improvement in depressive symptoms following SSRI treatment.

Taken together, these data indicate considerable differ-ential specificity for aspects of the 5-HT system involved in SSRI-induced recovery from depression and OCD. The lack of depressive symptom relapse in SSRI-treated pa-tients during catecholamine depletion, in contrast to the extreme sensitivity of NE uptake inhibitor treatments, in-dicates that there is significant specificity of the type of treatment and the monoamine system affected. More im-portantly within the 5-HT system it appears that mainte-nance of SSRI-induced recovery for depressive symptoms is dependent on immediate availability of 5-HT, but this is not the case for SSRI-induced recovery from OCD

symptoms. Clearly more complex different and specific 5-HT mechanisms are involved in SSRI treatment of de-pression and OCD than just a simple model where defi-cient 5-HT function is augmented equally by SSRI treat-ment in both conditions.

Serotonin Effects on the Vascular Wall Depend on the 5-HT Receptor Subtype and Location

Serotonin (''serum tonic factor'') was initially discov-ered through its vasoconstrictor actions (58). It has since been shown that 5-HT possess both vasoconstrictor and vasodilator properties. In Table 3, some of the mecha-nisms involved in the vasoconstrictor and vasodilator ac-tions of 5-HT are listed. The vasodilator properties of 5-HT are often unmasked following the use of 5-HT2 antagonists, and the net effect of 5-HT on the blood vessel wall can depend on (a) location of vessel studied, (b) the degree of activation of the vascular smooth muscle, (c) the integrity of the endothelium, and (d) many other mod-ulating factors such as local temperature, oxygen tension, blood pressure, and so on (69).

Exactly how these factors modify the complex array of the different types and diversity of 5-HT receptors on the vascular smooth muscle cells, the endothelial cells, and the adrenergic nerves is not precisely known. It is

TABLE 3. *Effects of 5-HT on the vascular wall[a]*

Vasoconstrictor	Vasodilator
S_2 receptor: Direct activation of vascular smooth muscle.	S_1 Receptor: Activation of endothelial cells which release endothelial derived relaxing factors.
Release of norepinephrine from adrenergic nerves.	S_1 receptor: Inhibition of adrenergic neurotransmission via action on prejunctional receptors.
Augmentation of other endogenous vasoconstrictors.	Release of other endogenous mediators. Direct inhibition of vascular smooth muscle.

[a] Adapted from ref. 69.

clear, however, that the known mechanisms are sufficient to account for the apparent discrepancies in 5-HT effects such as the observation that excess 5-HT is released only in painful areas during cluster headache attacks (2), while the 5-HT agonist, sumatriptan, is at the same time an effective treatment for cluster headaches (5,43,63).

Sumatriptan is active at the "5-HT1-like" receptor sites, and it binds with high affinity to those receptor sites that most closely resemble the 5-HT1D receptor. It also binds with lower affinity to 5-HT1A and 5-HT1B recognition sites. Sumatriptan does not significantly cross the blood–brain barrier. It produces vascular smooth muscle constriction within intracranial vessels and some extra cranial ones also. It also reduces neurogenic inflammation thought to be important in the pathogenesis of migraine, it has effects on the trigeminovascular nerves that transmit nociceptive information from the meninges, and it may be involved in blocking the effects of more central events on trigeminal nerve function (5,43,63).

Figure 6 illustrates the robust positive results from four studies of sumatriptan in headache (5). Its equal efficacy in cluster headache and migraine is illustrated, and the superiority of the subcutaneous administration over oral administration can also be seen. The 70% improvement rate following subcutaneous administration when the placebo response is 20% demonstrates a net 50% improvement. Thus, it is one of the most specific and efficacious of the available 5-HT-based treatments.

The specificity and efficacy of sumatriptan in the treatment of headache emphasizes the importance of the receptor location and the receptor subtype affected by the 5-HT-based treatments. Even though sumatriptan may be acting on several mechanisms at once (i.e., vascular smooth muscle contraction, reduction of neurogenic inflammation, and reduction of trigeminovascular nociceptive information), it is still one of the best examples of the importance of directing 5-HT-based treatments to specific locations and 5-HT subtypes. The strong positive clinical utility of sumatriptan in the treatment of headache illustrates not only how the development of drugs acting on specific 5-HT receptors can provide important new clinical treatments, but also that by understanding the drug mechanism of action, we can also add considerably to our understanding of the role of the 5-HT systems in general.

The Role of 5-HT Interactions with Other Neurotransmitter Systems: Ondansetron in the Treatment of Nausea and Emesis

The preclinical data on 5-HT indicate that the 5-HT systems are predominately modulatory and that most 5-HT effects interact with the ongoing status of the other involved neurotransmitter systems. At the clinical level, it is difficult, if not impossible, to ascribe an effect to

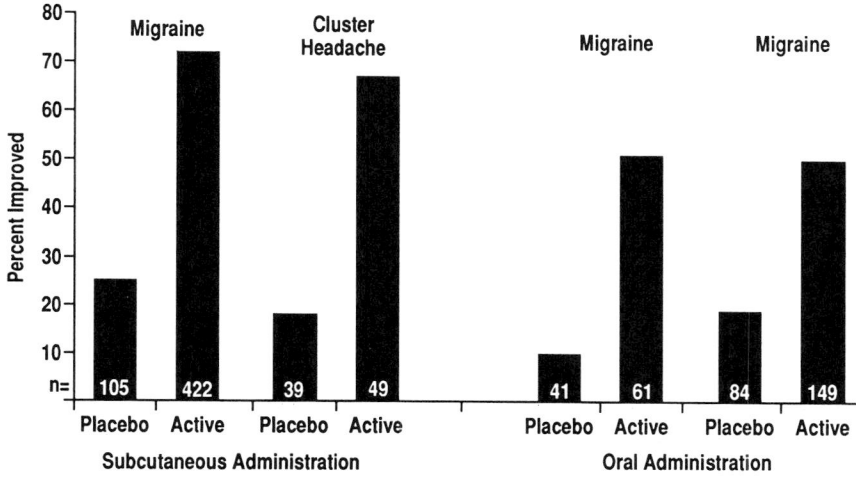

FIG. 6. Response rates of patients with headaches to sumatriptan in four separate placebo-controlled studies. Subcutaneous administration, 6 mg, migraine evaluated at 1 hr; subcutaneous administration, 6 mg, cluster headache evaluated at 15 min; oral administration, 100 mg, evaluated at 2 hr. (Adapted from ref. 5.)

TABLE 4. *Neurotransmitter systems involved in the control of emesis*

Emetic	Transmitter system	Receptor	Receptor location	Emetic antagonist
Cisplatin	Serotonin	5-HT3	Visceral afferents Area postrema	Ondansetron
Apomorphine	Dopamine	D_2	CTZ Area postrema	Metopimazine
Motion	Histamine	H_1	Vestibular afferents Area postrema	Meclizine
Motion	Acetylcholine	M_1 M_2	Vestibular apparatus Cortex	Scopolamine

a single mechanism because of these interactions. As a consequence of this highly interdependent interaction with other systems, the clinical effects of 5-HT treatments usually only result in partial symptomatic improvement. This contrasts with other clinical conditions where the clinical biochemical abnormality is primarily a deficiency of a single molecule that can be replaced. In these instances, a nearly complete symptomatic remission is seen (e.g., vitamin deficiencies, diabetes, hypothyroidism, etc.).

One of the systems involving 5-HT where some of the neurotransmitters and receptors are better understood involves the systems regulating the control of nausea and emesis (62). Table 4 lists four of the neurotransmitter systems where agonists produce nausea and emesis while antagonists prevent it. This system is one of the better examples of the interaction of 5-HT with other systems even though the neural circuits involved are complex in that the same receptors may be located at different points in the circuit and the interrelationships between the circuits of the neurotransmitter systems are not precisely known (62). Ondansetron is a 5-HT3 receptor antagonist that appears to act on the 5-HT3 receptors located in the area postrema and in the gastrointestinal tract (27,30,62). Ondansetron by itself has a moderate efficacy in reducing nausea and emesis (left half of Fig. 7). However, when a D2-receptor-blocking drug metopimazine is added to the treatment, significant improvement in efficacy is observed (right half of Fig. 7). This illustrates an additive effect of other treatments with 5-HT drug action that is also seen in many other clinical situations. It is important to note that in the same type of patients and with the same type of chemotherapy where ondansetron and metopimazine were additive, ondansetron alone was less effective than a combination of dexamethasone and metoclopramide (37). Thus, in the clinical situation considerable testing will be necessary before optimal combinations and doses can be arrived at. In those instances where the pathophysiologic role of 5-HT is more direct, specific targeted treatments should be more effective. It is of interest in this regard that ondansetron produced an "impressive response" in the treatment of symptoms of the carcinoid syndrome (50).

Given the prevailing view that the 5-HT systems are primarily modulatory, it is not surprising that in the clinical situation most 5-HT-based treatments result in only a partial symptomatic improvement and that there are strong interactive effects with other treatments. The neuroanatomy of the 5-HT system suggest that up to 60% or more of 5-HT released may not be at synapses (15). Thus, 5-HT effects would not be expected to be highly anatomically localized or to demonstrate the properties associated with systems that more directly mediate neurotransmission. The modulatory nature of the 5-HT systems can be seen at the clinical level through interactions with other neurotransmitter systems.

There Is a Wide Spectrum of Symptomatic Response to SSRI Treatments in Different Disorders

The increased availability of SSRIs for clinical use has led to treatment trials in a wide variety of different clinical conditions. Even though the availability of new drug treatments often stimulates overly optimistic published case reports of beneficial treatment response, in the case of SSRIs a number of randomized placebo-controlled studies have been conducted in several disorders other than depression, the primary indication for SSRI treatment. Placebo-controlled studies have demonstrated positive results of SSRI treatment in OCD (7), panic disorder, premenstrual syndrome (71), bulimia nervosa (17), autistic disorder (22), diabetic neuropathy (41,57), and diabetic obesity (24) (see Chapters 81, 102, 109, 110, 113, and 142, *this volume*). The nature and magnitude of the symptomatic responses reported in several other clinical conditions suggests that they will eventually be found to be reliable also. Table 5 lists the wide spectrum of different clinical conditions that have been reported to demonstrate a beneficial symptomatic response following SSRI treatment. It can be seen that even though a common factor such as anxiety may underlie some disorders (e.g., panic disorder, social phobia, and post-traumatic stress disorder) or a repetitive behavior in others (e.g., OCD, trichotillomania, and onychophagia), it is not possible to reduce the divergence of the clinical effects of SSRI treatment to any simple holistic scheme. Instead, the diversity of treatment responses to SSRIs suggests that the 5-HT system is more like a chameleon; that is, in each instance it reflects different properties each one strongly influenced by the system that it is modulating.

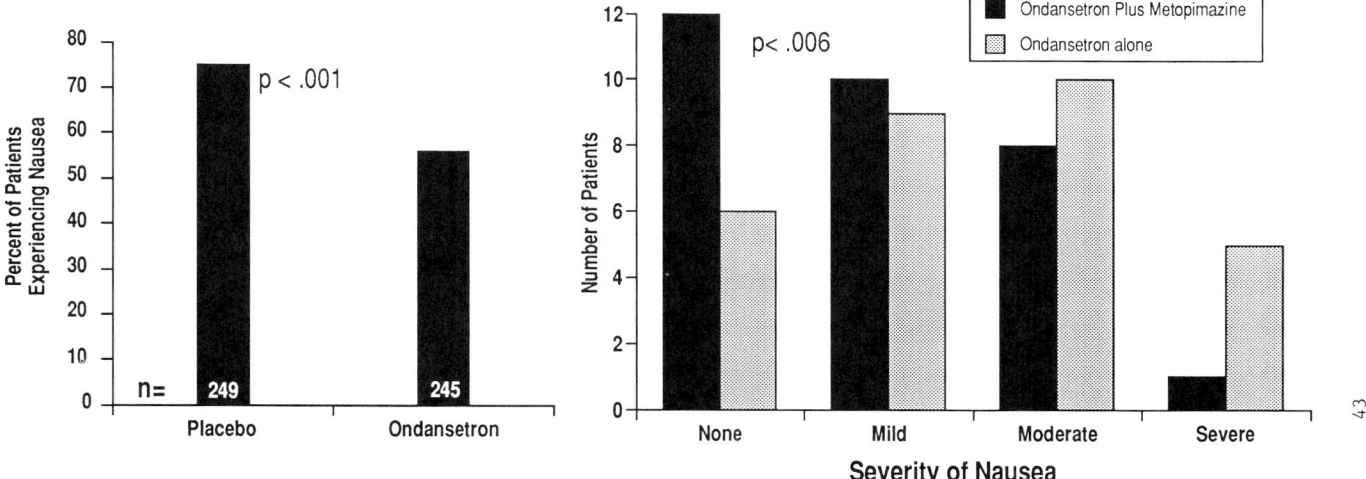

FIG. 7. Left: Percent of patients in each treatment group who experienced nausea in the first 24 hr after recovery from anesthesia for major gynecological surgery. Ondansetron 8 mg was given 1 hr before anesthesia, and then again 8 and 16 hr later. (Adapted from ref. 30.) **Right:** Treatment dosage was ondansetron 8 mg twice a day with 30 mg. metopimazine 4 times a day or ondansetron 8 mg twice a day with placebo 4 times a day. Chemotherapy was given after the first dose. Data are for ratings of nausea over the first day of treatment. (Adapted from ref. 27.)

The wide diversity of effects following SSRI treatment would be consistent with the complexity of the 5-HT system. This includes: the multiple 5-HT receptor subtypes, the different cellular groups containing 5-HT that project widely throughout the central nervous system (CNS), the relative abundance of nonjunctional varicosities containing secretory vesicles, the complex microcircuits involving different 5-HT receptors on pre- and post-synaptic elements, and the predominantly modulatory nature of the 5-HT systems relative to other neurotransmitter systems. This relative lack of specificity has major implications for the evaluation of new 5-HT-based treatments (66). On the positive side, the widespread involvement of 5-HT in many physiologic systems offers many opportunities for the development of new treatments. However, because of the complexity, it will not be possible to predict the clinical conditions and the quality of response to the new treatments with reasonable consistency. The degree of clinical improvement may be limited in many instances, and 5-HT-based treatments may work

TABLE 5. *Clinical conditions reported to have some symptomatic improvement following SSRI treatment*

Major depression[a]	Paraphilias and sexual addictions (29,32,60)
Dysthymia[a]	Migraine prophylaxis (1)
Obsessive–compulsive disorder[b]	Diabetic neuropathy (41,58)
Panic disorder[c]	Chronic abdominal pain (16)
Post-traumatic stress disorder (44)	Diabetic obesity (24,34)
Social phobia (38,65)	Weight gain in smokers (51)
Borderline personality disorder (9)	Alcoholism (23,45)
Depersonalization syndrome (28)	Emotional lability following brain injury (46)
Body dysmorphic syndrome (48)	Sleep paralysis (31)
Premenstrual syndrome (71)	Pathologic jealousy (25,35)
Postpartum obsessive–compulsive disorders (56)	Chronic schizophrenia (19)
Bulemia nervosa (17,18)	Self-injurious behavior (40)
Autistic disorder (8,22)	Arthritis (47)
Attention deficit hyperactivity disorder (4)	Raynaud's phenomenon (6)
Tourette's syndrome (33)	Upright tilt syncope (26)
Trichotillomania (61)	Intention myoclonus (67)
Onychophagia (36)	Neuroendocrine regulation (49,52,64)
Prader–Willi syndrome (70)	

[a] See Chapter A.—Serotonin and Depression
[b] See Chapter B.—Treatment of OCD
[c] See Chapter C.—Serotonin and anxiety

best when combined with other treatments because of the predominantly modulatory nature of the 5-HT systems. An area of considerable promise involves the development of more specific 5-HT receptor agonists and antagonists, and this will allow more targeted and effective therapies as exemplified by the use of sumatriptin in migraine.

An additional area where understanding the properties of the 5-HT systems might help clarify 5-HT effects at the clinical level involves the dual 5-HT projections to the forebrain and their differential sensitivity to neurotoxic amphetamine derivatives. The cerebral cortex in many mammals is innervated by two morphologically distinct classes of 5-HT axon terminals. Fine axons with small varicosities arise from the dorsal raphe nuclei, and beaded axons with large spherical varicosities arise from the median raphe nuclei. These two types of axons have different regional and laminar distributions and are differentially sensitive to neurotoxic effects of certain amphetamine derivatives, which include 3,4-methylenedioxymethamphetamine (ecstasy) (MDMA). The fine axons are much more sensitive to neurotoxic effects than the beaded axons, and the loss of fine axons lasts for months whereas the beaded axons remain unaffected following neurotoxic drug treatment (39). Individuals using MDMA utilize doses approaching those shown to be neurotoxic in nonhuman primates, and indeed a 26% decrease in 5-hydroxy indoleacetic acid (5-HIAA) in cerebrospinal fluid was found in MDMA users (53), providing evidence of lost 5-HT turnover—presumably in the fine axon system. Thus, the study of MDMA users could provide information on the selective effects of loss of the fine axon system in humans. Unfortunately, these studies have been difficult to conduct because of the difficulty in controlling for other drug use and subject selection bias. It is of interest, however, that when subjects retrospectively compared their MDMA experience *after* taking fluoxetine (which is known to block the neurotoxic effects of MDMA) to their experience *before* taking fluoxetine, the euphoric and positive interpersonal effects of MDMA were reported to be unchanged (42). Although this might suggest a differential role for the fine and beaded axon systems in explaining the effects of MDMA and the role of 5-HT in reward systems, additional data will clearly be needed to clarify this interesting question.

SUMMARY

Following the discovery of the "serum tonic" factor, 5-HT, in 1948 (see Chapter 58, *this volume*), the exponentially increasing amount of information on the molecular biology, biochemistry, pharmacology, anatomy, physiology, and behavior of the 5-HT system has led to a wide array of clinical applications. Probes of 5-HT turnover in CNS and peripheral tissue have demonstrated alterations in 5-HT metabolism to be associated with a wide number of clinical conditions, and many drugs such as antidepressants, antipsychotics, and anxiolytics have been shown to alter 5-HT function in several disorders. The development and widespread use of SSRIs has demonstrated that the 5-HT systems are involved is a diverse array of very different clinical conditions. In contrast, the development of specific 5-HT receptor agonists and antagonists has led to more specific targeted therapeutic interventions such as (a) the use of the 5-HT agonist, sumatriptin, in migraine and cluster headache and (b) the use of 5-HT3 antagonist ondansetron in the control of nausea and emesis.

At present, a simple holistic view of the 5-HT systems role in clinical disorders cannot be advocated. Rather, a more empirical experimental but optimistic approach would be proposed. The widespread involvement of the 5-HT systems in modulating the physiologic functions of a large number of different and important biologic systems, coupled with the rapid progress of the molecular biologic approach in discovering new 5-HT receptor subtypes, should foster increased research activity directed at the development of clinically applicable and specific 5-HT receptor subtype agonists and antagonists. These new drugs can then be studied alone and in combination with other treatments in order to clarify the parameters of drug use for the clinical effect. By comparing and contrasting the optimal clinical effect of a drug to the proven effects of the drug on the specific 5-HT system involved, it will be possible in the future to more clearly specify the role of the specific 5-HT system in the pathogenesis and treatment of the particular clinical disorder.

ACKNOWLEDGMENTS

This work was supported, in part, by USPHS grants MH362290 and MH25642.

REFERENCES

1. Adly C, Straumanis J, Chesson A. Fluoxetine prophyaxis of migraine. *Headache* 1992;2:101–104.
2. Aubineau P, Cunin G, Brochet B, Louvet-Giendaj C, Henry P. Release of serotonin only in painful area during cluster headache attacks. *Lancet* 1992;339:1294–1295.
3. Barr LC, Goodman WK, McDougle CJ, et al. Tryptophan depletion in obsessive compulsive disorder patients responding to serotonin reuptake inhibitors. *Arch Gen Psychiatry* 1994;51:304–317.
4. Barrickman L, Noyes R, Kuperman S, Schumacher E, Verda M. Treatment of ADHD with fluoxetine: a preliminary trial. *J Am Acad Child Adolesc Psychiatry* 1991;30:762–767.
5. Bateman DN. Sumatriptan. *Lancet* 1993;341:221–224.
6. Bolte MA, Avery D. Case of fluoxetine-induced remission of Raynaud's phenomenon—a case report. *Angiology* 1993;2:161–163.
7. Clomipramine Collaborative Study Group. Comipramine in the treatment of patients with obsessive compulsive disorder. *Arch Gen Psychiatry* 1991;48:730–738.
8. Cook EM, Rowlett R, Jaselskis C, Leventhal BL. Fluoxetine treatment of children and adults with autistic disorder and mental retardation. *J Am Acad Child Adolesc Psychiatry* 1992;31:739–745.
9. Cornelius JR, Soloff PH, Perel JM, Ulrich RF. A preliminary trial of

fluoxetine in refractory borderline patients. *J Clin Psychopharmacol* 1991;2:116–120.

10. Delgado PL, Charney DS, Price LH, Aghajanian GK, Landis H, Heninger GR. Serotonin function and the mechanism of antidepressant action. Reversal of antidepressant induced remission by rapid depletion of plasma tryptophan. *Arch Gen Psychiatry* 1990;47:411–418.

11. Delgado PL, Miller HL, Salomon RM, et al. Monoamines and the mechanism of antidepressant action: effects of catecholamine depletion on mood of patients treated with antidepressants. *Psychopharmacol Bull* 1993;3:389–395.

12. Delgado PL, Miller HM, Salomon RM, Licinio J, Krystal JH, Heninger GR, Charney DS. Tryptophan depletion challenge in depressed patients treated with desipramine or fluoxetine: implications for the role of serotonin in the mechanism of antidepressant action. Submitted for publication.

13. Delgado PL, Price LH, Miller HL, et al. Rapid serotonin depletion as a provocation challenge test for patients with major depression: relevance to antidepressant action and the neurobiology of depression. *Psychopharmacol Bull* 1991;27:321–330.

14. Delgado PL, Price LH, Miller HL, Salomon RM, Aghajanian GKJ, Heninger GR, Charney DS. Serotonin and the neurobiology of depression: effects of tryptophan depletion in drug-free depressed patients. *Arch Gen Psychiatry* 1994;[in press].

15. Descarries L, Audet MA, Doucet G, et al. Morphology of central serotonin neurons: brief review of quantified aspects of their distribution and ultrastructural relationships. In: Whitaker-Azmitia PM, Peroutka SJ, eds. *The neuropharmacology of serotonin.* New York: New York Academy of Sciences, 1990;81–92.

16. Eisendrath SJ, Kodama KT. Fluoxetine management of chronic abdominal pain. *Psychosomatics* 1992;2:L227–L229.

17. Fluoxetine Bulimia Nervosa Collaborative Study Group. Fluoxetine in the treatment of bulimia nervosa. A multicenter, placebo-controlled, double-blind trial. *Arch Gen Psychiatry* 1992;49:139–147.

18. Goldbloom DS, Olmsted MP. Pharmacotherapy of bulimia nervosa with fluoxetine: assessment of clinically significant attitudinal change. *Am J Psychiatry* 1993;5:770–774.

19. Goldman MB, Janecek HM. Adjunctive fluoxetine improves global function in chronic schizophrenia. *J Neuropsychiatry Clin Neurosci* 1990;4:429–431.

20. Goodman WK, Price LH, Delgado PL, et al. Specificity of serotonin reuptake inhibitors in the treatment of obsessive–compulsive disorder. Comparison of fluvoxamine and desipramine. *Arch Gen Psychiatry* 1990;47:577–585.

21. Goodwin FK, Jamison KR. *Manic depressive illness.* New York: Oxford University Press, 1990;416–447.

22. Gordon CT, State RC, Nelson JE, Hamburger SD, Rapoport JL. A double-blind comparison of clomipramine, desipramine, and placebo in the treatment of autistic disorder. *Arch Gen Psychiatry* 1993;50:441–447.

23. Gorelick DA, Paredes A. Effect of fluoxetine on alcohol consumption in male alcoholics. *Alcoholism* 1992;16:261–265.

24. Gray DS, Fujioka K, Devine W, Bray GA. A randomized double-blind clinical trial of fluoxetine in obese diabetics. *Int J Obesity* 1992;4:S67–S72.

25. Gross MD. Treatment of pathological jealousy by fluoxetine [Letter]. *Am J Psychiatry* 1991;148:683–684.

26. Grubb BP, Wolfe DA, Samoil D, Temesy-Armos P, Hahn H, Elliott L. Usefulness of fluoxetine hydrochloride for prevention of resistant upright tilt induced syncope. *Pacing Clin Electrophysiol* 1993;3:458–464.

27. Herrstedt J, Sigsgaard T, Boesgaard M, Jensen T, Domernowsky P. Ondansetron plus metopimazine compared with ondansetron alone in patients receiving moderately emetogenic chemotherapy. *N Engl J Med* 1993;328:1076–1080.

28. Hollander E, Liebowitz MR, DeCaria C, Fairbanks J, Fallon B, Klein DF. Treatment of depersonalization with serotonin reuptake blockers. *J Clin Psychopharmacol* 1990;10:200–203.

29. Kafka MP, Prentky P. Fluoxetine treatment of nonparaphilic sexual addictions and paraphilias in men. *J Clin Psychiatry* 1992;10:351–358.

30. Kenny GN, Oates JL, Leeser J, et al. Efficacy of orally administered ondansetron in the prevention of postoperative nausea and vomiting: a dose ranging study. *Br J Anaesth* 1992;68:466–470.

31. Koran LM, Raghavan S. Fluoxetine for isolated sleep paralysis. *Psychosomatics* 1993;2:184–187.

32. Kruesi MJ, Fine S, Valladares L, Phillips RA Jr, Rapoport JL. Paraphilias: a double-blind crossover comparison of clomipramine versus desipramine. *Arch Sexual Behav* 1992;21(6):587–593.

33. Kurlan R, Como PG, Deeley C, McDermott M, McDermott MP. A pilot controlled study of fluoxetine for obsessive compulsive symptoms in children with Tourette's syndrome. *Clin Neuropharmacol* 1993;16:167–172.

34. Kutnowski M, Daubresse JC, Friedman H, et al. Fluoxetine therapy in obese diabetic and glucose intolerant patients. *Int J Obesity* 1992;16:S63–S66.

35. Lane RD. Successful fluoxetine treatment of pathologic jealousy. *J Clin Psychiatry* 1990;51:345–346.

36. Leonard HL, Lenane MC, Swedo SE, Retew DC, Rapoport JL. A double-blind comparison of clomipraimine and desipramine treatment of severe onychophagia (nail biting). *Arch Gen Psychiatry* 1991;48(9):821–827.

37. Levitt M, Warr D, Yelle L, et al. Ondansetron compared with dexamethasone and metoclopramide as antimetics in the chemotherapy of breast cancer with cyclophosphamide, methotrexate, and fluorouracil. *N Engl J Med* 1993;328:1081–1084.

38. Liebowitz MR, Schneier FR, Hollander E, et al. Treatment of social phobia with drugs other than benzodiazepines. *J Clin Psychiat* 1991;52:10–15.

39. Mamounas LA, Mullen CA, O'Hearn E, Molliver ME. Dual serotonergic projections to forebrain in the rat: morphologically distinct 5HT axon terminals exhibit differential vulnerability to neurotoxic amphetamine derivatives. *J Comp Neurol* 1991;314:558–586.

40. Markowitz PI. Effect of fluoxetine on self-injurious behavior in the developmentally disabled: a preliminary study. *J Clin Psychopharmacol* 1992;12:27–31.

41. Max MB, Lynch SA, Muir J, Shoaf SE, Smoller B, Dubner R. Effects of desipramine, amitriptyline, and fluoxetine on pain in diabetic neuropathy. *N Engl J Med* 1992;19:1250–1256.

42. McCann UD, Ricaurte GA. Reinforcing subjective effects of ($\pm$) 3,4-methylenedioxymethamphetamine (ecstasy) may be separable from its neurotoxic actions: clinical evidence. *J Clin Psychopharmacol* 1992;13:214–217.

43. Moskowitz MA, Cutrer FM. Sumatriptan: a receptor-targeted treatment for migraine. *Annu Rev Med* 1993;44:145–154.

44. Nagy LM, Morgan CA, Southwick SM, Charney DS. Open prospective trial of fluoxetine for post-traumatic stress disorder. *J Clin Psychopharmacol* 1993;13:107–113.

45. Naranjo CA, Kadlec KE, Sanheuza P, Woodley-Remus D, Sellers EM. Fluoxetine differentially alters alcohol intake and other consummatory behaviors in problem drinkers. *Clin Pharmacol Ther* 1990;47:490–498.

46. Panzer MJ, Mellow AM. Antidepressant treatment of pathologic laughing or crying in elderly stroke patients. *J Geriatr Psychiatry Neurol* 1992;4:195–199.

47. Petitto JM, Mundle LB, Nagy BR, Evans DL, Golden RN. Improvement of arthritis with fluoxetine. *Psychosomatics* 1992;3:338–341.

48. Phillips KA, McElroy SL, Keck PE, Pope HG, Hudson JI. Body dysmorphic disorder: 30 cases of imagined ugliness. *Am J Psychiatry* 1993;150:302–308.

49. Pijl H, Kippeschaar HP, Willekens FL, Frolich M, Meinders AE. The influence of serotonergic neurotransmission on pituitary hormone release in obese and non-obese females. *Acta Endocrinol* 1993;4:319–324.

50. Platt AJ, Heddle RM, Rake MO, Smedley H. Ondansetron in carcinoid syndrome. *Lancet* 1992;339:1416.

51. Pomerleau OF, Pomerleau CS, Morrell EM, Lowenberg JM. Effects of fluoxetine on weight gain and food intake in smokers who reduce nicotine intake. *Psychoneuroendocrinology* 1991;16:433–440.

52. Potter BJ, Radder JK, Frolich M, Krans HM, Zwinderman AH, Meinders AE. Fluoxetine increases insulin action in obese nondiabetic and in obese non-insulin-dependent diabetic individuals. *Int J Obesity* 1992;2:79–85.

53. Ricaurte GA, Finnegan KT, Irwin I, Langston JW. Aminergic metabolites in cerebrospinal fluid of humans previously exposed to MDMA: preliminary observations. In: Whitaker PM, Peroutka SJ, eds. *The neuropharmacology of serotonin.* New York: New York Academy of Sciences, 1990;699.

54. Shopsin B, Friedman E, Gershon S. Parachlorophenylalanine reversal of tranylcypromine effects in depressed patients. *Arch Gen Psychiatry* 1976;33:811–819.

55. Shopsin B, Gershon S, Goldstein M, Friedman E, Wilk S. Use of synthesis inhibitors in defining a role of biogenic amines during imipramine treatment in depressed patients. *Psychopharmacol Commun* 1975;1:239–249.

56. Sichel DA, Cohen LS, Dimmock JA, Rosenbaum JF. Postpartum obsessive compulsive disorder: a case series. *J Clin Psychiatry* 1993;54:156–159.

57. Sindrup SH, Bjerrfe U, Dejgaard A, Brosen K, Aaes-Jorgensen T, Gram LF. The selective serotonin reuptake inhibitor citalopram relieves the symptoms of diabetic neuropathy. *Clin Pharmacol Ther* 1992;547–552.

58. Sjoerdsma A, Palfreyman MG. History of serotonin and serotonin disorders. In: Whitaker-Azmitia PM, Peroutka SJ, eds. *The neuropharmacology of serotonin.* New York: New York Academy of Sciences, 1990;1–8.

59. Smith SE, Pihl RO, Young SN, Ervin FR. A test of possible cognitive and environmental influences on the mood lowering effect of tryptophan depletion in normal males. *Psychopharmacology* 1987;91:451–457.

60. Stein DJ, Hollander E, Anthony DT, et al. Serotonergic medications for sexual obsessions, sexual additions, and paraphilias. *J Clin Psychiatry* 1992;8:267–271.

61. Swedo SE, Leonard HL, Rapoport JL, Lenane MC, Goldberger EL, Cheslow DL. A double-blind comparison of clomipramine and desipramine in the treatment of trichotillomania (hair pulling). *N Engl J Med* 1989;321(8):497–501.

62. Takeda N, Morita M, Hasegawa S, Horii A, Kubo T, Matsunaga T. Neuropharmacology of motion sickness and emesis. *Acta Otolaryngol (Stockh)* 1993;501:10–15.

63. Tansey M, Pilgrim A, Lloyd K. Sumatriptan in the acute treatment of migraine. *J Neurol Sci* 1993;114:109–116.

64. Urban RJ, Veldhuis JD. A selective serotonin uptake inhibitor, fluoxetine hydrochloride, modulates the pulsatile release of prolactin in postmenopausal women. *Am J Obstet Gynecol* 1991;64:147–152.

65. Van Ameringen M, Mancini C, Streiner DL. Fluoxetine efficacy in social phobia. *J Clin Psychiatry* 1993;54:27–32.

66. Van Praag HM, Asnis GM, Kahn RS, et al. Nosological tunnel vision in biological psychiatry: a plea for a functional psychopathology. In: Whitaker-PM, Peroutka SJ, eds. *The neuropharmacology of serotonin.* New York: New York Academy of Sciences, 1990;501.

67. Van Woert MH, Rosenbaum D, Chung E. Fluoxetine in the treatment of intention myoclonus. *Clin Neuropharmacol* 1983;1:49–54.

68. Van Woert MH, Rosenbaum D, Howieson J, Bowers MB Jr. Long-term therapy of myoclonus and other neurologic disorders with L-5-hydroxytryptophan and carbidopa. *N Engl J Med* 1977;296:70–75.

69. Vanhoutte PM. Serotonin and the vascular wall. *International J Cardiol* 1987;14:189–203.

70. Warnock JK, Kestenbaum T. Pharmacologic treatment of severe skin-picking behaviors in Prader–Willi syndrome. Two case reports. *Arch Dermatol* 1992;128:1623–1625.

71. Wood SH, Mortola JF, Chan YF, Moossazadeh F, Yen SS. Treatment of premenstrual syndrome with fluoxetine: a double-blind placebo-controlled, crossover study. *Obstet Gynecology* 1992;3:339–344.

72. Young SN, Ervin FR, Pihl RO, Finn P. Biochemical aspects of tryptophan depletion in primates. *Psychopharmacology* 1989;98:508–511.

73. Young SN, Pihl RO, Ervin FR. The effect of altered tryptophan levels on mood and behavior in normal human males. *Clin Neuropharmacol* 1988;11:(Suppl 1):S207–S215.

Psychopharmacology: The Fourth Generation of Progress, edited by Floyd E. Bloom and David J. Kupfer. Raven Press, Ltd., New York © 1995.

CHAPTER 43

General Overview of Neuropeptides

Tomas G. M. Hökfelt, Marie-Noëlle Castel, Patrizia Morino, Xu Zhang, and Åke Dagerlind

The development of the neuropeptide field was covered in several chapters in the last two volumes of this series (65,72); (see also refs. 11,36,39,57, and 88). In the second volume (65), 11 chapters out of 149 dealt with neuropeptides. In the third volume (72), 6 chapters discussed basic aspects on peptides, and in 11 chapters the possible involvement of peptides in various diseases, including schizophrenia and Alzheimer's disease, was considered. In the concluding chapter by Bloom (9) peptides were also discussed, suggesting that peptides have secured a position in the field of psychopharmacology. However, these 18 chapters only constituted about 10% of the total number of the contributions to the volume (184 chapters). This seems reasonable because, although many interesting concepts and hypotheses have been advanced with regard to the functional role of peptides both in experimental animals and in humans, there has been no major breakthrough in terms of a causal relation between a peptide and a disease or with regard to the use of peptide drugs for treatment of central nervous system (CNS) disorders. In this chapter, due to limited space, essentially only references from 1987 and later have been included.

NEW METHODOLOGICAL APPROACHES

There is reason to believe that over the next few years decisive data will emerge with regard to the involvement of peptides in various CNS functions, in one or the other direction, that is to confirm or refute existing theories. The basis for this cautious optimism is that several major advancements have been made since the previous volume was published in 1987. Thus, novel techniques for studies

of peptides have been employed. The histochemical approach has benefited in particular from various in situ hybridization procedures (125). Based on molecular biological methods, a number of peptide receptors have been cloned, including all three types of opioid receptors (see ref. 76 and Table 1). Furthermore, after the introduction of the first peptide antagonists, which all were modified peptide molecules, there is now available a second generation of compounds which are small molecules of nonpeptide nature and which pass the blood–brain barrier (Table 2). As indicated in Table 2, the development of these antagonists has occurred within the framework of the pharmaceutical companies, whereby various types of approaches have been taken. Thus, major screening efforts have resulted in lead compounds which have been modified into powerful and specific antagonists, but also rational drug design starting out from the peptide molecule itself has been employed (see ref. 43). Clearly, the resources of the industry and their commitment provide hope for further antagonists which can be available for studying the role of peptides in experimental animals and, hopefully, for testing them in various disorders. Finally, an alternative approach to explore the functional role of peptides is the use of antisense probes. Thus over the last few years numerous studies have been published in which oligonucleotide probes complementary to a sequence of a certain peptide mRNA have been used to block or attenuate translation of mRNA into protein. Interestingly, successful results have been obtained not only in in vitro studies but also, for example, after intraventricular administration (116). Moreover, it is considered that such oligonucleotides may become useful as therapeutic agents (104) (see also Chapters 47, 48, 52, and 158, *this volume*).

COEXISTENCE OF MESSENGERS

When discussing the role of peptides it is important to note that in virtually all systems they coexist with at

---

T. G. M. Hökfelt, M.-N. Castel, P. Morino, X. Zhang, and Å. Dagerlind: Department of Neuroscience, Karolinska Institutet, S-171 77 Stockholm, Sweden.

TABLE 1. *Cloned neuropeptide receptors*[a]

Receptor	Species	References
Substance K	Bovine	70
Substance P	Rat	124
	Rat	37
	Rat	110
Neuromedin K	Rat	99
Neurotensin	Rat	111
NPY	Rat	23
NPY/PYY	Human	58
NPY	Human	38
NPY	Bovine	90
Angiotensin II	Rat	94
	Bovine	84
Bombesin	Rat	115
	Swiss 3T3 cells	5
TRH	Mouse	106
	Rat	19
CCK$_A$	Rat	119
CCK$_B$/gastrin	Canine	56
Oxytocin	Human	52
Somatostatin SSR-14	Rat	77
	Human, murine	122
Somatostatin SSR-28	Rat	78
Vasopressin V1, V2	Rat, human	7
		66
		82
VIP	Human	44
	Rat	103
Opioid peptides, δ receptor	Rat	25
	Rat	51
	Mouse	12
Opioid peptides, μ receptor	Rat	118
Opioid peptides, κ receptor	Mouse	123

[a] Expanded from ref. 76.

least one classic transmitter (39). Most attention has been focused on colocalization with biogenic amines and acetylcholine. There is, however, immunohistochemical evidence that, in addition, they may express an amino acid transmitter, such as gamma-aminobutyric acid (GABA) (6) or glutamate (48,86). In fact, using triple-staining methodology, evidence for coexpression of glutamate-, 5-hydroxytryptamine- and substance P-like immunoreac-

tivities in bulbospinal neurons has been presented (87). In an elegant in vitro study, Johnson (47) has recently shown co-release of serotonin and glutamate from rat mesopontine neurons. In the peripheral nervous system, certain neurons may release ATP, noradrenaline and neuropeptide tyrosine (NPY) (50,101). Thus, neurons may release a "cocktail" of messenger molecules providing a spectrum of biological actions, including different temporal information (fast, intermediate, and slow signaling).

An important issue will be to understand the mechanisms underlying the release of these different classes of messenger molecules. There is early evidence that the release of classic transmitter and peptide can be differential and dependent on frequency and patterns of firing, presumably due to different subcellular storage sites. Verhage et al. (113) have analyzed this question on isolated nerve endings, providing evidence that neuropeptide release is triggered by small elevations in the Ca^{2+} concentration in the bulk cytoplasm, whereas secretion of amino acids requires higher elevations, as produced in the vicinity of Ca^{2+} channels—that is, near the active zone at synapses.

NEUROPEPTIDE RECEPTORS

The existence of neuropeptide receptors remained obscure for a long period, in spite of the fact of many serious attempts were made to biochemically purify and to clone such receptors, particularly with regard to the opioid receptors. Thus, in spite of the early demonstration of multiple types of binding sites for various opioid peptides as well as the strong evidence from many ligand binding studies, the receptor proteins were elusive. In fact, since peptides frequently seem to coexist with classic transmitters, it could not be excluded that binding sites for peptides were located on the receptor molecules of classic transmitters. It was therefore important to establish the nature of peptide receptors, and this was first achieved for members of the tachykinin family.

In 1987 the isolation of a cDNA clone for a bovine substance K receptor from a stomach cDNA library was reported (70), and this first cloned peptide receptor belonged to the family of G-protein-coupled receptors with

TABLE 2. *Nonpeptide antagonists*

Receptor	Code name	Drug company	References
Cholecystokinin A	L-364,718	MSD	24
	LY 219057	Eli Lilly	42
Cholecystokinin B	L-356,260	MSD	10
	CI 988	Parke-Davis	43
	LY 262691	Eli Lilly	4
Neurokinin 1	CP 96345	Pfizer	102
	RP 67580	Rhône-Poulenc	27
	WIN 51708	Sterling Winthrop	2
Neurokinin 2	SR 48968	Sanofi	1
Neurotensin	SR 48692	Sanofi	34

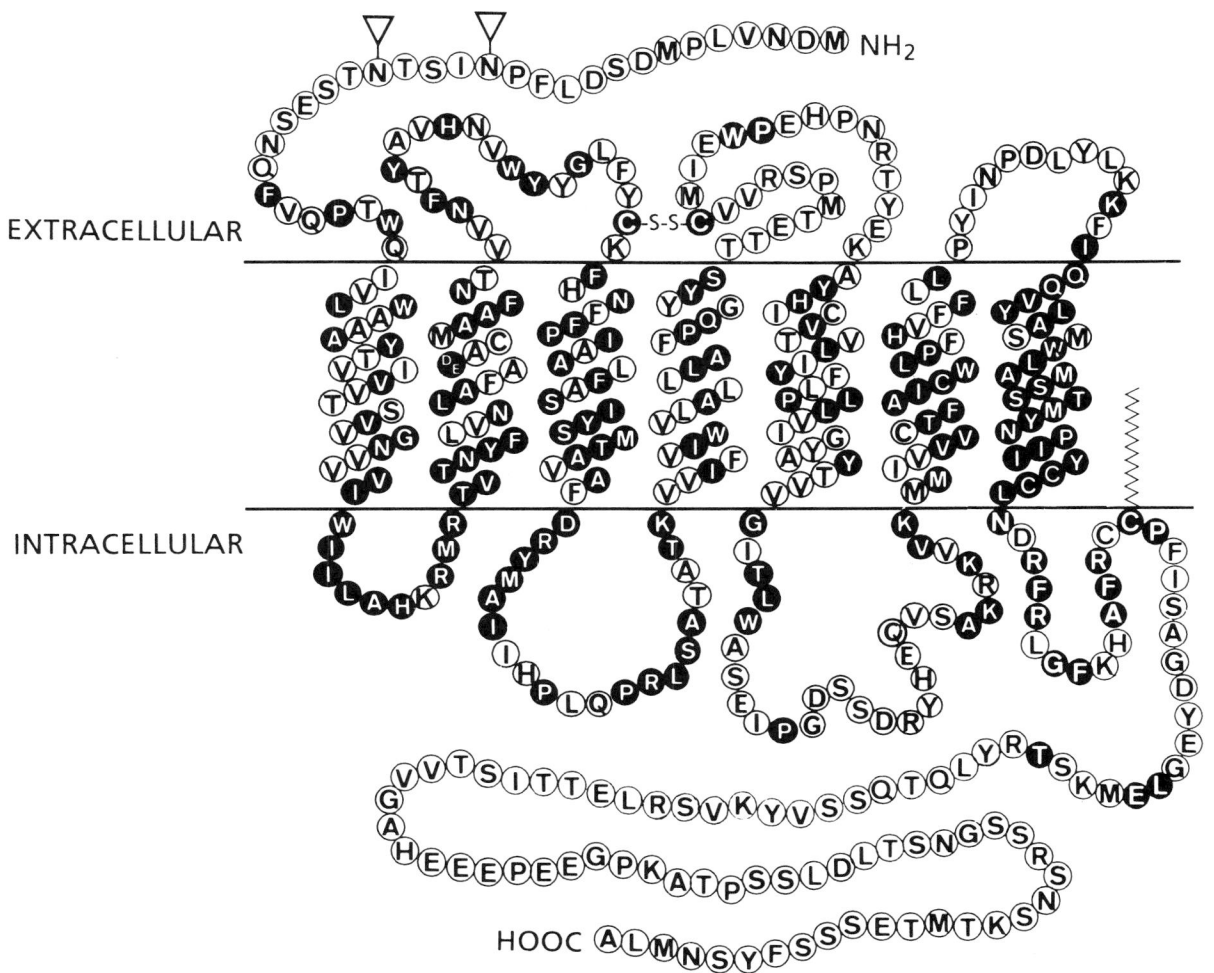

FIG. 1. The substance P receptor. (Drawing provided by Professor S. Nakanishi. From ref. 124.)

seven membrane-spanning segments. Subsequently the neuronal substance P (Fig. 1) and substance K (37,124) and the neurotensin (111) receptors were cloned and shown to belong to the G-protein-coupled receptors. Subsequent work has demonstrated that so far all neuropeptide receptors are of this type, including the recently cloned δ, μ, and κ opioid receptors (76) (Table 1).

The cloning of various peptide receptors allows studies of their regulation and of the distribution of cell bodies producing these receptors using in situ hybridization. The information from the cloning studies can also be used to produce antibodies against specific portions of the receptor protein, either raised against a short, unique peptide sequence or against longer peptides produced in various expression systems. For example, antibodies against the substance P receptor have been produced and used for analysis of distribution in the rat striatum (49,98). Also the δ opioid receptor protein has been analyzed with immunohistochemistry (18).

NEW PEPTIDES

In the 1970s the hunt for new peptides was intense, and an ever-growing list could be compiled. However, it seems that the pace of appearance of novel peptides on the scene has slowed down. Since the publication of the latest volume in this series (72), some important peptides are the atrial natriuretic factor and the endothelins which have corresponding family members in the brain with interesting distribution patterns (31,100,107). In 1993 secretoneuron, a 33-amino-acid cleavage product from secretogranin II (or chromogranin C), was identified (53). This peptide has interesting distribution patterns both in the rat (68) and human (69) brain, as well as potent biological effects, causing (for example) release of dopamine from striatal slices (93). These recent studies strengthen earlier knowledge that the large peptide precursor molecules may hide interesting biological activities, and they suggest that further analysis of precursors may yield other peptides, as has been repeatedly shown (for example) in other studies on the opioid peptide precursors.

TROPHIC EFFECTS OF PEPTIDES

As described above, it is likely that peptides participate in signaling at nonsynaptic and synaptic sites, primarily

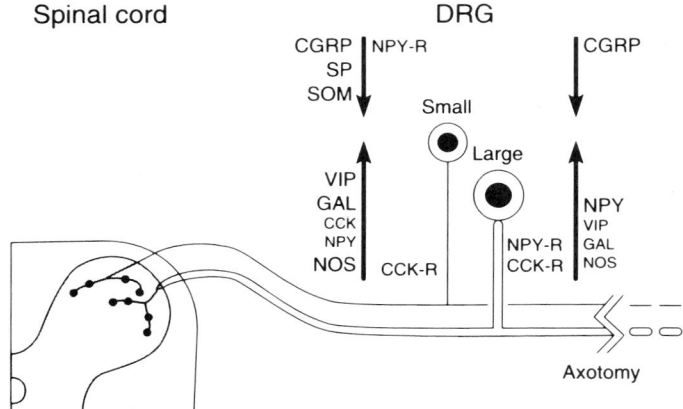

Spinal cord   DRG

FIG. 2. Schematic drawing of a small and a large primary sensory neuron in a dorsal root ganglion (DRG) sending a central branch to the dorsal horn of the spinal cord and with peripheral branches that have been sectioned (axotomy). The changes occurring in levels of peptides and of mRNAs for peptides and peptide receptors are indicated by *arrows.* Thus, in small DRG neurons calcitonin gene-related peptide (CGRP), substance P (SP), somatostatin (SOM), and the neuropeptide tyrosine (NPY) Y1-receptor mRNA are down-regulated, whereas vasoactive intestinal polypeptide (VIP), galanin (GAL), cholecystokinin (CCK), NPY, nitric oxide synthase (NOS), and the CCK$_B$ receptor mRNA are up-regulated. In the large neurons CGRP is down-regulated, whereas NPY, VIP, GAL, and NOS, as well as the mRNAs for the NPY and CCK receptors, are up-regulated. Large letters indicate pronounced changes, whereas smaller letters denote modest changes. R, receptor. (From ref. 41.)

in slow signaling. However, more recent evidence indicates that they also exert trophic actions (39,105). Although most results on the latter effects have been obtained in the periphery, it is probable that similar peptide actions also occur in the CNS. To mention a few recent studies, vasoactive intestinal peptide (VIP) has a dramatic effect on growth of whole fetuses in vitro (33) and calcitonin gene-related peptide (CGRP) may represent an anterograde factor which, after release at the motor end-plate, regulates gene expression of acetylcholine receptors (26). In another model system, CGRP has been reported to induce a dopaminergic phenotype in olfactory bulb neurons, thus mimicking the olfactory epithelium neurons and perhaps representing a differentiation factor for dopamine neurons (20).

PLASTICITY IN PEPTIDE EXPRESSION

Studies both in the periphery and in the CNS have demonstrated that peptide levels may vary considerably during different conditions, including endogenous variations and after experimental manipulations. This is not surprising per se, because peptides in general are assumed to be produced ribosomally and because replacement after

release only seems to occur via new synthesis in cell bodies (however, see below). This is in marked contrast to, for example, catecholamines which can be locally synthesized in nerve endings and also be replaced by efficient reuptake mechanisms. Moreover, the rate of catecholamine synthesis can also be regulated by phosphorylation of synthetic enzymes. Thus, it is possible to keep classic transmitter levels constant under various conditions. The quite dramatic regulation of peptide synthesis has been particularly evident when using the in situ hybridization technique (see ref. 125) for analysis of peptide mRNA levels in neuronal somata under various experimental conditions. Here we will focus on two systems, namely, primary sensory neurons and neurons in the rat striatum. We are convinced that similar regulations occur in many other systems, which are important from psychopharmacological point of view. We include primary sensory neurons because they represent, just as the striatum, an easily accessible model system.

Primary Sensory Neurons and the Dorsal Horn

Primary sensory neurons were one of the first systems to be shown to contain substantial amounts of peptides (Fig. 2) in the mid-1970s and have ever since represented a model for analysis of peptidergic mechanisms. It is now clear that peptides in primary sensory neurons can be divided into two groups (41). The first group consists of peptides which are present in substantial amounts under normal circumstances and which in all probability facilitate transmission in the dorsal horn. They include substance P, CGRP, and somatostatin. In contrast, the second group consists of peptides such as VIP/peptide histidine isoleucine (PHI), galanin, and NPY, which are normally expressed at low levels or cannot be detected at all, but which are dramatically increased after experimental manipulation, especially axotomy (Fig. 2) (40,96,117). There is also an impressive regulation of the mRNAs for cholecystokinin (CCK)$_B$ (127) and NPY (128) receptors in dorsal root ganglion neurons after axotomy (Fig. 2). Provided that the increase or decrease in mRNA levels results in corresponding changes in receptor protein and incorporation into the neuronal membrane, these findings suggest that changes in sensitivity to a certain peptide represent a further principle to adapt to a lesion. Although the exact role of these peptides and their receptors is unclear, they may exert modulating effects and, particularly after axotomy, suppress spinal excitability. Taken together, it therefore seems as if primary sensory neurons following peripheral nerve injury change their phenotype with regard to both messengers and function, the implications being that dorsal root ganglion neurons adapt to the new situation by suppressing excitatory transmitters and perhaps promoting survival and regeneration and enhance inhibitory mechanisms. This is in agreement with the general view of the reaction of neurons in response to injury, mainly based on studies on motoneurons, emphasizing that the synthetic machinery of the neuron is converted from transmitter synthesis to production of molecules of importance for survival and recovery. Here we will not continue to deal with the functional significance and possible effects of these regulations but will refer to, for example, some recent review articles (41,121).

Peptide Regulation in the Rat Striatum

The striatum occupies a central position in basal ganglia, partially due to its rich dopaminergic innervation and its relation to several serious CNS disorders such as Parkinson's disease and Huntington's chorea. Although much interest has been focused on dopamine and its functional role, it has become clear that also neuropeptides play an important role in this system (see refs. 28 and 32). In addition to the fact that many dopamine neurons themselves contain peptides such as CCK, several neuron populations in the striatum express peptides at higher or lower levels. Two major populations exist, one of which contains substance P and dynorphin; these neurons project to the substantia nigra zona reticulata, whereas enkephalin-immunoreactive neurons mainly seem to project to the globus pallidus (28,32). Double-staining techniques have demonstrated that many of these peptide neurons have GABA as their principal transmitter (89).

There is now strong evidence that the three peptides mentioned above—enkephalin, substance P, and dynorphin—are regulated by the dopaminergic input from the substantia nigra. Thus, various manipulations attenuating dopamine transmission in the striatum—for example, treatment with 6-hydroxydopamine or dopamine receptor antagonists—result in increased expression of enkephalin, as well as a decrease in dynorphin and substance P, whereas dopamine agonists increase levels of dynorphin and substance P but not enkephalin (see ref. 30).

More recent studies suggest the existence also of another peptide neuron population in the striatum which is dopaminergic-regulated. This peptide is neurotensin, which has been shown to have both interesting clinical and behavioral interactions with dopamine (54,85). Although early mapping studies provided little evidence for neurotensin neurons in the striatum, it could later be shown that drugs that attenuate dopamine transmission, such as haloperidol, 6-hydroxydopamine, and reserpine, reveal many neurotensin-positive cell bodies in the rat striatum (see ref. 21). This up-regulation seems to be mediated via D2 receptors, but also *increased* dopamine receptor stimulation with methamphetamine causes up-regulation of neurotensin in basal ganglia, in this case via a D1 receptor (3,63,73–75,114).

Studies using combined immunohistochemistry, in situ hybridization, and radioimmunoassay have provided

some more insight into this apparent discrepancy. Thus, it has been demonstrated that methamphetamine causes a marked increase in neurotensin-like immunoreactivity in the zona reticulata (i.e., the projection area for striatal neurons), as well as a rapid up-regulation of neurotensin mRNA in the striatum; both effects can be blocked by a D1, but not a D2, antagonist (14–17). In contrast, the neurotensin neurons projecting to the globus pallidus seem to be regulated by D2 receptors (15). All of these studies summarized in Fig. 3, are in agreement with the general view that striatonigral neurons are mainly under the control of the D1 receptors and that the striatopallidal neurons contain D2 receptors (29,35,59,60,91,92).

In situ hybridization studies have revealed that these two neurotensin neuron populations are only partly overlapping, suggesting that striatopallidal and striatonigral neurotensin neurons are separate systems and have different territories in the striatum (14). Interestingly, there is some evidence that combined injection of methamphetamine and sulpiride has a stronger effect on neurotensin-like immunoreactivity in the globus pallidus than does sulpiride alone, suggesting that a population of neurons may respond to both D1 and D2 receptor activation (15). This is in agreement with a recent report showing that several striatal cells coexpress the D1 and D2 receptor mRNAs (62,108,120). Interestingly, Schiffmann and Vanderhaeghen (95) have recently demonstrated up-regulation of neurotensin mRNA in the striatum after chronic injection of caffeine. This neuron population is located in the most lateral aspect of the striatum and does not overlap with any of the above-mentioned neurotensin neurons, suggesting further subpopulations of neurotensin expressing neurons in the striatum (14).

These distinct drug-induced changes in neurotensin are interesting, because methamphetamine is known to induce psychotic symptoms in humans similar to those associated with schizophrenia and also because it has been proposed that neurotensin systems may be involved in mental disorders (85). It is also possible that neurotensin could be associated with the extrapyramidal side effects seen after chronic treatment with neuroleptics. To pursue these questions it will, however, be necessary to analyze to what extent neurotensin is regulated by dopamine also in the human brain (see also Chapter 51, *this volume*).

mRNA IN AXONS

It has been a dogma that peptide synthesis is ribosomal with packaging in the Golgi apparatus and thus confined to the cell soma (97). However, in addition to studies with nonradioactive in situ hybridization showing neuropeptide-encoding mRNAs in neuronal processes beyond the perikaryon (8), over the last few years there has been evidence that oxytocin and vasopressin mRNAs can be detected in the posterior lobe of the pituitary and in

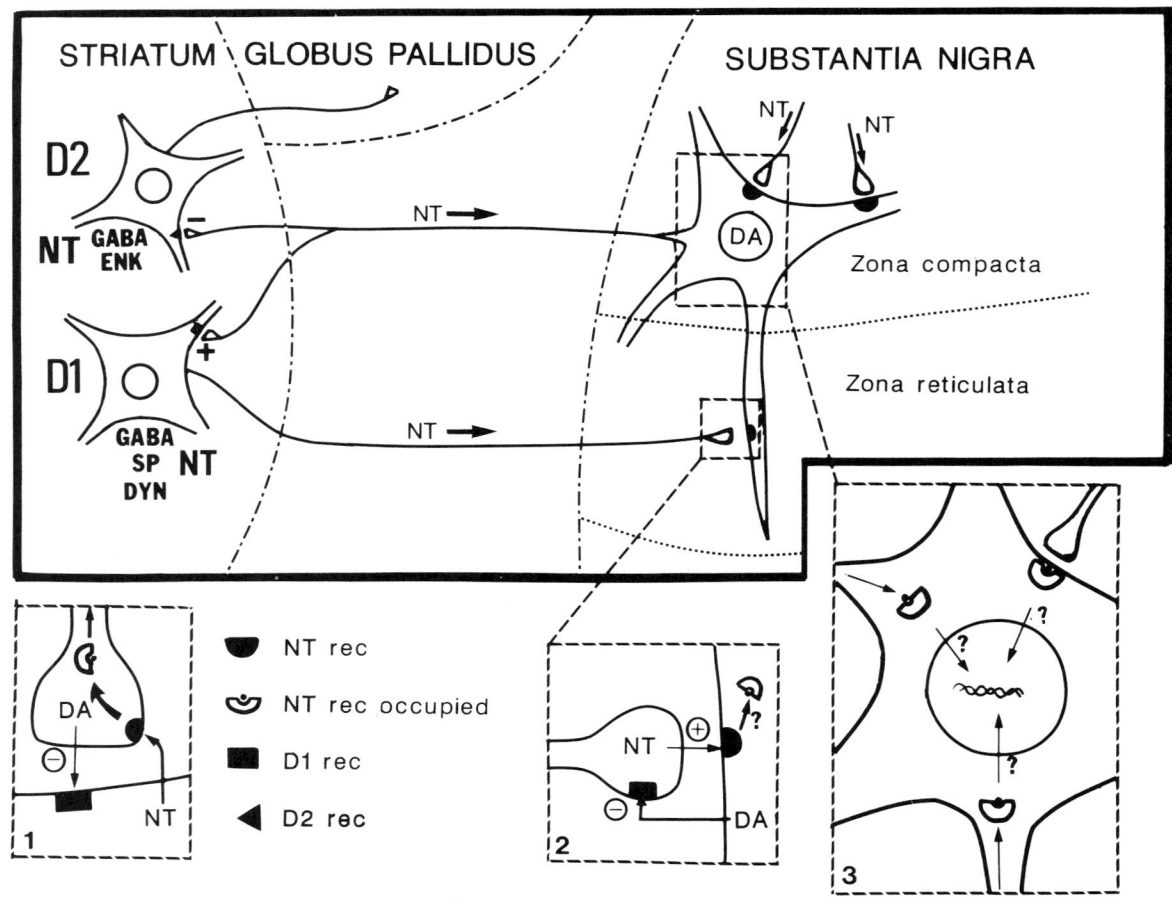

FIG. 3. Schematic drawing of neurotensin neurons related to basal ganglia. After up-regulation, neurotensin is detectable in at least two neuron populations in the striatum projecting to, respectively, globus pallidus and substantia nigra zona reticulata. The former is regulated by D2 receptors and may, in addition, contain GABA and enkephalin. The second population is D1-sensitive and contains GABA, substance P, and dynorphin. After internalization into dopaminergic nerve endings in the striatum, neurotensin may also be retrogradely transported to reach the dopamine neurons in the zona compacta and perhaps influence tyrosine hydroxylase synthesis (13). The dopamine neurons in the zona compacta are surrounded by many neurotensin nerve endings and have abundant neurotensin receptors (22,109,126). (Adapted from ref. 16.)

the median eminence—that is, the projection areas of the magnocellular hypothalamic neurosecretory neurons producing these two peptides (45,61,64,71,79–81,83). The methodologies underlying these observations have been the polymerase chain reaction, Northern blotting, and radioactive and nonradioactive in situ hybridization. Moreover, evidence has been presented for uptake and expression of exogenous vasopressin mRNA after injection into the lateral hypothalamus of vasopressin-deficient Brattleboro rats (46), and it has been shown that exogenous vasopressin mRNA can transiently correct diabetes insipidus in such rats (67). In a recent study using a newly developed in situ hybridization technique with improved sensitivity, Trembleau et al. (112) have analyzed in more detail the subcellular compartmentalization of vasopressin mRNA. Thus, in addition to its localization in discrete areas of the rat endoplasmic reticulum, vasopressin

mRNA was also observed in a subset of axonal swellings in the internal layer of the median eminence and in the posterior lobe of the pituitary. This was particularly evident in salt-loaded animals—that is, a paradigm where vasopressin synthesis is markedly up-regulated. The function of mRNA within the axonal compartment still remains to be elucidated, but these findings raise several interesting questions concerning role(s) of mRNA and site of synthesis of peptides (see also Chapter 47, *this volume*).

CONCLUSION

Major progress has been made in the field of neuropeptides since the publication of *Psychopharmacology: The Third Generation of Progress* (72). The peptides have found their receptors, powerful drugs have been developed, and novel insights into the regulation of peptide synthesis have been obtained, including the provocative finding of mRNA in axonal processes. Still, the physiological roles of neuropeptides not well-defined, and both transmitter-like functions, modulation, and trophic actions have to be considered. With the improved tools now available, it should be possible to clarify many of these open questions. The use of peptide agonists and antagonists should help to elucidate the function of neuropeptides in systems of importance for psychopharmacology.

ACKNOWLEDGMENTS

These studies were supported by the Swedish MRC (04X-2807), the NIMH (MH43230), and Marianne and Marcus Wallenbergs Stiftelse. We thank Professor S. Nakanishi of Kyoto Prefectural University for providing Fig. 1.

REFERENCES

1. Advenier C, Rouissi N, Nguyen QT, Emonds-Alt X, Breliere JC, Neliat G, Naline E, Regoli D. Neurokinin A (NK2) receptor revisited with SR 48968, a potent non-peptide antagonist. *Biochem Biophys Res Commun* 1992;184:1418–1424.
2. Appell KC, Fragale BJ, Loscig J, Singh S, Tomczuk BE. Antagonists that demonstrate species differences in neurokinin-1 receptors. *Mol Pharmacol* 1992;4:772–778.
3. Augood SJ, Kiyama H, Faull RLM, Emson PC. Differential effects of acute dopaminergic D1 and D2 antagonists on proneurotensin mRNA expression in rat striatum. *Mol Brain Res* 1991;9:341–346.
4. Barrett JE, Linden MC, Holloway HC, Yu MJ, Howbert JJ. Anxiolytic-like effects of the CCK-B antagonists LY262691, LY262684, and LY247348 on punished responding of squirrel monkeys. *Soc Neurosci Abstr* 1991;17:1063.
5. Battey JF, Way JM, Corjay MH, Shapira H, Kusano K, Harkins R, Wu JM, Slattery T, Mann E, Feldmann RJ. Molecular cloning of the bombesin/gastrin-releasing peptide receptor from Swiss 3T3 cells. *Proc Natl Acad Sci USA* 1991;88:395–399.
6. Belin MF, Nanopoulos D, Didier D, Aguera M, Steinbusch H, Verhofstad A, Maitre M, Pujol JF. Immunohistochemical evidence for the presence of gamma-aminobutyric acid and serotonin in one nerve cell. A study on the raphe nuclei of the rat using antibodies to glutamate decarboxylase and serotonin. *Brain Res* 1983;275:329–339.
7. Birnbaumer M, Seibold A, Gilbert S, Ishido M, Barberis C, Antaramian A, Brabet P, Rosenthal W. Molecular cloning of the receptor for human antidiuretic hormone. *Nature* 1992;357:333–335.
8. Bloch B, Guitteny AF, Normand E, Chouham S. Presence of neuropeptide messenger RNAs in neuronal processes. *Neurosci Lett* 1990;109:259–264.
9. Bloom FE. Future directions and goals in basic psychopharmacology and neurobiology. In: Meltzer HY, eds. *Psychopharmacology: the third generation of progress.* New York: Raven Press, 1987;1685–1689.
10. Bock MG, DiPardo RM, Evans BE, Rittle KE, Whitter WL, Veber DE, Anderson PS, Freidinger RM. Benzodiazepine gastrin and brain cholecystokinin receptor ligands: L-365,260. *J Med Chem* 1989;32:13–16.
11. Burbach JPH, de Wied D, eds. *Brain functions of neuropeptides. A current view.* Carnforth, NY: The Parthenon Publishing Group, 1993.
12. Bzdega T, Chin H, Kim H, Jung HH, Kozak CA, Klee WA.

13. Castel M-N, Malgouris C, Blanchard J-C, Laduron PM. Retrograde axonal transport of neurotensin in the dopaminergic nigrostriatal pathway in the rat. *Neuroscience* 1990;36:425–430.
14. Castel MN, Morino P, Dagerlind Å, Hökfelt T. Upregulation of neurotensin mRNA in the rat striatum after acute methamphetamine treatment. *Eur J Neurosci* 1994;6:646–656.
15. Castel MN, Morino P, Frey P, Terenius L, Hökfelt T. Immunohistochemical evidence for a neurotensin striatonigral pathway in the rat. *Neuroscience* 1993;55:833–847.
16. Castel MN, Morino P, Hökfelt T. Modulation of the neurotensin striato-nigral pathway by D1 receptors. *Neuroreport* 1993;5:281–284.
17. Castel M-N, Morino P, Nylander I, Terenius L, Hökfelt T. Differential dopaminergic regulation of the neurotensin striato-nigral and striato-pallidal pathways in the rat. *Eur J Pharmacol* 1994;[in press].
18. Dado RJ, Lay PY, Loh HH, Elde R. Immunofluorescent identification of a delta (γ)-opioid receptor on primary afferent nerve terminals. *Neuroreport* 1993;5:341–344.
19. De la Pena P, Delgado LM, Del Camino D, Barros F. Cloning and expression of the thyrotropin-releasing hormone receptor from GH3 rat anterior pituitary cells. *Biochem J* 1992;15:891–899.
20. Denis-Donini S. Expression of dopaminergic phenotypes in the mouse olfactory bulb induced by the calcitonin gene-related peptide. *Nature* 1989;339:701–703.
21. Deutch AY, Zahm DS. The current status of neurotensin-dopamine interactions. *Ann NY Acad Sci* 1992;668:232–252.
22. Elde R, Schalling M, Ceccatelli S, Nakanishi S, Hökfelt T. Localization of neuropeptide receptor mRNA in rat brain: initial observation using probes for neurotensin and substance P receptors. *Neurosci Lett* 1990;120:134–138.
23. Eva C, Keinänen K, Monyer H, Seeburg P, Sprengel R. Molecular cloning of a novel G protein-coupled receptor that may belong to the neuropeptide receptor family. *FEBS Lett* 1990;271:81–84.
24. Evans BE, Bock MG, Rittle KE, DiPardo RM, Whitter WL, Veber DF, Anderson PS, Freidinger RM. Design of potent, orally effective, nonpeptidal antagonists of the peptide hormone cholecystokinin. *Proc Natl Acad Sci USA* 1986;83:4918–4922.
25. Evans CJ, Keith DEJ, Morrison H, Magendzo K, Edwards RH. Cloning of a delta opioid receptor by functional expression. *Science* 1992;258:1952–1955.
26. Fontaine B, Klarsfeld A, Changeux J-P. Calcitonin gene-related peptide and muscle activity regulate acetylcholine receptor alpha-subunit mRNA levels by distinct intracellular pathways. *J Cell Biol* 1987;105:1337–1342.
27. Garret C, Carruette A, Fardin V, Moussaoui S, Peyronel J-F, Blanchard J-C, Laduron PM. Pharmacological properties of a potent and selective nonpeptide substance P antagonist. *Proc Natl Acad Sci USA* 1991;88:10208–10212.
28. Gerfen CR. The neostriatal mosaic: multiple levels of compartmental organization. *Trends Neurosci* 1992;15:133–139.
29. Gerfen CR, Engber PM, Mahan LC, Susel Z, Chase TN, Monsma FJJ, Sibley DR. D1 and D2 dopamine receptor-regulated gene expression on striatonigral and striatopallidal neurons. *Science* 1990;250:1429–1432.
30. Gerfen CR, McGinty JF, Young WSI. Dopamine differentially regulates dynorphin, substance P, and enkephalin expression in striatal neurons: in situ hybridization histochemical analysis. *J Neurosci* 1991;11:1016–1031.
31. Giaid A, Gibson SJ, Ibrahim BN, Legon S, Bloom SR, Yanagisawa M, Masaki T, Varndell IM, Polak JM. Endothelin 1, an endothelium-derived peptide, is expressed in neurons of the human spinal cord and dorsal root ganglia. *Proc Natl Acad Sci USA* 1989;86:7634–7638.
32. Graybiel AM. Neurotransmitters and neuromodulators in the basal ganglia. *Trends Neurosci* 1990;13:244–254.
33. Gressens P, Hill JM, Gozes I, Fridkin M, Brenneman DE. Growth factor function of vasoactive intestinal peptide in whole cultured mouse embryos. *Nature* 1993;362:155–158.
34. Gully D, Canton M, Boigegrain R, Jeanjean F, Molimard J-C, Poncelet M, Gueudet C, Heaulme M, Leyris R, Brouard A, Pelaprat D, Labbé-Jullié C, Mazella J, Soubrié P, Maffrand J-P, Ros-

tène W, Kitabgi P, Le Fur G. Biochemical and pharmacological profile of a potent and selective nonpeptide antagonist of the neurotensin receptor. *Proc Natl Acad Sci USA* 1993;90:65–69.

35. Harrison MB, Wiley RG, Wooten GF. Selective localization of striatal D_1 receptors to striatonigral neurons. *Brain Res* 1990;528:317–322.

36. Herbert J. Peptides in the limbic system: neurochemical codes for coordinated adaptive responses to behavioural and physiological demand. *Prog Neurobiol* 1994;41:723–791.

37. Hershey AD, Krause JE. Molecular characterization of a functional cDNA encoding the rat substance P receptor. *Science* 1990;247:958–962.

38. Herzog H, Hort YJ, Ball HJ, Hayes G, Shine J, Selbie LA. Cloned human neuropeptide Y receptor couples to two different second messenger systems. *Proc Natl Acad Sci USA* 1992;89:5794–5798.

39. Hökfelt T. Neuropeptides in perspective: the last ten years. *Neuron* 1991;7:867–879.

40. Hökfelt T, Wiesenfeld-Hallin Z, Villar M, Melander T. Increase of galanin-like immunoreactivity in rat dorsal root ganglion cells after peripheral axotomy. *Neurosci Lett* 1987;83:217–220.

41. Hökfelt T, Zhang X, Wiesenfeld-Hallin Z. Messenger plasticity in primary sensory neurons following axotomy and its functional implications. *Trends Neurosci* 1994;17:22–30.

42. Howbert JJ, Lobb KL, Brown RF, Reel JK, Neel DA, Mason NR, Mendelsohn LG, Hodgkiss JP, Kelly JS. A novel series of nonpeptide CCK and gastrin antagonists: medicinal chemistry and electrophysiological demonstration of antagonism. In: Dourish CT, Cooper SJ, Iversen SD, Iversen LL, eds. *Multiple cholecystokinin receptors in the CNS*. Oxford: Oxford University Press, 1992;p 28–37.

43. Hughes J, Boden P, Costall B, Domeney A, Kelly E, Horwell DC, Hunter JC, Pinnock RD, Woodruff GN. Cholekinoid antagonists, a new class of potent and specific CCK-B ligands having potent anxiolytic activity. *Proc Natl Acad Sci* 1990;87:6728–6732.

44. Ishihara T, Shigemoto R, Mori K, Takahashi K, Nagata S. Functional expression and tissue distribution of a novel receptor for vasoactive intestinal polypeptide. *Neuron* 1992;8:811–819.

45. Jirikowski GF, Sanna PP, Bloom FE. mRNA coding oxytocin is present in axons of the hypothalamo-neurohypophyseal tract. *Proc Natl Acad Sci USA* 1990;87:7400–7404.

46. Jirikowski GF, Sanna PP, Maciejewski-Lenoir D, Bloom FE. Reversal of diabetes insipidus in Brattleboro rats: intrahypothalamic injection of vasopressin mRNA. *Science* 1992;255:996–998.

47. Johnson MD. Synaptic glutamate release by postnatal rat serotonergic neurons in microculture. *Neuron* 1994;12:433–442.

48. Kaneko T, Akiyama H, Nagatsu I, Mizuno N. Immunohistochemical demonstration of glutaminase in catecholaminergic and serotonergic neurons of rat brain. *Brain Res* 1990;507:141–154.

49. Kaneko T, Shigemoto R, Nakanishi S, Mizuno N. Substance P receptor-immunoreactive neurons in the rat neostriatum are segregated into somatostatinergic and cholinergic aspiny neurons. *Brain Res* 1993;631:297–303.

50. Kasakov L, Ellis J, Kirkpatrick K, Milner P, Burnstock G. Direct evidence for concomitant release of noradrenaline, adenosine 5'-triphosphate and neuropeptide Y from sympathetic nerve supplying the guinea-pig vas deferens. *J Auton Nerv Syst* 1988;22:75–82.

51. Kieffer BL, Befort K, Gaveriaux-Ruff C, Hirth CG. The δ-opioid receptor: Isolation of a cDNA by expression cloning and pharmacological characterization. *Proc Natl Acad Sci USA* 1992;89:12048–12052.

52. Kimura T, Tanizawa O, Mori K, Brownstein MJ, Okayama H. Structure and expression of a human oxytocin receptor. *Nature* 1992;356:526–529.

53. Kirchmair R, Hogue-Angeletti R, Gutierrez J, Fischer-Colbrie R, Winkler H. Secretoneurin—a neuropeptide generated in brain, adrenal medulla and other endocrine tissues by proteolytic processing of secretogranin II (chromogranin C). *Neuroscience* 1993;53:359–366.

54. Kitabgi P. Neurotensin modulates dopamine neurotransmission at several levels along brain dopaminergic pathway. *Neurochem Int* 1989;14:111–119.

55. Kluxen F-W, Bruns C, Lübbert H. Expression cloning of a rat brain somatostatin receptor cDNA. *Proc Natl Acad Sci USA* 1992;89:4612–4622.

56. Kopin AS, Lee YM, McBride EW, Miller LJ, Lu M, Lin HY, LF, K, Beiborn M. Expression cloning and characterization of the canine parietal cell gastrin receptor. *Proc Natl Acad Sci USA* 1992;89:3605–3609.

57. Kupfermann I. Functional studies of cotransmission. *Physiol Rev* 1991;71:683–732.

58. Larhammar D, Blomqvist AG, Yee F, Jazin E, Yoo H, Wahlestedt C. Cloning and functional expression of a human neuropeptide Y/peptide YY receptor of the Y1 type. *J Biol Chem* 1992;267:10935–10938.

59. Le Moine C, Normand E, Bloch B. Phenotypical characterization of the rat striatal neurons expressing the D_1 dopamine receptor gene. *Proc Natl Acad Sci USA* 1991;88:4205–4209.

60. Le Moine C, Normand E, Guitteny AF, Fouque B, Teoule R, Bloch B. Dopamine receptor gene expression by enkephalin neurons in the rat forebrain. *Proc Natl Acad Sci USA* 1990;87:230–234.

61. Lehman E, Hanze J, Pauschinger M, Ganten D, Lang RE. Vasopressin mRNA in the neurolobe of the rat pituitary. *Neurosci Lett* 1990;111:170–175.

62. Lester J, Fink S, Aronin N, DiFiglia M. Colocalization of D1 and D2 dopamine receptors mRNAs in striatal neurons. *Brain Res* 1993;621:106–110.

63. Letter AA, Merchant K, Gibb JW, Hanson GR. Effect of methamphetamine on neurotensin concentrations in rat brain regions. *J Pharmacol Exp Ther* 1987;241:443–447.

64. Levy A, Lightman SL, Carter DA, Murphy D. The origin and regulation of posterior pituitary vasopressin ribonucleic acid in osmotically stimulated rats. *J Neuroendocrinol* 1990;2:329–334.

65. Lipton MA, DiMascio A, Killam KF, eds. *Psychopharmacology: a generation of progress*. New York: Raven Press, 1978.

66. Lolait S, O'Carroll A-M, McBride OW, Konig M, Morel A, Brownstein MJ. Cloning and characterization of a vasopressin V2 receptor and possible link to nephrogenic diabetes insipidus. *Nature* 1992;357:336–339.

67. Maciejewski-Lenoir D, Jirikowski GF, Sanna PP, Bloom FE. Reduction of exogenous vasopressin RNA poly(A) tail length increases its effectiveness in transiently correcting diabetes insipidus in the Brattleboro rat. *Proc Natl Acad Sci USA* 1993;90:1435–1439.

68. Marksteiner J, Kirchmair R, Mahata SK, Mahata M, Fischer-Colbrie R, Hogue-Angeletti R, Saria A, Winkler H. Distribution of secretoneurin, a peptide derived from secretogranin II, in rat brain. An immunocytochemical and radioimmunological study. *Neuroscience* 1993;54:923–944.

69. Marksteiner J, Saria A, Kirchmair R, Pycha R, Benesch H, Fischer-Colbrie R, Haring C, Maier H, Ransmay G. Distribution of secretoneurin-like immunoreactivity in comparison with substance P- and enkephalin-like immunoreactivities in various human forebrain regions. *Eur J Neurosci* 1993;5:1573–1585.

70. Masu Y, Nakayama K, Tamaki H, Harada Y, Kuno M, Nakanishi S. cDNA cloning of bovine substance-K receptor through oocyte expression system. *Nature* 1987;329:836–838.

71. McCabe JT, Lehman E, Chastrette N, Hanze J, Lang RE, Ganten D, Pfaff DW. Detection of vasopressin mRNA in the neurointermediate lobe of the rat pituitary. *Mol Brain Res* 1990;8:325–329.

72. Meltzer H, ed. *Psychopharmacology: the third generation of progress*. New York: Raven Press, 1987.

73. Merchant KM, Bush LG, Gibb JW, Hanson JR. Neurotensin–dopamine interactions in the substantia nigra of the rat brain. *J Pharmacol Exp Ther* 1990;255:775–780.

74. Merchant KM, Gibb JW, Hanson GR. Role of dopamine D-1 and D-2 receptors in the regulation of neurotensin systems of the neostriatum and the nucleus accumbens. *Eur J Pharmacol* 1989;160:409–412.

75. Merchant KM, Letter AA, Gibb JW, Hanson GR. Changes in the limbic neurotensin systems induced by dopaminergic drugs. *Eur J Pharmacol* 1988;153:151–154.

76. Meyerhof W, Darlison MG, Richter D. The elucidation of neuropeptide receptors and their subtypes through the application of molecular biology. In: Hucho F, ed. *Neurotransmitter receptors*, vol 25. Amsterdam: Elsevier, 1993;335–353.

77. Meyerhof W, Paust HJ, Schönrock C, Richter D. Cloning of a

cDNA encoding a novel putative G-protein-coupled receptor expressed in specific rat brain regions. *DNA Cell Biol* 1991;10:689–694.

78. Meyerhof W, Wolfsen I, Schönrock C, Fehr S, Richter D. Molecular cloning of a somatostatin-28 receptor and comparison of its expression pattern with that of a somatostatin-14 receptor in rat brain. *Proc Natl Acad Sci USA* 1992;89:10267–10271.

79. Mohr E, Fehr S, Richter D. Axonal transport of neuropeptide encoding mRNAs within the hypothalamo-hypophyseal tract of rats. *EMBO J* 10:2419–2424.

80. Mohr E, Richter D. Diversity of mRNAs in the axonal compartment of peptidergic neurons in the rat. *Eur J Neurosci* 1992;4:870–876.

81. Mohr E, Zhou A, Thorn NA, Richter D. Rats with physically disconnected hypothalamo-pituitary tracts no longer contain vasopressin–oxytocin gene transcripts in the posterior pituitary lobe. *FEBS Lett* 1990;263:332–336.

82. Morel A, O'Caroll A-M, Brownstein MJ, Lolait SJ. Molecular cloning and expression of a rat VIa arginine vasopressin receptor. *Nature* 1992;356:523–526.

83. Murphy D, Levy A, Lightman S, Carter D. Vasopressin mRNA in the neural lobe of the pituitary: dramatic accumulation in response to salt-loading. *Proc Natl Acad Sci USA* 1989;86:9002–9005.

84. Murphy TJ, Alexander RW, Griendling KK, Runge MS, Bernstein KE. Isolation of a cDNA encoding the vascular type-1 angiotensin II receptor. *Nature* 1991;351:233–236.

85. Nemeroff CB. The interaction of neurotensin with dopaminergic pathways in the central nervous system: basic neurobiology and implications for the pathogenesis and treatment of schizophrenia. *Psychoneuroendocrinology* 1986;11:15–37.

86. Nicholas AP, Cuello AC, Goldstein M, Hökfelt T. Glutamate-like immunoreactivity in medulla oblongata catecholamine/substance P neurons. *Neuroreport* 1990;1:235–238.

87. Nicholas AP, Pieribone VA, Arvidsson U, Hökfelt T. Serotonin-, substance P- and glutamate/aspartate-like immunoreactivities in medullospinal pathways of rat and primate. *Neuroscience* 1992;48:545–559.

88. Otsuka M, Yoshioka K. Neurotransmitter functions of mammalian tachykinins. *Physiol Rev* 1993;73:229–308.

89. Penny GR, Afsharpour S, Kitai ST. The glutamate decarboxylase-, leucine enkephalin-, methionine enkephalin- and substance P-immunoreactive neurons in the neostriatum of the rat and cat: evidence for partial population overlap. *Neuroscience* 1986;17:1011–1045.

90. Rimland J, Xin W, Sweetnam P, Saijoh K, Nestler EJ, Duman RS. Sequence and expression of a neuropeptide Y receptor cDNA. *Mol Pharmacol* 1991;40:869–875.

91. Robertson GS, Vincent SR, Fibiger HC. Striatonigral projection neurons contain D1 dopamine receptor-activated c-fos. *Brain Res* 1990;523:288–290.

92. Robertson HA. Dopamine receptor interactions: some implications for the treatment of Parkinson's disease. *Trends Neurosci* 1992;15:201–206.

93. Saria A, Troger J, Kirchmair R, Fischer-Colbrie R, Hogue-Angeletti R, Winkler H. Secretoneurin releases dopamine from rat striatal slices: a biological effect of a peptide derived from secretogranin II (chromogranin C). *Neuroscience* 1993;54:1–4.

94. Sasaki K, Yamano Y, Bardhan S, Iwai N, Murray JJ, Hasegawa M, Matsuda Y, Inagami T. Cloning and expression of a complementary DNA encoding a bovine adrenal angiotensin II type-1 receptor. *Nature* 1991;351:230–233.

95. Schiffmann SN, Vanderhaeghen JJ. Caffeine regulates neurotensin and cholecystokinin messenger RNA expression in the rat striatum. *Neuroscience* 1993;54:681–689.

96. Shehab SA, Atkinson ME. Vasoactive intestinal polypeptide (VIP) increases in the spinal cord after peripheral axotomy of the sciatic nerve originate from primary afferent neurons. *Brain Res* 1986;372:37–44.

97. Sherman TG, Akil H, Watson SJ. The molecular biology of neuropeptides. *Disc Neurosci* 1989;6:1–58.

98. Shigemoto R, Nakaya Y, Nomura S, Ogawa-Meguro R, Ohishi H, Kaneko T, Nakanishi S, Mizuno N. Immunocytochemical local-

99. Shigemoto R, Yokota Y, Tsuchida K, Nakanishi S. Cloning and expression of a rat neuromedin K receptor cDNA. *J Biol Chem* 1990;265:623–628.

100. Shinmi O, Kimura S, Yoshizawa T, Sawamura T, Uchiyama Y, Sugita Y, Kanazawa I, Yanagisawa M, Goto K, Masaki T. Presence of endothelin-1 in porcine spinal cord: isolation and sequence determination. *Biochem Biophys Res Commun* 1989;162:340–346.

101. Sneddon P, Westfall DP. Pharmacological evidence that adenosine triphosphate and noradrenaline are cotransmitters in the guinea-pig vas deferens. *J Physiol* 1984;347:561–580.

102. Snider RM, Constantine JW, Lowe IJ, Longo KP, Lebel WS, Woody HA, Drozda SE, Desai MC, Vinick FJ, Spencer RW, Hess H-J. A potent nonpeptide antagonist of the substance P (NK1) receptor. *Science* 1991;251:435–437.

103. Sreedharan SP, Robichon A, Peterson KE, Goetzl EJ. Cloning and expression of the human vasoactive intestinal peptide receptor. *Proc Natl Acad Sci USA* 1991;1:4986–4990.

104. Stein CA, Cheng Y-C. Antisense oligonucleotides as therapeutic agents. Is the bullet really magical? *Science* 1993;261:1004–1012.

105. Strand FL, Rose KJ, Zuccarelli LA, Kume J. Neuropeptide hormones as neurotrophic factors. *Physiol Rev* 1991;71:1017–1037.

106. Straub RE, Frech GC, Joho RH, Gershengorn MC. Expression cloning of a cDNA encoding the mouse pituitary thyrotropin-releasing hormone receptor. *Proc Natl Acad Sci USA* 1990;87:9514–9518.

107. Sudoh T, Kangawa K, Minamino N, Matsuo H. A new natriuretic peptide in porcine brain. *Nature* 1988;332:78–81.

108. Surmeier DJ, Reiner A, Levine MS, Ariano MA. Are neostriatal dopamine receptors co-localized? *Trends Neurosci* 1993;16:299–305.

109. Szigethy E, Beaudet A. Correspondence between high affinity ^{125}I-neurotensin binding sites and dopaminergic neurons in the rat substantia nigra and ventral tegmental area: a combined radioautographic and immunohistochemical light microscopic study. *J Comp Neurol* 1989;279:128–137.

110. Takeda Y, Chou KB, Takeda J, Sachais BS, Krause JE. Molecular cloning, structural characterization and functional expression of the human substance P receptor. *Biochem Biophys Res Commun* 1991;179:1232–1240.

111. Tanaka K, Masu M, Nakanishi S. Structure and functional expression of the cloned rat neurotensin receptor. *Neuron* 1990;4:847–854.

112. Trembleau A, Morales M, Bloom FE. Aggregation of vasopressin mRNA in a subset of axonal swellings of the median eminence and posterior pituitary: light and electron microscopic evidence. *J Neurosci* 1994;14:39–53.

113. Verhage M, McMahon HT, Ghijsen WEJM, Boomsma F, Scholten G, Wiegant VM, Nicholls DG. Differential release of amino acids, neuropeptides, and catecholamines from isolated nerve terminals. *Neuron* 1991;6:517–524.

114. Wachi M, Okuda M, Togashi S, Miyashita O, Wakahoi T. Effects of methamphetamine administration on brain neurotensin-like immunoreactivity in rats. *Neurosci Lett* 1987;78:222–226.

115. Wada E, Way J, Shapira H, Kusano K, Lebacq-Verheyden AM, Coy D, Jensen R, Battey J. cDNA cloning, characterization, and brain region-specific expression of a neuromedin-B-preferring bombesin receptor. *Neuron* 1991;6:421–430.

116. Wahlestedt C. Antisense oligonucleotide strategies in neuropharmacology. *Trends Pharmacol Sci* 1994;151:42–46.

117. Wakisaka S, Kajander KC, Bennett GJ. Increased neuropeptide (NPY)-like immunoreactivity in rat sensory neurons following peripheral axotomy. *Neurosci Lett* 1991;124:200–203.

118. Wang JB, Imai Y, Eppler CM, Gregor P, Spivak CE, Uhl GR. μ opiate receptor: cDNA cloning and expression. *Proc Natl Acad Sci USA* 1993;90:10230–10234.

119. Wank SA, Harkins R, Jensen RT, Shapira H, De Weerth A, Slattery T. Purification, molecular cloning, and functional expression of the cholecystokinin receptor from rat pancreas. *Proc Natl Acad Sci USA* 1992;89:3125–3129.

120. Weiner DM, Levey AI, Sunahara RK, Niznik HB, O'Dowd BF,

izatoin of rat substance P receptor in the striatum. *Neurosci Lett* 1993;153:157–160.

Seeman P, Brann MR. D_1 and D_2 dopamine receptor mRNA in rat brain. *Proc Natl Acad Sci USA* 1991;88:1859–1863.

121. Wiesenfeld-Hallin Z, Bartfai T, Hökfelt T. Galanin in sensory neurons in the spinal cord. *Front Neuroendocrinol* 1992;13:319–343.

122. Yamada Y, Post SR, Wang K, Tager HS, Bell GI, Seino S. Cloning and functional characterization of a family of human and mouse somatostatin receptors expressed in brain, gastrointestinal tract, and kidney. *Proc Natl Acad Sci USA* 1992;89:251–255.

123. Yasuda K, Raynor K, Kong H, Breder C, Takeda J, Reisine T, Bell GI. Cloning and functional comparison of κ and δ opioid receptors from mouse brain. *Proc Natl Acad Sci USA* 1993;90:6736–6740.

124. Yokota Y, Sasai Y, Tanaka K, Fujiwara T, Tsuchida K, Shigemoto R, Kakizuka A, Ohkubo H, Nakanishi S. Molecular characterization of a functional cDNA for rat substance P receptor. *J Biol Chem* 1989;264:17649–17652.

125. Young WSI. In situ hybridization histochemistry. In: Björklund A, Hökfelt T, Wouterlood FG, Van den Pol AN, eds. *Handbook of chemical neuroanatomy, vol 8. Analysis of neuronal microcircuits and synaptic interactions.* Amsterdam: Elsevier, 1990;481–512.

126. Young WSI, Kuhar MJ. Neurotensin receptor localization by light microscopic autoradiography in rat brain. *Brain Res* 1981;206:273–285.

127. Zhang X, Dagerlind Å, Elde RP, Castel M-N, Broberger C, Wiesenfeld-Halin Z, Hökfelt T. Marked increase in cholecystokinin B receptor messenger RNA levels in rat dorsal root ganglia after peripheral axotomy. *Neuroscience* 1993;57:227–233.

128. Zhang X, Wiesenfeld-Hallin Z, Hökfelt T. Effect of peripheral axotomy on expression of neuropeptide Y receptor mRNA in rat lumbar dorsal root ganglia. *Eur J Neurosci* 1994;6:43–57.

129. Zhao D, Yang J, Jones KE, Gerald C, Suzuki Y, Hogan PG, Chin WW, Tashijian AHJ. Molecular cloning of a complementary deoxyribonucleic acid encoding the thyrotropin-releasing hormone receptor and regulation of its messenger ribonucleic acid in rat GH cells. *Endocrinology* 1992;130:3529–3536.

Psychopharmacology: The Fourth Generation of Progress, edited by Floyd E. Bloom and David J. Kupfer. Raven Press, Ltd., New York © 1995.

CHAPTER **44**

Thyrotropin-Releasing Hormone

Focus on Basic Neurobiology

George A. Mason, James C. Garbutt, and Arthur J. Prange, Jr.

In 1969, a group led by Guillemin (7) and another by Schally (5), having worked competitively for many years, announced that the hypothalamic substance that causes the anterior pituitary gland to release thyrotropin (thyroid-stimulating hormone, TSH) is L-pyroglutamyl-L-histidyl-L-prolineamide (L-pGlu-L-His-L-ProNH$_2$). This tripeptide is now called thyrotropin-releasing hormone (TRH) (Fig. 1).

The discovery of the chemical identity of TRH verified the venerable theory that the brain can influence the anterior pituitary gland by means of hormones. It validated the discipline of neuroendocrinology: If neurons secrete hormones, they can properly be regarded as transducers between two of the great communication systems of the organism. The discovery revived interest in the role of peptides in the nervous system. Guillemin and Schally each received one-quarter of the 1977 Nobel Prize for Physiology or Medicine. Half the prize was awarded to Yalow for her contribution to the development of the radioimmune assay as a system for the detection of minute amounts of biological substances, including peptides.

TRH was not the first peptide found in the central nervous system (CNS). In 1931, von Euler and Gaddum (86) discovered substance P, though its identity as an undecapeptide was not revealed until later. In any case,

there was little interest in peptidology until an endocrine target for the brain (the anterior pituitary) was posited and until the chemical nature of brain hormones could reasonably be considered to be peptidergic. Furthermore, neither Guillemin nor Schally was the first to propose that the hypothalamus might regulate the anterior pituitary by secreting substances into the portal venous system that connects them. Others had made such suggestion; among them, the physiologist Geoffrey Harris is usually credited with formulating the concept. Attempting to prove its accuracy became his life's work (24).

The discovery of TRH led quickly to the discovery of other small peptides that regulate the secretion by the anterior pituitary of its tropic hormones. Such regulation is usually accomplished by increasing or decreasing stimulation. However, growth hormone appears mainly to be regulated by increasing or decreasing inhibition, though a growth-hormone-releasing factor has been identified (55). The peptide substances of which TRH was the first to be identified are often grouped as hypothalamic hypophysiotropic hormones. This term, while accurate, is insufficient. Many of the substances are found outside the hypothalamus. If activity follows anatomy, then they may be expected to exert nonhypophysiotropic functions. Indeed, this is the case (63).

DISTRIBUTION

The distribution of TRH has been studied extensively in the mammalian central nervous system and some peripheral tissues (see ref. 27 for review). Provided here is a brief description of the distribution of TRH in the rat; however, in some structures considerable species-specific variation exists.

G. A. Mason and A. J. Prange, Jr.: Department of Psychiatry, University of North Carolina School of Medicine, Chapel Hill, North Carolina 27599; and Brain and Development Research Center, University of North Carolina School of Medicine, Chapel Hill, North Carolina 27599.

J. C. Garbutt: Department of Psychiatry, University of North Carolina School of Medicine, Chapel Hill, North Carolina 27599; and Clinical Research Unit, Dorothea Dix Hospital, Raleigh, North Carolina 27603.

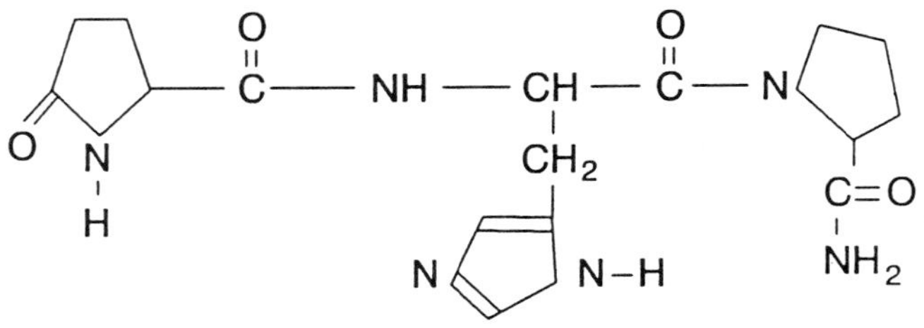

FIG. 1. Thyrotropin-releasing hormone.

TRH-immunoreactive cell bodies are distributed throughout the CNS of the rat (27). They are prominently clustered in the glomerular layer of the olfactory bulbs, piriform and entorhinal cortices, hippocampus, amygdala, nucleus accumbens, and olfactory tubercle. TRH-positive cells are scattered in the corpus striatum, the bed nucleus of the stria terminalis, the septohypothalamic nucleus, and the bed nucleus of the diagonal band of Broca. More caudally, TRH neurons are concentrated in the parvocellular portion of the paraventricular nucleus and in the periventricular area. Such neurons are also found above the optic chiasm, in the preoptic area, the lateral aspects of the anterior hypothalamic nucleus, the perifornical area, the supraoptic nucleus, and, less prominently, in other hypothalamic nuclei. Numerous TRH-positive cell bodies occur in the periaqueductal central gray; fewer are found in the substantia nigra, the ventrolateral lemniscal nucleus, and the roots of the trigeminal nerve. In the medulla, TRH cells occur in various raphe nuclei, the external cuneate nucleus, the dorsal vagal complex, and the area postrema. They are also prominent in lamina II–III of the dorsal horn of the spinal cord. In addition, major fiber tracts are located in the lateral septum, hypothalamus, the subiculum–amygdalohippocampal area, and the ventral horn of the spinal cord.

Outside the CNS, TRH immunoreactivity is observed in pancreatic beta cells, but levels decline sharply after birth, except in hypothyroidism (27). It appears that TRH may have an important prenatal function in pancreas. TRH is also present in various parts of the gastrointestinal tract, where it affects motility, acid secretion, and absorption of sugars.

INTRANEURONAL COLOCALIZATION

Of recent interest are immunohistochemical and immunocytochemical studies demonstrating coexistence of TRH in neurons with one or more other neuroactive substances including serotonin, substance P, the enkephalins, dopamine, neuropeptide Y, histamine, and growth hormone (see Table 1).

The coexistence in certain neurons of gamma-aminobutyric acid (GABA) (35), cholecystokinin (54), and proctolin (27) with serotonin, which has been shown to coexist with TRH (27,68) in a large portion of medullary bulbospinal neurons, suggests that these neuropeptides may also coexist with TRH in some neuronal populations. The coexistence of various neurotransmitters and neuromodulators is of great theoretical interest. It is clear that the presence in the same synapse of one or more neuromodulators with one or more acknowledged transmitters could provide additional pre- and postsynaptic mechanisms for the regulation of neuronal signaling (34). However, the effects of these interactions and their underlying cellular mechanisms are virtually unknown.

Colocalization is not limited to the nervous system. Evidence indicates that TRH and cholecystokinin coexist in a portion of gastrin-secreting cells located in the central mucosa of guinea-pig stomach (27). The importance of the relationship between these two peptides with regard to feeding behaviors and digestive processes has not been determined.

BIOSYNTHESIS

Mechanisms

In the decade that followed the announcement of its chemical identity, it was uncertain whether TRH was formed by a nonribosomal enzymatic mechanism or by post-translational processing of a larger precursor protein in ribosomes (28). By 1981, opinion strongly favored the post-translational processing hypothesis because convincing evidence could be adduced only for this alternative. For example, it was demonstrated that a high-molecular-

TABLE 1. Intraneuronal colocalization of TRH with other neuroactive substances

Neuroactive substance	Site of colocalization with TRH	References
Serotonin	Medullary raphe	27
	Spinal cord (ventral horn)	27, 68
Substance P	Medullary raphe	27
	Spinal cord (ventral horn)	27, 68
Neuropeptide Y	Hypothalamus (periacqueductal gray)	27
Enkephalin	Hypothalamus (perifornical area)	27, 58
Dopamine	Olfactory bulb (periglomerular layer)	27
Histamine	Hypothalamus (tuberomammillary neurons)	1
Human growth hormone-like peptide	Hypothalamus medullary raphe	27, 43

weight protein from frog brain, after chemical and enzymatic treatment, could yield TRH.

A post-translational enzymatic mode of TRH synthesis in amphibians was confirmed using molecular techniques (28). It was determined that frog DNA contained a segment of 478 nucleotides that coded for the amino-terminal region of pro-TRH, a 123-amino-acid precursor containing three copies of the progenitor sequence of TRH (Gln-His-Pro-Gly) flanked by paired dibasic residues and a fourth incomplete copy lacking the C-terminal glycine. A mammalian pro-TRH molecule was later identified in rat hypothalamus as a 255-amino-acid protein containing five copies of the amino acid sequence of the TRH progenitor (28). Human pro-TRH contains six copies (91).

The biosynthesis of TRH is essentially a five-step process (see Fig. 2), beginning with transcription of DNA of the TRH gene to TRH mRNA within the cell nucleus. Transcription is followed by translation of the TRH mRNA to the pro-TRH peptide on the ribosome. The post-translational processing of TRH begins with excision of the progenitor peptides by the action of carboxy peptidases. This is followed by amidation of proline by peptidyl glycine alpha-amidating monooxygenase, the amide moiety being donated by the C-terminal glycine (28). Finally, cyclization of the N-terminal glutamine by glutaminyl cyclase is accomplished (28). Post-translational processing of TRH appears to be restricted to the neuronal perikarya because of lack of TRH progenitor immunore-

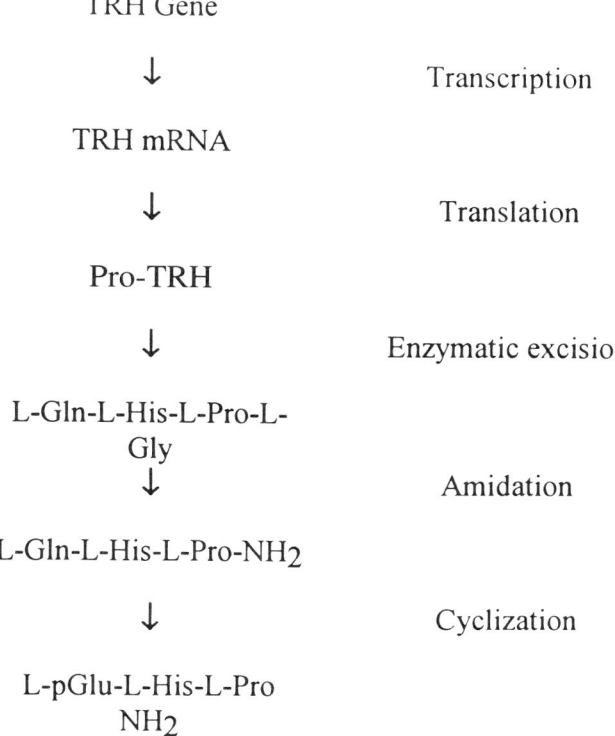

TRH Gene

↓   Transcription

TRH mRNA

↓   Translation

Pro-TRH

↓   Enzymatic excision

L-Gln-L-His-L-Pro-L-Gly

↓   Amidation

L-Gln-L-His-L-Pro-NH$_2$

↓   Cyclization

L-pGlu-L-His-L-Pro NH$_2$

FIG. 2. Biosynthesis of TRH, a five-step process from gene to tripeptide.

activity in axons or terminals of the median eminence or spinal cord (29).

The post-translational processing of pro-TRH also gives rise to a number of other peptides that may have behavioral or physiological activity (6).

Regulation

The steps of biosynthesis of TRH are similar, if not the same, throughout the CNS. Regulation of synthesis, however, may be more discrete. TRH levels in secretory cells of the hypothalamus must be maintained at concentrations sufficient to ensure functional integrity of the hypothalamic–pituitary–thyroid (HPT) axis, whereas extrahypothalamic levels of the peptide are likely to be responsive to other behavioral and physiological demands.

In the rat, thyroid hormones can regulate hypothalamic TRH production at the transcriptional level by negative feedback. An inverse relationship exists between thyroid hormone status and TRH mRNA levels in medial parvocellular tuberoinfundibular TRH neurons (44); however, this relationship is not observed in other hypothalamic or in extrahypothalamic sites. Thyroid hormones may also regulate *translation* of the TRH message (44). Whether the effects of altered thyroid states on the transcriptional or translational aspects of TRH synthesis are mediated by intracellular factors such as thyroid hormone receptors or by extracellular neural input is still unclear. It is of interest, however, that a small sequence of DNA flanking the TRH gene is homologous to a sequence of the DNA to which the L-triiodothyronine (T$_3$) receptor binds (45). This sequence is identical to a sequence of DNA near the gene for the beta subunit of TSH, the expression of which is regulated by T$_3$, but is unlike the sequence mediating T$_3$ regulation of growth hormone transcription. On the other hand, it has been shown that the 5′-deiodinase, which converts thyroxine (T$_4$) to T$_3$, its more active congener, is absent in the periventricular nucleus. This, together with evidence of synaptic connections between axons of epinephrine-containing neurons and perikarya of TRH neurons in the periventricular nucleus, suggests that thyroid hormones may regulate TRH biosynthesis indirectly via central catecholamine pathways (44). For example, cold exposure, which raises central catecholamine levels, elevates cellular TRH mRNA in the paraventricular nucleus even in the presence of elevated thyroid hormone levels (93). This effect on TRH mRNA synthesis is specifically blocked by ethanol; however, ethanol apparently does not block the *release* of TRH (94).

Regulation of post-translational processing of TRH has not been studied extensively even though it may be rate-limiting for TRH biosynthesis (13). It may also vary by cell type.

The regulation of TRH biosynthesis in extrahypothalamic areas of the CNS is poorly understood. However, it is well established that levels of TRH and TRH mRNA in these areas are not controlled by thyroid hormones (44). TRH biosynthesis varies in different brain areas (6,44), probably in accordance with specific neuronal stimuli. For example, TRH and TRH mRNA levels are markedly elevated in the hippocampus, amygdala, and pyriform cortex (but not in hypothalamus) after seizures induced by kindling or electroconvulsive shock (42,72), whereas acute administration of cocaine reduces TRH mRNA in the amygdala and hippocampus (77).

RELEASE

TRH is released into the hypophyseal portal circulation from axonal terminals whose cell bodies are found in the parvocellular division of the paraventricular nucleus (44). *Synaptic* release of TRH occurs in many parts of the brain. In addition, TRH is co-released with serotonin and substance P from projections of medullary raphe neurons that impinge primarily on cells of the ventral horn and sympathetic lateral column of the spinal cord and perhaps the dorsal horn (27). Similar events may occur in other areas of the CNS (27).

The release of TRH for maintenance of pituitary–thyroid axis homeostasis is regulated by T_3, as is TRH synthesis (see above). However, there is provision for override of this negative feedback system (93), probably by central noradrenergic input (30). Furthermore, serotonin (60) and probably GABA (84), somatostatin (49), and corticotropin-releasing factor (49) inhibit hypothalamic TRH release. Dopamine, acting through D_2 receptors, appears to produce a general stimulatory effect on the median eminence, eliciting release of both TRH and somatostatin (47). However, dopamine can also directly inhibit TSH secretion (see below and Chapters 8, 18, and 43, *this volume*).

Synaptic release of TRH in brain has not been studied extensively. It is a complex process, influenced by a variety of neurochemical signals that mediate behavioral and physiological responses to internal and external stimuli. It has been shown that histamine will release TRH from hypothalamic slices whereas somatostatin will do so in brainstem synaptosomes (22). More recently it was demonstrated that the muscarinic agonist pilocarpine will release TRH from slices of the preoptic area of the hypothalamus (17).

TRH is released from cells in the stomach wall into gastric juice by histamine (62) and serotonin (36). Whether these transmitters also release cholecystokinin, which is thought to be colocalized with TRH in some gastrin-secreting cells of stomach (27), has not been resolved.

RECEPTORS

Receptors for TRH are found on thyrotroph and mammotroph cells of the anterior pituitary and on neurons throughout the CNS (26,78). The structural and functional properties of both pituitary and central TRH receptors have been characterized in detail and shown to be similar in structure, binding characteristics, and mechanisms of signal transduction (26,78). TRH receptors belong to a class of G-protein-coupled receptors with seven membrane-spanning domains and an extracellular N-terminal region containing *N*-glycosylation sites (81) (see also Chapters 27 and 38, *this volume*).

Anterior Pituitary

Anterior pituitary TRH receptors have been studied extensively in cultured tumor cells originating from thyrotrophs and mammotrophs (26) and more recently in cells transfected with and expressing TRH receptor cDNA (11,18,48). All pituitary TRH receptors appear to be structurally identical, though there may be subtle differences in the transduction of hormone secretion between normal anterior pituitary cells and tumor cell models (74).

Pituitary TRH receptors contain saturable, noninteracting, high-affinity binding sites that exhibit strict structural specificity for TRH at all three amino acid positions. The affinity and rate of dissociation of the TRH receptor for its endogenous ligand are highly temperature-dependent: TRH binds with lower affinity and dissociates more rapidly at higher temperatures (26). The rate of dissociation for TRH is also directly related to the length of time of receptor occupancy and may reflect ligand-induced binding site aggregation or receptor internalization (26).

The turnover rate of the pituitary TRH receptor is slow, providing explanation for its equally slow homologous down-regulation (26). The number of pituitary TRH receptors is reversibly decreased by thyroid hormones and increased by estrogen and glucocorticoids. TRH receptors are down-regulated by drugs that elevate cAMP, while receptor affinity is generally reduced by agents that activate protein kinase C (26).

Central Nervous System

Central TRH receptors exhibit binding characteristics for both ^{3}H-TRH and the high-affinity synthetic TRH analogue ^{3}H-(3-methyl-His^2)TRH that are almost identical to those of the pituitary TRH receptor, including the time-dependent biphasic dissociation kinetics indicative of a ligand-induced affinity shift (78). Although heterogeneity of central TRH receptors has been reported, the bulk of evidence, including studies of solubilized highly purified receptors, indicates a single population of high-affinity receptors that are saturable and noninteracting (78).

TRH receptors in all mammals studied thus far, including the human (53), are heterogeneously distributed throughout the CNS. Nevertheless, specific patterns are evident that appear to correlate with species-specific physiological differences (78). Central TRH receptor number seems to be regulated in a conventional way—that is, diminished by TRH and its agonist analogues. It has been shown that dissimilar drugs, including ethanol, delta-9-tetrahydrocannabinol and chlordiazepoxide, also affect TRH receptor binding (79).

ENZYMATIC INACTIVATION

Regulation of both the peripheral and central actions of TRH involve intracellular and extracellular enzymatic inactivation of the peptide. In vitro studies have identified several TRH-degrading enzymes, including histidyl-proline imidopeptidase, prolylendopeptidase, pyroglutamyl aminopeptidase I and II, and thyroliberinase; however, it is generally acknowledged that thyroliberinase and pyroglutamyl aminopeptidase II are primarily responsible for removal of TRH in vivo (65).

TRH released into the hypophyseal portal circulation is degraded rapidly to His-Pro NH_2 by thyroliberinase, a highly specific serum peptidase (65). The activity of TRH released into synapses of the CNS is thought to be terminated primarily by pyroglutamyl aminopeptidase II, a high-specificity synaptosomal membrane ectoenzyme (65). Because this enzyme is specific for TRH, a drug (were one available) that would inhibit only this enzyme would elevate the levels of TRH and not the levels of other peptides. Such an indirect TRH agonist might also have diminished endocrine effects. Phorbol ester might appear promising in this regard because it inhibits pyroglutamyl aminopeptidase II, by stimulating protein kinase C-mediated phosphorylation of the enzyme, without blocking its cytosolic counterpart (82). However, the lack of specificity of this reaction would probably limit the use of phorbol ester as an indirect TRH agonist.

The enzymatic breakdown of TRH by cultured cells from the anterior pituitary is regulated by estrogen and thyroid hormones (4). However, the TRH-degrading activity of cultured brain cells is not affected by T_3 (4). TRH may inhibit its own enzymatic removal by enhancing translocation of protein kinase C from cytosol to plasma membrane, where it can inactivate pyroglutamyl peptidase II by phosphorylation of the enzyme.

ANTERIOR PITUITARY FUNCTION

The unequivocal endocrine function of TRH is to stimulate the synthesis and release of TSH from thyrotroph cells of the anterior pituitary gland. Thus, TRH, in concert with thyroid hormones and the inhibitory influences of dopamine and somatostatin from the hypothalamus, controls pituitary TSH synthesis and release (75). T_3 decreases hypothalamic TRH and the density of pituitary

TRH receptors (see above); it also inhibits TSH subunit gene expression (90) and TSH secretion (75). Dopamine acts directly on anterior pituitary cells through D_2 receptors negatively coupled to adenylate cyclase to inhibit TSH synthesis and secretion, while somatostatin likewise reduces TSH release via membrane receptors that modulate adenylate cyclase or voltage-dependent potassium channels (75). TSH initiates the synthesis and triggers the secretion of thyroid hormones, and TRH itself may directly stimulate the thyroid gland to release T_4 (2).

TRH stimulates prolactin (PRL) release, but evidence that it is a major physiologic PRL-releasing factor is either species-specific or controversial (46). TRH actions on growth hormone and adrenocorticotropic hormone (ACTH) secretion are complex, being virtually absent in normal subjects and occurring to varying degrees in different pathophysiologic states (75). TRH may exhibit a weak stimulatory effect on follicle-stimulating hormone (FSH) secretion in humans (75).

The basic cellular mechanisms of TRH actions on TSH (87) and PRL (19) secretion have been investigated using cultured pituitary tumor cells. The biphasic secretion of these two hormones has recently been shown to involve G-protein-coupled stimulation of inositol phospholipid turnover. The initial phase of hormone secretion is thought to result from inositol trisphosphate-mediated release of Ca^{2+} from intracellular stores; the second and more sustained phase results from influx of extracellular Ca^{2+} via voltage-sensitive channels activated by protein kinase C, which is induced by 1,2-DG (48). Stimulation of TRH receptors on thyrotroph tumor cells also induces the release of arachidonic acid metabolites that may act as additional intracellular messengers (34). In addition to stimulating TSH and PRL release, TRH regulates the transcription of PRL (61) and the post-translational glycosylation of TSH (50) (see also Chapter 62, *this volume*).

CENTRAL ACTIONS

The central actions of TRH are myriad, affecting brain chemistry, physiology, and behavior. It has been shown that these centrally induced effects are not mediated by the endocrine effects of TRH but may be harmonious with those endocrine effects (64) and dependent upon the behavioral/physiologic state of the organism (63). As a neuromodulator of several different neurotransmitters, including most prominently dopamine, serotonin, acetylcholine, and the opiates, TRH affects the actions of many drugs that themselves affect these and other neurotransmitters (22,63).

TRH has been shown to arouse hibernating animals, through a hippocampal mechanism, and to antagonize the sedation, motor impairment, and hypothermia produced by ethanol and other CNS depressants (63). However, unlike other agents that counteract the effects of ethanol such as the GABA antagonists (20), TRH has anticonflict properties, alone and in concert with ethanol and sedative-hypnotic drugs, and may protect against rather than induce seizures (42,92). The anxiolytic effects of TRH may also be involved in the recently reported attenuating effect of a TRH analogue on alcohol preference in a rodent model of human alcoholism (71). The anticonvulsive actions of TRH and its analogues may prove beneficial in ameliorating alcohol withdrawal symptoms.

TRH counteracts the hypothemia or poikilothermia produced by various drugs and several endogenous neuropeptides, including neurotensin, bombesin, and beta-endorphin (22,63). Its effects alone on body temperature are variable: TRH produces hypothermia in some species, hyperthermia in others, and in some it has no effect. Similarly, TRH produces only weak species-specific effects on nociception but is a potent antagonist of the antinociceptive effect of neurotensin (63).

TRH stimulates locomotor activity by activation of the mesolimbic dopamine system (9,22,63). The tripeptide also produces profound stimulation of the cardiovascular and respiratory systems (22,63) and induces increases in gastrointestinal motility and the volume and acidity of gastric secretion (21) while often suppressing the intake of both food and water (63). These gastrointestinal effects of TRH may play a role in the ulcerogenic actions of TRH, demonstrated in the cold-restraint stress paradigm (21).

The actions of TRH are generally short-lived because of rapid inactivation or biotransformation to less active metabolites (22). In any case, most (if not all) of the CNS effects of TRH can be achieved even when the endocrine targets of the tripeptide have been removed. With peripheral administration, high doses of TRH are required to produce CNS effects because of poor penetration into brain and rapid peripheral inactivation. These limiting properties of the native tripeptide have prompted synthesis of more stable agonist analogues. Analogues with high CNS receptor affinity and greater behavioral, as opposed to endocrine, effects would be desirable; however, the similarity of central and pituitary receptor binding characteristics has made the design of such drugs difficult. Nevertheless, some TRH analogues have been tested as therapeutic agents for disorders of the nervous system (see below).

USE IN DIAGNOSTIC TESTS

In Endocrine Disorders

Initial studies of the effects of TRH as a hypothalamic releasing factor revealed both expected and unanticipated results. Expected findings were as follows: (a) TRH is a potent releaser of TSH in both men and women, with release of TSH occurring at a whole-body threshold dose of 6.25 μg and peak response increasing linearly to a dose of 400 μg TRH (80); (b) the effect of TRH is transient, with peak TSH response occurring about 30 min after administration (80); and (c) the TSH response to TRH is reduced in hyperthyroidism and augmented in hypothyroidism, reflecting the net effect of the potent inhibitory actions of thyroid hormones on TSH release and synthesis (see above). Unexpected findings were as follows: (a) TRH is a potent releaser of PRL in both men and women (32) and (b) women have much greater PRL and slightly greater TSH responses than men.

With the establishment of the basic parameters of the pituitary response to TRH, the development of standardized TRH tests was possible. Two strategies emerged to test the TSH response: In one a submaximal dose of 200 μg TRH is used; in the other a supramaximal dose of 500 μg TRH is given. Probably for historical reasons the 500 μg TRH test became the standard for psychiatric studies. In its simplest version the TRH test requires that a baseline sample of TSH be drawn and then TRH is infused intravenously during 1 min. A second TSH sample is drawn 30 min later. This protocol produces results that are closely correlated with results from more frequent and prolonged sampling (76).

While the TRH test has been a mainstay for providing complete testing of the HPT axis for many years, recent advances in the analytical qualities of TSH assays have reduced its use. The increased sensitivity of TSH assays has enabled detection of hyperthyroid as well as hypothyroid states. Comparison of basal TSH to TRH-induced TSH values has revealed a high correlation between the two measures and raised the question of what role the TRH test should play in HPT axis evaluation (40).

In Behavioral Disorders

Soon after the advent of the TRH test in endocrinology came the discovery of a blunted TSH response to TRH in some patients with mental depression. This observation, reported in 1972 by Prange et al. (70) and Kastin et al. (37), that the TRH-induced TSH response is reduced in some depressed men and women compared to control subjects, has been replicated by many groups and has become an accepted biological marker in depression (51). Over the past 20 years the significance of this marker has been investigated on several fronts: (a) diagnostic and phenomenological associations, (b) relationship to treatment and prognosis, (c) status as a risk marker, and (d) pathophysiological basis. (For a review of these issues see ref. 51.)

As data accrued it became clear that a blunted TSH response occurs in 25–30% of patients with DSM-III- or RDC-defined major depression. What remains unclear is whether this 25–30% of depressed patients represents a distinct subgroup or the lower end of a single population.

TRH testing of many psychiatric patients led to several findings. First, as additional diagnostic groups were studied it became apparent that patients with certain other psychiatric disorders also had significantly higher prevalences of a blunted TSH response than did control populations (57). For example, blunted TSH responses have consistently been reported in patients with alcoholism (15). Less consistent have been reports of blunted TSH responses in patients with borderline personality disorder or panic disorder. Given these findings, it became apparent that the specificity of the blunted TSH response to TRH for depression was poor. This, combined with its low sensitivity, prevented the use of the TRH test as a screening tool for depression.

Separate from standard diagnostic categories, psychopathological features reported to be associated with a blunted TSH response have included suicidality, agitation, and panic (10). However, these findings have not been sufficiently replicated to establish them as reliable correlates of the blunted TSH response.

Another potential area of clinical application for the TRH test is in planning treatment and assessing prognosis. No consistent findings have emerged regarding the use of the TRH test to select treatment. However, there is some evidence that, in depressed patients, those whose TSH responses increase during the process of clinical recovery are less likely to relapse (38).

An important question is whether the blunted TSH response to TRH *precedes* psychiatric illness. Is it a risk marker for illness or is it a consequence? No studies have adequately addressed this question in depression, but several studies have been completed in individuals who, because of family history, are at high risk for alcoholism. These studies have adduced preliminary evidence of increased prevalence of a blunted TSH response in the nonalcoholic sons of alcoholic fathers (15). If confirmed, this finding would open a new area of investigation for the TRH test as a risk marker for certain psychiatric disorders.

Since the initial reports of a blunted TSH response in depression, the nature of the pathophysiological basis for the fault has been sought. The simplest explanation would be that the blunted TSH response results from increased feedback inhibition by thyroid hormones. Overt hyperthyroidism is uncommon in depression, though transient increases in thyroid hormones are frequent (52,83) and could account for some instances of blunting (8). The mechanism of the transient hyperthyroxinemia syndrome in depression is unknown; it has been hypothesized to derive from CNS activation either directly to the thyroid gland via sympathetic monoaminergic neurons (56) or indirectly via increased TRH release. In depression, hyperthyroxinemia is usually transient; the blunted TSH response may persist.

Another possible explanation for the blunted TSH response in depression is the hypercortisolemia commonly observed. Cortisol is known to inhibit TSH release, and if this were the cause of a blunted TSH response the phenomenon would unite a pathophysiological change in the HPT axis with one in the hypothalamic–pituitary–adrenal axis. However, a dissociation between these two endocrine faults generally has been found, militating against hypercortisolism as more than an occasional cause of the blunted TSH response (39).

A leading hypothesis to explain a blunted TSH response in depression is hypersecretion of hypothalamic TRH, which should lead to desensitization of pituitary TRH receptors. This hypothesis is attractive because activation of TRH neurons in the periventricular nucleus could be produced by monoaminergic neurons (45,93) that are thought to be dysfunctional in depression. In support of the hypersecretion hypothesis are reports that TRH is increased in cerebrospinal fluid (CSF) of patients with major depression compared to neurological controls or medically healthy controls (3). However, in neither of these studies was a correlation found between TRH in CSF and the TRH-induced TSH response. The increases in CSF TRH in depression may be related to attempts to compensate for the illness (67).

One study has examined TRH in CSF of abstinent alcoholics and healthy controls and reported no differences between the two groups (73). This suggests that changes in CSF TRH are not simply a function of nonspecific psychopathology.

At present the two leading hypotheses to explain a blunted TSH response in depression are transient hyperthyroxinemia and hypersecretion of hypothalamic TRH. However, it is probable that other factors at the level of the brain or pituitary are also involved in causing the abnormal response (31).

While a blunted TSH response to TRH occurs in some depressed patients, an exaggerated response occurs in others. This latter phenomenon supports the concept of an association of depression with subclinical hypothyroidism. Patients with subclinical hypothyroidism show neither classical signs and symptoms nor reductions in levels of thyroid hormones. The diagnosis depends upon either an elevated basal TSH or an exaggerated TSH response to TRH. It has been reported that 5–15% of depressed patients meet criteria for subclinical hypothyroidism (23), but whether these rates are significantly different from an age- and gender-matched population is uncertain (23). Preliminary data suggest that depressed patients with subclinical hypothyroidism have more cognitive impairment, resistance to antidepressants, and, if bipolar, a greater likelihood of rapid cycling (23).

Finally, it should be mentioned that much of the work on the TRH test in depression occurred prior to the development of highly specific and sensitive TSH assays. Two points need to be made with this in mind. First, it will be important to examine the relationship between basal TSH and TRH-induced TSH release in psychiatric patients to determine if basal TSH can provide sufficient information to obviate the need for the TRH test. Second, definitions of a blunted TSH response that were derived from less specific and sensitive radioimmunoassays are not valid when new TSH assay methods are employed (16).

USE AS A THERAPEUTIC AGENT

In Neurological Disorders

As described above, shortly after its discovery as a hypothalamic hypophysiotropic hormone, TRH was found to be distributed in many extrahypothalamic sites in brain, in spinal cord, and in other organ systems. The neuroanatomical location and neurochemical actions of TRH suggested that it could be utilized as a therapeutic agent in neurological and psychiatric disorders.

TRH receptors occur in the ventral horn area of the spinal cord. For this reason and because TRH excites anterior motor horn cells, therapeutic trials were initiated in amyotrophic lateral sclerosis (ALS) (12), a disorder characterized by loss of innervation to the anterior horn cells. These studies provided the impetus to administer TRH or its analogues in high doses. Although clear, albeit brief, improvement has been reported in patients with ALS, the application of TRH and its analogues in this disorder is still tentative. TRH has been tried in spinal–cerebellar degeneration, spinal cord injury, and disturbances in consciousness (66). Its efficacy in these conditions is unclear at this time.

In Behavioral Disorders

The blunted TSH response to TRH in depression occurred while investigating possible therapeutic effects. The initial studies of Prange et al. (70) and Kastin et al. (37) reported that, unlike saline, 500 μg of TRH administered intravenously to unipolar depressed women produced significant improvement in depression ratings that were apparent within 24 hr of administration. Since these initial reports about 30 studies have evaluated the antidepressant efficacy of TRH. Two generalizations seem justified: The number of positive and negative reports is about equal; even in the positive studies, the effects of TRH tend to be short-lived. The reasons for these inconsistent therapeutic effects of TRH are unclear. Preclinical behavioral studies have demonstrated that the peptide, like most antidepressants, potentiates L-DOPA-induced motor activity and decreases immobility in the Porsolt swim test. However, unlike most of its effects on central neurotransmission, which are compatible with an antidepressant-like action, TRH potently enhances cholinergic activity (22,63), which is, theoretically at least, depressogenic (33). The inconsistency in therapeutic effects, the transient nature of the effects, the lack of availability of TRH analogues for clinical use, and the availability of alternative treatments have delayed further study of TRH as an antidepressant.

In several of the early studies of TRH in depressed patients, improvement was noted in anxiety as well as in depressed mood. The possibility that TRH might have anxiolytic effects also derived support from animal studies indicating that TRH enhances the anticonflict effects of benzodiazepines, barbiturates, and ethanol and, in high doses, produces anticonflict actions itself (85,89). Very little work has been completed on a clinical anxiolytic effect for TRH. Reductions in tension in nonclinical populations have been reported (88), but studies of patients with a primary anxiety disorder are lacking.

Because of the observation that TRH enhances acetylcholine transmission, high doses of the tripeptide have been tested for possible therapeutic action in Alzheimer's disease. As in depression and ALS, several statistically significant effects were found but with little sustained benefit (57).

TRH is a potent antagonist of the sedation caused by drugs such as barbiturates and ethanol (63) even while potentiating their anticonflict effects. Unlike other sedative–hypnotic antagonists, TRH does not cause seizures and is not anxiogenic; indeed, as noted, it has anxiolytic properties. Because of this unique pharmacological profile, TRH has been studied as an ethanol antagonist in humans. Three studies have been published: two have found evidence that TRH counteracts some of the behavioral actions of ethanol and one that it slightly enhances intoxication (14).

Recently it was reported that an analogue of TRH, TA-0910, produces a reduction in ethanol intake in alcohol-preferring rats (71). The possibility exists that TRH or an analogue would reduce alcohol consumption or alcohol craving, but no relevant clinical data have been reported.

SYNTHESIS

Clearly TRH plays a regulatory role in an elaborately regulated system, the HPT axis. Just as clearly it can directly affect behavioral and physiological events outside that system. Phylogenetically, its functions outside the axis may have developed earlier (30), though they are less thoroughly understood. Given such considerations, how can one conceptualize the diverse functions of TRH?

Elsewhere (64), one of us, with Nemeroff, posited a theory of harmony between the behavioral effects and the endocrine effects of the hypothalamic hypophysiotropic hormones. We illustrated this with several examples, none of which is more striking than that pertaining to luteinizing-hormone-releasing hormone (LHRH). LHRH releases luteinizing hormone and FSH, which stimulate the gonads. LHRH also facilitates mating behavior. TRH lends itself to this general formulation. Through TSH, it causes the synthesis and release of thyroid hormones, which, in turn, not only increase metabolic rate but potentiate the action of ergotropic neurotransmitter activity. TRH, as noted above, exerts a variety of alerting effects. Indeed, it was this array of effects that prompted Kruse (41) and then Metcalf and Dettmar (59) to describe TRH as an ergotropic substance. This notion resonated with the earlier ergotropic–thyrotropic formulation of Hess (25). In this scheme, the organism is always oriented both internally and to its environment somewhere on a spectrum between two extremes. In a complete ergotropic state, the organism is totally engaged in the environment—alert, physically active, and maximally using energy. In a complete trophotropic state, by contrast, the organism is at rest, relatively inattentive to the environment, and restoring itself through the many processes that together are anabolic. In developing this concept, Hess emphasized two points that have become increasingly important. First, recuperation is not merely the absence of excitation; it is an active process. Second, the CNS, prominently the hypothalamus, orchestrates whatever balance of ergotropism–trophotropism may obtain at any time.

Following the concept described above and noting that TRH (and certain other peptides) abbreviated pentobarbital-induced sleep in mice while the tridecapeptide neurotensin (NT) extended it, our group formulated NT as a trophotropic hormone, in balance with the ergotropic tendencies of TRH (63). This concept was later developed in more detail and in the perspective of recent findings (69).

It would appear that the functions of TRH have been conserved during the evolution of simple species to complex ones. Its behavioral role may be older phylogenetically than its role as a regulator of thyroid function. Behaviorally it seems to be an ergotrophic substance (there are probably others) in dynamic balance with trophotropic substances such as NT. The ergotropic behavioral activity of TRH appears to be harmonious with the endocrine actions for which it was named.

ACKNOWLEDGMENTS

This work was supported by grants from the National Institute of Alcohol Abuse and Alcoholism, AA07809 (GAM) and AA08448 (JCG), and from the National Institute of Mental Health, MH33127 (AJP) and MH22536 (AJP).

REFERENCES

1. Airakinen MS, Alanen S, Szabat E, Visser TJ, Panula P. Multiple neurotransmitters in the tuberommillary nucleus: comparison of rat, mouse, and guinea pig. *J Comp Neurol* 1992;323:103–116.
2. Attali JR, Valensi P, Darnis D, Perret G, Sebaoun J. Evidence of direct thyroid stimulating action of thyrotropin releasing hormone (TRH) by perifusion of rat thyroid fragments. *Endocrinology* 1985;116:561–566.
3. Banki CM, Bissette G, Arato M, Nemeroff CB. Elevation of immunoreactive CSF TRH in depressed patients. *Am J Psychiatry* 1988;145:1526–1531.
4. Bauer K, Carmeliet P, Schulz M, Baes M, Denef C. Regulation and cellular localization of the membrane-bound thyrotropin-releasing hormone-degrading enzyme in primary cultures of neuronal, glial and adenohypophyseal cells. *Endocrinology* 1990;127:1224–1233.
5. Boler J, Enzmann F, Folkers K, Bowers CY, Schally AV. The identity of chemical and hormone properties of the thyrotropin releasing hormone and pyroglutamyl-histidyl-prolineamide. *Biochem Biophys Comm* 1969;37:505–510.
6. Bulant M, Delfour A, Vaudry H, Nichol P. Processing of thyrotropin-releasing hormone prohormone (Pro-TRH) generated Pro-TRH-connecting peptides. *J Biol Chem* 1988;263:17189–17196.
7. Burgus R, Dunn TF, Desiderio DM, Ward DN, Vale W, Guillemin R. Biological activity of synthetic polypeptide derivatives related to the structure of hypothalamic TRF. *Endocrinology* 1970;86:573–582.
8. Calloway SP, Dolan RI, Fonagy VFA, De Souza VF, Wakeline A. Endocrine changes and clinical profiles in depression. II. The thyrotropin-releasing hormone test. *Psychol Med* 1984;14:759–765.
9. Collu M, D'Aquila PS, Gessa GL, Serra G. TRH activates mesolimbic dopamine system: behavioural evidence. *Behav Pharmacol* 1992;3:639–641.
10. Corrigan MHC, Gillette GM, Quade D, Garbutt JC. Panic, suicide, and agitation: independent correlates of the TSH response to TRH in depression. *Biol Psychiatry* 1992;31:984–982.
11. de la Pena P, Delgado L, del Camino D, Barros F. Cloning and expression of the thyrotropin-releasing hormone receptor from GH3 rat anterior pituitary cells. *Biochem J* 1992;284:891–899.
12. Engel WK, Siddique T, Nicoloff JT. Effect on weakness and spasticity in amyotrophic lateral sclerosis of thyrotropin-releasing hormone. *Lancet* 1983;2:73–75.
13. Fuse Y, Polk DH, Lam RW, Fisher DA. Distribution of thyrotropin-releasing hormone (TRH) and precursor peptide (TRH-Fly) in adult rat tissue. *Endocrinology* 1990;127:2501–2505.
14. Garbutt JC, Hicks RE, Clayton CJ, Andrews RT, Mason GA. Behavioral and endocrine interactions between thyrotropin-releasing hormone and ethanol in normal human subjects. *Alcoholism: Clin Exp Res* 1991;15:1045–1049.
15. Garbutt JC, Loosen PT, Prange AJ Jr. Inter-relationships between the hypothalamic–pituitary–thyroid axis and alcoholism. In: Joffey RT, Levitt AJ, eds. *The thyroid and psychiatric disorders*. Washington, DC: American Psychiatric Press, 1993;279–296.
16. Garbutt JC, Mayo JP Jr, Mason GA, Quade D, Loosen PT, Prange AJ Jr. Interpretation of the thyrotropin (TSH) response to thyrotropin-releasing hormone (TRH): implications of an improved TSH assay system. *Biol Psychiatry* 1991;29:718–720.
17. Garcia SI, Dabsys SM, Santajuliana D, Delorenzi A, Finkielman S, Nahmod VE, Pirola CJ. Interaction between thyrotropin-releasing hormone and the muscarinic cholinergic system in rat brain. *J Endocrinol* 1992;134:215–219.
18. Gershengorn MC. Mechanism of thyrotropin releasing hormone stimulation of pituitary hormone secretion. *Annu Rev Physiol* 1986;48:515–526.
19. Gershengorn MC, Thaw CN. Regulation of thyrotropin-releasing hormone receptors is cell type specific: comparison of endogenous pituitary receptors and receptors transfected into non-pituitary cells. *Endocrinology* 1991;128:1204–1206.
20. Givens BS, Breese GR. Site-specific enhancement of γ-aminobutyric acid-mediated inhibition of neural activity of ethanol in the rat medial septal area. *J Pharmacol Exp Ther* 1990;254:528–538.
21. Glavin GB, Murison R, Overmier JB, Pare WP, Bakke HK, Henke PG, Hernandez DE. The neurobiology of stress ulcer. *Brain Res Rev* 1991;16:301–343.
22. Griffiths EC. Thyrotropin releasing hormone: endocrine and central effect. *Psychoneuroendocrinology* 1985;10:225–235.
23. Haggerty JJ Jr, Garbutt JC, Evans DL, Simon JS, Nemeroff CB. Subclinical hypothyroidism: a review of neuropsychiatric aspects. *Int J Psychiatry Med* 1990;20:193–208.

24. Harris GW. *Neural control of the pituitary gland.* London: Edward Arnold, 1955.
25. Hess WR. Die functionelle organization des vegetativen nerven systems. Basel: Schwabe, 1948.
26. Hinkle PM. Pituitary TRH receptors. *Ann NY Acad Sci* 1989;553: 176–187.
27. Hökfelt T, Tsuruo Y, Ulfhake B, Cullheim S, Arvidsson U, Foster GA, Schultzberg M, Schalling M, Arborelius L, Freedman J, Post C, Visser T. Distribution of TRH-like immunoreactivity with special reference to coexistence with other neuroactive compounds. *Ann NY Acad Sci* 1989;553:76–105.
28. Jackson IMD. Thyrotropin-releasing hormone. *N Engl J Med* 1982;306:145–155.
29. Jackson IMD. Controversies in TRH biosynthesis and strategies towards the identification of a TRH precursor. *Ann NY Acad Sci* 1989;553:7–13.
30. Jackson IMD, Wu P, Lechan RM. Immunohistochemical localization of the precursor for thyrotropin releasing hormone (PRO-TRH) in the rat brain. *Science* 1985;229:1097–1099.
31. Jacobowitz DM. Multifactorial control of pituitary hormone secretion: the "wheels" of the brain. *Synapse* 1988;2:186–192.
32. Jacobs LS, Snyder PJ, Utiger RD, Daughaday WH. Prolactin response to thyrotropin-releasing hormone in normal subjects. *J Clin Endocrinol Metabol* 1973;36:1069–1073.
33. Janowsky DS, El-Yousef MK, Davis JM, Sekerke HJ. A cholinergic–adrenergic hypothesis of mania and depression. *Lancet* 1972; 2:6732–6735.
34. Judd AM, MacLeod RM. Thyrotropin-releasing hormone and lysine-bradykinin stimulate arachidonate liberation from rat anterior pituitary cells through arachidonate liberation from rat anterior pituitary cells through different mechanisms. *Endocrinology* 1992;131: 1251–1260.
35. Kachidian P, Poulat P, Marlier L, Privat A. Immunohistochemical evidence for the coexistence of substance P, thyrotropin-releasing hormone, GABA, methionine-enkephalin, and leucine-enkephalin in the serotonergic neurons of the caudate raphe nuclei: a dual labelling in the rat. *J Neurosci Res* 1991;30:521–530.
36. Kaneko H, Mitsuma T, Morise K, Uchida K, Furusawa A, Maeda Y, Nakada K, Adachi K. Effect of serotonin on the immunoreactive thyrotropin-releasing hormone concentrations of the rat stomach. *Digestion* 1992;53:149–156.
37. Kastin AJ, Ehrensing RH, Schalch DS, Anderson MS. Improvement in mental depression with decreased thyrotropin response after administration of thyrotropin-releasing hormone. *Lancet* 1972;ii:740–742.
38. Kirkegaard C. The thyrotropin response to thyrotropin-releasing hormone in endogenous depression. *Psychoneuroendocrinology* 1981;6:189–212.
39. Kirkegaard C, Carroll BJ. Dissociation of TSH and adrenocortical disturbances in endogenous depression. *Psychiatry Res* 1980;3: 253–264.
40. Klee GC, Hay ID. Assessment of sensitive thyrotropin assays for an expanded role in thyroid function testing: proposed criteria for analytical performance and clinical utility. *J Clin Endocrinol Metab* 1987;64:461–471.
41. Kruse H. Thyrotropin releasing hormone interaction with chlorpromazine in mice, rats and rabbits. *J Pharmacol (Paris)* 1975;6:249–268.
42. Kubak MJ, Low WC, Sattin A, Morzorati SL, Meyerhoff JL, Larsen SH. Role of TRH in seizure modulation. *Ann NY Acad Sci* 1989;553:286–303.
43. Lechan RM, Molitch ME, Jackson MD. Distribution of immunoreactive human growth hormone-like material and thyrotropin-releasing hormone in the rat central nervous system: evidence for their coexistence in the same neurons. *Endocrinology* 1983; 112:877–884.
44. Lechan RM, Segerson TP. Pro-TRH gene expression and precursor peptides in rat brain: observations by hybridization analysis and immunocytochemistry. *Ann NY Acad Sci* 1989;553:29–59.
45. Lee SL, Sevarino K, Roos BA, Goodman RH. Characterization and expression of the gene-encoding rat thyrotropin-releasing hormone (TRH). *Ann NY Acad Sci* 1989;553:14–28.
46. Leong DA, Frawley LS, Neill JD. Neuroendocrine control of prolactin secretion. *Annu Rev Physiol* 1983;45:109–127.

47. Lewis BM, Dieguez C, Lewis MD, Scanlon MF. Dopamine stimulates release of thyrotrophin-releasing hormone from perfused intact rat hypothalamus via hypothalamic D_2 receptors. *J Endocrinol* 1887;115:419–424.
48. Li P, Thaw CN, Sempowski GD, Gershengorn MC, Hinkle PM. Characterization of the calcium response to thyrotropin-releasing hormone (TRH) in cells transfected with TRH receptor complementary DNA: importance of voltage-sensitive calcium channels. *Mol Endocrinol* 1992;6:1393–1402.
49. Liao N, Vaudry H, Pelletier G. Neuroanatomical connection between corticotropin-releasing factor (CRF) and somatostatin (SRIF) nerve endings and thyrotropin-releasing hormone (TRH) neurons in the paraventricular nucleus of rat hypothalsmus. *Peptides* 1992;13:677–680.
50. Lippman SS, Amr S, Weintraub BD. Discordant effects of thyrotropin (TSH)-releasing hormone on pre- and posttranslational regulation of TSH biosynthesis in rat pituitary. *Endocrinology* 1986;119: 343–348.
51. Loosen PT. The TRH-induced TSH response in psychiatric patients: a possible neuroendocrine marker. *Psychoneuroendocrinology* 1985;10:237–260.
52. Maes M, Vandewoude M, Maes L, Schotte C, Cosyns P. A revised interpretation of the TRH test results in female depressed patients. Part I: TSH responses. Effects of severity of illness, thyroid hormones, monoamines, age, sex hormonal, corticosteroid and nutritional state. *J Affect Dis* 1989;16:203–213.
53. Manaker S, Eichen A, Winokur A, Rhodes CH, Rainbow TC. Autoradiographic localization of thyrotropin releasing hormone receptors in human brain. *Neurology* 1986;36:641–646.
54. Mantyh PW, Hunt SP. Evidence for cholecystokinin-like immunoreactive neurons in the rat medulla oblongata which project to the spinal cord. *Brain Res* 1984;291:49–54.
55. Meister B, Hökfelt T. The somatostatin and growth hormone-releasing factors systems. In: Nemeroff CB, ed. *Neuroendocrinology.* Boca Raton, FL: CRC Press, 1992;219–278.
56. Melander A, Westgren U, Ericson L, Sundler F. Influence of the sympathetic nervous system on the secretion and metabolism of thyroid hormone. *Endocrinology* 1976;101:1228–1237.
57. Mellow AM, Sunderland T, Cohen RM, Lawlor BA, Hill JL, Newhouse PA, Cohen MR, Murphy DL. Acute effects of high-dose thyrotropin releasing hormone infusions in Alzheimer's disease. *Psychopharmacology* 1989;98:403–407.
58. Merchenthaler I. Co-localization of enkephalin and TRH in perifornical neurons of the rat hypothalamus that project to the lateral septum. *Brain Res* 1991;544:177–180.
59. Metcalf G, Dettmar PW. Is thyrotropin releasing hormone an endogenous ergotropic substance in the brain? *Lancet* 1981;i:586–589.
60. Morley JE, Brammer GL, Sharp B, Yamada T, Yuwiler A, Hershman JM. Neurotransmitter control of hypothalamic-pituitary-thyroid functions in rats. *Eur J Pharmacol* 1981;70:263.
61. Murdoch GH, Franco R, Evans RM, Rosenfeld MG. Polypeptide hormone regulation of gene expression: TRH rapidly stimulates both transcription of the prolactin gene and phosphorylation of a specific nuclear protein. *J Biol Chem* 1983;258:15329–15335.
62. Nakada K, Mitsuma T, Furusawa A, Maeda Y, Morise K. The effect of histamine on the concentration of immunoreactive thyrotropin-releasing hormone in the stomach and hypothalamus in the rat. *Gastroenterol Jpn* 1990;25:425–431.
63. Nemeroff CB, Kalivas PW, Golden RN. Behavioral effects of hypothalamic hypophysiotropic hormones, neurotensin, substance P and other neuropeptides. *Pharmacol Ther* 1984;24:1–56.
64. Nemeroff CB, Prange AJ Jr. Peptides and psychoneuroendocrinology: a perspective. *Arch Gen Psychiatry* 1978;35(8):999–1010.
65. O'Cuinn G, O'Conner B, Elmore M. Degradation of thyrotropin-releasing hormone and luteinizing hormone by enzymes of brain tissue. *J Neurochem* 1990;54:1–13.
66. Ogashiwa M, Takenchi K. Clinical studies of thyrotropin-releasing hormone tartrate (TRH-T) as a direct stimulant to the central nervous system. *Int J Clin Pharmacol Biopharm* 1979;17:145–151.
67. Post RM, Weiss SRB. Endogenous biochemical abnormalities in affective illness: therapeutic versus pathogenic. *Biol Psychiatry* 1992;32:469–484.
68. Poulat P, Marlier L, Ryaofetra N, Privat A. 5-hydroxytryptamine, substance P and thyrotropin-releasing hormone synapses in the in-

termedrolateral cell column of the rat thoracic spinal cord. *Neurosci Lett* 1992;136:19–22.

69. Prange AJ Jr. The manifold actions of neurotensin, a trophotropic agent. *Ann NY Acad Sci* 1992;668:298–306.

70. Prange AJ Jr, Wilson IC, Lara PP, Alltop LB, Breese GR. Effects of thyrotropin releasing hormone in depression. *Lancet* 1972;ii:999–1002.

71. Rezvani AH, Garbutt JC, Shimoda K, Garges PL, Janowsky DS, Mason GA. Attenuation of alcohol preference in alcohol-preferring rats by a novel TRH analogue, TA-0910. *Alcoholism: Clin Exp Res* 1992;16:326–330.

72. Rosen JB, Cain CJ, Weiss RB, Post RM. Alterations in mRNA of enkephalin, dynorphin and thyrotropin releasing hormone during amygdala kindling: an in situ hybridization study. *Mol Brain Res* 1992;15:247–255.

73. Roy A, Bissette G, Nemeroff CB, DeJong J, Ravitz B, Adinoff B, Linnoila M. Cerebrospinal fluid thyrotropin-releasing hormone concentrations in alcoholics and normal controls. *Biol Psychiatry* 1990;28:767–772.

74. Sato N, Wang X, Greer MA. An acute release of Ca^{2+} from sequestered intracellular pools is not the primary transduction mechanism causing the initial burst of PRL and TSH secretion induced by TRH in normal rat pituitary cells. *Cell Calcium* 1992;13:173–182.

75. Scanlon MF. Neuroendocrine control of thyrotropin secretion. In: Braverman LE, Utiger RD, eds. *The thyroid: a fundamental and clinical text.* 6th ed. Philadelphia: JB Lippincott, 1991;230–256.

76. Schlesser MA, Rush AJ, Fairchild C, Crowley G, Orsulak P. The thyrotropin-releasing hormone stimulation test: a methodological study. *Psychiatry Res* 1983;9:59–67.

77. Sevarino KA, Primus RJ. Cocaine regulation of brain preprothyrotropin-releasing hormone mRNA. *J Neurochem* 1993;60:1151–1154.

78. Sharif NA. Quantitative autoradiography of TRH receptors in discrete brain regions of different mammalian species. *Ann NY Acad Sci* 1989;553:147–175.

79. Shimoda K, Mason GA, Walker CH, Garbutt JC, Prange AJ Jr. Administration of chlordiazepoxide affects [^{3}H] [3-methyl-histidyl$_2$] thyrotropin releasing hormone binding in rat brain. *Peptides* 1991;12:199–202.

80. Snyder PJ, Utiger RD. Response to thyrotropin-releasing hormone (TRH) in normal man. *J Clin Endocrinol* 1972;34:380–385.

81. Straub RE, Frech GC, Joho RH, Gershengorn MC. Expression cloning of a cDNA encoding the mouse pituitary thyrotropin-releasing hormone receptor. *Proc Natl Acad Sci* 1990;87:9514–9518.

82. Suen CS, Wilk S. Inhibition of pyroglutamyl peptidase II synthesis by phorbal ester in the Y-79 rat retinoblastoma cell. *Endocrinology* 1991;128:2169–1974.

83. Unden F, Ljunggren J-G, Kjellman BF, Beck-Friis J, Wetterberg L. Twenty-four hour serum levels of T_4 and T_3 in relation to decreased TSH serum levels and decreased TSH response to TRH in affective disorders. *Acta Psychiatr Scand* 1986;73:358–365.

84. Vijayan E, McCann SM. Effects of intraventricular injection of gamma-aminobutyric acid (GABA) on plasma growth hormone and thyrotropin on conscious rats. *Endocrinology* 1978;103:1888.

85. Vogel RA, Frye GD, Wilson JH, Kuhn CM, Mailman RB, Mueller RA, Breese GR. Attenuation of the effects of punishment by ethanol: comparison with chlordiazepoxide. *J Pharmacol Exp Ther* 1980;212:153–161.

86. von Euler US, Gaddum JH. An unidentified depressor substance in certain tissue extracts. *J Physiol (Lond)* 1931;72:74–81.

87. Winicov I, Gershengorn MC. Receptor density determines secretory response patterns mediated by inositol lipid-derived second messengers. Comparison of thyrotropin-releasing hormone and carbamylcholine actions in thyroid-stimulating hormone-secreting mouse pituitary tumor cells. *J Biol Chem* 1989;264:9438–9443.

88. Winokur A, Amsterdam JD, Mihailovic V, Caroff SN. Improvement in ratings of tension after TRH administration in healthy women. *Psychoneuroendocrinology* 1982;7:239–244.

89. Witkin JM, Sickle J, Barrett JE. Potentiation of the behavioral effects of pentobarbital, chlordiazepoxide and ethanol by thyrotropin-releasing hormone. *Peptides* 1984;5:809–813.

90. Wondisford FE, Magner JA, Weintraub BD. Chemistry and biosynthesis of thyrotropin. In: Braverman LE, Utiger RD, eds. *The thyroid: a fundamental and clinical text.* 6th ed. Philadelphia: JB Lippincott, 1991;257–276.

91. Yamada M, Rudovick S, Wondisford FE, Nakayama Y, Weintraub BD, Wilber JF. Cloning and structure of human genomic DNA and hypothalamic cDNA encoding human preprothyrotropin-releasing hormone. *Mol Endocrinol* 1990;4:551–556.

92. Yatsugi S, Yamamoto M. Anticonvulsive properties of YM-14673, a new TRH analogue, in amygdaloid-kindled rats. *Pharmacol Biochem Behav* 1991;38:669–672.

93. Zoeller RT, Kabeer N, Albers HE. Cold exposure elevates cellular levels of messenger ribonucleic acid encoding thyrotropin-releasing hormone in paraventricular nucleus despite elevated levels of thyroid hormones. *Endocrinology* 1990;127:2955–2962.

94. Zoller RT, Rudeen PK. Ethanol blocks the cold-induced increase in thyrotropin-releasing hormone mRNA in paraventricular nuclei but not the cold-induced increase in thyrotropin. *Mol Brain Res* 1992;13:321–330.

Psychopharmacology: The Fourth Generation of Progress, edited by Floyd E. Bloom and David J. Kupfer. Raven Press, Ltd., New York © 1995.

CHAPTER 45

Corticotropin-Releasing Factor

Physiology, Pharmacology, and Role in Central Nervous System and Immune Disorders

Errol B. De Souza and Dimitri E. Grigoriadis

HISTORICAL PERSPECTIVES

The concept that the hypothalamus plays a primary role in the regulation of the pituitary–adrenocortical axis was first proposed by Sir Geoffrey Harris in 1948. Subsequently, during the 1950s the teams of Guillemin and Rosenberg and of Saffran and Schally observed independently the presence of a factor in hypothalamic extracts [termed *corticotropin-releasing factor* (CRF)] that could stimulate the release of adrenocorticotropic hormone (ACTH, corticotropin) from anterior pituitary cells in vitro. Although CRF was the first hypothalamic hypophysiotropic factor to be recognized, its chemical identity remained elusive for a variety of reasons. The presence in hypothalamic extracts of other, weaker secretagogues of ACTH secretion such as vasopressin, catecholamines, and angiotensin II, along with their synergistic effects with CRF on ACTH secretion in combination with the relative lack of specificity of the in vitro bioassays, hindered the purification of the peptide. Furthermore, the close proximity in sizes of ACTH (39 amino acids) and CRF (41 amino acids) did not allow for easy separation of the peptides by liquid chromatography. The development of radioimmunoassays for ACTH and quantitative in vitro methods for assaying hypophysiotropic substances, along with the utilization of ion-exchange and high-performance liquid chromatographic techniques, led to the successful purification of CRF from sheep hypothalamic extracts. In 1981, Wylie Vale and colleagues at

the Salk Institute reported the isolation, characterization, synthesis, and in vitro and in vivo biological activities of a 41-amino-acid hypothalamic ovine CRF (61).

This chapter will provide an overview of CRF rather than a comprehensive review. More detailed and comprehensive information on CRF is available in recent reviews (22,40) and books (10,19) on the topic (see Chapter 83, *this volume*).

CHARACTERISTICS OF THE CRF PEPTIDE AND GENE SEQUENCES

Amino Acid Sequence and Structure of CRF

The sequence of CRF has been determined in a variety of species, including sheep, humans, rats, pigs, goats, and cows. In all species, CRF is a 41-amino-acid-residue single-chain polypeptide (Fig. 1). Rat and human CRF are identical to one another and differ from ovine CRF by seven amino acid residues. All three CRFs have close amino acid homology and share some biological properties with sauvagine, a 40-amino-acid peptide that exists in frog skin, and urotensin I, a 41-amino-acid peptide derived from fish urophysis. Caprine and ovine CRF are identical and differ from bovine CRF by one amino acid. Porcine CRF more closely resembles rat/human CRF. CRF and related peptides are amidated at their carboxy terminal; CRF COOH-terminal-free acid has less than 0.1% of the potency of native CRF, suggesting the importance of amidation to biological activity of the peptide. Studies to determine the solution structure of CRF using

E. B. De Souza and D. E. Grigoriadis: Neurocrine Biosciences, Inc., San Diego, California 92121.

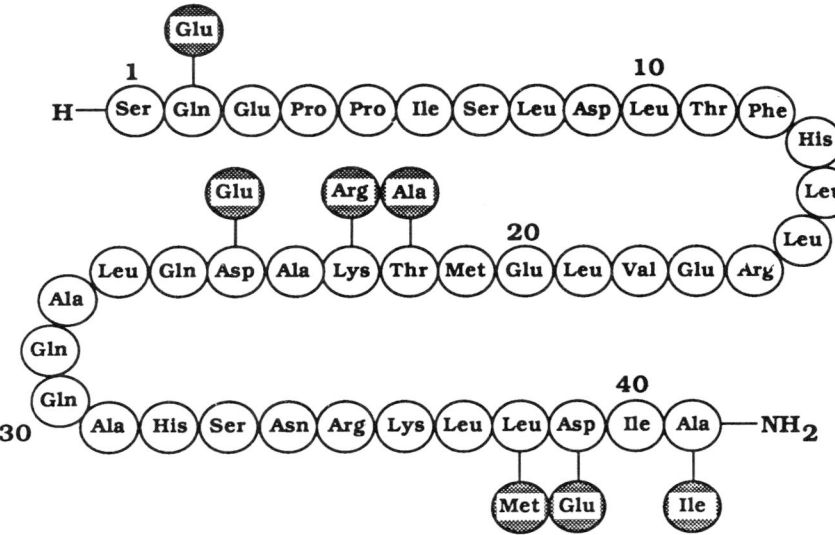

FIG. 1. Amino acid sequences of ovine and rat/human corticotropin-releasing factor (CRF). The amino acid sequence of ovine CRF is denoted by the *open circles*. Rat CRF and human CRF are identical and differ from ovine CRF by seven amino acid residues which are denoted by the *shaded circles*. Both peptides are amidated at the carboxy terminus, and the amidation is essential for biological activity.

proton nuclear magnetic resonance suggest that human CRF comprises an extended N-terminal tetrapeptide connected to a well-defined α-helix between residues 6 and 36 (48). An α-helical ovine CRF(9-41) has been demonstrated to be an antagonist of CRF receptors (47), which underscores the necessity of the α-helical conformation for receptor binding and biological activity.

Organization of the CRF Gene and Protein Precursor

The nucleotide sequences encoding ovine and rat CRF cDNA precursors as well as the human, rat, and ovine CRF genes have been determined (33,59). The locus of the CRF gene is on chromosome 8q13 in the human. The CRF genes are quite similar to one another, containing two exons separated by an intervening intron 686–800 base pairs long. The first exon encodes most of the 5'-untranslated region of the mRNA while the second exon encodes the entire prepro CRF precursor polypeptide, which is 187–196 amino acids long; the carboxy end of the precursor contains the 41-amino-acid peptide sequence. The high incidence of homology between species suggests that the gene has been highly conserved through evolution.

As previously demonstrated for other systems, the 5'-flanking DNA sequences are most likely to contain the DNA sequence elements responsible for glucocorticoid, cAMP, and phorbol ester regulation, tissue-specific expression, and enhancer activity. While a consensus cAMP response element, located 200 base pairs upstream from the major transcription initiation site, has been identified, no obvious glucocorticoid response elements or activation protein (AP)-1-binding elements are present. A potential AP-2 binding site which may mediate the responses to

protein kinase A and C is present 150 base pairs upstream from the major start site.

ANATOMY OF CRF

Distribution in the Central Nervous System

The distribution and localization of CRF mRNA in the central nervous system (CNS) have been evaluated using Northern blot analysis and in situ hybridization histochemistry, respectively. Radioimmunoassay and immunohistochemical studies have been critical in the determination of the neuroanatomical organization of CRF immunoreactive cells and fibers in the CNS. Overall, there is good concordance between studies demonstrating a widespread distribution of CRF cell bodies and fibers in the CNS. Detailed descriptions of the organization of CRF-immunoreactive cells and fibers in rat brain have been published (41,51,57). A schematic of the distribution of CRF-containing cell bodies and fibers in rat brain is shown in Fig. 2.

Morphological data clearly indicate that the paraventricular nucleus of the hypothalamus (PVN) is the major site of CRF-containing cell bodies that influence anterior pituitary hormone secretion. These neurons originate in the parvocellular portion of the PVN and send axon terminals to the capillaries of the median eminence. CRF is also present in a small group of PVN neurons that project to the lower brainstem and spinal cord; this group of neurons may be involved in regulating autonomic nervous system function. Other hypothalamic nuclei that contain CRF cell bodies include the medial preoptic area, the dorsomedial nucleus, the arcuate nucleus, the posterior hypothalamus, and the mammillary nuclei.

The neocortex contains primarily CRF interneurons with bipolar, vertically oriented cell bodies predominantly

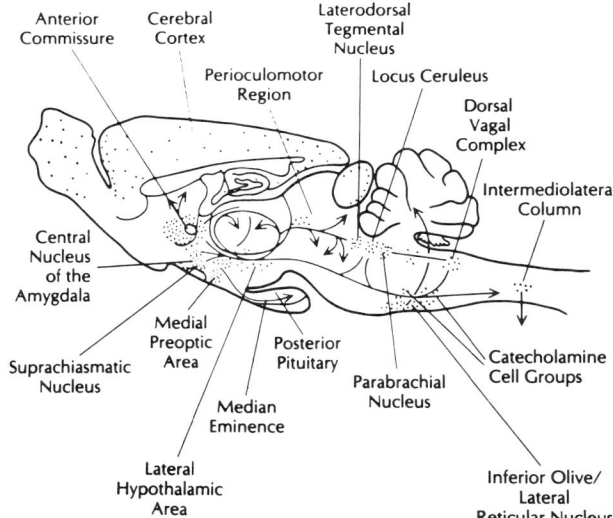

FIG. 2. Major groups of CRF-producing neuronal perikarya (*dots*) and their fiber systems (*arrows*) are shown in a sagittal view of the rat brain. (Adapted from ref. 51.)

localized to the second and third layers of the cortex and fiber projections to layers I and IV. In addition, scattered cells are present in the deeper layers and appear to be pyramidal cells. Although CRF-containing neurons are found throughout the neocortex, they are found in higher densities in the prefrontal, insular, and cingulate areas. CRF neurons in the cerebral cortex appear to be important in several behavioral actions of the peptide, including effects on cognitive processing. Furthermore, dysfunction of these neurons may contribute to many CNS disorders (see section entitled ''Role for CRF in Neuropsychiatric Disorders and Neurodegenerative Diseases,'' below).

Large and discrete populations of CRF perikarya are present in the central nucleus of the amygdala, the bed nucleus of the stria terminalis, and the substantia innominata. CRF neurons in the central nucleus of the amygdala project to the parvocellular regions of the PVN and to the parabrachial nucleus of the brainstem and thus may influence both neuroendocrine and autonomic function in addition to behavioral activity. CRF neurons originating in the bed nucleus of the stria terminalis send terminals to brainstem areas such as the parabrachial nuclei and dorsal vagal complex, which coordinate autonomic activity. CRF fibers also interconnect the amygdala with the bed nucleus of the stria terminalis and hypothalamus. Scattered CRF cells with a few fibers are also present in telencephalic areas such as regions of the amygdala, the central nucleus, the septum, the diagonal band of Broca, the olfactory bulb, and all aspects of the hippocampal formation, including the pyramidal cells, the dentate gyrus, and the subiculum.

Several groups of CRF cell bodies are present throughout the brainstem. In the midbrain, CRF perikarya are present in the periaqueductal gray, the Edinger–Westphal

nucleus, the dorsal raphe nucleus, and the ventral tegmental nucleus. Projections from the dorsal–lateral tegmental nucleus to a variety of anterior brain areas such as the medial frontal cortex, the septum, and the thalamus have also been described. In the pons, CRF cell bodies are localized in the locus coeruleus, the parabrachial nucleus, the medial vestibular nucleus, the paragigantocellular nucleus, and the periaqueductal gray. CRF neurons originating in the parabrachial nucleus project to the medial preoptic nucleus of the hypothalamus. In the medulla, large groups of cell bodies are present in the nucleus of the solitary tract and the dorsal vagal complex with ascending projections to the parabrachial nucleus. Scattered groups of cell bodies are also present in the medullary reticular formation, the spinal trigeminal nucleus, the external cuneate nucleus, and the inferior olive. The inferior olive gives rise to a well-defined olivocerebellar CRF pathway with projections to the Purkinje cells of the cerebellum. No CRF cell bodies are present in the cerebellar formation.

Within the spinal cord, CRF cell bodies are present in laminae V to VII and X and in the intermediolateral column of the thoracic and lumbar cord. CRF fibers originating in the spinal cord form an ascending system terminating in the reticular formation, the vestibular complex, the central gray, and the thalamus. This ascending CRF system may play an important role in modulating sensory input. In addition, spinal cord CRF neurons may represent preganglionic neurons that modulate sympathetic outflow.

Distribution in Peripheral Tissues

In addition to its CNS distribution, CRF has been localized in a variety of peripheral tissues (see ref. 40). CRF-like immunoreactive fibers are present in the intermediate lobe of the pituitary; these fibers originate in the hypothalamus. A physiological role has been proposed for CRF in regulating pro-opiomelanocortin (POMC)-derived peptide secretion from the intermediate pituitary. CRF has also been localized in the adrenal medulla and has been reported to be increased following stimulation of the splanchnic nerve and hemorrhagic stress. CRF-like immunoreactivity and CRF mRNA have been detected in lymphocytes, where they may play a role in regulating immune function (see section entitled ''CRF Regulation of Immune Function,'' below). Other tissues in which CRF has been localized include the testis (Leydig cells and advanced germ cells), pancreas, stomach and small intestine. While CRF is not detected in the circulation under normal circumstances, very high levels have been measured in the plasma of pregnant women; the source of CRF in pregnancy appears to be the placenta (see section entitled ''CRF-Binding Protein,'' below).

CRF RECEPTORS

Pharmacological Characteristics

The radioligand binding characteristics of CRF receptors in brain, endocrine, and immune tissues have been described in numerous publications (2,15,18,26,63). CRF receptors fulfill all of the criteria for bona fide receptors. The kinetic and pharmacological characteristics of CRF receptors are comparable in brain, pituitary, and spleen. The binding of [^{125}I]CRF in tissue homogenates is dependent on time, temperature, and tissue concentration, and it is saturable, reversible, and of high affinity, with K_D values of 200–400 pM. The pharmacological rank order profile of these receptors from various tissues has been compared using closely related analogues of CRF. Bioactive analogues of CRF have high affinity for [^{125}I]CRF binding sites, whereas biologically inactive fragments of the peptide and unrelated peptides are all without inhibitory binding activity in brain, endocrine, and immune tissues.

CRF receptors exhibit the typical properties of neurotransmitter receptors linked to the adenylate cyclase system through a guanine-nucleotide-binding protein. In in vitro radioligand binding studies, divalent cations (e.g., magnesium ions) have been shown to enhance agonist binding to receptors coupled to guanine-nucleotide-binding proteins by stabilizing the high-affinity form of the receptor–effector complex. In contrast, guanine nucleotides have the ability to selectively decrease the affinity of agonists for their receptors by promoting the dissociation of the agonist high-affinity form of the receptor. Consistent with CRF receptors being coupled to a guanine-nucleotide-regulatory protein, the binding of [^{125}I]CRF to pituitary, brain, and spleen homogenates is reciprocally increased by divalent cations such as Mg^{2+} and decreased by guanine nucleotides. (See also Chapters 27 and 38 for more details of these G-protein coupled receptors.)

Biochemical Characteristics

The molecular weight and biochemical characteristics of the CRF receptor have been determined using chemical-affinity cross-linking techniques and the bifunctional cross-linking reagent disuccinimidyl suberate to covalently attach [^{125}I]CRF to the CRF-receptor complex in central and peripheral tissues (18,26,63). Using this procedure, it has been demonstrated that the molecular weight of the CRF receptor as defined by sodium dodecyl sulfate–polyacrylamide gel electrophoresis (SDS-PAGE) is approximately 75,000 daltons in the pituitary and spleen, whereas CRF cross-linked to its receptor in brain appears to label a protein with an apparent molecular weight of 58,000 daltons. The pharmacological specificity of covalent labeling is typical of the CRF binding site,

because both the brain- and pituitary- or spleen-labeled proteins (i.e., 58,000- and 75,000-dalton proteins, respectively) exhibit the appropriate pharmacological rank order profiles characteristic of the CRF receptor.

The biochemical characteristics of CRF receptors have been further elucidated by utilizing selective lectins and enzymes that interact with specific carbohydrate moieties on receptor proteins. Adsorption of affinity cross-linked CRF receptors to the lectins concanavalin A and wheat-germ agglutinin demonstrate that CRF receptors in brain and pituitary are both glycosylated. Although both the central and peripheral CRF receptors demonstrate extensive glycosylation, the types of carbohydrate groups are clearly distinct as evidenced by the differential effects of the glycosidases in these tissues. The endoglycosidase N-glycanase, which deglycosylates all N-linked carbohydrate moieties, reduces both the central and peripheral CRF receptor to a single polypeptide band with an apparent molecular weight of 40,000–45,000 daltons, indicating that the ligand-binding subunits of the brain and pituitary CRF receptors most likely reside on similar proteins. Additional studies evaluating the effects of treatment of cross-linked CRF receptors with exo- and endoglycosidases demonstrate marked differences in the extent and nature of glycosylation between brain and peripheral (i.e., pituitary and splenic) CRF receptors. Thus, although both receptor forms are glycosylated with predominantly N-linked sugars, the extent to which they are glycosylated and the type of carbohydrate residues involved are different, suggesting that CRF receptors in brain and periphery undergo differential post-translational modification.

Distribution in Pituitary, CNS, and Spleen

Many studies to date have described the distribution of CRF receptors in various tissues, including the pituitary, brain, and spleen (2,18,26,63). An example of the autoradiographic distribution of [^{125}I]CRF binding sites in mouse pituitary, brain, and spleen is shown in Fig. 3.

The autoradiographic localization of CRF receptors in the anterior pituitary demonstrates a clustering of binding sites that corresponds to the distribution of corticotrophs (Fig. 3A). The intermediate lobe shows a more uniform distribution of binding sites characteristic of the homogeneous population of POMC-producing cells in this lobe. Overall, the distribution pattern of CRF receptors within the pituitary supports the functional role of CRF as the primary physiological regulator of POMC-derived peptide secretion from the anterior and intermediate lobes of the pituitary.

Receptor autoradiography and binding studies in discrete areas of the CNS demonstrate that, in general, the highest concentration of CRF binding sites is distributed in brain regions involved in cognitive function (cerebral cortex), in limbic areas involved in emotion and stress

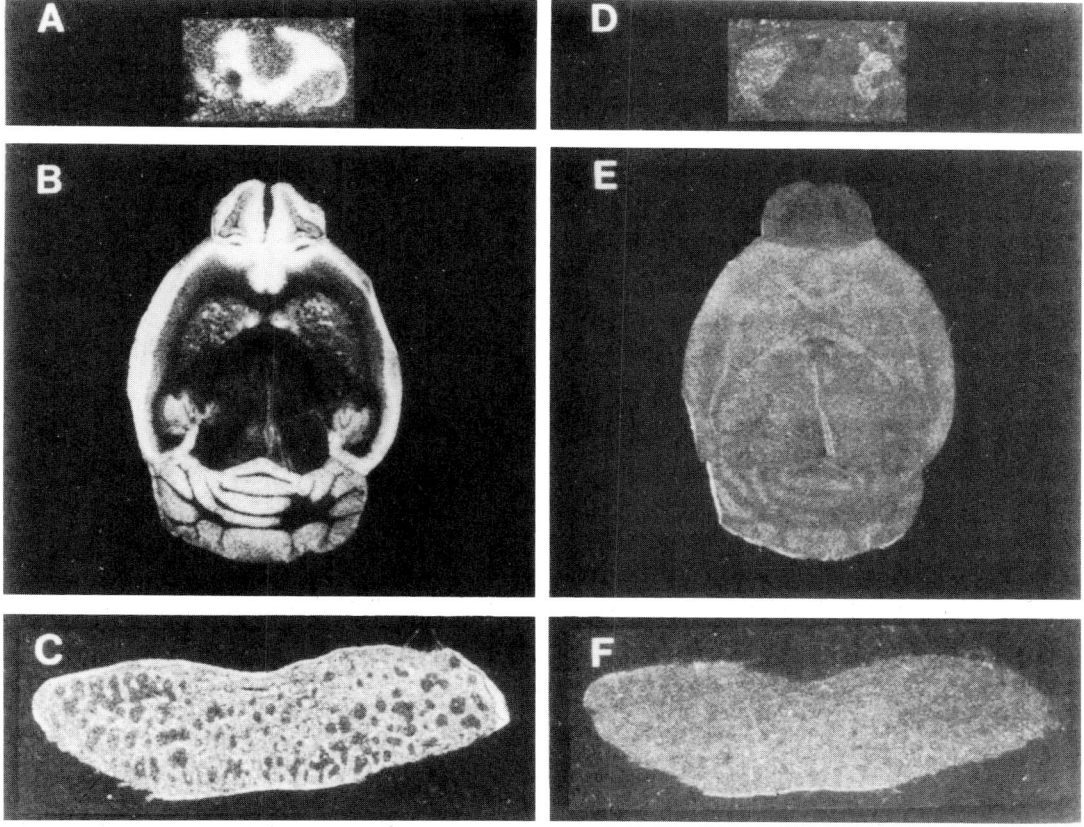

FIG. 3. Distribution of CRF receptors in the brain–pituitary–immune axis. **A–C:** Dark-field photomicrographs demonstrating the total distribution of $[^{125}I]Tyr^0$-oCRF binding sites in mouse pituitary, brain, and spleen, respectively. In dark-field illumination, the *bright areas* represent high densities of CRF receptors. In **A** (horizontal section of pituitary), note the higher density of CRF receptors in the intermediate lobe of the pituitary compared to the anterior lobe, and also note the conspicuous absence of CRF binding sites in the posterior lobe. In **B** (horizontal section of brain), note the higher densities of binding sites in cerebral cortex, olfactory bulb, and cerebellum, as well as in a variety of limbic areas. In **C** (sagittal section of spleen), note the diffuse density of CRF binding sites that are localized to the red pulp regions and also note the high density of CRF binding sites in the marginal zone surrounding the white pulp zone. There was a notable absence of CRF binding in the white pulp regions, which contain high concentrations of T and B lymphocytes. **D–F:** Dark-field photomicrographs showing the absence of specific binding in adjacent sections of all three tissues in which 1 μM unlabeled rat/human CRF was included in the incubation medium.

responses (amygdala, nucleus accumbens, and hippocampus), in brainstem regions regulating autonomic function (locus coeruleus and nucleus of the solitary tract), and in olfactory bulb (Fig. 3B). In addition, there is a high density of CRF binding sites in the molecular layer of the cerebellar cortex and in the spinal cord, where the highest concentrations are present in the dorsal horn.

CRF receptors in spleen are primarily localized to the red pulp and marginal zones (Fig. 3C). The localization of $[^{125}I]CRF$ binding sites in mouse spleen to regions known to have a high concentration of macrophages suggests that CRF receptors are present on resident splenic macrophages. The absence of specific $[^{125}I]CRF$ binding sites in the periarteriole and peripheral follicular white pulp regions of the spleen suggests that neither T nor B lymphocytes have specific high-affinity CRF receptors

comparable to those localized in the marginal zone and red pulp areas of the spleen or in the pituitary and brain.

Second Messengers Coupled to CRF Receptors

Radioligand binding studies have demonstrated that CRF receptors in the brain–endocrine–immune axis are coupled to a guanine-nucleotide-regulatory protein. In all of these tissues, the primary second messenger system involved in transducing the actions of CRF is stimulation of cAMP production (2,4,18,26,63). CRF initiates a cascade of enzymatic reactions in the pituitary gland beginning with the receptor-mediated stimulation of adenylate cyclase which ultimately regulates POMC-peptide secretion and possibly synthesis. POMC-derived peptide secretion mediated by the activation of adenylate cyclase in the anterior and neurointermediate lobes of the pituitary is dose-related and exhibits appropriate pharmacology. Similarly in the brain and spleen, the pharmacological rank order profile of CRF-related peptides for stimulation of adenylate cyclase is analogous to the profile seen in pituitary and is in keeping with the affinities of these compounds for receptor binding. In addition, the putative CRF-receptor antagonist α-helical ovine CRF(9-41) inhibits CRF-stimulated adenylate cyclase in brain and spleen homogenates.

In addition to the adenylate cyclase system, other signal transduction mechanisms may be involved in the actions of CRF. For example, CRF has been shown to increase protein carboxylmethylation and phospholipid methylation in AtT-20 corticotroph cells (27). Preliminary evidence suggests that CRF may regulate cellular responses through products of arachidonic acid metabolism (1). Furthermore, although the evidence in anterior pituitary cells suggests that CRF does not directly regulate phosphotidylinositol turnover or protein kinase C activity (1), stimulation of protein kinase C either directly or by specific ligands (vasopressin or angiotensin II) enhances CRF-stimulated adenylate cyclase activity, increases ACTH release, and inhibits phosphodiesterase activity (1). Thus, the effects of CRF on anterior pituitary cells and possibly in neurons and other cell types expressing CRF receptors are likely to involve complex interactions among several intracellular second messenger systems.

CRF-BINDING PROTEIN

CRF and Its Binding Protein in Human Plasma

Under normal conditions, the plasma levels of CRF remain low. However, CRF levels are markedly elevated in plasma during the late gestational stages of pregnancy (31,32,55). The source of the pregnancy-associated CRF is most likely the placenta, because previous studies have demonstrated that the human placenta synthesizes CRF (52). The CRF in the maternal plasma is bioactive in releasing ACTH from cultured pituitary cells (32). In spite of the high levels of CRF in the maternal plasma, there is no evidence of markedly increased ACTH secretion or hypercortisolism in pregnant women (31). A plausible explanation for this paradoxical situation could be the presence of a binding protein in the plasma of pregnant women which inhibits the biological actions of CRF (32,55). This hypothesis was recently validated by the isolation of a CRF-binding protein (CRF-BP) from human plasma and its subsequent cloning and expression (see below).

cDNA and Amino Acid Sequences

The CRF-BP was first isolated and purified to near homogeneity for sequencing and generation of oligonu-

cleotide probes (5). Screening a human liver cDNA library using probes generated from the original amino acid sequence revealed a full-length cDNA containing a 1.8-kb insert that codes for a novel protein of 322 amino acids (44). A single putative N-linked glycosylation site found at amino acid 203 agrees with the previous observation of the presence of asparagine-linked sugar moieties on the native protein (56). Subsequent screening of a rat cerebral cortical cDNA library revealed the presence of a single clone containing a 1.85-kb insert predicting a protein of 322 amino acids which was 85% identical to the human CRF-BP. The putative glycosylation site seems to be conserved between the rat and human sequences (44). The CRF binding profile of these proteins appears to be similar in both the rat and human binding proteins, because all of the proteins have high affinity for the rat/human CRF ($K_D \approx 0.2$ nM) and very low affinity for the ovine form of CRF ($K_D \approx 250$ nM). Although there may be some similarities in the binding domains of the CRF-BP and the CRF receptor, these are distinct proteins, each with unique characteristics and distributions.

Distribution in Brain and Pituitary

Although the human and rat forms of the CRF-BP are homologous, there is a somewhat different anatomical distribution pattern in the two species. The human form of the binding protein has been found abundantly in tissues such as liver, placenta, and brain, whereas levels of mRNA for the binding protein in the rat have only been localized in the brain and pituitary (44). Peripheral expression of the binding protein may have its greatest utility in the modulation and control of the elevated circulating levels of CRF induced by various normal physiological conditions (see above). In addition, expression of this binding protein in the brain and pituitary offers additional mechanisms by which CRF-related neuronal or neuroendocrine actions may be modulated.

CRF-binding protein has been localized to a variety of brain regions, including neocortex, hippocampus (primarily in the dentate gyrus), and olfactory bulb. In the basal forebrain, mRNA is localized to the amygdaloid complex with a distinct lack of immunostained cells in the medial nucleus. CRF-binding protein immunoreactivity is also present in the brainstem (particularly in the auditory, vestibular, and trigeminal systems), the raphe nuclei of the midbrain and pons, and the reticular formation (45). In addition, high expression levels of binding protein mRNA are seen in the anterior pituitary, predominantly restricted to the corticotrope cells. Expression of this protein in the corticotropes strongly suggests that the CRF-BP is involved in the regulation of neuroendocrine functions of CRF by limiting and/or affecting the interactions of CRF with its receptor, which is also known to reside on corticotropes. However, the detailed role of the binding protein in regulating pituitary–adrenal function remains to be elucidated.

CRF REGULATION OF NEUROENDOCRINE FUNCTION

Regulation of Pituitary Hormone Secretion

CRF is the major physiologic regulator of synthesis and the basal and stress-induced release of ACTH, β-endorphin, and other POMC-derived peptides from the anterior pituitary (for reviews see refs. 22, 40, and 60). CRF stimulates the release of POMC-derived peptides in anterior pituitary cells in culture and in vivo; these actions of CRF can be antagonized by the CRF-receptor antagonist α-helical ovine CRF(9-41) or by immunoneutralization with an anti-CRF antibody. Several other lines of evidence support a critical role for endogenous CRF in regulating ACTH secretion. For example, increases in CRF in the hypophyseal portal blood are observed following application of stress. Administration of CRF antisera or the CRF-receptor antagonist results in attenuation of stress- or adrenalectomy-induced ACTH secretion, further substantiating a role for CRF in regulating ACTH secretion from the anterior pituitary. In addition to effects in the anterior pituitary, CRF has also been reported to stimulate POMC-derived peptide secretion from the intermediate lobe of the pituitary gland.

Central administration of CRF inhibits the secretion of luteinizing hormone (LH) and growth hormone without any major effects on follicle-stimulating hormone, thyroid-stimulating hormone, or prolactin secretion (see refs. 22 and 40). The effects of CRF to inhibit LH secretion appear to be mediated at the hypothalamic level through effects of CRF to inhibit gonadotropin-releasing hormone secretion. CRF-induced inhibition of LH secretion may also involve endogenous opioids, because the effects are attenuated by administration of naloxone or antiserum to β-endorphin (see refs. 22 and 40, and Chapters 62 and 67, *this volume*).

Regulation of Hypothalamic CRF Release

Comprehensive reviews of the neurotransmitter regulation of hypothalamic CRF release are provided by Plotsky et al. (42) and by Owens and Nemeroff (39,40). Most studies demonstrate stimulatory effects of cholinergic and serotonergic neurons on CRF release. The muscarinic and/or nicotinic cholinergic receptor subtypes involved in the stimulatory effects of acetylcholine on CRF secretion remain to be precisely elucidated. The effects of serotonin (5-hydroxytryptamine, 5-HT) to stimulate CRF release appear to be mediated by a variety of receptor subtypes, including 5-HT$_2$, 5-HT$_{1A}$, and 5-HT$_{1C}$ receptors. The ef-

fects of catecholamines and opioids on hypothalamic CRF release are less well defined. Norepinephrine has been reported to have both stimulatory and inhibitory effects on CRF release that may be a consequence of the dose administered as well as the receptor subtype involved. For example, in studies sampling hypophyseal portal concentrations of CRF, Plotsky et al. (42) noted that low doses of norepinephrine stimulated CRF release via α1-adrenergic receptors and inhibited CRF release at high doses via β-adrenergic receptors. Similarly, opioids have been reported to either inhibit or stimulate CRF release, depending on the nature of the opioid tested, the dose utilized, and the receptor specificity (mu versus kappa) involved. Drugs acing at the gamma-aminobutyric acid (GABA)–benzodiazepine–chloride ionophore complex are potent inhibitors of CRF secretion.

Stress is a potent general activator of CRF release from the hypothalamus. The extent and time course of changes in CRF in the paraventricular nucleus and median eminence of the hypothalamus following application of stress are highly dependent on the nature of the stressor as well as the state of the animal. The effects of stress to increase the release and synthesis of CRF are mediated by many of the neurotransmitter systems described above.

Glucocorticoids, which are involved in the negative feedback regulation of the hypothalamic–pituitary–adrenocortical axis, are potent inhibitors of CRF release. Conversely, the absence of glucocorticoids following adrenalectomy results in marked elevations in the synthesis and release of CRF. The actions of glucocorticoids to inhibit CRF release are mediated directly at the level of the paraventricular nucleus of the hypothalamus as well as indirectly through actions on receptors in other brain areas such as the hippocampus.

Modulation of Pituitary CRF Receptors

Stress (2,3,18,26) or adrenalectomy (2,18,26) result in hypersecretion of CRF and a consequent down-regulation of receptors in the anterior pituitary. The adrenalectomy-induced decreases in anterior pituitary receptors can be prevented by glucocorticoid replacement with corticosterone or dexamethasone (2,18,26). In addition, chronic administration of corticosterone has been reported to cause dose-dependent decreases in anterior pituitary CRF receptor number (2,18,26). An age-related decline in anterior pituitary CRF receptors has also been reported (28). In contrast, lesions of the paraventricular nucleus which result in dramatic reductions in hypothalamic CRF secretion have been reported to increase the density of pituitary CRF receptors (40). Thus, CRF receptors in the anterior pituitary appear to be reciprocally regulated by hypothalamic CRF release.

CRF REGULATION OF CNS ACTIVITY

Electrophysiological Effects

CRF stimulates the electrical activity of (a) neurons in various brain regions that contain CRF and CRF receptors, including locus coeruleus (22,40,62), hippocampus (22,40,53), cerebral cortex, and hypothalamus, and (b) motor neurons in the lumbar spinal cord (22,40). In contrast, CRF has inhibitory actions in the lateral septum, thalamus, and hypothalamic PVN (22,40). The electrophysiological effects of CRF on spontaneous and sensory-evoked activity of locus coeruleus neurons is well-documented (22,40,62). Activation of the locus coeruleus, a brainstem nucleus consisting of noradrenergic cells, results in arousal and increased vigilance. Furthermore, dysfunction of this nucleus has been implicated in the pathophysiology of depression and anxiety. Centrally administered CRF increases the spontaneous discharge rate of the locus coeruleus in both anesthetized and unanesthetized rats, while decreasing evoked activity in the nucleus (62). Thus, the overall effect of CRF in the locus coeruleus is to decrease the signal-to-noise ratio between evoked and spontaneous discharge rates.

The effects of CRF on electroencephalographic (EEG) activity have been reviewed in detail (22,23,40). CRF causes a generalized increase in EEG activity associated with increased vigilance and decreased sleep time. At CRF doses below those affecting locomotor activity or pituitary–adrenal function, rats remain awake and vigilant and display decreases in slow-wave sleep compared to saline-injected controls (23). Higher doses of the peptide, on the other hand, cause seizures activity that is indistinguishable from seizures produced by electrical kindling of the amygdala, further confirming the role of CRF in brain activation (see also Chapters 33 and 34, *this volume*).

Autonomic Effects

A great deal of anatomical, pharmacological, and physiological data support the concept that CRF acts within the CNS to modulate the autonomic nervous system (see refs. 8,22,24, and 40). For example, central administration of CRF results in activation of the sympathetic nervous system, resulting in stimulation of epinephrine secretion from the adrenal medulla and noradrenergic outflow to the heart, kidney, and vascular beds. Other consequences of central administration of CRF include increases in the mean arterial pressure and heart rate. These cardiovascular effects of CRF can be blocked by the ganglionic blocker chlorisondamine, underscoring the sympathetic actions of the peptide. In contrast, CRF acts in brain to inhibit parasympathetic nervous system activity (for review see ref. 24). Peripheral administration of CRF

causes vasodilation and hypotension in a variety of species, including humans (see refs. 8,22,24, and 40). The physiological role of CRF in regulating the autonomic nervous system is supported by data demonstrating central effects of the CRF receptor antagonist, α-helical ovine CRF(9-41), to attenuate adrenal epinephrine secretion resulting from stressors such as insulin-induced hypoglycemia, hemorrhage, and exposure to ether vapor (8). Overall, these data substantiate a major role for CRF in coordinating the autonomic responses to stress.

Gastrointestinal Effects

Studies examining the gastrointestinal effects of CRF have determined that CRF modulates gastrointestinal activity by acting at central and possibly peripheral sites and that these effects are qualitatively similar to those observed following exposure to various stressors (for reviews see refs. 22,40, and 58). CRF inhibits gastric acid secretion, gastric emptying, and intestinal transit while stimulating colonic transit and fecal excretion in a dose-dependent manner when administered centrally or systemically to dogs or rats. CRF is equipotent in inhibiting gastric emptying following both central and peripheral routes of administration. The central effects of CRF on gastric acid secretion do not appear to be due to leakage of the peptide into peripheral blood because following injection of CRF into the third ventricle of the dog, measurable quantities of CRF are not present in the circulation. Furthermore, an intravenous injection of anti-CRF serum completely abolishes the peripheral, but not the central, effect of CRF on gastric acid secretion. These data strongly implicate CRF in the mechanisms through which various stressors alter gastrointestinal function and are consistent with its proposed role in integrating the autonomic nervous system's response to stress.

Behavioral Effects

The behavioral effects of CRF in the CNS have been reviewed extensively (see refs. 22,30, and 40). The effects of CRF on behavior are dependent on both the dose of peptide administered and the specific conditions under which the tests are performed. In a familiar or ''home'' environment, central administration of CRF produces a profound increase in locomotor activity. Although very low doses of CRF produce locomotor activation when tested in an open field test, higher doses produce a dramatic decrease in locomotor activity. CRF administered intracerebrally also produces additional behavioral effects, including increases in sniffing, grooming, and rearing in a familiar environment, increased ''emotionality'' and assumption of a freeze posture in a foreign environment, decreased feeding and sexual behavior, and increased conflict behavior. The behavioral effects of CRF are not an indirect consequence of actions of the peptide to activate pituitary–adrenocortical hormone secretion, because they are not seen following peripheral administration of CRF or following pretreatment with doses of dexamethasone that adequately block pituitary–adrenal activation. Of critical importance is the observation that these effects of CRF can all be blocked by central administration of the peptide antagonist α-helical ovine CRF(9-41), strongly supporting a specific CRF-receptor-mediated event in these behaviors. Furthermore, the CRF-receptor antagonist by itself attenuates many of the behavioral consequences of stress, underscoring the role of endogenous peptide in mediating many of the stress-related behaviors (see Chapters 67 and 83, this volume).

CRF REGULATION OF IMMUNE FUNCTION

Evidence for Autocrine/Paracrine Actions of CRF

CRF plays a significant role in integrating the stress-related and inflammatory response to immunological agents such as viruses, bacteria, or tumor cells through its coordinated actions in the nervous, endocrine, and immune systems (see refs. 7,22,40, and 63). CRF has direct effects on immune function and inflammatory processes. CRF induces the secretion of POMC-derived peptides such as ACTH and β-endorphin in human peripheral blood and mouse splenic leukocytes. Furthermore, CRF stimulates the secretion of interleukin-1 (IL-1) and interleukin-2 (IL-2), lymphocyte proliferation, and IL-2 receptor expression in peripheral blood leukocytes. These actions of CRF are mediated through functional receptors which are present on resident macrophages in mouse spleen and on human peripheral blood monocytes. Several sources of endogenous CRF may be important in regulating immune function. Immunoreactive CRF and CRF mRNA are expressed in human peripheral blood leukocytes. CRF immunoreactivity is also present in primary sensory afferent nerves and in the dorsal sensory and sympathetic intermediolateral columns of the spinal cord (see section entitled "Distribution in Pituitary, CNS, and Spleen," above); sensory afferents and sympathetic efferent nerve fibers strongly influence inflammatory responses.

Pro- and Anti-inflammatory Properties of CRF

Recent data provide evidence for a direct pro-inflammatory action of CRF in rat models of inflammation and arthritis. Carrageenin, a seaweed polysaccharide, elicits a chemical inflammatory response in rats. In this acute model of inflammation, increased levels of immunoreactive CRF are detected in the inflamed area but not in the systemic circulation (29). Furthermore, immunoneutralization of CRF reduces both the volume and cellularity of the exudate in the carrageenin model, indicating that CRF has pro-inflammatory actions (29). The anti-inflammatory effects of the anti-CRF antibody are comparable to the anti-inflammatory effects of an anti-tumor necrosis factor-α antibody (29). Recent studies in experimental rat models of arthritis further substantiate the pro-inflammatory paracrine and/or autocrine effects of peripheral CRF. CRF expression is markedly increased in the joints and surrounding tissues of arthritis-susceptible Lewis (LEW/N) rats with streptococcal cell wall (SCW)- and adjuvant-induced arthritis, but it is not increased in similarly treated Fisher (F344/N) arthritis-resistant rats and is only transiently increased in congenitally athymic nude LEW.rnu/rnu rats (14). CRF mRNA and CRF receptors are present in inflamed synovia of LEW/N rats, and increases in CRF markers parallel increases in other pro-inflammatory peptides such as substance P (14). A very recent clinical study examined synovial fluids and tissues from patients with rheumatoid arthritis (RA) or osteroarthritis (OA) and normal individuals in order to determine the role of CRF in human inflammatory arthritis (13). There is enhanced expression of immunoreactive CRF in situ in synovium from patients, which is significantly greater in RA than in OA; the extent and intensity of immunostaining correlates significantly with the intensity of mononuclear cell infiltration (13). Furthermore, the concentrations of CRF are approximately sixfold higher in RA than in OA synovial fluids (13). Overall, these data substantiate an important autocrine/paracrine pro-inflammatory role for CRF at the inflammatory site in arthritis and suggest that therapies directed at inactivation of CRF or blocking the effects of CRF may represent novel anti-inflammatory agents.

CRF also has potent indirect actions on immune function through its pituitary–adrenocortical effects, resulting in increased glucocorticoid secretion; glucocorticoids have potent anti-inflammatory effects through generalized suppression of immune cell recruitment and inhibition of inflammatory mediators such as the cytokines. A role has also been postulated for hypothalamic CRF in the pathogenesis of chronic autoimmune inflammatory disease. Experimental evidence demonstrates that arthritis-susceptible LEW/N rats have a deficient hypothalamic CRF response to a variety of inflammatory and non-inflammatory stimuli, whereas the arthritis-resistant F344/N strain of rats have normal increases in CRF, ACTH, and corticosterone secretion in response to the same stimuli (9,54). In addition, recent clinical data demonstrate that patients with active RA have an abnormality of the hypothalamic–pituitary–adrenal axis response to immune/inflammatory stimuli which may reside in the hypothalamus (11).

ROLE FOR CRF IN NEUROPSYCHIATRIC DISORDERS AND NEURODEGENERATIVE DISEASES

Major Depression and Anxiety Disorders

Many patients with major depression are hypercortisolemic and exhibit an abnormal dexamethasone suppression test. Given the primary role of CRF in stimulating pituitary–adrenocortical secretion, the hypothesis has been put forth that hypersecretion/hyperactivity of CRF in brain might underlie the hypercortisolemia and symptomatology seen in major depression. The concentration of CRF is significantly increased in the cerebrospinal fluid (CSF) of drug-free individuals (17,38,40), and a significant positive correlation is observed between CRF concentrations in the CSF and the degree of post-dexamethasone suppression of plasma cortisol (49). Furthermore, the observation of a decrease in CRF binding sites in the frontal cerebral cortex of suicide victims compared to controls is consistent with the hypothesis that CRF is hypersecreted in major depression (37). The elevated CSF concentrations of CRF seen in depressed individuals are decreased following treatment with electroconvulsive therapy (36). In addition, a blunted ACTH response to intravenously administered ovine or human CRF is observed in depressed patients when compared to normal controls (25,40). The blunted ACTH response to exogenous CRF seen in depressed patients may be due to the intact negative feedback of cortisol on the corticotrophs, due to a compensatory decrease in CRF receptors subsequent to chronic hypersecretion of the peptide and/or desensitization of the pituitary corticotrophs to respond to CRF (see Chapters 83 and 84, *this volume*).

A number of studies suggest that anxiety-related disorders (such as panic disorder and generalized anxiety disorder) and depression are independent syndromes which share both clinical and biological characteristics. The role that has been proposed for CRF in major depressive disorders, along with preclinical data in rats demonstrating effects of CRF administration to produce several behavioral effects characteristic of anxiogenic compounds (22,30,40), has led to the suggestion that CRF may also be involved in anxiety-related disorders. A role for CRF in panic disorder has been suggested by observations of blunted ACTH responses to intravenously administered CRF in panic disorder patients when compared to controls (50). The blunted ACTH response to CRF in panic disorder patients most likely reflects a process occurring at or above the hypothalamus, resulting in excess secretion of endogenous CRF (see Chapters 34, 84, and 111, *this volume*).

Anorexia Nervosa

Anorexia nervosa is an eating disorder characterized by a tremendous weight loss in the pursuit of thinness. There is similar pathophysiology in anorexia nervosa and in depression, including the manifestation of hypercortisolism, hypothalamic hypogonadism, and anorexia. Furthermore, the incidence of depression in anorexia nervosa patients is high. Like depressed patients, anorexics show a markedly attenuated ACTH response to intravenously

administered CRF (17,25,40). When underweight anorexic subjects are studied after their body weight had been restored to normal, their basal hypercortisolism, increased levels of CRF in the CSF, and diminished ACTH response to exogenous CRF all return to normal at varying periods during the recovery phase (17,25,40). CRF potently inhibits food consumption in rats, which further suggests that the hypersecretion of CRF may be responsible for the weight loss observed in anorexics (22,40). In addition, the observation that central administration of CRF diminishes a variety of reproductive functions (17,22,40) lends relevance to the clinical observations of hypogonadism in anorexics (see Chapter 136, *this volume*).

Alzheimer's Disease

Several studies have provided evidence in support of alterations in CRF in Alzheimer's disease (AD) (see refs. 6,16,17,20,21, and 40). There are decreases in CRF content and reciprocal increases in CRF receptors in cerebral cortical areas affected in AD, such as the temporal, parietal, and occipital cortex (see Fig. 4). The reductions in CRF and increases in CRF receptors are all greater than 50% of the corresponding control values. The upregulation in cerebral cortical CRF receptors in AD under conditions in which the endogenous peptide is reduced suggests that CRF-receptive cells may be preserved in the cortex in AD. The reduction in cortical CRF content may be due to selective degeneration of CRF neurons intrinsic to the cerebral cortex, or it could be due to dysfunction of CRF neurons innervating the cortex from other brain areas. Additional evidence for a role for CRF in AD is provided by observations of (a) decreases in CRF in other brain areas, including the caudate (6), and (b) decreased concentrations of CRF in the CSF (34,35). Furthermore, a significant correlation is evident between CSF CRF and the global neuropsychological impairment ratings, suggesting that greater cognitive impairment is associated with lower CSF concentrations of CRF (43).

Immunocytochemical observations demonstrating morphological alterations in CRF neurons in AD complement the studies described above. In AD, swollen, tortuous CRF-immunostained axons, termed *fiber abnormalities,* are clearly distinguishable from the surrounding normal neurons and are also seen in conjunction with amyloid deposits associated with senile plaques (46). Furthermore, the total number of CRF-immunostained axons is reduced in the amygdala of Alzheimer's patients (46). Interestingly, the expression of CRF antigen in neurons is not globally reduced in Alzheimer's patients. CRF immunostaining of perikarya and axons located in the hypothalamic paraventricular nucleus is much more intense in AD than in controls (46). Increased immunostaining of the paraventricular neurons in AD, if truly representative

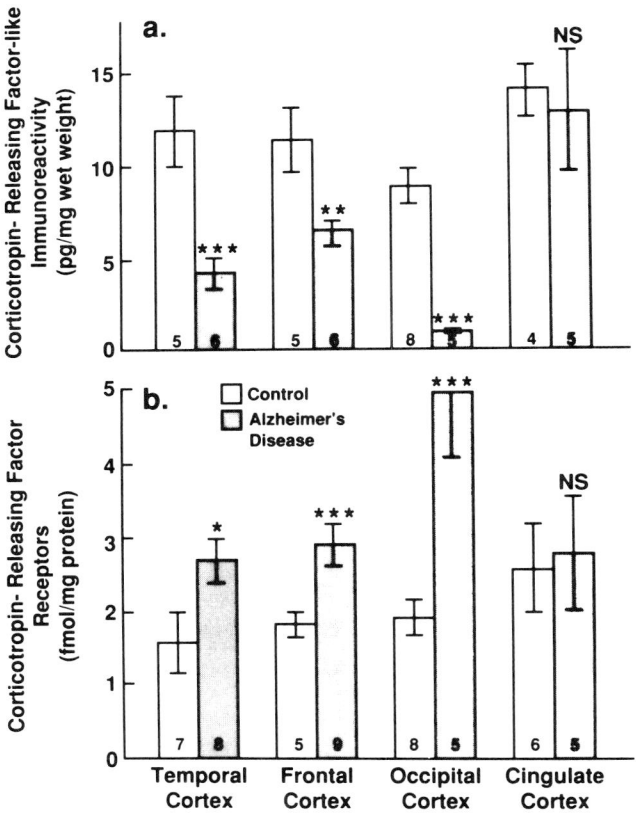

FIG. 4. CRF-like immunoreactivity (**a**) and CRF-receptor binding (**b**) in discrete regions of the cerebral cortex of Alzheimer's patients and controls. All values are means ± SEM. The number of subjects in each group is given at the bottom of each histogram. Significant differences from control group at $p < 0.05$, $p < 0.025$, and $p < 0.005$ are denoted by *, **, and ***, respectively. NS, nonsignificant.

of increased content of CRF, could be related to increased amounts of CRF mRNA in these cells or increased translation of available mRNA. The increased expression and/or release of CRF from the paraventricular nucleus of the hypothalamus would provide a reasonable explanation for the hypercortisolemia often seen in Alzheimer's patients.

At present, the cerebral cortical cholinergic deficiency seems to be the most severe and consistent deficit associated with AD. Reductions in cerebral cortical CRF correlate with decreases in choline acetyl transferase (ChAT) activity (20). In AD, there are significant positive correlations between ChAT activity and reduced CRF in the frontal, temporal, and occipital lobes. Similarly, significant negative correlations exist between decreased ChAT activity and increased number of CRF receptors in the three cortices. These data suggest that the reported reciprocal changes in pre- and postsynaptic markers in CRF in cerebral cortex of patients with AD may be, in part, a consequence of deficits in the cholinergic projections to the cerebral cortex. Additional studies are necessary to determine the functional significance of the interaction

between CRF and cholinergic systems (see Chapter 118, *this volume*).

Other Neurological Disorders

Alterations in brain concentrations of CRF have been reported in other neurological diseases. For example, in cases of Parkinson's disease with dementia that also show pathological features of AD, CRF content is decreased and shows a pattern similar to that of those cases exhibiting the pathology of AD alone (16,64). Specimens from patients with Parkinson's disease who did not have the histopathology characteristic of AD also demonstrate reductions of CRF content, although the reductions are less marked than in cases of combined AD and Parkinson's disease. Normal levels of CRF have been reported in the hypothalamus in Parkinson's disease (12), suggesting that the loss of CRF in the cerebral cortex is not generalized. CRF is decreased to approximately 50% of the control values in the frontal, temporal, and occipital lobes of patients with progressive supranuclear palsy (16,64), a rare neurodegenerative disorder that shares certain clinical and pathological features with AD.

The similarity of the changes in CRF found in the context of the three neurological diseases associated with Alzheimer-type pathology raises the possibility that cerebral cortical reduction is nothing more than a nonspecific sequela of the disease process. In Huntington's disease, a neurological disorder in which minimal cerebral cortical pathology is present, the CRF content in the frontal, temporal, parietal, occipital, and cingulate cortices and in the globus pallidus is not significantly different from that seen in neurologically normal controls (21). However, the CRF content in the caudate nucleus and putamen of the basal ganglia (brain areas that are severely affected in the disease) is less than 40% of the CRF concentrations seen in controls (21). The localization of the CRF changes to only affected brain regions in the four neurodegenerative disorders described suggests that CRF has an important role in the pathology of these dementias.

SUMMARY AND CONCLUSIONS

Corticotropin-releasing factor is the key regulator of the organism's overall response to stress. CRF has hormone-like effects at the pituitary level to regulate ACTH secretion, which, in turn, coordinates the synthesis and secretion of glucocorticoids from the adrenal cortex. CRF also functions as a bona fide neurotransmitter in the CNS. CRF neurons and receptors are widely distributed in the CNS and play a critical role in coordinating the autonomic, electrophysiological, and behavioral responses to stress. More recent data suggest that CRF can have direct, local effects in peripheral tissues, where it acts in a paracrine manner. Some of the paracrine effects include cytokine-like actions on the immune system.

Recent clinical data implicate CRF in the etiology and pathophysiology of various endocrine, psychiatric, neurologic, and inflammatory illnesses. Hypersecretion of CRF in brain may contribute to the symptomatology seen in neuropsychiatric disorders such as depression, anxiety-related disorders, and anorexia nervosa. Furthermore, overproduction of CRF at peripheral inflammatory sites such as synovial joints may contribute to autoimmune diseases such as rheumatoid arthritis. In contrast, deficits in brain CRF are apparent in neurodegenerative disorders such as Alzheimer's disease, Parkinson's disease, and Huntington's disease because they relate to dysfunction of CRF neurons in brain areas affected in the particular disorder. Strategies directed at developing CRF-related agents may hold promise for novel therapies for the treatment of these various disorders.

REFERENCES

1. Abou-Samra A-B, Harwood JP, Catt KJ, Aguilera G. Mechanisms of action of CRF and other regulators of ACTH release in pituitary corticotrophs. *Ann NY Acad Sci* 1987;512:67–84.
2. Aguilera G, Millan MA, Hauger RL, Catt KJ. Corticotropin-releasing factor receptors: distribution in brain, pituitary and peripheral tissues. *Ann NY Acad Sci* 1987;512:48–66.
3. Anderson SM, Kant GJ, De Souza EB. Effects of chronic stress on anterior pituitary and brain corticotropin-releasing factor receptors. *Pharmacol Biochem Behav* 1993;44:755–761.
4. Battaglia G, Webster EL, De Souza EB. Characterization of corticotropin-releasing factor receptor-mediated adenylate cyclase activity in the rat central nervous system. *Synapse* 1987;1:572–581.
5. Behan DP, Linton EA, Lowry PJ. Isolation of the human plasma corticotrophin-releasing factor-binding protein. *J Endocrinol* 1989;122:23–31.
6. Bissette G, Reynolds GP, Kilts CD, Widerlov W, Nemeroff CB. Corticotropin-releasing factor-like immunoreactivity in senile dementia of the Alzheimer type. *JAMA* 1985;254:3067–3069.
7. Blalock JE. A molecular basis for bidirectional communication between the immune and neuroendocrine systems. *Physiol Rev* 1989;69:1–32.
8. Brown MR, Fisher LA. Regulation of the autonomic nervous system by corticotropin-releasing factor. In: De Souza EB, Nemeroff CB eds. *Corticotropin-releasing factor: basic and clinical studies of a neuropeptide*. Boca Raton, FL: CRC Press, 1990;291–298.
9. Calogero AE, Sternberg EM, Bagdy G, et al. Neurotransmitter-induced hypothalamic–pituitary–adrenal axis responsiveness in inflammatory disease-susceptible Lewis rats: in vivo and in vitro studies suggesting a global defect in CRH secretion. *Neuroendocrinology* 1992;55:600–608.
10. Chadwick DJ, Marsh J, Ackrill K, eds. *Corticotropin-releasing factor*. Chichester: John Wiley & Sons, 1993.
11. Chikanza IC, Petrou P, Kingsley G, Chrousos G, Panayi GS. Defective hypothalamic response to immune and inflammatory stimuli in patients with rheumatoid arthritis. *Arthritis Rheum* 1992;35:1281–1288.
12. Conte-Devolx B, Grino M, Nieoullon A, et al. Corticoliberin, somatocrinin and amine contents in normal and parkinsonian human hypothalamus. *Neurosci Lett* 1985;56:217–222.
13. Crofford LJ, Sano H, Karalis K, et al. Corticotropin-releasing hormone in synovial fluids and tissues of patients with rheumatoid arthritis and osteoarthritis. *J Immunol* 1993;151:1587–1596.
14. Crofford LJ, Sano H, Karalis K, et al. Local secretion of corticotropin-releasing hormone in the joints of Lewis rats with inflammatory arthritis. *J Clin Invest* 1992;90:2555–2564.
15. De Souza EB. Corticotropin-releasing factor receptors in the rat central nervous system: Characterization and regional distribution. *J Neurosci* 1987;7:88–100.
16. De Souza EB. CRH defects in Alzheimer's and other neurologic diseases. *Hosp Pract* 1988;23:59–71.
17. De Souza EB. Role of corticotropin-releasing factor in neuropsychiatric disorders and neurodegenerative diseases. In: Seamon KB, ed. *Annual reports in medicinal chemistry*. San Diego: Academic Press, 1990;215–224.
18. De Souza EB. Corticotropin-releasing hormone receptors. In: Bjorklund A, Hokfelt T, Kuhar MJ, eds. *Handbook of chemical neuroanatomy. Neuropeptide receptors in the CNS, part III*. Amsterdam: Elsevier, 1992;145–185.
19. De Souza EB, Nemeroff CB, eds. *Corticotropin-releasing factor: basic and clinical studies of a neuropeptide*. Boca Raton, FL: CRC Press, 1990.
20. De Souza EB, Whitehouse PJ, Kuhar MJ, Price DL, Vale WW. Reciprocal changes in corticotropin-releasing factor (CRF)-like immunoreactivity and CRF receptors in cerebral cortex of Alzheimer's disease. *Nature* 1986;319:593–595.
21. De Souza EB, Whitehouse PJ, Price DL, Vale WW. Abnormalities in corticotropin-releasing hormone (CRH) in Alzheimer's disease and other human disorders. *Ann NY Acad Sci* 1987;512:237–247.
22. Dunn AJ, Berridge CW. Physiological and behavioral responses to corticotropin-releasing factor administration: is CRF a mediator of anxiety of stress responses? *Brain Res Rev* 1990;15:71–100.
23. Ehlers CL. CRF effects on EEG activity: implications for the modulation of normal and abnormal brain states. In: De Souza EB, Nemeroff CB eds. *Corticotropin-releasing factor: basic and clinical studies of a neuropeptide*. Boca Raton, FL: CRC Press, 1990;233–252.
24. Fisher LA. Corticotropin-releasing factor: endocrine and autonomic integration of responses to stress. *Trends Pharmacol Sci* 1989;10:189–193.
25. Gold PW, Loriaux DL, Roy A, et al. Responses to corticotropin-releasing hormone in the hypercortisolism of depression and Cushing's disease. *N Engl J Med* 1986;314:1329–1334.
26. Grigoriadis DE, Heroux JA, De Souza EB. Characterization and regulation of corticotropin-releasing factor receptors in the central nervous, endocrine and immune systems. In: Chadwick DJ, Marsh J, Ackrill K, eds. *Corticotropin-releasing factor*. Chichester: John Wiley & Sons, 1993;85–101.
27. Heisler S, Hook VYH, Axelrod J. Corticotropin-releasing factor stimulation of protein carboxylmethylation in mouse pituitary tumor cells. *Biochem Pharmacol* 1983;32:1295–1299.
28. Heroux JA, Grigoriadis DE, De Souza EB. Age-related decreases in corticotropin-releasing factor (CRF) receptors in rat brain and anterior pituitary gland. *Brain Res* 1991;542:155–158.
29. Karalis K, Sano H, Redwine J, Listwak S, Wilder RL, Chrousos GP. Autocrine or paracrine inflammatory actions of corticotropin-releasing hormone in vivo. *Science* 1991;254:421–423.
30. Koob GF, Britton KT. Behavioral effects of corticotropin-releasing factor. In: De Souza EB, Nemeroff CB, eds. *Corticotropin-releasing factor: basic and clinical studies neuropeptide*. Boca Raton, FL: CRC Press, 1990;253–266.
31. Laatikainen T, Virtanen T, Raisanen I, Salminen K. Immunoreactive corticotropin-releasing factor and corticotropin in plasma during pregnancy, labour and puerperium. *Neuropeptides* 1987;10:343–353.
32. Linton EA, Wolfe CDA, Behan DP, Lowry PJ. A specific carrier substance for human corticotropin-releasing factor in late gestational maternal plasma which could mask the ACTH-releasing activity. *Clin Endocrinol* 1988;28:315–324.
33. Majzoub JA, Emanuel R, Adler G, Martinez C, Robinson B, Wittert G. Second messenger regulation of mRNA for corticotropin-releasing factor. In: Chadwick DJ, Marsh J, Ackrill K, eds. *Corticotropin releasing factor*. Chichester: John Wiley & Sons, 1993;30–43.
34. May C, Rapoport SI, Tomai TP, Chrousos GP, Gold PW. Cerebral spinal fluid concentrations of corticotropin-releasing hormone (CRH) and corticotropin (ACTH) are reduced in Alzheimer's disease. *Neurology* 1987;37:535–538.
35. Mouradian MM, Farah JM Jr, Mohr E, Fabbrini G, O'Donohue

TL, Chase TN. Spinal fluid CRF reduction in Alzheimer's disease. *Neuropeptides* 1986;8:393–400.

36. Nemeroff CB, Bissette G, Akil H, Fink M. Neuropeptide concentrations in the cerebrospinal fluid of depressed patients treated with electroconvulsive therapy: corticotropin-releasing factor, β-endorphin and somatostatin. *Br J Psychiatry* 1991;158:59–63.

37. Nemeroff CB, Owens MJ, Bissette G, Andorn AC, Stanley M. Reduced corticotropin-releasing factor receptor binding sites in the frontal cortex of suicide victims. *Arch Gen Psychiatry* 1988; 45:577–579.

38. Nemeroff CB, Widerlov E, Bissette G, et al. Elevated concentration of CSF corticotropin-releasing factor-like immunoreactivity in depressed patients. *Science* 1984;226:1342–1344.

39. Owens MJ, Nemeroff CB. Neurotransmitter regulation of the CRF secretion in vitro. In: De Souza EB, Nemeroff CB, eds. *Corticotropin-releasing factor: basic and clinical studies of a neuropeptide.* Boca Raton, FL: CRC Press, 1990;107–114.

40. Owens MJ, Nemeroff CB. Physiology and pharmacology of corticotropin-releasing factor. *Pharmacol Rev* 1991;43:425–473.

41. Petrusz P, Merchenthaler I. The corticotropin-releasing factor system. In: Nemeroff CB, ed. *Neuroendocrinology.* Boca Raton, FL: CRC Press, 1992;129–184.

42. Plotsky PM, Cunningham ET Jr, Widmaier EP. Catecholaminergic modulation of corticotropin-releasing factor and adrenocorticotropin secretion. *Endocr Rev* 1989;10:437–458.

43. Pomara N, Singh RR, Deptula D, et al. CSF corticotropin-releasing factor (CRF) in Alzheimer's disease: its relationship to severity of dementia and monoamine metabolites. *Biol Psychiatry* 1989; 26:500–504.

44. Potter E, Behan DP, Fischer WH, Linton EA, Lowry PJ, Vale WW. Cloning and characterization of the cDNAs for human and rat corticotropin-releasing factor-binding proteins. *Nature* 1991; 349:423–426.

45. Potter E, Behan DP, Linton EA, Lowry PJ, Sawchenko PE, Vale WW. The central distribution of a corticotropin-releasing factor (CRF)-binding protein predicts multiple sites and modes of interaction with CRF. *Proc Natl Acad Sci USA* 1992;89:4192–4196.

46. Powers RE, Walker LC, De Souza EB, et al. Immunohistochemical study of neurons containing corticotropin-releasing factor in Alzheimer's disease. *Synapse* 1987;1:405–410.

47. Rivier J, Rivier C, Vale W. Synthetic competitive antagonist of corticotropin-releasing factor: effect on ACTH secretion in the rat. *Science* 1984;224:889–891.

48. Romier C, Bernassau J-M, Cambillau C, Darbon H. Solution structure of human corticotropin releasing factor by ^{1}H NMR and distance geometry with restrained molecular dynamics. *Prot Eng* 1993;6:149–156.

49. Roy A, Pickar D, Paul S, Doran A, Chrousos GP, Gold PW. CSF corticotropin-releasing hormone in depressed patients and normal control subjects. *Am J Psychiatry* 1987;143:896–899.

50. Roy-Byrne PP, Uhde T, Post R, Gallucci W, Chrousos GP, Gold PW. The corticotropin-releasing hormone stimulation test in patients with panic disorder. *Am J Psychiatry* 1986;143:896–899.

51. Sawchenko PE, Swanson LW. Organization of CRF immunoreactive cells and fibers in the rat brain: immunohistochemical studies. In: De Souza EB, Nemeroff CB, eds. *Corticotropin-releasing factor: basic and clinical studies of a neuropeptide.* Boca Raton, FL: CRC Press, 1990;29–52.

52. Shibasaki T, Odagiri E, Shizume K, Ling N. Corticotropin-releasing factor like activity in human placental extract. *J Clin Endocrinol Metab* 1982;55:384–386.

53. Siggins GR. Electrophysiology of corticotropin-releasing factor in nervous tissue. In: De Souza EB, Nemeroff CB, eds. *Corticotropin-releasing factor: basic and clinical studies of a neuropeptide.* Boca Raton, FL: CRC Press, 1990;205–216.

54. Sternberg EM, Young III WS, Bernardini R, et al. A central nervous system defect in biosynthesis of corticotropin-releasing hormone is associated with susceptibility to streptococcal cell wall-induced arthritis in Lewis rats. *Proc Natl Acad Sci USA* 1989;86:4771–4775.

55. Suda T, Iwashita M, Tozawa F, et al. Characterization of CRH binding protein in human plasma by chemical cross-linking and its binding during pregnancy. *J Clin Endocrinol Metab* 1988;67:1278–1283.

56. Suda T, Sumitomo T, Tozawa F, Ushiyama T, Demura H. Corticotropin-releasing factor-binding protein is a glycoprotein. *Biochem Biophys Res Commun* 1989;165:703–707.

57. Swanson LW, Sawchenko PE, Rivier J, Vale WW. Organization of ovine corticotropin-releasing factor immunoreactive cells and fibers in the rat brain: an immunohistochemical study. *Neuroendocrinology* 1983;36:165–186.

58. Tache Y, Gunion MM, Stephens R. CRF: central nervous system action to influence gastrointestinal function and role in the gastrointestinal response to stress. In: De Souza EB, Nemeroff CB, eds. *Corticotropin-releasing factor: basic and clinical studies of a neuropeptide.* Boca Raton, FL: CRC Press, 1990;299–308.

59. Thompson RC, Seasholtz AF, Douglass JO, Herbert E. Cloning and distribution of expression of the rat corticotropin-releasing factor (CRF) gene. In: De Souza EB, Nemeroff CB, eds. *Corticotropin releasing factor: basic and clinical studies of a neuropeptide.* Boca Raton, FL: CRC Press, 1990;1–12.

60. Vale W, Rivier C, Brown MR, et al. Chemical and biological characterization of corticotropin-releasing factor. *Rec Progr Horm Res* 1983;39:245–270.

61. Vale W, Spiess J, Rivier C, Rivier J. Characterization of a 41-residue ovine hypothalamic peptide that stimulates secretion of corticotropin and β-endorphin. *Science* 1981;213:1394–1397.

62. Valentino RJ. Effects of CRF on spontaneous and sensory-evoked activity of locus coeruleus neurons. In: De Souza EB, Nemeroff CB, eds. *Corticotropin-releasing factor: basic and clinical studies of a neuropeptide.* Boca Raton, FL: CRC Press, 1990;217–232.

63. Webster EL, Grigoriadis DE, De Souza EB. Corticotropin-releasing factor receptors in the brain–pituitary–immune axis. In: McCubbin JA, Kaufmann PG, Nemeroff CB, eds. *Stress, neuropeptides, and systemic disease.* San Diego: Academic Press, 1991;233–260.

64. Whitehouse PJ, Vale WW, Zweig RM, et al. Reduction in corticotropin-releasing factor-like immunoreactivity in cerebral cortex in Alzheimer's disease, Parkinson's disease, and progressive supranuclear palsy. *Neurology* 1987;37:905–909.

Psychopharmacology: The Fourth Generation of Progress, edited by Floyd E. Bloom and David J. Kupfer. Raven Press, Ltd., New York © 1995.

CHAPTER **46**

Neuropharmacology of Endogenous Opioid Peptides

John J. Wagner and Charles I. Chavkin

Interest in the physiologic and pharmacologic actions of the endogenous opioid peptides spans the full range of neuroscience research. Investigative approaches ranging from whole-animal/behavioral studies to the molecular study of opioid action are being employed to gather data at the preclinical level. The principal goal of these studies is to define the role of the endogenous opioid neuropeptides in brain function. Ultimately, information concerning the normal actions of this neuropeptide transmitter system can be related to clinical topics such as opiate tolerance and dependence, respiratory and cardiovascular regulation, learning and memory processes, analgesia and nociception, and epileptogenesis and seizure pathology, to name a few.

Following the biochemical purification and characterization of the three endogenous opioid peptide families (the enkephalins, the endorphins, and the dynorphins; see ref. 1), much progress has been made in mapping the specific locations of opioid peptides and their binding site distributions throughout the brain (49,56). Pharmacological studies have shown that multiple types (mu, delta, kappa) of opioid receptors exist, and they have indicated that subtypes (i.e., mu_1, mu_2, $kappa_1$, $kappa_2$, $delta_1$, $delta_2$, etc.) are also likely to occur (75). Exogenous application of opiates and opioid peptides has been used to study drug actions down to the molecular level of ion channel modulation and enzymatic regulation (12,19,69,73). As a model system of putative neurotransmitter peptides, the study of endogenous opioids has the advantage of a relatively extensive list of pharmacologic tools (selective agonists and antagonists) compared to the

other peptidergic systems. Despite this significant advantage, two general areas of opioid research have lagged behind. First, receptor purification and cloning has been slow, and results leading to the cDNA and amino acid sequence for the opioid receptors has only recently been obtained, some 18 years after the endogenous ligands were discovered (31,50). Second, elucidation of the specific actions of opioid peptides released from endogenous stores has also been only recently described (11,95,97) in the central nervous system (CNS). Recent and continuing advances in these general areas should ensure a prominent place for opioids in future neuropharmacological research.

In this chapter, we review the evidence addressing the properties of opioid peptides as neurotransmitters in the CNS. Opioid peptide processing, opioid receptor heterogeneity, opioid involvement in seizures/excitotoxicity, and mechanisms regarding opiate tolerance and addiction are areas which are covered elsewhere in this volume (see Chapters 61, 65, 66, and 148, *this volume*) or in other reviews (1,39,86). Here, we will be discussing the pharmacologic actions (i.e., of exogenously applied opiates and opioid peptides) and the physiologic actions (i.e., of endogenously released opioid peptides) of opioids in the mammalian CNS, with an emphasis placed on investigations done using hippocampal tissue when appropriate.

The principal thesis of this chapter is that recent studies of endogenous opioid action in the hippocampus have provided a better understanding of how these peptides normally function as transmitters. The key questions about the nature of the opioid peptide synapse concern the *anatomical* aspects (where are the sites of release and sites of action?), the *physiological* aspects (what are the kinetics of opioid action and the effects on the neural circuitry?), and the *molecular* aspects (which receptors and signal transduction mechanisms are involved?). Our

J. J. Wagner: Department of Physiology, University of Maryland, Baltimore, Maryland 21201.
C. I. Chavkin: Department of Pharmacology, University of Washington, Seattle, Washington 98195.

current understanding can be summarized as follows: (a) Opioid peptides are stored in dense-core vesicles in specific neurons which also contain a classical fast-acting transmitter such as glutamate; the opioids thus act as co-transmitters serving to modulate the actions of the primary transmitter. (b) The opioids are released into the extracellular space following prolonged depolarization of the neuronal membrane; thus, opioids modulate synaptic transmission only under conditions of intense afferent input. (c) The structure of the opioid peptide synapse may be larger than that of the fast-acting amine transmitters because the peptides may diffuse some distance from their sites of release to their sites of action; this is evident from the slow kinetics of the opioid peptide action (seconds until onset of effects, minutes until termination of the effect). A wider radius of action from the release site follows from the considerably higher affinities the opioids have for their receptors than the amine transmitters have for theirs. (d) Opioids activate a variety of signal transduction processes; different mechanisms are evident in different cell types. Evidence supporting each of these assertions is presented below. This model of neuropeptide function is clearly consistent with earlier ideas based on actions of neuropeptides in the peripheral nervous system (45,54), and recent work has provided an increasingly detailed description of the unique properties of neuropeptide transmitters. (Reproductive actions of opioids are described in Chapter 65, *this volume*.)

ACTIONS AT THE MOLECULAR LEVEL

Opioid Binding Sites are G-Protein-Coupled Receptors

The modulation of opioid ligand binding by physiologic salts, guanosine phosphates, and regulation of GTPase and adenylate cyclase activities by opioids has been extensively reviewed (see refs. 19,38,53, and 75). We wish to briefly summarize the results derived using in vitro assays which suggest that opioid receptors are likely to be members of the G-protein-coupled "superfamily" of receptors. The binding of ligands to all of the three well-accepted types of opioid receptors (mu, delta, and kappa) is modulated by the addition of GTP to radioligand binding assays. GTP significantly decreases the affinity of binding sites for opioid agonists without greatly affecting the binding of antagonists. Similarly, sodium also differentially decreases agonist binding, an effect which is additive with that of GTP. Mu, delta, and kappa agonists have all been shown to stimulate GTPase activity in a naloxone-sensitive manner. Opioid agonists inhibit the activity of adenylate cyclase, an effect which is GTP-dependent and pertussis-toxin-sensitive. The ability of antisera selective for various G proteins to inhibit opioid binding, GTPase activity, and the inhibition of adenylate

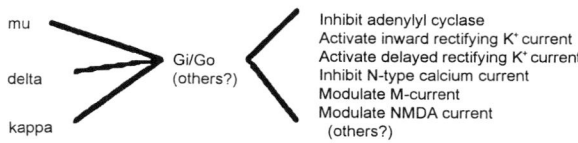

FIG. 1. The pharmacologically defined opioid receptor types activate a diverse group of heterotrimeric GTP-binding proteins which in turn regulate a variety of signal transduction proteins. The specific events depend on the cell-type.

cyclase activity is also consistent with opioid receptors being coupled to G proteins (see ref. 19).

The question of which G proteins are activated is still extensively debated (see ref. 91). Opioid receptor effects have been shown to be pertussis-toxin-sensitive, implicating members of the Gi or Go type in mediating opioid action (see ref. 19). However, a cholera-toxin-sensitive activation of adenylate cyclase in a neuroblastoma cell line by mu or delta receptors was also recently shown (26), suggesting that activation of Gs may mediate opioid effects in some cells. In addition, whether the alpha subunit of the G-protein complex acts alone or whether the beta/gamma subunits contribute to the signal transduction process has not been resolved.

An elusive goal of many research groups has been to achieve the purification or cloning of an opioid receptor protein (see ref. 86). This information would convincingly determine the validity of the hypothesis that opioid binding sites are G-protein-coupled receptors. The cloning and amino acid sequence has recently been obtained for delta opioid receptors (31,50), and related mu and kappa clones, isolated by hybridization screening, have also been reported recently (18,105). The sequences of the cloned opioid receptors supports the hypothesis that these are also members of the G-protein-coupled receptor superfamily.

The list of molecular targets of the activated G proteins is extensive (Fig. 1). Opioids have well-defined effects on adenylate cyclase activity and ion channel conductance mediated by G-protein activation (see below). In addition to the well-known inhibition of adenylate cyclase, some evidence has indicated that an opioid-mediated enhancement of this activity can also be demonstrated at low agonist concentrations (25,36). Evidence describing opioid regulation of additional second messenger systems has also been reported. In particular, kappa agonists affect the turnover of phosphatidylinositol (PI). Both positive (76) and inhibitory (64) effects on PI turnover have been reported in the hippocampus and cerebellum, respectively. A biphasic modulation of PI turnover has been studied in rat brain cell cultures (3). In 7-day-old cultures, PI formation was inhibited by kappa agonists, whereas in 21-day-old cultures, PI formation was enhanced. It is clear from this description that a unitary mechanism of opioid receptor signal transduction is unlikely. (Also see Chapters 11, 27, and 38 for additional details of G-protein coupled receptors.)

Inhibition of Transmitter Release

Opioids primarily act as inhibitory agents in the neural circuit (although examples of excitation are noted below). Opiates and opioid peptides have been shown to inhibit the release of a wide range of neurotransmitters from many brain regions in neurochemical release assays (69). These studies usually involve measuring the release either by preloading neuronal stores with radiolabeled transmitter or by specific radioimmunoassays of the perfusate. Electrical or chemical depolarization of the preparation is then performed in the absence and presence of applied opioid compounds. In the hippocampus, mu agonists have been shown to inhibit the release of norepinephrine and acetylcholine (43,44,98). Kappa agonists have also been shown to inhibit the release of both norepinephrine and acteylcholine (43,44,98). Delta agonists may be effective in inhibiting the release of norepinephrine in guinea pigs (98) but not in rats (43,44,69). Using a mossy fiber synaptosomal preparation, very high concentrations of kappa agonist could inhibit both dynorphin and glutamate release (35).

A series of studies describing biphasic effects of low and high concentrations of opioids on enkephalin release from the guinea-pig myenteric plexus illustrates the potential for diversity of opioid actions (36). Low concentrations (<10 nM) of mu, delta, or kappa agonists enhanced stimulated release, whereas higher concentrations (>10 nM) inhibit the stimulated release of enkephalin. Importantly, the inhibitory and enhancing effects could be dissociated based on the class of G protein coupled to the respective effects. Pertussis toxin, which inactivates Gi and Go classes of G proteins, could block the inhibitory effects of high opioid concentrations, leaving the enhancement by low concentrations uneffected. The converse was true when cholera toxin treatment was used to decrease Gs activity. Enhancement of release by low concentrations of opioids was blocked by cholera toxin, whereas the inhibitory effects of higher opioid concentrations was unaffected (36).

These studies have provided clear examples of the effectiveness of exogenously applied opiates and opioid peptides in the various preparations, but only a few examples of an electrophysiological correlate of these actions for endogenously released opioids have been reported (11,95,97; see below). One recent paper has described the ability of endogenously released opioids to inhibit the release of endogenous NE in hippocampal tissue (85). The methods of the study involved the use of an in vitro competition slice binding assay, which allows the release of endogenous transmitters to be quantified (70). The distinction between the effects of exogenously applied opioids and effects of endogenously released opioid peptides is important, because it is not necessarily true that a given population of receptors occupied by bath-applied drug are relevant targets for opioid peptides released from endogenous stores.

PHARMACOLOGIC ACTIONS AT THE CELLULAR LEVEL

Ionic Basis of Opioid Actions

In this section, we discuss the effects of exogenously applied opioids on neuronal activity. The regulation of ion channels by opioids has been intensely studied by several laboratory groups in various neuronal preparations (see refs. 12 and 60). We will be emphasizing the more recent advances in this area. In general, opioids have been found to inhibit neuronal excitability via two mechanisms: inhibition of calcium conductances and enhancement of potassium conductances (4,73). Initially, reports indicated that mu and delta receptors modulated potassium currents, whereas kappa receptors modulated calcium currents. The simplicity of this arrangement was nullified by the findings that delta agonists could inhibit calcium currents in cultured NG-108 cells (90) and that mu agonists could inhibit calcium currents in spinal ganglion neurons (82). Thus far, a clear example of kappa modulation of a potassium current has not been reported; however, it seems likely that this will eventually be shown.

The characterization of the potassium current enhanced by opioids in the locus coeruleus has indicated that the opioid-coupled current is of the inward rectifying type (100). This potassium current is blocked by cesium and is resistant to cadmium and tetrodotoxin. It is also barium-sensitive, and cAMP does not seem to be involved in opioid receptor modulation of the current. Instead, a direct, G-protein-coupled arrangement is suggested by single-channel studies (65,83). Being an inward rectifier, the opioid-induced conductance is much greater at potentials below E_K. The increase in potassium conductance has been shown to directly hyperpolarize and inhibit the firing frequency of locus coeruleus neurons.

Another potassium current, which is kinetically distinct from the inward rectifier, has been characterized in nonpyramidal hippocampal neurons (101). This one is a voltage-gated potassium current activated at positive potentials relative to the resting membrane potential and was insensitive to barium. In addition, cAMP application blocked the opioid-induced current, suggesting that a protein kinase mechanism may be involved in the modulation of this potassium current (102). It is interesting to note that this type of potassium current, unlike an inward rectifier, is not expected to affect firing threshold or frequency. Instead, by activating at depolarized potentials, the delayed rectifier would enhance the repolarization phase and reduce the duration of a firing burst and may thus change the firing pattern of these nonpyramidal cells.

Complex effects of opioids on a third type of potassium conductance (I_M) have also been observed by Siggins and co-workers (67) in CA3 pyramidal cells. Kappa agonists [U50488h and micromolar concentrations of dynorphin A(1-17)] increase the amplitude of this potassium current in a norbinaltorphimine sensitive way; whereas, delta agonists and low concentrations (20–100 nM) of dynorphin A(1-17) reduce I_M.

In addition to these actions, one group reported concentration-dependent, biphasic effects of opioids on potassium and calcium currents in sensory neurons (25). In these studies, low concentrations of opioid agonist (<10 nM) had the converse effect (i.e., inhibition of potassium current or enhancement of calcium current) with respect to the typical effect of higher concentrations (>10 nM, enhancement of potassium current or inhibition of calcium current). Pertussis-toxin-sensitive G proteins were shown to be involved in the inhibitory actions, whereas a cholera-toxin-sensitive G protein mediated the excitatory actions of low opioid concentrations (25). As with the release studies of Gintzler and Xu (36) discussed above, these results point out the potential for complex variations in the mechanisms of endogenous opioid actions. No analogous, direct excitatory action of opioids in the hippocampus has yet been described.

A novel mechanism of mu opioid action involving regulation of the N-methyl-D-aspartate (NMDA) receptor was reported in trigeminal cells (17). In this study, a mu agonist prolonged and enhanced the NMDA-receptor-mediated current. The opioid effect was blocked by protein kinase C inhibitors and mimicked by protein kinase C activation, suggesting that mu effects are coupled to protein kinase C activity in this preparation. This work provides a clear example of a mechanism by which direct, excitatory actions of mu agonists could occur. Such a mechanism could potentially be important for opioid involvement in synaptic plasticity and excitotoxicity, processes in which NMDA currents are known to be involved. A second example of an interaction between mu opioids and NMDA currents was shown in acutely dissociated rat spinal dorsal horn neurons; here mu receptor activation first depressed then potentiated the effects of applied NMDA (80). The mechanisms of these complex effects were not determined. A similar suppression of NMDA-induced responses was seen in the dentate gyrus of the rat hippocampus (104). In the latter report, application of a mu agonist decreased the synaptic NMDA-mediated excitatory postsynaptic current (EPSC) evoked by perforant path stimulation. The nature of the interaction was not characterized, but because non-NMDA EPSCs were not affected by mu agonist, a presynaptic action of inhibition of glutamate release (as discussed for kappa agonists below) did not appear likely. Although the mechanistic basis for the interactions between opioid and NMDA responses is not clear, the observed phenomena suggest that opioid receptors may indirectly modulate responses to other transmitters by activating other, less-well-defined systems. (See Chapter 5, *this volume,* for a review of these ion channels and their regulation.)

Hippocampal Mechanisms

Predominantly inhibitory actions of exogenously applied opioids on neuronal activity and transmitter release are found throughout the CNS (30). The hippocampal region is one exception to this general finding, because pyramidal neuron excitability is increased following opioid application (71). (Fig. 2) It is important to note that no direct effects of opioids on CA1 pyramidal cells themselves have been reported (72,84). This paradoxical effect was explained via a mechanism of "disinhibition" in which opioids were acting directly to inhibit inhibitory interneurons, resulting in excitation of the pyramidal neurons (55,107). This basic mechanism of opioid action in the hippocampus has been investigated by a number of researchers, and their findings have been summarized (12,16). In an extension of this work, recent studies have provided evidence that opioid receptors are specifically

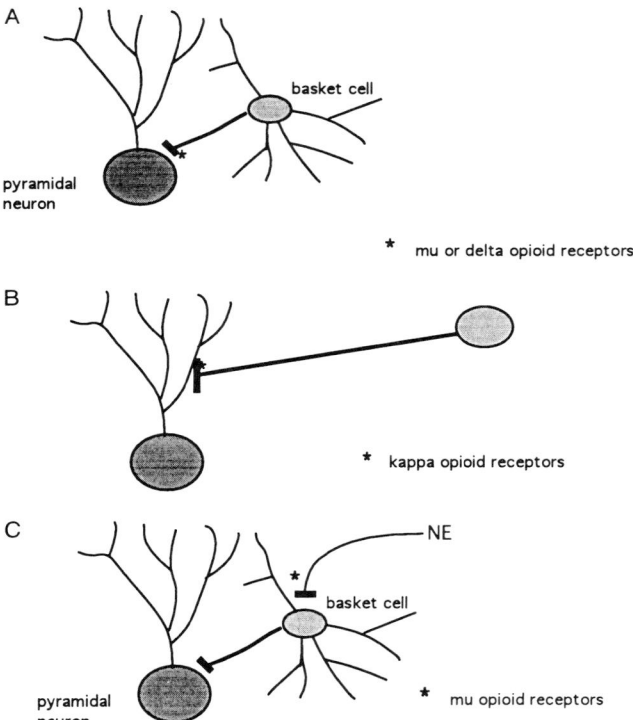

FIG. 2. Demonstrated actions of endogenously released opioid peptides in the hippocampus. **A:** Opioids inhibit GABA release from axon terminals of CA1/CA3 basket cells. **B:** Opioids inhibit glutamate release from perforant path axon terminals in the dentate gyrus and mossy fiber terminals in stratum lucidum. **C:** Opioids inhibit norepinephrine release from terminals of locus ceruleus afferents.

present on the terminals of interneurons, acting to inhibit gamma-aminobutyric acid (GABA) release. Lambert et al. (51) monitored pharmacologically isolated, monosynaptic inhibitory postsynaptic potentials (IPSPs) recorded from CA1 pyramidal cells following mu agonist application. Mu agonist application close to the recording site inhibited IPSPs, and application near the site of stimulation in the radiatum was ineffective. This indicated that the relevant mu receptors involved in inhibition of the IPSPs were located very near to the pyramidal cell bodies—that is, on GABAergic terminals. This report also found that barium application was not able to inhibit this opioid effect. This is of interest because evidence from the locus coeruleus region suggested that GABA$_B$ and opioid agonists modulated the same potassium conductance (20). The GABA$_B$-coupled potassium current is blocked by extracellular barium, so it would appear that the same potassium conductance is not involved in the mu effects observed by Lambert et al. (51). Two other groups have studied the effects of opioid application on tetrodotoxin (TTX)-insensitive spontaneous miniature IPSPs and found a decrease in the frequency of these events (22,79). Baclofen, which is known to hyperpolarize interneurons (55), did not affect the frequency of these action potential-independent IPSPs. Therefore, the decrease in IPSP frequency is consistent with the opioid acting at the interneuron terminal, not at the soma (22). This is not to say that opioid actions at the level of the interneuron soma may not be important for disinhibition, but somatic hyperpolarization is unlikely to be the only site of opioid action on interneurons.

In addition to disinhibition resulting from the reduction of GABA release, electrophysiological evidence for opioid inhibition of glutamate release has also been recently described. Kappa opioid agonists were found to inhibit excitatory synaptic transmission at the perforant path–granule cell synapse in guinea-pig hippocampal slices (94,95). In contrast to the mu and delta agonist effects described above, kappa agonists had no effect on inhibitory synaptic potentials, indicating that the kappa action was not mediated via interneurons. No changes in the membrane properties of the postsynaptic cell were observed, so a direct inhibition of the granule cells was unlikely. Excitatory synaptic potentials elicited by stimulation in the molecular layer were, however, significantly inhibited. Excitatory postsynaptic potentials (EPSPs) elicited from hilar stimulation were not significantly affected, arguing against a change in the postsynaptic response to endogenously released glutamate (95). The sum of these results argues that kappa receptors are located on perforant path terminals and act presynaptically to inhibit glutamate release in the dentate molecular layer of guinea-pig hippocampal slices. A similar presynaptic mechanism for kappa opioid action in the locus coeruleus has been described (60,77). Pharmacologic activation of mu receptors was similarly shown to inhibit excitatory amino acid

release from primary afferent fibers in rat spinal cord (48). Thus, opioid receptor regulation of excitatory transmission may be a very general mechanism of opioid action.

Because of the dense opioid (largely dynorphin) immunoreactivity localized to dentate granule cell axons, the mossy fiber–CA3 pyramidal cell synapse has long been thought to be a likely site for endogenous opioid action. Defining an effect of kappa ligands in the CA3 region has been enigmatic, because excitatory, inhibitory, nonopioid, and opioid-mediated actions have all been reported by various groups (2,10,42,66,96).

DO ENDOGENOUS OPIOIDS ACT AS NEUROTRANSMITTERS?

Up to this point, we have only been considering the actions of exogenously applied opioids and opioid peptides in various neurochemical and neurophysiological assays, the rationale being that endogenously released opioid peptides are likely to act via similar mechanisms. A key question is, How closely do the neurotransmitter actions of endogenous opioid peptides resemble pharmacologically applied opioids? Under what physiologic conditions are the peptides released? Once released, given the large variety of actions of opioids described above, what will the "net" effect of opioid action be on neuronal activity? Answering these questions has not been a simple exercise. Much of the anatomical data concerning the relationship between opioid peptide and binding site localization in the hippocampus suggest that endogenous opioids are not likely to act in a classical synaptic manner, and the nonclassical properties are only just being defined. The evidence that opioid peptides can act as neurotransmitters from several studies done using hippocampal tissue and employing a wide range of techniques will be summarized below.

Anatomical Studies

Endogenous opioid peptide distribution in the hippocampal formation has been described in several studies using immunohistochemical techniques (32,49,62). The results have shown that enkephalin-immunoreactivity is present in the lateral perforant path and the mossy fiber pathways, as well as in scattered interneurons. Dynorphin-immunoreactivity is restricted to the dentate granule cells (most prominently in their axonal projection to CA3, the mossy fibers) and a few interneurons in the dentate molecular layer. The distribution of opioid binding sites, which represents the locations of putative opioid receptors, is much more complex (56). The anatomical "mismatch" between localization of opioid peptides and their binding sites is contrary to what would be expected for a classical transmitter such as glutamate, suggesting that they may act in a neurohumoral manner (63). Much of the added complexity concerning binding site distributions is due to the large species variations evident when comparing rat and guinea pigs, for example (63). In addition to the endogenous opioid peptides and their binding sites, discrete localization of degradative enzymes thought to possibly be involved in the termination and/or spatial restriction of opioid peptide action has also been described (78).

Release Studies

Enkephalin and dynorphin peptides and peptide-immunoreactivity have been shown to be present in hippocampal tissue as measured with specific radioimmunoassays and high-pressure liquid chromatography (HPLC) assays (13,14). These assay methods have been used to measure the relative concentrations present and the amount of peptide released in response to chemically induced depolarization of the tissue. As one would expect for a neurotransmitter, the release of opioid peptides was calcium-dependent (13,14).

A radioligand displacement assay in which endogenously released opioids compete for opioid binding sites provided a means by which endogenous transmitter release occurring in a single in vitro hippocampal slice could be measured (70). This study also provided autoradiographic evidence suggesting that endogenously released opioids could diffuse to distant sites of action. While using mu- or kappa-selective opioid radioligands, focal electrical stimulation of the slice was utilized to demonstrate the release of endogenous opioids from specific opioid-containing fiber tracts in response to physiologic stimulation paradigms (92,93). High-frequency trains (>1 Hz) of stimulation were found to be most effective in eliciting opioid peptide release (11,92). This observation is similar to the requirements for the release of neuropeptide Y (NPY) and teleost luteinizing-hormone-releasing hormone (tLHRH) described in the peripheral nervous system and may represent a common characteristic of neuropeptide release (45,54).

Autoradiography of kappa$_1$ binding sites in the guinea pig revealed a population of putative kappa receptors which were restricted to the molecular layer of the dentate gyrus (93). High-frequency stimulation of regions containing either the perforant path or mossy fibers elicited the release of endogenous kappa opioids able to compete for kappa$_1$ binding. Importantly, application of a glutamate receptor antagonist could block the effects of perforant path stimulation, but not of the commissural/associational fibers. This result was consistent with granule cells being the likely endogenous source of kappa ligands. Experiments in which dynorphin antisera were found to be effective in blocking the effects of mossy fiber stimulation supported the hypothesis that dynorphin peptides released from granule cells were reaching kappa receptors in the molecular layer (93). These observations indicated that dynorphins could act as negative feedback transmitters on the perforant path afferents, modulating incoming excitatory transmission in the dentate gyrus (93,94).

PHYSIOLOGIC ACTIONS AT THE CELLULAR LEVEL

Synaptic Actions of Endogenously Released Opioids

Synaptic effects of endogenously released opioids were first demonstrated in the CA3 region of the hippocampus (11). Using the stimulation parameters previously characterized in the radioligand slice binding assay (92), the stimulated release of opioid peptides was found to control IPSP amplitudes measured CA3 pyramidal cells (11). The actions of the released opioids were blocked by naloxone [but not the inactive stereoisomer (+)naloxone] and were pathway-specific (i.e., only high-frequency stimulation of the perforant path had an effect on CA3 IPSPs) (11). Interestingly, the response to opioid release was extremely slow and prolonged, and the onset and duration were in the range of minutes following peptide release. The mechanism of the opioid effect was likely mediated by an effect on norepinephrine release (rather than a direct effect on GABA release) because the effects on IPSP amplitudes were sensitive to propranolol, a beta-adrenergic receptor antagonist (11), and the same stimulation parameters were also shown to directly reduce norepinephrine release in guinea-pig hippocampal slices (85). These results provide an example whereby one extrinsic afferent of the hippocampus (the perforant path) could regulate the actions of another extrinsic afferent (the norepinephrine projection from the locus coeruleus).

A more direct mechanism of endogenous opioid action has been characterized in the dentate gyrus of the guinea pig (95). The approach was based on the findings of two previous studies describing the effects of exogenously applied kappa opioids on EPSPs at the dentate granule cell–perforant path synapse (94) and the effects of high-frequency stimulation-induced release of dynorphins as measured in the ''in vitro slice'' binding assay (93). Therefore, an attempt to electrophysiologically measure the effects of endogenously released dynorphin on perforant path excitation was made by recording both whole-cell voltage clamp or extracellular population spike responses of dentate granule cells (95). Synaptic responses were monitored before and after a high-frequency stimulus train was given in the hilus. Following granule cell activation via antidromic stimulation, excitatory transmission at the perforant path synapse was reduced. This effect of hilar stimulation was blocked by a kappa-selective antagonist or by a cocktail of dynorphin antisera. Thus, a particular family of endogenous opioid peptides (i.e., the dynorphins) was identified, as well as a specific type of opioid receptor (i.e., the kappa receptor; see ref. 95).

Although granule cells contain the vast majority of dynorphin-immunoreactivity found in the hippocampus, the specific site of dynorphin release was not determined. Release either from recurrent collaterals or from dendrites of the granule cells is possible. Functionally, as the postsynaptic cell is the source of a molecule acting on the presynaptic terminal, dynorphin is acting as a retrograde transmitter. This inhibitory modulation of synaptic transmission mediated by dynorphin may be important in the pathophysiology of the hippocampus, because kappa opioids have been shown to be neuroprotective in excitotoxicity studies (39). In this role, endogenously released dynorphin could be acting in a compensatory manner to limit hyperexcitability existing during seizure activity (89). Consistent with this hypothesis is the phenomena of mossy fiber sprouting which occurs in human temporal lobe epilepsies (40). Contrary to expectations, the time course of this proliferation of mossy fiber recurrent collaterals into the inner molecular layer following a kindling paradigm could not be correlated with an increase in granule cell excitability (87). Rather, a recovery of inhibition was seen, which is consistent with the inhibitory influence of dynorphin as we have described above. Thus endogenous dynorphin modulation of synaptic activity in the dentate gyrus region may have a prominent role in the pathological and physiological function of the hippocampus.

A recent study (97) has also described an inhibitory presynaptic mechanism for kappa opioid actions in the CA3 region of the guinea-pig hippocampus, similar to the results of Wagner et al. (95) in the dentate gyrus. As well as the results described above for the perforant path synapse, this report also showed that the response to locally applied exogenous glutamate was not affected by kappa agonist, lending further support for the presynaptic site of action. Additionally, paired pulse facilitation, thought to be a presynaptic phenomena in origin, was enhanced by kappa agonists. Thus the net effect of kappa opioid application in both the CA3 and dentate gyrus regions of the guinea-pig hippocampus was a decrease in excitation of the principal neuron, rather than the net excitation of principal cells described previously (95,97). In this case, the endogenous dynorphins act to inhibit transmitter release from the same mossy fibers releasing the peptide (autoinhibition) as well as from adjacent mossy fibers (heterosynaptic depression).

Thus it would appear that several of the commonly listed criteria for classifying a molecule as an authentic neurotransmitter have been met in the hippocampus specifically and the CNS in general: (a) Opioid peptides are synthesized in, and localized to, specific neuronal populations. (b) Enzymatic means for degradation of the peptide has been described. (c) These peptides are released in a calcium-dependent manner from neuronal tissue. (d) Specific binding sites, representing putative opioid receptors, have been localized throughout the brain. (e) Phar-macologic effects have been described in response to exogenous application of the endogenous opioid peptides. (f) These effects can be mimicked by opioid agonists and reversed by antagonists. The principal differences between the actions of opioid transmitters and the more classical transmitters in this region are the relatively slow kinetics of opioid action and the larger radius of action. The functional implications of endogenous opioid action will be considered next.

Long-Term Potentiation Studies

We will begin our discussion by reviewing studies which have described the effects of naloxone application on physiologic responses assayed in the hippocampus. The most extensive body of evidence implicating endogenous opioids as having an active part in synaptic physiology concerns the effect of naloxone on the phenomena of long-term potentiation (LTP) in certain hippocampal pathways (7). LTP can be described simply as a long-lasting enhancement of synaptic response following an appropriate "inducing stimuli" (5,7,47). LTP is typically induced following a high-frequency (>10 Hz) tetani of the pathway of interest, conditions which we have described above as also likely to favor the release of endogenous opioids. Consistent with the excitatory effects of pharmacologically applied opioids in the hippocampus, many studies have demonstrated that LTP induction in the mossy fibers and the lateral perforant path (both of which contain endogenous opioids) is blocked in the presence of naloxone (8,9,28,29,41,57,103). The ability of naloxone to alter LTP induction is in marked contrast to the lack of naloxone effects on single-pulse, low-frequency synaptic events measured in the same opioid-containing pathways (15,28,29,52,103).

In the mossy fiber pathway, previous studies of both the population spike in slice preparations (41,57) and the field EPSP response in vivo (28,29) have demonstrated naloxone block of mossy fiber LTP, while LTP induction at a separate pathway (the commissural/associational fibers) is unaffected. The use of selective opioid receptor antagonists has provided evidence indicating that mu receptors are involved (29). Naloxone had no effect on LTP maintenance or expression when applied after LTP induction has occurred (28). Additionally, dynorphin application augmented mossy fiber LTP (81). Therefore, it was surprising that a recent study has failed to reproduce the naloxone-sensitivity of mossy fiber LTP induction, and in fact showed that a kappa-selective antagonist could facilitate LTP induction under their conditions (97). Interestingly, consistent with an inhibitory effect of endogenously released opioids on synaptic transmission in this region, the study also showed that naloxone blocked the phenomena of heterosynaptic depression (6), which accompanies mossy fiber LTP. The work of Weisskopf and co-workers involved measuring field EPSPs in the stratum lucidum in response to stimulation in the granule cell layer to evoke mossy fiber synaptic potentials in guinea-pig hippocampal slices. Although two prior groups had also used guinea pigs, the CA3 population spike response was monitored in the CA3 pyramidal cell layer (41,57). This seemingly subtle point could potentially be a basis for the discrepancy, because a dissociation of opioid effects on LTP induction monitored in the molecular layer field EPSPs and the granule cell population spike response has been described in the rat dentate gyrus (9,103; see below). An additional complication is that the dentate gyrus–CA3 area contains rather complex circuitry, making it very important (and difficult) to isolate and characterize the pathway being studied (21).

The LTP of the lateral perforant path (LPP) has been shown to be blocked by naloxone both in vivo (8,9) and when using the in vitro slice preparation (103), while LTP of the medial perforant path is unaffected. The potential for delta receptor involvement in lateral perforant path LTP was shown with the use of a delta-selective antagonist to selectively block the field EPSP enhancement without affecting the population spike response increase (9). Conversely, mu receptors were implicated by the ability of a mu-selective agonist to facilitate LTP of the population spike response without significantly affecting the field EPSP (103). Thus both studies revealed a dissociation of opioid effects on population spike and field EPSP LTP induced by lateral perforant path stimulation, and each provided evidence for a specific type of opioid receptor as being responsible.

The mechanism by which the facilitation of LTP induction in the mossy fibers by mu receptors and in the LPP by mu and delta receptors has not been determined, but several hypotheses exist. Based on the large amount of evidence indicating that exogenously applied opioids have disinhibitory effects, it is tempting to assume that is the case for LTP induction as well. Indeed it is well known that disinhibition caused by $GABA_A$ antagonists facilitates LTP induction (99). Disinhibition has been proposed to be the underlying mechanism by which mu receptors facilitate LTP of the lateral-perforant-path-evoked population spike (103). This mechanism has not been favored in the case of delta-mediated effects on lateral perforant path LTP (7,9), and a direct excitatory action at perforant path terminals was proposed (7), but a recent report in which naloxone had no effect on lateral perforant path in the presence of $GABA_A$ antagonists suggests that a disinhibitory mechanism may be relevant after all (37). Because the underlying locus of change in mossy fiber LTP appears to be presynaptic (106) and due to mu antagonist effects on the presynaptic phenomena of post tetanic potentiation, it has been suggested that a direct effect on mossy fiber presynaptic terminals is the underlying mechanism of action for opioids at this synapse (29). As reviewed above, however, there is no currently known

example of opioids exerting a direct, excitatory effect in the hippocampus that this hypothesis would require to explain the enhancement of LTP induction.

In contrast to the mu- and delta-mediated facilitory effects described above, and consistent with the kappa effects described by Weisskopf et al. (97) in the CA3, we have demonstrated that kappa opioids can have an inhibitory effects on LTP induction in the dentate gyrus of guinea pig (88,95). Either application of a kappa agonist or high-frequency (50 Hz) stimulus trains delivered in the hilus to induce dynorphin release from dentate granule cells was effective in blocking LTP of the population spike response. Blocking either the transmitter (by prior application of dynorphin-selective antisera) or the receptor (by kappa-selective antagonist) was effective in reversing the effects of hilus stimulation on LTP induction. As discussed previously, exogenously applied kappa agonists act in a manner consistent with presynaptic inhibition. Therefore, we hypothesize that a presynaptic inhibition of glutamate release underlies the ability of endogenously released or exogenously applied kappa agonists to block LTP induction at the perforant path–dentate granule cell synapse.

In summary, numerous studies have described opioid-mediated actions on LTP induction in the two opioid-containing pathways in the hippocampal formation. Although discrepancies among reports have occurred, it can be noted once again that endogenous opioid actions are correlated with high-frequency stimulation events. If one assumes that the phenomena of LTP is representative of learning and/or memory mechanisms, then by analogy with their interactions with LTP, endogenous opioids should potentially affect these processes as well.

PHYSIOLOGIC ACTIONS AT THE ORGANISMAL LEVEL

Opiate antagonists typically facilitate learning and memory, suggesting that endogenous opioids negatively affect these processes (61). Unfortunately, most of the studies have involved systemic application of opioids and opiate compounds, rather than local application to specified regions within the CNS. Thus although it is possible to distinguish between peripheral and CNS-mediated effects by utilizing opiate antagonists which do not cross the blood–brain barrier, the specific site of opioid action remains obscure. Studies done testing both peripheral and central administration of agonists and antagonists indicate that peripheral endogenous opioid systems are important in some forms of conditioning (58). Because we have been emphasizing work done in the hippocampus, the discussion in this section will be limited to the effects of opioid antagonists and the effects of stimulating opioid-containing pathways in experimental paradigms likely to involve hippocampal function.

The hippocampus has been identified as a brain structure necessary for the performance of certain spatial memory tasks (68,74). Once the maze procedure is learned, the animal relies on spatial cues to make the correct procedural choices in a given trial to obtain the reward. Post-training peripheral naloxone administration has been shown to enhance the acquisition of novel information presented when the spatial cues surrounding the maze apparatus are altered (33,34). This enhancement appears to be task-specific because post-training naloxone treatment does not enhance acquisition during the initial training of the animal (27,34). The endogenous opioids do not appear to be implicated in procedural memory (i.e., "learning how" to navigate the maze efficiently), but they do alter declarative memory (i.e., "learning where" the reward is) for a given trial. In addition to studies involving opioid antagonists, direct electrical stimulation of the hippocampal formation also affects spatial memory performance (23,24). High-frequency stimulation (60 Hz) of the dentate cell layer retrogradely impairs the performance of spatial memory tasks, an effect that is blocked by pretreatment with systemic application of naloxone. Interestingly, stimulation in the CA3 or CA1 layers (cells which do not contain endogenous opioids) did not retrogradely affect declarative memory (24). Given the information concerning opioid peptide localization and release parameters described above, a hypothesis in which dynorphins are released from granule cells following high-frequency stimulation and then act to impair spatial memory is easily supported. This hypothesis gains further support from a study done comparing the spatial memory performance and dynorphin content in young, middle-aged, and aged rats (46). In this study, the dynorphin content in the hippocampal formation was significantly elevated in middle-aged and aged rats compared to young animals. Importantly, animals exhibiting impaired spatial memory performance had significantly higher dynorphin A(1-8) levels than did their unimpaired, age-matched cohorts. Thus elevated dynorphin predicted impaired spatial memory performance in middle-aged and aged animals (46), and electrical stimulation of dynorphin-containing cells in young animals also impaired spatial memory (23,24).

CONCLUDING REMARKS

In the years since their first discovery, extensive progress has been made in the characterization of the transmitter properties of the endogenous opioid peptides. The clearest results are at the cellular and molecular level where the inhibitory mechanisms activated by opioids are best described. Less well defined is the modulatory role of opioids in the neural circuit where questions about the physical dimensions of the "opioid peptide synapse" and the kinetics of endogenous opioid action should be re-solved to provide a clearer insight to the role of these neuropeptides in synaptic function. Ultimately, new high-resolution techniques must be developed to define the roles of the opioid peptides in the whole animal. But clearly, considering the prevalence of peptides present in the brain, an understanding of how neuropeptides function in the control of behavior is essential to the description of complex neural function.

REFERENCES

1. Akil H, Watson SJ, Young E, Lewis ME, Khachaturian H, Walker JM. Endogenous opioids: biology and function. *Annu Rev Neurosci* 1984;7:223–255.
2. Alzheimer C, ten Bruggencate G. Nonopioid actions of the kappa-opioid receptor agonists, U 50488H and U69593, on electrophysiologic properties of hippocampal CA3 neurons in vitro. *J Pharmacol Exp Ther* 1990;255:900–905.
3. Barg J, Belcheva MM, Rowinski J, Coscia CJ. Kappa-opioid agonist modulation of [³H]thymidine incorporation into DNA: evidence for the involvement of pertussis toxin-sensitive G-protein-coupled phosphoinositide turnover. *J Neurochem* 1993;60:1505–1511.
4. Bean BP. Neurotransmitter inhibition of neuronal calcium currents by changes in Ca channel voltage dependence. *Nature* 1989; 340:153–156.
5. Bliss TVP, Collingridge GL. A synaptic model of memory: long-term potentiation in the hippocampus. *Nature* 1993;361:31–39.
6. Bradler JE, Barrioneuvo G. Heterosynaptic correlates of long-term potentiation induction in hippocampal CA3 neurons. *Neuroscience* 1990;35:265–271.
7. Bramham CR. Opioid receptor dependent long-term potentiation: peptidergic regulation of synaptic plasticity in the hippocampus. *Neurochem Int* 1992;20:441–455.
8. Bramham CR, Errington ML, Bliss TVP. Naloxone blocks the induction of long-term potentiation in the lateral but not in the medial perforant pathway in the anesthetized rat. *Brain Res* 1988;449:352–356.
9. Bramham CR, Milgram NW, Srebro B. Delta opioid receptor activation is required to induce LTP of synaptic transmission in the lateral perforant path in vivo. *Brain Res* 1991;567:42–50.
10. Caudle RM, Chavkin C. Mu opioid receptor activation reduces inhibitory postsynaptic potentials in hippocampal CA3 pyramidal cells of rat and guinea pig. *J Pharmacol Exp Ther* 1990;252:1361–1369.
11. Caudle RM, Wagner JJ, Chavkin C. Endogenous opioids released from perforant path modulate norepinephrine actions and inhibitory postsynaptic potentials in guinea pig CA3 pyramidal cells. *J Pharmacol Exp Ther* 1991;258:18–26.
12. Chavkin C. In: Pasternak GW, ed. *The opiate receptors.* Clifton, NJ: Humana Press, 1988;273–303.
13. Chavkin C, Bakhit C, Weber E, Bloom F. Relative contents and concomitant release of prodynorphin/neoendorphin-derived peptides in rat hippocampus. *Proc Natl Acad Sci USA* 1983;80:7669–7673.
14. Chavkin C, Shoemaker W, McGinty J, Bloom FE. Characterization of the prodynorphin and proenkephalin neuropeptide systems in rat hippocampus. *J Neurosci* 1985;5:808–816.
15. Chavkin C, Bloom FE. Opiate antagonists do not alter neuronal responses to stimulation of opioid-containing pathways in rat hippocampus. *Neuropeptides* 1985;7:19–22.
16. Chavkin C, Neumaier JF, Swearengen E. Opioid receptor mechanisms in the rat hippocampus. In: McGinty J, Friedman D, eds. *NIDA research monograph,* vol. 82. Washington, DC: US Government Printing Office 1988;94–117.
17. Chen L, Huang L-YM. Sustained potentiation of NMDA receptor-mediated glutamate responses through activation of protein kinase C by a mu opioid. *Neuron* 1991;7:319–326.
18. Chen Y, Mestek A, Liu J, Hurley JA, Yu L. Molecular cloning

and functional expression of a mu-opioid receptor from rat brain. *Mol Pharmacol* 1993;44:8–12.

19. Childers SR. Opioid receptor-coupled second messenger systems. *Life Sci* 1991;48:1991–2003.

20. Christie MJ, North RA. Agonists at mu-opioid, M2-muscarinic and GABA receptors increase the same potassium conductance in rat lateral parabrachial neurones. *Br J Pharmacol* 1988;5:896–902.

21. Claiborne BJ, Xiang Z, Brown TH. Hippocampal circuitry complicates analysis of long-term potentation in mossy fiber synapses. *Hippocampus* 1993;115–122.

22. Cohen GA, Doze VA, Madison DV. Opioid inhibition of GABA release from presynaptic terminals of rat hippocampal interneurons. *Neuron* 1992;9:325–335.

23. Collier TJ, Routtenberg A. Selective impairment of declarative memory following stimulation of dentate gyrus granule cells: a naloxone-sensitive effect. *Brain Res* 1984;310:384–387.

24. Collier TJ, Quirk GJ, Routenberg A. Separable roles of hippocampal granule cells in forgetting and pyramidal cells in remembering spatial information. *Brain Res.* 1987;409:316–328.

25. Crain SM, Shen K-F. Opioids can evoke direct receptor-mediated excitatory effects on sensory neurons. *Trends Pharmacol* 1990;11:77–81.

26. Cruciani RA, Dvorkin B, Morris SA, Crain SM, Makman MH. Direct coupling of opioid receptors to both stimulatory and inhibitory guanine nucleotide-binding proteins in F-11 neuroblastoma-sensory neuron hybrid cells. *Proc Natl Acad Sci USA* 1993;90:3019–3023.

27. Decker MW, Introini-Collison IB, McGaugh JL. Effects of naloxone on Morris water maze learning in the rat: enhanced acquisition with pretraining but not posttraining administration. *Psychobiology* 1989;17:270–275.

28. Derrick BE, Weinberger SB, Martinez JL. Opioid receptors are involved in an NMDA receptor-independent mechanism of LTP induction at hippocampal mossy fiber–CA3 synapses. *Brain Res Bull* 1991;27:219–223.

29. Derrick BE, Rodriguez SB, Lieberman DN, Martinez JL. Mu opioid receptors are associated with the induction of hippocampal mossy fiber long-term potentiation. *J Pharmacol Exp Ther* 1992;263:725–733.

30. Duggan AW, North RA. Electrophysiology of opioids. *Pharmacol Rev* 1984;35:219–281.

31. Evans CJ, Keith DE, Morrison H, Magendzo K, Edwards RH. Cloning of a delta opioid receptor by functional expression. *Science* 1992;258:1952–1955.

32. Gall C, Brecha N, Karten HJ, Chang K-J. Localization of enkephalin-like immunoreactivity to identified axonal and neuronal populations of the rat hippocampus. *J Comp Neurol* 1981; 198:335–350.

33. Gallagher M, King RA, Young NB. Opiate antagonists improve spatial memory. *Science* 1983;221:975–976.

34. Gallagher M, Bostock E, King RA. Effects of opiate antagonists on spatial memory in young and aged rats. *Behav Neural Biol* 1985;44:374.

35. Gannon RL, Terrian DM. U-50,488H inhibits dynorphin and glutamate release from guinea pig hippocampal mossy fiber terminals. *Brain Res* 1991;548:242–247.

36. Gintzler AR, Xu H. Different G proteins mediate the opioid inhibition or enhancement of evoked [5-methionine]enkephalin release. *Proc Natl Acad Sci USA* 1991;88:4741–4745.

37. Hanse E, Gustafsson B. Long-term potentiation and field EPSPs in the lateral and medial perforant paths in the dentate gyrus in vitro: a comparison. *Eur J Neurosci* 1992;4:1191–1201.

38. Harris HW, Nestler EJ. Opiate regulation of signal transduction pathways. In: Hammer RP, ed. *The neurobiology of opiates.* England: CRC P, 1993;301–331.

39. Hong JS, McGinty JF, Lee PHK, Xie CW, Mitchell CL. Relationship between hippocampal opioid peptides and seizures. *Prog Neurobiol* 1993;40:507–528.

40. Houser CR, Miyashiro JE, Walsh GO, Rich JR, Delgado-Escueta AV. Altered patterns of dynorphin immunoreactivity suggest mossy fiber reorganization in human hippocampal epilepsy. *J Neurosci* 1990;10:267–282.

41. Ishihara K, Katsuki H, Sugimura M, Kaneko S, Satoh M. Different

42. Iwama T, Ishihara K, Takagi H, Satoh M. Possible mechanism involved in the inhibitory action of U-50, 488H, an opioid kappa agonist, on guinea pig hippocampal CA3 pyramidal neurons in vitro. *J Pharmacobiodyn* 1987;10:564–570.

43. Jackisch R, Geppert M, Brenner AS, Illes P. Presynaptic opioid receptors modulating acetylcholine release in the hippocampus of the rabbit. *Naunyn Schmiedebergs Arch Pharmacol* 1986;332: 156–162.

44. Jackisch R, Geppert M, Illes P. Characterization of opioid receptors modulating noradrenaline release in the hippocampus of the rabbit. *J Neurochem* 1986;46:1802–1810.

45. Jan LY, Jan YN. Peptidergic transmission in sympathetic ganglia of the frog. *J Physiol (Lond)* 1982;327:219–246.

46. Jiang H-K, Owyang V, Hong J-S, Gallagher M. Elevated dynorphin in the hippocampal formation of aged rats: relation to cognitive impairment on a spatial learning task. *Proc Natl Acad Sci USA* 1989;86:2948–2951.

47. Johnston D, Williams S, Jaffe D, Gray R. NMDA-receptor-independent long-term potentiation. *Annu Rev Physiol* 1992;54:489–505.

48. Kangraga I, Randic M. Outflow of endogenous aspartate and glutamate from the rat spinal dorsal horn in vivo by activation of low- and high-threshold primary afferent fibers. Modulation by mu-opioids. *Brain Res* 1991;553:347–352.

49. Khachaturian H, Lewis ME, Schafer MK-H, Watson SJ. Anatomy of the CNS opioid systems. *Trends Neurosci* 1985;8:111–119.

50. Kieffer BL, Befort K, Gaveriaux-Ruff C, Hirth CG. The delta-opioid receptor: isolation of a cDNA by expression cloning and pharmacological characterization. *Proc Natl Acad Sci USA* 1992;9:12048–12052.

51. Lambert NA, Harrison NL, Teyler TJ. Evidence for mu opiate receptors on inhibitory terminals in area CA1 of rat hippocampus. *Neurosci Lett* 1991;124:101–104.

52. Linseman MA, Corrigall WA. Effects of morphine on CA1 versus dentate hippocampal field potentials following systemic administration in freely moving rats. *Neuropharmacology* 1981;21:361–366.

53. Loh HH, Smith AP. Molecular characterization of opioid receptors. *Annu Rev Pharmacol Toxicol* 1990;30:123–147.

54. Lundberg JM, Rudehill A, Sollevi A, Theodorsson-Norheim E, Hamberger B. Frequency- and reserpine-dependent chemical coding of sympathetic transmission: differential release of noradrenaline and neuropeptide V from pig spleen. *Neurosci Lett* 1986;63:96–100.

55. Madison DV, Nicoll RA. Enkephalin hyperpolarizes interneurones in the rat hippocampus. *J Physiol (Lond)* 1988;398:123–130.

56. Mansour A, Khachaturian H, Lewis ME, Akil H, Watson SJ. Anatomy of CNS opioid receptors. *Trends Neurosci* 1988;11:308–314.

57. Martin MR. Naloxone and long-term potentiation of hippocampal CA3 field potentials in vitro. *Neuropeptides* 1983;4:45–50.

58. Martinez JL, Janak PH, Weinberger SB, Schulties G, Derrick BE. In: Erinoff L, ed. *NIDA research monograph,* vol 97. Washington, DC: US Government Printing Office, 1990;48–78.

59. McFadzean I. The ionic mechanisms underlying opioid actions. *Neuropeptides* 1988;11:173–180.

60. McFadzean I, Lacey MG, Hill RG, Henderson G. Kappa opioid receptor activation depresses excitatory synaptic input to rat locus coeruleus neurons in vitro. *Neuroscience* 1987;20:231–239.

61. McGaugh JL. Involvement of hormonal and neuromodulatory systems in the regulation of memory storage. *Annu Rev Neurosci* 1989;12:255–287.

62. McGinty J, Henricksen S, Goldstein A, Terenius L, Bloom FE. Dynorphin is contained within hippocampal mossy fibers: immunochemical alterations after kainic acid administration and colchicine-induced neurotoxicity. *Proc Natl Acad Sci USA* 1983; 80:589–593.

63. McLean S, Rothman R, Jacobson A, Rice K, Herkenham M. *J Comp Neurol* 1987;255:497–510.

64. Misawa H, Ueda H, Satoh M. Kappa-opioid agonist inhibits phospholipase C, possibly via an inhibition of G-protein activity. *Neurosci Lett* 1990;112:324–327.

65. Miyake M, Christie MJ, North RA. Single potassium channels opened by opioids in rat locus ceruleus neurons. *Proc Natl Acad Sci USA* 1989;86:3419–3422.

66. Moises HC, Walker JM. Electrophysiological effects of dynorphin peptides on hippocampal pyramidal cells in rat. *Eur J Pharmacol* 1985;108:85–98.

67. Moore SD, Madamba SG, Schweitzer P, Siggins GR, Voltage dependent effects of opioid peptides on hippocampal CA3 pyramidal neurons in vitro. *J Neurosci* 1994;14(2):809–820.

68. Morris RGM, Garrud P, Rawlins JNP, O'Keefe J. Place navigation is impaired in rats with hippocampal lesions. *Nature* 1982;297: 681–683.

69. Mulder AH, Schoffelmeer ANM. Multiple opioid receptors and presynaptic modulation of neurotransmitter release in the brain. *Handbook Exp Pharmacol* 1993;104:125–144.

70. Neumaier JF, Chavkin C. Release of endogenous opioid peptides displaces [³H]diprenorphine binding in rat hippocampal slices. *Brain Res* 1989;493:292–302.

71. Nicoll RA, Siggins GR, Ling N, Bloom FE, Guillemin, R. Neuronal actions of endorphins and enkephalins among brain regions: a comparative microiontophoretic study. *Proc Natl Acad Sci USA* 1977;74:2584–2588.

72. Nicoll RA, Alger BE, Jahr CE. Enkephalin blocks inhibitory pathways in the vertebrate CNS. *Nature* 1980;287:22–25.

73. North RA. Opioid actions on membrane ion channels. *Handbook Exp Pharmacol* 1993;104:773–797.

74. Olton DS, Becker JT, Handelmann GE. Hippocampus, space and memory. *Behav Brain Sci* 1979;2:313–365.

75. Pasternak GW. Opioid receptors. In: Meltzer HY, ed. *Psycopharmacology: the third generation of progress.* New York: Raven Press, 1987;281–288.

76. Periyasamy S, Hoss W. Kappa opioid receptors stimulate phosphoinositide turnover in rat brain. *Life Sci* 1990;47:219–225.

77. Pinnock RD. A highly selective kappa-opioid receptor agonist, CI-977, reduces excitatory synaptic potentials in the rat locus coeruleus in vitro. *Neuroscience* 1992;47:87–94.

78. Pollard H, Bouthenet ML, Moreau J, Souil E, Verroust P, Ronco P, Schwartz, JC. Detailed immunoautoradiographic mapping of enkephalinase (EC 3.4.24.11) in rat central nervous system: comparison with enkephalins and substance P. *Neuroscience* 1989;30:339–376.

79. Rekling JC. Effects of met-enkephalin on GABAergic spontaneous miniature IPSPs in organotypic slice cultures of the rat hippocampus. *J Neurosci* 1993;13:1954–1964.

80. Ruskin KI, Randic M. Modulation of NMDA-induced currents by mu-opioid receptor agonist DAGO in acutely isolated rat spinal dorsal horn neurons. *Neurosci Lett* 1991;124:208–212.

81. Satoh M, Ishihara K, Katsuki H, Sugimura M. *Adv Biosci* 1989;75:193–196.

82. Schroeder JE, Fischbach PS, Zheng D, McClesky EW. Activation of mu opioid receptors inhibits transient high- and low-threshold Ca²⁺ currents, but spares a sustained current. *Neuron* 1991;6:13–20.

83. Shen KZ, North RA, Surprenant A. Potassium channels opened by noradrenaline and other transmitters in excised membrane patches of guinea-pig submucosal neurones. *J Physiol (Lond)* 1992;445:581–599.

84. Siggins GR. Zieglgansberger W. Morphine and opioid peptides reduce inhibitory synaptic potentials in hippocampal pyramidal cells in vitro without alteration of membrane potential. *Proc Natl Acad Sci USA* 1981;78:5235–5239.

85. Simmons ML, Wagner JJ, Caudle RM, Chavkin C. Endogenous opioid regulation of norepinephrine release in guinea pig hippocampus. *Neurosci Lett* 1992;141:84–88.

86. Simon EJ. Opioid receptors and endogenous opioid peptides. *Med Res Rev* 1991;11:357–374.

87. Sloviter RS. Possible functional consequences of synaptic reorganization in the dentate gyrus of kainate-treated rats. *Neurosci Lett* 1992;137:91–96.

88. Terman GW, Wagner JJ, Chavkin C. Endogenous dynorphin blocks induction of LTP in the guinea pig hippocampal dentate gyrus. *Soc Neurosci Abstr* 1993;19:1158.

89. Tortella FC. Endogenous opioid peptides and epilepsy: quieting the seizing brain? *Trends Pharmacol* 1988;9:366–372.

90. Tsunoo A, Yoshii M, Narahashi T. Block of calcium channels by enkephalin and somatostatin in neuroblastoma–glioma hybrid NG108-15 cells. *Proc Natl Acad Sci USA* 1986;83:9832–9836.

91. Ueda H, Nozaki M, Satoh M. Multiple opioid receptors and GTP-binding proteins. *Comp Biochem Physiol C* 1991;98:157–169.

92. Wagner JJ, Caudle RM, Neumaier JF, Chavkin C. Stimulation of endogenous opioid release displaces mu receptor binding in rat hippocampus. *Neuroscience* 1990;37:45–53.

93. Wagner JJ, Evans CJ, Chavkin C. Focal stimulation of the mossy fibers releases endogenous dynorphins that bind k1-opioid receptors in guinea pig hippocampus. *J Neurochem* 1991;57:333–343.

94. Wagner JJ, Caudle RM, Chavkin C. Kappa-opioids decrease excitatory transmission in the dentate gyrus of the guinea pig hippocampus. *J Neurosci* 1992;12:132–141.

95. Wagner JJ, Terman GW, Chavkin C. Endogenous dynorphins inhibit excitatory neurotransmission and block LTP induction in the hippocampus. *Nature* 1993;363:451–454.

96. Walker J, Moises H, Coy D, Baldrighi G, Akil H. Nonopiate effects of dynorphin and des-tyr-dynorphin. *Science* 1982;218: 1136–1138.

97. Weisskopf MG, Zalutsky RA, Nicoll RA. The opioid peptide dynorphin mediates heterosynaptic depression of hippocampal mossy fibre synapses and modulates long-term potentiation. *Nature* 1993;362:423–427.

98. Werling LL, Brown SR, Cox BM. Opioid receptor regulation of the release of norepinephrine in brain. *Neuropharmacology* 1987;26:987–996.

99. Wigstrom H, Gustafsson B. Facilitated induction of hippocampal long-lasting potentiation during blockade of inhibition. *Nature* 1983;301:603–604.

100. Williams JT, North RA, Tokimasa T. Inward rectification of resting and opiate-activated potassium currents in rat locus coeruleus neurons. *J Neurosci* 1988;8:4299–4306.

101. Wimpey TL, Chavkin C. Opioids activate both an inward rectifier and a novel voltage-gated potassium conductance in the hippocampal formation. *Neuron* 1991;6:281–289.

102. Wimpey TL, Chavkin C. 8-Bromo-cAMP blocks opioid activation of a voltage-gated potassium current in isolated hippocampal neurons. *Neurosci Lett* 1992;137:137–140.

103. Xie C-W, Lewis DV. Opioid-mediated facilitation of long-term potentiation at the lateral perforant path-dentate granule cell synapse. *J Pharmacol Exp Ther* 1991;256:289–296.

104. Xie C-W, Morrisett RA, Lewis DV. Mu opioid receptor-mediated modulation of synaptic currents in dentate granule cells of rat hippocampus. *J Neurophysiol* 1992;68:1113–1120.

105. Yasuda K, Raynor K, Kong H, Breder CD, Takeda J, Reisine T, Bell GI. Cloning and functional comparison of kappa and delta opioid receptors from mouse brain. *Proc Natl Acad Sci USA* 1993;90:6736–6740.

106. Zalutsky RA, Nicoll RA. Comparison of two forms of long-term potentiation in single hippocampal neurons. *Science* 1990;248: 1619–1624.

107. Zieglgansberger W, French ED, Siggins GR, Bloom FE. Opioid peptides may excite hippocampal pyramidal neurons by inhibiting adjacent inhibitory interneurons. *Science* 1979;205:415–417.

Psychopharmacology: The Fourth Generation of Progress, edited by Floyd E. Bloom and David J. Kupfer. Raven Press, Ltd., New York © 1995.

CHAPTER 47

Vasopressin and Oxytocin in the Central Nervous System

Linda Rinaman, Thomas G. Sherman, and Edward M. Stricker

The closely related peptides arginine vasopressin (AVP) and oxytocin (OT), found exclusively in mammals, were originally identified as hormones secreted from the neurohypophysis into the systemic circulation. The neurohypophyseal hormones are synthesized by separate populations of magnocellular neurons whose perikarya primarily occupy the supraoptic (SON) and paraventricular (PVN) nuclei of the hypothalamus, and whose axons terminate within the posterior lobe of the pituitary gland. A smaller number of neurons that synthesize AVP or OT and project to the neurohypophysis are located within the anterior commissural nucleus of the hypothalamus, and others are clustered within magnocellular accessory nuclei scattered between the PVN and SON.

AVP, the antidiuretic hormone, is secreted primarily under circumstances of dehydration. A rise in extracellular solute concentration is one of the most effective stimuli for AVP release, with as little as 2% elevation in plasma osmolality causing a two- to threefold increase in peripheral AVP levels. The kidneys are exquisitely sensitive to AVP, thus enabling adaptive renal water conservation during dehydration. AVP also is a vasoconstrictor agent (hence its name) and is secreted in relatively large amounts during hypovolemia and hypotension, in the absence of changes in plasma osmolality. Only such large amounts of AVP are sufficient to produce vasoconstriction; approximately 40 times more AVP is needed for a pressor response than for antidiuresis.

OT is structurally similar to AVP, presumably reflecting their common evolutionary derivation from the amphibian pituitary hormone, vasotocin (1) (Fig. 1). During labor, sensory signals from the uterus and birth canal

stimulate neurohypophyseal OT neurons, and the OT released into the bloodstream binds to uterine OT receptors to facilitate parturition by contracting the smooth muscle. Pituitary secretion of OT also is enhanced by signals related to suckling in lactating mammals. OT receptors are located on myoepithelial cells that are concentrated around the milk ducts and alveoli in the mammary glands; when OT binds to these receptors, the myoepithelial cells contract and stored milk is ejected.

These two familiar functions of systemic OT obviously apply only to sexually mature females. However, a third potent stimulus for pituitary OT secretion, plasma hyperosmolality, has recently been identified in both male and female rats. The OT secretory response to hyperosmolality is adaptive because OT promotes natriuresis in rats. Indeed, OT receptors in renal tissue are just as sensitive to OT as a sodium-excreting hormone as renal AVP receptors are to AVP as a water-retaining hormone. However, there is no evidence that OT has a comparable natriuretic function in other species, and there is in fact evidence that it does not in humans.

This chapter does not further address issues related specifically to neurohypophyseal AVP and OT. Instead, we focus on the roles of these peptides as neurotransmitter or neuromodulatory agents within the central nervous system. The fact that AVP and OT are released from axon terminals within distinct areas of the brain and spinal cord did not gain widespread appreciation until the early 1980s, but during the last decade an impressive amount of research has been performed on the neuroanatomy, neurobiology, and the possible functions of centrally projecting AVP and OT neurons (that is, neurons containing immunocytochemically detectable AVP or OT). This chapter will summarize some of the most firmly established findings that have emerged from these investigations (see also Chapters 43 and 65, *this volume*).

L. Rinaman, T. G. Sherman, and E. M. Stricker: Department of Behavioral Neuroscience, University of Pittsburgh, Pittsburgh, Pennsylvania 15260.

Arginine Vasopressin

Cys-Tyr-*Phe*-Gln-Asn-Cys-Pro-*Arg*-Gly(NH₂)
(prototherian, metatherian, and eutherian mammals)

Oxytocin

Cys-Tyr-*Ile*-Gln-Asn-Cys-Pro-*Leu*-Gly(NH₂)
(prototherian and eutherian mammals)

Vasotocin

Cys-Tyr-*Ile*-Gln-Asn-Cys-Pro-*Arg*-Gly(NH₂)
(nonmammalian vertebrates)

FIG. 1. Sequence similarities between the peptides AVP, OT, and vasotocin. Only the italicized amino acids differ between the three peptides. (Adapted from ref. 1.)

NEUROBIOLOGY OF CENTRAL VASOPRESSIN AND OXYTOCIN

Chromosomal Linkage of AVP and OT Genes

In recent years there has been a very rapid increase in the number of studies examining the structure and function of the AVP and OT genes, as well as studies on the transcriptional regulation of these genes as a function of neuronal secretory activity and physiological manipulation (8,78). From this work it is clear that AVP and OT are synthesized as portions of large precursor proteins from which AVP and OT are subsequently cleaved. Other portions of the precursor proteins, the neurophysin polypeptides, are also present in the dendritic, somatic, and axonal cytoplasm of AVP and OT neurons and are secreted from their axon terminals. There are separate pre-cursors for AVP and its associated neurophysin and for OT and its associated neurophysin, but these precursors are encoded by a pair of genes that share many similarities in structure and sequence. The high degree of DNA sequence identity and exon–intron distribution between the AVP and OT genes strongly suggests that these genes arose via a duplication event from an ancestral gene. It was of great interest, therefore, when it was determined that the human AVP and OT genes are linked on chromosome 20, separated by less than 12 kb of intervening DNA sequence (65) (see Fig. 2). This chromosomal domain undoubtedly represents the remnants of a gene duplication and inversion event that preceded the establishment of two genes with independent transcriptional regulation and cell-specific expression patterns, regulating distinct physiological systems. Despite occasional claims that neuropeptide hormones related to AVP or OT, such as vasotocin, may be expressed in mammals, careful examination of the human genome have failed to identify other genes with significant similarity to AVP and OT (41).

The results of molecular analyses of human and rat OT promoters have been described in detail (2,41). Similarly detailed analyses of the AVP promoter have not yet been performed, however. In contrast, studies using transgenic animals to examine the AVP gene are ongoing in several laboratories (3,28), whereas no similar studies on the OT gene have yet been reported.

Axonal Transport of AVP and OT mRNAs

Two novel mechanisms involving AVP and OT mRNAs have been observed recently in the hypothalamic–neurohypophyseal system. First, the mRNAs for AVP and OT are actively transported towards the posterior pituitary in the axons of magnocellular neurons (35).

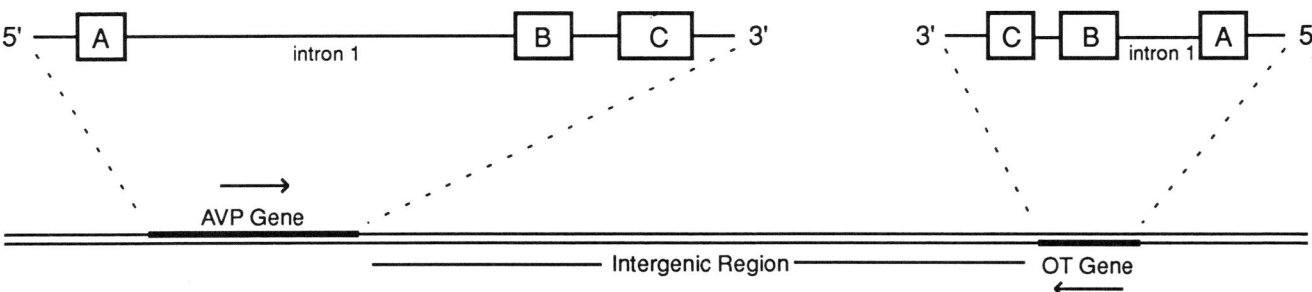

FIG. 2. The AVP and OT genes are localized on human chromosome 20 and are separated by only 8–12 kb of intervening DNA sequence. This DNA domain undoubtedly results from the genomic duplication of a progenitor gene (i.e., the vasotocin gene), an event estimated to have occurred 350–450 million years ago. The transcriptional orientations of the two genes are inverted (depicted by the *arrows* in the **lower diagram**) such that the promoter region for each gene lies within the flanking regions of the duplication domain. The more detailed schematic of the AVP and OT genes, shown in the **upper portions** of the figure, depicts the highly conserved exon–intron structures. Each gene is comprised of three exons (*lettered boxes*) separated by two intervening sequences (intron 2 is not labeled). Exon B of the AVP gene is the location for several mutations found to cause inherited forms of autosomal dominant hypothalamic diabetes insipidus.

The functional significance of AVP and OT mRNA axonal transport is unclear, and whether mRNA transport also occurs in AVP and OT neurons with central axonal projections remains an important question. Second, AVP mRNA injected into the hypothalamus of homozygous Brattleboro rats (which cannot produce AVP due to a genetic defect) is specifically taken up and expressed by magnocellular neurons, resulting in partial amelioration of their diabetic insipidus phenotype (64). Other studies found that AVP mRNAs with short poly(A) tails are taken up more effectively and are transported both retrogradely and anterogradely (43). It is possible that these capabilities are unique to neurohypophyseally projecting AVP and OT neurons, but they also may apply to neurons with central axonal projections.

Neuroanatomy of Centrally Projecting AVP and OT Neurons

The large majority of AVP and OT neurons with central axonal projections occupy the caudal portion of the PVN in rodents and primates, including humans (68,72). These neurons are called "parvocellular" because they are usu-

ally smaller than the magnocellular neurons that innervate the posterior lobe of the pituitary gland. Although parvocellular AVP and OT neurons that occupy the PVN do form intrahypothalamic projections, their axons terminate primarily outside of the hypothalamus (see Fig. 3). The density of their fibers within different termination areas varies considerably, from single isolated fibers in the frontal cortex to very dense innervation in the dorsal vagal complex in rats. The ratio of AVP to OT fibers also varies widely in different areas. Quantitative differences in the numbers of fibers present in certain brain areas have been noted in different species, including humans, but qualitatively the distribution of fibers appears to be quite similar. Limbic structures such as the lateral septum and the amygdala are particularly heavily innervated by AVP fibers, whereas OT fibers are predominant in the brainstem and spinal cord.

Other Central AVP and OT Systems

Not all centrally projecting AVP and OT neurons are located within the PVN. In rodents and in primates, including humans, immunoreactive neurons also occupy the

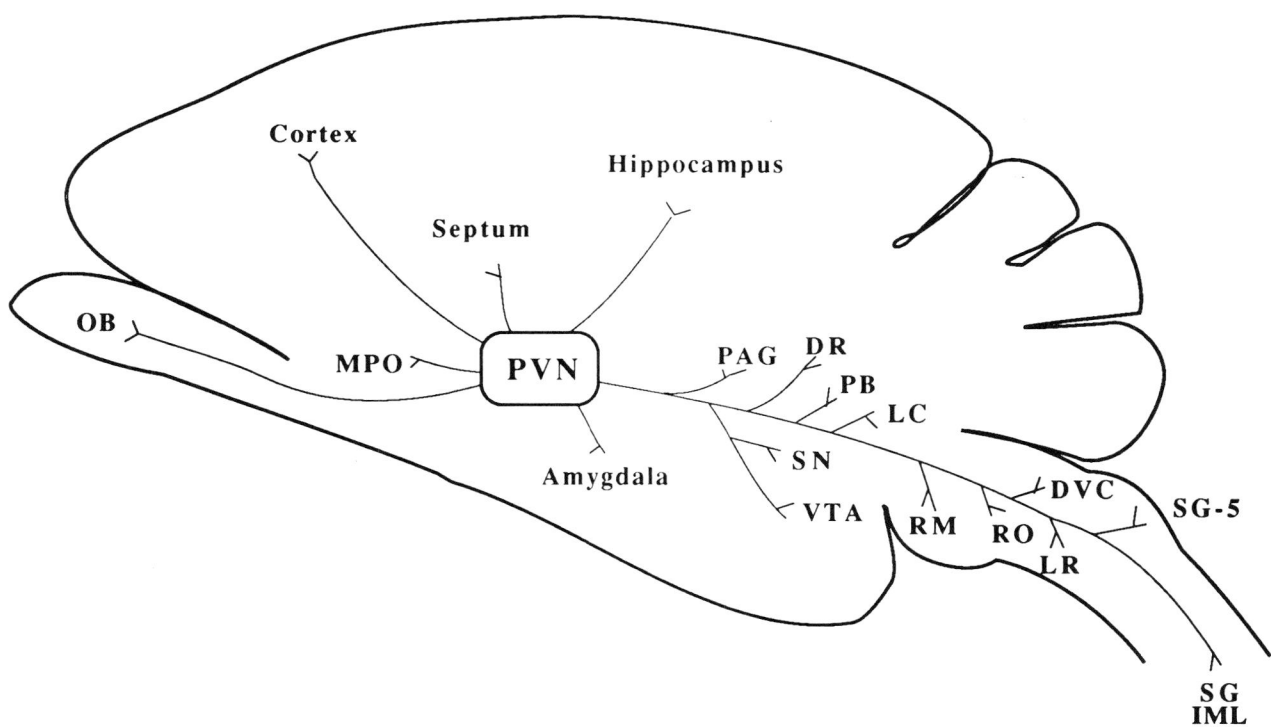

FIG. 3. Parvocellular AVP and OT neurons in the PVN give rise to axons that terminate in a variety of extrahypothalamic areas, depicted schematically in this figure. A subset of these AVP and OT projections may arise from neurons in the bed nucleus of the stria terminalis (see text). DR, dorsal raphe; DVC, dorsal vagal complex; IML, intermediolateral cell column of the spinal cord; LC, locus coeruleus; LR, lateral reticular nucleus; MPO, medial preoptic area; OB, olfactory bulb; PAG, periaqueductal gray; PB, parabrachial nucleus; PVN, paraventricular nucleus of the hypothalamus; RM, raphe magnus; RO, raphe obscurus; SG, substantia gelatinosa of the spinal cord; SG-5, substantia gelatinosa of the trigeminal nucleus; SN, substantia nigra; VTA, ventral tegmentum.

medial posterior region of the bed nucleus of the stria terminalis (AVP and OT), the medial preoptic area (OT), the dorsomedial suprachiasmatic nucleus (AVP), the septal region (AVP), the medial amygdala (AVP), and the locus coeruleus (AVP; not observed in humans) (34,61,72). The central projections of many of these neurons have been identified. In rodents, AVP neurons in the suprachiasmatic nuclei innervate the subparaventricular zone and dorsomedial nucleus of the hypothalamus, the medial and lateral preoptic areas, and midline thalamic nuclei (82). AVP neurons in the bed nucleus of the stria terminalis innervate the lateral habenular nucleus, the lateral septum, the medial amygdala, and the periaqueductal central gray (15). AVP neurons in the medial amygdala project to the ventral hippocampus (11). OT immunoreactivity in the locus coeruleus, raphe nuclei, and periaqueductal gray remains unaffected after extensive ablation of the PVN in rats, suggesting that OT fibers in these areas may originate outside of the PVN (29).

Differential Afferent Regulation of AVP and OT Neurons

Because different populations of AVP and OT neurons project to the neurohypophysis and to central brain areas, stimuli that elicit pituitary secretion of AVP and/or OT need not provoke the release of these peptides within the central nervous system, although they often do. Just as neurohypophyseal secretion of AVP and OT can occur independently of each other, central release of AVP and OT can occur independently of each other and also can differ from region to region. For example, suckling is well known to stimulate magnocellular OT neurons. PVN neurons that contain OT and project to the dorsal vagal complex apparently do not respond to suckling, but they do respond to dehydration, hemorrhage, and exogenous cholecystokinin (30,39). OT neurons projecting to the amygdala do not respond to suckling or hemorrhage, but do respond to dehydration (39), which also stimulates both AVP and OT magnocellular neurons. These and other data illustrate the selective and differential afferent control of AVP and OT neurons that have specific central projections.

Little is known about the chemical coding of afferent pathways that might differentially stimulate AVP and OT neurons in the PVN. The afferent innervation of the PVN is exceedingly complex, with most inputs appearing to innervate more than one PVN region (67,72). In many cases these connections have been confirmed by both anterograde and retrograde neural tract tracing and/or by electrophysiological recording. However, it seldom is known whether the neurons of some extrahypothalamic cell group synapse upon AVP or OT neurons, or both, or whether the postsynaptic targets are magnocellular or parvocellular. One exception is a recently identified projection arising from neurons in the caudal medulla. A small number of neurons in the nucleus of the solitary tract and in the region ventrolateral to it coexpress β-inhibin and somatostatin, and these neurons appear to preferentially innervate OT neurons in the PVN and SON (66). The SON targets obviously are magnocellular, but it is not known whether the PVN targets are magnocellular, parvocellular, or both. The β-inhibin/somatostatin projection is distinct from the well-documented, dense noradrenergic projection from the caudal medulla that innervates both magnocellular and parvocellular populations of AVP and OT neurons (67).

AVP and OT in the Cerebrospinal Fluid

Under normal physiological conditions, AVP and OT are present within the cerebrospinal fluid (CSF) in concentrations slightly higher than those in plasma. The separate regulation of AVP and OT in the blood and CSF is sustained by the blood–brain barrier, which prevents appreciable amounts of these peptides from entering the CSF after their secretion into the systemic circulation; that which does enter is presumed to do so through circumventricular structures, where the blood–brain barrier is absent (12). This arrangement does not exclude a possible central contribution of AVP and OT from neurons with neurohypophyseal projections, because peptide exocytosis occurs not only from their terminal boutons in the posterior pituitary but also along their perikarya, axons, and dendrites within the hypothalamus (51).

It is generally presumed that AVP and OT released into brain extracellular fluid will readily diffuse into the CSF, and vice versa, although the extent to which this is true is uncertain. It has been suggested that AVP and OT also may be released directly into the CSF, because AVP- and OT-immunoreactive processes have been observed in the ependymal lining of the third ventricle (12). The purpose of OT in the CSF remains unclear, but AVP is believed to play an important role in the regulation of blood flow to the choroid plexus and the rate of CSF production (12,44). Just as circulating catecholamines secreted from the adrenal glands supplement norepinephrine released from postganglionic sympathetic neurons, one could speculate that AVP and OT released into the CSF might supplement AVP and OT released into central synaptic clefts, thereby supporting the various central functions of these neuropeptides that are discussed below.

AVP and OT Receptors in the Central Nervous System

The available evidence suggests that the affinity and ligand selectivity of OT receptors in the brain do not differ from those in the mammary gland or uterus. Thus, central OT receptors bind both OT and AVP with high affinity (16,73,75). The reported maximal binding capacities for central OT receptors are relatively small (30–44 fmol/mg protein). The transduction mechanism triggered when OT binds to its receptors in the brain has not yet been ascertained, although central OT receptors appear not to be linked to either adenylate cyclase or to phosphoinositide breakdown (70).

AVP acts on three receptor subtypes: V_{1a}, V_{1b}, and V_2. Only the V_{1a} (vascular) subtype has been found in the central nervous system (6,75), although some evidence for central V_2-type (renal) receptors has been reported (16). The maximal binding capacities for central V_{1a} receptors also are small (20–80 fmol/mg protein) (6). AVP receptors in the anterior pituitary are classified as V_{1b} on the basis of different antagonist displacement profiles of [^{3}H]AVP binding compared with classical V_{1a} or V_2 receptors (33). Activation of both V_{1a} and V_{1b} receptors results in phosphoinositide breakdown (70).

cDNAs encoding the human OT receptor (37) and the rat V_{1a} receptor (50) were recently cloned. They are prototypic G-protein-coupled receptors, with seven putative transmembrane domains. They are more closely related to each other than to any other known G-protein-coupled receptors, perhaps accounting for the high affinity of AVP for OT receptors and (to a much lesser extent) vice versa. However, recent studies indicate that the central distribution of OT receptors is quite distinct from that of AVP receptors (42,75). Whenever present in the same general area, AVP and OT binding sites appear to be located in different parts of the structure. For example, AVP binding sites in the rat hippocampus are located mainly in the inner and outer blade of the dentate gyrus and in a subregion of the CA1 field, whereas OT binding sites are located in the subiculum and in a different part of the CA1 field. AVP binding sites in the rat dorsal vagal complex are concentrated in the nucleus of the solitary tract and the area postrema, whereas OT binding sites are concentrated in the dorsal motor nucleus of the vagus. Collectively, such data provide a structural basis for observations that AVP and OT differentially influence centrally regulated brain functions (below).

Most of the neural target areas that contain AVP- and/or OT-immunoreactive axon terminals have been shown to also contain AVP and/or OT binding sites (putative receptors) in rodents, monkeys, and humans (42,75), and the presence of AVP or OT binding sites is consistently associated with AVP or OT neuronal responsiveness (18,19,75,77). Comparison of electrophysiological recordings obtained from guinea-pig brain and rat brain have shown that species differences in OT receptor binding correlate positively with differences in OT neuronal sensitivity, suggesting that binding sites detected in the brains of other species also represent functional receptors (18,75). However, when immunocytochemical data are compared with receptor autoradiographic data, some discrepancies appear. For example, binding sites for OT are

abundant in the suprachiasmatic nuclei in rats, where very few or no OT-immunoreactive axons appear to be present. It remains to be established whether these observations reflect the technical limits of receptor autoradiography or immunocytochemistry, or whether they reveal authentic peptide–receptor mismatches suggestive of central paracrine-like effects of AVP and OT following their release in remote locations.

Pharmacological Analogues of AVP and OT

AVP and OT agonists are categorized primarily on the basis of the type of receptors they bind to. As stated above, most studies indicate that central AVP receptors are of the V_{1a} type, whereas central OT receptors appear pharmacologically identical to OT receptors in the uterus and mammary gland. The central binding characteristics and receptor-mediated effects of various analogues of AVP and OT are similar to their performance in peripheral tissues. Thus, agents that act as AVP agonists in vascular smooth muscle also mimic many of the central effects attributed to AVP (see below), and agents that act as agonists of OT in the uterine myometrium appear similarly effective on OT receptors within the central nervous system. However, because marked differences in rat, monkey, and human V_{1a} peripheral receptors have been demonstrated (55), and species differences may also exist in central AVP (and OT) receptors, the published pharmacological data for AVP and OT analogues serve as a useful guide only in that species for which data are reported.

The ring structure of the AVP molecule is an absolute requirement to elicit agonist responses (73), and no known compound displays higher V_1 agonist activity than AVP itself. Many centrally acting AVP agonists display selective binding to V_1 rather than V_2 receptors, but AVP analogues with high V_1 agonist activity and reduced affinity for OT receptors have not been reported. Central OT receptors bind both AVP and OT with high affinity; they also bind the agonist HO[Thr^4, Gly^7]OT (TGOT) with high affinity (16). In fact, TGOT is more selective for OT receptors than is OT itself, and is effective in smaller doses than OT in certain behavioral tests in rats (52), although it has a lower efficacy than OT in causing neuronal excitation in vitro (74).

The known antagonists of AVP and OT fall into four classes: (a) related cyclic peptides, (b) linear peptides, (c) cyclic peptides of bacterial origin, and (d) nonpeptides. A potent cyclic antagonist of central V_{1a} receptors is d(CH$_2$)^{5}Tyr(Me)AVP. It is the most widely used V_{1a} antagonist, and it is 100-fold more potent as a V_{1a} antagonist than as an OT antagonist in rats (45). Many linear V_{1a} antagonists are similarly potent, but most have not yet been evaluated for their specificity with regard to OT receptors (45). Substantial gains in both anti-OT potency and selectivity have been made; one recently reported OT antagonist has an anti-OT/anti-V_{1a} potency ratio of 17:1 (55).

AVP and OT as Neurotransmitters

The electrophysiological actions of AVP and OT on target neurons have been well studied in several brain areas, including hippocampus, septum, and dorsal vagal complex (75,77). There is strong evidence supporting physiological roles for both peptides as neurotransmitter substances in the descending pathway from the PVN to the dorsal vagal complex in rats, which contains high-affinity receptors for AVP and OT (75). Electron microscopy has revealed that AVP- and OT-immunoreactive axon terminals synapse on dendrites within motor and sensory subnuclei of the dorsal vagal complex (81). Both peptides are released in the dorsal vagal complex in a Ca^{2+}-dependent and K^+-stimulated manner (9), and their concentrations increase there following electrical stimulation of the PVN (38). Microinjection of low concentrations of AVP (5 nM) or OT (100–500 fmol) into the rat dorsal vagal complex both in vitro and in vivo potently enhances the spontaneous activity of responsive neurons in a receptor-mediated, dose-related, reversible, postsynaptic, TTX-resistant, and voltage-dependent manner (18,19,47).

The onset of neuronal responses to AVP or OT in the dorsal vagal complex occurs between 15 sec and 2 min after injection, and lasts from 30 sec to 20 min (18,19,47). The relatively slow onset and long duration of neuronal responses to AVP and OT are consistent with the possibility that these neuropeptides produce their effects by activating a postsynaptic second messenger cascade. This possibility also is consistent with the G-protein-coupled nature of the central AVP and OT receptors (37,50) (for detailed discussion of receptor structure–function relationships, see Chapters 11, 27, 38, and 46, *this volume*). Because the currents generated by AVP or OT do not show pronounced time-dependent inactivation, they might contribute to persistent depolarizing membrane potentials that could modify the repetitive firing properties of their target neurons. By virtue of their voltage dependence, these currents could participate in regulating other synaptic inputs by causing preferential amplification of excitatory postsynaptic potentials (18,47). Some of the functions attributed to central AVP and OT have been postulated to involve modifications of synaptic transmission, and they are consistent with the electrophysiological effects of these neuropeptides within the dorsal vagal complex. These functional correlates are considered in the next section.

PHYSIOLOGICAL AND BEHAVIORAL ACTIONS OF CENTRAL AVP AND OT

The physiological and behavioral effects of central AVP and OT usually have been studied by direct injection of these neuropeptides into the cerebroventricular system. Although it cannot be determined what concentrations are achieved subsequently at critical synapses, many of the reported effects are produced only when the administered doses are in the high (microgram) range. The acute effects of such large central doses of AVP and OT often resemble each other (e.g., barrel rotation, seizures, or ataxia), and they may reflect the cross-reactivity of AVP and OT with each other's receptors and/or the toxic effects of large doses. Bearing this in mind, we have focused our current discussion on results that have been corroborated by studies using more refined techniques such as stereotaxically localized injections and specific receptor antagonists.

The various putative functions of central AVP and OT that we review briefly do not represent an exhaustive survey, but are intended to reflect those areas in which the most significant recent progress has been made. Most of the experiments demonstrating central effects of AVP or OT have been performed in rats and cannot be extended with assurance to humans. Nevertheless, the distribution of AVP and OT neurons, fibers, and binding sites in experimental animals closely resembles their distribution in humans, thus encouraging speculation that functional similarities exist as well.

Hypophysiotropic Effects of AVP and OT on ACTH Secretion

AVP released from axon terminals in the median eminence enters the portal blood system and is carried to the anterior lobe of the pituitary gland, where it acts as a secretagogue for adrenocorticotropic hormone (ACTH) by binding to V_{1b} receptors (4). The parvocellular system containing corticotropin-releasing hormone (CRH) is a probable source of portal AVP. AVP and CRH occupy the same secretory vesicles in terminals that contain both peptides, and AVP potentiates CRH-induced ACTH secretion. Two approximately equal subsets of CRH perikarya occupy the medial parvocellular subdivision of the PVN, those that express pro-AVP peptides and those that do not (69). Because the two populations of CRH neurons have different topographical distributions, they may be regulated differentially.

The precise role of OT on the hypothalamic–hypophyseal–adrenal system remains controversial, but its effect seems to be limited to controlling ACTH release only in some instances (26,34,61). OT immunoreactivity is colocalized in many of the AVP-negative, CRH-positive neurons in the PVN (69). Although OT-positive fibers are rare in the median eminence, large amounts of OT are present in the hypophyseal portal blood of the rat (26) and rhesus monkey (58), and high-affinity receptors for OT have been reported in the anterior pituitary of the rat (4). OT is less potent than AVP in enhancing ACTH release, but passive immunoneutralization of OT blunts the ACTH response to some types of stress in rats (26). In contrast, OT appears to inhibit rather than to stimulate ACTH release in primates, including humans, under certain conditions such as physical exercise (34).

AVP and OT in Memory

The extensive research examining the effects of central AVP and OT on memory has been reviewed elsewhere (7,16). Intracerebroventricular (i.c.v.) injections of very small (picogram) doses of AVP or the AVP derivative [pGlu^4,Cyt^6]AVP-(4-8) (a natural proteolytic fragment of AVP) induce long-lasting facilitation of learned passive avoidance behavior in rats. In contrast, OT and its natural derivative [pGlu^4,Cyt^6]OT-(4-8) hasten the extinction of learned avoidance responses, and central antagonism of AVP or OT can attenuate or facilitate, respectively, these conditioned avoidance behaviors (16). AVP appears also to have facilitating effects on "social memory" (the tendency of rodents to investigate unfamiliar conspecifics more intensely than familiar ones), a perhaps more ethologically relevant model with which to investigate learning and memory in rats (13).

Studies using stereotaxic microinjections of AVP and OT to alter passive avoidance behaviors have supported distinct sites of action for the two peptides. The dorsal septal nucleus and the ventral hippocampus are most sensitive to AVP, whereas the hippocampal dentate gyrus and the dorsal raphe nucleus are most sensitive to OT (5). In addition to directly stimulating hippocampal neurons, very low doses of AVP or OT also modify catecholamine turnover in the midbrain–limbic areas where they are believed to induce their effects on memory. Specifically, AVP increases and OT decreases alpha-methyl-p-tyrosine-induced disappearance of catecholamines in these areas, suggesting that changes in catecholamine activity might be involved in the behavioral effects of AVP and OT (5). Other recent data support a modulatory role of AVP on the activity of central nicotinic mechanisms that are critical for memory retrieval (21).

The relevance of these findings to human memory is uncertain. Inconsistent effects of AVP on human memory in various experimental paradigms have been reported (22). Nevertheless, clinical researchers have sought to determine whether the severe memory disturbance characteristic of Alzheimer's disease might be attributed, at least in part, to alterations in central endogenous AVP or OT. Patients with Alzheimer's disease were found to have abnormal levels of AVP and OT in the CSF and in certain brain areas (42,46,61). The control of pituitary AVP release is impaired in patients with Alzheimer's disease, and AVP levels in the brain and CSF also are reduced (83). Conversely, a 35% increase in the concentration of hippocampal OT has been measured in men with Alzheimer's disease (46). Although these data appear to be consistent with the effects of AVP and OT in memory tests, clinical trials have not yet shown any beneficial effect of AVP analogues given chronically to patients with Alzheimer's disease (83; see also Chapter 120, *this volume*).

AVP in Thermoregulation

Central injections of AVP decrease body temperature in rabbits, guinea pigs, cats, rats, and sheep. Most studies examining the role of AVP in thermoregulation focus on its antipyretic effect in animals with experimentally induced fever, but a few studies have investigated the effect of AVP on basal body temperature. These latter studies have shown a marked decrease in body temperature, lasting up to 30 min after i.c.v. injection of only 30 ng of AVP (17). Conversely, low doses of a V$_1$ receptor antagonist (10 ng, i.c.v.) produce hyperthermia in euthermic, conscious, unrestrained rats, and they block the effect of exogenous AVP (up to 100 ng, i.c.v.) to attenuate induced fever. The antipyretic effects of AVP appear similar to those of indomethacin or aspirin; moreover, central blockade of V$_1$ receptors eliminates the antipyretic effects of peripherally administered indomethacin (36).

The ventral septal area, which is thought to mediate the antipyretic effects of AVP, contains both AVP binding sites and AVP-immunoreactive terminals derived from the bed nucleus of the stria terminalis (36,75). Electrical stimulation of the bed nucleus produces antipyresis, and this effect is blocked by V$_1$ receptor antagonists in the ventral septal area (36). The ventral septal area contains neurons that receive synaptic input transmitted from temperature sensors in the body, and these neurons alter their glutamate sensitivity in response to local application of AVP. Push–pull perfusion of the ventral septal area in sheep and rabbits reveals a direct relation between AVP levels and rising or falling body temperatures. These data have been interpreted to suggest that endogenously released AVP acts as a "brake" on febrile increases in body temperature (36). Because physiological stimuli that release AVP peripherally (such as plasma hyperosmolality) are antipyretic in rats and in guinea pigs, it was proposed that concurrent central release of AVP by these stimuli might mediate their effects on body temperature. Recent data have supported this hypothesis (57,63).

AVP in Cardiovascular Regulation

In conscious, unrestrained rats, low doses of AVP given i.c.v. induce tachycardia, whereas higher doses cause tachycardia preceded by significant bradycardia (17). Injection of a V_1 receptor antagonist i.c.v. increases heart rate, but this effect could be secondary to the behavioral activation that also results. Changes in both sympathetic and parasympathetic nervous outflow have been reported to underlie the central cardiovascular effects produced by i.c.v. injections of AVP, but conflicting data have been obtained along with marked interspecies variability (10,17).

Smaller doses of AVP and AVP antagonists injected into the caudal medulla have provided data that can be interpreted more easily. AVP-immunoreactive terminals derived from neurons in the PVN form synaptic contacts with dendrites in both the dorsal vagal complex (81) and the lateral reticular nucleus (27) in rats. Injection of AVP antagonists into the dorsal vagal complex reduces the pressor and tachycardic responses elicited by electrical stimulation of the PVN (59). Microinjections of as little as 1 pmol of AVP into the lateral reticular nucleus produces dose-related increases in arterial pressure and heart rate, and injections of AVP into the dorsal vagal complex have a similar but somewhat smaller effect (27). Bilateral microinjections of a specific AVP antagonist into the lateral reticular nucleus following acute, small hemorrhage in rats produces a decrease in arterial pressure, whereas neither the AVP antagonist nor the hemorrhage alone alters arterial pressure. These data have been interpreted to suggest that under conditions (such as hemorrhage) demanding increased sympathetic drive to maintain arterial pressure, a functional AVP receptor mechanism in the caudal medulla may be activated to help restore normal blood pressure (27). One conjecture is that AVP may enhance the sympathoinhibitory influence over the vagally mediated arterial baroreflex (10,59).

OT in Vagally Mediated Gastric Motility and Acid Secretion

Injecting OT into the dorsal vagal complex in rats increases gastric acid secretion and reduces gastric motility; these effects are eliminated by vagotomy (62). The OT innervation of the dorsal vagal complex arises from the PVN (68), and electrical stimulation of the PVN increases gastric secretion and has a biphasic effect on gastric motility, with a strong increase followed by a weaker decrease. OT antagonists injected into the dorsal vagal complex prior to PVN stimulation block the increase in gastric secretion and suppress the inhibitory phase of gastric motility, whereas central OT antagonism alone or acute PVN lesions increase baseline gastric motility (24,62). These data suggest that the PVN exerts a tonic, OT-mediated influence on the activity of vagal gastric motor neurons in rats.

Stimulation of gastric vagal sensory fibers affects gastric secretion and motility in a manner similar to that of central OT. Vagal sensory information is transmitted

directly to the PVN by ascending neural pathways (67). Gastric vagal stimulation excites OT neurons in the PVN (60), some of which project to the dorsal vagal complex in a reciprocal manner (53). Because microinjections of OT in the rat dorsal vagal complex specifically increase the excitability of neurons that receive mechanoreceptive gastric vagal sensory input (47), long-loop reciprocal pathways between the dorsal vagal complex and OT neurons in the PVN may enhance the efficiency of certain gastric vagal reflexes in rats. Whether OT plays a similar role in other species remains to be examined. In particular, OT binding sites are not discernible in the dorsal vagal complex of guinea pigs, and vagal neurons in guinea pigs are unresponsive to OT in vitro (77). These data caution against generalizing the gastric (and other) effects of central OT demonstrated in rats to other species.

OT in Ingestive Behavior

Pituitary secretion of OT in rats is elicited by a variety of treatments that also inhibit ingestion of food and NaCl, including plasma hyperosmolality or hypotension, gastric distension, and systemic administration of cholecystokinin or lithium chloride (79,80). Each of these treatments also stimulates parvocellular OT neurons with central axonal projections, resulting in increased central release of OT. Peripheral administration of OT or OT antagonists does not affect food or NaCl ingestion, mitigating against a role of systemic OT in these behavioral effects. In contrast, central administration of OT or a specific OT agonist reduces or completely eliminates ingestion of food or NaCl, and central injection of specific OT receptor antagonists blunts the ability of many treatments to inhibit food or NaCl intake (80). The inhibition of food and NaCl intake produced by treatments that stimulate central and systemic release of OT may reflect a coordinated effort to reduce solute concentrations in the body, because circulating OT derived from neurohypophyseal secretion increases urinary Na^+ excretion in rats (80).

Physiological or pharmacological treatments that inhibit feeding also inhibit gastric motility and emptying in rats (25,48). This association may be mediated by central OT systems, because OT acts in the dorsal vagal complex to inhibit gastric motility (discussed above). The inhibition of gastric motility may prolong or enhance gastric distension produced by food in the stomach, and thereby inhibit further food intake. It is likely that many of the chemical agents that potently stimulate central and pituitary OT secretion and inhibit gastric motility and food intake in rats also generate an aversive sensation such as nausea, because those agents produce strong learned taste aversions (79). However, as discussed above, activation of central OT transmission seems to hasten the extinction of other learned avoidance behaviors in rats. It remains to be determined whether anorexigenic/nauseogenic stimuli in rats enhance release of OT in the limbic forebrain regions that have been associated with memory. Similarly, although nauseogenic stimuli induce pituitary secretion of AVP rather than OT in several other species examined, including humans (49) (which could fit the "AVP-memory" hypothesis more neatly), it is not known whether central release of AVP rather than OT is stimulated in these species.

OT in Maternal Behavior

The triggering of maternal behavior in mammals is linked to endocrine changes that accompany the end of gestation and parturition. Considerable evidence now implicates central OT release in the initiation of maternal behavior during the immediate postpartum period. Parturition has been proposed to activate central OT release in addition to OT secretion from the pituitary, to provide coordinated maternal responses that could contribute to the survival of the young as well as to their birth. Many studies have provided support for this attractive hypothesis. Central injections of OT induce the rapid onset of maternal behaviors (i.e., retrieval, grooming, and nursing of the young) in steroid-primed virgin female rats in a dose-related manner (54). Central antagonism of OT transmission or PVN lesions each inhibit the onset of maternal behavior in postparturient rats (20). The site(s) of central action at which OT might act to stimulate maternal behavior has been localized variously to the ventral tegmentum, olfactory bulb, amygdala, midbrain, bed nucleus of the stria terminalis, and preoptic area; the reports are controversial, with some investigators seeing no effect of central OT at all (61). It seems likely that no one particular brain site is solely responsible for maternal behavior, but rather several sites that each facilitate different components of this complex behavior.

AVP and OT in Other Complex Social Behaviors

The proposed role of central OT in certain aspects of male and female sexual behavior is discussed elsewhere in this volume (see chapter by Pfaus and Everitt).

Central AVP may play a role in the control of male territorial displays and aggression. Studies of the golden hamster implicate an AVP-responsive region in the preoptic area of the anterior hypothalamus that is important in flankmarking (scent marking), a critical element in the behavioral repertoire associated with establishing and maintaining social dominance in males of this species (23). Flankmarking behavior is stimulated by intrahypothalamic administration of AVP and is inhibited by AVP antagonists. These site-specific effects are regulated by testosterone, which increases the presynaptic AVP innervation of the preoptic area (76).

It has been suggested that natural differences in AVP

and OT receptor distribution may be functionally associated with species-typical patterns of social organization in mice and in voles (31). For example, voles that are monogamous and highly parental have very different distributions of central AVP and OT receptors than do voles that are polygamous and minimally parental, and these species differences are associated with pronounced differences in the behavioral responses to exogenous AVP and OT. There is some evidence that AVP and OT may be involved in the process of pair bonding in monogamous species. OT infused centrally (10–100 ng/hr) confers striking partner preferences in monogamous female voles, whereas infusion of AVP (50–100 ng) in male monogamous voles markedly increases aggression towards all conspecifics except the mate (31). Because partner preferences and aggression in monogamous voles are normally reinforced by mating, mating may release endogenous central AVP and/or OT in these species. Data showing that central administration of a specific AVP antagonist (50 pg to 500 ng) blocks the aggressive behavior that normally follows mating in male monogamous voles support this idea, but it remains to be seen whether OT antagonism blocks the formation of partner preferences in monogamous female voles (31).

SUMMARY AND CONCLUSIONS

In addition to their release into the systemic circulation, AVP and OT act as neurochemicals within the central nervous system to modulate neuronal activity through receptor-mediated mechanisms. Centrally released AVP and OT derive largely (but not exclusively) from PVN neurons that have central axonal projections. It seems unlikely that neurohypophyseal and central secretion of AVP and OT are generally coordinated under basal conditions. However, certain stimuli (i.e., parturition, dehydration, toxins) induce pronounced secretion of AVP and/or OT from the neurohypophysis as well as from axon terminals in discrete brain regions, and in such situations the peripheral and central actions of AVP and OT may be complementary in function. Identification of the physiological stimuli that induce central release of AVP or OT, and the functional consequences of such release, is an area of increasing investigation.

Given the broad array of complex behaviors that are affected by supplementing or blocking central AVP and OT in experimental animals, there is understandably considerable interest regarding the central functions of these neuropeptides in humans, especially in humans with neurological and psychiatric disorders. There are many speculations but few findings relating changes in central AVP and OT systems to human psychopathology. Alterations in CSF levels of AVP and/or OT have been observed in patients with schizophrenia, anorexia, obesity, clinical depression, alcoholism, Alzheimer's disease, or Parkinson's disease (14,40,46), but the functional significance of these observations is unknown.

AVP and OT systems are anatomically and functionally linked with catecholaminergic systems (67). Roles for both peptides as "stress hormones" have been considered (32,34), consistent with their ability to alter ACTH secretion and thereby influence the adrenomedullary response to stress. In addition to their activation in situations of stress (71), many other functional and structural aspects of the central AVP and OT systems also are reminiscent of the central and peripheral catecholaminergic systems. For example, AVP and OT neurons are localized in discrete brain regions that receive afferent information from literally dozens of different cell groups, and they have axonal projections that extend throughout the central nervous system from the cerebral cortex to the spinal cord. Furthermore, AVP and OT may have effects on brain function that extend beyond classically defined (e.g., synaptic) limits, similar to what has already been proposed for centrally released catecholamines (71). These characteristics would permit the small, localized groups of AVP and OT neurons to influence neuronal events in many parts of the central nervous system, much as peripherally released catecholamines act on sympathetic targets throughout the periphery. A further similarity between the AVP, OT, and catecholamine systems is their demonstrated ability to modulate the responsiveness of their target neurons to other inputs. These influences often are exerted not over milliseconds but rather over minutes or hours, presumably due to receptor-mediated activation of second messenger systems. The diversity of physiological and behavioral effects that have been attributed to central AVP and OT supports the idea that these neuropeptides play a general role in modulating neural activity in hypothalamic, limbic, and autonomic circuits, and that the complexity of their effects arises from the complexity of the circuits in which they operate.

REFERENCES

1. Archer R. Principles of evolution: the neural hierarchy model. In: Krieger DT, Brownstein MJ, Martin JB, eds. *Brain peptides.* New York: John Wiley & Sons, 1983;135–163.
2. Adan RA, Cox JJ, Beischlag TV, Burbach JP. A composite hormone response element mediates the transactivation of the rat oxytocin gene by different classes of nuclear hormone receptors. *Mol Endocrinol* 1993;7:47–57.
3. Ang HL, Carter DA, Murphy D. Neuron-specific expression and physiological regulation of bovine vasopressin transgenes in mice. *EMBO J* 1993;12:2397–2409.
4. Antoni FA. Vasopressinergic control of pituitary adrenocorticotropin secretion comes of age. *Front Neuroendocrinol* 1993;14:76–122.
5. Argiolas A, Gessa GL. Central functions of oxytocin. *Neurosci Biobehav Rev* 1991;15:217–231.
6. Barberis C, Audigier S, Durroux T, Elands J, Schmidt A, Jard S. Pharmacology of oxytocin and vasopressin receptors in the central and peripheral nervous system. *Ann NY Acad Sci* 1992;652:39–45.
7. Bohus B, Borrell J, Koolhaas JM, Nyakas C, Buwalda B, Compaan JC, Roozendaal B. The neurohypophysial peptides, learning, and memory processing. *Ann NY Acad Sci* 1993;689:285–299.
8. Brooks PJ, McCarthy MM, Pfaff DW. Novel approaches to the study of oxytocin neurotransmission in the rat brain. *Reg Peptides* 1993;45:159–163.
9. Buijs RM, van Heerikhuize JJ. Vasopressin and oxytocin release in the brain—a synaptic event. *Brain Res* 1982;252:71–76.
10. Buwalda B, Koolhaas JM, Bohus B. Behavioral and cardiac responses to mild stress in young and aged rats: effects of amphetamine and vasopressin. *Physiol Behav* 1992;51:211–216.
11. Caffé AR, Holstege JC, van Leeuwen FW. Vasopressin immunoreactive fibers and neurons in the dorsal pontine tegmentum of the rat, monkey and human. *Prog Brain Res* 1991;88:227–240.
12. Coombes JE, Robinson ICAF, Antoni FA, Russell JA. Release of oxytocin into blood and into cerebrospinal fluid induced by naloxone in anaesthetized morphine-dependent rats: the role of the paraventricular nucleus. *J Neuroendocrinol* 1991;3:551–561.
13. Dantzer R, and Bluthé R-M. Vasopressin and behavior: from memory to olfaction. *Regul Pept* 1993;45:121–125.
14. Demitrack MA, Lesem MD, Brandt HA, Pigott TA, Jimerson DC, Altemus M, Gold PW. Neurohypophyseal dysfunction: implications for the pathophysiology of eating disorders. *Psychopharmacol Bull* 1989;25:439–443.
15. De Vries GJ, Duetz W, Buijs RM, Van Heerikhuize J, Breeburg JTM. Effects of androgens and estrogens on the vasopressin and oxytocin innervation of the adult rat brain. *Brain Res* 1986;399:296–302.
16. de Wied D, Elands J, Kovács G. Interactive effects of neurohypophyseal neuropeptides with receptor antagonists on passive avoidance behavior: mediation by a cerebral neurohypophyseal hormone receptor? *Proc Natl Acad Sci USA* 1991;88:1494–1498.
17. Diamant M, de Wied D. Differential effects of centrally injected AVP on heart rate, core temperature, and behavior in rats. *Am J Physiol* 1993;264:R51–R61.
18. Dreifuss JJ, Raggenbass M. Oxytocin-responsive cells in the mammalian nervous system. *Regul Pept* 1993;45:109–114.
19. Dubois-Dauphin M, Raggenbass M, Widmer H, Tribollet E, Dreifuss JJ. Morphological and electrophysiological evidence for postsynaptic localization of functional oxytocin receptors in the rat dorsal motor nucleus of the vagus nerve. *Brain Res* 1992;575:124–131.
20. Fahrbach SE, Morrell JI, Pfaff DW. Possible role for endogenous oxytocin in estrogen-facilitated maternal behavior in rats. *Neuroendocrinology* 1985;40:526–532.
21. Faiman CP, de-Erausquin GA, Baratti CM. Modulation of memory retrieval by pre-testing vasopressin: involvement of a central cholinergic nicotinic mechanism. *Methods Find Exp Clin Pharmacol* 1992;14:607–613.
22. Fehm-Wolfsdorf G, Born J. Behavioral effects of neurohypophyseal peptides in healthy volunteers: 10 years of research. *Peptides* 1991;12:1399–1406.
23. Ferris CF, Axelson JF, Shinto LH, Albers HE. Scent marking and the maintenance of dominant/subordinate status in male golden hamsters. *Physiol Behav* 1987;40:661–664.
24. Flanagan LM, Dohanics J, Verbalis JG, Stricker EM. Gastric motility and food intake in rats after lesions of hypothalamic paraventricular nucleus. *Am J Physiol* 1992;263:R39–R44.
25. Flanagan LM, Verbalis JG, Stricker EM. Effects of anorexigenic treatments on gastric motility in rats. *Am J Physiol* 1989;256:R955–R961.
26. Gibbs DM. Immunoneutralization of oxytocin attenuates stress-induced corticotropin secretion in the rat. *Regul Pept* 1986;12:273–277.
27. Gomez RE, Cannata MA, Milner TA, Anwar M, Reis DJ, Ruggiero DA. Vasopressinergic mechanisms in the nucleus reticularis lateralis in blood pressure control. *Brain Res* 1993;604:90–105.
28. Grant FD, Reventos J, Gordon JW, Kawabata S, Miller M, Majzoub JA. Expression of the rat arginine vasopressin gene in transgenic mice. *Mol Endocrinol* 1993;7:659–667.
29. Hawthorn J, Ang VTY, Jenkins JS. Effects of lesions in the hypothalamic paraventricular, supraoptic and suprachiasmatic nuclei on vasopressin and oxytocin in rat brain and spinal cord. *Brain Res* 1985;346:51–57.
30. Helmreich DL, Thiels E, Sved AF, Verbalis JG, Stricker EM. Effect

of suckling on gastric motility in lactating rats. *Am J Physiol* 1991;261:R38–R43.

31. Insel TR, Winslow JT, Williams JR, Hastings N, Shapiro LE, Carter CS. The role of neurohypophyseal peptides in the central mediation of complex social processes—evidence from comparative studies. *Regul Pept* 1993;45:127–131.

32. Iványi T, Wiegant VM, de Wied D. Differential effects of emotional and physical stress on the central and peripheral secretion of neuro-hypophysial hormones in male rats. *Life Sci* 1991;48:1309–1316.

33. Jard S, Gaillard RC, Guillon G, Marie J, Schoenenberg P, Muller AF, Manning M, Sawyer WH. Vasopressin antagonists allow demonstration of a novel type of vasopressin receptor in the rat adenohypophysis. *Mol Pharmacol* 1986;30:171–180.

34. Jenkins JS, Nussey SS. The role of oxytocin: present concepts. *Clin Endocrinol* 1991;34:515–525.

35. Jirikowski GF, Sanna PP, Maciejewski-Lenoir D, Bloom FE. Reversal of diabetes insipidus in Brattleboro rats: intrahypothalamic injection of vasopressin mRNA. *Science* 1992;255:996–998.

36. Kasting NW. Criteria for establishing a physiological role for brain peptides. A case in point: the role of vasopressin in thermoregulation during fever and antipyresis. *Brain Res Rev* 1989;14:143–153.

37. Kimura T, Tanizawa O, Mori K, Brownstein MJ, Okayama H. Structure and expression of a human oxytocin receptor. *Nature* 1992;356:526–529.

38. Landgraf R, Malkinson T, Horn T, Veale WL, Lederis K, Pittman QJ. Release of vasopressin and oxytocin by paraventricular stimulation in rats. *Am J Physiol* 1990;258:R155–R159.

39. Lawrence D, Pittman QJ. Response of rat paraventricular neurones with central projections to suckling, haemorrhage or osmotic stimuli. *Brain Res* 1985;341:176–183.

40. Legros J-J, Ansseau M, Timsit-Berthier M. Neurohypophyseal peptides and psychiatric diseases. *Regul Pept* 1993;45:133–138.

41. Lopes da Silva S, De Bree FM, Evans DA, Van Leeuwen FW, Burbach JP. Structure and expression of the vasopressin gene: analysis of mutations, novel genes, and gene products. *Ann NY Acad Sci* 1993;689:492–503.

42. Loup F, Tribollet E, Dubois-Dauphin M, Dreifuss JJ. Localization of high-affinity binding sites for oxytocin and vasopressin in the human brain. An autoradiographic study. *Brain Res* 1991;555:220–232.

43. Maciejewski-Lenoir D, Jirikowski GF, Sanna PP, Bloom FE. Reduction of exogenous vasopressin RNA poly(A) tail length increases its effectiveness in transiently correcting diabetes insipidus in the Brattleboro rat. *Proc Natl Acad Sci USA* 1993;90:1435–1439.

44. Maktabi MA, Elbokl FF, Faraci FM, Todd MM. Halothane decreases the rate of production of cerebrospinal fluid. Possible role of vasopressin V1 receptors. *Anesthesiol* 1993;78:72–82.

45. Manning M, Chan WY, Sawyer WH. Design of cyclic and linear peptide antagonists of vasopressin and oxytocin: current status and future directions. *Regul Pept* 1993;45:279–283.

46. Mazurek MF, Beal MF, Bird ED, Martin JB. Oxytocin in Alzheimer's disease—postmortem brain levels. *Neurology* 1987;37:1001–1003.

47. McCann MJ, Rogers RC. Oxytocin excites gastric-related neurons in rat dorsal vagal complex. *J Physiol* 1990;428:95–108.

48. McCann MJ, Verbalis JG, Stricker EM. LiCl and CCK inhibit gastric emptying and feeding and stimulate OT secretion in rats. *Am J Physiol* 1989;256:R463–R468.

49. Miaskiewicz SL, Stricker EM, Verbalis JG. Neurohypophyseal secretion in response to cholecystokinin but not meal-induced gastric distention in humans. *J Clin Endocrinol Metabol* 1989;68:837–843.

50. Morel A, O'Carroll A-M, Brownstein MJ, Lolait SJ. Molecular cloning and expression of a rat V1a arginine vasopressin receptor. *Nature* 1992;365:523–526.

51. Morris JF, Pow DV. Widespread release of peptides in the central nervous system: quantification of tannic acid-captured exocytoses. *Anat Rec* 1991;231:437–445.

52. Olson BR, Drutarosky MD, Chow M-S, Stricker EM, Hruby VJ, Verbalis JG. Oxytocin and an oxytocin agonist administered centrally decrease food intake in rats. *Peptides* 1991;12:113–118.

53. Olson BR, Hoffman GE, Sved A, Stricker EM, Verbalis JG. Cholecystokinin induces c-*fos* expression in hypothalamic oxytocinergic neurons projecting to the dorsal vagal complex. *Brain Res* 1992;569:238–248.

54. Pedersen CA, Ascher JA, Monroe YL, Prange AJ. Oxytocin induces maternal behavior in virgin female rats. *Science* 1982;216:648–649.

55. Pettibone DJ, Clineschmidt BV, Bock MG, Evans BE, Freidinger RM, Veber DF, Williams PD. Development and pharmacological assessment of novel peptide and nonpeptide oxytocin antagonists. *Regul Pept* 1993;45:289–293.

56. Pietrowsky R, Braun D, Fehm HL, Pauschinger P, Born J. Vasopressin and oxytocin do not influence early sensory processing but affect mood and activation in man. *Peptides* 1991;12:1385–1391.

57. Pittman QJ, Malkinson TJ, Kasting NW, Veale WL. Enhanced fever following castration: possible involvement of brain arginine vasopressin. *Am J Physiol* 1988;254:R513–R517.

58. Plotsky PM. Regulation of hypophysiotropic factors mediating ACTH secretion. *Ann NY Acad Sci* 1987;512:205–217.

59. Raggenbass M, Goumaz M, Sermasi E, Tribollet E, Dreifuss JJ. Vasopressin generates a persistant voltage-dependant sodium current in a mammalian motoneurone. *J Neurosci* 1991;11:1609–1616.

60. Renaud LP, Tang M, McCann MJ, Stricker EM, Verbalis JG. Cholecystokinin and gastric distension activate oxytocinergic cells in rat hypothalamus. *Am J Physiol* 1987;253:R661–R665.

61. Richard P, Moos F, Freund-Mercier M-J. Central effects of oxytocin. *Physiol Rev* 1991;71:331–370.

62. Rogers RC, Hermann GE. Central regulation of brainstem gastric vago-vagal control circuits. In: Ritter S, Ritter RC, Barnes CD, eds. *Neuroanatomy and physiology of abdominal vagal afferents.* Boca Raton, FL: CRC Press, 1992;99–114.

63. Roth J, Schulze K, Simon E, Zeisberger E. Alteration of endotoxin fever and release of arginine vasopressin by dehydration in the guinea pig. *Neuroendocrinology* 1992;56:680–686.

64. Sanna PP, Jirikowski GF, Maciejewski-Lenoir D, Bloom FE. Expression of exogenous vasopressin mRNA by magno-cellular neurons of the supraoptic and paraventricular nuclei in Brattleboro rats. *Ann NY Acad Sci* 1992;652:462–465.

65. Sausville E, Carney D, Battey J. The human vasopressin gene is linked to the oxytocin gene and is selectively expressed in a cultured lung cancer cell line. *J Biol Chem* 1985;260:10236–10241.

66. Sawchenko PE, Arias C, Bittencourt JC. Inhibin β, somatostatin, and enkephalin immunoreactivities coexist in caudal medullary neurons that project to the paraventricular nucleus of the hypothalamus. *J Comp Neurol* 1990;291:269–280.

67. Sawchenko PE, Swanson LW. The organization of noradrenergic pathways from the brainstem to the paraventricular and supraoptic nuclei in the rat. *Brain Res Rev* 1982;4:275–325.

68. Sawchenko PE, Swanson LW. Immunohistochemical identification of neurons in the paraventricular nucleus of the hypothalamus that project to the medulla or to the spinal cord in the rat. *J Comp Neurol* 1982;205:260–272.

69. Sawchenko PE, Swanson LW, Vale W. Corticotropin releasing factor: co-expression within distinct subsets of oxytocin-, vasopressin-, and neurotensin-immunoreactive neurons in the hypothalamus of the adult male rat. *J Neurosci* 1984;4:1118–1129.

70. Stephens LR, Logan SD. Arginine vasopressin stimulates inositol phospholipid metabolism in rat hippocampus. *J Neurochem* 1986;46:649–651.

71. Stricker EM, Zigmond MJ. Brain monoamines, homeostasis, and adaptive behavior. In: Mountcastle VB, Bloom FE, Geiger SR, eds. *Handbook of physiology, section 1: the nervous system.* Bethesda, MD: American Physiological Society, 1986;677–700.

72. Swanson LW. The hypothalamus. In: Björklund A, Hökfelt T, Swanson LW, eds. *Handbook of chemical neuroanatomy.* New York: Elsevier, 1987;5:1–124.

73. Thibonnier M. Vasopressin agonists and antagonists. *Horm Res* 1990;34:124–128.

74. Tolchard S, Ingram CD. Electrophysiological actions of oxytocin in the dorsal vagal complex of the female rat in vitro: changing responsiveness during the oestrous cycle and after steroid treatment. *Brain Res* 1993;609:21–28.

75. Tribollet E. Vasopressin and oxytocin receptors in the rat brain. In: Björklund A, Hökfelt T, Kuhar MJ, eds. *Handbook of chemical neuroanatomy.* New York: Elsevier, 1992;11:289–320.

76. Tribollet E, Audigier S, Dubois-Dauphin M, Dreifuss JJ. Gonadal

steroids regulate oxytocin receptors but not vasopressin receptors in the brain of male and female rats. An autoradiographical study. *Brain Res* 1990;511:129–140.

77. Tribollet E, Dubois-Dauphin M, Dreifuss JJ. Oxytocin receptors in the central nervous system. Distribution, development, and species differences. *Ann NY Acad Sci* 1992;652:29–38.

78. Van Tol HH, Burbach JP. Quantitation of vasopressin and oxytocin messenger RNA levels in the brain. *Methods Enzymol* 1989; 168:398–413.

79. Verbalis JG, McCann MJ, McHale CM, Stricker EM. Oxytocin secretion in response to cholecystokinin and food: differentiation of nausea from satiety. *Science* 1986;232:1417–1419.

80. Verbalis JG, Blackburn RE, Olson BR, Stricker EM. Central oxyto-cin inhibition of food and salt ingestion: a mechanism for intake regulation of solute homeostasis. *Regul Pept* 1993;45:149–154.

81. Voorn P, Buijs RM. An immuno-electronmicroscopical study comparing vasopressin, oxytocin, substance-P and enkephalin containing nerve terminals in the nucleus of the solitary tract of the rat. *Brain Res* 1983;270:169–173.

82. Watts AG, Swanson LW. Efferent projections of the suprachiasmatic nucleus. 1. Studies using anterograde transport of phaseolus vulgaris leucoagglutinin in the rat. *J Comp Neurol* 1987;258:230–252.

83. Wolters EC, Riekkinen P, Lowenthal A, Van der Plaats JJ, Zwart JMT, Sennef C. DGAVP (Org 5667) in early Alzheimer's disease patients: an international double-blind, placebo-controlled, multicenter trial. *Neurology* 1990;40:1099–1101.

Psychopharmacology: The Fourth Generation of Progress, edited by Floyd E. Bloom and David J. Kupfer. Raven Press, Ltd., New York © 1995.

CHAPTER **48**

Neuropeptide Y and Related Peptides

Claes Wahlestedt and Markus Heilig

THE NPY FAMILY OF PEPTIDES

NPY and Related Peptides

Avian pancreatic polypeptide (PP) was initially discovered as a by-product of insulin isolation (41), and was subsequently isolated from many other species. Although perhaps of little physiological significance, PP served as a predecessor of neuropeptide Y (NPY) and peptide YY (PYY). Using a technique to isolate peptides with C-terminal α-amide groups, Tatemoto and Mutt (62) reported that porcine brain and gut contained large amounts of a peptide resembling PP. The PP-like peptide isolated from gut was named peptide YY (PYY) because of its N- and C-terminal tyrosine (Y being the abbreviation for tyrosine in the single-letter amino acid code). At first PYY (61) was also thought to be the PP-like peptide in the brain but subsequent work showed the (predominant) brain peptide to differ from PYY, and because of its occurrence in brain, it was named neuropeptide Y (NPY) (63). Finally, a fourth nonmammalian 37-amino-acid, nonamidated member of the peptide family, pancreatic peptide Y (PY), was found in fish which showed 64% sequence identity to both NPY and PYY (5).

NPY, PYY, and PP are often said to belong to the "pancreatic polypeptide family." However, because of the fact that NPY has been much more conserved during evolution and also exhibits much greater biological activity when compared to PP, this peptide family should more appropriately be called the NPY family (43) (see also Chapters 18, 30, and 43, *this volume*).

C. Wahlestedt: Department of Neurology and Neuroscience, Cornell University Medical College, New York, New York; *current address* Astra Pain Research Unit, Laval, Quebec, H7V4A7 Canada.
M. Heilig: Department of Psychiatry and Neurochemistry, University of Göteborg, S-431 80 Mölndal, Sweden.

NPY Is Highly Conserved Through Evolution

Porcine NPY and PYY have 69% sequence homology and activate most NPY-responsive receptors with similar potencies as described below. In contrast, PP shows low efficacy and potency compared to NPY and PYY.

Currently, over 50 sequences of peptides belonging to the NPY family are available (43). Sequence comparison data indicate that NPY is one of the most highly conserved neuroendocrine peptides known; for example, human NPY is 92% identical to torpedo NPY (43). Many investigators have suggested that such a remarkable conservation of NPY would imply an important functional role(s) for this peptide, perhaps one or several of those described below.

Certain Structural Features Are Common to NPY Family Members

A characteristic tertiary structure is observed in NPY (as well as in PYY and PP) which consists of an N-terminal polyproline helix (residues 1–8) and an amphiphilic α-helix (residues 15–30), connected with a β-turn, creating a hairpin-like loop (see ref. 21). This domain has been identified from the crystal structure of avian PP, and nuclear magnetic resonance (NMR) studies also agree well with this three-dimensional configuration. The helices are kept together by hydrophobic interactions. The amidated C-terminal end (residues 30–36) projects away from the hairpin loop (4).

NPY Is Widely Distributed in the Body

Central Nervous System

Neurons displaying NPY-like immunoreactivity are abundant in the central nervous system (CNS), most nota-

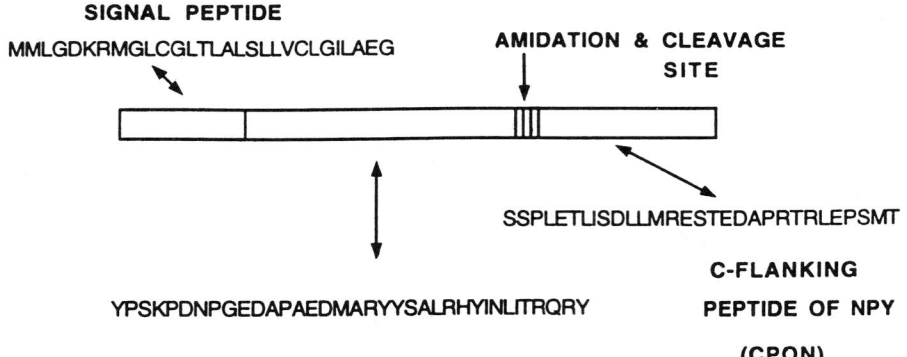

SIGNAL PEPTIDE

MMLGDKRMGLCGLTLALSLLVCLGILAEG

AMIDATION & CLEAVAGE SITE

SSPLETLISDLLMRESTEDAPRTRLEPSMT

C-FLANKING PEPTIDE OF NPY (CPON)

YPSKPDNPGEDAPAEDMARYYSALRHYINLITRQRY

NEUROPEPTIDE Y

FIG. 1. Schematic representation of the predicted precursor for rat NPY. The amino acids are shown in single-letter code. (Adapted from ref. 3.)

bly in the so-called limbic structures (14,34). Immunohistochemical studies indicate that NPY is present within very similar neurons throughout the cerebral cortex and forebrain nuclei, but is contained in a variety of neurons in the hypothalamus, brainstem, and spinal cord. Coexistence with somatostatin and NADPH-diaphorase/nitric oxide synthase is common in cortex and striatum. Although NPY neurons in the latter brain regions receive few inputs, they make numerous contacts with dendrites, including GABAergic neurons. NPY is also extensively colocalized with GABA in the cortex, but not in the striatum (6).

Many studies (reviewed in ref. 34) have demonstrated the occurrence of NPY in a variety of brainstem monoaminergic neurons—that is, arguing coexistence of the peptide with (i) norepinephrine (the A1 group in the ventrolateral medulla, the A2 group of the dorsal medulla and the locus coeruleus), (ii) epinephrine (C1 and C2 groups and solitary nucleus), or (iii) serotonin (nucleus raphe pallidus). It is sometimes overlooked that NPY occurs also in nonmonoaminergic brainstem cranial nerve nuclei.

Unlike the case of NPY, PYY-containing neurons are few in brain and are primarily confined to the brainstem and the cervical spinal cord (10,16). Finally, PP-positive neurons have not been found in the CNS.

Peripheral Nervous System

The existence of NPY in most sympathetic nerve fibers, particularly around blood vessels (i.e., perivascular fibers), has generated much interest (66). There are dense plexuses of NPY-like immunoreactivity (NPY-LI) found in vascular beds throughout the body. In addition, NPY also occurs in nonadrenergic perivascular, enteric, and cardiac nonsympathetic and parasympathetic nerves (60,66).

In contrast, PYY occurs primarily in endocrine cells of the lower gastrointestinal tract. However, low amounts of PYY immunoreactivity are also found in certain sympathetic fibers. PP is predominantly located in endocrine cells of the pancreatic islets (60).

NPY Gene Expression Is Tightly Regulated

Human NPY cDNA was originally cloned from a pheochromocytoma (48), a tumor of the adrenal medulla known to often contain high levels of NPY. The corresponding mRNA contained a single open reading frame that predicted a fairly simple precursor for NPY, consisting of 97 amino acids. The predicted precursor (Fig. 1) contains a hydrophobic 28-amino-acid signal peptide that is required for entry into the lumen of the endoplasmic reticulum (ER) and thus, entry into the secretory compartment of the cell. The signal peptide is then cleaved, and the resulting prohormone is 69 amino acids in length. There is no peptide flanking the N-terminus of NPY, as in several other peptides. However, in the prohormone, mature NPY (36 amino acids) is flanked at its C-terminus by 33 amino acids, three of which are the glycine–lysine–arginine motif, necessary for NPY amidation (a feature that is critical for all known actions of NPY with the exception of mast cell degranulation; see ref. 55). The peptide formed by the remaining 30 amino acids of the precursor has been named CPON (C flanking peptide of NPY). Although CPON has been found to be highly conserved (not to the same extent as NPY, but at a level comparable to that of insulin; see ref. 43), its function remains unknown. As expected, CPON is found in every cell that produces NPY, and the two peptides are consequently co-released (4,59).

The NPY gene is expressed in cells derived from the neural crest, and several factors are involved in its regulation. Consensus sequences for a number of DNA-binding proteins that could act as regulatory factors are contained within the NPY gene. These include five potential GC-rich SP-1 binding sites: two CCCCTC sites, a partial CAAT box, and one AP-1 binding site (3). Additional factors regulating NPY gene expression include activators of cyclic AMP and calcium- or phospholipid-dependent protein kinases (3,53).

NPY RECEPTORS

NPY Receptors Are Widely Distributed

Similar to "classical" neurotransmitters (e.g., its frequent coexistence partner, norepinephrine), NPY seems to have a wide range of effects on peripheral (blood vessels, heart, airways, gastrointestinal tract, kidney, pancreas, thyroid gland, platelet, mast cells, and sympathetic, parasympathetic and sensory nerves) and central (effects on pituitary hormone release, behavior, central autonomic control, and other neurotransmitter mechanisms) targets (reviewed in refs. 66 and 69). A number of these actions appear to be exerted by NPY per se, whereas others occur as a result of modulatory interactions with other agents—for example, norepinephrine and glutamate (66,69). In any case, it is likely that NPY (as well as its related peptides) acts upon membrane receptors that are linked to G proteins (66,69). When radioreceptor ligand studies employing radiolabeled NPY or PYY were conducted, binding sites in brain and peripheral organs—including vasculature, heart, kidney, spleen, and uvea—were detected (e.g., see refs. 66 and 74).

NPY Receptors Are Heterogeneous

Y1 and Y2 Receptors

Based on studies of sympathetic neuroeffector junctions, it was first proposed that there was heterogeneity among NPY/PYY receptors, specifically Y1 and Y2 receptor subclasses (73); this was later corroborated in other cell types and experimental systems (reviewed in refs. 66 and 69). Already by the mid-1980s, three types of NPY effects at sympathetic neuroeffector junctions were known: (i) a direct postjunctional response, (e.g., vasoconstriction manifested in certain vascular beds), (ii) a postjunctional potentiating effect on norepinephrine-evoked vasoconstriction, and (iii) a prejunctional suppression of stimulated norepinephrine release (73). [The two latter phenomena are probably reciprocal; thus, norepinephrine may affect NPY mechanisms similarly (69).] In principle, long C-terminal amidated fragments of NPY and PYY are essentially inactive in the assays for postjunctional activity (direct as well as potentiating effect), while retaining their efficacy prejunctionally (inhibition of transmitter release). On the basis of the selective prejunctional effect of C-terminal NPY (or PYY) fragments, it was thus proposed that NPY/PYY receptor subtypes may exist (73). The nomenclature Y1 and Y2 was introduced to denote the receptor that required the entire NPY (or PYY) molecule for activation (Y1), and the other receptor subtype which was selectively stimulated by the long C-terminal NPY (or PYY) fragments (Y2) (68). In the neuromuscular preparations, the postjunctional receptors were thus (predominantly) of the Y1-subtype.

Y3 Receptors

It has become apparent in recent years that some actions of NPY cannot be mimicked by PYY. This has been the

major argument supporting the existence of an exclusively NPY-responsive Y3-type receptor. This receptor is likely to be present in, for example, adrenal medulla, heart, and brainstem (21).

Features of the Y1 Receptor

Presence on Vascular Smooth Muscle Cells

Initial bioactivity studies suggested that the Y1 receptor is postjunctional at the vascular sympathetic neuroeffector junction (73) and is the sole mediator of pressor responses to NPY (66). The recent cloning of the Y1 receptor cDNA has provided strong evidence (see ref. 42) that fully supports the concept that vascular smooth muscle cells express the Y1 receptor.

Restricted Brain Distribution of the Y1 Receptor

Autoradiography studies using [Pro[34]]NPY, a Y1 receptor agonist, on frozen sections of rat brain have shown that Y1 receptors are discrete (being much less abundant than Y2 receptors) and mainly localized in distinct layers of the cerebral cortex, anterior olfactory nucleus, amygdala, and a few thalamic and hypothalamic nuclei (1,15,66). Furthermore, in situ hybridization with rat Y1 receptor cDNA (see below) has localized expression of this receptor protein in thalamus, cerebral cortex, dentate gyrus of hippocampus, and arcuate nucleus of hypothalamus (17,66).

In the CNS the Y1 receptor has been associated with a number of biological actions—for instance, with anxiolysis and stimulation of luteinizing-hormone-releasing hormone (LHRH) release (see refs. 66 and 69). However, it is possible that the pronounced effect of NPY on feeding (see below) is mediated through a receptor that is similar but not identical to Y1.

Requirement of Both N- and C-Termini for Y1 Receptor Activation

NPY and its related peptides are capable of retaining their distinct tertiary structure in solution, in contrast to most other small peptide messengers (64). There has been considerable interest in structure–function studies of NPY-related peptides in attempts to develop receptor-specific agonists and antagonists. These experiments were extensively examined using various NPY fragments and analogues both in receptor assays and different biological preparations. In general, PYY and NPY are equipotent and equally effective in all Y1 (and Y2) receptor assays studied (69). A characteristic of the Y1 receptor is that truncation of the first N-terminal residue Tyr[1] (NPY 2-36) results in a marked loss of biological activity or affinity (21). The hairpin loop of NPY is thought to present the N- and C-termini closely together for recognition at the Y1 receptor (21).

Molecular Biology of the Y1 Receptor

The Y1 receptor was first cloned as an "orphan" (unidentified) receptor candidate from a rat forebrain cDNA library by a technique that relied on its homology with already cloned members of the G-protein-coupled superfamily of receptors (17). The receptor was subsequently identified as Y1, and the human homologue was isolated (35;42).

Features of the Y2 Receptor

In the periphery, Y2 receptors are generally considered to be localized at prejunctional sites of autonomic fibers, where they suppress the release of transmitters (66).

Brain Distribution of Y2 Receptors

A differential localization of Y1 and Y2 receptors has been suggested by autoradiographic data from rat brain using radiolabeled PYY, displaced with Y1 or Y2 selective ligands (1,15). It appears that the Y2 receptor is the quantitatively predominant NPY/PYY receptor type in the rat brain (1,15,74).

There is a dense population of Y2 receptors in the hippocampus (1,15). Electrophysiological studies have suggested the existence of Y2 receptors on excitatory (glutamatergic) inputs to rat hippocampal CA1 neurons (13). NPY has been shown to affect memory processing in a complex manner, possibly reflecting a Y2-receptor-mediated action in the rostral part of the hippocampus (18). The presence of Y2 receptors, and associated inhibition of Ca^{2+} influx, has also been found in rat dorsal root ganglion neurons (9).

The C-terminus of NPY is sufficient to activate the Y2 receptor. Unlike the case of the Y1 receptor, NPY 2-36 is about equipotent with NPY or PYY, and N-terminally truncated NPY fragments from NPY 2-36 to 22-36 are rather potent.

Biochemistry/Molecular Biology of Y2 Receptors

The gene encoding the Y2 receptor has not yet been cloned. At present, several groups are pursuing its biochemical isolation using affinity labeling techniques to probe the structure of Y2 receptors from several species and tissues, notably hippocampus and kidney (see ref. 21).

Features of the Y3 Receptor

PYY Has Low Affinity to the Y3 Receptor

The pharmacological order of potency of NPY and its related peptides differs markedly from those of Y1/Y2 receptors in several binding and bioactivity studies on various tissues and cultured cells, which provides support for the existence of a Y3 receptor (66). The main characteristic of these Y3 receptors is that they recognize NPY, while PYY is several orders of magnitude less potent.

Functional Y3 Receptors in the Brain

Injections of NPY and related peptides into the nucleus of the solitary tract (NTS) were recently used to characterize the receptors mediating the evoked cardiovascular effects (22). The pharmacological profile of this response, which is associated with inhibition of glutamate, suggests that the Y3 receptor may be involved (22). These Y3 receptors may also be located in the hippocampus, because NPY, [Leu^{31},Pro^{34}]NPY, and NPY 13-36, but not PYY or PP, were found to potentiate the excitatory response to the glutamate-receptor agonist *N*-methyl-D-aspartate (NMDA) in CA3 neurons of rat hippocampus (49). However, a recent slice-patch study showed that NPY produced no changes in NMDA conductances in CA3 pyramidal neurons (47).

Do Additional Receptor Subtypes Exist?

Several lines of evidence have suggested further heterogeneity among the NPY receptors. First, and perhaps most important, it may be that food intake is mediated by a hypothalamic receptor that is similar, but not identical, to the Y1 receptor. Thus, central administration of NPY potently stimulates feeding behavior in rats, and this effect can be mimicked by the Y1 agonist [Leu^{31},Pro^{34}]-NPY, whereas the Y2 agonist NPY 13-36 is much less active. However, uncharacteristic of the Y1 receptor, NPY 2-36 is at least as potent as NPY itself (for references, see ref. 57). Second, although controversial, it has been proposed that NPY and PYY may bind to brain sigma and phencyclidine binding sites (52). Third, a drosophila NPY receptor was recently cloned (45), but it is not yet clear if mammalian homologues exist. Finally, it is unlikely that NPY-induced mast cell degranulation is mediated by any of the defined NPY receptor types, but rather may be the result of direct G-protein activation (55).

NPY Receptors Signal Through G Proteins

Inhibition of cAMP Accumulation

There is much evidence indicating that most, if not all NPY/PYY receptors are coupled to inhibition of adenylate cyclase and, consequently, decreased levels of cAMP (66).

Elevated Intracellular Ca²⁺

NPY has been observed to raise intracellular Ca^{2+} levels in many cell types (66). It is controversial whether NPY affects Ca^{2+} by stimulating phosphatidyl inositide (PI) turnover.

Second Messengers and NPY Receptor Subtypes

The study of second messenger systems may not be useful in distinguishing receptor subtypes because the Y1, Y2, and Y3 receptors appear to be capable of activating the same intracellular pathways in many systems, causing the reduction of cAMP accumulation and elevation of intracellular Ca^{2+} concentrations (66). Currently, it is not known if one or more G proteins (probably Gi and/or Go) mediate the coupling to cAMP and Ca^{2+}. This dual coupling is also a feature of the cloned Y1 receptor (35,42).

NPY IN BRAIN FUNCTION AND DYSFUNCTION

Some Hypothalamic Actions Suggest a Role of NPY in Psychiatric Illness

Among numerous actions of central NPY, the peptide exerts a profound influence on some hypothalamic systems which are thought to be dysregulated in depressive syndrome—for example, circadian rhythms, the hypothalamic–pituitary–adrenal (HPA) axis, and food intake.

NPY and Circadian Rhythms

NPY is present in a pathway from the thalamic ventrolateral geniculate to the hypothalamic suprachiasmatic nucleus (SCN), the major entraining pacemaker of the mammalian brain (50). When NPY (or avian PP) was injected into the SCN of hamsters kept under constant light, the free-running rhythm of the animals was shifted in a phase-dependent manner. The length of the activity phase was not affected. The effects resembled those of dark pulses and seemed to be highly localized, because they were not reproduced by intracerebroventricular (i.c.v.) injection of NPY (2).

NPY and the HPA Axis

NPY administered into the hypothalamic paraventricular nucleus (PVN) produced an increase in plasma adreno-corticotropic hormone (ACTH) and corticosterone (72). After i.c.v. administration, low NPY doses suppressed corticosterone secretion, whereas higher doses increased both ACTH and corticosterone levels (25). NPY fibers innervate corticotropin-releasing factor (CRF) cells of the PVN (46), and NPY administration increases hypothalamic CRF levels (23). The release of CRF seems to be stimulated by NPY (65). Mediation of this action through α_2-adrenoceptors has been suggested (24). Postsynaptic action of CRF seems also to be potentiated by NPY. In dog the ACTH response to NPY was partially blocked by a CRF antagonist, while a subthreshold dose of NPY potentiated the effects of exogenous CRF (36).

NPY and Feeding

When injected centrally with NPY (or PYY > PP), mammals eat excessively. This effect of NPY has been characterized in numerous elegant studies, recently reviewed in ref. 57. NPY's appetitive action is hypothalamically mediated, although the precise site within the hypothalamus is a matter of some debate. Several groups found the magnitude of NPY-induced feeding to be higher than that induced by any pharmacological agent previously tested, and also extremely long-lasting (e.g., see refs. 12,44, and 57). NPY-induced stimulation of feeding has been reproduced in a number of species (e.g., see ref. 57). Among the three basic macronutrients (fat, protein, and carbohydrate), the intake of carbohydrates was preferentially stimulated (57). Drinking was affected in a much less consistent manner, which, in addition, varied with species (e.g., see refs. 51 and 57). No tolerance was seen towards the orexigenic effect of NPY, and when administration of the peptide was repeated over 10 days, a marked increase in the rate of weight gain was observed (57). Following starvation, the concentration of NPY in the hypothalamic PVN increased with time, and it returned rapidly to control levels following food ingestion (54). This indicates that pharmacological effects of NPY on food intake may be representative of inherent physiological mechanisms. Such a conclusion is also directly supported by push–pull studies of hypothalamic NPY release and its inverse correlation with satiety (37). Because C-terminal fragments of NPY capable of activating Y2 receptors do not induce food intake, it has initially been assumed that the orexigenic action of NPY is mediated by Y1 receptors. Converging data from structure–activity studies (57,66) and from work with in vivo antisense blockade of Y1-receptor synthesis (see below) suggest, however, that an NPY receptor different from the cloned Y1 species may be involved.

The role of NPY in regulation of appetite may be of clinical relevance in itself. Elevated CSF content of NPY has been reported both in underweight amenorrheic anorectics and in the same amenorrheic patients restudied within 6 weeks after weight restoration. An inverse relationship between CSF NPY and caloric intake in healthy volunteer women was also found. Thus, the increase in CSF levels of NPY may be a secondary, compensatory response to decreased food intake. Also, because NPY regulates a number of endocrine parameters including the secretion of luteinizing hormone (LH), follicle-stimulating hormone (FSH), and ACTH, several symptoms of anorexia could be secondary to such an increase in NPY secretion (39,40).

NPY and Depressive Illness

What direct evidence is there then, to link NPY with the pathogenesis of any psychiatric illness? The levels of NPY-LI were decreased in the CSF of patients with major depression, compared to sex- and age-matched controls (77). The chromatography profiles of immunoreactive material differed between patients and controls (77). This seemed to indicate the processing of the NPY precursor to be altered in depression. Recently, marked reductions of tissue levels of NPY-LI were reported in suicide victims. Particularly dramatic reduction was seen in subjects with a verified diagnosis of major depression (76). The difficulties of purely descriptive radioimmunoassay (RIA)-based studies are however, illustrated by the fact that using an assay based on a different antibody, Berrettini et al. (8) did not find a decrease in CSF NPY-LI in depressed patients.

Increased levels of NPY-LI were found in rat brain tissue after chronic treatment with tricyclic antidepressants (TADs). The most consistent increases were seen in frontal cortical areas (32). Using assays with differing epitope-specificity as well as mRNA quantitation, variable results have been obtained by others, perhaps indicating an altered processing of NPY rather than increased synthesis as a result of TAD treatment (7,56). Another treatment known to be effective for depressive illness, electroconvulsive shocks (ECS), has yielded more consistent results. In several studies by different groups, ECS produced increased tissue levels of NPY-LI in frontal cortical and in hippocampal areas (58,67). Increased tissue levels can be due to increased synthesis or decreased utilization. Therefore, studies aimed at quantitating the actual level of transcription are needed. Interestingly, lithium was found to enhance NPY (but not proenkephalin) gene expression (75).

Olfactory bulbectomy has been suggested as an animal model of depression. Bulbectomized rats kill mice ("muricide behavior"). This behavior is inhibited by chronic treatment with antidepressant drugs, but also by injecting norepinephrine (NE) into the central nucleus of the amygdala. This "antidepressant" action of NE is markedly potentiated by NPY (38) (see also Chapter 84, this volume).

Cocaine withdrawal produces depressive symptoms, among which anhedonia (i.e., an inability to experience pleasure) is prominent. The anhedonia of cocaine withdrawal is closely related to that of "endogenous" depression and is effectively treated with conventional antidepressant therapy. Chronic cocaine administration to rats decreased levels of both NPY-LI and NPY mRNA in brain areas important for mechanisms of reward, such as the nucleus accumbens. The decrease persisted after cocaine administration was discontinued, possibly in parallel to the decrease in NPY-LI seen in the CSF and brain tissue of depressed patients. Transsynaptic mechanisms seem to be involved in cocaine's suppression of NPY synthesis, because lesions of medial prefrontal cortex prevented this action of the drug (70) (see also Chapters 66 and 145, this volume).

NPY and Anxiety

A lack of correlation between severity of depression and NPY-LI levels argued against a direct, causal relationship between the two. A strong negative correlation was however, seen between anxiety scores and NPY-LI levels in the CSF of depressed patients (28). Anxiety is a core component of the depressive syndrome, and the two psychopathological states may share a common biological basis because both respond to chronic TAD treatment. Shortly following its isolation, it was reported that i.c.v. administered NPY produced a synchronization of the electroencephalogram (19). As a behavioral correlate, a decrease of locomotor activity was seen both in a familiar environment (the home cage of the animal) and in a novel environment (open field) (27). These effects were dose-dependent and fully reversible. In other experiments, i.c.v. administration of NPY to a large extent prevented gastric ulceration induced by a strong stressor, water restraint (26). Thus, both electrophysiological and behavioral observations were compatible with a sedative/anxiolytic action of the peptide. In agreement with such a hypothesis, i.c.v. administration of nanomolar doses of NPY produced a marked anxiolytic-like action in several pharmacologically and ethologically validated animal models of anxiety, including Vogel's punished drinking test, the elevated plus-maze (31), and Geller-Seifter's operant punished responding test (30).

As mentioned above, i.c.v. administration of NPY is known to dramatically increase food intake. Control experiments indicated that the anxiolytic-like action of NPY was specific, and not related to the orexigenic properties of the peptide. In addition, the anxiolytic-like action of NPY was also present in the elevated plus-maze, and this exploratory anxiety model does not involve consummatory behaviors (31). It remained, however, a concern whether the apparent anxiolytic-like action of NPY was in some way related to NPY's effects on appetite. To address this issue, studies were performed to separate these two actions of NPY anatomically. The amygdala is a key structure in central integration of emotionally relevant information, and it seems to encode the stressful effect of aversive inputs. Local microinjections of NPY into the central nucleus of the amygdala reproduced the anxiolytic-like effect of i.c.v. injections with an ED_{50} of less than 50 pmol/side, but did not affect food intake (29). Thus, the actions of NPY on appetite and anxiety can be both anatomically and functionally separated, and seem to be independent of each other.

Mediation of NPY's action on anxiety by the central nucleus of the amygdala is also interesting in the context of NPY's ability to protect against stress-induced gastric ulcers (see above). The amygdala integrates autonomic responses associated with emotion, and the central nucleus in particular may be the point of output to areas controlling visceral responses to such information. The central nucleus receives a dense NPY-ergic innervation (11) which innervates neurons projecting to the dorsal vagal complex (20). Interactions between NPY and NE may be of importance for NPY's stress protective action. NPY-positive terminals in the central nucleus originate largely from cell bodies in the NTS, in a majority of which NPY is colocalized with NE (50).

With possible drug design in mind, a crucial question was which type of NPY receptors mediate the actions of the peptide on anxiety. After i.c.v. administration, intact NPY was "anxiolytic", whereas a C-terminal fragment with relative preference for the Y2-receptor, NPY 13-36, was not (31,33). This suggested the effects of NPY on anxiety to be mediated by Y1 receptors. Subsequently, local injections of NPY receptor agonists into the amygdala showed that NPY itself and the highly selective Y1-receptor agonist [Leu^{31},Pro^{34}]NPY were roughly equipotent with respect to their anxiolytic-like action. The fragment NPY 13-36 produced only marginal effects (29). The accumulated evidence thus suggests the anxiolytic-like action of NPY to be mediated by Y1 receptors in the amygdala.

The strongest evidence for a Y1 mediation of NPY's anxiolytic-like action is supplied by experiments performed to address a related question. While an anxiolytic-like action of exogenously administered NPY seems to be well established and highly specific, it does not constitute conclusive evidence for a similar action of the endogenous transmitter. Similar to the situation with most peptide mediators, the lack of specific receptor antagonists has made it difficult to establish such a role for endogenous NPY. We have attempted to circumvent this difficulty by a novel approach. Short antisense oligonucleotides complementary to a specific mRNA can be taken up through receptor-mediated endocytosis, and they inhibit the translation of a specific message into functional protein. We administered an 18-mer antisense oligonucleotide targeted at the Y1-receptor message using repeated

i.c.v. injections. This led to a 60% decrease in the B_{max} of Y1-type binding, without affecting Y2 receptors. The decrease in Y1 receptors was accompanied by marked signs of anxiety in one of our standard animal models, the elevated plus-maze, in which NPY itself is markedly "anxiolytic" (71). This provides evidence that endogenous NPY acts in an anxiolytic-like manner by activating Y1 receptors, and that disturbed NPY transmission leads to symptoms of anxiety.

It can be noted that no effects were seen on food intake after the antisense blockade of Y1 receptor synthesis. While not conclusive, this observation suggests that hypothalamic NPY receptors involved in food intake regulation may differ from the cloned Y1 receptor (see above). On the basis of differing pharmacological profiles, this has independently been suggested by others (reviewed in ref. 66; also see Chapter 111, *this volume*).

NPY-Containing Neurons Are Relatively Unaffected by Neurodegenerative Disorders

While it deserves mention that NPY-containing neurons show a potential to survive even advanced cases of neurodegenerative disorders (i.e., Huntington's, Alzheimer's, and Parkinson's disease), it is difficult to conceive that NPY plays any unique role in these disorders and, consequently, that potential NPY-ergic drugs may significantly benefit such patients.

CONCLUDING REMARKS: POTENTIAL USE OF NPY-RELATED DRUGS IN NEUROPSYCHIATRIC DISORDERS

No NPY antagonists, in the classical pharmacological meaning, with reasonable potency and/or receptor selectivity have yet gained full acceptance. Moreover, no nonpeptide agonist has been described (66).

First, a centrally acting Y1 agonist will most certainly have anxiolytic properties. Conversely, a Y1 receptor antisense oligodeoxynucleotide, administered directly into the brain of rats, was shown to be markedly anxiogenic, implying that endogenous NPY mechanisms act to tonically relieve anxiety (71). A nonpeptide (and nonbenzodiazepine) anxiolytic drug that mimics NPY at Y1 receptors might find a place in the treatment of affective disorders, including major depression as well as the clinically similar condition that often follows psychostimulant (e.g., cocaine) withdrawal. The latter syndromes have been associated with reduced brain NPY synthesis and, quite often, with severe anxiety.

Second, many investigators work towards the development of a centrally acting NPY antagonist effectively suppressing feeding elicited by (endogenous) NPY. Interestingly, several lines of evidence have recently pointed to the possibility that an "atypical" (not Y1, Y2, or Y3) hypothalamic receptor is involved in this robust feeding response. Hence, in theory it might be possible to find an antagonist capable of suppressing food intake, with specific affinity to the "atypical" hypothalamic NPY receptor, and thereby to avoid possible side effects associated with Y1, Y2, or Y3 receptors.

REFERENCES

1. Aicher SA, Springston M, Berger SB, Reis DJ, Wahlestedt C. Receptor-selective analogs demonstrate NPY/PYY receptor heterogeneity in rat brain. *Neurosci Lett* 1990;130:32–36.
2. Albers HE, Ferris CF, Leeman SE, Goldman BD. Avian pancreatic polypeptide phase shifts hamster circadian rhythms when microinjected into the suprachiasmatic region. *Science* 1984;223:833–835.
3. Allen JM, Balbi D. Structure and expression of the neuropeptide Y gene. In: Colmers WF, Wahlestedt C, eds. *The biology of neuropeptide Y and related peptides.* Totowa, NJ: Humana Press, 1993;43–64.
4. Allen J, Novotny J, Martin J, Heinrich G. Molecular structure of mammalian neuropeptide Y: analysis by molecular cloning and computer-aided comparison with crystal structure of avian homologue. *Proc Natl Acad Sci USA* 1987;84:2532–2536.
5. Andrews PC, Hawke D, Shively JE, Dixon JE. A nonamidated peptide homologous to porcine peptide YY and neuropeptide YY. *Endocrinology* 1985;116:2677–2681.
6. Aoki C, Pickel VM. Neuropeptide Y in cortex and striatum: ultrastructural distribution and coexistence with classical neurotransmitters and neuropeptides. *Ann NY Acad Sci* 1990;611:186–205.
7. Bellmann R, Sperk G. Effects of antidepressant drug treatment on levels of NPY or prepro-NPY-mRNA in the rat brain. *Neurochem Int* 1993;22:183–187.
8. Berrettini WH, Doran AR, Kelsoe J, Roy A, Pickar D. Cerebrospinal fluid neuropeptide Y in depression and schizophrenia. *Neuropsychopharmacology* 1987;1(1):81–83.
9. Bleakman D, Colmers WF, Fournier A, Miller RJ. Neuropeptide Y inhibits Ca²⁺ influx into cultured dorsal root ganglion neurones of the rat via a Y2 receptor. *Br J Pharmacol* 1991;103:1781–1789.
10. Brommé M, Hökfelt T, Terenius L. Peptide YY (PYY)-immunoreactive neurons in the lower brainstem and spinal cord of the rat. *Acta Physiol Scand* 1985;125:340–352.
11. Chronwall BM, DiMaggio DA, Massari VJ, Pickel VM, Ruggiero DA, O'Donohue TL. The anatomy of neuropeptide-Y-containing neurons in rat brain. *Neuroscience* 1985;15:1159–1181.
12. Clark JT, Kalra PS, Crowley WR, Kalra SP. Neuropeptide Y and human pancreatic polypeptide stimulate feeding behavior in rats. *Endocrinology* 1984;115:427–429.
13. Colmers WF, Klapstein GJ, Fournier A, St-Pierre S, Treherne KA. Presynaptic inhibition by neuropeptide Y in rat hippocampal slice in vitro is mediated by a Y2 receptor. *Br J Pharmacol* 1991;102:41–44.
14. De Quidt ME, Emson PC. Distribution of neuropeptide Y-like immunoreactivity in the rat central nervous system. II. Immunohistochemical analysis. *Neuroscience* 1986;18:545–618.
15. Dumont Y, Fournier A, St Pierre S, Quirion R. Comparative characterization and autoradiographic distribution of neuropeptide Y receptor subtypes in the rat brain. *J Neurosci* 1993;13:73–86.
16. Ekman R, Wahlestedt C, Böttcher G, Håkanson R, Panula P. Peptide YY-like immunoreactivity in the central nervous system of the rat. *Regul Pept* 1986;16:157–168.
17. Eva C, Keinänen K, Monyer H, Seeburg P, Sprengel R. Molecular cloning of a novel G protein-coupled receptor that may belong to the neuropeptide receptor family. *FEBS Lett* 1990;271:80–84.
18. Flood JF, Morley JE. Dissociation of the effects of neuropeptide Y in feeding and memory: evidence for pre- and postsynaptic mediation. *Peptides* 1989;10:963–966.
19. Fuxe K, Agnati LF, Härfstrand A, Zini I, Tatemoto K, Pich EM, Hökfelt T, Mutt V, Terenius L. Central administration of neuropeptide Y induces hypotension, bradypnea and EEG synchronization in the rat. *Acta Physiol Scand* 1983;118:189–192.
20. Gray TS, O'Donohue TL, Magnuson DJ. Neuropeptide Y innervation of amygdaloid and hypothalamic neurons that project to the dorsal vagal complex in rat. *Peptides* 1986;7:341–349.
21. Grundemar L, Sheikh SP, Wahlestedt C. Characterization of receptor types for neuropeptide Y and related peptides. In: Colmers WF, Wahlestedt C, eds. *The biology of neuropeptide Y and related peptides.* Totowa, NJ: Humana Press, 1993;197–239.
22. Grundemar L, Wahlestedt C, Reis DJ. Neuropeptide Y acts at an atypical receptor to evoke cardiovascular depression and to inhibit glutamate responsiveness in the brainstem. *J Pharmacol Exp Ther* 1991;258:633–638.
23. Haas DA, George SR. Neuropeptide Y administration acutely increases hypothalamic corticotropin-releasing factor immunoreactivity: lack of effect in other rat brain regions. *Life Sci* 1987;41:2725–2731.
24. Haas DA, George SR. Neuropeptide Y-induced effects on hypothalamic corticotropin-releasing factor content and release are dependent on noradrenergic/adrenergic neurotransmission. *Brain Res* 1989;498:333–338.
25. Härfstrand A, Eneroth P, Agnati L, Fuxe K. Further studies on the effects of central administration of neuropeptide Y on neuroendocrine function in the male rat: relationship to hypothalamic catecholamines. *Regul Pept* 1987;17:167–179.
26. Heilig M, Murison R. Intracerebroventricular neuropeptide Y protects against stress-induced gastric erosion in the rat. *Eur J Pharmacol* 1987;137:127–129.
27. Heilig M, Murison R. Intracerebroventricular neuropeptide Y suppresses open field and home cage activity in the rat. *Regul Pept* 1987;19:221–231.
28. Heilig M, Widerlöv E. Neuropeptide Y: an overview of central distribution, functional aspects, and possible involvement in neuropsychiatric illnesses. *Acta Psychiatr Scand* 1990;82:95–114.
29. Heilig M, McLeod S, Brot M, Heinrichs SC, Menzaghi F, Koob GF, Britton KT. Anxiolytic-like action of neuropeptide Y: mediation by Y1 receptors in amygdala, and dissociation from food intake effects. *Neuropsychopharmacology* 1993;8(4):357–363.
30. Heilig M, McLeod S, Koob GK, Britton KT. Anxiolytic-like effect of neuropeptide Y (NPY), but not other peptides, in an operant conflict test. *Regul Pept* 1992;41:61–69.
31. Heilig M, Söderpalm B, Engel JA, Widerlöv E. Centrally administered neuropeptide Y (NPY) produces anxiolytic-like effects in animal anxiety models. *Psychopharmacology* 1989;98:524–529.
32. Heilig M, Wahlestedt C, Ekman R, Widerlöv E. Antidepressant drugs increase the concentration of neuropeptide Y (NPY)-like immunoreactivity in the rat brain. *Eur J Pharmacol* 1988;147:465–467.
33. Heilig M, Wahlestedt C, Widerlöv E. Neuropeptide Y (NPY)-induced activity suppression in the rat: evidence for NPY receptor heterogeneity and for interaction with α-adrenergic receptors. *Eur J Pharmacol* 1988;157:205–213.
34. Hendry JHC. Organization of neuropeptide Y neurons in the mammalian central nervous system. In: Colmers WF, Wahlestedt C, eds. *The biology of neuropeptide Y and related peptides.* Totowa, NJ: Humana Press, 1993;65–156.
35. Herzog H, Hort YJ, Ball HJ, Hayes G, Shine J, Selbie LA. Cloned human neuropeptide Y receptor couples to two different second messenger systems. *Proc Natl Acad Sci USA* 1992;89:5794–5798.
36. Inoue T, Inui A, Okita M, Sakatani N, Oya M, Morioka H, Mizuno N, Oimomi M, Baba S. Effect of neuropeptide Y on the hypothalamic–pituitary–adrenal axis in the dog. *Life Sci* 1989;44:1043–1051.
37. Kalra SP, Dube MG, Sahu A, Phelps CP, Kalra PS. Neuropeptide Y secretion increases in the paraventricular nucleus in association with increased appetite for food. *Proc Natl Acad Sci USA* 1991;88:10931–10935.
38. Kataoka Y, Sakurai Y, Mine K, Yamashita K, Fujiwara M, Niwa M, Ueki S. The involvement of neuropeptide Y in the antimuricide action of noradrenaline injected into the medial amygdala of olfactory bulbectomized rats. *Pharmacol Biochem Behav* 1987;28:101–103.
39. Kaye WH, Berrettini WH, Gwirtsman HE, Gold PW, George DT, Jimerson DC, Ebert MH. Contribution of CNS neuropeptide (NPY, CRH, and beta-endorphin) alterations to psychophysiological abnor-

malities in anorexia nervosa. *Psychopharmacol Bull* 1989;25:433–438.

40. Kaye WH, Berrettini W, Gwirtsman H, George DT. Altered cerebrospinal fluid neuropeptide Y and peptide YY immunoreactivity in anorexia and bulimia nervosa. *Arch Gen Psychiatry* 1990;47:548–556.

41. Kimmel JR, Hayden LJ, Pollock HG. Isolation and characterization of a new pancreatic polypeptide hormone. *J Biol Chem* 1975;250:9369–9376.

42. Larhammar D, Blomqvist AG, Yee F, Jazin E, Yoo H, Wahlestedt C. Cloning and functional expression of a human neuropeptide Y/peptide YY receptor of the Y1-type. *J Biol Chem* 1992;267:10935–10938.

43. Larhammar D, Söderberg C, Blomqvist AG. Evolution of the neuropeptide Y family of peptides. In: Colmers WF, Wahlestedt C, eds. *The biology of neuropeptide Y and related peptides.* Totowa, NJ: Humana Press, 1993;1–41.

44. Levine AS, Morley JE. Neuropeptide Y: a potent inducer of consummatory behavior in rats. *Peptides* 1984;5:1025–1029.

45. Li X-J, Wu Y-N, North A, Forte M. Cloning, functional expression, and developmental regulation of a neuropeptide Y receptor from *Drosophila melanogaster. J Biol Chem* 1992;267:9–12.

46. Liposits Z, Sievers L, Paull WK. Neuropeptide-Y and ACTH-immunoreactive innervation of corticotropin releasing factor (CRF)-synthesizing neurons in the hypothalamus of the rat. An immunocytochemical analysis at the light and electron microscopic levels. *Histochemistry* 1988;88:227–234.

47. McQuiston AR, Colmers WF. Neuropeptide Y does not alter NMDA conductances in CA3 pyramidal neurons: a slice-patch study. *Neurosci Lett* 1992;138:261–264.

48. Minth CD, Bloom SR, Polak JM, Dixon JE. Cloning, characterization, and DNA sequence of a human cDNA encoding neuropeptide tyrosine. *Proc Natl Acad Sci USA* 1984;81:4577–4581.

49. Monnet FP, Debonnel G, Fournier A, de Montigny C. Neuropeptide Y potentiates *N*-methyl-D-aspartate response in the CA$_3$ dorsal hippocampus. II. Involvement of a subtype of *sigma* receptor. *J Pharmacol Exp Ther* 1992;263:1219–1225.

50. Moore RY, Card JP. Visual pathways and the entrainment of circadian rhythms. *Ann NY Acad Sci* 1985;453:123–133.

51. Morley JE, Flood JF. The effect of neuropeptide Y on drinking in mice. *Brain Res* 1989;494:129–137.

52. Roman FJ, Pascaud X, Duffy O, Vauche D, Martin B, Junien JL. Neuropeptide Y and peptide YY interact with rat brain σ and PCP binding sites. *Eur J Pharmacol* 1989;174:301–302.

53. Sabol SL, Higuchi H. Transcriptional regulation of the neuropeptide Y gene by nerve growth factor. *Mol Endocrinol* 1990;4:384–392.

54. Sahu A, Kalra PS, Kalra SP. Food deprivation and ingestion induce reciprocal changes in neuropeptide Y concentrations in the paraventricular nucleus. *Peptides* 1988;9:83–86.

55. Shen SH, Grundemar L, Zukowska-Grojec Z, Håkanson R, Wahlestedt C. C-terminal neuropeptide Y fragments are mast cell-dependent vasodepressor agents. *Eur J Pharmacol* 1991;204:249–256.

56. Smialowska M, Legutko B. Influence of imipramine on neuropeptide Y immunoreactivity in the rat brain. *Neuroscience* 1991;41:767–771.

57. Stanley BG. Neuropeptide Y in multiple hypothalamic sites controls eating behavior, endocrine, and autonomic systems for body energy balance. In: Colmers WF, Wahlestedt C, eds. *The biology of neuropeptide Y and related peptides.* Totowa, NJ: Humana Press, 1993;457–509.

58. Stenfors C, Theodorsson E, Mathé AA. Effect of repeated electroconvulsive treatment on regional concentrations of tachykinins, neu-

rotensin, vasoactive intestinal polypeptide, neuropeptide Y, and galanin in rat brain. *J Neurosci Res* 1989;24:445–450.

59. Suburo AM, Gibson SJ, Moscoso G, Terenghi G, Polak JM. Transient expression of neuropeptide Y and its C-flanking peptide immunoreactivities in the spinal cord and ganglia of human embryos and fetuses. *Neuroscience* 1992;46:571–584.

60. Sundler F, Böttcher G, Ekblad E, Håkanson R. PP, PYY and NPY—occurrence and distribution in the periphery. In: Colmers WF, Wahlestedt C, eds. *The biology of neuropeptide Y and related peptides.* Totowa, NJ: Humana Press, 1993;157–196.

61. Tatemoto K. Isolation and characterization of peptide YY (PYY), a candidate gut hormone that inhibits pancreatic exocrine function. *Proc Natl Acad Sci USA* 1982;79:2514–2518.

62. Tatemoto K, Mutt V. Isolation of two novel candidate hormones using a chemical method for finding naturally occurring polypeptides. *Nature* 1980;285:417–418.

63. Tatemoto K, Carlquist M, Mutt V. Neuropeptide Y—a novel brain peptide with structural similarities to peptide YY and pancreatic polypeptide. *Nature* 1982;296:659–660.

64. Tonan K, Kawata Y, Hamaguchi S. Conformations of isolated fragments of pancreatic polypeptide. *Biochemistry* 1990;29:4424–4429.

65. Tsagarakis S, Rees LH, Besser GM, Grossman A. Neuropeptide-Y stimulates CRF-41 release from rat hypothalami in vitro. *Brain Res* 1989;502:167–170.

66. Wahlestedt C, Reis DJ. Neuropeptide Y-related peptides and their receptors: are the receptors potential therapeutic drug targets? *Annu Rev Pharmacol Toxicol* 1993;32:309–352.

67. Wahlestedt C, Blendy JA, Kellar KJ, Heilig M, Widerlov E, Ekman R. Electroconvulsive shocks increase the concentration of neocortical and hippocampal neuropeptide Y (NPY)-like immunoreactivity in the rat. *Brain Res* 1990;507:65–68.

68. Wahlestedt C, Edvinsson L, Ekblad E, Håkanson R. Effects of neuropeptide Y at sympathetic neuroeffector junctions: existence of Y1- and Y2-receptors. In: Nobin A, Owman C, Arneklo-Nobin B, eds. *Neuronal messengers in vascular function.* Amsterdam: Elsevier, 1987;231–241.

69. Wahlestedt C, Grundemar L, Håkanson R, Heilig M, Shen GH, Zukowska-Grojec Z, Reis DJ. Neuropeptide Y receptor subtypes, Y1 and Y2. *Ann NY Acad Sci* 1990;611:7–26.

70. Wahlestedt C, Karoum F, Jaskiw G, Wyatt RJ, Larhammar D, Ekman R, Reis DJ. Cocaine-induced reduction of brain neuropeptide Y synthesis dependent on medial prefrontal cortex. *Proc Natl Acad Sci USA* 1991;88:2078–2082.

71. Wahlestedt C, Pich EM, Koob GF, Yee F, Heilig M. Modulation of anxiety and neuropeptide Y-Y1 receptors by antisense oligodeoxynucleotides. *Science* 1993;259:528–531.

72. Wahlestedt C, Skagerberg G, Ekman R, Heilig M, Sundler F, Håkanson R. Neuropeptide Y (NPY) in the area of the hypothalamic paraventricular nucleus activates the pituitary–adrenocortical axis in the rat. *Brain Res* 1987;417:33–38.

73. Wahlestedt C, Yanaihara N, Håkanson R. Evidence for different pre- and postjunctional receptors for neuropeptide Y and related peptides. *Regul Pept* 1986;13:307–318.

74. Walker MW, Miller MJ. ^{125}I-neuropeptide Y and ^{125}I-peptide YY bind to multiple receptor sites in rat brain. *Mol Pharmacol* 1988;34:779–792.

75. Weiner ED, Mallat AM, Papolos DF, Lachman HM. Acute lithium treatment enhances neuropeptide Y gene expression in rat hippocampus. *Mol Brain Res* 1992;12:209–214.

76. Widdowson PS, Ordway GA, Halaris AE. Reduced neuropeptide Y concentrations in suicide brain. *J Neurochem* 1992;59:73–80.

77. Widerlöv E, Lindström LH, Wahlestedt C, Ekman R. Neuropeptide Y and peptide YY as possible cerebrospinal markers for major depression and schizophrenia, respectively. *J Psychiatr Res* 1988;22(1):69–79.

Psychopharmacology: The Fourth Generation of Progress, edited by Floyd E. Bloom and David J. Kupfer. Raven Press, Ltd., New York 1995.

CHAPTER **49**

Somatostatin in the Central Nervous System

David R. Rubinow, Candace L. Davis, and Robert M. Post

Early efforts to screen hypothalamic extracts for growth hormone (GH)-releasing activity inadvertently resulted in the discovery in 1968 of an inhibitor of GH release, the biological activity of which was localized to the median eminence and anterior hypothalamus. This inhibiting factor, somatostatin (SS, SRIF), was subsequently isolated and structurally characterized in 1973 and was found to be identical to an insulin inhibitor described in 1969. The discovery of SS, for which Guillemin received the Nobel prize in 1977, established both (a) the dual regulation of anterior pituitary peptides by hypothalamic releasing and release-inhibiting factors and (b) the existence of "brain-gut" peptides, present in both the central nervous system (CNS) and gastrointestinal system.

While the anatomical distribution of SS is widespread, it is particularly concentrated in the central and peripheral nervous systems and in the gastrointestinal (GI) tract (including the pancreas), the major source of circulatory SS. In the GI tract, SS is localized in the D cells of the stomach and islets of Langerhans, the small intestine, and the vagal neurons of the myenteric and submucosal plexuses. SS secreted from these sites acts both locally (paracrine) and distally (endocrine) to modulate nutrient homeostasis through regulation of endocrine and exocrine secretions of the stomach, intestine, and pancreas as well as regulation of motor activity of the stomach and intestine. As described below, SS is widely but discretely distributed throughout the CNS, where its range of neuroregulatory effects has expanded far beyond its originally discovered role.

STRUCTURE

While the originally identified hypothalamic GH release inhibitor is a tetradecapeptide (SS-14), SS now re-

fers to a family of peptides that are cleavage products of a larger precursor, prepro-somatostatin (116 amino acids) (35). After removal of a leader sequence, the 92-amino-acid prohormone (pro-SS) is cleaved at monobasic or dibasic sites to yield the different molecular forms of SS (see Fig. 1). SS-14 is the C-terminal fragment of the prohormone and may be directly cleaved from pro-SS or from the SS-14 N-terminal extension fragment, SS-28, the other major bioactive product (see Fig. 2). SS-14 and SS-28 are secreted in different amounts by SS-containing cells and appear in a variety of proportions in different tissues. SS-14 is the predominant form appearing in neural tissue and the exclusive form in the retina and peripheral nerves, pancreas, and stomach. The mucosal cells of the gut secrete mainly SS-28, which represents 20–30% of SS-like immunoreactivity in the brain (35).

LOCALIZATION/DISTRIBUTION

SS-containing nerve fibers are densely but selectively distributed throughout the brain, appearing in the median eminence (the source of anterior pituitary regulation), the posterior pituitary, the limbic system, the cortex, and the hypothalamus and hypothalamic projections to the brainstem and spinal cord. SS-containing cell bodies have similarly been identified in diverse brain regions including the neocortex, all limbic structures, the hypothalamus (particularly the anterior periventricular region but also the paraventricular, arcuate, and ventromedial nuclei), the striatum, the periaqueductal gray, the nucleus accumbens, the locus coeruleus, and the septal nuclei (48). SS neurons also appear at the synapses of the major sensory systems (somatosensory, visual, auditory, and olfactory) (35). While SS is most concentrated in the hypothalamus, it is most abundant in the cortex, which accounts for approximately 49% of brain SS. Spinal cord (30%), brainstem (12%), hypothalamus (7%), olfactory lobe (1%), and cerebellum (1%) represent the other major SS-containing

D. R. Rubinow, C. L. Davis, and R. M. Post: National Institute of Mental Health, NIH, Bethesda, Maryland 20892.

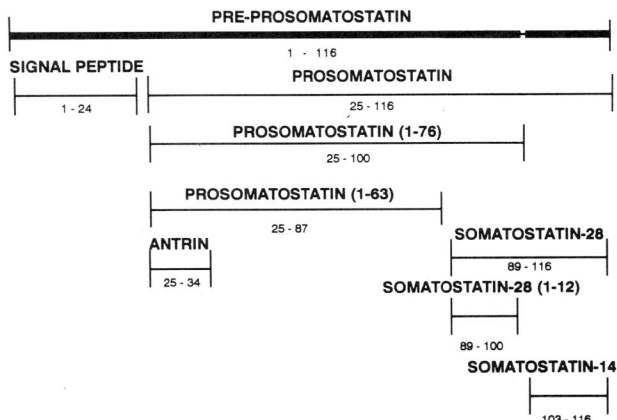

FIG. 1. SS-14 and related cleavage products of prepro-SS. (Adapted from ref. 48, with permission.)

brain regions (35). Postmortem studies in humans have revealed a distribution of SS neurons and fibers similar (although not identical) to that seen in rodents. Several CNS SS pathways have been identified (48). The periventricular nucleus is the primary source of somatostinergic input to the median eminence, while the SS-containing nerve terminals of the anterior hypothalamic nuclei and lateral and ventromedial hypothalamus originate in the amygdala. Periventricular hypothalamic somatostatinergic fibers travel in a variety of pathways, including short-distance projections to hypothalamic nuclei (e.g., suprachiasmatic, arcuate, and preoptic nuclei), long-distance rostral and ascending projections to many limbic structures (e.g., stria terminalis, amygdala, and arcuate nucleus), and caudal projections into the brainstem and spinal cord.

ACTIONS

In parallel with its widespread distribution, SS displays multiple regulatory effects in a variety of tissues. The general processes that are regulated are neurotransmission, glandular secretion, smooth muscle contractility, and cell proliferation (35). Electrophysiologic studies have demonstrated both inhibitory and excitatory effects of SS on neuronal activity. These ostensibly contradictory findings may reflect regional specificities as well as dose–response and time-course characteristics. Intracellular recording studies have revealed a biphasic dose-related neuronal response to SS, with low doses increasing and high doses inhibiting, or not affecting, action potential generation (48). More recent studies have consistently demonstrated the ability of SS to hyperpolarize CA1 pyramidal and solitary tract neurons, with both pharmacologic and voltage-clamp evidence for SS-induced m-current (a voltage-dependent outward potassium conductance) activation as the mechanism for this hyperpolarization (48). Stimulatory and inhibitory effects of SS have been ob-

served in the cortex [increased dopamine (DA), norepinephrine (NE); decreased histamine (HS)], hippocampus [increased acetylcholine (ACh), DA, serotonin (5-HT); decreased HS], striatum (increased DA, decreased glutamate), and hypothalamus (decreased NE, HS; increased 5-HT) (16,48). The effects of SS on the secretion of an array of hormones and neuropeptides is so uniformly inhibitory that McCann suggested that SS be called "panhibin" (32). SS is clearly involved in the physiologic regulation of GH and thyroid-stimulating hormone (TSH), inhibiting both their basal and stimulated secretion (38). While SS has no effect on luteinizing hormone (LH), follicle-stimulating hormone (FSH), prolactin, or adrenocorticotropic hormone (ACTH) in normal subjects, contradicting reports exist regarding SS-induced suppression of elevated ACTH levels in patients with Addison's disease or Nelson's syndrome (3,35). While the reported ability of SS to suppress stimulated ACTH secretion from mouse pituitary tumor (AtT-20) cells was not confirmed in pituitary cell culture, intracerebroventricular (i.c.v.) SS-28 was noted to inhibit stress-induced corticotropin-releasing factor (CRF) secretion in rats (48). Furthermore, SS infusion in humans was observed to blunt insulin-induced hypoglycemia-stimulated elevations of β-endorphin, β-lipotropin, and cortisol (48). Similarly, while SS has no effect on basal prolactin levels in normal subjects, it decreases elevated prolactin levels in acromegaly and inhibits both basal and TRH-stimulated prolactin secretion in vitro and in an estrogen-dependent fashion in rats (16,64). All of the diverse actions of SS appear to be mediated by SS binding to high-affinity membrane-bound receptors.

SS RECEPTORS

The existence of SS receptor subtypes was suggested (6) on the basis of different patterns of desensitization after exposure to SS or SS analogues (homologous desensitization). Further support for receptor heterogeneity was derived from observations of pharmacologically distinct receptors displaying different affinities for SS agonists, regional distributions, functions, and linkage to transduc-

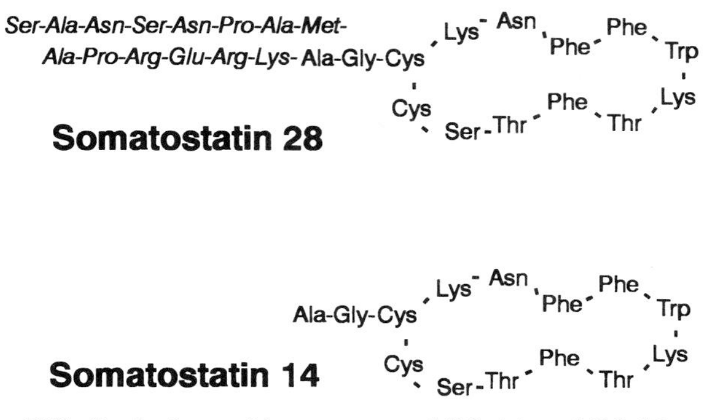

Ser-Ala-Asn-Ser-Asn-Pro-Ala-Met-
Ala-Pro-Arg-Glu-Arg-Lys- Ala-Gly-Cys   Lys⁻ Asn   Phe⁻ Phe   Trp

Cys   Phe   Lys

Somatostatin 28   Cys   Ser-Thr⁻   Thr

Ala-Gly-Cys   Lys⁻ Asn   Phe⁻ Phe   Trp

Somatostatin 14   Cys   Phe   Lys
   Ser-Thr⁻   Thr

FIG. 2. Amino acid sequence of SS-14 and SS-28.

tion systems (see ref. 6 for review). The SRIF1 receptor is a G-protein-coupled receptor that is expressed in high concentration in the dentate gyrus of the hippocampus, neostriatum, locus coeruleus, and inner layers of the cerebral cortex and is highly sensitive to homologous desensitization (6). In contrast, the SRIF2 receptor is not coupled to G proteins, is localized in the CA1 region of the hippocampus and diffusely throughout the cerebral cortex, and is resistant to homologous desensitization (6). As reviewed by Bell and Reisine (6), three SS receptors have recently been cloned and sequenced. The three receptors, SSTR1, SSTR2, and SSTR3, consist of 391, 369, and 428 amino acids, respectively, and display approximately 50% homology. Like other G-protein-coupled receptors, they appear to have seven membrane-spanning segments, with the transmembrane regions showing the most extensive sequence identity. The receptor sequences are highly conserved across species: human and mouse SSTR1, SSTR2, and SSTR3 show 99%, 94%, and 85% amino acid identity, respectively. SSTR1 messenger ribonucleic acid (mRNA) is expressed in high levels in the human GI tract, but not in the cerebral cortex, despite the presence of high levels of transcripts in the mouse and rat brain. In contrast, high levels of SSTR2 transcripts are present in human brain and kidney, and SSTR3 transcripts are present only in the brain. In situ hybridization studies confirm the expression of all three receptor transcripts in mouse brain, displaying distinct but overlapping distributions, particularly in the cortex, hippocampus, and amygdala (6).

In their selective affinities for SS analogues and in their expression patterns in mouse brain, SSTR1 and SSTR2 resemble the SRIF2 and SRIF1 receptors, respectively (10,30). SSTR3 displays a different pattern of pharmacologic properties and thus is not explained by the original classification. The differential effects of SS-14 and SS-28 on target cells (16) (e.g., SS-28 more potently inhibits hypothalamic CRF, GH, and TSH, while SS-14 more effectively inhibits electrical activity in the cortex) (35), as well as tissue-specific differences in binding potency (SS-14 greater in brain, SS-28 greater in pituitary) and distinct labeling patterns in brain, lent empiric support to the early notion of receptor heterogeneity (35,36). While SSTR1, SSTR2, and SSTR3 bind SS-14 and SS-28 with similar high affinities, a fourth recently cloned receptor, SSTR4, has higher affinity for SS-28 (6). Even more recently, the gene for a fifth human receptor, SSTR5, has been localized to chromosome 20, in contrast to the localization of SSTR1, SSTR2, and SSTR3 to human chromosomes 14, 17, and 22, respectively (63). Many of the known and proposed mechanisms of action of SS can be linked to and mediated by distinct properties of the five cloned receptors.

Ligand binding to SS receptors modulates one of five different cellular effector systems: adenylyl cyclase, K^+ channels, Ca^{2+} channels, exocytosis, and tyrosine phosphatase (6). Activation of the SS receptor decreases intra-cellular cyclic adenosine monophosphate (cAMP) by inhibiting adenylyl cyclase (through coupling with Gia1) and decreases intracellular Ca^{2+} by activating the voltage-dependent outward potassium conductance or m current (possibly through Gia3) and by inhibiting Ca^{2+} channel activity (possibly through Goa) (24,55). SS also blocks hormone secretion at a step distal to either cAMP formation or Ca^{2+} mobilization as evidenced by the ability of SS to block stimulated secretion by cAMP, adenylate cyclase stimulation or phosphodiesterase inhibition, inositol triphosphate or diacylglycerol, or elevation of intracellular Ca^{2+} with calcium ionophores (35). This action of exocytosis inhibition also appears to involve coupling to a G protein (36). The mechanism by which SS stimulates tyrosine phosphatase is currently unclear, although the effect is believed to underlie an observed antiproliferative effect on pancreatic and breast cancer (6,54,61).

As reviewed by Bell and Reisine (6), only SSTR3 is coupled to Gia1 and inhibits adenyl cyclase activity. (It is not established whether SSTR4 is linked to G protein, although it, too, appears to mediate SS inhibition of cAMP generation.) SSTR2 is coupled to Gia3 and Goa2, through which it may alter K^+ and Ca^{2+} channel activity, respectively. The actions of SSTR1 are not G-protein-dependent and may include regulation of Na^+/H^+ ion exchange and, conceivably, tyrosine phosphatase stimulation. Availability of the cloned SS receptors will no doubt considerably advance attempts to precisely define the molecular events underlying the remarkable range of effects of SS.

SS GENE EXPRESSION

While two separate genes code for either SS-14 or SS-28 in fish, a single gene codes for both in mammals (35). This gene consists of two exons (238 and 367 base pairs) separated by an intron (621 base pairs). Between two 5' upstream promoters (TATA and CAAT boxes) lies an enhancer, the cAMP response element (CRE), which was first discovered in the SS gene (20). Among the myriad factors (nutrients, neurotransmitters, neuropeptides, hormones, second messengers, growth factors) that influence SS secretion, often in a tissue-specific fashion, many have been shown as well to enhance SS genomic transcription (see Table 1). For example, SS secretion is stimulated by dopamine (via the D2 receptor), acetylcholine (muscarinic), glutamate (NMDA), growth hormone, neurotensin, CRF, insulin, insulin-like growth factor-1 (IGF-1), interleukin 1 (IL-1), and tumor necrosis factor (TNF) (7,35,48). In addition to stimulating secretion, the following also increase SS mRNA: NMDA agonists (cortex), GH (hypothalamus), testosterone and estradiol (hypothalamus), glucocorticoids (hypothalamus, cortex), and IL-1 and TNF (diencephalic culture) (4,35,64). The mechanism by which these factors alter SS genomic expression is unknown, although in some cases it will most likely in-

TABLE 1. *Modulators of SS secretion and gene expression[a]*

Modulator	↑ Secretion	↑ SS mRNA	↓ Secretion
Dopamine (D2)	+ (H[b])	+ (H)	
Acetylcholine (muscarinic)	+ (H, cortex)		
Glutamate (NMDA)	+ (H)	+ (cortex)	
Quinolinic acid	+ (cortical culture, striatum—low dose)	+ (cortical culture, striatum—low dose)	− (striatum—high dose)
GABA			− (H, cortex)
Norepinephrine	+ (H-α, amygdala-B)		
Growth hormone	+ (H)	+ (H)	
Thyroid hormone (T3, T4)	+ (H, cortical culture—low dose)		− (H, cortical culture—high dose)
Neurotensin	+ (H, cortex)		
VIP	+ (cortex)		− (H)
CRF	+ (cortex)		
Testosterone	+ (H)	+ (H)	
Estradiol	+ (H)	+ (H)	
Glucocorticoids	+ (cortex—low dose)	+ (cortex, H)	− (cortex—high dose)
Insulin	+ (H)		
Bombesin	+ (H)		
IL-1	+ (diencephalic culture)	+ (diencephalic culture)	
IL-6	+ (diencephalic culture)	+ (diencephalic culture)	
TNF	+ (diencephalic culture)	+ (diencephalic culture)	
IGF-1	+ (pituitary, H)		

[a] See text for references. For reviews see refs. 16, 35, 38, and 44.
[b] H, hypothalamus.

volve stimulation of cAMP, which increases both SS secretion and SS genomic transcription through the CRE. Several hormones and neuroregulators have been found to inhibit SS secretion or to regulate it in a dose-related or highly tissue-specific fashion. Gamma-aminobutyric acid (GABA) is almost uniformly inhibitory, ACTH inhibits secretion in the hypothalamus, vasoactive intestinal polypeptide (VIP) is inhibitory in the hypothalamus but stimulatory in the neocortex, and glucocorticoids are stimulatory at low doses and inhibitory at high doses (35,48).

SS: ROLE IN BEHAVIOR AND NEUROPSYCHIATRIC DISORDERS

Behavioral Effects

An important potential role for SS in CNS activity is suggested by many studies in which alterations of central SS levels result in the modulation of a variety of vegetative and related functions (48). Early studies reported decreased total, slow-wave, and rapid-eye-movement (REM) sleep following intracerebral or i.c.v. administration of SS. A more recent report observed (a) significant increases in REM sleep in rats following i.c.v. SS and (b) suppression of REM sleep following i.c.v. administration of cysteamine, a depletor of SS. No effect on electroencephalographic measures of sleep was seen, however, following intravenous infusion of SS in a study of 11 normal men by Kupfer et al. (27).

Effects of SS on hunger and locomotor activity appear to vary with the dose employed (48). Increased or dose-

related biphasic food consumption have both been reported to accompany intracerebral or i.c.v. SS. Chronic i.c.v. administration of the SS analogue octreotide increased daily food intake, whereas SS antiserum significantly decreased food intake. Antagonism of CRF-induced anorexia by SS in starved rats has also been demonstrated. As reviewed by Vecsei and Widerlov (58), SS influences locomotor activity, the nature of the response being dependent upon the SS analogue, the dose, and the behavioral measure employed.

In both animals and humans, analgesia is seen following intrathecal administration of SS (48). Several SS analogues display high affinity at the mu-opiate receptor, and SS colocalizes with methionine enkephalin in neurons of the raphe nucleus and nucleus gigantocellularis (48). However, because the analgesic effects of intrathecal SS in humans are not reversed by naloxone, a non-opiate-mediated mechanism is suggested (25). Finally, a series of studies by Vecsei and Widerlov (58) and Walsh et al. (60) show that SS may enhance learning and reverse induced learning deficits, whereas SS depletion (with cysteamine) diminishes performance.

Neuropsychiatric Disease-Related Alterations

Disease-related alterations in SS levels in the cerebrospinal fluid (CSF) were first reported by Patel et al. in 1977 (37). They described increased levels of SS in several inflammatory or destructive neurologic disorders (cerebral tumor, meningitis, spinal cord disease, nerve root compression, metabolic encephalopathy). These findings

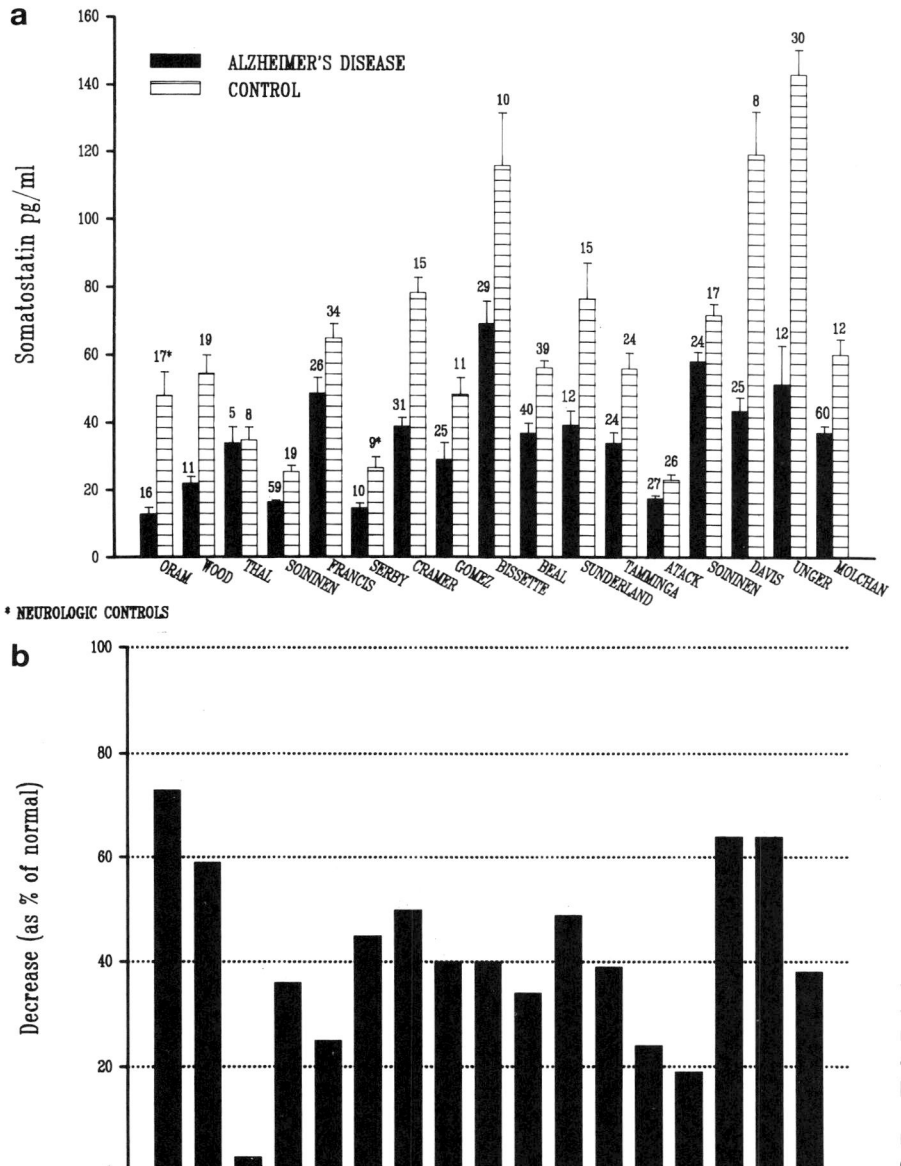

a

Somatostatin pg/ml

■ ALZHEIMER'S DISEASE
□ CONTROL

(bars labeled along x-axis): ORAM, WOOD, THAL, SOININEN, FRANCIS, SERBY, CRAMER, GOMEZ, BISSETTE, BEAL, SUNDERLAND, TAMMINGA, ATACK, SOININEN, DAVIS, UNGER, MOLCHAN

* NEUROLOGIC CONTROLS

b

Decrease (as % of normal)

(bars labeled along x-axis): ORAM, WOOD, THAL, SOININEN, FRANCIS, SERBY, CRAMER, GOMEZ, BISSETTE, BEAL, SUNDERLAND, TAMMINGA, ATACK, SOININEN, DAVIS, UNGER, MOLCHAN

FIG. 3. Summary of 17 studies of CSF SS in Alzheimer's disease. (**a**) Absolute SS levels in patients and controls. The numbers of subjects and controls appear above the standard error bars. Studies are presented in chronological order. *Asterisks* indicate neurological rather than normal controls. (**b**) The percentage decrease in CSF SS in Alzheimer's disease in the same studies. (Adapted from ref. 48, with permission.)

were subsequently replicated by other investigators (48). While these elevated CSF SS levels presumably reflected neuronal damage, the decreased CSF SS levels seen in several neuropsychiatric disorders suggested more functional neuronal alterations. These disorders include Parkinson's disease, delirium, Alzheimer's disease, depression, and multiple sclerosis (MS) during relapse (48). Su et al. (53) recently confirmed decreased SS in progressive MS, in contrast to the findings of Rosler et al. (46). Su et al. further demonstrated a significant decrease in SS in serial CSF samples over 2 years in a small group of medication-free patients with MS who manifested neurological deterioration during this interval. Three groups have reported significantly decreased SS in multi-infarct dementia patients, with nonsignificant decreases reported by a fourth group (48). Decreased CSF SS has also been observed in patients with ACTH-dependent Cushing's

syndrome (25). Finally, both decreased and normal levels of SS have been reported in patients with Huntington's disease (25,48). Postmortem studies have demonstrated decreased SS concentrations in the brains of patients with Alzheimer's disease (see below) and Parkinson's disease (cortex and hippocampus) (48) and increases in the basal ganglia, locus coeruleus, and frontal and temporal cortex of patients with Huntington's disease (5) (presumably due to selective neuronal sparing) (42) (see also Chapters 118 and 126, *this volume*).

ALZHEIMER'S DISEASE

Reports of low CSF SS in senile dementia and Alzheimer's disease have been remarkably uniform (48) (see Fig. 3). Human postmortem studies also demonstrate decreased SS concentrations in a variety of cortical and subcortical sites in Alzheimer's disease (48). The amount of the reduction and the brain region most clearly affected differ across studies. These differences may reflect a number of factors including postmortem changes, molecular heterogeneity of SS-like immunoreactivity, or decreases in SS masked by the loss of non-SS tissue volume (11). Additionally, Lowe et al. (29) attributed reported discrepancies to differences in the length and severity of the disease, consistent with the observation that studies with a greater representation of severely ill patients report greater decreases in brain SS than are seen in other studies. Nonetheless, SS concentrations are widely (but not without exception) reported as reduced to 21–61% of control values in the temporal cortex, with similar reductions seen in the frontal and parietal but not occipital or cingulate cortex (29).

Decreased brain and CSF SS levels in Alzheimer's disease have been observed with remarkable consistency. The clinical relevance of these findings is suggested by the following: (a) reports of correlations between the degree of cognitive impairment and reduction of SS levels in brain and CSF; (b) reports of the colocalization of SS-like immunoreactivity with senile plaques and neurofibrillary tangles; (c) observation of a correlation between the loss of SS and disease severity as determined by plaque density; (d) the demonstration that the brain areas showing the greatest reduction in SS are those that are most markedly hypometabolic as determined by positron emission tomography (PET) scan; and (e) the observation of relative increase in CSF SS concentration in association with a reversal of dementia symptoms in patients with Alzheimer's disease exposed to intensive environmental stimulation (see ref. 48 for review). This last finding is of interest given the presumption that the changes in brain SS in Alzheimer's disease reflect neuronal degeneration. It is further noteworthy given the lack of therapeutic success associated with attempts to manipulate pharmacologically central SS levels [by administering an SS analogue to patients with Alzheimer's disease or an SS-depleting agent, (i.e., cysteamine) to patients with Huntington's disease] (48). The extent to which these treatments produced changes in central SS levels is uncertain (see also Chapter 118, *this volume*).

DEPRESSION AND OTHER PSYCHIATRIC DISORDERS

Among the psychiatric disorders studied, the clearest evidence of abnormal central SS levels or activity is in depression. Seven studies document significantly decreased CSF SS in depression compared with controls (48) (see Fig. 4). Additionally, significantly lower CSF levels were seen in patients with a major depressive disorder compared with other psychiatric patients (56) and in a group of depressed patients studied during their worst

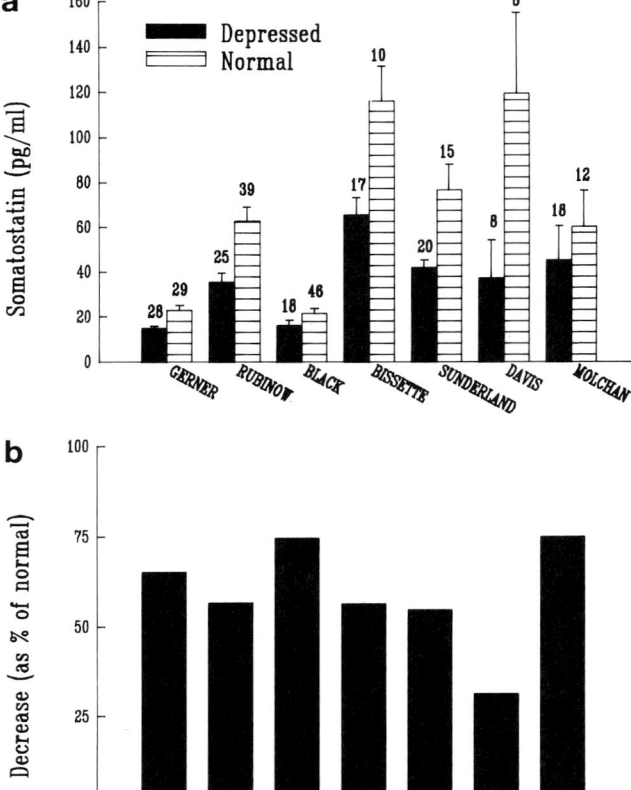

FIG. 4. Summary of seven studies showing decreased CSF SS in depression. (**a**) Absolute SS levels in patients and controls. The studies are presented in chronological order. The data in the Sunderland study have been slightly extended in the study by Molchan. The numbers of subjects and controls appear above the standard error bars. (**b**) The percentage decrease in CSF SS in depression in the same studies. (Adapted from ref. 48, with permission.)

week of depression compared with a group of depressed patients studied more than 2 months after their most depressed week (1). In addition to these decreased levels observed in depression, Molchan et al. (33) found a significant negative correlation between CSF SS levels and the degree of depressed mood in 60 patients with Alzheimer's disease, as well as significantly lower CSF SS levels in the depressed Alzheimer's patients compared with the nondepressed patients. Longitudinal examination of patients in different affective states demonstrated that SS values obtained during depression were significantly lower than those obtained during either the manic or improved states (47). Decreased CSF SS levels, therefore, appear to be state-related and to normalize with recovery from depression, similar to the restoration of normal CSF SS levels in MS patients during clinical remission (51).

Studies of CSF SS in samples of patients with psychiatric disorders other than depression have yielded conflicting or as yet unconfirmed results (48). Both increased and normal SS levels have been observed in manic patients. Both decreased and normal SS levels have been reported in patients with schizophrenia and anorexia nervosa (8,15,23). Kaye et al. (23) described a small but significant increase in CSF SS in patients with bulimia during abstinence from bingeing compared with the same patients when actively bingeing. Normal levels of CSF SS in patients with panic disorder were reported by Vecsei and Widerlov (57), who also noted normal SS levels in the premenstrual syndrome (PMS) as well as no effect of menstrual cycle phase on SS in either PMS patients or controls. Kruesi et al. (26) observed significantly higher SS levels in 10 children with obsessive–compulsive disorder (OCD) compared with 10 age- and sex-matched children with conduct disorder. Despite the absence of a normal control group in this study, these findings are of particular interest given the recent report by Altemus et al. (2) of significantly elevated CSF SS levels in adult patients with OCD relative to controls. The elevated SS levels in OCD are particularly intriguing in light of the recent demonstration in rat brain of decreased SS following administration of serotonergic agents, the treatment of choice for OCD (21).

Relatively few postmortem studies of brain SS have been performed in patients with psychiatric illness. Several early studies demonstrated no consistent abnormality in the brains of patients with schizophrenia (48). Charlton et al. (12) observed no difference in SS concentration or SS receptor affinity and binding capacity in the temporal or occipital cortex in nine primarily medicated depressed patients compared with controls. These investigators also found no difference in SS immunoreactivity in the frontal cortex in depressed patients (17) or in the frontal, motor, parietal, or temporal cortex of 12 suicide victims compared with controls (13). Significantly decreased SS content has also been observed in the temporal pole and pars opercularis of the frontal lobe (but not in other brain regions examined) in seven depressed and previously medicated patients (9). Finally, no differences in SS content were noted in the frontal cortex, amygdala, or caudate in a small series of schizophrenic ($n = 13$) or affectively ill suicide victims ($n = 9$) compared with accident victim controls ($n = 24$) (Davis et al., *unpublished data*) (see also Chapters 83 and 84, *this volume*).

SEIZURE DISORDERS

Although the precise role of SS in depression and other neuropsychiatric disorders is currently unknown, the potential relevance of alterations in SS secretion to CNS activity and seizure development is increasingly apparent. The following supportive observations (see ref. 48) exemplify the as yet undocumented mechanisms by which somatostatinergic neurons may be involved in other neuropsychiatric disorders:

1. Long-term (but not permanent) increases in SS in selective brain regions (amygdala and sensorimotor, piriform, and entorhinal cortex; striatum) following kindling (an animal model of epilepsy in which daily subictal stimuli result in progressively more intense brain activity culminating in generalized seizures) or prekindling [rats injected with pentylenetetrazol (PTZ) but not fulfilling the criteria of kindling].
2. A 200% increase in SS precursor and 60% and 80% increases in SS-14 and SS-28, respectively, in the frontal cortex after both PTZ-kindled and kainic-acid-stimulated seizures.
3. Long-lasting increases (30 days) in prepro-somatostatin mRNA in the frontal cortex and hippocampus (but not striatum or substantia nigra) following kainic-acid-induced seizures.
4. Selective increases in SS and prepro-somatostatin mRNA (but not glutamic acid decarboxylase (GAD or GAD mRNA) in the striatum and neocortex (34,48) in stage 5 kindled rats.
5. Increases of SS in stage 3 kindled rats (forelimb clonus) and in stage 5 kindled rats (generalized seizures, rearing and falling), with the elevation in the latter observed 1 hr after the seizure and persisting up to 2 weeks following the last seizure.
6. Significant increases in SS mRNA after stage 5 kindling in hippocampus (CA1, CA2, dentate gyrus), cingulate cortex, olfactory tubercle, and rostral cortex compared with increases seen following a single electrical stimulation or control conditions (50).
7. Increases in SS-14 in focal (epileptic) compared with nonfocal (nonepileptic) regions of the temporal cortex in 33 of 35 patients with intractable seizures.
8. Precipitation of atypical seizures following i.c.v. or intracerebral injection of SS.
9. Inhibition of kindled seizures following administration of cysteamine or SS antiserum.
10. Reversal of the inhibitory effects of cysteamine by i.c.v. infusion of SS.
11. Selective loss of SS neurons in the hilus of the dentate gyrus after kainic-acid-induced seizures (52) and in human temporal lobe epilepsy (45).
12. Inhibition of kainic acid or quinolinic-acid-induced seizures (in the hippocampus) by a peptidase-resistant somatostatin analogue (59).
13. Enhancement of hippocampal kindling after infusion of SS antiserum (34).
14. Reversible decreases in SS during acute seizures stimulated by PTZ (and presumed to be related to seizure-related increased release) (48,52).
15. Kindling-related downregulation of SS receptors in the hippocampus.
16. Periventricular SS release following electrical stimulation of several limbic sites.

Despite the conclusions of the authors of two additional studies that changes in SS may not be relevant to the development of seizures (14,40), further support for a potential role of SS in seizure susceptibility or activity is

TABLE 2. *SS: paradigmatic neuropeptide in neuropsychiatric illness*

SS	Functional Depression	Neurological MS	Neurological Kindling	Neurological Kainic acid	Neurodegenerative Alzheimer's disease
Cell death				$++^a$	$++$
Plaques and tangles					$++$
Long-term decreases				$++$	
Long-term increases			$++$		
Transient decreases	$++$	$++$			

^{a} Sustained epileptic seizure model (52).

provided by reports (described below) of the effects on SS of several anticonvulsants. The precise role of SS in seizure modulation remains to be documented but is particularly intriguing in relation to long-lasting increases of SS in some seizure models, such as kindling, but losses in others, such as kainate-precipitated seizures (see Table 2).

EFFECTS OF PSYCHOPHARMACOLOGIC AGENTS—POSTULATED MECHANISMS

Decreased CSF SS levels have been observed in humans following administration of several different anticonvulsants including diphenylhydantoin and carbamazepine. This effect of carbamazepine has been observed in patients with affective disorder as well as in patients with temporal lobe epilepsy (48). Lower CSF SS levels have also been observed in rats 2 hr after intraperitoneal administration of carbamazepine (48). This effect of carbamazepine on CSF SS most likely reflects the ability of carbamazepine to alter many of the neurotransmitters involved in SS regulation (dopamine, GABA, acetylcholine, norepinephrine) (41). Carbamazepine modulation of GABA, an inhibitor of SS secretion, appears particularly relevant (48). Carbamazepine decreases GABA turnover, perhaps involving a GABA agonist mechanism. Additionally, the action of carbamazepine at the trigeminal nucleus may be mediated via baclofen-like or GABA-B receptor mechanisms. Furthermore, the ability of midazolam to inhibit SS secretion from diencephalic and cerebral cultures is postulated to occur via stimulation of the GABA-B receptor. Finally, SS appears to act presynaptically in the CA1 region of the hippocampus to dramatically depress GABA-mediated inhibitory postsynaptic potentials. Sharfman and Schwartzkroin (49) speculated that the SS-related inhibition of GABA-induced hyperpolarization might render the hippocampus hyperexcitable, facilitating the induction of long-term potentiation (LTP). While SS has been reported to facilitate LTP in CA3 (but not CA1) (31), it also may hyperpolarize CA1 neurons, which, by itself, would dampen excitability (62). Excitability of brain regions such as the hippocampus (in which SS and GABA colocalize) (62) may thus reflect the reciprocal (albeit complicated) inhibitory regulatory effects of

GABA and SS. Therefore, the anticonvulsant effects of carbamazepine may in part result from carbamazepine-induced decreases in SS activity. This hypothesis is supported by several observations: (a) Carbamazepine blunts kindling-induced increases of SS in the frontal, temporal, and occipital cortex and amygdala (but not hippocampus), and (b) acute and chronic high-dose carbamazepine administration results in decreased SS and increased GABA levels in several (primarily limbic) brain regions (48). Several other studies, however, suggest that the effects of carbamazepine on basal SS concentrations in the brains of nonkindled rats are only slight or absent (28,48).

The effects of other psychopharmacologic agents on SS have been examined in several studies. The neuroleptic fluphenazine decreased SS in the CSF of a group of schizophrenic patients (15), and the neuroleptic haloperidol decreased SS in several brain regions (striatum and nucleus accumbens) and decreased SS receptors in the rat cerebral cortex and hippocampus (39). One additional study reported an increase in CSF SS in a small group of patients during treatment with haloperidol (18). No significant effects of desmethylimipramine, piribedil, or lithium carbonate were observed on CSF SS (48), nor were there effects of imipramine, maprotilline, or mianserin on SS concentrations in rat brain (22). However, Kakigi et al. (21,22) did observe (a) significant decreases in SS concentrations in a variety of brain regions following repeated administration of serotonergic agents (clomipramine, zimelidine, 5-hydroxytryptophan) and (b) increased concentrations following treatment with a serotonin synthesis inhibitor or neurotoxin. As noted above, these latter findings are of interest given the selective efficacy of serotonergic agents in the treatment of OCD, a disorder characterized by elevated CSF SS levels. Finally, in contrast to the ability of several psychopharmacologic agents to decrease CSF SS, nimodipine, a calcium channel antagonist employed in the treatment of several cyclic mood disorders, significantly increased CSF SS in eight patients with affective disorder (*unpublished data*).

CONCLUSIONS

Many of the questions raised by the observation in 1977 of alterations in SS levels in neuropsychiatric disorders still remain: What are the determinants, and what are the consequences of altered SS levels and function? What are the mechanisms by which SS regulates behavior, and what is the range of behavioral functions that it can modulate? What is the regulatory relevance of the differential effects of pro-somatostatin-derived peptides? It seems reasonable to conclude at present that the decrease in brain and CSF SS that are uniformly observed in Alzheimer's disease appear to reflect neuronal degeneration, while the decreased CSF SS seen in depression, which, like that in MS, is transient and reversible, perhaps reflects functional alterations in SS secretion and/or metabolism. While alterations in CNS SS in neuropsychiatric disorders may merely be epiphenomenal to more etiologically relevant upstream neuroregulatory disturbances, the central role played by SS in sensory processing and complex integrated behaviors suggests that, at the very least, disturbances of SS function will influence the phenomenology of disorders in which SS dysregulation occurs. For example, the possible contribution of SS dysregulation to cognitive impairment is suggested by the following: SS administration facilitates learning and memory; cognitive impairment characterizes the neuropsychiatric disorders associated with decreased SS (Alzheimer's disease, depression, MS, Parkinson's disease, and Cushing's disease); and the extent of the decrease in CSF or brain SS has been reported by some (but not all) to be significantly correlated with the degree of cognitive impairment in patients with Alzheimer's disease and Parkinson's disease (48). Distinct roles for the SS-related peptides in neuropsychiatric disorders cannot be assigned at present, although several authors (19,43) have suggested that abnormal processing of SS precursors may contribute to abnormal levels observed as well as influence syndromal characteristics. To the extent that dysregulation of SS may contribute to neuropsychiatric disorder-related symptomatology, therapeutic benefits may accompany successful efforts to increase brain SS activity, whether through intrathecal administration of SS, development of analogues or drug transport mechanisms that circumvent the blood–brain barrier, modulation of SS metabolism, or selective enhancement of SS gene expression.

The availability of five cloned high-affinity SS receptors offers the promise of an explosion of information about SS in the next decade. Identification of the characteristics of these receptors—including pharmacologic profile, physiologic effects, and intracellular effector systems—will permit precise definition of the consequences of alterations in specific SS fragments or receptor subtypes. The development of specific agonists and antagonists for SS receptor subtypes will not only facilitate the physiologic and pharmacologic dissection of the SS system, but may also result in the development of a new generation of therapeutically successful SS analogues. A mere 20 years after its identification, we are on the verge of understanding not only the role of SS in CNS function,

but also the consequences of dysregulation of the expression of SS and its receptors.

REFERENCES

1. Agren H, Lundqvist G. Low levels of somatostatin in human CSF mark depressive episodes. *Psychoneuroendocrinology* 1984;9:233–248.
2. Altemus M, Pigott T, L'Heureux F, Davis CL, Rubinow DR, Murphy DL, Gold PW. CSF somatostatin in obsessive-compulsive disorder. *Am J Psychiatry* 1993;150:460–464.
3. Ambrosi B, Bochicchio D, Fadin C, Colombo P, Faglia G. Failure of somatostatin and octreotide to acutely affect the hypothalamic–pituitary–adrenal function in patients with corticotropin hypersecretion. *J Endocrinol Invest* 1990;13:257–261.
4. Argente J, Chowen-Breed JA, Steiner RA, Clifton DK. Somatostatin messenger RNA in hypothalamic neurons is increased by testosterone through activation of androgen receptors and not by aromatization to estradiol. *Neuroendocrinology* 1990;52:342–349.
5. Beal MF, Mazurek MF, Ellison DW, Swartz KJ, McGarvey U, Bird ED, Martin JB. Somatostatin and neuropeptide Y concentrations in pathologically graded cases of Huntington's disease. *Ann Neurol* 1988;23:562–569.
6. Bell GI, Reisine T. Molecular biology of somatostatin receptors. *Trends Neurosci* 1993;16:34–38.
7. Benyassi A, Tapia-Arancibia L, Arancibia S. Glutamate peripherally administered exerts somatostatin-releasing actionin the conscious rat. *J Neuroendocrinol* 1991;3:429–432.
8. Bissette G, Widerlov E, Walleus H, Karlsson I, Eklund K, Forsman A, Nemeroff CB. Alterations in cerebrospinal fluid concentrations of somatostatin-like immunoreactivity in neuropsychiatric disorders. *Arch Gen Psychiatry* 1986;43:1148–1151.
9. Bowen DM, Najlerahim A, Procter AW, Francis PT, Murphy E. Circumscribed changes of the cerebral cortex in neuropsychiatric disorders of later life. *Proc Natl Acad Sci USA* 1989;86:9504–9508.
10. Breder CD, Yamada Y, Yasuda K, Seino S, Saper CB, Bell GI. Differential expression of somatostatin receptors subtypes in brain. *J Neurosci* 1992;12:3920–3934.
11. Candy JM, Gascoigne AD, Biggins A, et al. Somatostatin immunoreactivity in cortical and some subcortical regions in Alzheimer's disease. *J Neurol Sci* 1985;71:315–323.
12. Charlton BG, Leake A, Wright C, Fairbairn AF, McKeith IG, Candy JM, Ferrier IN. Somatostatin content and receptors in the cerebral cortex of depressed and control subjects. *J Neurol Neurosurg Psychiatry* 1988;51:719–721.
13. Charlton BG, Wright C, Leake A, Ferrier IN, Cheetham SC, Horton RW, Crompton MR. Somatostatin immunoreactivity in postmortem brain from depressed suicides [Letter]. *Arch Gen Psychiatry* 1988;45:597.
14. Cottrell GA, Robertson HA. Prevention of cysteamine-induced myoclonus blocks the long-term inhibition of kindled seizures. *Brain Res* 1987;412:161–164.
15. Doran AR, Rubinow DR, Wolkowitz OM, Roy A, Breier A, Pickar D. Fluphenazine treatment reduces CSF somatostatin in patients with schizophrenia: correlations with CSF HVA. *Biol Psychiatry* 1989;25:431–439.
16. Epelbaum J. Somatostatin receptors in the central nervous system. In: Weil C, Muller EE, Thorner MO, eds. *Somatostatin: basic and clinical aspects of neuroscience,* vol 4. Berlin: Springer-Verlag, 1992;17–28.
17. Ferrier IN, McKeith IG, Charlton BG, et al. Postmortem investigations of serotonergic and peptidergic hypotheses of affective illness. In: Lerer B, Gershon S, eds. *New directions in affective disorders.* New York: Springer-Verlag, 1989;60–63.
18. Gattaz WF, Rissler K, Gattaz D, Cramer H. Effects of haloperidol on somatostatin-like immunoreactivity in the CSF of schizophrenic patients. *Psychiatry Res* 1986;17:1–6.
19. Gomez S, Davous P, Rondot P, Faivre-Bauman A, Valade D, Puymirat J. Somatostatin-like immunoreactivity and acetylcholinesterase activities in cerebrospinal fluid of patients with Alzheimer disease and senile dementia of the Alzheimer type. *Psychoneuroendocrinology* 1986;11:69–73.

20. Goodman RH, Rehfuss RP, Verhave M, Ventimiglia R, Low MJ. Somatostatin gene regulation: an overview. *Metabolism* 1990;39 (Suppl 2):2–5.
21. Kakigi T, Maeda K. Effect of serotonergic agents on regional concentrations of somatostatin- and neuropeptide Y-like immunoreactivities in rat brain. *Brain Res* 1992;599:45–50.
22. Kakigi T, Maeda K, Kaneda H, Chihara K. Repeated administration of antidepressant drugs reduces regional somatostatin concentrations in rat brain. *J Affective Disord* 1992;25:215–220.
23. Kaye WH, Rubinow DR, Gwirtsman HE, George DT, Jimerson DC, Gold PW. CSF somatostatin in anorexia nervosa and bulimia: relationship to the hypothalamic pituitary–adrenal cortical axis. *Psychoneuroendocrinology* 1988;13:265–272.
24. Kleuss C, Hescheler J, Ewel C, Rosenthal W, Schultz G, Wittig B. Assignment of G protein subtypes to specific receptors inducing inhibition of calcium currents. *Nature* 1991;353:43–48.
25. Kling MA, Rubinow DR, Doran AR, et al. Cerebrospinal fluid somatostatin immunoreactive somatostatin concentrations in patients with Cushing's disease and major depression: relationship to indices of corticotropin-releasing hormone and cortisol secretion. *Neuroendocrinology* 1993;57:79–88.
26. Kruesi MJP, Swedo S, Leonard H, Rubinow DR, Rapoport JL. CSF somatostatin in childhood psychiatric disorders: a preliminary investigation. *Psychiatry Res* 1990;33:277–284.
27. Kupfer DJ, Jarrett DB, Ehlers CL. The effect of SRIF on the EEG sleep of normal men. *Psychoneuroendocrinology* 1992;17:37–43.
28. Lahtinen H, Pitkanen A, Tuomisto L, Riekkinen P. Effect of antiepileptic drugs on somatostatin release in vitro. *Neuropeptides* 1990;17:29–34.
29. Lowe SL, Francis PT, Procter AW, Palmer AM, Davison AN, Bowen DM. Gamma-aminobutyric acid concentration in brain tissue at two stages of Alzheimer's disease. *Brain* 1988;111:785–799.
30. Martin JL, Chesselet MF, Raynor K, Gonzales C, Reisine T. Differential distribution of somatostatin receptor subtypes in rat brain revealed by newly developed somatostatin analogs. *Neuroscience* 1991;41:581–593.
31. Matsuoka N, Kaneko S, Satoh M. Somatostatin augments long-term potentiation of the mossy fiber–CA3 system in guinea pig hippocampal slices. *Brain Res* 1991;553:188–194.
32. McCann SM. Physiology and pharmacology of LHRH and somatostatin. *Annu Rev Pharmacol Toxicol* 1982;22:491–515.
33. Molchan SE, Lawlor BA, Hill JL, et al. CSF monoamine metabolites and somatostatin in Alzheimer's disease and major depression. *Biol Psychiatry* 1991;29:1110–1118.
34. Monno A, Rizzi M, Samanin R, Vazzani A. Anti-somatostatin antibody enhances the rate of hippocampal kindling in rats. *Brain Res* 1993;602:148–152.
35. Patel YC. General aspects of the biology and function of somatostatin. In: Weil C, Muller EE, Thorner MO, eds. *Basic and clinical aspects of neuroscience,* vol 4. Berlin: Springer-Verlag, 1992;1–16.
36. Patel YC, Murthy KK, Escher EE, Banville D, Spiess J, Srikant CB. Mechanism of action of somatostatin: an overview of receptor function and studies of the molecular characterization and purification of somatostatin receptor proteins. *Metabolism* 1990;39(Suppl 2):63–69.
37. Patel YC, Rao K, Reichlin S. Somatostatin in human cerebrospinal fluid. *N Engl J Med* 1977;296:529–533.
38. Patel YC, Srikant CB. Somatostatin mediation of adenohypophysial secretion. *Annu Rev Physiol* 1985;48:551–567.
39. Perez-Oso E, Lopez-Ruiz MP, Arilla E. Effect of haloperidol withdrawal on somatostatin level and binding in rat brain. *Biosci Rep* 1990;10:15–22.
40. Pitkanen A, Jolkkonen J, Riekkinen P. β-endorphin, somatostatin, and prolactin levels in cerebrospinal fluid of epileptic patients after generalised convulsion. *J Neurol Neurosurg Psychiatry* 1987;50:1294–1297.
41. Post RM, Ballenger JC, Uhde TW, Bunney WE. Efficacy of carbamazepine in manic–depressive illness: implications for underlying mechanisms. In: Post RM, Ballenger JC, eds. *Neurobiology of mood disorders.* Baltimore: Williams & Wilkins, 1984;777–816.
42. Qin Y, Soghomonian J, Chesselet M. Effects of quinolinic acid on messenger RNAs encoding somatostatin and glutamic acid decarboxylases in the striatum of adult rats. *Exp Neurol* 1992;115:200–211.
43. Rissler K, Cramer H, Schaudt D, Strubel D, Gattaz WF. Molecular size distribution of somatostatin-like immunoreactivity in the cerebrospinal fluid of patients with degenerative brain disease. *Neurosci Res* 1986;3:213–225.
44. Robbins RJ. Regulation of hypothalamic somatostatin secretion. In: Reichlin S, ed. *Somatostatin: basic and clinical status.* New York: Plenum Press, 1987;149–156.
45. Robbins RJ, Brines ML, Kim JH, et al. A selective loss of somatostatin in the hippocampus of patients with temporal lobe epilepsy. *Ann Neurol* 1991;29:325–332.
46. Rosler N, Reuner C, Geiger J, Rissler K, Cramer H. Cerebrospinal fluid levels of immunoreactive substance P and somatostatin in patients with multiple sclerosis and inflammatory CNS disease. *Peptides* 1990;11:181–183.
47. Rubinow DR. Cerebrospinal fluid somatostatin and psychiatric illness. *Biol Psychiatry* 1986;21:341–365.
48. Rubinow DR, Davis CL, Post RM. Somatostatin in neuropsychiatric disorders. In: Weil C, Muller EE, Thorner MO, eds. *Somatostatin: basic and clinical aspects of neuroscience,* vol 4. Berlin: Springer-Verlag, 1992;29–42.
49. Scharfman HE, Schwartzkroin PA. Selective depression of GABA-mediated IPSPs by somatostatin in area CA1 of rabbit hippocampal slices. *Brain Res* 1989;493:205–211.
50. Shinoda H, Nadi NS, Schwartz JP. Alterations in somatostatin and proenkephalin mRNA in response to a single amygdaloid stimulation versus kindling. *Mol Brain Res* 1991;11:221–226.
51. Sorensen KV, Christensen SE, Dupont E, Hansen AP, Pedersen E, Orskov H. Low somatostatin content in cerebrospinal fluid in multiple sclerosis. *Acta Neurol Scand* 1980;61:186–191.
52. Sperk G, Marksteiner J, Gruber B, Bellmann R, Mahata M, Ortler M. Functional changes in neuropeptide Y- and somatostatin-containing neurons induced by limbic seizures in the rat. *Neuroscience* 1992;50:831–846.
53. Su T, Hauser P, Rubinow DR, et al. CSF somatostatin (SRIF), mood, and cognition in multiple sclerosis. In: *Abstracts of the twenty-first congress of the ISPNE,* 1990;81.
54. Tahiri-Jouti N, Cambillau C, Viguerie N, Vidal C, Saint Laurent N, Vaysse N, Susini C. Characterization of a membrane tyrosine phosphatase in AR42J cells: regulation by somatostatin. *Am J Physiol* 1992;262:G1007–G1014.
55. Tallent M, Reisine T. Gi alpha 1 selectively couples somatostatin receptors to adenylyl cyclase in pituitary-derived AtT-20 cells. *Mol Pharmacol* 1992;41:452–455.
56. Traskman-Bendz L, Ekman R, Regnell G, Ohman R. HPA-related CSF neuropeptides in suicide attempts. *Eur Neuropsychopharmacol* 1992;2:99–106.
57. Vecsei L, Widerlov E. Brain and CSF somatostatin concentrations in patients with psychiatric or neurological illness: an overview. *Acta Psychiatr Scand* 1988;78:657.
58. Vecsei L, Widerlov E. Effects of somatostatin-28 and some of its fragments and analogs on open-field behavior, barrel rotation, and shuttle box learning in rats. *Psychoneuroendocrinology* 1990;15:139–145.
59. Vezzani A, Serafini R, Stasi MA, Vigano G, Rizzi M, Samanin R. A peptidase-resistant cyclic octapeptide analogue of somatostatin (SMS 201-995) modulates seizures induced by quinolinic and kainic acids differentially in the rat hippocampus. *Neuropharmacology* 1991;30:345–352.
60. Walsh TJ, Emerich DF, Winokur A, Banki C, Bissette G, Nemeroff CB. Intrahippocampal injection of cysteamine depletes somatostatin and produces cognitive impairments in the rat. *Neurosci Abstr* 1985;11:621.
61. Weckbecker G, Tolcsvai L, Liu R, Bruns C. Preclinical studies on the anticancer activity of the somatostatin analogue octreotide (SMS 201-995). *Metabolism* 1992;41(Suppl 2):99–103.
62. Xie Z, Sastry BR. Actions of somatostatin on GABA-ergic synaptic transmission in the CA1 area of the hippocampus. *Brain Res* 1992;591:239–247.
63. Yasuda K, Espinosa R III, Davis EM, LeBeau MM, Bell GI. Human somatostatin receptor genes: localization of SSTR5 to human chromosome 20p11.2. *Genomics* 1993;17:785–786.
64. Zorrilla R, Simard J, Rheaume E, Labrie F, Pelletier G. Multihormonal control of pre-pro-somatostatin mRNA levels in the periventricular nucleus of the male and female rat hypothalamus. *Neuroendocrinology* 1990;52:527–536.

*Psychopharmacology: The Fourth
Generation of Progress,* edited by
Floyd E. Bloom and David J. Kupfer.
Raven Press, Ltd., New York © 1995.

CHAPTER 50

Galanin

A Neuropeptide with Important Central Nervous System Actions

Tamas Bartfai

Galanin is a neuropeptide which is not a member of any known family of neuropeptides, despite repeated efforts to discover related peptides. Its actions are mediated via G_i-protein-coupled receptors and ion channels, usually producing inhibition of secretion of a transmitter or hormone in the nervous and endocrine system. In many respects, these inhibitory actions of galanin remind us of those of gamma-aminobutyric acid (GABA) and of neuropeptide Y (NPY). Galanin coexists with GABA, noradrenaline, 5-hydroxytryptamine (5-HT), and NPY in several regions of the brain.

Its central nervous system (CNS) actions—and in particular its proposed role in Alzheimer's disease—have helped to fuel interest in galanin. The galanin literature is now numbering over 1200 papers. The late introduction of specific, high-affinity galanin antagonists in 1991 made it possible to study the role of endogenous galanin—which often appears as a strong tonic inhibitor of neuronal actions, a feature studied best by use of antagonists. Several excellent reviews (6,57,73) have appeared on different aspects of galanin actions, and these can provide more detail than this short overview. This chapter is devoted to the central actions and central neuroanatomy of galanin and galanin receptors. The literature on galanin actions on the pancreas, heart, and gut is abundant and rapidly increasing. We have, however, chosen to concentrate on the CNS actions of galanin which may underlie a role of galanin receptor ligands in therapy of Alzheimer's disease, depression, and eating disorders, respectively (see also Chapters 8, 30, 43, 83, 84, 118, and 136, *this volume*).

T. Bartfai: Arrhenius Laboratories of Natural Sciences, Department of Neurochemistry and Neurotoxicology, Stockholm University, S-106 91 Stockholm, Sweden.

BIOSYNTHESIS OF GALANIN AND GALANIN-MESSAGE-ASSOCIATED PEPTIDE (GMAP)

Structure of Galanin–GMAP mRNA

The mRNA encoding the galanin is composed of a 5' portion encoding a signal sequence, followed by a Lys-Arg cleavage site, then the 29-amino-acid-long galanin peptide followed by Gly-Lys-Arg at the C-terminal containing the amide donor Gly and the cleavage site Lys-Arg (63,72). Both the signal sequence and the galanin sequence show a very high degree of homology (>85%) between the rat, mouse, porcine, bovine, and human sequences (see Table 1). The galanin-encoding portion of the mRNA is followed by 180 bases encoding a 60-amino-acid-long peptide, named the *galanin-message-associated peptide* (GMAP). Several homology regions (some with homology up to 97%) of 15–20 amino acids within the GMAP in rat, mouse, bovine, porcine, and human sequences have been examined so far. The biological significance of GMAP as a neurohormone or precursor to neurohormones is not yet known.

Galanin Gene Expression Is Regulated by Steroids, Nerve Growth Factor, and Nerve Injury

Galanin mRNA levels rise in the pituitary during pregnancy, and they are also present in the placenta (72). During the estrous cycle of the rat, pituitary galanin mRNA levels vary 30-fold! Estrogen treatment induced changes (two- to threefold) in several hypothalamic nuclei. The pituitary galanin mRNA levels are controlled

TABLE 1. *Endogenously occurring galanin sequences*

	1 5 10 15	16 20 25	30
Man	G W T L N S A G Y L L G P H A	V G N H R S F S D K	N G L T S**
Pig	G W T L N S A G Y L L G P H A	I D N H R S F H D K	Y G L A*
Cow	G W T L N S A G Y L L G P H A	L D S H R S F Q D K	H G L A*
Rat	G W T L N S A G Y L L G P H A	I D N H R S F S D K	H G L T*
Mouse	G W T L N S A G Y L L G P H A	I D N H R S F S D K	H G L T*
Sheep	G W T L N S A G Y L L G P H A	I D N H R S F H D K	H G L A*
Chicken	G W T L N S A G Y L L G P H A	V D N H R S F N D K	H G F T*

* C-terminal amide.
** C-terminal free acid.
Boldface denotes amino acids which are not conserved between species.

by thyroid hormones which appear to play a permissive role in galanin expression (40), an effect which may relate to galanin-mediated regulation of the secretion of thyrotropin (60). In human pituitary tumors a very high (67–100%) correlation between expression of galanin and ACTH was found (39). These tumors are also carrying galanin receptors in most cases. Galanin is found in the human adrenals, and pheochromocytoma show elevated levels of galanin-like immunoreactivity (galanin-LI) (8). In the rat PC12 pheochromocytoma cells, nerve growth factor (NGF) induces transcription of the galanin gene (40). The regulation of the galanin gene and of the tissue levels of galanin in the pituitary, as well as the regulation of circulating galanin levels, are under strong estrogen control in the female rat. The galanin mRNA is very strongly up-regulated by chronic estrogen treatment in an estrogen-induced pituitary tumor and in the female rat anterior pituitary (75). The interactions between the components of the hypothalamic–pituitary–adrenal axis involve and affect the expression of galanin, but nowhere as dramatically as in the anterior pituitary (60,75).

Regulation of the galanin gene expression under conditions of axotomy of sensory neurons has also been observed (39). The increase in galanin-LI and galanin mRNA is dramatic (up to 100-fold). It appears that destruction of the axons and/or terminal fields of central galaninergic neurons also leads to a similar up-regulation of the galanin mRNA and galanin-LI in the cell bodies (17).

DISTRIBUTION OF GALANIN- AND GMAP-LI AND COEXISTENCE SITUATIONS

Distribution of Galanin-LI in the Rat CNS

In the rat, the highest densities of galanin-LI are found in more ventral structures such as the amygdaloid complex, the hypothalamus, and the brainstem (12,56,66,67).

In contrast, neocortical areas and cerebellum have considerably lower numbers of galanin-LI-positive fibers and cells (54). Galanin-immunoreactive cell bodies are observed in the *telencephalon,* including the bed nucleus of the stria terminalis, the nucleus of the diagonal band

continuing into the medial septum, and the medial aspects of the central amygdaloid nucleus. In the *diencephalon* the only thalamic positive cell bodies are seen in the anterior dorsal and periventricular nuclei. The hypothalamus contains a large number of galanin-positive cell groups such as the medial and lateral preoptic nuclei, the arcuate nucleus, the periventricular nucleus, the dorsomedial nucleus, the lateral hypothalamus/medial forebrain bundle area, the tuberal, caudal, accessory supraoptic and paraventricular magnocellular nuclei, and the area lateral to the mamillary recess. In the *mesencephalon/ pons,* large midline cell groups that are galanin-positive include the dorsal raphe nuclei. Many neurons in the locus coeruleus and dorsal raphe nucleus contain galanin-LI.

Coexistence of Galanin with Other Neurotransmitters

Galanin is present in neurons which express classical transmitters such as catecholamines and amino acids as well as other peptides (53,55). Many such coexistence situations have been identified for galanin. In the *ventral forebrain,* galanin is present in a population of the large cholinergic neurons projecting to cortical areas (43,63). These cells are present in the diagonal band nucleus extending into the medial septum but not in the basal nucleus of Meynert. In the rat they project especially to the hippocampal formation.

The hypothalamus is particularly rich in coexistence situations: In the arcuate nucleus, galanin coexists with tyrosine hydroxylase as well as with the GABA-ergic marker glutamic acid decarboxylase (GAD) (55), and with neurotensin-LI, growth-hormone-releasing-factor (GRF)-LI, and choline acetyltransferase-LI (25). The main signal substances in the latter neurons is presumably GRF, which is the stimulating factor for growth hormone release. A large proportion of the magnocellular and many parvocellular neurons in the paraventricular nucleus have galanin, which here coexists mainly with vasopressin-, dynorphin-, and cholecystokinin (CCK)-LI. The tuberomamillary nucleus has many galanin-positive neurons which also in part contain GAD-, histamine-, adenosineaminase-, and monoaminoxidase-LI, and these neurons also have the property of 5-hydroxytryptophan up-take (42). More recently the coexistence of galanin and luteinizing-hormone-releasing hormone (LHRH) has been demonstrated. In the *lower brainstem* a large proportion of the noradrenergic cell bodies of the locus coeruleus are strongly galanin-positive (37).

Coexistence is shown between galanin and 5-HT, both at the dorsal raphe nuclei and at the medullary raphe nuclei. Furthermore, nucleus raphe pallidus, obscurus, and magnus contain GAL-LI.

Galanin-LI in the Primate Brain

Several earlier studies addressed the distribution of galanin-LI in primate brain. Kordower et al. (41) have published a comprehensive distributional study on adult Cebus monkey, baboon, and human brains, demonstrating in the monkey that *telencephalon* galanin-positive cell bodies apparently have a wider spread than in the rat. Positive cell bodies are found in the anterior olfactory nucleus, the basal forebrain, the endopiriform nucleus, the hippocampus, and the bed nucleus of the stria terminalis. The caudate nucleus and putamen contained galanin-positive cell bodies, a location which so far has not been described conclusively in the rat. As in the rat, numerous *hypothalamic nuclei* were galanin-positive, including those in the medial preoptic area, the periventricular, suprachiasmatic, paraventricular, and arcuate areas, and the lateral hypothalamic area. No cell bodies were observed in the thalamus or mesencephalon, but small numbers of fibers could be seen in various nuclei, including the ventral tegmental area. In the *lower brainstem* the medial vestibular nucleus, nucleus prepositus, and the solitary tract and hypoglossal nuclei contained galanin-positive cell bodies. With regard to fibers, dense networks were observed in the spinal trigeminal nucleus, the solitary tract nucleus, the dorsal vagal motor nucleus, and the dorsal horn of the *spinal cord*. Of particular interest is the distribution of galanin-LI in the basal forebrain, in part because of its possible relation to Alzheimer's disease and because of apparent species differences. While galanin in the rat is restricted to the septal diagonal band complex, these cells have an apparently wider distribution in the monkey basal forebrain where also the nucleus basalis is included. So far it has not been possible to demonstrate galanin-LI or galanin mRNA in the human magnocellular basal forebrain, with the exception of some medium-sized neurons described by Chan-Palay (13,14).

CHEMISTRY AND PHARMACOLOGY OF GALANIN RECEPTOR AGONISTS AND ANTAGONISTS

Galanin Receptor Agonists

Structure–Activity Relationships

The sequence of galanin from six species is known, including the human galanin sequence (Table 1). The galanin peptides show a complete sequence homology in the N-terminal 15 amino acids, suggesting that this portion of the peptide is of importance for recognition by the galanin receptors and for exerting agonist activity. Furthermore, the 100% homology of the N-terminal half of the peptide suggests that galanin from any species will be recognized by galanin receptors in any other species (at least among these six known species), which is indeed the experimental observation. Despite some sequence variability in the C-terminal 16-29/30 portion of the peptide, the galanin molecules bind with the same high affinity ($K_d = 0.8$ nM) to receptors in any species tested so far (see ref. 45).

It is noteworthy that human galanin consists of 30 amino acids (24) and that the C-terminus is a free carboxylic acid, whereas all other known types of galanin are composed of 29 amino acids (69) and carry a C-terminal amide (i.e., the preprogalanin has 30 amino acids, but the 30th glycine is the amide donor).

The amino acid residues of importance for binding and for biological activity were studied most extensively in three preparations: rat hippocampus and hypothalamus and mouse pancreatic islets or in the Rin m5F rat insulinoma cells.

In the hippocampal test system, intracerebroventricularly (i.c.v.) injected galanin inhibits the hippocampal acetylcholine release measured by microdialysis technique (28). In the ventral hippocampus, rat galanin appears to be the most potent known endogenous inhibitor of the evoked acetylcholine release (experimentally induced by intraperitoneal injection of scopolamine 2 mg/kg). Galanin injected i.c.v. or into the paraventricular nucleus (PVN) of the hypothalamus causes a robust stimulation of food intake. In the mouse pancreatic islets, galanin potently inhibits the glucose-induced insulin release; and in Rin m5F cells, which possess an exceptionally high number of galanin receptors (2,4,31,35) (~4000–20,000/cell), galanin also inhibits forskolin-stimulated cAMP accumulation. Thus in these systems the binding and biological effects of galanin, galanin analogues, and fragments were evaluated by two research groups (2,30), with the following results:

1. Intact N-terminus: Gly^1-Trp^2-Thr^3-Asn^4 is required for high affinity and for hippocampal inhibition of acetylcholine release and for pancreatic inhibitory action on cAMP accumulation and insulin release.
2. The N-terminal 1-15 or 1-16 fragment is a high-affinity ($K_d = 8$ nM) full agonist, whereas the 17-29 C-terminal fragment has very low affinity $K_d > 1$ mM) and no agonist effect.
3. The shortest galanin fragment with documented agonist activity is galanin(1-9) in the hippocampal system, and galanin(1-10) on smooth muscle.
4. The most important amino acid residues for the high-affinity binding of galanin(1-16) were identified by subsequent L-alanine substitutions, and it was found

TABLE 2. *Galanin receptor antagonists reverse the effects of galanin upon i.cv, PVN, or in vitro application[a]*

	Galanin effects reversed							
Antagonist	Lowered spinal excitability	Inhibition of insulin release	Stimulation of feeding	Cognitive impairment	Inhibition of ACh release	Stimulation of growth hormone release	Stimulation of prolactin release	Vagal attenuation
M15	++	++	++	nt	++	++	+	++
M35	++	++	+	+	++	nt	nt	
M40	+	No effect	++		++	nt	nt	

[a] Some data are from ref. 6. nt, not tested. ++, reversal of galanin effect at equimolar dose. +, reversal of galanin effect at 10-fold or higher excess of the antagonist.

that glycine[1], tryptophan[2], asparagine[5], and tyrosine[9] were among these for binding important amino acids and thus may be the pharmacophores in galanin receptor agonists (46).

Degradation and Biological Half-Life of Galanin

The agonist action of galanin and of its N-terminal fragments is terminated by their degradation at the N-terminus by enzymes which cleave the first or the first two residues, with G-W yielding the inactive 3-29/30 and 3-16 fragments—as studied in the spinal cord and hypothalamus (44; Bedecs et al., *in preparation*). Preliminary data suggest that these diaminoacylpeptidases which cleave and inactivate galanin may belong to the class of metalloproteases because chelating agents afford some inhibition of the degradation of galanin by cerebrospinal fluid (CSF) and by spinal cord membranes.

The biological half-life of galanin upon incubation with rat CSF or with hypothalamic membranes is about 60 min, which is almost 10-fold longer than that of the equal-sized peptide vasoactive intestinal peptide. The long half-life may enable galanin to exert paracrine actions.

Galanin agonists with peptidase-resistant N-terminus are currently being synthesized and tested.

Among the galanin receptor agonists, one should mention two endogenously occurring, minor galanin isoforms isolated in small amounts (~1% of the amount of galanin-LI) from the porcine adrenal: galanin(7-29) and galanin(9-29) (8,11). Whether or not these N-terminally elongated forms of galanin occur in human tissues is not known. In the rat spinal cord these N-terminally elongated forms of galanin bind with a 100-fold lower affinity than galanin and have commensurately weak agonist effect on the spinal flexor reflex (Wiesenfeldt et al., *in preparation*).

Galanin Receptor Antagonists

Recently a series of galanin receptor antagonists have been synthesized and tested in a variety of in vivo and in vitro models of galanin action (6).

The first galanin receptor antagonists are chimeric, bire-

ceptor recognizing peptides composed of the N-terminal 1-12 fragment of galanin followed by proline[13] and a sequence corresponding to the recognition sequence of another neuropeptide whose recognition and activity are dependent on its C-terminus (5). Thus M 15 or galantide is galanin(1-12)-pro-substance P(5-11) (5,49), M 32 is galanin(1-12)-pro-neuropeptide Y(25-36), M 35 is galanin(1-12)-pro-bradykinin(2-9) (36,79), and C 7 carries a substance P antagonist (i.e., spantide)—rather than an agonist—as its C-terminus: galanin(1-12)-pro-spantide. Finally M 40 and its analogues carry a C-terminal sequence with no known receptor: galanin(1-12)-(Pro)$_3$-(Ala-Leu)$_2$Ala amide (19).

The key to the usefulness of these antagonists lies in their very high affinity ($10^{-10} - 10^{-9}$ M) (6), making possible their use in vivo. The use of these galanin receptor antagonists, barely a year after their introduction, is widespread and will lead to definition of even more effects of endogenous galanin in the nervous and endocrine system. All of these antagonists have been tested in numerous models of galanin actions in the periphery and CNS (see Table 2). Their action in most systems is that of an antagonist. However, M 40 appears to distinguish between pancreatic and CNS galanin receptors (cf. receptor subtypes).

The major drawbacks of these antagonists are (a) their peptide nature which prevents their passage through blood–brain barrier, (b) their possible peptidase sensitivity, and (c) that when applied in very high concentration they may exhibit agonist-like effects due to their intact N-terminus. Because the galanin receptor antagonists hold considerable pharmacological potential, several large-scale screening programs are underway to identify nonpeptide galanin receptor antagonists.

GALANIN RECEPTORS, SUBTYPES, AND SIGNAL TRANSDUCTION

Galanin Receptors

Structure

The galanin receptor(s) has not yet been sequenced despite purification (15), solubilization, cross-linking (2), and cDNA cloning efforts. We know that it belongs to the class of G-protein-coupled receptors, and in particular to the G_i/G_o-protein-coupled receptor subclass, because all actions of galanin at membrane (3), cellular (21), and in vivo levels in the hippocampus of freely moving rats (16) were abolished by pretreatment with pertussis toxin. Thus the receptor is assumed to be coupled via a pertussis toxin ADP-ribosylable G protein. There have been suggestions that the inhibitory action of galanin on the release of numerous signal substances would be exerted at a G protein directly involved in the release apparatus (65).

Galanin Receptor Subtypes

In the absence of sequence data on different galanin receptor proteins, definitions of galanin receptor subtypes have been proposed based on pharmacological studies with agonists and antagonists. The pancreatic and the CNS galanin receptors appear to accept the N-terminal 1-15/16 fragment as a full agonist (18,27,77), while it is suggested that smooth muscle galanin receptors have a structural requirement for both the N- and the C-termini of galanin (62). In addition, it has been suggested that the anterior pituitary of the rat expresses a specific galanin receptor which recognizes galanin(3-29) (76), whereas all other galanin receptors have an absolute requirement for the intact N-terminus of galanin.

Classification of galanin receptor subtypes proposed by the present authors is based on the observation that the antagonist M 40 blocks the galanin effects on feeding and also blocks acetylcholine release in the hippocampus but does not antagonize the galaninergic inhibition of the glucose-induced insulin release, suggesting that pancreatic galanin receptors may be different from CNS galanin receptors (Bartfai et al., *in preparation*).

Second Messenger Systems Coupled to the Galanin Receptors via G_i/G_o Proteins

Galanin-Mediated Opening of K^+ Channels

Galanin has been reported to hyperpolarize neurons in a number of central and peripheral preparations. This hyperpolarization is brought about in some systems by opening of K^+ channels. This has been demonstrated in pancreatic β cells (20,21), as well as in noradrenergic cells in the locus coeruleus. In the Rin m5F rat insulinoma cells the galanin-mediated hyperpolarization appears to involve opening of an ATP-sensitive K^+ channel (20).

Galanin Effects on Intracellular Ca^{2+} Concentrations and on L- and N-Type Ca^{2+} Channels

Galanin is a potent inhibitor of the release of a number of neurotransmitters and hormones, including acetylcho-

line, dopamine, insulin, and gastrin. Its actions in some systems have been shown to involve a decrease in the cytosolic Ca^{2+} concentration (1,58). This may be the consequence of the hyperpolarization brought about by opening of galanin-receptor-coupled K^+-channels (see above), or it may be a result of the galanin-receptor-mediated closure of some Ca^{2+} channels—or of a combination of galanin effects on K^+-channel opening and Ca^{2+}-channel closure. In the hippocampus, pharmacological experiments using ω-conotoxin suggested that closure of an N-type Ca^{2+} channel is part of the galanin action (61). In the Rin m5F cells, pharmacological and electrophysiological (patch clamp) experiments suggest that the involvement of an L-type Ca^{2+} channel in the inhibitory galanin effect (38) on insulin release.

Galanin-Mediated Inhibition of Adenylate Cyclase and of cGMP Accumulation

Galanin has been shown to inhibit the β-noradrenergic stimulation of adenylate cyclase in the rat cerebral cortex (59), and forskolin stimulated the accumulation of cAMP in the Rin m5F insulinoma cells (3). These effects could be abolished by pretreatment with pertussis toxin, indicating that the galanin receptor acts via a pertussis-toxin-sensitive G protein.

In tissue slices from the lumbar spinal cord the K^+-depolarization-mediated rise in cGMP levels is partially inhibited by galanin in a dose-dependent manner (10). This observation is in line with the restriction of Ca^{2+} entry by galanin, because Ca^{2+} entry is a prerequisite for the full activity of the guanylate cyclase.

Galanin also diminishes the muscarinic-cholinergic-receptor-mediated stimulation of phospholipase C, resulting in less inositol triphosphate (IP_3) production in the presence of galanin than by the muscarinic agonist alone (61). This interaction probably reflects a postsynaptic antagonism between acetylcholine and galanin released from the same septal afferent and acting probably on the same hippocampal cells, because it was previously shown that muscarinic stimulation of phospholipase C is a predominantly postsynaptic effect in the hippocampus.

The effects of galanin on nitric oxide synthesis have not yet been studied.

Galanin Inhibits the Protein-Kinase-C-Catalyzed Phosphorylation of Hippocampal Proteins

The phorbol-ester-stimulated (and therefore probably protein kinase-C-catalyzed) phosphorylation of two hippocampal proteins of 20 and 41 kD is inhibited in the presence of galanin (47). The galanin effect could be blocked by galanin receptor antagonists M 15 and M 35. The identity of the two proteins whose phosphorylation is inhibited is not yet known.

CELLULAR EFFECTS OF GALANIN IN THE CNS

Locus Coeruleus

Galanin hyperpolarizes the noradrenergic neurons in the locus coeruleus and reduces the rate of spontaneous firing (5,64). These effects are probably brought about by opening some non-ATP-sensitive K+ channels. The hyperpolarizing effects of galanin are long-lasting, dose-dependent, and fully reversible. Specific galanin receptor antagonists block this effect of galanin (5). The galaninergic control of firing rate is particularly interesting because locus coeruleus neurons contain large amounts of galanin in coexistence with noradrenaline. It is possible that dendritic release of galanin occurs within the structure and contributes to the overall regulation of noradrenergic activity in the CNS (see also Chapter 33, *this volume*).

Hippocampus

Galanin inhibits the slow muscarinic postsynaptic potential, especially in the hippocampus (23), by a presynaptic inhibition of the release of acetylcholine from the septal afferents, as demonstrated also by in vivo microdialysis studies (26). Galanin also inhibits the evoked release of the excitatory amino acids glutamate and asparate, while not affecting the release of GABA under the same conditions (78). By virtue of its pre- and postsynaptic effects on K+ and Ca^{2+} conductances, galanin is a hyperpolarizing agent in the hippocampus; galanin receptor antagonists accordingly lower the seizure threshold for picrotoxin-induced seizures, for example.

Galanin appears to affect the binding affinity of serotonin to serotonin receptors (5-HT$_{IA}$) in the diencephalic and telencephalic areas. Galanin applied i.c.v. strongly reduces 5-HT metabolism in the hippocampus and frontoparietal cortex of the rat (29).

Hypothalamus and Pituitary

Galanin inhibits dopamine release from the median eminence and strongly stimulates the release of prolactin and growth hormone in humans and in rats (7,9,32,33). In humans, intravenous injections of galanin cause substantial release of growth hormone, while reduction of the plasma levels of insulin, glucagon, somatostatin, and gastrin is also observed (7,9,32,33). The galanin receptor antagonist M 15 has been shown to inhibit the amplitude of growth hormone release while not affecting the periodicity of the pulsatile release (30). The coexistence of dopamine, galanin, and GRF-LIs in hypothalamic nerve endings and neurons (53) may thus give rise to complex inhibitory and disinhibitory patterns in control of growth hormone and prolactin release.

BEHAVIORAL EFFECTS OF GALANIN

Food Intake

Galanin, both applied i.c.v. and when injected into the PVN (18,42) in a dose-dependent manner, stimulates feeding behavior—in particular the intake of fat. The increase induced by galanin is highly significant: 200% above baseline. Several galanin receptor antagonists have been shown to antagonize the stimulatory effects of galanin (48).

It should be noted that among the prominent peripheral actions of galanin is its inhibitory effect on the glucose-induced insulin release, making galanin a hyperglycemic substance (52). The present assumption is that galanin—which coexists with noradrenaline in the sympathetic nerves which innervate the pancreas—mediates the stress-induced inhibition of insulin release (22). Galanin appears to regulate both fat and glucose levels by its central and peripheral actions.

Pain Threshold

Galanin appears to act as a physiological antagonist of substance P in several types of pain, and intrathecal application of galanin in a dose-dependent manner reduces pain sensation (74). Intrathecal application of galanin receptor antagonists to rats with only superficial cuts caused a pronounced autotomy, demonstrating the important analgesic effects of endogenous galanin in peripheral nerve injury (70). These observations are in line with the exceptionally high increases in galanin and galanin mRNA in dorsal root ganglia upon axotomy (71) and suggest that one of the functions of galanin at nerve injury is to control pain.

Cognitive Performance

Galanin (i.c.v.) impairs the performance of rats in the Morris swim maze (68) and in a one trial reward learning task (50). Galanin impairs working memory when injected into medial septal area (34). Furthermore, galanin antagonizes the acetylcholine-injection (i.c.v.)-produced improvements in cognitive performance of basal forebrain-lesioned rats (51). Galanin antagonist M 35, on the other hand, has been shown to improve performance of rats in the Morris swim maze (79). This improvement probably involves enhanced acquisition and, to a lesser extent, improved retention.

PHARMACOLOGICAL PERSPECTIVES OF GALANIN RECEPTOR LIGANDS

Galanin has numerous peripheral and central effects which are well worth exploiting. Accordingly, several groups in the industry as well as in the academic community work on specific, high-affinity, nonpeptide agonists and antagonists which will act as galanin receptors. Development of receptor-subtype-specific ligands will even further increase the usefulness of the galanin receptors as pharmacological targets.

Potential of Galanin Receptor Agonists

CNS Use: Prevention of Anoxic Damage

It is argued by several groups that galanin receptor agonists may be useful in preventing anoxic damage because these ligands do not suppress GABA release or the release of the excitatory amino acids glutamate and aspartate (78). Thus the galanin receptor agonists would have an advantage over Ca^{2+}-channel blockers, which, in general, suppress release. It is envisaged that under the conditions of open heart surgery (for example), galanin receptor agonists would be useful in preventing oxidative damage.

Neuroendocrinology

Galanin receptor agonists enhance the release of growth hormone without affecting the diurnal rhythm of this process and therefore appear as attractive agents to increase growth hormone secretion in humans (7,9,32,33).

Galanin receptors seem to control prolactin release from pituitary adenomas and are considered as targets for endocrine manipulation of these tumors.

Analgesia

Galanin, although not a potent analgesic agent on its own, appears to prolong the morphine analgesia four- to eightfold. Application of CCK_b antagonists together with morphine and galanin produced remarkable prolongation of the morphine effects and may therefore contribute to reduction of morphine doses needed to manage chronic pain (75).

Potential Use of Galanin Receptor Antagonists

Alzheimer's Disease: Improvement of Cholinergic Function

Immunohistochemical data on autopsy samples from Alzheimer's-afflicted brains suggest that galaninergic fibers hyperinnervate the nucleus basalis cholinergic cells (13,14). This may have a consequence similar to that found in the rat locus coeruleus—that is, that the cells are hyperpolarized by galanin and lower their firing rate (64). This would further deepen the hippocampal cholinergic deficit arising from the death of many cholinergic

cells in this nucleus. Thus a galanin receptor antagonist may improve cholinergic function by enhancing the firing rate of surviving cholinergic neurons.

In the hippocampus, at the level of the cholinergic nerve endings it was shown by in vivo microdialysis that galanin suppresses the per-pulse release of acetylcholine in the ventral hippocampus of rats (28). Galanin receptor antagonists reverse this presynaptic inhibition (5). Thus galanin receptor antagonists may improve cholinergic function both at the level of the cell body by enhancing firing and at the cholinergic nerve terminal by enhancing the per-pulse release.

At the level of the hippocampal cholinoreceptive cell, galanin also opposes the slow depolarizing action of acetylcholine at muscarinic receptors because it reduces the muscarinic stimulation of IP_3 production (61); thus, even at these cholinoreceptive cells, galanin receptor antagonists may contribute to the overall enhancement of cholinergic transmission.

Experiments with normal rats receiving galanin receptor antagonist M 35 have already shown an enhanced cognitive function (79). These studies are now being extended to old rats and to lesion models of Alzheimer's disease. Galanin receptor antagonists today appear as one of the more interesting new approaches to enhance cholinergic function (see Chapter 118, *this volume*).

Antidepressants

Galanin is colocalized with both serotonin in the raphe nucleus and with noradrenaline in the locus coeruleus. In the latter structure, sufficient amount of data have been collected to suggest that galanin receptor antagonists enhance firing of noradrenergic neurons probably by reversing the tonic galanin-mediated inhibition/hyperpolarization (5). In addition, it is known that galanin also suppresses 5-HT metabolism (29). The strategic localization of both galanin and galanin receptors in the raphe nucleus and in the locus coeruleus, along with the neuronal-activity-enhancing effects of galanin receptor antagonists in the monoamine systems, argues for their potential as antidepressant agents (see Chapters 83 and 84, *this volume*).

Feeding Disorders

Because galanin antagonists suppress fat intake specifically (19,48) but do not suppress all kinds of food intake, these compounds are interesting agents for development of drugs in the area of eating disorders.

ACKNOWLEDGMENTS

This chapter summarizes the work carried out in collaboration with the following individuals: Dr. Thomas Hökfelt, Karolinska Institute; Dr. Sylvana Consolo, Mario Negri Institute; Dr. Jacqueline Crawley, NIMH, Dr. Zsuzsanna Wisenfeld-Hallin, Huddinge Hospital; and Dr. Ülo Langel, Stockholm University. The study was supported by the National Institute of Aging, Drug Discovery Programme, Swedish Medical Research Council, and Riksbankens Jubileumsfond.

REFERENCES

1. Ahrén B, Arkhammar P, Berggren P-O, Nilsson T. Galanin inhibits glucose-stimulated insulin release by a mechanism involving hyperpolarization and lowering of cytoplasmic free Ca^{2+} concentration. *Biochem Biophys Res Commun* 1986;140:1059–1063.

2. Amiranoff B, Lorinet AM, Laburthe M. Galanin receptor in the rat pancreatic beta-cell line Rin m5F—molecular characterization by chemical cross-linking. *J Biol Chem* 1989;264:20714–20717.

3. Amiranoff B, Lorinet AM, Lagny-Pourmir I, Laburthe M. Mechanism of galanin-inhibited insulin release. Occurrence of a pertussis-toxin-sensitive inhibition of adenylate cyclase. *Eur J Biochem* 1988;177:147–152.

4. Amiranoff B, Servin AL, Rouyer-Fessard C, Couvineau A, Tatemoto K, Laburthe M. Galanin receptors in a hamster pancreatic β-cell tumor: identification and molecular characterization. *Endocrinology* 1987;121:284–289.

5. Bartfai T, Bedecs K, Land T, et al. M-15—high-affinity chimeric peptide that blocks the neuronal actions of galanin in the hippocampus, locus coeruleus, and spinal cord. *Proc Natl Acad Sci USA* 1991;88:10961–10965.

6. Bartfai T, Fisone G, Langel Ü. Galanin and galanin antagonists—molecular and biochemical perspectives. *Trends Pharmacol Sci* 1992;13:312–317.

6a. Bartfai T, Langel Ü, Bedecs K, Andell S, Land T, Gregersen S, Ahrén B, Girotti P, Consolo S, Corwin R, Crawley J, Xu XJ, Wiesenfeld-Hallin Z, Hökfelt T. Galanin-receptor ligand M40 peptide distinguishes between putative galanin-receptor subtypes. *Proc Natl Acad Sci USA* 1993;90:11287–11291.

7. Bauer FE, Ginsberg L, Venetikou M, MacKay DJ, Burrin JM, Bloom SR. Growth hormone release in man induced by galanin, a new hypothalamic peptide. *Lancet* 1986;2:192–194.

8. Bauer FE, Hacker GW, Terenghi G, Adrian TE, Polak JM, Bloom SR. Localization and molecular forms of galanin in human adrenals: elevated levels in pheochromocytomas. *J Clin Endocrinol Metab* 1986;63:1372–1378.

9. Bauer FE, Zintel A, Kenny MJ, Calder D, Ghatei MA, Bloom SR. Inhibitory effect of galanin on postprandial gastrointestinal motility and gut hormone release in humans. *Gastroenterology* 1989;97:260–264.

10. Bedecs K, Langel Ü, Bartfai T, Wiesenfeld-Hallin Z. Galanin receptors and their second messengers in the lumbar dorsal spinal cord. *Acta Physiol Scand* 1992;144:213–220.

11. Bersani M, Thim L, Rasmussen TN, Holst JJ. Galanin and galanin extended at the N-terminus with seven and nine amino acids are produced in and secreted from the porcine adrenal medulla in almost equal amounts. *Endocrinology* 1991;129:2693–2698.

12. Ch'ng JLC, Christofides ND, Anand P, et al. Distribution of galanin immunoreactivity in the central nervous system and the responses of galanin-containing neuronal pathways to injury. *Neuroscience* 1985;16:343–354.

13. Chan-Palay V. Neurons with galanin innervate cholinergic cells in the human basal forebrain and galanin and acetylcholine coexist. *Brain Res Bull* 1988;21:465–472.

14. Chan-Palay V. Hyperinnervation of surviving neurons of the human basal nucleus of Meynert by galanin in dementias of Alzheimer's and Parkinson's disease. *Alzheimer's Dis* 1990;51:253–255.

15. Chen YH, Couvineau A, Laburthe M, Amiranoff B. Solubilization and molecular characterization of active galanin receptors from rat brain. *Biochemistry* 1992;31:2415–2422.

16. Consolo S, Bertorelli R, Girotti P, et al. Pertussis toxin-sensitive G-protein mediates galanin's inhibition of scopolamine-evoked acetylcholine release in vivo and carbachol-stimulated phosphoinosi-

tide turnover in rat ventral hippocampus. *Neurosci Lett* 1991;126:29–32.

17. Cortés R, Villar MJ, Verhofstad A, Hökfelt T. Effects of central nervous system lesions on the expression of galanin—a comparative in situ hybridization and immunohistochemical study. *Proc Natl Acad Sci USA* 1990;87:7742–7746.

18. Crawley J, Austin MC, Fiske SM, et al. Activity of centrally administered galanin fragments on stimulation of feeding behaviour and on galanin receptor binding in the rat hypothalamus. *J Neurosci* 1990;10:3695–3700.

19. Crawley JN, Robinson JK, Langel Ü, Bartfai T. Galanin receptor antagonist-M40 and antagonist-C7 block galanin-induced feeding. *Brain Res* 1993;600:268–272.

20. de Weille J, Schmid-Antomarchi H, Fosset M, Lazdunski M. ATP-sensitive K^+-channels that are blocked by hypoglycemia-inducing sulfonylureas in insulin-secreting cells are activated by galanin, a hyperglycemia-inducing hormone. *Proc Natl Acad Sci USA* 1988;85:1312–1316.

21. Dunne MJ, Bullett MJ, Li GD, Wollheim CB, Petersen OH. Galanin activates nucleotide-dependent K^+ channels in insulin-secreting cells via a pertussis toxin-sensitive G-protein. *EMBO J* 1989;8:413–417.

22. Dunning BE, Karlsson S, Ahrén B. Contribution of galanin to stress-induced impairment of insulin secretion in swimming mice. *Acta Physiol Scand* 1991;143:145–152.

23. Dutar P, Lamour Y, Nicoll RA. Galanin blocks the slow cholinergic EPSP in CA1 pyramidal neurons from ventral hippocampus. *Eur J Pharmacol* 1989;164:355–360.

24. Evans H, Shine J. Human galanin: molecular cloning reveals a unique structure. *Endocrinology* 1991;129:1682–1684.

25. Everitt BJ, Meister B, Hökfelt T, et al. The hypothalamic arcuate nucleus-median eminence complex: immunohistochemistry of transmitters, peptides and DARPP-32 with special reference to coexistence in dopamine neurons. *Brain Res Rev* 1986;11:97–155.

26. Fisone G, Bartfai T, Nilsson S, Hökfelt T. Galanin inhibits the potassium-evoked release of acetylcholine and the muscarinic receptor-mediated stimulation of phosphoinositide turnover in slices of monkey hippocampus. *Brain Res* 1991;568:279–284.

27. Fisone G, Berthold M, Bedecs K, et al. N-Terminal galanin-(1-16) fragment is an agonist at the hippocampal galanin receptor. *Proc Natl Acad Sci USA* 1989;86:9588–9591.

28. Fisone G, Wu CF, Consolo S, et al. Galanin inhibits acetylcholine release in the ventral hippocampus of the rat: histochemical, autoradiographic, in vivo, and in vitro studies. *Proc Natl Acad Sci USA* 1987;84:7339–7343.

29. Fuxe K, Ögren S-O, Jansson A, Cintra A, Hårfstrand A, Agnati LF. Intraventricular injections of galanin reduces 5-HT metabolism in the ventral limbic cortex, the hippocampal formation and the fronto-parietal cortex of the male rat. *Acta Physiol Scand* 1988;133:579–581.

30. Gabriel SM, Rivkin A, Mercado J. The galanin antagonist, M-15, inhibits growth hormone release in rats. *Peptides* 1993;14:633–636.

31. Gallwitz B, Schmidt WE, Schwarzhoff R, Creutzfeldt W. Galanin—structural requirements for binding and signal transduction in Rin m5F insulinoma cells. *Biochem Biophys Res Commun* 1990;172:268–275.

32. Ghigo E, Maccario M, Arvat E, et al. Interactions of galanin and arginine on growth hormone, prolactin, and insulin secretion in man. *Metabolism* 1992;41:85–89.

33. Giustina A, Girelli A, Bodini C, et al. Comparative effect of porcine and rat galanin on growth hormone secretion in normal adult men. *Horm Metab Res* 1992;24:90–91.

34. Givens BS, Olton DS, Crawley JN. Galanin in the medial septal area impairs working memory. *Brain Res* 1992;582:71–77.

35. Gregersen S, Hermansen K, Lindskog S, et al. Galanin-induced inhibition of insulin secretion from rat islets: effects of rat and pig galanin and galanin fragments and analogues. *Eur J Pharmacol* 1991;203:111–114.

36. Gregersen S, Lindskog S, Land T, Langel Ü, Bartfai T, Ahren B. Blockade of galanin-induced inhibition of insulin secretion from isolated mouse islets by the non-methionine containing antagonist-M35. *Eur J Pharmacol* 1993;232:35–39.

37. Holets VR, Hökfelt T, Rökaeus A, Terenius L, Goldstein M. Locus coeruleus neurons in the rat containing neuropeptide Y, tyrosine hydroxylase or galanin and their efferent projections to the spinal

cord, cerebral cortex and hypothalamus. *Neuroscience* 1988; 24:893–906.

38. Homaidan FR, Sharp GWG, Nowak LM. Galanin inhibits a dihydropyridine-sensitive Ca^{2+} current in the Rin m5F cell line. *Proc Natl Acad Sci USA* 1991;88:8744–8748.

39. Hulting A-L, Meister B, Grimelius L, Wersäll J, Änggård A, Hökfelt T. Production of a galanin-like peptide by a human pituitary adenoma: immunohistochemical evidence. *Acta Physiol Scand* 1990;137:561–562.

40. Kaplan LM, Hooi SC, Abraczinkas DR, et al. Neuroendocrine regulation of galanin gene expression. In: Hökfelt T, Bartfai T, Jacobowitz D, Ottoson D, eds. *Galanin: a new multifunctional peptide in the neuro-endocrine system.* London: McMillan Press, 1991;43–65.

41. Kordower JH, Le HK, Mufson EJ. Galanin immunoreactivity in the primate central nervous system. *J Comp Neurol* 1992;319:479–500.

42. Köhler C, Ericson H, Watanabe T, et al. Galanin immunoreactivity in hypothalamic histamine neurons: further evidence for multiple chemical messengers in the tuberomammillary nucleus. *J Comp Neurol* 1986;250:58–64.

43. Lamour Y, Senut MC, Dutar P, Bassant MH. Neuropeptides and septo-hippocampal neurons: electrophysiological effects and distributions of immunoreactivity. *Peptides* 1988;9:1351–1359.

44. Land T, Langel Ü, Bartfai T. Hypothalamic degradation of galanin(1-29) and galanin(1-16): identification and characterization of the peptidolytic products. *Brain Res* 1991;558:245–250.

45. Land T, Langel Ü, Fisone G, Bedecs K, Bartfai T. Assay for galanin receptor. *Methods Neurosci* 1991;5:225–234.

46. Land T, Langel Ü, Löw M, Berthold M, Undén A, Bartfai T. Linear and cyclic N-terminal galanin fragments and analogs as ligands at the hypothalamic galanin receptor. *Int J Peptide Protein Res* 1991;38:267–272.

47. Laporta C, Bianchi R, Sozzani S, Bartfai T, Consolo S. Galanin reduces PDBu-induced protein phosphorylation in rat ventral hippocampus. *FEBS Lett* 1992;300:46–48.

48. Leibowitz SF, Kim T. Impact of a galanin antagonist on exogenous galanin and natural patterns of fat ingestion. *Brain Res* 1992; 599:148–152.

49. Lindskog S, Ahrén B, Land T, Langel Ü, Bartfai T. The novel high affinity antagonist galantide blocks the galanin mediated inhibition of glucose-induced insulin secretion. *Eur J Pharmacol* 1992; 210:183–188.

50. Malin DH, Novy BJ, Lettbrown AE, et al. Galanin attenuates retention of one-trial reward learning. *Life Sci* 1992;50:939–944.

51. Mastropaolo J, Nadi NS, Ostrowski NL, Crawley JN. Galanin antagonizes acetylcholine on a memory task in basal forebrain-lesioned rats. *Proc Natl Acad Sci USA* 1988;85:9841–5.

52. McDonald TJ, Dupre J, Tatemoto K, Greenberg GR, Radziuk J, Mutt V. Galanin inhibits insulin secretion and induces hyperglycemia in dogs. *Diabetes* 1985;34:192–196.

53. Meister B, Hökfelt T. Peptide- and transmitter-containing neurons in the mediobasal hypothalamus and their relation to GABA-ergic systems: possible roles in control of prolactin and growth hormone secretion. *Synapse* 1988;2:585–605.

54. Melander T, Hökfelt T, Rökaeus Å. Distribution of galanin-like immunoreactivity in the rat central nervous system. *J Comp Neurol* 1986;248:475–517.

55. Melander T, Hökfelt T, Rökaeus Å, et al. Coexistence of galanin-like immunoreactivity with catecholamines, 5-hydroxytryptamine, GABA and neuropeptides in the rat CNS. *J Neurosci* 1986;6:3640–3654.

56. Melander T, Hökfelt T, Roa⁻aeus Å, Fahrenkrug J, Tatemoto K, Mutt V. Distribution of galanin-like immunoreactivity in the gastrointestinal tract of several mammalian species. *Cell Tissue Res* 1985;239:253–270.

57. Merchentaler ILFJ, Negro-Vilar A. Anatomy and physiology of central galanin containing pathways. *Prog Neurobiol* 1993;40:711–769.

58. Nilsson T, Arkhammar P, Rorsman P, Berggren PO. Suppression of insulin release by galanin and somatostatin is mediated by a G-protein. An effect involving repolarization and reduction in cytoplasmic free Ca^{2+} concentration. *J Biol Chem* 1989;264:973–980.

59. Nishibori M, Oishi R, Itoh Y, Saeki K. Galanin inhibits noradrenaline-induced accumulation of cyclic AMP in the rat cerebral cortex. *J Neurochem* 1988;51:1953–1955.

60. Ottlecz A, Snyder GD, McCann SM. Regulatory role of galanin in control of hypothalamic–anterior pituitary function. *Proc Natl Acad Sci USA* 1988;85:9861–9865.

61. Palazzi E, Felinska S, Zambelli M, Fisone G, Bartfai T, Consolo S. Galanin reduces carbachol stimulation of phosphoinositide turnover in rat ventral hippocampus by lowering Ca^{2+} influx through voltage-sensitive Ca^{2+}-channels. *J Neurochem* 1991;56:739–747.

62. Rossowski WJ, Rossowski TM, Zacharia S, Ertan A, Coy DH. Galanin binding sites in rat gastric and jejunal smooth muscle membrane preparation. *Peptides* 1990;11:333–338.

63. Senut MC, Menetrey D, Lamour Y. Cholinergic and peptidergic projections from the medial septum and the nucleus of the diagonal band of Broca to dorsal hippocampus, cingulate cortex and olfactory bulb: a combined wheatgerm agglutinin–apohorseradish peroxidase–gold immunohistochemical study. *Neuroscience* 1989; 30:385–403.

64. Seutin V, Verbanck P, Massotte L, Dresse A. Galanin decreases the activity of locus coeruleus neurons in vitro. *Eur J Pharmacol* 1989;164:373–376.

65. Sharp GW, Le M, Brustel Y, et al. Galanin can inhibit insulin release by a mechanism other than membrane hyperpolarization or inhibition of adenylate cyclase. *J Biol Chem* 1989;264:7302–7309.

66. Skofitsch G, Jacobowitz DM. Immunohistochemical mapping of galanin-like neurons in the rat central nervous system. *Peptides* 1985;6:509–546.

67. Skofitsch G, Jacobowitz DM. Quantitative distribution of galanin-like immunoreactivity in the rat central nervous system. *Peptides* 1986;7:609–613.

68. Sundström E, Melander T. Effects of galanin on 5-HT neurons in the rat CNS. *Eur J Pharmacol* 1988;146:327–329.

69. Tatemoto K, Rökaeus Å, Jörnvall H, McDonald TJ, Mutt V. Galanin—a novel biologically active peptide from porcine intestine. *FEBS Lett* 1983;164:124–128.

70. Verge VMK, Xu XJ, Langel Ü, Hökfelt T, Wiesenfeld-Hallin Z, Bartfai T. Evidence for endogenous inhibition of autotomy by galanin in the rat after sciatic nerve section—demonstrated by chronic intrathecal infusion of a high affinity galanin receptor antagonist. *Neurosci Lett* 1993;149:193–197.

71. Villar MJ, Cortés R, Theodorsson E, et al. Neuropeptide expression in rat dorsal root ganglion cells and spinal cord after peripheral nerve injury with special reference to galanin. *Neuroscience* 1989;33:587–604.

72. Vrontakis ME, Schroedter IC, Cosby H, Friesen HG. Expression and secretion of galanin during pregnancy in the rat. *Endocrinology* 1992;130:458–464.

73. Vrontakis ME, Torsello A, Friesen HG. Galanin. *J Endocrinol Invest* 1991;14:785–794.

74. Wiesenfeld-Hallin Z, Villar MJ, Hökfelt T. Intrathecal galanin at low doses increases spinal reflex excitability in rats more to thermal than mechanical stimuli. *Exp Brain Res* 1988;71:663–666.

75. Wiesenfeld-Hallin Z, Xu XJ, Hughes J, Horwell DC, Hökfelt T. PD134308, a selective antagonist of cholecystokinin type-B receptor, enhances the analgesic effect of morphine and synergistically interacts with intrathecal galanin to depress spinal nociceptive reflexes. *Proc Natl Acad Sci USA* 1990;87:7105–7109.

76. Wynick D, Smith DM, Ghatei M, et al. Characterization of a high-affinity galanin receptor in the rat anterior pituitary: absence of biological effect and reduced membrane binding of the antagonist M15 differentiate it from brain/gut receptor. *Proc Natl Acad Sci USA* 1993;90:4231–4235.

77. Yanaihara N, Mochizuki T, Iguchi K, et al. Structure–function relationships of galanin. In: Hökfelt T, Bartfai T, Jacobowitz D, Ottoson D, eds. *Galanin: a new multifunctional peptide in the neuro-endocrine system.* London: McMillan Press, 1991;185–196.

78. Zini S, Roisin MP, Langel Ü, Bartfai T, Benari Y. Galanin reduces release of endogenous excitatory amino acids in the rat hippocampus. *Eur J Pharmacol Mol Pharmacol* 1993;245:1–7.

79. Ögren S-O, Hökfelt T, Kask K, Langel Ü, Bartfai T. The galanin antagonist M 35 facilitates acquisition in the Morris swim maze. *Neuroscience* 1992;51:1–5.

Psychopharmacology: The Fourth Generation of Progress, edited by Floyd E. Bloom and David J. Kupfer. Raven Press, Ltd., New York © 1995.

CHAPTER 51

The Neurobiology of Neurotensin

Garth Bissette and Charles B. Nemeroff

NEUROBIOLOGY OF NEUROTENSIN

The last iteration of this ACNP-sponsored volume, *Psychopharmacology: The Third Generation of Progress,* did not have a chapter devoted exclusively to neurotensin (NT). Our chapter (65) on neuropeptides in schizophrenia provided a brief overview of the data promulgating the hypothesis of NT as an endogenous, neuroleptic-like peptide. However, NT has a variety of actions on the endocrine and gastrointestinal systems that appear to be unrelated to these putative antipsychotic-like central nervous system (CNS) effects. Unfortunately, the scope of this present chapter does not allow even a cursory review of these peripheral effects. The effects of NT within the CNS are also quite diverse; in this review we attempt to briefly survey these areas with emphasis on current avenues of research.

As in the case of most of the endogenous neuropeptides, the majority of the early information concerning the putative physiological roles of NT were derived from studies in which the peptide was exogenously administered. Because NT_{1-13} does not cross the blood–brain barrier in quantities sufficient to increase concentrations at CNS receptor sites, it must be administered directly into the CNS in pharmacologic doses. This usually requires previous surgical cannulation of the CNS target site or the additional complication of anesthesia. Specific NT-receptor antagonists are just now being developed that promise to allow determination of what physiological effects would ensue from diminished NT-receptor activity. However, even in the face of these impediments to progress, much has been learned about the role of NT

in the CNS and a remarkably rich literature has now accumulated.

The second international conference on the neurobiology of NT generated the latest compendium of CNS neurotensin research fronts, and the proceedings were published in 1992 (67). This volume contains a considerably more comprehensive treatment of many of the topics addressed in this review. Whenever possible, we have chosen to cite the most current reference available for a particular topic under discussion rather than re-cite the original archival literature.

Discovery

Although the history of NT only covers some 20 years since Carraway and Leeman's (17) initial isolation of NT from bovine hypothalamic extracts, it has proven to be one of the more remarkable neuropeptide discoveries outside of the classic hypothalamic releasing factors. The tridecapeptide structure of NT (pGlu-Leu-Tyr-Glu-Asn-Lys-Pro-Arg-Arg-Pro-Tyr-Ile-Leu-OH) places it among the intermediate-sized neuropeptides. The midportion of the NT molecules, being highly enriched in basic amino acids, likely confers some of its unusual properties. Once synthetic NT became commercially available in 1973, a variety of NT-induced effects were discovered in addition to the early description of hypotension and cyanosis after NT was injected intravenously in mice. Most of the panoply of CNS effects of exogenously administered NT were discovered only after direct CNS application and, like the peripheral effects, require integrity of the C-terminal region of NT. Thus, one of the first CNS effects of NT was discovered during routine screening of a variety of peptides to determine their effects on the sedation and hypothermia produced by a fixed-dose of pentobarbital. Neurotensin was the only one of 48 neuropeptides tested (8) that markedly potentiated the narcosis and hypother-

G. Bissette: Departments of Psychiatry and Pharmacology, Duke University Medical Center, Durham, North Carolina 27710.

C. B. Nemeroff: Department of Psychiatry and Behavioral Sciences, Emory University School of Medicine, Atlanta, Georgia 30322.

mia produced by pentobarbital, and this was associated with decreased metabolism of pentobarbital in brain, liver, and blood of mice. This effect was only observed after intracisternal (IC) injection of NT and led to the discovery of the potent hypothermic effect of NT in a variety of mammals (7) which is accentuated by low ambient temperatures. The inability of drugs acting on cholinergic, serotonergic, and noradrenergic systems to alter this effect, in contrast to its potentiation by agents reducing dopaminergic neurotransmission, served as the initial impetus for launching an intensive investigation aimed at testing the hypothesis that NT acts as an endogenous neuroleptic (63).

Shortly after the discovery of the hypothermic effects of NT, several investigators noted the potent analgesic effects of centrally administered NT which, along with the hypothermic effects, were regionally mapped (46). This NT-induced analgesia is not blocked by opiate receptor antagonists. Direct injection of NT into the central periaqueductal gray (PAG) region produces a long-lasting analgesia which is associated with increases in the firing rate of the majority of PAG neurons to which it is applied. These, in turn, inhibit the response of spinal cord neurons to noxious stimuli using a neuronal circuit which includes cells of the rostral ventral medulla. Williams and Beitz (96) reported induction of NT–neuromedin-N (NMN) mRNA expression in the caudal portion of the PAG in the acute pain phase followed by induction in adjacent midbrain tegmental nuclei in the adaptive phase of three models of chronic pain (arthritis, sciatic nerve ligation, and paw inflammation).

The ontogeny of NT has been studied in the rat. Neurotensin immunoreactivity is detectable by gestational day 18 and generally exhibits increases in regional CNS concentrations during the first 10–20 days of life before returning to adult levels by 60 days of age. Aged rats (22 months) have greatly reduced concentrations of NT in the striatum and substantia nigra compared to 3-month-old controls (24), whereas the relative concentrations in the nucleus accumbens of aged rats are only mildly decreased. Evidence for a trophic effect of NT in CNS growth and development include the fact that NT and NT receptors have been reported to be transiently expressed in some rat brain regions during development, that NT receptors are present in meningioma's (72), and that NT is found in high concentrations in cerebrospinal fluid (CSF) from human infants (38). Interestingly, NT-like immunoreactivity has been described in all species of mammalian CNS examined thus far, and C-terminally directed NT antisera have shown positive immunoreactivity to extracts of lobster and all other animal phyla, including species of Porifera and Protozoa.

NMN is a hexapeptide (H-Lys-Ile-Pro-Tyr-Ile-Leu-OH) which has significant C-terminal sequence similarity with NT and is contained in the pro-hormone precursor NT molecule, where it is separated from the NT sequence by a single pair of dibasic amino acids (26). NMN shares many properties with NT and binds to the NT receptor with similar affinity, but is less potent and apparently more easily degraded than NT. The post-translational processing of NMN exhibits some regional differences, but, thus far, agents that increase NT synthesis also increase NMN synthesis. Another neuropeptide derived from extracts of frog skin that shares some sequence homology with NT is xenopsin (pGlu-Gly-Lys-Arg-Pro-Trp-Ile-Leu-OH), and two NT-related, structurally homologous peptides (p-Glu-Leu-His-Val-Asn-Lys-Ala-Arg-Arg-Pro-Tyr-Ile-Leu-OH and H-Lys-Asn-Pro-Tyr-Ile-Leu-OH) from chicken intestinal extracts have also been described.

Molecular Biology

The tools of molecular biology have now been applied to NT systems in the CNS. Both the NT–NMN prohormone and the NT–NMN receptor genes have now been successfully cloned and sequenced. The rat gene for NT spans 10.2 kb of DNA and consists of four exon sequences separated by three intervening introns (50). Exon 4 contains one copy of the sequence for NT and one for NMN, separated by a sequence coding for a single pair of basic amino acids. Production of the 170-amino acid pro-hormone from either 1.5- or 1.0-kb messenger RNAs is regulated by elements that are cis-responsive to nerve growth factor, cyclic nucleotides, glucocorticoids, and, possibly, lithium, upstream of the pro-hormone sequence. This NT–NMN gene sequence is highly conserved, as comparison between dog, bovine, rat, and human species has demonstrated. Expression of NT mRNA in neurons where NT message was previously absent is seen after either pharmacologic stimuli such as antipsychotic drugs (60,100) or exposure to chronic pain (96). Other known inducers of NT–NMN messenger RNA are caffeine (79), staurosporine (85) sigma receptor antagonists (55) and osmotic stimulation (92). Drugs such as haloperidol that induce NT synthesis also induce NMN in the same regions and in similar proportions (see Fig. 1). The reported regional disparities in the molar ratio of NT to NMN are thought to be caused by post-translational processing differences in prohormone cleavage, as well as by regional product degradation differences.

The rat NT–NMN receptor is comprised of a 424-amino-acid protein with the seven-membrane-spanning domains characteristic of G-protein-coupled receptors. It has a somewhat lower-than-expected sequence homology (18–24%) with other members of this receptor superfamily (82). The human NT–NMN receptor has also now been cloned and found to contain 418 amino acids with 84% sequence homology to the rat NT–NMN receptor (88). Both of these receptors are thought to represent the high-affinity form of the NT receptor that is revealed in the presence of the antihistamine agent, levocabastine,

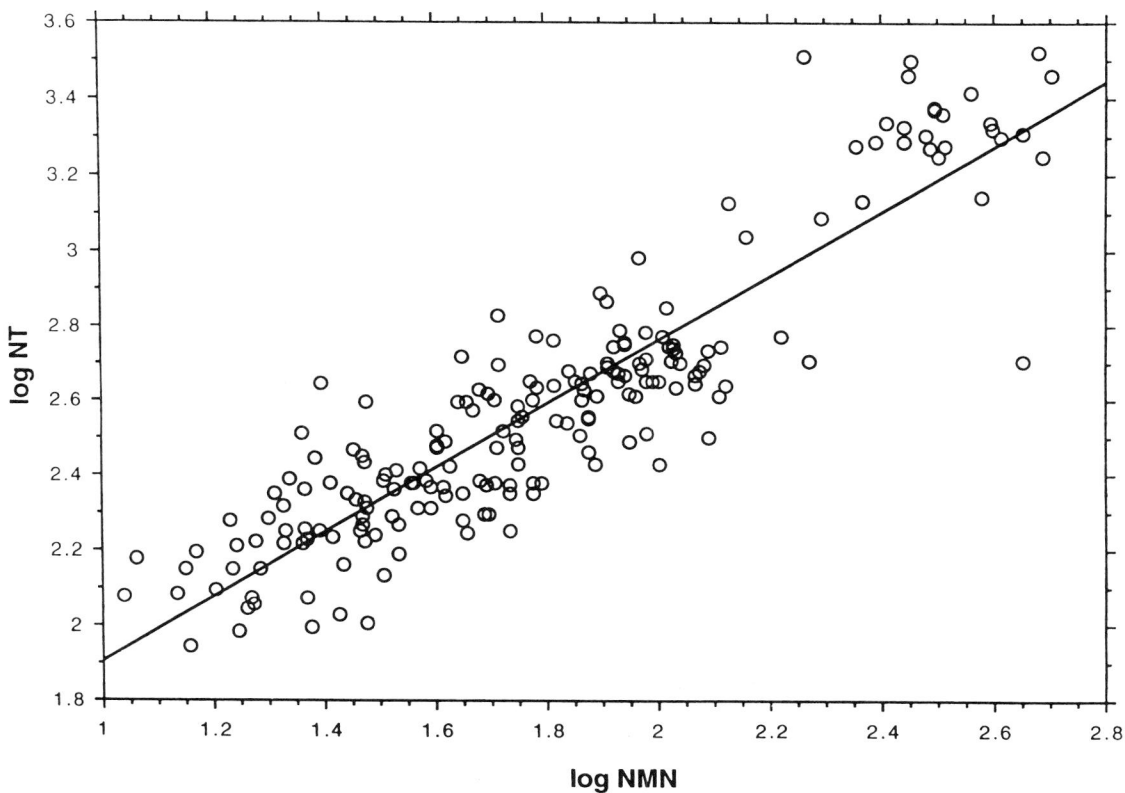

FIG. 1. Graph demonstrating that the relationship between NT and NMN concentration increases in the caudate nucleus, nucleus accumbens, and olfactory tubercles of rats after 2 weeks of daily intraperitoneal injection of haloperidol (1 or 2 mg/kg). The correlation is highly statistically significant ($r \le 0.001$). (From ref. 22, with permission.)

which binds to an apparent low-affinity NT site in brain membrane receptor preparations. Both the rat and human NT–NMN-receptor clones exhibit sequence similarities with other G-protein receptors that use inositol phosphate as a second messenger transducer. The rat NT-receptor sequence, when expressed in oocytes, is linked to this second messenger, but the human NT-receptor sequence has multiple base-pair differences compared to the rat in the third cytoplasmic loop sequence known to mediate second messenger linkage. Evidence for NT receptor linkage to a G protein which stimulates adenylate cyclase in the rat ventral tegmental area (VTA) is also available (48) (see also Chapters 11, 27, and 38, *this volume*).

Localization

Many immunohistochemical and radioimmunoassay distribution studies in a variety of species have revealed that NT is distributed heterogeneously among the various anatomic regions of the brain. More recently, in situ hybridization studies of NT prohormone mRNA have been added to the growing list of techniques used to visualize endogenous NT neurons. Highest brain levels of NT are found in the hypothalamus, with the greatest concentra-

tion in the posterior hypothalamus and mammillary body regions. The substantia nigra, ventral tegmental area, and central nucleus of the amygdala, as well as the dorsal hippocampus, nucleus accumbens, septum, and globus pallidus, also contain significant amounts of NT in micropunched rat brain regions (49). Neuronal cell bodies containing NT are found in most of these regions, along with high densities of NT-containing nerve terminals. Interestingly, few NT cell bodies are found in the striatum of normal, non-drug-treated animals. A particularly wide band of NT cells arises from the medial anterior hypothalamus and courses through the medial preoptic area to the bed nucleus of the stria terminalis/diagonal band area and on to the lateral aspects of the anterior septum. Immunohistochemical studies have also shown NT and NT mRNA to be present within the anterior pituitary gland.

Hökfelt et al. (40) originally described NT colocalization in tyrosine hydroxylase-containing dopamine (DA) neurons of the VTA and the arcuate nucleus of the hypothalamus. Since then, NT in rat brain has been shown to be colocalized with cholecystokinin in VTA DA neurons, within subsets of corticotropin-releasing factor (CRF) neurons in the hypothalamus, with growth-hormone-releasing factor in the arcuate nucleus of the hypothalamus (68), and with calcitonin gene-related peptide in the bed nucleus of the stria terminalis (45) as well as in the central nucleus of the amygdala (99). The caveat of species-specificity in these findings is emphasized by the apparent lack of NT colocalization within human midbrain DA neurons that project to the cerebral cortex (34). The anatomic colocalization of NT and DA has considerable implications for the understanding of NT interactions with DA systems.

Several putative pathways have been described in rat brain (see ref. 53 for review). Projections from cell bodies in the arcuate nucleus to the median eminence provide NT to the hypothalamic hypophyseal portal system. Projections from NT cell bodies in the central nucleus of the amygdala to the bed nucleus of the stria terminalis (86) and midbrain parabrachial nucleus have also been mapped. A hippocampal NT pathway from the subiculum to the alveus and fimbria regions and from the dorsal hippocampus to the adjacent cortex (75) have been described. A projection from the nucleus tractus solitarii to the nucleus accumbens has now been reported. Other NT pathways include a projection from piriform cortex to the anterior olfactory nucleus (41) and from cell bodies in the PAG region (4) and parabrachial nucleus (70) to terminals in the nucleus raphe magnus. However, the most extensively characterized NT pathway is a mesolimbicocortical projection of NT-containing neurons from the VTA to the frontal cortex and nucleus accumbens. The former target contains an appreciable component of colocalized NT and dopamine and some cholecystokinin, whereas the latter is thought to be predominantly NT without dopamine (47).

The pattern of distribution of NT receptors depends partly upon whether $[^3H]$-NT or $[^{125}I]$-NT is used, though NT receptor distribution generally agrees well with immunohistochemical localization of NT-containing nerve terminals. Autoradiographic studies of brain NT binding sites have been conducted in rat, pigeon, guinea pig, monkey, and human brain as well as in transgenic mice overexpressing the gene for superoxide dismutase (15). High concentrations of putative NT receptors are found in the substantia nigra (pars compacta) and VTA and their terminal projections to the caudate, nucleus accumbens, and cortex. NT numbers are greatly diminished by 6-hydroxydopamine (6-OHDA) destruction of the DA neurons, where these receptors are predominately located (14). However, many NT terminals synapse on non-DA neurons in these regions (97). Moderate densities of NT receptors are also seen in the other components of the striatum, ventral hippocampus, PAG matter, superior colliculus, and dorsal raphe nucleus. Cerebral cortex in nonhuman primates and in humans contains higher densities of NT binding sites in the deep cortical layers than does rat brain (42). Recent evidence indicates that after NT binds to the NT receptor, a portion of the resulting receptor–NT complexes (19) is internalized through the postsynaptic membrane (58) and is subsequently transported

to the postsynaptic neuron's nucleus (18), where it may regulate tyrosine hydroxylase activation via protein kinase C (6) or, possibly, regulate NT-receptor synthesis. If the tyrosine hydroxylase regulation by NT (13) is confirmed, this would provide another mechanism by which NT regulates DA neurons. There is good agreement that the predominant second messenger systems linked to the activated NT receptor are the inisitol triphosphate/diacyl glycerol and the cyclic guanosine monophosphate (cGMP) signal transduction systems. The rapid desensitization of NT receptors after continued application of NT has been demonstrated in a neuroblastoma cell line by Richelson and co-workers (25,98). This phenomena is apparently due to NT-receptor down-regulation associated with a decrease in receptor number without changes in affinity.

Peptidases are the enzymes directed toward specific amino acid sequences that degrade neuropeptides. Several such enzymes have been identified that cleave NT, including endopeptidases 24.11, 24.15, and 24.16 (see chapter by Kitabgi in ref. 67). Their biological significance can be appreciated by the profound potentiation of CNS effects of NT observed after administration of specific peptidase inhibitors. Thiorphan, which inhibits endopeptidase 24.11 cleavage of NT on either side of the Tyr'' moiety, and bestatin, which inhibits the aminopeptidase that cleaves NMN between Lys^1 and Ile^2, both potentiate the hypothermia and analgesia observed after intracerebral injection of NT or NMN, respectively. Differential processing of the NT–NMN precursor protein by trypsin-like enzymes have been implicated in the regional differences in NT/NMN ratios reported by various research groups, while the reduced potency of NMN in evoking NT-like responses is thought to be due to its relatively unprotected amino terminus.

CNS PHYSIOLOGY AND PHARMACOLOGY

Endocrine

The effects of NT on the release of anterior pituitary hormones depend upon whether NT is injected peripherally or centrally, whether NT is applied alone or after stimulation by other peptides or pharmacologic agents, whether the experimental animal is awake or anesthetized, male or female, and, if female, whether they are ovariectomized (OVX) and/or whether they are estrogen-primed. Thus, NT injected into the third ventricle of conscious rats reduces plasma concentrations of prolactin and luteinizing hormone, increases plasma growth hormone, and has no effect on thyrotropin (TSH) or follicle-stimulating hormone plasma levels (see chapter by McCann and Vijayan in ref. 67). This direct hypothalamic effect of NT in reducing prolactin secretion is thought to be mediated by DA release into the portal system, because blockade of dopamine receptors in lactotrophs prevents NT from acting. However, NT, when injected intravenously in conscious rats and acting directly on the adenohypophysis, elevates plasma TSH and prolactin while not having much effect on the other pituitary hormones. Intravenous injection of antiserum to NT in conscious, OVX female rats, which would remove endogenous NT from pituitary circulation, decreases plasma levels of prolactin and TSH and increases growth hormone in plasma. Thus NT may play a physiologic role in the secretory regulation of these anterior pituitary hormones. Alexander and colleagues (see chapter in ref. 67) have shown that NT neurons in the medial preoptic anterior hypothalamus contain estrogen receptors and that NT may physiologically regulate the preovulatory surge of luteinizing hormone in female rats. Direct injection of NT antiserum to OVX, estrogen-primed rats, in the afternoon before a proestrus-like surge in the secretion of luteinizing hormone, prevented this surge. Others (39) have shown these neurons to be devoid of tyrosine hydroxylase, cholecystokinin, or luteinizing-hormone-releasing hormone.

Interactions with Centrally Active Agents

Interactions of NT with CNS-active drugs can be divided into two components: (i) effects of exogenous NT on the actions of certain drugs and (ii) the effects of certain classes of drugs on endogenous NT systems. We have already described the ability of centrally administered NT to potentiate the sedation and hypothermia induced by pentobarbital in rodents. This potentiation of sedative effects extends to other CNS depressants such as alcohol in both mice and rats (32). While reduction of the rate of pentobarbital metabolism may be partly responsible for the effects of NT on barbiturate, this is not the case for ethanol. The site within the CNS where NT elicits these effects remains unknown. However, Erwin and Jones (29) have reported that, in mice bred for long (LS) or short (SS) sleep after ethanol treatment, SS mice had higher densities of high-affinity NT receptors in the entorhinal and frontal cortex and striatum and exhibited greater sensitivity to the NT-induced potentiation of ethanol narcosis.

This potentiation of sedatives, along with the hypothermic and analgesic effects of centrally administered NT, led to our original "endogenous neuroleptic" hypothesis (63). Soon after this hypothesis was first promulgated, Govoni et al. (36) demonstrated the ability of clinically efficacious antipsychotic drugs to increase the concentrations of endogenous NT in brain regions where projections of midbrain DA neurons terminated—that is, the nucleus accumbens, caudate nucleus, and olfactory tubercles. This effect is seen within 16 hr after a single injection of haloperidol and does not exhibit tachyphylaxis to repeated doses over several months (73). A wide variety of

classical and atypical (54) antipsychotic drugs have now been studied. Classical antipsychotics such as haloperidol, pimozide, chlorpromazine, and butaclamol increase NT concentrations in both the caudate nucleus and nucleus accumbens. In contrast, atypical antipsychotic drugs, such as clozapine, which are devoid of extrapyramidal side effects or tardive dyskinesia liability, produce increases in NT concentrations in the nucleus accumbens, but not in the striatum (55). Thus NT increases in the striatum may predict extrapyramidal liability. Another recent dichotomy between the effects of haloperidol and clozapine is the report that haloperidol, but not clozapine, increases NT-receptor mRNA levels in the substantia nigra (90). Recent work has shown that NT mRNA is increased by antipsychotic drugs such as haloperidol within 2 hr after a single dose in the dorsolateral striatum and the shell region of the nucleus accumbens of rats (60). In contrast, neurotensin mRNA expression is increased only in the nucleus accumbens after clozapine treatment (61). The dorsolateral striatal NT–NMN mRNA increase is immediately preceded by c-fos gene activation (59), but this is not seen in the accumbal shell region's NT–NMN mRNA induction (see Fig. 2). Recently, both Robertson (*personal communication*) and Dorsa (*personal communication*) have shown that injection of antisense probes to c-fos blocks the antipsychotic drug-induced increases in NT synthesis. The increase in NT synthesis following the administration of antipsychotic drugs is not altered by blockade or stimulation of cholinergic muscarinic or D_2 DA receptors (60). Thus, these drugs increase NT concentrations by increasing the synthesis of NT relative to effects on release and degradation, though these processes require further study. The steroisomers of butaclamol, (+)- and (−)-butaclamol, which share all effects on adrenergic, serotonergic, and histaminergic systems, have also been investigated for NT-system interactions. Only (+)-butaclamol (10) is able to increase NT concentrations in

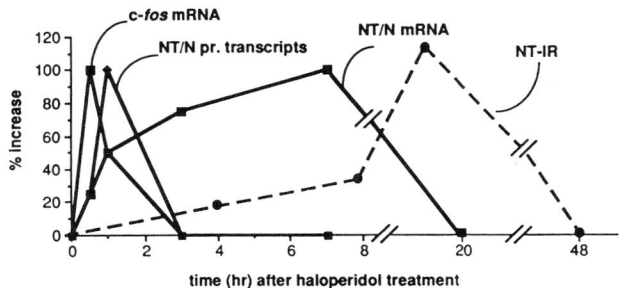

FIG. 2. Graph portraying the time course of the cellular and molecular events occurring after a single exposure of rat dorsolateral striatal neurons to haloperidol. Activation of c-fos mRNA production immediately precedes production of NT–NMN primary transcripts. This is followed by a steady increase over 7 hr in cytoplasmic mRNA for NT and NMN, which does not result in peak immunoreactive concentrations until around 16 hr after the initial haloperidol exposure. (From ref. 62, with permission.)

the caudate nucleus and nucleus accumbens, and only the (+)-isomer blocks D_2 receptors and has antipsychotic efficacy. A variety of other drugs have also been studied for their effects on NT systems. Tricyclic antidepressants, benzodiazepines, and antihistamines do not alter NT concentrations in the striatum or nucleus accumbens.

Surprisingly, the psychostimulant indirect DA agonists, such as cocaine, methylphenidate, and amphetamine, are able to reverse NT-induced hypothermia, yet in high doses these drugs increase NT concentrations in DA terminal regions. Within 8–24 hr after several high doses of cocaine or after chronic cocaine administration in moderate doses, NT production is apparently induced in these DA terminal regions. This results in increased NT concentrations (16) and decreased NT-receptor binding in the VTA (71), during both chronic treatment and 10 days after withdrawal of chronic cocaine. Recent work in our laboratory (22) has extended this finding to the relatively specific D_2-receptor agonist, quinelerone, which increased NT concentrations in caudate and nucleus accumbens, similar to haloperidol. The ability of centrally administered NT to release dopamine from mesolimbic terminal regions (94) has been extensively documented using increasingly elegant techniques, such as microdialysis (20) and in vivo chronoamperometry (12), and is thought to be due to direct NT effects on mesencephalic DA neurons. The ability of these drugs to release NT in colocalized prefrontal cortical DA terminal regions has recently been documented by During et al. (28), while Rivest et al. (74) reported that the effect of NT on dopamine release is of greater magnitude in the nucleus accumbens than the striatal response.

However, using the specific D_2 and D_1 DA-receptor agonists and antagonists, differential regional CNS effects on NT systems have been observed. Singh et al. (81) reported that D_2 antagonists increase striatal NT concentrations whereas D_2 agonists decrease NT concentrations in this region. Both nucleus accumbens and striatal NT concentrations are increased by D_1 agonists, and N-methyl-D-aspartate (NMDA) receptor blockade completely blocks this D_1 agonist effect. Taylor et al. (84) have reported that D_1 antagonists decrease NT concentrations in the striatum. Fuxe et al. (33) ascribe these striatal effects to an NT–DA-receptor interaction that reduces the affinity of D_2 pre- and postsynaptic receptors while enhancing D_1-receptor sensitivity; cholecystokinin exerts a synergistic effect (83). Recent theories have postulated that NT and dopamine may form a chemical complex (1), thereby attenuating dopamine's ability to activate dopamine receptors. Attempts to replicate the initial evidence for this complex have not been successful (69,80), however.

Haloperidol not only has a high affinity for D_2 DA receptors, but also has a high affinity for sigma receptors. In fact, extant data suggest that the ability of antipsychotic drugs to increase NT concentrations may reside in the ability to act at both D_2- and sigma-receptor sites. Selective sigma antagonists, such as BMY-14802, increase NT–NMN mRNA (56) and NT (55) concentrations in the nucleus accumbens and the caudate nucleus, but produce a decrease in frontal cortical NT concentrations. Previous studies have only observed a decrease in NT in the micropunch-dissected medial prefrontal cortex after chronic haloperidol and clozapine (49). Conceivably, sigma-receptor and D_2-receptor blockade may regulate NT neurons together. However, the inability of (−)-butaclamol, a sigma, but not D_2 DA, receptor antagonist, to alter NT concentrations (10) indicates that more than sigma-receptor blockade is required to induce NT production. Another sigma-receptor ligand, SR 31742A, has been reported to selectively increase NT in the nucleus accumbens, but not in the striatum (52), which is similar to the anatomic selectivity of clozapine for producing NT effects.

Currently, two schools of thought exist about the anatomic relationship of these DA and sigma receptors and the NT receptive neurons mediating the neuroleptic-like effects of NT. Destruction of DA neurons by 6-OHDA does not prevent haloperidol from increasing NT concentrations in the nucleus accumbens and caudate nucleus, indicating a postsynaptic location of the relevant D_2 DA or sigma receptor on, or immediately adjacent to, the resident NT neurons. However, Fuxe et al. (33) argue for a presynaptic effect of NT in decreasing the affinity of D_2 DA receptors, which is postulated to result in decreased DA activity.

Electrophysiology

The electrophysiological effects of exogenously applied NT depends upon the regional cell population under study, whether brain slices or in vivo recording sites are used and the concentration of NT applied. Until recently, the lack of specific NT receptor antagonists precluded any definitive conclusion as to whether these effects of NT were due to the direct activation of NT receptors or due to indirect effects. Most of the brain regions where NT has been applied respond with excitation of the majority of neurons tested. Two exceptions to this general statement are the locus coeruleus and the nucleus accumbens (see chapter by Shi and Bunney in ref. 67). The application of NT or NMN to midbrain DA neurons produces an increase in firing rates and DA release at the terminal DA projections. DA-induced inhibition of the firing rate of DA neurons through autoreceptor activation is also attenuated by NT application. This effect is not produced by cholecystokinin, which, like NT, is colocalized in a sizable proportion of midbrain DA neurons. Fuxe and co-workers have conducted a series of experiments which present convincing evidence that these effects of NT are mediated by NT-receptor-induced disinhibition of DA-autoreceptor activation through a direct NT-receptor–DA-receptor interaction (89). Thus, midbrain DA neurons respond to NT with effects that are similar to the effect of the DA-receptor antagonists such as haloperidol. This similarity does not extend to the frontal cortex, however, because NT effects following application to this region resemble those of DA. Interestingly, this region also responds to neuroleptic drug administration with decreases in NT concentrations rather than the increases seen in the striatum or nucleus accumbens.

Behavioral Effects

The behavioral effects of NT also depend upon the site of application within the CNS. Intraventricularly administered NT decreases spontaneous and psychostimulant-induced locomotor activity in rats and mice. This effect is likely mediated by actions of the peptide in the nucleus accumbens, because similar results are obtained when NT is microinjected directly into this brain region. However, NT administered into the VTA increases locomotor activity and rearing behavior in rats that can be blocked by pretreatment with antipsychotic drugs. In fact, the increase in locomotion induced by intra-VTA neurotensin can be blocked by intra-accumbens NT. Thus, NT can block the behavioral effects of DA at either end of this circuit. When DA agonists are used to produce penile erection or yawning behavior (44), NT administered intracerebroventricularly blocks these responses without altering the increase in sniffing stereotypies.

The intra-VTA administration of NT exhibits rewarding properties as measured by place-preference (35) and self-administration paradigms, but it decreases the response for food rewards in an operant paradigm. This latter effect may be due in part to NT's role in gut endocrinology, as NT is increased in hypothalamus by fatty meals (3) and may be responding to the cascade of gut hormones that are thought to induce satiety. When rats are cannulated with stimulating electrodes in the posterior lateral hypothalamus or PAG matter, the self-stimulation rate of bar presses is decreased by NT injection into the VTA (77), suggesting that NT applied to this region is reinforcing. Cholecystokinin application into the VTA has the opposite effect (76). Both NT (31) and NMN (30) decrease self-stimulation when injected into the medial prefrontal cortex, indicating possible reinforcing properties of NT and NMN in this circuit.

NEUROCHEMICAL PATHOLOGY

Schizophrenia

The primary evidence for NT involvement in the pathogenesis of schizophrenia rests on several clinical studies. Our group has repeatedly observed decreased group mean NT concentrations in CSF in drug-free schizophrenic patients compared to normal, healthy, sex- and age-matched volunteers (57,95). This observation is consistent with the hypothesis of reduced NT availability in schizophrenia. We have shown that NT concentrations increase in CSF after antipsychotic drug treatment, an effect similar to that observed in the laboratory animal studies. Obviously, the presence of some period of antipsychotic drug pretreatment in almost all of the patients studied thus far is a potential confound for assessing NT involvement in the primary pathology of schizophrenia. The four published studies (see ref. 11 for review) in which NT concentrations have been measured in postmortem brain tissue from schizophrenic patients are encumbered by the same potential confound, although antipsychotics are usually withdrawn relatively early in the terminal phases of illness. Of the seven cortical regions examined among all of these studies, only Brodmann's area 32 from the schizophrenic tissue exhibited any group mean change in NT concentrations, an increase relative to controls (64). None of the seven total subcortical regions examined thus far have shown any group mean differences in NT concentrations, including two studies using nucleus accumbens (51) and one with caudate nucleus tissue (64). Thus, the schizophrenic postmortem tissue data do not confirm the expectations engendered by the CSF studies, where decreases in NT have been observed. A recent study of NT–NMN messenger RNA expression and genomic sequence in ventral midbrain neurons from schizophrenic patients compared to controls did not find any differences (2). Kleinman and colleagues (*personal communication*), using autoradiography, have not found differences between schizophrenics and controls as regards NT-receptor density. However, Watson et al. (91) have found evidence of polymorphisms in the NT-receptor mRNA sequences from human CNS tissue. Whether similar polymorphisms are present in schizophrenia and what the functional implications of such differences would represent await future studies (see also Chapters 70, 75, and 100, *this volume*).

In Parkinson's disease, NT receptors residing on DA neurons in the substantia nigra are reduced in number (78,87) as these neurons degenerate over the disease course. However, group mean NT concentrations is postmortem Parkinson's disease brain regions are generally not found to be different from age- and sex-matched controls, including the caudate nucleus, nucleus accumbens, and VTA (9). A decrease in hippocampal NT concentrations in Parkinson's disease patients relative to controls that was reported by our group has not been confirmed by others. This finding in Parkinson's disease is similar to the lack of effect on NT concentrations in the rat brain in response to 6-OHDA-induced destruction of DA neurons—except in regions such as the medial prefrontal cortex, where NT and DA are extensively colocalized. Interestingly, in an animal model of Parkinson's disease using 6-OHDA, Jolicoeur et al. (43) found that intraventricular NT administration would reduce the tremor and rigidity of rats (see also Chapter 126, *this volume*).

Alzheimer's Disease

In Alzheimer's disease, there have been four postmortem tissue reports where regional NT concentration changes were sought. Our group reported a decrease in amygdala NT concentrations in Alzheimer's patients relative to controls (66), and this has been confirmed by Benzing et al. (5) using immunohistochemical methods. No other brain regions have been reported to exhibit alterations in NT systems in Alzheimer's disease.

Others

Patients with Huntington's chorea have also been investigated for postmortem regional alterations in NT concentrations. Increases in NT concentrations in the caudate nucleus and in the globus pallidus have been reported (64).

Two groups have reported alterations in NT systems in the CNS of infants dying of sudden infant death syndrome (SIDS). Coquerel et al. (23) described increased NT concentrations in CSF of SIDS patients relative to control children and adults and measured NT in brainstem regions of SIDS patients. Because no controls were used in the brainstem studies, the results are difficult to interpret, but the SIDS brainstem NT concentrations are much higher than previously reported adult concentrations. The second study measured high-affinity NT receptors in SIDS brainstem sections and compared them to age-matched, non-SIDS controls (21). They observed increased densities of NT binding sites in the nucleus tractus solitarius, but no differences were found in other brainstem regions. Another study using SIDS brainstem tissue reported a transient increase in GTP-sensitive, high-affinity NT receptors over the first month of life, with levels decreasing to near adult values by 15 months of age (101). The transient increase of NT receptors at 1 month in SIDS tissue was interpreted as putative evidence for NT playing a role in brainstem development and points to possible disruption of this process in SIDS.

Rett's syndrome is a progressive neurological disorder in female children characterized by decelerated brain and body growth, cortical atrophy, and severe mental deficiency. Stereotypical "hand washing" movements are often present, and this syndrome is now considered to be an X-linked dominant mutation that is lethal to males. An investigation (93) into several neurochemical systems thought to be involved in the resulting neuropathology of Rett's syndrome found no changes in NT concentrations in CSF nor in NT-receptor numbers in postmortem brain tissue despite evidence that both dopaminergic and cholinergic systems are targets of Rett's syndrome neuropathology.

DRUGS TARGETED TOWARD NT RECEPTORS

Antagonists

The goal of availability of agonists and antagonists at the NT–NMN receptor has begun to be realized. Recently described nonpeptide NT-receptor antagonists (37), such as the polycyclic compound SR-48692, promise to afford the long-awaited opportunity to block the actions of endogenous NT, hopefully providing information on the physiological role(s). This compound, in particular, promises to be extremely useful because it is lipophilic and penetrates into the CNS after peripheral administration.

Agonists

One of the obvious tests of the endogenous neuroleptic hypothesis of NT would be the administration of an NT-receptor agonist to symptomatic schizophrenic patients to determine if the NT-receptor agonist would possess antipsychotic properties. Previously, substituted peptide NT analogues (27) required direct CNS injection to produce effects. However, this goal may soon be possible, because a C-terminal NT analogue linked to a small, CNS accessible molecule has recently been observed to potentiate pentobarbital sedation and produce hypothermia in a dose-dependent manner after intraperitoneal injection (Bissette and Richelson, *personal communication*). Should this compound prove nontoxic at useful doses, clinical trials will be subsequently initiated.

DISCUSSION

Whether NT is truly an endogenous neuroleptic or not, the past 20 years of research have certainly shown it to be one of the most interesting peptides investigated to date. At present, NT is definitely implicated in the physiological regulation of luteinizing hormone and prolactin release and a variety of CNS dopaminergic systems. The involvement of NT systems in the clinical neuropathology of several neurologic and psychiatric diseases is adumbrated by the available data; in most cases, however, independent verification has been difficult, probably because of the relatively modest populations sampled thus far. The close relationship between NT and dopaminergic systems in the CNS, combined with the extra-opioid analgesia mediated by NT, would be enough to sustain interest in NT apart from the tantalizing possibility of NT systems mediating some of the psychopathology of schizophrenia. The future development of positron emission tomography ligands to directly image NT-receptor density in humans will be a major advance in the NT research field. Given the explosion of knowledge in the past two decades, even the most grandiose visions of NT may be fully realized in the next several years.

ACKNOWLEDGMENTS

This work was supported by NIMH MH-39415. We are grateful for the expert assistance of Andrea Laws in the preparation of this manuscript.

REFERENCES

1. Adachi DK, Kalivas PW, Schenk JO. Neurotensin binding to dopamine. *J Neurochem* 1990;54:1321–1328.
2. Bean AJ, Dagerlind A, Hokfelt T, Dobner PR. Cloning of human neurotensin/neuromedin N genomic sequences and expression in the ventral mesencephalon of schizophrenics and age/sex matched controls. *Neuroscience* 1992;50:259–268.
3. Beck B, Krongtad AS, Burlet A, Nicolas J, Burlet C. Changes in hypothalamic neurotensin concentrations and food intake in rats fed a high diet. *Int J Obes* 1991;16:361–366.
4. Beitz AJ. The sites of origin of brain stem neurotensin and serotonin projections to the rodent nucleus raphe magnus. *J Neurosci* 1982;2:829–842.
5. Benzing WC, Mufson EJ, Jennes L, Armstrong DM. Reduction of neurotensin immunoreactivity in the amygdala in Alzheimer's disease. *Brain Res* 1990;537:298–302.
6. Berry SA, Gudelsky GA. Evidence for protein kinase-C mediation of the neurotensin-induced activation of tyrosine hydroxylase in tuberoinfundibular dopaminergic neurons. *Endocrinology* 1992;131:1207–1211.
7. Bissette G, Nemeroff CB, Loosen PT, Prange AJ, Jr., Lipton MA. Hypothermia and intolerance to cold induced by the intracisternal administration of the hypothalamic peptide neurotensin. *Nature* 1976;262:607–609.
8. Bissette G, Nemeroff CB, Loosen PT, Breese GR, Burnette GN, Lipton MA, Prange AJ. Modification of pentobarbital-induced sedation by natural and synthetic peptides. *Neuropharmacology* 1978;17:229–237.
9. Bissette G, Nemeroff CB, Decker MW, Kizer JS, Agid Y, Javoy AF. Alterations in regional brain concentrations of neurotensin and bombesin in Parkinson's disease. *Ann Neurol* 1985;17:324–328.
10. Bissette G, Dauer WT, Kilts CD, O'Connor L, Nemeroff CB. The effect of stereoisomers of butaclamol on neurotensin concentrations in discrete regions of the rat brain. *Neuropsychopharmacology* 1988;1:329–335.
11. Bissette G, Levant B, Nemeroff CB. Neurotensin and its possible significance in the pathophysiology of schizophrenia. In: Fuxe K, Agnati LF, eds. *Volume transmission in the brain: novel mechanisms for neural transmission.* New York: Raven Press, 1991;549–556.
12. Blaha CD, Phillips AG. Pharmacological evidence for common mechanisms underlying the effects of neurotensin and neuroleptics on in vivo dopamine efflux in the rat nucleus accumbens. *Neuroscience* 1992;49:867–877.
13. Burgevin MC, Castel D, Quarteronet T, Chevet, Laduron PM. Neurotensin increases tyrosine hydroxylase messenger RNA-positive neurons in substantia nigra after retrograde axonal transport. *Neuroscience* 1992;49:627–633.
14. Cadet JL, Kayoko K, Przedborski S. Bilateral modulation [³H]-neurotensin binding by unilateral intrastriatal 6-hydroxydopamine injections: evidence from a receptor autoradiographic study. *Brain Research* 1991;564:37–44.
15. Cadet JL, Kayoko K, Carlson E, Epstein CJ. Autoradiographic distribution of [³H]neurotensin receptors in the brains of superoxide dismutase transgenic mice. *Synapse* 1993;14:24–33.
16. Cain ST, Griff D, Joyner CM, Ellinwood EH, Nemeroff CB. Chronic continuous or intermittent infusion of cocaine differentially alter the concentration of neurotensin-like immunoreactivity in specific rat brain regions. *Neuropharmacology* 1993;8:259–265.
17. Carraway RE, Leeman SE. The isolation of a new hypotensive peptide, neurotensin, from bovine hypothalami. *Biol Chem* 1973;248:6854–6861.
18. Castel MN, Wang WX, Laduron PM, Beaudett A. Light and electron microscopic localization of retrogradely transported neurotensin in rat nigrostriatal dopaminergic neurons. *Neuroscience* 1992;50:269–282.
19. Chabry J, Gaudriault G, Vincent JP, Mazella J. Implication of various forms of neurotensin receptors in the mechanism of internalization of neurotensin in cerebral neurons. *J Biol Chem* 1993;268:17138–17144.
20. Chapman MA, See RE, Bissette G. Neurotensin increases extracellular striatal dopamine levels in vivo. *Neuropeptides* 1992;22:175–183.
21. Clement R, Griff D, Banks B, Nemeroff CB, Kitabgl P, Bissette G. The effects of haloperidol, quinelorane and lithium on regional neurotensin/neuromedin N concentrations: further evidence for neurotensin/neuromedin N-dopamine interactions. *Synapse* 1994; [in press].
22. Chigr F, Jordan D, Najimi M, Denoroy L, Sarrieau A, de Broca A, Rostene W, Epelbaum J, Kopp N. Quantitative autoradiographic study of somatostatin and neurotensin binding sites in medulla oblongata of SIDS. *Neurochem Int* 1992;20:113–118.
23. Conquerel A, Buser M, Tayot J, Pfaff F, Matray F, Proust B. Beta-endorphin and neurotensin in brainstem and cerebrospinal fluid in the sudden infant death syndrome. *Neurochem Int* 1991;20:97–102.
24. DeCeballos ML, Boyce S, Taylor M, Jenner P, Marsden CD. Age-related decreases in the concentration of met- and leu-enkephalin and neurotensin in the basal ganglia of rats. *Neurosci Lett* 1987;75:113–117.
25. Di Paola ED, Cusack B, Yamada M, Richelson E. Desensitization and down-regulation of neurotensin receptors in murine neuroblastoma clone N1E-115 by [D-Lys⁸] neurotensin. *J Pharmacol Exp Ther* 1992;264:1–5.
26. Dobner PR, Barber DL, Komaroff LV, Mckiernan C. Cloning and sequence analysis of cDNA for the canine neurotensin/neuromedin N precursor. *Proc Natl Acad Sci USA* 1987;84:3516–3523.
27. Dubuc I, Costentin J, Doulut S, Rodriguez M, Martinez J, Kitabgi P. JMV 440: a pseudopeptide analogue of neurotensin-(8-13) with highly potent and long-lasting hypothermic and analgesic effects in the mouse. *Eur J Pharmacol* 1992;219:327–329.
28. During MJ, Bean AJ, Roth RH. Effects of CNS stimulants on the *in vivo* release of the colocalized transmitters, dopamine and neurotensin, from rat prefrontal cortex. *Neurosci Lett* 1992;140:129–133.
29. Erwin VG, Jones BC. Genetic correlations among ethanol-related behaviors and neurotensin receptors in long sleep (LS) × short sleep (SS) recombinant inbred strains of mice. *Behav Genet* 1993;23:191–196.
30. Ferrer JMR, Sabater S, Saez JA. Neuromedin N decreases self-stimulation of the medial prefrontal cortex. *NeuroReport* 1992;3:1027–1029.
31. Ferrer JMR, Sabater S, Saez JA. Neurotensin participates in self-stimulation of the medial prefrontal cortex in the rat. *Eur J Pharmacol* 1992;231:39–45.
32. Frye GD, Luttinger D, Nemeroff CB, Vogel RA, Prange AJ Jr, Breese GR. Modification of the actions of ethanol by centrally active peptides. *Peptides* 1981;99–106.
33. Fuxe K, O'Connor W, Antonelli T, Osborne PG, Tanganelli S, Agnati LF, Ungerstedt U. Evidence for a substrate of neuronal plasticity based on pre- and postsynaptic neurotensin–dopamine receptor interactions in the neostriatum. *Proc Natl Acad Sci USA* 1992;89:5591–5595.
34. Gaspar P, Berger B, Febvret A. Neurotensin innervation of the human cerebral cortex: lack of colocalization with catecholamines. *Brain Res* 1990;530:181–195.

35. Glimcher PW, Margolin DH, Giovino AA, Hoebel BG. Neurotensin: a new "reward peptide". *Brain Res* 1984;291:119–124.
36. Govoni S, Hong JS, Yang H-YT, Costa E. Increase of neurotensin content elicited by neuroleptics in nucleus accumbens. *J Pharmacol Exp Ther* 1980;215:413–417.
37. Gully D, Canton M, Boigergrain R, Jeanjean F, Molimard JC, Poncellet M, Gueudet C, Heaulme M, Leyris R, Brouard A, Pelaprat D, Labre-Jullie C, Mazella J, Soubrie P, Maffrand JP, Rostene W, Kitabgi P, LeFur G. Biochemical and pharmacological profile of a potent and selective nonpeptide antagonist of the neurotensin receptor. *Proc Natl Acad Sci USA* 1993;90:65–69.
38. Hedner J, Hedner T, Lundell KH, Bissette G, O'Connor L, Nemeroff CB. Cerebrospinal fluid concentrations of neurotensin and corticotropin-releasing factor in pediatric patients. *Biol Neonate* 1989;55:260–267.
39. Herbison AE, Theodosis DT. Localization of oestrogen receptors in preoptic neurons containing neurotensin but not tyrosine hydroxylase, cholecystokinin or luteinizing hormone-releasing hormone in the male and female rat. *Neuroscience* 1992;50:283–298.
40. Hökfelt T, Everitt BJ, Theodorsson-Norheim E, Goldstein M. Occurrence of neurotensin-like immunoreactivity in subpopulations of hypothalamic, mesencephalic, and medullary catecholamine neurons. *J Comp Neurol* 1984;222:543–559.
41. Inagaki S, Shinoda K, Kubota Y, Shiosaka S, Marsuzaki T, Tohyama M. Evidence for the existence of a neurotensin-containing pathway from the endopiriform nucleus and the adjacent prepiriform cortex to the anterior olfactory nucleus and nucleus of diagonal band (Broca) of the rat. *Neuroscience* 1983;8:487–493.
42. Jansen KLR, Faull RLM, Dragunow M, Leslie RA. Distribution of excitatory and inhibitory amino acid, sigma, monoamine, catecholamine, acetylcholine, opioid, neurotensin, substance P, adenosine and neuropeptide Y receptors in human motor and somatosensory cortex. *Brain Res* 1991;566:225–238.
43. Jolicoeur FB, Rivest R, St Pierre S, Drumheller A. Antiparkinson-like effects of neurotensin in 6-hydroxydopamine lesioned rats. *Brain Res* 1991;538:187–192.
44. Jolicoeur FB, Gagne MA, Rivest R, Drumheller A, St-Pierre S. Atypical neuroleptic-like behavioral effects of neurotensin. *Brain Research Bulletin* 1993;32:487–491.
45. Ju G. Calcitonin gene-related peptide-like immunoreactivity and its relation with neurotensin- and corticotropin-releasing hormone-like immunoreactive neurons in the bed nuclei of the stria terminalis in the rat. *Brain Res Bull* 1991;27:617–624.
46. Kalivas PW, Jennes L, Nemeroff CB, Prange AJ Jr. Neurotensin: topographic distribution of brain sites involved in hypothermia and antinociception. *J Comp Neurol* 1992;210:225–238.
47. Kalivas PW, Miller JS. Neurotensin neurons in the ventral tegmental area project to the medial nucleus accumbens. *Brain Res* 1984;300:157–160.
48. Kalivas PW. Neurotransmitter regulation of dopamine neurons in the ventral tegmental area. *Brain Res Rev* 1993;18:75–113.
49. Kilts CD, Anderson CM, Bissette G, Ely TD, Nemeroff CB. Differential effects of antipsychotic drugs on the neurotensin concentration of discrete rat brain nuclei. *Biochem Pharmacol* 1988;37:1547–1554.
50. Kislauskis E, Bullock B, McNeil D, Dobner PR. The rat gene encoding neurotensin and neuromedin N: structure, tissue-specific expression, and evaluation of exon sequences. *J Biol Chem* 1988;263:4963–4968.
51. Kleinman JE, Iadorola M, Govoni S, Hong J, Gillin JC, Wyatt RJ. Post-mortem measurements of neuropeptides in human brain. *Psychopharmacol Bull* 1983;19:375–377.
52. Labie C, Keane PE, Soubrie P, LeFur G. The σ receptor ligand SR 31742A increases neurotensin in the nucleus accumbens but not in the caudate-putamen of the rat. *Eur J Pharmacol* 1993;231:465–467.
53. Levant B, Nemeroff CB. The psychobiology of neurotensin. *Neuroendocrinology* 1988;8:232–262.
54. Levant B, Bissette G, Widerlov E, Nemeroff CB. Alterations in regional brain neurotensin concentrations produced by atypical antipsychotic drugs. *Regul Pept* 1991;32:193–201.
55. Levant B, Nemeroff CB. Further studies on the modulation of regional brain neurotensin concentrations by antipsychotic drugs: focus on haloperidol and BMY 14802[1]. *J Pharmacol Exp Ther* 1992;262:348–355.
56. Levant B, Merchant KM, Dorsa DM, Nemeroff CB. BMY 14802, a potential antipsychotic drug, increases expression of proneurotensin mRNA in the rat striatum. *Mol Res* 1992;12:279–284.
57. Lindstrom LH, Widerlov E, Bissette G, Nemeroff CB. Reduced CSF neurotensin concentration in drug-free schizophrenic patients. *Schizophr Res* 1988;1:55–59.
58. Mazella J, Leonard K, Chabry J, Kitabgi P, Vincent JP, Beaudet A. Binding and internalization of iodinated neurotensin in neuronal cultures from embryonic mouse brain. *Brain Res* 1991;564:249–255.
59. Merchant KM, Dorsa DM. Differential induction of neurotensin and c-fos gene expression by typical versus atypical antipsychotics. *Proc Natl Acad Sci USA* 1993;90:3447–3451.
60. Merchant KM, Miller MA, Ashleigh EA, Dorsa DM. Haloperidol rapidly increases the number of neurotensin mRNA-expressing neurons in neostriatum of the rat brain. *Brain Res* 1991;540:311–314.
61. Merchant KM, Dobner PR, Dorsa DM. Differential effects of haloperidol and clozapine on neurotensin gene transcription in rat neostriatum. *J Neurosci* 1992;12(2):652–663.
62. Merchant KM, Dobie DJ, Dorsa DM. Expression of the proneurotensin gene in the rat brain and its regulation by antipsychotic drugs. In: Nemeroff CB, Kitabgi P, eds. *The neurobiology of neurotensin. Annals of the New York Academy of Sciences*, vol 668. New York: New York Academy of Sciences, 1992;54–69.
63. Nemeroff CB. Neurotensin: perchance an endogenous neuroleptic? *Biol Psychiatry* 1980;15:283–302.
64. Nemeroff CB, Youngblood WW, Manberg PJ, Prange AJ Jr, Kizer JS. Regional brain concentrations of neuropeptides in Huntington's chorea and schizophrenia. *Science* 1983;221:972–975.
65. Nemeroff CB, Berger PA, Bissette G. Peptides in schizophrenia. In: Meltzer HY, ed. *Psychopharmacology*. New York: Raven Press, 1987;727–744.
66. Nemeroff CB, Kizer JS, Reynolds GP, Bissette G. Neuropeptides in Alzheimer's disease: a postmortem study. *Regul Pept* 1989;25:123–130.
67. Nemeroff CB, Kitabgi P, eds. *The neurobiology of neurotensin. Annals of the New York Academy of Sciences*, vol 668. New York: New York Academy of Sciences, 1992.
68. Niimi M, Takahara J, Sato M, Kawanishi K. Neurotensin and growth hormone-releasing factor-containing neurons projecting to the median eminence of the rat: a combined retrograde tracing and immunohistochemical study. *Neurosci Lett* 1991;133:183–186.
69. Nouel D, Costentin J, Lugrin D, Kitabgi P, Ple N, Davoust D. Investigations about a direct neurotensin–dopamine interaction by nuclear magnetic resonance study, synaptosomal uptake of dopamine, and binding of neurotensin to its receptors. *J Neurochem* 1992;59:1933–1936.
70. Petrov T, Jhamandas JH, Krukoff TL. Characterization of peptidergic efferents from the lateral parabrachial nucleus to identified neurons in the rat dorsal raphe nucleus. *Chem Neuroanat* 1992;5:367–373.
71. Pilotte NS, Mitchell M, Sharpe LG, DeSouza EB, Dax EM. Chronic cocaine administration and withdrawal of cocaine modify neurotensin binding in rat brain. *Synapse* 1991;9:111–120.
72. Przedborski S, Levivier M, Cadet JL. Neurotensin receptors in human meningiomas. *Ann Neurol* 1991;30:650–654.
73. Radke JM, MacLennan AJ, Beinfeld MC, Bissette G, Nemeroff CB, Vincent SR, Fibiger HC. Effects of short- and long-term haloperidol administration and withdrawal on regional brain cholecystokinin and neurotensin concentrations in the rat. *Brain Res* 1989;480:178–183.
74. Rivest R, St Pierre S, Jolicoeur FB. Structure-activity studies of neurotensin on muscular rigidity and tremors induced by 6-hydroxydopamine lesions in the posterolateral hypothalamus of the rat. *Neuropharmacology* 1991;30:47–52.
75. Roberts GW, Crow TJ, Polak JM. Neurotensin: first report of a cortical pathway. *Peptides* 1981;2:37–43.
76. Rompré P, Bauco P, Gratton A. Facilitation of brain stimulation reward by mesencephalic injections of neurotensin-(1-13). *Eur J Pharmacol* 1992;211:295–303.
77. Rompré PP, Boye SM. Opposite effects of mesencephalic microin-

jections of cholecystokinin octapeptide and neurotensin-(1-13) on brain stimulation reward. *Eur J Pharmacol* 1993;232:299–303.

78. Sadoul JL, Checler F, Kitabgi P, Rostene W, Javoy-Agid F, Vincent JP. Loss of high affinity neurotensin receptors in substantia nigra from parkinsonian subjects. *Biochem Biophys Res Commun* 1984;125:395–404.

79. Schiffmann SN, Vanderhaeghen JJ. Caffeine regulates neurotensin and cholecystokinin messenger RNA expression in the rat striatum. *Neuroscience* 1993;54:681–689.

80. Shi WX, Bunney BS. Effects of neurotensin on midbrain dopamine neurons: Are they mediated by formation of a neurotensin-dopamine complex? *Synapse* 1991;9:157–164.

81. Singh NA, Bush LG, Gibb JW, Hanson GR. Role of *N*-methyl-D-aspartate receptors in dopamine D₁-, but not D₂-, mediated changes in striatal and accumbens neurotensin systems. *Brain Res* 1992;571:260–264.

82. Tanaka K, Masu M, Nakanishi S. Structure and functional expression of the cloned rat neurotensin receptor. *Neuron* 1990;4:847–854.

83. Tanganelli S, Li XM, Ferraro L, von Euler G, O'Connor WT, Bianchi C, Beani L, Fuxe K. Neurotensin and cholecystokinin octapeptide control synergistically dopamine release and dopamine D₂ receptor affinity in rat neostriatum. *Eur J Pharmacol* 1992;230:159–166.

84. Taylor MD, De Ceballos ML, Jenner P, Marsden CD. Acute effects of D-1 and D-2 dopamine receptor agonist and antagonist drugs on basal ganglia [Met⁵]- and [Leu⁵]-enkephalin and neurotensin content in the rat. *Biochem Pharmacol* 1991;41:1385–1391.

85. Tischler AS, Ruzicka LA, Dobner PR. A protein kinase inhibitor, staurosporine, mimics nerve growth factor induction of neurotensin/neuromedin N gene expression. *J Biol Chem* 1991;266:1141–1146.

86. Uhl GR, Snyder SH. Neurotensin: a neuronal pathway projecting from amygdala through stria terminalis. *Brain Res* 1979;161:522–526.

87. Uhl GR, Whitehouse PJ, Price DL, Tourtelotte WW, Kuhar MJ. Parkinson's disease: depletion of substantia nigra neurotensin receptors. *Brain Res* 1984;308:186–190.

88. Vita N, Laurent P, Lefort S, Chalon P, Dumont X, Kaghad M, Gully D, LeFur G, Ferrara P. Cloning and expression of a complementary DNA encoding a high affinity human neurotensin receptor. *FEBS Lett* 1993;317:139–142.

89. von Euler G. Biochemical characterization of the intramembrane interaction between neurotensin and dopamine D₂ receptors in the rat brain. *Brain Res* 1991;561:93–98.

90. Watson CB, Watson AW, Murray KD, Isackson PJ, Richelson

91. Watson M, Makker M, Isackson P, Yamada M, Yamada M, Cusak B, Richelson E. Identification of a polymorphism in the human neurotensin receptor gene. *Mayo Clin Proc* 1993;68:1043–1048.

92. Watts AG. Osmotic stimulation differentially affects cellular levels of corticotropin-releasing hormone and neurotensin/neuromedin N mRNAs in the lateral hypothalamic area and central nucleus of the amygdala. *Brain Res* 1992;581:208–216.

93. Wenk GL, O'leary M, Nemeroff CB, Bissette G, Moser H, Naidu S. Neurochemical alterations in Rett syndrome. *Dev Brain Res* 1993;74:67–72.

94. Widerlov E, Kilts CD, Mailman RB, Nemeroff CB, McCown TJ Jr, Breese GR. Increase in dopamine metabolites in rat brain by neurotensin. *J Pharmacol Exp Ther* 1982;222:1–6.

95. Widerlov E, Lindstrom LH, Besev G, Manberg PJ, Nemeroff CB, Breese GR, Kizer JS, Prange AJ Jr. Subnormal CSF levels of neurotensin in a subgroup of schizophrenic patients: normalization after neuroleptic treatment. *Am J Psychiatry* 1982;139:1122–1126.

96. Williams FG, Beitz AJ. Chronic pain increases brainstem proneurotensin/neuromedin-N mRNA expression: a hybridization histochemical and immunohistochemical study using three different rat models for chronic nociception. *Brain Res* 1993;611:87–102.

97. Woulfe J, Beaudet A. Neurotensin terminals form synapses primarily with neurons lacking detectable tyrosine hydroxylase immunoreactivity in the rat substantia nigra and ventral tegmental area. *J Comp Neurol* 1992;321:163–176.

98. Yamada M, Yamada M, Richelson E. Further characterization of neurotensin receptor desensitization and down-regulation in clone N1E-115 neuroblastoma cells. *Biochem Pharmacol* 1993;45:2149–2154.

99. Yamano M, Hillyard CJ, Girgis S, Emson PC, MacIntyre I, Tohyama M. Projection of neurotensin-like immunoreactive neurons from the lateral parabrachial area to the central amygdaloid nucleus of the rat with reference to the coexistence with calcitonin gene-related peptide. *Exp Brain Res* 1988;71:603–610.

100. Zahm DS. Subset of neurotensin-immunoreactive neurons revealed following antagonism of the dopamine-mediated suppression of neurotensin immunoreactivity in the rat striatum. *Neuroscience* 1992;46:335–350.

101. Zsurger N, Chabry J, Coquerel A, Vincent JP. Ontogenesis and binding properties of high-affinity neurotensin receptors in human brain. *Brain Res* 1992;586:303–310.

E. Haloperidol but not clozapine increases neurotensin receptor mRNA levels in rat substantia nigra. *J Neurochem* 1993;61:1141–1143.

Psychopharmacology: The Fourth Generation of Progress, edited by Floyd E. Bloom and David J. Kupfer. Raven Press, Ltd., New York © 1995.

CHAPTER 52

Cholecystokinin/Gastrin

Margery C. Beinfeld

DISCOVERY OF CHOLECYSTOKININ (CCK)/GASTRIN, ITS CHEMISTRY, AND MOLECULAR FORMS

Discovery of CCK/Gastrin in the Brain and Its Identification as CCK 8

The discovery of the hormone which would eventually be called CCK dates to the beginning of the 20th century and culminated with the sequencing of CCK 33 by Mutt and Jorpes (39) in the 1960s. The name CCK/gastrin originated with the discovery of this material in brain. Vanderhaeghen et al. (53), using a gastrin antisera which cross-reacts strongly with CCK, detected abundant gastrin-like material in the brains of several vertebrate species, including man. The discovery of CCK in the brain in 1975 was part of the mini-revolution that was taking place at that time in our thinking about biologically active peptides. The fact that it wasn't until 1975 that anyone even considered looking for CCK in the brain is indicative of the prevailing view that the peptides in brain and gut were fundamentally different: It was though that the brain contained hypothalamic releasing factors and that the gut contained gastrointestinal hormones. The discovery of the abundance and wide distribution of vasoactive intestinal peptide (VIP) and CCK (6) in the brain, along with the presence of somatostatin in the gut and pancreas, soon changed that view.

Based on its chromatographic behavior and biological activity, and finally amino acid sequence analysis (17), it was soon clear that this material was mainly the carboxyl-terminal amidated peptide CCK 8. The sequences of CCK 8, gastrin, and caerulein (a CCK-like peptide from the skin of the frog *Hyla caerulea*) are shown in Table 1.

M. C. Beinfeld: Department of Pharmacological and Physiological Science, St. Louis University Medical Center, St. Louis, Missouri 63104.

Small amounts of authentic gastrin have been detected in the brain and pituitary of several species, although the significance of this has never been established (see also Chapter 43, *this volume*).

Molecular Cloning of CCK and the Chemistry of pre-pro-CCK

Our knowledge of the chemistry of pre-pro-CCK was greatly enhanced by the cloning of the cDNA for the rat sequence (15). This was followed in rapid succession by the cloning of the porcine and human cDNAs. The human CCK gene is found on the third chromosome, whereas the gastrin gene is on the 17th (32). The transcription unit spans 7 kb and is interrupted by two introns. The promoter region is within 144 bases 5′ to the transcription start site (14).

Not much is known about the regulation of CCK gene expression. The promoter region contains putative cAMP and phorbol ester response elements. As described in the section of release, the cAMP element appears to be active, because treatment of most CCK-secreting endocrine cells in culture with forskolin elevate CCK secretion and increase CCK mRNA expression. Treatment of some endocrine cells with phorbol esters does increase their CCK mRNA levels, but a similar secretory response to phorbol esters has not been observed. Short-term treatment of brain slices with forskolin or phorbol esters causes increases in potassium-evoked CCK release, although it is not known whether a concomitant increase in CCK mRNA levels occurs. Little is known about the regulation of CCK gene expression in the brain in intact animals. This has proven somewhat difficult to study, because minor surgical manipulations are sufficient to induce large transient increases in CCK mRNA levels.

CCK has a long evolutionary history, and it is thought that CCK and gastrin probably evolved from a common

TABLE 1. *Structure of CCK-related peptides*[a]

CCK 8:	Asp-Tyr*-Met-Gly-Trp-Met-Asp-Phe-NH$_2$
Gastrin:	Pro-Trp-Leu-Glu-Glu-Glu-Glu-Glu-Ala-Tyr-Gly-Trp-Met-Asp-Phe-NH$_2$
Caerulein:	pGlu-Gln-Asp-Tyr*-Thr-Gly-Trp-Met-Asp-Phe-NH$_2$

[a] An asterisk indicates a sulfated tyrosine residue.

ancestral protein. The sequence of CCK 8 is highly conserved across mammalian species.

Rat pre-pro-CCK is shown schematically in Fig. 1 with the known cleavage sites (inferred from products isolated and sequenced from brain and intestine). In the lower portion of the figure, a model of the temporal cleavages which produce CCK 8 is presented.

The Molecular Forms of CCK in Brain

CCK displays an unusually high degree of tissue heterogeneity, and this heterogeneity appears to be somewhat species-dependent. The major tissue difference is between the way pro-CCK is processed in brain and gut.

The major carboxyl-terminal amidated peptide in brain is CCK 8, whereas in gut the larger forms such as CCK 22, 33, 39, and 58 are more abundant than CCK 8. The determination of the major form of CCK in tissue is confounded by the low cross-reactivity of large forms of CCK (e.g., CCK 58) for antisera generated against CCK 8. The major forms of CCK in plasma appear to reflect the forms present in the gut. Larger forms such as CCK 33, 39, and 58 have also been identified in brain, as have their amino-terminal peptides minus CCK8. Small amounts of carboxyl-terminally extended peptides have been identified in brain; of these, CCK 33 and CCK 8 predominate. Human anterior pituitary and the cerebelli of several species appear to be unable to completely process pro-CCK to CCK 8.

Plasma levels of CCK are low, and their measurement by radioimmunoassay (RIA) is complicated by the cross-reactivity of many of the CCK antisera with circulating gastrin. A sensitive and specific bioassay has been developed which has been used successfully to document changes in plasma CCK levels under normal and pathological situations (31).

DISTRIBUTION OF CCK IN THE CENTRAL NERVOUS SYSTEM

CCK Distribution

CCK is very abundant in the brain, more abundant than in the gut. To date, the only neuropeptide which is more abundant than CCK is neuropeptide Y (NPY).

CCK levels are very high (>4 ng CCK/mg protein) in cerebral cortex, caudate-putamen, hippocampus, and amygdala, whereas in thalamus, hypothalamus, and olfactory bulb they are lower (1–2 ng/mg protein). The pons, medulla, and spinal cord have even lower levels (<1 ng/mg protein), while CCK is barely detectable in the cerebellum (6).

The anatomy of central CCK-ergic projections is very complex and has been the subject of intense investigation since its discovery. Even so, every year brings new insights into important neuronal projections which contain CCK.

The ability to visualize CCK mRNA has provided much

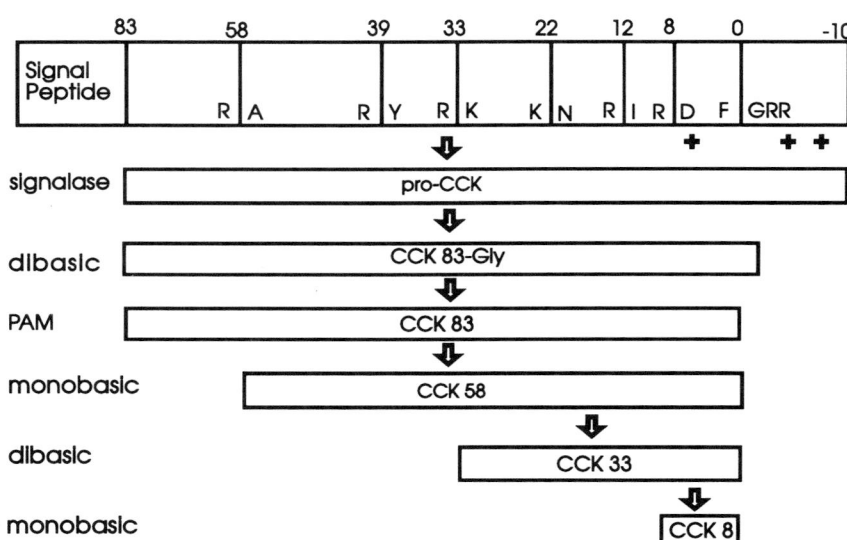

FIG. 1. Structure of rat pre-pro-CCK. The *vertical lines* indicate the location of cleavage sites, and the *single amino acid code* shows the amino acids flanking these sites. The *numbers at the top* indicate the location of the different carboxyamidated forms of CCK. The *plus signs* mark the location of the sulfated tyrosine residues. The **lower portion** of the figure shows a proposed model of the temporal order of cleavages in the processing of pre-pro-CCK, and the class of enzyme responsible for the cleavage is indicated on the *left*.

additional information about the location of CCK cell bodies, because it appears to be much more sensitive than peptide staining. The reasons for this difference are unclear but probably reflect different distribution and/or abundance of CCK mRNA transcripts and processed peptides.

Many brain regions contain both CCK-positive interneurons and a mixture of afferent and/or efferent cells and terminals. Certain regions such as the striatum, nucleus accumbens, and olfactory tubercle have abundant CCK terminals, but few CCK-positive cells.

Description of some of the Major CCK-ergic Projections

A number of major CCK-ergic projections have been identified:

1. *Cortico-striatal.* The striatum contains very few CCK-positive cells, although the level of immunoreactive CCK peptides is among the highest in the brain. Lesion studies indicated that the bulk of this CCK originates outside the striatum. Although CCK is present in some dopamine cells in the substantia nigra which project to the striatum, these cells provide very little of this CCK. Subsequent experiments have indicated that a significant amount of the immunoreactive CCK in the striatum originates in cerebral cortical cells (36). This has been verified by retrograde tracing and CCK in situ hybridization. Some of the CCK-containing cells in the nigra also project to the amygdala.

2. *Mesolimbic.* CCK cells in the ventral tegmental area, some of which also contain dopamine (26) and neurotensin, project to specific subdivisions of the nucleus accumbens, olfactory tubercle, and prefrontal cortex.

3. *Thalamo-cortical and thalamo-striatal.* The thalamus has moderate levels of CCK immunoreactivity, but relatively few peptide-positive cells are visualized. With hybridization, many neurons are identified which contain CCK transcripts, from 100% in the medial geniculate or ventral lateral nucleus to none in the ventrolateral geniculate. A high percentage of the cells [which are thought to be non-gamma-aminobutyric acid (GABA)-ergic] appear to be efferent and project topographically to sites in the cortex and striatum (9). Some of the CCK neurons which project to cortex are also VIP-ergic.

4. *Ascending visceral sensory.* CCK neurons project from the dorsal medial nucleus tractus solitarius and the outer rim of the area postrema to the parabrachial nucleus (25). From the parabrachial nucleus, an additional set of CCK neurons project to the ventromedial nucleus of the hypothalamus (59).

5. *Ascending visual auditory.* CCK is abundant in amacrine cells in the retinas of some species and also has been found in retinal ganglion cells. CCK neurons in the

TABLE 2. *Neurotransmitters colocalized with CCK*

Co-transmitter	Brain region
Dopamine/and or neurotensin	Substantia nigra and vta[a]
VIP/GABA	Cortex, hippocampus
NPY/GABA	Cortex, hippocampus
VIP	Thalamus
Substance P	Medulla
5-Hydroxytryptamine	Medulla
Oxytocin	Hypothalamus
CRF	Hypothalamus
Enkephalin	Cortex, thalamus

[a] vta, ventral tegmental area (A10).

dorsal lateral geniculate project to visual cortex, and other cells in the inferior olive project to the inferior colliculus.

6. *Hippocampal-septal.* Lesions of the fornix caused a significant decrease in CCK levels in the lateral septum, bed nucleus of the stria terminalis, mamillary bodies, anteroventral nucleus of the thalamus, and subiculum (24). These results suggest that there is a significant efferent CCK-ergic projection from the hippocampus.

7. *Magnocellular/parvocellular hypothalamic-hypophyseal.* CCK-containing neurons in the paraventricular nucleus, some which contain oxytocin and some corticotropin-releasing factor (CRF) (37), project to the median eminence and posterior lobe of the pituitary (42).

8. *Descending projections to spinal cord.* CCK neurons in the periaqueductal gray, Edinger–Westphal nucleus, and ventral medulla project to the spinal cord.

9. *Spinal cord.* The use of mRNA hybridization has also revealed small-to-medium cells in layers II, III, and X of Rexed and motoneurons in layer IX of cervical, thoracic, and lumbrosacral spinal cord (48). The ability to localize CCK mRNA specifically should help resolve any remaining questions concerning the identity of the CCK-like material in spinal cord. Previous cross-reactivity between CCK and CGRP of some antisera used for immunostaining had complicated the analysis.

CCK Colocalization

CCK has been found to be colocalized with a number of "classical transmitters" and other neuropeptides with a distinct distribution. This is summarized in Table 2 (see also Chapter 18, *this volume*).

BIOSYNTHESIS AND PROCESSING OF CCK

An Overview of CCK Processing.

CCK biosynthesis takes place in the context of the regulated secretory pathway. Drugs which disrupt the Golgi (Brefeldin) or alter acidification of secretory granules (ammonium chloride) drastically reduce or eliminate completely the pool of processed CCK available for secretion. After insertion into the endoplasmic reticulum (ER) and removal of the signal peptide, pro-CCK assumes its correct three-dimensional structure. From there it is probably not further modified until it reaches the *trans*-Golgi. Pro-CCK has no consensus sequence(s) for N- or O-linked glycosylation, and there is no indication that it is glycosylated. In the *trans*-Golgi, three out of four of its tyrosine residues are sulfated by a specific membrane-bound tyrosine sulfotransferase (40). One of the tyrosine residues (in CCK 8) is important for biological activity at CCK A receptors. Recent evidence suggests that sulfation of the tyrosines in pro-CCK is important for correct sorting and/or processing of pro-CCK (5). This may also be true for gastrin. In the *trans*-Golgi network, sulfated pro-CCK is sorted into secretory granules with other material destined for the regulated secretory pathway.

Based on the products isolated from brain and intestine, the most probable model of the processing of pro-CCK is depicted in Fig. 1 and involves the following steps: signal peptide cleavage and removal of the carboxyl-terminal extension, followed by conversion of the carboxyl-terminal glycine to an amide, thereby producing CCK 83 (18). CCK 83 is then cleaved at a number of sites, thereby producing CCK 58, CCK 39, CCK 33, CCK 22, and CCK 8. The ability to engineer endocrine tumor cells to express high levels of CCK mRNA and to correctly process it to CCK 8 will undoubtedly permit us to elucidate this process.

The significance of the presence of low levels of COOH-terminal extended peptides coexisting with the full-length carboxy-amidated peptides is not clear. It has been suggested that within a single tissue, different population of cells may utilize different pro-CCK processing pathways (46). The presence of elevated levels of carboxyl-terminal extended peptides in endocrine tumor cells which fail to correctly process pro-CCK implies that the dibasic and/or amidating enzymes are down-regulated or are unable to completely process the pro-CCK produced by these cells. The failure of previous pulse-chase studies to clearly demonstrate a precursor–product relationship between large carboxy-amidated forms and CCK 8 implies that there is no unique order of cleavages. In this case, once amidated CCK 83 is produced, the remaining mono- and dibasic cleavages can occur in any order.

The processing of pro-CCK is somewhat unusual because most of the cleavage sites occur at single Arg residues. Although the enzyme(s) responsible for the monobasic cleavages has not been definitively identified, a serine protease which will cleave CCK 33 to produce CCK 8 has been extensively purified from rat brain synaptosomes (55). This enzyme will also cleave CCK 33 at the single lysine residue, generating CCK 22. It has a very broad pH optimum with a maximum at 8 and is highly specific, requiring the sulfated tyrosine or a suitably charged residue in the same position in CCK 8 for cleavage. Whether this enzyme makes the other monoba-

sic cleavages in pro-CCK is under investigation. The cloning of this enzyme is in progress.

The enzyme(s) responsible for the dibasic cleavages in pro-CCK have not been identified. Among the recently cloned subtilisin-like enzymes (52), the most likely candidate for the dibasic cleavages in pro-CCK is PC2. Experiments are underway to evaluate this possibility.

The turnover of CCK 8 in rat brain in vivo has been measured by intraventricular injection of labeled amino acids or sulfate followed by high-pressure liquid chromatography (HPLC) analysis of the labeled products. The peak of incorporation of label into CCK 8 occurs after about 4 hr. The half-life of turnover of labeled CCK 8 in this model is about 16 hr (35).

The enzyme(s) responsible from the degradation of CCK 8 after it is released has not been definitely identified. There is no evidence that desulfation is the route of degradation, because little nonsulfated CCK 8 has been isolated from brain. Studies of the degradation of CCK 8 are complicated by the general lack of knowledge of which among the myriad of cellular proteases that might have the right catalytic activity are located in the synaptic cleft. Early experiments indicated that enkephalinase (E.C. 3.4.11.7) may be involved in the degradation of both enkephalin and CCK (16). This is a logical candidate because it has been localized to pre- and postsynaptic membranes (4). More recent studies have disputed this claim and have indicated that either a thiol (34) or a serine protease (47) in concert with an aminopeptidase is responsible.

Studies with Endocrine Cells and Recombinant Cells in Culture

A number of different neural and endocrine tumor cells which express CCK mRNA have been identified. Some of them (some rat thyroid medullary carcinoma cells, mouse At-T20 pituitary cells, human small-cell lung carcinoma cells, and RIN5F rat insulinoma cells) process pro-CCK like the brain, producing mainly CCK 8, whereas some (neuroepithelioma, neuroblastomas, acoustic neuromas, Ewing sarcomas, rhabdomyosarcomas, human gastric carcinomas, and some insulinoma cells) appear to be unable to completely process pro-CCK to CCK 8. A human cortical cell line from a patient with unilateral megalencephaly has been reported to express CCK immunoreactivity, but whether this material is correctly processed to CCK 8 has not been reported.

Subclones of the mouse pro-opiomelanocortin (POMC)-secreting pituitary AtT20 cell line which express barely detectable amounts of CCK (0.2 ng CCK/mg protein) when stably transfected with the rat CCK cDNA produce and correctly process pro-CCK to CCK 8 (30). When the expression of the CCK cDNA is driven by a strong viral promoter, it is possible to boost the production of CCK peptides by over 300-fold. Preliminary studies with these engineered cells indicate that the turnover of CCK 8 is similar to that observed in rat brain in vivo.

REGULATION OF CCK RELEASE

In Vivo and In Vitro Studies

The release of CCK is relatively easy to study because of its abundance in most brain regions. The majority of studies have focused on release of CCK from brain slices in vitro. A few early studies have utilized synaptosomes, and more recently some push–pull and microdialysis studies have appeared. Although it is feasible to measure CCK peptides released into a push–pull cannula, the low recovery of CCK peptides using microdialysis has prevented many studies using this technology.

Like other neuropeptides, the release of CCK can be elicited by stimulation by potassium, veratridine, or an electrical field. Unlike the catecholamines, CCK requires a relatively strong stimulus for release: 40–60 mM potassium, as compared to 25 mM for dopamine.

The fractional release of CCK from brain slices varies depending upon the brain region studied. The cortex and hippocampus release about 2% of their CCK upon a strong stimulation, whereas the caudate-putamen releases less than 1%. This has been attributed to the tonic inhibition of an unknown substance which is released by a calcium-dependent mechanism along with CCK from a number of brain regions, but whose effect is most apparent in the caudate-putamen (23).

Studies of the effect of different pharmacological agents on the release of CCK from brain slices have yielded conflicting results, but they do indicate that the modulation of CCK release is regionally specific. Depending upon the study, dopamine agonists, dopamine antagonists, and depletion of endogenous dopamine has been reported to either decrease or increase CCK release from caudate or cortex. Most of the recent studies find that dopamine stimulates CCK release from the caudate (8). Psychotomimetic drugs such as phencyclidine have been reported to inhibit CCK release (2). Delta opiates have been reported to increase CCK release from the substantia nigra and spinal cord, whereas mu opiates decrease CCK release from these tissues. The results on the effect of GABA and excitatory amino acids on release have been contradictory.

A few studies have evaluated the effect of alteration of intracellular mediators on CCK release. Incubation with phorbol esters causes a two- to threefold increase in potassium-evoked release from cortex, hippocampus, and caudate-putamen (1). Paradoxically, a 40-min preincubation with 10 mM lithium also increases potassium-evoked CCK release from caudate-putamen (22). Incubation with forskolin + IB isobutylmethylxanthine (which activates

adenylate cyclase) also increases potassium-evoked CCK release from cerebral cortical, but not caudate, slices. A similar result was seen with primary cortical cells in culture.

CCK RECEPTORS

The Cloning of the CCK A and CCK B Receptors

A vast literature exists on the pharmacology and physiology of CCK. By the early 1980s it was clear that based on the ability of different CCK receptors to recognize sulfated versus unsulfated CCK, that two major subtypes of CCK receptors exist. The CCK_A subtype, typically found in the pancreas, is relatively specific for sulfated CCK peptides, whereas unsulfated peptides are two to three orders of magnitude less potent. For the CCK_B subtype, the difference in potency between sulfated and unsulfated peptides is about one order of magnitude. The CCK_B subtype closely resembles the gastrin receptor.

In April 1992 in the same issue of the *Proceedings of the National Academy of Sciences,* the cloning of the rat pancreatic CCK_A receptor (56) and the canine parietal gastrin receptor (29) were reported. Both appear to be classical seven-membrane-spanning domain receptors which are homologous to the β-adrenergic receptor. The CCK_A and B receptors are 48% identical to each other and code for a protein of about 450 amino acids. They contain potential sites for N-linked glycosylation and serine phosphorylation (see also Chapters 11, 27, and 38, *this volume*).

Subsequently, it was found that the gastrin receptor in the stomach is the same as the CCK_B receptor found in brain and that the CCK_B receptor is also found in the pancreas, gallbladder, and bowel. Unlike other neurotransmitter receptor systems such as acetylcholine, serotonin, and somatostatin, the CCK system with only two receptor subtypes appears to be a model of simplicity.

The CCK_B receptor expressed in COS-7 cells responds to the addition of CCK by mobilizing internal calcium, suggesting that CCK's effect is mediated by the activation of phospholipase C (29). This mechanism has been previously established in the pancreas. Similar results have been observed in cultured striatal neurons, also using fura-2 and calcium imaging (38).

In the pancreas, it appears that there are both very-high-affinity (70 pM) and very-low-affinity (10 nM) CCK_A receptors, which explains the biphasic, concentration-dependent effect of CCK 8 on amylase secretion. An artificial CCK peptide agonist CCK-JMV-180 (Boc-Tyr$_{(SO_3)}$-Nle-Gly-Trp-Nle-Asp-2-phenylethyl ester) is an agonist at the high-affinity site and an antagonist at the low-affinity site (51). It has been suggested that CCK binding to the low-affinity site regulates pancreatic calcium mobilization. Whether any

TABLE 3. *Inhibitor constants of high-affinity subtype-specific CCK antagonists*

Antagonist	IC$_{50}$ for receptor	
	CCK$_A$	CCK$_B$
A-65186	5 nM	4 μM
CI988	3 μM	2 nM
L-364,718	1 nM	300 nM
L-365,260	300 nM	1 nM
LY262691	10 μM	30 nM

A-65186 (54), CI988 = PD134308 (27), L-364,718 = MK329 = devazepide (10), L-365,260 (7), LY262691 (45).

of the physiological effects of CCK in the brain can be explained by a similar mechanism is not yet clear.

The Distribution of CCK Receptor Subtypes in the Brain

The distribution of the CCK$_A$ and CCK$_B$ subtypes in brain is species-dependent. In general, the CCK$_B$ receptor predominates in the brain, although a significant number of physiological effects of CCK in the brain are mediated by CCK$_A$ receptors. By receptor autoradiography, CCK$_A$ receptors are most abundant in the nucleus tractus solitarius, area postrema, interpeduncular nucleus, posterior hypothalamus, and nucleus accumbens.

Specific CCK Agonists and Antagonists

The development of a number of selective, potent antagonists, some of which penetrate the blood–brain barrier, has greatly enhanced our understanding of the pharmacology and physiology of CCK. The discovery of asperlicin (11), a potent nonpeptide benzodiazepine-like metabolite of *Aspergillus alliaceus,* set the stage for the new round of discovery. These antagonists have been derived from cyclic nucleotides, amino acids, CCK and gastrin, benzodiazepines, quinazolinone, and diphenyl-pryzolidinone derivatives (44). The pace of development of new CCK agonists and antagonists appears to have quickened recently. Given all the possible physiological effects of CCK,· there is ample therapeutic rationale for their development. The affinities of some of these antagonists for CCK$_A$ and B receptors are summarized in Table 3.

PHARMACOLOGY AND PHYSIOLOGY OF CCK

Overview

The pharmacology and physiology of CCK have been studied in detail. This review will deal solely with the physiology and pharmacology of CCK in the brain. CCK is well established as a gastrointestinal hormone. Determination of the precise role of CCK in the brain has been more elusive.

Porcine CCK 33 isolated by Vitkor Mutt was the first material available for studies of the biological activity of CCK. The chemical synthesis of sulfated CCK 12 was reported by Ondetti et al. (41) at Squibb in 1970. They provided synthetic CCK 8 to investigators for years until it became commercially available in the early 1980s. The synthesis of CCK is complicated by the difficulty and low efficiency of the addition of the sulfate group to the tyrosine after conventional peptide synthesis with *t*-boc (*t*-butyloxycarbonyl) amino acids. Recent improvements in peptide synthesis in which the sulfated tyrosine is incorporated into the peptide backbone as an FMOC (9-fluorenyl-methoxycarbonyl) amino acid has allowed the synthesis of human and porcine CCK 33 (43) and canine CCK 58.

Exogenously applied CCK produces a wide variety of effects. It is still not entirely clear whether these effects are purely pharmacological, or whether they are physiologically relevant. The amount of CCK that is released under physiological conditions appears to be too small to account for many of the observed effects of CCK. In these studies, CCK is administered intraperitonealy, subcutaneously, intrathecally, intraventricularly, and so on, and it is not clear how much CCK is reaching its site of action, be it central or peripheral. It is also not clear what measurements of circulating or released CCK really mean. All of the release paradigms are relying on measurement of overflow or release into circulation and are detecting that amount of CCK which has been released and which manages to pass out of the tissue into the vessel, bath, probe, and so on. It is unclear how efficient this process is, and there is no way of determining the concentration of CCK in the synaptic cleft or how much reaches CCK receptors in their sites in the periphery. On the other hand, because CCK is reasonably abundant the actual amount of CCK that is potentially available for release may be substantial.

Some of the effects of CCK are thought to be centrally mediated, whereas others are peripherally mediated. When CCK acts peripherally, it activates CCK receptors whose message is delivered to the brain by the vagus. Higher doses administered centrally will produce the same effect, but this is probably due to some of the peptide passing into peripheral circulation. When CCK is acting centrally, administration of much lower doses into cerebral ventricle or in specific nuclei in the brain will produce the same effect as peripheral administration. In some cases, CCK appears to have both a peripheral and central site of action, which complicates the situation considerably. The ability to inhibit the effect of endogenous CCK acting at either A- or B-type receptors by peripheral administration of specific antagonists has greatly advanced our knowledge of the physiology of CCK.

Neurotransmitter Properties

CCK fulfills many of the standard criteria for a neurotransmitter:

1. *Subcellular localization and biosynthesis.* CCK is located exclusively in neurons in the brain. CCK is synthesized, processed, and packaged into vesicles in neurons. Subcellular fractionation studies have indicated that it is enriched in crude mitochondrial and microsomal fractions and even more highly enriched in synaptic vesicle preparations.

2. *Release.* CCK is released from isolated brain synaptosomes or brain slices by depolarization with high potassium or with veratridine, or by electrical stimulation. The release by potassium and electrical stimulation are calcium-dependent.

3. *Effect on neurons.* CCK is a potent excitatory agent when applied to a number of neuronal preparations. A number of investigators have reported that it excites neurons in the hippocampus. It depolarizes oxytocin containing neurons in the supraoptic nucleus of the hypothalamus via a B type receptor. Serotonin containing neurons in the dorsal raphe nucleus are excited via an A-type receptor. CCK appears to be able to modulate the effect of dopamine on midbrain neurons.

4. *Receptors.* As described above, two specific high-affinity receptors have been identified for CCK.

5. *Degradation.* As described above, CCK is rapidly degraded after it is released.

Pharmacological and Behavioral Effects of CCK

Role of CCK in Analgesia

The effect of CCK on opiate analgesia appears to be dependent on dose (3). At pharmacologic doses (minimum effective dose 50–750 μg/kg, i.p.), CCK acting through CCK$_A$ receptors is an analgesic agent which is 700- to 8000-fold more potent than morphine. This effect is opiate-mediated and is blocked by low doses of naloxone. At this dose, CCK does not alter morphine tolerance. This analgesic effect is likely to be centrally mediated, because much lower doses are required when administered directly into the brain (28).

At lower, more physiological doses (as little as 1 μg/kg, i.p.), CCK acting again through CCK$_A$ receptors antagonizes opiate analgesia (19). Much lower doses of CCK (as little as 3.6 ng) administered intrathecally antagonized front paw shock (opiate-mediated) analgesia. Treatment with a CCK$_A$ antagonist increases the peak effect and duration of morphine analgesia and prevents the development of tolerance but not dependence to morphine. Experimental evidence has been presented that the release of CCK in the spinal cord is the mechanism by which environmental stimuli (safety clues) mediate physiological anti analgesia (57). CCK$_A$ antagonists by themselves are not analgesic. The results suggest that CCK$_A$ antagonists could be useful clinically in enhancing morphine analgesia and in preventing the development of tolerance to morphine.

Role of CCK in Satiety

CCK released after a meal from the duodenum is thought to be a physiological regulator of food intake (49). This effect of CCK was first reported in 1973, before the discovery of brain CCK (21). Peripheral CCK appears to act additively with other hormones such as bombesin, somatostatin, calcitonin, and glucagon and with absorbed nutrients to produce termination of a meal and the intermeal interval. The precise mechanism by which CCK elicits satiety is not known, but decreased gastric emptying, production of hyperglycemia, and antagonism of the opiate feeding system are just a few possibilities. This "peripheral" action of CCK is thought to be mediated by CCKA-type receptors located in the stomach, because sectioning of the gastric vagus prevents the satiety effect of peripherally administered CCK (50). Studies of the role of CCK in satiety have been confounded by significant species and experimental paradigm differences.

Central administration of CCK is reported to cause satiety, although these results appear to be somewhat controversial and are species-dependent.

CCK, at doses which produce the same circulating levels of CCK observed after a meal, does cause decrease in food intake in experimental animals and in humans. The use of CCK to treat obesity or bulimia has met with limited success to date (see also Chapter 136, *this volume*).

Role of CCK in Memory

Feeding mice following a training session has been shown to increase memory. This effect is mimicked by injection of CCK 8 and is blocked by cutting the vagus (20) and by administration of a CCK$_A$ antagonist.

Interaction Between CCK and Dopamine

The discovery that CCK and dopamine are colocalized in the mesolimbic and mesocortical systems has inspired many studies of the interaction of these two transmitters. Numerous studies have examined their ability to alter each other's release, receptor binding, and pharmacology. By and large, these results have been conflicting, although technical differences between how the experiments were performed makes direct comparison of results difficult. An additional complication is caused by the anatomical and perhaps also functional microheterogeneity of the nucleus accumbens (NAC) and by the presence of the two different subtypes of CCK receptors which appear to cause opposite effects. Despite all of these shortcomings, some common themes do emerge.

The midbrain neurons containing both CCK and dopamine which project mainly to the NAC have a distinct topology. They terminate mainly in the medial and posterior NAC (58), whereas the anterior and lateral NAC contain mainly non-colocalized terminals. In contrast, although there are some CCK neurons containing dopamine which project to the caudate-putamen, the bulk of the CCK neurons which are thought to originate mainly in the cerebral cortex do not contain dopamine (36).

A number of studies have indicated that this anatomical difference has functional consequences, because the interaction between CCK and dopamine in the anterior, lateral nucleus is different from that in the posterior, medial NAC. CCK increased dopamine release from the posterior NAC through CCK_A receptors, whereas in the anterior NAC, CCK acting through CCK_B receptors inhibited dopamine release (33). Most studies indicate that dopamine release from the caudate is inhibited by CCK, although the opposite has also been reported.

Other studies support the functional microheterogeneity of CCK's actions in the nucleus accumbens. CCK acting through CCK_A receptors in posterior NAC potentiated dopamine-induced hyperlocomotion, whereas CCK_B receptors in the anterior NAC inhibit it (12). CCK potentiates reward (intracranial self-stimulation) when injected into posterior NAC, whereas in the anterior NAC it inhibits reward. CCK 8 acting through A-type receptors in the posterior NAC decreased the number of open-arm entries in an elevated plus-maze test (a measure of anxiety), whereas in the anterior NAC it had no effect on this behavior. CCK increases dopamine-induced adenylate cyclase activity in posterior NAC, whereas it inhibits it in the anterior NAC. Medial NAC neurons were excited by CCK, whereas lateral NAC neurons were not. That there is a distinctly different pharmacology which correlates with this projection does imply that coexistence may have some functional significance. Whether these effects are pharmacological or physiological is not entirely clear, because the CCK antagonists by themselves rarely seem to alter basal activity.

The effect of CCK agonists and antagonists on midbrain dopamine neurons have been somewhat contradictory, although most studies indicate that CCK potentiates the inhibitory action of dopamine agonists (see also Chapters 15 and 21, *this volume*).

Role of CCK in Anxiety

A number of animal studies on the possible involvement of CCK in anxiety have been inspired by several human studies which showed that administration of CCK 4 or CCK 5 to panic attack patients or normal volunteers (13) evoked panic-like attacks which were blocked by the benzodiazepine anxiolytic lorazepam. Panic attack patients were more sensitive than normal volunteers to the effect of CCK 4, and preadministration of the CCK_B receptor antagonist was shown to inhibit the effect of CCK 4. That CCK 8 did not induce similar attacks may be due to its poor central nervous system penetration, because CCK 8 administered directly into the NAC of rats displays anxiogenic activity in one behavioral test of anxiety.

Animals studies support the observation that CCK induces panic-like attacks, whereas CCK antagonists are anxiolytic. Which CCK receptor is involved appears to depend on the behavioral test utilized. The CCK_A-type antagonists appear to be active in the black–white box and elevated plus-maze test. In a rat conditioned suppression of drinking model and the "call-box" mouse model, the CCK_B antagonists were more active than the CCK_A antagonists. These results certainly suggest that CCK antagonists might prove to be useful anxiolytic drugs (see also Chapter 111, *this volume*).

Neuroendocrine Role of CCK

CCK causes secretion of both vasopressin and oxytocin from isolated neural lobes of the rat and is known to stimulate oxytocin secretion from intact rats. Hypothalamic CRF and pituitary adrenocorticotropic hormone (ACTH) secretion are stimulated in intact rats by CCK acting through A receptors. CCK has been reported to stimulate ACTH release and to act additively with vasopressin and CRF in stimulating ACTH release from isolated rat pituitaries and mouse pituitary tumor cells in culture.

Role of CCK in Neuroprotection/Stroke

CCK at submicromolar concentrations, acting through CCK_B receptors, protects neuronal cells in culture from glutamate or NMDA cytotoxicity. It has been suggested that this effect of CCK is caused by an inhibition of nitric oxide formation.

Other Physiological Effects of CCK

CCK antagonizes seizures caused by picrotoxin. It increases respiratory tidal volume and decreases body temperature, an effect which is abolished by pretreatment with capsaicin. Activation of CCK_B receptors increases release of excitatory amino acids in spinal cord, hypothalamus, and striatum, whereas it decreases acetylcholine release from the striatum but not cortex.

ACKNOWLEDGMENT

This work was supported in part by NIH NS18667.

REFERENCES

1. Allard LR, Beinfeld MC. Phorbol esters stimulate the potassium-induced release of cholecystokinin from slices of cerebral cortex, caudato-putamen, and hippocampus incubated in vitro. *Biochem Biophys Res Commun* 1988;153:372–376.
2. Allard LR, Brog JS, Viereck JC, et al. Inhibition of potassium-evoked release of cholecystokinin (CCK) from rat caudato-putamen, cerebral cortex, and hippocampus incubated in vitro by phencyclidine (PCP) and related compounds. *Brain Res* 1990;522:224–226.
3. Baber NS, Dourish CT, Hill DR. The role of CCK, caerulein, and CCK antagonists in nociception. *Pain* 1989;39:307–328.
4. Barnes K, Turner AJ, Kenney AJ. Membrane localization of endopeptidase-24.11 and peptidyldipeptidase A (antiotensin converting enzyme) in the pig brain: a study using subcellular fractionation and electron microscopic immunocytochemistry. *J Neurochem* 1992;58:2088–2096.
5. Beinfeld MC. Inhibition of pro-cholecystokinin sulfation by treatment with sodium chlorate alters its processing and decreases cellular content and secretion of CCK 8. *Neuropeptides* 1994;26:195–200.
6. Beinfeld MC, Meyer DK, Eskay RL, Jensen RT, Brownstein MJ. The distribution of cholecystokinin in the central nervous system of the rat as determined by radioimmunoassay. *Brain Res* 1981;212:51–57.
7. Bock MG, DePardo RM, Evans BE, et al. Benzodiazepine gastrin and brain cholecystokinin receptor ligands: L-365,260. *J Med Chem* 1989;32:13–16.
8. Brog JS, Beinfeld MC. Cholecystokinin release from the rat caudate-putamen, cortex, and hippocampus is increased by activation of the D1 dopamine receptor. *J Pharmacol Exp Ther* 1992;260:343–348.
9. Burgunder J-M, Young WS, III. The distribution of thalamic projection neurons containing cholecystokinin mRNA, using in situ hybridization histochemistry and retrograde labeling. *Mol Brain Res* 1988;4:179–189.
10. Chang RSL, Lotti VJ. Biochemical and pharmacological characterization of an extremely potent and selective nonpeptide cholecystokinin antagonist. *Proc Natl Acad Sci USA* 1986;83:4923–4926.
11. Chang RSL, Lotti VJ, Monaghan RL, et al. A potent nonpeptide cholecystokinin antagonist selective for peripheral tissues isolated from aspergillus alliaceus. *Science* 1985;230:177–180.
12. Crawley JH. Subtype-selective cholecystokinin receptor antagonists block cholecystokinin modulation of dopamine-mediated behaviors in the rat mesolimbic pathway. *J Neurosci* 1992;12:3380–3391.
13. deMontigny C. Cholecystokinin tetrapeptide induces panic-like attacks in healthy volunteers. *Arch Gen Psychiatry* 1989;46:511–517.
14. Deschenes RJ, Haun RS, Funckes CL, Dixon JE. A gene encoding rat cholecystokinin. *J Biol Chem* 1985;260:1280–1286.
15. Deschenes RJ, Lorenz LJ, Haun RS, Roos BA, Collier KJ, Dixon JE. Cloning and sequence analysis of a cDNA encoding rat precholecysotokinin. *Proc Natl Acad Sci USA* 1984;81:726–730.
16. Deschodt-Lanckman M, Strosberg AD. In vitro degradation of the c-terminal octapeptide of cholecystokinin by "enkephalinase A". *FEBS Lett* 1983;152:109–113.
17. Dockray GJ, Gregory RA, Hutchinson JB. Isolation, structure, and biological activity of two cholecystokinin octapeptides from sheep brain. *Nature* 1978;264:568–570.
18. Eberlein GA, Eysseling VE, Davis MT, et al. Patterns of prohormone processing. Order revealed by a new procholecystokinin derived peptide. *J Biol Chem* 1992;267:1517–1521.
19. Faris PL, Komisaruk BR, Watkins LR, Meyer DJ. Evidence for the neuropeptide cholecystokinin as an antagonist of opiate analgesia. *Science* 1983;219:310–312.
20. Flood JF, Smith GF, Morley JE. Modulation of memory processing by cholecsytokinin: dependence on the vagus nerve. *Science* 1987;236:832–834.
21. Gibbs J, Young RC, Smith GP. Cholecystokinin decreases food intake in rats. *J Comp Physiol Psychol* 1973;84:488–495.
22. Gysling K, Allard LR, Beinfeld MC. Lithium preincubation stimulates the potassium-induced release of cholecystokinin from slices of cerebral cortex and caudato-putamen incubated in vitro. *Brain Res* 1987;413:365–367.
23. Gysling K, Beinfeld MC. The regulation of cholecystokinin release from rat caudato-putamen in vitro. *Brain Res* 1987;407:110–116.
24. Handelmann G, Beinfeld MC, O'Donohue TL, Nelson JB, Brenneman DE. Extra-hippocampal projections of CCK neurons of the hippocampus and subiculum. *Peptides* 1983;4:331–334.
25. Herbert H, Saper CB. Cholecystokinin-, galanin-, and corticotropin-releasing factor-like immunoreactive projections from the nucleus of the solitary tract to the parabrachial nucleus in the rat. *J Comp Neurol* 1990;293:581–598.
26. Hokfelt T, Rehfeld JF, Skirboll L, Ivemark B, Goldstein M, Markey K. Evidence for coexistence of dopamine and CCK in mesolimbic neurons. *Nature* 1980;285:474–478.
27. Hughes J, Boden P, Costall B, et al. Development of a class of selective cholecystokinin type B receptor antagonists having potent anxiolytic activity. *Proc Natl Acad Sci USA* 1990;87:6728–6732.
28. Jurna I, Zetler G. Antinociceptive effects of centrally administered caerulein and cholecystokinin (CCK). *Eur J Pharmacol* 1981;73:323–331.
29. Kopin AS, Lee Y-M, McBride EW, et al. Expression cloning and characterization of the canine parietal cell gastrin receptor. *Proc Natl Acad Sci USA* 1992;89:3605–3609.
30. Lapps W, Eng J, Stern AS, Gubler U. Expression of porcine cholecystokinin cDNA in a murine neuroendocrine cell line. Proteolytic processing, sulfation, and regulated secretion of cholecystokinin peptides. *J Biol Chem* 1988;263:13456.
31. Liddle RA, Goldfine ID, Williams JA. Bioassay of plasma cholecystokinin in rats: effects of food, trypsin inhibitor and alcohol. *Gastroenterology* 1984;87:542–549.
32. Lund T, Geurts van Kessel AHM, Haun RS, Dixon JE. The genes for human gastrin and cholecystokinin are located on different chromosomes. *Hum Genet* 1986;73:77–80.
33. Marshall FH, Barnes S, Hughes J, Woodruff GN, Hunter JC. Cholecsytokinin modulates the release of dopamine from the anterior and posterior nucleus accumbens by two different mechanisms. *J Neurochem* 1991;56:917–922.
34. McDermott JR, Dodd PR, Edwardson JA, Hardy JA, Smith AI. Pathway of inactivation of cholecystokinin (CCK-8) by synaptosomal fractions. *Neurochem Int* 1983;5:641–647.
35. Meek JL, Iadarola MJ, Giorgi O. Cholecystokinin turnover in brain. *Brain Res* 1983;276:375–378.
36. Meyer DK, Beinfeld MC, Brownstein MJ. Origin of cholecystokinin containin fibers in the rat caudatoputamen. *Science* 1982;215:187–188.
37. Mezey E, Reisine TD, Skirboll LR, Beinfeld MC, Kiss JZ. Role of cholecystokinin in corticotropin release: Coexistence with vasopressin and corticotropin-releasing factor in cells of the rat hypothalamic paraventricular nucleus. *Proc Natl Acad Sci USA* 1986;83:3510–3512.
38. Miyoshi R, Kito S, Nomoto T. Cholecystokinin increases intracellular calcium concentration in cultured striatal neurons. *Neuropeptides* 1991;18:115–119.
39. Mutt V, Jorpes JE. Structure of porcine cholecystokinin pancreozymin I. Cleavage with thrombin and with trypsin. *Eur J Biochem* 1968;6:156–162.
40. Niehrs C, Huttner WB. Purification and characterization of tyrosylprotein sulfotransferase. *EMBO J* 1990;9:35.
41. Ondetti MA, Pluscec J, Sabo EF, Sheehan JT, Williams N. Synthesis of cholecystokinin-pancreozymin. I. The c-terminal dodecapeptide. *J Am Chem Soc* 1970;92:195–199.
42. Palkovits M, Kiss JZ, Beinfeld MC, Brownstein MJ. Cholecystokinin in the hypothalamus–hypophyseal system. *Brain Res* 1984;299:186–189.
43. Penke B, Nyerges L. Solid-phase synthesis of porcine cholecystokinin-33 in a new resin via FMOC—strategy. *Pept Res* 1991;4:289–295.

44. Presti M, Gardner JD. Receptor antagonists for gastrointestinal peptides. *Am J Physiol* 1993;264:G399–G406.
45. Rasmussen K, Stockton ME, Czachura JF, Howbert JJ. Cholecystokinin (CCK) and schizophrenia: the selective CCK b antagonist LY262691 decreases midbrain dopamine unit activity. *Eur J Pharmacol* 1991;209:135–138.
46. Rehfeld JF, Hansen HF. Characterization of precholecystokinin products in the porcine cerebral cortex. *J Biol Chem* 1986; 261:5832–5840.
47. Rose C, Camus A, Schwartz JC. Protection by serine peptidase inhibitors of endogenous cholecystokinin released from brain slices. *Neuroscience* 1989;29:583–594.
48. Schiffmann SN, Teugels E, Halleux P, Menu R, Vanderhaeghen J-J. Cholecystokinin mRNA detection in rat spinal cord motoneurons but not in dorsal root ganglia neurons. *Neurosci Lett* 1991;123:123–126.
49. Silver AJ, Morley JE. Role of CCK in regulation of food intake. *Prog Neurobiol* 1991;36:23–34.
50. Smith GP, Jerome C, Cushin BJ, Eterno R, Simansky KJ. Abdominal vagotomy blocks the satiety effect of cholecystokinin in the rat. *Science* 1981;213:1036–1037.
51. Stark HA, Sharp CA, Sutliff VE, Martinez J, Jensen RT, Gardner JD. CCK-JMV-180: a peptide that distinguishes high affinity cholecystokinin receptors from low-affinity cholecystokinin receptors. *Biochim Biophys Acta* 1989;1010:145–150.
52. Steiner DF, Smeekens SP, Ohagi S, Chan SJ. The new enzymology of precursor processing endoproteases. *J Biol Chem* 1992; 267:23435–23438.
53. Vanderhaeghen JJ, Signeau JC, Gepts LO. New peptide in the vertebrate CNS reacting with gastrin antibodies. *Nature* 1975;257:604–605.
54. Vickroy TW, Bianchi BR, Kerwin JF, Kopecka H, Nadzan AM. Evidence that type A CCK receptors facilitate dopamine efflux in rat brain. *Eur J Pharmacol* 1988;152:371–372.
55. Viereck JC, Beinfeld MC. Purification and characterization of an endoprotease from rat brain synaptosomes which generates CCK 8 from CCK 33. *J Biol Chem* 1992;267:19475–19481.
56. Wank SA, Harkins R, Jensen RT, Shapira H, DeWeerth A, Slattery T. Purification, molecular cloning, and functional expression of the cholecystokinin receptor from rat pancreas. *Proc Natl Acad Sci USA* 1992;89:3125–3129.
57. Wierteleak EP, Maier SF, Watkins LR. Cholecystokinin antianalgesia: safety cues abolish morphine analgesia. *Science* 1992;256:830–833.
58. Zaborsky L, Alheid GF, Beinfeld MC, Eiden LE, Heimer L, Palkovits M. Cholecystokinin innervation of the ventral striatum: a morphological and radioimmunological study. *Neuroscience J* 1985; 14:427–453.
59. Zaborsky L, Beinfeld MC, Palkovits M, Heimer L. Brainstem projection to the hypothalamic ventromedial nucleus in the rat: CCK-containing long ascending pathway. *Brain Res* 1984;303:225–232.

Psychopharmacology: The Fourth Generation of Progress, edited by Floyd E. Bloom and David J. Kupfer. Raven Press, Ltd., New York 1995.

CHAPTER 53

Arachidonic Acid

Daniele Piomelli

A TALE OF TWO ROLES

When a neurotransmitter binds to its receptor on the membrane of a target neuron, it triggers the formation of second messengers, responsible for translating receptor occupation into cellular responses. For example, the binding of dopamine to D_1-type receptors stimulates the activity of adenylyl cyclase, which catalyzes the conversion of ATP into cyclic AMP. This second messenger, in turn, binds to and activates a specific protein kinase, protein kinase A, which puts inorganic phosphate on select intracellular proteins. Phosphorylation modifies the biological activity of these proteins and constitutes the basis for many physiological effects of dopamine in the central nervous system (CNS) (see Chapters 11 and 27, *this volume*).

This model of transmembrane signaling assumes that the range of action of a second messenger is confined to the intracellular environment. In agreement with this view, most "classical" signaling systems—cyclic AMP, cyclic GMP, Ca^{2+}, inositol trisphosphate, and diacylglycerol—produce their effects by binding to protein receptors located within the cell, whether they be protein kinases, protein phosphatases, Ca^{2+}-binding proteins, or ion channels. Such a model is not likely to account, however, for all known transduction pathways. Examples of more complex scenarios include the arachidonic acid cascade, examined in the present chapter, and nitric oxide, outlined in Chapter 54 (*this volume*).

A schematic picture of the ways in which arachidonic acid and its metabolites may act in regulating neuronal activity is shown in Fig. 1. Arachidonic acid is released from phospholipids in cells stimulated by many first messengers, including neurotransmitters, neuromodulators, and neurohormones. The free fatty acid has, as such, a short lifespan, during which it may interact with and affect the activity of ion channels and protein kinases within the cell. Alternatively, it may be transformed to a family of metabolites—the eicosanoids—which may also produce important effects on intracellular targets. In both cases, the arachidonic acid cascade affects neuronal excitability by fulfilling the primary criteria defining a second messenger system—that is, receptor-dependent formation and intracellular site of action.

Where the eicosanoids differ from "classical" second messengers is in their ability to cross the cell membrane, diffuse through the extracellular space, and interact with high-affinity receptors located on neighboring neurons (Fig. 1). Eicosanoid receptors have been characterized in the brain and have been shown to be linked to second messengers, such as cyclic AMP, very much like the receptors recognized by dopamine, noradrenaline, and so on. Therefore, thanks to the ability to branch at the same time within and without a cell, the arachidonic acid cascade may give rise both to intracellular second messengers and to local mediators, bridging the gap between transmembrane and transcellular communication. This two-pronged role may be important in integrating the responses of postsynaptic neurons with the activity of presynaptic terminals and of other contacting cells.

AN OVERVIEW OF THE ARACHIDONIC ACID CASCADE

In resting cells, arachidonic acid is stored within the cell membrane, esterified to glycerol in phospholipids (Fig. 2). A receptor-dependent event, requiring a transducing G protein, initiates phospholipid hydrolysis and releases the fatty acid into the intracellular medium. Three

D. Piomelli: Unité de Neurobiologie et Pharmacologie, Institut National de la Santé et Recherche Médicale, Paris 75014, France.

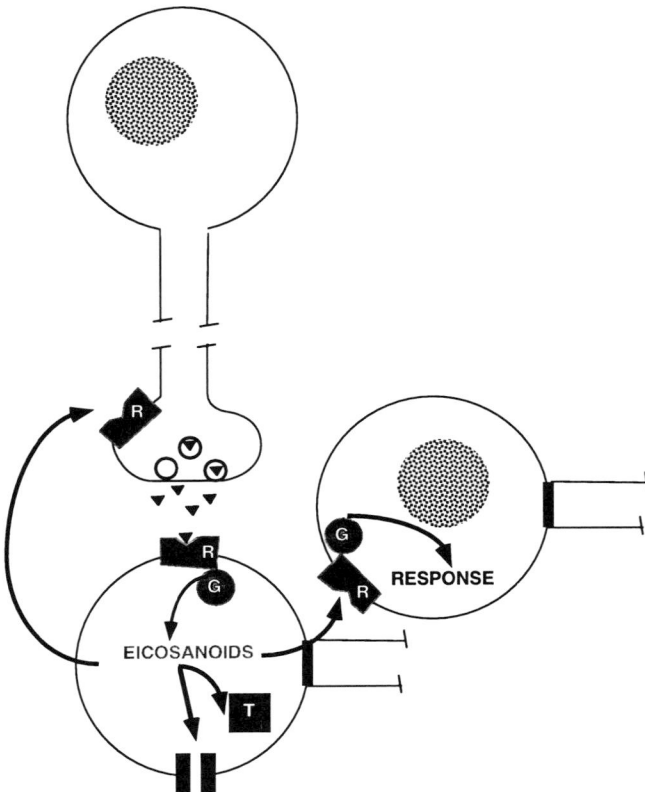

FIG. 1. Possible mechanisms of action of arachidonic acid and its metabolites (eicosanoids) in regulating neuronal activity. For a detailed description, see text. On the postsynaptic cell at bottom, the intracellular formation of eicosanoids can consequently act on a target enzyme (T) such as protein kinase C, or on ion channels.

enzymes may mediate this deacylation reaction: phospholipase A₂ (PLA₂), phospholipase C (PLC), and phospholipase D (PLD), whose different sites of attack on the phospholipid backbone are shown in Fig. 2 (inset). PLA_2 catalyzes the hydrolysis of phospholipids at the sn (stereospecific numbering)-2 position. Therefore, this enzyme can release arachidonate in a single-step reaction. By contrast, PLC and PLD do not release free arachidonic acid directly. Rather, they generate lipid products containing arachidonate (diacylglycerol and phosphatidic acid, respectively), which can be released subsequently by diacylglycerol- and monoacylglycerol-lipases (Fig. 2).

Once released, free arachidonate has three possible fates: reincorporation into phospholipids, diffusion outside the cell, and metabolism. Metabolism is carried out by three distinct enzyme pathways expressed in neural cells: cyclooxygenase, lipoxygenases, and cytochrome P_{450}. Several products of these pathways act within neurons to modulate the activities of ion channels, protein kinases, ion pumps, and neurotransmitter uptake systems. The newly formed eicosanoids may also exit the cell of

origin and act at a distance, by binding to G-protein-coupled receptors present on nearby neurons or glial cells. Finally, the actions of the eicosanoids may be terminated by diffusion, uptake into phospholipids, or enzymatic degradation.

HOW IS ARACHIDONIC ACID PROVIDED TO NEURONS?

Neurons can take up preformed arachidonic acid, but they cannot synthesize it ex novo, as other cells do, by elongation and desaturation of dietary linoleic acid. Yet, neuronal lipids are highly enriched in arachidonate, raising the question as to how does the fatty acid get there. The liver is a major source, via the circulation, but two types of cells in the CNS appear also to play an important role: cerebral endothelium and astrocytes. These cells accumulate circulating linoleate, use it to synthesize arachidonic acid, and secrete the latter into the interstitial medium, making it available to neurons (45,46).

FREE ARACHIDONIC ACID IS RAPIDLY STORED IN NEURONAL PHOSPHOLIPIDS

Neurons take up free arachidonic acid and store it rapidly by esterifying it to membrane phospholipids (10,26). As a result, only trace levels of free arachidonate may be found in resting cells. Such tight control, justified both by the signaling role of this lipid and by its potential toxicity, is exerted by two concerted enzymatic activities, arachidonoyl-coenzyme A (CoA) synthetase and arachidonoyl-CoA:lysophospholipid transferase (note that a lysophospholipid lacks one of the two phospholipid acyl chains).

Arachidonoyl-CoA synthetase catalyzes the ATP- and Mg^{2+}-dependent formation of arachidonoyl-CoA, using fatty acid and reduced CoA as substrates (35,48,83,88). Next, the activated fatty acid is incorporated into lysophospholipid by arachidonoyl-CoA:lysophospholipid transferase (11). After ultracentrifugation of brain extracts, both enzymes are found in the particulate fraction, and indirect evidence suggests that they may be organized in a multienzyme complex on the intracellular aspect of the neuronal membrane (77).

ARACHIDONIC ACID IS RELEASED FROM PHOSPHOLIPIDS BY RECEPTOR STIMULATION

Several neuromodulators stimulate the deacylation of phospholipids, causing release of free arachidonate. These include excitatory amino acids (such as glutamate), biogenic amines (such as serotonin and histamine), and pep-

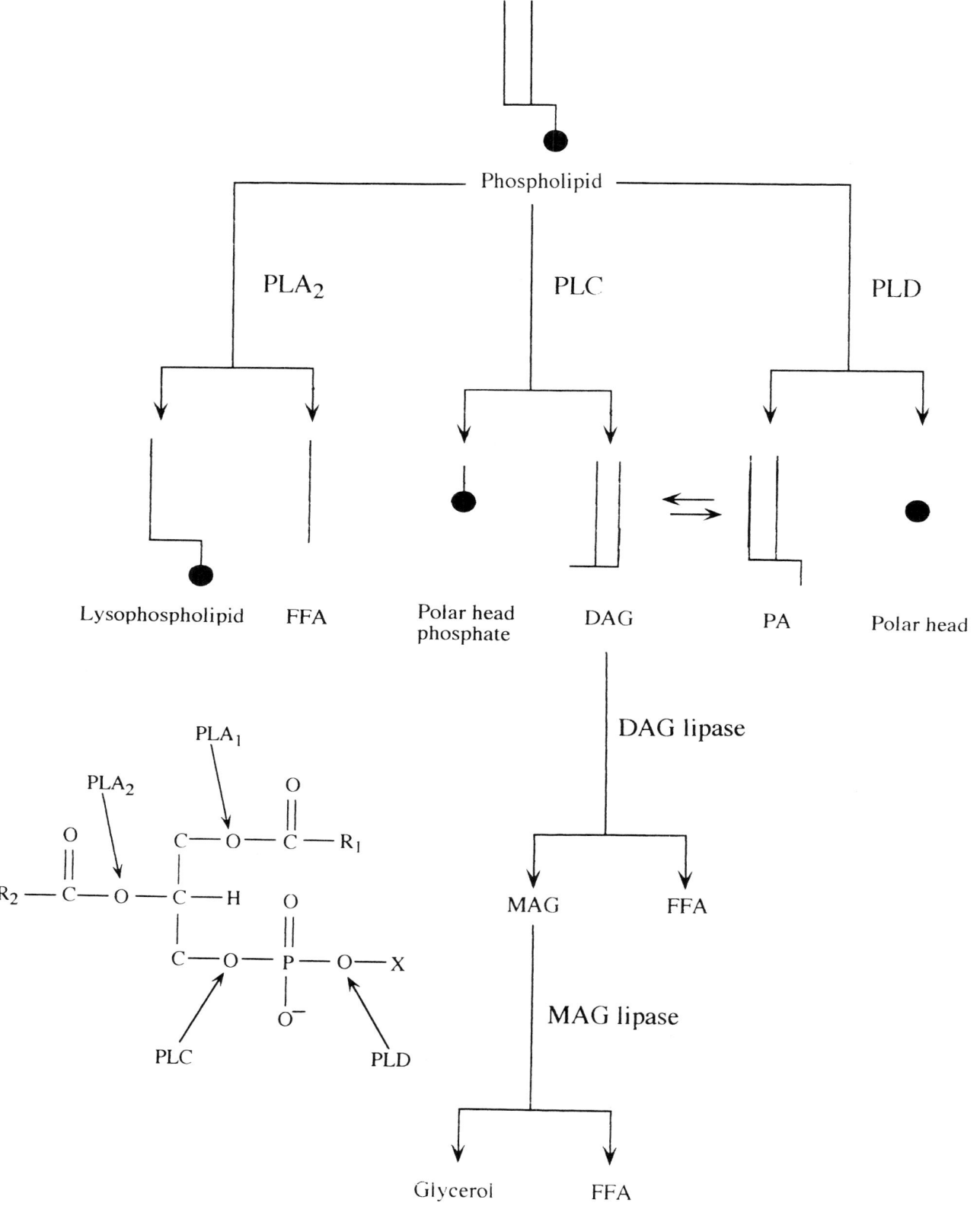

FIG. 2. Pathways of arachidonic acid release. DAG, diacylglycerol; FFA, free fatty acids; MAG, mono-acylglycerol; PA, phosphatidic acid; PL, phospholipase.

tides (such as bradykinin) (1,14,17,30,36,57–60). Even though the final effect of these various substances on arachidonate turnover is similar, they may use different mechanisms to achieve it. As we have seen above, at least three distinct phospholipases are thought to generate free arachidonic acid, either directly or indirectly: PLA_2, PLC, and PLD. Recent studies have shown that all of them may be activated by neurotransmitters.

Julius Axelrod and his colleagues at the National Institutes of Health have used primary cultures of hippocampal neurons to study the effect of serotonin on arachidonic acid release (17). They labeled neuronal phospholipids by prolonged incubation with [^{3}H]arachidonic acid, and then exposed the neurons to serotonin or to drugs acting at select serotonin (5-HT) receptors. They discovered that stimulating the 5-HT_2 receptor, a subtype known to be linked to transducing G proteins, resulted in the accumulation of unesterified radioactive fatty acid. Which phospholipase activity mediated this effect? To answer this question, Axelrod and his colleagues examined the ability of serotonin to stimulate the formation of lysophosphatidylcholine, which (as shown in Fig. 2) is produced selectively by PLA_2 activity, but not by PLC or PLD. Using a radiolabeled precursor, they found that the quantity of radioactive lysophospholipid in the membrane was increased by serotonin, strongly arguing for a participation of PLA_2 in the response (17). These results, and those obtained in several other laboratories using different experimental preparations (30,64), support the idea that PLA_2 may play a widespread role in receptor-dependent release of arachidonic acid. Despite these progresses, important information on the mechanism of activation of PLA_2 in neurons is still lacking. For example, most researchers believe that a G protein ensures the coupling of receptors with PLA_2. This convinction is based on the ability of pertussis toxin (a *Bordetella* toxin which inactivates two families of G proteins, G_i and G_o) to prevent receptor-stimulated arachidonate release, as well as on the ability of nonhydrolyzable GTP analogues to evoke it (7). The precise identity of the G protein(s) involved remains, however, unknown, because the existing pharmacological tools do not allow us to discriminate among the various members of the G_i and G_o families. Likewise, recent findings indicate that multiple PLA_2s may be expressed in neurons and in other cells (8,12,82,92). Do these different isoforms couple selectively to different receptors? Or rather, do they serve distinct functions? And if so, which functions? Answering these questions will require the development of new classes of PLA_2 inhibitors, more specific and more potent than those available at present. We have seen above that—in addition to PLA_2—arachidonic acid release may also proceed from the sequential activation of PLC, diacylglycerol-lipase and monoacylglycerol-lipase. The reactions carried out by these enzymes, which were discovered in the labora-

tory of Philip Majerus (5), are shown in Fig. 2: PLC cleaves the polar heads of phospholipids, thereby forming diacylglycerol, which is then hydrolyzed to glycerol and free fatty acids by diacylglycerol- and monoacylglycerollipases (16). Recently, Pierre Morell and colleagues, at the University of North Carolina, were able to show that, in primary cultures of sensory neurons, bradykinin may evoke arachidonic acid release by activating selectively this enzyme pathway. Neurons obtained from the spinal cord of embryonic rats were labeled by incubation with various radioactive lipid precursors and were exposed to bradykinin. Application of the neuroactive peptide raised the levels of unesterified arachidonate, but had no effect on lysophospholipids, arguing against an involvement of PLA_2. By contrast, appearance of the free fatty acid was preceded by a transient increase in diacylglycerol content, likely caused by PLC activation, which took place within a few seconds of exposure to bradykinin. In addition, arachidonate release could be prevented by an inhibitor of diacylglycerol lipase, the compound RG 80267 (1).

In contrast with PLA_2 and PLC, participation of PLD in receptor-dependent arachidonic acid release has not been demonstrated yet. However, one of the products of its activity, phosphatidic acid (the other is a phospholipid head-group, such as choline or inositol), is dephosphorylated to diacylglycerol, which, as we have seen, enters the diacylglycerol-lipase pathway yielding free arachidonate (Fig. 2) (15). In addition, the ability of some neurotransmitters to stimulate PLD activity adds further support to the possibility that this lipase may participate in receptor-mediated arachidonate release (15).

SOME NEUROTRANSMITTER RECEPTORS INHIBIT ARACHIDONIC ACID RELEASE

Nonhydrolyzable GTP analogues, such as GTP-γ-S, have been very useful to determine the role of G proteins in transmembrane transduction. As a rule, their ability to produce a certain response is taken as good evidence for the presence of a G-protein-mediated coupling mechanism. By using GTP analogues, Carol Jelsema and Julius Axelrod have provided the first evidence of an inhibitory control by G proteins over the activity of PLA_2. While studying signaling events in retinal photoreceptors, they observed that flashing light on dark-adapted rod outer segments (ROS) enhanced PLA_2 activity. However, when the ROS were exposed to light after incubation with GTP-γ-S, this increase was significantly smaller. They concluded that an unidentified G protein, which could be activated by the GTP analogue, exerted an inhibitory action on the activity of retinal PLA_2 when this enzyme was stimulated by light (27,28).

Do neurotransmitter receptors link to inhibition of arachidonate release? Experiments carried out on a heterologous expression system, in the laboratory of Jean-Charles Schwartz in Paris, suggest this possibility (78). Chinese hamster ovary (CHO) cells were transfected with a plasmid vector directing expression of histamine H_2-type receptor, which is known to be positively coupled to adenylyl cyclase via a G_s protein. CHO cells were no exception to this rule, and the transfected receptor was found to be very effective in evoking cyclic AMP formation when stimulated with an H_2 agonist. Unexpectedly, in addition to this response, H_2-receptor occupation was also found to reduce the release of arachidonic acid evoked by raising intracellular Ca^{2+} levels (a stimulus for PLA_2). The mechanism underlying this effect has been only partially uncovered, but the evidence collected allows us to draw a few conclusions. First, inhibition of arachidonate release was independent of the rises in cAMP produced by stimulating the H_2 receptor, because membrane-permeant cAMP analogues did not mimic the response. Second, inhibition was not secondary to a reduction in Ca^{2+} entry, because H_2-receptor stimulation had no effect on either basal or stimulated Ca^{2+} levels. The results, therefore, support the possibility that transfected H_2 receptors in CHO cells are directly coupled to inhibition of PLA_2 activity (78). It remains to be determined whether a similar response occurs in neurons or in other cells expressing this receptor constitutively.

A THIRD GROUP OF RECEPTORS FACILITATES ARACHIDONIC ACID RELEASE, BUT DOES NOT STIMULATE IT DIRECTLY

Several structurally different neurotransmitter receptors—including D_2-dopaminergic and α_2-adrenergic— share the ability to reduce adenylyl cyclase activity and to lower cAMP levels in cells, through the intermediate of an "inhibitory" G protein (G_i). When transfected in CHO cells, receptors of this group produce, in addition, what appears to be a "silent" facilitation of arachidonic acid release. Namely, receptor activation has no effect, per se, on arachidonate release, but, if release is triggered by a second agent—for example, by stimulation of a different receptor or by a Ca^{2+} ionophore—it will greatly potentiate it (18,63). This novel form of regulation involves, like adenylyl cyclase inhibition, a G_i protein, as shown by the ability of pertussis toxin to inhibit the response, and of GTP-γ-S to mimic it (63).

ARACHIDONIC ACID METABOLISM IN THE BRAIN

The three pathways of arachidonic acid metabolism discovered in most animal tissues—lipoxygenases,

cyclooxygenase, and cytochrome P_{450}—have been also described in brain (Fig. 3).

LIPOXYGENASES

Lipoxygenases are a family of enzymes which catalyze the oxygenation of arachidonic acid, each lipoxygenase forming a distinct hydroperoxy-eicosatetraenoic acid (HPETE) (90). HPETEs may undergo a series of metabolic transformations—what is referred to as a *lipoxygenase pathway*. Here, we will focus our attention on the two lipoxygenases whose presence in the CNS has been best characterized: 12- and 5-lipoxygenase (Fig. 3). 12-Lipoxygenase converts arachidonic acid into 12(S)-HPETE (containing a -OOH group on the chiral carbon 12), which may be further metabolized into four distinct products: an alcohol [12(S)-hydroxy-eicosatetraenoic acid, 12(S)-HETE], a ketone (12-keto-eicosatetraenoic acid, 12-KETE), or two epoxy alcohols (hepoxilin A_3 and B_3) (54,55,60,61).

The sequence of reactions initiated by 5-lipoxygenase is more complex. To become active, 5-lipoxygenase requires three cofactors: Ca^{2+}, ATP, and an integral membrane protein called *five lipoxygenase-activating protein* (FLAP). Inactive 5-lipoxygenase binds Ca^{2+} and ATP and translocates onto the membrane, where it anchors to FLAP. Membrane translocation activates 5-lipoxygenase, which carries out two sequential reactions: First, it converts arachidonic acid into 5(S)-HPETE; second, it dehydrates 5(S)-HPETE to yield the epoxide, leukotriene A_4 (LTA_4). The newly formed leukotriene leaves the active site of 5-lipoxygenase but, being itself quite short-lived, is rapidly metabolized to form, by hydrolysis, LTB_4 (via an LTA_4-hydrolase) or, by addition of glutathione, LTC_4 (via a glutathione-S-transferase) (68).

Brain 12-lipoxygenase was purified, and a complementary DNA encoding it was cloned (51,86). Immunohistochemical studies revealed the occurrence of this enzyme in neurons (particularly in hippocampus, striatum, and olivary nucleus), as well as in glial and in cerebral endothelial cells (50). In agreement with these findings, 12-lipoxygenase metabolites are among the most abundant eicosanoids produced by nervous tissue, as first shown by Lidia Sautebin and co-workers, at the University of Milan (69).

5-Lipoxygenase activity in the CNS was demonstrated by Samuelsson and his colleagues at the Karolinska Institut in Stockholm and was confirmed by further studies (32,39,68,75). Even though several of the products formed have been identified (notably, LTC_4 and LTB_4), little is known on the distribution in the CNS of 5-lipoxygenase, FLAP, and glutathione-S-transferase. The laboratory of Takao Shimizu in Tokyo has shown that LTA_4-hydrolase is expressed in virtually all regions of the brain,

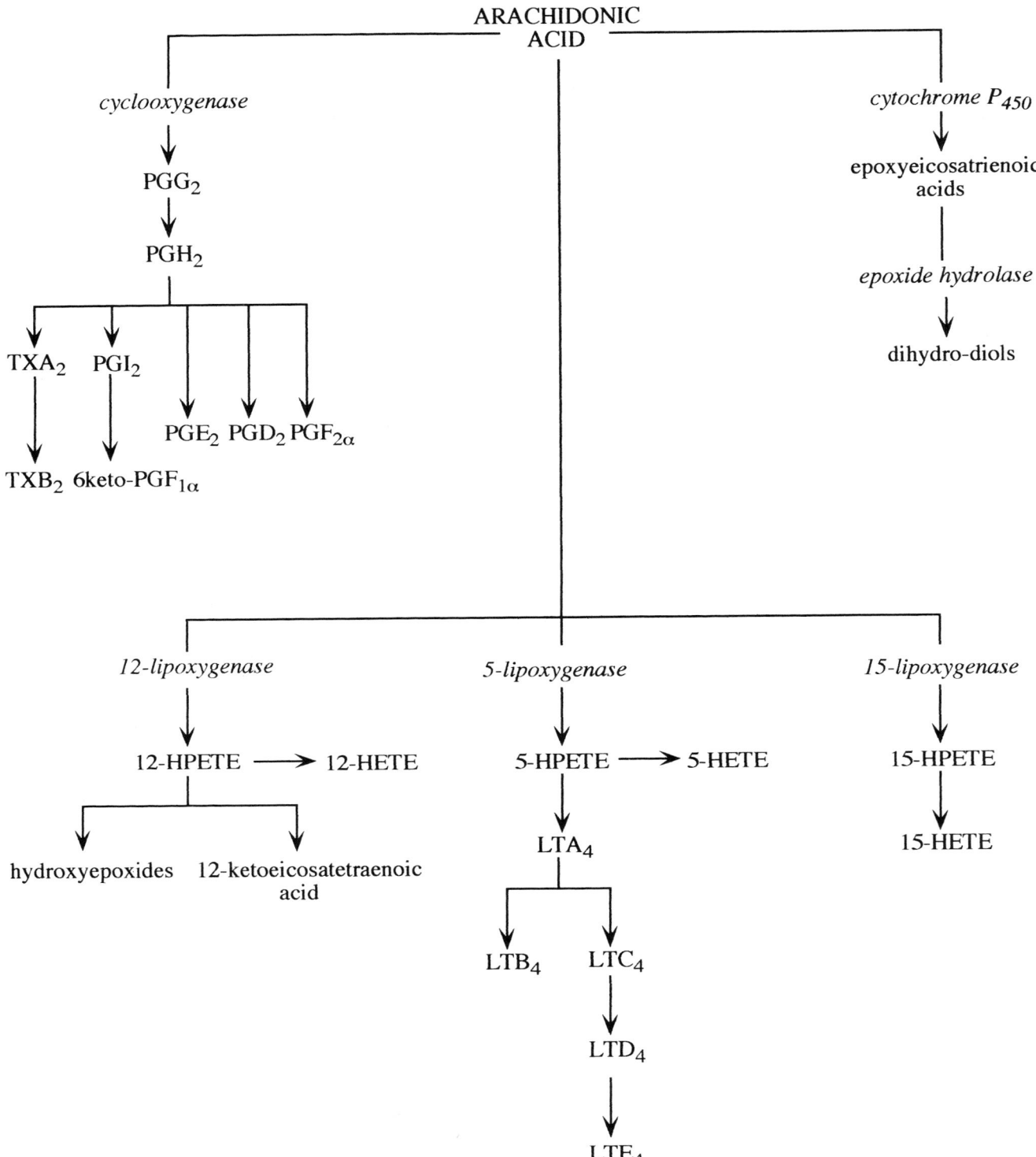

FIG. 3. Pathways of arachidonic acid metabolism. H(P)ETE, hydro(per)oxy-eicosatetraenoic acid; LT, leukotriene; PG, prostaglandin; TX, thromboxane.

suggesting that—in addition to converting LTA_4 into LTB_4—this enzyme may serve more general functions, possibly unrelated to arachidonic acid metabolism (75).

CYCLOOXYGENASE

Cyclooxygenase (prostaglandin G/H synthase) cata-lyzes the stepwise conversion of arachidonic acid into two short-lived intermediates, prostaglandin G (PGG) and prostaglandin (PGH). The latter is metabolized to PGs, prostacyclin (PGI_2), and thromboxane A_2 (TXA_2) by the activity of specific enzymes: prostaglandin isomerases for the various PGs, prostacyclin synthase for PGI_2, and thromboxane synthase for TXA_2 (Fig. 3).

Since the pioneering work of Bengt Samuelsson (at the Karolinska Institut) and Leonard Wolfe (at the Hospital for Sick Children in Toronto), three most prominent cyclooxygenase products have been identified in nervous tissue ($PGF_{2\alpha}$, PGD_2, and PGE_2), and the enzymes in-volved in their biosynthesis have been purified and char-acterized (22,31,52,79,89). Immunohistochemical stud-ies, carried out primarily by Osamu Hayaishi and his colleagues (80) have established the presence of these enzymes in both neurons and glia. These studies have been supported by experiments demonstrating that pri-mary cultures enriched in either neurons or glial cells have the ability to synthesize prostaglandins (72,81).

CYTOCHROME P_{450}

Cytochrome P_{450}, the microsomal enzyme complex par-ticipating in drug metabolism, may also act on endoge-nous arachidonic acid, catalyzing its conversion into epoxy-eicosatrienoic acids (EETs). The epoxide ring of these EETs may be cleaved by the action of epoxide hydrolases, to yield the corresponding vicinal diols. In addition, cytochrome P_{450} has been shown to produce a family of HETEs by hydroxylation (monooxygenation) of arachidonic acid (Fig. 3) (41).

Even though mammalian brain tissue contains very low levels of cytochrome P_{450}, several isoforms of this enzyme were detected in both neural and glial cells by immunohis-tochemistry, and biosynthesis of arachidonate metabolites via the cytochrome P_{450} pathway has been reported (2,29,84).

ANANDAMIDE, AN ENDOGENOUS CANNABINOID SUBSTANCE

A novel arachidonic acid derivative was recently iso-lated from brain and was identified as the ethanolamide of arachidonic acid (Fig. 4). This compound was shown to (a) inhibit the specific binding of a radiolabeled agonist

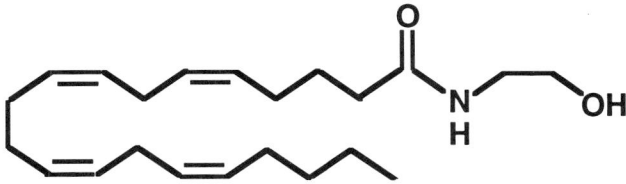

FIG. 4. Chemical structure of anandamide, a putative en-dogenous cannabinoid substance.

to the cannabinoid receptor and (b) produce inhibition of the twitch response in mouse vas deferens, a typical response to cannabinoids. These properties have led to the suggestion that arachidonoylethanolamide (dubbed "anandamide" after the sanskrit word for bliss, "an-anda") may act as the endogenous ligand for brain canna-binoid receptors (13). The pathways leading to the biosyn-thesis and the degradation of anandamide in the CNS are not known.

IN SEARCH OF A FUNCTION

The arachidonic acid cascade is arguably the most elab-orate signaling system neurobiologists have to deal with. Not only can it generate multiple messenger molecules (at least 16, according to a conservative estimate limited to the brain), but these molecules may act both within and without the neuron, bringing into play intracellular as well as extracellular targets. To help find our way in this complex network, it may be helpful, rather than list-ing all known neuronal actions of the eicosanoids, to discuss in greater depth a few examples representative of the roles of these lipids as either intracellular second messengers or transcellular mediators.

INTRACELLULAR SECOND MESSENGERS OF PRESYNAPTIC INHIBITION?

The potential role of arachidonic acid in mediating K^+ channel modulation and presynaptic inhibition of neuro-transmitter release—our first example of a second mes-senger role for the eicosanoids—was first suggested by experiments carried out in the laboratory of James Schwartz at Columbia University, using the simple ner-vous system of the marine mollusk, *Aplysia californica*. *Aplysia* has large, easily identifiable and well-character-ized neurons, which can be dissected out individually and maintained in culture for several days. When these neurons were stimulated with the neurotransmitter, hista-mine, they released both 12- and 5-lipoxygenase products (58). Histamine is known to exert inhibitory actions on identified *Aplysia* neurons, causing membrane hyperpo-larization and reducing neurotransmitter release at specific synapses. This clue led to the idea that arachidonic acid metabolites may be involved in inhibitory responses, and it prompted the study of a neurotransmitter with better-defined electrophysiological effects. FMRF-amide, a neuroactive tetrapeptide, hyperpolarizes *Aplysia* sensory neurons and inhibits neurotransmitter release at sensory–motor synapses, by increasing the activity of a subclass of K^+ channels termed S-K^+ channels. To determine whether arachidonic acid metabolites participate in the effects of FMRF-amide, a series of biochemical, pharmacological, and electrophysiological experiments were carried out. First, application of FMRF-amide to sensory cells resulted in the formation of 12- and 5-lipoxygenase metabolites. Next, drugs that inhibit PLA_2 and lipoxygenase activities prevented the electrophysiological actions of FMRF-amide on sensory neurons, whereas cyclooxygenase inhibitors had no effect. Finally, applications of arachidonic acid or 12-HPETE mimicked the effects of FMRF-amide on both S-K^+ channels and transmitter release. By contrast, 12-HETE, 5-HPETE and 5-HETE had no effect (59).

In subsequent studies, it was shown that the actions of 12-HPETE on S-K^+ channel activity required metabolism of the hydroperoxyacid via an enzymatic activity sensitive to cytochrome P_{450} inhibitors (4). The results support the possibility that a 12-lipoxygenase metabolite, possibly a hepoxilin, acts as a second messenger in mediating the effects of FMRF-amide on K^+ channels and neurotransmitter release (Fig. 5).

FMRF-amide is a modulatory neurotransmitter, and its effects on K^+ channels occur within seconds of its application and last as long as the application lasts. Repeated administrations of FMRF-amide may result, however, in long-term changes in neuronal excitability. Samuel Schacher and his colleagues at Columbia University found that prolonged exposure of *Aplysia* sensory neurons to FMRF-amide (2 hr), produced a depression in synaptic transmission that lasted for several days and was accompanied by a significant reduction in the number of varicosities on sensory neuron dendrites. As with the short-term modulation discussed above, this form of long-term depression may be mediated by arachidonic acid. In agreement, the number of varicosities was significantly reduced 24 hr after a 2-hr application of arachidonic acid to sensory neurons. This effect is likely to involve gene expression and protein synthesis, because it could be prevented by protein synthesis inhibitors (43,44).

Actions of the eicosanoids similar to those described in *Aplysia* have also been found in mammalian brain. For example, 12-lipoxygenase products were shown to inhibit glutamate release from hippocampal mossy fiber nerve endings (19), whereas 5-lipoxygenase metabolites were found to increase the activity of muscarine-inactivated M-K^+ channels in rat hippocampal CA1 neurons (71). K^+ channel modulation by lipoxygenase products has also

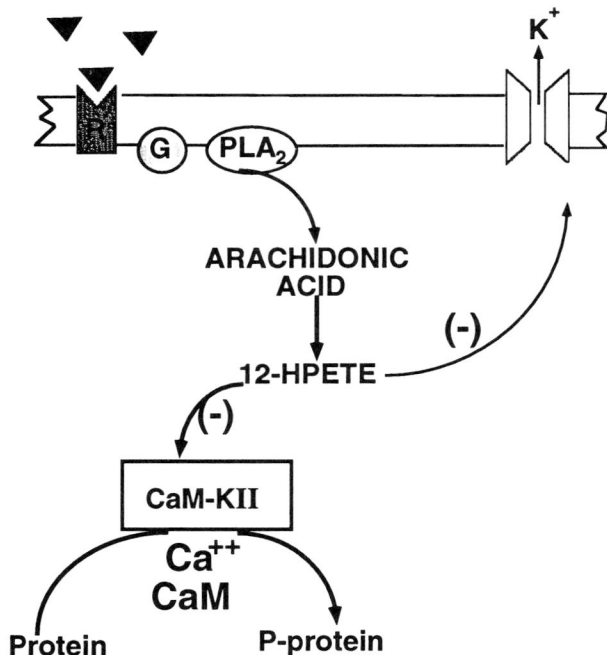

FIG. 5. Hypothetical mode of action of 12-lipoxygenase metabolites in producing presynaptic inhibition of neurotransmitter release. For a detailed description, see text. CaM, calmodulin; CaMKII, Ca^{2+}/calmodulin-dependent protein kinase II; G, G protein; 12-HPETE, 12-hydroperoxy-eicosatetraenoic acid; PLA_2, phospholipase A_2; P-protein, phosphoprotein.

been reported in a number of non-neural cells, including heart myocytes (33,34).

Phosphorylation of specific proteins in the presynaptic nerve terminal may participate, together with ion channel modulation, in regulating neurotransmitter release. The state of phosphorylation of the synaptic-vesicle-associated protein, synapsin I, is thought to regulate the availability of synaptic vesicles for exocytosis. In its dephosphorylated state, synapsin I may cross-link synaptic vesicles to the surrounding cytoskeletal lattice. According to this model, when synapsin I is phosphorylated on its "tail"-region by Ca^{2+}/calmodulin-dependent protein kinase II, its interaction both with synaptic vesicles and with cytoskeletal elements is reduced, resulting in dissociation of the vesicles from the cytoskeleton. This would, in turn, increase the number of vesicles available for exocytosis. Therefore, reducing the state of phosphorylation of synapsin I may be a way to reduce synaptic strength independent of, and possibly parallel to, ion channel modulation (see Chapter 5, *this volume*).

Arachidonic acid and its metabolites may regulate neurotransmitter release partly through such a phosphorylation-dependent mechanism. In agreement, experiments carried out in Paul Greengard's laboratory at the Rockefeller University showed that lipoxygenase-derived eicosanoids are potent and selective inhibitors of purified

Ca^{2+}/calmodulin-dependent protein kinase II. 12-HPETE inhibited activity of this protein kinase with a half-maximal effect at a concentration of 0.7 μM. By contrast, the eicosanoid has no effect on the activities of protein kinase C, cAMP-dependent protein kinase, Ca^{2+}/calmodulin-dependent protein kinase I and III, or the Ca^{2+}/calmodulin-activated phosphatase, calcineurin (62).

The effects of the eicosanoids on K^+ channels and on Ca^{2+}/calmodulin-dependent protein kinase II may be integrated in a model, shown in Fig. 5, for the role played by these lipids in presynaptic inhibition. Free arachidonic acid, produced as a result of receptor activation, is metabolized by 12-lipoxygenase to form 12-HPETE. The hydroperoxyacid may, on the one hand, modulate the activity of K^+ channels and, on the other, inhibit Ca^{2+}/calmodulin-dependent protein kinase II, reducing Ca^{2+}-evoked protein phosphorylation. These two parallel effects might be synergistic in decreasing synaptic strength.

ARACHIDONIC ACID, A SECOND MESSENGER ACTIVATOR OF PROTEIN KINASE C?

In addition to these actions mediated by the eicosanoids, arachidonic acid and other fatty acids may regulate neuronal excitability directly, by mechanisms that do not involve metabolism or intervention of other second messenger pathways. For example, fatty acids may modify the activity of a variety of ion channels, possibly by interacting with hydrophobic binding sites within the channel protein (like local anesthetic or antiarrhythmic drugs). The interested reader is referred to a recent review on this topic (53). In this section, I will examine instead an additional potential role of unsaturated fatty acids—that of second messengers in the receptor-dependent stimulation of protein kinase C (PKC) activity.

PKC, which was originally described as a Ca^{2+}- and phospholipid-dependent protein kinase activated by diacylglycerol, is now recognized to consist of a family of at several related isoenzymes with different properties and distribution in the brain. Nishizuka and his colleagues (47,73) have recently shown that low concentrations of unsaturated fatty acids (1–10 μM), which are likely to be attained in stimulated cells, activate with high selectivity a single PKC isoform, type I, in the absence of Ca^{2+} and phospholipid.

What is the physiological significance of this stimulation, and how does it relate to the well-characterized ability of diacylglycerol to activate PKC? To address these questions, David Linden and collaborators (in John Connor's laboratory at the Roche Institute) have carried out a series of electrophysiological experiments on primary cultures of rat cerebellar neurons (38). In rat cerebellum, type I and type II PKC are segregated: Type I is expressed in Purkinje cells, whereas type II is expressed in granule cells. The application of phorbol esters, which causes a nonselective stimulation of all PKC isoforms, reduced voltage-gated K^+ currents equally in both neurons. By contrast, the administration of unsaturated fatty acids affected K^+ currents selectively in Purkinje cells, not in granule cells. The findings suggest that, in neurons expressing type I PKC, activation of this protein kinase isoform may result from the receptor-dependent stimulation of PLA_2 activity and from the generation of free arachidonic acid (as well as other fatty acids) (38).

TRANS-SYNAPTIC ACTIONS OF THE EICOSANOIDS

The examples discussed thus far illustrate one possible role played by the eicosanoids—that of intracellular second messengers. We will examine now the alter ego of the arachidonic acid cascade: its ability to act as a transcellular (or trans-synaptic) signaling system.

Diffusible signals may exert important neurophysiological functions. Neurons in the CNS are organized as interconnected groups of functionally related cells (e.g., in sensory systems). A diffusible factor released from a neuron into the interstitial fluid, and able to interact with membrane receptors on adjacent cells, would be ideally used to "synchronize" the activity of an ensemble of interconnected neural cells. Furthermore, during development and in certain forms of learning, postsynaptic cells may secrete regulatory factors which diffuse back to the presynaptic component, determining its survival as an active terminal, the amplitude of its sprouting, and its efficacy in secreting neurotransmitters—a phenomenon known as *retrograde regulation*. The participation of arachidonic acid metabolites in retrograde signaling and in other forms of local modulation of neuronal activity has been proposed.

RETROGRADE MESSENGERS OF LONG-TERM POTENTIATION?

Long-term potentiation of synaptic transmission (LTP) is a mammalian model of synaptic plasticity and information storage. LTP is believed to consist of two phases: induction and maintenance. Induction is initiated by the postsynaptic entry of Ca^{2+}, which occurs through glutamate N-methyl-D-aspartate (NMDA)-type receptor channels. Maintenance appears to be produced at least partly by presynaptic mechanisms. To bridge postsynaptic induction with presynaptic maintenance, the existence of a diffusible retrograde messenger was proposed (6).

Arachidonic acid was suggested as a potential candidate for this role (59). In agreement, stimulation of glutamate receptors evokes arachidonic acid release from a variety of neural cell preparations (14,36). In addition, nonselective PLA$_2$ inhibitors (such as *p*-bromophenacyl-bromide) prevent induction of LTP, while application of arachidonic acid (or other unsaturated fatty acids) to hippocampal slices causes a slow-onset enhancement of synaptic transmission that resembles LTP (37,87). The mechanism of action of arachidonic acid in enhancing neurotransmission remains to be established, and several potential targets have been proposed. The fatty acid may increase glutamate release from hippocampal nerve terminals, block glutamate uptake, or potentiate NMDA receptor current (41,93). Alternatively, it may act by enabling presynaptic glutamate receptors to produce enhanced glutamate release (25).

RETROGRADE MESSENGERS AT THE DEVELOPING SYNAPSE?

Orna Harish and Mu-Ming Poo at Columbia University have provided evidence suggesting that a 5-lipoxygenase metabolite of arachidonic acid may act as a retrograde messenger at the developing neuromuscular synapse (21) (Fig. 6). Using primary cultures of innervated muscle cells from *Xenopus,* they found that injections of GTP-γ-S into the myocyte caused an increase in the frequency of spontaneous synaptic currents (SSCs), an indication that acetylcholine release from presynaptic terminals was enhanced. They concluded that a G-protein-driven signal was released from the muscle cell, crossed the synaptic cleft, and acted on the presynaptic neuron to modulate transmitter secretion. To determine the nature of this diffusible signal, they injected drugs that activate cAMP-dependent protein kinase or PKC, but found no effect. However, when they loaded arachidonic acid into the myocyte, a significant increase in SSC frequency occurred, an effect which could be prevented by the selective 5-lipoxygenase inhibitor, AA861. In agreement with an involvement of 5-lipoxygenase-mediated metabolism, the postsynaptic application of 5-HPETE, but not of 12-HPETE, resulted in an increase in the spontaneous synaptic events (21).

PROSTAGLANDINS AND LEUKOTRIENES AS NEUROMODULATORS

After the discovery of the PGs in the CNS, much attention has been given to the roles these eicosanoids may play in modulating neurotransmission, by interacting with presynaptic or with postsynaptic PG receptors. The existence of such receptors is well-demonstrated, and, in the brain, high-affinity binding sites have been described for both PGE$_2$ and PGD$_2$ (65,66,74,85,91). Peripheral PGE$_2$ receptors are subdivided into three subtypes—EP$_1$, EP$_2$ and EP$_3$—characterized by distinct pharmacological

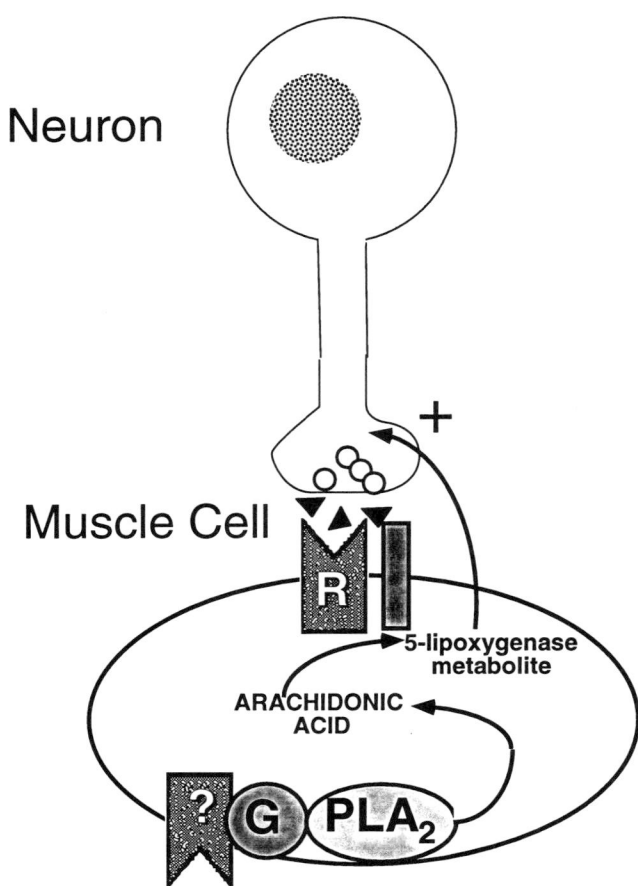

FIG. 6. Possible role of 5-lipoxygenase metabolites in retrograde enhancement of acetylcholine release in *Xenopus* nerve–muscle cultures. For a detailed description, see text. G, G protein; PLA$_2$, phospholipase A$_2$; R, a nicotinic acetylcholine receptor. The question mark indicates an unknown receptor linked to the activation of arachidonic acid release.

properties and intracellular signaling systems (9). EP$_1$ receptors are coupled to phosphoinositide-specific PLC activity, while EP$_2$ and EP$_3$ receptors stimulate and inhibit, respectively, adenylyl cyclase activity. Recently, a cDNA encoding an EP$_3$-type PGE$_2$ receptor was isolated and characterized, and expression of its mRNA in brain tissue was demonstrated by Northern blot. Sequence analysis of EP$_3$-type receptor cDNA revealed the presence in this molecule of seven putative transmembrane domains, characteristic of G-protein-coupled receptors (76).

Presynaptic PG receptors have been often, but not always, linked to inhibition of neurotransmitter release. For example, PGE$_2$ (as well as its analogue, PGE$_1$) inhibits noradrenaline release in a variety of nervous tissue preparations (20,23,24,67). This inhibitory role is by no means universal, however. For example, in dorsal root ganglion neurons in culture, PGE$_2$ was shown to increase Ca^{2+} conductance and to stimulate release of substance P (49). Such an effect may be related to the sensitizing and hyperalgesic properties of this PG, and it might mediate the hyperalgesia produced, in the spinal cord, by the stimulation of glutamate and substance P receptors (40).

The receptor-dependent effects produced by lipoxygenase products in brain have been poorly characterized thus far, even though the existence of a high-affinity binding site for the leukotriene, LTC_4, was reported (70). Both LTC_4 and LTB_4 were shown to evoke the rapid release of luteinizing hormone (LH), when applied at picomolar concentrations in primary cultures of anterior pituitary cells (32). Because gonadotropin-releasing hormone was shown to stimulate leukotriene biosynthesis, it is possible that the leukotrienes play a role in LH secretion.

Cerebellar Purkinje neurons display a remarkable response to the iontophoretic administration of LTC_4. The leukotriene was found to cause a slowly developing increase in the firing rate of these cells, which could last for up to 1.5 hr after application. The lack of effect of LTB_4, along with the ability of a leukotriene-receptor antagonist, the compound FPL 55712, to prevent this response, indicates the selective participation of LTC_4 receptors (56). The physiological significance of this intriguing response remains unknown.

REFERENCES

1. Allen AC, Gammon CM, Ousley AH, McCarthy KD, Morell P. Bradykinin stimulates arachidonic acid release through the sequential actions of an sn-1 diacylglycerol lipase and a monoacylglycerol lipase. *J Neurochem* 1992;58:1130–1139.
2. Amruthesh SC, Falck JR, Ellis EF. Brain synthesis and cerebrovascular action of epoxygenase metabolites of arachidonic acid. *J Neurochem* 1992;58:503–510.
3. Barbour B, Szatkowski M, Ingledew N, Attwell D. Arachidonic acid induces a prolonged inhibition of glutamate uptake into glial cells. *Nature* 1989;342:918–920.
4. Belardetti F, Campbell WB, Falck JR, Demontis G, Rosolowsky M. Products of heme-catalyzed transformation of the arachidonate derivative 12-HPETE open S-type K^+ channels in *Aplysia*. *Neuron* 1989;3:497–505.
5. Bell RL, Kennerly DA, Stanford N, Majerus PW. DG lipase: a pathway for arachidonate release from human platelets. *Proc Natl Acad Sci USA* 1979;76:3238–3241.
6. Bliss TVP, Collingridge GL. A synaptic model of memory: long-term potentiation in the hippocampus. *Nature* 1993;361:31–39.
7. Burch RM. G protein regulation of phospholipase A_2. *Mol Neurobiol* 1989;3:155–171.
8. Clark JD, Lin L-L, Kriz RW, Ramesha CS, Sultzman LA, Lin AY, Milona N, Knopf JL. A novel arachidonic acid-selective cytosolic PLA_2 contains a Ca^{2+}-dependent translocation domain with homology to PKC and GAP. *Cell* 1991;65:1043–1051.
9. Coleman RA. Methods in prostanoid receptors classification. In: Benedetto C, McDonald-Gibson RG, Nigam S, Slater T, eds. *Prostaglandins and related substances. A practical approach.* Oxford: IRL Press, 1987;267–303.
10. De George JJ, Noronha JG, Bell J, Rapoport SI. Intravenous injection of (^{14}C) arachidonate to examine regional brain lipid metabolism in unanesthetized rat. *J Neurosci Res* 1989;24:413–423.
11. Deka N, Sun GY, MacQuarrie R. Purification and properties of acyl-CoA:1-acyl-*sn*-glycero-3-phosphocholine-*O*-acyltransferase from bovine brain microsomes. *Arch Biochem Biophys* 1986;246:554–563.
12. Dennis EA. *Phospholipases.* In: Abelson JN, Simon MI, eds. *Methods in enzymology.* San Diego: Academic Press, 1991.
13. Devane WA, Hanus L, Breuer A, Pertwee RG, Stevenson LA, Griffin G, Gibson D, Mandelbaum A, Etinger A, Mechoulam R. Isolation and structure of a brain constituent that binds to the cannabinoid receptor. *Science* 1992;258:1946–1949.
14. Dumuis A, Sebben M, Haynes L, Pin JP, Bockaert J. NMDA receptors activate the arachidonic acid cascade system in striatal neurons. *Nature* 1988;336:68–70.
15. Exton JH. Signaling through phosphatidylcholine breakdown. *J Biol Chem* 1990;265:1–4.
16. Farooqui AA, Taylor WA, Horrocks LA. Characterization and solubilization of membrane bound diacylglycerol lipases from bovine brain. *Int J Biochem* 1986;18:991–997.
17. Felder CC, Kanterman RY, Ma AL, Axelrod J. Serotonin stimulates phospholipase A_2 and the release of arachidonic acid in hippocampal neurons by a type 2 serotonin receptor that is independent of inositolphospholipid hydrolysis. *Proc Natl Acad Sci USA* 1990;87:2187–2191.
18. Felder CC, Williams HL, Axelrod J. A transduction pathway associated with receptors coupled to the inhibitory guanine nucleotide binding protein Gi that amplifies ATP-mediated arachidonic acid release. *Proc Natl Acad Sci USA* 1991;88:6477–6480.
19. Freeman EJ, Damron DS, Terrian DM, Dorman RV. 12-Lipoxygenase products attenuate the glutamate release and Ca^{2+} accumulation evoked by depolarization of hippocampal mossy fiber nerve endings. *J Neurochem* 1991;56:1079–1082.
20. Gustafsson LE. Mechanisms involved in the action of prostaglandins as modulators of neurotransmission. In: Barkai AI, Bazan NG, eds. *Arachidonic acid metabolism in the nervous system. Annals of the New York Academy of Sciences,* vol 559. New York: New York Academy of Sciences, 1989;178–191.
21. Harish OE, Poo M-M. Retrograde modulation at developing neuromuscular synapses: involvement of G protein and arachidonic acid cascade. *Neuron* 1992;9:1201–1209.
22. Hayaishi H, Fuji Y, Watanabe K, Hayaishi O. Enzymatic formation of prostaglandin $F_{2\alpha}$ in human brain. *Neurochem Res* 1990;15:385–392.
23. Hedqvist P, Brundin J. Inhibition by prostaglandin E_1 of noradrenaline release and of effector response to nerve stimulation in the cat spleen. *Life Sci* 1969;8:389–395.
24. Hedqvist P. Basic mechanisms of prostaglandin action on autonomic neurotransmission. *Annu Rev Pharmacol Toxicol* 1977;17:259–279.
25. Herrero I, Miras-Portugal MT, Sanchez-Prieto J. Positive feedback of glutamate exocytosis by metabotropic presynaptic receptor stimulation. *Nature* 1992;360:163–165.
26. Horrocks LA. Sources for brain arachidonic acid uptake and turnover in glycerophospholipids. In: Barkai AI, Bazan NG, eds. *Arachidonic acid metabolism in the nervous system. Annals of the New York Academy of Sciences,* vol 559. New York: New York Academy of Sciences, 1989;17–24.
27. Jelsema CL. Light activation of phospholipase A_2 in rod outer segments of bovine retina and its modulation by GTP-binding proteins. *J Biol Chem* 1987;262:163–168.
28. Jelsema CL, Axelrod J. Stimulation of phospholipase A_2 activity in bovine rod outer segment by the $\beta\gamma$ subunits of transducin and its inhibition by the α subunit. *Proc Natl Acad Sci USA* 1987;84:3625–3627.
29. Junier MP, Dray F, Blair I, Capdevila J, Dishman E, Falck JR, Ojeda S. Epoxygenase products of arachidonic acid are endogenous constituents of the hypothalamus involved in D_2 receptor-mediated, dopamine-induced release of somatostatin. *Endocrinology* 1990;126:1534–1540.
30. Kanterman RY, Felder CC, Brenneman DE, Ma AL, Fitzgerald S, Axelrod J. α_1-Adrenergic receptor mediates arachidonic acid release in spinal cord neurons independent of inositol phospholipid turnover. *J Neurochem* 1990;54:1225–1232.
31. Keller M, Jackisch R, Seregi A, Hertting G. Comparison of prostanoid forming capacity of neuronal and astroglial cells in primary culture. *Neurochem Int* 1985;7:655–665.
32. Kiesel L, Przylipiak AF, Habenicht AJR, Przylipiak MS, Runnebaum B. Production of leukotrienes in gonadotropin-releasing

hormone-stimulated pituitary cells: potential role in luteinizing hormone release. *Proc Natl Acad Sci USA* 1991;88:8801–8805.

33. Kurachi Y, Ito H, Sugimoto T, Shimizu T, Miki I, Ui M. Arachidonic acid metabolites as intracellular modulators of the G protein-gated cardiac K⁺ channel. *Nature* 1989;337:555–557.

34. Kurachi Y, Ito H, Sugimoto T, Shimizu T, Miki I, Ui M. α-Adrenergic activation of the muscarinic K⁺ channel is mediated by arachidonic acid metabolites. *Pflugers Arch* 1989;414:102–104.

35. Laposata M, Reich EL, Majerus PW. Arachidonoyl-CoA synthetase. Separation from non-specific acyl-CoA synthetase and distribution in various cells and tissues. *J Biol Chem* 1985;260:11016–11020.

36. Lazarewicz JW, Wroblewki JT, Palmer ME, Costa E. Activation of N-methyl-D-aspartate-sensitive glutamate receptors stimulates arachidonic acid release in primary cultures of cerebellar granule cells. *Neuropharmacology* 1988;27:765–769.

37. Linden DJ, Sheu F-S, Murakami K, Routtemberg A. Enhancement of long-term potentiation by cis-unsaturated fatty acid: relation to protein kinase C and phospholipase A₂. *J Neurosci* 1987;7:3783–3792.

38. Linden DJ, Smeyne M, Sun SC, Connor JA. An electrophysiological correlate of protein kinase C isozyme distribution in cultured cerebellar neurons. *J Neurosci* 1992;12:3601–3608.

39. Lindgren JA, Hökfelt T, Dahlén SE, Patrono C, Samuelsson B. Leukotrienes in the rat central nervous system. *Proc Natl Acad Sci USA* 1984;81:6212–6216.

40. Malmberg AB, Yaksh TL. Hyperalgesia mediated by spinal glutamate or substance P receptor blocked by spinal cyclooxygenase inhibition. *Science* 1992;257:1276–1279.

41. McGiff JC. Cytochrome P₄₅₀ metabolism of arachidonic acid. *Annu Rev Pharmacol Toxicol* 1991;31:339–369.

42. Miller B, Sarantis M, Traynelis SF, Attwell D. Potentiation of NMDA receptor currents by arachidonic acid. *Nature* 1992;355:722–725.

43. Montarolo PG, Kandel ER, Schacher S. Long-term heterosynaptic inhibition in *Aplysia. Nature* 1988;333:171–174.

44. Montarolo PG, Glanzman DL, Kandel ER, Schacher S. cAMP and arachidonic acid induce opposite morphological changes with long-term presynaptic facilitation and inhibition in the sensory neurons of *Aplysia. Soc Neurosci Abstr* 1991;17:1591.

45. Moore SA, Yoder E, Spector AA. Role of the blood–brain barrier in the formation of long-chain ω-3 and ω-6 fatty acids from essential fatty acid precursors. *J Neurochem* 1990;55:391–402.

46. Moore SA, Yoder E, Murphy S, Dutton GR, Spector AA. Astrocytes, not neurons, produce docosahexaenoic acid (22:6 ω-3) and arachidonic acid (20:4 ω-6). *J Neurochem* 1991;56:518–524.

47. Naor Z, Shearman MS, Kishimoto A, Nishizuka Y. Calcium-independent activation of hypothalamic type I protein kinase C by unsaturated fatty acids. *Mol Endocrinol* 1988;2:1043–1048.

48. Neufeld EJ, Sprecher H, Evans RW, Majerus P. A mutant HSDM1C1 fibrosarcoma line selected for defective eicosanoid precursor uptake lacks arachidonate-specific acyl-CoA synthetase. *J Biol Chem* 1984;259:1986–1992.

49. Nicol GD, Klingberg DK, Vasko MR. Prostaglandin E₂ increases calcium conductance and stimulates release of substance P in avian sensory neurons. *J Neurosci* 1992;12:1917–1927.

50. Nishiyama M, Okamoto H, Watanabe T, Hori T, Hada T, Ueda N, Yamamoto S, Tsukamoto H, Watanabe K, Kirino T. Localization of arachidonate 12-lipoxygenase in canine brain tissues. *J Neurochem* 1992;58:1395–1400.

51. Nishiyama M, Watanabe T, Ueda N, Tsukamoto H, Watanabe K. Arachidonate 12-lipoxygenase is localized in neurons, glial cells and endothelial cells of the canine brain. *J Histochem Cytochem* 1993;41:111–117.

52. Ogorochi T, Ujiara M, Narumiya S. Purification and properties of prostaglandin H-E isomerase from the cytosol of human brain: identification as anionic forms of glutathione transferase. *J Neurochem* 1987;48:900–909.

53. Ordway RW, Singer JJ, Walsh JV. Direct regulation of ion channels by fatty acids. *Trends Neurosci* 1991;14:96–100.

54. Pace-Asciak CR, Granström E, Samuelsson B. Arachidonic acid epoxides. Isolation and structure of two hydroxy epoxide intermediates in the formation of 8,11,12- and 10,11,12-trihydroxyeicosatrienoic acids. *J Biol Chem* 1983;258:6835–6840.

55. Pace-Asciak CR. Formation and metabolism of hepoxilin A₃ by the rat brain. *Biochem Biophys Res Commun* 1988;151:493–498.

56. Palmer MR, Palmer MR, Hoffer BJ, Murphy RC. Electrophysiological response of cerebellar Purkinje neurons to leukotriene D₄ and B₄. *J Pharmacol Exp Ther* 1981;219:91–96.

57. Partington CR, Edwards MW, Daly JW. Regulation of cAMP formation in brain tissue by α-adrenergic receptors: requisite intermediacy by prostaglandins of the E-series. *Proc Natl Acad Sci USA* 1980;77:3024–3028.

58. Piomelli D, Shapiro E, Feinmark SJ, Schwartz JH. Metabolites of arachidonic acid in the nervous system of *Aplysia:* possible mediators of synaptic modulation. *J Neurosci* 1987;7:3675–3686.

59. Piomelli D, Volterra A, Dale N, Siegelbaum SA, Schwartz JH, Belardetti F. Lipoxygenase metabolites of arachidonic acid as second messengers for presynaptic inhibition in *Aplysia* sensory cells. *Nature* 1987;328:38–43.

60. Piomelli D, Feinmark SJ, Shapiro E, Schwartz JH. Formation and biological activity of 12-keto-eicosatetraenoic acid in the nervous system of *Aplysia. J Biol Chem* 1988;263:16591–16596.

61. Piomelli D, Shapiro E, Zipkin R, Schwartz JH, Feinmark SJ. Formation and action of 8-hydroxy-11,12-epoxy-5,9,14-icosatrienoic acid in *Aplysia:* a possible second messenger in neurons. *Proc Natl Acad Sci USA* 1989;86:1721–1725.

62. Piomelli D, Wang JKT, Shires TS, Nairn AC, Czernik AJ, Greengard P. Inhibition of Ca²⁺/calmodulin-dependent protein kinase II by arachidonic acid metabolites. *Proc Natl Acad Sci USA* 1989;86:8550–8554.

63. Piomelli D, Pilon C, Giros B, Sokoloff P, Martres MP, Schwartz JC. Dopamine activation of the arachidonic acid cascade as a basis for D₁/D₂ receptor synergism. *Nature* 1991;353:164–167.

64. Ponzoni M, Montaldo PG, Cornaglia-Ferraris P. Stimulation of receptor-coupled phospholipase A₂ by interferon-γ. *FEBS Lett* 1992;310:17–21.

65. Pralong E, Vesin M-F, Droz B. Prostaglandin E₂ receptors in the chicken spinal cord. 1. Biochemical characterization. *Eur J Neurosci* 1990;2:897–903.

66. Pralong E, Vesin M-F, Droz B. Prostaglandin E₂ receptors in the chicken spinal cord. 2. Autoradiographic localization. *Eur J Neurosci* 1990;2:904–908.

67. Rump LC, Wilde K, Schollmeyer P. Prostaglandin E₂ inhibits noradrenaline release and purinergic pressor responses to renal nerve stimulation at 1 Hz in isolated kidneys of young spontaneously hypertensive rats. *J Hypertens* 1990;8:897–908.

68. Samuelsson B. Leukotrienes: mediators of immediate hypersensitivity reaction and inflammation. *Science* 1983;220:568–575.

69. Sautebin L, Spagnuolo C, Galli C, Galli G. A mass fragmentographic procedure for the simultaneous determination of HETE and PGF₂α in the central nervous system. *Prostaglandins* 1977;16:985–988.

70. Schalling M, Neil A, Terenius L, Lindgren JA, Miamoto T, Hökfelt T, Samuelsson B. Leukotriene C₄ binding sites in the rat central nervous system. *Eur J Pharmacol* 1986;122:251–257.

71. Schweitzer P, Madamba S, Siggins GR. Arachidonic acid metabolites as mediators of somatostatin-induced increase in neuronal M-current. *Nature* 1990;346:464–467.

72. Seregi A, Keller M, Hertting G. Are cerebral prostanoids of astroglial origin? Studies on the prostanoid forming system in developing rat brain and primary cultures of rat astrocytes. *Brain Res* 1987;404:113–120.

73. Shearman MS, Naor Z, Sekiguchi K, Kishimoto A, Nishizuka Y. Selective activation of the γ-subspecies of protein kinase C from bovine cerebellum by arachidonic acid and its lipoxygenase metabolites. *FEBS Lett* 1989;243:177–182.

74. Shimizu T, Yamashita A, Hayaishi O. Specific binding of prostaglandin D₂ to rat brain synaptic membrane. Occurrence, properties, and distribution. *J Biol Chem* 1982;257:13570–13575.

75. Shimizu T, Takusagawa Y, Izumi T, Ohishi N, Seyama Y. Enzymic synthesis of leukotriene B₄ in guinea pig brain. *J Neurochem* 1987;48:1541–1546.

76. Sugimoto Y, Namba T, Honda A, Hayashi Y, Negishi M, Ichikawa A, Narumiya S. Cloning and expression of a cDNA for mouse prostaglandin receptor EP₃ subtype. *J Biol Chem* 1992;267:6463–6466.

77. Sun GY, MacQuarry RA. Deacylation-reacylation of arachidonoyl groups in cerebral phospholipids. In: Barkai AI, Bazan NG, ed. *Arachidonic acid metabolism in the nervous system. Annals of the New York Academy of Sciences,* vol 559. New York: New York Academy of Sciences, 1989;37–55.

78. Traiffort E, Ruat M, Arrang J-M, Leurs R, Piomelli D, Schwartz J-C. Expression of a cloned rat histamine H_2 receptor mediating inhibition of arachidonate release and activation of cAMP accumulation. *Proc Natl Acad Sci USA* 1992;89:2649–2653.

79. Urade Y, Fujimoto N, Hayaishi O. Purification and characterization of rat brain prostaglandin D synthetase. *J Biol Chem* 1985;260:12410–12415.

80. Urade Y, Fujimoto N, Kaneko T, Konishi A, Mizuno N, Hayaishi O. Postnatal changes in the localization of prostaglandin D synthetase from neurons to oligodendrocytes in the rat brain. *J Biol Chem* 1987;262:15132–15136.

81. Vesin MF, Barakat-Walter I, Droz B. Preferential synthesis of prostaglandin D_2 by neurons and prostaglandin E_2 by fibroblasts and nonneuronal cells in chick dorsal root ganglia. *J Neurochem* 1991;57:167–174.

82. Waite M. The phospholipases. In: Hanahan DJ, ed. *Handbook of lipid research,* vol. 5. New York: Plenum Press, 1987.

83. Waku K. Origins and fates of fatty acyl-CoA esters. *Biochim Biophys Acta* 1992;1124:101–111.

84. Warner M, Köhler C, Hansson T, Gustafsson J-A. Regional distribution of cytochrome P-450 in the rat brain: spectral quantitation and contribution of P-450b,e and P-450c,d. *J Neurochem* 1988;50:1057–1065.

85. Watanabe Y, Tokumoto H, Yamashita A, Narumiya S, Mizuno N, Hayaishi O. Specific bindings of prostaglandin D_2, E_2 and $F_{2\alpha}$ in postmortem human brain. *Brain Res* 1985;342:110–116.

86. Watanabe Y, Watanabe Y, Hamada K, Bommelaer-Bayt MC, Dray F, Kaneko T, Watanabe T, Medina JF, Haeggstrom JZ, Radmark O, Samuelsson B. Molecular cloning of a 12-lipoxygenase from rat brain. *Eur J Biochem* 1993;212:605–612.

87. Williams JH, Errington ML, Lynch MA, Bliss TVP. Arachidonic acid induces a long-term activity-dependent enhancement of synaptic transmission in the hippocampus. *Nature* 1989;341:739–742.

88. Wilson DB, Prescott SM, Majerus PW. Discovery of an arachidonoyl coenzyme A synthetase in human platelets. *J Biol Chem* 1982;257:3510–3515.

89. Wolfe LS, Pellerin L. Arachidonic acid metabolites in the rat and human brain. In: Barkai AI, Bazan NG, ed. *Arachidonic acid metabolism in the nervous system. Annals of the New York Academy of Sciences,* vol 559. New York: New York Academy of Sciences, 1989;74–83.

90. Yamamoto S. Mammalian lipoxygenases: molecular structure and functions. *Biochim Biophys Acta* 1992;1128:117–131.

91. Yamashita A, Watanabe Y, Hayaishi O. Autoradiographic localization of a binding protein(s) specific for prostaglandin D_2 in rat brain. *Proc Natl Acad Sci USA* 1983;80:6114–6118.

92. Yoshihara Y, Watanabe Y. Translocation of phospholipase A_2 from cytosol to membranes in rat brain induced by calcium ions. *Biochem Biophys Res Commun* 1990;170:484–490.

93. Yu ACH, Chan PH, Fishman RA. Arachidonic acid inhibits uptake of glutamate and glutamine but not of GABA in cultured granule cells. *J Neurosci Res* 1987;424–427.

Psychopharmacology: The Fourth Generation of Progress, edited by Floyd E. Bloom and David J. Kupfer. Raven Press, Ltd., New York © 1995.

CHAPTER 54

Nitric Oxide and Related Substances as Neural Messengers

Solomon H. Snyder and Ted M. Dawson

The history of neurotransmission is full of surprises. A reasonable person would assume that the brain could make do with few, perhaps only two, neurotransmitters—one excitatory and one inhibitory. For most of the 20th century this appeared to be the case, because between the 1920s (when acetylcholine was appreciated) and the late 1960s only a handful of molecules were accepted as neurotransmitters, specifically biogenic amines and amino acids. Research on opiate receptors and enkephalins spurred interest into peptides, and, within a few years, up to 50 or more neuropeptides had been characterized. Though differing markedly in many properties, amines, amino acids, and peptides follow closely the conventional neurotransmitter dogma. They are stored in synaptic vesicles which release their contents by exocytosis involving fusion with the plasma membrane and expulsion. They diffuse to closely adjacent cells, where they interact reversibly with membrane protein receptors which influence cellular events through the mediation of intracellular second messenger molecules or by influencing ion permeation. Inactivation either by enzymes or by reuptake pumps is also a crucial factor in regulating the duration of transmitter action.

The discovery of nitric oxide (NO) as a neurotransmitter has radically altered our thinking about synaptic transmission. Being a labile, free radical gas (though in most biological situations NO is in solution), NO is not stored in synaptic vesicles. Instead it is synthesized as needed by NO synthase (NOS) from its precursor L-arginine.

S. H. Snyder: Departments of Neuroscience, Pharmacology and Molecular Sciences, and Psychiatry and Behavioral Sciences, Johns Hopkins University School of Medicine, Baltimore, Maryland 21205.

T. M. Dawson: Departments of Neuroscience and Neurology, Johns Hopkins University School of Medicine, Baltimore, Maryland 21287.

Rather than exocytosis, NO simply diffuses from nerve terminals. It does not react with receptors but diffuses into adjacent cells. In place of reversible interactions with targets, NO forms covalent linkages to a multiplicity of targets which may be enzymes, such as guanylyl cyclase (GC) or other protein or nonprotein targets. Inactivation of NO presumably involves diffusion away from targets as well as covalent linkages to an assortment of small or large molecules such as superoxide and diverse proteins.

DEVELOPMENT OF EVIDENCE FOR NO AS A BIOLOGICAL MESSENGER

While the neurosciences have been markedly influenced by new insights into NO in the nervous system, NO was first appreciated in mammalian systems associated with inflammatory responses and blood vessel reactivity. In the early 1980s, studies of nitrosamines as carcinogens led to the demonstration that endogenous nitrates can be produced, because germ-free rats excrete large amounts of nitrates as do humans, whose excretion rises markedly during infections (54). Clever detective work led to the finding that the nitrates in the urine arise from macrophages through oxidation of the guanidine nitrogen of L-arginine, giving rise to L-citrulline and a reactive substance subsequently shown to be NO. The ability of macrophages to kill tumor cells and fungi depended upon external arginine, whose effects were blocked by arginine derivatives which also blocked the formation of nitrite, leading to identification of NO as the active substance (48).

A role of NO in blood vessels derives from work in the 1970s implicating NO as the active metabolite of nitroglycerin and other organic nitrates in dilating blood vessels by stimulating cGMP formation through activa-

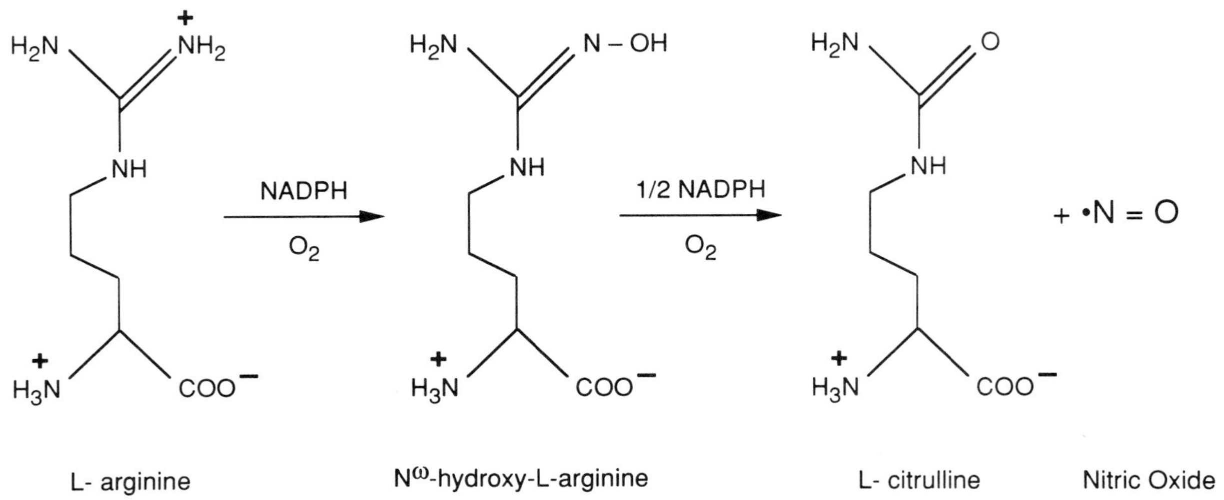

FIG. 1. Biosynthesis of nitric oxide. A guanidino nitrogen of L-arginine undergoes a five-electron oxidation via an *N*-omega-hydroxyl-L-arginine intermediate to yield NO.

tion of GC (1). Meanwhile, Furchgott and Zawadzki (23) had shown that blood vessel relaxation in response to acetylcholine and other substances requires the endothelial lining which releases a labile substance that diffuses to the adjacent smooth muscle. The active agent was identified as NO (35,52).

A role in the brain for NO first came from observations that brain cells in culture stimulated by excitatory amino acids release a substance with the properties of NO (25,26). A definitive involvement of NO was demonstrated by the ability of NOS inhibitors, such as nitroarginine and methyl arginine, to block the pronounced stimulation of cGMP in brain slices that is elicited by the excitatory transmitter glutamate acting at *N*-methyl-D-aspartate (NMDA) subtype receptors (4,5,15).

NO BIOSYNTHESIS

Because NO cannot be stored by conventional means nor inactivated after synaptic release, its biosynthesis constitutes the only means for regulating NO levels. Not surprisingly, NOS is one of the most regulated enzymes in biology. NOS oxidizes the guanidine group of L-arginine in a process that consumes five electrons and results in the formation of NO with stoichiometric formation of L-citrulline (Fig. 1). Initial efforts to purify the enzyme were unsuccessful because of a rapid loss of enzyme activity upon purification. The discovery that calmodulin is required for NOS activity in the brain permitted a simple purification of brain NOS to homogeneity (3). Based on this scheme, other groups purified brain NOS; and macrophage and endothelial NOS proteins were purified as well (4,5,15,49). Molecular cloning of the cDNA for brain, endothelial, macrophage, and nonmacrophage inducible forms of NOS has considerably clarified

NOS function (5,15,45,49) (Fig. 2). The structure of NOS as well as biochemical features elucidated in numerous studies reveal a remarkable multiplicity of regulatory mechanisms.

Oxidative enzymes generally employ an electron donor. NOS is unprecedented in employing five. Cloned NOS displays recognition sites for NADPH, flavin mononucleotide (FMN), and flavin adenine dinucleotide (FAD). Direct biochemical analysis shows FAD and FMN bound stoichiometrically to NOS (5,49). The only other mammalian enzyme that possesses recognition sites for both FMN and FAD as well as NADPH is cytochrome P-450 reductase (CPR) (Fig. 2). CPR is the electron donor for the liver's drug-metabolizing cytochrome P-450 enzymes. The carboxyl half of NOS displays about 60% amino acid identity to CPR. Presumably, early in evolution, CPR donated electrons for NOS, and at some point a fusion between CPR and NOS took place. Indeed, when the N-terminal and C-terminal halves of NOS are expressed separately and mixed together, one obtains NOS catalytic activity (D. S. Bredt and S. H. Snyder, *unpublished observations*). NOS also utilizes tetrahydrobiopterin as an electron-transferring cofactor (5,49). Recently, several groups showed that NOS contains bound heme which reacts with CO to form a species absorbing at 450 nm, indicating that NOS itself is a cytochrome P-450 enzyme (5,49). It is likely that the mechanism of electron transfer is similar to that of the P-450 enzymes—namely, that NADPH reduces FAD, which reduces FMN, which, in turn, transfers electrons to the ferric heme promoting the interaction with molecular oxygen. The exact role of tetrahydrobiopterin is not clear but probably involves a stabilization of the enzyme (5,49).

NOS enzymes can be discriminated as inducible or constitutive. The brain and endothelial forms are constitutive in that stimuli for NO formation do not typically result in new enzyme protein synthesis. Instead, in the brain a stimulus (such as glutamate) acting at NMDA receptors triggers Ca^{2+} influx which binds to calmodulin, thereby activating NOS. This mode of activation explains the ability of glutamate neurotransmission to stimulate NO formation in a matter of seconds. In blood vessels, acetylcholine acting at muscarinic receptors on endothelial cells activates the phosphoinositide cycle to generate Ca^{2+}, which stimulates NOS. Thus, constitutive NOS accounts for the role of NO in mediating rapid events such as neurotransmission and blood vessel dilatation. New synthesis of constitutive brain NOS can take place, because neuronal damage in the spinal cord is associated with the appearance of NADPH-diaphorase staining or newly immunoreactive NOS neurons and the induction of mRNA for brain NOS in dorsal root ganglia (5,15). New synthesis of endothelial NOS in the brain also occurs following middle cerebral artery occlusion (72).

The inducible NOS of macrophages and nonmacrophage sources is not stimulated by Ca^{2+}. Surprisingly, inducible NOS enzymes possess calmodulin recognition sites (Fig. 2). Nathan and colleagues (10) have shown that calmodulin is very tightly bound to inducible NOS, with the binding unaffected by Ca^{2+}, whereas calmodulin cannot bind to neuronal NOS unless Ca^{2+} is present. The fact that calmodulin binds so tightly to inducible NOS that it can be considered an enzyme subunit accounts for the resistance of inducible NOS to Ca^{2+} activation (54).

Under normal circumstances, macrophages possess no detectable NOS protein. Stimuli such as interferon-γ and lipopolysaccharide (LPS) elicit new NOS protein synthesis over 2–4 hr, mediating the NO responses to inflammatory stimuli. It was first thought that macrophages contained the only form of inducible NOS. Following endotoxin treatment, inducible NOS activity has been demonstrated in a great diversity of animal tissues lacking

macrophages (54). The hepatocyte inducible NOS which has been recently cloned (27) might represent the prototype for nonmacrophage inducible NOS. Conceivably the ubiquitous distribution of this form of inducible NOS reflects a primitive sort of immune response. The simplicity of the NO system might have sufficed to repel invading microorganisms early in evolution.

NOS can also be regulated by phosphorylation. Consensus sequences for phosphorylation by cAMP-dependent protein kinase are evident in neuronal and endothelial NOS and hepatic inducible NOS (Fig. 2). These are not as obvious in the macrophage form of NOS. Consensus sites for phosphorylation by other kinases have not been characterized in detail. However, biochemical studies indicate that neuronal NOS can be phosphorylated by cAMP-dependent protein kinase, protein kinase C, cGMP-dependent protein kinase, and Ca^{2+}/calmodulin-dependent protein kinase (5,15). Phosphorylation by all of these enzymes decreases enzyme catalytic activity (5,15; J. L. Dinerman, J. P. Steiner, T. M. Dawson, and S. H. Snyder, *in preparation*). This provides for multiple levels of enzyme regulation. For instance, Ca^{2+}-calmodulin can directly activate the enzyme and, by phosphorylation through Ca^{2+}/calmodulin-dependent protein kinase, inhibit enzyme activity. Ca^{2+}, together with lipids, also activates protein kinase C, whose actions would also inhibit NOS. NO stimulates GC to form cGMP, which, via cGMP-dependent protein kinase, can inhibit NOS.

For inducible NOS one would expect the regulatory region of the gene to determine the rate of synthesis of enzyme protein. Characterization of the promoter region of the gene for macrophage inducible NOS (macNOS) reveals a pattern for complex regulation (44,70). There appear to be two distinct regulatory regions upstream of the TATA box, which is 30 base pairs upstream of the transcription start site. One of these, region 1, lies about

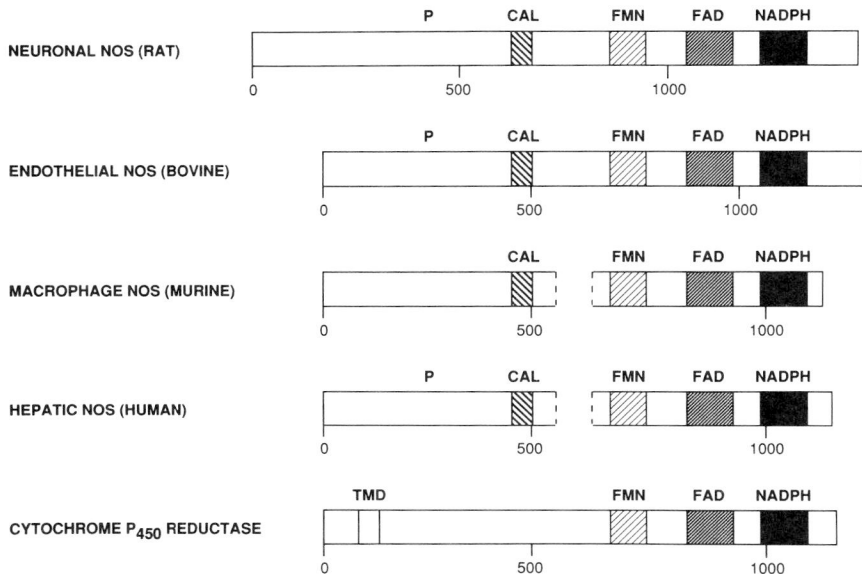

FIG. 2. Molecular isoforms of NOS. Diagrammatic representation of the structure of cloned isoforms of NOS and cytochrome P-450 reductase. P, consensus sequence for phosphorylation by cAMP-dependent protein kinase; CAL, calmodulin binding site; FMN, flavin mononucleotide; FAD, flavin adenine dinucleotide; NADPH, reduced form of nicotinamide adenine dinucleotide phosphate; TMD, transmembrane domain.

50–200 base pairs upstream of the start site. Region 1 contains LPS-related response elements such as the binding site for NF-IL6 and the KB binding site for NFKB, indicating that this region regulates the LPS-induced expression of macNOS. Region 2, which is about 900–1000 bases upstream of the start site, does not itself directly regulate NOS expression, but provides a 10-fold increase above the 75-fold increase in NOS expression provided by region 1. Region 2 contains motifs for interferon-γ-related transcription factors and thus is presumably responsible for interferon-γ-mediated regulation. In sum, LPS- and interferon-γ-responsive elements occur in two distinct regulatory genes: LPS directly stimulates macNOS expression, whereas interferon-γ acts only in the presence of LPS.

This unique organization of gene enhancers may explain important aspects of inflammation. In sepsis, LPS is released from gram-negative bacterial cell walls and circulates throughout the body to stimulate inflammatory responses. By contrast, interferon-γ is released locally and serves to augment inflammatory responses in specific cell populations close to its release. LPS alone stimulates macrophages only to a limited extent. Interferon-γ elaborated by infiltrating lymphocytes can prime the macrophages for a maximal response to LPS. Thus maximal production of NO is restricted to those cells needed to kill the invader, thereby minimizing damage to adjacent tissue.

The NOS proteins are fairly large proteins. Neuronal NOS, the largest, has a molecular weight of 160 kD and occurs as a dimer. Endothelial and the inducible NOS enzymes are in the range of 130 kD and also function as dimers. Neuronal and macrophage NOS have been characterized largely as soluble proteins, though subcellular fractionation reveals a substantial amount of particulate neuronal NOS which is not readily solubilized by high salt concentrations (D. S. Bredt and S. H. Snyder, *unpublished observations*) and a particulate neuronal NOS has been purified from rat cerebellum (32). Endothelial NOS is predominantly particulate (56). Molecular cloning of endothelial NOS reveals no obvious transmembrane-spanning regions (5,15,45,49). However, there is a consensus motif for N-terminal myristoylation, whose deletion in mutagenesis experiments renders NOS soluble (9). Moreover, [³H]myristate is directly incorporated into endothelial NOS (9). Insertion of the myristoyl group in the plasma membrane presumably accounts for the enzyme's particulate location.

NO IN NEURONAL FUNCTION

With any neurotransmitter, major insight into function comes with information about localization. Purification of neuronal NOS permitted the development of antibodies for immunohistochemical staining (4). Throughout the brain, neuronal NOS occurs only in neurons. In many areas such as the cerebral cortex, hippocampus, and corpus striatum, NOS neurons comprise only about 2% of all the cells. They are scattered in no obvious pattern and display morphologic properties of medium-to-large aspiny neurons. In the hippocampus, none of the pyramidal cells contain NOS, but granule cells of the dentate gyrus have abundant NOS. In the corpus striatum, NOS occurs in both the cell bodies and terminals of the medium aspiny neurons. In most areas, NOS-containing cells are prominent, whereas in the islands of Callejae, NOS staining is confined to a dense fiber bundle.

In striking contrast to the pattern in the cerebral cortex, in the cerebellum NOS occurs in a high proportion of certain cell types. For instance, NOS is abundant in all granule cells and all basket cells, but in no Purkinje cells. This pattern explains how glutamate influences cGMP in the cerebellum. Endogenous cGMP is selectively concentrated in Purkinje cells, which receive input from terminals of granule and basket cells. Granule and basket cells possess NMDA receptors. Presumably, stimulation of the NMDA receptors on basket and granule cells triggers formation of NO which diffuses to Purkinje cells to activate GC.

While GC is clearly a target for NO in the cerebellum, this link may not be universal throughout the brain. If NO transmission occurred exclusively through GC and if all the GC in the brain were associated with NO transmission, then GC and NOS localizations should be closely similar. However, they differ markedly, indicating that NO may act through other targets than GC and/or GC may be the target for other transmitters besides NO.

Many, if not all, neurons in the brain contain more than one neurotransmitter. There does not appear to be a specific pattern for NOS. Thus, in the cerebellum NOS occurs in the glutamate-containing granule cells as well as in the gamma-aminobutyric acid (GABA)-containing basket cells. Many of the cerebral cortical NOS neurons also contain GABA. In the corpus striatum all NOS neurons stain for somatostatin and neuropeptide Y, but in areas such as the pedunculopontine nucleus of the brainstem, NOS neurons lack somatostatin and neuropeptide Y but stain for choline acetyltransferase (13).

What are the normal functions of these NOS neurons? One answer is that NO is responsible for cGMP generation. This answer leads to another question, namely, What is the role of cGMP? Though cGMP has been studied in the brain for well over 30 years, its exact functions remain obscure.

NO appears to influence neurotransmitter release. In several model systems, NOS inhibitors such as nitroarginine block the release of neurotransmitters (15). In brain synaptosomes the release of neurotransmitter evoked by stimulation of NMDA receptors is blocked by nitroarginine (33), whereas release elicited by potassium depolarization is not affected (33). Presumably, glutamate acts at NMDA receptors on NOS terminals to stimulate the formation of NO, which diffuses to adjacent terminals to enhance neurotransmitter release, so that blockade of NO formation inhibits release. Potassium depolarization will release transmitter from all terminals so that any effect of NO would be masked.

PC12 cells, which develop neuronal properties in the presence of nerve growth factor, provide a valuable system linking NO to transmitter release. Rogers and colleagues (59,60) showed that the release of acetylcholine in response to depolarization is markedly enhanced after 8 days of nerve growth factor application. NOS staining and NOS catalytic activity, which are absent in untreated PC12 cells, do not appear until 8 days, coincident with marked enhancement of neurotransmitter release. Release of both acetylcholine and dopamine from the cells is blocked by NOS inhibitors and reversed by excess L-arginine (33).

Direct evidence for specific neurotransmitter functions of NO comes from studies in the peripheral autonomic nervous system. NOS neurons occur in the myenteric plexus throughout the gastrointestinal pathway (2,13). Depolarization of myenteric plexus neurons is associated with relaxation of the smooth muscle associated with peristalsis. The blockade of this process by NOS inhibitors indicates that NO is the transmitter (5,52,54).

In blood vessels, besides localizations in the endothelium, NOS occurs in autonomic nerves in the outer, adventitial layers of various large blood vessels (2,55). In the cerebral cortex and the retina these neurons derive from cells in the sphenopalatine ganglia at the base of the skull (55). Approximately 40% of the NOS neurons contain the neuropeptide vasoactive intestinal polypeptide (VIP) (55). NOS neurons are prominent in penile tissue, specifically the pelvic plexus and its axonal processes that form the cavernous nerve as well as the nerve plexus in the adventitia of the deep cavernosal arteries and the sinusoids in the periphery of the corpora cavernosa (8). Electrical stimulation of the cavernous nerve in intact rats produces prominent penile erection which is blocked by low doses of intravenously administered NOS inhibitors (8). Nerve-stimulation-induced relaxation of isolated corpus cavernosum strips is also blocked by NOS inhibitors (58). These findings establish that NO is the transmitter of these nerves which regulate penile erection.

In the adrenal gland, NOS occurs in discrete ganglion cells and fibers in the medulla (2,13). Splanchnic nerve stimulation augments both blood flow and catecholamine secretion from the adrenal medulla, with nitroarginine blocking the blood flow but not catecholamine secretion (7). NOS is also prominent in fibers and terminals in the posterior pituitary gland (2,13), but its relation to function has not yet been established.

NO has been implicated in long-term potentiation (LTP) in the hippocampus. Nitroarginine application to hippocampal slices blocks LTP formation. Injection of nitroarginine into pyramidal cells of the hippocampus also inhibits LTP, suggesting that NO might act as a retrograde messenger for LTP passing from pyramidal cells to Schaffer collateral terminals (4,5,15). However, neuronal NOS is not yet demonstrable in these pyramidal cells (4).

NO IN NEUROTOXICITY

While NO mediates normal synaptic transmission, excess levels of NO may be neurotoxic. Evidence has accumulated for a number of years that glutamate released in excess, acting via NMDA receptors, mediates neurotoxicity in the focal ischemia of vascular stroke (11) which is blocked by NMDA antagonists (50). Glutamate neurotoxicity may also contribute to dysfunction in neurodegenerative diseases such as Alzheimer's and Huntington's diseases. Because glutamate, via NMDA receptors, stimulates NO formation, one might expect excess NMDA receptor stimulation to destroy NOS neurons. Surprisingly, NOS neurons are resistant to NMDA neurotoxicity (17). This conclusion derives from the demonstration that NOS neurons are identical to those that stain for NADPH-diaphorase (13,34). Diaphorase staining reflects a blue precipitate obtained with tetrazolium dyes in the presence of NADPH (5,15). Numerous studies have demonstrated that diaphorase-staining neurons are notably resistant to destruction in Huntington's and Alzheimer's diseases, in vascular stroke, and in NMDA neurotoxicity (15). We were struck with the close similarity in localizations of diaphorase- and NOS-staining neurons. Transfection of neuronal NOS cDNA into human kidney 293 cells lacking NOS or diaphorase results in staining of the cells for diaphorase and NOS in exactly the same proportions as neurons in the brain (13). Because diaphorase derives from any NADPH oxidative activity, most diaphorase in brain homogenates is unrelated to NOS, but a discrete portion represents NOS (34).

If NMDA stimulates NOS neurons to make NO, but these cells are themselves resistant to neurotoxicity, could the released NO damage other cells? Exposure of cerebral cortical cultures to NMDA kills 60–90% of neurons, with NOS-diaphorase cells being undamaged (17,37). Treatment with nitroarginine or other NOS inhibitors or removal of arginine from the media block this neurotoxicity (17,18). The toxicity is also prevented by flavoprotein and calmodulin inhibitors. Superoxide dismutase attenuates neurotoxicity. Because this enzyme removes superoxide which interacts with NO to form the toxic radical peroxynitrite, NO presumably kills via peroxynitrite. NO has been implicated in NMDA neurotoxicity in a variety of models, including hippocampal slices, striatal slices, and several culture systems (5,15). Others have failed to show that NO is involved in NMDA neurotoxicity (15), and NO may be neuroprotective (38). NO may exert both neurodestruction and neuroprotection, depending on its oxidation–reduction status (40), with NO⁻ being neuro-destructive and NO⁺ being neuroprotective (40). If NMDA neurotoxicity is responsible for neuronal damage in vascular stroke, then NOS inhibitors should be neuroprotective. Administration of low doses of nitroarginine blocks neural damage following middle cerebral artery occlusion in mice, rats, and cats (15). High doses of NOS inhibitors exacerbate the damage following occlusion of the middle cerebral artery (15), presumably through decreased cerebral blood flow.

Why are NOS neurons resistant to NMDA toxicity? One possibility arises from findings of Michel et al. (51) regarding translocation of NOS in endothelial cells. Phosphorylation of NOS translocates the enzyme from membrane to soluble fractions. Because phosphorylated NOS is catalytically inactive, NO will not be generated within the cytoplasm. Instead, catalytically active, nonphosphorylated NOS is localized to the plasma membrane, where it presumably generates NO that is released into the extracellular environment. While neuronal NOS has been thought to be predominantly soluble, about 50% of NOS activity in brain homogenates is particulate and cannot be solubilized even with strong salt treatment (D. S. Bredt and S. H. Snyder, *unpublished observations*). Thus, in neurons as well as blood vessels the active form of NOS may be the unphosphorylated enzyme localized to the plasma membrane to release NOS to the exterior. Presumably, NO is never released in the interior of NOS cells, which accordingly are resistant to NO damage.

NO can mediate other forms of neurotoxicity. The pathophysiology of acquired immunodeficiency syndrome (AIDS) dementia has been a puzzle, because little human immunodeficiency virus (HIV) virus is detected in neurons in the brain. Instead, the gp120 coat protein appears to mediate some of the toxicity. Extremely low,

picomolar concentrations of gp120 kill neurons in primary cortical cultures (6,21). The killing is absolutely dependent upon the presence of glutamate acting through NMDA receptors (19,41). We showed that this toxicity requires NO, being absent in arginine-free medium and blocked by various inhibitors of NOS (19). The gp120 neurotoxicity also requires the presence of macrophages and/or astrocytes (39). These cells produce cytokines and arachidonic acid metabolites which can potentiate NMDA receptor currents. Conceivably, gp120 elicits release of arachidonic acid metabolites and cytokines from macrophages and glia, which synergize with glutamate to activate NMDA receptors, in turn triggering the formation of NO (Fig. 3).

Neuroprotection can derive from indirect means of NOS inhibition. Gangliosides are neuroprotective in animal models of neural damage and in patients with spinal cord injury (46,62). Based on observations that gangliosides bind calmodulin (30,31), we showed that a series of gangliosides inhibit NOS activity and prevent glutamate toxicity in neuronal cultures with potencies closely paralleling their affinities for calmodulin and their ability to inhibit NOS (14).

Immunosuppressants such as FK506 and cyclosporin A bind to small soluble receptor proteins. The drug-receptor complex in turn binds to the Ca^{2+} activated phosphatase calcineurin to inhibit calcineurin activity (42). Thus, treatment with these immunosuppressant drugs leads to accumulation of phosphorylated substrates of calcineurin (64). We observed that NOS is a calcineurin substrate and that phosphorylated NOS levels are enhanced by FK506 and cyclosporin A (16). Because phosphorylated NOS is catalytically inactive, treatment with the immunosuppressants should be equivalent to treatment with NOS inhibitors. Indeed, both FK506 and

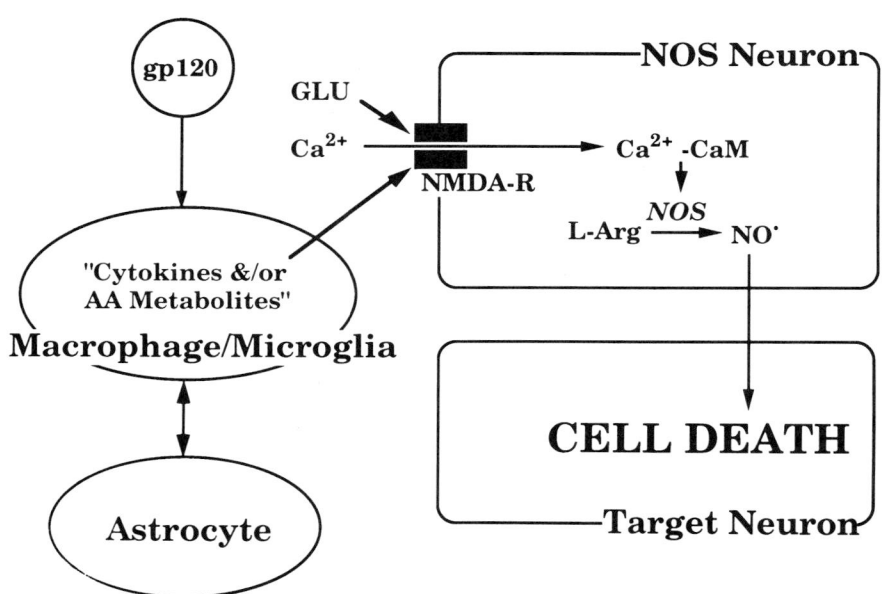

FIG. 3. Mechanism of gp120-induced neurotoxicity. gp120, the HIV-1 coat protein, may elicit neurotoxicity by interacting with macrophage/microglia and astrocytes to release cytokines and/or arachidonic acid metabolites. Glutamate then interacts with the cytokines and/or arachidonic acid metabolites to activate NMDA receptors, which increases intracellular calcium levels. NOS is subsequently activated, and excessive formation of NO kills adjacent neurons. (From ref. 16.)

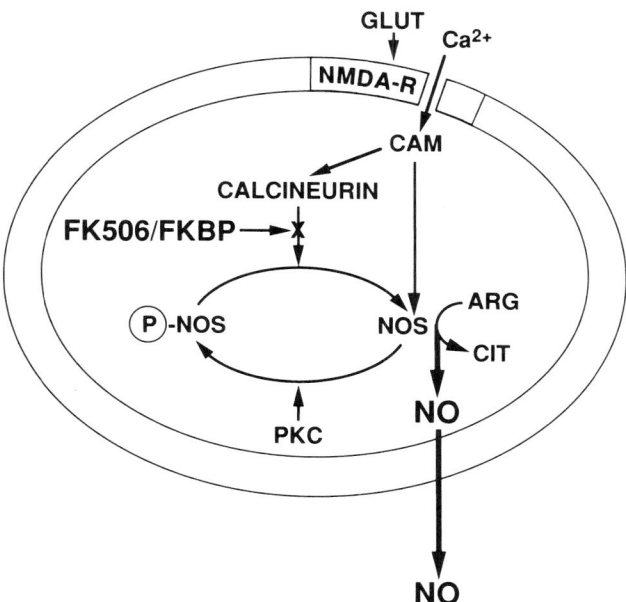

FIG. 4. Mechanism of the regulation of the phosphorylation state and catalytic activity of NOS. NMDA receptor activations increase intracellular Ca^{2+} levels which subsequently activate NOS and calcineurin via calmodulin. With excessive NMDA receptor stimulation, large quantities of NO are produced and adjacent neurons die. NOS catalytic activity is inhibited by protein kinase C (PKC)-mediated phosphorylation as well as by cAMP- and cGMP-dependent protein kinases and Ca^{2+}/calmodulin-dependent protein kinase. Ca^{2+} entry activates calcineurin, which dephosphorylates and activates NOS. FK506, complexed to FKBP, binds to calcineurin and inhibits its phosphatase activity. This prevents the dephosphorylation of NOS, thus decreasing NOS catalytic activity. NO production is subsequently lowered, and adjacent neurons remain viable. (From ref. 19.)

cyclosporin A block NMDA neurotoxicity in cortical cultures at very low concentrations (Fig. 4). The neuroprotective effect of FK-506 may have clinical relevance. FK506 and cyclosporin A have been employed extensively in organ transplant surgery. FK506 penetrates readily into the brain, whereas cyclosporin A does not. In a study of liver transplantation, 7 of 14 patients receiving cyclosporin A showed global cerebral ischemia, whereas none of the 14 patients receiving FK506 showed such alterations (43). Furthermore, cyclosporin A reduces infarct volume following middle cerebral artery infarction in rats (61).

NO TARGETS

While activation of GC accounts for some of the synaptic activities of NO, it cannot account for neurotoxicity, because inhibitors of GC do not block neurotoxicity (15,17). Moreover, 8-bromo cGMP, which penetrates readily into cells, is not neurotoxic. Identifying the molecular target for neurotoxicity is difficult, because when a

cell is killed, all of its biochemistry deteriorates. Numerous candidates for the toxic actions of NO have been investigated.

NO activates GC by binding to iron in the heme which is at the active site of the enzyme, altering the enzyme's conformation to activate it. NO can bind to nonheme iron in numerous enzymes such as NADH-ubiquinone oxidoreductase, NADH:succinate oxidoreductase, and *cis*-aconitase, all iron–sulfur enzymes (54). NO can bind to the iron in ferritin, an iron storage protein, thereby liberating the iron, which could cause lipid peroxidation (54). NO also binds to the nonheme iron of ribonucleotide reductase to inhibit DNA synthesis (54). Its ability to bind iron enables NO to influence iron metabolism. Iron metabolism is regulated post-transcriptionally by specific mRNA–protein interactions between iron-regulatory factor (IRF) and iron-responsive elements (IREs) which occur in the untranslated regions of the mRNA transcripts for the erythroid form of 5-aminolevulinate synthase, the transferrin receptor and ferritin (36,53). Weiss et al. (68) recently showed that NO formed by macrophages augments the IRE binding activity of IRF which causes translational repression of IRE containing messenger RNA.

NO can stimulate the *S*-nitrosylation of numerous proteins (63). NO also stimulates the auto-ADP-ribosylation of glyceraldehyde-3-phosphate dehydrogenase (5,15). This ADP-ribosylation takes place at the cysteine which is at the active site of the enzyme, hence inhibiting its activity and potentially depressing glycolysis.

How is one to ascertain which of these actions is responsible for neurotoxicity? Recent studies provide evidence that DNA damage is central to NO neurotoxicity (71). NO, like other free radicals, can damage DNA by base deamination (69). DNA damage stimulates the activity of poly(ADP ribose) synthetase (PARS). PARS is a nuclear enzyme which utilizes NAD as a substrate to catalyze the attachment of 50–100 ADP-ribose units to nuclear proteins such as histones and, most prominently, to PARS itself (20). In brain homogenates incubated with [^{32}P]NAD, NO stimulates the poly-ADP-ribosylation of PARS (71). NMDA neurotoxicity in cortical cultures is blocked by a series of PARS inhibitors with potencies closely paralleling their potencies in inhibiting PARS. These observations implicate the following series of events in NO neurotoxicity (Fig. 5). NO damages DNA to activate PARS. Massive activation of PARS depletes the cell of NAD and ATP, because four high-energy phosphate bonds, the equivalent of four molecules of ATP, and one of NAD are consumed in the activation of PARS and the regeneration of NAD, respectively. Considering that PARS is a particularly abundant protein and that catalytic activity involves the addition of up to 100 ADP-ribose units to a single protein molecule, it is not surprising that depletion of energy sources takes place when PARS is activated. The resulting cell death accordingly can be blocked by PARS inhibitors. With lesser degrees

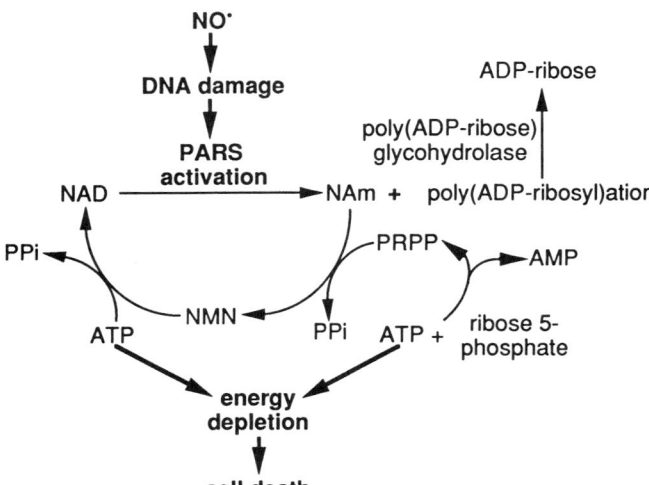

FIG. 5. Mechanism of NO-mediated neurotoxicity. DNA damaged by NO activates PARS, which depletes cells of NAD by poly-ADP-ribosylating nuclear proteins. Poly(ADP-ribose) is rapidly degraded by poly(ADP-ribose) glycohydrolase. This futile cycle continues during the prolonged PARS activation. It takes an equivalent of four ATPs to resynthesize NAD from nicotinamide (NAm) via nicotinamide mononucleotide (NMN), a reaction that requires phosphoribosyl pyrophosphate (PRPP) and ATP. The depletion of energy ultimately leads to cell death. (From ref. 71.)

of DNA damage, PARS activation is thought to facilitate DNA repair (24) (see Chapters 101, 120, 132, and 134, *this volume*).

CARBON MONOXIDE AS A NEURAL MESSENGER

The dramatic properties of NO suggested that it may not be the only gaseous, labile small molecule transmitter. CO is an additional candidate. There are several resemblances between NO and CO disposition. Electrons for NO synthesis are donated by a CPR-like activity of NOS. CPR itself donates electrons to heme oxygenase, the enzyme that makes CO. Heme oxygenase cleaves the heme ring into CO and biliverdin, which is rapidly reduced to bilirubin. Also like NO, CO can bind to the iron in heme, accounting for CO's lethality because hemoglobin can no longer deliver oxygen to tissues. CO can bind to the heme in GC to activate cGMP formation (47). In cultures of olfactory neurons, we showed that CO is responsible for maintaining endogenous cGMP levels, because potent, selective inhibitors of heme oxygenase deplete cGMP, whereas nitroarginine is ineffective (67). Also, as with NOS, heme oxygenase displays discrete localizations. Our in situ hybridization studies demonstrated selective localizations with high levels in the pyramidal cells of the hippocampus and dentate gyrus (67). In the cerebellum, high concentrations are evident in the granule and

Purkinje cells layers, while the pontine nuclei are also heavily labeled. Large densities of heme oxygenase 2 (HO2) are also observed in the piriform cortex, tenia tecta, olfactory tubercle, and islands of Callejae. Highest densities in the brain are in the neurons of the olfactory epithelium and in the neuronal and granule cell layers of the olfactory bulb. Somewhat similar localizations are evident in immunohistochemical studies of enzyme protein (22) (J. L. Dinerman and S. H. Snyder, *unpublished observations*).

Like NO, there are two systems for CO generation. An inducible heme oxygenase (HO1) is responsible for the destruction of heme in aging red blood cells (12,66). New HO1 protein is formed in response to heme as well as numerous oxidative stressors. In contrast, the constitutive form of the enzyme, HO2, is not inducible. HO1 is concentrated in peripheral tissues such as the spleen and liver, while particularly high densities of HO2 occur in the brain (66,67).

Though only recently identified in the brain, CO already has been implicated in various functions. Because HO2 is concentrated in hippocampal pyramidal cells, CO might be a candidate for the retrograde messenger of LTP. Zinc protoporphyrin IX (ZnPP-9) blocks the induction of LTP in the CA1 region of hippocampal slices (73). Application of CO to slices produces a long-lasting increase in the size of evoked synaptic potentials when applied at the same time as a weak tetanic stimulation (65).

Just as NO mediates certain glutamate actions at NMDA receptors, CO may be responsible for glutamate effects via metabotropic receptors. Glaum and Miller (28) showed that metabotropic receptor activation in the solitary tract nucleus of the brainstem regulates a specific channel conductance through a cGMP mechanism. NO synthase inhibitors fail to alter the conductance, but ZnPP-9 and related agents block effects of receptor stimulation in proportion to their potencies as inhibitors of heme oxygenase.

CO also appears to be involved in the regulation of carotid body sensory activity. The chemosensors of the carotid body are regulated by molecular oxygen and inhibited by CO (29). HO2 activity is readily demonstrable in the carotid body (J. L. Dinerman, N. R. Prabhakar, and S. H. Snyder, *unpublished observations*), and ZnPP-9 markedly enhances the chemosensory discharge of the carotid body (57).

SUMMARY

In a remarkably brief period of time, NO and CO have been recognized as putative neurotransmitters. Their unexpected properties have revolutionized thinking about criteria for a chemical's candidacy as a neurotransmitter and about how synaptic transmission takes place. The involvement of NO and CO in several important areas of neuronal function suggests that agents influencing the disposition of NO and CO may have therapeutic relevance. Whether other gases and free radicals will join NO and CO as transmitters is an open question.

REFERENCES

1. Ahlner J, Andersson RGG, Torfgard K, Axelsson KL. Organic nitrate esters: clinical use and mechanisms of actions. *Pharmacol Rev* 1991;43:351–423.
2. Bredt DS, Hwang PM, Snyder SH. Localization of nitric oxide synthase indicating a neural role for nitric oxide. *Nature* 1990; 347:768–770.
3. Bredt DS, Snyder SH. Isolation of nitric oxide synthetase, a calmodulin-requiring enzyme. *Proc Natl Acad Sci USA* 1990; 87:682–685.
4. Bredt DS, Snyder SH. Nitric oxide, a novel neuronal messenger. *Neuron* 1992;8:3–11.
5. Bredt DS, Snyder SH. Nitric oxide: a physiologic messenger molecule. *Annu Rev Biochem* 1994;[in press].
6. Brenneman DE, Westbrook GL, Fitzgerald SP, Ennist DL, Elkins KL, Ruff MR, Pert CB. Neuronal cell killing by the envelope protein of HIV and its prevention by vasoactive intestinal peptide. *Nature* 1988;335:639–642.
7. Breslow MJ, Tobin JR, Bredt DS, Ferris CD, Snyder SH, Traystman RJ. Role of nitric oxide in adrenal medullary vasodilation during catecholamine secretion. *Eur J Pharmacol* 1992;87:682–685.
8. Burnett AL, Lowenstein CJ, Bredt DS, Chang TSK, Snyder SH. Nitric oxide: a physiologic mediator of penile erection. *Science* 1992;257:401–403.
9. Busconi L, Michel T. Endothelial nitric oxide synthase. N-terminal myristoylation determines subcellular localization. *J Biol Chem* 1993;268:8410–8413.
10. Cho HJ, XIE Q-W, Calaycay J, Mumford RA, Swiderek KM, Lee TD, Nathan C. Calmodulin as a tightly bound subunit of calcium-, calmodulin-independent nitric oxide synthase. *J Exp Med* 1992;176:599–604.
11. Choi DW. Glutamate neurotoxicity and diseases of the nervous system. *Neuron* 1988;1:623–634.
12. Cruse I, Maines MD. Evidence suggesting that the two forms of heme oxygenase are products of different genes. *J Biol Chem* 1988;263:3348–3353.
13. Dawson TM, Bredt DS, Fotuhi M, Hwang PM, Snyder SH. Nitric oxide synthase and neuronal NADPH diaphorase are identical in brain and peripheral tissues. *Proc Natl Acad Sci USA* 1991;88:7797–7801.
14. Dawson TM, Hung K, Dawson VL, Steiner JP, Snyder SH. Neuroprotective effects of gangliosides may involve inhibition of nitric oxide synthase. *Ann Neurol* 1994;[in press].
15. Dawson TM, Snyder SH. Gases as biological messengers: nitric oxide and carbon monoxide in the brain. *J Neurosci* 1993;in press.
16. Dawson TM, Steiner JP, Dawson VL, Dinerman JL, Uhl GR, Snyder SH. The immunosuppressant, FK506, enhances phosphorylation of nitric oxide synthase and protects against glutamate neurotoxicity. *Proc Natl Acad Sci USA* 1993;90:9808–9812.
17. Dawson VL, Dawson TM, Bartley DA, Uhl GR, Snyder SH. Mechanisms of nitric oxide mediated neurotoxicity in primary brain cultures. *J Neurosci* 1993;13:2651–2661.
18. Dawson VL, Dawson TM, London ED, Bredt DS, Snyder SH. Nitric oxide mediates glutamate neurotoxicity in primary cortical culture. *Proc Natl Acad Sci USA* 1991;88:6368–6371.
19. Dawson VL, Dawson TM, Uhl GR, Snyder SH. Human immunodeficiency virus type 1 coat protein neurotoxicity mediated by nitric oxide in primary cortical cultures. *Proc Natl Acad Sci USA* 1993;90:3256–3259.
20. de Murcia G, Menissier-de Murcia J, Schreiber V. Poly(ADP-ribose) polymerase: molecular biological aspects. *BioEssays* 1991;13:455–462.
21. Dreyer EB, Kaiser PK, Offermann JT, Lipton SA. HIV-1 coat protein neurotoxicity prevented by calcium channel antagonists. *Science* 1990;248:364–367.
22. Ewing JF, Maines MD. In situ hybridization and immunohistochemical localization of heme oxygenase-2 mRNA and protein in normal rat brain: differential distribution of isozyme 1 and 2 cell. *Mol Cell Neurosci* 1992;3:559–570.
23. Furchgott RF, Zawadzki JV. The obligatory role of endothelial cells in the relaxation of arterial smooth muscle by acetylcholine. *Nature* 1980;288:373–376.
24. Gaal JC, Smith KR, Pearson CK. Cellular euthanasia mediated by a nuclear enzyme: a central role for nuclear ADP-ribosylation in cellular metabolism. *Trends Biol Sci* 1987;12:129–130.
25. Garthwaite J. Glutamate, nitric oxide and cell–cell signalling in the nervous system. *Trends Neurol Sci* 1991;14:60–67.
26. Garthwaite J, Charles SL, Chess-Williams R. Endothelium-derived relaxing factor release on activation of NMDA receptors suggests role as intercellular messenger in the brain. *Nature* 1988;336:385–388.
27. Geller DA, Lowenstein CJ, Shapiro RA, Nussler AK, Di Silvio M, Wang SC, Nakayama DK, Simmons RL, Snyder SH, Biliar TR. Molecular cloning and expression of inducible nitric oxide synthase from human hepatocytes. *Proc Natl Acad Sci USA* 1993;90:3491–3495.
28. Glaum SR, Miller RJ. Zinc protoporphyrin-IX blocks the effects of metabotropic glutamate receptor activation in the rat nucleus tractus solitarii. *Mol Pharmacol* 1993;43:965–969.
29. Gonzalez C, Almaraz L, Obeso A, Rigual R. Oxygen and acid chemoreception in the carotid body chemoreceptors. *Trends Neurosci* 1992;15:146–153.
30. Higashi H, Omori A, Yamagata T. Calmodulin, a ganglioside-binding protein. Binding of gangliosides to calmodulin in the presence of calcium. *J Biol Chem* 1992;267:9831–9838.
31. Higashi H, Yamagata T. Mechanism for ganglioside-mediated modulation of a calmodulin-dependent enzyme. Modulation of calmodulin-dependent cyclic nucleotide phosphodiesterase activity through binding of gangliosides to calmodulin and the enzyme. *J Biol Chem* 1992;267:9839–9843.
32. Hiki K, Hattori R, Kawai C, Yui Y. Purification of insoluble nitric oxide synthase from rat cerebellum. *J Biochem* 1993;111:556–558.
33. Hirsch DB, Steiner JP, Dawson TM, Mammen A, Hayek E, Snyder SH. Neurotransmitter release regulated by nitric oxide in PC-12 cells and brain synaptosomes. *Curr Biol* 1993;3:749–754.
34. Hope BT, Michael GJ, Knigge KM, Vincent SR. Neuronal NADPH diaphorase is a nitric oxide synthase. *Proc Natl Acad Sci USA* 1991;88:2811–2814.
35. Ignarro LJ. Biosynthesis and metabolism of endothelium-derived nitric oxide. *Annu Rev Pharmacol Toxicol* 1990;30:535–560.
36. Klausner RD, Rouault TA. A double life: cytosolic aconitase as a regulatory RNA binding protein. *Mol Biol Cell* 1993;4:1–5.
37. Koh J-Y, Peters S, Choi DW. Neurons containing NADPH-diaphorase are selectively resistant to quinolinate toxicity. *Science* 1986;234:73–76.
38. Lei SZ, Pan ZH, Aggarwal SK, Chen HSV, Hartman J, Sucher NJ, Lipton SA. Effect on nitric oxide production on the redox modulatory site of the NMDA receptor–channel complex. *Neuron* 1992;8:1087–1099.
39. Lipton SA. Requirement for macrophages in neuronal injury induced by HIV envelope protein gp120. *NeuroReport* 1992;3:913–915.
40. Lipton SA, Choi YB, Pan Z-H, Lei SZ, Vincent Chen H-S, Sucher NJ, Loscalzo J, Singel DJ, Stamler JS. A redox-based mechanism for the neuroprotective and neurodestructive effects of nitric oxide and related nitroso-compounds. *Nature* 1993;364:626–632.
41. Lipton SA, Sucher NJ, Kaiser PK, Dreyer EB. Synergistic effects of HIV coat protein and NMDA receptor-mediated neurotoxicity. *Neuron* 1991;7:111–118.
42. Liu J, Farmer JD Jr, Lane WS, Friedman J, Weissman I, Schreiber SL. Calcineurin is a common target of cyclophilin-cyclosporin A and FKBP-FK506 complexes. *Cell* 1991;66:807–815.
43. Lopez OL, Martinez AJ, Torre-Cisneros J. Neuropathologic findings in liver transplantation: a comparative study of cyclosporine and FK506. *Transplant Proc* 1991;23:3181–3182.
44. Lowenstein CJ, Alley EW, Raval P, Snowman AM, Snyder SH, Russell SW, Murphy WJ. Macrophage nitric oxide synthase gene:

two upstream regions mediate induction by interferon-gamma and lipopolysaccharide. *Proc Natl Acad Sci USA* 1993;90:9730–9734.

45. Lowenstein CJ, Snyder SH. Nitric oxide, a novel biologic messenger. *Cell* 1992;70:705–707.

46. Mahadik Sahebarao P. Gangliosides: new generation of neuroprotective agents. In: Malangos PJ, Lal H, eds. *Emerging strategics in neuroprotection.* Boston: Birkhäuser, 1992;187–223.

47. Marks GS, Brein JF, Nakatsu K, McLaughlin BE. Does carbon monoxide have a physiological function. *Trends Pharmacol Sci* 1991;12:185–188.

48. Marletta MA. Nitric oxide: biosynthesis and biological significance. *Trends Biochem Sci* 1989;14:488–492.

49. Marletta MA. Nitric oxide synthase structure and mechanism. *J Biol Chem* 1993;268:12231–12234.

50. Meldrum B, Garthwaite J. Excitatory amino acid neurotoxicity and neurodegenerative disease. *Trends Pharmacol Sci* 1990;11:379–387.

51. Michel T, Li GK, Busconi L. Phosphorylation and subcellular translocation of endothelial nitric oxide synthase. *Proc Natl Acad Sci USA* 1993;90:6252–6256.

52. Moncada S, Palmer RMJ, Higgs EA. Nitric oxide: physiology, pathophysiology and pharmacology. *Pharmacol Rev* 1991;43:109–142.

53. Munro H. The ferritin genes: their response to iron status. *Nutr Rev* 1993;51:65–73.

54. Nathan C. Nitric oxide as a secretory product of mammalian cells. *FASEB J* 1992;6:3051–3064.

55. Nozaki K, Moskowitz MA, Maynard KI, Koketsu N, Dawson TM, Bredt DS, Snyder SH. Possible origins and distribution of immunoreactive nitric oxide synthase-containing nerve fibers in rat and human cerebral arteries. *J Cereb Blood Flow Metab* 1993;13:70–79.

56. Pollock JS, Forstermann U, Mitchell JA, Warner TD, Schmidt HHHW, Nakane M, Murad F. Purification and characterization of particulate endothelium-derived relaxing factor synthase from cultured and native bovine aortic endothelial cells. *Proc Natl Acad Sci USA* 1991;88:10480–10484.

57. Prabhakar NR, Agani FH, Dinerman JL, Snyder SH. Endogenous carbon monoxide (CO) and carotid body sensory activity. *Soc Neurosci Abstr* 1993;19:1402.

58. Rajfer J, Aronson WJ, Bush PA, Dorey FJ, Ignarro LJ. Nitric oxide as a mediator of the corpus cavernosum in response to nonadrenergic noncholinergic transmission. *N Engl J Med* 1992;326:90–94.

59. Sandberg K, Berry CJ, Eugster E, Rogers TB. A role for cGMP during tetanus toxin blockade of acetylcholine release in the rat

pheochromocytoma (PC12) cell lines. *J Neurosci* 1989;9:3946–3954.

60. Sandberg K, Berry CJ, Rogers TB. Studies on the intoxication pathway of tetanus toxin in the rat pheochromocytoma (PC12) cell line. *J Biol Chem* 1989;264:5679–5686.

61. Shiga Y, Onodera H, Matsuo Y, Kogure K. Cyclosporin A protects against ischemia-reperfusion injury in the brain. *Brain Res* 1992;595:145–148.

62. Skaper SD, Leon A. Monosialogangliosides, neuroprotection, and neuronal repair processes. *J Neurotrauma* 1992;9:S506–S516.

63. Stamler JS, Simon DI, Osborne JA, Mullins ME, Jaraki O, Michel T, Singel DJ, Loscalzo J. S-Nitrosylation of proteins with nitric oxide: synthesis and characterization of biologically active compounds. *Proc Natl Acad Sci USA* 1992;89:444–448.

64. Steiner JP, Dawson TM, Fotuhi M, Glatt CE, Snowman AM, Cohen N, Snyder SH. High brain densities of the immunophilin FKBP colocalized with calcineurin. *Nature* 1992;358:584–587.

65. Stevens CF, Wang Y. Reversal of long-term potentiation by inhibitors of haem oxygenase. *Nature* 1993;364:147–148.

66. Sun Y, Rotenberg MO, Maines MD. Developmental expression of heme oxygenase isozymes in rat brain. Two HO-2 mRNAs are detected. *J Biol Chem* 1990;265:8212–8217.

67. Verma A, Hirsch DJ, Glatt CE, Ronnett GV, Snyder SH. Carbon monoxide, a putative neural messenger. *Science* 1993;259:381–384.

68. Weiss G, Goossen B, Doppler W, Fuchs D, Pantopoulos K, Werner-Felmayer G, Wachter H, Hentze MW. Translational regulation via iron-responsive elements by the nitric oxide/NO-synthase pathway. *EMBO J* 1993;12:3651–3657.

69. Wink DA, Kasprzak KS, Maragos CM, Elespuru RK, Misra M, Dunams TM, Cebula TA, Koch WH, Andrews AW, Allen JS, Keefer LK. DNA deaminating ability and genotoxicity of nitric oxide and its progenitors. *Science* 1991;254:1001–1003.

70. Xie QW, Whisnant R, Nathan C. Promoter of the mouse gene encoding calcium-independent nitric oxide synthase confers inducibility by interferon gamma and bacterial lipopolysaccharide. *J Exp Med* 1993;177:1779–1784.

71. Zhang J, Dawson VL, Dawson TM, Snyder SH. Poly(ADP-ribose) synthetase activation by nitric oxide damaged DNA may mediate neurotoxicity. *Science* 1994;263:687–689.

72. Zhang ZG, Chopp M, Zaloga C, Pollock JS, Forstermann U. Cerebral endothelial nitric oxide synthase expression after focal cerebral ischemia in rat. *Stroke* 1993;24:2016–2021.

73. Zhuo M, Small SA, Kandel ER, Hawkins RD. Nitric oxide and carbon monoxide produce activity-dependent long-term synaptic enhancement in hippocampus. *Science* 1993;260:1946–1950.

Psychopharmacology: The Fourth Generation of Progress, edited by Floyd E. Bloom and David J. Kupfer. Raven Press, Ltd., New York © 1995.

CHAPTER 55

Neuronal Growth and Differentiation Factors and Synaptic Plasticity

Paul H. Patterson

There is a growing realization that mechanisms and molecules that regulate the development of circuits in the embryonic nervous system can also influence the flow of synaptic information in maturity. This is done both by modifying the efficacy of transmission at established connections and by regulating the rearrangement of such connections. It is now well known that neuronal survival and growth in the embryo is controlled in part by proteins and steroids that act as trophic (Greek for nourishment) factors. These factors can govern the number of neurons that innervate a target cell in a retrograde fashion, through secretion of the factors by the target cell. Trophic factors can also act anterogradely, allowing a neuron to influence its targets, as well as more globally, either through the circulation or via glial or immune cells. In addition to controlling life, death, and growth, these and other families of factors can act instructively, to direct neurons to adopt one or another phenotype. For example, a noradrenergic neuron can be converted to the cholinergic phenotype by such a differentiation factor. In fact, this switch in phenotype is known to occur during the normal development of a subpopulation of sympathetic neurons when they contact their particular target cell type, the sweat gland. Dramatic changes in transmitter and associated neuropeptide systems like these are due to the ability of instructive neuronal differentiation factors to direct gene expression (see Chapters 59, 60, and 98, *this volume*).

It is less well appreciated that these phenomena of plasticity in growth and gene expression persist into maturity. There is evidence implicating growth and differentiation factors in synaptic plasticity and particular behaviors. The implications of this plasticity are threefold: (i) The adult system is metastable, representing a balance between

growth and withdrawal, gene induction, and repression; (ii) neuronal trophic and differentiation factors are required for maintenance of the mature system; and (iii) these proteins and hormones could therefore be used for therapeutic intervention. Thus, growth and differentiation factors are potent and highly specific tools, not only for the rescue of dying neurons, but also for changing the balance of transmitter and neuropeptide systems, thereby modifying behavior (see Chapter 60, *this volume*).

TROPHIC FACTORS

The classic trophic factor is, of course, nerve growth factor (NGF). Its best known activity is the rescue of particular sets of embryonic neurons from death. In many parts of the nervous system, 50% of the neurons produced during embryogenesis die during subsequent development, and the target tissues that neurons innervate can play a major role in controlling how many neurons survive (125). This survival effect of targets is mediated in part by trophic factors such as NGF. The family of NGF-related survival factors is now composed of at least four members [the *neurotrophins:* NGF, brain-derived neurotrophic factor (BDNF), neurotrophins 3 and 4/5 (NT-3, NT-4/5); see Table 1] (135). The neurotrophins are not only required for survival, but they enhance growth of neuronal cell bodies and processes in a dose-dependent manner.

The neurotrophins act on partially overlapping populations of neurons in both the central nervous system (CNS) and peripheral nervous system (PNS) (61). Responsivity to the various family members is determined by which neurotrophin receptor is expressed on a neuron's surface. The high-affinity receptors for this family belong to the *trk* family of transmembrane protein kinases (21). The

P. H. Patterson: Biology Division, California Institute of Technology, Pasadena, California 91125.

TABLE 1. *Neuronal differentiation and growth factors*[a]

Neurotrophins
NGF (nerve growth factor)
BDNF (brain-derived neurotrophic factor)
NT-3, NT-4/5 (neurotrophins 3 and 4/5)

Neuropoietic factors
CDF/LIF (cholinergic differentiation factor/leukemia inhibitory factor)
CNTF (ciliary neurotrophic factor)
OSM (oncostatin M)
GPA (growth-promoting activity)
SGF (sweat gland factor)
IL-6, IL-11 (interleukins 6 and 11)

TGF family
EGF (epidermal growth factor)
TGF-α, TGF-β (transforming growth factors α and β)
GDNF (glial-cell-line-derived neurotrophic factor)
Activin A

FGF family
aFGF, bFGF (acidic and basic fibroblast growth factors)
FGF-5

Insulin-like growth factors
Insulin
IGF (insulin-like growth factors)

Platelet-derived growth factors
PDGF

[a] This list includes only those cytokines discussed in this chapter and is therefore not complete.

basal forebrain cholinergic neurons, well known because of their potential role in learning and memory and their loss in Alzheimer's disease, are the most intensively characterized neurotrophin-sensitive cells in the CNS. Of particular clinical interest are studies demonstrating that administration of NGF to rats with lesioned CNS cholinergic neurons enhances the survival of these neurons as well as performance in spatial memory tasks (29). Similar results were obtained with unlesioned but impaired, aged rats (38). Moreover, BDNF mRNA is decreased in the hippocampus of Alzheimer brains, relative to other mRNAs assayed (96). BDNF is also implicated in motor neuron disease and its potential treatment. This protein prevents the death of motor neurons after nerve section (60, 121,150), and its mRNA is expressed at the appropriate stages in the embryonic spinal cord and in the limb bud for it to act on spinal neurons during development (48). NT-3 and NT-4/5 also share this expression pattern and can rescue motoneurons in culture (48). In addition, two proteins belonging to a different cytokine family, the neuropoietic factors cholinergic differentiation factor/leukemia inhibitory factor (CDF/LIF) and ciliary neurotrophic factor (CNTF) (discussed below), also promote motor neuron survival (73,88). Moreover, CNTF prevents the degeneration of motor neurons in a mutant mouse model of progressive motor neuronopathy (122). For these reasons, CNTF is currently being tested in clinical trials with amyotrophic lateral sclerosis (ALS) patients.

Other trophic factors active on CNS neurons include insulin and insulin-like growth factors [IGFs (56,65); also being tested on ALS patients], fibroblast growth factors [FGFs (51,139); FGF-5 is also a good candidate as the motor neuron trophic factor (51)], platelet-derived growth factors (23,52), and members of the transforming growth factor superfamily [TGFs (78,98)]. Of particular interest is the recent discovery of a trophic factor for midbrain dopamine neurons, called glial-cell-line-derived neurotrophic factor [GDNF (68)]. A member of the TGFβ superfamily, GDNF is more selective in its action on midbrain cultures than other factors that enhance survival of dopaminergic cells such as IGF-I and II, epidermal growth factor (EGF), aFGF and bFGF, and BDNF. It will be of interest to see the results of tests of the utility of GDNF in Parkinson's disease models.

DIFFERENTIATION FACTORS

In addition to neuronal survival and growth, target tissues can also control the phenotype of the neurons that innervate them. Phenotypic traits regulated qualitatively by targets in vivo include (a) the neuron's transmitter and neuropeptide profile (62) and (b) the type of synapses the neuron receives on its dendrites. That is, targets encountered by a neuron's axons in the periphery can influence the connections made on that neuron's dendrites in the CNS (reviewed in ref. 39). A classic example of the presumptive ability of a postsynaptic cell to control the phenotype of its presynaptic input is the type of synapses formed by the various branches of single auditory nerve fibers. When these axons contact neurons in one region of the cochlear nucleus, they form the very large end bulbs of Held; when collateral branches of the same axons encounter neurons in other regions of the nucleus, they form small boutons (102). Qualitative control of this order can be regulated by the neuronal differentiation factors, and such effects can be distinguished from the classical NGF survival and growth activities. Differentiation factors characteristically alter neuronal gene expression and phenotype without changing neuronal survival or growth (90).

The most intensively studied family of instructive differentiation factors is termed the *neuropoietic cytokines,* named for their effects on both the nervous and hematopoietic systems. Unlike the neurotrophins, this group of proteins does not share an extensive degree of amino acid sequence identity. The neuropoietic family members are linked by (a) the many biological activities they have in common (36,59,93), (b) the protein structure they are predicted to share in common with growth hormone (14,111), and (c) their promiscuous use of common receptor subunits (28,41).

Five of the neuropoietic cytokines [CDF/LIF, CNTF, OSM (oncostatin M), GPA (growth-promoting activity), and SGF (sweat gland factor; not yet cloned)] evoke nearly identical changes in gene expression when added to cultured sympathetic neurons, while the somewhat more distantly related family members, interleukins 6 and 11 (IL-6 and IL-11), evoke a subset of these changes (36,104,116). There is a striking overlap in the activities of CDF/LIF, IL-6, and IL-11 on other types of cells such as hepatic and myeloid cells, however (59). The molecular basis for this apparent functional redundancy is the sharing of common subunits in the receptor complexes for these cytokines (28,41). Not only can some of these cytokines displace others at high-affinity ligand binding sites, but the receptor complexes can all employ the same transducing subunit (129). Presumably, a shared signal transducer ensures an identical set of effects on gene expression in the target cells. While there are a number of inconsistencies in this current picture (41), the sharing of receptor subunits is a major chapter in the story of this family.

Initially surprising, redundancy in ligand activity and promiscuity in the use of receptor subunits has also become a theme of cytokine action in the hematopoietic system (85). Moreover, it occurs in the neurotrophin family (21). One possibility is that other, more selective and nonoverlapping receptors may be discovered in the future. This would allow the members of the cytokine family to evoke unique as well as overlapping effects, leading to interesting combinatorial possibilities. Another parallel between the generation of cell diversity in the hematopoietic and nervous systems lies in the pyramidal structures of their lineages. It appears that multipotential stem cells generate progenitors committed to particular pathways, each of which may yield multiple phenotypes (8). Moreover, proliferation and differentiation at each of these steps can be influenced by cytokines that are shared between the hematopoietic and nervous systems (82,93).

Not all intercellular signals that direct neuronal gene expression belong to the neuropoietic family. Activin A, a member of the TGF superfamily, induces a different, but partially overlapping, set of genes when compared to the neuropoietic cytokines in the cultured sympathetic neurons (36). Activin A can also mimic a target-derived factor that induces expression of the neuropeptide somatostatin (SOM) in cultured ciliary ganglion neurons (25). Moreover, activin A mRNA is found in cells cultured from this target (the choroid; see ref. 24).

What is the role of these differentiation factors in the nervous system? In the adult, evidence is emerging that these proteins can serve interesting functions in the response to injury (see below). In development, attention has focused on a possible role for the neuropoietic cytokines in the switch in phenotype that sympathetic neurons undergo when they contact the sweat glands. Landis (62) demonstrated that noradrenergic sympathetic neurons switch their transmitter phenotype to cholinergic when their axons contact sweat glands, even if this target tissue

is placed in ectopic locations. The change in gene expression that occurs in this switch is very similar to that evoked in cultured sympathetic neurons when either CDF/LIF, CNTF, GPA, or OSM are added. Studies on the cholinergic differentiation factor extracted from rat sweat glands suggest that it is a unique protein, resembling CNTF (103,110). There is, in fact, good evidence that CDF/LIF can convert noradrenergic sympathetic neurons to the cholinergic phenotype in vivo. A transgenic mouse line was created in which an insulin transcriptional promoter was used to ectopically express CDF/LIF in pancreatic islet cells. The result is an induction of cholinergic properties in the sympathetic innervation of the pancreas (R. Palmiter, *unpublished data*). Recent experiments have further demonstrated that labeled CDF/LIF can be taken up by the endings of sympathetic neurons and retrogradely transported back to the neuronal cell body (49).

It is now clear that the same protein can act instructively as a differentiation factor or permissively as a growth factor, depending on the responsive cell population. CDF/LIF, for instance, can act as a survival factor, enhancing the growth of embryonic sensory and motor neurons (44,73,80). CNTF and GPA can act as trophic factors for ciliary neurons, and GPA is expressed in chick eye during the period of naturally occurring cell death for ciliary neurons that innervate eye muscles (66). CNTF can also prevent axotomy-induced death in the CNS (22). By the same token, the trophic factor BDNF can selectively induce the expression of the neuropeptides SOM and neuropeptide Y (NPY) in cultures of rat cortical neurons, without affecting neuronal survival in this population (83). Similarly, NGF can selectively induce the expression of particular neuropeptides in sensory neurons (70).

ANTEROGRADE CONTROL OF GENE EXPRESSION

The discussion to this point has emphasized the role of target tissues in the control of neuronal survival and gene expression. It is clear that anterograde effects, from neurons to their targets, can be another major mechanism in development and in maturity. Anterograde influences can be mediated by small molecules or by proteins. In the former class are the neurotransmitters and neuropeptides released by the presynaptic terminal. These signaling agents evoke changes in ion fluxes and intracellular messengers in the postsynaptic cell that have long been known to up-regulate transmitter biosynthesis in many types of neurons. This transsynaptic effect is an effective way for the stimulated postsynaptic neuron to replenish its transmitter stores that are transiently depleted by its newly elevated rate of activity and consequent release rates. When stimulation is prolonged, transsynaptic induction of mRNAs for the transmitter biosynthetic enzymes and neuropeptide precursors is elicited, thereby chronically elevating transmitter and neuropeptide production (10,42,153). Evoked activity can also influence the choice of which transmitter is to be produced. For instance, depolarization of cultured sympathetic and sensory neurons blocks their responses to certain differentiation factors (CDF/LIF but not CNTF; see ref. 105). There are also numerous examples of regulation of neuropeptide as well as neuronal trophic factor expression by activity (see refs. 16,32, and 55). It is also important to note that there is evidence that neurotransmitters themselves can regulate cell proliferation and differentiation (63).

More novel is the notion that proteins may also act as anterograde trophic or differentiation signals. While not known to be a neuronal differentiation or trophic factor, the protein agrin is a good example of signal that can act in an anterograde fashion. Motor neurons in the spinal cord can produce agrin, transport it anterogradely to their synaptic endings, and release it (108,113). Agrin then binds to the muscle cell and evokes clustering of several different muscle surface proteins under the synaptic endings (114).

Neurons also anterogradely transport known cytokines. In addition to acting as a trophic factor for many types of neurons in culture, bFGF has been shown to be anterogradely transported by retinal ganglion neurons to their target sites in the lateral geniculate body and the superior colliculus (37). FGF is also known to be synthesized and released by retinal cells in vivo (45). There is also evidence that the neurotransmitter vesicles of adrenal chromaffin cells contain bFGF (97,144). Moreover, preliminary reports indicate that neurotrophic activity is released from these cells when they are depolarized (138). Chromaffin cells also contain several TGF-βs and a CNTF-like trophic factor (138,140). Because chromaffin cells resemble neurons in many respects, and neurons themselves produce neurotrophic factors (see refs. 34,119, and 145), it seems highly likely that these factors are used in the nervous system in both the antero- and retrograde directions. There is ample evidence that anterograde influences can regulate neuronal survival and gene expression during development (42,87).

A key feature of cytokines acting in retrograde and anterograde pathways is that these transsynaptic actions make use of the exceedingly complex circuitry that underlies nervous system function. This is important for two reasons. First, because the circuitry is designed for discrete, cell-to-cell interactions, cytokines can regulate neuronal survival and gene expression with the same degree of precision that is inherent in the wiring. This allows for unique differentiation decisions by individual neurons within layers or large groups of cells. Such small, minority populations are, in fact, a common feature of many parts of the nervous system. Second, using circuitry to control gene expression will help ensure that the phenotypes of neurons linked in a given pathway are functionally appropriate. Postsynaptic receptors must match transmitters released presynaptically, for example. If the genes for these proteins are regulated in part by interactions between the synaptic partners, phenotype need not be completely preprogrammed earlier in development. Moreover, phenotypic decisions can be reversed at very late stages, because axons encounter distinct synaptic partners in postnatal life (62) (see also Chapters 63 and 132, this volume).

GROWTH AND DIFFERENTIATION FACTORS IN THE ADULT NERVOUS SYSTEM

Growth and differentiation factors are known to act in the normal, undamaged, adult nervous system, and they play a role in the response to injury as well. There is considerable evidence in the older literature that the adult system, while seemingly very stable, is actually in a state of dynamic equilibrium (99). For example, it has been known for many decades that denervation of skeletal muscle causes a series of changes in the myotubes that can be viewed as a return to an embryonic, preinnervation state. When nerves subsequently reinnervate the myotubes, a sequence of changes that were seen in development unfolds once again, producing a mature muscle. Thus, the nerve controls the state of differentiation of the muscle. Much of the influence of the nerve is mediated through synaptic transmission; that is, it is based on activity. Indeed, many of the changes observed in denervation can be prevented by electrically stimulating the muscle after cutting the nerve.

Similar phenomena are observed in the nerve fibers when imbalances are introduced experimentally. If only part of the muscle is denervated, the remaining, intact axons are observed to sprout and innervate the denervated myotubes. An activity-based mechanism can be invoked here as well, because sprouting can also be induced by blocking nerve–muscle transmission or paralyzing the muscle, and electrical stimulation of the muscle prevents sprouting induced by partial denervation. These and other experiments illustrate the state of dynamic balance that the mature nerve–muscle system represents. Similar phenomena have been repeatedly observed in neuron–neuron synapses. In fact, contemporary imaging methods are sufficiently sensitive that they have demonstrated that even in intact, undisturbed neuron–neuron and neuron–muscle synapses, small axonal sprouts are constantly arising, parts of postsynaptic gutters are being vacated, and new contacts are being formed (100,146). Moreover, sprouting from intact synapses can be evoked by administration of trophic factors such as IGF-2 and CNTF (18,44).

These and other observations suggest that neurotrophic and differentiation factors may participate in the regulation of synaptic circuitry in the intact adult system. Consistent with this hypothesis is the evidence that neuronal activity can control the transcription of the genes for these factors. For example, the balance between the activity of the glutaminergic and γ-aminobutyric acid systems can regulate the level of BDNF and NGF mRNA in the adult rat hippocampus (151). In the visual system, physiological variations in sensory stimulation can elicit dramatic changes in neurotrophin expression. One hour of exposure to light after a period in the dark can nearly double the levels of BDNF mRNA in adult rat visual cortex (20). Because light-evoked activity can control the growth and sprouting of axons in the visual cortex, it was also of interest to test the effects of neurotrophin administration on this phenomenon. In fact, NGF can prevent the shift in ocular dominance normally observed in monocularly deprived rats and cats (72).

The neuropoietic cytokines may also be involved in such regulatory events. For instance, CDF/LIF mRNA levels are highest in the visual cortex and hippocampus, reaching maximal values in adulthood (77,91,149). The same conclusions hold for the CDF/LIF receptor (11). Moreover, mice in which the CDF/LIF gene has been disrupted by homologous recombination display severe alterations in the hippocampus and visual cortex (94). It is not yet known, however, whether these alterations occur during development or in maturity. It is now clear that the adult sensory cortex is capable of enormous plasticity, making very large changes in sensory maps exceedingly quickly (35). It will be of great interest to see what role the trophic and differentiation factors play in these remarkable changes in wiring. Another very promising area is that of gene expression in the adult CNS. There is evidence that continual presence of differentiation factors such as CDF/LIF is required for maintenance of neuropeptide expression in peripheral sensory neurons, for instance (82).

Another key group of trophic and differentiation factors active in the CNS are the *steroid hormones.* In addition to their organizational effects on the embryonic brain (17), gonadal steroids can direct neuropeptide expression in the adult CNS independently of effects on neuronal survival and growth. Estrogen regulates the expression of cholecystokinin (CCK) and substance P (SP) mRNAs differentially in a sexually dimorphic pathway in the amygdala (123). The selectivity of this control is particularly striking because these two neuropeptides are co-expressed in the same neurons. The hormonal influence is exerted during normal physiological events as indicated by the fact that the number of CCK-expressing neurons varies over the estrous cycle (89). The variation in CCK content makes it likely that the character of the synaptic transmission between this subset of estrogen-sensitive neurons in the amygdala and their target cells in the preoptic area is altered during the estrous cycle. Such alterations have been termed "chemical switching" of transmission by these cells (128). Another striking example of this phenomenon is the differential regulation of galanin (GAL)

and luteinizing-hormone-releasing hormone (LHRH) in neurons that express both neuropeptides simultaneously. In female rats, such neurons in the medial preoptic area and their axons in the median eminence contain higher levels of GAL during proestrus than during estrus, while the number of neurons expressing LHRH is unaffected by the hormonal state of the organism (76).

These examples of hormonal regulation are especially interesting because the presence of a co-expressed neuropeptide that does not change with hormonal fluctuations serves as a good control for true trophic effects. Thus, the steroid effects described here are "activational," altering gene expression in the mature brain rather than (or in addition to) guiding the morphological organization of the system during development. Such activational alterations in gene expression have been observed in several other areas of the brain and PNS that subserve reproductive behaviors (30,46,115). Also worth noting is that the changes in neuropeptide expression represent only part of this story. Estrogen may also regulate neurotransmitter and steroid receptor levels (5,9). Finally, estradiol can alter neuronal circuitry on a very rapid time scale. In the 24-hr period between proestrus and estrus, for example, synaptic density in the CA1 region of the hippocampus declines about a third (147), a result consistent with changes in synaptic density evoked by experimental manipulations in hormone levels.

Glucocorticoids instruct neuropeptide and neurotransmitter expression in several systems. The corticotropin-releasing factor (CRF)-containing neurons of the paraventricular nucleus of the hypothalamus express at least eight different transmitters/peptides simultaneously. Glucocorticoid exerts a selective, negative feedback on the expression of CRF and vasopressin (VP), without affecting levels of enkephalin and neurotensin (see ref. 128). CRF mRNA levels follow the diurnal surge in corticosterone, and adrenalectomy results in higher CRF and a massive increase in VP (54,143). Independent control of the many neuropeptides in these neurons is likely to reflect the fact that these neurons are thought to form various synapses with different functions as their axons traverse the hypothalamus, median eminence, and anterior pituitary (128). The three physiological conditions of chronically low, medium, and high circulating corticosterone would yield paraventricular neurons of three distinct chemical states with discrete functional consequences. This steroid, in its neuronal differentiation factor role, thereby alters synaptic function in an anatomically stable circuit that is the final common pathway for mediating the pituitary–adrenal response to stress, on a minute-to-minute time scale (see ref. 54). In addition, there is evidence that VP/CRF co-expression is enhanced in response to behavioral stress paradigms in the absence of adrenal glands (J. Barrett, A.-J. Silverman, and D. Kelly, *personal communication*).

Glucocorticoids may also act indirectly to alter neuronal gene expression. For example, corticosterone (as well as testosterone) can regulate NGF expression in neurons and astrocytes (12,69). This hormone can also inhibit the production of CDF/LIF by heart cells and non-neuronal cells of sympathetic ganglia (40,47,75). This inhibition can thereby affect the phenotype of neurons cultured with such non-neuronal cells.

Another aspect of cytokine action in the adult nervous system is the response to injury. Wounds in the CNS or severing a peripheral nerve results in the up-regulation of many growth and differentiation factors, including CDF/LIF, NGF, TGF-β1, and glial maturation factor β (see ref. 95). Tumor necrosis factor α (TNF-α), IL-1α, FGF, and EGF have also been implicated in the response to nerve injury (13,26,33,112,132). Although the interplay of these signaling agents with neurons, glia, and immune cells is not well understood, there is evidence that damaged neurons may participate in feedback loops involving neuronal differentiation factors in the injury response. For example, transecting postganglionic nerves, or culturing sympathetic ganglia for 24 hr, causes a dramatic increase in the neuropeptides vasoactive intestinal polypeptide (VIP), SP, and GAL (53,106,107,154). This is of interest in the context of the neuropoietic cytokines because these agents can induce the same peptides in sympathetic neurons. Moreover, cutting these nerves or isolating the ganglia in culture causes an enormous rise in CDF/LIF mRNA (11). Tying these observations together is the recent finding that ganglia from CDF/LIF-deficient mice (produced by disrupting this gene by homologous recombination) do not display this striking increase in VIP and GAL expression upon explanation to culture or axotomy (107). Thus, CDF/LIF mediates a major part of the neuropeptide induction that occurs in response to injury.

Why is the neuropeptide phenotype altered when sympathetic neurons are damaged? One possibility is that the neuropeptides play a trophic role. Tissue injury and inflammation, for instance, alter neuronal gene expression through enhanced nociceptor (pain receptors) activity, and the induced neuropeptides and excitatory amino acids are thought to be involved in the axonal sprouting and plasticity associated with these injuries and with nerve damage (31,127). A novel possibility in the case of sympathetic neurons is that it may be important to change the neuropeptides the neurons are producing. Release of CDF/LIF could induce the particular neuropeptides that are known to attract immune cells and activate them (VIP and SP) (reviewed in ref. 95). There is evidence that sympathetic axons participate in the inflammation associated with arthritis (67). A role for CDF/LIF in the nervous system injury response fits nicely with its proposed functions in the hematopoietic and hepatic responses to infection (59) (see also Chapters 45, 50, and 62, this volume).

BEHAVIOR AND SYNAPTIC PLASTICITY

A major, and perhaps unexpected, feature of the studies discussed thus far is that dynamic alterations in transmitter/neuropeptide expression can occur in postnatal, fully functional neurons. This can occur as a response to normal fluctuations in neuronal activity or hormone levels, or in response to injury or other insults to the system. Because these alterations in neuronal gene expression can entail qualitative changes in the mode of synaptic transmission (e.g., chemical switching), it is worth asking how many higher functions/behaviors may be influenced by instructive differentiation factors in the normal organism. As discussed in the prior section, the behaviors associated with the estrous cycle are clearly higher functions that can be included in this context. A second example is the circadian rhythms that drive many different behaviors.

In mammals, daily rhythms such as the sleep–wake cycle are controlled by a circadian clock located in the suprachiasmatic nucleus (SCN) of the anterior hypothalamus. Ablation of the SCN disrupts the daily rhythm of locomotor activity (125), and implantation of an SCN drives the circadian rhythm of the host animal according to the clock of the donor (64,101). The SCN contains two major neuronal populations, one containing VIP and the other containing arginine-VP (142). Neuropeptide mRNAs, neuropeptide levels, and neuropeptide release vary precisely with the circadian cycle (6,86,137). The importance of the SCN peptides in controlling the rhythm is shown by the ability of injected VIP and peptide histidine isoleucine to shift the cycle (7).

What drives the cyclic changes in SCN neuropeptide mRNAs? Neuronal activity from visual afferents presumably regulates VIP expression, because its mRNA levels are influenced by light (86). In contrast, the diurnal change in VP mRNA and peptide is not influenced by visual inputs or endocrine products (19). Moreover, the diurnal cycle of VP release is retained by SCN explants in vitro, and it is also observed in dissociated neurons in long-term cell cultures (79). These observations suggest that the SCN can serve as a circadian pacemaker independently of exogenous neural and endocrine regulation. Possible mechanisms include cell autonomous oscillations and oscillations in the interactions among cells within the SCN, including potential variations in paracrine/autocrine cytokine release or action. There is evidence to support both of these mechanisms (79,130).

There is also evidence that oscillations in paracrine/autocrine factors could play a role. Levels of the neurotrophic cytokine S100β exhibit circadian variation in the SCN and visual cortex (141). In addition, there is correlative evidence that S100β may be involved in the development of serotonin neurons in the CNS (4,81,136). Thus, it is possible that the diurnal variations in S100β in the SCN could contribute to the variations in neuropeptide expression there. Although there is presently only circumstantial evidence implicating cytokines in circadian rhythms, these systems are rich areas for investigation.

Alterations in synaptic transmission are also believed

to be central to the complex events comprising learning and memory. Long-term potentiation (LTP) of synaptic efficacy is one of the most intensively studied mechanisms in this regard (see ref. 126). Is there a role for cytokines in LTP and similar types of synaptic plasticity? It is clear that expression of neurotrophins such as NGF and BDNF can be regulated by neuronal activity in a time scale of hours (55,71,151). As discussed above, cytokines can be transported anterogradely to synaptic endings and can be released by depolarization, and they can act retrogradely as well. In fact, tetanic stimulation of intact neocortex releases heat-labile factors that enhance neurite outgrowth from PC12 cells (a sympathetic neuron-like line) as well as induce LTP in slices of hippocampus (117). The LTP-inducing factors do not appear to influence resting membrane potential or input resistance. The LTP-inducing activities in the cortical superfusate are heterogeneous in size, ranging from <3 to >50 kD (148). The high-molecular-weight fraction induces LTP soon after its application, whereas the smaller fractions require 50 min to induce potentiation. These results suggest that diverse molecules and mechanisms are involved. It is also worthwhile examining known factors; a stimulus paradigm used to induce LTP in hippocampal slices produces enhanced levels of BDNF and NT-3 mRNAs (92).

The complementary type of experiment—testing known cytokines and their antagonists in LTP paradigms—is also informative. In hippocampal slices, EGF and FGF enhance potentiation of the population spike amplitude and field excitatory postsynaptic potential slope in the CA1 region after tetanic, but not low-frequency, stimulation (133,134). These effects have been reproduced in several laboratories, and they are significant at 6–60 ng/ml of cytokine (1). The action of the two cytokines is distinguishable: Enhancement of LTP by EGF is more obvious in the earlier phase, whereas the effect of FGF is more significant in the later phase (1,134). Such time periods correspond to the induction versus the maintenance phases of LTP. Cytokine administration is also effective in the living animal. EGF and FGF, but not NGF, increase the magnitude and probability of LTP induction in the dentate gyrus of the intact hippocampus (57). Moreover, differences have been observed between the actions of aFGF and bFGF on LTP induction in fasted versus nonfasted rats (50). The mechanism of LTP facilitation by EGF is being pursued in dissociated hippocampal neurons. Using the fura-2 assay, EGF and bFGF are found to significantly enhance the intracellular calcium increase induced by N-methyl-D-aspartate (NMDA; a glutamate analogue) (2,3). These results suggest that both proteins selectively enhance NMDA-receptor-mediated responses in hippocampal neurons, an effect that could contribute to the facilitation of LTP by these cytokines.

In contrast to the effects of EGF and FGF, IL-1β induces synaptic inhibition in rat hippocampal pyramidal neurons (152). This result could be due to the inhibitory function of SOM, which can be induced by IL-1β in the cortex (118). Other cytokines are active in such assays; interferon and IL-2 can suppress previously established LTP, as well as inhibit its induction in the hippocampus (15,27). TNF-α can affect LTP an hour after its addition to hippocampal slices (131).

The relatively rapid effects of the cytokines suggest that they could influence intercellular signaling directly, rather than through the alteration of gene expression. Many cytokine receptors have tyrosine kinase domains (120), and electrophysiological and genetic evidence implicate protein kinases in LTP (see ref. 126). Thus, it is entirely possible that cytokines could act directly as neuromodulators or neurotransmitters. It is also possible, however, that cytokine-driven changes in gene expression may be involved in learning and memory. For example, long-term changes in synaptic efficacy involve RNA and protein synthesis, and there is evidence that some aspects of LTP may also require new protein synthesis (124). In fact, cytokines can induce major changes in neuropeptide expression rather quickly; 20-fold increases in SP and VIP mRNAs were observed in sympathetic ganglia within 24 hr (109). Thus, the instructive actions of cytokines could be involved in relatively short-term synaptic plasticity, as well as in the consolidation phase of memory or its conversion from short- to long-term storage. An intriguing correlation in this respect is the recent finding that one of the genes induced in the hippocampal dentate gyrus by the glutamate analogue kainate is MyD118, a gene that is also induced by CDF/LIF and IL-6 in myeloid cells (84). If nothing else, this finding suggests common signaling pathways for cytokine action and activity involved in long-term plasticity.

Another point at which cytokines could influence learning is in the morphological changes that can accompany learning and related behavioral paradigms. It is now clear that anatomical connections are continually remodeled in adult as well as developing nervous systems, and some of these changes can be linked directly to learning (see refs. 43 and 95). A particularly intriguing example in this context are the structural changes that accompany long-term synaptic facilitation in *Aplysia*. In this case, growth of presynaptic processes requires the presence of the postsynaptic neuron, suggesting the action of a retrogradely acting trophic factor (74). Once more, the suggestion is that same developmental mechanisms employed to set up the wiring system can be used in the mature brain to modify these connections (58).

PERSPECTIVES

It is clear that cytokines can act as neuronal differentiation factors, and that these agents are probably utilized in both the retrograde and anterograde directions. There are newly emerging families of cytokines and receptors that, along with other superfamilies, are likely to be involved in the following: (i) the response to injury, as well as the feedback between the immune and nervous systems; (ii) the ongoing daily and monthly biological rhythms of the organism; (iii) the changes in synaptic plasticity involved in learning and memory; and (iv) synaptic transmission directly. The ability to regulate neuropeptide expression, both quantitatively and qualitatively, adds another dimension to the plasticity and capacity for change that is becoming clear from experimental manipulations of cortex. This regulation can dramatically alter synaptic function, both rapidly (in short-term physiological assays) or over the course of a day or month. These changes in synaptic function appear to contribute in key ways to complex animal behaviors, such as estrus, the stress response, and possibly circadian rhythms. While evidence is accumulating that cytokines may be involved in experimental paradigms of learning and memory, it is not yet clear if this involvement is in the context of neurotransmitter/neuropeptide regulation, through physical rearrangement of synaptic contacts, or through direct action on membrane tyrosine kinases and signal cascades. Another frontier is the potential use of cytokines in the treatment of pathological conditions in the nervous system. Clinical trials are underway to test the efficacy of these agents in the neurotrophic context where neurons are dying, but they could also prove useful in the manipulation of transmitter/neuropeptide imbalances in mental disorders. Moreover, genetic testing for predisposition to particular conditions could open the way for early, prophylactic intervention with these factors.

ACKNOWLEDGMENTS

I thank Floreen Rooks-Les Pierre for help in preparing the manuscript, and I also thank Herman Govan and Ming-ji Fann for their helpful comments on the text.

REFERENCES

1. Abe K, Xie F, Saito H. Epidermal growth factor enhances short-term potentiation and facilitates inductions of long-term potentiation in rat hippocampal slices. *Brain Res* 1991;547:171–174.
2. Abe K, Saito H. Epidermal growth factor selectively enhances NMDA receptor-mediated increase of intracellular Ca^{2+} concentration in rat hippocampal neurons. *Brain Res* 1992;587:102–108.
3. Abe K, Saito H. Selective enhancement by basic fibroblast growth factor of NMDA receptor-mediated increase of intracellular Ca^{2+} concentration in hippocampal neurons. *Brain Res* 1992;595:128–132.
4. Akbari HM, Whitaker-Azmitia PM, Azmitia EC. Prenatal cocaine exposure alters hippocampal serotonin, 5-HT1A receptor, and S-100β immunoreactivity in the neonatal rat. *Soc Neurosci* 1992;18:340.4.
5. Akesson TR, Mantyh PW, Matt DW, Micevych PE. Estrous cyclicity of ^{125}I-cholecystokinin octapeptide binding in the ventromedial hypothalmic nucleus. *Neurendocrinology* 1987;45:257–262.
6. Albers HE, Stopa EG, Zoeller RT, et al. Day-night variation in preprovasoactive intestinal peptide/peptide histidine isoleucine mRNA within the rat suprachiasmatic nucleus. *Mol Brain Res* 1990;7:85–89.
7. Albers HE, Liou S-Y, Stopa EG, Zoeller RT. Interaction of colocalized neuropeptides: functional significance in the circadian timing system. *J Neurosci* 1991;11:846–851.
8. Anderson DJ. The neural crest cell lineage problem; neuropoiesis? *Neuron* 1989;3:1–12.
9. Attardi B. Facilitation and inhibition of the estrogen-induced luteinizing hormone surge in the rat by progesterone: effects on cytoplasmic and nuclear estrogen receptors in the hypothalamus-preoptic area, pituitary, and uterus. *Endocrinology* 1981;108:1487–1496.
10. Bading H, Ginty DD, Greenberg ME. Regulation of gene expression in hippocampal neurons by distinct calcium signaling pathways. *Science* 1993;260:181–186.
11. Banner LR, Patterson PH. Tissue distribution, developmental expression and response to injury of rat CDF/LIF and its receptor. *Soc Neurosci* 1993;19:6.
12. Barbany G, Persson H. Regulation of neurotrophin mRNA expression in the rat brain by glucocorticoids. *Eur J Neurosci* 1992;4:396–403.
13. Bartfai T, Schultzberg M. Cytokines in neuronal cell types. *Neurochem Int* 1993;22:435–444.
14. Bazan JF. Neuropoietic cytokines in the hematopoietic fold. *Neuron* 1991;7:197–208.
15. Bindoni M, Perciavalle V, Berretta S, Belluardo N, Diamanstein T. Interleukin 2 modifies the bioelectric activity of some neurosecretory nuclei in the rat hypothalamus. *Brain Res* 1988;462:10–14.
16. Black IB, Adler JE, Dreyfus CF, Friedman WF, LaGamma EF, Roach AH. Biochemistry of information storage in the nervous system. *Science* 1987;236:1263–1268.
17. Breedlove SM. Sexual dimorphism in the vertebrate nervous system. *J Neurosci* 1992;12:4133–4142.
18. Caroni P, Grandes P. Nerve sprouting in innervated adult skeletal muscle induced by exposure to elevated levels of insulin-like growth factors. *J Cell Biol* 1990;110:1307–1317.
19. Carter DA, Murphy D. Diurnal rhythm of vasopressin mRNA species in the rat suprachiasmatic nucleus: independence of neuroendocrine modulation and maintenance in explant culture. *Mol Brain Res* 1989;6:233–239.
20. Castren E, Zafra F, Thoenen H, Lindholm D. Light regulates expression of brain-derived neurotrophic factor mRNA in rat visual cortex. *Proc Natl Acad Sci USA* 1992;89:9444–9448.
21. Chao MV. Neurotrophin receptors: a window into neuronal differentiation. *Neuron* 1992;9:583–593.
22. Clatterbuck RE, Price DL, Koliatsos VE. Ciliary neurotrophic factor prevents retrograde neuronal death in the adult central nervous system. *Proc Natl Acad Sci USA* 1993;90:2222–2226.
23. Collarini EJ, Richardson WD. Growth factors for myelinating glial cells in the central and peripheral nervous systems. In: Loughlin SE, Fallon JH, eds. *Neurotrophic factors.* San Diego: Academic Press, 1993;489–508.
24. Coulombe JN, Nishi R. Stimulation of somatostatin expression in developing ciliary ganglion neurons by cells of the choroid layer. *J Neurosci* 1991;11:553–562.
25. Coulombe JN, Schwall R, Parent AS, Eckenstein FP, Nishi R. Induction of somatostatin immunoreactivity in cultured ciliary ganglion neurons by activin in choroid cell-conditioned medium. *Neuron* 1993;10:899–906.
26. Cunningham ET Jr, De Souza EB. Interleukin 1 receptors in the brain and endocrine tissues. *Immunol Today* 1993;14:171–176.
27. D'Arcangelo G, Grassi F, Ragozzino D, Santoni A, Tancredi V, Eusebi F. Interferon inhibits synaptic potentiation in rat hippocampus. *Brain Res* 1991;564:245–248.
28. Davis S, Aldrich TH, Stahl N, et al. LIFRβ and gp130 as heterodimerizing signal transducers of the tripartite CNTF receptor. *Science* 1993;260:1805–1808.
29. Dekker AJ, Gage FH, Thal LJ. Delayed treatment with nerve growth factor improves acquisition of a spatial task in rats with lesions of the nucleus basalis magnocellularis: evaluation of the involvement of different neurotransmitter systems. *Neuroscience* 1992;48:111–119.

30. DeVries GJ. Sex differences in neurotransmitter systems. *J Neuroendocrinol* 1990;2:1–13.

31. Dubner R, Ruda MA. Activity-dependent neuronal plasticity following tissue injury and inflammation. *Trends Neurosci* 1992;15:96–103.

32. Dugich-Djordjevic MM, Tocco G, Willoughby DA, et al. BDNF mRNA expression in the developing rat brain following kainic acid-induced seizure activity. *Neuron* 1992;8:1127–1138.

33. Eckenstein FP, Shipley GD, Nishi R. Acidic and basic fibroblast growth factors in the nervous system: distribution and differential alteration of levels after injury of central versus peripheral nerve. *J Neurosci* 1991;11:412–419.

34. Ernfors P, Wetmore C, Olson L, Persson H. Identification of cells in rat brain and peripheral tissues expressing mRNA for members of the nerve growth factor family. *Neuron* 1990;5:511–526.

35. Eysel UT. Remodelling receptive fields in sensory cortices. *Curr Biol* 1992;2:389–391.

36. Fann M-J, Patterson PH. New members of the neuropoietic cytokine family and activin A regulate the phenotype of cultured sympathetic neurons. *Proc Natl Acad Sci USA* 1994;[in press].

37. Ferguson IA, Schweitzer JB, Johnson EM Jr. Basic fibroblast growth factor: receptor-mediated internalization, metabolism, and anterograde axonal transport in retinal ganglion cells. *J Neurosci* 1990;10:2176–2189.

38. Fischer W, Bjorklund A, Chen K, Gage FH. NGF improves spatial memory in aged rodents as a function of age. *J Neurosci* 1991;11:1889–1906.

39. French KA, Kristan WB Jr. Target influences on the development of leech neurons. *Trends Neurosci* 1992;15:169–174.

40. Fukada K. Hormonal control of neurotransmitter choice in sympathetic neurone cultures. *Nature* 1980;287:553–555.

41. Gearing DP. The leukemia inhibitory factor and its receptor. *Adv Immunol* 1993;53:31–58.

42. Goodman RH. Regulation of neuropeptide gene expression. *Annu Rev Neurosci* 1990;13:111–127.

43. Greenough WT, Bailey CH. The anatomy of a memory: convergence of results across a diversity of tests. *Trends Neurosci* 1988;11:142–147.

44. Gurney ME, Yamamoto H, Kwon Y. Induction of motor neuron sprouting in vivo by ciliary neurotrophic factor and basic fibroblast growth factor. *J Neurosci* 1992;12:3241–3247.

45. Hageman GS, Kirchoff-Rempe MA, Lewis GP, Fisher SK, Anderson DH. Sequestration of basic fibroblast growth factor in the primate retinal interphotoreceptor matrix. *Proc Natl Acad Sci USA* 1991;88:6706–6710.

46. Hammill RW, Schroeder B. Hormonal regulation of adult sympathetic neurons: the effects of castration on neuropeptide Y, norepinephrine, and tyrosine hydroxylase activity. *J Neurobiol* 1990;21:731–742.

47. Hart RP, Shadiack AM, Jonakait GM. Substance P gene expression is regulated by interleukin-1 in cultured sympathetic ganglia. *J Neurosci Res* 1991;29:282–291.

48. Henderson CE, Camu W, Mettling C, et al. Neurotrophins promote motor neuron survival and are present in embryonic limb bud. *Nature* 1993;363:266–270.

49. Hendry IA, Murphy M, Hilton DJ, Nicola NA, Bartlett PF. Binding and retrograde transport of leukemia inhibitory factor by the sensory nervous system. *J Neurosci* 1992;12:3427–3434.

50. Hisajima H, Saito H, Abe K, Nishiyama N. Effects of acidic fibroblast growth factor on hippocampal long-term potentiation in fasted rats. *J Neurosci Res* 1992;31:549–553.

51. Hughes RA, Sendtner M, Goldfarb M, Lindholm D, Thoenen H. Evidence that fibroblast growth factor 5 is a major muscle-derived survival factor for cultured spinal motoneurons. *Neuron* 1993;10:369–377.

52. Hutchins J, Jefferson V. Developmental distribution of platelet-derived growth-factor in the mouse central-nervous-system. *Dev Brain Res* 1992;67:121–135.

53. Hyatt-Sachs H, Schreiber RC, Bennett TA, Zigmond RE. Phenotypic plasticity in adult sympathetic ganglia in vivo: effects of deafferentation and axotomy on the expression of vasoactive intestinal peptide. *J Neurosci* 1993;13:1642–1653.

54. Imaki T, Nahan J-L, Rivier C, Sawchenko PE, Vale W. Differential regulation of corticotropin-releasing factor mRNA in rat brain regions by glucocorticoids and stress. *J Neurosci* 1991;11:585–599.

55. Isackson PJ, Huntsman MM, Murray KD, Gall CM. BDNF mRNA expression is increased in adult rat forebrain after limbic seizures: temporal patterns of induction distinct from NGF. *Neuron* 1991;6:937–948.

56. Ishii DN. Neurobiology of insulin and insulin-like growth factors. In: Loughlin SE, Fallon JH, eds. *Neurotrophic factors*. New York: Academic Press, 1992;415–442.

57. Ishiyama J, Saito H, Abe K. Epidermal growth factor and basic fibroblast growth factor promote the generation of long-term potentiation in the dentate gyrus of anesthetized rats. *Neurosci Res* 1991;12:403–411.

58. Kandel ER, O'Dell TJ. Are adult learning mechanisms also used for development? *Science* 1992;258:243–245.

59. Kishimoto T, Akira S, Taga T. Interleukin-6 and its receptor: a paradigm for cytokines. *Science* 1992;258:593–597.

60. Koliatsos VE, Clatterbuck RE, Winslow JW, Cayouette MH, Price DL. Evidence that brain-derived neurotrophic factor is a trophic factor for motor neurons in vivo. *Neuron* 1993;10:359–367.

61. Korsching S. The neurotrophic factor concept: a reexamination. *J Neurosci* 1993;13:2739–2748.

62. Landis SC. Target regulation of neurotransmitter phenotype. *Trends Neurosci* 1990;13:344–350.

63. Lauder JM. Neurotransmitters as growth regulatory signals: role of receptors and second messengers. *Trends Neurosci* 1993;16:233–240.

64. Lehman MN, Silver R, Gladstone WR, Kahn RM, Gibson M, Bittman EL. Circadian rhythmicity restored by neural transplant: immunocytochemical characterization of the graft and its integration with the host brain. *J Neurosci* 1987;7:1626–1636.

65. LeRoith D, Roberts CT Jr., Werner H, Bondy C, Raizada M, Adamo M. Insulin-like growth factors in the brain. In: Laughlin SE, Fallon JH, eds. *Neurotrophic factors*. New York: Academic Press, 1992;391–414.

66. Leung DW, Parent AS, Cachianes G, et al. Cloning, expression during development, and evidence for release of a trophic factor for ciliary ganglion neurons. *Neuron* 1992;8:1045–1053.

67. Levine JD, Dardick SJ, Roizen MF, Helms C, Basbaum AI. Contribution of sensory afferents and sympathetic efferents to joint injury in experimental arthritis. *J Neurosci* 1986;6:3423–3429.

68. Lin L-FH, Doherty DH, Like JD, Bektesh S, Collins F. GDNF: a glial cell line-derived neurotrophic factor for midbrain dopaminergic neurons. *Science* 1993;260:1130–1132.

69. Lindholm D, Castren E, Hengerer B, Zafra F, Berninger-Benedikt B, Thoenen H. Differential regulation of nerve growth factor (NGF) synthesis in neurons and astrocytes by glucocorticoid hormones. *Eur J Neurosci* 1992;4:404–410.

70. Lindsay RM, Harmar AJ. Nerve growth factor regulates expression of neuropeptide genes in adult sensory neurons. *Nature* 1989;337:362–364.

71. Lu B, Yokoyama M, Dreyfus CF, Black IB. Depolarizing stimuli regulate nerve growth factor gene expression in cultured hippocampal neurons. *Proc Natl Acad Sci USA* 1991;88:6289–6292.

72. Maffei L, Berardi N, Domenici L, Parisi V, Pizzorusso T. Nerve growth factor (NGF) prevents the shift in ocular dominance distribution of visual cortical neurons in monocularly deprived rats. *J Neurosci* 1992;12:4651–4662.

73. Martinou J, Martinou I, Kato AC. Cholinergic differentiation factor (CDF/LIF) promotes survival of isolated rat embryonic motoneurons in vitro. *Neuron* 1992;8:737–744.

74. Mayford M, Barzilai A, Keller F, Schacher S, Kandel ER. Modulation of an NCAM-related adhesion molecule with long-term plasticity in *Aplysia*. *Science* 1992;256:638–644.

75. McLennan IS, Hill CE, Hendry IA. Glucocorticoids modulate transmitter choice in developing superior cervical ganglion. *Nature* 1980;283:206–207.

76. Merchenthaler I, Lopez FJ, Lennard DE, Negro-Vilar A. Sexual differences in the distribution of neurons co-expressing galanin and luteinizing hormone-releasing hormone in the rat brain. *Endocrinology* 1991;129:1977–1986.

77. Minami M, Kuraishi Y, Satoh M. Effects of kainic acid on messenger RNA levels of IL-1β, IL-6, TNFα and LIF in the rat brain. *Biochem Biophys Res Commun* 1991;176:593–598.

78. Morrison R. Epidermal growth factor: structure, expression, and functions in the central nervous system. In: Laughlin SE, Fallon JH, eds. *Neurotrophic factors.* New York: Academic Press, 1992;339–358.

79. Murakami N, Takamure M, Takahashi K, Utunomiya K, Kuroda H, Etoh T. Long-term cultured neurons from rat suprachismatic nucleus retain the capacity for circadian oscillation of vasopressin release. *Brain Res* 1991;545:347–350.

80. Murphy M, Reid K, Brown MA, Bartlett PF. Involvement of leukemia inhibitory factor and nerve growth factor in the development of dorsal root ganglion neurons. *Development* 1993;117:1173–11182.

81. Naruse I, Kato K, Asano T, Suzuki F, Kameyama Y. Developmental brain abnormalities accompanied with the retarded production of S-100b protein in genetic polydactyly mice. *Dev Brain Res* 1990;51:253–258.

82. Nawa H, Yamamori T, Le T, Patterson PH. Generation of neuronal diversity: analogies and homologies with hematopoiesis. *Cold Spring Harbor Symp Quant Biol* 1990;55:247–253.

83. Nawa H, Bessho Y, Carnahan J, Nakanishi S, Mizuno K. Regulation of neuropeptide expression in cultured cerebral cortical neurons by BDNF. *J Neurochem* 1993;60:772–775.

84. Nedivi E, Hevroni D, Naot D, Israeli D, Citri Y. Numerous candidate plasticity-related genes revealed by differential cDNA cloning. *Nature* 1993;363:718–722.

85. Nicola NA, Metcalf D. Subunit promiscuity among hemopoietic growth factor receptors. *Cell* 1991;67:1–4.

86. Okamoto S, Okamura H, Miyake M, et al. A diurnal variation of vasoactive intestinal peptide (VIP) mRNA under a daily light–dark cycle in the rat suprachiasmatic nucleus. *Histochemistry* 1991;95:535–528.

87. Oppenheim RW. Cell death during development of the nervous system. *Annu Rev Neurosci* 1991;14:453–501.

88. Oppenheim RW, Prevette D, Qin-Wei Y, Collins F, MacDonald J. Control of embryonic motoneuron survival in vivo by ciliary neurotrophic factor. *Science* 1991;251:1616–1618.

89. Oro AE, Simerly RB, Swanson LW. Estrous cycle variations in levels of cholecystokinin immunoreactivity within cells of three interconnected sexually dimporphic forebrain nuclei. *Neuroendocrinology* 1988;47:225–235.

90. Patterson PH. Environmental determination of autonomic neurotransmitter functions. *Annu Rev Neurosci* 1978;1:1–17.

91. Patterson PH, Fann M-J. Further studies of the distribution of CDF/LIF mRNA. *Ciba Foundation Symp* 1992;167:125–140.

92. Patterson PH, Grover LM, Schwartzkroin PA, Bothwell M. Neurotrophin expression in rat hippocampal slices—a stimulus paradigm inducing LTP in CA1 evokes increases in BDNF and NT-3 messenger-RNAs. *Neuron* 1992;9:1081–1088.

93. Patterson PH. The emerging neuropoeitic cytokine family: first CDF/LIF, CNTF and IL-6; next ONC, MGF and GCSF? *Curr Opin Neurobiol* 1992;2:94–97.

94. Patterson PH, Bugga L, Stewart CL. CDF/LIF-deficient mice display an altered complement of neuronal phenotypes in the CNS. *Soc Neurosci* 1993;19:710.

95. Patterson PH, Nawa H. Neuronal differentiation factors/cytokines and synaptic plasticity. *Cell* 1993;72:123–137.

96. Phillips HS, Hains JM, Armanini M, Laramee GR, Johnson SA, Winslow JW. BDNF mRNA is decreased in the hippocampus of individuals with Alzheimer's disease. *Neuron* 1991;7:695–702.

97. Presta M, Rifkin DB. Immunoreactive basic fibroblast growth factor-like proteins in chromaffin granules. *J Neurochem* 1991;56:1087–1088.

98. Puolakkainen P, Twardzik DR. Transforming growth factors alpha and beta. In: Loughlin SE, Fallon JH, eds. *Neurotrophic factors.* San Diego: Academic Press, 1993;359–389.

99. Purves D, Lichtman JW. *Principles of neural development.* Sutherland, MA: Sinauer Associates, 1985.

100. Purves D, Hadley RD, Voyvodic JT. Dynamic changes in the dendritic geometry of individual neurons visualized over periods up to three months in the superior vervical ganglion of living mice. *J Neurosci* 1986;6:1051–1060.

101. Ralph MR, Foster RG, Davis FC, Menaker M. Transplanted suprachiasmatic nucleus determines circadian period. *Science* 1990;247:975–978.

102. Ramon y Cajal S. *Histologie du système de l'homme et des vertèbres* (1952 reprint). Madrid: Instituto Ramon y Cajal, Consejo Superior de Investigaciones Scientifique, 1909.

103. Rao MS, Patterson PH, Landis SC. Multiple cholinergic differentiation factors are present in footpad extracts: comparison with known cholinergic factors. *Development* 1992;731–744.

104. Rao MS, Symes A, Malik N, Shoyab M, Fink JS, Landis SC. Oncostatin M regulates VIP expression in a human neuroblastoma cell line. *Neuroreport* 1992;3:865–868.

105. Rao MS, Tyrrell S, Landis SC, Patterson PH. Effects of ciliary neurotrophic factor (CNTF) and depolarization on neuropeptide expression in cultured sympathetic neurons. *Dev Biol* 1992;150:281–293.

106. Rao MS, Sun Y, Vaidyanathan U, Landis SC, Zigmond RE. Regulation of Substance P is similar to that of vasoactive intestinal peptide after axotomy or explanation of the rat superior cervical ganglion. *J Neurobiol* 1993;24:571–580.

107. Rao MS, Sun Y, Escary JL, Perreau J, Tresser S, Patterson PH, Zigmond RE, Brulet P, Landis SC. Leukemia inhibitory factor mediates an injury response but not a target-directed developmental transmitter switch in sympathetic neurons. *Neuron* 1994;11:1175–1185.

108. Reist NE, Werle MJ, McMahan UJ. Agrin released by motor neurons induces the aggregation of acetylcholine receptors at neuromuscular junctions. *Neuron* 1992;8:865–868.

109. Roach A, Adler JE, Black IB. Depolarizing influences regulate preprotachykinin mRNA in sympathetic neurons. *Proc Natl Acad Sci USA* 1987;84:5078–5081.

110. Rohrer H. Cholinergic neuronal differentiation factors: evidence for the presence of both CNTF-like and non-CNTF-like factors in developing rat footpad. *Development* 1992;114:689–698.

111. Rose TM, Bruce AG. Oncostatin M is a member of a cytokine family that includes leukemia-inhibitory factor, granulocyte colony-stimulating factor, and interleukin 6. *Proc Natl Acad Sci USA* 1991;88:8641–8645.

112. Rothwell NJ, Relton JK. Involvement of cytokines in acute neurodegeneration in the CNS. *Neurosci Biobehav Rev* 1993;17:217–227.

113. Ruegg MA, Tsim KWK, Horton SE, et al. The agrin gene codes for a family of basal lamina proteins that differ in function and distribution. *Neuron* 1992;8:691–699.

114. Rupp F, Hoch W, Campanelli JT, Kreiner T, Scheller RH. Agrin and the organization of the neuromuscular junction. *Curr Opin Neurobiol* 1992;2:88–93.

115. Rydhstrom H, Walles B, Owman C. Effects of oophorectomy, sympathetic denervation and sex steroids on uterine norepinephrine content and myometrial contractile response to norepinephrine in the guinea pig. *Neuroendocrinology* 1990;52:332–336.

116. Saadat S, Sendtner M, Rohrer H. Ciliary neurotrophic factor induces cholinergic differentiation of rat sympathetic neurons in culture. *J Cell Biol* 1989;108:1807–1816.

117. Sastry BR, Chirwa SS, May PBY, Maretic H. Substances released during tetanic stimulation of rabbit neocortex induce neurite growth in PC-12 cells and long-term potentiation in guinea pig hippocampus. *Neurosci Lett* 1988;91:101–105.

118. Scarborough DE, Lee SL, Dinarello CA, Reichlin S. Interleukin-1β stimulates somatostatin biosynthesis in primary cultures of fetal rat brain. *Endocrinology* 1989;124:549–551.

119. Schecterson LC, Bothwell M. Novel roles for neurotrophins are suggested by BDNF and NT-3 mRNA expression in developing neurons. *Neuron* 1992;9:449–463.

120. Schlessinger J, Ullrich A. Growth factor signaling by receptor tyrosine kinases. *Neuron* 1992;9:383–391.

121. Sendtner M, Kreutzberg GW, Thoenen H. Ciliary neurotrophic factor prevents the degeneration of motor neurons after axotomy. *Nature* 1990;345:440–441.

122. Sendtner M, Schmalbruch H, Stockil KA, Carroll P, Kreutzberg GW, Thoenen H. Ciliary neurotrophic factor prevents degeneration of motor neurons in mouse mutant progressive motor neuronopathy. *Nature* 1992;358:502–504.

123. Simerly RB. Hormonal control of neuropeptide gene expression in sexually dimorphic olfactory pathways. *Trends Neurosci* 1990;13:104–110.

124. Stanton PK, Sarvey JM. Blockade of long-term potentiation in

rat hippocampal CA1 region by inhibitors of protein synthesis. *J Neurosci* 1984;4:3080–3088.

125. Stephan FK, Zucker I. Circadian rhythms in drinking behavior and locomoter activity of rats eliminated by hypothalmic lesions. *Proc Natl Acad Sci USA* 1972;69:1583–1586.

126. Stevens CF. Quantal release of neurotransmitter and long-term potentiation. *Cell* 1993;72:55–63.

127. Strand FL, Rose KJ, Zuccarelli LA, et al. Neuropeptide hormones as neurotrophic factors. *Physiol Rev* 1991;71:1017–1046.

128. Swanson LW. Biochemical switching in hypothalamic circuits mediating responses to stress. *Prog Brain Res* 1991;87:181–200.

129. Taga T, Kishimoto T. Cytokine receptors and signal transduction. *FASEB J* 1992;6:3387–3396.

130. Takahashi JS. Cellular basis of circadian rhythms in the avian pineal. In: Hiroshige T, Honma K, eds. *Comparative aspects of circadian clocks*. Tokyo: Hokkaido University Press, 1987;3–15.

131. Tancredi V, D'Arcangelo G, Grassi F, et al. Tumor necrosis factor alters synaptic transmission in rat hippocampal slices. *Neurosci Lett* 1992;146:176–178.

132. Tchelingerian J-L, Quinonero J, Booss J, Jacque C. Localization of TNFα and IL-1α immunoreactivities in striatal neurons after surgical injury to the hippocampus. *Neuron* 1993;10:213–224.

133. Terlau H, Siefert W. Influence of epidermal growth factor on long-term potentiation in the hippocampal slice. *Brain Res* 1989;484:352–356.

134. Terlau H, Siefert W. Fibroblast growth factor enhances long-term potentiation in the hippocampal slice. *Eur J Neurosci* 1990;2:973–977.

135. Thoenen H. The changing scene of neurotrophic factors. *Trends Neurosci* 1991;14:165–170.

136. Ueda S, Gu XF, Azmitia EC. Serotonergic fibers are not developed in the hippocampus and neocortex in the S-100β retarded mutant mouse (*Polydactyly nagoya*). *Soc Neurosci* 1992;18:340.9.

137. Uhl GR, Reppert SM. Suprachiasmatic nucleus vasopressin messenger RNA: circadian variation in normal and Brattleboro rats. *Science* 1986;232:390–393.

138. Unsicker K, Bieger S, Blottner D, et al. The trophic cocktail made by chromaffin cells. *Res Neurol Neurosci* 1992;4:174.

139. Unsicker K, Grothe C, Ludecke G, Otto D, Westermann R. Fibroblast growth factors: their roles in the central and peripheral nervous system. In: Laughlin SE, Fallon JH, eds. *Neurotrophic factors*. New York: Academic Press, 1992;313–338.

140. Unsicker K, Gehrke D, Stogbauer F, Westermann R. Trophic factors from chromaffin granules promote survival of peripheral and central nervous system neurons. *Exp Neurol* 1993;123:167–173.

141. Vaidya U, Morin L, Wells MR. Circadian variation in S100 protein in hamster CNS. *Soc Neurosci* 1992;18:511.14.

142. Vandesande F, Dierick K, De Mey J. Identification of the vasopressin/neurophysin producing neurons of the rat suprachiasmatic nuclei. *Cell Tissue Res* 1975;156:377–380.

143. Watts AG, Swanson LW. Diurnal variations in the content of preprocoticotropin-releasing hormone messenger ribonucleic acids in the hypothalamic paraventricular nucleus of rats of both sexes as measured by in situ hybridization. *Endocrinology* 1989;125:1734–1738.

144. Westermann R, Johannsen M, Unsicker K, Grothe C. Basic fibroblast growth factor (bFGF) immunoreactivity is present in chromaffin granules. *J Neurochem* 1990;55:285–292.

145. Wetmore C, Cao Y, Petterson RF, Olson L. Brain-derived neurotrophic factor: subcellular compartmentalization and interneuronal transfer as visualized with anti-peptide antibodies. *Proc Natl Acad Sci USA* 1991;88:9843–9847.

146. Wigston DJ. Remodeling of neuromuscular junctions in adult mouse soleus. *J Neurosci* 1989;9:639–647.

147. Woolley CS, McEwen BS. Estradiol mediates fluctuation in hippocampal synapse density during the estrous cycle in the adult rat. *J Neurosci* 1992;12:2549–2554.

148. Xie Z, Morishita W, Kam T, Maretic H, Sastry BR. Studies on substances that induce long-term potentiation in guinea-pig hippocampal slices. *Neuroscience* 1991;43:11–20.

149. Yamamori T. Localization of cholinergic differentiation factor/leukemia inhibitory factor mRNA in the rat brain and peripheral tissues. *Proc Natl Acad Sci USA* 1991;88:7298–7302.

150. Yan Q, Elliott J, Snider WD. Brain-derived neurotrophic factor rescues spinal motor neurons from axotomy-induced cell death. *Nature* 1992;360:753–755.

151. Zafra F, Castren E, Thoenen H, Lindholm D. Interplay between glutamate and γ-aminobutyric acid transmitter systems in the physiological regulation of brain-derived neurotrophic factor and nerve growth factor synthesis in hippocampal neurons. *Proc Natl Acad Sci USA* 1991;88:10037–10041.

152. Zeise ML, Madamba S, Siggins GR. Interleukin-1β increases synaptic inhibition in rat hippocampal pyramidal neurons in vitro. *Regul Pept* 1992;39:1–7.

153. Zigmond RE, Schwarzschild MA, Rittenhouse AR. Acute regulation of tyrosine hydroxylase by nerve activity and by neurotransmitters via phosphorylation. *Annu Rev Neurosci* 1989;12:415–461.

154. Zigmond RE, Hyatt-Sachs H, Baldwin C, et al. Phenotypic plasticity in adult sympathetic neurons: changes in neuropeptide expression in organ culture. *Proc Natl Acad Sci USA* 1992;89:1507–1511.

Psychopharmacology: The Fourth Generation of Progress, edited by Floyd E. Bloom and David J. Kupfer. Raven Press, Ltd., New York © 1995.

CHAPTER 56

Proto-Oncogenes

Beyond Second Messengers

James I. Morgan and Thomas E. Curran

THE IMMEDIATE-EARLY GENE RESPONSE AND ITS RELEVANCE TO NEUROBIOLOGY

The interaction of extracellular ligands with their receptors on the plasma membrane elicits the flow of information into the cytoplasm via numerous signal transduction pathways. Historically, this information flow was considered to bring about rapid alterations in cellular functions by modifying the activity of existing proteins. However, it is now clear that signal transduction cascades do not terminate in the cytoplasm but rather extend to the nucleus where they are capable of bringing about alterations in gene expression (Fig. 1). This provides a mechanism whereby a cell can adapt to alterations in the extracellular milieu by changing the levels, or patterns, of gene expression (see Chapter 2, *this volume*).

Oncogenes are defined as any genetic element that can cause cellular transformation, and proto-oncogenes are the normal cellular genes from which the oncogenes are derived. Historically, oncogenes were first described as the transforming elements present in some retroviruses. Therefore, the viral oncogene was designated v-*onc* to distinguish it from its normal cellular counterpart (the proto-oncogene), c-*onc*. By convention, most genes or their messenger ribonucleic acids (mRNAs) are referred to by three letter names in lower case that are italicized, whereas their protein products are not italicized and use upper case. For example, v-*src* is the viral oncogene (or its mRNA) that encodes the protein v-Src. Proto-oncogenes can be activated to become oncogenes by

many other mechanisms besides capture by retroviruses (which is actually relatively rare). Such processes include mutation, rearrangement, or amplification (reviewed in ref. 34). In these cases, the c- prefix is not used, because no viral homolog exists. Many proto-oncogenes encode proteins that fulfill a role in signal transduction pathways; these functions include extracellular growth factors, membrane receptors, cytoplasmic and membrane-associated protein kinases, guanosine triphosphate (GTP) -binding proteins, and transcription factors. A generic signaling pathway is depicted in Fig. 1 that shows the flow of information from the extracellular milieu to the cytoplasm and finally into the nucleus. In this cascade of events, there is a further distinction between events that require a nuclear response (long-term cellular responses) and those that are protein-synthesis independent (short-term cellular responses). Examples of specific proto-oncogenes are given within the framework of this general signal transduction pathway to illustrate the range of their biochemical and cellular properties (see Chapters 27, 51, and 61, *this volume*).

A more detailed list of proto-oncogenes with their functions (where known) is provided in Table 1. Proto-oncogenes can be conveniently classified by the role they play in signal transduction. In Table 1, we have arranged specific proto-oncogenes into various general classes such as receptor ligands and membrane receptor tyrosine kinases. The order of presentation is designed to indicate the stage in the signal transduction pathway that particular proto-oncogenes act starting in the extracellular milieu, moving to the membrane, through the cytoplasm, and into the nucleus. Where it is known, we have indicated the specific function of particular proto-oncogenes. For

J. I. Morgan and T. E. Curran: Roche Institute of Molecular Biology, Roche Research Center, Nutley, New Jersey 07110.

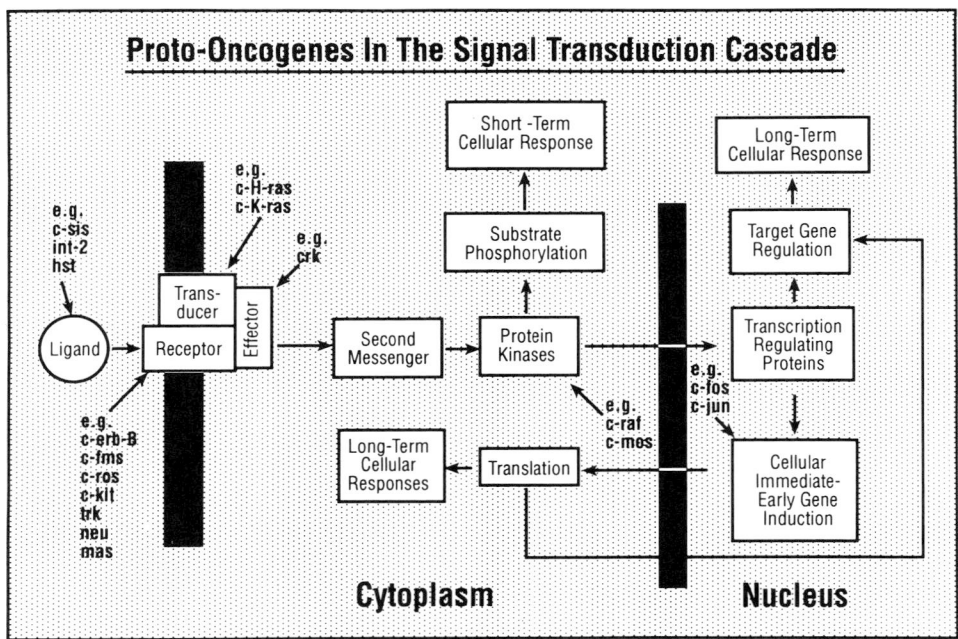

FIG. 1. Proto-oncogenes in the signal transduction cascade. (Reproduced with permission from *Discussions in Neuroscience*, Vol. VII, no. 4, August 1991. Elsevier Science Publishers B.V.)

example, the proto-oncogene c-*sis* encodes the B chain of platelet-derived growth factor. In many cases, proto-oncogenes belong to a gene family in which the function of one member is known. In this case we refer to the proto-oncogene function as -like. For example, the proto-oncogene *int*-2, encodes a protein that is related to basic fibroblast growth factor.

As our knowledge of stimulus–transcription coupling has grown it has begun to reveal the molecular basis of a number of neurobiological processes. Some of these processes were already known to be protein-synthesis dependent and, therefore, likely to have a transcriptional component. However, in other instances the finding of rapid alterations in gene expression was quite unexpected and has lead to a reexamination of the molecular basis of these responses. From the neuropharmacological perspective, two types of studies involving gene expression in the nervous system are relevant. First, monitoring gene expression can provide insights into which cells are involved in particular neurobiological or neuropathological responses. Second, the molecules that couple second messengers to gene expression, as well as the products of these genes, offer new substrates for potential neuropharmacological intervention. Although there is considerable interest in developing therapeutics that act on gene transcription, this is a field still in its infancy. Therefore, this chapter will deal with methods of studying neurobiological and neuropharmacological responses by assessing immediate-early gene (IEG) expression.

Much of what we know concerning stimulus–transcrip-

tion coupling in the nervous system has its origins in studies of cancer biology. One critical discovery was the recognition that most proto-oncogenes, the normal cellular homologs of oncogenes, encoded proteins involved in signal transduction (see Fig. 1 for details) (34). (Oncogenes are defined as being any genetic element that can cause cellular transformation.) Furthermore, and somewhat surprisingly at the time, some proto-oncogenes (e.g., *erb*A, c-*myb*, c-*myc*, and c-*fos*) encoded nuclear proteins that, with the exception of *erb*A (the thyroid hormone receptor), did not fit into any conventional signal transduction pathway. It was supposed that the products of these genes should act as transcription factors, although little direct evidence existed for this assumption at the time. Subsequently it was discovered that addition of serum to quiescent fibroblasts resulted in a rapid and transient induction of several of these proto-oncogenes (4,12,27,36), the best known being c-*fos*, c-*jun*, and c-*myc*. Therefore, it was postulated that these inducible proto-oncogenes might encode transcription factors that could act as nuclear "third messengers," coupling second messenger-mediated events to subsequent alterations in gene expression (5,33). In the meantime a considerable body of evidence has accumulated to support this view, although the entire picture is still far from clear.

Although rapidly inducible proto-oncogenes, such as *fos*, were studied primarily in the context of mitogenesis and transformation, it soon became clear that they could be induced by stimuli that had no influence on cell proliferation (6,11). Indeed, they could be activated by depolar-

TABLE 1. *Functional classification of proto-oncogenes*[a]

Class	Proto-oncogene nomenclature	Homolog
Receptor ligand	c-*sis*	PDGF B chain
	int-2	Basic-FGF-like
	hst	FGF-like
Transmembrane tyrosine kinases	c-*erb*B	EGF receptor
	c-*fms*	CSF-1 receptor
	neu (c-*erb*B-2)	EGF receptor-like
	*trk, trk*B, *trk*C	Neurotrophin receptors
	c-*met*	Insulin receptor-like
	c-*kit*	w locus gene
	c-*ros*	Insulin receptor-like
	c-*sea*	Insulin receptor-like
Membrane-associated tyrosine kinases	c-*src*	
	hck	
	c-*abl*	
	c-*yes*-1 and -2	
	c-*fgr*	
	c-*lck*	
	c-*fps/fes*	
	fer	
	flk	
	flk	
	c-*syn*	
	c-*lyn*	
	c-*slk*	
	fyn	
Nontyrosine kinase receptors	*mas*	Angiotensin receptor
Serine/threonine kinases	c-*raf*-1	
	c-*mos*	
	pim-1	
G-protein-like	c-Ha-*ras*	
	c-Ki-*ras*	
	c-N-*ras*	
	rab (1-4)	
	ypt-1	
	rho	
	smg	
Signal transduction enzymes	*crk*	Phospholipase C-like
Nuclear proteins	c-*ski*	
	c-*erb*A	Thyroid hormone receptor
	*sno*A and B	
	ets-1 and -2	
	c-*myb*	Related to NFkB
	*myb*A and B	
Zinc finger proteins	*gli*	Related to krueppel
	gr-1 and -2	Related to krueppel
Leucine zipper protein	c-*fos*	
	fra-1 and -2	AP-1 complexes
	*fos*B	
	c-*jun*, -B, -D	
Helix-loop-helix	c-*myc*	
	N-*myc*	
	L-*myc*	

[a] Reproduced with permission from *Discussions in Neuroscience,* vol. VII, no. 4, August 1991. Elsevier Science Publishers B. V.

ization of neurons (32), cells that are not even competent for mitosis. Therefore, it was thought that the signal transduction pathways utilizing inducible proto-oncogenes should be involved in many biological processes and would be used as ubiquitously as any of the more conventional second-messenger systems (5,33).

In parallel with the quest for the function of proto-oncogenes, other studies were designed to identify genes that were activated by serum treatment of quiescent fibroblasts. These investigations identified a range of inducible genes; some were proto-oncogenes, others were structurally related to known proto-oncogenes (i.e., members of gene families such as *fos*B and *jun*B) yet others had no obvious homology to known proto-oncogenes and encoded proteins that were either of unknown function or that were involved in signal transduction (e.g., tyrosine phosphatases and cytokinelike molecules). Therefore, the view arose of a much more global transcriptional response to stimulation that involved whole families of genes whose products might contribute to signal transduction both within and between cells.

It was subsequently found that many of the genes that were activated immediately after serum addition were transcriptionally induced even if protein synthesis was blocked. Indeed, they were superinduced in the presence of agents such as cycloheximide and anisomycin. This unifying property lead to the definition of these genes as constituting the cellular IEG class (5,26). This name was adopted from the IEGs of viruses, which are expressed promptly upon infection of a host cell even in the absence of protein synthesis. The property of protein synthesis independence is taken to mean that all of the signaling and regulatory molecules necessary to elicit the transcriptional response of this class of genes are already present in the unstimulated cell. Furthermore, since the function of IEGs of viruses is to control the expression of early genes and progression of the viral replication cycle, so the cellular IEGs (cIEGs) were postulated to control the expression of genes necessary for subsequent adaptive programs. As noted above, not all cIEGs encode transcription factors. Thus the cellular immediate-early response should be viewed as an integrated biological process involving transcriptional changes and modification of signal transduction pathways in the stimulated cell and dissemination of the response to adjacent cells and tissues (Fig. 2) (for reviews see refs. 5,17,30,31, and 43).

Cellular responses to extracellular stimuli can be divided into those that are dependent upon protein synthesis and those that are not. In general, transcription-independent responses tend to be rapid events that are mediated by second messenger molecules that control the posttranslational modification of preexisting substrates such as ion channels, membrane receptors, and cytoskeletal proteins. Such changes result in alterations in the properties of the substrates that might include alterations in

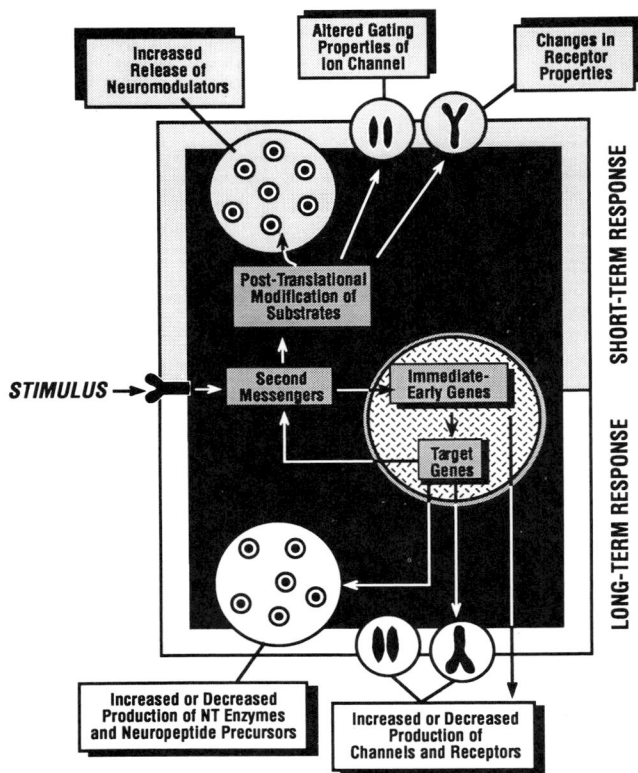

FIG. 2. Hypothetical model of immediate-early gene function in neurons.

ion gating or changes in secretion of neurotransmitters. This type of process is referred to as the short-term response to stimulation. The cell also mounts a delayed, but more protracted, response to stimulation that is referred to as the long-term response. This involves second-messenger molecules altering gene expression. The example shown in Fig. 2 focuses on the immediate-early genes, although second messengers (and some ligands such as retinoids and steroids) can act to alter expression of many other classes of genes. Immediate-early genes frequently encode transcription factors that control the expression of further, so-called target, genes. In the hypothetical scheme in Fig. 2, it is supposed that target genes might be those encoding neurotransmitter synthesizing enzymes and receptors, neuropeptide precursors, and ion channels. In addition, some immediate-early genes encode secreted proteins or enzymes involved in second-messenger metabolism. These can be viewed as molecules that disseminate the response to other cells and alter the coupling efficiency of the signal transduction pathway. It should be emphasized, however, that this scheme is hypothetical and grossly oversimplified. No target genes for particular cellular immediate-early gene products have been identified in neurons, and it is most unlikely that the regulation of any individual gene is controlled by a single transcription factor or class of factors, but rather involves complex

STIMULUS - TRANSCRIPTION COUPLING

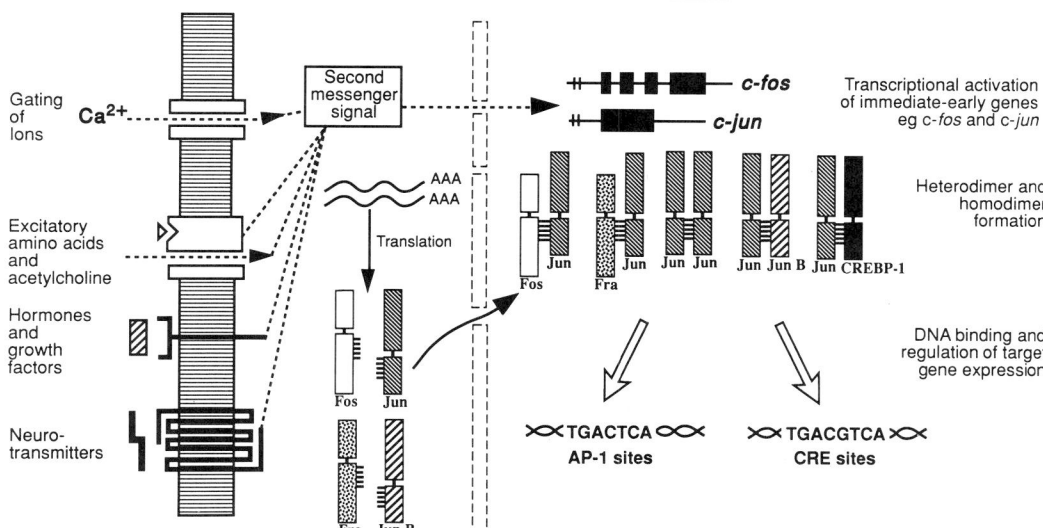

FIG. 3. Stimulus–transcription coupling in the nervous system. (Reproduced with permission from *Cold Spring Harbor Symposium on Quantitative Biology*, vol. 55, Cold Spring Harbor Press, 1990;225–234.

combinatorial interactions between resident and inducible proteins.

Fos, Jun, and Activator Protein-1

Many of the applications of cIEG expression in neuropharmacological investigations stem from the properties of two prototypic members of this gene class, c-*fos* and c-*jun*. Both of these inducible proto-oncogenes encode nuclear phosphoproteins (Fos and Jun) that physically associate with one another through an amphipathic α-helical domain containing a heptad repeat of leucine residues that has been termed a leucine-zipper (25). Both Fos and Jun, as well as all other members of the *fos* and *jun* gene families (i.e., *fos*B, *fra*1, *fra*2, *jun*B, and *jun*D), possess leucine zippers. All members of the *fos* family of proteins can form heterodimers with any member of the *jun* family. In addition, proteins of the *jun* family can form hetero- and homodimers among themselves, a property that is not shared by Fos or its family members (Fig. 3) (for reviews see refs. 7 and 23).

Subsequent to dimerization, the various homo- and heterodimeric complexes bind to a specific deoxyribonucleic acid (DNA) sequence, TGACTCA (7,24,37). Independently, this sequence was identified as the canonical binding site for the transcription factor activator protein 1 (AP-1) and is essential for both basal and stimulated transcription from several genes (reviewed in ref. 7). Subsequently, AP-1 was shown to be comprised of Fos and Jun as well as several Fos- and Jun-related proteins. Binding of deoxyribonucleic acid is largely confirmed by regions

in Fos and Jun that are rich in basic amino acids. Each member of the dimer contributes a half-site for DNA binding. Whereas all dimeric combinations of AP-1 interact with the same, or similar, DNA sequences, it is to be expected that there must be dimer-specific differences in the details of binding and/or the consequences for transcription. Indeed, distinctions can be detected with DNA binding and transactivation assays. For example, Fos–Jun heterodimers bend DNA in a different direction to Jun–Jun homodimers (23). Such an effect might account for why some combinations of AP-1 dimers promote transcription from a particular target gene whereas others inhibit expression.

Both leucine zipper and basic DNA-binding domains have been detected in other families of transcription factors, such as the activating transcription factors (ATFs) and cyclic adenosine monophosphate response element binding proteins (CREBs). This led to the coining of the term basic-zipper protein to describe the members of a superfamily of transcription factors that includes the Fos and Jun families of proteins as well as CREBs and ATFs (24). Furthermore, various members of this superfamily are capable of cross-family dimerization (15). For example, Jun may dimerize with CREBP1, giving rise to a heterodimer that binds to the cyclic adenosine monophosphate (cAMP) response element (CRE, TGAGCTCA) rather than the AP-1 site (TGACTCA). Thus, the use of the term AP-1 to describe Jun, is a misnomer, since its DNA-binding specificity (and possibly transactivating potential) is a function of its partner in the dimer. One other point should be noted here, namely that many members of the basic-zipper superfamily are not inducible genes. In fact, *jun*D, a member of the *jun* family, is a constitutively expressed transcription factor. Therefore, a more accurate view of the immediate-early response as it applies to members of the basic-zipper family is one in which there is a varied and complex pattern of dimer formation between both inducible and constitutively expressed transcription factors. Although not extensively investigated, it is supposed that the precise details of this pattern are a function of the cell type and the stimulus used. Likewise, it is postulated that the genomic targets for these dimers and the consequences for transcription will also be dictated to some degree by cell type and stimulus.

Diverse types of extracellular stimuli, via second messenger molecules, elicit the rapid transcriptional activation of cellular IEGs such as c-*fos* and c-*jun*. Both c-*fos* and c-*jun* belong to gene families whose products in turn share general structural features with other transcription factors that together constitute a superfamily, termed *basic-zipper* proteins. Further families of basic-zipper proteins include the CREBs (cyclic AMP response element binding proteins), ATFs (activating transcription factors) and the Maf proteins. These proteins all form homo- and heterodimers by way of a leucine-zipper structure, shown in Fig. 3 as four horizontal bars. These dimeric complexes then show relatively specific binding to short DNA elements that is mediated by domains rich in basic amino acids. In the case of Fos–Jun heterodimers, DNA binding is to the AP-1 (activator protein-1) consensus site (TGACTCA). The binding of the dimeric complex is then believed to contribute to the transcription of genes bearing such sites in their promoters. Although many members of the *fos* and *jun* gene families are IEGs (e.g. *fra*-1, *fos*B, *jun*B) others, such as *jun*D, are constitutively expressed as are many members of the basic-zipper superfamily, such as CREBP1 in the example shown. Furthermore, these additional families of basic-zipper proteins can form intra- and interfamily dimers that can interact with other consensus DNA-binding sites. Thus, a more realistic picture of the IEG response as applied to the basic-zipper family is one in which inducible and constitutive proteins interact in a temporally dynamic manner to control transcription of target genes. DNA binding specificity is determined by the precise composition of the complex. In the example shown in Fig. 3, Fos–Jun dimers bind at the AP-1 site, whereas Jun-CREBP1 dimers bind at a CRE site. However, it is now known that other consensus sequences exist for other dimer configurations. Obviously this situation provides for enormous diversity, and it is presumed that the phenotype of the cell and the nature of the stimulus must determine the net genomic response.

When *fos* and *jun* expression was investigated in the nervous system, a further property of AP-1 dimer formation emerged. Seizures result in a transient induction of c-*fos* and c-*jun* messenger ribonucleic acid (mRNA) in the brain (49). However, when gel retardation and immunoblot analyses were carried out on nuclear extracts from brains of mice that had received seizures, a paradox emerged (47). Although *fos* mRNA and protein appeared and disappeared in the brain within 3 to 4 hr of a seizure, AP-1 DNA-binding activity was elevated for 8 to 17 hr (depending on the type of seizure). This was explained by the fact that there was a delayed, but protracted, induction of several proteins that cross-reacted with the Fos-antiserum that could also participate in AP-1 complexes. That is, there was a staggered appearance and disappearance of Fos and several Fos-related proteins that can all contribute to AP-1-like complexes. Thus, the composition of AP-1 alters in a dynamic and reproducible manner with time after seizure (30,47). Therefore, when analyzing components of the immediate-early gene response, time is a critical variable.

Immediate-Early Gene Expression in the Nervous System

Even though the study of immediate-early gene expression in the nervous system has burgeoned in recent years, basically only two types of experiments have been performed. The large majority of the studies have involved the monitoring of one or another IEG product (usually Fos) as a surrogate marker of neuronal activation. These investigations range from the analysis of IEG expression in cell culture to measurements of IEG levels and distribution in the brain following the application of many types of physiological, pharmacological, and behavioral stimuli. These studies are now so numerous (in excess of 500) that it would be inappropriate to elaborate them here and the interested reader is directed to a number of reviews on the subject (30,31,43). However, specific examples are used to illustrate particular methods or approaches in IEG research. A lesser number of investigators have tried to establish the roles that IEG products might play in particular neurobiological processes by trying to perturb their expression or activity.

Mapping, studies have utilized a range of techniques that include, Northern and Western blotting, immunohistochemistry, in situ hybridization, and gel retardation assays, as well as transgenic animal and DNA transfection technologies. Investigations of IEG function have proven much more difficult and have involved a range of approaches such as in vitro transcription assays, transfection analyses, antisense, and gene knockout methods, as well as transgenic mouse experiments utilizing targeted overexpression of particular IEGs or inhibitors (e.g., transdominant suppressors). Given the preponderance of the mapping type of study, most of the methodological details and critique elaborated in this chapter are focused on this type of analysis. In addition, a novel approach is presented for IEG mapping that employs transgenic *fos–lacZ* reporter mice. These animals represent a model in which one can rapidly and unambiguously follow IEG expression with single-cell resolution.

MAPPING OF IMMEDIATE-EARLY GENE EXPRESSION IN THE NERVOUS SYSTEM

Biochemical Analyses

The least ambiguous and simplest measure of IEG expression involves Northern transfer and hybridization (28,49). This method has the advantage of clearly identifying the transcript, it is quantifiable, and it can be applied to multiple IEGs in the same sample. Its principal limitation is that it lacks cellular resolution and requires a substantial amount of tissue. Although a polymerase chain reaction (PCR) may circumvent the sample size problem, thereby permitting a finer regional localization, this method is notoriously nonquantitative and should, in any case, be confirmed by Northern analysis. In terms of sensitivity, RNAase protection assays lie between Northern blots and PCR, and they can be made quantitative. However, the method is far less routine than the other two and conditions need to be worked out for each IEG transcript. Finally, Northern blots, RNAse protection, and PCR may not necessarily reflect the level of the cognate protein, because mRNA for IEGs can accumulate to high levels in the absence of protein synthesis. This is not a facile point, because a number of neuropathological situations, such as cerebral ischemia, may be associated with a block of translation. This is known to have produced confusing, and sometimes contradictory, results in studies of IEG expression in animal models of stroke (13,14,21,22).

To circumvent the issue of extrapolating alterations in mRNA levels to changes in protein levels, a number of investigators have used immunoblotting to assess IEG expression (e.g., 47). This procedure still has the limitation of lacking cellular resolution, but it has proven useful in establishing the time frame of changes in the expression of some IEGs. However, this approach does have additional complications. First, sample preparation becomes a significant issue, because some authors have found that crude nuclear extracts must be prepared from brain to obtain adequate Western blots for some IEGs. Second, the validity of the data relies solely on the specificity and affinity of the antisera or antibodies used. Because many of the IEGs belong to gene families, some antisera are known to cross-react with related proteins and reveal bands of the incorrect size in immunoblots (47). Unfortunately, few of the investigators using this approach run authentic (i.e., recombinant) protein standards.

A further biochemical approach for investigating IEG expression takes advantage of the fact that many of their products bind to specific DNA sequences. Thus their levels can been determined in a semiquantitative manner by so-called gel retardation or mobility shift assays (47). In this procedure protein extracts are mixed with radioactively labeled double-stranded oligonucleotides that contain the consensus-binding sequence for particular IEG transcription factors. These complexes are then run on a nondenaturing gel, which separates bound from free probe. The bound and unbound species can be detected subsequently by autoradiography. This strategy has proven very useful in analysis of AP-1 levels in both mouse and rat brains following a number of challenges, including seizures and chronic administration of drugs of abuse (see Chapter 61, this volume). In addition, by using other consensus sites, it has proven possible to analyze binding of CREB proteins in brain extracts.

In our hands, gel retardation analysis is most reproducible when using crude nuclear brain extracts rather than whole homogenates. This nuclear preparation has the added advantage that it is amenable to assay by immunoblotting, which can be performed in parallel with the gel shift and provides a further level of information concerning the composition of the complexes (47). The analysis of the components of particular complexes can be extended by the use of commercial antisera to many components of the CREB, ATF, and AP-1 families. These are useful not only for immunoblots but also gel shifts. Conventionally, one pretreats the nuclear extracts for from a few hours up to a day (in some cases) before adding the labeled oligonucleotide and performing the gel shift. Active antisera may either supershift the complex (by contributing to its mass and further slowing the probe's migration) or destroy its DNA binding activity. A further proof of specificity relies on appropriate patterns of displacement of radiolabeled probe binding by unlabeled oligonucleotides. In many cases, investigators have used unlabeled cognate probe and an irrelevant oligonucleotide. However, it is now apparent that such controls for specificity are incomplete. Just because a complex forms on an AP-1 site does not necessarily mean that it will not bind as well or better to other consensus sites. For example, complexes that bind to AP-1 sites often bind just as well to CRE sites. Thus competition curves should be performed for various canonical binding sites and to sequences containing point mutations that destroy biological activity.

One advantage of the gel shift method is that it involves the assay of an intrinsic biological property of a protein(s) and, therefore, requires neither prior knowledge of the composition of the complex nor specific reagents. Thus it nicely complements the other biochemical methods that rely exclusively on hybridization of specific copy DNA (cDNA) probes or reaction with specific antisera. However, like other bulk methods, gel shifts do not provide

cellular resolution. Another limitation is that they are notoriously sensitive to the incubation conditions. Indeed,
there are a number of fundamentally different sets of
incubation conditions for gel shift analysis. For example,
some workers use low ionic strength buffers, whereas
others use high ionic strength. Another example specifically relates to AP-1 binding. It is known that recombinant
Fos and Jun do not bind the AP-1 consensus site with high
affinity unless they are in a highly reducing environment;
usually 5 mM diothiothreitol (DTT) (1). The molecular
basis for this effect has been elucidated and involves the
reduction of a single cysteine residue that appears to spontaneously oxidize to an uncharacterized intermediate (e.g.,
sulfinic acid derivative). These redox-driven changes on
cysteine do not involve disulfide bond formation. A cellular protein, Ref-1, has been cloned that is able to reduce
the partially oxidized cysteine present in both Fos and Jun
to the sulfhydryl form (51). Therefore, details of tissue
preparation and reducing capacity are especially critical
when determining AP-1-like DNA binding activity. Nevertheless, some studies still employ 1 mM DTT, which
is normally insufficient to maintain the cysteine in Fos in
its sulfhydryl (DNA-binding) form. Unfortunately, these
disparate assay conditions often make it difficult or impossible to directly compare results obtained in different
laboratories.

Anatomical Methods

The fundamental limitation of the preceeding methods
is that they all lack cellular resolution. That is, they cannot
reveal precisely which cells are expressing particular IEG
products. Conventionally, two methods have been used
to investigate the cellular localization of IEG products:
namely, in situ hybridization and immunohistochemistry.
These are the anatomical homologs of Northern and Western blots, respectively, and have the same limitations regarding their dependence on the availability of specific
reagents. Nevertheless, both of these techniques have
been widely applied as neuroanatomical mapping techniques. Indeed, their use has burgeoned with the availability of commercial sources of antisera to Fos and several
other IEG products (31).

Initially, immunohistochemistry for Fos was limited by
the fact that most antisera were supplied by individual
researchers and several of these reagents were known to
cross-react with other inducible proteins (10,19,29,41).
Indeed, one of the most commonly used antisera revealed
a composite picture of Fos-like immunoreactivity (FLI)
that included Fos, FosB and two unidentified inducible
proteins of approximately 35 and 46 kDa, respectively
(47). In the unstimulated brain, the predominant contributor to FLI is an unidentified 35-kDa Fos-related antigen
(FRA 35K). During the first 2 hr after application of a

convulsant stimulus, the predominant contributor to FLI
is Fos itself. Subsequently Fos levels wane, and by far
the major components of FLI are the FRA-35K and FRA-
46K. The latter component can be detected 18 to 48 hr
following certain types of seizures (48).

Fos immunohistochemistry has been used to determine
the pattern of activation of neurons in many situations.
Administration of many types of neuropharmacologically
active substances induce FLI. It would be impossible to
document all the examples of these applications, because
it would reduce this chapter to little more than a catalog
of drugs and effects on FLI. Likewise, the constraint on
citations precludes exhaustive referencing. Therefore, in
the absence of any current reviews we have listed a number of more recent papers that provide a more detailed
literature base. Thus, FLI has been used to investigate
the pharmacology of dopamine D_1 and D_2 receptors (see
Chapter 19, this volume), nicotinic (39) and muscarinic
(18) cholinergic receptors, serotonin (40) and catecholaminergic (50) systems, as well as N-methyl-D-aspartate
(NMDA) and non-NMDA glutamate receptors (2). It has
also been used to study more complex neural processes
such as long-term potentiation (8), circadian rhythmicity
(38), and behavioral phenomena such as kindling (10)
and learning (3).

Studies with antisera to the Jun family of proteins are
now beginning to reveal interesting patterns of expression
in a number of neurobiologically relevant situations
(16,20). Like c-fos, both c-jun and junB are activated by
numerous types of stimuli in a characteristic spatial and
temporal manner in the brain. Although many of these
sites and situations are the same as those in which FLI
is detected, some unique patterns of expression have been
observed. A notable example is the persistent expression
of Jun (but not Fos) following axotomy (16,20). A further
family member, junD, appears to be expressed continuously and at relatively high levels in the brain. Although
junD is not an IEG, sensu stricto (it is not superinduced
by cycloheximide treatment), some reports have indicated
localized and delayed increases in its expression in the
nervous system (e.g., 16). However, in our hands, expression of junD mRNA is constant in several seizure models
in rats and mice.

Published protocols for immunohistochemistry are diverse, although generally the most reproducible and convincing results have been obtained on floating cryostat
sections. Many of the references cited above for the application of Fos mapping in the brain contain details of
successful immunohistochemical protocols. In most all
instances, FLI is nuclear and one observes exclusion from
the nucleolus and its associated heterochromatin (35). A
number of studies have shown cytoplasmic staining using
anti-Fos antisera, although the only case for which there
is any evidence of Fos being present outside of the nucleus
involves cell death. Thus, when showing cytoplasmic FLI,

an independent confirmation is required (e.g., in situ hybridization or a biochemical characterization), and one should consider the likelihood that a cross-reacting material is being detected.

The major limitation of in situ hybridization is not so much specificity (although this may be a concern with closely related gene products or where nucleotide sequences are based upon cDNAs from other species) but rather the fact that it does not measure directly the level of IEG proteins. In addition, there may be problems with detection limits and quantitation. Like immunohistochemistry, this approach has been quite rewarding and is especially useful when combined with immunohistochemistry for IEG products or other proteins (e.g., neuropeptides or cell-specific markers).

Because immunohistochemistry and in situ hybridization are methods that are generally slow and prone to ambiguity, we have developed a completely novel approach to neuroanatomical mapping of IEG products. The strategy has been to introduce a readily detectable reporter gene (bacterial β-galactosidase) into the IEG of interest in such a way as to retain all natural regulatory elements of the gene (42). Furthermore, these constructs generate a fusion protein between the enzyme and the IEG protein that still translocates to the nucleus. Thus, this fusion gene drives expression of nuclear β-galactosidase, which can be readily detected in frozen sections by routine histochemistry. The nuclear localization was chosen, because it provides a more useful anatomical marker that discriminates pre- from postsynaptic elements. In addition, it concentrates the signal, thereby improving the signal-to-noise ratio.

We have used such fusion genes to construct cell lines (42) and transgenic mice (45) that accurately recapitulate expression of several IEGs (28,44,45,46). This method provides excellent cellular resolution; it is relatively rapid compared to both immunohistochemistry and in situ hybridization; it can be made quantitative; it does not require specialized (and often expensive) reagents; it is nonradioisotopic; and there is no ambiguity with regard to the gene that has been activated. Using trangenic mice, one can obtain complete maps of *fos–lacZ* expression following administration of various types of stimuli to the central nervous system (45). Furthermore, primary neural cultures can be generated from the mice that permit analysis of gene expression in vitro following administration of classical neurotransmitters and neuropeptides, as well as neuropharmacological agonists and antagonists (45). In addition, permanent cell lines harboring the fusion gene can be grown in microtiter plates so that they can be treated, lysed, incubated with substrate, and assayed for β-galactosidase by a multiwell reader (42). This assay has a rapid throughput, it is quantitative, and it is particularly useful in screening for agents that interact with ion channels or neurotransmitter receptors.

The obvious caveat of this transgenic approach is that one must firmly establish that the transgene faithfully reflects the expression of the endogenous gene (although for some applications this may be irrelevant). To some degree this can be achieved by ensuring that the transgene is expressed under all of the same circumstances that have been reported in the literature for the cognate IEG. At least to a first approximation, this is true, and those differences that do exist are likely to reflect shortcomings in antibody specificity and/or species differences (most analyses of IEG expression have been performed on the rat). Thus both basal and inducible sites of Fos–lacZ expression are coincident with that observed using antibodies and oligonucleotides probes.

Another word of caution should be raised here regarding variability in expression between independent lines of mice harboring a particular gene construct. When embarking on this type of approach, one needs to be aware that rarely are two lines identical in their expression properties. Typically, there is great variability in the absolute level of expression. Thus for practical reasons we select lines that have robust expression. In addition, with *fos–lacZ* constructs we have noted that the induced patterns of expression are incomplete in some lines. That is, one observes induced expression but only in a subset of cells or tissues. Therefore, we apply a second selection criteria: namely that the overall pattern of expression should match, as far as we can determine it, the normal expression profile of the endogenous gene. For this reason, we always attempt to confirm novel sites of Fos–lacZ expression by some independent means such as immunohistochemistry or Northern blot (28). Based on our experience with over 20 lines of *fos–lacZ* rodents, one needs to derive a minimum of five independent founder lines to obtain one that fulfills both selection criteria of robust and faithful expression.

The half-life of the Fos–lacZ fusion protein is somewhat longer than that of Fos (42), although it is still relatively short-lived. The greater half-life of the fusion protein lengthens the time window in which expression can be detected (which is often an advantage for Fos), and it also improves the detection limits of the method. Despite the altered protein half-life, the transgene is induced and repressed with the same kinetics as *fos*. Like c-*fos*, the mRNA for the transgene is short-lived, a property that is conferred by inclusion of 3' untranslated sequences from c-*fos* in the fusion construct. A minor technical caveat is that the histochemical method can detect endogenous galactosidases, which makes working with tissues that are rich in these enzymes more difficult. Even though the brain is not among these tissues, we have, nevertheless, refined the fixation and incubation conditions to such a point that most tissues can now be studied. We should also point out that since the Fos–lacZ carries a nuclear localization signal, it is readily distinguished from artifactual staining which is invariably extra- or perinuclear.

A number of novel features of IEG expression have emerged from studies of these transgenic mice. Besides the well-documented induction of *fos* and *jun* by various stimuli, we found many tissues that either constitutively expressed these genes in the adult or that spontaneously expressed them during development (28,44–46). In some instances the continuous expression of Fos–lacZ was associated with cells that were undergoing terminal differentiation, particularly where this culminated in cell death within a period of a few days to a week (45,46). Examples of this in the adult animal included the skin and hair follicle, hypertrophic chondrocytes of the bone and follicular cells within atretic follicles of the ovary. Similarly a number of cell populations that are eliminated during development spontaneously expressed Fos–lacZ, such as interdigital web cells and cells of the periderm and the heart valve cushion. In other instances of *fos–lacZ* expression during development, the cells appear to undergo complex processes that include programmed cell death, migration, or transdifferentiation. Examples here include, the medial edge epithelium of the palate, the ureteric bud of the kidney, and developing bronchioles of the lung (28,46). A number of examples of Fos–lacZ expression were also found in the developing nervous system (44). For instance, Fos–lacZ was noted in some of the cranial and dorsal root ganglia at a time when programmed cell death is known to occur. Other instances of naturally occuring Fos–lacZ expression appeared to be related to maturation of certain neuronal pathways and may be a reflection of plasticity. Thus in the perinatal brain, spontaneous Fos–lacZ expression is associated with cells in the olfactory tract, limbic system, and thalamus (44). This expression is more consistent with the acquisition of behaviors involving chemosensory, exploratory, and motor processing. It is now interesting to examine whether the transgene can be used to map the maturation of functional circuitry in the nervous system.

The circumstantial association of Fos–lacZ expression with programmed cell death, both in the nervous system and elsewhere, suggested that the transgene might have utility in following the demise of neurons under pathological conditions. This notion has been tested in three models of neuronal death. The first involved crossing the *fos–lacZ* transgenic mice onto the *weaver* mutation, which exhibits degeneration of cerebellar granule cells in the immediate postpartum period and neurons of the substantia nigra in the adult. In both cases, inappropriate expression of Fos–lacZ was observed in the affected neuronal populations (46).

In a second paradigm, the sciatic nerve was transected in the neonatal *fos–lacZ* mouse. This results in the degeneration of sensory neurons in the dorsal root ganglia and α-motor neurons in the ventral spinal cord. Once again,

both populations of cells exhibited inappropriate expression of Fos–lacZ, suggesting that death triggered by growth factor deprivation results in an activation of the IEG cascade (46).

Finally, transgenic mice were exposed to the excitatory neurotoxin, kainic acid, which resulted in the delayed death of pyramidal neurons in CA1 and CA3 of the hippocampus as well as neurons within the amygdala. Again, all of these cells expressed Fos–lacZ while the death process was going on. Indeed, in this case, there were two phases of transgenic expression. There was an initial, transient, global phase of expression associated with the seizures elicited by kainic acid and a subsequent reexpression of Fos–lacZ some 4 to 7 days later only in the vulnerable neuronal populations. Furthermore, a hallmark of this delayed expression was that the LacZ was detected both in the nucleus and cytoplasm of the neurons (46). This may be because the cells were deteriorating and loosing nuclear integrity or simply were metabolically compromised and could not traffic the protein adequately. Alternatively, it may be that elevated proteolysis associated with the treatment results in the cleavage of some proportion of the LacZ from Fos, thereby removing the nuclear localization sequences. Whatever the reason, the presence of cytoplasmic Fos seems to be a harbinger of neuronal death. The key issue now is to determine what role, if any, the IEGs play in promoting or combating neuronal death in vivo.

The transgenic approach has one unique advantage over all other conventional neuroanatomical mapping techniques: namely, it can provide information regarding the signaling pathways operating in given neurobiological responses in vivo. The promoter of c-*fos* (and many other IEGs) contains a series of response elements that confer inducibility by various intracellular signaling pathways (reviewed in refs. 31 and 43). For example, experiments involving transient transfection in cell culture have established that nerve growth factor and NMDA induction of c-*fos* requires an intact serum response element (SRE). In contrast, depolarizing stimuli, or agents that act by elevating intracellular cAMP levels, act through a quite distinct site, the calcium-cAMP–response element (CARE). This situation affords the possibility of dissecting these pathways in vivo by introducing point mutations into one or another of the responsive elements in the context of *fos–lacZ* transgenes.

Transgenic mice have been generated that carry a number of mutated *fos* promoter constructs driving *lacZ* expression. These mice reveal a number of properties of *fos* expression that provide insights into the cellular and biochemical mechanisms involved in neurophysiological and neuropharmacological responses. For example, some mutations eliminate both basal and stimulated expression of the transgene. In other cases, basal and continuous sites of expression are lost, but the gene is perfectly inducible in the brain. Yet other mutations reveal a heterogeneity among neuronal populations with regard to their response to a given stimulus. For example, with the unmutated promoter, all CA1 and CA3 pyramidal neurons of the hippocampus are induced for *fos-lacZ* by kainic acid, whereas one promoter mutation shows normal (if not better) induction in CA1 but no expression in CA3 following administration of the same stimulus. One would conclude, therefore, that the signaling pathways linking a single type of stimulant, kainic acid, to IEG expression is distinct in CA1 and CA3 neurons. Thus this genetic dissection approach offers a unique potential for furthering our understanding of information processing in specific neuronal populations.

We have now generated a series of transgenic mice and rats that harbor various fusion constructs between IEGs and *lacZ*. These animals provide a unique and novel resource for studying IEG expression in vivo. The approach can be extended by crossing the mice onto various neurologically mutant backgrounds or by using promoter mutations that can reveal subtleties in neuronal signaling that could not be inferred from any other known method. We feel that these animals represent merely the first generation of such constructs and that we have not yet begun to tap the real potential of this type of methodology. For example, parallel strategies might be to use the IEG promoters to drive inducible expression of engineered forms of IEGs that interfere with the function of the cognate proteins. Such transdominant suppressors might thereby provide a means by which one could establish whether individual IEG products contributed to particular neurobiological processes. Indeed, it now seems most likely that the emphasis in the field will shift from simple mapping studies to those involving function.

REFERENCES

1. Abate C, Patel L, Rauscher FJ III, Curran T. Redox regulation of Fos and Jun DNA binding activity in vitro. *Science* 1990;249:1157–1161.
2. Berreta S, Robertson HA, Graybiel AM. Dopamine and glutamate agonists stimulate neuron-specific expression of Fos-like protein in the striatum. *J Neurophysiol* 1992;68:767–777.
3. Castro-Alamancos MA, Borrell J, Garcia-Segura LM. Performance in an escape task induces *fos*-like immunoreactivity in a specific area of the motor cortex of the rat. *Neuroscience* 1992;49:157–162.
4. Cochran BH, Reffel AC, Stiles CD. Molecular cloning of gene sequences regulated by platelet-derived growth factor. *Cell* 1983;33:939–947.
5. Curran T, Morgan JI. Memories of Fos. *BioEssays* 1987;7:255–258.
6. Curran T, Morgan JI. Superinduction of *fos* by nerve growth factor in the presence of peripherally active benzodiazepines. *Science* 1985;229:1265–1268.
7. Curran T, Franza BR Jr. Fos and Jun: the AP-1 connection. *Cell* 1988;55:395–397.
8. Demmer J, Dragunow M, Lawlor PA, et al. Differential expression of immediate early genes after hippocampal long-term potentiation in awake rats. *Mol Brain Res* 1993;17:279–286.
9. Dragunow M, Faull R. The use of c-*fos* as a metabolic marker in neuronal pathway tracing. *J Neurosci Meth* 1989;29:261–265.
10. Dragunow M, Robertson HA. Kindling stimulation induces c-*fos* protein(s) in granule cells of the dentate gyrus. *Nature* 1987;329:441–442.
11. Greenberg ME, Greene LA, Ziff EB. Nerve growth factor and epidermal growth factor induce rapid transient changes in proto-oncogene transcription in PC12 cells. *J Biol Chem* 1985;260:14101–14110.
12. Greenberg ME, Ziff EB. Stimulation of 3T3 cells induces transcription of the *fos* proto-oncogene. *Nature* 1984;311:433–438.
13. Gubits RM, Burke RE, Casey-MacIntosh G, Bandele A, Munell F. Immediate-early gene induction after neonatal hypoxia-ischemia. *Mol Brain Res* 1993;18:228–238.
14. Gunn AJ, Dragunow M, Faull RLM, Gluckman PD. Effects of hypoxia-ischemia and seizures on neuronal and glial-like c-*fos* protein levels in the infant rat. *Brain Res* 1990;531:105–116.
15. Hai T, Curran T. Cross-family dimerization of transcription factors Fos/Jun and ATF/CREB alters DNA binding specificity. *Proc Natl Acad Sci USA* 1991;88:1–5.
16. Herdegen T, Fiallos-Estrada CE, Schmid W, Bravo R, Zimmermann M. The transcription factors c-JUN, JUN D and CREB, but not FOS and KROX-24, are differentially regulated in axotomized neurons following transection of rat sciatic nerve. *Mol Brain Res* 1992;14:155–165.
17. Hilbush BS, Curran T, Morgan JI. (1994) Cellular immediate-early genes in the nervous system: genes for all reasons? In: Fuxe K, Leon A, Ottoson D, eds. *Trophic regulation in the basal ganglia. Focus on dopamine neurons.* New York: Pergamon Press, 1994; [*in press*].
18. Hughes P, Dragunow M. Muscarinic receptor-mediated induction of FOS protein in rat brain. *Neurosci Lett* 1993;150:122–126.
19. Hunt SP, Pini A, Evan G. Induction of c-*fos* like protein in spinal cord neurons following sensory stimulation. *Nature* 1987;328:632–634.
20. Jenkins R, Hunt SP. Long term increase in the levels of c-*jun* mRNA and Jun protein-like immunoreactivity in motor and sensory neurons following axon damage. *Neurosci Lett* 1991;129:107–110.
21. Jorgenson M, Deckert J, Wright D, Gehlert D. Delayed c-*fos* proto-oncogene expression in the rat hippocampus induced by transient global cerebral ischemia: an in situ hybridization study. *Brain Res* 1989;484:393–398.
22. Keissling M, Stumm P, Xie Y, Gass P. Differential transcription and translation of immediate-early genes after global ischaemia in gerbil brain. *J Cereb Blood Flow* 1993;13(Suppl 1):S465.
23. Kerppola T, Curran T. Fos-Jun heterodimers and Jun homodimers bend DNA in opposite orientations: implications for transcription factor cooperativity. *Cell* 1992;66:317–326.
24. Kerppola T, Curran T. Transcription factor interactions: basics on zippers. *Curr Opin Struct Biol* 1991;1:71–79.
25. Landshultz WH, Johnson PF, McKnight SL. The leucine zipper: a hypothetical structure common to a new class of DNA binding proteins. *Science* 1988;240:1759–1764.
26. Lau LF, Nathans D. Expression of a set of growth-related immediate-early genes in BALB/c 3T3 cells: coordinate regulation with c-*fos* or c-*myc*. *Proc Natl Acad Sci USA* 1987;84:1182–1186.
27. Lau LF, Nathans D. Identification of a set of genes expressed during the G0/G1 transition of cultured mouse cells. *EMBO J* 1985;4:3145–3151.
28. Molinar-Rode R, Smeyne RJ, Curran T, Morgan JI. Regulation of proto-oncogene expression in adult and developing lungs. *Mol Cell Biol* 1993;13:3213–3220.
29. Morgan JI, Cohen DR, Hempstead JL, Curran T. Mapping patterns of c-*fos* expression in the central nervous system after seizure. *Science* 1987;237:192–197.
30. Morgan JI, Curran T. Stimulus-transcription coupling in neurons: role of cellular immediate-early genes. *Trends Neurosci* 1989;12:259–462.
31. Morgan JI, Curran T. Stimulus-transcription coupling in the nervous system: involvement of the inducible proto-oncogenes *fos* and *jun*. *Annu Rev Neurosci* 1991;14:421–451.
32. Morgan JI, Curran T. The role of ion flux in the control of c-*fos* expression. *Nature* 1986;322:552–555.

33. Morgan JI, Curran T. Calcium as a modulator of the immediate-early gene cascade in neurons. *Cell Calcium* 1988;9:303–311.
34. Morgan JI. *Proto-oncogene expression in the nervous system.* (vol. 7). Magistretti JP, ed; *Discussion in neuroscience, FESN;* Amsterdam: Elsevier; 1991.
35. Mugnaini E, Berrebi A, Morgan JI, Curran T. *fos*-like immunoreactivity induced by seizure is specifically associated with euchromatin in neurons. *Eur J Neurosci* 1989;1:46–52.
36. Muller R, Bravo R, Burckhardt J, Curran T. Induction of c-*fos* gene and protein by growth factors precedes activation of c-*myc*. *Nature* 1984;312:716–720.
37. Rauscher FJ III, Sambucetti LC, Curran T, Distel RJ, Spiegelman BM. A common DNA binding site for Fos protein complexes and transcription factor AP-1. *Cell* 1988;52:471–480.
38. Rea MA. Light increases Fos-related protein immunoreactivity in the rat suprachiasmatic nuclei. *Brain Res Bull* 1989;23:577–581.
39. Ren T, Sagar SM. Induction of c-*fos* immunostaining in the rat brain after systemic administration of nicotine. *Brain Res Bull* 1992;29:589–597.
40. Richard D, Rivest S, Rivier C. The 5-hydroxytryptamine agonist fenfluramine increases Fos-like immunoreactivity in the brain. *Brain Res* 1992;594:131–137.
41. Sagar SM, Sharp FR, Curran T. Expression of c-*fos* protein in brain: metabolic mapping at the cellular level. *Science* 1988;240:1328–1331.
42. Schilling K, Luk D, Morgan JI, Curran T. Regulation of a *fos-lacZ* fusion gene: a paradigm for quantitative analysis of stimulus-transcription coupling. *Proc Natl Acad Sci USA* 1991;88:5665–5669.
43. Sheng M, Greenberg ME. The regulation and function of c-*fos* and other immediate-early genes in the nervous system. *Neuron* 1990;4:477–485.
44. Smeyne RJ, Curran T, Morgan JI. Temporal and spatial expression of a *fos-lacZ* transgene in the developing nervous system. *Mol Brain Res* 1992;16:158–162.
45. Smeyne RJ, Schilling K, Robertson L, et al. Fos-lacZ transgenic mice: mapping sites of gene induction in the central nervous system. *Neuron* 1992;8:13–23.
46. Smeyne RJ, Vendrell M, Hayward M, et al. Continuous c-*fos* expression precedes programmed cell death in vivo. *Nature* 1993;363:166–169.
47. Sonnenberg JL, Macgregor-Leon PF, Curran T, Morgan JI. Dynamic alterations occur in the levels and composition of transcription factor AP-1 complexes after seizure. *Neuron* 1989;3:359–365.
48. Sonnenberg JL, Mitchelmore C, Macgregor-Leon PF, Hempstead JL, Morgan JI, Curran T. Glutamate receptor agonists increase the expression of Fos, Fra and AP-1 DNA binding activity in the mammalian brain. *J Neurosci Res* 1989;24:72–80.
49. Sonnenberg JL, Rauscher FJ III, Morgan JI, Curran T. Regulation of proenkephalin by proto-oncogenes *fos* and *jun*. *Science* 1989;246:1622–1625.
50. Tsujino J, Sano H, Kubota Y, et al. Expression of FOS-like immunoreactivity by yohimbine and clonidine in the rat brain. *Eur J Pharmacol* 1992;226:69–78.
51. Xanthoudakis S, Miao G, Feng W, Pan Y-CE, Curran T. Redox activation of Fos–Jun DNA binding activity is mediated by a DNA repair enzyme. *EMBO J* 1992;11:3323–3335.

Psychopharmacology: The Fourth Generation of Progress, edited by Floyd E. Bloom and David J. Kupfer. Raven Press, Ltd., New York © 1995.

CHAPTER 57

Purinoceptors in Central Nervous System Function

Targets for Therapeutic Intervention

Michael Williams

The seminal observation of Drury and Szent-Gyorgi in 1929 that adenosine (Fig. 1) and its nucleotide congener, adenosine monophosphate (AMP), caused central nervous system (CNS) sedation, reduced cardiac contractility, and increased coronary vasodilation, thus lowering blood pressure in the intact animal has provided the basis for a wealth of studies targeted to elucidating the role(s) of adenosine and adenine nucleotides in mammalian tissue function. It is now well established that both adenosine triphosphate (ATP) and adenosine function as distinct neuromodulatory agents acting through discrete cell-surface receptors (see Chapter 5, *this volume*).

Neuromodulators differ from neurotransmitters in that their effects are generally more global and longer lasting than the effects of the latter (4). Although the function(s) of neuromodulators continue to be refined as more is learned regarding the dynamics of nervous tissue function, the dividing line between neurotransmitters and neuromodulators, autocrine agents and homeostatic modulators, autocrine and paracrine has become increasingly imprecise, especially when neurotransmitters, acting via early-response gene activation, have effects on neuronal and glial phenotypes (38) (see also Chapters 56, 58, and 59, *this volume*).

Adenosine has been described as the "prototypic neuromodulator" (69) acting as a homeostatic agent that probably preceeds the peptide neuromodulators in evolutionary terms. Adenosine triphosphate responses have been recorded in amoeba, annelids, molluscs, coelenter-

ates, crustacea, and insects (8), whereas the adenosine nucleotide, cyclic AMP (cAMP) is a well-established chemoattractant agent in *Dictyostelium discoidium* acting via cell-surface recognition sites (42). Adenosine and ATP, the endogenous agonists active at purinoceptors, are the primary cellular constituents involved in nearly all aspects of cell function, both as metabolic cofactors and as building blocks for nucleic acids and proteins. Therefore the concept that these entities might function as neuromodulators in the synaptic cleft was a subject of controversy for a considerable period of time (3,69). In the last decade, however, with the development of selective ligands for the various receptor subtypes and the isolation of the genes that code for both adenosine and ATP receptors, definitive evidence has been obtained for the existence of purinoceptors.

RECEPTOR NOMENCLATURE

In 1978, Burnstock described two classes of purinoceptors based on pharmacologic criteria. At P_1 receptors, adenosine and its analogs were agonists (Table 1) and their effects could be blocked by various xanthines and other nonxanthine heterocycles. P_2 receptors were activated by ATP and other purine and pyrimidine nucleotides. Proposed antagonists for P_2 receptors have not proven to be sufficiently robust and selective to function as tools for the assessment of receptor function.

The P_1/P_2 nomenclature has undergone continuous refinement as new receptor subclasses have been identified on the basis of pharmacologic and molecular structural

M. Williams: Neuroscience Research, Pharmaceutical Products Division, Abbott Laboratories, Abbott, Illinois 60064.

PURINOCEPTOR AGONISTS

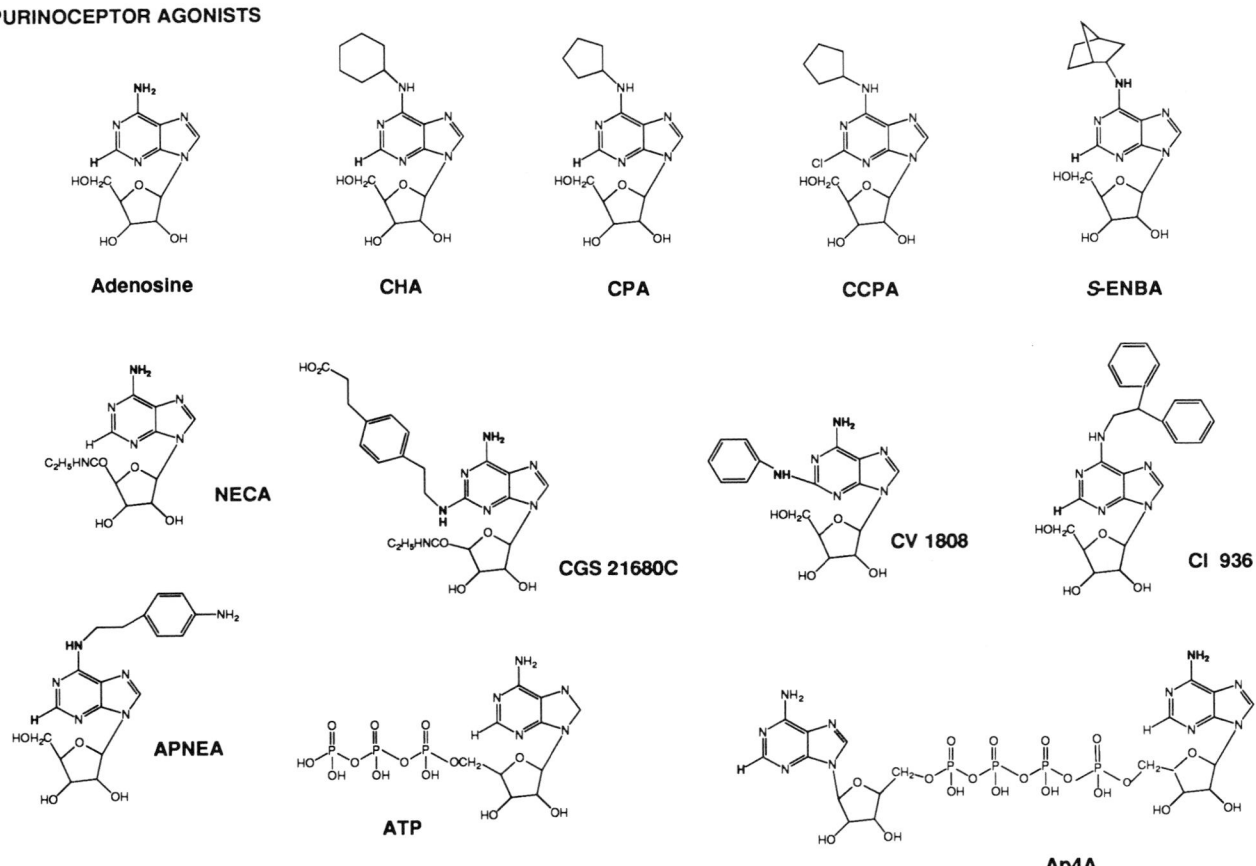

FIG. 1. Structures of purinoceptor ligands.

studies. Nonetheless, the nomenclature has stood the test of time and is the basis of the IUPHAR Committee on Purinoceptor Nomenclature recommendations (2,25).

ADENOSINE P₁ PURINOCEPTORS

The P₁ purinoceptor family is a G-protein coupled receptor (GPCR) superfamily that can be further subdivided into A₁, A₂ₐ, A₂ᵦ, A₃, and A₄ subclasses, the A prefix referring to the agonist activity of adenosine (Table 1). A₁, A₂ₐ, and A₂ᵦ receptors are blocked by xanthines. The A₃ and A₄ receptors, however, are functionally insensitive to xanthines, negating one of the original criteria for establishing an adenosine receptor-mediated response.

The A₁ receptor was defined originally on the basis of the ability of adenosine agonists to inhibit adenylate cyclase activity. This response is blocked by the prototypic adenosine antagonists, caffeine and theophylline, as well as by a variety of more potent and selective 8-phenyl substituted xanthines (cyclopentylxanthine, CPX; cyclopentyltheophylline, CPT; xanthine amine congener, XAC) (Fig. 1) most of which are selective for the A₁ receptor. The A₁ receptor is coupled to Gᵢ and Gₒ proteins

(25). A₁ receptors are also linked to stimulation of potassium conductance, inhibition of N-channel mediated calcium conductance, stimulation of phospholipase C production, and modulation of nitric oxide production (8,24,30).

Structure–activity relationships at the A₁ receptor have shown that adenosine analogs substituted in the N⁶ position in general have greater selectivity for the A₁ receptor than for the A₂ receptor (34). N⁶-cyclohexyl (CHA) and N⁶-cyclopentyl adenosine (CPA) (Fig. 1) are 400- to 800-fold selective for the A₁ receptor. N⁶-2-chloroCPA (CCPA) and N⁶-endonorborn-2-yladenosine (S-ENBA) are 1500- and 4700-fold selective, respectively (Fig. 1).

Four of the five P₁ purinoceptor subclasses have been cloned. The canine A₁ receptor RDC7 was identified from a group of orphan GPCRs cloned from canine thyroid (39). Like other GPCRs, RDC7 is a seven helical transmembrane receptor (34). Degenerate concensus primers from RDC7 allowed the cloning of A₁ receptors from cow, rat, and human brain, all of which, like RDC7, encode proteins of 326 amino acids. The human receptor is 94% homologous at the amino acid level with the dog, cow, and rat A₁ receptors differing by 20, 19, and 18 amino acids, respectively (39). These differences may

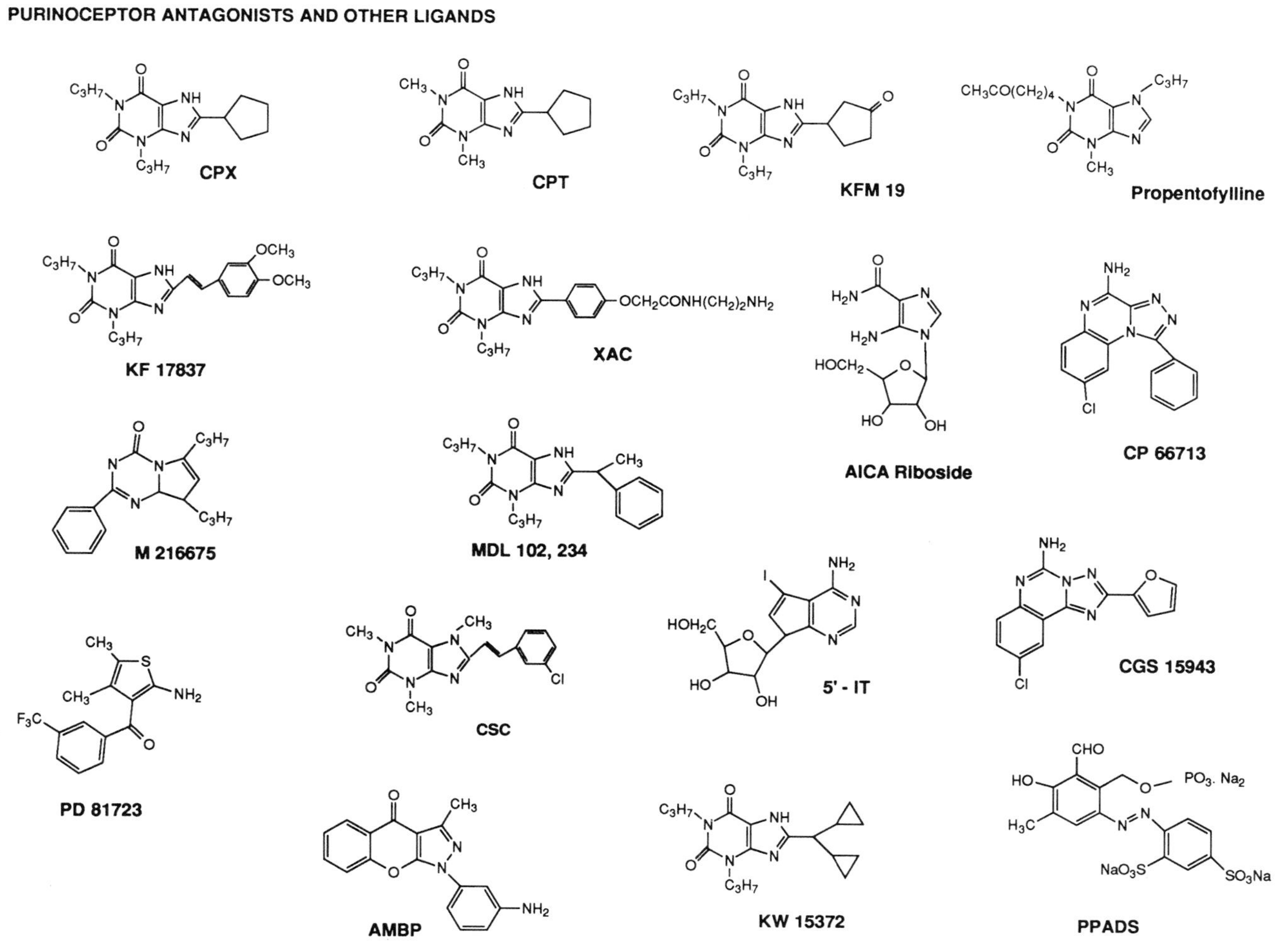

PURINOCEPTOR ANTAGONISTS AND OTHER LIGANDS

FIG. 1. *Continued.*

underlie the reported species differences in the pharmacology of A₁ receptors (69).

The A₂ receptor, originally classified on the basis of its ability to stimulate cAMP formation, can be further subdivided into A₂ₐ and A₂ᵦ subclasses on the basis of pharmacology, functional activity, tissue distribution, and cloning (34,39).

Early studies related to the A₂ receptor involved the use of 5′N-ethylcarboxamido adenosine (NECA) (Fig. 1), a nonselective adenosine agonist that while potent (Ki ~ 10 nM) is equiactive at both A₁ and A₂ receptors. Until the discovery of A₂ₐ-selective agonists in the late 1980s, responses to NECA were thus mistakenly classified as being due to the functional activation of A₂ receptors. The 2-substituted adenosine analog, CV 1808 (2-phenylamino adenosine; Fig. 1), was the first A₂ₐ-selective agonist. It was relatively weak at A₂ₐ receptors (Ki = 100 nM) and was only fivefold selective as compared to its activity at A₁ receptors. Extensive structure–activity studies targeted at the A₂ receptor resulted in the identification of the N⁶-substituted adenosine analog, CI936 (Fig. 1) as the first potent (Ki = 7 nM) A₂ₐ receptor agonist, although

the compound was only fourfold selective. CGS 21680C, a 2-substituted NECA analog was the first potent (Ki = 22 nM) and selective (141-fold) A₂ₐ receptor agonist identified (34). In the absence of selective A₂ₐ receptor antagonists, CGS 21680C has been used to define A₂ₐ responses.

The majority of the published data on the function of the A₂ receptor has been generated using NECA and consequently has not distinguished between A₂ₐ- and A₂ᵦ-mediated events. Additional studies using compounds like CGS 21680C may be anticipated to better define A₂ₐ- and A₂ᵦ-mediated responses. There are currently no known selective ligands for the A₂ᵦ receptor, the lower affinity form of the A₂ receptor identified in fibroblasts and brain slices (34).

Agonist activity at both A₂ receptor subclasses is blocked by theophylline and various 8-phenyl substituted xanthines. The 8-styrylxanthines, KF 17837 (59) and (8-(3-chlorylstyryl) caffeine (CSC) 35) are A₂ₐ receptor selective. A series of nonxanthine heterocycles (Fig. 1) including the triazoloquinazolines (e.g., CGS 15943A), the triazoloquinoxalinamines (e.g., CP 66713), the imidazo-triazinones (e.g., M216675 ZD4398) and the benzopy-

TABLE 1.

Receptor type	Agonists	Antagonists	Transductional Systems	Amino Acids	Clone
P₁ (adenosine)					
A1	CCPA, CPA, CHA	CPX, CPT, XAC, CGS 15943A	Decrease in adenylate cyclase activity Increase in IP3 production Increase in calcium flux Decrease in potassium flux	326	Human, rat, cow, dog
A$_{2a}$	CGS 21680, CHEA, APEC	KF 17867, CGS 15943A, CSC	Increase in adenylate cyclase activity	410–412	Human, rat, dog
A$_{2b}$	NECA	CPX, 8-PT	Increase in adenylate cyclase activity	332	Rat, dog
A3	APNEA N^6-benzylNECA	None yet identified	Decrease in adenylate cyclase activity	320	Rat, human[b]
A4	CV1808	CGS 15943A	Increase in potassium conductance	Not yet cloned	
P₂ (ATP) Receptors[a]					
P$_{2X}$ (p$_{2X1-3}$)	α,β-MeATP	Seramin, ANAPP3, PPADS	Ion channel-linked superfamily	Not yet cloned	
P$_{2Y}$ (P$_{2Y1}$)	2MeSATP	Suramin, reactive blue 2	G-protein-linked superfamily	P$_{2Y1}$ cloned, 318	Chick
P$_{2U}$/P$_{2N}$ (P$_{2Y2}$)	UTP ≥ ATP	None yet identified	G-protein linked	373	Mouse neuroblastoma
P$_{2T}$ (P$_{2Y3}$)	2-ADP	FPL 66096	Not determined	Not yet cloned	
P$_{2Z}$	ATP^{4-}	None yet identified	Nonselective ion pore	Not yet cloned	
P$_{2D}$ (P$_{2Y7}$)	Ap4A	None yet identified	G-protein linked	Not yet cloned	
P₂	ATP	None yet identified	G-protein linked	Not yet cloned	

[a] For the P₂ receptor the P$_{2d}$, P$_{2i}$, P$_{2u}$/P$_{2n}$, P2t, and P2z subtypes may be more readily classified as members of the P$_{2x}$ and P$_{2y}$ superfamilies. See ref. 1 for further discussion. The proposed classification of Abbracchio and Burnstock (1) is shown in parentheses in the first column.

[b] The human and sheep A3 receptors have recently been cloned by J. Linden and colleagues and unlike the rat A3 receptor are xanthine-sensitive (38a,54a).

ranopyrazolones (e.g., AMBP) are moderately selective and potent as A$_{2a}$ receptor antagonists (70).

The orphan canine thyroid GPCR clone, RDC8, was identified as the dog A$_{2a}$ receptor having 67% homology with RDC7 encoding for a protein of 412 amino acids. The cloned human brain A$_{2a}$ receptor, the cyclic deoxyribonucleic acid (cDNA) for which a protein of 412 amino acids encodes, differs by 28 amino acids from RDC8, which has 93% homology with the canine receptor. The cloned rat A$_{2a}$ receptor differs from RDC8 by 71 amino acids and has 82% homology with the canine A$_{2a}$ receptor (39).

The adenosine A$_{2b}$ receptor has been cloned from rat and human brain cDNAs that encode a protein of 332 amino acids (39). The human A$_{2b}$ receptor has 46% and 58% homology with the human A1 and A$_{2a}$ receptors, respectively, and 86% homology with the rat A$_{2b}$ receptor; this reflects a difference of 48 amino acids between the two species all but 9 of which are outside the transmembrane domains. The A$_{2b}$ receptor has also been cloned

from human hippocampus and encodes for 328 amino acids (39).

The A3 receptor is a novel adenosine receptor initially cloned (73) from a rat brain cDNA library that has 58% sequence homology with the RDC7 and RDC8 receptors. The rat A3 clone, R226, encodes a protein of 320 amino acids and is negatively coupled to adenylate cyclase in transfected CHO cells. R226 is homologous to the GPCR, *tgpcrl*, and is present in the cerebral cortex, striatum, and olfactory bulb, with the highest concentrations in the testis. N^6-2-(4-aminophenyl) ethyladenosine (APNEA) (Fig. 1) has a high affinity (Kd = 17 nM) for the A3 receptor although N^6-benzyl-NECA is the most selective A3 agonist yet identified (70). Xanthine adenosine antagonists are without effect at the rat A3 receptor (73). In the pithed rat, APNEA has hypotensive actions (27) via activation of the xanthine-insensitive adenosine A3 receptor. This receptor is also involved in mast cell mediator release (52). Adenosine A3 receptors have also been cloned and expressed from sheep (38a) and human (54a) cDNA libraries. In contrast to the rat A_3 receptor, these are xanthine-sensitive.

The A_4 receptor (11) was identified in rat striatum using [^{3}H]CV1808 (Fig. 1) as a radioligand. It has not yet been cloned. Like the A_3 receptor, the A_4 receptor is not blocked by xanthine adenosine antagonists but it is blocked by triazolopyrimidines like CGS15943A. The A_4 receptor is linked to potassium channels in aortic smooth muscle cells (11) (see also Chapters 11, 27, and 38, *this volume,* for related receptors).

ADENOSINE TRIPHOSPHATE (P_2) PURINOCEPTORS

The P_2 receptor family can be divided into two major subclasses; the P_{2X}, an ATP receptor superfamily coupled to ligand-gated ion channels (LGIC); and the P_{2Y}, an ATP GPCR superfamily (1,2). The initial classification of P_2 receptors was based on the rank order potency of a limited series of ATP analogs. P_{2D}, P_{2I}, P_{2T}, P_{2S}, P_{2N}, P_{2U}, and P_{2Z} receptors sensitive to purine nucleotides have also been described (Table 1) (25,33). These have been designated in a somewhat random alphabetical manner and may represent subclasses of either of the two major classes of P_2 receptor (1). The P_{2U} receptor, defined by its sensitivity to uridine triphosphate (UTP), is potentially a pyrimidine rather than a purine receptor (2) but is probably a P_2 receptor subtype that recognizes uridine phosphates in addition to ATP. The P_{2T} receptor on platelets is most sensitive to adenosine diphosphate (ADP). The diadenosine polyphosphates (Ap(n)A) are another group of adenine nucleotides that via the activation of cell-surface receptors serve an as yet unknown neuromodulatory role that may be related to stress (31). The Ap(n)As are known to be intimately involved in the regulation of intracellular events at the nucleic acid and mitochondrial levels (32). Receptors for diadenosine tetraphosphate (Ap4A) (Fig. 2) have been identified by radioligand binding with highest densities found in the heart (80). The latter receptor has a Kd value of 710 nM (31). In the rat brain, two Ap4A binding sites with Kd values of 100 pM and 570 nM have been identified. The former has been designated as the P_{2D} receptor (49) and is involved in the modulation of neurotransmitter release. Although amphetamine can elicit Ap4A release in vivo (49), the factors involved in regulating its appearance in the extracellular milieu remain to be determined.

A number of compounds including PPADS (Fig. 1, Table 1), reactive blue 2, Coumassie blue, apamin, suramin, and ANAPP$_3$ have been described as selective ATP receptor antagonists (2,25), but their potency and selectivity is controversial. The lack of antagonists has limited P_2 receptor subtyping and the delineation of their function. FPL66069 has been recently reported as a selective P_{2T} receptor antagonist with a pKB of 8.74 (P. Leff, personal communication) A recent analysis (1) of the P_2 receptor literature has resulted in the P_{2Y} receptor being subclassified into P_{2Y1-3} subtypes and the P_{2X} receptor being subdivided into seven subtypes designated P_{2X1-7} (Table 1).

A GPCR that binds ATP has been cloned and expressed from a chick brain cDNA library (66). This receptor designated as the P_{2Y1} receptor is a polypeptide of 362 amino acids that has only 27% homology with other known GPCRs. It is present in the brain, spinal cord, GI tract, spleen, and muscle but not in the heart, liver, lung, stomach, or kidney. Its function is unknown at this time. Another P_2 GPCR has been expression cloned from mouse neuroblastoma cells (40). This is a polypeptide of 373 amino acids and pharmacologically resembles the P_{2U} receptor in that, when transfected into ooctyes, UTP was able to increase intracellular calcium levels.

ALLOSTERIC MODULATION OF P_1 RECEPTOR ACTIVITY

Although it is a member of the GPCR superfamily with the seven transmembrane helical structure based on bacteriorhodopsin, the A_1 receptor can be allosterically modulated by compounds that do not directly interact at the receptor binding site. The benzoylthiophene, PD81723 (Fig. 1) does not bind to the A_1 receptor but selectively enhances A_1 radioligand binding and function (34,44).

ADENOSINE AND ADENOSINE TRIPHOSPHATE AVAILABILITY

The factors governing the extracellular availability of adenosine and ATP in nervous tissue have been controversial. Microdialysis studies have shown that adenosine is normally present in the extracellular space at concentrations between 0.02 and 1 mM, the levels being dependent on the metabolic activity of the adjacent tissues.

Under basal conditions, adenosine levels in the extracellular milieu are tightly regulated by ongoing metabolic activity. Adenosine formed intracellularly from ATP and transported to the extracellular milieu via nucleoside transporters represents a major source (29,61). The purine can also be formed extracellularly from ATP via ecto-nucleotidase activity. Bidirectional nucleoside transporters, adenosine deaminase (ADA) and adenosine kinase (AK), regulate the removal of adenosine from the extracellular space (61). Under hypoxic or ischemic conditions, extracellular adenosine levels are markedly increased in response to the increased metabolic demand. Adenosine has accordingly been termed a "retaliatory metabolite" (34) acting to regulate the energy supply/demand balance in a given tissue in response to changes in blood flow and energy availability (7). Reductions in oxygen or glucose availability due to tissue trauma as occurs during stroke, epileptogenic activity, and reduced cerebral blood flow lead to the breakdown of ATP with the sequential formation of ADP, AMP, and adenosine. Thus the normal homeostatic role of extracellular adenosine can be locally amplified severalfold resulting in an enhanced protective role to prevent further traumatic insult to affected tissues (19).

Evidence for a potential role for ATP as a cotransmitter has been obtained from studies in the peripheral nonadrenergic, noncholinergic (NANC) nervous system where ATP is coreleased with norepinephrine and acetylcholine (8). Depolarization-dependent ATP release has been demonstrated in the CNS (8) and ATP has direct effects as an excitatory neurotransmitter in the brain (18,22).

ADENOSINE POTENTIATION

Therapeutic agents acting via purinoceptor receptors may be divided into two classes; (i) conventional ligands that are agonist, partial agonist or antagonist in nature; and (ii) compounds that act to potentiate the actions of endogenously produced purinoceptor ligands. At present, the latter class of agents is exclusively targeted toward adenosine receptor-mediated events, which again is a reflection of the paucity of knowledge related to ATP receptor function.

Adenosine potentiating agents include the allosteric modulators already discussed; inhibitors of ADA and AK, the enzymes that facilitate the removal of adenosine from the extracellular space by deamination and phosphorylation respectively; and inhibitors of the nucleoside transporters that mediate both the uptake and release of adenosine. The uptake process is linked to AK-dependent phosphorylation, such that, when AK is inhibited, the increased intracellular adenosine levels inhibit the nucleoside transporter gradient.

Studies with a limited number of ADA and AK inhibitors have shown that inhibition of AK is physiologically more relevant in increasing extracellular adenosine availability than ADA inhibition (36,58,72). The prototypic AK inhibitor, 5'-iodotubercin (5'-IT) (Fig. 1), has potent anticonvulsant activity (72) and can increase cerebral blood flow (58).

The effects of compounds that act to potentiate the actions of endogenous adenosine are theoretically more pronounced in those areas where tissue trauma results in an increased production of extracellular adenosine, for example, in stroke, reperfusion injury, or epilepsy. The term "site and event specific" has been used to describe compounds that potentiate adenosine responses under such conditions (19) and are typified by AICA riboside (Fig. 1) a compound with an unknown mode of action that has clinical efficacy in myocardial reperfusion injury (45).

ADENOSINE AND ADENOSINE TRIPHOSPHATE IN THE CENTRAL NERVOUS SYSTEM

At the mechanistic level, adenosine is a potent inhibitor of dopamine, γ-aminobutyric acid (GABA), glutamate, acetylcholine, serotonin, and norepinephrine release acting via presynaptic A$_1$ receptors (24). The purine nucleoside preferentially affects excitatory as opposed to inhibitory neurotransmitter release (50,71) thus implying some degree of specificity in regard to its effects on neuronal function. Postsynaptically, adenosine modulates neuronal excitability via both A$_1$ and A$_2$ receptor mechanisms causing hyperpolarization of the postsynaptic membrane (24).

Adenosine is a potent CNS depressant decreasing locomotor activity and at high doses inducing ataxia and catalepsy (23) and adenosine agonists can decrease schedule-controlled behavior in both rodents and primates, effects that are mediated via A$_2$ receptor activation. Conversely, the adenosine antagonist, caffeine, is a motor stimulant, acting via A$_2$ receptors (23).

Adenosine A$_1$ receptors are widely distributed in the CNS, with the highest densities in the hippocampus, striatum, and neocortex (34). A$_{2a}$ receptors show a more limited distribution, being localized to the substantia nigra, nucleus accumbens, globus pallidus, and olfactory tubercule (34). A$_{2b}$ receptors have a wider distribution in brain tissue as deduced by the activation of adenylate cyclase by adenosine agonists in brain regions distinct from those containing A$_{2a}$ receptors. Little is currently known regarding the distribution of A$_3$, A$_4$, or any of the classes of P$_2$ receptor in nervous tissue.

Immunocytochemical and ADA immunohistochemical studies have demonstrated discrete adenosinergic pathways in the brain (5,46) and adenosine release in the CNS occurs following depolarization and in response to morphine and glutamate (69). Yet the factors regulating adenosine availability in the synaptic cleft are unknown. From what is known regarding the use of caffeine in beverage form, most tissues are bathed in adenosine reflecting the homeostatic role of the purine (69). The physiologic factors regulating ATP and Ap4A release are unknown.

THERAPEUTIC POTENTIAL OF PURINOCEPTOR LIGANDS IN NERVOUS TISSUE

Considerable interest has focused on the neuromodulatory role(s) of adenosine in the CNS and cardiovascular system with a view to the development of novel therapeutic agents that act via purinoceptor mechanisms. Extensive data exists to suggest that CNS adenosine systems are involved in the actions of a wide variety of CNS drugs including analgesics, antipsychotics, antidepressants, anxiolytics, nootropics/cognition enhancers, and agents potentially effective in stroke-related CNS damage. These data have been derived from studies involving test paradigms in which either the effects of CNS drugs on adenosine responses have been evaluated or, alternatively, the effects of adenosine agonists or antagonists on the effects of prototypic CNS agents were assessed. In the latter studies, single, somewhat high, concentrations of a limited number of compounds were often used to draw conclusions related to a complete class of psychotherapeutic agent often with no negative control data. This represents a somewhat reductionistic, and necessarily preliminary, approach to delineating the role of adenosine in drug actions. Thus while the purine has been implicated in the mechanism of action of a wide variety of CNS-active agents, much of this data must be viewed as potentially interesting, subject to more rigorous evaluation using newer purinoceptor ligands.

ADENOSINE AND ANXIETY

The prototypic adenosine antagonist, caffeine, is a widely consumed CNS stimulant with potential anxiogenic activity. The seminal anxiolytic agents, the benzodiazepines (BZs) inhibit adenosine uptake (69) leading to potentiation of the effects of the purine. Inosine, the deamination product of adenosine, was identified as a potential ligand for the central BZ receptor complex. Inosine had weak activity (Ki = 1 mM) and with the discovery of the β-carbolines as nanomolar ligands for the BZ receptor, interest in purines as BZ receptor modulators–effectors diminished (69). The reported relationships between the BZ receptor and adenosine receptor ligands may therefore occur at the functional, rather than molecular, level.

ADENOSINE IN STROKE

The reduction in blood flow and oxygen supply resulting from the interruption of the cerebral circulation results in a marked increase in extracellular adenosine from, in part, the breakdown in ATP as tissue energy supplies are depleted (53). There is also a massive release of the excitatory amino acids (EAAs), glutamate and aspartate. The EAAs are neurotoxic due to their disruption of neuronal calcium homeostasis (53).

The increased availability of adenosine during stroke can act to both inhibit the release of EAAs and block their excitotoxic actions by preventing the opening of voltage-dependent Ca^{2+} channels as well as removing the voltage-dependent Mg^{2+} blockade of N-methyl-D-aspartate (NMDA) channels (53). Increased glutamate release during hypoxia may also contribute to an increase in extracellular adenosine since purine levels in nervous tissue are reduced when a glutamate antagonist is present.

The colocalization of A_1 receptors with NMDA receptors in the hippocampal CA_1 region, an area especially vulnerable to ischemic damage, further supports a functional relationship between the purine and EAA effects. Adenosine can increase cerebral blood flow (58) and, acting via neutrophil A_{2a} receptors, inhibit neutrophil-dependent superoxide formation (12). 2-Chloroadenosine, R-PIA, and CHA, like many other classes of CNS-active agent, reduce the stroke related death and neurodegeneration occurring in the hippocampus (21,64). Data on selective A_{2a} receptor agonists has not yet been reported. The effects of adenosine in the sequelae of an ischemic episode are thus potentially multifaceted and offer significant potential in the treatment of stroke-related neuronal injury (53,70). The potentially beneficial effects are, however, confounded by their side effects most notably depression of cardiac conduction, decreased blood pressure, and altered plasma renin angiotensin activity (34).

As might be anticipated, adenosine antagonists have been shown to increase ischemic damage by enhancing glutamate release (53). An exception to this is the 1-substituted xanthine, propentofylline (HWA 285) (Fig. 1), which is a weak, micromolar-activity adenosine antagonist and can also inhibit adenosine transport (26). Propentofylline has antiischemic activity in a gerbil model of stroke that may involve a decrease in glutamate release (43).

ADENOSINE IN EPILEPSY

Adenosine levels increase markedly in the brain following the hypoxia resulting from seizure activity leading to the proposal that adenosine acts as an endogenous anticonvulsant (16), under normal conditions providing a tonic effect to maintain a high seizure threshold. Hippocampal microdialysis probes in patients with intractable complex partial epilepsy have shown a 6- to 31-fold increase in extracellular adenosine levels that reach a level of 65 μM consistent with the concentrations required in vitro to depress epileptiform activity (17). Anticonvulsant effects of a variety of adenosine agonists have been described in audiogenic, electrical, chemical, and kindling-induced seizure models (16). Consistent with the potential anticonvulsant role of adenosine agonists, adenosine antagonists are well known as proconvulsant and convulsant agents (16) and can produce status epilepticus in humans (17).

The anticonvulsant actions of the tricyclic agent, carbamazepine, have been attributed to an effect on A_1 receptor-mediated responses that produce the functional supersensitivity associated with chronic carbamazepine treatment (63). AK inhibitors are potent anticonvulsant agents (72) when administered into the prepiriform cortex, an area of the brain involved in seizure initiation and expression. Given that the mechanism of action of most clinically effective anticonvulsant agents has yet to be elucidated, making it difficult to target the beneficial actions of such agents while reducing their side-effect liabilities, a CNS-selective adenosine agonist or adenosine potentiating agent like an AK inhibitor may represent a novel approach to anticonvulsant therapy.

ADENOSINE AND NEURODEGENERATION

The molecular events of epilepsy and stroke-related nerve cell death may be considered as part of a continuum that also includes the process of neurodegeneration that occurs with aging. Thus the nerve cell death that occurs following excess EAA release may reflect an acute manifestation of the more subtle and more chronic phenomenon of neurotoxicity. Accordingly, agents effective in treating stroke may also have potential in arresting or reversing the neurodegeneration occuring in Alzheimer's Disease (AD) and Parkinson's Disease (PD).

The adenosine antagonist caffeine is a well-known cognition enhancer. KW15372, KFM19, and MDL102234 (Fig. 1) are 8-substituted xanthines with selective A_1 receptor antagonist activity that are currently being evaluated as cognition-enhancing agents (34,70) for potential use in AD and other age-related dementias. Compounds of this type have the potential to function primarily as palliative agents, restoring some aspects of normal brain function without arresting or reversing the neurodegenerative process. Propentofylline, which has been shown to have beneficial effects in animal models of stoke, has been reported to modulate nerve growth factor availability in vitro (43). The compound can also ameliorate the changes in muscarinic receptor density that result from basal forebrain lesioning in rats, indicating a potentially beneficial effect on presynaptic function in this animal model of AD-related cholinergic dysfunction (28). Hippocampal A_1 receptor binding, but not function, is reduced in AD brains (62). Such findings must be viewed, however, within the context of the almost universal disruption of neurotransmitter systems and binding sites in the AD brain (see also Chapters 118 and 126, *this volume*).

The putative role of adenosine in the processes underlying neurodegeneration suggests potential benefits for both agonist and antagonist ligands. Agonists can reduce the neurotoxic events that can lead to neuronal death, and antagonists can produce a cognitive enhancement most probable involving a disinhibition of the inhibitory effects of adenosine on excitatory neurotransmission (50,71). Clearly if CNS-selective purinoceptor ligands are proven to be effective in ameliorating some aspects of the cognitive decline associated with the aging process, it will be necessary to achieve an equilibrium between the neuroprotective and neurostimulatory actions of this class of compound reflecting the homeostatic role of the purine.

A final aspect of the role of purinoceptor-mediated pro-

cesses in neurodegeneration relates to the potential antiinflammatory actions of adenosine agonists (12). The latter are of interest within the context of the recent finding that amyloid-β-protein ($A\beta$) may elicit nerve cell death in AD by activation of the classical complement cascade via an immunoglobulin-independent mechanism (41). This finding and epidemiologic data indicating that aged individuals with rheumatoid arthritis who consume large quantities of antiinflammatory agents have a reduced incidence of AD suggests an additional neuroprotective role for adenosine over and above beneficial effects related to neurotransmitter-mediated neuronal events (11b).

ADENOSINE AND DOPAMINERGIC FUNCTION

Since 1974, a considerable body of data has accumulated demonstrating the effects of adenosine receptor ligands in animal models of CNS dopamine malfunction. The adenosine antagonists, caffeine and theophylline, enhanced the actions of L-dopa and dopamine agonists in the classical unilaterally lesioned rat model of PD (23). The relationship between central dopaminergic and adenosine systems has been substantiated by further work. It has also been established that adenosine agonists can block the behavioral effects of dopamine via activation of an A_{2a} receptor, whereas they can enhance the actions of dopamine in the striatum. As already noted, adenosine A_{2a} receptors are highly localized in the striatum, nucleus accumbens, and olfactory tubercule brain regions that also have high densities of dopamine D_1 and D_2 receptors (23).

In the basal ganglia messenger ribonucleic acids (mRNAs) for adenosine A_{2a} and D_2 receptors are colocalized in GABAergic-enkephalin striatopallidal neurons (23,39). These neurons represent an indirect pathway from the striatum to the globus pallidus, the dysfunction of which may be involved in the etiology of Huntington's chorea as well as the movement disorders associated with PD. In this context, it is noteworthy that Huntington's chorea is associated with a decrease in adenosine A_2 receptors associated with a loss of medium-sized spiny neurons in the striatum (23).

The indirect pathway arising from the GABA-enkephalinergic neurons in the striatum interacts through GABAergic relays with a glutaminergic pathway arising in the subthalamic nucleus. This, in turn can activate the internal segment of the pars reticulata which, through a pars reticulata–thalamic GABAergic pathway, can inhibit the thalamic/cortical glutaminergic pathway (Fig. 2). A direct dopamine pathway involving D1 receptors also arises from the striatum from GABA-substance P-dynorphinergic neurons, which, through a GABAergic pathway, also inhibits the internal segment of the pars reticulata to disinhibit the ascending thalamic glutaminergic pathway. The balance between the direct (cortical-activating) and indirect (cortical-inhibiting) striatal do-paminergic pathways can then tonically regulate normal motor activity. Dopaminergic inputs arising from the pars compacta (Fig. 2) can facilitate motor activity, inhibiting the indirect pathway by activation of D_2 receptors and activating the direct pathway via activation of D_1 receptors.

These findings have led to the hypothesis that adenosine systems in the striatum, specifically those involving A_{2a}-receptor-related events, may be involved in neurologic disorders involving basal ganglia malfunction. Adenosine A_1 agonists have neuroprotective effects in the mouse MPTP model of PD (27), whereas KW17837, an antagonist at A_{2a} receptors, is reportedly effective in mouse models of dopamine hypofunction. This compound is being targeted as a novel therapeutic approach to PD (59).

Adenosine agonists conversely mimic both the biochemical and behavioral actions of dopamine antagonists in animal models, effects that also involve A_{2a} receptor activation (23). Mechanistically adenosine agonists inhibit dopamine release, attenuate dopamine transductional processes, and decrease dopamine synthesis, actions that contribute to a diminution in dopaminergic neurotransmission (23). Adenosine receptor agonists can thus act as functional dopamine antagonists (69). At the behavioral level, adenosine agonists are psychomotor depressants, decrease schedule-controlled behavior, and can elicit ataxia and catalepsy (23).

CI936, an N^6-substituted adenosine analog with potent A_{2a} receptor activity (34) had a preclinical profile similar to that observed for classical dopamine receptor antago-

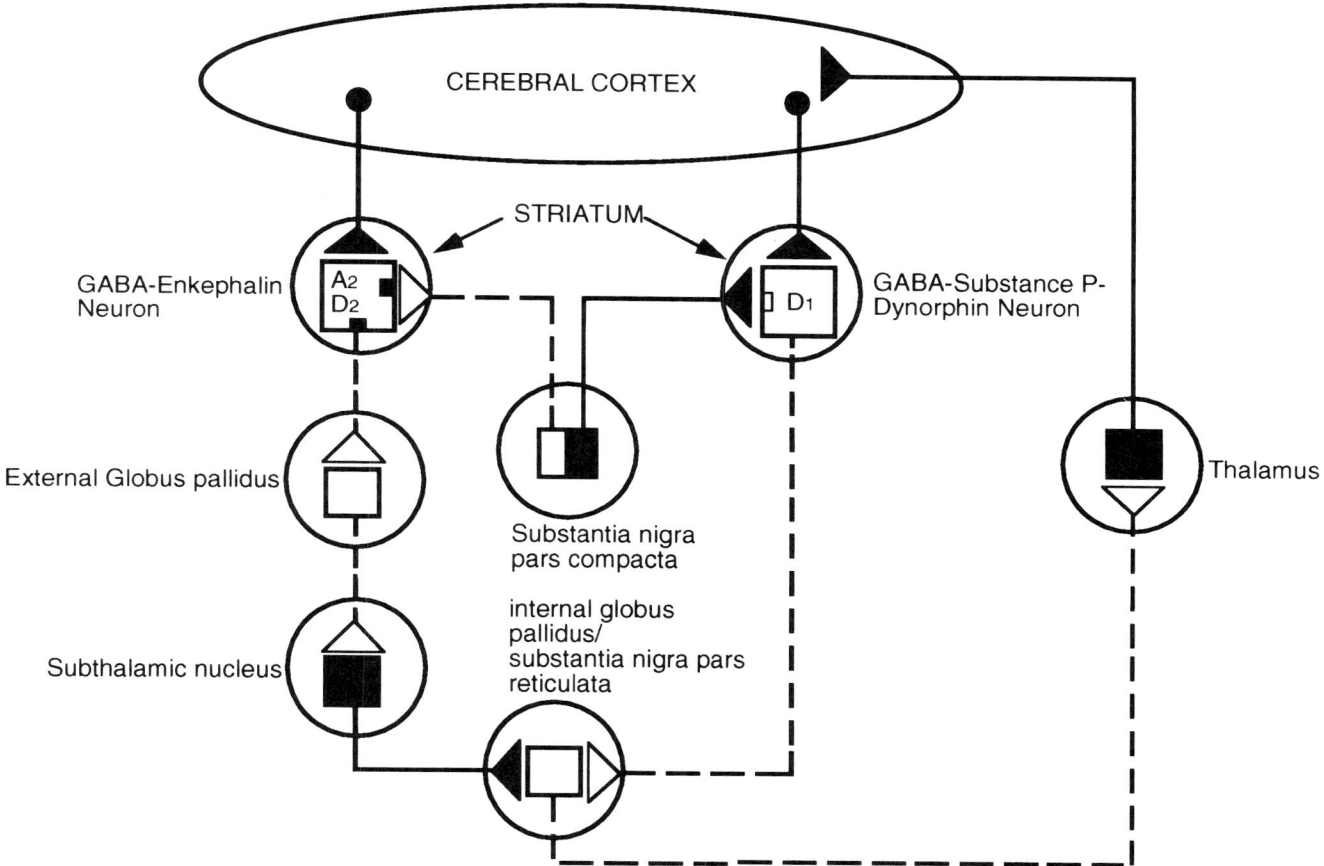

FIG. 2. Dopamine–adenosine interactions in the substantia nigra. An indirect dopaminergic pathway arises from the striatal GABA-enkephalinergic dopaminergic neurons on which both dopamine D1 and adenosine A2a receptors are colocalized. Via a GABAergic interneuron originating in the external globus pallidus, the indirect pathway connects with a glutaminergic pathway arising in the subthalamic nucleus. This, in turn can activate the internal segment of the pars reticulata and, through another GABA pathway, inhibit ascending glutaminegic neurons arising from the thalamus that innervate the cortex. The direct pathway arises from striatal GABA-substance P-dynorphinergic neurons that inhibit via a GABAergic relay the internal segment of the pars reticulata to disinhibit the ascending thalamic/cortical glutaminergic pathway. The balance between the direct (activating) and indirect (inhibitory) striatal dopaminergic pathways can then tonically regulate normal motor activity. Dopaminergic inputs arising from the substantia nigra pars compacta can facilitate motor activity, inhibiting the indirect pathway by activation of D_2 receptors and activating the direct pathway via D_1 receptor activation. Adapted from Ferre et al. (23).

nists. The compound entered clinical trials as an antipsychotic but was withdrawn due to unspecified side effect problems. The selective A_{2a} receptor agonist, CGS 21680, can decrease the affinity of the D_2 receptor agonist, N-propylnorapomorphine (NPA) at D_2 receptors in rat neostriatum without affecting D_1 receptor binding, an effect that is more pronounced in denervated striata (23).

The relationship between A_{2a} and D_2 receptors has also been postulated to underlie the CNS stimulant effects of caffeine and other adenosine antagonists (23) and to play a role in self-mutilation behaviors like Lesch-Nyhan syndrome (69). The demonstrated effects of adenosine ligands on dopaminergic systems in the mammalian brain at both the molecular and behavioral levels offers the opportunity to develop indirect dopamine receptor agonists (adenosine antagonists) and antagonists (adenosine agonists) that may avoid the side-effect liabilities seen with the currently available dopamine agonists and antagonists used, respectively, for the treatment of Parkinson's disease and schizophrenia (see also Chapters 24, 100, and 126, *this volume*).

ADENOSINE AND SLEEP

The hypnotic and sedative effects of adenosine are well documented (3,51) as are the CNS stimulatory activities of adenosine antagonists like caffeine (3,23,69). Direct administration of adenosine into the brain elicits an EEG profile similar to that seen in deep sleep, manifested as an increase in REM sleep with a reduction in REM sleep latency that results in an increase in total sleep (51). Caffeine, on the other hand, supresses REM sleep and decreases total sleep time. Sleep deprivation has been reported to increase adenosine A_1 receptor density in the cortex and corpus striatum (51). The effects of selective A_{2a} receptor agonists on sleep processes have yet to be reported.

ADENOSINE AND STRESS

Sustained exposure to footshock, restraint, or sleep deprivation can upregulate A_1 receptors in the rat hypothalamus (69). Stomach ulcers induced by chronic restraint stress can be reduced by A_1 receptor agonists via a central purinoceptor mechanism (67). Adenosine systems may also be involved in the modulation of the pituitary–adrenocortical axis in response to stress (57), whereas Ap4A receptors may be involved in generalized stress-related responses (31).

ADENOSINE AND DEPRESSION

In early studies, it was found that tricyclic antidepressants could potentiate the CNS depressant actions of aden-

osine and that certain tricyclic antidepressants were weak inhibitors of adenosine uptake (69). Furthermore, chronic electroconvulsive shock therapy (ECT), a commonly used treatment for depression can upregulate A_1 receptors.

A series of adenosine receptor (both A_1 and A_{2a}) antagonists typified by CP66713 (Fig. 1) were identified as antidepressants by screening in animal models. These agents entered clinical trials but were withdrawn for unknown reasons. Conceptually, however, the anticipated increase in transmitter release resulting from the administration of adenosine antagonists has the potential to reverse neuronal depression that may be clinically manifested as depression. Thus the potential use of CNS selective purinoceptor ligands in the treatment of depression still remains an interesting hypothesis (69).

ADENOSINE AND NOCIOCEPTION

Considerable evidence supports a role for both P_1 and P_2 receptor ligands in pain processing (36,55,56) although these data appear to be highly dependent on the site of administration of such agents. Adenosine has antinociceptive activity when administered systemically or intrathetically but when given peripherally can induce pain. The purine may also mediate the antinociceptive actions of morphine and α-adrenoceptor agonists in the spinal cord (55). Such effects are mediated through A_2 receptors with NECA being 10 to 100 times more active than A_1 agonists. AK inhibitors, but not ADA inhibitors, act antinociceptively (36). These antinociceptive effects can be blocked by methylxanthines. ATP is released in response to capcasin treatment and may have antinociceptive actions (56). A_1-receptor-mediated modulation of spinal substance P and CGRP release reflect additional purinoceptor-mediated intervention points in the nociceptive process (11a,70).

ADENOSINE AND SUBSTANCE ABUSE

The potential role of central purinoceptor systems in the molecular aspects of substance abuse—the consumption of CNS-active agents like the opiates, cocaine, the amphetamines, alcohol, and caffeine—has been suggested by various studies, although much of the evidence remains circumstantial. Caffeine is an addictive substance and can be self-administered and shows withdrawal in humans (69). An initial report of the stereoselective antagonism of phencyclidine discrimination by adenosine agonist treatment (6) proved to be a pharmacodynamic rather than pharmacologic interaction. Adenosine appears to be involved in the actions of ethanol in the CNS (13,15). Ethanol acts as a noncompetitive inhibitor of adenosine uptake, an effect that disappears upon chronic exposure to ethanol. Lymphocytes from alcoholics were found to be more sensitive to the effects of alcohol and also showed abnormalities in adenosine transductional processes. Adenosine agonists, like the opiates and clonidine, cause a novel form of dependence in the guinea pig ileum (9). Adenosine agonists can also attenuate the dependence associated with the anxiolytic, alprazolam (10). These data, although somewhat inconclusive suggest an involvement of purinergic systems in substance abuse (see also Chapters 152 and 154, *this volume*).

LIMITATIONS TO CNS-SELECTIVE THERAPEUTIC AGENTS

Although there are a number of potential CNS therapeutic targets for agents acting at purinoceptors, the ligands currently available are limited by their degree of receptor and tissue selectivity and brain bioavailability. Adenosine is a ubiquitous neuromodulatory agent with effects on nearly every organ system (34,69). Currently available adenosine agonists and antagonists may thus be anticipated to produce a multitude of effects when administered in vivo. A_1 agonists targeted as antihypertensive agents also cause CNS sedation, whereas A_1 antagonists effective in enhancing cognitive performance also have the potential to act as cardiotonic agents and

increase renal output. To circumvent these issues, it will be necessary to either develop ways of selectively targeting purinoceptor ligands to the CNS or hope that purinoceptors will show some element of tissue selectivity. Work on CNS targeting has been limited to in vitro models in which adenosine, by increasing cAMP, can increase penetration of the blood–brain barrier (54) and to studies on nucleoside transporters in the blood–brain barrier (48). The involvement of the blood–brain barrier in antagonist pharmacokinetics has had limited study. Some evidence for tissue selectivity in adenosine receptors has come from the use of monoclonal antibodies that demonstrate differences in adenosine A_{2a} receptors from dog striatum and liver (47).

Tolerance is another issue related to adenosine agonist therapy. Implantation of minipumps containing the A_{2a} agonist, CGS 21680 for 2 weeks leads to a decrease in brain A_{2a} receptors and a complete loss of the hypotensive actions of the compound (65). In contrast, chronic administration of A_1 and A_{2a} agonists via the more conventional systemic route for 21 days leads to a tolerance to A_1 but not A_{2a} agonists (8a). The pharmacokinetics for minipumps thus differs markedly from traditional methods for bolus administration. Nonetheless, the contrast in the findings from these two chronic studies need not preclude strategies using purinoceptor agonists directed towards acute situations (stroke), or the development of partial agonists, antagonists, and indirectly acting agents as therapeutic entities.

THE PURINERGIC CASCADE

The metabolic pathways that link ATP, ADP, AMP, and adenosine and the potential for each of these purines to interact with cell-surface recognition sites represents a potential pharmacologic cascade comparable to that seen in blood clotting and in the complement cascade. Adenosine triphosphate released as a cotransmitter can lead to the sequential formation of ADP, AMP, and adenosine, each of which can interact with distinct membrane recognition sites (Fig. 3). Thus, exogenous ATP can conceptually activate the various classes of P_2 purinoceptors as it undergoes dephosphorylation. ADP interacts with the platelet P_{2T} receptor and can enhance its own availability. Diadenosine tetraphosphate, in addition to interacting with the P_{2D} receptor can be degraded to ATP and ADP.

Adenosine interacts with A_1, A_{2a}, A_{2b}, A_3, and A_4 receptors. A_1- or A_{2a}-receptor activation can lead to a physiologically relevant inhibition of ATP availability. Further interactions among the components of the proposed purinergic cascade are outlined in the legend to Fig. 3. The proposed purinergic cascade is an elegant and complex system for the regulation of cell-to-cell communication that in physiological terms will be dependent on the dynamics of the local milieu in which ATP is made available

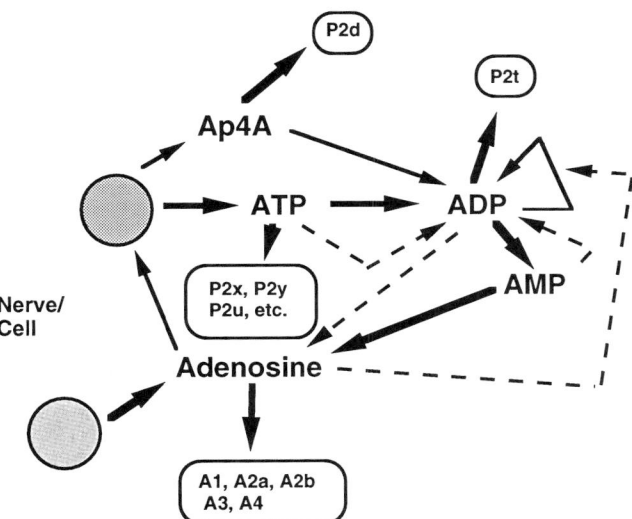

FIG. 3. The purinergic cascade. ATP, Ap4A, or adenosine are released into the extracellular milieu from nerves or cells where they can interact to form a purinergic cascade. Ap4A can activate P_{2D} receptors and has the potential to be hydrolyzed to ADP. ATP acts at a variety of P_2 receptors (see text) and is sequentially degraded to ADP and AMP by ectonucleotidase activity. ADP interacts with P_{2t} receptors. AMP gives rise to adenosine, which can interact with the various P_1 receptors (A_1, A_{2a}, A_{2b}, A_3, A_4). Adenosine can also be formed by intracellular 5′-nucleotidase activity. Heavy lines indicate metabolic routes, dotted lines indicate feedback inhibitory pathways. The solid line from ADP to ADP indicates a facilitation of ADP availability. Receptors are indicated in rounded boxes. See text for further discussion.

thus reflecting the purinoceptor phenotype of the tissue, ectonucleotidase activities, and ADA, AK, and nucleoside transporter activity.

FUTURE PROSPECTS

With the tremendous advances in the molecular biology of purinoceptors that will lead to a better understanding of the functional role(s) of the various subtypes of P_1 and P_2 receptors and concomitant efforts in medicinal chemistry, it may be anticipated that purinoceptor ligands will be important therapeutic agents in the 21st century in line with the concept that adenosine specifically, and purines in general, represent the "signal of life" (20).

ACKNOWLEDGMENTS

This chapter is dedicated to the memory of Henry McIlwain whose vision provided some of the crucial biochemical data to support the concept of a role for adenosine and ATP in CNS function. The author thanks Mark Holladay for assistance with the chemical structures. Because of space limitations, the number of references was kept to a minimum. The author apologizes to those researchers whose work has only been cited through review articles.

REFERENCES

1. Abbracchio MP, Burnstock G. Purinoceptors: are there superfamilies of P2x and P2y purinoceptors? *Pharmacol Ther* 1994 [*in press*].
2. Abbracchio MP, Cattabeni F, Fredholm BB, Williams M. Purinoceptor nomenclature: a status report. *Drug Dev Res* 1993;28:207–213.
3. Barraco RA. Behavorial actions of adenosine and related substances. In Phillis JW, ed. *Adenosine and Adenine Nucleotides as Regulators of Cellular Function.* Boca Raton, FL: CRC Press; 1991:339–366.
4. Bloom FE. Neurotransmitters: past, present and future. *FASEB J* 1988;2:32–41.
5. Brass K, Newby AC, Wilson VS, Snyder SH. Adenosine-containing neurons in the brain localized by immunocytochemistry. *J Neurosci* 1986;6:547–553.
6. Browne RG, Welch WM. Stereoselective antagonism of phencyclidine's discriminative properties by adenosine receptor agonists. *Science* 1982;217:1157–1158.
7. Bruns RF. Role of adenosine in energy supply/demand balance. *Nucleoside Nucleotides* 1991;10:931–943.
8. Burnstock G. Physiological and pathological roles of purines: an update. *Drug Dev Res* 1993;28:195–206.
8a. Casatri C, Monopoli A, Dionisotti S, Zocchi C, Bonizzoni E, Ongini E. Repeated administration of selective adenosine A_1 and A_2 receptor agonists in the spontaneously hypertensive rat: tolerance develops to A_1-mediated hemodynamic effects. *J Pharmacol Exp Ther* 1994;268:1506–1511.
9. Collier HOJ, Tucker JF. Novel form of drug-dependence—on adenosine in guinea pig ileum. *Nature* 1983;302:618–621.
10. Contreras E, Germany A. Adenosine analogs attenuate tolerance-dependence on alprazolam. *Gen Pharmacol* 1991;22:637–641.
11. Cornfield LJ, Hu S, Hurt SD, Sills MA. [³H] 2-Phenylaminoadenosine ([³H] CV1808) labels a novel adenosine receptor in rat brain. *J Pharmacol Exp Ther* 1992;363:552–561.
11a. Correia-de-Sá P, Riberio JA. Potentiation by tonic A_{2a}-adenosine receptor activation of CGRP-facilitated [³H]-ACh release from rat motor nerve endings. *Br J Pharmacol* 1994;111:582–588.
11b. Cronstein BN. Adenosine, an endogenous anti-inflammatory agent. *J Appl Physiol* 1994;76:1–13.
12. Cronstein BN, Daguma L, Nichols D, Hutchison AJ, Williams M. The adenosine/neutrophil paradox resolved: human neutrophils possess both A_1 and A_2 receptors that promote chemotaxis and inhibit O^{2-}, respectively. *J Clin Invest* 1990;85:1150–1157.
13. Dar MS, Clark M. Tolerance to adenosine's accentuation of ethanol-induced motor incordination in ethanol-tolerant mice. *Alcoholism* 1992;16:1138–1146.
14. DeLander GE, Hopkins GJ. Behavior induced by putative nociceptive neurotransmitters us inhibited by adenosine or adenosine analogs coadministered intrathecally. *J Pharmacol Exp Ther* 1988;246:565–670.
15. Diamond I, Nagy L, Mochly-Rosen D, Gordon A. The role of adenosine and adenosine transport in ethanol-induced cellular tolerance and dependence. Possible biologic and genetic markers of alcoholism. *Ann NY Acad Sci* 1991;625:473–487.
16. Dragunow M. Adenosine and epileptic seizures. In Phillis JW, ed. *Adenosine and Adenine Nucleotides as Regulators of Cellular Function.* Boca Raton, FL: CRC Press; 1991:367–379.
17. During MJ, Spencer DD. Adenosine: a potential mediator of seizure arrest and postictal refractoriness. *Ann Neurol* 1992;32:618–624.
18. Edwards FA, Gibb AJ, Colquhoun D. ATP receptor-mediated synaptic currents in the central nervous system. *Nature* 1992;359:144–147.
19. Engler R. Consequences of activation and adenosine-mediated inhibition of granulocytes during myocardial ischemia. *Fed Proc* 1987;46:2407–2412.
20. Engler R. Adenosine: the signal of life? *Circulation* 1991;84:951–954.
21. Evans MC, Swan JH, Meldrum BS. An adenosine analogue, 2-chloroadenosine, protects against long term development of ischemic cell loss in the rat hippocampus. *Neurosci Lett* 1987;78:295–300.
22. Evans RJ, Derkach V. Suprenant A. ATP mediates fast synaptic transmission in mammalian neurons. *Nature* 1992;357:505–507.
23. Ferre S, Fuxe K, Von Euler G, Johansson B, Fredholm BB. Adenosine–dopamine interactions in the brain. *Neuroscience* 1992;51:501–512.
24. Fredholm BB, Dunwiddie TV. How does adenosine inhibit transmitter release? *Trends Pharmacol Sci* 1988;9:130–134.
25. Fredholm BB, Abbracchio MP, Burnstock G, Daly JW, Hardin TK, Jacobson KA, Left P, Williams M. Nomenclature and classification of purinoceptors: a report from the IUPHAR Subcommittee. *Pharmacol Rev* 1994;46:143–156.
26. Fredholm BB, Fastbom J, Kvanta A, Gerwins P, Parkinson F. Further evidence that propentofylline (HWA285) influences both adenosine receptors and adenosine transport. *Fund Clin Pharmacol* 1992;6:99–111.
27. Fozard JR, Carruthers AM. Adenosine A_3 receptors mediate hypotension in the angiotensin-II supported circulation of the pithed rat. *Br J Pharmacol* 1993;109:3–5.
28. Fuji K, Hiramatsu M, Hayashi S, Kameyama T, Nabeshima T. Effects of propentofylline, a NGF synthesis stimulator, on alterations in muscarinic cholinergic receptors induced by basal forebrain lesion in rats. *Neurosci Lett* 1993;150:99–102.
29. Geiger JD, Nagy JI. Adenosine deaminase and [³H]-nitrobenzylthioinosine as markers of adenosine metabolism and transport in central purinergic systems. In: Williams M, ed. *Adenosine and Adenosine Receptors.* Clifton, NJ: Humana; 1990:225–288.
30. Gerwins P, Fredholm BB. ATP and its metabolite adenosine act synergistically to mobilize intracellular calcium via the formation of inositol 1,4,5-triphosphate in a smooth muscle cell line. *J Biol Chem* 1992;267:16081–16087.
31. Hilderman RH, Martin M, Zimmerman JK, Pivorun EB. Identification of a unique membrane receptor for adenosine 5′, 5‴-P_1 P_4 tetraphosphate. *J Biol Chem* 1991;266:6915–6918.
32. Hoyle CHV. Pharmacological actions of adenine dincleotides in the periphery; possible receptor classes and transmitter function. *Gen Pharmacol* 1990;21:827–831.

33. Illes P, Norenberg W. Neuronal ATP receptors and their mechanism of action. *Trends Pharmacol Sci* 1993;14:50–54.
34. Jacobson KA, van Galen PJM, Williams M. Adenosine receptors: pharmacology, structure–activity relationships, and therapeutic potential. *J Med Chem* 1992;35:407–415.
35. Jacobson KA, Gallo-Rodriguez C, Melman N, et al. Structure–activity relationships of 8-styrylxanthines as A$_2$ selective adenosine antagonists. *J Med Chem* 1993;36:1333–1342.
36. Keil II GJ, DeLander G. Spinally-mediated nocioception is induced in mice by an adenosine kinase—but not by an adenosine deaminase—inhibitor. *Life Sci* 1992;51:PL171–PL176.
37. Lau Y-S, Mouradian MM. Protection against acute MPTP-induced dopamine depletion in mice by adenosine A$_1$ agonist. *J Neurochem* 1993;60:768–771.
38. Lauder JM. Neurotransmitters as growth regulatory signals. Role of receptors and second messengers. *Trends Neurosci* 1993;16:233–240.
38a. Linden J, Taylor HE, Robeva AS, Tucker AL, Stehle JH, Rivkees SA, Fink JS, Reppert SM. Molecular cloning and functional expression of a sheep A$_3$ adenosine receptor with widespread tissue distribution. *Mol Pharmacol* 1993;44:524–532.
39. Linden J, Jacobson MA, Hutchins C, Williams M. Adenosine receptors. In: Peroutka SJ, ed., *G Protein-Linked Receptors*. Boca Raton, FL: CRC Press; 1994:29–44 (*Handbook of Receptors and Channels*: vol 1).
40. Lustig KD, Shaiu AK, Brake AJ, Julius D. Expression cloning of an ATP receptor from mouse neuroblastoma cells. *Proc Natl Acad Sci USA* 1993;90:5113–5117.
41. McGeer PL, Rogers J. Anti-inflammatory agents as a therapeutic approach to Alzheimer's Disease. *Neurology* 1992;42:447–449.
42. Milne JL, Devreotes PN. The surface cyclic AMP receptors, cAR1, cAR2 and cAR3 promote Ca^{2+} influx in *Dictyostelium discoidium* by a Ga2-independent mechanism. *Mol Biol Cell* 1993;4:283–292.
43. Miyashita K, Nakajima T, Ishikawa A, Miayatake T. An adenosine uptake blocker, propentofylline, reduces glutamate release in gerbil hippocampus following transient forebrain ischemia. *Neurochem Res* 1992;17:147–150.
44. Mudumbi RV, Montamat SC, Bruns RF, Vestal RE. Cardiac functional responses to adenosine by PD 81,723, an allosteric enhancer of the adenosine A1 receptor. *Am J Physiol Heart Circ Physiol* 1993;246:H1017–H1022.
45. Mullane KM, Young M. Acadesine: prototype adenosine regulating agent for treating myocardial ischemia-reperfusion injury. *Drug Dev Res* 1993;28:336–343.
46. Nagy JI, LaBella LA, Buss M, Daddona D. Immunohistochemistry of adenosine deaminase: implication for adenosine neurotransmission. *Science* 1984;224:166–168.
47. Palmer TM, Jacobson KA, Stiles GL. Immunological identification of A$_2$ adenosine receptors by two antipeptide antibody preparations. *Mol Pharmacol* 1992;42:391–397.
48. Parridge WM, Yoshikawa T, Kang Y-S, Miller LP. Blood–brain barrier transport and brain metabolism of adenosine and adenosine analogues. *J Pharmacol Exp Ther* 1994;268:14–18.
49. Pintor J, Porras A, Mora F, Miras-Portugal MT. Amphetamine-induced release of diadenosine phosphates—Ap4A and Ap5A—from caudate putamen of conscious rat. *Neurosci Lett* 1993;150:13–16.
50. Prince DA, Stevens CF. Adenosine decreases neurotransmitter release at central synapses. *Proc Natl Acad Sci USA* 1992;89:8586–8590.
51. Radulovacki M. Adenosine and sleep. In Phillis JW, ed. *Adenosine and Adenine Nucleotides as Regulators of Cellular Function* Boca Raton, FL: CRC Press; 1991:381–390.
52. Ramkumar V, Stiles GL, Beaven MA, Ali H. The A$_3$AR is the unique adenosine receptor which facilitates release of allergic mediators in mast cells. *J Biol Chem* 1993;268:16887–16890.
53. Rudolphi K, Schubert P, Parkinson FE, Fredholm BB. Neuroprotec-

tive role of adenosine in cerebral ischemia. *Trends Pharmacol Sci* 1992;13:439–445.
54. Rubin L, Porter S, Horner H, Yednock T. Blood–brain barrier model. *Patent Pub* 1991;WO91/05038.
54a. Salvatore CA, Jacobson MA, Taylor HE, Linden J, Johnson RG. Molecular cloning and characterization of the human A$_3$ adenosine receptor. *Proc Natl Acad Sci USA* 1993;90:10365–10369.
55. Sawynok J, Sweeney MI. The role of purines in nociception. *Neuroscience* 1989;32:557–569.
56. Sawynok J, Downie JW, Reid AR, Cahill CM, White TD. ATP release from dorsal spinal cord synaptosomes: characterization and neuronal origin. *Brain Res* 1993;610:32–38.
57. Schettini G, Landolfi E, Meucci O, et al. Adenosine and its analogue (−)-N^6-phenylisopropyladenosine modulate anterior pituitary adenylate cyclase activity and prolactin secretion in the rat. *J Mol Endocrinol* 1990;5:69–76.
58. Sciotti VM, Van Wylen DGL. Increases in interstitial adenosine and cerebral blood flow with inhibition of adenosine kinase and adenosine deaminase. *J Cerebral Blood Flow Metab* 1993;13:201–207.
59. Shimada J, Suzuki F, Nonaka H, Ishii A, Ichikawa S. (E)-1,3,dialkyl-7-methyl-8-(3,4,5-trimethoxystyryl) xanthines: potent and selective adenosine A$_2$ antagonists. *J Med Chem* 1992;35:2342–2345.
60. Shinoda I, Furukawa Y, Furukawa S. Stimulation of nerve growth factor synthesis/secretion by protentofylline in cultured mouse astroglial cells. *Biochem Pharmacol* 1990;39:1813–1816.
61. Stone TW, Newby AC, Lloyd HGE. Adenosine release. In *Adenosine and Adenosine Receptors* Williams M, ed. Clifton, NJ: Humana; 1990:173–223.
62. Ulas J, Brunner LC, Nguyen L, Cotman CW. Reduced density of adenosine A$_1$ receptors and preserved coupling of adenosine A$_1$ receptors to G proteins in Alzheimer's Disease: a quantitative autoradiographic study. *Neuroscience* 1993;52:843–854.
63. van Calker D, Steber R, Klotz K-N, Greil W. Carbamazepine distinguishes between adenosine receptors that mediate different second messenger responses. *Eur J Pharmacol (Mol Pharmacol Sect)* 1991;206:285–290.
64. von Lubitz DKJE, Dambrosai JM, Kempski O, Redmond DJ. Cyclohexyl adenosine protects against neuronal death following ischemia in the CA3 region of gerbil hippocampus. *Stroke* 1988;19:1133–1139.
65. Webb RL, Sills MA, Chovan JP, Peppard JV, Francis JE. Development of tolerance to the antihypertensive effects of highly selective adenosine A$_2$ agonists upon chronic administration. *J Pharmacol Exp Ther* 1993;267:287–295.
66. Webb TE, Simon J, Krishek BJ, et al. Cloning and functional expression of a brain G-protein coupled ATP receptor. *FEBS Lett* 1993;324:219–225.
67. Westerberg VS, Geiger JD. Central effects of adenosine analogs on stress-induced gastric ulcer formation. *Life Sci* 1987;41:2201–2205.
68. White TD, Hoehn K. Release of adenosine and ATP from nervous tissue. In Stone TW, ed. *Adenosine in the Nervous System* London: Academic Press; 1991:173–195.
69. Williams M. Adenosine: the prototypic neuromodulator. *Neurochem Inter* 1989;14:249–264.
70. Williams M. Progress towards purinoceptor based therapeutics. *Curr Opinion Invest Drugs* 1993;2:1105–1117.
71. Yoon KW, Rothman SM. Adenosine inhibits excitatory but not inhibitory synaptic transmission in the hippocampus. *J Neurosci* 1991;11:1375–1380.
72. Zhang G, Franklin PH, Murray TF. Manipulation of endogenous adenosine in the rat prepiriform cortex modulates seizure susceptibility. *J Pharmacol Exp Ther* 1993;264:1415–1424.
73. Zhou FQ-Y, Olah ME, Li C, Johnson RA, Stiles GA, Civelli O. Molecular cloning and characterization of a novel adenosine receptor: the A$_3$ adenosine receptor. *Proc Natl Acad Sci USA* 1992;89:7432–7436.

Psychopharmacology: The Fourth Generation of Progress, edited by Floyd E. Bloom and David J. Kupfer. Raven Press, Ltd., New York © 1995.

CHAPTER 58

Brain Energy Metabolism

An Integrated Cellular Perspective

Pierre J. Magistretti, Luc Pellerin, and Jean-Luc Martin

The development of a felted sheath of neuroglia fibers in the ground-substance immediately surrounding the blood vessels of the Brain seems therefore . . . to allow of the free passage of lymph and metabolic products which enter into the fluid and general metabolism of the nerve cells.
— W. L. ANDRIEZEN (ref. 1)

Glucose is the obligatory energy substrate for brain and it is almost entirely oxidized to CO_2 and H_2O. This simple statement summarizes, with few exceptions, over four decades of careful studies of brain energy metabolism at the organ and regional levels, extensively reviewed elsewhere (e.g., 10,60,61). To reflect the focus of this book, and to include recent observations made in several laboratories including our own, we provide in this chapter a key for reinterpreting brain energy metabolism with a cellular perspective. This key relies primarily on the cytological relationships and chemical interactions among the various cell types of the brain. The view that emerges from this cellular and molecular analysis is a cell-specific sequence of processes that eventually leads to the almost complete oxidation by the brain of blood-borne glucose, which is in accordance with the introductory statement. The proposed model relies on already available data; it can further be tested experimentally, and it provides an explanation for some recent unexpected data obtained by positron emission tomography (PET) and functional magnetic resonance imaging (MRI) studies in humans (14,40,49).

P. J. Magistretti, L. Pellerin, and J.-L. Martin: Institut de Physiologie, Faculté de Médecine, Université de Lausanne, CH 1005 Lausanne, Switzerland.

ENERGY METABOLISM AT THE ORGAN LEVEL

Although the brain represents only 2% of the body weight, it receives 15% of the cardiac output, 20% of total body oxygen consumption, and 25% of total body glucose utilization. With a global blood flow of 57 ml/ 100 g·min, the brain extracts approximately 50% of oxygen and 10% of glucose from the arterial blood. Hence, the glucose utilization of the brain, as assessed by measuring the arterial–venous difference (22), is 31 μmol/100 g·min. Oxygen consumption is 160 μmol/100 g·min; because CO_2 production is almost identical, the respiratory quotient (RQ) of the brain is nearly 1, indicating that carbohydrates are the substrates for oxidative metabolism (60). Given a theoretical stoichiometry of 6 μmol of oxygen consumed for each μmole of glucose, glucose utilization by the brain should in theory be 26.6 μmol/100 g·min. As indicated earlier, the measured glucose utilization is 31 μmol/100 g·min, indicating that an excess of 4.4 μmol/100 g·min of glucose follows other metabolic fates. Glucose can produce metabolic intermediates, such as lactate and pyruvate, which do not enter necessarily in the tricarboxylic acid cycle but rather can be released and removed by the circulation. Glucose can be incorporated into lipids, proteins, and glycogen, and it is also the precursor of certain neurotransmitters such as γ-aminobutyric acid (GABA), glutamate, and acetylcholine (10,60).

Numerous studies have been performed to identify molecules that could substitute for glucose as an alternative substrate for brain energy metabolism. Among the vast array of molecules tested, mannose is the only one that can sustain normal brain function in the absence of glucose (59). Mannose crosses the blood–brain barrier and in two enzymatic steps is converted to fructose-6-phosphate, a physiological intermediate of the glycolytic pathway. However, mannose is not normally present in the blood and cannot therefore be considered a physiological substrate for brain energy metabolism. Lactate and pyruvate can sustain synaptic activity in vitro (36,55). Because of their limited permeability across the blood–brain barrier, they cannot substitute for plasma glucose to maintain brain function (43). However, if formed inside the brain parenchyma, they are useful metabolic substrates for neural cells (66). Under particular conditions, such as starvation, diabetes, or in breast-fed neonates, plasma levels of the ketone bodies acetoacetate and D-3-hydroxybutyrate increase markedly (41). Under these conditions, acetoacetate and D-3-hydroxybutyrate can be used by the brain as metabolic substrates (41).

As a corollary to these studies, steady-state arterial–venous (A–V) differences provide indirect evidence that a substance can be either used as a substrate by the brain (a positive A–V difference) or produced by the brain (a negative A–V difference) from a particular substrate such as glucose. Thus, in ketotic states, positive A–V differences have been measured for acetoacetate and D-3-hydroxybutyrate, indicating net utilization under these particular conditions. Net release of lactate and pyruvate (a negative A–V difference) is occasionally measured in normal individuals and more frequently in aged subjects or during convulsions (21).

ENERGY METABOLISM AT THE REGIONAL LEVEL

Whole-organ studies, which allowed the determination of the substrate requirements for the brain, failed to provide the appropriate level of resolution to appreciate two major features of brain energy metabolism: (a) its regional heterogeneity and (b) its tight relationship with the functional activation of specific pathways. The autoradiographic 2-deoxyglucose method (2-DG) developed by Sokoloff and colleagues afforded a sensitive means to measure local rates of glucose utilization (LCMRglu) with a spatial resolution of approximately 50 to 100 μm (61). The method is based on the fact that tracer amounts of radioactive 2-DG are taken up by glucose transporters and phosphorylated by hexokinase with kinetics that are similar to those for glucose; however, unlike glucose-6-phosphate, 2-deoxyglucose-6-phosphate cannot be metabolized further and therefore accumulates intracellularly, thus providing, after appropriate corrections (61), an accurate measurement of the amount of glucose utilized. For a detailed description of the method, the reader is referred to the original articles by Sokoloff and colleagues (60,61). Using this method, LCRMglu have been determined in virtually all structurally and functionally defined brain structures in various physiological and pathological states

including sleep, seizures, and dehydration, and following a variety of pharmacological treatments (10). Furthermore, the increase in glucose utilization following activation of pathways subserving specific modalities, such as visual, auditory, olfactory, or somatosensory stimulations, as well as during motor activity, has been revealed in the pertinent brain structures (10).

Basal glucose utilization of the grey matter as determined by the 2-DG technique varies, depending on the brain structure, between 50 and 150 μmol/100 g wet weight·min in the rat (61). If a protein content of 10% of wet weight is assumed, a value of 5 to 15 nmol/mg protein·min is obtained. These values are approximately 50% lower in the primate brain (10). Physiological activation of specific pathways results in a 1.5 to 3-fold increase in lCMRglc as determined by the 2-DG technique (38).

With the advent of PET and the use of positron-emitting isotopes such as ^{18}F, local glucose utilization has been studied in humans with 2-(^{18}F)fluoro-2-deoxyglucose (52) (see also Chapter 76, *this volume*). Similarly, local oxygen consumption and changes in blood flow can be studied in humans by PET using $^{15}O_2$ and $H_2^{15}O$ (15,53). Earlier studies had already demonstrated changes in local cerebral blood flow during activation of relevant brain regions by specific modalities (27).

In summary, changes in local brain energy metabolism can now be studied in humans with PET by monitoring alterations in glucose utilization, oxygen consumption, and blood flow during activation of specific areas. As we discuss below, recent studies in which these three parameters have been analyzed during activation of a given modality have yielded unexpected results, which suggest provocative hypotheses. Thus, an uncoupling between glucose uptake and oxygen consumption was observed during activation, since the increase in blood flow and in glucose utilization in the activated cortical area was not matched by an equivalent increase in oxygen consumption (13,14). This observation raises the puzzling possibility that, at least during the early stages of activation, the increased energy demand is met by glycolysis rather than by oxidative phosphorylation.

Glycolysis and Oxidative Phosphorylation

Glycolysis (Embden-Meyerhof pathway) is the metabolism of glucose to pyruvate and lactate (Fig. 1). It results in the net production of only 2 mol of adenosine triphosphate (ATP)/mol of glucose as well as in the regeneration of reducing equivalents (the oxidized form of nicotinamide-adenine dinucleotide, NAD$^+$) through the conversion of pyruvate into lactate. Alternatively, pyruvate can enter the tricarboxylic acid (TCA) cycle (or the Krebs cycle) and produce 30 mol of ATP/mol of glucose via the mitochondrial oxidative phosphorylation cascade (Fig. 2). The energetic value of oxidative phosphorylation over

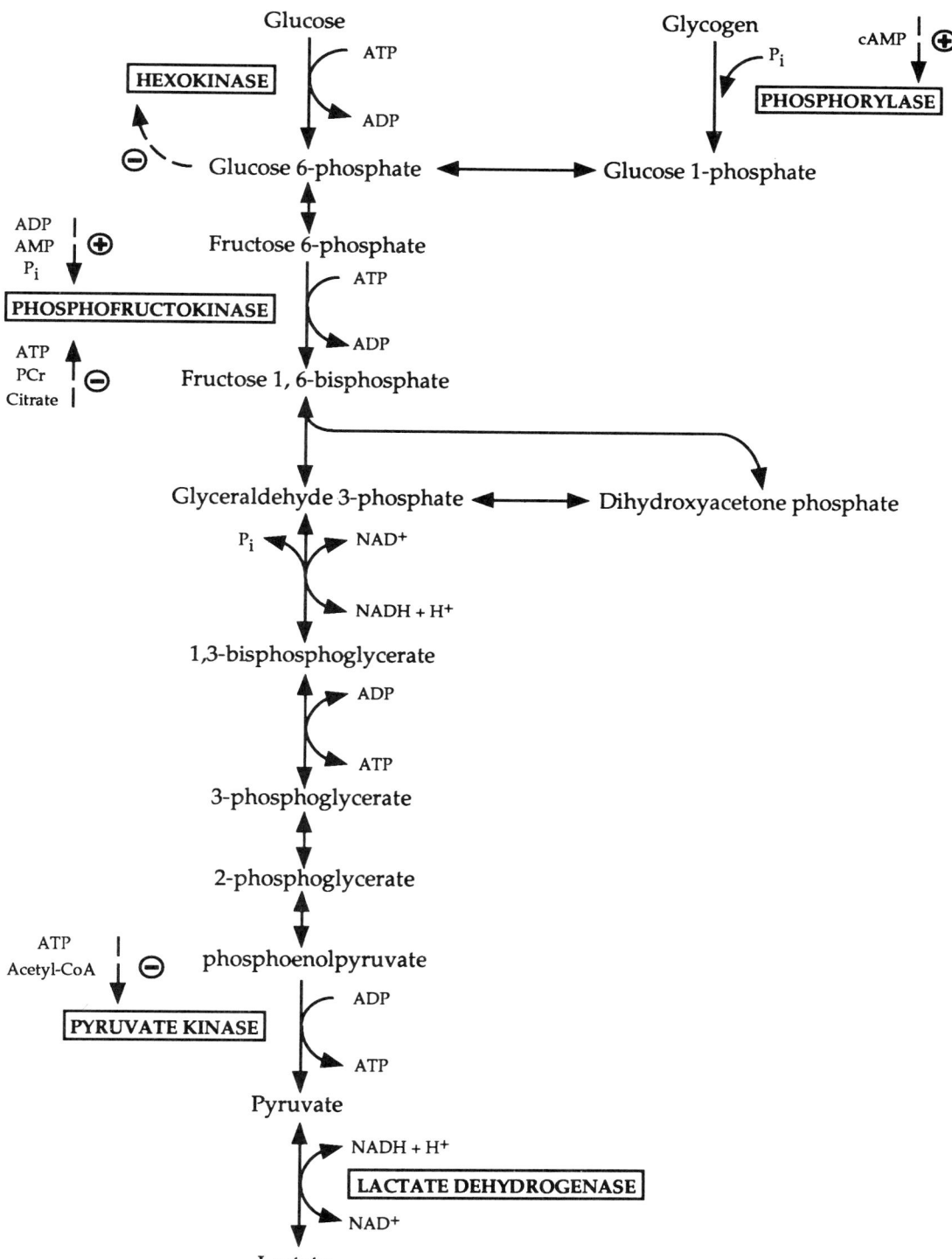

FIG. 1. Glycolysis—the Embden-Meyerhof pathway. Glucose entry is regulated by hexokinase, an enzyme inhibited by glucose-6-phosphate. Two other important points of regulation of glycolysis are phosphofructokinase and pyruvate kinase. Their activities are controlled by the levels of high-energy phosphates as well as of citrate and acetyl-CoA. Pyruvate, via lactate dehydrogenase, is in dynamic equilibrium with lactate; this reaction is essential to regenerate NAD$^+$ residues. *PCr,* phosphocreatine.

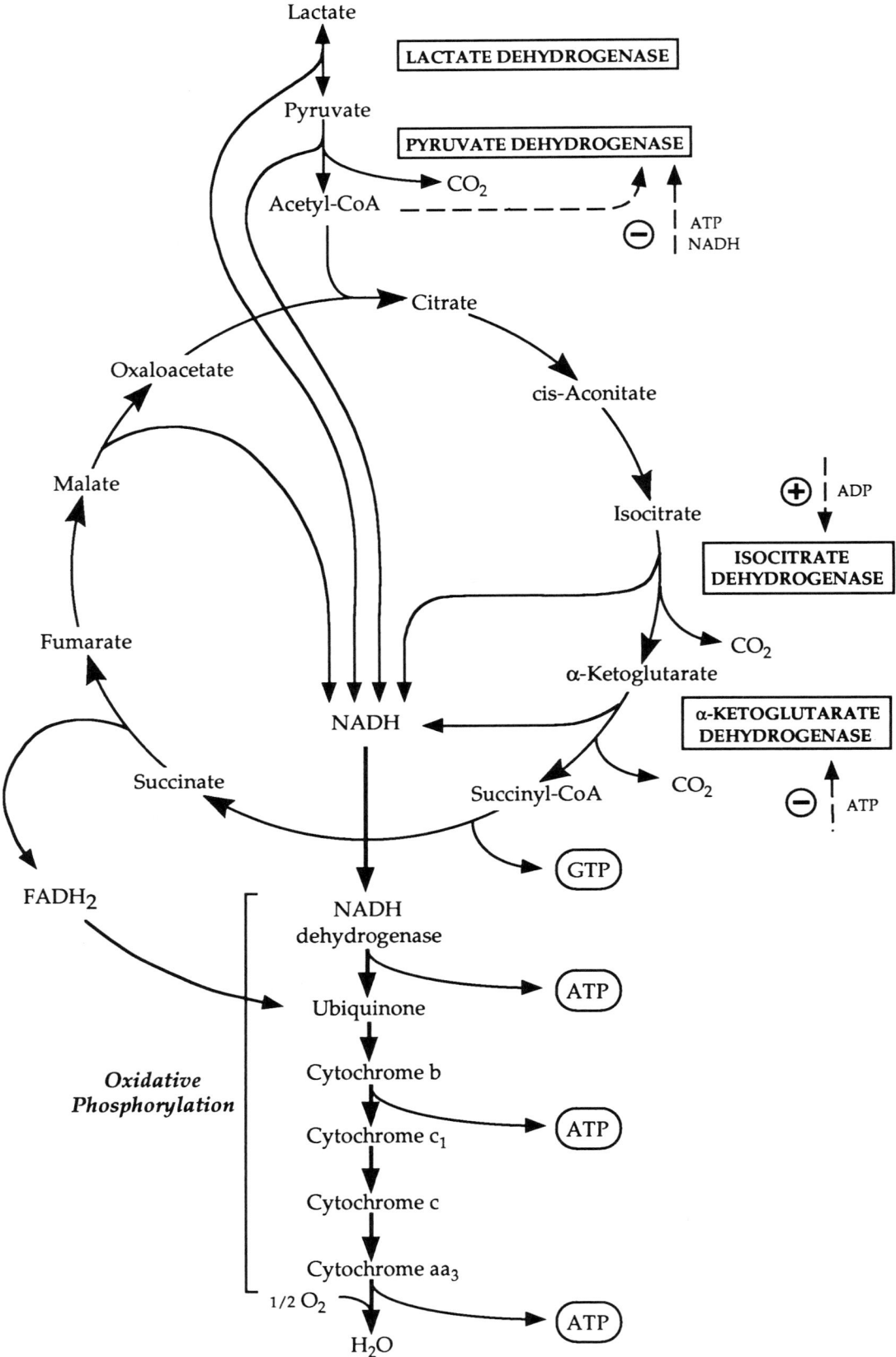

FIG. 2. Tricarboxylic acid cycle (the Krebs cycle) and oxidative phosphorylation. Pyruvate entry into the cycle is controlled by pyruvate dehydrogenase activity, which is inhibited by the levels of ATP and NADH. Two other regulatory points of the cycle are isocitrate and α-ketoglutarate dehydrogenases, which are influenced by the levels of high-energy phosphates.

glycolysis is thus obvious. The only positive A–V differences consistently observed in the human brain are those of glucose and oxygen (except for ketotic states), and the respiratory quotient of the brain is virtually 1; therefore, the question of whether glycolysis or oxidative phosphorylation play a significant role in brain energy metabolism seems superfluous. As noted earlier, at most an excess of 5 μmol/100 g·min (i.e., 20% of total utilized glucose) is not oxidized completely to CO_2 and H_2O, and only a portion of it will yield pyruvate and lactate. Therefore, based on these whole-organ studies (i.e., A–V differences), at best less than 20% of glucose may eventually be utilized glycolytically. However, an array of recent data, obtained from studies both in vitro and in vivo raise the provocative question of a key role of glycolysis in brain energy metabolism. Consistent with the PET studies indicating an uncoupling between glucose uptake and oxygen consumption during activation (13,14), rises in lactate have been monitored by ^{1}H MRI spectroscopy in the primary visual cortex of humans following appropriate photic stimulation (49,54). Lactate levels are increased in the rat somatosensory cortex following forepaw stimulation (68). When lactate was measured in vivo by microdialysis in freely moving rats, similar increases in hippocampus and striatum following somatosensory stimulation were demonstrated (11). Interestingly, the rate of lactate clearance from the extracellular space was markedly slowed in the presence of tetrodotoxin, a specific blocker of the neuronal voltage-sensitive sodium channels responsible for the generation of action potentials (11). This latter observation implies that during activation, lactate may normally be taken up by neurons as an energy fuel. It should be remembered that, after conversion to pyruvate, lactate can enter the TCA cycle with the potential to generate a total of 36 mol of ATP/mol of glucose (Fig. 2).

These in vivo data reveal a previously unrecognized prevalence of glycolysis over oxidative phosphorylation during activation. In fact, estimates of enzyme capacities indicate that glucose oxidation is already nearly maximal under basal conditions, implying that the activation-induced increases in energy demands are to be met primarily by glycolysis (69). One of the possible roles for activation-induced glycolysis may be to provide ATP to fuel energy-dependent ion transport, in particular the Na^+/K^+-ATPase, which represents the main energy-consuming process in neural cells (58). In fact, for the activity of the Na^+/K^+-ATPase, a preferential role of ATP derived from glycolysis has been recognized in various tissues (44,50), including the brain (29). Other energy-consuming processes in the nervous system appear to preferentially use glycolytically derived ATP (51).

In summary, the analysis of brain energy metabolism at the regional level, afforded by the autoradiographic 2-DG method and by the development of PET-based analyses of glucose utilization, oxygen consumption, and blood flow, have clearly established a relationship between functional activity ("brain work") and energy metabolism. The PET and MRI studies in humans (13,14,40,49,54) have also revealed a previously unexpected role of glycolysis during activation of discrete and functionally defined areas, in the face of indisputable evidence from whole-brain steady-state A–V differences indicating that glucose is almost entirely oxidized to CO_2 and H_2O. How can these apparently opposite results be reconciled? As we discuss below, in vitro analyses of brain energy metabolism at the cellular level, and in particular of the flux of metabolic substrates between neurons and astrocytes, provide clues that may be useful in resolving this controversy.

ENERGY METABOLISM AT THE CELLULAR LEVEL

Most of the information on energy metabolism at the cellular level has been obtained from cellularly homogeneous, purified preparations enriched in astrocytes, neurons, or vascular endothelial cells. Currently, most studies are conducted in primary cultures prepared from neonatal or embryonic rodent brain tissue. A cautionary note is always necessary when attempting to extrapolate results obtained in vitro to in vivo situations. It is, however, generally accepted that important insights may be gained from these cellularly homogeneous preparations.

Brain energy metabolism is often considered to reflect predominantly, if not exclusively, neuronal energy metabolism. However, it is now clear that other cell types, namely neuroglia and vascular endothelial cells not only consume energy but also can play an active role in the flux of energy substrates to neurons. First, there is a quantitative consideration; although it is arduous to provide a definitive ratio between neurons and nonneuronal cells given the variability in figures obtained in various species, brain areas, and developmental ages using methods that are not easily comparable, it is clear that neurons contribute at most 50% of cerebral cortical volume (23). In addition there is clear evidence indicating that the astrocyte-to-neuron ratio increases with increasing brain size (67); this is an important consideration when approaching the study of the cellular bases of brain energy metabolism in humans. It is therefore clear that glucose reaching the brain parenchyma through the circulation should provide energy substrates to a variety of cell types, only a portion of which are neurons.

Astrocytes as the Site of Glucose Uptake Following Neuronal Activation

Some structural relationships between astrocytes and other elements of nervous tissue are of particular relevance in this discussion of brain energy metabolism at

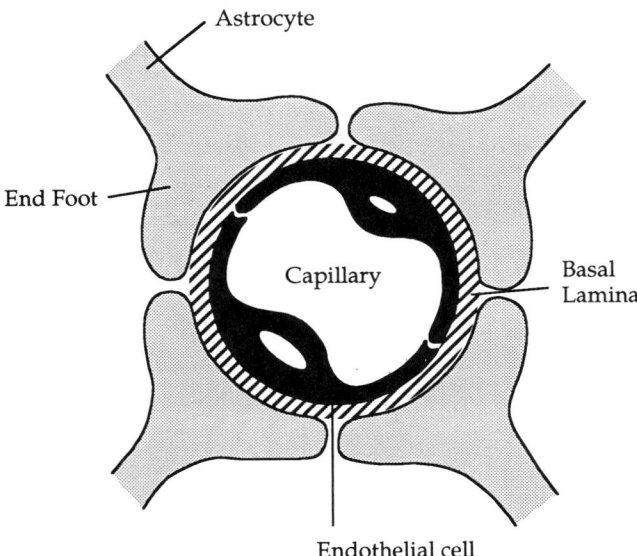

FIG. 3. Astrocytic end-feet abutting on a capillary. Redrawn from ref. 4.

the cellular level. Astrocyte processes are wrapped around synaptic contacts, whereas particular astrocytic profiles, the end-feet, surround intraparenchymal capillaries, and provide a cellular zone interposed between the blood-stream and other elements of the brain parenchyma (46) (Fig. 3). This latter structural feature has long been suggested as evidence indicating a role of astrocytes in the transit of substances from blood to other brain cells (1) (Fig. 4). A review of the physiological functions of astrocytes, which are only beginning to be elucidated, is beyond the scope of this article; however, their relationship to the structural features outlined above provides a background to the discussion of metabolic fluxes between cell types of the brain.

Two well-established functions of astrocytes are to maintain extracellular K^+ homeostasis (3,46) and to ensure the reuptake of neurotransmitters (17,46). Neuronal activity results both in increases in extracellular K^+ concentration and, at least at excitatory synapses, in augmented glutamate levels in the synaptic cleft (for the purpose of this discussion it should be borne in mind that glutamate is the major excitatory neurotransmitter in the brain, see ref. 12). One of the proposed mechanisms for the clearance of K^+ from the extracellular milieu is by spatial buffering through the astrocytic syncytium (3). The potassium ion can also accumulate in astrocytes through inwardly rectifying K^+ conductances (3). The activity of the Na^+,K^+-ATPase, which by hydrolyzing ATP to adenosine diphosphate (ADP) extrudes $3Na^+$ against $2K^+$, has also been shown to contribute to K^+ homeostasis (24). In this latter case, maintaining K^+ homeostasis is an energy-consuming process. Accordingly, 2-DG uptake into primary astrocyte cultures is

markedly inhibited by ouabain, an inhibitor of the Na^+,K^+-ATPase (5).

On the other hand, recent results in our laboratory have indicated that glutamate also increases 2-DG uptake in cultured astrocytes (Table 1), with an EC_{50} of approximately 100 μM. This effect is blocked by the specific glutamate uptake inhibitor THA and by ouabain. This latter finding indicates that glutamate uptake into astrocytes, which occurs through a cotransport with Na^+, results in the activation of Na^+,K^+-ATPase, probably by an increase in the intracellular concentration of Na^+ (24). In fact, there appears to exist in astrocytes a large reserve of Na^+,K^+-ATPase activity, which can be stimulated by Na^+ entry (24), resulting in a two- to threefold increase in 2-DG uptake (71). In the present context, it is important to note that the main mechanism that links energy metabolism and functional activity as determined by 2-DG uptake is represented by the activation of the Na^+,K^+-ATPase (35).

In vitro observations indicate (a) that astrocytes utilize glucose (5,48) at a basal rate of 5 to 10 nmol/mg·min (5,71,72), a rate similar to that determined in whole-animal studies with the 2-DG autoradiographic method (61); (b) that two physiological functions of astrocytes linked to increased synaptic activity, that is, K^+ and glutamate clearance from the extracellular space, markedly stimulate in a ouabain-sensitive manner 2-DG uptake; and finally (c) that the activation of Na^+,K^+-ATPase represents the coupling mechanism between the increase in glucose utilization and functional activity of the nervous tissue, raise the possibility that glucose utilization, as determined by PET in humans and by autoradiography in laboratory animals, reflects primarily the uptake of glucose by astrocytes rather than by neurons.

These considerations, based on in vitro studies and on the actual cytological relationships between astrocytic and neuronal processes, are in fact substantiated by results obtained in animal or human studies with the 2-DG method. It is now well established that the increases in 2-DG uptake linked to functional activation occur in the neuropil, that is, in regions that are enriched in axon terminals, dendrites and synapses ensheathed by astrocytic processes and not where neuronal perikarya are located (18). For example, when the sciatic nerve of anesthetized rats is stimulated, a frequency-dependent

TABLE 1. *Effects of glutamate and ouabain on 2-DG uptake by astrocytes[a]*

	^3H–2-DG uptake (fmol/mg protein·20 min)
Basal	1157 ± 94
Glutamate 500 μM	2144 ± 119
Ouabain 1 mM	657 ± 60
Ouabain + Glutamate 500 μM	615 ± 61

[a] Results are the mean ± SEM of triplicate determinations.

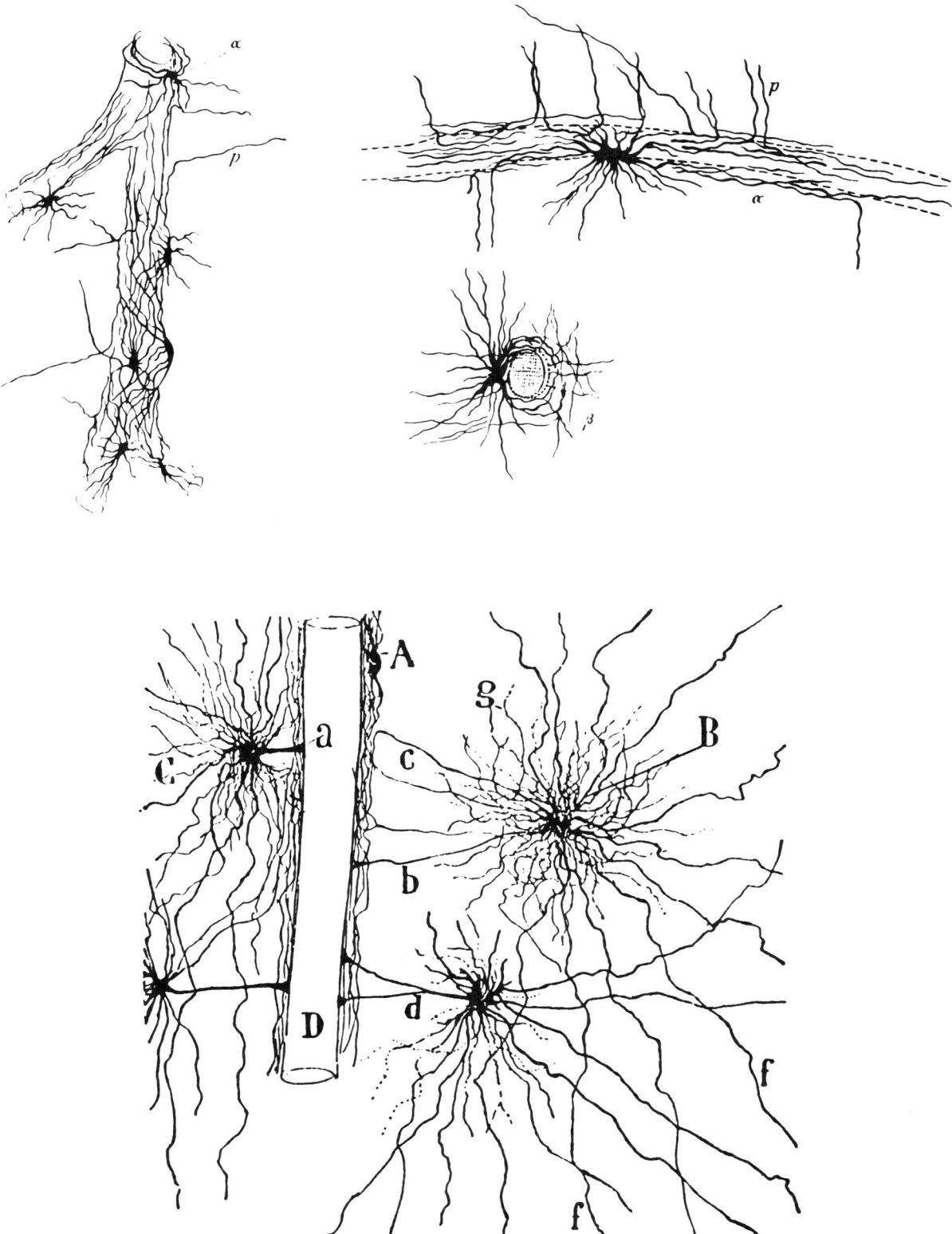

FIG. 4. Cytological relations between astrocytes and intraparenchymal microvessels. **Top Left:** Several neuroglia fiber cells (intrinsic) forming a sheath (perivascular) of fibers interwoven into a feltwork. α, An encircling cell; all the other are elongated cells. p, A fiber entering the sheath at right angle from a distant (extrinsic) cell. Chromate of silver staining. **Top Right:** α, A vessel indicated by dotted lines. An elongated cell is seen giving longitudinal and oblique fibers (intrinsic); p also several (extrinsic) fibers entering the sheath at right angles (human brain). β, Cross-section of a vessel (*dotted*), surrounded by a transverse cell (intrinsic). A few fibers are seen entering the feltwork perpendicularly. Drawing and legend for both left and right from ref. 1. **Bottom:** A, Flat perivascular neuroglial cell; B, another neuroglial cell with long processes; C, neuroglial cells with pedicles; D, capillary; a, pedicle fixed on the vascular endothelium. From ref. 6, legend translated.

increase in 2-DG uptake occurs in the dorsal horn of the spinal cord (where afferent axon terminals make synaptic contacts with second order neurons) but not in the dorsal root ganglion, where the cell body of the sensory neurons is localized (18). As another example, increases in glucose utilization in the well-laminated monkey primary visual cortex elicited by appropriate visual stimuli are most pronounced in layer IV, which is poor in perikarya but in which the terminals of axons projecting from the lateral geniculate engage in synaptic contacts (20). In addition, activation studies of specific functional pathways using PET determination of cerebral blood flow indicate that the increases in energy demands occur in the projection areas, that is, where axon terminals are found (73).

The resolution of the 2-DG autoradiographic method does not allow us to determine whether the increase in 2-DG uptake occurs in axon terminals, dendrites, or the astrocytes that surround these elements. However, the observations on glucose utilization as determined by the 2-DG autoradiographic method, taken together with the fact that a rate of 2-DG uptake very similar to that observed in vivo can be demonstrated in pure astrocyte preparations is strongly suggestive of the fact that a large proportion of the glucose uptake that occurs during activation of modality-specific circuits is localized in astrocytes rather than in neurons. Other in vitro observations support this view. Reports have indicated that the rate of glucose uptake in cultured neurons is lower than in astrocytes (16,30). In addition, glucose as the sole energy substrate cannot support neuronal survival in vitro (39,56); other substrates such as pyruvate, glutamine, and lactate are needed (36,39,56).

To summarize, in vivo and in vitro data indicate that glucose utilization occurs at synaptic sites, not at neuronal perikarya, and that astrocytes are the likely cells where glucose uptake occurs during activation.

Metabolic Trafficking between Astrocytes and Neurons

If glucose is taken up predominantly by astrocytes and if glucose alone cannot support the survival of neurons in vitro, then energy substrates other than glucose must be released by astrocytes. As indicated earlier, lactate and pyruvate are adequate substrates for brain tissue in vitro (36,55,66). In fact, synaptic activity can be maintained in cerebral cortical slices with only lactate or pyruvate as a substrate (36,55). Thus a metabolic compartmentation whereby glucose taken up by astrocytes is metabolized glycolytically to lactate or pyruvate (Fig. 5), which are then released in the extracellular space to be utilized by neurons, is consistent with the available biochemical and electrophysiological observations. In particular, in vitro studies indicate that quantitatively lactate is the main metabolic intermediate released by astrocytes at a rate of 15

to 30 nmol/mg of protein·min (9,70). This rate of release correlates well with the rate of glucose uptake by the grey matter (61) or by astrocytes in culture (71,72), which is between 5 and 15 nmol/mg of protein·min. Other, quantitatively less important intermediates released by astrocytes are pyruvate (approximately 10 times less than lactate), α-ketoglutarate, citrate, and malate (56,57,62). Furthermore, fluxes of endogenous lactate between astrocytes and neurons have been quantified in vitro (26), and an avid lactate uptake has been demonstrated in neurons (8,26). In addition, cytological evidence also supports this view. First, immunohistochemical data on the localization of the glucose transporter (GT) protein and of the pyruvate dehydrogenase (PDH) complex indicate that GT is primarily localized at the neuropil, that is, where axon terminals, dendrites, and the astrocytic processes that ensheath them are localized, whereas PDH [the enzyme that catalyzes the entry of pyruvate in dynamic equilibrium with lactate through the action of lactate dehydrogenase (Fig. 1) in the TCA cycle] is localized predominantly in the neuronal perikaryon (2,37). In the adult rat cerebellum, an analogous differential distribution of key enzymes of energy metabolism exists (19). Thus, although Purkinje cells contain a high PDH activity, Bergman glia surrounding them is enriched in hexokinase, implying a high glucose phosphorylating activity (19).

The functional cytology of astrocytes provides a second set of arguments to support the existence of such metabolic compartmentation and trafficking. Astrocytes derive their name from the numerous processes that emerge from their cell-body conferring on them a star-shaped morphology. In addition, astrocytes are connected between them through gap junctions, thus giving rise to what is called the astrocytic syncytium (46). A critical role has been shown for such an astrocytic syncytium in the spatial buffering of K^+ (3), whereby potassium ions flow through the syncytium from sites of high K^+ extracellular concentration (Ke) brought about by increased neuronal activity, to sites where Ke is lower, thus maintaining Ke within the physiological range. The astrocytic syncytium appears to be equally suited to maintain energy metabolism homeostasis. Thus, specialized astrocytic processes, the endfeet surround intraparenchymal microvessels, which are the source of glucose; whereas other astrocytic processes surround the synapses, where the energy-consuming uptake of glutamate, and to a lesser extent of K^+, coupled to synaptic activity occurs. Release of lactate and pyruvate is likely to occur at yet other sites, that is, at astrocytic processes that surround neuronal perikarya, where PDH, the enzyme complex for which pyruvate (or lactate through the action of LDH) is a substrate, is preferentially localized (2,37) (Fig. 6).

These observations on the metabolic trafficking between astrocytes and neurons as well as on the cellular compartmentalization of enzymes that regulate glucose uptake and glycolysis versus oxidative phosphorylation

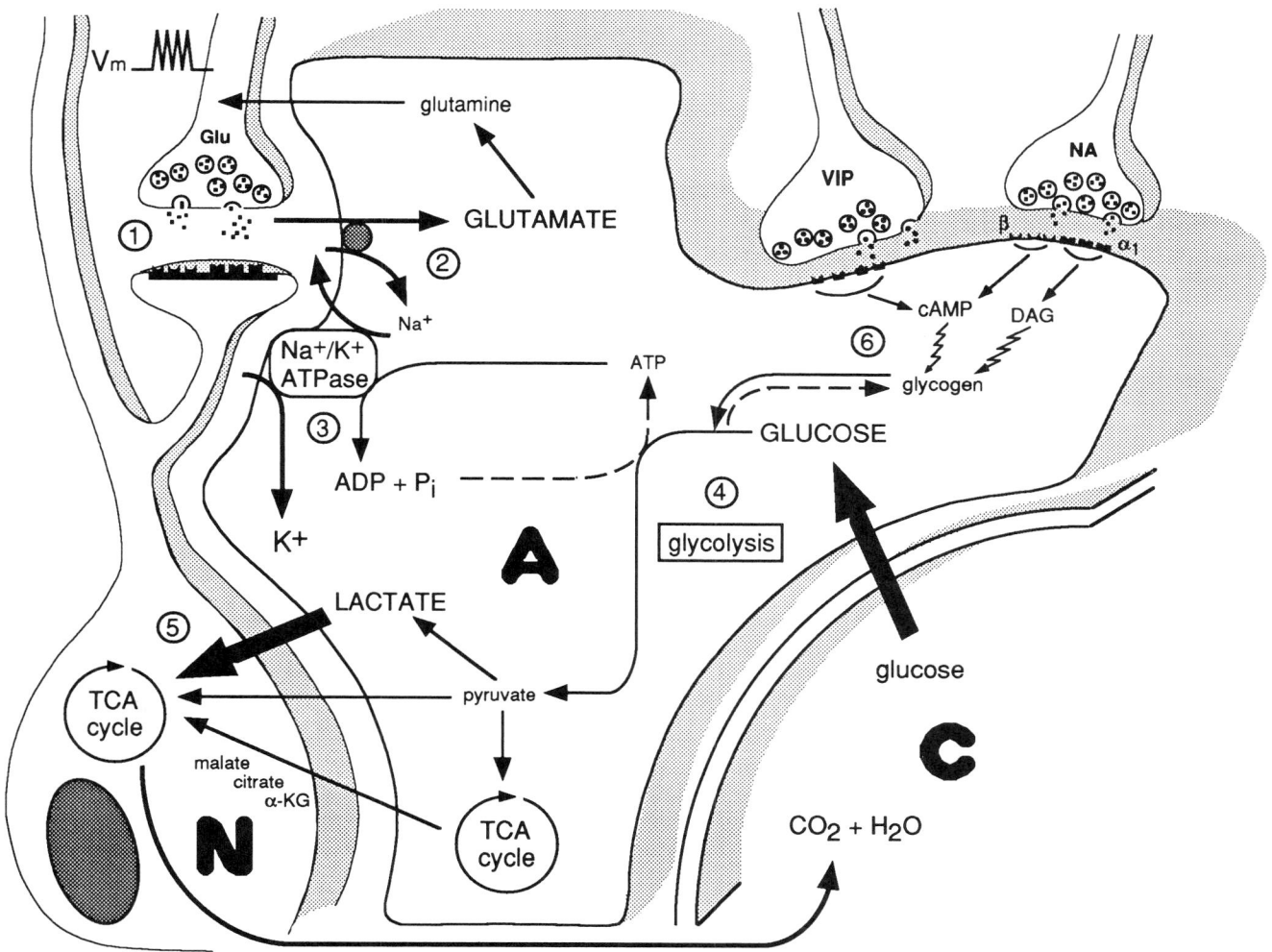

FIG. 5. Metabolic trafficking between astrocytes and neurons. ①: Synaptic activity causes an accumulation of glutamate in the synaptic cleft. ②: An astrocytic glutamate transporter ensures removal of glutamate from the synaptic cleft. ③: The entry of Na^+ cotransported with glutamate activates the Na^+,K^+-ATPase hence decreasing ATP levels. ④: The decrease in ATP levels activates the glycolytic flux (see Fig. 1) hence stimulating glucose uptake from the capillaries. ⑤: Lactate, the major end product of glycolysis, is released by astrocytes and taken up by neurons where it can enter the TCA cycle. Other metabolic intermediates such as pyruvate and the TCA cycle intermediates malate, citrate, and α-ketoglutarate, although quantitatively less significant, may also be released. ⑥: Certain neurotransmitter systems such as those containing NE and VIP promote glycogenolysis hence supplying further glycosyl residues for glycolysis. N, Neuron; A, astrocyte, C, capillary; Glu, glutamate; α-KG, α-ketoglutarate; DAG, diacylglycerol; Vm, depolarization of glutamate-containing terminal.

support the fact that glucose, taken up by astrocytic processes is metabolized glycolytically to lactate and pyruvate, which are then released as substrates for oxidative phosphorylation in neurons (Fig. 5).

REGULATION OF ENERGY METABOLISM BY NEUROTRANSMITTERS: A CELLULAR PERSPECTIVE

Local energy metabolism, in particular blood flow, has been viewed until recently as being regulated by products that accumulate following neuronal activity, such as adenosine and K^+, as well by changes in extracellular pH and pCO_2 (25,45). This mechanistic view of events implies a post-hoc regulation of energy metabolism, that is, adenosine, K^+, pCO_2, and pH are the coupling factors between neuronal activity and blood flow (25,45). One of the lines of research of our laboratory during the last 10 years has been aimed at testing the hypothesis that energy metabolism may be controlled by specific neurotransmitter systems that function in parallel with, or possibly even in anticipation of, those that act by releasing fast-acting neurotransmitters, such as glutamate and GABA, and convey

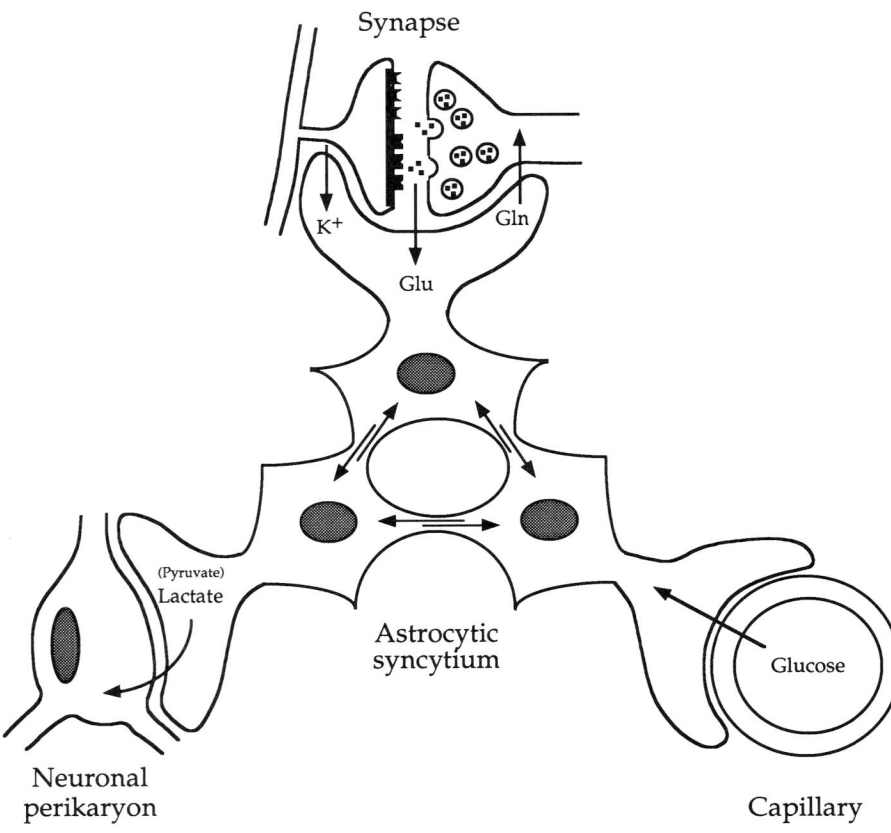

FIG. 6. Metabolic polarity of the astrocytic syncytium. Astrocytes have various processes that make contact either with capillaries, neuronal perikarya, or synapses. In addition, they are connected with each other at gap junctions; through these junctions small molecules (MW < 1000) can be exchanged. These properties endow the astrocytic syncytium with the capacity to ensure the transfer of metabolic intermediates from areas of production to areas of demand. *Glu,* Glutamate; *Gln,* glutamine.

rapid, point-to-point information within the brain. Experimental evidence indicates that the neuronal systems that contain norepinephrine (NE) and vasoactive intestinal peptide (VIP) may play such a homeostatic function within the cerebral cortex.

Regulation of Glycogen Metabolism in Astrocytes by Norepinephrine and Vasoactive Intestinal Peptide

Within the brain, glycogen is primarily stored in astrocytes, although ependymal and choroid plexus cells, as well as certain large neurons in the brainstem contain the polysaccharide (see ref. 34 for review). Glycogen levels in brain are low compared to liver and muscle; however, the glycogen turnover rate is very rapid; its synthesis and breakdown are regulated by the two key enzymes glycogen phosphorylase and synthase (34). Glycogen levels are tightly coupled to synaptic activity as illustrated by the fact that during anesthesia they rise sharply (47); furthermore, reactive astrocytes, which develop in areas in which neuronal activity is decreased or absent as a consequence of injury, contain high amounts of glycogen (34 and the refs. therein). Approximately a decade ago, we showed that VIP, a then recently discovered peptide contained in a homogeneous population of bipolar, radially oriented neurons (33), could promote a cyclic adenosine monophosphate (cAMP) dependent glycogenolysis

in mouse cerebral cortical slices (31). In view of the morphology and arborization pattern of VIP-containing neurons (Fig. 7), we proposed that these cells could regulate the availability of energy substrates locally, within cortical columns (31,33). A similar effect had been previously described for NE, serotonin, and histamine (34). The noradrenergic system is organized according to principles strikingly different from those of VIP neurons: The cell bodies of NE-containing neurons are localized in the locus coeruleus in the brainstem from which axons project to various brain areas including the cerebral cortex. Here, they enter the rostral end and progress caudally with a predominantly horizontal trajectory, across a vast rostro-caudal expanse of cortex (33). Given these morphological features, we suggested that, in contrast to VIP-containing intracortical neurons, the noradrenergic system could regulate energy homeostasis globally, spanning across functionally distinct cortical areas (31,33) (Fig. 7).

The glycogenolytic effect of VIP and NE is exerted in astrocytes, as indicated by studies in primary astrocyte cultures (32,63) as well as by the fact that glycogen is primarily localized in this cell type (46). Thus VIP and NE promote a concentration- and time-dependent glycogenolysis in astrocytes, with EC_{50} of 3 and 20 nM, respectively (32,63). The effect of NE is mediated by both β and α_1 receptors. The initial rate of glycogenolysis is between 5 and 10 nmol/mg protein·min (63), a value that

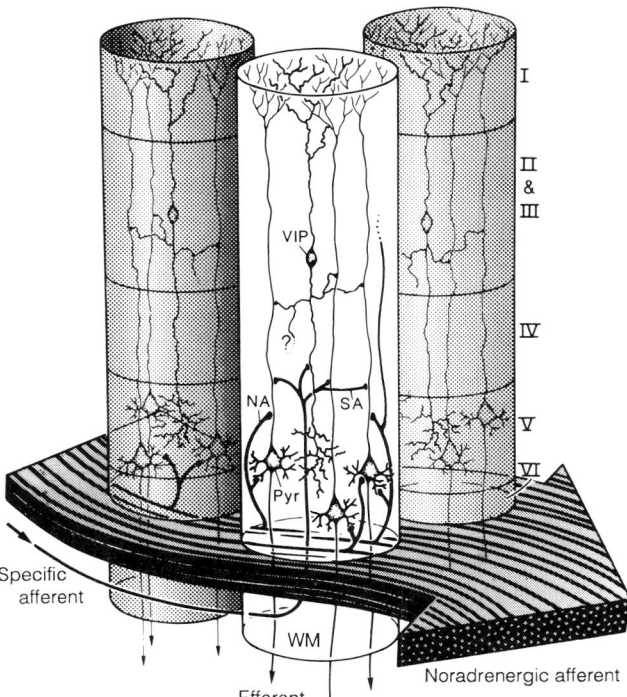

FIG. 7. Diagrammatic representation of the anatomic substrate for the metabolic actions of NE and VIP. *VIP*, VIP-containing bipolar neuron; *NA*, noradrenergic afferent; *Pyr*, pyramidal cell furnishing major efferent projection; *SA*, specific afferent (i.e., from thalamus or from other cortical areas); *WM*, subcortical white matter. Cortical layers denoted in roman numerals. Note the tangential orientation of NA fibers and the radially restricted domain of VIP-containing neurons. From ref. 33.

is remarkably close to glucose utilization of the grey matter as determined by the 2-DG autoradiographic method (61). This correlation indicates that the glycosyl units mobilized in response to the two glycogenolytic neurotransmitters can provide quantitatively adequate substrates for the energy demands of the brain parenchyma.

Another action of NE on energy metabolism is the marked stimulation of 2-DG uptake in primary astrocyte cultures (72). This action is functionally coordinated with glycogenolysis, because the same extracellular signal (NE) results in an increased availability of glycosyl units for ATP production in astrocytes. In contrast to NE, VIP does not influence glucose uptake by astrocytes (72).

Glycogenolysis and Neuronal Activity

Glycogenolysis, revealed by a newly developed autoradiography technique for glycogen, has also been demonstrated in vivo following physiological activation of a modality-specific pathway (64). Thus, repeated stimulation of the vibrissae resulted in a marked decrease in the density of glycogen-associated autoradiographic grains in

the somatosensory cortex of rats (barrel field) as well as in the relevant thalamic nuclei (64). These observations indicate that the physiological activation of specific neuronal circuits results in the mobilization of glial glycogen stores.

As noted earlier, systemic administration of general anesthetics increases brain glycogen levels (47). Interestingly however, they do not increase the glycogen content of cultures exclusively containing astrocytes (65); this observation indicates that the in vivo action of general anesthetics on astrocytic glycogen is due to the inhibition of neuronal activity, further stressing the existence of a tight coupling between neuronal activity and astrocytic glycogen.

In view of the foregoing, it appears that astrocytic glycogen represents a metabolic buffer under the dynamic control of neuronal activity, which can be mobilized in the early stages of activation. Evidence supporting such a role of astrocytic glycogen has been provided by the hippocampal slice preparation. Electrical stimulation of the slice resulted in an immediate and marked increase in NADH fluorescence, an index for the activation of glycolysis (28). This increase in NADH fluorescence was observed in a well-oxygenated medium containing adequate supplies of glucose and occurred at the onset of synaptic activity. However, the signal disappeared when the glycogen content of the slices was depleted by dibutyryl cAMP (28). This observation further suggests that an activation of glycogenolysis occurs at the onset of synaptic activity.

What is the metabolic fate of the glycosyl units mobilized from glycogen? As noted earlier, lactate is the main metabolic intermediate released by astrocytes (9,70). No glucose is released from astrocyte cultures, even when glucose is absent from the medium (9), consistent with the view that brain glucose-6-phosphatase activity is very low or not measurable (61). Blockade of oxidative phosphorylation by azide or cyanide doubles the release of lactate by astrocytes (9) indicating that part of the glycosyl units mobilized from glycogen are oxidized by astrocytes rather than being exported as lactate.

Homeostatic Functions of NE and VIP

The foregoing observations support the notion that energy metabolism at the cellular level is regulated by specific neurotransmitter systems, such as those containing VIP and NE. These neurotransmitter systems could be viewed as the CNS counterparts of the autonomic nervous system that maintains cellular homeostasis in peripheral tissues. At this stage, it appears that astrocytes are the preferred targets for the homeostatic functions exerted by VIP and NE. However, immunohistochemical and more recently ultrastructural evidence provides strong support for the existence of interactions between various neurotransmitter systems, including those containing VIP, NE, serotonin, and acetylcholine, with endothelial cells of intraparenchymal microvessels in the rodent cerebral cortex (7,10). In further support of the existence of interactions between certain neurotransmitter systems and vascular endothelial cells, specific recognition sites for a variety of neurotransmitters including VIP, NE, serotonin, and acetylcholine, have been demonstrated in various preparations of intraparenchymal microvessels (42). In addition, most of these recognition sites represent functional receptors, because they are coupled to conventional signal transduction pathways (42).

There is little doubt that in the coming years the interactions between neurotransmitters and nonneuronal cells of the brain will provide new insights into brain functions and open fertile areas for pharmacological developments.

AN INTEGRATED VIEW

The preceding sections of this chapter have attempted to provide an overview of brain energy metabolism at the organ, regional, and cellular levels. The claim is not to have been exhaustive, rather the challenge has been to try to provide an integrated perspective for well-accepted experimental evidence spanning from in vivo studies to cellular and molecular analyses. As a means to provide a synthesis of the features that we consider salient and conceptually novel, we should look at the fate of a molecule of glucose from blood to neurons (Fig. 5).

Glucose is avidly taken up by astrocytes in vitro, at a rate that is similar to brain glucose utilization as determined with the 2-DG autoradiographic method. In vivo, the activation-induced increase in glucose uptake is visualized in the neuropil, that is, where synapses ensheathed by astrocytes are present, and not at the level of the neuronal perikarya. Furthermore, astrocyte end-feet surround intraparenchymal blood vessels. From this and other evidence previously reviewed, it can be inferred that most of the activation-induced glucose uptake in the brain parenchyma, notably as visualized by the PET (^{18}F)2-DG technique, occurs in astrocytes. In vivo as well as in vitro studies indicate that the physiological stimulation of a given brain region triggers a rapid activation of glycogenolysis (proven to be exclusively astrocytic) and glycolysis, which in turn result in the release of lactate.

Lactate, which has the potential of providing 36 ATP molecules through oxidative phosphorylation can be taken up and oxidized by neurons (actually 1 mol of lactate yields 18 mol of ATP; however, since 1 mol of glucose provides 2 mol of lactate, the overall ATP flux from glucose-derived lactate is 36 mol). Supporting this view is the fact, among other evidence, that synaptic activity in vitro can be maintained when lactate is the only metabolic substrate present. The bookeeping of energy metabolism provided by the A–V differences showing complete oxidation of glucose is consistent with this view: Glucose enters the brain from the arterial side and is predominantly taken up by astrocytes, which then transform it to lactate. Lactate exchange occurs with neurons, which oxidize it to CO_2 and H_2O drained by the venous blood. The increase in lactate levels measured in vivo by ^{1}H MRI spectroscopy or by microdialysis as well as the uncoupling between oxygen consumption and glucose uptake revealed by PET at the early stages of activation, can be interpreted in light of the proposed cellular compartmentation of lactate fluxes between astrocytes and neurons. Thus, because phosphofructokinase (PFK) activity is one of the rate-limiting steps for glycolysis (Fig. 1), activation-induced glycolysis implies a disinhibition of PFK and an increase in the levels of the metabolic intermediates that are downstream to it, notably lactate. A delay in the entry of lactate in the TCA cycle is likely to occur, because it takes place in another cell type (neurons), resulting in a temporary overflow of lactate linked to an absence of increase in oxygen consumption (uncoupling).

Several questions remain open to further investigation. To list a few: What are the molecular mechanisms of the coupling between neuronal activation and astrocytic glycolysis? Because ATP inhibits PFK activity, a decrease in the energy charge of astrocytes following activation is a likely possibility. What is the relative role of other metabolic substrates (such as citrate, α-ketoglutarate, or malate) that have been shown to be shuttled from astrocytes to neurons? Glycolysis and oxidative phosphorylation are not strictly compartmentalized between astrocytes and neurons, respectively. Clearly, some glucose oxidation occurs in astrocytes, and moderate release of lactate can be demonstrated from cultured neurons; mechanisms that regulate the relative activity of these two metabolic pathways in neurons and astrocytes are likely to exist and still need to be elucidated. The flux of metabolic substrates within the astrocytic syncytium provides yet another level of regulation to be studied (Fig. 6).

One can hope that, in addition to offering an accurate view of physiological brain energy metabolism, further elucidation of the cell-specific molecular mechanisms of energy metabolism regulation will provide useful clues to probe, with cellular and molecular specificity, the physiopathological processes that underlie the expression of certain neurological and psychiatric disorders.

ACKNOWLEDGMENTS

Research in the laboratory of PJM is supported by a grant from Fonds National Suisse de la Recherche Scientifique (31-26427.89). The authors are grateful to Ms. M. Emch for expert secretarial help.

REFERENCES

1. Andriezen WL. On a system of fibre-like cells surrounding the blood vessels of the brain of man and mammals, and its physiological significance. *Int Monatsschr Anat Physiol* 1893;10:532–540.
2. Bagley PR, Tucker SP, Nolan C, et al. Anatomical mapping of glucose transporter protein and pyruvate dehydrogenase in rat brain: an immunogold study. *Brain Res* 1989;499:214–224.
3. Barres BA. New roles for glia. *J Neurosci* 1991;11:3685–3694.
4. Bignami A. *Discussions in neuroscience*. vol. VIII, no. 1. Amsterdam: Elsevier, 1991;1–45.
5. Brookes N, Yarowsky PJ. Determinants of deoxyglucose uptake in cultured astrocytes: the role of the sodium pump. *J Neurochem* 1985;44:473–479.
6. Cajal RS. *Histologie du système nerveux de l'homme et des vertébrés*. Paris: Maloine, 1909;11.
7. Chédotal A, Umbriaco D, Descarries L, Hartman BK, Hamel E. Light and electron microscopic immunocytochemical analysis of neurovascular relationships of choline-acetyltransferase and vasoactive intestinal peptide nerve terminals in rat cerebral cortex. *J Comp Neurol* 1994;343:57–71.
8. Dringen R, Wiesinger H, Hamprecht B. Uptake of L-lactate by cultured rat brain neurons. *Neurosci Lett* 1993;163:5–7.
9. Dringen R, Gebhardt R, Hamprecht B. Glycogen in astrocytes: possible function as lactate supply for neighboring cells. *Brain Res* 1993;623:2208–2214.
10. Edvinsson L, MacKenzie ET, McCulloch J. *Cerebral blood flow and metabolism*. New York: Raven Press, 1993.
11. Fellows LK, Boutelle MG, Fillenz M. Physiological stimulation increases nonoxidative glucose metabolism in the brain of the freely moving rat. *J Neurochem* 1993;60:1258–1263.
12. Fonnum F. Glutamate: a neurotransmitter in mammalian brain. *J Neurochem* 1984;42:1–11.
13. Fox PT, Raichle ME. Focal physiological uncoupling of cerebral blood flow and oxidative metabolism during somatosensory stimulation in human subjects. *Proc Natl Acad Sci USA* 1986;83:1140–1144.
14. Fox PT, Raichle ME, Mintun MA, Dence C. Nonoxidative glucose consumption during focal physiologic neural activity. *Science* 1988;241:462–464.
15. Frackowiak RSJ, Lenzi GL, Jones T, Heather JD. Quantitative measurement of regional cerebral blood flow and oxygen metabolism in man using ^{15}O and positron emission tomography: theory, procedure, and normal values. *J Comput Assist Tomogr* 1980;4:727–736.
16. Heidenreich KA, Gilmore PR, Garvey WT. Glucose transport in primary cultured neurons. *J Neurosci Res* 1989;22:397–407.
17. Hösli E, Hösli L, Schousboe A. Amino acid uptake. In: Fedoroff S, Vernadakis A, eds. *Astrocytes. Biochemistry, physiology, and pharmacology of astrocytes*. Vol. 2. Orlando: Academic Press, 1986;133–153.
18. Kadekaro M, Crane AM, Sokoloff L. Differential effects of electrical stimulation of sciatic nerve on metabolic activity in spinal cord and dorsal root ganglion in the rat. *Proc Natl Acad Sci USA* 1985;82:6010–6013.
19. Katoh-Semba R, Keino H, Kashiwamata S. A possible contribution by glial cells to neuronal energy production: enzyme-histochemical studies in the developing rat cerebellum. *Cell Tissue Res* 1988;252:133–139.
20. Kennedy C, Des Rosiers MH, Sakurada O, et al. Metabolic mapping of the primary visual system of the monkey by means of the autoradiographic [^{14}C]deoxyglucose technique. *Proc Natl Acad Sci USA* 1976;73:4230–4234.
21. Kety SS. The general metabolism of the brain in vivo. In: Richter D, ed. *The metabolism of the nervous system*. London: Pergamon Press, 1957;221–237.
22. Kety SS, Schmidt CF. The nitrous oxide method for the quantitative determination of cerebral blood flow in man: theory, procedure, and normal values. *J Clin Invest* 1948;27:476–483.
23. Kimelberg HK, Norenberg MD. Astrocytes. *Sci Am* 1989;260:44–52.
24. Kimelberg HK, Jalonen T, Walz W. Regulation of the brain microenvironment: transmitters and ions. In: Murphy S, ed. *Astrocytes: pharmacology and function*. San Diego: Academic Press, 1993;193.
25. Kuschinsky W, Wahl M. Local chemical and neurogenic regulation of cerebral vascular resistance. *Physiol Rev* 1978;58:656–689.
26. Larrabee MG. Extracellular intermediates of glucose metabolism: fluxes of endogenous lactate and alanine through extracellular pools in embryonic sympathetic ganglia. *J Neurochem* 1992;59:1041–1052.
27. Lassen NA, Ingvar D, Skinhoj E. Brain function and blood flow. *Sci Am* 1978;239:62–71.
28. Lipton P. Effects of membrane depolarization on nicotinamide nucleotide fluorescence in brain slices. *Biochem J* 1973;136:999–1009.
29. Lipton P, Robacker K. Glycolysis and brain function: [K$^+$]$_0$ stimulation of protein synthesis and K$^+$ uptake require glycolysis. *FASEB J* 1983;42:2875–2880.
30. Lopes-Cardozo M, Larsson OM, Schousboe A. Acetoacetate and glucose as lipid precursors and energy substrates in primary cultures of astrocytes and neurons from mouse cerebral cortex. *J Neurochem* 1986;46:773–778.
31. Magistretti PJ, Morrison JH, Shoemaker WJ, Sapin V, Bloom FE. Vasoactive intestinal polypeptide induces glycogenolysis in mouse cortical slices: a possible regulatory mechanism for the local control of energy metabolism. *Proc Natl Acad Sci USA* 1981;78:6535–6539.
32. Magistretti PJ, Manthorpe M, Bloom FE, Varon S. Functional receptors for vasoactive intestinal polypeptide in cultured astroglia from neonatal rat brain. *Regul Pept* 1983;6:71–80.
33. Magistretti PJ, Morrison JH. Noradrenaline- and vasoactive intestinal peptide-containing neuronal systems in neocortex: functional convergence with contrasting morphology. *Neuroscience* 1988;24:367–378.
34. Magistretti PJ, Sorg O, Martin JL. Regulation of glycogen metabolism in astrocytes: physiological, pharmacological, and pathological aspects. In: Murphy S, ed. *Astrocytes: pharmacology and function*. San Diego: Academic Press, 1993;243.
35. Mata M, Fink DJ, Gainer H, et al. Activity-dependent energy metabolism in rat posterior pituitary primarily reflects sodium pump activity. *J Neurochem* 1980;34:213–215.
36. McIlwain H, Bachelard HS. In: *Biochemistry and the central nervous system*. Edinburgh: Churchill Livingstone, 1985;54–83.
37. Milner TA, Aoki C, Sheu RKF, Blass JP, Pickel VM. Light microscopic immunocytochemical localization of pyruvate dehydrogenase complex in rat brain: topographical distribution and relation to cholinergic and catecholaminergic nuclei. *J Neurosci* 1987;7:3171–3190.
38. Miyaoka M, Shinohara M, Batipps M, Pettigrew KD, Kennedy C, Sokoloff L. The relationship between the intensity of the stimulus and the metabolic response in the visual system of the rat. *Acta Neurol Scand Suppl* 1979;60:16–17.
39. Müller HW, Beckh S, Seifert W. Neurotrophic factor for central neurons. *Proc Natl Acad Sci USA* 1984;81:1248–1252.
40. Ogawa S, Tank DW, Menon R, et al. Intrinsic signal changes accompanying sensory stimulation: functional brain mapping with magnetic resonance imaging. *Proc Natl Acad Sci USA* 1992;89:5951–5955.
41. Owen OE, Morgan AP, Kemp HG, Sullivan JM, Herrera MG, Cahill GF Jr. Brain metabolism during fasting. *J Clin Invest* 1967;46:1589–1595.
42. Owman C, Hardebo JE, eds. *Neural regulation of brain circulation*. Amsterdam: Elsevier, 1986.
43. Pardridge WM, Oldendorf WH. Transport of metabolic substrates through the blood–brain barrier. *J Neurochem* 1977;28:5–12.
44. Paul RJ, Hardin DC, Raeymaekers L, Wuytack F, Casteels R. Vascular smooth muscle: aerobic glycolysis linked to sodium and potassium transport processes. *Science* 1979;206:1414–1416.
45. Paulson OB, Newman EA. Does the release of potassium from astrocyte endfeet regulate cerebral blood flow? *Science* 1987;237:896–898.
46. Peters A, Palay SL, Webster HD, eds. *The fine structure of the nervous system: the neurons and supporting cells*. 2nd ed. Philadelphia: W. B. Saunders, 1991.
47. Phelps CH. Barbiturate-induced glycogen accumulation in brain. An electron microscopic study. *Brain Res* 1972;39:225–234.
48. Poitry-Yamate CL, Tsacopoulos M. Glucose metabolism in freshly

isolated Müller glial cells from a mammalian retina. *J Comp Neurol* 1992;320:257–266.

49. Prichard J, Rothman D, Novotny E, et al. Lactate rise detected by ^{1}H NMR in human visual cortex during physiologic stimulation. *Proc Natl Acad Sci USA* 1991;88:5829–5831.

50. Proverbio F, Hoffman JF. Membrane compartmentalized ATP and its preferential use by the Na^+-K^+ ATPase of human red cell ghosts. *J Gen Physiol* 1977;69:605–632.

51. Raffin CH, Rosenthal M, Busto R, Sick TJ. Glycolysis, oxidative metabolism and brain potassium ion clearance. *J Cereb Blood Flow Metab* 1992;12:34–42.

52. Raichle ME. Quantitative in vivo autoradiography with positron emission tomography. *Brain Res Rev* 1979;1:47–68.

53. Raichle ME, Martin WRW, Herscovitch P, Mintun MA, Markham J. Brain blood flow measured with intravenous $H_2^{15}O$. II. Implementation and validation. *J Nucl Med* 1983;24:790–798.

54. Sappey-Marinier D, Calabrese G, Fein G, Hugg JW, Biggins C, Weiner MW. Effect of photic stimulation on human visual cortex lactate and phosphates using ^{1}H and ^{31}P magnetic resonance spectroscopy. *J Cereb Blood Flow Metab* 1992;12:584–592.

55. Schurr A, West CA, Rigor BM. Lactate-supported synaptic function in the rat hippocampal slice preparation. *Science* 1988;240:1326–1328.

56. Selak I, Skaper SD, Varon S. Pyruvate participation in the low molecular weight trophic activity for central nervous system neurons in glia-conditioned media. *J Neurosci* 1985;5:23–28.

57. Shank RP, Leo GC, Zielke HR. Cerebral metabolic compartmentation as revealed by nuclear magnetic resonance analysis of D-[1-13C]glucose metabolism. *J Neurochem* 1993;61:315–323.

58. Siesjö BK. *Brain energy metabolism.* New York: John Wiley, 1978;42–43.

59. Sloviter HA, Kamimoto T. The isolated, perfused rat brain preparation metabolizes mannose but not maltose. *J Neurochem* 1970;17:1109–1111.

60. Sokoloff L. Circulation and energy metabolism of the brain. In: Siegel G, Agranoff B, Albers RW, and Molinoff P, eds. *Basic neurochemistry: molecular, cellular, and medical aspects.* 4th ed. New York: Raven Press, 1989.

61. Sokoloff L, Reivich M, Kennedy C, et al. The [14C]deoxyglucose method for the measurement of local cerebral glucose utilization: theory, procedure, and normal values in the conscious and anesthetized albino rat. *J Neurochem* 1977;28:897–916.

62. Sonnewald U, Westergaard N, Krane J, Unsgård G, Petersen SB, Schousboe A. First direct demonstration of preferential release of citrate from astrocytes using [13C]NMR spectroscopy of cultured neurons and astrocytes. *Neurosci Lett* 1991;128:235–239.

63. Sorg O, Magistretti PJ. Characterization of the glycogenolysis elicited by vasoactive intestinal peptide, noradrenaline and adenosine in primary cultures of mouse cerebral cortical astrocytes. *Brain Res* 1991;563:227–233.

64. Swanson RA, Morton MM, Sagar SM, Sharp FR. Sensory stimulation induces local cerebral glycogenolysis: demonstration by autoradiography. *Neuroscience* 1992;51:451–461.

65. Swanson RA, Yu ACH, Sharp FR, Chan PH. Regulation of glycogen content in primary astrocyte culture: effect of glucose analogues, phenobarbital, and methionine sulfoximine. *J Neurochem* 1989;52:1359–1365.

66. Teller DN, Banay-Schwartz M, Deguzman T, Lajtha A. Energetics of amino acid transport into brain slices: effects of glucose depletion and substitution of Krebs' cycle intermediates. *Brain Res* 1977;131:321–334.

67. Tower DB, Young OM. The activities of butyrylcholinesterase and carbonic anhydrase, the rate of anaerobic glycolysis, and the question of a constant density of glial cells in cerebral cortices of various mammalian species from mouse to whale. *J Neurochem* 1973;20:269–278.

68. Ueki M, Linn F, Hossmann KA. Functional activation of cerebral blood flow and metabolism before and after global ischemia of rat brain. *J Cereb Blood Flow Metab* 1988;8:486–494.

69. Van den Berg C. In: Hockey GRJ, Gaillard AWK, Coles MGH, eds. *Energetics and Human Information Processing.* Boston: Nijhoff, 1986;131–135.

70. Walz W, Mukerji S. Lactate release from cultured astrocytes and neurones: a comparison. *Glia* 1988;1:366–370.

71. Yarowsky PJ, Wierwille R, Brookes N. Effect of monensin on deoxyglucose uptake in cultured astrocytes: energy metabolism is coupled to sodium entry. *J Neurosci* 1986;6:859–866.

72. Yu N, Martin JL, Stella N, Magistretti PJ. Arachidonic acid stimulates glucose uptake in cerebral cortical astrocytes. *Proc Natl Acad Sci USA* 1993;90:4042–4046.

73. Zeki S, Watson JDG, Lueck CJ, Friston KJ, Kennard C, Frackowiak RSJ. A direct demonstration of functional specialization in human visual cortex. *J Neurosci* 1991;11:641–649.

Psychopharmacology: The Fourth
Generation of Progress, edited by
Floyd E. Bloom and David J. Kupfer.
Raven Press, Ltd., New York © 1995.

CHAPTER 59

Molecular and Cellular Mechanisms of Brain Development

David A. Morilak, Matthew H. Porteus, and Roland D. Ciaranello

Researchers and clinicians concerned with severe psychiatric disorders are focusing increasing attention on brain development. There are several reasons for this, including an increasing recognition that exogenous or endogenous disruptions in brain development may play an important etiologic role in psychiatric disorders, particularly such severe disturbances as infantile autism and schizophrenia. There has also been a veritable explosion in our knowledge of developmental neurobiology, that area of neuroscience that focuses on factors regulating the development of neurons, neural circuitry, and the complex regional organization of systems in the brain. Finally, the application of molecular genetics to neurologic disease has enabled us for the first time to understand the genetic bases of certain diseases without requiring foreknowledge of the underlying biochemical abnormalities.

It is difficult, if not impossible, to overstate the importance of this last point. We know virtually nothing about the biologic substrates of the severe neurodevelopmental disorders, despite years of intensive study. The same statement can be made about psychiatric diseases in adults, where an even greater, more prolonged research endeavor has failed to disclose even a single consistent biologic deficit which can guide the diagnosis or treatment of any psychiatric disorder. Until recently, this lack of knowledge was a major obstacle to progress in psychiatric research. Although this remains a formidable impediment today, the ability to identify defective genes without a priori knowledge of their protein products or underlying pathophysiology has contributed recently to breathtaking advances in medicine, and there is every reason to believe

that such advances also hold great hope for breakthroughs in psychiatric diseases, and in particular for the developmental disorders.

This chapter attempts to guide the reader through the basic principles of neuronal and brain development. The relatively new discipline of developmental neurobiology draws, as one might expect, from many other disciplines, including neuroanatomy, neurophysiology, neuropharmacology, endocrinology, and genetics, as well as molecular biology, and derives its clinical sustenance from pediatrics, neurology, and psychiatry. This chapter is organized so as to provide the reader with a basic understanding of the genetic, metabolic, and cellular processes underlying brain development before considering how disruptions in these processes might lead to disturbances in brain maturation and ultimately to disturbances in behavior and social functioning (see also Chapters 2, 56, 60, and 62, *this volume*).

FUNDAMENTALS OF MAMMALIAN BRAIN DEVELOPMENT

This section summarizes what is known about mammalian brain development at a molecular level in a four-part way. The first gives a broad overview of the basic embryology of the developing brain. This is intended as a review and to establish a common ground from which further discussion will emanate. The second outlines certain cell biological events and concepts that are important in brain development. The third part addresses the possible molecular bases underlying some of these developmental processes. Finally, in the fourth part, we speculate about the future focus of molecular brain research as it relates to issues in developmental neurobiology. In this section, we emphasize the emergence of new and power-

D. A. Morilak, M. H. Porteus, and R. D. Ciaranello: Nancy Pritzker Laboratory of Developmental and Molecular Neurobiology, Department of Psychiatry and Behavioral Sciences, Stanford University School of Medicine, Stanford, CA 94305.

ful techniques and approaches that are just starting to contribute to our general understanding of the molecular basis for development (for related issues and discussion, see Chapters 2, 56, 60, and 98, *this volume*). One point that will become obvious from this overview is that there is not yet a comprehensive picture of mammalian brain development; many hypotheses have been derived from experiments in other developmental systems and remain to be confirmed or repudiated in the mammalian brain.

Elements of Neuroembryology

Neurogenesis begins with the formation of the neural plate, a thickening of ectodermal cells on the dorsal aspect of the developing embryo. Ridges form at the lateral edges of the plate, curling up to meet at the dorsal midline to form the neural tube. The internal cavity created by the tube is called the ventricle. Initially, the neural plate appears uniform along its entire axis. However, even as closure of the neural tube is occurring, specialized regions of the nervous system begin to emerge through differential cell division and migration. Major subdivisions include the mylencephalon and metencephalon (giving rise to the medulla, pons, and cerebellum), the mesencephalon, and the prosencephalon, which matures into the diencephalon and telencephalon. Through this process, the subdivision of the developing brain lays the foundation for regional specialization in the mature brain.

The development of the laminar organization of the neocortex (see Fig. 1) presents a salient example of many of the issues discussed in this chapter. Excellent and detailed reviews of this process can be found in refs. 1, 34, 44, and 45. First, the ventricular zone forms. This is a layer of ectodermal pseudostratified neuroepithelial cells lining the ventricle of the neural tube. Ventricular zone cells are small round mitotically active cells that eventually give rise to all of the cell types, including both neurons and glia, in the mature brain. Thus, the ventricular zone is also known as the germinal zone. After ventricular zone cells stop dividing, becoming terminally postmitotic, they migrate to their target destination, which is remote from the ventricular zone, where they differentiate and mature.

As proliferation of precursor cells in the germinal layer of the primordial cortex progresses, a second layer of mitotic cells emerges above the ventricular zone, called the subependymal or subventricular zone. A third layer then forms above it, called the intermediate zone. Cells in this region have undergone their final mitosis and have begun to migrate upward to what will become the cerebral cortex. Throughout development, the intermediate zone represents a region of transition and cell migration, as well as a staging area, where cells begin to extend processes and attain specific orientation. This process determines the direction of their migration. The next layer to

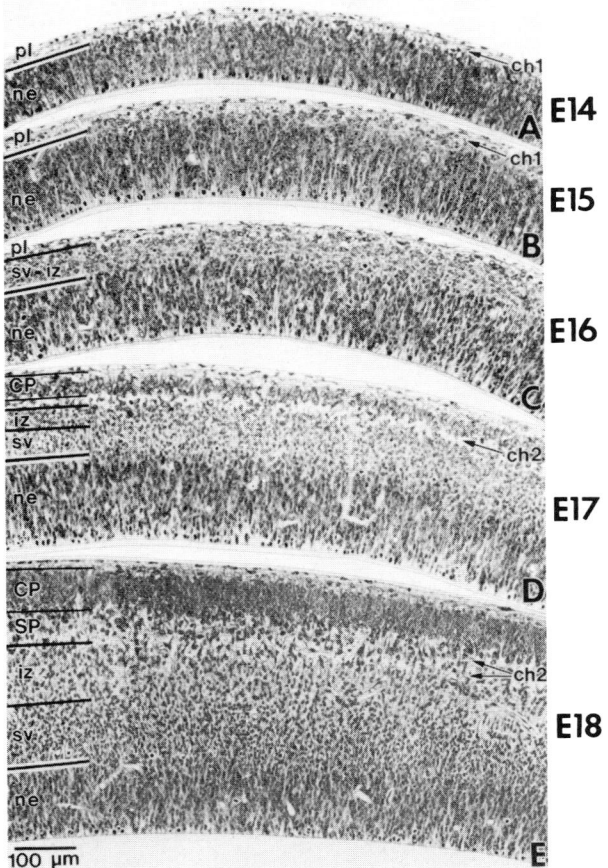

FIG. 1. Sagittal sections of the dorsal neocortex in the embryonic rat illustrating the successive emergence of developing cortical layers. Toluidine blue stain, 3-μm methacrylate sections. Abbreviations: ch1, extracellular channel 1; ch2, extracellular channel 2; CP, cortical plate; iz, intermediate zone; ne, neuroepithelium; pl, primordial plexiform layer; SP, cortical subplate; sv, subventricular zone. Reprinted with permission from Bayer and Altman (1; p. 26).

form in the developing cortex is the primordial plexiform layer, formed by the first neurons to arrive in the cortex. As more neurons are born (i.e., undergo final mitosis) and migrate, the plexiform layer is split by the new arrivals into two layers, the marginal zone and the subplate. The marginal zone becomes layer I in the adult cortex, a superficial, cell-sparse zone underlying the pial surface. The cortical subplate lies under the newly arriving cortical neurons. Cells in the subplate are the targets of early afferent fibers from subcortical structures. This innervation is a transient phenomenon and may serve an organizational or coordinating function in the formation of the developing cortex and in establishing appropriate mature contacts with subcortical afferents. Finally, the neurons of the cortical gray matter are born and migrate up through the intermediate zone and subplate to reside in the cortical plate.

There is a radial inside–out gradient of neurogenesis, such that the earliest born neurons occupy the deepest layers of the cortex. Successive generations of cortical neurons migrate up through the already established layers to reside in the next most superficial layer until all layers VI–II have been established. The timing of the passage of migrating neurons through the subplate seems to coincide precisely with the gradients of innervation of the cortex by the major subcortical afferent systems, including specific thalamic inputs, noradrenergic innervation from the locus coeruleus, serotonergic innervation from the raphe nuclei, dopaminergic innervation from the ventral tegmental region, and cholinergic innervation from the basal forebrain.

The proliferation, organization, and specialization of the brain at a regional level subsumes a variety of cell biological processes unique to development, including division, migration, differentiation, and the establishment of appropriate synaptic connectivity. These, and related developmental cellular processes, are addressed in the next two sections.

Basic Issues in Brain Development

In this section, we describe research relating to five important developmental questions: i) What is the cell lineage of neurons in the brain? ii) How do cells migrate to their appropriate destinations? iii) How do neurons make the correct axonal connections? iv) How do cells and regions differentiate? v) How plastic is the developmental process? These issues are based on the decisions that an undifferentiated ventricular zone cell must make to become a functionally mature neuron. Moreover, these issues take on added significance for understanding human psychopathology, as presumed abnormalities in these developmental processes of migration, differentiation, cell death and regression, and formation of appropriate circuit connections are hypothesized to play a role in the etiology of certain neuropsychiatric disorders, especially schizophrenia (see Chapter 98, *this volume*).

Cell Lineage

To summarize what is known about cell lineage of neurons in the brain, we focus on three types of experiments: birthdating studies, transplantation studies, and retroviral tracing experiments. Birthdating studies can reveal if the final destination of a cell is related to the time at which it undergoes final mitosis. These studies are done by giving a pulse of tritiated thymidine to animals in utero. When cells replicate, they then incorporate tritiated thymidine into their DNA and become radiolabeled. If a cell continues to divide from that point, the label will dilute among its daughter cells and become undetectable by autoradiography. Thus, the most intensely labeled cells are those that will have divided only once (final mitosis) after the thymidine pulse. After a period of maturation, usually when the animal has become an adult, the brain

is sectioned, and the location of the radiolabeled cells are determined. By varying the time during development at which the thymidine pulse is delivered, the distribution in the mature brain of cells that underwent their final mitoses together can be determined. Conversely, the different times at which neurons in a particular location became terminally postmitotic can be established.

It was through such birthdating studies that the timing and developmental gradients of cortical neogenesis described in the preceding section were established. Similar studies have been conducted in other regions of the brain, including those with a nuclear, rather than laminar, pattern of organization. For example, cells in the neostriatum are organized into clumps, or patches, surrounded by more loosely arranged matrix cells; birthdating studies have shown that patch cells become postmitotic at a distinctly earlier time than matrix cells (54). Thus, both the cerebral cortex and the striatum are examples in which there is a temporal determinant to the final cell location.

However, even though birthdating studies have shown that the layers of the cortex develop in a sequential manner, such studies do not show whether the cells migrate to appropriate layers in response to specific signals in the surrounding environment or if their destination is predetermined. Transplantation studies have revealed some complex answers to this question. For example, thymidine-labeled ventricular zone cells that normally would have migrated to layer 6 were transplanted into a ventricular zone that was making layer 2/3 cells (32). If the cells underwent final mitosis while in the layer 6 environment, they still migrated to layer 6 when placed in the new environment. However, if they incorporated labeled thymidine while temporarily placed in culture, they responded to the new environment and migrated to layer 2/3. Thus there is a complicated relationship between the time at which the cell becomes postmitotic, the environment in which it undergoes its final DNA synthesis, and the layer to which it will eventually migrate.

Retroviral lineage studies are designed to determine whether a given ventricular zone cell gives rise to different cell types or to cells of a single cell type. These studies are carried out by infecting ventricular zone cells with a small number of disabled retroviruses bearing a genetic marker. The retrovirus inserts itself into the host cell genome during DNA replication and gives the cell a novel genetic marker, but is unable to infect other cells. Thus, once in the genome, that marker is passed on uniquely to all of the infected cell's progeny, and all the cells that show the marker are clonally related to the single original cell that was infected. These studies can address whether cells within a clonal population are restricted in their final destination and whether cells within a clonal population are restricted in their mature phenotype.

Retroviral lineage studies in the cerebral cortex have shown that early in brain development any given ventricular zone cell can give rise to every cell type in the brain.

However, at later stages of development, the multipotency of ventricular zone cells becomes restricted. An early split in lineage occurs between the astrocytes of the grey matter and other cells of the brain (41). Some studies suggest that certain germinal cells become restricted to only generating neurons (29). Germinal cells appear able to give rise to cells of all cortical layers within a vertical column. On the other hand, some ventricular zone cells can generate offspring cells separated widely in the horizontal plane (41,56). These studies highlight the fact that we are only beginning to understand the process that determines the lineage of cells in the brain.

Cell Migration

Once a cell becomes postmitotic, how does it get from the ventricular zone to its final destination? In cortex, as neurons begin to migrate out of the germinal zone, the beginnings of process formation occur. An apical dendrite extends vertically toward the pial surface, and this defines the path along which the cell will migrate. These processes are in close association with radial glial cells, which themselves extend processes that are anchored at both the pial and ventricular surfaces. These glia form a scaffold through the developing cortex and act as guide wires along which radial migration occurs into and through the cortical plate (17,44,45). With the electron microscope, putatively migrating cells can be seen in close apposition to radial glial fibers and appear to be creeping up the fiber. Real-time video microscopy shows that cerebellar neurons in vitro move along Bergmann glial cells and resemble the migrating brain cells that are seen in the electron microscope (17). It has been suggested that migration along these radial glia forms the developmental basis for the vertical, columnar organization of functional cortical modules in the mature brain.

Genetic mouse mutants that show defects of neuronal migration highlight the importance of the interaction between migrating neurons and radial glia. In the *weaver* mutant, migrating cerebellar granule cells are unable to attach to the glia and do not migrate correctly, ultimately leading to the death of the granule cells (4,17). In the *reeler* mutant, the cerebral cortex develops outside–in rather than inside–out, but there is no cell death (4,17). In this mutation, it seems that the migrating cells are unable to detach from the radial glia cell and thus form a roadblock for the migration of subsequent waves of neurons.

As the primitive neurons traverse the intermediate zone, there is often a pause in their migration, during which their orientation and their direction of movement may adjust, to be resumed again in a vertical direction just below their final cortical destinations. During this sojourn, axons begin to emerge, and the temporary shifts in orientation may in part determine the direction in which axons are initially extended.

Axon Outgrowth and Pathway Formation

The mechanisms are vaguely understood for establishing a neural pathway in the brain, sometimes over a very long and circuitous route. Axons grow toward a successive series of intermediate targets, like signposts, along the route to their final destinations. Along the way, a striking degree of organizational specificity is attained by the establishment of appropriate axonal connections over long distances and, equally important, by the omission and preclusion of a myriad of potentially inappropriate connections.

This process represents a complex interaction between cell-surface proteins, extracellular matrix proteins, and diffusible attractant and repellant factors secreted by target regions in the brain (reviewed in refs. 6 and 51). Axons emanating from any general region adhere to each other, forming a pathway or bundle (fasciculation) from the interaction of surface proteins expressed on the axons. Similarly, they adhere to and migrate along the extracellular matrix and along cell-to-matrix boundaries by virtue of interactions between surface proteins and proteins on the surface of other cells or in the matrix itself.

The most studied example of axonal pathfinding is the developing visual system. In the mammalian visual system, retinal ganglion cells form synapses with neurons in the lateral geniculate nucleus (LGN), which then project to layer 4 of the visual cortex. A striking aspect of this pathway is the organization and maintenance of a precise retinotopic map in both the LGN and visual cortex. One strategy by which such organization is believed to develop is by the initial projections of pioneer neurons from target regions, which then serve as a template upon which the mature pathway is established. The concept of pioneer neurons was first proposed in the developing grasshopper (2), and it has been proposed that cells in the cortical subplate act as pioneer neurons in the cerebral cortex (31). Subplate cells are present only in development and are among the first cells to become postmitotic in the developing cortex. As determined in dye tracing studies, the cortifugal subplate neurons make connections with the LGN even before layer 4 cells are born. Moreover, these studies suggested that LGN axons dock on the subplate cells of the visual cortex. The LGN axons then wait in the subplate until layer 4 cells, the mature targets of LGN axons, are born and migrate into place before the axons themselves grow into layer 4 to form synapses (13). If the subplate cells beneath the developing visual cortex were removed, the LGN axons grew past the visual cortex and never found a place to dock. Although such studies point out the importance of a transient cellular scaffold in guiding axons as they approach their final targets, they do not address how the LGN axons got to the subplate or how the pioneer subplate axons got to the LGN in the first place.

At the tips of developing axons are specialized, enlarged structures called growth cones. These exhibit a highly active, ameboidlike array of filamentous processes that extend and retract continuously. The direction of outgrowth of these processes determines the direction of axon extension and hence the direction of axon pathway formation. Whereas axon fasciculation and adherence is mediated by surface proteins, growth cone motility and hence the direction of pathway formation is influenced by diffusible attractant or repellant substances secreted by their intermediate or final destinations. A chemoaffinity hypothesis, proposed by Sperry in the 1940s, suggests that axons follow such chemical gradients to find their correct destination (43). Specific secretion of diffusible factors establishes gradients to which the growth cones respond by either extending and growing toward (an attractant gradient) or retracting and turning from (a repellant gradient). Coculture experiments show that axons preferentially grow toward appropriate neural target tissue and not toward other tissues (19). Even in the early stages of axon formation, the floor plate of the developing neural tube releases a substance that attracts axons to the midline (6). When the floor plate is prevented from forming by removing the notochord, axons fail to migrate to the midline.

In development of cortical connections, there is an overabundance of synapse formation and more neurons than in the adult. Thus, an important part of cortical development and connectivity is the retraction and elimination of excess cells and exuberant synaptic contacts (reviewed in ref. 9). As many as 25% to 50% of the maximal number of cortical neurons seen during development in a given layer ultimately die and are eliminated in the early postnatal period (10,37,58). These regressive processes serve to refine the cortical circuitry and again are not well understood. Cell death may result from competition for limited supplies of neurotrophic growth factors (see below) or from a failure to establish a functional synaptic connection with a target region, leading to a reduced availability of such factors for uptake and transport.

Differentiation and Regional Specification

Cell differentiation is the process by which a cell changes from an immature, pluripotent phenotype to a more mature, specialized one. This process encompasses cell lineage, cell migration, axonal outgrowth, and plasticity, as well as the establishment of such specific neuronal characteristics as neurotransmitter content and interneuronal patterns of synaptic connectivity and responsivity. These processes, occurring at the cellular level, also reflect a higher level of organization resulting in the specification of particular regions of the brain as cells within those regions mature. Regional specification is thus the process by which a part of the brain takes on, through characteristic patterns of cellular phenotype, organization,

and connectivity, a functional identity that distinguishes it from other regions. The question of regional specification is one of the most actively studied and debated areas in developmental neurobiology. There are two fundamental views of regional specification: (i) that it is an intrinsic, genetically controlled process or (ii) that it is an extrinsic, environmentally controlled process.

Cell transplantation has been used to explore this question. Cells are transplanted from one environment to another, and then they are examined as to whether the transplanted cells have adopted the phenotype of the donor environment or of the acceptor environment. For example, part of the developing occipital cortex has been transplanted into the developing somatosensory cortex. The transplanted tissue adopted the organizational and connectivity characteristics of the acceptor environment. Occipital donor tissue, which normally does not project through the pyramidal tract, established a pyramidal projection when transplanted into the rostral neocortex, an area that normally maintains such a projection (36). In another experiment, transplanted occipital cortex cells formed "barrels," a functional architectural feature unique to the somatosensory cortex (46). Thus, based on these results, local environment does play an important role in specifying morphologic and functional phenotype. However, the retroviral tracing and transplantation studies described earlier highlight the importance of timing in interpreting these results. If the transplantations had been performed later in development, after some critical period had passed, the donor tissue may not have taken on host tissue characteristics, and the interpretation could have been that environment had no influence. A more serious concern is the issue of selective attrition; it is possible that only the tissue that was capable of assuming host characteristics could survive the transplantation. Thus, the experiment may have selected for tissue that could adapt, rather than revealing the differentiation potential of the donor tissue. Nevertheless, it seems certain that the local environment does play an important role in differentiation, although exactly what the local environment contributes is not known.

Another approach has been to alter the input to a particular region of the cerebral cortex. One way of altering the input to the visual cortex is to study an anophthalmic animal. Rakic (45) showed that the visual cortex of an anophthalmic mouse maintained its correct topography and connections. This suggests that the visual cortex does not need environmental cues to develop correctly. A second way to alter the input to the visual cortex was to enucleate an eye of an embryonic animal. This caused cell death in the lateral geniculate nucleus and a corresponding decrease in the number of thalamic inputs to the visual cortex. The visual cortex of such an animal appeared biochemically and cytologically normal (45). There was a decrease in the size of the visual cortex that was attributable to a decrease in the number of columns. But each column seemed functionally normal, despite the lack of normal input. A third type of experiment was to reroute retinal ganglionic afferents to the medial geniculate nucleus, the thalamic auditory relay center (45). After such an alteration, what would normally have been the auditory cortex became capable of processing visual information. Thus, the functional specificity of a cortical region was altered by changing its functional input.

Plasticity

The final developmental phenomenon we wish to discuss is the plasticity of the developing brain. The immature brain shows an amazing ability to adapt to changes in its environment and to fine tune its connections during development. Again, the visual system provides the best example to illustrate plasticity. The mature visual cortex consists of a series of alternating columns that respond preferentially to one eye or the other, called ocular dominance columns. When a radioactive tracer is injected into one eye or the other, it is retrogradely transported back to the visual cortex, revealing a series of alternating stripes corresponding to the ocular dominance columns (21). This organization is created by the axonal arborization of LGN neurons, which are driven by one eye or the other, with the projections of a given LGN neuron limited to a single column. During development, however, the axon terminals of LGN neurons that are driven by opposite eyes overlap in the cortex. It is only by subsequent pruning that the ocular dominance columns are formed. If activity from one eye is blocked, either pharmacologically or physically, during a particular time called the critical period, the normal ocular dominance columns do not form (47). Instead, the stripes corresponding to the blocked eye become narrower and the stripes corresponding to the unblocked eye get wider. The unblocked eye seems to take over the columns normally controlled by the blocked eye. It has been proposed that the organization into ocular dominance columns is, therefore, the result of some sort of activity-dependent competition among neurons. In the next section, we discuss a possible molecular mechanism for this competition. Moreover, this activity-dependent competition has a temporal profile (47). If activity is blocked after a critical period, there is no effect, and if the block is removed before the critical period, there is also no effect. The block has to span a specific period of time during development to affect the organization of ocular dominance columns.

Molecular Aspects of Brain Development

The techniques of molecular biology allow scientists to study individual genes and gene products in a unique and powerful way. Only recently, however, have those techniques been applied to the study of mammalian brain development. Thus, our knowledge of possible molecular mechanisms underlying the developmental phenomena described in the previous two sections is just beginning to accumulate.

Cell Division

An important decision for ventricular zone cells is when to divide and when to stop dividing. It appears that, as a cell progresses through the sequential steps of the cell cycle, it must pass certain checkpoints, without which further division and proliferation will not occur. A long-standing issue in developmental biology has been what determines the initiation of cell division, the progression to a new cycle of division, and the cessation of division. Recent molecular studies have indicated the importance of specific gene products or factors that are involved in regulating certain aspects of the cell cycle and the sequential passage of a dividing cell through its various stages. For example, studies in yeast have shown that the product of the *cdc*2 gene, called p34^{cdc2}, must be phosphorylated for the cell to pass from the G1 into the S phase (27). The mammalian homolog of the *cdc*2 gene also appears to serve such a checkpoint function (27). Phosphorylated p34^{cdc2} is itself an active protein kinase. A number of genes have been isolated that regulate the state of phosphorylation of p34^{cdc2} in both yeast and vertebrates (27). However, although it is likely that the division of neuronal precursors in the brain are also regulated by a similar mechanism, there is little data on what gene products are present in ventricular zone cells that may regulate the cell cycle. Moreover, there is presently no molecular data on what triggers a neuron to become terminally postmitotic.

Migration

As discussed previously, cells are thought to migrate to their final destination along radial glia cells. Understanding neuronal migration will require knowledge about the molecular relationship between the radial glial cell and the migrating neuron. Cloning of the genes involved in mouse mutants, for instance reeler and weaver mutants, that show migration defects might be a first step in understanding that relationship. One molecule that is missing or defective in weaver mouse granule cells is astrotactin. Antibodies against astrotactin, but not against other cell-adhesion molecules such as L1 or NCAM, were able to block the adherence of granule cells to radial glia in culture (17). Thus, astrotactin is possibly involved in neuron–glia interactions.

Axon Outgrowth and Pathway Formation

A number of substances that play important roles in axonal outgrowth have been identified. In Drosophila, certain genetic mutants show axonal path-finding defects, either choosing the wrong tract to follow or simply not growing (16). The genes encoding the cell-adhesion proteins neuroglian and the fasciclins-1, -2, and -3 were shown to underly some of the path-finding mutations (3,16,50,60). Biochemical analyses showed that these proteins engage in homophilic adhesion; that is, the surface protein binds to itself on the surface of another cell. Axons may find the correct tract by matching the homophilic adhesion molecule on its surface with the tract that expresses the same homophilic adhesion molecule.

In the vertebrate spinal cord, certain axons must cross the midline. The floor plate is thought to release a substance that causes the axon to grow toward the midline. These axons express the cell adhesion molecule Tag-1 on their surface while they are on the same side of the spinal cord as the parent cell body. After crossing the midline, however, the axons no longer express Tag-1. Instead, they express another cell-adhesion molecule called L1. Both Tag-1 and L1 promote neurite outgrowth (6), suggesting that these molecules act as site-specific guides for axonal pathway formation.

Another class of substances that are important in the establishment and maintenance of appropriate patterns of cell growth and connectivity in the brain are the so-called target-derived neurotrophic growth factors, the most extensively studied of which is nerve growth factor (NGF) (see reviews in refs 8, 52, and 55 and also the chapter by Patterson, this volume). Related members of the NGF family are brain-derived neurotrophic factor (BDNF), neurotrophin-3 (NT-3), NT-4, and NT-5. These substances are secreted by the innervated targets of nerve fibers, taken up into the terminal via a receptor-mediated process and transported retrogradely to the cell body, where they serve multiple functions to promote the survival, growth, and differentiation of neurons. The synthesis and secretion of neurotrophic substances is influenced by many factors, but the effect of afferent activity is of particular interest. In cells that secrete NGF, expression is increased by excitation of the cells and is decreased by neural inhibition. Excitatory inputs to a target cell will thus activate NGF secretion and promote the survival of other afferents to the same cell. Likewise, the activity of a cell that is dependent on NGF will itself influence the production of NGF in its target, and thereby promote its own survival. This may explain in part the observation that neuronal activity promotes survival and the need for a cell to establish functional synaptic connections to survive. The various NGF-like substances, although related, show a great deal of specificity in that they are differentially distributed, influence different populations of neurons, and interact with different receptors.

Differentiation and Regional Specification

In terms of molecular mechanisms, the maturational transitions that take place during differentiation at either the cell or regional level can be attributed in part to both cell-autonomous (i.e., intracellular) and nonautonomous (i.e., intercellular) factors. Gene transcription factors are an example of cell-autonomous agents, whereas cell-to-cell signaling molecules and morphogens are examples of nonautonomous factors.

In the development of the Drosophila nervous system, there is a cluster of genes, called proneural genes, that when mutated cause an alteration in the number of sensory neurons in the periphery (14,22). This set of genes codes for a class of transcriptional regulatory proteins that contain a common domain called the "basic-helix-loop-helix" (bHLH) domain. Studies of these and other bHLH proteins have shown that they are intimately involved in specifying particular cell fates (57). For example, when MyoD (a mammalian muscle determination gene) is induced in myoblasts, the myoblasts mature into multinucleate muscle cells. Two mammalian homologs of the Drosophila genes have been cloned and have been found to be expressed in many parts of the nervous system during development (23,28). These are likely to control some aspect of cell differentiation in the mammalian nervous system during development.

Also in Drosophila, there is a class of genes that play a role in body segmentation and in specification of body parts. These genes share a common 180 nucleotide motif called a homeobox that encodes a 60 amino acid protein "homeodomain" (12). Homeodomain-containing proteins mediate their developmental effects by regulating the transcription of many target genes, and are expressed with an orderly regional or segmental distribution. There have been over 30 mammalian homologs of homeobox genes cloned, and there is evidence that these mammalian homeogenes play similar developmental roles as their counterparts in flies, controlling the identity of particular segments (25,24). A subset of mammalian homeobox genes show a distribution of expression that parallels specific organizational patterns in the nervous system (20,25), such as layer-specific expression in the cerebral cortex (18), or differential dorsal-ventral expression in the developing forebrain and diencephalon (40,42). These genes may thus participate in the regional differentiation of the developing brain.

Cells can also differentiate based on nonautonomous factors, such as secreted proteins. During early neural development, the notochord, a mesodermal derivative, induces the overlying neural plate, an ectodermal derivative, to form nervous tissue. Transplantation studies have shown that the notochord induces the floor plate to release a diffusable factor, that has not yet been identified, which causes the overlying spinal cord to form cells of the appropriate types, such as motoneurons (38,59). Other factors are important later in development. For instance, a homozygous null mutation in the Wnt-1 gene, which codes for a secreted protein that is normally expressed in the hindbrain, led to abnormal hindbrain development in mice

(33,53). It is likely, therefore, that this and other related Wnt gene products are important in cell determination via their intercellular signaling properties in the developing brain.

Certain substances can induce differential patterns of morphologic maturation depending on a spatial concentration gradient. Retinoic acid (RA) or its metabolites are thought to act as such morphogens in vertebrate development. The receptor for RA belongs to the steroid receptor superfamily of genes (15), which alter the transcription of target genes after binding their appropriate ligand. In cell culture, different concentrations of RA can have different effects on the expression of certain homeobox genes (48). During development of the chick wing bud, RA can cause a mirror duplication of wing structures in a concentration-dependent manner (49) and causes anteroposterior transformations in the frog nervous system and in the mouse vertebral column (7,26). The concept of a graded morphogen is an important one in mammalian developmental biology, and even though RA is a likely candidate, it is not a proven one, and there are few, if any, others.

Plasticity

Plasticity of neurons and their connections have been studied in many systems. The molecular studies of desensitization and sensitization in the invertebrate sea slug Aplysia are likely to have important ramifications in our understanding of brain development. However, we focus on the role of correlated activity as an important determinant during brain development. Tetrodotoxin (TTX), a toxin from puffer fish, blocks the sodium channel in axons and thereby blocks action potentials. When TTX is injected into the pathway of the developing visual system, the normal segregation of the LGN into eye-specific layers and the visual cortex into ocular dominance columns is blocked (47). At a cellular level, TTX prevents the normal pruning of the extensive axonal arborizations that are present during development.

The N-methyl-D-aspartate (NMDA) receptor is a glutamate neurotransmitter receptor. When activated, it allows Na^+, K^+, and Ca^{2+} to flow through its channel. It is the only known glutamate-gated channel that allows Ca^{2+} to pass, eliciting a host of calcium-dependent effects, some of which may be involved in the molecular aspects of plasticity. However, activation of the NMDA receptor is dependent both on binding of glutamate and on the prior depolarization of the cell. Thus, Ca^{2+} only enters the cell if the receptor is activated in a correlated manner with another excitatory input. This property of the NMDA channel suggests that it may be involved in strengthening inputs that are temporally coactivated. If NMDA receptor antagonists are used to treat developing or regenerating visual system pathways, the normally precise retinotopic maps are disrupted (47). This disruption may be the result of the cell being unable to correlate normally synchronous inputs. The recent cloning of the NMDA receptor will help to unravel the role it plays in the normally developing brain (35) (see also Chapters 7 and 55, *this volume*).

In this section, we have sketched the characteristics of various neurotrophic factors, transcription factors, cell signaling molecules, morphogens, cell adhesion molecules, and neurotransmitter receptors to show how brain development is beginning to be understood at a molecular level. In the next section, we speculate about the future directions of molecular research in brain development (see also Chapter 62, *this volume,* for a discussion of gender-dependent brain development).

Future Directions of Molecular Developmental Neurobiology

In the immediate future, new approaches will lead to a better understanding of the function of developmentally important genes that have been and will continue to be cloned and identified. There are now techniques for studying and manipulating mammalian genes transgenically. Transgenic mouse technology gives the ability to put an altered copy of a gene back into the genome, and, in the last few years, gene targeting by homologous recombination has allowed the generation of mice that have null mutations in specific genes (30). In the previous section, we discussed how null mutations in two Hox genes and one Wnt gene have helped underscore their importance in development. In the future, many mouse mutants will be created by gene-targeting approaches, and mammalian brain development can be understood more directly at a genetic level.

We believe that a major focus of future molecular research in brain development will be on the higher order relationship between the genome and the developing brain. The classic genetic code translates nucleotide sequence into amino acid sequence. However, this is but one level of genetic understanding. Higher order processes are involved in translating the genome, with all of its associated structure, into an organism. Understanding of these higher order processes requires, but is by no means limited to, characterizing regulatory elements and interactions of specific genes, characterizing the signals for alternative splicing of a gene, characterizing how chromatin is folded and bent to make certain regions transcriptionally active or unactive, and characterizing the role that DNA modifications, such as methylation, have in gene expression.

Researchers estimate there are approximately 100,000 different genes in higher mammals, perhaps 30% to 60% of which are uniquely expressed in the brain. At present only 5% have been cloned. The nature of cloning suggests that this 5% is skewed toward the most abundantly expressed genes. Thus, there are 95,000 genes that still remain to be cloned; these genes are likely to control the subtle aspects of brain development. The use of subtractive hybridization (39), which isolates genes based on their preferential expression in one tissue over another, and enhancer/promoter traps (11), which identify genes by trapping the regulatory elements of that gene using a marker transgene, are promising methods to isolate genes involved in brain development.

BRAIN DEVELOPMENT AND DEVELOPMENTAL PSYCHOPATHOLOGY

At the outset of this chapter we expressed our conviction that advances in developmental and molecular neurobiology could provide important new insights into the mechanisms underlying developmental psychopathology. We believe the following issues are pertinent to this discussion: (i) the relative importance of environmental and genetic factors in brain development; (ii) the need for fresh conceptualizations of developmental disorders, and (iii) the importance of biologic markers to researchers in this field.

First, we have learned that the normal development of the nervous system unfolds as a series of timed genetic events, the coordinated expression of which depends on appropriate environmental stimuli. We also know that the degree to which this genetic programming can be influenced by environmental events varies greatly across cell types, brain regions, and time periods. Deprived of light, the visual cortex will not develop properly, even though the genetic information for normal development is not affected. In rat pups deprived of maternal tactile stimulation, important metabolic enzymes are not activated, even though their structural genes are perfectly intact. Indeed such genetic–environmental interactions should be considered the norm rather than the exception.

Second, we believe a new approach is required to understand how perturbations of normal brain development can lead to severe childhood psychopathology, such as infantile autism. Autism is a devastating clinical disorder characterized by extreme social dysfunction, stereotypic behaviors, failure to develop normal language, and, in most cases, mild to moderate mental retardation. It begins in infancy; both its temporal course and outcome suggest it is a disorder of CNS development. But with few exceptions, no structural neurologic or neuropathologic deficits have been found in the brains of autistic children, and those that have been found are inconsistent and inadequate to explain the clinical deficits.

What new concepts emerging from basic research in developmental neurobiology can increase our understanding of disorders such as autism? One is the notion of the transient expression of important developmental factors or functions, either at the gene or cellular level, at critical time points in ontogeny, examples of which we have described in the sections above. Certain genes are actively expressed only during certain times in development, and we currently know the most about the class of transiently expressed transcription factors that themselves regulate the expression of other genes and are critical to normal nervous system development. Similarly, certain neurons in the developing subplate exist only transiently, helping developing cortical neurons establish appropriate connections, and then disappear. Both examples suggest a potentially important point regarding developmental disorders: despite their clinical severity, their underlying neuropathology must be very subtle, because we do not observe gross abnormalities with existing research methodologies (5). Aberrations in the developmental processes of migration and differentiation, establishing appropriate synaptic connectivity, axonal pruning, dendritic arborization, neurite regression, and programmed cell death all could give rise to considerable neurologic impairment (see chapter by Weinberger, this volume), but may not be obvious on autopsy or microscopic examination. Defects in developmentally transient processes could be even more subtle and less likely to be detected with current methodologies. However, specific hypotheses derived from basic models in developmental neurobiology could be applied to the understanding of clinical developmental disorders. For instance, in the case of transiently expressed factors, there are several candidate genes, derived from research in flies and mice, that could be tested for mutations in children with developmental disorders. Even though such a gene may no longer be expressed, mutations can still be identified using the standard techniques of molecular biology.

This brings us to the third point, the need for reliable and consistent biological markers that can be used to unambiguously classify developmental disorders. Clinically, rather than being single, defined syndromes, these disorders typically represent clusters of heterogenous and overlapping entities classified by sets of diagnostic criteria. Attempts to differentiate among them along such symptomatologic criteria, however refined and sophisticated, do not substitute for objective and conclusive biologic markers. Decades of biologic psychiatric research have failed to identify a single marker that can be used to diagnose, plan treatment, or predict the outcome of any psychiatric disorder. The lack of reliable, objective markers greatly hinders our ability to frame testable hypotheses that could lead to important advances. As new findings emerge from basic cellular, genetic, and developmental biologic research, it will be essential to incorporate these findings into a better clinical understanding of the neurodevelopmental bases of psychiatric disorders.

ACKNOWLEDGMENTS

This work was supported by a program-project grant from the National Institute of Mental Health (MH 39437), by a Research Scientist Award (RDC) from the National Institute of Mental Health (MH 00219), by the endowment fund of the Nancy Pritzker Laboratory, and by the Spunk Fund, the Meyer Fund, the John Merck Fund, the Rebecca and Solomon Baker Fund, and the Edward and Marjorie Gray Endowment Fund (DAM).

REFERENCES

1. Bayer SA, Altman J. *Neocortical Development.* New York: Raven Press; 1991.
2. Bentley D, Keshishian H. Pathfinding by peripheral pioneer neurons in grasshoppers. *Science* 1982;218:1082–1088.
3. Bieber AJ, Snow PM, Hortsch M, et al. Drosophila neuroglian: a member of the immunoglobulin superfamily with extensive homology to the vertebrate adhesion molecule L1. *Cell* 1989;59:447–460.
4. Caviness VSJ, Rakic P. Mechanisms of cortical development: a view from mutations in mice. *Annu Rev Neurosci* 1978;1:297–326.
5. Ciaranello RD, VandenBerg SR, Anders TF. Intrinsic and extrinsic determinants of neuronal development: relations to infantile autism. *J Autism Devel Disorders* 1982;12:115–146.
6. Dodd J, Jessell TM. Axon guidance and the patterning of neuronal projections in vertebrates. *Science* 1988;242:692–699.
7. Durston AJ, Timmermans JPM, Hage WJ, et al. Retinoic acid causes an anteroposterior transformation in the developing central nervous system. *Nature* 1989;340:140–144.
8. Ebendal T. Function and evolution in the NGF family and its receptors. *J Neurosci Res* 1992;32:461–470.
9. Ferrer I, Soriano E, Del Rio JA, Alcantara S, Auladell C. Cell death and removal in the cerebral cortex during development. *Prog Neurobiol* 1992;39:1–43.
10. Finlay BL, Slattery M. Local differences in the amount of early cell death in neocortex predict adult local specializations. *Science* 1983;219:1349–1351.
11. Friedrich G, Soriano P. Promoter traps in embryonic stem cells: a genetic screen to identify and mutate developmental genes in mice. *Genes Devel* 1991;5:1513–1523.
12. Gehring W. Homeo boxes in the study of development. *Science* 1987;236:1245–1252.
13. Ghosh A, Antonini A, McConnell SK, Shatz CJ. Requirement for subplate neurons in the formation of thalamocortical connections. *Nature* 1990;347:179–181.
14. Ghysen A, Dambly-Chaudiere C. From DNA to form: the achaete-scute complex. *Genes Devel* 1988;2:495–501.
15. Giguere V, Ong ES, Segui P, Evans RM. Identification of a receptor for the morphogen retinoic acid. *Nature* 1987;330:624–629.
16. Harrelson AL, Goodman CS. Growth cone guidance in insects: fasciclin II is a member of the immunoglobulin superfamily. *Science* 1988;242:700–708.
17. Hatten ME. Riding the glial monorail: a common mechanism for glial-guided neuronal migration in different regions of the developing mammalian brain. *Trends Neurosci* 1990;13:179–184.
18. He X, Treacy MN, Simmons DM, Ingraham HA, Swanson LW, Rosenfeld MG. Expression of a large family of POU-domain regulatory genes in mammalian brain development. *Nature* 1989;340:35–42.
19. Heffner CD, Lumsden AGS, O'Leary DDM. Target control of collateral extension and directional axon growth in the mammalian brain. *Science* 1990;247:217–220.
20. Holland PWH, Hogan BLM. Expression of homeobox genes during mouse development: a review. *Genes Devel* 1988;2:773–782.
21. Hubel DH, Wiesel TN. Shape and arrangement of columns in cat's striate cortex. *J Physiol* 1963;165:559–568.
22. Jimenez F, Campos-Ortega JA. Defective neuroblast commitment in mutants of the achaete-scute complex and adjacent genes of D. melanogaster. *Neuron* 1990;5:81–89.
23. Johnson JE, Birren SJ, Anderson DJ. Two rat homologues of Drosophila achaete-scute specifically expressed in neuronal precursors. *Nature* 1990;346:858–861.
24. Kessel M, Balling R, Gruss P. Variations of cervical vertebrae after expression of a Hox-1.1 transgene in mice. *Cell* 1990;61:301–308.
25. Kessel M, Gruss P. Murine developmental control genes. *Science* 1990;249:374–379.
26. Kessel M, Gruss P. Homeotic transformations of murine vertebrae and concomitant alteration of Hox codes induced by retinoic acid. *Cell* 1991;67:89–104.
27. Lee M, Nurse P. Cell cycle control genes in fission yeast and mammalian cells. *TIG* 1988;4:287–290.
28. Lo L, Johnson JE, Wuenschell CW, Saito T, Anderson DJ. Mammalian achaete-scute homolog 1 is transiently expressed by spatially restricted subsets of early neuroepithelial and neural crest cells. *Genes Devel* 1991;5:1524–1537.
29. Luskin MB, Pearlman AL, Sanes JR. Cell lineage in the cerebral cortex of the mouse studied in vivo and in vitro with a recombinant retrovirus. *Neuron* 1988;1:635–647.
30. Mansour SL, Thomas KR, Capecchi MR. Disruption of the proto-oncogene int-2 in mouse embryo-derived stem cells: a general strategy for targeting mutations to nonselectable genes. *Nature* 1988;336:348–352.
31. McConnell SK, Ghosh A, Shatz CJ. Subplate neurons pioneer the first axon pathway from the cerebral cortex. *Science* 1989;245:978–982.
32. McConnell SK, Kaznowski CE. Cell cycle dependence of laminar determination in developing neocortex. *Science* 1991;254:282–285.
33. McMahon AP, Bradley A. The Wnt-1 (int-1) proto-oncogene is required for development of a large region of the mouse brain. *Cell* 1990;62:1073–1085.
34. Moore KL. *The Developing Human: Clinically Oriented Embryology.* Philadelphia: W.B. Saunders; 1988.
35. Moriyoshi K, Masu M, Ishii T, Shigemoto R, Mizuno N, Nakanishi S. Molecular cloning and characterization of the rat NMDA receptor. *Nature* 1991;354:31–37.
36. O'Leary DDM, Stanfield BB. Selective elimination of axons extended by developing cortical neurons is dependent on regional locale: Experiments utilizing fetal cortical transplants. *J Neuroscience* 1989;9:2230–2246.
37. Pallas SL, Gilmour SM, Finlay BL. Control of cell number in the developing neocortex. I. Effects of tectal ablation. *Dev Brain Res* 1988;43:1–11.
38. Placzek M, Tessier-Lavigne M, Yamada T, Jessell T, Dodd J. Mesodermal control of neural cell identity: floor plate induction by the notochord. *Science* 1990;250:985–988.
39. Porteus MH, Brice EJ, Bulfone A, Usdin TB, Ciaranello RD, Rubenstein JLR. Isolation and characterization of a library of cDNA clones that are preferentially expressed in the embryonic telencephalon. *Mol Brain Res* 1992;12:7–22.
40. Porteus MH, Bulfone A, Ciaranello RD, Rubenstein JLL. Isolation and characterization of a novel cDNA clone encoding a homeodomain that is developmentally regulated in the ventral forebrain. *Neuron* 1991;7:221–229.
41. Price J, Thurlow L. Cell lineage in the rat cerebral cortex: a study using retroviral-mediated gene transfer. *Development* 1988;104:473–482.
42. Price M, Lemaistre M, Pischetola M, DiLauro R, Duboule D. A mouse gene related to distal-less shows a restricted expression in the developing forebrain. *Nature* 1991;351:748–751.
43. Purves D, Lichtman JW. *Principles of Neural Development.* Sunderland, MA: Sinauer Associates; 1985.
44. Rakic P. Neuronal migration and contact guidance in the primate telencephalon. *Postgrad Med J* 1978;54(Suppl. 1):25–37.
45. Rakic P. Specification of cerebral cortical areas. *Science* 1988;241:170–176.
46. Schlagger BL, O'Leary DDM. Potential of visual cortex to develop an array of functional units unique to somatosensory cortex. *Science* 1991;252:1556–1560.
47. Shatz CJ. Impulse activity and the patterning of connections during CNS development. *Neuron* 1990;5:745–756.
48. Simeone A, Acampora D, Arcioni L, Andrews P, Boncinelli E, Mavilio F. Sequential activation of Hox2 homeobox genes by retinoic acid in human embryonal carcinoma cells. *Nature* 1990;346:763–766.
49. Smith SM, Pang K, Sundin O, Wedden SE, Thaller C, Eichele G. Molecular approaches to vertebrate limb morphogenesis. *Development* 1989;(Suppl):121–131.

50. Snow PM, Bieber AJ, Goodman CS. Fasciclin III: a novel homophilic adhesion molecule in Drosophila. *Cell* 1989;59:313–323.
51. Tessier-Lavigne M, Placzek M, Lumsden AGS, Dodd J, Jessell TM. Chemotropic guidance of developing axons in the mammalian central nervous system. *Nature* 1988;336:775–778.
52. Thoenen H. The changing scene of neurotrophic factors. *Trends Neurosci* 1991;14:165–170.
53. Thomas KR, Capecchi MR. Targeted disruption of the murine int-1 protooncogene resulting in severe abnormalities in midbrain and cerebellar development. *Nature* 1990;346:847–850.
54. Van der Kooy D, Fishell G. Neuronal birthdate underlies the development of striatal compartments. *Brain Res* 1987;401:155–161.
55. Vantini G, Skaper SD. Neurotrophic factors: from physiology to pharmacology? *Pharmacol Res* 1992;26:1–15.
56. Walsh C, Cepko CL. Clonally related cortical cells show several migration patterns. *Science* 1988;241:1342–1345.
57. Weintraub H, Davis R, Tapscott S, et al. The myoD gene family: Nodal point during specification of the muscle cell lineage. *Science* 1991;251:761–766.
58. Windrem MS, Jan de Beur S, Finlay BL. Control of cell number in the developing neocortex. II. Effects of corpus callosum section. *Dev Brain Res* 1988;43:13–22.
59. Yamada T, Placzek M, Tanaka H, Dodd J, Jessell TM. Control of cell pattern in the developing nervous system: polarizing activity of the floor plate and notochord. *Cell* 1991;64:635–647.
60. Zinn K, McAllister L, Goodman CS. Sequence analysis and neuronal expression of fasciclin I in grasshoppers and Drosophila. *Cell* 1988;53:577–587.

*Psychopharmacology: The Fourth
Generation of Progress,* edited by
Floyd E. Bloom and David J. Kupfer.
Raven Press, Ltd., New York © 1995.

CHAPTER 60

The Development of Brain and Behavior

Thomas R. Insel

In the course of a few months of gestation, the human central nervous system (CNS) changes from a microscopic band of embryonic neuroblasts to a 350 g mass with more than 10^9 interconnected highly differentiated neurons in the cortex alone. By age 5, the human brain reaches 90% of its adult weight (1.3 Kg) and the density of synapses in the cortex has already peaked and is beginning to decline. How this extraordinary growth with its intricate connectivity results in sensorimotor, cognitive, affective, and behavioral development is one of the great mysteries of biology. Developmental neurobiologists have begun to discover some of the mechanisms by which neurons migrate to their correct position, send efferents to the appropriate targets, and receive afferents from distant and adjacent sources. As various neurotransmitters and growth factors as well as specific pharmacologic treatments affect these processes, the insights of developmental neurobiology have recently become important for neuropharmacology. In addition, abnormalities of neuronal migration or differentiation might underlie various behavioral disorders, offering the hope that developmental approaches might prove important for understanding psychopathology and possibly offer new strategies for treatment.

This chapter is a brief summary of some of the major findings in recent studies of both neural and behavioral development. This is not a comprehensive review nor is it a careful critique of new findings. The intent here is to provide an organizational context with which the reader can approach more focused parts of this volume or from which the reader can search in other books on development to find in-depth coverage. Accordingly, three major perspectives are provided. First, some of the basic princi-

ples and recent directions in neuroanatomic development are summarized. Any reader interested enough to read through this section should know that two superb texts, one by Jacobson (1) and a second by Purves and Lichtman (2), will prove enormously helpful guides to developmental neurobiology, even for the non-anatomically minded neuropharmacologist. Next, aspects of neurochemical development are described. There are fewer general references here, although several focused reviews on the development of monoaminergic or neuropeptide systems are now available (3,4). Finally, some recent new directions in behavioral development are noted (see ref. 5 for further reading).

After summarizing the anatomic, chemical, and behavioral approaches, this chapter addresses the epigenetic questions of how drugs (or other environmental influences) affect neural development, and conversely, how the stage of development alters drug response. These areas of research are of critical importance, not only for the practical therapeutic questions of how drugs work in children, but more fundamentally for determining how early experience can have longterm consequences for neural organization and behavior. The study of neural and behavioral development is one of the growth industries of modern neuroscience. Hopefully, this review will provide some impetus to search further into this exciting literature (see also Chapters 59, 98, 141, 142, and 144, *this volume*).

NEUROANATOMIC DEVELOPMENT

The course of neural development can be traced through four overlapping processes: cell birth (neurogenesis), migration, formation of connectivity (including elaboration of processes, synapse formation, cell death, and axonal regression), and myelination (Fig. 1). In mammals, there are important species differences in the duration of each of these processes as well as their timing

T. R. Insel: Laboratory of Neurophysiology, National Institute of Mental Health, National Institutes of Health, Poolesville, Maryland 20837; *current address*: Yerkes Regional Primate Research Center and Department of Psychiatry, Emory University, Atlanta, Georgia 30322.

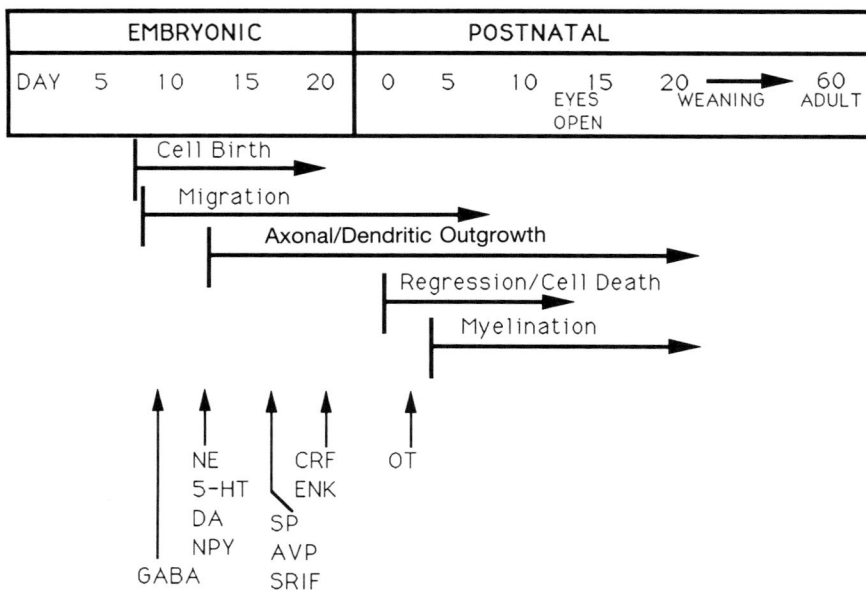

FIG. 1. The timing of various processes of neural development in the rat brain (birth occurs on day 22 of gestation). In general, the first postnatal week of rat development is analogous to the third trimester of human gestation (although there are many exceptions to this generalization). Diagram also provides approximate dates for immunocytochemical appearance of several neurotransmitters: norepinephrine (NE), serotonin (5-HT), dopamine (DA), neuropeptide Y (NPY), substance P (SP), vasopressin (AVP), somatostatin (SRIF), luteinizing hormone releasing hormone (LHRH), corticotropin releasing hormone (CRF), enkephalin (ENK), oxytocin (OT).

with respect to birth. In all mammalian species, however, the basic pattern of neural development involves exuberant production of neural elements followed by widespread elimination of neurons or regression of some of their axon collaterals.

Neurogenesis

It has long been known that the nervous system originates from embryonic ectoderm, but identifying the transition from ectoderm to neural precursor cells has never been easy. The identification of several neuron-specific proteins, such as the neural cell adhesion molecules (N-CAMs), has provided a clearer picture of when and where the CNS originates. This has been most elegantly demonstrated in frog embryos, where N-CAM can be detected as early as the 128-cell stage, 2.5–3 hours after the beginning of gastrulation (6). This initial differentiation of ectoderm into the neural plate occurs largely under the inductive influence of the underlying mesoderm which is believed to release some diffusible factor (possibly a steroid or peptide hormone or growth factor). Soon after the emergence of neuroblasts, the CNS begins to develop at a phenomenal rate with an orderly progression of cell birth and differentiation.

The time when specific neurons are born can now be detected with great precision using ^{3}H-thymidine autoradiography (reviewed in ref. 1). These studies, in which labeled thymidine is permanently incorporated into the DNA of dividing cells, have suggested several basic principles of neurogenesis in rodents which are relevant to all mammals: (a) there is an orderly pattern of development with littermates injected at the same time showing nearly identical patterns of ^{3}H-thymidine labeling; (b) in laminar structures (e.g., cerebral cortex) there is a characteristic "inside-out" pattern of origin—that is, neurons that are born later migrate past those born earlier to attain the most peripheral location; and (c) in a given region, large neurons are produced before small neurons, motor nuclei are born before sensory nuclei (at the same level of the neuraxis), and cells in phylogenetically older regions are born before cells in regions that are more recently evolved (e.g., ventral thalamus before dorsal thalamus).

It should also be noted that although neurogenesis is predominantly a prenatal event, in some regions neurons are generated postnatally in the mammalian brain. Granule cells continue to be produced in the olfactory bulb and dentate gyrus through postnatal development (7) and even into adulthood in some species (8).

Migration

The mechanisms by which neurons born in the ventricular zone reach their final position in either cortical or sub-cortical structures have been the focus of intense study recently. Early stages of migration to the cortex may occur rapidly in a relatively unguided fashion, but as the distance increases and new cells have to migrate through layers of older cells, the journey becomes more complex. Rakic has described the importance of radial glia for the normal guidance of cells born in the ventricular zone to reach their appropriate destination in the cortical mantle (9). Radial glia are found only during a distinct period of development and appear to differentiate later into fibrillary astrocytes. This mechanism for cell migration may account for the columnar organization of the neocortex which has been recognized with both functional and anatomic mapping. In addition, considerable attention has recently focused on the cortical subplate (10,11), a transient band of cells that appears to (a) serve as a staging ground for arriving afferents, (b) provide a chemically-rich matrix through which cortical cells must migrate, and (c) offer an "axonal scaffold" for early cortical efferents. The cells in this cortical subplate disappear early in postnatal life, but may be essential for the appropriate organization of cortical architecture during the early phases of development.

It now appears that some forms of migration even occur in the adult brain. The cell adhesion molecules (especially the neuron specific N-CAM) are important for neural migration as well as neural induction. During development, N-CAM changes from a highly sialylated form to several isoforms with less sialic acid. In a recent study, Theodosis et al. demonstrated the persistence of the highly sialylated form of N-CAM in the adult brain, specifically in parts of the hypothalamus known to undergo a remarkable form of reorganization in adulthood (12). During lactation, magnocellular neurons in this region of the hypothalamus reversibly change their orientation due to retraction of the intervening glia and migration of neural processes to permit synchronous depolarization. This embryonic isoform of N-CAM is found specifically in the processes of magnocellular neurons in the adult hypothalamus.

The discovery of ectopic cells and migratory arrests in post-mortem tissue from patients with dyslexia, autism, schizophrenia, and fetal alcohol syndrome have suggested the hypothesis that abnormal migration may be of pathophysiologic importance (reviewed in ref. 13). In fact, migration shows considerable individual variation and the functional significance of even severely disordered migration remains uncertain. Studies of the reeler mutant mouse have been particularly instructive in this regard. This mouse shows extensive disorganization of laminar structures due to widespread deficits in neuronal migration, yet connectivity of hippocampal and neocortical neurons is generally intact (14). Pathology within the late-developing cerebellum is probably responsible for the tremor, hypotonia, and ataxia characteristic of the reeler mutant (see also Chapters 59, 98, 142, and 154, *this volume*).

Connectivity

Most research in developmental neurobiology over the past three decades has been focused on the mechanisms of how axons find their targets and how the mature pattern of synapses forms. Although much has been learned about axonal growth, heralded by studies of the axonal growth cone and its unique protein markers such as GAP-43, the mechanisms by which axons find their targets remain mysterious. Axonal outgrowth from cortical neurons is a surprisingly early event, beginning even before a neuron has finished migrating and often reaching the appropriate target even when migration is obstructed (15).

It is clear that the brain produces many axons that ultimately are eliminated, but the reason for this ostensibly inefficient strategy is still a puzzle. Three examples of this phenomena are worth noting. Initially, there is a diffuse connection between cortical fields via the corpus callosum. In the monkey, these axon collaterals are eliminated in late fetal life (about one month before birth) to result in the adult pattern in which each cortical neuron sends a single axon to a specific contralateral region (16). Within a hemisphere there are multiple cortical–cortical connections that are eliminated about the same time (17). Perhaps most remarkable, layer V neurons in the visual cortex transiently send axons via the pyramidal tract to the spinal cord (18). In each of these cases, the neurons survive, but axons to some targets are retracted while others are preserved. It should be noted that all of these studies require the injection of retrograde tracers into a presumed target site several days prior to examining the animal for cortical cells of origin. As a result, we still know very little about the development of circuitry in the human brain. The development of the carbocyanine dye, DiI, that can be used as a retrograde tracer in post-mortem tissue might allow for similar studies in the developing human brain (see e.g., ref. 19), but this technique is slow and may be of limited usefulness for long pathways or tract-tracing in the more mature brain (20).

Axonal regression has been attributed to trophic factors at the target, trophic factors in the region of the cell body, or activity dependent changes which favor some projections over others. The existence of soluble growth factors, such as NGF, has been known for many years. Recently, several new protein growth factors, such as BDNF, CNTF, and IGF-1 have been identified (reviewed in ref. 21). Perhaps of greatest interest is the identification and cloning of a novel factor, glial cell-line derived neurotrophic factor, GDNF, which is not only a highly potent growth factor, but one that thus far appears specific for dopamine cells in dissociated cell cultures from rat midbrain (22). One might predict that the discovery of related specific growth factors (and their receptors) for other neuronal phenotypes, such as serotonin, GABA, and glutamate, will have an enormous impact on our understanding of neural development as well as offering a new class of potential therapeutic agents for degenerative diseases of the nervous system (see Chapter 55, *this volume*).

The process of over-production followed by elimination occurs for neurons as well as their axons. In some regions of the rat brain, as many as 50% of neurons die before birth (23). Studies of cell lineage have been done most extensively in the transparent nematode *Caenorhabditis elegans,* which consists of 1090 postmitotic somatic cells of which 959 survive into adulthood (24). The developmental death of 131 cells (including 20% of all presumptive neural cells) is surprisingly invariant, suggesting that early death is destined or programmed for specific cells. It is now clear that "programmed" cell death is characteristic of vertebrates as well as invertebrates and occurs in many organs including the brain. Of course, the problem with studying this phenomenon is recognizing which cells will die before the terminal event.

Almost two decades ago, Kerr et al. described specific morphologic changes that precede death, such as cell shrinkage, condensation of chromatin, and changes in membrane morphology (25). They called these highly predictable changes *apoptosis* (Greek for "a flower losing its petals"). More recently, various investigators have identified those genes that are expressed with apoptosis to examine the molecular basis of programmed cell death during development. It is now clear from studies in *C. elegans* that there is a family of genes associated with cell death (*ced-3* and *ced-4*) and another associated with survival (*ced-9*). Recently, the oncogene *bcl-2* has been hypothesized to function in mammalian neurons as a homologue to *ced-9* of the nematode. Although there are still questions about the extent to which cell death within the mammalian CNS is "programmed," one can imagine how normal development might be altered by changes in the expression of genes for either cell death or survival. Conversely, the possibility that oncogenic transformation is initiated by the failure of genes normally associated with apoptosis may prove of great therapeutic significance.

In addition to increased numbers of neurons and axons, synaptic density is higher during development than adulthood. Synaptogenesis begins very early in development (as soon as axons reach postsynaptic cells) and continues well into postnatal life. In the human visual cortex, the peak of synaptic density is at age 8 to 11 months with a gradual decrease to adult levels by puberty (26). Changes in synaptic density, while ostensibly impressive, may be neither ubiquitous nor informative. Neurons which receive only a single afferent axon (such as cells within the submandibular ganglion) show a gradual ontogenetic increase in the number of synapses although the number of axons innervating each cell decreases (27). In cortical neurons, where hundreds of axons innervate a given neuron with its extensive dendritic arbor, changes in synaptic density involve several different processes, including elimination of some axonal input, increased numbers of synaptic boutons on surviving axons, and developmental elaboration of the dendritic arbor (28). Synaptic density is thus a consequence of many different changes in connectivity, and interpretation of changes in density depends on which specific aspect of afferent input is altered.

Myelination

With the current emphasis on regressive events in brain development, it is easy to forget that the brain is undergo-ing tremendous growth during postnatal life. The human brain weighs 350 g at birth and nearly 1.2 Kg at 5 years of age (29). This growth can be attributed partly to increased neuropil from the elaboration of dendrites, but also to increased myelin formation by oligodendrocytes. In the rat, myelin formation begins after the period of cellular proliferation and migration and extends into adulthood. Jacobson estimates that myelin content increases 1500% between 15 days and 6 months after birth in the rat brain (1). In the human brain, myelination continues at least through the first decade of life, with some phylogenetically recent structures only appearing fully myelinated in the second decade (30). Although the time course of myelination suggests that this phase of neural development would be most vulnerable to postnatal environmental influences, little is known about either the influence of epigenetic factors on myelin formation or the functional consequences of subtle changes in either retarded or reduced myelination.

NEUROCHEMICAL DEVELOPMENT

Concurrent with the dramatic morphologic changes of neural development, neurotransmitters and their receptors fluctuate, in some cases markedly, during ontogeny. Indeed, for certain neurochemical systems, the changes in regional expression that occur normally in development dwarf any changes that are observed with experimental manipulations in adulthood. Phenotypic plasticity, that is the capacity of a cell to shift from one neurochemical phenotype to another, has been known in sympathetic neurons (which shift from noradrenergic to cholinergic) and adrenomedullary cells (which shift from noradrenergic to adrenergic), but now appears to occur within the CNS as well (31). As a first approach to this broad area, the development of neurotransmitters, their receptors, and their effectors in the brain will be briefly summarized.

Neurotransmitters

Monoaminergic neurons are born early in the course of CNS development (Fig. 1). Serotonin, norepinephrine, and dopamine are detectable in nuclear groups by E13 in the rat brain (prior to the peak of cortical neurogenesis) (32). Monoaminergic cells from the brainstem send off processes quickly and are among the first afferents to colonize the cortex, migrating to the wall of the telencephalon (33). Norepinephrine has long been implicated in cortical development not only because of this early invasion of the cortex [E18 in the rat (34) and E70 in the monkey (33)] but because of several different forms of experimental evidence linking noradrenergic input to synaptic plasticity in the visual system (reviewed in ref. 1). Serotonergic fibers also invade the cortex early and have been implicated as trophic for the developing cortical architecture (reviewed in ref. 32). Serotonin in the early postnatal neocortex is present at roughly twice the adult concentration (35). Autoradiographic labeling of serotonin uptake sites has demonstrated the transient appearance of serotonin terminals specifically in the barrel fields of the developing somatosensory cortex (36). While the function of this highly specific distribution has not yet been demonstrated, the timing and the distribution of these transient fibers suggest a role in the organization of the arriving thalamocortical axons.

The ontogeny of amino acid neurotransmitters such as GABA and glutamate appears somewhat different from the picture with monoamines. Glutamate has been detected mostly postnatally in the rat brain, reaching adult concentrations by postnatal day 15 (37). Remarkably, careful immunocytochemical studies for glutamate in the embryonic brain have not been published. In the rat visual cortex, GABA immunocytochemically-identified cells appear to be born from E14 to E20, concurrent with the appearance of the pyramidal cells that they innervate (33). GABA immunoreactivity can be detected even earlier in less differentiated neural elements. Indeed, GABA may be the earliest neurotransmitter to emerge in the CNS, although its role as a developmental signal may turn out to be quite different from its traditional role as a fast, inhibitory neurotransmitter.

Acetylcholine, as detected by ChAT immunoreactivity, appears relatively late in development. In the cortex, most ChAT-positive cells are not observed until the second or third post-natal week (38,39). However, a transient expression of ChAT-positive cells has been noted in the cortex as early as E17, disappearing by P1. Acetylcholine, like norepinephrine has been implicated in visual cortical plasticity (40).

Neuropeptides during development are also expressed in a unique distribution in several brain regions, although some, like oxytocin, are not fully processed until the first postnatal week. In the cortex of the embryonic macaque, for instance, proenkephalin, tachykinin, and somatostatin appear transiently (41). It is not clear if the cells expressing these peptides change phenotype or if these cells are eliminated during cortical development (see also Chapters 12, 24, 32, 39, and 43, *this volume*).

Receptors

Given the concurrent reorganization in both axonal and dendritic branching, it is not surprising that the distribution of receptors in development might appear quite different from the patterns observed in adulthood. Even in developing muscle where cholinergic receptors can be detected before the arrival of cholinergic innervation, the distribution of α-bungarotoxin binding is initially widespread, migrating in the membrane to the point of innervation (42). Although monoaminergic receptors and amino

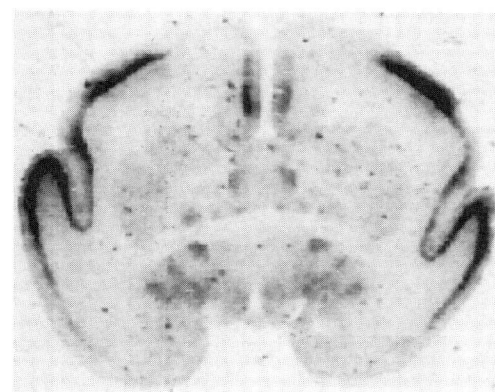

1251-OTA BINDING

MARMOSET

DAY 1

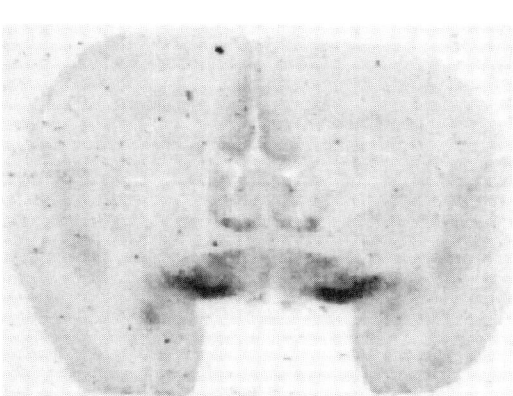

ADULT

FIG. 2. Increased expression of neuropeptide receptors is shown for oxytocin. **A:** Binding of an iodinated selective analogue to oxytocin receptors is evident in several regions of neocortex in the one day old marmoset. **B:** Under identical conditions, binding of the same ligand is not detectable in cortex, but appears in the ventral pallidum at the same level of the adult marmoset brain. ac, anterior commissure. (Autoradiograms from Moody, Newman, and Insel, *unpublished data*.)

acid receptors show some local differences, receptor binding in these systems generally develops monotonically with an overshoot (relative to adult levels of binding) in the second or third postnatal week of the rat. For 5-HT$_2$ and 5-HT$_{1c}$ receptors, the developmental changes in binding have been associated with concurrent changes in mRNA levels, suggesting that binding increases represent increased receptor synthesis (43). In the case of peptide receptors, particularly in the cortex, the degree of overshoot is far more dramatic, amounting to severalfold increases relative to adult concentrations (Figs. 2 and 3).

The function of these transient receptors remains unclear. Indeed, these receptors may not be functional in the sense of being linked to an intracellular effector, but nevertheless may serve some other role as cell surface markers. In any case, three general rules should be appreciated: (a) receptor binding may develop independently of innervation; (b) the pattern of receptor binding is remarkably diverse with specific brain regions often showing intense binding transiently in the first through third postnatal weeks (in the rat); and (c) the expression of binding precedes receptor-effector coupling (45).

Effectors

In addition to the unique patterns of receptor distribution, one also finds patterns of coupling to second-messengers during development which are absent or less obvious in the adult brain. For instance, a 5-HT receptor (5-HT$_4$) in the superior colliculus coupled to adenylate cyclase was first described in the neonate (46). Similarly the high levels of phosphoinositol generated in the first three postnatal weeks in rat hippocampal slices exposed to glutamate provided the first recognition of a metabotropic receptor distinct from the channel-linked site originally thought to be the only form of glutamate receptor in the adult brain (47).

The developmental patterns of second messengers, such as various G proteins, is of note independent of their coupling to receptors. Figure 4 shows the developmental pattern of stimulation of cyclase in the rat brain. Clearly, the capacity for neurotransmitters to function will depend on the maturation of their respective intracellular effectors (see also Chapters 11, 27, 38, and 61, *this volume*).

BEHAVIORAL DEVELOPMENT

Although the most dramatic discoveries in development have been in the realm of neuroscience, research into how behavior becomes organized in development has also undergone some major conceptual shifts in the past decade. Three new areas of research should be noted by neuropharmacologists.

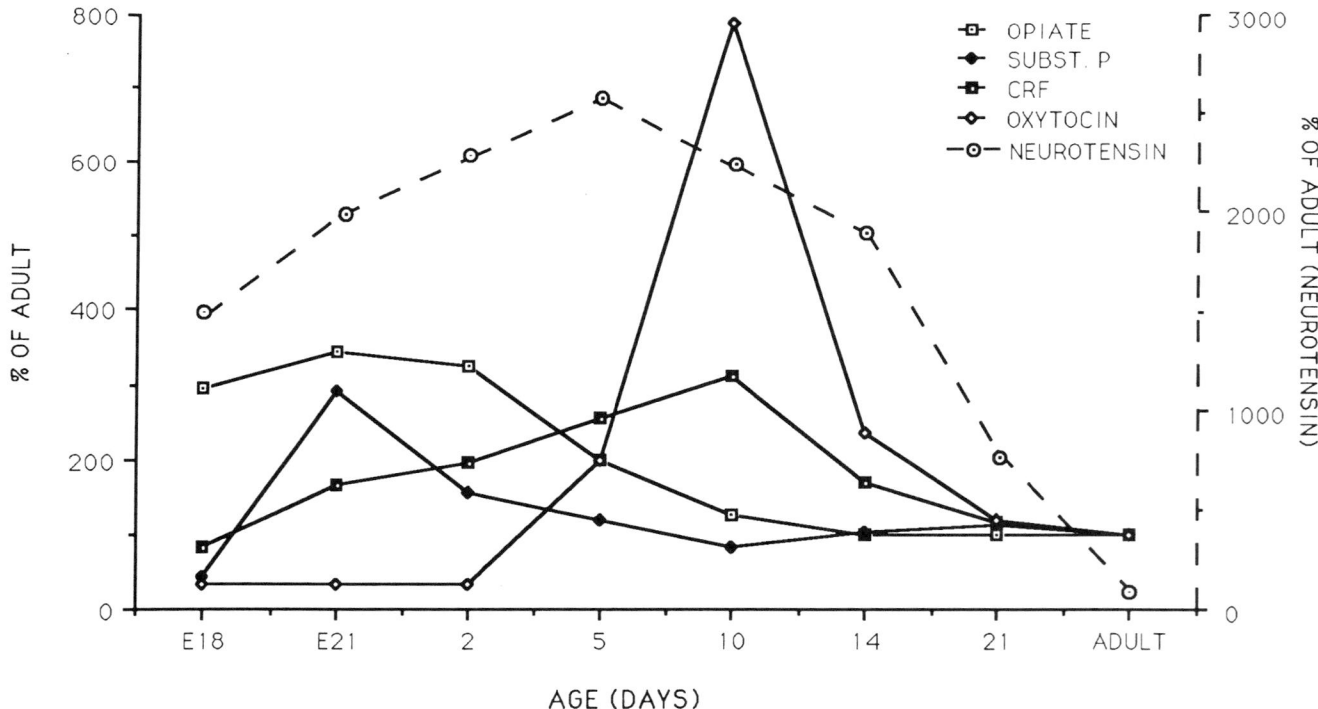

FIG. 3. A pattern of transient increased receptor binding has been previously shown for several neuropeptides in the rat cortex. Neurotensin receptors are increased by more than 2000% above levels observed in the adult and therefore are shown on a separate axis. Note that binding does not necessarily imply function. (From ref. 44.)

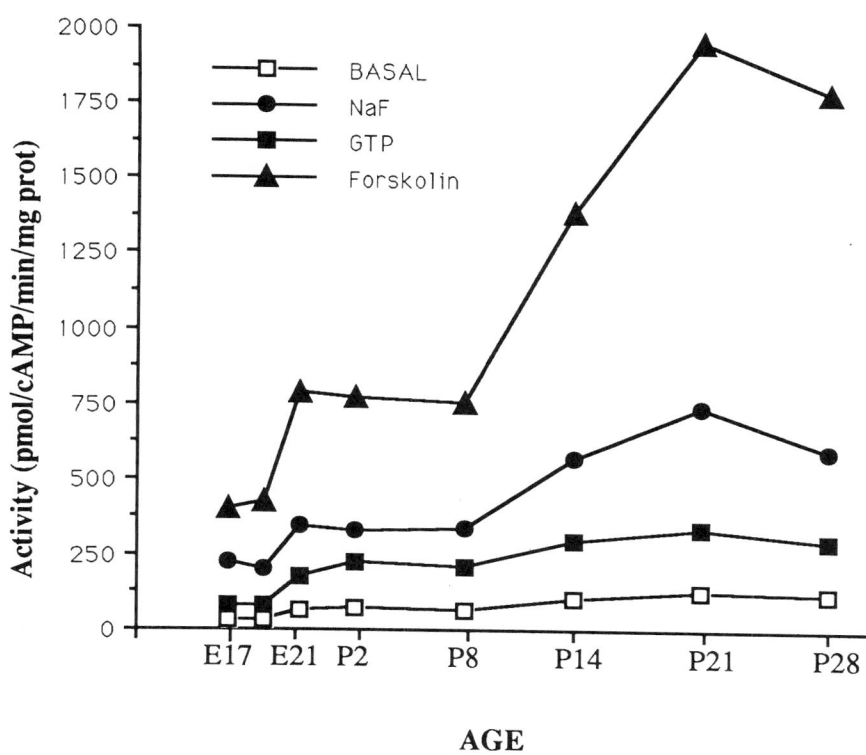

FIG. 4. Functional development of guanine nucleotide binding protein (G_s) and catalytic subunit from embryonic day 17 to postnatal day 28 in whole rat brain homogenates, expressed as percentage of day 28 values. Basal rate of cAMP formation represents the unstimulated level. Sodium fluoride (NaF) and forskolin, believed to activate the G_s and catalytic subunit, respectively, show increasing stimulatory effects through development, roughly in parallel with the basal level. (Data from ref. 48.)

Prenatal Learning

Viktor Hamburger, who is arguably the father of modern developmental neurobiology, became in his later years, a student of behavioral development. In classic studies carried out in the 1960s, Hamburger showed that motor development in the embryonic chick precedes sensory stimulation (49). Recently, Smotherman and Robinson have begun to follow Hamburger's lead by studying fetal behavior in mammals (50). Studies in the exteriorized rat fetus have demonstrated a surprising capability for rapid associative learning, at least some of which is mediated by opioid peptides.

Temperament

A major shift in developmental psychology has been led by the work of Kagan and colleagues (51). These investigators have demonstrated the relatively consistent expression of specific clusters of personality traits (i.e., temperaments) across development. One cluster, labeled as behavioral inhibition, is operationally defined as a tendency to be shy, timid, and constrained in novel situations provided in a laboratory setting. Children who appear inhibited at 21 months and who remain inhibited at age 7.5 years show increased rates of anxiety disorders and have parents with increased rates of anxiety disorders. The focus on temperament, as opposed to manifest symptoms, provides an opportunity to study vulnerability to various mental disorders. Moreover, the search for spe-

cific genes that predispose to mental illness may ultimately find that the phenotype is not a specific psychiatric disorder, but a more general temperamental predisposition to develop a form of psychopathology.

Attachment/Separation vs. Hidden Regulators

The field of attachment theory, which has been at the center of ego psychology for the past three decades, has undergone an important conceptual shift from a focus on a single process that affects the infant to a focus on the interaction of caregiver and infant. Hofer has described a number of "hidden regulators" which maintain this dyad at a physiological as well as behavioral level (52). The concept is that the caregiver provides several different forms of comfort—nutritional, tactile, thermal, and olfactory—each of which regulates a specific aspect of the infant's physiology (Table 1). As a result, withdrawal of one aspect of care (as opposed to the more global concept of "loss") could lead to dysregulation of a specific physiologic response (53). For instance, Levine and colleagues have described how normal maternal contact regulates the infant rat's hypothalamic-pituitary-adrenal axis. With prolonged (i.e., 24 hours) separation from maternal contact (in the presence of warmth, nutrition, and maternal odors), plasma corticosterone increases severalfold (54).

EPIGENETIC CONSIDERATIONS

For the neuropharmacologist (as for the psychobiologist), the two major questions provoked by this generation

TABLE 1. *Maternal "hidden regulators" of infant physiology and behavior*[a]

Maternal stimulus	Infant response	Reference
Passive contact (olfactory/thermal)	Increase activity, decrease corticosterone, vocalization	54
Tactile stimulation (vigorous stroking)	Increase growth hormone, ODC, decrease activity	52,53
Ingestion (milk)	Increase sucking, heart rate, O_2 consumption	52

[a] Modified from ref. 1.
ODC, ornithine decarboxylase.

of studies in development are: (1) How do environmental events (hormones, drugs, stressors, infection) affect neural development? and (2) How does the stage of neural development affect the response to environmental events? In fact, neither question admits to a satisfactory answer, but there are useful data for consideration in both cases.

Environmental Influences on Neural Development

Activity-Dependent Plasticity

Many of the processes of neuroanatomic and neurochemical development described above are modified by activity in the developing CNS. The formation of ocular dominance columns in the cat visual system (55), somatosensory representations of both the thalamus and the cortex (56), and the alignment of auditory and visual maps in the bird's optic tectum (57) are perhaps the most intensively studied forms of experience-dependent plasticity in development. The period during which experience can alter the neural representation defines the *sensitive period*. In the case of the owl's visual-auditory maps, Knudsen and Knudsen have defined the sensitive period by elegant experiments in which either visual or auditory input is altered (58). The *critical period*, which is often used interchangeably with the sensitive period, is more strictly defined as the developmental interval during which normal maps can be restored following a period of deprivation.

Neurophysiologic and anatomic studies in kittens by Hubel et al. (59), Singer (55), and Spinelli et al. (60) have demonstrated that monocular deprivation leads to lasting changes in ocular dominance columns in the cortex and to smaller neurons in the lateral geniculate nucleus. Remarkably, experience confers a selective advantage for a particular aspect of vision. For instance, in the normal kitten visual cortex, virtually all neurons respond to visual orientation, with a roughly equal number showing preference for horizontal, vertical, and oblique patterns. When a kitten is reared in an environment that restricts vision to a single orientation, the majority of cells adopt preference for this orientation, apparently through the repeated excitation of the circuits subserving this pattern, with the consequent elimination of connections for the other visual orientations (60,61). Within this specific sensitive period, certain connections within the mammalian CNS develop

in an experience-dependent fashion with lasting morphologic and behavioral consequences.

Similar conclusions might be drawn from a literature on the influence of the complexity of the environment on neural development. Studies in primates as well as rodents have described a variety of morphologic effects resulting from rearing animals in a complex rather than simple environment. These effects include cortical thickening, alterations in cortical dendritic branching, increases in the number of spines per dendrite, and changes in the morphology of synaptic contacts (reviewed in ref. 62).

How experience sculpts the developing neural circuitry is one of the most intriguing questions in developmental neurobiology. D. O. Hebb, in his classic volume, *The Organization of Behavior*, formulated the concept that neural activity in some way reinforces specific circuits, so that when cell A excites cell B some change takes place in both cells to increase A's efficiency at firing B (63). In this way, synapses that are active become more efficient and synapses that are inactive might be ultimately eliminated. This basic idea has been elaborated in a number of ways to suggest that competition for some trophic factor, bursts of asynchronous activity, or changes in the stability of membrane bound receptors mediate the effects of neural activity on synaptic survival (see ref. 2) for a more detailed discussion). These mechanisms may not be mutually exclusive—all of them recognize the importance of competition, of the timing of activity, and of the remarkable magnitude of the effects in an organ where as many as 50% of the cells may be eliminated during a brief period of development. Norepinephrine, acetylcholine, NMDA, and GABA have all been implicated in this process (see above).

Organizational Effects

Just as stimulation of the visual system at a sensitive period of development appears essential for subsequent vision, exposure to gonadal steroids at particular phases of development is essential for the subsequent expression of normal adult sexual behavior. This concept was first introduced by experiments 40 years ago demonstrating that testosterone administration in developing guinea pigs could alter sex behavior in adulthood (64). Similar results have been reported in various species from frogs to primates, leading to the well-accepted notion that steroids, which functionally resemble growth factors, may have effects in development that are quite distinct from their effects in adulthood (65). These long-term effects of gonadal steroid exposure in development have been termed organizational effects as exposure appears to organize the system for later responsiveness. For instance, androgens administered to female rat pups in the first week of postnatal life confer an altered sensitivity to subsequent physiologic levels of gonadal steroids such that masculinization (enhancement of mounting behavior) and defeminization (reduced capacity for lordosis) are manifested after puberty (66). The first postnatal week is normally associated with a transient increase in hypothalamic receptors for gonadal steroids, possibly providing for this sensitive period (67). An analogous "feminization" of adult sexual behavior is evident in males that are not exposed to adequate levels of testosterone prenatally (66). Prenatal stress is also associated with subsequent feminized sexual behavior in male offspring, an effect which may be mediated by stress-induced decreases in testosterone concentrations in fetal plasma (68,69).

Although there is little question that gonadal steroids in development can have longterm consequences for adult behavior, the mechanisms for these organizational effects are not entirely elucidated. Some of these effects may be related to trophic actions, as estrogen induces neurite outgrowth in hypothalamic cells in vitro (70). In addition, androgens appear to reduce cell loss from certain targets during the normal period of neuronal elimination (71). Gonadal steroids appear essential for the full development of the sexually dimorphic area in the preoptic region of the hypothalamus—an area which appears markedly more cellular in the male brain (reviewed in ref. 72). Although the functional role of this sexually dimorphic area remains unclear, analogous dimorphisms are also found in the human hypothalamus (73,74) and may also be sensitive to neonatal sex steroid levels in man. The reader should note that in spite of a considerable literature on the functional consequences of increases or decreases in gonadal steroids in development, at present there is little evidence that gonadal steroids have cellular or molecular effects in the infant distinct from their effects in the adult (75).

Chemical Imprinting

Recent evidence suggests that gonadal steroids are not the only compounds to have longterm effects on the organization of neural systems: various neurotransmitters and neuromodulators appear to have similar properties during development. In addition, the interaction of neurotransmitters with their receptors may have different consequences in development. In adulthood, administration of an agonist for a neurotransmitter receptor generally leads to a compensatory downregulation and administration of an antagonist may lead to upregulation of receptor num-

ber. These changes are usually rapid (reflecting either local changes such as membrane internalization of the receptor or genetic changes in receptor transcription) and reversible, suggesting that the cell has some homeostatic control over receptor sensitivity. Several studies have demonstrated that during ontogeny, when receptor number (i.e., genetic control), receptor regulation (i.e., the presumed homeostat), and second messenger or channel coupling are incompletely developed, exposure to agonists or antagonists may have effects which are paradoxical and enduring. For instance, offspring of mothers treated with haloperidol show lasting decreases in dopamine receptors (76). Curiously, exposure to haloperidol in the early postnatal period results in increased not decreased numbers of dopamine receptors (76). As another example, morphine given to rat pups from day 1 until day 7 confers a lasting increase in mu opiate receptors as well as behavioral analgesia (77).

Similar longterm consequences of neonatal drug administration have been reported for several compounds including neuroleptics, antidepressants, substance P, vasopressin, benzodiazepines, and corticotropin releasing hormone (reviewed in ref. 44). These actions, which have been variously described as organizational (78) or chemical imprinting (44) effects, all suggest that exposure to an agonist during the neonatal period induces enduring functional increases in receptor responsiveness. As noted above, receptors for many of these systems show a profound "overshoot" during development, but it is not clear that this is causally related to these "imprinting" effects.

While the data are still lacking, reasonable hypotheses for the chemical imprinting effects include increases in survival of post-synaptic cells with a given receptor (79), increases in processes on those cells that do survive (80,81), and increases in coupling to a second messenger or ion channel (48). Whatever the mechanism, it appears that classical neurotransmitters might function as neurotrophic factors in development with organizational effects similar to what has been previously reported with gonadal steroids.

DEVELOPMENTAL INFLUENCES ON DRUG EFFECTS

Protective Effects Against Lesions

Although infants are uniquely sensitive to certain environmental insults, they are either relatively spared or show enhanced recovery from others. Kennard was perhaps the first to demonstrate behavioral sparing following lesions to the motor cortex in neonatal monkeys (82). Certain excitotoxins, such as quinolinate, which cause marked neurodegeneration in the adult rat hippocampus and striatum, have little effect when injected during the first two post-natal weeks (83). Neonatal administration of the catecholamine neurotoxin, 6-hydroxydopamine, causes an enduring depletion of norepinephrine and dopamine associated with locomotor hyperactivity, but several behavioral consequences observed in lesioned adults are not seen when the toxin is given to developing rats (84). And rat pups with extensive depletion of serotonin following the selective neurotoxin methyl,diethylmethamphetamine (MDMA) show virtually no change in thermoregulation, weight gain, or locomotor activity (85). In each case, the targeted system is still developing and one might assume, as with structural lesions, that plasticity persists through this period of development. Plasticity however is a description, not a mechanism. How these systems adapt remains an open question (86). How the adult organism might be induced to adapt similarly to neurochemical insults is clearly an exciting future focus for research.

Developmental Specificity of Drug Response

The developing organism responds in a unique fashion not only to neurotoxins, but also to various psychopharmacologic agents. The α-2 adrenergic agonist clonidine provides one of the most remarkable examples of a developmentally determined drug response. In the rat, clonidine increases locomotor activity from Day-1 to Day-14 postnatal and dramatically decreases locomotor activity thereafter (87). Both the stimulating and the suppressant effects are dose-dependent and both are blocked by yohimbine (author's *unpublished data*). This apparent reversal of clonidine's locomotor effects may be attributed to the late development of α-2 receptors in motor pathways (approximately Day-21 postnatal) (88). The early stimulatory effects of clonidine have not been fully explained. Destruction of presynaptic α-2 receptors potentiates both the stimulatory and the inhibitory effects on locomotion (89). The transient expression of α-1 receptors in the globus pallidus of the rat during the first two postnatal weeks matches the temporal course of the stimulatory effect of clonidine, but this correlation may be only coincidental (90).

Similar developmental patterns have been described with a number of drugs, emphasizing the importance of age on the "normal" pharmacologic response. In addition to the ontogeny of receptors and their effectors, metabolic enzymes and the blood-brain barrier are maturing postnatally, ensuring very different pharmacokinetic profiles during development (91). While this point is generally appreciated by neuropharmacologists, there has been less recognition of these developmentally idiosyncratic responses as "experiments of nature" providing an opportunity for studying the mechanisms of drug response. For example, the study of how adrenergic receptor expression and coupling in discrete brain regions changes between days 14 and 21 should provide important insights into those pathways that mediate the locomotor suppressant effects of clonidine.

SUMMARY

As the research base grows, the fields of developmental neurobiology and developmental psychobiology seem to grow further apart. We have begun to address phenotypic plasticity and regressive events with more powerful cellular and molecular techniques, but unfortunately, the functional importance of these events has become less of a focus of inquiry. Similarly, the problems of how behavioral patterns are organized through development has been remarkably uninformed by the rapid advances in developmental neurobiology.

Neuropharmacology may provide one of the bridges to link these two disciplines. For instance, studying the neurochemical events that underlie experience-dependent changes and determining the range of functions of neurotransmitters in development are important goals for neuropharmacology that should advance our understanding of both the neurobiological and behavioral aspects of development. Moreover, the immature organism provides a unique opportunity for investigating the mechanisms of drug action. By a careful choice of ages, the investigator can study receptor gene expression, receptor-effector coupling, and cellular consequences of activation in tissues in which various aspects of cellular machinery are developmentally modulated. Finally, the investigator interested in the pathophysiology of major mental illnesses may find abnormalities in one or more of the aspects of neural development which ultimately result in the emergence of pathological behavior—an observation that will bridge the behavioral and anatomic aspects of development.

REFERENCES

1. Jacobson M. *Developmental Neurobiology.* New York: Plenum Press, 1991.
2. Purves D, Lichtman JW. *Principles of Neural Development.* Sunderland: Sinauer Associates, 1985.
3. Parnavelas JG, Papadopoulos GC, Cavanagh ME. Changes in neurotransmitters during development. In: Peters A, Jones EG, eds. *Cerebral Cortex,* New York: Plenum Press, 1988;177–205.
4. Zagon IS, McLaughlin PJ. *Receptors in the Developing Nervous System. Growth Factors and Hormones,* New York: Chapman & Hall, 1993.
5. Shair HN, Barr GA, Hofer MA. *Developmental Psychobiology: New Concepts and Changing Methods,* New York: Oxford University Press, 1991.
6. Jacobson M, Rutishauser U. Induction of neural cell adhesion molecule (NCAM) in *Xenopus* embryos. *Dev Biol* 1986;116:524–531.
7. Altman J. Autoradiographic and histological studies of postnatal neurogenesis. II. A longitudinal investigation of the kinetics, migration and transformation of cells incorporating tritiated thymidine in infant rats, with special reference to postnatal neurogenesis in some brain regions. *J Comp Neurol* 1966;128:431–474.
8. Kaplan MS, Hinds JW. Neurogenesis in the adult rat: electron microscopic analysis of light radioautographs. *Science* 1977; 197:1092–1094.
9. Rakic P. Neuronal-glial interaction during brain development. *Trends Neurosci* 1981;4:184–187.
10. McConnell SK, Ghosh A, Shatz CJ. Subplate neurons pioneer the

first axon pathway from the cerebral cortex. *Science* 1989;245:978–982.

11. Shatz CJ, Chun JJM, Luskin MB. The role of the subplate in the development of the mammalian telencephalon. In: Jones EG, ed. *The Cerebral Cortex*, New York: Plenum Press, 1988;35–58.

12. Theodosis DT, Rougon G, Poulain DA. Retention of embryonic features by an adult neuronal system capable of plasticity: polysialylated neural cell adhesion molecule in the hypothalamoneurohypophysial system. *Proc Natl Acad Sci USA* 1991;88:5494–5498.

13. Nowakowski RS. Genetic disturbances of neuronal migration: some examples from the limbic system of mutant mice. In: Mednick SA, Cannon TD, Barr CE, Lyon M, eds. *Fetal Neural Development and Adult Schizophrenia*, New York: Cambridge University Press, 1991;69–96.

14. Stanfield BB, Caviness VS Jr., Cowan WM. The organization of certain afferents to the hippocampus and dentate gyrus in normal and reeler mice. *J Comp Neurol* 1979;185:461–484.

15. Floeter MK, Jones EG. Transplantation of fetal postmitotic neurons to rat cortex: survival, early pathway choices and long-term projections of outgrowing axons. *Dev Brain Res* 1985;22:19–38.

16. Killackey HP, Chalupa LM. Ontogenetic change in the distribution of callosal projection neurons in the postcentral gyrus of the fetal rhesus monkey. *J Comp Neurol* 1986;244:331–348.

17. Innocenti GM, Clarke S. Bilateral transitory projections to visual areas from auditory cortex in kittens. *Dev Brain Res* 1984;14:143–148.

18. Stanfield BB, O'Leary DD, Fricks C. Selective collateral elimination in early postnatal development restricts cortical distribution of rat pyramidal tract neurons. *Nature* 1982;298:371–373.

19. Burkhalter A, Bernardo KL. Organization of corticocortical connections in human visual cortex. *Proc Natl Acad Sci USA* 1989;86:1071–1075.

20. Godement P, Vanselow J, Thanos S, Bonhoeffer F. A study in developing visual system with a new method of staining neurones and their processes in fixed tissue. *Development* 1987;101:697–713.

21. Korsching S. The neurotrophic factor concept: a reexamination. *J Neurosci* 1993;13:2739–2748.

22. Lin L-FH, Doherty DH, Lile JD, Bektesh S, Collins F. GDNF: a glial cell line-derived neurotrophic factor for midbrain dopaminergic neurons. *Science* 1993;260:1130–1132.

23. Cowan WM, Fawcett JW, O'Leary DDM, Stanfield BB. Regressive events in neurogenesis. *Science* 1984;225:1258–1265.

24. Sulston JE. Postembryonic cell lineages of the nematode *Caenorhabditis elegans*. *Dev Biol* 1976;56:110–156.

25. Kerr JFR, Wyllie AH, Currie AR. Apoptosis: a basic biological phenomenon with wide-ranging implications in tissue kinetics. *Br J Cancer* 1972;26:239–257.

26. Huttenlocher PR. Synaptic density in human frontal cortex—developmental changes and effects of aging. *Brain Res* 1979;163:195–205.

27. Lichtman JW, Purves D. The elimination of redundant preganglionic innervation to hamster sympathetic ganglion cells in early postnatal life. *J Physiol* 1980;301:213–228.

28. Purves D, Lichtman JW. Elimination of synapses in the developing nervous system. *Science* 1980;210:153–157.

29. Jerison H. Brain size. In: Adelman G, ed. *Encyclopedia of Neuroscience*, Boston: Birkhauser, 1985;168–170.

30. Yakovlev PI, Lecours A-R. The myelogenetic cycles of regional maturation of the brain. In: Minkowski A, ed. *Regional Development of the Brain in Early Life*, Oxford: Blackwell, 1967.

31. Black IB. Stages of neurotransmitter development in autonomic neurons. *Science* 1982;215:1198–1204.

32. Lauder JM, Krebs H. Do neurotransmitters, neurohumors, and hormones specify critical periods? In: Greenough WT, Juraska JM, eds. *Developmental Neuropsychobiology*, New York: Academic Press, 1986;119–174.

33. Jones EG. The development of the primate neocortex—an overview. In: Mednick SA, Cannon TD, Barr CE, Lyon M, eds. *Fetal Neural Development and Adult Schizophrenia*, New York: Cambridge University Press, 1991;40–65.

34. Levitt P, Moore RY. Development of the noradrenergic innervation of neocortex. *Brain Res* 1979;162:243–259.

35. Hohman CF, Hamon R, Batshaw ML, Coyle JT. Transient postnatal elevation of seotonin levels in mouse neocortex. *Dev Br Res* 1988;43:163–166.

36. D'Amato RJ, Blue ME, Largent BL. Ontogeny of the serotonergic projection to rat neocortex: Transient expression of a dense innervation to primary sensory areas. *Proc Natl Acad Sci USA* 1987;84:4322–4326.

37. Kvale I, Fosse VM, Fonnum F. Development of neurotransmitter parameters in lateral geniculate body, superior colliculus and visual cortex of the albino rat. *Dev Brain Res* 1983;7:137–145.

38. Coyle JT, Yamamura HI. Neurochemical aspects of the ontogenesis of cholinergic neurons in the rat brain. *Brain Res* 1976;118:429–440.

39. Dori I, Parnavelas JG, Eckenstein F. The postnatal developmental of the cholinergic system in the rat visual cortex. *Neurosci Lett [Suppl]* 1985;22:S354.

40. Bear MF, Singer W. Modulation of visual cortical plasticity by acetylcholine and noradrenaline. *Nature* 1986;320:172–176.

41. Huntley GW, Hendry SHC, Killackey HP, Chalupa LM, Jones EG. Temporal sequence of neurotransmitter expression by developing neurons of fetal monkey visual cortex. *Dev Brain Res* 1988;43:69–96.

42. Goldfarb J, Cantin C, Cohen MW. Intracellular and surface acetylcholine receptors during normal development of a frog skeletal muscle. *J Neurosci* 1990;10:500–507.

43. Roth BL, Hamblin MW, Ciaranello RD. Developmental regulation of $5\text{-}HT_2$ and $5\text{-}HT_{1C}$ mRNA and receptor levels. *Dev Brain Res* 1991;58:51–58.

44. Insel TR. Long-term neural consequences of stress during development: Is early experience a form of chemical imprinting? In: Carroll BJ, Barrett JE, eds. *Psychopathology and the Brain*, New York: Raven Press, 1991;133–152.

45. Milligan G, Streaty R, Gierschik P, Spiegel AM, Klee WE. Development of opiate receptors and GTP-binding regulatory proteins in neonatal rat brains. *J Biol Chem* 1987;262:8626–8630.

46. Enjalbert A, Bourgoin S, Hamon M, Adrien J, Bockaert J. Postsynaptic serotonin-sensitive adenylate cyclase in the central nervous system. *Mol Pharmacol* 1978;14:2–10.

47. Nicoletti F, Iadorola MJ, Wroblewski JT, Costa E. Excitatory amino acid recognition sites couples with inositol phospholipid metabolism: developmental changes and interaction with alpha-1 adrenoreceptors. *Proc Natl Acad Sci USA* 1986;83:1931–1935.

48. Insel TR, Battablia G, Fairbanks DW, De Souza EB. The ontogeny of brain receptors for corticotropin-releasing factor and the development of their functional association with adenylate cyclase. *J Neurosci* 1988;8:4151–4158.

49. Hamburger V, Wenger E, Oppenheim R. Motility in the chick embryo in the absence of sensory input. *J Exp Zool* 1966;162:133–160.

50. Smotherman WP, Robinson SR. Accessibility of the rat fetus for investigation. In: Shair HN, Barr GA, Hofer MA, eds. *Developmental Psychobiology: New Concepts and Changing Methods*, New York: Oxford University Press, 1991;148–163.

51. Kagan J, Snidman N. Temperamental factors in human development. *Am Psychol* 1991;46:856–862.

52. Hofer MA. Relationships as regulators: a psychobiologic perspective on bereavement. *Psychosom Med* 1984;46:183–197.

53. Kuhn CM, Pauk J, Schanberg SM. Endocrine responses to mother-infant separation in developing rats. *Dev Psychobiol* 1990;23:395–410.

54. Stanton ME, Levine S. Inhibition of infant glucocorticoid stress response: specific role of maternal cues. *Dev Psychobiol* 1990;23:411–426.

55. Singer W. Neuronal activity as a shaping factor in postnatal development of visual cortex. In: Greenough WT, Juraska JM, eds. *Developmental Neuropsychobiology* Orlando: Academic Press, 1986;271–293.

56. Kaas J, Merzenich MM, Killackey HP. The reorganization of somatosensory cortex following peripheral nerve damage in adult and developing animals. *Ann Rev Neurosci* 1983;6:325–356.

57. Knudsen E. Experience alters the spatial tuning of auditory units in the optic tectum during a sensitive period. *J Neurosci* 1985;5:3094–3109.

58. Knudsen E, Knudsen P. The sensitive period for auditory localiza-

tion in barn owls is limited by age, not experience. *J Neurosci* 1986;6:1918–1924.

59. Hubel DH, Wiesel TN, LeVay S. Plasticity of ocular dominance columns in monkey genesis. *Phil Trans R Soc Lond* 1977;278.
60. Spinelli DN, Hirsch HVB, Phelps RW, Metzler J. Visual experience as a determinant of the response characteristics of cortical receptive fields in cats. *Exp Brain Res* 1972;15:289–304.
61. Blakemore C, Cooper GF. Development of the brain depends on the visual environment. *Nature* 1970;228:477–478.
62. Greenough WT. What's special about development? Thoughts on the basis of experience-psychobiology. In: Greenough WT, Juraska JM, eds. *Developmental Neuropsychobiology,* Orlando: Academic Press, 1986;387–407.
63. Hebb DO. *The Organization of Behavior.* New York: John Wiley & Sons, 1949.
64. Phoenix CH, Gor RW, Gerall AA, Young WC. Organizing action of prenatally administered testosterone propionate on the tissues mediating mating behavior in the guinea pig. *Endo* 1959;65:369–382.
65. MacLusky NJ, Naftolin F. Sexual differentiation of the central nervous system. *Science* 1981;211:1294.
66. Goy RW, McEwen BS. *Sexual Differentiation of the Brain.* Cambridge: MIT Press, 1980.
67. MacLusky NJ, Chaptal C, McEwen BS. The development of estrogen receptor systems in the rat brain and pituitary: postnatal development. *Brain Res* 1979;178:143–160.
68. Ward IL. Prenatal stress feminizes and demasculinizes the behavior of males. *Science* 1972;175:82–84.
69. Ward IL, Weisz J. Maternal stress alters plasma testosterone in fetal males. *Science* 1980;207:328–329.
70. Toran-Allerand CD, Gerlach JL, McEwen BS. Autoradiographic localization of [³H] estradiol related to steroid responsiveness in cultures of the newborn mouse hypothalamus and preoptic area. *Brain Res* 1980;184:517–522.
71. Wright LL, Smolen AJ. The role of neuron death in the development of the gender difference in the number of neurons in the rat superior cervical ganglion. *Int J Dev Neurosci* 1987;5:305–311.
72. Diamond MC. Sex differences in the rat forebrain. *Brain Res* 1987;12:235–240.
73. Allen LS, Hines M, Shryne JE, Gorski RA. Two sexually dimorphic cell groups in the human brain. *J Neurosci* 1989;9:497–506.
74. Swaab DF, Fliers EA. A sexually dimorphic nucleus in the human brain. *Science* 1985;228:1112–1115.
75. Arnold AP, Breedlove SM. Organizational and activational effects of sex steroids on brain and behavior: a reanalysis. *Horm Behav* 1985;19:469–498.
76. Rosengarten H, Friedhoff AJ. Enduring changes in dopamine receptor cells of pups from drug administration to pregnant and nursing rats. *Science* 1979;203:1133–1135.
77. Handelmann GE. A developmental role of neuropeptides. *J Physiol* 1985;80:268–274.
78. Boer GJ, Swaab DF. Neuropeptide effects on brain development to be expected from behavioral teratology. *Peptides* 1985;6:21–28.
79. Meriney SD, Gray DB, Pilar G. Morphine-induced delay of normal cell death in the avian ciliary ganglion. *Science* 1985;228:1451–1453.
80. Bardo MT, Schmidt RH, Bhatnagar RK. Effects of morphine on sprouting of locus coeruleus fibers in the neonatal rat. *Dev Brain Res* 1985;22:161–168.
81. Hauser KF, McLaughlin PJ, Zagon IS. Endogenous opioids regulate dendritic growth and spine formation in developing rat brain. *Brain Res* 1987;416:157–161.
82. Kennard M. Reorganization of motor function in the cerebral cortex of monkeys deprived of motor and premotor areas in infancy. *J Neurophysiol* 1938;1:477–496.
83. Keilhoff G, Wolf G, Stastny F, Schmidt W. Quinolinate neurotoxicity and glutamatergic structures. *Neuroscience* 1990;34:235–242.
84. Weihmuller FB, Bruno JP. Age-dependent plasticity in the dopaminergic control of sensorimotor development. *Behav Br Res* 1989;35:95–109.
85. Winslow JT, Insel TR. Serotonergic modulation of rat pup ultrasonic vocal development: Studies with 3,4-methylenedioxymethamphetamine. *J Pharmacol Exp Ther* 1990;254:212–220.
86. Almli CR, Finger S. *Early Brain Damage,* Orlando: Academic Press, 1984.
87. Reinstein DK, Isaacson RL. Clonidine sensitivity in the developing rat. *Brain Res* 1977;135:378–382.
88. Hartley EJ, Seeman P. Development of receptors for dopamine and noradrenaline in rat brain. *Eur J Pharmacol* 1983;91:391–397.
89. Smythe JW, Pappas BA. Neonatal 6-hydroxydopamine potentiates clonidine's locomotor effects throughout maturation in the rat. *Pharmacol Biochem Behav* 1985;22:1075–1078.
90. Sargent Jones L, Gauger LL, Davis JN, Slotkin TA, Bartolome JV. Postnatal development on brain alpha₁-adrenergic receptors: in vitro autoradiography with [¹²⁵I]heat in normal rats and rats treated with alpha-difluoromethylornithine, a specific, irreversible inhibitor of ornithine decarboxylase. *Neurosci* 1985;15:1195–1202.
91. Saunders NR, Mollgard K. Development of the blood-brain barrier. *J Dev Physiol* 1984;6:45–57.

Psychopharmacology: The Fourth Generation of Progress, edited by Floyd E. Bloom and David J. Kupfer. Raven Press, Ltd., New York © 1995.

CHAPTER 61

Intracellular Messenger Pathways as Mediators of Neural Plasticity

Eric J. Nestler and Ronald S. Duman

Previous chapters have described the postreceptor, intracellular messenger pathways that mediate signal transduction in the brain (see chapters by Aghajanian, Duman and Nestler, Piomelli, and Sanders-Bush and Canton, this volume). These pathways serve three major functions in signal transduction. First, they mediate certain short-term aspects of synaptic transmission; those rapid actions of neurotransmitters on ion channels that do not involve ligand-gated channels are achieved through intracellular messengers. Second, they play the central role in mediating other actions of synaptic transmission: Virtually all other effects of neurotransmitters on target neuron functioning, both short-term and long-term, are achieved through intracellular messengers (see Chapters 11, 27, and 38, *this volume*). This includes those long-term actions of neurotransmitters that are mediated through alterations in neuronal gene expression. This role for intracellular messengers is not limited to the actions of neurotransmitters mediated by G-protein-linked receptors. Although activation of ligand-gated ion channels leads to initial changes in membrane potential independent of intracellular messengers, activation of ligand-gated ion channels also leads to numerous additional (albeit slower) effects that are mediated by intracellular messengers. Third, by virtue of numerous interactions among various intracellular messenger pathways, these pathways play the central role in coordinating a myriad of neuronal processes and adjusting neuronal function to environmental cues (24).

The short- and long-term modulatory effects that neurotransmitters exert on their target neurons by regulating

intracellular messenger pathways can be viewed as the basis of neural plasticity. Environmental factors of virtually every type produce long-term changes in brain function by influencing these processes. In this chapter, we demonstrate how psychotropic drugs can serve as unique tools to study the mechanisms by which the brain adapts to chronic environmentally induced perturbations in its signaling pathways. This is because drugs provide bridges between preclinical and clinical situations. Indeed, because most types of psychotropic drugs must be given for several weeks before their therapeutic effects are apparent and because drugs of abuse induce addiction gradually and progressively with continued drug exposure, the clinically relevant actions of most psychotropic drugs can be considered drug-induced neural plasticity. We present evidence that the brain's intracellular messenger pathways are themselves targets of long-term regulation and contribute prominently to drug-induced neural plasticity. In addition, the role of intracellular messengers as general mediators of neural plasticity is discussed.

GENERAL MODEL OF DRUG-INDUCED NEURAL PLASTICITY

A model of drug-induced neural plasticity is shown in Fig. 1. According to this scheme, drugs produce acute and short-term changes in brain function by influencing the brain's signal transduction pathways. This includes drug regulation of the amount of neurotransmitter available at the synapse and of neurotransmitter activation of plasma membrane receptors and postreceptor signaling pathways (e.g., second messengers and protein phosphorylation). (These short-term processes are discussed in greater detail in Chapters 27 and 38, *this volume*.) This is true regardless of whether the drug interacts initially

E. J. Nestler and R. S. Duman: Laboratory of Molecular Psychiatry, Departments of Psychiatry and Pharmacology, Yale University School of Medicine and Connecticut Mental Health Center, New Haven, Connecticut 06508.

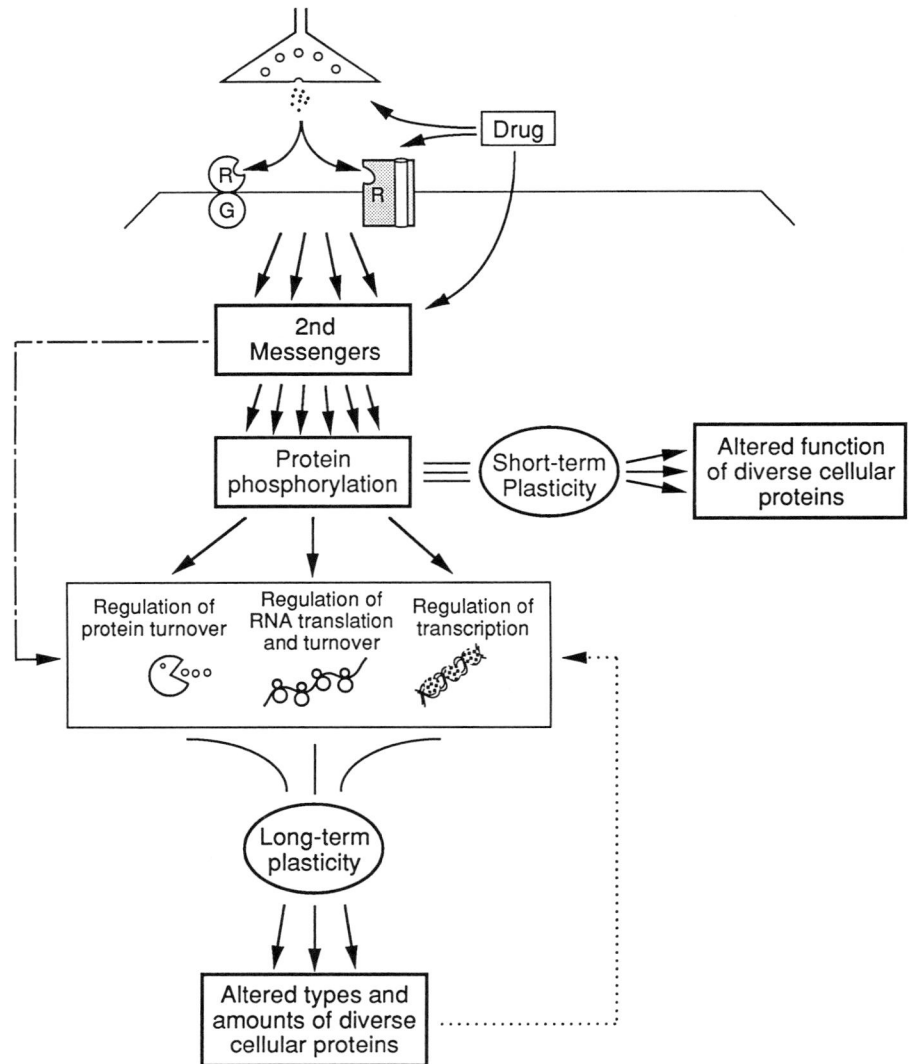

FIG. 1. Scheme illustrating general mechanisms of drug-induced neural plasticity. Psychotropic drugs induce prolonged alterations in brain function (i.e., neural plasticity) by influencing the brain's signal transduction pathways. This occurs regardless of whether the drugs interact initially with proteins involved in presynaptic neurotransmitter function (e.g., cocaine and tricyclic antidepressants as inhibitors of monoamine reuptake transporters), postsynaptic neurotransmitter function [e.g., morphine as an agonist at the opioid receptor (*R*) which is G-protein (*G*) coupled, or nicotine as an agonist at the nicotinic acetylcholine receptor (*R'*) which is a ligand-gated channel], or post-receptor signal transduction pathways (e.g., lithium on the cAMP and phosphatidylinositol pathways). The single most important molecular mechanism of neural plasticity is protein phosphorylation. Although neural plasticity is mediated in some situations by other mechanisms of covalent and noncovalent modification (*dot–dash line*), protein phosphorylation is a unique mechanism because of its ubiquity: the number and diversity of neural proteins and processes regulated and the cell types involved. By regulating the phosphorylation state of virtually every type of neural protein, short-term drug exposure produces relatively rapid, usually short-lived effects on diverse aspects of neuronal function. This includes initial drug effects on processes (regulation of protein turnover, RNA translation and turnover, and gene transcription) that determine the types and amounts of proteins present in neurons. With chronic drug exposure, these changes in protein levels lead to long-term neural plasticity as they accumulate and become functionally important. Among the many aspects of drug-induced, long-term neural plasticity are permissive effects, a process whereby chronic drug treatment alters the type, as opposed to the level, of responsiveness of a neuron to the drug itself or other stimuli (*dotted line*). For example, chronic drug treatment, by inducing the expression of a novel transcription factor, can change the genomic responses elicited by subsequent exposure to the drug or to other acute perturbations (21).

with proteins located extracellularly or intracellularly, presynaptically or postsynaptically. While these transient and readily reversible effects occur in response to drug treatment, drug perturbation of signal transduction pathways is also initiating longer-term effects, which involve altered levels and altered types of proteins expressed in target neurons. These changes build up gradually over time in response to continued exposure to the drug and eventually become quantitatively significant, leading to long-term changes in brain function.

There are three types of mechanisms by which a drug could alter levels of a protein: regulation of gene transcription, regulation of ribonucleic acid (RNA) translation and turnover, or regulation of protein turnover (Fig. 1). Most attention to date has focused on drug regulation of gene expression. This attention is based on the many demonstrated cases of equivalent drug-induced changes in various proteins and their messenger RNAs (mRNAs), and of drug regulation of transcription factors (24). Transcription factors are proteins that bind to specific sequences of deoxyribonucleic acid (DNA) contained within the regulatory regions of certain genes and thereby increase or decrease the rate at which those genes are transcribed (see Chapter 56, this volume). Most genes contain binding sites for multiple types of transcription factors, such that their transcriptional rates are probably determined by unique combinations of transcription factors that interact cooperatively.

Studies of drug regulation of gene expression to date have focused almost exclusively on two families of transcription factors: cyclic adenosine monophosphate (cAMP) response element binding protein (CREB) and related proteins mediate many of the effects of cAMP and probably Ca^{2+} on gene expression (24,33). Primarily, CREB's transcriptional activity is regulated by its phosphorylation by cAMP- and Ca^{2+}-dependent protein kinases. Increasing evidence demonstrates that psychotropic drug treatments can regulate CREB function in the brain, presumably by influencing these intracellular pathways. Although CREB expression is believed to be constitutive and not subject to physiologic regulation, recent evidence challenges this view (40).

c-Fos, c-Jun, and products of related immediate early genes (IEGs) are regulated in the brain by diverse types of stimuli, including numerous drug and other treatments (36; see also Chapters 41, 46, 56, and 57, this volume). Extracellular stimuli are thought to regulate these transcription factors primarily by regulating their expression, possibly mediated by the cAMP- or Ca^{2+}-dependent phosphorylation of CREB or CREB-like proteins. However, Fos- and Jun-like proteins are also known to be phosphorylated by many protein kinases, and this serves to further regulate their transcriptional activity.

Although there is little doubt that these transcription factors play an important role in mediating the effects of certain drugs and other extracellular signals on gene expression, there is also little doubt that the effects of a drug on gene expression are probably mediated through regulation of enumerable transcription factors, with different mechanisms operating in different neuronal cell types. Moreover, proteins that control the packaging of chromatin and the accessibility of certain genes to transcription factors are also highly regulated and possibly subject to drug effects (16).

Current emphasis on gene expression as a long-term target of drug action should not detract from the likely importance of posttranscriptional mechanisms of drug-induced neural plasticity. Indeed, increasing evidence indicates that RNA processing, transport to the cytoplasm, assembly into polysomes, stability, and rate of translation are also highly regulated in neurons (20,49). More attention should be given in future studies to drug regulation of these parameters. Similarly, more attention should be given to regulation of protein turnover, including rates, and possibly sites, of proteolysis, subcellular trafficking, and association with specific cellular organelles and macromolecular complexes. Changes in the processing and degradation of the β-adrenergic receptor induced by long-term exposure to agonists (see Chapter 27, this volume) emphasize the probable importance of posttranslational regulatory mechanisms in drug effects on the nervous system. Finally, it should be emphasized that regulation of levels of a particular protein often involves all three of the processes shown in Fig. 1, as the cell gradually adapts to drug exposure or other environmental inputs.

EXAMPLES OF DRUG-INDUCED NEURAL PLASTICITY

The complexity of these regulatory systems makes it exceedingly difficult to delineate the precise mechanisms underlying neural plasticity. However, studies of drugs permit investigation of these regulatory mechanisms within a functional context by studying drug action in anatomically well-defined brain regions known from behavioral pharmacologic studies to mediate important effects of the drugs. The goal of such studies is threefold: (i) to identify molecular and cellular adaptations that drugs induce in those regions; (ii) to relate the altered biochemical phenotype of cells in those regions to the altered electrophysiologic phenotype of the cells and to the altered behavioral phenotype of the organism; and (iii) to elaborate the detailed molecular mechanisms by which the drugs produce the altered biochemical and electrophysiologic phenotypes. One experimental system in which this approach has been used with considerable success is opiate action in the locus coeruleus (LC).

Studies of Opiate Addiction in the Locus Coeruleus

The LC is the major noradrenergic nucleus in the brain, located on the floor of the fourth ventricle in the rostral

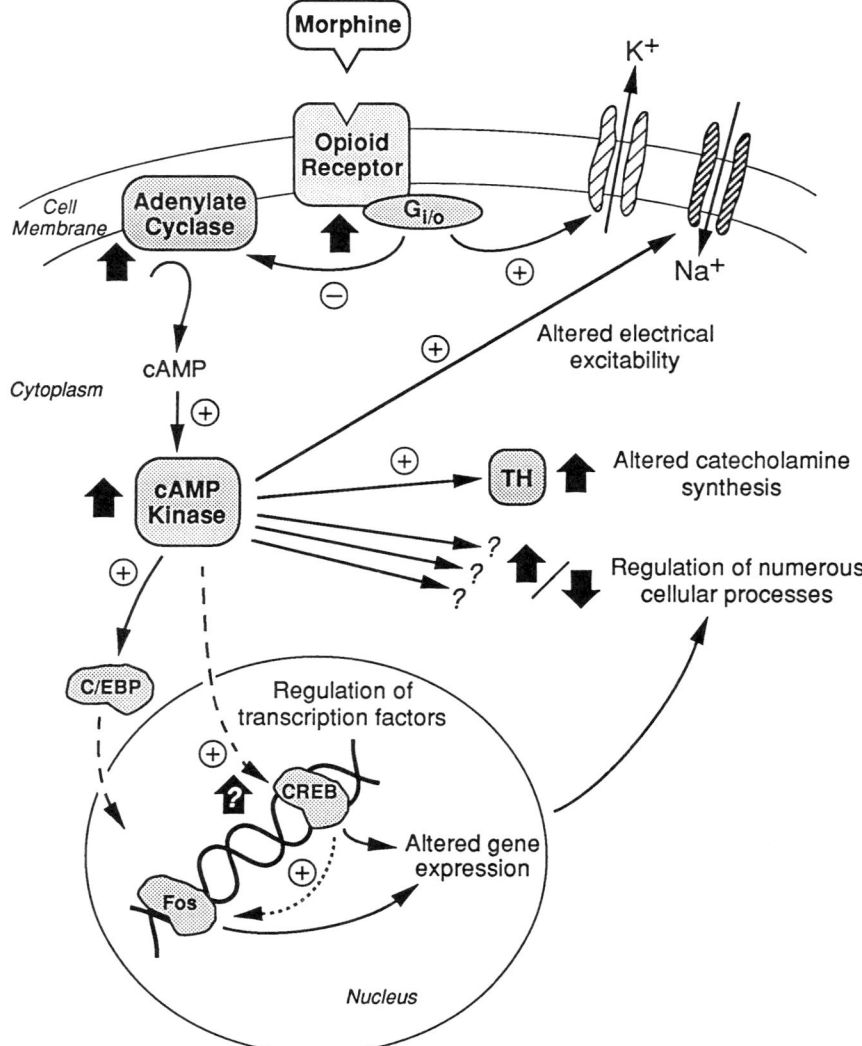

FIG. 2. Scheme illustrating opiate actions in the LC. Opiates acutely inhibit LC neurons by increasing the conductance of a K$^+$ channel (*light cross-hatch*) via coupling with subtypes of Gi and/or Go, and by decreasing a Na$^+$-dependent inward current (*dark cross-hatch*) by coupling with Gi/o and the consequent inhibition of adenylyl cyclase. Reduced levels of cAMP decrease cAMP-dependent protein kinase activity and the phosphorylation of the responsible channel or pump (or closely-associated protein). Inhibition of the cAMP pathway also decreases phosphorylation of numerous other proteins and thereby affects many additional processes in the neuron. In addition to reducing firing rates, for example, inhibition of the cAMP pathway decreases catecholamine synthesis by reducing phosphoryla-tion of TH and initiates alterations in gene expression by regulating transcription factors [e.g., reduced phosphorylation of CREB (associated with reduced nuclear translocation of the protein kinase catalytic subunit); reduced expression of c-fos and other IEGs (possibly mediated by CREB, *dotted line*); and reduced activation and nuclear translocation of C/EBP, CCAAT-enhancer binding protein(s)]. *Dashed lines* indicate nuclear translocation of a protein.

Upward bold arrows summarize effects of chronic morphine in the LC. Chronic morphine increases levels of Giα and Goα, adenylyl cyclase, cAMP-dependent protein kinase, and several phosphoproteins including TH. These changes contribute to the altered phenotype of the drug-addicted state. For example, the intrinsic excitability of LC neurons is increased by enhanced activity of the cAMP pathway and Na$^+$-dependent inward current, which contributes to the tolerance, dependence, and withdrawal exhibited by these neurons. Another example is the capacity of the neurons to synthesize catechol-amines, which is increased by induction of TH. This altered phenotypic state may be maintained in part by persisting changes in transcription factors (e.g., CREB, c-Fos, C/EBP). From Nestler et al. (40).

pons. A variety of pharmacologic and behavioral studies have demonstrated that regulation of LC neuronal excitability plays an important role in physical aspects of opiate addiction, namely, physical dependence and withdrawal (28,37).

Acute Opiate Action

The electrophysiologic effects of opiates in the LC are well-established (Fig. 2). Acutely, opiates inhibit LC neurons by activation of an inward-rectifying K$^+$ channel and inhibition of a Na$^+$-dependent inward current (3,5,41). Both actions are mediated by pertussus toxin-sensitive G-proteins (i.e., subtypes of Giα and/or Goα). It is believed that activation of the K$^+$ channel occurs through direct coupling of the opioid receptor to the channel by a G-protein. In contrast, inhibition of the Na$^+$-dependent current appears to be indirect. The current is normally activated by cAMP-dependent protein kinase through the phosphorylation of the responsible channel or pump itself, or some associated protein (4). Opiate inhibition of the current appears to be mediated by reduced levels of cAMP and of activated cAMP-dependent protein kinase. Biochemical studies have confirmed that opiates acutely inhibit adenylyl cyclase activity in the LC, as seen in many other brain regions, as well as inhibit cAMP-dependent protein phosphorylation (37,40).

Chronic Opiate Action

Chronically, LC neurons develop tolerance to these acute inhibitory actions as neuronal firing rates recover toward control levels. The neurons also become dependent on opiates after chronic exposure because abrupt cessation of opiate treatment, for example, through administration of an opiate receptor antagonist, leads to a marked elevation in LC firing rates above control levels in vivo and in vitro (1,26,45).

Because G-proteins and the cAMP pathway play a role in the acute actions of opiates on the LC, we investigated whether long-term adaptations in these intracellular messengers could be involved in the tolerance, dependence, and withdrawal that occurs with chronic opiate exposure. Indeed, over the past several years, chronic administration of opiates has been shown to increase LC levels of Giα and Goα, adenylyl cyclase, cAMP-dependent protein kinase, and several phosphoprotein substrates for the protein kinase, including tyrosine hydroxylase (TH), the rate-limiting enzyme in the biosynthesis of catecholamine neurotransmitters (Fig. 2) (37,40). Up-regulation of the cAMP pathway occurs in the absence of alterations in several other major protein kinases (e.g., Ca^{2+}/calmodulin-dependent protein kinases, protein kinase C, protein tyrosine kinases) in this brain region (53).

Evidence for a Functional Role of an Up-regulated cAMP Pathway in Opiate Addiction in the LC

Up-regulation of adenylyl cyclase and cAMP-dependent protein kinase can be viewed as a compensatory, homeostatic response of LC neurons to persistent opiate inhibition of the cells (Fig. 2) (37). According to this view, up-regulation of the cAMP pathway increases the intrinsic excitability of LC neurons and thereby accounts, at least in part, for opiate tolerance, dependence, and withdrawal. In the opiate-dependent state, the combined presence of the opiate and the up-regulated cAMP pathway would return LC firing rates to control levels. Removal of the opiates would leave the up-regulated cAMP pathway unopposed, which would lead to withdrawal activation of the neurons. This scheme is similar to the one proposed previously based on studies of cAMP levels in cultured neuroblastoma × glioma cells (48).

There is now direct evidence for a role of the up-regulated cAMP pathway in opiate dependence and withdrawal: First, the spontaneous firing rate of LC neurons is dependent on the activity of the cAMP protein phosphorylation pathway and of the Na$^+$-dependent inward current activated by this pathway (4). Second, the spontaneous firing rate of LC neurons from morphine-dependent rats in brain slices where most synaptic connections of the neurons have been severed is more than twice the rate of neurons from control rats and shows a greater maximal excitatory response to cAMP analogs (26). Third, excitation of LC neurons during withdrawal is both necessary and sufficient for producing many of the behavioral signs of physical opiate withdrawal (28,31,37,45). Finally, the time course by which the up-regulated cAMP pathway reverts to normal during opiate withdrawal parallels the time course by which withdrawal activation of LC neurons, and various behavioral signs of withdrawal, recover (45). Taken together, these findings indicate that up-regulation of the cAMP pathway is a likely mechanism of opiate dependence in the LC. Although there may be many other mechanisms of opiate dependence in the LC and elsewhere, up-regulation of the cAMP pathway represents one of the few examples where a behavioral manifestation of neural plasticity (in this case physical opiate dependence) can be linked to electrophysiologic and biochemical adaptations that occur in specific neurons.

The mechanisms underlying tolerance remain less certain but probably overlap with those underlying dependence (Fig. 3). The up-regulated cAMP system may contribute to tolerance by making it more difficult for opiates to inhibit the Na$^+$-dependent inward current by inhibition of the cAMP system. It is also possible that the up-regulated cAMP system, through phosphorylation of the opioid receptor, could result in greater levels of receptor desensitization. This possibility is based on recent observations that brief exposure to met-enkephalin desensitizes the μ-opioid receptor in the LC (2,19) and the evidence

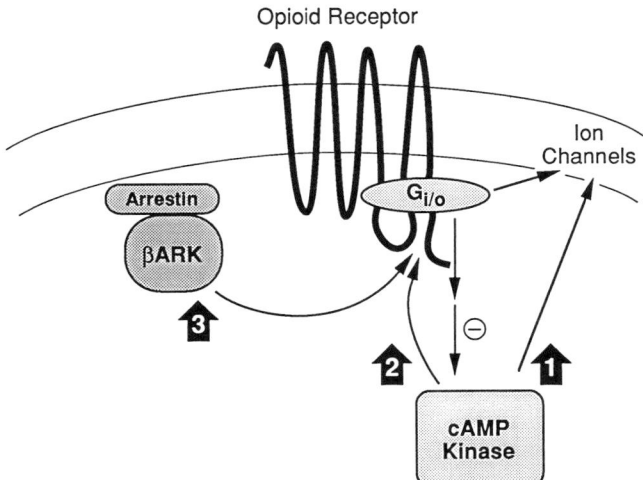

FIG. 3. Scheme illustrating possible mechanisms of opiate tolerance in the LC. Chronic opiate administration produces tolerance—a relative decrease in the ability of μ-opiate agonists to regulate K^+ channels and a Na^+-dependent inward current in LC neurons. Although the mechanisms underlying tolerance have not yet been established, three types of mechanisms are proposed. *Arrow 1:* The up-regulated cAMP system in the LC would contribute to tolerance by making it more difficult for opiates to acutely inhibit the Na^+-dependent inward current via inhibition of the cAMP system. *Arrow 2:* It is possible that the up-regulated cAMP system also contributes to tolerance in LC neurons by enhancing desensitization of the μ-opioid receptor. This is based on the observation that the cAMP pathway promotes desensitization of the receptor (possibly by receptor phosphorylation) induced by short-term enkephalin exposure under control conditions. This mechanism is consistent with the ability of cAMP-dependent protein kinase to phosphorylate and desensitize other G-protein-linked receptors. *Arrow 3:* Based on the evidence that several G-protein-linked receptors are also phosphorylated and desensitized by βARK and associated proteins (e.g., β-arrestin), it is possible that the chronic morphine-induced increase in βARK levels in LC neurons contributes to opiate tolerance. From Nestler et al. (40).

that those agents that activate the cAMP pathway promote this desensitization (2). The up-regulated cAMP system in the tolerant state, by promoting desensitization, could lead to a reduced ability of opiates to activate G-proteins and subsequently regulate the K^+ channel and Na^+-dependent inward current regulated by opiates acutely.

Chronic opiate-induced alterations in β-adrenergic receptor kinases (βARKs), or other protein components of this system (e.g., the β-arrestins), could also conceivably be involved in tolerance. This possibility is based on the role of βARKs and β-arrestins in mediating ligand-induced desensitization of other G-protein-coupled receptors (see Chapter 27, *this volume*). This is believed to occur via the following scheme: Ligand binding to the receptor renders it a good substrate for βARK; phosphorylation of the receptor then triggers its binding to β-arrestin, which inhibits coupling of the receptor to its G-protein. Consistent with a role for βARK in opioid

tolerance is the recent finding that chronic morphine increases levels of one form of βARK in the LC (53), which might be expected to increase opioid receptor desensitization. Cloning and biochemical characterization of the μ-opioid receptor expressed in LC neurons is needed to study these various possibilities directly.

Molecular Mechanisms of Opiate Action in the Locus Coeruleus

Regulation of gene expression may be involved in opiate up-regulation of the cAMP pathway in the LC. Up-regulation of the individual protein components of this pathway is associated with equivalent changes in their mRNAs. In addition, recent studies in transgenic mice have shown that chronic morphine increases the expression of the chloramphenicol acetyltransferase gene fused to 4.8 kb of $5'$ regulatory sequence of the TH gene (40).

As a first step in understanding how opiates might alter the genetic expression of these proteins, a systematic investigation of opiate regulation of transcription factors in the LC has been undertaken in recent years. To date, short- and long-term opiate exposure, and precipitation of opiate withdrawal, have been shown to influence CREB phosphorylation and the DNA-binding activity of this and other cAMP-regulated transcription factors (e.g., CCAATT-enhancer binding proteins) and expression and DNA-binding activity of Fos and Jun-like proteins (40).

Although still preliminary and phenomenologic, these studies highlight the utility of the LC as a model system in which to study the mechanisms underlying molecular plasticity to psychotropic drugs. In this system, altered expression of specific target genes has been shown to have physiologically important consequences. The next step in these studies is to relate regulation of a specific transcription factor to altered expression of a specific target gene and to a functional effect in LC neurons. Such studies, although very difficult methodologically, will gradually delineate the precise steps by which long-term exposure to opiates induces addiction in these neurons.

Studies of Other Psychotropic Drugs

Studies of chronic opiate action in the LC have the unique advantage that the behavioral consequences of such action, for example, physical opiate dependence and withdrawal, can be readily and accurately quantified in laboratory animals. This is much more complicated for most other psychotropic drugs, where the target behavior (e.g., anxiolysis, mood elevation, reduction in psychosis) cannot be studied in animals in a straightforward manner. Nevertheless, recent studies of neural plasticity induced by some other psychotropic drugs have been promising.

Drug Reinforcement

The rewarding properties of drugs of abuse, thought to be a core feature of their addictiveness, are also amenable to detailed molecular investigations. This is because it is possible to quantify aspects of drug reward in laboratory animals by use of various experimental procedures, such as drug self-administration and conditioned place preference (27). This makes it possible to identify brain areas that mediate drug reward and to study the functional relevance of molecular events that occur in those areas in response to chronic exposure to drugs of abuse. Most attention to date has been given to dopaminergic neurons in the ventral tegmental area and their various projection regions, such as the nucleus accumbens and the medial prefrontal cortex. Recent studies have provided increasing evidence that adaptations in G-proteins and other intracellular messenger proteins contribute to the long-term effects of drugs of abuse in these brain-reward pathways. This work has been reviewed recently and is not presented in detail here (27,37,40,47,52).

Antidepressant Drugs

Until recently, studies of antidepressant drugs have focused almost exclusively on drug regulation of the metabolism of monoamine neurotransmitters and of binding sites of monoamine receptors in various brain regions. More recent studies have extended this work by attempting to identify the molecular basis of drug-induced changes in monoamine metabolism and receptor binding, as well as characterization of other molecular actions of antidepressant treatments.

Antidepressant regulation of catecholamine levels has been related to long-term changes in the phosphorylation and expression of TH in the LC and other brain regions (29,39). Decreased expression of TH in the LC by chronic antidepressant treatment is accompanied by down-regulation of cAMP-dependent protein kinase and decreased firing rates of LC neurons (32). Antidepressant regulation of TH and cAMP-dependent protein kinase could represent a compensatory response to antidepressant-induced augmentation of noradrenergic function in projection areas such as cerebral cortex.

Antidepressant treatments are also known to regulate β-adrenergic and 5HT$_2$-serotonin receptor-binding sites in the cerebral cortex and other brain regions, but the mechanisms underlying regulation of these receptors have remained elusive. Recent studies demonstrate that regulation of receptor-binding sites is associated with regulation of receptor mRNA levels (8,23). Although the regulation of receptor mRNA is sometimes associated with an equivalent change in the levels of binding sites, in other cases regulation of receptor mRNA is opposite that observed for receptor binding. This suggests that the turnover of either receptor mRNA and/or protein is influenced by these treatments (23). The complex mechanisms by which antidepressants regulate the β-adrenergic and other receptors is highlighted by the many ways in which the receptor is regulated by long-term exposure to agonists in cultured cells, with alterations seen in receptor affinity for ligand, receptor coupling to G-proteins, receptor sequestration from the plasma membrane, receptor degradation, and receptor synthesis (see Duman and Nestler, this volume). Antidepressant regulation of these various processes must now be investigated.

The mechanisms by which antidepressant treatments regulate mRNA expression of the β-adrenergic and 5-HT$_2$ receptors in brain have not been identified. However, studies in cultured cells indicate that agonist regulation of β-adrenergic receptor mRNA is mediated by the cAMP system (12,18,22). In vivo studies have shown that chronic antidepressant treatments induce an apparent nuclear translocation of cAMP-dependent protein kinase (38), as well as a change in its enzymatic activity (44), in cerebral cortex. Acute and long-term antidepressant treatment has also been reported to influence Fos and related IEG transcription factors in this and other brain regions (15,21,51,54). Antidepressant regulation of the protein kinase and of these and other transcription factors could conceivably be related to altered expression of the β-adrenergic receptor (βAR).

In addition to changes in the expression of the βAR, antidepressant-induced nuclear translocation of the protein kinase and regulation of transcription factors would be expected to result in altered expression of many additional target genes in the brain, that would underlie many of the long-term consequences of antidepressant exposure. Such target genes are only now beginning to be identified. Chronic antidepressant administration has been shown to alter the expression and functional activity of specific G-protein subunits and adenylyl cyclase in brain (11,30,42), changes that would further influence βAR- and other receptor-mediated signal transduction. Antidepressants have been reported to alter the expression of glucocorticoid receptors in cultured cells in vitro (43). If replicated in vivo, this action could contribute to the ability of antidepressants to influence the brain's responses to stress. Preliminary studies demonstrate that antidepressants increase the expression of neurotrophin mRNA in limbic brain regions (35). Increased expression of neurotrophins could contribute to antidepressant-induced plasticity in the brain and to some of the drugs' long-term actions. Future studies will undoubtedly identify many additional target genes of antidepressant treatments.

One critical obstacle in studies of antidepressant drugs is that no specific target brain area has been identified as the major substrate of antidepressant action. This results, in part, from the fact that it is exceedingly difficult to assay clinically relevant effects of the drugs in laboratory animals. This limitation also makes it difficult to study the functional importance of drug-induced adaptations in the brain's signal transduction pathways at the behavioral level. However, antidepressant regulation of the expression of specific genes provides functional endpoints by which drug-induced effects in the brain can be assessed for the first time at the molecular and cellular levels.

GENERAL MECHANISMS OF NEURAL PLASTICITY

Mechanisms underlying drug-induced neural plasticity may be representative of general ways in which neural systems adapt to physiologic and behavioral stimuli. Adaptations that drugs and other stimuli induce in the brain can often be classified into two broad categories: negative- or positive-feedback mechanisms.

Negative feedback can be defined as up- or down-regulation of a system that compensates for, respectively, decreased or increased stimulation of the system. One example is the up-regulation of the cAMP pathway in the LC in response to chronic opiate exposure, as outlined above. Another example is agonist-induced down-regulation of the β-adrenergic receptor, which involves agonist regulation of the receptor at many levels, as mentioned above and covered in detail by Duman and Nestler (*this volume*). It is likely that similar mechanisms operate for other neurotransmitter receptor systems.

Positive feedback can be defined as enhanced responsiveness of a system to the same stimulus. One example is long-term potentiation, characterized by enhanced synaptic efficacy (postsynaptic potentials) elicited by high-frequency stimulation of a presynaptic pathway. Another example is locomotor sensitization (increased locomotor activation), which has been observed in response to repeated administration of cocaine or other stimulants. The mechanisms underlying these sensitization phenomena have not yet been established with certainty but appear to involve presynaptic and postsynaptic adaptations: increased presynaptic release of the stimulating neurotransmitter as well as increased responsiveness of the receptor–intracellular signal transduction pathways for the stimulating neurotransmitter (7,25).

In addition to negative- and positive-feedback processes, certain chronic perturbations can result in different types of responses to the original stimulus not just up- or down-regulation. In other words, chronic peturbation could produce qualitative, as well as quantitative, changes in the brain's signaling pathways. One example is the ability of chronic electroconvulsive seizures or cocaine to alter the types (not just the amounts) of Fos-like proteins expressed in the brain (21). Altered Fos-like proteins in the acute versus chronic state would be expected to mediate different types of effects of a seizure or cocaine on neural gene expression.

A critical need is to identify the factors that determine whether a negative- or positive-feedback response, or different response, will occur following a particular perturbation. This depends not only on the stimulus but also on the specific receptor systems, intracellular messenger pathways, and nuclear regulatory mechanisms active in a cell at a given point in time. Such adaptations are the subject of tremendous interest, because these types of mechanisms at the molecular and cellular level presumably accumulate and interact to form the basis of complex forms of learning and memory at the behavioral level.

Such neural plasticity processes are in constant operation as the brain receives external stimuli via neuronal pathways as well as endocrine and cytokine substances in the circulation. These inputs influence multiple signal-transduction pathways, which ultimately control the function and activity of the neural pathways that make up the brain. Other than drug-induced neural plasticity, the ways in which these processes could operate in response to environmental changes have been best studied for stress.

Stress-induced Neural Plasticity

Numerous studies have documented the effects of short- and long-term exposure to stress on the brain. Particular attention has been given to the hypothalamic–pituitary–adrenal axis, which controls glucocorticoid secretion, and to each of the major monoamine-neurotransmitter systems in brain. Many neurotransmitter and neuropeptide systems in the brain are known to be influenced by acute and chronic stress, and more recent studies have begun to extend this work by examining stress-induced adaptations in intracellular messenger pathways.

The influence of stress on the brain's catecholamine systems is one of the most studied and is discussed here for illustrative purposes. Similar types of adaptations to stress probably occur in many other brain neurotransmitter systems. Acute stress leads to activation of LC neurons in part by activation of corticotropin-releasing hormone (CRH) pathways that innervate the LC (possibly from the paraventricular nucleus of the hypothalamus). Chronic stress leads to a sustained activation of LC neurons and to increased expression of TH, adenylyl cyclase, and cAMP-dependent protein kinase (32,46). Up-regulation of the cAMP pathway may contribute to the increased firing of these neurons in response to chronic stress by mechanisms similar to those discussed above for opiate addiction. These biochemical adaptations to stress, which can be viewed as a positive-feedback mechanism, could result from stress-induced activation of LC neuronal firing and the increased demand for norepinephrine. Increased firing could also be driven by a combination of sustained positive inputs, such as CRH activation, and loss of negative inputs, such as α_2-adrenergic autoreceptor feedback inhibition, both of which would contribute to increased activation in the cAMP system.

Chronic stress also leads to adaptations of norepinephrine-stimulated cAMP formation and related signal transduction pathways in the cerebral cortex. This effect is mediated in part by sustained elevation of adrenal glucocorticoids in response to stress (14,34,50). Norepinephrine-stimulated cAMP formation in cerebral cortical brain slices is mediated by β-adrenergic receptors, which directly couple to adenylyl cyclase, and α_1-adrenergic receptors, which alone have little effect but enhance direct-acting agonists. Chronic stress decreases norepinephrine activation of cAMP formation by decreasing the α_1-adrenergic enhancement of β-adrenergic receptor action. The exact mechanism for α_1-adrenergic receptor enhancement is not known, but depends on extracellular Ca^{2+} and may involve activation of protein kinase C or release of free G protein $\beta\gamma$ subunits which can activate certain forms of adenylate cyclase (see Chapter 61, *this volume*).

Chronic stress probably alters the expression of specific genes in the brain. Altered levels of TH, AMP-dependent protein kinase, and receptor function could be mediated, at least in part, at the transcriptional level. Indeed, acute stress has been shown by several groups to induce the expression of c-fos and related IEG transcription factors in specific brain regions, including the LC, mesolimbic dopamine system, amygdala, hippocampus, and certain layers of cerebral cortex (6,9,10,13,15,17). Interestingly, repeated application of the stressful stimulus leads to down-regulation of the c-fos response, whereas exposing an animal to a neutral stimulus previously associated with stress leads to IEG induction (9). Stress regulation of these and other transcription factors, which could mediate some of the long-term effects of stress on brain function, provides novel tools with which to investigate the detailed effects of stress on the nervous system (see also Chapters 33, 34, and 67, *this volume*).

REFERENCES

1. Aghajanian GK. Tolerance of locus coeruleus neurons to morphine and suppression of withdrawal response by clonidine. *Nature* 1978;267:186–188.
2. Aghajanian GK, Alreja M. Cyclic AMP promotes desensitization of the μ opioid response in locus coeruleus (LC) neurons—evidence for heterologous desensitization. *Soc Neurosci Abstr* 1992;18:21.
3. Aghajanian GK, Wang YY. Common alpha-2 and opiate effector mechanisms in the locus coeruleus: intracellular studies in brain slices. *Neuropharmacology* 1987;26:789–800.
4. Alreja M, Aghajanian GK. Pacemaker activity of locus coeruleus neurons: whole-cell recordings in brain slices show dependence on cAMP and protein kinase A. *Brain Res.* 1991;556:339–343.
5. Alreja M, Aghajanian GK. Opiates suppress a resting sodium-dependent inward current in addition to activating an outward potassium current in locus coeruleus neurons. *J Neurosci* 1993;13:3525–3532.
6. Bing G, Filer D, Miller JC, Stone EA. Noradrenergic activation of immediate early genes in rat cerebral cortex. *Mol Brain Res* 1991;11:43–46.
7. Bliss TVP, Collingridge GL. A synaptic model of memory: long-term potentiation in the hippocampus. *Nature* 1993;361:31–39.
8. Butler MO, Morinobu S, Duman RS. Chronic electroconvulsive seizures increase the expression of serotonin2 receptor mRNA in rat frontal cortex. *J Neurochem* 1993;61:1–7.
9. Campeau S, Hayward MD, Hope BT, Rosen JB, Nestler EJ, Davis M. Induction of the c-fos proto-oncogene in rat amygdala during acute and chronic stress. *Brain Res* 1991;565:349–352.
10. Ceccatelli S, Villar MJ, Goldstein M, Hokfelt T. Expression of c-fos immunoreactivity in transmitter-characterized neurons after stress. *Proc Natl Acad Sci USA* 1989;86:9569–9573.
11. Colin SF, Chang H-C, Mollner S, et al. Chronic lithium regulates the expression of adenylate cyclase and Giα in rat cerebral cortex. *Proc Natl Acad Sci USA* 1991;88:10634–10637.
12. Collins S, Bouvier M, Bolanowski MA, Caron MG, Lefkowitz RJ. cAMP stimulates transcription of the β_2-adrenergic receptor gene in response to short-term agonist exposure. *Proc Natl Acad Sci USA* 1989;86:4853–4857.
13. Deutch AY, Lee MC, Gillham MH, Cameron DA, Goldstein M, Iadarola MJ. Stress selectively increases Fos protein in dopamine neurons innervating the prefrontal cortex. *Cerebral Cortex* 1991; 1:273–292.
14. Duman RS, Strada SJ, Enna SJ. Effect of imipramine and adrenocorticotropin administration on the rat brain norepinephrine-coupled cyclic nucleotide generating system: alterations in alpha and beta adrenergic components. *J Pharm Exp Ther* 1985;234:409–414.
15. Knapp DJ, Johnson KB, Breese GR, Criswell HE, Duncan GE. Comparison of topographic patterns of Fos induction by different stress paradigms: forced swim, footshock, and ethanol withdrawal. *Soc Neurosci Abstr* 1993;19:86.
16. Felsenfeld G. Chromatin as an essential part of the transcriptional mechanism. *Nature* 1992;355:219–224.
17. Gubits RM, Smith TM, Fairhurst JL, Yu H. Adrenergic receptors mediate changes in c-fos mRNA levels in brain. *Mol Brain Res* 1989;6:39–45.
18. Hadcock JR, Malbon CC. Agonist regulation of gene expression of adrenergic receptors and G proteins. *J Neurochem* 1993;60:1–9.
19. Harris GC, Williams JT. Transient homologous μ-opioid receptor desensitization in rat locus coeruleus neurons. *J Neurosci* 1991; 11:2574–2581.
20. Hentze MW. Determinants and regulation of cytoplasmic mRNA stability in eukaryotic cells. *Biochim Biophys Acta* 1991;1090:281–292.
21. Hope BT, Kelz M, Duman RS, Nestler EJ. Chronic administration of ECS produces a long-lasting AP-1 complex in rat cerebral cortex of altered composition and characteristics. *J Neurosci* 1994; [*in press*].
22. Hosoda K, Feussner G, Fishman PH, Duman RS. Agonist and cyclic AMP mediated regulation of β_1-adrenergic receptor mRNA and gene transcription in rat C6 glioma cells. *J. Neurochem* 1994;[*in press*].
23. Hosoda K, Duman RS. Regulation of β_1-adrenergic receptor mRNA and ligand binding by antidepressant treatments and norepinephrine depletion in rat frontal cortex. *J Neurochem* 1993;60:1335–1343.
24. Hyman SE, Nestler EJ. *The Molecular Foundations of Psychiatry.* Washington, DC: American Psychiatric Press; 1993.
25. Kalivas PW, Stewart J. Dopamine transmission in the initiation and expression of drug- and stress-induced sensitization of motor activity. *Brain Res Rev* 1991;16:223–244.
26. Kogan JH, Nestler EJ, Aghajanian GK. Elevated basal firing rates and enhanced responses to 8-Br-cAMP in locus coeruleus neurons in brain slices from opiate-dependent rats. *Eur J Pharmacol* 1992;211:47–53.
27. Koob GF. Drugs of abuse: anatomy, pharmacology and function of reward pathways. *Trends Pharmacol Sci* 1992;13:177–184.
28. Koob GF, Maldonado R, Stimus L. Neural substrates of opiate withdrawal. *Trends Neurosci* 1992;15:186–191.
29. Leviel V, Fayada C, Guibert B, et al. Short- and long-term alterations of gene expression in limbic structures by repeated electroconvulsive-induced seizures. *J Neurochem* 1990;54: 899–904.
30. Li PP, Tam Y-K, Young T, Warsh JJ. Lithium decreases Gs, Gi-1 and Gi-2 α-subunit mRNA levels in rat cortex. *Eur J Pharmacol* 1991;206:165–166.
31. Maldonado R, Koob GF. Destruction of the locus coeruleus de-

creases physical signs of opiate withdrawal. *Brain Res* 1993;605: 128–138.

32. Melia KR, Rasmussen K, Terwilliger RZ, Haycock JW, Nestler EJ, Duman RS. Coordinate regulation of the cyclic AMP system with firing rate and expression of tyrosine hydroxylase in the rat locus coeruleus: effects of chronic stress and drug treatments. *J Neurochem* 1992;58:494–502.

33. Meyer TE, Habener JF. Cyclic adenosine 3',5'-monophosphate response element binding protein (CREB) and related transcription-activating deoxyribonucleic acid-binding proteins. *Endocrine Rev* 1993;14:269–290.

34. Mobley PL, Sulser F. Adrenal corticoids regulate the sensitivity of noradrenergic receptor coupled adenylate cyclase in brain. *Nature* 1980;286:608–609.

35. Morinobu S, Duman RS. Induction of BDNF mRNA by electroconvulsive seizure (ECS) and antidepressants in rat frontal cortex. *Soc Neurosci Abstr* 1993;19:499.

36. Morgan JI, Curran T. Stimulus-transcription coupling in the nervous system. *Annu Rev Neurosci* 1991;14:421–452.

37. Nestler EJ. Molecular mechanisms of drug addiction. *J Neurosci* 1992;12:2439–2450.

38. Nestler EJ, Terwilliger RZ, Duman RS. Chronic antidepressant administration alters the subcellular distribution of cyclic AMP-dependent protein kinase in rat frontal cortex. *J Neurochem* 1989;53:1644–1647.

39. Nestler EJ, McMahon A, Sabban EL, Tallman JF, Duman RS. Chronic antidepressant administration decreases the expression of tyrosine hydroxylase in the rat locus coeruleus. *Proc Natl Acad Sci USA* 1990;87:7522–7526.

40. Nestler EJ, Hope BT, Widnell KL. Drug addiction: a model for the molecular basis of neural plasticity. *Neuron* [in press]. 1993; 11(6):995–1006.

41. North RA, Williams JT, Suprenant A, Christie MJ. Mu and delta receptors belong to a family of receptors that are coupled to potassium channels. *Proc Natl Acad Sci USA* 1987;84:5487–5491.

42. Ozawa H, Rasenick MM. Chronic electroconvulsive treatment augments coupling of the GTP-binding protein Gs to the catalytic moiety of adenylyl cyclase in a manner similar to that seen with chronic antidepressant drugs. *J Neurochem* 1991;56:330–338.

43. Pepin M-C, Beaulieu S, Barden N. Antidepressants regulate glucocorticoid receptor messenger RNA concentrations in primary neuronal cultures. *Mol Brain Res* 1989;6:77–83.

44. Perez J, Tinelli D, Brunello N, Racagni G. cAMP-dependent phosphorylation of soluble and crude microtubule fractions of rat cerebral cortex after prolonged desmethylimipramine treatment. *Eur J Pharmacol* 1989;172:305–316.

45. Rasmussen K, Beitner-Johnson D, Krystal JH, Aghajanian GK, Nestler EJ. Opiate withdrawal and the rat locus coeruleus: behavioral, electrophysiological, and biochemical correlates. *J Neurosci* 1990;10:2308–2317.

46. Richard F, Faucon-Biguet N, Labatut R, Rollet D, Mallet J. Modulation of tyrosine hydroxylase gene expression in rat brain and adrenals by exposure to cold. *J Neurosci Res* 1988;20:32–37.

47. Self DW, Terwilliger RZ, Nestler EJ, Stein L. Regulation of cocaine and heroin self-administration by pertussis toxin administration into the nucleus accumbens. *J Neurosci* 1994; [in press].

48. Sharma SK, Klee WA, Nirenberg M. Dual regulation of adenylate cyclase accounts for narcotic dependence and tolerance. *Proc Natl Acad Sci USA* 1975;72:3092–3096.

49. Steward O, Banker GA. Getting the message from the gene to the synapse: sorting and intracellular transport of RNA in neurons. *Trends Neurosci* 1992;15:180–185.

50. Stone EA, Platt JE, Herrera AS, Kirk KL. Effect of repeated restraint stress, desmethylimipramine or adrenocorticotropin on the alpha and beta adrenergic components of the cyclic AMP response to norepinephrine in rat brain slices. *J Pharmacol Exp Ther* 1986; 237:702–707.

51. Strausbaugh HJ, Morinobu S, Duman RS. Modulation of c-fos expression by electroconvulsive seizure (ECS) and antidepressants in rat frontal cortex. *Soc Neurosci Abstr* 1993;19:499.

52. Striplin CD, Kalivas RW. Correlation between behavioral sensitization to cocaine and G protein ADP-ribosylation in the ventral tegmental area. *Brain Res* 1992;579:181–186.

53. Terwilliger RZ, Ortiz J, Guitart X, Nestler EJ. Chronic morphine administration increases levels of βARK in the rat locus coeruleus. *Soc Neurosci Abstr* 1993;19:500.

54. Winston SM, Hayward MD, Nestler EJ, Duman RS. Chronic electroconvulsive seizures down regulate expression of the c-fos proto-oncogene in rat cerebral cortex. *J Neurochem* 1990;54:1920–1925.

Psychopharmacology: The Fourth
Generation of Progress, edited by
Floyd E. Bloom and David J. Kupfer.
Raven Press, Ltd., New York © 1995.

CHAPTER 62

Neuroendocrine Interactions

Bruce S. McEwen

One of the key problems in biology is understanding the connection between genetic (nature) and environmental (nurture) influences. During the past hundred years, there have been many debates as to which is more important in explaining the origins of the traits of individuals, nature or nurture. Neither side has been able to win such arguments, because the dispute itself reflects a fundamental misunderstanding, namely, a failure to acknowledge that genes are continually being regulated by the external environment from conception throughout life. Modern cell and molecular biology is elucidating this fact at an accelerating pace. One of the purposes of this chapter is to provide a sense of what is meant by hormonal regulation of gene expression in the brain and how it relates to behavior and pathophysiology.

The discussion will focus on circulating hormones, because endocrine secretions represent one of the principal links between the environment and the genes (see Fig. 1). Hormone secretion is controlled by the brain acting through the hypothalamus, and it is coordinated by or, in some cases, triggered by the external environment. Furthermore, hormones act on many tissues and cells, including the brain, to promote appropriate responses to environmental change. Illustrative examples include the coordination by gonadal hormones of reproductive processes with reproductive behavior during reproductive cycles that are synchronized to diurnal or seasonal rhythms; and the synchronization by adrenal steroids of energy metabolism with food-seeking behavior and cognitive alertness during the diurnal sleep−wake cycle. Another important example of hormone involvement is the adaptive responses of the organism to stressful environmental challenges, which are mediated principally by epinephrine and adrenal glucocorticoids.

Besides these cyclic or otherwise reversible processes, hormones also mediate important permanent developmental events, such as sexual differentiation and the growth-coordinating effects of thyroid hormone. Furthermore, stressful experiences early in life can have long-lasting effects on emotionality.

Not all of the actions of hormones are beneficial to the organism, and pathophysiological changes are also an important component of environmental influences on the adult and developing organism. In some cases, irreversible changes ensue, such as neural damage that results from severe chronic stress. In other cases, stress exacerbates existing pathophysiology in the form of atherosclerosis or worsening of diabetes, gastrointestinal pathology, or asthma. The genetic constitution plays an important role by providing certain individuals with systems that are vulnerable to the impact of external forces in promoting a disease process. Studies of various diseases in identical twins reveal that it is rare for concordances to be higher than 50% (42), indicating that there is considerable latitude for exerting external control and even prevention when we can only know the underlying mechanisms.

This chapter therefore discusses a full range of topics concerning hormone action on the nervous system, beginning with cellular mechanisms and ending with a discussion of how hormone effects may culminate in individual differences in brain function and malfunction (see also Chapters 5, 43, 55, 67, 83, and 84, *this volume*).

CELLULAR MECHANISMS OF ACTION OF NEUROACTIVE HORMONES

The brain is a target for the actions of circulating hormones and is the principal controller of hormone secretion. Hormones act on brain cells as they do on other cells, through receptors that mediate both cell-surface

B. S. McEwen: Laboratory of Neuroendocrinology, Rockefeller University, New York, New York 10021.

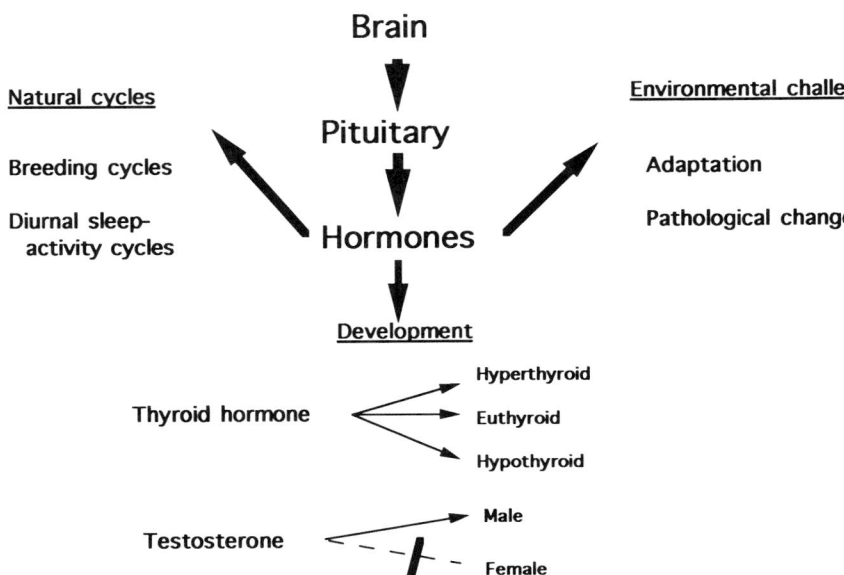

Brain

Natural cycles

Breeding cycles

Diurnal sleep-
    activity cycles

Pituitary

Hormones

Environmental challenge

Adaptation

Pathological change

Development

Thyroid hormone
→ Hyperthyroid
→ Euthyroid
→ Hypothyroid

Testosterone
→ Male
→ Female

FIG. 1. Overview of hormone actions on brain. Hormones secreted under control of natural cycles coordinate reproductions and sleep–wake functions, whereas hormones secreted in response to stressors promote adaption but also pathologic changes. Hormones secreted in development have long-lasting effects on neural development.

phenomena and intracellular events, including gene expression. Steroid hormones and thyroid hormone act via intracellular receptors that bind to deoxyribonucleic acid (DNA) and regulate gene expression (48). In some cases, steroid hormones also act via cell-membrane receptor sites (see Fig. 2) (33).

The brain also produces some steroids from cholesterol, notably pregnenolone, and it can convert pregnenolone to dehydroepiandrosterone. Such steroids have been called neurosteroids (see Fig. 3) (7,8). It is important to distinguish between *neurosteroids,* meaning steroids produced in the brain, and the broader class of *neuroactive steroids,* which includes any steroid with actions upon neural tissue. It should also be emphasized that the term neuroactive steroids is not restricted to any one cellular mechanism of action.

Intracellular steroid hormone receptors were the first proteins recognized to be capable of regulating gene expression by binding to specific nucleotide sequences in the promotor region of various genes. Such proteins are called *transacting factors.* Since their discovery, many other DNA-binding proteins have been identified. Some of these are regulated in their ability to bind to the DNA site (called a *response element*) by phosphorylation in a number of different second messenger systems; others, such as the immediate early genes, are induced by second-messenger-system activation, and they then promote or inhibit the transcription of other genes by binding to response elements located in the promotor regions of some genes. A schematic diagram of some of these interactions is presented in Figure 4.

There are two types of response elements: simple and composite (48). Simple response elements bind only one transacting factor, whereas composite response elements bind one of several types: for example, a steroid receptor

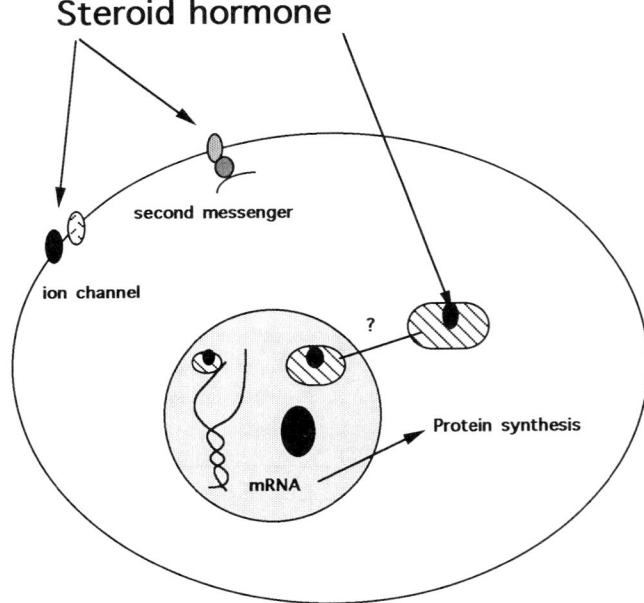

Steroid hormone

second messenger

ion channel

?

mRNA

Protein synthesis

FIG. 2. Diagram of steroid hormone actions showing that they exert both genomic and nongenomic effects on a variety of cells in the brain and throughout the body. Cell-surface actions of steroids include effects on receptors with ion channels and on receptors coupled to second messengers via G proteins. *Question mark* denotes uncertainty as to how much intracellular steroid hormones receptors reside in the cytoplasm or in the nucleus in the absence of hormone. In the presence of hormone, these intracellular receptors are found in the cell nuclei where they regulate transcription leading to mRNA production and protein synthesis.

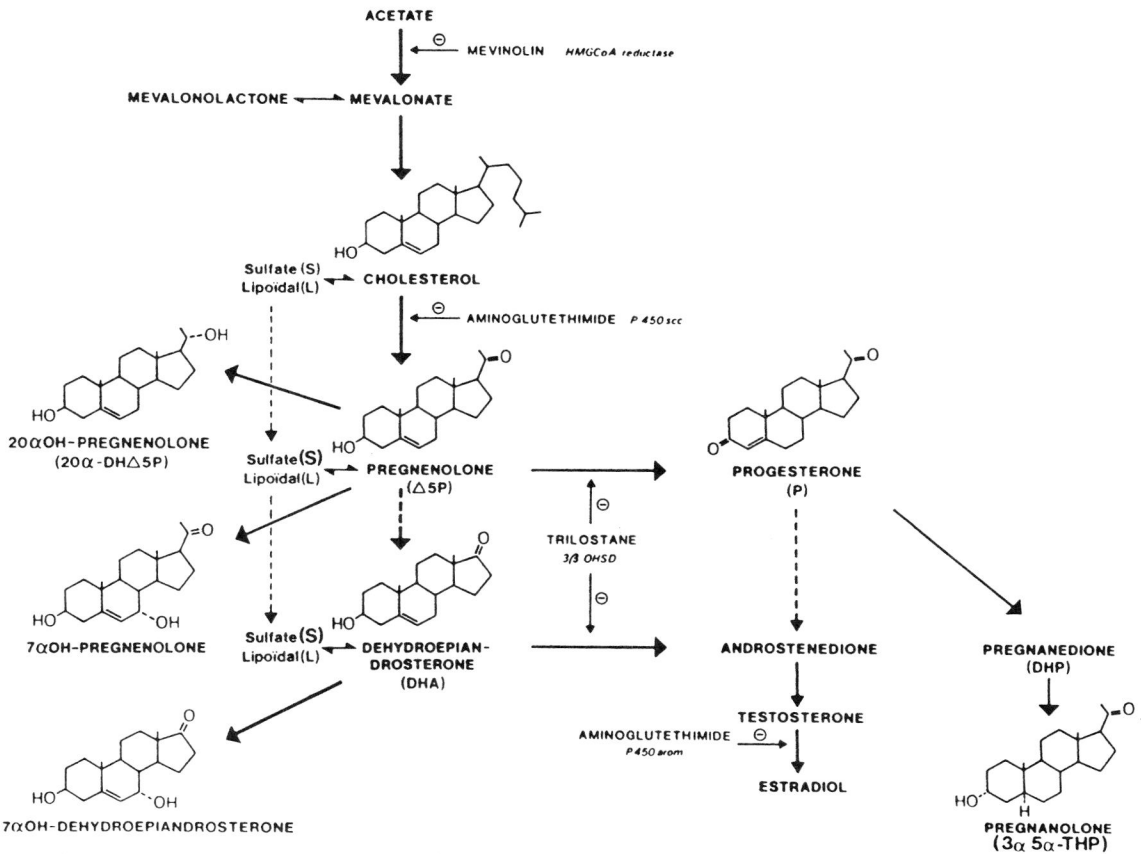

FIG. 3. Neurosteroids are defined as steroid produced in the brain from cholesterol. Some products include dehydroepiandrosterone (DHA), progesterone, and pregnanolone, which is active on the GABAa receptor chloride channel. From Baulieu (8) with permission.

and a transacting factor, such as CREB, which is phosphorylated by second messenger systems. An alternative mode of interactions between transacting factors is that they sometimes bind to each other, and, in so doing, inactivate each others ability to bind to the DNA response element.

Membrane actions of steroid hormones are not as well characterized as those mediated by the intracellular genomic receptors. Representative nongenomic effects of steroids (38) are listed below:

1. *GABAa receptor.* A-ring reduced metabolites of progesterone and deoxycorticosterone facilitate opening of chloride channel; this is a property of a variety of combinations of GABAa receptor subunits expressed in cells that normally do not express such receptors (23).
2. *Corticosterone receptor.* A G-protein coupled membrane site in the newt brain is linked to rapid inhibition of sexual behavior (52,53).
3. *Progesterone receptor.* A membrane progesterone receptor mediates mobilization of calcium stores in spermatozoa, leading to capacitation of the sperm (11).

4. *Aldosterone receptor.* Monocytes respond to aldosterone in altering ionic balance via a receptor distinct from the intracellular Type I adrenal steroid receptor (80).
5. *Estrogen receptor.* Estradiol rapidly facilitates non-NMDA excitatory amino acid effects on hippocampal CA1 neurons (84).

Binding studies have been successful in only one case, namely, a corticosteroid receptor present in the forebrain of a newt that is coupled to a G-protein and appears to mediate a rapid inhibition of sexual behavior. The other well-characterized steroid site is on the γ-aminobutyric acid a (GABAa) receptor, specifically the site to which A-ring–reduced steroids (see Fig. 3) bind and facilitate opening of the chloride channel. This site is recognized for its functional activity rather than its binding, and its existence on the GABA receptor has been demonstrated by showing that GABAa receptors have such steroid response sites when they are expressed from DNA in cells that normally do not express the GABAa receptor. Inferences about other membrane receptors for steroids come from the actions of various steroids on membrane-based

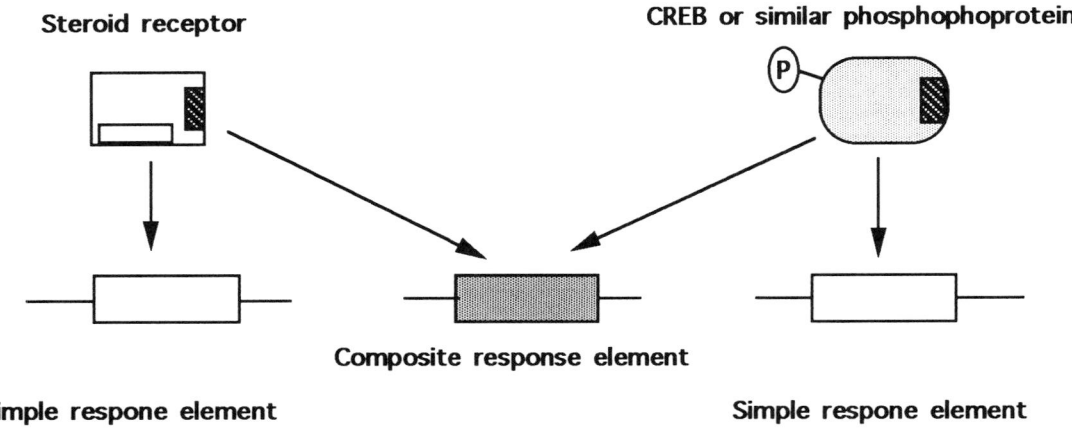

Steroid receptor

CREB or similar phosphophoprotein

Composite response element

Simple respone element

Simple respone element

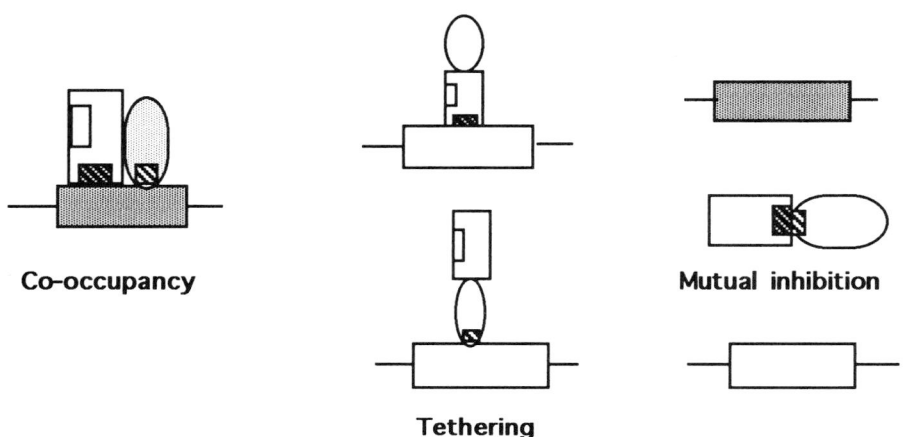

Co-occupancy

Mutual inhibition

Tethering

FIG. 4. Regulation of gene expression by DNA-binding proteins. Steroid hormones bind to receptors that interact with simple response elements in promoter regions of certain genes and with composite response elements in promoter regions of other genes. Composite response elements require CREB or another DNA-binding protein that does not bind steroids. Complex response elements involve cooccupancy by two different DNA binding proteins, but these proteins can also interact with each other, including tethering or mutual inhibition. Adapted from Miner and Yamamoto (48).

events: for example, the facilitation of non-N-methyl-D-aspartate (non-NMDA) receptor activity by estradiol in hippocampal neurons; the promotion of calcium mobilization by progesterone in spermatozoa.

From these and other examples, it appears that membrane actions of steroids may be quite common. Nevertheless, there are also actions of steroids on neural excitability that are rapid and yet which may be mediated genomically. For example, androgens act on muscle cells to increase acetylcholine-activated ion channels (17), whereas estradiol and progesterone act on myometrial cells to increase potassium and calcium currents (63,78); these effects require hours or days of exposure and are blocked by antagonists of intracellular steroid receptors. Moreover, adrenal steroids have rapid actions (within a

number of minutes) to modulate excitability of hippocampal pyramidal neurons and dentate gyrus granule neurons (30,41). These effects are antagonized by steroid antagonists of the intracellular type I and type II adrenal steroid receptors, implying that they involve a genomic mechanism.

CIRCULATING HORMONES AS MEDIATORS OF CHANGE IN ADULT BRAIN

One of the most important roles of circulating hormones is to coordinate cellular and organ responses during cyclic processes such as reproduction and daily sleep–wake activity by synchronizing neural activity and behavior with processes throughout the body. Circulating hormones complement the actions of neural connections and release of neurotransmitters, although neural actions are rapid, hormone actions have longer lasting influences and can affect tissues independently of whether they are innervated, provided that they have hormone receptors. Gonadal hormones act both in the brain and peripherally to coordinate the timing of mating with the optimal chance for pregnancy, and adrenal hormones play a key role both peripherally and centrally in coordinating energy metabolism with food-seeking behavior and cognitive alertness.

Reproductive Behavior

The capacity for reproduction is usually tied to cycles: seasonal in some species, monthly in humans and primates, and on the order of a few days in rats and mice. The ovarian cycle of the female is the key for successful reproduction. For the rat, synchronizing the time of ovulation with the time of behavioral sexual receptivity and preparation of the reproductive tract for pregnancy is the function of circulating estradiol and progesterone. Although many aspects of reproduction have been intensively investigated by endocrinologists, reproductive behavior has been the province of behavioral scientists, that is, until the past two decades, when behavioral neuroscience has emerged and moved ever closer to the cellular, molecular, anatomical, and neurophysiological aspects of neuroscience and to cellular and molecular endocrinology. Studies of the rat have been particularly useful in elucidating brain mechanisms underlying reproductive behavior (60).

The 4- or 5-day estrous cycle of the female rat is tightly coupled to the diurnal clock, and increasing levels of estradiol during the initial phase of the cycle serve to amplify a diurnal peak of luteinizing hormone (LH) secretion so that, on the afternoon of proestrus, this peak becomes the LH surge, which is the immediate stimulus for ovulation. The LH surge also stimulates a surge of ovarian progesterone release; the progesterone synergizes with the prior secretion of estradiol to trigger neural mechanisms subserving the mating response of the female rat, namely, lordosis behavior (60).

What makes the rat particularly advantageous for the study of brain mechanisms underlying reproductive behavior is the importance of a pair of hypothalamic nuclei for the hormonal control of lordosis. Lordosis behavior is primed by estradiol acting in various neural sites, principally the ventromedial nuclei (VMN) of the hypothalamus. Estradiol priming acts via genomic receptors in the cell nuclei of VMN neurons to induce a number of fundamental changes in these cells (39):

Cellular Processes in Ventromedial Nuclei Regulated by Estradiol and Progesterone in Relation to Lordosis Behavior

1. *Rapid increase of RNA synthesis.* Within 2 h after estradiol, VMN neurons increase their capacity to make proteins by making more ribosomal RNA (45).
2. *Rapid increase in new synapses.* In the ensuing 24 h to 48 h, these neurons produce new synaptic contacts with as yet unknown afferent neurons; the production of new synapses and their postsynaptic structures, including spines on dendrites, must require some of the new protein synthetic capability of the VMN neurons. However, these new synaptic contacts disappear rapidly during the 24-h period following proestrus and after the progesterone surge, and thus they appear and disappear cyclically during the estrous cycle (20).
3. *Induction of oxytocin receptors.* Concurrently with item 2. above, estradiol also induces VMN neurons to make new oxytocin receptors, and oxytocin appears to be an important neurotransmitter that helps to trigger the lordosis behavior (69).
4. *Induction of progesterone receptors.* Concurrently with these changes, estradiol induced VMN neurons to make more progesterone receptors, and these receptors play a key role in the acute triggering of lordosis behavior by rapid induction of as-yet unidentified proteins (46).
5. *Nongenomic actions of progesterone.* Progesterone also plays another important role in the triggering of lordosis through nongenomic mechanisms: in the VMN, it acts at the membrane level to activate oxytocin receptors and make them functionally active in the right place within the ventromedial hypothalamus (69); and in the midbrain, progesterone produces a nongenomic facilitation of the mating response (122).
6. *Mating activates c-fos expression.* The mating stimulus by the male activates oxytocin-containing neurons in two other hypothalamic regions, the paraventricular nucleus (PVN) and the bed nuclei of the stria terminalis. This activation can be seen by the induction of the protooncogene transcription factor, c-*fos*, in the small (parvocellular) oxytocin neurons of the PVN (18).
7. *Shutdown of lordosis after proestrus.* Following the proestrus occurrence of ovulation and mating, the lordosis system shuts down, and the progesterone surge is believed to play a major role in this event. Progesterone administration produces, sequentially, facilitation and then inhibition of lordosis responding, and protein synthesis inhibitors were shown to block both phases of action (56). A possible correlate of the inhibition is clearance of synapses formed as a result of estrogen

secretion, and recent evidence indicates that progesterone plays an active role in synaptic down-regulation during the estrous cycle (86).

These changes illustrate the types of cellular responses that may characterize the response of other neuronal systems to circulating hormones of the adrenals, gonads, and thyroid gland.

Coordination of Food-seeking, Metabolism, Salt Intake, and Cognition

Adrenal steroid secretion provides an important coordinating mechanism for the sleep–wake transition and for behavior and brain function associated with the waking state. The peak of endogenous adrenocortical secretion precedes the daily waking period in rats and humans— in the early morning for humans and in the late afternoon for nocturnally active rats. Endogenous adrenocortical activity is driven by two largely independent entrainable clocks: one located in the suprachiasmatic nuclei (SCN) is synchronized by the light–dark cycle; the other, whose location is unknown, is entrained by the availability of food (73). When food is available for a restricted time of each day, corticosterone levels anticipate the appearance of food and appear to act as a wake-up signal. When food becomes available continuously, the anticipatory corticosterone (CORT) peak disappears, and the normal light-entrainable rhythm emerges without any evidence of phase shifting (73).

Adrenal steroids are of two types, glucocorticoids, such as corticosterone and cortisol, and mineralocorticoids, such as aldosterone, because of actions to promote gluconeogenesis and sodium retention, respectively. A summary of the effects of adrenal steroids on brain function (43,44) are listed below:

Behavioral and Neurologic Effects

1. Stimulates food intake, especially at the beginning of the waking period.
2. Promotes obesity in genetically prone or brain-lesioned animals.
3. Biphasically modulates hippocampal long-term potentiation and primed-burst potentiation.
4. Increases salt hunger and biphasically regulates blood pressure.

Structural Effects

1. Stabilizes dentate gyrus granule neurons - prevents increased cell death and de novo neurogenesis.
2. Facilitates atrophy of dendrites of hippocampal CA3 pyramidal neurons.

3. Promotes pyramidal neuronal loss during aging and as a result of chronic stress.
4. Promotes hippocampal CA1 and subiculum damage after ischemia.

However, in spite of their names, both classes of steroids play an important role in stimulating food intake as well as facilitating salt intake and regulating blood pressure. Glucocorticoids also promote food intake and metabolism leading to obesity in genetically obese-prone rats and mice, as well as in rodents with hypothalamic lesions that cause obesity. Adrenalectomy markedly reduces the body weight gain and obesity in both situations (for review, see ref. 44). Finally, adrenal steroids play a role in promoting neural activity that optimizes waking cognitive function. Synaptic activity and long-term potentiation in the hippocampus, a brain region involved in learning and memory, are greatest during the waking period of the light–dark cycle in squirrel monkeys and in rats, and bilateral adrenalectomy abolishes this dark–light difference in rats (43). Adrenal steroids exert a biphasic influence on the magnitude of long-term potentiation (LTP) and primed-burst potentiation (PBP), two neurophysiologic processes related to learning: low levels of adrenal steroid potentiate the response, whereas high levels of adrenal steroids inhibit LTP and PBP (14). Two types of adrenal steroid receptors are involved in these effects. The adrenal steroid potentiation of the LTP–PBP response is blocked by an inhibitor of intracellular type I adrenal steroid receptors, whereas the adrenal steroid inhibition of the LTP–PBP response is blocked by an inhibitor of intracellular type II adrenal steroid receptors (41). The symptoms of jet lag may be a consequence, at least in part, of the failure of adrenal steroid secretion to rise at the time of day that would be appropriate to the time zone in which the traveler finds him or herself; as a result, the normal stimulation of metabolism and cognitive function that results from the diurnal cortisol rise early in the morning does not take place until later in the day (see also Chapters 5, 46, and 55, this volume, for related LTP issues).

Steroids Regulate Neuronal Morphology and Neuronal Survival

Adrenal and gonadal steroids exert surprising effects during adult life on the formation and destruction of synapses and on survival of certain nerve cell types and damage to neurons produced by chronic stress, transient ischemia or aging (see the above listing).

Type I adrenal steroid receptors, which are important in regulating LTP, also play an important role in stabilizing the neuronal population of the dentate gyrus, since adrenalectomy has been found to cause death of granule neurons and aldosterone replacement of adrenalectomized rats blocks this neuronal death (for review, see ref. 25). When adrenalectomy stimulates granule neuron death it also accelerates the process of neurogenesis in the dentate gyrus of the adult rats, and new granule neurons are born (25). The functional significance of the neuronal birth and death in the dentate gyrus of the adult rat is presently obscure, but it is conceivable that it is part of a seasonal or even diurnal mechanism by which the number of neurons is changed (72).

The actions of adrenal steroids on dentate gyrus granule neurons are but one example of hormone effects on neuronal morphology. Another example is the regulation of synapse formation by estradiol and progesterone, not only in the VMN in connection with lordosis behavior, but also in the CA1 region of the hippocampus (85,86). Estradiol promotes formation of new excitatory spine synapses on dendrites of CA1 pyramidal neurons, and progesterone actively stimulates the rapid disappearance of these synapses after ovulation; and it does this via intracellular progesterone receptors that are blockable using Ru38486 (86).

Yet another example of morphological plasticity is the damaging effect of adrenal steroids on hippocampal pyramidal neurons. Loss of pyramidal neurons in the hippocampus was first described during aging in the rat. After it was shown that it could be attenuated by adrenalectomy in midlife (33,40), glucocorticoid treatment for 12 weeks was shown to produce pyramidal neuron loss in the hippocampal formation of young adult rats (30). Prolonged social stress was later shown to produce hippocampal neuronal loss in vervet monkeys and tree shrews, and it has been tempting to conclude that stress-induced secretion of glucocorticoids is to blame (see refs. 40 and 43 for review).

However, the probable mechanism for hippocampal neuronal loss is a good deal more complicated. This was first indicated by the finding that neuronal damage produced by the excitotoxin, kainic acid, was potentiated by endogenous and exogenous glucocorticoids. Likewise, ischemic damage to the hippocampus, which also involves excitatory amino acids, is potentiated by glucocorticoids, and excitotoxic effects on hippocampal neurons in cell culture are exacerbated by glucocorticoids in the medium acting at type II glucocorticoid receptors (67).

There are also important regional differences within the hippocampal formation, namely, that ischemic damage is worse in CA1 pyramidal neurons and subiculum, whereas age- and stress-related damage are more pronounced in the CA3 pyramidal layer. One difference between these two regions is that the CA3 neurons receive the mossy fiber input from the dentate gyrus as well as a direct perforant pathway input from the entorhinal cortex, whereas CA1 neurons do not receive the Schaeffer collateral input from the CA3 neurons.

The CA3 neurons are known to be very susceptible to seizure-induced damage. The CA3 neurons also respond to several weeks of repeated restraint stress or to repeated injections of corticosterone by showing atrophy of the apical dendrites of the long-shaft pyramidal neurons. This atrophy does not occur in the basal dendrites and there is no indication of neuronal death. The stress-induced atrophy can be blocked by several types of treatments: (i) interference with release and action of excitatory amino acids by phenytoin; (ii) enhancement of serotonin reuptake by tianeptine, an atypical tricyclic antidepressant drug (36); and (iii) inhibition of adrenal steroid synthesis in response to stress (41). The atrophy of dendrites of CA3 pyramidal neurons may represent the first stage of the degenerative process, or, alternatively, it may represent an adaptive mechanism that is intended to protect the CA3 neurons from overstimulation. Further research is needed to distinguish between these possibilities, but it is clear that the hippocampus is a vulnerable brain structure and that permanent damage can result from severe and prolonged stress, as well as from seizures and ischemia.

Impact of Stressful Experience on the Brain

Another important function of circulating hormones is to mediate responses to external challenges that are frequently stressful to the organism. Natural disasters, manmade disasters such as transportation accidents, military combat, rape, physical trauma, and stressful life events such as job loss, divorce, and death of a loved-one are all occurrences that are not cyclic and produce a huge impact on those who experience them (81).

One of the main roles of hormonal responses to stressful situations is to protect the organism from further damage. The secretion of epinephrine and adrenocortical hormones are the most general hormonal features of the stress response, whereas epinephrine secretion is a rapid reaction and is involved in the fight-or-flight reaction, the role of adrenal steroids is as a second line of defense, helping to restore and repair systems and also preventing the primary reactions, such as epinephrine secretion, from gaining the upper hand. Both inflammation and primary immune responses are examples of rapid reactions to insults to the body, and glucocorticoids contain and counterregulate these actions (50).

Neurochemical systems in the brain follow a similar pattern of primary response to stressors, and glucocorticoids are involved in mediating effects of repeated stress on the brain, which often take the form of a counterregulation of the primary effects of stressful stimulation (see Fig. 5) (43). The production and secretion of corticotropin releasing hormone is a primary response mechanism to stressors, leading to behavioral activation and to the secretion of adrenocorticotropic hormone (ACTH), as well as

Stress Effect   **Glucocorticoid Effect**

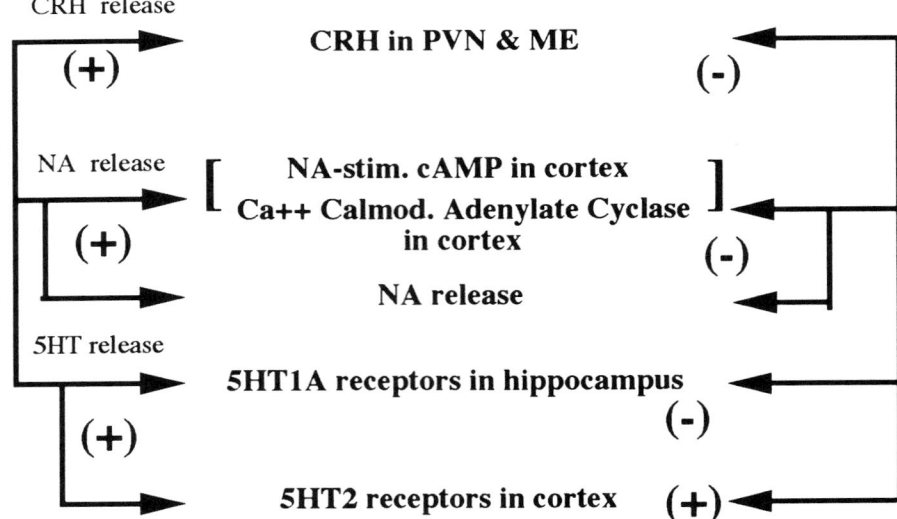

FIG. 5. Scheme for glucocorticoid involvement in mediating or counter-regulating effects of stress on the brain.

immunosuppressive effects. Yet glucocorticoid secretion counterregulates part of this system, particularly the hypothalamic production of corticotropin-releasing hormone (CRH), and keeps this part of the CRH system in check. Likewise, norepinephrine (NE) is released from the locus coeruleus system in response to arousing and stressful stimuli. Repeated stress induces a progressively greater capacity to produce and release NE, because it induces increased production of the rate-limiting enzyme, tyrosine hydroxylase. Glucocorticoids keep this system in check by inhibiting release of catecholamines (55) and by reducing the postsynaptic response to released NE via a suppression of the adenylate cyclase response to NE (see Figure 5) (65). The adenylate cyclase effect is accomplished by at least two mechanisms: (i) a suppression of the α-1 adrenergic receptor-effector system that works cooperatively with beta adrenergic receptors to regulate cyclic adenosine monophosphate (cAMP) production (76); (ii) a suppression of calcium-calmodulin adenylate cyclase activity by a mechanism that does not involve reducing messenger ribonucleic acid (mRNA) production but does involve the actions of glucocorticoids (43).

Another example of adrenal steroid involvement in the effects of repeated stress involves serotonin (5HT). The serotonergic system is turned on by stressful events, and glucocorticoid feedback counterregulates the 5HT1A receptors in the hippocampus (36), but it also up-regulates the 5HT2 receptor in the cerebral cortex (32,43).

As noted above for CRH, 5HT, and NE, adrenal steroid regulation and counterregulation of neurochemical systems occurs in some brain areas and not in others, re-

sulting in an altered balance of various neurotransmitter systems. For example, there are a number of groups of neurons making CRH outside of the hypothalamus that are not counterregulated by glucocorticoids (29,77). Likewise, the counterregulation of cAMP production and adenylate cyclase activity is more pronounced in the cerebral cortex than in the hippocampus (43). On the other hand, the counterregulation of 5HT1A receptors by glucocorticoids is found only in the hippocampus and not in the cerebral cortex, whereas the up-regulation of 5HT2 receptors is found in the cerebral cortex (32,43).

We have also noted that not all aspects of glucocorticoid action involve counterregulation. Acute actions of corticosteroids facilitate the stress-induced activity of the serotonergic system (6) and also potentiate the activity of GABAa-benzodiazepine receptors (57). Both of these effects may be produced by nongenomic actions of steroids (Fig. 2). Whereas the mechanism for activating serotonin formation remains a mystery, the activation of GABAa-benzodiazepine receptors is known to involve the generation of metabolites of desoxycorticosterone, a steroid released by the adrenal cortex during stress, and the interaction of the metabolite, tetrohydrodesoxycorticosterone (THDOC), with a specific site on the chloride channel of the GABAa-benzodiazepine receptor complex to facilitate chloride flux (57).

Thus the interactions of glucocorticoids with the neurochemical systems described above represent an interlocking and carefully balanced system that modulates arousal and excitation and prevents any of these systems from overresponding to stressful stimuli. The protective role of adrenal steroids in relation to behavioral consequences of stress is illustrated by the finding that glucocorticoids, which are anxiolytic, suppress the development of learned helplessness in rats in response to inescapable shock (15). Insofar as learned helplessness is a putative animal model of depressive illness, these results suggest that depression may be regarded as a failure of normal adapation in the face of stressful experiences, in which any one of many neurochemical systems becomes disregulated in relation to other systems (43) (see also Chapters 33, 34, and 39, *this volume,* for related issues).

HORMONES AS MEDIATORS OF DEVELOPMENTAL TRAJECTORIES

Hormone actions in the adult brain are often reversible, as in the case of cyclic changes and adaptive responses to stressors, but they can also be irreversible, as exemplified by the neuronal damage after prolonged stress or repeated elevation of glucocorticoids. Some developmental effects of hormones are permanent, and they are characteristically actions that program the organism to respond in a certain way or within certain limits when it is mature. The actions of thyroid hormone and testosterone on brain development illustrate this important class of hormone effects.

Thyroid Hormone

Thyroid hormone action early in life plays a key role in determining the normal timing of neural development. Either excess or insufficiency of thyroid hormone during early development leads to abnormalities in brain structure. For example, neonatal hyperthyroidism in rats causes hypertrophied development of pyramidal neurons of the CA3 region of hippocampus and of astroglial cells within the hippocampus and basal forebrain (26). The basal forebrain cholinergic system is also permanently increased by transient postnatal hyperthyroidism (82). In contrast, hyperthyroidism in adulthood causes a totally different alteration, namely, a *reduction* in dendritic spine density in the CA1 region of the hippocampus (26).

In spite of hypertrophied CA3 pyramidal neurons and elevated levels of cholinergic neurons in the basal forebrain, developmentally hyperthyroid rats are actually less efficient in learning a spatial maze (58). In contrast, there is a mouse strain in which thyroid hormone treatment at birth improves cognitive performance (70); it may be that this strain suffers from a congenital insufficiency of thyroid hormone at birth, which is counteracted by the transient treatment with thyroid hormone at birth.

Having less thyroid hormone during postnatal life decreases neuronal number in the CA1 pyramidal cell layer of the hippocampus but not in CA3 region (70), although the dendritic and glial morphology of the hippocampus and basal forebrain have so far not been investigated in relation to postnatal hypothyroidism. Based on the effects of hyperthyroidism summarized above, one would predict opposite effects.

Sexual Differentiation

Sexual differentiation of the brain, reproductive tract, and secondary sex characteristics is another major developmental event in which hormones play a determining role. Nurture triumphs over nature, in the sense that testosterone can turn a genetic female into a phenotypic male (see Fig. 6). In mammals, the principle role of the Y chromosome is to determine that the presumptive gonad differentiates into a testis, whereas the presence of two X chromosomes means that ovaries will develop. The testes then secrete testosterone during a specific period of embryonic or neonatal life, whereas the ovary does not secrete any hormones during this time. As a result of the actions of testosterone on a variety of tissues, including the brain, the masculine phenotype becomes differentiated (1).

In the developing human man, there are three phases of testosterone secretion during early life: a testosterone peak at midgestation (12 to 20 weeks), which masculinizes the reproductive tract and probably also the hypothalamus; a second testosterone surge within the first year after birth, which may act on the developing cerebral hemispheres; and a third testosterone elevation at the time of puberty. In the rat, the first two peaks are fused into one, since the rat is born in an immature state; however, there are important distinctions between what happens prenatally and postnatally. Prenatally, testosterone secretion masculinizes the reproductive tract and begins to masculinize the brain, particularly those aspects that govern male sexual and aggressive behavior. Some of the testosterone can reach females in utero. In litters of rats, females lying between two males in utero have greater anogenital distance, indicating exposure to testosterone; in litters of mice, females lying between two males in utero have higher levels of aggressive behavior. However, these females are not sterile and still show sexual behavior and ovulation. Thus, the process of defeminization, which is designed to suppress both sexual behavior and ovulation, has been programmed to occur postnatally to protect females in utero from sterilization (37).

How do we know that the brain undergoes sexual differentiation? Until the late 1960s, the brain was not regarded as different between males and females, but then studies using light microscopy revealed effects of neonatal hormonal manipulations on the size of hypothalamic neurons (59). Then in 1971, a landmark paper was published by Geoffrey Raisman and Pauline Field who used

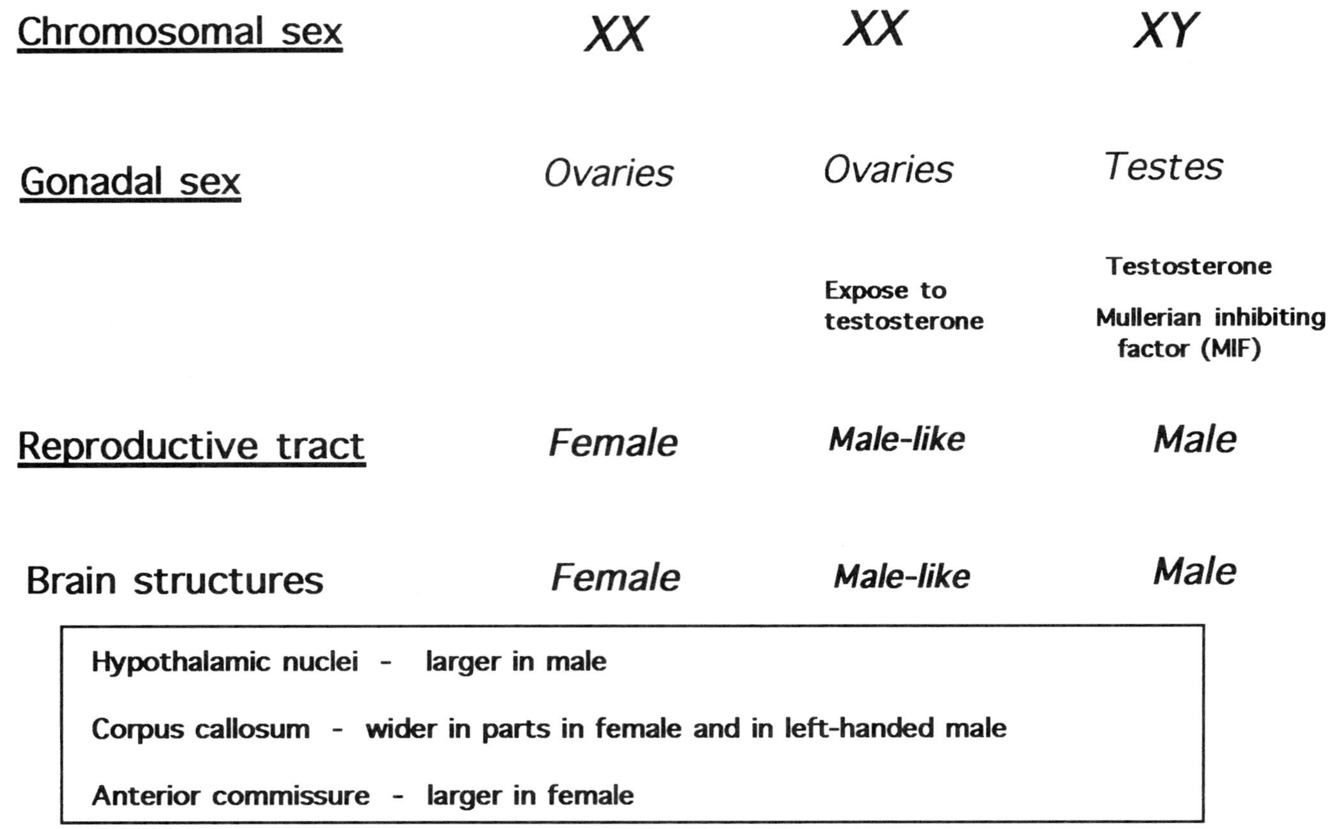

Chromosomal sex	XX	XX	XY
Gonadal sex	Ovaries	Ovaries	Testes
		Expose to testosterone	Testosterone Mullerian inhibiting factor (MIF)
Reproductive tract	Female	Male-like	Male
Brain structures	Female	Male-like	Male

> Hypothalamic nuclei - larger in male
>
> Corpus callosum - wider in parts in female and in left-handed male
>
> Anterior commissure - larger in female

FIG. 6. Diagram of sexual differentiation of gonadal sex, the reproductive tract, and the brain, showing how gonadal sex is determined by genetic sex, but the rest is mediated by the presence or absence of testosterone.

an electron microscope to show morphologic sex differences that are developmentally programmed by testosterone early in postnatal life (61). This study opened the floodgates on light microscopic and neurochemical studies that established numerous sex differences in the brains of rats, songbirds, and other species, including humans (9,75). One of the earliest examples of a morphologic sex difference for mammals was the finding by Gorski et al. (24) that the nucleus of the preoptic areas is sexually dimorphic; Nottebohm and Arnold (51) described sex differences in vocal control areas of the songbird brain. Another important study (19) concerns the sexual dimorphism of the spinal nucleus of the bulbocavernosus muscle, which innervates the penis and is present only in males. The retention of this nucleus during early development is promoted by the presence of androgens, which promote survival of the muscle and of the motor neurons that innervate them; an important question is whether the androgen is acting on the muscle, on the motor neurons, or on both.

Many of the morphologic sex differences have functional correlates (9). In songbirds, the size of brain nuclei that control the production of song are larger in males than in females in accordance with the greater and more complex song production by males. In rats and other species, the male has a spinal motor control nucleus, which innervates the penis; as noted, this nucleus is absent in females (19). In humans, the size of parts of the corpus callosum, as well as the anterior commissure, both of which connect the two cerebral hemispheres, are on the average greater in women than in men (2,4,83). This feature correlates with, and may eventually help to explain, the greater ability of women to overcome congenital defects or brain damage to one cerebral hemisphere by using the other cerebral hemisphere to compensate (28).

Brain sex differences arise through the developmental actions of testosterone (or its metabolite, estradiol) on developing neuronal systems at intracellular androgen and estrogen receptors (9,40). During pre- or early postnatal development, depending on the species, these receptors are expressed permanently in the hypothalamus, preoptic area, and pituitary and transiently in the cerebral cortex and hippocampus (37). The developmental actions of these hormones are the subject of intensive investigation. Neuronal migration and survival are among the processes influenced by hormones that give rise to morphologic sex differences. Hormones also promote differentiation of specific programs of response of neuronal systems when they are mature. For example, the ability of estradiol to induce cyclic synaptogenesis in the ventromedial hypothalamus of the adult female rat is suppressed early in life by the defeminizing actions of testosterone in the male (39).

Brain sex differences have been detected in the human species as differences in size of cell groupings, or nuclei at the hypothalamic level as well as in the size and shape of the corpus callosum and anterior commissure, leading to the conclusion that the process of sexual differentiation operates on the human brain much as it does in lower mammalian species (3,75). However, it is not clear whether the midgestation testosterone peak or the postnatal testosterone elevation is responsible for producing these sex differences.

Moreover, it is difficult to specify the behavioral or neurologic traits that are associated with morphologic sex differences. Play behavior of children has been studied with regard to boy–girl differences in energy level and choice of play styles and toys, by analogy with studies in rhesus monkeys and rats showing that males engage in more rough-and-tumble play (16). However, attribution of sex differences in behavior to developmental hormonal influences is virtually impossible owing to the many social factors that contribute to play behavior in children. A more objective endpoint has been spatial learning, as in the mental rotation of figures test. Here, men outperform women significantly. However, just as there is overlap in brain morphologic traits between men and women, so is there overlap in test scores on the mental rotation test, so that sex differences in mean measures should not obscure the fact that there is much overlap between the sexes (32). Nevertheless, some data show a developmental endocrine influence on this test. In the adrenogenital syndrome (AGS), genetic females with an enzyme defect in adrenal steroid production produce androgens that masculinize the fetus; normally the masculinized genitalia of AGS girls is surgically corrected at birth and these individuals are raised as girls (16). Nevertheless, there is clearcut data showing a mean performance by AGS girls on mental rotation of figures tests that approximates that of normal males (79).

Evidence for normal sex differences in human brain morphology led three research groups to examine the brains of homosexual men who had died of AIDS for evidence of differences from heterosexual men. The first study revealed that the suprachiasmatic nucleus of homosexual men was larger than that of heterosexual men, even though there was not a marked sex difference in the SCN volume (74). The second study showed that homosexual men have a smaller interstitital nucleus of the anterior hypothalamus (INAH3) than heterosexual men, resembling the size of this nucleus in women (34). The third study showed that homosexual men have a larger anterior commissure than heterosexual men, which even exceeds the somewhat larger area found in women. In none of the three studies did AIDS appear to affect the results, since heterosexual individuals who died of AIDS showed the same size of these structures typical of their sex (5). It is not possible to say what behavioral features these differences in three brain structures may serve, but the existence of such differences between the brains of homosexual and heterosexual men raise the interesting possibility that a biological substrate exists for the differences in sexual preference and lifestyle. Needless to say, the results must be taken provisionally until other investigators have confirmed the essential findings on other groups of brains.

EMERGING CONCEPTS

Having covered specific information concerning the major types of hormone effects on the brain, it is time to note some of the concepts that these examples illustrate. First, it is evident from studies of hormone action that *the brain changes all the time, not just during early development, but also in adult life.* Cyclic changes, within the 4- to 5-day-estrous cycle of the female rat, in synaptogenesis in hypothalamus and CA1 neurons of hippocampus, controlled by estradiol and progesterone, are a dramatic illustration of reversible alterations. Other examples of irreversible changes are those produced by stress on the hippocampus or the increased cell death of dentate gyrus granule neurons following adrenalectomy. These structural changes, together with reversible induction and down-regulation of neurotransmitter and peptide systems and their receptors by hormones and by other agents, illustrate the dynamic nature of the brain.

It is evident from the analysis of hormone effects on brain that *many of these actions differ across developmental stage as well as among brain regions.* Estrogen actions during early postnatal development mediate the effects of testosterone on brain sexual differentiation, and one of the consequences of sexual differentiation of the rat hypothalamus is the reprogramming of how the adult hypothalamus will respond to estradiol in adult life; for example, the ability of estradiol to induce progesterone receptors or to elicit synapse formation in the adult hypothalamus is markedly suppressed in the male. An example of brain regional differences in hormone action is the protective action of adrenal steroids on dentate gyrus neurons, blocking programmed cell death, whereas neighboring hippocampal pyramidal neurons are not affected in this way by the presence or absence of adrenal steroids. Both dentate gyrus granule neurons and hippocampal pyramidal neurons have both types of adrenal steroid receptors, so one cannot predict what effect the relevant hormone will have simply on the basis of what hormone receptors are present.

We have also seen that *developmental effects often bias or determine an adult response.* One example, already cited above, is how the process of sexual differentiation suppresses the ability of the adult hypothalamus to respond to estradiol in showing progesterone receptor induction and synaptogenesis. Another illustration is how developmental hyperthyroidism alters not only basal forebrain and hippocampal morphology but also compromises the efficiency of radial maze learning in adult life (58).

Finally, it is possible to suggest that *hormones participate in the expression of individual as well as group differences.* The thyroid hormone example cited above shows, in principle, how deviations in normal thyroid hormone levels during early development can help to determine not only morphology but also learning ability on an individual basis. Likewise, the effects of prenatal stress (21) and postnatal handling (47) have shown long-term influences on emotionality (21) as well as the rate at which the hippocampus ages (47). There is evidence in infrahuman primates that prenatal stress can lead to impairments in motor coordination and attention span and that adrenal steroids may participate in these effects (69). Finally, sex hormones play a major role in determination of sex (i.e., group) differences in brain structure, neurochemistry, and certain features of behavior, and there is the intriguing possibility that sexual orientation, which can be regarded as an individual trait but also as a subgroup of human sexual behavior, may also involve a combination of hormonal, genetic, and experiential factors (see also Chapters 55, 59, and 60, *this volume*).

CONCLUSIONS

A final question remains, namely, what is the relevance of hormone actions on the brain to human and animal pathophysiology and, in particular, to nervous and mental disorders? We consider these in order of some of the major types of hormone effects: cyclic processes, sex differences, and the effects of stress.

Cyclic disorders include catamenial epilepsy, premenstrual tension, and jet lag. Catamenial epilepsy varies according to the menstrual cycle, with the peak frequency of occurrence corresponding to the lowest ratio of progesterone to estradiol during the cycle (12,27). Bearing in mind that there is some genetic and/or developmental predisposition to express seizures, there may be at least three types of hormone actions involved in the cyclic occurrence of epilepsy: (i) estrogen induction of excitatory synapses in hippocampus, leading to decreased seizure thresholds (85); (ii) progesterone actions via the steroid metabolites that act via the GABAa receptor to decrease excitability (38); and (iii) hormone actions on

the liver to increase clearance rates of antiseizure medication (27).

Premenstrual tension is a cyclic mood disorder, which is referred to as premenstrual syndrome (PMS) in its most severe form, and it symptoms are eliminated by arresting the menstrual cycle (13). However, specific hormonal causes are unknown (65). Although there are indications that high luteal-phase estrogen and progesterone levels may exacerbate symptoms of PMS, the administration of a gonadotropin-releasing hormone agonist along with low amounts of estradiol and progesterone to prevent ovarian hormone deficiency has been reported to alleviate symptoms of PMS (13).

As far as jet lag is concerned, one of the causal factors for malaise and cognitive dysfunction may be that cortisol is secreted according to the time zone of origin rather than the time zone of destination, that is, until the diurnal clock is entrained to the local light–dark cycle (43). The diurnal cycle involves shifting thresholds of vulnerability, as, for example, with an increased frequency of heart attacks occurring in the morning hours (42). Moreover, shift work alters risk factors for cardiovascular disease as well as the sense of well-being (54).

Sex differences play a significant role in the occurrence of diseases. Besides the well-known predominance of cardiovascular disease in men over premenopausal women, men also have more frequent developmental learning disorders (28). Also mental disorders differ in occurrence between the sexes according to type: Anxiety disorders and depression are more common in women; substance abuse and antisocial behavior are more prevalent in men (62). Schizophrenia, however, is equally prevalent in men and women (62), but estrogens play an important role in containing dopaminergic function and reducing the severity of symptoms in younger women (10). Moreover, different doses of neuroleptic drugs are required for treating schizophrenia in women and men, depending on the presence of circulating estrogens, and there are sex differences in the type and severity of symptoms and response to treatment (71). Likewise, Parkinson's disease is more severe in women with circulating estrogens, reflecting antidopaminergic actions of estradiol in the face of dopaminergic hypofunction (10). One of the important lessons of these examples is that men and women must be studied separately for the actions of psychotropic drugs, including antidepressants as well as antipsychotics and benzodiazepines, because differences in circulating hormone levels or intrinsic, developmentally programmed sex differences may bias the mechanisms by which these pharmaceutical agents act on the brain.

In addition to the cardiovascular system, the brain also may be differentially vulnerable to severe stress in men and women. Both severe social stress in vervet monkeys (79) and cold swim stress in rats (49) damage the hippocampus of males but not of females. Again, it may be differences in circulating hormone levels or intrinsic sex differences that will explain these sex differences.

Stress is a factor in exacerbating symptoms of a number of diseases, such as atherosclerosis, asthma, diabetes, gastrointestinal disorders, as well as resistance to viral infections and metastasis of tumors (42,81). However, it is not always clear what aspects of stressful experience contribute to the pathological process, and it is likely that both chronic and acute stress is involved. For example, chronic stress appears to facilitate development of atherosclerotic plaques (36), whereas acute stress may precipitate myocardial infarction (42).

We have made the point several times throughout the article that hormones participate in determining the expression of individual differences, possibly by regulating the expression of genetic factors that contribute to or determine the vulnerability to a disease. This attractive notion remains hypothetical; support for it requires the elucidation of specific mechanisms by which hormones affect normal brain function as well as mechanisms by which the endocrine system participates in the development of pathologic states. This chapter has provided glimpses into specific mechanisms for sex, stress, and thyroid hormone actions on diverse neural mechanisms and structural changes, which can provide guidelines for future investigations.

ACKNOWLEDGMENT

Research in the author's laboratory for work described in this chapter is supported by NIH Grants NS 07080, MH 41256, and MH 43787.

REFERENCES

1. Adkins-Regan E. Early organizational effects of hormones. In: Adler NT, ed. *Neuroendocrinology of reproduction.* New York: Plenum Press; 1981:159–228.
2. Allen L, Richey M, Chai Y, Gorski R. Sex differences in the corpus callosum of the living human being. *J Neurosci* 1991;11:933–942.
3. Allen L, Hines M, Shryne J, Gorski R. Two sexually dimorphic cell groups in the human brain. *J Neurosci* 1989;9:497–506.
4. Allen L, Gorski R. Sexual dimorphism of the anterior commissure and massa intermeida of the human brain. *J Comp Neurol* 1991; 312:97–104.
5. Allen L, Gorski R. Sexual orientation and the size of the anterior commissure in the human brain. *PNAS* 1992;89:7199–7202.
6. Azmitia E, McEwen BS. Adrenocortical influence on rat brain tryptophan hydroxylase activity. *Brain Res* 1974;78:291–302.
7. Baulieu EE. Steroid hormones in the brain: several mechanisms? In: Fuxe K, ed. *Steroid hormone regulation of the brain.* Oxford and New York: Pergamon Press; 1981:3–14.
8. Baulieu EE. Neurosteroids: a function of the brain In: Costa E, Paul SM, eds. *Neurosteroids and brain function,* New York: Thieme; 1991:63–73.
9. Becker J, Breedlove SM, Crews D, eds. *Behavioral endocrinology.* MIT Press:Cambridge; 1992:574.
10. Bedard P, Langelier P, Villeneuve A. Oestrogens and extrapyramidal system. *Lancet* 1977;24, 31:1367–1368.
11. Blackmore PF, Neulen J, Lattanzio F, Beebe SJ. Cell surface

12. Bonuccelli U, Melis GB, Paoletti AM, Fioretti P, Murri L, Muratoria A. Unbalanced progesterone and estradiol secretion in catamenial epilepsy. *Epilepsy Res* 1989;3:100–106.
13. DeVane GW. Editorial: premenstrual syndrome. *J Clin Endocrinol Metab.* 1991;72:250–251.
14. Diamond DM, Bennet MC, Fleshner M, Rose GM. Inverted-U relationship between the level of peripheral corticosterone and the magnitude of hippocampal primed burst potentiation. *Hippocampus* 1992;2:421–430.
15. Edwards E, Harkins K, Wright G, Henn F. Effects of bilateral adrenalectomy on the induction of learned helplessness behavior. *Neuropsychopharmacology* 1990;3:109–114.
16. Ehrhardt AA. Behavioral sequellae of prenatal hormonal exposure in animals and man. In: Lipton MA, DeMascio A, Killam KF, eds. *Psychopharmacology: a generation of progress.* New York: Raven Press; 1978:531–539.
17. Erulkar SD, Wetzel DM. 5 alpha dihydrotestosterone has nonspecific effects on membrane channels and possible genomic effects on ACh-activated channels. *J Neurophysiol* 1989;61:1036–1052.
18. Flanagan L, Pfaus J, Pfaff D, McEwen, BS. Induction of fos immunoreactivity in oxytocin neurons after sexual activity in female rats. *Neuroendocrinology* 1993;58:352–358.
19. Forger NG and Breedlove SM. Steroid influences on a mammalian neuromuscular system. *Seminars Neurosci* 1991;3:459–468.
20. Frankfurt M, Gould E, Woolley CS, McEwen BS. Gonadal steroids modify dendritic spine density in ventromedial hypothalamic neurons: a Golgi study in the adult rat. *Neuroendocrinology* 1990;51: 530–535.
21. Fride E, Dan Y, Feldon J, Halevy G, Weinstock M. Effects of prenatal stress on vulnerability to stress and prepubertal and adult rats. *Physiol Behav* 1986;37:681–687.
22. Frye CA, Mermelstein PG, DeBold JF. Evidence for a non-genomic action of progestins on sexual receptivity in hamster ventral tegmental area but not hypothalamus. *Brain Res* 1992;578:87–93.
23. Gee K. Steroid modulation of the GABA/benzodiazepine receptor-linked chloride ionophore. *Mol Neurobiol* 1988;2:291–317.
24. Gorski RA, Gordon JH, Shryne JE, Southam AM. Evidence for a morphological sex differences within the medial preoptic area of the rat brain. *Brain Res* 1978;148:333–346.
25. Gould E, McEwen BS. Neuronal birth and death. *Curr Opin Neurobiol* 1993;3:676–682.
26. Gould E, Woolley C, McEwen BS. The hippocampal formation: morphological changes induced by thyroid, gonadal and adrenal hormones. *Psychoneuroendocrinology* 1991;16:67–84.
27. Herzog AG. Reproductive endocrine considerations and hormonal therapy for women with epilepsy. *Epilepsy* 1991;62(Suppl.6): S27–S33.
28. Hier D. Sex differences in hemispheric specialization: hypothesis for the excess of dyslexia in boys. *Bull Orton Soc* 1979;29:74–83.
29. Imaki T, Nahan J, Rivier C, Sawchenko P, Vale W. Differential regulation of corticotrophin-releasing factor mRNA in rat brain regions by glucocorticoids and stress. *J Neurosci* 1991;11:585–599.
30. Joels M, DeKloet ER. Control of neuronal excitability by corticosteroid hormones. *Trends Neurosci* 1992;15:25–30.
31. Kimura D. Sex differences in the brain. *Sci Amer* 1992;267: 119–125.
32. Kuroda Y, Mikuni M, Ogawa T, Takahashi K. Effect of ACTH, adrenalectomy and the combination treatment of the density of 5-HT2 receptor binding sites in neocortex of rat forebrain and 5-HT2 receptor-mediate wet-dog shake behaviors. *Psychopharmacology* 1992;108:27–32.
33. Landfield P. Modulation of brain aging correlates by long-term alterations of adrenal steroids and neurally-active peptides. *Prog Brain Res* 1987;72:279–300.
34. LeVay S. A difference in hypothalamic structure between heterosexual and homosexual men. *Science* 1991;253:1036–1038.
35. Madeira M, Sousa N, Lima-Andrade M, Calheiros F, Cadete-Leite A, Paula-Barbosa M. Selective vulnerability of the hippocampal pyramidal neurons to hypothyroidism in male and female rats. *J Comp Neurol* 1992;322:501–518.
36. Manuck SB, Kaplin JR, Adams MR, Clarkson TB. Studies of psy-

binding sites for progesterone mediate calcium uptake in human sperm, *J Biol Chem* 1990;199:1266:18655.

chosocial influences on coronary artery atherosclerosis in cynomolgus monkeys. *Health Psychol* 1988;7:113–124.

37. McEwen BS. Actions of sex hormones on the brain: "organization" and "activation" in relation to functional teratology. *Prog Brain Res* 1988;73:121–134.

38. McEwen BS. Non-genomic and genomic effects of steroids on neural activity. *TIPS* 1991;112:141–147.

39. McEwen BS. Our changing ideas about steroid effects on an everchanging brain. *Seminars Neurosci* 1991;3:497–507.

40. McEwen BS. Re-examination of the glucocorticoid hypothesis of stress and aging. *Prog Brain Res* 1992;93:365–383.

41. McEwen BS, Cameron H, Chao HM, Gould E, Luine VN, Magarinos A-M, Pavlides C, Spencer RL, Watanabe Y, Woolley C. Resolving a mystery: progress in understanding the function of adrenal steroid receptors in hippocampus. *Prog Brain Res* 1994;100:[*in press*].

42. McEwen BS, Stellar E. Stress and the individual: mechanisms leading to disease. *Arch Intern Med.* 1993;153:2093–2101.

43. McEwen B, Angulo J, Cameron H, et al. Paradoxical effects of adrenal steroids on the brain: protection versus degeneration. *Biol Psychiatry* 1992;31:177–179.

44. McEwen BS, Spencer RL, Sakai RR. Adrenal steroid actions upon the brain: versatile hormones with good and bad effects. In: Schulkin J, ed. *Hormonally induced changes in mind and brain*, New York: Academic Press, 1993.

45. McEwen BS, Jones KJ, Pfaff DW. Hormonal control of sexual behavior in the female rat: molecular, cellular and neurochemical studies. *Biol Reprod* 1987;36:37–45.

46. McEwen BS, Biegon A, Davis P, Krey L, Luine V, McGinnis M, Paden C, Parsons B, Rainbow T. Steroid hormones: humoral signals which alter brain cell properties and functions. *Recent Progr Hormone Res* 1982;38:41–92, New York: Academic Press.

47. Meaney M, Mitchell J, Aitken D, et al. The effects of neonatal handling on the development of the adrenocortical response to stress: implications for neuropathology and cognitive deficit later in life. *Psychoneuroendocrinology* 1991;16:85–103.

48. Miner J, Yamamoto K. Regulatory crosstalk at composite response elements. *TIBS* 1991;16:423–426.

49. Mizoguchi K, Kunishita T, Chui D-H, Tabira T. Stress induces neuronal death in the hippocampus of castrated rats. *Neurosci Lett* 1992;138:157–160.

50. Munck A, Guyre P, Holbrook N. Physiological functions of glucocorticoids in stress and their relation to pharmacological actions. *Endocrin Rev* 1984;5:25–44.

51. Nottebohm F, Arnold AP. Sexual dimorphism in vocal control areas of the songbird brain. *Science* 1976;194:211–213.

52. Orchinik M, Murray TF, Moore FL. A corticosteroid receptor in neuronal membranes. *Science* 1991;252:1848.

53. Orchinik M, Murray TF, Franklin PH, Moore FL. Guanyl nucleotides modulate binding to steroid receptors in neuronal membranes. *Proc Natl Acad Sci USA* 1992;89:3830.

54. Orth-Gomer K. Intervention on coronary risk factors by adapting a shift work schedule to biologic rhythmicity. *Psychosom Med.* 1983;45:407–415.

55. Pacak K, Kvetnansky R, Palkovits M, Fukuhara K, Yadid G, Kopin IJ, Goldstein DS. Adrenalectomy augments in vivo release of norepinephrine in the paraventricular nucleus during immobilization stress. *Endocrinology* 1993;133:1404–1410.

56. Parsons B, McEwen BS. Sequential inhibition of sexual receptivity by progesterone is prevented by a protein synthesis inhibitor and is not causally related to decreased levels of hypothalamic progestin receptors in the female rat. *J. Neurosci* 1981;1:527.

57. Paul S, Purdy R. Neuroactive steroids. *FASEB J* 1992;6:2311–2322.

58. Pavlides C, Westlind-Danielsson A, Nyborg H, McEwen BS. Neonatal hyperthyroidism disrupts hippocampal LTP and spatial learning. *Exp Brain Res* 1991;85:559–564.

59. Pfaff DW. Morphological changes in the brains of adult male rats after neonatal castration. *J Endocrinol* 1966;36:415–416.

60. Pfaff DW. *Estrogens and brain function*. New York: Springer-Verlag; 1980.

61. Raisman G, Field P. Sexual dimorphism in the preoptic area of the rat. *Science* 1971;173:731–733.

62. Regier DA, Boyd JH, Burke JD, et al. One-month prevalence of mental disorders in the United States. *Arch Gen Psychiatry* 1988;45:977–986.

63. Rendt JM, Toro L, Stefani E, Erulkar SD. Progesterone increases Ca currents in myometrial cells from immature and nonpregnant adult rats. *Am J Physiol* 1992;262:C293–C301.

64. Resnick S, Gottesman I, Berenbaum S, Bouchard T. Early hormonal influences on cognitive functioning in congenital adrenal hyperplasia. *Dev Psychol* 1986;22:191–198.

65. Rubinow DR. The premenstrual syndrome: new views. *JAMA* 1992;268:1908–1912.

66. Sapolsky R, Krey L, McEwen BS. Prolonged glucocorticoid exposure reduces hippocampal neuron number: implications for aging. *J Neurosci* 1985;5:1222–1227.

67. Sapolsky R. *Stress, the aging brain and the mechanisms of neuron death.* Cambridge, MA: The MIT Press; 1992:423.

68. Schneider ML, Coe CL, Lubach GR. Endocrine activation mimics the adverse effects of prenatal stress on the neuromotor development of the infant primate. *Devel Psychobiol* 1992;25:427–439.

69. Schumacher M, Coirini H, Pfaff DW, McEwen BS. Behavioral effects of progesterone associated with rapid modulation of oxytocin receptors. *Science* 1990;250:691–694.

70. Schwegler H, Crusio WE, Lipp H-P, Brust I, Mueller GG. Early postnatal hyperthyroidism alters hippocampal circuitry and improves radial-maze learning in adult mice. *J Neurosci* 1991;11:2102–2106.

71. Seeman MV, Lang M. The role of estrogens in schizophrenia gender differences. *Schizophrenia Bull* 1990;16:185–194.

72. Sherry DF, Jacobs LF, Gaulin SJ. Spatial memory and adaptive specialization of the hippocampus. *Trends Neurosci* 1992;15:298–303.

73. Stephan F. Coupling between feeding- and light-entrainable circadian pacemakers in the rat. *Physiol Behav* 1986;38:537–544.

74. Swaab D, Hofman M. An enlarged suprachiasmatic nucleus in homosexual men. *Brain Res* 1990;537:141–148.

75. Swaab D, Gooren L, Hofman M. The human hypothalamus in relation to gender and sexual orientation. *Prog Brain Res* 1992;93:205–219.

76. Stone E, McEwen B, Herrera, Carr K. Regulation of alpha and beta components of noradrenergic cyclic AMP responses in cortical slices. *Eur J Pharmacol* 1987;141:347–356.

77. Swanson LW, Simmons DM. Differential steroid hormone and neural influences on peptide mRNA levels in CRH cells of the paraventricular nucleus: a hybridization histochemical study in the rat. *J Comp Neurol* 1989;285:413–435.

78. Toro L, Stefani E, Erulkar SD. Hormonal regulation of potassium currents in single myometrial cells. *Proc Nat Acad Sci USA* 1990;87:2892–2895.

79. Uno H, Ross T, Else J, Suleman M, Sapolsky R. Hippocampal damage associated with prolonged and fatal stress in primates. *J Neurosci* 1989;9:1705–1711.

80. Wehling M, Christ M, Thiesen K. Membrane receptors for aldosterone: a novel pathway for mineralocorticoid action. *Am J Physiol* 1992;263:E974.

81. Weiner H. *Perturbing the organism: the biology of stressful experience.* Chicago: University of Chicago Press; 1992:35.

82. Westlind-Danielsson A, Gould E, McEwen BS. Thyroid hormone causes sexually distinct neurochemical and morphological alterations in rat septal-diagonal band neurons. *J Neurochem* 1990;56:119–128.

83. Witelson S. Hand and sex differences in the isthmus and genu of the human corpus callosum. *Brain* 1989;112:799–835.

84. Wong M, Moss RL. Long-term and short-term electrophysiological effects of estrogen on the synaptic properties of hippocampal CA1 neurons. *J Neurosci* 1992;12:3217.

85. Woolley C, McEwen BS. Estradiol mediates fluctuation in hippocampal synapse density during the estrous cycle in the adult rat. *J Neurosci* 1992;12:2549–2554.

86. Woolley C, McEwen BS. Roles of estradiol and progesterone in regulation of hippocampal dendritic spine density during the estrous cycle in the rat. *J Comp Neurol* 1993;336(2):293–306.

Psychopharmacology: The Fourth Generation of Progress, edited by Floyd E. Bloom and David J. Kupfer. Raven Press, Ltd., New York © 1995.

CHAPTER **63**

Interactions Between the Nervous System and the Immune System

Implications for Psychopharmacology

Adrian J. Dunn

Interaction between the nervous and immune systems provides a physiological basis for psychosomatic medicine. In approximately 200 AD, the Greek author Galen wrote that melancholic women are more susceptible to breast cancer than sanguine women. Since then, a wealth of anecdotal evidence has convinced physicians of the importance of psychological factors in the prognosis of disease. This belief is now bolstered by substantial evidence that nervous system output can indeed modulate immune function. However, the interactions are not unidirectional. The immune system can also have powerful influences on the nervous system. This should not be surprising to anyone who has ever felt sick. Anomalies of immune system function can certainly cause diseases of the nervous system, and this may be manifest in psychiatric disease. It is clear that effective defense against infections requires a complex coordination of the activities of the nervous and immune systems, and that abnormalities in the relationships between the two systems can cause disease (see also Chapters 43, 55, 84, and 85, *this volume*).

EVIDENCE FOR INTERACTIONS BETWEEN THE NERVOUS AND IMMUNE SYSTEMS

The interactions of the nervous system and the immune system have been the subject of a number of critical reviews (e.g., 20) and several books, of which the most recent comprehensive text is that edited by Ader et al. (2).

A. J. Dunn: Department of Pharmacology and Therapeutics, Louisiana State University Medical Center, Shreveport, Louisiana 71130.

The experimental evidence for nervous system–immune system interactions can be summarized:

1. Alterations in immune responses can be conditioned.
2. Electrical stimulation or lesions of specific brain sites can alter immune function.
3. Stress alters immune responses and the growth of tumors and infections in experimental animals.
4. Activation of the immune system is correlated with altered neurophysiological, neurochemical, and neuroendocrine activities of brain cells.

This evidence is discussed below, but it is pertinent to consider first what the potential links between the nervous and immune systems might be. Classical medical teaching leaves little scope for interactions between the nervous and immune systems, but with the benefit of hindsight we can postulate a number of specific mechanisms by which the nervous system might affect immune function. These include glucocorticoids secreted from the adrenal cortex, catecholamines secreted from sympathetic nerve terminals and the adrenal medulla, other hormones secreted by the pituitary and other endocrine organs, and peptides (including endorphins) secreted by the adrenal medulla and autonomic nerve terminals. The network includes not only the autonomic nervous system and classical neuroendocrine mechanisms, but involves an endocrine function of the immune system. A variety of immune system products (e.g., cytokines,[1] peptides, and

---

[1] The cytokines are a large group of proteins that were originally identified as products of immune cells that functioned as chemical messengers between cells of the immune system. They are now known to be synthesized by a variety of different cell types in the body and can have a very wide range of actions on many organ systems. The cytokines include the interleukins (of which there are at least 13), the interferons, tumor necrosis factors, and a variety of cell growth-stimulating factors.

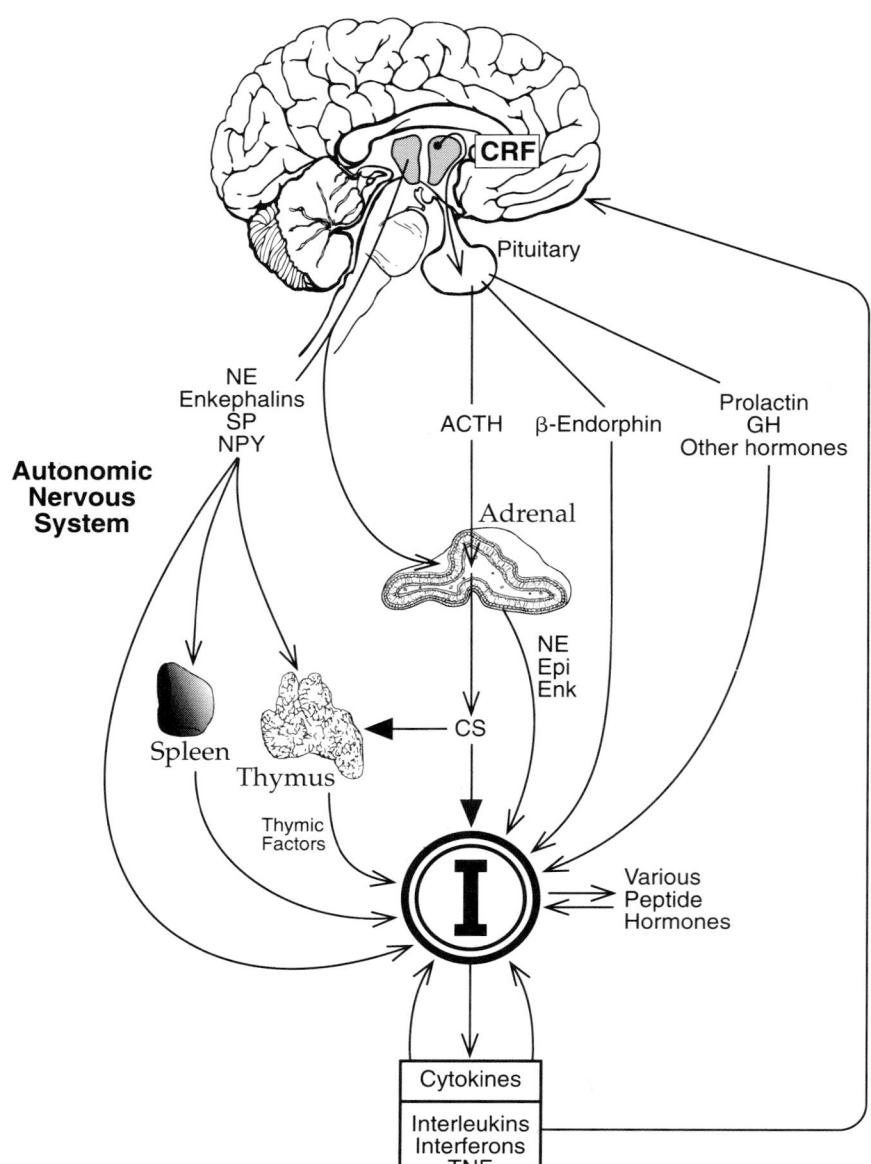

FIG. 1. A schematic diagram of the interactions between the brain and components of the endocrine and immune systems. The ability of the brain to alter immune system function by a variety of endocrine pathways and the autonomic nervous system is emphasized, and the effects of peptides and cytokines produced by the immune system on immune cells and the brain is indicated. Abbreviations: CRF, corticotropin-releasing factor; CS, corticosteroids; Enk, enkephalins; Epi, epinephrine; GH, growth hormone; I, immunocytes; NE, norepinephrine; NPY, neuropeptide Y; SP, substance P; TNF, tumor necrosis factor.

other factors) that function to coordinate the immune response may also provide important signals for the nervous system. Thus chemical messengers can account for a variety of interactions between the nervous system and the immune system. Figure 1 provides a schematic of the most well-known interactions between the nervous system and components of the endocrine and immune systems.

CONDITIONING OF THE IMMUNE RESPONSE

Compelling evidence for an influence of the nervous system on the immune system arises from studies that indicate that behavioral conditioning can modify immune responses. Many early observations suggested this, but more recent studies have provided strong experimental support (see ref. 1). A landmark study by Ader and Cohen published in 1975 found that after the immunosuppressive drug, cyclophosphamide, had been paired with the taste of saccharin, subsequent ingestion of the saccharin prevented the production of antibodies in response to sheep red blood cell (SRBC) administration (1). These findings were not greeted with universal enthusiasm; many immunologists were reluctant to accept the notion that immune system function could be regulated by the brain. However, the original findings were replicated and extended by the original authors and others. The technique has been used to prolong the lives of mice with the autoimmune disease lupus erythematosus. Thus far, there have only been reports of conditioned augmentation of immune activity from one research group, and the effects have been small. There can be little doubt that conditioning can alter immune responses, but the immunological specificity of the effects is not clear, and the mechanisms are as yet unknown. It is possible that at least some of the immunosuppressive effects are from a conditioning of hormone and neurotransmitter secretion (e.g., glucocorticoids or catecholamines).

EFFECTS OF BRAIN LESIONS ON IMMUNE FUNCTION

Although many studies have indicated that brain lesions have an effect on immunity, the literature is exceptionally fragmented and complex (see ref. 70). Effective lesions are most commonly located in the hypothalamus and are generally inhibitory. Lesions in other limbic areas may also be effective, notably in the septum, hippocampus, and amygdala. Some studies have indicated that cortical lesions can affect immune responses and that the effects depend upon the laterality of the lesion. Renoux et al. have reported evidence that lesions of the left cortex, but not the right, produced pronounced immune deficits in spleen cell number, lymphocyte proliferation, and natural killer (NK) cell activity (68). The lateral specificity indicates that the effect cannot be from nonspecific effects of the lesion, and it could account for the greater number of left-handed individuals who exhibit diseases of the immune system. Lesions of the central noradrenergic systems have also been shown to impair various aspects of the immune response.

EFFECTS OF STRESS ON THE IMMUNE SYSTEM

Everybody knows that stress impairs the immune system, but the truth is probably much more complicated. Certainly chronic stress is unhealthy, but the mechanisms involve much more than a depression of immune function. The dogma that stress suppresses immunity is to some extent based on the well-established immunosuppressive effects of glucocorticoids. However, the supraphysiological doses of the steroids used in most of the studies do not allow simple extrapolation to the normal physiological state. In fact, endogenous glucocorticoids at physiological doses are not universally immunosuppressive and actually may enhance immune function (see below). Furthermore, glucocorticoids may not even be the major mechanism by which stress suppresses immune function.

Experimental data from both animal and human studies have confirmed the immunosuppressive effect of stress (1,43,49). However, it is important to emphasize that there is considerable evidence to suggest that stress may also enhance immune function (1). Common human experiences suggest that under acute stress conditions (approaching examinations, grant deadlines, etc.) an impending infection can be held at bay, but resistance collapses when the pressure is relieved. Some animal experiments also suggest that mild acute stressors may actually enhance measures of immunity (e.g., see ref. 92; for a more complete review, see ref. 1; see also Chapters 62 and 67, *this volume*).

The Role of the Adrenal

Adrenalectomy has been shown to prevent the immunosuppressive effects of stress in some animal studies (20,43), but many other studies have found that stress-induced changes in immunity persist in adrenalectomized animals (8). Adrenalectomy appears to be effective in studies that have examined acute responses to brief stressors (for which the immunosuppressive effects are rapidly reversed), but may be less important for the effects of chronic stress (20,43). Adrenalectomy does not permit a distinction among the effects of steroids, catecholamines, or even of neuropeptides secreted by the adrenal gland. More recent studies have suggested an important role for the circulating catecholamines, derived from the sympathetic nervous system and adrenal medulla, in the chronic studies (see below).

The choice of immune parameters measured may also influence the results. Earlier studies relied heavily on mitogen-stimulated proliferation assays, which assess the responsivity [i.e., cell division measured by deoxyribonucleic acid (DNA) synthesis] to lectin mitogens [such as concanavalin A (Con A), phytohemagglutinin (PHA), lipopolysaccharide (LPS), or pokeweed mitogen] in vitro. The interpretation of such assays is questionable, because the results are susceptible to a large number of extraneous influences, and the assays are conducted after several days of in vitro incubation separated from normal physiological influences (55). Also, the data typically display high variability. A measure used more often recently has been that for NK cells. There is good evidence that NK cells are involved in the rejection of tumors (4), and therefore at least one of their immunophysiological functions is clear. Stressful treatments have been shown to suppress NK cell function in both animal and human studies (45,77). The major effector for the stress-induced effects on NK cell function appears to be opiates (77) and catecholamines through β-adrenergic receptors (84).

Because most of the studies of stress on immune function have used ex vivo procedures (i.e., stress in vivo, immune assays in vitro), another important factor is whether or not the population of cells sampled may be altered by the in vivo treatment. Cell trafficking, the movement of lymphocytes around the body, is known to be regulated by hormones and other secretions, including those secreted during stress, and it is likely, therefore, that the stressful treatments alter the population of cells harvested for the in vitro studies (see below).

The Role of Glucocorticoids

The best known mechanism for an influence of the nervous system on the immune system is circulating glucocorticoid hormones secreted by the adrenal cortex. Glucocorticoids have long been known to have immunosuppressive effects (13,88). The data derive in part from the medical practice of using glucocorticoids postsurgically to decrease tissue inflammation and the rejection of transplanted tissues. However, considerable experimental data suggest that the effects of glucocorticoids are not exclusively immunosuppressive (47,88).

Although it is well established, it is too often forgotten that glucocorticoids are essential for normal immune responses. Extensive experimental data from animal and human studies indicates that adrenally compromised individuals are more susceptible to infections and that the adrenal cortex is more important than the medulla in this respect (47). Replacement studies clearly implicate a major role for the corticosteroids in immune defense mechanisms. Of particular importance is the work of Kass (see ref. 47), who showed that an optimal concentration of corticosteroids was essential for normal recovery from infections in adrenalectomized animals.

Nevertheless, the extensive evidence for the immunosuppressive effects of glucocorticoids should not be ignored. It should, however, be viewed in the light that most of the data were generated using high doses of synthetic glucocorticoids, such as prednisolone, triamcinolone, or dexamethasone, which are considerably more potent than the native steroids. The concentrations of these compounds used clinically can cause lysis of immune cells, especially immature ones. The more careful studies have used natural steroids at doses in the normal physiological range; these have noted stimulatory effects of steroids at lower doses (see ref. 88). Inhibitory effects occur at higher doses, typically 10^{-6} M, which is close to the maximum concentration of free corticosterone or cortisol found in stressed animals after correcting for that bound by corticosteroid-binding globulins (20). It is also important that elevations of plasma glucocorticoids following acute stressors are short-lived.

Although there are direct effects of glucocorticoids on immune cells in vitro, there may also be indirect ones in vivo. One of the oldest known physiological correlates of stress is the involution of the thymus. This involution, which can decrease thymus weight by more than half, occurs largely because lymphocytes that normally reside there are driven out to the periphery. Stress-induced thymic involution is prevented by adrenalectomy and can be induced by administration of glucocorticoids (13). Thus glucocorticoids can alter the body's distribution of lymphocytes, which may in itself be an important factor mar-

shalling the immune response to infection. Moreover, as mentioned above, the population of lymphocytes derived by harvesting tissues from animals subjected to experimental treatments may be altered by the redistribution of cells due to glucocorticoid secretion. This should be an important consideration in interpreting the results of ex vivo data.

The Role of Catecholamines

Lymphocytes bear both α- and β-adrenergic receptors. Catecholamines appear in the circulation from both the adrenal medulla [norepinephrine (NE) and epinephrine] and from sympathetic terminals (NE). In addition, lymphocytes may be exposed more directly to neuronal secretions while they are resident in the thymus, spleen, and lymph nodes. Anatomical studies have clearly demonstrated a sympathetic innervation of immune structures, such as the bone marrow, thymus, spleen, and lymph nodes (28). Thus lymphocytes could be exposed to high local concentrations of catecholamines, as well as neuropeptides. A parasympathetic (i.e., cholinergic) innervation of these organs, has not been confirmed (see ref. 28).

In vitro studies have revealed adrenergic effects on lymphocytes. Early studies suggested separate α- and β-adrenergic effects; β-adrenergic receptors were largely inhibitory, whereas α-adrenergic receptors were stimulatory (35). This generalization has endured to some extent, but the detailed results are very complex. There appear to be separate α- and β-adrenergic stimulatory effects on antibody production in vitro (71), whereas NK cell activity appears to be inhibited by β-adrenergic stimulation.

The results of in vivo studies have been bewilderingly complex. Depending on the parameters used, sympathectomy has been shown to impair, enhance, or not change immune responses (54). In general, sympathectomy in adult animals depresses immune reactivity, but there are also paradoxical effects on lymphocyte proliferation and B cell differentiation. Among the confounding factors that may contribute to the complexity are compensatory increases in adrenomedullary output, redistribution of lymphocytes, compensatory changes in the number and kind of adrenergic receptors, and the coexistence in sympathetic terminals of peptides, such as neuropeptide Y (NPY).

Several recent studies have suggested that a major mechanism by which NK cell activity is regulated in vivo involves catecholamines released by the sympathetic nervous system. For example, the inhibitory effect of intracerebroventricular corticotropin-releasing factor (CRF) on NK activity is blocked by the ganglionic blocker, chlorisondamine (44), as is the immunosuppressive effect of icv interleukin-1 (IL-1) (83). There is also direct evidence that β-adrenergic receptor blockade can prevent stress-induced effects on NK cell activity (16).

The Role of Peptides

Sympathetic terminals contain not only NE, but also neuropeptides, including endorphins, which may act on the immune system. Felten et al. described the presence of NPY, substance P (SP), and vasoactive intestinal polypeptide (VIP) in the thymus spleen and lymph nodes, as well as calcitonin gene-related peptide (CGRP) in the thymus and lymph nodes, enkephalin and somatostatin in the spleen, tachykinin in the thymus, and peptide histidine isoleucine in lymph nodes (28).

It has been shown that lymphocytes can synthesize and secrete certain peptides. The spectrum of peptides reported to be synthesized is large, and includes many of the known peptide hormones, as well as the hypophysiotropic factors. The peptides include adrenocorticotropin hormone (ACTH), CRF, growth hormone, thyrotropin (TRH), prolactin, human chorionic gonadotropin, the endorphins, enkephalins, SP, somatostatin, and VIP (11,34). The quantities of the peptides produced are typically very small, and their biochemical characterization has often been perfunctory. Sometimes their existence has been inferred only from the results obtained in the very sensitive assays used to detect their messenger ribonucleic acids (mRNAs), which should not be construed as unequivocal evidence for the presence of the peptides themselves. More careful analyses have not always substantiated the original claims, especially for the endorphins (76). There is probably considerable variability in the ability of lymphocytes from different sources to produce a specific peptide, but this issue has received no serious attention in the literature.

The physiological significance of this production of peptides is not at all clear. Because in many cases lymphocytes display receptors for these same peptides, they may function as chemical messengers within the immune system. However, Blalock has suggested that the peptides may also have systemic functions, for example, ACTH could activate the adrenal cortex. Although there is no good experimental support for this specific example (see below), it is possible that there may be a local bidirectional communication between lymphocytes and other cells. One example of this communication may be in the spleen, where CRF appears to be present in the innervating neurons and CRF-receptors are present on resident macrophages (91). Another example involves endorphins; β-endorphin produced by lymphocytes in an area of inflammation may exert an analgesic action directly on sensory nerve terminals (79). Such a mechanism is attractive, because the concentrations of the peptides produced locally may be adequate to exert such effects, and the metabolic lability of peptides would ensure that the effect was localized.

The principal known actions of peptides not covered elsewhere in this chapter on immune function can be summarized briefly. Substance P is a potent stimulator of cellular proliferation and cytokine [IL-1, IL-6, and tumor necrosis factor (TNF)] production (60). Its proinflammatory properties may be important in rheumatoid arthritis and inflammatory bowel disease. Vasoactive intestinal polypeptide may be involved in the regulation of lymphocyte migration (66). The interested reader is referred to reviews of this very complex topic (2,78).

Other Hormones of the Hypothalamic–Pituitary–Adrenocortical Axis

Many other hormones are known to affect the immune system. Firstly, there are the hormones of the hypothalamic–pituitary–adrenocortical (HPA) axis, each of which has been reported to affect immune function: CRF, ACTH, and the endorphins.

Corticotropin-releasing factor itself has been reported to have a variety of effects. The reported direct effects of CRF on immune cells have generally been stimulatory. For example, CRF has been shown to stimulate B cell proliferation and NK activity, as well as IL-1, IL-2, and IL-6 production (52). Receptors for CRF have been found on immune cells (91), providing a mechanism for these effects. Although it seems unlikely that CRF in the general circulation ever achieves concentrations high enough to stimulate these receptors, it is possible that local actions may occur, for example, in the spleen (91). By contrast, CRF injected intracerebroventricularly (icv) has largely inhibitory effects on immune function. A major effect of icv CRF is evident on NK cell activity and appears to be mediated through the sympathetic nervous system (44). The footshock-induced reduction of NK activity appears to be mediated by cerebral CRF, because an antibody to CRF injected icv but not peripherally prevented the shock-related response (46).

Although, ACTH has been shown to have some direct effects on immune function, including an inhibition of antibody production and modulation of B cell function (38), the effects have not been striking. On the other hand, the endorphins have been shown to exert a plethora of effects on immune function (10,38). Lymphocytes possess binding sites for opiates, but at least some of these are not sensitive to the opiate antagonist, naloxone (see the review by Carr in ref. 10). Interestingly, binding sites have been found for N-acetyl-β-endorphin, which is the commonest form of β-endorphin secreted from the anterior pituitary and has no opiate activity (75). β-Endorphin and other opioid peptides can exert effects on lymphocytes in vitro (10). By and large, the effects are facilitatory. Such effects have been observed on NK activity as well as on proliferative responses (38). Opioid peptides are also chemoattractants for lymphocytes. By contrast with the enhancing effects in vitro, in vivo opiates are largely inhibitory, especially on NK activity. This apparent contradiction can be explained, because, at least in the case of morphine, the site of opiate action appears to be in the central nervous system (CNS) (see ref. 90).

Moreover, the effects appear to be mediated by the adrenal gland, most probably by catecholamines (4).

Other Hormones

Perhaps the most interesting effect of a pituitary hormone on the immune system is that of prolactin. As summarized by Bernton et al. (5), its effects are largely stimulatory. Reduction of pituitary prolactin secretion (e.g., by dopaminergic agonists or opiate antagonists) impairs immune function and increases susceptibility to infections, such as *Listeria monocytogenes,* whereas stimulation of prolactin secretion (e.g., by D2 dopaminergic antagonists or opiates) can enhance it. Bernton et al. postulate that prolactin may be the counter-regulatory hormone to glucocorticoids, and opposing interactions between these two hormones on immune function can be demonstrated in vivo (5). Direct effects of prolactin on lymphocyte function have been difficult to demonstrate, but prolactin antibodies do impair proliferative responses in vitro. Lymphocytes can produce a prolactinlike protein, although its identity with prolactin has not been demonstrated. Thus it appears that prolactin is yet another example of a multifunctional peptide produced by both the pituitary and the lymphocytes.

IMMUNE SYSTEM SIGNALING OF THE BRAIN

Infection as a Stressor

Few would challenge the notion that sickness is stressful. In his autobiography, Hans Selye indicates that it was the common characteristics of sickness regardless of the underlying disease "the syndrome of just being sick" that first interested him in stress research and led him to advance his much maligned proposal of the *nonspecificity* of stress (74). That the HPA axis is activated following infections has long been known. During World War I, it was noted that fatalities from infections were associated with striking morphological changes in the adrenal cortex (47). It was later discovered that endotoxin (lipopolysaccharide, LPS), a potent stimulator of the immune system, stimulated the HPA axis. Subsequently, it was shown that infection of rats with *Escherichia coli* increased the secretion of ACTH.

The concept was expanded considerably when Besedovsky et al. showed that increases of plasma corticosterone accompanied the appearance of cells producing antibodies to such commonly used antigens as SRBCs. The observation, replicated by Besedovsky et al. and Saphier (see review in ref. 72), complemented earlier Russian observations of the electrophysiological activation of cells in the medial hypothalamus accompanying an immune response. Besedovsky also showed that SRBC inoculation

changed the apparent turnover of NE in the hypothalamus.

There now seems to be a consensus that the primary physiological responses in stress are the activation of the HPA axis and of peripheral and central catecholamines. To the extent that infections and immune challenges exert the same physiological effects, they can be regarded as stressful (Table 1).

Immune Activation and the HPA Axis

The foregoing has indicated that infections and immune challenges can activate the HPA axis, but is this a specific response or merely the reaction of the organism to a disturbance of its homeostasis? Work by Besedovsky and others implicates cytokines produced by the immune system as mediators of the HPA response, which suggests that it is specific. The initial observation was that supernatants of immune cells challenged in vitro with mitogens, such as Con A, had the ability to activate the HPA axis. The active factor synthesized and secreted in response to the mitogens was suggested to be IL-1, because the supernatants of Newcastle disease virus- (NDV-) treated lymphocytes could be neutralized with an antibody to IL-1, and because injection of purified recombinant human IL-1β was found to be a potent stimulator of the HPA axis (6). It is notable that IL-1 is a considerably more potent activator of ACTH and glucocorticoid secretion than CRF itself. A scheme for this arrangement is depicted in Fig. 2.

It is important to distinguish the HPA activation that occurs at different stages in the immune response. The HPA activations related to treatment with SRBC and other antigens occurred 5 to 8 days following treatment and coincided with the peak production of antibody. Similar observations have been noted by others with myelin basic protein (53) or keyhole limpet hemocyanin (81). However, there is also an acute HPA response to immune

TABLE 1. *Comparison of physiological responses to physical and behavioral stressors to those to infections and immune challenges*

	Physical and behavioral stressors	Immune stimulation
HPA axis (plasma CRF, ACTH, β-endorphin, and CS)	↑[a]	↑
Sympathetic system (plasma NE)	↑	↑
Adrenal medulla (plasma epinephrine + NE)	↑	↑
Brain NE (MHPG)	↑	↑
Brain DA (DOPAC)	↑	0/+[b]
Brain 5-HT (5-HIAA)	↑	↑
Brain tryptophan	↑	↑

[a] ↑, increased.
[b] 0/+, unchanged or increased.

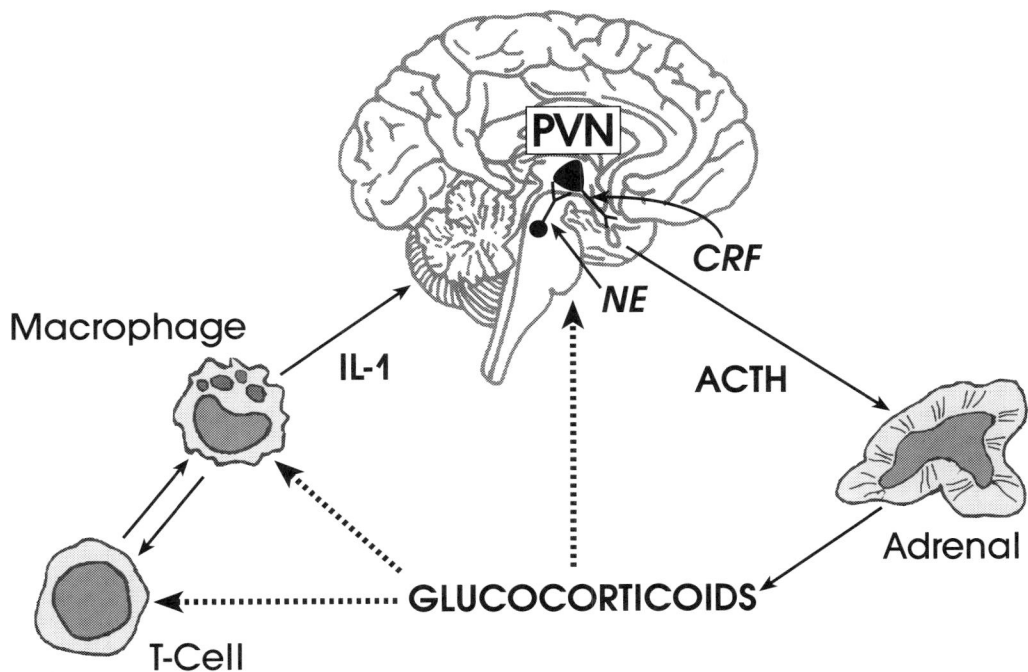

FIG. 2. A schematic diagram of the relationship between the brain, the HPA axis, and immune cells. Interleukin-1 (IL-1) produced by lymphocytes during the immune response activates noradrenergic (NE) projections for the brainstem to the hypothalamic paraventricular nucleus (PVN). This input activates the hypothalamic-pituitary-adrenocortical (HPA) axis, stimulating the release of corticotropin-releasing factor (CRF) in the median eminence region of the hypothalamus, which in turn stimulates the secretion of ACTH from the anterior lobe of the pituitary, which then activates the adrenal cortex to synthesize and secrete glucocorticoid hormones. The glucocorticoids in turn provide a negative feedback on cytokine production by lymphocytes.

stimulation that occurs within the first few hours. This acute response is observed following LPS and NDV administration (22,81). It seems likely that this early response is related to cytokine secretion (see below), but whether cytokines are responsible for the later response is not known.

The mechanism of the activation of the HPA axis by immune stimuli has been the subject of intense investigation. Speculation has largely centered on the role of IL-1. However, Blalock (7) has suggested that lymphocytes may synthesize and secrete their own ACTH following immune stimulation and that this ACTH may be sufficient to activate the adrenal cortex. This mechanism has been excluded because rigorous hypophysectomy prevents the responses to NDV (26). Evidence exists for IL-1-induced activation of the axis at every level. However, the bulk of the evidence strongly favors the need for hypothalamic CRF. Deafferentation of the hypothalamus and lesions of the paraventricular nucleus (PVN) prevent the ACTH response to IL-1, and hypophysectomy prevents the effect of IL-1 and LPS (24). Moreover, antibodies to CRF attenuate or block the ACTH and corticosterone responses to IL-1 (e.g., ref. 89). The data that conflict with this are largely based on in vitro studies, which are notoriously subject to artifact. For example, although several authors

have reported that IL-1 can stimulate hormone release from the pituitary in vitro, the results are remarkably inconsistent (see ref. 21), and, in general, prolonged incubation in vitro is necessary to observe such responses. Similar considerations apply to the in vitro studies on adrenal tissue.

Neurochemical Correlates of Immune Activation

As indicated above, Besedovsky first reported changes in cerebral NE metabolism associated with immune activation (see ref. 26). Injection of SRBCs caused an apparent decrease in NE turnover as determined following blockade of synthesis with α-methyl-p-tyrosine. This change coincided in time with the peak antibody response at 5 to 8 days. Subsequent studies have confirmed changes in NE metabolism associated with immune stimulation, but in all cases the changes have suggested increased rather than decreased metabolism (26). Administration of SRBCs decreased the NE content of the PVN 4 days, but not 2 or 6 days, later. The decrease in NE in the PVN could reflect increased NE release. Subsequent postmortem neurochemical studies using a variety of different challenges have demonstrated acute increases in cerebral NE catabolites to challenges such as NDV (26) and LPS

(22,40). These neurochemical changes are greatest in the hypothalamus; changes in other brain regions are significantly smaller. Dopamine (DA) metabolism is affected to a lessor extent and only by LPS (22). Thus the changes contrast with those typically observed for behavioral stressors, which cause similar changes in NE metabolism in most brain regions and exhibit a pronounced activation of dopaminergic systems, especially in the prefrontal cortex. The latter is rarely observed following immune stimulation. The increases in biogenic amine catabolites (accompanied in a few cases by decreases in the parent amines) suggest increased synaptic release; studies with in vivo microdialysis reinforce this possibility. Like the HPA responses, those in the catecholamines have been best characterized after acute stimulation, but some studies suggest that similar changes occur later during the primary immune response, and this has been confirmed by studies of metabolites following SRBC administration (94).

The neurochemical changes are not confined to the catecholamines; indolamine metabolism is also affected. Decreases of 5-HT have been observed in the paraventricular and supraoptic hypothalamic nuclei. Increases in the serotonin catabolite, 5-hydroxyindolacetic acid (5-HIAA) were observed acutely following NDV (26). These increases in 5-HIAA accompany increases in tryptophan (22,40). Interestingly, the catecholaminergic and serotonergic responses can be distinguished. In contrast to the hypothalamic emphasis of the noradrenergic responses, the indolamine responses have no apparent regional specificity (22). Moreover, they follow different time courses; the increases in DA and NE catabolism peak after 2 hours, whereas the indolaminergic ones are much slower, reaching a peak at approximately 8 hours (22,40). Interestingly, these changes in brain tryptophan and 5-HIAA appear to be dependent upon the sympathetic nervous system, because ganglionic blockade with chlorisondamine prevents changes in these neurochemicals normally induced by IL-1 or LPS (27).

Recently, we have demonstrated a complete dissociation in the responses to LPS. Endotoxin-resistant mice (C3H/HeJ strain) do not exhibit significant noradrenergic responses (in parallel with the diminished HPA response), but do exhibit normal indolaminergic ones; however, nitric oxide synthase inhibitors can block the indolaminergic responses without affecting the noradrenergic (or HPA) responses.

Administration of IL-1 mimics the neurochemical responses to LPS and NDV very closely. The increased NE metabolism is focused on the hypothalamus, with a regionally nonspecific increase in tryptophan and in 5-HT metabolism (19,22). The only distinction is that LPS exerts a modest effect on DA. Thus the neurochemical data complement the HPA data implicating IL-1 as a mediator of the responses.

Because NE is considered to be a major regulator of CRF secretion, it is reasonable to ask whether NE is involved in the response to IL-1. Studies in rats lesioned with 6-hydroxydopamine (6-OHDA) suggest that the ventral noradrenergic bundle input to the hypothalamus is indeed necessary for HPA responses to IL-1 (12), but studies with adrenergic blockers have been less successful in demonstrating adrenergic control of the HPA response to IL-1 (69), although we have observed a partial blockade of the HPA response to IL-1 by the α_1-adrenergic antagonist, prazosin, but not by α_2- or β-adrenergic receptor antagonists.

Significance of HPA Effects on the Immune System

The activation of the HPA axis associated with immune responses has been interpreted to indicate that the immune system can act as a sensory system, signaling the brain to indicate the presence of a threat from the external environment and triggering a classical stress response (7). The role of the HPA activation has been suggested to be a negative-feedback mechanism provided by the immunosuppressive activity of the glucocorticoids. The inhibitory activity of the glucocorticoids limits inflammatory responses and prevents the immune system from overreacting and causing autoimmunity (6,62). Consistent with this result, adrenal corticosteroids have been shown to play a critical role in the recovery from experimental allergic encephalomyelitis (EAE). Rats treated with myelin basic protein produce antibodies to this protein 11 to 14 days after immunization, at the same time that paralysis of the tail and hind limbs appears and plasma corticosterone is appreciably elevated (53). Intact rats normally recover within a few days, but the spontaneous recovery does not occur in adrenalectomized rats, unless glucocorticoid replacement therapy is instituted.

Conversely, a decreased responsivity of the HPA axis is associated with the susceptibility to arthritis in Lewis rats. Lewis rats show an arthritic response that mimics human rheumatoid arthritis in response to administration of a streptococcal cell wall peptidoglycan polysaccharide (SCW), whereas the histocompatible Fischer rats do not. The arthritic response in Lewis rats can be prevented by dexamethasone and can be induced in Fischer rats by the glucocorticoid-receptor antagonist RU 486 (82). The deficit in Lewis rats appears to be associated with a deficient activation of the HPA axis to SCW, IL-1, and CRF (compared to Fischer rats), and may be associated with an inappropriate regulation of the CRF gene. These two examples indicate the physiological significance of the glucocorticoid feedback on the immune response.

Cytokines as Immunotransmitters

The most likely messengers from the immune system to the nervous system are the cytokines. In this sense, cytokines, the hormones of the immune system are immunotransmitters. Although the cytokines play a major role in coordinating the immune response, they also have substantial effects on other tissues, including the nervous system. A large number of cytokines has been identified, including thirteen interleukins, several interferons, and a variety of other factors. Those currently known to have the most relevance for the nervous system are IL-1, IL-6, TNFα, and the interferons, but many others may soon be recognized. Shortly following most immunological challenges, macrophages produce TNFα, followed closely by IL-1 and then IL-6 (95). Surprisingly, each of these three cytokines is capable of inducing the others, so that IL-1 administration induces TNFα synthesis and vice versa (18); IL-1 and TNFα induce IL-6, and so on.

All of the interferons (IFNα, IFNβ, and IFNγ) are secreted by lymphocytes in response to viruses and RNA (IFNβ_2 has been renamed IL-6). Each of them has a variety of immunological effects that are regarded as antiviral. They include inhibition of T-cell proliferation, enhancement or suppression of antibody synthesis, and enhancement of NK activity (30).

These cytokines have a plethora of effects, many of which are related to the physiology of infections. Interleukin-1 is not the only cytokine that can affect the HPA axis; other cytokines, such as IL-6 and TNFα, can have similar effects (58), although they are significantly less potent (23). Interestingly, the production of TNFα and IL-1 is inhibited by glucocorticoids, so that the HPA activation elicited by the cytokines provides feedback regulation of cytokine synthesis (95). Also, IFNα affects the HPA axis, its effects being largely inhibitory and apparently mediated through opiate receptors. Interleukin-1 and -6 have a variety of other endocrine effects (21) and along with TNFα are each pyrogenic (18).

Interferon α is used therapeutically as an antiviral agent, although its utility has often been limited by its neurological and psychiatric side effects. It can cause an opiate-like euphoria, polyneuropathies, and behavioral and motor deficits and can alter the electroencephalogram (EEG) (61). The neurotoxic effects of both IFNα and IFNγ have been postulated to depend on the altered metabolism of tryptophan. This effect may be mediated largely by an induction of indolamine 2,3-dioxygenase, a catabolic enzyme for tryptophan (39), so that plasma concentrations of tryptophan are reduced, for example, in patients with autoimmune deficiency syndrome (AIDS) (31). There is also increased metabolism of tryptophan to kynurenine and quinolinic acid (39). Quinolinic acid is a potent neurotoxin, which may be involved in neurodegenerative disorders of the CNS. Its presence in the brain is correlated with inflammatory responses from a variety of sources, including viral infections (41). The potential effects of the IFNs on serotonin and its functions are largely unknown.

Both IL-1 and IFNα are electrophysiologically active and can alter the EEG (72). Many of the effects of IFNα

are prevented by naloxone, suggesting an interaction with opiate receptors.

The cytokines are also behaviorally active. Thus, IL-1 and TNFα are somnogenic (65); IL-1, TNFα, and IFNα are anorexic (15,59); locomotor activity is decreased by IL-1 (67) and IFNα (15); and IL-1 decreases exploratory activity (25). In most cases, these responses can be elicited by both central and peripheral administration, and some may be mediated by CRF (25). Each of these responses is characteristic of sickness, and a case can be made that IL-1, perhaps in combination with other cytokines, accounts for many if not most of the physiological and behavioral responses to infections. These responses can clearly be rationalized in terms of what has been termed "sickness behavior" (37,48). The fever may be instrumental in fighting invading organisms, and the behavioral responses (sleep, anorexia, hypomotility) may cause the animal to hide and thus escape predators (37).

The immunotransmitter activity of cytokines has been tested to some extent with antagonists. Thus, the IL-1 receptor antagonist (the IL-1ra, a naturally occurring polypeptide often synthesized and secreted along with IL-1) can prevent the HPA-activating and neurochemical effects of some immune challenges, such as NDV (24). The IL-1ra also blocked the effects of LPS on social behavior in rats but not the anorexia (48) or the HPA activation (23). Thus, IL-1 may not be the only factor mediating responses to LPS. A TNFα antibody was also ineffective against LPS, even in combination with IL-1ra (23). Because immune challenges produce a "cocktail" of cytokines, it seems likely that differences in these cocktails account for the different patterns of responses to different immune stimuli. As more suitable cytokine antagonists become available, this hypothesis can be tested.

Site of Action of Interleukin 1 in the Brain

An important question is the mechanism by which IL-1 activates the HPA axis. Given that activation of CRF-containing neurons in the hypothalamus appears to be required, does IL-1 penetrate the brain and directly activate CRF-containing neurons in the PVN or are other intermediates involved? The answer to this apparently simple question may be quite complex. When injected directly into the brain, IL-1 does indeed activate the HPA axis; thus it is possible that IL-1 acts directly in the brain. However, a number of observations are not consistent with a direct action of peripherally administered IL-1 on the hypothalamus: IL-1 is a relatively large protein (molecular weight 17,500) so that it is unlikely that it readily penetrates the blood–brain barrier, although it could act on one or other circumventricular organs, such as the median eminence (ME) or the organum vasculosum laminae terminalis (OVLT) that lack a blood–brain barrier. Moreover, studies of IL-1 binding in the brain have not been encouraging. In the rat, there has been no clear demonstration of cerebral binding sites for IL-1, except for those in the capillary endothelium and choroid plexus (36,85). Messenger RNA for IL-1 receptors has been demonstrated in some studies but not in others, and the presence of mRNA does not necessarily indicate the existence of functional receptors. In the mouse brain, binding studies with IL-1 indicate very few, if any, receptors in the hypothalamus, especially in the PVN (36,85). In addition, although lower doses of IL-1 are necessary to activate the HPA axis when administered icv compared to those effective when administered peripherally, the concentrations may be higher than those likely to reach the hypothalamus after intraperitoneal (ip) or subcutaneous (sc) injections. Lastly, the time course of the HPA response to icv IL-1 is quite slow; maximal plasma concentrations of ACTH and corticosterone are reached only after 2 hours, like the response to peripheral injections. Such a slow response seems unlikely to reflect a direct action of IL-1 on receptors within the medial hypothalamus.

Nevertheless, several groups of researchers have reported that IL-1 can stimulate release of CRF from hypothalamic tissue in vitro (87). Although this response is observed at very low doses of IL-1 (10^{-13} M), the relationship of this in vitro stimulation of CRF release to that observed following peripheral injections of IL-1 is unclear for the reasons mentioned above: the lack of IL-1 receptors in the hypothalamus and the slow response to intracerebral administration of IL-1. It may be that the HPA responses to peripheral and intracerebral IL-1 occur by different mechanisms.

A specific brain uptake system for IL-1 has been proposed, based on the accumulation of radioactively labeled IL-1 in excised brain tissue (3). However, it has not been proven that the IL-1 is taken up into brain tissue, and it is possible that the apparent accumulation occurs because the IL-1 binds to sites in the capillary endothelium and choroid plexus, which are known to be rich in IL-1 binding sites (36,85). A careful study in cats was unable to detect IL-1 in the cerebrospinal fluid (CSF) of normal cats before or after the peripheral injection of high doses of IL-1 (14), suggesting that IL-1 from the periphery does not readily cross the blood–brain barrier.

It has been suggested that IL-1 from the periphery acts directly on the OVLT. In the OVLT, IL-1 stimulates the synthesis of prostaglandin E_2 (PGE_2), which in turn may elicit CRF release by stimulating PVN neurons. This hypothesis is consistent with the observations that intravenous IL-1β administration increases hypothalamic concentrations of PGE_2 as determined by microdialysis (51), that hypothalamic infusions of PGE_2 can stimulate the HPA axis, and that prostaglandin synthesis inhibitors, such as indomethacin, can prevent the IL-1-induced HPA activation. An alternative hypothesis is that IL-1 acts directly on CRF-containing terminals in the ME (57). When injected directly into this region, IL-1 elicits CRF release,

as indicated by increases of plasma ACTH, and these effects can be prevented by local administration of IL-1ra (56). Interestingly, this effect appears to be indirect because icv administration of 6-OHDA prevents this response to IL-1, suggesting that noradrenergic neurons in the ME normally regulate the release of CRF. Consistent with this, local (ME) injection of phenoxybenzamine or propranolol can prevent the IL-1-induced elevation of plasma ACTH (57).

Whether or not IL-1 is present in normal brain is controversial. Fontana first showed that glial cells can produce an IL-1-like substance, and showed that it was a potent growth factor for astrocytes. Several studies have suggested the presence of IL-1 in normal brain using immunohistochemical techniques, but the results have varied markedly, especially in the anatomical distributions and intensities described (see ref. 73). Moreover, to date, no study using rigorous biochemical purification and analysis has unequivocally identified IL-1 in normal brain. There is little doubt that IL-1 appears in the brain in pathological circumstances, such as following endotoxin administration (14,29,42) or damage such as caused by insertion of cannulae or microdialysis probes (42,86,93). Thus it is possible that the reports of IL-1 in normal brain reflect an unrecognized pathology in the subjects studied. Whether or not the IL-1 is present in neurons is also controversial, but, whereas the immunohistochemical studies have suggested that it might be, most believe that IL-1 is found primarily in microglia (32). An attractive hypothesis is that when the brain is infected or lesioned, the blood–brain barrier is breached. This allows invasion of macrophages from the periphery, which then proliferate in the CNS as microglia. The microglia synthesize IL-1, which acts as a potent growth factor for astroglia, causing them to proliferate, sealing off the lesion, and restoring the damaged blood–brain barrier (33). The IL-1 (and possibly other factors produced by the microglia) may also play other roles in the repair mechanisms and also activate the HPA axis. This schema attributes a major role to IL-1 in a classical pathological mechanism for protection of the brain.

CONCLUDING REMARKS

Communication Between the Nervous and Immune Systems

The foregoing indicates that there is now substantial evidence for bidirectional communications between the nervous and immune systems. Communication occurs via chemical messengers, just as it does within the nervous and immune systems. Many of the messengers are already familiar as hormones, neurotransmitters, and cytokines, but presently the messages are poorly understood. Certain messengers from the neuroendocrine system appear to facilitate or inhibit the functions of immune cells, but the specificity remains to be elucidated. Cytokines, such as IL-1, are clearly potent activators of the HPA axis, but also exert a variety of other physiological effects. In all likelihood, many other messengers remain to be discovered.

Although our current understanding of the system is primitive, it may be important to distinguish local from systemic effects. Whereas circulating concentrations of catecholamines and steroids are probably adequate to exert physiological effects, and this also appears to be true for cytokines, the role of the peptides is less clear. Their systemic concentrations are very low and are unlikely to be sufficient to modulate immune system function in a general way. However, it is possible that peptides secreted by nerve terminals in the thymus, spleen, and lymphoid tissue may achieve local concentrations sufficient to affect immune cells. Such effects may also be possible locally in tissue at sites of inflammation.

Messengers that can travel more readily and are more stable metabolically may be active systemically, whereas the less stable peptides may be confined to local actions. The chemical nature of the messengers may be suited to their functions. As lipophilic molecules, the glucocorticoids can readily penetrate membrane barriers and affect cells in all bodily tissues, whereas the hydrophilic catecholamines are more labile and their action may be limited to the circulatory systems. Our present knowledge indicates that the glucocorticoids and catecholamines predominantly inhibit immune responses, whereas the peptides are largely facilitatory. When the organism is threatened, the systemic activity of the glucocorticoids to limit immune responses may be important to depress immune activity to prevent undesirable autoimmune actions. By contrast, peptides could facilitate immune responses in small areas close to the site of their release, for example, in an area of inflammation induced by infection or tissue damage. Catecholamines may occupy an intermediate position, existing in sufficient concentrations to have systemic actions but not having broad access to tissues and having relatively short durations of action, except when chronically elevated. Such an arrangement would permit focusing of the activation of immune response in local areas of inflammation, while preventing potentially damaging autoimmune actions that could be triggered by widespread activation.

Psychiatry and Immunity

There is an ongoing and growing literature suggesting abnormalities of immune function in the mentally ill and gnawing suggestions of a viral etiology in both psychoses and affective disorders (see ref. 50). The psychiatric implications of interactions between the brain and the immune system can be posed as two questions: to what extent can brain dysfunction alter immune function, and can immune effects cause psychiatric disease?

The literature contains a variety of reports to indicate that deficits in immunity are associated with psychiatric disease. The most consistent data have been obtained related to depression. Decreased immune function has been reported in depressed patients as measured by mitogenic stimulation and NK cytotoxicity (9,80). Given that there is a strong association between depression and elevations of plasma cortisol, it is natural to suggest that the immune deficits may be related to the hypercortisolemia, however, a causal relationship has yet to be documented. Depression has also been correlated with a hyperactivity of noradrenergic systems. Thus either cortisol or NE could be responsible for the immunosuppression. The work of Irwin et al. indicating that icv CRF administration in rats decreases immunity (44), coupled with the observations that CSF CRF is elevated in major depression (64), suggests a potential mechanism. To the extent that the animal model is valid, it may be that the immunosuppressive effect of depression is related to the catecholamines rather than the glucocorticoids. Regardless of the mechanism, the chronic elevation of these humors that occurs in depression may add immunosuppression to the patients' other woes.

Evidence for deficits in immune function in other psychiatric diseases has been less consistent. Early studies found evidence of reduced immune function in schizophrenics, but this has not been substantiated in most recent studies (9). It was suggested that the deficits in some of the studies may have been due to neuroleptic medication. A recent analysis suggests increased incidence of schizophrenia following major epidemics of influenza (63), but the mechanism for this effect is unknown.

If immune-stimulated HPA activation provides a regulatory feedback mechanism, the balance between the nervous system and the immune system may be very delicate. Hyperactivity of the HPA axis to immune stimulation would impair immune defense mechanisms, and hypoactivity would run the risk of autoimmune disease. An example of the latter may be arthritis, which is associated with a hyperactive inflammatory and immune response. As discussed above, the susceptibility to arthritis in Lewis rats may be caused by a hyposensitivity of the HPA axis to normal stressful stimuli, so that the antiinflammatory effects of the glucocorticoids are diminished (82). Another example may be chronic fatigue syndrome (CFS), which has been likened to a glucocorticoid insufficiency because of the debilitating fatigue, the feverishness, arthralgias, myalgias, adenopathy, postexertional fatigue, exacerbation of allergic responses, and disturbances of mood and sleep (17). If, as postulated, CFS follows a chronic viral infection, it is possible that the infection may have caused sustained activation of the HPA axis, desensitizing the normal glucocorticoid response. Consistent with this, abnormalities of the HPA axis have been detected in CFS patients (17) (see also Chapters 85, 98, and 118, *this volume*).

REFERENCES

1. Ader R, Cohen N. Psychoneuroimmunology: conditioning and stress. *Annu Rev Psychol* 1993;44:53–85.
2. Ader R, Felten DL, Cohen N. *Psychoneuroimmunology.* 2nd ed. San Diego: Academic Press; 1991.
3. Banks WA, Ortiz L, Plotkin SR, Kastin AJ. Human interleukin (IL)1α, murine IL-1α and murine IL-1β are transported from blood to brain in the mouse by a shared saturable mechanism. *J Pharmacol Exp Therapeut* 1991;259:988–1007.
4. Ben-Eliyahu S, Page GG. In vivo assessment of natural killer cell activity in rats. *Prog NeuroEndocrinImmunol* 1992;5:199–214.
5. Bernton EW, Bryant HU, Holaday JW. Prolactin and immune function. In: Ader R, Felten DL, Cohen N, eds. *Psychoneuroimmunology.* 2nd ed. San Diego: Academic Press; 1991:403–428.
6. Besedovsky HO, del Rey A, Sorkin E, Dinarello CA. Immunoregulatory feedback between interleukin-1 and glucocorticoid hormones. *Science* 1986;233:652–654.
7. Blalock JE, Smith EM. A complete regulatory loop between the immune and neuroendocrine systems. *Fed Proc* 1985;44:108–111.
8. Bonneau RH, Sheridan JF, Feng NG, Glaser R. Stress-induced modulation of the primary cellular immune response to herpes simplex virus infection is mediated by both adrenal-dependent and independent mechanisms. *J Neuroimmunol* 1993;42:167–176.
9. Caldwell CL, Irwin M, Lohr J. Reduced natural killer cell cytotoxicity in depression but not in schizophrenia. *Biol Psychiatry* 1991;30:1131–1138.
10. Carr DJJ. The role of endogenous opioids and their receptors in the immune system. *Proc Soc Exp Biol Med* 1991;198:710–720.
11. Carr DJJ, Blalock JE. Neuropeptide hormones and receptors common to the immune and neuroendocrine systems: bidirectional pathway of intersystem communication. In: Ader R, Felten DL, Cohen N, eds. *Psychoneuroimmunology.* 2nd ed. San Diego: Academic Press; 1991:573–588.
12. Chuluyan H, Saphier D, Rohn W, Dunn AJ. Noradrenergic innervation of the hypothalamus participates in the adrenocortical responses to interleukin-1. *Neuroendocrinology* 1992;56:106–111.
13. Claman HN. How corticosteroids work. *J Allergy Clin Immunol* 1975;55:145–151.
14. Coceani F, Lees J, Dinarello CA. Occurrence of interleukin-1 in cerebrospinal fluid of the conscious cat. *Brain Res* 1988;446:245–250.
15. Crnic LS, Segall MA. Behavioral effects of mouse interferon-α and interferon-γ and human interferon-α in mice. *Brain Res* 1992;590:277–284.
16. Cunnick JE, Lysle DT, Kucinski BJ, Rabin BS. Evidence that shock-induced immune suppression is mediated by adrenal hormones and peripheral β-adrenergic receptors. *Pharmacol Biochem Behav* 1990;36:645–651.
17. Demitrack MA, Dale JK, Straus SE, et al. Evidence for impaired activation of the hypothalamic-pituitary-adrenal axis in patients with chronic fatigue syndrome. *J Clin Endocrinol Metab* 1991;73:1224–1234.
18. Dinarello CA. Interleukin-1 and its related cytokines. In: Sorg C, ed. *Macrophage-Derived Cell Regulatory Factors: Cytokines.* Basel: Karger; 1989:105–150.
19. Dunn AJ. Systemic interleukin-1 administration stimulates hypothalamic norepinephrine metabolism parallelling the increased plasma corticosterone. *Life Sci* 1988;43:429–435.
20. Dunn AJ. Psychoneuroimmunology for the psychoneuroendocrinologist: a review of animal studies of nervous system-immune system interactions. *Psychoneuroendocrinology* 1989;14:251–274.
21. Dunn AJ. Interleukin-1 as a stimulator of hormone secretion. *Prog NeuroEndocrinImmunol* 1990;3:26–34.
22. Dunn AJ. Endotoxin-induced activation of cerebral catecholamine and serotonin metabolism: comparison with interleukin-1. *J Pharmacol Exp Therapeut* 1992;261:964–969.
23. Dunn AJ. The role of interleukin-1 and tumor necrosis factor α in the neurochemical and neuroendocrine responses to endotoxin. *Brain Res Bull* 1992;29:807–812.
24. Dunn AJ. Role of cytokines in infection-induced stress. *Ann NY Acad Sci* 1993;697:189–202.
25. Dunn AJ, Antoon M, Chapman Y. Reduction of exploratory behavior by intraperitoneal injection of interleukin-1 involves brain corticotropin-releasing factor. *Brain Res Bull* 1991;26:539–542.
26. Dunn AJ, Powell ML, Moreshead WV, Gaskin JM, Hall NR. Effects of Newcastle disease virus administration to mice on the metabolism of cerebral biogenic amines, plasma corticosterone, and lymphocyte proliferation. *Brain Behav Immun* 1987;1:216–230.
27. Dunn AJ, Welch J. Stress- and endotoxin-induced increases in brain tryptophan and serotonin metabolism depend on sympathetic nervous system activation. *J Neurochem* 1991;57:1615–1622.
28. Felten SY, Felten DL. Innervation of lymphoid tissue. In: Ader R, Felten DL, Cohen N, eds. *Psychoneuroimmunology.* 2nd ed. San Diego: Academic Press, 1991;27–61.
29. Fontana A, Weber E, Dayer JM. Synthesis of interleukin 1/endogenous pyrogen in the brain of endotoxin-treated mice: a step in fever induction? *J Immunol* 1984;133:1696–1698.
30. Friedman RM, Vogel SN. Interferon with special emphasis on the immune system. *Adv Immunol* 1983;34:97–140.
31. Fuchs D, Forsman A, Hagberg L, et al. Immune activation and decreased tryptophan in patients with HIV-1 infection. *J Interferon Res* 1990;10:599–603.
32. Giulian D, Baker TJ, Shih L-CN, Lachman LB. Interleukin-1 of the central nervous system is produced by ameboid microglia. *J Exp Med* 1986;164:594–604.
33. Giulian D, Lachman LB. Interleukin-1 stimulation of astroglial proliferation after brain injury. *Science* 1985;228:497–499.
34. Goetzl EJ, Turck CW, Speedharan SP. Production and recognition of neuropeptides by cells of the immune system. In: Ader R, Felten DL, Cohen N, eds. *Psychoneuroimmunology.* 2nd ed. San Diego: Academic Press, 1991;263–282.
35. Hadden JW, Hadden EM, Middleton E. Lymphocyte blast transformation—1. Demonstration of adrenergic receptors in human peripheral lymphocytes. *Cell Immunol* 1970;1:583–595.
36. Haour F, Ban E, Marquette C, Milon G, Fillion G. Brain interleukin-1 receptors: mapping, characterization and modulation. In: Rothwell NJ, Dantzer RD, eds. *Interleukin-1 in the Brain.* Oxford: Pergamon Press; 1992:13–25.
37. Hart BL. Biological basis of the behavior of sick animals. *Neurosci Biobehav Rev* 1988;12:123–137.
38. Heijnen CJ, Kavelaars A, Ballieux RE. Corticotropin-releasing hormone and proopiomelanocortin-derived peptides in the modulation of immune function. In: Ader R, Felten DL, Cohen N, eds. *Psychoneuroimmunology.* 2nd ed. San Diego: Academic Press; 1991:429–446.
39. Heyes MP. Relationship between interferon-γ, indoleamine-2,3-dioxygenase and tryptophan. *FASEB J* 1991;5:3003–3004.
40. Heyes MP, Quearry BJ, Markey SP. Systemic endotoxin increases L-tryptophan, 5-hydroxyindoleacetic acid, 3-hydroxykynurenine and quinolinic acid content of mouse cerebral cortex. *Brain Res* 1989;491:173–179.
41. Heyes MP, Saito K, Crowley JS, et al. Quinolinic acid and kynurenine pathway metabolism in inflammatory and non-inflammatory neurological disease. *Brain* 1992;115:1249–1273.
42. Higgins GA, Olschowka JA. Induction of interleukin-1β mRNA in adult rat brain. *Molec Brain Res* 1991;9:143–148.
43. Irwin J, Livnat S. Behavioral influences on the immune system: stress and conditioning. *Prog Neuro-Psychopharmacol Biol Psychiatry* 1987;11:137–143.
44. Irwin M, Hauger RL, Jones L, Provencio M, Britton KT. Sympathetic nervous system mediates central corticotropin releasing factor induced suppression of natural killer cytotoxicity. *J Pharmacol Exp Ther* 1990;255:101–107.
45. Irwin M, Patterson T, Smith TL, et al. Reduction of immune function in life stress and depression. *Biol Psychiatry* 1990;27:22–30.
46. Irwin M, Vale W, Rivier C. Central corticotropin-releasing factor mediates the suppressive effect of stress on natural killer cytotoxicity. *Endocrinology* 1990;126:2837–2844.
47. Jefferies WM. Cortisol and immunity. *Med Hypoth* 1991;34:198–208.
48. Kent S, Bluthé R-M, Kelley KW, Dantzer R. Sickness behavior as a new target for drug development. *TIPS* 1992;13:24–28.
49. Kiecolt-Glaser JK, Glaser R. Stress and immune function in humans. In: Ader R, Felten DL, Cohen N, eds. *Psychoneuroimmunology.* 2nd ed. San Diego: Academic Press; 1991;849–867.
50. King DJ, Cooper SJ. Viruses, immunity and mental disorder. *Brit J Psychiatry* 1989;154:1–7.
51. Komaki G, Arimura A, Koves K. Effect of intravenous injection

of IL-1β on PGE2 levels in several brain areas as determined by microdialysis. *Endocrinol Metab* 1992;25:E246–E251.

52. Leu S-JC, Singh VK. Stimulation of interleukin-6 production by corticotropin-releasing factor. *Cell Immunol* 1992;143:220–227.

53. MacPhee IAM, Antoni FA, Mason DW. Spontaneous recovery of rats from experimental allergic encephalomyelitis is dependent on regulation of the immune system by endogenous adrenal corticosteroids. *J Exp Med* 1989;169:431–445.

54. Madden KS, Livnat S. Catecholamine action and immunologic reactivity. In: Ader R, Felten DL, Cohen N, eds. *Psychoneuroimmunology*. 2nd ed. San Diego: Academic Press; 1991:283–310.

55. Maier SF, Laudenslager ML. Inescapable shock, shock controllability and mitogen stimulated lymphocyte proliferation. *Brain Behav Immun* 1988;2:87–91.

56. Matta SG, Linner KM, Sharp BM. Interleukin-1-α and interleukin-1-β stimulate adrenocorticotropin secretion in the rat through a similar hypothalamic receptors(s): effects of interleukin-1 receptor antagonist protein. *Neuroendocrinology* 1993;57:14–22.

57. Matta SG, Singh J, Newton R, Sharp BM. The adrenocorticotropin response to interleukin-1β instilled into the rat median eminence depends on the local release of catecholamines. *Endocrinology* 1990;127:2175–2182.

58. Matta SG, Weatherbee J, Sharp BM. A central mechanism is involved in the secretion of ACTH in response to IL-6 in rats: comparison to and interaction with IL-1β. *Neuroendocrinology* 1992;56:516–525.

59. McCarthy DO, Kluger MJ, Vander AJ. Effect of centrally administered interleukin-1 and endotoxin on food intake of fasted rats. *Physiol Behav* 1986;36:745–749.

60. McGillis JP, Mitsuhashi M, Payan DG. Immunologic properties of substance P. In: Ader R, Felten DL, Cohen N, eds. *Psychoneuroimmunology*. 2nd ed. San Diego: Academic Press; 1991:209–223.

61. Meyers CA, Scheibel RS, Forman AD. Persistent neurotoxicity of systemically administered interferon-alpha. *Neurology* 1991;41:672–676.

62. Munck A, Guyre P. Glucocorticoid physiology, pharmacology and stress. *Adv Exp Med Biol* 1986;196:81–96.

63. Murray RM, Jones P, O'Callaghan E, Takei N, Sham P. Genes, viruses and neurodevelopmental schizophrenia. *J Psychiatr Res* 1992;26:225–235.

64. Nemeroff CB, Widerlöv E, Bissette G, et al. Elevated concentrations of CSF corticotropin-releasing factor-like immunoreactivity in depressed patients. *Science* 1984;226:1342–1344.

65. Opp MR, Kapas L, Toth LA. Cytokine involvement in the regulation of sleep. *Proc Soc Exp Biol Med* 1992;201:16–27.

66. Ottaway CA. Vasoactive intestinal peptide and immune function. In: Ader R, Felten DL, Cohen N, eds. *Psychoneuroimmunology*. 2nd ed. San Diego: Academic Press, 1991;225–262.

67. Otterness IG, Seymour PA, Golden HW, Reynolds JA, Daumy GO. The effects of continuous administration of murine interleukin-1α in the rat. *Physiol Behav* 1988;43:797–804.

68. Renoux G, Biziere K. Neocortex lateralization of immune function and of the activities of imuthiol, a T-cell-specific immunopotentiator. In: Ader R, Felten DL, Cohen N, eds. *Psychoneuroimmunology*. 2nd ed. San Diego: Academic Press; 1991:127–147.

69. Rivier C, Vale W, Brown M. In the rat, interleukin-1α and -β stimulate adrenocorticotropin and catecholamine release. *Endocrinology* 1989;125:3096–3102.

70. Roszman TL, Cross RJ, Brooks WH, Markesbery WR. Neuroimmunomodulation: effects of neural lesions on cellular immunity. In: Guillemin R, Cohn M, Melnechuk T, eds. *Neural modulation of immunity*. New York: Raven Press; 1985:95–109.

71. Sanders VM, Munson AE. Norepinephrine and the antibody response. *Pharmacol Rev* 1985;37:229–248.

72. Saphier D. Neurophysiological and endocrine consequences of immune activity. *Psychoneuroendocrinology* 1989;14:63–87.

73. Schultzberg M. Location of interleukin-1 in the nervous system. In: Rothwell NJ, Dantzer RD, eds. *Interleukin-1 in the brain*. Oxford: Pergamon Press; 1992:1–11.

74. Selye H. *The stress of my life*. 2nd ed. New York: Van Nostrand Reinhold; 1979.

75. Shahabi NA, Peterson PK, Sharp BM. β-Endorphin binding to

naloxone-insensitive sites on a human mononuclear cell line (U937): effects of cations and guanosine triphosphate. *Endocrinology* 1990;126:3006–3015.

76. Sharp B, Linner K. What do we know about the expression of proopiomelanocortin transcripts and related peptides in lymphoid tissue? *Endocrinology* 1993;133:1921–1922.

77. Shavit Y, Lewis JW, Terman GW, Gale RP, Liebeskind JC. Opioid peptides mediate the suppressive effect of stress on natural killer cell cytotoxicity. *Science* 1984;223:188–190.

78. Spadaro F, Dunn AJ. Effects of neuropeptides on cells of the immune system. *Clin Immun Newslett.* 1991;11:105–111.

79. Stein C, Hassan AHS, Przewlocki R, Gramsch C, Peter K, Herz A. Opioids from immunocytes interact with receptors on sensory nerves to inhibit nociception in inflammation. *Proc Natl Acad Sci USA* 1990;87:5935–5939.

80. Stein M, Miller AH, Trestman RL. Depression and the immune system. In: Ader R, Felten DL, Cohen N, eds. *Psychoneuroimmunology*. 2nd ed. San Diego: Academic Press; 1991;897–930.

81. Stenzel-Poore M, Vale WW, Rivier C. Relationship between antigen-induced immune stimulation and activation of the hypothalamic-pituitary-adrenal axis in the rat. *Endocrinology* 1993;132:1313–1318.

82. Sternberg EM, Young WS, Bernardini R, et al. A central nervous system defect in biosynthesis of corticotropin-releasing hormone is associated with susceptibility to streptococcal cell wall-induced arthritis in Lewis rats. *Proc Natl Acad Sci USA* 1989;86:4771–4775.

83. Sundar SK, Cierpial MA, Kilts C, Ritchie JC, Weiss JM. Brain IL-1-induced immunosuppression occurs through activation of both pituitary-adrenal axis and sympathetic nervous system by corticotropin-releasing factor. *J Neurosci* 1990;10:3701–3706.

84. Takamoto T, Hori Y, Koga Y, Toshima H, Hara A, Yokoyama MM. Norepinephrine inhibits human natural killer cell activity in vitro. *Int J Neurosci* 1991;58:127–131.

85. Takao T, Tracey DE, Mitchell WM, De Souza EB. Interleukin-1 receptors in mouse brain: characterization and neuronal localization. *Endocrinology* 1990;127:3070–3078.

86. Tchelingerian JL, Quinonero J, Booss J, Jacque C. Localization of TNFα and IL-1α immunoreactivities in striatal neurons after surgical injury to the hippocampus. *Neuron* 1993;10:213–224.

87. Tsagarakis S, Gillies G, Rees LH, Besser M, Grossman A. Interleukin-1 directly stimulates the release of corticotrophin releasing factor from rat hypothalamus. *Neuroendocrinology* 1989;49:98–101.

88. Tsokos GC, Balow JE. Regulation of human cellular immune responses by glucocorticosteroids. In: Plotnikoff NP, Faith RE, Murgo AJ, Good RA, eds. *Enkephalins and endorphins: stress and the immune system*. New York: Plenum Press; 1986:159–171.

89. Uehara A, Gottschall PE, Dahl RR, Arimura A. Interleukin-1 stimulates ACTH release by an indirect action which requires endogenous corticotropin releasing factor. *Endocrinology* 1987;121:1580–1582.

90. Weber RJ, Pert A. The periaqueductal gray matter mediates opiate-induced immunosuppression. *Science* 1989;245:188–190.

91. Webster EL, Tracey DE, Jutila MA, Wolfe SA, De Souza EB. Corticotropin-releasing factor receptors in mouse spleen: identification of receptor-bearing cells as resident macrophages. *Endocrinology* 1990;127:440–452.

92. Wood PG, Karol MH, Kusnecov AW, Rabin BS. Enhancement of antigen-specific humoral and cell-mediated immunity by electric footshock stress in rats. *Brain Behav Immun* 1993;7:121–134.

93. Woodroofe MN, Sarna GS, Wadhwa M, et al. Detection of interleukin-1 and interleukin-6 in adult rat brain, following mechanical injury, by in vivo microdialysis: evidence of a role for microglia in cytokine production. *J Neuroimmunol* 1991;33:227–236.

94. Zalcman S, Shanks N, Anisman H. Time-dependent variations of central norepinephrine and dopamine following antigen administration. *Brain Res* 1991;557:69–76.

95. Zuckerman SH, Shellhaas J, Butler LD. Differential regulation of lipopolysaccharide-induced interleukin-1 and tumor necrosis factor synthesis: effects of endogenous and exogenous glucocorticoids and the role of the pituitary-adrenal axis. *Eur J Immunol* 1989;19:301–305.

Psychopharmacology: The Fourth Generation of Progress, edited by Floyd E. Bloom and David J. Kupfer. Raven Press, Ltd., New York © 1995.

CHAPTER **64**

Adaptive Processes Regulating Tolerance to Behavioral Effects of Drugs

Alice M. Young and Andrew J. Goudie

This chapter surveys major adaptive learning processes involved in development, expression, and maintenance of tolerance to behavioral effects of drugs. A prevailing view of drug tolerance is that sustained or repeated administration of a drug initiates multiple adaptive processes that reduce the acute effects of an initial drug dose and increase the dose or concentration needed to produce effects of a given magnitude. Higher intensities of drug treatment may also decrease the maximal effects that can be produced by any dose. Adaptations may occur by biochemical, cellular, and behavioral processes triggered by the initial effects of a drug. The specific adaptations recruited by repeated drug treatment are determined by the type of drug administered chronically; its dose, frequency, and duration of administration; and the functional demands placed on the biological system. Tolerance to behavioral effects of drugs in vivo is also determined by an individual's experiences during chronic treatment, that is, by learning processes. Unfortunately, there has been little interaction among researchers working on different levels of tolerance, and a major challenge for future research in this area is to link behavioral adaptations to those occurring at biochemical and cellular levels (see also Chapters 6, 61, 62, and 66, *this volume*).

Tolerance is an acquired decrease in sensitivity to a particular effect of a drug that results from exposure to that or a related drug. A distinction is often made between *acute tolerance,* decreases in sensitivity that develop during a single drug exposure, and *chronic tolerance,* decreases in sensitivity that develop from repeated exposure. A distinction is also made between tolerance to a specific

drug, to related drugs (selective or homologous cross-tolerance), or to drugs from unrelated drug classes (heterologous cross-tolerance). The definition of tolerance carries no implications about specific processes. Potential processes are commonly divided into two groups: (a) dispositional or pharmacokinetic processes, which reduce the concentration of a drug or its duration of action in a target system; and (b) pharmacodynamic or functional processes, which reduce the sensitivity of drug-sensitive systems to a given drug concentration. *Dispositional tolerance* describes changes in sensitivity that arise from changes in absorption, distribution, metabolism, or excretion that diminish concentrations of a drug at effector sites; these processes are surveyed elsewhere (e.g., 27). In contrast, *pharmacodynamic tolerance* describes changes in sensitivity that result from adaptive changes in drug-sensitive systems that diminish the initial effects of a drug.

Two general models have been advanced to account for pharmacodynamic tolerance. Although multiple mechanisms are involved in the development of tolerance (reviewed in refs. 4,12,19,22,38,51,56), they can be grouped into two logical classes (4,32). One class of models postulates that tolerance results from a reduction in the drug signal or stimulus, as a result of adaptations that reduce activity of a drug at its receptors. Such a reduction would of course occur in dispositional tolerance but may also result from adaptive pharmacodynamic processes, such as receptor down-regulation or desensitization, that reduce the intensity of the drug-induced biological signal. These could include changes in affinity, coupling, distribution, or number of target receptors. A second class of models postulates that signal intensity is constant (i.e., that the interaction between a drug and its receptors is unchanged), and that initial acute effects of the drug are opposed or counteracted by homeostatic changes in bio-

A. M. Young: Department of Psychology, Wayne State University, Detroit Michigan 48202.

A. J. Goudie: Department of Psychology, University of Liverpool, Liverpool, L69 3BX, England

chemical, cellular, and effector systems that mediate primary drug effects or in systems changed by these effects. For individual drugs or drug classes, these might include changes in postreceptor signal transduction; intraneuronal signaling pathways; neuronal architecture, connections, or sensitivity to transmitters; neurotransmitter synthesis or distribution; or functioning of effector systems themselves. Behavioral accounts of tolerance generally are of this type, postulating that conditioning of coordinated homeostatic behavioral responses reduces the initial response to a constant biological signal.

Different models make different predictions about the types of adaptive processes that are recruited by chronic drug treatment and about activity of drug-sensitive systems after treatment ends. Littleton and Little (32) have referred to the two basic models of tolerance as decremental and oppositional, respectively. Decremental pharmacodynamic models focus on processes that change the number or properties of drug-sensitive receptor populations and make no predictions about changes in the functioning of other posttransductional processes. In this scheme, termination of drug treatment would be followed by a delayed recovery of initial sensitivity. Oppositional models postulate that continued drug treatment recruits processes that oppose the initial acute effects of a drug or of receptor alterations. When drug treatment ends, these processes may operate unopposed for some period, resulting in appearance of withdrawal signs, followed by readaptation to the drug-free state. For example, increased activity in an intraneuronal signaling pathway normally inhibited by a drug could produce both tolerance (because a greater fractional inhibition of activity, and thus a higher drug dose, would be needed to produce inhibition equivalent to that produced initially in nontreated tissue) and withdrawal after treatment ends (because removal of the drug would be followed for a time by activity above basal levels in the drug-sensitive pathway). A recent extension of these models (22) distinguishes between adaptations occurring within a drug-sensitive neuronal system and those occurring between systems. In the case of within-system adaptations, repeated drug treatment would elicit opposing activity in the system through which a drug induces its primary pharmacological actions. For example, Nestler and Duman (this volume) review evidence indicating that, in the locus coeruleus, opioid tolerance involves up-regulation of cyclic adenosine monophosphate (cAMP) systems that oppose an initial sustained opioid-induced inhibition of adenylyl cyclase. In the case of between-system adaptations, initial changes in primary drug-sensitive neurons would trigger adaptations in biochemical, cellular, or behavioral pathways different from those directly involved in the initial pharmacological actions of a drug. Such between-systems adaptations may be implicated, for example, in the apparently pervasive role of N-methyl-D-aspartate receptors in modulating tolerance to opiates and other drugs (e.g., 55,56).

For many drugs, emerging accounts of tolerance incorporate features of both logical classes, albeit often from studies conducted at different levels of analysis. Hypotheses about the mechanisms involved in drug tolerance can be usefully organized in terms of general principles of biological regulation at behavioral, cellular, and biochemical levels. Integration of information across studies requires parametric studies to link changes occurring at one level with those studied at another level. Although such studies are only beginning to emerge, several features of descriptive studies of tolerance to behavioral effects of a drug can improve their usefulness as bases for inferences about mechanisms. Among these are systematic variations of pharmacological and behavioral parameters, concurrent or matched measures of multiple endpoints, and independent verification of potential mechanisms. At the most basic level, useful studies assess the occurrence and magnitude of any decreases in the potency and/or maximal effects of a repeatedly administered drug. Unfortunately, studies of tolerance to behavioral effects of drugs frequently assess changes in effects of only one or two doses of a drug. Although this approach can demonstrate loss of an initial drug effect, it cannot assess either the magnitude of decreased sensitivity or the ability of a tolerant system to express the initial effect. Information of the latter sort is critical for full characterization of adaptive processes underlying diminished drug effects. Additional useful information is provided by explorations of how changes in the potency and/or maximal effects of a drug change as a function of a variety of pharmacological and behavioral factors. Useful pharmacological information is provided by manipulations of the dose, frequency, and duration of repeated drug administrations; studies of whether adaptive changes are reversed after discontinuation of treatment; and studies of the pharmacological selectivity of tolerance. As will be reviewed more fully below, useful behavioral information is provided by manipulation of the learning conditions encountered during repeated treatment.

INFLUENCES OF LEARNING PROCESSES ON TOLERANCE TO BEHAVIORAL EFFECTS OF DRUGS

It is well established that development of tolerance to complex behavioral effects of drugs can depend on an individual's experiences in the drugged state. Such contingent tolerance is illustrated by a study by Chen (3), in which one group of rats received three doses of 1.2 g/kg ethanol before running a circular maze every fourth day, and a second group received the same doses of ethanol after running the maze. In the critical test of tolerance, all rats received their fourth dose of ethanol before running the maze. All rats displayed tolerance to sedative effects of ethanol, but only those rats that had always received ethanol before running the maze displayed tolerance to its error-enhancing effects. Because the groups differed only in whether rats had previously run the maze while intoxicated, such selective tolerance probably arose from intoxicated practice.

Several learning processes appear to play key roles in the acquisition, expression, or retention of tolerance to behavioral effects of drugs from numerous pharmacological classes (11,12,64). A number of terms have been used to describe behavioral influences, including associative tolerance, behavioral tolerance, behaviorally augmented tolerance, conditioned tolerance, contingent tolerance, environment-dependent tolerance, and learned tolerance. Although these multiple terms highlight situations in which different learning processes may operate to regulate tolerance, they also impede recognition of situations in which common processes operate. As with biochemical and cellular influences on tolerance, the learning processes that are likely to operate in a particular situation are those that normally govern the behaviors affected by a drug. In the case of complex learned behaviors, these learning processes are involved in their acquisition, maintenance, or adaptability. To date, the most important processes appear to be classical and instrumental conditioning. In the sections that follow, we review how these learning processes influence tolerance to behavioral effects of drugs (see also Chapters 6, 66, and 68, *this volume*).

INFLUENCES OF CLASSICAL CONDITIONING AND HABITUATION ON TOLERANCE

The classical conditioning account of tolerance derives largely from empirical studies initiated by Siegel in 1975 (44), although it has been recognized for many years that classical conditioning processes may modulate drug effects (52,63). Additionally, Solomon (50) independently developed a general opponent process theory of motivation that accounts for much of the data that support the classical conditioning theory of tolerance.

Procedures for the study of tolerance frequently involve repeated drug administrations and repeated testing. Such procedures are essentially classical conditioning trials. The drug acts as an unconditional stimulus (UCS) that elicits unconditional responses (UCRs). Almost inevitably, the drug UCS will be consistently paired with distinctive environmental stimuli (e.g., handling procedures or the environment in which drug is administered). After repeated pairings, such environmental stimuli may become conditional (drug-predictive) stimuli (CSs) that when presented alone elicit, as conditional responses (CRs), drug effects previously seen only as UCRs. Under such circumstances, one might expect conditioning of drug-like CRs. Siegel noted, however, that in many studies drug UCSs have been reported to elicit drug-opponent

or compensatory CRs. Siegel proposed that tolerance develops when a drug UCS elicits two opposing responses in drug-experienced subjects: a constant UCR and a compensatory CR that grows with repeated treatments. Over repeated treatments (i.e., reiterated conditioning trials), the sum of the constant UCR and the increasing compensatory CR should progressively reduce the net drug effect, resulting in tolerance. This theoretical account of tolerance is logically similar to biochemical and cellular accounts of pharmacodynamic tolerance that emphasize recruitment of adaptive homeostatic processes.

The key postulate of the conditioning theory of tolerance is the compensatory CR, which counteracts the initial effects of the drug. In contrast, a drug-like CR should produce sensitization, that is, a decrease in the dose of a drug required for effect and/or an increase in the maximal effect obtained. Both drug-like and drug-compensatory CRs have been observed, however (45), raising questions about behavioral and pharmacological requirements for conditioning of adaptive responses. Stewart and colleagues have suggested that many drug effects are biphasic (e.g., an initial drug-induced hypothermia followed by hyperthermia). It is thus possible that development of compensatory CRs may involve conditioning of the secondary responses. As conditioning proceeds, the CS may elicit these opponent responses coincidentally with the initial drug effect, diminishing the effects of a constant drug dose (see ref. 8 for a detailed discussion of this issue).

If compensatory CRs mediate tolerance, a number of predictions follow from classical conditioning theory. The most obvious is that tolerance should be situation-specific; that is, it should be greater in the presence of CSs eliciting compensatory CRs than in the absence of such CSs. Tolerance to various effects of numerous drugs can show situation specificity in laboratory animals and humans (see ref. 45 for review). In a typical experimental demonstration of situation specificity, subjects are treated with drug in one environment and vehicle in a different environment. The environments differ in their lighting, sound, smell, and so on. After repeated pairings, drug effects are tested in both environments. Typically, more tolerance is seen in the drug-predictive environment than in the vehicle-predictive environment, due presumably to the fact that the compensatory CR is elicited only in the former environment.

Situation specificity of tolerance has been studied most extensively for antinociceptive effects of μ-opiates, although animal studies provide evidence for considerable pharmacological and behavioral generality of the phenomenon (10,45). Situation-specific tolerance has been reported with pentobarbital, ethanol, haloperidol, nicotine, midazolam, and scopolamine. The response systems supporting situation-specific tolerance include those involved in regulation of temperature, pain, drinking, motor activity, and catalepsy. Situation specificity has also been reported in human opiate addicts, who show tolerance to self-administered heroin but not to heroin administered by the experimenter, suggesting that drug-taking rituals become CSs that induce tolerance (7). Perhaps the most striking example of the dynamic manner in which environmental CSs modulate sensitivity to drug effects is provided by situation-specific tolerance to the lethal effects of heroin. Rats that receive a large dose of heroin in a drug-predictive environment suffer lower mortality than rats tested in an environment not previously paired with heroin (47). Siegel (45) suggested that so-called accidental opiate overdose deaths, which occur when addicts take a dose they have previously tolerated, are due to some critical change in the stimuli surrounding drug administration, such that the compensatory CR is not recruited and the full drug UCS is reinstated with dramatic adverse effects.

A further prediction from conditioning theory is that presentations of drug-predictive CSs in the absence of the drug UCS should leave the compensatory CR unopposed and thus detectable as a drug-opponent response. Furthermore, because withdrawal signs are typically drug-opposite, such compensatory CRs may resemble withdrawal signs. Thus, if subjects show situation-specific tolerance, they may also show situation-specific withdrawal. Studies do suggest that situation-specific withdrawal can be elicited by cues repeatedly associated with drug administration (9,20,24). Studies to identify biochemical or cellular correlates of situation-specific withdrawal should provide very interesting information about the pharmacological specificity of such changes.

Conditioning theory makes a number of other predictions about tolerance. Tolerance should be extinguished by repeated presentations of a drug-predictive CS in the absence of a drug UCS. This prediction has been validated. Morphine antinociception can be reinstated in previously tolerant animals by repeated exposure to a hot-plate test and placebo injections (44). The case for conditioning theory is strengthened further by demonstrations that tolerance displays other critical features of classical conditioning, including partial reinforcement, latent inhibition, sensory preconditioning, overshadowing, blocking, and external inhibition (see ref. 11 for a review). The phenomenon of conditional inhibition is particularly vivid. According to conditioning theory, if a CS is presented so that it predicts the absence of the UCS, it should become a conditional inhibitor that will retard subsequent conditioning. That is, if CS/UCS pairings are subsequently introduced, the rate of CR acquisition will be lower than in naive subjects. Siegel et al. (46) demonstrated conditional inhibition of tolerance to morphine-induced antinociception. Rats were kept in darkened cages for most of the day, so that a light CS could be presented for 1 hr/day. The conditional inhibition group was given explicitly unpaired morphine exposures, such that the light CS was presented 4 hr before the morphine

UCS. Various control groups were exposed to the light CS alone, morphine alone, or no treatment. Subsequently, all rats received repeated tests on a hot plate in the presence of morphine and the light. Tolerance developed more slowly in the conditional inhibition group than in all other groups, including the morphine-alone group, which was drug-experienced at the start of hot-plate testing. Thus, exposure to morphine in a conditional inhibition procedure retards acquisition of tolerance to antinociceptive effects of morphine, making a strong case for the influence of classical conditioning processes.

The classical conditioning account of tolerance is supported by an impressive body of data. The theory is not without problems, however. Most specifically, attempts to demonstrate the compensatory CR, the central theoretical idea of the theory, have met with mixed success. A number of studies have reported marked situation-specific tolerance without a clear compensatory CR (e.g., refs. 21,34,43). The presence of situation-specific tolerance in such studies implies that the absence of a compensatory CR was not due merely to low salience of the experimental CS. In other studies, however, evidence exists for compensatory CRs (e.g., ref. 23,28). Relatively recent studies in humans have also reported the presence of compensatory CRs in alcoholics (35) and opiate addicts (7). The compensatory CR remains, therefore, an intriguing enigma in empirical studies.

The significance attributed to failures to detect compensatory CRs varies among researchers. Negative results may be of less significance than positive ones, as it is possible to explain the absence of the compensatory CR in a post-hoc fashion (37). There are a number of reasons why compensatory CRs may be difficult to detect (45). First, they may be difficult to detect in specific assays. For example, hyperalgesia may be detectable with a hot-plate but not with a tail-flick assay, due to the very low response latency in latter assay (23). Second, compensatory CRs may be difficult to detect after placebo treatment, because, in the absence of the drug UCR (which the CR is designed to counteract), normal homeostatic responses may be recruited to counteract the developing compensatory CR. Finally, drug onset cues themselves may become an essential feature of the CS complex. When drug is administered, a reliable predictor of a specific dose will inevitably be a lower dose. Thus low dose CSs may be a critical part of the overall compound CS, and tests for the CR after placebo may fail.

Siegel (45) and others (33) also suggest that the compensatory CR mediating tolerance may be unobservable under certain circumstances. For example, King et al. (21) found situation-specific tolerance to sedative effects of midazolam, but only weak evidence for conditional hyperactivity. They suggested that the CR mediating tolerance was conditional adrenocorticotropic hormone (ACTH) secretion, which antagonized midazolam's effects. Similarly, Melchior and Tabakoff (36) suggested that situation-specific ethanol tolerance may be mediated by conditional metabolism, because brain ethanol levels in a drug-predictive environment were lower than those in a non-drug-predictive environment. There may well be a strong case for extending the theory beyond CRs that are readily observable to promote studies of the biochemical and cellular bases of adaptive compensatory CRs. Extending the theory to unobserved CRs may weaken it, however, because it cannot be readily refuted unless the nature of the compensatory CR is specified explicitly. For example, if situation-specific tolerance is observed in the absence of an observable compensatory CR, it is possible to explain away the absence of the CR by assuming that tolerance was induced by an hypothetical unobservable compensatory CR. Such a theory is empirically irrefutable. There are obvious dangers in inferring that tolerance is mediated by an unobservable compensatory CR in the absence of any evidence that such a CR was present!

Failures to detect reliably compensatory CRs have resulted in accounts of classical conditioning of tolerance that do not make recourse to compensatory CRs. The most influential classical conditioning account of tolerance that denies a role for compensatory CRs is Baker and Tiffany's (1) habituation theory, which is based upon Wagner's (59) model of habituation to exteroceptive stimuli. There is a formal similarity between habituation to environmental stimuli, in which repeated exposures to a novel stimulus produce progressively smaller behavioral responses, and tolerance, in which repeated exposures to a drug stimulus produce smaller pharmacological responses. Baker and Tiffany's (1) theory assumes that the extent to which a drug stimulus elicits a response depends upon the extent to which the stimulus surprises the subject, which in turn depends upon the degree to which the stimulus is primed in short-term memory (STM). If a drug stimulus is not primed, its presentation surprises the subject and elicits a response. A drug stimulus can be primed in two ways: either by recent presentations of the drug or by recent presentations of drug-predictive stimuli. In both conditions the drug will elicit no response (tolerance will be observed) because the subject is not surprised by the drug. This psychological account of tolerance explains the evidence implicating classical conditioning processes in tolerance by assuming that habituation also involves conditioning processes by which drug-predictive stimuli prime STM and thus induce tolerance.

In contrast to compensatory CR theory, Baker and Tiffany's (1) theory assumes that there are two kinds of tolerance: classically conditioned or associative tolerance, which results from priming by drug-predictive stimuli and is thus situation-specific, and nonassociative, which results from priming by recent drug presentations and is situation-independent. Habituation theory makes predictions about conditions under which these two types of tolerance will be observed. It predicts that infrequent administrations of high doses will lead to situation-specific

(associative) tolerance, whereas frequent administrations of the same doses will produce situation-independent (nonassociative) tolerance that will, in turn, disrupt development of situation-specific tolerance. This prediction follows from the idea that frequent administrations of high doses will continuously "prime" the drug stimulus in STM and therefore block associations between drug stimuli and environmental stimuli. Recent studies support the prediction that situation-independent tolerance retards development of situation-specific tolerance. Tiffany and Maude-Griffin (54), using doses of 30 mg/kg morphine given at different interdose intervals, showed that only situation-specific tolerance is seen at a 96-hr interdose interval, whereas situation-independent tolerance predominates at a 24-hr interdose interval, accompanied by a decline in situation-specific tolerance.

Similarly, Dafters and Odber (5) found that situation specificity of morphine tolerance is maximal at long interdose intervals, whereas high doses of morphine given at short interdose intervals produce situation-independent tolerance. Tiffany et al. (53) also showed that long interdose intervals produce situation-specific tolerance to antinociceptive effects of morphine, which is retained over a 30-day period. At short interdose intervals, tolerance is situation independent and rapidly lost. Again, conditions (large drug doses at short interdose intervals) that facilitate situation-independent tolerance inhibit situation-specific tolerance, supporting Baker and Tiffany's (1) theory. Such data are predicted uniquely by habituation theory. Compensatory CR theory, which deals only with situation-specific tolerance, makes no predictions about interactions between situation-specific and situation-independent tolerance. However, habituation theory is not without problems. First, unlike compensatory CR theory, habituation theory has nothing to say about the possible relationship between tolerance and dependence. Second, it is difficult to comprehend how habituation theory can account for the finding that procedures that induce situation-specific tolerance may also induce situation-specific withdrawal (see above). Finally, habituation theory cannot account for demonstrations of compensatory CRs other than by assuming that such phenomena are simply artifacts (34). However, as described above, many drugs have biphasic effects with acute effects being followed by rebound phenomena. The notion that it is possible to condition secondary drug-compensatory effects has intrinsic appeal, as conditioning of such responses would prepare the organism for a forthcoming toxin. The time is clearly ripe for an attempt to resolve the controversies between habituation theory and compensatory CR theory. This will not prove easy, however, because, as noted above, recent formulations of compensatory CR theory are vague in their definitions of compensatory CRs.

The links between behavioral habituation or compensatory conditioning and cellular or biochemical processes are largely unexplored. It is possible to condition activity of neurochemical systems (57). There is therefore reason to suppose that the habituation or classical conditioning processes involved in tolerance act at various levels of neuronal organization. For example, Liljequist et al. (31) reported situation-specific tolerance to ethanol's sedative actions accompanied by situation-specific tolerance to ethanol's action in stimulating dopamine metabolism. As noted above, Nestler and Duman (this volume) review evidence suggesting that tolerance to inhibitory effects of morphine on locus coeruleus neurons involves compensatory up-regulation of the cAMP system, producing responses that oppose the actions of morphine. As such responses are, almost by definition, compensatory responses, it is possible that such intraneuronal responses can be conditioned, although empirical studies have not yet addressed this important issue. Integration of work at different levels of analysis represents a substantial challenge for the future.

Finally, it is worth commenting on these approaches to tolerance in so far as they relate to the question of whether tolerance involves a change in the drug stimulus during tolerance acquisition. Habituation theory assumes that the stimulus that causes tolerance is present at a constant intensity throughout treatment. If this were not the case, priming of STM would be reduced and tolerance would be lost. The conditions most favorable for priming of STM, and induction of tolerance, are drug presentations at high doses and short interdose intervals. However, induction of the drug stimulus presumably requires activation of appropriate receptor populations. It appears likely that these are precisely the conditions that might, for some drugs and treatment regimens, favor receptor down-regulation or desensitization, a decline in the drug stimulus and the resulting appearance of pharmacodynamic tolerance. Thus habituation theory requires that there be a constant drug stimulus during chronic treatment to induce tolerance, whereas some forms of pharmacodynamic tolerance may involve a diminishing drug stimulus. As regards conditioning theory, reduced stimulus strength (reduction in the magnitude of the UCS) should retard conditioning, which is positively related to UCS magnitude. Thus any biochemical or cellular processes that progressively diminish a drug stimulus should retard acquisition of tolerance mediated by habituation or classical conditioning. Clearly, it is a matter of considerable importance to attempt to dissect out differences between changes in sensitivity acquired as a result of conditioning or habituation processes and those involving other adaptive processes (see also Chapters 66, 68, and 148, this volume).

INFLUENCES OF INSTRUMENTAL CONDITIONING ON TOLERANCE

Many behavioral effects of drugs are changes in instrumental behaviors, behaviors whose topography, temporal pattern, and persistence are shaped by their consequences. Complex instrumental behaviors emerge from undifferentiated behavior through reinforcement of successive changes in form and temporal patterning. When an individual encounters regular scheduling arrangements between instrumental behaviors and their reinforcing or punishing consequences, predictable steady-state performances emerge. Although stable over time, these steady-state performances remain sensitive to changes in the probability or scheduling of their antecedents and consequences. If a drug initially disrupts instrumental performances, the persistence of such disruptions can be modified by their consequences. Current evidence implicates at least two instrumental learning processes, reinforcement and stimulus control, in tolerance to effects on instrumental behaviors of a wide range of drugs, including behavioral stimulants, anxiolytics and sedative-hypnotics, cannabinoids, and opiates (11,58,64).

Tolerance to disruptive effects of drugs on instrumental behaviors can depend on performing the behaviors during intoxication or, alternatively, experiencing behavioral disruptions that change the consequences of behavior. The general principles can be illustrated by studies with ethanol. LeBlanc et al. (29,30) studied rats negotiating a circular maze for food or traversing a moving belt above an electrified grid. Ethanol initially impairs performance in either task, decreasing the frequency of food delivery or increasing contact with electric shock. Rats allowed to execute their task while intoxicated, and therefore to experience the consequences of ethanol-induced impairment, develop tolerance to effects of a daily dose of ethanol faster than rats given the same daily dose but allowed to execute the task while intoxicated only at intervals of several days. Later work by Wenger et al. (60,61) showed that removing interpolated intoxicated test sessions prevents development of tolerance to ataxic effects of ethanol over at least 3 weeks of exposure. Recent studies by Holloway and colleagues have shown that, under various schedules of food reinforcement, consequences of intoxicated performances can shift the full dose-effect curve for ethanol, so that higher doses are required for both rate-increasing and rate-decreasing effects. Rats given ascending daily doses of ethanol before experimental sessions develop greater tolerance to both effects than rats given the same doses after daily sessions or while testing is suspended (2,14,17). Presession ethanol produces greater tolerance than postsession ethanol when administered either daily (2,14,17) or at intervals of several days (16). Control experiments showed that such differential tolerance requires both performance while intoxicated and some minimal exposure to ethanol.

Several features suggest that the greater tolerance after presession ethanol arises from instrumental reinforcement processes. The magnitude of tolerance to initial effects of ethanol varies directly with the number of opportunities for intoxicated practice (18,30) and can be retained for long periods after chronic treatment ends (see refs. 2,14,17,26). Moreover, differential tolerance does not appear to arise from differences in ethanol distribution or metabolism, age-related factors, or sensitivity to drug-induced disruptions in general (14,16,25). Tolerance developed through reinforcement processes is, in turn, modulated by the dose and duration of ethanol treatment (26,62). Interestingly, reinforcement processes also modulate development of within-session tolerance to ethanol (25), suggesting rapid recruitment of adaptive processes.

The strongest evidence that immediate consequences of drug-induced behavior can regulate development of tolerance comes from studies demonstrating differential tolerance to effects that differentially alter how successfully behavior meets local requirements for reinforcement. Schuster et al. (42) introduced what has come to be called the reinforcement density or reinforcement loss hypothesis to account for differential tolerance to stimulant effects of d-amphetamine that have different effects on the likelihood of reinforcement. Schuster et al. studied performances under two schedules of food reinforcement: one in which responses were reinforced only when a pre-specified time interval elapsed between successive responses, and a second in which responses during a pre-specified interval had no effect and the first response at the end of the interval produced reinforcement. The two schedules alternated several times within short daily sessions. Both schedules generated fairly low rates of responding, and a dose of 1.0 mg/kg d-amphetamine initially increased response rates under both. When d-amphetamine was administered daily, tolerance developed rapidly to rate increases that forfeited reinforcers under the first type of schedule, but not to comparable rate increases that did not forfeit reinforcers under the second type. Because the two reinforcement schedules, and their corresponding tolerant or nontolerant behaviors, alternated within sessions, differential tolerance probably did not arise from dispositional sources. Under other conditions, no tolerance developed to rate-increasing effects of d-amphetamine that improved shock avoidance performances. A common interpretation of such outcomes is that reinforcement processes determine both tolerance to drug effects that produce costly behavioral outcomes and lack of tolerance to effects that improve or do not change the likelihood of reinforcement.

Multiple lines of evidence suggest that dynamics of local reinforcement processes modulate development of tolerance to behavioral effects of not only d-amphetamine and other behavioral stimulants, but also anxiolytics and sedative-hypnotics, opiates, cannabinoids, and other drugs (11,58,64). The most common, albeit indirect, evidence comes from studies showing that tolerance to drug-induced changes in instrumental behaviors develops when drug is administered chronically before daily experimental sessions, and fails to develop when the same doses are administered postsession. More direct evidence for

control of tolerance by drug-induced changes in the interactions of behavior with its consequences comes from demonstrations that tolerance develops to initial effects that decrease reinforcer deliveries, but may not develop, or develops to a lesser degree, to similar initial effects that do not change reinforcer deliveries under other schedules of reinforcement. Such differences are particularly powerful when they occur in the same subjects sequentially within the same experimental session (42,58,64), because such sequences minimize the possibility that differential tolerance arises from unsuspected differences in drug disposition. In the case of some drugs, particularly d-amphetamine, control experiments have also ruled out certain other nonlearning processes, such as differential food deprivation or altered body weight set point, as mechanisms for differential tolerance to effects on food-reinforced behaviors (6).

Reinforcement loss is only one behavioral influence on tolerance to drug effects on instrumental behaviors. Tolerance to the effects of drugs on instrumental behaviors can come under the stimulus control of environmental cues, so that tolerance to behavioral effects in one environment may not transfer to similar behavioral effects associated with distinctly different environments or task demands (49). Tolerance is also modulated by strength of stimulus control of behavior (39); amount of work, or effort, required for reinforcement (13); relative number of reinforcement opportunities (18); mental rehearsal of task components (58); and context of reinforcement loss (48). With respect to the latter factor, costly initial effects of a drug may diminish later drug effects only when the drug-induced loss is large relative to total available reinforcers. One challenge for future research will be to delineate how stimulus control and reinforcement loss interact with other controls on instrumental behavior to modulate tolerance development. Another will be to define the boundary conditions, especially the dosing conditions, under which these learning processes modulate tolerance, and to identify factors responsible for reported exceptions (see ref. 64).

Although there is considerable evidence that tolerance to behavioral effects of numerous drugs can be controlled by the dynamics of local reinforcement and/or stimulus control processes, many unanswered questions remain. One concerns how reinforcement processes operate. Reinforcement processes may (a) reestablish instrumental repertoires that have been disrupted by novel effects of a drug, (b) establish new instrumental repertoires that incorporate initially incompatible responses elicited by a drug, or (c) establish new repertoires that incorporate responses that compensate for or oppose initial effects of a drug (37,64). As an example of the second possibility, Wolgin and Kinney (65) suggested that reinforcement processes shape the stereotyped head movements originally elicited by d-amphetamine into a new instrumental response topography that meets requirements for reinforcement in a milk drinking task. As an example of the third possibility, Holloway and King (15) reported that development of tolerance to initial rate-decreasing effects of ethanol in food-reinforced tasks that favor rapid responding may be accompanied by compensatory rate-increasing effects, as revealed by changes in performances in tasks that favor paced responding. A second question concerns how variations in pharmacological parameters affect the influence of instrumental learning. Of particular importance, few studies have examined how, or whether, the dose, frequency, or duration of drug treatment constrains the operation of instrumental learning processes; whether tolerance modulated by learning processes is retained over long drug-free intervals (2,42); whether it is accompanied by homologous or heterologous cross-tolerance (14,40,41,66); or whether instrumental learning processes can modulate biochemical or cellular adaptations. With respect to this latter point, it is unclear whether instrumental learning processes operate primarily to modulate effects of a constant drug signal (as might be expected at low doses that do not recruit other homeostatic adaptive processes), or whether they can operate in concert with biochemical or cellular adaptations that reduce the initial behavioral effects of a drug.

Finally, few studies have examined whether differential tolerance to behavioral effects of drugs is accompanied by differential changes in their cellular or biochemical effects. Such studies are becoming technically feasible, and their results may provide challenging information about interactions of adaptive changes at multiple levels of analysis. For example, Sannerud and colleagues (40) compared behavioral and biochemical effects following pre- or postsession administration of chlordiazepoxide. Repeated doses of 18 mg/kg chlordiazepoxide produced tolerance to behavioral effects of chlordiazepoxide only when administered presession. Cross-tolerance developed to midazolam in all rats, but was greater in rats treated with presession chlordiazepoxide. Pre- or postsession treatment produced comparable sensitization to the inverse agonist FG 7142 and did not change sensitivity to various nonbenzodiazepines. Repeated treatment also produced a significant increase in γ-aminobutyric acid (GABA) -stimulated Cl^- uptake in both cortical and cerebellar tissue. Differences between rats treated pre- or postsession with chlordiazepoxide appeared only in cerebellar tissue, with a smaller increase in GABA sensitivity following presession treatment, suggesting a complex relation among learning processes, changes in functional states of the GABA/benzodiazepine receptor complex, and changes in sensitivity to behavioral effects of chlordiazepoxide.

CONTRIBUTIONS OF MULTIPLE PROCESSES TO DEVELOPMENT OF TOLERANCE

Behavior is an activity of living organisms, not a passive transmitter of drug effects. The lasting effects of a repeatedly encountered drug are jointly determined by properties of the drug and its specific receptor and effector systems, properties of predrug behavior, and learning processes that govern the expression and plasticity of behavior during drug exposure. We have reviewed some of the behavioral adaptations that may be initiated by repeated drug administration and stressed that these adaptations can be organized in terms of general principles of behavior, specifically classical and instrumental conditioning processes. A key challenge for future research will be to define boundary conditions for operation of specific behavioral adaptations. For instance, recruitment of behavioral adaptations may be critically dependent on chronic dosing regimens. Low doses given infrequently may favor classical or instrumental learning processes, whereas higher doses may favor other homeostatic adaptations or receptor regulation processes that decrease signal intensity. Although some theoretical accounts of tolerance to behavioral effects of drugs argue that oppositional and decremental adaptive processes are mutually exclusive (i.e., 1,37), it remains an empirical question as to whether such processes operate concurrently and under what conditions they do so.

Progress in understanding the influences of these behavioral adaptations complements progress in understanding biochemical and cellular adaptations to repeated drug administrations. In our view, a major challenge for the future is to identify the cascades of adaptations involved in tolerance to behavioral effects of major psychoactive drugs. A useful perspective holds that these adaptive processes are triggered by the acute initial effects of a drug and can be organized in terms of general principles of biological regulation at biochemical, cellular, and behavioral levels. To date, however, few studies have linked adaptive changes at a behavioral level with adaptations studied at biochemical or cellular levels. Studies of behavioral factors in drug tolerance have rarely included detailed examinations of changes in drug disposition or kinetics, or of changes in biochemical or cellular effects of the drug of interest. Similarly, studies of biochemical or cellular factors in tolerance have rarely explored how relevant processes are modulated by environmental factors known to modulate changes in sensitivity to behavioral effects in living organisms. Progress in understanding the consequences of repeated drug administration will require iterative parametric work to organize information within and across levels of analysis.

ACKNOWLEDGMENTS

We thank the editors of this volume and the following colleagues for critical comments on a prior version of this chapter: F. C. Colpaert, M. Emmett-Oglesby, F. A. Holloway, C. A. Sannerud, J. B. Smith, S. T. Tiffany, and D. L. Wolgin. Preparation of this chapter was supported in part by U.S. Public Health Service grant DA03796 from the National Institute of Drug Abuse to A. M. Young, who is recipient of NIDA Research Scientist Development Award K02 DA00132.

REFERENCES

1. Baker TB, Tiffany ST. Morphine tolerance as habituation. *Psychol Rev* 1985;92:78–108.
2. Bird DC, Holloway FA. Development and loss of tolerance to the effects of ethanol on DRL performance of rats. *Psychopharmacology* 1989;97:45–50.
3. Chen C. A study of the alcohol-tolerance effect and an introduction of a new behavioural technique. *Psychopharmacologia* 1968;12:433–440.
4. Cox BM. Drug tolerance and physical dependence. In: Pratt WB, Taylor P, eds. *Principles of drug action: the basis of pharmacology.* 3rd ed. New York: Churchill Livingston, 1990;639–690.
5. Dafters R, Odber J. Effects of dose, interdose interval and drug-signal parameters on morphine analgesic tolerance: implications for current theories of tolerance. *Behav Neurosci* 1989;103:1082–1090.
6. Demellweek C, Goudie AJ. Behavioural tolerance to amphetamine and other psychostimulants: the case for considering behavioral mechanisms. *Psychopharmacology* 1983;80:287–307.
7. Ehrman R, Ternes J, O'Brien CP, McLellan AT. Conditioned tolerance in human opiate addicts. *Psychopharmacology* 1992;108:218–224.
8. Eikelboom R, Stewart J. Conditioning of drug-induced physiological responses. *Psychol Rev* 1982;89:507–528.
9. Falls WA, Kelsey JE. Procedures that produce context-specific tolerance to morphine in rats also produce context-specific withdrawal. *Behav Neurosci* 1989;103:842–849.
10. Goudie AJ. Conditioned opponent processes in the development of tolerance to psychoactive drugs. *Prog Neuro psychopharmacol Biol Psychiatry* 1990;14:675–688.
11. Goudie AJ, Demellweek C. Conditioning factors in drug tolerance. In: Goldberg SR, Stolerman IP, eds. *Behavioural approaches to drug dependence.* New York: Academic Press, 1986;225–285.
12. Goudie AJ, Emmett-Oglesby MW, eds. *psychoactive drugs: tolerance and sensitization.* Clifton NJ: Humana Press, 1989.
13. Hoffman SH, Branch MN, Sizemore GM. Cocaine tolerance: acute versus chronic effects as dependent upon fixed-ratio size. *J Exp Anal Behav* 1987;47:363–376.
14. Holloway FA, Bird DC, Holloway JA, Michaelis RC. Behavioral factors in development of tolerance to ethanol's effects. *Pharmacol Biochem Behav* 1988;29:105–113.
15. Holloway FA, King DA. Parallel development of ethanol tolerance and operant compensatory behaviors in rats. *Pharmacol Biochem Behav* 1989;34:855–861.
16. Holloway FA, King DA, Bedingfield JB, Gauvin DV. Role of context in ethanol tolerance and subsequent hedonic effects. *Alcohol* 1992;9:109–116.
17. Holloway FA, King DA, Michaelis RC, Harland RD, Bird DC. Tolerance to ethanol's disruptive effects on operant behavior in rats. *Psychopharmacology* 1989;99:479–485.
18. Holloway FA, Michaelis RC, Harland RD, Criado JR, Gauvin DV. Tolerance to ethanol's effects on operant performance in rats: role of number and pattern of intoxicated practice opportunities. *Psychopharmacology* 1992;106:112–120.
19. Johnson SM, Fleming WW. Mechanisms of cellular adaptive sensitivity changes: applications to opioid tolerance and dependence. *Pharmacol Rev* 1989;41:435–488.
20. Kelsey JE, Aranow JS, Matthews RT. Context-specific withdrawal in rats: duration and effects of clonidine. *Behav Neurosci* 1990;104:704–710.
21. King DA, Bouton MA, Musty RE. Associative control of tolerance to the sedative effect of a short acting benzodiazepine. *Behav Neurosci* 1987;101:104–114.
22. Koob GF, Bloom FE. Cellular and molecular mechanisms of drug dependence. *Science* 1988;242:715–723.
23. Krank MD. Conditioned hyperalgesia depends on the pain sensitivity measure. *Behav Neurosci* 1987;101:854–857.
24. Krank MD, Perkins WL. Conditioned withdrawal signs elicited by contextual cues for morphine administration. *Psychobiology* 1993;21:113–119.
25. Lê AD, Kalant H. Influence of intoxicated practice on the development of acute tolerance to the motor impairment effect of ethanol. *Psychopharmacology* 1992;106:572–576.
26. Lê AD, Kalant H, Khanna JM. Roles of intoxicated practice in the development of ethanol tolerance. *Psychopharmacology* 1989;99:366–370.
27. Lê AD, Khanna JM. Dispositional mechanisms in drug tolerance and sensitization. In: Goudie AJ, Emmett-Oglesby MW, eds. *Psychoactive drugs: tolerance and sensitization.* Clifton NJ: Humana Press, 1989:281–351.
28. Lê AD, Poulos CX, Cappell H. Conditioned tolerance to the hypothermic effects of ethyl alcohol. *Science* 1979;206:1109–1110.
29. LeBlanc AE, Gibbins RJ, Kalant H. Behavioral augmentation of tolerance to ethanol in the rat. *Psychopharmacologia* 1973;30:117–122.
30. LeBlanc AE, Kalant H, Gibbins RJ. Acquisition and loss of behaviorally augmented tolerance to ethanol in the rat. *Psychopharmacology* 1976;48:153–158.
31. Liljequist S, Ekman A, Snape B, Söderpalm B, Engel JA. Environment-dependent effects of ethanol on DOPAC and HVA in various brain regions of ethanol-tolerant rats. *Psychopharmacology* 1990;102:319–324.
32. Littleton JM, Little HJ. Adaptation in neuronal calcium channels as a common basis for physical dependence on central depressant drugs. In: Goudie AJ, Emmett-Oglesby MW, eds. *Psychoactive drugs: tolerance and sensitization.* Clifton NJ: Humana Press, 1989:461–518.
33. Mackintosh NJ. Neurobiology, psychology and habituation. *Behav Res Therap* 1987;25:81–97.
34. Maude-Griffin PM, Tiffany ST. Associative morphine tolerance in the rat: examinations of compensatory responding and cross-tolerance with stress-induced analgesia. *Behav Neural Biol* 1989;51:11–33.
35. McCaul M, Turkhan JS, Stitzer ML. Conditioned opponent responses: effects of placebo challenge in alcoholic subjects. *Alcoholism: Clinic Exp Res* 1989;13:613–635.
36. Melchior CL, Tabakoff B. Features of environment dependent tolerance to ethanol. *Psychopharmacology* 1985;87:94–100.
37. Poulos CX, Cappell H. Homeostatic theory of drug tolerance: a general model of physiological adaptation. *Psychol Rev* 1991;98:390–408.
38. Pratt J, ed. *The biological bases of drug tolerance and dependence.* San Diego: Academic Press, 1991.
39. Rees DC, Wood RW, Laties VG. Stimulus control and the development of behavioral tolerance to daily injections of *d*-amphetamine in the rat. *J Pharmacol Exp Ther* 1987;240:65–73.
40. Sannerud CA, Marley RJ, Serdikoff SL, Alastra AJG, Cohen C, Goldberg SR. Tolerance to the behavioral effects of chlordiazepoxide: pharmacological and biochemical selectivity. *J Pharmacol Exp Ther* 1993;267:1311–1320.
41. Sannerud CA, Young AM. Modification of morphine tolerance by behavioral variables. *J Pharmacol Exp Ther* 1986;237:75–81.
42. Schuster CR, Dockens WS, Woods JH. Behavioral variables affecting the development of amphetamine tolerance. *Psychopharmacologia* 1966;9:170–182.
43. Shapiro NR, Dudel BC, Rosellini RA. The role of associative factors in tolerance to the hypothermic effects of morphine in mice. *Pharmacol Biochem Behav* 1983;19:327–333.
44. Siegel S. Evidence from rats that morphine tolerance is a learned response. *J Comp Physiol Psychol* 1975;89:498–506.
45. Siegel S. Pharmacological conditioning and drug effects. In: Goudie AJ, Emmett-Oglesby MW, eds. *Psychoactive drugs: tolerance and sensitization.* Clifton NJ: Humana Press, 1989:115–180.
46. Siegel S, Hinson RE, Krank MD. Morphine-induced attenuation of morphine tolerance. *Science* 1981;212:1533–1534.
47. Siegel S, Hinson RE, Krank MD, McCully J. Heroin "overdose" death: contribution of drug-associated environmental cues. *Science* 1982;216:436–437.
48. Smith JB. Effects of chronically administered *d*-amphetamine on

spaced responding maintained under multiple and single-component schedules. *Psychopharmacology* 1986;88:296–300.

49. Smith JB. Situational specificity of tolerance to effects of phencyclidine on responding of rats under fixed-ratio and spaced-responding schedules. *Psychopharmacology* 1991;103:121–128.

50. Solomon RL. An opponent-process theory of acquired motivation: The affective dynamics of addiction. In: Maser JD, Seligman MEP, eds. *Psychopathology: experimental models.* San Francisco: Freeman, 1977:124–145.

51. Stewart J, Badiani A. Tolerance and sensitization to the behavioral effects of drugs. *Behav Pharmacol* 1993;4:289–312.

52. Subkov AA, Zilov GN. The role of conditioned reflex adaptation in the origin of hyperergic reactions. *Bull Biol Med Exp* 1937;4:294–296.

53. Tiffany ST, Drobes DJ, Cepeda-Benito A. Contribution of associative and nonassociative processes to the development of morphine tolerance. *Psychopharmacology* 1992;109:185–190.

54. Tiffany ST, Maude-Griffin PM. Tolerance to morphine in the rat: associative and nonassociative effects. *Behav Neurosci* 1988;102:534–543.

55. Tiseo PJ, Inturrisi CE. Attenuation and reversal of morphine tolerance by the competitive N-methyl-D-aspartate receptor antagonist LY274614. *J Pharmacol Exp Ther* 1993;264:1090–1096.

56. Trujillo KA, Akil H. Opiate tolerance and dependence: recent findings and synthesis. *New Biologist* 1991;3:915–923.

57. Turkhan JS. Classical conditioning: the new hegemony. *Behav Brain Sci* 1989;12:121–179.

58. Vogel-Sprott M, Sdao-Jarvie K. Learning alcohol tolerance: the contribution of response expectancies. *Psychopharmacology* 1989;98:289–296.

59. Wagner AR. Priming in STM: an information processing mechanism for self-generated or retrieval-generated depression in performance. In: Tighe TJ, Leaton RN, eds. *Habituation: perspectives from child development, animal behavior and neurophysiology.* Hillsdale NJ: Lawrence Erlbaum, 1976:95–128.

60. Wenger JR, Berlin V, Woods SC. Learned tolerance to the behaviorally disruptive effects of ethanol. *Behav Neural Biol* 1980;28:418–430.

61. Wenger JR, Tiffany TM, Bombardier C, Nicholls K, Woods SC. Ethanol tolerance in the rat is learned. *Science* 1981;213:575–577.

62. Wigell AH, Overstreet DH. Acquisition of behaviourally augmented tolerance to ethanol and its relationship to muscarinic receptors. *Psychopharmacology* 1984;83:88–92.

63. Wikler A. Recent progress in research on the neurophysiological basis of morphine addiction. *Am J Psychiatry* 1948;105:329–338.

64. Wolgin DL. The role of instrumental learning in behavioral tolerance to drugs. In: Goudie AJ, Emmett-Oglesby MW, eds. *Psychoactive drugs: tolerance and sensitization.* Clifton NJ: Humana Press, 1989:17–114.

65. Wolgin DL, Kinney GG. Effect of prior sensitization of stereotypy on the development of tolerance to amphetamine-induced hypophagia. *J Pharmacol Exp Ther* 1992;262:1232–1241.

66. Young AM, Walton MA, Carter TL. Selective tolerance to discriminative stimulus effects of morphine or d-amphetamine. *Behav Pharmacol* 1992;3:201–209.

Psychopharmacology: The Fourth Generation of Progress, edited by Floyd E. Bloom and David J. Kupfer. Raven Press, Ltd., New York © 1995.

CHAPTER **65**

The Psychopharmacology of Sexual Behavior

James G. Pfaus and Barry J. Everitt

The history of research into the effects of drugs on human sexual behavior has been concerned primarily with the search for an aphrodisiac. More recently, psychoactive drugs used in the treatment of psychiatric and neurological disorders have been seen to have (usually unwanted) side effects that include impaired libido in men and women or, occasionally, increases in sexual interest that have been much publicized in the press (e.g., the effects of L-dopa in Parkinsonian patients in the 1960s). Although modern medical and scientific opinion has tended to dismiss the idea of chemical stimulation of sexuality as improbable, at least as far as human sexuality is concerned, there has in recent years been a resurgence of interest in the development of such drugs within the pharmaceutical industry. This has in part resulted from the medicalization of male sexual dysfunction, which has emerged over the past 10 years with the widespread involvement of urology and vascular surgery in this clinical field, and with the discovery that injection of various smooth-muscle-relaxing drugs into the corpora cavernosa of the penis is effective in producing erection. The development of a drug that could be taken by mouth that would enhance sexual responses without other undesirable side effects would have major clinical as well as commercial consequences.

In men with sexual dysfunction, dopamine agonists and α_2-adrenoceptor antagonists are currently being explored as therapeutic agents, a development based largely on the effects of such drugs on animal, in particular rodent, sexual behavior. This brings into focus the question concerning the relevance of such observations to human sexuality, since the behavioral parameters measured in rats, such as mounting and intromission latencies, have no obvious counterpart in men.

Recently, there have been new conceptual developments in the analysis of rodent sexual behavior and its neurochemical determinants (19,52,57), which, as a result of their relative sophistication, may more effectively address issues of importance in understanding the neural and neurochemical basis of human sexuality. In particular, these methods allow distinctions to be made between the psychological processes underlying appetitive and consummatory elements of sexual behavior and thereby the more effective study of their neural basis. To date, such methods have been developed mainly for male sexual behavior, although similar methods for females are emerging. They include (a) instrumental behavior of male rats maintained by sexual reinforcement (the opportunity to copulate with a female in heat) presented under a second-order schedule of reinforcement (19,20); (b) conditioned level changing in a bilevel chamber (44); (c) conditioned place preference acquired by allowing sexual interaction in a distinctive environment (19,52); (d) sexual partner preference, that is, the preference of a male for an estrous versus an anestrous female, or a female for an active or inactive male (see ref. 19). These procedures allow appetitive, or incentive motivational, components of sexual behavior to be studied independently of the ability to copulate and thereby represent a useful development in dissecting the neurochemical basis of sexual motivation and performance (19) (see also Chapters 6 and 68, *this volume*).

The comparable attempts to produce models of human sexuality have been fundamentally different. In particular, they have focused not on patterns of behavior, such as mounting, intromission, or lordosis, but on patterns of physiological response, in particular genital responses and other manifestations of arousal. This in part reflects the assumption that, for the human subject, lying between a physiological state of arousal and a behavioral response is a largely imponderable complex of cognitive processes, with a wide variety of psychosocial influences. More concretely, it can be said that, whereas there are very specific

J. G. Pfaus: Center for Studies in Behavioural Neurobiology, Department of Psychology, Concordia University, Montreal, Quebec, H3G 1M8, Canada.

B. J. Everitt: Department of Experimental Psychology, University of Cambridge, Cambridge, CB2 3EB United Kingdom. Address for correspondence.

behavioral or motor patterns involved in animal, especially rodent, sexual behavior (such as mounting, intromission, or lordosis, some of which are clearly reflexive and hormonally determined), there are no comparably predictable motor patterns in the human repertoire. There is certainly no human (or primate) counterpart of lordosis. The nearest measure of a predictable mounting pattern is the semivoluntary tendency to pelvic thrusting which is a feature of human sexual arousal, but which in fact has been largely ignored in the human literature.

In addition, the measurement of physiological responses in a sexual situation, at least within a laboratory setting, is technically much more feasible in human subjects. In fact, the animal, and in particular the rodent literature has not to date considered genital responses or other physiological parameters of arousal, with the exception of the specific reflexive erections of the male rat, which are frequently elicited in a nonsexual context and which have very uncertain relevance to their normal sexual behavior (see ref. 68 for discussion). Bancroft (6) has suggested that a complex set of processes be considered in the context of human sexual response, involving cognition, some form of central arousability of a specifically sexual kind, peripheral physiological manifestations of this state, and a variety of behaviors (see ref. 21). For example, in the case of a mans' sexual response, in a cognitive domain, self-ratings of frequency of sexual thoughts and associated excitement have been obtained. Behaviorally, assessment of the frequency and quality of various sexual acts, such as sexual intercourse or masturbation, has proved useful, whereas two principle psychophysiological methods have been employed: the measurement of spontaneous erections during sleep, or nocturnal penile tumescence (NPT), and the measurement of erectile responses to various types of erotic stimuli, recorded in a laboratory setting in a more or less standardized fashion.

The number of chemical transmitters, including neuropeptides, that have been implicated in the neurobiology of sexual behavior has grown exponentially since the first demonstration of cholinergic and monoaminergic effects on masculine and feminine sexual behavior in rats and humans. In this chapter, we consider some recent data on the monoaminergic neurotransmitters dopamine (DA), norepinephrine (NE), and serotonin (5-hydroxytryptamine or 5-HT), as well as some neuropeptides and other agents reported to affect sexual behavior, referring where appropriate to relevant studies in humans. The review is not intended to be exhaustive, but to illustrate advances based on the development of behavioral and neural methodologies.

MONOAMINES

Dopamine

Masculine Sexual Behavior

Apomorphine, a mixed D_1 and D_2 dopamine receptor agonist, increases the likelihood of spontaneous erections in normal human volunteers and men with psychogenic erectile dysfunction (32,67). The D_2 side effects of such agonists, such as nausea or vestibular disturbance, make such positive drug effects difficult to elicit. Thus, whereas agonists, such as bromocriptine, are effective in reducing prolactin levels and increasing sexual desire in men with hyperproplactinemia, they are highly likely to produce overpowering side effects in men with normal prolactin levels (21). Recently, a new dopamine agonist, shown to be effective in enhancing sexual behavior in male rats, has been evaluated in the treatment of human male sexual dysfunction. However, D_2 side effects were frequent and often severe (Bancroft, *unpublished*).

Systemic treatment with a range of dopaminergic drugs has long been known to affect profoundly the display of sexual behavior in rodents. Recently, it has become apparent that these effects of dopamine receptor blockade are not simple; with more careful attention to differential effects on D_1 and D_2 receptors as well as dosage, discrete effects on precopulatory behaviors have been demonstrated. For example, in male rats all neuroleptic drugs decreased rates of conditioned level changing, and atypical neuroleptics delayed dose-dependently the initiation of copulation, but had little effect on copulatory behavior once it was initiated (58). Metoclopramide, on the other hand, reduced dose-dependently the number of intromissions to ejaculation but had no effect on initiation latencies, whereas the typical neuroleptics haloperidol and pimozide both prolonged mount and intromission latencies and also altered the number of intromissions preceding ejaculation (58). The different behavioral effects of these drugs may be interpreted in the light of recent in vivo neurochemical data indicating the differential release of dopamine in the preoptic area and the dorsal and ventral striatum that is correlated with relatively discrete epochs of sexual interaction (see below). Thus, those dopaminergic antagonists that more or less selectively block dorsal–striatal (i.e., caudate–putamen) dopamine receptors affect only copulatory responses; in fact, they may actually decrease the ejaculation threshold in terms of the number of intromissions required to reach it. By contrast, those drugs that predominantly affect ventral–striatal dopamine receptors, such as the atypical neuroleptics (e.g., clozapine), delay the initiation of copulation with no other behavioral effects. In other words, appetitive rather than copulatory elements of sexual behavior are primarily affected.

The special sensitivity of such precopulatory responses to dopaminergic blockade was further demonstrated in experiments utilizing a second-order schedule of sexual reinforcement. Thus, the mixed D_1/D_2 dopaminergic receptor antagonist, α-flupenthixol, dose-dependently decreased in response to a receptive female. The drug also prolonged mount and intromission latencies, although at doses slightly greater than those that decreased instrumental responses. More importantly, these effects on appetitive or precopulatory behavior were achieved at doses of the drug that had no significant effect on mounts or intromissions. Only at the highest doses tested were all measures of sexual behavior affected, when the majority of males did not intromit or ejaculate (19).

It is important to consider the neural site of action of these behavioral effects of dopaminergic drugs. However, a number of investigators have also explored actions within the medial preoptic area (mPOA). Infusion of dopamine receptor agonists into this area selectively enhanced measures of copulatory behavior, such as intromission rates and efficiency, but did not affect latencies to mount and intromit (8). Dopaminergic receptor antagonists, or presynaptic doses of the agonists, tended to have opposite effects. All these effects were suggested to depend upon alterations in the autonomic control of penile reflexes, for example, lengthening the latency to erection. This demonstrates the often neglected importance (at least in animal studies) of genital changes in mediating the apparent motivational effects of drugs when measured only as alterations in initiation latencies.

It is evident that the marked changes in appetitive aspects of masculine sexual behavior that follow systemic (8,58,19) or intracerebroventricular (icv) infusion (8) of dopaminergic drugs do not obviously follow direct intrahypothalamic treatment, although infusions of haloperidol into the mPOA reduced rates of conditioned level changing (58), an appetitive response that does not appear to depend upon alterations in penile responsiveness. Clearly, sites of action outside the hypothalamus must mediate these effects of dopaminergic drugs on noncopulatory measures of sexual activity, the striatum being an obvious candidate.

Manipulating dopamine in the ventral striatum affects appetitive sexual responses, but not copulation itself. Thus, infusing the dopamine releaser d-amphetamine into the nucleus accumbens dose-dependently increased instrumental responding for access to an estrous female, reduced latencies to mount and intromit, but did not alter copulatory responses (such as mounts, intromissions and ejaculation), hit rate, or ejaculation latency (Fig. 1) (19). Conversely, lesioning the dopaminergic innervation of the ventral striatum by infusing the neurotoxin 6-hydroxydopamine (6-OHDA), significantly lengthened mount and intromission latencies, also without altering copulatory performance (19). Similarly, infusing the predominantly D_2-receptor antagonist, haloperidol, into the ventral striatum reduced rates of conditioned level changing but did not affect measures of copulation (58).

The impact of these manipulations on incentive motivational processes in a sexual context was further demonstrated by a procedure that effectively devalued as sexual incentives the receptive females with which neuroleptically treated males were interacting. This was achieved by injecting hormone-primed females systemically with the neuroleptic, α-flupenthixol. This treatment selectively abolishes the female's proceptive soliciting responses but actually enhances her display of immobile lordosis pos-

tures (18). In this condition, mounts and intromissions only occur if the male initiates them and, even in normal males, this results in prolonged mount and intromission latencies (19). Males infused into the ventral striatum with the D_2-dopamine receptor antagonist, raclopride, were markedly affected by this coincident treatment of females with α-flupenthixol, such that latencies to mount and intromit were more than doubled (Fig. 1). Some males were so affected by this relative immobilization of females, that mounting and intromitting were actually prevented, even though males treated in this way showed only modest increases in their latencies to mount and intromit when with untreated females who were actively soliciting (19). These data demonstrate the importance of the dopaminergic innervation of the ventral striatum in the display of appetitive responses to sexual incentive stimuli.

Feminine Sexual Behavior

The ability of estrogen to stimulate DA release and to augment DA release and behavior in response to amphetamine has been well established (reviewed in ref. 7). Thus it would appear that brain DA systems are influenced by estrogens, and this may be one mechanism underlying the control of female sexual behavior, although this has been difficult to establish. Systemic administration of DA agonists can facilitate or inhibit lordosis behavior in ovariectomized rats primed with estrogen and progesterone or estrogen alone (18). Paradoxically, systemic administration of a range of doses of DA antagonists also facilitates lordosis, although the behavioral signature of the effect is different. Whereas DA agonists can increase lordosis quotients and proceptivity counts, DA antagonists increase lordosis quotients and the duration that female rats hold the lordosis posture, but abolish proceptive behavior (18). These latter effects have led to the suggestion that DA facilitates the active behavioral components of female sexual behavior, that is, proceptivity, but inhibits the passive components, that is, lordosis (10). Alternatively, the effects of DA antagonists could be viewed as decreasing the ability of the female to disengage from lordosis once it is initiated or to switch between lordosis and proceptive pacing, two mutually exclusive behavioral sequences.

Both the facilitatory and inhibitory effects of DA agonists and antagonists appear to occur through an action on D_2 receptors, as selective D_1 agonists and antagonists do not affect measures of sexual proceptivity or receptivity in female rats (23,24). However, there is little agreement concerning the involvement of pre- and postsynaptic DA receptors. Few studies have examined the central sites of action of DA in female sexual behavior. Neurochemical lesions of the mesolimbic DA pathways with 6-OHDA facilitate lordosis behavior in ovariectomized, estrogen-primed rats (66), suggesting that DA release in the nucleus accumbens or other projection regions

(A) Effects of intra-accumbens raclopride on males' ejaculations with un- or α–flupenthixol-treated females

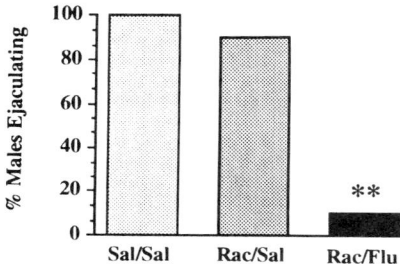

(B) Effects of intra-accumbens raclopride on mount & intromission latencies with un- or α–flupenthixol-treated females

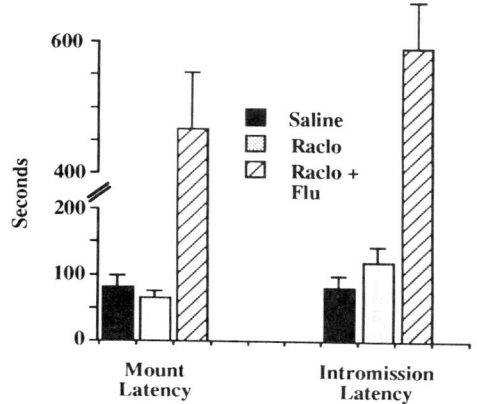

(C) Effects of intra-accumbens d-amphetamine on responding for an oestrous female under a second-order schedule

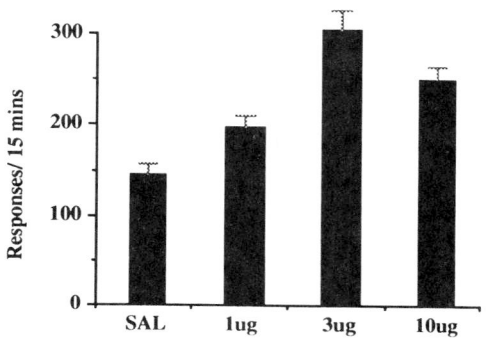

(D) Effects of intra-accumbens d-amphetamine on mount and intromission latencies

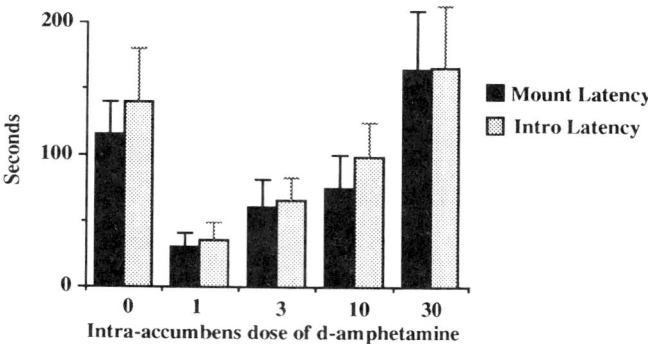

FIG. 1. The effects of dopaminergic drugs on masculine sexual behavior. **A:** The effects of intraaccumbens infusions of the D_2 receptor antagonist raclopride on sexual behavior (% males ejaculating). On its own, raclopride (Rac) has little effect compared with saline (sal) treated males. However, when females are treated with α-flupenthixol to decrease their proceptive behavior, raclopride-treated males rarely copulate to ejaculation. **B:** Mount and intromission latencies of males in the same experiment as in A. Note how mount and intromission latencies are greatly lengthened only when females are not initiating copulation, that is, when mounting behavior only occurs if the males initiate it (see ref. 22). **C:** Intraaccumbens infusions of *d*-amphetamine dose-dependently increase responding for females in heat presented under a second-order schedule of reinforcement (see ref. 22). **D:** Intraaccumbens infusions of *d*-amphetamine dose-dependently reduce mount and intromission latencies, but have no effect on performance measures of sexual behavior (mounts, intromissions, or the rates at which they occur).

of this pathway are inhibitory to lordosis. However, others have found no effect of mesolimbic 6-OHDA lesions on lordosis or proceptive behaviors following a similar level of depletion of DA and its acid metabolites (25). No studies have yet examined the effect of DA agonists or antagonists in other regions of the brain or on other forms of appetitive sexual responding in females.

Norepinephrine

Masculine Sexual Behavior

Yohimbine, an α2 receptor antagonist, has long been regarded as an aphrodisiac. Recently, a number of place-

bo-controlled studies of its effects on erectile dysfunction have been reported (65,74). Although each study has certain methodological problems, the consistency of the results suggests a positive effect, at least in a subgroup of men with erectile dysfunction. Equally important has been the striking lack of side effects in contrast to comparable attempts to evaluate dopamine agonists. The main problem in evaluating this evidence is that there was no underlying rationale for using the drug. In each case, men with erectile dysfunction were involved resulting in heterogeneous groups. It was assumed that the drug would enhance erectile response, but no consideration of the type of erectile response or circumstances relevant to the response were taken into account (see ref. 21). Recent studies, however, have confirmed the potential of α_2 receptor antagonists, especially in a younger group of men with psychogenic impotence (Bancroft, *unpublished*).

In rodents, there are marked effects of α_2 adrenoceptor agonists and antagonists on measures of masculine sexual behavior. For example, yohimbine increased the proportion of sexually naive male rats that mounted, intromitted, and ejaculated and decreased latencies to initiate copulation (14,15). Idazoxan, enhanced copulatory rate and decreased ejaculation latency (15). Agonists at the α_2 receptor had essentially opposite effects (15) that were interpreted as being mediated by changes in sexual arousal.

However, the sexual specificity of the effect remains unclear. It seems unlikely that a drug interacting with diffuse, noradrenergic projection systems that innervate the entire neuraxis are having an effect exclusively on sexual behavior. Furthermore, changes in sexual responsiveness may be mediated by spinal and/or peripheral autonomic effects. Nevertheless, as indicated above, positive effects on sexual responsiveness in men have been obtained with minimal side effects.

Feminine Sexual Behavior

There is considerable evidence that the hormonal changes that underlie lordosis behavior and certain neuroendocrine reflexes, such as the preovulatory luteinizing hormone (LH) surge and pseudopregnancy, are associated with altered norepinephrine transmission. Systemic treatment with α and β receptor agonists and antagonists clearly modulate feminine sexual behavior, but no clear picture emerges (22,43). Central effects of adrenergic treatments on female sexual behavior have not been studied in detail. Infusion of the α_1 antagonist prazocin into the ventromedial hypothalamus (VMH), but not the mPOA, inhibited lordosis (22,17), whereas infusions of the α_2 antagonist idazoxan or the β antagonist metoprolol into the VMH had only a small inhibitory effect in some animals (17). In contrast, infusions of metoprolol into the mPOA inhibited lordosis in most rats (17). Together, these results have been suggested to indicate that stimulation of α_1 receptors in the VMH plays some part in the hormonal facilitation of lordosis behavior, whereas stimulation of β receptors in the mPOA, and to a lesser extent in the VMH, appears to inhibit lordosis. Nothing is known about the role of norepinephrine in other forms of appetitive sexual responding in female rats.

Serotonin

Masculine Sexual Behavior

There is minimal methodologically-sound evidence on the effects on human sexuality of manipulating the serotoninergic system. Ware et al. (76) compared the effects of trazadone, which inhibits serotonin reuptake and decreases 5-HT$_2$ receptor binding, with trimipramine and placebo in six normal volunteers. Trazadone had an enhancing effect on NPT that was independent of any direct effect on rapid-eye-movement (REM) sleep, but no effect on waking erections was reported. Otherwise, there are only anecdotal reports of patients taking serotoninergic drugs such as fluoexetine, trazadone, and fenfluramine, which suggest both negative and positive effects on sexual arousal and performance measures (see ref. 67).

The long history of facilitative effects on masculine sexual behavior of impairing serotonin transmission have been complemented recently by the observation that the selective 5-HT$_{1A}$ receptor agonist, 8-OH-DPAT, markedly facilitated sexual behavior when given systemically to male rats (1,27). The effect is a dramatic one; treated subjects were seen to ejaculate after only one or two intromissions, rather than the more usual ten or twelve. The apparently paradoxical effect of this drug, namely that a 5-HT receptor agonist has a facilitatory effect on copulatory behavior similar to, or even greater than, global 5-HT depletion while being opposite to the effects of other direct, or indirect, nonspecific 5-HT agonists has yet fully to be explored. However, it has been convincingly demonstrated that the facilitatory effects of 8-OH-DPAT depend upon actions at the 5-HT$_{1A}$ autoreceptor on midbrain raphé serotonin neurons resulting in the inhibition of their activity (27) (see also Chapters 14, 26, 37, and 38, *this volume*).

Feminine Sexual Behavior

An extensive literature suggests both inhibitory and facilitatory effects of serotoninergic transmission on feminine sexual behavior, depending on the receptor subtype involved, for example, activity at 5-HT$_{1A}$ and possibly 5-HT$_3$ receptors inhibits, whereas activity at either 5-HT$_{1B}$, 5-HT$_{1C}$, or 5-HT$_2$ receptors facilitates, lordosis (45). However, Mendelson (45) has suggested that there is little reason to suspect that the powerful effects of serotonergic drugs on lordosis reflect a physiological role of brain serotonin systems in this behavior.

BRAIN NEUROPEPTIDE SYSTEMS

Opiates and Opioid Peptides

Masculine Sexual Behavior

Experimentally, morphine generally inhibits mounting, intromissions, and ejaculation in male rats, whereas naloxone given systemically (often in high doses which are not selective for opiate receptors) tends either to have no effect, or to facilitate aspects of sexual behavior, for example in sexually sluggish rats (see ref. 53). These effects of predominantly μ-receptor agonist and antagonist treatments have also been studied using some of the methods described above (instrumental behavior, conditioned place preference, and partner preference), initially by assessing the effects of naloxone given both systemically and into the medial preoptic/anterior hypothalamic area (mPOA) as well as the effects of the endogenous opioid peptide, β-endorphin, infused within the mPOA. The mPOA was studied both because of its well established, central importance in the neural system underlying masculine sexual behavior and also because of its relatively rich innervation by proopiomelanocortin (POMC) containing neurons of the ventral hypothalamus (19,20).

Infused bilaterally into the mPOA, β-endorphin dose-dependently inhibited sexual behavior (Fig. 1). Mounts and intromissions eventually ceased to occur and the latencies to mount, intromit, and ejaculate were prolonged, eventually to the duration of the 15-min test session or even longer (29,30). Subsequent experiments explored the nature of this effect, especially assessing whether males lose interest in females as a result of the treatment. Careful observation of precopulatory, investigative responses revealed that males infused with β-endorphin actively investigated and pursued females and, to some extent, made abortive mounting attempts (29); changes in behavior that were seen in a more emphatic way following lesions of the mPOA (20). Analysis of the behavioral sequence revealed that when a treated male and female first made contact, the pattern of interaction was not significantly different from that seen with control males, but that the sequence broke down at the point when investigative responses usually switched to the copulatory responses of mounting and intromitting; thus, β-endorphin infused into the preoptic area appears not to affect sexual interest or arousal, but instead the transition between investigative and copulatory responses of mounting and intromitting (29,72). These males also showed evidence of thwarting a motivated response tendency in that irrelevant behaviors, such as scratching and grooming, emerged at very high rates in β-endorphin-treated males who could not copulate (29). In addition, these sexually inhibited males now showed a release of the drinking of a preferred sweet solution, which is normally suppressed in the presence of a receptive female with which the male would usually copulate (29).

Infusion of β-endorphin into the mPOA had no effect on instrumental responding for a receptive female presented under a second-order schedule of sexual reinforcement, nor on the expression of a place preference conditioned by sexual interaction with such a female. However, the same treatment rapidly abolished a male's preference for a receptive, over an unreceptive, female tethered in either side of the place preference apparatus (Fig. 2) (30,19).

A further dimension to the analysis of the effects of β-endorphin followed its infusion into the mPOA after an intromission, rather than before interaction with a female had begun. The peptide no longer had an inhibitory effect on mounting, intromission, or ejaculation. Furthermore, the inhibitory effects of β-endorphin were lost or reduced even if a delay of 2 hr or so was interposed between a single intromission and the infusion, provided the male was retested with the same female with which he had intromitted previously. If a different female was placed with the male following intromission, then the inhibitory effect on copulatory behavior of β-endorphin reappeared (72). These results clearly suggest that β-endorphin does not simply act to prevent copulation, because, if the male is allowed to begin interacting sexually with an individual female, the otherwise inhibited behavior can be emitted normally and ejaculation will occur.

Taken together, the results of these experiments reveal the remarkable behavioral specificity of the effects of β-endorphin infused into the mPOA. The peptide does not, apparently, influence appetitive aspects of sexual behavior nor reward-related processes, so far as these are assessed in the place preference procedure. Instead, intrahypothalamic β-endorphin appears to prevent the display of the copulatory reflexes, which together form the consummatory elements of the sexual response sequence. However, even here the effects of the peptide are not absolute, because if the male is allowed to engage sexually with a female, then the inhibitory effects of the peptide are themselves inhibited. The impaired preference for a receptive female that follows β-endorphin infusion appears to be related to the failure to initiate the copulatory sequence—presumably only if the peptide is infused prior to an intromission, although this has not been tested explicitly by studying its effects on preference when infused after an intromission.

Therefore, a neural mechanism may exist in the mPOA that allows the appropriate behavioral responses of mounting and intromitting to be matched to a relevant sexual incentive stimulus, and this is what is impaired in the β-endorphin-treated male rat. This may suggest a particular relationship between the intrinsic sensory properties of a receptive female and the species-specific motor output of copulatory reflexes, since acquired motor responses (e.g., bar-pressing or conditioned approach) for conditioned incentives, such as a light CS or the properties of the preferred place, are completely unaffected by the same β-endorphin manipulation of the mPOA. The behavior of a rat in the operant and place preference procedures may, therefore, be controlled by the same mechanisms that underlie unconditioned appetitive or preparatory responses, and these appear not to reside within the mPOA, because lesions of the structure are also without effect on these parameters (19,20). Reduced preference for an estrous female after β-endorphin infusions, however, may be related more to the switch from sexual to ingestive responses, which is seen to follow manipulations of testosterone or hypothalamic β-endorphin in male rats (29).

The effects of naloxone on sexual behavior have also been studied using a number of these behavioral proce-

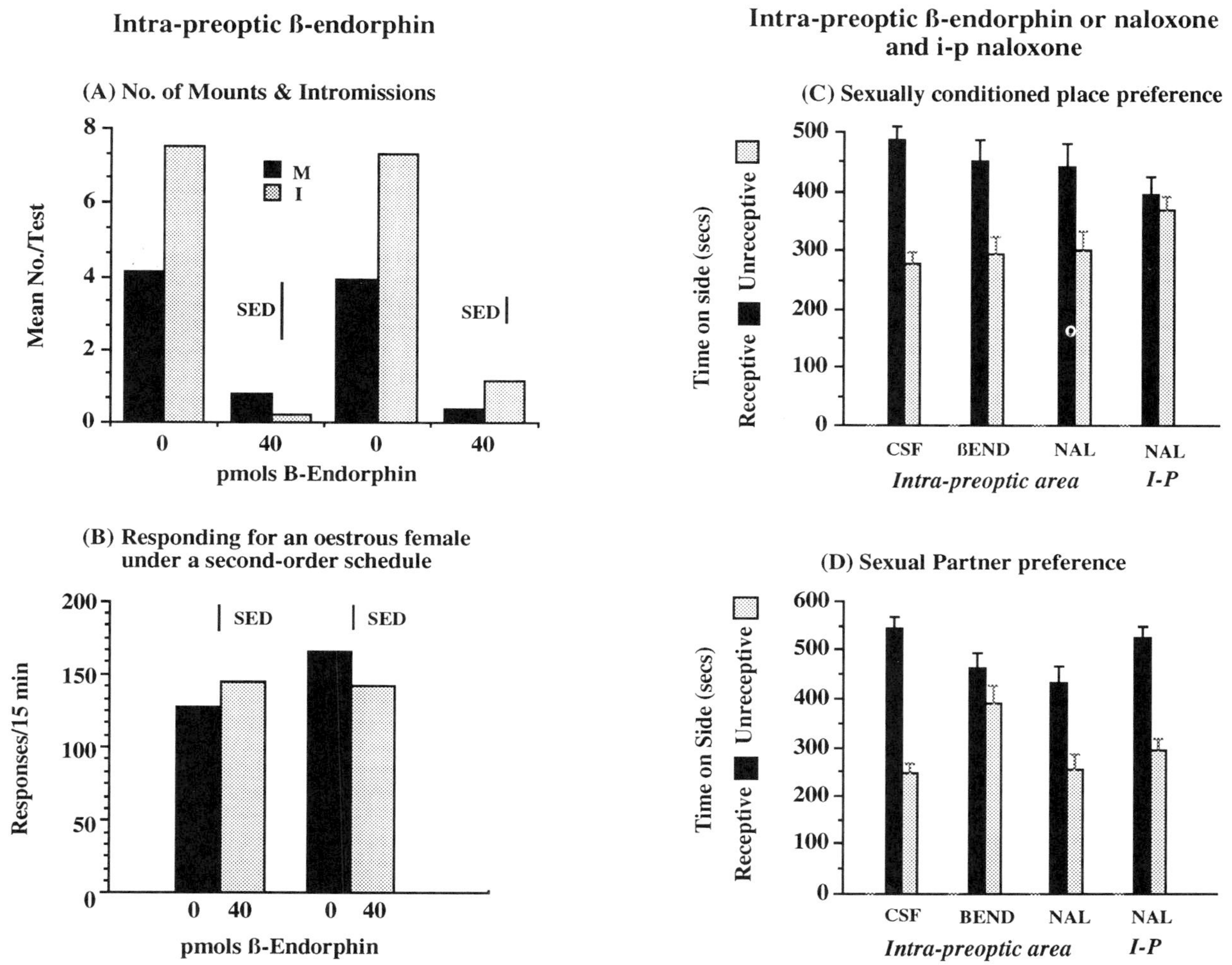

Intra-preoptic ß-endorphin

(A) No. of Mounts & Intromissions

(B) Responding for an oestrous female under a second-order schedule

Intra-preoptic ß-endorphin or naloxone and i-p naloxone

(C) Sexually conditioned place preference

(D) Sexual Partner preference

FIG. 2. The effects of β-endorphin or naloxone on measures of masculine sexual behavior. **A**: Infusions of β-endorphin into the preoptic area virtually abolish mounts and intromissions, but in **B**: it can be seen that they have no effect on responding for a female under a second-order schedule. **C**: Neither β-endorphin (β-END) nor naloxone (NAL) when infused into the preoptic area affect a sexually conditioned place preference, however naloxone abolishes such a place preference when given systemically (ip). **D**: Intra-preoptic β-endorphin abolishes a male's preference for an estrous over an anestrous female, but naloxone given ip or into the preoptic area has no effect on this measure.

dures, and the results also indicate the complexities underlying the superficially simple effects of the systemically administered opioid antagonist. Systemic naloxone may, in some circumstances, facilitate sexual behavior in male rats (see above), but if given to intact, sexually active males these effects are vanishingly small (29). However, the same treatment reduced instrumental responses for a female presented under a second-order schedule of reinforcement, promptly abolished a previously acquired conditioned place preference, but had no effect on partner preference (19,31). Infusing naloxone bilaterally into the mPOA resulted in a powerful facilitation of copulatory behavior; males required fewer intromissions to ejaculate with a much reduced latency, yet had no effect on instrumental behavior or a conditioned place preference. Partner preference was seen to be reduced following this treatment, but analysis of the data revealed this to be an

epiphenomenon of the increased sexual activity, since males spent more of the test period in a state of refractoriness and therefore away from both females in the neutral compartment of the choice apparatus (19,20,31).

It is clear from these results that opioid mechanisms within the POA do not seem primarily to be involved with incentive motivational responses to sexual stimuli but are more involved with consummatory sexual responses. However, more interesting, perhaps, is the indication that such incentive, or reward-related, responses are sensitive to systemic naloxone. In addition, it has been shown that this sensitivity is much greater in animals that were recently castrated (41,46). Because castration also profoundly affected a sexually conditioned place preference (19,31) and instrumental sexual responses (19), whereas mPOA lesions, as well as intra-mPOA opioid manipulations, were without effect on these measures, opioid involvement in sexual reward-related processes may both be sex-hormone-dependent and involve extra-hypothalamic substrates (20). The ventral–tegmental area dopaminergic system innervating ventral–striatal and limbic structures is an obvious focus for experiments investigating this problem.

Indeed, in a particularly interesting series of experiments, Mitchell and Stewart (48,49) have demonstrated that infusions into the ventral–tegmental area of morphine and dynorphin$_{1-13}$ increased the number of males that mounted and showed female-directed behavior (47). Morphine, but not dynorphin$_{1-13}$, increased DA metabolism in the nucleus accumbens, indicating that the effects of these opioid peptides infused into the A10 region may have DA-dependent and DA-independent actions on sexual behavior. In addition, it was demonstrated that masculine sexual behavior was facilitated when males were placed in an environment that previously had been associated with systemic injections of morphine (49). This important observation demonstrates that the conditioned reinforcers established through the pairing of a previously arbitrary constellation of cues with the positive incentive effects of morphine can significantly affect, in this case facilitate, sexual behavior that is under the control of the conditioned and unconditioned incentive properties of an estrous female.

Infusion of another member of the POMC peptide family, melanocyte-stimulating hormone (MSH), into the mPOA results in a markedly different pattern of effects than those seen following infusions of β-endorphin. This peptide facilitates, rather than inhibits, sexual behavior: ejaculation and intromission latencies, as well as the post-ejaculatory interval are shortened, ejaculation occurs after fewer intromissions, and the number of ejaculations occurring within a 15-min test is increased (29). Although this same treatment has no direct effects on place or partner preference, it results in a small, but significant, increase in responding under the second-order schedule of sexual reinforcement.

Systemic administration of the κ-receptor agonist U-50,488H, decreased sexual behavior in male rats, and this effect was prevented by systemic naloxone or intracranial infusions of a κ-receptor antagonist, nor-binaltorphimine (NBNI). The latter compound markedly facilitated female-directed behavior and also prevented the effects of systemically administered U-50,488H when infused either into the ventral–tegmental area or the mPOA (33).

From these results, it is apparent that there are quite complex opioid influences on sexual behavior and that the sites of action of μ- and κ-receptor agonists and antagonists determine markedly different effects on sexual behavior, some of which may require interactions with DA neurons in the ventral–tegmental area. What remains unclear are the circumstances under which these opioid systems are activated so as to modulate the neural systems underlying sexual behavior. One possibility is that they come into play, especially the POMC-containing neurons of the hypothalamus, under conditions of stress to mediate the inhibition of reproductive function (26).

Feminine Sexual Behavior

Systemic administration of opiate agonists, such as morphine or heroin, inhibits the sexual behavior of female monkeys, dogs, and rodents (reviewed in ref. 53). In female rats, acute systemic morphine decreases lordosis quotients and reflex scores, and abolishes proceptive pacing and solicitation. These effects are reversible with naloxone or naltrexone. However, there have been no consistent reports of an effect of systemically administered opioid antagonists on female sexual behavior, suggesting that endogenous opioids do not exert a tonic inhibitory influence, at least not in females that display full receptivity and proceptivity.

In contrast to an exclusive inhibitory effect of systemic morphine, centrally administered opioid agonists may inhibit or facilitate the sexual behavior of female rats depending upon the receptor type and brain area stimulated. For example, β-endorphin can inhibit or facilitate lordosis behavior following infusion of comparable doses into the third ventricle (79) or lateral ventricles (54), respectively. However, low doses of β-endorphin and the μ-selective agonist morphiceptin inhibit lordosis, whereas high doses of these agonists facilitate lordosis following infusion into the lateral ventricles (54). Lateral ventricular infusions of the μ-selective agonist D-Ala^2-MePhe^4-Gly-ol^5-enkephalin (DAMGO) inhibit lordosis in rats primed with estrogen and progesterone, but not in rats primed with estrogen alone (54,59), suggesting that progesterone enhances the ability of μ agonists to exert their inhibitory effects. Infusions of morphine to the ventromedial hypothalamus or mesencephalic central grey inhibit lordosis behavior (75), as do infusions of β-endorphin into the medial preoptic area, VMH, mesencephalic central gray (MCG), or mesencephalic reticular formation (71,79). The inhibitory effect of β-endorphin and morphiceptin may occur through an interaction with high-affinity μ_1 receptors, as the selective μ_1 antagonist naloxazone can reverse the inhibitory effect of these peptides (54,79). However, unlike μ agonists, central infusions of the ∂-selective agonists D-Ser^2-Leu^5-Thr^6-enkephalin (DSTLT) and D-Pen^2-D-Pen^5-enkephalin (DPDPE) into the lateral ventricles facilitate lordosis behavior (54,59), as do infusions of the κ-selective agonists U50-488 and leumorphin (59). Infusions of DPDPE into the lateral ventricles also facilitate proceptive behaviors (59).

Central administration of opioid antagonists also facilitates or inhibits female sexual behavior depending upon the brain area and hormonal state of the animal. For example, infusions of naloxone intrathecally or into the mesencephalic central grey can facilitate lordosis in female rats primed with estrogen alone (71,77), whereas infusions of naloxone into the lateral ventricles inhibit lordosis in females primed with estrogen and progesterone (34). Although naloxone binds with highest affinity to μ receptors, an effect on other receptors cannot be ruled out. The effects of selective opioid receptor antagonists have not been examined in females.

It is difficult at present to incorporate these effects of opioid drugs on feminine sexual behavior within a clear conceptual framework, in marked contrast, therefore, to the situation in males.

Oxytocin

Oxytocin is a nonapeptide secreted by the posterior pituitary, but it is also released into the brain from the terminals of neurons located in the supraoptic and paraventricular hypothalamus, the latter of which projects axons *inter alia* to the ventrolateral regions of the VMH, lateral septum, brainstem and spinal cord autonomic regions (see Rinaman et al., *this volume*). Both estrogen and testosterone stimulate the synthesis of oxytocin binding sites, and recent evidence links oxytocin with the facilitation of sexual behavior in both male and female rats, and perhaps with the stimulation of sexual desire and arousal in humans (see also Chapter 47, *this volume*).

Masculine Sexual Behavior

Systemic injections of oxytocin, either intravenous (iv) or intraperitoneal (ip), reduce the number of intromissions required for ejaculation, decrease the ejaculation latency, and increase the number of ejaculations in a timed test (5,73). Central infusions of oxytocin into the ventricles also produce a syndrome of yawning and penile erections in male rats that is displayed even in the absence of a receptive female (2). The effects of icv infusions of oxytocin on male sexual behavior seem to be of a dual nature depending upon the dose and brain area. Very low doses of oxytocin infused into the lateral ventricles stimulate male sexual behavior by decreasing both the ejaculation latency and postejaculatory interval (2,4). In contrast, higher doses infused into the third ventricle increased the mount and intromission latencies and the postejaculatory interval (73). The infusion of lower doses into the third ventricle did not affect sexual behavior. Infusion of very low doses of the oxytocin antagonist $d(CH_2)_5Tyr(Me)$-[Orn^8]-vasotocin dramatically and dose-dependently inhibited penile erections and copulatory behavior in sexually experienced male rats (2,3). This antagonist also prevented the induction of the yawning and penile erection syndrome by icv infusions of oxytocin. These data suggest that endogenous oxytocin serves to facilitate certain components of sexual arousal and copulatory behavior. Hughes et al. (28) demonstrated that oxytocin levels in cerebrospinal fluid (CSF) more than doubled after 5 min of copulatory behavior and more than tripled 20 min

after an ejaculation. However, although lesions of the lateral and posterior paraventricular hypothalamus prevented the rise in CSF oxytocin levels during copulation, and produced a small but significant increase in the mount and intromission latencies, those lesions had little effect on copulatory behavior once it was initiated. Moreover, those lesions decreased the postejaculatory interval. Thus, it remains to be established whether endogenous oxytocin release is necessary or sufficient for male sexual behavior. The effect of oxytocin on measures of conditioned sexual arousal in male rats is not yet known.

Systemic or intracranial infusions of oxytocin in male prairie voles (*Microtus ochrogaster*) inhibit copulation (80). However, this may be the result of a concomitant increase in social affiliative behaviors (e.g., side-by-side contact). Although oxytocin agonists and antagonists have not been tested on human subjects, exposure to erotic stimuli and masturbation to orgasm in men leads to an increase in plasma oxytocin levels (13).

Feminine Sexual Behavior

Oxytocin and its receptor are highly regulated in different brain regions during the estrous cycle, an effect that is likely due to changes in estrogen and progesterone. Numbers of oxytocin immunoreactive cells, and levels of oxytocin receptor mRNA, are stimulated by estrogen and enhanced by progesterone. Estrogen stimulates the transcription of oxytocin binding sites in the VMH, and progesterone quickly modifies the effect of estrogen by spreading the active oxytocin receptor sites laterally to innervate oxytocin terminal regions (69). This suggests that estrogen and progesterone may act to synchronize the availability of endogenous oxytocin with its receptor.

Lordosis behavior is facilitated dramatically by oxytocin. Systemic injections of the nonapeptide increase the frequency of lordosis responding in estrogen-primed females (5,11). Similarly, icv infusions increase lordosis behavior in rats treated chronically with estrogen or treated with estrogen and progesterone, suggesting that progesterone may exert a permissive effect on the actions of exogenous oxytocin (11). Caldwell (12) identified the mPOA as an important site for the regulation of lordosis behavior by oxytocin in female rats. Infusions of the nonapeptide into the mPOA increased lordosis quotients in rats treated with estrogen and given multiple tests of copulation. Most importantly, this facilitation occurred at doses that were ineffective in other sites, such as the third ventricle, VMH, ventral–tegmental area, or the mesencephalic central grey. However, a recent study provided evidence that oxytocin in the mPOA and VMH contribute to different aspects of lordosis behavior in rats primed with estrogen and progesterone. Infusions of very low doses into the VMH facilitated the duration of each lordosis, without affecting the lordosis frequency, whereas infusions of higher doses into the mPOA facilitated the lordosis frequency but not the duration of each lordosis (70). Additionally, oxytocin infusions into the VMH of estrogen-primed female prairie voles reduced rates of aggression and increased the amount of physical contact that females made with males, although it led to a faster termination of estrus (81). Nothing is known about the possible effects of oxytocin on appetitive aspects of sexual behavior in female rats.

Sexual stimulation during copulation increases plasma oxytocin levels in female rats, as does vaginal distention or vaginocervical stimulation. In human females, masturbation to orgasm also increases plasma oxytocin levels (13). Thus, taken together, the data in males and females suggest that oxytocin may form part of a neurochemical axis that participates in the desire to affiliate with a sexual partner, to engage in sexual contact, and to achieve sexual satiety after extended matings.

OTHER DRUGS

Alcohol

The effects of alcohol on sexual behavior are of interest for at least two reasons. First, alcohol consumption has been repeatedly implicated in the etiology of various sexual disorders and dysfunctions in humans, such as inhibited sexual desire, erectile failure, delayed ejaculation, and inhibited orgasm. Second, alcohol has long been associated with sexual disinhibition and has been reported to enhance sexual arousal and behavior in some individuals with preexisting sexual dysfunctions, such as premature ejaculation, inhibited sexual desire, or inhibited orgasm.

Only two published experiments exist in which the effects of alcohol on human sexual behavior have been examined directly, one in men (38) and one in women (39). In both studies, the effects of a range of doses of alcohol were examined on the ability of subjects to masturbate to orgasm while viewing a sexually explicit film. In men, alcohol dose-dependently delayed ejaculation, reduced the intensity of orgasm, and decreased both physiological and subjective measures of sexual arousal. Nearly identical effects were observed in women, although alcohol increased, rather than decreased, their subjective levels of sexual arousal. These reports generally support clinical observations that alcohol can disrupt sexual activity; however, their relevance to other forms of sexual behavior is unclear. Furthermore, it has been difficult to find unambiguous evidence of the disinhibition of sexual arousal commonly associated with low-to-moderate doses of alcohol (see also Chapters 149 and 154, *this volume*).

Masculine Sexual Behavior

The effects of a range of doses of alcohol, administered ip, on the copulatory behavior of sexually active male rats were studied by Pfaus and Pinel (55). Low doses of alcohol increased the mount, intromission, and ejaculation latencies, and reduced the percentage of rats that achieve ejaculation in a 30-min test (55). A moderate dose intensified these effects further and increased the postejaculatory interval, whereas a high dose abolished all copulatory activity. No disinhibitory effect was observed at any dose. However, sexually active rats do not show evidence of sexual inhibition; therefore, a second study was conducted in rats that had learned to suppress their copulatory advances toward sexually nonreceptive females. Sexually active males were given sequential access to sexually receptive and nonreceptive females at 48-hr intervals. Although all males attempted to mount the nonreceptive females in the first training session, none attempted to do so by the sixth and subsequent sessions, despite being fully sexually active during interspersed sessions with receptive females.

The effects of low and moderate doses of alcohol in these males were examined in two tests following this training period, one during exposure to receptive females, and one during exposure to nonreceptive females. As in the first experiment, both doses of alcohol disrupted sexual behavior when males were exposed to receptive females. However, the low dose dramatically released mounting behavior and subsequent ejaculations from inhibition during the test with nonreceptive females, despite vigorous defensive and rejection responses made by the females and despite the fact that none of the males gained vaginal intromission. The moderate dose did not produce any disinhibition of sexual behavior during this test. These data indicate that alcohol can produce a disinhibition of sexual behavior in the male rat but only under conditions in which the rat's behavior is already inhibited.

Another critical feature of alcohol's effects on male sexual behavior is that tolerance may accrue to its disruptive effects. Although empirical reports are sparse in the clinical literature, tolerance to a variety of effects of alcohol have been noted in the animal literature, including its anticonvulsive effects and its disruption of balance and motor coordination. Such tolerance is said to be contingent, that is, its development depends largely upon the occurrence of some experience or behavior during periods of drug exposure.

The development of tolerance to alcohol's disruptive effect on sexual behavior has been examined in male rats (63). Rats were administered a moderate dose of alcohol either before or after they engaged in a 30-min test of sexual behavior with receptive females. The control group received an equal volume of saline. Tests were conducted every 4 days, to approximate the normal estrous cycle of the female. This dose of alcohol increased the mount, intromission, and ejaculation latencies and increased the postejaculatory interval in the alcohol-before group on the first tolerance-development trial, although these disruptive effects became progressively less pronounced in subsequent trials. By the fifth trial, these measures were indistinguishable from control values and from the animals' own no-drug baseline values. No lingering effect of this dose of alcohol was observed on the sexual behavior of the alcohol-after group. On the final test, this dose of alcohol was administered to rats in the three groups before the test of sexual behavior. Significant increases in the mount, intromission, and ejaculation latencies, and in the postejaculatory intervals, were observed in rats of the saline control and alcohol-after groups, but not in rats of the alcohol-before group, thus demonstrating that contingent tolerance to alcohol's disruptive effects had occurred. These results suggest that some of the variability and inconsistency in the magnitude and nature of alcohol's disruptive effect on human sexual behavior may be attributed to differences in the frequency with which individuals have previously engaged in sexual activity while intoxicated.

Feminine Sexual Behavior

Very little work has been done to examine the effects of alcohol on female sexual behavior. In both female hamsters and rats, moderate-to-high doses of alcohol inhibited receptive and proceptive behaviors (62). However, in the latter study, a low dose of alcohol facilitated proceptive behavior in ovariectomized female rats who normally display a small amount of proceptive behavior following treatment with estrogen and a moderate dose of progesterone. Thus, alcohol may have synergistic effects with progesterone in the disinhibition of proceptive behaviors.

NEW VISTAS

In Vivo Measurement of Transmitter Release during Sexual Behavior

The analysis of drug effects on behavior gives rise to hypotheses concerning transmitter activity during ongoing behavior. Although ex vivo studies, which rely on postmortem tissue analysis of transmitter levels using high-performance liquid chromatography (HPLC) with electrochemical detection (ED), have provided suggestive data in this regard, they do not permit a clear resolution of which behaviors contribute to the increases or decreases in transmitter levels. The more recent development of techniques to monitor extracellular concentrations of neurotransmitters in vivo, most notably microdialysis and voltammetry, has moved us closer to resolving these issues. Often, however, these techniques provide information that in some ways underscores the limits of the pharmacological approach (see Chapter 31, this volume).

Microdialysis has been used to examine extracellular concentrations of DA, its acid metabolites DOPAC and homovanillic acid (HVA), and the serotonin metabolite 5-hydroxyindoleacetic acid (5-HIAA) during preparatory

and consummatory aspects of sexual activity in male rats. Recall that DA antagonists are capable of reducing rates of conditioned level changing in male rats at doses that do not affect the initiation and subsequent performance of copulatory behavior (58). This led us to suggest that, as with feeding, preparatory sexual behavior is highly dependent upon the functional integrity of brain DA systems, whereas consummatory sexual behavior is less dependent (50). Accordingly, we predicted that DA release would be more pronounced during preparatory sexual behavior compared to copulation. Exactly the opposite occurred. Dialysates from the nucleus accumbens of sexually active male rats revealed a small increase in DA and its metabolites during the preparatory phase, but a dramatic and sustained increase during active copulation (Fig. 3) (56). In contrast, dialysates from the dorsal striatum revealed a small and progressive increase in DA and its metabolites throughout the test session that was not correlated with any particular aspect of copulation (Fig. 3). Subsequent work established that the increases were not due to general locomotor activity, nor were they due to the novelty of the testing chamber (16), and that the increased DA transmission in the nucleus accumbens during these phases of sexual activity did not require sexual experience (40,78). These results suggest another interpretation of the role of DA in sexual behavior. Given that DA receptor antagonists bind competitively with DA for occupancy at DA receptors, the greater sensitivity of preparatory behaviors to the disruptive effects of these drugs may reflect the lower concentration of extracellular DA that is available to compete with the drug. In contrast, consummatory behaviors may be less susceptible to disruption by DA antagonists because DA release is high during such behavior. However, to date consummatory elements of masculine sexual behavior have not been seen to be disrupted following DA receptor antagonist infusions into, or 6-OHDA-induced lesions of the dopaminergic innervation of the ventral striatum.

The use of in vivo voltammetry has further enhanced our understanding of the role of DA in male sexual behavior. This technique has shown a small phasic rise in DA oxidation current in the nucleus accumbens that is of short duration during the preparatory phase, but a larger and sustained increase during copulation (Fig. 3) (61). However, the DA oxidation current declines precipitously after ejaculation, during the absolute refractory period, but rises again before the male reinitiates another copulatory series (Fig. 3). The dynamic nature of DA transmission in the nucleus accumbens contrasts with that of the dorsal striatum, which, as observed with microdialysis, showed a small but progressive increase throughout the test that was not correlated with any specific phase of sexual behavior. The DA oxidation current in the nucleus accumbens of male rats also appears to be sensitive to olfactory or pheromonal cues provided by estrous females (47), although the increases observed during the presentation of estrous vaginal secretions on a glass slide are less

Nucleus accumbens

Striatum

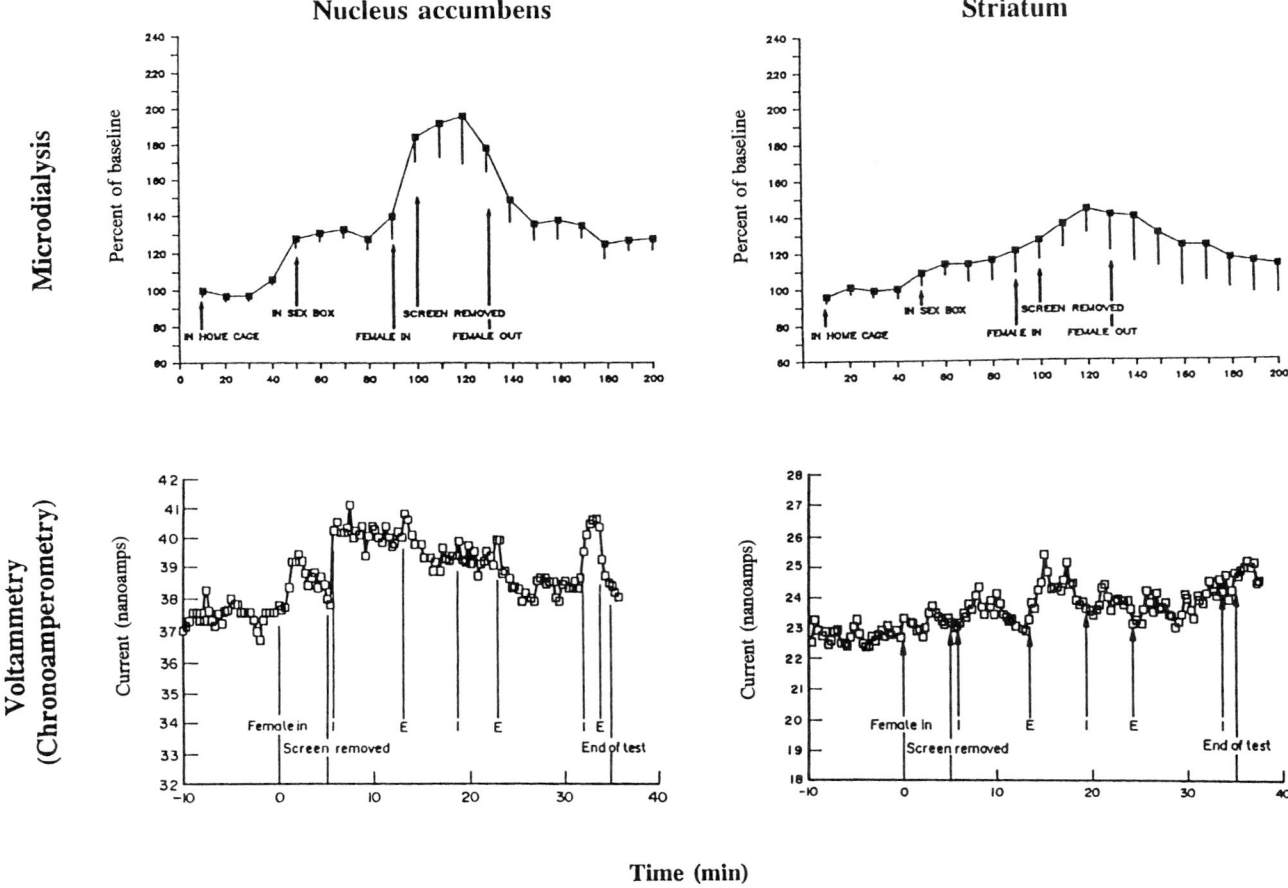

Time (min)

FIG. 3. Changes in dopamine measured by dialysis (*top panels*) in the nucleus accumbens (*left panels*) and dorsal striatum (*right panels*) in male rats prior to and during sexual interaction.

than those obtained during the presentation of an estrous female (61). In contrast, DA oxidation currents did not increase in the dorsal striatum during the presentation of sexually relevant stimuli.

In females, DA antagonists facilitate lordosis but inhibit proceptivity, suggesting that DA is inhibitory with respect to lordosis, but may facilitate proceptive behaviors. In contrast, NE may facilitate lordosis without affecting proceptive behaviors. Dialysis samples have been taken from the nucleus accumbens and dorsal striatum during ongoing sexual behavior in ovariectomized rats fully primed with estrogen and progesterone (Pfaus, Wenkstern, and Fibiger, *unpublished data*). Dopamine transmission increased comparably in both regions during sexual behavior, although the effect in the nucleus accumbens seemed to be related to the incentive quality of the stimulus male, whereas the effect in the striatum seemed to be related to the ability of the female to pace the copulatory contact (50). Increases in DA transmission have also been reported during sexual behavior in female Syrian hamsters, who assume the lordosis posture for very long durations (42). Both DA and norepinephrine transmission increase in the VMH of female rats during sexual behavior (75). These latter results are easier to interpret, as both DA and

noradrenergic agonists are reported to facilitate lordosis following infusion into the VMH.

In summary, in vivo techniques are fast becoming a major experimental tool, one which can provide direct assessments of neurotransmitter activity during behavior and which can refine our understanding of pharmacological manipulations.

Use of Antisense Oligonucleotides

One of the most exciting techniques to come from the revolution in molecular biology is the use of antisense oligonucleotides to halt the transcription of particular genes (see Chapter 2, *this volume* and ref. 37). Antisense to mRNA for glutamic acid decarboxylase (GAD), the enzyme that converts glutamate to GABA, was shown to inhibit lordosis behavior in ovariectomized female rats made continuously receptive with chronic estrogen implants (35). The effect was maximal 24 hr after infusions into either the hypothalamus or the MCG, and took between 4 and 6 days to recover. Control animals that received the same nucleotides, but in a scrambled order, did not show a reduction in lordosis behavior following infusion. These results are similar to those obtained following infusion of GABA receptor antagonists to those regions. In contrast, infusion of GAD antisense to the mPOA did not affect lordosis behavior, a finding consistent with the fact that GABA in this region does not affect lordosis. Thus, the inhibition observed following infusion of antisense was predictable, site-specific, and reversible. Successful modulation of female sexual behavior was also accomplished by infusion of antisense to progesterone receptor mRNA to the VMH of ovariectomized female rats primed with estrogen and progesterone (51,64). Antisense infusions reduced lordosis behavior and blocked the induction of proceptive behaviors following progesterone treatment. Infusion of the scrambled control sequence had little effect. Finally, McCarthy et al. (36) demonstrated that infusions of estrogen receptor (ER) mRNA antisense into the hypothalamus protected neonatal females from the masculinizing effects of neonatal androgen treatment, including the masculinization of their sexual behavior, locomotion, and volume of sexually dimorphic brain nuclei. In contrast, infusions of ER mRNA antisense to the hypothalamus of neonatal males demasculinized their physical appearance (i.e., they had shorter anogenital distances) and disrupted their ability to show male sexual behavior 60 days after antisense treatment.

Antisense technology, although still in its formative stage, shows much promise in providing us with the ability to limit or halt gene expression selectively within discrete brain regions in vivo. As more and more genes that encode specific proteins in the brain are cloned and sequenced, the causal relationship between their expression and their effects on sexual behavior can be explored, rather than inferred from the administration of relatively nonselective drugs.

SYNTHESIS

There has been substantial progress in defining the consequences for the sexual behavior of males and females of manipulating monoamine, amino acid, and peptide transmitters in the CNS. However, the conceptual framework within which these data exist is unclear in many instances. This is in part from limitations in behavioral methods and because only some aspects of reproductive behavior have been studied. For example, in females, the lordosis reflex has been investigated to the virtual exclusion of any other aspect of feminine sexual behavior. Such limitations make between-sex and, especially, between-species comparisons very difficult indeed, and this is one reason for the slow progress in developing clinically viable drugs with which to treat disorders of sexual arousal and performance.

At a neural level of analysis, there is also a problem of interpretation of such psychopharmacological data which concerns the nature of the neural system that underlies the expression of sexual behavior. A common interpretation of drug effects on sexual behavior is as follows: receptor-binding drug x enhanced behavior y (e.g., mounting/lordosis), thus indicating that transmitter z has an inhibitory role in the control of this parameter of sexual behavior. This argument, that the action of the drug defines the (opposite, in this case) functional significance of the affected transmitter as an element of a neural system is, of course, both circular and flawed. Furthermore, experiments involving lesions and hormonal implantation in the CNS that have defined critical elements of the neural system underlying sexual behavior in males and females have not generally mapped onto the neurochemically defined systems with any degree of consistency. Nor is it clear whether the functions subserved by monoaminergic, peptidergic, or amino acid-containing neurons are related to hormone-sensitive mechanisms, to the sensory systems defined by lesion studies as critical for sexual behavior, or to more general processes such as arousal, reward (often called incentive motivation), or attention (see refs. 5,19).

A relatively novel method that has successfully revealed the parts of the brain that are engaged during sexual interaction is the immunocytochemical visualization of the protein product of the immediate-early gene, c-fos (6; see also Chapter 56, this volume). In these experiments, it was demonstrated that neurons in the mPOA are activated during sexual interaction in male rats and that this activation, revealed as increases in Fos-immunoreactivity in many neurons, depends upon the relay of olfactory information via the medial amygdala (in which c-fos was also induced by appropriate olfactory sexual stimuli, similarly the bed nucleus of the stria terminalis) and genital somatosensory information relayed via the midbrain central tegmental field (in which c-fos was induced by intromissions). Lesions of each of these structures comprising nodes in the system severely impair copulation, but do not affect appetitive responses to sexual stimuli (e.g., ref. 19). By contrast, exposure to conditioned cues (i.e., previously neutral stimuli reliably paired with copulation) strongly increased the expression of c-fos in neurons in the nucleus accumbens and basolateral amygdala, but not in those diencephalic and midbrain structures activated following copulation itself (Everitt and Baum, unpublished). Manipulations of these latter structures have little or no effect on copulation, but profoundly affect appetitive sexual responses. It seems a similar system is activated by coitus and/or cervical stimulation in female rats, although the analysis has not extended beyond this to other aspects of sexual behavior (60). How do the neurochemical systems addressed by drug treatments that have been reviewed here interface with these critical neural structures revealed by other experimental approaches to be essential for the display of discrete patterns of sexual response?

In large part, this is the challenge of the next generation of progress. In the case of DA and the ventral striatum, real progress has been made in integrating the effects of dopaminergic drugs on sexual behavior in male rats with theories of incentive motivation and reward (19,61). This is much less the case for noradrenergic and serotoninergic systems. The effects of neuropeptides on sexual behavior are difficult in most cases to relate to hypothalamic or related limbic mechanisms underlying sexual behavior. Herbert (26) has argued that the high information content of peptide molecules and their preferential distribution in limbic structures indicate a chemical code of behavior and that given peptides have coordinated central and peripheral roles that have been conserved through evolution. But in terms of sexual behavior, this claim is far from secure. For example, LH releasing hormone (LHRH) clearly controls the gonadal axis, but the function of central LHRH neurons in sexual behavior in males is virtually unknown, and it is still unclear whether, despite early interest, LHRH neurons in females are necessary or sufficient for lordosis to occur, even though the peptide influences the occurrence of this response.

The list of drugs and peptides that affect the display of lordosis is enormous and growing. Is it the case that all of the chemically identified neurons, monoaminergic, peptidergic, and more, with which such drugs and peptides interact are really to be considered as part of a single neural system that is normally engaged during the display of a simple, hormone-dependent reflex such as lordosis? Can the same conclusion be drawn concerning the neural basis of sexual behavior in males, which is also profoundly affected by a similarly wide range of compounds? If so, then it becomes crucial to identify the contexts in which each chemically defined unit is brought into play. Not only are we a long way from such an endpoint, but it seems unlikely to be a generally fruitful task. In the case of peptide neurons, there is no doubt that part of the problem in establishing their functional *role* within such a neural network is greatly limited by the lack of selective tools with which to manipulate them, especially receptor antagonists. Antisense technology is likely to be especially important in this regard. In the case of monoamines, attempts to integrate drug effects on sexual behavior within prevailing theories of the functions of such systems are more advanced, but there are still wide gaps in our understanding.

The neural tools and behavioral approaches with which to make such advances are increasingly available. The next phase must concern itself more with hypothesis testing and less with the phenomenology of drug effects on sexual behavior, dramatic though they are.

REFERENCES

1. Ahlenius S. Larsson K. Evidence for a unique pharmacological profile of 8-OH-DPAT by evaluation of its effects on male rat sexual behaviour. In: Dourish CT, Ahlenius S, Hutson PH, eds. *Pharmacology of central 5-HT1A receptors*. Chichester: Ellis Horwood, 1987;185–198.
2. Argiolas A, Melis MR, Gessa GL. Intraventricular oxytocin induces yawning and penile erection in rats. *Eur J Pharmacol* 1985;117: 395–396.
3. Argiolas A, Collu M, Gessa, GL, Melis MR, Serra G. The oxytocin antagonist d(CH2)5Tyr(Me)-Orn8-vasotocin inhibits male copulatory behavior in rats. *Eur J Pharmacol* 1988;149:389–392.
4. Arletti R, Benelli A, Bertolini A. Oxytocin involvement in male and female sexual behavior. *Ann NY Acad Sci* 1992;652:180–193.
5. Bancroft J. *Human sexuality and its problems*. 2nd ed. Edinburgh: Churchill Livingstone, 1989.
6. Baum MJ, Everitt BJ. Increased expression of c-*fos* in the medial preoptic area after mating in the male rat: role of afferent inputs from the medial amygdala and midbrain central tegmental field. *Neuroscience* 1992;50:627–646.
8. Becker JB. Hormonal influences on extrapyramidal sensorimotor function and hippocampal plasticity. In: Becker JB, Breedlove SM, Crews D, eds. *Behavioral endocrinology* Cambridge, MA: MIT Press, 1992;325–356.
8. Bitran D, Hull EM. Pharmacological analysis of male rat sexual behavior. *Neurosci Biobehav Rev* 1987;11:365–389.
9. Blackburn JR, Pfaus JG, Phillips AG. Dopamine function in appetitive and defensive behaviors. *Prog Neurobiol* 1982;39:247–279.
10. Caggiula AR, Herndon JG, Scanlon R, Greenstone D, Bradshaw W, Sharp D. Dissociation of active from immobility components of sexual behavior in female rats by central 6-hydroxydopamine: implications for CA involvement in sexual behavior and sensorimotor responsiveness. *Brain Res* 1979;172:505–520.
11. Caldwell JD, Prange AJ, Pedersen CA. Oxytocin facilitates the sexual receptivity of estrogen-treated rats. *Neuropeptides* 1986;7: 175–189.
12. Caldwell JD, Jirikowski, GF, Greer ER, Pedersen CA. Medial preoptic area oxytocin and female sexual receptivity. *Behav Neurosci* 1989;103:655–662.
13. Carmichael MS, Humbert R, Dixen J, Palmisano G, Greenleaf W, Davidson JM. Plasma oxytocin increases in the human sexual response. *J Clin Endocrinol Metab* 1987;64:27–31.
14. Clark JT, Smith ER, Davidson JM. Enhancement of sexual motivation in male rats by yohimbine. *Science* 1984;225:847–849.
15. Clark JT, Smith ER, Davidson JM. Evidence for the modulation of sexual behavior by alpha adrenoceptors in male rats. *Neuroendocrinology* 1985;41:36–43.
16. Damsma G, Pfaus JG, Wenkster D, Phillips AG, Fibiger HC. Sexual behavior increases dopamine transmission in the nucleus accumbens and striatum of male rats: comparison with novelty and locomotion. *Behav Neurosci* 1992;106:181–191.
17. Etgen AM. Intrahypothalamic implants of noradrenergic antagonists disrupt lordosis behavior in female rats. *Physiol Behav* 1990;48:31–36.
18. Everitt BJ, Fuxe K, Hokfelt T, Jonsson G. Role of monoamines in the control by hormones of sexual receptivity in the female rat. *J Comp Physiol Psychol* 1975;89:556–572.
19. Everitt BJ. Sexual motivation: a neural and behavioural analysis of the mechanisms underlying appetitive and copulatory responses of male rats. *Neurosci Biobehav Rev* 1990;14:217–232.
20. Everitt BJ. Neuroendocrine and psychological mechanisms underlying masculine sexual behaviour. In: Archer T, Hansen S, eds. *Biological psychology: neuroendocrine axis*. Hillsdale, New Jersey: Lawrence Erlbaum, 1991;111–122.
21. Everitt BJ, Bancroft J. Of rats and men: the comparative approach to male sexuality. In: Bancroft J, Davis CM, Ruppel HJ Jr., eds. *Annual review of sex research*. Vol. II. Society for the Scientific Study of Sex, 1991;77–118.
22. Fernandez-Guasti A, Larsson K, Beyer C. Potentiative action of α- and β-adrenergic receptor stimulation in inducing lordosis behavior. *Pharmacol Biochem Behav* 1985;22:613–617.
23. Foreman MM, Hall JL. Effects of D2-dopaminergic receptor stimulation on the lordotic response of female rats. *Psychopharmacology* 1987;91:96–100.
24. Grierson JP, James MD, Pearson JR, Wilson CA. The effect of selective D1 and D2 dopaminergic agents on sexual receptivity in the female rat. *Neuropharmacology* 1988;27:181–189.
25. Hansen S, Harthon C, Wallin E, Löfberg L, Svensson K. Mesotelencephalic dopamine system and reproductive behavior in the female rat: effects of ventral tegmental 6-hydroxydopamine lesions on maternal and sexual responsiveness. *Behav Neurosci* 1991;105:588–598.
26. Herbert J. Peptides in the limbic system: neurochemical codes for

co-ordinated adaptive responses to behavioural and physiological demand. *Prog Neurobiol* 1993;41:723–791.

27. Hillegart V. Functional topography of brain serotonergic pathways in the rat. *Acta Physiol Scand* 1991;142(Suppl 598):1–180.

28. Hughes AM, Everitt BJ, Lightman SL, Todd K. Oxytocin in the central nervous system and sexual behavior in male rats. *Brain Res* 1987;41:133–137.

29. Hughes AM, Everitt BJ, Herbert J. Selective effects of β-endorphin infused into the hypothalamus, preoptic area and bed nucleus of the stria terminalis on the sexual and ingestive behavour of male rats. *Neuroscience* 1987;23:1063–1073.

30. Hughes AM; Everitt BJ, Herbert J. The effects of simultaneous or separate infusions of some pro-opiomelanocortin-derived peptides (β-endorphin, melanocyte stimulating hormone and corticotrophin-like intermediate polypeptide) and their acetylated derivatives upon sexual and ingestive behavior of male rats. *Neuroscience* 1988; 2:689–698.

31. Hughes AM, Herbert J, Everitt BJ. Comparative effects of preoptic area infusions of opioid peptides, lesions and castration on sexual behavior in male rats: studies of instrumental behavior, conditioned place preference and partner preference. *Psychopharmacology* 1990;102(2):243–256.

32. Lal S, Ackman D, Tharundayil JX, Kiely ME, Etienne P. Effects of apomorphine, a dopamine receptor agonist, on penile tumescence in normal subjects. *Prog Neurpsychopharmacol Biol Psychiatry* 1984;8:695–699.

33. Leyton M, Stewart J. The stimulation of central κ-opioid receptors decreases male sexual behavior and locomotor activity. *Brain Res* 1992;594:56–74.

34. Lindblom C, Forsberg G, Södersten P. The effect of naloxone on sexual behavior in female rats depends on the site of injection. *Neurosci Lett* 1987;70:97–100.

35. McCarthy MM, Schwartz-Giblin S, Pfaff DW. Intracerebral administration of glutamic acid decarboxylase (GAD) antisense oligodeoxynucleotide reduces lordosis behavior in the rat. *Soc Neurosci Abstr* 1991;17:497.

36. McCarthy MM, Schlenker E, Pfaff DW. Neonatal intracerebral infusion of antisense DNA to estrogen receptor mRNA alters estrogen-dependent parameters in adult rats. *Soc Neurosci Abstr* 1992; 18:893.

37. McCarthy MM, Brooks PJ, Pfaus JG, et al. Antisense oligodeoxynucleotides in behavioral neuroscience. *Neuroprotocols* 1993;2:67–74.

38. Malatesta VJ, Pollack RH, Wilbanks WA, Adams HE. Alcohol effects on the orgasmic-ejaculatory response in human males. *J Sex Res* 1979;15:101–107.

39. Malatesta VJ, Pollack RH, Crotty TD, Peacock LJ. Acute alcohol intoxication and female orgasmic response. *J Sex Res* 1982;18:1–17.

40. Mas M, Gonzalez-Mora J, Louilot A, Sole C, Guadalupe T. Increased dopamine release in the nucleus accumbens of copulating male rats as evidenced by in vivo voltammetry. *Neurosci Lett* 1990;110:303–308.

41. Mehrara BJ, Baum MJ. Naloxone disrupts the expression but not the acquisition by male rats of a conditioned place preference response for an oestrous female. *Psychopharmacology* 1990;101: 118–125.

42. Meisel RL, Cam DM, Robinson TE. A microdialysis study of ventral striatal dopamine during sexual behavior in female Syrian hamsters. *Behav Brain Res* 1990;55:151–157.

43. Mendelson SD, Gorzalka BB. Stimulation of β-adrenoreceptors inhibits lordosis behavior in the female rat. *Pharmacol Biochem Behav* 1988;29:717–723.

44. Mendelson SD, Pfaus JG. Level searching: a new assay of sexual motivation in the male rat. *Physiol Behav* 1989;45:337–341.

45. Mendelson SD. A review and reevaluation of the role of serotonin in the modulation of lordosis behavior in the female rat. *Neurosci Biobehav Rev* 1992;16:309–350.

46. Miller RL, Baum MJ. Naloxone inhibits mating and conditioned place preference for an estrous female in male rats soon after castration. *Pharmacol Biochem Behav* 1987;26:781–789.

47. Mitchell JB, Gratton A. Opioid modulation and sensitization of dopamine release elicited by sexually relevant stimuli: a high-speed chronoamperometric study in freely-behaving rats. *Brain Res* 1991;551:20–27.

48. Mitchell JB, Stewart J. Facilitation of sexual behaviors in the male

49. Mitchell JB, Stewart J. Facilitation of sexual behaviors in the male rat in the presence of stimuli previously paired with systemic injections of morphine. *Pharmacol Biochem Behav* 1990;35:367–372.

50. Murmelstein PG, Becker JB. Increased extracellular dopamine in the nucleus accumbens and striatum of the female rat during paced copulatory behavior. *J Neurosci* [*in press*].

51. Ogawa S, Olazabel UE, Pfaff DW. Effects of hypothalamic administration of antisense DNA for progesterone receptor mRNA on lordosis behavior and progesterone receptor immunoreactivity. *Soc Neurosci Abstr* 1992;18:893.

52. Oldenburger WP, Everitt BJ, De Jonge FH. Conditioned place preference induced by sexual interaction in female rats. *Horm Behav* 1992;26:214–228.

53. Pfaus JG, Gorzalka BB. Opioids and sexual behavior. *Neurosci Biobehav Rev* 1987;11:1–34.

54. Pfaus JG, Gorzalka BB. Selective activation of opioid receptors differentially affects lordosis behavior in female rats. *Peptides* 1987;8:309–317.

55. Pfaus JG, Pinel JPJ. Alcohol inhibits and disinhibits sexual behavior in the male rat. *Psychobiology* 1989;17:195–201.

56. Pfaus JG, Damsma G, Nomikos GG, et al. Sexual behavior enhances central dopamine transmission in the male rat. *Brain Res* 1990;530:345–348.

57. Pfaus JG, Mendelson SD, Phillips AG. A correlational and factor analysis of anticipatory and consummatory measures of sexual behavior in the male rat. *Psychoneuroendocrinology* 1990;15:329–340.

58. Pfaus JG, Phillips AG. Role of dopamine in anticipatory and consummatory aspects of sexual behavior in the male rat. *Behav Neurosci* 1991;105:727–743.

59. Pfaus JG, Pfaff DW. μ-, α-, and κ-opioid receptor agonists selectively modulate sexual behaviors in the female rat: differential dependence on progesterone. *Horm Behav* 1992;26:457–473.

60. Pfaus JG, Wenkstern D, Fibiger HC. Sexual activity increases dopamine transmission in the nucleus accumbens and striatum of female rats. [submitted].

61. Phillips AG, Pfaus JG, Blaha CD. Dopamine and motivated behavior: insights provided by in vivo analyses. In: Willner P, Scheel-Kruger J, eds. *The mesolimbic dopamine system: from motivation to action.* London: Wiley, 1991:199–224.

62. Pinel JPJ, Pfaus JG. Effects of alcohol on the sexual behavior of female rats. *Soc Neurosci Abstr* 1988;14:41.

63. Pinel JPJ, Pfaus JG, Christensen BK. Contingent tolerance to the disruptive effects of alcohol on the copulatory behavior of male rats. *Pharmacol Biochem Behav* 1991;41:133–137.

64. Pollio G, Xue P, Zanisi M, Nicolin A, Maggi A. Antisense oligonucleotide blocks progesterone-induced lordosis behavior in ovariectomized rats. *Molec Brain Res* 1993;19:135–139.

65. Riley AJ, Goodman RE, Kellet JM, Orr R. Double-blind trial of yohimbine hydrochloride in the treatment of erection inadequacy. *Sex Marital Ther* 1989;4:17–26.

66. Robbins TW, Everitt BJ. Functional studies of the central catecholamines. *Int Rev Neurobiol* 1982;23:303–365.

67. Rosen RC. Alcohol and drug effects on sexual response: human experimental and clinical studies. In: Bancroft J, Davis CM, Ruppel HJ Jr. *Annual Review of Sex Research.* Vol. II. Society for the Scientific Study of Sex, 1991:119–180.

68. Sachs BD, Meisel RL. The physiology of male sexual behavior. In: Knobil E, Neill J. et al. eds. *The physiology of reproduction.* New York: Raven Press, 1988:1393–1486.

69. Schumacher M, Coirini H, Pfaff DW, McEwen BS. Behavioral effects of progesterone associated with rapid modulation of oxytocin receptors. *Science* 1990;250:691–694.

70. Schulze HG, Gorzalka BB. Oxytocin effects on lordosis frequency and lordosis duration following infusion into the medial pre-optic area and ventromedial hypothalamus of female rats. *Neuropeptides* 1991;18:99–106.

71. Sirinathsinghji DJS. Modulation of lordosis behavior of female rats by naloxone, β-endorphin, and its antiserum in the mesencephalic central grey: possible mediation via GnRH. *Neuroendocrinology* 1984;39:222–230.

72. Stavy M, Herbert J. Differential effects of β-endorphin infused into the hypothalamic preoptic area at various phases of the male rat's sexual behavior. *Neuroscience* 198;30:433–442.

73. Stoneham MD, Everitt BJ, Hansen S, Lightman SL, Todd K. Oxytocin and sexual behavior in the male rat and rabbit. *J Endocrinol* 1985;107:97–106.

74. Susset JG, Tessier CD, Wincze J, Bansal S, Malhotra C, Schwacha MG. Effect of yohimbine hydrochloride on erectile impotence: a double-blind study. *J Urol* 1989;141:1360–1363.

75. Vathy I, van der Plas J, Vincent PA, Etgen AM. Intracranial dialysis and microinfusion studies suggest that morphine may act in the ventromedial hypothalamus to inhibit female sexual behavior. *Horm Behav* 1991;25:354–366.

76. Ware JC, Pittard JT, Nadig PW, Morrison JL, Quinn JB. Trazodon: its effects on nocturnal penile tumescence. *Sleep Res* 1987;16:157.

77. Wiesenfeld-Hallin Z, Södersten P. Spinal opiates affect sexual behavior in rats. *Nature* 1984;309:257–258.

78. Wenkstern D, Pfaus JG, Fibiger HC. Dopamine transmission increases in the nucleus accumbens of male rats during their first exposure to sexually receptive female rats. *Brain Res* 1993;618:41–46.

79. Wiesner JB, Moss RL. A psychopharmacological characterization of the opioid suppression of sexual behaviour in the female rat. In: Dyer RG, Bicknell RJ, eds. *Brain opioid systems in reproduction.* Oxford: Oxford University Press; 1989:187–202.

80. Williams JR, Carter CS. Oxytocin inhibited sexual behavior and facilitated social behavior in male prarie voles. *18th annual conference on reproductive behavior,* Atlanta. 1990.

81. Witt DM, Carter CS, Walton DM. Central and peripheral effects of oxytocin administration in prarie voles (*Microtus ochrogaster*). *Pharmacol Biochem Behav* 1990;37:63–69.

Psychopharmacology: The Fourth Generation of Progress, edited by Floyd E. Bloom and David J. Kupfer. Raven Press, Ltd., New York © 1995.

CHAPTER 66

Animal Models of Drug Addiction

George F. Koob

DEFINITIONS AND VALIDATION OF ANIMAL MODELS

Definitions of Drug Addiction

Two characteristics are common to definitions of dependence and addiction: a compulsion to take the drug with a loss of control in limiting intake and a withdrawal syndrome that results in physical as well as motivational signs of discomfort when the drug is removed. The concept of reinforcement or motivation is a crucial part of both of these characteristics. A *reinforcer* can be defined operationally as "any event that increases the probability of a response." This definition can also be used to signify a definition for *reward,* and the two words are often used interchangeably. However, reward often connotes some additional emotional value such as pleasure.

Most models and definitions of drug dependence also involve the development of tolerance and dependence, which appear to onset and decay with a similar time course. The concepts of tolerance and dependence are integral parts of the hypothesis that adaptive processes are initiated to counter the acute effects of a drug. These processes persist long after the drug has cleared from the brain, thus leaving opposing processes unopposed during abstinence. Such conceptualizations have been explored at all levels of drug-dependence research from the behavioral to the molecular (40). Motivational hypotheses, involving central nervous system "counter-adaptive changes" (70), have been generated that have particular relevance to dependence phenomena.

Multiple sources of reinforcement can be identified during the course of drug dependence. Based on Wikler's extensive work with opiate drugs and his innovative conceptualizations about dependence (70), the primary phar-

macological effect of a drug was hypothesized to produce a direct effect through positive or negative reinforcement as a process (e.g., self-medication) and/or can produce an indirect motivational effect through drug-engendered dependence (relief from aversive abstinence signs). The secondary pharmacological effects of the drug can also have motivating properties. Again, direct effects can be obtained through conditioned reinforcement (e.g., pairing of previously neutral stimuli with acute reinforcing effects of drugs) or indirect effects through removal of the conditioned negative reinforcing effects of conditioned abstinence. Recently, attempts have been made to explore the neurobiological bases for both the acute positive reinforcing effects of drugs and also the negative reinforcing effects imparted by the dependent state (42) (see also Chapters 6, 61, 69, and 145–152, *this volume*).

Validation of Animal Models of Addiction

An animal model can be viewed as an experimental preparation developed for the purpose of studying phenomena found in humans. Animal models are constructed to study selected parts of human syndromes (48). Two criteria appear to be necessary and sufficient for validating an animal model: reliability and predictive validity (see Chapter 68, *this volume*). Where possible, the animal models discussed below are evaluated in terms of these two criteria.

ANIMAL MODELS FOR THE POSITIVE REINFORCING PROPERTIES OF DRUGS

In recent conceptualizations of drug reinforcement, the positive reinforcing properties of drugs have been thought to play an important role in drug dependence (70,74). It is amply clear that animals and humans will readily self-administer drugs in the nondependent state and that drugs

G. F. Koob: Department of Neuropharmacology, The Scripps Research Institute, La Jolla, California 92037.

TABLE 1. *Drugs that are self-administered by rats or monkeys*

Psychomotor Stimulants	Barbiturates
Cocaine	Amobarbital
d-Amphetamine	Secobarbital
Methamphetamine	Pentobarbital
Phenmetrazine	Hexobarbital
Methylphenidate	Benzodiazepines
Diethylpropion	Chlordiazepoxide
Opiates	Diazepam
Morphine	Others
Meperidine	Ethanol
Codeine	Nicotine
Pentazocine	Phencyclidine
Heroin	

have powerful reinforcing properties in that animals will perform many different tasks to obtain drugs. The drugs that have positive reinforcing effects correspond well with the drugs that have high abuse potential in humans (7,10,35,43,59,60) (see Table 1). Much earlier work focused on operant paradigms in primates; however, studies in the last few years have illustrated that many of these same paradigms can be utilized in rodent models, and the new work in rodent models has provided a major benefit to studies focusing on the neurobiology of addiction (40,41).

Operant Intravenous Drug Self-Administration

Drugs of abuse are readily self-administered intravenously by animals, and, in general, drugs that are self-administered correspond to those that have high abuse potential (10,60). Indeed, this relationship is so strong that intravenous drug self-administration is considered an animal model that is predictive of abuse potential (10) and has been suggested to be used as part of a battery for the preclinical assessment of the abuse liability of new agents (35).

Some typical patterns of cocaine self-administration in a rat maintained on a simple fixed-ratio schedule are shown in Fig. 1. Within the range of doses that maintain stable responding, animals increase their self-administration rate as the unit dose is decreased, apparently compensating for decreases in the unit dose. Conversely, animals reduce their self-administration rate as the unit dose is increased. Thus, pharmacological manipulations, which increase the self-administration rate on this fixed-ratio schedule resemble decreases in the unit dose, causing a shift to the right of the dose effect function (a decrease in the reinforcing potency of cocaine). As would be predicted by the unit dose–response model, low to moderate doses of dopamine receptor antagonists increase cocaine self-administration maintained on this schedule in a manner similar to decreasing the unit dose of cocaine (Fig. 1), suggesting that partial blockade of dopamine

receptors by competitive antagonists reduces the reinforcing potency of cocaine. Conversely, dopamine agonists decrease cocaine self-administration in a manner similar to increasing the unit dose of cocaine, suggesting that the effects of dopamine agonists together with cocaine self-administration can be addictive, perhaps due to their mutual activation of the same neural substrates (5).

Schedules of Reinforcement

The use of different schedules of reinforcement in intravenous self-administration can provide important control manipulations for nonspecific motor and motivational actions. For example, fixed-interval schedules of self-administration can be designed to measure response rate independently of frequency of reinforcement. An extended discussion of these schedules of reinforcement can be found elsewhere (25,30,36,37,73; see also Chapter 6, *this volume*).

Simple Schedules

In a simple fixed-ratio schedule, the number of responses required for an infusion of drug is set at a fixed number. In rats, these fixed-ratio schedules will generally not maintain stable responding below a certain unit dose, and, within the range of doses that do maintain stable responding, the self-administration rate is inversely related to dose.

Second-order Schedules

Second-order schedules are different from fixed-ratio schedules with regard to the unit dose–response function. In a second-order schedule, completion of an individual component (or part) of the schedule produces the terminal event (drug infusion) according to another overall schedule (25). In contrast to simple fixed-interval schedules, response rates in second-order schedules have been shown to increase with increasing drug doses (36,37). Further increases in dose lead to a decrease or leveling off of response rates and a sigmoidal or inverted-U-shaped dose–response function. Dose–response relationships have been observed in dose preference measures in both animals and humans where higher doses are preferred over lower doses (17,34). However, it should be noted that, although there is generally a good correlation between cocaine self-administration and its subjective "positive" and stimulant effects, there are areas where these measures are different (17). For example, humans will self-administer doses that do not produce subjective effects (17).

Such inverted-U-shaped unit dose–response functions are sensitive to pharmacological manipulations. In a re-

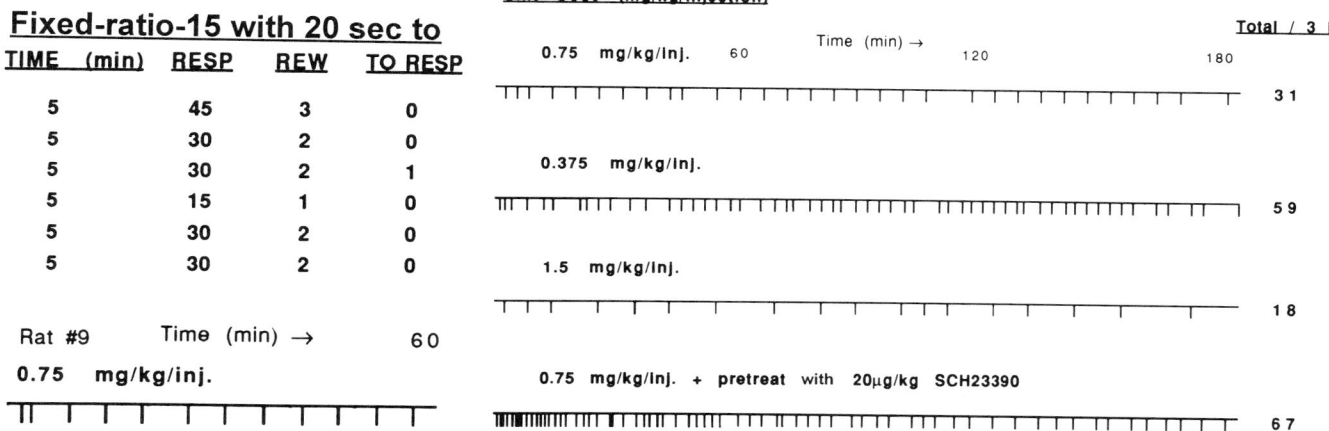

FIG. 1. Left: Actual response record of a rat maintained on a fixed-ratio 15 schedule of cocaine self-administration at a unit dose of 0.75 mg/kg. The *columns* represent the total number of responses in sequential 5-min periods when the lever is active (*RESP*) and during the time-out periods (*TO RESP*) when the lever is inactive. The total number of injections received is indicated in (*REW*). The *bottom* record shows the response record over time and *each mark* represents the delivery of a cocaine injection. From Caine et al. (6) with permission. **Right:** Typical patterns of cocaine substance abuse in the rat as a function of unit dose, and following pretreatment with a dopamine-receptor antagonist. The *abscissa* represents time in minutes, and *each mark* denotes delivery of a cocaine injection. From Caine et al. (6) with permission.

cent study of cocaine self-administration in squirrel monkeys, a complete inverted-U-shaped unit dose–response function was entirely shifted to the right by dopamine receptor antagonists in some monkeys (2). This study elegantly demonstrated that dopamine receptor antagonists increase or decrease cocaine-maintained behavior depending upon the unit dose, but both alterations represent an attenuation of the effects of self-administered cocaine by these agents.

Multiple Schedules

A procedure controlling for nonselective effects of treatments on drug reinforcement is to incorporate self-administration into a multiple component schedule with other reinforcers. Behavior maintained by food or cocaine alternately in the same test session and with identical reinforcement requirements has been reported for various species (6). These schedules may be used to evaluate the selectivity of manipulations that apparently reduce the reinforcing efficacy of cocaine.

Progressive Ratio Schedules

Progressive ratio schedules have been used to evaluate the reinforcing efficacy of the self-administered drug by increasing the response requirements for each successive reinforcement and determining the *breaking point*, the point at which the animal will no longer respond (30,56). A variety of evidence supports the hypothesis that this schedule is effective in determining the rank-order rein-

forcing effectiveness for different reinforcers including drugs. Increasing the unit dose of self-administered drugs increases the breaking point on a progressive ratio schedule (30,56), and dopamine receptor antagonists have been shown to decrease the breaking point for cocaine self-administration (56).

Intravenous drug self-administration in animals has both reliability and predictive validity. The dependent variable is very reliable as a measure of the motivation to obtain drugs (the amount of work an animal will perform to obtain the drug) or, in an alternative framework, in demonstrating that drugs are powerful reinforcers. Where assessed with the appropriate operant schedules, the motivation or the reinforcing efficacy to obtain drugs changes with the type of drug, the dose, and the induction of drug dependence. Performance maintained by drugs as reinforcers is stable from session to session and can be altered predictably by drug antagonists.

Intravenous drug self-administration also has predictive validity, because drugs and doses having high reinforcement potential in animals are reported to have reinforcing effects in humans as measured by both operant and subjective reports (17,35,44,60). The correspondence between subjective reports of euphoria and operant responding for drugs in humans is not perfect, but then subjective reports are clearly under different contingencies than drug-seeking behaviors (17,44). Intravenous self-administration of a given drug is also predictive of abuse potential because of the high correspondence between the ability of various drugs to support operant responding for intravenous injection and their abuse by humans (10).

Brain Stimulation Reward

Electrical self-stimulation of certain brain areas is rewarding for animals and humans as demonstrated by the fact that subjects will readily self-administer the stimulation (52). The powerful nature of the reward effect produced by intracranial self-stimulation (ICSS) is indicated by the behavioral characteristics of the ICSS response, which include rapid learning and vigorous execution of the stimulation-producing behavior (for a review, see ref. 19). The high reward value of ICSS has led to the hypothesis that ICSS directly activates neuronal circuits that are activated by conventional reinforcers (for example, food, water, sex). In bypassing much of the input side of these neuronal circuit(s), ICSS provides a unique tool in neuropharmacological research to investigate the influence of various substances on reward and reinforcement processes. Intracranial self-stimulation differs significantly from drug self-administration in that, in this procedure, the animal is working to directly stimulate presumed reinforcement circuits in the brain and the effects of the drugs are assessed on these reward thresholds. Drugs of abuse decrease thresholds for ICSS, and there is a good correspondence between the ability of drugs to decrease ICSS thresholds and their abuse potential (43).

Many ICSS procedures have been developed over the years (for a review, see ref. 63), but an important methodological advance has been the development of procedures to provide a valid measure of reward threshold unconfounded by influences on motor and performance capability. Two ICSS procedures that have been used extensively to measure the changes in reward threshold produced by drugs are the rate-frequency, curve-shift procedure and the discrete-trial, current-intensity procedure (43,47). These two procedures are widely used in ICSS research because they have been validated experimentally, but other valid ICSS procedures are available. (For a review of the procedures and a detailed description of the methodology employed in the rate-frequency and discrete-trial procedure, see ref. 47.)

Rate-Frequency Procedure

The rate-frequency procedure involves the generation of a stimulation input-output function and provides a frequency threshold measure (19,50). Rate-frequency curves are collected by allowing the rats to press a lever for an ascending series of pulse frequency stimuli, delivered through an electrode in the medial forebrain bundle or other rewarding brain site. A runway apparatus can also be used with running speed as the dependent measure (19). Frequencies can also be presented in a descending or random order or in alternating descending and ascending series and are changed in 0.05 or 0.1 log-unit steps. Two measures are obtained.

The locus of rise (LOR) refers to the "location" (that is, the frequency) at which the function rises from zero to an arbitrary criterion-of-performance level and is presumed to be a measure of ICSS reward threshold (19). The most frequently used criterion is 50% of maximal rate. The behavioral maximum (MAX) measure is the asymptotic maximal response rate, and changes in MAX are thought to reflect motor or performance effects.

Validation studies indicate that changes in the reward efficacy of the stimulation (i.e., intensity manipulations) shift the rate-frequency functions laterally, which translates into large changes in the LOR value but produce no alterations in the asymptote or in the shape of the function (19). In contrast, performance manipulations (for example, weight on the lever, curare, etc.), including changes in motivation (that is, priming), alter the MAX value and the shape of the function (19,50). However, the effects of a manipulation on self-stimulation of LOR smaller than 0.2 log-units must be interpreted carefully because studies indicate that the effects of performance manipulations on the LOR can be as high as 0.2 log-units (19).

Discrete-trial Threshold Procedure

The discrete-trial procedure is a modification of the classical psychophysical method of limits and provides a current-intensity-threshold measure (43,47). This procedure consists of a series of discrete trials in which the subject is expected to emit a single response to receive the electrical stimulus, the current intensity of which is varied between trials. At the start of each trial, rats receive a noncontingent, experimenter-administered electrical stimulus and then have 7.5 sec to turn a wheel manipulandum to obtain a contingent stimulus identical to the previously delivered noncontingent stimulus (positive reinforcer) (see refs. 43 and 47 for details). The threshold value is defined as the midpoint in microamperes between the current intensity level at which the animal makes two or more positive responses out of the three stimulus presentations and the level at which the animal makes less than two positive responses at two consecutive intensities. Response latency is defined as the time in seconds that elapses between the delivery of the noncontingent electrical stimulus (end of the stimulus) and the animal's response on the wheel.

Again, lowering the thresholds can be interpreted as an increase in the reward value of the stimulation, whereas increases in threshold reflect decreases in reward value. Increases in response latency can be interpreted as a motor or performance deficit, but decreases in response latencies in the procedure are difficult to induce, because response latencies are already very short (1.5 to 2.0 sec) under control conditions. In general, the discrete-trial threshold procedure is designed to minimize behavioral response requirements. Therefore, the procedure is not expected to be sensitive to manipulations that indicate motor and performance deficits (47).

Place Preference

Place preference or place conditioning is not an explicitly operant procedure that has been used for assessing the reinforcing efficacy of drugs using, in effect, a Pavlovian conditioning procedure. In a simple version of the place preference paradigm, animals experience two distinct neutral environments that are subsequently paired spatially and temporally with distinct drug states (the unconditioned stimuli, UCS). The animal is later given an opportunity to choose to enter and explore either environment, and the time spent in either environment is considered an index of the reinforcing value of the drug (the UCS). The animal's choice to spend more time in an environment is assumed to be an expression of the positive reinforcing experience within that environment. With a positive reinforcing UCS, the previously neutral stimuli become secondary positive reinforcers. Of course, the opposite can also occur, an aversive experience becomes a secondary negative reinforcer (see below). Perhaps one of the earliest demonstrations of place preference was the observation by Olds and Milner (52) that rats stimulated through an intracranial electrode would return to the location in which they received the stimulation.

Two-choice Procedures

The simple version of the place-conditioning paradigm involves allowing an animal to freely explore and experience two distinct environments for 10 to 20 min to obtain a pretest preference. Subsequently, the animals are restricted to one of the environments under the drug condition and the other environment under the nondrug or placebo condition. Subsequent posttraining tests are performed in the drug-free state, again with a choice of freely exploring both environments (for details see ref. 69).

There are a number of critical independent and dependent variables that can affect place conditioning dramatically. Dependent variables include the duration of the posttraining testing, the method for calculating preference (difference score, percentage of pretraining, etc.), and the actual measures used (number of entries, mean duration of time per entry). A critical independent variable is the use of a biased or unbiased training schedule. In the *biased* design, animals are first tested for their baseline preference, and the animals may show a significant preference for a given environment. Pairings are made during training with the least-preferred environment. Clearly, one could have, instead of a true place preference, simply a reversal of a place aversion. In the *unbiased* design, a

manipulation of the stimuli comprising the environments is made such that there is no preference. Other independent variables are numerous and include housing of the animals, age of the animals, familiarity with the training environment, and physical structure of the training and testing environment. Detailed discussion of these issues is beyond the scope of this chapter (for more information see refs. 7, 65, 68, and 69).

Multiple-choice Procedures

The multiple-choice procedure simply adds additional environmental choices, such as three distinct environments (31), or multiple spatial locations, such as on an elevated radial maze (49). In either case, an additional choice allows for additional controls for nonspecific effects and permits easier balancing between two locations being used for subsequent pairings. (For details of two types of apparati and procedures, see refs. 49 and 66).

Drug Discrimination

Drug discrimination in animals is based on the hypothesis that the same components of a drug's action subserve discriminative stimulus effects in animals and subjective effects in humans (32). Even more importantly, the similarity of the subjective effects of a given drug to the subjective effects produced by a known drug of abuse such as amphetamine can predict abuse potential. Drug discrimination procedures developed in animals have provided a powerful tool for identifying the relative similarity of the discriminative stimulus effects of drugs and, by comparison with known drugs of abuse, the generation of hypotheses regarding the abuse potential of these drugs (32).

Drug discrimination typically involves training an animal to produce a particular response in a given drug state for a food reinforcer and to produce a different response in the placebo or drug-free state. The interoceptive cue state (produced by the drug) controls the behavior as a discriminative stimulus or cue that informs the animal to make the appropriate response in order to gain reinforcement. The choice of response that follows administration of an unknown test compound can provide valuable information about the similarity of that drug's interoceptive cue properties to those of the training drug.

Fixed-ratio Operant Procedures

Some of the original drug discrimination procedures utilized a T-shaped maze escape procedure (53). However, high drug doses are required and the T-shaped maze is not easily automated. More commonly, an appetitively motivated operant procedure is used where the rat has access to two levers (11). Responding on one lever (e.g., left lever) is reinforced on a fixed-ratio 10 schedule for food following injection of the training drug; the other lever is reinforced on a fixed-ratio 10 schedule for food in sessions that follow the injection of the drug vehicle (for details see ref. 32). Schedules of reinforcement other than fixed-ratios and species other than rats, such as rhesus and squirrel monkeys, are used in drug discrimination procedures. However, according to recent trends, rats and fixed-ratio schedules are most commonly employed (67).

Tests of generalization to a novel drug can be interspersed among the training sessions once performance has stabilized. Such tests are often conducted once or twice each week. Alternatively, an entire drug generalization function can be generated in a few hours of a single day using a cumulative dosing method where animals are tested in a series of short sessions with a time-out between each short session (3).

In tests of stimulus generalization, data are often collected only until the delivery of the first reinforcer, which eliminates the influence of reinforcement on subsequent choice responding (which would effectively place the animal in a new training situation). Alternatively, the sessions can be conducted as extinction sessions in which no reinforcers are delivered or can be conducted when responses on both levers are reinforced.

Discrete-trials Procedure

An alternative drug discrimination training procedure used extensively by Holtzman and colleagues in both rats and squirrel monkeys (32) involves a discrete-trials procedure using avoidance or escape from shock. Here, animals are trained to lever press on one of two levers to avoid or escape electric shocks that are delivered intermittently to the grid floor of the cage. A trial is signaled by the illumination of a house light. A third lever (called the observing lever) must be pressed before the choice is made to prevent the rat from perseverating on the appropriate choice lever. A major advantage of this aversively maintained responding is that no food restriction is necessary and there is no confound from the anorexic effects of the drug in question (32). Another advantage is that higher doses of the drug can be tested, which may reveal important aspects of the pharmacology of the test drugs (62).

Advantages and Disadvantages of Animal Models for the Positive Reinforcing Properties of Drugs

The advantages of intravenous self-administration and drug discrimination as animal models for the reinforcing effects of drugs are numerous. Drug self-administration has high sensitivity to low doses of drugs, it has potential utility in studying both the positive and negative reinforc-

ing actions of drugs, drug reinforcement can be tested in drug-free conditions, and it allows precise control over the interaction of environmental cues with drug administration. As described above, both procedures have predictive validity and are reliable. Another major advantage of these procedures is that they lend themselves to within-subjects designs, limiting the number of subjects required. Indeed, once an animal is trained, full dose–effect functions can be generated for different drugs, and the animal can be tested for weeks and months. Pharmacological manipulations can be conducted with standard reference compounds to validate any effects. In addition, a rich literature on the experimental analysis of behavior is available for exploring the hypothetical constructs of drug action as well as for modifying drug reinforcement by modifying the history and contingencies of reinforcement.

The advantage of the ICSS paradigm as a model of drug effects on motivation and reward is that by directly stimulating the putative reward systems, one presumably bypasses the input side of the system and eliminates the nonspecific effects of consummatory behaviors, such as feeding, that can complicate data interpretation. Also, the behavioral threshold measure provided by ICSS procedures is easily quantifiable, because ICSS threshold estimates are very stable over periods of several months (for a review, see ref. 63). Another considerable advantage of the ICSS technique is the high reliability with which it predicts the abuse liability of drugs. For example, there has never been a false positive with the discrete-trials threshold technique (43).

The advantages of place conditioning as a model for evaluating drugs of abuse are similar to those of drug self-administration and include (a) a high sensitivity to low doses of drugs, (b) the potential utility in studying both sides of hedonic valence (e.g., both positive and negative reinforcement), (c) the fact that testing for drug reinforcement is done under drug-free conditions, and (d) the allowance for precise control over the interaction of environmental cues with drug administration (7,69).

The disadvantages of intravenous self-administration and ICSS are largely technical, that is, the procedures require survival surgery as well as reasonably sophisticated testing apparati. Special skills and procedures are required to implement and maintain a chronic catheter preparation, and success in maintaining viable catheter preparations in rodent studies can be poor, particularly over periods of 6 weeks or more (for details of the technical issues and procedures, see ref. 6).

Disadvantages of drug discrimination are that subjects receive numerous doses of the training drug, and any neuropharmacological changes caused by such phenomenon as sensitization cannot be measured; in fact, they may be masked by the training and testing procedure. The other disadvantage is that the predictive validity of the procedure is indirect (e.g., the ability to predict abuse potential) and is based on knowledge of the class to which the previously unknown compound generalizes.

The major disadvantage of place conditioning is the enormous cost, effort, and time required to generate meaningful results. Each dose requires 8 to 12 rats in an independent (between-subjects) design, and each animal must be trained and tested numerous times yet yields only one independent data point. Contributing to these enormous costs are all the control experiments required to address issues such as state dependency, familiarity, hyperactivity, and biased initial preferences. Because only a limited number of animals can be trained at one time, even with automated apparati, the paradigm becomes time consuming as well.

ANIMAL MODELS OF THE NEGATIVE REINFORCING PROPERTIES OF DRUG WITHDRAWAL

Drug withdrawal from chronic drug administration is usually characterized by responses opposite to the acute initial actions of the drug. Many of the overt physical signs associated with withdrawal from drugs (e.g., alcohol and opiates) can be easily quantified. However, motivational measures of abstinence have proven to be more sensitive measures of drug withdrawal and powerful tools for exploring the neurobiological bases for the motivational aspects of drug dependence. Animal models for the motivational effects of drug withdrawal have included operant schedules, place aversion, ICSS, the elevated plus maze, and drug discrimination. Although some of these models may reflect more general malaise than others, each of these models can be considered to address a different hypothetical construct associated with a given motivational aspect of withdrawal.

Operant Drug Self-Administration in Drug-dependent Animals

Drug self-administration can easily be conducted in drug-dependent animals, and the procedures are very similar to those discussed above regarding drug self-administration in nondependent rats. However, some evidence suggests that the reinforcing efficacy of a drug can increase with dependence. Monkeys made dependent on morphine showed increases in their progressive ratio performance compared to their performance in the nondependent state (75). Also, baboons in a discrete-trials choice procedure for food and heroin showed significant behavioral elasticity when allowed access to heroin or food periodically in a nondependent state (15). In the dependent state, one would hypothesize that the animals would be much less likely to respond for food, even if the cost of heroin in terms of response requirements was dramatically increased. Thus, the reinforcing value of drugs may

change with dependence. The neurobiological basis for such a change is only beginning to be investigated (42), but much evidence has been generated to show that drug dependence itself can produce an aversive or negative motivational state that is manifested by changes in a number of behavioral measures, such as response disruption, changes in reward thresholds, and place aversions.

Operant Schedules for Nondrug Reinforcers in Dependent Animals

Several operant schedules have been used to characterize the response–disruptive effects of drug withdrawal (13,22,33,42), providing a readily quantifiable measure of withdrawal (e.g., response rate). These include high rate schedules, such as fixed ratios (22), and a stable, but low, steady-state rate of responding, such as the differential reinforcement of low rates of responding (DRL) (13). However, response disruption can be caused by any number of variables from motor problems to malaise and decreases in appetite, and thus other measures must be used to rule out nonspecific effects (see below).

Place Aversion

Place aversion has been used to measure the aversive stimulus effects of withdrawal (31,42,66). Here, in contrast to the place-preference conditioning discussed above, rats exposed to a particular environment while undergoing withdrawal will spend less time in the withdrawal-paired environment when subsequently presented with a choice between that environment and one and two possible unpaired environments. Naloxone itself will produce a place aversion in non-opiate-dependent rats, but the threshold dose required to produce a place aversion decreases significantly in dependent rats (31) (see Fig. 2). Hypothetically, identical studies could be performed in dependent rats undergoing spontaneous withdrawal. The challenge would be to find a discrete period of sufficient unconditioned stimulus value (aversive state) to be associated with a previously neutral conditioned stimulus.

Brain Stimulation Reward

Intracranial self-stimulation thresholds have been used to assess changes in systems mediating reward and reinforcement processes during the course of drug dependence. Although no actual negative reinforcement is measured using this technique, it is included in this section because it constitutes a model of the aversive motivational state associated with the negative reinforcement of drug abstinence in dependent animals. Acute administration of psychostimulant drugs lowers ICSS threshold (i.e., in-

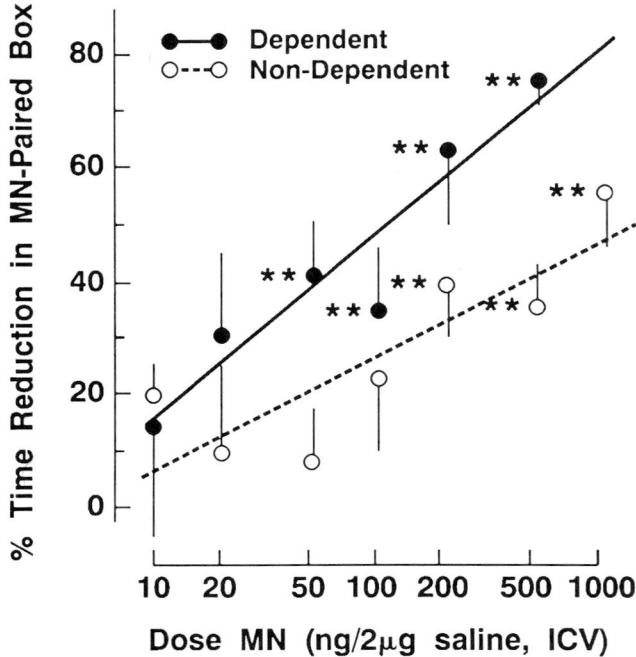

FIG. 2. Conditioned place aversions following a 6-day conditioning regimen with i.c.v. methylnaloxonium (MN) in naive vs. morphine-dependent rats, presented as group mean with standard errors (**p < 0.01). *Ordinate* shows the percent reduction in time spent in the MN-paired compartment (1 − test time/preconditioning time × 100%). *Abscissa* shows the dose of i.c.v. MN applied before conditioning sessions. From Hand et al. (31) with permission.

creases ICSS reward) (for reviews see refs. 43, and 63, and withdrawal from chronic administration of these same drugs elevates ICSS thresholds (i.e., decrease ICSS reward) (39,45,46) (see Fig. 3). Similar results have been observed with precipitated withdrawal in opiate-dependent rats (58). Rats trained in the discrete-trials threshold procedure showed dramatic increases in ICSS thresholds to naloxone injections that occurred in a dose-related manner and at doses below which obvious physical signs of opiate withdrawal were manifest. These doses of naloxone had no effect on reward thresholds in this dose range in nondependent animals.

Drug Discrimination

Drug discrimination can be used to characterize both specific and nonspecific aspects of withdrawal. Generalization to an opiate antagonist provides a more general nonspecific measure of opiate withdrawal intensity and time course (18,21). Examples of a more specific aspect of withdrawal are animals that have been trained to discriminate pentylenetetrazol, an anxiogenic-like substance, from saline in ethanol-, diazepam-, and opiate-dependent animals. During withdrawal, generalization to the pentyl-

enetetrazol cue has suggested an anxiogenic-like component to the withdrawal syndrome (16,20).

Advantages and Disadvantages of Animal Models of the Negative Reinforcing Properties of Drugs

These motivational measures of drug withdrawal have most of the same advantages and disadvantages as do the positive reinforcing effects of drugs. To summarize, intravenous drug self-administration is a direct measure of the reinforcing effects of drugs, ICSS threshold procedures have high predictive validity for changes in reward valence, disruption of operant responding during drug abstinence is very sensitive, place aversion implies an aversive unconditioned stimulus, and drug discrimination

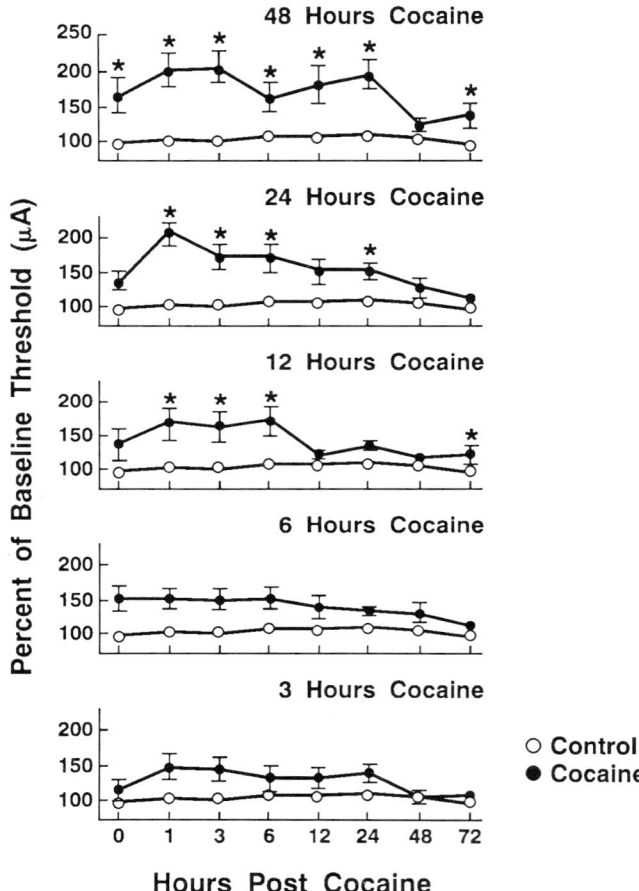

FIG. 3. Intracranial self-stimulation thresholds following 0, 3, 6, 12, 24, and 48 hr of cocaine self-administration at several time points postcocaine (0, 1, 3, 6, 12, 24, 48, and 72 hr). The results are expressed as percent change from baseline threshold levels. The mean ± SEM baseline threshold for the experimental group was 37.414 ± 2.516 µA and for the control group 35.853 ± 3.078 µA. The *asterisks* indicate statistically significant differences ($p < 0.05$) between control and experimental groups with Dunnett's tests after a significant group spent x hours interaction in the ANOVA. From Markou and Koob (46) with permission.

allows a powerful and sensitive comparison to other drug states.

The disadvantages of each of these dependent variables are also similar to those described above for the positive reinforcing effects of drugs. Intravenous self-administration and ICSS have numerous technical challenges, disruption of operant responding is subject to non-specific effects and is difficult to interpret in isolation, place aversion is costly because of the large number of subjects that are necessary for between-subject designs, and drug discrimination is weak on predictive validity. Clearly, each of these dependent variables in isolation has weaknesses, but when combined can provide a powerful insight into the motivational effects of drug abstinence.

ANIMAL MODELS OF THE CONDITIONED REINFORCING PROPERTIES OF DRUGS

Some of the earliest evidence for the ability of drug-paired stimuli to function as conditioned reinforcing stimuli was provided by a study in which an anise-flavored solution of etonitazene (an opiate agonist), was provided as the sole drinking solution to non-opiate-dependent rats (72). Several months later, in a two-bottle choice situation, the animals consumed twice as much anise-flavored water as control rats. Furthermore, opiate-dependent rats that were given access to the anise-flavored etonitazene solution during morphine withdrawal, several months later consumed twice as much anise-flavored water as the rats with similar anise-flavored etonitazene experience that were never opiate-dependent. These results suggest that previously neutral stimuli can acquire reinforcing properties when paired with reinforcing drugs and that the development of dependence and the amelioration of withdrawal can also contribute to the motivational efficacy of such secondary reinforcers.

Extinction with and without Cues Associated with Drug Self-Administration

Extinction procedures can provide measures of the incentive or motivational properties of drugs by assessing the persistence of drug-seeking behavior in the absence of response-contingent drug availability. Extinction testing sessions are identical to training sessions for drug self-administration, except that no drug is delivered after completion of the response requirement.

Measures provided by an extinction paradigm reflect the degree of resistance to extinction and include the duration of extinction responding and the total number of responses emitted during the entire extinction session. The probability of reinitiating responding under extinction conditions with drug-paired stimuli or even stimuli previously paired with drug withdrawal can be explored

at a later time after successful extinction of the self-administrative behavior.

In this type of paradigm both stimulant and opiate self-administration have been consistently reinstated following extinction in animals with systemic or intracerebral noncontingent drug infusions (e.g., priming) (23,64). Responding for a conditioned reinforcer contingency in rats that is extinguished can also be reinstated by noncontingent drug infusions (12). The effectiveness of compounds in reinstating drug self-administration decreases as their discriminative stimulus similarity to the training drug decreases (23,64).

This specificity of drug priming is consistent with the specificity of conditioned responses in human drug users. An experimental study in human drug users indicated that cocaine-related stimuli were effective in eliciting conditioned physiological responses and self-reported cocaine craving in cocaine users, but not in opiate or nondrug users, but neutral stimuli were ineffective in eliciting any conditioned responses (14). In addition to general physiological responses, conditioned stimuli associated with drug administration also induce the psychological phenomenon of drug craving in humans, even after a period of abstinence (9).

Positive Reinforcing Properties of Cues Associated with Drug Self-Administration

A conditioned reinforcer can be defined as any neutral stimulus that acquires reinforcing properties through association with a primary reinforcer. In a conditioned reinforcement paradigm, subjects are usually trained in an operant box containing two levers by which responses on one lever result in presentation of a brief stimulus followed by a drug injection (active lever), whereas responses on the other lever have no consequences throughout the experiment (inactive lever) (12,61). Previously neutral stimuli can also acquire conditioned reinforcing properties when the drug administration is not contingent on the animal's behavior, as long as the stimulus precedes the drug injection (12). Subsequently, the ability of the previously neutral, drug-paired stimuli to maintain responding in the absence of drug injections provide a measure of the reinforcing value of these stimuli. Psychomotor stimulants also potentiate conditioned reinforcement to nondrug reinforcers (55), and the neural substrate for these effects appears to be the release of dopamine to the nucleus accumbens (38).

Second-order schedules can also be used as a measure of the conditioned reinforcing properties of drugs. As described above, completion of the first component or unit of the schedule, rather than an individual response, produces the terminal event according to another overall schedule (25). In some versions of a second-order schedule, completion of the first component or unit produces a stimulus (2-sec light) and then completion of a fixed number of first components produces the light and drug.

Manipulation of the stimuli that are part of the second-order schedule can alter acquisition, maintenance, resistance to extinction, and recovery from extinction in second-order schedules (25). To assess the effects of conditioned reinforcement, the number of responses with the paired stimulus can be compared to the number of responses with a nonpaired stimulus. For example, substitution of drug-paired stimuli with non-drug-paired stimuli can actually decrease response rates (36). This maintenance of performance in second-order schedules with drug-paired stimuli appears to be analogous to the maintenance and reinstatement of drug seeking in humans with the presentation of drug-paired stimuli (9).

The conditioned place preference paradigm also provides a measure of conditioned reinforcement that is conceptually similar to the measures provided by the operant paradigms. Several extensive reviews have been written on the place preference paradigm (7,65,68,69); also see above.

Conditioned Negative Reinforcing Effects of Withdrawal—Cues Conditioned to the Motivational Effects of Drug Abstinence

The motivation for maintenance of compulsive drug use requires more than just positive reinforcement; negative reinforcement also has been hypothesized to play a role in that drug self-administration relieves the aversive affects of abstinence from chronic drug administration. These motivational aspects of withdrawal can be conditioned, and conditioned withdrawal has been repeatedly observed in opiate-dependent animals and humans. Patients, even detoxified subjects, report signs and symptoms resembling opiate abstinence when returning to environments similar to those associated with drug experiences. In a more direct demonstration performed in opiate addicts maintained on methadone, naloxone injections were repeatedly paired with a compound stimulus of a tone and a peppermint smell (51). Following these pairings, presentation of only the tone and odor elicited both subjective reports of sickness and discomfort and objective physical signs of withdrawal.

In early animal studies, rats made dependent by gradually increasing daily doses of morphine were exposed to a distinct environment each evening while experiencing the gradual and progressive onset of morphine abstinence. After 6 weeks of such pairings, rats exposed to this same distinct environment showed somatic signs of withdrawal up to 155 days after the last morphine injection (70,71).

In addition to somatic signs of withdrawal, motivational signs of withdrawal have also been conditioned in animals. Morphine-dependent rhesus monkeys, trained to lever press for food on a fixed-ratio 10 schedule, showed an immediate suppression of food-maintained responding in addition to clear physical signs of withdrawal after injection of the opiate-mixed agonist/antagonist nalorphine (27,28, see also ref. 24). Presentation of the conditioned stimuli resulting from repeated pairings of a light or tone with the nalorphine injection also produced a complete suppression of this food responding (27,28). Similar results have now been observed with rats (1). Four pairings of a compound stimulus of a tone and smell with an injection of naloxone in morphine-dependent rats trained to lever press for food on a fixed-ratio 15 schedule resulted in a reduction in operant responding in response to the tone and smell alone, and this conditioned response persisted for 1 month, even after pellet removal (see Fig. 4). The animals showed no obvious conditioned physical signs of withdrawal. These results suggest that a conditioned stimulus can acquire aversive stimulus effects that persist even in the absence of opiate occupancy of receptors and that motivational signs of conditioned withdrawal can occur in the absence of withdrawallike somatic symptoms.

The motivational significance of conditioned withdrawal was provided in a series of elegant operant studies by Goldberg and colleagues (26,29). After repeated pairings of nalorphine and the light in monkeys self-administering morphine intravenously 24 hr/day, presentation of the light alone (with injection of saline) resulted in a conditioned increase in responding for morphine, presumably to avoid the onset of withdrawal (29). An even more compelling demonstration of the negative reinforcing properties of conditioned withdrawal was provided by a study in which opiate-dependent monkeys were given daily 2-hr sessions in which a green light signaled an intravenous infusion of nalorphine or naloxone (26). Lever-pressing by the monkey terminated the green light and prevented the injections of opiate antagonists for 60 sec. Initially, most responses occurred after the onset of injection, but with repeated pairings of the light cue and the antagonist, most of the responding occurred during the period when the light cue was illuminated, but before the antagonist infusion. These results are a powerful demonstration of the negative reinforcing properties of antagonist-precipitated drug withdrawal.

Advantages and Disadvantages of Animal Models of the Conditioned Reinforcing Properties of Drugs

The advantage of the extinction paradigm as a model for the conditioned reinforcing effects of drugs is that it can be a reliable indicator of the ability of conditioned stimuli to reinitiate drug-seeking behavior and thus have predictive validity as a measure of drug relapse. The conditioned-reinforcement paradigm has the advantage of assessing the reinforcing value of a drug infusion in the absence of acute effects of the self-administered

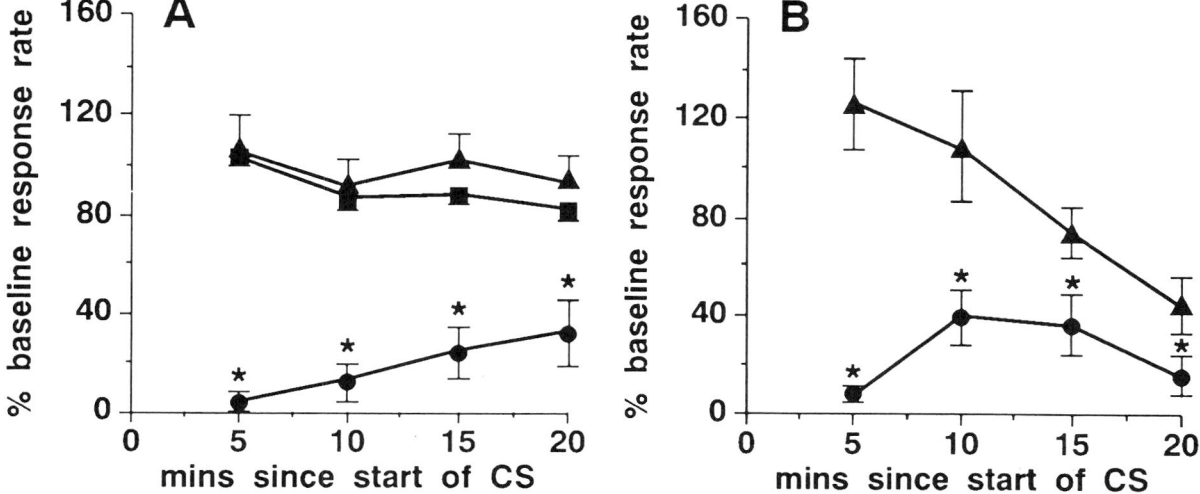

FIG. 4. Left: Test for conditioned withdrawal in morphine-dependent rats. Values are mean ± SEM percentages of baseline rate of lever pressing/minute. Mean ± SEM pretreatment baseline response rates on the test day were as follows: paired group = 60.0 ± 8.4, unpaired group = 74.7 ± 8.1, saline controls = 95.1 ± 8.7 lever presses/minute. Asterisks indicate results significantly different from the unpaired group and saline controls ($p < 0.05$). (●, paired group; ▲, unpaired group; ■, saline controls). From Baldwin and Koob (1) with permission. **Right:** Test for conditioned withdrawal in postdependent rats. Values are mean ± SEM percentages of baseline rate of lever pressing/minute. Mean ± SEM pretreatment baseline response rates on the test day were as follows: paired group = 66.0 ± 10.8, unpaired group = 81.9 ± 9.3 lever presses/minute. Asterisks indicate results significantly different from the unpaired group ($p < 0.05$). (●, paired group; ▲, unpaired group). From Baldwin and Koob (1) with permission.

drug that could influence performance or other processes that interfere with reinforcing functions. For example, nonspecific effects of manipulations administered before the stimulus drug pairings do not directly affect the assessment of the reinforcing value of the conditioned stimuli because the critical test can be conducted several days after the stimulus drug pairings. Also, the paradigm contains a built-in control for nonspecific motor effects of a manipulation by its assessment of the number of responses on an inactive lever.

One of the advantages of second-order schedules is that they reliably maintain high rates of responding in a variety of species (thousands of responses per session in monkeys) and extended sequences of behavior before any drug administration (25,36). Thus, potentially disruptive nonspecific acute drug and treatment effects on response rates can be minimized. High response rates can be maintained even for doses that decrease rates during a session on a regular fixed-ratio schedule, indicating that performance on the second-order schedule can be less affected by those acute effects of the drug that disrupt operant responding (36). However, there can still be disruption in response rates under second-order schedules at high doses per injection, unless all the injections occur at the end of the session. These schedules have predictive validity of drug abuse potential, because performance in second-order schedules is maintained by injections (intravenous, intramuscular, or oral) of a variety of drugs that

are abused by humans, with the animals exhibiting similar behavioral patterns in second-order schedules that terminate in drug injections.

Similar advantages can be observed for the models of conditioned negative reinforcing effects of withdrawal. These paradigms are reliable measures of the negative reinforcing effects of drug dependence and may have predictive validity as measures of protracted abstinence. Future studies will be required to establish this relationship. In addition, in all of these procedures the stimuli have taken on secondary reinforcing properties and as such can profit from much of what is known about the experimental analysis of behavior as it relates to primary reinforcers.

The disadvantages of all of these procedures is that they involve extensive training procedures and significant learning. Thus, treatments or manipulations that affect acquisition of new associations will disrupt the development of the conditioned reinforcing effects of drugs. The challenge of future behavioral design will be to explore means of separating these hypothetical constructs, both at the behavioral and the neurobiological levels of analysis.

ANIMAL MODELS OF ACQUISITION OF DRUG-SEEKING BEHAVIOR

The focus of this chapter has been on the animal models for established drug dependence and more specifically on recent studies in rodent models. However, there are numerous models for studying the acquisition of drug seeking behavior that involve many of the paradigms and procedures used in studying the acquisition of responding for other reinforcers. Significant success has been obtained in studying the acquisition of stimulant self-administration using smaller doses and in rodents, a nose poke response that has a high baseline frequency of emission (54).

Acquisition of drug self-administration also recruits variables covered in other chapters of this volume that can contribute to vulnerability for drug-seeking behavior, such as drug tolerance, drug sensitization (57), environmental variables (8), and genetic variables (see Chapters 61, 64, and 145–154, *this volume*).

SUMMARY AND CONCLUSIONS

Significance of Animal Models of Addiction

The importance of animal models of drug addiction is the assumption that findings observed in the animal models will have relevance to the social problems of drug abuse and addiction in man (60). Certainly, animal models of drug addiction can predict abuse potential (see the next section). However, the value of these animal models goes far beyond just the capacity to predict abuse potential. Animal models of drug addiction can provide a means of studying both the behavioral and biological basis of drug addiction. Factors involved in acquisition, maintenance, extinction, and reinstatement of drug reinforcement can carefully be extracted in laboratory-controlled situations. The neurobiological mechanisms involved in the positive reinforcing effects of drugs and the negative reinforcing effects of drug abstinence can and are being elucidated. Perhaps even more importantly, the environmental, behavioral, and neurobiological factors that contribute to individual differences in vulnerability to drug addiction can be explored with animal models. Finally, studies of the antecedents, mechanisms, and consequences of drug addiction using animal models provides a window on the antecedents, mechanisms, and consequences of other hypothetical constructs, such as emotions, that have long intrigued behavioral biologists (4).

Validity of Existing Animal Models

Most of the animal models discussed above appear to have predictive validity and are reliable. For the positive reinforcing effects of drugs, drug self-administration, ICSS, and conditioned place preference have been shown to have predictive validity for abuse potential of drugs. Drug discrimination has predictive validity for abuse potential of drugs indirectly through generalization to the training drug. Animal models of conditioned drug effects are successful in predicting the potential for conditioned drug effects in humans. In a limited number of examples, the negative reinforcing properties of drug abstinence appear to have predictive validity for the negative reinforcing properties of abstinence in humans. Predictive validity is more problematic for such concepts as craving, largely due to the inadequate formulation of the concept of craving in humans to date (48). Virtually all of the measures described here, with the possible exception of place preference and place aversion, have demonstrated reliability. Consistency and stability of the measures, small within-subject and between-subject variability, and reproducibility of the phenomenon is a characteristic of most of the measures employed in animal models of dependence.

Future Research

Most of the experimental work on the aversive motivational effects of drugs have been focused on the opiate model, but abstinence from opiates, stimulants, and alcohol result in aversive motivational states characterized by increases in behavioral responsiveness to stressors in animal models of anxiety, increases in reward thresholds, disruptions in motivated behavior, and conditioned place aversions. This (presumably aversive) motivational state serves as a dysregulator of motivational homeostasis and thus provides a mechanism for a negative-reinforcement process in which the organism administers the drug to alleviate the aversive withdrawal state.

Clearly, much remains to be explored about the neurobiological mechanisms of the unconditioned positive and negative motivational state(s), and in particular the conditioned positive and negative motivational state(s) associated with drug use and withdrawal. The study of the changes in the central nervous system that are associated with these homeostatic dysregulations may provide not only the key to drug dependence, but also the key to the etiology of psychopathologies associated with anxiety and affective abnormalities. The animal models described above provide a basis to begin such studies; however, a rich behavioral literature exists from which to draw even more creative and innovative models of the behavioral processes that form the syndrome of drug dependence.

REFERENCES

1. Baldwin HA, Koob GF. Rapid induction of conditioned opiate withdrawal. *Neuropsychopharmacology* 1993;8:15–21.
2. Bergman J, Kamien JB, Spealman RD. Antagonism of cocaine self-administration by selective dopamine D1 and D2 antagonist. *Behav Pharmacol* 1990;1:355–363.
3. Bertalmio AJ, Herling S, Hampton RY, Winger G, Woods JH. A procedure for rapid evaluation of the discriminative stimulus effects of drugs. *J Pharmacol Exp Ther* 1982;141:289–299.
4. Brady JV. Emotion revisited. *J Psychiatr Res* 1971;8:363–384.
5. Caine SB, Koob GF. Modulation of cocaine self-administration in

the rat through D-3 dopamine receptors. *Science* 1993;260:1814–1816.

6. Caine SB, Lintz R, Koob GF. Intravenous drug self-administration techniques in animals. In: Sahgal A, ed. *Behavioral neuroscience: a practical approach.* New York: Oxford University Press; 1993:93–115.

7. Carr GD, Fibiger HC, Phillips AG. Conditioned place preference as a measure of drug reward. In: Liebman JM, Cooper SJ, eds. *The neuropharmacological basis of reward.* New York: Oxford University Press; 1989:264–319.

8. Carroll ME, Lac TL, Nygaard SL. A concurrently available nondrug reinforcer prevents the acquisition or decreases the maintenance of cocaine-reinforced behavior. *Psychopharmacology* 1989;97:23–29.

9. Childress AR, McLellan AT, Ehrman R, O'Brien CP. *Classically conditioned responses in opioid and cocaine dependence: a role in relapse?* NIDA Research Monograph 84. Rockville, MD: Department of Health and Human Services; 1988:25–43.

10. Collins RJ, Weeks JR, Cooper MM, Good PI, Russell RR. Prediction of abuse liability of drugs using IV self-administration by rats. *Psychopharmacology* 1984;82:6–13.

11. Colpaert FC, Lal H, Niemegeers CJE, Janssen PAJ. Investigations on drug produced and subjectively experienced discriminative stimuli. 1. The fentanyl cue, a tool to investigate subjectively experienced narcotic actions. *Life Sci* 1975;16:705–716.

12. Davis WM, Smith SG. Role of conditioned reinforcer in the initiation, maintenance and extinction of drug-seeking behavior. *Pavlov J Biol Sci* 1976;11:222–236.

13. Denoble U, Begleiter H. Response suppression on a mixed schedule of reinforcement during alcohol withdrawal. *Pharmacol Biochem Behav* 1976;5:227–229.

14. Ehrman RN, Robbins SJ, Childress AR, O'Brien CP. Conditioned responses to cocaine-related stimuli in cocaine abuse patients. *Psychopharmacology* 1992;107:523–529.

15. Elsmore TF, Fletcher GV, Conrad DG, Sodetz FJ. Reduction of heroin intake in baboons by an economic constraints. *Pharmacol Biochem Behav* 1980;13:729–731.

16. Emmett-Oglesby MW, Mathis DA, Moon RTY, Lal H. Animal models of drug withdrawal symptoms. *Psychopharmacology* 1990;101:292–309.

17. Fischman MW. Relationship between self-reported drug effects and their reinforcing effects: studies with stimulant drugs. In: Fischman MW, Mello NK, eds. *Testing for abuse liability of drugs in humans.* NIDA Research Monograph 92. Rockville, MD: Department of Health and Human Services; 1989:211–230.

18. France CP, Woods JH. Discriminative stimulus effects of naltrexone in morphine-treated rhesus monkeys. *J Pharmacol Exp Ther* 1989;250:937–943.

19. Gallistel CR. Self-stimulation. In: Deutsch JA, ed. *The physiological basis of memory.* New York: Academic Press; 1983:73–77.

20. Gauvin DV, Holloway FA. Cue dimensionality in the 3-choice pentylenetetrazole-saline-chlordiazepoxide discrimination task. *Behav Pharmacol* 1991;2:417–428.

21. Gellert VF, Holtzman SG. Discriminative stimulus effects of naltrexone in the morphine-dependent rat. *J Pharmacol Exp Ther* 1979;211:596–605.

22. Gellert VF, Sparber SB. A comparison of the effects of naloxone upon body weight loss and suppression of fixed-ratio operant behavior in morphine-dependent rats. *J Pharmacol Exp Ther* 1977;201:44–54.

23. Gerber GJ, Stretch R. Drug-induced reinstatement of extinguished self-administration behavior in monkeys. *Pharmacol Biochem Behav* 1975;3:1055–1061.

24. Goldberg SR. Stimuli associated with drug injections as events that control behavior. *Pharmacol Rev* 1976;27:325–340.

25. Goldberg SR, Gardner ML. Second-order schedules: extended sequences of behavior controlled by brief environmental stimuli associated with dosing administration. In: Thompson T, Johanson CE, eds. *Behavioral pharmacology of human drug dependence.* NIDA Research Monograph No. 37, DHEW Publication No. (ADM) 81-1137, Washington, DC: U.S. Government Printing Office; 1981:241–270.

26. Goldberg SR, Hoffmeister F, Schlichting V, Wolfgang W. Aversive properties of nalorphine and naloxone in morphine-dependent rhesus monkeys. *J Pharmacol Exp Ther* 1971;179:268–276.

27. Goldberg SR, Schuster CR. Suppression by a stimulus associated with nalorphine in morphine-dependent monkeys. *J Exp Anal Behav* 1967;10:235–242.

28. Goldberg SR, Schuster CR. Conditioned nalorphine-induced abstinence changes: persistence in post morphine-dependent monkeys. *J Exp Anal Behav* 1970;14:33–46.

29. Goldberg SR, Woods JH, Schuster CR. Morphine: conditioned increases in self-administration in rhesus monkeys. *Science* 1969;166:1306–1307.

30. Griffiths RR, Brady JV, Snell JD. Progressive ratio performance maintained by drug infusions: comparison of cocaine, diethylpropion, chlorphentermine, and fenfluramine. *Psychopharmacology* 1978;56:5–13.

31. Hand TH, Koob GF, Stinus L, Le Moal M. Aversive properties of opiate receptor blockade are centrally mediated and are potentiated by previous exposure to opiates. *Brain Res* 1988;474:364–368.

32. Holtzman SG. Discriminative stimulus effects of drugs: relationship to potential for abuse. In: *Modern methods in pharmacology. Vol. 6. Testing and evaluation of drugs of abuse.* New York: Wiley-Liss; 1990:193–210.

33. Holtzman SG, Villarreal JE. Operant behavior in the morphine-dependent rhesus monkey. *J Pharmacol Exp Ther* 1973;184(3):528–541.

34. Johanson CE. Pharmacological and environmental variables affecting drug preference in rhesus monkeys. *Pharmacol Rev* 1976;27:343–355.

35. Johanson CE, Balster RL. A summary of the results of a drug self-administration study using substitution procedures in rhesus monkeys. *Bull Narc* 1978;30:43–54.

36. Katz JL, Goldberg SR. Second-order schedules of drug injection: implications for understanding reinforcing effects of abused drugs. In: Mello NK, ed. *Advances in substance abuse.* vol. 4. London: Jessica Kingsley Publishers; 1991:205–223.

37. Kelleher RT. Characteristics of behavior controlled by scheduled injections of drugs. *Pharmacol Rev* 1975;27:307–323.

38. Kelley AE, Delfs JM. Amphetamine and conditioned reinforcement. II. Contrasting effects of amphetamine microinjection into the nucleus accumbens with peptide microinjection into the ventral tegmental area. *Psychopharmacology* 1991;103:197–203.

39. Kokkinidis L, McCarter BD. Postcocaine depression and sensitization of brain stimulation reward: analysis of reinforcement and performance effects. *Pharmacol Biochem Behav* 1990;36:463–471.

40. Koob GF, Bloom FE. Cellular and molecular mechanisms of drug dependence. *Science* 1988;242:715–723.

41. Koob GF, Goeders N. Neuroanatomical substrates of drug self-administration. In: Liebman JM, Cooper SJ, eds. *Neuropharmacological basis of reward,* Vol. 6. New York: Oxford University; 1989:214–264.

42. Koob GF, Markou A, Weiss F, Schulteis G. Opponent process and drug dependence: Neurobiological mechanisms. *Semin Neurosci* 1993;5:351–358.

43. Kornetsky C, Esposito RU. Euphorigenic drugs: effects on reward pathways of the brain. *Fed Proc* 1979;38:2473–2476.

44. Lamb RJ, Preston KL, Schindler CW, et al. The reinforcing and subjective effects of morphine in post-addicts: a dose–response study. *J Pharmacol Exp Ther* 1991;259:1165–1173.

45. Leith NJ, Barrett RJ. Amphetamine and the reward system: evidence for tolerance and post-drug depression. *Psychopharmacologia* 1976;46:19–25.

46. Markou A, Koob GF. Post cocaine anhedonia. An animal model of cocaine withdrawal. *Neuropharmacology* 1991;4:17–26.

47. Markou A, Koob GF. Intracranial self-stimulation thresholds as a measure of reward. In: Sahgal A, ed. *Behavioral neuroscience: a practical approach.* New York: Oxford University Press; 1993:93–115.

48. Markou A, Weiss F, Gold LH, Caine SB, Schulteis G, Koob GF. Animal models of drug craving. *Psychopharmacology* 1993;112:163–182.

49. McDonald RJ, White NM. A triple dissociation of memory systems: hippocampus, amygdala, and dorsal striatum. *Behav Neurosci* 1993;107(1):3–22.

50. Milliaressis E, Rompre PP, Laviolette P, Philippe L, Coulombe D. The wave-shift paradigm in self-stimulation. *Physiol Behav* 1986;37:85–91.

51. O'Brien CP, Jesta J, O'Brien TJ, Brady JP, Wells B. Conditioned narcotic withdrawal in humans. *Science* 1977;195:1000–1002.
52. Olds J, Milner P. Positive reinforcement produced by electrical stimulation of septal area and other regions of rat brain. *J Comp Physiol Psychol* 1954;47:419–427.
53. Overton DA. Experimental methods for the study of state-dependent learning. *Fed Proc* 1974;33:1800–1813.
54. Piazza PV, Deminiere J-M, LeMoal M, Simon H. Factors that predict individual vulnerability to amphetamine self-administration. *Science* 1989;245:1511–1513.
55. Robbins TW. The potentiation of conditioned reinforcement by psychomotor stimulant drugs: a test of Hill's hypothesis. *Psychopharmacologia* 1975;45:103–114.
56. Roberts DCS, Loh EA, Vickers G. Self-administration of cocaine on a progressive ratio schedule in rats: dose–response relationship and effect of haloperidol pretreatment. *Psychopharmacology* 1989;97:535–538.
57. Robinson TE, Berridge KC. The neural basis of drug craving: an incentive-sensitization theory of addiction. *Brain Res Rev* 1993;18:247–291.
58. Schulteis G, Carrera R, Markou A, Gold LH, Koob GF. Motivational consequences of naloxone-precipitated opiate withdrawal: a dose-response analysis. *Neurosci Abstr* 1993;19:1247.
59. Schuster CR, Johanson CE. Relationship between the discriminative stimulus properties and subjective effects of drugs. In: Colpaert FC, Balster RL, eds. *Transduction mechanisms of drug stimuli.* Berlin: Springer-Verlag, 1988;161.
60. Schuster CR, Thompson T. Self-administration and behavioral dependence on drugs. *Annu Rev Pharmacol Toxicol* 1969;9:483–502.
61. Schuster CR, Woods JH. The conditioned reinforcing effects of stimuli associated with morphine reinforcement. *Int J Addict* 1968;3:223–230.
62. Shannon HE. Pharmacological analysis of the phencyclidine-like discriminative stimulus properties of narcotic derivatives in rats. *J Pharmacol Exp Ther* 1982;222(1):146–151.
63. Stellar JR, Stellar E. *The neurobiology of reward and motivation,* New York: Springer-Verlag, 1985.
64. Stewart J, deWit H. Reinstatement of drug-taking behavior as a method of assessing incentive motivational properties of drugs. In:

Bozarth MA, ed. *Assessing the reinforcing properties of abused drugs.* New York: Springer-Verlag; 1987:211–227.
65. Stewart J, Eikelboom R. Conditioned drug effects. In: Iversen LI, Iversen SD, Snyder SH, eds. *New directions in behavioral pharmacology.* Vol 19. New York: Plenum Press; 1987:1–57.
66. Stinus L, Le Moal M, Koob GF. The nucleus accumbens and amygdala as possible substrates for the aversive stimulus effects of opiate withdrawal. *Neuroscience* 1990;37:767–773.
67. Stolerman IP, Rasul F, Shine PJ. Trends in drug discrimination research analysed with a cross-indexed bibliography, 1984–1987. *Psychopharmacology* 1989;73:1–19.
68. Swerdlow NR, Gilbert D, Koob GF. Conditioned drug effects on spatial preference. In: Boulton AB, Baker GB, Greenshaw AJ, eds. *Neuromethods.* Vol 13. Clifton, NJ: The Humana Press, 1989;399–446.
69. van der Kooy D. Place conditioning: a simple and effective method for assessing the motivational properties of drugs. In: Bozarth MA, ed. *Methods of assessing the reinforcing properties of abused drugs.* New York: Springer-Verlag; 1987:229–240.
70. Wikler A. Dynamics of drug dependence: implications of a conditioning theory of research and treatment. *Arch Gen Psychiatry* 1973;28:611–616.
71. Wikler A, Pescor FT. Classical conditioning of a morphine abstinence phenomenon, reinforcement of opioid-drinking behavior and "relapse" in morphine addicted rats. *Psychopharmacologia* 1967;10:255–284.
72. Wikler A, Pescor FT, Miller D, Norrell H. Persistent potency of a secondary (conditioned) reinforcer following withdrawal of morphine from physically dependent rats. *Psychopharmacology* 1971;20:103–117.
73. Winger G, Woods JH. Comparison of fixed-ratio and progressive-ratio schedules of maintenance of stimulant drug-reinforced responding. *Drug Alcohol Depend* 1985;15:123–130.
74. Wise R. The neurobiology of craving: implications for the understanding and treatment of addiction. *J Abnorm Psychol* 1988;97:118–132.
75. Yanagita T. An experimental framework for evaluations of dependence liability of various types of drugs in monkeys. *Bull Narc* 1973;25:57–64.

Psychopharmacology: The Fourth Generation of Progress, edited by Floyd E. Bloom and David J. Kupfer. Raven Press, Ltd., New York © 1995.

CHAPTER 67

Stress

Huda A. Akil and M. Inés Morano

Stress, though a nebulous concept, is often evoked as an important trigger in the expression of several psychiatric illnesses, including major depression, anxiety disorders, and schizophrenia. The term generally refers to any physical or psychological change that disrupts the organism's balance or homeostasis. Psychological stressors are typically emphasized as key elements in psychiatric illness, although physical stressors (e.g. viral infections, autoimmune disorders) are becoming increasingly recognized as potential triggers.

Stress activates many systems in the body, including the adrenal medulla and the autonomic nervous system. It was first proposed by Cannon as the integrator of fight-or-flight responses (15). Of particular interest, however, is the role of the brain in orchestrating responses to stress. The interface between the emotional or limbic system and the stress control circuits may indeed represent the site(s) of interaction between the control of stress and the expression of various psychiatric diseases. In the following sections, we focus on some of the major actors that participate in the expression and termination of stress responses at the level of the brain and briefly summarize what is known about the circuits involved. We also describe what is currently known about aging and the stress system, both because the aged animal has been proposed as a model of a somewhat dysregulated stress system and because, in clinical studies, there appears to be an interaction between aging, indices of dysregulation of the stress axis, and some psychiatric illnesses such as severe depression. Finally, we present a brief overview of current research on the relationship between stress and depression, as an example of one psychiatric illness whose relationship to stress has been extensively investigated. This discussion also illustrates the impact of the basic science findings

on the choice of clinical research approaches. The overview in the last section attempts to emphasize the conceptual and integrative questions at the interface between stress biology and affective disorders (see also Chapters 33, 34, 62, 83, and 84, *this volume*).

THE STRESS AXIS

All organisms, from bacteria to humans, have evolved mechanisms to deal with significant changes in their external or internal environments, that is, stressors. In mammals, this function is carried out, in part, by the limbic–hypothalamo–pituitary–adrenal (LHPA) axis. This system integrates various inputs indicative of stress, converging on a final common path in the brain, the neurons of the medial parvocellular division of the paraventricular nucleus of the hypothalamus (mpPVN). These neurons synthesize corticotropin-releasing hormone (CRH) and arginine vasopressin (AVP), and project to the external layer of the median eminence (86). Activation by stressors leads to release of the peptides into the portal blood, carrying these secretagogues to the anterior pituitary. In turn, CRH and AVP receptors on the anterior pituitary corticotropes are responsible for the release into the total circulation of adrenocorticotropin hormone (ACTH) and related peptides derived from the common precursor pro-opiomelanocortin (POMC). ACTH activates the biosynthesis and release of glucocorticoids, corticosterone in rodents, and cortisol in primates by the cells of the adrenal cortex. These steroids possess extremely broad actions mediated by specialized receptors affecting expression and regulation of genes throughout the body, and readying the organism for the changes in energy and metabolism required for coping (60).

Corticotropin-releasing hormone is a 41-residue peptide that plays the major role in regulation of pituitary

H. A. Akil and M. I. Morano: Mental Health Research Institute, The University of Michigan, Ann Arbor, Michigan 48109.

corticotrope trophic activity (34), POMC gene transcription (10), and ACTH secretion (8). In addition to CRH, various other factors have also been shown to induce ACTH secretion during stress. These intrinsically weaker secretagogues include AVP, oxytocin (OT), angiotensin II, cholecystokinin, vasoactive intestinal peptide (VIP), and catecholamines (11). However, most of them have been shown to depend upon the presence of CRH for their modulatory action in LHPA axis activation. Among these other secretagogues, the physiological importance of AVP in the regulation of the stress response should be highlighted, because of the colocalization and corelease of CRH and AVP in mpPVN (86) and because of the synergistic effects of both peptides on the corticotropes. Although AVP is a weak ACTH stimulator by itself, it markedly potentiates the effect of CRH (8).

The CRH-stimulation of ACTH secretion, POMC transcription, and POMC mRNA levels in the corticotropes is thought to be mediated by cyclic adenosine monophosphate- (cAMP) coupled CRH receptors. In contrast, the corticotrope AVP receptors are thought to be coupled to phosphatidyl inositol turnover (8) and to mediate primarily effects on ACTH secretion. Moreover, AVP does not further affect CRH-induced POMC transcription or messenger ribonucleic acid (mRNA) expression (53).

Proopiomelanocortin (POMC) is one of the three opioid peptide precursor genes. This precursor encodes, not only the stress hormone ACTH, but also the opioid peptide β-endorphin 1–31 and three copies of the active core of melanocortin (α, β, and γMSH). Although the major site of expression of the POMC gene is the pituitary gland, it is also expressed in several brain regions and peripheral tissues. In the pituitary, it is expressed in anterior lobe (AL) corticotropes, and in every cell of the intermediate lobe (1). The precursor POMC undergoes an orderly series of enzymatically mediated posttranslational processing steps to produce its tissue-specific final products. In the corticotropic cells, the cleavage of double basic residues converts POMC into equimolar amounts of a carboxy-terminal glycopeptide termed 16K, ACTH 1-39, and β-LPH. Approximately one-third of β-LPH molecules are further processed in these cells to produce the opioid active β-endorphin 1–31. By contrast, in the intermediate lobe, all of the β-LPH is converted to β-endorphin and, ACTH, β-endorphin, and 16K undergo further posttranslational modifications to produce highly altered final products. In particular, ACTH is converted to αMSH and CLIP (1).

NEGATIVE FEEDBACK

Specifically because of their potency and their range of action, glucocorticoids have to be maintained within an optimal range—either too little or too much is deleterious to the organism (60). Therefore, the LHPA is well controlled to produce rapid and optimal responses, which terminate promptly upon cessation of stress. This is achieved by multiple, nested, negative-feedback loops, primarily mediated by the steroids themselves (47). These mechanisms differ in terms of their timing, their underlying mechanisms, as well as their sites of action. The most rapid mechanism is the so-called rate-dependent fast feedback, which occurs within minutes of activation, that is, as soon as steroid levels begin to rise. This mechanism monitors the rate of rise of steroids in the circulation, rather than their absolute level, and serves to turn off CRH/AVP secretion. The exact receptors mediating this feedback are unknown, but the site of action is thought to be suprapituitary (47), at hypothalamic or possibly suprahypothalamic levels (25,45). At the other extreme, is a genomically mediated negative feedback with a much slower time course, whereby glucocorticoid receptors, which are in fact transacting factors, negatively control gene expression, decreasing rates of transcription of critical genes such as POMC. Indeed, the negative regulation starts immediately upon receptor activation by steroids, but its consequences on the cell, in terms of mRNA and peptide levels take hours or even days to manifest, because of their intrinsic kinetics and the presence of large reserves. This genomic feedback operates at the level of the pituitary corticotrope by controlling POMC gene expression (10) as well as at the brain level. Finally, there is an intermediate feedback, with a time course between the fast and the genomic, that remains ill-understood (47). In a living organism, all these mechanisms are probably activated simultaneously, but they come into play in different time domains; fast feedback is likely to set the magnitude and duration of each response, whereas genomic feedback sets the range of stress responsiveness of an organism. In addition, these feedback mechanisms can be seen as different lines of defense, involving a hierarchy in time and space, with fast feedback being more sensitive, rapid and brain mediated, and genomic feedback being slower but having more profound effects at multiple levels of the axis.

Brain steroid receptors are thought to mediate negative feedback upon the axis, but the relative role of the various elements is not fully delineated. What is known is that glucocorticoids inhibit CRH and AVP mRNA levels (82), probably from reduced gene transcription, which would lead to diminished biosynthetic capacity and possibly result in decreased peptide release. These inhibitory effects are amplified at the level of the anterior pituitary. When steroid levels are high, the pituitary POMC cell is simultaneously under reduced secretory drive and under direct genomic inhibition, both of which dramatically inhibit biosynthesis. Conversely, when corticosteroids are removed (e.g., by adrenalectomy or steroid synthesis inhibitors), CRH and AVP mRNA expression is significantly induced in the hypothalamic neurons. These presumably fire more actively, releasing their contents. In turn, corticotropic cells receive the combined influence of increased activation by secretagogues, which is known to induce POMC biosynthesis, and of the absence of steroid feedback, leading to an overall tenfold increase in POMC mRNA levels (10). An important question is: Are the effects of steroids on CRH neurons direct or indirect? The hypothalamus is rich in steroid receptors (68) and the steroid effects could be direct. Indeed, glucocorticoid implants within the hypothalamus have been shown to suppress CRH/AVP peptide expression (48). However, negative regulation may also be mediated by neuronal pathways that are sensitive to steroids and that modulate the firing of CRH/AVP neurons. The fact that the hippocampus is the brain area richest in corticosteroid receptors (40,68) strengthens the notion that negative steroid feedback does not reside exclusively in the PVN. The specific role of the hippocampus in negative feedback remains unclear, but the existence of an indirect hippocampal–PVN pathway that modulates CRH/AVP expression is suggestive of a circuit that plays a role in negative regulation of the LHPA (see below).

TWO CORTICOSTEROID RECEPTORS IN THE BRAIN

Two steroid receptors mediate negative feedback in the CNS. Why two? remains an interesting questions, as the field attempts to understand their similarities and differences at a molecular and functional level. DeKloet and his colleagues (68) using steroid receptor binding and autoradiography first described the existence of two binding sites in the hippocampus that recognize corticosteroids. These were termed type I and type II and have different pharmacological profiles in vivo: Type I has higher affinity to cortisol/corticosterone than type II, whereas type II recognizes dexamethasone with higher affinity than type I. More recently, these receptors have been cloned and identified as the glucocorticoid receptor (GR), which subserves type II binding (42), and mineralocorticoid receptor (MR), which in the kidney recognizes aldosterone and in brain corresponds to type I binding (9,64). Both receptors have a broad distribution; although both are particularly enriched in the hippocampus, the PVN region appears to express predominantly GR or type II receptors (40).

Both receptors belong to the steroid receptor family, which has a well-known topology. The carboxy terminal domain is the ligand-binding domain and subsumes the specific recognition site for ligands. In the middle is the DNA-binding domain, which contains so-called cysteine-rich zinc fingers critical for DNA interactions, and the amino terminal domain, which is thought to be important for transcriptional modulation. These domains appear to be functionally separable, and numerous chimeras have been constructed to retain appropriate binding selectivities and DNA recognition properties (36,78). Glucocorticoid and mineralocorticoid receptors are very similar in the ligand-binding domain, which is reasonable given their recognition of common ligands. However, they have interesting differences that reflect their possible unique functions in the context of the stress axis.

In the absence of steroids, the majority of GR- and MR-binding sites reside in the cytoplasm and appear to be associated with a protein complex that involves several heat-shock proteins including hsp-90 (22,23). Association with this complex is thought to be critical to the ability of the corticoid receptors to bind ligand; GR and MR in the absence of hsp-90 lose their binding affinity to glucocorticoids (143). In the presence of glucocorticoids, hormone-receptor interaction takes place in the cytoplasm. This cytoplasmic interaction, which can also be seen in cell-free systems, results in both the dissociation of the receptor–hsp-90 complex and an increased affinity of the receptor for deoxyribonucleic acid (DNA). This represents the initial step necessary for the nuclear translocation and activation of the receptor to its final, DNA-bound state. Recent work from our laboratory (Morano et al., *unpublished*), using GRs mutated in the hsp-90 binding region, suggests that the receptor/hsp-90 interaction is required not only for hormone binding but also for its activation to a transcriptionally functional DNA-binding form. Thus the hsp-90 association is a critical aspect of the cell cycle of these receptors, and, along with the steroids themselves, determines the state of activity of these transacting factors. This is in contrast to other members of the steroid family (e.g., thyroid hormone receptor) that dwell in the nucleus and are not complexed with a heat-shock protein.

In addition to the multiplicity of receptor types, there is heterogeneity within the MR family. We have shown that there are at least three types of mRNAs for MR, termed α, β, and γ, which harbor the same protein coding domain but differ in their 5′ untranslated regions (5′UT) (50,64). These variants appear to be the result of alternative splicing of a single MR gene, are differentially expressed in various brain regions and other tissues, have unique developmental patterns, and are differentially regulated (50).

Steroid receptors exert their effect on DNA by binding to specific stretches of DNA or recognition elements. The glucocorticoid recognition element (GRE) consists of 15 base pairs of DNA and is a motif found in numerous genes. Receptors of other classes of steroid hormones, progestins, and androgens, can also modulate genomic activity by binding this element (36). In the best studied cases, binding of the GR to the GRE causes an increase in transcription. This positive regulation is predominant.

However, all the known genes of the stress axis—POMC, CRH, AVP—appear to be negatively regulated by glucocorticoids. If this regulation is direct (as opposed to being neuronally or secretion mediated), then these genes must possess a negative GRE. Indeed, GRE-like elements have been identified in the POMC promoter (27) and there are several examples of negative GRE's in nonstress system genes (70). However, other hypotheses exist suggesting that negative regulation by steroid receptors may be due to proteins preventing activation by another transacting factor, either because the DNA elements overlap or through protein–protein interactions with other transacting factors such as c-fos/c-jun (27,87). An interesting synthesis was offered in a paper by Yamamoto and his colleagues (26) showing that a single element could be either positive or negative depending on the cellular milieu and the recent history of activation of the gene.

The question of gene regulation is even more difficult with regard to the mineralocorticoid receptor (MR or type I). No specific MRE has yet been defined. Evans and his colleagues (9) have shown that MR can activate a positive GRE-containing gene (MMTV) but is weak (5%) compared to GR activation. They suggested that MR may share the same DNA recognition site as GR but be weaker at transactivation. Given that MR has a higher affinity for natural corticosteroids, this receptor would represent a lower threshold, but be a low-efficiency mediator of steroid actions, whereas GR would represent a higher threshold but be a higher efficacy element. This is an interesting hypothesis, which remains to be tested.

Recently, Yamamoto's group analyzed the activities of GR and MR at a composite response element to which both the steroid receptors and the transcription factor AP1 can bind. In this case, under conditions in which GR repressed AP1-stimulated transcription, MR was inactive (66) suggesting that the differential interactions of nonreceptor factors with specific receptor domains at composite response elements may explain distinct physiological effects of MR and GR. Under this model, one can see MR, not only as a weak GR but also as a potential GR antagonist, binding to the same DNA elements but failing to produce a transcriptional effect (33,66).

The Evans hypothesis along with the findings of Yamamoto's laboratory on the composite element, raise several interesting questions: For example, does MR work exclusively through GREs or are there unique MREs that may mediate its effects? Are both receptors equally likely to interact with other transacting factors? Even if MR is acting at a GRE, is the potency of MR relative to GR always low, regardless of the target gene? In particular, what happens for negatively regulated genes? Are some more sensitive to MR than to GR? An intriguing example is the case of AVP in CRH neurons. This gene appears to be quite sensitive to adrenal steroids, as indicated by the low basal level of AVP expression in control rats.

Following removal of steroids by adrenalectomy, AVP mRNA is dramatically induced (eightfold) (77). On the other hand, the CRH gene in the same neurons, is expressed actively in the unstressed rat, and is only induced two- to threefold by adrenalectomy (77). This suggests that steroid levels in the basal circadian range (i.e., levels that primarily activate MR, see below) are sufficient to inhibit AVP but not CRH expression. Yet when dexamethasone (a GR agonist) is administered in supraphysiological doses, CRH mRNA levels are dramatically reduced. Thus, it is likely that AVP may be more MR-responsive than is CRH, suggesting that different genes, even in the same tissue, may exhibit different responses to the two types of steroid receptors.

THE TWO RECEPTORS AND THE CIRCADIAN RHYTHM

One of the characteristics of basal steroid levels is that they oscillate in a circadian fashion. The levels are correlated with the rest–activity cycle of the animal, rather than the light cycle. Thus, in man, steroids begin to rise in the early morning hours, peak around awakening, and then fall throughout the day. In nocturnal animals such as rats, the converse pattern is seen, whereby levels peak in late evening and are at a nadir in early morning. Connections between this cycle and rest–activity, sleep, and feeding behavior have been made. The effects of stress, then, are superimposed on the basal rhythmicity, and there is evidence that stress responsiveness and the effectiveness of negative feedback may also oscillate across the cycle. Thus, at the trough of the rhythm, animals appear to be more sensitive to both stress activation and inhibition by glucocorticoids, suggesting that at this time, the axis is exquisitely responsive (21). The drive to the axis prior to awakening appears to be initiated by the suprachiasmatic nucleus (SCN), leading to enhanced tone of CRH, and resulting in increased activity throughout the LHPA (49). Interestingly, the basal levels of steroids at the peak are thought to be sufficiently high to occupy a majority of the type I or MR receptors (estimates vary from 60% to 90%) but only occupy a small proportion of type II or GR (~10%) (68). Thus, there may be elements of the axis (e.g., AVP in mpPVN) that are particularly sensitive to circadian drive and are modulated by MR, whereas others are particularly stress responsive and only modulated by GR or by both receptors.

In addition, the circadian rhythmicity of the system needs to be kept in mind as one examines the anatomy and function of various stress-related circuits. It is important to recognize that both stress activation and stress termination mechanisms might either modulate or be modulated by this daily rhythmicity. In addition, manipulations, whether they are surgical or pharmacological, intended to look at the stress circuits might alter the rhythm. Such an interplay may also prove important in aging, which is known to alter sleep, rest–activity, and stress responsiveness. Thus circadian rhythmicity is an intrinsic feature of this system, having molecular, anatomical and integrative implications.

NEGATIVE REGULATORY CIRCUITS

As we discussed above, negative feedback, which is critical to the termination of the stress response as well as to establishing the overall set point of the axis, may be mediated both directly at the level of gene regulation and by neuronal circuits. The presence of high levels of both GR and MR in the hippocampus led to the notion that it may play a key role in negative feedback (c.f., 25,45). Previous work has demonstrated that hippocampal lesions elevate circulating levels of glucocorticoids, both basally and poststress (30). Our group (Watson, Akil, and coworkers) was therefore interested in investigating the possible existence of a hippocampo–hypothalmic pathway that may play a role in negative control of the axis. We used lesions as our tool and examined CRH and AVP mRNAs and, ACTH and corticosteroid plasma levels. Our reasoning was as follows: if a brain site is critical to inhibiting the tone of the LHPA, its destruction should result in an increase in that tone, as evidenced by a chronic increase in circulating stress hormones (ACTH, corticosteroids). If steroids only have direct effects on CRH/AVP in the PVN, then the high steroid levels resulting from these lesions should lead to down regulation of the CRH/AVP message. However, if steroid feedback works in part through our target site, then lesioning that site should not only increase secretion but also prevent steroid-induced down-regulation, and actually lead to the unusual condition of increased circulating hormones, and increased CRH/AVP.

To date we have studied multiple regions of the hippocampus and have shown that, indeed, hippocampal lesions result in this unusual combination of elevated glucocorticoids and elevated levels of secretagogues (41). Although several hippocampal sites participate in controlling basal CRH expression, only very discrete regions appear involved in the termination of the stress response (Herman et al., *unpublished*). Lesions of the latter sites result in stress response patterns where activation appears normal but termination appears slow, a pattern seen in aged animals (see below). What are the neural pathways mediating these effects? Interestingly, the hippocampus apparently lacks significant direct projections to the PVN, suggesting the existence of one or more relays. Extensive anatomical studies in our laboratory have suggested that these are multiple redundant pathways, which connect the hippocampus to the PVN through various relays points, includ-

ing one in the bed nucleus of the striaterminalis (BNST) (19). These pathways may play a role in controlling various aspects of the stress response or may serve other distinct functions (Fig. 1).

POSITIVE REGULATORY CIRCUITS

Even less is known about the neuronal circuits involved in the initiation of the stress response (Fig. 1). We, of course, know the final common path in the mpPVN, and we also know that brainstem nuclei are likely to play an important role in stress detection, for example, locus coereleus and nucleus of the solitary tract. A number of afferent inputs have been shown to participate in the activation of the HPA axis. In particular, noradrenergic and adrenergic neurons of the A2 region in the caudal medulla are known to send direct inputs to the mpPVN (20) and their modulation clearly alters the tone of the CRH neuron, presumably by a_1 adrenoceptors (4,58,18). The nucleus tractus solitarius, which is partly catecholaminergic, has been shown to be critical in inducing ACTH release in response to hypotension (24). Similarly, serotonergic cell groups (dorsal raphe and raphe magnus) project to the parvocellular PVN (76) and appear involved in stress responsiveness (31) and circadian rhythmicity (83). The amygdala has also been implicated in stress responsiveness (3,12) as has the medial BNST (28). More rostrally, stimulation of the preoptic area and frontal cortex can excite PVN neurons that project to median eminence (71).

Different types of stressors (physical vs. psychological, painful vs. nonpainful) are likely to engage the system from different starting points. But at what level do they converge? Is it only at the level of the CRH/AVP neuron in the parvocellular PVN? Or do they do so more proximally, for example in limbic sites, which then lead to the mpPVN? A major stumbling block for these experiments has been the need to develop a strategy for detecting stress activation in the CNS. This is a prerequisite to carrying out lesion studies to disrupt the pathway and begin to delineate its components. One can, of course, measure peripheral indices of stress—corticosterone and ACTH increases in plasma. However, the ability to monitor CNS correlates of acute activation by various stressors is critical to discerning the existence of unique pathways as well as common elements. The measure has to be rapid enough to detect the activation before negative steroid feedback dampens or even reverses the response. Several recent studies have been undertaken in an effort to map brain regions activated by various stressors, using immediate early genes (IEGs) such as c-fos, c-jun, and zif/268 as markers for early neuronal activity. To date we have examined IEG responses following restraint stress and swim stress (Cullinan et al., *unpublished*). The results suggest

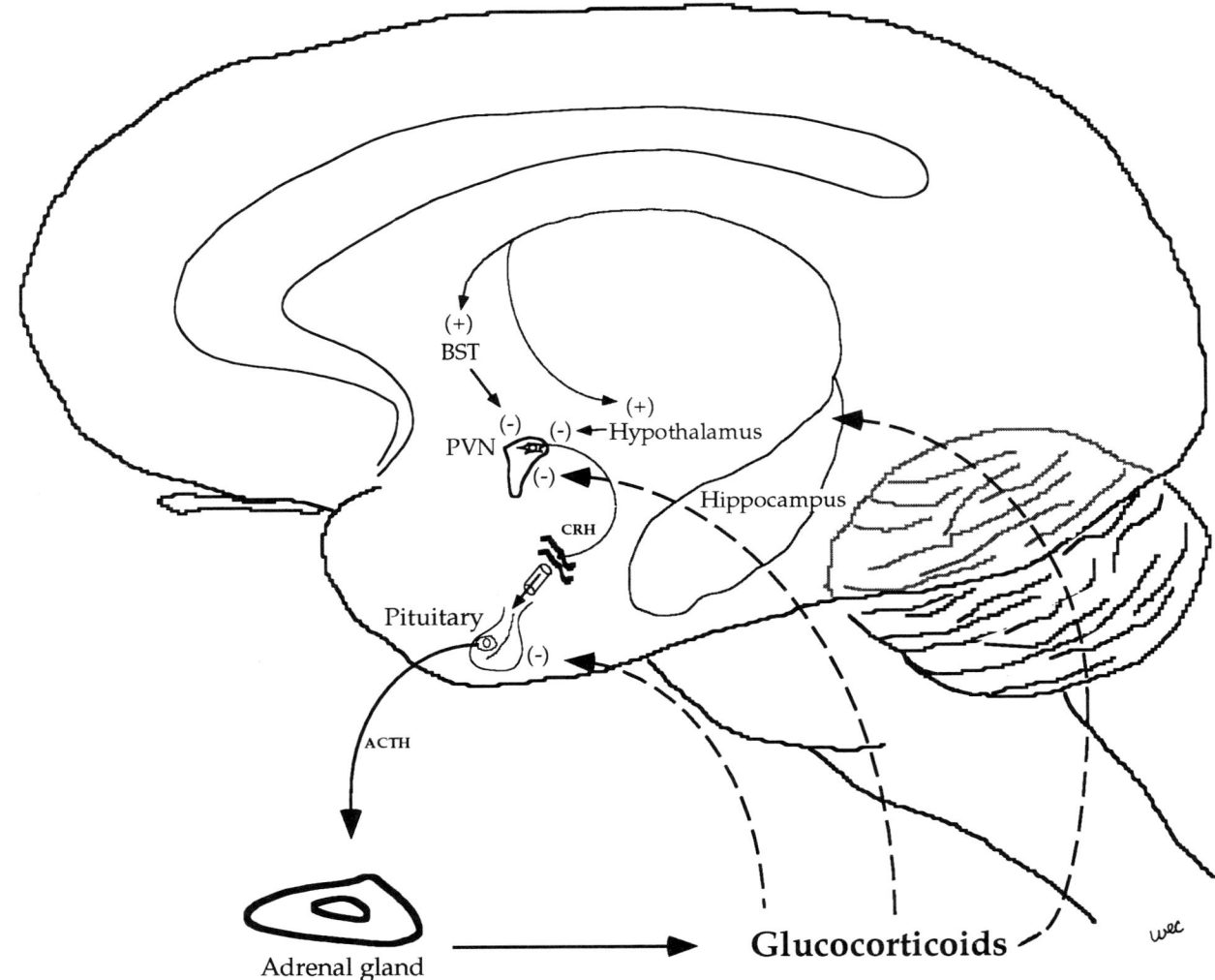

FIG. 1. Stress-related inputs converge upon the neurons of the medioparvocellular division of the PVN. These cells release CRH and other secretagogues into the portal plasma, which are then carried to the anterior pituitary, stimulating the synthesis and release of ACTH (and other POMC-derived peptides) from corticotropes into the systemic circulation. These events culminate in the ACTH-induced release of glucocorticoids from the adrenal cortex. Glucocorticoids exert inhibitory feedback effects at multiple levels, including the pituitary, PVN, and other brain sites, possibly including the hippocampus. Hippocampal effects on the PVN may be mediated through neuronal relays, including the BST and various hypothalamic nuclei. Abbreviations: BST, bed nucleus of the stria terminalis; CRH, corticotropin-releasing hormone; PVN, hypothalamic paraventricular nucleus. Drawing courtesy of W. E. Cullinan.

that in addition to activation of the mpPVN, a core set of cortical and subcortical limbic brain areas are activated following both stressors, as are certain brainstem nuclei (e.g., catecholaminergic cell groups) implicated in HPA activation. However, various stress-specific areas of IEG induction were also encountered. Current studies examining very early time points after stress should provide insight into the sequence of this neuronal activation.

THE AGED RAT: A DISRUPTED LHPA

Aging offers a model for studying the way in which the LHPA axis can become mildly dysregulated and the manner in which the multiple elements can interact to establish the most optimal homeostasis in the face of mild but persistent damage (see Table 1). The findings on aging are particularly relevant here, because they parallel in many ways some of the patterns of dysregulation observed in clinical conditions, such as severe depression (see below). Sapolsky and his collaborators (72,74) first described an abnormality in the stress axis related to aging: whereas aged animals responded normally to restraint stress, they failed to terminate the stress response in a timely fashion, suggesting an aberrant feedback mechanism. This has led to speculations regarding the

TABLE 1. *Comparing HPA Profiles in Aged Rats and Depressed Humans*

	Aging	Chronic stress	Major depression
Hippocampal GR/MR	↓	−↓	?
Hypothalamic CRH mRNA	−	↑	?
Hypothalamic CRH secretion	↑	−↑	↑
CRH pituitary responsiveness	↓	↓	↓−
Peripheral cort. levels at rest	Unchanged or elevated at nadir	Unchanged or elevated at nadir	Unchanged or elevated at nadir
Drive (metyrapone test)	?	?	↑
Cort. levels following stress	Delayed turn off to some stressors	−↑	?
Fast-feedback	↓	↓	↓
Dexamethasone feedback	↓	↓	↓
Pituitary POMC mRNA	Decreased but increased translatability	↑	↑

↑ shows an increase, ↓ shows a decrease, — indicates no change, ? indicates unknown effect.

role of various brain sites, including the hippocampus, in this aberrant pattern (45,52,73). Although there are many controversies in this area, it appears clear that aged animals do have a decreased number of corticosteroid receptors in their hippocampi (29,44,72, and our own work).

However, the possible consequences or even correlates of this alteration on other levels of the LHPA are not well established. Therefore, we have examined in the same group of aged animals every level of the LHPA, looking at the expression and regulation of each of the key molecules in the system (Morano and Akil, *in preparation*). Our findings can be briefly summarized as follows: GR and MR receptors are decreased in the hippocampus, both at the mRNA and at the protein-binding levels (59). It might be expected that this receptor loss would result in an upregulation of CRH mRNA at the level of the PVN (41); however, we were unable to detect such a change, suggesting that control at this level may require the massive drop in receptor numbers induced by hippocampal lesions. On the other hand, we have obtained clear evidence of increased CRH secretion from the median eminence and of increased releasability of this peptide by NE. That such an increase in CRH tone does take place in these aged rats is further supported by our finding that these same animals, when compared to young controls, exhibit hyporesponsiveness of CRH receptors at the level of the pituitary, whereas their AVP responsiveness remains unaltered. This decreased CRH receptor tone leads, as expected, to a decrease in POMC mRNA levels. Interestingly, however, this is compensated for by an improvement in the translational efficiency of the POMC message.

Surprisingly, this series of compensatory changes at each level of the axis is associated with completely normal basal tone or circadian rhythmicity in these aged animals, as well as normal initial responses to stress, with the only evident functional defect being the aberrant termination of stress. These findings allow us to draw several conclusions: (1) The loss of hippocampal receptors must be primary, rather than being secondary to high circulat-

ing levels of glucocorticoids as has been previously suggested. This idea is supported by our finding of completely normal circadian patterns in the face of profound decreases in hippocampal receptors. (2) The system is capable of using a remarkable range of mechanisms to control basal and stress responsiveness at the level of circulating glucocorticoids, even when the tone of each of the individual elements is altered. (3) It may be difficult to detect even complex and extensive alterations in the axis by simply examining peripheral steroid levels. Designing appropriate challenge paradigms is of paramount importance to examining the brain elements of the axis. This will become relevant to our discussion of the stress axis dysregulation in depression (below).

CHRONIC STRESS: EFFECTS AT MULTIPLE LEVELS OF THE LHPA

Another model that has been extensively utilized to study the interplay of the various components of the stress axis has been repeated or chronic stress. This model offers the opportunity to examine the plasticity of the system, uncover the various ways in which it can adapt to continue to achieve an optimal circadian basal tone, and maintain its exquisite responsiveness to stressors. In addition, chronic stress has been proposed by Sapolsky and colleagues as a model for what happens during aging. Finally, thinking about chronic stress appears particularly relevant to thinking about the changes seen during psychiatric illnesses, as these are usually chronic and unquestionably stressful.

We shall not detail here the body of research describing the consequences of repeated stress. The effects vary based on the nature of the stressor, the duration of the regimen, the lag time between when stress is administered and the LHPA evaluated, and the age of the animal. Few laboratories have examined the entire LHPA profile in a single animal, as we have done for the aged Fisher rat.

Thus, it is often difficult to make direct comparisons between studies. Nevertheless, there are some findings that appear often enough to be thought hallmarks of a chronically stressed LHPA. These have been recently summarized by Dallman (21) and are highlighted in Table 1. Note that many of the changes seen in chronic stress parallel those seen in aging. Some notable differences include the fact that CRH mRNA is elevated in chronically swum animals (López et al., *unpublished*), an effect not seen in aged rats. In addition, certain chronic stressors, such as footshock, increase POMC mRNA in the pituitary (80), whereas POMC mRNA in the aged rat appears decreased, although its translatability is more efficient (Morano et al., *in preparation*). Finally, some studies have not been carried out in exactly the same fashion in aged versus chronically stressed rats. For example, we have shown changes in the pituitary responsiveness to dexamethasone following chronic stress (89), but are unaware of parallel studies in the aged animals. Similarly, while studies on aging have focused on the natural time course of stress termination as an indicator of fast feedback, chronic stress studies have looked at the effect of preinjection with corticosterone to test fast feedback (88).

The two models described above show that repeated or long-term demands on the stress axis can certainly alter it, resulting in some aberrant responses, such as defects in feedback mechanisms or in circadian rhythmicity. However, these defects are relatively limited, and the axis can function adequately to maintain both its basal tone and it ability to respond to stress, thanks to the intricate checks and balances that it possesses. Such a pattern of partial dysregulation, with changes in set points in key brain and peripheral structures, may also take place in humans following conditions of chronic stress or in patients suffering from certain types of psychiatric illnesses.

AN EXAMPLE OF STRESS AXIS INTERACTION WITH PSYCHIATRIC ILLNESS: THE CASE OF MAJOR DEPRESSION

There are numerous indications of HPA axis dysregulation in a number of psychiatric syndromes, including eating disorders, anxiety and panic disorders (see Chapters 83 and 84, *this volume*). However, the best studied case of a stress axis interface with a psychiatric illness is that of major depressive disorder (MDD). Although a detailed description of this interaction is beyond the scope of this chapter (see Chapter 84, this volume), we shall briefly describe how an understanding of the HPA axis has informed the study of this syndrome and how it can continue to suggest new avenues for exploring the causes and sequelae of depression.

There is little question that the stress axis is somehow altered in major depression, at least in a significant number of patients suffering from this illness. However, there is little agreement beyond this point. Is the dysregulation of the axis primary to the disease or is it secondary to the stress of being profoundly disturbed emotionally? Is this simply a state-dependent dysregulation, or is it an underlying imbalance exacerbated when the patient is in episode? Do all patients with MDD manifest disturbances in their LHPA axis, or is this a problem seen in a subset of the subjects? If the latter is true, then can they be distinguished on the basis of clinical diagnosis or symptomatology (manic–depressive illness, melancholia, etc.), course and history of the illness, or individual variables such as age, sex, or severity of the episode? Finally, if a defect does exist, regardless of its primacy, does it reside in the periphery, the pituitary or even the adrenal, or in the brain, perhaps the hypothalamus or the limbic system?

The correlation between stress and depression has face validity, not only because being profoundly depressed is unquestionably stressful, but because external stressful events often precipitate depressive episodes (67). Epidemiological studies strongly suggest a role for both genetic factors and psychosocial stressors in unipolar depression. For example, adverse life events are likely to occur around the onset of affective illness (65) and the presence of psychosocial stressors is associated with poor outcome in depressed patients (75). Even in cases where no precipitating events may be apparent, the occurrence of a depressive episode in itself can lead to substantial psychosocial stress, secondary to the disruption of family and work relations.

A brief historical overview of research on LHPA axis and depression reveals an interesting course. The association between stress and depression has led to studies of peripheral indices of the stress axis in depressed subjects. The assumption appeared to be that the defect being sought is certainly within the brain, but that studying the pituitary–adrenal components offers a window into the brain. Thus began a number of studies that described cortisol levels in depressed subjects using either urinary free cortisol or plasma cortisol levels during the course of the day (15,16,39). Carroll and his colleagues introduced the Dexamethasone Suppression Test (DST) in the mid-1970s (15). The 1980s were marked by a move toward hormonal challenges that focused more clearly on the peripheral elements of the axis. Implicitly or explicitly, these studies recognized that "the window into the brain" was a complex set of organs (adrenal and pituitary) that needed to be studied in their own right, in an attempt to discern their biological status in MDD subjects. This led to challenge studies with ACTH and with CRH, and these have revealed abnormalities at both the adrenal and pituitary levels (see Chapters 83 and 84, this volume).

While this brief overview underscores the recent tendency to be more analytical about the individual components of the axis, it also points out that these studies have not directly tackled the role of the brain elements of the axis in the dysregulation. This is of course very difficult to do, as we only have access to peripheral or indirect measures of brain activity. Nevertheless, armed with knowledge about the basic biology of the stress axis in animals, it may be possible to devise and validate more brain-related paradigms for studying the axis in normal and depressed human subjects.

As described above, the CRH and AVP neuron (in the mpPVN) is the final brain integrator of numerous inputs which determine stress-responsiveness. The amount and frequency of release of the secretagogues by the mpPVN neurons represents a balance between positive forces that increase synthesis and activate secretion and negative or restricting forces that limit their biosynthesis and inhibit secretion. Numerous factors have been identified that perform these activating functions (e.g., serotonin, acetylcholine) or the inhibitory controls (e.g., glucocorticoids, GABA). In considering the dysregulation of the LHPA axis in depression, we can conceive of an increase in drive, or a decrease in inhibition, or both, as contributing to the disturbance.

Another feature of the axis—its circadian rhythmicity—is also important to consider in depression. Recall that circulating cortisol is highest in humans as they awaken, and falls throughout the day, reaching a nadir in the late evening. Glucocorticoids begin to rise again by 2 a.m. to 3 a.m. moving toward their peak. While MDD subjects have a normal looking rhythm or circadian pattern of steroid secretion (albeit more active) they may exhibit more subtle disruptions and differential responsiveness to stress across the course of the day. The above notions of altered drive, altered restraint, and their interaction with daily rhythm need to be kept in mind when considering major depression.

Several lines of evidence, each with its own limitations, have converged to suggest that there is increased drive in the LHPA of MDD subjects. The first is the work of Nemeroff and his colleagues (61) showing that CRH levels are high in the CSF of depressed patients, although not all workers have confirmed this observation (69). In a collaborative study with Nemeroff and Fink, we have found that both β-endorphin (derived from brain sources) and CRH are elevated in the CSF of depressed subjects and become significantly reduced following electroconvulsive therapy (62). Although there are many CRH cell groups in the brain beyond the PVN that may contribute to the observed increase in CSF CRH, it is thought that these groups may also contribute to stress perception and responsiveness. This is based on behavioral and physiological studies suggesting that CRH mediates many behavioral and autonomic symptoms of stress and negative effect (c.f. Chapters 45, 83, and 84, this volume). Thus, the notion that brain CRH systems are overly active in depression has face validity. A second line of evidence

pointing to increased central drive derives from our postmortem studies on the pituitaries of suicides and controls showing an increase in POMC mRNA and peptides (55). This is consistent with changes observed in animals that have been exposed to increased central drive or chronic stress (80). Finally, our metyrapone studies have been revealing in this regard. Metyrapone alone given to normal controls does not alter release of POMC products in the evening; however, the same treatment in MDD subjects results in a significant increase in POMC products in the blood. This suggests that at the nadir of the rhythm, MDD subjects have an actively driven axis which is being restrained by circulating glucocorticoids (Young et al., *unpublished*). Whether this increased drive can be seen at the peak of the rhythm is currently being tested. In addition, the type of steroid receptor(s) that keep this increased drive in check is of interest.

Although an increase in CRH/AVP drive is a viable hypothesis in depression, it is unclear whether this is due to an increase in the activating forces or a decrease in the restraining forces on this stress axis. Yet, a great deal is known about one of the factors that inhibits the LHPA both basally, across the circadian rhythm, and upon stress, that is, glucocorticoids acting via their receptors. We have described above multiple-feedback mechanisms that work together to maintain an optimal state of readiness and responsiveness of the axis. The coordination between multiple elements occurs in time and in space, using different mechanisms and monitoring different indices. It may be helpful to conceive of the fast, rate-dependent, brain-mediated feedback as the more sensitive mechanism, working against a background of slower, multilevel genomic control that constrains the overall tone of the system. It is therefore quite possible for these differing mechanisms to be dysregulated separately, to manifest this disruption more clearly under certain specific conditions (e.g., specific points on the daily rhythm or following stress) but to have consequences on the functioning of the entire axis. The classical DST is carried out in such a way that it is difficult to discern which level of feedback is being tested. The time delay between dexamethasone administration and HPA testing (approximately 14 to 24 hours) is too long for fast feedback but may not be long enough to fully reveal genomic feedback mechanisms. Recently, we have focused on studying mechanisms of fast feedback in normal and MDD subjects (90). Our results to date suggest that mechanisms of fast feedback are dysregulated in MDD subjects. However, our tests so far have examined the effect of rapidly rising cortisol levels on basal secretion. The question remains as to whether MDD subjects exhibit evidence of altered fast feedback following an acute stressor. These studies are of interest because control of rate-dependent feedback is thought to occur at suprapituitary levels, thus bringing us closer to studying brain rather than peripheral mechanisms. It should be noted however that not all fast feedback is rate dependent and that we have other results showing that the human anterior pituitary can indeed respond rapidly to a glucocorticoid stimulus. Thus, the rate-dependent nature of the challenge needs to be ascertained, if one is to use the paradigm as a probe of more central aspects of the stress axis.

The specific nature of the receptors involved in these feedback mechanisms is of interest; such information could help us ascertain the site of dysregulation in various patient populations, and inform us as to whether the dysfunction resides in the control of basal circadian rhythmicity, stress responsiveness or both. As described above, basic studies suggest an important role of MR in the control of circadian rhythmicity and a critical role of GR in controlling the magnitude and duration of responses to stress. However, these notions have not been specifically tested in humans, nor do we know whether major depressive disorders involve a dysregulation of MR-mediated feedback (hence the increased basal tone throughout the day?), GR-mediated feedback (exaggerated responses to stress?), or both. It will be necessary to employ GR-specific and MR-specific ligands (agonist and antagonists) to determine which receptors contribute to rate-dependent feedback either under basal or stress-induced conditions in normal subjects. These paradigms can then be extended to the study of the possible dysregulation of negative feedback mediated by one or both of these elements in MDD subjects. These studies are currently underway in our laboratory.

We have been discussing MDD subjects as a group; however, it is evident that a great deal of heterogeneity can exist in terms of the status of the LHPA axis in depression. We have concerned ourselves in the past with several sources of possible variance. We have seen differences between males and females (2) and we and others have reported profound differences between older and younger MDD subjects (2,3,38,54,63). Beyond issues of age and sex, it is clear that there may be multiple profiles of dysregulation of the LHPA axis among depressed subjects. For example, although most researchers agree that CRH challenge results in pituitary hyporesponsiveness in MDD subjects (6,37,43,91), we have pointed out that this may not be easily explained on the basis of pre-CRH cortisol levels (91). It is true that a subpopulation of the subjects does exhibit high resting cortisol, but another has, in fact, subnormal resting levels of cortisol and yet a very weak pituitary responsiveness to CRH, indicating a very different status of the LHPA axis. Similar heterogeneity can be seen following dexamethasone, metyrapone, or cortisol administration. The weight of the evidence suggests that there are a number of ways that the LHPA axis can become dysregulated, all of which are seen in depression. Thus, adrenal hypertrophy in the face of a normal-appearing pituitary is one possibility, and another

may be increased drive throughout the axis, or faulty negative feedback at the brain and/or pituitary level. The challenge before us is twofold: (a) to describe these patterns as fully as possible by carrying out multiple measures at the various levels of the axis across multiple time points and (b) to try to understand whether some of these patterns are related and represent different stages of dysregulation, for example, is adrenal hypertrophy a late stage of the increased drive pattern? Factors, such as the history of the patient, and the number and frequency of past episodes need to be considered to ascertain the possible relationship between a given LHPA profile captured at a certain point in time and the overall course of dysregulation across the lifetime of an individual.

One variable that has consistently emerged as an important source of heterogeneity is age (2,3,38,54,88). Whereas this may well represent an "end stage" dysregulation following repeated episodes and may also reflect changes in hormonal status in postmenopausal women (2), it may also result from interesting changes in the brain specifically related to mechanisms of fast feedback. We have described above a body of research in rats that suggests that aging is accompanied by significant changes in the LHPA axis. Interestingly, not all aged rats exhibit the disruption in negative feedback nor do they all exhibit the loss of pyramidal cells. The work of Meaney and his colleagues (44) has suggested an interesting correlation between hippocampal damage and feedback abnormality. In addition, Meaney et al. (57) have shown that stress early in life may be protective, decreasing the likelihood of hippocampal damage in aging. It is also interesting to note that the aged animals with the most clear-cut feedback aberration also exhibit clear-cut memory deficits (44). The above observations are extremely suggestive, especially that age alone does not appear to be sufficient to produce the damage; rather, a combination of factors (e.g., a certain developmental history and a history of repeated stress interacting with aging) needs to occur for the damage to become apparent. This is of particular relevance to the study of depression. Whereas normal aged subjects may have normal basal rhythms of steroids (Tiongco et al., *personal communication*) and normal patterns of turn off following a stressor (although this latter has not been tested), it is possible that older MDD patients would exhibit aberrations in the LHPA axis, particularly in the stress-termination response. If this were the case, and if indeed it were due to a loss of corticosteroid receptors in the hippocampus, then this disruption would not be state dependent. Rather, we would expect to detect altered patterns of turn-off to the stressor even when the elderly subject is euthymic. Here again, basic LHPA studies would lead us to design specific paradigms of relevance to understanding the nature of the dysregulation in depression, in this case in the aged depressed population.

OVERVIEW AND SPECULATION

We hope that we have provided the reader with a sense of the richness and plasticity of the LHPA axis and the impressive body of information we currently possess about it. Although much remains to be learned, we are in the enviable position of knowing, at the molecular level, many of the key elements involved in the control of the axis. We can also describe the broad integrative features of the system and are beginning to delineate the neuronal circuits that participate in orchestrating the molecules into an exquisitely tuned and responsive physiological system. It is against this background that we can begin to understand how the stress axis copes, or fails to cope, with extreme demands placed upon it, be they exposure to repeated stress, aging, or physical and psychiatric illnesses. Possibly the two main features we would emphasize about the system are (a) the multiple levels of control from the hippocampus (and possibly above) to the adrenal gland, and (b) the constant interplay of activation and inhibition to set optimal levels of circulating glucocorticoids, both at rest and following stress. The existence of multiple levels of control throughout the axis should explain the difficulties in pinpointing a single dysregulation to be observed in chronic stress, aging, or psychiatric disorders.

There are some hints of fascinating interfaces that we have not really fully explored, either in this chapter or in terms of research efforts in the field. One of them is the functional significance of the hippocampus in this axis. Although research has focused on the role of the hippocampus in basal control or in stress termination, only a few studies have addressed the question: why the hippocampus? The work of Levine and coworkers (18) and more recently DeKloet and his colleagues (25) and Meaney and his colleagues (57) points to an intricate interface between stress and learning and memory. Given what we know about the general functions of this structure, it may be more reasonable for us to view the hippocampus, not simply as a major controller of the stress axis, but as a critical structure that integrates information from all sources, attributing salience to it, and determining its relevance to general information processing at any one time. In this context, it would be reasonable for the hippocampus to both monitor (possibly through the steroid receptors) and modulate the status of the stress axis. This view becomes particularly plausible if one thinks of the stress axis not simply as an emergency system but also as a constant monitor of internal and external events, a function it needs to perform routinely to detect emergencies and to allocate priorities to maintenance functions (e.g., eating, drinking, reproduction) versus fight-or-flight. That this is a reasonable concept of this system is supported by the intricate controls we have alluded to not only on regulating stress responsiveness but on regulating the basal tone of the LHPA axis. To function adequately as a monitor or detector, the stress system needs to access historical information regarding any past encounters of the organism with

a given stimulus (i.e., memory) and the valence or affect associated with the stimulus. The hippocampus, along with other limbic structures, would thus play a key role in determining the very assignment of a stimulus as stressful or nonstressful. In turn, whether or not a stimulus or a situation are coded as stressful would be critical to hippocampal processing in the course of learning and remembering.

Such a view of the stress axis and its interface with both metabolic and cognitive functions, may bring this system to a more central position in our concept of the biology of major depression. Of course the interface between stress and depression may be simply the result of the fact that depression is a chronic stressor. However, it may also be possible to conceive of a disruption in stress control as a critical feature in the development and/or maintenance of depression. This idea may entail a slight reframing of the standard view of major depression. Although severe depression is certainly defined by negative affect as its major feature, it can also be construed as involving a dramatic imbalance in the assignment of salience and valence to internal and external stimuli. Severely depressed people not only experience unpleasant emotions, but attend to them very strongly; their feelings appear to take precedence over other social, emotional, cognitive, or even metabolic functions. The substantial disruptions in appetetive activities, such as sleep, eating, and sex, is indicative of a dramatic shift in the priorities of the organism. Although we do not mean to imply that a dysregulation in the LHPA axis is necessarily at the root of depression, it appears reasonable to propose that a disruption in the stress axis may represent a necessary feature of severe depression. Such a disruption may represent the loss of a key control mechanism that allows humans to keep their biological and psychological priorities in working order. In someone who is vulnerable to affective disorders, an adequately functioning stress axis may serve as a break to reset matters on a more physiologically and psychologically balanced course, whereas a loss of the ability to cope or assign priorities to the various demands on the system may represent the very trigger necessary for progressing from sadness and negative affect to a serious depressive episode. Beyond that point, it is easy to envision the establishment of a vicious cycle, whereby the depressive episode further dysregulates the axis, and this, in turn would make the next episode more likely. The genetic, environmental, molecular, and neurobiological antecedents of a resilient stress axis are far from understood, and this area may represent the next challenge for both basic and clinical investigation.

REFERENCES

1. Akil H, Watson SJ, Young EA, Lewis ME, Kachaturian H, Walker JM. Endogenous opioids: biology and function. *Annu Rev Neurosci* 1984;7:223–255.

2. Akil H, Haskett RF, Young EA, et al. Multiple HPA profiles in endogenous depression: effect of age and sex on cortisol and beta-endorphin. *Biol Psychiatry* 1993;33:73–85.

3. Alexopoulos GS, Young RC, Kocsis JH, Brockner N, Butler TA, Stokes PE. Dexamethasone suppression test in geriatric depression. *Biol Psychiatry* 1984;19:1567–1571.

4. Alonso G, Szafarczyk A, Balmefrezol M. Immunocytochemical evidence for stimulatory control by the ventral noradrenergic bundle of parvocellular neurons of the paraventricular nucleus secreting corticotropin releasing hormone and vasopressin in rats. *Brain Res* 1986;397:297–307.

5. Amsterdam JD, Winokur A, Abelman E, Lucki I, Richels K. Cosyntropin (ACTH alpha 1-24) stimulation test in depressed patients and healthy subjects. *Am J Psychiatry* 1983;140:907–909.

6. Amsterdam JD, Maislin G, Winokur A, Kling M, Gold P. Pituitary and adrenocortical responses to ovine corticotropin releasing hormone in depressed patients and healthy volunteers. *Arch Gen Psychiatry* 1987;44:775–781.

7. Amsterdam JD, Marinelli DL, Arger P, Winokur A. Assessment of adrenal gland volume by computed tomography in depressed patients and healthy volunteers: a pilot study. *Psychiatry Res* 1987; 21:189–198.

8. Antoni FA. Hypothalamic control of adrenocorticotropin secretion: advances since the discovery of 41-residue CRF. *Endocrine Rev* 1986;7:351–378.

9. Arriza JL, Weinberger C, Cerelli G, et al. Cloning of the human mineralocorticoid receptor complementary DNA; structural and functional kinship with the glucocorticoid receptor. *Science* 1987; 237:268–275.

10. Autelitano DJ, Blum M, Lopingco M, Allen RG, Roberts JL. CRF differentially regulates anterior and intermediate pituitary lobe pro-opiomelanocortin gene transcription, nuclear precursor RNA and mature mRNA in vivo. *Neuroendocrinology* 1990;51:123–130.

11. Beato M. Gene regulation by steroid hormones. *Cell* 1989;56:335–344.

12. Beaulieu S, DiPoalo T, Barden N. Control of ACTH secretion by the central nucleus of the amygdala: implications of the serotinergic system and its relevance to the glucocorticoid delayed negative feedback mechanism. *Neuroendocrinology* 1986;44:247–254.

13. Caamaño CA, Morano MI, Patel PD, Watson SJ, Akil HA. Bacterially expressed mineralocorticoid receptor is associated in vitro with the 90-kDA heat shock protein and shows typical hormone- and DNA-binding characteristics. *Biochemistry* 1993;32:8589–8595.

14. Cannon W. *The wisdom of the body.* New York: Norton; 1932.

15. Carroll BJ, Curtis GC, Mendels J. Neuroendocrine regulation in depression I. Limbic system-adrenocortical dysfunction. *Arch Gen Psychiatry* 1976;33:1039–1044.

16. Carroll BJ, Feinberg M, Greden JF. A specific laboratory test for the diagnosis of melancholia: standardization, validation and clinical utility. *Arch Gen Psychiatry* 1981;38:15–22.

17. Cascio CS, Shinsako J, Dallman MF. The suprachiasmatic nuclei stimulate evening ACTH secretion in the rat. *Brain Res* 1987; 423:173–178.

18. Coover GD, Goldman L, Levine S. Plasma corticosterone levels during extinction of a lever-press response in hippocampectomized rats. *Physiol Behav* 1971;7:727–732.

19. Cullinan WE, Herman JP, Watson SJ. Ventral subicular interaction with the hypothalamic paraventricular nucleus: evidence for a relay in the bed nucleus of the stria terminalis. *J Comp Neurol* 1993; 332:1–20.

20. Cunningham ETJ, Bohn MC, Sawchenko PE. Organization of adrenergic inputs to the paraventricular and supraoptic nuclei of the hypothalamus in the rat. *J Comp Neurol* 1990;292:651–657.

21. Dallman MF, Akana SF, Scribner KA, et al. Stress, feedback and facilitation in the hypothalamo-pituitary-adrenal axis. *J Neuroendocrinol* 1991;4:517–526.

22. Dalman FC, Bresnick EH, Patel PD, Perdew GH, Watson SP, Pratt WB. Direct evidence that the glucocorticoid receptor binds to hsp90 at or near termination of receptor translation in vitro. *J Biol Chem* 1989;264:19815–19821.

23. Dalman FC, Scherrer LC, Taylor LP, Akil H, Pratt WB. Localization of the hsp90 binding site within the hormone binding domain of the glucocorticoid receptor by peptide competition. *J Biol Chem* 1991;266:3482–3490.

24. Darlington DN, Shinsako J, Dallman MF. Medullary lesions eliminate ACTH responses to hypotensive hemorrage. *Am J Physiol* 1986;251:R106–115.

25. DeKloet ER. Brain, corticosteroid receptor balance and homeostatic control. *Front Neuroendocrinol* 1991;12:95–164.

26. Diamond MI, Miner JN, Yoshinaga SK, Yamamoto KR. Transcription factor interactions: selectors of positive or negative regulation from a single DNA element. *Science* 1990;249:1266–1272.

27. Drouin J, Trifiro MA, Plante RK, Nemer M, Eriksson P, Wrange O. Glucocorticoid receptor binding to a specific DNA sequence is required for hormone-dependent repression of proopiomelanocortin gene transcription. *Molec Cell Biol* 1989;9:5305–5314.

28. Dunn JD, Whitener J. Plasma corticosterone responses to electrical stimulation of the amygdaloid complex: cytoarchitectonic specificity. *Neuroendocrinology* 1986;42:211–217.

29. Eldridge JC, Brodish A, Kute TE, Landfield PW. Apparent age-related resistence of type II hippocampal corticosteroid receptors to down-regulation during chronic escape training. *J Neurosci* 1989; 9:3237–3242.

30. Feldman S, Conforti N. Participation of the dorsal hippocampus in glucocorticoid negative feedback effect on adrenocortical activity. *Neuroendocrinology* 1980;30:52–55.

31. Feldman S, Conforti N. Modifications of adrenocortical responses following frontal cortex stimulation in rats with hypothalamic de-afferentations and medial forebrain bundle lesions. *Neuroscience* 1985;15:1045–1047.

32. Ferraguti F, Zoli M, Aronsson M, et al. Distribution of glutamic acid decarboxylase messenger RNA-containing nerve cell populations of the male rat brain. *J Chem Neuroanat* 1990;3:377–396.

33. Funder JW. Mineralocorticoids, glucocorticoids, receptors, and response elements. *Science* 1993;259:1132–1133.

34. Gertz BJ, Contreras LN, McComb DJ, Kovacs K, Tyrell JB, Dallman MF. Chronic administration of corticotropin-releasing factor increases pituitary corticotroph number. *Endocrinology* 1987;120:381–388.

35. Gibson A, Hart SL, Patel S. Effects of 6-hydroxydopamine-induced lesions of the parventricular nucleus, and prazosin, on the corticosterone response to restraint in rats. *Neuropharmacology* 1986; 25:257–260.

36. Godowski PJ, Picard D, Yamamoto KR. Signal transduction and transcriptional regulation by glucocorticoid receptor-LexA fusion proteins. *Science* 1988;241:812–816.

37. Gold PW, Loriaux DL, Roy A, et al. Response to corticotropin-releasing hormone in the hypercortisolism of depression and Cushing's disease. *New Engl J Med* 1986;314:1329–1335.

38. Halbreich U, Asnis GM, Zurrnoff B, Nathan RS. The effect of age and sex on cortisol secretion in depressives and normals. *Psychiatry Res* 1984;13:221–229.

39. Halbreich U, Asnis GM, Schindledecker R, Zurnoff B, Nathan RS. Cortisol secretion in endogenous depression I. Basal plasma levels. *Arch Gen Psychiatry* 1985;42:909–914.

40. Herman JP, Patel PD, Akil H, Watson SJ. Localization and regulation of glucocorticoid and mineralocorticoid receptor messenger RNAs in the hippocampal formation of the rat. *Mol Endocrinol* 1989;3:1886–1894.

41. Herman JP, Schafer MK-H, Young EA, et al. Evidence for hippocampal regulation of neuroendocrine neurons of the hypothalamo-pituitary-adrenocortical axis. *J Neurosci* 1989;9:3072–3082.

42. Hollenberg SM, Weinberger C, Ong ES, et al. Primary structure and expression of a functional human glucocorticoid receptor cDNA. *Nature* 1985;318:635–641.

43. Holsboer F, Bardeleden U, Gerken A. Blunted corticotropin and normal cortisol response to human corticotropin-releasing factor in depression. *New Engl J Med* 1984;311:1127.

44. Issa AM, Rowe W, Gauuthier S, Meaney MJ. Hypothalamic-pituitary-adrenal activity in aged, cognitively impaired and cognitively unimpaired rats. *J Neurosci* 1990;10(10):3247–3254.

45. Jacobson L, Sapolsky R. The role of the hippocampus in feedback regulation of the hypothalamic-pituitary-adrenocortical axis. *Endocrine Rev* 1991;12:118–134.

46. Jaeckle RS, Kathol RG, Lopez JF, Meller WH, Krummel SJ. Enhanced adrenal sensitivity to exogenous ACTH 1-24 stimulation in major depression; relationship to dexamethasone suppression test results. *Arch Gen Psychiatry* 1987;44:233–240.

47. Keller-Wood ME, Dallman F. Corticosteroid inhibition of ACTH secretion. *Endocrine Rev* 1984;5:1–24.

48. Kovacs K, Kiss JZ, Makar GB. Glucocorticoid inplants around the hypothalamic paraventricular nucleus prevent the increase of corticotropin-releasing factor and arginine vasopressin immunostaining induced by adrenalectomy. *Neuroendocrinology* 1986;44: 229–234.

49. Kwak SP, Morano MI, Young EA, Watson SJ, Akil H. Diurnal CRH mRNA rhythm in the hypothalamus: decreased expression in the evening is not dependent on endogenous glucocorticoids. *Neuroendocrinology* 1993;57:96–105.

50. Kwak SP, Patel PD, Thompson RC, Akil H, Watson SJ. 5′heterogeneity of the mineralocorticoid receptor mRNA: differential expression and regulation of splice variants within the rat hippocampus. *Endocrinology* 1993;133:2344–2350.

51. Lamberts SW, Verleun T, Oosterom R. Corticotropin-releasing factor (ovine) and vasopressin exert a synergistic effect on adrenocorticotropin release in man. *J Clin Endocrinol Metab* 1984;298–303.

52. Landfield P, Waymire J, Lynch G. Hippocampal aging and adrenocorticoids: quantitative correlations. *Science* 1978;202:1098–1102.

53. Levin N, Blum M, Roberts JL. Modulation of basal and corticotropin-releasing factor-stimulated proopiomelanocortin gene expression by vasopressin in rat anterior pituitary. *Endocrinology* 1989;125: 2957–2966.

54. Lewis DA, Pfohl B, Schlecte J, Coryell W. Influence of age on the cortisol response to dexamethasone. *Psychiatry Res* 1984;13:213–220.

55. López JF, Palkovits M, Arato M, Mansour A, Watson SJ. POMC and glucocorticoid receptor gene expression in the pituitaries of suicide victims. *Neuroendocrinology* 1992;56:491–501.

56. Maquire KP, Schweitzer I, Biddle N, Bridge S, Tiller JWG. The dexamethasone suppression test: importance of dexamethasone concentrations. *Biol Psychiatry* 1987;22:957–967.

57. Meaney MJ, Aitken DH, Bhatnagar S, VanBerkel C, Sapolsky RM. Postnatal handling attenuates neuroendocrine, anatomical and cognitive impairments related to the aged hippocampus. *Science* 1988; 238:766–768.

58. Mezey E, Kiss JZ, Skirboll LR. Increase of corticotropin-releasing factor staining in rat paraventricular nucleus neurons by depletion of hypothalamic adrenaline. *Nature* 1984;310:140–141.

59. Morano MI, Akil H. Age-related changes in the POMC stress axis in the rat. In: Van Ree JM, Mulder AH, Wiegant VM, van Wimersma Greidanus TB, eds. *New leads in opioid research.* Amsterdam: Excerpta Medica; 1990:9–11.

60. Munck A, Guyre PM, Holbrook NJ. Physiological functions of glucocorticoids in stress and their relation to pharmacological actions. *Endocrine Rev* 1984;5:25–55.

61. Nemeroff CB, Widerlov E, Bisette G, et al. Elevated concentrations of CSF corticotropin-releasing-factor-like immunoreactivity in depressed patients. *Science* 1984;226:1342–1344.

62. Nemeroff CB, Bissette G, Akil H, Fink M. Cerebrospinal fluid neuropeptides in depressed patients treated with ECT: Corticotropin-releasing factor, beta-endorphin and somatostatin. *Br J Psychiatry* 1991;158:59–63.

63. Oxenkrug GF, Pomara N, McIntrye IM, Branconnier RJ, Stanley M, Gershon S. Aging and cortisol resistance to suppression by dexamethasone: a positive correlation. *Psychiatry Res* 1983;10: 125–130.

64. Patel PD, Sherman TG, Goldman DJ, Watson SJ. Molecular cloning of a mineralocorticoid receptor cDNA from rat hippocampus. *Mol Endocrinol* 1989;3:1877–1885.

65. Paykel ES. Life events and early environment. In: Paykel ES, ed. *Handbook of affective disorders.* Edinburg: Churchill Livingstone; 1982:146–161.

66. Pearce D, Yamamoto KR. Mineralocorticoid and glucocorticoid receptor activities distinguished by nonreceptor factors at a composite response element. *Science* 1993;259:1161–1165.

67. Post RM. Transduction of psychosocial stress into the neurobiology of recurrent affective disorder. *Am J Psychiatry* 1992;149:999–1010.

68. Reul JM, DeKloet ER. Two receptor systems for corticosterone receptors in rat brain: microdistribution and differential occupation. *Endocrinology* 1985;117:2505–2511.

69. Roy A, Pickar D, Paul S, Doran A, Ghrousos GP, Gold PW. CSF corticotropin-releasing hormone in depressed patients and normal control subjects. *Am J Psychiatry* 1987;144:641–5.

70. Sakai DD, Helms S, Carlstedt-Duke J, Gustafsson JA, Rottm FM, Yamamoto KR. Hormone-mediated repression: a negative glucocorticoid response element from the bovine prolactin gene. *Genes Dev* 1988;2:1144–1154.

71. Saphier D, Feldman S. Effects of neural stimuli on paraventricular nucleus neurons. *Brain Res Bull* 1985;14:401–407.

72. Sapolsky RM, Krey LC, McEwen BS. The adrenocortical stress-response in the aged male rat: impairment of recovery from stress. *Exp Gerontol* 1983;18:55–64.

73. Sapolsky RM, Krey LC, McEwen BS. Prolonged glucocorticoid exposure reduces hippocampal neuron number: implications for aging. *J Neurosci* 1985;5:1222–1227.

74. Sapolsky RM, Krey LC, McEwen BS. The neuroendocrinology of stress and aging: the glucocorticoid cascade hypothesis. *Endocrine Rev* 1986;7:284–301.

75. Sargeant JK, Bruce ML, Florio LP, Weissman MM. Factors associated with 1-year outcome of major depression in the community. *Arch Gen Psychiatry* 1990;47:519–526.

76. Sawchenko PE, Swanson LW, Steinbusch HWM. The distribution and cells of origin of serotonin inputs to the paraventricular and supraoptic nuclei of the rat. *Brain Res* 1983;277:355–360.

77. Schafer MK, Herman JP, Watson SJ. *In situ* hybridization analysis of gene expression in the HPA stress axis: regulation by glucocorticoids. *Wenner-Grenn International Symposium Series: Visualization of brain function.* 1990, 11–22.

78. Scherrer LC, Picard D, Massa E, et al. Evidence that the hormone binding domain of steroid receptors confers hormonal control on chimeric proteins by determining their hormone-regulated binding to heat-shock protein 90. *Biochemistry* 1993;32:5381–5386.

79. Selye H. The diseases of adaptation. *Rec Prog Horm Res* 1953; 8:117.

80. Shiomi H, Watson S, Kelsey J. Pretranslational and posttranslational mechanisms for regulating beta-endorphin/ACTH cells: Studies in anterior lobe. *Endocrinology* 1986;119:1793–1799.

81. Sutton RE, Koob GF, LeMoal M, Rivier J, Vale W. Corticotropin releasing factor produces behavioural activation in rats. *Nature* 1982;297:331–333.

82. Swanson LW, Simmons DM. Differential steroid hormone and neural influences on peptide mRNA levels in CRH cells of the paraventricular nucleus: a hybridization histochemical study in the rat. *J Comp Neurol* 1989;285:413–435.

83. Szafarczyk A, Hery M, Laplante E. Temporal relationships between the circadian rhythmicity in plasma levels of pituitary hormones and in hypothalamic concentrations of releasing factors. *Neuroendocrinology* 1980;30:376.

84. Szafarczyk A, Guillaume V, Conte-Devolx B. Central catecholaminergic system stimulates secretion of CRH at different sites. *Am J Physiol* 1988;255:E463–E468.

85. Walaas I, Fonnum F. Biochemical evidence for glutamate as a transmitter in hippocampal efferents to the basal forebrain and hypothalamus in the rat brain. *Neuroscience* 1980;5:1691–1698.

86. Whitnall MH, Smyth D, Gainer H. Vasopressin coexists in half of the corticotropin-releasing factor axons present in the external zone of the median eminence in normal rats. *Neuroendocrinology* 1987;45:420–424.

87. Yang-Yen HF, Chambard JC, Sun YL, et al. Transcriptional interference between c-Jun and the glucocorticoid receptor: mutal inhibition of DNA binding due to direct protein-protein interaction. *Cell* 1990;62:1205–1215.

88. Young EA, Akana S, Dallman MF. Decreased sensitivity to glucocorticoid fast feedback in chronically stressed rats. *Neuroendocrinology* 1990;51:536–542.

89. Young EA, Akil H. Changes in releasability of ACTH and beta-endorphin with chronic stress. *Neuropeptides* 1985;5:545–548.

90. Young EA, Haskett RF, Murphy-Weinberg V, Watson SJ, Akil H. Loss of glucocorticoid fast feedback in depression. *Arch Gen Psychiatry* 1991;48:693–699.

91. Young EA, Watson SJ, Kotun J, et al. Beta-lippotropin-beta-endorphin response to low dose ovine corticotropin releasing factor in endogenous depression. *Arch Gen Psychiatry* 1990;47:449–57.

Psychopharmacology: The Fourth Generation of Progress, edited by Floyd E. Bloom and David J. Kupfer. Raven Press, Ltd., New York © 1995.

CHAPTER 68

Animal Models of Psychiatric Disorders

Mark A. Geyer and Athina Markou

This chapter critically discusses the process of developing, validating, and working with animal models relevant to psychiatric disorders. A model is defined as any experimental preparation developed for the purpose of studying a condition in the same or different species. Typically, models are animal preparations that attempt to mimic a human condition, including human psychopathology. In developing and assessing an animal model, it is critical to consider the explicit purpose intended for the model, because the intended purpose determines the criteria that the model must satisfy to establish its validity. Hence, before discussing the criteria by which the validity of an animal model might be assessed, it is important to consider the variety of purposes for which an animal model may be used to promote our knowledge of a psychiatric disorder (see also Chapters 6, 61, 65, 66, and 98, *this volume*).

PURPOSES OF AN ANIMAL MODEL

At one extreme, one can attempt to develop an animal model that mimics a psychiatric syndrome in its entirety. To do so, one must establish homology between the behavior of the affected animal and the syndrome being modeled. Typically, the signs and symptoms that are characteristic of the particular syndrome in humans are identified and enumerated. The ability of the experimental manipulation to induce homologous changes in the behavior of the test animal is then determined. In the early years of neuropsychopharmacology, the term *animal model* often denoted such an attempt to reproduce a psychiatric disorder in a laboratory animal. As will be illustrated, this approach is fraught with difficulty, in part because it com-

monly relies upon arguments of apparent similarities (i.e., face validity) that are difficult to defend and in part because the symptoms that define a given disorder are often defined in subjective terms. Furthermore, the defining symptoms of psychiatric disorders and even the diagnostic categories themselves are continuously being revised and redefined. It is not uncommon for diagnostic categories to be split into multiple new entities or combined into a new category as clinical experience reveals the limitations of previous categorizations (see Chapter 71, *this volume*).

At the other extreme, one more limited purpose for an animal model is to provide a way to systematically study the effects of potential therapeutic treatments. In such a case, the model may or may not mimic the actual psychiatric disorder. Rather, the behavior of the model is only intended to reflect the efficacy of known therapeutic agents and thus lead to the discovery of new pharmacotherapies. Because the explicit purpose of the model is to predict treatment efficacy, the principle guiding this approach has been termed "pharmacological isomorphism" (53). As illustrated below and discussed elsewhere (53,63), the fact that such models are developed and validated by reference to the effects of known therapeutic drugs frequently limits their ability to identify new drugs having different chemical structures or novel mechanisms of action. Similarly, an inherent limitation of this approach is that it is not designed to identify new therapeutics that might treat those symptoms of the disorder that are refractory to current treatments. An extreme case of such a limitation is found in the use of drug-discrimination paradigms used to identify new treatment compounds. In these paradigms, the animal is trained to recognize the drug state induced by a prototypical drug. Typically, the animal is required to press either the right or left lever, depending upon whether it had been treated with saline or the training drug. Potential new therapeutics are then identified by their ability to substitute for the

M. A. Geyer: Department of Psychiatry, School of Medicine, University of California, San Diego, La Jolla, California 92093.
A. Markou: Department of Neuropharmacology, The Scripps Research Institute, La Jolla, California 92037.

prototypical drug on which the animal was trained. Because these paradigms rely only on the drug-induced cue to which each animal responds and not on any endpoint that can be validated by reference to other behaviors in animals or humans, they can only identify drugs having a similar effect on some unknowable dimension.

Because of the complexity and evolving nature of diagnostic categories in psychiatry, another approach to the development of animal models relies on mimicking only specific signs or symptoms associated with psychopathologic conditions, rather than mimicking an entire syndrome. In such cases, specific observables that have been identified in psychiatric populations provide a focus for study in experimental animals. The particular behavior being studied may or may not be pathognomonic for or even symptomatic of the disorder, but must be defined objectively and observed reliably. Thus, even phenomena that are found in more than one diagnostic entity may be studied in animals using this approach. It is important to emphasize that the reliance of such a model on specific observables minimizes a fundamental problem plaguing animal models of psychopathology designed to model diagnostic syndromes. Specifically, the number of definitive clinical findings with which one can validate an animal model have been limited by the difficulties inherent in conducting experimental studies of psychiatric populations. As illustrated below, the validation of any animal model can be only as sound as the information available in the relevant clinical literature (63). With this approach, the investigator may generate more definitive information related to a more circumscribed domain of psychopathology. By limiting the purpose of the animal model, one can increase the confidence in the cross-species validity of the model. The narrow focus of this approach generally leads to pragmatic advantages in the conduct of mechanistic studies addressing the neurobiological substrates of the behavior in question. By contrast, in models intended to reproduce entire syndromes, the need for multiple simultaneous endpoints makes it relatively difficult to apply the invasive experimental manipulations that are typically required to establish underlying mechanisms.

Another approach to the development of animal models is more theoretically based on psychological constructs that are thought to be affected by the psychiatric disorder under investigation. Such an identification of what has been termed psychological processes or behavioral dimensions (53,63) involves the definition of a hypothetical construct and subsequent establishment of operational definitions suitable for the experimental testing of the validity of the construct. This approach is fruitful when conceptually related experiments are undertaken in both the relevant patient population and in the putative animal model. That is, studies of appropriate patients are needed to establish the operational definitions of the hypothetical construct and the construct's relevance to the particular disorder. In concert, parallel studies of the theoretically homologous construct, process, or dimension are required to determine the similarity of the animal model to the human phenomena. An important and advantageous aspect of this approach is that the validation of the hypothetical construct and its cross-species homology can be established by studies of normal humans and animals, in addition to psychiatrically disordered patients or experimentally manipulated animals. Thus, this approach adds to and benefits from the psychological and neuroscientific literature relevant to the hypothetical construct on which the model is based. In a sense, this approach explicitly recognizes that the experimental study of the disorder in humans requires as much modeling as does the study of the disorder in an animal model.

CRITERIA FOR EVALUATING ANIMAL MODELS

In evaluating animal models, the ultimate need for reliance on predictive validity must be stressed. Validation criteria are general standards that are relevant to the evaluation of any model. Over the years, several reviews have discussed criteria for the evaluation of animal models (e.g. refs. 36,52–54,63). Most of these discussions are based on an assumption that is not always explicit. Namely, it is commonly assumed that there is a homology, or at least analogy, between the physiological and behavioral characteristics of various species; hence, extrapolations can be made from animals to humans (61). If we accept this postulate, the necessary and sufficient validation criteria for any animal model remains a question. In general, as mentioned above, the validity of a model refers to the extent to which a model is useful for a given purpose. In neurobiological research, the purpose of a model is, most commonly, to promote our understanding of a human condition that is expressed behaviorally by elucidating the neurobiological mechanisms underlying the human condition. In the following sections, we argue that there are only two criteria that a model must satisfy to establish its value in basic neurobiological research: reliability and predictive validity (52). The satisfaction of other criteria, such as construct or discriminant validity, may have heuristic value; however, it is not essential.

Reliability

Reliability refers to the consistency and stability with which the variable of interest is observed. This consistency should be evident in (a) the ability to measure the variable objectively; (b) its small within-subject variability; (c) its small between-subject variability; (d) the reproducibility of the phenomenon under similar conditions; and (e) the reproducibility of the effects of manipulations (52). Having a reliable and reproducible experimental system is essential to scientific study. Nevertheless, although small within- and between-subject variability is usually desirable, there are cases in which the study of the variability of the model system could lead to a better understanding of the phenomenon. Variability cannot always be considered as error.

Validity

Many different types of validity have been described and defined (3,13,16,22,56), including predictive, construct, concurrent or convergent, discriminant, etiological, and face validity. Depending on the nature and the desired purpose of the test, different types of validity are relevant. The primary purpose of animal models is to enhance our understanding of a human phenomenon. Thus, the question of what are the criteria for evaluating the usefulness of models is equivalent to the philosophical question of what scientific understanding is. As formalized by the logical positivists of the Vienna circle, scientific understanding is the ability to predict (10). A phenomenon is defined by its correlations with antecedent or consequent phenomena (5). Logical positivism takes the position that the only valid scientific observables are correlations (i.e., one event preceding the other always in the same order), whereas causality is an inference that is beyond the evidence and can never be shown to be true or false (38). Hence, the only meaningful evaluating criterion for an animal model is the model's ability to lead to accurate predictions. That is, the evaluating criterion is whether the model has predictive validity. Even though other types of validity, such as construct, etiological, convergent, discriminant, and face validity, are relevant to animal models, predictive validity and reliability are the only necessary and sufficient criteria for the evaluation of any animal model. The arguments for this position will be made in the following sections as the other types of validity are defined and discussed in relation to animal models. It should be noted, however, that the process of construct, etiological, convergent, and discriminant validation of an animal model are integral components of scientific theory development and testing.

Predictive Validity

Predictive validity is generally defined as the ability of a test to predict a criterion that is of interest to the investigator (16). For animal models, the criterion is the human phenomenon. Thus, an animal model has predictive validity to the extent that it allows one to make predictions about the human phenomenon based on the performance of the model. Therefore, an important factor that influences the predictive validity of a model is the reliability of measurement, which must be considered not only for the model but also for the clinical phenomena. Thus,

development of animal models requires parallel development of clinical measures to allow meaningful comparisons.

In animal models of human psychopathology, the term predictive validity is often used in a narrow sense to refer to the model's ability to identify drugs with potential therapeutic value in humans (i.e., pharmacological isomorphism) (53,79). Although this use of the term is not incorrect, it is limited, because it ignores other important ways in which a model can lead to successful predictions (63). For example, the identification of any variables that influence both the animal model and the modeled phenomenon in similar ways can enhance one's understanding of the phenomenon.

Construct Validity

Construct validity of a test is commonly defined as the accuracy with which the test measures what it is intended to measure (16). Although construct validity is considered by investigators in a variety of fields as the most important property of a test (16,22,79,89), it can be very rarely established. The process of construct validation of a test is not different in any essential way from the general scientific procedure for developing and testing theories (16) and thus for developing animal models. Conceptions about what a test is supposed to measure or a model is supposed to mimic are constantly changing as scientific theories and theoretical constructs are modified. Thus, a model's usefulness, and hence its overall validity, cannot be determined by the degree of construct validation that it has. Nevertheless, the process of construct validation is valuable in the neverending process of further development and refinement of the model. As new experimental and observational evidence accrues from both the animal model and the clinical conditions, the model is refined and therefore enables more accurate predictions.

Etiological Validity

The concept of etiological validity is closely related to the concept of construct validity. A model has *etiological validity* if the etiologies of the phenomenon in the animal model and the human condition are identical. When etiological validity can be established, the model can become extremely useful in the development of treatments. The limitations of treatment-oriented models based on pharmacological isomorphism, alluded to above, can be overcome if an etiologically based model is found. Unfortunately, the etiologies of psychiatric disorders are seldom known. Hence, etiological validity in this context is generally limited to speculations or hypotheses regarding a possible etiology. Indeed, the purpose for the development of animal models is often to identify the etiology or to test a hypothesis about the etiology of the disease.

In such an instance, one could not require that a model has etiological validity for the model to be valid. Like construct validation, the process of etiological validation is a fundamental component of scientific investigation.

Convergent and Discriminant Validity

A model or a test has convergent (or concurrent) and discriminant validity only in relation to other models, tests, or measures. *Convergent validity* is the degree to which a test correlates with other tests that attempt to measure the same construct (13). *Discriminant validity* is the degree to which a test measures aspects of a phenomenon that are different from other aspects of the phenomenon that other tests assess (13). Discriminant validity is indicated by low correlations between the measures provided by the various models. Thus, a model is invalid to the extent that it is highly correlated with other models from which it was intended to differ. Both convergent and discriminant validity are required for the establishment of construct validity. It has been argued that convergent operationalism (also called converging measures) should replace single operationalism in behavioral sciences (13). Convergent operationalism refers to the process of defining a construct by a multiplicity of methods or operations. The concern is that a single operation might not measure what one wishes to measure and therefore would lead to erroneous conclusions. With convergent operationalism, one could better approximate the measurement of the construct of interest. The evaluation of convergent validity is central to the approach described above in which a model is theoretically based on a psychological process or behavioral dimension that is hypothesized to be affected in a psychiatric disorder.

Face Validity

Face validity refers to the phenomenological similarity between the behavior exhibited by the animal model and the specific symptoms of the human condition (56). Although face validity appears to be a desirable and is certainly an intuitively appealing criterion (20,80), such a criterion is actually not necessary, can be misleading, and is difficult to defend rigorously. Because most models involve a species other than the one whose condition we are trying to mimic, it is unrealistic to expect the two species to exhibit similar symptoms or phenomenology, even in cases in which the etiology of the condition is known (53,63). In contrast, similarities between certain aspects of the behavior or physiology of animals and humans do not necessarily implicate similar etiology (2,36). Moreover, establishing the face validity of a model objectively is impossible. Face validity may provide a heuristic starting point for the development of an animal model, but it cannot be used to establish the validity of

the model. The claim for face validity of a model almost invariably involves subjective arbitrary arguments (see ref. 79 for examples of models with proposed face validity). Thus, the face validity of most models of human psychopathology is difficult to establish objectively and is irrelevant to the potential usefulness of the model in understanding the disease. It should be understood that face validity refers to the superficial similarity in symptomatology between the model and the disorder (e.g., changes in appetite or activity levels) and can be distinguished from construct validity, which relies on similarities in underlying processes (e.g., hypothetical constructs specifying the mechanisms that lead to changes in appetite or activity levels). Thus, although face validity does not detract from an animal model, it simply does not provide scientific support for a model.

ANIMAL MODELS

In the following sections, selected examples of animal models used in the contexts of depression and schizophrenia are discussed. These discussions offer neither a compendium of current animal models, nor thorough reviews of the selected models. Rather, selected aspects of these models are discussed to illustrate the principles, approaches, and concerns that should be contemplated in developing and validating a model.

Animal Models of Depression

The Learned Helplessness and Behavioral Despair Models of Depression

One of the most widely used animal models of depression is the learned helplessness model. This model is based on the observation that exposure to uncontrollable stress produces performance deficits in subsequent learning tasks that are not seen in subjects exposed to identical stressors under the subjects' control (47). This paradigm is an example of a model intended to reproduce a psychiatric syndrome in its entirety, in which claims of face validity and pharmacological isomorphism are offered as the principal support.

It has been argued that the model has good face validity, because there is similarity between the behavioral characteristics of learned-helpless animals and signs of depression in humans (for critical reviews, see refs. 79 and 80). For example, learned-helpless animals exhibit loss of appetite and weight, decreased locomotor activity, and poor performance in both appetitively and aversively motivated tasks. These behavioral characteristics of learned-helpless animals are considered equivalent to loss of appetite and weight, psychomotor retardation, and anhedonia, respectively, demonstrated by depressed humans (DSM-III-R). As discussed above, however, symptom similarity (i.e., face validity) does not necessarily imply homology (36). Thus, these claims for the model's face validity do not address the question of whether the model has any utility.

The predictive validity in terms of pharmacological isomorphism of the model is indicated by the fact that pharmacological treatments clinically effective in depression, such as tricyclics, monoamine oxidase inhibitors, atypical, antidepressants, and electroconvulsive shock therapy, are effective in reducing the behavioral and physical abnormalities seen in animals exposed to uncontrollable stress (79,80). Thus, the model appears to have good predictive validity in terms of identifying potentially useful pharmacotherapies for depression. Nevertheless, the model's predictive and discriminant validity might be limited because false positives have also been reported (79).

The model's predictive and construct validity, and thus its potential to further our understanding of the neurobiology of depression, depends on the validity of two assumptions that have been extensively debated (80): The first assumption is related to the process that is assumed to occur while the animals are exposed to uncontrollable stressors, namely, that animals learn that they have no control and therefore become helpless. Alternatively, subjects might learn to become inactive (32). Evidence suggests that both learned helplessness and inactivity might be learned by animals in these paradigms (46). Because these two processes are confounded in most learned helplessness experiments (i.e., a lack of construct and discriminant validity) (80), this paradigm might not be the best procedure to investigate either of these two processes. The second assumption of the model is that learned helplessness is exhibited by depressed individuals. However, very little evidence supports this assumption (9). Clinical observations describing depressed patients as exhibiting behavioral despair or negative cognitive sets do not constitute experimental evidence for the existence of the specific psychological process of learned helplessness on which the model is based. The absence of explicit support for the occurrence of this process in depressed humans seriously questions the construct validity of the paradigm as a model of depression. Furthermore, the fact that presumably normal humans do not unambiguously develop learned helplessness under conditions of uncontrollable stress (11), and only 10% to 50% of rats develop this syndrome (19), disputes the reliability of the phenomenon and its generality across species. In summary, the learned helplessness paradigm's usefulness as a model of depression is severely limited by the potential lack of reliability in either human or infrahuman species and by the lack of evidence that learned helplessness is a behavioral process characterizing depressed individuals (i.e., a lack of predictive and construct validity). The advantage of the model is its pharmacological isomorphism, which suggests some limited predictive validity.

Another version of the learned helplessness model is the behavioral despair paradigm. In this model, mice or rats are forced to swim in a confined environment. The animals initially swim around and attempt to escape, and eventually assume an immobile posture. On subsequent tests, the latency to immobility is decreased. In a modification of this paradigm, animals are first exposed to uncontrollable stress before the swim test (76). These paradigms are conceptually similar to the learned helplessness paradigm in assuming that animals have learned to despair (i.e., they acquired learned helplessness). As such, the model has the potential of providing convergent evidence about the process(es) of learned helplessness. Unfortunately, studies of subjects tested in both paradigms indicated a lack of cross-predictability (i.e., a lack of convergent validity), which suggests that the two models may assess processes mediated by separate neuromechanisms (19,58). Furthermore, the interpretation of the immobility observed during forced swimming as reflecting failure to cope has been questioned. Instead the immobility might reflect a successful strategy that conserves energy and allows the animal to float for prolonged periods of time, thus surviving longer (77). Furthermore, some evidence suggests that the effect of tricyclics on reducing the immobility might be, at least partly, attributed to altered learning-consolidation memory processes, and not to reduced despair (18,77). Nevertheless, the behavioral despair model has one of the highest degrees of pharmacological isomorphism (i.e., predictive validity) in terms of identifying antidepressants (79). As with learned helplessness, however, the degree of pharmacological isomorphism is limited by false positives. Under certain circumstances, even saline acts as a false positive (17), which constitutes a failure to demonstrate good discriminant validity. More generally, the ability of acute antidepressants to effectively reverse the immobility when only chronic antidepressant treatment is effective in humans represents a failure to demonstrate good predictive validity. In summary, the degree of overall predictive validity of the behavioral despair paradigm as a model of depression appears rather small.

One common aspect of the two models discussed above that could potentially furnish them with construct, etiological, and predictive validity is the fact that behavioral and neurochemical changes are produced by exposing subjects to chronic unpredictable stress. The behavioral changes have been described above. The neurochemical changes involve dysfunctions of the noradrenergic system (76), the neurotransmitter system on which classical antidepressants have their primary pharmacological action (34). Extensive neuropharmacological investigations indicated that in chronically stressed animals the locus coeruleus, from which most noradrenergic projections to the forebrain originate, is disinhibited, probably through a functional blockade of α_2-noradrenergic autoreceptors (76). Therapeutic doses of typical or atypical antidepressants and electroconvulsive shock therapy downregulate

β-adrenergic receptors (34), presumably normalizing the dysregulated function of noradrenergic neurotransmission that has been hypothesized to be one of the neurotransmitter imbalances mediating depression (34). Even though the exact parameters of stress (e.g., frequency, severity, duration, repetitiveness) necessary to induce the behavioral and neurochemical syndromes of interest have not been investigated systematically, the etiology of the syndrome in animals might be the same as the etiology of some types of depression in humans. It has been hypothesized that stress predisposes humans to depression (35). Even though some human data support this hypothesis (15,35), well-controlled clinical investigations are needed to more extensively and unambiguously define the role of stress in depression. Such clinical investigations would assist significantly in the development and validation of animal models related to human depression.

Intracranial Self-stimulation Model

The intracranial self-stimulation (ICSS) paradigm provides an operational measure of anhedonia, a core feature of depression. Anhedonia in humans is defined as "the markedly diminished interest or pleasure in all, or almost all, activities most of the day, nearly every day" (DSM-III-R). Because the anhedonia experienced by depressed patients suggests that these individuals might exhibit alterations in reward processes, the ICSS paradigm has been proposed as a model of this symptom of depression. The ICSS paradigm requires that animals be prepared with intracranial electrodes aimed at specific brain sites. Because brief electrical stimulation of these sites is reinforcing, animals will work to electrically stimulate parts of their own brains. Both the rate of response for ICSS and the psychophysically defined threshold(s) for ICSS have been used as measures of the reward value of the stimulation (49). Substantial evidence suggests that ICSS thresholds are reliable measures of reward (49) that reflect the whole continuum from hedonia to anhedonia. Because it appears that ICSS acts directly on some of the same neuronal substrates that mediate the rewarding effects of natural reinforcers such as food and water (45), it is considered to be a valuable tool for the investigation of brain-reward systems (see also Chapter 66, *this volume*).

Investigations of brain stimulation reward without any prior manipulations have not provided a satisfactory model of depression for two reasons. First, one would expect that depressed individuals exhibit alterations in brain-reward mechanisms, and thus the study of reward processes in normal organisms, although informative, does not mimic any aspect of depression. Second, neither acute nor chronic treatments with tricyclic antidepressants affect ICSS behavior per se (e.g., ref. 51), unless thresholds have been elevated through some manipulation (see below). Even when effects of tricyclics on ICSS behavior

have been observed (23), they have not been large or consistent (51).

By contrast, the study of the neurosubstrates of ICSS behavior following experiential or pharmacological manipulations promises to promote our understanding of reward mechanisms that seem to be altered in several psychiatric disorders, including depression and schizophrenia (DSM-III-R). Two manipulations have been used to produce an anhedonic state in animals, as operationally defined by decreases in ICSS response rates or elevations of thresholds: (a) exposure to uncontrollable stress (83) and (b) withdrawal from long-term exposure to psychomotor stimulants (43,48). In the first of these procedures, mice exposed to either swim stress or uncontrollable footshock exhibit protracted decreases in the reward value of ICSS (72). These stress-induced alterations in ICSS behavior were reversed with repeated treatment with the tricyclic antidepressant, desmethylimipramine (83), indicating some predictive validity in terms of pharmacological isomorphism of the model. This model also appears to have considerable construct validity insofar as it addresses a specific process that appears to be impaired in depressed individuals and enables the investigation of the neurobiology of this phenomenon. Potentially, the paradigm may have good etiological validity by inducing an anhedonic state through a mechanism (i.e., exposure to uncontrollable stress) that has been hypothesized to play a critical role in inducing depression in humans (35).

Converging evidence for dysfunctions in reward processes induced by stress is provided by another paradigm intended to measure the hedonic value of stimuli. Here, rats are exposed chronically to a series of mild stressors and their consumption of a sweet solution is monitored. Stressed animals tend to consume less sweet solution than controls (81), suggesting an induction of a mild anhedonic state by stress. This effect of stress was reversed by chronic antidepressant treatment (81). Thus, there is converging evidence that stress induces abnormalities in reward processes. As discussed above, the relevance of such stress-induced abnormalities to depressive illnesses in humans needs to be established to validate these effects as models of depression.

The second procedure for inducing an elevation in ICSS thresholds involves withdrawal from prolonged exposure to psychomotor stimulants, such as cocaine (48) or amphetamine (43). For example, when rats were withdrawn after being allowed to self-administer cocaine for prolonged periods of time, their thresholds for ICSS reward were elevated in proportion to the amount of cocaine consumed during the cocaine binge (48). Because the paradigm allowed rats to self-administer cocaine at doses and patterns that were reinforcing rather than aversive or stressful, the subsequent anhedonia cannot be attributed to the effects of uncontrollable stress but instead appears attributable to the pharmacological effects of cocaine. The use of the self-administration paradigm mimicks human cocaine-binging episodes. Similar elevations in ICSS thresholds or decreases in response rates have also been observed following repeated treatment with experimenter-administered cocaine (42) or amphetamine (43), suggesting good reliability of the phenomenon. Evidence for the predictive validity of this model derives from the finding that the postcocaine elevation in thresholds was reversed by either the dopamine (DA) agonist bromocriptine (50) or repeated administration of the tricyclic antidepressant desmethylimipramine (51). Both these compounds have been used in the treatment of stimulant-induced withdrawal and dependence (25,30). Tricyclics also appear to be effective in reversing the effects of withdrawal from amphetamine on ICSS (43). Thus, although many more studies are needed, the evidence to date suggests that the ICSS model has good construct and etiological validity and exhibits pharmacological isomorphism (i.e., predictive validity) as a model for the drug-induced anhedonia. Nevertheless, it is not known at this point what the relationship is between drug-induced and non-drug-induced depressions in humans. Thus, although it is promising, the possible etiological validity of the ICSS paradigm as a model of non-drug-induced depression remains unclear. It has been argued that withdrawal from psychomotor stimulants induces most of the signs and symptoms typical of non-drug-induced depression in humans (73). Future clinical and preclinical research needs to address this issue further.

Animal Models of Schizophrenia

The vast majority of animal models related to schizophrenia have been based on the induction of abnormal behaviors by drugs such as hallucinogens or psychostimulants. It is important to recognize, however, that drug-induced states in humans have similarities with the early stages of a range of psychotic disorders but not necessarily with the diagnostic syndrome of schizophrenia (40,63). Most recently, research efforts have emphasized parallel studies of potentially homologous behavioral phenomena in both patients and animals, with the abnormalities in animals being induced by a variety of drugs or other experimental manipulations.

The Hallucinogen Model

Soon after the discovery of the psychoactive properties of lysergic acid diethylamide (LSD) 50 years ago, researchers began to explore the suggestion that the class of drugs represented by LSD might appropriately be called psychotomimetics or even psychotogens. This initial effort was engendered by the apparent face validity of the effects of LSD on perception and affective lability as being similar to the symptoms of the early stages of psychoses such as schizophrenia (6). Although many similar-

ities were noted between the effects of the drugs in humans and the symptoms of schizophrenia (37,74), two major differences prompted the widely accepted, but not necessarily justified, conclusion that this class of drugs does not provide a useful model of schizophrenia. First, tolerance was found to develop rapidly to the subjective effects of LSD-like drugs, whereas the symptoms of schizophrenia persist for a lifetime (74). Second, the hallucinations produced by LSD and related drugs are typically in the visual modality, whereas those characteristic of schizophrenia are in the auditory modality (37). These two observations weaken the predictive validity of the hallucinogen model as a model of the syndrome of schizophrenia.

Initial interest in hallucinogens was spurred by the possibility that abnormalities of normal biochemistry might lead to the endogenous production of such compounds and hence be responsible for some psychotic symptomatology. The transmethylation hypothesis in particular posited that serotonin (5-HT) could provide a substrate for the endogenous production of hallucinogens similar to N,N-dimethyltryptamine (DMT) (74). Initially, this etiologically based model was dismissed because of the rapid tolerance associated with traditional hallucinogens such as LSD and mescaline. More recent studies indicating that tolerance may not occur to the subjective and behavioral effects of DMT (31) suggest that DMT may differ from other hallucinogens and that this model may still be viable. Indeed, different mechanisms may be involved in the various actions of the different hallucinogenic drugs, as suggested by the lack of cross-tolerance to DMT in human subjects made tolerant to LSD (60). Hence, further studies are warranted to provide the objective evidence needed to adequately evaluate the model of psychosis based on the hypothesis of an endogenous psychotogen.

Furthermore, it remains possible that these drugs may be psychotomimetic without being psychotogenic. That is, the study of hallucinogen effects in animals may have relevance as models of some aspects of psychotic episodes in humans. Recent suggestions of serotonergic abnormalities in schizophrenia (41) and 5-HT₂ receptor contributions to the clinical efficacy of antipsychotics (55) have revitalized interest in this possibility. For example, hallucinogens are now believed to produce their characteristic subjective effects by acting as 5-HT₂ agonists (33). Many of the newer atypical antipsychotic drugs appear to be potent antagonists at 5-HT₂ receptors (55). Furthermore, if one seeks to model a specific abnormality exhibited by schizophrenic patients rather than the syndrome of schizophrenia, evidence suggests that the study of hallucinogenic action may provide a fruitful line of investigation. For example, both schizophrenic and schizotypal patients are known to exhibit deficits in the habituation of the startle response (4,12,26). Hallucinogenic 5-HT₂ agonists such as LSD or mescaline produce similar deficits in the homologous behavior in animals (26). Conversely, opposite behavioral effects are produced by 5-HT$_2$ antagonists (26,71), some of which are thought to be effective in the treatment of schizophrenia (55). Hence, the effects of hallucinogens in animals have some degree of predictive validity for specific abnormalities exhibited by schizophrenic patients and the effects of antipsychotic drugs. In addition, as discussed below, such a model has been argued to have construct validity based on the widespread evidence that both the symptoms of schizophrenia and the effects of hallucinogens reflect exaggerated responses to sensory and cognitive stimuli due theoretically to failures in normal processes of sensorimotor gating, such as habituation (26,63).

The Psychostimulant Model

The most widely studied class of drug-induced models of schizophrenia is based on the behavioral effects of psychostimulant drugs such as amphetamine in animals. Much of the impetus for this group of models derives from the similarities between the effects of amphetamine in humans and the symptoms of schizophrenia (face validity) or at least the broadly defined early stages of psychotic disorders (40). The prevailing view that schizophrenia reflects a hyperactivity of brain dopaminergic systems (potential etiological validity) has also encouraged the use of this group of models. A wide range of behaviors has been studied in this context, using a variety of species. Typically, rodent studies have focused on increases in locomotor activity or stereotypy, whereas studies of infrahuman primates have examined both motor effects and alterations in social interactions induced by amphetaminelike drugs (20). Many reviews have evaluated these models in great detail (e.g., ref. 14); therefore, we do not review them again here. Suffice it to say that these models have a considerable degree of predictive validity, particularly in predicting the results of pharmacological treatments for schizophrenia. That is, the drugs used to treat schizophrenia are typically DA antagonists and effectively block the effects of DA agonists in animals. Cogent attempts have also been made to argue that some of these models exhibit construct validity as well (see below).

One aspect of predictive validity that has received considerable attention involves the necessary dosage regimens needed for amphetamine or related drugs to produce psychoticlike behavior in psychiatrically normal humans. Because of the widespread belief that amphetamine-induced psychosis was produced only by repeated or so-called chronic exposure to the drug (21), many preclinical researchers have directed their attention toward the behavioral effects of amphetamine that are augmented or sensitized by repeated drug administrations. A thorough review of the available clinical literature, however, strongly indicates that chronic exposure is not required and that psychotic episodes can be produced by acute administrations of amphetamine or related drugs (64). The complex and limited nature of the clinical data seems to have led to mistaken interpretations, which have inordinately influenced a large proportion of the basic research in this area. Although it is clear that tolerance does not occur to the psychosis-inducing effects of amphetamine in humans, it is not clear that sensitization is required for these effects. Hence, even though an animal model based on the effects of chronic amphetamine could be invalidated if tolerance were observed, the development of sensitization does not provide evidence supporting a model's relevance to schizophrenia. Indeed, it appears that the animal models having the greatest amount of predictive validity are those based on the effects of the psychostimulant evident after acute administrations (14,64).

Arguments for the construct and etiological validity of the psychostimulant models are a bit more convoluted and derive largely from the fundamental DA hypothesis of schizophrenia, as reviewed elsewhere (14,63). Among the first observations that led to these models was the apparent similarity (i.e., face validity) of the effects of high doses of amphetamine in presumably normal humans to the symptoms exhibited by schizophrenic patients (21). Cross-species studies in animals treated with psychostimulants revealed striking stereotyped or perseverative behaviors, which were seen as having face validity for the stereotyped behavior induced by amphetamine in humans (14,20,21). Despite the fact that stereotyped behavior was not seen as a key feature of schizophrenia, subsequent studies in rodents have focused on the stereotypies produced by high doses or repeated administrations of psychostimulants. Although the models that evolved from this approach demonstrated considerable predictive validity in terms of pharmacological isomorphism, current thinking now indicates that the original appearance of face validity was actually misleading, and constitutes another example of the limited value of face validity. In recent years, the DA hypothesis of schizophrenia has evolved into the narrower hypothesis that the mesolimbic DA system, as distinct from the nigrostriatal DA system, is most relevant to schizophrenic disorders. The mesolimbic system, in particular, appears to mediate the locomotor-activating effects of relatively low doses of amphetamine and not the stereotypies that predominate at higher doses (14). The nigrostriatal DA system is seen as more relevant to the dyskinetic side effects of antipsychotic treatments and is believed to subserve the stereotypy induced by amphetamine in animals. Thus, the animal behavior proposed to have the most face validity for the human condition now appears to be more closely linked neurobiologically to phenomena that are considered side effects of the clinical treatments. Because schizophrenic patients are not generally considered to be motorically hyperactive, the amphetamine-induced hyperactivity that is mediated by what is believed to be the most relevant neurobiological substrate has seldom been considered to have face validity as a model of the human disorder. Note that the failure of the model to have face validity has in no way weakened its utility in neurobiological research, which is based on its etiological and predictive validity. Nevertheless, virtually any of the behavioral effects of amphetamine in rodents, including either locomotor hyperactivity or stereotypy, have high degrees of pharmacological isomorphism, a form of predictive validity, as models for the efficacy of clinical treatments for schizophrenia (14,64) (see also Chapters 70, 98, and 100, *this volume*).

The Sensorimotor Gating Model

Theories describing the group of schizophrenias often conceptualize the fundamental disorder as involving one or more of several possible deficits in the mechanisms that enable normal individuals to filter or gate most of the sensory stimuli they receive. Collectively, this class of mechanisms is referred to as sensorimotor gating (7,26). Theoretically, impairments in gating lead to sensory overload and cognitive fragmentation. The hypothetical construct of sensorimotor gating has been operationalized and explored in both human and animal studies. For example, numerous studies have examined habituation deficits in schizophrenic patients (e.g., ref. 26), which may reflect failures of sensory filtering that could lead to disorders of cognition. As mentioned above, such quantifiable abnormalities in the behavior of schizophrenic patients are mimicked when the homologous behavior is examined in rats treated with hallucinogenic 5-HT agonists (26) or phencyclidine hydrochloride (PCP) -like N-methyl-D-aspartate (NMDA) antagonists (29). The convergent validity of this gating construct has been further assessed using other operational measures, such as the prepulse inhibition (PPI) of startle and the gating of P_{50} event-related-potentials (ERPs). Like the habituation model, both of these paradigms take advantage of the fact that very similar experiments can be conducted in humans and animals when homologous behaviors have been identified. The PPI paradigm is based on the fact that weak prestimuli when presented 30 to 500 msec before a startling stimulus reduce (or gate) the amplitude of the blink reflex component of the startle response. The generality and reliability of this robust phenomenon is indicated by the fact that PPI is observed in many species; PPI is evident both within and between multiple sensory modalities using a variety of stimulus parameters; PPI does not require learning or comprehension of instructions; and several laboratories have reported PPI deficits in schizophrenic, schizotypal, and presumably psychosis-prone subjects (8,12,65,82).

In the P_{50} sensory gating paradigm, two acoustic clicks are presented in rapid succession, usually 500 msec apart.

In normal individuals, the P_{50} ERP to the second click is reduced or gated relative to the ERP to the first click. Schizophrenic patients and their first-degree relatives exhibit less of this sensory gating (24). The demonstration that schizophrenic patients exhibit conceptually linked deficits in habituation, PPI, and P_{50} gating provides strong support (i.e., convergent validity) for the hypothetical construct that schizophrenia involves disturbances in the filtering of sensory and cognitive information (i.e., construct validity). A recent study of individual differences further tested the convergent validity of the hypothetical construct of gating. In a group of normal subjects, P_{50} gating was strongly correlated with the amount of startle habituation and only weakly with PPI (62), despite the fact that P_{50} gating appears to be more similar phenomenologically to PPI than to habituation (is this another failure of face validity?). Further support for the convergence of these different operational measures of the gating construct is that the amount of habituation was positively correlated with the amount of PPI. Although a failure to obtain significant correlations using this approach can result from the restricted range of many measures in normal populations, significant correlations provide persuasive evidence for the convergent validity of the hypothetical construct. Thus, the suggestion that gating deficits characterize schizophrenia has considerable construct validity by virtue of a number of converging lines of evidence.

Animal models that address the gating deficits seen in schizophrenic patients involve studies of very similar behavioral phenomena in rodents. Studies of the N_{40} ERP in rats have been used successfully as an animal analog of the P_{50} sensory gating paradigm in humans (24). Pharmacological treatments, such as amphetamine and PCP, which are thought to produce psychosis-like symptoms in humans (21,39), produce deficits in the sensory gating of the N_{40} ERP that appear similar to the gating deficits in schizophrenic patients (1). Similarly, studies of the PPI of startle responses in rats have provided extensive support for the predictive, construct, and convergent validity of sensorimotor gating deficits as an animal model of the demonstrated gating deficits in schizophrenic patients. The apparent homology between the human and animal behaviors assessed in the PPI paradigm is supported not only by evidence of parametric similarities of startle responses across species but also by the many studies confirming the cross-species comparability in the specific features of PPI. Thus, this literature constitutes much of the fundamental predictive validity supporting this animal model as being relevant to the human condition. In rats, disruptions in PPI similar to those observed in schizophrenic patients are produced by either direct or indirect DA agonists and by PCP and other noncompetitive NMDA antagonists (27). As in studies of schizophrenic patients, the effects are observed with both intramodal and cross-modal presentations of the prepulse and startle stimuli (8,27). In keeping with the corresponding model of psychoses in humans, the DA agonist effects are blocked by neuroleptics, and the NMDA antagonist effects are not (27). Indeed, impressive correlations have been found between the clinical efficacy of antipsychotic drugs in patients and their ability to reduce the disruptive effects of the DA agonist apomorphine on PPI (68). Even the ability of the atypical antipsychotic clozapine to block the effects of a DA agonist in this paradigm is predictive of its clinical efficacy (68). Furthermore, with appropriate test parameters, clozapine can improve PPI in otherwise untreated rats (70). This result parallels the preliminary finding that clozapine treatment tends to normalize PPI deficits in schizophrenic patients (82). Thus, the model has considerable predictive validity, in addition to construct and convergent validity (20,68). In this case, the predictive validity of the model is derived from both parametric similarities and pharmacological isomorphism.

There are two respects in which the model could be considered to have failed to exhibit discriminant validity. First, one could require that the model discriminate abnormalities in schizophrenia from other psychiatric disorders. Such a requirement would not be met by the model because deficits in PPI have also been found in disorders such as obsessive–compulsive disorder (67). Nevertheless, this model is a theoretically derived model that purports to investigate an abnormality in a neuropsychological process that is not necessarily specific to schizophrenia. The lack of discriminant validity in terms of currently accepted psychiatric diagnoses does not invalidate the usefulness of the model for the study of sensorimotor gating. Similarly, one could ask that the model discriminate the effects of DA agonists and NMDA antagonists from other drugs that do not appear to produce psychotic symptoms in humans. Evidence that 5-HT_{1A} and other 5-HT agonists disrupt PPI in rats (59,66) speaks against such discriminant validity for the model. Furthermore, extensive studies of the neurobiological substrates that modulate PPI in rats have revealed that multiple neurotransmitter systems influence this form of sensorimotor gating, including dopaminergic, serotonergic, glutamatergic, γ-aminobutyric acid-ergic (GABAergic), and cholinergic pathways (27,59,69). Similarly, the animal version of the ERP sensory gating model is reportedly sensitive to dopaminergic, noradrenergic, and cholinergic manipulations (1,24). Hence, if one evaluates the gating models strictly with respect to the prevailing DA hypothesis of schizophrenia, the models appear to be overinclusive. Alternatively, it has been suggested that the multiple determinants of PPI in rats may ultimately be related to the multiple subtypes of schizophrenia (26) and that the observation of gating deficits in nonschizophrenic patients may reflect abnormalities in different parts of the limbic–striatal circuitry that work in concert to enable the appropriate filtering of sensory and cognitive events (69). The viability of such possibilities illustrates why discriminant

validity is seldom required of an animal model of psychopathology intended to explore a hypothetical construct.

The above animal models of gating disturbances all relied on pharmacological treatments to produce the deficit observed in patient populations. Accordingly, they derive much of their support from high degrees of pharmacological isomorphism. Some newer models relevant to schizophrenia have sought to avoid this reliance on behaviors induced by drugs. For example, deficits in PPI of startle have been demonstrated to result from socially isolating rats from weaning until after puberty (28). Social isolation of rats in early stages of development has been used to produce a variety of behavioral abnormalities that have been related to both schizophrenia and depression (44). Recent studies have shown that 6 to 8 weeks of social isolation during development, but not during adulthood (78), produces deficits in PPI that are at least partially reversible by the administration of a DA antagonist (28). Because schizophrenia commonly emerges in early adulthood, developmental factors have provided the basis for some etiological hypotheses (57,75). Hence, further study of the gating deficits produced by isolation rearing of rats may establish a nonpharmacological and developmentally relevant animal model of the gating deficits observed in schizophrenic patients. Potentially, in contrast to the drug-induced models of gating deficits, such a model might have etiological validity and might be sensitive to antipsychotic drugs having novel mechanisms of action.

CONCLUSIONS

Even though there may be no perfect animal models, it is clear that each model has strengths and limitations that need to be recognized in order to use the model effectively in the investigation of psychiatric disorders. Therefore, multiple animal models are needed for each psychiatric disorder to allow investigation of the various aspects of the disease and to provide convergent validation of the research findings. Furthermore, each model is useful for a specific purpose, for example, the identification of potential pharmacotherapies or the investigation of a specific hypothetical construct. The validation criteria that each model has to meet to demonstrate its usefulness in neurobiological research are determined by the defined purpose of the model. Ultimately, however, the degree to which the performance of the model allows accurate predictions to be made about the human condition, or predictive validity, is the only necessary and scientifically meaningful criterion for the validation of any animal model. As a result, it is critical that objectively defined abnormalities characteristic of the disorder in question be identified to provide the focus for the development of animal models. Thus, the process of developing and validating animal models must work in concert with the process of identifying reliable measures of the human phenomenology.

ACKNOWLEDGMENTS

This work was supported by a Research Scientist Development Award from the National Institute of Mental Health to MAG (MH00188) and an Individual NRSA Fellowship from the National Institute on Drug Abuse to AM (DA05444).

REFERENCES

1. Adler LE, Rose G, Freedman R. Neurophysiological studies of sensory gating in rats: effects of amphetamine, phencyclidine, and haloperidol. *Biol Psychiatry* 1986;21:787–798.
2. Ahlenius S. The "Clever Hans" phenomenon in animal models of schizophrenia, or homology as an important factor in comparing behavioral functions across species. *Persp Biol Med* 1991;34:219–225.
3. American Psychological Association. *Technical recommendations for psychological tests and diagnostic techniques.* Washington, DC: APA; 1954.
4. Bolino F, Manna V, DiCicco L. Startle reflex habituation in functional psychoses: a controlled study. *Neurosci Lett* 1992;145:126–128.
5. Boring EG. The use of operational definitions in science. *Psychol Rev* 1945;52:243–245.
6. Bowers MB, Freedman DX. "Psychedelic" experiences in acute psychoses. *Arch Gen Psychiatry* 1966;15:240–248.
7. Braff DL, Geyer MA. Sensorimotor gating and schizophrenia: human and animal model studies. *Arch Gen Psychiatry* 1990;47:181–188.
8. Braff DL, Grillon C, Geyer MA. Gating and habituation of the startle reflex in schizophrenic patients. *Arch Gen Psychiatry* 1992;49:206–215.
9. Brewin CR. Depression and causal attributions: what is their relation? *Psychological Bull* 1985;98:297–309.
10. Bridgman PW. Some general principles of operational analysis. *Psychol Rev* 1945;52:246–249.
11. Buckwald AM, Coyne JC, Cole CS. A critical evaluation of the learned helplessness model of depression. *J Abnorm Psychol* 1978;87:180–193.
12. Cadenhead KS, Geyer MA, Braff DL. Impaired startle prepulse inhibition and habituation in schizotypal patients. *Am J Psychiatry* 1993;150:1862–1867.
13. Campbell DT, Fiske DW. Convergent and discriminant validation by the multitrait-multimethod matrix. *Psychol Bull* 1959;56:81–105.
14. Creese I, ed. *Stimulants: neurochemical, behavioral, and clinical perspectives.* New York: Raven Press; 1983.
15. Cornell DG, Milden RS, Shimp A. Stressful life events associated with endogenous depression. *J Nerv Ment Dis* 1985;173:470–476.
16. Cronbach LJ, Meehl PE. Construct validity in psychological tests. *Psychol Bull* 1955;52:281–302.
17. DePablo JM, Ortiz-Caro J, Sanchez-Santed F, Guillamon A. Effects of diazepam, pentobarbital, scopolamine, and the timing of saline injection on learned immobility in rats. *Physiol Behav* 1991;50:895–899.
18. DePablo JM, Parra A, Segovia S, Guillamon A. Learned immobility explains the behavior of rats in the forced swimming test. *Physiol Behav* 1989;46:229–237.
19. Drugan RC, Skolnick P, Paul SM, Crawley JN. A pretest procedure reliably predicts performance in two animal models of inescapable stress. *Pharmacol Biochem Behav* 1989;33:649–654.
20. Ellenbroek BA, Cools AR. Animal models with construct validity for schizophrenia. *Behav Pharmacol* 1990;1:469–490.
21. Ellinwood EH, Sudilovsky A, Nelson L. Evolving behavior in the clinical and experimental amphetamine (model) psychoses. *Am J Psychiatry* 1973;130:1088.
22. Embretson (Whitely) S. Construct validity: construct representation versus nomothetic span. *Psychol Bull* 1983;93:179–197.
23. Fibiger HC, Phillips AG. Increased intracranial self-stimulation in rats after long-term administration of desipramine. *Science* 1981;214:683–685.
24. Freedman R, Mirsky AF. Event-related potentials: exogenous components. In: Steinhauer SR, Gruzelier JH, Zubin J, eds. *Handbook of schizophrenia. Volume 5: neuropsychology, psychophysiology and information processing.* Amsterdam: Elsevier Science Publishers, 1991;71–90.
25. Gawin FH, Kleber HD. Cocaine abuse treatment. Open pilot trial with desipramine and lithium carbonate. *Arch Gen Psychiatry* 1984;41:903–909.
26. Geyer MA, Braff DL. Startle habituation and sensorimotor gating in schizophrenia and related animal models. *Schizophr Bull* 1987;13:643–668.
27. Geyer MA, Swerdlow NR, Mansbach RS, Braff DL. Startle response models of sensorimotor gating and habituation deficits in schizophrenia. *Brain Res Bull* 1990;25:485–498.
28. Geyer MA, Wilkinson LS, Humby T, Robbins TW. Isolation rearing of rats produces a deficit in prepulse inhibition of acoustic startle similar to that in schizophrenia. *Biol Psychiatry* 1993;34:361–372.
29. Geyer MA, Segal DS, Greenberg BD. Increased startle responding in rats treated with phencyclidine. *Neurobehav Toxicol Terat* 1984;6:1–4.
30. Giannini AJ, Folts DJ, Feather JN, Sullivan BS. Bromocriptine and amantadine in cocaine detoxification. *Brain Res* 1989;29:11–16.
31. Gillin JC, Cannon E, Magyar R, Schwartz M, Wyatt RJ. Failure of *N,N*-dimethyltryptamine to evoke tolerance in cats. *Biol Psychiatry* 1973;7:213–220.
32. Glazer HI, Weiss JM. Long-term interference effect: an alternative to "learned helplessness". *J Exp Psychol Anim Behav Proc* 1976;2:201–213.
33. Glennon RA, Titeler M, McKenney JD. Evidence for 5-HT₂ involvement in the mechanism of action of hallucinogenic agents. *Life Sci* 1984;24:2505–2511.
34. Green AR. Evolving concepts on the interactions between antidepressant treatments and monoamine neurotransmitters. *Neuropharmacology* 1987;26:815–822.
35. Hammen CL, Cochran SD. Cognitive correlates of life stress and depression in college students. *J Abnorm Psychol* 1981;90:23–27.
36. Hinde RA. The use of differences and similarities in comparative psychopathology. In: G Serban and A Kling, eds. *Animal models in psychobiology.* New York: Plenum Press; 1976:187–202.
37. Hollister LE. *Chemical psychoses: LSD and related drugs.* Springfield, IL: Charles Thomas, 1968.
38. Hume D. *Hume selections,* CW Hendel, Jr, ed. Amsterdam: Charles Scribner's Sons, 1955.
39. Javitt DC, Zukin SR. Recent advances in the phencyclidine model of schizophrenia. *Am J Psychiatry* 1991;148:1301–1308.
40. Joyce EM. The amphetamine model of schizophrenia: a critique. *Anim Models Psychiatr Disord* 1988;2:89–100.
41. Joyce JN, Shane A, Lexow N, Winokur A, Casanova MF, Kleinman JE. Serotonin uptake sites and serotonin receptors are altered in the limbic system of schizophrenics. *Neuropsychopharmacology* 1993;8:315–336.
42. Kokkinidis L, McCarter BD. Postcocaine depression and sensitization of brain-stimulation reward: analysis of reinforcement and performance effects. *Pharmacol Biochem Behav* 1990;36:463–471.
43. Kokkinidis L, Zacharko RM, Predy PA. Post-amphetamine depression of self-stimulation responding from the substantia nigra: reversal by tricyclic antidepressants. *Pharmacol Biochem Behav* 1980;13:379–383.
44. Kornetsky C, Markowitz R. Animal models of schizophrenia. In: Lipton MA, DiMascio A, Killam KF, eds. *Psychopharmacology: a generation of progress.* New York: Raven Press; 1978:583–593.
45. Liebman JM, Cooper SJ. *The neuropharmacological basis of reward.* Oxford: Clarendon Press; 1989.
46. Maier SF, Testa TJ. Failure to learn to escape by rats previously exposed to inescapable shock is partly produced by associative interference. *J Comp Physiol Psychol* 1975;88:554–564.

47. Maier SF, Seligman MEP. Learned helplessness: theory and evidence. *J Exp Psychol (Gen)* 1976;1:3–46.
48. Markou A, Koob GF. Postcocaine anhedonia: an animal model of cocaine withdrawal. *Neuropsychopharmacology* 1991;4:17–26.
49. Markou A, Koob GF. Construct validity of a self-stimulation threshold paradigm: effects of reward and performance manipulations. *Physiol Behav* 1992;51:111–119.
50. Markou A, Koob GF. Bromocriptine reverses the elevation in intracranial self-stimulation thresholds observed in a rat model of cocaine withdrawal. *Neuropsychopharmacology* 1992;7:213–224.
51. Markou A, Hauger RL, Koob GF. Desmethylimipramine attenuates cocaine withdrawal in rats. *Psychopharmacology* 1992;109:305–314.
52. Markou A, Weiss F, Gold LH, Caine SB, Schulteis G, Koob GF. Animal models of drug craving. *Psychopharmacology* 1993;112:163–182.
53. Matthysse S. Animal models in psychiatric research. *Prog Brain Res* 1986;65:259–270.
54. McKinney WT, Bunney WE. Animal model of depression. *Arch Gen Psychiatry* 1969;21:240–248.
55. Meltzer HY, Matsubara S, Lee JC. Classification of typical and atypical antipsychotic drugs on the basis of dopamine D-1, D-2 and serotonin2 pKi values. *J Pharmacol Exp Ther* 1989;251:238–246.
56. Mosier CI. A critical examination of the concepts of face validity. *Educ Psychol Measurement* 1947;7:191–205.
57. Murray RM, Lewis SW. Is schizophrenia a neurodevelopmental disorder? *Br Med J* 1987;295:681–682.
58. O'Neil KA, Valentino D. Escapability and generalization: effect on 'behavioral despair.' *Eur J Pharmacol* 1982;78:379–380.
59. Rigdon GC, Weatherspoon J. 5HT1A receptor agonists block prepulse inhibition of the acoustic startle reflex. *J Pharmacol Exp Ther* 1992;263:486–493.
60. Rosenberg DE, Isbell H, Miner EJ, Logan CR. The effect of N,N-dimethyltryptamine in human subjects tolerant to lysergic acid diethylamide. *Psychopharmacologia* 1964;5:217–227.
61. Russell RW. *The comparative study of behavior.* London: HK Lewis; 1951.
62. Schwarzkopf SB, Lamberti JS, Smith DA. Concurrent assessment of acoustic startle and auditory P50 evoked potential measures of sensory inhibition. *Biol Psychiatry* 1993;33:806–814.
63. Segal DS, Geyer MA. Animal models of psychopathology. In: Judd LL, Groves PM, eds. *Psychobiological foundations of clinical psychiatry.* Philadelphia: JB Lippincott; 1985: Chap. 45.
64. Segal DS, Geyer MA, Schuckit A. Stimulant-induced psychosis: an evaluation of animal models. In: Youdim MBH, Lovenberg W, Sharman DF, Lagnado JR, eds. *Essays in neurochemistry and neuropharmacology,* Vol. 5. New York: John Wiley; 1981:95–130.
65. Simons RF, Giardina BD. Reflex modification in psychosis-prone young adults. *Psychophysiology* 1992;29:8–16.
66. Sipes TA, Geyer MA. Multiple serotonin receptor subtypes modulate prepulse inhibition of the startle response in rats. *Neuropharmacology* 1994;33:441–448.
67. Swerdlow NR, Benbow CH, Zisook S, Geyer MA, Braff DL. A preliminary assessment of sensorimotor gating in patients with obsessive compulsive disorder. *Biol Psychiatry* 1993;33:298–301.
68. Swerdlow NR, Braff DL, Taaid N, Geyer MA. Assessing the validity of an animal model of deficient sensorimotor gating in schizophrenic patients. *Arch Gen Psychiatry* 1994;51:139–154.
69. Swerdlow NR, Caine SB, Braff DL, Geyer MA. Neural substrates of sensorimotor gating of the startle reflex: preclinical findings and their implications. *J Psychopharmacol* 1992;6:176–190.
70. Swerdlow NR, Geyer MA. Clozapine and haloperidol in an animal model of sensorimotor gating deficits in schizophrenia. *Pharmacol Biochem Behav* 1993;44:741–744.
71. Swerdlow NR, Keith VA, Braff DL, Geyer MA. The effects of spiperone, SCH 23390 and clozapine on apomorphine-inhibition of sensorimotor gating of the startle response in the rat. *J Pharmacol Exp Ther* 1991;256:530–536.
72. Valentino DA, Dufresne RL, Riccitelli AJ. Effects of a single inescapable swim on long-term brain stimulation reward thresholds. *Physiol Behav* 1990;48:215–219.
73. Weddington WW, Brown BS, Haertzen CA, et al. Changes in mood, craving, and sleep during short-term abstinence reported by male cocaine addicts. *Arch Gen Psychiatry* 1990;47:861–868.
74. Weil-Malherbe H, Szara SI. *The biochemistry of functional and experimental psychoses.* Springfield, IL: Charles Thomas; 1971.
75. Weinberger DR. Implications of normal brain development for the pathogenesis of schizophrenia. *Arch Gen Psychiatry* 1987;44:660–669.
76. Weiss JM, Simson PE. Neurochemical and electrophysiological events underlying stress-induced depression in an animal model. *Adv Exp Med Biol* 1988;245:425–440.
77. West AP. Neurobehavioral studies of forced swimming: the role of learning and memory in the forced swim test. *Prog Neuropsychopharmacol Biol Psychiatry* 1990;14:863–877.
78. Wilkinson LS, Killcross AS, Humby T, et al. Social isolation produces developmentally specific deficits in prepulse inhibition of the acoustic startle response but does not disrupt latent inhibition. *Neuropsychopharmacology* 1994;10:61–72.
79. Willner P. The validity of animal models of depression. *Psychopharmacology* 1984;83:1–16.
80. Willner P. Validation criteria for animal models of human mental disorders: learned helplessness as a paradigm case. *Prog Neuropsychopharmacol Biol Psychiatry* 1986;10:677–690.
81. Willner P, Towell A, Sampson D, Sophokleous S, Muscat R. Reduction of sucrose preference by chronic unpredictable mild stress, and its restoration by a tricyclic antidepressant. *Psychopharmacology* 1987;93:358–364.
82. Wu JC, Potkin SG, Ploszaj DI, Lau V, Telford J, Richmond G. Clozapine improves sensory gating more than haldol. *APA Abstr* 1992;156.
83. Zacharko RM, Bowers WJ, Kelley MS, Anisman H. Prevention of stressor-induced disturbances of self-stimulation by desmethylimipramine. *Brain Res* 1984;321:175–179.

*Psychopharmacology: The Fourth
Generation of Progress*, edited by
Floyd E. Bloom and David J. Kupfer.
Raven Press, Ltd., New York © 1995.

CHAPTER 69

Genetic Strategies in Preclinical Substance Abuse Research

John C. Crabbe, Jr. and Ting-Kai Li

It is increasingly accepted that there may be a genetic predisposition to abuse drugs. This is clearest for alcoholism, where recent studies suggest that two (or more) diagnostically distinct forms of alcoholism may be influenced by different patterns of inheritance (17). As this review indicates, genetic control probably extends to other drugs of abuse as well. However, predispositions are not inherited; rather, one inherits *genes,* and the number and identity of genes whose gene products increase susceptibility to drugs remain unknown.

The expense and limitations inherent in human genetic research have led to a great increase in the use of genetic animal models to elucidate the pathways from genes to behavior. This chapter deals with preclinical research and almost entirely with genetic animal models. The intent is not to review existing data exhaustively, as in a recent volume (21). Rather, we wish to indicate strategies that have been fruitfully employed in recent years, and highlight future applications in this area. Data exist indicating genetic influences on responses to virtually all drugs of abuse. In roughly declining order with respect to the amount and quality of interpretable genetic research, responses to drugs of abuse from these classes have been shown to have substantial genotypic determinants: ethanol, opiates, and nicotine; psychostimulants and depressants; benzodiazepines; caffeine, hallucinogens, and organic solvents. We draw informative examples, generally from studies with drugs of the first group. A recent review has addressed studies of nicotine, cocaine, and opiates (60; see also Chapters 66, 153, and 155, *this volume*).

J. C. Crabbe, Jr.: Departments of Medical Psychology and Pharmacology, Oregon Health Sciences University, and VA Medical Center, Portland, Oregon 97201.

T-K. Li: Departments of Medicine and Biochemistry, Indiana University School of Medicine, Indianapolis, Indiana 46202.

The primary question these studies attempt to address is are there inheritable predispositions to abuse drugs? This general question can better be approached by considering some of its elements. Relevant responses to be considered in analyzing genetic determinants of drug sensitivity include at least the following: innate (first-dose) sensitivity, which operationally often includes the development of within-session tolerance; chronic (2 doses or more) tolerance; dependence (i.e., withdrawal severity); reinforcing efficacy; and metabolism. For any given component response, there are several aspects of genetic influence we must distinguish. First, we need to ascertain how many genes are involved. Although biomedical disorders where a single gene is sufficient to induce disease have yielded to experimental dissection, the apparent situation in psychopharmacology is considerably more complex, and multiple genes are likely operative. Next, we need to ascertain the function of their protein products. Knowledge of their genomic location is also desirable for two reasons. This may allow the identification of markers of drug susceptibility, even if the function of that marker gene is not important for a drug abuse outcome. Second, mapping drug susceptibility genes may lead one to a chromosome region where an apparent candidate gene is located, which may then lead to an understanding of function. We also would like to determine how these susceptibility genes are regulated, and how they are modulated by environmental conditions. If strictly genetic therapies are unlikely, such knowledge may allow therapeutic interventions at levels higher than the genome.

The current state of the art in psychopharmacogenetics provides no clear and shining example that can be traced from a single gene to a drug-related behavioral endpoint, with all the questions posed above answered. Nonetheless, significant advances have been made, and new approaches offer great promise that this outcome will be achieved.

TWO STANDARD METHODS IN GENETIC ANIMAL MODEL RESEARCH

Artificial selection for traits of relevance to understanding drug abuse represents a major historical contribution of genetic animal model research. Lines of mice and rats have been systematically mated to respond characteristically to drugs of abuse using essentially the same techniques as those employed to breed animals for desired agricultural or esthetic characteristics. The genetic result of this procedure is to increase the frequencies of most genes affecting drug response positively in a high-response line, whereas those genes leading to low responsiveness become more frequent in a line bred for low

TABLE 1. *Lines selected for drug abuse-related traits*

Line/species	Selection phenotype	Replicates?[a]	Source[b]
Withdrawal Seizure Prone/Resistant mice (WSP/WSR)	Handling-induced convulsions after ethanol vapor inhalation	Yes	1
High/Low Ethanol Withdrawal mice (HW/LW)	Handling-induced convulsions after ethanol vapor inhalation	Yes	2
Preferring/Nonpreferring rats (P/NP)	Preference for drinking 10% ethanol	No	3
High/Low Alcohol Drinking rats (HAD/LAD)	Preference for drinking 10% ethanol	Yes	3
ALKO Alcohol/Nonalcohol rats (AA/ANA)	Preference for drinking 10% ethanol	No	4
Low/High ethanol consuming rats (UChA/UChB)	Preference for drinking 10% ethanol	No	5
Sardinian Preferring/Nonpreferring Rats (sP/sNP)	Preference for drinking 10% ethanol	No	6
High/Low Alcohol Preference mice (HAP/LAP)	Preference for drinking 10% ethanol	Yes	3
ALKO tolerant/nontolerant rats (AT/ANT)	Ethanol impairment of tilting-plane performance	No	4
Long/Short Sleep mice (LS/SS)	Duration of loss of righting reflex after ethanol	No	2
High/Low Alcohol Sensitive rats (HAS/LAS)	Duration of loss of righting reflex after ethanol	Yes	7
COLD/HOT mice	Acute ethanol hypothermia	Yes	1
FAST/SLOW mice	Ethanol-stimulated open-field activity	Yes	1
High/Low Alcohol Functional Tolerance mice (HAFT/LAFT)	Acute ethanol functional tolerance on stationary rod balancing	Yes	2
High/Low Analgesic Response mice (HAR/LAR)	Levorphanol analgesia in the hot-plate test	No	1
High/Low Stress-Induced Analgesia (HA/LA)	Analgesia induced by cold water swim stress	No	8
Diazepam Sensitive/Resistant mice (DS/DR)	Diazepam-induced rotarod ataxia	No	1
Diazepam High/Low Responders (DHR/DHL)	Diazepam-induced rotarod ataxia	Yes	1
High/Low Diazepam Sensitive mice	Diazepam-induced loss of righting reflex	No	9
Flinders Sensitive/Resistant rats (FS/FR)	Diisopropylflurophosphate hypothermia	No	10
Neuroleptic Responder/Nonresponder mice (NR/NNR)	Haloperidol-induced catalepsy	Yes	11

[a] Replicates? The existence of genetically distinct duplicate selected lines. Thus, there are two WSP (WSP-1 and WSP-2) and two WSR (WSR-1 and WSR-2) lines. Adapted and updated from ref. 20a.

[b] Sources for selected lines:

1. Animal Research Facility, Research Service (151Z), VA Medical Center, Portland, OR, 97201.
2. Institute for Behavioral Genetics, University of Colorado, Box 447, Boulder, CO, 80309.
3. Department of Medicine, Indiana University, Emerson Hall 421, 545 Barnhill Drive, Indianapolis, IN, 46202.
4. ALKO Research Laboratories, PO Box 350, SF-10100 Helsinki 10, Finland.
5. Departamento de Farmacologia, Universidad de Chile, PO Box 70.000, Santiago 9, Chile.
6. Department of Experimental Biology, University of Cagliari, Via Palabanda 12, Cagliari, Italy 09123.
7. Department of Pharmacology (C-236), Univ. Colorado Health Sciences Ctr., 4200 E. Ninth Avenue, Denver, CO, 80262.
8. Department of Psychology, University of California-Los Angeles, Los Angeles, CA 91024.
9. Department of Pharmacology, Faculty of Medicine, National Univ. of Singapore, Singapore 0511.
10. Center for Alcohol Studies, University of North Carolina, Chapel Hill, North Carolina, 27514.
11. Department of Psychiatry, State University of New York, Stony Brook, NY, 11794.

response. In contrast, the other standard method is to examine multiple existing inbred strains of animals. An inbred strain results after more than 20 generations of brother-sister matings. After inbreeding, all members of an inbred strain are genetically identical, and, for each gene, a single allele has been fixed homozygous. Which particular alleles are fixed in a given inbred strain is the result of chance, in contrast to selected lines. More than one hundred inbred strains of mice and rats are commercially available. Uses of these techniques are complementary, and will be discussed in turn.

Selective Breeding

The successful development of selected lines provides a population in which tests for genetically correlated traits can be performed. To the extent that several stringent criteria are approached (see ref. 28), any other difference between a pair of selected lines is presumed to be due to the common influence, or pleiotropism, of the genes determining the selected response. Selective breeding has been most widely used to select for ethanol-related traits, but has also been employed for opioids, benzodiazepines, and other psychoactive drugs. Lines that are no longer maintained have been bred for sensitivity to barbiturates, nicotine, and cocaine. Table 1 summarizes the currently available lines selectively bred for traits related to drug abuse. In most cases, lines have been bred for acute sensitivity of naive animals to a particular drug or for ethanol preference drinking.

Although the technique of selective breeding is extremely powerful for pharmacological analyses, it also has limitations. These studies are expensive to perform with appropriate controls; without them, the results can be very difficult to interpret. Guidelines for use and interpretation of data derived from selected lines have been suggested elsewhere (28). There are two principal limitations of interpreting studies with selected lines. One is that they are available for only some responses. For example, no lines are currently available that have been bred successfully for enhanced or attenuated drug tolerance (although a selection for and against acute functional ethanol tolerance is underway (Dr. V. G. Erwin, *personal communication*). A second caveat is that older sets of selected lines were often not produced under ideal genetic conditions: they were typically not duplicated (replicated), and relatively small numbers were maintained, which led to high levels of random inbreeding at genes unrelated to the selected trait. These deficiencies lead to an increased risk of false-positive findings in the search for other genetically related traits differentiating the lines. When lines are replicated, frequently a difference is found only between one of a pair of replicate lines; this suggests that the genetic difference underlying this seemingly cor-

related response may have arisen by chance fixation of some alleles due to inbreeding. Newer sets of selected lines are usually being developed with greater recognition of these problems, which has increased their interpretability. The best solution is to verify differences between selected lines using other pharmacogenetic methods, such as studies with inbred strains (see the next section), but few investigators have taken the trouble and expense to do this. Some insights gained from the study of three sets of selected lines for which there are fairly extensive data will be reviewed.

Withdrawal Seizure-Prone and -Resistant Mouse Lines

One animal model has been developed for differential genetic susceptibility to ethanol withdrawal (22). Chronic exposure to ethanol vapor for 3 days was followed by assessment of withdrawal for 24 hours, using the handling-induced convulsion. Each generation, Withdrawal Seizure-Prone (WSP) mice with the most severe withdrawal scores were mated to form the next generation, whereas Withdrawal Seizure-Resistant (WSR) mice with the lowest scores were similarly mated *inter se* to produce the WSR line. There are two WSP and two WSR lines. In a direct comparison of WSP and WSR mice from selected generation S_{25}, there was no overlap between the two pairs of selected lines (22).

Several interesting results have emerged in studies of these lines. Although WSP and WSR mice were selected strictly for differences in alcohol withdrawal severity, WSP mice have more severe withdrawal than WSR mice after chronic intoxication with diazepam, phenobarbital, and nitrous oxide (7,22). WSP mice have become so sensitive to withdrawal that a single intraperitoneal injection of ethanol (4 g/kg) produced a rebound exacerbation of the handling-induced convulsion, which reached maximum several hours after injection, and WSP and WSR mice are differentially sensitive to acute withdrawal from pentobarbital, diazepam, acetaldehyde, or tertiary butanol (25). Together, these results strongly suggest that a group of genes acts to influence drug withdrawal severity, not only to ethanol but also to a number of other depressants. Corroborative experiments are discussed in a later section.

Other studies with WSP and WSR mice have illuminated several neurochemical features of the ethanol withdrawal reaction; these have recently been reviewed (13,22). Chronic ethanol treatment has been found to produce a large increase in the number of dihydropyridine-sensitive calcium channel binding sites in whole-brain homogenates from WSP mice, versus a much smaller increase in WSR mice. Untreated WSP mice have dorsal hippocampal mossy fiber zinc content that is reduced by 70% as compared with WSR mice. The threshold sensitivity to seizures induced by tail-vein infusion of a number of convulsants is approximately 10% lower in WSP than in WSR mice (Kosobud and Crabbe, *unpublished*). A potentially important exception to this finding is the excitatory amino acid agonist, *N*-methyl-D-aspartate, which is more effective in WSR mice (51). WSP mice show enhanced sensitivity to excitatory amino acid receptor agonists and antagonists during acute ethanol withdrawal (26); these results support other indications that excitatory amino acid receptor-coupled ion channels are important regulators of ethanol withdrawal severity (40,41). Other studies implicate the γ-aminobutyric acid (GABA) system in the neuroadaptive responses accompanying ethanol dependence and withdrawal (1,12–14).

A striking finding in the WSP and WSR mice has been the genetic independence of the many different responses to ethanol (22). Withdrawal Seizure-Prone and -Resistant mice do not differ in sensitivity to ethanol's locomotor stimulant, hypnotic, or hypothermic effects. More surprisingly, after several doses of ethanol, WSP and WSR mice developed tolerance to the same degree. Ethanol withdrawal and preference drinking are probably largely unrelated at the genetic level in mice (52). In addition, WSP (but not WSR) mice develop a conditioned preference for a location paired with ethanol injections; thus two-bottle choice preference drinking and conditioned place preferences may not tap the same underlying substrate (presumably, reward) in mice (27). Deitrich and Spuhler (30) have discussed the strength of selected line models for excluding common mechanisms in cases where no correlated response to selection is found.

This pattern of results has made it clear that the genetic factors controlling ethanol sensitivity, tolerance, dependence, and drinking are independent. In turn, this strongly suggests that they are maintained to a significant degree by nonoverlapping neurobiological mechanisms. A replication of the WSP/WSR selection is underway (V. Gene Erwin, *personal communication*).

Rats Exhibiting Preference and Nonpreference for Ethanol and High and Low Alcohol Drinking

Rats were developed for preference and nonpreference, respectively, for 10% ethanol versus water. This is one of the older selection experiments in psychopharmacology, and it has recently been replicated through the development of two High Alcohol Drinking (HAD) and two Low Alcohol Drinking (LAD) lines (56). There are also several other sets of rodent lines developed using similar paradigms, including a set of mouse lines (HAP and LAP) under development (see Table 1). Thus, there is the opportunity for achieving convergent validity in the search for genetic correlates of ethanol drinking. This has been pursued most vigorously by the Indiana group. We

largely confine our discussion to major findings in the P/NP and HAD/LAD rat lines. Studies with ALKO Alcohol/Nonalcohol, (AA/ANA), Sardinian Preferring/Nonpreferring (sP/sNP), and low/high ethanol-consuming (UChA/UChB) rat lines have been reviewed elsewhere (32,72,79, and see Table 1).

Rats from the P line voluntarily drink 10% to 30% ethanol solutions in quantities that produce pharmacologically meaningful blood alcohol concentrations (59). With chronic drinking, both metabolic and neuronal tolerance, and physical withdrawal signs develop in the P rats. The P but not the NP rats will perform an operant response (bar-pressing) to obtain ethanol in concentrations as high as 30% for reasons other than the caloric value, taste, or smell of the ethanol solutions (66), and will self-administer substantial doses of ethanol (62,83). The difference in self-administration is not absolute, for NP rats will maintain substantial levels of self-administration of ethanol after initiation (e.g., by initial adulteration with sucrose, followed by fading of sucrose until only ethanol is self-administered). The pattern of self-administration, however, is clearly quite different for the P and NP rats (74), and these selected lines clearly differ in their avidity for ethanol.

Comparison of P and NP rats has revealed several other differences. The P rats are more sensitive to stimulation by low doses of ethanol and are less affected by sedative-hypnotic doses of ethanol. They are less sensitive to ethanol's aversive properties and develop tolerance to ethanol's ataxic properties more quickly; this tolerance persists for a much longer period of time in P than NP rats (56). The P rats have lower levels of serotonin (5-HT) and dopamine (DA) in some brain regions (67), particularly the nucleus accumbens (68). Densities of 5-HT receptors in some regions (cerebral cortex and hippocampus) have been found to be higher in P rats; in addition, immunocytochemical studies reveal fewer 5-HT fibers in the affected regions of P than NP rats (56).

Ethanol drinking in the P rats is suppressed by 5-HT uptake inhibitors, DA agonists, DA uptake inhibitors, the GABA inverse agonist Ro 15-4513, and opioid receptor antagonists (56,63). Thus, although the most obvious neuroanatomical/neurochemical difference between the P and NP lines appears to involve 5-HT neurons, other neurotransmitter systems, perhaps through interaction with the 5-HT and DA pathways of the limbic-forebrain system, are also important in regulating alcohol self-administration.

Initial sensitivity to locomotor stimulant effects of ethanol, and within-session or acute tolerance to ethanol ataxia, are by far the most generalizable and robust responses to ethanol found in association with ethanol preference. The P, HAD, and AA rats exhibit increased spontaneous locomotor activity with low dose ethanol, and are more able to develop tolerance with exposure to a single sedative/hypnotic dose of ethanol, in contrast with NP, LAD, and ANA rats (54,56). Tolerance and preference were also correlated in eight inbred rat strains (80), and in individual HS/Ibg heterogenous stock mice with high and low ethanol preference (33). However, alcohol-preferring C57BL mice are insensitive to ethanol stimulation, and alcohol-nonpreferring DBA mice are very sensitive to this response, which is inconsistent with the rat studies, and studies of their relative propensities to develop tolerance to ethanol's ataxic effects have been variable (72). Both P and AA rats also exhibit a greater preference for oral consumption of sweet solutions than the NP and ANA rats.

Relatively low brain contents of 5-HT have been reported for alcohol-preferring C57BL inbred mice and Fawn-Hooded rats, and HAD rats have lower contents of 5-HT and DA in the limbic forebrain regions of their brains than respective alcohol nonpreferrers (56), but the AA and ANA lines apparently do not differ in brain 5-HT content (50). Both the P and sP rats are more sensitive than are the NP, Wistar, and sNP rats in ethanol-stimulated DA release from the nucleus accumbens. Both P and sP rats also have fewer dopamine D2 receptors in various limbic-forebrain regions than the NP and sNP rats (61,81). Clearly, more systematic study of the selected lines (and the HAP and LAP mouse lines when they are ready) for associated behavioral and neurobiological traits can provide important understanding of the underlying mechanisms of ethanol reinforcement.

Long/Short Sleep Mice and High/Low Alcohol Sensitive Rats

The Long Sleep (LS) and Short Sleep (SS) mice were among the first selected lines in pharmacogenetics. The LS and SS mice differ markedly in response to the hypnotic effects of ethanol (64), and well over one hundred papers now report differences between these lines in behavioral, physiological, pharmacological, and biochemical traits. In the same way that the success of the P/NP selection led to its replication with HAD/LAD rats, interest in the LS/SS mice has been followed by the production of replicated pairs of high alcohol-sensitive (HAS) and low alcohol-sensitive (LAS) rats differing in an equivalent response. The LS/SS mice have also been frequently studied for their nicotine responsiveness (see ref. 18). Studies with LS and SS mice have recently been comprehensively reviewed (21), and studies relating GABA function to ethanol's sedative effects are discussed in a later section.

Other Selected Lines

Many other lines have been selected for drug-related traits. Reasonably comprehensive reviews of their use

may be found (21). High analgesic response (HAR) and low analgesic response (LAR) lines have been bred for high and low sensitivity to levorphanol using the hot-plate assay of analgesia (4). After more than 15 generations of selective breeding, the two lines differed by approximately sevenfold in their analgesic sensitivity to intraperitoneal (ip) levorphanol or morphine, and about 67-fold to intracerebroventricular (icv) [D-Ala^2-,NMePhe^4,Gly-ol^5]-enkephalin (DAMGO), a specific μ-opioid receptor agonist. These lines differ predominantly for μ receptor-mediated responses, but differ relatively little in response to κ or δ agonists on the hot-plate assay (4). Receptor autoradiographic studies reveal a 150% to 200% greater [^{3}H]DAMGO binding density in HAR mice in the dorsal raphé nucleus, but only small differences (16%) were seen in the periaqueductal gray, an area more traditionally associated with pain sensitivity (8).

Diazepam-sensitive (DS) mice, bred for sensitivity to the rotarod ataxia induced by diazepam, are responsive to about tenfold lower doses than the diazepam-resistant (DR) line (36). Studies with these lines have been reviewed (34), and development of a replicated pair of diazepam-sensitive (DLP) and resistant (DHP) lines is underway (E. Gallaher, *personal communication*).

Summary

A number of selective breeding studies have thus revealed both the power of the approach to address psychopharmacological problems and a number of pitfalls to be avoided in future research. The theoretical importance of the hedonic properties of drugs in determining human susceptibility to drug abuse has variously been described as failure to avoid, or uncontrollable tendency to approach, the drug. Animal models for reinforcing properties are notoriously difficult to work with, but the success of studies with oral self-administration suggests that it might be timely to undertake a selection project to develop rodent lines differing in sensitivity to the hedonic properties of drugs. A number of choices exist (e.g., stimulated or sensitized open-field activity; conditioned place preference and aversion; effects of drug on threshold for intracranial self-stimulation; and conditioned taste aversion). Since most data support a prominent role for DA systems in reinforcement mechanisms (see Koob, ref. 48), a set of mouse lines selected for their sensitivity to haloperidol catalepsy may prove to be useful (43). A number of differences have been documented between Neuroleptic Responder and Nonresponder (NR/NNR) mice in dopaminergic and cholinergic systems of the basal ganglia (44).

Psychopharmacological agents of abuse typically have a biphasic effect, that is, they are positively reinforcing at lower doses but becoming aversive at high doses.

Hence, it is believed that the development of acute and chronic tolerance to the aversive actions of the drug is an important, if not essential, feature to model. If needed, tandem selection could be employed to develop a model that manifests both high reinforcing responses to the drug and tolerance development to the aversive effects of the drug. Selecting for ethanol preference, however, appears to have accomplished this goal in some of the developed lines (e.g., the P and NP lines). To what extent the other selected lines (e.g., HAD and LAD) behave similarly in magnitudes of responsiveness remains to be established.

No models currently exist for a number of other interesting behavioral traits. For example, drug-induced aggression is not modeled, nor are the potential anxiolytic effects of drugs. Finally, it might be of interest to develop genetic animal models that recapitulate particular factors thought to enhance risk to abuse drugs, such as impulsivity. In this regard, the finding of Schuckit and colleagues (75) that sensitivity to an alcohol challenge in humans can predict future alcohol abuse/dependence suggests that this direction of research will be fruitful.

Inbred Strains

Because each member of an inbred strain is genetically identical to all other members of that strain, if the variation in means among the inbred strain exceeds that within strains (which is essentially nongenetic), this demonstrates the presence of significant genetic control of the trait. Genetic influence has been demonstrated for all drug responses studied (for reviews, see refs. 21, 60, 78). Such findings imply that other genetic methods such as selective breeding may be fruitfully applied to study drug-related traits.

A second use of inbred strains is to estimate the strength of genetic correlation. For example, strains showing a high degree of initial sensitivity to ethanol-induced hypothermia also tend to develop tolerance to this effect when ethanol is chronically administered. Patterns of correlation among inbred strains for a number of alcohol-related traits have revealed a pattern of genetic codetermination of sensitivity to some traits (e.g., hypnosis, depression of locomotor activity), and a fair degree of genetic independence of different groups of responses (20,23). The genetic stability of inbred strains (across laboratories and across time) offers an enormous advantage to the experimenter. Data sets on a common battery of standard inbred strains are cumulative, and allow the pooled expertise and resources of multiple laboratories to accrue a common data base. For three inbred strains of mice (C57BL/6, BALB/c, and DBA/2), a rather large data base has been accrued for many responses to drugs of abuse, and these have been recently reviewed (21). A recent collaborative effort has undertaken to characterize several responses

to ethanol, diazepam, pentobarbital, phenobarbital, and morphine in a panel of 15 mouse strains. Sensitivity to morphine hypothermia and morphine-induced depression of activity were found to be correlated (10). In contrast, several responses to diazepam were genetically uncorrelated (35). Preference drinking of ethanol and morphine were genetically correlated across strains, but preference for diazepam solutions was unrelated to either (5,6). Acute withdrawal severity between ethanol and pentobarbital was correlated, as was that between pentobarbital and diazepam, but the diazepam and ethanol withdrawal severities were unrelated (65).

In general, such studies offer evidence for common genetic determination of specific clusters of drug response variables and provide insight into neurobiological mechanisms underlying mechanisms of action. Inbred strain studies and studies with selected lines offer two independent methods for assessing genetic correlations, and the use of both methods is increasing.

FUTURE DIRECTIONS

Candidate Gene Approaches

The GABA$_A$-Benzodiazepine Receptor-Coupled Chloride Channel

Recent advances in molecular biology are of great potential importance for exploiting existing genetic animal models. The wealth of pharmacological and behavioral data available on some model systems has suggested areas where particular genes appear to be good candidates for further study. For example, recent reviews summarize a great deal of work implicating the GABA-benzodiazepine receptor complex as potentially important for mediating several effects of ethanol (1,13). Thus, there is a candidate gene family (those genes coding for GABA$_A$ receptor complex proteins) for molecular biological investigation.

Pharmacological manipulations with GABA agonists and antagonists affect ethanol sensitivity, and LS mice were more sensitive to such manipulations than were SS mice. This suggested that ethanol might produce depression in part by augmenting GABA's stimulant effects on chloride flux. Brain membrane preparations from LS (and HAS) strains were shown to be more sensitive than those from SS (and LAS) strains to ethanol-potentiated muscimol-stimulated chloride flux (13). Furthermore, the insensitivity to ethanol of GABA-activated chloride channels from SS mice can be seen in *Xenopus* oocytes in which mRNA has been expressed; this finding is also apparent in HAS and LAS. Studies with oocytes expressing different combinations of cloned GABA$_A$ receptor subunits showed that ethanol sensitivity in this preparation specifically requires the presence of the γ_{2L} subunit, which differs from the alternative γ_{2S} subunit by only eight amino acids. This region contains a consensus phosphorylation site for protein kinase C. However, molecular biological analyses of α and γ subunit compositions have not as yet identified critical differences between LS and SS mice that could explain their differential sensitivity to ethanol potentiation (for discussion, see ref. 84).

With chronic ethanol, alterations in levels of mRNA for specific GABA$_A$ subunits are seen (84), and ethanol chronically administered to oocytes alters receptor function (14). In other studies, chronic feeding of ethanol to WSP and WSR mice also led to changes in mRNA expression for specific GABA$_A$ receptor subunits, which may be important to the development of withdrawal hyperexcitability (12).

This ion channel is also influenced by binding sites recognizing barbiturates and benzodiazepines. The Alcohol Nontolerant (ANT) selected line of rats is known to be sensitive to ataxia induced by benzodiazepine injection, and a recent investigation found that this line of rats possessed a mutant α_6 subunit due to a point mutation in the gene (49), which may be related to behavioral sensitivity to this cerebellar motor response (82, but see also ref. 42).

Together, these studies suggest that GABA plays an important role in modulating some effects of ethanol and benzodiazepines. Genetic analysis with selectively bred lines and inbred strains have made a major contribution to clarifying these relationships. Similar studies in other candidate gene systems are addressing other drug response systems and will likely prove fruitful (see Chapters 4, 5, 6, and 66, *this volume*).

Enzymes of Alcohol Metabolism

In humans, genetic variants of the principal enzymes of alcohol metabolism, alcohol dehydrogenase (ADH) and mitochondrial aldehyde dehydrogenase (ALDH2) have been shown to influence alcohol drinking behavior and rates of alcoholism (70). The enzyme variants that are associated with lowered consumption and decreased rate of alcohol dependence are found in a large percentage of Chinese, Japanese, Koreans, and Vietnamese (37). The specific alleles that confer this protective effect on abusive drinking are *ADH2*2* (which produces a high activity β_2-ADH form) and *ALDH2*2* (which produces a low activity ALDH2 enzyme). The net result is that acetaldehyde, a highly toxic substance, is produced more rapidly by the β_2-ADH variant and is metabolized less rapidly by the low-activity ALDH2 variant, producing the alcohol-flush syndrome. Alcoholic patients can develop this response if they drink when they are being treated with disulfiram, which is an inhibitor of aldehyde dehydrogenase.

To discern whether *ADH* and *ALDH2* might be candidate genes in the rat lines selected for alcohol preference, variants of *ADH* and *ALDH2* were sought in the P/NP and AA/ANA lines. An *ALDH2* cDNA polymorphism was discovered in the P and NP rats that would code for either a glutamine or an arginine residue at position 67 of the *ALDH2* protein. The P rats were found to have a higher frequency (0.82) of the glutamine variant (allele *ALDH2^Q*) whereas the NP rats had a higher frequency (0.63) of the arginine variant (allele *ALDH2^R*) (ref. 16). Because ANA rats are known to be less able to metabolize acetaldehyde compared with AA rats, the frequency of the *ALDH2* polymorphism was examined in these lines. Although both male and female ANA rats had higher hepatic acetaldehyde levels in liver than AA rats after ethanol challenge, and female ANA rats had lower *ALDH2* activity than female AA rats ($\mu m/mg$ protein), both lines had allele frequencies of 0.75 for *ALDH2^R* and 0.25 for *ALDH2^Q* (47). Thus, this polymorphism in the ALDH2 gene does not explain the difference in acetaldehyde metabolism and the difference in alcohol drinking behavior of these lines. In support of this conclusion, the purified isoforms of this enzyme from the P and NP rats do not differ significantly in their catalytic properties.

Enzymes of Synthesis and Degradation of Monoaminergic Neurotransmitters and Their Receptors

With the identification of involvement of 5-HT and DA systems in drug and ethanol reinforcement, genes for tyrosine and tryptophan hydroxylase, rate-limiting enzymes of DA and 5-HT synthesis, respectively, and monoamine oxidase become obvious candidates for molecular biological study. Genes for receptors and transporters are other targets. The approach would be to compare messenger ribonucleic acid (mRNA) abundance in specific brain regions using the cloned deoxyribonucleic acid of the candidate genes and to analyze the promoter regions of the candidate genes for differences. For example, with the discovered neurobiological differences in some of the alcohol-preferring and alcohol-nonpreferring rat lines, exploration of differences in the promoter regions of the tryptophan hydroxylase and dopamine D2 receptor genes, and the regulation of their tissue specificity and expression, would be of interest. (See Chapter 2, *this volume*, for background issues.)

Subtractive Techniques

Another molecular biological technique that could be applied to the study of drug sensitivity responses is the use of subtractive hybridization. Procedures based on cross-hybridization can be used for directly comparing the DNA or RNA of two groups to identify regions of similarity.

Although these methods have not been used in the context of drug-response studies to our knowledge, such a technique could be used to analyze two lines selectively bred for differences in sensitivity to a drug response, or two strains with differential responsiveness. With repeated subtraction, one might be able to eliminate large regions of genetic similarity, leaving only those regions that differ between genotypes.

Subtractive techniques may be applied to DNA, which would identify differences in gene sequence. They are more usually applied to RNA to identify differences limited to those genes actively being expressed. Recent innovations suggest that improvements in detection power will continue to be developed. For example, a peptide specific to sensory neurons of *Aplysia* was recently identified by a differential screening procedure based on the polymerase chain reaction (11), and a method capable of identifying and cloning individual mRNAs has recently been reported (57). A variant of subtractive hybridization called representational difference analysis (RDA) may allow identification of the relatively small proportion of differences between the complex genomes represented by selected lines or inbred strains (58).

Whether the genetic differences important for mediating drug sensitivity differences between selectively bred lines or among inbred strains reside in DNA sequences (e.g., mutations), or in patterns of regulation and expression of genes, or both, is currently unknown. Subtractive methods would be expected to have more difficulty in detecting DNA signal from a background of genetic differences unrelated to the drug response of interest. Three potential starting points seem promising, and potentially able to overcome this problem. First, congenic strains are inbred strains that are so closely related that they differ only in a small percent of their DNA. Many mutations are placed for maintenance purposes on the C57BL/6J inbred background using this scheme. Congenics have been successfully used to map multiple genes influencing such polygenic traits as autoimmune, insulin-dependent diabetes mellitus. A single locus can have demonstrable effect on drug responses: two studies have shown that congenic C57BL/6J strains bearing several different mutations differ from wild-type C57BL/6J in response to morphine (4). A related, promising possibility is afforded by the C57BL/6J and C57BL/6By sublines, which were developed by separate inbreeding from a common ascestor and now differ by about 0.2% of their genome, or probably fewer than 50 loci. The B6J subline is substantially less sensitive to morphine analgesia, and has fewer [^{3}H]dihydromorphine binding sites than the B6By subline (78). Subtractive hybridization of these sublines would seem likely to identify one or more genes from the relatively small number of differences that would be important in determining the analgesic response.

Coupling this technique to quantitative trait loci (QTL)

analysis (see next section) is a second potential use of the subtractive procedure, which is more speculative. Mapping by QTL is capable of identifying a small region of a particular chromosome as the location of a gene influencing the drug response trait. If such a region could be isolated and amplified using polymerase chain reaction (PCR) to provide sufficient starting material, subtraction might allow rapid isolation of the relevant gene. Finally, selected lines offer an enriched population of genes influencing the selected trait. If selected lines were first inbred (after selection) to reduce the genetic noise (i.e., unselected, heterozygous loci), comparisons of replicated lines in various combinations might allow identification of the particular subtraction products important for the drug response differences between lines. This line of research is being pursued with P and NP inbreds.

Transgenics and Related Techniques

The production of transgenic mice that either overexpress or have deleted specific gene sequences by retroviral infection of embryos, manipulation of embryonic stem cells, or direct microinjection of fertilized mouse eggs is an increasingly routine procedure in neurobiology. To date, no transgenic mice have been produced, to our knowledge, with the express intent of manipulating a candidate gene thought to influence drug responses (but the basics of the methods and their potential are discussed in ref. 2). Altered sensitivity to ethanol has been found in mice with the protooncogene, *c-fos*, deleted, so transgenic animals can clearly differ in sensitivity to drugs (71). It may be feasible to target such knockouts more discretely, so that a neurotransmitter receptor or transporter gene, or one coding for particular receptor subunit proteins, could be deleted (or enhanced) in specific brain areas. For example, Ledent et al. (55) coupled a canine A2 adenosine receptor with the promoter sequence for bovine thyroglobulin. Expression of the receptor was functional, and seen only in thyroid.

Introduction of genes into a target tissue to study their function may be accomplished in ways other than insertion into the genome or deletion. For example, purified mRNAs from normal rat hypothalami (or synthetic copies of vasopressin mRNA) were injected into the hypothalami of Brattleboro rats, which lack a functional gene for hypothalamic vasopressin. These molecules were apparently taken up by neurons and retrogradely transported to magnocellular neurons, where they transiently expressed vasopressin and normalized the diabetes insipidus of the mutant rats for up to 5 days. Others have used an adenovirus to transfect rat nerve cells (as well as glia and astrocytes) by intracerebral injection with the reporter gene, β-galactosidase (69).

Quantitative Trait Loci Gene Mapping

Use of this technique in psychopharmacological studies has depended upon the analysis of drug responses in recombinant inbred (RI) strains. The RI strains are derived from two inbred strains by inbreeding from their F_2 (genetically heterogeneous) cross. They are called RI strains because the parental chromosomes are recombined several times per chromosome during their development, resulting in a unique pattern of recombinations of the parental chromosomes in each RI strain. Each RI strain thus represents a random sample of the genetic variability available in the two parent strains. Like any other inbred strain, all members of each RI strain are genetically identical, and each RI must have inherited any given allele from one of the two parents. The power of RI analysis lies in the existence of many strain distribution patterns identifying the genetic map location of previously typed genes.

When both parents and a battery of their RIs are tested for a drug response trait under controlled environmental conditions, strains will differ due to their unique genotypes. The strain means can then be referred to the pattern of previously mapped marker loci (3,39). Recently, methods have been developed to detect the influence of genes with relatively small influences on such responses and then to assign a tentative map location (53). These genes are known as minor gene loci, or quantitative trait loci (QTL). When a significant association is found between strain mean patterns and a pattern for a previously mapped locus, this suggests linkage between a QTL affecting the trait of interest and the marker.

Of the several sets of RI strains, the best studied in psychopharmacology is the BXD RI series, derived from the C57BL/6 and DBA/2 parent strains. The BXD RI strains have a relatively large number of loci (nearly 800) that have been previously mapped. An early study found that DBA/2J hyperthermia was much greater than that seen in C57BL/6J mice after amphetamine administration. A QTL analysis revealed a very strong association with the *Lamb-2* locus on chromosome 1, with a correlation of 0.96 (r^2 of 0.92). This suggests close linkage between *Lamb-2* and a gene with a major influence on amphetamine hyperthermia (76).

Such pronounced major gene effects are exceptional for drug response traits. Most drug responses appear to be determined by several QTL, as several recent studies have shown for morphine, ethanol, and amphetamine sensitivity (9,39,73). In an analysis of three ethanol-related traits in the BXD RI battery, 15 significant QTL associations were found for low-dose locomotor stimulation, 17 for acceptance of ethanol solutions, and 7 for withdrawal seizure severity (39). These QTL were located on several regions of several chromosomes: multiple regression analyses indicated that together, the QTL identified ac-

counted for 43% of the variability in activation, 95% of that in acceptance, and 62% of that in withdrawal. An important result was the finding that some chromosomal hot-spots were associated with multiple traits. Furthermore, the QTL markers, *Car-2* and *Ly-9*, on chromosomes 3 and 1, respectively, were significantly correlated with both amphetamine hyperthermia and ethanol withdrawal severity (39,76). When protein polymorphisms were studied for several polypeptides known to display allelic charge variants in mouse brain, one QTL for ethanol acceptance could also be tentatively mapped to a region on chromosome 1, where it apparently is identical or closely linked to the gene, *Ltw-4*. This association was verified in a panel of 20 inbred strains (38).

One area of interest has been the possibility that susceptibility to withdrawal from different drugs of abuse may have common genetic determinants. Results discussed earlier with WSP and WSR mice, and inbred strains, indicate substantial genetic commonality of influence on withdrawal from multiple drugs of abuse. During the past year, six QTL candidates possibly influencing the severity of acute ethanol withdrawal have been identified (9). For one of these candidate sites, the *Pmv-7* locus (a proviral RFLP) on chromosome 2, confirmation was sought using F_2 mice derived from C57 and DBA parental crosses. If an influential gene were on chromosome 2, genetic markers from this region should predict withdrawal severity in individual mice. By use of PCR amplification of the allelic status of individual mice for four linked polymorphic markers, a significant association of acute ethanol withdrawal intensity with the very closely linked (4 cM distance) PCR marker locus, *D2Mit9*, was found but not with the other markers on chromosome 2. This confirmation of the BXD findings in an independent, genetically segregating population is important to rule out a chance association, and established that there is a QTL in the *Pmv-7/D2Mit9* region of chromosome 2 accounting for about 40% of the total genotypic variance in acute ethanol withdrawal (15). These results are even more interesting, because data for chronic ethanol withdrawal severity (24) and the severity of nitrous oxide withdrawal also suggest the influence of the same QTL on chromosome 2, suggesting that some specific genes may be found that confer susceptibility to withdrawal from multiple drugs of abuse (9,65).

After these first two steps, the association was also verified by examining the allelic status of the WSP and WSR selected mouse lines, which provided independent verification that a gene closely linked to the *D2Mit9* locus has a marked influence on withdrawal severity (15). This region is syntenic (i.e., has homologous markers) with a large region of human genome and suggest the existence of a human equivalent to this QTL near human chromosome 2q24-q37. Candidate genes near *D2Mit9* include *Gad-1*, coding for glutamic acid decarboxylase, the rate-limiting enzyme catalyzing synthesis of the inhibitory neurotransmitter, GABA. Other candidate genes to consider include a cluster of genes (*Scn1a, Scn2a,* and *Scn3a*) for the α (major) subunit of brain voltage-dependent sodium channels, responsible for the rapid rising phase of the action potential in a variety of excitable cells, including neurons.

These results emphasize the utility of QTL analysis as a powerful hypothesis-generating approach to identify genes influencing drug sensitivity, both in animal models and humans. Furthermore, identification of candidate genes may indicate their more general role in CNS excitability and seizure susceptibility.

The principles of RI analysis can also be used in RIs developed from selectively bred lines. This application of RIs to detect single genes is strengthened by the fact that the parental stocks differ markedly on the traits analyzed (because they were specially bred to have those differences). On the other hand, such RIs have the limitation that they are almost completely uncharacterized with regard to marker loci. A recent project is undertaking to analyze responses in RIs developed from the LS and SS selected lines of mice. Use of rapid genotyping methods based on PCR will be required to develop a substantially dense genetic map for simple sequence length polymorphisms in the RIs. For some regions, a sufficiently dense map has been produced to allow detection of significant QTL affecting alcohol-induced loss of righting reflex (46).

A comparative linkage map of the mouse and human genomes has been published estimating that at least 61%, and possibly as much as 80%, of the linked regions in the mouse are conserved in humans (19). The genetic map of the rat is rudimentary compared with that of the mouse. Nonetheless, recent developments stemming from the interests stimulated by Lander and others in QTL analysis of complex traits (53) has led to the founding of a large collection of polymorphic markers (simple sequence repeats) that were first used to identify a gene, *Bp1*, that has a major effect on blood pressure (45). The gene is closely linked to that for the angiotensin-converting enzyme (ACE). The study employed F_2 progeny of a cross between the selectively bred SHRSP rat (spontaneously hypertensive rat, stroke prone) and the normal control WKY (Wistar-Kyoto) rats. More recently, a rat gene-mapping study using PCR-analyzed microsatellites was published (77). One hundred seventy-four loci that contain short tandem repeat sequences were identified from existing data bases and used to define primers for PCR amplification of the microsatellite regions. One hundred and thirty-four of the sequence-tagged microsatellite sites (STMSs) have been assigned to specific chromosomes, and length variation of the STMSs were visualized at 85 of 107 loci examined among eight inbred rat strains. Currently, 126 STMSs and primer pairs are available

commercially. This resource will enable a beginning for gene mapping of alcohol and drug related traits in rats by use of the QTL approach. A program has been initiated to examine the inbred P and NP rats and their F_2 progeny.

Other New Approaches

Innovation at the level of molecular biology is paralleled by the application of more finely tuned genetic techniques at the level of behavior. One example is the notion of creating new congenic lines based on phenotypic differences thought to be controlled by one or two genes. Two such projects are currently underway. Dudek and Underwood (31) found that C57BL/6J mice, which are not behaviorally stimulated by ethanol, and DBA/2J mice, which are markedly stimulated, probably differ in this response due to one or two genes. By analyzing the responses of individual mice from specific genetic crosses, and by repetitive backcrossing to the opposite parental strain, they are moving the genes responsible for sensitivity from the DBA/2J background onto the C57BL/6J strain, and vice versa. This will result in DBA/2J mice congenic to wild type DBA/2J except for the few very small chromosomal regions bearing the alcohol-sensitivity genes. A similar project is in progress in Colorado, where Dr. V. Gene Erwin (*personal communication*) is creating congenic DBA/2J mice that drink alcohol solutions, and parallel C57BL/6J mice that do not.

In studies following up the QTL analysis identifying a locus on chromosome 2 influencing drug withdrawal severity, Belknap, Buck, and their colleagues (*personal communication*) are developing genetically selected mouse strains from F_2 crosses between C57 and DBA inbred mice. Individual animals genotyped by PCR to be C57 homozygotes at the *D2Mit9* marker locus will be crossed repeatedly with DBA parents, until a congenic strain based on genotyping will be developed. Parallel strains will be created on the C57 background by introgressing the DBA allele responsible for elevating withdrawal. As Plomin and McClearn have suggested (73), it should be possible to breed selectively in this way for animals bearing specific genotypes, such as a collection of several QTL demonstrated to affect a drug response. Finally, the use of cryogenic techniques to preserve embryos from different generations during development of selected lines will allow retrospective questions to be entertained regarding behavior, pharmacology, and genetics during the course of development of genetic differences in drug responses (29).

CONCLUSIONS

The studies discussed above represent only a small fraction of the available pharmacogenetic data related to abused substances. Some reasonably firm conclusions may be offered based on earlier work and some predictions for the future ventured. There is a considerable amount of evidence for a heritable contribution to drug sensitivity for all drugs of abuse studied thus far. All potentially important pharmacological features of drug action appear to be influenced by genes, including acute sensitivity, tolerance development, dependence liability, and the tendency to be reinforced by the drug. Increasingly, evidence suggests that there are commonalities of genetic influence among drugs of abuse. In particular, some genotypes appear to be susceptible to dependence on multiple drugs of abuse. There are also individual genes that appear to predispose to particular drug responses or to multiple drug responses. Some have been roughly mapped to particular locations on the mouse genome. Given the similarity between mouse and human genomes, this is likely to result in rapid identification of the analogous site in humans.

Most progress in the analysis of genetic determinants of drug sensitivity to date has been derived from behavioral and biochemical-pharmacological levels of analysis. For the future, more molecularly based techniques are likely to be on the leading edge of progress. As candidate genes are identified as having important functions in mediating the biological effects of drugs, the tools of molecular biology will allow the genetic diversity underlying their expression and function to be exploited to better and better effect. The recent advances in genetic mapping strategies, such as QTL mapping, are especially promising, because they suggest that the beginnings of a merger of molecular biological techniques and use of genetic animal models is beginning to occur. The interface of these methods in the study of drugs of abuse seems likely to lead this new field, because of the long history in drug abuse research of the use of genetic animal models.

ACKNOWLEDGMENTS

We thank Dr. Kris Wiren for her comments. Some of the studies reviewed in this chapter were supported by a grant from the Department of Veterans Affairs and by NIH Grants AA08621, DA05228, AA06243, AA05828, AA07611, and AA08553.

REFERENCES

1. Allan AM, Harris RA. Neurochemical studies of genetic differences in alcohol actions. In Crabbe JC, Harris RA, eds. *The genetic basis for alcohol and drug actions.* New York: Plenum; 1991:105–152.
2. Barondes SH. Basic concepts and techniques of molecular genetics. This volume.
3. Belknap JK, Crabbe JC. Chromosome mapping of gene loci affecting morphine and amphetamine responses in BXD recombinant inbred mice. *Ann NY Acad Sci* 1992;654:311–323.
4. Belknap JK, O'Toole LA. Studies of genetic differences in response to opioid drugs. In Crabbe JC, Harris RA, eds. *The genetic basis for alcohol and drug actions.* New York: Plenum; 1991:225–252.
5. Belknap JK, Crabbe JC, Young ER. Voluntary consumption of ethanol in 15 inbred mouse strains. *Psychopharmacology* 1993;112:503–510.
6. Belknap JK, Crabbe JC, Young ER, Riggan J, O'Toole LA. Voluntary consumption of morphine in 15 inbred mouse strains. *Psychopharmacology* 1993;112:352–358.
7. Belknap JK, Laursen SE, Danielson PW, Crabbe JC. Ethanol and diazepam withdrawal convulsions are extensively codetermined in WSP and WSR mice. *Life Sci* 1989;44:2075–2080.
8. Belknap JK, Laursen SE, Sampson KE, Wilkie A. Where are the mu opioid receptors that mediate analgesia? An autoradiographic study in HAR and LAR mice. *J Addict Dis* 1991;10:29–44.
9. Belknap JK, Metten P, Helms ML, et al. QTL applications to substances of abuse: Physical dependence studies with nitrous oxide and ethanol. *Behav Genet* 1993;23:211–220.
10. Belknap JK, Riggan J, Young ER, Crabbe JC. Genetic determinants of morphine activity and thermal responses in inbred mice. *Psychopharmacology* 1994; [in press].
11. Brunet J-F, Shapiro E, Foster SA, Kandel ER, Iino Y. Identification of a peptide specific for *Aplysia* sensory neurons by PCR-based differential screening. *Science* 1991;252:856–859.
12. Buck KJ, Hahner L, Sikela J, Harris RA. Chronic ethanol treatment alters brain levels of γ-aminobutyric acidₐ receptor subunit mRNAs: relationship to genetic differences in ethanol withdrawal seizure severity. *J Neurochem* 1991;57:1452–1455.
13. Buck KJ, Harris RA. Neuroadaptive responses to chronic ethanol. *Alcohol Clin Exp Res* 1991;15:460–470.
14. Buck KJ, Harris RA. Chronic ethanol exposure of *Xenopus* oocytes expressing mouse brain mRNA reduces GABA receptor-activated current and benzodiazepine receptor ligand modulation. *Molec Neuropharmacol* 1991;1:59–64.
15. Buck KJ, Metten P, Glenn D, Belknap JK, Crabbe JC. Genetic mapping of quantitative trait loci modulating withdrawal neuroexcitability in the mouse. [Submitted.]
16. Carr L, Mellencamp B, Crabb D, Weiner H, Lumeng L, Li T-K. Polymorphism of the rat liver mitochondrial aldehyde dehydrogenase cDNA. *Alcohol Clin Exp Res* 1991;15:753–756.
17. Cloninger CR. Neurogenetic adaptive mechanisms in alcoholism. *Science* 1987;236:410–416.
18. Collins AC, Marks MJ. Genetic studies of nicotinic and muscarinic agents. In Crabbe JC, Harris RA, eds. *The genetic basis for alcohol and drug actions.* New York: Plenum; 1991:323–352.
19. Copeland NG, Jenkins NA, Gilbert DJ, et al. A genetic linkage map of the mouse: current applications and future prospects. *Science* 1993;262:57–66.
20. Crabbe JC. Sensitivity to ethanol in inbred mice: genotypic correlations among several behavioral responses. *Behav Neurosci* 1983;97:280–289.
20a. Crabbe JC, Belknap JK. Genetic approaches to drug dependence. *Trends Pharmacol Sci* 1992;13:212–219.
21. Crabbe JC, Harris RA, eds. *The genetic basis of alcohol and drug actions.* New York: Plenum; 1991.
22. Crabbe JC, Phillips TJ. Selective breeding for alcohol withdrawal severity. *Behav Genet* 1993;23:169–175.
23. Crabbe JC, Gallaher ES, Phillips TJ, Belknap JK. Genetic determinants of sensitivity to ethanol in inbred mice. *Behav Neurosci* 1994;108:186–195.
24. Crabbe JC, Kosobud A, Young ER, Janowsky JS. Polygenic and single-gene determination of responses to ethanol in BxD/Ty recombinant inbred mouse strains. *Neurobehav Toxicol Teratol* 1983;5:181–187.
25. Crabbe JC, Merrill CD, Belknap JK. Acute dependence on depressant drugs is determined by common genes in mice. *J Pharmacol Exp Ther* 1991;257:663–667.
26. Crabbe JC, Merrill CM, Belknap JK. Effect of acute alcohol withdrawal on sensitivity to pro- and anti-convulsant treatments in WSP mice. *Alcohol Clin Exp Res* 1994;17:1233–1239.
27. Crabbe JC, Phillips TJ, Cunningham CL, Belknap JK. Genetic determinants of ethanol reinforcement. *Ann NY Acad Sci* 1992;654:302–310.
28. Crabbe JC, Phillips TJ, Kosobud A, Belknap JK. Estimation of

genetic correlation: Interpretation of experiments using selectively bred and inbred animals. *Alcohol Clin Exp Res* 1990;14:141–151.

29. Crabbe JC, Schneider U, Hall JW, Mazur P. Invited commentary: cryopreservation as a tool for the study of selectively bred lines in rodent behavioral genetics. *Behav Genet* 1993;24(4):307–312.

30. Deitrich RA, Spuhler K. Genetics of alcoholism and alcohol actions. In Smart RG, Cappell HD, Glazer FB, et al., eds. *Research advances in alcohol and drug problems*, Vol 8. New York: Plenum; 1984:47–98.

31. Dudek BC, Underwood KA. Selective breeding, congenic strains, and other classical genetic approaches to the analysis of alcohol-related polygenic pleiotropisms. *Behav Genet* 1993;23:179–189.

32. Eriksson K, Rusi M. Finnish selection studies on alcohol-related behaviors: general outline. In McClearn GE, Deitrich RA, Erwin VG, eds. *Development of animal models as pharmacogenetic tools*. Washington: NIAAA Research Monograph No. 6; 1981:87–145.

33. Erwin VG, McClearn GE, Kuse AR. Interrelationships of alcohol consumption, actions of alcohol and biochemical traits. *Pharmacol Biochem Behav* 1980;13:297–302.

34. Gallaher EJ, Crabbe JC. Genetics of benzodiazepines, barbiturates and anesthetics. In Crabbe JC, Harris RA, eds. *The genetic basis of alcohol and drug actions*. New York: Plenum; 1991:253–272.

35. Gallaher EJ, Belknap JK, Jones G, Cross SJ, Crabbe JC. Genetic determinants of sensitivity to diazepam in inbred mice. [*Submitted*.]

36. Gallaher EJ, Hollister LE, Gionet SE, Crabbe JC. Mouse lines selected for genetic differences in diazepam sensitivity. *Psychopharmacology* 1987;93:25–30.

37. Goedde HW, Agarwal DP, Fritze G, et al. Distribution of ADH₂ and ALDH2 genotypes in different populations. *Hum Genet* 1992; 88:344–346.

38. Goldman D, Lister RG, Crabbe JC. Mapping of a putative genetic locus determining ethanol intake in the mouse. *Brain Res* 1987; 420:220–226.

39. Gora-Maslak G, McClearn GE, Crabbe JC, Phillips TJ, Belknap JK, Plomin R. Use of recombinant inbred strains to identify quantitative trait loci in psychopharmacology. *Psychopharmacology* 1991;104:413–424.

40. Grant KA, Snell LD, Rogawski MA, Thurkauf A, Tabakoff B. Comparison of the effects of the uncompetitive *N*-methyl-D-aspartate antagonist (±)-5-aminocarbonyl-10,11-dihydro-5H-dibenzo-[a,d]cyclohepten-5,10-imine (ADCI) with its structural analogs dizocilpine (MK-801) and carbamazepine on ethanol withdrawal seizures. *J Pharmacol Exp Ther* 1992;260:1017–1022.

41. Gulya K, Grant KA, Valverius P, Hoffman PL, Tabakoff B. Brain regional specificity and timecourse of changes in the NMDA receptor-ionophore complex during ethanol withdrawal. *Brain Res* 1991;547:129–134.

42. Harris RA. Alcohol sensitivity [Letter] *Nature* 1990;348:589.

43. Hitzemann R, Dains K, Bier-Langing CM, Zahniser NR. On the selection of mice for haloperidol response and nonresponse. *Psychopharmacology* 1991;103:244–250.

44. Hitzemann R, Qian Y, Hitzemann B. Dopamine and acetylcholine cell density in the neuroleptic responsive (NR) and neuroleptic nonresponsive (NNR) lines of mice. *J Pharmacol Exp Ther* 1993; 266:431–438.

45. Jacob HJ, Lindpaintner K, Lincoln SE, et al. Genetic mapping of a gene causing hypertension in the stroke-prone spontaneously hypertensive rat. *Cell* 1991;67:213–224.

46. Johnson TE, DeFries JC, Markel PD. Mapping quantitative trait loci for behavioral traits in the mouse. *Behav Genet* 1992;22:635–653.

47. Koivisto T, Carr LG, Li T-K, Eriksson CJP. Mitochondrial aldehyde dehydrogenase (ALDH2) polymorphism in AA and ANA rats: lack of genotype and phenotype line differences. *Pharmacol Biochem Behav* 1993;45:215–220.

48. Koob GF. Drugs of abuse: anatomy, pharmacology and function of reward pathways. *Trends Pharmacol Sci* 1992;13:177–184.

49. Korpi ER, Kleingoor C, Kettenmann H, Seeburg PH. Benzodiazepine-induced motor impairment linked to point mutation in cerebellar GABAₐ receptor. *Nature* 1993;361:356–359.

50. Korpi ER, Sinclair JD, Kaheinen P, Viitamaa T, Hellevuo K, Kiianmaa K. Brain regional and adrenal monoamine concentrations

and behavioral responses to stress in alcohol-preferring AA and alcohol-avoiding ANA rats. *Alcohol* 1988;5:417–425.

51. Kosobud AE, Crabbe JC. Sensitivity to NMDA-induced convulsions is genetically associated with resistance to ethanol withdrawal seizures. *Brain Res* 1993;610:176–179.

52. Kosobud A, Bodor AS, Crabbe JC. Voluntary consumption of ethanol in WSP, WSC and WSR selectively bred mouse lines. *Pharmacol Biochem Behav* 1988;29:601–607.

53. Lander ES, Botstein D. Mapping Mendelian factors underlying quantitative traits using RFLP linkage maps. *Genetics* 1989;121: 185–199.

54. Lê AD, Kiianmaa K. Characteristics of ethanol tolerance in alcohol drinking (AA) and alcohol avoiding (ANA) rats. *Psychopharmacology (Berl)* 1988;94:479–483.

55. Ledent C, Dumont JE, Vassart G, Parmentier M. Thyroid expression of an A₂ adenosine receptor transgene induces thyroid hyperplasia and hyperthyroidism. *EMBO J* 1992;11:537–542.

56. Li T-K, Lumeng L, Doolittle DP. Selective breeding for alcohol preference and associated responses. *Behav Genet* 1993;23:163–170.

57. Liang P, Pardee AB. Differential display of eukaryotic messenger RNA by means of the polymerase chain reaction. *Science* 1992; 257:967–971.

58. Lisitsyn N, Lisitsyn N, Wigler M. Cloning the differences between two complex genomes. *Science* 1993;259:946–951.

59. Lumeng L, Li T-K. The development of metabolic tolerance in the alcohol preferring P rats: comparison of forced and free-choice drinking of ethanol. *Pharmacol Biochem Behav* 1986;25:1013–1020.

60. Marley RJ, Elmer GI, Goldberg SR. The use of pharmacogenetic techniques in drug abuse research. *Pharmacol Ther* 1992;53:217–237.

61. McBride WJ, Chernet E, Dyr W, Lumeng L, Li T-K. Densities of dopamine D₂ receptors are reduced in CNS regions of alcohol-preferring P rats. *Alcohol* 1993;10(5):387–390.

62. McBride WJ, Murphy JM, Gatto GJ, et al. CNS mechanisms of alcohol self-administration. *Alcohol Alcohol* 1993;28[Suppl 1]:463–467.

63. McBride WJ, Murphy JM, Lumeng L, Li T-K. Serotonin, dopamine and GABA involvement in alcohol drinking of selectively bred rats. *Alcohol* 1990;7:199–205.

64. McClearn GE, Kakihana R. Selective breeding for ethanol sensitivity: short-sleep and long-sleep mice. In McClearn GE, Deitrich RA, Erwin VG, eds. *Development of animal models as pharmacogenetic tools*. Washington: NIAAA Research Monograph No. 6, 1981:147–159.

65. Metten P, Crabbe JC. Common genetic determinants of severity of acute withdrawal from ethanol, pentobarbital and diazepam in mice. *Behav Pharmacol* 1994; [*in press*].

66. Murphy JM, Gatto GJ, McBride WJ, Lumeng L, Li T-K. Operant responding for oral ethanol in the alcohol-preferring P and alcohol-nonpreferring (NP) lines of rats. *Alcohol* 1989;6:127–131.

67. Murphy JM, McBride WJ, Lumeng L, Li T-K. Regional brain levels of monoamines in alcohol-preferring and -nonpreferring lines of rats. *Pharmacol Biochem Behav* 1982;16:145–149.

68. Murphy JM, McBride WJ, Lumeng L, Li T-K. Contents of monoamines in forebrain regions of alcohol-preferring (P) and -nonpreferring (NP) lines of rats. *Pharmacol Biochem Behav* 1987;26:389–392.

69. Neve RL. Adenovirus vectors enter the brain. *Trends Neurosci* 1993;16:251–253.

70. Ohmori T, Koyama T, Chen C-C, Yeh E-K, Reyes BV, Yamashita I. The role of aldehyde dehydrogenase isozyme variance in alcohol sensitivity, drinking habits formation and the development of alcoholism in Japan, Taiwan and the Philippines. *Prog Neuro Psychopharmacol Biol Psychiatry* 1986;10:229–235.

71. Paylor R, Johnson RS, Cao W, et al. Increased ethanol sensitivity and reduced tolerance in c-fos mutant mice. [*Submitted*.]

72. Phillips TJ, Crabbe JC. Behavioral studies of genetic differences in alcohol action. In Crabbe JC, Harris RA, eds. *The genetic basis for alcohol and drug actions*. New York: Plenum; 1991:25–104.

73. Plomin R, McClearn GE. Quantitative trait loci (QTL) analyses and alcohol-related behaviors. *Behav Genet* 1993;23:197–211.

74. Samson HH, Tolliver GA, Lumeng L, Li T-K. Ethanol reinforcement in the alcohol nonpreferring rat: initiation using behavioral techniques without food restriction. *Alcohol Clin Exp Res* 1989; 13:378–385.

75. Schuckit MA. Low level of response to alcohol as a predictor of future alcoholism. *Am J Psychiat* 1994;151:184–189.

76. Seale TW, Carney JM, Johnson P, Rennert OM. Inheritance of amphetamine-induced thermoregulatory responses in inbred mice. *Pharmacol Biochem Behav* 1985;23:373–377.

77. Serikawa T, Kuramoto T, Hilbert P, et al. Rat gene mapping using PCR-analyzed microsatellites. *Genetics* 1992;131:701–721.

78. Shuster L. Pharmacogenetics of drugs of abuse. *Ann NY Acad Sci* 1989;562:56–73.

79. Sinclair JD, Lê AD, Kiianmaa K. The AA and ANA rat lines, selected for differences in voluntary alcohol consumption. *Experientia* 1989;45:798–805.

80. Spuhler K, Deitrich RA. Correlative analysis of ethanol-related phenotypes in rat inbred strains. *Alcohol Clin Exp Res* 1984;8:480–484.

81. Stefanini E, Frau M, Garau MG, Garau B, Fadda F, Gessa GL. Alcohol preferring rats have fewer dopamine D_2 receptors in the limbic system. *Alcohol Alcohol* 1992;27:127–130.

82. Uusi-Oukari M, Korpi ER. Diazepam sensitivity of the binding of an imidazobenzodiazepine, [^{3}H]Ro 15-4513, in cerebellar membranes from two rat lines developed for high and low alcohol sensitivity. *J Neurochem* 1990;54:1980–1987.

83. Waller MB, McBride WJ, Gatto GJ, Lumeng L, Li T-K. Intragastric self-infusion of ethanol by ethanol-preferring and -nonpreferring lines of rats. *Science* 1984;225:78–80.

84. Zahniser NR, Buck KJ, Curella P, et al. GABA$_A$ receptor function and regional analysis of subunit mRNAs in long-sleep and short-sleep mouse brain. *Molec Brain Res* 1992;14:196–206.

Psychopharmacology: The Fourth Generation of Progress, edited by Floyd E. Bloom and David J. Kupfer. Raven Press, Ltd., New York © 1995.

CHAPTER 70

Introduction to Clinical Neuropsychopharmacology

David J. Kupfer

One of the major goals of this volume is both to demonstrate and to emphasize the growing linkages between basic preclinical science research, clinical neuroscience, and clinical therapeutics. We believe that a major aspect of recent advances in neuropsychopharmacology and, thus, the basis for the *Fourth Generation* has been to establish such linkages and to exemplify various strategies that are being used to achieve a new level of integration. As may be obvious to most readers, the role of drugs and drug development essentially is to provide clinicians with the ability to treat psychopathology and aberrant behavior and their concomitant levels of dysfunctioning—primarily central nervous system (CNS) dysfunctioning. To treat the psychopathology in the most rational and empirical manner, one would like not only to understand the mechanisms of action of drugs used for treatment, but also to utilize drug treatment findings to learn more about the pathogenesis and pathophysiology of the underlying disorders. In this manner, the integration of brain and behavior becomes a key objective and motivates our scientific pursuits toward a basic science thrust and cellular and molecular research that can inform and guide important strands of clinical research activity. In these pursuits, we need to appreciate the broad dimensions of normal development and behavior and how the emerging and developing CNS interacts with changes in behavior over the early periods of the life cycle, as well as across the entire life span. Advances in the past 5 years on neuronal development and plasticity have rekindled a focus on the interaction between neuronal activity and behavior. As a consequence of this increasing interest in developmental neurobiology, considerable opportunity now exists to understand more about pathological or abnormal development in the central nervous system, as well as about parallel developments in behavior "going astray." As we proceed to integrate what we know about normal and pathological development, it thus is our mission also to utilize the tools of neuropsychopharmacology to consolidate these linkages and to provide improved clinical treatments for individuals who suffer from either syndromes or symptoms we generally characterize as neuropsychiatric disorders.

ORGANIZATION OF THE CLINICAL SECTION

This chapter serves to introduce the clinical sections of the *Fourth Generation of Progress*. It will provide an overview, especially for those individuals with limited experience in clinical science of the chapters contained in this section. Initial attention is paid to the principal methods that are used in clinical psychopharmacology and how data are obtained and analyzed (chapters on the critical analysis of methods).

The next group of chapters spans those serious neuropsychiatric disorders that represent the target disorders of clinical psychopharmacology. Considerable effort has been devoted to documenting the range of mental disorders that affect over 22% of the population in any given year with 9% demonstrating significant dysfunction. Of these disorders, the most severe illnesses (e.g., schizophrenia and unipolar and bipolar recurrent disorders) affect some 5 million American adults (2.8% of the adult population) causing considerable suffering to patients and their families. In addition to pain experienced by those afflicted with these disorders and their families, they also result in considerable economic cost, reflecting lost productivity, disability and social service payments, and increased morbidity and mortality.

D. J. Kupfer: Department of Psychiatry, University of Pittsburgh, School of Medicine, Western Psychiatric Institute and Clinic, Pittsburgh, Pennsylvania 15213.

For each of these disorders covered in the chapters on psychobiology and treatment, the extent of coverage is related to advances made since the last volume. Differential coverage highlights differential advances made in certain disorders. The more extensive coverage devoted to mood disorders and schizophrenia reflects their continuing prominence in our field as the most serious, chronic disorders. It is interesting to note, however, that anxiety disorders are also well represented. Considerable advances have occurred in the geriatric disorders, which is reflected in the broadening range of coverage devoted to them. It is noteworthy that a greater level of attention is also devoted to so-called neurological disorders. Brief updates are included on personality, eating and sleep disorders. Although we continue to remain optimistic concerning psychopharmacological intervention in childhood disorders, progress has not been dramatic since the last edition. The final group of disorders is concerned with substance abuse. This interesting area is covered in ten chapters devoted to use of abuse of different substances. Finally, although methods have been discussed throughout the clinical section, we wish to redirect our attention to genetics, strategies for multimodality research, and specific methodological and statistical approaches. One of the major objectives of these sections will be the translation of new knowledge derived from preclinical science into the design of psychobiological and therapeutic investigations. It is expected that this overall format can provide greater ease for the reader in reviewing the clinical sections of the volume and, perhaps more importantly, facilitate the utilization of specific chapters from the preclinical section. As we discuss different changes and advances that have occurred and how they are integrated through our increasing knowledge of preclinical science, we hope the reader will be able to make use of the entire volume.

OVERVIEW OF THE CLINICAL SECTION

As discussed earlier, four strategies are used to analyze the neuroscientific substrates of neuropsychological phenomena: molecular, cellular, multicellular (or systems), and behavioral (see Chapter 1, *this volume*). These four terms constitute the minimal approach to a complex hierarchical ensemble that have been used to characterize the principle methods of neuroscience research (1). A major concept is that "drugs which influence behavior and improve the functional status of patients with neurologic or psychiatric diseases, act by enhancing or blunting the effectiveness of chemical transmission at the sites of principal interneuronal communication, the specialized chemical junctions termed *synapses*" (see Chapter 1, *this volume*).

The emphasis of the clinical section is placed on the interaction of psychopharmacology and behavior (the fourth hierarchical level). In this area, the relationship of normative behavior and its threshold or transition into psychopathology is a central, perplexing, conceptual, as well as pragmatic problem, which clinicians continue to address. At this time, we have not yet achieved a level of hierarchical thresholds at the clinical surface comparable to what has been described for the preclinical realm.

For the preclinical scientist the nosology of psychiatric disorders may appear to be somewhat bewildering, both in terms of complexity and language. There has been considerable debate concerning the definition and classification of mental disorders and the determination of various thresholds that have been utilized to reflect impairment. It is important, however, to realize that specific behaviors in isolation of their related impact on functioning does not necessarily connote a mental disorder. In our clinical approaches we have sought to design operational clinical criteria for disorders that can be discriminated from each other in a number of ways. Indeed, to accomplish validity of a diagnosis numerous authors have proposed strategies involving an iterative process with five phases: clinical description, laboratory studies, delineation from other disorders, follow-up study, and family study (2). More recently, the possibility of more direct genetic approaches rather than the more traditional descriptive approaches have been proposed as methods to discriminate groups of patients with neuropsychiatric disorders and to differentiate subtypes (see Chapter 155, *this volume*). Basic to all these approaches, however, is whether an individual suffers from a disorder or symptom cluster in such a way that the behavior leads to dysfunction in work, school, family and other aspects of the individual's life, since it is the degree of this dysfunction that often prompts an individual and family to seek treatment and that usually leads our society to diagnose deviant behavior that is not of "psychotic" dimension. The interaction between behavioral symptoms and functioning represents the clinician's dilemma in diagnosis and treatment. Part of this difficulty is that the diagnosis of these disorders is quite complex unless there are drastic behavior manifestations, such as obvious delusional thoughts and hallucinations, or profound mood disturbances where individuals display severe manic or depressive behavior. Nevertheless, advances in clinical diagnosis and treatment have encouraged scientists to search for neurobiological correlates and to develop animal models that might mimic human psychopathology and allow us to examine the brain bases of certain syndromes. Chapters in this volume, in both the preclinical and clinical sections, devote considerable attention to potential linkages between neurotransmitters and brain circuitry, which, in turn, can link molecules to brain systems and behavior. Recent changes in our treatment strategies are now allowing us to follow the longitudinal course of schizophrenia, major depression, and manic–depressive disorders providing methods for discrimination of these disorders from each other and the testing of specific long-term treatments. The delineation of specific treatments, their efficacy, as well as the definition of criteria for remission and recovery, have, in turn, provided stimulus to both preclinical and clinical scientists to examine with increased vigor how the clinical pathophysiology and treatment of specific disorders affect the functioning of the CNS and vice-versa.

Several alternative strategies were available for organizing the clinical sections. One approach would have been to discuss normal development and behavior and place them in the context of gender and development across the life span. Using such a mode of organization, one would have proceeded from normal development to symptom formation and the concomitant dysfunctioning in behavior, interpersonal relationships, and interactions with the environment. This represents a dimensional approach to psychopathology which has inherent advantages over a categorical one in that it allows us to build conceptual models on the emergence and longitudinal course of mental disorders and to establish tentative relationships to CNS functioning and even potentially CNS neuroanatomy. However, as is discussed in one of the methodological chapters (see Chapter 71, *this volume*), the use of syndromes and what is considered a more descriptive psychiatric approach remains the hallmark of our level of organization of psychopathology and represents the most successful approach to date. The use of a categorical approach has inherent advantages as well, most importantly in that it represents a more pragmatic attempt to cope with various ''consumers'' and providers of medical care. However, although the use of syndromes facilitates communication, it often fails to capture fully the rich relationships between brain and behavior and also does not lend itself to conveying the pathways in and out of illness that can be observed in many patients. Thus, other strategies are needed to provide a more dynamic longitudinal, even developmental perspective on psychiatric symptoms and syndromes and to provide the framework for understanding relationships between neuropsychopharmacology and behavior over time. In such an approach, notions relating to state (episodic) versus trait (persistent) characteristics of disorders gain a prominent position, since they are most important in examining the psychobiological aspects of a disorder. This emphasis provides an opportunity to compare individuals across time as they may go in and out of episodes of illness, as well as to compare individuals with a particular disorder to healthy controls.

Regardless of the overall approach that one takes to the classification of psychopathology, the major task for the authors of this volume is to provide a road map in which CNS functioning and CNS neurochemistry can be related and correlated with behavior. The exciting advances of the last 6 to 7 years provide a new set of tools, such as functional neuroimaging to examine brain–behavior relationships in a more dynamic functional manner than previously available. For example, both position

emission tomography (PET) with its possibilities of neuroreceptor strategies and nuclear magnetic resonance (NMR) with its capability for both structural and functional analysis are most important in providing new leads for the next 10 years. We have elected to provide in most ''disease areas'' chapters that specialize on psychobiology and others that focus primarily on treatment. In some areas where fewer advances have occurred, a single chapter provides both the psychobiological and therapeutic update.

Finally, an area that has received some attention in past editions but requires increasing concentration of efforts over the next decade is that of genetics and the integration of genetic neurodevelopmental science with the existing knowledge base on onset of psychopathology (see Chapters 2 and 155, *this volume*). Not only do we have new tools for genetic research, but combining such tools with a neurodevelopmental approach will provide important opportunities to understand how schizophrenia, for example, develops (see Chapter 98, *this volume*). These strategies may also be useful in developing treatment interventions for schizophrenia, as well as for autism and other disorders.

In short, the work currently ongoing in both preclinical and clinical neuroscience provides the theater in which clinical therapeutics and the application of new and more traditional neuropsychopharmacological agents can occur. The play itself is becoming more interesting, where previously it represented a one-act play with a small cast, it is now possible to conceptualize both one-act and three-act plays within the context of intervention (short-term and long-term) but also ones that include not only the traditional actors and actresses, but an extended cast, with new roles designed specifically for the particular play. The advances in preclinical science are providing the basis for the design of new psychopharmacological agents (see Chapter 158, *this volume*), but they also help us to use our current armamentarium in more imaginative ways. The aim of the chapters on critical analysis of methods is designed with the above concept in mind. In a similar fashion, the chapters on integrative concepts represent attempts to provide a greater degree of vertical integration with the remaining sections of the clinical set of chapters which are syndrome driven.

CRITICAL METHODS

As in the preclinical science arena, our choice of chapters covering critical methods represent those viewed as the most promising and essential tools used in clinical science and neuropsychopharmacology. These chapters are not meant to provide exhaustive coverage of the entire array of methods used in clinical psychopharmacology. Rather, they reflect advances that have occurred since the last *Generation* and strategies and methods which are likely to be used increasingly over the next 5 to 10 years. The first such tool has already been alluded to and essentially represents the need to classify psychopathology in order to conduct both clinical trials and to understand the efficacy and effectiveness of neuropsychopharmacological agents. Chapter 71 by Frances et al. (*this volume*) is concerned with the development of the current classification system for psychiatric disorders, DSM-IV, and points to several key areas and their limitations important to our current psychopharmacological research efforts. Key issues in psychiatric nosology, such as reliability, generalizability, and validity are highlighted, as are several of the newer approaches taken in the preparation of DSM-IV. These include reanalyses of data sets collected on psychopathology but, more interestingly, also a number of field trials conducted to outline both the promises and descriptive limitations of the DSM-IV nosology. The descriptive limitations of the criteria sets raise issues of reliability and validity discussed extensively by Kraemer in the subsequent integrative chapter (Chapter 157). Although the DSM-IV will continue to provide a necessary common language for study and practice, issues of thresholds and categorical versus dimensional approaches remain very much of central interest, and an improved categorical classification system certainly does not represent the only manner in which advances in this area will continue to occur.

The next set of methods described represent a range of issues related to clinical study design (see Chapter 72). The critical issues discussed include issues pertaining to the traditional randomized controlled trials (RCTs) as well as involved specialized trial designs (cross-over, longitudinal, dose–response, and concentration control studies). The emphasis in this chapter is also on documentation and a greater attention to biostatistical approaches throughout the design data collection and data analysis phases of RCTs. In the section of this chapter highlighting future directions, the authors point to changes that have occurred since the last *Generation* was produced, including increased emphasis on documentation of research data, adequate informed consent, and audit procedures. Other issues highlighted are greater emphasis on longer term studies and the resulting push to improve our study designs for long-term trials. This change, in turn, also raises the need for continuing efforts to define those methods that should be used for evaluation and outcome comparison of appropriate therapeutic alternatives. Increased emphasis on longer term trials also reflects the importance of issues concerning research on cost effectiveness and of health economic methodologies, which will need to be applied more extensively (see Chapter 161).

The need for improved clinical design methodologies is also reflected in the discussion concerning short-term and long-term psychopharmacological treatment strategies (see Chapter 73). In this methods chapter, the authors have set out to establish a rationale for longer term medi-cation strategies and how "treatment strategies" need to play an increasing role in our psychopharmacological research and practice. Using three disorders as examples (schizophrenia, depression, and anxiety disorders), they demonstrate how short-term and long-term strategies have common principles for these serious disorders and how the effective psychopharmacological management of these disorders requires adequate dosages and duration of treatments, including phases of long-term maintenance treatment. The authors argue that this approach represents a paradigm shift in our treatment strategies for psychiatric disorders (see also Chapter 156, *this volume*).

The need to understand more about our psychopharmacological approaches is reflected also in the next chapter on pharmacokinetics and pharmacodynamics (see Chapter 74). In this discussion we receive an essential update on the methods now available in both pharmacokinetics and pharmacodynamics to examine sensitivity and specificity of treatments. Pharmacokinetics utilizes mathematical models to describe and predict the time course of drug concentrations in body fluids. With improved measurement methods and by applying pharmacokinetic models, the level of sophistication in therapeutic drug monitoring has increased significantly. For example, these techniques are extremely useful in quantitating drug toxicity. Pharmacodynamics, which is the study of time course and intensity of drug effects on the organism, has also experienced major advances, especially increasing our capacity to measure long-term drug effects. The thrust of this methods chapter is to help us understand individual variability in drug response, a theme developed further in later sections of the volume (see Chapter 162).

The next methods chapter heightens our appreciation of new tools that were not previously available. In a brief chapter on neuropathology we are treated to an introductory set of principles on methods of neuropathology likely to play a role in our understanding of CNS alterations and serious psychiatric disorders (see Chapter 75). Our research strategies for investigating CNS (structural and neurochemical) abnormalities in psychiatric disorders will be aided tremendously by a greater concentrated effort in neuropathology spanning both animal models and human work. Much has already been gained in studies on Huntington's disease and Parkinson's disease, in which the study of postmortem human brain tissue has improved our overall understanding of behavioral manifestations. The application of these techniques to specific forms of psychopathology is likely to drive progress in our understanding of their brain bases.

The chapter just reviewed should be put in the context of the subsequent three chapters, which demonstrate collectively the major advances made concerning tools for understanding the living CNS and brain functioning. The first of these chapters represents a primer on both positive emission tomography (PET) and single photon emission computerized tomography (SPECT) (see Chapter 76). As the authors indicate, these contemporary brain imaging methods allow and offer exciting opportunities to study CNS function in vivo. The major principles of PET and SPECT are described, as well as their current limitations. All consumers now know that these imaging techniques are methods of high sensitivity in which the injection of radioactively labelled drugs can provide measures of local neuronal activity, in vivo neurochemistry, or in vivo pharmacology. Thus, they provide an interesting window to examine in vivo brain functioning and drawing upon advances in preclinical science, and opportunity to integrate them with clinical research (see Chapters 87, 99, 109, and 119, *this volume*). Given the high cost and technical complexity of these research methods, however, they will certainly require multidisciplinary collaboration and considerable further research to provide more opportunity for clinical research and to be applied in clinical trials of neuropsychopharmacological agents.

The next chapter, also part of the functional imaging array of contemporary developments, deals more directly with in vivo structural brain assessment (see Chapter 77). Here the technical improvements have allowed us within a very few years to make major improvements in the acquisition and processing of structural imaging data, utilizing primarily magnetic resonance imaging (MRI) with its superior tissue contrasts and resolution. Improved differentiation of white from gray matter and a much improved flexibility to view and measure specific structures represent major advances. Because it is likely that most of the structural changes in psychiatric disorders will be subtle, opportunities to have systematic and reliable quantification techniques are vital to further progress. The use of MRI will also allow us to give greater attention to normal developmental and aging effects, variations in normative distribution of size and tissue loss, as well as provide the opportunity to do longitudinal studies despite their greater complexity. Finally, MRI also promises to open avenues of functional brain imaging, which may eventually replace some of the current PET and SPECT work.

The last chapter in this section on new tools to assess CNS functioning is an update on electrophysiological techniques currently available to the clinical researcher (see Chapter 78). This discussion deals with the methodological issues that are involved in both event-related brain potential and magnetic field studies. The discussion of newer electrophysiological techniques, particularly those involved in a spacial localization of brain processes, highlights several advances over and above what we have examined with respect to event-related potentials (ERPs) in the past. It is now possible to elicit event-related magnetic fields (ERFs) in a fashion time-locked to specific events and analogous to ERPs. Magnetoencephalogram (MEG) and ERFs definitely convey different information than EEG and ERPs and in this manner offer new strategies for testing information processing, complex behav-

ior, and cognitive processing not as easily available with other systems of functional imaging. As the methodologies for evoked brain potential and magnetic field studies continue to develop technologically, the coordination of EEG and MEG data with data from MRI, PET, and SPECT scans will be necessary. The integration of findings across different forms of functional brain imaging and processing may very well represent the uses and promising strategy to obtain comprehensive sets of data on both normals and individuals with neuropsychiatric disorders.

INTEGRATIVE THEMES

In the three chapters dealing with integrative themes, perspectives on genetics, strategies for multimodality research, and methodological and statistical advances in psychiatric clinical research are discussed. These three areas represent important integrative arenas in which much of the clinical neuropsychopharmacological research occurs. Chapter 155 on genetics seeks to provide an integrative discussion to demonstrate that the advances in human genetics and recombinant DNA technology, as well as those relating the explosion of knowledge on the human genome are very important for psychiatry. Progress in understanding the human genome is also paralleled by developments in genetic research in rodents and other species of relevances as potential animal models. The implications for psychiatry are obvious. Currently, many of the major disorders covered in our volume are examined in collaborative efforts to determine and explore the potential genetic linkages that contribute to schizophrenia, the mood, disorders, Alzheimer's disease, and alcoholism. The data derived from molecular genetic strategies and genetic epidemiology will ultimately have a major influence on psychopharmacological approaches to treating these disorders (see Chapter 153). Current research activities in mood disorders, schizophrenia, Tourette's syndrome, panic disorder, and alcoholism are briefly reviewed as representative examples of the ongoing work in psychiatry (see Chapter 141). These research activities are contrasted with those on several other neuropsychiatric disorders, notably fragile X syndrome and Huntington's disease. The chapter represents not only a primer for genetics but an integrated review of approaches that can be placed in the context of other sections throughout the clinical portion of the volume which relate to genetics.

This leads us directly into the next chapter offering an extensive discussion of strategies for multimodality research (see Chapter 156). Given the likelihood that treatment outcome research will increasingly involve both pharmacotherapeutic and psychotherapeutic treatment modalities, we must realize that combination treatment will need to play an important role in our treatment strategies for various disorders and both for short and long-term treatment (see Chapters 91 and 107). This chapter is reminiscent of a chapter in the earlier methods sections which focused on strategies for acute and long-term treatment (see Chapter 73), but goes one step further to include psychotherapeutic approaches to specify a more complex set design, such as that need to deal with combination treatments issues relating to the types of trials, duration, dosages, and comparability across treatments; and the utility of assessing psychosocial variables.

The last integrative chapter (Chapter 157) is one that revisits many of the topics that have been discussed throughout the clinical chapters and relate to fundamental questions underlying psychopharmacological research. The sections on diagnosis, longitudinal research, and specific applications of mathematical models seek to integrate discussions on clinical treatment issues. The author raises a series of cautionary and provocative questions, which have become increasingly important as we conduct more research applying DSM-IV criteria for short and long-term clinical trials (see Chapters 71, 72, and 73).

SPECIFIC DISORDERS

We have discussed several of the key issues relating to critical analysis of methods and integrative concepts for the clinical sections; however, it may be useful to also highlight changes both in coverage or emphasis that reflect advances made in major disorders since the last edition. In the area of mood disorders a total of ten chapters deal with issues relating to the psychobiology of mood disorders. These chapters encompass a series of detailed reviews concerning specific neurotransmitters (see Chapters 79, 80, 81, and 82) presented in the basic section; specific aspects of neuroendocrinology and neuropeptide alterations in mood disorders (see Chapters 83 and 84); advances in psychoimmunology (see Chapter 85) and mood disorders; as well as an extensive chapter on biological rhythms in mood disorders. This latter chapter (Chapter 86), as is true of some of the earlier chapters in the psychobiology of mood disorders, presents interesting links to the preclinical sections reviewing neurotransmitter systems, neuroendocrine interactions (see Chapter 62), and neuroimmune interactions (see Chapter 63). The remaining two chapters in the portion on the psychobiology of mood disorders deal with areas important to the diagnosis, pathophysiology, and treatment of mood disorders. The chapter on brain imaging in mood disorders (Chapter 87) represents an application of earlier approaches discussed in the section on critical methods. The chapter on gender issues and cycle effects (see Chapter 88) is important, since it ties together with the earlier clinical chapter on biological rhythms (see Chapter 86).

Treatment approaches in mood disorders are covered by nine chapters reflecting the current state-of-the-art in the entire range of clinical therapeutics. One of the major

changes since the last edition is a greater emphasis on a longitudinal approach to the treatment of mood disorders, as well as the introduction of newer compounds (SSRIs). Thus, the chapter on SSRIs for acute treatment (see Chapter 89) is juxtaposed with a chapter on standard treatment approaches (see Chapter 90) and followed by a chapter on the long-term treatment of mood disorders (see Chapter 91). Recognition that mood disorders, despite overall gains in treatment efficacy, are still faced with a great degree of treatment resistance has led to the inclusion of a separate chapter on treatment-resistant depression (see Chapter 92). Several subsequent chapters highlight treatment approaches for particular subgroups of mood disorder patients. Advances in the use of lithium and anticonvulsants, primarily but not exclusively applied in bipolar disorder are discussed in Chapter 93. The increasing understanding that psychosocial factors may play an important role in treatment outcome is then reflected in a further chapter (see Chapter 94) which followed by two chapters dealing with new (old) approaches to the treatment of affective disorders, including a review of the role of electroconvulsive therapy (see Chapter 95) and of novel pharmacological approaches (see Chapter 96). The final chapter in the treatment section reviews our current understanding of treatment resistance in bridging neurobiology and preclinical science (see Chapter 97).

The section on schizophrenia is also divided into psychobiology and treatment chapters. In the eight chapters devoted to the psychobiology of schizophrenia, attention is now being paid to the neurodevelopmental perspectives on schizophrenia (see Chapter 98), which are also reflected in a subsequent chapter providing an introduction to developmental neurobiology and a review of other direct applications from the preclinical area (see Chapter 59). We hope that the clinical scientist will again utilize the sections on critical analysis of integrative concepts in the preclinical section to appreciate the full impact of the advances made over the past 7 years in understanding the psychobiology of schizophrenia. The second chapter on schizophrenia deals with functional brain imaging (Chapter 99), which recaptures the emphasis placed in the new functional neuroimaging methods discussed earlier. Although attention is paid to particular neurotransmitters, notably the effect of dopamine on schizophrenia (see Chapters 100 and 103), the roles of other neurotransmitters potentially involved in schizophrenia are discussed. This is reflected in Chapter 101 on glutamate in schizophrenia as well as in a review of the potential role of serotonin in schizophrenia (Chapter 102). Importantly, our improved understanding of the symptomatology of schizophrenia is leading us to a broader appreciation of the neurocognitive and neurophysiological aspects of the disorder, as reflected in two subsequent chapters on neurocognitive functioning in patients with schizophrenia (see Chapter 105). A final chapter reviews the current state of neurophysiological and psychophysiological approaches to schizophrenia (see Chapter 104).

Treatment approaches for schizophrenia have also improved over the last 7 years, based on numerous studies that address both acute and long-term treatment. These areas are reviewed in the respective chapters on the acute treatment of schizophrenia (see Chapter 106) and on maintenance drug treatments (see Chapter 107). The final chapter on the treatment of schizophrenia is concerned with atypical antipsychotics and emphasizes recent opportunities and gains made in using atypical antipsychotics for selected patients with schizophrenia (see Chapter 108).

The next section is devoted to anxiety disorders, with four chapters covering the psychobiology of anxiety disorders and two reviewing treatment approaches. Not surprisingly, in the sections dealing with psychobiology the important role of functional neuroimaging in improving our basic understanding of the pathophysiology of anxiety disorders is highlighted (see Chapter 109). Chapter 110 on the 5-HT1A receptor compliments the chapters that deal with this topic in the preclinical sections, particularly those chapters on indoleamines (see Chapters 37 and 42). Although discussed in chapters on mood disorders and schizophrenia, the use of psychopharmacological challenges and "probes" for anxiety disorders is highlighted in the next chapter (Chapter 111). The final chapter in the psychobiology section deals with environmental factors in the etiology of anxiety disorders, issues that have become increasingly important in understanding the long-term pathway of the development, onset, and maintenance of anxiety states (Chapter 112). The two treatment chapters highlight the need to appreciate that anxiety disorder is a disorder with an often chronic persistent course (see Chapter 73). A specific chapter on issues of long-term treatment (see Chapter 114) is complimented by a chapter on acute treatment strategies (see Chapter 113).

The section on geriatric disorders has changed rather dramatically from the previous edition, as is reflected in the seven chapters devoted to Alzheimer's disease alone. The first two chapters deal with aspects of genetics (see Chapter 115) and a subsequent one with amyloid development in Alzheimer's disease and the use of animal models (see Chapter 116). A review follows of cognitive and memory changes that occur in Alzheimer's disease, including a discussion of appropriate assessment (see Chapter 117). Although our understanding of Alzheimer's disease is moving rapidly in the direction of developing pharmacological approaches for treatment intervention, we need to address the probability of using biological correlates in assessing treatment outcome in this disorder. The chapter on biological markers (see Chapter 118) is followed by one on anatomic and functional brain imaging in Alzheimer's disease (Chapter 119), a chapter demonstrating once more the pervasive impact of newer functional neuroimaging techniques. Even though thera-

peutic interventions for Alzheimer's disease are sparse, reflecting a long unsuccessful history with such endeavors, two chapters review experimental treatments for Alzheimer's disease (see Chapter 120) and the treatment of noncognitive behavioral abnormalities (see Chapter 121).

One set of chapters in the geriatric section relate to specific characteristics of psychotic disorders occurring in the elderly. The first chapter in this section focuses on paraphrenia and other related late-life psychoses and reviews both diagnostic and treatment issues (see Chapter 122). The next chapters deals very specifically with advances made over the past 7 years on the characterization of the cognitive impairment in geriatric schizophrenia patients including postmortem data (see Chapters 75 and 123). A final set of issues relates to specialized psychopharmacological interventions in this age group. Chapters outline specific issues relating to psychotropic drug distribution in the elderly (see Chapter 124) and the principles of treatment for depression in late life (see Chapter 125).

The next chapters in the clinical section are concerned with "neurologic disorders" and highlight a set of approaches and descriptions which again represent major advances since the last edition. After a chapter on Parkinson's disease (see Chapter 126), several interrelated chapters discuss key issues relating to tardive dyskinesia. Since the tardive dyskinesias represents a public health problem, we have devoted a chapter to their epidemiological and clinical presentation (Chapter 127), followed by an update on the pathophysiology of tardive dyskinesia (Chapter 128) and completed by a chapter on treatment approach (Chapter 129). Several other CNS disorders are included in this section to gain a fuller appreciation of both the major changes that have occurred since the last edition, but also to highlight new opportunities to explore the psychopathology and psychopharmacology of these disorders. A chapter on multiinfarct dementia (see Chapter 130) is followed by one on Prion diseases (see Chapter 131). Current advances in Huntington's disease and amyotrophic lateral sclerosis are reviewed (see Chapter 132).

Although not a section of the previous *Generation of Progress*, it is clear that the AIDS epidemic as part of its clinical picture and pathological manifestations, has important aspects relating to clinical psychopathology and dysfunctioning. We have now devoted two chapters to this area; one reviewing neuropsychiatric manifestations of HIV infection (Chapter 133) and the second potential mechanism of neurological dysfunction in HIV infection (Chapter 134).

The following section on personality disorders includes a comprehensive chapter on the neuropsychopharmacology of personality disorder (see Chapter 135). Advances in eating disorders are captured in the subsequent sections. Three chapters cover the psychopharmacology of anorexia nervosa, bulimia, and binge eating (Chapter 136); an update on obesity, fat intake and chronic disease

(Chapter 137); and finally a basic biological overview of this set of disorders (Chapter 138). A comprehensive updated review on selected sleep disorders follows (Chapter 139).

Childhood disorders are the exclusive focus of the following section of five chapters. They review our current state of knowledge on selected childhood disorders with a neuropsychopharmacological component. The first chapter focuses on early-onset mood illness (Chapter 140), followed by a chapter on attention deficit–hyperactive disorder dealing with the interface of neurochemistry, genetics and neuroimaging (Chapter 141). The remaining portion of this section includes a chapter on autism (Chapter 142), a review of current work on tic disorders (Chapter 143) and finally a specific chapters on eating disorders in childhood (Chapter 144).

Research advances in substance abuse and psychopharmacology are reviewed in an expanded major section. The reader is first referred to several chapters on integrative concepts in the preclinical section (see Chapters 66 and 69). In ten chapters, an attempt is made to provide comprehensive coverage of specific areas of substance use and abuse with each chapter providing both an overview and a specific set of treatment approaches. The first few chapters deal with cocaine, caffeine, tobacco, and opioids (Chapters 145, 146, 147, and 148). These are followed by chapters on alcoholism, marijuana, phencyclidine, and benzodiazepines abuse (Chapters 149, 150, 151, and 152). Chapter 153 in this section deals with genetic influences in drug abuse and the final chapter in this section emphasizes the use of behavioral treatments in this set of disorders (Chapter 154).

FUTURE DIRECTIONS

Since the *Third Generation of Progress* was published, there has been a wealth of advances in various areas affecting neuropsychopharmacology. It has been the major aim of this volume to demonstrate how these advances link together and can provide the foundation for further advances in clinical therapeutics and basic neuropsychopharmacology.

In the final section on future directions, we review under "Special Topics" several areas of interest we have chosen, since we believe they will play an increasingly important role in neuropsychopharmacology. These topics include new drug design, bioethics, the economics of drug development, the economic evaluation of drug treatment, ethnic and cultural aspects of psychopharmacology and, finally, violence and aggression.

A first chapter deals with the impact of molecular biology, new drug design based on the cloning of receptor molecules, and other advances in molecular biology in which new drug candidates will be developed by rational design from three-dimensional structures of target molecules (see Chapter 158). As the authors review this particular approach, they indicate how the improved precision of drug design will force a certain perspective and impact on molecular design and discovery within the pharmaceutical industry. The second chapter highlights a set of current bioethical issues confronting clinical and basic researchers associated with genetic screening and testing, gene therapy and scientific conduct (see Chapter 159). The authors review the impact of the human genome project and current developments in genetic counseling. They propose a proactive approach and preventive ethics, which will necessitate new specific codes of conduct. They point to the example of the presymptomatic Huntington's disease testing program as one model of dealing with genetic counseling, bioethics, and the impact of a partnership with "patients" on the likelihood as prospective disease.

In the next chapter, the development of psychotropic drugs is placed in the context of other drug development strategies (Chapter 160). The authors demonstrate that psychotropic drug development in the United States has been lengthier and economically riskier than average and that these factors have led to above-average costs for psychotropics. However, this needs to be placed in the context of strongly growing markets and the extreme lucrativeness of new psychotropic drugs with demonstrable effectiveness. The authors point to several dilemmas impeding the search and timing for new psychotropic drugs, akin to some of the same problems discussed in an earlier chapter on drug design (see Chapter 158). This discussion of the economics of drug development leads directly into a subsequent chapter on economic evaluation of drug treatment for selected psychiatric disorders (Chapter 161). The authors provide specific examples of what has been collected traditionally to assess outcome and discuss how such measures are inappropriate for economic evaluations of drug treatments in the psychiatric disorders. They describe several techniques and types of data that should be utilized in clinical trials for economic evaluation and also provide recommendations for the integration of data from clinical trials, clinical practice, and post-market studies.

The next chapter in this section deals with ethnicity and psychopharmacology (see Chapter 162), a topic related directly to the methodological chapter on pharmacokinetics and pharmacodynamics (see Chapter 74). The authors review the influence of ethnicity on psychotropic responses and point to the new field of pharmacogenetics in which it was found that ethnic differences in drug responses may be genetically determined. The case is reviewed in different classes of psychotropics, as is the role of these parameters in relationship to ethnic concerns. The authors suggest that cross-ethnic research designs will represent a powerful tool for psychopharmacological research in the future.

The final chapter in the critical analysis section is concerned with issues relating to violence and aggression

(Chapter 163). Although these issues do not concern every one of the disorders discussed throughout the clinical section, it is noteworthy that there are a number of disorders in which both outwardly directed aggression as well as internally directed aggression (suicidal behavior) have played a role in long-term prognosis. The author reviews a number of key issues, models of aggression, as well as self-injurious behavior in animals. The linkage between the neurobiology of aggression and suicidal behavior is important as one thinks of the potential serotonergic influences on much of the psychopharmacological discussion with respect to mood disorders and schizophrenia. Furthermore, this chapter ties in with the preclinical discussion on the neurobiology of neurotransmitters.

As we indicated earlier, the volume is not meant to be encyclopedic, but comprehensive in highlighting advances in neuropsychopharmacology over the last 7 years.

While one could anticipate a number of advances that will no doubt be covered in the next edition, we believe that the present volume includes most seminal developments and can represent a specialized set of reviews useful for both the clinical investigator and the basic neuroscientist. In this manner, we hope it will facilitate and accelerate the further integration of basic and clinical research in neuropsychopharmacology.

REFERENCES

1. Bloom FE. Neurohumoral transmission and the central nervous system, In Gilman AG, Rall TW, Nies AS, Taylor P, eds. *Goodman and Gilman's The pharmacological basis of therapeutics*. New York: Pergamon Press, 1990;244–268.
2. Robins E, Guze SB. Establishment of diagnostic validity in psychiatric illness: application to schizophrenia. *Am J Psychiatry* 1970; 126:107–111.

Psychopharmacology: The Fourth
Generation of Progress, edited by
Floyd E. Bloom and David J. Kupfer.
Raven Press, Ltd., New York © 1995.

CHAPTER 71

The DSM-IV Classification and Psychopharmacology

Allen Frances, Avram H. Mack, Ruth Ross, and Michael B. First

During the past 25 years, the DSM system and psychopharmacology have ''grown up'' together and have had a strong influence upon one another. The psychopharmacological revolution required that there be a method of more systematic and reliable psychiatric diagnosis. This provided the major impetus for the development of the structured assessments and the research diagnostic criteria that were the immediate forerunners of DSM-III (30). In turn, the availability of well-defined psychiatric diagnoses stimulated the development of specific treatments and increasingly sophisticated psychopharmacological studies. We expect that DSM-IV will continue to influence, and future revisions to be influenced by, the next steps in the advance of psychopharmacology. This chapter discusses the development of DSM-IV and the ways in which several issues in psychiatric nosology (e.g., descriptive diagnosis, reliability, generalizability, validity, and the heuristic value of the current classification) interact with psychopharmacological research. We suggest that DSM-IV is likely to be a useful tool in psychopharmacological research, but one with numerous limitations that must be understood if this research effort is to have optimal value (see Chapter 157, *this volume*).

PREPARATION OF DSM-IV

The major innovation in the development of DSM-IV was the careful three-stage process of empirical review that informed all decisions (33). The three stages included (a)

A. Frances, A. H. Mack, and R. Ross: Department of Psychiatry, Duke University Medical Center, Durham, North Carolina 27710.
M. B. First: Columbia University College of Physicians and Surgeons, New York State Psychiatric Institute, New York, New York 10032.

comprehensive and systematic reviews of the published literature, (b) reanalyses of already collected but previously unanalyzed data sets, and (c) field trials. Each stage was carefully documented and the results will be published in the detailed five volume DSM-IV *Sourcebook* (5).

The Work Groups generated 150 literature reviews on questions most crucial to the development of DSM-IV. A standard format was used to insure that these reviews would be methodical, objective, and comprehensive (17,34). Each review began with an explicit statement of the issues and a discussion of their significance for clinical practice and research. This was followed by a summary of the literature gathered from as many sources as possible. Finally, there was a discussion of the advantages and disadvantages of the various possible options proposed for DSM-IV. The reviews were then carefully critiqued by Work Group members and advisors to ensure balance and cohesiveness. This process ensured that everyone involved in making decisions was working from a commonly accepted data base, which facilitated agreement among individuals who sometimes began with widely differing positions and orientations. It was hoped that the DSM-IV decisions would reflect the conclusions of an ideal ''consensus scholar'' and not be unduly influenced by the preconceptions of the participants (9). In some cases, the literature reviews provided enough information to resolve questions. In others, they indicated the need for further investigation in the subsequent two stages of the review process. The specific options for change in criteria resulting from the literature reviews were presented to the Task Force and to the mental health field in the DSM-IV *Options Book* (3).

The data reanalyses, funded by the John A. and Catherine D. MacArthur Foundation, were designed to resolve a number of important diagnostic questions for which incomplete answers were available in the published literature. A method was developed for reanalyzing data previously collected in a variety of settings, but not yet analyzed in a way that was useful for answering the Work Group's questions (33). This enabled the Work Groups to develop and refine suggested new criteria that could then be studied in field trials.

We conducted twelve field trials to examine questions that the first two stages had been unable to resolve, which served to bridge the clinical research literature and clinical practice. Each field trial compared alternative DSM-III, DSM-III-R, ICD-10, and proposed DSM-IV options at 5 to 10 sites with approximately 100 subjects at each site. The field trials [sponsored by the National Institute of Mental Health (NIMH) in conjunction with the National Institute on Drug Abuse (NIDA) and the National Institute on Alcohol Abuse and Alcoholism (NIAA)] studied: Antisocial Personality Disorder, Autism and related Pervasive Developmental Disorders, Disruptive Behavior Disorders, Insomnia, Major Depression and Dysthymia, Mixed Anxiety-Depression, Panic Disorder, Obsessive-Compulsive Disorder, Posttraumatic Stress Disorder, Schizophrenia, Somatization Disorder, and Substance Use Disorders (33).

The DSM-IV Task Force was very conservative in making changes from DSM-III-R. A major reason for this was to enable researchers to generalize from data gathered using the different DSMs. A conservative approach also reduces discontinuities in assessment and creates minimal disruption to studies in progress.

The first two stages (i.e., literature reviews and data reanalyses) depended heavily on the published and unpublished results of psychopharmacological studies. In many instances, the diagnostic information that was the most useful for the purposes of the literature reviews emerged from the diagnostic findings that have accumulated over the years as part of clinical trials. There were many advantages and also very serious limitations to the information thus obtained. It was extremely useful to have the extensive pool of data available from clinical trials, especially because the information generally had been carefully collected by skilled investigators under conditions that ensured very high reliability. The Work Groups also had to be cautious about generalizing from pharmacological trials to more general populations, because the results were most often drawn from patient samples after a highly selective screening process. There was a considerable effort to balance data obtained from pharmacological trials with data obtained from other types of clinical research and from epidemiological studies.

In a similar fashion, the reanalyses also used previously unpublished data drawn from many samples collected in pharmacological trials. These trials provided an extremely valuable pool of information and enabled the Work Groups to base deliberations on a much larger empirical base than would otherwise have been possible. As with the literature reviews, however, the Work Groups had to

balance data reanalyses from pharmacological trials with data gathered in other clinical settings and from epidemiological samples to ensure generalizability.

The field trials provided a bridge between clinical research (including pharmacological trials) and more general clinical practice. They used methods that more closely approximated general practice than would the method of a typical, more rigorously controlled clinical trial (13). Consecutive patients were evaluated to eliminate the sampling bias inherent in the application of inclusionary and exclusionary criteria for treatment outcome studies. Patients were selected using a diversity of representative sites that sampled different socioeconomic, cultural, and ethnic groups in many different geographic locations and, in some instances, included randomly selected general community samples. Finally, reliability was not established as a precondition to beginning the formal portion of the study as is done routinely in pharmacological trials. Rather the field trial interviewers were given only limited training to approximate more closely the conditions that are obtained in general clinical practice.

DESCRIPTIVE APPROACH

Throughout the history of psychiatric nosology, there has been a back and forth alternation between systems that were based more on theories of etiology and those that were based more exclusively on descriptive observation. The ancient systems of psychiatric classification developed by Hippocrates, Galen, and Rhazes were anchored in etiological explanations (e.g., for Hippocrates, mental health or illness depended upon the balance or imbalance of the four humours: blood, phlegm, black bile, yellow bile) (24,10). Modern psychopharmacology has continued the search for more meaningful humours, using vastly more powerful instruments of study. With the Renaissance came an increasing emphasis on descriptive classification. The English physician Sydenham (1624–1663 A.D.) assumed that because nature is "uniform" and "consistent," the same symptoms and signs "that you would observe in the sickness of a Socrates you would observe in the sickness of a simpleton" (31). Sydenham's emphasis on careful descriptive observation influenced the taxonomies of Linnaeus and Boissier de Sauvages. The latter developed perhaps the most extensive psychiatric classification in history, listing 2400 different "species" of mental disorders. Descriptive methods were also used by the early nineteenth century psychiatrists Pinel and Esquirol (18).

Explanatory, etiological models were soon offered to replace these superficial descriptive systems. Cabanis wrote that the excessive reliance on description would lead science to "lose itself in the multitude of facts gathered" (18). The physicians Gall and Broussais declared that to classify by symptoms was arbitrary and instead emphasized the value of brain dissection performed at autopsy (1). In this environment, the descriptive classification of Pinel and Esquirol was "now forgotten, [and] the neuropsychiatric perspective . . . took a leading position" (25). Many etiological models of mental illness have since been offered, ranging from phrenology to psychoanalytic theory, but more recently most have been based upon the attempt to determine the specific structure and function of the brain abnormalities that are closely associated with mental disorders.

Kraepelin's careful descriptive classification provided the inspiration, and much of the content, for the assertively descriptive approach used in DSM-III (7). Perhaps the most cogent (and still totally current) defense for the descriptive approach was offered by a contemporary of Kraepelin, the nineteenth century American psychiatrist, Pliny Earle, who said, "In the present state of our knowledge, no classification of insanity can be erected upon a pathological basis, for the simple reason that, with but slight exceptions, the pathology of the disease is unknown . . . we are forced to fall back upon the symptomatology of the disease" (19). The descriptive system has been extremely valuable both to psychiatric classification and to psychopharmacology because it increases reliability and promotes communication across all of the various psychiatric orientations (7). Nonetheless the user of the DSM-IV must also understand that any descriptive approach is only an unsatisfactory and limited step along the way toward a system of classification that is based on etiological understanding.

DSM-IV provides no more, but also no less, than a descriptive heuristic for discovery of underlying pathogenesis in the same way as descriptive systems in other disciplines have suggested eventually explanatory models (e.g., the role of Mendeliev's periodic table in chemistry and of Linneaus's taxonomy of species in furthering the theory of evolution). New findings, much of them drawn from psychopharmacological research, will hopefully help us gradually to replace our current descriptive system with one that is based on a much deeper knowledge of underlying etiology. In effect, DSM-IV provides the useful descriptions that will hopefully facilitate our moving away from, and beyond, the descriptive approach (14).

Another, more immediate, limitation of the DSM-IV descriptive system arises from the way in which the criteria sets have been generated. For the most part, the definitions of the individual DSM-IV disorders are based upon the covariation of symptoms (descriptive validity) and without any clear gold standards for choosing items or setting thresholds based on other forms of validity. Many (if not most) of the DSM-IV disorders are heterogeneous, lack clear boundaries with near neighbors, and could as well have been defined with alternative items or thresholds that had essentially equal claims to validity. We must, therefore, avoid reifying the existing DSM-IV cate-

gories, thresholds, or definitional items. It is possible that with greater understanding, new disorders and new combinations will emerge and that many of the descriptively defined DSM-IV disorders will cease to stand on their own. Many DSM-IV categories that now appear as separate disorders may be reunited when eventually it is determined that they have a shared etiology or pathogenesis. Other DSM-IV descriptive categories may be divided further based on discoveries about their etiological heterogeneity. There is no reason to assume that the current descriptive classification follows nature with any degree of precision.

There is also the misunderstood issue of comorbidity. We cannot assume that so-called comorbid disorders necessarily have separate and independent pathogeneses. Many disorders that appear to be comorbid may instead be no more than the split descriptive parts of a more complex syndrome or may reflect a definitional artifact resulting from the fact that many items appear in more or less equivalent form in the definitions of more than one disorder. There are five factors inherent in the DSM system that enhance (and perhaps artifactually elevate) comorbidity: (a) the narrowly defined criteria sets, (b) the large number of distinct diagnoses, (c) the explicit diagnostic criteria, (d) the use of structured interviews, and (e) the removal of diagnostic hierarchies. Ever since DSM-III, our system of classification has been a splitter's dream. However, we can expect a gradual return to the lumping together of at least some descriptive categories once we know more about shared etiology (16,12).

RELIABILITY AND GENERALIZABILITY

Before DSM-III, the reliability of psychiatric diagnosis was limited by the lack of widely accepted and standardized diagnostic criteria and assessment instruments (8,27,29). Low reliability made it difficult to interpret (and impossible to generalize) the results of psychopharmacological trials. The development of explicit and reliable diagnostic criteria sets in the Feighner criteria (11), the Research Diagnostic Criteria (RDC) (28), and DSM-III (2) was a necessary prerequisite for the development of meaningful psychopharmacological research. The DSM-IV reliance upon carefully conducted field trials to select item sets with optimal demonstrable reliability represents one further step in the process of enhancing the reliability of psychiatric diagnosis.

Despite these achievements, we must be aware of certain limitations. There has been a considerable controversy regarding the claims made for the reliability that can be achieved using the DSM system. Kirk and Kutchins (23) have argued that the DSM-III field trials were performed and reported in an inconsistent manner that did not truly document the reliability of the DSM-III criteria sets. Moreover, they have correctly pointed out that the reliability achieved has been much greater when measured for the wider DSM sections (e.g., mood disorder or anxiety disorder) than for the more specific disorders contained in those sections (e.g., dysthymic disorder or generalized anxiety disorder).

The Kirk and Kutchins critique is much more germane to reliability measured in general clinical practice (i.e., the conditions that were approximated in the DSM-III field trials) than to the reliability measured in psychopharmacological studies. In the carefully controlled, somewhat "hot house" environment of a typical treatment outcome study, highly selected patients are evaluated by expert and highly trained interviewers who are very familiar with the diagnosis being studied and with one another and are using systematic and standardized assessment instruments. Under these conditions, it is almost always possible within any given site and/or any given diagnosis to achieve satisfactory to excellent reliability using the DSM system.

The more difficult issue for psychopharmacology is the degree of generalizability of the reliability achieved in one site to multiple sites or to more general clinical practice. For multisite studies, it is necessary to provide cross-site training and reliability testing (often using videotapes) as a means of ensuring that the reliability in any given site is not merely home grown. This problem has generally received insufficient attention in the implementation and reporting of multisite trials and certainly should be built into every multisite design and report of methods. An even tougher question is whether results generated in the very specific conditions of a clinical trial are generalizable to the rough and tumble of everyday clinical practice. One possible implication of this issue is the importance of measuring reliability in health services research studies and in Phase IV clinical trials that can be conducted in a wide variety of settings that more closely approximate the conditions in which patients are routinely seen.

VALIDITY

Whereas a low reliability certainly sets the ceiling on our ability to determine validity, a high reliability by no means implies that we are engaged in making valid, or even interesting, distinctions. Kendell points out that "reliability can be very high while validity remains trivial and in such a situation high reliability is of very limited value" (21). An excessive devotion to reliability may in fact distract us from the more fundamental and meaningful validity questions if we focus too exclusively on polishing our methodological lenses rather than looking through them. We must therefore move forward in applying our more or less reliable diagnostic system to those research questions that will further our understanding of etiology and pathogenesis.

There is also an urgent need to understand more about the performance characteristics, beyond the descriptive level, of the DSM-IV items, thresholds, and disorders. It must be admitted that, despite the accumulating literature, there are very few diagnoses for which there are meaningful gold standards of validity. We often have little evidence to determine what is, and what is not, predicted by the various descriptive diagnoses. In conducting the three-stage process of empirical review for DSM-IV, we became aware of how relatively few data were available to guide the choice between alternative options regarding the specific definitional items that should be chosen for the criteria sets or the possible alternative thresholds to determine the presence or absence of a disorder. There is an important lesson in this for psychopharmacological research. In designing projects, we should avoid giving too much weight to the DSM-IV system as it now stands and take a broader overview. Although the DSM-IV is extraordinarily useful, it certainly does not deserve reification and we must avoid premature closure. This suggests three precautions that might inform the design and implementation of clinical trials: (a) Researchers should cast a much wider net of items in their assessment batteries beyond the items contained in the DSM-IV criteria sets and should not assume that the DSM-IV items provide the only useful predictor variables (additional items may be drawn from the Associated Features section of the text for each disorder). (b) The prediction of outcome and determination of indications can be improved by assessing for the comorbid near-neighbor symptoms or disorders that may one day become known as part of the disorder within a more complex syndrome. (c) Finally, efforts at data analysis should begin by using the DSM-IV algorithms but should also proceed in an exploratory fashion to test different possible thresholds and different defining items. To the degree that psychopharmacological research is limited to the DSM-IV approach, there will be numerous delays in learning more about how to improve it.

HEURISTIC ISSUES

The preparation of DSM-IV helped us to identify any number of gaps in our knowledge base and suggested many areas of future research. These are indicated in the various sections that comprise the DSM-IV *Sourcebook* (5). The proposals that were made for the possible inclusion of new diagnoses in DSM-IV are of particular relevance to the search for new indicators that is so important in psychopharmacological research. The conservative mandate to the DSM-IV Task Force caused it to hold the line against the proliferation of new disorders (26). The Task Force accepted for official classification only a handful of the more than 100 suggested new diagnoses. Many of the new suggestions had been based on interesting clinical observation and/or preliminary research findings but were without sufficient empirical data on the descriptive characteristics and validity of the proposed categories to warrant inclusion. Appendix B of DSM-IV provides a list (see Table 1) of the Suggested New Diagnoses and Criteria Sets that did not yet have sufficient documentation to warrant inclusion in the classification but did show potential for further study.

Many of the suggested new categories are conditions that are subthreshold to existing DSM-IV categories. Including these conditions as official mental disorders would have had the effect of widening the definition of caseness and the sensitivity of the DSM-IV diagnostic system (thus decreasing false negatives) but at the cost of decreasing the specificity of the system and increasing false positives. Until there are many additional systematic studies to determine how the suggested subthreshold disorders respond to treatment, we cannot accurately measure the relative utility costs of false negatives versus those of false positives. It seems likely that the psychopharmacological community will benefit from studying at least some of these potential diagnoses and psychiatric classification will benefit from accumulated knowledge

TABLE 1. *Criteria sets and axes provided for further study*

Asperger's disorder
Postconcussional disorder
Mild cognitive disorder
Caffeine withdrawal
Postpsychotic depression of schizophrenia
Simple schizophrenia
Minor depressive disorder
Recurrent brief depressive disorder
Premenstrual dysphoric disorder
Mixed anxiety-depressive disorder
Facticious disorder by proxy
Dissociative trance disorder
Telephone scatalogia
Binge eating disorder
Depressive personality disorder
Passive agressive personality disorder
Medication-induced movement disorders
   Neuroleptic-induced Parkinsonism
   Neuroleptic malignant syndrome
   Neuroleptic-induced acute dystonia
   Neuroleptic-induced acute akathisia
   Neuroleptic-induced tardive dyskinesia
   Neuroleptic-induced postural tremor
Axis for defense mechanisms
GARF (Global assessment of relational functioning scale)
SOFAS (Social and occupational functioning assessment scale)

This table is a reprint of Appendix B from DSM-IV (4) and contains a number of proposals for new categories and axes that were suggested for possible inclusion in DSM-IV. The DSM-IV Task Force and Work Groups subjected each of these proposals to a careful empirical review and invited wide commentary from the field. The Task Force determined that there was insufficient information to warrant inclusion of these proposals as official categories in DSM-IV.

regarding treatment response. Some such studies are indeed in progress.

We summarize briefly the status of three proposed new categories (minor depression, brief recurrent depression, and mixed anxiety depression) that are particularly important to consider as potential new indications in clinical trials. The thresholds for severity and duration of major depression established in DSM-III and DSM-III-R were necessarily arbitrary and not based on any strong validation. It is therefore not surprising that a number of studies, particularly those performed in primary care and community settings, report that many patients who fall short of the DSM thresholds for mood disorder nonetheless exhibit clinically significant impairment as measured by functional disability and health care utilization. Three different types of subthreshold depression have been identified. Minor Depression is subthreshold in symptom severity to Major Depressive Disorder (22,32). Brief Recurrent Depressive Disorder is subthreshold to Major Depressive Disorder with regard to duration and consists of many episodes in a year, each meeting the full symptom severity criteria of Major Depressive Disorder but lasting for only a few days (6). Mixed Anxiety Depression is characterized by a combination of dysphoric symptoms of anxiety and depression in individuals who fail to meet syndromal criteria for any specific anxiety disorder or depressive disorder (20).

There were several reasons that minor depressive disorder, brief recurrent depressive disorder, and mixed anxiety/depressive disorder were not included as official categories, but rather in the Appendix for Criteria Sets and Axes Provided for Further Study (Table 1): (a) Their inclusion might result in unnecessary treatment for the false positives. (b) Subthreshold categories may trivialize the construct of mental disorder and artificially inflate prevalence rates. (c) The evidence suggesting that subthreshold conditions are associated with significant impairment is difficult to interpret because the subthreshold diagnosis may have resulted from inadequate assessments. (d) The research on these conditions is incomplete and there are virtually no treatment studies. Indeed, at least some of the patients with subthreshold diagnoses might have met the criteria for major depression or an anxiety disorder were they diagnosed more carefully. On the other hand, it must be noted that the treatment implications of the proposed categories are unknown. We may be depriving patients of effective treatment by not recognizing the given category and/or we may be protecting the individuals from unnecessary and ineffective treatment. The suggestions for these subthreshold categories raise the fundamental question of how best to define the boundary between psychopathology and normality.

CONCLUSION

DSM-III was an innovative system. Unlike DSM-II, it focused on descriptive diagnosis and provided explicit diagnostic criteria (7,30). In many ways this aided, and was aided by, the knowledge derived from psychopharmacology. To avoid disrupting research, DSM-IV has chosen to be a conservative system and changes were made only when convincing empirical evidence could be marshalled (26). Pharmacological research will play an important role in gradually replacing the DSM descriptive system with one that is increasingly based on etiology. This will occur through studies that expand our knowledge of treatment response and underlying mechanisms. DSM-IV provides a necessary common language for current study and practice, but should not be subject to reification or promote premature closure. Our knowledge will be enhanced to the degree that we also study additional definitional items, thresholds, and diagnoses that have not been included in DSM-IV. The diagnostic system and psychopharmacology will continue to mature with one another.

REFERENCES

1. Ackernecht, *A Brief History of Medicine.* Baltimore: Johns Hopkins; 1982.
2. American Psychiatric Association. *Diagnostic and statistical manual of mental disorders.* 3rd ed. Washington, DC: 1980.
3. American Psychiatric Association. *Diagnostic and statistical manual of mental disorders.* 4th ed. *Options Book.* Washington, DC: 1991.
4. American Psychiatric Association. *Diagnostic and statistical manual of mental disorders.* 4th ed. Washington, DC: 1994.
5. American Psychiatric Association. *Diagnostic and statistical manual of mental disorders.* 4th ed. *Sourcebook.* Washington, DC: 1994.
6. Angst J, Merikangas K, Scheidegger P, Wicki W. Recurrent brief depression: a new subtype of affective disorder. *J Affect Disord* 1990;19:87–98.
7. Blashfield RK. *The classification of psychopathology.* New York: Plenum; 1984.
8. Blashfield RK, Draguns JG. Evaluative criteria for psychiatric classification. *J Abnormal Psychol* 1976;85:140–150.
9. Cooper HM. *The integrative research review. A systematic approach.* Vol. 2. Beverly Hills: Sage; 1984.
10. Dodds ER. *The Greeks and the irrational.* Berkeley: University of California Press; 1951.
11. Feighner J, Robins E, Guze S, et al. Diagnostic criteria for use in psychiatric research. *Arch Gen Psychiatry* 1972;26:57–63.
12. First M, Spitzer R, Williams J. Exclusionary principles and comorbidity of psychiatric diagnoses: a historical review and implications for the future. In Maser JD, Cloninger CR, eds. *Comorbidity of mood and anxiety disorders.* Washington, DC: American Psychiatric Press, 1990.
13. Frances A, Davis WW, Kline M, et al. The DSM-IV field trials: moving towards an empirically derived classification. *Eur Psychiatry* 1991;6:307–314.
14. Frances A, First M, Pincus H. An introduction to DSM-IV. *Hosp Commun Psychiatry* 1990;41:493–494.
15. Frances A, Pincus H, Widiger T, et al. DSM-IV: Work in progress. *Am J Psychiatry* 1990;147:1439–1448.
16. Frances AJ, Widiger TA, Fyer M. The influence of classification methods on comorbidity, In Maser JD, Cloninger CR, eds. *Comorbidity of mood and anxiety disorders.* Washington, DC: American Psychiatric Press; 1990.
17. Frances A, Widiger TA, Pincus H. The development of DSM-IV. *Arch Gen Psychiatry* 1989;46:373–375.
18. Goldstein J. *Console and classify: the French psychiatric profession in the nineteenth century.* New York: Cambridge University Press; 1988.
19. Grob G. *Mental Illness and American Society, 1875–1940.* Princeton: Princeton University Press, 1983.
20. Katon W, Roy-Burne P. Mixed anxiety and depression, In *DSM-IV Sourcebook.* Washington, DC: American Psychiatric Press; 1991.
21. Kendell RE. *The Role of Diagnosis in Psychiatry.* London: Blackwell; 1975.
22. Klerman GL. Depressive disorders: further evidence for increased medical morbidity and impairment of social functioning. *Arch Gen Psychiatry* 1989;46:856–858.
23. Kirk S, Kutchins H. *The selling of DSM: the rhetoric of science in psychiatry.* New York: Aldine de Gruyter; 1992.
24. Menninger K. *The vital balance.* New York: Viking; 1963.
25. Pichot P. Basis and theories of classification in psychiatry, In Freedman A, Silverman I, Brotman R, Hutson D, eds. *Issues in psychiatric classification.* New York: Human Sciences Press; 1986.
26. Pincus HA, Frances AJ, Davis WW, et al. DSM-IV and new diagnostic categories: holding the line on proliferation. *Am J Psychiatry* 1992;149:112–117.
27. Rosenhan DL. The contextual nature of psychiatric diagnosis. *J Abnormal Psychol* 1975;84:462–472.
28. Spitzer RL, Endicott J, Robins E. *Research diagnostic criteria (RDC) for a selected group of functional disorders.* 3rd ed. New York: Biometrics Research Division, New York State Psychiatric Institute; 1978.
29. Spitzer RL, Fleiss JL. A re-analysis of the reliability of psychiatric diagnosis. *Br J Psychiatry* 1974;125:341–347.
30. Spitzer RL, Williams JBW, Skodol AE. DSM-III: the major achievements and an overview. *Am J Psychiatry* 1980;137:151–164.
31. Sydenham T. Preface to the third edition of *Observationes Medicae.* In Latham RG, trans. *The works of Thomas Sydenham.* Vol. 3. London: The Sydenham Society, 1682.
32. Wells KB, Stewart A, Hays RD, et al. The functioning and well being of depressed patients: results from the medical outcomes study. *JAMA* 1988;262:914–919.
33. Widiger T, Frances A, Pincus H, et al. Toward an empirical classification for the DSM-IV. *J Abnormal Psychol* 1991;100:280–288.
34. Widiger T, Frances A, Pincus H, Davis WW. The DSM-IV literature reviews: rationale, process, and limitations. *J Psychopathol Behav Assess* 1990;12:189–202.

Psychopharmacology: The Fourth Generation of Progress, edited by Floyd E. Bloom and David J. Kupfer. Raven Press, Ltd., New York 1995.

CHAPTER **72**

Clinical Study Design

Critical Issues

Donald S. Robinson and Robert F. Prien

This chapter on study design focuses on methodological issues of importance in designing a study to evaluate the treatment effects of psychotropic drugs. Critical choices facing the clinical investigator in planning trials of approved and investigational drugs are discussed, and recommendations are given for enhancing the reliability and validity of experiments. For a comprehensive review of clinical methodology in psychopharmacology, the reader is referred to the recent volume on clinical evaluation of psychotropic drugs jointly sponsored by the National Institute of Mental Health and the American College of Neuropsychopharmacology (43).

Prior to approval, new drugs undergo stringent clinical testing in studies whose design, analysis, and method of reporting in a New Drug Application (NDA) are shaped to a large extent by U.S. Food and Drug Administration (FDA) guidelines (12,13). The clinical experience gained during phase I, II, and III trials is limited to a few thousand patients who receive the agent before it becomes available for use in practice. Therefore, much of the important information about a new drug is gained under typical practice conditions in postmarketing clinical studies, which are subject to fewer regulatory restrictions. The underlying principles governing clinical evaluation of psychotherapeutic agents, however, apply to all investigations, whether conducted during development of a drug or following its approval.

D. S. Robinson: CNS Clinical Research, Bristol-Meyers Squibb Company, Melbourne, Florida 32940.
R. F. Prien: Clinical Treatment Research Branch, National Institute of Mental Health, Rockville, Maryland 20857.

BASIC DESIGN ELEMENTS OF CLINICAL DRUG STUDIES

Controlled and Uncontrolled Studies

Clinical psychopharmacology, perhaps more than most other fields, is subject to a degree of inherent experimental variability that can tax the skills of the most careful and experienced investigator. Effect sizes tend to be modest and variance is substantial. In concert, these factors can make it difficult to show a treatment effect, highlighting the critical importance of observing sound clinical methodology in psychotropic drug trials.

In psychopharmacology, hypothesis-testing experiments must be well controlled (35). Because of the length of treatment (typically weeks or months) and the variable course of most psychiatric disorders, this generally mandates a double-blind, placebo-controlled study of parallel groups. Experiments involving more than one control treatment (typically, a standard drug and a placebo treatment) can be the most informative for several reasons. Such designs provide another standard for evaluating efficacy, quantify drug treatment effect, and serve to reduce experimental bias. Another advantage is that they increase the probability that a patient will receive an active treatment, which can have several advantages: among these are easier recruitment of patients to a study and improved blinding from the more active treatments.

Acquiring the most definitive data on the dose–response relationship for a psychotropic drug also requires well-controlled trials. Because a single experiment can address only a limited number of questions or hypotheses, complete understanding of how to use a drug therapeutically, especially dosing, requires a body of knowledge gained from many different controlled trials, many conducted after the introduction of a drug into clinical practice.

Uncontrolled studies in clinical psychopharmacology have value for some purposes, often as exploratory trials. Preliminary assessment of a new drug's efficacy, in addition to evaluating its safety and tolerability, may be possible early in phase II using an open-trial design (however, one can place more confidence in a finding of no benefit than in one of possible efficacy). Uncontrolled, nonblind studies are also useful to generate supplementary information about a drug, for example, the effects in special populations such as the elderly or chronically ill. These patients are difficult to recruit for controlled trials. Well-controlled trials are still required for more definitive dose–response and efficacy data in special populations and generally require more time to complete than other studies.

Standard Clinical Trial Paradigms

Randomized controlled trials (RCTs) remain the mainstay of studies intended to define a drug's safety, efficacy, and dose–response relationships. Placebo-controlled, double-blind designs, with randomized assignment to treatment, and usually three (or more) treatment arms, represent the methodological standard (35). This basic study paradigm has many variations, depending on the objectives and the specific properties of the drug being studied (30).

Once the study objectives have been set and the patient sample, entry criteria, and statistical power specified, a particularly critical design decision is whether to stratify randomization based on some characteristic of the target population. Although stratification adds complexity to a trial, it can have methodological advantages that offset this disadvantage (25). It may be crucial to safeguard against a chance (but critical) baseline imbalance in treatment groups that would limit inferences to be drawn about the results of a trial. Sometimes, employing a matching or stratification strategy in protocol design can enhance statistical power, if the matching variable is itself an important independent predictor of outcome (25,39). The crucial factor in the decision to stratify randomization is to identify the variables that are expected to have the foremost role on the outcome of the trial. Because of the complexities of stratification for sample size, recruitment of patients, and overall administration of the study (which increases with each additional stratum), patients should be stratified based on the smallest number of variables possible, and only on those for which there is evidence of prognostic value for the type of treatment being studied. Using a stratification design complicates drug packaging and procedures for assigning treatments, especially for multisite studies, and data analyses become more complex. Therefore, it should be clear that the statistical advantages outweigh the logistical and other disadvantages of the more complicated design.

Under ideal circumstances, an RCT should be conducted as a single-site study, although frequently this is not practical. Addition of sites to a study inevitably increases variance as well as logistical complexity. Minimizing site variability is a major consideration in the planning of a multicenter psychopharmacology study. Critical concerns are ensuring intersite reliability and uniformity of protocol implementation. Testing for treatment-by-site interactions sometimes can remedy an aberrant outcome involving one of the sites in analyzing a multicenter study. However, the ability to test for site by treatment interactions is impaired if there are numerous sites, because statistical power to conclusively show an interaction is restricted.

Alternatives to Parallel Group Placebo Controls

There is no completely satisfactory alternative for a concurrent placebo control in evaluating the efficacy of a psychopharmacological agent. However, if a placebo is inappropriate for ethical or other reasons, a well-designed, multiple fixed-dose study may be a useful option. This approach involves the comparison of fixed high and low doses of the test drug. A significant difference in efficacy between doses is interpreted as evidence of the drug's efficacy. This is an economical approach, because it generates dose-ranging data as well as efficacy information. However, it may produce an unacceptably high risk of false-negative errors because of uncertainty in defining a priori what constitutes fully effective and less effective dose levels. If there is no significant difference between doses (or alternatively, plasma levels), no inference can be made regarding therapeutic effect. Also, the purposeful selection of a low dose outside the therapeutic range, or a dose that is marginally effective, raises the same ethical concerns that apply to use of placebo.

Another option is to compare the test drug against a standard drug. However, as is the case with the multiple fixed-dose control, it may be difficult to interpret a finding of no significant difference because of the difficulty in controlling for factors that are not drug specific, such as natural fluctuations in the course of illness, insensitive outcome measures, investigator or patient bias or expectations, and strong therapeutic benefits of the treatment setting and support systems. There is also the possibility that one is inadvertently using a treatment-resistant population. The test drug may appear as effective as the reference drug because neither is working. Another disadvantage is that it may require a very large sample to test the statistical hypothesis of no true difference between the test and reference drug.

A third option is to use a historical placebo control (29). With this option, a standard placebo response is established for a given investigator and study design and is then applied to subsequent trials involving the same investigator and protocol but a different drug. With this strategy, it has been suggested that a smaller placebo treatment arm be included in the protocol to enhance the blinding of ratings and to see if the pattern of placebo response corresponds to past experience. Major drawbacks to this approach include the statistical inadequacies of the placebo control group and the fact that factors affecting placebo response often do not remain static over time even with the same investigator using the same protocol. Also, there may be ethical concerns about the use of the small placebo sample, in part because it would not be scientifically conclusive.

Longitudinal drug studies sometimes include periods of single-blind placebo treatment to determine whether the drug is active and how long it needs to be continued. This approach is often used to obtain preliminary information regarding efficacy, dose management, and required duration of treatment as a prelude to definitive randomized parallel group studies.

Specialized Trial Designs

Crossover Designs

A balanced, randomized, crossover design has theoretical appeal because it factors out interindividual variability, enhances statistical power, and enables a study of much smaller sample size to detect a treatment effect. Unfortunately, this design is rarely appropriate for a therapeutic trial. Carryover effects from the first period of treatment generally complicate or preclude valid statistical analyses of outcomes beyond initial treatment.

A crossover design may be applicable for studies dealing with chronic, stable conditions where within-subject variability is less than between-subject variability and where patients return to the baseline condition after therapeutic intervention. The crossover paradigm is also an appropriate design for phase I normal volunteer studies, where the primary focus is on pharmacokinetics and safety assessments and carryover effects are not an issue.

A variation of the crossover study design is the so-called N-of-one study (19), where a subject undergoes several alternating courses of drug and placebo, preferably under double-blind conditions. This study design presupposes that a patient returns to baseline condition following each course of treatment (as for a crossover experiment of balanced design). Because of the obvious limitations with respect to generalizability of a single-patient study, proponents of the N-of-one study design generally advocate that a series of patients be studied,

with each crossing over treatment three or four times. Despite the limitations of this design for psychopharmacological applications, there may be occasional circumstances involving special populations where intensive observation of a single patient by a skilled investigator is a preferred (or the only possible) approach, for example, if the target disorder is extremely rare or difficult to study (28,30).

Longitudinal Study Designs

There is a growing interest in, and importance of, evaluations of an entire therapeutic course of treatment, as opposed to trials establishing acute efficacy. Studies to assess long-term benefits and risks of treatment are designed differently than those used for short-term trials and pose difficult and complex methodological issues that have not been fully resolved. (Study designs in this category are also discussed in the last section of this chapter on ''Future Directions in Clinical Psychopharmacology Trials.'') It is reasonable for clinicians and health agencies to seek valid comparative data about long-term treatment alternatives, because this information can be critical in making judgments about managed care and drug formularies. This interest has been generated, in part, by the discipline of pharmacoeconomics and its evolving role in the evaluation of mental health therapy and care programs.

Treatment response of most psychiatric disorders follows an indolent and highly variable course. Schizophrenia, obsessive compulsive disorder, and the mood disorders are typical examples. Drug treatments can effectively control many of the acute symptoms of these disorders, but relapse and/or recurrence frequently occur when acute medication is withdrawn and unless medication is continued for periods of months to years. Although it seems to be true that drugs having established short-term benefit show continued therapeutic benefit with ongoing treatment, longitudinal studies complement acute treatment studies and are important to gaining a full understanding of how a drug should be used in practice. These studies are also useful for acquiring long-term safety data (a requirement of many regulatory agencies for drug approval of marketing).

A frequently used design for evaluating the efficacy of long-term treatment is a placebo-substitution paradigm, by which patients who have been successfully treated and remain in treatment, are randomly assigned to either continue their study medication or receive a placebo. This design can be used for evaluating treatments for the prevention or attenuation of relapse, recurrence, or a chronic state. Most of these studies admit patients during the acute phase of illness and require that patients attain adequate control of symptoms before they are randomized to long-term treatments. Therefore, this is a form of enrichment design. The attrition from the time of admission into the acute phase to the randomization to long-term treatment often reaches 50% or more. A large part of the attrition stems from failure to stabilize the patient on assigned acute treatments. This heavy loss can produce samples that are not representative of the population defined by study intake criteria.

Relatively few study reports provide data on the difference between the sample entering the acute phase of the study and the subset of survivors that are subsequently randomized to the long-term treatment. Furthermore, many studies fail to consider the loss of patients prior to long-term treatment as it may affect proper interpretation and generalizibility of the findings. Although this is a problem generic to therapeutic studies in general, it is particularly critical for long-term, multiphasic trials where prerandomization attrition may significantly skew the study sample (32).

Another problem with multiphase studies is that prerandomization attrition may favor one treatment over another in the long-term phase of the study (18). Various efforts to deal with this problem have been proposed (34): For example, the patients could enter the study during an interepisode period rather than during an acute episode. Patients receiving long-term treatment are taken off whatever therapy they are receiving and are randomly assigned to study treatments. There are disadvantages to this design. Patients who have been episode-free for a significant period of time may be reluctant to participate in a study where they might receive a different drug, or worse, a placebo. Obviously, recruitment of patients in this setting has practical difficulties. One long-term study that attempted this approach with patients receiving treatment for recurrent mood disorders fell far short of obtaining the requisite sample (44).

Another type of design used to evaluate long-term treatment is the single-blind, longitudinal trial in which the study treatment is periodically discontinued and/or replaced by a placebo. A similar type of longitudinal study is the mirror-image trial in which the course of illness during study treatment is compared to the course of illness during an equivalent period preceding the treatment. Both provide useful information on long-term efficacy of treatment. A major advantage of these designs is that they require a smaller sample than studies with a concurrent control treatment. However, there are several problems. There is no control for relevant nonspecific factors, such as the variable fluctuations in the natural course of illness, the effects of treatment setting (e.g., formal or informal medical support systems), and observer and physician expectations regarding the test drug.

Overall, none of the designs for evaluating long-term treatment are flawless; all have methodological problems. However, in well-conducted studies, these problems usu-

ally are not sufficiently serious to preclude implementation. Nonetheless, it is important that the difficulties and limitations of these approaches be recognized in undertaking such studies and in the interpretation and generalization of results.

Long-term treatment strategies are discussed in other chapters in this volume (see Chapters 73, 91, and 157, *this volume*).

Dose–Response Studies

Accurate dose-response data provide essential prescribing information for a new drug and is a condition for drug approval in many countries. Because no single study design can address all aspects of the dose–response relationship, these data must be generated from a number of different trials. Although the composite safety data base from all of the phase I, II, and III studies provides some assessment of how dose relates to safety and side effects, well-controlled trials can provide additional safety information of value. Multiple-dose RCT design can furnish vital dose–response data, both for efficacy and safety purposes. Studies of this design provide direct comparisons of concurrent treatments at different dose levels of the test drug.

Defining how dose and efficacy are related requires a rigorous experimental approach, primarily from placebo-controlled studies. A minimum effective dose of a new drug and its therapeutic dose range need to be established. It is desirable to know the optimal doses or optimal dose range of a new drug. Study designs with several treatment arms that compare either different fixed doses, or different dose ranges, of a drug constitute one experimental approach to obtaining such information (7). As we discussed in the earlier section on alternatives to placebo controls, a variation of the multiple-dose RCT design involves substituting a marginally active (low) dose of the drug for placebo. This has been proposed as a way to obviate ethical and logistical concerns about placebo treatment. Incorporating a low-dose treatment arm in a study protocol presupposes preexisting knowledge of the dose–response relationship. An incorrect choice for the low dose arm could be a costly error if it does not discriminate from other doses. Beyond this concern, including a placebo treatment arm in a dose–response study has the clear advantage of permitting the drug treatment to be quantified.

Fixed-dose studies with multiple treatment arms have gained popularity for investigating dose–response relationships. Although this study design yields valuable information, it does not characterize the response to a drug as it will be used in clinical practice. First-pass metabolism and systemic bioavailability vary substantially among individuals for most drugs, particularly the psychotherapeutic agents (52). To optimize therapeutic benefit during clinical management of a patient, the drug dose should be titrated within a defined range based on observed effects. Dose-titration studies where dose is individualized, as opposed to fixed-dose studies, more closely approximate actual practice conditions and arguably are a better assessment of the relationship of dosage to therapeutic benefit.

Concentration-controlled Studies

A modification of the standard RCT design has been proposed by Peck (40). This concentration-controlled study design has been advocated as a more cost-effective and efficient way to investigate the clinical pharmacology and efficacy of a new drug, especially in early development (49). This methodological approach is predicated on the assumption that the plasma concentration of a drug correlates better with clinical response than does dosage (30). In psychopharmacology, except for a few drugs, such as lithium, this has not proven to be the case (41,54). The low predictive value for efficacy of plasma drug levels is understandable, given that centrally active drugs tend to be highly lipophilic with a large brain-plasma concentration ratio. Plasma levels, therefore, constitute an indirect index of target tissue (brain) concentrations and have proven to have limited use for optimizing therapeutic response of most psychotherapeutic agents.

The concentration-controlled study design has several practical drawbacks as well. Implementation requires significant modification of the standard RCT design in a way that may be counter to sound research design. Compromising the blind is risked because of the requirement to adjust dose based on drug level monitoring. An elaborate procedure would be required to allow regulating the plasma concentration of a patient, if indicated based on the drug level. Evidence is lacking that this experimental paradigm can be adapted successfully to RCTs, especially pivotal psychopharmacological studies. It is unclear whether the logistics would be manageable for drug development purposes in psychopharmacology. More experience is necessary to establish the practicality and utility of this approach for clinical research (37).

Degrees of Blinding

Rigorous blinding procedures for RCTs are essential in psychopharmacology, because outcome measures are principally based on subjectively rated items (17). The original double-blind design has undergone modification to guard against possible experimental bias. An example of such bias would be cues about treatment assignment inferred by study personnel from the real or perceived side effects of the treatments (15). It is important to instruct study personnel to resist drawing inferences about a patient's treatment assignment as they assess outcome. All research staff need to be encouraged to maintain objectivity, by observing a standard approach in eliciting information and making ratings.

Another concern is the possibility that outcomes of patients enrolled early in a trial may bias results of subsequent patients, if the clinician becomes aware of treatment assignment as each patient completes the study. Emerging patterns of adverse experiences and/or clinical responses associated with one or more of the treatments could affect clinicians in their ratings and decision making as a trial proceeds. This is undesirable from a research standpoint and could be a source of bias that is hard to detect or to quantify.

A third concern is that knowing the randomization of completing patients increases the likelihood that unplanned interim analyses will be done. This can also introduce bias as a study proceeds, in addition to being a cause for statistical concern because of multiple (and unscheduled) probability testing. The pressure to publish interim results to enhance curricula vitae should be resisted. For all of these reasons, many now advocate that key RCTs be implemented in a triple-blind mode, that is, neither the clinical nor the research staff (including the trial sponsor) have access to the randomization code until the clinical phase is completed, and all data have been entered into a verified data base. Emergency codebreaking for safety reasons for an individual, when necessary, is routinely provided in such protocols.

Consideration can be given to setting up an independent safety-monitoring committee for high-risk treatments, or for extremely large or protracted studies where there are compelling reasons for periodic review of some of the data. It is more or less the standard within the pharmaceutical industry to conduct placebo-controlled RCTs in psychopharmacology as triple-blind studies, especially if considered potentially pivotal in a regulatory sense. There are some disadvantages to this approach. Imposing triple-blind conditions on a trial adds to the complexity and cost of the study. It delays review and analysis of data, usually until all clinical portions of the study have been completed. In drug development, where studies are sequential, this delay in access to clinical data creates inefficiencies in the already costly development process. It may also be disadvantageous to the patient. There can be a compelling need to know what drug was given to a patient so that continuing therapy can be planned by the clinician. One approach to this dilemma, which insures continuity of care, has been to allow double-blind continuation treatment for patients on completion of the initial efficacy phase of an RCT, if the treating clinician feels the patient would benefit (2). This avoids disrupting effective therapy, protects the blinding, and potentially can generate valuable additional data about a drug's long-term effectiveness.

Occasionally, it may not be feasible, or ethical, to conduct a clinical evaluation of an agent where all of the treatment providers are blind to the therapy being given. In this circumstance, it has been common practice to either have all formal ratings made by a blind rater, who is unaware of treatment assignment, or else to give a supervising clinician access to the clinical data, with all others remaining blind. The latter approach is necessary, for example, with the concentration-controlled study design and could potentially introduce experimental bias.

Any design variations that might compromise the integrity of a double-blind protocol should be approached with the greatest caution and only after careful consideration. Alternatives should be explored that preserve the blinding of an RCT. A degree of skepticism from reviewers and regulators is to be expected if there are deviations from strict protocol-defined maintenance of blind.

Treatment Outcome Measures

Standard Rating Instruments

Many existing psychometric rating instruments have been used for decades in evaluating psychotropic agents. Although this underscores the validity of such scales, it does not follow that they are necessarily the optimal or the most sensitive scales for certain applications. Many rating scales do not adequately reflect our current understanding of the phenomenology of disorders, or they omit core symptoms (30). It is unfortunate that more resources are not allocated to scale development in clinical psychopharmacology. This could facilitate drug discovery, as well as promote clinical research in the field.

To improve and validate a scale or to develop a new one is a daunting task that often exceeds the capacity of the individual investigator. The industrial sponsor of a new drug is similarly limited in ability to create an outcome measure that might be more optimal for developing a novel agent. Proven instruments are required in a New Drug Application (NDA) so that outcome data from a new rating scale are regarded as supplemental. The emphasis that regulatory agencies place on the use of standard instruments, although understandable, has drawbacks for development of a new scale. For a novel compound, standard scales may be insensitive to or biased against detection of a useful therapeutic action (30).

Another dilemma, perhaps unique to psychotropic drugs, is that many of the symptoms of psychiatric disorders overlap treatment-emergent side effects of psychoactive drugs. This could result in a new therapeutic agent being disadvantaged compared to a standard or placebo treatment if the efficacy rating instrument subsumes adverse drug experiences.

Another potential bias of existing instruments is apparent in the case of the universally used Hamilton scales for depression (20) and anxiety (21). These scales were developed during the era of tricyclic antidepressants and benzodiazepines, when assay sensitivity to the effects of these drugs served as one measure of scale validity. Greater latitude in the use of modified and new rating instruments in drug evaluations seems indicated to avoid overlooking useful properties of newer agents.

Choice of Outcome Measures

In assessing efficacy, it is desirable to measure both change in symptoms and change in global functioning (48). The number of primary outcome measures, specified in the protocol, should be held to a minimum, primarily for statistical reasons, to avoid a penalty for testing multiple hypotheses. An overabundance of scales can also intrude on the clinical interview and may adversely affect the quality of ratings. A well-validated symptom rating scale and global improvement scale constitute appropriate primary outcome measures for efficacy evaluation in RCTs.

With the recent emphasis on clinical services, effectiveness research as opposed to clinical therapeutic efficacy research, quality of life (51), functional capacity, cost effectiveness (8,53), and other dimensions of outcome deserve consideration for incorporation in a protocol when planning an RCT. Scales in these domains are relatively untested, especially in psychopharmacology. Increasingly, health authorities and formulary committees require cost-effectiveness data during the approval process for drug registration and reimbursement. For this reason, clinical evaluations are shifting focus to include data on long-term outcome and costs, ideally in comparison to a standard treatment (19). These types of studies are still at a rudimentary design stage for psychotropic drugs. Ancillary measures of a drug's effectiveness should be considered in the planning of an RCT.

Safety Outcome Measures

Collection of safety data is a key element of all clinical drug studies, whether the prime objective of a protocol is to evaluate efficacy, to conduct biological or pharmacokinetic measurements, or to accrue safety and tolerability data. Methods for assessing side effects in RCTs are much less advanced than are those for measuring efficacy (4,31). It is essential as part of a drug trial to capture all adverse experiences, either on a symptom rating scale or adverse event (AE) form.

Although structured AE rating instruments are available, it is usual practice to elicit AEs by general questioning or by voluntary report from the patient. A standard glossary of AE dictionary terms can be supplied to each investigator as a supplement to the study protocol. This can improve the quality and precision of safety data collection and allows for more meaningful analyses when consolidating safety results across studies (31).

A comprehensive but lengthy interview such as SAFTEE (36) can be time-consuming, limiting how frequently it can be administered. A leading concern has been generation of many more AEs than with an unstructured approach to elicitation. In their methodological comparison study, Rabkin et al. (45) concluded that general elicitation of AEs is appropriate and more practical for routine clinical trials than is SAFTEE. Abbreviated versions of SAFTEE have been successfully adapted for use in specialized research applications, for example, phase I tolerability studies. Structured safety instruments are also valuable for assessing extrapyramidal symptoms and tardive dyskinesia in antipsychotic drug studies and withdrawal symptoms in antianxiety drug trials.

Most health authorities agree on the regulatory definition of AEs regarded as serious in nature and requiring special reporting. Adverse events in this category include any event within 30 days of exposure to the suspect drug that is life threatening or fatal, as well as hospitalizations, overdoses, cancer, congenital abnormalities, or permanent disability. Regulations require that the appropriate regulatory agencies and institutional review boards be promptly notified of such an occurrence if there is a reasonable possibility that the AE could be from the drug (and the AE is unexpected, i.e., not in the investigational brochure or in the labeling of a drug). In the case of marketed drugs, suspected drug reactions in this category should be brought to the attention of the manufacturer by an investigator or practitioner, and/or it may be directly reported to the FDA.

Rare serious AEs, that is, those with an incidence of less than one per 1,000 are generally difficult to detect during preapproval development of a new drug, because the number of patients treated is too few (31). Spontaneous reports of AEs when a drug comes into wider clinical use remain the mainstay for detection of rare, although toxic, occurrences. The spontaneous AE reporting network serves as an important early alerting system providing valuable information to the drug's sponsor and regulatory agencies.

Several approaches to the postmarketing surveillance of new psychotropic drugs have been taken with uneven success (22). Creation of an FDA center for the assessment of pharmaceutical effectiveness to collect postapproval data from clinicians has been advocated (46). A promising study design relies on telephone queries of pharmacy-based cohorts of patients who agree to report on their response to a psychotropic agent, using another standard drug as a concurrent comparator (14). However, overall, psychotherapeutics has suffered from a paucity of postmarketing studies, no doubt in part from the cost and methodological and logistical complexities of such studies. In psychopharmacology, formal postmarketing surveillance studies so far have failed to detect unsuspected AEs and toxicities of clinical importance (22).

STUDY IMPLEMENTATION, MONITORING, AND DOCUMENTATION

Industry-sponsored Trials

Today drug discovery and development are heavily influenced by good laboratory and clinical practice guidelines that have been adopted by regulatory agencies worldwide (24). These guidelines clarify the responsibilities of both individual investigators and drug sponsors undertaking pharmaceutical research. In addition to requiring peer review and informed consent, clinical guidelines specify the importance of adherence to the study protocol and stress the need to promptly report any unexpected, serious AEs. Furthermore, drug supplies must be accounted for and research records maintained until 2 years after an NDA is approved or the investigation of a new drug (IND) is discontinued.

Most industry sponsors of drug trials have adopted standard operating procedures, which includes a requirement for preinvestigation visits to investigators to ensure that they fully understand the protocol and their obligations as required by the regulations (23). Investigators' meetings and frequent monitoring of studies by research sponsors should be standard practices. In psychotherapeutic studies, interrater reliability training and ongoing monitoring during the progress of the study are critical, especially for multisite trials.

Documentation of Clinical Trials

Clinical research, whether sponsored or unsponsored, requires attention to quality control through proper documentation. An RCT protocol should specify objectives, state hypotheses, define response criteria, and present the statistical power calculations and proposed methods of data analyses. Any subsequent protocol changes should be kept to a minimum, with protocol amendments furnished to the appropriate institutional review committees, regulatory agencies, and research sponsors.

Other research documentation is required as a necessary supplement to the research case report forms and the study protocol. For example, an overall research plan should summarize an overall project, providing relevant background information, stating major hypotheses (both a priori and exploratory), and describing the overall research strategy. A individual study log is essential to record day-to-day activities of a trial. Some method of cross-referencing research records to clinical records should be provided for audit purposes. The goal of comprehensive research documentation is to support and provide the justification for conclusions drawn, or claims made, about the drug(s) based on the research.

REPORTING RESULTS OF TRIALS

Results of RCTs are reported in different ways depending on the purpose and intended audience. Federally sponsored research is generally summarized in progress reports, usually annually. Often, ongoing trial results and interim analyses are included in progress reports. Results of industry-sponsored trials are reported periodically to regulatory authorities. Regulations require a degree of detail in these reports that exceeds what would be appropriate for publication, but is necessary to regulatory oversight.

How clinical research results should be disseminated by publication has been addressed by Kupfer et al. (26,27). These authors and others have pointed out how the resistance of journal editors to overly long and detailed presentations of study results imposed by space limitations runs counter to the readers' need for better and more detailed documentation of methods, problems encountered, and so on (5,34,38). Sufficient details of study design, a priori hypotheses, statistical power, study conduct, and data analyses should be included to allow one to form judgements about the authors' conclusions. Documentation of the quality of the measurement procedures and adequate justification of statistical tests should be provided. Information should also be provided about patients excluded as well as those entered into the study, and "intent-to-treat" patient sample data should be given in addition to other data analyses.

Authors should discuss possible compromises to the scientific validity of the conclusions of the study, either from decisions during the planning stages or from lack of compliance of either the patients or the investigators with the protocols of the study. Kupfer and colleagues (26) point out that even in the most carefully designed and executed studies, unanticipated problems and accidents happen, and when these affect the results of a study, they *must* be reported. As Mosteller et al. (38) state, "We must encourage authors to report and editors to publish work that includes a thoughtful discussion of mistakes and difficulties encountered in the research. . . . Without more systematic reporting of problems encountered in clinical trials, we will be unable to do much about them."

Many authors (e.g., 1,6,10,26,33) have admonished editors and reviewers to focus on proper description of the methods and reporting of results of the protocol-defined experiment. Editors should resist the requests of some referees for authors to address ancillary issues that the study was not designed to test, no matter how intriguing. A common problem that readers experience is lack of a clear distinction between what were the confirmatory and what were the exploratory aspects of a study.

Presentations of results need to be made more informative, for example, using confidence intervals and box and whisker plots (47,50). Improved presentation of data allows the reader to better judge whether the findings of a clinical trial are justified by the study design and methodology employed. Equally important, improved display of data can provide a better basis for the reader to judge a trial's results in terms of clinical rather than merely statistical significance.

More complete and informative reporting of an RCT's findings in a published report is necessary to allow a thorough evaluation of a psychotropic drug's effects. To accomplish this, both investigators and editors must appreciate that adequate description and critique of a clinical study's design and implementation, in addition to presenting outcomes, is essential to the scientific evaluation process and should receive space and attention in reporting the research.

FUTURE DIRECTIONS IN CLINICAL PSYCHOPHARMACOLOGY TRIALS

The past decade has seen important changes in methodologies. Good clinical practice guidelines has led to greater emphasis on documentation of research data, adequate informed consent, and audit procedures (24). More critical and conservative statistical treatment of RCT results have evolved to minimize possible bias and to avoid type I errors (e.g., requiring protocol-defined samples to be analyzed, primary outcome measures to be employed, and safety definitions to be used in defining AEs. It is evident that the proper conduct of a clinical drug evaluation is a sophisticated and demanding, but necessary, process for acquisition of safety and efficacy data of an existing or entirely new drug. Rigorously controlled trials form the basis for deciding that a new drug warrants clinical development and how best to use a marketed drug in practice.

Efforts to make the clinical evaluation of a psychotropic drug more efficient are currently being pursued. The discovery and development of a new agent is a time-consuming and costly process that has implications for the cost of health care. More efficient clinical development programs can cut costs by truncating the length of phase II and III programs. The concentration-controlled clinical trial design proposed by Sanathanan and Peck et al. (49) requires careful study as a means to improve the efficiency of RCTs, especially in phase II, where rapid efficacy answers could greatly facilitate the discovery process. The stated advantages of this approach in psychopharmacology await practical demonstration before it can be recommended.

The recent emphasis on longer term studies to assess the risks and benefits of a course of treatment indicates the need for enhanced methodological research to develop appropriate study designs. Sample enrichment and dropout issues pose particularly difficult problems in improving the design of long-term psychopharmacology trials. The pressing need for long-term efficacy and safety data on most psychotropic drugs calls for continuing efforts to refine research methods for evaluating and comparing outcomes of therapeutic alternatives.

Health economics has given rise to cost-effectiveness research that will continue to play an increasing role in funding decisions by the health care field. A distinction is made between a drug's efficacy (i.e., an outcome based on controlled studies in a population with a well-defined disorder) and its clinical effectiveness (i.e., how well the treatment works in everyday practice and across settings). The latter can be variously defined depending on the health care services research question, such as the cost to the health care system of a particular drug treatment, functional capacity, quality of life years gained, work productivity, and so on. Many of these evaluations can be obtained in association with, or immediately following, controlled clinical trials (9). Increasingly, clinical investigators will be asked to consider incorporating additional outcome measures, such as health care costs, functional capacity, and quality of life (3,51,53), into drug trials. Inevitably, this will add to the intricacy of clinical studies, whereas health economics methodologies are still in their infancy and remain largely unvalidated. Although these methods are imperfect for quantifying overall treatment effects and costs for drugs, such studies at least will provide a basis for critical thinking about the therapeutic choices that need to be made in health care planning. The coming years will see increasing emphasis on evaluating a drug's effectiveness and cost, as well its efficacy (11; also see Chapters 160 and 161, *this volume*).

REFERENCES

1. Altman DG, Dore CJ. Randomization and baseline comparisons in clinical trials. *Lancet* 1990;335:149–153.
2. Anton SF, Robinson DS, Roberts DL, et al. Long-term treatment with nefazodone. *Psychopharmacol Bull* 1994;30:[in press].
3. Banta HD. Quality of life. Perspectives. *Pharm World Sci* 1993;15:45–49.
4. Castle WM. Problems in assessing drug safety: a plea for improved methodology and a possible route. *Drug Info J* 1986;20:323–326.
5. Chalmers I. Underreporting research is scientific misconduct. *JAMA* 1990;263:1405–1408.
6. Chalmers I, Adams M, Dickersin K, et al. A cohort study of summary reports of controlled trials. *JAMA* 1990;263:1401–1405.
7. D'Amico F, Roberts DL, Robinson DS, et al. Placebo-controlled dose-ranging trial designs in phase II development of nefazodone. *Psychopharmacol Bull* 1990;26:147–150.
8. Drummond M, Stoddart G, Labelle R, Cushman R. Health economics: an introduction for clinicians. *Ann Intern Med* 1987;107:89–92.
9. Drummond MF, Stoddart GL, Torrance GW. *Methods for the economic evaluation of health care programmes.* Oxford: Oxford University Press, 1987.
10. Ekstrom D, Quade D, Golden RN. Statistical analysis of repeated measures in psychiatric research. *Arch Gen Psychiatry* 1990;47:770–772.
11. Eddy DM. Cost-effectiveness analysis. *JAMA* 1992;267:1669–1675.
12. Food and Drug Administration. *General considerations for the clinical evaluation of drugs.* HEW Publ No. 77-3040. Washington, DC: Government Printing Office; 1977.
13. Food and Drug Administration. Guidelines for the clinical evaluation of psychotropic drugs—antidepressant and antianxiety drugs. *Psychopharmacol Bull* 1978;14:45–63.
14. Fisher S, Bryant SG, Kent J. Post-marketing surveillance by patient self-monitoring: trazodone versus fluoxetine. *J Clin Psychopharmacology* 1993;13:235–242.
15. Fisher S, Greenberg RP. How sound is the double-blind design for evaluating psychotropic drugs? *J Nerv Ment Dis* 1993;186:345–350.
16. Gardner MJ, Bond J. An exploratory study of statistical assessment of papers published in the British Medical Journal. *JAMA* 1990;263:1355–1357.
17. Glynn JR. A question of attribution. *Lancet* 1993;342:530–532.
18. Greenhouse JP, Stangl D, Kupfer DJ, Prien RF. Methodologic issues in maintenance therapy in clinical trials. *Arch Gen Psychiatry* 1991;48:313–318.
19. Guyatt GH, Heyting A, Jaeschke R, et al. N of 1 randomized trials for investigating new drugs. *Controlled Clin Trials* 1990;11:88–100.
20. Hamilton M. Development of a rating scale for primary depressive illness. *Br J Soc Clin Psychol* 1967;6:278–296.
21. Hamilton M. Diagnosis and rating of anxiety. *Br J Psychiatry* 1969;3:76–79.
22. Hollister LE, Jones JK, Fisher S. Post-marketing surveillance of drugs. In: Prien RF, Robinson DS, eds. *Clinical evaluation of psychotropic drugs: principles and guidelines.* New York: Raven Press; 1994.
23. Kartzinel R, Lisook AB, Rulls B, et al. Clinical trial implementation. In: Prien RF, Robinson DS, eds. *Clinical evaluation of psychotropic drugs: principles and guidelines.* New York: Raven Press; 1994.
24. Kelsey FO. Good clinical practices in the US: impact of European guidelines. *Drug Info J* 1992;26:125–132.
25. Kraemer HC. To increase power in randomized clinical trials without increasing sample size. *Psychopharmacol Bull* 1991;27:217–224.
26. Kupfer DJ, Kraemer HC, Bartko JJ. Documenting and reporting study results of a randomized clinical trial. In: Prien RF, Robinson DS, eds. *Clinical evaluation of psychotropic drugs: principles and guidelines.* New York: Raven Press; 1994.
27. Kupfer DJ, Rush AJ. Recommendations for depression publications. *Arch Gen Psychiatry* 1983;40:1031.
28. Larson EB, Ellsworth AJ, Oas J. Randomized clinical trials in single patients during a 2-year period. *JAMA* 1993;270:2708–2712.
29. Laska EM. Epilogue, prologue, and a bayesian approach. In: Levine J, ed. *Coordinating clinical trials in psychopharmacology: planning, documentation, and analysis.* Washington, DC: Government Printing Office, 1979.
30. Laska EM, Klein DF, Lavori PW, et al. Design issues for the clinical evaluation of psychotropic drugs. In: Prien RF, Robinson DS, eds. *Clinical evaluation of psychotropic drugs: principles and guidelines.* New York: Raven Press; 1994.
31. Laughren TP, Levine J, Levine J, Thompson WL. Premarketing safety evaluation of psychotropic drugs. In: Prien RF, Robinson DS, eds. *Clinical evaluation of psychotropic agents: principles and guidelines.* New York: Raven Press; 1994.
32. Lavori P. Statistical issues: sample size and dropout. In: Benkert

O, Maier W, Rickels K, eds. *Methodology of the evaluation of psychotropic drugs.* Berlin: Springer-Verlag, 1990; 91–104.

33. Lavori P. ANOVA, MANOVA, my black hen. Comments on repeated measures. *Arch Gen Psychiatry* 1990; 47:775–778.

34. Lavori P. Clinical trials in psychiatry: should protocol deviation censor patient data? *Neuropsychopharmacology* 1992; 6:39–48.

35. Leber P. Is there an alternative to the randomized controlled trial? *Psychopharmacol Bull* 1991; 27:3–8.

36. Levine J, Schooler N. Strategies for analysing side effects data from SAFTEE. *Psychopharmacol Bull* 1986; 22:343–381.

37. Levy G. Concentration-controlled versus concentration-defined clinical trials. *Clin Pharm Ther* 1993; 53:385–388.

38. Mosteller F, Gilbert JP, McPeek B. Reporting standards and research strategies for controlled trials. *Controlled Clin Trials* 1980; 1:37–58.

39. Overall JE, Ashby B. Baseline corrections in experimental and quasi-experimental clinical trials. *Neuropsychopharmacology* 1981; 4:273–281.

40. Peck CC. The randomized concentration-controlled clinical trial: an information rich alternative to the randomized placebo-controlled trial. *Clin Pharm Ther* 1990; 47:126.

41. Preskorn SH, Mac DS. The implication of concentration/response studies of tricyclic antidepressants for psychiatric research and practice. *Psychiatr Dev* 1984; 11:210–222.

42. Prien RF. Methods and models for placebo use in pharmacotherapeutic trials. *Psychopharmacol Bull* 1988; 24:4–8.

43. Prien RF, Robinson DS, eds. *Clinical evaluation of psychotropic drugs: principles and guidelines.* New York: Raven Press; 1994.

44. Quitkin FM, Kane J, Rifkin A, et al. Prophylactic lithium with and without imipramine for bipolar I patients. *Arch Gen Psychiatry* 1981; 38:902–907.

45. Rabkin JG, Markowitz JS, Ocepek-Welikson K, Wager SS. General versus systematic inquiry about emergent clinical events with SAFTEE: Implications for clinical research. *J Clin Psychiatry* 1992; 12:3–10.

46. Ray CC, Griffin MR, Avorn J. Evaluating drugs after their approval for clinical use. *New Engl J Med* 1993; 329:2029–2032.

47. Rothman KJ. Significance questing. *Ann Intern Med* 1986; 105:445–447.

48. Rush AJ, Raskin A, Kellner R, Bartko JJ. Assessment and measurement of clinical change. In: Prien RF, Robinson DS, eds. *Clinical evaluation of psychotropic drugs: principles and guidelines.* New York: Raven Press; 1994.

49. Sanathanan LP, Peck CC. The randomized concentration-controlled trial: an evaluation of its sample size efficiency. *Controlled Clin Trials* 1991; 12:780–794.

50. Simon R. Confidence intervals for reporting results of clinical trials. *Ann Intern Med* 1986; 105:420–435.

51. Spilker B, ed. *Quality of life assessments in clinical trials.* New York: Raven Press; 1990.

52. Tam YK. Individual variation in first-pass metabolism. *Clin Pharmacokinetics* 1993; 4:300–328.

53. Wells KB, Steward A, Hayes RD. The functioning and well-being of depressed patients: results from the Medical Outcomes Study. *JAMA* 1989; 262:914–919.

54. Wilson JF, Tsanaclis LM, Williams J, et al. External quality assurance of tricyclic antidepressant measurements in serum: eight years of progress? *Ther Drug Monit* 1989; 11:196–199.

Psychopharmacology: The Fourth Generation of Progress, edited by Floyd E. Bloom and David J. Kupfer. Raven Press, Ltd., New York © 1995.

CHAPTER 73

Short- and Long-Term Psychopharmacological Treatment Strategies

Ira D. Glick, David L. Braff, and David S. Janowsky

In the previous three volumes, there were no chapters on strategies of treatment. Now that it has been convincingly established that psychiatric illness can be defined and treated as effectively as most other medical illnesses, the question is no longer whether psychotropic medications *should* be prescribed? In our opinion, the clinical issue is when medication is prescribed, and is effective, under what circumstances should the dosage be reduced or the medication be discontinued for each specific disorder?'' This strategic issue bears on both short-term acute and continuation phases as well as long-term maintenance phases.

Why has this set of very different treatment questions arisen in the past decade? First, many active episodes of Axis I disorders have been found to have relatively long durations (e.g., 6 to 12 months for mood disorders and 6 to 18 months for schizophrenia) and many, if not most, Axis I disorders evolve into a chronic vulnerability for repeated episodes or assume a smoldering subsyndromal course. By way of contrast, conventional wisdom in the 1960s stated that most episodes of depression were short-lived, self-limited, and would not recur if psychotherapeutic or psychoanalytic treatment was successful or even if no treatment was given. Second, some Axis I disorders have been found to recur more frequently and become more severe over time probably because neurobiological mechanisms induce potentiation or sensitization of underlying neural deficits (e.g., in bipolar disorder). Third, there is some data to suggest that, for the prevention or recur-

rence phase, once a patient goes off medication, if recurrence occurs, a previously effective medication may no longer be as effective (e.g., the case of lithium treatment of bipolar disorder) (27). Finally, there may be a direct correlation between adequate psychopharmacological treatment and outcome; for many, but not all patients, poor outcome can be easily avoided by adequate treatment. The outcome of treatment affects not only the patients but also their families and society in general.

We review here the general rationale and guidelines for short- and long-term psychopharmacological treatment strategies and specifically discuss three important Axis I disorders by way of illustrating current models: schizophrenic, mood, and anxiety disorders. We synthesize some of the best current controlled and experiential data to integrate information about a disorder and its course (e.g., schizophrenia), treatment (e.g., neuroleptics), side effects (e.g., tardive dyskinesia), family variables (e.g., expressed emotion), and societal attitudes (e.g., stigmatization of mental illness) as these factors bear on treatment strategies. We do not cover issues more properly associated with ''treatment'' (e.g., specific drug selection or the detailed biological deficits of disorders) as they are reviewed in the separate chapters on schizophrenia, mood disorder, and anxiety disorder. Rather, our focus is on strategies of treatment as such (see Chapters 156 and 157, *this volume*).

RATIONALE FOR LONGER TERM MEDICATION STRATEGIES

Regardless of the disorder, after the acute episode, a major clinical task is not just to reduce symptoms and prevent relapse, but also to raise the level of social and vocational functioning as close as possible to preepisode

I. D. Glick: Department of Psychiatry and Behavioral Sciences, Stanford University School of Medicine, Stanford, California 94305.
D. L. Braff: Department of Psychiatry, University of California at San Diego, LaJolla, California 92093.
D. S. Janowsky: Psychiatry Department, University of North Carolina, Medical School, Chapel Hill, North Carolina 27599.

levels. A concept that is generally unappreciated is that in some cases and in certain disorders, for example, schizophrenia, this may take as long as 18, 24, or even 36 months. Furthermore, it is unclear whether the best treatment or treatment strategy is drugs alone or drugs plus family or individual interventions. It is also not well accepted by treating clinicians, patients, or their families, that each episode of a disorder may lead to lower future social, vocational, and symptomatic functioning (38). For example, each episode of schizophrenia can lower function by as much as 50%.

Even among some mental health professionals, the concept of long-term medication strategies may seem extreme and evokes concerns about giving the patients and families pessimistic messages about progress and about the potential for negative side-effects. Because these concerns can be ameliorated via educational strategies, we base our recommendations regarding length of treatment solely on the follow-up literature and our knowledge of the natural course of these disorders. There is a wealth of experimental and naturalistic data suggesting that cognitive impairment is enduring, even after an episode resolves. Furthermore, cognitive deficits worsen with time as suggested by Altshuler for bipolar disorder (2), by Waddington et al. for schizophrenic disorder (45), and by Faravelli and Albanesi for anxiety disorders (9). More broadly, untreated psychotic symptoms have a detrimental effect on subsequent course and outcome (48). The point is that "these mechanisms underlying the expression of psychosis (as distinct from its neurodevelopmental origin) may contribute to apparent progression of the illness" (39).

Needless to say, the challenge in schizophrenic, mood, and anxiety disorders is to identify which patients do not need longer term medication. Unfortunately, there are little data on this question, in part, because we lack definitive data on the natural history and underlying neurobiological deficits and etiology of the disorders. Thus, our recommendation is to discuss alternatives with the patient and with the family (see below). In general, the clinician should explain that the more chronic the illness is, the more likely is the possibility of relapse, and that these factors should weigh heavily in deciding whether to continue maintenance treatment.

As a general principle, the most important distinction is to establish whether a patient has a recurrent or chronic fixed condition. The clinician must also decide when an acute episode has resolved and the condition is in full rather than partial remission. If this is the first episode, then the clinician should discuss the probability of recurrence (and its consequences) versus the consequences of maintenance medication. A reasonable general strategy for many disorders is to maintain medication for a first episode patient for 6 months after remission. If the condition is established as recurrent, the scale is weighed toward staying on medication for a significantly longer period of time. As a general rule in our experience, patients,

and even more strongly their families, when given the choice, prefer the side effects of maintenance medications to the consequences of recurrence of schizophrenia, mood disorders, or anxiety disorders (16). Some recurrent patients prefer to try tapering or stopping drugs after 3 to 5 years of treatment-associated remission, whereas others prefer the prophylaxsis of maintenance therapy and will not risk a discontinuation strategy with its associated increased risk of relapse.

SCHIZOPHRENIA

The short- and long-term goals of the treatment of schizophrenia include the use of antipsychotic medications as well as psychosocial therapy. Although schizophrenia is frequently a chronic and deteriorating illness, it is important to note that poor outcome is not inevitable for all patients globally and on all axes, that is, the social, vocational, and symptomatic axes of outcome (38). We focus here on the medication domain, although mention must be made of the synergistic effects of psychosocial therapies when combined with antipsychotic medications.

In the short-term, the primary goal of antipsychotic medication therapy is to reduce the dramatic (usually positive) symptoms of psychosis such as hallucinations, delusions, agitation, and the general fragmentation of thought and behavior. There remains some ambiguity about whether low-dose or high-dose antipsychotic therapy is most appropriate even for short-term therapy. Specifically, it is clear that, in the short-term, relatively high doses of medication may not be needed for many psychotic patients (18). Unfortunately, even if 10% to 20% of schizophrenic patients require a higher dose, there is no effective way to now identify this subgroup. Large numbers of patients are thus frequently committed to the higher doses of neuroleptics (31), which may have superior initial therapeutic effects but also may have increased side-effects such as dystonias, the extrapyramidal syndromes and general dysphoria that correlate with poor compliance and poor long-term outcome (44).

There is general consensus that long-term therapy should be used for schizophrenic patients who have received short-term medication regimens and have relapsed on one or more occasions. In addition, many clinicians would start long-term maintenance treatment with a patient who has had even one psychotic episode, in order to prevent relapse. These patients are then committed to long-term therapy with a primary goal of restoring them to the highest level of functioning along social, vocational, and symptomatic axes, described by Strauss and Carpenter (38). While attempting to get to the highest level of long-term functioning it is very important to have a good baseline assessment of how the patient functioned premorbidly in these three domains, because frequently the best possible long-term outcome is not good in absolute terms, but represents a restoration of functioning to marginal premorbid levels.

Although the clinician attempts to minimize symptoms and the risk of relapse, it is also important to minimize long-term neurotoxicity, especially tardive dyskinesia. Two major strategies have been employed in this respect: First, Carpenter and colleagues (5) have utilized an intermittent or targeted drug strategy, which necessitates careful longitudinal monitoring where medications are withdrawn and then reintroduced at the first symptomatic signs of the onset of psychosis (8). Unfortunately, this strategy, as assessed by the Treatment Strategies in Schizophrenia (TSS) collaborative study, results in a high level of relapse (42). Still, this type of approach is humanely and intuitively appealing to many clinicians. An alternative is to use a fixed low dose antipsychotic strategy (19,23). It should be emphasized that, in the long-run, these latter strategies may provide some very important benefits, but they also require a higher level of psychosocial monitoring and assessment on a continuing basis and are therefore more expensive. They also may increase the risk of relapse (4). Therefore, a standard dose of antipsychotic medication continues widely to be the treatment of choice. The use of lower doses or intermittent strategies may reduce side effects, but also increases vulnerability to the potentially devastating effects of relapse (36,42).

Short-term Strategies

Acutely, the choice of a drug can be made most easily when a patient has a history of a positive response to a previous specific antipsychotic drug regimen. Also, an aliphatic phenothiazine (e.g., chlorpromazine) may be chosen for its high levels of sedation. Thus, as in most areas of psychopharmacology, previous response or patterns of familial response to antipsychotics is a critical domain. Usually, a therapeutic response with lessening of acute positive psychotic symptoms is observed in a few days to 3 or 4 weeks but some may take up to 12 weeks even on a good dose. When such improvement is lacking on an acute basis, ancillary or augmentation strategies, including the use of lithium, benzodiazepines, and other agents are used, to minimize exposure to acute high dose antipsychotics that sometimes need to be employed when the patient's symptoms are refractory in the short-run (6). It appears that both benzodiazepines and lithium are efficient at augmenting antipsychotic medications, although the current predominant strategy is to use benzodiazepines (that may have intrinsic dopaminergic antagonistic properties) first and on an acute basis (47) and lithium on for a longer-term. Many clinicians use sequential trials of different antipsychotic medications before using ancillary or augmentation strategies. There is currently no clear consensus about which path is more efficient and specific outcome studies should be con-

ducted. Because little is known about the effects of switching drugs, when to do it, how to do it, timing, and indications remain an area of art in psychopharmacology and one for which no clear recommended critical pathways have been identified.

The problem of short-term compliance has long been mentioned in the literature. It appears that initial side effects such as dysphoria tend to correlate with poorer outcome. Whether this is because the patient experiences dystonias and other extrapyramidal symptoms and is therefore less likely to take medications or (perhaps syntonically) whether the patient's initial side effects are dictated by a different neurobiological substrate remains unclear. While using these compounds a cognitive/educational framework should be employed, both with the patient and the family, to create the best psychosocial environment for the use of these medications (13,16). Some clinicians (a minority) use intramuscular preparations to alleviate the issue of noncompliance to oral medications.

A new generation of atypical neuroleptic drugs such as clozapine (22) and respiradone are being developed that takes advantage of the antiserotonergic properties of some of these drugs and also effects new classes of dopamine receptors (i.e., D_3 or D_4 dopamine blockade). In general, on an acute basis, these antipsychotic medications have been traditionally viewed as being relatively more effective in treating patients with positive symptoms, such as hallucinations and delusions, than those with negative symptoms, such as anhedonia and withdrawal. Even this widely accepted idea has been recently challenged as some investigators have reported good therapeutic results with atypical antipsychotic compounds on negative symptoms (see below).

Long-term Strategies

The major issues with the long-term pharmacological treatment of schizophrenia is the prevention of relapse, disability, and the need to avoid tardive dyskinesia. There is also the issue of whether recurrent psychotic episodes somehow kindle or facilitate certain neural substrates, as has been posited for mood disorders (27) and thereby increase symptom severity and decrease psychosocial functioning over the long term. The long-term objective is to prevent (multiple) episodes that may kindle or potentiate the neural circuit dysfunction basis of schizophrenia and lead to a poorer future course. Maintenance therapies raise multiple issues of dose range and the time that patients should be exposed to antipsychotic medications (18,36). A major issue, once the patient has had multiple episodes and a chronic form of schizophrenia, is how to best manage the patient. Drug therapy should probably be continuous and at the lowest effective dosage; as mentioned previously, the strategy of drug holidays or strategies that include intermittent drug therapy, although of interest, have not been effective (42) for most patients. Long-acting depot mechanisms will effectively address some but not all compliance issues.

A patient's individual history is critical. A patient, who cannot tolerate drug withdrawal for more than a month or so, should be committed to longer term drug therapy to avoid the devastating neurobiological and psychosocial consequences of repeated exacerbations. The current consensus is that fully remitted patients may be withdrawn from antipsychotic medications, at least on one occasion after 6 months or more, to see if they can tolerate being off antipsychotic medications. However, it should be recognized that this strategy makes patients vulnerable to increased psychotic symptoms. There is also the issue of low- versus high-dose maintenance therapy. The benefits and risks must be discussed with the patient and the patient's family or guardian, where appropriate.

The advent of a new generation of atypical antipsychotic medications, such as clozapine, is critically important. These new medications may act through non-D$_2$ receptor mechanisms (e.g., D$_4$ or 5-HT receptors) and thus do not create the neurotoxicity of tardive dyskinesia seen with primary D$_2$ blockers (24). Although many clozapine studies are negatively loaded with a skewed distribution of patients in the more chronic and drug refractory groups, the drug still offers significant advantages to at least a significant subgroup of schizophrenic patients who are refractory to other therapies. New studies employing clozapine as a first choice drug need to be fitted into the tableau of the antipsychotic drug response literature. Still, it seems clear that clozapine, operating at least partially or mainly through serotonergic and adrenergic as well as selective efficacy and non-D$_2$ mechanisms offers a major advantage in terms of reducing neurotoxicity (25). To employ this medication, educating the patient and the patient's family is absolutely necessary because serial (currently weekly) blood counts must be obtained to minimize the chance of white blood cell suppression and its potential devastating effects. The addition of respiradone to our therapeutic armamentarium will undoubtedly offer new advantages and opportunities. Likewise, the use of anticonvulsants as adjuncts to standard treatment have been tried if lability or impulsivity with sustained changes in mood are a prominent part of the symptom picture. SSRIs have been used if persistent depressive symptoms are present—but such symptoms must be carefully differentiated from demoralization and/or the psychomotor retardation secondary to standard antipsychotics.

Many investigators have presented data suggesting that the psychosocial family environment may either potentiate or decrease the level of symptomatology of patients (16). The family that is highly expressive of emotion does not create schizophrenia but certainly can exacerbate symptomatology. Specifically, sending a patient with schizophrenia home to an environment filled with conflict, critical comments, and highly charged emotions may act as a stressor, much as challenges with low-dose stimulants act as a probable stressor in the laboratory. It is also important to recognize that the family does not cause schizophrenia, but that any family with a schizophrenic member may undergo a profound reorganization and the other family members may feel confusion, guilt, responsibility, and shame. It is thus critically important that the psychopharmacological approach to schizophrenia be combined with family education. For a substantial number of patients, a lot of creative work has been done by combining antipsychotic medications and intervention in the social environment of the patient. Educational family therapy can facilitate better patient outcome and reduce the frequency, duration, and (possibly) medication dosage required to stabilize the patient on a long-term basis.

Ultimately, when studying the outcome of schizophrenia, ongoing short- and long-term trials are critically important for designing rational drug therapy combined with psychosocial therapy for patients with schizophrenic disorders. The reader should also refer to Chapter 107 on Maintenance Treatment of Schizophrenia in this volume for further details.

MOOD DISORDERS

Short-term Strategies

The primary goal of short-term antidepressant therapy should be to rapidly decrease affective symptoms and to return the patient to his or her original level of functioning or as near to that as is possible. With respect to attaining this goal, several new directions, innovations, and reappraisals have evolved over the past several years. The first involves a consideration of how long antidepressants should be given acutely before deciding to change drugs having an inadequate effect. The evidence continues to accumulate that antidepressants as a class require from nearly a week to several weeks to begin to exert their effects. Recently, it has been reported that a 6- to 8-week trial of full-dose antidepressants increases the yield of responding patients; this is a change from the earlier consensus that a 3- to 4-week trial is adequate to see if efficacy is likely to occur (21).

It has become accepted dogma in psychopharmacological circles that the choice of an antidepressant should in large part be made on the basis of side effects. To that end, a drug's anticholinergic, hypotensive, sedating/soporific, gastrointestinal, overdose toxicity in suicidal patients, and other side effects should determine choice. Strategically, the clinician needs to carefully consider the patient's biology and psychology, respectively, and this process is not always formally done. There needs to be careful attention to predicting patients' cardiovascular, prostatic, ophthalmological, and cerebrovascular status, as well as other responses to specific drugs before administering a given drug, which probably necessitates a comprehensive history and physical examination. Conversely, the clinicians should consider the advantages of a given medication's side effects to a specific patient. For example an agitated an insomniac depressed patient may require a sedating antidepressant (34,41).

Another choice based on side effects is whether to use those drugs that have appeared most recently on the market, and are thus being heavily advertised or drugs that are "tried and true" and whose advantages and disadvantages have become known over time. With the recent advent of selective serotonin reuptake inhibitors (SSRIs), such as fluoxetine, sertraline, and paroxetine, and the dopaminergic-activating antidepressant bupropion, a predictable shift in utilization has occurred, especially by primary care physicians. The newer serotonergic agents generally have less cardiovascular and anticholinergic side effects, and they are less toxic in an overdose than the conventional older antidepressants. However, the SSRIs are more prone to cause gastrointestinal side effects, (which can be avoided by starting at a low dose), and to precipitate insomnia, agitation, and psychostimulation, and bupropion may cause relatively more epileptic seizures, although this is not firm.

The treating physician also needs to carefully consider the financial implications of prescribing a particular drug. In spite of differences in side effects, it is important to note that the SSRIs and other new antidepressants show similar efficacies in depressed patients and similar degrees of symptom alleviation as do the older conventional antidepressants. However, they usually cost considerably more than do generic and even conventional brand compounds. Some authorities have suggested using the newer antidepressants as second-line treatments except in exceptional cases, whereas others have advocated utilizing SSRIs and other new antidepressants initially. In general, however, the practicing community, especially primary care physicians, have shifted their prescribing patterns to use the SSRIs, in part because they are more clearly "broad spectrum" than the TCAs and that is a real plus.

Related to the issue of prescribing novel or newer antidepressants for refractory or partially refractory cases of depression is the question of what should be done if a patient is nonresponsive or only partially responsive to a given drug. Such simple measures as raising the dose of a drug or measuring blood levels to see if therapeutic norms are being attained or if compliance is occurring are obvious first strategies, which should precede switching drugs. In addition, in recent years a variety of augmentation strategies and drug-switching strategies have developed. For example, the addition of lithium and/or thyroid hormones to antidepressants in refractory or partially refractory depressed patients has become widely accepted and can increase treatment efficacy. In addition, there is considerable evidence that there is a genetic component to the efficacy of specific antidepressant drugs, so that if one member of a family has responded well to a specific drug, the chances are high that a positive response will occur in a relative of the index patient. Similarly, an efficacious antidepressant drug in a specific individual will be more likely to be effective when used during subsequent episodes. Finally, there appears to be some selective advantage over conventional antidepressants to the utilization of monoamine oxidase inhibitors (MAOIs), such as phenelzene and tranylcypromine, in patients with atypical depression or in patients with variants of bipolar disorder and possibly in the elderly. Use of MAOIs probably should be a second line (SSRIs being the first line) of treatment, even in cases of atypical depression, and the MAOIs must be used with caution in older patients due to the hypotensive effects.

Lithium, used in relatively high doses and with relatively high serum levels, is indicated in acute mania, as is the addition of an antipsychotic drug when psychotic symptoms are present. As symptoms remit, the antipsychotic drug should be lowered. In patients refractory or non-responsive to lithium, carbamazepine and valproate are considered alternative treatments (12,17,29). Alternatively there is growing evidence that the addition of carbamazepine and valproate to lithium non-response is a viable strategy usable instead of adding an antipsychotic drug to the acute regimen. Others use valproate as a first choice based on the rationale that lithium and valproate are at least equivalent in efficacy and valproate is easier to manage.

Short-term treatment strategies also involve the art, as well as the science, of pharmacotherapy. The treating physician should be thought of as part of the treatment mix. For example, it is important for the prescribing clinician to maintain close and frequent contact with the patient and the patient's family to monitor side effects and to assure compliance. This is especially true when drugs are initially started or the dose is changed. Several times weekly, or even more frequent contact, either in person or by telephone, is indicated in the early phases of pharmacotherapy. In addition, the fear of stigma and the embarrassment often experienced by patients who are prescribed psychotropic drugs may lead to the patient discontinuing these agents, a phenomena that needs to be explored and discussed openly with the patient. Similarly, there is a compelling need to discuss the potential side effects of the various antidepressants and antimanic drugs prospectively, and over time as the patient remains in psychopharmacologic treatment.

By tradition, the relationship of the patient with his or her therapist has been an insular one. This is especially true in dynamically oriented psychotherapy, which has traditionally been of a one-to-one nature and has usually excluded family members. However, treatments of patients with mood disorders of a severity requiring pharmacotherapy often need to involve family members or significant others as coparticipants (14,15). This is accomplished best by bringing them in for the initial interview as sources of information, which gets them on your SIVC immediately. For patients requiring medication, family members should be advised in depth about the nature of the prescribed medication and its side effects. In addition, family members can and should be incorporated as helpers in undercutting resistance to taking medications, making sure medications are taken regularly, and monitoring side effects. Finally, the impacts of the patients' illness and the medications and their side effects on the patients' family need to be considered and appropriately handled.

It is worth noting that a number of drugs originally used for other medical purposes have been incorporated into the psychopharmacologist's armamentarium as treatments for depression and mania. There is good evidence that used alone or in combination with lithium, carbamazepine or valproate is efficacious in the treatment of mania. Carbamazepine appears especially efficacious in the treatment of rapidly cycling mania. Thus, the prescribing physician needs to remain cognizant of the utilization of nonpsychiatric drugs as effective treatments for mood disorders and at the same time to be aware of the role of these agents in causing affective symptoms (27).

In any discussion of short-term strategies for utilizing antidepressant and antimanic medications, it is important to step back and consider the strategy of not prescribing medications in a given case. Approximately 30% to 40% of patients with major depression, maintained in placebo controlled outpatient trials of antidepressant drugs, respond to the placebo treatment with significant alleviation of their symptoms. These patients often, but not always, tend to have episodes that are associated with stress, that is, the episodes have been precipitated by obvious social causes and are less likely to relapse over time. Thus, an important and difficult to employ strategy for the prescribing physician is to monitor the patient with social/psychotherapeutic treatment only, and to see if symptoms significantly decrease over a period of 3 to 6 weeks. This strategy is often difficult for the patient and the prescribing physician, because there is usually a great pressure to "do something." However, used judiciously, as in the fairly acute short-term nonsevere case may avoid the costs and side effects of antidepressants.

Finally, it is important to note that several antidepressant psychotherapies have shown efficacy in the treatment of mild depression (37), and a combination of psychotherapy and pharmacotherapy possibly may be more effective than either treatment used alone (3,32).

Long-term Strategies

In contrast to the major goal of short-term treatment of mood disorders, which is essentially to reestablish mood and functioning to relative normalcy, the goal of long-term antidepressant treatment is to maintain the previously depressed patient at the best level of functioning possible, and, most importantly, to prevent relapse. In the past few years, several studies have demonstrated that the risk of rapid relapse from a given episode of major depression is high if less than 4 to 6 months of continuing and full-dose antidepressant therapy are given following apparent symptomatic remission. In addition, it appears from several studies that antidepressants should be continued in full doses during the entire period that a patient is receiving them. Similarly, lithium should be given for 4 to 6 months following a manic episode, although in this case a decrease in serum levels is acceptable (21,28,30).

The latter suggestions for relatively long-term treatment of affective disorders represent a major shift in the strategy for treating affective episodes over time. In the past, the alleviation of a depressive or manic episode was often followed by the physician rapidly decreasing or terminating medications. Knowledge that the frequency of relapse is high in the short run after an affective episode would indicate a 4- to 6-month drug treatment phase for virtually all patients started on antidepressant drugs or antimanic drugs. Furthermore, until relatively recently, many clinicians considered it good clinical practice to taper medications once remission had occurred, because the risk of side effects would intuitively appear lower with lower doses of medication. Such a strategy apparently has been successful for a small number of patients in the treatment of schizophrenia with antipsychotic drugs and possibly in the treatment of mania. However, knowledge that tapering of antidepressant drugs leads to a higher relapse rate suggests that a full-dose strategy be used in patients with mood disorders in the acute phases and beyond (7,10,11).

After a 4- to 6-month period of active antidepressant (or antimanic) treatment has been completed, a decision needs to be made as to how much longer treatment should continue. Again, conventional wisdom previously suggested that in most cases drug treatment can be stopped, at least until a subsequent episode occurs. To this end, the patient's individual history needs to be considered. Stopping medications may be indicated in a patient who has had a complete remission, and has had no previous episodes. In patients with a history of recurrent episodes of depression, or mania, or both, (i.e., three or more episodes), there is good evidence that chronic treatment lasting for several years or even longer will decrease partial and complete relapses (40). Also, many patients with only partial remission of symptoms require ongoing treatment. The lethality of even one previous suicide episode should also be considered when weighing the advantages of continuing medications, because the severity and existence of previous attempts by a patient when depressed to no small extent predicts similar future attempts, as should be the disruptiveness of prior episodes. Thus, the earlier strategy of stopping medication in patients with a mood disorder after several months and resuming treatment if and when signs of relapse reappear may be ill advised. The strategy employing chronic, open-ended medication administration in at least a subgroup of patients with mood disorders appears indicated, as there appears to be many patients who have significant interepisode subsyndromal depression (7,10,20,40). Also, there is suggestive evidence that many patients, who were once responsive to either antidepressants for unipolar depression or to lithium for bipolar disorder, and have gone off medication, are no longer responsive when restarted on the same (previously effective) medication (27).

Conversely, however, there are some disadvantages to open ended antidepressant and antimanic therapy. As described with respect to short-term strategies, psychiatric patients, and especially patients with mood disorders often feel embarrassed to be taking psychotropic medications. These patients may believe that the consumption of these psychotropic medications is a sign of weakness. They may wish to deny that they have been ill and, in the case of bipolar patients, may even wish to experience the ''high'' of mania. In addition, there is some epidemiological evidence that TCAs, given chronically, may induce increases in cardiac arrhythmias, leading to statistically significant increases in mortality in patients with preexisting arrhythmias. In addition, antidepressant drugs exert significant withdrawal effects if withdrawn too quickly, and these symptoms may mimic the primary illness. Finally, the plethora of potential interactions between antidepressants and other drugs increases as the patient ages and is placed by a physician on increasing numbers of psychotropic and nonpsychotropic drugs. This can be considered to be a drawback to open-ended continuation of therapy. Indeed, it may be considered as an indication for withholding or stopping drug therapy. Nevertheless, at least for the patient with a history of frequent relapses, there are now indications that chronic and continuing maintenance treatment for depression, as well as for mania, is strategically indicated.

In any case, if an antidepressant drug is withdrawn after a period of continuation therapy, and if symptoms recur, rapid reinstitution of the drug is indicated. With respect to the recurrence of symptoms which occur when the patient is still receiving antidepressants or antimanic drugs, a strategy of checking for drug compliance, raising the dosage of drug, and checking for medical or pharmacodynamic influences is indicated.

Several additional strategies exist to deal with manic patients treated prophylactically or who are on continuation therapy with lithium who relapse. Conventional wisdom would suggest the addition of an antipsychotic agent is temporarily indicated if such a relapse occurs. This should occur along with a raising of the lithium serum level to acute treatment levels if the patient is receiving lithium. Alternatively, augmentation of the lithium treatment with a mood stabilizer such as carbamazepine or sodium valproate, with ongoing continuation of these drugs is indicated. This augmentation may be done in combination with the short term administration of a benzodiazepine such as clonazepam or lorazepam for sleep and antimanic effects. The latter strategy avoids the risks of giving an antipsychotic drug with such side effects as development of tardive dyskinesia, dysphoria, and dystonia.

Finally, as with the patient with acute mood disorder, there is good reason to involve family members in the treatment of patients on continuing medications. During chronic or continuing treatment, visits to the physician occur less frequently, and with time the patients' wish not to use (what he perceives to be) a crutch blends with the fading memory of the pain of the episode to greatly increase the risk of treatment noncompliance. It is at this time that the patient's family needs to be involved, to undercut its own resistance to medication treatment and to help the patient to continue needed therapy.

The issues discussed in this section are similar to those in Chapter 91 and the reader is referred to this chapter for further information.

ANXIETY DISORDERS

In this section, we focus on panic disorder, but also mention agoraphobia, and generalized anxiety disorder (GAD). For each, we comment on strategies of when to initiate treatment, which drugs to use (although a full discussion of this issue is outside the scope of this chapter), and when to discontinue treatment, that is, long-term strategies. All of the anxiety disorders can be effectively treated with pharmacological agents, which have a variety of serotonergic and noradrenergic actions. In addition, recent work suggests abnormal dopaminergic function might be involved in the etiology of anxiety disorders (26). As with mood disorders, the major therapeutic aim is to interrupt kindling and potentiation of these disorders for reasons discussed earlier in this chapter.

Short-term Strategies

The goal of acute treatment is remission of symptoms and return to normal levels of psychosocial function. As to when to initiate treatment, the first issue is to decide if the anxiety disorder is primary or secondary to another disorder, like chronic alcoholism or depression. If secondary, that disorder must be treated first. The next issue is to take a careful history of the nature, frequency, and severity of the attacks. In this context, it should be noted that a very high placebo response rate has been seen clinically and in some panic disorder studies. Perhaps even more true than in depression, if a patient has had one or two panic attacks, the clinician may want to temporize for a few weeks. One attack in 4 years is quite different than four attacks in 1 year, but the dramatic impact of even one episode can precipitate a disproportionately strong response. Once the diagnosis of the subclass of anxiety disorder (panic disorder, GAD, obsessive–compulsive disorder, etc.) is made the appropriate medication trials should be started.

After the episode has remitted, we recommend continuation for several months. At that point, a medication should be tapered (slowly, over months) in an attempt to minimize withdrawal and rebound symptoms. Contrary to conventional wisdom, the data do not show differences in gradual withdrawal between high-potency benzodiazepines, such as lorazepam or alprazalam, and low-potency diazepines, such as diazepam. As Schatzberg (35) has pointed out, "all available pharmacological treatments may pose some problem with respect to maintenance and discontinuation," specifically MAOIs may cause weight gain, hypertensive crises, hyperpyrexic reactions, and rebound mania. Tricyclic antidepressants (TCAs) may cause weight gain, rebound mania, and increased blood pressure, whereas benzodiazepines may cause cognitive impairment, ataxia (elderly), dependence, and withdrawal (35).

It is important to emphasize that patients with chronic anxiety who are effectively treated do not escalate their dose and that they remain relatively symptom free. Furthermore, if they do become noncompliant, their clinical picture usually worsens.

Agoraphobia, even when it occurs without panic, can be extraordinarily disabling, severely limiting daily activities. In any case imipramine, alprazolam, and phenelzine have all been found to be effective. General anxiety disorder is most commonly treated with benzodiazepines, but TCAs have also been shown to be effective although slower in onset. Post-traumatic Stress Disorder (PTSD) has not been well studied, but both imipramine and phenelzine will reduce symptoms. The new SSRIs are also being tried. Medication should be combined with family or individual psychotherapy as appropriate to each clinical situation.

Long-term Strategies

Many recent studies suggest that all of the anxiety disorders (GAD, panic disorders, OCD, and the phobias) are both very disabling and have chronic courses, rather than being limited to a single episode (9,33):

It is well documented that the life time prevalence rate for all the anxiety disorders in Europe and North American is approximately 14% of those over the age of 18 years. In addition, such disorders are often associated with other types of mental illness such as depression, alcoholism and drug abuse. Despite the high prevalence of anxiety disorders and sleep disorders which may accompany such conditions, the seriousness of such disorders is often underestimated by the media and by society in general. It

has been established, for example, that of those patients with anxiety disorders one-third recover but in the remainder the symptoms persist throughout their lives (39).

Thus, the cost of anxiety disorders to the individual and to the society is considerable and frequently underestimated. In fact "in a detailed study of over 3000 patients with 'pure' anxiety in Sweden, the risk of suicide was found to be as high as in those with depression or other diagnoses that require in-patient care" (1). In part, the high suicide rate is thought be related to the demoralization that is associated with the day-by-day symptoms in untreated or partially treated patients.

Accordingly, the strategies we advocate are based in part upon data showing that there is severe morbidity in panic disorder as manifested by depressive symptoms, suicidal behavior, alcohol abuse, and social and vocational function deterioration (46). Accordingly, a Task Force of the Collegicum Internationale Neuro-Psychopharmacologicum (CINP) has noted:

It is well established that the long-term use of anxiolytics and hypnotics can cause dependence in some individuals. However, a significant number of patients suffering from chronic anxiety and insomnia require continuous treatment for periods exceeding the 4 to 6 weeks usually recommended by regulatory authorities. Such long-term treatments may together with other health measures improve the quality of life of such patients and there is no clear evidence that the efficacy of long-term medication diminishes with time or that escalation of the dose may occur in such a way that it may create a clinical or public health problem (39).

As to which classes of drugs to use for the anxiety disorders, we suggest two possible strategies. The first, older strategy is the use of benzodiazepines. The efficacy and safety of these drugs has been well documented. Most importantly these drugs offer large comparative advantages to the classic alternatives (barbiturates, meprobamate, etc.) or to no treatment, which if relapse occurs increases the likelihood of great individual and social cost (as mentioned above). The second, newer strategy is the use of antidepressants. We include here the use of tricyclics, MAOs, and the newer SSRIs. Which medication for which subcategory of anxiety disorders will be discussed in the chapters on treatment (of anxiety disorder). Here, in the context of discussing strategies, the relevant issues are that antidepressants are an effective alternative to benzodiazepines, but have greater untoward effects (mostly anticholinergic effects) and a longer onset of action (43). They do, however, have a lower risk of dependence. Until controlled head-to-head comparisons are made, more definitive strategies cannot be suggested.

As to when to stop therapy, we recommend considering discontinuation after six months of sustained improvement. If no relapse or recurrence is observed, then periodic visits and contact with the patient and the patient's family seem sensible. If symptoms exacerbate, then treatment for another year may be a serviceable guideline. We do not as yet know which percentage of patients will require maintenance treatment, but our guess is that it may be 40% of those who initially present with DSM-III-R criterion for panic disorder.

In summary, Schatzberg (35) has well delineated the issues: overall, the risk of anxiety disorders causing morbidity and becoming chronic appears to be much higher than the risk of a treatment being injurious to patients. Given the responsiveness of the disorder to currently available therapies, the overall risk-to-benefit ratio for treating panic disorder patients weighs in favor of treatment.

SUMMARY OF THE NEW MODEL OF PSYCHOPHARMACOLOGICAL TREATMENT STRATEGIES

The following is a summary of some of the new and most important guidelines for pharmacological strategies. They are based on the assumptions that discreet diagnostic entities can be identified, that effective medication treatments exist, that most of the Axis I and II disorders are life long or represent life-long vulnerabilities, and that, most importantly, exacerbations and recurrences are often disastrous to patients, their families, and the societies in which they live.

In the short term, the goals are to reduce symptoms as rapidly as possible; build an alliance for long-term management; educate the patients and their families about the illness, its treatment, and its course (treated and untreated); and lay the groundwork for as maximal a return to premorbid function as possible. Effective strategies include the use of adequate dosage for each medication, adequate duration before abandoning a trial, avoiding polypharmacy where possible, combining medication with psychotherapeutic strategies (*almost always,* for both patients and their families), and providing systematic (and repetitive) psychoeducation for patients and their families. Almost all acute treatments should continue for at least 6 months, and with disorders like schizophrenia may take 18 months, until symptom remission. Further, we recommend a discrete, 6-month period of remission before starting to taper therapeutic medications.

In the long term, that is, during the prevention phase of treatment, we recommend the primary goal of minimizing the risk of relapse, because, for most patients and their families, relapse means marked impairment in social and vocational function, as well as symptom exacerbation. In our experience, many patients and families prefer the consequences of staying on medication for life, rather than the consequences of discontinuing medication. Therefore, we recommend the strategies of (a) staying on medication in the minimal effective dose, (b) frequent monitoring of side effects and life circumstances, and (c) frequent contact with families to maximize compliance and reduce the burden of living with chronic psychiatric illness. We recognize that keeping patients on medication for a lifetime is costly. But we believe the cost is worth it, as there are long-term benefits for the individual, the family, and society. In fact, a Swedish study has shown that initially putting patients on expensive psychotropics saves money in the long-run, because they lower relapse and rehospitalization rates (22).

SUMMARY

In conclusion, we have presented a rationale and a model for the psychopharmacological treatment of acute and chronic psychiatric illness. The data suggests that (a) patients and their families prefer treatment to no treatment because of the devastating effects of recurrence and relapse; (b) if practitioners choose to treat, it must be utilizing an adequate (i.e., effective) dose and an adequate duration of treatment (often lifelong). However, there must be a continual search for the minimal dose that yields a treatment with maximal efficacy and safety. More data from controlled studies is needed to define more precisely treatment strategies over time (i.e., the life course, rather than only for acute episodes). The last four generations of psychopharmacology have seen enormous progress toward developing rational treatment strategies for mental illness based on controlled double-blind studies rather than on theoretical biases. We are confident that this trend will continue.

REFERENCES

1. Allgulander A, Lavori PW. Excess mortality among 3302 patients with ''panic'' anxiety neurosis. *Arch Gen Psychiatry* 1991;48:599–602.
2. Altshuler L. Bipolar disorder: Are repeated episodes associated with neuroanatomic and cognitive change. *Biol Psychiatry* 1993;33:563–565.
3. Blackburn IM, Eunson KM, Bishop S. A two-year naturalistic follow-up of depressed patients treated with cognitive therapy, pharmacotherapy and combination of both. *J Affect Disord* 1986;10:67–75.
4. Braff DL. Reply to cognitive therapy and schizophrenia. *Schizophr Bull* 1992;18:37–38.
5. Carpenter WT, Jr, Heinrichs D. Early intervention, time limited, targeted pharmacotherapy of schizophrenia. *Schizophr Bull* 1983;9:533–542.
6. Christison GW, Kirch DG, Wyatt RJ. When symptoms persist: choosing among alternative somatic treatments for schizophrenia. *Schizophr Bull* 1991;17:217–245.
7. Depression Guideline Panel. *Depression in primary care; Vol. I. Treatment of major depression. Clinical practice guideline.* Rockville, MD: U.S. Department of Health and Human Services, Public Health Service, Agency for Health Care Policy and Research; 1993. AHCPR Publication No. 93-0551.
8. Docherty JP, Van Kammen DP, Siris SG, Marder SR. Stages of onset of schizophrenic psychosis. *Am J Psychiatry* 1978;135:420–426.
9. Faravelli C, Albanesi G. Agoraphobia with panic attacks; one-year prospective follow-up. *Compr Psychiatry* 1987;28:481–487.
10. Frank E, Kupfer DJ, Perel C, et al. Three-year outcomes for mainte-

nance therapies in recurrent depression. *Arch Gen Psychiatry* 1990;47:1093–1099.

11. Frank E, Johnson S, Kupfer DJ. Psychological treatments in the prevention of relapse. In: Montgomery S, Rouillon F, eds. *Long-term treatment of depression.* New York: John Wiley; 1992:187–228.

12. Gelenberg AJ, Kane JM, Keller MB. Comparison of standard and low serum levels of lithium for maintenance treatment of bipolar disorder. *N Engl J Med* 1989;321:1489–1493.

13. Goldstein MJ, Strachau AM. The family and schizophrenia. In: Jacob T, ed. *Family interaction and psychopathology: theories, methods, and findings.* New York: Plenum Press; 1989:481–508.

14. Glick ID, Burti L, Suzuki K, Sacks M. Effectiveness in psychiatric care: I. A cross-national study of the process of treatment and outcomes of major depressive disorder. *J Nerv Ment Disease* 1991;179:55–63.

15. Glick ID, Burti L, Suzuki K, Sacks M. Effectiveness in psychiatric care: IV. Achieving effective medication management for major affective disorder. *Psychopharmacol Bull* 1992;28:257–259.

16. Glick ID, Clarkin JF, Haas GL, Spencer JH. Clinical significance of inpatient family intervention: VII. Conclusions from the clinical trial. *Hosp Commun Psychiatry* 1993;9:869–873.

17. Goodwin FK, Jamison KR. *Manic-depressive illness.* New York: Oxford Press; 1990.

18. Kane JM, Marder SR. Psychopharmacologic treatment of schizophrenia. *Schizophr Bull* 1993;19:287–302.

19. Kane JM, Woerner MG, Sarantakos S. Depot neuroleptics: a comparative review of standard, intermediate, and low dose regiments. *J Clin Psychiatry* 1986;47:30–33.

20. Keller MB, Shapiro RW, Lavori PW, Wolfe N. Relapse in major affective disorders. *Arch Gen Psychiatry* 1982;39:911–915.

21. Kupfer DJ, Frank E. The minimum length of treatment for recovery. In: Montgomery S, Rouillon F, eds. *Long-term treatment of depression.* New York: John Wiley; 1992:33–52.

22. Lewander T, Westerberg SE, Morrison D. Clinical profile of remoxipride—A combined analysis of a comparative double-blind multicenter trial programme. *Acta Psychiatrica Scandinavica* 1990;82:92–98.

23. Marder SR, Van Putten T, Mintz J, Lebell M, McKenzie J, May PR. Low and conventional dose maintenance therapy with fluphenazine decanoate: two-year outcome. *Arch Gen Psychiatry* 1987;44:510–517.

24. Meltzer HY. The mechanism of action of novel antipsychotic drugs. *Schizophr Bull* 1991;17:263–287.

25. Pickar D, Owen RR, Litman RE, Konicki PE, Gutierrez R, Rapaport MH. Clinical and biological response to clozapine in patients with schizophrenia: crossover comparison with fluphenazine. *Arch Gen Psychiatry* 1992;49:345–353.

26. Pitchot W, Ansseau M, Moreno Ag, Hansenne M, Jon Frenckell R. Dopaminergic function in panic disorder: comparison with major and minor depression. *Biol Psychiatry* 1992;32:1004–1011.

27. Post RM. Anticonvulsants and novel drugs. In: Paykel ES, ed. *Handbook of affective disorders.* London: Churchill Livingstone; 1992:387–417.

28. Prien RF, Kupfer DJ. Continuation drug therapy for major depressive episodes: how long should it be maintained? *Am J Psychiatry* 1986;143:18–23.

29. Prien RF, Gelenberg AJ. Alternatives to lithium for preventive treatment of bipolar disorder. *Am J Psychiatry* 1989;840–848.

30. Prien RF. Maintenance therapy. In: Paykel E, ed. *Handbook of affective disorders.* London: Churchill Livingston; 1992:419–435.

31. Reardon GT, Rifkin A, Schwartz A, Myerson A, Siris SH. Changing pattern of neuroleptic dosage over a decade. *Am J Psychiat* 1989;146:726–729.

32. Reynolds CF, Frank E, Perel J, et al. Combined pharmacotherapy and psychotherapy in the acute and continuation treatment of elderly patients with recurrent major depression: a preliminary report. *Am J Psychiatry* 1992;149:1687–1691.

33. Robins LN, Reiger DA, eds. *Psychiatric disorders in America: the epidemiologic catchment area study.* New York: Free Press; 1991.

34. Rouillon F. Unwanted effects of long-term treatment. In: Montgomery S, Rouillon F, eds. *Long-term treatment of depression.* New York: John Wiley; 1992:81–112.

35. Schatzberg AF, Ballenger JC. Decisions for the clinicians in the treatment of panic disorder: when to treat, which treatment to use and how long to treat. *J Clin Psychiatry* 1991;52:26–31.

36. Schooler NR. Maintenance medication for schizophrenia: strategies for dose reduction. *Schizophr Bull* 1991;17:311–324.

37. Shea MT, Elkin I, Imber SM, et al. Course of depressive symptoms over follow-up: findings from the National Institute of Mental Health Treatment of Depression Collaborative Research Program. *Arch Gen Psychiatry* 1992;49:782–787.

38. Strauss J, Carpenter W. The prognosis of schizophrenia: rationale for a multidimensional concept. *Schizophr Bull* 1978;4:56–67.

39. Task Force of the Collegium Internationale Neuro-Psychopharmacologicum (CINP). Impact of neuropharmacology in the 1990's—treatment strategies for anxiety disorders and insomnia. *Eur Neuro Psychopharmacol* 1992;2:167–169.

40. Thase ME. Long-term treatments of recurrent depressive disorders. *J Clin Psychiatry* 1992;53(Suppl):32–44.

41. Tollefson GD. Adverse drug reaction/interactions in maintenance therapy. *J Clin Psychiatry* 1993;54(Suppl):48–58.

42. Treatment Strategies in Schizophrenia (TSS). *Proceedings of the American College of Neuropsychopharmacology.* Nashville: American College of Neuropsychopharmacology; 1992:62–63.

43. Tyrer P, Hallstrom C. Antidepressants in the treatment of anxiety disorder. *Psychiat Bull* 1993;17:75–76.

44. Van Putten T, Marder SR, Mintz J. A controlled dose comparison of haloperidol in newly admitted schizophrenic patients. *Arch Gen Psychiatry* 1990;47:754–758.

45. Waddington JL, Weller MP, Crow TJ, Hirsch SR. Schizophrenia, genetic retrenchment, and epidemiologic renaissance. *Arch Gen Psychiatry* 1992;49:990–994.

46. Weissman MM. Panic disorder: Impact on quality of life. *J Clin Psychiat* 1991;52(Suppl):6–8.

47. Wokowitz CM, Pickar D. Benzodiazepines in the treatment of schizophrenia: a review and reappraisal. *Am J Psychiatry* 1991;148:714–726.

48. Wyatt RJ. Neuroleptics and the natural course of schizophrenia. *Schizophr Bull.* 1991;17:325–351.

Psychopharmacology: The Fourth Generation of Progress, edited by Floyd E. Bloom and David J. Kupfer. Raven Press, Ltd., New York © 1995.

CHAPTER **74**

Pharmacokinetics and Pharmacodynamics

David J. Greenblatt, Jerold S. Harmatz, Lisa L. von Moltke, and Richard I. Shader

Pharmacokinetics is a discipline that uses mathematical models to describe and predict the time-course of drug concentrations in body fluids. During the last 30 years, our ability to apply pharmacokinetic principles to clinical psychiatry and psychopharmacology has undergone major advances. Important improvements in analytical chemistry techniques partly explain this progress. Methods for quantitation of drug concentrations in plasma and tissues are now highly sensitive and specific. For almost all drugs used to treat mental disorders, techniques such as gas chromatography, liquid chromatography, and mass spectroscopy can be used to quantitate serum or plasma concentrations of these agents and their pertinent metabolites after single therapeutic doses or during chronic therapy. These improved measurement methods have facilitated the application of pharmacokinetic models and have increased the role of therapeutic drug monitoring in clinical psychopharmacology. For some psychotropic drugs, ranges of therapeutic and potentially toxic plasma concentrations are reasonably well established; for others, such ranges are tentatively established or postulated, and research is ongoing. Clinicians are also increasingly familiar not only with how plasma drug concentrations can be helpful, but also with the potential pitfalls of therapeutic monitoring (11).

The discipline of pharmacokinetics has also been advanced by the general availability of iterative computer methods for nonlinear regression analysis. In the precomputer era, only the simplest modeling problems could be solved by approximation, usually after data transformation or linearization. Now, complex problems involving

simultaneous determination of a number of clinically relevant pharmacokinetic variables can be rapidly solved, including numerical estimates of the statistical strength of the solution.

Pharmacodynamics, the study of the time course and intensity of drug effects on the organism, also has undergone major advances, largely due to technological advances in our capacity to measure drug effects. Kinetic–dynamic modeling uses mathematical methods to link drug concentrations directly to clinical effects. Iterative nonlinear regression procedures expeditiously solve the problems of fitting theoretical models to actual data (see Chapter 124, *this volume*).

PHARMACOKINETICS

Approaches to Pharmacokinetic Modeling

Lipid-soluble psychotropic drugs generally do not behave as if the body were a single homogeneous space. The two-compartment model resolves the living organism into two distinct mathematical spaces, thereby enhancing the precision of describing and predicting drug behavior (Fig. 1). The assumptions of this model are as follows: (a) Intravenously administered medications are introduced directly into the "central" compartment, which consists of the circulating blood as well as other high-flow tissues such as brain, heart, lung, liver, and endocrine organs. (b) Irreversible drug elimination, either by hepatic biotransformation or renal excretion, takes place only from the central compartment. (c) Reversible distribution occurs between central and peripheral compartments, with a finite time (usually between 30 min and 6 hr after intravenous dosage) required for distribution equilibrium to be attained. (d) The peripheral compartment is usually

D. J. Greenblatt, J. S. Harmatz, L. L. von Moltke, and R. I. Shader: Department of Pharmacology and Experimental Therapeutics, Tufts University School of Medicine, and the Division of Clinical Pharmacology, New England Medical Center Hospital, Boston, Massachusetts 02111.

I.V. DOSE

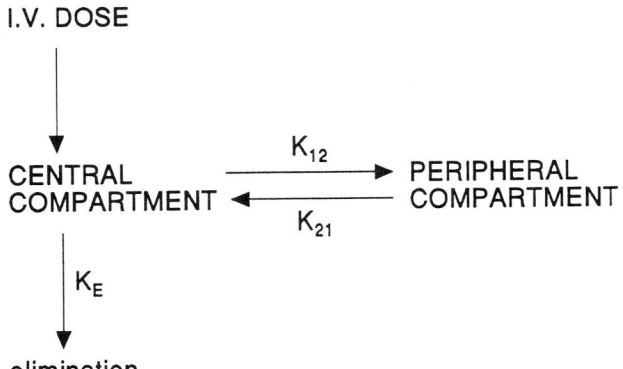

elimination

FIG. 1. Schematic diagram of the two-compartment open model. It is assumed that intravenously-administered medications are given directly into the central compartment. Irreversible elimination (via hepatic biotransformation or renal excretion) only occurs via the central compartment; K_E is the first-order elimination rate constant. Reversible distribution occurs between central and peripheral compartments, with first-order distribution rate constants of K_{12} and K_{21}.

inaccessible to direct measurement and is not a site of drug elimination or clearance (13,18,20,43).

This model predicts that rapid intravenous drug administration will yield a profile of drug disappearance from serum or plasma that is consistent with a linear sum of exponential terms.

$$C = Ae^{-\alpha t} + Be^{-\beta t} \qquad [1]$$

In this equation, C is the plasma drug concentration at time t after rapid intravenous injection. A and B are intercept terms having units of concentration, and α and β are exponents having units of reciprocal time. The exponents α and β are related to, but are not equal to, the intrinsic rate constants associated with the two-compartment model (Fig. 1).

A real clinical study typically yields a series of concentration-time data points, which, when plotted on a logarithmic concentration axis, appears biphasic (Fig. 2). The investigator's task is to determine the parameters A, B, α, and β from Eq. 1 which yield the best fit to the data points. This is done by computer using iterative least-squares regression methods (29,33). The function of best fit can then be used to calculate clinically useful pharmacokinetic parameters (Fig. 3).

The biphasic profile of drug disappearance following rapid intravenous injection of lipid-soluble psychotropic drugs has important clinical implications. In physiological terms, the initial phase of rapid drug disappearance is attributable mainly to distribution, whereas the slower phase that follows is largely due to elimination or clearance. Distribution, elimination, and duration of action are interdependent. A drug's elimination half-life refers to the apparent half-life of disappearance in the post-distributive elimination phase. This half-life value does not necessarily correspond to its duration of action, which actually is

determined by the relation of the actual plasma concentration to a minimum effective concentration. Drug action may be terminated during the distribution phase and have little to do with the value of the elimination half-life measured in the postdistributive phase (21,22). The absolute size of the dose is also of critical importance, since a proportional change in dose will produce corresponding changes in all plasma concentrations, which in turn may disproportionately increase duration of action (Fig. 4). The same principles are also applicable following oral drug administration, although the mathematics becomes more complex.

Refinements in computerized techniques for nonlinear least-squares regression now allow distinct but interdependent sets of data points to be analyzed simultaneously. An example is the plasma drug concentration–time relationship during and after zero-order (constant-rate) intravenous infusion for a drug having a kinetic profile consistent with a two-compartment model. During the infusion, plasma concentrations (C) are related to time after the start of the infusion (t) as follows:

$$C = \frac{Q}{CL}(1 - X_1 e^{-\alpha t} - X_2 e^{-\beta t}) \qquad [2]$$

After the infusion, the relationship is

$$C = \frac{Q}{CL}X_1(1 - e^{-\alpha \cdot T_{inf}})e^{-\alpha(t - T_{inf})}$$

$$+ \frac{Q}{CL}X_2(1 - e^{-\beta \cdot T_{inf}})e^{-\beta(t - T_{inf})} \qquad [3]$$

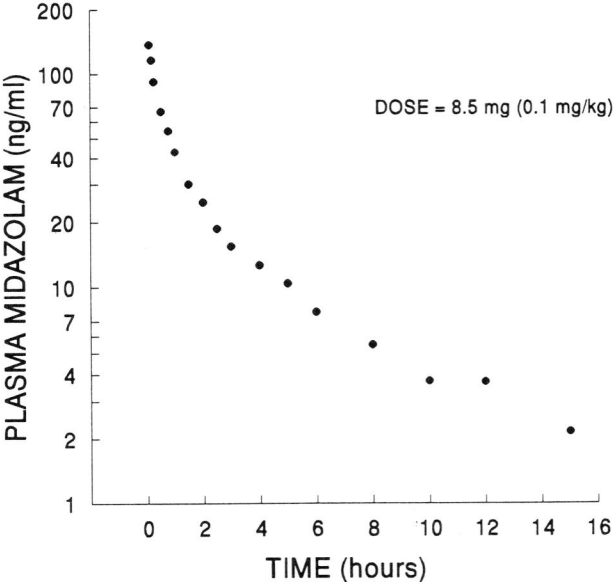

FIG. 2. Plasma midazolam concentrations following a 0.1 mg/kg intravenous dose of midazolam administered to a healthy male volunteer by continuous (zero-order) infusion over a period of 1 min. (The plasma level of 381 ng/ml just at the end of the infusion is not shown.)

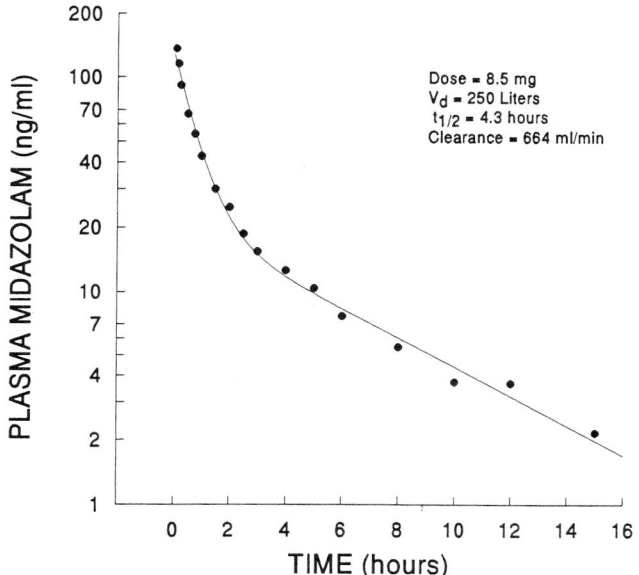

Dose = 8.5 mg
V_d = 250 Liters
$t_{1/2}$ = 4.3 hours
Clearance = 664 ml/min

FIG. 3. The same data points as in Fig 2. The *solid line* is the pharmacokinetic function, consistent with Eq. 1, which was fitted to the data points by computer using nonlinear least-squares regression. Coefficients and exponents from the fitted function were used to calculate the kinetic variables as indicated on the figure.

In these equations, α and β again are exponents having units of reciprocal time, T_{inf} is the duration of the infusion, Q is the infusion rate, and CL is the drug's metabolic clearance. The coefficients X_1 and X_2 are related to α, β, and K_E. Equation 2, which represents an ascending function, is applicable during the time that the infusion is ongoing ($0 \leq t \leq T_{inf}$). The infusion ends at $t = T_{inf}$, at which time Eq. 3 becomes applicable ($t \geq T_{inf}$); this equation represents a descending function. Taken together, Eqs. 2 and 3 are continuous at all points in time, but at $t = T_{inf}$, the change point, the collective function does not have a first derivative.

Physiologically, the pharmacokinetic properties of a particular drug should be unique and constant for a particular individual subject, as long as no intervening factors alter drug distribution or clearance in that individual. Under this assumption, the same values of α, β, K_e, and CL should be applicable both during and after an intravenous infusion. Accordingly, Eq. 2 is fitted to concentration–time points measured *during* the infusion, simultaneous with fitting Eq. 3 to points measured *after* the infusion (Fig. 5). The result is a single set of parameters (α, β, K_e, and CL) that are consistent with the drug's behavior both during and after the infusion.

The same approach can be extended to circumstances in which the same drug is given to the same individual on different occasions. Figure 6 shows actual, measured concentration–time points, along with functions of best fit as consistent with Eqs. 2 and 3, in a three-way cross-

over study of the benzodiazepine derivative midazolam. A fixed total dose of midazolam (0.1 mg/kg) was administered to a healthy volunteer on three separate occasions by zero-order infusion. The rates of infusion differed across the three trials as follows: 1 min, 1 hr, and 3 hr. Assuming that pharmacokinetic parameters for midazolam in this particular subject are constant from trial to trial, Eqs. 2 and 3 can be fitted to all sets of data points simultaneously, with values of Q and T_{inf} appropriately adjusted to correspond to the duration of infusion for each trial. The result is a single set of pharmacokinetic parameters that is consistent with drug behavior during and after each of the infusions across the three trials (Fig. 6).

Stable Isotopes in Clinical Pharmacokinetics

Techniques in synthetic chemistry allow the preparation of drug entities labeled with nonradioactive "heavy" isotopes of carbon or nitrogen, differing from the natural isotopes by as little as one molecular weight unit. If one carbon or nitrogen atom in a drug's customary structure is replaced by a heavy isotope of the same atom, the result

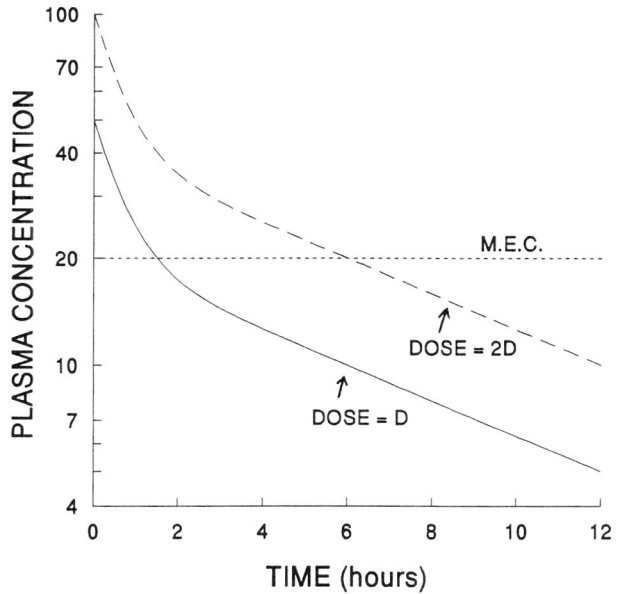

FIG. 4. The *solid line* is the pharmacokinetic function consistent with a two-compartment model (Eq. 1) after rapid intravenous injection of a hypothetical drug (dose = D). The elimination half-life in the post-distributive phase is 6 hr. The *horizontal dotted line* represents the minimum effective concentration (M.E.C.), below which the drug has no clinical activity. Note that the duration of activity of the drug is short (less than 2 hr) because the plasma concentration falls below the M.E.C. during the distribution phase. The *dashed line* represents the function corresponding to an administration of the same drug at twice the dose (dose = 2D). Note that doubling the dose disproportionately prolongs the duration of action.

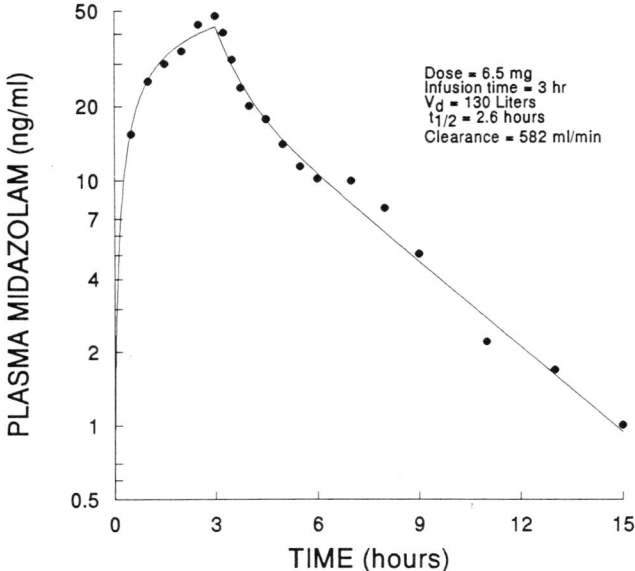

FIG. 5. Plasma midazolam concentrations in a healthy volunteer who received a 0.1 mg/kg intravenous dose by constant-rate (zero-order) infusion over a period of 3 hr. The *solid lines* are the pharmacokinetic functions determined by simultaneous fitting of Eqs. 2 and 3 to data points during and after the infusion, respectively. Pharmacokinetic variables based on the fitted functions are indicated on the figure.

is a nonradioactive stable-isotope-labeled (SIL) drug. The customary and SIL drug forms are identical, except that the SIL form differs by one atomic mass unit. These two forms cannot be distinguished using analytical techniques such as high-pressure liquid chromatography or gas chromatography, since the change in molecular weight by itself does not cause a measurable change in retention time. However, the customary drug form can be distinguished from the SIL form by gas chromatography (GC)/ mass spectroscopy (MS), because one molecular weight unit will separate the corresponding fragments of the two drug forms (38).

Assuming that the customary and SIL drug forms have identical pharmacokinetic properties in vivo, SIL methodology can substantially extend the power of clinical pharmacokinetics (4–6). Bioequivalence studies traditionally require a cross-over design, in which the same drug is administered to the same individual on separate occasions. One trial involves dosage with the ''reference'' compound; in the other trial, the dosage form being tested is administered. Plasma drug concentrations are measured at multiple time points after drug administration in each trial, and bioequivalence is evaluated by comparison of variables such as peak plasma concentration (C_{max}), time of peak concentration (T_{max}), elimination half-life, and area under the plasma concentration curve (AUC). A similar crossover design is used to compare the rate and completeness of drug absorption after oral or intramuscular administration relative to intravenous dosage. With SIL methodology, bioequivalence studies can be done with a

single exposure trial per subject. One dosage form is the conventional drug; the other is the SIL form. Both are administered at the same time. The GC/MS analytical procedure can simultaneously quantitate concentrations of each drug form in each plasma sample. This approach saves time and reduces drug exposure and blood sampling requirements for human volunteers. It also reduces variance due to sequence effects. After oral administration, for example, C_{max} and T_{max} may vary within the same individual when the same dosage form of the same drug is administered on different occasions. AUC may also vary from time to time due to subtle changes in clearance, regardless of dosage form or rate of administration.

Stable-isotope-labeled methodology can also be used to study definitively the single-dose pharmacokinetics of a drug in a patient already receiving the same drug on a chronic basis. Under conventional circumstances, the dosing rate divided by the steady-state plasma concentration yields an estimate of clearance, assuming complete absorption of each oral dose. However, elimination half-life and volume of distribution cannot be determined unless the drug is discontinued. A single intravenous dose of SIL drug can be used to determine all pharmacokinetic parameters without interfering with ongoing therapy and with no assumptions about drug absorption.

SIL methodology has drawbacks as well as benefits. Substantial synthetic and medicinal chemistry resources are needed to prepare SIL drugs and formulate them for

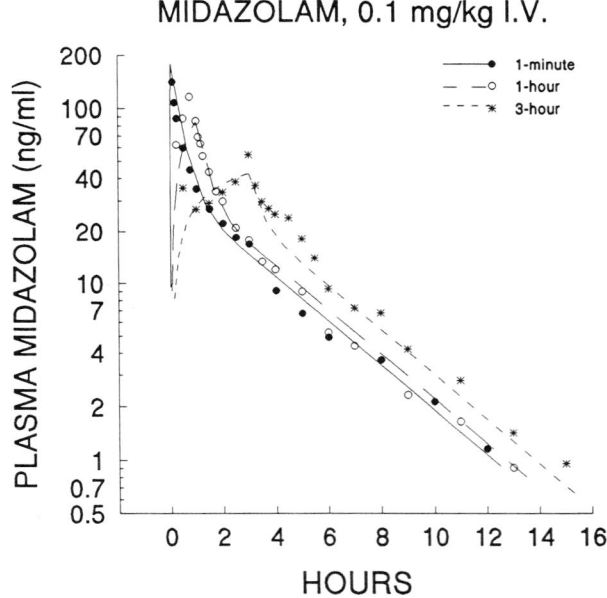

FIG. 6. A healthy male volunteer received 0.1 mg/kg of midazolam intravenously by constant rate (zero-order) infusion on three occasions separated by at least 1 week. The durations of infusion in the three trials were 1 min, 1 hr, and 3 hr. Equations 2 and 3 were fitted to the data points for all three trials simultaneously. Kinetic variables were volume of distribution, 121 L; elimination half-life, 2.4 hr; clearance, 584 ml/min.

human administration. GC/MS facilities must be available for analysis of all biological samples. These analyses are much more difficult and expensive than usual high-performance liquid chromatographic and GC procedures.

Mathematical Modeling of Drug Interactions In Vitro

The serotonin-specific reuptake inhibitor (SSRI) antidepressants, of which fluoxetine is the prototype, are now prescribed extensively in clinical practice. The class of SSRIs has the secondary pharmacologic property of reversibly inhibiting the activity of hepatic drug-metabolizing enzymes. Following the introduction of fluoxetine, experimental and clinical reports of drug interactions began to appear, in which coadministration of fluoxetine caused decreased clearance and elevated plasma concentrations of certain other coadministered medications (8). Some of these interactions have been of clinical importance. The various SSRIs (and their metabolites) that are now available, and those under investigation, are not equivalent in their capacity to inhibit drug metabolism, nor is the metabolism of every drug equally affected by SSRI coadministration.

Literally hundreds of clinical pharmacokinetic studies would be needed to delineate which drugs will interact with SSRIs, the extent of the interactions, and whether they can be safely coadministered under usual clinical circumstances. However, recent advances in the field of cytochrome chemistry have made it possible to study drug interactions using in vitro models, thereby making at least some clinical pharmacokinetic studies unnecessary (2,3, 14,15,26,27,42). Using ultracentrifugation techniques, the microsomal drug-metabolizing component of human liver tissue can be isolated (41). When mixed with appropriate reaction cofactors, human liver microsomes will metabolize drugs in vitro much as happens in vivo.

Nonlinear least-squares regression techniques are applied to enzyme kinetics in much the same way as in clinical pharmacokinetics. In a typical in vitro enzyme kinetic study, varying concentrations of a drug substrate (S) are incubated with human liver microsomes for a fixed period of time. The amount of metabolic product generated is quantitated in the reaction mixture, and converted to a normalized reaction velocity (V), usually in units of nanomoles of product per minute per milligram of microsomal protein. In most cases the relation of V to S is consistent with the following equation:

$$V = \frac{V_{max} \cdot S}{S + K_m} \qquad [4]$$

where V_{max} is the maximum reaction velocity and K_m is the substrate concentration at which V is 50% of V_{max}. Linearizing transformations of data, with their inherent

distorting effects, were commonly used in the pre-computer era to estimate values of V_{max} and K_m from experimental data. However, current computerized methods allow direct analysis of untransformed data by nonlinear regression. Reliable analysis of in vitro metabolic inhibition studies likewise is dependent on nonlinear regression methods. If a metabolic inhibitor is added to a reaction mixture, the reaction velocity will be depressed depending on the concentration of substrate, the concentration of inhibitor (I), and an inhibition constant (K_i) which reflects the inhibiting "potency" of the inhibiting compound. Numerical values of K_i reciprocally reflect inhibiting potency; that is, low values of K_i indicate high inhibiting potency.

If competitive inhibition is the mechanism of the inhibiting effect, the variables described above are related as follows:

$$V = \frac{V_{max} \cdot S}{S + K_m \cdot (1 + I/K_i)} \qquad [5]$$

A typical in vitro study will measure V at varying concentrations of S and I. V_{max}, K_m, and K_i can be determined using linearizing transformations of data, but these have the potential to distort the relationships (1). Computerized nonlinear regression can simultaneously analyze all data points without transformation, and provide best-fit estimates of V_{max}, K_m, and K_i.

In vitro drug interaction studies have provided data directly useful to clinical decision making. Coadministration of the SSRI fluoxetine with the cyclic antidepressant desipramine (DMI) impairs metabolic clearance of DMI and significantly elevates steady-state plasma levels of DMI in humans (35). The biotransformation of DMI involves hydroxylation by the hepatic microsomal system, yielding 2-hydroxy-desipramine (2-OH-DMI). This reaction is mediated by Cytochrome P450-2D6, of which fluoxetine and its principal metabolite, norfluoxetine, are competitive inhibitors. In vitro studies using human liver microsomes, based on methods described above, provide K_i estimates for fluoxetine and norfluoxetine with regard to their capacity to inhibit formation of 2-OH-DMI from DMI (40) (Fig. 7). Based on steady-state plasma concentrations of fluoxetine and norfluoxetine measured in humans, the expected partitioning of these two drugs between plasma and liver, and K_i values measured in vitro, impairment of DMI clearance in vitro during coadministration of fluoxetine can be qualitatively and quantitatively predicted (40). Similar methods correctly predict that the SSRI paroxetine also will strongly impair DMI clearance in vivo. In contrast, the SSRI sertraline, its metabolite desmethylsertraline, and the SSRI fluvoxamine are weak inhibitors of DMI clearance in vivo (35), and weak inhibitors of 2-OH-DMI formation from DMI in vitro (40).

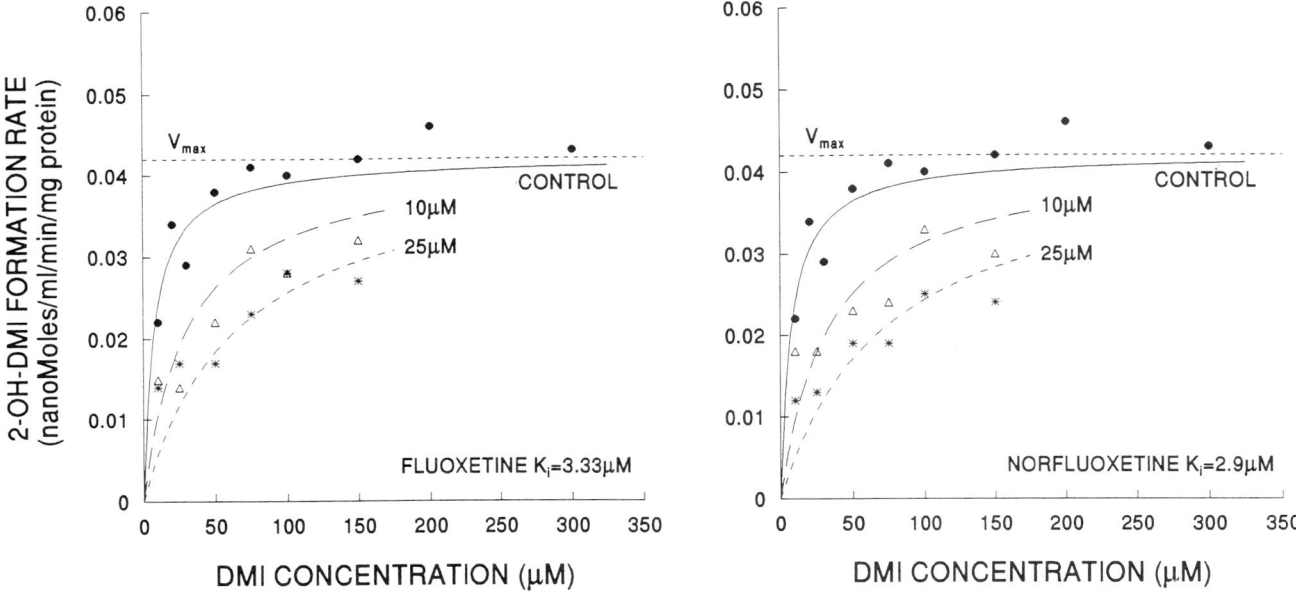

FIG. 7. Rates of formation of 2-OH-DMI following incubation of human liver microsomes with varying concentrations of desipramine (DMI). Closed circles represent reaction velocities in the control condition, with no inhibitors added. The other points represent reaction rates with coaddition of 10 μM or 25 μM of fluoxetine (FLU), **left,** or norfluoxetine (NOR), **right.** Lines were determined by fitting of Eq. 5 to the data points by nonlinear least-squares regression. The resultant K_i values were 3.33 μM for fluoxetine and 2.90 μM for norfluoxetine.

PHARMACODYNAMICS

After a single dose of a psychotropic medication, its plasma concentrations and clinical effects will increase, reach a maximum, and then decline with time. Pharmacokinetics deals with the time-course of drug concentration, whereas the discipline of pharmacodynamics refers to the time-course and intensity of drug action or response. The capacity to understand and predict individual differences in drug response is of critical importance in psychopharmacology, since the objective of drug treatment is to produce therapeutic benefit while minimizing side-effects. Advances in the clinical applications of pharmacodynamics are due to improved precision and objectivity in methods for measuring human drug response, and the emergence of the discipline of kinetic–dynamic modeling, in which drug concentration is used as a direct predictor of response.

Methods of Measurement

Each class of psychotropic drugs produces unique pharmacodynamic effects, as well as problems with measurement. Pharmacodynamic studies of sedative–anxiolytic drugs serve to illustrate available approaches to quantitation, and the limitations associated with each (24,31).

Benzodiazepine derivatives, and other γ-aminobutyric acid (GABA)-benzodiazepine receptor agonists, produce clinical sedation as a final common pathway of action

(16,28). However, the clinical consequences of benzodiazepine agonist action depend on the therapeutic objective and the setting of drug administration. Antianxiety–antipanic effects, enhancement of sleep, and reduction of seizure activity are usually described as primary therapeutic actions. Typical side-effects include excessive or persistent sedation, drowsiness, ataxia, incoordination, slowed reaction time, or slowed psychomotor performance. Some clinical actions are ambiguous; impaired memory, for example, may be desirable in the context of premedication before general anesthesia or sedation prior to endoscopy or cardioversion, but undesirable in other circumstances. Benzodiazepines also produce some effects whose direct link to clinical efficacy or side-effects are not directly established. These include: increased beta activity on the electroencephalogram (EEG), reduced saccadic eye movement velocity, increased postural sway, elevated concentrations of plasma growth hormone, and reduced plasma concentrations of cortisol and ACTH.

Measurement of the pharmacodynamic effects of benzodiazepine agonists becomes more reliable and objective as the effects become more removed from the primary therapeutic action. The time-course and intensity of primary therapeutic effects are the most difficult to measure. Clinical anxiolytic or sedative properties can be quantitated using global assessments by patients or trained observers, or by rating instruments targeted to specific symptoms or symptom groups. These measurement approaches have been extremely useful in clinical psychopharmacology, but have limitations. They are subjective ratings, and can be influenced by the outlook, expectation, and experience of the patient as well as the observer. Quantitative drug effects must be evaluated as change scores relative to both the pretreatment baseline condition and, to inactive placebo. If special populations (such as the elderly) have a unique way of interpreting rating scale items or describing drug effects, this further complicates the methodology.

Procedures quantitating secondary effects of benzodiazepine agonists generally focus on aspects of psychomotor performance, such as measures of reaction time, speed, and accuracy of task performance, and the capacity for information acquisition and recall. These measures are only partly objective, although they provide numeric results. Again, change scores are the most meaningful; drug effects must be compared to pre-dose baseline performance, and to effects of placebo. Psychomotor performance procedures are influenced by practice—subjects' performance will progressively improve if they repeatedly perform a task in the absence of medication. This can complicate interpretation of drug-associated changes, and must be accounted for in the experimental design. The study of special populations (such as the elderly) is also affected by baseline performances that differ from that of the control group. It is not clear how best to incorporate differences in baseline performance when comparing drug effects (25). The relation of drug effects on laboratory performance tasks to effects on real life tasks is not clearly established. Even for complex and seemingly realistic laboratory tasks such as simulated automobile operation, the consequences of error are negligible in the laboratory, but potentially lethal on the road.

Fully objective measures of pharmacodynamic effects of benzodiazepines are of increasing interest. Computerized analysis of the EEG can directly quantitate benzodiazepine effect, either by evaluation of activity in the beta frequency band by fast-Fourier transform, or by aperiodic analysis (12,21–23,32,37,39). In addition to being completely objective, these measures are unresponsive to placebo, and are not altered by practice or experience. No theoretical basis is yet established to link EEG changes to changes in therapeutic effects or psychomotor side effects. Empirical data, however, demonstrate that the pharmacodynamic profile of EEG changes following benzodiazepine agonist administration closely intercorrelates with other measures of drug activity (12,23).

Kinetic–Dynamic Modeling

Kinetic–dynamic modeling procedures directly evaluate the relation of drug concentrations (C) to drug effect (E), with the objective of determining how much variability in drug effect is attributable to measurable drug concentrations (9,10,12,30,32,36,37). The Sigmoid-E_{max} rela-

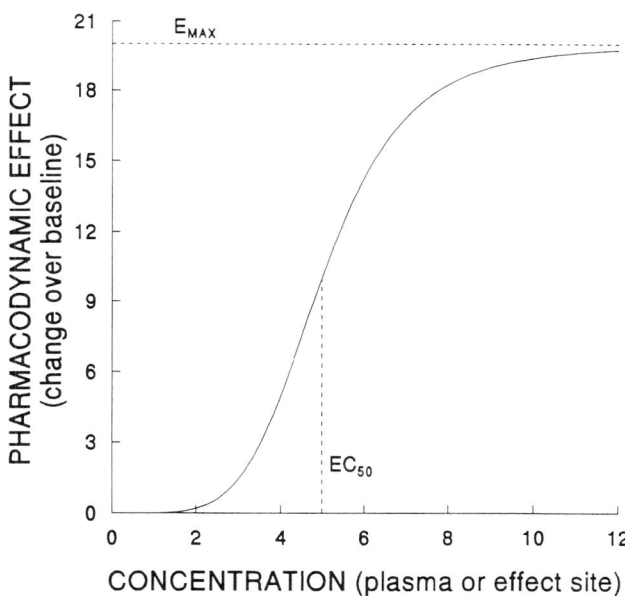

FIG. 8. Graphical representation of the Sigmoid-E_{max} model, consistent with Eq. 6 (see text). In this hypothetical situation $E_{max} = 20$, $EC_{50} = 5$, and $A = 5$.

tionship is commonly used in kinetic–dynamic modeling. When this model fits the data, investigators are reassured about the concentration–effect relationship, since many drug-receptor interactions fit the same model. The linkage is described by the following equation:

$$E = \frac{E_{max} \cdot C^A}{C^A + EC_{50}^A} \qquad [6]$$

E_{max} is the maximum drug effect (relative to baseline), which cannot be exceeded no matter how high the drug concentration; EC_{50}, is the concentration at which the drug effect is 50% of E_{max}; A is an exponent of unknown biological significance related to the "steepness" of the curve in its linear phase (Fig. 8). When applicable, this model allows quantitation of individual differences in sensitivity to a given drug, relative potencies of drugs having the same mechanism of action, and the quantitative and qualitative effects of pharmacologic potentiators or antagonists. However, not all data sets are consistent with the Sigmoid-E_{max} model, and it may be inappropriate or even misleading to "force" this model on data which it does not fit (17). In many cases, data from kinetic–dynamic studies can be described by an exponential function such as:

$$E = B \cdot C^A \qquad [7]$$

or by a linear function such as:

$$E = m \cdot C + b \qquad [8]$$

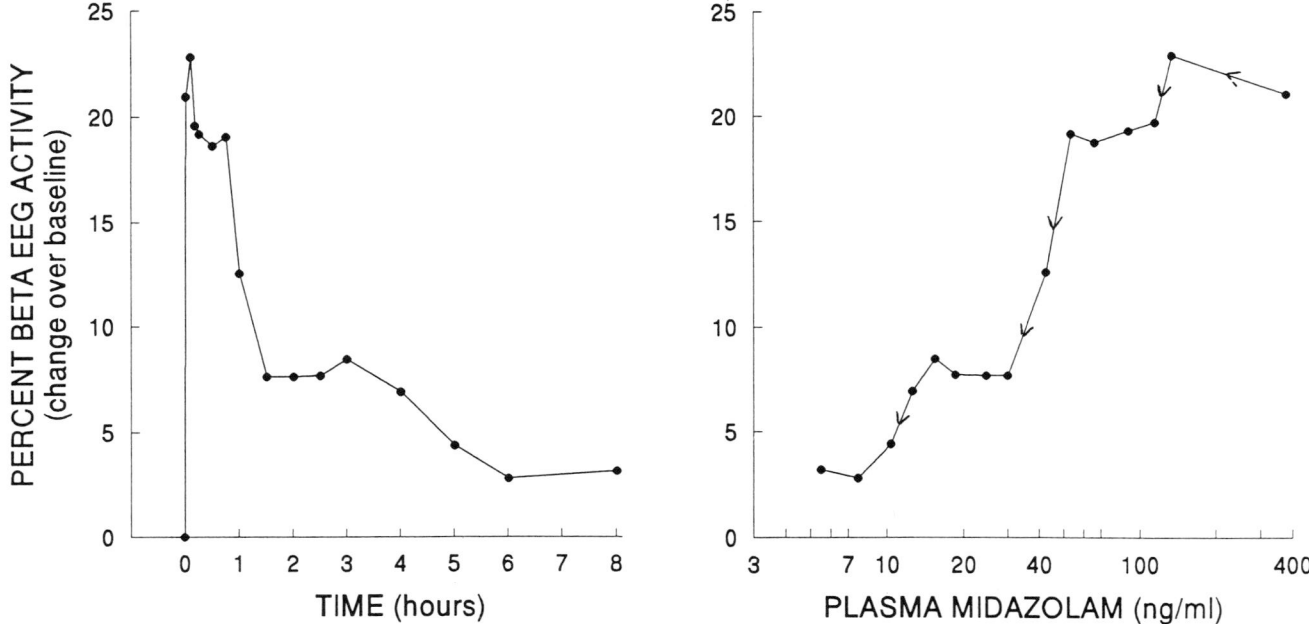

FIG. 9. Left: For the subject referred to in Figures 2 and 3, the EEG was monitored prior to and for 8 hr after the intravenous dose of midazolam. The EEG signal was analyzed by computer to determine the relative activity in the 13–30 cps range, also termed the beta range. The maximum EEG change was not attained immediately after the end of the infusion, but rather at *five* minutes after completion of the infusion. **Right:** A plot of plasma midazolam concentrations (*x* axis, logarithmic scale) versus EEG change (*y* axis) shows that the maximum EEG change does not correspond to the maximum plasma concentration. Arrows indicate the direction of increasing time.

Plasma Concentration Versus Effect-Site Concentration

The use of plasma drug concentration as the independent variable in kinetic–dynamic modeling procedures (Eqs. 6, 7, and 8) assumes that equilibration of drug between plasma and the site of action (effect-site) in brain is very rapid, such that plasma concentrations are proportional to concentrations at the effect site. This assumption may need modification in some circumstances. For the subject described in Figs. 2 and 3, maximum change over baseline in EEG beta activity is delayed following completion of the infusion of midazolam (Fig. 9). A kinetic–dynamic plot of EEG effect versus plasma concentration reveals "counterclockwise hysteresis," in which the maximum effect does not correspond to the maximum plasma concentration. This may be explained by the time necessary for midazolam to equilibrate between plasma and effect site (19). To account for this delay, the model is modified to include the hypothetical effect site (Fig. 10). Effect-site concentrations, as opposed to plasma concentrations, are presumed to determine pharmacodynamic effects (9,36,37). The first-order rate constant K_{EO} governs the exit of drug from the hypothetical effect site, and also determines the observed equilibration of drug between plasma and effect-site. K_{EO} can be used to calculate a half-life of equilibration ($t_{1/2KEO}$). If K_{EO} is incorporated

as a variable in the iterative analysis, the resulting plot of effect-site concentration versus EEG effect eliminates the hysteresis and yields data points that are consistent with Eq. 7 (Fig. 11).

COMMENT

The major challenge for health care professionals involved in clinical psychopharmacology is to understand

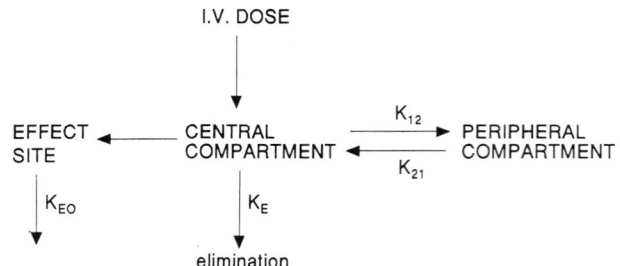

FIG. 10. Modification of the kinetic–dynamic model to incorporate an effect-site, presumed to correspond to the site of pharmacologic activity. The first-order rate constant for drug exit from the effect-site (K_{EO}) is effectively the rate constant determining the time necessary for drug equilibration between plasma and effect-site. Kinetic–dynamic linkage models are then applied to hypothetical effect-site concentrations rather than plasma concentrations.

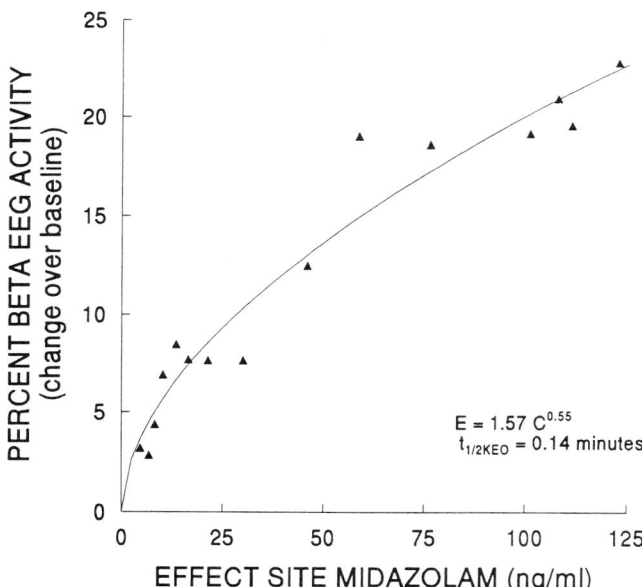

FIG. 11. For the subject referred to in Figs. 2, 3, and 9, EEG data were analyzed using the pharmacokinetic parameters shown in Fig. 3, together with the model shown in Fig. 10. Nonlinear regression yielded K_{EO} = 4.95/min, or $t_{1/2KEO}$ = 0.14 min. The relation between midazolam concentrations at the presumed effect site versus EEG change now fits a kinetic–dynamic model consistent with Eq. 7.

and compensate for individual variations in drug response. Why does a given dose of a given psychotropic medication produce different clinical responses among individuals comprising a population of patients? When the same dose produces different plasma concentrations in different individuals, the variance is pharmacokinetic. When the same concentration produces different responses in different individuals, the variance is pharmacodynamic. The principles described in this chapter, as they become increasingly available to and used by clinicians, should enhance our ability to deliver effective drug treatment with minimal side effects.

ACKNOWLEDGMENTS

This work was supported in part by grant MH-34223 from the Department of Health and Human Services. Dr. von Moltke is the recipient of an Abbot Laboratories Fellowship in Clinical Pharmacology.

The authors are grateful for the collaboration and assistance of Drs. Bruce L. Ehrenberg and Lawrence G. Miller.

REFERENCES

1. Barlow RB. Effects of "rogue" points on non-linear fitting. *TIPS* 1993;14:399–403.
2. Birkett DJ, MacKenzie PI, Veronese ME, Miners JO. In vitro approaches can predict human drug metabolism. *TIPS* 1993;14:292–294.
3. Brosen K. Recent developments in hepatic drug oxidation: implications for clinical pharmacokinetics. *Clin Pharmacokinet* 1990;18:220–239.
4. Browne TR. Stable isotopes in clinical pharmacokinetic investigations. Advantages and disadvantages. *Clin Pharmacokinet* 1990;18:423–433.
5. Browne TR. Stable isotopes in pharmacology studies: present and future. *J Clin Pharmacol* 1986;26:485–489.
6. Browne TR, Szabo GK. New pharmacokinetic methods for the study of antiepileptic medications of the 1990s. *Epilepsia* 1991;32[Suppl 5]:S66–S73.
7. Cholerton S, Daly AK, Idle JR. The role of individual human cytochromes P450 in drug metabolism and clinical response. *TIPS* 1992;13:434–439.
8. Ciraulo DA, Shader RI. Fluoxetine drug-drug interactions. *J Clin Psychopharmacol* 1990;10:48–50, 213–217.
9. Colburn WA. Simultaneous pharmacokinetic and pharmacodynamic modeling. *J Pharmacokinet Biopharmaceut* 1981;9:367–388.
10. Dingemanse J, Danhof M, Breimer DD. Pharmacokinetic–pharmacodynamic modeling of CNS drug effects: an overview. *Pharmacol Ther* 1988;38:1–52.
11. Friedman H, Greenblatt DJ. Rational therapeutic drug monitoring. *JAMA* 1986;256:2227–2233.
12. Friedman H, Greenblatt DJ, Peters GR, et al. Pharmacokinetics and pharmacodynamics of oral diazepam: effect of dose, plasma concentration, and time. *Clin Pharmacol Ther* 1992;52:139–150.
13. Gibaldi M, Perrier D. *Pharmacokinetics*. New York: Marcel Dekker; 1975.
14. Gonzalez FJ. Human cytochromes P450. *TIPS* 1992;13:346–352.
15. Gonzalez FJ. In vitro systems for prediction of rates of drug clearance and drug interactions. *Anesthesiology* 1992;77:413–415.
16. Goodchild CS. GABA receptors and benzodiazepines. *Br J Anaesth* 1993;71:127–133.
17. Greenblatt DJ, Harmatz JS. Kinetic-dynamic modeling in clinical psychopharmacology. *J Clin Psychopharmacol* 1993;13:231–234.
18. Greenblatt DJ, Koch-Weser J. Clinical pharmacokinetics. *N Engl J Med* 1975;293:702–705, 964–970.
19. Greenblatt DJ, Sethy VH. Benzodiazepine concentrations in brain directly reflect receptor occupancy: studies of diazepam, lorazepam, and oxazepam. *Psychopharmacology* 1990;102:373–378.
20. Greenblatt DJ, Shader RI. *Pharmacokinetics in clinical practice*. Philadelphia: WB Saunders; 1985.
21. Greenblatt DJ, Ehrenberg BL, Gunderman J, et al. Pharmacokinetic and electroencephalographic study of intravenous diazepam, midazolam, and placebo. *Clin Pharmacol Ther* 1989;45:356–365.
22. Greenblatt DJ, Ehrenberg BL, Gunderman J, et al. Kinetic and dynamic study of intravenous lorazepam: comparison with intravenous diazepam. *J Pharmacol Exp Ther* 1989;250:134–140.
23. Greenblatt DJ, Harmatz JS, Gouthro TA, Locke J, Shader RI. Distinguishing a benzodiazepine agonist (triazolam) from a non-agonist anxiolytic (buspirone) by electroencephalography: kinetic-dynamic studies. *Clin Pharmacol Ther* 1994;56:110–111.
24. Greenblatt DJ, Harmatz JS, Shader RI. Clinical pharmacokinetics of anxiolytics and hypnotics in the elderly: therapeutic considerations. *Clin Pharmacokinet* 1991;21:165–177, 262–273.
25. Greenblatt DJ, Harmatz JS, Shapiro L, Engelhardt N, Gouthro TA, Shader RI. Sensitivity to triazolam in the elderly. *N Engl J Med* 1991;324:1691–1698.
26. Guengerich FP. Bioactivation and detoxication of toxic and carcinogenic chemicals. *Drug Metab Disp* 1993;21:1–6.
27. Guengerich FP. Human cytochrome P-450 enzymes. *Life Sci* 1992;50:1471–1478.
28. Haefely WE. The GABA$_A$-benzodiazepine receptor: biology and pharmacology. In: Burrows GD, Roth M, Noyes Jr R, eds. *Handbook of Anxiety, Vol 3, The Neurobiology of Anxiety*. Amsterdam: Elsevier; 1990:165–188.
29. Harmatz JS, Greenblatt DJ. A SIMPLEX procedure for fitting nonlinear pharmacokinetic models. *Comp Biol Med* 1987;17:199–208.
30. Holford NHG, Sheiner LB. Kinetics of pharmacologic response. *Pharmacol Ther* 1982;16:143–166.
31. Hommer DW, Matsuo V, Wolkowitz O, et al. Benzodiazepine sensi-

tivity in normal human subjects. *Arch Gen Psychiatry* 1986;43:542–551.

32. Mandema JW, Danhof M. Electroencephalogram effect measures and relationships between pharmacokinetics and pharmacodynamics of centrally acting drugs. *Clin Pharmacokinet* 1992;23:191–195.

33. Motulsky HJ, Ransnas LA. Fitting curves to data using nonlinear regression: a practical and nonmathematical review. *FASEB J* 1987;1:365–374.

34. Murray M. P450 enzymes: inhibition mechanisms, genetic regulation and effects of liver disease. *Clin Pharmacokinet* 1992;23:132–146.

35. Preskorn SH, Alderman J, Chung M, Harrison W, Messig M, Harris S. Pharmacokinetics of desipramine coadministered with sertraline or fluoxetine. *J Clin Psychopharmacol* 1994;14:90–98.

36. Sheiner LB, Stanski DR, Vozeh S, Miller RD, Ham J. Simultaneous modeling of pharmacokinetics and pharmacodynamics: application to d-tubocurarine. *Clin Pharmacol Ther* 1979;25:358–371.

37. Stanski DR. Pharmacodynamic modeling of anesthetic EEG drug effects. *Annu Rev Pharmacol Toxicol* 1992;32:423–447.

38. Szabo GK, Browne TR. Mass spectrometry: preparation of biologic specimens. *J Clin Pharmacol* 1986;26:400–405.

39. van Steveninck AL, Mandema JW, Tuk B, et al. A comparison of the concentration-effect relationships of midazolam for EEG-derived parameters and saccadic peak velocity. *Br J Clin Pharmacol* 1993;36:109–115.

40. von Moltke LL, Greenblatt DJ, Cotreau-Bibbo MM, Duan SX, Harmatz JS, Shader RI. Inhibition of desipramine hydroxylation in vitro by serotonin-reuptake-inhibitor antidepressants, and by quinidine and ketoconazole: a model system to predict drug interactions in vivo. *J Pharmacol Exp Ther* 1994;268:1278–1283.

41. von Moltke LL, Greenblatt DJ, Harmatz JS, Shader RI. Alprazolam metabolism in vitro: studies of human, monkey, mouse, and rat liver microsomes. *Pharmacology* 1993;47:268–276.

42. von Moltke LL, Greenblatt DJ, Harmatz JS, Shader RI. Cytochromes in psychopharmacology. *J Clin Psychopharmacol* 1994;14:1–4.

43. Wagner JG. *Fundamentals of clinical pharmacokinetics.* Hamilton, IL: Drug Intelligence Publications; 1975.

Psychopharmacology: The Fourth Generation of Progress, edited by Floyd E. Bloom and David J. Kupfer. Raven Press, Ltd., New York 1995.

CHAPTER 75

Methodological Issues in the Neuropathology of Mental Illness

Joel E. Kleinman, Thomas M. Hyde, and Mary M. Herman

Although schizophrenia has been referred to as "the graveyard of neuropathology" (1), there has been a renaissance of postmortem studies in mental illness. This rebirth has been fueled by advances in neuroimaging that have allowed for in vivo neuropathology and new techniques in neuropathology such as immunocytochemistry, autoradiography, computerized neuronal morphometrics, and in situ hybridization. In point of fact, the "graveyard" quote was never meant to discourage neuropathological research, but to encourage the use of more advanced techniques. Most of this new research has involved schizophrenia and suicide, but drug addictions and specific affective disorders will probably follow suit. Although there have been numerous findings to date, many have unfortunately not been replicable or have failed to lead to significant advances. Therefore, a review of methodology in this area may prove useful.

One place to start this review is with a success story. One obvious success involves Parkinson's Disease. The discovery of reduced dopamine concentrations in the nigrostriatal pathway of patients with Parkinson's Disease (2) led to the L-Dopacarbidopa replacement treatment strategy (3), a modern neuroscience/neuropathology triumph. This success was based in large part by knowing where to look in the brain of Parkinson's Disease patients, a fact made more obvious by the loss of pigment in the substantia nigra (4). Advances in neurochemistry, such as assays to measure dopamine in fresh-frozen specimens, was also essential to this clinical research advance.

Neuropathological studies of mental illnesses have a number of issues that are not found in neurological diseases. A number of these problems are discussed in the

first section, Neuropsychiatric Issues. The next two sections, Neuroanatomic Issues and Neuropathological Issues, cover issues that are probably relevant to all brain diseases.

NEUROPSYCHIATRIC ISSUES

Collection

The rate-limiting step in neuropathological studies of mental illnesses is the collecting of sufficient numbers of brain specimens to allow for a scientific study. There are at least five proven sources, which include medical examiners' offices, Veteran's Administration hospitals, state psychiatric hospitals, hospices, and brain banks. Each of these sources has advantages and disadvantages that must be considered.

Medical examiners' offices are the source of choice for the study of suicide. Most states have laws dictating that autopsies be performed by medical examiners on victims of suicide. This source of tissue offers the advantages of specimens from younger subjects who are also more likely to fall into the purview of the medical examiner. For the study of schizophrenia, this advantage may be offset by relatively less psychiatric history, which makes an accurate diagnosis more difficult. A second confound in medical examiner cases, substance abuse, can be mitigated by toxicological screening of urine, blood, or brain. The medical examiner's office provides two other major advantages: relatively short postmortem intervals and a source of normal controls from the same facility, which may reduce the effects of postmortem artifacts in the collection, resulting from factors such as ambient temperatures, which vary with the season of the year, delays in refrigeration, mode of death, and so on.

J. E. Kleinman, T. M. Hyde, and M. M. Herman: Clinical Brain Disorders Branch, Intramural Research Programs, NIMH Neuroscience Center at St. Elizabeths, Washington, DC 20032.

A second major source of brain specimens involves the Veteran's Administration hospitals. Along with medical examiners' offices this source is an excellent place to study alcoholism and other drug addictions. This source offers the advantages of relatively easy accessibility to medical records essential to an accurate diagnosis. Unfortunately, the large percentage of patients with dual diagnoses such as manic–depressive illness and alcoholism is a major problem in doing research in this system. Normal controls can also be obtained in these hospitals.

The state psychiatric hospital offers the most promise for prospective studies. Large numbers of schizophrenic patients who have not been placed in the community make prospective studies in the state and Veteran's Administration Hospitals feasible. The obvious advantages of this approach is that psychiatric diagnosis can be made with greater accuracy in living patients. The disadvantage of this approach is that the subjects collected in this fashion have the confound of advanced age, which may be associated with enlarged ventricles, brain atrophy, and dementia. Careful neuropathological examination for strokes and Alzheimer's Disease is a necessity in this type of study. A second major problem in this setting is that normal controls must be obtained from another source.

The hospice has been used with considerable success for the study of illnesses where death is imminent, such as from Alzheimer's Disease or other dementias. This approach is ideal for short postmortem intervals. It is of limited value for most traditional psychiatric illnesses since psychiatric patients rarely die in a hospice. Although nonpsychiatric disease controls can be obtained from this source, the patients usually have a severe debilitating systemic disease such as cancer or AIDS.

Lastly, for those researchers who do not have access to one of the aforementioned sources, brain banks at UCLA and Harvard are funded by the NIMH. Brain banks obtain tissues from any of the above sources in a standardized fashion. They have the disadvantages of obtaining tissues from great distances and multiple sources, limiting to some degree their abilities to satisfy the diverse needs of their users. The resourcefulness of their respective leaders, Drs. Wallace Tourtelotte and Edward Bird, have allowed the banks to assist numerous researchers despite their limited financial resources.

Diagnosis

The second major problem after collection is diagnosis. This can be accomplished with prospective studies or after death using medical records, family interviews, and police reports. As mentioned previously, prospective studies are frequently confounded by age. Establishing a diagnosis after death can be difficult. The NIMH experience is that approximately a third of possible schizophrenic cases cannot be confirmed by existing records or interviews or can be confounded by alcoholism or substance abuse. Accurate psychiatric diagnosis of suicides may be even more difficult. Both of these seem simple next to determining an accurate history on substance abusers. For the most part, the latter are described by their toxicological screens. Attempts to better characterize their history by systematic use of segmental hair analysis is a possibility that has yet to become routine.

Controls

The need for proper controls is a third major issue. A good example of the problems may be a typical NIMH study. Schizophrenics collected through the medical examiner's office may involve half of the subjects dying by suicide. For this reason, a nonpsychotic suicide control group is used to control for manner of death. The confound of prior neuroleptic treatment can be met by using those schizophrenics who do not satisfy diagnostic criteria, or other neuroleptic treated patients (manic–depressive patients, psychotic depressed patients or the like). The two NIMH funded brain banks at Harvard and UCLA frequently use Alzheimer's and Huntington's Disease patients who have been treated with neuroleptics. Lastly, a group of normal controls is used as well. Each of these groups needs to be matched for age, gender, race, postmortem interval, and storage time. Controlling for socioeconomic status and intelligence is not feasible at this point in time. Tests for toxicology of urine and blood can be routinely performed, but routine brain toxicology has not been employed as of yet. Recently, testing for HIV has become routine.

Other Issues

A major impediment to postmortem research in mental illness has been medicolegal-ethical issues, which require family consent for brain tissue donations. Many mentally ill subjects do not have families available to donate brain tissue. Donor cards are rarely sufficient "evidence" for pathologists. Lastly, society has not been well educated to the public health benefits of neuropathological research. The need for other tissues (pituitary gland, pineal gland, adrenal gland, and the like) is also not appreciated by the public.

Despite these obstacles, this research area continues to grow. Two final methodological considerations are worth mentioning. If one collects enough tissue to match for all the relevant variables, a computerized inventory is a "must." Lastly, maintaining strict double-blind between the collectors and the biochemist or molecular biologist is an essential last step toward a good study.

NEUROANATOMICAL ISSUES

Gross Neuroanatomy

The first consideration in neuroanatomical localization lies at the macroscopic or gross level. The central nervous system (CNS) is exceedingly complex, composed of innumerable cortical areas and subcortical nuclei. Random sampling of cerebral structures, like the proverbial hunt for a needle in a haystack, is unlikely to be productive. Research should be driven by hypotheses, and neuroanatomical investigations are especially in need of such an orientation. Specific regions of interest should be identified and selected on the basis of scientific evidence. This task is complicated by the subtle neuropathological basis of neuropsychiatric disorders. Brains from patients with well-recognized psychiatric disorders have been studied for more than 100 years, with comparatively little to show from this effort until very recently. The paucity of meaningful findings reflects less about the abilities of the researchers and more about the subtlety of the abnormalities. Gross inspection of the brain is a valuable screen for such comorbid conditions as tumor or infarct. In research, gross examination is useful in the assessment of subtle volumetric changes in large structures, such as the hippocampus (5).

Microscopic Exams

Microscopic analyses of brain tissue probably will prove to be more valuable than macroscopic analyses in the investigations of psychiatric disorders. Recently, microscopic cytoarchitectural studies have led to a number of exciting findings in the brains of patients with schizophrenia. In the mesial temporal lobe, driven in part by data from in vivo neuroimaging studies (6), cytoarchitectural investigations have reported a subtle disarray in the entorhinal cortex (7,8). Large structures in the brain often vary in neuronal type and arrangement regionally, in both the anterior–posterior dimension as well as the dorsal–ventral domains. This holds true for the six-layered neocortex and the more primitive palleocortex. For example, the entorhinal cortex is characterized by clusters of neurons in layer two in its more rostral aspects, with a normal disappearance of these clusters caudally (9). It is incumbent to study the same level of entorhinal cortex in affected individuals, to make the appropriate comparison with normal controls.

Subcortical structures also have a great deal of often unrecognized anatomical complexity at the microscopic level. The patch-matrix pattern of the striatum reflects a heterogeneous distribution of neurons and neurotransmitters, and differing patterns of connectivity (10). The many nuclei of the thalamus, hypothalamus, and brainstem have been subdivided into subnuclei, differing in neuronal type,

neurotransmitters, and patterns of connectivity. The nucleus of the solitary tract (NTS) in the brainstem illustrates these concepts. The rostral third receives gustatory input, and the posterior two-thirds receives input from a variety of chemoreceptors and mechanoreceptors associated with the viscera. Within the visceral NTS, there are ten distinct subnuclei (11). Input from one class of pulmonary receptors project primarily to just one, the ventrolateral subnucleus, whereas gastric afferents project to at least two different subnuclei (12,13). Receptor distribution is also inhomogenous in this structure, with 5-HT3 receptors restricted largely to one subnucleus (14). Therefore, careful consideration of subtle neuropathological changes must take into account these levels of complexity.

Other Issues

In addition to anatomical heterogeneity in brain structures, there also is functional heterogeneity. For example, in many cortical and subcortical structures, there is a topographic organization that corresponds to specific parts of the body or of the visual fields. In the striatum, there is a complicated yet well-understood somatotopy, which should be considered in any investigations involving this structure (15). Therefore, investigations involving the striatum should involve anatomically identical regions across subjects.

Connectivity also plays a role. Neuronal networks are important in the generation and modulation of complicated behaviors. Neuropathological analyses must account for the primary and secondary changes in the neural network disrupted in the disorder. For example, pathological changes in the mesial temporal lobe could cause profound but secondary neurochemical changes in the frontal lobe. Secondary abnormalities may explain many of the clinical manifestations in a disorder, such as deficits in executive function in schizophrenia (16).

Neuropathology studies must also consider the normal cellular constituency of a structure under investigation. There can be a selective loss of one subset of neurons within a structure, with relative preservation of other neuronal subtypes. Within the striatum, there are multiple neuronal subtypes. In Huntington's Disease, there is a primary loss of Golgi type II neurons, with a relative sparing of larger neurons (17). Clarification of the pathophysiology of Huntington's Disease is now focusing on the neurobiological characteristics of the Golgi type II neurons. These principles may be applicable to psychiatric disorders as well.

When fresh brain specimens are obtained, the initial handling of the tissue will dictate how the aforementioned principles of anatomic inquiry can be applied. Blocks of tissue, taken in a preselected and uniform plane of section, allow consideration of many of the concepts outlined above, including issues of precise localization and cytoarchitectural configuration. Precise localization of pathology to cortical lamina, subcortical subnuclei, and neuronal subtype requires this type of tissue. Autoradiography for both receptors and in situ hybridization are best performed on tissue blocks that preserve the normal anatomy and landmarks. The immediate dissection of fresh tissue into smaller blocks can make detailed anatomical analysis difficult if not impossible. However, immediate dissection facilitates rapid neurochemical analyses resulting in, for example, the characterization of receptors using grind-and-bind techniques or measurement of neurotransmitter levels. Micropunch methodology can be applied to large tissue blocks, allowing more precise anatomical localization while rapidly accessing tissue for detailed neurochemical analyses.

Two other issues must be considered in human postmortem studies. The first issue is lateralization of function, which is important in cortical structures, and may be a consideration with subcortical structures as well. In right-handed individuals, regions within the left temporal and frontal lobes are the primary repositories of language function. Damage to analogous structures in the contralateral hemisphere produces a completely different, and much more subtle set of behavioral abnormalities. Lateralization of function is often tied to handedness. Unfortunately, handedness is rarely a consideration in many postmortem studies, and should be considered when studying structures whose function is lateralized. A second important issue is that of normal intersubject variability. There is a great deal of variation between individuals in brain size and configuration. Any conclusion of atrophy must consider normal variations. Variations in gyral patterns and sizes are another illustration of this principle. Lateralization of function, handedness, which is often linked to lateralization, and the normal amount of individual variability must be considered in any anatomical study of human brain tissue.

In summary, the anatomical complexity of the CNS must be recognized in the postmortem study of human brain tissue in behavioral disorders. Uniform selection of regions of interest, chosen on the basis of precise hypotheses, must then be studied using methods that take into account the macroscopic and microscopic characteristics of the structure. Consideration must be given to cytoarchitectural, laminar, and/or subnuclear divisions. Finally, lateralization of function, handedness, and normal intersubject variability cannot be ignored. Although these precepts are daunting in scope, rigorous application will improve the quality of human postmortem research into neuropsychiatric disorders, and increase the value of the findings from these investigations.

An often repeated phrase that compares neurology to real estate also holds true for neuropsychiatry: in the end, all that matters is location, location, location. Lesion localization, whether within an isolated site or more widely distributed throughout the cerebrum, holds the key to deciphering neuropsychiatric disorders.

NEUROPATHOLOGICAL ISSUES

Case Selection

The difficulties involved in this type of research make almost every brain desirable. These are some exceptions, however. These include respirator brains, decomposed brains, and some (but not all) gunshot wounds to the head. Although brains of HIV subjects may be used, they present obvious risks to neuropathology personnel and potential confounds for research. A common misconception involves the refusal to use brains after some arbitrary postmortem interval. To be certain, death and prolonged postmortem intervals are not good for the brain. However, time from death to refrigeration is probably a more meaningful variable than postmortem interval; however, this measure is more difficult to obtain and is rarely reported.

At the time of opening the thoracic cavity, cardiac blood is obtained for HIV, toxicology, or other testing. During removal of the brain, the calvarium is carefully sectioned to avoid saw blade marks on the cerebrum. The cerebral dura is reflected dorsally and the brain is carefully freed up, using a sharp scalpel for the cranial nerves and spinal nerve roots and a curved scissors for the tentorium cerebelli and vertebral arteries. A deep cut is made in the foramen magnum to obtain all of the medulla and as much as possible of the upper cervical cord. After the brain is completely freed, it is gently delivered from the skull, weighed, put in a plastic bag, and held on wet ice, which should surround the bag as much as possible. Traction must be avoided in order not to tear the cerebral peduncles or other brainstem structures. The pineal remains with the brain if the cerebral dura and proximal tentorium are kept attached to the brain. The pituitary is removed by carefully breaking the posterior clinoid processes and pulling them caudally. The gland is then dissected out with the tip of a sharp scalpel blade, leaving its capsule intact. The pituitary and additional segments of the cervical cord, if not obtained with the initial brain removal, are placed in a plastic bag on ice.

After returning to the laboratory, the pituitary and pineal are frozen separately before beginning to section the brain. If the pineal is not accessible at this point, it can be dissected out following the rostral midbrain section. Samples of dura and vessels from the base of the brain can also be frozen at this time. A flat section is made through the rostralmost midbrain, above the oculomotor nerves, to remove the brainstem and cerebellum, taking care not to damage the inferior medial temporal lobes (entorhinal cortex and hippocampus) in the process. After bisecting the cerebrum through the corpus callosum, the brain is frozen using 1- to 1.5-cm coronal sections. The portions of the brain that are not frozen immediately continue to be held in a plastic bag on wet ice. Where laterality is the principle research issue, bissection should be avoided if possible.

Throughout all procedures of brain removal and dissection, face masks, eye glasses or goggles, durable gloves (preferrably N-Dex Nitrile gloves, which are more resistant to accidental cuts), sleeve protectors and an apron should be worn. After the procedure is completed, all surfaces and instruments should be cleaned with a 10% solution of freshly prepared household bleach (Clorox) by submersion for a minimum of 20 min. This is done to protect personnel from potential infectious organisms such as hepatitis, tuberculosis, HIV, and other agents.

The coronal sections of the cerebrum are labelled left or right and sequentially, level one (being the most rostral) through the most caudal level. The coronal sections are arranged so that the second or third section begins at the rostralmost tip of the temporal pole. As sectioning proceeds, the neuropathologist examines each piece for pathological changes and takes sections for formalin-fixation and histology from any questionable areas.

The cerebellum is separated from the brainstem by cutting through the cerebral peduncles and is then bissected into two pieces in the horizontal plane. A small section is made in both pieces, in order to examine the dorsal cerebellar vermis, still leaving both hemispheres attached in the midline. The brainstem is cut in sections perpendicular to its long axis, with at least two levels of midbrain, two of pons, three of medulla, and one or two of cervical cord. Thus tissue will be available for more than one study at each level. The levels can be indicated on the bag as to upper, middle, and lower levels. The brainstem should not be cut through the midline as this will destroy midline structures.

Fixation

Although modern approaches have employed fresh-frozen tissue, there is still a place for fixed tissue. Formaldehyde-fixed specimens are essential for ruling out conditions such as cerebrovascular disease and Alzheimer's Disease. Moreover, this approach is especially useful for determining the size of brain structures. It is important when using this approach to control for storage time, because this will influence brain shrinkage. Formaldehyde should be changed regularly to maintain a 10% concentration, thus preventing tissue decomposition or growth of deep-seated bacteria because of lack of potency of the fixative. Lastly, electron microscopic studies for viral particles or the like may require glutaraldehyde as a primary fixative.

Formalin-fixed tissue can also be used for immunocytochemistry and in situ hybridization studies. Routine stains are hematoxylin-eosin and the Bielschowsky method for axons, adapted for paraffin sections.

Freezing

Brain specimens can be frozen in a number of ways. Rapid freezing prevents ice artifacts, which are a major enemy of autoradiography and in situ hybridization studies. Rapid freezing can be accomplished by freezing 1- to 1.5-cm-thick coronal sections with a mixture of powdered dry ice and isopentane or between metal plates immersed in liquid nitrogen. Samples are then placed in airtight plastic bags and stored in $-70°C$ freezers with either carbon dioxide or liquid nitrogen tanks as a backup.

Neuropathological Screening

Ruling out concurrent Alzheimer's Disease, cerebrovascular disease and tumors is essential, especially if the cases involve the elderly. Alzheimer's cases require sections from the frontal temporal/parietal, occipital cortex, and/or the amygdala/hippocampal region. The presence of cerebrovascular disease, hemorrhage, trauma, or tumors are screened by inspection and confirmed by appropriate sections from suspected areas. Inspection and sections of the locus coeruleus and substantia nigra are also necessary to rule out Parkinson's Disease and related disorders. A piece of dorsal cerebellar vermis is necessary to evaluate ethanol-induced atrophy, and sections of the cerebellar hemisphere with dentate nucleus and hippocampus and other cortical areas aid in the evaluation of anoxic/hypoxic alterations.

Further Dissection Issues

Fresh tissue is difficult to accurately dissect as the tissue is quite soft. Frozen tissue poses equally difficult problems with fogging from early thawing and the danger that thawing can lead to protein denaturation. Motor driven saws are especially problematic, because their heat may denature tissues in their immediate contact. Techniques such as autoradiography and in situ hybridization can be especially helpful in avoiding these problems as they lend themselves well to half or whole coronal 14- to 20-μm-thick sections that can be made from frozen coronal blocks by use of a cryostat. Both small structures, such as the locus coeruleus, and large structures, such as the cerebral cortex, are ideal for this approach.

SUMMARY

Although the tasks may seem daunting, the rewards can be great. Neuropathological research is not for the faint of heart. It is not easy and it is not cheap. Any startup budget involves freezers ($10,000/freezer with backup and racks) and a cryostat ($10,000 to $70,000, depending on the model). Personnel ideally would include a neuroanatomist, a neuropathologist, a psychiatrist (preferrably two) and a minimum of two technicians. The potential, however, is great. When the infamous bank robber, Willie Sutton, was asked "why do you rob banks?" he responded, "that's where the money is." Such is the promise of neuropathological research for mental illness.

REFERENCES

1. Plum F. Prospects for research on schizophrenia. 3. Neuropsychology. Neuropathological findings. *Neurosci Res Prog Bull* 1972; 10:384–388.
2. Ehringer H, Hornykiewicz O. Verteilung von noradrenalin und dopamin (3-hydroxytyramine) im gehirn des menschen und ihr verhalten bei erkrankungen des extrapyramidalen systems. *Klin Wschr* 1960;38:1236–1239.
3. Cotzias GC, Van Woert MH, Schiffer LM. Aromatic amino acids and modification of parkinsonism. *N Engl J Med* 1967;276:374–379.
4. Foix MC. Les lesions anatomiques de la maladie de Parkinson. *Rev Neurolog* 1921;28:593–600.
5. Bogerts B, Meertz E, Schönfeldt-Bausch R. Basal ganglia and limbic system pathology in schizophrenia. *Arch Gen Psychiatry* 1985;42:784–791.
6. Suddath RL, Casanova MF, Goldberg TE, et al. Temporal lobe pathology in schizophrenia: a quantitative magnetic resonance imaging study. *Am J Psychiatry* 1989;146:464–472.
7. Jakob H, Beckmann H. Prenatal developmental disturbances in the limbic allocortex in schizophrenics. *J Neural Transm* 1986;65:303–326.
8. Arnold SE, Hyman BT, Van Hoesen GW, Damasio AR. Some cytoarchitectural abnormalities of the entorhinal cortex in schizophrenia. *Arch Gen Psychiatry* 1991;48:625–632.
9. Hyde TM, Krimer LS, Saunders RC. The entorhinal cortex in humans: a cytoarchitectonic and comparative study with non-human primates. [*Submitted*].
10. Semba K, Fibiger HC, Vincent SR. Neurotransmitters in the mammalian striatum: neuronal circuits and heterogeneity. *Can J Neurol Sci* 1987;14:386–394.
11. Hyde TM, Miselis RR. The subnuclear organization of the human caudal nucleus of the solitary tract. *Brain Res Bull* 1992;29:95–109.
12. Kalia M, Mesulam M-M. Brainstem projections of sensory and motor components of the vagus complex in the cat. *J Comp Neurol* 1980;193:435–465.
13. Kalia M, Sullivan JM. Brainstem projections of sensory and motor components of the vagus nerve in the rat. *J Comp Neurol* 1982; 211:248–264.
14. Ohuoha DC, Knable ME, Wolf SS, Kleinman JE, Hyde TM. 5-HT$_3$ receptor distribution in the dorsal vagal complex of the human medulla: a quantitative autoradiographic study. *Brain Res* 1994; 637:222–223.
15. Young AB, Penney JB. Neurochemical anatomy of movement disorders. *Neurol Clinics* 1982;2:417–433.
16. Goldberg TE, Gold JM, Braff DL. Neuropsychological functioning and time-linked information processing in schizophrenia. In: Tasman A, Goldfinger SM, eds. *Review of psychiatry*. Washington, DC: American Psychiatric Press; 1991:10:60–78.
17. Dom R, Baro F, Brucher JM. A cytometric study of the putamen in different types of Huntington's chorea. In: Barbeau A, Chase TN, Paulson GW, eds. *Advances in neurology. Vol. 1: Huntington's chorea 1872–1972*. New York: Raven Press; 1973:369–385.

Psychopharmacology: The Fourth Generation of Progress, edited by Floyd E. Bloom and David J. Kupfer. Raven Press, Ltd., New York © 1995.

CHAPTER 76

Positron and Single Photon Emission Tomography

Principles and Applications in Psychopharmacology

Robert T. Malison, Marc Laruelle, and Robert B. Innis

Modern brain imaging methods now afford unprecedented opportunities for the in vivo study of central nervous system (CNS) function. Within the field of psychopharmacology, interest in two radiotracer techniques, positron emission tomography (PET) and single-photon emission computed tomography (SPECT), has been particularly avid. Much of these methods' appeal derives from their conceptual relatedness to existing preclinical tools, including homogenate receptor binding, in vitro autoradiography, and radioimmunoassay. More compelling to clinical researchers, however, is the ability of PET and SPECT to provide noninvasive measurements of local neuronal activity, neurochemistry, and pharmacology in the living human brain. Despite their tremendous potential, these nascent technologies are as technically complex as they are promising. Thus, this chapter initially emphasizes the salient physical principles and intrinsic limitations of these methodologies before proceeding to a discussion of their specific applications in psychopharmacology (see Chapters 99, 109, and 119, *this volume*).

PRINCIPLES OF PET AND SPECT

PET and SPECT are imaging techniques in which a radionuclide is synthetically introduced into a molecule

R. T. Malison: Department of Psychiatry, Yale University School of Medicine, Connecticut Mental Health Center, New Haven, Connecticut 06508.
M. Laruelle and R. B. Innis: Department of Psychiatry, Yale University School of Medicine, West Haven Veteran Affairs Medical Center, West Haven, Connecticut 06516.

of potential biological relevance and administered to a patient. Depending on the nature of the so-called radiopharmaceutical, it may be inhaled, ingested, or, most commonly, injected intravenously. The subsequent brain uptake of the radiotracer is measured over time and used to obtain information about the physiological process of interest. Because of the high-energy (γ-ray) emissions of the specific isotopes employed and the sensitivity and sophistication of the instruments used to detect them, the two-dimensional distribution of radioactivity within a brain slice may be inferred from outside of the head. Thus, PET and SPECT are both emission and tomographic (from the Greek *tomos* for cut) techniques. Both features distinguish these modern imaging modalities from more conventional radiographic methods, like a chest X ray, where an external source of radiation is transmitted through the subject to create a planar silhouette of the body's organs and cavities. Whereas PET and SPECT rely on similar principles to produce their images, important differences in instrumentation, radiochemistry, and experimental applications are dictated by inherent differences in their respective physics of photon emission.

Positron and Single-Photon Emission

Unstable nuclides that possess an excess number of protons may take one of two approaches in an effort to reduce their net nuclear positivity. In one radioactive decay scheme, a proton is converted to a neutron and a particle called a positron (denoted e^+ or β^+) is emitted (33,69). Of identical mass but opposite charge, positrons

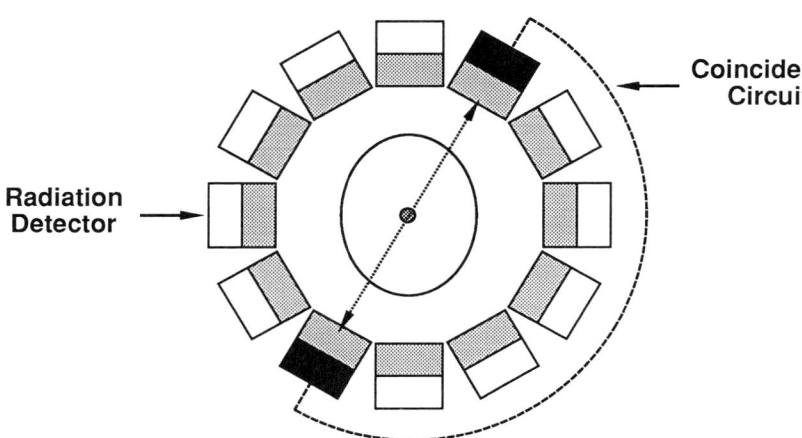

Coincidence Circuit

Radiation Detector

FIG. 1. A PET scanner consists of a ring of radiation detectors designed to detect the simultaneously emitted, characteristically back-to-back (180° apart) dual photons that are created by the annihilation of a positron and an electron. Opposing detectors are electronically coupled to form a coincidence circuit. Thus, when separate scintillation events in paired detectors coincide, an annihilation event is presumed to have occurred at some point along an imaginary line connecting the two. This information is registered by a computer and later used to reconstruct images using the principles of computed tomography.

are the antimatter equivalent of electrons. When ejected from the nucleus, a positron collides with an electron, resulting in the annihilation of both particles and the release of energy. The principles of conservation of mass and momentum dictate that two γ photons (rays) are produced, each of equivalent energy (511 keV) and exactly opposite trajectory (180° apart). For this reason, PET is sometimes referred to as dual photon emission tomography. Among the most commonly used positron-emitting nuclides in PET are included 11-carbon (^{11}C), 13-nitrogen (^{13}N), 15-oxygen (^{15}O), and 18-fluorine (^{18}F).

The unique spatial signature of back-to-back photon paths is cleverly exploited by PET scanners in locating the source of an annihilation event, a method known as *coincidence detection* (Fig. 1) (33,50). A PET scanner may be conceptualized as a ringlike camera that surrounds the head. Instead of using photographic film, however, PET (and SPECT) scanners employ highly sensitive scintillation detectors made of dense crystalline materials (e.g., bismuth germanium oxide, sodium iodide, or cesium fluoride) which capture the invisible, high-energy γ rays and convert them to visible light. This brief flash of light is converted into an electrical pulse by an immediately adjacent photomultiplier tube (PMT). The crystal and PMT together make up a radiation detector. Rather than using individual detectors in isolation, a PET camera is constructed such that opposing detectors are electronically connected. Thus, when separate scintillation events in paired detectors coincide (to within 3 to 10 nsec for practical purposes), an annihilation event is presumed to have occurred at some point along an imaginary line between the two. This information is registered by a computer and later used to reconstruct images using the principles of computed tomography (vide infra). Conversely, single events are ignored. Although it is conceivable that two unrelated photons from spatially separate annihilation events might reach opposing detectors in unison, these accidental coincidences are much less frequent than true ones. In fact, coincidence detection is a very efficient

technique and contributes to PET's superior sampling rates and sensitivity. Nevertheless, random coincidences constitute one source of background noise in PET images (32,33,50).

One intrinsic limitation of PET derives from the nature of positron decay and the principle of coincidence detection. Specifically, PET recognizes the site of positron annihilation and not the site of radioactive decay. Since a positron must generally come to rest in tissues before being able to collide with an electron, annihilation often occurs some distance away from the positron's origin. The distance separating these two events, decay and annihilation, depends on the average kinetic energy of the positron as it leaves the nucleus, and varies according to the specific isotope involved (62) (Table 1). For ^{11}C decay, this range is roughly 2 mm. In addition, if the positron is not entirely at rest at annihilation, photons will be emitted at an angle slightly different than 180°. Taken together, remote positron annihilation and photon noncolinearity place a theoretical limit on PET's achievable spatial resolution, which is estimated at 2–3 mm (50).

In an alternative scheme to positron emission, certain proton-rich radionuclides may instead capture an orbiting

TABLE 1. *Decay characteristics of commonly used PET and SPECT radionuclides*

Radionuclide	Maximum positron energy	$T_{1/2}$	Photon energy
Positron emitters			
^{15}Oxygen	1.72 MeV	2.1 min	511 keV
^{13}Nitrogen	1.19 MeV	10.0 min	511 keV
^{11}Carbon	0.96 MeV	20.3 min	511 keV
^{18}Fluorine	0.64 MeV	109.0 min	511 keV
Single-photon emitters			
^{99m}Technetium	—	6.0 hr	140 keV
^{123}Iodine	—	13.0 hr	159 keV
^{133}Xenon	—	5.3 days	80 keV

electron, once again transforming a proton to a neutron (69). The resulting daughter nucleus often remains residually excited. This metastable arrangement subsequently dissipates, thereby achieving a ground state and producing a single γ photon in the process. Isotopes that decay by electron capture and/or γ emission are used in SPECT, and include both 123-iodine (^{123}I) and the long-lived metastable nuclide 99m-technetium (^{99m}Tc). Because γ rays are emitted directly from the site of decay, no comparable theoretical limit on spatial resolution exists for SPECT. However, the emission of a single photon means that instrumentation in SPECT must be intrinsically different from that in PET. Instead of coincidence detection, SPECT utilizes a technique known as *collimation* (Fig. 2)(39). A collimator may be thought of as a lead block containing many tiny holes that is interposed between the subject and the radiation detector. The holes are sufficiently long and narrow so as to permit only photons of essentially parallel trajectory to pass through the collimator and reach the detector. Given knowledge of the orientation of a collimator's holes, the original path of a detected photon is linearly extrapolated. In contrast to parallel photons, γ rays, which deviate slightly are absorbed by the lead and go undetected (Fig. 2). As might be imagined, collimation is less efficient than coincidence

detection, because many potentially informative photons are filtered out (6). Although collimation is less sensitive than PET, advances in collimator design and radiation detection have made SPECT sufficiently sensitive for routine use in nearly all of the same applications (17,39).

Computed Tomography

Although the physical principles relating to photon emission and detection are different, the means by which PET and SPECT translate information about photon paths into cross-sectional brain images are largely the same (5,15,59). Because only information about a photon's direction, not depth, is known, views of photon trajectories from multiple angles around the entire head are required. A set of measurements from a given angle or viewpoint is referred to as a *projection*. In PET, multiple projections are obtained by a ring of essentially contiguous radiation detectors (Fig. 1), whereas SPECT cameras typically use several detector heads that rotate around the subject in synchrony and collect data over an entire 360° (Fig. 2). After recording many thousands of trajectories from multiple projections, a picture of the distribution of radioactivity within a given brain slice is created by retracing or

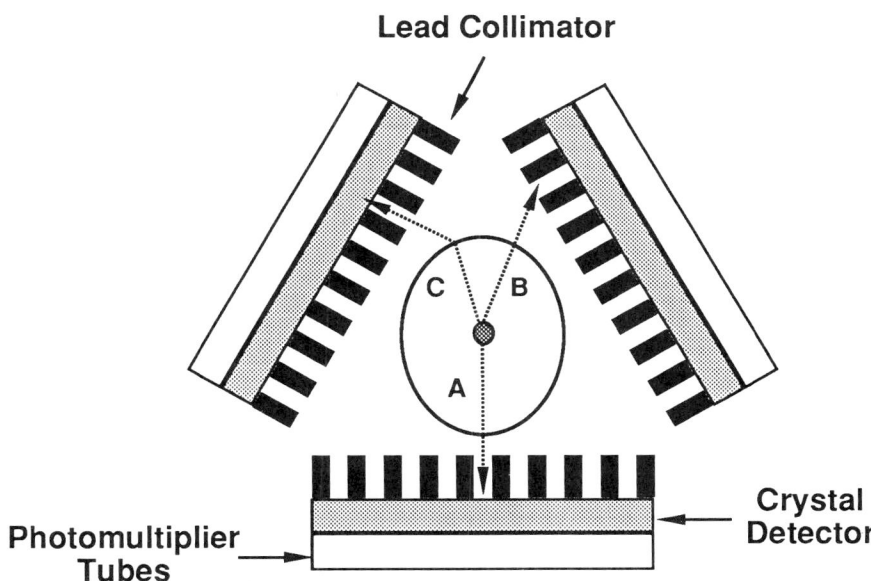

FIG. 2. SPECT scanners utilize the principle of collimation to determine the trajectory of γ rays produced by single-photon emitting nuclides. A collimator is a lead block containing many tiny holes that is interposed between the subject and the radiation detector. The holes are sufficiently long and narrow so as to permit only photons of essentially parallel trajectory to pass through the collimator and reach the detector (**A**). Given knowledge of the orientation of a collimator's holes, the original path of a detected photon is linearly extrapolated. In contrast to parallel photons, γ rays that deviate slightly are absorbed by the lead and go undetected (**B**). Compton scattering (**C**) causes γ rays to deviate from their original trajectory and may result in the false interpretation of a photon's path and origin. In contrast to PET scanners, SPECT radiation detectors typically rotate around the subject's head in synchrony, thus acquiring multiple views or projections from many imaging angles over an entire 360°.

"backprojecting" the trajectories of γ rays across the field of view for every imaging angle. The method of backprojection, although complex, is conceptually analogous to the simple childhood puzzle in which numbers in a square grid are inferred from their sums along each row. However, PET and SPECT images consist of much larger matrices (e.g., 128×128 or 256×256 elements) of radiation density values. Thus, fast computer coprocessors and efficient mathematical algorithms (fast Fourier transformations) are required to handle the enormous amounts of data and the intensive calculations involved. Once their radiation values are determined, individual matrix elements are assigned corresponding shades of color and displayed as picture elements or pixels on a video terminal. In this manner, a PET or SPECT image of the distribution of radioactivity within the brain is produced (Fig. 3).

In practice, the method of simple backprojection is rarely used for reconstructing images today. Rather a modified technique known as filtered backprojection is nearly universally applied (33,39). The reason for filtering relates to quantitative imaging artifacts introduced by the method of backprojection itself, even in the absence of other sources of statistical noise (*vide infra*). In retracing a photon's path, the actual point of decay is indeterminate. Thus, the backprojection algorithm is forced to assume an equal probability of radioactive decay, and hence radiation value, for every point along the line of trajectory. Areas of the brain that have high concentrations of radioactivity will standout as many trajectories from multiple projections are superimposed and their probability values summed. However, areas that contain no radioactivity will bear the residual imprint of the algorithm's statistical guess, and small, but finite, values are ascribed to areas where none should exist. Although this problem decreases with increased spatial sampling and greater numbers of projections (8,36), a filter is still required to restore quantitative accuracy by subtracting spurious values from the images. Multiple filtering techniques have been developed (e.g., Ramp, Butterworth, Hanning, etc.) (59), and the considerations involved in choosing one, although important, are beyond the scope of this chapter. However, suffice it to say that trade-offs between filters exist with respect to their relative impact on spatial resolution and noise amplification. Thus, filter selection depends on the imaging context.

Physical Constraints on Quantitation

Several physical factors affect the quantitative accuracy of PET and SPECT, including the statistics of radioactive decay, attenuation, scatter, limited spatial resolution, and partial volume effects (33,50,69).

Statistics of Radioactive Decay

The process of radioactive decay can be mathematically described by an exponential curve (69). The radioactive half-life, or $T_{1/2}$ value, is the measure most commonly used to quantify the decay rate, and refers to the time required for half of the radioactive atoms to undergo transformation. Values of $T_{1/2}$ vary between species, and can be determined for a given nuclide by taking multiple measurements of an isotopically pure sample over time. The characteristic $T_{1/2}$ values of several commonly used PET and SPECT isotopes are listed in Table 1.

Although the half-life of an isotopic species is characteristically constant, the process of radioactive decay is fundamentally statistical. In other words, if one were to measure a radioisotope of essentially infinite half-life (i.e., infinitely constant radioactivity) over identical intervals of time, variations in individually recorded values would be observed. From the average of many values, the true radioactivity could be inferred. Importantly, this variation in sampling is independent of detection method and instead derives from the intrinsic probabilistic nature (as described by the Poisson distribution) of radioactive decay and the random fluctuation in individual decay events from moment to moment. The spatial equivalent of this temporal variation in sampling is a mottled appearance to images obtained from a container (or phantom) having a uniform concentration of radioactivity. Thus, the statistical nature of radioactive decay itself accounts for random inconsistencies in both PET and SPECT images. This statistical noise is inversely related to the square root of the counts acquired (7) and is easily reduced in images by collecting more counts. Longer sampling times and greater instrument sensitivity are the two principle ways in which PET and SPECT improve counting statistics. Depending on which approach is taken, however, improvements in statistical noise are generally traded for sacrifices in either temporal or spatial resolution, respectively. For example, larger collimator holes in SPECT allow greater numbers of events to be counted, albeit at the expense of including slightly less than parallel photons.

Attenuation

A significant number of high-energy γ photons escape detection by PET and SPECT scanners as a result of their interactions with surrounding tissues. Two major types of interactions exist, Compton scattering and photoelectric absorption (69), and together they result in only a fraction of an internal radioactive signal reaching external radiation detectors. The physical basis for these attenuation effects derives from the interaction of γ rays with atomic electrons. In Compton scattering, a γ photon is deflected from its original trajectory after colliding with an electron

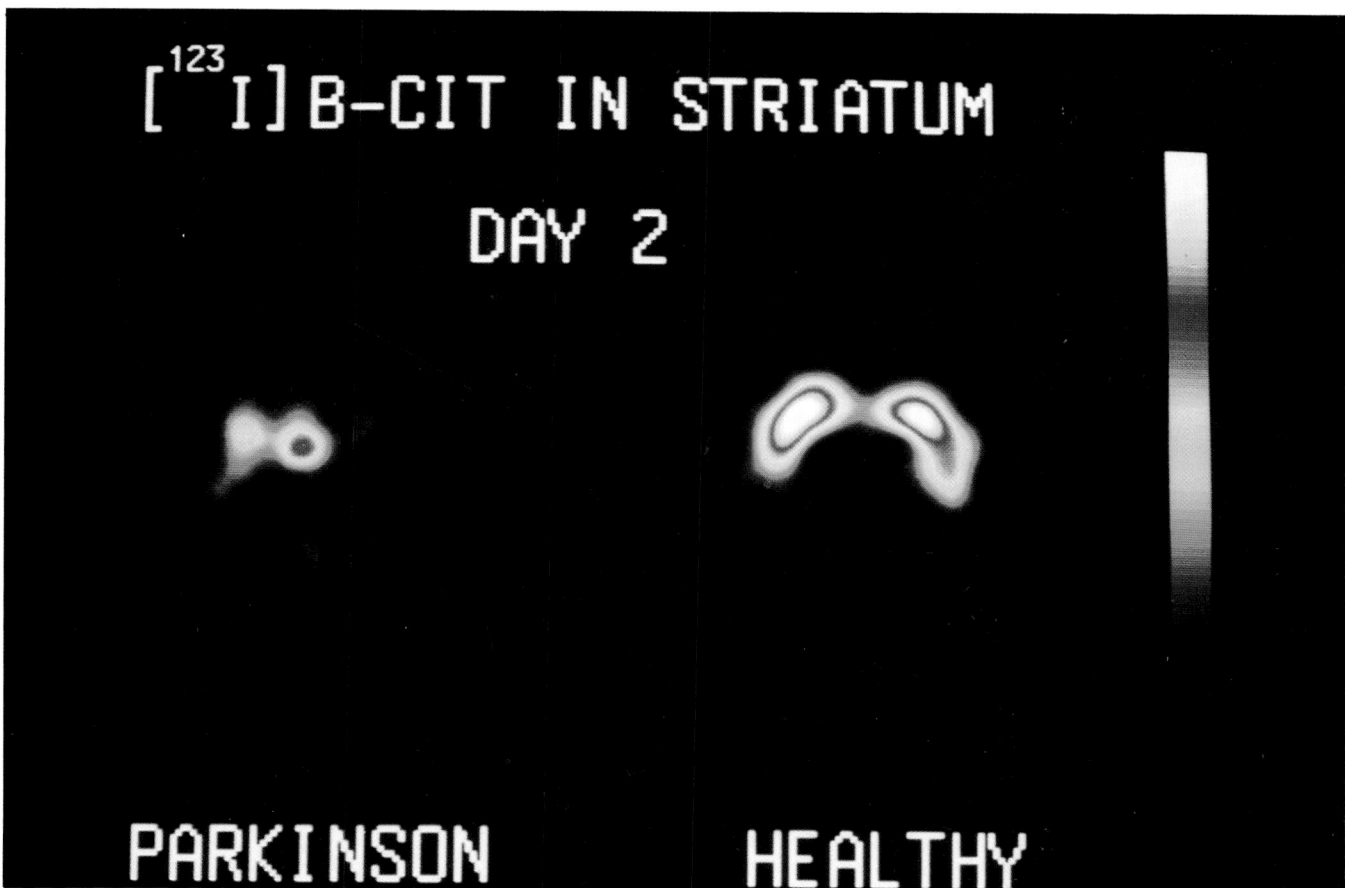

FIG. 3. SPECT images of the distribution of [^{123}I]β-CIT in a healthy subject and a patient with Parkinson's Disease. [^{123}I]β-CIT is a radiolabeled cocaine analog and is a probe of dopamine transporters in the striatum. These transporters are located presynaptically on terminals of dopamine neurons projecting from the substantia nigra to the striatum. These transverse images show a high density of DA transporters in striatum and a marked reduction of these sites in an age- and sex-matched patient with idiopathic Parkinson's Disease. The transporters are lost, because the entire neuron (including its terminal projections) degenerate in this disorder.

and loses a fraction of its original energy in the process. Alternatively, collision may instead result in the complete absorption of a photon's energy. In the latter instance, the imparted kinetic energy is generally sufficient to eject the electron from the atom, and thus γ radiation is said to be ionizing.

Because a photon's chances of being scattered or absorbed become greater as the distance a photon must travel increases, attenuation is said to be depth dependent and results in a progressive underestimation of radioactivity, which is greatest at the brain's center. The diminishment in signal strength can be significant, or roughly 4 to 5 times greater for deep as compared to superficial structures (39,50). Accurately compensating for undetected photons is therefore critical for comparing levels of radioactivity in different regions of the brain (35). The most rigorous attenuation correction approaches utilize a preceding transmission study. In a manner exactly analogous to a CT scan, an individualized attenuation map of the entire head is produced by directing radiation from an external ring source through the subject. Such an approach is generally optimal since the size and shape of patients' heads vary and because the attenuation properties of bone, tissue, fluid, and air differ. Although most PET scanners currently employ this technique, SPECT cameras have only recently implemented transmission scanning in research applications.

Photon attenuation is less problematic for PET than for SPECT. Since photons in PET have higher energies (i.e., 511 keV) than those in SPECT (typically 80–160 keV), they are less prone to attenuation (Table 1). Moreover, linear attenuation is largely depth independent in PET because of coincidence detection. More simply explicated, the probability that dual photons will be detected is equal for all such pairs along a given trajectory because the combined distance traveled by each pair is identical. As a result, a less rigorous, mathematical estimation is often reasonable in PET brain imaging. This first-order approximation involves fitting an ellipse to images of the brain and uniformly assigning a single attenuation value (typically equal to that of water) to all points within the ellipse (14). At present, most commercially available SPECT cameras utilize this second approach, despite uncertainties as to the precise levels of error incurred. Thus, estimating the error associated with algorithmic approximations, and correcting for these, whether by instrumentation or reconstruction techniques, is currently an area of active research, and should help to improve the quantitative potential of SPECT.

Scatter

Accurate reconstruction in PET and SPECT depends on the detection of high-energy photons that travel in a straight path. However, Compton effects cause photons to deviate from their original trajectories. Since many scattered photons retain a sufficient degree of energy to escape from the brain, the detection of scattered events leads to the misinterpretation of photon trajectories (Fig. 2) and produces errors in image reconstruction. The net effect of such errors is similar to that of accidental coincidences, namely an increase in background noise that compromises image contrast.

Current methods of correcting for scatter most commonly rely on the loss of energy incurred by photons as a result of their interactions with electrons. PET and SPECT cameras are routinely equipped to measure the energy spectrum of photons, a range that not only includes the primary photopeak of unaffected γ rays but also the lower energy components that constitute scattered events. Accurately discriminating between true and scattered photons is often difficult, however, since the energy resolution of current PET and SPECT scanners is limited and photopeak energies are normally distributed. Thus, scatter and photopeak windows inevitably overlap. Algorithms for subtracting the scatter fraction from the photopeak window can partially compensate for this problem. As noted above, however, Compton scattering is a depth-dependent phenomenon and occurs in proportion to the electron density of the medium traversed. Hence, the development of more sophisticated correction methods to address regional differences in scatter and incorporate a priori information about brain structure is among the most active areas of research in image reconstruction (39).

Spatial Resolution and Partial Volume Effects

Immediately apparent to the first-time observer of PET and SPECT images is a fuzzy or blurred quality to the pictures. This impressionistic appearance, although permitting a general sense of gross anatomical features, hinders discrimination of finer structures. In fact, this subjective sense of imprecision in visual detail is the qualitative consequence of emission tomography's limited spatial resolution. Less readily recognized, yet more critically important, are the quantitative implications of finite resolution and their influence on the measured radioactivity in individual brain regions (33,50). The opposite side of the same conceptual coin, partial volume effects specifically denote the latter repercussions and require a more objective understanding of spatial resolution and its definition.

Definitions of spatial resolution in PET and SPECT derive from the desire to specify that distance by which two objects must be separated to perceive them as discrete (Fig. 4). In an ideal detection device, an infinitely small isotopic source might be rendered graphically as a vertical line whose infinitely narrow width reflected perfect spatial resolution. When viewed in an actual PET or SPECT scanner, however, radioactivity from such a point source is spread-out and appears as a Gaussian curve. This so-called point (or line) spread function characterizes a camera's resolving capacity and reflects the degree of spatial diffusion of imaged radioactivity. The full-width-at-half-maximum (FWHM), or the width of the Gaussian at half of the curve's peak activity, is the parameter most commonly used to define resolution. When two points are separated by the distance equal to the FWHM, the peaks of both sources begin to be distinguishable.

Apart from theoretical limitations arising from positron range (62), image resolution is principally determined by instrumentation and physical factors, such as the precision of collimation, the number and size of detectors, and the accuracy in localizing scintillation events within the crystalline elements. Although rapid advances in instrumentation may make these published numbers obsolete, resolution currently averages 5 to 6 mm and 6 to 8 mm FWHM for PET and SPECT scanners, respectively. However, researchers have already developed a single-slice PET instrument that approaches theoretical limits of accuracy (3 mm FWHM; University of California at Berkeley), and improvements in collimation and detector technology are likely to lead to similar advances for future SPECT instruments.

One type of partial volume effect arises intuitively from the apparent spatial diffusion of activity created by limited

scanner resolution. Much as the ambient light in that part of a room distant from two lamps depends on the relative brightness and closeness of each, so too the measured radioactivity in a given brain region reflects the relative activity and geometric relationship of neighboring structures. Thus, brain regions having relatively lower concentrations of radioactivity will appear "hotter" in PET and SPECT images as imaged activity spills over from adjacent (more active) areas. Conversely, as the physical dimensions of a relatively more active region become less than 2 to 3 times the FWHM resolution, the measured concentration of radioactivity is effectively diluted, as averaging with adjacent (less active) areas from within the overall field of resolution occurs (31,43). Brain regions of identical radioactivity therefore appear to have differing concentrations based on their relative sizes (53). By visual analogy, the combined effects of partial voluming result in sharp peaks and steep canyons of brain radioactivity being rendered as short hills and shallow valleys in PET and SPECT images.

Several methods are currently available for dealing with errors due to limited spatial resolution and partial volume effects. In one approach, errors created by partial voluming are simulated in a plastic model or phantom. Models typically consist of cavities that are filled with radioactivity and approximate the actual distribution of tracer in the brain. For example, finely machined, polycarbonate brain phantoms are commercially available to recreate the geometry of gray and white matter. By imaging such phantoms, regionally specific correction factors, or recovery coefficients, are derived that may be applied when imaging human subjects. Although this method is convenient, it is unable to account for pathological and nonpathological variations in brain anatomy. As a result, investigators have increasingly utilized structural (e.g., CT, or MRI) scans from individual subjects. Once acquired, an MR or CT scan is aligned with a subject's own functional (i.e., PET or SPECT) study using one of a variety of computer-assisted, image coregistration techniques, thereby creating an individualized brain atlas of matching anatomical relationship (52,61). Anatomical areas can be identified on the high-resolution structural image, and a redirected region of interest template can be applied to the high-sensitivity functional data. In addition, anatomical information may be combined with a priori functional (e.g., relative blood flow ratios in gray and white matter) and physical information (e.g., a PET or SPECT camera's three-dimensional point spread function) to mathematically correct for partial volume errors (55). Thus, in conditions where changes in brain anatomy are likely to accompany changes in brain physiology (e.g., cortical atrophy in Alzheimer's disease), the latter approach will be highly desirable and will help to tease apart the relative structural and functional contributions to imaging abnormalities.

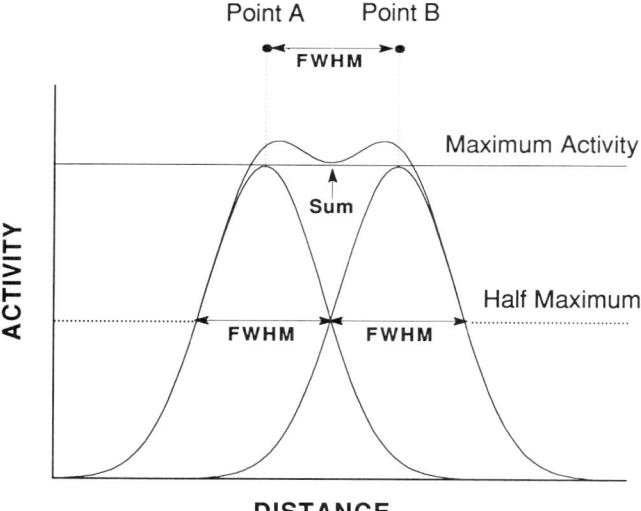

FIG. 4. The limited resolution of PET and SPECT scanners blurs activity from two discrete point sources (**A** and **B**), resulting in the apparent spatial diffusion of activity into regions with no radioactivity. Viewed in one dimension, the activity distribution from each source appears as a Gaussian curve referred to as the point spread function. Camera resolution is defined as the full width of the point spread function at half of its maximum activity (FWHM). When separated by a distance equal to the FWHM, two point sources of identical activity begin to demonstrate a modest decrease at the midpoint of their summed activities, suggesting that the original source consisted of two points rather than one.

Radiochemistry

With limited exceptions, an ideal radiopharmaceutical is one that can be synthesized in high chemical purity, in high radioactive yield, and in small mass quantities. These requirements, namely high purity and high specific activity (expressed in units of radioactivity per chemical quantity; e.g., Ci/mmol), help to insure that the specific biological system of interest is adequately measured, yet unperturbed, by the tracer. However, the physical nature of radioactive decay and the short half-lives of most suitable radionuclidic species (Table 1) work against these radiochemical goals. For example, although chemical yield generally improves with increasing reaction times, radioactivity diminishes with decay (16). As a result, optimal activities require a balanced synthetic scheme to maximize chemical yields, minimize unwanted reaction by-products, and still enable prompt purification of the compound. For both PET and SPECT, specific activities of greater than 2000 Ci/mmol are generally desirable and achievable. Although a limited number of radiochemical syntheses are now automated and performed in robotically controlled hot cells (e.g., [18F]-2-fluoro-2-deoxyglucose; [18F]FDG), most radiopharmaceuticals are still manually prepared by radiochemists racing against the clock of a nuclide's decay.

The particularly narrow radiochemical window for positron-emitting radionuclides has special implications for the construction of PET-imaging facilities. Specifically, the most commonly used PET isotopes include ^{15}O, ^{13}N, ^{11}C, and ^{18}F, which have half-lives of 2, 10, 20, and 109 min, respectively. Because of their extremely rapid decay, essentially all PET isotopes must be produced on the premises. One exception is ^{18}F, whose nearly 2-hr half-life could conceivably permit a regional facility to produce quantities for a large or nearby metropolitan center. Nevertheless, most PET centers have an on-site cyclotron, which generates radionuclides for real-time utilization. In contrast, SPECT isotopes, like ^{123}I, have a sufficiently long half-life (13 hr) to enable centralized production at distant (>3000 miles) commercial reactors and to allow delivery via express mail. Alternatively, ^{99m}Tc ($T_{1/2}$ = 6 hr) may be obtained from inexpensive molybdenum generators located in most hospital radiopharmacies. A cyclotron is expensive (typically $1 to $2.5 million) and requires a highly skilled staff for its operation and maintenance. Hence, the cost associated with PET is a significant disadvantage relative to SPECT.

The chemical nature of a radiotracer depends upon the physiological process to be studied. For example, the measurement of regional cerebral blood flow relies on relatively nonspecific diffusable tracers, which may be foreign to biological systems (e.g., the gaseous tracer ^{133}Xe). Most neurochemical processes in the brain require greater biochemical selectivity. As a result, PET and SPECT radiotracers typically are naturally occurring substances, structural analogs, or pharmaceuticals that selectively label target sites in the brain. PET radiochemistry offers significant versatility here, because ^{11}C can be relatively easily substituted for ^{12}C in existing organic molecules without altering their chemical properties. Even though fluorine is not commonly found in human biochemistry, native hydrogen moieties may frequently be replaced by ^{18}F without significant isotopic effects (e.g., [18F]FDG) (16). Thus, even though their half-lives are a liability, the chemical nature of PET radionuclides eases the radiochemist's task. In contrast, SPECT nuclides are not intrinsic to most neurotransmitters or biological substrates. The metallic nature and multiple valence states of ^{99m}Tc necessitate bulky complexing groups for its molecular stabilization. These barriers have thus far limited the use of ^{99m}Tc to nonselective processes (e.g., the blood flow agent [^{99m}Tc]-hexamethyl propyleneamine oxime; [^{99m}Tc]HMPAO). On the other hand, rapid advances in iododemetallation procedures and increasing knowledge of the structure–activity relationships of pharmacologically active compounds have fueled the development of ^{123}I-containing tracers. For example, iodinated radioligands now permit SPECT imaging of several neurotransmitter receptors (38,42,45,56) and uptake sites (57). In fact, the lipophilic nature of ^{123}I may actually facilitate transfer across the blood–brain barrier and, in some instances, improve affinity of the parent compound at its site of action (46).

Many useful in vitro radioligands may be entirely useless in vivo because of their handling by human physiology. For example, an ideal radiopharmaceutical must easily enter the brain. Hence, tracer binding to plasma proteins must be readily reversible, and its transport across the blood–brain barrier must be favorable. Except for tracers with facilitated carriers (e.g., [18F]-FDG), the latter necessitates that a ligand be sufficiently lipid-soluble to permit its passive diffusion into the brain. Equally important, and a counterbalancing factor in this regard, is the signal-to-noise properties of a tracer. Namely, measurable specific binding is often compromised for highly lipophilic tracers by high levels of nonspecific binding. Thus, lipophilicity as well as affinity are both important factors influencing an imaging agent's signal-to-noise ratio (42). Additionally, peripheral metabolism of the tracer must not be too rapid, or central availability will be secondarily reduced. Moreover, metabolites should either be hydrophilic, so that they do not cross the blood–brain barrier, or if lipophilic, be non–radioactive so as to prevent extraneous sources of central radioactivity from confounding central measurements.

Modeling

Although PET and SPECT images provide measures of regional radioactivity, tracer concentrations in the brain are frequently influenced by processes other than the one of physiological interest, like the peripheral clearance of tracer from plasma and the regional cerebral blood flow. As a result, model-based methods are required to distill from imaging data that component of activity that reflects purely the process under study. Although such models are extremely important for analyzing PET and SPECT measurements, the complexity of such modeling techniques is beyond the scope of this chapter. A general introduction to basic concepts with a focus on neuroreceptor binding may nonetheless provide a basis for understanding more comprehensive discussions (10,11,30).

Empirical Versus Model-Based Methods

Approaches for quantitating physiological processes can be broadly divided into empirical ratio and model-based methods (12). Empirical ratio methods use the ratio of activity in a region of interest (ROI) compared to that in either the whole brain or a region of reference (e.g., a region devoid of receptors) as outcome measures. The principle advantage of this approach is simplicity, since multiple image acquisitions and multiple plasma measurements are not required. However, a major limitation of ratio methods is their inability to account for variations in regional radioactivity, which may arise from differences in blood flow, nonspecific binding, or peripheral clearance of the tracer. Hence, the impact of nonspecific factors on empirical methods must be first evaluated with model-based methods.

Model-based methods relate the observed concentration of activity in a brain ROI to that in the arterial circulation through a defined model. As opposed to empirical methods, model-based methods may require multiple measurements of both brain and arterial, metabolite-corrected, tracer concentration over time in order to derive quantitative physiological parameters (e.g., receptor density, B_{max}; receptor affinity, $1/K_D$). Even though model-based methods are technically difficult to perform and less suited to routine clinical applications, they are needed to validate simpler empirical methods.

Reversible and Irreversible Binding

The type of physiological parameters that can be derived from a PET or SPECT study depends on whether equilibrium is reached during the experiment. For neuroreceptor binding, equilibrium is reached when the rate of association and dissociation to and from the receptors are equal. At equilibrium, the relationship between the specifically bound (B_e) and the intracerebral level of free tracer (F) satisfies the Michaelis-Menten equation

$$B_e = \frac{B_{max}F}{(K_D + F)}$$

During the initial phase following a bolus injection of tracer (uptake phase), the rate of association to receptors is higher than the rate of dissociation (Fig. 5), and specific binding (B) increases. This phase will last as long as B is lower than its calculated equilibrium value (B_e). After variable periods of time (ranging from a few minutes to more than 24 hr), the specific binding reaches equilibrium ($B = B_e$ and the association is equal to the dissociation). Equilibrium is momentary, however, because F is continually falling due to peripheral clearance of the radioligand. As a result, B exceeds B_e, dissociation increases relative to association, and B decreases as tracer leaves the brain (washout phase).

The time at which equilibrium occurs depends on several factors, including peripheral clearance, blood flow, tracer mass, association (k_{on}) and dissociation (k_{off}) rate constants, and receptor density (B_{max}). For some ligands,

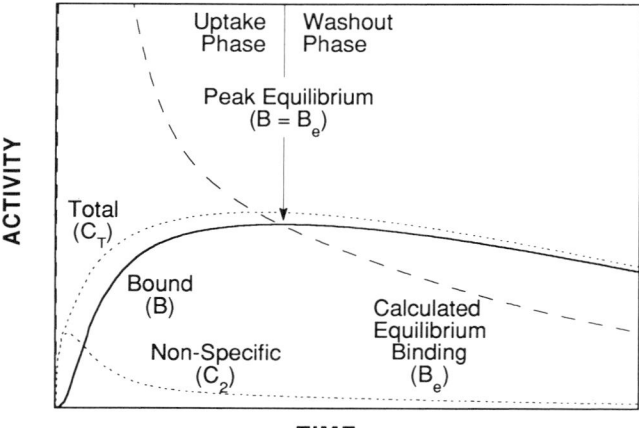

FIG. 5. A diagram of the kinetics of regional brain activity for a radioligand over time, including curves depicting the concentrations of total regional (C_T), free and nonspecifically bound (C_2), and specifically bound (B) activities. The calculated equilibrium binding (B_e) is defined as the concentration of bound that satisfies the Michaelis-Menten equation: $B_e = (B_{max} \cdot \text{Free})/(K_D + \text{Free})$, where $\text{Free} = C_2 * f_2$ and f_2 is the fraction of free tracer in the compartment. During the initial phase following a bolus injection of tracer, $B < B_e$, so association is greater than dissociation, and the activity in the brain increases (*uptake phase*). At the point in time when specific binding (B) peaks (*arrow*), $B = B_e$, association is equal to dissociation, and equilibrium conditions are satisfied. Because free tracer concentrations will fall as a result of peripheral clearance from the plasma, immediately after peak, $B > B_e$, dissociation is greater than association, and brain activity decreases (*washout phase*). The time to reach equilibrium varies and depends upon blood flow, brain extraction, receptor affinity and density, and peripheral clearance. When equilibrium is not achieved during the time-frame of the experiment, only the uptake phase is observed, and the ligand's binding is said to be irreversible.

several hours are required to reach equilibrium, and only the association phase is observed during the time frame of the experiment (typically 1 to 2 hr). From the standpoint of modeling, binding is sometimes referred to as *irreversible* under these circumstances. Conversely, when equilibrium occurs during the experiment, binding is said to be *reversible*. This distinction is important and determines the physiological parameters that can be derived from an experiment. For reversible ligands, the outcome measure of experiments performed at tracer doses (high specific activity) is the binding potential (BP) or equilibrium volume of distribution (V_3; *vide infra*), which equals the product of receptor density and affinity (B_{max}/K_D) (54). For irreversible ligands, the outcome measure is the association rate (usually referred to as k_3, *vide infra*). Experiments involving the administration of pharmacological (i.e., nontracer) doses are needed to obtain separate estimations of B_{max} and K_D. These parameters have been measured with paired tracer and pharmacological dose experiments for both reversible (19,34) and irreversible ligands (70,71).

Compartments, Fractional Rate Constants, and Distribution Volume

Most model-based methods rely on the notion of a compartment. A compartment is a physiological or biochemical space in which the tracer concentration is assumed to be homogeneous at all times. A model consists of a given compartmental configuration and forms the basis for a mathematical description of a tracer's behavior in a biological system. One of the most general configurations for describing a neuroreceptor ligand's behavior is depicted in Fig. 6 (24,25,54). For brain regions with specific binding sites (i.e., receptors), a capillary compartment (C_1), an intracerebral compartment (C_2) in which the tracer is free, a nonspecifically bound compartment (C_2'), and a specifically bound compartment (C_3) are specified. The transfer of a tracer between compartments is governed by a corresponding set of fractional rate constants (i.e., k_1 to k_6). A fractional rate constant defines the direction and the rate of transfer between compartments, expressed as a fraction of the concentration in the originating compartment per unit of time. Thus, the change in tracer concentration in any given compartment can be expressed in mathematical terms as the amount of tracer entering and leaving per unit time.

In practice, the four-compartment model described above is difficult to implement for reasons of mathematical and experimental complexity, and circumstances generally require simplification of the model. The model depicted in Fig. 7 represents a more workable model for PET and SPECT experiments. The parameters K_1 and k_2 describe the exchange of tracer across the blood–brain barrier and are dependent on blood flow and extraction (diffusion). Compartments C_2 and C_2' are combined to form a single, *nondisplaceable* compartment. Pooling these compartments assumes that the rate of nonspecific binding in the brain is rapid relative to the rate of other processes measured in the experiment. The ratio of free-to-total tracer concentration in the arterial compartment (C_a) is designated f_1; similarly, the ratio of free-to-total tracer in C_2 is designated f_2. Both f_1 and f_2 are assumed to be constant over time. Thus, k_3 corresponds to the bimolecular process of receptor association [$k_{on}(B_{max} - B)f_2$] and k_4 represents the dissociation rate constant (k_{off}).

In a PET or SPECT experiment, the arterial concentration of free tracer is experimentally measured over time [$f_1C_a(t)$]. Simultaneously, the activity in a brain ROI

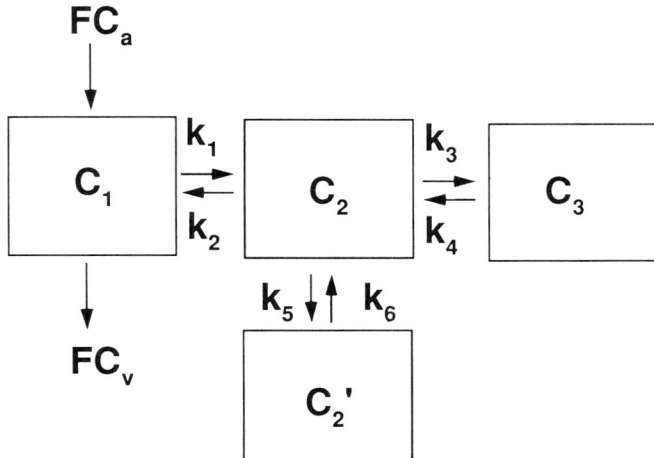

FIG. 6. A general four-compartment model of radiotracer behavior in the brain; F is the cerebral blood flow; C_a is the arterial concentration; C_v is the venous concentration; C_1 is the capillary concentration; C_2 is the intracerebral free concentration; C_2' is the intracerebral nonspecifically bound concentration; C_3 is the specifically bound concentration; k_1–k_6 are fractional rate constants that describe the direction and rate of tracer exchange between compartments.

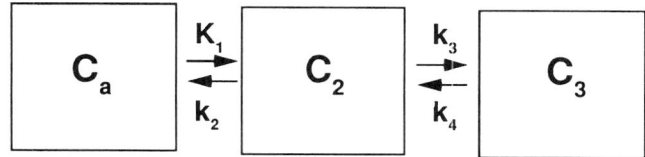

FIG. 7. A simplified three-compartment model that is more practically implemented for PET and SPECT experiments: C_a is the total tracer concentration in arterial plasma; C_2 is the intracerebral tracer concentration, including free and nonspecifically bound tracer; C_3 is the concentration of receptor-bound tracer; K_1 is the rate of extraction of tracer from the plasma into the brain; k_2–k_4 are fractional rate constants governing tracer exchange between compartments. The current model describes the behavior of a reversible ligand. Under conditions of ligand irreversibility, k_4, the dissociation rate constant, is considered negligible and is set equal to zero.

$[C_{\text{ROI}}(t)]$ is also measured. Thus, the activity measured in a brain ROI is the sum of activities in the second and third compartments $[C_{\text{ROI}}(t) = C_2(t) + C_3(t)]$, after subtracting the amount of activity present in brain vasculature. The ratio of these two measures, namely the ratio of tissue to free arterial tracer, at time t is known as the tissue distribution volume $[V_a(t)]$. A conceptual or virtual volume, $V_a(t)$ denotes the volume of tissue in which the tracer would be distributed were the tissue concentration equal to that of free tracer in plasma. The equilibrium distribution volume (V) of a compartment is the corresponding ratio at equilibrium, that is, when no net transfer occurs between the plasma and tissue compartments $(V_i = C_i/f_1C_a)$. For example, V_2 and V_3 are the equilibrium distribution volumes of the nondisplaceable and receptor compartments, respectively, and the total tissue equilibrium volume of distribution equals their sum (i.e., $V_T = V_2 + V_3$). Thus, the binding potential may be expressed in several ways based on the following mathematical relationship.

$$BP = \frac{B_{\max}}{K_D} = \frac{k_{\text{on}} B_{\max}}{k_{\text{off}}} = \frac{k_3}{k_4 f_2} = \frac{K_1 k_3}{k_2 k_4 f_1} = V_3$$

Kinetic, Graphical, and Equilibrium Methods

Several model-based methods exist for quantitating receptors and can be divided into kinetic (54), graphical (51,60), and equilibrium (19) approaches. Kinetic and graphical methods can be applied to both reversible and irreversible ligands, whereas equilibrium methods can be used only for reversible ligands.

The kinetic method yields quantitative information about receptors from the estimation of individual fractional rate constants (54). The rate constants are usually estimated by a least-squares procedure that minimizes the difference between the measured and modeled values of ROI activity. The modeled values of ROI activity are obtained from the arterial time–activity curve and the mathematical description of the system. In the corresponding mathematical language of signal processing, modeled values of ROI activity are said to derive from the convolution of the input and impulse response functions, respectively. The latter is generally defined by a sum of n exponential equations, where n is the number of observed compartments in the ROI.

In the graphical approach, the relationship between brain and blood activity data is linearized by various techniques, and the parameters of interest are obtained by linear regression (51,60). Such techniques have the relative advantage of computational simplicity. For example, in the case of reversible ligands, the total tissue volume of distribution, V_T, can be determined graphically by plotting $\int \text{ROI}(t)/\text{ROI}(t)$ versus $\int \text{ROI}(t)/C_a(t)$ (51). The slope of the linear portion of this graph is V_T in a region with

receptors. In a region of reference (i.e., devoid of receptors), the slope is equal to the nonspecific tissue distribution volume, V_2. Assuming equal nonspecific binding in both regions, and given that $V_T = V_2 + BP$ (vide supra), BP is easily obtained. Graphical methods for analyzing irreversibly bound tracers (e.g., $[^{18}F]FDG$) have also been developed (29,60). The ability of the latter methods to provide information about receptor density requires careful evaluation, however, because the relative ratio of k_2 to k_3 will determine whether linear regression provides information primarily about receptor density, blood flow, or a combination of both.

Equilibrium methods derive receptor parameters from the analysis of the activity distribution at equilibrium (19). The *peak* equilibrium method provides a measure of V_T at peak uptake (Fig. 5). At this single point in time, a ratio of ROI activity (C_{ROI}) to free arterial tracer concentration $[f_1C_a(t)]$ yields V_T. One difficulty associated with this method is the proper identification of the time of peak brain activity. Since plasma tracer concentration falls rapidly after bolus administration, errors in the estimation of the time of peak can lead to errors in the estimation of V_T. To overcome these difficulties, a tracer may instead be administered as a bolus followed by a constant infusion (13,48). Under these conditions, equilibrium will be *sustained*, and V_T is measured directly from the ratio of ROI and plasma activities. As before, BP may be calculated if V_2 is known, as determined either from a region of reference or as the ROI activity remaining after injection of a receptor-saturating dose of a nonradioactive competitor (48).

APPLICATIONS IN PSYCHOPHARMACOLOGY

The uses of PET and SPECT brain imaging can be roughly divided into measurements of local neuronal activity, neurochemistry, or in vivo pharmacology.

Local Neuronal Activity

Local neuronal activity is associated with energy consumption and can be measured with glucose metabolism which itself is usually positively coupled with blood flow. Thus, PET tracers for measurement of local neuronal activity include $[^{18}F]FDG$ (glucose metabolism) and $[^{15}O]H_2O$ (blood flow). On the other hand, SPECT does not have a comparable tracer for glucose metabolism but does have ^{99m}Tc- and ^{123}I-labeled agents, as well as ^{133}Xe to provide measures of blood flow.

Neuronal metabolic demands are felt to primarily reflect terminal rather than cell body activity. That is, in any given volume of brain, the majority of $[^{18}F]FDG$ uptake is thought to be in terminals rather than cell bodies, a conclusion that is based upon a limited number of studies in which the cell bodies are anatomically distant from their terminals (41,65). Whether this applies to cortical regions is unknown but may be a moot point if the majority of terminals in any region primarily derive from local circuit neurons. However, metabolic rate does not distinguish activity of excitatory and inhibitory neurons. Although increased [^{18}F]FDG uptake is usually interpreted as increased functional activity of a region, it may, in fact, reflect an overall decreased activity based upon increased firing of inhibitory interneurons.

The clinical uses of PET and SPECT imaging to measure local neuronal activity are largely restricted to neurological disorders and include localization of both cerebral ischemia and epileptic focus and distinguishing radiation necrosis from tumor growth. In at least the latter two conditions, imaging results can directly impact clinical care. For example, the neurosurgical treatment of patients with medication refractory epilepsy critically depends upon accurate localization of the seizure focus, which is often distant from the surface of the brain and poorly localized by scalp electrode electroencephalogram (EEG). In the interictal period, the seizure focus is hypometabolic and has decreased blood flow. PET and SPECT imaging has been used either as a primary means of localization or confirmation of other diagnostic tests to select the portion of the brain that is subsequently resected. In the ictal period, the seizure focus is associated with increased metabolism and increased blood flow and may have a greater likelihood of showing positive localization than interictal imaging.

Using [^{15}O]H$_2$O, PET imaging has been elegantly combined with neuropsychological activation studies to localize cognitive functions, including reading, speaking, and word associations. The short half-life of ^{15}O (T$_{1/2}$ of 2 min) allows multiple (often 8 to 10) bolus injections of the tracer in one experimental session. Thus, both baseline scans and those following neuropsychological tasks can be repeated and averaged.

Recently developed techniques in functional MRI offer great promise to provide measures of local neuronal activity similar to those from PET and SPECT imaging. The primary signal from functional MRI is believed to derive from the concentration of deoxyhemoglobin (58). Functional MRI is superior to PET and SPECT in that it involves no radiation exposure and has greater temporal (<1 sec) and spatial (<1 mm) resolutions. If these methods are fully developed with adequate quantitation, they may largely supplant PET and SPECT for measures of local neuronal activity.

Neurochemistry

Two major attributes of both PET and SPECT, high sensitivity and chemical selectivity, make these methods particularly well suited for in vivo neurochemical measurements. The sensitivity of PET and SPECT to detect radiotracers is less than 10^{-12} M, which is orders of magnitude greater than the sensitivity of MRI (10^{-3} to 10^{-5} M). In a manner exactly analogous to nonradioactive drugs, radiotracers can be developed to label specific target sites in the brain. These specific tracers can, thereby, provide measures of multiple neurochemical pathways in the brain, including synthesis and release of transmitters, receptors, reuptake sites, metabolic enzymes, and possibly even second messenger systems. Of these multiple neurochemical systems in the brain, the greatest effort has been devoted to imaging of dopaminergic transmission, and this system is now briefly summarized as an example of the types of measurements provided by these methods.

Synthesis

6-[^{18}F]Fluoro-L-3,4-dihydroxyphenylalanine ([^{18}F]-FDOPA) has been successfully used in animal and human studies to provide a measure of dopamine (DA) terminal innervation of the striatum (27). These studies have demonstrated decreased striatal uptake in Parkinsonian patients compared to healthy subjects (9). Furthermore, these studies have questioned the widely held notion that symptoms develop only after 85% to 90% depletion of endogenous DA levels. Imaging studies of patients with early signs of the disorder suggest symptoms may begin with only a 50% to 60% decrease in striatal DA terminal innervation (49).

Following injection of [^{18}F]FDOPA in primates, the majority of striatal activity represents a combination of [^{18}F]fluorodopamine and the metabolite [^{18}F]fluoro-3-methoxydopamine (28). Thus, quantitation of the imaging results is not definitive, in part because of the presence of radiolabeled metabolites in striatum.

After conversion to [^{18}F]fluorodopamine by aromatic L-amino acid decarboxylase, the striatal activity is believed to be largely trapped in the brain during the time of a typical PET experiment. Based upon studies in animals under normal physiological conditions, conversion of [^{18}F]fluorodopamine to radiometabolites that leave the brain is considered negligible. However, DA turnover (measured as the ratio of metabolite to the transmitter) is typically increased in animals with nigrostriatal lesions and in postmortem Parkinsonian brain (40). A result of this enhanced turnover is that an increased proportion of radiometabolites may leave the brain of Parkinsonian patients compared to healthy subjects and thereby exaggerate the deficits in these patients measured with [^{18}F]FDOPA.

Release

A potential method for the measurement of transmitter release involves the displacement of receptor radiotracers by the endogenous transmitter. On first consideration, this displacement may seem impossible, since the endogenous transmitter tends to have a much lower affinity than the tracer for the receptor. For example, [^{11}C]raclopride has an IC_{50} value (which is inversely related to affinity) for the dopamine D_2 receptor of approximately 1 nM, whereas the IC_{50} value for dopamine itself may be as high as 1 μM (66). How then could dopamine effectively compete with [^{11}C]raclopride for binding to the D_2 receptor? This potentially confusing question can be more simply understood by considering equilibrium and dynamic conditions. In an equilibrium state, if the displacer (in this case, dopamine) is present at a concentration equal to its IC_{50} value, then 50% of the receptors will be occupied by the drug and 50% of the radioligand (which is associated with negligible receptor occupancy) will be displaced. Viewed in this more straightforward manner, the real questions of feasibility will be determined by physiological concentrations of DA in the synapse, the in vivo inhibition constant (K_i) of DA for the receptor, and whether adequate time has elapsed to establish equilibrium-binding conditions. Several investigators have provided evidence from in vivo labeling studies in rodents that both the resting levels of synaptic DA and stimulant-induced DA release are associated with significant D_2 receptor occupancy, which is mirrored by comparable displacement of radiotracer from the receptor (63,64,73). Furthermore, recent PET and SPECT dopamine D_2 receptor imaging studies in humans and monkeys support this notion and may in the future provide quantitative measures of DA release (18,37).

Receptors

Receptor studies have probably received the greatest effort among the various targets of neurochemical imaging. If a receptor is selectively altered in a specific disease, then imaging of this site may provide diagnostic information about the disorder. For the DA receptor system, the Johns Hopkins PET group has reported that drug-naive schizophrenic patients have a 2.5-fold elevation of dopamine D_2 receptor density in the striatum using the virtually irreversible tracer [^{11}C]N-methylspiperone and kinetic modeling (72). In contrast, the PET group at the Karolinska Institute, Sweden have reported normal levels of D_2 receptor densities in drug-naive schizophrenic patients using the reversible radiotracer [^{11}C]raclopride and an equilibrium approach (21). Reasons for these disparate results have received significant scrutiny but remain elusive (1,66,67). The use of different tracers and data-analyzing methods are presently being examined by each group using the probe developed at the other institution.

Transporters

Several radiotracers for the DA transporter have been developed: [^{11}C]cocaine, [^{11}C]nomifensine, [^{11}C]CFT

(also designated WIN 35,428), [^{123}I]β-CIT (also designated RTI-55), and [^{18}F]GBR 13119 (2,23,44,57,68). [^{18}F]GBR 13119 and [^{11}C]nomifensine have relatively high nonspecific uptake. Radiolabeled cocaine may be particularly useful for studying the pharmacokinetics of the parent compound but has the limitations of relatively high nonspecific binding and rapid uptake and clearance from the brain. In comparison to cocaine, the analogs CFT and β-CIT have higher affinity (approximately 10- and 150-fold, respectively), lower nonspecific binding, and slower brain kinetics.

The transporter is located presynaptically on terminals of dopamine projections from substantia nigra to striatum. Thus, the transporter is a marker for DA terminal innervation, which is decreased in patients with idiopathic Parkinson's disease. The striatal uptake of both [^{11}C]CFT (26) and [^{123}I]β-CIT (38) have recently been shown to be markedly decreased in patients with Parkinson's disease in comparison to healthy subjects of similar mean age (Fig. 3). Imaging with these tracers may be a useful research tool for early diagnosis and for monitoring the progression of the disorder.

Metabolism

Metabolism of a neurotransmitter can be studied by injection of selective inhibitors of the catabolic enzymes. For example, deprenyl is an irreversible inhibitor of monoamine oxidase type B (MAO-B), and imaging with ^{11}C-labeled deprenyl has been reported to provide a measure of regional enzyme activity in the brain (3,22). With [^{11}C]deprenyl, PET scanning may provide useful dose–response measurements in patients treated with MAO inhibitors (47). Furthermore, reversible MAO inhibitors like [^{11}C]Ro19-6327 may have advantages relative to the irreversible agents in terms of data analysis and ease of performing in vivo occupancy studies (4).

In Vivo Pharmacology

Since receptors are frequently the targets of therapeutic medications, several investigators have argued that receptor imaging may be used to more accurately monitor drug treatment than is possible with measurement of plasma levels of the medications. For example, a nonresponding patient might have normal or even elevated levels of a medication that does not cross the blood–brain barrier and reach its target site in brain. In this case, neuroreceptor imaging would certainly demonstrate the lack of significant receptor occupancy. However, such a hypothetical clinical situation would appear to represent an essential abnormality in the patient's blood–brain barrier. Such a defect would presumably be associated with nonresponsiveness to a variety of centrally active medications and has not been clearly shown to exist.

Several pharmaceutical companies and academic researchers have begun to explore the role of receptor imaging in new drug development. The two basic methods are the radiolabeling of the target compound (e.g., with ^{11}C) or the in vivo screening of the effects of the intravenously administered nonradioactive compound with previously developed radiotracers. The first method is probably better suited to PET radiochemistry, which can more easily provide a pharmacologically identical radiolabeled form of the target compound than SPECT, which would likely use an iodinated analog. However, the second method may be equally well performed with PET or SPECT provided that an appropriate radiotracer has been developed for each method.

Brain imaging studies of antipsychotic medications provide an example of advantages and limitations of both these methods. Several pharmaceutical companies are trying to develop atypical medications like clozapine, which would have superior efficacy and fewer side effects than typical antipsychotic medications. Studies with [11C]-clozapine have been relatively disappointing because of the high nonspecific uptake of the radioactivity. In fact, these results may prove to be typical, since only a small percentage of potential compounds prove to be useful in vivo radiotracers with low nonspecific binding. On the other hand, studies of nonradioactive antipsychotic medications with established and selective receptor tracers have provided valuable information on both the receptor occupancy profiles and the pharmacokinetics of brain uptake. For example, Farde and coworkers (20) have shown that, in comparison to several typical neuroleptic medications, clozapine is associated with a disproportionately high occupancy of D_1 relative to D_2 receptors. Novel therapeutic compounds could be examined for both the pharmacokinetics of entry into the brain and their receptor occupancy profiles, which will provide the combined effect of the parent compound and any active metabolites. Although the authors are not aware of any therapeutic compound whose development has been significantly enhanced with neuroreceptor imaging, this potential application is receiving growing attention.

CONCLUSIONS

PET and SPECT imaging are methods of high sensitivity in which the injection of radioactively labeled drugs are used to provide measures of local neuronal activity, in vivo neurochemistry, or in vivo pharmacology. These methods are particularly attractive to clinical researchers, because they can be applied to the living human brain. The γ-ray emissions pass directly through the skull, and the camera measurements truly provide a window on the brain. Perhaps the two greatest barriers to wider application of these research methods are their high cost and technical complexity. With regard to cost, further devel-

opment and validation of SPECT is justified in the reasonable expectation that tracers and paradigms will be developed that are adequate for clinical research studies. With regard to technical complexity, both PET and SPECT will continue to require multidisciplinary collaboration from the fields of drug development, radiochemistry, instrumentation physics, pharmacology, compartmental modeling, radiation health physics, and the basic and clinical neurosciences. This field will require additional training and orientation by all members of the research group, and this chapter has reviewed several of the important methodological aspects of functional imaging that may be useful to those entering this exciting research field.

REFERENCES

1. Andreasen NC, Carson R, Diksic M, et al. Workshop on schizophrenia, PET, and dopamine D2 receptors in the human neostriatum. *Schizophrenia Bull* 1988;14:471–484.
2. Aquilonius SM, Bergstrom K, Eckernas SA, et al. In vivo evaluation of striatal dopamine reuptake sites using ^{11}C-nomifensine and positron emission tomography. *Acta Neurol Scand* 1987;76:283–287.
3. Arnett CD, Fowler JS, MacGregor RR, et al. Turnover of brain monoamine oxidase measured in vivo by positron emission tomography using L-[11C]deprenyl. *J Neurochem* 1987;49:522–527.
4. Bench CJ, Price GW, Lammerstma AA, et al. Measurement of human cerebral monoamine oxidase type B (MAO-B) activity with positron emission tomography (PET): a dose ranging study with the reversible inhibitor Ro 19-6327. *Eur J Clin Pharmacol* 1991; 40:169–173.
5. Brooks RA, DiChiro G. Theory of image reconstruction in computed tomography. *Radiology* 1975;117:561.
6. Budinger TF. Physical attributes of single-photon tomography. *J Nucl Med* 1980;21:579–592.
7. Budinger TF, Derenzo SE, Greenberg WL, Gullberg GT, Huesman RH. Quantitative potentials of dynamic emission computed tomography. *J Nucl Med* 1978;19:309–315.
8. Budinger TF, Derenzo SE, Gullberg GT, Greenberg WL, Huesman RH. Emission computer assisted tomography with single-photon and positron annihilation photon emitters. *J Comput Assist Tomogr* 1977;1:131–145.
9. Calne DB. PET after MPTP: observations relating to the cause of Parkinson's disease. *Nature* 1985;317:246–248.
10. Carson RE. Parameter estimation in positron emission tomography. In: Phelps ME, Mazziotta JC, Schelbert HR, eds. *Positron emission tomography. Principles and applications for the brain and the heart.* New York: Raven Press; 1986:347–390.
11. Carson RE. The development and application of mathematical models in nuclear medicine. *J Nucl Med* 1991;32:2206–2208.
12. Carson RE. Precision and accuracy considerations of physiological quantification in PET. *J Cereb Blood Flow Metab* 1991;11:A45–A50.
13. Carson RE, Channing MA, Blasberg RG, et al. Comparison of bolus and infusion methods for receptor quantification: application to [18F]-cyclfoxy and positron emission tomography. *J Cereb Blood Flow Metab* 1992;13:24–42.
14. Chang LT. A method for attenuation correction in radionuclide computed tomography. *IEEE Trans Nucl Sci* 1978;25:638.
15. Coffman JA. Computed tomography. In: Andreasen NC, eds. *Brain imaging: applications in psychiatry.* Washington, DC: American Psychiatric Press; 1989:1–66.
16. Dannals RF, Ravert HT, Wilson AA. Radiochemistry of tracers for neurotransmitter receptor studies. In: Frost JJ, Wagner HN, eds. *Quantitative imaging: neuroreceptors, neurotransmitters, and enzymes.* New York: Raven Press; 1990:19–35.
17. Devous MD. Imaging brain function by single-photon emission computer tomography. In: Andreasen NC, eds. *Brain imaging: ap-*

plications in psychiatry. Washington, DC: American Psychiatric Press; 1989:147–234.

18. Dewey SL, Logan J, Wolf AP, et al. Amphetamine induced decreases in (18F)-*N*-methylspiroperidol binding in the baboon brain using positron emission tomography (PET). *Synapse* 1991;7:324–327.

19. Farde L, Hall H, Ehrin E, Sedvall G. Quantitative analysis of D2 dopamine receptor binding in the living human brain by PET. *Science* 1986;231:258–261.

20. Farde L, Nordstrom AL, Wiesel FA, Pauli S, Halldin C, Sedvall G. PET analysis of central D1 and D2 dopamine receptor occupancy in patients treated with classic neuroleptics and clozapine—relationship to extrapyramidal side effects. *Arch Gen Psychiatry* 1992;49:538–544.

21. Farde L, Wiesel FA, Stone-Elander S, et al. D2 dopamine receptors in neuroleptic-naive schizophrenic patients. *Arch Gen Psychiatry* 1990;47:213–219.

22. Fowler JS, MacGregor RR, Wolf AP, et al. Mapping human brain monoamine oxidase A and B with ^{11}C-labeled suicide inactivators with PET. *Science* 1987;235:481–485.

23. Fowler JS, Volkow ND, Wolf AP, et al. Mapping cocaine binding sites in human and baboon in vivo. *Synapse* 1989;4:371–377.

24. Frey KA, Hichwa RD, Ehrenkaufer RLE, Agranoff BW. Quantitative in vivo receptor binding III: tracer kinetic modeling of muscarinic cholinergic receptor binding. *Proc Natl Acad Sci USA* 1987;82:6711–6715.

25. Frost JJ, Douglass KH, Mayberg HS, et al. Multicompartimental analysis of ^{11}C-carfentanil binding to opiate receptors in human measured by positron emission tomography. *J Cereb Blood Flow Metab* 1989;9:398–409.

26. Frost JJ, Rossier AM, Reich S, et al. PET imaging of dopamine reuptake sites in Parkinson's disease by C-11-WIN 35,428 and PET. *J Nucl Med* 1993;34:31P(abstr.).

27. Garnett ES, Firnau G, Nahmias C. Dopamine visualized in the basal ganglia of living man. *Nature* 1983;305:137–138.

28. Garnett ES, Firnau G, Nahmias C, Chirakal R. Striatal dopamine metabolism in living monkeys examined in positron emission tomography. *Brain Res* 1983;280:169–171.

29. Gjedde A. High- and low-affinity transport of D-glucose from blood to brain. *J Neurochem* 1981;36:1463–1471.

30. Gjedde A, Wong DF. Modeling neuroreceptor binding of radioligands in vivo. In: Frost JJ, Wagner HN Jr, eds. *Quantitative imaging: neuroreceptors, neurotransmitters, and enzymes.* New York: Raven Press; 1990:51–79.

31. Hoffman EJ, Huang SC, Phelps ME. Quantitation in positron emission computed tomography: 1. Effect of object size. *J Comput Assist Tomogr* 1979;3:299–308.

32. Hoffman EJ, Huang SC, Phelps ME, Kuhl DE. Quantitation in positron emission computed tomography: 4. Effect of accidental coincidences. *J Comput Assist Tomogr* 1981;5:391–400.

33. Hoffman EJ, Phelps ME. Positron emission tomography: principles and quantitation. In: Phelps M, Mazziotta J, Schelbert H, eds. *Positron emission tomography and autoradiography: principles and applications for the brain and heart.* New York: Raven Press; 1986:237–286.

34. Huang SC, Bahn MM, Barrio JR, et al. A double-injection technique for in vivo measurement of dopamine D2-receptor density in monkeys with 3-(2'-[18F] Fluoroethyl)spiperone and dynamic positron emission tomography. *J Cereb Blood Flow Metab* 1989;9:850–858.

35. Huang SC, Hoffman EJ, Phelps ME, Kuhl DE. Quantitation in positron emission computed tomography: 2. Effects of inaccurate attenuation correction. *J Comput Assist Tomogr* 1979;3:804–814.

36. Huang SC, Hoffman EJ, Phelps ME, Kuhl DE. Quantitation in positron emission computed tomography: 3. Effect of sampling. *J Comput Assist Tomogr* 1980;4:819–826.

37. Innis RB, Malison RT, Al-Tikriti M, et al. Amphetamine-stimulated dopamine release competes in vivo for ^{123}I]IBZM binding to the D2 receptor in nonhuman primates. *Synapse* 1992;10:177–184.

38. Innis RB, Seibyl JP, Wallace E, et al. SPECT imaging demonstrates loss of striatal dopamine transporters in Parkinson's disease. *J Nucl Med* 1993;34:31P (abst.)

39. Jaszczak RJ. SPECT: state-of-the-art scanners and reconstruction strategies. In: Diksic M, Reba RC, eds. *Radiopharmaceuticals and brain pathology studied with PET and SPECT.* Boca Raton: CRC Press; 1991:93–118.

40. Jenner P, Marsden CD. MPTP-induced parkinsonism as an experimental model of Parkinson's disease. In: Jankovic J, Tolosa E, eds. *Parkinson's disease and movement disorders.* Baltimore: Urban and Schwarzenberg; 1988:37–48.

41. Kadekaro M, Crane AM, Sokoloff L. Differential effects of electrical stimulation of sciatic nerve on metabolic activity in spinal cord and dorsal root ganglion in the rat. *Proc Natl Acad Sci USA* 1985;82:6010–6013.

42. Kessler RM, Ansari MS, dePaulis T, et al. High affinity dopamine D2 receptor radioligands. 1. Regional rat brain distribution of iodinated benzamides. *J Nucl Med* 1991;32:1593–1600.

43. Kessler RM, Ellis JR, Eden M. Analysis of emission tomographic scan data: limitations imposed by resolution and background. *J Comput Assist Tomogr* 1984;8:514–522.

44. Kilbourn MR, Haka MS, Mulholland GK, Jewett DM, Kuhl DE. Synthesis of radiolabeled inhibitors of presynaptic monoamine uptake systems: [18F]GBR 13119 (DA), [11C]nisoxetine (NE), and [11C]fluoxetine (5-HT). *J Lab Compd Radiopharm* 1989;26:412.

45. Kung HF, Alavi A, Chang W, et al. In vivo SPECT imaging of CNS D-2 dopamine receptors: initial studies with iodine-123 IBZM in humans. *J Nucl Med* 1990;31:573–579.

46. Kung HF, Pan S, Kung MP, et al. In vitro and in vivo evaluation of [123I]IBZM: a potential CNS D-2 dopamine receptor imaging agent. *J Nucl Med* 1989;30:88–92.

47. Lammertsma AA, Bench CJ, Price GW, et al. Measurement of cerebral monoamine oxidase B activity using [11C]deprenyl and dynamic positron emission tomography. *J Cereb Blood Flow Metab* 1991;11:545–556.

48. Laruelle M, Abi-Dargham A, Rattner Z, et al. SPECT measurement of benzodiazepine receptor number and affinity in primate brain: a constant infusion paradigm with [123I]iomazenil. *Eur J Pharmacol* 1993;230:119–123.

49. Leenders KL, Salmon EP, Tyrrell P, et al. The nigrostriatal dopaminergic system assessed in vivo by PET in healthy volunteer subjects and patients with Parkinson's disease. *Arch Neurol* 1990;47:1290–1298.

50. Links JM. Physics and instrumentation of positron emission tomography. In: Frost JJ, Wagner HN, eds. *Quantitative imaging: neuroreceptors, neurotransmitters, and enzymes.* New York: Raven Press; 1990:37–50.

51. Logan J, Fowler J, Volkow ND, et al. Graphical analysis of reversible radioligand binding from time-activity measurements applied to [*N*-11C-methyl]-(−)-cocaine PET studies in human subjects. *J Cereb Blood Flow Metab* 1990;10:740–747.

52. Malison RT, Miller EG, Greene R, McCarthy G, Charney DS, Innis RB. Computer-assisted coregistration of multislice SPECT and MR brain images by fixed external fiducials. *J Comput Assist Tomogr* 1993;17(6):952–960.

53. Mazziotta JC, Phelps ME, Plummer D, Kuhl DE. Quantitation in positron emission computed tomography: 5. Physical-anatomical effects. *J Comput Assist Tomogr* 1981;5:734–743.

54. Mintun MA, Raichle ME, Kilbourn MR, Wooten GF, Welch MJ. A quantitative model for the in vivo assessment of drug binding sites with positron emission tomography. *Ann Neurol* 1984;15:217–227.

55. Muller-Gartner HW, Links JM, Prince JL, et al. Measurement of radiotracer concentration in brain gray matter using positron emission tomography: MRI-based correction for partial volume effects. *J Cereb Blood Flow Metab* 1992;12:571–583.

56. Muller-Gartner HW, Wilson AA, Dannals RF, Wagner HN, Frost JJ. Imaging muscarinic choinergic receptors in human brain in vivo with SPECT, [123I]-iododexetimide, and [123I]-iodolevetimide. *J Cereb Blood Flow Metab* 1992;12:562–570.

57. Neumeyer JL, Wang S, Milius RA, et al. [123I]-2-β-Carbomethoxy-3-β-(4-iodophenyl)-tropane (β-CIT): high affinity SPECT radiotracer of monoamine reuptake sites in brain. *J Med Chem* 1991;34:3144–3146.

58. Ogawa S, Lee TM, Nayak A, Glynn P. Oxygenation-sensitive contrast in magnetic resonance image of rodent brain at high magnetic fields. *Magn Reson Med* 1990;14:68–78.

59. Parker JA. *Image reconstruction in radiology,* Boca Raton: CRC Press; 1990.

60. Patlak CS, Balsberg RG, Fenstermacher JD. Graphical evaluation of blood to brain transfer constants from multiple time uptake data. *J Cereb Blood Flow Metab* 1983;3:1–7.
61. Pelizzari CA, Chen GTY, Spelbring DR, Weichselbaum RR, Chen CT. Accurate three-dimensional registration of CT, PET, and MR images of the brain. *J Comput Assist Tomogr* 1989;13:20–26.
62. Phelps ME, Hoffman EJ, Huang SC, Ter-Pogossian MM. Effect of positron range on spatial resolution. *J Nucl Med* 1975;16:649–652.
63. Ross SB. Synaptic concentration of dopamine in the mouse striatum in relationship to the kinetic properties of the dopamine receptors and uptake mechanism. *J Neurochem* 1991;56:22–29.
64. Ross SB, Jackson DM. Kinetic properties of the in vivo accumulation of ^{3}H-(−)-*N-n*-propylnorapomorphine in mouse brain. *Naunyn-Schmied Arch Pharmacol* 1989;340:13–20.
65. Schwartz WJ, Smith CB, Davidsen L, Savaki H, Sokoloff L. Metabolic mapping of functional activity in the hypothalamo-neurohypophysial system of the rat. *Science* 1979;205:723–725.
66. Seeman P, Guan H-C, Niznik HB. Endogenous dopamine lowers the dopamine D2 receptor density as measured by ^{3}H-raclopride: implications for positron emission tomography of the human brain. *Synapse* 1989;3:96–97.
67. Seeman P, Niznik HB, Guan H-C. Elevation of dopamine D2 receptors in schizophrenia is underestimated by radioactive raclopride. *Arch Gen Psychiat* 1990;47:1170–1172.
68. Shaya EK, Scheffel U, Dannals RF, et al. In vivo imaging of dopamine reuptake sites in the primate brain using single photon emission computed tomography (SPECT) and iodine-123 labeled RTI-55. *Synapse* 1992;10:169–172.
69. Sorenson JA, Phelps ME. *Physics in nuclear medicine*, 2nd ed. Philadelphia: W.B. Saunders; 1987.
70. Wong DF, Gjedde A, Wagner HN. Quantification of neuroreceptors in the living human brain. I. Irreversible binding of ligand. *J Cereb Blood Flow Metab* 1986;6:137–146.
71. Wong DF, Gjedde A, Wagner HNJ, et al. Quantification of neuroreceptors in the living brain. II. Inhibition studies of receptor density and affinity. *J Cereb Blood Flow Metab* 1986;6:147–153.
72. Wong DF, Wagner HN Jr., Tune LE, et al. Positron emission tomography reveals elevated D2 dopamine receptors in drug naive schizophrenics. *Science* 1986;234:1558–1563.
73. Young LT, Wong DF, Goldman S, et al. Effects of endogenous dopamine on kinetics of [^{3}H]raclopride binding in the rat brain. *Synapse* 1991;9:188–194.

Psychopharmacology: The Fourth Generation of Progress, edited by Floyd E. Bloom and David J. Kupfer. Raven Press, Ltd., New York 1995.

CHAPTER **77**

In Vivo Structural Brain Assessment

Kelvin O. Lim, Margaret Rosenbloom, and Adolf Pfefferbaum

Over the past few years, technical improvements in the acquisition and processing of structural neuroimaging data, particularly with magnetic resonance imaging (MRI), have provided vivid visual representations of the human brain both as two-dimensional slices through the brain and as three-dimensional views of the external surface and internal structures of the brain. In the years since computerized tomography (CT) first provided in vivo evidence of gross brain morphological abnormalities in schizophrenia (32), there have been many CT reports of an increase in cerebrospinal fluid (CSF) filled spaces, both centrally (ventricles), and peripherally (sulci) in a variety of psychiatric patients (58). Magnetic resonance imaging, with its superior tissue contrast for differentiation of white matter from gray matter, and greater flexibility in acquiring, or reslicing images in orientations best suited for viewing and measuring specific structures, now promises additional capabilities for uncovering both generalized and regionally specific brain abnormalities associated with schizophrenia and other mental disorders (50). Patients with psychiatric disorders generally manifest brain abnormalities that are of a subtle and/or diffuse nature, and thus may best be characterized by systematic and reliable quantification techniques, rather than qualitative assessments.

Numerous approaches to characterize the size, tissue composition, and shape of different cortical or subcortical neuroanatomic structures with a view to better understanding possible etiology, pathophysiology, and course of different mental disorders have been and continue to be developed. These measures of brain morphology need to be carefully interpreted in the context of other brain and biological features, as well as the clinical and demographic characteristics of the patient, before they can provide insight into the pathophysiology of psychiatric disorders. The goal of this chapter is to provide an overview of the capabilities and limitations of current in vivo structural neuroimaging acquisition and quantification techniques. We identify some of the important technical and methodological issues connected with acquiring, measuring, and interpreting MRI data and provide a point of reference from which to evaluate the large number of neuroimaging studies now appearing in the literature (see Chapters 76, 87, 99, 109, and 119, *this volume*).

ACQUISITION OF MAGNETIC RESONANCE IMAGES

Mechanisms of Tissue Contrast: Pulse Sequences

One of the strengths of MRI is that investigators can manipulate the amount of contrast between different biological tissues by varying elements of the image acquisition sequence. A highly simplified outline of the principle of MRI is provided here to orient the reader to how these acquisition elements can be varied. More detailed descriptions can be found elsewhere (48). Atomic nuclei with an odd number of nucleons (protons plus neutrons) behave as spinning tops with an electric charge, and thus they produce a magnetic field, oriented along the axis of rotation of the nucleus. Under normal circumstances, the spin axes of these nuclei are randomly oriented so that the sum of all magnetic fields is zero. However, when these nuclei are exposed to a strong external magnetic field, they align either parallel or antiparallel with the field in an equilibrium state, that is either in a high- or low-energy state, with a slight preponderance of the high-energy state. These aligned atomic nuclei rotate around their axes at a

K. O. Lim, M. Rosenbloom, and A. Pfefferbaum: Department of Psychiatry and Behavioral Sciences, Stanford University, Stanford, California 94305; and Psychiatry Service, Department of Veterans Affairs Medical Center, Palo Alto, California 94304.

characteristic frequency, also dependent on the strength of the magnetic field. Electromagnetic radiofrequency (RF) pulses, applied at the appropriate frequency perpendicular to the main magnetic field, excite the spinning nuclei, knocking them out of equilibrium. When the radio waves are turned off, the nuclei return to equilibrium. Magnetic resonance imaging employs appropriately tuned radiofrequency coils to detect the radio signals given off as the nuclei return to equilibrium and localize them using magnetic gradients in the three orthogonal axes.

Hydrogen atoms (protons) are the most abundant element in biological tissue, primarily in the form of water. Proton MRI thus records signals arising predominantly from free water (i.e., water not biochemically bound in complex molecules), but there is also a measurable but much lesser contribution from protons in fat. Proton density (PD), based on the number of nuclei stimulated, and the relaxation times, T_1 and T_2, which reflect the chemical environment of the tissue stimulated, determine the image intensity of the different tissues. The time T_1 is an exponential time constant, which represents the time taken for excited nuclei to return to equilibrium after the RF pulse has been turned off, and T_2 is an exponential time constant describing the time it takes for the excited nuclei to lose signal, mainly from dephasing in the transverse plane. The time between radiofrequency pulses (T_R), and the amount of time after the pulse for which the signal is acquired (echo time, or T_E), determine the contribution of PD, T_1 and T_2, and vary the contrast between different biological substances in the resulting images. For example, a long T_R (2 to 3 sec), spin echo sequence with a long T_E (80 msec) provides a heavily T_2-weighted image in which CSF appears bright (CSF has a long T_2) whereas brain parenchyma is darker and homogeneous. In contrast, T_1 weighting, which optimizes contrast between gray matter and white matter is typically achieved by using relatively short T_R (200 to 400 msec), short T_E (20 msec), spin echo or inversion recovery sequences. In T_1-weighted images, tissue with shorter T_1s are brighter, whereas in T_2-weighted images, tissues with longer T_2s are brighter. For brain imaging, the choice of T_1- or T_2-weighted images presents a trade-off between obtaining high contrast between gray matter and white matter or obtaining high contrast between CSF and brain parenchyma. Although T_1-weighted spin-echo and inversion recovery sequences provide excellent white-gray contrast and have been used extensively for morphometric studies, they are limited by their poor definition of CSF/skull margins for reliably measuring intracranial volume. Thus, there is no single correct MR brain sequence, but rather a range of options, with the optimal selection determined by the questions being asked.

Two-dimensional Multislice and Three-dimensional Imaging

Two-dimensional images are acquired in a defined orthogonal plane, typically in axial, sagittal, and coronal orientations (Fig. 1). Image orientation is defined by use of selective RF pulse excitations of the appropriate magnetic gradients in the three orthogonal axes. Each orientation provides a different view of the brain with optimal visualization of different structures. For example, midsagittal images provide clear delineation of the prefrontal cortex and the corpus callosum, coronal images provide views of the hippocampus and limbic structures over several sections or slices (in this chapter, the terms section and slice are used interchangeably) and axial images provide a good view of basal ganglia structures such as the putamen, globus pallidus, caudate, and substantia nigra, as well as the lateral ventricular system. One limitation of two-dimensional image acquisition is that only selected slices of specified thickness are excited and imaged.

Three-dimensional volume acquisition protocols encompass the entire brain and are amenable to postacquisition reformatting in any plane subject to the limitations imposed by the resolution of the original data. This approach takes a relatively short period of time compared to two-dimensional image acquisition and minimizes the need for standardizing slice selection angles between individuals during image acquisition. Three-dimensional MRI has the potential to reduce measurement errors related to head misalignment in all three orientations between subjects, or within a subject in a longitudinal study. Three-dimensional images are acquired by exciting a broad volume of tissue with a nonslice selective RF pulse (3). Additional magnetic gradients are then used to spatially encode within the excited region. After the raw images have been collected, a Fourier transform decodes the section positions from the entire data set. These section data are further reconstructed with a two-dimensional Fourier transform into the final image. Limitations in post scan analysis of three-dimensional data sets are discussed in more detail in the section on image analysis below.

Most published MRI data on brain morphology in psychiatric patients is based on images acquired in the two-dimensional mode. In this mode, it is critical that the orientation of the selected slices be standardized across subjects, so comparisons can be made, especially for studies where asymmetry of brain structures is of interest. External skull or scalp landmarks, such as the canthomeatal line, have been used but are not optimal for this task, as considerable variation may exist in the relationship of such external landmarks to internal brain structures (28). Internal cerebral landmarks provide a more reproducible guide for image orientation. The anterior and posterior commissures provide two such internal landmarks, and serve to define a plane passing through them, perpendicular to the sagittal plane (72). Once defined, this plane, which corresponds to the plane used in some anatomical atlases (70), can be used to standardize both axial (parallel) and coronal (perpendicular) imaging orientations. However, even when the acquisition plane is

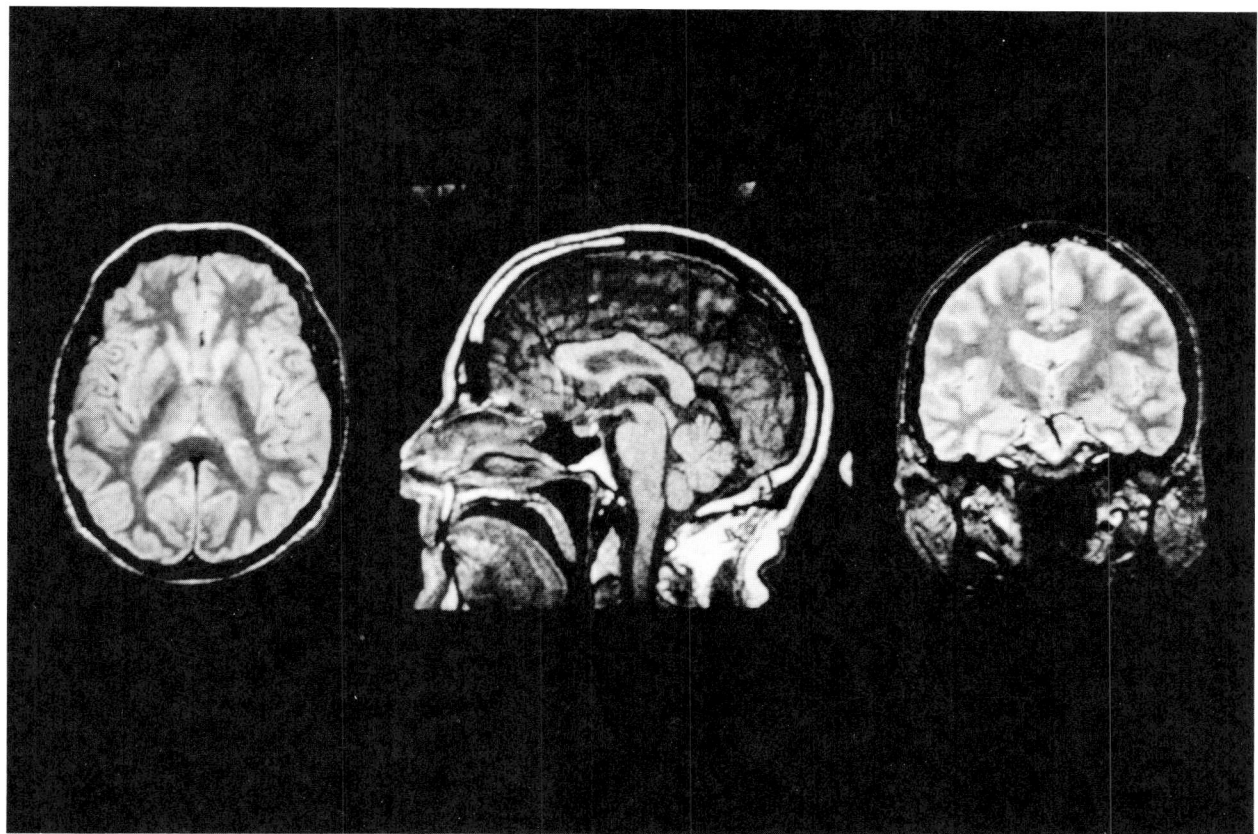

FIG. 1. MRI scans acquired in axial (*A*), coronal (*B*), and sagittal (*C*) planes. All images were acquired with a field of view of 24 cm, NEX = 1, and 256 × 256 matrix. **Left:** Axial image, 5-mm thick, passing through the lateral ventricles and basal ganglia. The image was acquired in an oblique plane parallel to a line connecting anterior and posterior commissures (AC-PC) line using a spin-echo sequence, gated to achieve an effective T_R of >2400 msec with one excitation for each of 256 phase encodes and a T_E of 20 msec. **Center:** Midsagittal image, 3 mm thick, acquired using a single-echo pulse sequence (T_R = 600 msec; T_E = 20 msec), collected without using internal anatomical landmarks. The image highlights the corpus callosum, brainstem, and cerebellum. **Right:** Coronal image, 3 mm thick, passing through lateral ventricles and temporal lobes. The image was acquired in a plane perpendicular to the AC-PC line using a multiecho, flow-compensated, cardiac gated pulse sequence (T_E = 40 msec; effective T_R ≈ 2800 msec).

located relative to internal landmarks, bias in the plane of acquisition can still occur.

Image Resolution, Signal-to-Noise Ratio, and Section Thickness

An image is composed of a grid (usually 256 × 256) of two-dimensional picture elements (pixels). The resolution of the image is affected both by in-plane resolution and by section thickness. An in-plane resolution of 1 mm means that each pixel in the image matrix represents 1 mm^2. However, the 5-mm section, typical of many two-dimensional MRI protocols, means that each image pixel actually represents a three-dimensional volume element (voxel), which in this case is 5 mm deep, and thus the

voxel volume is 5 mm^3. Partial volume effects are present when the tissue comprising a voxel represents some combination of CSF, white matter, or gray matter. The thicker the slice, the more likely that voxels will manifest partial volume effects, rather than be fully volumed, that is, represent a homogenous brain tissue type. To optimize quantitative volumetric measurements and reduce partial voluming, high in-plane resolution and thin sections are used. However, technical factors, such as gradient strength and the amount of RF energy used to excite the object, limit the thinness effectively available. In addition the signal-to-noise ratio (SNR) per voxel will be lower because there is less material producing the signal in a thin section (a typical voxel size in three-dimensional images is 1.5 × 0.9 × 1.2 mm = 1.6 mm^3) than in a thicker section (a typical voxel size in a two-dimensional spin-echo axial sequence is 5 ×

$0.94 \times 0.94 = 4.4$ mm^3). Thus, although the resolution may be finer, there will be more noise and less signal per pixel. Unlike CT data, magnetic resonance data voxels cannot be simply added together to enhance SNR. Thin sections also require increased in-plane sampling and thus longer scanning time to encompass an equivalent volume of the brain, with the attendant disadvantages of requiring subjects to remain still in the scanner.

Section thickness using the standard two-dimensional selective excitation methods is generally limited to 3 mm because of RF power and gradient strength limitation. Section profiles (the shape of the slice viewed on edge) are not perfectly rectangular but have broad shoulders that may extend each edge by as much as 25%. If adjacent sections are too close to each other, their profiles can overlap, resulting in a mixing of signals from one section into another, an artifact called crosstalk. The most common way to avoid crosstalk is to leave a half-section thick gap between sections. The disadvantage is that up to 33% of the portion of the brain being imaged is excluded from the data set. An alternative technique is section interleaving in which data is first collected from the odd-numbered sections and then collected from the intervening even-numbered sections, on a second pass. The disadvantage is that the imaging time is doubled.

Artifact

Magnetic resonance images are susceptible to various types of artifact, some of which can be minimized during image acquisition and others that can only be remedied during data analysis.

Hardware-induced Artifact

The RF coil's sensitivity is not homogeneous across all dimensions of the imaging plane, which often introduces a low-frequency gradient of signal intensity across a given image. Although the human visual system can maintain contrast detection in the face of this artifact, most automated thresholding techniques assume a constant baseline level and require the RF inhomogeneity to be corrected before the image can be processed. A variety of solutions have been proposed to this problem, including filtering (40), bifeature thresholding (35), and line-by-line inversion of the slope of the pixel values within each section (14).

Effects of CSF and Blood Pulsation and Subject Movement

Physiological sources of artifact include pulsation of blood and CSF through regions of the brain being imaged.

The limbic system is particularly vulnerable to this artifact because of its vascularization pattern and relationship to the ventricular system. Cardiac-gating (18) and flow-compensated pulse sequences (57) help reduce these sources of movement artifact, although not without cost. Because more gradients are used with flow compensation, the minimum echo time is lengthened and the maximum number of slices that can be acquired is reduced. Voluntary or involuntary gross head movements are another source of artifact. Head restraints provide one solution (34). A complementary approach, adopted by some research groups, involves administering a sedative hypnotic, adequate to calm the subject or put him to sleep. Despite its advantage of a shorter image acquisition time, three-dimensional image acquisition with short T_Rs (approximately 25 msec) is more sensitive to head movement during scanning, because movement will affect a greater proportion of the collected data.

Need for Phantoms

The accuracy and reproducibility of image data is directly related to the stability of the imaging hardware, especially the magnetic field gradient systems, the main magnetic field, and the RF pulse system. Routine imaging of a quality-assurance phantom permits monitoring the scanner's stability over time. Direct comparison of data collected in different scanners can be facilitated if standardized phantoms are used in the different scanners.

Tradeoffs

A recurring theme in any discussion of MRI data acquisition for clinical studies is the constant tradeoff an investigator must make between resolution of the image, its SNR, and the length of time the subject is in the scanner. Optimal image acquisition parameters for specific studies need to be determined empirically and will vary depending on the structure being imaged, the scanner hardware, and the clinical characteristics of the subjects being studied. The high cost of MRI scanning time, along with limitations in patient tolerance, combine to favor short acquisition sessions. However, if two-dimensional images are acquired in more than one orientation, thin sections are interleaved, and cardiac gating and flow compensation techniques are employed, the entire acquisition session can easily exceed an hour. Reductions in scanning time may be at the cost of poorer image resolution and contrast or sampling less of the brain. Even with cooperative and relaxed subjects, involuntary head movements during a lengthy scan session can be a problem. Although the currently popular Spoiled Gradient Recalled Acquisition (SPGR) three-dimensional protocol provides a strong advantage in its brevity, it may not provide the same contrast between fluid and tissue as standard spin-echo two-dimensional images and may require different approaches to image analysis (41).

ANALYSIS OF MAGNETIC RESONANCE BRAIN IMAGES

Automated computerized analysis of many elements or characteristics of an image is becoming increasingly feasible and accessible to investigators. These approaches offer considerable advantages of flexibility and efficiency, although there are limitations of image resolution and distortions from artifacts in data collection that need to be guarded against. Most analyses combine both automated and interactive approaches. Clinical reading or qualitative scoring of MRI brain data, still widely used by neuroradiologists, serves as a useful complement to quantification, particularly for assessment of image features not readily subject to reliable quantification such as white matter lucencies (e.g., ref. 13) or gross abnormalities in brain morphology (39).

Resolution Issues

Resolution is limited by parameters of the data collection protocol, including in-plane resolution and slice thickness. Generally, two-dimensional data are analyzed as acquired with a known in-plane resolution and slice thickness. In contrast, three-dimensional data sets offer the opportunity for reformatting images in user-defined planes in any orientation and slice thickness. This provides greater flexibility in optimizing the view of specific structures. However, reslicing is bound, not only by the hardware and software constraints of the acquisition parameters but also by constraints of the object space (i.e., the defined plane and thickness) of the original images. The effective thickness of a user-defined slice depends on the orientation of the slice in the three-dimensional volume. For example, with an isotropic data set (i.e., each voxel is a true cube with side length, L) where resolution in the x, y, and z axes is equal, reconstructing a slice in a plane normal to a line going from one corner of the cube to the opposite corner will have an effective slice thickness of $\sqrt{3}*L$. This orientation-dependent effective slice thickness needs to be kept in mind when analyzing such data. This problem is compounded further when the data set is anisotropic, as are most.

Measurement of Gross Morphology

Magnetic resonance imaging provides great flexibility in acquiring a number of different visual representations of the human brain, each designed to enhance contrast between different tissue types, highlight abnormalities within a tissue type, or provide an optimal view of a specific lobar region or subcortical neuroanatomical structure. Techniques for morphometric analysis rely to varying degrees on user interaction with a visual representation of the brain image, displayed on film or a computer console, and automated algorithms applied to the matrix of numerical values representing each pixel in the image. Issues of validity are applicable to both interactive and automated approaches. To the extent that any technique involves human input, issues of reliability acquire a particular salience, given the complexity and individual variability of each human brain. Whereas fully automated methods provide a standardized approach and are less labor intensive, their output needs to be validated against the original image before further analysis is performed.

Volumetric and Area Measures

The size of structures of the brain can be estimated using linear, area, or volumetric measurements. In the early CT literature, planimetric (area) measures were most commonly used and applied to one or two best-view sections. This approach was accessible to investigators without computerized image processing facilities but was vulnerable to sampling error (60) and sacrificed volumetric information. With the advent of magnetic resonance and increasing availability of computerized analysis, volumetric analysis has become the norm.

Volumetric estimates of brain morphology are derived from two-dimensional images by summing areas over successive slices, and extrapolating over interslice gaps, if necessary. Volumetric assessments of manually defined regions of interest can prove labor intensive and motivate the development of automated analysis techniques, as well as stereological techniques, which allow unbiased sampling (24) for estimating volumes of designated neuroanatomic structures. The stereological approach has recently been used to assess the volume of midbrain (16), cerebellum (19), and caudate nuclei (36) by counting the number of intersections of a 1.0 mm × 1.0 mm grid laid over the structures of interest. Another advantage of the stereological approach is that it provides a statistical basis for estimating the degree of error in a measure based on slice thickness and the size and shape of the structure.

Volumetric measurements are particularly important for studying left–right asymmetry of structures (75). Relatively small brain structures may not be located in a perfectly parallel position relative to one another in each hemisphere. The section where a given structure appears largest on one side of the brain may not be the section in which the contralateral structure also appears largest. This applies to both axial and coronal sections. For irregularly shaped brain structures, there is little reason to expect that the asymmetry measured on a given section is representative of overall asymmetry of that structure. A volumetric measurement of the entire structure in each hemisphere can compensate for any bias in selection of imaging plane, or apparent asymmetries due to head placement.

Cerebrospinal Fluid and Tissue Differentiation

In vivo estimates of brain size are usually based on estimates of the total volume of brain tissue and CSF, including both ventricular and subarachnoid fluid. Measuring brain size from MRI scans involves certain assumptions and estimations and is complicated by the fact that bone can easily be confused with CSF and tissue in many MRI acquisition sequences, especially those designed to enhance contrast between white matter and gray matter. Late echo images in which CSF has a long T_2 and thus a higher signal than bone, provide the sharp transition in image intensity values necessary for automatically identifying subarachnoid fluid margins. One automatic approach is to identify pixels external to the peripheral CSF, representing meninges, skull, and scalp, and strip them away from the image. The resulting information about these boundary locations can then be transferred to images obtained with sequence parameters on which contrasts of CSF and tissue and of white and gray matter are optimized (40).

Two commonly used approaches to identifying CSF and tissue on MRI scans are edge detection and thresholding. Edge detection, for example, of the outer margin of the brain or of the ventricles, can be done manually, by tracing outlines on a computer display. Algorithms that identify pixels whose value differs sufficiently from neighboring pixels to qualify them as boundary pixels can speed the process (5,21). Automated edge detection works well when contrast is high and structures to be outlined are of a relatively simple shape. Low contrast, or partial voluming can contribute to failure of the algorithm and need for manual intervention. Thresholding involves classifying pixels according to image intensity values as representative of CSF or tissue. A variety of approaches have been described, some of which take advantage of the different contrasts obtained by different pulse sequences or echo times, by sampling analogous pixels acquired with different pulse sequences (e.g., refs. 11 and 35) or subtracting one image from another to enhance the contrast between CSF and tissue (26,40). Automated assessments may employ discriminant functions based on ranges of pixel values representing known tissue and fluid samples (14,30). Interactive assessments are made by comparing a two-bit image to its full gray scale representation until a pixel value is identified that differentiates CSF from tissue (40). Approaches that in-

volve setting a single threshold for a whole MRI section need to ensure that bias from radiofrequency artifact has been minimized by prior filtering. Validation of all techniques needs to include measuring phantoms of known shape and size, demonstrating that CSF and tissue volumes, computed using the same algorithms, bear a relationship to some well-established variable such as age.

Segmentation of Cerebrospinal Fluid, Gray Matter, and White Matter

Although certain MRI pulse sequences provide images with marked visual contrast between white and gray matter, many clinical studies differentiating white from gray matter for quantitative analysis still rely heavily on user-interactive techniques. As with CSF/tissue differentiation, two commonly used approaches to differentiating CSF and white and gray matter on MRI scans are edge detection (21) and thresholding (14,30,40). With edge detection, operator-defined bridges and barriers can be used to help delineate more complex shapes (5). Thresholding involves classifying pixels as CSF, white matter, or gray matter, with some models recognizing additional compartments such as white matter lucencies (WML) and a variety of other types of tissue pathology (30). Models for tissue segmentation that work well on healthy young brains may fail when applied to patient populations with greater tissue pathologies (e.g., Pfefferbaum et al. (52). Estimates of cortical gray matter volume have been used with greater confidence than those of white matter, especially in studies of aging and Alzheimer's disease (30,31) primarily because of the effect of WMLs on segmentation algorithms. Furthermore, assessments of subcortical gray matter volume using thresholding algorithms can be affected by variations in tissue iron content, which shortens T_2, and has been shown to change over the life span and in basal ganglia disorders, particularly in the substantia nigra and globus pallidus (56). In addition, some subcortical structures are composed of mixed gray and white matter elements that are difficult to differentiate.

An important challenge still facing neuroimaging studies is to develop segmentation algorithms that work well in the face of focal abnormalities such as gliosis, edema, demyelination, and ischemia: processes that alter the properties of tissue water and produce changes in white and gray matter signal intensity.

Defining Anatomical Structures and Regions of Interest for Measurement

Although much can be inferred from global measures of the brain as a whole, specific brain regions and subcortical structures are seen to be of particular interest in characterizing the pathophysiology of psychiatric disorders (8). Most investigators seek ways to identify and measure these regions and structures, often attempting to relate image data to structures as shown on neuroanatomical atlases. Direct interpolation from magnetic resonance images to postmortem specimens or neuroanatomical atlases can be problematic, however, because of resolution and partial voluming issues described above, as well as discrepancies in planes of view. Furthermore, the sheer quantity of in vivo brain images now available for study have greatly expanded recognition of the range of normal variability, especially in such major landmarks as the Sylvian fissure and planum temporale (66). Delineation of the topography of functional brain regions onto MRIs, using sulcal boundaries can be challenging. For example, although the central sulcus provides the boundary separating frontal lobes from parietal lobes, its configuration varies between individuals and each cerebral hemisphere. To some extent, the collection parameters of the MRI, and the plane of view will determine the ease with which these landmarks can be identified. Estimates of frontal lobes have been made from sagittal (1,2), coronal (7), or axial (74) images, but the anatomical landmarks distinguishing the frontal regions are more obscure on coronal sections. Some investigators outline the putative boundaries of designated ROIs (63,68), and others have developed a stereotactic approach which combines anatomical landmarks with a priori geometric rules (30,74). Definition of more specific frontal brain areas, such as the motor strip, remain hampered by difficulties in identifying specific sulcal boundaries on MRI.

Measures of temporal lobe and limbic structures used in studies of patients with various mental disorders are not standardized and may encompass quite a variety of different portions of these structures. This is particularly evident in some recent studies of MRI studies of the temporal lobe in schizophrenia (6,63,68,75), which have adopted varying boundary criteria. Anatomical criteria for defining the extent and boundaries of the temporal lobes have been proposed (29); however, rules for defining specific regions and structures such as the superior temporal gyrus (STG), planum temporale, hippocampus, and amygdala are still being developed, and their specifics are mandated in many cases by the resolution and plane of view available to the investigator. For example, Barta (6) measured the STG in three anterior 3-mm sections at the level of the amygdala, whereas Shenton (63) also included posterior portions of the STG in their measurements from 1.5-mm sections.

At this point, no standardized approach to defining either broad-based ROIs, or even specific anatomical structures, has been established for generalized use by investigators. As in image acquisition, where tradeoffs need to be made between the length of time a subject spends in the scanner and optimizing image resolution, tissue contrast, and range of structures visualized, so in image analysis there are tradeoffs to be made between labor-intensive, interactive delineation of boundaries, and automated or geometrically based boundary drawing algorithms, which may not fully encompass all elements.

Shape Analysis

In addition to the assessment of structural size (e.g., volume, area, length, width), shape analysis is another morphometric method to examine focal characteristics of a structure that are independent of variations in size. For example, shape analysis of a structure such as the hippocampal formation might attempt to quantify morphological distortion by measuring the number, size, and variability of convexities and concavities along a structural boundary using Fourier or wavelet analysis. Boundary length, the shape of contours within a boundary, the compactness of a structure, or the topological relationships between various regions on a boundary to one another or to a neighboring structure are the parameters amenable to quantification. As with volumetric assessments, shape analysis can be vulnerable to the confounding effects of partial voluming in low-resolution images.

Shape analysis techniques are used commonly in digital image analysis applications such as robotics. In brain morphology, they have been used to assess cortical surface area and complexity from pathological samples in animals (43), but they have not yet been applied comprehensively to in vivo assessments of brain morphometry from MRI data. Although the pathophysiological significance of any changes in shape parameters has not yet been established, quantitative shape analyses of the temporal and prefrontal lobes and corpus callosum in schizophrenic patients and controls (9) suggest that nonspecific disease-related structural distortions may be present in schizophrenia.

Surface Rendering

Until recently, a three-dimensional representation of the brain structure from which a two-dimensional image is sliced could only be visualized in the investigator's imagination. The development of three-dimensional volumetric MRI acquisition and the extrapolation of these images from two-dimensional data sets now make it possible to generate three-dimensional images of brain in living subjects, startlingly similar to the appearance of the postmortem brain. Neurosurgeons and neurologists have lead the way in the clinical application of these techniques for localizing lesions and vasculature before neurosurgery (15,17,37) and for characterizing the normal surface anatomy of the brain (73). The availability of three-dimensional images provides an exciting new dimension to the in vivo assessment of normal brain anat-

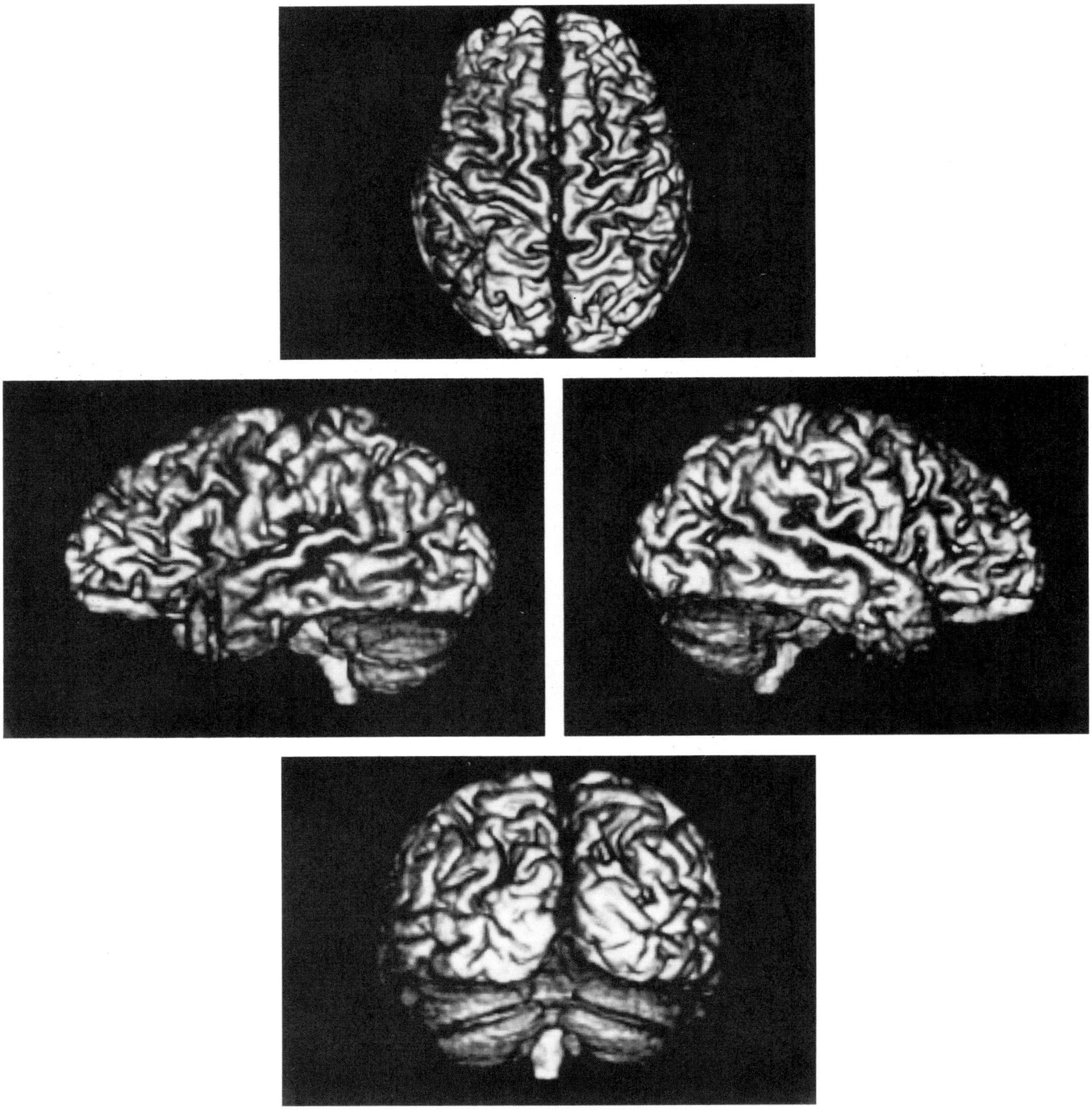

FIG. 2. Three-dimensional renderings of MRI dataset presenting images of the brain as if viewed from above (**top**), left and right, and behind (**bottom**). (Courtesy of Patrick Barta, NIMH.)

omy as well as of brain dysmorphology in a variety of psychiatric disorders. A three-dimensional brain image in which surface rendering software has been combined with a knowledge base in which each voxel has been coded by various attributes, including its location, function, and the arterial system supplying it (71), has recently been published as a teaching tool. Such an atlas enables stu-

dents the opportunity to explore the structure and function of the brain in virtual reality.

Creation of three-dimensional images employs a range of rapidly evolving computer graphics software and hardware methods (22), including both surface and volume-rendering techniques. In surface rendering, a surface is defined within the three-dimensional data set using an algorithm to distinguish the desired surface from its surroundings (10). Different viewpoints and lighting sources may also be used to create images of the object as seen from varying viewpoints (12) (Fig. 2). In volume rendering, each voxel from the three-dimensional dataset is rendered starting from a point farthest from the viewer to create successive views through the brain. Although visually compelling, these rendered images may contain distortions introduced by the viewing model and image preprocessing used to generate the surface. These must be taken into account before quantitative analysis is made of the rendered image (35). Despite these limitations, rendering techniques are beginning to find some quantitative use, for example, to identify and measure specific sulci to aid in anatomical localization for neurosurgery (73).

Coregistration with Other In Vivo Neuroimages

The relatively poor in-plane resolution and wide sections of images from functional imaging techniques such as positron emission tomography (PET) and proton or phosphorus magnetic spectroscopic imaging (MRS) limits anatomic localization. Interpretation of data from these imaging modalities can be enhanced when structural information from magnetic resonance images is available. Indeed, this anatomical localization of functional data is important to its proper interpretation, especially in research applications. Structural brain images can provide an anatomically accurate overlay for localizing observed functional activity, such as glucose metabolism obtained by PET (46) and the distribution of putative markers of neuronal viability and metabolic activity inferred from proton and phosphorus MRS. Since voxels obtained with MRI are generally considerably smaller than those obtained in MRS or PET, imaging coregistration of MRI and PET or MRS images can potentially allow correction for regional or group differences in CSF, gray matter, and white matter composition of the partially volumed functional voxel (44,45). Such corrections are computationally challenging, but eventually they will allow much greater precision in assessing functional activity.

The simplest case of coregistration is when both data sets have been collected on the same imaging hardware without moving the subject (Fig. 3). A recent MRI/MRS study used morphometric information on whole slice CSF and tissue volumes to calculate phosphorus metabolite concentrations relative to brain tissue (46). For PET scanning, differences in hardware and time of scan are unavoidable. Several different approaches to image acquisition to facilitate subsequent matching of acquired PET and MRI images have been developed. These include use of external landmarks, or fiducials, consistently placed and of a size and property to be adequately imaged by both modalities (20), and head holders to stabilize and

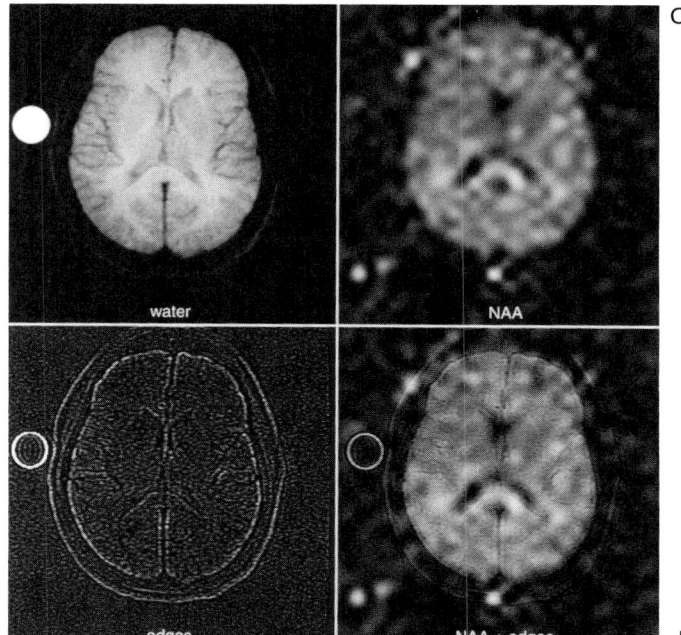

FIG. 3. Coregistration of structural MRI and proton MRS images, acquired in the same scan session from a healthy young control. **A:** Unprocessed axial water-based structural image; **B:** the edge-detected version. **C:** Proton inversion recovery MRS image of *N*-acetylaspartic acid (NAA) distribution in the axial plane; **D:** a linear combination of NAA distribution and structural edges providing neuroanatomic definition without obscuring spectroscopic data. (Courtesy of Daniel Spielman, Department of Radiology, Stanford University.)

standardize head position between scanners (34). Varying levels of sophistication have been applied to postacquisition computerized registration. A simple analytical approach can be used to compute a transformation matrix between two sets of images (33). Iterative matching of brain surfaces (38,51) or projections (67) have also been developed (Fig. 4). Postacquisition approaches can also be combined with use of fiducial markers (20).

INTERPRETATION OF MAGNETIC RESONANCE BRAIN IMAGES

Neuroimaging findings in some mental disorders can be elusive. The true effect is small, and brain morphology is strongly affected by several variables that are relatively independent of disease, such as age, sex, and somatic size, as well as those that might be associated with mental disorder, for example, alcohol consumption, socioeconomic status, and handedness. These variables must be taken into consideration and appropriate controls implemented before inferences about the pathophysiology of various mental disorders can be properly drawn.

Selection of Appropriate Controls

When CT was the prevailing technology, medical patients with normal scans were frequently used as controls in imaging studies of psychiatric patients—a practice motivated, to some extent, by reluctance to expose healthy subjects to unwarranted radiation. Whether or not this practice contributed to observed group differences was never fully resolved (59,65). With MRI scanning, this radiation concern is not relevant. However, the prospective recruitment of control samples for any neuroimaging studies of psychiatric disorder requires attention not only to excluding cases with psychiatric disorders (64) but also to including subjects who match the educational and ethnic status of the patients (61). In addition to comparisons with normative data, comparisons between pathological groups are also valuable, especially between different diagnostic groups with documented abnormalities in common anatomical region(s). For example, comparisons between patients with temporal lobe epilepsy and schizophrenia are appropriate for studies investigating the role of limbic structures in these disorders.

Accounting for Normal Developmental and Aging Effects

Schizophrenia is typically a disease with onset in late adolescence or early adulthood, a period during which cortical gray matter undergoes significant reduction, but cortical white continues to increase in volume (53). Its course coincides with a period of stable white matter volume, but gradual reduction in gray matter and increase in CSF (30,47,53) (Fig. 5). These normal developmental and aging effects need to be taken into account when interpreting observed brain dysmorphology in schizophrenia. Studies of Alzheimer's disease, Parkinson's disease, and other diseases which typically make their appearance after middle age, likewise need to take into account not only the escalation of normal age-related changes occurring at this point in the life span, but also the greater variability in brain tissue volumes found among the healthy elderly than the healthy young (30,31).

Accounting for Normal Variations in Somatic Size

Given the existence of a wide range of body and head sizes among the population, it is important to demonstrate that any size difference of a specific brain structure is independent of such nondisease-relevant differences. In general, large people will have larger heads and larger brains than small people. In most research contexts, this variability constitutes a form of noise which investigators need to minimize in order to compare the volume of a particular brain region or structure between individuals

and groups. Head size correction is particularly appropriate when gender differences in brain morphology are under investigation (25).

The most common approach for head-size correction has been the use of a ratio, such as the ventricle brain ratio (VBR) (69), which was developed to provide an index of ventricular enlargement relative to the size of the total brain. Other correction approaches have included proportions, where the size of a structure, or the amount of tissue or CSF in a ROI, is divided by an estimate of the intracranial volume (e.g., ref. 30), and regression analysis which partials out the components of quantitative brain measures attributable to headsize variation (e.g., ref. 53).

Concern that the ratio or proportion approaches to head size correction could introduce error or obscure the complexity of underlying relationships has lead some investigators to warn against their use and to advocate regression or multifactorial approaches as necessary to parse out contribution of nonspecific variables (4). Others (42) have demonstrated that a regression approach to head-size correction removes irrelevant true-score variance, which reduces reliability and improves the correlation with validity criteria such as age and diagnostic status. Linear regression of specific ROIs against estimated head-size in a sample of normal control subjects highlighted the fact that different parts of the brain bear different relationships to overall brain size and suggests that ROI-specific correction factors should be applied (42).

While head-size correction is appropriate in some contexts, in others, such as developmental studies (53), it may not be. For such studies, absolute volumes of particular brain regions rather than head-size corrected values should be used. Because investigators have described reduced intracranial volume in patients with schizophrenia (49), the issue has become more complicated. If schizophrenia affects the brain before it has completed its growth, leading to diminished brain size and as a result diminished skull size, the correction of all structural brain measures for intracranial volume could obscure pathologically relevant information. Regardless of possible disease-related reduction in head size, however, an investigator asking whether particular brain structures are disproportionately reduced, must control for differences in intracranial volume.

Accounting for Generalized Tissue Loss

Generalized morphological differences in the brains of psychiatric patients compared to controls should be taken into account before assessing smaller structures. For instance, schizophrenia appears to be characterized by generalized ventricular and cortical sulcal enlargement (49,55) as well as a diffuse loss of gray matter (27,74).

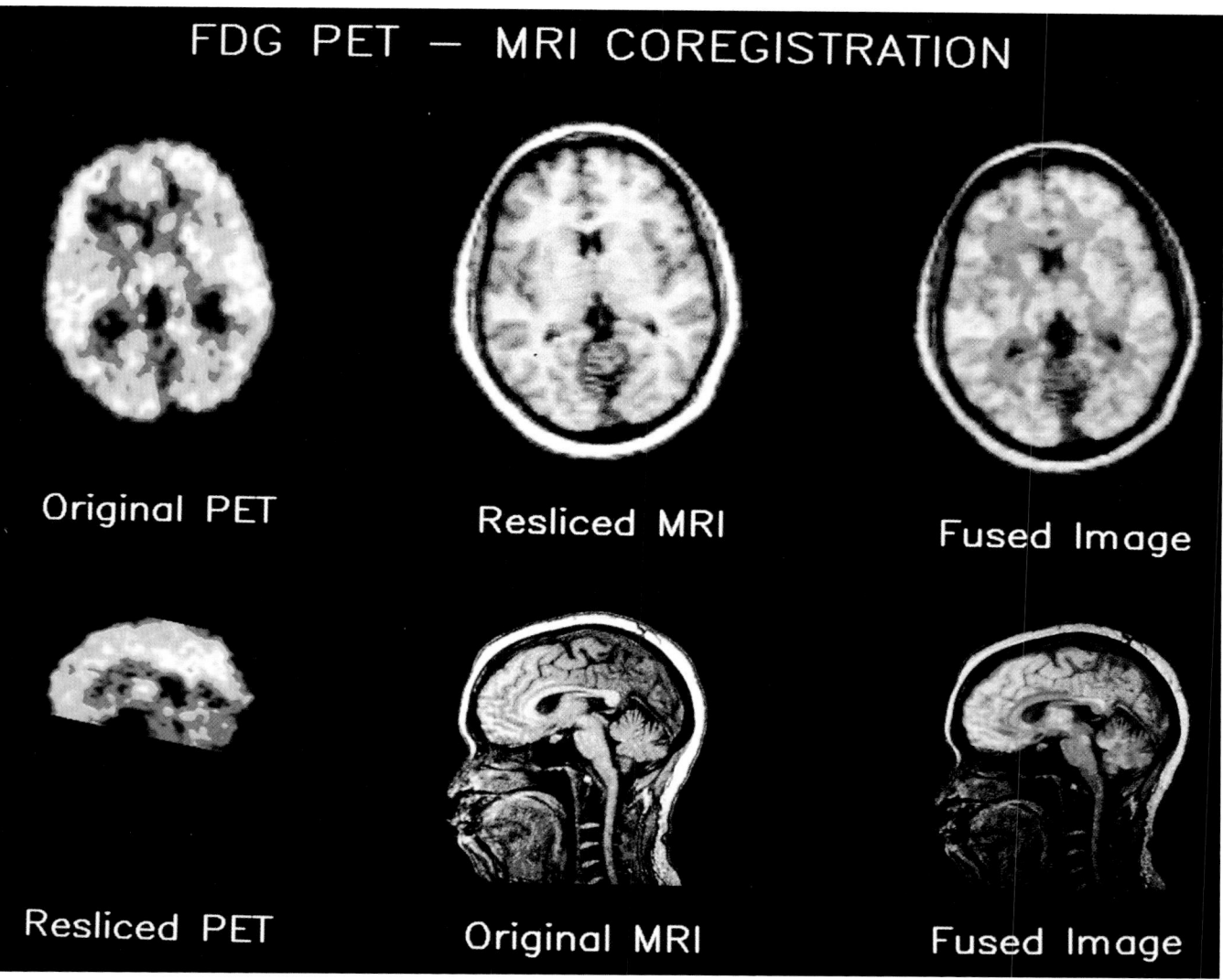

FIG. 4. Reslicing and coregistration of structural MRI and fluorodeoxyglucose (FDG) PET images of glucose metabolism from a 39-year-old healthy female control. The original MRI was acquired in the sagittal plane and the original FDG PET in the axial plane. Surface-matching (Analyze) software enabled images in each modality to be resliced to match the orientation of the other modality, and then fused to provide anatomical definition for functional image. The PET scan was obtained on a 7-slice Scanditronix PC1024-7B dedicated head scanner with an in-plane resolution of 5.2 mm and an axial resolution of 11 mm. The tracer was 5 mCi of FDG. There were four transmission scans (one for each frame) with a rotating Ge/Ga pin source. The subject had a hexalite head holder and eye-patches on and performed an auditory continuous performance task for 30 minutes and was then scanned for 30 minutes (four frames of seven slices to yield 28 interleaved slices). The interslice distance is 13.75 mm for the seven original slices and hence 3.4375 mm for the 28 slices resulting from the four interleaved frames. The PET image resliced in the sagittal plane clearly shows the brainstem, cerebellum, and fourth ventricle. The sagittally acquired MRI was obtained on a Picker 0.5T scanner. Slice thickness 2.5 mm, acquired with two repetitions. 256 × 256 pixels × 64 slices. It is a T_1 weighted field echo scan with $T_R = 36$, $T_E = 6$, flip angle = 30 degrees. (Courtesy of T. Ketter, NIH.)

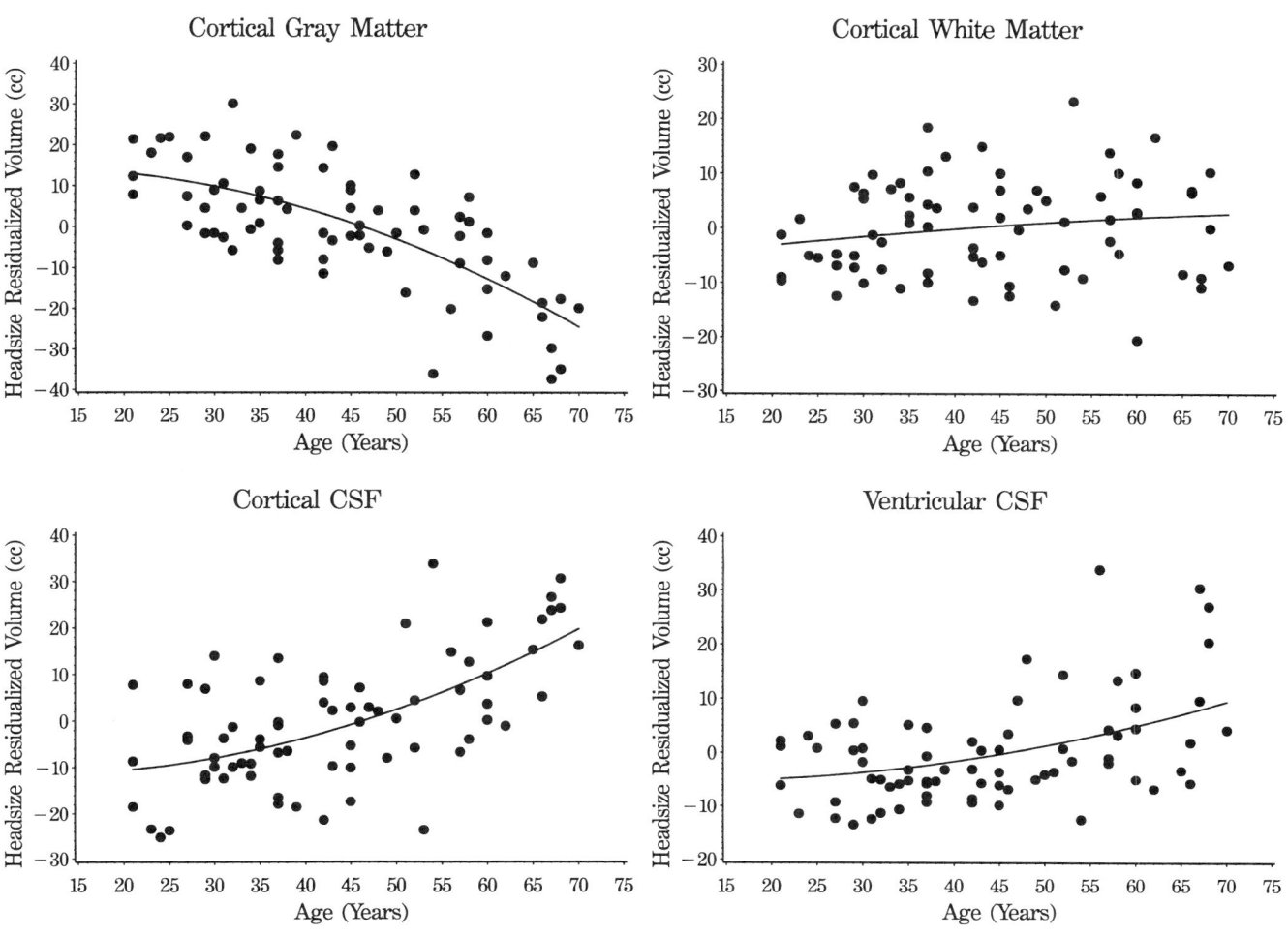

FIG. 5. Volumetric measurements of cortical gray matter, cortical white matter, cortical CSF, and ventricular CSF from 73 healthy men, aged 21 to 70 years old plotted as a function of age. The regression line is a weighted constrained quadratic function. Weighting was used to take into account the heteroscedasticity (increased variance in older age) of the data. Brain measures (expressed in cc) were first regressed against an estimate of head size volume. Residual values were then calculated for each subject by subtracting their predicted score for each ROI, based on head size, from the observed score. Cortical gray matter volume showed an average decrease of 0.7 cc per year, whereas cortical white matter remained stable across the five decades. Cortical CSF increased 0.6 cc per year, and ventricular CSF 0.3 cc per year.

Therefore, it is necessary to demonstrate a disproportionate loss of localized tissue before concluding that a specific brain structure is uniquely affected by the disease. For example, before being able to interpret the MRI findings of reduced gray matter volume in the hippocampus or in the temporal lobe, it is critical to determine whether similar gray matter reduction exists in other cortical areas.

LONGITUDINAL STUDIES

An important question regarding brain dysmorphology in any psychiatric disorder is the extent to which any abnormalities observed preceded the onset of the disease (e.g., schizophrenia), progress at a faster rate than the changes of normal aging (e.g., Alzheimer's disease), or even reverse with improvements in clinical status, (e.g., with abstinence in alcoholism). Whereas cross-sectional studies of patients with different lengths of illness, or remission, can provide clues to answer such questions, longitudinal designs with repeated measures are preferable. Longitudinal studies, particularly using neuroimaging, pose a number of methodological challenges. One of these is the impact of evolving technology on comparability of measures obtained with successive generations of imaging devices. Even when imaging devices and protocol remain constant, another challenge is to ensure replicability of alignment relative to internal neuroanatomical landmarks over successive scans. Even a small misalignment can contribute variance greatly exceeding that expected with disease progression or reversal (23).

Standardizing Measures in the Face of Changing Technology

As neuroimaging methods advance and new imaging techniques are used, it is necessary to understand how morphometric methods are affected by differences in imaging methods. A major transition in the past 10 years has been the replacement of CT scanning with MRI scanning. Although MRI adds much information, particularly from its enhanced soft-tissue resolution, to that provided by CT, it also provides similar information on CSF-filled spaces, particularly ventricular enlargement, which has been a hallmark of CT studies. Thus MRI values can potentially offer continuity for longitudinal studies in which a transition was made from CT to MRI.

A recent study compared CT- and MRI-derived estimates of ventricular and sulcal CSF volume obtained within 2 weeks of each other in patients meeting Research Diagnostic Criteria criteria for alcohol dependence (54) and found them to be highly correlated. However, although CT estimates of absolute ventricular volume were comparable to those obtained with MRI, CT considerably underestimated cortical sulcal volume as compared with MRI. Several factors probably contributed to this difference. The spectral shift artifact in CT is generally larger than the low frequency noise (probably RF inhomogeneity) seen in MRI, and uncorrected spectral shift artifact will always bias CSF into the tissue compartment in the CT analysis. Also, the actual acquired slice thickness of MRI was half that of CT in this comparison, allowing the resolution of more sulci with MRI than CT. This finding counsels against directly comparing cortical CSF volumes across modalities, but suggests that data on ventricular volume may, with caution, be compared across modalities.

Magnetic resonance three-dimensional image acquisition and analysis techniques now enable the collection of whole-brain data sets which can be subsequently resliced in any orientation to match slices obtained in a two-dimensional acquisition protocol. Thus replacing lengthy axial and coronal acquisition sequences with a brief three-dimensional acquisition sequence is an attractive possibility if issues of comparability with earlier data collected in the two-dimensional mode can be resolved. In a pilot study, we tested the comparability of CSF, gray matter, and white matter measures made from three-dimensional SPGR images to those acquired using a T_2-weighted axial spin-echo protocol (41). Images obtained by SPGR were reconstructed and resliced to match the axial spin-echo images. Three compartment segmentation was applied to both sets of images. Although there was a high degree of correlation between the two sets of CSF, white matter, and gray matter values, there was relatively greater white matter and less CSF and gray matter in SPGR compared to spin-echo images, suggesting that there are systematic differences between the methods. This preliminary analysis indicates that results from studies using different acquisition methods should be compared with caution, because the differences in tissue contrast, SNRs, and slice profiles will affect the results of morphometric measures.

Longitudinal Measurement Error

Even when software protocols are identical, differences in head positioning between scans can contribute measurement error in studies involving repeat scans (23). The acquisition of three-dimensional images offer enhanced potential for postacquisition realignment according to anatomical landmarks so that differences in head placement between scans are irrelevant. However, the transformations, interpolations, and other manipulations performed on three-dimensional MRI data can potentially result in subtle measurement error. A longitudinal CT study on patients with Alzheimer's disease, reported a technique to assess method error (62), which could be applicable to any neuroimaging modality from which accurate estimates of head size can be made. The assumption behind this method is that, at least in mature adults, total cranial volume (CSF plus tissue) should be unchanged between scans. The data, however, revealed an apparent intraindividual change in total cranial volume between first and second scans ranging from −60.5 to 89.5 cc, which correlated significantly, but differentially with several of the ROI change scores. This head size difference provided an estimate of the longitudinal method error and was used to derive a specific correction factor for each ROI change score, which removed at least part of the error variance. Procedures to reduce head positioning error appear to be important for improving the sensitivity of longitudinal studies.

CONCLUSIONS

The superior resolution and greater flexibility of MRI offer the hope that this modality will enable identification of any regionally specific brain abnormalities that might be associated with various psychiatric disorders. New developments in acquisition and image processing software continue to expand the possibilities available to investigators, not only for visual presentation, but also for quantitative analyses. Although there continue to be important methodological and technical issues to attend to, investigators are becoming increasingly sophisticated in using appropriate techniques and adopting strategies to ensure the reliability and validity of the data being produced. It continues to be important that data are collected and analyzed in such a way that specific hypotheses about particular regions of the brain can be tested within the context of the brain as a whole.

ACKNOWLEDGMENT

Preparation of this chapter was made possible by support from the Department of Veterans Affairs, and research grants from NIH (MH30854, AG11427, and AA05965).

REFERENCES

1. Andreasen N, Nasrallah A, Dunn V, et al. Structural abnormalities in the frontal system in schizophrenia. *Arch Gen Psychiatry* 1986;43:136–144.
2. Andreasen NC, Ehrhardt JC, Swayze VW, Alliger RJ, Yuh WTC, Cohen G, Ziebell S. Magnetic resonance imaging of the brain in schizophrenia: the pathophysiologic significance of structural abnormalities. *Arch Gen Psychiatry* 1990;47:35–44.
3. Andrew ER, Bydder G, Friffiths J, Iles R, Styles P. *Clinical magnetic resonance: imaging and spectroscopy.* New York: John Wiley, 1990.
4. Arndt S, Cohen G, Alliger RJ, Swayze VW, Andreasen NC. Problems with ratio and proportion measures of imaged cerebral structures. *Psychiatry Res Neuroimag* 1991;40:79–90.
5. Ashtari M, Zito J, Gold BI, Lieberman JA, Borenstein MT, Herman PG. Computerized volume measurement of brain structure. *Invest Radiol* 1990;25:798–805.
6. Barta PE, Pearlson GD, Powers RE, Richards SS, Tune LE. Auditory hallucinations and smaller superior temporal gyral volume in schizophrenia. *Am J Psychiatry* 1990;147:1457–1462.
7. Buchanan RW, Breier A, Kirkpatrick B, et al. Structural abnormalities in deficit and nondeficit schizophrenia. *Am J Psychiatry* 1993; 150:59–65.
8. Buchsbaum MS. The frontal lobes, basal ganglia, and temporal lobes as sites for schizophrenia. *Schizophr Bull* 1990;16:379–389.
9. Casanova MF, Goldberg TE, Suddath RL, et al. Quantitative shape analysis of the temporal and prefrontal lobes of schizophrenic patients: a magnetic resonance image study. *J Neuropsychiatry Clin Neurosci* 1990;2:363–372.
10. Cline HE, Dumoulin HR, Hart HR, Lorensen WE, Ludke S. 3D reconstruction of the brain from magnetic resonance images using a connectivity algorithm. *Magn Reson Imag* 1987;3:345–352.
11. Cline HE, Lorensen WE, Kikinis R, Jolesz F. Three-dimensional segmentation of MR images of the head using probability and connectivity. *J Comput Assist Tomogr* 1990;14:1037–1045.
12. Cline HE, Lorensen WE, Ludke S, Crawford CR, Teeter BC. Two algorithms for the three-dimensional reconstruction of tomograms. *Med Phys* 1988;15:320–327.
13. Coffey CE, Wilkinson WE, Weiner RD, et al. Quantitative cerebral anatomy in depression: a controlled magnetic resonance imaging study. *Arch Gen Psychiatry* 1993;50:7–16.
14. Cohen G, Andreasen NC, Alliger R, et al. Segmentation techniques for the classification of brain tissue using magnetic resonance imaging. *Psychiatry Res Neuroimag* 1992;45:33–51.
15. Damasio H, Frank R. Three-dimensional in vivo mapping of brain lesions in humans. *Arch Neurol* 1992;49:137–143.
16. Doraiswamy PM, Na C, Husain MM, et al. Morphometric changes of the human midbrain with normal aging: MR and stereologic findings. *Am J Neuroradiol* 1992;13:383–386.
17. Ehricke H-H, Laub G. Integrated 3D display of brain anatomy and intracranial vasculature in MR imaging. *J Comput Assist Tomogr* 1990;14:846–852.
18. Enzmann DR, Rubin JB, O'Donohue D, et al. Use of cerebrospinal fluid gating to improve T2-weighted images. II: temporal lobes, basal ganglia and brain stem. *Radiology* 1987;162:768–773.
19. Escalona PR, McDonald WM, Doraiswamy PM, et al. In vivo stereological assessment of human cerebellar volume: effects of gender and age. *Am J Neuroradiol* 1991;12:927–929.
20. Evans AC, Marrett S, Torrescorzo J, Ku S, Collins L. MRI-PET correlation in three dimensions using a volume-of-interest (VOI) atlas. *J Cer Blood Flow Metab* 1991;11:A69–A78.
21. Filipek PA, Kennedy DN, Caviness VS, Rossnick SL, Spraggins TA, Starewicz PM. Magnetic resonance imaging-based brain morphometry: development and application to normal subjects. *Ann Neurol* 1989;25:61–67.
22. Foley JD, van Dam A, Feiner SK, Hughes JF. *Computer graphics: principles and practice.* 2nd ed. Reading, MA: Addison-Wesley, 1990.
23. Goodkin DE, Vanderburg-Medendorp S, Ross J. The effect of repositioning error on serial magnetic resonance imaging scans. *Arch Neurol* 1993;50:569–570.
24. Gundersen HJG, Jensen EB. The efficiency of systematic sampling in stereology and its prediction. *J Microsc* 1987;147:229–263.
25. Gur RC, Mozley PD, Resnick SM, et al. Gender differences in age effect on brain atrophy measured by magnetic resonance imaging. *Proc Natl Acad Sci USA* 1991;88:2845–2849.
26. Harris GJ, Rhew EH, Noga T, Pearlson GD. User-friendly method for rapid brain and CSF volume calculation using transaxial MRI images. *Psychiatry Res Neuroimag* 1991;40:61–68.
27. Harvey I, Ron M, du Bouley G, Wicks D, Lewis S, Murray RM. Reduction of cortical volume in schizophrenia on magnetic resonance imaging. *Psychol Med* 1993;23:591–604.
28. Homan RW, Herman J, Purdy P. Cerebral location in international 10–20 system electrode placement. *Electroenceph Clin Neurophysiol* 1987;66:376–382.
29. Jack CRJ, Gehring DG, Sharbrough FW, et al. Temporal lobe volume measurement from MR images: accuracy and left–right asymmetry in normal persons. *J Comput Assist Tomogr* 1988;12:21–29.
30. Jernigan TL, Press GA, Hesselink JR. Methods for measuring brain morphologic features on magnetic resonance images: validation and normal aging. *Arch Neurol* 1990;47:27–32.
31. Jernigan TL, Salmon DP, Butters N, Hesselink JR. Cerebral structure on MRI .2. specific changes in Alzheimer's and Huntington's diseases. *Biol Psychiatry* 1991;29:68–81.
32. Johnstone EC, Crow TJ, Frith DC, Husband J, Kreel L. Cerebral ventricular size and cognitive impairment in schizophrenia. *Lancet* 1976;2:924–926.
33. Kapouleas I, Alavi A, Alves WM, Gur RE, Weiss DW. Registration of three-dimensional MR and PET images of the human brain without markers. *Radiology* 1991;181:731–739.
34. Kearfott KJ, Rottenberg DA, Knowles RJR. A new headholder for PET, CT, and NMR imaging. *J Comput Assist Tomogr* 1984;8: 1217–1220.
35. Kohn MI, Tanna NK, Herman GT, et al. Analysis of brain and cerebrospinal fluid volumes with MR imaging. 1. methods, reliability, and validation. *Radiology* 1991;178:115–122.
36. Krishnan KR, Husain MM, McDonald WM, et al. In vivo stereological assessment of caudate volume in man: effects of normal aging. *Life Sci* 1990;47:1325–1329.
37. Levin DN, Hu X, Tan KK, et al. The brain: integrated three-dimensional display of MR and PET images. *Radiology* 1989; 172:783–789.
38. Levin DN, Pelizzari CA, Chen GTY, Chen C-T, Cooper MD. Retrospective geometric correlation of MR, CT and PET images. *Radiology* 1988;169:817–823.
39. Lieberman J, Bogerts B, Degreef G, Ashtari M, Lantos G, Alvir J. Qualitative assessment of brain morphology in acute and chronic schizophrenia. *Am J Psychiatry* 1992;149:784–794.
40. Lim KO, Pfefferbaum A. Segmentation of MR brain images into cerebrospinal fluid spaces, white and gray matter. *J Comput Assist Tomogr* 1989;13:588–593.
41. Marsh L, Lim KO, Pfefferbaum A. Measurement of cerebral spinal fluid, gray and white matter in MRI in psychiatric disorders: a

comparison of SPGR and spin-echo acquisition. *Biol Psychiatry* 1992;31:121A (abst.).

42. Mathalon DH, Sullivan EV, Rawles JM, Pfefferbaum A. Correction for head size in brain imaging measurements. *Psychiatry Res Neuroimag* 1993;50:121–139.

43. Mayhew TM, Mwamengele GLM, Dantzer V. Comparative morphometry of the mammalian brain: estimates of cerebral volumes of cortical surface areas obtained from macroscopic slices. *J Anat* 1990;172:191–200.

44. Meltzer CC, Leal JP, Mayberg HS, Wagner HN, Frost JJ. Correction of PET data for partial volume effects in human cerebral cortex by MR Imaging. *J Comput Assist Tomogr* 1990;14:561–570.

45. Muller-Gartner HW, Links JM, Prince JL, et al. Measurement of radiotracer concentration in brain gray matter using positron emission tomography—MRI-based correction for partial volume effects. *J Cer Blood Flow Metab* 1992;12:571–583.

46. Murphy DGM, Bottomley PA, Salerno JA, et al. An in vivo study of phosphorus and glucose metabolism in Alzheimer's disease using magnetic resonance spectroscopy and PET. *Arch Gen Psychiatry* 1993;50:341–349.

47. Murphy DGM, DeCarli C, Schapiro MB, Rapoport SI, Horwitz B. Age-related differences in volumes of subcortical nuclei, brain matter, and cerebrospinal fluid in healthy men as measured with magnetic resonance imaging. *Arch Neurol* 1993;49:839–845.

48. Oldendorf WH, Oldendorf WJ. *Basics of magnetic resonance imaging*. Boston: Martinus Nijhoff Publishing, 1988.

49. Pearlson GD, Kim WS, Kubos KJ, et al. Ventricle-brain ratio, computed tomographic density and brain area in 50 schizophrenics. *Arch Gen Psychiatry* 1989;46:690–697.

50. Pearlson GD, Marsh L. Magnetic resonance imaging in psychiatry. In: Oldham JM, Riba MB, Tasman A, eds. *Annual review of psychiatry*. Vol 12. Washington, DC: American Psychiatric Association Press; 1993:347–382.

51. Pelizzari CA, Chen GTY, Spelbring DR, Weichselbaum RR, Chen C-T. Accurate three-dimensional registration of CT, PET and/or MR images of the brain. *J Comput Assist Tomogr* 1989;13:20–26.

52. Pfefferbaum A, Lim KO, Zipursky RB, et al. Brain gray and white matter volume loss accelerates with aging in chronic alcoholics: a quantitative MRI study. *Alcohol Clin Exp Res* 1992;16:1078–1089.

53. Pfefferbaum A, Mathalon DH, Sullivan EV, Rawles JM, Zipursky RB, Lim KO. A quantitative MRI study of changes in brain morphology from infancy to late adulthood. *Arch Neurol* [in press].

54. Pfefferbaum A, Sullivan EV, Rosenbloom MJ, Shear PK, Mathalon DH, Lim KO. Increase in brain CSF volume is greater in older than younger alcoholics: a replication study and CT/MRI comparison. *Psychiatry Res Neuroimag* 1993;50:257–274.

55. Pfefferbaum A, Zipursky RB, Lim KO, Zatz LM, Stahl SM, Jernigan TL. Computed tomographic evidence for generalized sulcal and ventricular enlargement in schizophrenia. *Arch Gen Psychiatry* 1988;45:633–640.

56. Pujol J, Junque C, Vendrell P, et al. Biological significance of iron-related magnetic resonance imaging changes in the brain. *Arch Neurol* 1992;49:711–717.

57. Quencer RM, Hinks RS, Pattany PH, Horen M, Post MJD. Improved MR imaging of the brain by using compensated gradients to suppress motion-induced artifacts. *Am J Neuroradiol* 1988;9:431–438.

58. Raz S, Raz N. Structural brain abnormalities in the major psychoses: a quantitative review of the evidence from computerized imaging. *Psychol Bull* 1990;108:93–108.

59. Raz S, Raz N, Bigler ED. Ventriculomegaly in schizophrenia: is the choice of controls important? *Psychiatry Res* 1988;24:71–77.

60. Raz S, Raz N, Weinberger DR, et al. Morphological brain abnormalities in schizophrenia determined by computed tomography: a problem of measurement? *Psychiatry Res* 1987;22:91–98.

61. Resnick SM. Matching for education in studies of schizophrenia [Letter]. *Arch Gen Psychiatry* 1992;49:246.

62. Shear PK, Sullivan EV, Mathalon DH, et al. Longitudinal volumetric CT analysis of regional brain changes in normal aging and Alzheimer's disease. *Arch Neurol* [in press].

63. Shenton ME, Kikinis R, Jolesz FA, et al. Abnormalities of the left temporal lobe and thought disorder in schizophrenia—a quantitative magnetic resonance imaging study. *New Eng J Med* 1992;327:604–612.

64. Shtasel DL, Gur RE, Mozley PD, et al. Volunteers for biomedical research—recruitment and screening of normal controls. *Arch Gen Psychiatry* 1991;48:1022–1025.

65. Smith GN, Iacono WG, Moreau M, Tallman K, Beisser M, Flak B. Choice of comparison group and findings of computerized tomography in schizophrenia. *Br J Psychiatry* 1988;153:667–674.

66. Steinmetz H, Ebeling U, Huang Y, Kahn T. Sulcus topography of the parietal opercular region: an anatomic and MR study. *Brain Lang* 1990;38:515–533.

67. Steinmetz H, Huang YX, Seitz RJ, et al. Individual integration of positron emission tomography and high-resolution magnetic resonance imaging. *J Cer Blood Flow Metab* 1992;12:919–926.

68. Swayze VW, Andreasen NC, Alliger RJ, Yuh WTC, Ehrhardt JC. Subcortical and temporal structures in affective disorder and schizophrenia—a magnetic resonance imaging study. *Biol Psychiatry* 1992;31:221–240.

69. Syneck V, Reuben JR. The ventricular-brain ratio using planimetric measurement of EMI scans. *Br J Radiol* 1976;49:233–237.

70. Talairach J, Szikla G. *Atlas of stereotaxic anatomy of the telencephalon. Anatomo-radiological studies*. Paris: Masson; 1967.

71. Tiede U, Bomans M, Hohne KH, et al. A computerized three-dimensional atlas of the human skull and brain. *Am J Neuroradiol* 1993;14:551–559.

72. Vanier M, Ethier R, Clark J, Peters TM, Olivier A, Melanson D. Anatomical interpretation of MR scans of the brain. *Magn Reson Med* 1987;4:185–188.

73. Vannier MW, Brunsden BS, Hildebolt CF, et al. Brain surface cortical sulcal lengths—quantification with three-dimensional MR imaging. *Radiology* 1991;180:479–484.

74. Zipursky RB, Lim KO, Sullivan EV, Brown BW, Pfefferbaum A. Widespread cerebral gray matter volume deficits in schizophrenia. *Arch Gen Psychiatry* 1992;49:195–205.

75. Zipursky RB, Marsh L, Lim KO, et al. Volumetric MRI assessment of temporal lobe structures in schizophrenia. *Biol Psychiatry* [in press].

*Psychopharmacology: The Fourth
Generation of Progress,* edited by
Floyd E. Bloom and David J. Kupfer.
Raven Press, Ltd., New York 1995.

CHAPTER 78

Methodological Issues in Event-Related Brain Potential and Magnetic Field Studies

Walton T. Roth, Judith M. Ford, Adolf Pfefferbaum, and Thomas R. Elbert

Psychiatry in its search for the roots of abnormal thoughts, feelings, and behavior has again turned its attention to the human brain and is trying to apply the methods of the many scientific disciplines that have cast light on normal brain functioning—disciplines such as neuroanatomy and histology, biochemistry and molecular biology, and electrophysiology. This chapter concentrates on ways of maximizing what can be learned from noninvasive electrophysiology, a technique that is singular in its ability to record millisecond-by-millisecond changes in the brain following repeated external or internal events. Although the triggering events are often simple sensory stimuli, the cognitive processes that follow them and leave their trace in fluctuating voltage or magnetic fields can be quite complex. In the last decade competing noninvasive techniques such as positron emission tomography (PET) have challenged the preeminence of electrophysiology, particularly in spatial localization of brain processes. This challenge has stimulated a number of technological and methodological developments in acquiring, analyzing, and presenting brain electrical and magnetic data. But before we review these developments, we remind you of some basic principles and give examples of their relevance to psychiatry (see also Chapters 4, 5, and 29, *this volume,* for related discussion).

SOME BASIC PRINCIPLES

Nerve cells generate extracellular current flow by fluctuations in the slower changing membrane potentials of

W. T. Roth, J. M. Ford, and A. Pfefferbaum: Psychiatry Service, Department of Veterans Affairs Medical Center, Palo Alto, California 94304; and Department of Psychiatry and Behavioral Sciences, Stanford University School of Medicine, Stanford, California 94305.
T. R. Elbert: Institut für Experimentelle Audiologie, Westfälische Wilhelms-Universität, DH48129 Münster, Germany.

dendrites and cell bodies. Postsynaptic potentials cause an outflow of negative (excitatory) or positive (inhibitory) ionic charges into extracellular fluid, which are then pumped back into the cell. This current flow, when summated, results in volume-conducted potentials recorded at the scalp as the electroencephalogram (EEG). Event-related potentials (ERPs) are EEG changes that are time-locked to sensory, motor, or cognitive events. They have provided a way to evaluate brain functioning in mental disorders and the effects of psychoactive drugs. Recent conceptual and technical developments have greatly expanded our capability to understand and document the mechanisms underlying surface recordings. Particular attention has been paid to identifying the location, orientation, and distribution of current dipoles (pairs of opposite charges) that may be the sources of scalp-recorded electrical activity.

Nerve cells also generate intracellular current flow from dendrites to cell body. This flow results in a magnetic field that can be detected at the scalp as a magnetoencephalogram (MEG), even though it is a billionfold less intense than the earth's magnetic field. Event-related magnetic fields (ERFs) can be elicited and time-locked to specific events and are analogous to ERPs. Magnetoencephalograms and ERFs convey different information than EEG and ERPs. This is because voltage fields on the surface of a sphere, which the skull enclosing the brain approximates, are produced equally well by dipoles oriented radially and tangentially with respect to a radius of the sphere. In contrast, 90% of the magnetic field at the skull can be ascribed to tangential dipoles alone. This is a consequence of the geometrical orientation of masses of nerve cells and of magnetic sensors. Figure 1 illustrates how dipole orientation can be either correlated or random for different gyri and sulci. Parallel dipoles lying tangentially on sulcal walls contribute much more to the MEG than random dipoles or dipoles lying radially along the crowns of gyri.

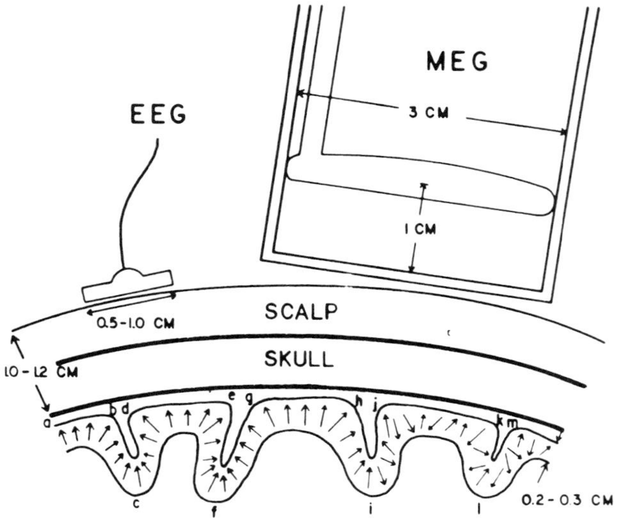

FIG. 1. An EEG is most sensitive to a similarly oriented dipole layer in the gyri (*ab*, *de*, *gh*), less sensitive to a similarly oriented dipole layer in the sulcus (*hi*), and insensitive to an opposing dipole layer in sulci (*bcd*, *efg*) and to a random dipole layer (*ijklm*). A MEG is most sensitive to a similarly oriented dipole layer in the sulcus (*hi*) and much less sensitive to all others. The latest MEG sensors are smaller than the one shown. From Nunez (47).

EVENT-RELATED POTENTIALS AND MAGNETIC FIELDS IN PSYCHIATRY

Why are the methodological issues that this chapter addresses relevant to psychiatrists and psychologists? First, ERPs and ERFs are theoretically relevant because they provide ways of testing theories of abnormal brain functioning that no other methods can offer. For example, unlike ordinary behavioral tests of cognitive processing, ERPs give an index of the processing of task-irrelevant events, distracting stimuli, or events subjects have been told to ignore. The topographic distribution of ERPs and ERFs gives clues as to what parts of the brain are active during a particular cognitive activity. Second, ERPs and to a less extent ERFs have been demonstrated empirically to be relevant. ERP abnormalities have been repeatedly observed in psychiatric disorders, notably in the P300 and P50 components. The P or N signifies positive or negative and the number is the mean peak latency in milliseconds. Thus, the P300 component is a positive potential that occurs approximately 300 msec after a stimulus that is infrequent and in some way relevant. The most venerable and consistent psychiatric ERP finding is that of reduced P300 amplitude in schizophrenics (60), although this is not specific to schizophrenia (see refs. 59 and 22 for reviews). For instance, a longitudinal study demonstrated that lower P300 amplitude at age 15 was predictive of poorer global personality functioning at age 25 (66). Latency at P300 is generally greater in patients with dementia than in normals or in patients with schizophrenia or

depression (28,54). Recently, psychiatric attention has been directed to P50, an ERP component to auditory stimuli whose amplitude is suppressed if the eliciting stimulus is paired with another that precedes it by one-half second. Schizophrenics show less P50 suppression than controls (25) as indicated by smaller amplitude ratios (P50 to the second stimulus of a pair divided by P50 to the first), although again this finding is not limited to schizophrenia (4).

Abnormalities of ERPs in psychiatric patients can be interpreted in light of a considerable amount of knowledge that has accumulated about the significance of certain ERP components in normal human information processing. For example, P300 is known to reflect the categorization of events, depending jointly on stimulus probability, stimulus significance, and the information value of the event (36). Probably, P300 has multiple, partially asynchronous generators (58). Components occurring 60 to 100 msec after onset of auditory stimuli, including N100, have been shown to reflect selective attention to auditory stimulus channels (42). In contrast, auditory ERPs with latencies less than 10 msec are insensitive to attention effects but give a unique assessment of the intactness of brainstem circuitry (32).

The literature on ERFs in normal subjects is quite extensive although magnetic recording techniques have been available only a relatively short time. Much of that literature has documented the existence of ERF components that parallel those established by invasive and noninvasive ERP recording. However, to date, most clinical MEG studies have been done in neurological rather than psychiatric patients, although that is likely to change in the near future. Reite et al. (57) recorded ERFs in six medicated, paranoid schizophrenic patients and six normal controls. The M100 component (analogous to the N100 of the ERP) showed less interhemispheric asymmetry in schizophrenics and had different source orientations in the left hemisphere. Tiihonen et al. (68) compared the M100 component in two schizophrenic patients when they were experiencing auditory hallucinations and when they were not. During hallucinations, M100 peaked approximately 20 msec later, an effect similar to that of external masking noise in normals.

We now turn to methodological trends that are transforming ERP and ERF research. Specific topics include data acquisition, signal averaging, ocular artifact, choice of reference electrodes, digital filtering, measuring components including dipole modeling, and statistical and diagnostic considerations.

DATA ACQUISITION

Electroencephalogram Systems

Older electroencephalographic tube-based amplifiers have been completely replaced with high impedance solid-state amplifiers with electronically controlled amplification and filter settings. In many laboratories, pen-chart recorders have been replaced with electronic data storage and display systems, but paper records are still widely used for visual analysis of diagnostic EEGs and sleep. Laboratory computers are constantly evolving toward faster, cheaper, and more powerful models. New storage media based on tape or magnetic or optical disks permit archiving of data from many subjects in an easily retrievable form. As welcome as these advances have been, they have generated difficult new choices for researchers. Should they buy commercial EEG and ERP hardware and software systems or develop their own? Which commercial systems or routes to laboratory-program development are satisfactory? Commercial systems tend to be limited in flexibility, details of data analysis may be a trade secret (which is unacceptable scientifically), and access to raw data for special analyses may be difficult. Laboratory-developed systems require deciding among manifold hardware and software possibilities, and then allocating many hours to programming. As will be learned from this chapter, methodologically up-to-date ERP analysis requires much more than eye-movement artifact rejection and signal averaging.

Whereas the conventional 10–20 system of Jasper (35) used 19 electrodes with a typical distance of 6 cm between them, some investigators have greatly expanded the electrode arrays in order to record more of the spatial detail present in the EEG. Thus arrays of 124, or even 256 electrodes, which yield interelectrode distances of 2.25 and 1.6 cm, are now being advocated (27) and have been shown to enhance localization. The application of multiple electrodes is a lengthy, labor-intensive process, which requires care in scalp preparation and accuracy in electrode placement. For localization studies relating EEG or MEG data to brain structures visualized by magnetic resonance imaging (MRI), it is important that electrodes be aligned correctly according to skull landmarks, and fiducial markers visible in MRI scans are used. (Vitamin E capsules are easily available and the right size.)

Electrode application entails a potential health risk to both subject and technician if the intactness of the scalp is compromised by procedures to reduce electrical resistance between electrode and scalp or by skin lesions. Acquired immunodeficiency syndrome and hepatitis B can both be transmitted by this route, so it is absolutely essential that proper precautions be taken. Putnam et al. (56) give recommendations for disinfecting reusable electrodes and for protecting the technician.

Magnetoencephalogram Systems

The recording of the MEG has been made practical by the development of superconducting quantum interference devices (SQUIDs) that are sensitive to minute magnetic fields. The MEG technology is much more expensive than the EEG technology. Not only are the SQUIDs themselves expensive, but they require provision for liquid helium at 4.2°K to cool them, and a recording room shielded with a high-permeability material against magnetic fields and with aluminum against eddy currents. The liquid helium is kept in a vacuum-insulated container called a dewar. Locating magnetic sources requires recording from multiple sites, preferably simultaneously. Otherwise, separate stimulation runs must be made, moving sensors from one location to another between runs. More runs take more recording time and increase the likelihood that the subject's mental state will change, altering the sources. A MEG system with over 30 channels costs approximately $3,000,000, 100 times more than the same number of EEG channels. Because MEG prices reflect the cost of research and development more than construction of the apparatus, the price per unit would drop if more units were sold. In one system, 37 sensors are placed 2.2 cm apart to cover a single hemisphere (12).

An advantage of MEG sensors is that they do not touch the head, so transmission of infectious agents is of less concern. Fixation of head position is critical so that sensors can be aligned according to skull landmarks. Modern SQUID technology allows recording of signals that vary slowly over a minute, undisturbed by electrode drift. A new method for recording even slower or static magnetic fields converts such fields to more rapidly changing fields by having the subject lie on a mechanically driven platform that executes a circular movement of a few centimeters at 0.2 Hz (26). Auditory and visual stimulation cannot be given by conventional earphones or CRT displays because of their magnetic properties. Instead, sounds have to be delivered from outside the testing chamber through hollow tubes and visual stimuli projected through a window in the magnetic shield or delivered fiber optically.

SIGNAL AVERAGING

Both ERPs and ERFs benefit greatly from signal averaging to enhance their signal-to-noise ratio (SNR). Data are generally digitized at a fixed rate to fill a data array, and a stimulus or other synchronizing event defines the time epoch of interest within this array. The event is repeated (each repetition is called a trial), and a time-locked signal (ensemble) average is calculated across trials epochs for each time point of the epoch. If $X_j(t)$ is the electrical potential (voltage) or magnetic field strength at some electrode or sensor location at time t and trial j, the signal average is defined as

$$\bar{X}_t = \frac{1}{J} \sum_{j=1}^{J} X_{jt}$$

If X_{jt} is considered the sum of true signal μ_t and random noise N_{jt} (background EEG and measurement error), signal averaging improves the SNR. Unbiased estimates of signal power $\hat{\sigma}_S^2$, noise power $\hat{\sigma}_N^2$, and SNR can be calculated as follows (71).

$$\hat{\sigma}_S^2 = \frac{1}{T} \sum_{t=1}^{T} \bar{X}_t^2 - \frac{1}{J} \hat{\sigma}_N^2$$

$$\hat{\sigma}_N^2 = \frac{1}{T(J-1)} \sum_{j=1}^{J} \left(\sum_{t=1}^{T} (X_{jt} - \bar{X}_t)^2 \right) \approx \text{Variance } \bar{X}_t$$

$$\text{SNR} = \hat{\sigma}_S^2 / \hat{\sigma}_N^2$$

One of the assumptions of signal averaging is that the signal is invariant across trials. This assumption is violated when the amplitude of the ERP component of interest habituates or when its latency varies from trial to trial, as is clearly the case for components related to certain cognitive processes, such as the P300. One way of dealing with component latency variability is to locate the signal on each trial and align the trials on these signals rather than on the eliciting stimulus. Woody (75) proposed an iterative procedure (an adaptive filter) that located the signal on each single trial by moving a template (initially the signal average) by time increments along the trial to find the latency of maximum correlation. A new average was then formed by aligning trials on the identified signal latencies, and the new average was used as a new template. If the SNR is too low, this procedure produces results that simply reflect random noise. Gratton et al. (31) tested the procedure with simulated signals and background EEG noise and demonstrated that iterations (up to three) were important only when the original template had a wavelength on the order of two times longer than the signal.

Roth et al. (61) used this procedure to analyze ERPs elicited from schizophrenics and controls performing an auditory choice reaction time paradigm in order to test whether P300 amplitude reduction in schizophrenics could be attributed to latency variability. They found that individual trial P300 latency was indeed more variable in schizophrenics but that schizophrenic P300 amplitude was still smaller than control amplitude after latency adjustment. To reduce distortions due to noise, Pfefferbaum and Ford (53) modified the procedure by only including trials whose covariance is greater in the part of the epoch where signal is expected than in the part where noise is expected, and whose correlation with the template (initially a half-sine wave) exceeds a set threshold. Using this modified procedure, Ford et al. (23) replicated the Roth et al. (61) finding that schizophrenic P300 remained smaller. Furthermore, schizophrenics had more trials that did not pass the covariance–correlation screen than controls. Trials that did not qualify for latency adjustment had longer reaction times, showing that they were deviant behaviorally as well as electrophysiologically. In addition, Ford et al. calculated for each subject the covariance of P300 signal average across trials with that subject's EEG in single signal epochs and in single nonsignal epochs. The ratio of mean signal covariance to mean noise covariance was significantly smaller in the schizophrenics. Because trials were filtered with a bandpass of 0.5 to 4.4 Hz, noise was EEG activity in the frequency range of P300 rather than higher frequency like α, β, or muscle activity.

Another assumption of signal averaging is that background EEG noise is random noise. This is only an approximation to the truth, as a study of event-related spectral perturbation indicates (41). In normal subjects, auditory tone pips reliably produced momentary increases in spectral power in the 2- to 8-Hz and 10- to 40-Hz bands.

EYE MOVEMENT AND BLINK ARTIFACT

Eye movement and blinks produce electrical potentials and magnetic fields that are often much larger than those deriving from brain sources. The magnetic fields are more restricted to the vicinity of the eye than are the electrical fields and for this reason are less troublesome if unsynchronized with events of experimental interest. Synchronized eye artifact can cause major errors in peak measurement or source localization. Attempts to control this artifact by instructing subjects to fixate their gaze on a point or not to blink are often ineffective, particularly if the subject is psychotic or cognitively impaired. Thus methods for removing eye artifact from the ERP or ERF need to be applied. Many are based on determining the coefficients A_k in the equation

$$V(k,t) = A_k * \text{EOG}(t) + \text{EEG}(k,t)$$

where $V(k,t)$ is the voltage observed in lead k at time t, and $\text{EOG}(t)$ and $\text{EEG}(k,t)$ are the true EOG and EEG voltage contributions at that time.

Spatial-temporal dipole models of eye movements and blinks make it clear that the same correction cannot be used for both (6). Thus eye-correction procedures should include at a minimum the following steps: (a) Separate blinks from movements on the basis of their temporal properties, (b) calculate separate linear regressions for the propagation of artifacts from each, and (c) correct EEG leads by the amount predicted by the regression coefficients. Gratton et al. (29), whose method has been used by a number of investigators, adds an additional step of subtracting signal averages from individual trials to avoid distortions resulting from ERP effects in both EEG and EOG records. A computerized implementation of this procedure that adjusts for both a vertical and a horizontal EOG channel, has been developed (43). Although certain technical issues in implementing EOG corrections remain unresolved—the proper number and position of EOG electrodes, the error attendant upon assuming a linear relationships between the EOG signal and EEG artifacts, the implications of the presence of EEG artifacts in EOG leads, how to deal with overlapping eye movement and blinks, and instability of individual propagation factors between sessions and even between tasks within a session (19)—the use of such off-line procedures have greatly increased the number of trials available for analysis in clinical studies.

REFERENCE ELECTRODES

Whereas MEG sensors detect the absolute magnetic field at a given location in space and need no reference in the body, the EEG must be measured as voltage differences between two points on or in the organism. Ideally one point should be close to the biological voltage source under investigation, and the other should be a reference point with constant voltage or at least a voltage not correlated with the source voltage. Traditional references for human ERP have been linked mastoids, linked ears, or the nose; unfortunately none of these is unaffected by brain sources. Special disadvantages of linked ear references include the possibility that shorting can reduce asymmetry if resistance is low, and the possibility that artifactual spatial asymmetry will result if resistances at the two ears are not equal (48). Shorting is not a serious consideration as long as skin-electrode resistance at each ear is greater than 5 kΩ, because in that case scalp path resistance is reduced less than 5% (44). Resistance at the two ears can be balanced with a potentiometer, or one ear (say A1) can be used as a reference and recorded as a separate channel. Then a linked ear reference for say Cz, a scalp electrode in the 10–20 system, can be created algebraically, $(Cz - A1) - (A2 - A1)/2 = Cz - (A1 + A2)/2$.

To avoid active reference electrodes on the head, some investigators have turned to noncephalic (e.g., sternovertebral) electrodes (67). Unfortunately these electrodes are liable to pick up heart activity even when adjusted to be at right angles to the main vector of voltage during the cardiac cycle, since cardiac depolarization and repolarization vectors do not maintain a perfectly constant direction over the cycle.

Another solution is to use an average reference. At each time point, an average reference defines zero over C electrodes in a data array A as

$$\sum_{c=1}^{C} A_c = 0$$

A limitation of the average reference is that when electrodes are not densely and equally spaced around the brain, for example, there are none at the bottom of the head (69), the sum in the formula above is generally different from true zero. For example, Desmedt et al. (16) have shown that P14 of the somatosensory evoked response, which is present with a linked ears reference, disappears when a zero reference based on 27 scalp electrodes is applied, becoming surrounded by ''ghost'' negativities. A linked-ear reference reflects more accurately the medial lemniscal volley that is the presumed basis of P14. In addition, local changes can be mistaken for global changes with a zero reference. These distortions are less likely to affect tangential than radial dipoles.

In conclusion, there is no perfect reference for all cases. As a general principle, a known local source should be referred to an electrode distant from it.

FILTERING

Before measurements are made on ERPs or ERFs, it is useful to apply SNR-enhancing filters that incorporate assumptions about frequency, timing, and spatial distribution of the component of interest. For example, the ERP P300 component may be expected from experiments in the literature to have a frequency lower than 2 Hz (30), to peak in a range of 280 to 400 msec (in a simple auditory choice reaction time task in young adults) and to be maximal at Pz, another electrode in the 10–20 system. Though signal averaging attenuates unsynchronized noise at every frequency as it improves SNR, frequency filters are commonly applied prior to component measurement. These filters are useful whenever the frequency of the noise is different from that of the signal.

Digital Filters

Digital frequency filters (11) have the advantage over analog filters of being able to operate without introducing distorting phase shifts into the signal. The most commonly used digital filter has been the moving average or boxcar filter, in which each point of the signal is replaced by an average of that point and a certain number of prior and subsequent points. This is only possible for stored data, because it makes use of future time points to calculate current output. Farwell et al. (20) have shown that a simple moving average filter does not prepare average and single-trial waveforms as well for P300 peak-picking as does a filter designed by an optimizing algorithm. Such an algorithm determines a set of weights that are able to reduce deviations (ripple or ringing) in the passband and stopband of the filter. Optimized filters have less tendency to reduce P300 amplitude or distort shape and, in the case of averages, gave more stable latency measurements. For P300, the authors recommend that the optimum filter have a passband cut-off frequency of 6 Hz, a stopband cut-off frequency of 8 or 8.5 Hz, and use $490/n$ points, where n is the sampling interval in milliseconds. It should be emphasized that analog filters still have a place in data acquisition prior to digital filtering—a low-pass analog filter with a half-power frequency below but close to half the sampling rate prevents aliasing, and, for P300 recording, a high-pass analog filter with a half-power frequency of less than 0.16 Hz minimizes irrelevant baseline shifts (20).

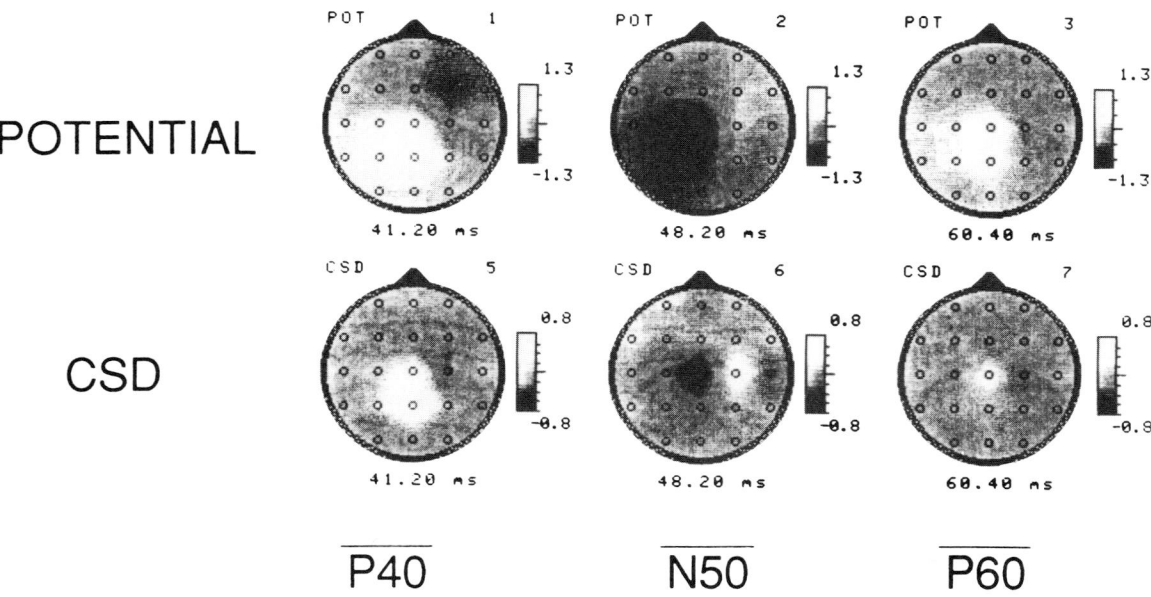

FIG. 2. Potential (voltage) and current source density (CSD) maps of the somatosensory evoked response (SER) following left (*lt*) tibial nerve (*N*) stimulation. Data are based on averages of responses to 500 to 1,000 electrical stimuli delivered at a rate of 2.1/sec to a healthy man. Maps are given for P40, N50, and P60 components (P or N signify positive and negative, and the number is the mean peak latency in msec). Lighter shading is more positive. Note that localization of components is better in CSD maps than in potential maps. Adapted from Nagamine et al. (46).

Spatial Filters

Current source density maps (also called surface Laplacian or radial current estimate maps) act as spatial filters emphasizing localized components with a high spatial frequency. For this to work well of course, electrodes must be placed with a high spatial frequency. Maps can be made of unaveraged activity such as epileptic spikes or of signal averages. Sensory ERP components show a more localized distribution using this approach than in voltage maps. For example, Nagamine et al. (46) compared voltage and current source density maps on the scalp ERPs obtained by tibial nerve stimulation. The results for a single subject presented in Fig. 2 demonstrate better localization for P40, N50, and P60 for the current source density map. The equation for calculating current source density is $I = \rho(\delta^2 V/\delta x^2 + \delta^2 V/\delta y^2)$, where V is the voltage, x and y the surface location on the x–y plane, and ρ the charge density. In addition, $\rho = k * d^2$, where d is the distance between electrodes and k is a constant for all electrodes within a subject. The Laplacian operator can give limits for finding equivalent dipoles. It has a physical interpretation—local radial current flow from the brain into the scalp and vice versa—but it is different from dipole modeling (described below) and is free of dipole modeling's ambiguities.

In the Laplacian calculation, surface contours can be generated by a method called spherical spline interpolation, which is based on physical principles for minimizing the deformation energy of a thin sphere constrained to pass through known points (51). This produces a smooth surface running through the data values and filling in between them, even when electrodes are irregularly placed on the scalp. Spherical splines have advantages over plate splines, which are based on deformation of an infinite thin plate. As might be expected from the fact that interpolated values at any point are derived from data from other locations, coherence (a measure of covariation) is inflated by interpolation. Nearest-neighbor interpolations are less smooth and inferior for locating extrema (peaks and troughs must lie on an electrode site) but do not inflate coherence.

Gevins et al. (27) have demonstrated a method of current source density mapping they call *finite element model deblurring* that they believe is superior to the Laplacian method. Mathematically, it is a less computationally demanding version of dipole modeling known as spatial deconvolution, which assumes that all dipoles are located on a cortical surface. Gevins et al. use the subject's head MRI to provide information about conducting volumes between scalp and cortical surfaces.

A simpler spatial filter, the vector filter (30), has been used for component measurement. Its output is the weighted sum of data points at different electrodes. Conceptually, measuring a component at one lead is the same as applying a vector filter with weight 1 assigned to values at that lead and weight 0 to values at all other leads. Vector filtering assumes that the distribution of the component to be measured is constant despite changes in amplitude or latency. The crux of the procedure is how to specify the weights: using three 10–20 system scalp electrodes, Fz, Cz, and Pz, weights of 0.15 for Fz, −0.53 for Cz, and 0.83 for Pz were found to produce optimal discrimination in an oddball paradigm between rare trials, which contain substantial P300s, and frequent trials, which do not (30). Thus, optimum weights do not necessarily correspond to component distribution, because P300 is larger at Cz than at Fz. Dipole modeling, which is described below, can act as both a spatial and temporal filter.

MEASURING COMPONENTS

Measurement Methods

A component can be defined as electrical or magnetic activity associated with a specific neurological or psychological process, for example, a motor act such as moving one's finger, a sensory process such as the reaction to a light flash, or a cognitive process such as categorizing a stimulus as target or nontarget. In a statistical sense a component explains experimental variance. The details of the experimental method are part of the operational definition of a component. As more experiments are done, theoretical expectations about components develop into generalizations. For example, many experiments in which subjects performed a fixed foreperiod reaction time task have resulted in a parietal–central negative shift prior to the button press. A natural generalization is that the parietal–central shift represents preparation for a motor act. Furthermore, because the source of the recorded data is a physical location within the brain, the ultimate description of a component must include reference to the specific brain structures activated. Some leads or sensors will pick up activity from those structures better than others, particularly when sources are multiple with overlapping influences. In the case of ERPs, the choice of voltage reference influences how electrical activity from a source appears in the EEG recording.

Measurement procedures include peak picking, area measurement, waveform subtraction, principal components analysis, template correlation, and dipole modeling. *Peak picking* means finding maxima or minima in specified latency ranges and determining peak latency and amplitude with respect to a prestimulus baseline. This is the simplest method of component evaluation, but can be biased when latency ranges are selected after an inspection of the data, and is perhaps unduly restricted in that it considers only peaks among other waveform features. In addition, it is often based on only one point, which may be influenced by noise or overlapping components. With multiple leads, another limitation of peak picking becomes obvious: what appears by shape to be a single component has maxima at different time points in different leads, and it is not clear how best to resolve the

discrepancies. Furthermore, the choice of reference electrodes can determine when peaks and troughs appear.

Area measurement is sometimes used when the component is believed to be more rectangular than peaked. Area is measured in a specified latency range, and is thus based on multiple points, but area measurement, like peak picking, can be biased and is influenced by overlapping components.

Waveform subtraction can be used before peak picking or area measurement to reduce the effects of component overlap. For example, consider a paradigm where tones of two pitches are given in an unpredictable sequence and one occurs less frequently and is designated as the target of some task. The ERP to the rare tone can be considered a combination of the sensory effects of the tone and the cognitive effects of the tone being a rare target. By subtracting the ERP to the frequent tones from the ERP to the infrequent tones, the sensory effects are removed leaving behind the cognitive effects. This assumes that the sensory responses to the two tones are identical and that cognitive and sensory effects are additive, an assumption that is not always warranted. For example, frequency-specific temporal recovery of the auditory N100, a non-cognitive effect, makes the response of N100 to frequents smaller than the response of N100 to rares.

Principal components analysis (PCA) is another approach to ERP component measurement, which uses the time points on waveforms from different subjects, different electrodes, and different experimental conditions to define components. In statistical terms PCA identifies orthogonal axes of maximal variance in a multidimensional space defined by the variables. Generally these axes are rotated according to the varimax procedure. Less arbitrary than peak picking, PCA makes no assumption about the latency range in which specific components will be found but only that they have a fixed latency across conditions and subjects. It has some ability to separate overlapping components. However, PCA is not completely free from arbitrariness. First, PCA solutions are not unique. Many rotations of the factors are possible. Second, results depend to a certain extent on what experimental conditions are chosen and how many leads are included. Variance from electrodes, subjects, conditions, and correlated noise are all treated the same. Furthermore, each experiment gives slightly different factor structures, and there is no established criterion for deciding whether these differences are significant or not. Thus, it is uncertain how many statistical components to interpret, and how to identify these components with ones previously described.

Template correlation assesses the similarity of a template of the component to the waveform to be evaluated. The template may be based on prior knowledge of the component shape or on signal averages (see the iterative Woody filter procedure described above). The template is usually compared to waveforms at specified intervals over a designated latency range to identify the latency of maximum correlation (or in one variation, maximum

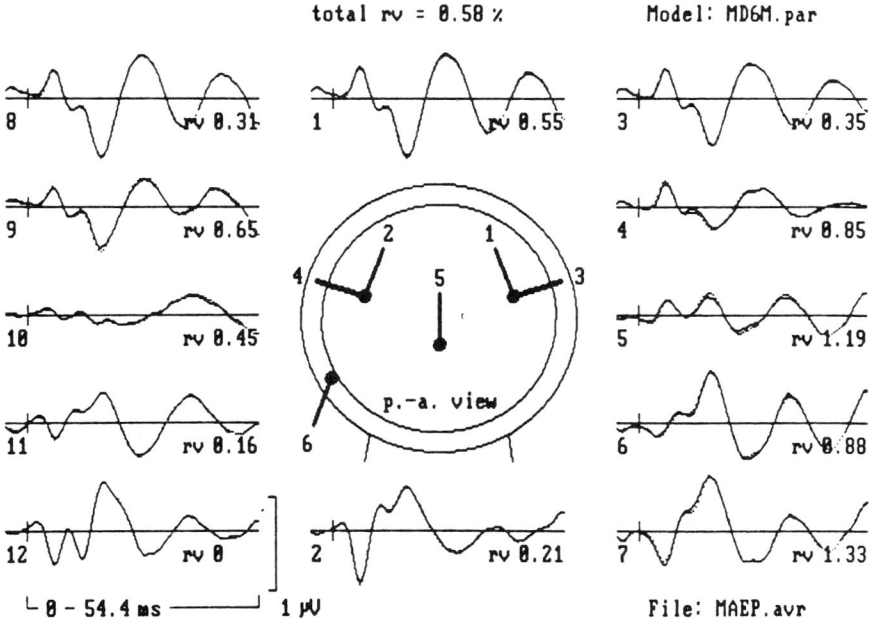

FIG. 3. Coronal ERP scalp distribution to clicks in a 38-year-old man. He was presented with 2,000 trials of 70-dB HR right ear clicks at 60-msec intervals. On a head model viewed from the front are drawn the six dipoles that were found by modeling to account for the most variance in the most anatomically plausible way. From Scherg (63).

covariance). This time point is defined as the peak. The sum of cross products at this time point or the difference between amplitude at this point and a baseline can define amplitude.

Interpreting latency data under different experimental conditions can be difficult when multiple leads are involved. Latency may vary at different leads and topography may vary under different conditions, implying different components whose latency cannot be compared. To solve these problems, Brandeis et al. (8) spatially generalized the Woody filter procedure using an average reference map, and applying a measure they call global field power (GFP) defined by the following formula for an array A consisting of data from C electrodes:

$$GFP(A) = \left[\frac{1}{C} \sum_{c=1}^{C} A_c^2 \right]^{1/2}$$

Further, global dissimilarity (GD) is defined as the root mean square (rms) power of the difference maps calculated by subtracting two normalized GFP maps. The procedure is as follows: (a) Grand averages are used to form template GFP maps, from which component model maps at single latencies near 100, 200, and 400 msec are derived, corresponding to P1, N1, and P3 (see ref. 8 for details). (b) Component model maps are moved in specified latency ranges around the latency of each model's component. The minimum of GD multiplied by sequential dissimilarity (GD between current and previous map: a stability constraint) is calculated, and the minimum of this function (best fit) is defined as the map latency for that component. (c) In an iteration, the average of all normalized maps at their latencies of best fit is used as a new model, and the search window is set around the new mean latency. The results show that components can be identified by topography alone, without respect to ampli-

tude or time. However, this method does not take into account possible overlapping components and would fail if such components influenced topographies. Furthermore, average references for P300, which is widely distributed on the top of the head, may be inferior to a noncephalic reference.

Dipole modeling is a method for reducing data from multilead EEG or multisource MEG by deducing the dipole sources that may have produced them. Although the forward problem (calculating scalp distribution from known dipoles) has a unique solution whose accuracy is limited only by the approximations of skull geometry and conductivities, the inverse problem has multiple mathematically valid solutions as was pointed about by Helmholz more than a century ago (33). The reason is that a single scalp distribution can be produced by different numbers of dipoles in different combinations of locations and orientations. Thus, various constraints on the number of sources allowed and their approximate location must be applied to reach a solution. Sometimes these constraints are so severe as to specify that the source be a single dipole located somewhere in the brain.

At an abstract level, dipole modeling is like PCA in that an equation $U = C * S$ must be solved where U is an array of k electrodes at t times that represents the linear superimposition of the array S of m sources at t times multiplied by C weighing coefficients at k electrodes for m sources (62). Whereas PCA determines C and S from mathematical constraints, dipole modeling assumes that C depends on volume conduction from j dipoles at certain locations, assuming $C_{kj} = f(r_j, o_j, e_k)$, where f is a nonlinear function of the electrode location vector e_k and of the geometry of the source and the head. The dipole has a location vector r_j and the orientation vector o_j. Equations defining a 3-shell sphere model of the head with differing

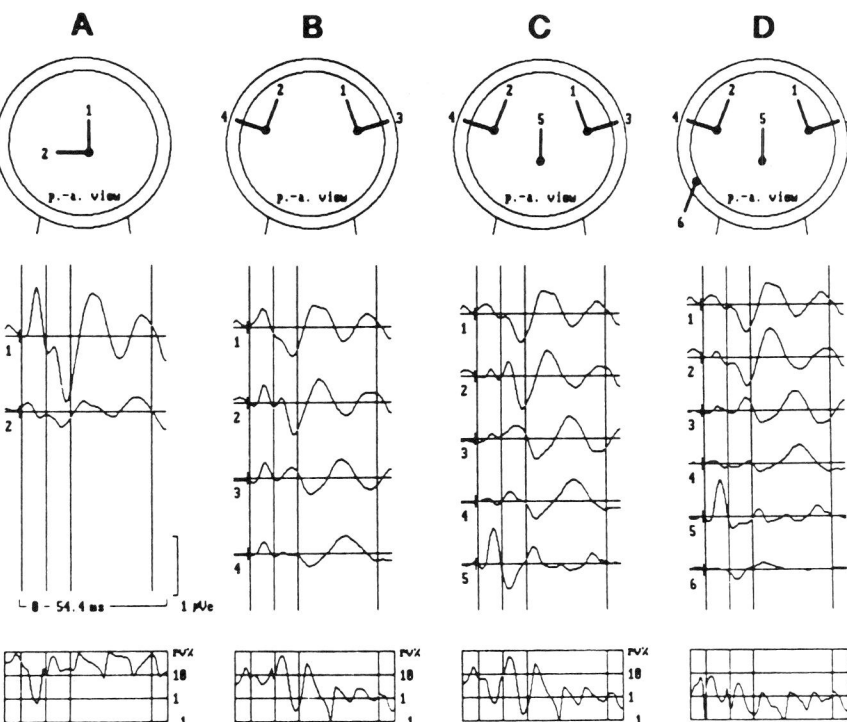

FIG. 4. Dipole source potentials and residual variance (RV) as evaluated from the data in Fig. 3 by hypothetical models A to D. *Vertical bars* mark the latency intervals 1–10 msec, 10–19 msec, and 19–49 msec. **A** shows that a central source is necessary to account for activity in the first interval as seen by a dip in RV. **B** shows that bilateral temporal pole sources account for considerable variance in the second interval, and **D** that adding a unilateral scalp source (due to myogenic reflex activity) gives a better solution than **C**, which is based on the results of A and B together. From Scherg (63).

conductivities for scalp, skull, and brain are found in the appendix to this chapter. Using these equations to model dipoles at various depths, Pfefferbaum (52) demonstrated how increasing the thickness of the superficial extrasulcal subarachnoid layer of cerebrospinal fluid (CSF) or skull thickness might affect scalp ERP amplitudes and topographic distributions.

One procedure for the dipole modeling of ERPs was developed by Scherg and Berg (64). Their software is available commercially as brain electrical source analysis (BESA, from Neuroscan, Inc.). It models a window of points, assuming a finite number of equivalent dipoles with fixed location and orientation. In its recent version, it does not assume a parametric dipole magnitude function (like the decaying sinusoid of ref. 70) but computes a varying magnitude function over the window of points for each dipole. The BESA model is applied iteratively, calculating at each step the residual variance (percentage of recorded data not explained by the model). The first step looks for the inverse solution by calculating parameters of a plausible dipole from an EEG or MEG data map. Then forward solutions calculate resultant EEG or MEG maps from those dipoles. Hundreds of iterations may take place, stopping when the change in residual variance is less than some criterion, such as 0.001%. When more than one dipole is modeled, some may be fixed in position (but not in amplitude) while a new dipole is optimized. The results of these procedures depend among other things on the starting location and other parameters of a dipole. An iterative procedure may find topographically local optima that would not be optima if all locations and orientations were tested. Scherg and Berg (64) explained that multiple-source solutions are less arbitrary if spatial

and temporal constraints are added. For example, two sources may be required to have a symmetry between hemispheres, radial and tangential dipoles, or lie in the supratemporal plane. How this method works is illustrated in Figs. 3 and 4. Figure 3 shows ERPs to clicks and resultant dipoles that were inferred from these ERPs. Figure 4 shows how well four models account for the data. The model that explains the greatest amount of the variance (99.4%) and corresponds best to anatomic reality assumes six dipoles: one central, two bilaterally symmetrical pairs, and one unilateral, coming from the postauricular muscle. Of course, some of the 99.4% may be noise rather than signal.

Other procedures are possible. Turetsky et al. (70) developed a method called the dipole components model, which simultaneously fits multilead data from a time window in multiple averages, pooling noise estimates. It assumes that the component shape is a decaying sinusoid and that the skull is a sphere of homogeneous conductivity. Turetsky et al. (70) applied it to P300 elicited in an auditory oddball paradigm and found four dipoles in two dimensions, three of which varied with experimental conditions. Cardenas et al. (9) applied it to the P50 suppression paradigm in the reliability study described below.

A single dipole modeled at brief intervals can mathematically generate a moving trajectory of loci. The two main alternatives to single dipole modeling are multiple dipole models and fully distributed models (34). For the second, a probability density is generated for widely distributed current sources. In addition, cylinders rather than points may be modeled. A distinction between a point source and a region can only be made if the region is of a size comparable to the distance between sensors.

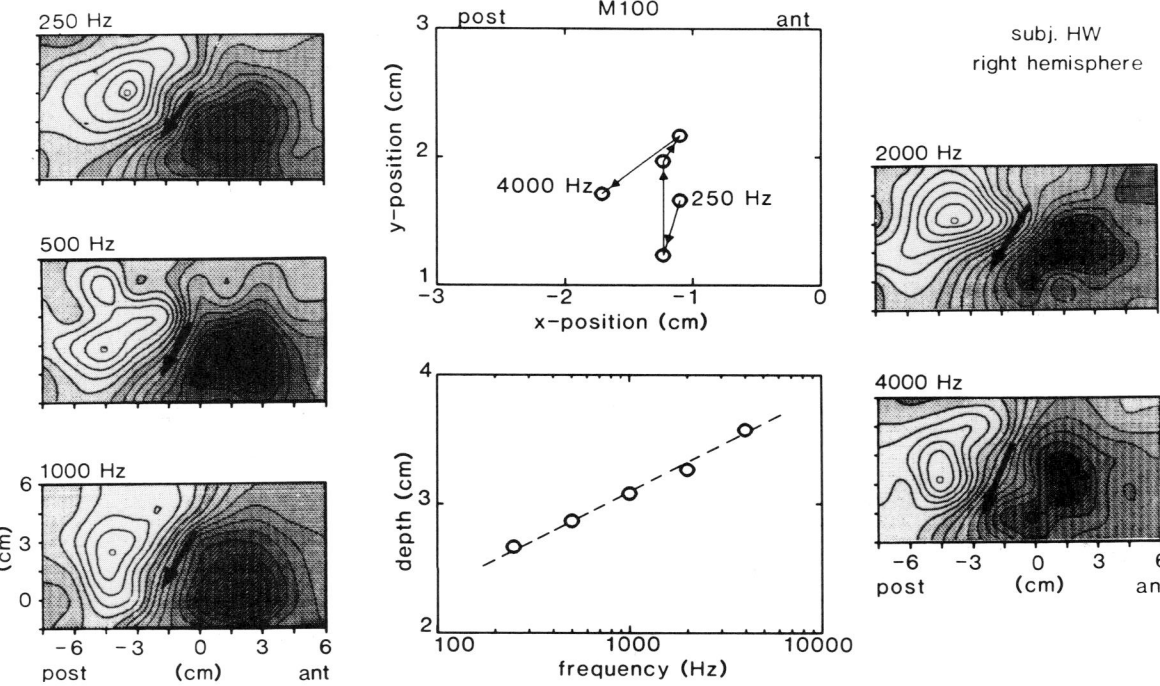

FIG. 5. Isofield right hemisphere ERF plots at a latency of 88 msec for four tone pitches in a left-handed subject. 500-msec, 60-dB HL tones were presented to the left ear at 4-sec intervals. Field strength is encoded with a gray scale (*dark,* outgoing flux; *light,* ingoing flux). In the middle column are the positions of the current dipoles associated with each tone. The *dark arrow* indicates the location and orientation of the current dipoles, their length proportional to the dipole moment. The origin of the coordinate system is T4. From Pantev et al. (50).

For a MEG, it is not necessary to employ a layer model because magnetic permeability is unaffected by variations in conductivity. In practice only the radial component of the field is measured because it is convenient to place pickup coils parallel to the scalp (reviewed in ref. 39). Although generally it is assumed that the source is composed of similarly oriented and concurrently active neurons, this simplification is clearly wrong in certain cases, such as the folds of the visual cortex, which are better modeled by a cross-shaped arrangement of dipoles. The strength of the resultant dipole detected at the scalp depends very much on the symmetry. Synchronization (as with the appearance of α waves) may actually be a periodic breaking of symmetry of activation of the component dipoles (39).

Often, ERF analyses use peak data to model the dipole, because the SNR is likely to be highest there. An example of a dipole analysis in which the results were coordinated with MRI scan data is the work of Pantev et al. (50). They analyzed ERFs elicited by auditory tones of varying pitches and based on at least 96 trials for each pitch from each of 60 measuring positions at the M100 peak (in this case at 88 msec) for a single current dipole source. Figure 5 shows isofield contour plots of the ERF at 88 msec for a single subject and the positions of the dipoles associated with each pitch. Figure 6 shows the coronal MRI section with the dipole locations for that subject. They lie just

below the surface of the transverse temporal gyrus (Heschl), the assumed location of the primary auditory cortex, and are ordered in depth by pitch. Modeling before and after the peak may give somewhat different dipoles, but it is hard to exclude the possibility that they are spurious. To accentuate the onset of activation of weak secondary dipoles, Moran et al. (45) calculated dipoles associated with auditory ERFs on the basis of differences in magnetic fields in 4-msec intervals between 0 and 300 msec. This interval selects for components of a frequency high enough to change during it. Using this method, the authors found evidence for a source spatially separate from N1m but coactive with it. A distributed source in Heschl's gyrus and adjacent areas could also produce such a result.

The number of sensors (SQUIDs or electrodes) is important. For ERFs we need to know $n * 5$ parameters if n is the number of sources and, for ERPs, $n * 6$ (65). For ERPs, this means a minimum of $(n * 6) + 1$ electrodes. Thus, the conventional 19 electrodes allow only 1 or 2 generators to be determined. The results of dipole modeling can be ambiguous in that substantially different models provide only trivially inferior fits. It is more important to analyze the number of sources and their gross location than their exact location. A good initial approximation escapes local minima in residual (unexplained) variance but begs the question. Noise, particularly if it is spatiotem-

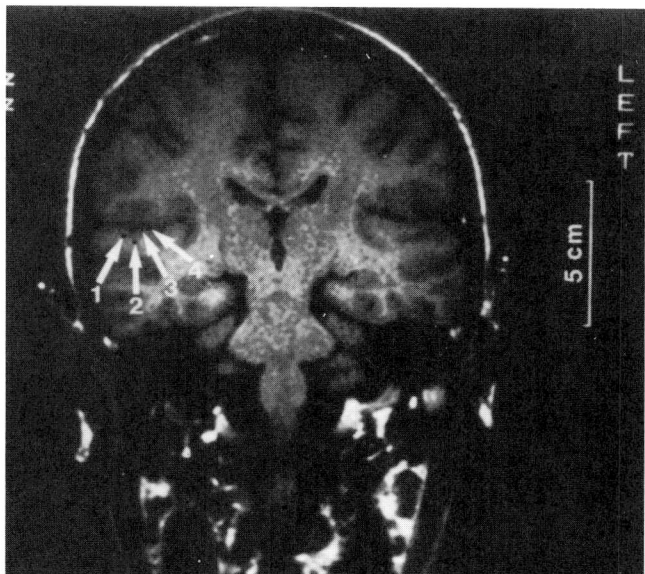

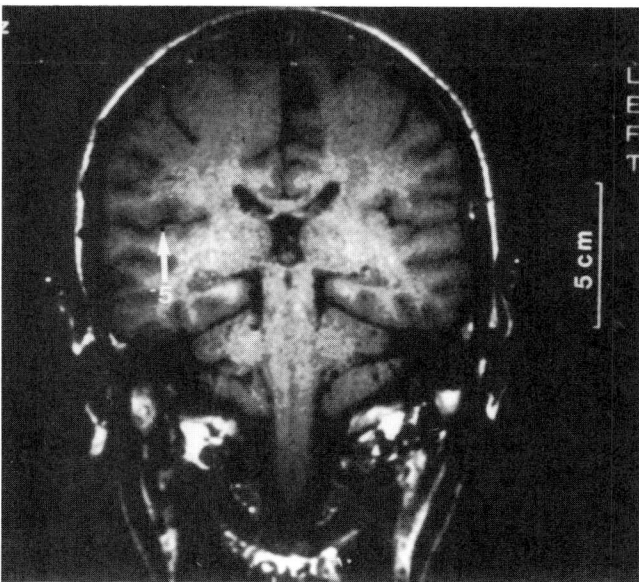

FIG. 6. Coronal MRI tomogram of the subject whose data are presented in Figure 5. Locations of the current dipoles are marked by black dots at the tips of the arrows. From Pantev et al. (50).

Witt et al. (74) applied dipole modeling to brainstem auditory evoked potentials (BAEPs). These authors recorded simultaneously from 12 electrodes constituting three three-channel bipolar montages. Data from all montages were transformed to fit the same central dipole. The authors concluded that a tetrahedral montage equivalent to Einthoven's Triangle for the EKG is adequate for clinical work, although it is slightly inaccurate because the dipole is known to move over time.

In an investigation of a nonsensory ERF, Elbert et al. (17) measured the magnetic field prior to button response in a go–no-go reaction time task. With this task, the EEG shows a negative shift prior to the button press called the contingent negative variation (CNV). The magnetic equivalent, which they called the contingent magnetic variation (CMV), was larger for go than no-go conditions, but a moving single dipole model accounted for less than 80% of the variance in four of eight subjects. The authors conclude that the later parts of the CMV are particularly dependent on distributed sources in motor, sensory, and association areas. Another component that is likely to have multiple sources is P300 (37). Turetsky et al. (70) applied their dipole model to model electrical P300 in 18 subjects using data from the oddball two-tone choice reaction time task. Using four dipoles in the midsaggital plane, they could explain approximately two-thirds of the total variance across subjects, conditions, and electrodes.

An unsolved problem with dipole estimation is how to decide if dipoles are equivalent. For example, experimenters may want to statistically compare dipoles modeled from individual subjects to draw general conclusions valid for a group, yet each dipole will vary somewhat in its location and orientation from every other. In the approach of Turetsky et al. (70), a single solution encompasses all subjects and conditions in an experiment, but it is still important to be able to compare dipoles between experiments. A related problem is how many of the multiple component dipoles generated in a given application of a model should be considered valid. This is analogous to the problem of how many PCA components to accept in a given analysis.

Measurement Reliabilities

The reliability and accuracy of certain computerized methods for measuring P300 has been assessed for averages and single trials. Reliability of automated measurement is a function of two factors that are often difficult to untangle: the stability of the underlying component being measured over time and the effects of electrical sources other than the component (background EEG and muscle and eye artifact). Whatever its cause, unreliability reduces a measure's usefulness.

Recent parametric studies have illuminated some of the variables underlying unreliability. Fabiani et al. (19) found that P300 latency estimates of averages had split-

porally organized, can distort solutions by creating local minima. Achim et al. (1) created simulations and used a variety of procedures to analyze them. By using several initial approximations (rather than simply reinitializing with a previous solution) and a multiplicity of optimizations, they managed largely to escape local minima. Precise localization is prevented by the presence of background EEG noise. Errors ranged from 2.5% to 13% of sphere radius. The authors developed a residual orthogonality test for testing the presence of signal in residues after modeling.

Sensory ERPs and ERFs are more likely to be amenable to dipole modeling than more complex cognitive ones.

half reliabilities between 0.63 and 0.88, and in most paradigms was rather similar for peak picking and template correlation. Amplitude estimates of P300 were most reliable (between 0.90 and 0.96) when based on covariance with a full-cycle 2-Hz cosinusoidal wave. Making measurements at Pz alone was almost as good as using the output of a vector filter based on Fz, Cz, and Pz. Subtracting averages of frequent trials from infrequent trials led to more reliable measurement of the probability effect than when the two types of trials were measured separately. Test–retest reliabilities of both amplitude and latency were lower between than within sessions, probably because of changes in P300 over time. Gratton et al. (31) did a simulation study of P300 single-trial latency estimation, embedding known signals in noise from actual EEG records adjusted to give various SNRs. Peak picking and several methods of template correlation were compared after data were prepared by frequency filtering with various lowpass parameters (in some comparisons, 6.29 to 2.38 Hz) and sometimes by vector filtering. Accuracy of latency estimation increased exponentially with the template SNR. Regardless of the SNR, template crosscorrelation was better than peak picking. Vector filtering helped, but with lower lowpass frequencies, the differences were rather small (in one comparison, the optimum lowpass cutoff was 1.76 Hz). Vector filtering was most useful when overlapping components of different distributions were simulated.

P50 is a more difficult component to measure than P300 because its amplitude is 10% to 25% that of P300. Typically measurements have been made by human observers picking peaks from averages of 32 trials. The ratio of P50 amplitudes to paired conditioning (S1) and testing (S2) stimuli is calculated. Ratios are less reliable than measurement of the numerator or denominator alone because ratios combine the statistically independent noise of both measures (3,9). Two studies have found the reliabilities of P50 amplitude ratios to be less than 0.15 (7,38). Freedman (24) has emphasized the importance of using only moderate intensity clicks and recording with the subject in a supine position for minimizing muscle artifact. Cardenas et al. (9) showed that the reliability of S2/S1 could be improved by applying the dipole modeling method of Turetsky et al. (70) to averages of 110 to 120 trials filtered with a 10- to 50-Hz bandpass. Even though reliability for peak picking was only 0.27 (interclass correlation of 6 repetitions), it was 0.63 for a model that fit a single source simultaneously to P50s evoked by S1 and S2. One caveat about reliabilities from dipole modeling is that complex computational methods can achieve results that turn out to be artifactual in simulations. These checks have yet to be made.

Accuracy of Source Localization

To accurately locate brain sources a number of known error sources must be controlled. Electrodes or magnetic sensors must be accurately placed in relation to the skull. A precise alignment of dipole and structural brain images must be made and the SNR must be enhanced. Assumptions of mathematical models for computing the dipole must be met, including assumptions about sphericity, conductivity (in the case of an EEG), and the temporal stability of sources. The size of the error made by the assumption of a spherical head shape was explored by Law and Nunez (40). Using a three-dimensional digitizer, they located 62 positions on an electrode cap. An ellipsoidal shape fit the electrode positions better than a sphere. Law and Nunez described a method for determining by tape measure the three axes of the shape conforming best to the head of an individual subject.

One presumed advantage of a MEG over an EEG was that the former affords more precise localization of sources. Controversy about this point, stimulated by a report by Cohen et al. (10), reached the news section of the magazine Science (12). Cohen et al. created an artificial source by passing subthreshold current through depth electrodes implanted in three patients for seizure monitoring. The exact locations of the electrodes could be determined from roentgenographs, and these locations were compared to those calculated for dipoles based on MEG and EEG recordings, each from 16 head locations. The average error for a MEG was 8 mm and for an EEG, 10 mm, thus showing no significant advantage for the MEG. In a follow-up study from the same research group, Cuffin et al. (13) calculated additional EEG dipoles using the same method and found an average localization error of 11 mm.

The studies above used artificial sources. Baumann et al. (5) tested the between-session reliability of dipole parameters from the P1m (50 msec), N1m (100 msec), and P2m (165 msec) components of an auditory ERF. Spatial parameters had an absolute difference of 3 to 10 mm. Errors were attributed to changes in attention, SNR, and local asymmetries in head shape. The sizes of sources detected by MEG after sensory stimulation have been estimated by Williamson and Kaufman (73) to be between 40 and 400 mm^2. These are intermediate in size between macrocolumns of the visual cortex and a full sensory area, which can be several square centimeters.

A consensus statement by a group of scientists (2) pointed out that EEG and MEG should be considered complementary, because their different sensitivity to dipoles of different direction and depth gives valuable information about neural organization. The MEG is most sensitive to activity in fissures of the cortex where currents flow tangentially and to superficial sources, whereas the EEG is sensitive to both radial and tangential currents and is more sensitive than the MEG to deep sources, since in the MEG there is minimal magnetic field spreading by volume condition. The MEG has the advantage of being independent of inhomogeneities in concentric conductivities, whereas localization by an EEG depends on how accurately these conductivities can be approximated. Information from MRI and models of the real geometry of the head are needed. Additional advantages of the MEG are that it requires no electrode placement and permits very slow frequencies to be measured. On the other hand, it is not portable and is sensitive to ambient noise. Until recently, the MEG has had a limited number of channels, and its sensors have been relatively large, with diameters of 3 cm or more positioned at least 1 cm from the scalp.

EEG and MEG localization is comparable to the best ^{15}O positron emission tomography (PET) resolution (6 to 100 mm), but both EEGs and MEGs have certain advantages over PET: the sample time of O^{15}PET is 45 to 60 sec in contrast to the millisecond resolution of an EEG or MEG, PET requires administration of radioactive materials, and PET facilities are much more expensive than even MEG facilities (27). In addition, important neural events may not be concentrated enough to increase blood flow regionally. For example, Eulitz et al. (18) had subjects respond to nouns every 6 sec by silently articulating related verbs. Subjects repeated the task during separate sessions of MEG recording and PET imaging. In two regions, one in Wernicke's area and one in Broca's area, cerebral blood flow was increased on PET. Analysis of the MEG showed that during the first 200 msec of the 6-sec interval, a single current dipole was present in the primary cortex, but thereafter multiple dipoles appeared that were not confined to the regions of increased blood flow. Of course, it is somewhat misleading to cast PET and EEG/MEG as direct competitors because the two methods are most valid in different realms. Only PET assesses blood flow, disturbances of which are often the primary cause of brain dysfunction.

A framework for combining from EEG, MEG, and MRI data has been provided by Dale and Sereno (15). Such a combination of data makes possible the identification of plausible multiple cortical sources with a spatial resolution as good as PET but with a much finer temporal resolution. When available, PET and functional MRI data, can be added to the reconstruction.

STATISTICAL CONSIDERATIONS

Modern multichannel EEG and MEG recording have expanded many fold the amount of data recorded from each subject, leading to problems of statistical inference. This can be seen graphically, for example, when the probability of statistical difference between two groups is plotted across electrode sites (this has been called significance probability mapping). Groups usually differ by at least one electrode, and if they differ at one electrode, they tend to differ at adjacent electrodes, creating regions of significant difference. Of course, because there are multiple electrodes and because data at adjacent electrodes tend to correlate, the extent of significant difference often appears greater than it is. For correct statistical inference, the number of variables must somehow be reduced. Be-

cause data between time points and between topographic locations are often highly correlated, breakdown into components, factors, or dipoles as outlined above is possible. Even then, too many variables may remain for the number of subjects that can be tested.

The best way to avoid type I errors (rejecting the null hypothesis when it is true) is by replication of initial findings on a second data set, distinguishing between exploratory and confirmatory data analysis. In the exploratory phase of research, it would be foolish to limit data collection to a few variables chosen to test definitively a few a priori hypotheses. For clinical studies, the second data set needs to come from an independent clinical sample. Less satisfactory than the two-step approach of confirmation of exploratory findings is the application to a single data set of Bonferroni corrections or leave-one-out (jackknifing) methods. The latter sequentially leaves out one subject from the data set and determines how well a discriminant function based on the other subjects classifies the one. The cost of the Bonferroni correction is high, since it increases the likelihood of type 2 errors (accepting the null hypothesis when it is false). It should be noted that demonstrations of statistically significant replicability do not guarantee that significant neural events have been observed—artifact can be highly replicable too.

DIAGNOSTIC CONSIDERATIONS

The application of evoked MEG and EEG tests to clinical diagnosis has the same requirements as for other clinical tests. To establish the usefulness of a test, well-accepted standards should be used to define the disease, the test should be evaluated on a population different from the one used to derive the test, and the test should have a low false-positive rate, or if it is meant to exclude a diagnosis, a low false-negative rate (49). A few definitions need to be kept in mind: a true positive (TP) is a positive test in a patient with the disease, whereas a false positive (FP) is a positive test in a patients without the disease. A true negative (TN) is a negative test in a person without the disease, and a false negative (FN) is a negative test in a person with the disease. Sensitivity = TP/(TP + FN) and specificity = TN/(TN + FP). Positive predictive power = TP/(TP + FP) and negative predictive power = TN/(TN + FN).

In psychiatric contexts, ERPs have generally been considered a way to investigate cognitive or biological differences between already-diagnosed patients and controls, rather than a way to make a diagnosis. This has been the case even for the most replicable ERP findings such as P300 amplitude reduction in schizophrenia and P300 latency prolongation in dementia. Occasionally, the diagnostic usefulness of ERPs in psychiatry has been debated as in the pair of articles discussing the pros (28) and cons (54) of P300 latency in assessing dementia. Goodin (28) points out that in neurology, brainstem auditory ERPs are very sensitive in diagnosing cerebellopontine angle tumor, with a false-negative rate of less than 3%. The EEG is useful in diagnosing suspected epileptics, although its sensitivity is only 52% because it is 96% specific. However, P300 latency is limited for diagnosing dementia because its sensitivity in some studies is less than 60%, but since its false-negative rate is low, a negative result can give valuable information in some contexts. Of course P300's usefulness presumes that it can be elicited reliably in the population to be tested, which some studies affirm (more than 95% of subjects had adequate P300s) and one denies (less than 20% had adequate P300s) (54).

Pfefferbaum et al. (54) argue that better discrimination between demented and nondemented patients can be made if the effects of age itself are taken into account by regression analysis. They point out that the sensitivity and specificity of a test depends on the cutoff used to define abnormality and the prevalence of the disease in the population. The trade-offs between sensitivity and specificity at various cutoffs can be depicted in a receiver operating-characteristics graph. In the data of Pfefferbaum et al. (54) a statistically optimal cutoff for discrimination between demented and nondemented neurological and psychiatric patients yielded a specificity of 93% and a sensitivity of 38%. Thus, P300 latency is unsuitable for screening because of the low sensitivity, but might be more useful for confirmation of diagnosis because of its higher specificity. In a low-risk population, however, the specificity of P300 is likely to be even lower. A fundamental problem in dementia testing with P300 is that the paradigm used so far to elicit P300 requires the subject to perform a task that severely demented patients may be unable to do, or do in a way that results in P300s with low SNRs. ERP or ERF components less dependent on subject cooperation may play a greater role in clinical assessment in the future.

Ford et al. (21) did a sensitivity–specificity (receiver operating characteristics) analysis of the utility of P300 in diagnosing schizophrenia. Using data originally reported in Pfefferbaum et al. (55) they expressed P300 amplitudes of 20 schizophrenics, 34 depressed, 37 demented, and 9 nondemented patients as age-corrected z-scores based on P300 data from 115 control subjects. Diagnosis of schizophrenia on the basis of P300 amplitude was less successful than the diagnosis of dementia on the basis of P300 latency: a specificity of 90% corresponded to a sensitivity of only 15%. However, P300 amplitude could be used to rule out schizophrenia in certain cases: no patient with a z-score above 1.6 was schizophrenic.

FUTURE PROSPECTS

The methodology of evoked brain potential and magnetic field studies is in a phase of rapid technical evolu-

tion. A 122-channel MEG system is already on-line in Finland (72). In the future more and more studies will coordinate EEG and MEG data with data from MRI, PET, and SPECT scans. The claims of analysis methods to identify actual brain sources will be tested. Electrical and magnetic localization and other imaging methods will vie with each other in precision. Not just the sources of ERP and ERF components to simple stimuli will be localized, but also those reflecting more complex cognitive processes. The application of these new methods, particularly magnetic field measurement, to psychiatric disorders has hardly begun. We hope and expect that this situation will change in the near future.

APPENDIX

To calculate the potential on the surface of a sphere, the following equations must be satisfied (14). For a P_x dipole located along the radial projection at distance f from the center of a sphere

$$V = \frac{P_x\cos\phi}{4\pi\sigma_4 R^2}\sum_{n=1}^{\infty}\frac{(2n+1)^4 f^{n-1}(cd)^{2n+1}P_n^1(\cos\theta)}{n\Gamma}$$

For a P_y dipole located along the radial projection at distance f from the center of a sphere

$$V = \frac{P_y\sin\phi}{4\pi\sigma_4 R^2}\sum_{n=1}^{\infty}\frac{(2n+1)^4 f^{n-1}(cd)^{2n+1}P_n^1(\cos\theta)}{n\Gamma}$$

For a P_z dipole located along the radial projection at distance f from the center of a sphere

$$V = \frac{P_z}{4\pi\sigma_4 R^2}\sum_{n=1}^{\infty}\frac{(2n+1)^4 f^{n-1}(cd)^{2n+1}P_n(\cos\theta)}{\Gamma}$$

where P_n and P_n^1 are Legendre polynomials and for $n = 1$ to 30 iterations

$$\begin{aligned}\Gamma = {}& d^{2n+1}\{b^{2n+1}n(k_1-1)(k_2-1)(n+1)\\ &+ c^{2n+1}(k_1 n+n+1)(k_2 n+n+1)\}\\ &\times\{(k_3 n+n+1)+(n+1)(k_3-1)d^{2n+1}\}\\ &+ (n+1)c^{2n+1}\{b^{2n+1}(k_1-1)(k_2 n+k_2+n)\\ &+ c^{2n+1}(k_1 n+n+1)(k_2-1)\}\\ &\times\{n(k_3-1)+(k_3 n+k_3+n)d^{2n+1}\}\end{aligned}$$

and where

R = radius of head in centimeters
b = radial thickness of brain parenchyma
c = radial thickness of superficial CSF
d = radial thickness of skull
$\sigma_1 = \sigma_4 = 3.3\times10^{-3}$ mho/cm; $\sigma_2 = 10^{-2}$ mho/cm;
$\quad \sigma_3 = 4.2\times10^{-5}$ mho/cm
$k_1 = \sigma_1/\sigma_2$; $k_2 = \sigma_2/\sigma_3$; $k_1 = \sigma_3/\sigma_4$

ACKNOWLEDGMENTS

Preparation of this chapter was supported by the National Institute of Mental Health, grants MH30854 and MH40052, and by the Department of Veterans Affairs. We thank Margaret J. Rosenbloom for her critical comments.

REFERENCES

1. Achim A, Richer F, St-Hilaire JM. Methodological considerations for the evaluation of spatio-temporal source models. *Electroenceph Clin Neurophysiol* 1991;79:227–240.
2. Anogianakis G, Badier JM, Barrett G, et al. A consensus statement on the relative merits of EEG and MEG. *Electroenceph Clin Neurophysiol* 1991;82:317–319.
3. Arndt S, Cohen G, Alliger RJ, Swayze VW, Andreasen NC. Problems with ratio and proportion measures of imaged cerebral structures. *Psychiatry Res: Neuroimaging* 1991;40:79–90.
4. Baker N, Adler L, Franks R, et al. Neurophysiological assessment of sensory gating in psychiatric inpatients: comparison between schizophrenia and other diagnoses. *Biol Psychiatry* 1987;22:603–617.
5. Baumann SB, Rogers RL, Papanicolaou AC, Saydjari CL. Intersession replicability of dipole parameters from three components of the auditory evoked magnetic field. *Brain Topography* 1990;3:311–319.
6. Berg P, Scherg M. Dipole models of eye movements and blinks. *Electroenceph Clin Neurophysiol* 1991;79:36–44.
7. Boutros NN, Overall J, Zouridakis G. Test-retest reliability of the P50 mid-latency auditory evoked response. *Psychiatry Res* 1991;39:181–192.
8. Brandeis D, Naylor H, Halliday R, Callaway E, Yano L. Scopolamine effects on visual information processing, attention, and event-related potential map latencies. *Psychophysiology* 1992;29:315–336.
9. Cardenas VA, Gerson J, Fein G. The reliability of P50 suppression as measured by the conditioning/testing ratio is vastly improved by dipole modeling. *Biol Psychiatry* 1993;33:335–344.
10. Cohen D, Cuffin BN, Yunokuchi K, et al. MEG versus EEG localization test using implanted sources in the human brain. *Ann Neurol* 1990;28:811–817.
11. Cook EW, Miller GA. Digital filtering: background and tutorial for psychophysiologists. *Psychophysiology* 1992;29:350–367.
12. Crease RP. Images of conflict: MEG vs. EEG. *Science* 1991;253:374–375.
13. Cuffin BN, Cohen D, Yunokuchi K, et al. Tests of EEG localization accuracy using implanted sources in the human brain. *Ann Neurol* 1991;29:132–138.
14. Cuffin NB, Cohen D. Comparison of magnetoencephalogram and electroencephalogram. *Electroenceph Clin Neurophysiol* 1979;47:640–644.
15. Dale AM, Sereno MI. Improved localization of cortical activity by combining EEG and MEG with MRI cortical surface reconstruction: a linear approach. *J Cogn Neurosci* 1993;5:162–176.
16. Desmedt JE, Chalklin V, Tomberg C. Emulation of somatosensory evoked potential (SEP) components with the 3-shell dead model and the problem of ghost potential fields when using an average reference in brain mapping. *Electroenceph Clin Neurophysiol* 1990;77:243–258.
17. Elbert T, Rockstroh B, Hampson S, Pantev C, Hoke M. The contingent magnetic variation (CMV). *Electroenceph Clin Neurophysiol* 1994;92:262–272.
18. Eulitz C, Elbert T, Bartenstein P, et al. Brain activity during a verb generation task evaluated by PET and MEG. In: Deecke L, Baumgartner C, Stroink G, et al., eds. *Advances in Biomagnetism.* Amsterdam: Elsevier [in press].
19. Fabiani M, Gratton G, Karis D, Donchin E. Definition, identification, and reliability of measurement of the P300 component of the event-related brain potential. *Adv Psychophysiol* 1987;2:1–78.
20. Farwell LA, Martinerie JM, Bashore TR, Rapp PE, Goddard PH.

Optimal digital filters for long-latency components of the event-related brain potential. *Psychophysiology* 1993;3:306–315.
21. Ford J. Event-related potentials in the psychophysiology of schizophrenia. *Psychophysiology* 1990;27:S4(abst.).
22. Ford JM, Roth WT, Pfefferbaum A. P3 and schizophrenia. In: Friedman D, Bruder G, eds. *Psychophysiology and experimental psychopathology: a tribute to Sam Sutton.* New York: New York Academy of Sciences; 1992:146–162.
23. Ford JM, White P, Lim KO, Pfefferbaum A. Schizophrenics have fewer and smaller P300s: a single-trial analysis. *Biol Psychiatry* 1993;35:96–111.
24. Freedman R. Evoked response to repeated auditory stimuli. *Biol Psychiatry* 1990;28:1065–1080.
25. Freedman R, Adler L, Gerhardt G, et al. Neurobiological studies of sensory gating in schizophrenia. *Schiz Bull* 1987;13:669–678.
26. Gardner-Medwin AR, Swithenby SJ, Fiaschi K, Elbert T, Kowalik Z. Direct measurement of the slow field changes with light adaptation. *Ninth International Conference on Biomagnetism* 1993 (abst.).
27. Gevins A, Le J, Brickett P, Reutter B, Desmond J. Seeing through the skull: advanced EEGs use MRIs to accurately measure cortical activity from the scalp. *Brain Topography* 1991;4:125–131.
28. Goodin DS. Clinical utility of long latency "cognitive" event-related potentials (P3): the pros. *Electroenceph Clin Neurophysiol* 1990;76:2–5.
29. Gratton G, Coles MGH, Donchin E. A new method for off-line removal of ocular artifact. *Electroenceph Clin Neurophysiol* 1983;55:468–484.
30. Gratton G, Coles MGH, Donchin E. A procedure for using multielectrode information in the analysis of components of the event-related potential. *Psychophysiology* 1989;26:222–232.
31. Gratton G, Kramer AF, Coles MGH, Donchin E. Simulation studies of latency measures of components of the event-related brain potential. *Psychophysiology* 1989;26:233–248.
32. Hackley SA. An evaluation of the automaticity of sensory processing using event-related potentials and brain-stem reflexes. *Psychophysiology* 1993;30:415–428.
33. Helmholz H. Über einigen Gesetze der Verteilung elektrischer Ströme in körperlichen Leitern mit Anwendung auf die tierelektrische Versuche. *Poggendorffsche Ann Phys Chem* 1853;29:211–233.
34. Ioannides AA, Muratore R, Balish M, Sato S. In vivo validation of distributed source solutions for the biomagnetic inverse problem. *Brain Topography* 1993;5:263–273.
35. Jasper HH. The ten–twenty electrode system of the International Federation. *Electroenceph Clin Neurophysiol* 1957;10:371–375.
36. Johnson R Jr. A triarchic model of P300 amplitude. *Psychophysiology* 1986;23:367–384.
37. Johnson R Jr. Developmental evidence for modality-dependent P300 generators: a normative study. *Psychophysiology* 1989;26:651–667.
38. Kathmann N, Engel RR. Sensory gating in normals and schizophrenics: a failure to find strong P50 suppression in normals. *Biol Psychiatry* 1990;27:1216–1226.
39. Kaufman L, Kaufman JH, Wang JZ. On cortical folds and neuromagnetic fields. *Electroenceph Clin Neurophysiol* 1991;79:211–226.
40. Law SK, Nunez PL. Quantitative representation of the upper surface of the human head. *Brain Topography* 1991;3:365–371.
41. Mekeig S. Auditory event-related dynamics of the EEG spectrum and effects of exposure to tones. *Electroenceph Clin Neurophysiol* 1993;86:283–293.
42. Michie PT, Bearpark HM, Crawford JM, Glue LCT. The nature of selective attention effects on auditory event-related potentials. *Biol Psychol* 1990;30:219–250.
43. Miller GA, Gratton G, Yee CM. Generalized implementation of an eye movement correction procedure. *Psychophysiology* 1988;25:241–243.
44. Miller GA, Lutzenberger W, Elbert T. The linked-reference issue in EEG and ERP recording. *Psychophysiology* [in press].
45. Moran JE, Tepley N, Jacobson GP, Barkely GL. Evidence for multiple generators in evoked responses using finite difference field mapping: auditory evoked fields. *Brain Topography* 1993;5:229–240.
46. Nagamine T, Kaji R, Suwazono S, Hamano T, Shibasaki H, Kimura J. Current source density mapping of somatosensory evoked responses following median and tibial nerve stimulation. *Electroenceph Clin Neurophysiol* 1992;84:248–256.

47. Nunez PL. Towards a physics of neocortex. In: Marmarelis VZ, ed. *Advanced methods of physiological system modeling*, Vol 2. New York: Plenum; 1989:241–259.

48. Nunez PL, Pilgreen KL, Westdorp AF, Law SK, Nelson AV. A visual study of surface potentials and Laplacians due to distributed neocortical sources: computer simulations and evoked potentials. *Brain Topography* 1991;4:151–168.

49. Nuwer MR. On the controversies about clinical use of EEG brain mapping. *Brain Topography* 1990;3:103–111.

50. Pantev C, Hoke M, Lehnertz K, Lutkenhoner B, Fahrendorf G, Stober U. Identification of sources of brain neuronal activity with high spatiotemporal resolution through combination of neuromagnetic source localization (NMSL) and magnetic resonance imaging (MRI). *Electroenceph Clin Neurophysiol* 1990;75:173–184.

51. Perrin F, Pernier J, Bertrand O, Echallier JF. Spherical splines for scalp potential and current density mapping. *Electroenceph Clin Neurophysiol* 1989;72:184–187; corrigendum of interpolation formula in ibid., 1990, 76:565.

52. Pfefferbaum A. Model estimates of CSF and skull influences on scalp-recorded ERPs. *Alcohol* 1990;7:479–482.

53. Pfefferbaum A, Ford JM. ERPs to stimuli requiring response production and inhibition: the effects of age, probability and visual noise. *Electroenceph Clin Neurophysiol* 1988;71:55–63.

54. Pfefferbaum A, Ford JM, Kraemer HC. Clinical utility of long latency "cognitive" event-related potentials (P3): the cons. *Electroenceph Clin Neurophysiol* 1990;76:6–12.

55. Pfefferbaum A, Wenegrat B, Ford J, Roth WT, Kopell BS. Clinical application of the P3 component of event-related potentials: II. Dementia, depression and schizophrenia. *Electroenceph Clin Neurophysiol* 1984;59:104–124.

56. Putnam L, Johnson R Jr, Roth WT. Guidelines for reducing the risk of disease transmission in the psychophysiology laboratory. *Psychophysiology* 1992;29:127–141.

57. Reite M, Teale P, Goldstein L, Whalen J, Linnville S. Late auditory magnetic sources may differ in the left hemisphere of schizophrenic patients. A preliminary report. *Arch Gen Psychiatry* 1989; 1989:565–572.

58. Rockstroh B, Elbert T, Canavan A, Lutzenberger W, Birbaumer N. *Slow Brain Potentials and Behaviour*, Baltimore: Urban & Schwarzenberg, 1989.

59. Roth WT. Electrical brain activity in psychiatric disorders. In: Melzer H, ed. *Psychopharmacology: the third generation of progress*. New York: Raven Press; 1987:793–801.

60. Roth WT, Cannon EH. Some features of the auditory evoked response in schizophrenics. *Arch Gen Psychiatry* 1972;27:466–471.

61. Roth WT, Pfefferbaum A, Horvath TB, Berger PA, Kopell BS. P3 reduction in auditory evoked potentials of schizophrenics. *Electroenceph Clin Neurophysiol* 1980;49:497–505.

62. Scherg M. Separation and identification of event-related potential components by brain electric source analysis. Presented at Noordwijk, The Netherlands, Ninth International Conference on Event-Related Potentials of the Brain (EPIC)., 1989.

63. Scherg M. Fundamentals of dipole source potential analysis. *Advances in Audiology* 1990;6:40–69.

64. Scherg M, Berg P. Use of prior knowledge in brain electromagnetic source analysis. *Brain Topography* 1991;4:143–150.

65. Snyder AZ. Dipole source localization in the study of EP generators—a critique. *Electroenceph Clin Neurophysiol* 1991;80:321–325.

66. Squires-Wheeler E, Friedman D, Skodol AE, Erlenmeyer-Kimling L. A longitudinal study relating P3 amplitude to schizophrenia spectrum disorders and to global personality functioning. *Biol Psychiatry* 1993;33:774–785.

67. Stephenson WA, Gibbs FA. A balanced non-cephalic reference electrode. *Electroenceph Clin Neurophysiol* 1951;3:237–240.

68. Tiihonen J, Hari R, Naukkarinen H, Rimon R, Jousmaki V, Kajola M. Modified activity of the human auditory cortex during auditory hallucinations. *Am J Psychiatry* 1992;149:255–257.

69. Tomberg C, Noel P, Ozaki I, Desmedt JE. Inadequacy of the average reference for the topographic mapping of focal enhancements of brain potentials. *Electroenceph Clin Neurophysiol* 1990;77:259–265.

70. Turetsky B, Raz J, Fein G. Representation of multi-channel evoked potential data using a dipole component model of intracranial generators—application to the auditory P300. *Electroenceph Clin Neurophysiol* 1990;76:540–556.

71. Turetsky BI, Raz J, Fein G. Noise and signal power and their effects on evoked potential estimation. *Electroenceph Clin Neurophysiol* 1988;71:310–318.

72. Wikswo JP, Gevins A, Williamson SJ. The future of the EEG and MEG. *Electroenceph Clin Neurophysiol* 1993;87:1–9.

73. Williamson SJ, Kaufman L. Evolution of neuromagnetic topographic mapping. *Brain Topography* 1990;3:113–127.

74. Witt JC, Towle VL, Bolaños J, Spire J-P. Tetrahedral recording of 3-D BAEPs: evidence for the centered dipole model. *Electroenceph Clin Neurophysiol* 1991;80:551–560.

75. Woody CD. Characterization of an adaptive filter for the analysis of variable latency neuroelectronic signals. *Med Biol Eng Comp* 1967;5:539–553.

Psychopharmacology: The Fourth
Generation of Progress, edited by
Floyd E. Bloom and David J. Kupfer.
Raven Press, Ltd., New York © 1995.

CHAPTER 79

Recent Studies on Norepinephrine Systems in Mood Disorders

Alan F. Schatzberg and Joseph J. Schildkraut

That the catecholamine (CA), norepinephrine, may play a pivotal role in the mechanism of action of antidepressant drugs and the pathophysiology of depressive disorders was hypothesized nearly 30 years ago (66). Since that time, research on various aspects of these hypotheses has provided us with much important information about the biology and treatment of depressive disorders. However, many questions remain about the exact role this neurotransmitter plays in depression. In this chapter, we review where we are today and provide a framework for approaching future studies of this important CA system.

Norepinephrine (NE) is synthesized in a variety of peripheral and central sites, including the sympathetic nervous system, adrenal glands, and brain (locus coeruleus). There are limitations in studying this system in man, since most studies of NE or its metabolites in patients and controls involve at best indirect measures of central activity. For example, although metabolite levels in urine or blood may give us important information about central activity, they are still heavily derived from the periphery. Neuroendocrine challenges, such as growth hormone response to clonidine, can also provide potentially important information concerning brain NE activity, but they too are only indirect assessments of NE physiology. The limitations of such approaches has led to debate about the significance of NE in depression, a state of affairs common to research on all other neurotransmitter and neuromodulator systems in psychiatric disorders. The use of postmortem brain tissue can provide useful information, but here too such methodological issues of when

and how the tissue was obtained, subjects' diagnoses, drug exposure, and so on, limit what one can truly conclude from such investigations. Ultimately, molecular biology and brain imaging may provide more powerful strategies in this area and could help to clarify the significance of data obtained from current clinical research strategies (see also Chapters 32 and 34, *this volume*).

NOREPINEPHRINE AND METABOLITES AS DIAGNOSTIC DISCRIMINATORS

Urinary 3-Methoxy-4-hydroxyphenylglycol

The study of CA physiology in mood disorders was given a major boost when the metabolite 3-methoxy-4-hydroxyphenylglycol (MHPG) was found to be present in both brain and in the periphery and the proportion of urinary MHPG that was derived from central sources was found to be substantial. There has been a great deal of investigation on 24-hr urinary MHPG levels, because they provide a view of NE function over a full day, and early investigators could more easily and reliably determine MHPG in urine than in blood. Although the exact proportion of urinary MHPG that derives from brain is still in debate, some 20% appears to derive from central NE pools (43).

Early case studies demonstrated that in bipolar patients, urinary MHPG levels were lower during the depressed phase and higher during the manic phase than during periods of euthymia (61). These earliest reports did not attempt to control for the nonspecific effects of activity. Subsequently, we and others reported that urinary MHPG levels were significantly lower in bipolar depressives than in unipolar depressions or control subjects (7,17,60,63). Differences between bipolars and control subjects did not

A. F. Schatzberg: Department of Psychiatry and Behavioral Sciences, Stanford University School of Medicine, Stanford, California 94305.

J. J. Schildkraut: Department of Psychiatry, Harvard Medical School, Boston, Massachusetts 02115.

appear to be caused by differences in relative retardation, agitation, or anxiety (65). Generally, these studies included small samples such that the effects of age (and to some extent, sex) were not well explored.

In more recent years, the use of CA measures to distinguish between unipolar and bipolar depressed patients has continued to be a major focus of study. After our group again reported that bipolar depressed patients demonstrate significantly lower urinary MHPG levels than do unipolar nonendogenous subjects (54), several, but not all, recent studies have supported this finding (2,23,38,57). A comparison of these four studies indicates that the nature of the patient's bipolar history (hypomania vs. mania) may be an important variable in determining urinary MHPG levels in bipolar depressed patients. The development of more comprehensive classifications of bipolar disorders, in part on the basis of severity of manic episodes (i.e., bipolar I vs. bipolar II), has aided greatly in this area. In the Depression Collaborative Study, significant differences in catecholamine excretion were not observed when unipolar and bipolar depressives were compared (23). In that study, bipolar patients were not further classified into bipolar I and bipolar II subtypes. In a Swedish study (2), significant differences were also not observed between unipolar and bipolar depressives, but, in that study, over 80% of the bipolar patients appeared to have a bipolar II disorder. In an National Institute of Mental Health (NIMH) intramural study, Muscettola and colleagues (38) reported that patients with bipolar I depressions demonstrated significantly lower urinary MHPG levels than did patients with unipolar depressions. In contrast, significant differences were not observed between bipolar II and unipolar subjects. Similarly, our group (57) reported that bipolar I, but not bipolar II, depressives excreted lower mean 24-hr urinary MHPG levels than did unipolar depressed patients. Thus, the degree of bipolarity may play a crucial role in determining relative urinary MHPG excretion. Unfortunately, the study of bipolar I depressed patients today is difficult since the majority of such patients are on thymoleptic agents and the withdrawal of such agents poses great ethical and medical dilemma.

Plasma Norepinephrine and 3-Methoxy-4-hydroxyphenylglycol

Plasma NE levels have been reported to be higher in depressives in the supine position than in healthy controls (11,42,46). Using orthostatic challenges, unipolar and bipolar patients both demonstrate greater increases in plasma NE after moving to the upright position than do controls (49,51). In the studies from the NIMH intramural program, heart rate and blood pressure did not change in parallel with plasma NE fashion, but those investigators have suggested that some depressed patients demonstrate insufficient NE tone, that is they require greater changes in NE levels to maintain homeostasis (2,51).

Plasma NE and MHPG levels also have been compared in unipolar and bipolar patients. Plasma NE levels have been reported to be significantly lower in bipolar patients with a history of melancholia than in their unipolar counterparts who had significantly greater NE levels than control subjects (49). Similar differences between unipolars and bipolars were reported on plasma MHPG measures (47). Degree of bipolarity was not reported in these studies.

Integrated Measures

Several groups, including our own, have explored the potential application of measures of CAs and other metabolites, in addition to MHPG, to help discriminate among subtypes of depression. In the Depression Collaborative Study, Koslow et al. (23) reported that compared to healthy control subjects, depressed patients demonstrated significant elevations in urinary levels of both NE and epinephrine (E) as well as their metabolites with the exception of MHPG. They suggested that total body CA turnover may provide more salient information about CA dysregulation than does urinary MHPG alone. Increased levels were interpreted as reflecting increased sympathetic nervous system and adrenal activity. In this study, urinary NE levels were significantly higher in unipolar than in bipolar depressed patients.

Maas et al. of the Depression Collaborative Study (26) have reported that the individual ratios of NE to NE plus metabolites or E to E plus metabolites may provide better estimates of CA metabolism than are obtained using individual amine or metabolite data alone. Specifically, they noted that the ratios of NE to NE plus metabolites and E to E plus metabolites were significantly higher in depressed patients than in control subjects. In contrast, the ratio of MHPG to NE plus metabolites was lower in depressives than in controls. They argued that there was a relative increase in CAs and a relative decrease in MHPG in depression. Moreover, they noted that the relative increases in NE and epinephrine were largely due to differences between unipolars and controls. These data not only point to the use of CA measures to help discriminate unipolars from controls but also again suggest such patients may be characterized as having increased sympathetic and adrenal activity.

A number of years ago we reported on the use of discriminant function analysis of 24-hr urinary CAs and metabolites [so-called Depression (D)-type scores] to provide better separation between bipolar manic–depressive from unipolar nonendogenous patients than do urinary MHPG levels alone (62). In a more recent study (57), we reported that bipolar I patients demonstrated both significantly lower MHPG levels and D-type scores than did unipolar nonendogenous patients. However, D-type scores provided greater sensitivity and specificity for

TABLE 1. *Sensitivity and specificity of lowest quartile measures for separating bipolar/schizoaffective from unipolar nonendogenous depressed patients*

Measure	Sensitivity	Specificity
D-type score	0.85	0.93
NE + Metabolites	0.31	0.73
MHPG	0.54	0.80
VMA	0.08	0.67
NMN	0.38	0.73
NE	0.54	0.80

Adapted from Schatzberg et al. (57).

separating bipolar I depressions from unipolar nonendogenous depressions (as well as all other subtypes of depressions) than did urinary levels of MHPG, NE, normetanephrine (NMN), vanillylmandelic acid (VMA), or the sum of NE plus its metabolites (see Table 1). In contrast, bipolar II and unipolar depressed patients could not reliably be separated using MHPG or any of the other measures. In this study, age, sex, hospital status, anxiety, and overall severity did not account for differences in D-type scores between bipolar I and unipolar patients. These data suggest that urinary CAs can be used to discriminate among subtypes of depressed patients, particularly those with bipolar I and unipolar subtypes; however, merely summing NE and its metabolites does not provide as powerful discrimination as does using discriminant function analysis of CAs and their metabolites.

The pathophysiological significance of D-type scores remains to be elucidated. It is possible that the equation is correcting for that proportion of urinary MHPG that is not derived from brain. Alternatively, such analysis may be incorporating relevant data provided by measures of urinary NE or its other metabolites. The application of such equations by others will require each laboratory standardizing their assays and determining either specific coefficients or their own equations (42,44).

HETEROGENEITY OF UNIPOLAR DEPRESSIONS

In the 1970s, we noted in a preliminary sample that unipolar patients were more heterogeneous with regard to urinary MHPG excretion than were bipolar subjects (63). In the early 1980s, we reported in a larger sample that unipolar patients were relatively heterogeneous in their excretion of urinary MHPG, with some patients demonstrating relatively low values (similar to bipolar patients) others demonstrating very high values, and still others demonstrating midrange values (54). In contrast to bipolar and control comparisons, the mean urinary MHPG level did not differ significantly when unipolar patients and healthy controls were compared. Bipolar and control differences were not due to apparent age or sex effects. At that time, we suggested that unipolar depressives with

low or high urinary MHPG levels might represent two different forms of CA dysregulation—the former a low output state and the latter a high output state secondary to either noradrenergic receptor subsensitivity or increased acetylcholine (ACh) activity that could result in increased 24-hr urinary CA and metabolite levels. [More recent studies suggest that elevations in MHPG and cortisol could be due to increased corticotropin-releasing factor (CRF) activity (see below).] The midrange subgroup was viewed as having a dysfunction of another neurotransmitter system. As indicated above, other groups have also reported higher NE and metabolite levels in unipolar depressed patients than in control subjects.

CATECHOLAMINE LEVELS AND RESPONSE TO ANTIDEPRESSANTS

Urinary 3-Methoxy-4-hydroxyphenylglycol as a Predictor of Antidepressant Response

A number of early studies suggested that 24-hr urinary MHPG levels could predict response to antidepressant agents (25,64). The earliest of these studies reported that patients with low urinary MHPG levels responded to imipramine (25). Subsequently, many studies have reported that low MHPG patients respond significantly more robustly to treatment with tricyclic and tetracyclic agents (imipramine, nortriptyline, and maprotiline) that exert pronounced effects on norepinephrine reuptake than do patients with high urinary MHPG levels (19,27,55). In a recent review, Garvey et al. (15) concluded the data were most compelling for MHPG predicting imipramine response. Still, studies have not reported on which drug strategies might prove particularly effective in patients with high MHPG excretion who fail to respond to these agents.

Three nontricyclic antidepressants have been recently studied with respect to relative efficacy in low and high MHPG output depressions. Pretreatment urinary MHPG levels did not predict response to the monoamine oxidase inhibitor, phenelzine, in a group of 38 unipolar patients (67). In another study, our group reported that patients with high urinary MHPG levels responded significantly better to alprazolam, a triazolobenzodiazepine, than did patients with low MHPG levels (36). High, baseline CA excretion in these patients was associated with agonist nonspecific heterologous desensitization of the platelet receptor–G-protein–adenylate cyclase complex (see below). In a recent study, our group has observed that patients with low MHPG levels responded more robustly to treatment with fluoxetine, a selective serotonin reuptake inhibitor, than did patients with high MHPG levels (59).

Longitudinal Effects on Norepinephrine and Metabolites

The three studies above (36,59,67) also explored the effects of treatment on urinary NE or MHPG excretion.

In all three, significant reduction in CA or metabolite levels were observed in both responders and nonresponders to all agents, and thus reductions did not appear to correlate with treatment response (36,59,67). However, in a previous report of the Depression Collaborative Study, amitriptyline and imipramine decreased 24-hr urinary MHPG levels in both unipolar responders and nonresponders, but responders demonstrated greater reductions in MHPG excretion than did nonresponders (5). In our study on alprazolam, the reduction in CA and metabolite excretion in high CA patients was associated with normalization of the desensitized platelet receptor–G-protein–adenylate cyclase complex (36). These data suggest response to treatment with alprazolam may require both a decrease in CA and metabolite output and receptor–G-protein–adenylate cyclase reregulation. Taken together, these studies suggest that reductions in CA and metabolite excretion may be necessary, but not sufficient, for response to antidepressants (see the section below on "Norepinephrine Measures and Mania").

Although in our hands both desipramine and fluoxetine resulted in significant decreases in NE metabolite excretion, longitudinal biochemical data suggest the two agents exert different effects on NE excretion (59). Desipramine was associated with significant reductions in urinary MHPG and VMA by 6 weeks but with significant increases in NE excretion, in keeping with its effects on blocking NE reuptake. In contrast, although fluoxetine resulted in significant decreases in MHPG, VMA, and NMN excretion (albeit for MHPG and VMA less than were seen with desipramine), NE excretion was not increased. These data suggest fluoxetine affects NE excretion through mechanisms that do not involve norepinephrine reuptake blockade. Other studies have reported that selective serotonin reuptake inhibitors reduce levels of NE or metabolites (43), although, not all studies agree (21).

Combining data from our study comparing desipramine (DMI) and fluoxetine with those of other studies, we have noted that the desipramine-induced decrease in urinary MHPG excretion at 4 and 6 weeks was observable after one week of treatment (Schildkraut et al., *unpublished data*). In contrast, NE and NMN levels demonstrate a more variable response. At 1 week, they are decreased, but, at weeks 4 and 6, they are increased over baseline. These data indicate that response to DMI involves a complex reregulation of NE metabolism over time.

Karege et al. (22) reported that dividing of plasma MHPG levels into three ranges may provide more useful longitudinal information than using group mean values or dividing the sample into high and low subgroups. Low and high plasma MHPG patients who responded to imipramine or desipramine demonstrated "normalization" of their values (i.e., low values increased into normal midrange and high values decreased into the midrange). In contrast, in the overall group, mean MHPG levels were

found to decrease with treatment with little relationship to treatment response. These data suggest that changes in MHPG levels may indeed be important for treatment response and that analysis of overall group data may provide less meaningful information than dividing the sample into biochemical subgroups. Further studies on larger samples are required to determine the effectiveness of this strategy.

D-type Scores as Predictors of Response

Mooney et al. (37) have compared urinary MHPG levels and D-type scores to discriminate between responders and nonresponders to alprazolam or imipramine. Patients with low MHPG levels responded better to imipramine than did high MHPG subjects; as indicated above, the converse was true for alprazolam. However, D-type scores provided significantly better discrimination between responders and nonresponders to both drugs than did MHPG levels. These data further suggest that more useful clinical data may be derived from analysis of CAs and their various metabolites than can be obtained using urinary MHPG levels alone (see above).

CATECHOLAMINE DEPLETION STUDIES

In the 1970s, Shopsin et al. (68) reported on the potential use of CA depleters to reverse antidepressant responses. This approach has been readapted in recent years by Delgado and colleagues (8). In a series of studies, tryptophan depletion reversed the antidepressant response in patients who had been treated with selective serotonin reuptake inhibitors. Patients who were treated with desipramine were not similarly affected (9).

In a later study, this group administered α-methyl-para-tyrosine (AMPT) to patients treated with desipramine or SSRIs(8). This study involved limited samples; however, data suggest AMPT produces relapses into depression in patients treated with desipramine but not with SSRIs. In contrast to earlier studies in which AMPT may by itself exacerbate depressive symptoms in depressed patients, this group has reported that AMPT does not worsen depressive symptoms (34). Taken together, these data suggest that maintaining NE tone or levels is necessary for sustaining antidepressant responses to potent noradrenergic agents as does maintaining 5-HT levels for sustaining antidepressant responses to SSRIs. They also suggest that these systems play important roles in mediating antidepressant responses.

CATECHOLAMINE MEASURES AND SYMPTOMS

A number of studies have attempted to correlate clinical characteristics to NE measures. Samson and colleagues

(52) recently reported that psychomotor retardation was correlated linearly with MHPG excretion in a group of nonbipolar I depressed patients. In contrast, sleep disturbance [as measured using the Hamilton Depression Rating Scale (HDRS) ratings] was highest in patients with low or high MHPG values. Patients with midrange values demonstrated less sleep disturbance than did low or high MHPG subjects. When data were analyzed dividing the sample into low and high MHPG subgroups, meaningful relationships were not observed between sleep and MHPG excretion. These data further suggest that there may be three biochemical subgroups that can be defined using MHPG levels.

In another study, Samson et al. (53) reported that depressed patients with high MHPG levels were also characterized by perceptions of powerlessness. These findings in depressed patients appear to parallel studies on lower animals relating learned helplessness to depression. The findings of Roy et al. (17) that plasma MHPG correlates significantly and positively with anxiety suggest a possible triad of a sense of powerlessness, anxiety, and elevated MHPG excretion in depressed patients. Further studies of larger samples are required to explore the relationship between symptoms and measures of CA activity.

NOREPINEPHRINE MEASURES AND CORTISOL ACTIVITY

In the early 1980s, three groups reported on significant positive relationships between measures of CAs and cortisol activity. Stokes et al. (71) reported significant positive correlations between urinary MHPG and plasma cortisol in depressed patients and our group reported significant positive relationships between urinary MHPG and urinary free cortisol (UFC) levels (45). Jimerson et al. (20) reported significant positive relationships between plasma MHPG levels and dexamethasone suppression test (DST) nonsuppression. These results were initially quite surprising since CAs were then thought to act primarily as tonic inhibitors of the hypothalamic–pituitary–adrenal (HPA) axis. Subsequent to these early reports, a number of studies have replicated these initial observations (15,50,77), although not all studies agree (24).

Other studies have explored NE, epinephrine, and metabolites other than MHPG in an effort to determine whether CA–HPA axis relationships reflect increased peripheral, sympathetic or adrenal activity. For example, Roy et al. (48) reported significant positive correlations between a number of CA and metabolite measures in several tissues [cerebrospinal fluid (CSF), urine, and blood] and cortisol measures in blood. Similarly, Stokes et al. (72) reported significant, positive correlations between 24-hr levels of epinephrine and cortisol, as measured in urine. Taken together, these studies point to activation of peripheral CA systems in depressed patients

with pronounced HPA axis activity. The MHPG–cortisol relationships, however, still suggest a relationship between increased activity of both the HPA axis and central NE systems.

Maes and colleagues (28) reported that the significant, positive correlations between 24-hr MHPG and cortisol levels in urine were lost when the effects of 24-hr urinary volume and creatinine were taken out. Our group has performed similar analyses on a large group of unipolar depressives. In our hands, significant positive correlations between urinary MHPG and urinary free cortisol were still present after any possible effects of urinary volume and creatinine were taken out (58). Similarly, we failed to observe any effects for severity. This area warrants further study, although, data from our studies and those of others using measures in blood and CSF suggest that the MHPG–cortisol relationships are not merely due to nonspecific effects of kidney function.

The biological significance of this CA–HPA axis relationship also remains to be determined. One possibility is that the simultaneous elevation of these measures reflects increased adrenal and sympathetic nervous system activity, perhaps indicative of general stress. Another possibility is that elevated CRF activity centrally could result in simultaneous elevation of both systems (28). Such simultaneous elevation could also reflect increased central cholinergic activity, which could result in increased epinephrine, MHPG, and cortisol levels and which has been hypothesized as playing a role in depression. In addition, β-adrenergic agonists have been reported to increase adrenocorticotropin (ACTH) secretion from the pituitary suggesting adrenergic hyperactivity could lead to or exacerbate HPA axis overactivity (28).

PLATELET MONOAMINE OXIDASE ACTIVITY AND CORTISOL MEASURES

Monoamines are metabolized by monoamine oxidase (MAO). The platelets contain MAO of the B form, which primarily metabolizes dopamine and phenylethylamine. However, we have reported a significant correlation between platelet MAO activity and the ratio of NMN plus MN to VMA, and others have reported that infusion of epinephrine results in increased MAO activity. These data suggest MAO activity could provide information relevant to CA activity.

Several studies have reported on significant positive correlations between platelet MAO activity and cortisol measures. Agren and Oreland (1) initially reported significant positive correlations between platelet MAO activity and UFC in a group of unipolar patients. In that study, MAO activity correlated significantly with insomnia ratings. Subsequently, our group reported that patients with high platelet MAO activity were more likely to fail to suppress when challenged with dexamethasone than were their low MAO counterparts (56). Similar results were noted in both men and women, even though women had higher MAO activity than men. A significant positive correlation was observed between platelet MAO activity and 4 pm post-dexamethasone cortisol levels. Total HDRS scores and ratings of insomnia correlated significantly and positively with both platelet MAO activity and 4 pm post-dexamethasone cortisol levels. These data suggest overall severity and insomnia may be related to elevations in MAO and cortisol measures.

Significant positive relationships between MAO activity and post-dexamethasone cortisol measures have now been replicated by several groups (32,39). The finding appears to be more robust in unipolar than in bipolar subjects and to not be present in healthy controls or schizophrenic patients (39). The significance of these findings in unipolar subjects is unclear. One possibility is that high platelet MAO activity may be a genetically based risk factor for DST nonsuppression if and when patients become depressed. A second explanation is that elevated, circulating CA levels, that are associated with increased HPA axis activity may result in increased platelet MAO activity (56). Still another is that elevated MAO activity could result in low serotonin levels and resultant supersensitive serotonin receptor activity, which could play a role in increased glucocorticoid activity (32). To date, the underlying pathophysiology that accounts for this curious relationship has not been elucidated.

NOREPINEPHRINE MEASURES AND MANIA

A number of studies in the past decade have examined CA levels in patients with mania. In one longitudinal study, bipolar patients during manic episodes demonstrated significantly higher plasma NE and epinephrine levels than they did when depressed or when in euthymia (29). Plasma CA levels were also higher during mania than they were in control subjects. In that study, patients were on lithium carbonate during the study raising questions concerning a possible confound, although, these findings are quite reminiscent of much earlier studies (see above).

In the Depression Collaborative Study, CSF levels of MHPG and urinary levels of NE were both significantly higher in manic than in depressed patients or controls (74). Significant correlations were observed between these biochemical measures and severity of mania. Manic patients also demonstrated lower ratios of urinary MHPG to total NE plus metabolites and higher ratios of urinary NE to total NE plus metabolites than did control subjects. Although individual pretreatment CA and metabolite values did not differ between responders and nonresponders to lithium carbonate, responders demonstrated significantly lower ratios of MHPG to total NE plus metabolites and higher ratios of VMA to total NE plus metabolites

than did nonresponders. Nonresponder values were similar to controls. Lithium significantly reduced NE turnover in responders and nonresponders, leading the investigators to argue that reduction in NE turnover may be necessary but not sufficient for antimanic effects of lithium carbonate. Reductions of CA and metabolite measures were not merely due to reductions in agitation.

In a later report from the Depression Collaborative Study, Swann et al. (75) noted that environmental sensitivity had a significant effect on urinary NE excretion. Manic patients whose episodes were reported to be "environmentally sensitive" demonstrated elevated NE excretion; in contrast, manic patients with autonomous episodes did not. As indicated above, elevated NE activity in manic patients has also been reported to be a positive predictor of lithium response. These data suggest that the elevated NE activity in mania may be related to the effects of external stressors. In the future it would be of interest to simultaneously explore the effects of stress, perceived sense of powerlessness, and CA metabolite measures in both manic and depressed subjects (see above).

NORADRENERGIC RECEPTOR ACTIVITY

α_2-Receptors

Considerable attention has been paid to α_2-noradrenergic receptors in depression since presynaptic α_2-receptors control release of NE from central neurons. Several approaches have been used to study α_2-receptor activity in patients with depression. Binding by agonists, such as clonidine, has generally been reported to be increased in the platelets of depressed patients (13,40), although this finding has not been consistent across studies (16). Differences in population demographics, extent of drug washout, assay used, and so on, may help to explain these inconsistencies. Binding studies using yohimbine, an α_2-antagonist, have failed to show differences in α_2-receptor numbers between patients and controls (42). These data suggest that clonidine as an antagonist may provide more important information regarding α_2-receptor activity than is obtained using antagonists. However, recent findings indicate that agents with putative α_2-adrenergic receptor activity may bind intensely to nonadrenergic sites on platelets (33), suggesting that clonidine binding data may not merely reflect α_2-receptor activity (42).

Another approach has been to explore functional aspects of α_2 receptors, for example, by determining epinephrine suppression of adenylate cyclase (AC) activity in platelets or α_2-agonist induced platelet aggregation. Several studies have reported that CA inhibition of prostaglandin E_1 stimulation of AC is reduced in depressed patients (69), although not all studies agree (14). Mooney et al. (36) have reported a blunting of such suppression, which correlated with increased excretion of both NE and epinephrine in urine. However, elevated NE and epinephrine excretion were also associated with blunting of both prostaglandin and NaF stimulation of AC activity suggesting blunted α_2-receptor activity reflected agonist non-specific or heterologous desensitization of the platelet receptor–G-protein–AC complex. Garcilla-Sevilla et al. (14) have reported that α_2-agonist-induced platelet aggregation in depressed patients is increased in depressed patients. The discrepancy between increased responses in platelet aggregation and blunted adenylate cyclase responses to clonidine has been thought to be difficult to reconcile (42). These findings do require further study to understand the underlying physiology.

Growth Hormone Responses to Clonidine

Hypothalamic α_2-receptors control release of growth hormone releasing hormone (GHRH) and subsequently release of growth hormone (GH). Clonidine, stimulates GH release in man. In depressed patients, blunted GH responses to clonidine have been observed in many but not all studies (3,70). Negative studies have frequently used relatively low doses of clonidine (6). Blunted GH responses to desipramine have been reported in both unipolar and bipolar depressives as well as in patients with mania and panic disorder (4,61). Of particular interest is the observation that the blunted GH response to clonidine may be a trait marker which persists in depressed patients after recovery (35).

Although the blunted GH response to clonidine has been inferred to reflect postsynaptic α_2-receptor down-regulation there is also considerable controversy regarding the mechanisms that underlie these observations (6). Clonidine stimulates both pre and postsynaptic α_2 receptors, which produce opposite effects on GH release. Moreover, GH release is also controlled by somatomedins and somatostatin, which have been reported to be altered in some depressed patients. Still, the blunted response to clonidine has been a consistent finding in many studies on depressed patients.

β Receptors

Generally, β receptors are postsynaptic. Early reports by Sulser and colleagues (73) noted that in the rat chronic administration of known antidepressants results in down-regulation of β_1 receptors in brain. These observations have been pursued in two ways in man. One approach has been to explore β receptors in the cortex of suicide victims. This approach has yielded conflicting results. Some studies have reported higher β-receptor density in suicide victims than in controls (31), whereas other studies have failed to replicate this finding (10). Psychiatric diagnoses, radioligand used, and previous exposure to

antidepressants may be key variables that need to be considered when interpreting studies done to date.

The other approach has been to measure either the number of or functional activity of β receptors in lymphocytes or leukocytes. Although there are numerous reports that there are fewer β receptors in the lymphocytes or leukocytes of depressed patients than in healthy controls, many studies have failed to find similar differences (12,18). As in α_2-receptor studies, there are a number of possible methodological explanations for these disparate results.

Functional activity of beta receptors may be measured by exploring adenylate cyclase responses to specific agonists. Several studies have reported relatively decreased responses of adenylate cyclase activity to β agonists in depressed patients as compared with healthy controls (12,76). These responses appear to normalize with treatment (30). Potter and colleagues (42) have reported that desensitized β receptors may be inversely correlated to certain measures of NE activity, suggesting that blunted β-receptor activity may reflect or be due to increased circulating NE levels (42). Taken together with the findings of Mooney et al. (36), these studies point to the need to simultaneously measure CA output or turnover and receptor activity to better interpret receptor studies.

RELATIONSHIPS TO OTHER MONOAMINE SYSTEMS

Data reviewed suggest that disturbances in NE physiology in depression may occur in conjunction with disruption in homeostasis of other neurotransmitters or peptides. In this section, we briefly review three possible interactions. As indicated above, the simultaneous elevation in measures of CA and HPA axis activity could reflect an increase in ACh activity. Increased ACh activity has long been thought to play a role in the pathophysiology of depression. Early on, Janowsky and colleagues hypothesized that depression represented a relative increase in ACh activity and a decrease in NE activity. In contrast, mania represented a relative increase in NE activity and a decrease in ACh activity. A number of lines of evidence suggest elevated ACh activity is involved in depression; however, data from a number of groups suggest elevated ACh activity is associated with both increased NE and HPA axis activity. For example, administration of physostigmine, a procholinergic agent, increases plasma cortisol, plasma epinephrine and CSF MHPG levels.

Similarly, the simultaneous elevation in NE and cortisol activity could reflect increased CRF activity (28). Several studies have reported that CRF is elevated in the CSF of severely depressed patients, and CRF has been reported to increase NE activity in the locus coeruleus. Thus, the simultaneous increase in NE and HPA axis activity might involve this key neurotransmitter or neuromodulator. However, we recently observed in normal controls that administration of ovine CRH results in a significant increase in plasma homovanillic acid (HVA) but not in plasma MHPG. (Posener, Schildkraut, and Schatzberg, *unpublished data*). Further studies are required to assess the relationships between CRH and NE activity.

γ-Aminobutyric acid (GABA) is a third neurotransmitter that may play a role in NE disturbances in depression. Although this widely expressed neurotransmitter has been thought to exert a tonic inhibitory effect on NE systems, recent data suggest that this is not the case. Although GABA may exert an inhibitory effect on NE in some brain regions, recent data from Petty et al. (41) suggest that GABA may in fact facilitate NE activity. They reported that plasma GABA levels are relatively reduced in depressed patients. The role of GABA in mood disorders and its interactions with NE systems is worthy of further study.

SUMMARY

In reviewing the recent literature several findings appear to emerge with reasonable consistency.

1. Bipolar I–but not bipolar II–depressed patients can be separated from unipolar patients on the basis of urinary MHPG levels as well as other catecholamine and metabolite measures.
2. At least some unipolar depressed patients are characterized by elevated catecholamine and metabolite measures.
3. In depressed patients, increased levels of CAs and metabolites as well as elevated platelet MAO activity are associated with increased levels of cortisol or DST nonsuppression.
4. Patients with low urinary MHPG levels respond more robustly to imipramine (and perhaps to fluoxetine) than do patients with high MHPG levels.
5. Depressed patients demonstrate blunted GH responses to clonidine during both periods of depression and remission.
6. Depressed patients demonstrate decreased responsiveness of β receptors to challenges with specific agonists.
7. Manic patients demonstrate elevated CA and metabolite levels.
8. Treatment of depressed and manic patients, with antidepressants and lithium carbonate, respectively, results in a decrease in NE turnover.

The significance and explanation of these findings remains to be determined. Although they point to alterations in CA activity in affectively ill patients, it is difficult to determine the relative peripheral and central contributions of these findings, the exact roles that receptor activity and CA synthesis play, and the specific biological dysfunctions that may account for these findings. Alternative approaches need to be developed further to move along research in this area; imaging studies may help to define the key loci of CA activity both for underlying pathophysiology and clinical biological characteristics. Furthermore, the development of animal models with such biological hallmarks as increased NE and HPA axis activity (particularly in response to stress and behavioral sequelae) would enable one to assess the primacy of one or another system in the pathogenesis of depression on their relative contributions. Molecular biological studies of CA regulation are needed to define normative and maladaptive processes and their possible genetic underpinnings. Such studies can be done in both lower animals and in man.

ACKNOWLEDGMENTS

This work was supported in part by grants MH15413 and MH38671 from the National Institute of Mental Health as well as by grants from the Poitras Charitable Foundation and the Karen Tucker Fund.

We also would like to thank Marsha D. Wallace for her assistance in the preparation of this manuscript.

REFERENCES

1. Agren H, Oreland L. Early morning awakening in unipolar with higher levels of platelet MAO activity. *Psychiatry Res* 1982;7:245–254.
2. Agren H. Depressive symptom patterns and urinary MHPG excretion. *Psychiatry Res* 1982;6:185–196.
3. Amsterdam JD, Maislin G, Skolnick B, et al. Multiple hormonal responses to clonidine in depressed patients and volunteers. *Biol Psychiatry* 1989;26:265–278.
4. Annseau M, Von Frenckell R, Cerfontaine JL, et al. Neuroendocrine evaluation of catecholaminergic transmission in mania. *Psychiatry Res* 1987;22:193–206.
5. Bowden CL, Koslow S, Maas JW, et al. Changes in urinary catecholamines and their metabolites in depressed patients treated with amitriptyline or imipramine. *J Psychiatr Res* 1987;21:111–128.
6. Coupland N, Glue P, Natt DJ. Challenge tests: assessment of the noradrenergic and GABA systems in depression and anxiety disorders. *Mol Aspects Med* 1992;13:221–247.
7. De leon-Jones FD, Maas JW, Dekirmenjian H, et al. Diagnostic subgroups of affective disorders and their urinary excretion of catecholamine metabolites. *Am J Psychiatry* 1975;132:1141–1148.
8. Delgado PL Miller HL, Salomon RM, et al. Monoamines and the mechanism of antidepressant action: effects of catecholamine depletion on mood of patients treated with antidepressants. *Psychopharmacol Bull* 1993;29:389–396.
9. Delgado PL, Charney DS, Price LH, et al. Serotonin function and the mechanism of anti-depressant action: reversal of antidepressant induced remission by rapid depletion of plasma tryptophan. *Arch Gen Psychiatry* 1990;47:411–418.
10. DeParmentier F, Cheetham SC, Crompton MR, et al. Brain β-adrenoreceptor binding sites in antidepressant-free depressed suicide victims. *Brain Res* 1990;525:71–77.
11. Esler M, Turbott JT, Schwartz R, et al. The peripheral kinetics of norepinephrine in depressive illness. *Arch Gen Psychiatry* 1982;39:295–300.
12. Extein I, Tallman J, Smith CC, et al. Changes in lymphocyte beta-adrenergic receptors in depression and mania. *Psychiatry Res* 1979;1:191–197.
13. Garcia-Sevilla JA, Guimon J, Garcia-Vallejo P, et al. Biochemical and functional evidence of supersensitive platelet α_2-adrenorecep-

tors in major affective disorder: effect of long-term lithium carbonate treatment. *Arch Gen Psychiatry* 1986;43:51–57.

14. Garcia-Sevilla JA, Pardo D, Giralt MT, et al. α_2-Adrenoreceptor-mediated inhibition of platelet adenylate cyclase and induction of aggregation in major depression: effect of long-term antidepressant drug treatment. *Arch Gen Psychiatry* 1990;47:125–132.

15. Garvey MJ, Hollon S, Evans M, DeRubeis RJ, Tuason VB, et al. The association of MHPG to dexamethasone suppression test status. *Psychiatry Res* 1988;24:223–230.

16. Georgotas A, Schwertzer J, McCue RE, et al. Clinical and treatment effects on 3-H-clonidine and 3-H-imipramine binding in elderly depressed patients. *Life Sci* 1987;40:2137–2143.

17. Goodwin FK, Post RM. Studies of amine metabolites in affective illness and in schizophrenia: a comparative analysis. In: Freedman DX, ed. *Biology of the major psychoses.* New York: Raven Press; 1975:299–232.

18. Healy D, Halloran AO, Carney PA, et al. Peripheral adrenoreceptors and serotonin receptors in depression; changes associated with response to treatment with trazodone or amitriptyline. *J Affect Dis* 1985;9:285–296.

19. Hollister LE, David KL, Berger PA. Subtypes of depression based on excretion of MHPG and response to nortriptyline. *Arch Gen Psychiatry* 1980;37:1107–1110.

20. Jimerson DC, Insel TR, Reus VI, Kopin IJ. Increased plasma MHPG in dexamethasone-resistant depressed patients. *Arch Gen Psychiatry* 1983;40:173–176.

21. Johnson MR, Lydiard RB, Morton WA, et al. Effect of fluvoxamine, imipramine and placebo on catecholamine function in depressed outpatients. *J Psychiatr Res* 1993;27:161–172.

22. Karege F, Bovier PH, Gaillard JM, Tissot R. Plasma MHPG and AMDP depression relations, evolution and drug effect in a follow-up study of depressed patients. *Hum Psychopharmacol* 1991;6:11–17.

23. Koslow SH, Maas JW, Bowden CL, et al. CSF and urinary biogenic amines and metabolites in depression and mania. *Arch Gen Psychiatry* 1983;40:999–1010.

24. Loo H, Poirier MF, Dennis T, et al. Lack of correlation between DST results and urinary MHPG in depressed inpatients. *J Neural Transm* 1988;72:121–130.

25. Maas JW, Fawcett JA, Dekirmenjian H. Catecholamine metabolism, depressive illness, and drug response. *Arch Gen Psychiatry* 1972;26:252–262.

26. Maas JW, Koslow SH, David J, et al. Catecholamine metabolism and disposition in healthy and depressed subjects. *Arch Gen Psychiatry* 1987;44:337–344.

27. Maas JW, Koslow SH, Katz MM, et al. Pretreatment neurotransmitter metabolite levels and response to tricyclic antidepressant drugs. *Am J Psychiatry* 1984;141:10:1159–1171.

28. Maes M, Minner B, Suy E, et al. Coexisting dysregulations of both the sympathoadrenal system and hypothalamic-pituitary-adrenal-axis in melancholia. *J Neural Transm* [Gen Sect] 1991;85:195–210.

29. Maj M, Ariano MG, Arena F, Kemali D. Plasma cortisol, catecholamine and cyclic AMP levels, response to dexamethasone suppression test and platelet MAO activity in manic-depressive patients. *Neuropsychobiology* 1984;11:168–173.

30. Mann JJ, Mahler JC, Wilner RJ, et al. Normalization of blunted lymphocyte N-adrenergic responsivity in melancholic inpatients by a course of electroconvulsive therapy. *Arch Gen Psychiatry* 1990;47:461–464.

31. Mann JJ, Stanley M, McBride PA, et al. Increased serotonin$_2$ and β-adrenergic receptor binding in the frontal corties of suicide victims. *Arch Gen Psychiatry* 1986;43:954–969.

32. Meltzer HY, Lowry MT, Locascio JL. Platelet MAO activity and the cortisol response to dexamethasone in depression. *Biol Psychiatry* 1988;24:129–142.

33. Michel MC, Regan JW, Gerhardt MA, et al. Noradrenergic [³H]idazoxan binding sites are physically distinct from alpha-2 adrenergic receptors. *Mol Pharmacol* 1990;37:65–68.

34. Miller HL, Delgado PL, Salomon RM, et al. Alpha-methyl-para-tyrosine in drug-free depressed patients. Presented at the 146th annual meeting of the American Psychiatric Association. *New Res Abst* 1993;476.

35. Mitchell PB, Bearn JA, Corn TH, Checkley SA. Growth hormone response to clonidine after recovery in patients with endogenous depression. *Br J Psychiatry* 1988;152:34–38.

36. Mooney JJ, Schatzberg AF, Cole JO, et al. Rapid antidepressant response to alprazolam in depressed patients with high catecholamine output and heterologous desensitization of platelet adenylate cyclase. *Biol Psychiatry* 1988;23:543–559.

37. Mooney JJ, Schatzberg AF, Cole JO, et al. Urinary 3-methoxy-4-hydroxyphenylglycol and the depression-type score as predictors of differential responses to antidepressants. *J Clin Psychopharmacol* 1991;11:339–343.

38. Muscettola G, Potter WZ, Pickard D, et al. Urinary 3-methoxy-4-hydroxyphenylglycol and major affective disorders. *Arch Gen Psychiatry* 1984;41:337–342.

39. Pandey GN, Sharma RP, Janicak PH, Davis JM. Monoamine oxidase and cortisol response in depression and schizophrenia. *Psychiatry Res* 1992;44:1–8.

40. Pandey GN, Janicak PG, Javaid JI, et al. Increased 3-H-clonidine bindings in the platelets of patients with depressive and schizophrenic disorders. *Psychiatry Res* 1989;28:73–88.

41. Petty F, Kramer GL, Hedricksen W. GABA and depression. In: Mann JJ, Kupfer DJ, eds. *Biology of depressive disorders, part A: a systems perspective.* New York: Plenum Press; 1993:79–108.

42. Potter WZ, Grossman F, Rudoerfer MV. Noradrenergic function in depressive disorders. In: Mann JJ, Kupfer DJ, eds. *Biology of depressive disorders, part A: a systems perspective.* New York: Plenum Press; 1993:1–27.

43. Potter WZ, Karoum F, Linnoila M. Common mechanism of action of biochemically ''specific'' antidepressants. *Prog Neuropsychopharmacol Biol Psychiatry* 1984;8:153–161.

44. Potter WZ, Linnoila M. Biochemical classifications of diagnostic subgroups and D-type scores. *Arch Gen Psychiatry* 1989;46:269–271.

45. Rosenbaum AH, Maruta T, Schatzberg AF, et al. Toward a biochemical classification of depressive disorders. VII: urinary free cortisol and urinary MHPG in depressions. *Am J Psychiatry* 1983;140:314–318.

46. Rothschild AJ, Schatzberg AF, Langlais PJ, Lerbinger JE, Miller MM, Cole JO. Psychotic and nonpsychotic depressions. I: Comparison of plasma catecholamines and cortisol measures. *Psychiatry Res* 1987;20:143–153.

47. Roy A, Jimerson DC, Pickar D. Plasma MHPG in depressive disorders and relationship to the dexamethasone suppression test. *Am J Psychiatry* 1986;143:7:846–851.

48. Roy A, Pickar D, De Jong J, et al. Norepinephrine and its metabolites in cerebrospinal fluid, plasma, and urine. *Arch Gen Psychiatry* 1988;45:849–857.

49. Roy A, Pickar D, Linnoila M, et al. Plasma norepinephrine level in affective disorders. *Arch Gen Psychiatry* 1985;42:1181–1185.

50. Rubin AL, Price LH, Charney DS, Heninger GR. Noradrenergic function and the cortisol response to dexamethasone in depression. *Psychiatry Res* 1985;15:5–15.

51. Rudorfer MV, Ross RS, Linnoila M, et al. Exaggerated arthostatic responsivity of plasma norepinephrine in depression. *Arch Gen Psychiatry* 1985;42:1186–1192.

52. Samson JA, Mirin SM, Griffin M, et al. Urinary MHPG and clinical symptoms in unipolar depressed patients. *Psychiatry Res* [in press].

53. Samson JA, Mirin SM, Hauser SJ, et al. Learned helplessness and urinary MHPG levels in unipolar depression. *Am J Psychiatry* 1992;149:806–809.

54. Schatzberg AF, Orsulak PJ, Rosenbaum AH, et al. Toward a biochemical classification of depressive disorders. V: heterogeneity of unipolar depressions. *Am J Psychiatry* 1982;139:471–475.

55. Schatzberg AF, Rosenbaum AH, Orsulak PJ, et al. Toward a biochemical classification of depressive disorders. III: pretreatment of urinary MHPG levels as predictors of response to treatment with maprotiline. *Psychopharmacology* 1981;75:34–38.

56. Schatzberg AF, Rothschild AJ, Gerson B, et al. Toward a biochemical classification of depressive disorders. IX: DST results and platelet MAO activity. *Br J Psychiatry* 1985;146:633–637.

57. Schatzberg AF, Samson JA, Bloomingdale KL, et al. Toward a biochemical classification of depressive disorders. X: urinary catecholamines, their metabolites, and D-type scores in subgroups of depressive disorders. *Arch Gen Psychiatry* 1989;46:260–268.

58. Schatzberg AF, Samson JA, Schildkraut JJ, et al. Relationships

between catecholamine and cortisol measures in depressed patients. Presented at the American College of Neuropsychopharmacology Annual Meeting. Maui, Hawaii, 1989.

59. Schatzberg AF, Bowden CL, Rosenbaum AH, Schildkraut JJ. Prediction of response to fluoxetine versus desipramine. *CME Syllabus and Proceedings Summary,* 145th Annual Meeting. Washington, DC: American Psychiatric Association; 1992:44 (No. 25D).

60. Schildkraut JJ, Keeler BA, Grab EL, et al. MHPG excretion and clinical classification in depressive disorders. *Lancet* 1973;1:1251–1252.

61. Schildkraut JJ, Keeler BA, Rogers MP, et al. Catecholamine metabolism in affective disorders: a longitudinal study of a patient treated with amitriptyline and ECT. *Psychosom Med* 1973;34:470 and 35:274 (abst).

62. Schildkraut JJ, Orsulak PJ, LaBrie RA, et al. Toward a biochemical classification of depressive disorders. II: application of multiariate discriminant function analysis of data on urinary catecholamines and metabolites. *Arch Gen Psychiatry* 1978;35:1436–1439.

63. Schildkraut JJ, Orsulak PJ, Schatzberg AF, et al. Toward a biochemical classification of depressive disorders. I: differences in urinary excretion of MHPG and other catecholamine metabolites in clinically defined subtypes of depressions. *Arch Gen Psychiatry* 1978;35:1427–1433.

64. Schildkraut JJ. Norepinephrine metabolites as biochemical criteria for classifying depressive disorders and predicting response to treatment. Preliminary findings. *Am J Psychiatry* 1973;130:695–699.

65. Schildkraut JJ. Catecholamine metabolism and affective disorders: studies of MHPG excretion. In: Usdin E, Snyder S, eds. *Frontiers in catecholamine research.* New York: Pergamon Press; 1973:1165–1171.

66. Schildkraut, JJ. The catecholamine hypothesis of affective disorders: a review of supporting evidence. *Am J Psychiatry* 1965;122:509–522.

67. Sharma RP, Janicak PG, Javaid JI, et al. Platelet MAO inhibition, urinary MHPG, and leukocyte beta-adrenergic receptors in depressed patients treated with phenelzine. *Am J Psychiatry* 1990;147:1318–1321.

68. Shopsin B, Gershon S, Goldstein M, et al. Use of synthesis inhibitors in defining a role for biogenic amines during imipramine treatment in depressed patients. *Psychopharmacol Commun* 1975; 2:239–249.

69. Siever LJ, Kafka MS, Targum SM, et al. Platelet alpha adrenergic binding and biochemical responsiveness in depressed patients and controls. *Psychiatry Res* 1984;11:287–302.

70. Siever LJ, Uhde TW, Jimerson DC, et al. Differential inhibitory noradrenergic responses to clonidine in 25 depressed patients and 25 normal control subjects. *Am J Psychiatry* 1984;141:733–741.

71. Stokes PE, Frazer A, Casper R. Unexpected neuroendocrine-transmitter relationships. *Psychopharmacol Bull* 1981;17:72–75.

72. Stokes PE, Maas JW, Davis JM, et al. Biogenic amine and metabolite levels in depressed patients with high versus normal hypothalamic–pituitary–adrenocortical activity. *Am J Psychiatry* 1987;144:7:868–872.

73. Sulser F, Vetulani J, Mobley PL. Mode of action of antidepressant drugs. *Biochem Pharmacol* 1978;27:257–271.

74. Swann AC, Koslow SH, Katz MM, et al. Lithium carbonate treatment of mania. *Arch Gen Psychiatry* 1987;44:345–354.

75. Swann AC, Secunda SK, Stokes PE, et al. Stress, depression, and mania; relationship between perceived role of stressful events and clinical and biochemical characteristics. *Acta Psychiatr Scand* 1990;81:389–397.

76. Westiuk ES, Steiner M, Burns T. Studies on leukocyte β-adrenergic receptors in depression: A critical appraisal. *Life Sci* 1990;47:85–105.

77. Zhou D, Shen Y, Shu L, Lo H. Dexamethasone suppression test and urinary MHPG—SO$_4$ determination in depressive disorders. *Biol Psychiatry* 1987;22:883–891.

Psychopharmacology: The Fourth Generation of Progress, edited by Floyd E. Bloom and David J. Kupfer. Raven Press, Ltd., New York © 1995.

CHAPTER 80

Dopaminergic Mechanisms in Depression and Mania

Paul Willner

Traditional accounts of the biochemical basis of depression have focused largely on norepinephrine (NE) and serotonin (5-HT), and although most of the evidence that coalesced into the catecholamine hypothesis of depression does not distinguish clearly between NE and dopamine (DA), the potential role of DA was at first overlooked. Following two influential reviews that drew attention to this oversight (67,88), there has been an upsurge of interest in the possible involvement of DA in affective disorders. In fact, as will be seen below, there is little in the recent clinical evidence to justify this change of fashion; the pressure to reconsider the role of DA in depression arises almost entirely from preclinical developments. One is the now substantial body of work (reviewed below) demonstrating that antidepressant drugs enhance the functioning of mesolimbic DA synapses. However, the major driving force has undoubtedly been the massive research effort around the involvement of DA systems in motivated behavior (see Chapter 26, *this volume*).

It is important at the outset to recognize that neurotransmitters operate in the brain within well-defined projection systems that may subserve discrete functions. Of the two major forebrain DA projections, the larger nigrostriatal pathway is involved primarily in extrapyramidal motor functions, whereas the smaller mesocorticolimbic system, which innervates limbic structures such as the nucleus accumbens, amygdala, ventral hippocampus, and prefrontal cortex, supports a variety of behavioral functions related to motivation and reward (91); the third major DA pathway, the tuberoinfudibular projection, subserves neuroendocrine functions. The behavioral functions of the mesocorticolimbic DA system make this pathway an obvious candidate for investigation in relation to mood disorders. However, this focus on a specific pathway, which contains a relatively small proportion of forebrain DA neurons, creates a very real risk that changes in DA activity relevant to the psychopathology of mood could be obscured, in studies that employ global measures of brain DA function or apply anatomically nonspecific interventions.

Two phases can be distinguished in the development of a theoretical perspective on the role of the mesocorticolimbic DA system in motivated behavior. The first was the formulation by Wise and colleagues of the DA hypothesis of reward, which proposed that rewarding events, irrespective of their modality, shared the common property of activating the mesocorticolimbic DA system; conversely, inactivation of DA function would lead to anhedonia, the inability to experience pleasure (92). More recently, this research perspective has broadened to include consideration of the wider brain circuitry within which the mesocorticolimbic DA system is embedded. In this approach, the major focus shifts to the role of DA in gating the flow of information through the nucleus accumbens, which serves as the major interface through which information in limbic structures gains access to motor output systems. The major nondopaminergic afferent projections to the nucleus accumbens, which represent the major output pathways of the limbic system, are from the amygdala, hippocampus, and prefrontal cortex. Each of these three structures is itself innervated by the mesocorticolimbic DA system, and their projections to the nucleus accumbens overlap with one another and with the mesoaccumbens DA afferents (91). It is noteworthy that all of these structures afferent to the nucleus accumbens are implicated in mood psychopathology.

Although the hypothesis that the mesoaccumbens DA projection functions as a reward pathway (92) remains controversial, it is now indisputable that this pathway

P. Willner: Department of Psychology, University College of Swansea, Swansea SA2 8PP, Wales, United Kingdom.

plays a crucial role in the selection and orchestration of goal-directed behaviors, particularly those elicited by incentive stimuli (91). These properties make a hypofunction of the mesocorticolimbic DA system a prime candidate to mediate the inability to experience pleasure (anhedonia) and loss of motivation (lack of interest) that lie at the heart of major depressive disorder. [Conversely, manic hyperexcitability could readily result from a DA hyperfunction; this possibility has long been recognized (67).] This hypothesis differs somewhat from earlier biochemical theories in that it not only proposes a relationship between a biochemical entity (DA) and a mental disorder (depression or mania), but also defines explicitly the nature of the relationship, in terms of the functional properties of the relevant DA neurons. The hypothesis also defines certain boundary conditions; it involves a limited set of DA projections (the mesocorticolimbic system) and a limited set of depressive symptoms (anhedonia and lack of interest). This chapter critically reviews the recent clinical and preclinical evidence pertaining to the DA hypothesis of mood disorders, with particular reference, where possible, to the DA innervation of the nucleus accumbens. The three sections of the review deal with attempts to measure DA function in patients with mood disorders, the effects of pharmacological manipulations of DA function in human subjects, and preclinical evidence that antidepressant drugs increase transmission through mesolimbic DA synapses. The emphasis is on recent developments, and in particular, on issues not covered in detail by earlier reviews, which are frequently used in place of references to the older literature (12,38,67,88).

DOPAMINE FUNCTION IN MOOD DISORDERS

Dopamine Turnover

Numerous studies have attempted to assess forebrain DA function in depressed patients by measuring levels of the DA metabolite homovanillic acid (HVA) in cerebrospinal fluid (CSF). In some studies, patients were pretreated with probenecid to block the transport of HVA out of the CSF; this procedure, which measures the accumulation of HVA, is considered to give a better estimate of DA turnover. Most studies have tended to report a decrease in CSF HVA in depressed patients, and this relationship holds strongly in studies using the probenecid technique. Decreases in CSF HVA are particularly pronounced in patients with marked psychomotor retardation. In fact, a 1983 review of this area concluded that "The consistent finding of decreased post-probenecid CSF HVA accumulation in depressed patients, particularly those with psychomotor retardation, is probably the most firmly established observation in the neurochemistry of depression" (88). More recent studies have not altered this conclusion (12,38,68). There are also many reports

of decreased CSF HVA in depressed suicide attempters (12). Consistent with these findings, a recent study reported a decrease in 24-hr urinary excretion of HVA and DOPAC in depressed suicide attempters (71). As abnormalities of DA metabolism are not observed in nondepressed suicide attempters (12), these data provide further evidence that decreased DA turnover is a correlate of depression.

Nevertheless, the interpretation of these data is far from straightforward. Although one study has reported that CSF HVA was lower in melancholic than in nonmelancholic patients (72), this relationship is probably explained by the association between low CSF HVA and psychomotor retardation (12,88), which is a prominent feature of melancholia. In fact, low CSF HVA has been associated with psychomotor slowing (bradyphrenia) not only in depressed patients, but also in Parkinson's disease and Alzheimer's disease (93). In agitated patients, however, CSF HVA levels are normal or slightly elevated (88). Levels of CSF HVA [as well as plasma DA (74)] are also elevated in delusional patients (88). Again, this finding may reflect psychomotor change: in a study of psychotic patients, CSF HVA levels were elevated in those with delusions and agitation, but normal in those with delusions but no agitation (87). Levels of CSF HVA are usually found to be elevated in mania (38). These data suggest that CSF HVA levels may reflect motor activity rather than mood, and further raise the problem of whether a reduction in HVA level is the primary cause or a secondary reflection of psychomotor retardation. This latter problem has lain dormant since an early study in which a group of depressed patients were asked to simulate mania: the exercise did increase DA turnover but also elevated mood (62).

It is hardly surprising that CSF HVA levels are associated with level of motor activity, since CSF HVA derives largely from the caudate nucleus, on account of its large size and its periventricular location. In schizophrenic patients, decreased CSF HVA concentrations are associated with ventricular enlargement (18), which is equally common in major depressive disorder (37). Indeed, PET imaging studies have reported hypometabolism of the head of the caudate nucleus in unipolar and bipolar depressed patients, which may reflect a decreased DA activity in this structure (6). However, the contribution to CSF HVA of DA release in mesolimbic structures such as the nucleus accumbens and frontal cortex is relatively minor. There is therefore no reason to expect that changes in mesolimbic DA function would be apparent in studies measuring HVA levels in lumbar CSF; it is far more likely that any such changes would be obscured by alterations in nigrostriatal DA function associated with changes in motor output. Thus, although most reviewers have tended to interpret the HVA data as evidence for a DA dysfunction in depression (36,67,88), these data are actually silent with respect to the important question of the state of activity in the mesocorticolimbic DA system.

In one series of studies, increased levels of DA itself were observed in the CSF of melancholic patients, with higher concentrations occurring more frequently in patients who were delusional (29). In depressed patients, CSF DA levels have been found to correlate with extraversion (40). However, the proportion of DA in lumbar CSF that originated in the forebrain is unknown.

Dopamine Receptors

There have as yet been very few studies of DA receptors in patients with mood disorders. Studies using PET imaging suggest that D_2 receptor numbers may be elevated in manic but not in nondelusional depressed patients (94,95). However, a recent single-photon emission computed tomographic (SPECT) study of a relatively large group of depressed patients ($n = 21$), most of them drug free for at least 3 weeks, reported a bilateral increase in D_2 receptor binding in the basal ganglia (25). This finding is compatible with a decrease in DA turnover, but is subject to similar problems of interpretation: the relative contributions of mood and motor activity and the inability of current techniques to image the nucleus accumbens independently of the dorsal striatum. One PET study of D_1 receptors has reported a decrease in D_1 receptor binding in the frontal cortex, but not the striatum, of bipolar patients ($n = 6$ euthymic, $n = 3$ manic, and $n = 1$ depressed). However, the ligand used in this study (SCH-23390) also binds to 5-HT$_2$ receptors (83).

Although there is strong evidence for a genetic contribution to bipolar mood disorder, molecular genetic studies have so far provided no evidence that bipolar disorder is associated with abnormalities of the genes coding for the D_1 (49,53), D_2 (14,35,49,53), or D_3 (69,78) receptors.

Neuroendocrine Studies

The tuberoinfundibular DA system has neuroendocrine functions, inhibiting the release of prolactin and stimulating the release of growth hormone (GH). Thus, basal levels of these hormones have been examined as potential markers of DA function in mood disorders, and their responses to DA agonists have been used to evaluate DA receptor responsiveness. These studies suffer two serious limitations: the inability to generalize any conclusions to the forebrain DA systems, and the involvement of many other neurotransmitters in neuroendocrine regulation; in particular, a stimulatory role of 5-HT in prolactin secretion and a stimulatory role of α-adrenergic receptors in GH secretion.

Abnormal prolactin levels have frequently been reported in depressed patients, but there is no consistency in the direction of change; low, normal, and high values

have been reported in different studies (12,38,88). Prolactin levels are reported to be normal in mania (39,108). Prolactin responses were also normal in depressed patients following DA agonist (12,38) or antagonist (2) challenges. However, two recent studies have reported a decrease in prolactin levels in seasonal affective disorder (SAD), which was seen in both unipolar and bipolar patients, and was present during both winter depression and summer euthymia (23,24). This apparent trait abnormality in SAD patients is consistent either with increased DA function or with decreased 5-HT function. The former interpretation is supported by the observation that SAD patients also showed a seasonally independent increase in spontaneous eye blinking: this behavior is thought to be under dopaminergic control, being increased by D_2 agonists and suppressed by D_2 antagonists (23,24).

Studies of GH are similarly inconclusive. Basal GH levels have been reported to be decreased (11), normal (4), or increased (48) in major depression; no changes were seen in mania (38). A recent study reported a blunting of the GH response to apomorphine in major depression, relative to patients with minor depression or normal controls (4), but no differences were observed in many earlier studies, using either a slightly higher dose of apomorphine (0.75 vs. 0.5 mg), or L-dopa (38,88). The group reporting blunted GH responses to apomorphine have reported a difference between major and minor depressives in two further studies (3,59) and have also reported blunted responses in manic patients (3) and in suicide attempters (60). The same group also reported that blunted apomorphine responses in depressed patients were associated with low introversion and anxiety scores on the MMPI but not with severity of depression (61); others have reported a negative correlation between GH response and severity of delusions (47). Together, these observations suggest that there may be some subsensitivity to apomorphine in a subgroup of depressed patients. If these findings are confirmed, the question remains of whether they reflect DA receptor subsensitivity, or a more general decrease in GH responsivity [it is well established that the GH response to α-adrenergic challenges is subsensitive in major depression (79)]. The relevance of GH changes for forebrain DA function also remains to be determined.

MOOD EFFECTS OF DOPAMINE AGONISTS AND ANTAGONISTS

Psychostimulants

The psychostimulants amphetamine and methylphenidate cause activation and euphoria in normal volunteers. Although these drugs enhance activity at both DA and noradrenergic synapses, the psychostimulant effects are mediated at DA synapses, since they are antagonized by

DA receptor blockers but not by adrenergic receptor blockers (36,55,56). The euphoric effects of low doses of psychostimulants at low doses closely parallel the symptomatology of hypomania, whereas high doses, particularly when taken repeatedly or chronically, can cause grandiosity, delusions, dysphoria, and all the other symptoms of a full-blown manic episode (36,63).

Single doses of amphetamine or methylphenidate also cause a transient mood elevation in a high proportion (more than 50%) of depressed patients (43); the response in depressed patients appears similar, in size and in the proportion of subjects responding, to that seen in nondepressed volunteers (15,55). Following an initial report by Fawcett and Siomopoulos (27), a number of studies have used the acute mood response to psychostimulants to predict the clinical response to chronic antidepressant therapy. A recent review of this literature confirmed that the response to antidepressants was well predicted by the result of an amphetamine challenge (85% improvement in responders versus 43% in nonresponders), but questioned the predictive value of a methylphenidate challenge (66% improvement in responders versus 68% in nonresponders) (43). However, the amphetamine and methylphenidate studies differ in that the amphetamine studies involved mainly patients treated with imipramine and desipramine, whereas the methylphenidate studies also included a high proportion of patients treated with serotonergic antidepressants. A reanalysis of the same literature showed that the acute response to methylphenidate does predict antidepressant efficacy, provided that the analysis is restricted to patients treated with noradrenergic antidepressants (34).

Psychostimulants are not themselves considered to be efficacious as antidepressants. In early trials, the catecholamine precursor L-dopa produced a modest global improvement, primarily in retarded patients, but the effect was largely one of psychomotor activation with little effect on mood; in bipolar patients, dopa frequently caused a switch into hypomania (32). These data have been interpreted as evidence against a prominent role for DA in depression. However, the effects of dopa were greatest in patients with the lowest pretreatment CSF HVA levels (86), which suggests that the effect of dopa might primarily be to increase DA release in the caudate nucleus, perhaps causing motor side effects that could mask any potentially therapeutic effects of an increase in mesolimbic DA release. It is now known that low doses of amphetamine preferentially release DA within the nucleus accumbens (26). Despite the absence of clinical trial data, amphetamine continues to find widespread, if little publicized, use in the treatment of depression (5).

Dopamine-active Antidepressants

More convincing antidepressant effects have been reported with the directly acting DA agonists piribedil and bromocriptine. These were largely open trials, but there are also controlled studies, including a double-blind trial showing piribedil to be superior to placebo, particularly in patients with low pretreatment CSF HVA, and two large trials, which found no difference in antidepressant efficacy between bromocriptine and imipramine (88). The antidepressant response to bromocriptine may be greater in bipolar patients (80), and one study suggests a preferential effect of bromocriptine on emotional blunting (1). Hypomanic responses during bromocriptine therapy have been reported (39,80). In a particularly interesting development, Mouret and colleagues have described striking and rapid therapeutic effects of piribedil in previously nonresponsive patients whose sleep EEG showed signs characteristic for Parkinson's disease; in patients not showing these signs, piribedil was ineffective (50).

Trials of DA agonists in depression are not currently fashionable, but it is notable that DA uptake inhibition is a prominent feature of a number of newer antidepressants, including nomifensine, buproprion, and amineptine (12). Amineptine, which is a relatively selective DA uptake inhibitor, was more efficacious than clomipramine and had a faster onset of antidepressant action in a double-blind trial in retarded patients; another dopaminomimetic agent, minaprine, was also more effective than clomipramine in retarded patients (66).

Contrary to expectations, given the antidepressant effects of DA agonists, there is also clear evidence that under certain circumstances, neuroleptics, which are DA receptor antagonists, are also active as antidepressants (52,70). One potential resolution of this apparent paradox (which will be discussed below) is that neuroleptics may act as antidepressants only at low doses that act preferentially as DA autoreceptor antagonists, and so increase DA turnover. This hypothesis has been advanced in particular in relation to certain atypical antidepressants, such as sulpiride, which are said to have activating properties. Antidepressant effects of sulpiride are seen in a dose range of 50 to 150 mg/day, which is considerably lower than the typical antipsychotic dose of 800 to 1,000 mg/day. A DA-activating effect of sulpiride at low doses is supported by the finding that low doses of sulpiride antagonized the sedative actions of apomorphine in human subjects (77).

Antidepressant effects have also been reported for roxindole, a putatively selective DA autoreceptor agonist. In an open trial, roxindole caused rapid improvements in 8 of 12 patients suffering from a major depressive episode, as well as reducing depression and anergia in schizophrenic patients (8). Roxindole possesses 5-HT uptake-inhibiting and 5-HT$_{1A}$ agonist actions, both of which could contribute to an antidepressant effect, but neuroendocrine data [suppression of prolactin secretion (8)] suggest that DA agonism is the predominant action of this drug. If, as claimed, roxindole is a selective autoreceptor agonist, the effect should be to decrease DA function.

However, it is questionable whether roxindole is antidepressant by virtue of decreasing DA function; the drug also appears to be effective in negative schizophrenia (8), which is compatible with a DA-activating effect.

Neuroleptic-induced Depression

Depression is frequently encountered as a side effect of neuroleptic therapy in schizophrenia (67,82). There are strong grounds for believing that the effect is caused by antagonism of DA receptors, but it is difficult to exclude the possibility that by bringing schizophrenic symptoms under control, neuroleptics unmask a preexisting depression. Conversely, neuroleptic drugs decrease manic symptomatology. Although classical neuroleptics act at a variety of receptor sites, antimanic effects are also observed with drugs that act relatively specifically as DA receptor antagonists (38). In normal volunteers, neuroleptics induce feelings of dysphoria, paralysis of volition, and fatigue (7).

Based on a series of reports in the 1950s, it is still widely believed that the catecholamine-depleting drug reserpine causes depression, despite the findings of Goodwin et al. (31), on reanalysis of these data, that the great majority of reserpine depression patients had been incorrectly diagnosed. Patients treated with reserpine tended to display a pseudodepression characterized by psychomotor slowing, fatigue, and anhedonia but lacking cognitive features of depression such as hopelessness or guilt. Only a small proportion of patients (5% to 9%) showed symptoms analogous to major depression, and these patients usually had a prior history of mood disorders (31). It remains unclear whether the doses of reserpine administered in the reserpine depression studies were sufficient to decrease DA function. However, it may be significant that in the Goodwin et al. reanalysis, major depression was considered to be the correct diagnosis in almost 50% of patients who developed marked psychomotor retardation (31).

Parkinson's Disease

More convincing evidence of an association between DA depletion and depression is seen in the high incidence of depression in Parkinson's disease (36,67, cf. 84). At the level of symptomatology, there is substantial overlap between Parkinsonian akinesia and depressive psychomotor retardation (9,84). It is difficult to determine whether Parkinsonian depression should be considered a secondary response to loss of motor function, rather than a direct consequence of DA depletion. There is no agreement in the literature as to whether the severity of depression is correlated with the extent of physical impairment. However, Parkinsonian depression is more severe than would be expected from the physical symptoms alone, and the onset of depression can precede the physical disabilities (33).

It is now recognized that Parkinson's disease is in no sense a pure DA deficiency syndrome: NE, 5-HT, acetylcholine (ACh), somatostatin, and neurotensin are also abnormal (58). Nevertheless, there are good reasons to relate the symptoms of Parkinsonian depression to DA depletion. In one well-designed study, depressed Parkinsonian patients showed profound attenuation of the euphoric response to methylphenidate, relative to nondepressed Parkinsonian patients, depressed non-Parkinsonian patients, and normal controls (15). The antidepressant effect of dopa in Parkinson's disease (1,32,67) also points toward a dopaminergic substrate of Parkinsonian depression. In some cases, there is clear evidence that mood improvement precedes the improvement in physical symptoms (51), suggesting that the antidepressant effect cannot simply be explained away as secondary to an improvement in physical symptoms. Antidepressant effects of bupropion (30) and bromocriptine (39) have also been reported in Parkinsonian patients.

Neuroleptics as Antidepressants

The clinical pharmacology literature reviewed in this section is broadly consistent with the hypothesis that increases in DA function elevate mood and decreases in DA function induce symptoms of depression. However, not all of the data are compatible with this formulation. In particular, the fact that neuroleptics are used to treat depression (52,70) strikes at the heart of the dopamine–anhedonia–depression hypotheses. This phenomenon therefore requires careful consideration.

One hypothesis, discussed above, is that neuroleptics are administered in depression at low doses that interact selectively with presynaptic autoreceptors. However, while an autoreceptor hypothesis might explain some of the data, particularly those pertaining to sulpiride, it is not necessarily the case that low doses are used when neuroleptics are prescribed as antidepressants. Doses below the antipsychotic range have usually been prescribed in studies of mild, nonendogenous depression; however, in delusional depression, neuroleptics are more commonly prescribed at normal antipsychotic doses (52). However, it is not certain that DA antagonism is the mechanism of antidepressant action. Indeed, in one study, antidepressant effects of cis-flupenthixol were negatively correlated with increase in serum prolactin levels, suggesting that DA blockade might actually antagonize the antidepressant effect (70). In a similar vein, antidepressant effects on withdrawal of neuroleptics are well documented, although the evidence tends to arise from case reports rather than from formal studies (67). In a recent trial, Del Zompo et al. (21) treated depressed patients with a haloperidol/chlorimipramine cocktail and reported marked improvement, relative to a group treated with chlorimipramine alone, when the haloperidol component was withdrawn after 3 weeks treatment. It was assumed that the improvement resulted from the unmasking of DA receptors rendered supersensitive by chronic neuroleptic treatment. Clearly, more trials of this kind are needed, and the proposed mechanism of action requires confirmation.

It is also questionable whether neuroleptics are truly antidepressant, and examination of the pattern of symptomatic improvement may provide the clearest resolution to the paradox of the antidepressant action of neuroleptics: in brief, there is no evidence that neuroleptics can improve either psychomotor retardation or anhedonia, the core symptom of depression most closely associated with the DA hypothesis. The antidepressant potential of neuroleptics is most firmly established in delusional depression, which responds well to combined therapy with a neuroleptic and a tricyclic, but responds poorly if at all to tricyclics alone. However, neuroleptics alone are also ineffective in delusional depression; they produce a substantial global improvement, but this arises almost entirely from a decrease in agitation and delusional thinking; motor retardation, lack of energy, and anhedonia do not respond to neuroleptic treatment and indeed, may become worse (52). In endogenous depressions, although neuroleptics have been claimed to be as effective as tricyclics, or nearly so, this appearance may be spurious, insofar as the studies in question may have seriously underestimated the true effectiveness of tricyclics (owing to a failure to attain adequate plasma drug levels and other factors) (52). On the basis of the findings in delusional depression, it seems likely that the global improvement seen in endogenous depressives treated with neuroleptics results from the preponderance in these studies of agitated and delusional patients (52,70). This analysis of the place of neuroleptics in the treatment of depression implies that retardation and delusions are mediated by different sets of DA terminals, which may be activated independently (28). In support of this assumption, it is well established that different components of the mesocorticolimbic DA projection are differentially regulated (81).

DOPAMINERGIC MECHANISMS OF ANTIDEPRESSANT ACTION

Dopamine Autoreceptor Desensitization

Most antidepressant drugs have little effect on DA function following acute administration; in particular, tricyclic antidepressants do not act as potent DA uptake inhibitors (88), in contrast to their well-known effects at adrenergic and serotonergic synapses [although some data suggest that antidepressants may cause significant inhibition of DA uptake within the nucleus accumbens and frontal cortex (16,19)]. Nevertheless, there is now consid-

erable evidence that antidepressants do enhance dopaminergic function following chronic administration.

In one of the earliest studies to demonstrate an antidepressant-induced increase in DA function, Serra et al. (75) reported that imipramine, amitriptyline, and mianserin all decreased the sedative effect of a low dose of apomorphine. Because this latter effect was assumed to be mediated by stimulation of DA autoreceptors, the results were interpreted as a decrease in autoreceptor sensitivity. However, the evidence that antidepressants desensitize DA autoreceptors is equivocal in the extreme. There are a number of supportive studies, using a variety of techniques, but also, there have been failures to replicate all of these data (88). Some studies have reported that clear evidence of DA autoreceptor subsensitivity was not present until 3 to 7 days following withdrawal from chronic antidepressant treatment (73,85). Another reason to question the relevance of DA autoreceptor desensitization for the clinical action of antidepressants is that these data were obtained in normal rats; rats exposed to chronic mild stress, which has been proposed as an animal model of depression, show evidence of DA autoreceptor desensitization similar to that sometimes seen following chronic antidepressant treatment in normal animals (90). Finally, changes in apomorphine-induced sedation do not necessarily imply changes in DA autoreceptor function. High doses of apomorphine cause locomotor stimulation, so a decrease in apomorphine-induced sedation might equally well indicate an increase in postsynaptic responsiveness rather than autoreceptor subsensitivity.

Sensitization of D_2/D_3 Receptors

In fact, a substantial body of literature now demonstrates that following chronic treatment, antidepressants do increase the responsiveness of postsynaptic D_2/D_3 receptors in the mesolimbic system; these effects are seen irrespective of the primary neurochemical action of the drug (44,89). The majority of studies have examined the locomotor stimulant response to moderate doses of apomorphine or amphetamine; these responses are consistently elevated following chronic administration of antidepressants. Similar effects were observed using the specific D_2/D_3 agonist quinpirole (44). There are well-known pharmacokinetic interactions between antidepressants and amphetamine. However, antidepressants also increased the psychomotor stimulant effect when amphetamine, or DA itself, was administered directly to the nucleus accumbens (44), confirming a true pharmacodynamic interaction. Furthermore, these effects were present within a short time (2 hr) of the final antidepressant treatment, confirming that, unlike DA autoreceptor desensitization, the increase in responsiveness of postsynaptic D_2/D_3 receptors is not simply a withdrawal effect. The potentiation of D_2/D_3 receptor function by chronic antidepressant treatment is confined to mesolimbic terminal regions; antidepressants do not increase the intensity of behavioral stereotypes caused by high doses of amphetamine, which are mediated by DA release within the dorsal striatum (89). Neither did chronic antidepressant treatment potentiate a DA-mediated neuroendocrine response (64).

With two exceptions, receptor-binding studies have consistently failed to detect any alterations in the binding parameters of D_2/D_3 receptors that would explain the increased functional responses. The majority of these studies are of limited relevance, because they assayed DA receptors in samples of dorsal striatum. Nevertheless, no change was detected in D_2/D_3 receptor binding, even in the nucleus accumbens (42,46). In contrast to these negative data in normal animals, a recent study found that a decrease in the D_2/D_3 receptor numbers in the limbic forebrain of rats subjected to chronic mild stress was completely reversed by chronic treatment with imipramine (57). It has also been reported that D_2/D_3 receptors in the limbic forebrain (but not the dorsal striatum) have an increased affinity for the agonist ligand, quinpirole, following chronic antidepressant administration to rats (42). [α_1-Adrenergic receptors show a similar increase in agonist affinity after chronic antidepressant treatment, with no changes in binding parameters as assessed using antagonist ligands (89).]

In addition to increasing the agonist affinity of the D_2/D_3 receptors, antidepressants also decrease the number of D_1 receptors, following chronic treatment (19,20,42). This effect is associated with a decrease in the ability of DA to stimulate adenyl cyclase (19,20) and a decreased behavioral response (grooming) to D_1 receptor stimulation (45), which is consistent with the binding data. A role for D_1 receptor changes in the sensitization of D_2/D_3 receptors has been proposed (76), but this seems unlikely, as the down-regulation of D_1 receptors is species specific: D_1 receptors were down-regulated by chronic imipramine in rats but not in mice (54). Furthermore, D_1 receptors were not down-regulated by chronic imipramine in chronically stressed rats, which did show D_2/D_3 receptor up-regulation (57). In both of these studies, functionally relevant behavioral effects of chronic antidepressant treatment were seen in the absence of D_1 receptor changes (54,57).

Role of Mesolimbic Dopamine in Animal Models of Depression

Although these data confirm that antidepressants change the functional status of DA receptors in the nucleus accumbens, they give little insight into the role that these changes play in the clinical action of antidepressants. Animal models of depression provide one means of addressing this question, albeit indirectly. The mecha-

nisms by which antidepressants act have been analyzed most extensively in the Porsolt swim test. In this model, rats or mice are required to swim in a confined space, and antidepressants prolong the period in which the animal displays active escape behavior. Immobility in the swim test may be reversed not only by antidepressants, but also by D_2/D_3 receptor agonists, applied systemically or to the nucleus accumbens (10). Conversely, a number of studies have reported that antidepressant effects in the swim test were reversed by DA antagonists (10); these include studies in which antidepressants were administered chronically (22,65). The effects of chronically administered tricyclic antidepressants were reversed by the administration of sulpiride in the nucleus accumbens but not in the dorsal striatum (17). Despite these positive findings, Borsini and Meli urge caution in accepting that the data demonstrate a dopaminergic mechanism of antidepressant action in the swim test and suggest that the effects of intraaccumbens sulpiride could be related to the presence in the mesolimbic system of nondopaminergic sulpiride binding sites that also bind antidepressants (10). The swim test has been criticized on a number of counts, most prominently, that it responds to acute administration of antidepressants, unlike the clinical situation, which requires chronic treatment. This criticism is not entirely justified, because the test only responds acutely to extremely high drug doses but becomes slowly more sensitive with repeated treatment (89). However, the validity of the test as a model of depression is extremely weak.

Mechanisms of antidepressant action have also been analyzed in the chronic mild stress procedure, which represents a more valid and realistic animal model of depression than the swim test (90). In this procedure, rats are exposed chronically (weeks or months) to a variety of mild unpredictable stressors. This causes a generalized decrease in responsiveness to rewards (anhedonia), which can be reversed by chronic administration of tricyclic or atypical antidepressants (90). These behavioral changes are accompanied by a decrease in D_2/D_3-receptor binding in the nucleus accumbens (57) and a pronounced functional subsensitivity to the rewarding and locomotor stimulant effects of the D_2/D_3 agonist quinpirole, administered systemically or within the nucleus accumbens (90). In animals successfully treated with antidepressants (including tricyclics, specific 5-HT or NE uptake inhibitors, or mianserin), behavioral recovery was reversed by acute administration of D_2/D_3 receptor antagonists, at low doses that were without effect in nonstressed animals or in untreated stressed animals (90). Chronic stress also causes an antidepressant reversible decrease in aggressive behavior, and this effect of chronic antidepressant treatment was also reversed by acute administration of DA antagonists (96). These data argue strongly that an increase in D_2/D_3 receptor responsiveness may be responsible for the therapeutic action of antidepressants in this model.

CONCLUSIONS

Outstanding Issues

The data reviewed in the preceding section present a strong case that elevation of DA transmission in the nucleus accumbens may represent a final common pathway responsible for at least part of the spectrum of behavioral actions of antidepressant drugs. The mechanisms by which antidepressants sensitize DA transmission are unknown, but the best guess at present is that the effects are indirectly mediated by primary actions at NE or 5-HT terminals. The evidence supporting a dopaminergic mechanism of antidepressant action is almost entirely preclinical: clinical studies evaluating the role of DA mechanisms in the action of classical antidepressants have yet to be carried out. Nevertheless, the preclinical studies suggest that D_2/D_3 receptors in the nucleus accumbens might represent a potential target for antidepressant action, and it is likely that this receptor population will serve as a focus for novel drug development strategies. The value of this approach remains to be determined. However, the initial clinical studies of the antidepressant potential of D_2/D_3 agonists and DA autoreceptor antagonists are promising.

It remains the case that the preclinical evidence for enhancement of DA transmission following chronic treatment with antidepressant drugs provides the strongest support for the DA hypothesis of mood disorders. The strongest evidence against the DA hypothesis comes from the clinical use of neuroleptics in depression. As discussed above, there are a number of potential resolutions of this troublesome paradox, including the possibility of autoreceptor-selective actions of neuroleptics at low doses, the possibility that neuroleptics control delusions but actually worsen depressive symptoms, and the possibility that DA hypofunction in some terminal fields coexists with DA hyperfunction in other regions (28,52). [The latter hypothesis has also been advanced to explain the coexistence of negative and positive symptoms in schizophrenia (18,28).] There has been little research directed specifically at understanding the place of neuroleptics in the treatment of depression: more is urgently needed.

Setting aside the question of neuroleptics as antidepressants, the effects of pharmacological interventions, in human subjects, lead broadly to the conclusion that inhibiting DA transmission is therapeutic in mania and induces depressive symptomatology in normal volunteers, whereas stimulation of DA transmission has antidepressant effects and induces manic symptoms. However, the extent of overlap between these pharmacological effects and clinical changes is far from complete. Although the effects of psychostimulants provide a good match to the symptoms of mania, the primary effects of neuroleptics or reserpine in normal subjects are fatigue, apathy, and dysphoria (7,31). Conversely, while L-dopa readily induces hypomania in depressed patients, there is little evidence of mood improvement (32). Thus, the pharmacological evidence for DA involvement appears rather stronger in mania than in depression. However, this conclusion overlooks the anatomical nonspecificity of these drugs: They are of limited value as research tools for evaluating whether depression is associated with a dysfunction of mesolimbic DA specifically. In contrast to L-dopa, directly acting DA agonists do appear to be effective antidepressants, although the number of controlled trials remains unacceptably low. The clinical efficacy of these agents may reflect a preferential action within the nucleus accumbens, but it is not yet possible to evaluate this hypothesis in human subjects.

Similarly, the inability to measure DA activity within the nucleus accumbens seriously limits the value of virtually all of the correlative studies of DA function in depression and mania. The fact that there are no reliable neuroendocrine changes in patients with mood disorders simply tells us that there are no generalized abnormalities of D_2/D_3 receptors, not that such abnormalities are absent within the nucleus accumbens specifically. Similarly, we have no useful information on the release of DA from mesocorticolimbic terminals in human subjects. The clearest evidence implicating DA in depression, the decrease in CSF HVA concentrations in retarded depression, is intriguing, but appears to relate primarily to changes in motor function. Discovering the direction of causality in this relationship remains an important objective. However, the priority for understanding the role of DA in depression must be to redress the imbalance between the preclinical and the clinical evidence. This requires the development of research tools for human use with sufficient anatomical precision to evaluate DA function within distinct terminal fields.

Syndromes or Symptoms?

As noted in the introduction to this chapter, our emerging understanding of the behavioral functions of forebrain DA systems suggests that the involvement of DA in affective disorders might profitably be analyzed at the level of symptoms rather than syndromes. The clinical literature contains a number of findings that support this position. Thus, there is some evidence that emotional blunting responds more rapidly and more completely than other symptoms in depressed patients treated with bromocriptine (1), and that DA-uptake inhibiting antidepressants may be superior to tricyclics in retarded patients (66). Conversely, Parkinsonian or pre-Parkinsonian (50) depressions, which respond to treatment with DA agonists (1,50,67), are characterized by decreased motivation and drive, but not by feelings of guilt, self-blame and worthlessness (13); these characteristic depressive cognitions are also conspicuously absent from descriptions of neuroleptic- or reserpine-induced depressive states (7,31).

From a psychobiological standpoint, it seems obvious that the major psychiatric syndromes are likely to involve multiple neurotransmitter systems that contribute to different syndromes to differing degrees. An obvious research strategy is to investigate, as a first step, the involvement of specific pathways in specific behavioral processes, which need not, on a priori grounds, bear any obvious relationship to nosological boundaries. It is clear that features of what might be termed a DA-deficiency syndrome, involving low CSF HVA, anhedonia, psychomotor slowing, and a good response to DA agonist treatment, are characteristic not only of depression, but also of Parkinson's disease (9,84,87,93), and negative schizophrenia (8,28,41,87). At the other extreme, there is considerable overlap in symptoms between positive schizophrenia and mania, and these common symptoms are reliably reproduced in psychostimulant-induced psychoses (28,63). The extent to which these similar functional outcomes reflect common underlying mechanisms remains to be determined, and represents a major challenge for future research. However, the difficulties of pursuing a research agenda that cuts across DSM-IV diagnostic categories should not be underestimated.

REFERENCES

1. Ammar S, Martin P. Modelisation des effets des agonistes dopaminergiques en psychopharmacologie: vers une homothetie clinique et experimentale. *Psychol Franc* 1991;36:221–232.
2. Anderson IM, Cowen PJ. Prolactin response to the dopamine antagonist, metoclopramide, in depression. *Biol Psychiatr* 1991;30:313–316.
3. Ansseau M, von Frenckell R, Cerfontaine JL, et al. Neuroendocrine evaluation of catecholaminergic neurotransmission in mania. *Psychiatr Res* 1987;22:193–206.
4. Ansseau M, von Frenckell R, Cerfontaine JL, et al. Blunted response of growth hormone to clonidine and apomorphine in endogenous depression. *Br J Psychiatry* 1988;153:65–71.
5. Ayd FJ Jr., Zohar J. Psychostimulant (amphetamine or methylphenidate) therapy for chronic and treatment-resistant depression. In: Zohar J, Belmaker RH, eds. *Treating resistant depression.* New York: PMA Corp. 1987:343–355.
6. Baxter LR, Schwartz JM, Phelps ME, et al. Reduction of prefrontal cortex glucose metabolism common to three types of depression. *Arch Gen Psychiatry* 1989;46:243–250.
7. Belmaker RH, Wald D. Haloperidol in normals. *Br J Psychiatry* 1977;131:222–223.
8. Benkert O, Brunder G, Wetzel H. Dopamine autoreceptor agonists in the treatment of schizophrenia and major depression. *Parmacopsychiatry* 1992;25:254–260.
9. Bermanzohn PC, Siris G. Akinesia: a syndrome common to Parkinsonism, retarded depression and negative symptoms of schizophrenia. *Compr Psychiatry* 1992;33:221–232.
10. Borsini F, Meli A. The forced swimming test: its contribution to the understanding of the mechanisms of action of antidepressants. In: Gessa GL, Serra G, eds. *Dopamine and mental depression.* Oxford: Pergamon Press; 1990;63–76.
11. Boyer P, Davila M, Schaub C, Nassiet J. Growth hormone response to clonidine stimulation in depressive states. Part I. *Psychiatr Psychobiol* 1986;1:189–195.
12. Brown AS, Gershon S. Dopamine and depression. *J Neural Transm* 1993;91:75–109.
13. Brown RG, MacCarthy B, Gotham A-M, Der GJ, Marsden CD. Depression and disability in Parkinson's disease: a follow-up of 132 cases. *Psychol Med* 1988;18:49–55.
14. Byerley W, Leppert M, O'Connell P, et al. D2 dopamine receptor gene not linked to manic-depression in three families. *Psychiatr Genet* 1990;1:55–62.
15. Cantello R, Aguggia M, Gilli M, et al. Major depression in Parkinson's disease and the mood response to intravenous methylphenidate: possible role of the "hedonic" dopamine synapse. *J Neurol Neurosurg Psychiatry* 1989;52:724–731.
16. Carboni E, Tanda GL, Frau R, Di Chiara G. Blockade of the noradrenaline carrier increases extracellular dopamine concentrations in the prefrontal cortex. Evidence that dopamine is taken up in vivo by noradrenergic terminals. *J Neurochem* 1990;55:1067–1070.
17. Cervo L, Samanin R. Repeated treatment with imipramine and amitriptyline reduces the immobility of rats in the swimming test by enhancing dopamine mechanisms in the nucleus accumbens. *J Pharm Pharmacol* 1988;40:155–156.
18. Davis KL, Kahn RS, Ko G, Davidson M. Dopamine in schizophrenia: a review and reconceptualization. *Am J Psychiatry* 1991; 148:1474–1486.
19. De Montis MG, Devoto P, Gessa GL, Porcella A, Serra G, Tagliamonte A. Possible role of DA receptors in the mechanism of action of antidepressants. In: Gessa GL, Serra G, eds. *Dopamine and mental depression.* Oxford: Pergamon Press; 1990;147–157.
20. De Montis MG, Gambarana C, Meloni D, Taddei I, Tagliamonte A. Long-term imipramine effects are prevented by NMDA receptor blockade. *Brain Res* 1993;606:63–67.
21. Del Zompo M, Boccheta A, Bernardi F, Corsini GU. Clinical evidence for a role of dopaminergic system in depressive syndromes. In: Gessa GL, Serra G, eds. *Dopamine and mental depression.* Oxford: Pergamon Press; 1990:177–184.
22. Delina-Stula A, Radeke E, van Riezen H. Enhanced functional responsiveness of the dopaminergic system: the mechanism of anti-immobility effects of antidepressants in the behavioural despair test in the rat. *Neuropharmacology* 1988;27:943–947.
23. Depue RA, Arbisi P, Krauss S, et al. Seasonal independence of low prolactin concentration and high spontaneous eye blink rates in unipolar and bipolar II seasonal affective disorder. *Arch Gen Psychiatry* 1990;47:356–364.
24. Depue RA, Arbisi P, Spoont MR, Krauss S, Leon A, Ainsworth B. Seasonal and mood independence of low basal prolactin secretion in premenopausal women with seasonal affective disorder. *Am J Psychiatry* 1989;146:989–995.
25. D'haenen H, Bossuyt A. Dopamine D2 receptors in the brain measured with SPECT. *Biol Psychiatry* 1994;35:128–132.
26. Di Chiara G, Tanda G, Frau R, Carboni E. On the preferential release of dopamine in the nucleus accumbens by amphetamine: further evidence obtained by vertically implanted concentric probes. *Psychopharmacology* 1993;112:398–402.
27. Fawcett J, Siomopoulos V. Dextroamphetamine response as a possible predictor of improvement with tricyclic therapy in depression. *Arch Gen Psychiatry* 1971;25:247–255.
28. Fibiger HC. The dopamine hypotheses of schizophrenia and depression: contradictions and speculations. In: Willner P, Scheel-Kruger J, eds. *The mesolimbic dopamine system: from motivation to action.* Chichester: John Wiley; 1991:615–637.
29. Gjerris A, Werdelin L, Rafaelson OJ, Alling C, Christensen NJ. CSF dopamine increased in depression: CSF dopamine, noradrenaline and their metabolites in depressed patients and in controls. *J Affect Disord* 1987;13:279–286.
30. Goetz CG, Tanner CM, Klawans HL. Bupropion in Parkinson's disease. *Neurology* 1984;34:1092–1094.
31. Goodwin FK, Ebert MH, Bunney WE. Mental effects of reserpine in man: a review. In: Shader RI, ed. *Psychiatric complications of medical drugs.* New York: Raven Press; 1972:73–101.
32. Goodwin FK, Sack RL. Central dopamine function in affective illness: evidence from precursors, enzyme inhibitors, and studies of central dopamine turnover. In: Usdin E, ed. *Neuropsychopharmacology of monoamines and their regulatory enzymes.* New York: Raven Press; 1974:261–279.
33. Guze BH, Barrio JC. The etiology of depression in Parkinson's disease patients. *Psychosomatics* 1991;32:390–394.
34. Gwirtsman HE, Guze BH. Amphetamine, but not methylphenidate, predicts antidepressant response. *J Clin Psychopharmacol* 1989; 9:453.
35. Holmes DS, Brynjolfsson J, Brett P, et al. No evidence for a suscep-

tibility locus predisposing to manic depression in the region of the dopamine (D2) receptor gene. *Br J Psychiatry* 1991;158:635–641.

36. Jacobs D, Silverstone T. Dextroamphetamine-induced arousal in human subjects as a model for mania. *Psychol Med* 1988;16:323–329.

37. Jeste DV, Lohr JB, Goodwin FK. Neuroanatomical studies of major affective disorders: a review and suggestions for future research. *Br J Psychiatry* 1988;153:444–59.

38. Jimerson DC. Role of dopamine mechanisms in the affective disorders. In: Meltzer HY, ed. *Psychopharmacology: The third generation of progress.* New York: Raven Press, 1987;515–511.

39. Jouvent R, Abensour P, Bonnet AM, Widlocher D, Ajid Y, Lhermitte F. Antiparkinson and antidepressant effects of high doses of bromocriptine. *J Affect Disord* 1983;5:141–145.

40. King RJ, Mefford IN, Wang C, Murchison A, Caligari EJ, Berger PA. CSF dopamine levels correlate with extraversion in depressed patients. *Psychiatr Res* 1986;19:305–310.

41. Kirkpatrick B, Buchanan RW. Anhedonia and the deficit syndrome of schizophrenia. *Psychiatr Res* 1990;31:25–30.

42. Klimek V, Maj J. The effect of antidepressant drugs given repeatedly on the binding of ^{3}H-SCH 23390 and ^{3}H-spiperone to dopaminergic receptors. In: Gessa GL, Serra G, eds. *Dopamine and mental depression.* Oxford: Pergamon Press, 1990;159–166.

43. Little KY. Amphetamine, but not methylphenidate, predicts antidepressant response. *J Clin Psychopharmacol* 1988;8:177–183.

44. Maj J. Behavioral effects of antidepressant drugs given repeatedly on the dopaminergic system. In: Gessa GL, Serra G, eds. *Dopamine and mental depression.* Oxford: Pergamon Press, 1990;139–146.

45. Maj J, Papp M, Skuza G, Bigajska K, Zazula M. The influence of repeated treatment with imipramine, (+)- and (−)-oxaprotiline on behavioural effects of dopamine D-1 and D-2 agonists. *J Neural Transm* 1989;76:29–38.

46. Martin-Iverson M, Leclere JF, Fibiger HC. Cholinergic-dopaminergic interactions and the mechanisms of action of antidepressants. *Eur J Pharmacol* 1983;94:193–201.

47. Meltzer HY, Kolakowska T, Fang VS, et al. Growth hormone and prolactin response to apomorphine in schizophrenia and major affective disorders. Relation to duration of illness and affective symptoms. *Arch Gen Psychiatry* 1984;41:512–519.

48. Mendlewicz J, Linkowski P, Kerkhofs M, et al. Diurnal hypersecretion of growth hormone in depression. *J Clin Endocrinol Metab* 1985;60:505–512.

49. Mitchell P, Selbie L, Waters B, et al. Exclusion of close linkage of bipolar disorder to dopamine D_1 and D_2 receptor gene markers. *J Affect Disord* 1992;25:1–11.

50. Mouret J, LeMoine P, Minuit M-P. Marqueurs polygraphiques, cliniques et therapeutiques des depressions dopamino-dependantes (DDD). *Confront Psychiatr* 1989;(Special Issue):430–437.

51. Murphy DL. L-Dopa, behavioral activation and psychopathology. *Res Publ Ass Res Nerv Ment Dis* 1972;50:472–493.

52. Nelson JC. The use of antipsychotic drugs in the treatment of depression. In: Zohar J, Belmaker RH, eds. *Treating resistant depression.* New York: PMA Corp. 1987:131–146.

53. Nothen MM, Erdmann J, Korner J, et al. Lack of association between dopamine D_1 and D_2 receptor genes and bipolar affective disorder. *Am J Psychiatry* 1992;149:199–201.

54. Nowak G, Skolnick P, Paul IA. Downregulation of dopamine$_1$ (D_1) receptors is species-specific. *Pharmaol Biochem Behav* 1991;39:769–771.

55. Nurnberger JJ Jr., Gershon ES, Simmons S, et al. Behavioral, biochemical and neurochemical responses to amphetamine in normal twins and "well-state" bipolar patients. *Psychoneuroendocrinology* 1982;7:163–176.

56. Nurnberger JJ Jr., Simmons-Alling S, Kessler L, et al. Separate mechanisms for behavioral, cardiovascular and hormonal responses to dextroamphetamine in man. *Psychopharmacology* 1984;84:200–204.

57. Papp M, Klimek V, Willner P. Parallel changes in dopamine D2 receptor binding in limbic forebrain associated with chronic mild stress-induced anhedonia and its reversal by imipramine. *Psychopharmacology* [in press].

58. Perry EK. Cortical neurotransmitter chemistry in Alzheimer's disease. In: Meltzer HY, ed. *Psychopharmacology: the third generation of progress.* New York: Raven Press, 1987;887–895.

59. Pitchot W, Ansseau M, Gonzalez Moreno A, Hansenne M, von Frenckell R. Dopaminergic function in panic disorder: comparison with major and minor depression. *Biol Psychiatry* 1992;32:1004–1011.

60. Pitchot W, Hansenne M, Gonzalez Moreno A, Ansseau M. Suicidal behavior and growth hormone response to apomorphine test. *Biol Psychiatry* 1992;31:1213–1219.

61. Pitchot W, Hansenne M, Gonzalez Moreno A, von Frenckell R, Ansseau M. Psychopathological correlates of dopaminergic disturbances in major depression. *Neuropsychobiology* 1990;24:169–172.

62. Post RM, Kotin J, Goodwin FK, Gordon E. Psychomotor activity and cerebrospinal fluid metabolites in affective illness. *Am J Psychiatry* 1973;130:67–72.

63. Post RM, Weiss SRB, Pert A. Animal models of mania. In: Willner P, Scheel-Kruger J, eds. *The mesolimbic dopamine system: from motivation to action.* Chichester: John Wiley; 1991;443–472.

64. Przegalinski E, Budziszewska B, Blaszcztnska E. Repeated treatment with antidepressant drugs and/or electroconvulsive shock (ECS) does not affect the quinpirole-induced elevation of serum corticosterone concentration in rats. *J Psychopharmacol* 1990;4:198–203.

65. Pulverenti L, Samanin R. Antagonism by dopamine, but not noradrenaline receptor blockers of the antiimmobility activity of desipramine after different treatment schedules in the rat. *Pharmacol Res Commun* 1986;18:73–80.

66. Rampello L, Nicoletti G, Raffaele R. Dopaminergic hypothesis for retarded depression: a symptom profile for predicting therapeutical responses. *Acta Psychiatr Scand* 1991;84:552–554.

67. Randrup A, Munkvad I, Fog R, et al. Mania, depression and brain dopamine. In: Essman WB, Valzelli L, eds. *Current developments in psychopharmacology* Vol. 2. New York: Spectrum Press; 1975:206–248.

68. Reddy PL, Khanna S, Subhash MN, Channabasavanna SM, Sridhara Rama Rao BS. CSF amine metabolites in depression. *Biol Psychiatry* 1992;31:112–118.

69. Rietschel M, Nothen MM, Lannfelt L, et al. A serine to glycine substitution at position 9 in the extracellular *N*-terminal part of the dopamine D3 receptor protein: No role in genetic predisposition to bipolar affective disorder. *Psychiatr Res* 1993;46:253–259.

70. Robertson MM, Trimble MR. Neuroleptics as antidepressants. *Neuropharmacology* 1981;20:1335–1336.

71. Roy A, Karoum F, Pollack S. Marked reduction in indexes of dopamine transmission among patients with depression who attempt suicide. *Arch Gen Psychiatry* 1992;49:447–450.

72. Roy A, Pickar D, Linnoila M, Doran AR, Ninan P, Paul SM. Cerebrospinal fluid monoamine and monoamine metabolite concentrations in melancholia. *Psychiatr Res* 1985;15:281–290.

73. Scavone C, Aizenstein ML, De Lucia R, Da Silva Planeta C. Chronic imipramine administration reduces apomorphine inhibitory effects. *Eur J Pharmacol* 1986;132:263–267.

74. Schatzberg AF, Rothschild AJ. The roles of glucocorticoid and dopaminergic systems in delusional (psychotic) depression. *Ann NY Acad Sci* 1988;537:462–471.

75. Serra G, Argiolas A, Fadda F, Melis MR, Gessa GL. Chronic treatment with antidepressants prevents the inhibitory effect of small doses of antidepressants on dopamine synthesis and motor activity. *Life Sci* 1979;25:415–424.

76. Serra G, Collu M, D'Aquila PS, de Montis GM, Gessa GL. Possible role of dopamine D_1 receptor in the behavioural supersensitivity to dopamine agonists induced by chronic treatment with antidepressants. *Brain Res* 1990;527:234–243.

77. Serra G, Forgione A, D'Aquila PS, Collu M, Fratta W, Gessa GL. Possible mechanism of antidepressant effect of L-sulpiride. *Clin Neuropharmacol* 1990;13(Suppl. 1):76–83.

78. Shaikh S, Ball D, Craddock N, et al. The dopamine D3 receptor gene: no association with bipolar affective disorder. *J Med Genet* 1993;30:308–309.

79. Siever LJ, Uhde TW. New studies and perspectives on the noradrenergic receptor system in depression: effects of the alpha$_2$-adrenergic agonist clonidine. *Biol Psychiatry* 1984;19:131–156.

80. Silverstone T. Response to bromocriptine distinguishes bipolar from unipolar depression. *Lancet* 1984;1:903–904.

81. Simon H, LeMoal M. Mesencephalic dopamine neurons: role in the

general economy of the brain. In: Kalivas PW, Nemeroff CB, eds. *The mesocorticolimbic dopamine system.* New York: New York Academy of Sciences; 1988;235–253.

82. Siris S. Diagnosis of secondary depression in schizophrenia. Implications for DSM-IV. *Schizophr Bull* 1991;17:75–98.

83. Suhara T, Nakayama K, Inoue O, et al. D_1 dopamine receptor binding in mood disorders measured by positron emission tomography. *Psychopharmacology* 1992;106:14–18.

84. Taylor AE, Saint-Cyr JA. Depression in Parkinson's disease: reconciling physiological and psychological perspectives. *Neuropsychiatr Pract Opin* 1990;2:92–98.

85. Towell A, Willner P, Muscat R. Behavioural evidence for autoreceptor subsensitivity in the mesolimbic dopamine system during withdrawal from antidepressant drugs. *Psychopharmacology* 1986;90:64–71.

86. Van Praag HM, Korf J. Central monoamine deficiency in depression: causative or secondary phenomenon. *Pharmacopsychiatry* 1975;8:321–326.

87. Van Praag HM, Korf J, Lakke JPWF, Schut T. Dopamine metabolism in depression, psychoses, and Parkinson's disease: the problem of specificity of biological variables in behavior disorders. *Psychol Med* 1975;5:138–146.

88. Willner P. Dopamine and depression: a review of recent evidence. *Brain Res Rev* 1983;6:211–246.

89. Willner P. Sensitization to antidepressant drugs. In: Emmett-Oglesby MV, Goudie AJ, eds. *Psychoactive drugs: tolerance and sensitization.* Clifton, NJ: Humana Press; 1989;407–459.

90. Willner P, Muscat R, Papp M. Chronic mild stress-induced anhedonia: a realistic animal model of depression. *Neurosci Biobehav Rev* 1992;16:525–534.

91. Willner P, Scheel-Kruger J, eds. *The mesolimbic dopamine system: from motivation to action.* Chichester: John Wiley; 1991.

92. Wise RA. Neuroleptics and operant behaviour: the anhedonia hypothesis. *Behav Brain Sci* 1982;5:39–88.

93. Wolfe N, Katz DI, Albert ML, et al. Neuropsychological profile linked to low dopamine: in Alzheimer's disease, major depression, and Parkinson's disease. *J Neurol Neurosurg Psychiatry* 1990;53:915–917.

94. Wong DF, Pearlson G, Ross C, et al. In vivo measurement of dopamine receptor abnormalities in drug naive and drug free manic-depressive patients. *Soc Neurosci Abstr* 1987;13:216.

95. Wong DF, Wagner HN Jr., Pearlson G, et al. Dopamine receptor binding of C-11-3-N-methyl-spiperone in the caudate of schizophrenic and bipolar disorder: a preliminary report. *Psychopharmacol Bull* 1985;21:595–598.

96. Zebrowska-Lupina I, Ossowska G, Klenk-Majewska B. The influence of antidepressants on aggressive behavior in stressed rats: the role of dopamine. *Pol J Pharmacol Pharm* 1992;44:325–335.

*Psychopharmacology: The Fourth
Generation of Progress*, edited by
Floyd E. Bloom and David J. Kupfer.
Raven Press, Ltd., New York © 1995.

CHAPTER 81

The Serotonin Hypothesis of Major Depression

Michael Maes and Herbert Y. Meltzer

The serotonin (5-HT) hypothesis of major depression has been formulated in three distinct ways. One version of this hypothesis is that a deficit in serotonergic activity is a proximate cause of depression. A second theory is that a deficit in serotonergic activity is important as a vulnerability factor in major depression. A third hypothesis, now of historical interest only, attributed increased vulnerability to major depression to enhanced serotonergic activity (51).

The last review of these hypotheses in this series (51) concluded that the available data on the role of 5-HT in major depression favored the hypothesis that a deficiency in brain serotonergic activity increases vulnerability to major depression. This review (51) summarized the following evidence: (a) Disorders in serotonergic activity could contribute to many of the symptoms of major depression, for example, mood, appetite, sleep, activity, suicide, sexual, and cognitive dysfunction. (b) Interference with 5-HT synthesis or storage may induce depression in some vulnerable individuals. (c) Abnormalities in serotonergic activity in depression could occur at one or more of several levels, for example, diminished availability of L-tryptophan (L-TRP), the precursor of 5-HT, impaired 5-HT synthesis, release, reuptake, or metabolism, or 5-HT postsynaptic receptor abnormalities. (d) Finally, antidepressant drugs may act, in part, by enhancing central serotonergic activity.

Since that review, there have been numerous developments shedding further light on the role of 5-HT in depression. This chapter reviews the highlights of serotonergic research in major depression since 1987, aiming to elucidate the role of 5-HT activity in the pathogenesis or pathophysiology of that illness. Because of limitations on refer-

ences, secondary sources were frequently cited and some sources were left out entirely (see Chapters 41 and 42, *this volume*).

This chapter discusses new findings on the role of 5-HT in the pathogenesis or pathophysiology of major depression and the mechanism of action of antidepressant drugs. Clinical studies of 5-HT metabolism in major depression that provide evidence for an abnormality of the 5-HT system are reviewed. New evidence that the availability of L-TRP, the rate-limiting step in the synthesis of 5-HT, is an important factor in the pathophysiology of depression and the response of antidepressant drugs are discussed. The evidence for abnormalities in the 5-HT uptake system in major depression as well as abnormalities in some of the numerous types of postsynaptic 5-HT receptors are reviewed. The 5-HT$_{1A}$ and 5-HT$_2$ postsynaptic receptors appear to be of particular importance. Cooperative and competitive interactions may be important to the function of the 5-HT system and abnormalities in this regard are possible factors in the pathophysiology of major depression. The function of these postsynaptic receptors in depression has been assessed with a variety of pharmacological probes as well as postmortem studies. The evidence that antidepressants may act via their long-term ability to modulate pre- and postsynaptic serotonergic function is discussed. The important relationships between serotonergic activity and the hypothalamic–pituitary–adrenal (HPA) axis are reviewed. The possibility that disorders in the functional relationships between both systems and gender differences in 5-HT function may be involved in the pathophysiology of major depression are also discussed. Finally, the importance of studying interactions among 5-HT and other neurotransmitter systems in depression is stressed. Indeed, it seems doubtful that any one neurotransmitter is entirely responsible for the pathogenesis or pathophysiology of depression because of the extensive interactions between neurotrans-

M. Maes and H. Y. Meltzer: Department of Psychiatry, Laboratory of Biological Psychiatry, Case Western Reserve University School of Medicine, Cleveland, Ohio 44106.

mitters at the levels of cell bodies as well as terminal regions. Nevertheless, 5-HT appears to be the most important monoamine relevant to the pathophysiology of depression and the action of antidepressant drugs (see Chapters 36–42, *this volume*, for related discussion and background).

THE AVAILABILITY OF L-TRYPTOPHAN

Total or free L-TRP and the ratio of L-TRP to the sum of competing amino acids (CAA), known to compete for the same cerebral uptake mechanism, provide measures of the availability of L-TRP to the brain and hence for 5-HT synthesis in the brain (42). There are several reports that plasma L-TRP availability is significantly lower in subjects with major depression than in normal controls or subjects with minor depression (42,51). The data suggest that a lower plasma L-TRP/CAA ratio in depression is related to decreased concentrations of plasma L-TRP rather than to increases in CAA (42). Plasma L-TRP levels following ingestion of large oral doses of L-TRP or intravenous L-TRP have been reported to be lower in depressed patients (15,28).

One hypothesis to explain lower plasma L-TRP concentrations and altered L-TRP pharmacokinetics in depression is enhanced catabolism of L-TRP in the liver by induction of pyrrolase, the first rate-limiting enzyme of the kynurenine-nicotinamide pathway (39). The activity of this pathway can be quantified by measuring 24-hr urinary excretion of xanthurenic acid after loading with 5 g of L-TRP (25,39). In depression, L-TRP–induced xanthurenic acid excretion was significantly and negatively related to plasma L-TRP concentrations (39). The above findings lend support to the hypothesis that increased activity of this pathway may contribute to the lower plasma L-TRP concentrations and increased clearance in major depression (39).

Recent studies suggest that a reduction of dietary L-TRP can induce depressive symptomatology under some circumstances. In normal men, lowering of plasma L-TRP by dietary means has been reported to cause an acute lowering of mood, which was inversely related to postingestion plasma L-TRP levels (75). In recently remitted depressed patients receiving selective 5-HT reuptake inhibitors (SSRIs), acute L-TRP depletion coupled with ingestion of large concentrations of CAA led to a rapid clinically significant return of depressive symptoms, such as depressed mood, terminal insomnia, decreased appetite, loss of energy, loss of interest, anhedonia, decreased concentration, ruminative thinking, and a sense of worthlessness (16,23). Remitted depressed patients maintained with tricyclic antidepressants, however, were less prone to a depressive relapse following L-TRP depletion. Because SSRIs enhance central presynaptic 5-HT activity (see the

section below on neuroendocrine probes and antidepressive treatments), the findings strongly suggest that the synthesis of 5-HT from plasma L-TRP is necessary for the maintenance of remission induced by those drugs. Decreased plasma L-TRP concentrations are most likely related to lower central presynaptic 5-HT activity, because diets causing a decrease in plasma L-TRP availability also reduce cerebrospinal fluid (CSF) levels of 5-hydroxyindoleacetic acid (5-HIAA) in humans. Therefore, the behavioral and cognitive changes observed may be due to a deficiency in central presynaptic 5-HT elements, which may result from lower plasma L-TRP availability. The above results are consistent with the findings that anorexia, anergy, sleep disorders, cognitive disturbances, and depressed mood are psychopathological correlates of lowered L-TRP availability in depression (43). However, it is noteworthy that unmedicated depressed patients do not worsen following L-TRP depletion. The lack of worsening by further interference with 5-HT synthesis may suggest that decreased serotonergic activity is not the limiting factor in the severity of depression in untreated major depression. This is consistent with the hypothesis of diminished serotonergic activity as a vulnerability factor in depression.

Møller et al. (56) reported that the plasma ratio of L-TRP/CAA was inversely related to the response to antidepressive treatment, such as L-TRP, imipramine, amitryptiline, and lithium + L-TRP, and that major depressed subjects with lower L-TRP availability responded preferentially to treatment with SSRIs, such as citalopram and paroxetine. These results suggest that (a) plasma L-TRP availability may influence the therapeutic response to antidepressive treatment and may predict a favorable response to SSRIs; (b) lower plasma L-TRP availability may be related to lower central 5-HT activity; and (c) that antidepressive treatment with serotonergic drugs (L-TRP, L-TRP + lithium, SSRIs) may compensate for this deficit.

INDICES OF PRESYNAPTIC SEROTONERGIC NEURON FUNCTION

Blood Platelets

Blood platelets are able to take up, store, and release 5-HT by mechanisms that are sufficiently similar to those of central 5-HT neurons to render platelets a model for the 5-HT neuron (50). Several dozen studies of platelet 5-HT uptake in major depression have been published between 1971 and 1992; approximately 65% to 75% have reported significantly lower V_{max} values in patients with major depression than in normal controls (50). However, studies on platelet 5-HT uptake lack specificity and sensitivity for clinical use on their own. The question of whether lower platelet 5-HT uptake indicates lower 5-HT uptake in the brain remains elusive.

There are now several reports on lower imipramine binding (B_{max}) in platelets of depressed patients compared to normal controls (50). However, ^{3}[H]imipramine binding is rather heterogeneous since this substance labels two separate binding sites: one high-affinity binding site that corresponds to the 5-HT uptake site and one low-affinity site that is unrelated to the 5-HT transporter (49). Paroxetine is a potent and selective inhibitor of 5-HT uptake in platelets and brain. Paroxetine is a superior ligand for labeling the 5-HT transporter in both platelets and brain compared to imipramine, because ^{3}[H]paroxetine labels the 5-HT transporter more selectively than does ^{3}[H]-imipramine, while exhibiting a higher affinity (49). Several groups were unable to find significant differences in platelet paroxetine binding between depressed patients and controls (31).

5-Hydroxyindoleacetic Acid in Cerebrospinal Fluid

Concentrations of 5-HIAA, the major 5-HT metabolite, in CSF have been extensively studied in depressed subjects, both in basal conditions and after blockade of its reabsorption by probenecid treatment (51). Meltzer and Lowy (51) concluded that it is very difficult to draw any valid conclusions on 5-HT turnover in depression on the basis of CSF 5-HIAA data. Several papers published after their 1987 review were also unable to find significant differences in CSF 5-HIAA between major depressed subjects and normal controls (63). In fact, there is more evidence that low CSF 5-HIAA levels are related to (violent) suicidal behavior and to violence-impulsivity rather than to depression per se (17).

Plasma or Platelet Serotonin Contents

The possibility that peripheral abnormalities in 5-HT metabolism occur in melancholic patients has been further investigated by the study of the 5-HT content of plasma and platelets. Platelet 5-HT is considered to represent a reserve pool of peripheral 5-HT (64). Plasma 5-HT has a turnover rate considerably higher than the platelet pool and represents the equilibrium between 5-HT secretion, 5-HT catabolism (by monoamine oxidase enzyme activity in liver and lung), and platelet uptake mechanisms (64). Lowered plasma and platelet 5-HT contents in depression have been reported by several groups (64). Celada et al. (7) reported that chronic treatment with fluvoxamine decreased platelet 5-HT content and that responders had significantly lower platelet 5-HT content pretreatment. These authors suggest that SSRIs may be most useful in patients with low platelet 5-HT. The significance of

the above findings for central serotonergic activity is unknown.

Indices of Serotonin Presynaptic Function Obtained from Postmortem Samples

Reports of 5-HT and 5-HIAA concentrations in the brain of suicide victims have yielded conflicting results: some found decreased levels or no changes in 5-HIAA concentrations in the brain of depressed suicides, whereas others reported increased 5-HIAA levels in the hippocampus or amygdala of (depressed) suicide victims (10). Taken together, the above results offer little support that 5-HT turnover is reduced in depressed subjects who have committed suicide. Moreover, the effect of drug treatments, substance abuse, glucocorticoid elevations, and receptor sensitivity alterations make it difficult to interpret the results.

Brain Serotonin Uptake Transporter

Some, but not all, groups described a reduction in imipramine binding in the frontal cortex of suicides (20). The latter group also found an increase in imipramine binding sites in the hippocampus of suicide victims. No significant differences in paroxetine binding sites of several brain areas could be detected between normal controls and suicide victims in whom a diagnosis of depression was made (30). Leake et al. (32) found lower ^{3}[H]citalopram binding in the brains from depressed subjects.

POSTSYNAPTIC SEROTONIN RECEPTORS

5-HT$_2$ Receptors

Three studies of 5-HT$_2$ binding in the blood platelets of depressed patients and normal controls, found increased 5-HT$_2$ binding (B_{max}) in the former, but one study did not (2). Increased 5-HT$_2$ binding (B_{max}) in depressed patients is also supported by the increased 5-HT$_2$ receptor functional response as measured by phophoinositide turnover and 5-HT–induced platelet aggregation (55). Mikuni et al. (55) reported that the effects of 5-HT to increase intracellular calcium in platelets was greater in depressed patients than in controls, which is consistent with the hypothesis of 5-HT$_2$ receptor up-regulation in depression.

A new and original method to assess central 5-HT$_2$ function is the assessment of slow-wave sleep (SWS) after challenge with 5-HT$_2$ receptor antagonists. Blockade of 5-HT$_2$ receptors is normally accompanied by an increase in SWS (69). Sharpley et al. (67) found that the normal increase in SWS following treatment with cyproheptadine, a nonspecific 5-HT receptor antagonist, was absent in major depressed patients maintained on tricyclic antidepressants. Staner et al. (69) found that ritanserin enhanced SWS stage 3 in normal controls and depressed subjects, but the latter group showed significantly lower SWS in stage 4. These findings are consistent with 5-HT$_2$ receptor up-regulation in patients with major depression (69).

There are now several reports of increased 5-HT$_2$ receptor-binding sites in the frontal cortex of (depressed) suicide victims or depressed subjects who died from natural causes (1,2). Other laboratories found a trend toward or a significant decline in 5-HT$_2$ binding in membrane homogenates from the prefrontal cortex of suicide victims (11). However, differences among the above studies may be due to drug effects (treatment with antidepressants and antipsychotic agents reducing 5-HT$_2$ binding), use of different ligands, the postmortem interval, or the heterogeneity of psychiatric illnesses (e.g., schizophrenia, alcoholism) and personality (e.g., borderline and antisocial) disorders associated with suicide.

5-HT$_1$ Receptors

Increased 5-HT$_{1A}$ binding in the prefrontal cortex of nonviolent suicides compared to violent suicides and controls has been reported (48). Several other studies reported no significant differences in the number or affinity of 5-HT$_1$ binding sites in the frontal or temporal cortex between drug-free depressed suicide victims and controls (12). The number of 5-HT$_1$ binding sites was significantly lower in hippocampus, whereas the affinity of 5-HT$_1$ binding sites was significantly lower in the amygdala (12). These results may provide some evidence of increased cortical 5-HT$_1$ receptors in (depressed) suicides, and decreased density of 5-HT$_1$ receptors in the hippocampus and amygdala of depressed subjects. These findings need to be further explored using more specific ligands, autoradiography, and with attention to variables such as type and severity of depression, concomitant alcoholism or other drug abuse, the effects of suicide per se, and so on.

THE NEUROENDOCRINE STRATEGY

One strategy to assess central serotonergic neurotransmission in vivo is the measurement of HPA-axis hormone, prolactin, growth hormone, and other responses following the administration of 5-HT precursors and direct or indirect 5-HT agonists (38,54). Secretion of these hormones is, in part, regulated by 5-HT inputs, and their responses to the acute administration of 5-HT agents are mediated at least in part by 5-HT mechanisms (54).

There is strong evidence suggesting that 5-HT$_{1A}$, 5-HT$_{1C}$, and 5-HT$_2$ receptors may stimulate cortisol and prolactin secretion in man (52). Various neuroendocrine

(behavioral and electrophysiological) studies with 5-HT agonists and antagonists have provided evidence for important interactions between 5-HT$_{1A}$ and 5-HT$_{2/1C}$ receptors (52). In rats, there is some evidence that 5-HT$_2$/5-HT$_{1C}$ receptors may modulate 5-HT$_{1A}$-related behaviors. 5-HT$_{1A}$ receptors may provide inhibitory effects on 5-HT$_2$ receptor-mediated functions. These findings suggest the possibility of a signal transduction from 5-HT$_{1C}$/5-HT$_2$ to 5-HT$_{1A}$ receptors in the expression of 5-HT$_{1A}$-mediated behaviors, together with an inhibitory effect of 5-HT$_{1A}$ receptors on 5-HT$_2$-mediated functions. Cooperation among those receptors has important implications for the interpretation of neuroendocrine challenge studies with serotonergic agents (52). In particular, our laboratory has provided some evidence that blunted prolactin responses to challenge with 5-HT precursors or agonists may be due to diminished 5-HT$_{1A}$ or 5-HT$_{1C}$/5-HT$_2$ receptor sensitivity, whereas enhanced cortisol responses might be from increased sensitivity of 5-HT$_{1C/2}$ receptors which would be unaffected by 5-HT$_{1A}$ receptor subsensitivity (52).

5-HT$_{1A}$ Agonists

Ipsapirone administration significantly increases HPA-axis hormone secretion in normal men and rodents (34). Major depressed subjects show blunted HPA-axis hormone [adrenocorticotropic hormone (ACTH) or cortisol] responses following ipsapirone challenge compared to normal controls (34; also Meltzer and Maes, *unpublished*). Therefore, these attenuated responses may be interpreted to indicate that major depression is characterized by a down-regulation or hyporesponsivity of postsynaptic 5-HT$_{1A}$ receptors.

Buspirone is another azapirone which is a partial agonist at 5-HT$_{1A}$ receptors; its acute administration evokes dose-related HPA-axis and prolactin responses (53). The prolactin response is blocked by pindolol, suggesting it is 5-HT$_{1A}$-mediated. Our laboratory found no significant differences in buspirone-induced cortisol or prolactin responses between major depressed subjects and normal controls. The reason for the discrepancy between the cortisol responses to ipsapirone and buspirone in major depression requires further study. It is possible that differences in the intrinsic activity as partial 5-HT$_{1A}$ agonist may be relevant. It is likely that the prolactin response to buspirone is mediated by DA$_2$-receptor blockade rather than 5-HT$_{1A}$ agonism. Further efforts to employ buspirone-induced cortisol or prolactin responses as probes of 5-HT$_{1A}$ function in depression appear to be of limited value.

Precursors of Serotonin

Intraperitoneal or oral administration of high doses of 5-HT precursor (5-HTP) causes a marked increase in corticosterone secretion in rodents, whereas the effects of oral 5-HTP on HPA-axis hormone secretion in humans are somewhat more variable in studies using lower doses of the racemic mixture (D, L) and/or enteric coated tablets (52). There is now evidence that 200 mg L-5-HTP, in nonenteric coated tablets, reliably stimulates HPA-axis hormones and prolactin secretion in normal humans, and that 5-HTP-induced activation of both HPA-axis and prolactin secretion are probably related to 5-HT mechanisms (52). Significantly higher 5-HTP (D, L: 200 mg; L: 125 to 200 mg) -induced cortisol responses were observed in major depressed subjects than in normal controls or minor depressed subjects (38,54). The use of 5-HTP as a 5-HT probe was challenged, because administration of very high doses of 5-HTP in rodents may lead to 5-HT synthesis in central catecholaminergic neurons and may increase synthesis of catecholamines (73). The dose of L-5-HTP used in human studies, however, is much lower than that needed to increase catecholamine turnover in animal studies. Because 5-HT$_{1A}$ postsynaptic receptors are probably down-regulated in major depression, the above findings may be explained either by supersensitive 5-HT$_2$ or 5-HT$_{1C}$ receptors. Since several types of studies (reviewed here) indicate increased 5-HT$_2$ receptor binding or disorders in 5-HT$_2$–related behaviors in major depression or suicide, whereas there is no specific evidence as yet for 5-HT$_{1C}$ receptor supersensitivity in depression, it may be suggested that the results of the studies with 5-HTP as challenger are compatible with up-regulation or supersensitivity of 5-HT$_2$ postsynaptic receptors (52).

Administration of L-TRP reliably increases prolactin secretion (58). Several papers reported blunted prolactin responses to intravenous L-TRP in depression (15,28). The blunted prolactin responses to L-TRP may reflect abnormalities in the synthesis of 5-HT from L-TRP, its release or reuptake, or decreased responsivity of postsynaptic 5-HT receptors that may mediate the serotonergic influence on prolactin secretion (e.g., 5-HT$_{1A}$ postsynaptic receptors). There is as yet no evidence from studies with direct-acting 5-HT agonists for a blunted prolactin response in depression.

Higher doses of L-TRP also increase corticosterone secretion in rodents (18). Our laboratory has reported significantly increased 24-hr urinary free cortisol (UFC) secretion in melancholic subjects than in normal controls or minor depressed patients after loading with L-TRP (2 or 5 g orally) (46). This finding is consistent with hyperresponsivity of 5-HT$_2$ postsynaptic receptors.

However, the use of L-TRP as a 5-HT probe was challenged: (a) One study found that, after controlling for differences in L-TRP plasma concentrations, the differences in prolactin responses between depressed subjects and normal controls disappeared (28). Thus, blunted TRP-induced prolactin responses, in fact, may result from disorders in L-TRP disposition in major depression.

(b) L-Tryptophan may be acting nonspecifically, that is, not via 5-HT (73). Indeed, administration of 2 to 5 g of L-TRP significantly decreased various indices of catecholaminergic turnover (26,46,73). This may be explained by the capacity of L-TRP to decrease L-tyrosine availability to the brain and the transport of tyrosine through the blood–brain barrier, which may cause a decrease in brain noradrenergic turnover (46). (c) Finally, administration of L-TRP produces only small increases in 5-HT formation but very important increments in metabolites of the nicotinamide pathway, which may exert pharmacological actions (26,27).

Indirect and Direct Serotonin Agonists

D,L-Fenfluramine promotes a rapid release of 5-HT, inhibits its reuptake, and may function as an indirect 5-HT receptor agonist. In rats and humans, D,L-fenfluramine produces a dose-dependent increase in prolactin secretion. Most but not all laboratories (36,41) have reported significantly blunted D,L-fenfluramine-induced prolactin responses in major depressed subjects compared with controls. However, because the L-isomer may block striatal DA receptors and increase DA turnover, a combination of serotonergic and dopaminergic effects could account for blunted D,L-fenfluramine–induced prolactin responses in major depression (58).

D-Fenfluramine stimulates the serotonergic system more specifically than the racemic mixture; D-fenfluramine–induced prolactin secretion may be mediated via 5-HT$_{1A}$ receptors as well as 5-HT$_2$/5-HT$_{1C}$ receptors. Maes et al. (41) were unable to detect any significant differences in post–D-fenfluramine (45 mg orally) prolactin responses between healthy controls and major depressed subjects. O'Keane and Dinan (60), on the other hand, found that plasma prolactin responses after D-fenfluramine (30 mg orally) were significantly lower in major depressed patients than in control groups. In conclusion, there is some agreement that prolactin responses to D,L- and D-fenfluramine administration may be blunted in major depressed subjects compared to normal controls. These findings could be explained by a combination of decreased availability of 5-HT, increased inactivation or diminished 5-HT$_{1A}$ postsynaptic receptor sensitivity.

The clomipramine probe assesses central 5-HT activity through the assay of prolactin responses following acute, intravenous challenge with clomipramine. There are now several publications reporting blunted clomipramine-induced prolactin responses in major depressed subjects compared to healthy controls (19). Blunted prolactin responses to clomipramine are not attributable to diminished prolactin secretory capacity in anterior pituitary, because prolactin responses to thyrotropin-releasing hormone, which acts directly on the pituitary to release prolactin, were normal in those patients. In conclusion, the clomipramine-challenge findings are in agreement with the blunted prolactin responses after challenge with L-TRP, D,L-fenfluramine, or D-fenfluramine.

SEROTONIN AND ANTIDEPRESSIVE TREATMENTS

Neuroendocrine Probes in Relation to Antidepressive Treatments

Enhanced prolactin responsivity to TRP challenge has been found following various antidepressive treatments, for example, amitriptyline, desipramine, fluvoxamine, clomipramine, tranylcypromine, and tricyclics with lithium (9). Fenfluramine-induced prolactin responses were significantly increased following therapy with imipramine, clomipramine, and amitryptiline or fluoxetine (61). Electroconvulsive therapy may or may not (61) enhance the prolactin responses to fenfluramine. Prolactin responses to clomipramine were significantly enhanced by short-term lithium treatment. Shapira et al. (66) and Upadhyaya et al. (72) provided some evidence that this enhancement of serotonergic function by antidepressive treatments represents a true correction of an underlying serotonergic deficit and not a continued effect of antidepressant treatment or a manifestation of medication withdrawal. In conclusion, it appears that various antidepressive treatments share the capacity to enhance central pre- or postsynaptic 5-HT activity.

Effects of Antidepressive Treatments at 5-HT$_2$ Receptors

Several studies have shown that long-term treatment with tricyclic antidepressants or monoamine oxidase inhibitors leads to down-regulation in the number of 5-HT$_2$ receptor binding sites in the brains of rodents (13). A further observation is that the time course of this 5-HT$_2$ receptor down-regulation following antidepressive treatment is similar to that of clinical response in depressed patients. Some, but not all (e.g., citalopram) SSRIs produce adaptive changes that manifest themselves by a decreased responsiveness of 5-HT$_2$ receptors (35). Chronic treatment with 5-HT$_{1A}$ agonists also may induce 5-HT$_2$ receptor down-regulation (35). Electroconvulsive therapy, on the other hand, has been shown to increase the number of 5-HT$_2$ binding sites in the brain (33). Most antidepressant drugs reduce 5-HT$_2$ receptor mediated behaviors in the rodent (e.g., head-twitch response), whereas electroconvulsive therapy may increase 5-HT$_2$-related behavior (13). One study has shown that increased 5-HTP–induced cortisol responses in depressed patients were normalized after chronic antidepressive treatment (54). It

may be argued that the above effects of antidepressives on 5-HT$_2$ receptors are probably due to rapid desensitization or down-regulation following agonist stimulation or to the 5-HT$_2$ receptor-blocking properties of some antidepressive drugs (35).

Effects of Antidepressive Treatments at 5-HT$_{1A}$ Receptors

Effects of antidepressive treatments on 5-HT$_1$–receptor binding or functioning are rather conflicting. Chronic treatment with some monoamine oxidase inhibitors, SSRIs, typical antidepressants or electroconvulsive therapy may decrease 5-HT$_1$ binding sites, responsiveness of 5-HT$_{1A}$ presynaptic receptors, or 5-HT$_{1A}$ postsynaptic receptor-mediated behaviors (47,70). Hayakawa et al. (22) found that repeated treatment with electroconvulsive therapy causes an upregulation of postsynaptic 5-HT$_{1A}$ receptors in the hippocampus. Chronic treatment with desipramine or amitryptiline resulted in a functional upregulation of 5-HT$_{1A}$-receptor-mediated behaviors in rats or increased postsynaptic 5-HT$_{1A}$ receptor binding in the hippocampus (37,74).

Electrophysiological Changes in the 5-HT System Induced by Antidepressive Treatments

Blier and colleagues (3) have thoroughly investigated the effects of short- and long-term treatment with various antidepressants on pre- and postsynaptic electrophysiological properties of 5-HT neurons. Long-term treatment with tricyclic antidepressants and electroconvulsive therapy appears to increase the sensitivity of postsynaptic 5-HT receptors, although no long-term effects on basal firing rate or autoreceptor-induced inhibition of 5-HT turnover are observed. Postsynaptic sensitization to 5-HT occurs probably in the hippocampus, suprachiasmatic nucleus, and somatosensory cortex (3). Blier et al. (3) have provided some evidence that this postsynaptic sensitization to 5-HT is, at least in part, attributable to the increased number of 5-HT$_{1A}$ binding sites in the hippocampus, cerebral cortex, and septum. Moreover, the time course for developing sensitization to 5-HT is consistent with the delayed activity of tricyclic drugs in relieving the symptoms of depression (3). Administration of monoamine oxidases and SSRIs appear to enhance 5-HT release per impulse from desensitization of the terminal autoreceptor (probably the 5-HT$_{1B}$ in rodents or the 5-HT$_{1D}$ receptor in humans). In conclusion, rodent studies indicate that various antidepressive treatments induce a gradual development of increased 5-HT activity; the mechanisms by which this enhancement is achieved may be different for these treatments.

RELATIONSHIPS BETWEEN SEROTONIN AND HYPOTHALAMIC–PITUITARY–ADRENAL AXIS FUNCTION IN MAJOR DEPRESSION

Hypothalamic–Pituitary–Adrenal Axis Hyperactivity in Major Depression

Increased activity of the HPA-axis has been consistently reported in severe depression. There is converging evidence from various studies that major depression is characterized by a moderately increased spontaneous HPA-axis function and by a failure to suppress plasma intact ACTH (the 1–39 sequence) and cortisol with the 1 mg dexamethasone suppression test (DST) (45). It is assumed that the above disorders are related to (a) central corticotropin releasing hormone (CRH) hypersecretion; (b) potentiating effects of increased arginine vasopressin (AVP) secretion on CRH-induced ACTH secretion; and (c) subsensitivity in negative feedback by glucocorticoids, which may be related to down-regulation of glucocorticoid receptors (GR) or mineralocorticoid receptors (MR) in the hippocampus, which, in turn, may be induced by sustained exposure to high concentrations of glucocorticoids.

Glucocorticoids and Plasma L-Tryptophan Levels

One major hypothesis to relate the HPA axis to serotonergic dysfunction in depression is that lowered plasma L-TRP availability may be related to activation of the kynurenine-nicotinamide pathway in the liver due to induction of liver pyrrolase by glucocorticoids (42). This hypothesis is supported by the following findings: in depression there is a significant inverse relationship between plasma L-TRP or L-TRP/CAA values and post-DST cortisol values (44); in rats, administration of a cortisol suppression dose of dexamethasone results in significantly augmented liver pyrrolase activity and a decreased availability of L-TRP to the brain (57); dexamethasone (1 mg, orally) administration also significantly reduces L-TRP plasma levels in normal controls and minor and major depressed subjects (42).

Glucocorticoids and Serotonin Turnover

The hippocampus has been demonstrated to be a site of serotonergic innervation associated with CNS control of the HPA-axis. A good correlation exists between the concentrations of cellular receptors for 5-HT and glucocorticoids. There is now compelling evidence that glucocorticoids may accelerate 5-HT synthesis and turnover in the brain of rodents (8). Increased central 5-HT turnover is, in part, caused by glucocorticoid or CRH-mediated induction of tryptophan hydroxylase (68). In humans, glu-

cocorticoids may also augment central 5-HT turnover; some groups found that TRP-induced prolactin responses were significantly higher after dexamethasone administration and found increased levels of CSF 5-HIAA after administration of dexamethasone in a group of psychiatric patients (71).

Glucocorticoids and 5-HT$_{1A}$ Receptors

It has been suggested that glucocorticosteroid hypersecretion in major depressed subjects may down-regulate the sensitivity of postsynaptic 5-HT$_{1A}$ receptor signal transduction or of the 5-HT$_{1A}$ receptor itself (15,34, Meltzer and Maes, *unpublished*). Increased baseline cortisol secretion was shown to be related to diminished ipsapirone-induced cortisol responses (34, Meltzer and Maes, *unpublished*). Hypercortisolemia may also explain the impaired D,L-fenfluramine and L-TRP–induced prolactin responses (15,61). This hypothesis is supported by experimental data showing that chronic exposure to glucocorticoids may alter 5-HT$_{1A}$ receptor-mediated functions or behaviors in rodents and that adrenalectomy may increase the number of 5-HT$_{1A}$ binding sites (8).

Glucocorticoids and 5-HT$_2$ Receptors

It has been shown that both ACTH and corticosterone administration may increase the number of 5-HT$_2$ receptors in the neocortex of forebrain and 5-HT$_2$–mediated behavioral responses in rodents (29,62). These findings suggest that HPA-axis hyperactivity in depression may contribute to upregulated 5-HT$_2$ receptor density in the prefrontal cortex (29).

Effects of Serotonin on Hypothalamus–Pituitary–Adrenal Axis Function

The role of 5-HT in stimulating the HPA axis encompasses effects on CRH by activation of 5-HT$_{1A}$ and 5-HT$_2$/5-HT$_{1C}$ receptors and on AVP by activation of 5-HT$_2$ receptors (5,18). Recently, it has been demonstrated that serotonergic structures may modify glucocorticoid negative-feedback effects on HPA-axis function. Seckl and Fink (65) found that depletion of 5-HT in hippocampal structures may attenuate the negative-feedback effects of glucocorticoids on the HPA axis through reduced expression of GR or MR. In depression, a significant negative correlation between plasma L-TRP availability and baseline cortisol-adjusted post-DST cortisol values was found, suggesting that lower presynaptic 5-HT activity is related to escape of negative-feedback inhibition (44). This suggests the possibility that a diminished central 5-HT neurotransmission in major depression may attenuate the hippocampal negative-feedback control over the HPA axis, thus inducing excessive corticosteroid secretion. Treatment with L-TRP (3.5 to 7 g/day) for 1 to 2 weeks has been shown to improve DST nonsuppression in depressed subjects (59). Therefore, it may be hypothesized that TRP treatment may have restored the serotonergic deficit in the hippocampus, thus increasing the negative feedback over the HPA axis. Treatment with fluoxetine and imipramine may also increase the level of MR messenger ribonucleic acid (mRNA), thus increasing the efficacy of the negative feedback on hypothalamic CRH mRNA (4). Other results may indicate that up-regulation of postsynaptic 5-HT$_2$ receptors in major depression is related to escape of ACTH/cortisol secretion from negative-feedback effects; compared with patients who had minor depression, those with a diagnosis of major depression exhibited a significant enhancing effect of L-5-HTP (125 to 200 mg) on post-DST ACTH or cortisol values, although L-5-HTP converted DST cortisol or ACTH suppression into nonsuppression in some major depressed subjects (40).

GENDER DIFFERENCES IN PERIPHERAL AND CENTRAL SEROTONIN ACTIVITY

There are several reports suggesting that there are gender differences in peripheral and central 5-HT metabolism. Preclinical data suggest that female rats have a higher activity of 5-HT synthesizing enzymes, a greater storage capacity for 5-HT in brain 5-HT neurons, a more pronounced 5-HT behavioral syndrome in response to 5-HT agonists, and higher brain and CSF levels of TRP, 5-HT, and 5-HIAA compared to males (6). Animal data show that female rats exhibit a larger prolactin response to 5-HT$_{1A}$ receptor agonists than male rats (21).

Significantly lower fasting plasma L-TRP levels are found in female control subjects (42). Delgado et al. (16) found that males maintained their plasma free and total TRP levels closer to baseline values in response to TRP depletion. Our laboratory found that buspirone evoked a significantly greater prolactin response in women than in men (53). Delgado et al. (16) found that males demonstrated smaller prolactin responses to L-TRP infusion than did female subjects.

In depression, plasma total L-TRP levels tend to be more reduced in female than in male patients (42). In female major depressed subjects, but not in males, there is a significant negative correlation between self-rated depression and plasma levels of total L-TRP (42). Depressed females show significantly higher xanthurenic acid excretion following L-TRP loading than depressed males (39). Major depressed females exhibit significantly higher L-5-HTP-induced cortisol responses than male major depressed subjects (38).

Some of these gender related differences in 5-HT metabolism may perhaps be explained by the fact that liver pyrrolase activity is greater in women and that 5-HT receptors appear to be estrogen sensitive. Curzon's group (14) found that female rats, as opposed to male rats, failed to adapt to repeated restraint stress. Maladaption in female rats was associated with greater corticosterone response and defects in 5-HT$_{1A}$ receptor-mediated behavior.

THE SEROTONIN HYPOTHESIS OF MAJOR DEPRESSION

The above review has provided some evidence that among the biological factors predisposing a person to major depression, alterations in presynaptic 5-HT activity, alterations in postsynaptic 5-HT$_2$ and 5-HT$_{1A}$ receptors in the brain, and reciprocal relationships between dysfunctions in these systems and the HPA axis may be of special importance. Table 1 summarizes the various findings on peripheral and central and pre- and postsynaptic 5-HT activity in major depression.

There are several arguments to support a deficient 5-HT presynaptic activity: lower availability of plasma L-TRP to the brain; induction of depressive symptomatology by L-TRP depletion techniques; the relationship between lower L-TRP levels and positive response to serotonergic antidepressive treatments; lower L-TRP, 5-HT, and 5-HIAA in postmortem tissues of some depressed suicide victims; blunted L-TRP, D,L-fenfluramine, D-fenfluramine, or clomipramine-induced prolactin responses; antidepressive-treatment−induced increases in L-TRP-, D,L-fenfluramine-, or electroconvulsive-therapy−stimulated prolactin responses; and antidepressive-treatment−induced increments in presynaptic 5-HT activity.

Major depression is characterized by an increased number, affinity, or responsivity of central postsynaptic 5-HT$_2$ receptors. This evidence comes from higher 5-HT$_2$ receptor binding in platelets of major depressed subjects and in the prefrontal cortex of depressed suicide victims; lower 5-HT2 antagonist-induced SWS; increased HPA-axis responses to L-TRP and (L)-5-HTP; and antidepressive-treatment−induced decrements in 5-HT$_2$ binding and 5-HT$_2$-related behavioral or hormonal responses.

Major depression is accompanied by down-regulated or desensitized postsynaptic 5-HT$_{1A}$ receptors. This hypothesis is corroborated by attenuated ipsapirone-induced HPA-axis hormone responses; lower hippocampal 5-HT$_1$ receptor binding in postmortem brain; blunted prolactin responses to L-TRP, fenfluramine, or clomipramine; and sensitization or up-regulation of 5-HT$_{1A}$ postsynaptic receptors by chronic antidepressive treatment with tricyclic antidepressants and electroconvulsive therapy.

At present, it is difficult to conclude whether presynap-

TABLE 1. *Summary of serotonergic findings in major depression*

Serotonergic marker	Replication A[a]	Replication B[b]	Putative serotonergic mechanism
Lower plasma L-TRP and L-TRP/CAA	S	−/+++	Lowered availability of L-TRP
Higher plasma TRP clearance after TRP loading	S	−/++	Lowered availability of L-TRP through excessive peripheral catabolism
Higher urinary xanthurenic acid excretion after TRP loading	S	−/+	Induction of liver pyrrolase−nicotinamide pathway
Lower plasma TRP in relation to clinical response to serotonergic antidepressants	IS	+++	Lower TRP availability predicts favorable outcome to serotonergic drugs
Induction of depressive symptoms by TRP depletion techniques	S	++	Lowered TRP availability is related to depressive phenomenology
Lower platelet 5-HT uptake	S	−−/++	Indicative of lower 5-HT transporter
Lower platelet imipramine binding	S	−−/+++	Indicative of lower 5-HT transporter
Lower platelet paroxetine binding	S	−−	No indication of abnormal 5-HT transporter
Lower platelet or plasma 5-HT levels	S	+	Indicative of lower 5-HT storage or release
Lower postmortem brain TRP, 5-HT, 5-HIAA	S	−/+	Lower central 5-HT turnover/activity
Lower CSF 5-HIAA concentrations	S	−−−/++	Lower central 5-HT turnover/activity
Higher platelet 5-HT$_2$ receptor binding	S	++	Indicative of up-regulated (central?) 5-HT$_2$ receptors
Higher postmortem brain 5-HT$_2$ receptor binding	S	−/+++	Up-regulated central 5-HT$_2$ receptors (prefrontal cortex)
Lower 5-HT$_2$ antagonist-induced slow wave sleep	S	+	Up-regulated central 5-HT$_2$ receptors
Lower postmortem brain 5-HT$_{1A}$ receptor binding	S	−/++	Down-regulated central 5-HT$_{1A}$ receptors/hippocampus
Lower TRP-induced prolactin	S	−/+++	Indicative of lower central presynaptic 5-HT activity or postsynaptic receptor responsivity
Higher TRP-induced cortisol	S	−/++	Indicative of up-regulated central 5-HT$_2$ receptors
Higher 5-HTP-induced cortisol	S	−/+++	Indicative of up-regulated central 5-HT$_2$ receptors
Lower fenfluramine-induced prolactin	S	−/+++	Indicative of lower central presynaptic 5-HT activity or postsynaptic receptor responsivity
Lower clomipramine-induced prolactin	S	++	Indicative of lower central presynaptic 5-HT activity or postsynaptic receptor responsivity
Lower buspirone-induced cortisol/production		−	
Lower ipsapirone-induced cortisol	S	++	Indicative of downregulated central 5-HT$_{1A}$ receptors
Higher TRP, fenfluramine, or clomipramine-induced prolactin responses to ADT[c]	S	++	ADT increase brain 5-HT activity (pre- or postsynaptic)
Lower 5-HTP-induced cortisol to ADT	I	0	ADT may desensitize 5-HT$_2$ receptors

[a] A is the number of laboratories that have investigated the listed marker: 1, only one lab; S, several labs; IS, one principal investigator in various collaborative studies.

[b] B is the degree of replication: 0, no attempts were made to replicate; −/+ ratios reflect the approximate ratio of negative versus positive reports.

[c] ADT: antidepressive treatments.

tic 5-HT hypoactivity and changes in 5-HT$_2$ or 5-HT$_{1A}$ postsynaptic receptor function are causally related. First, lesioning of serotonergic neurons has been reported to enhance, not decrease, certain responses of 5-HT$_{1A}$ receptors (24). Second, there are now several data that suggest that an increase in 5-HT$_2$ binding does not represent a compensatory up-regulation of postsynaptic elements in response to deficiencies in the presynaptic neurons innervating cortical targets (29,35). It may be hypothesized that desensitized postsynaptic 5-HT$_{1A}$ receptors could diminish the 5-HT$_{1A}$−mediated inhibition of 5-HT$_2$ receptor responsivity, leading to an augmentation of 5-HT$_2$ receptor responsivity. In addition, the decrease in presynaptic 5-HT activity may be a factor preventing the restoration of normal 5-HT$_2$ receptor responsivity.

Disorders in both peripheral and central 5-HT metabolism and HPA-axis hyperactivity may be interrelated phenomena, which participate in the pathophysiology of major depression. Diminished central hippocampal serotonergic activity may result in elevated central and peripheral HPA-axis activity due to lowered hippocampal negative feedback by GR or MR on hypothalamic CRH. Increased CRH secretion may stimulate HPA-axis activity and increased glucocorticoid levels may be involved in further down-regulation of GR or MR, defective 5-HT$_{1A}$ postsynaptic receptor signaling pathways and maybe up-regulation of 5-HT$_2$ receptors. Supersensitive 5-HT$_2$ receptors in limbic structures or in the hypothalamus may sustain 5-HT−related HPA-axis hyperactivity, through stimulatory effects on CRH and AVP secretion and an enhanced negative-feedback breakthrough secretion of pituitary ACTH. Increased cortisol secretion may further compromise central serotonergic activity, by lowering L-TRP availability through induction of the liver-pyrrolase pathway. Other putative effects of HPA-axis hormones may be regarded as compensatory mechanisms that try to restore a lowered central presynaptic 5-HT activity, for example, increased 5-HT turnover. The latter could also explain the more conflicting results on central presynaptic 5-HT activity in major depression.

The gender-related differences in peripheral and central 5-HT metabolism, together with the greater susceptibility of 5-HT and HPA-axis systems to environmental stressors in females, could contribute to the higher incidence of major depression in females.

FUTURE RESEARCH

Although much has been learned about serotonergic dysfunction in major depression since 1987, it is clear that there is no simple answer to the question of whether altered 5-HT activity is directly related to the pathogenesis or pathophysiology of major depression or whether it acts as a vulnerability factor in that illness. Future research on serotonergic activity in depression might focus on the following issues.

The availability of L-TRP to the brain, which may be the rate-limiting factor in the synthesis of 5-HT in patients with major depression remains an important issue. Further study is needed of the conversion of a TRP load to 5-HT versus the products of the kynurenine-nicotinamide pathway. The transport of L-TRP into the brain needs to be studied. The findings of Møller (56) of a low-plasma L-TRP to CAA ratio predicting clinical response to serotonergic antidepressive drugs needs confirmation. The basis for the failure of L-TRP depletion to exacerbate major depression in untreated patients should be clarified.

Further studies are needed of postmortem indices of 5-HT function, such as brain 5-HT and 5-HIAA concentrations; 5-HT_{1A}, 5-HT_{1C}, and 5-HT_2 receptor binding; and second messenger systems in depressed patients who died of natural as well as suicide causes. They must control for gender, age, drug treatment, substance use or abuse, seasonality in 5-HT function, comorbidity with, for example, anxiety, personality, or impulse control disorders, and glucocorticoid elevation.

There are only a few studies using single photon emission computed tomography (SPECT) or positron emission tomography (PET) with serotonergic markers in depression (e.g., ^{125}I-ketanserin). The results of these studies are difficult to interpret for a variety of reasons. More SPECT or PET scan studies with ligands that are relatively specific for $5\text{-HT}_2/5\text{-HT}_{1C}$ or 5-HT_{1A} sites and the 5-HT transporter in depressed patients prior to and after remission are needed.

Until now, there have been few neuroendocrine studies using direct agonists at $5\text{-HT}_2/5\text{-HT}_{1C}$ sites (e.g., MK-212, mCPP) in major depression. The finding of hyporesponsiveness of cortisol to the 5-HT_{1A} agonist ipsapirone needs further replication. More research should be focused on the possible cooperation between 5-HT2/5-HT1C and 5-HT1A receptors. One strategy to investigate this cooperation between 5-HT receptors in major depression is neuroendocrine challenge (HPA-axis hormone and prolactin assays) after administration of L-5-HTP in depressed patients and normal controls pretreated with pindolol or ritanserin.

The relationships between HPA-axis hyperactivity and peripheral and central 5-HT turnover in major depression await further elucidation. More information on the following topics is needed to fully delineate the 5-HT/HPA-axis hypothesis: effects of glucocorticoids on L-TRP transport through the blood–brain barrier, and the uptake of 5-HT, and imipramine and paroxetine binding to blood platelets. Additionally, the effects of glucocorticoids at 5-HT_{1A} and $5\text{-HT}_2/5\text{-HT}_{1C}$ receptor sites need further exploration through neuroendocrine or imaging studies.

Finally, comprehensive studies of the relevant monoamine systems, such as norepinephrine and dopamine, and γ-aminobutyric acid which may interact with 5-HT and each other to cause depression, must be studied using the techniques described above.

Because multiple variables must be measured, large sample sizes and multiple cooperating laboratories will be needed. This could be the goal of a national or international collaboration.

REFERENCES

1. Arango V, Underwood MD, Mann JJ. Alterations in monoamine receptors in the brain of suicide victims. *J Clin Psychopharmacology* 1992;12:8–12.
2. Arora RC, Meltzer HY. Increased serotonin 2 (5-HT2) receptor binding as measured by 3H-lysergic acid diethylamide (3H-LSD) in the blood platelets of depressed patients. *Life Sci* 1989;44:725–734.
3. Blier P, de Montigny G, Chaput Y. A role for the serotonin system in the mechanism of action of antidepressant treatments: preclinical evidence. *J Clin Psychiatry* 1990;51:14–20.
4. Brady LS, Gold PW, Herkenham M, Lynn AB, Whitfield HJ Jr. The antidepressants fluoxetine, idazaxan and phenelzine alter corticotropin-releasing hormone and tyrosine hydroxylase mRNA levels in rat brain: therapeutic implications. *Brain Res* 1992;572:117–125.
5. Calogero AE, Bagdy G, Moncada ML, D'Agata R. Effect of selective serotinin agonists on basal, corticotropin-releasing hormone-induced and vasopressin-induced ACTH release in vitro from rat pituitary cells. *J Endocrinology* 1993;136:381–387.
6. Carlsson M, Svensson K, Ericksson E, Carlsson A. Rat brain serotonin: biochemical and functional evidence for a sex difference. *J Neural Transm* 1985;63:297–313.
7. Celada P, Dolera M, Alvarez E, Artigas F. Effects of acute and chronic treatment with fluvoxamine on extracellular and platelet serotonin in the blood of major depressive patients. Relationships to clinical improvement. *J Affect Disord* 1992;25:243–250.
8. Chaouloff F. Physiopharmacological interactions between stress

hormones and central serotonergic systems. *Brain Res Rev* 1993; 18:1–32.
9. Charney DS, Delgado PL. Current concepts of the role of serotonin function in depression and anxiety. In: Langer SZ, Brunello N, Racagni G, Mendlewicz J, eds. *Serotonin receptor subtypes: pharmacological significance and clinical implication.* Basel: Karger, 1992;89–104.
10. Cheetham SC, Crompton MR, Czudek C, Horton RW, Katona CL, Reynolds GP. Serotonin concentrations and turnover in brains of depressed suicides. *Brain Res* 1989;502:332–340.
11. Cheetham SC, Crompton MR, Katona CLE, Horton RW. Brain 5-HT$_2$ receptor binding sites in depressed suicide victims. *Brain Res* 1988;443:272–280.
12. Cheetham SC, Crompton MR, Katona CLE, Horton RW. Brain 5-HT1 binding sites in depressed suicides. *Psychopharmacology* 1990;102:544–548.
13. Cowen PJ. A role for 5-HT in the action of antidepressant drugs. *Pharmacol Ther* 1990;46:43–51.
14. Curzon G. 5-Hydroxytryptamine and corticosterone in an animal model of depression. *Prog Psychopharmacol Biol Psychiatry* 1989; 13:305–310.
15. Deakin JF, Pennell I, Upadhyaya AJ, Lofthouse R. A neuroendocrine study of 5HT function in depression: evidence for biological mechanisms of endogenous and psychosocial causation. *Psychopharmacology* 1990;101:85–92.
16. Delgado PL, Charney DS, Price LH, Landis H, Heninger GR. Neuroendocrine and behavioral effects of dietary tryptophan restriction in healthy subjects. *Life Sci* 1990;45:2323–2332.
17. Faustman WO, King RJ, Faull KF, Moses JA Jr, Benson KL, Zarcone VP, Csernansky JG. MMPI measures of impulsivity and depression correlate with CSF 5-HIAA and HVA in depression but not schizophrenia. *J Affect Disord* 1991;22:235–239.
18. Fuller RW. The involvement of serotonin in regulation of pituitary-adrenocortical function. *Front Neuroendocrinol* 1992;13:250–270.
19. Golden RN, Ekstrom D, Brown TM, Ruegg R, Evans DL, Haggerty JJ Jr, Garbutt JC, Pedersen CA, Mason GA, Browne J. Neuroendocrine effects of intravenous clomipramine in depressed patients and healthy subjects. *Am J Psychiatry* 1992;149:1168–1175.
20. Gross-Isseroff R, Israeli M, Biegon A. Autoradiographic analysis of initiated imipramine binding in the human brain post-mortem: effects of suicide. *Arch Gen Psychiatry* 1989;46:237–241.
21. Haleem DJ, Kennett GA, Whitton PS, Curzon G. 8-OH-DPAT increases corticosterone but not other 5-HT1A receptor-dependent responses more in females. *Eur J Pharmacol* 1989;164:435–443.
22. Hayakawa H, Yokota N, Shimizu M, Nishida A, Yamawaki S. Repeated treatment with electroconvulsive shock increases numbers of serotonin-1A receptors in the rat hippocampus. *Biog Amine* 1993;4:295–306.
23. Heninger GR, Delgado PL, Charney DS, Price LH, Aghajanian GK. Tryptophan-deficient diet and amino acid drink deplete plasma tryptophan and induce a relapse of depression in susceptible patients. *J Chem Neuroanatomy* 1992;5:347–348.
24. Hensler JG, Kovachich GB, Frazer A. A quantitative autoradiographic study of serotonin 1A receptor regulation. Effect of 5,7-dihydroxytryptamine and antidepressant treatments. *Neuropharmacology* 1991;25:563–576.
25. Hoes MJAJM, Sijben N. The clinical significance of disordered renal excretion of xanthurenic acid in depressive patients. *Psychopharmacology* 1981;75:346–349.
26. Huether G, Hajak G, Reimer A, Poeggeler B, Blomer M, Rodenbeck A, Ruther E. The metabolic fate of infused L-tryptophan in men: possible clinical implications of the accumulation of circulating tryptophan and tryptophan metabolites. *Psychopharmacology* 1992;109:422–432.
27. Jhamandas K, Boegman RJ, Beninger RJ, Bialik M. Quinolinate-induced cortical cholinergic damage: modulation by tryptophan metabolites. *Brain Res* 1990;529:185–191.
28. Koyama T, Meltzer HY. A biochemical and neuroendocrine study of the serotonergic system in depression. In: Hippius H., ed. *New results in depression research,* Berlin-Heidelberg: Springer-Verlag; 1986:169–188.
29. Kuroda Y, Mikuni M, Ogawa T, Takahashi K. Effect of ACTH, adrenalectomy and the combination treatment on the density of 5-HT2 receptor binding sites in neocortex of rat forebrain and 5-HT2 receptor-mediated wet-dog shake behaviors. *Psychopharmacology* 1992;108:27–32.
30. Lawrence KM, DePaermentier F, Cheetham SC, Crompton MR, Katona CLE, Horton RW. Brain 5-HT uptake sites, labelled with [^{3}H]paroxetine, in antidepressant-free depressed suicides. *Brain Res* 1990;526:17–22.
31. Lawrence KM, Falkowski J, Jacobson RR, Horton RW. Platelet 5-HT uptake sites in depression—3 concurrent measures using ^{3}H-imipramine and ^{3}H-paroxetine. *Psychopharmacology* 1993;110:235–239.
32. Leake A, Fairbairn AF, McKeith IG, Ferrier IN. Studies on the serotonin uptake binding site in major depressive disorder and control port-mortem brain: neurochemical and clinical correlates. *Psychiatr Res* 1991;39:155–165.
33. Lerer B. Neurochemical and other neurobiological consequences of ECT: implications for the pathogenesis and treatment of affective disorders. In: Meltzer HY, ed. *Psychopharmacology: the third generation of progress.* New York: Raven Press, 1987:577–588.
34. Lesch K-P, Mayer S, Disselkamp-Tietze J, Hoh A, Wiesmann M, Osterheider M, Schulte HM. 5-HT1A receptor responsivity in unipolar depression: evaluation of ipsapirone-induced ACTH and cortisol secretion in patients and controls. *Biol Psychiatry* 1990;28:620–628.
35. Leysen JE. 5-HT2 receptors: location, pharmacological, pathological and physiological role: In: Langer SZ, Brunello N, Racagni G, Mendlewicz J, eds. *Serotonin receptor subtypes: pharmacological significance and clinical implication.* Basel: Karger, 1992:31–43.
36. Lichtenberg P, Shapira B, Gillon D, Kindler S, Cooper TB, Newman ME, Lerer B. Hormone responses to fenfluramine and placebo challenge in endogenous depression. *Psychiatr Res* 1992;43:137–146.
37. Lund A, Mjellem-Jolly N, Hole K. Desipramine, administered chronically, influences 5-hydroxytryptamine 1A-receptors, as measured by behavioral tests and receptor binding in rats. *Neuropharmacology* 1992;31:25–32.
38. Maes M, De Ruyter M, Claes R, Bosma G, Suy E. The cortisol responses to 5-hydroxytryptophan, orally, in depressive inpatients. *J Affect Disord* 1987;13:23–30.
39. Maes M, De Ruyter M, Suy E. The renal excretion of xanthurenic acid following L-tryptophan loading in depressed patients. *Human Psychopharmacology* 1987;2:231–235.
40. Maes M, D'Hondt P, Martin M, Claes M, Schotte C, Vandewoude M, Blockx P. L-5-hydroxytryptophan stimulated cortisol escape from dexamethasone suppression in melancholic patients. *Acta Psychiatr Scand* 1991;83:302–306.
41. Maes M, D'Hondt P, Suy E, Minner B, Vandervorst C, Raus J. HPA-axis hormones and prolactin responses to dextro-fenfluramine in depressed patients and healthy controls. *Prog Neuro-Psychopharmacol Biol Psychiatry* 1991;15:781–790.
42. Maes M, Jacobs M-P, Suy E, Minner B, Leclercq C, Christiaens F, Raus J. Suppressant effects of dexamethasone on the availability of plasma L-tryptophan and tyrosine in healthy controls and in depressed patients. *Acta Psychiatr Scand* 1990;81:19–23.
43. Maes M, Maes L, Schotte C, Vandewoude M, Martin M, D'Hondt P, Blockx P, Scharpé S, Cosyns P. Clinical subtypes of unipolar depression, part III: Quantitative differences in various biological markers between the cluster analysis-generated non-vital and vital depression classes. *Psychiatr Res* 1990;34:59–75.
44. Maes M, Minner B, Suy E. The relationships between the availability of L-tryptophan to the brain, the spontaneous HPA-axis activity, and the HPA-axis responses to dexamethasone in depressed patients. *Amino Acids* 1991;1:57–65.
45. Maes M, Vandervorst C, Suy E, Minner B, Raus J. A multivariate study on the simultaneous urinary free cortisol, plasma cortisol, adrenocorticotropic hormone and β-endorphin escape from suppression by dexamethasone in melancholic patients. *Acta Psychiatr Scand* 1991;83:480–491.
46. Maes M, Vandevelde R, Suy E. Influences on cortisol and noradrenergic turnover of healthy controls and depressed patients during L-tryptophan loading. *J Affect Disord* 1989;17:173–182.
47. Maj J, Moryl E. Effects of sertraline and citalopram given repeatedly

on the responsiveness of 5-HT receptor subpopulations. *J Neural Transm* 1992;88:143–156.

48. Matsubara S, Arora RC, Meltzer HY. Serotonergic measures in suicide brain: 5-HT1A binding sites in frontal cortex of suicide victims. *J Neural Transm* 1991;85:181–194.

49. Mellerup ET, Plenge P, Engelstoft M. High affinity binding of ^{3}H-paroxetine and ^{3}H-imipramine to human platelet membranes. *Eur J Pharmacology* 1983;96:303–309.

50. Meltzer HY, Arora RC. Platelet serotonin studies in affective disorders: evidence for a serotonergic abnormality. In: Sandler M, Coppen A, Harnett S, eds. *5-Hydroxytryptamine in psychiatry: a spectrum of ideas.* New York: Oxford University Press, 1991:50–89.

51. Meltzer HY, Lowy MT. The serotonin hypothesis of depression. In: Meltzer HY, ed. *Psychopharmacology: the third generation of progress.* New York: Raven Press, 1987:513–526.

52. Meltzer HY, Maes M. Effect of pindolol on the L-5-HTP-induced increase in plasma prolactin and cortisol concentrations in man. *Psychopharmacology* 1993;[in press].

53. Meltzer HY, Maes M. Effects of buspirone on cortisol and prolactin secretion in major depression. *Biol Psychiatry* 1994;35:316–323.

54. Meltzer HY, Wiita B, Robertson A, Tricou BJ, Lowy M, Perline R. Effect of 5-hydroxytryptophan on serum cortisol levels in major affective disorders: enhanced response in depression and mania. *Arch Gen Psychiatry* 1984;41:366–374.

55. Mikuni M, Kagaya A, Takahashi K, Meltzer HY. Serotonin but not norepinephrine-induced calcium mobilization of platelets is enhanced in affective disorders. *Psychopharmacology* 1992;106:311–314.

56. Møller SE, Bech P, Bjerrum H, Bøjholm S, Butler B, Folker H, Gram LF, Larsen JK, Lauritzen L, Loldrup D, Munk-Andersen E, Odum K, Rafaelson OJ. Plasma ratio tryptophan/neutral amino acids in relation to clinical response to paroxetine and clomipramine in patients with major depression. *J Affect Disord* 1990;18:59–66.

57. Morgan CJ, Badawy AA-B. Effects of a suppression test dose of dexamethasone on tryptophan metabolism and disposition in the rat. *Biol Psychiatry* 1989;25:360–362.

58. Nash JF, Meltzer HY. Neuroendocrine studies in psychiatric disorders: the role of serotonin. In: Brown S-L, van Praag HM, eds. *The role of serotonin in psychiatric disorders.* New York: Brunner/Mazel, 1991:57–90.

59. Nuller JL, Ostroumova MN. Resistance to inhibiting effect of dexamethasone in patients with endogenous depression. *Acta Psychiatr Scand* 1980;61:169–177.

60. O'Keane V, Dinan TG. Prolactin and cortisol responses to d-fenfluramine in major depression: evidence for diminished responsivity of central serotonergic function. *Am J Psychiatry* 1991;148:1009–1015.

61. O'Keane V, McLoughlin D, Dinan TG. D-fenfluramine-induced prolactin and cortisol release in major depression: response to treatment. *J Affect Disord* 1992;26:143–150.

62. Pranzatelli MR, Eng B. Chronic ACTH treatment: influence on 5-HT2 receptors and behavioral supersensitivity induced by 5,7-dihydroxytryptamine lesions. *Peptides* 1989;10:5–8.

63. Reddy PL, Khanna S, Subhash MN, Channabasavanna SM, Rao BS. CSF amine metabolites in depression. *Biol Psychiatry* 1992;31:112–118.

64. Sarrias MJ, Artigas F, Martinez E, Gelpi E, Alvarez E, Udina C, Casas M. Decreased plasma serotonin in melanchoic patients: a study with clomipramine. *Biol Psychiatry* 1987;22:1429–1438.

65. Seckl JR, Fink G. Use of in situ hybridization to investigate the regulation of hippocampal corticosteroid receptors by monoamines. *J Steroid Biochem Mol Biol* 1991;40:685–688.

66. Shapira B, Cohen J, Newman ME, Lerer B. Prolactin response to fenfluramine and placebo challenge following maintenance pharmacotherapy withdrawal in remitted depressed patients. *Biol Psychiatry* 1992;33:531–535.

67. Sharpley AL, Gregory CA, Solomon RA, Cowen PJ. Slow wave sleep and 5-HT2 receptor sensitivity during maintenance tricyclic antidepressant treatment. *J Affect Disord* 1990;19:273–277.

68. Singh VB, Hao-Phan T, Corley KC, Boadle-Biber MC. Increase in cortical and midbrain tryptophan hydroxylase activity by intracerebroventricular administration of corticotropin releasing factor: block by adrenalectomy, by RU 38486 and by bilateral lesions to the central nucleus of the amygdala. *Neurochem Int* 1991;20:81–92.

69. Staner L, Kempenaers C, Simonnet M-P, Fransolet L, Mendlewicz J. 5-HT2 receptor antagonism and slow-wave sleep in major depression. *Acta Psychiatr Scand* 1992;86:133–137.

70. Stockmeier CA, Wingenfeld P, Gudelsky GA. Effects of repeated electroconvulsive shock on serotonin 1A receptor binding and receptor mediated hypothermia in the rat. *Neuropharmacology* 1992;31:1089–1094.

71. Traskman-Bendz L, Haskett RF, Zis AP. Neuroendocrine effects of L-tryptophan and dexamethasone. *Psychopharmacology* 1986;89:85–88.

72. Upadhyaya AK, Pennell I, Cowen PJ, Deakin JF. Blunted growth hormone and prolactin responses to L-tryptophan in depression, a state-dependent abnormality. *J Affect Disord* 1991;21:213–218.

73. van Praag HM, Lemus C, Kahn R. Hormonal probes of central serotonergic activity: do they really exist? *Biol Psychiatry* 1987;22:86–98.

74. Welner SA, de Montigny C, Desroches J, Desjardins P, Suranyi-Cadotte BE. Autoradiographic quantification of serotonin 1A receptors in rat brain following antidepressant drug treatment. *Synapse* 1989;4:347–352.

75. Young SN, Smith SE, Pihl R, Ervin FR. Tryptophan depletion causes a rapid lowering of mood in normal males. *Psychopharmacology* 1985;87:173–177.

Psychopharmacology: The Fourth Generation of Progress, edited by Floyd E. Bloom and David J. Kupfer. Raven Press, Ltd., New York © 1995.

CHAPTER 82

The Role of Acetylcholine Mechanisms in Mood Disorders

David S. Janowsky and David H. Overstreet

Considerable information suggests a role for mono-aminergic-cholinergic balance in the pathogenesis of mood disorders. As proposed by Janowsky et al. (27), depression may be a manifestation of a central cholinergic predominance, whereas mania, conversely, may be due to a relative monoaminergic (i.e., adrenergic) predominance. This chapter on cholinergic mechanisms in the affective disorders summarizes research findings from both animal and human studies that suggest that central muscarinic and possibly nicotinic mechanisms are likely to contribute to the psychopathology of the affective disorders (see Chapters 10 and 11, *this volume*).

BEHAVIORAL EFFECTS OF CHOLINOMIMETIC DRUGS IN ANIMAL MODELS OF DEPRESSION

It has long been recognized that cholinergic effects in animals are mediated by both muscarinic and nicotinic mechanisms. However, muscarinic mechanisms have been the focus of most investigations into the potential role of the central cholinergic system in affective psychopathology, and indeed muscarinic mechanisms are the major focus of this review. Nevertheless, as a part of this review, we also consider a potential role of nicotinic mechanisms in the etiology of affective disorders.

Many preclinical animal behavioral models of depression have been developed, including the self-stimulation model, the hypoactivity model, the learned helplessness

model, the chronic stress model, the behavioral despair or forced swim model, and the HPA axis activation model (20,43,46). Significantly, increasing central cholinergic tone with such centrally active cholinomimetic agents as physostigmine, arecoline, and oxotremorine usually induces or enhances the behavioral analogs of depression in such models of depression. Thus, centrally acting cholinomimetic drugs consistently produce behavioral inhibitory effects including lethargy and hypoactivity, activation of the HPA axis, decreases in self-stimulation (27), increases in behavioral despair in the forced swim test, and decreases in saccharin preference. These cholinergically induced phenomena are generally reversible with centrally active sympathetic agents and antimuscarinic drugs, thus supporting evidence of a balance between adrenergic and muscarinic cholinergic factors in their regulation (27). Several animal species, developed by selective breeding, have demonstrated differentially enhanced responses to cholinergic agonists; these animals appear to represent genetic animal models of depression. The psychogenetically selected Roman low avoidance (RLA) rats, which do not effectively learn avoidance responses, are relatively more sensitive to cholinergic agonists (41) and have been considered to be an animal model for anxiety/depression (70). The hypercholinergic Flinders sensitive line (FSL) of rats, which were selectively bred to have differentially increased responses to the anticholinesterase agent diisopropylfluorophosphate (DFP), as compared to control Flinders resistant line (FRL) rats, which are differentially sensitive to other muscarinic agonists (46,55). Overstreet and colleagues have proposed that, like the RLA rats, the FSL rats are an animal model of depression (46).

Similarities between FSL rats and depressed humans include reduced body weight, learning difficulties, reduced general activity and locomotion, increased REM

D. S. Janowsky: Department of Psychiatry, University of North Carolina Medical School, Chapel Hill, North Carolina 27599.
D. H. Overstreet: Department of Psychiatry, Center for Alcohol Studies, University of North Carolina, Chapel Hill, North Carolina 27599.

sleep and reduced REM sleep latency, and exaggerated HPA axis activation (i.e., corticosterone release) after cholinomimetic administration (46). The FSL rats also demonstrate a greater reduction in saccharin preference than do control FRL rats during exposure to chronic mild stress (47), the latter suggesting a greater degree of stress induced anhedonia.

In addition to possessing a number of characteristics that parallel those of depressed humans (46), FSL rats also have baseline exaggerated immobility in the forced swim test, a test commonly used to screen for antidepressant drugs (6), and considered by some also to be an animal model of depression. This exaggerated immobility is not unexpected; there is literature indicating that cholinergic agonists accentuate and cholinergic antagonists reduce swim test immobility (6). Hasey and Hanin (21) recently confirmed the acute depressive effects of cholinergic agonists (i.e., physostigmine) on swim test immobility. These investigators also reported that these cholinergic effects could be partially counteracted by noradrenergic manipulations, and they proposed a balance model reminiscent of the original adrenergic/cholinergic balance model of affective disorders (27).

EFFECTS OF CHOLINOMIMETICS ON MANIC SYMPTOMS

If an aberrant mood is from an imbalance between adrenergic and cholinergic factors, it is logical to expect that increases in central cholinergic activity might decrease manic symptoms. Several studies have shown that centrally active cholinergic agonists and cholinesterase inhibitors possess antimanic properties. In a seminal study by Rowntree et al. (cited in Chapter 53 of ref. 43a), the centrally active cholinesterase inhibitor DFP was given to manic–depressive patients and normals. The normal subjects and remitted manic–depressives developed irritability, lassitude, depression, apathy, and slowness and/or poverty of thoughts. Two patients who were hypomanic at the time of the study improved with DFP and continued euthymic after its administration. One hypomanic patient became less manic and was minimally depressed after each of two courses of DFP, but relapsed upon DFP withdrawal.

Janowsky et al. (27,28) found that the centrally active cholinesterase inhibitor physostigmine caused a dramatic but brief reduction in hypomanic and manic symptoms in bipolar patients. Neither placebo nor the noncentrally acting cholinesterase inhibitor neostigmine produced such changes, thus suggesting a central mechanism. After physostigmine administration, the manics became significantly less talkative, active, euphoric, happy, grandiose, and friendly, and showed a decrease in flight of ideas on the Beigel Murphy Mania Rating Scale. The effects of physostigmine lasted from 20 to 90 min. Modestin et al.

(cited in Chapter 53 of ref. 43a) subsequently also reported a lessening of manic symptoms following infusion of physostigmine, but not neostigmine, and Davis et al. (cited in Chapter 53 of ref. 43a) reported that physostigmine caused dramatic antimanic effects, particularly in patients with low levels of hostility and/or irritability. Carroll et al. (cited in Chapter 53 of ref. 43a) and Shopsin et al. (cited in Chapter 53 of ref. 43a) also reported a decrease in euphoria and mobility in manics after physostigmine infusion. More recently, Berger et al. (3) reported pilot data suggesting that RS86, a relatively specific muscarinic (M_1) agonist, has significant antimanic effects.

Although most data to date are supportive of cholinomimetic agents exerting an antimanic effect, some authors have reported effects only on the affective and motoric components of mania, and no effects on the cognitive aspects of mania such as grandiose thinking and expansiveness (ref. citations 4 and 58 in Chapter 53 of ref. 43a). Skeptics of the possibility that cholinomimetics exert antimanic effects have pointed out that manic patients, treated with centrally acting cholinomimetic drugs still continue to show grandiosity and to have manic delusions. In addition to the antagonism of motoric behaviors, there is evidence that when the central cholinergic system is activated, there may be a later compensatory and antagonistic activation of the adrenergic system. Fibiger et al. (cited in Chapter 53 of ref. 43a) demonstrated that the increase in cholinergic activity caused by the administration of physostigmine led to an eventual increase in locomotion in rats, as presumed adrenergic mechanisms began to exert effects. This activating effect became apparent as the cholinergic predominance induced by physostigmine decreased and was exaggerated if a centrally acting anticholinergic agent such as scopolamine was given at the beginning of the hyperactivity phase.

As with the work of Fibiger et al. (cited in Chapter 53 of ref. 43a), there is some evidence that a behavioral rebound following physostigmine infusion can also occur in humans. A case of rebounding into mania was noted by Rowntree et al. (cited in Chapter 53 of ref. 43a), and by Shopsin et al. (cited in Chapter 53 of ref. 43a), who demonstrated rebounding into hypermania in two of three manic patients given physostigmine. However, "rebounding" in humans has rarely been observed following physostigmine infusion.

RED BLOOD CELL CHOLINE IN MANIA

Although there is considerable evidence that centrally acting muscarinic cholinergic drugs can effectively decrease manic symptoms, at least acutely, few reliable direct markers of a cholinergic deficit have been noted in mania. One measure of such function may be reflected in the measurement of erythrocyte choline activity. Erythrocyte choline levels have been investigated as a biochemical marker of acetylcholine activity since choline is the major precursor, as well as a major metabolite of acetylcholine. Changes in central acetylcholine have been shown to affect cholinergic neurotransmission. Slight elevations in erythrocyte choline have been noted in patients with bipolar disorders (66) and have also been observed in schizophrenics and depressives (5,66). Stoll et al. (66) also noted that there exists an increased level of choline in a subgroup of manic bipolar patients at pretreatment. These patients had more severe illnesses at admission and a less desirous outcome at discharge. In addition, and of potential theoretical significance, bipolar patients with low concentrations of red blood cell choline had four times as many previous episodes of mania as they had episodes of depression. This contrasted with the finding in patients with high erythrocyte choline levels, who had similar numbers of manic and depressive episodes. Thus, those patients with low choline and presumably low central acetylcholine activity had a relatively greater predominance of manic episodes. Interestingly, these patients with low choline showed no depressive symptoms in their clinical presentation. If erythrocyte choline in any way reflects central brain choline and acetylcholine activity, the above findings may be consistent with high central acetylcholine levels causing depression.

MOOD DEPRESSING/DEPRESSION-INDUCING EFFECTS OF CHOLINOMIMETICS

Probably the most convincing evidence that acetylcholine is involved in the regulation of the affective disorders is the observation that centrally active cholinomimetic drugs rapidly induce depressed moods. In addition to observations of depression-induction caused by DFP (citation 57 in Chapter 53 of ref. 43a) and cholinomimetic insecticides (citation 21 in Chapter 53 of ref. 43a), Janowsky et al. found induction and/or intensification of depressive symptoms in actively ill bipolar manic patients given physostigmine, as well as a worsening of depression in groups of unipolar depressed and schizoaffective-depressed patients (29). Similarly, Davis et al. (cited in Chapter 53 of ref. 43a) and Modestin et al. (cited in Chapter 53 of ref. 43a) demonstrated an increase in depression in manic patients given physostigmine. In addition, Risch et al. (52,54) and Nurnberger et al. (cited in Chapter 53 of ref. 43a) found that depressed patients given the direct cholinergic agonist arecoline also developed depression and other forms of negative affect, including hostility and anxiety. Physostigmine also caused a depressed mood in a majority of euthymic bipolar patients maintained on lithium (citation 47 in Chapter 53 of ref. 43a). Risch et al. (51) found a statistically significant increase in self- and observer-rated negative affect on the Brief Psychiatric Rating Scale (BPRS), Profile of Mood

States (POMS), and the Activation-Inhibition Rating Scales in normals receiving intravenous physostigmine or arecoline. Likewise, Mohs et al. (cited in Chapter 53 of ref. 43a) reported severe depression occurring in Alzheimer's patients receiving the cholinergic agonist oxotremorine. El-Yousef et al. (15) reported that normals, having smoked marijuana, became profoundly depressed after receiving physostigmine, an effect that was atropine-reversible. Davis et al. (cited in Chapter 53 of ref. 43a) also noted severe depression induction in volunteers receiving physostigmine who had surreptitiously smoked marijuana before receiving physostigmine.

Evidence supportive of a role for acetylcholine in the phenomenology of affective disorders also comes from descriptions of the anergic-inhibitory behavioral effects, as opposed to the mood effects of centrally acting cholinesterase inhibitors and cholinergic agonists. These drugs induce a psychomotor retardation that is very similar to that occurring in endogenous depression. Thus, Rowntree et al. (cited in Chapter 53 of ref. 43a) and Modestin et al. (cited in Chapter 53 of ref. 43a), studying normals, depressives, and manics, and Gershon and Shaw (cited in Chapter 53 of ref. 43a), observing normals, all reported that cholinesterase inhibitors exerted anergic and behavioral-inhibitory effects, as did Janowsky et al. (25) in their physostigmine-treated subjects.

Depressed moods have also been observed in subjects receiving acetylcholine precursors, including deanol, choline, and lecithin. Davis et al. (cited in Chapter 53 of ref. 43a) and Tamminga et al. (cited in Chapter 53 of ref. 43a) found that depressive symptoms occurred in some schizophrenic patients who were treated with choline, a phenomenon that was atropine-reversible. In a subgroup of cases, it was noted that depressed mood was a side effect of choline and lecithin treatments employed to try to reverse the memory deficits of Alzheimer's Disease (citation 1 in Chapter 53 of ref. 43a). Also, Casey (citation 6 in Chapter 53 of ref. 43a) observed that a depressed mood and, in some cases, a paradoxical hypomania occurred in some deanol-treated tardive dyskinesia and other movement-disorder patients. Thus, precursors of acetylcholine may induce a depressed mood, a finding that is consistent with the adrenergic-cholinergic imbalance hypothesis.

SPECTROSCOPIC STUDIES

The vast majority of evidence suggesting that increasing central cholinergic activity can induce depression and supporting the validity of an adrenergic/cholinergic balance hypothesis of affective disorders has come from the utilization of cholinergic agonist/antagonist strategies. These strategies have proved promising in suggesting a cholinergic defect in the affective disorders. However, they are all indirect indicators.

Two more direct techniques support a role for increased acetylcholine in depression. The first is the measurement of red blood cell choline in manics and bipolars described previously (66). Clinical in vivo hydrogen magnetic resonance spectroscopy provides another means for more directly assessing human cholinergic function in vivo.

Magnetic resonance spectroscopy can measure choline-containing substances noninvasively in the brain. Charles et al. (7) have observed that there is a state-dependent increase in choline in the brains of patients with major depression, as compared to controls. This increase in choline reverted to normal after successful drug treatment of the patients' depression.

DIFFERENTIAL BEHAVIORAL EFFECTS OF CHOLINOMIMETICS IN AFFECT DISORDER PATIENTS

Patients with affective disorders appear to be more sensitive than normal subjects to the effects of cholinomimetics, and an inherent muscarinic receptor hypersensitivity has been proposed to underlie this hyperreactivity. With respect to the affect-inducing and behavioral inhibitory effects of cholinomimetics, Janowsky et al. (26,33) noted that those patients with depression, mania, or schizoaffective disorders, as compared to schizophrenics without a significant mood component to their illness, became significantly sadder and more depressed after receiving physostigmine.

Oppenheimer et al. (cited in Chapter 53 of ref. 43a) likewise observed that a significant percentage of euthymic bipolar patients receiving lithium developed a depressed mood after receiving physostigmine, whereas normal controls who received physostigmine alone did not become depressed. Furthermore, Janowsky et al. (26,33) found that rater-evaluated behavioral inhibition and self-rated anxiety, depression, hostility, confusion, and elation subscales of the POMS showed significantly greater increases in affect disorder patients than in other psychiatric patient groups or normals after physostigmine infusion. That physostigmine may differentiate behaviorally patients with affective disorder diagnoses from others has received further support from the work of Edelstein et al. (cited in Chapter 53 of ref. 43a). These investigators used physostigmine to differentiate schizophrenic patients who were responsive to lithium carbonate therapy from those who were not. They found that patients who responded to physostigmine with a clearing of psychotic symptoms were significantly more likely to respond to a trial of lithium, presumably because they represented an affective disorder variant. Similarly, Casey (cited in Chapter 53 of ref. 43a) noted that those tardive dyskinesia patients with a strong history of affective disorder selectively showed increased affective symptoms while receiving the presumed acetylcholine precursor deanol. Conversely, Silva

et al. (59) noted anergia, but no depressed mood after physostigmine infusion in a group of carefully screened normals.

Finally, Steinberg et al. (63) noted that increases in negative affect after physostigmine administration occurred selectively in those personality disordered patients with preexisting affectively unstable personalities (i.e., borderlines), as compared with those who were affectively stable. In contrast, those affectively unstable patients who reacted to physostigmine with negative affect did not show mood changes following noradrenergic, serotonergic, and placebo challenges.

Nevertheless, nonaffective disorder subjects and normals receiving physostigmine sometimes do develop depression and other negative affects after receiving cholinomimetic drugs, and the differences between affective disorder patients and controls are not profound. Furthermore, the observation by Nurnberger (cited in Chapter 53 in ref. 43a) that a differential behavioral sensitivity was not seen in a group of euthymic affective disorder patients is suggestive of the possibility that increased behavioral sensitivity to cholinomimetics is a state, rather than a trait phenomenon.

SUPERSENSITIVE CHOLINOMIMETIC EFFECTS ON SLEEP PARAMETERS

Although not as specific as previously believed, major depression is generally associated with a series of characteristic sleep changes, including decreased rapid eye movement sleep (REM) latency and increased REM density. In parallel with these characteristics of depression, such cholinergic agonists as arecoline, physostigmine, and pilocarpine cause a shortening of REM latency and an increase in REM density (4,61,62, and citation 3 in Chapter 53, ref. 43a). In addition, Sitaram et al. (61,62) have shown that induction of muscarinic up-regulation by the withdrawal of chronic scopolamine leads to a shortening of REM latency and an increase in REM density. Furthermore, Sitaram et al. (61,62) have found that REM latency shortened significantly more following arecoline infusion in patients with an affective disorder episode, a history of affective disorder, or a family history of affective disorder than in those with no such history (60). Similarly, Gillin et al. (18) recently replicated Sitaram's earlier work, showing enhanced cholinergic-induced REM latency shortening in depressives following arecoline infusion.

Berger et al. also found that a supershortening of REM latency in endogenous depressives occurred following administration of the long-acting oral muscarinic agonist, RS86 (3), when compared to normals and to eating disorder patients. Possibly related to all of the above findings, Berger et al. (cited in Chapter 53 of ref. 43a) also found that physostigmine-induced arousal and awakening from sleep more frequently occurred in affective disorder patients than in normals.

More recently, Gann et al. (17) investigated sleep electroencephalogram (EEG) profiles during placebo administration and after cholinergic stimulation with RS86 in patients with major depression, healthy subjects, and patients with anxiety disorders. Like arecoline's effects in previous studies, RS86 had a more profound impact in patients with major depression with respect to sleep onset REM episodes, shortening of REM latency, increasing REM density and REM duration. Significantly, patients with anxiety disorders and associated secondary depression did not show enhanced REM abnormalities following RS86 administration. Anxiety disorder patients in fact showed decreased REM density compared to controls. Similarly, Dube and coauthors (14) were able to show that the REM sleep response to cholinergic stimulation with arecoline was significantly more pronounced in cases of primary depression, compared to both patients with manic disorders and to those who constituted a mixed anxious/depressive group. Rapaport et al. (48) recently reported that panic disorder patients responded similarly to physostigmine as controls, supporting the concept of cholinergic supersensitivity being unrelated to anxiety disorders.

A controversy exists as to whether or not the supersensitivity to cholinomimetic agents demonstrated by enhanced REM shortening and increases in other REM parameters is a state or a trait phenomena. The work of Sitaram et al. (60) and Nurnberger et al. (44) would suggest the latter, because remitted bipolar's showed exaggerated REM latency shortening after receiving arecoline. In contrast, Berger et al. (3) noted exaggerated REM latency shortening following administration of RS86 only in actively depressed patients, and Lauriello (37) did not find a supersensitive REM latency shortening response to pilocarpine in mildly depressed patients, although a greater shortening of REM latency did occur in their most symptomatic depressed patients.

The presumed hypersensitivity of REM sleep parameters to cholinomimetics appears to be genetically linked, as noted in monozygotic twin studies in which arecoline was administered to paired twins (citation 46 in Chapter 53 of ref. 43a) and caused correlated changes on REM sleep parameters, and as observed in the recent work of Sitaram et al. in which affectively ill members of the families of affectively ill patients showed exaggerated shortening of REM latency after arecoline infusion (60). More recently, Schreiber et al. (57) has observed exaggerated shortening of REM latency and increased spontaneous sleep onset REM periods following RS86 administration in healthy first-degree relatives of patients with a DSM III diagnosis of major depression. These authors suggest that the phenomenon they observed may be from a lack of REM suppressing monoaminergic mechanisms, rather than cholinergic supersensitivity. In any case, their

data support a cholinergic/adrenergic balance hypothesis of affective disorders (27). In contrast to evidence supportive of cholinergic REM related supersensitivity in depression, Gillin et al. (18) noted that depressives, withdrawn from chronically administered scopolamine, did not show differential cholinergic rebound effects, as measured by sleep EEGs. Similarly, the muscarinic receptor blocker, biperiden was not capable of reversing the relapse of depression following napping which occurred in patients whose depression had been alleviated by sleep deprivation. (13)

HYPOTHALAMIC–PITUITARY–ADRENAL AXIS AND β-ENDORPHIN SUPERSENSITIVITY TO CHOLINOMIMETIC DRUGS IN AFFECT DISORDER PATIENTS

In humans, a major characteristic of depression is the apparent activation of the hypothalamic–pituitary–adrenal (HPA) axis. A variety of studies have shown that increased cortisol and adrenocorticotropic hormone (ACTH) release occurs in depressed patients, and that some depressed patients fail to suppress cortisol secretion after dexamethasone. As with behavioral and sleep parameters, there is evidence from a variety of studies that cholinomimetic drugs can release CRF and elevate serum ACTH and cortisol in animals, in normals, and in psychiatric patients (23, and see refs. 23 and 51). Also, physostigmine has been shown to reverse dexamethasone-induced suppression of cortisol in normals (12) and in depressives (cited in Chapter 53 of ref. 43a). Thus, it appears that physostigmine and other cholinomimetic-induced increases in HPA axis activity occur, and that these parallel other phenomena noted in endogenous depression, such as increased cortisol secretion, cortisol resistance to suppression by dexamethasone, and elevated ACTH levels.

The secretion of β-endorphin appears linked to the secretion of ACTH, probably by a common precursor, β-lipotropin. Like ACTH and cortisol, β-endorphin and β-lipotropin are often elevated in depressives, and like ACTH and cortisol, they are released by physostigmine (see Janowsky and Risch, ref. 23 for Risch et al., 1981). Furthermore, affective disorder patients have been found to show significantly greater increases in both ACTH and β-endorphin levels after physostigmine infusion (53), when compared to normal controls and to nonaffective psychiatric patients.

GROWTH HORMONE SUPERSENSITIVITY IN AFFECTIVE DISORDER PATIENTS

Acetylcholine can increase plasma growth hormone levels as well as β-endorphin, β-lipotropin, ACTH, and cortisol levels. As reviewed elsewhere (23,24; also see

Bruni and Meites, 1978, cited in ref. 23), pilocarpine, acetylcholine, and physostigmine all have been noted to increase growth hormone release in vivo in rats, and in vitro in rat pituitaries. However, this increase is prevented and reversed by the concurrent administration of atropine or methscopolamine. Likewise, piperadine, a nicotinic cholinergic receptor agonist, has been found to enhance growth hormone secretion in humans during sleep (see Mendelson, et al., 1981, cited in ref. 23), and methscopolamine, a non-centrally-active peripheral anticholinergic agent inhibits nocturnal growth hormone secretion in man (see Martin, et al., 1978, cited in ref. 23).

Work in humans by Janowsky et al. (29), Davis and Davis (cited in ref. 34), and Risch et al. (51) did not demonstrate statistically significant growth hormone increases after physostigmine infusion in subjects pretreated with peripheral anticholinergic agents such as probanthetine and methscopolamine. The very limited increase in growth hormone release following physostigmine administration in the latter studies may have been due to the peripheral muscarinic blocking effects of the anticholinergics given as a pretreatment; as noted above, a similar blockade occurs with sleep-induced growth hormone elevations after methscopolamine administration (see Mendelson et al., 1978, 1979, cited in ref. 23).

O'Keane et al. (45) have reported growth hormone release following administration of the cholinominotic agent pyridostigmine in depressed patients and normals, who were not pretreated with a peripheral anticholinergic drug. Their depressed patients showed an exaggerated release of growth hormone. This was especially true of male depressives who had high baseline cortisol levels. These authors note that acetylcholine exerts important influences on growth hormone release, probably causing its effects by acting through the muscarinic release of somatostatin. Thus, enhanced growth hormone release in depressives may have been due to a supersensitive cholinergic system or possibly an increase in basal cortisol levels. This finding suggests that there may be peripheral as well as central muscarinic supersensitivity in depressives. Lucey et al. (40) recently reported a similar finding in obsessive–compulsives.

SUPERSENSITIVE PUPILLARY RESPONSES TO PILOCARPINE

DeMet and Sokolski (11) have recently reported that the pupillary miotic response to the cholinergic agonist pilocarpine was exaggerated in patients with major depression. They suggest that a trait-dependent supersensitivity exists. These authors noted that they believe the supersensitive pupillary response to pilocarpine in depressives is probably mediated by M_3 muscarinic receptors, working through a G protein–phosphoinositol system. Thus, these data support the notion of both peripheral and central muscarinic supersensitivity in depressives.

ADRENOMEDULLARY AND CARDIOVASCULAR EFFECTS OF CHOLINOMIMETIC DRUGS

There is evidence that patients with major depressive disorder often have increased urinary epinephrine excretion and, to a lesser extent, increased norepinephrine excretion (see ref. 32). As with many parameters, physostigmine infusion causes effects in normals with respect to catecholamine release similar to those occurring in depressives. Administration of physostigmine to normals and affect disorder patients causes profound increases in serum epinephrine levels, and slight increases in serum norepinephrine levels (32). Furthermore, Janowsky et al. (32) have demonstrated a blunting of the epinephrine response to physostigmine in affective disorder patients, possibly from receptor down-regulation caused by chronically elevated epinephrine levels. Physostigmine and arecoline have both been shown to increase pulse rate and blood pressure levels in subjects treated with peripherally acting anticholinergic drugs. These changes can be profound and appear, as with cholinomimetic-induced increases in epinephrine release, to be due to muscarinic activation of centrally mediated sympathetic outflow (27,34).

CENTRAL MUSCARINIC REGULATION OF CHOLINOMIMETIC EFFECTS

Several studies have attempted to better understand the mechanisms by which the behavioral, cardiovascular, and neuroendocrine effects of cholinomimetic drugs occur. In early studies, Janowsky et al. (27) and Modestin et al. (citations 39 and 40 in Chapter 53 of ref. 43a) noted that in contrast to centrally acting physostigmine, the peripherally acting cholinesterase inhibitor, neostigmine, like the placebo, did not exert any behavioral effects. This indicated that the behavioral affects of physostigmine were probably central in origin. More recently, Janowsky et al. (31) noted that the increases in blood pressure, pulse rate, serum epinephrine, ACTH, cortisol, and prolactin, as well as the anergia and negative affect caused by physostigmine also occurred via a central mechanism, since no such changes occurred with neostigmine. Furthermore, Janowsky et al. (31) have noted that the behavioral, cardiovascular, and neuroendocrine effects of physostigmine can be blocked by the centrally acting anticholinergic drug scopolamine, but not by the noncentrally acting anticholinergic drug methscopolamine, again suggesting a central focus for the above effects.

MOOD EFFECTS OF CENTRALLY ACTIVE ANTICHOLINERGIC AGENTS

There is evidence that centrally active anticholinergic drugs have mood-elevating properties, although this evidence is generally anecdotal and mostly uncontrolled. As noted by Jellinec in 1981 and Smith in 1980, antiparkinsonian drugs used to treat drug-induced parkinsonian symptoms have been reported to cause feelings of euphoria associated with a sense of well-being, increased sociability, and a reversal of depressed mood (23). Furthermore, one report by Coid and Strang (see Janowsky and Risch, 1984 [reference 23] for Coid and Strang, 1982) suggested that the anticholinergic agent procyclidine caused a switch into mania in a bipolar patient.

In addition, several reports suggest that high doses of atropine and other anticholinergics such as ditran may alleviate depression, and one report suggests that a tricyclic-antidepressant-induced central anticholinergic syndrome may alleviate depression. Also, Jimerson et al. (cited in ref. 23) reported that trihexylphendyl may have antidepressant properties; and Kasper et al. (cited in Chapter 53 of ref. 43a) observed antidepressant effects with the anticholinergic drug biperiden, especially in patients with endogenous depression who had a nonsuppressing dexamethasone suppression test. In spite of the above-reviewed positive evidence, it must be stressed that many effective antidepressant medications, such as fluoxetine and related selective serotonin reuptake inhibitors, as well as mianserin and trazodone, lack significant muscarinic receptor-blocking properties and yet can alleviate depression. To address this incongruity, Janowsky et al. (24,31,32) have reviewed evidence suggesting that increased noradrenergic and dopaminergic activity occurring secondarily to tricyclic antidepressant administration may inhibit cholinergic neurotransmission via a presynaptic mechanism.

ANTICHOLINERGIC DRUG-WITHDRAWAL PHENOMENA

As noted by Dilsaver and Greden, in addition to the mood-depressing and inhibitory effects of centrally active cholinomimetics, antidepressant and antiparkinsonian agent-treated patients may develop some aspects of depression, including a depressed mood, anxiety, withdrawal, agitation, and insomnia soon after discontinuing these medications (cited in Chapter 53 of ref. 43a). These symptoms are preventable and/or reversible with anticholinergic treatment, and may represent the unmasking of muscarinic receptor hypersensitivity. This issue has been elaborated in detail by Dilsaver and Greden, who proposed the concept of "cholinergic overdrive," consisting of anxiety, nausea, agitation, and sometimes depression. Cholinergic overdrive is described as occurring after discontinuation of anticholinergic tricyclics and antiparkinsonian drugs and especially after anticholinergic drug withdrawal combined with marijuana intoxication. Dilsaver and Greden attribute cholinergic overdrive to the unmasking of up-regulated cholinergic receptors oc-

curring secondary to the withdrawal of muscarinic blockade, and propose that such overdrive may also activate noradrenergic receptors, leading to induction of arousal and manic symptoms in some cases.

MOOD EFFECTS OF ANTIADRENERGIC AGENTS

Several reports suggest that many sympatholytic-antihypertensive medications, including α-methyldopa, propranolol, clonidine, and reserpine can cause depression. These drugs also have significant cholinomimetic properties (27). In humans, the CNS side effects of reserpine and other antiadrenergic-cholinomimetic antihypertensives are similar to those of centrally active cholinergic agents, and include mood depression, vivid nightmares, lethargy, and sleepiness. With respect to antipsychotic drugs, Van Putten and May (cited in Chapter 53 of ref. 43a) have shown that these agents, which block central dopamine and increase acetylcholine turnover, can also cause some of the components of depression in selected patients, effects that can be reversed with centrally active anticholinergic medications.

MUSCARINIC RECEPTORS IN AFFECTIVE DISORDER PATIENTS

Several studies optimistically have suggested a difference among affective disorder and normal subjects with respect to muscarinic receptor binding. Nadi et al. (cited in Chapter 53 of ref. 43a) reported that fibroblasts grown in culture from affective disorder patients and their mood-disordered relatives had more muscarinic binding sites than controls, and Meyerson et al. (cited in Chapter 53 of ref. 43a) noted that samples from the frontal cortexes of individuals who committed suicide had more muscarinic receptor binding activity than from matched brains from people dying from accidents or murder. However, Kelsoe et al. (35) have not been able to replicate the fibroblast receptor findings described above, and others (citations 34 and 62 in Chapter 53 of ref. 43a) have not been able to find increased muscarinic binding in the brains of suicide victims. Generally, at present most evidence suggests that muscarinic binding in fibroblasts and brain is not altered in affective disorder patients. It should be pointed out, however, that the FSL rats previously mentioned as a cholinergic supersensitivity model of depression also do not exhibit changes in cortical muscarinic receptors (46), but do exhibit increases in such receptors in the hippocampus and striatum. It may be that previous workers have not examined the key regions of the human brain relevant to muscarinic receptor changes in depression.

MONOAMINE–ACETYLCHOLINE AND OTHER NEUROTRANSMITTER–ACETYLCHOLINE INTERACTIONS

A pharmacological–behavioral model for naturally occurring adrenergic and cholinergic regulation of mood may be found in the interactions and reciprocal effects of psychostimulants (which increase catecholaminergic activity) and cholinomimetics (which increase cholinergic activity). Methylphenidate-induced psychostimulation in rats and in humans is rapidly antagonized by physostigmine, but not by neostigmine, and, conversely, physostigmine's inhibitory-depressant effects can be reversed by methylphenidate (25,28). Possibly related to the ability of physostigmine to antagonize methylphenidate-induced psychostimulation is the observation that physostigmine caused a rapid, dramatic drop in the norepinephrine metabolite serum 3-methyoxy-4-hydroxyphenylglycol (MHPG) in a manic patient, presumably reflecting a drop in CNS noradrenergic activity. This phenomenon was associated with induction of a tearful depressed state and an improvement in the manic symptoms (citation 48 in Chapter 53 of ref. 43a).

Furthermore, a reciprocal relationship apparently may exist between a subject's response to a psychostimulant and his or her separate response to a cholinomimetic agent. A negative correlation was noted between amphetamine-induced behavioral excitation and the ability of arecoline, given on another occasion, to decrease REM latency (citation 44 in Chapter 53 of ref. 43a). Similarly, Siever et al. (58) showed that in a mixed group of affective disorder and normal subjects, those with the most dramatic physostigmine- and arecoline-induced anergy and negative affect showed a blunted growth hormone response to the noradrenergic agonist clonidine (presumably a reflection of decreased noradrenergic responsiveness).

Two recent studies have also provided evidence in support of the catecholamine–acetylcholine balance model of affective disorders. In a preclinical study, Hasey and Hanin (21) showed that the immobility-promoting effects of the anticholinesterase, physostigmine, could be modified by manipulating the β-noradrenergic system. Schittecatte et al. (56) have recently demonstrated that human depressives are subsensitive to the REM sleep-suppressing effects of clonidine, thereby supporting the α-adrenergic subsensitivity postulated to exist in depressives on the basis of neuroendocrine challenge studies (1). It is not clear at this stage whether the clonidine subsensitivity is a direct reflection of changes in the α-noradrenergic system or merely a consequence of the supersensitivity proposed to exist in the balancing cholinergic systems. It could be very illuminating to obtain both clonidine and cholinomimetic challenge data in the same subjects (58).

Acetylcholine also interacts with GABA and serotonin, but space does not permit a detailed consideration of these findings (see refs. 23 and 46 for details). Similarly, postsynaptic cholinergic effects may be mediated through a range of second-messenger systems, including phosphotidyl inositol, cyclic AMP, and calcium (42). There is growing interest in the possibility that an abnormality in one or more of these second-messenger systems may indeed contribute to the biochemical changes underlying depression (2,38). Such a revelation may help to reconcile the differing functional and biochemical results on muscarinic mechanisms, including the question of why functional muscarinic supersensitivity has been frequently reported, but changes in muscarinic receptors have not (23). An alteration in one or more of the second-messenger systems could account for the muscarinic supersensitivity observed in depressives and could occur without any obvious change in receptors.

ACETYLCHOLINE AND STRESS

Although virtually all the stress-sensitive neurohormones are released by centrally acting cholinomimetic drugs, and many can be decreased by anticholinergic drugs, a controversy exists as to the interpretation of these phenomena, especially with respect to human studies. Davis and Davis (cited in ref. 23) observed that in their normal subjects, serum prolactin, cortisol, and growth hormone levels did not increase after physostigmine infusion unless other unpleasant symptoms of the physostigmine response occurred, such as dizziness, nausea, or emesis. They suggested that cholinomimetic-induced increases in stress hormones may be due to nonspecific stress effects (i.e., feeling sick or distressed), rather than to a direct cholinergic mediation of stress. Kohl and Homick (cited in ref. 34) observed evidence that motion sickness, which appears quite similar to the physostigmine response at its extreme, and which includes nausea, dizziness, and vomiting, almost certainly involves central cholinergic mechanisms. Motion sickness is a potent stimulator of growth hormone, prolactin, and cortisol secretion.

However, contrary to the interpretation that nonspecific stress causes cholinomimetic-induced hormonal effects, Janowsky et al. (23,24) have reported the occurrence of increases in serum prolactin and cortisol in physostigmine-treated patients and in normals who manifested no nausea, emesis, or dizziness. In addition, Risch et al. (51) have observed that in arecoline-treated subjects in whom serum β-endorphin, ACTH, and cortisol levels significantly increased, a sizable proportion of subjects could not tell when active drug and when placebo had been administered. Furthermore, Janowsky et al. (30,31) reported that physostigmine's behavioral-anergic effects almost always precede its nauseating effects, and Raskind et al. (49) noted that increases in serum ACTH, epinephrine, and cortisol occurred in aged controls and in Alzheimer patients, whether or not nausea occurred. Finally, Hasey and Hanin (21) demonstrated that physostigmine caused significantly greater increases in cortisol release in rats than did neostigmine, even though the peripheral toxicity of both drugs was recorded to be severe and equal to one another. Thus, it is quite possible that the nauseating, behavioral, and neurohormonal effects of centrally acting cholinomimetic drugs occur at similar dose thresholds, and that they occur in parallel with each other, rather than causing each other.

Conversely, it is possible that acetylcholine actually moderates the body's stress responses. Stress is multidimensional, and includes gastrointestinal, cardiovascular, behavioral, analgesic, immunological, endocrinological, psychological-behavioral, and psychopathological changes (see Akiskal and McKinney, 1973; Anisman and Zacharko, 1982; and Weiss, 1971a,b,c, cited in ref. 23). Information from animal studies has accumulated suggesting that the manifestations of stress are likely to be mediated by complex alterations in central neurotransmitters, including norepinephrine, dopamine, serotonin, and gamma amino butyric acid (GABA) (see Janowsky and Risch, 1984 [reference 23] for Anisman and Zacharko, 1982). Acetylcholine, may also have a role in the mediation of the stress response, although such a role for this chemical has not been widely investigated (see Janowsky and Risch, 1984 [reference 23] for Anisman and Zacharko, 1982).

As with other neurotransmitters (see Anisman and Zacharko, 1982, cited in ref. 23), there is growing evidence that stressors can cause changes in central acetylcholine activity. Probably the most dramatic of these studies of stress-acetylcholine linkages is the work of Gilad et al. (cited in ref. 23), which shows that stress causes an increase in acetylcholine release and compensatory downregulation of muscarinic receptors. Gilad et al. also have shown that choline uptake, as well as the increase in acetylcholine release occurring after exposure to stress, is differentially exaggerated in stress-sensitive rats. Other investigators have shown that central levels of acetylcholine in rats are increased 1 hr after stress termination, and decreased acetylcholine turnover has been observed in the frontal cortex of rats 1 hr following exposure to restraint plus cold (see Costa, et al., 1980, cited in ref. 23). In the hypothalamus, acetylcholine turnover increases after 1, 4, or 24 hr of stress. Furthermore, central acetylcholine receptor sites are increased during uncontrollable stress (see Cherek, et al., 1980, cited in ref. 23), as are acetylcholine levels (see Karczmar, 1975, cited in ref. 23). Similarly, Hingtgen et al. (cited in ref. 23) have found that a conditioned stimulus increases central acetylcholine levels. Thus, there is considerable evidence that acute stress can alter central acetylcholine activity, although whether an increase or decrease occurs is not totally consistent between experiments.

The cholinomimetic agents physostigmine, neostigmine, and arecoline, and the anticholinergic agents, atropine, scopolamine, and methscopolamine, have been used to explore an acetylcholine hypothesis of stress. As described above, cholinomimetic drugs cause many of the same effects as do naturally occurring stressors. These include increases in negative affect, the induction of affective symptoms, increases in stress-sensitive neuroendocrines including ACTH, cortisol, β-endorphin, growth hormone, prolactin, epinephrine, and possibly norepinephrine, increases in blood pressure and pulse rate, and increases in analgesia. These cholinomimetic effects, combined with the effect of stress on central acetylcholine activity, suggest a stress-acetylcholine linkage.

Although it has been hypothesized that increases in acetylcholine activity are fundamental to the multiple manifestations of acute stress, acetylcholine does not exert its effects in a vacuum. It is likely that the final manifestations of stress involve complex, multiple interactions involving inhibitory and excitatory neurotransmitters, such as norepinephrine, serotonin, and the opioid polypeptides, which are impacted upon by acetylcholine. Also, the possibility exists that acetylcholine may be a secondary, rather than a primary, mediator of stress. However, it is probably significant that there is little or no evidence that any neurotransmitter or neuromodulator other than acetylcholine is simultaneously able to activate the cardiovascular, sympathetic, adrenal-medullary, behavioral-affective, analgesic, and neuroendocrine systems involved in the stress response. Thus, a primary role for acetylcholine in the modulation of stress is possible, and even likely, and this possibility is worthy of further investigation.

CIGARETTE SMOKING AND DEPRESSION

Although the vast majority of observations linking the cholinergic nervous system to affective disorders have focused on muscarinic mechanisms, there is also evidence that nicotinic cholinergic mechanisms may also be linked to depression. As described previously, the cholinesterase inhibitor, physostigmine and cholinergic agonists such as oxotremorine produce a range of behavioral and physiological effects in animals. Reduction in locomotor activity is commonly seen after physostigmine, oxotremorine, and arecoline administration and these changes are generally thought to be muscarinic in nature. In contrast, nicotine has biphasic effects, stimulating locomotor behavior at lower doses and depressing it at higher doses (64). On the other hand, nicotinic and muscarinic compounds both produce dose-dependent decreases in core body temperature and may enhance memory under the appropriate experimental conditions (39). These drugs also have fairly similar neuroendocrine effects, particularly with respect to a stimulation of the HPA axis leading to cortisol and ACTH release.

One of the questions about the behavioral and physiological effects of nicotine is whether they are the consequence of a direct interaction of nicotine on postsynaptic nicotinic receptors or due to an indirect interaction with presynaptic nicotinic receptors leading to stimulation of (i.e., disinhibition of) the release of acetylcholine onto muscarinic receptors. The antinociceptive and hypothermic effects of nicotine (22,46) have been attributed, at least in part, to the latter mechanism. Some of the other effects of nicotine, such as locomotor stimulation and nicotine's reinforcing effects have been proposed to be from nicotine-induced release of dopamine or other neurotransmitters (9,65). With respect to nicotine's effects in humans, Glassman's (19) extensive review indicates that a high rate of cigarette smoking is associated with current major depression and current depressive symptoms. He also noted that a lifetime history of major depression, even if not active at the time that a person starts to smoke, increases the chances of a person trying nicotine and becoming addicted to it and has a significant negative impact on smoking cessation efforts. This latter deleterious effect appears more pronounced in women than in men. There is also evidence that in predisposed individuals with a history of major depression, smoking cessation may precipitate severe depressive symptoms, which also appear to counteract smoking cessation efforts. Of course, the linkage between cigarette addiction, smoking, and emotional disorders is not exclusive for depression, since there are observed linkages between smoking and alcoholism, anxiety disorders, and especially schizophrenia.

Another interesting linkage between smoking and depression has been noted. Using monozygotic and dyzygotic twin pair data, Kendler et al. (36) have found that smoking and depression are indeed linked, but that smoking doesn't necessarily cause depression, and that depression doesn't necessarily cause smoking. It appears that the association of depression and smoking are linked through genetic factors that influence vulnerability to both conditions.

Although, as noted above, nicotine's effects on dopaminergic reward mechanisms have been offered as an explanation for why depressives, as well as schizophrenics, smoke and have more trouble stopping smoking (19), it is also possible that a relationship between muscarinic and nicotinic mechanisms may be important in causing nicotine addiction. Obviously, a common neurotransmitter, acetylcholine, underlies muscarinic and nicotinic behavioral and physiological effects. It is conceivable that stress and/or depression, by activating muscarinic mechanisms leads to an overall muscarinic predominance. This may conceivably be overcome by nicotinic stimulation, leading to a relief of symptoms. Withdrawal from nicotine, allowing an unmasking of down-regulated nicotinic receptors, could lead to a muscarinic predominance and the induction of depression and dysphoria. Furthermore, there is evidence that activation of nicotinic receptors can lead to muscarinic outflow. Specifically, nicotine-induced changes in temperature and nociception can be blocked by the antimuscarinic agent, atropine (22,46). Therefore, it is possible that nicotinic stimulation could lead to muscarinic activation, which would become the predominant effect when nicotine administration was stopped. A logical adjunct to utilization of nicotine replacement therapy would thus be the addition of a centrally acting anticholinergic drug to the treatment.

SUMMARY

As reviewed above, considerable evidence suggests that the cholinergic nervous system, alone or acting in concert with other neurotransmitters, may have an important role in the regulation of affect. Nevertheless, as with all currently proposed biological hypotheses of the etiology of affective disorders, there exist alternative explanations, as well as some data that are inconsistent with the cholinergic hypothesis.

One question concerns the specificity of the cholinergic alterations: Are they confined to patients with affective disorder? A number of studies have failed to detect any evidence for cholinergic supersensitivity among patients with anxiety disorders (14,48). In contrast, several studies suggest an involvement of cholinergic mechanisms in schizophrenia. Early investigators used cholinesterase inhibitors to treat schizophrenia (8,10). Others proposed a dopaminergic/cholinergic balance model for schizophrenia (16). More recently, it has been suggested that cholinergic overactivity may underlie the negative symptoms of schizophrenia, such as affective flattening, anhedonia, asociality, and apathy (67,68,69). A reduced REM sleep latency has also been observed in schizophrenics (50). Thus, symptoms of schizophrenia that bear some similarity to key symptoms of depression may also be mediated by cholinergic overactivity.

It is possible that pharmacologically induced changes in acetylcholine may cause perturbations in depression-relevant systems other than the cholinergic nervous system. Pharmacologically induced acetylcholine alterations could cause a "model depression" by perturbing other potential governing neurotransmitters (for example, GABA, serotonin, dopamine, or norepinephrine) or second messengers in affect disorder patients. Furthermore, obviously, the fundamental biochemical changes in depression could be due to a relatively low level of central norepinephrine or serotonin activity, a situation that could explain all of the above observations under the scope of a balance hypothesis. It is also conceivable that the cholinergic supersensitivity observed in many depressives may be a reflection of altered second messengers, including G proteins (2,38).

However, even if cholinomimetics can only cause a "model depression" (with such components as low mood; psychomotor depression; elevated ACTH, cortisol, β-endorphin, and epinephrine levels; as well as sleep architecture changes and increased pulse rates and blood pressure), understanding how this presumed pharmacological phenomenon occurs may ultimately offer a window into understanding the pathophysiology of affective disorders and may have useful treatment implications. Thus, at the least, understanding the future implications of the mood-depressant and other depression like effects of cholinomimetics may give clues as to the actual neurobiology of affective disorders. Alternatively, it is not beyond possibility that acetylcholine actually is directly involved in the etiology and the expression of the affective disorders, alone or acting through other relevant neurotransmitters and/or second messengers.

ACKNOWLEDGMENTS

We wish to thank Barbara Munden for her expert secretarial assistance and the following investigators for sending recently published papers: K. K. R. Krishnan, R. Tandon, A. Glassman, M. Berger, J. C. Gillin, E. M. DeMet, I. Hanin, and L. J. Siever.

REFERENCES

1. Amsterdam JD, Maislin G, Skolnick B, Berwish N, Winokur A. The assessment of abnormalities in hormonal responsiveness at multiple levels of the hypothalamic-pituitary-adrenocortical axis in depressive illness. *Biol Psychiatry* 1989;26:265–278.
2. Avissar S, Schreiber G. Muscarinic receptor subclassification and G-proteins: significance for lithium action in affective disorders and for the treatment of extrapyramidal side effects of neuroleptics. *Biol Psychiatry* 1989;26:113–130.
3. Berger M, Riemann D, Hochli D, Spiegel R. The cholinergic rapid eye movement sleep induction test with RS-86. *Arch Gen Psychiatry* 1989;46:421–428.
4. Berkowitz A, Sutton L, Janowsky DS, Gillin JC. Pilocarpine, an orally active muscarinic cholinergic agonist, induces REM sleep and reduces delta sleep in normal volunteers. *Psychiatry Res* 1990;33:113–119.
5. Bidzinski A, Puzynski S, Mrozek S. Choline transport in erythrocytes of healthy controls and patients with endogenous major depression. *New Trends Exp Clin Psychiatry* 1989;5:179–185.
6. Borsini F, Meli A. Is the forced swimming test a suitable model for revealing antidepressant activity? *Psychopharmacology* 1984;94:147–160.
7. Charles HC, Lazeyras F, Krishnan KRR, Boyko OB, Payne M, Moore D. Brain choline in depression: in vivo detection of potential pharmacodynamic effects of antidepressant therapy using hydrogen localized spectroscopy. *Prog Neuro-Psychopharmacol Biol Psychiatry* [in press].
8. Cohen LH, Thale T, Tissenbaum MJ. Acetylcholine treatment of schizophrenia. *Arch Neurol Psychiatry* 1944;51:171–175.
9. Clarke PBS, Fu DS, Jakubovic A, Fibiger HC. Evidence that mesolimbic dopaminergic activation underlies the locomotor stimulant action of nicotine in rats. *J Pharmacol Exp Ther* 1988;246:701–708.
10. Collard J, Lecoq R, Demaret A. Un essai de therapeutique pathogenique de la schizophrenei par un acetylcholine: l'oxotremorine. *Acta Neurol Psychiat Belg* 1946;65:122–127.
11. DeMet EM, Sokolski KA. Pupillary response to pilocarpine in depression. Presented at Seattle meeting of West Coast College of Biological Psychiatry, 1993.
12. Doerr P, Berger M. Physostigmine-induced escape from dexamethasone suppression in normal adults. *Biol Psychiatry* 1983;18:261–268.
13. Dressing H, Riemann D, Gann H, Berger M. The effects of biperiden on nap sleep after sleep deprivation in depressed patients. *Neuropsychopharmacology* 1992;7:1–5.
14. Dube S, Kuman N, Ettedgui A, Pohl R, Jones D, Sitaram N. Cholinergic REM induction response: separation of anxiety and depression. *Biol Psychiatry* 1985;20:408–418.
15. El-Yousef M, Janowsky DS, Davis JM, Rosenblatt JE. Induction of severe depression in marijuana intoxicated individuals. *Br J Addict* 1973;68:321–325.
16. Friedhoff AJ, Alpert M. A dopaminergic-cholinergic mechanism in production of psychotic symptoms. *Biol Psychiatry* 1973;6:165–169.
17. Gann H, Riemann D, Hohagen F, Dressing H, Muller WE, Berger M. The sleep structure of patients with anxiety disorders in comparison to that of healthy controls and depressive patients under baseline conditions and after cholinergic stimulation. *J Affect Dis* 1992;26:179–190.
18. Gillin JC, Sutton L, Ruiz C, et al. The cholinergic rapid eye movement induction test with arecoline in depression. *Arch Gen Psychiatry* 1991;48:264–270.
19. Glassman AH. Cigarette smoking: implications for psychiatric illness. *Am J Psychiatry* 1993;150:546–553.
20. Goldman ME, Erickson CK. Effects of acute and chronic administration of antidepressant drugs on the central cholinergic system. Comparison with anticholinergic drugs. *Neuropharmacology* 1983;22:1215–1222.
21. Hasey G, Hanin I. The cholinergic-adrenergic hypothesis of depression reexamined using clonidine, metoprolol, and physostigmine in an animal model. *Biol Psychiatry* 1991;29:127–138.
22. Iwamoto ET. Antinociception after nicotine administration into the mesopontine tegmentum of rats: evidence for muscarinic actions. *J Pharmacol Exp Ther* 1989;251:412–421.
23. Janowsky DS, Risch SC. Cholinomimetic and anticholinergic drugs used to investigate an acetylcholine hypothesis of affective disorder and stress. *Drug Dev Res* 1984;4:125–142.
24. Janowsky DS, Risch SC. Role of acetylcholine mechanisms in the affective disorders. In: Meltzer HY, ed. *Psychopharmacology. The third generation of progress.* New York: Raven Press; 1987:527–534.
25. Janowsky DS, El-Yousef MK, Davis JM. Antagonistic effects of physostigmine and methylphenidate in man. *Am J Psychiatry* 1973;130:1370–1376.
26. Janowsky DS, El-Yousef MK, Davis JM. Acetylcholine and depression. *Psychosom Med* 1974;36:248–257.
27. Janowsky DS, El-Yousef MK, Davis JM, Sekerke HJ. A cholinergic-adrenergic hypothesis of mania and depression. *Lancet* 1972;2:632–635.
28. Janowsky DS, El-Yousef MK, Davis JM, Sekerke HJ. Parasympathetic suppression of manic symptoms by physostigmine. *Arch Gen Psychiatry* 1973;28:542–547.
29. Janowsky DS, Risch SC, Judd LL, Huey LY, Parker DC. Cholinergic supersensitivity in affect disorder patients: behavioral and neuroendocrine observations. *Psychopharmacol Bull* 1981;17:129–132.
30. Janowsky DS, Risch SC, Judd LL, Huey LY, Parker DC. Brain cholinergic systems and the pathogenesis of affective disorders. In: Singh MM, Warburton DM, Lal H, eds. *Central cholinergic mechanisms and adaptive dysfunction.* New York: Plenum; 1985:309–353.
31. Janowsky DS, Risch SC, Kennedy B, Ziegler M, Huey LY. Central muscarinic effects of physostigmine on mood, cardiovascular function, pituitary, and adrenal neuroendocrine release. *Psychopharmacology* 1986;89:150–154.
32. Janowsky DS, Risch SC, Huey LY, Kennedy B, Ziegler M. Effects of physostigmine on pulse, blood pressure and serum epinephrine levels. *Am J Psychiatry* 1985;142:738–740.
33. Janowsky DS, Risch SC, Parker D, Huey LY, Judd LL. Increased vulnerability to cholinergic stimulation in affect disorder patients. *Psychopharmacol Bull* 1980;16:29–31.
34. Janowsky DS, Risch SC, Ziegler M, Kennedy B, Huey L. Cholinomimetic model of motion sickness and space adaptation syndrome. *Aviat Space Eng* 1984;55:692–696.

35. Kelsoe JJr, Gillin J, Janowsky DS, Brown J, Risch SC, Lumkin B. Failure to confirm muscarinic receptors on skin fibroblasts. *N Engl J Med* 1985;312:861–862.

36. Kendler K, Nenale MC, MacLean CL, Heath AC, Eaves LJ, Kessler RC. Smoking and major depression: a causal analysis. *Arch Gen Psychiatry* 1993;50:36–43.

37. Lauriello J, Kenny WM, Sutton L, et al. The cholinergic REM sleep induction test with pilocarpine in mildly depressed patients and normal controls. *Biol Psychiatry* 1993;33:33–39.

38. Lesch KP, Manji HK. Signal-transducing G proteins and antidepressant drugs: evidence for modulation of alpha subunit gene expression in rat brain. *Biol Psychiatry* 1992;32:549–579.

39. Levin E. Nicotinic systems and cognitive function. *Psychopharmacology* 1992;108:417–431.

40. Lucey JV, Butcher G, Clare AW, Dinan TG. Elevated growth hormone responses to pyridostigmine in obsessive-compulsive disorder: evidence of cholinergic supersensitivity. *Am J Psychiatry* 1993;150:961–962.

41. Martin JR, Driscoll P, Gentsch C. Differential response to cholinergic stimulation in psychogenetically selected rat lines. *Psychopharmacology* 1984;83:262–267.

42. McKinney M, Richelson E. The coupling of the neuronal muscarinic receptor to responses. *Annu Rev Pharmacol Toxicol* 1984;24:121–146.

43. McKinney WT. Animal models of depression: An overview. *Psychiatr Dev* 1984;2:77–96.

43a. Meltzer HY, ed. *Psychopharmacology. The third generation of progress.* New York: Raven Press; 1987.

44. Nurnberger JL, Berrettini W, Mendelson WB, Sack B, Gershon ES. Measuring cholinergic sensitivity: I. Arecoline effects in bipolar patients. *Biol Psychiatry* 1989;25:610–617.

45. O'Keane V, O'Flynn K, Lucey J, Dinan TG. Pyridostigmine-induced growth hormone responses in healthy and depressed subjects—evidence for cholinergic supersensitivity in depression. *Psychol Med* 1992;22:55–60.

46. Overstreet DH. The Flinders sensitive line rats: a genetic animal model of depression. *Neurosci Biobehav Rev* 1993;17:51–68.

47. Pucilowski O, Overstreet DH, Rezvani AH, Janowsky DS. Chronic mild stress-induced anhedonia: greater effect in a genetic rat model of depression. *Physiol Behav* 1993;54:1215–1220.

48. Rapaport MH, Risch SC, Gillin JC, Golshan S, Janowsky D. The effects of physostigmine infusion on patients with panic disorder. *Biol Psychiatry* 1991;29:658–664.

49. Raskind MA, Peskind ER, Veith RC, et al. Neuroendocrine response to physostigmine in Alzheimer's Disease. *Arch Gen Psychiatry* 1989;46:535–540.

50. Riemann D, Gann H, Fleckenstein R, Hohagen F, Olbrich R, Berger M. Effect of RS86 on REM latency in schizophrenia. *Psychiatry Res* 1991;38:84–92.

51. Risch SS, Kalin NH, Janowsky DS. Cholinergic challenge in affective illness: behavioral and neuroendocrine correlates. *J Clin Psychopharmacol* 1981;1:186–192.

52. Risch SC, Cohen PM, Janowsky DS, Kalin NH, Insel TR, Murphy DL. Physostigmine induction of depressive symptomatology in normal human subjects. *Psychiatry Res* 1981;4:89–94.

53. Risch SC, Janowsky DS, Kalin NH, Cohen RM, Aloi JA, Murphy DL. Cholinergic beta endorphin hypersensitivity associated with depression. In: Hanin I, Usdin E, eds. *Biological markers in psychiatry and neurology.* Oxford: Pergamon Press; 1982:269–278.

54. Risch SC, Siever LJ, Gillin JC, et al. Differential mood effects of arecoline in depressed patients and normal volunteers. *Psychopharmacol Bull* 1983;19:696–698.

55. Schiller GD, Overstreet DH. Selective breeding for increased cholinergic function: preliminary study of nicotinic mechanisms. *Med Chem Res* 1993;2:578–583.

56. Schittecatte M, Charles G, Machowsky R, Garcia J, Medlewicz J, Wilmotte J. Reduced clonidine rapid eye movement suppression in patients with primary major affective illness. *Arch Gen Psychiatry* 1992;49:637–642.

57. Schreiber W, Lauer CJ, Krumrey K, Holsboer F, Krieg JC. Cholinergic REM sleep induction test in subjects at high risk for psychiatric disorders. *Biol Psychiatry* 1992;32:79–90.

58. Siever LJ, Risch SC, Murphy DL. Central cholinergic-adrenergic balance in the regulation of affective state. *Psychiatry Res* 1981;5:108–109.

59. Silva SG, Stern RA, Golden RA, Davidson EJ, Mason GA, Janowsky DS. The effects of physostigmine on behavioral inhibition, cognitive processes, mood state and neuroendocrine functioning in healthy males. *Biol Psychiatry* [submitted].

60. Sitaram N, Jones D, Dube S, et al. The association of supersensitive cholinergic REM-induction and affective illness within pedigrees. *J Psychiatr Res* 1987;21:487–497.

61. Sitaram N, Jones D, Dube S, Bell J, Rivard P. Supersensitive ACh REM-induction as a genetic vulnerability marker. *Int J Neurosci* 1985;32:777–778.

62. Sitaram N, Nurnberger J, Gershon ES, Gillin JC. Cholinergic regulation of mood and REM sleep. A potential model and marker for vulnerability to depression. *Am J Psychiatry* 1982;139:571–576.

63. Steinberg BJ, Weston S, Trestman RL, Temple J, Mitchell D, Siever LJ. Mood response to cholinergics in personality disorder patients. *Proceedings of the American Psychiatric Association Meeting,* San Francisco, CA, 1993;NR113:88.

64. Stolerman IP. Psychopharmacology of nicotine: stimulant effects and receptor mechanisms. In: Iversen LL, Iversen SD, Snyder SH, eds. *Handbook of psychopharmacology.* New York: Raven Press. 1987;421–465.

65. Stolerman IP, Reavill C. Primary cholinergic and indirect dopaminergic mediation of behavioural effects of nicotine. *Behav Brain Res* 1989;79:227–237.

66. Stoll A, Cohen BM, Hanin I. Erythrocyte choline concentrations in psychiatric disorders. *Biol Psychiatry* 1991;29:309–321.

67. Tandon R, Greden JF. Cholinergic hyperactivity and negative schizophrenic symptoms: a model of dopaminergic/cholinergic interactions in schizophrenia. *Arch Gen Psychiatry* 1989;46:745–753.

68. Tandon R, Greden JF, Silk KR. Treatment of negative schizophrenic symptoms with trihexyphenidyl. *J Clin Psychopharmacol* 1988;9:212–215.

69. Tandon R, Taylor S, Greden JF, Shipley JF, DeQuardo JR, Goodson J. The cholinergic system in schizophrenia reconsidered: anticholinergic modulation of sleep and symptom profiles. *Am J Psychiat* [in press].

70. Walker CD, Aubert ML, Meaney MJ, Driscoll P. Individual differences in the activity of the hypothalamus-pituitary-adrenocortical system after stress: use of psychogenetically selected rat lines. In: Driscoll P, ed. *Genetically defined animal models of neurobehavioral dysfunctions.* Boston: Birkhauser; 1992:276–296.

Psychopharmacology: The Fourth
Generation of Progress, edited by
Floyd E. Bloom and David J. Kupfer.
Raven Press, Ltd., New York © 1995.

CHAPTER 83

Neuroendocrinology of Mood Disorders

Florian Holsboer

The term *endocrinological psychiatry* was coined by Laignel-Lavastine, who first used it at a psychiatric congress in Dijon in 1908 when he was encouraging his colleagues to intensify research on the interaction between personality and the endocrine system. Later, Manfred Bleuler in Switzerland established a school, and it was here that psychopathological changes in endocrine diseases such as acromegaly, Graves' disease, Cushing's syndrome, and Addison's disease were first documented as being secondary to endocrinopathy.

These seminal works are still valid and continue to fertilize psychiatric research even today. From the early studies, we learned that the brain is an endocrine target and that compounds such as hormones and pharmaceutical agents that enter the brain can induce changes in mood and behavior. Thus, the concept of endocrinological psychiatry paved the way for attempts to influence brain function with drugs, although early hormone treatments of psychiatric disorders were not successful at all. Interest has now shifted from the mental symptoms associated with endocrine disorders to the other end of the continuum, the focus now being on the endocrinological symptoms that emerge as part of psychiatric disorders. The landmark works by Gibbons, Sachar, Stokes, Rubin, Prange and other pioneers have triggered an enormous number of studies explicitly describing the nature of neuroendocrinological changes under baseline conditions and after specific probes. The rapid progress in biotechnology has opened up the possibility of translating these observations into questions that can be readily pursued in basic research laboratories. Thus, experimental neuroendocrinological research in mood disorders encompasses both clinical and basic research strategies, which in tandem promise to narrow the gap between "bench and bedside." This chapter does not attempt to be exhaustive, but rather uses selected examples to illustrate this process (see

Chapters 44, 45, 62, 67, and 84, *this volume* for related topics).

RELATIONSHIP BETWEEN STRESS AND MOOD DISORDERS

The idea that those individuals with a genetic predisposition to a mood disorder who have also experienced life events are more likely to develop depression than those who have not dates back to Kraepelin, who also postulated that once triggered the disease may then progress independently of psychosocial stressors. More recently, epidemiological studies have corroborated this view; in addition a wealth of preclinical studies have emerged that have focused on acute and long-term consequences of psychosocial stress upon regulatory processes in specific brain circuitries that are commonly linked to the etiology of mood disorders.

Classically, stress is defined as a threatening of homeostasis to which the organism, in order to survive, responds with a large number of adaptive responses. According to work by Cannon, this mainly implicates the sympathetic nervous system and the hormones of the adrenal medulla. Selye was the first to suggest that neuroendocrine factors play a decisive role, and he considered the pituitary–adrenal system to be the major organizer of nonspecific responses to stress. Any type of emotional (cognitive) or physical (noncognitive, e.g., inflammatory) stressor sets into motion a cascade of processes that fine-tune the adaptive response according to specific demands. Centrally, sympathetic pathways are activated to allow for enhanced alertness and focused attention, whereas vegetative functions such as feeding, sleep, and sexual drive are decreased. Peripherally, the humoral and neural systems support the most pressing requirements by elevating heart rate, blood pressure, respiratory rate, and gluconeogenesis.

An integral part of adaptation to a stressor is the protec-

F. Holsboer: Clinical Institute, Max-Planck-Institute for Psychiatry, D-80804 Munich, Germany.

tion of the organism against an overreaction and curtailment of the response following termination of stress exposure. If the organism is incapable of terminating the response to stress at the end of stress exposure or if it is exposed to chronic stress, then the adaptive response can lead to pathological changes. The core hypothesis of this chapter is that counter-regulatory mechanisms are essential if overreaction is to be prevented, and that termination of the stress response is defunct in affective disorders. Defects in the counter-regulatory mechanisms may be either genetically encoded or acquired during premorbid life, or they may be a scar imprinted by previous disease episodes. Whatever their origin, there is plausible evidence that changes in stress-adaptive mechanisms are involved in the development, treatment, and prevention of mood disorders.

HYPOTHALAMIC–PITUITARY–ADRENOCORTICAL SYSTEM

Baseline Studies

Patients with depression exhibit increased hypothalamic–pituitary–adrenocortical (HPA) activity, as evidenced by an increase in the number of adrenocorticotropic hormone (ACTH) secretory episodes and an increase in the magnitude of cortisol secretory episodes. This HPA overactivity is further reflected in elevated urinary "free" cortisol (UFC) levels, which appear to be about twice as high in depressed patients as in normal controls, but lower than in patients with Cushing's syndrome. Furthermore, salivary and cerebrospinal fluid (CSF) concentrations of cortisol, which represent the free (i.e., unbound) fraction of cortisol, are reported to be elevated in depression. Finally, the group led by Nemeroff found that the concentration of corticotropin-releasing hormone (CRH) in the CSF is elevated in depressives, but decreases after electroconvulsive treatment (46).

Whereas clinical neuroendocrine studies and preclinical behavioral studies provide compelling evidence for a key role of elevated CRH in the development of mood disorders (30), it must be noted that the CRH levels in the CSF may not be an appropriate reflection of enhanced hypothalamic CRH drive during stress and depression. A study in which CRH concentrations in CSF were serially collected every 10 min for 4 hr showed decreased CRH levels in the presence of increased plasma ACTH and cortisol concentrations (22). The value of this study is perhaps limited by the small number of subjects ($n = 6$) and the failure of the subjects to exhibit pituitary adrenocortical characteristics typical for depression, but it points to a possible dissociation of the secretory activity of CRH, ACTH, and cortisol. Another example is the finding in primate CSF that CRH exhibits a peak preceding the cortisol peak by approximately 14 hr and is similarly uncoupled from peripheral HPA indices (21). A similar dissoci-

ation exists between plasma levels of ACTH and cortisol, where the degree of temporal association between the hormones is 50% to 60% (36).

There are several obvious explanations for this discrepancy. One is the specificity of the radioimmunoassay used in most studies. If other peptides are released in excess in depression or if the precursor molecule of ACTH, pro-opiomelanocortin (POMC), is cleaved differently, then the antibody might cross-react with some of these peptides, giving values for ACTH that are too high. Another caveat stems from equating immunoassayable ACTH with the adrenocortical-stimulating activity of ACTH. Poland et al. (51) showed that the amount of cortisol released from dispersed adrenocortical cells corresponds more closely to bioactive ACTH than to the immunoassayable amount of ACTH. One source of variance between plasma ACTH and cortisol levels in depression is the gradual development of adrenal hyperplasia during ongoing HPA overactivity, rendering the zona fasciculata of the adrenocortical gland hypersensitive to the tropic hormone ACTH. This hypothesis, derived by Amsterdam et al. (1) from testing with synthetic ACTH, was recently confirmed by Nemeroff et al. (47), who showed adrenal gland enlargement in major depression by computed tomography. Another possibility is the existence of non-ACTH mechanisms, perhaps involving neural sympathetic factors or humoral factors from the immune system. For example, interleukin-1 may activate the HPA system not only by increasing hypothalamic CRH and pituitary ACTH secretion but also by initiating a direct adrenocortical action, mediated by prostaglandin.

Recent studies with more sophisticated computer-aided deconvolution programs have revealed that the secretory pattern of pituitary hormone release is more complex than previously thought, and such techniques need to be employed in patients with major depression to describe more explicitly the changes in HPA-drive under baseline conditions (see Chapters 45, 67, and 84, *this volume*).

Dexamethasone Suppression Test

In healthy subjects, the release of ACTH and cortisol can be suppressed for approximately 24 hr by a single oral dose of 1 to 2 mg dexamethasone, a synthetic glucocorticoid. This suppressive action is less pronounced in patients with major depression, 50% to 70% of whom escape from dexamethasone suppression (72). The phenomenon is not merely a reflection of ACTH and cortisol hypersecretion, as one might infer from the analogy with Cushing's syndrome, and it occurs quite frequently among depressives with normal cortisol secretion at baseline. A number of studies by Carroll (12) concluded that nonsuppression on the dexamethasone suppression test (DST) is specific for the diagnosis of melancholia. Although this conclusion has since proven to be invalid, the use of the DST in psychiatric research still has considerable merit. For example, serial DST monitoring of depressed patients undergoing drug treatment showed that in treatment responders DST nonsuppression gradually turned into suppression. Patients whose DST remained abnormal or who were initially suppressors but became DST nonsuppressors during an observation period had a poorer prognosis. At a long-term follow-up, those depressed patients who were DST suppressors at baseline had a better outcome than the nonsuppressors (27).

The plasma dexamethasone concentrations are highly variable and were initially regarded as a major confounder after observation of a negative correlation between post-DST plasma cortisol and dexamethasone concentrations. However, pharmacokinetic studies of the test drug showed that plasma dexamethasone concentrations in the early biophase, which determine the pharmacodynamic effect, are identical in suppressors and nonsuppressors (26). Furthermore, when dexamethasone is administered intravenously to normal controls, the plasma dexamethasone levels are extremely low at the time when samples are drawn for measurements of plasma cortisol levels. Despite these low plasma dexamethasone levels, the cortisol concentrations are adequately suppressed (27). This set of studies indicates that the low plasma dexamethasone levels, measured at the conventional sampling times, in depressed patients do not account for DST nonsuppression.

Corticotropin-releasing Hormone Test

After CRH became available for clinical studies, several groups measured the ACTH and cortisol response following injections of this neuropeptide, and they consistently reported that the ACTH response was blunted regardless of whether ovine or human CRH was used (28). In some studies, an inverse relationship was found between baseline cortisol secretion and post-CRH ACTH secretion, and it was concluded that elevated baseline cortisol accounts for ACTH blunting via negative feedback. This view was substantiated by studies in which depressed patients were pretreated with metyrapone, which suppresses cortisol biosynthesis: the subjects had normalized ACTH output after CRH stimulation (30).

These data suggest that circulating cortisol is indeed the main determinant preventing an adequate ACTH response to a CRH challenge. Of course, other factors, such as CRH receptor desensitization of corticotropes, altered processing and storage of ACTH precursors, and alternative processing of POMC may also contribute to this phenomenon. For example, Rupprecht et al. (58) reported a dissociation of the ACTH and β-endorphin responses after CRH in depression. Another dissociation was observed at the adrenocortical level, where aldosterone but not cortisol release was found to be blunted in depression (30). The latter observation is in line with the finding that the ratio of ACTH to cortisol decreases with ongoing

HPA excess. The functional hyperplasia is apparently limited to the zona fasciculata of the target cell, which regresses after hypophysectomy, an effect that is counteracted by the injection of ACTH. Finally, endogenous CRH may enhance the adrenal response to endogenous and exogenous ACTH in rats, perhaps through a synergistic action on adrenal blood flow. The role of the intraadrenal CRH system may also be altered in mood disorders, resulting in altered ACTH-to-cortisol ratios. The dissociation between pituitary and adrenocortical suppression by dexamethasone has also been noted. Young et al. (82) found β-endorphin nonsuppression to be much more frequent than cortisol nonsuppression, which suggests faulty feedback at corticotropes that is not reflected in increased adrenocortical activity.

Combined Dexamethasone and Corticotropin-releasing Hormone Test

A surprising finding emerged when patients with depression were given a DST and were then challenged with CRH during the afternoon of the next day. One would expect that inadequately suppressed cortisol levels and dexamethasone together would be additive in blunting ACTH release. In fact, normal volunteers showed an ACTH and cortisol response to CRH that gradually decreased with increasing dosages of dexamethasone before CRH administration (27). In contrast, depressed patients showed a paradoxical pattern insofar as dexamethasone pretreatment resulted in increased ACTH and cortisol responses to CRH despite combined endogenous (elevated cortisol) and exogenous (dexamethasone) glucocorticoid levels (77). This abnormality disappears after successful antidepressant treatment (27,31). The mechanism underlying this phenomenon is not yet fully elucidated, but vasopressin appears to play a role as a possible synergizer of the CRH effects on corticotropic cells. In dexamethasone-pretreated normal controls even high dosages of CRH do not result in plasma ACTH and cortisol levels like those seen among depressed DST nonsuppressors who were not CRH-stimulated (30). This suggests that CRH alone may not account for DST nonsuppression in depressives. When dexamethasone-pretreated normal controls received vasopressin and CRH in combination, ACTH and cortisol secretory patterns emerged that strongly resemble those seen in depressives (30).

From these data and a vast number of preclinical investigations, suggesting a profound synergy between CRH and vasopressin at the pituitary level, the following hypothesis was derived: In depression as in chronic stress, there is a shift to a gradually intensifying vasopressinergic regulation of the pituitary adrenocortical system. Dexamethasone, which does not bind to corticosteroid-binding globulins, thus exerts its effect on the HPA system primarily at the level of the pituitary corticotropes and does not suppress hypothalamic CRH and vasopressin as effectively as endogenous corticosteroids. A transient cortico-steroid receptor desensitization gradually develops, and vasopressin expression, which reacts differently to changes in glucocorticoid concentration than does CRH expression, becomes less effectively suppressed than CRH by circulating corticosteroids. As a result, in a depressed dexamethasone-pretreated patient, secretion of ACTH in response to exogenous CRH would be greater than in a control because of the synergistic interaction of the administered CRH bolus with the larger amount of vasopressin present at corticotropes due to insufficient suppression by dexamethasone.

The idea that there is an increased vasopressinergic drive in depression is also indirectly supported by the observed effect of age upon plasma cortisol levels after a combined dexamethasone-CRH test (78). The older the patient, the more cortisol is released in response to a dexamethasone-CRH test, which agrees with findings that with increasing age vasopressin release is enhanced, possibly because of a gradually decreasing capacity of vasopressin receptors. This effect of age is amplified by excessive physical stress such as marathon running (25).

Recently, the above hypothesis received substantial support from preclinical studies showing that repeated stress activates hypothalamic CRH neurons, resulting in increased vasopressin stores and colocalization in CRH nerve terminals. In these parvocellular neurosecretory neurons of the hypothalamic paraventricular nucleus, repeated stress evokes increased CRH and vasopressin synthesis through afferent excitatory neuronal input overriding negative feedback of glucocorticoids upon CRH and vasopressin biosynthesis (13). Vasopressin and CRH are produced during stress, and depending on the severity and duration of stress more and more CRH neurons start to produce vasopressin. When, secondary to chronic stress in the rat or depression in humans, the enhanced vasopressinergic activity is no longer suppressed by dexamethasone, then a synergy with exogenous CRH may occur (30). Furthermore, additional functional changes in the interaction of glucocorticoid receptors with the regulatory elements of the POMC gene may occur.

Negative Hypothalamic–Pituitary–Adrenocortical Feedback Disturbance

Similarly, hypoglycemic stress induced by intravenous insulin results in a blunted ACTH response in depression. However, the amounts of ACTH released are much higher than in the CRH test and would never be achieved by CRH alone. Here again, a synergistic interaction between CRH and vasopressin at the corticotropes is likely to be involved. At present, there is no ready explanation for the depression-related blunted ACTH response to insulin, but this finding is certainly caused by a combination of many different factors. Taken together, the results from these and many other dynamic probes of the HPA system

support the view that negative feedback is disturbed in depression. By infusing cortisol in depressed patients and measuring the short-term effect upon β-endorphin and β-lipotropin (both are POMC cleavage products, as mentioned earlier) Young et al. (81) showed a decrease in β-endorphin and β-lipotropin release concomitantly with rapidly increasing plasma cortisol levels, indicating the presence of fast-feedback effects of cortisol upon β-endorphin and β-lipotropin. Such a fast feedback could not be demonstrated in depressed patients, which points to a defect at the level of the corticosteroid receptor-mediated inhibition of synthesis and release of ACTH secretagogues. It is presently not known exactly how glucocorticoids exert their suppressive effect upon the expression of genes coding for several proteins that are likely to be involved in negative feedback (65) at all the various levels. However, the data base established so far indicates clearly that negative feedback regulation is defunct at the level of the limbic rather than the pituitary–adrenocortical system.

What is not known is whether the disturbance is primary, at the level of a corticosteroid receptor whose function of fine-tuning ACTH secretion via CRH, vasopressin, and POMC regulation is disturbed, or whether other factors drive expression of CRH and vasopressin and their release into hypophyseal portal blood, resulting in an ACTH and cortisol excess that secondarily decreases corticosteroid receptor capacity and function. The pertinent question of whether the corticosteroid receptor disturbance is the cause or the consequence of a CRH hyperdrive that progresses into a combined CRH–AVP hyperdrive cannot yet be answered. Too many other factors that we are only beginning to identify are likely to play a role. One of these is the excitatory amino acids involved in a variety of physiological and pathophysiological processes and also in the neuroendocrine regulation of the HPA system. A further potential modulator of CRH in the hypothalamus is nitric oxide.

Another interesting aspect that has received renewed attention is the possibility of corticotropin-inhibiting factor (CIF) action. Recently, Kellner et al. (34) observed that atrial natriuretic factor (ANF) can suppress the CRH-elicited release of ACTH in normal human controls, providing further evidence for what had been suggested by animal studies (19). These clinical and basic studies demonstrating in vivo and in vitro inhibition of ACTH as well as the neuroanatomical evidence that ANF neurons project to the external layer of the median eminence suggest that ANF may indeed represent a physiologically relevant corticotropin-inhibiting factor.

Still another possible modulator is the recently discovered CRH-binding protein (53), which may modify the synaptic and hormonal actions of CRH at selected sites in the central nervous system and the pituitary. Such interactions may be relevant in the pituitary, where this binding protein is extensively expressed and where the effects of centrally released CRH may be blunted under certain conditions. Future pharmacological research should attempt to clarify whether CRH-binding protein can aid in designing peptides that are capable of blocking the action of CRH. Such compounds, as well as nonpeptidergic drugs, that mimic the ANF effects, would be of potential therapeutic significance. Finally, the recent cloning of the CRH receptor promises the design of drugs that inhibit the potentially anxiogenic effect of hypersecreted CRH.

THE BRAIN—A SITE OF CORTICOID ACTION

In response to stressful environmental signals processed by the nervous system, several hormonal adaptations occur that modify the function of specific brain areas. Two principal mechanisms, by which corticosteroids act on neurons, are involved: (a) genomic actions, where the steroid enters the nervous cell and binds to cognate receptors that transform into transcription factors, enhancing or suppressing expression of steroid hormone-regulated genes; and (b) nongenomic actions, where steroids bind to sites at synaptic membranes, affecting ion conductance. Steroids that exert their activity on neurons primarily at membrane sites are often called neuroactive steroids, although neuroactivity of steroids can be conferred through genomic actions, too (48).

The central role of corticosteroids in the maintenance of basic functions and in adaptation and survival under stressful conditions has led to the development of two distinct receptor systems, the mineralocorticoid receptors (MRs) and the glucocorticoid receptors (GRs) (14). The need for this dual system becomes evident if one considers that in a healthy individual plasma concentrations of cortisol may undergo circadian fluctuations from 0.5 nM to 50 nM, and under stressful conditions the maximum may well be above 150 nM. An adequate physiological response to such a wide range of hormone concentrations could not be achieved by a single receptor system only (18). However, two types of receptor, the MRs with high affinity to cortisol and the GRs with low affinity, provide sufficient control over tonic (MR) and stress response (GR) mechanisms in the hippocampus (20). Under baseline conditions the MRs are 90% occupied by cortisol (or corticosterone in the rat), whereas the GRs are only 50% occupied. In the early morning, when circadian HPA activation occurs, or following stress the GRs become more fully occupied in order to curtail HPA-activating mechanisms. Under pathological conditions, for example, severe major depression or Cushing's syndrome, continuing corticosteroid hypersecretion leads to overexposure of GRs and MRs which, in turn, are down-regulated. In nonhuman primates, the hippocampal formation plays an important role in the inhibition of the pituitary—adrenocortical system (61), and sustained stress results in progressive pyramidal neurodegeneration, mainly in the CA3 region. This morphological change results in neuroendocrine changes, because the decreased number of corticosteroid-receptor—bearing neurons in the hippocampus results in a weakened capacity to shut off stress-elevated plasma glucocorticoid levels, thus propelling forward the neurodegenerative effect in this brain area. It is important to note that glucocorticoids are not generally neurotoxic but rather create a condition that makes neurons less able to survive coincident insults such as hypoglycemia, hypoxia, and excitatory amino acids. Another hippocampal region, the granule cells of the dentate gyrus, needs the presence of corticosteroids to survive, underscoring the complexity of GR-neuronal interaction (64). Glucocorticoid receptor density in brain regions other than the hippocampus is also sensitive to chronic overexposure, and a fine-tuned mechanism maintains the capacity of the acute stress response even in the presence of chronic stress. The nature of this particular mechanism is still unknown but may involve a pathway proximal to the CRH–vasopressin neurons in the hypothalamus.

Behavioral Effects of Altered Corticosteroid Regulation

The implications of the dual corticosteroid receptor system for affective disorders are manifold. Administration of glucocorticoids to normal volunteers results in cognitive impairment, and, given the important role of the hippocampus in maximizing memory processes, it is tempting to speculate that excessive corticosteroid exposure decreases the effectiveness of the hippocampus in filtering out behaviorally irrelevant stimuli and maintaining selective attention. The inability to discriminate relevant, important information from irrelevant or unimportant information appears to be a common neuropsychological disturbance in various forms of hypercortisolemia, regardless of whether they are due to Cushing's syndrome or major depression. Yet no specific attribution of steroid effects on neuropsychological function is available. It is also of note that the hypercortisolemia in major depression is driven by central processes such as hypersecretion of CRH, vasopressin, and possibly other ACTH secretagogues. Effects of exogenously administered synthetic corticosteroids or of those corticosteroids secondary to Cushing's syndrome suppress these neuropeptides, which makes comparison of neuropsychological findings between drug-induced Cushing's syndrome, Cushing's disease, and major depression valuable only to a very limited extent.

Further evidence for a corticosteroid-receptor—mediated behavioral effect comes from sleep EEG studies with several corticosteroid probes. In general, these studies found that cortisol enhances slow-wave sleep (SWS) and suppresses rapid-eye-movement (REM) sleep, which suggests that GRs mediate REM sleep and MRs mediate SWS (8). The latter conclusion is derived from the SWS suppressive effect of canrenoate, an MR antagonist. It is not yet clear which mechanisms are involved, particularly because cortisol administration during sleep enhances GH release and suppresses central CRH and vasopressin by negative feedback. Corticotropin-releasing hormone suppresses SWS (29), vasopressin suppresses REM sleep (9), and growth hormone-releasing hormone (GHRH) stimulates SWS (68), suggesting that the effects found following steroid administration are mediated through their effects on the expression and release of neuropeptides, whose involvement in sleep regulation is firmly established (16).

In view of the evidence for hypercortisolism as the precipitator of affective symptoms in patients with Cushing's syndrome, it seems plausible to ask whether the overexposure of the brain to corticosteroids is causally related to the development of affective disorders. Corticosteroids have profound effects on the biochemistry and survival of neuronal brain cells, which may culminate in changes detectable by cranial computed tomography (CT) in HPA-altered depressives (62). If the total quantity of glucocorticoids released is enhanced and if the composition of various corticosteroids other than cortisol is profoundly altered, the pertinent question becomes whether suppression of corticosteroids would be a straightforward approach to treating depression. Some small exploratory studies suggest such a possibility (44). Because of the adverse effects of the drugs employed (metyrapone, aminogluthetionide, and the potentially dangerous drug ketoconazol) this approach cannot be recommended at present as either the sole or an adjunct treatment for depression.

The considerations regarding cortisol-suppressive therapies are based on the assumption that excessive corticosteroids precipitate mood disorders by cytosolic receptor-mediated effects. The cortisol-suppressive treatments used so far disturb the negative feedback, which then leads to enhanced secretion of CRH, vasopressin, and other ACTH secretagogues, all of which have behavioral and possibly anxiogenic or depressogenic effects of their own. The use of selective antagonists of MR and GR at the start of treatment with antidepressants (which later readjust the availability of these two corticosteroid receptors) appears to be the most promising approach for future studies.

Potential Role of Neuroactive Steroids in Mood Disorders

In addition to excessive total adrenocortical hormone output in major depression, changes in adrenocortical steroid metabolism have been reported repeatedly (44). These changes have attracted renewed interest because of the recently reported existence of nongenomic effects of a certain class of steroids, termed neuroactive steroids (40,48).

The first behavioral observations related to these steroids date back to Selye, who over 50 years ago reported

that progesterone and deoxycorticosterone (DOC) have a strong sedative action through their A-ring–reduced metabolites. These two steroids, termed allopregnanolone (THP) and allotetrahydrodeoxycorticosterone (THDOC), bind at γ-aminobutyric acid$_A$ (GABA$_A$) receptors to enhance GABA-induced chloride currents. In rats, THDOC and THP are elevated in cortical and hypothalamic tissue after stress (48), and they have been shown to be anxiolytic and hypnotic, respectively, as predicted by electrophysiology, where a benzodiazepine-like action was demonstrated. Administration of DOC to normal human controls did not evoke effects upon the sleep electroencephalogram (EEG) that would suggest a hypnotic effect after hepatic or central metabolization into THDOC (70). Furthermore, metyrapone treatments, which elevate DOC and THDOC by C-11 steroidhydroxylase inhibition, were not reported to be hypnotic.

Several other neuroactive steroids have the opposite effect. For example, the sulfated form of pregnenolone has been observed to be proconvulsant, as one would expect from electrophysiological experiments, where this steroid has been reported to antagonize GABA$_A$-receptor–mediated chloride currents by reducing the channel-opening frequency (40). Steiger et al. (69) administered pregnenolone to normal healthy controls and analyzed the sleep EEG changes. Pregnenolone increased SWS and decreased sigma power without altering delta power. These spectral analytical data and the absence of any in vivo or in vitro evidence for genomic effects of pregnenolone at GRs or MRs suggest that this steroid acts as a partial inverse agonist at the GABA receptor complex. If this holds true, several clinical implications emerge: Drugs with similar pharmacological profiles (e.g., β-carbolines) are currently being tested as potential memory enhancers, and pregnenolone has already been found to be memory-enhancing in mice (20). Furthermore, the group led by Baulieu (6) discovered a biosynthetic pathway of steroidal compounds in the central neurons and glial cells, possibly rendering the brain independent of peripheral sources. If the bioavailability of pregnenolone is endangered by other drugs such as centrally acting cholesterol synthesis inhibitors, then this might be an explanation for the frequently occurring mental disturbances in patients treated with such compounds.

Whereas it seems attractive to differentiate genomic from nongenomic actions upon neurons, a recent study by Rupprecht et al. (59) showed that transitions may exist between these two modes of action. Steroids that are believed to have limited effects at membrane sites, such as THP and THDOC, can be oxidized intracellularly and then exert genomic actions through progesterone receptors. Thus, the steroid molecule provides a rather flexible structure, which can be modified depending on the tissue to satisfy specific demands (see Chapter 8, *this volume*).

HYPOTHALAMIC–PITUITARY– ADRENOCORTICAL SYSTEM ACTIVITY AND ANTIDEPRESSANT ACTION

Longitudinal studies of patients with depression showed that not only psychopathology but also symptoms of HPA dysfunction respond to antidepressants, and there is a temporal association between changes in mood and hormones. Specifically, in DST nonsuppressors normalization of the suppression response is associated with good treatment response, whereas if plasma cortisol levels remain refractory to dexamethasone suppression this indicates either persistent depression or liability to relapse (27). Studies with more sensitive neuroendocrine function tests such as the combined dexamethasone–CRH challenge yielded similar results and showed that neuroendocrine changes precede psychopathological changes toward both remission and relapse (31). These findings suggested a causal role of HPA alterations in the pathogenesis of depression and challenged several research groups to investigate whether antidepressants elevate mood in depressives through their long-term effects on HPA regulation.

During chronic stress in animals and possibly also in patients with major depression secretion of CRH and the activity of the locus coeruleus (LC) are increased. Both systems are reciprocally innervated, since tyrosine hydroxylase- (TH-, the rate-limiting enzyme in the norepinephrine biosynthesis) positive cells and processes overlap CRH-immunoreactive fibers. This was functionally confirmed by Valentino et al. (74), who showed that CRH applied to LC neurons increases the spontaneous discharge rate of LC cells. This experiment and many others strongly suggested that noradrenergic fibers, projecting from the LC to the paraventricular nucleus (PVN), are stimulators of CRH, which in turn serves as a neurotransmitter to activate the LC. In fact, acute and chronic stress increase immunoreactivity to CRH in the PVN, and infusion of CRH directly into the LC increases catecholamine levels in the cerebral cortex, plasma cortisol levels, and certain stress-related behaviors (11). When rats were treated with imipramine (5 mg/kg i.p.) for 8 weeks, the CRH-mRNA levels were decreased by 37% in the PVN. Moreover, the induction TH was reduced in the LC. Thus, the mutual activation of the two brain centers (PVN and LC) that coordinate the response to stress is dampened through antidepressants. Reul et al. (56) studied the time course of corticosteroid receptor concentration changes in rats treated with amitriptyline or moclobemide (a reversible inhibitor of monoamine oxidase-A). They focused on both MRs and GRs, which, as detailed earlier, dually control HPA system activity and whose equilibrium is possibly defunct in mood disorders. Both amitriptyline and moclobemide transiently elevated hippocampal MR by 40% to 70% between 2 and 5 weeks after the start of treatment. At 7 weeks, the increments in MR had largely disappeared. Hypothalamic GR was increased by 20% to 25% at 5 weeks of treatment, suggesting that antidepressant-induced changes in brain corticosteroid capacity may underlie the observed decrease in circulating ACTH and corticosterone levels and the decreased adrenal size. Furthermore, when challenged by a stressor, rats treated with antidepressants showed a decreased ACTH and corticosterone response, which is understandable in terms of an attenuated LC-CRH response, possibly through enhanced effectiveness of negative corticosteroid feedback from reestablished GR and MR capacity (56).

To investigate more conclusively the hypothesis that antidepressants modulate GR, Barden's group first showed that different types of antidepressants alter GR mRNA levels, a process that appears to be unrelated to monoamine uptake because increased activity of GR gene transcription is seen in mouse fibroblast cells, which do not contain any catecholamines (49). Based on the hypothesis that the apparent lack of sensitivity to corticosteroids seen in the majority of depressives results in neuroendocrine changes, which are causally linked both to pathogenesis and to the therapeutic effectiveness of antidepressant drugs, Pepin et al. (50) created a transgenic mouse with precisely this neuroendocrine deficit. An antisense RNA complementary to the 3′ noncoding region of the GR mRNA was inserted into the mouse genome, producing an animal in which the GR gene expression is partially knocked out by formation of GR antisense RNA. These mice have increased HPA activity, a resistance to dexamethasone suppression, lethargy, and feeding disturbances, which support the idea that they are appropriate animal models for studying the neuroendocrine symptoms of depression. Treatment of these mice with antidepressants resulted in a partial reversal of enhanced ACTH and corticosteroid secretion and concurrently increased GR mRNA and steroid receptor binding. Moreover, the mRNA levels of hippocampal MR increase after long-term treatment with antidepressants (10).

The precise molecular mechanism of action of antidepressant drugs on corticosteroid receptor gene expression is unknown but may involve more basic mechanisms than synaptic transmission. For example, G-proteins, which play a key role in coupling receptors to intracellular effector systems, are targets of glucocorticoid action in the CNS. In the rat cortex, mRNA levels of stimulatory G-proteins ($G_{s\alpha}$) are increased and the level of the inhibitory subunit ($G_{i\alpha}$) is decreased (60). This may have implications for treatment with tricyclics, which decrease $G_{s\alpha}$ and, to a lesser extent, $G_{i\alpha}$ (38). Because corticosteroids modulate the actions of other transmitters that act through cyclic adenosine monophosphate (cAMP), they have been termed "permissive hormones." It is therefore very likely that the observed clinical effects upon psychopathological and neuroendocrine symptoms of depression and the involvement of these hormones at many antidepressant-induced levels of action (membrane sites, signal transduction, nuclear gene transcription) are functionally interrelated.

THE THYROID SYSTEM

The effect of thyroid hormones upon mood and behavior is documented by dysphoria, anxiety, fatigue, and irritability in hyperthyroidism and by impairment of cognitive functions in milder states of hypothyroidism. In psychiatric populations, regardless of specific diagnoses, thyroid dysfunction is more common than in the general population, and among patients with mood disorders 20% to 30% exhibit some form of hypothalamic–pituitary–thyroid (HPT) abnormality. The HPT system has a hierarchical structure similar to that of the HPA system, with thyrotropin-releasing hormone (TRH) as the hypothalamic master hormone that is released from nerve endings in the median eminence, from where it enters the anterior pituitary through the portal system. There, it induces synthesis and release of thyreotropin (TSH), which enters the circulation and causes the release of the two major thyroid hormones, triiodothyronine (T_3) and thyroxine (T_4). Thyroid hormones feed back at the hypothalamus to inhibit TRH release and at the anterior pituitary to inhibit TSH release. Of course, many other factors are involved in fine-tuning this circuit. Among these, somatostatin (SRIF) and HPA hormones play an important role as inhibitors of HPT activity.

In the aggregate, studies that employed a TRH stimulation test in depressed patients reported that the TSH response was blunted in approximately 25% of the cases in the presence of normal T_3, T_4, and TSH levels at baseline (55). When Duval et al. performed TRH tests with 200 μg TRH at both 8 a.m. and 11 p.m., they found that stimulation in the evening produced greater ΔTSH differences between patients and controls than stimulation in the morning (15). A parameter called $\Delta\Delta$TSH (which is defined as the difference between morning and evening TSH responses) proved to detect HPT abnormality at a sensitivity rate of 89% among patients with major depression. Another indication of altered TSH secretion is the loss of the nocturnal TSH rise, which usually occurs between midnight and 3 a.m. The absence of a nocturnal surge in TSH is believed to be a more sensitive indicator of an HPT abnormality than a blunted TSH response to TRH (5). One putative mechanism to explain the decreased TSH secretion would be chronic hypersecretion of hypothalamic TRH, which would decrease the number of pituitary TRH receptors. Such a hypothesis is consonant with the finding of increased TRH in the CSF of depressed patients. The possibility that SRIF antagonizes TRH effects can be ruled out because SRIF levels in the CSF were decreased rather than elevated (57). Also, a possible inhibitory effect of thyroid hormones is not likely because serum total and free thyroid levels were reduced rather than elevated among depressives (55). It is well known that glucocorticoids inhibit TSH secretion, and the mean 24-hr serum TSH levels were fully suppressed in response to dexamethasone. In depressives, nighttime plasma cortisol and TSH levels were inversely related (5)

and the TSH response to TRH was found to be linearly correlated with the ACTH response to CRH (28), suggesting that HPA activity is a modulator of spontaneous or specifically stimulated TSH surges, or both. Approximately 16% of depressed patients in remission show blunted TSH responses, but in the absence of TRH test results for premorbid patients it remains an enigma whether the TRH blunting is a true trait marker or a neuroendocrine scar acquired from preceding depressive episodes. Nevertheless, persistent TRH blunting appears to be associated with an increased likelihood of relapse (see also Chapter 44, *this volume*).

Interaction of Thyroid Hormones and Antidepressant Therapy

Several groups (7,33) found that antidepressant treatment reduced plasma T_4 levels and that responders had more pronounced reduction in plasma T_4 and free T_4 than nonresponders. Joffe and Singer (33) compared the potential clinical effects of T_3 and T_4 as adjuvants to treatment with antidepressants and found T_3 to be superior to T_4. Furthermore, patients with panic disorder who were treated with antidepressants appeared to profit from adjunctive T_3 treatment (71). The working hypothesis formulated by Joffe and Singer (33) is that the effect of antidepressants includes reduced exposure of central neurons to thyroid hormone. The observed amplification of treatment effects by T_3 does not contradict this hypothesis of a central hyperthyroidism in mood disorders. Brain cells utilize T_3, which is derived from T_4 by deiodination. Exogenous T_3 would increase plasma T_3, but, through negative feedback of T_3 upon TSH, secretion of both T_3 and T_4 would be decreased. Thus, T_3 administration would lead to decreased central bioavailability of T_4, the major source of neuronal thyroid demands, and central hyperthyroidism would be compensated in this way. The antidepressant effect and possibly also the prophylactic effect of carbamazepine involves an antithyroid effect, too, because peripheral T_3 and T_4 decrease under this drug, whereas TSH increases.

Subclinical Hypothyroidism

A substantial portion of patients with mood disorders have elevated TSH at baseline and following TRH stimulation tests, but normal thyroid hormone concentration. This condition defines subclinical hypothyroidism and represents a considerable risk for development of depression. Several early studies suggested that one underlying mechanism is a symptomless autoimmune thyroiditis. Nemeroff et al. (45) observed that 20% of depressed patients had antithyroid antibodies; in the normal population, the figure is only 5% to 10%. Patients with bipolar disorder have a higher rate of symptomless autoimmune thyroiditis than those with unipolar depression, and rapidly cycling bipolar patients have a particularly high rate of hypothyroidism.

Possible Mechanisms Involved

The discovery by Mason et al. (41) that endogenous T_3 is concentrated in presynaptic nerve terminals, where the cellular uptake is achieved and where the synthesis of T_3 by deiodination of T_4 takes place, points to a possible role of T_3 as a neurotransmitter. In addition, the possibility that T_3 neurotransmitter receptor regulation is defunct in patients with affective disorders needs to be considered. In attention-deficit hyperactivity disorder (characterized by impulsiveness, inattention, aggressiveness, intrusiveness, destructiveness, hyperactivity and purposeless motor behavior and formerly termed ''minimal brain damage'') such a thyroid hormone receptor deficit may be a causative factor. In a study by Hauser et al. (24), 50% of the patients with generalized resistance to thyroid hormones had an inherited (usually autosomal dominant) disorder caused by a mutation in the thyroid receptor β-gene and met the criteria for attention-deficit hyperactivity disorder as children. The mutant human thyroid receptors exert hormone resistance through a lower binding affinity and subsequently through a lower transcriptional activation of positive T_3 response elements than found in normal receptors.

In light of the many findings on changes in thyroid regulation in mood disorders, it seems plausible that disturbed thyroid receptor-mediated signal transduction, possibly in concert with corticosteroid receptor dysfunction, is involved in the causation of mood disorders. The antidepressant-induced changes in HPT support this conclusion.

THE SOMATOTROPIC SYSTEM

Baseline Studies and Studies with Pharmacological Probes

If healthy individuals are exposed to acute stressors they respond with increased secretion of growth hormone (GH), but if they are exposed to mild chronic stressors such as academic examinations this does not provoke continuous GH hypersecretion. In contrast, under testing conditions of mild stress patients with depression show GH secretory patterns that are clearly distinct from those of normal controls. The integrated 24-hr GH values appear to be increased in depression, whereas the GH surge around the time of sleep onset is decreased.

The use of neuropharmacological probes has made it possible to relate altered GH responses to specific neurotransmitter receptor alterations in depression. The most consistent findings have emerged from studies with clonidine, an α_2-adrenoceptor agonist, namely that this drug evokes less GH in depressed patients than in controls.

The original finding by Matussek et al. (42) prompted numerous studies, from which it was concluded that the reduced GH response to clonidine cannot be accounted for by drug treatment, age, or sex but may be an indicator of noradrenergic dysregulation in affective disorders (63). This view is amplified by the concomitantly decreased response of 3-methoxy-4-hydroxyphenylglycol (MHPG) and cortisol. Furthermore, a number of antidepressants that inhibit presynaptic monoamine transporters are potent GH stimuli, and some studies, but not all, demonstrated that depressed patients have a reduced GH response to these antidepressant drugs.

The earliest challenge test used in mood disorders was the insulin tolerance test, which documented a blunted GH response after insulin-induced hypoglycemia. Initially, this finding, too, was attributed to a disturbed adrenoceptor function in depressed patients. Although recent knowledge about the complex counter-regulatory humoral and neuronal responses to hypoglycemia calls into question a simple mechanistic interpretation of insulin-induced GH secretion in mood disorders, the insulin resistance of depressed patients remains a potentially interesting finding. Amsterdam and Maislin (2) have postulated that patients with bipolar disorders have GH responses to insulin that are distinct from those of unipolar patients and controls, which suggests different neuroendocrine alterations in different mood disorder subtypes.

With the clinical availability of GHRH, the hypothalamic-releasing factor specifically stimulating GH from somatotropic cells, a number of studies investigated the GH response to GHRH in mood disorders. Discordant results emerged: Whereas some studies found a reduced GH response to GHRH in depression (37), others (e.g., ref. 35) did not. One factor possibly confounding the GH response to GHRH and causing inconsistent findings is the level of circulating somatomedin C (SM-C), which is reported to be elevated in depression (37), perhaps as a result of elevated GH secretion. However, Voderholzer et al. (76) recently reported that the baseline level of GH secretory activity does not determine the amount of GH release following GHRH. Hence the question remains open whether blunted responses to GHRH are determined by the secretory activity of GH at baseline. In depressed patients and controls, positive correlations between the GH responses to α_2-adrenoceptor agonists and GHRH were reported and interpreted as evidence that the GH response to clonidine is mediated by GHRH. Suri et al. (73) noted that the GH response to GHRH depends on the GH secretory status during the hour prior to challenge. Specifically, the GHRH-induced GH peak was higher when GHRH was administered while plasma GH levels were increasing than while they were decreasing. In this study, clonidine-induced GH surges were not determined by spontaneous GH patterns. Furthermore, pretreatment with clonidine did not augment the peak GH response to GHRH, but pretreatment with GHRH attenuated the peak GH response to clonidine. In another study, clonidine pretreatment increased the number of GH pulses and the total amount of GH released (39). These findings suggest that the α_2-adrenoceptor agonist-induced GH stimulation occurs through pathways different from GHRH-induced GH stimulation.

Pathophysiology Underlying Altered Growth Hormone Regulation in Mood Disorders

The secretion of GH is regulated by an extremely complex system, in which GHRH, secreted from neurons in the arcuate nucleus, stimulates GH release from the pituitary and somatostatin (SRIF), secreted from neurons in the paraventricular nucleus, suppresses it. In turn, GH secretion stimulates transcription of the SRIF-encoding gene and SRIF secretion inhibits transcription of the GHRH-encoding gene and the release of GHRH into the portal system. However, pulse frequency and the amount of GH released per pulse are determined not only by these reciprocal effects; many other factors are also critically involved. For example, there are at least three receptors that enhance GH secretion from somatotropic cells. Ligands for these receptors are, besides GHRH, the natural but still unknown ligand through which the synthetic GH-releasing peptide (a hexapeptide, developed from an enkephalin analog) activates GH (32) and pituitary adenylate cyclase-activating peptide (PACAP). The latter peptide stimulates somatotropic activity and fulfills the requirement for a hypophysiotropic factor. It releases GH through a receptor system that can be expressed in five different splice variants, which differentially activate two distinct second messenger systems (66). Although somatostatin suppresses these effects, elevated somatostatin secretion is not likely to be the cause of the blunted GH response to GHRH because, as numerous studies have shown, somatostatin tends to be decreased in the CSF of depressed patients and to increase after clinical improvement (57). It is not known, however, whether these CSF findings reflect the secretory activity of hypothalamic somatostatin neurons.

In depression a predominance of CRH over GHRH may develop and as a result somatostatin may be suppressed by enhanced CRH in a pulsatile fashion during the daytime, giving rise to increased GH pulses during the daytime and decreased GH release at night (80). Sleep endocrinological studies provide further support for this hypothesis: when GHRH is centrally injected into rats or intravenously administered to humans in a pulsatile fashion it enhances SWS and suppresses cortisol, whereas CRH suppresses both GH and SWS and elevates ACTH and cortisol, thus mimicking some of the spontaneously occurring events seen in depression (16,29,68). These findings raise the possibility that alterations in GH secretion are a phenomenon secondary to enhanced HPA activity. Although cross-sectional correlations of cortisol with other hormones (e.g., thyroid hormones) at baseline or following specific probes render this unlikely, it is of note that the modulating effects of cortisol and other hormones are subject to different, and at least in humans largely unknown, time grids. Thus, cross-sectional correlations will fail to detect causal relationships. Acutely administered corticosteroids increased GH (80), whereas there were changes after 4 days in the secretion profile but not in the overall amount of GH released (54). The amount of GH released during the daytime was increased, whereas the nocturnal sleep-related GH surge was attenuated, resembling the situation seen in mood disorders (43,67) and after administration of cortisol pulses to healthy men (80). The decreased nocturnal GH secretion after glucocorticoid administration probably involves increased SRIF release and/or negative feedback by elevated plasma GH levels and induction of SM-C (54). In a recent study by Veldhuis et al. (75), a low dosage of dexamethasone (1.5 mg b.i.d.) was administered for 1 week and found to increase integrated 24-hr plasma GH concentrations 250% and SM-C 200%. This increase was achieved by an increase in the number of secretory GH bursts and an increase in the amount of GH released per burst.

Cortisol inhibits the GH response to GHRH acutely after prolonged administration, the latter effect and also being attributed to an increase in glucocorticoid-induced SRIF (79) because pyridostigmine, a suppressor of SRIF, reverses the steroid effects (23). In agreement with this interpretation is the finding that in adrenalectomized rats the number of SRIF receptors decreases, but it normalizes again after glucocorticoid replacement. However, in pituitary cell cultures glucocorticoids desensitize SRIF receptors. Taken together, these studies suggest that the HPA hyperactivity in depression strongly influences both basal and stimulated GH secretion, probably by modulating somatostatin effects. Basic studies document a direct corticosteroid receptor-mediated effect on GH gene expression, and GH gene expression is similarly affected through ligand-activated thyroid receptors (17). In addition to these transcriptional effects on the GH-encoding gene, glucocorticoids also increase the number of pituitary GHRH receptors. Direct proof of the clinical relevance of these findings was provided by Barbarino et al. (4), who injected CRH in combination with GHRH and showed that CRH is capable of suppressing GHRH-elicited GH release, at the same time corroborating a study in which the spontaneous sleep-related GH surge was decreased by CRH administration (29) in a way similar to that seen in depressed patients with hypercortisolemia in the absence of exogenous CRH (68).

GH secretion declines with increasing age, which is best reflected by the near absence of nocturnal GH surges, accompanied by reduced SWS. Whether these effects are also secondary to increased HPA activity in the elderly is not known. In depressed patients, in whom ACTH and cortisol are enhanced and SWS and the associated GH secretion are reduced, GHRH administration does not rectify the endocrine pattern during sleep, although one would expect this from the SWS-enhancing and cortisol-suppressing effects of GHRH administration in healthy men (68).

The behavioral correlates of altered GH regulation in depression are difficult to reconcile. In patients with acromegaly, a number of cognitive and behavioral abnormalities have been noted. The best-documented effects are those on the sleep EEG. Exogenous administration of GH and pathologically hypersecreted GH (as is the case in acromegaly) attenuate SWS, most likely through suppression of GHRH, which is sleep-promoting (16,68). After surgical removal of the GH-secreting adenoma, the amount of SWS increases (3). Animal studies have linked CRH to anorectic behavior and GHRH to increased food intake. The hypothesized increased CRH-to-GHRH ratio in depression is in keeping with the loss of appetite and weight in these patients.

Studies in which GH is administered to elderly humans or to patients after hypophysectomy have not yet systematically elaborated the potential psychotropic effects of this hormone. Therefore, more such studies should be conducted. Also of interest would be investigations with GH-releasing peptide, which is a long-acting GH releaser acting at receptors different from those for GHRH and PACAP.

CONCLUSIONS

The focus of this brief and selective review has been on those clinical studies that provide input for basic research, ranging from animal behavior studies to cellular and molecular experiments. The neuroendocrinology of mood disorders has gone through numerous phases and currently hormonal alterations are considered to be neuroendocrine symptoms that may lead to a deeper understanding of pathogenesis. Clinically this conclusion is drawn from the concomitance of changes in mood and behavior and in hormonal activity. Basic studies strengthen this view by showing how environmental stimuli are translated into changes in neurohormonal activity and how this leads to altered expression of genes coding for proteins that are directly or indirectly involved in mediation of mood and behavior. Likewise, encoded vulnerability for the development of mood disorders is probably subclinically apparent in enhanced HPA responses to specific probes. This inherited sensitization is then further amplified by repeated episodes, thus providing a pathogenetic rationale for early intervention strategies (52). Antidepressants interfere at various levels of hormone regulation, and with the new technology available the hypothesis that they act clinically by rectifying the perturbed HPA system can now be tested. If additional evidence can be accumulated that neuroendocrine alterations are causally involved in mood disorders, this would provide a lead for the development of more efficacious drugs.

REFERENCES

1. Amsterdam JD, Winokur A, Abelman E, Lucki I, Rickels K. Cosyntropin (ACTH 1-24) stimulation test in depressed patients and healthy subjects. Am J Psychiatry 1983;140:907–909.
2. Amsterdam JD, Maislin G. Hormonal responses during insulin-induced hypoglycemia in manic-depressed, unipolar depressed, and healthy control subjects. J Clin Endocrinol Metab 1991;73:541–548.
3. Åström C, Christensen L, Gjerris F, Trojaborg W. Sleep in acromegaly before and after treatment with adenomectomy. Neuroendocrinology 1991;53:328–331.
4. Barbarino A, Corsello SM, della Casa S, et al. Corticotropin-releasing hormone inhibition of growth hormone-releasing hormone-induced growth hormone release in man. J Clin Endocrinol Metab 1990;71:1368–1374.
5. Bartalena L, Placidi GF, Martino E, et al. Nocturnal serum thyrotropin (TSH) surge and the TSH response to TSH-releasing hormone: dissociated behavior in untreated depressives. J Clin Endocrinol Metab 1990;71:650–655.
6. Baulieu EE, Robel P. Neurosteroids: a new brain function? J Steroid Biochem 1990;37:395–403.
7. Baumgartner A, Graf KK, Kerten I, Meinold H. The hypothalamic-pituitary-thyroid axis in psychiatric patients and healthy subjects: parts 1–4. Psychiatry Res 1988;24:271–332.
8. Born J, de Kloet ER, Wenz H, Kern W, Fehm HL. Gluco- and antimineralocorticoid effects on human sleep: a role of central corticosteroid receptors. Am J Physiol 1991;260:E183–E188.
9. Born J, Kellner C, Uthgenannt D, Kern W, Fehm HL. Vasopressin regulates human sleep by reducing rapid-eye-movement sleep. Am J Physiol 1992;262:E295–E300.
10. Brady LS, Whitfield HJ Jr, Fox RJ, Gold PW, Herkenham M. Long-term antidepressant administration alters corticotropin-releasing hormone, tyrosine hydroxylase, and mineralocorticoid receptor gene expression in rat brain. J Clin Invest 1991;87:831–837.
11. Butler PD, Weiss JM, Stout JC, Nemeroff CB. Corticotropin-releasing factor produces fear-enhancing and behavioral-activating effects following infusion into the locus coeruleus. J Neurosci 1990;10:176–183.
12. Carroll BJ. The dexamethasone suppression test for melancholia. Br J Psychiatry 1982;140:292–304.
13. de Goeij DCE, Jezova D, Tilders FJH. Repeated stress enhances vasopressin synthesis in corticotropin releasing factor neurons in the paraventricular nucleus. Brain Res 1992;577:165–168.
14. de Kloet ER. Brain corticosteroid receptor balance and homeostatic control. Front Neuroendocrinol 1991;12:95–164.
15. Duval F, Macher JP, Mokrani MC. Difference between evening and morning thyrotropin responses to protirelin in major depressive episode. Arch Gen Psychiatry 1990;47:443–448.
16. Ehlers CL, Reed TK, Henriksen SJ. Effects of corticotropin-releasing factor and growth hormone-releasing factor on sleep and activity in rats. Neuroendocrinology 1986;42:467–474.
17. Evans RM, Birnberg NC, Rosenfeld MG. Glucocorticoid and thyroid hormones transcriptionally regulate growth hormone gene expression. Proc Natl Acad Sci USA 1982;79:7659–7663.
18. Evans RM, Arriza JL. A molecular framework for the actions of glucocorticoid hormones in the nervous system. Neuron 1989;2:1105–1112.
19. Fink G, Dow RC, Casley D, et al. Atrial natriuretic peptide is a physiological inhibitor of ACTH release: evidence from immunoneutralization in vivo. J Endocrinol 1991;131:R9–12.
20. Flood JF, Morley JE, Roberts E. Memory-enhancing effects in male mice of pregnenolone and steroids metabolically derived from it. Proc Natl Acad Sci USA 1992;89:1567–1571.
21. Garrick NA, Hill JL, Szele FG, Tomai TP, Gold PW, Murphy DL. Corticotropin-releasing factor: a marked circadian rhythm in primate cerebrospinal fluid peaks in the evening and is inversely related to the cortisol circadian rhythm. Endocrinology 1987;121:1329–1334.
22. Geracioti TD Jr, Orth DN, Ekhator NN, Blumenkopf B, Loosen PT. Serial cerebrospinal fluid corticotropin-releasing hormone concentrations in healthy and depressed humans. J Clin Endocrinol Metab 1992;74:1325–1330.
23. Giustina A, Girelli A, Doga M, et al. Pyridostigmine blocks the inhibitory effect of glucocorticoids on growth hormone-releasing

hormone stimulated growth hormone secretion in normal man. *J Clin Endocrinol Metab* 1990;71:580–584.

24. Hauser P, Zametkin AJ, Martinez P, et al. Attention deficit-hyperactivity disorder in people with generalized resistance to thyroid hormone. *N Engl J Med* 1993;328:997–1001.
25. Heuser I, Wark HJ, Keul J, Holsboer F. Hypothalamic-pituitary-adrenal-axis function in elderly endurance athletes. *J Clin Endocrinol Metab* 1991;73:485–488.
26. Holsboer F, Wiedemann K, Boll E. Shortened dexamethasone half-life in depressed dexamethasone nonsuppressors. *Arch Gen Psychiatry* 1986;43:813–815.
27. Holsboer F. The hypothalamic-pituitary-adrenocortical system. In: Paykel ES, ed. *Handbook of Affective Disorders*. Edinburgh: Churchill Livingstone; 1992:267–287.
28. Holsboer F, Gerken A, von Bardeleben U, et al. Human corticotropin-releasing hormone in depression. *Biol Psychiatry* 1986;21:609–611.
29. Holsboer F, von Bardeleben U, Steiger A. Effects of intravenous corticotropin-releasing hormone upon sleep-related growth hormone surge and sleep EEG in man. *Neuroendocrinology* 1988;48:32–38.
30. Holsboer F, Spengler D, Heuser I. The role of corticotropin-releasing hormone in the pathogenesis of Cushing's disease, anorexia nervosa, alcoholism, affective disorders and dementia. *Prog Brain Res* 1992;93:385–417.
31. Holsboer-Trachsler E, Stohler R, Hatzinger M. Repeated administration of the combined dexamethasone/hCRH stimulation test during treatment of depression. *Psychiatry Res* 1991;38:163–171.
32. Huhn WC, Hartman ML, Pezzoli SS, Thorner MO. Twenty-four-hour growth hormone (GH)-releasing peptide (GHRP) infusion enhances pulsatile GH secretion and specifically attenuates the response to a subsequent GHRP bolus. *J Clin Endocrinol Metab* 1993;76:1202–1208.
33. Joffe RT, Singer W. The effect of tricyclic antidepressants on basal thyroid hormone levels in depressed patients. *Pharmacopsychiatry* 1990;23:67–69.
34. Kellner M, Wiedemann K, Holsboer F. ANF inhibits the CRH-stimulated secretion of ACTH and cortisol in man. *Life Sci* 1992;50:1835–1842.
35. Krishnan KRR, Manepalli AN, Ritchie CJ, et al. Growth hormone-releasing factor stimulation test in depression. *Am J Psychiatry* 1988;145:90–92.
36. Krishnan KRR, Ritchie JC, Saunders W, Wilson W, Nemeroff CB, Carroll BJ. Nocturnal and early morning secretion of ACTH and cortisol in humans. *Biol Psychiatry* 1990;28:47–57.
37. Lesch KP, Laux G, Pfüller H, Erb A, Beckmann H. Growth hormone (GH) response to GH-releasing hormone in depression. *J Clin Endocrinol Metab* 1987;65:1278–1281.
38. Lesch KP, Aulakh CS, Tolliver TJ, Hill JL, Murphy DL. Regulation of G proteins by chronic antidepressant drug treatment in rat brain: tricyclics but not clorgyline increase G$_{o\alpha}$ subunits. *Eur J Pharmacol* 1991;207:361–364.
39. Lima L, Arce V, Diaz MJ, Tresguerres JAF, Devesa J. Clonidine pretreatment modifies the growth hormone secretory pattern induced by short-term continuous GRF infusion in normal man. *Clin Endocrinol* 1991;35:129–135.
40. Majewska MD. Neurosteroids: endogenous bimodal modulators of the GABA$_A$ receptor. Mechanism of action and physiological significance. *Prog Neurobiol* 1992;38:379–395.
41. Mason GA, Walker CH, Prange AJ Jr. L-Triiodothyronine: is this peripheral hormone a central neurotransmitter? *Neuropsychopharmacology* 1993;8:253–258.
42. Matussek N, Ackenheil M, Hippius H, et al. Effect of clonidine on growth hormone release in psychiatric patients and controls. *Psychiatry Res* 1980;2:25–36.
43. Mendlewicz J, Linkowski P, Kerkhofs M, et al. Diurnal hypersecretion of growth hormone in depression. *J Clin Endocrinol Metab* 1985;60:505–517.
44. Murphy BEP. Steroids and depression. *J Steroid Biochem Mol Biol* 1991;38:537–559.
45. Nemeroff CB, Simon JS, Haggerty JJ, Evans DL. Antithyroid antibodies in depressed patients. *Am J Psychiatry* 1985;142:840–843.
46. Nemeroff CB, Bissette G, Akil H, Fink M. Neuropeptide concentrations in the CSF of depressed patients treated with electroconvulsive therapy. *Br J Psychiatry* 1991;158:59–63.
47. Nemeroff CB, Krishnan KRR, Reed D, Leder R, Beam C, Dunnick

R. Adrenal gland enlargement in major depression. *Arch Gen Psychiatry* 1992;49:384–387.
48. Paul SM, Purdy RH. Neuroactive steroids. *FASEB J* 1992;6:2311–2322.
49. Pepin MC, Beaulieu S, Barden N. Antidepressants regulate glucocorticoid receptor messenger RNA concentrations in primary neuronal cultures. *Mol Brain Res* 1989;6:77–83.
50. Pepin MC, Pothier F, Barden N. Impaired type II glucocorticoid-receptor function in mice bearing antisense RNA transgene. *Nature* 1992;355:725–728.
51. Poland RE, Hanada K, Rubin RT. Relationship of nocturnal plasma bioactive and immunoactive ACTH concentrations to cortisol secretion in normal men. *Acta Endocrinol (Copenh)* 1989;121:857–865.
52. Post M. Transduction of psychosocial stress into the neurobiology of recurrent affective disorder. *Am J Psychiatry* 1992;149:999–1010.
53. Potter E, Behan DP, Linton EA, Lowry PJ, Sawchenko PE, Vale WW. The central distribution of a corticotropin-releasing factor (CRF)-binding protein predicts multiple sites and modes of interaction with CRF. *Proc Natl Acad Sci USA* 1992;89:4192–4196.
54. Pralong FP, Miell JP, Corder R, Gaillard RC. Dexamethasone treatment in man induces changes in 24-hour growth hormone (GH) secretion profile without altering total GH released. *J Clin Endocrinol Metab* 1991;73:1191–1196.
55. Prange AJ Jr, Garbutt JC, Loosen PT. The hypothalamic-pituitary-thyroid axis in affective disorders. In: Meltzer HY, ed. *Psychopharmacology: the third generation of progress*. New York: Raven Press, 1987:629–636.
56. Reul JMHM, Stec I, Söder M, Holsboer F. Chronic treatment of rats with the antidepressant amitriptyline attenuates the activity of the hypothalamic-pituitary-adrenocortical system. *Endocrinology* 1993;133:312–320.
57. Rubinow DR, Gold PW, Post RM, et al. CSF somatostatin in affective illness. *Arch Gen Psychiatry* 1983;40:409–412.
58. Rupprecht R, Lesch KP, Müller U, Beck G, Beckmann H, Schulte HM. Blunted adrenocorticotropin but normal β-endorphin release after depression. *J Clin Endocrinol Metab* 1989;69:600–603.
59. Rupprecht R, Reul JMHM, Trapp T, et al. Progesterone receptor-mediated effects of neuroactive steroids. *Neuron* 1993;11:523–530.
60. Saito N, Guitart X, Hayward M, Tallman JF, Duman RS, Nestler EJ. Corticosterone differentially regulates the expression of G$_{s\alpha}$ messenger RNA and protein in rat cerebral cortex. *Proc Natl Acad Sci USA* 1989;86:3906–3910.
61. Sapolsky RM, Zola-Morgan S, Squire LR. Inhibition of glucocorticoid secretion by the hippocampal formation in the primate. *J Neurosci* 1991;11:3695–3704.
62. Schlegel S, von Bardeleben U, Wiedemann K, Frommberger U, Holsboer F. Computerized brain tomography measures compared with spontaneous and suppressed plasma cortisol levels in major depression. *Psychoneuroendocrinology* 1989;14:209–216.
63. Siever LJ, Trestman RL, Coccaro EF, et al. The growth hormone response to clonidine in acute and remitted depressed male patients. *Neuropsychopharmacology* 1992;6:165–177.
64. Sloviter RS, Valiquette G, Abrams GM, et al. Selective loss of hippocampal granule cells in the mature rat brain after adrenalectomy. *Science* 1989;243:535–538.
65. Spengler D, Rupprecht R, Phi Van L, Holsboer F. Identification and characterisation of a 3′,5′-cyclic adenosine monophosphate-responsive element in the human corticotropin-releasing hormone gene promoter. *Mol Endocrinol* 1992;6:1931–1941.
66. Spengler D, Waeber C, Pantaloni C, et al. Differential signal transduction patterns of five splice variants of the PACAP receptor. *Nature* 1993;365:170–175.
67. Steiger A, von Bardeleben U, Herth T, Holsboer F. Sleep-EEG and nocturnal secretion of cortisol and growth hormone in male patients with endogenous depression before treatment and after recovery. *J Affective Disord* 1989;16:189–195.
68. Steiger A, Guldner J, Hemmeter U, Rothe B, Wiedemann K, Holsboer F. Effects of growth hormone-releasing hormone and somatostatin on sleep EEG and nocturnal hormone secretion in male controls. *Neuroendocrinology* 1992;56:566–573.
69. Steiger A, Trachsel L, Guldner J, et al. Neurosteroid pregnenolone induces sleep-EEG changes in man compatible with inverse agonistic GABA$_A$ receptor modulation. *Brain Res* 1993;615:267–274.
70. Steiger A, Rupprecht R, Spengler D, et al. Functional properties of deoxycorticosterone and spironolactone: molecular characterization

and effects on sleep-endocrine activity. *J Psychiatr Res* 1993;27: 275–284.

71. Stein MB, Uhde TW. Triiodothyronine potentiation of tricyclic antidepressant treatment in patients with panic disorder. *Biol Psychiatry* 1990;28:1061–1064.

72. Stokes PE, Pick GR, Stoll PM, Nunn WD. Pituitary-adrenal function in depressed patients: resistence to dexamethasone suppression. *J Psychiatr Res* 1975;12:271–281.

73. Suri D, Hindmarsh PC, Brain CE, Pringle PJ, Brook CGD. The interaction between clonidine and growth hormone releasing hormone in the stimulation of growth hormone secretion in man. *Clin Endocrinol* 1990;33:399–406.

74. Valentino RJ, Foote SL, Aston-Jones G. Corticotropin-releasing factor activates noradrenergic neurons of the locus coeruleus. *Brain Res* 1983;270:363–367.

75. Veldhuis JD, Lizarralde G, Iranmanesh A. Divergent effects of short term glucocorticoid excess on the gonadotropic and somatotropic axes in normal men. *J Clin Endocrinol Metab* 1992;74:96–102.

76. Voderholzer U, Laakmann G, Hinz A, et al. Dependency of growth hormone (GH) stimulation following releasing hormones on the spontaneous 24-hour GH secretion in healthy male and female subjects. *Psychoneuroendocrinology* 1993;18:365–381.

77. von Bardeleben U, Holsboer F. Cortisol response to a combined dexamethasone-human corticotropin-releasing hormone challenge in patients with depression. *J Neuroendocrinol* 1989;1:485–488.

78. von Bardeleben U, Holsboer F. Effect of age on the cortisol response to human corticotropin-releasing hormone in depressed patients with dexamethasone. *Biol Psychiatry* 1991;29:1042–1050.

79. Wehrenberg WB, Janowski BA, Piering AW, Culler F, Jones KL. Glucocorticoids: potent inhibitors and stimulators of growth hormone secretion. *Endocrinology* 1990;126:3200–3203.

80. Wiedemann K, von Bardeleben U, Holsboer F. Influence of human corticotropin-releasing hormone and adrenocorticotropin upon spontaneous growth hormone secretion. *Neuroendocrinology* 1991;54:462–468.

81. Young EA, Haskett RF, Murphy-Weinberg V, Watson SJ, Huda A. Loss of glucocorticoid fast feedback in depression. *Arch Gen Psychiatry* 1991;48:693–699.

82. Young EA, Kotun J, Haskett RF, et al. Dissociation between pituitary and adrenal suppression to dexamethasone in depression. *Arch Gen Psychiatry* 1993;50:395–403.

Psychopharmacology: The Fourth Generation of Progress, edited by Floyd E. Bloom and David J. Kupfer. Raven Press, Ltd., New York © 1995.

CHAPTER 84

Neuropeptide Alterations in Mood Disorders

Paul M. Plotsky, Michael J. Owens, and Charles B. Nemeroff

The past several decades have witnessed an explosion of knowledge about the central nervous system (CNS). Dozens of peptide neurotransmitter and neuromodulator candidates have been identified and characterized, their CNS distributions mapped, and their genes cloned. Dale's principle of one neuron–one transmitter has been overturned (22) with numerous demonstrations of neurons containing multiple peptides or combinations of peptides and nonpeptides (32; see also Chapter 43, *this volume*). Additionally, the past ten years have yielded an embarrassment of riches in the form of neurotransmitter receptor diversity, diversity of receptor–effector coupling, and neurotransmitter transporters. These recent discoveries have not yet been fully integrated into our concepts of normal or aberrant CNS function, although dysfunction at any level could conceivably lead to neurological and cognitive disorders. Thus, although there are many choices for discussion, in this chapter, we have chosen to review three of the many peptide neurotransmitter systems: corticotropin-releasing factor (CRF), somatostatin (SRIF), and thyrotropin-releasing hormone (TRH). These have been selected on the basis of clinical interest in the potential consequences of dysregulation of these circuits for the pathophysiology of specific mood disorders. There has accumulated a considerable amount of basic and clinical research on these systems since the publication of the previous volume in 1987, but limitations of this volume prevent extensive citations of the original literature and, thus, the reader is referred to recent reviews.

CORTICOTROPIN-RELEASING FACTOR

After a search spanning three decades, CRF was isolated and characterized by Vale's group in 1981 as a 41-

amino acid peptide (83; see also Chapter 45, *this volume*). Corticotropin-releasing factor is a primary and an obligatory hypothalamic adrenocorticotropic hormone (ACTH) secretagogue in most species (61); it also appears to function as a putative neurotransmitter in a CNS network and may coordinate global responses to stressors. Along with its homologs, CRF represents an ancient family of peptides subserving numerous functions. In the higher organisms, including mammals, evidence supports the hypothesis that CRF plays a complex role in integrating the endocrine, autonomic, immunological, and behavioral responses of an organism to stress (20,58). Of particular concern in this chapter are the clinical ramifications drawn from the remerging evidence implicating dysregulation of central CRF circuits in association with mood and anxiety disorders, as well as anorexia nervosa and Alzheimer's disease, disorders also commonly associated with comorbid mood alterations. A more complete review of CRF neurobiology, with citations, is presented in Chapter 45 (*this volume*) and reviews by Dunn and Berridge (20) and Owens and Nemeroff (58).

Preclinical Studies

The Hypothalamic–Pituitary–Adrenal Axis

The synthesis and secretion of glucocorticoids represents the final step in a neuroendocrine cascade beginning in the CNS. Physical and psychological stressors, circadian drive, and humoral influences initiate the cascade by releasing multiple hypothalamic ACTH secretagogues into the hypophyseal–portal circulation (61). Elaborated by perikarya in the hypothalamic parvocellular paraventricular nuclei (pPVN), CRF plays an integral and obligatory role in the regulation of adenohypophyseal ACTH and β-endorphin production and secretion, as well as expression and synthesis of their precursor, proopiomelanocortin (POMC).

P. M. Plotsky, M. J. Owens, and C. B. Nemeroff: Department of Psychiatry and Behavioral Sciences, Emory University School of Medicine, Atlanta, Georgia 30322.

The negative feedback loop necessary for hypothalamic–pituitary–adrenal (HPA) axis regulation is completed by ACTH-induced glucocorticoid secretion (16). Many stressors have been shown to increase CRF messenger ribonucleic acid (mRNA) concentrations in the pPVN, whereas glucocorticoids negatively regulate CRF mRNA concentrations in the PVN. It has been suggested that the adaptive function of the HPA axis is critically dependent on glucocorticoid feedback mechanisms to dampen the stressor-induced activation of the HPA axis and to shut off further glucocorticoid secretion. In animal models, exogenous CRF or endogenous hypersecretion of CRF leads to reproductive failure, altered locomotor activity, reduced food intake, sleep disruption, hypercortisolemia, and dexamethasone resistance (20,58); these effects are similar to the changes observed in patients with major depression.

Preclinical studies by Meaney et al. (50) and Plotsky and Meaney (62) on the long-term consequences of the neonatal environment support the hypothesis that early, severe, or chronic stress may be transduced into neurobiological changes, which then increase an organism's probability of exhibiting clinically significant mood disorders (63,64). In animal models, chronic elevation of CRF secretion can lead to increased corticotrope numbers (26), which may underlie the observed increase of pituitary size in depressed patients (see ref. 43 for review). Furthermore, transgenic mice, which overproduce CRF (81) or lack glucocorticoid receptors (59) exhibit behavioral and endocrine signs consistent with major clinical depression. Hypersecretion of hypothalamic CRF is clearly associated with down-regulation of adenohypophyseal CRF receptor numbers (30), thus giving rise to a blunted ACTH and normal or exaggerated glucocorticoid responses to exogenous CRF administration (see ref. 68 for review).

Extrahypothalamic Corticotropin-Releasing Factor

Mapping of the distribution of CRF-like activity in the CNS using immunohistochemistry and radioimmunoassay revealed a wide extrahypothalamic distribution compatible with its involvement in stress responses, emotionality, and cognition. In particular, CRF activity has been reported in forebrain limbic areas and in autonomic and viscerosensory brainstem nuclei (see Chapter 45, *this volume*).

Consistent with its role as a putative neurotransmitter, central administration of CRF mimics many of the behavioral and autonomic aspects of the stress response (20,42,58). Conversely, pretreatment with a specific CRF antagonist attenuates many of the behavioral and autonomic components of the stress response. This may be interpreted as support for the hypothesis that endogenous CRF acts on extrahypophyseal targets to produce autonomic and behavioral components of stress responses. In

most, but not all, cases these effects have been demonstrated to be independent of the effects of CRF on HPA function. As reviewed in Dunn and Berridge (20) and Koob et al. (42), CRF has been found to: (a) increase the latency to begin eating in food-deprived animals provided food in a novel setting, (b) increase the acoustic startle response, and (c) decrease punished-responding. In each case, these effects are reversed by benzodiazapine treatment. The CRF receptor antagonist, α-helical CRF$_{9-41}$, although certainly not an anxiolytic drug, attenuates some, but not all, of the behavioral effects of stressors.

Clinical Studies in Mood Disorders

Dysregulation of the HPA axis in major depression remains one of the most consistent findings in biological psychiatry (reviewed in ref. 68). Since the association between HPA axis dysfunction and major depression was made, neuroendocrine function tests have served as a window into the brain in attempts to elucidate mechanisms that underlie the pathophysiology. A subset of patients fulfilling DSM-III-R criteria for major depression often present with a constellation of symptoms including hypercortisolemia, resistance of cortisol to suppression by dexamethasone, blunted ACTH responses to CRF challenge as compared to controls, and elevated CRF concentrations in the cerebrospinal fluid (CSF). The pathological mechanisms underlying HPA axis dysregulation in major depression and other affective disorders remain to be elucidated.

Administration of rat, human, or ovine CRF yields blunted ACTH, β-lipotropin, and β-endorphin secretion with a normal cortisol response in patients with major depression (3,28,33,44,85). Patients with posttraumatic stress disorder (79), 50% of whom also fulfill DSM-III criteria for major depression, and patients with panic disorder (70) also show blunted ACTH secretion in response to CRF challenge. In patients with major depression, a correlation appears to exist between DST nonsuppression and a blunted ACTH response to CRF challenge (44), suggesting that these features may represent state markers for depression. According to Amsterdam et al. (3), normalization of the ACTH response to CRF challenge occurs following clinical recovery.

Two hypotheses have been advanced to account for the observed blunting of ACTH secretion in response to CRF challenge that is associated with major depression: (a) down-regulation of adenohypophyseal CRF receptors occurs as a result of hypothalamic CRF hypersecretion, and (b) increased glucocorticoid-mediated negative feedback tone at the pituitary or CNS. Although the first hypothesis has not been directly tested in humans by measurement of postmortem hypothalamic CRF secretion or mRNA content or by the assessment of anterior pituitary CRF receptor function or mRNA levels, substantial support has accumulated favoring it. Animal studies (*vide supra*) show down-regulation of adenohypophyseal CRF receptors under conditions of chronic stress and/or elevated CRF. Postmortem measurements of CNS CRF receptors in the frontal cortex demonstrate down-regulation in suicide victims (56) who were, presumably, suffering from depression. Finally, preliminary data from our laboratory suggests the presence of increased CRF mRNA in the hypothalamus of suicide victims versus age- and sex-matched controls. Less data is available to support the second hypothesis. In all of these studies, neuroendocrine studies represent a secondary measure of CNS activity; pituitary ACTH responses reflect the activity of hypothalamic CRF rather than that of the corticolimbic circuits, which are likely to be involved in the pathophysiology of major depression.

A potentially more direct avenue for evaluation of extrahypothalamic CRF tone may be obtained from measurements of CRF in ventricular or lumbar CSF. A marked dissociation between CSF and plasma neuropeptide concentrations has been described, thus indicating that neuropeptides are secreted directly into CSF from brain tissue as opposed to being derived from plasma-to-CSF transfer (65). Evidence that CRF concentrations in CSF originate from nonhypophyseotropic CRF has been obtained from studies in which CRF concentrations in CSF were repeatedly measured over the course of the day. Moreover, CRF concentrations in rhesus monkey CSF are not entrained with pituitary–adrenal activity (24). The proximity of corticolimbic, brainstem, and spinal CRF neurons to the ventricular system suggests that these areas contribute to the CRF pool found in CSF.

In a series of studies, Nemeroff's group has demonstrated significant elevation of CRF in the CSF of drug-free patients with major depression or following suicide. In the initial study, CRF was measured in the CSF of 10 normal controls, 23 depressed patients, 11 schizophrenics, and 29 demented patients; CSF concentrations of CRF were elevated in the depressed patients compared to all of the other groups (57). In a larger study of CRF in the CSF of 54 depressed patients, 138 neurological controls, 23 schizophrenic patients, and 6 manic patients, the depressed patients exhibited a marked twofold elevation in CSF–CRF concentrations. Collection of postmortem cisternal CSF–CRF concentrations from postmoterm depressed suicide victims and sudden death controls also revealed elevated CRF concentrations in the depressed group (5). Risch et al. (67) have confirmed these findings of elevated CSF concentrations of CRF in depressed patients.

Elevation of CSF concentrations of CRF has also been reported in patients with anorexia nervosa (38) and reverts to the normal range as these patients approach normal body weight. No alterations of CSF concentrations of CRF appear to be associated with other psychiatric disorders including mania, panic disorder, and somatization disorders as compared to controls (8,36).

More critically, Nemeroff et al. (53) have shown that the elevated CRF concentrations in the CSF of depressed patients (versus normal controls) are significantly decreased 24 hr after final electroconvulsive therapy (ECT) treatment indicating that CSF–CRF concentrations, like hypercortisolemia, represent a state rather than a trait marker. Other recent studies have confirmed this normalization of CRF concentrations in the CSF following successful therapeutic intervention. Banki et al. (9) demonstrated significant reduction of elevated CRF in the CSF of 15 female patients with major depression who remained depression-free for at least 6 months following antidepressant treatment as compared to little significant treatment effect on CRF in the CSF of nine patients who relapsed in this 6-month period. The authors suggest that elevated or increasing CSF concentrations of CRF during antidepressant treatment may indicate lack of normalization in major depression despite symptomatic improvement and, thus may predict early relapse. Treatment of depressives with fluoxetine (18) is also reported to reduce CRF concentrations in CSF.

Increased central drive to the pituitary–adrenal axis is associated with an increase in the number and volume of corticotropes as well as adrenal gland hypertrophy (16,76). Recently, Krishnan (43) reviewed magnetic resonance imaging (MRI) and computed tomography (CT) studies of changes in human pituitary and adrenal cross-sectional area and volume in patients with mood disorders. Two studies reported enlargement of the pituitary gland in depressed patients as compared to age- and sex-matched controls. Furthermore, a significant correlation existed between pituitary gland enlargement and post-dexamethasone cortisol concentrations. In a study of postmortem tissue, Zis and Zis (86) observed adrenal gland enlargement in suicide victims versus controls, a result first observed in an early CT study (4). This has been confirmed in a study comparing adrenal volume by CT in depressed and age- and sex-matched normal controls (55); however, adrenal volume did not correlate with dexamethasone suppression test results, patient age, or the severity or duration of the depressive episode. A study by Rubin et al. (71) confirmed the finding of adrenal enlargement and presented evidence of the state dependency of this change. Correlation of these depression-associated changes in pituitary and adrenal size with the results of CRF stimulation tests and CRF concentrations in CSF would be welcome.

Summary

In the relatively short span of a decade, the putative role of CRF has expanded from that of a classical hypophysiotropic factor participating in the regulation of pituitary–adrenal drive to that of a central neurotransmitter implicated in organization of counterregulatory responses to a variety of stressors. This expanded role was first suggested by immunohistochemical mapping studies, which identified a unique extrahypothalamic distribution of CRF and was further supported by electrophysiological, pharmacological, and behavioral work in animals and, subsequently, in clinical studies. From these studies, it is clear that dysfunction of central CRF systems is associated with selected mood disorders. However, neither the exact nature of these dysfunctions nor whether they represent primary or secondary defects is yet clear.

Functional alterations in the HPA axis and central CRF systems have been studied most extensively in patients with major depression. Current evidence leads to the hypothesis of CRF hypersecretion of either hypothalamic or extrahypothalamic origin. Evidence of a hypersecretory state in depression may be inferred from basic and clinical observations of down-regulation of CRF receptors in the adenohypophysis and frontal cortex, increased CRF concentrations in CSF, blunted ACTH response to a standard CRF stimulation test, and enlarged pituitary and adrenal areas and volumes as assessed by MRI or CT scans. Many, if not all, of these abnormalities revert to normal after successful treatment of depression. Therefore, in major depressive illness, the neuroendocrine system serves as a window into the brain, with abnormalities reflecting a state, rather than a trait marker of depression. Interpretation of the cerebrocortical reductions in CRF concentration in brains from patients with Alzheimer's disease is unclear. Enhanced receptor numbers in these brains support the hypothesis of reduced CRF secretion; however, no direct demonstration of degeneration of CRF-containing neurons in this disorder has been reported. Furthermore, as in depression, little work has been performed at the molecular level. Although extrahypothalamic CRF circuits are increasingly accepted as participating in cognitive processes, it is unclear which, if any, symptoms of Alzheimer's disease are secondary to the pathological involvement of CRF neurons in this disease.

Overall, then, many important research avenues remain open with respect to the role of CRF in mood disorders. Postmortem studies of CNS tissue from these patients at the molecular level are in progress in our laboratory and at numerous other sites; the results from these studies are bound to lead to new insights into the pathophysiology of these diseases. However, it will be important to examine tissue from numerous control groups drawn from age- and sex-matched disease-free populations as well as from populations representative of other neurological disease states. The recent cloning of the CRF-binding protein and the CRF receptor provides new tools, both specific molecular probes and antisera, for assessing changes in these entities in various disease states. On the basis of the considerable pharmacological and behavioral work cited above, it is clear that one of the most exciting areas

will be the development of long-acting, CNS-potent CRF-like agents. One exciting prospect would be the possibility of using a CRF antagonist or CRF-binding protein analog for the treatment of depression and/or anxiety disorders. Perhaps the recent cloning of the CRF-binding protein and the CRF receptor will aid in the elucidation of the active portion of the peptide or the active site on the receptor. These discoveries may lead to the rational design of lipophilic drugs that will be clinically useful. Finally, design of appropriate ligands for PET scanning would permit evaluation of CRF receptor distribution and, perhaps, affinity during the course of these diseases.

SOMATOSTATIN

Somatostatin (somatotropin release-inhibiting factor, SRIF), like a number of other neuropeptides, was serendipitously discovered during attempts to purify growth hormone-releasing factor (GRF). As the name implies, somatostatin inhibits the release of growth hormone from the anterior pituitary. Since its structural identification 20 years ago, somatostatin has been unequivocally shown to be the major inhibitory influence on endocrine growth hormone secretion. Additionally, and perhaps of more interest, somatostatin fulfills a number of criteria for status as a neurotransmitter within the CNS. The acceptance of somatostatin's role as a neurotransmitter has led to its investigation in a number of psychiatric and neurological diseases. As will be discussed below, nonendocrine somatostatin neurons may play a role in a number of illnesses including, but not limited to, depression, dementia, and epilepsy (see also Chapter 49, *this volume*).

Preclinical Studies

Prior to discussion of somatostatin's role in mood disorders, we briefly review several aspects of basic somatostatin neurobiology. Interested readers will find a detailed description of somatostatin neurobiology and preclinical pharmacology in Chapter 49 (*this volume*).

Radioimmunoassay and immunocytochemical studies reveal that somatostatin-containing neurons are heterogenously distributed throughout the CNS. High concentrations of somatostatin are found in the hypothalamus and median eminence, amygdala, hippocampus, cerebral cortex, medial preoptic area, and nucleus accumbens. Cell bodies are most numerous in the preoptic and periventricular nuclei of the hypothalamus, although they are present in significant amounts in cortical and limbic regions as well. As is increasingly the case with many neurotransmitter systems, somatostatin is colocalized within a number of other monoamine- or neuropeptide-containing neurons. Moreover, like many neuropeptide systems, the distribution of somatostatin neurons in humans is similar, but not identical, to that observed in rodents. Of the two major forms of somatostatin present in the body (somatostatin$_{1-14}$ and somatostatin$_{1-28}$), somatostatin$_{1-14}$ is the major form found in the brain (70% to 80%).

Studies have shown that pharmacologically distinct somatostatin receptor subtypes exist in the CNS with different affinities for somatostatin analogs, differential localization, differential coupling to second messenger systems, and functional responses. These have been termed SRIF$_1$ and SRIF$_2$ receptors of which the SRIF$_1$ subtype is most predominant. Recently, four distinct somatostatin receptors (SSTR$_1$–SSTR$_4$) have been cloned. The receptor sequences appear to be highly conserved across species and are members of the G-protein coupled family of receptors.

Electrophysiological experiments have revealed both excitatory and inhibitory actions of somatostatin. Central administration of somatostatin has been observed to alter cholinergic, dopaminergic, noradrenergic, and serotonergic neurotransmission. Moreover, not only does somatostatin regulate growth hormone release from the anterior pituitary, somatostatin can also inhibit the secretion of a number of other hormones, particularly TSH, and CRF-stimulated ACTH secretion.

Like many other neuropeptide transmitters, central administration of somatostatin produces a variety of behavioral and physiological effects. Briefly, the peptide can produce a nonopioid-mediated analgesia in animals and man. Changes in sleep patterns, food consumption, locomotor activity and memory are also altered by somatostatin administration. This wide spectrum of effects of somatostatin led to investigation of its involvement in a number of psychiatric and neurological disorders. Of particular interest is the fact that the above changes in sleep, eating, activity, and anterior pituitary hormone secretion are all altered in depression.

Clinical Studies in Mood Disorders

The greatest number of clinical studies with somatostatin have focused on its involvement in neurological disorders. Consistent decreases in tissue and CSF concentrations of somatostatin are observed in senile dementia, Alzheimer's disease, Parkinson's disease, and multiple sclerosis during relapse. Somatostatin neurons have been found to be a major source of the observed plaques and tangles associated with Alzheimer's pathology. In contrast to the decrements in central somatostatin measures, elevated CSF concentrations of somatostatin, presumably reflecting leakage from neuronal damage, are observed in patients suffering from a number of inflammatory or destructive neurological disorders including spinal cord compression, destructive cerebral disease, meningitis, and metabolic encephalopathy.

Preclinical studies showing that central administration of somatostatin can alter sleep patterns, appetite, locomo-

tor activity, and cognition have created interest in investigating somatostatin's role in mood disorders. The clearest evidence for involvement of somatostatin in psychiatric illness has come from studies of major depression. A consistent decrease has been reported in CSF somatostatin concentrations in depressed individuals. In primates, CSF somatostatin has been reported to undergo circadian variation, with concentrations varying 10% over 24 hr with the highest concentrations observed at night (6). Although the reported differences between depressed and normal patients are substantially greater than 10%, this circadian variation emphasizes the need for attempts at CSF sampling at uniform times. Although Rubinow et al. (72) did not find any time-of-day differences in patients, he did note large differences (increases and decreases) in subjects who were sampled in both morning and evening. Research over the past 15 years on a number of neuropeptides in CSF have revealed that they are almost exclusively of central origin, although the actual sites are unclear (65,66). Decreases in CSF somatostatin concentrations are proposed to be the result of decreased neuronal synthesis and release. Whether this is a primary or secondary effect of the illness is unknown (see below).

Gerner and Yamada (25) first reported CSF somatostatin changes in psychiatric patients. In their study, medication-free patients with either depression or anorexia nervosa had decreased somatostatin concentrations versus either normal controls or healthy young women, respectively. This was replicated shortly thereafter in a large study by Rubinow and colleagues (73). Although there was considerable overlap, CSF somatostatin was significantly decreased in depressed patients, whether unipolar or bipolar. Moreover, whereas CSF somatostatin levels did not correlate with severity of depression, CSF values in clinically improved patients rose toward concentrations in normal subjects. In nine bipolar patients followed longitudinally, CSF somatostatin concentrations were significantly lower during the depressed state than during improved or manic states. In this study, CSF somatostatin concentrations were similar in men and women as well as across age in the subjects. Following the addition of a number of patients to his original study, Rubinow (72) again reported lower levels CSF somatostatin in depressed patients than in normal subjects, improved depressed patients, manics, dysthymics, or schizophrenics. No correlations between somatostatin and age among the depressed patients, severity of depression, or time of day were observed. In a large study lacking controls, Ågren and Lundqvist (1) reported significant correlations between severity of depression and CSF somatostatin concentrations. Moreover, CSF somatostatin was significantly lower in patients studied during their worst week of depression compared to those studied more than two months following their most severe week of depression. Black et al. (13) also reported decreased ventricular CSF somatostatin concentrations in medicated depressed patients referred for cingulotomy compared with lumbar CSF from normal controls. Bissette et al. (12) have also observed decreased CSF somatostatin in depressed patients. Like the patients of Ågren and Lundqvist (1), CSF somatostatin concentrations were not correlated to post-dexamethasone cortisol concentrations.

In contrast to this finding, Doran et al. (19) reported a significant negative correlation between post-dexamethasone plasma cortisol concentrations and CSF somatostatin concentrations in depressed patients. Kling et al. (41) have also reported decreased CSF somatostatin concentrations in depressed patients. Rather than a simple linear relationship, these investigators observed an inverted U-shape relationship between post-dexamethasone cortisol and CSF somatostatin concentrations in the depressed patients, suggesting a complicated relationship between central somatostatin neurons and hypothalamic CRF neurons. As we noted earlier in the chapter, neuropeptide systems, many of which we are more familiar with as hypothalamic releasing factors involved in behavior, are likely to be of both extrahypothalamic and hypothalamic origin. Sunderland et al. (82) reported similar decreases in CSF somatostatin in older depressed patients with no correlation between CSF concentrations and severity of depression. Davis et al. (17) also observed decreased CSF somatostatin concentrations in older depressed patients versus elderly controls. Molchan et al. (51) observed similar findings in elderly depressed and control populations. Moreover, CSF somatostatin from depressed Alzheimer's disease (AD) patients was significantly lower than the already low nondepressed Alzheimer's population. Although CSF 5-hydroxyindole acetic acid (5-HIAA) did not differ among diagnostic categories, CSF somatostatin and 5-HIAA were positively correlated among both AD and non-AD depressed groups (i.e., the lower the 5-HIAA concentrations, the lower the somatostatin concentrations). Whether these are related or separate results and/or causes of depression is unclear, although a number of monoamine transmitter systems can alter somatostatin neuronal activity (see Chapter 49, this volume).

Somatostatin concentrations in CSF have also been examined in several other psychiatric disorders. Kaye et al. (39) found no differences in anorexics, but observed a small increase in CSF somatostatin concentrations in normal weight bulimics when they stopped binging. Berrettini et al. (11) found no differences in CSF somatostatin between controls, unmedicated euthymic bipolar patients, and lithium-treated bipolar patients. Altemus et al. (2) reported significantly higher CSF somatostatin concentrations in patients with obsessive–compulsive disorder (OCD) compared to controls. Although a normal control group was lacking, Kruesi et al. (45) also reported an increase in CSF somatostatin levels in a small group of children with OCD versus a group of children with conduct disorder.

Few postmortem studies of CNS somatostatin in de-

pressed patients have been reported to date. Charlton et al. (15) found no differences in temporal or occipital cortex somatostatin concentrations or somatostatin receptor affinity or number in a small group of controls (N = 7) versus depressed patients who died of coincidental physical illness while inpatients at a psychiatric hospital (N = 9). In another study of seven depressed patients and twelve controls, Bowen et al. (14) measured somatostatin concentrations in the pars opercularis and orbital gyrus of the frontal lobe, the parahippocampal gyrus and pole of the temporal lobe, and postcentral gyrus and superior lobule of the parietal lobe. Significant decreases (30%) in somatostatin concentrations were observed only in the pole of the temporal lobe. Although these studies are complicated by wide ranges of postmortem delay until sampling and freezing of the tissue and further complicated by the finding that somatostatin concentrations decrease within the first 6 hr following death (80), studies of this nature are exceptionally useful and sorely needed.

As mentioned in Chapter 49 (this volume), preclinical studies show that a variety of neurotransmitter systems can alter CNS somatostatin neurons. Of the centrally active drugs used clinically, serotonin-selective uptake inhibitors increase somatostatin concentrations in rat brain (37). In a group of depressed patients, carbamazepine was found to produce a significant decrease in CSF somatostatin concentrations (74). The same study found that the selective serotonin (5-HT) uptake inhibitor, zimelidine, significantly increased CSF somatostatin in five of five patients. In a small group of patients, neither desipramine nor lithium had any effect on CSF somatostatin concentrations. The further reductions in CSF somatostatin produced by carbamazepine were not correlated to worsening or improvement of symptoms. This finding suggests that (a) somatostatin may be implicated in the anticonvulsant mechanism of action of carbamazepine, and (b) together with the neurological disorders characterized by decreased CSF somatostatin concentrations without necessarily having concomitant changes in mood, decreases in CSF somatostatin are not responsible for the changes in affect seen in depression.

Summary

Although the data is still relatively limited, an overview of the extant literature suggests that decreases in CSF somatostatin are a consistent state-dependent finding of depression. Indeed, next to the hypercortisolemia associated with depression, this may be one of the more consistent findings in biological psychiatry. However, it probably does not possess any diagnostic usefulness, because similar changes are observed in a number of neurological disorders without psychiatric comorbidity. However, it appears to be associated with impairment in cognitive function. Evidence is beginning to appear to suggest that the decrease in CSF somatostatin may be related to the overactivity of the HPA axis seen in depression. Whether one is responsible for the other or both are responses to dysregulation of other neurotransmitter systems associated with depression is unknown. Finally, somatostatin-active drugs may not be of therapeutic usefulness as changes in CSF somatostatin apparently do not affect mood. Nevertheless, rational design of peptide- or nonpeptide-based drugs selectively active at different receptor subtypes will certainly aid in understanding somatostatin's role in behavior and may lead to therapeutic benefits.

THYROTROPIN-RELEASING HORMONE

The early availability of adequate tools (i.e., assays, synthetic peptides) coupled with observations that primary hypothyroidism can cause depressive symptomatology ensured extensive investigation of the involvement of the hypothalamic–pituitary–thyroid (HPT) axis in mood disorders (see ref. 48 for a review). Interested readers will find a detailed description, along with citations, of TRH neurobiology and preclinical pharmacology in Chapter 44 (this volume). Thyrotropin releasing hormone, a pyroglutamylhistidylprolinamide tripeptide, was the first of the hypothalamic releasing hormones to be isolated and characterized. In its role as a hypophysiotropic factor, TRH is released from hypothalamic nerve endings in the median eminence into the primary capillary plexus of the hypophyseal–portal circulatory system where it is transported to thyrotropes in the adenohypophysis. Then, TRH diffuses out of these capillaries and binds to specific membrane receptors to facilitate the release and synthesis of thyroid-stimulating hormone (TSH). Circulating TSH acts at the thyroid gland to evoke release of L-triiodothyronine (T_3) and thyroxine (T_4).

Early studies established the hypothalamic and extrahypothalamic distribution of TRH (reviewed in ref. 52). This extensive extrahypothalamic presence of TRH quickly led to speculation that TRH might function as a neurotransmitter or neuromodulator. Subsequent studies established the necessary foundation required to seriously consider TRH in such a role. Thyrotropin-releasing hormone is concentrated in nerve terminal regions and presumably stored in synaptic vesicles. Enzymes were identified in the CNS which inactivate TRH and, thus, could curtail its action following release. Specific, high-affinity TRH receptors were characterized and found to be widely and selectively distributed throughout the CNS. Electrophysiological studies provided evidence that TRH directly altered neuronal activity. Thus, a large body of evidence supports the involvement of TRH as a hypophysiotropic factor and as a neurotransmitter or neuromodulator.

Preclinical Studies

Administration of exogenous TRH is associated with a variety of physiological and behavioral effects including alterations in cardiovascular function, respiratory rate, body temperature, gastric secretion, colonic motility, and electroencephalographic activity (52; see also Chapter 44, this volume). Interest in putative CNS actions of TRH were stimulated by studies of the thyroid axis and depression by Prange and colleagues (see Chapter 44, this volume). Utilizing the mouse L-dopa potentiation test to screen for putative antidepressant effects, Plotnikoff et al. (60) found that TRH produced enhancement of motor activity, a behavioral marker of compounds possessing putative antidepressant efficacy. Indeed, the effects of TRH in this test were similar to those observed in imipramine-treated mice, suggesting that TRH might act as an antidepressant compound. Importantly, TRH was equally effective in intact and hypophysectomized mice, thus indicating that the observed effects were not dependent upon activation of the HPT axis but instead reflected a direct CNS action of TRH.

Profound increases in CNS activity evoked by electroconvulsive shock (ECS) administered on an alternate-day schedule for 5 days (46) produced pronounced increases in TRH concentration in limbic regions, including the amygdala and hippocampus. Neither administration of a single ECS treatment nor administration of a subconvulsant electrical current altered TRH in any region assayed, indicating that the induction of a seizure was essential to produce effects on TRH. Other observations suggest that the efficacy of TRH or analogs in the treatment of seizure disorders is an area ripe for further evaluation. In summary, these animal studies have highlighted the wide range of physiological and behavioral effects exerted by TRH. One may speculate on the possibility that limbic system TRH-containing circuits may mediate, in part, the antidepressant actions of ECT and may be involved in the pathophysiological mechanisms of seizure disorders. The potential clinical implications of these studies include the possible utility of TRH in treating overdoses of sedatives or hypnotics and in treating certain forms of epilepsy.

Learned helplessness, an animal model of depression (31), can be reversed by many clinically effective antidepressants and by ECT. Interestingly, when these animals are rendered hypothyroid they exhibit resistance to the effects of tricyclic antidepressants and treatment with thyroid hormone reverses the antidepressant resistance. Over a decade ago, Whybrow and Prange (84) hypothesized that thyroid function was integral to the pathogenesis of, and recovery from, mood disorders because of the copious interactions among thyroid hormones, catecholamines, and adrenergic receptors in the central nervous system. Overall, these studies suggest a role for thyroid dysfunction in refractory depression and are consonant with clinical studies suggesting the existence of an increased rate of hypothyroidism among patients with refractory depression. Furthermore, animal and clinical studies suggest that depressive symptoms in hypothyroid patients may, in part, be determined by thyroid function before the onset of depression (reviewed in ref. 34).

Clinical Studies in Mood Disorders

The use of TRH as a provocative agent for assessment of thyroid-axis function evolved rapidly after its isolation and synthesis. A relatively standard protocol involves measurement of basal plasma TSH concentrations followed by intravenous administration of exogenous TRH (200 to 500 μg) with subsequent measurement of plasma TSH concentrations at 30-min intervals for a period of 2 to 3 hr (77). Clinical use of the TRH stimulation test to assess hypothalamic–pituitary–thyroid (HPT) axis function revealed blunting of the TSH response in approximately 25% of euthyroid patients with major depression, as reviewed by Loosen (48), Nemeroff (52), and Howland (34). These data have been widely confirmed, and it has been proposed that decreased nocturnal plasma TSH concentration may be a sensitive marker of depression (10). Using a modified TRH stimulation test in which the peptide (200 μg) is administered intravenously at 8 a.m. and at 11 p.m. Duval et al. (21) claimed a diagnostic specificity of 95% and a diagnostic sensitivity of 89%. The difference in the TSH response between the 11 p.m. and 8 a.m. tests appears to be markedly reduced in depressed patients as compared to controls. Recently, Shelton et al. (78) reported that among outpatients with major depression, 26% percent showed some abnormality of thyroid hormone concentrations; the majority of these were normalized by antidepressant treatment. Even though antidepressants did not exhibit a statistically significant effect on thyroid hormone concentrations when tested across the whole group, it must be noted that patients in this study did not exhibit a high frequency of TSH blunting to TRH. Overall, this study implies that subpopulations of the more severely depressed patients may be more likely to exhibit TSH blunting and elevations of T_4 prior to therapy. The relevance of TRH to psychiatric disorders has recently been reviewed by Nemeroff (52).

The observed blunting of TSH in depressed patients does not appear to be the result of excessive negative feedback from secretion of either thyroid hormone or somatostatin hypersecretion. In fact, as noted above in detail, depressed patients exhibit reduced CSF concentrations of SRIF. It is possible, although unlikely, that the blunting is a reflection of pituitary TRH receptor downregulation as a result of median eminence hypersecretion of endogenous TRH (65). The observation that lumbar CSF concentrations of TRH are higher in depressed patients than in controls supports a hypothesis of TRH hy-

persecretion but does not elucidate the origin of this tripeptide (7). The Banki study consisted of 16 control subjects (12 patients diagnosed as having only peripheral neurological disease and 4 patients having a DSM-III diagnosis of somatization disorder) and 17 patients with major depression. None of the subjects had been treated with psychotropic medications for at least 2 weeks prior to start of the study. The mean CSF concentration of TRH for the combined control group was 4.4 ± 1.8 pg/ml, whereas the concentration in the depressed group was 12.8 ± 5.7 pg/ml. In animal models, chronic administration of TRH for 2 to 3 weeks results in of the TSH response to TRH, and decreased circulating concentrations of TSH, T_3, and T_4 (54). Furthermore, repeated administration of TRH in humans also produces a blunted TSH response to TRH (49). Finally, these elevations of TRH concentration in CSF may be relatively specific to depression, as no such alteration has been reported in patients with Alzheimer's disease, anxiety disorders, or alcoholism (23,69). Clearly, further studies for which CSF test concentrations are measured are needed.

Although the majority of depressed patients readily respond to treatment with antidepressants, approximately 15% to 30% of depressed patients are treatment refractory (75). Approximately 15% of depressed patients display Grade III hypothyroidism, characterized by normal T_3, T_4, and TSH concentrations and an exaggerated TSH response to the TRH stimulation test, and almost 60% of these patients have detectable antimicrosomal and/or antithyroglobulin antibodies in their circulation (27). Interestingly, approximately 50% of depressed patients who are DST nonsuppressers exhibit exaggerated TSH (29). Overall, the rate of asymptomatic autoimmune thyroiditis (SAT) in depressed patients is greater than would be expected in the general population (34,52). It may be postulated that the development of autoimmune thyroiditis gives rise to hypersecretion of hypothalamic TRH as a compensatory mechanism to maintain normal plasma T_3 and T_4 concentrations. A considerable literature, recently reviewed by Joffee et al. (35), exists regarding interactions between the HPT axis and mood disorders.

Summary

Preclinical studies have added to our current understanding of the physiological and behavioral effects exerted by TRH. However, clinical studies of TRH in depression have yielded mixed results with no definitive role for TRH in the pathophysiology or treatment of any psychiatric disorder. Thus, despite the initial promise offered by early preclinical and clinical studies of TRH, many subsequent investigations have yielded equivocal results. At present, the diagnostic validity of the TRH stimulation test remains open to question with respect to depression. However, several investigators have suggested that this test demonstrates prognostic value in predicting treatment responses. For instance, Langer et al. (47) presented evidence to suggest that a change in the TSH response from blunted to normal predicts a positive response to antidepressant therapy, whereas Kirkegaard (40) suggested that the TSH response to a TRH challenge appears to be of value in predicting long-term clinical outcome (remission or relapse) following completion of therapy. Obviously, additional studies are required to clarify the potential clinical utility of the TRH stimulation test in the diagnosis and treatment of depression.

Thus despite years of study, considerable gaps in our knowledge remain. Many avenues for future experimentation are available. A concerted effort should be made to perform postmortem measurements of regional brain TRH concentrations, mRNA levels of TRH, pituitary and brain TRH receptor kinetics, and mRNA concentrations of TRH, as well as postreceptor signal transduction in tissues obtained from depressed suicide victims and well-matched controls. Furthermore, studies of CSF concentrations of TRH and rhythms should be performed in populations of depressed patients, those with autoimmune thyroiditis, and well-matched controls. Finally, the synthesis of a long-acting TRH analog as well as development of a lipophilic TRH radioligand permitting PET/SPECT visualization of TRH receptor density in the CNS and pituitary would be of great utility in assessing the importance of the interaction between the HPT axis and mood disorders.

FUTURE DIRECTIONS

Significant progress has been made over the past decade, and many new tools have entered the basic and clinical scientist's armamentarium. Application of the RNase protection assay and of in situ hybridization will permit detection and mapping of specific mRNAs in experimental animal CNS and in human postmortem CNS tissue. Widespread use of these methods will yield a picture of the concentrations and distributions of CRF, SRIF, and TRH in mRNAs and their receptor mRNAs in normal subjects, those with mood disorders, and those with other disorders. For those mRNAs of particularly low abundance, in situ hybridization or RNase protection assays may be preceded with polymerase chain reaction (PCR) amplification of the target mRNA. Studies to assess postmortem stability of the mRNAs of interest will be necessary and might be most easily accomplished using CNS tissue removed during neurosurgical procedures and then subject to controlled processing delays. A more accurate determination of transcriptional activity may be derived by measurement of heteronuclear RNA (hnRNA) using intronic antisense hybridization probes in RNase protection or in situ hybridization protocols. However, the rapid turnover time and small pool size of nuclear hnRNA will necessitate rigid control of the postmortem delay and studies of hnRNA stability after death.

With our advancing knowledge of potential peptidinergic circuit or peptide receptor dysfunction contributing to the pathophysiology of mood disorders, the development of animal models will assume increasing importance. This may be most readily accomplished using transgenic overexpression or knock-out models or by the use of stereotaxic microinjection of sense or antisense RNA directly or carried by adenovirus or modified herpes virus vectors. Using these models, the consequences of hypo- or hyperactivity of each of these neuropeptides or receptor systems may be assessed at the neurobiological and behavioral levels, and potential therapeutic approaches may be developed.

Another exciting development is the ability to image CNS tissue using MRI, PET, and variants of these methods. It is becoming possible to monitor CNS circuits in action in healthy and diseased CNS tissue using metabolic markers and to assess receptor distribution using labeled ligands. As these techniques are refined with increases in sensitivity and resolution, they should have a major positive impact on both basic and clinical studies of the CNS mechanisms underlying mood disorders.

ACKNOWLEDGMENTS

We would like to thank Jan Fowler for assistance in preparation of this manuscript and the support of the National Institute of Mental Health through grants MH39415, MH42088, MH40524, and MH45216, and the National Institutes of Health through grant DK33093.

REFERENCES

1. Ågren H, Lundqvist G. Low levels of somatostatin in human CSF mark depressive episodes. *Psychoneuroendocrinology* 1984;9:233–248.
2. Altemus M, Pigott T, L'Heureux F, et al. CSF somatostatin in obsessive-compulsive disorder. *Am J Psychiatry* 1993;150:460–464.
3. Amsterdam JD, Maislin G, Winokur A, Berwish N, Kling M, Gold P. The oCRH test before and after clinical recovery from depression. *J Affect Dis* 1988;14:213–222.
4. Amsterdam JD, Marinelli DL, Arger P, Winokur A. Assessment of adrenal gland volume by computed tomography in depressed patients and healthy volunteers: a pilot study. *Psychiatry Res* 1987; 21:189–197.
5. Arato M, Banki CM, Bissette G, Nemeroff CB. Elevated CSF CRF in suicide victims. *Biol Psychiatry* 1989;25:355–359.
6. Arnold MA, Reppert SM, Rorstad OP, et al. Temporal patterns of somatostatin immunoreactivity in the cerebrospinal fluid of the rhesus monkey: effect of environmental lighting. *J Neurosci* 1982; 2:674–680.
7. Banki CM, Bissette G, Arato M, Nemeroff CB. Elevation of immunoreactive CSF TRH in depressed patients. *Am J Psychiatry* 1988; 145:1526–1531.
8. Banki CM, Karmacsi L, Bissette G, Nemeroff CB. Cerebrospinal fluid neuropeptides in mood disorder and dementia. *J Affect Dis* 1992;25:39–45.
9. Banki CM, Karmacsi L, Bissette G, Nemeroff CB. CSF corticotro-

pin-releasing hormone and somatostatin in major depression: response to antidepressant treatment and relapse. *Eur Neuropsychopharmacol* 1992;2:107–113.

10. Bartalena L, Placidi GF, Martino E, et al. Nocturnal serum thyrotropin (TSH) surge and the TSH response to TSH-releasing hormone: dissociated behavior in untreated depressives. *J Clin Endocrinol Metab* 1990;71(3):650–655.

11. Berrettini WH, Nurnberger JL Jr, Zerbe RL, Gold PW, Chrousos GP, Tomai T. CSF neuropeptides in euthymic bipolar patients and controls. *Br J Psychiatry* 1987;150:208–212.

12. Bissette G, Widerlöv E, Walléus H, et al. Alterations in cerebrospinal fluid concentrations of somatostatinlike immunoreactivity in neuropsychiatric disorders. *Arch Gen Psychiatry* 1986;43:1148–1151.

13. Black PMcL, Ballantine HT Jr, Carr DB, Beal MF, Martin JB. Beta-endorphin and somatostatin concentrations in the ventricular cerebrospinal fluid of patients with affective disorder. *Biol Psychiatry* 1986;21:1075–1077.

14. Bowen DM, Najlerahim A, Procter AW, Francis PT, Murphy E. Circumscribed changes of the cerebral cortex in neuropsychiatric disorders of later life. *Proc Natl Acad Sci USA* 1989;86:9504–9508.

15. Charlton BG, Leake A, Wright C, et al. Somatostatin content and receptors in the cerebral cortex of depressed and control subjects. *J Neurol Neurosurg Neuropsychiatry* 1988;51:719–721.

16. Dallman MF. Regulation of adrenocortical function following stress. In: Brown MR, Koob GF, Rivier C, eds. *Stress neurobiology and neuroendocrinology*. New York: Marcel Dekker; 1991:173–192.

17. Davis KL, Davidson M, Yang R-K, et al. CSF somatostatin in Alzheimer's disease, depressed patients, and control subjects. *Biol Psychiatry* 1988;24:710–712.

18. DeBellis MD, Gold PW, Geracioti TD, Listwak S, Kling MA. Fluoxetine significantly reduces CSF CRH and AVP concentrations in patients with major depression. *Am J Psychiatry* 1993;150:656–657.

19. Doran AR, Rubinow DR, Roy A, Pickar D. CSF somatostatin and abnormal response to dexamethasone administration in schizophrenic and depressed patients. *Arch Gen Psychiatry* 1986;43:365–369.

20. Dunn AJ, Berridge CW. Physiological and behavioral responses to corticotropin-releasing factor administration: is CRF a mediator of anxiety or stress responses? *Brain Res Rev* 1990;15:71–100.

21. Duval F, Macher JP, Mokrani MC. Difference between evening and morning thyrotropin response to protirelin in major depressive episode. *Arch Gen Psychiatry* 1990;47:443–448.

22. Eccles J. Chemical transmission and Dale's principle. In: Hökfelt T, Fuxe K, Pernow B, eds. *Progress in Brain Research*. Amsterdam: Elsevier; 1986:3–13.

23. Fossey MD, Lydiarel RB, Larara MT, Bissette G, Nemeroff CB, Balleyer JC. CSF thyrotropin-releasing hormone in patients with anxiety disorders. *Biol Psychiatry* 1990;27(Suppl):167A.

24. Garrick NA, Hill JL, Szele FG, Tomai TP, Gold PW, Murphy DL. Corticotropin-releasing factor: a marked circadian rhythm in primate cerebrospinal fluid peaks in the evening and is inversely related to the cortisol circadian rhythm. *Endocrinology* 1987;121:1329–1334.

25. Gerner RH, Yamada T. Altered neuropeptide concentrations in cerebrospinal fluid of psychiatric patients. *Brain Res* 1982;238:298–302.

26. Gertz BJ, Cantreras LN, McComb DJ, Kovacs K, Tyrrell JB, Dallman MF. Chronic administration of corticotropin-releasing factor increases pituitary corticotroph number. *Endocrinology* 1987;120:381–388.

27. Gold MS, Pottash AL, Extein I. Hypothyroidism and depression. Evidence from complete thyroid function evaluation. *JAMA* 1981;245(19):919–922.

28. Gold PW, Loriaux DL, Roy A, et al. Responses to corticotropin-releasing hormone in the hypercortisolism of depression and Cushing's disease. Pathophysiologic and diagnostic implications. *New Engl J Med* 1986;314:1329–1335.

29. Haggerty JJ Jr, Garbutt JC, Evans DL, Simon JS, Nemeroff CB. Subclinical hypothyroidism: a review of neuropsychiatric aspects. *Int J Psychiatry Med* 1990;20:193–208.

30. Hauger RL, Lorang M, Irwin M, Aguilera G. CRF receptor regulation and sensitization of ACTH responses to acute ether stress during chronic intermittent immobilization stress. *Brain Res* 1990;532:34–40.

31. Henn FA, McKinney WT. Animal models in psychiatry. In: Meltzer HY, ed. *Psychopharmacology: the third generation*. New York: Raven Press; 1987:687–696.

32. Hökfelt T. Neuropeptides in perspective: the last ten years. *Neuron* 1991;7:867–879.

33. Holsboer F, Gerken A, Stalla GK, Muller OA. Blunted aldosterone and ACTH release after human corticotropin-releasing factor administration in depressed patients. *Am J Psychiatry* 1987;144:229–231.

34. Howland RH. Thyroid dysfunction in refractory depression: implications for pathophysiology and treatment. *J Clin Psychiatry* 1993;54:47–54.

35. Joffee RT, Sokolov TH. Thyroid hormones, the brain, and affective disorders. *Crit Rev Neurobiol* 1994;8:45–63.

36. Jolkkonen J, Lepola U, Bissette G, Nemeroff CB, Riekkinen P. CSF corticotropin-releasing factor is not affected in panic disorder. *Biol Psychiatry* 1993;33:136–138.

37. Kakigi T, Maeda K, Kaneda H, Chihara K. Repeated administration of antidepressant drugs reduces regional somatostatin concentrations in rat brain. *J Affect Dis* 1992;25(4):215–220.

38. Kaye WH, Gwirtsman HE, George DT, et al. Elevated cerebrospinal fluid levels of immunoreactive corticotropin-releasing hormone in anorexia nervosa; relation to state of nutrition, adrenal function, and intensity of depression. *J Clin Endocrinol Metab* 1987;64:203–208.

39. Kaye WH, Rubinow D, Gwirtsman HE, George DT, Jimerson DC, Gold PW. CSF somatostatin in anorexia nervosa and bulimia: relationship to the hypothalamic pituitary-adrenal cortical axis. *Psychoneuroendocrinology* 1988;13:265–272.

40. Kirkegaard C. The thyrotropin response to thyrotropin-releasing hormone in endogenous depression. *Psychoneuroendocrinology* 1981;6:189–212.

41. Kling MA, Rubinow DR, Doran AR, et al. Cerebrospinal fluid immunoreactive somatostatin concentrations in patients with Cushing's disease and major depression: relationship to indicies of corticotropin-releasing hormone and cortisol secretion. *Neuroendocrinology* 1993;57:79–88.

42. Koob GF, Heinrichs SC, Pich EM, et al. The role of CRF in behavioral responses to stress. In: Chadwick DJ, Marsh J, Ackrill K, eds. *CIBA Foundation Symposium #172*. New York: John Wiley; 1993:277–295.

43. Krishnan KRR. Pituitary and adrenal changes in depression. *Psychiatric Ann* 1993;23:671–675.

44. Krishnan KRR, Rayasam K, Reed DR, et al. The corticotropin-releasing factor stimulation test in patients with major depression: relationship to dexamethasone suppression test results. *Depression* 1993;1:133–136.

45. Kruesi MJP, Swedo S, Leonard H, Rubinow DR, Rapoport JL. CSF somatostatin in childhood psychiatric disorders: a preliminary investigation. *Psychiatry Res* 1990;33:277–284.

46. Kubek MJ, Sattin A. Effect of electroconvulsive shock on the content of thyrotropin-releasing hormone in rat brain. *Life Sci* 1984;34:1149–1152.

47. Langer G, Koinig G, Hatzinger R, et al. Response of thyrotropin to thyrotropin-releasing hormone as predictor of treatment outcome. *Arch Gen Psychiatry* 1986;43:861–868.

48. Loosen PT. Pituitary-thyroid axis in affective disorders. In: Meltzer HY, ed. *Psychopharmacology: the third generation*. New York: Raven Press; 1987:629–636.

49. Maeda K, Yoshimoto Y, Yamadori A. Blunted TSH and unaltered PRL responses to TRH following repeated administration of TRH in neurologic patients: a replication of neuroendocrine features of major depression. *Biol Psychiatry* 1993;33:277–283.

50. Meaney MJ, Mitchell JB, Aitken DH, et al. The effects of neonatal handling on the development of the adrenocortical response to stress: implications for neuropathology and cognitive deficits in later life. *Psychoneuroendocrinology* 1991;16:85–103.

51. Molchan SE, Lawlor BA, Hill JL, et al. CSF monoamine metabolites and somatostatin in Alzheimer's disease and major depression. *Biol Psychiatry* 1991;29:1110–1118.

52. Nemeroff CB. The relevace of thyrotropin-releasing hormone to psychiatric disorders. In: Nemeroff CB, ed. *Progress in psychiatry, neuropeptides and psychiatric disease.* Washington DC: American Psychiatric Association Press; 1990:15–28.

53. Nemeroff CB, Bissette G, Akil H, Fink M. Neuropeptide concentrations in the cerebrospinal fluid of depressed patients treated with electroconvulsive therapy: corticotropin-releasing factor, β-endorphin and somatostatin. *Br J Psychiatry* 1991;158:59–63.

54. Nemeroff CB, Bissette G, Martin JB, et al. Effect of chronic treatment with thyrotropin-releasing hormone (TRH) or an analog of TRH (linear β-alanine TRH) on the hypothalamic-pituitary-thyroid axis. *Neuroendocrinology* 1980;30:193–199.

55. Nemeroff CB, Krishnan KRR, Reed D, Leder R, Beam C, Dunnick NR. Adrenal gland enlargement in major depression: a computed tomography study. *Arch Gen Psychiatry* 1992;49:384–387.

56. Nemeroff CB, Owens MJ, Bissette G, Andorn AC, Stanley M. Reduced corticotropin-releasing factor (CRF) binding sites in the frontal cortex of suicides. *Arch Gen Psychiatry* 1988;45:577–579.

57. Nemeroff CB, Widerlov E, Bissette G, et al. Elevated concentrations of CSF corticotropin-releasing factor-like immunoreactivity in depressed patients. *Science* 1984;226:1342–1344.

58. Owens MJ, Nemeroff CB. The physiology and pharmacology of corticotropin releasing factor. *Pharmacol Rev* 1992;43:425–473.

59. Pepin MC, Pothier F, Barden N. Antidepressant drug action in a transgenic mouse model of the endocrine changes seen in depression. *Mol Pharmacol* 1992;42(6):991–995.

60. Plotnikoff NP, Prange AJ Jr, Breese GR, Anderson MS, Wilson IC. Thyrotropin releasing hormone: enhancement of DOPA activity by a hypothalamic hormone. *Science* 1972;178:417–418.

61. Plotsky PM. Pathways to the secretion of ACTH: a view from the portal. *J Neuroendocrinol* 1991;3:1–9.

62. Plotsky P, Meaney M. Early postnatal experience alters hypothalamic corticotropin-releasing factor (CRF) mRNA, median eminence CRF content, and stress-induced release in adult rats. *Mol Brain Res* 1993;18:195–200.

63. Post RM. Transduction of psychosocial stress into the neurobiology of recurrent affective disorder. *Am J Psychiatry* 1992;149(8):999–1010.

64. Post PM. Models for the impact of affective illness on gene expression. *Clin Neurosci* 1993;1:129–138.

65. Post RM, Gold P, Rubinow DR, Ballenger JC, Bunney WE, Goodwin FK. Peptides in cerebrospinal fluid of neuropsychiatric patients: an approach to central nervous system peptide function. *Life Sci* 1982;31:1–15.

66. Post RM, Weiss SRB. Endogenous biochemical abnormalities in affective illness: therapeutic versus pathogenic. *Biol Psychiatry* 1992;32:469–484.

67. Risch SC, Lewine RJ, Jewart RD, et al. Relationship between cerebrospinal fluid peptides and neurotransmitters in depression. In: Risch SC, ed. *Central nervous system peptide mechanisms in stress and depression.* Washington DC: American Psychiatric Press; 1991:93–103.

68. Rothschild AJ. The dexamethasone suppression test in psychiatric disorders. *Psychiatric Ann* 1993;23:662–670.

69. Roy A, Bissette G, Nemeroff CB. Cerebrospinal fluid thyrotropin-releasing hormone concentrations in alcoholics and normal controls. *Biol Psychiatry* 1990;28:767–772.

70. Roy-Byrne PP, Uhde TW, Post RM, Gallucci W, Chrousos GP, Gold PW. The corticotropin-releasing hormone stimulation test in patients with panic disorder. *Am J Psychiatry* 1986;143:896–899.

71. Rubin RT, Phillips JJ. Adrenal gland enlargement in major depression [letter]. *Arch Gen Psychiatry* 1993;50:833–835.

72. Rubinow DR. Cerebrospinal fluid somatostatin and psychiatric illness. *Biol Psychiatry* 1986;21:341–365.

73. Rubinow DR, Gold PW, Post RM. CSF somatostatin in affective illness. *Arch Gen Psychiatry* 1983;40:409–412.

74. Rubinow DR, Post RM, Gold PW, Ballenger JC, Reichlin S. Effects of carbamazepine on cerebrospinal somatostatin. *Psychopharmacology* 1985;85:210–213.

75. Russ MJ, Ackerman SH. Antidepressant treatment response in depressed hypothyroid patients. *Hosp Community Psychiatry* 1989;40:954–956.

76. Sapolsky RM, Plotsky PM. Hypercortisolism and its possible neural basis. *Biol Psychiatry* 1990;27:937–952.

77. Schlesser MA, Rush AJ, Fairchild C, Crowley G, Orsulak P. The thyrotropin-releasing hormone stimulation test: a methodological study. *Psychiatry Res* 1983;9:59–67.

78. Shelton RC, Winn S, Ekhatore N, Loosen PT. The effects of antidepressants on the thyroid axis in depression. *Bio! Psychiatry* 1993;33:120–126.

79. Smith MA, Davidson J, Ritchie JC, et al. The corticotropin-releasing hormone test in patients with post-traumatic stress disorder. *Biol Psychiatry* 1989;26:349–355.

80. Sorensen KV. Rapid post-mortem decomposition of the somatostatin cells in human brain. An immunohistochemical examination. *Biomed Pharmacother* 1984;38:458–461.

81. Stenzel-Poore MP, Cameron VA, Vaughan J, Sawchenko PE, Vale W. Development of Cushing's syndrome in corticotropin-releasing factor transgenic mice. *Endocrinology* 1992;30(6):3378–3386.

82. Sunderland T, Rubinow DR, Tariot PN, et al. CSF somatostatin in patients with Alzheimer's disease, older depressed patients, and age-matched control subjects. *Am J Psychiatry* 1987;144:1313–1316.

83. Vale W, Spiess J, Rivier C, Rivier J. Characterization of a 41 residue ovine hypothalamic peptide that stimulates secretion of corticotropin of β-endorphin. *Science* 1981;213:1394–1397.

84. Whybrow PC, Prange AJ. A hypothesis of thyroid-catecholamine receptor interaction. *Arch Gen Psychiatry* 1981;38:106–113.

85. Young EA, Watson SJ, Kotun J, et al. β-lipotropin/β-endorphin response to low-dose ovine corticotropin releasing factor in endogenous depression. *Arch Gen Psychiatry* 1990;47:449–457.

86. Zis KD, Zis A. Increased adrenal weight in victims of violent suicide. *Am J Psychiatry* 1987;144:1214–1215.

Psychopharmacology: The Fourth Generation of Progress, edited by Floyd E. Bloom and David J. Kupfer. Raven Press, Ltd., New York 1995.

CHAPTER 85

Psychoneuroimmunology of Depression

Michael Irwin

The central nervous system is hypothesized to have a role in the modulation of immune function. This chapter provides an overview of the association between psychological factors and immunity, concentrating on the immunological alterations of depression. In addition, experimental evidence is reviewed of the neural and endocrine mechanisms that have been proposed to alter immune function in depression. Finally, because psychological distress has recently been associated with an increased susceptibility to infectious disease and possibly risk of cancer, the possible health implications of depression or stress-associated immune changes are discussed. Before describing the interactions between the brain, behavior, and immunity, a brief overview of the immune system is provided (see Chapter 63, *this volume*).

THE IMMUNE SYSTEM

The immune system functions to discriminate "self" from "nonself" cells, protecting the organism from invasion by pathogens, such as viruses and bacteria, or from abnormal internal cells such as cancer cells. These functions are closely regulated and performed without damage to the host, although an overresponsive immune system is purported to lead to autoimmune disease in which the organism's own tissues are attacked.

The organs of the mammalian immune system include the thymus, spleen, and lymph nodes. The working cells of the immune system are represented by three distinct populations: T cells, B cells, and natural killer (NK) cells. Immune responses are typically divided into two important components: cellular immunity and humoral responses. There is evidence that T cells and B cells interact and cooperate in many cellular immune responses and in

most humoral immune responses, although cellular immunity is thought to be mediated primarily by T lymphocytes and humoral responses by B lymphocytes and their soluble products.

The T lymphocytes develop from stem cells in the bone marrow and migrate to the thymus, where they mature into several subsets including the cytotoxic T cell, T helper cell, and T suppressor cell. These T cells circulate into the periphery and are found in the lymph nodes, blood vessels and spleen. Briefly, the cytotoxic T cell is characterized by its ability to seek out and destroy either cells infected with viruses or tumor cells that have acquired foreign nonself antigens. In the development of the cytotoxic T cell response, a foreign antigen is first encountered and incorporated onto the surface of an antigen-presenting cell such as a macrophage. After the antigen is presented to the T cell, is recognized, and is bound by a specific receptor on the T cell, then the T cell multiplies and becomes capable of attacking any cell that presents that specific foreign surface antigen. Other types of T lymphocytes, such as the T helper cells, secrete interleukin-2 (IL-2) and regulate the proliferative response of the T cell to antigenic stimulation. Reexposure of the cytotoxic T cell to an antigen produces a more rapid and extensive reaction than that found upon initial presentation.

Interacting with the T helper and T suppressor cell, the B cell is primarily involved in the humoral response. Like the T cell, the B cell arises from a precursor stem cell in the bone marrow, although in humans its site of maturation remains unknown. Following initial antigen processing by the macrophage, the antigen–major histocompatibility complex (MHC) on the accessory cell surface engages the receptors of an appropriate T helper cell antigen and the macrophage releases interleukin-1 (IL-1). Thus stimulated the T helper cell proliferates by forming a clone and secretes factors, such as IL-2, that stimulate T-cell and B-cell growth. The activated B cell proliferates

M. Irwin: Department of Psychiatry, University of California, San Diego, and San Diego VA Medical Center, San Diego, California 92161.

and differentiates to antibody secreting status, switching with the help of interleukin-4 (IL-4) from immunoglobulin M (IgM) secretion to synthesis of other classes of antibodies such as immunoglobulin G (IgG).

In addition to the T and B cells, a distinct subpopulation of lymphocytes comprised of NK cells has been described. The NK cell is immunologically nonspecific and does not require sensitization to specific antigens to perform its cytotoxic activity. Thus, the NK cell responds to a variety of cell surface markers, as long as the markers differ from ''self'' markers, and lyses a wide variety of cell types. Although the role of the NK cell in tumor surveillance remains controversial, substantial evidence has demonstrated the importance of the NK cell in the control of herpes and cytomegalovirus infections in man and animals.

Regulation of immune responses involves the secretion of cellular factors or lymphokines. These lymphokines together form a network of regulatory signals that show considerable overlap in activity and patterns of synergism as well as antagonism. For example, the lymphokine IL-1 is produced by nearly all immunological cell types including NK cells, T and B lymphocytes, brain astrocytes, microglia, and macrophages. Interleukin-1 acts mainly as an endogenous adjuvant serving as a cofactor during lymphocyte activation, inducing the synthesis of other lymphokines and the activation of resting T cells. For example, IL-1 stimulates T lymphocytes to synthesize and release IL-2, and IL-1 further acts on NK cells to induce the expression of the IL-2 receptor. Binding of IL-2 by its receptor on the NK cell is a crucial step in activating such cytotoxic cells (predominantly large granular lymphocytes) to form lymphokine-activated killers that are able to lyse a wide range of target cells in a non-MHC-restricted manner.

MEASURES OF IMMUNE FUNCTION

The immune system can be evaluated by measures that assess the *number* of different cell types as well as the *function* of various components of cellular and humoral immunity. To quantitate the number of cells in various subpopulations, specific monoclonal antibodies are available that bind to unique surface markers on cell types such as T helper, T suppressor, and NK cells. Whereas enumeration of cell types reveals the balance of different cell types needed for the optimal immune response, numbers of different cell types do not necessarily correlate with functional capacity, and changes of cell numbers in the peripheral circulation may merely reflect a redistribution of cell types from various immune compartments (60).

Measurement of the *function* of the immune system can involve in vivo and in vitro techniques. One in vivo assay of immunity includes measurement of the delayed-type hypersensitivity (DTH) response following administration of skin tests. This in vivo technique provides valuable data about the physiological response of the organism to an antigenic challenge and has been proposed to be more relevant in the clinical assessment of immunocompetence than in vitro measures of immune function (32). For the assessment of the DTH response, a series of antigens (i.e., tetanus, diphtheria, streptococcus, tuberculin, candida, trichophyton, proteus) and a glycerin control are applied in a standardized fashion to the forearm. The induration response at each site of antigen exposure is measured typically after 48 hr and the number of antigenic responses and size of induration at each site is recorded. Cutaneous anergy is indicated by the absence of an induration response to any of the seven test antigens.

Immunization with a novel antigen and evaluation of antibody response is another technique that has been used to assess immune function in vivo. For example, Glaser et al. (27) have used the hepatitis B recombinant vaccine and quantitated rates of seroconversion by assaying serum antibody titers to the hepatitis B surface antigen. In addition to the use of well-recognized vaccines such as hepatitis B or pneumovax, the use of a novel protein antigen (keyhole limpet hemocyanin) has also been proposed to evaluate in vivo the kinetics and magnitude of this biologically important response (33).

An indirect in vivo assessment of cellular immune function includes the measurement of antibody titers to latent viruses. The cellular immune response is thought to be important in controlling latent viral infections, and reactivation of viruses, such as herpes viruses, can occur during conditions in which cellular immunity is compromised. In turn, synthesis of virus or viral proteins is increased and elevations in antibody titers are detected in the serum.

Two in vitro correlates of cellular immune function, mitogen-induced lymphocyte proliferation and NK cell activity, have been widely used to assess the cell-mediated immune system of depressed patients. Both of these assays evaluate the function of cells ex vivo outside the body. Mitogen-induced lymphocyte stimulation determines the proliferative capacity of lymphocytes following activation in vitro either with plant lectins such as concanavalin A (Con A) or phytohemagglutinin (PHA) which predominantly activate the T lymphocyte to divide or with pokeweed mitogen that induces proliferation of B cells. The proliferative response is quantitated by the cellular incorporation of radioactively labeled thymidine or idoxuridine into newly synthesized deoxyribonucleic acid (DNA). The other frequently used in vitro assessment of cellular immunity involves measurement of NK activity. Assay of NK lytic activity is carried out by the coincubation of isolated effector lymphocytes with radioactively labeled target tumor cells. The release of radioactivity by the lysed target cells is proportionate to the activity of the effector NK cells.

Assay of levels of lymphokines (IL-1, IL-2, and interferon) in the plasma or following lymphocyte stimulation has been employed recently to quantitate possible alterations in the regulation of these cellular factors, which are important in humoral and cellular immune responses (26). Interleukin-1 promotes lymphocyte differentiation via increased expression of IL-2 receptors, whereas IL-2 provides a signal for the proliferation and differentiation of immune cells. Assay of these lymphokines is proposed to provide information about the immunological mechanisms that may be related to changes in ex vivo measures such as lymphocyte proliferation or NK activity (26,55).

STRESS AND IMMUNITY: ANIMAL MODELS OF DEPRESSION

Effects of Stress on Cellular Immune Responses

Behavioral responsiveness to inescapable aversive stimulation has provided an animal model to investigate clinical depression. Administration of aversive stressors, including sound, rotation, intermittent shock, and forced immobilization, have been found to alter in vitro correlates of cellular immunity (i.e., lymphocyte responses to mitogen stimulation and/or NK activity) in a manner that depends on dose- and time-response profiles. For example, using either an audiogenic stressor or intermittent footshock repeated at daily intervals, several studies showed that acute immune suppression occurred after only one or two exposures to the stressor and was followed by an increase or enhancement of lymphocyte proliferation or natural cytotoxicity if the stressor was repeated or prolonged (41,42). The dose of the stressor is also associated with the degree of immune change; a progressive decrease of PHA-induced proliferation is found in animals that receive an increasing severity of stress from low- and high-level electric tail shock (46).

Cellular in vivo immune responses show a similar reduction of function following the administration of aversive stressors. Delayed hypersensitivity reactions are decreased in mice exposed to heat stress, and the graft-versus-host response is suppressed in animals subjected to limited feeding, an effect that is independent of adrenocortical levels (see also Chapters 62, 63, and 67, *this volume,* for related discussions).

Stress and Humoral Immune Responses

Studies of the effects of stress on the immune system have recently suggested the importance of measuring immune function in vivo, rather than by assay of in vitro parameters of cellular immunity (56). For example, in vivo assessment of an antibody response to a novel antigen reveals the integrated action of the intact immune system, which can not be fully evaluated when multiple parameters of cellular immune function are separately assayed in vitro (56). In addition, measurement of an in vivo response is carried out within the internal milieu, providing a model that can test the physiological role of neurotransmitters and neuroendocrine hormones in the modulation of immune function during stress.

Administration of aversive stressors such as tail shock, footshock, or social status change has been found to produce a reliable suppression of a specific IgG antibody response following immunization with the T-cell–dependent antigen keyhole limpet hemocyanin (KLH). Likewise, following intraperitoneal administration of sheep red blood cells (SRBC), the plaque-forming cell response was reduced in monkeys exposed to aversive stimuli, in mice housed in high- versus low-density group-housing, and in mice subjected to changes in housing condition (either from individual to group housing or from a group to an individual cage).

A critical period exists during which the humoral response is vulnerable to the effects of stress, although disparate results have been reported. Restraint produced a significant reduction in antibody response to SRBC only if the stress is applied before, but not after, immunization; rotational stress depressed antibody-forming cell responses to SRBC when administered 24 hr after immunization but not at the time of immunization, whereas a critical period extending up to 72 hr following immunization was described for footshock. Because inescapable shock has been found to alter mesenteric lymph node lymphocyte subpopulations as well as specific antibody responses in a time-dependent manner (changes occurring immediately following stress become absent 48 hr after stress), the temporal profile of stress-induced immune suppression could be due to the differential effects of stressor on the alteration of lymphocyte subpopulations as reflected by an increased T helper/T suppressor/cytotoxic lymphocyte ratio.

The effects of stress on antibody response is also antigen-dose dependent. In other words, the effects of stress such as footshock are found only when the amount of antigen used is close to a physiological concentration not when suprathreshold amounts of antigen are used to evoke an exaggerated, rapid response (33).

Stress Alterations of Accessory Cell Function

Accessory cells, such as macrophages, which are essential for the modulation of immune responses including lymphocyte proliferation and antibody responses by release of IL-1 and prostaglandins, are likely to play a role in stress-induced alterations of immune responses. During an antibody response, the macrophage expresses class II MHC gene products, processes and presents antigen, and facilitates activation of T helper cells. To evaluate whether macrophage function might be a target of stress and lead to suppression of antigen-specific T-helper-cell function, we have used irradiated spleen cells from either amphetamine-stressed or control animals to present antigen to antigen-specific T-cell hybridomas. Interleukin-2 production by T-cell hybridomas was abolished when antigen-presenting cells from amphetamine-stressed animals were used, suggesting that stress-induced defect in antigen-specific proliferation and/or IL-2 production may be at the level of antigen presentation by the macrophage. Other recent data have further demonstrated that stress produces a dysregulation of macrophage function as measured by enhanced IL-1 and prostaglandin E_2 production and diminished interferon-induced class II MHC gene product expression. Diminished class II MHC expression is thought to compromise antigen presentation and T-helper-cell activation.

Stress Alterations in Immune Cell Second-messenger Systems

Although data have supported the hypothesis that macrophage function may be impaired by stress, the possibility of some additional defect in T-cell function cannot be excluded. Activation of lymphocytes as measured by lymphocyte proliferation is a multistep process, and thus stress-induced suppression of this immune activity might also be mediated by alterations of discrete intracellular biochemical events that occur immediately after mitogen binding. For example, mitogen binding to the T-cell receptor is transducted via a bifurcating pathway from the hydrolysis of phosphatidyl inositol biphosphate (PIP_2) into inositol triphosphate (IP_3) and diacylglycerol (DAG). IP_3 in turn elevates free calcium while DAG activates protein kinase C (PKC). Finally, activation of calcium-dependent proteins increases synthesis of the IL-2 receptor and the lymphokine IL-2 (26).

Because of the important role of the early activating biochemical steps in the proliferative response of lymphocytes to mitogens, initial studies have begun to explore whether the effects of stress on lymphocyte function are mediated by alterations in calcium mobilization or calcium-dependent biochemical mechanisms. Indeed, both acute and chronic restraint stress have been found to suppress mitogen-stimulated increases in calcium, suggesting that stress induces an inhibition of calcium mobilization in lymphocytes and attenuates this obligatory signal for certain signal-transduction pathways. However, other data suggest that stress-induced defects in T-cell proliferation are not solely due to alterations in free-calcium mobilization but rather may be due to intracellular biochemical changes in addition or subsequent to early events driven by calcium release. For example, diminished lymphocyte responses following stimulation with either calcium ionophores (i.e., ionomycin or A23187 that releases free intracellular calcium) or tetradecanoylphor-

bol acetate (TPA) which activates PKC are found in stressed animals. Together, these data suggest that stress may induce some defect in surface-receptor signal transduction, but that an additional intracellular defect is present at a site beyond the action of calcium or PKC, possibly in the synthesis of IL-2 and IL-2 receptors. Interestingly, a stress-induced suppression of IL-2 production with PHA has not been demonstrated, and the addition of IL-2 failed to correct stress-related suppression of blastogenesis.

Psychological Predictors of Stress-induced Immune Alterations

Stressor Predictability and Controllability

Stressor characteristics, such as severity and type of stressor and/or time response, partly determine alterations of a wide range of cellular and/or humoral immune parameters. However, the psychological state of the animal in response to the stressor has also been related to the immunological consequences of the stress. Maier and Laudenslager (56) found that rats exposed to inescapable, uncontrollable electric tail shock have reduced lymphocyte activity, whereas animals that received the same total amount of shock but were able to terminate it did not show altered immunity. Furthermore, stress predictability, such as a warning stimulus preceding inescapable footshock, completely reverses the shock-induced suppression of lymphocytes. Finally, consistent with the hypothesis that fear ultimately determines the amount of immunosuppression induced by aversive stimuli, a nonaversive stimulus that is associated with electric shock can be conditioned to impair lymphocyte proliferation independent of any physical effects of aversive stimulation.

Role of Early Life Experiences

Premature maternal separation produces alterations in a number of measures of immune function, such as lymphocyte proliferation, macrophage responses, decreased levels of complement proteins and immunoglobulins, an inhibited capacity to mount antibody responses to the bacteriophage ×174, increased hemolytic complement activity, and greater delayed hypersensitivity responses to dinitrochlorobenzene (8). In addition to the acute effects of maternal separation on immune function in the infant animal, these immune alterations persist into adulthood, leading to changes of the immune system and possibly of host resistance to infectious disease in the adult animal (52).

Role of Affiliative Social Behavior

The impact of psychosocial stress on immune function may also be buffered by social environment and/or the social behavior of the animal at the time of exposure to the stressor. Administration of a chronic (2 years) social stressor involving housing either in a stable or in a changing social group produces a decrement of cellular immune responses in monkeys that is consistent with the effects of other social stressors. Of unique interest, those animals who showed affiliative behaviors while undergoing social stress had greater values of lymphocyte proliferation as compared to less affiliative animals. In other words, social behaviors that are affiliative may serve to protect animals from the immunosuppressive effects of chronic social stress.

STRESS AND IMMUNITY: CLINICAL FINDINGS RELEVANT TO DEPRESSION

Life stressors such as bereavement, marital separation, academic examinations, or the stress of Alzheimer spousal caregiving have all been shown to have effects on immune function. Individuals undergoing bereavement show alterations of cellular immunity including suppression of lymphocyte responses to mitogenic stimulation, reduction of NK cell activity, and alterations of T-cell subpopulations. Consistent with the observation that severity of depressive symptoms is a reliable negative correlate of altered immunity in depressed patients (as described below), psychological response to bereavement, not merely the event, appears to contribute to the immune changes in severe life stress. Likewise, using various measures of humoral and cell-mediated immunity, reduced lymphocyte responses to the mitogen PHA were found in bereaved subjects who had high depression scores but not in those bereaved subjects who had few signs of depression as compared to controls. Similar to the effects of conjugal bereavement, marital disruption in women and in men is associated with a suppression of proliferative lymphocyte responses to Con A and PHA and with increased antibody titers to Epstein-Barr virus (EBV). These immune alterations in separated and divorced individuals are correlated with depressive symptoms and measures of psychological attachment.

Psychological stress during relatively minor aversive events such as academic examinations is also temporally associated with higher white blood cell counts, an increased absolute lymphocyte count, a reduction of lymphocyte proliferation and NK activity, and alterations in the regulation of IL-2 and IL-2 receptor on peripheral blood lymphocytes (26). Furthermore, these alterations of cellular immunity in medical students undergoing examination stress have been hypothesized to be of health significance since antibody titers to EBV, cytomegalovirus (CMV), and herpes simplex virus (HSV) are significantly increased during the first day of examination as compared to either the month before examination or upon return from summer vacation. Finally, Glaser et al. (27) has

further demonstrated that medical students who are less stressed and anxious are more likely to show a shorter time to seroconversion following vaccination with the hepatitis B vaccine.

Chronic stressors that last over periods of one or more years not only increase the risk for depression but also are likely to result in alterations of immune function. As compared to age-matched controls, family caregivers of Alzheimer patients are more likely to be psychologically distressed and to have significantly higher antibody titers to EBV and reduced percentages of total T lymphocytes and T helper cells. Additional observations have found higher rates of syndromal depressive disorders and impairment of cellular immunity (i.e., increased EBV titers and poorer lymphocyte proliferation to PHA and Con A) in spousal caregivers (47). An important clinical implication of these findings has suggested that these immunological alterations are longitudinally associated with more days of infectious illness, primarily upper respiratory tract infections (47).

DEPRESSION AND IMMUNE CHANGES

Summary of Findings

Studies of immunity in depression have been concerned primarily with the evaluation of enumerative (numbers of circulating white blood cells or lymphocyte subsets) and/or in vitro correlates of cellular immune function (lymphocyte responses to mitogens and NK activity). Because of the disparate results from several dozen studies conducted since 1978, three comprehensive reviews have recently been published (31,71,76), although the conclusions reached from these reviews using overlapping studies are not in agreement. For example, Stein et al. (71) used a tabular summary of the findings from 22 studies and concluded that "the findings have been inconsistent and inconclusive." Enumerative measures do not distinguish depressed patients from controls and "... no consistent or reproducible alterations of functional measures of lymphocytes" have been reported. In contrast, Weisse (76) evaluated 18 studies using similar vote-counting methods and concluded that "indexes of immunocompetence [as reflected in lymphocyte responses to mitogen proliferation] are lower among the clinically depressed." Finally, Herbert and Cohen (31) evaluated essentially the same series of studies (of the 36 studies reviewed by Herbert and Cohen, 18 overlapped with Weisse and 22 with those reviewed by Stein et al.) and concluded using a metaanalytical approach that "clinical depression is reliably associated with decreases in all of the measures of lymphocyte function" including NK activity and responses to PHA, Con A, and pokeweed mitogen. Furthermore, in an analysis of 15 methodologically restricted studies that assessed depression using diagnostic criteria, included a comparison control group, and fulfilled several other criteria of methodological rigor (i.e., age and gender of depressed and control subjects indicated, age and gender matching of depressed patient–controls or statistical control for age and gender, drug-free assessment of depressed patients, and psychological and physical health of controls), effects sizes increased and were "particularly robust" ranging from −0.24 to −0.45 (31).

The following summary further reviews alterations of cellular immune function in depression but is restricted to those studies published since 1978 that have employed several methodological strengths (31) and used interassay controls to evaluate and/or control the effects of data variance in the measurement of mitogen responses or NK activity (71). Briefly, because of the essential importance of diagnostic homogeneity as well as control for confounding influences of medication, age, and gender in the interpretation of immune alterations in depression, the present review includes those studies that have evaluated samples of depressed patients who fulfilled diagnostic criteria (either DSM-III or Research Diagnostic Criteria) for major depression, were assessed while psychotropic medication free for at least one week, and were compared with healthy age- and gender-matched comparison controls. In addition, because of the recognized variability of functional immune assays and the need for interassay controls (71), this summary only includes those studies that have been conducted using a matched subject–control pair design and/or laboratory controls with one or more cryopreserved standards. Of the 38 studies evaluating lymphocyte proliferation or NK activity in depression, 12 studies (16,17,18,34,35,38,40,50,62,65,66,67) fulfill these methodological criteria. With the addition of Irwin et al. (34) and Darko et al. (17), the 38 studies reviewed herein overlap with those 36 publications reviewed by Herbert and Cohen (31); 22 overlap with those reviewed by Stein et al. (71); and 18 with Weisse et al. (76).

Mitogen-induced lymphocyte proliferation was assessed in five (16,17,65,66,67) of the 12 depression-immune studies fulfilling the specified stringent methodological criteria. Of these five studies, one study has found a reduction of PHA-, Con-A-, and pokeweed mitogen-induced lymphocyte proliferative responses in depressed patients (67). The other four studies found no group difference in this immune response between depressed patients and controls, although Schleifer et al. (65) found that severity of depression was associated with suppression of proliferative responses within the depressed sample.

For the measurement of NK activity, eight studies published since 1978 (18,34,35,38,40,50,61,65) have employed interassay controls in addition to fulfilling the other important methodological criteria of diagnostic homogeneity, medication-free status, and age and gender

matching with control comparison subjects. Of these eight studies, seven have reported a reduction of NK activity in depressed patients as compared to controls (18,34,35,38,40,50,61). Although the one study by Schleifer et al. (65) failed to find a reduction of NK activity in the depressives, a modest trend was evident between the severity of depressive symptoms and NK activity (Keller, *personal communication*).

Methodological Issues

Several factors such as sample differences in age, gender, hospitalization stress, concurrent life stress in either the depressed patients or controls, comorbidity in the depressives, or severity of depressive symptoms are likely to increase the immune variability in depressives and contribute to different results even in series that are restricted to those carefully controlled studies. For example, immune decrements occur in aged individuals (34), and depressed patients who are older may be more vulnerable to the effects of depression (33). Schleifer et al. (65) have shown that depressed people show decreased proliferative responses to mitogens with advancing age, whereas controls appeared to show increases. Furthermore, metaanalytical techniques have demonstrated that the effect size of depression-related reduction of immune function is reliably stronger in older clinically depressed people than in young subjects (31). However, in the 12 studies reviewed here, subjects were on the average middle-aged, and cellular immune measures often do not show either increased variability or declines in persons who are younger than aged 65 years (34).

Gender appears to have a striking influence on depression-related reduction of NK activity. Many studies have focused only on men and typically found a reduction of NK activity (34,35,38,40) whereas the largest study that was conducted using predominantly female subjects found no difference in cellular immunity (65). Evans et al. (18) have separately compared gender differences for NK activity and NK cell counts and reported that depressed men exhibit significant reduction in these immune measures. Female depressed patients have similar levels of NK activity as well as NK numbers compared to female controls, suggesting the possibility that major depression has differential effects on NK cell function in male and female subjects. Indeed, *increased* NK activity was reported in female depressives which was speculated to be due to direct effects of progesterone, or possibly progesterone-mediated antagonism of glucocorticoid suppression on cellular immune function (57).

Hospitalization stress has been proposed to exacerbate the relationship between depression and immunity, although this relationship may be due to increased severity of depressive symptoms in hospitalized depressives (66). However, hospitalization status was not found to statistically contribute to mitogen-induced lymphocyte proliferation or NK activity (65), and schizophrenic patients undergoing the stress of hospitalization failed to show a reduction of cellular immune function even though a group of similarly hospitalized depressed inpatients did show such a reduction of immunity. Together, these data suggest that the effects of depression on immunity are probably not from nonspecific effects of hospitalization.

Considerable evidence has found that life stress can alter immune function. Depressed patients often undergo increased numbers of life events secondary to their affective illness and depression-related reduction of cellular immunity could possibly be a result of the effects of life stress, not depression (35). Conversely, approximately 10% of control subjects who volunteer for clinical research and are free of any psychiatric diagnosis are found to be undergoing severe life stress as identified by structured life event interviews (38). Failure to assess life stress in depressed patients and controls could lead either to the inclusion of depressed patients who show a reduction of immunity secondary to life stress or alternatively to the enrollment of stressed controls who show stress-related reduction of immune function. To evaluate the relative contribution of stress to depression-related immune decreases as well as to strengthen the methodological rationale for assessing life stress by structured interviews in controls, one study of immune function in depression has rated severity of life stress in depressed patients and controls and demonstrated that both depression and life stress have independent, but not interactive effects on NK activity (38). In other words, depressed patients who were not severely stressed had a similar reduction of NK activity as that found in depressed patients who were also stressed. Psychiatric controls who are undergoing stress also show reduced immunity similar to depressed patients even though these controls reported no significant depressive symptoms. Important for the design of further clinical studies, inclusion of such normal controls in the comparison group could potentially obscure immunological differences between the depressed and control groups.

Increased use of tobacco and/or alcohol might worsen depression-related immune changes; depressed patients increase their tobacco smoking and over 30% escalate their alcohol drinking during a depressive episode. Despite the potential importance of alcohol and tobacco smoking to immune alterations in depression, evaluation of the contribution of either substance to altered immunity during depression is essentially limited to a few studies. In one study (38), smoking was found to be a strong predictor of the increased number of circulating neutrophils and lymphocytes in the depressives, but cigarette use did not affect the association between depression and NK activity. Indeed, others have found that depressed patients who are smokers have higher levels of lytic activity than tobacco smoking controls (23).

The effects of current alcohol intake and past long-term alcohol abuse on immune function in depressed patients has also been evaluated (35,38). Although alcohol consumption in the 6 months prior to immune assessment was a significant predictor of total leukocyte and neutrophil cell counts similar to the effects of smoking, histories of recent alcohol use were not associated with NK activity (35). Past heavy alcohol consumption as reflected by histories of alcohol abuse and alcohol dependence however, did produce a graded decrement of NK activity beyond the effects of depression alone (35). Nevertheless, depression had an effect on NK activity independent of the effect of past alcoholism.

In addition to careful assessment of substance comorbidity, psychoimmunological studies of psychiatric patients with mood disorders need to evaluate comorbidity for other psychiatric disorders and the potential influence of this comorbidity on immune function. For example, Andreoli et al. (1) investigated the contribution of the additional presence of panic disorder to the variability of lymphocyte proliferation in depressed patients and found that depression with simultaneous panic disorder had a greater number of T cells and PHA mitogen responses than depressed patients without comorbid panic disorder.

Severity of depressive symptoms is a correlate of immunity and may be a more important determinant of altered immunity than depression diagnostic classification per se. For example in Schleifer et al. (65) depressed patients had similar levels of lymphocyte proliferation compared to controls, yet severity of depressive symptoms was associated with suppression of mitogen proliferation. Furthermore, Schleifer et al. (66) suggested that ambulatory depressives have similar levels of immune function compared to controls due to their modest symptom severity. In our studies of NK activity in depression, severity of depressive symptoms has been reliably associated with a reduction of NK activity (35,38,65), a finding that has been replicated by Evans et al. (18) and strengthened by the metaanalysis reported by Herbert and Cohen (31). Finally, Irwin and colleagues used a longitudinal case control design and found that NK activity increases when symptom severity resolves following clinical psychopharmacological treatment (37).

To extend these findings regarding symptom severity and to evaluate the effects of diagnostic subtype on immune function, Hickie et al. (32) have assessed delayed-type hypersensitivity (DTH) response and PHA-induced lymphocyte proliferation in 57 patients with major depression as compared to age and gender matched controls. Patients with melancholic depression had a higher rate of abnormally reduced DTH induration diameter when compared with both nonmelancholic patients and with age- and gender-matched controls; this difference could not be accounted for by age, severity of depressive symptoms, hospitalization status, or weight loss. A similar pattern of results was found for in vitro assessment of immunity by PHA lymphocyte proliferation in that melancholic depressed patients showed impaired blastogenic response when compared with those with nonmelancholic depressive disorder. The significance of diagnosis of melancholia in determining impaired cellular immunity as measured by mitogen responsiveness is supported by two previous studies (54).

Finally, in an effort to broaden immunological assessment and to explore whether mediators important in the regulation of cellular immune responses are altered in melancholic depression, production of IL-1β and soluble IL-2 receptors in PHA culture supernatants has been determined in depressed patients with melancholic subtype (55). Depressed melancholic patients showed higher accumulation of IL-1β and possibly IL-2 receptors. Furthermore, dexamethasone suppressed IL-1β and IL-2 receptor production in controls but failed to alter responses in depressives. These findings, together with evidence of an increased number of pan T, pan B, and T-suppressor/cytotoxic cells in melancholics, have suggested to Maes et al. (55) that melancholics exhibit a systemic immune activation. Contrary to the hypotheses that blunted lymphocyte responses or NK activity are mediated through a deficit in T helper cells and/or lymphokine stimulation (65) or by inhibiting effects of various neuroendocrine signals (34), Maes et al. hypothesized that lower ex vivo mitogen responses may be due to immune activation in vivo, which leads to increased in vivo production of soluble IL-2 receptors inducing a state of relative deficiency of IL-2, which is necessary for proliferation.

MECHANISMS OF DEPRESSION-RELATED IMMUNE ALTERATIONS

Behavioral Factors

Sleep

A link between sleep and immune-related activity has been demonstrated by the ability of immune mediators to alter sleep activity in animals. For example, several cytokines such as IL-1, interferon-α_2, and tumor necrosis factor have the capacity to enhance slow-wave sleep, and a growing body of evidence suggests that IL-1 is directly involved in sleep regulation in humans and animals (51). Antibodies to IL-1 reduce sleep in normal rabbits and the specific IL-1 receptor antagonist blocks the somnogenic effects of IL-1, inhibiting IL-1–induced increases of non-REM sleep without reversing IL-1 induced suppression of REM sleep. Additional data from Krueger (51), and colleagues have suggested that IL-1 may have a physiological role in sleep regulation since the IL-1 receptor antagonist transiently reduces non-REM sleep in rabbits. Studies have further demonstrated a wide distribution of IL-1 mRNA in the brain (19), the presence of IL-1 immunoreactivity in neurons of the human hypothalamus, and

the secretion of IL-1 into the CSF and plasma during sleep–wake cycles (58).

In addition to the likely direct effects of IL-1 on sleep regulation, IL-1 may be involved in the regulation of other substances that either enhance or inhibit normal sleep. For example, IL-1 enhances the release of corticotropin-releasing factor (CRF) and CRF, in turn, inhibits normal sleep and IL-1–induced sleep (51). Less information is available concerning sleep regulation by other cytokines. However, both tumor necrosis factor and interferon are somnogenic after intracerebroventricular administration (51).

Not only are immune response modifiers capable of altering sleep, but it is also possible that sleep processes and sleep–wake activity may mediate changes of cellular immunity, possibly by producing changes in the nocturnal secretion of immune response modifiers such as interleukins. Indeed, Moldofsky et al. (58) have reported a temporal association between the onset of slow-wave sleep and the secretion of IL-1 and IL-2, two lymphokines that are known to stimulate or activate NK cells. Other data in normal controls have shown that sleep deprivation alters immunity. Palmblad et al. (63) found that 48 hr of sleep deprivation reduced lymphocyte proliferative responses to phytohemagglutinin as compared to baseline levels, and Moldofsky and colleagues (58) found a decline in NK activity following 40 hr of wakefulness. Finally, our group has shown that even modest amounts of sleep disturbance, such as either early (sleep time 3 a.m. to 7 a.m.) or late-night (sleep time 11 p.m. to 3 a.m.) partial sleep deprivation produces a 30% to 50% transient decrease in NK activity.

The effects of sleep deprivation on immune function suggest that insomnia and sleep disturbance, which occur during life stress and depression may be associated with depression-related alterations of immunity. To test whether sleep disturbance accounts for the reliable association between depressive symptoms and reduced immunity, correlational analyses have shown that insomnia is negatively correlated with NK activity in bereaved women, individuals undergoing other severe life stress (35), patients with major depression (40), and patients comorbid for depression and alcoholism (35). Together, these data are consistent with the hypothesis that specific symptom profiles contribute to the reduction of NK activity found in depression, and further implicate the severity of insomnia in depression-related suppression of NK activity.

Insomnia or subjective sleep disturbance is characterized objectively by disturbances of several sleep EEG continuity measures including increased sleep latency and decreased total sleep time and sleep efficiency. To extend the correlational findings between insomnia and NK activity, Irwin and colleagues (37) predicted that EEG measures of sleep continuity would also be associated with NK activity. Indeed, in depressed patients, EEG measures of total sleep time, sleep efficiency, duration of non-REM sleep and Stage 2 sleep were positively correlated with lytic activity. Furthermore, these relationships between sleep amounts and continuity measures were independent of the presence of a mood disorder because similar correlations between lytic activity and total sleep time, sleep efficiency, and duration of non-REM sleep were found in nondepressed control subjects. It appears that sleep amounts and/or quality, whether assessed by objective or subjective methods, are associated with immune function.

Further studies are needed to examine the mechanisms underlying an association between sleep disturbance and reduced NK activity in depression, although sleep-related changes in lymphokines or neuroendocrine signals are hypothesized. For example, a decrease in amounts of slow-wave sleep occurs in depression, and Moldofsky et al. (58) have reported a temporal association between the onset of slow-wave sleep and the secretion of IL-1 and IL-2, two lymphokines that are known to stimulate or activate NK cells. Alternatively, sleep is associated with decreased sympathetic outflow, and disturbance of total sleep time or loss of sleep efficiency has been proposed to elevate sympathetic activity and in turn reduce cellular immunity.

Activity

Changes in physical activity in depressed patients might also contribute to the reduction of cellular immunity. In our laboratory, assessment of psychomotor retardation and/or agitation by the Hamilton Depression Scale has shown that ratings of retardation negatively correlate with values of NK activity, whereas agitation is positively associated with lymphocyte proliferative responses (17). Separate from the study of depressed patients, a reduction of physical activity such as induced bed rest or immobilization in humans has been found to produce a reduction of immune function as measured by decreased antibody response to specific antigens. Conversely, acute physical exercise sharply increases NK activity (60) as well as circulating levels of interferon and IL-1, and exercise training of sedentary subjects also yields an increase in basal levels of cytotoxicity as compared to nonexercise controls. Finally, given the possible role of NK cells in immune surveillance, it is of interest that increased levels of physical activity are associated with a decrease in the incidence of certain tumors in animals.

Neuroendocrine-immune Interactions

This section focuses on those neuroendocrine hormones that are altered in depression and/or hypothesized to have a role in depression-related immune changes. Anatomical and in vitro evidence will be reviewed that indicates a direct influence of the hormone on immune cells. Discus-

sion of the in vivo regulation of immune function will then be described with a review of clinical studies that have evaluated the relationship between regulation of neuroendocrine function and immunity in depression (see also Chapters 62, 63, and 67, *this volume*).

Adrenal Axis

The secretion of corticosteroid has long been considered as the mechanism of stress-induced and/or depression-related suppression of immune function (14, 59). Specific intracytoplasmic corticosteroid receptors have been identified in normal human lymphocytes, and these receptors bind corticosteroids and appear to play a role in the regulation of cellular function through modulation of cyclic adenosine monophosphate (cAMP) levels. Indeed, in vitro studies have demonstrated that glucocorticoids inhibit IL-1 and IL-2 production at the level of cytokine gene transcription with resulting suppression of lymphocyte responses to mitogenic stimulation and NK cell activity (antibody-dependent cytotoxicity is relatively refractory to glucocorticoids) (14).

Glucocorticoids also have numerous in vivo effects on immune function. Serum levels of IgG, IgA, and IgM are suppressed by pharmacological doses of glucocorticoids in vivo (14). In addition, glucocorticoids affect the distribution of circulating lymphocytes, potently inhibit cellular cytotoxicity, and suppress mitogen-induced T-cell proliferation in vivo (14). B-cell proliferation is relatively resistant to glucocorticoids. Together these data demonstrate that glucocorticoids pharmacologically modulate cellular and humoral immune responses.

The role of in vivo physiological elevations of glucocorticoids in mediating alterations of immune function following stress has not been as conclusively demonstrated as the pharmacological effects of glucocorticoids. For example, in rats, acute administration of either forced immobilization (24), audiogenic stress, or isolation produces an activation of adrenal steroid secretion but does not alter cellular immune function. Likewise with repeated exposure to the stressor, pituitary adrenal activation is dissociated from a reduction in cytotoxicity. Furthermore, stress-induced suppression of lymphocyte function and/or NK activity following inescapable aversive stress occurs in either adrenalectomized or hypophysectomized animals (46). Finally, antagonism of stress-induced activation of the pituitary adrenal axis by the peripheral preadministration of an antiserum to corticotropin-releasing hormone (CRH) fails to alter stress-induced suppression of NK activity even though the release of ACTH and corticosterone is inhibited (41).

Consistent with these animal studies, clinical research has found no relationship between adrenocortical activity and immunity in depressed patients and in stressed persons. In depressed patients, decreased lymphocyte responses to mitogens were not correlated with circulating levels of adrenal cortical hormones (16,65) increased excretion rates of urinary free cortisol (49) or dexamethasone nonsuppression. Furthermore, in bereavement in which a reduction of NK activity has been demonstrated, we have found that this immunological change occurs even in subjects who had plasma cortisol levels comparable to control subjects. Miller and colleagues (57) also found no association between hypercortisolemia and NK activity in depressed patients. In contrast with these findings, Maes et al. found that baseline cortisol, urinary free cortisol, and postdexamethasone β-endorphin values explained up to 45% of the variance in lymphocyte proliferation, although in these studies lymphocyte function was inversely related to baseline cortisol but positively correlated with urinary free cortisol excretion.

It is alternatively hypothesized that lymphocytes of depressed patients may be even less sensitive to the effect of glucocorticoids (53). Following chronic exposure to glucocorticoids, adrenal steroid receptors expressed in immune tissues exhibit down regulation. Furthermore, dexamethasone-induced inhibition of T-cell blastogenesis is inversely correlated with plasma concentrations of cortisol (77), suggesting the possibility that elevated activity of the adrenal axis down-regulates the lymphocyte glucocorticoid receptor axis in depressed patients and decreases the sensitivity of lymphocytes to pharmacological as well as physiological concentrations of glucocorticoids.

Opioid Peptides

Pharmacological evidence has shown that opiate receptors are located on lymphocytes and macrophages, although few studies have reported on the saturability or stereospecificity of these binding sites (68). Nevertheless, opioid binding on immune cells is suggested by the finding that nanomolar concentrations of opiates affects active rosetting of human T lymphocytes. Morphine inhibits rosetting, whereas *met*-enkephalin stimulates it and both effects are blocked by naloxone. Using radiolabeling techniques, specific opioid binding on human phagocytic leukocytes (19), platelets, and lymphocytes has been demonstrated. Finally, Carr et al. (6) utilized antibodies to recognize opiate receptors on lymphocytes.

In vitro studies have found that opioid agonists alter a number of immune functions with both inhibitory and immunoenhancing effects described. Johnson et al. (43) found that α-endorphin, *met*-enkephalin, and *leu*-enkephalin (all with approximately equal potency) decrease the proliferation and antibody production of splenocytes in the plaque-forming assay, an effect that is blocked by naloxone. Confirming these results, (*des-tyr*)-β-endorphin is also active in suppressing the plaque-forming cell response. Proliferation induced by PHA is affected by opioid peptides, although both stimulatory

and inhibitory effects have been reported. Opioid agonist enhancement of mitogen-induced lymphocyte proliferation and IL-2 production are not blocked by the specific opiate antagonist naloxone. Also, NK activity is modulated by opiate agonists; very low concentrations of β-endorphin (10 fM) increase NK cell activity, an effect that is naloxone reversible. Interestingly, β-endorphin induced change of NK activity has been reported to have an inverted U-shaped dose–response curve, and enkephalins and selective opiate agonists also show bidirectional effects on human NK activity; subjects with "low" (below the median) NK activity show stimulation with enkephalin whereas the cytolytic activity of cells from the "high" group is inhibited by similar doses of enkephalin. Recent evidence suggested that endorphins modulate NK activity through the (6–9) amino acid region, that is, the α-helix portion of β-endorphin.

Peripheral administration of opioid agonists in vivo also alters cellular immune function as reflected by suppression of mitogen-induced lymphocyte proliferation, in vivo lymphocyte proliferation in a graft–host reaction (5), production of IL-2 and interferon, delayed-type hypersensitivity response (5), and NK activity. In contrast, induction of humoral immune responses to bacterial or viral antigens is not altered by chronic morphine.

The suppressive effects of peripherally administered opioid agonists has been proposed to be due to an indirect influence of opiates by CNS activation of either the hypothalamic-pituitary-adrenal (HPA) axis or the sympathetic nervous system. For example, the suppressive effects of morphine on the graft–host assay are less pronounced in adrenalectomized mice (5) and acute morphine suppression of NK activity is mediated by both α- and β-adrenergic pathways (6).

Nevertheless, direct peripheral effects of opioid agonists on the immune system are also possible, because opioid agonists bind on specific receptors on cells of the immune system. Indeed, experimental and correlative evidence suggest that peripheral increases of endogenous circulating concentrations of β-endorphin stimulate NK activity, similar to the findings generated in vitro. In the rat, release of β-endorphin into the plasma following acute exposure to forced immobilization are correlated with immediate, poststress *increases* of splenic NK activity. Likewise, clinical research has found exercise-induced enhancement of NK cytotoxicity is completely antagonized by the preadministration of the opiate antagonist naloxone (22). Finally, plasma levels of β-endorphin are *positively* correlated with NK activity in depressed patients (15).

Adrenocorticotropic Hormone

A receptor for ACTH has been identified on lymphocytes, also raising the possibility that some aspects of altered lymphocyte function in depression are regulated by this peptide. In vitro studies have shown that ACTH inhibits the antibody response at an early state in the antibody response (43). In regards to cellular immunity, the effects of ACTH administered in vitro and in vivo on NK cell function have been evaluated. Exogenous, peripheral administration of ACTH at physiological concentrations increases both NK activity and IL-2 stimulated NK cytotoxicity compared to levels in saline controls. Because in vitro doses of ACTH have no effect on NK activity, the action of this peptide in vivo is likely by an indirect mechanism, that is, alteration of leukocyte traffic or suppression of central CRH. In depressed patients, no association between plasma concentrations of ACTH and lymphocyte proliferation has been demonstrated, although the effects of ACTH on NK activity has not yet been evaluated.

Prolactin

A direct involvement of prolactin in the regulation of the immune system has been proposed. Prolactin receptors have been found on T and B lymphocytes, and prolactin induces a marked enhancement of NK activity. In hypophysectomized rats, as well as animals treated with bromocriptine, a dopamine agonist drug that inhibits prolactin secretion, impairment of both humoral and cell-mediated immune response has been demonstrated that can be reversed by treatment with exogenous, physiological doses of prolactin (3). In addition, antibodies to prolactin have been reported to inhibit lymphocyte proliferation (28). Preliminary observations by Darko and colleagues (16) have found that plasma levels of prolactin positively correlated with T-cell mitogen proliferation, although Clodi et al. (7) failed to show any immune alteration as reflected by serum concentrations of immunoglobulin, IL-1, soluble IL-2 receptor, lymphocyte subsets, and NK activity in patients with prolactinomas. Possibly chronic prolactin elevations lead to adaptive changes such that the immunomodulatory effects of prolactin are abolished.

Growth Hormone

Growth hormone is a polypeptide that plays a pivotal role in growth and development. In addition to its endocrine and metabolic effects, growth hormone is likely to have significant effects on the immune system, particularly T-cell development. In growth hormone-deficient mouse strains, hematopoietic, and B-cell progenitor deficiencies, marked atrophy of the cortical region of the thymus and an impairment of cell-mediated immunity have been found that can be reversed by treatment with growth hormone. In contrast to these observations, Cross and colleagues (11) indicated that hypopituitary mice lag behind heterozygous littermates with respect to development of immunocompetence but that normal immune responsiveness does fully develop. Exploratory clinical studies in depression have failed to identify any relationship between growth hormone and immune function (16), although the numbers of depressed subjects studied is small.

Serotonin

Substantial evidence has demonstrated that serotonergic systems are altered in depression, and recent in vitro data have shown that serotonin modulates lymphocyte proliferation and NK activity. For example, serotonin suppresses lymphocyte response to PHA in vitro, whereas the addition of serotonin to mononuclear cells enriched for NK activity induces a twofold dose-dependent enhancement of NK activity, similar to the stimulation induced by IL-2 (30). The induction of NK activity is monocyte dependent and is likely mediated by specific binding of serotonin at the 5-HT$_1$ receptor on the monocyte; the enhancing properties of serotonin are mimicked by the 5-HT$_1$ specific receptor agonist 8-OH DPAT and completely antagonized by the serotonin receptor antagonist cyproheptadine. Clinical studies have not yet characterized whether expression and regulation of the 5-HT$_{1A}$ receptor on monocytes is altered in depressed patients, and it is not known whether monocyte 5-HT$_{1A}$ activity has a role in the reduction of NK activity in depression (see also Chapter 37, *this volume*).

Autonomic Nervous System

Anatomical studies have revealed an extensive presence of autonomic fibers in both primary and secondary lymphoid organs (21), innervating both the vasculature and the parenchyma of the tissues and serving as one pathway for communication from the brain to cells of the immune system. Immunohistochemical studies of splenic tissue have demonstrated that nervous fibers containing norepinephrine, substance P or neuropeptide Y branch into the parenchyma (21) where lymphocytes (primarily T cells) reside. These postganglionic sympathetic fibers are not only adjacent to T cells but, at the electron microscopic level, end in synapticlike contacts with lymphocytes in the spleen (21).

In the adult animal, norepinephrine appears to act as a neurotransmitter in the spleen. Norepinephrine is likely released within the spleen; early studies found that splenic nerve stimulation yields a release of norepinephrine. Furthermore, in vivo dialysis techniques documented a 1-μM concentration of norepinephrine in the rat spleen (21); a concentration that is more than 100-fold higher than that in blood suggesting local release of norepinephrine within the spleen.

Lymphocytes have been found to receive signals from the sympathetic neurons by adrenoreceptor binding of norepinephrine, epinephrine, and dopamine. These β-receptors are linked to adenylate cyclase and have a functional role in the modulation of cellular immunity. In vitro incubation of lymphocytes with varying concentrations of either norepinephrine or epinephrine decreases NK activity and mitogenic responses, an effect that is reversed by a β-receptor antagonist. Additional in vitro studies have found that neuropeptide Y, a sympathetic neurotransmitter present in peripheral sympathetic nerves, also acts to inhibit NK activity (61).

In vivo studies have shown that the sympathetic nervous system has a role in the modulation of immune function. Either surgical denervation of the spleen or chemical sympathectomy using the neurotoxin 6-hydroxydopamine produces an augmented antibody response to thymus-dependent antigens such as SRBCs, an enhanced plaque-forming cell response to thymus-independent antigens, increased macrophage phagocytosis, and enhanced T- and B-cell responsiveness to mitogen stimulation that is strain specific. Conversely, infusion of adrenergic agonists such as isoproterenol in rats and in humans results in a down-regulation of β-adrenergic receptors in circulating mononuclear cells and a dose-dependent, transient decrement in mitogen responses that is likely mediated by a redistribution of circulating lymphocyte subpopulations via β_2 adrenergic mechanisms (60). In addition to sympathetic-induced alterations of nonspecific immune function, sympathetic neurotransmitters also suppress antigen-specific lymphocyte proliferation by inhibiting macrophage antigen processing and presentation and, indirectly, T-helper responses.

Acute, stress-induced elevations of sympathetic activity is one pathway that likely plays a role in stress-induced suppression of cellular and humoral immune responses. For example, in animals exposed to aversive stress or central doses of neuropeptides such as CRH that activate sympathetic outflow, suppression of cellular immunity or in vivo specific antibody responses is completely antagonized by either autonomic blockade, chemical sympathectomy, or β-receptor antagonism (13,36).

Chronic elevation of sympathetic tone has also been found to mediate a reduction of immunity (34). For example, in animals, induction of a chronic hyperadrenergic state (experimental congestive heart failure or 2-week infusion of the β-agonist isoproterenol) reduces NK activity, in vivo antibody responses, and lymphocyte proliferation. Similar to findings following acute stress, the immunosuppressive effect of chronic increased sympathetic tone is completely antagonized by β-receptor blockade. In humans, chronic elevated sympathetic tone, as reflected by circulating concentrations of neuropeptide Y, may also contribute to the modulation of immune function during severe life stress and depression (34). Neuropeptide Y is present in peripheral sympathetic nerves and is released following emotional stress potentiating the effects of vasoactive catecholamines and other pressor substances. Irwin et al. (34) have shown that plasma concentrations of neuropeptide Y are elevated in depressed patients as well as in aged individuals and persons undergoing severe Alzheimer caregiver stress. Furthermore, activation of the sympathetic nervous system and release of neuropeptide Y is associated with a reduction of natural cytotoxicity in depression and life stress. Additional findings also support the hypothesis that elevated sympathetic activity in depression is associated with immune alterations. In depressed patients, excretion of 3-methoxy-4-hydroxyphenylglycol (MHPG) has been used as an index of total body noradrenergic turnover or sympathetic activity, and MHPG excretion was inversely related with lymphocyte proliferative responses in depressed patients (54). Together, these data suggest that elevated sympathetic tone in patients with major depressive disorder and/or in persons undergoing life stress is inversely correlated with cellular immune function.

Central Nervous System

Central Lesion Studies

Much evidence exists that the brain coordinates autonomic nervous system and neuroendocrine outflow, which has been shown in separate studies to mediate immune function. To evaluate the role of the brain in the neural modulation of immunity, early experiments placed electrolytic or other destructive lesions in the CNS and demonstrated alterations in lymphoid tissue architecture, either impairment or enhancement of lymphoid cell activation, impairment of delayed-type hypersensitivity, and suppression of NK cell activity. Furthermore, hemispheric lateralization of immune control is evident, since partial ablation of the left hemisphere cortex, which results in a relative right-sided activation, produces significant decreases in the number of T lymphocytes and NK activity. Comparable lesions in the right cortex either have no effect or increase immune responses, although some investigations have found that right as compared to left decortication of mice produced a greater reduction of natural cytotoxic activity (2). In an effort to extend these preclinical observations of hemispheric lateralization of immune modulation, patterns of hemispheric activation in the frontal scalp region have been related to immune responses in women who show extreme differences in the asymmetry of frontal cortex activation (44). Consistent with animal studies, women with extreme right frontal activation had lower levels of NK activity than did left frontally activated individuals. Measure of lymphocyte proliferation and T-cell subsets did not differ.

Central Catecholamines

Additional studies have further evaluated the role of the brain in modulation of immunity and tested whether central catecholamine activity is associated with immune function. Injection of the neurotoxin 6-hydroxydopamine into the cisterna magna depletes CNS catecholamines and impairs the primary antibody immune response by inducing T-suppressor-cell activity (12). Further studies have evaluated the relationship between stress-induced central catecholamine alterations and changes in splenic NK activity and found positive correlations between mesocortical dopamine and dihydroxyphenylacetic acid (DOPAC) and NK activity but no relation between catecholamines and NK activity, possibly due to the limited number of brain regions, the large tissue samples assayed, and assay of catabolic products rather than in vivo release.

Central Opiates

Opiate-induced modulation of NK cytotoxicity is mediated in part by the CNS. Injection of methionine enkephalin directly into the cisterna magna results in an enhancement of NK cell activity. As well, opiate-mediated pathways in the brain produce polyinosinic:polycytidilic acid (poly I:C) conditioned-enhancement of NK activity. In contrast with these observations, NK activity is suppressed when a dose of morphine is given into the cerebral ventricle, an effect that is likely mediated by central opiate receptors since the effective central dose is a thousand times smaller than that required when given systemically. Moreover, peripheral administration of low doses of a morphine analog (one that does not cross the blood–brain barrier to enter the CNS) is not effective in altering NK activity. Finally, intracerebral infusion of morphine into the periaqueductal gray, but not other brain regions, produces a suppression of splenic NK activity (74). Use of selective μ, κ, and δ agonists microinjected into the lateral ventricle have further shown that central opiate-induced suppression of NK activity is mediated primarily through μ-type opioid receptors.

Central Interleukin-1β

Interleukin-1, a cytokine originally detected in the macrophage, has been preliminarily shown to be increased in the peripheral circulation of depressed patients (55). In addition to its biological effects peripherally, this cytokine when introduced into the brain induces slow-wave sleep, releases hypothalamic CRH, and produces increased circulating concentrations of ACTH. Because IL-1 plays a crucial role in regulating a number of immunological responses, Sundar et al. (73) and Brown et al. (4) have investigated whether central administration of IL-1 would affect immunity and demonstrated that central doses of IL-1 (3.1 to 12.4 fmol) rapidly reduces ex vivo cellular immune responses such as NK cell activity, lymphocyte proliferative response to PHA, IL-2 production, and macrophage IL-1 secretion. Importantly, the effects of central IL-1 on immune function are blocked by the administration of an antibody to CRH, indicating that IL-1β likely mediates immunosuppression by central release of CRH (64,73). Consequently, the pathways by which IL-1 regulates peripheral immune function are similar to mechanisms involved in central CRH suppression of immunity. Administration of a ganglionic blocker abrogates the effects of IL-1 (73) similar to observations that autonomic and sympathetic nervous mechanisms mediate CRH-induced suppression of NK activity (36).

Central Corticotropin Releasing Hormone

Depressed patients show elevated concentrations of cerebrospinal fluid CRH and this neuropeptide has been postulated to be a physiological CNS regulator that integrates biological responses to stress. Relevant to depression-related reduction of cellular immunity, central CRH has indeed been found to have a physiological role in mediating stress-induced suppression of immunity (41,42). Antiserum to CRH when given centrally into the lateral ventricle prior to foot shock stress completely abrogated stress-induced suppression of cellular immunity. In contrast, peripheral administration of antiserum to CRH failed to attenuate suppression of immunity following foot shock even though stress-induced release of ACTH and corticosterone was significantly antagonized. Further observations have supported the hypothesis that brain CRH coordinates immune function. Central administration of CRH, at doses known to act at extrahypothalamic sites to induce an increase in the firing rate of the locus coeruleus and activate autonomic outflow, produces a dose-dependent suppression of NK activity, in vivo specific antibody responses (33), and lymphocyte proliferation. In contrast, peripheral administration of CRH fails to suppress either cellular or humoral immune responses, even though such doses activate the pituitary adrenal axis. Finally, coadministration of the CRH antagonists immediately prior to a central dose of CRH has been found to antagonize central CRH-induced suppression of immune function, indicating that CRH coordinates reduction of immunity in a receptor-mediated manner in the brain, possibly at stress sites such as the locus coeruleus or central nucleus of the amygdala (33).

As reviewed above, considerable evidence has shown that noradrenergic projections to lymphoid tissue have a role in the modulation of immune function, and central CRH is crucial in coordinating sympathetic outflow. Neuroimmunological data have demonstrated that CRH activation of the sympathetic nervous system is essential in mediating the link between the brain and immune function. Either ganglionic blockade, sympathetic denervation, or β-adrenergic receptor antagonism completely abrogates CRH-induced suppression of cellular immunity (36). Again, CRH-induced modulation of immune function is dissociated from circulating levels of ACTH and corticosterone.

The health implications of these data are not known. However, it has recently been proposed that older depressed persons who have been shown to have increased morbidity and mortality are also more vulnerable to depression-related immune decline. To test the hypothesis of increased vulnerability of the aged to stress-related immune decline, CRH has been used as a neuropeptide probe and sympathetic and immune responses of aged rats to central CRH were compared to responses in young animals. Central CRH has been found to induce an exaggerated sympathetic activation and a greater suppression of NK activity in the aged rats as compared to responses in young animals, suggesting an increased responsivity or vulnerability of the aged to stress-induced immune suppression. Further data showing that central CRH modulates in vivo specific antibody responses (33) suggest that, under conditions in which CRH is released, such as stress or possibly depression in humans, the immune response may be down-regulated, leading to a delay in the synthesis of adequate levels of antibodies and failure of the immunological protection of the host to an infectious agent. Indeed, Glaser et al. (27) have shown that the immunological defense that is assumed to follow a vaccination may not be fully operative if the immunization occurs during times of stress. Consistent with these findings that CRH-induced immune modulation may have health implications, decreases in the central secretion of CRH have been associated with pathological increases of immune function. Lewis rats show a defect in CNS biosynthesis of CRH and these rats exhibit an increased susceptibility to streptococcal cell-wall-induced inflammatory arthritis (72).

Whereas endogenous brain CRH has been found to have a role in the in vivo suppression of immunity, additional data have suggested that CRH might also have local direct effects on immune processes, interacting with immune cells by paracrine mechanisms to provide a peripheral counterbalance in the regulation of the immune response. For example, CRH is contained in T lymphocytes, and PHA stimulation induces an increase in CRH mRNA levels. In vitro studies have reported both stimulatory (69) and inhibitory effects of CRH on cellular immune function, whereas peripheral injections of CRH have been found to promote several immune functions. For example, peripheral in vivo administration of CRH binds at receptors on macrophage (75), enhances macrophage secretion of IL-1, and increases secretion of β-endorphin from lymphocytes leading to stimulation of the antibody response when the control response was low (29). Karalis et al. (45) have also shown that CRH pro-

duced by immune cells has autocrine inflammatory action, such that in vivo administration of antiserum to CRH caused suppression of both inflammatory exudate volume and cell concentration. These data regarding the peripheral direct effect of CRH on immune function suggest that CRH is capable of acting on immune cells in a manner that is antithetical to that of hypothalamic CRH (see also Chapters 45 and 84, *this volume*).

HEALTH IMPLICATIONS OF DEPRESSION-RELATED IMMUNE ALTERATIONS

The clinical importance of altered cellular immunity in depressed patients is not yet known. Although substantial evidence has been found for an association between stress or depression and increased illness (10), the association between psychological stress and immune-related disease remains limited to several studies. In regard to infectious illness, Cohen et al. (9) have recently shown that psychological stress was associated in a dose–response manner with an increased risk of acute infectious respiratory illness. Importantly, this association was due to increased rates of infection rather than to an increased frequency of symptoms after infection. Measures of cellular immune function were not obtained in this study. Other studies, but not all, have found that stressful events increase the risk of verified acute respiratory illness. Depressed patients have been found to show a higher incidence and higher titers of herpes simplex virus antibodies, but again no study has yet delineated a causal chain showing that severe life stress or a particular psychological state such as depression produced an immunological response, which then resulted in an altered clinical outcome.

The findings of increased cancer incidence in clinically depressed patients are consistent with a ''null or weak relationship'' (25). Although several prospective follow-up studies have demonstrated a relationship between mood disorders and clinical depression and increased cancer morbidity and mortality particularly in male patients over age 40 who had primary diagnoses of mood disorders, small case numbers indicate that these results should be cautiously interpreted. Likewise, epidemiological studies on the role of depression in cancer have been inconclusive. Depressed mood as measured by the Minnesota Multiphasic Personality Inventory depression scale was found to be a significant risk factor for cancer incidence and mortality over 20 years of follow up. However, subsequent studies have failed to replicate the observation that depression is associated with an increase in the relative risk of cancer. However, other factors such as smoking or alcohol use have been proposed to interact with depressive symptoms to increase the risk of cancer, and an increased risk of cancer has been reported in persons with depressed mood who are smokers when compared with persons who are never smokers without depressed mood.

Furthermore, there was a dose–response effect of cigarette smoking on the depressed mood–cancer relationship in the smokers.

The promise of recent investigations has suggested that psychiatric interventions that reduce psychological distress may have beneficial effects on cancer survival. Spiegel et al. (70) found that group psychotherapy of breast cancer patients improved quality of life and extended life expectancy for patients with metastatic breast cancer, and Fawzy et al. (20) showed that other types of cancer patients improve both psychologically as well as immunologically with psychosocial group therapy. The psychoneuroimmunological link between depression and psychological stress and the outcome of immune-related medical disorders will be refined by further research that addresses the role of depressive symptoms, such as sleep disturbance, in the modulation of immunity and defines the neurobiological paths that underlie the interaction between the brain, behavior, and immunity.

ACKNOWLEDGMENTS

This work was supported in part by VA Merit Review, NIMH Grant MH44275, MH46867, 5-T32 MH183999, and MH30914; and the General Clinical Research Center (M01RR00827).

REFERENCES

1. Andreoli A, Keller SE, Rabaeus M, Zaugg L, Garrone G, Taban C. Immunity, major depression, and panic disorder comorbidity. *Biol Psychiatry* 1992;31:896–908.
2. Belluardo N, Mudo G, Cella S, Bindoni M. Effect of cerebral hemisphere decortication on the cytotoxic activity of natural killer and natural cytotoxic lymphocytes in the mouse. *Brain Res* 1990;524:297–302.
3. Bernton E, Meltzer M, Holaday JW. Suppression of macrophage activation and T-lymphocyte function in hypoprolactinemic mice. *Science* 1988;239:401–404.
4. Brown R, Li Z, Vriend CY, et al. Suppression of splenic macrophage interleukin-1 secretion following intracerebroventricular injection of interleukin-1β: evidence for pituitary–adrenal and sympathetic control. *Cell Immunol* 1991;132:84–93.
5. Bryant HU, Roudebush RE. Suppressive effects of morphine pellet implants on in vivo parameters of immune function. *J Pharm Exp Ther* 1990;255(2):410–414.
6. Carr DJJ, Gebhardt BM, Paul D. Alpha adrenergic and Mu-2 opioid receptors are involved in morphine-induced suppression of splenocyte natural killer activity. *J Pharm Exp Ther* 1993;264(3):1179–1186.
7. Clodi M, Svoboda T, Kotzmann H, et al. Effect of elevated serum prolactin concentrations on cytokine production and natural killer cell activity. *Neuroendocrinology* 1992;56:775–779.
8. Coe CL, Rosenberg LT, Levine S. Immunological consequences of psychological disturbance and maternal loss in infancy. In: Rovee-Collier C, Lipsitt LP, eds. *Advances in infancy research*. Norwood, OH: Ablex Publishing; 1985:98–136.
9. Cohen S, Tyrrell DA, Smith AP. Psychological stress and susceptibility to the common cold. *New Engl J Med* 1991;325(9):606–656.
10. Cohen S, Williamson G. Stress and infectious disease in humans. *Psychol Bull* 1991;109(1):5–24.
11. Cross RJ, Bryson JS, Roszman TL. Immunologic disparity in the hypopituitary dwarf mouse. *J Immunol* 1992;148(5):1347–1352.
12. Cross RJ, Roszman TL. Central catecholamine depletion impairs in vivo immunity but not in vitro lymphocyte activation. *J Neuroimmunol* 1988;19:33–45.
13. Cunnick JE, Lysle DT, Kucinski BJ, Rabin BS. Evidence that shock-induced immune suppression is mediated by adrenal hormones and peripheral β-adrenergic receptors. *Pharmacol Biochem Behav* 1990;36:645–651.
14. Cupps TR, Fauci AS. Corticosteroid-mediated immunoregulation in man. *Immunol Rev* 1982;65:133–155.
15. Darko D, Irwin M, Risch SC, Gillin JC. Plasma beta-endorphin and natural killer cell activity in patients with major depression. *Psychiatry Res* 1992;43:111–119.
16. Darko DF, Gillin JC, Risch SC, et al. Mitogen-stimulated lymphocyte proliferation and pituitary hormones in major depression. *Biol Psychiatry* 1989;26:145–155.
17. Darko DF, Wilson NW, Gillin JC, Golshan S. A critical appraisal of mitogen-induced lymphocyte proliferation in depressed patients. *Am J Psychiatry* 1991;148(3):337–344.
18. Evans DL, Folds JD, Petitto JM, et al. Circulating natural killer cell phenotypes in men and women with major depression. *Arch Gen Psychiatry* 1992;49:388–395.
19. Farrar WL, Hill JM, Harel-Bellan A, Vinocour M. The immunological brain. *Immunol Rev* 1987;100:361–377.
20. Fawzy FI, Kemeny ME, Fawzy NW, et al. A structured psychiatric intervention for cancer patients. II. Changes over time in immunological measures. *Arch Gen Psychiatry* 1990;47(8):729–735.
21. Felten DL, Felten SY, Bellinger DL, et al. Noradrenergic sympathetic neural interactions with the immune system: structure and function. *Immunol Rev* 1987;100:225–260.
22. Fiatarone MA, Morley JE, Bloom ET, Benton D, Solomon GF, Makinodan T. The effects of exercise on natural killer cell activity in young and old subjects. *J Gerontol* 1989;44:M37–M45.
23. Fischler B, Bocken R, DeWaele M, Thielemans K. Major depressive disorder, endogenicity and natural killer cell numbers and activity. *Int J Neurosci* 1990;51:357–358.
24. Flores CM, Hernandez MC, Hargreaves KM, Bayer BM. Restraint stress-induced elevations in plasma corticosterone and β-endorphin are not accompanied by alterations in immune function. *J Neuroimmunol* 1990;28:219–225.
25. Fox BH. Depressive symptoms and risk of cancer. *JAMA* 1989;262:1231–1231.
26. Glaser R, Kennedy S, Lafuse WP, et al. Psychological stress-induced modulation of interleukin-2 receptor gene expression and interleukin-2 production in peripheral blood leukocytes. *Arch Gen Psychiatry* 1990;47:707–712.
27. Glaser R, Kiecolt-Glaser JK, Bonneau RH, Malarkey W, Kennedy S, Hughes J. Stress-induced modulation of the immune response to recombinant hepatitis B vaccine. *Psychosom Med* 1992;54:22–29.
28. Hartmann DP, Holaday JW, Bernton EW. Inhibition of lymphocyte proliferation by antibodies to prolactin. *FASEB J* 1989;3:2194–2202.
29. Heijnen CJ, Kavelaars AK, Ballieux RE. β-Endorphin: cytokine and neuropeptide. *Immunol Rev* 1991;119:41–63.
30. Hellstrand K, Hermodsson S. Role of serotonin in the regulation of human natural killer cell cytotoxicity. *J Immunol* 1987;139(3):869–875.
31. Herbert TB, Cohen S. Depression and immunity: a meta-analytic review. *Psychosom Med* 1993;55:364–379.
32. Hickie I, Hickie C, Lloyd A, Silove D, Wakefield D. Impaired in vivo immune responses in patients with melancholia. *Br J Psychiatry* 1993;162:751–757.
33. Irwin M. Brain corticotropin releasing hormone and interleukin-1β induced suppression of specific antibody production. *Endocrinology* 1993;133:1352–1360.
34. Irwin M, Brown M, Patterson T, Hauger R, Mascovich A, Grant I. Neuropeptide Y and natural killer cell activity: findings in depression and Alzheimer caregiver stress. *FASEB J* 1991;5:3100–3107.
35. Irwin M, Caldwell C, Smith TL, Brown S, Schuckit MA, Gillin JC. Major depressive disorder, alcoholism, and reduced natural killer cell cytotoxicity: role of severity of depressive symptoms and alcohol consumption. *Arch Gen Psychiatry* 1990;47:713–719.
36. Irwin M, Hauger RL, Jones L, Provencio M, Britton KT. Sympathetic nervous system mediates central corticotropin-releasing factor

induced suppression of natural killer cytotoxicity. *J Pharmacol Exp Ther* 1990;255(1):101–107.

37. Irwin M, Lacher U, Caldwell C. Depression and reduced natural killer cytotoxicity: a longitudinal study of depressed patients and control subjects. *Psychol Med* 1992;22:1045–1050.
38. Irwin M, Patterson T, Smith TL, et al. Reduction of immune function in life stress and depression. *Biol Psychiatry* 1990;270:22–30.
39. Irwin M, Smith TL, Gillin JC. Electroencephalographic sleep and natural killer activity in depressed patients and control subjects. *Psychosom Med* 1992;54:10–21.
40. Irwin M, Smith TL, Gillin JC. Reduced natural killer cytotoxicity in depressed patients. *Life Sci* 1987;41:2127–2133.
41. Irwin MR, Vale W, Rivier C. Central corticotropin releasing factor mediates the suppressive effect of stress on natural killer cytotoxicity. *Endocrinology* 1990;126(6):2837–2844.
42. Jain R, Zwickler D, Hollander CS, et al. Corticotropin-releasing factor modulates the immune response to stress in the rat. *Endocrinology* 1991;128:1329–1336.
43. Johnson HM, Downs MO, Pontzer CH, Blalock JE. Neuroendocrine peptide hormone regulation of immunity. *Neuroimmunoendocrinol Chem Immunol* [Basel] 1992;2:49–83.
44. Kang DH, Davidson RJ, Coe CL, Wheeler RE, Tamarken AJ. Frontal brain asymmetry and immune function. *Behav Neurosci* 1991;105(6):860–869.
45. Karalis K, Sano H, Redwine J, Listwak S, Wilder RL, Chrousos GP. Autocrine or paracrine inflammatory actions of corticotropin-releasing hormone in vivo. *Science* 1991;254:421–423.
46. Keller SE, Schleifer SJ, Liotta AS, Bond RN, Farhoody N, Stein M. Stress-induced alterations of immunity in hypophysectomized rats. *Proc Natl Acad Sci USA* 1988;85:9297–9301.
47. Kiecolt-Glaser JK, Dura JR, Speicher CE, Trask OJ, Glaser R. Spousal caregivers of dementia victims: longitudinal changes in immunity and health. *Psychosom Med* 1991;53:345–362.
48. Kronfol Z, House JD. Depression, hypothalamic–pituitary adrenocortical activity and lymphocyte function. *Psychopharmacol Bull* 1985;21:476–478.
49. Kronfol Z, Hover JD, Silva J, et al. Depression, urinary free cortisol excretion, and lymphocyte function. *Br J Psychiatry* 1986;148:70–73.
50. Kronfol Z, Nair M, Goodson J, Goel K, Haskett R, Schwartz S. Natural killer cell activity in depressive illness: a preliminary report. *Biol Psychiatry* 1989;26:753–756.
51. Krueger JM, Karnovsky ML. Sleep and the immune response. *Ann NY Acad Sci* 1987;496:510–516.
52. Laudenslager M, Capitanio JP, Reite M. Possible effects of early separation experiences on subsequent immune function in adult macaque monkeys. *Am J Psychiatry* 1985;142(7):862–864.
53. Lowy MT, Reder AT, Gormley GJ, Meltzer HY. Comparison of in vivo and in vitro glucocorticoid sensitivity in depression: relationship to the dexamethasone suppression test. *Biol Psychiatry* 1988;24:619–630.
54. Maes M, Bosmans E, Suy E, Minner B, Raus J. Impaired lymphocyte stimulation by mitogens in severely depressed patients a complex interface with HPA axis hyperfunction, noradrenergic activity and the ageing process. *Br J Psychiatry* 1989;155:793–798.
55. Maes M, Bosmans E, Suy E, Vandervorst C, deJonckheere C, Raus J. Depression-related disturbances in mitogen-induced lymphocyte responses and interleukin-1β and soluble interleukin-2 receptor production. *Acta Psychiatr Scand* 1991;84:379–386.
56. Maier SF, Laudenslager ML. Inescapable shock, shock controllability, and mitogen stimulated lymphocyte proliferation. *Brain Behav Immun* 1988;2:87–91.
57. Miller AH, Asnis GM, Lackner C, Halbreich U, Norin AJ. Depres-

58. sion, natural killer cell activity, and cortisol secretion. *Biol Psychiatry* 1991;29:878–886.
59. Moldofsky H, Lue FA, Davidson JR, Gorczynski R. Effects of sleep deprivation on human immune function. *FASEB J* 1989;3:1972–1977.
60. Munck A, Guyre PM, Holbrook NJ. Physiological functions of glucocorticoids in stress and their relation to pharmacologic actions. *Endocrine Rev* 1984;5:25–44.
61. Murray DR, Irwin M, Rearden CA, Ziegler M, Motulsky H, Maisel AS. Sympathetic and immune interactions during dynamic exercise: mediation via a β2-adrenergic dependent mechanism. *Circulation* 1992;86:203–213.
62. Nair MPN, Schwartz SA, Wu K, Kronfol Z. Effect of neuropeptide Y on natural killer activity of normal human lymphocytes. *Brain Behav Immun* 1993;7:70–78.
63. Nerozzi D, Santoni A, Bersani G, et al. Reduced natural killer cell activity in major depression: neuroendocrine implications. *Psychoneuroendocrinology* 1989;14:295–302.
64. Palmblad J, Petrini B, Wasserman J, Akerstedt T. Lymphocyte and granulocyte reactions during sleep deprivation. *Psychosom Med* 1979;41(4):273–278.
65. Saperstein A, Brand H, Audhya T, et al. Interleukin 1β mediates stress-induced immunosuppression via corticotropin-releasing factor. *Endocrinology* 1992;30(1):152–158.
66. Schleifer SJ, Keller SE, Bond RN, Cohen J, Stein M. Major depressive disorder and immunity: role of age, sex, severity, and hospitalization. *Arch Gen Psychiatry* 1989;46:81–87.
67. Schleifer SJ, Keller SE, Meyerson AT, Raskin MJ, Davis KL, Stein M. Depression and immunity: lymphocyte function in ambulatory depressed patients, hospitalized schizophrenic patients, and patients hospitalized for herniotheraphy. *Arch Gen Psychiatry* 1985;42:129–133.
68. Schleifer S, Keller SE, Meyerson AT, Raskin MD, Davis KL, Stein M. Lymphocyte function in major depressive disorder. *Arch Gen Psychiatry* 1984;41:484–486.
69. Sibinga NES, Goldstein A. Opioid peptides and opioid receptors in cells of the immune system. *Ann Rev Immunol* 1988;6:219–249.
70. Singh VK. Stimulatory effect of corticotropin-releasing neurohormone on human lymphocyte proliferation and interleukin-2 receptor expression. *J Neuroimmunol* 1989;23:257–262.
71. Spiegel D, Bloom J, Kraemer HC, Gottheil E. The beneficial effect of psychosocial treatment on survival of metastatic breast cancer patients: a randomized prospective outcome study. *Lancet* 1989;10/14:888–891.
72. Stein M, Miller AH, Trestman RL. Depression, the immune system, and health and illness. *Arch Gen Psychiatry* 1991;48:171–177.
73. Sternberg EM, Young WS III, Calogero AE, et al. A central nervous system defect in biosynthesis of corticotropin-releasing hormone is associated with susceptibility to streptococcal cell wall-induced arthritis in Lewis rats. *Proc Natl Acad Sci USA* 1989;86:4771–4775.
74. Sundar SK, Cierpial MA, Kilts C, Ritchie JC, Weiss JM. Brain IL-1-induced immunosuppression occurs through activation of both pituitary-adrenal axis and sympathetic nervous system by corticotropin-releasing factor. *J Neurosci* 1990;10(11):3701–3706.
75. Weber RJ, Pert A. The periaqueductal gray matter mediates opiate-induced immunosuppression. *Science* 1989;245:188–190.
76. Webster EL, Tracey DE, Jutila MA, Wolfe SAJr, DeSouza EB. Corticotropin-releasing factor receptors in mouse spleen: identification of receptor-bearing cells as resident macrophages. *Endocrinology* 1990;127:440–452.
77. Weisse CS. Depression and immunocompetence: a review of the literature. *Psychol Bull* 1992;111(3):475–489.
78. Wodarz N, Rupprecht R, Kornhuber J, et al. Normal lymphocyte responsiveness to lectins but impaired sensitivity to in vitro glucocorticoids in major depression. *J Affect Disord* 1991;22:241–248.

Psychopharmacology: The Fourth Generation of Progress, edited by Floyd E. Bloom and David J. Kupfer. Raven Press, Ltd., New York © 1995.

CHAPTER 86

Biological Rhythms in Mood Disorders

Anna Wirz-Justice

Evolution has provided us with a day within, an endogenous template that anticipates the demands of the day without—the circadian system. If temporal order is essential for health, as the appropriate timing of psychological, behavioral, physiological, and hormonal rhythms with respect to the external day–night cycle imply, then temporal disorder should have clinical sequelae. Indeed, it is now well established that certain sleep disorders, such as delayed- or advanced-sleep-phase syndrome, arise from inappropriate phasing of the endogenous circadian clock with respect to normal sleep times. These rhythm disturbances are generally not accompanied by any psychiatric illness. Other sleep disorders, such as those related to shift work and transmeridian flight, arise from sudden shifts of the sleep–wake cycle without concomitant synchronization of the endogenous circadian component. Here there appears to be a closer link with mood disorders.

The remarkable episodic nature of some forms of affective illness as a manifestation of abnormal rhythmicity was first described in detail by German psychiatrists at the beginning of the century. The patterns of periodic recurrence, links with time of year or hormonal cycles, characteristic sleep disturbances, or diurnal mood fluctuations, later stimulated very specific hypotheses, beginning with the original studies of Curt Richter in the 1950s (49). The question as to whether the observed disturbances of biological rhythms in mood disorders reflect an underlying disorder of the biological clock is as yet unresolved. The last decade has seen an unprecedented growth into this aspect of depression research. The circadian system provides an integrative framework for concepts of affective illness involving psychopathological changes, sleep regulation, and neuroendocrine and neurotransmitter mechanisms.

A. Wirz-Justice: Psychiatric University Clinic, CH-4025 Basel, Switzerland.

PERIODICITY IN PSYCHOPATHOLOGY

The rare clinical observation of precise periodicity in psychopathology has provided certain clues to an underlying aberration of normal physiological rhythms. What mechanisms could explain the extraordinary stability, unaffected by any drug treatment, of the manic–depressive cycles documented for over 35 years in a single patient (Fig. 1A) (40)? Is there a causal link between rapid cycling and the circadian system? How are mood changes in women susceptible to affective illness linked with the menstrual cycle and the postpartum period? (See Chapter 88, *this volume.*) And most remarkably, how can depressive phases be triggered by time of year? A new diagnostic subgroup of depressive disorders with seasonal pattern (seasonal affective disorder, SAD) has been successfully treated with bright light (51). Prospective weekly depression self-ratings in a SAD patient over three consecutive cycles document this replicable seasonality of recurrence in autumn (Fig. 1B). Without treatment, the depressive phase lasted until spring. Light therapy administered toward the end of the depressive phase in January induced remission, light therapy administered at the beginning of the depressive phase in November prevented its evolution. Light therapy can be considered the most successful clinical application of circadian rhythm concepts in psychiatry to date.

DIURNAL VARIATION OF MOOD

The most extensively described, yet still least understood, rhythmic phenomenon in depression is the so-called classic melancholic symptom of diurnal variation of mood (DV) (see ref. 21 for a review). In the last few years, a number of studies have documented that DV is a frequent phenomenon, but not specific for endogenous depression (DV is also found, for example, in reactive

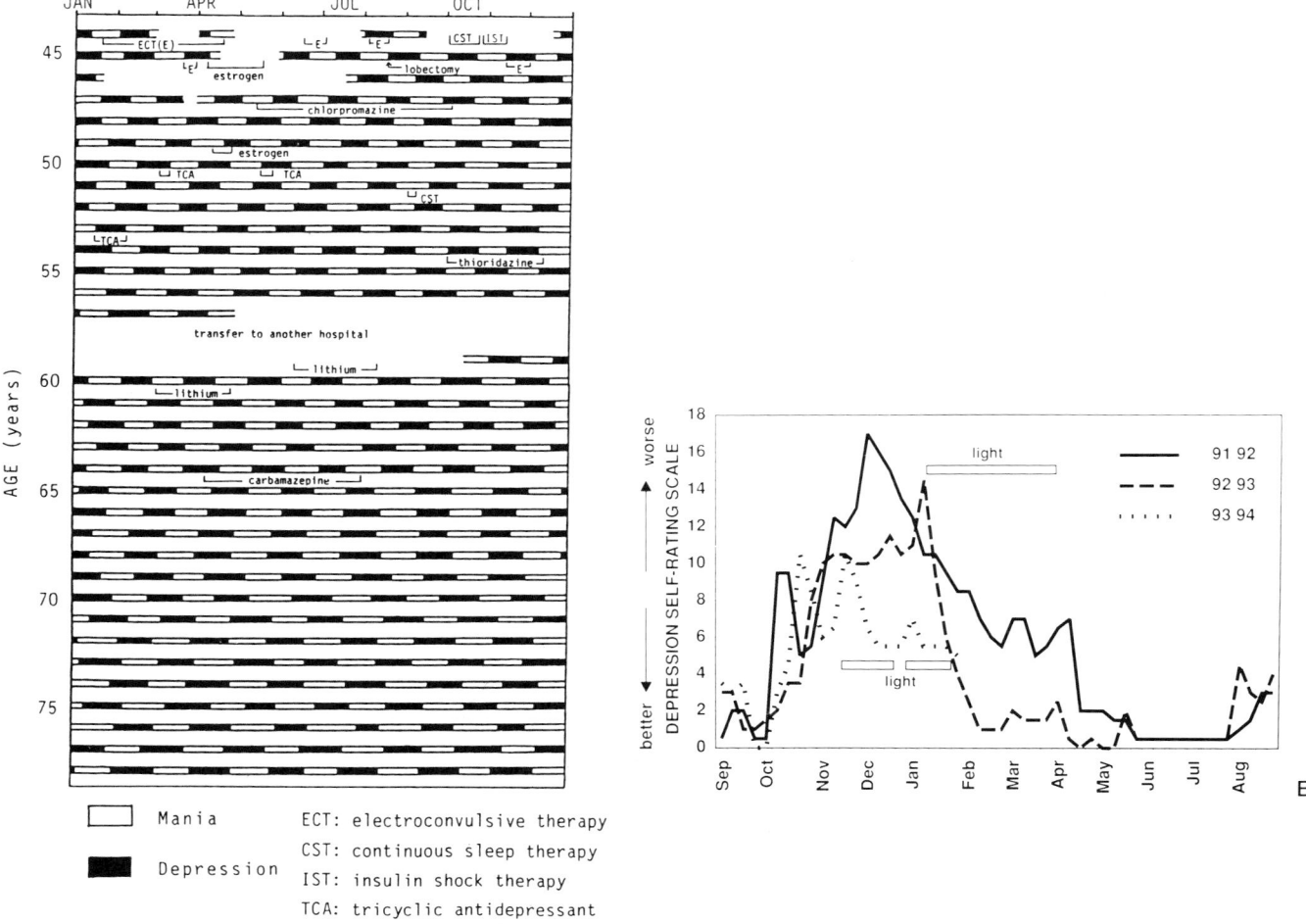

FIG. 1. **A:** Clinical records (35 years) of a rapid-cycling manic-depressive woman were analyzed. The precision of cycling was within 2—4 days. No drug treatment affected the periodicity. However the manic—depressive cycles showed a positive correlation with age, beginning with a length of 21 days at 50 years and extending to 28 days at 80 (0.27 days/year). The number of manic days in summer tended to be longer than in the other three seasons. Reprinted with permission from ref. 40. **B:** Long-term prospective weekly self-ratings (von Zerssen scale, ratings higher than 6 document increasing depressive symptoms) in a diagnosed SAD patient (52-year-old woman) following successful participation in a light therapy trial in 1990 (study summarized in ref. 74). In the winter of 1991—1992 she had no treatment of any kind. Thus the onset of depression in October and the spontaneous remission in April represents the natural time course of the illness. In the winter of 1992—1993 she decided late in the season to initiate light therapy. This induced rapid amelioration and shortened the depressive phase by approximately 2 months. In the winter of 1993—1994 she initiated light therapy at the onset of depression in autumn, which prevented the appearance of a major depressive episode. Wirz-Justice et al., *unpublished data.*

depression, or in SAD). It is not even specific for depression, because it occurs in healthy subjects and in other psychiatric illnesses. The presence of DV is not consistent throughout the course of depression: the type of DV (morning low, evening low, indifferent pattern) can change from day to day in a given patient. In short, DV is surprisingly variable when one considers its prominent position in established diagnostic systems.

There is poor agreement between daily mood self-ratings and retrospective judgement of DV. Diurnal variation of mood is not dependent on clinical state (e.g., depth

of depression, or season in SAD patients). There is no systematic relationship between the type of DV and melancholic or atypical depressive symptoms.

New long-term prospective documentation of hospitalized patients by the Groningen research group show that every pattern of DV can be documented (2). The underlying potential for manifestation of DV may be present, but DV is not expressed on all days. The patterns in two individual patients, one predominantly with, and one without significant DV during a 90-day period of gradual clinical improvement, are shown in Fig. 2. This list of

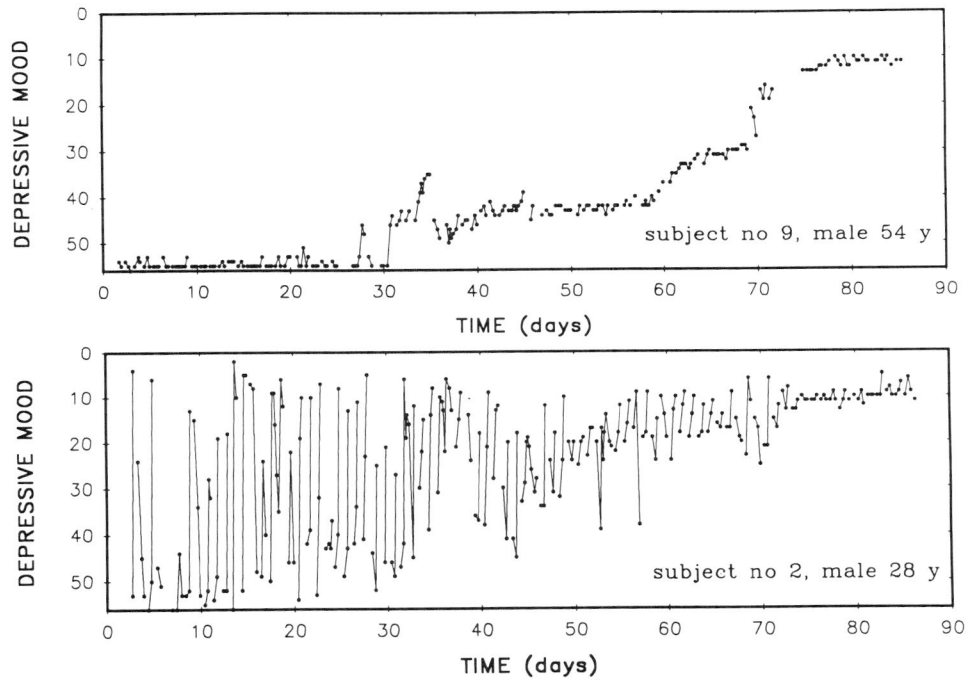

FIG. 2. Longitudinal registration of self-ratings of depressed mood using the Adjective Mood Scale (this method is described in ref. 2) three times daily, at 9 a.m., 5 p.m., and 10 p.m. in major depressive patients throughout their entire hospitalization period. Two extreme examples of data-sets are (*top*) a patient without any large fluctuations of mood but a slow and steady improvement, and (*bottom*), a similar long-term improvement at the end of a long period of large diurnal mood swings. In this patient, most of the days were characterized by severe depression in the morning and euthymia in the evening. Reprinted with permission from Gordijn et al. (*in preparation*).

rather negative observations leads to the moot question as to the relevance of the phenomenon. Clinically, there remain certain consistencies that underline its importance. One of these is that the propensity to produce DV, and in particular, DV with morning low, is a good predictor for sleep deprivation response.

In recent studies of the circadian rhythm of mood during controlled 40-hr sleep deprivation (the constant routine protocol), we have been able to document the kinetics of mood change very precisely (11,74) (Fig. 3). The subjects are kept sitting in bed without temporal input during this study, and thus mood ratings are not influenced by outside daily events. It can be seen that on the first day, the depressed patients (SAD in winter) show low morning mood that increases slightly in the afternoon, but that during the night, mood declines again. The minimum at 5 to 6 a.m. appears to be the switch point. There is an almost linear improvement after this time. However, the pattern on the second day is more complex, since an afternoon dip is noticeable, with mood improving again before sleep. From these data, it is clear that measurement of mood at two or three time points each day, under normal conditions, may give misleading information as to the presence of DV. Given that the circadian rhythm of mood is individually somewhat different in its timing adds to the potential variance. However, the sleep-deprivation–induced mood improvement is very clear. This pattern can be contrasted with that of control subjects, whose mood is much higher than that of depressed patients throughout the entire experiment, but whose mood rather declines after sleep deprivation. In summary, these studies provide the first data documenting a circadian rhythm in mood (as opposed to diurnal variation).

The extent of DV has been suggested to predict later response to conventional antidepressant drugs. As a working hypothesis, it has been proposed that the presence of DV (or greater variability) is a symptom signaling the propensity for change, that is, the potential for improvement, and preliminary findings do support this concept (21).

SLEEP AND SLEEP DEPRIVATION IN DEPRESSION

Sleep disturbances are inextricably linked with depressive illness (3,4,65; see also Chapter 139, *this volume*). Insomnia with early morning awakening is most characteristic. However, hypersomnia is also found (e.g., in bipolar patients or in atypical depression with or without seasonal pattern). That the interrelation of sleep and mood in major depression is not an epiphenomenon, is most clearly demonstrated by the rapid and dramatic, albeit usually short-lasting, improvement after total sleep deprivation first described by Schulte more than 20 years ago (56), and found in about 60% of depressed patients (3,4,32,34,53,65,67,70,75). The equally rapid return of depressive symptoms after subsequent recovery sleep again suggests a crucial role for sleep regulatory mechanisms in the clinical manifestation of depression. The therapeutic response to sleep deprivation is found independent of diagnostic categories, whether endogenous or reactive, psychotic or nonpsychotic, unipolar or bipolar, late luteal phase dysphoric disorder, schizoaffective or seasonal depression. There is evidence that a propensity for diurnal variation of mood with amelioration in the

MOOD IN WINTER

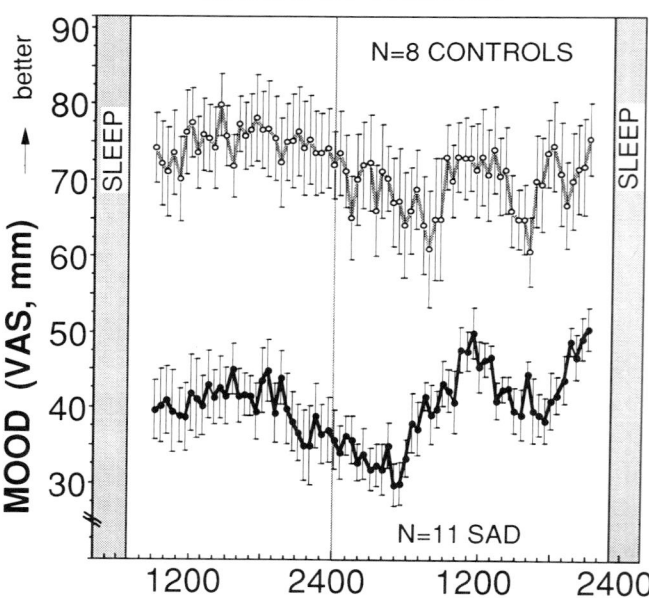

FIG. 3. Circadian rhythm of half-hourly self-ratings of mood (Visual Analogue Scale, VAS, mean ± sem): 0 mm = extremely depressed mood; 50 mm = euthymia; 100 mm = extremely good mood) throughout a total sleep deprivation during a 40-hr constant routine protocol (see ref. 74 for details). The subjects slept in the laboratory before and after the constant routine. The vertical line is anchored at midnight. Two groups of women were studied in winter, in the follicular phase of their menstrual cycle, when present: patients diagnosed as SAD, N = 11, aged 46.5 ± 3.9 years (Hamilton Depression Scale score = 13.9 ± 1.5) and matched nondepressed controls, N = 8, aged 50.4 ± 4.4 years. ANOVA for repeated measures was carried out using 1.5 hourly averages. This showed that (a) controls had higher mood ratings than SAD {$F_{(1,17)}$ = 58.6, p = 0.0001}; (b) both groups showed a circadian rhythm {$F_{(23,391)}$ = 2.8, p = 0.0001}; (c) the time course of mood change was different in the two groups. SAD showed a mood improvement with sleep deprivation, controls rather a decline: {interaction term $F_{(23,391)}$ = 1.7, p = 0.026} (Wirz-Justice et al., *unpublished data*).

evening predicts sleep deprivation response (summarized in ref. 21).

Other sleep manipulations that have positive effects are partial sleep deprivation in the second half of the night, rapid-eye-movement (REM) sleep deprivation, or phase advance of the sleep–wake cycle. The variety of these sleep manipulations and their temporal course are summarized in Table 1. These experimental results suggest that the depressive process is sleep dependent and requires that sleep coincide with a sleep-sensitive early morning circadian phase (70). The switch out of depression (and into hypomania and mania) often occurs after a spontaneous sleep deprivation. The time when this switch is most likely to occur is also the second half of the night (67). In the rapid cycler above (Fig. 1A), 81% of 64 switches

into mania observed over a 10-year period occurred between 11 p.m. and 8 a.m. half of these between 2 a.m. and 8 a.m. (40).

The phenomenon of relapse after recovery sleep has been studied using naps at different times of day, of different duration and sleep architecture. Although a nap in the morning induced relapse more often than an afternoon nap (suggesting a circadian-dependent factor), no clock time has been found where relapse cannot occur, nor is a depressogenic nap predominantly associated with REM- or non-REM sleep (nap studies are summarized in ref. 4).

Preliminary studies suggest that sleep deprivation can potentiate long-term drug treatment and may even predict it. Conversely, there have been attempts to prolong the sleep deprivation response with adjuvant antidepressants, lithium, or thyroid hormones, repeated partial sleep deprivations, or most recently phase advance of the sleep–wake cycle (4).

In order to consider putative mechanisms underlying these clinical observations, the concepts of circadian physiology and sleep regulation need first to be described.

CIRCADIAN RHYTHMS AND SLEEP REGULATION

Mammalian circadian rhythms are driven by a central pacemaker located in the suprachiasmatic nuclei (SCN) of the anterior hypothalamus. The SCN is the only pacemaker in mammalian systems for which convincing evidence exists (neural mechanisms of the mammalian circadian system are reviewed in ref. 25). There may be a second, coupled circadian pacemaker in the retina actively gating the transduction of photic information (48).

The endogenous rhythms generated by the SCN (whose periodicity is slightly different from 24 hr) are synchronized (entrained) to the 24-hr day by "zeitgebers" (regular recurring environmental signals). Light is the major, but not unique zeitgeber, entraining the circadian clock to 24 hr as well as providing information about daylength or photoperiod. Two visual pathways mediate entrainment. First, light stimuli reach the SCN through a direct retinohypothalamic tract (RHT) from specific ganglion cells in the retina. Glutamate is a probable neurotransmitter of the RHT. The second visual pathway is the geniculohypothalamic tract. Neurons of the intergeniculate leaflet of the lateral geniculate complex, which contain γ-aminobutyric acid (GABA) and neuropeptide Y, also receive light stimuli from the same retinal ganglion cells and project to the zone of the SCN receiving RHT input (Fig. 4).

An important neural pathway leads from the SCN to the pineal gland, via the paraventricular nucleus (PVN). The pineal hormone melatonin is considered to act as a hormonal transducer of the light–dark (LD) cycle to the rest of the organism. The pineal gland is not a circadian

TABLE 1. *Time course of sleep-wake interventions in affective illness*

	Latency to therapeutic effect	Duration of therapeutic effect
Total sleep deprivation	hours	usually only 1 day
Partial sleep deprivation in the 2nd half of the night	hours	usually only 1 day, longer if repeated
Phase advance of the sleep–wake cycle	3–7 days	1–2 weeks
REM sleep deprivation	2–3 weeks	months
Temporal isolation	3–14 days	changes with reentrainment
Total sleep deprivation followed by phase advance	1 day	several days?
Comparison Treatments		
Light therapy	3–4 days	1 or more weeks
Antidepressant drugs	10–30 days	months

pacemaker in mammals; its major output, melatonin, feeds back on to melatonin receptors in the SCN (25) (Fig. 4). Locomotor activity also feeds back on the SCN, although these mechanisms are still being elucidated (42). Serotonin (5-HT) is the putative neurotransmitter of this nonphotic entrainment pathway from the raphé nuclei via the intergeniculate leaflet. The neural substrates of additional zeitgebers, such as food availability and social factors, and the putative central oscillators on which they may act are not yet known (25).

There are two classical techniques to establish whether a stimulus affects the mammalian circadian clock in the SCN. First, the endogenous circadian period of the rest-activity cycle can be documented under constant conditions without time cues (called free running). Second, the susceptibility to stimuli can be mapped as a phase response curve (PRC). When a stimulus is administered, the subsequent direction and amount of phase shift that occurs is dependent on the time at which the stimulus was given. The PRC to light in nocturnal rodents shows phase delays to light pulses given around dusk and early in the night, and phase advances to light pulses given late in the night and around dawn. The PRC to light in humans is similar, although the timing is somewhat different: phase delays occur when light is administered before the circadian temperature minimum near 5 a.m., and advances when light pulses are given after the temperature minimum (11,39).

In rodents, administration of a dark pulse yields a PRC with nearly inverse pattern to that of a light pulse. Similar PRCs result from locomotor activity pulses induced by a variety of behavioral methods (e.g., novel situations) or drugs (summarized in refs. 25 and 52). There is, as yet, little data for an activity PRC in humans (64). The PRC to melatonin in rodents shows only a narrow sensitive circadian time in the early evening where phase advances can be induced (25). However, a PRC to melatonin application in humans appears to show nearly opposite patterns to that for a light pulse (36).

These stringent techniques, which yield information about pacemaker characteristics, are difficult to apply in humans. Thus, a compromise must be made to at least attempt to measure phase and amplitude (indirect information about pacemaker characteristics) under optimal conditions. A given overt measured rhythm is modified by many internal and external (masking) factors. Sleep, for example, reduces body temperature and suppresses TSH secretion; this is called internal masking. Food or stress stimulate cortisol secretion, and bright light suppresses, whereas supine position diminishes, melatonin: these are examples of external masking. Masking effects, as evoked physiological responses, are thus superimposed upon the expression of the true endogenous circadian rhythm and may give misleading information. Only recently have adequate methods been established to study unmasked circadian rhythms in humans. These important methodological advances provide the techniques for testing circadian hypotheses of affective illness, for example, dim light to measure the precise timing of melatonin onset (35) or the constant routine protocol to measure amplitude and phase of the core temperature rhythm (11).

The above techniques can provide information about circadian rhythm parameters. The circadian pacemaker also regulates aspects of sleep, and, to investigate the etiopathological role of sleep disturbances in depression, the two-process model of sleep regulation has proved a useful framework (5). In this model, the timing, duration, and architecture of sleep are considered to be determined by the interaction of the circadian pacemaker process C with a homeostatic process S dependent solely on prior wakefulness. The level of process S increases during waking and declines exponentially during sleep. Sleep deprivation augments process S even further (Fig. 5). The level of process S is considered to be an indicator of sleep intensity. The time course of the decline in process S is based on electroencephalogram (EEG) slow-wave activity in non-REM sleep. Process C is assumed to modulate thresholds that define the time of sleep onset and termination.

Given these models, we can consider the evidence for disturbances in rhythmic processes underlying mood disorders in very specific terms, whether of the circadian

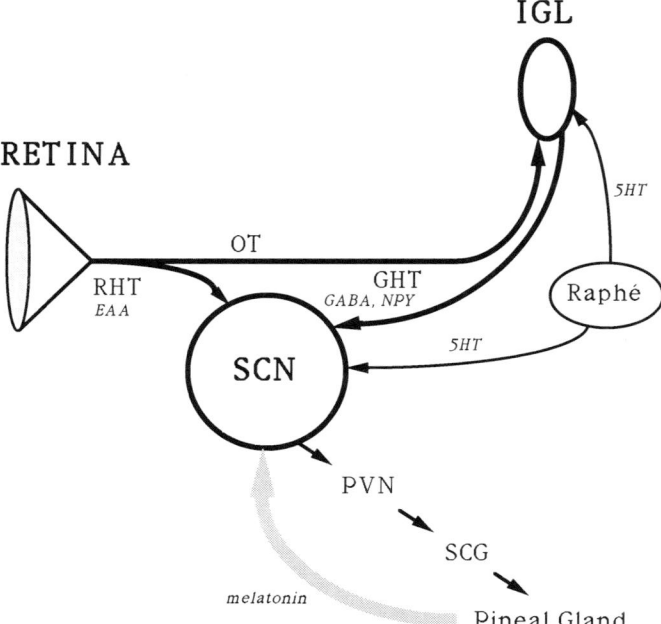

FIG. 4. Schematic representation of the major neural components of the mammalian circadian system (based on information in ref. 25). Light information is transduced by the retina and reaches the suprachiasmatic nuclei (SCN) directly via the retinohypothalamic tract (RHT), and indirectly via the optic tract (OT) to the intergeniculate leaflet (IGL), and then via the geniculohypothalamic tract (GHT) to the SCN. The raphé nuclei project to both the IGL and SCN. An important efferent pathway from the SCN leads to the paraventricular nucleus (PVN), and an important subparaventricular zone. This pathway projects to the intermediolateral nucleus of the spinal cord and passes to preganglionic adrenergic fibers of the sympathetic nervous system, and thus to the superior cervical ganglion (SCG) which provides final sympathetic input to the pineal gland. The hormonal feedback of melatonin on melatonin receptors in the SCN is indicated by the dotted line. Putative neurotransmitters for each neuronal tract are identified as: *EAA*, excitatory amino acids; *NPY*, neuropeptide Y; *5HT*, serotonin; *GABA*, γ-aminobutyric acid.

pacemaker (i.e., process C), whether of a sleep regulatory process S, and/or of the sensory systems transducing information from the external environment to the organism. Since there are multiple zeitgebers, the mechanisms of entrainment are quite complex. Not only may a given zeitgeber have multiple entrainment pathways, but such an external stimulus can have direct masking effects. Thus the circadian system is vulnerable to disturbance at many different levels.

RHYTHM HYPOTHESES OF MOOD DISORDERS

In a remarkably prescient review in 1975, Papoušek was the first to integrate rhythm disturbances in mood disorders within a contemporary framework of circadian

rhythm regulation. The risk of a depressive episode was considered in terms of a *tempora minoris resistentiae*, that is, depression could arise out of those temporal constellations that disturb outer and/or inner synchronization in predisposed individuals (44). This concept was later reformulated; in terms of an "internal coincidence" model, depression occurs when sleep (and its concomitant physiological and endocrine changes) occurs at a certain susceptible circadian phase (70), and, in terms of an "external coincidence" model, the susceptible circadian phase is linked with sensitivity to external stimuli such as light (30). More specifically, a phase advance of circadian rhythms was proposed to be pathognomonic for major depression (70). The circadian models proposed in the 1980s were straightforward in their simplicity, and could elegantly explain much of the then available clinical data. The data supporting these hypotheses have been extensively reviewed (1,10,20,53,67) and this chapter does not reiterate these reviews nor the individual studies but focuses on conceptual approaches. However, at that time there was no information about unmasked human rhythms in depression, nor was the complexity of the circadian system with its multiple entrainment pathways yet recognized. For this reason we are now at a critical stage with respect to circadian hypotheses: the following brief summaries indicate their present status and suggest directions for further research.

Critique of Methods Used to Study Circadian Rhythms

Under nychthemeral conditions, the expression of the circadian pacemaker is masked to varying degrees (depending on the "hand of the clock" that is measured) by activity, sleep, meals, light, and ambient temperature. For this reason, the constant routine (CR) protocol (as first designed by Mills and refined by Czeisler in ref. 11) is considered the best method to measure circadian rhythm amplitude and phase in humans. In the constant routine protocol, patients who are studied in a laboratory controlled for temperature, humidity, and light are given regular small isocaloric meals and remain awake in a sitting position for 25 to 40 hours. This method minimizes exogenous effects and unmasks circadian amplitude and phase. In control subjects, certain parameters (e.g., core body temperature) have been validated as markers of the biological clock (11).

The constant routine is only just being adapted for use in depressive patients. One major drawback exists—and it remains an unresolvable paradox. A total sleep deprivation is intrinsic to the constant routine. Sleep deprivation may alleviate depression, so the very method used to analyze a putative circadian disorder changes the clinical state during the course of study. Thus, the uncertainty principle precludes precise attribution of any modification

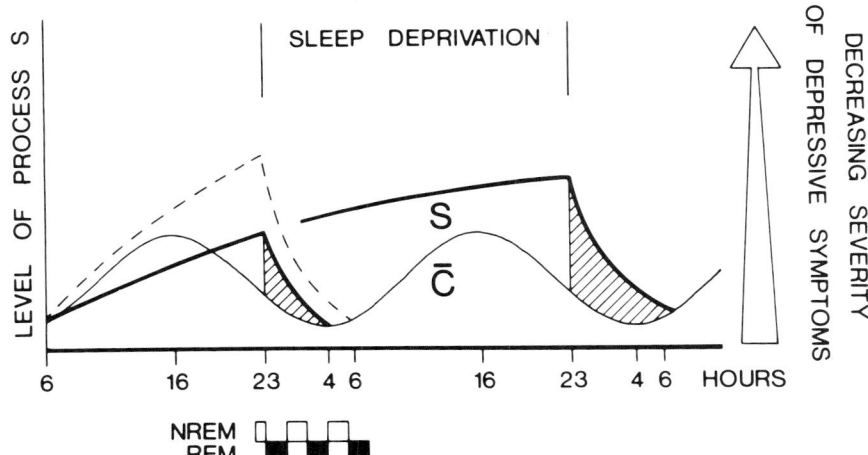

FIG. 5. The two-process model of sleep regulation and its application to depression and sleep deprivation response. Process C (the circadian pacemaker) and process S (the homeostatic component) in a healthy subject (*dotted curve*) and in a depressive patient (*continuous curve*) plotted for a regular sleep–wake cycle followed by total sleep deprivation. The sleep periods of the depressive patient are indicated by shading. Due to the deficiency of Process S, sleep propensity and the amount of slow-wave sleep are reduced, and the sleep period shortened. The deficiency of Process S leads to disinhibition of the REM sleep controlling process in the first part of sleep. Consequently, the latency to the first REM sleep periods is shortened and its duration increased (black and white rectangles represent the REM–non-REM cycles). Sleep deprivation normalizes not only the depressive sleep architecture, but induces a remission of depressive symptomatology (*arrow on right ordinate*). Reprinted with permission from ref. 5.

of the circadian system to a neurobiological correlate of depression. A similar problem has been noted during the difficult free-running studies of depressive patients; in some patients, the release from external time cues and social zeitgebers induced a switch out of depression into hypomania, and thus the circadian period measured could not be unequivocally attributed to the depressive state (69).

One important circadian marker is not masked by the sleep–wake cycle. The major influence on the pineal hormone melatonin is its suppression by bright light (35,37). As an alternative to the constant routine, measurement of melatonin rhythms under dim light conditions does appear to provide a valid estimate of circadian phase in humans (35). However, the new findings that posture masks melatonin secretion (14) may require that previous findings in depressed patients be reevaluated with respect to posture during sample collection. It is not known to what extent immediate or long-term prior light exposure history modifies melatonin production, and how long these after-effects of light last. Because there is a wide individually determined range in melatonin secretion levels, it is often difficult to find significant (and functionally meaningful) interindividual differences that can be related to the illness being studied.

Disturbance in Process S

Sleep and mood are obviously interrelated in major depression (reviewed in refs. 3, 4, and 65; see also Chap-

ter 139, *this volume*). This is particularly evidenced by the rapid antidepressant effect of sleep deprivation and relapse after recovery sleep (3,4,32,34,53,65,67,70,75). Process S is hypothesized to be the link between sleep and depression, whereby the buildup of S during waking is impaired, but can be normalized by extending the length of wakefulness, as during sleep deprivation (Fig. 5) (5).

Process S is considered to be represented by the EEG slow-wave activity in non-REM sleep (5). Few studies have used spectral analysis of the EEG to estimate the time course of process S during sleep and after sleep deprivation in major depression, and the hypothesis is in need of stringent testing (reviewed in refs. 3–5).

Disturbance in Process C

If depression is a circadian disorder, this disturbance could occur at one or many levels: the SCN could have an abnormally short endogenous period or there could be abnormalities of zeitgeber input pathways (e.g., the retina, see Fig. 4) or coupling between circadian oscillatory systems. Very precise experimental protocols are required to differentiate potential mechanisms underlying disturbed overt rhythmic behavior.

Free-running Period

One of the very first hypotheses considered was that manic–depressive disorder arose as a beat phenomenon

between a free-running circadian rhythm and the entrained sleep–wake cycle (18). Very few individuals have
been studied over the long-term to detect such free-
running rhythmic components in an otherwise entrained
rhythm (31,46). These early findings have not yet been
replicated, probably for reasons of inadequate methodology. Such circadian pathology may be specific for extreme cases of rapid cycling (e.g., see ref. 40), but as
yet, evidence for this is lacking. Rather, this circadian
abnormality appears to be characteristic of certain blind
individuals with a periodically recurring sleep disorder:
the endogenous pacemaker free runs and cannot be synchronized to normal sleep times (54). There is, however,
no evidence in these blind subjects of concurrent periodically recurring mood changes.

The rare investigation of depressive subjects isolated
from time cues has not shown any consistent abnormally
short period (16,69). However, these difficult studies have
been made even more difficult to interpret by the fact that
the clinical state itself changed throughout the time the
subject was in temporal isolation.

Phase Advance

The phase advance hypothesis of major depression, first
proposed by Papoušek (44), was explicitly defined and
tested with an experiment of phase advancing the sleep–
wake cycle (70). The few replication studies have also
found an antidepressant effect (reviewed in ref. 4). A
novel experiment has facilitated the phase advance by
preceding it with a total sleep deprivation (4). If replicated, this method may be useful to sustain the antidepressant effect of sleep deprivation.

Phase-advanced rhythms in depressed patients have
been reviewed for a large number of neurochemical parameters (67), hormones (see Chapter 83, *this volume*),
and temperature (53). The most impressive data for a
correlation of phase position with clinical state come from
the long-term studies in rapid-cycling manic–depressive
patients, where, for example the most advanced phase
position of temperature and REM sleep is found just before the switch out of mania into depression (67).

One of the earliest and most consistent rhythm abnormalities in depression has been an early nadir and hypersecretion of plasma cortisol. A recent metaanalysis of
cortisol rhythms reiterates the validity of this finding (Van
Cauter, *personal communication*). Important, and new in
this metaanalysis, is the detailed differentiation of waveform characteristics. Interpretation is based on twin studies of cortisol rhythms that permit separation of these
specific circadian parameters into primarily genetically
controlled, or environmentally influenced. The timing of
the nocturnal nadir appears to be under genetic control, as
is the proportion of overall temporal variability associated
with pulsatility (38). The mean level of cortisol secretion

and the timing of the morning peak are environmentally
modified. The timing of the cortisol nadir is thus a robust
marker of circadian phase in humans. This differentiated
reevaluation of cortisol abnormalities in major depression
lends certain support to the phase-advance hypothesis,
albeit in a modified form.

Conversely, attempts have been made to induce depressive symptoms with a phase delay of the sleep–wake
cycle in healthy normal subjects. Modest but reliable
mood decrements have been induced. Certain individuals,
however, became noticeably depressed (e.g., two out of
ten in ref. 59). In the extreme case, a healthy subject
committed suicide after a phase-shift experiment (50). He
was found to have had abnormal and unstable circadian
phase relationships during the baseline period. This suggests that sudden circadian phase shifts can induce depressive symptoms in predisposed individuals. For example, subjects with a history of affective illness have
become depressed after a westbound flight, or manic after
an eastward shift over several time zones (24).

Phase Delay

The hypothesis that a phase-delayed circadian system
can be depressogenic has only been applied to winter
depression (discussed below). Phase-delayed rhythms are
often manifested in phase-delayed sleep, from the night-
owl behavior in students to the serious disorder of delayed
sleep phase syndrome. No augmented incidence of depression has been associated with this sleep disorder.

Unstable Phase Position Between Pacemaker and Light–Dark Cycle

It has been suggested that the pathophysiology of depression is characterized not by a specific decrease or
increase in neurotransmitter function (such as the monoamine hypothesis originally postulated), but by high variance and instability (57). Similarly, in longitudinal studies
of depressed patients, the characteristic rhythm disturbance appears to be instability of phase from day to day,
or a continuous shift in phase throughout the course of a
depressive or manic episode, not an abnormal phase position per se (46,67). Phase instability could arise through
a short endogenous circadian period too near to the 24-
hr external LD cycle to entrain properly, low circadian
amplitude, or weak coupling between pacemaker and the
LD cycle (e.g., low light perception, disturbed retinohypothalamic tract/geniculohypothalamic tract input).

There are few studies addressing this possibility. Two
deserve attention for using spectral analysis on longitudinal data. The diurnal rhythm of temperature was measured
in a large cohort of major depressed patients who showed
higher phase variability and decreased amplitude than
controls (63). Both depressive and manic fluctuations re-

duced circadian fit; instability of the diurnal rhythm was the main feature. Similarly, another large cohort of major depressed patients showed a normal or delayed phase of the temperature rhythm together with a lower amplitude than in controls (13). The 24-hr component was lower in power, with an increase in ultradian components. This suggests a possible weakening of the coupling processes between internal pacemakers and abnormal sensitivity to environmental information.

Diurnal variation of mood has also been used as a variable. A group of patients with major depression carried out hourly mood ratings throughout the day; they showed both greater mood variability and a higher amplitude of ultradian fluctuations than controls (19). In a group of SAD patients, mood rated six times a day during winter depression showed that DV was more unstable than in controls. Light treatment reduced or eliminated all group differences in both mean level and variability (28).

Amplitude Diminution

Comparison of multiple circadian rhythms during depression and after recovery have suggested that blunted amplitude is the main chronobiological abnormality (e.g., see refs. 10,58,66). However, the majority of studies have been carried out under normal nychthemeral conditions (i.e., masked conditions). Thus, the often-observed diminution of amplitude in the core body temperature rhythm may be a consequence of a disturbed sleep–wake cycle in depression and not of disturbed circadian clock function (58,66). This can be illustrated by a study of 24-hr heart rate in untreated major depressives; two groups of patients were distinguished, those with a low amplitude rhythm, and patients without any demonstrable 24-hr rhythm at all (61). This dichotomy may be more apparent than real, since the amplitude of a given rhythm probably lies on a continuum, resulting in a nonsignificant circadian frequency component below a given threshold. Additionally, heart rate is highly masked by activity, sleep, and stress. It is unclear how much of the reduced amplitude is an epiphenomenon of behavioral inhibition during the day and poor sleep at night.

Many measures, not reviewed here (but see e.g. refs. 1, 10, and 67) manifest lower amplitude of diurnal variation in major depression than in control subjects. However, to test the hypothesis of circadian amplitude reduction adequately, requires the methodology of the constant routine and validation of the measured variable as an adequate marker of circadian amplitude.

As yet, no studies have been published on circadian rhythms in major depression measured in a constant routine. The need for such studies are illustrated by data from a single severely depressed, hospitalized, nonseasonal patient (J. Anderson et al., unpublished data). The patient was diagnosed with recurrent major depression and was

therapy resistant; he was withdrawn from drug treatment 1 week before the study, and carried out two CR protocols prior to and following treatment for 1 month with light therapy alone. During 2 weeks, light was administered for 4 hr/day over midday (to augment amplitude); during the next 2 weeks light was administered in the evening (to delay phase). However, neither treatment regimen induced any amelioration of his depression, whereas during the sleep deprivation of the CR his depressive symptoms transiently improved. In both CRs, his temperature rhythm showed a robust amplitude for a 60-year-old man. A curious response was found on the second day of each CR after sleep deprivation, in that regulation of the temperature set-point appeared to go awry. Temperature increased markedly above normal values, as did heat production. The reproducibility of such temperature increases concomitant with sleep deprivation response remains to be further explored.

Of course, this example cannot define the role of circadian rhythm abnormalities in major depression. Although somewhat heroic for both patient and therapist, further studies using the constant routine in depressive patients may provide data that test these circadian hypotheses. Additionally, clues to the mechanism of the sleep-deprivation–induced mood elevation may also be found, because the timing of the switch can be narrowed very precisely under these controlled conditions and compared with the timing of psychophysiological events.

Most studies of depressed patients document a diminution in melatonin amplitude (e.g., refs. 10 and 58). However, it is not clear whether melatonin can be used as a marker of amplitude in depression, as opposed to being a validated marker of phase (35). This issue is illustrated by melatonin rhythms measured in the CR in two patients (J. Arendt et al., unpublished data). First, the above described major depressive patient had undetectable salivary melatonin secretion when depressed. After 4 weeks of a 4-hr daily midday light treatment, a melatonin rhythm was clearly present. Yet concomitantly, there was no change in depressed state. Second, an euthymic SAD patient in summer had undetectable saliva melatonin secretion. One week of 4-hr daily midday light treatment in summer also augmented melatonin secretion, but again without any change in clinical state. These examples suggest that light has a direct pharmacological effect to increase the level (and thus amplitude) of melatonin secretion. In the same SAD patient, euthymic after 6 weeks of treatment with the selective 5-HT uptake inhibitor citalopram, even higher melatonin levels were found. Thus three different levels of nocturnal melatonin secretion were present during three separate euthymic episodes in one patient, and two different levels of nocturnal melatonin secretion during two separate depressive episodes in the former patient. These data imply that melatonin levels (and thus amplitude) are genetically regulated but also pharmacologically modified. This also means that the amplitude of the melatonin peak has not been validated as a marker for circadian amplitude.

Ratio Between Activity and Rest Phase

In many species that have seasonal behaviors (e.g., in reproduction, migration, and hibernation), it is the duration of daylength (photoperiod) that initiates these seasonal changes. The circadian system responds with great precision to these changes in photoperiod, for example with expansion and reduction of the locomotor activity: rest ratio (α:ρ).

Although humans do indeed manifest a number of seasonal rhythms (reviewed in ref. 33), studies have usually been carried out under artificial lighting conditions, which obscure the natural signals of dawn and dusk. Only recently has a winter-time expansion of nocturnal duration of several parameters been documented in humans (decreased α:ρ from summer to winter) (68). This remarkable study simulated winter and summer photoperiods by controlling the nights: subjects remained in long or short nights of absolute darkness. Such a defined, completely dark phase is never experienced under normal urbanized conditions. Under these controlled photoperiodic conditions, sleep time, melatonin, and prolactin secretion expanded in winter. These data suggest that humans are indeed susceptible to independent shifts in the timing of dawn and dusk markers with season, that is, a change in the α:ρ ratio.

An analogy with depression was first made by Kripke (29), based on the extensive knowledge of seasonal mechanisms in rodents. The model of separate, but coupled, oscillators for the dawn and dusk signal was applied to circadian concepts of depressive pathophysiology. Instead of simply looking at circadian amplitude and phase (as in the phase-advance or amplitude diminution hypotheses), it becomes necessary to investigate characteristics of the wave form of a rhythm. It has been unambiguously demonstrated that in rodents, the onset and offset of melatonin secretion can shift independently (23). In women with premenstrual depression, the offset of the melatonin rhythm was earlier, reducing the duration of nocturnal secretion (increased α:ρ) (45). The metaanalysis of cortisol rhythms in depression indicated that a phase advance was specific for the nadir, not the peak, resulting in a longer duration of nocturnal cortisol secretion (decreased α:ρ ratio) (Van Cauter, *personal communication*). This permits an hypothesis that disturbances in the α:ρ ratio may underlie certain mood disorders. Conversely, in the photoperiod study of healthy subjects, one volunteer became severely suicidal after decrease of the α:ρ ratio (long nights), even though all the others felt remarkably well on this protocol (68).

Zeitgeber Coupling

Zeitgeber strength is a measure of the capacity of an external entraining agent to synchronize circadian rhythms. Zeitgeber strength is relative, being also dependent on the sensitivity of the system to the zeitgeber. Light is the major synchronizing agent. Additionally, the circadian timekeeping system in animals phase shifts in response to periodic locomotor activity (42). Food availability (6) and social cues can also entrain rhythms in certain species.

In the free running experiments in Andechs, where humans were deprived of time cues, social factors were considered the most important synchronizer (71). Later experiments indicated that light was also a major zeitgeber for human circadian rhythms (71,72). The two zeitgebers are not independent, because social behavior determines whether a person is exposed to the physical zeitgebers of light and temperature, and the timing of going to bed and waking up (which also gates light input via the retina).

Social factors, as social zeitgebers, have been formalized within a circadian hypothesis of mood disorders (17). This conceptual approach has the attractive feature of linking the biological hypotheses with psychosocial research. Social zeitgebers are personal relationships, jobs, social demands, or tasks that serve to entrain biological rhythms. They determine the timing of meals, sleep, and physical exercise. These social factors also have the potential to disrupt circadian rhythms. Some of the particular psychosocial precipitants of depressive disorder, such as life events, chronic stresses, or lack of appropriate social support systems, may be considered to act as precipitants by inducing rhythm disruptions (e.g., acute changes in the sleep–wake cycle, drop in activity level). Conversely, psychotherapy, as well as social interventions, may act to synchronize the circadian system. Perhaps they incidentally enhance exposure to physical zeitgebers such as light. Given the new knowledge about behavioral feedback on the circadian clock, social zeitgebers could be postulated to act through neural pathways related to arousal.

This phenomenon had been described in qualitative terms by Schulte more than 20 years ago (56): the absence of usual habits and sudden lack of duties, as well as changes in the usual social patterns requiring adaptative behavior, were considered potential precipitants of depressive episodes. He pointed out that depressed patients had two major predisposing factors: the chronicity of sleep disturbances, and their vulnerability to changing external conditions. This he interpreted as possibly resulting from insufficient mechanisms for circadian synchronization.

Experimental tests of social zeitgebers have been carried out using scales developed to quantify these daily social rhythms. For example, in the acute bereavement stage of recently widowed subjects, those individuals with highly disrupted social patterns had higher depression scores than those who maintained social routines (17). Overall social activity scores were negatively correlated with depression ratings in hospitalized major depressives and were lower than for a group of control subjects (60); similar correlations were found in the elderly (47). Remitted depressives showed no differences from controls, but enhanced variability (41), which suggests that low zeitgeber strength may be linked with a certain instability.

We now know that there are multiple zeitgebers for the circadian system, of different relative strengths, that act on and interact with different systems (25). It is not known how much social synchronization is actually related to augmented locomotor activity or increased arousal. If further confirmed, this more complex approach also suggests that a variety of zeitgebers could be used singly, or in combination, to achieve improved synchronization. Application has already been made to improve disordered or reversed sleep–wake cycles in demented patients, using both increased social interaction and bright light (43).

Disturbance in Retinal Processes

Circadian rhythm studies in depression have primarily measured output parameters. For example, the secretion of melatonin provides a measure of phase of the circadian pacemaker, as well as noradrenergic receptor sensitivity at the pinealocyte. Melatonin is suppressed by light given at night. Melatonin suppression has been used as an index of light sensitivity in depressed patients (e.g., ref. 37).

Measuring sensitivity to light via light suppression of melatonin is rather indirect. A novel, and little-used strategy, would be to measure retinal function itself. Although some aspects of retinal function have been investigated in depressive patients, particularly with respect to modification by drugs such as lithium, there is insufficient research on putative disturbances in retinal sensitivity. The retina is a part of the CNS that is directly accessible to measurement. The accumulating evidence that there is a circadian clock in the mammalian eye and that dopamine and melatonin are important neurotransmitters mediating light and dark, respectively (48), makes this approach all the more attractive.

Activity Feedback or Arousal Level

One of the tenets of circadian physiology has been that the biological clock is immutable. This is not so. Not only is circadian timekeeping modulated by changes in internal state (e.g., by reproductive and thyroid hormones), but also its own output can feed back on its function. This is now clear for the pineal hormone melatonin, because melatonin receptors are selective to the SCN (reviewed in ref. 25, Fig 4). More surprisingly, it appears

that the rest–activity cycle can, under certain conditions, feed back on the period and phase of the circadian clock. In hamsters, locomotor activity induced at particular circadian phases (by a drug such as triazolam, by a social stimulus such as an estrus female in the adjacent cage, by a novel situation such as changing the cage or a new running wheel) can phase shift the endogenous rhythm (42) and shorten free-running period in mice and rats (52). These findings lend credence to the idea that alterations in behavioral arousal state or activity level can lead to alterations in circadian period and phase.

Psychomotor disturbances are an important hallmark of depression and mania. The causal relationships between agitation and inhibition in depression and the circadian system are still unclear. Preliminary studies in humans suggest that high-level activity can phase shift circadian rhythms, although this is not yet certain (55,64). Enhanced activity has been used to test the hypothesis that increased zeitgeber strength could treat SAD patients (bright light also increases zeitgeber strength). Two hours of regular exercise in the early morning decreased depressive symptoms, together with a phase advance of the temperature minimum (26).

Not a Primary Clock Disturbance

Exogenous shifts in timing of the sleep–wake cycle in healthy subjects have been shown to induce dysphoric mood, poor performance, fatigue, and anorexia, as well as mimicking sleep patterns found in depressed patients (early morning awakening and short REM latency) (e.g., 59). After transmeridian travel, the incidence of hospitalization for depression was higher after westward than eastward flight, whereas hypomania occurred more often after eastward shifts (24). Some of the neuroendocrine abnormalities in depression may arise from alterations in circadian rhythm organization, as shown by blunting of evening prolactin and by thyrotropin responses to TRH after reversal of the sleep–wake cycle the response was similar to the normal low response to TRH when given in the morning hours (9).

Healy has postulated that mood-related cognitive and attributional disturbances are sequelae of shifting circadian rhythms (22). This clearly shifts the disruption from being innate to the circadian pacemaker itself, to a secondary level, that of subjective interpretation of internal temporal disorder. In a first test of this hypothesis, healthy student nurses undertaking night shift work for the first time were found to manifest enhanced psychosomatic complaints and negative perceptions of altered neurovegetative function, perceived criticism from others, and less sense of purpose and control (22). In this respect, a further point is important: subjects in free running experiments, whose circadian rhythms of temperature and sleep desynchronized, did not notice that this phenomenon had oc-

TABLE 2. *Biological and psychosocial factors relevant to circadian hypotheses of affective illness*

Factors	Biological	Psychosocial

	heredity
	intrauterine influences
		Developmental:
		  poor parental bonding
		  poor socialization
		  learned helplessness paradigm (uncontrollable stress)

PREDISPOSING	Pacemaker properties:
	  abnormal period
	  abnormal limits of entrainment
	  weak &/or altered coupling
	  altered sensitivity &/or
	  response to zeitgebers	

PRECIPITATING	maturation/aging
	hormonal state
	season
	primary sleep disorders
	physical trauma
		Changes in Temporal Order:
		  family, social, work, meal disruption
		  jet lag
		  shift work
		  unusual pattern of chosen behavior
		  breakdown/loss of social interactions
		  separation or death

PERPETUATING	Zeitgebers
	  absent or weak
	  phase shifts
	  change of photoperiod
		Stress:
		  symbolic significance of losses
		  learned helplessness paradigm
		  (uncontrollable stress)

PROTECTING	absence of predisposing factors
	lithium, tricyclics, MAOI's
	sleep–wake manipulations
	light exposure
		absence of predisposing factors
		  normal 24-hr social cues
		  activity scheduling
		  timing of treatments
		  stress management

Modified and reprinted with permission from ref. 20.

curred. They showed no decrement in mood or functioning; on the contrary, they felt rather well (71). This switch into positive mood on internal desynchronization has been used as a model for the switch out of depression into hypomania after sleep deprivation (67,70). Thus the depressive disturbances concomitant with shift work and jet lag in vulnerable subjects must result from external (i.e., with conflicting zeitgebers) and not from internal dysnchronization.

Predisposing and Precipitating Factors

Models of depression implicating predisposing and precipitating factors, such as genetic vulnerability, sex, age, chronic stress, the change of seasons, can equally be represented in circadian terms. Some of these biological and psychosocial phenomena relevant to circadian hypotheses of affective illness are summarized in Table 2 (see ref. 20 for details). The previous sections have delineated possible disturbances in temporal order according to the formal properties of the circadian system. To focus on practical application of these principles, the following section describes the example of light therapy, a treatment modality that arose out of circadian models of rhythm disorder.

LIGHT THERAPY

Seasonal Affective Disorder

Extensive research in the last decade has focused on a group of patients who indeed appear to fulfill the criteria of suffering from a rhythm disorder. Seasonal affective disorder (SAD) is characterized by recurrent episodes in autumn and winter of depression, hypersomnia, augmented appetite with carbohydrate craving and weight gain (51). Bright light (more than 2500 lux for more than 1 hr per day) reverses these symptoms within 3 to 4 days (51,62). We are still far from understanding the mechanisms underlying the pathophysiology of SAD and the therapeutic response to light. At last count, eight explicit hypotheses have been proposed, of which the majority are linked with circadian system abnormalities (reviewed in refs. 51 and 62). These hypotheses utilize the concepts presented above and are briefly summarized as follows:

1. The first theoretical basis for light treatment was that SAD symptoms are precipitated by the lengthening night in autumn and winter (decreased $\alpha{:}\rho$). Photoperiodic time measurement is mediated by melatonin. The long duration of melatonin secretion in winter can be suppressed by bright light given at dawn and dusk to simulate a summer day. Clinical improvement is considered to be a consequence of melatonin suppres-

sion. Evidence against this hypothesis comes from (a) light given at a time of day when melatonin is not suppressed is also therapeutic; (b) light does not have to be given at dawn and dusk to simulate a summer photoperiod—a single daily treatment is sufficient; (c) the reverse, administering melatonin to simulate winter night duration, does not reinstate depression.

2. The second hypothesis is that SAD is a consequence of abnormal phase position: the circadian system is delayed with respect to the sleep–wake or LD cycle. This would predict that only light given in the morning (which phase-advances circadian rhythms) should be therapeutic. The hypothesis is still controversial because (a) although the majority of studies find that the majority of SAD patients have phase-delayed melatonin rhythms, not all patients do; (b) light appears to be therapeutic at most times of day; and (c) even if a given patient has phase-delayed rhythms, this does not predict preferential response to morning light.

3. The third concept proposes flattened amplitude of circadian rhythms as responsible for the depressive symptoms of SAD. Such a circadian rhythm disturbance has also been proposed to underlie major depression. Light application during the day should thus act to increase circadian rhythm amplitude. Two constant routine studies on SAD patients (12, and Wirz-Justice et al., 74 and *unpublished data*) provide the first evidence refuting this hypothesis. Circadian amplitude of the rhythm of core body temperature was no different in SAD subjects than in controls, nor was the amplitude augmented by morning or midday light, both of which improved depressive symptoms.

4. A seasonal instability of phase control has also been invoked. At high latitudes the long winter nights or long summer days result in large day-to-day variability in the timing of the rest–activity cycle in animals. The circadian system is more vulnerable to instability under these extreme photoperiodic conditions. In this model, the role of bright light is to increase zeitgeber strength and thus stabilize synchronization.

5. Retinal deficiencies in SAD patients (either sub- or supersensitivity) may modify light input in winter. Bright light would thus act by directly modulating photoreceptor function.

6. In contrast to the previous circadian models, the photon-counting hypothesis (light as a drug) focuses solely on the amount of light received over time. A given individual threshold is postulated for the number of photons required by the retina and CNS to mediate the therapeutic effect of light. Data in favor of this theory are (a) the dose–response relationship to light therapy (either in terms of duration or intensity) and (b) the antidepressant effect of light at any time of day.

7. The medial hypothalamic syndrome hypothesis attempts to integrate the atypical vegetative symptoms characteristic of SAD patients (increased appetite, particularly for carbohydrates, weight gain, and hypersomnia) within a framework of known neurobiological mechanisms (27). In mammals, carbohydrate selection is primarily regulated by serotonergic and α_2-adrenergic mechanisms in the PVN and lateral hypothalamus. Neural input from the SCN to the PVN transduces circadian and seasonal information, thus implicating the PVN as a primary interface linking food selection and time of year. Since light therapy specifically and selectively suppresses carbohydrate intake in depressed SAD patients (27), this also provides a clue to possible serotonergic mechanisms underlying these relationships between mood, food, and season. These are supported by preliminary findings that SAD patients respond well to serotonergic antidepressant drugs, and that these concomitantly suppress carbohydrate intake (reviewed in ref. 62).

8. Similar to other models of depression, a dysregulation hypothesis focuses on the variance in mood regulation in SAD. Within-day variation and between-day variability in mood fluctuates more widely in SAD than in normal subjects and can be normalized by light therapy (28).

These various hypotheses are not mutually exclusive. Bright light acts directly on the circadian pacemaker and not on sleep-dependent processes. Thus successful treatment of SAD must act on mechanisms within known retinohypothalamic pathways. Conversely, SAD may result from failure of one or several mechanisms at different neuroanatomical foci to respond appropriately to decreasing daylength. In spite of being a relatively homogeneous group of depressed patients in symptomatology, SAD patients are not necessarily homogeneous in the etiology of their illness. Winter depression may arise from a disturbance in of any of the above hypothesized pathways. Thus, although light therapy was initially based on a specific seasonal hypothesis implicating melatonin suppression, this has been disproved.

Two hypotheses have been systematically addressed under the controlled conditions of the constant routine: whether SAD patients are phase-delayed in winter or whether their rhythm amplitude is diminished. In a 25-hr CR protocol, the circadian rhythm of body core temperature and melatonin onset in depressed SAD patients was phase-delayed in winter compared with age-matched controls (12). Morning light treatment phase-advanced these rhythms concomitant with alleviation of symptoms. In a 40-hr CR protocol in SAD patients, a midday light regimen induced antidepressant response (74). The effects of sleep deprivation and light on the circadian rhythm of mood have been detailed in Fig. 3. Depressed SAD patients showed a tendency for core body temperature rhythms in winter to be phase-delayed compared with controls, but there was no delay in melatonin. There was also no amplitude diminution during winter depression, nor did midday light augment it (Wirz-Justice et al., *unpublished data*).

Applications in Other Psychiatric Disorders

Since the discovery that light can treat winter depression, a number of further applications have been subjected to experimental testing (summarized in ref. 62). The success of light therapy in SAD has led to investigation of whether seasonal patterns in other psychiatric disorders could predict therapeutic response to light. Indeed, there appears to be wintertime exacerbation of symptoms in certain patients with bulimia, panic attacks, obsessive–compulsive disorder, and improvement with light treatment. In contrast, atypical depressive patients without seasonality did not show amelioration.

Light treatment studies in nonseasonal depression have been mainly negative (summarized in ref. 62). It may be that the intensity and duration of light application (1 to 2 hr of 2500 lux for 1 to 2 weeks) may not be a sufficiently high dose of light for a clinically relevant effect. Antidepressant drug trials in major depression, particularly in hospitalized patients, require at least 3 to 6 weeks of treatment before any statement about nonresponse can be made. Future studies will need such a conservative time course to adequately test the clinical efficacy of light in nonseasonal depression. In an open pilot study of hospitalized, untreated patients with major depression, 4 to 8 hr of 4000 lux light daily over a period of 10 days reduced depressive symptoms by more than 50% (Graw et al., *unpublished data*), suggesting the range of intensity and duration that should be tested in a longer controlled trial.

Sleep Disorders

Bright light has been employed as a treatment for certain sleep disorders associated with alterations in the circadian timing system (i.e., advanced- and delayed-sleep-phase syndrome, jet lag, and shift work) (15). Light has also a direct activating effect, which may interfere with sleep initiation (7), but also improves performance (e.g., 74). Another potential treatment group are the elderly. The age-related decrease of circadian rhythm amplitude, and phase advance of its timing has been suggested to cause, in part, the characteristic sleep disturbances associated with aging (8). Light therapy has been employed in nursing home populations (primarily demented patients) to manage the behavioral disorders and often reversed sleep–wake cycle (reviewed in ref. 8).

In contrast to the light PRC, melatonin induces phase advances when given in the late afternoon and phase delays when given in the early morning (36). This phase-shifting property of melatonin has been applied to treat jet lag and to advance the delayed-sleep-phase syndrome

in sighted and blind persons (e.g., see ref. 54). Melatonin has not been very successful in treating depressive symptoms, acting on alertness rather than on mood. Thus the future application of melatonin and its analogs appears to lie in certain sleep and not mood disorders (see also Chapter 139, *this volume*).

CIRCADIAN RHYTHM DISTURBANCE IN DEPRESSION: CAUSE OR EFFECT?

Rhythm disturbances in depression are heterogeneous. Of course, the heterogeneity of the depressive disorders is a basic classificatory problem in depression research. Yet even in the well-defined subgroup of SAD patients, circadian rhythm characteristics (such as melatonin phase) do not appear unitary and circadian phase is neither correlated with depth of depression nor with preferential response to morning or evening light (e.g., see ref. 73). Additionally, chronobiological characteristics may change throughout a depressive episode (see refs. 46 and 67). This renders many of the findings inconclusive, and contributes to the large variance often observed (patients with similar depths of depressive symptoms may be at different stages in the course of their illness). The necessity for individual long-term study is apparent, particularly to distinguish whether any of these rhythm abnormalities are state or trait dependent. It has not yet been possible to attribute a specific pathogenetic role to the circadian system in depression: a patient's prior history has not been known; the use of antidepressant medication at some stage itself impacts on rhythmic phenomena; the behavioral withdrawal during depression from social and physical zeitgebers augments vulnerability to rhythm disruption; and the majority of investigations have not been carried out under the requisite controlled conditions with adequate sampling intervals and validated markers.

Altered rhythmicity could be either a cause or an effect of altered affective state. Both could independently reflect abnormalities in a third system, such as psychomotor activity. The rhythmic phenomena in mood disorders could be largely a consequence of, rather than a cause of, behavioral depression and mania.

The previous summary of potential foci of rhythmic disturbances have been consciously separated for didactic purposes. Yet a single cause is unlikely. Additionally, a single observation of abnormal entrainment phase could arise from different causes: altered underlying period of the circadian pacemaker, diminished amplitude, the pacemaker's response to light, the strength of the zeitgeber, not to mention pacemaker-independent phenomena such as masking. Separating these causes require methods for determining amplitude and phase of good markers of the circadian system under longitudinal conditions (patients as their own state-dependent control). Yet given the multiplicity of zeitgebers, and the multiple CNS entrainment pathways, the intrinsic interactions may prove to be intransigent. A summary of these multiple foci and their putative role in affective illness has been summarized in Table 2. Not only is vulnerability to circadian dysfunction present at the genetic level, but this is modified during ontogeny, by sex and thyroid hormones, by situative factors such as arousal level and stress, and clinically by drugs.

Circadian rhythm and sleep research have provided the rationale for novel, nonpharmacological therapies of depression (sleep deprivation, light, social interaction). The remarkable temporal course of response and relapse after sleep deprivation (hours) and light therapy (days) is a clue to understanding mechanisms of therapeutic response. Sleep deprivation is antidepressant in all diagnostic subgroups. In contrast, light is antidepressant in SAD but appears to have little effect in other forms of depression. This would suggest that sleep deprivation is a more generalized intervention in the depressive process than light. In the two-process model of sleep regulation, sleep deprivation is postulated to act via process S, with little effect on the circadian pacemaker. In contrast, light acts directly on process C and not on sleep dependent processes. Thus further investigation of the neuroendocrinological and neurobiological changes around the switch out of depression (see Fig. 3), and during recovery sleep or depressogenic naps are required.

ANIMAL MODELS

A recent, excellent review of those animal models that purport to mimic features of depression, as well as involving dysregulation of circadian rhythms and monoaminergic and cholinergic neurotransmitter systems, is summarized here (see ref. 52 for references; also Chapter 68, *this volume*).

One of the most researched animal models of depression is that of stress-induced behavioral change. In rhythm studies, stress has resulted in failure to entrain to a light–dark cycle, 48-hr days, lengthening of free-running period, and long-term reductions in the 24-hr mean activity level. A second strategy yields findings suggesting that strains selected for specific behavioral or neurochemical properties also manifest altered circadian rhythmicity (e.g., the Flinders sensitive rat strain has both an upregulated cholinergic system and short circadian period and advanced phase of temperature and REM sleep). A third strategy analyzes circadian rhythm sequelae of specific lesions (e.g., olfactory bulbectomy in rats results in delayed entrainment phase and lengthening of free-running period).

In both depressed patients and experimental animal models, alterations in phase, period, amplitude, 24-hr mean, and coherence of rhythms have been documented, although cause-and-effect relationships have not been established. In depressed patients, both circadian rhythm phase advances and phase delays have been observed and, in experimental animal models, both lengthening and shortening of the free-running period. It is not clear what clinical or neurobiological characteristics distinguish these two groups, for example, psychomotor disturbances or anxiety. The situation becomes even more complex when comparing circadian period and locomotor activity level. Manipulations that diminish or augment activity do not induce predictable and parallel changes in free-running period.

It is often forgotten that even within nocturnal rodents, important species and even strain differences are present: for example, in drug metabolism, sensitivity to stress, or stability of the circadian system. In the course of evolution diverse mechanisms subserve the same phenomenon in different species. Thus any parallels with the human circadian system (and the human is not usually a nocturnal animal) require this caveat. To cite Zucker (76)

> The biological psychiatrist perusing physiology journals for a viable animal model of SAD, like the reader of fashion ads, is in danger of buying a bill of goods. The animal physiologist has available several thousand species for chronobiological investigation and can turn up specimens that manifest virtually any trait in exaggerated or muted form. Laboratory settings can be structured to produce uniform conditions and to yield reliable data that are simply unattainable in most human experimentation. The descendants of animals that respond in other than the normative fashion can be eliminated from subsequent studies, thereby creating a subject pool that shares many features with modal animals, but, like fashion models in advertisements, shows none of the scars associated with life in the woods.

The somatic factors of depression (changed appetite and weight, disturbed sleep and psychomotor activity, loss of interest in sex) are intrinsic to the illness. Nuclei in the hypothalamus regulate the physiological functions of sleep, reproduction, weight, food choice, and their daily and seasonal timing. Circadian and seasonal rhythms in sleep, weight, and appetite are intrinsically linked with energy expenditure and energy conservation. These symptoms can be explored and manipulated in both depressive patients and experimental animals in the search for mechanisms. In spite of the temptation to search for a global animal model of depression, it may be more realistic to focus on particular behaviors.

An example of this approach is the model of seasonal hibernation in hamsters, which provided the rationale for initiating light therapy in seasonal depression (51). Although this model does have certain face and predictive validity, it is oversimplified: traits, not individuals, are photoperiodic (76). It is not legitimate to use winter weight gain in hamsters as a model of seasonal weight gain in SAD patients, unless the functions of weight gain are similar in both species (76). Nevertheless, playing with these fruitful analogies is not forbidden! For example, we have focused on the specific SAD symptom of enhanced carbohydrate-rich food intake in autumn, and the gender differences in the incidence of SAD, to postulate a link with classic serotonergic hypotheses of mood disorder (27).

The most rapid rate of decreasing CNS 5-HT turnover occurs in autumn, and the most rapid rate of increasing 5-HT turnover occurs in spring (33). Carbohydrate selection is driven by 5-HT in the PVN and can be reversed by serotonergic agonists (27). In a variety of animal studies (e.g., in ref. 25), it has been shown that 5-HT release occurs in the dark phase; light can modify sensitivity of the SCN to 5-HT, and 5-HT can influence photic responsiveness of the SCN. When a hamster in a summer photoperiod is depleted of 5-HT, behavior is switched into the winter mode with a reduction of the α:ρ ratio (nocturnal activity onset occurs earlier). Chronic 5-HT depletion can modify entrainment, decrease amplitude, and increase irregularity of the rest–activity cycle. Finally, 5-HT function is modified by gonadal hormones. This brief summary provides hints for serotonergic mechanisms underlying the exaggerated seasonal rhythms in carbohydrate intake in SAD patients, as well as the vulnerability of women to suffer from winter depression.

NEUROPHARMACOLOGY OF CIRCADIAN RHYTHMS

Input and output pathways from the SCN suggest complex neuroanatomical feedback loops, mediated by a variety of neurotransmitters and neuropeptides (reviewed in ref. 25) (simplified in Fig. 4). Thus, there are multiple loci for circadian rhythm modification by psychopharmacological agents. Psychoactive drugs have become tools to dissect neurochemical substrates of circadian pacemaker function, define neurotransmitters coding for light entrainment, as well as to test hypotheses of circadian rhythm mechanisms mediating antidepressant drug action. The following summary is condensed from the review by Rosenwasser (52).

An emerging neuropsychopharmacology of circadian rhythms indicates that drug effects fall into two main categories of PRC: mimicking either the effects of a light pulse (carbachol, clonidine) or of a dark pulse (glutamate, neuropeptide Y, benzodiazepines, muscimol, serotonergic agonists, protein synthesis inhibitors). A variety of nonphotic and nonpharmacological stimuli also mimic the dark PRC, some mediated by increased activity.

Several antidepressant drugs have been given chronically to hamsters and rats to measure their effects on free-running circadian period and entrained phase position. The early studies on lithium indicated period lengthening and phase delay in most (but not all) species. Rolipram, putative antidepressant, also lengthened period. Rubidium, another alkali metal with antidepressant potential,

and valproate, used prophylactically in some bipolar patients, shortened circadian period. Later, clorgyline, an irreversible, selective monoamine oxidase-A (MAO-A) inhibitor, was extensively studied in hamsters, where it also lengthened period, delayed phase, and increased the α:ρ ratio.

A wide range of antidepressant drugs have been studied in this classical circadian paradigm, but they have failed to reveal a common action on the circadian clock. Imipramine, clomipramine, fluoxetine, citalopram, levoprotiline, and a selective MAO-B inhibitor were without systematic effect. Only desipramine (a selective norepinephrine uptake inhibitor) and moclobemide (a reversible and selective MAO-A inhibitor) shortened circadian period and increased overall locomotor activity and the circadian amplitude of the activity rhythm. This is consistent with the hypothesis that monoaminergic neurotransmitters play an important role in the control of behavioral state and circadian rhythmicity.

Delayed entrainment phase and marked lengthening of free-running period have been induced by chronic treatment with methamphetamine. Monoaminergic agents have also been shown to induce complex dissociations or splitting of free-running rhythms that may reflect weakening of coupling relationships within a network of mutually coupled circadian oscillators.

The effect of psychopharmacological drugs on retinal function requires mention. The retina, itself a part of the CNS, transduces light–dark information to the rest of the brain and may itself contain a circadian pacemaker; dopamine and melatonin are the putative neurotransmitters mediating light and dark signals (48). Thus a given drug can modify retinal sensitivity as well as circadian function: this has been most clearly shown for lithium, clorgyline, and methamphetamine (48).

Finally, a related application of circadian rhythm concepts not reviewed here is that of chronopharmacology. Studies that focus on the optimum time of day for giving the lowest dose, to provide maximum efficacy with minimum side effects are still rare, but may aid in strategies for therapy-resistant depression.

FUTURE DIRECTIONS

Circadian Neuroscience

The last decade has seen an unprecedented growth in circadian rhythm neuroscience (reviewed in ref. 25). Important has been the identification of the genetic basis of period. Mutations of period genes in *Drosophilia* result in long or short circadian period, or arrhythmic behavior. In the mutant hamster, circadian period can be transplanted. It is to be hoped that further knowledge of the molecular biology of the clock may lead to understanding mechanisms underlying putative clock disturbances in humans. For example, the use of immediate early gene expression (such as the protooncogene c-*fos*) as a very specific functional marker of neuronal activation, has been applied to the circadian timing system. This specificity is most remarkable light pulses induce c-*fos* expression only in those regions involved in the photic entrainment of circadian rhythms (the retina, SCN, and perhaps the intergeniculate leaflet), and only at those circadian times when light induces a phase advance or phase delay. Thus c-*fos* localization may be an important tool to localise pathways involved in photic entrainment, as well as phase shifts induced by activity pulses or drugs (25).

Methods and Strategies

The critique of methods has focused on the necessity for a new generation of circadian rhythm studies in affective illness. The importance of dim light and posture for correct interpretation of melatonin rhythm characteristics (as well as documentation of prior lighting history), has been emphasized. Prior light exposure probably also determines the amplitude and phase of other circadian rhythms, although this has not yet been systematically investigated. The majority of markers of the circadian pacemaker are highly vulnerable to masking effects, thus require a constant routine protocol for correct measurement. The blunted rhythm amplitude documented for many parameters in depressive patients cannot be considered more than an epiphenomenon of the activity–rest cycle unless replicated under stringently controlled conditions.

Validated markers now exist for the output of the circadian pacemaker in normal subjects under such controlled conditions (e.g., core body temperature). Different mathematical methods permit estimates of the timing of the temperature minimum and maximum and the rhythm amplitude (e.g., see ref. 11). Melatonin secretion can be measured under dim light conditions, and provide phase estimates of onset, peak, and offset, as well as duration of secretion and amplitude of the fitted peak (35,68). Cortisol nadir, onset of the nocturnal rise, peak timing, 24-hr mean and relative amplitude, as well as ultradian frequencies of pulsatile secretion, can also be differentiated (38). Thus simple description of a single parameter (e.g., phase advance of the temperature rhythm) is now insufficient to describe the complex changes that occur (e.g., phase advance of the nadir of the cortisol rhythm with increased pulsatility and change in $\alpha{:}\rho$ ratio).

We live in a world that is no longer dominated by the day–night cycle or seasonal rhythms. A 24-hr society impacts on circadian rhythm integrity through low exposure to adequate light levels or shift work schedules. A society that can choose its seasons (jet to tropical beaches to avoid the long dark winter nights) is no longer synchronized to the natural ebb and flood of daylength or tempera-

ture. Artificial light, a bonus for a dynamic consumer society, simulates a summer day throughout the year, yet this lighting is of insufficient intensity to truly synchronize. Too little is known of the sequelae of such irregular patterns of light and temperature exposure on a vulnerable circadian system, and how light or temperature could trigger or alleviate a depressive phase. Genetic predisposition, hormonal fluctuations, environmental stress, and altered light–dark cycles could all induce rhythm disturbances. Conversely, altered sleep, arousal, mood state could feed back on to the circadian system.

The heuristic value of basic animal research directed at understanding temporal organization in animals has been to provide paradigms for conceptualizing and manipulating human biological rhythms. ''The worst that can happen to a scientific hypothesis is that it is ignored'' (5). The field of chronobiology and related sleep research has stimulated innovative circadian rhythm models of depression and has provided novel, nonpharmacological therapies.

Postmodern eclecticism has also reached psychiatry. As in other neurotransmitter-based hypotheses, explanations in terms of single causes, linear function, and reductionist simplification have been replaced by interacting, nonlinear dynamical systems, vulnerability thresholds, and efforts toward a more sophisticated bridge linking intrinsic and external phenomena.

ACKNOWLEDGMENTS

Leave of absence at the University of Cambridge is gratefully acknowledged. I thank Alexander Borbély, Hans-Joachim Haug, Alan Rosenwasser, and Michael Terman for comments. The author's studies on SAD patients were supported by the Swiss National Science Foundation.

REFERENCES

1. Anderson J, Wirz-Justice A. Biological rhythms in the pathophysiology and treatment of affective disorders. In: Horton R, Katona C, eds. *Biological aspects of affective disorders.* London: Academic Press; 1991:223–269.
2. Beersma DGM, Reinink E, Gordijn MCM, Bouhuys AL, Van den Hoofdakker RH. Concepts in circadian rhythm research in relation to diurnal variations in depressed mood. In: Westenberg HGM, ed. *Stress, biological rhythms and psychiatric disorders.* Houten: Medidact; 1991:63–69.
3. Benca RM, Obermeyer WH, Thisted RA, Gillin JC. Sleep and psychiatric disorders: a meta-analysis. *Arch Gen Psychiatry* 1992;49:651–668.
4. Berger M, Riemann D. REM sleep in depression—an overview. *J Sleep Res* 1993;2:211–223.
5. Borbély AA, Wirz-Justice A. Sleep, sleep deprivation and depression. A hypothesis derived from a model of sleep regulation. *Hum Neurobiol* 1982;1:205–210.
6. Boulos Z, Terman M. Food availability and daily biological rhythms. *Neurosci Biobehav Rev* 1980;4:119–131.
7. Campbell SS. Alerting/activating effects of light. ASDA/SLTBR

Task Force on the Use of Light Therapy for Sleep Disorders. *LTBR Bull* 1993;6:19–21.

8. Campbell SS. Treatment stategies for age-related disturbance using timed exposure to bright light. ASDA/SLTBR Task Force on the Use of Light Therapy for Sleep Disorders. *LTBR Bull* 1993;6:9–12.

9. Caroff SN, Winokur A. Hormonal response to thyrotropin-releasing hormone following rest–activity reversal in normal men. *Biol Psychiatry* 1984;19:1015–1025.

10. Checkley S. The relationship between biological rhythms and the affective disorders. In: Arendt J, Minors DS, Waterhouse JM, eds. *Biological rhythms in clinical practice*. London: Butterworth; 1989:160–183.

11. Czeisler CA, Kronauer RE, Allan JS, et al. Bright light induction of strong (type O) resetting of the human circadian pacemaker. *Science* 1989;244:1328–1333.

12. Dahl K, Avery DH, Lewy AJ, et al. Dim light melatonin onset and circadian temperature during a constant routine in hypersomnic winter depression. *Acta Psychiatr Scand* 1993;88:60–66.

13. Daimon K, Yamada N, Tsujimoto T, Takahashi S. Circadian rhythm abnormalities of deep body temperature in depressive disorders. *J Affect Dis* 1992;26:191–198.

14. Deacon S, Arendt J. Posture influences melatonin concentrations in plasma and saliva in humans. *Neurosci Lett* 1994;167:191–194.

15. Dijk D-J. Effects of light on circadian rhythms and sleep: basic processes. ASDA/SLTBR Task Force on the Use of Light Therapy for Sleep Disorders. *LTBR Bull* 1994;6:35–64.

16. Dirlich G, Kammerloher A, Schulz H, Lund R, Doerr P, von Zerssen D. Temporal coordination of rest–activity cycle, body temperature, urinary free cortisol, and mood in a patient with 48-hr unipolar depressive cycles in clinical and time-cue-free environments. *Biol Psychiatry* 1981;16:163–179.

17. Ehlers CL, Frank E, Kupfer DJ. Social zeitgebers and biological rhythms: a unified approach to understanding the etiology of depression. *Arch Gen Psychiatry* 1988;45:948–952.

18. Halberg F. Physiologic considerations underlying rhythmometry with special reference to emotional illness. In: de Ajuriaguerra J, ed. *Cycles Biologiques et Psychiatrie*. Paris: Masson et Cie, 1968;73–126.

19. Hall Jr. DP, Sing HC, Romanoski AJ. Identification and characterization of greater mood variance in depression. *Am J Psychiatry* 1991;148:418–419.

20. Hallonquist JD, Goldberg MA, Brandes JS. Affective disorders and circadian rhythms. *Can J Psychiatry* 1986;31:259–272.

21. Haug H-J, Wirz-Justice A. Diurnal variation of mood in depression: important or irrelevant? *Biol Psychiatry* 1993;34:201–203.

22. Healy D, Minors DS, Waterhouse JM. Shiftwork, helplessness and depression. *J Affect Dis* 1993;29:17–25.

23. Illnerová H, Vanecek J, Hoffmann K. Different mechanisms of phase delays and phase advances of the circadian rhythm in rat pineal *N*-acetyltransferase activity. *J Biol Rhythms* 1989;4:187–200.

24. Jauhar P, Weller MPI. Psychiatric morbidity and time zone changes. *Br J Psychiatry* 1982;140:231–235.

25. Klein DC, Moore RY, Reppert SM, eds. *Suprachiasmatic nucleus: the mind's clock*. New York: Oxford University Press; 1991.

26. Köhler WK, Fey P, Schmidt KP, Pflug B. Zeitgeber und das circadiane System bei depressiven Patienten. In: Baumann P, ed. *Biologische Psychiatrie der Gegenwart*. Vienna: Springer-Verlag; 1993:233–237.

27. Kräuchi K, Wirz-Justice A. Seasonal patterns of nutrient intake in relation to mood. In: Anderson GH, Kennedy SH, eds. *The biology of feast and famine: relevance to eating disorders*. Orlando: Academic Press; 1992:157–182.

28. Krauss SS, Depue RA, Arbisi PA, Spoont M. Behavioral engagement level, variability, and diurnal rhythm as a function of bright light in bipolar II seasonal affective disorder: an exploratory study. *Psychiatry Res* 1992;43:147–160.

29. Kripke DF. Photoperiodic mechanisms for depression and its treatment. In: Perris C, Struwe G, Jansson B, eds. *Biological psychiatry 1981*. Amsterdam: Elsevier/North-Holland Biomedical Press; 1981:1249–1252.

30. Kripke DF. Critical interval hypotheses for depression. *Chronobiology Int* 1984;1:73–80.

31. Kripke DF, Mullaney DJ, Atkinson M, Wolf SR. Circadian rhythm disorders in manic–depressives. *Biol Psychiatry* 1978;13:335–351.

32. Kuhs H, Tölle R. Sleep deprivation therapy. *Biol Psychiatry* 1991;29:1129–1148.

33. Lacoste V, Wirz-Justice A. Seasonal variation in normal subjects: an update of variables current in depression research. In: Rosenthal NE, Blehar MC, eds. *Seasonal affective disorders and phototherapy*. New York: Guilford Press; 1989:167–229.

34. Leibenluft E, Wehr TA. Is sleep deprivation useful in the treatment of depression? *Am J Psychiatry* 1992;149:159–168.

35. Lewy AJ, Sack RL, Miller LS, et al. The use of plasma melatonin levels and light in the assessment and treatment of chronobiologic sleep and mood disorders. *J Neural Transm* 1986;Suppl. 21:279–289.

36. Lewy AJ, Saeeduddin A, Latham Jackson JM, Sack RL. Melatonin shifts human circadian rhythms according to a phase response curve. *Chronobiol Int* 1992;9:380–392.

37. Lewy AJ, Wehr TA, Goodwin FK, Newsome DA, Rosenthal NE. Manic–depressive patients may be supersensitive to light. *Lancet* 1981;1:383–384.

38. Linkowski P, Van Onderbergen A, Kerkhofs M, Bosson D, Mendlewicz J, Van Cauter E. A twin study of the 24-hour cortisol profile: evidence for genetic control of the human circadian clock. *Am J Physiol* 1993;264:E173–E181.

39. Minors D, Waterhouse JM, Wirz-Justice A. A human phase-response curve to light. *Neurosci Lett* 1991;133:36–40.

40. Mizukawa R, Ishiguro S, Takada H, Kishimoto A, Ogura C, Hazama H. Long-term observation of a manic–depressive patient with rapid cycles. *Biol Psychiatry* 1991;29:671–678.

41. Monk TH, Kupfer DJ, Frank E, Ritenour AM. The social rhythm metric (SRM): measuring daily social rhythms over 12 weeks. *Psychiatry Res* 1991;36:195–207.

42. Mrosovsky N, Reebs SG, Honrado GI, Salmon PA. Behavioral entrainment of circadian rhythms. *Experientia* 1989;45:696–702.

43. Okawa M, Mishima K, Hishikawa Y, Hozumi S, Hori H. Sleep disorder in elderly patients with dementia and trials of new treatments—enforcement of social interaction and bright light therapy. In: Kuman VM, Mallick HN, Nayar U, eds. *Sleep-wakefulness*. New Delhi: Wiley Eastern; 1993:128–132.

44. Papoušek M. Chronobiologische Aspekte der Zyklothymie. *Fortschr Neurol Psychiat* 1975;43:381–440.

45. Parry BL, Berga SL, Kripke DF, et al. Altered waveform of plasma nocturnal melatonin secretion in premenstrual depression. *Arch Gen Psychiatry* 1990;47:1139–1146.

46. Pflug B, Johnsson A, Martin W. Alterations in the circadian temperature rhythms in depressed patients. In: Wehr TA, Goodwin FK, eds. *Circadian rhythms in psychiatry*. Pacific Grove, CA: Boxwood Press; 1983:71–76.

47. Prigerson HG, Reynolds III CF, Frank E, Kupfer DJ, George CJ, Houck PR. Stressful life events, social rhythms, and depressive symptoms among the elderly: an examination of hypothesized causal linkages. *Psychiatry Res* 1994;51:33–49.

48. Remé C, Wirz-Justice A, Terman M. The visual input stage of the mammalian circadian pacemaking system: I. Is there a clock in the mammalian eye? *J Biol Rhythms* 1991;6:5–29.

49. Richter CP. *Biological clocks in medicine and psychiatry*. Springfield, IL: Charles C Thomas; 1965.

50. Rockwell DA, Winget CM, Rosenblatt LS, Higgins EA, Hetherington NW. Biological aspects of suicide: circadian disorganisation. *J Nerv Ment Dis* 1978;166:851–858.

51. Rosenthal NE, Blehar MC, eds. *Seasonal affective disorder and phototherapy*. New York: Guilford Press; 1989.

52. Rosenwasser AM. Circadian rhythms and depression: animal models? *LTBR Bull* 1992;4:35–39.

53. Sack DA, Rosenthal NE, Parry BL, Wehr TA. Biological rhythms in psychiatry. In: Meltzer HY, ed. *Psychopharmacology: the third generation of progress*. New York: Raven Press; 1987:669–685.

54. Sack RL, Lewy AJ, Blood ML, Keith D, Nakagawa H. Circadian rhythm abnormalities in totally blind people: incidence and clinical significance. *J Clin Endocrinol Metab* 1992;75:127–134.

55. Schmidt KP, Köhler WK, Fleissner G, Pflug B. Locomotor activity accelerates the adjustment of the temperature rhythm in shiftwork. *J Interdisc Cycle Res* 1990;21:243–245.

56. Schulte W. Zum Problem der Provokation und Kupierung von mel-

ancholischen Phasen. *Arch Neurol Neurochir Psychiatr* 1971;109: 427–435.

57. Siever LJ, Davis KL. Overview: toward a dysregulation hypothesis of depression. *Am J Psychiatry* 1985;142:1017–1031.

58. Souêtre E, Salvati E, Belugou J-L et al. Circadian rhythms in depression and recovery: evidence for blunted amplitude as the main chronobiological abnormality. *Psychiatry Res* 1989;28:263–278.

59. Surridge-David M, MacLean AW, Coulter ME, Knowles JB. Mood change following an acute delay of sleep. *Psychiatry Res* 1987;22:149–158.

60. Szuba MP, Yager A, Guze BH, Allen EM, Baxter LR. Disruption of social circadian rhythms in major depression: a preliminary report. *Psychiatry Res* 1992;42:221–230.

61. Taillard J, Sanchez P, Lemoine P, Mouret J. Heart rate circadian rhythm as a biological marker of desynchronization in major depression: a methodological and preliminary report. *Chronobiology Int* 1990;7:305–316.

62. Terman M, Terman JS. Seasonal affective disorder and light therapy: *Report to the Depression Guidelines Panel, Public Health Service Agency for Health Care Policy and Research.* New York: New York State Psychiatric Institute: 1991.

63. Tsujimoto T, Yamada N, Shimoda K, Hanada K, Takahashi S. Circadian rhythms in depression. Part II: Circadian rhythms in inpatients with various mental disorders. *J Affect Dis* 1990;18:199–210.

64. Van Cauter E, Sturis J, Byrne MM, et al. Preliminary studies on the immediate phase-shifting effects of light and exercise on the human circadian clock. In: Rusak B, Haddad G, eds. *J Biol Rhythms.* New York: Guilford Press; 1993:S99–S108.

65. Van den Hoofdakker RH, Beersma DGM. On the contribution of sleep wake physiology to the explanation and treatment of depression. *Acta Psych Scand (Suppl)* 1988;341:53–71.

66. von Zerssen D, Barthelms H, Dirlich G, et al. Circadian rhythms in endogenous depression. *Psychiatry Res* 1985;16:51–63.

67. Wehr TA, Goodwin FK. Biological rhythms in manic–depressive illness. In: Wehr TA, Goodwin FK, eds. *Circadian rhythms in psychiatry* Pacific Grove, CA: Boxwood Press; 1983:129–184.

68. Wehr TA, Moul DE, Barbato G, et al. Conservation of photoperiod-responsive mechanisms in humans. *Am J Physiol* 1993;265:R846–R857.

69. Wehr TA, Sack DA, Duncan WC, et al. Sleep and circadian rhythms in affective patients isolated from external time cues. *Psychiatry Res* 1985;15:327–339.

70. Wehr TA, Wirz-Justice A. Circadian rhythm mechanisms in affective illness and in antidepressant drug action. *Pharmacopsychiat* 1982;15:31–39.

71. Wever R. *The circadian system of man: results of experiments under temporal isolation.* New York: Springer Verlag; 1979.

72. Wever RA. Light effects on human circadian rhythms: a review of recent Andechs experiments. *J Biol Rhythms* 1989;4:161–185.

73. Wirz-Justice A, Graw P, Kräuchi K, et al. Light therapy in seasonal affective disorder is independent of time of day or circadian phase. *Arch Gen Psychiatry* 1993;50:929–937.

74. Wirz-Justice A, Graw P, Kräuchi K, Haug H-J, Leonhardt G, Brunner DP. Effect of light on unmasked circadian rhythms in winter depression. In: Wetterberg L, ed. *Light and biological rhythms in man.* Oxford: Pergamon Press; 1993:385–393.

75. Wu JC, Bunney WE Jr. The biological basis of an antidepressant response to sleep deprivation and relapse: review and hypothesis. *Am J Psychiatry* 1990;147:14–21.

76. Zucker I. Seasonal affective disorders: animal models *non fingo. J Biol Rhythms* 1988;3:209–223.

Psychopharmacology: The Fourth Generation of Progress, edited by Floyd E. Bloom and David J. Kupfer. Raven Press, Ltd., New York © 1995.

CHAPTER 87

Brain Imaging in Mood Disorders

Godfrey D. Pearlson and Thomas E. Schlaepfer

The ultimate aim of imaging studies is to define a neuroanatomy of mood disorders. The question that remains to be answered is whether there is a single such common change or set of changes associated with these diverse clinical syndromes.

Knowledge of the underlying pathobiology of mood disorders is still sketchy (39). Brain imaging is potentially able to shed useful light on pathophysiological changes associated with mood disorders. However, such a picture is only now beginning to emerge. There are several reasons for this. For example, in schizophrenia, neuropathological structural investigations have often initiated hypotheses later tested by brain imaging techniques. However, virtually no such neuropathological investigations of mood disorders have been carried out. Although schizophrenia is by no means a clinically uniform disorder, affective illness can appear bewilderingly diverse, a fact that has made brain imaging studies hard to plan and to interpret.

The logic for the use of neuroimaging studies in elucidating the pathophysiology of affective syndromes has been laid out by Cummings (18). Supportive evidence is first gathered from the study of affective patients with neuroimaging techniques and delineation of differences from healthy controls. Similar studies are also carried out in parallel in patients with mood changes occurring in the context of focal brain pathology, due to traumatic injury or disease processes of known location (for example, stroke, seizure disorders, Huntington's disease, and so on). Significant associations between the syndromes and regional deficits revealed on neuroimaging are then delineated. Commonalties in findings between the two types of studies are then examined, and further hypotheses generated.

Neuroimaging studies in mood disorders to date have been complicated by many factors, which are outlined here and discussed in more detail below. First, sample sizes have generally been small. Second, mood disorders are a remarkably diverse collection of entities. The heterogeneity of the disorder necessitates very careful descriptions of study populations; most investigations have not provided these. Kupfer and Rush (45) made recommendations for explicit description of populations of mood disorder patients studied in biological psychiatric reports. Such basic descriptive parameters and definitions have not been consistently employed in the majority of neuroimaging studies of affective disorders. Few studies have compared diagnostic subgroups directly; most look either at only one of many of subgroups or at a mixture. Inherent differences in the imaging methods used to study patients has made comparisons across different studies less than straightforward. Methods of analysis can differ widely between otherwise similar studies. Potential artifacts of analysis, for example those associated in blood flow with ratio methods must be addressed. With the need to study changes in neural systems as well as in localized regions, these considerations are especially important.

Phenomenologically, clinical symptoms can overlap among mood disorders, schizophrenia, anxiety disorders, and obsessive–compulsive disorder. By analogy, one might reasonably expect a similar overlap in associated disturbances of cerebral pathophysiology and hence findings on structural and functional neuroimaging. Therefore, diagnostic specificity is a key question.

State-versus-trait issues are also of great importance, given the episodic nature of most affective illness. Whether underlying neuroimaging abnormalities are detectable only during periods of illness or whether they exist independent of clinical status can only be addressed clearly through longitudinal studies. For example, it has been suggested that the hypercortisolemia often accompanying episodes of major depression could cause reversible

G. D. Pearlson and T. E. Schlaepfer: Department of Psychiatry, Johns Hopkins University School of Medicine, Baltimore, Maryland 21287-7362.

TABLE 1. *Subtypes of mood disorders*

(a) *Subtypes with possible relevance to neuroimaging*
Unipolar/bipolar
Psychotic/nonpsychotic
With cognitive impairment/without
Late onset/early onset
Family history positive/negative
Primary/secondary
Endogenous/non
Melancholic/non
DST suppression/nonsuppression
Psychomotor retarded/agitated
(b) *Other possible confounds*
Comorbid substance abuse
Cerebral effects of weight loss
Treatment status (medications, ECT)
Current clinical state
Gender
Age (current)
Episodic number, frequency, duration
Illness severity
Treatment responsiveness

cerebral atrophy. Progression of structural changes has been hypothesized to occur in concert with clinical episodic progression, in an analogy with Post's model of kindling (e.g., ref. 2).

Psychotropic medications and other treatments may cause significant changes in cerebral pharmacological receptors, neurotransmitters, blood flow, and metabolism. Treatment status of patients thus has the potential to confound many functional studies of mood disorder.

As shown in Table 1, mood disorder is clinically and phenomenologically heterogeneous. One could use neuroimaging techniques to "biotype" mood disorders. The potential advantages of doing so are to identify useful unitary putative markers for mood disorders that show relative specificity and to provide novel classification. Equally, potential disadvantages are of further blurring the picture, identifying changes of a relatively nonspecific nature (which are also seen in schizophrenia or obsessive–compulsive disorders), or changes that are highly specific, but closely associated with specific minor component symptoms of mood disorders. For example, global resting cerebral blood flow may well be influenced by the level of motor activity, so that agitated and retarded depressive patients could show opposite changes.

The population being imaged may well make an important difference if the corresponding underlying pathophysiology is nonuniform. The reality, however, is that most studies to date have included very diverse patient populations. There is preliminary evidence from several studies that studying patients with more homogeneous subtypes of mood disorder may help clarify associated biological changes. Several examples are provided. Drevets et al. (26) studied patients with familial pure depressive disorder, defined by Winokur's (78) relatively homogeneous clinical subtype of unipolar disorder. Using

positron emission tomography (PET) measurements, they determined that regional cerebral blood flow was increased in left prefrontal cortex, left amygdala, and left medial thalamus but reduced in the left medial caudate. These changes appeared fairly robust (replicated in an independent sample) but were in the opposite direction to many prior reported functional changes in less homogeneous mood disorder populations.

There is much to suggest that the distinction between early-in-life and late-in-life onset (early onset and late onset) depressive patients is meaningful. Additional evidence suggests an etiology (cerebral microvascular disease) associated with a proportion of late-onset cases. The two age-of-onset groups seem distinguishable on both structural and functional neuroimaging studies. Shima (68) demonstrated using computed tomography (CT) that late-onset depressive patients had larger ventricles than comparable early-onset patients. Dolan also showed that late-onset depressives had ventricular enlargement compared to age-appropriate normals, whereas early-life onset depressives did not (24). However, similar studies in young mood disorder patients did not find clear effects of age of onset (for example, see ref. 62). Using magnetic resonance imaging (MRI), Coffey et al. (14) found more white matter lesions in late-onset depressive patients and Figiel found that basal ganglia lesions were commoner in the late-onset depressive patients (31).

Targum et al. found that delusionally depressed patients had larger ventricles on CT than nondelusional comparison patients and specifically more delusional than nondelusional patients had values two standard deviations or more greater than the normal control mean (75). Saccetti et al. (63) found a similar effect in psychotic patients.

Other workers have examined the effects of duration of disorder on ventricular measures. This measure is confounded to some extent by age of onset. No effect of duration was demonstrable by Tanaka et al. (74). The severity of the most recent episode on ventricular enlargement was explored by Pearlson et al. (55) in bipolars, with no clear-cut relationship demonstrable. Other workers examined CT measures for differences between patients with and without family histories of mood disorders. No differences between these groups were discovered by Dolan et al. (24) or Jacoby and Levy (38). Saccetti demonstrated that family-history-negative patients tended to have larger ventricles (63).

Some depressed patients show reversible cognitive abnormalities. Pearlson et al. (56) compared in a CT study cognitively normal elderly patients with depression to similarly aged patients with a reversible dementia syndrome of depression. The depressed sample as a whole was intermediate on several measures between normal controls and patients with Alzheimer's disease. Relative to normal, demented depressed patients had larger ventricles and reduced CT brain attenuation numbers. Dupont et al. (27) demonstrated in younger bipolar patients that those with more white matter hyperintensities on MRI showed more cognitive abnormalities.

Finally, and separate from the question of state-versus-trait markers (which will be discussed below), some workers have investigated possible relationships between dexamethasone suppression test status and structural brain measures in patients with major depression. One hypothesis is that high circulating levels of endogenous steroids produce cortical atrophy and ventricular enlargement in a manner similar to that of indigenously administered cortisol. Kellner et al. (41) showed a relationship between lateral ventricular enlargement on CT and raised 24-hr free urinary cortisol measurements in depressed patients (41). Schlegel et al. (67) demonstrated a similar relationship between ventricular enlargement and average afternoon plasma cortisol values. Other investigators have shown no relationship between dexamethasone nonsuppression and the ventricle-to-brain ratio (VBR), including Schlegel et al. (67) and Targum et al. (75).

Overall, there appears to be convincing evidence of distinct subtypes of mood disorder that may be characterized by different constellations of neuroimaging changes.

STRUCTURAL FINDINGS

Biological research in mood disorders focused traditionally on the neurochemical basis of the disease. The neuroanatomical basis of these disorders has not been extensively studied until 10 years ago. At this time, radiological techniques allowing investigation of the living brain in health and disease became widely available. Structural abnormalities in mood disorders have first been investigated with CT. Later the more precise and less invasive methodology of MRI has been applied. Compared to the investigation of structural differences in patients with schizophrenia, relatively few data focusing on differences in patients with mood disorders have been obtained. Various types of structural abnormalities were described in schizophrenia, but the initial hope that these differences might turn out to be specific for schizophrenia was not realized, as similar abnormalities were reported in mood disorders. As discussed below, the most consistent finding of differences that are relatively specific for mood disorders are abnormalities of subcortical white matter and basal ganglia.

Structural Findings in Primary Depression

Increased Ventricle-to-Brain Ratio and Lateral Ventricular Enlargement

The most frequently reported structural difference in mood disorders is increase in the VBR and, more specifically, lateral ventricular enlargement. As discussed above, the drive to study structural abnormalities in patients with

mood disorders was first generated from neuropathological and imaging studies in schizophrenia. Patients with mood disorders were initially included in studies of structural changes in schizophrenia to control for the specificity of the findings. Computerized tomography studies show that patients with mood disorders tend to be quite similar to schizophrenic patients and significantly different from normal control subjects in VBR (39,67). These differences tended to be less pronounced in patients with mood disorders (77). However, a number of more recent studies were not able to confirm the findings of ventricular enlargement (15,46), and a more recent review of the literature suggested that the correlation between VBR and clinical measures was inconclusive (21). Of 19 studies focusing on VBR, only 3 reported data on patients with unipolar and bipolar depression separately (24,66). The other two studies found no differences for VBR in these two subtypes of mood disorders. Studying manic patients, several groups (51,58) found the lateral cerebral ventricle to be enlarged compared to normal controls. Other groups found enlargement only in the third ventricle (22,74). The reason for these inconsistencies is not clear (53), and it is difficult to compare these studies because of differences in the methodologies of image acquisition and processing and the inhomogeneity of patient populations. Important and often overlooked confounding factors could be comorbidity with substance abuse, medication, and lack of adequate matching of the control subjects. Alcohol use, for instance, even in socially accepted amounts, has been shown in a CT study to lead to brain atrophy (13).

Sulcal Widening

Another structural difference between normal subjects and patients with mood disorders is sulcal widening. Tanaka et al. described the widening of the interhemispheric and sylvian fissures as characteristic of older depressed patients (74). This finding was confirmed in younger manic patients (51). Others found sulcal widening particularly in frontal and temporal areas (e.g., see refs. 25 and 59). However, other studies failed to confirm sulcal widening both globally and in specific areas (22,66). As with ventricular enlargement, the data on the existence of this structural difference in mood disorders remains inconclusive and inconsistent.

Cerebellar Vermian Atrophy

The above observation is true also for a third structural difference reported in manic patients: cerebellar vermian atrophy. Atrophy of the cerebellum in both manic and depressed patients has been reported in several studies (52,77). No alterations of the cerebellum have been found in other studies (e.g., see ref. 58).

Basal Ganglia and Subcortical White Matter Abnormalities

Probably the most interesting and most consistent findings of structural abnormalities in patients with mood disorders came from the recent focus of interest on subcortical structures. Using CT, one study demonstrated increased radiodensity of the caudate head bilaterally in elderly depressed patients (7). Smaller volumes of caudate (44) and putamen nuclei have also been reported using MRI (37).

Recently several groups reported on the consistent finding of subcortical hyperintensities in patients with mood disorders using MRI (27,28,31,59). Dupont et al. for instance reported on these abnormalities in 8 of 14 young bipolar patients (28). He reported later, that patients with these unidentified bright objects tended to have more previous hospitalizations and tended to perform worse on neuropsychological tests than patients without these abnormalities (27). The abnormalities are areas of increased signal intensity (therefore, they appear as white spots) in T_2-weighted MRI images found to be located (a) as a rim periventricularly, (b) as patchy or confluent areas in subcortical white matter, and (c) in subcortical gray matter structures like the basal ganglia, thalamus, and pons. Almost two-thirds of elderly patients referred for electroconvulsive therapy (ECT) were found in one study (14). The authors suggested, that subcortical white matter changes might predispose to late-onset, treatment-resistant depression. It is important to note, that higher rates of subcortical hyperintensities have been reported in both young bipolar (31) and elderly depressed, mainly unipolar patient groups (59). There are currently no data on the existence of these abnormalities in younger bipolar patients. Like the structural changes discussed before, subcortical white matter changes are a nonspecific finding of unknown significance.

Abnormalities in Elderly Depressed Patients

Some studies have focused on an elderly population with a particular emphasis on depression, with late-onset compared to age-matched patients with early-onset depression. An association with greater sulcal widening and greater severity of subcortical white matter lesions has been reported in elderly depressives with late-onset depression (16), and these findings have recently been confirmed by Rabin et al. (59). Patients with late-onset depression have recently been reported to have more and larger white matter hyperintensities in the caudate than age-matched patients with early-onset depression suggesting that these structural changes may be involved in the etiology of late-onset depression in some patients (31). Elderly depressed patients were found to be similar to patients with dementia in regard to a decreased centrum

semiovale intensity on CT (54). Hyperintensities of deep gray matter structures such as the basal ganglia and the thalamus found in the elderly could not be detected in younger bipolar samples (31).

An MRI study in 29 normal volunteers and in 20 patients with major depression revealed particularly prominent shortened T_1 relaxation times in the hippocampus of elderly depressed patients suggesting that major depression in the elderly may be associated with tissue changes in the aging hippocampus (43).

Structural Findings in Secondary Depression

Considerably more data on secondary mood disorders following central nervous system (CNS) lesions have been obtained compared to primary mood disorders. In a review of affective symptoms following stroke, it was noted that depression was much more common than mania but that manic symptoms were more frequently observed in patients with a previous personal or familial history of mood disorders (69). Establishing a connection between site of lesion and depressive symptomatology has been tried in several studies. It has been demonstrated in a CT study of patients with closed-head injury that major depression developed more in patients with left basal ganglia and left dorsolateral frontal lesions (30). In a CT study, stroke patients with right temporal, right superior frontal, left inferior frontal, and left parietal occipital were found to have more sleep disturbance and greater dysphoria than patients with lesions in other areas of the brain (71). Lesions associated with depression and mania occur often in the temporal and frontal lobes, right-sided lesions tending to be associated with mania and left-sided lesions with depression (69).

Mood disorders are often associated with Huntington's disease. Because the disease has a fairly well documented neuropathology and correlations between the extent of the structural alterations and clinical abnormalities have been established, it is of particular interest for psychiatry. Approximately 40% of patients suffering from Huntington's disease develop symptoms of mood disorder over the course of their illness and approximately 10% have manic episodes (32). It is interesting that the affective symptoms associated with Huntington's sometimes precede the motor and cognitive symptoms for many years. A recent MRI study reported marked reduction of the volume of the putamen and the caudate nucleus in mild cases of Huntington's disease (33). The changes in putaminal size correlated, unlike that of the caudate, with neurological impairment.

FUNCTIONAL FINDINGS

Functional abnormalities in mood disorders have been assessed with the techniques of single photon emission computed tomography (SPECT) and PET. Both modalities provide data in a similarly useful way about cerebral blood flow (CBF) and cerebral metabolic rate (CMR), thus giving by quantification of physiological parameters insight in the biochemical basis of the disorder. Few mood disorder patients have been investigated in the manic phase, because of the difficulty of image acquisition in these patients without prior pharmacological treatment. Almost no studies have tracked patients longitudinally. Therefore most data have been obtained in patients with major depression or bipolar patients in the depressive phase of the disease. Results are interesting, but hardly unanimous, most likely due to wide differences in patient selection, choice of comparison populations, stimulus conditions, and image acquisitions and analysis methods.

Global Differences

Many functional imaging studies in mood disorders have initially focused on whether patients in acute affective episodes have abnormal global changes in blood flow or metabolic rates. A number of studies reported about decreased rates for both CBF and CMR in patients with various mood disorders compared to normal controls in a resting state (e.g., ref. 47). Other groups were not able to replicate the finding of reduced CBF in major depression (e.g., ref. 8), and one study even reported a global CBF elevation (61). In an activation study, global CMR of depressed patients, schizophrenic patients, and normal controls was investigated while they received unpleasant electrical stimuli. No differences were found in this study across groups in global brain metabolism, but a decreased anterior/posterior ratio was found in both mood disorder and schizophrenic patients (11). The same group found in another activation study a global increase of glucose metabolism in bipolar and unipolar patients (12).

It is not quite clear why these findings are so inconsistent. A probable source of error is the great heterogeneity of the patient groups included in the discussed studies. Unipolar, bipolar, young outpatients with mild depression, elderly severely depressed patients, patients with scores on the Hamilton depression rating scale (HRS-D) ranging from 15 to 35 have been studied. Furthermore image assessment and processing varied considerably between studies, resulting in partly incomparable data.

Lateral Asymmetries at the Cortical Level

Regional reduction of metabolic activity in frontal cortical regions, particularly the dorsolateral prefrontal cortex (DLPFC) in major depression have been suggested in PET studies (e.g., ref. 6). Most prominent was a decreased ratio of metabolic rate of the left DLPFC relative to the total metabolic rate of the left hemisphere. This ratio

correlated significantly with HRS-D scores. Anterior frontal hypometabolism mainly on the right side was reported in a sample of depressed patients (36). In an activation study using PET, depressed patients performing an attentional task showed a reduction of CMR in the medial frontal cortex (17). In a recent SPECT study using ^{123}I-labeled amphetamine (IMP) in patients with major depression an increased IMP activity in the right temporal lobe (3) was observed. Another SPECT study significantly decreased rates of cortical blood flow in the left hemisphere in bipolar patients (20). Only a few groups reported on the absence of regional abnormalities of CBF and CMR at rest (e.g., ref. 42).

In contrast to the relatively inconsistent findings about abnormalities of global CBF and CMR there are many observations of hypofrontality in major depression.

Differences in the Basal Ganglia

The possibility of an abnormal caudate-to-hemisphere ratio in major depression was raised by one group. Patients with unipolar depression showed a significantly lower ratio of the metabolic rate in the caudate nucleus, divided by that of the hemisphere as a whole, when compared with normal controls and patients with bipolar depression (4). Depressed patients with Parkinson's syndrome were found to have decreased metabolism in the caudate, suggesting that a lesion at the level of the basal ganglia might be associated with depression (50). This finding is particularly interesting in the light of the evidence of high prevalence of mood disorders in patients with lesions of the basal ganglia (70).

Treatment Responses

As discussed above, CBF and CMR changes in affective disorders have been found in specific brain regions including the limbic system, the basal ganglia, and both frontal and temporal cortex. Of great interest are changes in blood flow and metabolism in these regions induced by treatment. In a SPECT study using the tracer Tc-99m-hexamethylpropylenamineoxime (HMPAO) depressed patients before and after sleep deprivation were investigated. All patients showed relative hypoperfusion in the left anterolateral prefrontal cortex under both conditions. Only responders to the therapy showed relative hyperperfusion in parts of the limbic system and a reduction of blood flow in these regions after sleep deprivation (29).

Abnormalities at the Level of Neurotransmission

Biological hypotheses regarding the pathophysiology of mood disorders concentrated on abnormalities in neurochemical transmission with a particular emphasis on possible alterations in receptor physiology. Although both SPECT and PET are capable of examining binding of various ligands to receptors of neurotransmitters on a regional basis and thus having the potential to assess these hypotheses, relatively few imaging studies looking at receptor ligands have been performed. It is important to note that no hypothesis about the dysfunction of neurotransmission in mood disorders explains adequately all the assessed data.

A recent SPECT study in depressed patients using a ligand of the 5-HT$_2$ receptor demonstrated a higher uptake of the tracer in the parietal cortex and a higher right than left asymmetry in the inferior frontal region of the patients, suggesting changes in the serotonin (5-HT) receptor density (19). In six patients with histories of major depressive disorder, significantly lower uptake of [b-^{11}C]5-hydroxytryptophane (5-HTP) across the blood–brain barrier was reported in a PET study (1). These differences were observed mainly in the basal ganglia and in the prefrontal cortex. An other PET study demonstrated that patients with strokes of the right hemisphere had higher binding of (3-N-[11C]methyl)-spiperone to 5-HT$_2$ receptors in the right parietal and temporal cortex than a similar group of patients with strokes in the left hemisphere or normal subjects. The ratio of binding in the ipsilateral to binding in the contralateral cortex showed a negative correlation with severity of depression, suggesting a different biochemical response of the brain depending on the location of the injury and that some secondary depressions may be a consequence of insufficient up-regulation of 5-HT receptors after stroke (48). In another PET study, lower binding of a dopamine D$_1$ receptor ligand in the frontal cortex of bipolar patients than of normal controls was reported, suggesting abnormalities of the dopaminergic transmission in the ethiology of bipolar disorder (72).

Involvement of Functional Circuits

It is likely that mood disorder involves dysfunction of integrated neural circuits or networks, rather than individual brain regions. Four recent reviews discuss such involvement of neural circuits in mood disorders (21,26,49,73).

Drevets et al. (26) implicates two related loops: one involving the amygdala, mediodorsal thalamic nucleus, vertrolateral prefrontal cortex, and medial prefrontal cortex (PFC), and a second linking the striatum and ventral pallidum to the first circuit. Swerdlow and Koob (73) implicated the forebrain in dopaminegric circuits that affect limbic–thalamic–cortical loops, and are secondarily modulated by dopaminergic projections to the striatum, amygdala, and PFC.

Depue and Iacono (21) view mood disorder as a dysfunction of a behavioral facilitation system, which normally provides motor, affective, and motivational components to achieve environmental engagement or withdrawal. They implicate circuitry influencing locomotor activity and incentive/reward behaviors in two dopaminergic projections from the ventral tegmental area. The first of these is the mesolimbic projection to the nucleus accumbens and amygdala; the second is the neocortical efferent system to the motor cortex, dorsomedial PFC, anterior cingulate, and orbital and dorsolateral PFC. Mayberg (49) draws together evidence from neuroimaging studies of Huntington's disease, Parkinson's disease, and basal ganglia stroke, which are all related to depressive disorders. She feels that involvement of the paralimbic cortex (PLC) (i.e., orbital/cortical, inferior frontal, and anterior temporal cortex) is crucial. Two circuits are hypothesized to involve the PLC in this role; one orbitofrontal–basal ganglia–thalamic, and the second orbitofrontal–uncinate fasciculus–anterior temporal (the basotemporal–limbic circuit).

The reviews above implicate many of the same structures and circuits, most frequently those involving portions of the prefrontal cortex (especially orbital), basal ganglia, thalamus, and amygdala. Many of these circuits involve neurotransmitter interactions between dopamine (DA) and 5-HT.

DISCUSSION

The importance of the heterogeneity of mood disorder was stressed above. Other important issues include specificity of brain changes to mood disorder and major confounds in prior studies.

Specificity of Changes to Mood Disorder

Jeste et al. (39) stated that "in every area in which structural abnormalities have been found in neuroradiological studies of schizophrenia, abnormalities of similar magnitude have also been demonstrated in affective disorders." That this is the case could be true for several reasons. First, common pathophysiological mechanisms could underlie the two syndromes, as suggested, for example by Buchsbaum et al. (11) and Cohen et al. (17). Studies have seldom been designed to address these hypotheses directly. Mood disorder patients have often been studied only as a comparison group in primary studies of schizophrenic illnesses. Nevertheless, there are numerous illustrations of Jeste's comment. Schizophrenics and manics have been shown to be similar in multiple CT studies of sulcal widening (e.g., ref. 60), vermian cerebellar atrophy (e.g., ref. 77), and lateral ventricular enlargement (51,58). These studies generally have shown similar changes in mood disorder patients and schizophrenics as opposed to controls but are less marked in mood disorders. Some functional neuroimaging studies have reached similar conclusions. Buchsbaum et al. (11) demonstrated similar hypofrontality in schizophrenic and mood disorder patient samples compared to normals. Pearlson et al. (57) demonstrated analogous DA D_2 elevated B_{max} measurements in PET neuroreceptor studies of psychotic and schizophrenic patients compared to both normal controls and nonpsychotic mood disorder patients. Berman (9) examined the issue of specificity of altered cortical blood flow in schizophrenics and mood disorder patients. They examined 10 patients with schizophrenia, 10 depressed subjects, and 20 age- and sex-matched normal controls. Regional cerebral blood flow was separately measured at rest, during a simple number-matching task, and during performance of the Wisconsin Card Sorting Test, using inhaled radioactive Xenon. Schizophrenic patients demonstrated lower prefrontal regional cerebral blood flow only during performance of the Wisconsin Card Sorting Test. No differences in either regional or global flow were demonstrable between depressed patients and normals during any testing condition.

Overall then, although there is considerable overlap with other major psychiatric syndromes, especially schizophrenia, brain imaging changes in mood disorders exhibit some putatively specific findings.

Sensitivity of Changes to Illness Status

Ill-versus-well and state-versus-trait issues are especially relevant to neuroimaging studies of mood disorders, which by its nature tends to be episodic with return to normal functioning between episodes. Structural or functional neuroimaging changes could be seen only during periods of illness, with return to normal between episodes. Although this is harder to imagine for structural changes, the issue of possible reversible steroid-related structural alterations has already been mentioned. A second contrasting possibility is that neuroimaging changes represent trait markers of the illness and that differences from normal are present irrespective of whether an individual patient is ill or well at the time of testing. Dupont et al. (28) demonstrated state-independent white matter abnormalities in more than half of a sample of young bipolar individuals on MRI. Drevets et al. (26) showed that even though increased left prefrontal regional cerebral blood flow was seen only in depressed individuals, and appeared to be state-related, increased flow in left amygdala appeared in both ill and remitted patients. Thus, this episodic illness may have both state and trait markers, but supporting data are preliminary and need further confirmation. In particular, few or no studies have examined the same patients in the ill and remitted states.

Treatment Effects on Neuroimaging Data

This important issue is linked conceptually to state-versus-trait issues, as many studies of remitted patients examined those taking mood-altering medications or those suffering longer-term effects of physical treatment, such as electroconvulsive therapy (ECT). Few studies have attempted to resolve this issue. Also, very few human investigations have addressed effects of longer term lithium or antidepressant treatment given to normal volunteers. Coffey et al. (15) examined depressed elderly individuals before and during ECT treatment and demonstrated no structural MRI changes between the two conditions.

Some longitudinal studies that attempted to address state–trait issues have been complicated in their interpretation by possible treatment effects (e.g., refs. 36 and 47). Baxter et al. (4) demonstrated that in three unipolar depressed patients caudate metabolism on glucose PET increased concomitant with antidepressant treatment. Baxter showed treatment-related increases in glucose metabolism in the DLPFC (5). In cross-sectional studies, no effect of prior ECT was demonstrated on lateral ventricular enlargement in mood disorders by Dolan et al. (24) or Pearlson et al. (55). Similarly, no effect of prior medication treatment was demonstrable on lateral ventricular enlargement (24,55). Future studies need to account for treatment effects more regularly than has been the norm in much of the existing literature.

Progression of Changes

This is an important, but little-studied topic. Altshuler et al. (2) have argued recently for the possibility of progressive structural change in bipolar disorder. The major supporting evidence is of the cognitive abnormalities associated with the disorder, which may worsen with time (e.g., ref. 23), and the study of Vita et al. (76), suggesting increasing VBR over an average 3-year period in comparison to both normal controls and schizophrenia patients. If this effect is real, one possible mechanism to explain it could be the neurotoxic effects of hypercortisolemia. However intriguing, more evidence needs to be gathered to support or refute the notion of progression.

Predictive Value of Neuroimaging Changes in Mood Disorder

Theoretically, neuroimaging changes could be predictive in several senses. The previously mentioned associations with biological response (e.g., dexamethasone suppression test status) is one example. Imaging changes could also predict response to treatment of various sorts, be markers of relapse or recurrence, and conceivably predict treatment side effects or complications.

Jacoby and Levy (38) demonstrated in an outcome study that elderly depressed individuals with the greatest degree of ventricular enlargement on CT had excess mortality on follow-up. One question to determine is whether this observation is explained by a subpopulation of patients in whom depression is appearing early in the course of a neurodegenerative disease, (such as Alzheimer's or multiinfarct dementia). If this is the case, it is consistent with CT studies suggesting that elderly depressed patients with reversible cognitive changes have brain alterations intermediate between those of elderly depressed and Alzheimer patients (e.g., 54,56).

The area of prediction is one of great potential importance. Shima et al. (68) showed an association between ventricular enlargement on CT in depressed patients and treatment outcome. Coffey et al. (16) showed that the presence of white matter lesions in elderly depressed patients was associated with prior poor response to antidepressant treatment, better subsequent response to ECT, and a greater likelihood of ECT-linked delirium. Wu et al. (79) showed specific regional cerebral metabolic changes (elevations in amygdala and cingulate) in depressives predicted successful antidepressant response to sleep deprivation.

Review of the evidence here yields few definite conclusions. Nasrallah et al. (51) showed a lower frequency of hospital stays in manic patients with ventricular enlargement on CT. However, Pearlson et al. (55) demonstrated the opposite. Bird et al. (10) found that baseline ventricular enlargement in control subjects was associated with the later development of late-onset depression. Further follow-up studies are needed to clarify the area of prediction.

To return to the paradigm outlined by Cummings (18) and mentioned earlier, to what extent do neuroimaging findings in mood disorders provide clues as to the underlying pathophysiology of the illness?

Clinical and Biological Correlates of the Changes

The issue of heterogeneity was discussed above. Subtypes may be associated with neuroimaging differences. Examples include the reversible dementia of depression being associated with reduced CT white matter attenuation values (54,56) and an association of enlarged VBR on CT with increased urinary free cortisol (41). These studies also stress the need to examine structural and functional changes in the same patients.

One major hypothesis is that the neuroimaging changes in regional cerebral blood flow in elderly depressed patients on CT and MRI are a consequence of vascular disease. Coffey et al. (14) showed that many elderly patients with white matter lesions on MRI were at high risk for cerebrovascular disease (possessing multiple vascular risk factors) compared to controls. Pearlson et al. (54) showed reduced CT attenuation values in centrum semiovale of depressed patients. Rates in elderly depressed patients for MRI white matter hyperintensities are similar to those seen in multiinfarct dementia (e.g., ref. 35); this

topic was reviewed by Sackeim and Prohovnik (64). There is support from Sackeim et al. (65), whose perfusion studies showed similar changes in depressed elderly individuals and in nondepressed subjects with cerebrovascular disease.

The second major area of investigation involves the specific brain regions and neural circuits most likely involved in mood disorder.

It is possible that many of the metabolic and blood flow changes seen on functional neuroimaging in elderly depressed patients could be associated with regional atrophy. There is certainly some evidence on CT studies that patients with mood disorders have reduced temporal lobe area, relative to cerebral area (34), and reduced temporal lobe volume (2). However, Johnstone showed no differences in total brain or total temporal lobe area between mood disorder patients and controls (40). The area of clinical and biological associations of neuroimaging changes in mood disorders remains largely unexplored, but clear hypotheses are emerging, which have been briefly outlined above.

CONCLUSIONS

As reviewed, there are significant obstacles in documenting reproducible brain-imaging changes associated with mood disorder, including the nature of the syndrome and its associations. Important lessons have been learned in how best to study the disorder and potential pitfalls to avoid from these earlier endeavors, including the need to use standardized clinical assessments and instruments for adequate description and categorization of patient samples and adequately sized patient and control populations. Given the diversity of the syndrome and the nature of the investigations, especially of quantitative functional studies, this whole area of investigation must be regarded as potentially fruitful but in its early stages. The generation of hypotheses from neuropathologic studies in guiding the design of subsequent brain-imaging studies envisaged by Cummings (18) is gradually coming to pass.

Directions for future investigations need to include quantitative DA and 5-HT receptor PET/SPECT studies and both structural and functional investigations of circuits (rather than just regions) implicated in the pathology of mood disorders. These will include integrated cortical and subcortical studies of such circuits as the basotemporal–limbic loop.

REFERENCES

1. Ågren H, Reibring L, Hartvig P, et al. Low brain uptake of L-[11C]5-hydroxytryptophan in major depression: a positron emission tomography study on patients and healthy volunteers. *Acta Psychiatr Scand* 1991;83:449–455.
2. Altshuler LL, Conrad A, Hauser P, Li XM, Guze BH, Denikoff K. Reduction of temporal lobe volume in bipolar disorder: a prelimi-

nary report of magnetic resonance imaging. *Arch Gen Psychiatry* 1991;48:482–483.

3. Amsterdam JD, Mozley PD. Temporal lobe asymmetry with iofetamine (IMP) SPECT imaging in patients with major depression. *J Affect Disord* 1992;24:43–53.

4. Baxter L, Phelps M, Mazziotta J, et al. Cerebral metabolic rates for glucose in mood disorders. Studies with positron emission tomography and fluorodeoxyglucose F 18. *Arch Gen Psychiatry* 1985;42:441–447.

5. Baxter L, Schwartz J, Phelps M, et al. Reduction of prefrontal cortex glucose metabolism common to three types of depression. *Arch Gen Psychiatry* 1989;46:243–250.

6. Baxter LR. PET studies of cerebral function in major depression and obsessive-compulsive disorder. The emerging prefrontal cortex consensus. *Ann Clin Psychiatry* 1991;3:103–109.

7. Beats B, Levy R, Förstl H. Ventricular enlargement and caudate hyperdensity in elderly depressives. *Biol Psychiatry* 1991;30:452–458.

8. Bench CJ, Scott LC, Brown RG, Friston KJ, Frackowiak RSJ, Dolan RJ. Regional cerebral blood flow in depression determined by positron emission tomography. *J Cereb Blood Flow Metab* 1991;11(Suppl. 2):654.

9. Berman KF. Cortical "stress tests" in schizophrenia: regional cerebral blood flow studies. *Biol Psychiatry* 1987;22:1304–1326.

10. Bird J, Levy R, Jacoby R: Computed tomography in the elderly: changes over time in a normal population. *Br J Psychiatry* 1986;148:80–85.

11. Buchsbaum M, DeLisi L, Holcomb H, et al. Anteroposterior gradients in cerebral glucose use in schizophrenia and affective disorders. *Arch Gen Psychiatry* 1984;41:1159–1166.

12. Buchsbaum MS, Wu J, Delisi LE, et al. Frontal cortex and basal ganglia metabolic rates assessed by positron emission tomography with (18F)2-deoxyglucose in affective illness. *J Affect Disord* 1986;10:137–152.

13. Cala LA, Mastaglia FL. Computerized tomography in chronic alcoholics. *Alcoholism* 1981;5:283–294.

14. Coffey C, Figiel G, Djang W, Cress M, Saunders W, Weiner R. Leukoencephalopathy in elderly depressed patients referred for ECT. *Biol Psychiatry* 1988;24:143–161.

15. Coffey C, Wilkinson W, Weiner R, et al. Quantitative cerebral anatomy in depression. A controlled magnetic resonance imaging study. *Arch Gen Psychiatry* 1993;50:7–16.

16. Coffey CE, Figiel GS, Djang WT, Saunders WB, Weiner R. White matter hyperintensity on magnetic resonance imaging: clinical and neuroanatomic correlates in the depressed elderly. *J Neuropsychiatry Clin Neurosci* 1989;1:135–144.

17. Cohen RM, Semple WE, Gross M, et al. Evidence for common alterations in cerebral glucose metabolism in major affective disorders and schizophrenia. *Neuropsychopharmacology* 1989;2:241–254.

18. Cummings JL. The neuroanatomy of depression. *Psychiatr Times* 1993;37.

19. D'haenen H, Bossuyt A, Mertens J, Bossuyt-Piron C, Gijsemans M, Kaufman L. SPECT imaging of serotonin-2 receptors in depression. *Psychiatry Res* 1992;45:227–237.

20. Delvenne V, Delecluse F, Hubain PP, Schoutens A, De Maertelaer V, Mendlewicz J. Regional cerebral blood flow in patients with affective disorders. *Br J Psychiatry* 1990;157:359–365.

21. Depue R, Iacono W. Neurobehavioral aspects of major affective disorders. *Annu Rev Psychol* 1989;40:447–492.

22. Dewan MJ, Haldipur CV, Lane EE, Ispahani A, Boucher MF, Major LF. Bipolar affective disorder. I. Comprensive quantitative computed tomography. *Acta Psychiatr Scand* 1988;77:670–676.

23. Dhingra U, Rabins PV. Mania in the elderly: a 5–7 year follow-up. *J Am Geriatr Soc* 1991;39:581–583.

24. Dolan R, Calloway S, Mann A. Cerebral ventricular size in depressed subjects. *Psychol Med* 1985;15:873–878.

25. Dolan R, Calloway S, Thacker P, Mann A. The cerebral cortical appearance in depressed subjects. *Psychol Med* 1986;16:775–779.

26. Drevets W, Videen T, Price J, Preskorn S, Carmichael S, Raichle M. A functional anatomical study of unipolar depression. *J Neurosci* 1992;12:3628–3641.

27. Dupont RM, Jernigan TL, Butters N, et al. Subcortical abnormalities detected in bipolar affective disorder using magnetic resonance im-

aging: clinical and neuropsychological significance. *Arch Gen Psychiatry* 1990;47:55–59.

28. Dupont RM, Jernigan TL, Gillian JC, Butters N, Delise DC, Hesselink JR. Subcortical signal hyperintensities in bipolar patients detected by MRI. *Psychiatry Res* 1987;21:375–358.

29. Ebert D, Feistel H, Barocka A. Effects of sleep deprivation on the limbic system and the frontal lobes in affective disorders: a study with Tc-99m-HMPAO SPECT. *Psychiatry Res* 1991;40:247–251.

30. Fedoroff J, Starkstein S, Forrester A, et al. Depression in patients with acute traumatic brain injury. *Am J Psychiatry* 1992;149:918–923.

31. Figiel GS, Krishnan KR, Doraiswamy PM, Rao VP, Nemeroff CB, Boyko OB. Subcortical hyperintensities on brain magnetic resonance imaging: a comparison between late age onset and early onset elderly depressed subjects. *Neurobiol Aging* 1991;12:245–247.

32. Folstein SE, Chase GA, Wahl WE, McDonnell AM, Folstein MF. Huntington disease in Maryland: clinical aspects of racial variation. *Am J Hum Genet* 1987;41:168–179.

33. Harris GJ, Pearlson GD, Peyser CE, et al. Putamen volume reduction on magnetic resonance imaging exceeds caudate changes in mild Huntington's disease. *Ann Neurol* 1992;31:69–75.

34. Hauser P, Dauphinais ID, Berrettini W, Delisi LE, Gelernter J, Post RM. Corpus callosum dimensions measured by magnetic resonance imaging in bipolar affective disorder and schizophrenia. *Biol Psychiatry* 1989;26:659–668.

35. Hershey LA, Modic MT, Greenough PG, Jaffe DF. Magnetic resonance imaging in vascular dementia. *Neurology* 1987;37:29–36.

36. Hurwitz TA, Clark C, Murphy E, Klonoff H, Martin WR, Pate BD. Regional cerebral glucose metabolism in major depressive disorder. *Can J Psychiatry* 1990;35:684–688.

37. Husain M, McDonald W, Doraiswamy P, et al. A magnetic resonance imaging study of putamen nuclei in major depression. *Psychiatry Res* 1991;40:95–99.

38. Jacoby RJ, Levy R. Computed tomography in the elderly. 3: Affective disorder. *Br J Psychiatry* 1980;136:270–275.

39. Jeste DV, Lohr JB, Goodwin FK. Neuroanatomical studies of major affective disorders. A review and suggestions for further research. *Br J Psychiatry* 1988;153:444–459.

40. Johnstone EC, Owens DG, Crow TJ, et al. Temporal lobe structure as determined by nuclear magnetic resonance in schizophrenia and bipolar affective disorder. *J Neurol Neurosurg Psychiatry* 1989;52:736–741.

41. Kellner C, Rubinow D, Gold P, Post R. Relationship of cortisol hypersecretion to brain CT scan alterations in depressed patients. *Psychiatry Res* 1983;8:191–197.

42. Kling A, Metter E, Riege W, Kuhl D. Comparison of PET measurement of local brain glucose metabolism and CAT measurement of brain atrophy in chronic schizophrenia and depression. *Am J Psychiatry* 1986;143:175–180.

43. Krishnan K, Doraiswamy P, Figiel G, et al. Hippocampal abnormalities in depression. *J Neuropsychiatry Clin Neurosci* 1991;3:387–391.

44. Krishnan K, McDonald W, Escalona P, et al. Magnetic resonance imaging of the caudate nuclei in depression. Preliminary observations. *Arch Gen Psychiatry* 1992;49:553–557.

45. Kupfer DJ, Rush AJ. Recommendations for scientific reports on depression. *Am J Psychiatry* 1983;140:1327–1328.

46. Lewine R, Risch S, Risby E, et al. Lateral ventricle-brain ratio and balance between CSF HVA and 5-HIAA in schizophrenia. *Am J Psychiatry* 1991;148:1189–1194.

47. Martinot J, Hardy P, Feline A, et al. Left prefrontal glucose hypometabolism in the depressed state: a confirmation. *Am J Psychiatry* 1990;147:1313–1317.

48. Mayberg H, Robinson R, Wong D, et al. PET imaging of cortical S2 serotonin receptors after stroke: lateralized changes and relationship to depression. *Am J Psychiatry* 1988;145:937–943.

49. Mayberg HS. Neuroimaging studies of depression in neurologic disease. In: Starkstein SE, Robinson RG, eds. *Depression in neurologic disease.* Baltimore: Johns Hopkins University Press; 1993.

50. Mayberg HS, Starkstein SE, Sadzot B, et al. Selective hypometabolism in the inferior frontal lobe in depressed patients with Parkinson's disease. *Ann Neurol* 1990;28:57–64.

51. Nasrallah H, McCalley-Whitters M, Jacoby C. Cerebral ventricular

enlargement in young manic males. A controlled CT study. *J Affect Disord* 1982;4:15–19.

52. Nasrallah H, McCalley-Whitters M, Jacoby C. Cortical atrophy in schizophrenia and mania: a comparative CT study. *J Clin Psychiatry* 1982;43:439–441.

53. Nasrallah HA, Coffman JA, Olson SC. Structural brain-imaging findings in affective disorders: an overview. *J Neuropsychiatry Clin Neurosci* 1989;1:21–26.

54. Pearlson G, Rabins P, Burns A. Centrum semiovale white matter CT changes associated with normal ageing, Alzheimer's disease and late life depression with and without reversible dementia. *Psychol Med* 1991;21:31–328.

55. Pearlson GD, Garbacz DJ, Tompkins RH. Clinical correlates of lateral ventricular enlargement in bipolar affective disorder. *Am J Psychiatry* 1984;141:253–256.

56. Pearlson GD, Rabins PV, Kim WS, Speedie LJ, Mobers PJ, Bascom MJ, Burns A. Structural brain CT changes and cognitive deficits in elderly depressives with and without reversible dementia ('pseudodementia'). *Psychol Med* 1989;19:573–584.

57. Pearlson GD, Ross C, Wong DF, Links J, Dannals R, Tune LE. Increased PET DA D2 receptors across psychoses. In: A. P. Associon, ed. Presented at 142nd Annual Meeting of the American Psychiatric Association. San Francisco, CA; 1989:

58. Pearlson GD, Veroff AE. Computerised tomographic scan changes in manic-depressive illness. *Lancet* 1981;2:440.

59. Rabins P, Pearlson G, Aylward E, Kumar A, Dowell K. Cortical magnetic resonance imaging changes in elderly inpatients with major depression. *Am J Psychiatry* 1991;148:617–620.

60. Rieder RO, Mann LS, Weinberger DR, van Kammen DP, Post RM. Computed tomographic scans in patients with schizophrenia, schizoaffective, and bipolar affective disorder. *Arch Gen Psychiatry* 1983;40:735–739.

61. Rosenberg R, Vostrup S, Andersen A, Bolwig T. Effect of ECT on cerebral blood flow in melancholia assessed with SPECT. *Convulsive Ther* 1988;4:62–73.

62. Roy-Byrne P, Post R, Kellner C, Joffe R, Uhde T. Ventricular-brain ratio and life course of illness in patients with affective disorder. *Psychiatry Res* 1988;23:277–284.

63. Saccetti E, Vita A, Conte G. Brain morphology in major affective disorders: clinical and biological correlates. Milan, 1987.

64. Sackeim HA, Prohovnik I. Brain imaging studies of depressive disorders. In: Mann JJ, Kupfer D, eds. *The biology of depressive illness*. New York: Plenum Press; 1993.

65. Sackeim HA, Prudic J, Devanand DP, Decina P, Kerr B, Malitz S. The impact of medication resistance and continuation pharmacotherapy on relapse following electroconvulsive therapy in major depression. *J Clin Psychopharmacol* 1990;10:96–104.

66. Schlegel S, Kretzschmar K. Computed tomography in affective disorders. Part II. Brain density. *Biol Psychiatry* 1987;1:15–23.

67. Schlegel S, von Bardeleben U, Wiedemann K, Frommberger U, Holsboer F. Computerized brain tomography measures compared with spontaneous and suppressed plasma cortisol levels in major depression. *Psychoneuroendocrinology* 1989;14:209–216.

68. Shima S, Shikano T, Kitamura T, et al. Depression and ventricular enlargement. *Acta Psychiatr Scand* 1984;70:275–277.

69. Starkstein SE, Robinson RG. Affective disorders and cerebral vascular disease. *Br J Psychiatry* 1989;154:170–182.

70. Starkstein SE, Robinson RG, Berthier ML, Parikh RM, Price TR. Differential mood changes following basal ganglia vs. thalamic lesions. *Arch Neurol* 1988;45:725–730.

71. Stern RA, Bachmann DL. Depressive symptoms following stroke. *Am J Psychiatry* 1991;148:351–356.

72. Suhara T, Nakayama K, Inoue O, et al. D1 Dopamine receptor binding in mood disorders measured by positron emission tomography. *Psychopharmacology* 1992;106:14–18.

73. Swerdlow NR, Koob GF. Dopamine, schizophrenia, mania and depression: toward a unified hypothesis of cortico–striato–pallido–thalamic function. *Behav Brain Sci* 1987;10:197–245.

74. Tanaka Y, Hazama H, Fukuhara T, Tsutsui T. Computerized tomography of the brain in manic-depressive patients—a controlled study. *Fol Psychiatr Neurol Jpn* 1982;36:137–143.

75. Targum S, Rosen L, DeLisi L, Weinberger D, Citrin C. Cerebral ventricular size in major depressive disorder: association with delusional symptoms. *Biol Psychiatry* 1983;18:329–336.

76. Vita A, Sacchetti E, Cazzullo CL. A CT scan follow-up study of cerebral ventricular size in schizophrenia and major affective disorder. *Schizophr Res* 1988;1:165–166.

77. Weinberger D, DeLisi L, Perman G, Targum S, Wyatt R. Computed tomography in schizophreniform disorder and other acute psychiatric disorders. *Arch Gen Psychiatry* 1982;39:778–783.

78. Winokur G. The development and validity of familial subtypes in primary unipolar depression. *Pharmacopsychiatry* 1982;15:142–146.

79. Wu J, Gillin J, Buchsbaum M, Hershey T, Johnson J, Bunney WE Jr. Effect of sleep deprivation on brain metabolism of depressed patients. *Am J Psychiatry* 1992;149:538–543.

Psychopharmacology: The Fourth Generation of Progress, edited by Floyd E. Bloom and David J. Kupfer. Raven Press, Ltd., New York © 1995.

CHAPTER **88**

Mood Disorders Linked to the Reproductive Cycle in Women

Barbara L. Parry

In both medicine and psychiatry, there are gender-differentiated predispositions to certain illnesses. For example, men are at greater risk for developing cardiovascular disorders, alcoholism, and sociopathy, whereas women have a greater lifetime risk for thyroid disease, eating disorders, late-in-life schizophrenia, and depression (35,63). Sex differences in the prevalence of depression begin to appear after puberty and are maintained throughout the reproductive years (82). More recent evidence indicates that major depressive disorders are increasing with time, that the age of onset is becoming earlier, and that women continue to show an increased incidence of the disorder. Furthermore, female offspring of depressed patients have earlier onsets of depressive disorders (81).

WOMEN AND DEPRESSION

Women, as compared with men, have a greater lifetime risk for depression. They predominate with respect to unipolar depression (83), the depressive subtype of bipolar illness, and cyclical forms of affective illness such as rapid-cycling manic–depressive illness and seasonal affective disorder. In addition, events associated with the reproductive cycle are capable of provoking affective changes in predisposed individuals. Examples include depression associated with oral contraceptives (53), the luteal phase of the menstrual cycle (14), the postpartum period, and menopause. The fluctuation of gonadal steroids during specific phases of the reproductive cycle may bear some relationship to the particular vulnerability of women for affective changes. The reproductive hormones could exert their effects on mood directly or indirectly by their effect on neurotransmitter, neuroendocrine, or circadian systems, all of which have been implicated in the pathogenesis of affective illness.

Rapid-cycling Affective Illness

Several clinical models can be used to examine the role of reproductive hormones on affective illness in women. As most patients with rapid cycling manic-depressive illness are women, reviewing the factors that predispose women to the development of rapid cycles of mood may shed light on how reproductive hormones may influence the course of affective illness.

Rapid-cycling manic-depressive illness, defined as four or more affective episodes a year, predominates in women. Kraepelin (37), in describing patients with regular, daily fluctuations of periodic excitement noted "in contrast to other forms, in which there was a preponderance of men, two thirds of these patients were women in whom the periodicity of sexual life obviously favors this kind of development." In Kukopulos' (38) sample of rapid cyclers, 70% were women. In contrast, in the non-rapid cyclers, women represented 47% of the sample. Cowdry et al. (12) reported that women represented 83% of rapid cycling bipolar patients and 53% of nonrapid cyclers. A review by Wehr et al. (78) indicated that 92% of patients with rapid cycling and 64% with nonrapid cycling affective disorder were women.

Women's Risk Factors for Rapid-cycling Affective Illness

In addition to being a woman, two other factors appear to be associated with the rapid-cycling form of bipolar illness: (a) treatment with tricyclic and other antidepressants, and (b) hypothyroidism. Women, compared with

B. L. Parry: Department of Psychiatry, University of California at San Diego, La Jolla, California 92093.

men, show an increased incidence of both drug-induced rapid cycling and hypothyroidism (78).

Drug-induced Rapid Cycling

Of those patients whose rapid cycles of mania and depression have been induced by tricyclics, women predominate. Wehr and Goodwin (76) found that five patients, in whom rapid cycles developed, represented all but one of the bipolar women who had been maintained on antidepressant drugs. Rapid cycles did not develop in either of two bipolar male patients who were maintained on tricyclics. Wehr and Goodwin speculated that the female reproductive neuroendocrine axis, a generator of physiological rapid cycles, may have been instrumental in the expression of drug-induced cycling. Reproductive hormonal disturbances and treatments may have been predisposing factors in their patients' illnesses; all but one (four of five) of the women in their sample had irregular menses, amenorrhea, history of estrogen or progesterone treatment, or onset of the illness in the postpartum period.

In Kukopulos' (38) longitudinal study of the patients who developed rapid cycles after tricyclics, 70% were women. According to Kukopulos, "female sex, middle age, and menopause, along with anti-depressant drugs, contributed to the establishment of rapid cyclicity." Of the patients in his longitudinal study whose course of illness changed to rapid cycling, 87% were women, and in a third (25 of 77) of these women, the change in course coincided with menopause. Kukopulos also noted that the patients with depression and hypomania (bipolar II) were those most prone to rapid cycling.

Wehr and Goodwin (76) concluded that women have a higher risk of drug-induced mania and drug-induced rapid cycling than do men. In contrast, Kupfer et al. (39) report that women with recurrent depression are not more likely to switch into hypomania than men and Coryell et al. (11) deemphasize the effects of drug-induced rapid cycling.

Hypothyroidism and Rapid Cycling

In addition to female gender and antidepressant drugs, thyroid impairment may be associated with rapid cycling (12,78), and women are prone to thyroid disease. Studies that document sex differences indicate that almost all patients on lithium who develop hypothyroidism are female. In studies by Transbol et al. (73) and Cho et al. (9), 90% to 100% of bipolar patients with lithium-induced hypothyroidism were women.

As shown by Cowdry et al. (12), abnormalities of the thyroid axis, some of which may become apparent only during treatment with $LiCO_3$, are associated with rapid cycling. In a mood disorder clinic population, Cho et al. (9) found postlithium thyroid medication use was significantly higher among rapid-cycling women (32.2%) than

nonrapid cycling women (2.1%). Furthermore, thyroid dysfunction was primarily limited to women. Of those patients taking thyroid medication in addition to lithium, 92% were women. Five out of seven women with hypothyroidism had rapid cycling.

In a study by Cowdry et al. (12), overt hypothyroidism was found in 12 (51%) of 24 rapid-cycling patients and in none of the nonrapid cycling patients. Elevated TSH levels were present (and higher) in 92% of the rapid-cycling group as compared with 32% of the nonrapid cycling group. In this sample, women represented 83% of the rapid-cycling group and 53% of the nonrapid cyclers. In a study by Wehr et al. (78), 47% of women with rapid-cycling and 39% of women with nonrapid-cycling bipolar illness developed thyroid disease. Of those patients with thyroid disease, the thyroid disease emerged after the onset of affective illness in 90% of the patients and in the majority of cases it emerged during lithium treatment.

Transbol et al. (73) evaluated the prevalence of hypothyroidism in lithium-treated manic–depressive outpatients and found elevated TSH levels in 25% of the patients. Of these patients, 95% were women over 40 years of age. None of the men had elevated TSH levels. Rapid-cycling and nonrapid-cycling subgroups were not reported separately.

Reproductive status may affect the appearance of thyroid disease. There is a common appearance of goiter during puberty, pregnancy, and menopause. Women are particularly prone to develop hypothyroidism during the postpartum period (2). This type of hypothyroidism may represent an autoimmune phenomenon, as the extent of postpartum hypothyroidism correlates with traces of microsomal antibodies early in pregnancy (30). Women with isolated gonadotropin deficiency have blunted basal TSH, and TSH responses to TRH (71). Administration of estrogen restores the TSH response to that of normal controls, and cessation of estrogen treatment reduces the amount of releasable TSH. In hypogonadal men, TSH response to TRH is similar to normal men but increases with estrogen treatment. Oral contraceptives increase the TSH response to TRH (59). Thus, estrogens seem to be required to maintain, and may enhance, the normal TSH response to TRH in the female.

In summary, cyclic mood disorder in the form of rapid-cycling manic–depressive illness is more prevalent in women. Treatment with antidepressant drugs often precipates rapid mood cycles, particularly in women with bipolar II illness. Thyroid impairment, more prevalent in women, also is associated with the rapid cycling form of the illness. There is very little information available on the course of rapid cycling bipolar illness in men.

Clinical Psychopharmacological Treatment

Thyroid Treatment

Thyroid hormone has been used to treat both cyclic and noncyclic forms of mood disorders. Hypermetabolic thyroid treatment was first used by Gjessing in the 1930s to treat periodic catatonia and rapid-cycling mood disorder. Stancer and Persad (72) reported treatment of intractable rapid-cycling manic–depressive illness with levothyroxine. Five of the seven women, who developed rapid-cycling bipolar disorder with an onset during the postpartum or involutional period, responded to hypermetabolic doses of thyroid hormone. The effect of thyroid hormone had different effects in men and women: The treatment was unsuccessful in two men and one adolescent girl.

Prange et al. (56) reported triiodothyronine (T_3) enhanced the antidepressant effect of imipramine in women but not in men. Men responded to initial doses of imipramine in a shorter period of time than women. Women treated with imipramine and thyroid supplement responded as rapidly as men treated with imipramine alone. Later, Goodwin et al. (23) demonstrated that, among tricyclic nonresponders, men benefited from the addition of T_3 as often as women.

The mechanisms for thyroid enhancement of responses to antidepressants may be, as Whybrow and Prange (86) suggest, related to the capacity of thyroid hormone to alter the ratio of α- to β-2 adrenergic receptors and their sensitivity to noradrenergic neurotransmitters. Depressed women appear to be uniquely responsive to thyroid hormone. Women also are uniquely vulnerable to thyroid impairment.

Estrogen

Women also are sensitive to other hormonal treatments. Estrogen also has been used as a treatment in refractory depression. Klaiber et al. (36) used 5 to 25 mg of oral conjugated estrogen in cyclic doses to treat pre- and postmenopausal women. With estrogen, as compared with placebo, there was a significant drop in Hamilton scores, which correlated with reduction in previously elevated monoamine oxidase (MAO) levels. With inconsistent results, Prange (56) gave 25 and 50 mg estradiol to depressed patients already treated with imipramine. The higher estrogen dose was toxic. The lower dose was associated with reduction of Hamilton scores and improved sleep.

The mechanism by which estrogen exerts its possible antidepressant effect is unknown, but work by Kendall et al. (33) showed that estrogen is needed for reduction of serotonin receptor binding during imipramine treatment. Ovariectomy blocked the effect of imipramine on serotonin receptors, and estrogen treatment reinstituted it.

Estrogen may also induce rapid cycling or at least predispose to tricyclic-induced rapid cycling as reported by Oppenheim (46). Interestingly, we observed one male rapid-cycling patient who had low testosterone secondary to mumps orchitis. Progesterone, on the other hand, may suppress rapid cycles of mood (28).

Seasonal Affective Disorder

Like rapid-cycling mood disorder, seasonal affective disorder (SAD) is a cyclic mood disorder that occurs predominantly in women (80%). Thus, it also may serve as a model to understand the contribution of reproductive hormones to affective illness in women.

Patients with SAD who have recurrent winter depressions, have symptoms of major mood disorder with characteristic atypical features (such as hyperphagia, hypersomnia, and lethargy), which begin to develop each year in association with shortening of the daylength. A majority of these patients respond to high-intensity (2500 lux) light treatments, which artificially extend the daily photoperiod. Initially, bright light was thought to act in seasonal depression by suppressing melatonin, a hormone that is centrally involved in seasonal reproductive cycles in animals. This hypothesis since has been brought into question and a multitude of other hypotheses have been proposed (64,77).

A large proportion (70%) of women with SAD also have mood changes in association with the menstrual cycle. Some women with SAD report improvement in their premenstrual symptoms with light therapy. We identified a woman with a family history of bipolar illness who developed severe premenstrual depression with suicidal ideation only during the fall and winter and was relieved of premenstrual symptoms during the spring and summer (52). We found that light was an effective treatment for this patient with seasonal PMS and that its therapeutic effect could be blocked by the simultaneous administration of melatonin. Light also increased this patient's TSH. Propranolol and atenolol, beta blockers that inhibit the synthesis of melatonin, had a therapeutic effect similar to light. Light therapy also may benefit women with nonseasonal premenstrual syndrome (49,51).

In patients with SAD who have summer depression and winter hypomania, Wehr et al. (79) reported that 8 of 12 patients were women and suggested that temperature may influence these patients' clinical state.

It appears that certain women with genetic vulnerability for mood disorders may be at risk for developing other cyclic mood disorders, such as seasonal premenstrual disorders.

Applications of Rapid Cycling and Seasonal Affective Disorder to Postpartum and Premenstrual Affective Illness

Rapid-cycling bipolar illness and SAD are examples of cyclic forms of mood disorders that predominate in women. The interaction of reproductive hormones, particularly with thyroid hormones in rapid-cycling mood disorder and with melatonin in SAD, may provide clues to the pathogenesis of reproductive-related depressions. The increased incidence of hypothyroidism occurring postpartum (2) or in winter may in part account for rapidly cycling mood disorders and depression that may occur at these times, respectively. Another cyclic mood disorder that can be viewed as a form of rapid cycling is recurrent premenstrual depression, in which thyroid and melatonin disturbances also have been implicated (48,52). Melatonin may play a role not only in the pathogenesis of seasonal premenstrual syndrome (52) but also in nonseasonal forms of this disorder (48). Recent studies demonstrate that patients with premenstrual depression have circadian disturbances of melatonin secretion compared with normal controls and may respond to light treatment (48,49, 51). Similar studies of melatonin in postpartum mood disturbances are currently underway.

Postpartum Mood Disorders

The relative risk for developing a major psychiatric illness or psychosis requiring hospitalization is highest during the postpartum period and the lowest during pregnancy (34). First episodes of manic–depressive illness in women often have their onset in the postpartum period (20,60). Reich and Winokur (60) observed that not only is there a special risk for female manic–depressive patients to develop mania or depression in the postpartum period, but having a postpartum affective episode appears to predispose to subsequent postpartum affective episodes (an increased risk of 50%). Furthermore, a woman's initial risk for a postpartum psychosis is 1 in 500 (34). Once a woman has had a postpartum psychosis, her risk for psychosis following a subsequent pregnancy is 1 in 3 (34). Thus, in postpartum depression and psychosis, a previous episode sensitizes a woman to the development of future episodes with subsequent pregnancies.

Clinical Psychopharmacological Treatment

Before discussing specific treatment modalities, it needs to be emphasized that at this early stage of recognition of postpartum psychiatric syndromes by American psychiatry, a rational treatment plan for postpartum depression and psychosis cannot be developed from double-blind, placebo-controlled crossover trials of pharmacological or psychotherapeutic interventions. Because these illnesses can be so devastating to the individual and her family, treatment approaches have utilized whatever interventions have been immediately useful and available. In the literature, the majority of the scientifically rigorous treatment studies are confined to studies that utilize patients with maternity blues, that is, those individuals without severe disorders, as their study subjects. Therefore, by necessity, suggested treatment approaches discussed in this chapter reflect clinical experience more than information derived from research investigations.

There are several important principles in treating postpartum depression and psychoses. The first principle is that organic illnesses must be ruled out. An initial presentation of postpartum psychiatric illness may be caused by an underlying Sheehan's syndrome, thyrotoxicosis (if presenting as an acute psychosis in the first month after delivery), or as hypothyrodism (if presenting as major depression in the 4th to 5th month postpartum). All too often these medical emergencies are overlooked with disastrous consequences. Thus, one of the first crucial steps in the evaluation and treatment of postpartum disorders, as in other medical and psychiatric disorders, is a thorough history with a complete physical and laboratory examination.

The other important principle guiding treatment is that the earlier the symptoms are recognized and treated, the better the outcome. For example, postpartum psychosis may initially present with symptoms of depersonalization: the patient may feel distant from her child and from the situation at hand. She may feel as though she is just an onlooker (as portrayed in the film *Rosemary's Baby*). This phenomenon may be interpreted as a failure to bond but more likely represents the initial presentation of an emerging psychosis. Patients then may develop strange and bizarre sensations described as though their, or that of their child's head, is separate from their body. If treatment is instituted with small doses of an antipsychotic medication, these symptoms may resolve within a few days to a week. However, if not recognized and treated in its initial stages these symptoms may rapidly progress to paranoid delusions and a frank agitated psychosis, which may become more severe, more refractory to treatment, and more likely to recur over the next 6 months to a year. Without aggressive management and early detection, the symptoms may extend into the second and third year postpartum.

It also must be stressed that because of the changing nature of postpartum psychiatric illness, different treatments at different stages of the illness are indicated. For example, an early presentation of psychosis would best be treated with neuroleptic medication. However, this psychosis may resolve and the patient may develop symptoms of major depression later in the course of the illness that may require antidepressant medication. Furthermore, the initial presentation of the depression may appear in an agitated form with many anxious features and insomnia. Thus treatment with a more sedative antidepressant (e.g., imipramine, nortriptyline) would be indicated, whereas later the patient may present with symptoms of a retarded, anergic depression sometimes with obsessive–compulsive features in which a more activating compound (e.g., desimipramine, fluoxetine) may be indicated. As Post (55) suggests in the treatment of affective illness and psychosis, different treatment modalities may have different effects and efficacies depending upon when in the course of the illness these treatments are administered.

Specific issues related to the treatment of first postpartum psychosis and then postpartum depression are discussed below.

Postpartum Psychoses

One of the most important aspects of management of the postpartum psychoses are that the earlier they are recognized and treated, the more likely they are to respond to treatment and be associated with a more positive outcome and prognosis. Most postpartum psychoses have an acute onset within the first 2 weeks postpartum (generally not until after the 3rd day postpartum) and 80% of them occur within 1 month postpartum; therefore, clinicians should be on the alert for early signs of depersonalization, delusional thinking, mania, or bizarre behavior. Women with a previous history of postpartum psychiatric illness or affective illness are at particularly high risk. The clinician should have a low threshold for hospitalization in any patient with symptoms of an impending postpartum psychosis. Early hospitalization can prevent infanticide or suicide that may occur when mothers at risk are left at home alone to care for their infants, a frequent occurrence in modern culture. Often small (2 to 5 mg) doses of neuroleptics such as haloperidol (or if it contributes to extrapyramidal symptoms, perphenazine or loxapine) may decrease the symptomatology and prevent the development of a more severe psychosis. Neuroleptic medication also is efficacious in treating the symptoms of a postpartum psychotic depression (see below) without incurring the risks of tricyclic antidepressants. In the potentially hypothyroid postpartum state, antidepressants may induce rapid cycling and are not recommended in breast-feeding women. Risk factors for antidepressant-induced rapid cycling include being female, being in the postpartum state, and being hypothyroid. If the symptoms of an emerging postpartum psychosis are recognized and treated early, they may resolve within a week. Cases in which the symptoms are not recognized and treated in their initial stages may become refractory to treatment and take much longer to resolve. In general, however, the postpartum psychoses have a good prognosis, resolve in 2 to 3 weeks, and are amenable to treatment. Unfortunately postpartum psychosis is the condition under which women are most likely to commit infanticide. Of those women with postpartum psychoses, 4% may commit infanticide (20). This consequence generally does not occur unless the patient is psychotic. The tragedy of this occurrence is made all the more poignant by the recognition that this disorder is otherwise so amenable to treatment and thereby preventable.

Although dosages of neuroleptics can be reduced after the initial episode of psychosis is resolved, this process should be done gradually and cautiously. Women remain at risk for recurrences, particularly those women with a previous history of psychiatric illness, for at least 6 months, and often up to 12 months postpartum. Data from a large-scale epidemiological study in Edinburgh (34) suggested that there is an increased risk for psychiatric admissions for up to 2 years postpartum. Although it is not necessary to leave a patient on neuroleptic medication for this length of time, it is wise for the clinician to be on the alert for early signs of recurrence and to bear in mind that a patient who initially presents with symptoms of a postpartum psychosis within the first few weeks after delivery may develop symptoms of a postpartum depression later in the course of her illness (i.e., 4 to 5 months postpartum). For an early onset of psychoses, patients should probably remain on neuroleptics for at least six weeks postpartum. Neuroleptics are not contraindicated with breast-feeding.

As in other psychiatric illnesses, psychopharmacological intervention is most effective when combined with psychotherapeutic interventions. Particularly with regard to postpartum psychoses, pharmacological intervention is urgent to prevent the mother from becoming increasingly psychotic and potentially committing infanticide. At this point the patient cannot be cognitively and emotionally available to participate in a psychotherapeutic interaction until the medications help to reduce the hallucinations, delusions, and agitated behavior. However, as most clinicians and even psychotic patients appreciate, medications are most likely to be received and taken willingly when some sense of rapport, trust, and support is perceived by the patient and her family as coming from the physician.

Postpartum Depression

In contrast to postpartum psychosis in which there is an acute onset occurring early in the postpartum period, postpartum depression generally has a more insidious onset that occurs later, usually 4 to 5 months postpartum. Its severity may range from mild to moderate dysthymia and anxiety disorders to major melancholia. As with the postpartum psychoses, organic abnormalities need to be ruled out, particularly hypothyroidism, which occurs in 10% of women postpartum and has a peak incidence at 4 to 5 months postpartum (30). Transient hyperthyroidism may actually appear earlier in the postpartum course. Indications for the use of antidepressant medication are similar to those for other affective illnesses, and include the presence of neurovegetative signs. It is necessary to bear in mind that during the course of affective illness over time, and that of postpartum illness being no exception, untreated episodes tend to become more severe, more frequent, and often more refractory to treatment. These depressive episodes should be treated aggressively with both pharmacological and psychotherapeutic strategies early in the course to prevent untoward biological and psychological consequences. Since many of the depressions appear with obsessive–compulsive features, implicating serotonergic mechanisms, recent clinical experience suggests the efficacy of the serotonergic antidepressants, such as fluoxetine, sertraline, and paroxetine. However, side effects particularly of agitation from fluoxetine need to be monitored closely, and this drug should not be the first line of treatment in the anxious depressions often seen early in the postpartum state. For patients who present with symptoms of more agitated and anxious depressions, more sedative antidepressants such as imipramine or nortriptyline would be more appropriate. If agitated depressive symptoms occur early in the postpartum state, small doses of neuroleptics can be beneficial. Anxiolytics are best avoided because of their risk for the development of physiological dependence, withdrawal, paradoxical exacerbation of agitation, and their inadvisability of use in breast-feeding women. It also is best with the use of antidepressant medication to advise the cessation of breast-feeding, as some studies indicate that small amounts may be excreted into the breast milk. However, if the mother is reluctant to give up breast-feeding, and her depressive symptoms are severe enough to warrant pharmacological treatment, experience suggests that antidepressants such as nortriptyline or desimpramine are beneficial without long-term serious consequences. The clinician is advised if administering antidepressant drugs to a postpartum patient, to rule out hypothyroidism, to follow closely the course and timing of the mood changes of the patient, and to discontinue antidepressant medication if there is evidence of drug-induced rapid cycling. Recently, estrogen skin patches have been reported to be beneficial in severe postpartum depression. For postpartum dysphoria, Dalton (15) has recommended progesterone treatment (100 mg im for the first week postpartum and then 400 mg bid by suppository for two or more months postpartum). However, some clinicians and investigators find that progesterone may actually exacerbate depression. For severe or psychotic postpartum depression or mania refractory to pharmacotherapy, electroconvulsive therapy (ECT) remains the treatment of choice. Sleep deprivation has therapeutic efficacy in a majority of patients with major depressive disorders. The efficacy of sleep deprivation in postpartum nonpsychotic depression currently is under experimental investigation (Parry et al., *unpublished*). The relapse that may occur with recovery sleep after postpartum sleep deprivation potentially may be averted with lithium, in non-breast-feeding women.

Since the experience of a postpartum depression or psychosis can be very disruptive cognitively and emotionally for the woman and her family, these disorders, like other psychiatric disorders, are best treated with a combination of pharmacological and psychotherapeutic management with the aim of providing education, support, and cognitive structuring whereby these patients and their families can attempt to gain "some method out of the madness" to cope with this very confusing, disorienting, and emotionally traumatic cataclysm in their lives.

Anthropological studies indicate that other cultures have rituals allowing for 40-day rest periods for the mother after the birth of a baby in which the mother is mothered. During this time period, the focus is on allowing the mother time to rest, recuperate, eat, and sleep. Female relatives come to the home to prepare meals, do housework, and care for the infant. Thus, social support, education, child care services, and social recognition of the new motherhood status is ensured. Previously, a week hospital stay for the mother after delivery was required. Now, in modern cultures, the mother usually goes home a day after delivery, and often without extended family or neighbors to help with infant care. This isolated environment does not provide the supportive therapeutic care that would otherwise mitigate against the development or exacerbation of the spectrum of nonpsychotic depressions.

Maternity Blues

The maternity blues is not considered a disorder, because it occurs in 50 to 80% of women and because of the absence of major symptomatology. It is best treated with reassurance that the symptoms occur in a majority of women, and that they generally improve spontaneously within a week to 10 days. The fact that, in rare instances, the symptoms may progress to a more severe postpartum disorder stresses the necessity of making frequent follow-up visits. However, this progression is the exception rather than the rule. In contrast to postpartum psychosis, pharmacological intervention generally is not warranted for the maternity blues. Instead, psychotherapeutic intervention in the form of education, support, and reassurance has more import.

Prophylaxis

Given that there is a high recurrence rate for both postpartum psychosis (initial risk 1/500; subsequent risk 1/3) and postpartum depression (initial risk 1/10; subsequent risk 1/2), prophylactic treatment for women, particularly for those who have a previous history of affective illness, is an integral part of the management of these disorders. Patients with a previous history of nonpuerperal affective illness are three times more likely to develop postpartum mood disorders, particularly mania. Thus, one of the most effective prophylactic interventions in this group is lithium. Although lithium dosage should be halved about 1 week before delivery because of marked fluid and electrolyte changes occurring then, it can be restarted shortly thereafter. However, lithium, in contrast to neuroleptic medication, is contraindicated in breast-feeding women. Clinicians particularly should be on alert for lithium-induced hypothyroidism in postpartum women, because 90% of patients who develop hypothyroidism on lithium are women (9) and the postpartum period presents a particular risk factor for the development of hypothyroidism (2). Furthermore, postpartum hypothyroidism can induce rapid mood cycling.

Patients with a previous history of mood disorders may have an exacerbation of their illness during pregnancy. Although lithium is contraindicated during the first trimester because of the infant's risk for Ebsteins anomaly of the heart, in severe cases lithium may be administered cautiously, checking particularly for fluid and electrolyte changes, during the third trimester. For mania occurring during pregnancy, neuroleptics or ECT can be given without undue risk to the fetus.

Another prophylactic treatment that has received attention, but is still controversial, is progesterone (100 im after labor, daily for 7 days, then progesterone suppositories for 2 months or until the return of menstruation) (15). Since progesterone is essentially an anesthetic in animals, its use in humans is probably more effective for the agitated rather than the depressive symptomatology of postpartum psychiatric syndromes. It also may exacerbate depressive symptomatology.

Additional information contributes to the hypothesis that postpartum illnesses are unique and organic in etiology. There has been successful use of three different substances for prophylaxis in high-risk patients, that is, those patients who have had previous postpartum psychosis or depression. Administration of long-acting parenteral estrogen or progesterone has seemed to ward off recurrences.

In summary, the severity and recurrence of postpartum psychiatric disorders deserve early, aggressive, and innovative treatment approaches. Their presentation is often episodic and fluctuating, with different presentations of symptoms being more related to different stages of the illness than to different categories of the illness. Treatment requires longitudinal follow-up care. Because postpartum psychiatric disorders appear to exhibit a pattern consistent with a model of kindling and behavioral sensitization (as opposed to a model of tolerance), it is crucial in treatment strategies to interrupt this cycle using early and aggressive treatment and prophylactic management whether it is by ECT, lithium, hormonal, or chronobiological interventions such as sleep deprivation or phototherapy.

Premenstrual Depression

One clinical model for studying the relationship of gonadal hormones to affective illness is the affective changes associated with the menstrual cycle. Historically referred to as premenstrual syndrome (PMS), this condition has been more rigorously defined as late luteal phase dysphoric disorder (LLPDD) in the DSM-III-R and as premenstrual dysphoric disorder (PMDD) in the DSM-IV under mood disorders. For purposes of familiarity, the term PMS will be used in this chapter. In PMS, the mood and behavioral changes are recurrent and predictable and thus can be studied prospectively and longitudinally. Similar to winter in SAD and the postpartum period in affective illness, the late luteal phase of the menstrual cycle is a vulnerable time for the development of depressive mood changes. Studies indicate that PMS may be related

to major depressive disorders. In support of this hypothesis, patients with PMS and mood disorders, in contrast to patients with anxiety disorders (65), respond to sleep deprivation: Total and late-night partial sleep deprivation temporarily alleviate symptoms in a majority of patients with major mood disorders (67). We found that 80% of patients with premenstrual depression responded to a night of total sleep deprivation and that late-night partial sleep deprivation (in the second half of the night) was more effective than early-night partial sleep deprivation (in the first half of the night) (54). In a follow-up study, PMS subjects responded equally well to both early- and late-night partial sleep deprivations, but only after a night of recovery sleep (Parry et al., *unpublished data*). Sleep deprivation lowers prolactin (47) and increases TSH (68), although at least in one of the studies (32) these hormonal changes did not correlate with clinical response. An effective intervention with total or partial sleep deprivation in patients with PMS would be consistent with current theories that implicate prolactin and thyroid disturbances in the pathogenesis of PMS. Sleep reduction may also serve as a final common pathway in the genesis of mania in postpartum psychiatric illness (80). Thus, the interaction of sleep with a sensitive circadian phase of thyroid or prolactin secretion may be a common predisposing factor for the development of affective illness, premenstrual depression, and possibly postpartum mood disorders.

Clinical Psychopharmacological Treatment

Nutritional Supplements

Vitamin B_6 (pyridoxine) has been used to treat premenstrual mood symptoms because of its purported efficacy in treating oral-contraceptive–induced depressions (53). This effect is related to observations that estrogen may increase tryptophan metabolism via the kynurenine-niacin pathway and thus increase the requirements for vitamin B_6. A slight decrease in the excretion of tryptophan metabolites in women suffering from PMS symptoms has been found, although plasma levels of pyridoxal phosphate generally are not different in women with and without premenstrual symptoms. Controlled studies suggest mixed results for pyridoxine; some find vitamin B_6 to be better than placebo, whereas other controlled studies find it no better than placebo. Some of the studies affirming efficacy are confounded by women taking concomitant hormones, psychotropics, or diuretics, or by reported improvements not being specific to the premenstrual phase. Pyridoxine may have weak effects on global ratings, behavior, and social activities (87), although a significant amount of physical and mood symptomatology may remain. High and prolonged doses of pyridoxine may be associated with neurological toxicity. In PMS studies, very few of these symptoms have been noted in controlled studies. There has been no dose–response relationship evident for vitamin B$_6$ in reported studies; significant improvements have been reported at doses as low as 50 mg.

The evidence supporting vitamin E's efficacy over placebo is not presently convincing. Vitamin E has been studied for the treatment of premenstrual symptoms, with improvements in motor coordination reported. Significant improvements in premenstrual anxiety and depression found in earlier studies of women with fibrocystic breast disease, have not been replicated. For vitamin A, early uncontrolled studies are encouraging, but no placebo-controlled studies are available to support its use.

One recent controlled study indicates that oral magnesium is effective in relieving premenstrual mood changes (18). Magnesium deficiency may activate premenstrual symptoms through various means. Significant magnesium deficiency in red blood cells of PMS patients initially reported warrant further follow-up. Although magnesium supplements have been recommended, consistent reports linking treatment of low blood-magnesium levels with reduction of premenstrual symptoms have not been found.

Hormones

Theories of PMS often attribute symptoms to fluctuations of ovarian steroid hormones. Thus, several studies have tested hormonal treatments. Although some studies support low luteal progesterone, high estrogen, or low progesterone–estrogen ratios being etiological, other studies do not implicate high estrogen or low progesterone levels. Some studies support the possibility of an asynchrony between declining rates of progesterone and estrogen, early ovulation, or decreases in progesterone over time relative to estrogen.

Consistent with the studies suggesting that estrogen is high and progesterone is low, several investigators have treated PMS symptoms with progesterone or other progestin compounds. However, efficacy claims for the progestins are based primarily on uncontrolled studies. Although Dalton (13) reported good results with open progesterone administration and Dennerstein et al. (16) found beneficial trends during the first but not second month in a controlled study of oral progesterone, other studies have not found progesterone to be superior to placebo (19).

With synthetic progestins, several open or single-blind trials report improvement rates of 50% to 82%. When compared to placebo, however, the synthetic progestins are not found to be effective over placebo, including ethisterone, norethisterone, or, with some exceptions, medroxyprogesterone acetate, when given short of inhibiting ovulation. Ylostalo and colleagues (90) found norethisterone effective for breast tenderness.

Most of the evidence does not support either natural or synthetic progestins as effective treatments of premenstrual mood symptoms. It appears that the improvements attested to this treatment are likely attributable to a placebo effect, except perhaps where given in a manner sufficient to induce anovulation.

Ovarian steroid treatment studies using oral contraceptives have also yielded inconsistent results. Several studies suggest that premenstrual moodiness, irritability, fatigue, and depressed mood may be less commonly reported in women using various oral contraceptives than in women not using them. However, other studies have found little difference in premenstrual symptoms between oral contraceptive users and nonusers. The results suggest that suppression of ovulation is not curative of PMS, when gonadal steroids are yet present from exogenous administration. Given that steroids have psychological effects, it can be difficult to predict individual responses in different women. Some data, for example, suggest that the estrogen-dominated pills may adversely affect women with premenstrual irritability, whereas progesterone-dominated pills adversely affect women with premenstrual depression. More research is necessary to determine whether specific identified subgroups would reliably benefit from oral contraceptive treatment of premenstrual mood symptoms.

Gonadotropin-Releasing Hormone

At a more central level, interruption of hypothalamic–pituitary–ovarian cyclicity may relieve premenstrual symptoms by induction of amenorrhea. Gonadotropin-releasing hormone (GNRH) agonists, which with chronic administration down-regulate pituitary gonadotropin secretion, have been used with some success in several studies. Muse and colleagues reported that a GNRH agonist robustly attenuated both behavioral and physical symptoms in seven women over a 3-month period compared to placebo (44). In this study, GNRH effectively interrupted the menstrual cycle (reversibly) during a 3-month administration, with amenorrhea induced during the second and third cycles. There were no significant differences in behavioral symptoms between GnRH and placebo during the first cycle, although physical symptoms improved during the first cycle. Two subsequent studies have since used the intranasally administered form of GNRH agonist, buserelin. Bancroft et al. (4) found a total daily dose of 600 mg of buserelin prompted improvement in bloating and breast tenderness with less clear effects on mood in 10 of 20 women studied openly. The other 10 women suffered adverse effects, including worsening of their symptoms. Hammarback and Backstrom (26) found GNRH to be better than placebo for mood, swelling and breast tenderness, although 3 of 26 women experienced worsening of their symptoms at 400 mg/day. This form of treatment may be considered a medical ovariectomy (44) and the potential hazards for long-term use, such as increased cardiovascular morbidity and mortality and osteoporosis, have not been clarified. Estrogen supplementation will not reverse these effects (43).

Danazol

Danazol is another antigonadotropin that causes hypothalamic–pituitary–gonadotropin suppression as a synthetic androgenic derivative of ethisterone. Preliminary reports indicate that this steroid is better than placebo for negative affect, pain, and behavioral change at doses of 100 to 400 mg/day. Since then, two double-blind studies (69,75) indicate that danazol compared with placebo significantly lowers premenstrual symptoms of lethargy, irritability and anxiety. Side effects of nausea, giddiness, skin rash, flushing, vaginitis, musculoskeletal and breast pain, decreased breast size, weight gain, and mild hirsutism have been reported. Thus treatment with danazol should be considered only after other treatments fail and when symptoms are severe. It should not be considered in women contemplating pregnancy or nursing. As such, danazol's usefulness may be limited because of its androgenic properties in women of childbearing age. As a trend in these studies, the 200 mg/day dose appears to be better tolerated. Its efficacy is comparable to the 400 mg/day dose in most patients.

Prolactin Inhibition with Bromocriptine

Several studies have tested bromocriptine for treatment of premenstrual symptoms because of the observed increases in prolactin levels during the luteal phase. Although most studies do not find abnormalities in prolactin levels in women with premenstrual symptoms, most, but not all studies indicate bromocriptine to be effective primarily for the treatment of mastodynia.

Significant improvements in mood, depressive symptoms (17), and irritability (90) have been sporadically reported, in double-blind, and single-blind placebo-controlled studies, respectively. Limiting side effects have been noted in approximately 20% of women treated with bromocriptine; side effects can include nausea, headache, vomiting, dizziness, fatigue, and paroxysmal tachycardia.

Salt and Water Balance

Diuretics have been studied because fluctuations in capillary filtration rate and permeability to plasma proteins occurs premenstrually. Women with premenstrual symptoms also have a higher luteal body water–potassium ratio than controls. Early uncontrolled studies of diuretics indicated satisfactory results with various compounds, including ammonium chloride, chlorothiazide, chlorthalidone, and quinethazone. However, neither chlorthalidone or potassium chloride have been found to be better than placebo in double-blind placebo studies. For bloatedness, two studies (45,74) suggest the superior efficacy of spironolactone over placebo.

The sulfuramide diuretic, metolazone (1 to 5 mg/day) was found to be effective for irritability, tension, depression, headache, and water retention symptoms (84) in a placebo-controlled diuretic study that included only women with premenstrual weight gain. Excessive diuresis and weakness occurred occasionally with the 5 mg dose. Thus, some evidence supports diuretic or antimineralocorticoid efficacy. The efficacy of such interventions, however, may be limited to subgroups of women with premenstrual weight gain.

Prostaglandin System

Women with premenstrual symptoms have also been treated experimentally with compounds affecting prostaglandin (PG) metabolism. Prostaglandins are known to mediate dysmenorrheic somatic complaints and also have been investigated in women with premenstrual mood complaints. Linoleic acid, the main precursor for PGE_1, was elevated in women with premenstrual symptoms in one study (5), whereas the PGE_1 product was lower in these women in another study (29). One interpretation is that the conversion of linoleic acid to PGE_1 is impaired in symptomatic women.

Mefenamic acid, a prostaglandin synthesis inhibitor, has been found more effective than placebo for mood symptoms in some studies (41,89), although Gunston (24) found no significant benefit on mood for mefenamic acid over placebo. In this study, there were improvements in gastrointestinal symptoms. Budoff (7) suggests that mefenamic acid improves breast tenderness, ankle swelling, and abdominal bloating with little effect on mood symptoms of tension, lethargy, and depression. Overall, the effects of mefenamic acid on mood have been inconsistent in comparison to its effects on pain. Many of its effects on affective symptoms have been obscured by the inclusion of dysmenorrheic women in study populations. One methodologically sound study (41), however, that excluded dysmenorrheic subjects, did find positive effects on mood of active drug over placebo. Significant decreases in premenstrual water retention and arousal symptoms have been reported with a diet low in fat that reduces the availability of prostaglandin precursors (31).

Efamol (evening primrose oil), a prostaglandin synthesis precursor (containing linoleic acid precursors, gamma linoleic acid, and vitamin E) also has been tried as a strategy to augment PGE_1 from administration of these essential fatty acid precursors. Although more effective than placebo for depressive symptoms in one study (58), another study was unable to find significant differences between placebo and Efamol (8). Again, the results of the treatment effects on premenstrual mood symptoms, distinct from dysmenorrhea, are complicated by inclusion of women with dysmenorrheic symptoms.

Psychotropics

Because of the complex effects of the hypothalamic–pituitary–gonadal axis and CNS neurochemistry, some treatment studies have aimed to influence neurotransmitters or neuromodulators more directly. The central α_2-adrenergic presynaptic autoreceptor agonist properties of clonidine have been theorized to compensate for a putative excess of central noradrenergic activity by presynaptic noradrenergic inhibition. One placebo comparison of clonidine (21) indicated efficacy over placebo in reducing premenstrual psychiatric rating (BPRS) scores. Clonidine can decrease plasma renin activity and promote aldosterone secretion and has been used for the treatment of opiate withdrawal. The promising results from this initial controlled trial deserve further study to determine which specific symptoms may respond best to stimulation of this inhibitory autoreceptor that governs the release of serotonin as well as norepinephrine.

In a double-blind crossover study (10), naltrexone was recently employed in an attempt to discover whether an opiate antagonist, given before an expected midcycle rise and fall of β-endorphin, would inhibit the effects of a putative premenstrual endogenous opioid withdrawal. The naltrexone treatment was modestly, but significantly, better than placebo, with the largest improvements found in ability to concentrate, behavioral changes, and negative affect. It was given only on days 9 to 18 of the cycle, such that patients may have been in an opiate antagonist withdrawal state during the late luteal phase. These results suggest that either an increased luteal opiate receptor sensitivity or a blockade of midcycle agonist occupancy may be therapeutic for premenstrual dysphoria. More work is needed to determine replicability and if the dose or schedule could be optimized to augment the benefit or decrease the side effects of nausea, decreased appetite, and dizziness.

Lithium has been tried for premenstrual mood symptoms because of the thymoleptic action of the compound observed in patients with mood disorders. Rubinow and Roy-Byrne (66) reviewed lithium treatment in premenstrual tension, citing three open trials with positive results, which were not confirmed in two subsequent double-blind, placebo-crossover studies. For recurrent suicidal depressions, or rapid-cycling mood disorders linked to the menstrual cycle, lithium may well be the treatment of choice. Other authors have suggested that patients who respond to lithium may be those who meet diagnostic criteria for cyclothymic disorders. Glick and Stewart (22) reported lithium to be effective in open trials of three schizophrenic patients with premenstrual exacerbations of schizophrenia. However, even at low doses (600 to 900 mg/day), most patients may detect significant lithium-related side effects. Lithium's teratogenicity, of course, indicates caution in women of childbearing potential.

Alprazolam also has been found in two published reports to be more effective than placebo for mood symptoms and global improvement (27,70). The agreement between studies is encouraging and suggests that alprazolam may indeed be a useful treatment for premenstrual mood symptoms, although, some questions remain as to whether there is attribution secondary to the subjective effects of alprazolam. Longer term studies are now needed to determine whether dependence or withdrawal symptoms would be problematic over a longitudinally intermittent treatment regimen of luteal alprazolam and follicular drug withdrawal.

Given the overlap of premenstrual mood symptoms with that of depression or anxiety, recent studies have focused on the use of antidepressants. After open studies indicated encouraging pilot results with nortriptyline, clomipramine, and fluoxetine, double-blind trials indicate that fluoxetine, clomipramine, imipramine, and phenelzine may be effective. Although several lines of evidence suggest luteal fluctuations of monoamine oxidase (MAO) activity, there is little information available on MAO inhibitor trials. Antidepressants may be indicated for the more severe PMS mood symptoms, although premenstrual dysphoric changes and irritability may continue despite effective antidepressant treatment (91). A drug that selectively enhances serotonin-mediated neurotransmission, d-fenfluramine, compared to placebo, effectively relieved appetite, depression, and anxiety in one study of 17 women (6). Consistent with some studies that report premenstrual changes in the platelet serotonin-transport system, the authors of this study interpreted their findings as supporting the hypothesis that raphe serotonin neurons are implicated in premenstrual disturbances of mood and appetite (6).

The 5-HT$_{1A}$ partial agonist, buspirone, has also been used in the treatment of premenstrual mood symptoms. Rickels and colleagues (62) have shown that buspirone was significantly more effective than placebo for irritability, fatigue, pain, and social functioning in 34 patients treated with a mean daily dose of 25 mg for 12 days prior to menstruation. Buspirone can cause lightheadedness, headache, or gastrointestinal distress primarily when the dose is first being adjusted, but lacks apparent dependence potential. It is not known whether the therapeutic effects reported for fenfluramine, nortriptyline, clomipramine, fluoxetine, and buspirone might all be mediated through 5-HT$_{1A}$ receptor mechanisms.

Sleep Cycle Manipulation

Some nonpharmacological experimental treatments, based on chronobiological models, include sleep deprivation and light therapy. One night of total sleep deprivation during the symptomatic premenstrual phase of the menstrual cycle was found to alleviate PMS symptoms. Follow-up studies suggest only one night of partial sleep deprivation (sleep 9 p.m. to 1 a.m. or 3 a.m. to 7 a.m.) may be beneficial (54). Light therapy involves sitting in front of a box of lights for 2 hrs/day for 1 week. Although early studies suggested superior efficacy of evening (7 to 9 p.m.) bright light (>2500 lux, 5 times brighter than room light) (49), subsequent trials showed equal efficacy of bright evening, bright morning (6:30 to 8:30 a.m.) and dim (10 < lux) red evening light administered in the premenstrual phase to PMS patients (51). Although these treatments may show promise, further trials are needed before these interventions can be recommended for general clinical usage. These findings are interesting in comparison with recent evidence suggesting a seasonal variation in PMS with approximately 70% of the women experiencing fewer symptoms during the summer when the photoperiod is naturally longer.

RELATIONSHIP BETWEEN REPRODUCTIVE-RELATED DEPRESSIONS

A depression occurring in association with the reproductive cycle may sensitize a woman to future depressions. A previous history of psychiatric illness or of affective changes during pregnancy may predispose a woman to oral contraceptive-induced depressions (53). Severe premenstrual depression may predispose a woman to postpartum depression and, like affective illness, premenstrual depression may have its onset or be exacerbated after a postpartum depression. Alternatively, a major affective disorder may be exacerbated or precipitated during a premenstrual period. There are anecdotal reports that after treating cycles of bipolar illness with lithium, premenstrual and seasonal mood cycles persist or become more prominent. Price et al. (57) report patients with rapid-cycling disorders have an increased tendency to have more severe forms of PMS, although Wehr et al. (78) found no convincing relationship between manic–depressive cycles and menstrual cycles in their patients with rapid-cycling disorders.

Thus, the cyclicity of affective disorders in the form of rapidly cycling bipolar illness or SAD may be compounded by periodic affective change occurring in association with the premenstruum, with pregnancy, and the postpartum period, and with altered reproductive hormonal milieus induced by oral contraceptives or gonadal hormone treatments.

MECHANISMS OF REPRODUCTIVE-RELATED DEPRESSIONS

With the kindling model of depression in mind (55), one wonders whether such periodic reproductive-related depressions may sensitize women to future affective episodes. Most longitudinal studies to date have not specifically focused on gender-related differences in the course of illness. Sex differences in depression begin to appear after the onset of puberty in adolescence (82). There is a marked increase in major depression in female children at approximately 16 years of age. In contrast, male children exhibit a gradual increase in depression across all ages, with considerably lower absolute rates than in female children. Furthermore, the onset of major depression is

earlier (12 to 13 years of age) in both male and female offspring of depressed probands (81), and the risk for depression appears to increase with time (25,81,83).

How cyclic depressions related to reproductive events may affect other forms of cyclic mood disorders is unknown, but a relationship does seem to exist. Work in animals may provide models and possibly shed light on the mechanisms involved. For example, the predisposition of women with thyroid impairment to cyclic forms of depression has a parallel in an animal model. Richter (61) produced abnormal cycles of motor activity experimentally in female animals but not in male animals by partial thyroidectomy. As in rapidly cycling patients, treatment with thyroid extract abolished the abnormal behavioral cycles, which returned after cessation of treatment. Richter hypothesized that the abnormal, regular cycles of activity were produced by the effect of thyroid deficiency on homeostatic mechanisms controlling luteotropin (prolactin) release (possibly related to the effect of TRH on prolactin). He induced similar cycles by daily subcutaneous injections of prolactin. Such cycles were also produced by inducing pseudopregnancy. This condition stimulates pituitary secretion of prolactin, which acts on the ovary to produce persistent corpora lutea and the secretion of progesterone. Ovariectomy abolished running activity; estrogens increased it. Longer abnormal activity cycles were produced by giving the rats anhydrohydroxy progesterone. As occurs in affective illness, the abnormal activity cycles become shorter with time. Of relevance here is our clinical work demonstrating higher baseline prolactin levels (Parry et al., *unpublished data*) and increased prolactin response to TRH in women with rapid cycles of mood related to the menstrual cycle (PMS) (50).

Reproductive hormones modulate hormonal, neurotransmitter, and biological clock mechanisms that have each been the focus of hypotheses about the pathophysiology of mood disorders. Estrogen and progesterone can alter the biosynthesis, release, uptake, degradation, and receptor density of norepinephrine, dopamine, serotonin, and acetylcholine (40). The gonadal steroids also modulate other hormonal mechanisms (thyroid, cortisol, prolactin, and opiates) that also affect neurotransmitter systems.

Gonadal hormones affect biological clock mechanisms, which also have been implicated in the pathophysiology of mood disorders. Estrogen shortens the period of circadian activity in ovariectomized hamsters and rats (1,42). The onset of activity occurs earlier on days of the estrous cycle when endogenous titers of estradiol are high in intact hamsters. Progesterone delays the onset of activity in intact rats by antagonizing the effect of estrogen (3). Estrogen, in addition to shortening the free-running period and altering the phase relationship of the activity rhythm to the light–dark cycle, increases the total amount of activity and decreases the variability of day-to-day onsets of activity. These findings parallel clinical work by Wever (85) who found that the mean free-running period of the sleep–wake cycle is significantly shorter in women than in men (28 min). The wake episode is shorter (1 hr, 49 min) and the sleep episode longer (1 hr, 21 min) in women compared with men. Thus, the fraction of sleep is longer for women than men. The circadian temperature rhythm was similar in both sexes. According to Wirz-Justice et al. (88), women sleep longer than men at all times of the year. When in free-running conditions, women, compared with men, tend to become internally desynchronized, particularly in the summer, by shortening the period of their sleep–wake cycle.

Estrogen also serves to enhance coupling between different circadian pacemaker components (1). Ovariectomized female rodents develop rhythm desynchronies. Replacement with estrogen restores the normal coupling relationship between these disparate rhythms. This factor may be involved in some of its therapeutic effects.

Thus, the decline of ovarian hormones common to the premenstrual, postpartum, and menopausal periods and their inherent cyclicity may destabilize or sensitize neurotransmitter, neuroendocrine, and biological clock mechanisms, thereby setting the stage for the development of cyclic mood disorders.

Although the cyclicity of the endocrine milieu may increase the vulnerability to episodic depressions in women, it may protect against the development of many chronic illnesses, which, as previously mentioned, are more characteristic in men. The investigation of hormonal contributions to affective illness in women and the examination of the way in which the course of these illnesses is affected by reproductive events of the life cycle may increase our understanding of affective illness and potentially provide alternative treatment strategies.

SUMMARY

Women are at higher risk than men to develop depressive episodes during the reproductive years. Furthermore, women are vulnerable to depressions associated with oral contraceptives, abortion, the premenstrual period, the puerperium, and menopause. The phenomenology and the biological mechanisms involved in these illnesses should perhaps be viewed in the context of other manifestations of the link between depression and female reproductive functions. For example, women are especially vulnerable to a rapidly cycling form of affective illness and to hypothyroidism, an associated factor for this form of mood disorder. The postpartum period also is associated with impaired thyroid function, and there are reports of the induction of rapid cycles of mood following the termination of pregnancy. Thus, alterations in thyroid hormones may be a feature of both postpartum and rapid-cycling forms of mood disorder in women.

A previous history of a postpartum depression places a woman at a high risk for the development of a subsequent puerperal episode. Also, difficulties during pregnancy may predispose a woman to the development of other reproductive-related depressions. The role reproductive hormones play in this possible sensitization phenomenon should be examined to understand the relationship of depression to the female reproductive cycle. Appropriately timed clinical psychopharmacological interventions may serve to inhibit this sensitization phenomenon and benefit long-term prognosis.

REFERENCES

1. Albers EH, Gerall AA, Axelson JF. Effect of reproductive state on circadian periodicity in the rat. *Physiol Behav* 1981;26:21–25.
2. Amino N, More H, Iwatani Y, et al. High prevalence of transient postpartum thyrotoxicosis and hypothyroidism. *N Engl J Med* 1982;306:849–852.
3. Axelson JF, Gerall AA, Albers E. Effect of progesterone on the estrous activity cycle of the rat. *Physiol Behav* 1981;26:631–635.
4. Bancroft J, Boyle H, Warner P, Fraser HM. The use of an LHRH agonist, buserelin, in the long term management of premenstrual syndromes. *Clin Endocrinol* 1987;27:171–182.
5. Brush MG, Watson SJ, Horrobin DF, Manku MS. Abnormal essential fatty acid levels in plasma of women with premenstrual syndrome. *Am J Obstet Gynecol* 1984;150:363–366.
6. Brzezinski AA, Wurtman JJ, Wurtman RJ, Gleason R, Greenfield J, Nader T. *d*-Fenfluramine suppresses the increased calorie and carbohydrate intakes and improves the mood of women with premenstrual depression. *Obstet Gynecol* 1990;76:296–301.
7. Budoff PW. The use of prostaglandin inhibitors for the premenstrual syndrome. *J Reproductive Med* 1983;28:469–478.
8. Callender K, McGregor M, Kirk P, Thomas CS. A double-blind trial of evening primrose oil in the premenstrual syndrome: nervous symptom subgroup. *Hum Psychopharmacol* 1988;3:57–61.
9. Cho JT, Bone S, Dunner DL, et al. The effects of lithium treatment on thyroid function in patients with primary affective disorder. *Am J Psychiatry* 1979;136:115–116.
10. Chuong CJ, Coulam CB, Bergstrahl EJ, O'Fallon WM, Steinmetz GI. Clinical trial of naltrexone in premenstrual syndrome. *Obstet Gynecol* 1988;72:332–336.
11. Coryell W, Endicott J, Kuler M. Rapid cycling affective disorder: demographics, diagnosis, family history and course. *Arch Gen Psychiatry* 1992;49:126–131.
12. Cowdry RW, Wehr TA, Zis AP, Goodwin FK. Thyroid abnormalities associated with rapid cycling bipolar illness. *Arch Gen Psychiatry* 1983;40:414–420.
13. Dalton K. Progesterone, fluid and electrolytes in the premenstrual syndrome. *Br Med J* 1980;281:1008–1009.
14. Dalton K. Progesterone prophylaxis used successfully in postnatal depression. *Practioner* 1985;229:507–508.
15. Dalton K. *The premenstrual syndrome.* London: Heineman Medical; 1964.
16. Dennerstein L, Spencer-Gardener C, Gotts G. Progesterone and the premenstrual syndrome: a double-blind cross-over trial. *Br Med J* 1985;290:1617–1621.
17. Elsner CW, Buster JE, Schindler RA, Nessin SA, Abraham GE. Bromocriptine treatment of premenstrual tension syndrome. *Obstet Gynecol* 1980;56:723–726.
18. Facchinetti F, Borella P, Sances G, Fioroni L, Nappi RE, Genazzani AR. Oral magnesium successfully relieves premenstrual mood changes. *Obstet Gynecol* 1991;78:177–181.
19. Freeman E, Rickels K, Sondheimer SJ, Polansky M. Ineffectiveness of progesterone suppository treatment for premenstrual syndrome (see comments). *JAMA* 1990;264:349–353.
20. Garvey MJ, Tuason VB, Lumry AE, et al. Occurrence of depression in the postpartum state. *J Affect Dis* 1983;5:97–101.
21. Giannini AJ, Sullivan B, Sarachene J, Loiselle RH. Clonidine in the treatment of premenstrual syndrome: a subgroup study. *J Clin Psychiatry* 1988;49:62–63.
22. Glick ID, Stewart D. A new drug treatment for premenstrual exacerbation of schizophrenia. *Compr Psychiatry* 1980;21:281–287.
23. Goodwin FK, Prange AJ, Post RM, Muscettola G, Lipton MA.

Potentiation of antidepressant effects by 1-triiodothyronine in tricyclic nonresponders. *Am J Psychiatry* 1982;139:34–38.

24. Gunston KD. Premenstrual syndrome in Cape Town. Part II. A double-blind placebo-controlled study of the efficacy of mefenamic acid. *S Afr Med J* 1986;70:159–160.

25. Hagnell O, Lanke J, Roisman B, et al. Are we entering an age of melancholy? Depressive illness and prospective epidemiological study over 25 years. The Lundby Study, Sweden. *Psychol Med* 1982;12:279–289.

26. Hammarback S, Backstrom T. Induced anovulation as treatment of premenstrual tension syndrome. *Acta Obstet Gynecol Scand* 1988; 67:159–166.

27. Harrison WM, Endicott J, Rabkin JG, Nee JC, Sandberg D. Treatment of premenstrual dysphoria with alprazolam and placebo. *Psychopharmacol Bull* 1987;23:150–153.

28. Hatotani N, Nomara J. *Neurobiology of periodic psychoses.* Tokyo: Igaku-Shoin; 1983.

29. Jakubowicz DL, Godard E, Dewhurst J. The treatment of premenstrual tension with mefenamic acid: analysis of prostaglandin concentrations. *Br J Obstet Gynaecol* 1984;91:78–84.

30. Jansson R, Bernander S, Karlesson A, et al. Autoimmune thyroid depression in the postpartum period. *J Clin Endocrinol Metab* 1984;58:681–687.

31. Jones DY. Influence of dietary fat and on self-reported menstrual symptoms. *Physiol Behav* 1987;40:483–487.

32. Kasper S, Sack DA, Wehr TA, et al. Nocturnal TSH and prolactin secretion during sleep deprivation and prediction of antidepressant response in patients with major depression. *Biol Psychiatry* 1988;24:631–641.

33. Kendall DA, Stancel AM, Enna SJ: Imipramine: effect of ovarian steroids on modification in serotonin receptor binding. *Science* 1981;211:1183–1185.

34. Kendell RE, Chalmers JC, Platz C. Epidemiology of puerperal psychoses. *Br J Psychiatry* 1987;150:662–673.

35. Kendell RE, Hall DJ, Hailey A, Babigian M. The epidemiology of anorexia nervosa. *Psychol Med* 1973;3:200–203.

36. Klaiber EL, Broverman DM, Vogel W, et al. Estrogen therapy for severe persistent depressions in women. *Arch Gen Psychiatry* 1979;36:550–554.

37. Kraeplin E. *Manic depressive insanity and paranoia.* Edinburgh: Livingstone; 1921.

38. Kukopulos A, Reginaldi P, Laddomada GF, et al. Course of the manic depressive cycle and changes caused by treatments. *Pharmacopsychiatry* 1980;13:156–167.

39. Kupfer DJ, Carpenter LL, Frank E. Possible role of antidepressants in precipitating mania and hypomania in recurrent depression. *Am J Psychiatry* 1988;145:804–808.

40. McEwen BS, Parsons B. General steroid action on the brain: neurochemistry and neuropharmacology. *Annu Rev Pharmacol Toxicol* 1982;22:555–598.

41. Mira M, McNeil D, Fraser IS, Vizzard J, Abraham S. Mefenamic acid in the treatment of premenstrual syndrome. *Obstet Gynecol* 1986;68:395–398.

42. Morin LP, Fitzgerald KM, Zucker I. Estradiol shortens the period of hamster circadian rhythms. *Science* 1977;196:305–306.

43. Mortola JF, Girton L, Fischer U. Successful treatment of severe premenstrual syndrome by combined use of gonadotropin-releasing hormone agonist and estrogen/progesterone. *J Clin Endocrinol Metab* 1991;72:252A–252F.

44. Muse KN, Cetel NS, Futterman LA, Yen SSC. The premenstrual syndrome: effects of "medical ovariectomy." *New Engl J Med* 1984;311:1345–1349.

45. O'Brien PM, Craven D, Selby C, Symonds EM. Treatment of premenstrual syndrome by spironolactone. *Br J Obstet Gynaecol* 1979;86:142–147.

46. Oppenheim G. A case of rapid mood cycling with estrogen: implications for therapy. *J Clin Psychiatry* 1984;45:34–35.

47. Parker DC, Rossman LG, Vanderloom EF. Sleep related, nyctohemeral and briefly episodic variation on human plasma prolactin concentrations. *J Clin Endocrinol Metab* 1973;36:1119–1124.

48. Parry BL, Berga SL, Kripke DF, et al. Altered waveform of plasma nocturnal melatonin secretion in premenstrual depression. *Arch Gen Psychiatry* 1990;47:1139–1146.

49. Parry BL, Berga SL, Mostofi N, Sependa PA, Kripke DF, Gillin JC. Morning vs. evening bright light treatment of late luteal phase dysphoric disorder. *Am J Psychiatry* 1989;146:1215–1217.

50. Parry BL, Gerner RH, Wilkins JN, et al. CSF and endocrine studies of premenstrual syndrome. *Neuropsychopharmacology* 1991;5: 127–137.

51. Parry BL, Mahan AM, Mostofi N, Klauber MR, Lew GS, Gillin JC. Light therapy of late luteal phase dysphoric disorder: an extended study. *Am J Psychiatry* 1993;150:1417–1419.

52. Parry BL, Rosenthal NE, Tamarhin L, Wehr T. Treatment of a patient with seasonal premenstrual syndrome. *Am J Psychiatry* 1987;144:762–766.

53. Parry BL, Rush AJ. Oral contraceptives and depressive symptomatology: biologic mechanisms. *Compr Psychiatry* 1979;20: 347–358.

54. Parry BL, Wehr TA. Therapeutic effect of sleep deprivation in patients with premenstrual syndrome. *Am J Psychiatry* 1987; 144:808–810.

55. Post RM, Rubinow DR, Ballenger JC: Conditioning, sensitization and kindling: implications for the course of affective illness. In Post RM, Ballenger JC, eds. *Neurobiology of mood disorders.* Baltimore: Williams and Wilkins; 1984.

56. Prange AJ, Wilson IC, Rabon AM, et al. Enhancement of imipramine antidepressant activity by thyroid hormone. *Am J Psychiatry* 1969;126:457–469.

57. Price WA, Dimarzio L. Premenstrual tension syndrome in rapid-cycling bipolar affective disorder. *J Clin Psychiatry* 1986;47: 415–417.

58. Puolakka J, Makarainen L, Viinikka L, Ylikorkala O. Biochemical and clinical effects of treating the premenstrual syndrome with prostaglandin synthesis precursors. *J Reprod Med* 1985;30:149–153.

59. Ramey JN, Burrow GN, Polackwich RJ, Donabedian RK. The effect of oral contraceptive steroids on the response of thyroid stimulating hormone to thyrotropin releasing hormone. *J Clin Endocrinol Metab* 1975;40:712–714.

60. Reich T, Winokur G. Postpartum psychoses in patients with manic depressive disorder. *J Nerv Ment Dis* 1970;151:60–68.

61. Richter CP, Jones GS, Biswanger L. Periodic phenomena and the thyroid. *Arch Neurol Psychiatry* 1959;81:117–139.

62. Rickles K, Freeman E, Sondheimer S. Buspirone in treatment of premenstrual syndrome (Letter). *Lancet* 1989;1:777.

63. Robins LN, Helzer JE, Weissman MM, et al. Lifetime prevalence of specific psychiatric disorders in three sites. *Arch Gen Psychiatry* 1984;41:949–958.

64. Rosenthal NE, Sack DA, James SP, et al. Seasonal affective disorder and phototherapy. *Ann NY Acad Sci* 1985;453:260–269.

65. Roy-Byrne PP, Uhde TW, Post RM. Effects of one night's sleep deprivation on mood and behavior in panic disorder. *Arch Gen Psychiatry* 1986;43(9):895–900.

66. Rubinow DR, Roy-Byrne P. Premenstrual syndromes: overview from a methodologic perspective. *Am J Psychiatry* 1984;141:163–172.

67. Sack DA, Duncan W, Rosenthal NE, et al. The timing and duration of sleep in partial sleep deprivation therapy of depression. *Acta Psychiatr Scand* 1988;77:219–224.

68. Sack DA, James SP, Rosenthal NE, et al. Deficient nocturnal surge of TSH secretion during sleep and sleep deprivation in rapid cycling bipolar illness. *Psychiatry Res* 1988;23:179–191.

69. Sarno AP, Miller EJ, Lundblad EG. Premenstrual syndrome: beneficial effects of periodic, low-dose danazol. *Obstet Gynecol* 1987; 70:33–36.

70. Smith S, Rinehart JS, Ruddock VE, Schiff I. Treatment of premenstrual syndrome with alprazolam: results of a double-blind, placebo-controlled, randomized crossover clinical trial. *Obstet Gynecol* 1987;70:37–43.

71. Spitz IM, Zylber-Haran A, Trestian S. The thyrotropin (TSH) profile in isolated gonadotropin deficiency: a model to evaluate the effect of sex steroids on TSH secretion. *J Clin Endocrinol Metab* 1983;57:425–430.

72. Stancer HC, Persad E. Treatment of intractable rapid cycling manic depressive disorder with levothyroxine. *Arch Gen Psychiatry* 1982;39:311–312.

73. Transbol I, Christiansen C, Baastrup PC. Endocrine effects of lithium. *Acta Endocrinol* 1978;87:759–767.

74. Vellacott ID, Shroff NE, Pearce MY, Stratford ME, Akbar FA. A double-blind placebo evaluation of spironolactone in the premenstrual syndrome. *Curr Med Res Opin* 1987;10:450–456.

75. Watts JF, Butt WR, Logan Edwards R. A clinical trial using danazol

for the treatment of premenstrual tension. *Br J Obstet Gynecol* 1987;94:30–34.

76. Wehr TA, Goodwin FK. Rapid cycling in manic depressives induced by tricyclic antidepressants. *Arch Gen Psychiatry* 1979; 36:555–559.

77. Wehr TA, Sack DA, Jacobsen FM, et al. Phototherapy of seasonal affective disorder: time of day and suppression of melatonin are not critical for antidepressant effects. *Arch Gen Psychiatry* 1986; 43:870–875.

78. Wehr TA, Sack DA, Rosenthal NE. Rapid cycling affective disorder: contributing factors and treatment responses of 51 patients. *Am J Psychiatry* 1988;145:179–184.

79. Wehr TA, Sack DA, Rosenthal NE. Seasonal affective disorder with summer depression and winter hypomania. *Am J Psychiatry* 1987;144:1602–1603.

80. Wehr TA, Sack DA, Rosenthal NE. Sleep reduction as a final common pathway in the genesis of mania. *Am J Psychiatry* 1987; 144:201–204.

81. Weissman MM, Gammon D, John K, et al. Children of depressed parents: increased psychopathology and early onset of major depression. *Arch Gen Psychiatry* 1987;44:847–853.

82. Weissman MM, Klerman GL. Sex differences and the epidemiology of depression. *Arch Gen Psychiatry* 1977;34:98–111.

83. Weissman MM, Leaf PJ, Holzer CE, et al. The epidemiology of depression: an update on sex differences in rates. *J Affect Dis* 1984;7:179–188.

84. Werch A, Kane RE. Treatment of premenstrual tension with metolazone: a double-blind evaluation of a new diuretic. *Curr Therapeutic Res* 1976;19:565–572.

85. Wever RA. Properties of human sleep-wake cycles: parameters of internally synchronized free running rhythms. *Sleep* 1984;7:27–51.

86. Whybrow PC, Prange AJ. A hypothesis of thyroid-catecholamine receptor interaction. *Arch Gen Psychiatry* 1981;38:106–113.

87. Williams MJ, Harris RI, Dean BC. Controlled trial of pyridoxine in the premenstrual syndrome. *J Int Med Res* 1985;13:174–179.

88. Wirz-Justice A, Wever RA, Aschoff J. Seasonality in freerunning rhythms in man. *Naturwissenschaften* 1984;71:316–319.

89. Wood C, Jakubowicz D. The treatment of premenstrual symptoms with mefenamic acid. *Br J Obstet Gynaecol* 1980;87:627–630.

90. Ylostalo P, Kauppila A, Puolakka J, Ronnberg L, Janne O. Bromocriptine and norethisterone in the treatment of premenstrual syndrome. *Obstet Gynecol* 1982;59:292–298.

91. Yonkers KA, White K. Premenstrual exacerbation of depression: one process or two? *J Clin Psychiatry* 1992;53:289–292.

Psychopharmacology: The Fourth Generation of Progress, edited by Floyd E. Bloom and David J. Kupfer. Raven Press, Ltd., New York © 1995.

CHAPTER 89

Selective Serotonin Reuptake Inhibitors in the Acute Treatment of Depression

Stuart A. Montgomery

The impetus for the development of the selective serotonin reuptake inhibitors (SSRI) was the perceived need for antidepressants with an improved therapeutic profile compared with the traditional tricyclic antidepressants (TCA). The TCAs made a great contribution to giving depressed patients a better quality of life when they were introduced more than a generation ago, but they have many limitations (see Chapter 90, *this volume*).

The TCAs produce a wide range of pharmacological actions affecting a variety of neurotransmitters; many of these pharmacological effects produce unwanted and sometimes dangerous side effects without being of apparent therapeutic benefit for the depression. The need for drugs with an improved safety profile compared with the older TCAs was recognized early. The anticholinergic effects of the TCAs, for example, lead to worsening in concentration and memory and it has been suggested may worsen dementia. The TCAs have marked effects on cardiac function and can be cardiotoxic in therapeutic dosage as well as overdose (28). This limits their usefulness particularly in the elderly, who are at increased risk of undetected impaired cardiac function. They are toxic in overdose (12,49), and, in prescribing them a doctor may be providing patients with the means to harm themselves.

The older TCAs are poorly tolerated by patients, which contributes considerably to the therapeutic failure of these antidepressants due to poor compliance (33). Their well-known anticholinergic effects, such as dry mouth and blurred vision, are often cited by patients as the reason for withdrawing from treatment. The difficulty experienced in tolerating the unwanted side effects also prejudices the use of therapeutic doses. Even if treatment is initiated at low doses and increased slowly, it is sometimes difficult to reach the full therapeutic dose.

The need for better-tolerated, safer antidepressants than the TCAs is clear. It was hoped that the SSRIs, which act selectively on the serotonergic system and avoid activity on receptor systems that appear unrelated to antidepressant effect, would not be associated with the unwelcome side effects characteristic of the TCAs. This selectivity of pharmacological action was also expected to result in safer drugs particularly in cardiotoxicity and overdose toxicity.

SELECTIVITY OF ANTIDEPRESSANT EFFECT

Another reason for developing the SSRIs was the possibility that improved efficacy could be achieved by focusing the pharmacological activity on a specific neurotransmitter system. There is a considerable body of evidence to indicate the importance of serotonin in the pathophysiology of depression and to suggest the serotonergic pathway as the most closely involved with mood regulation. An antidepressant acting primarily on serotonin might therefore lead to an improved therapeutic effect. A second possibility might be that the SSRIs would be of particular benefit in a particular subgroup of depression (64). Asberg et al. (5) suggested that there was a bimodal distribution of 5-hydroxyindoleacetic acid (5-HIAA) in the cerebrospinal fluid (CSF) of depressed patients, which was a marker of a subgroup. Therefore, SSRIs might offer treatment for this subgroup of patients characterized by a dysfunction in serotonin metabolism. It appears, however, that SSRIs have similar efficacy to reference antidepressants and that the evidence for serotonin-specific depressions is weak.

The SSRIs were developed in response to the need for drugs that were less "pharmacologically dirty" than the

S. A. Montgomery: Academic Department of Psychiatry, St Mary's Hospital Medical School, London W21NY, United Kingdom.

TCAs. The selectively acting antidepressants that are the fruit of that development have provided a pharmacological tool for investigating the clinical effects of activity on specific neuronal systems as a means of unraveling the underlying mechanisms of antidepressant action.

ANTIDEPRESSANT EFFICACY OF SSRIs

The list of SSRIs that have reached the market or are in development is considerable. Several have been in clinical use for some years. This chapter discusses those SSRIs that have currently been licensed as antidepressants in the United States, Canada, or Europe, as well as their efficacy, side effects, and safety in the acute treatment of depression. The SSRIs currently available are citalopram (available in Europe since 1988), fluoxetine, fluvoxamine (available in Europe since 1983), paroxetine, and sertraline. Standard doses of these SSRIs are shown in Table 1.

The standards for assessing the efficacy of new antidepressants are more stringent than was formerly the case and as a result there is evidence from placebo-controlled studies on which to base a judgement. There are also studies that included both placebo and a reference comparator antidepressant, and these provide reassurance about the population of patients investigated and the size of effect observed.

Tables 2 to 5 summarize the efficacy studies of the different SSRIs. In some cases individual centers participating in multicenter studies have published separately. To avoid citing the same data twice these have been excluded.

Citalopram

Citalopram was developed initially using reference-controlled studies only. These have not all been published, but the antidepressant efficacy was suggested by Bech and Cialdella (9, see also refs. 3 and 59). A small, as yet unpublished, placebo-controlled study also suggested efficacy compared with placebo. This was later confirmed in two large multicenter placebo-controlled studies (see

TABLE 1. *Standard doses of selective serotonin reuptake inhibitors*

SSRI	Dose
Citalopram	20–40 mg/day
Fluoxetine	20 mg/day
Fluvoxamine	150 mg/day
Sertraline	50–150 mg/day
Paroxetine	20–40 mg/day

TABLE 2. *Placebo-controlled studies of citalopram*

Study	N	Result
Mendels et al. (39)	142	CIT > PLC
Montgomery et al. (50)	199	CIT 40 mg > PLC
		CIT 20 mg = PLC

CIT, citalopram; PLC, placebo.

Table 2). In the 142 patient study of Mendels et al. (39), which has not yet been fully published, citalopram in a dose of 20 mg to 80 mg was better than placebo. In the study of Montgomery et al. (50), which included 199 patients, 40 mg of citalopram was clearly effective compared with placebo but 20 mg was not.

Fluoxetine

Fluoxetine was the first SSRI to appear in the United States, although it was a latecomer in Europe. Its antidepressant efficacy is shown in its superiority compared with placebo demonstrated in three large studies and in three out of four smaller studies (25,29,52,56,60,67,68). The efficacy assessment was based on 834 patients treated with fluoxetine compared with 397 treated with placebo and 227 treated with TCAs (see Table 3). The number of patients included in the large multicenter studies was sufficiently large to justify comparison between response to fluoxetine and to the comparator, imipramine. The results suggest that fluoxetine has a very similar level of efficacy to the TCAs (41).

Fluvoxamine

Fluvoxamine is the longest available SSRI in Europe. The efficacy of fluvoxamine has been investigated in

TABLE 3. *Placebo-controlled studies of fluoxetine*

Study	N	Result
Placebo		
Wernicke et al. (68)	336	FLX 20 mg > PLC
		FLX 40 mg > PLC
		FLX 60 mg = PLC
Wernicke et al. (67)	354	FLX 5 mg > PLC
		FLX 20 mg > PLC
		FLX 40 mg > PLC
Fabre and Crimson (25)	37	FLX > PLC
Rickels et al. (56)	38	FLX = PLC
Fluoxetine + imipramine		
Stark and Hardison (60)	589	FLX = IMI > PLC
Heiligenstein et al. (29)	52	FLX > PLC
Placebo + mianserin		
Muijen et al. (52)	70	FLX > PLC + MIA

FLX, fluoxetine; PLC, placebo; IMI, imipramine; MIA, mianserin.

TABLE 4. *Placebo-controlled studies of fluvoxamine*

Study	N	Result
Placebo		
Conti et al. (16)	45	FLV > PLC
Placebo + imipramine		
Amin et al. (2)	481	FLV = IMI > PLC
Itil et al. (31)	69	FLV < IMI > PLC
Lydiard et al. (36)	52	FLV = IMI = PLC
Feighner et al. (26)	86	FLV > IMI = PLC
March et al. (37)	40	FLV > PLC = IMI
Placebo + desipramine		
Roth et al. (58)	90	FLV = DMI > PLC

FLV, fluvoxamine; PLC, placebo; IMI, imipramine; DMI, desipramine.

small placebo-controlled studies, some of which were positive and others negative (16,26,31,36,37,58). Confirmation of efficacy was provided by a collective analysis of the eight centers participating in two large multicenter placebo and reference-controlled studies (2). Four of the centers published their results separately (20,34,53). In the main analysis and in other reference-controlled studies, fluvoxamine was found to have very similar levels of efficacy to reference TCAs (see Table 4).

Two of the studies and two of the centers in the multicenter studies did not find a difference from placebo for either fluvoxamine or the active comparator (31,34, 36,53).

Paroxetine

A number of small studies conducted in Europe indicated the probable efficacy of paroxetine, which was later confirmed in two large studies, one placebo controlled and the other placebo and reference antidepressant controlled (see Table 5). Four studies following identical

TABLE 5. *Placebo-controlled studies of paroxetine*

Study	N	Result
Placebo		
Cohn	50	PAR = PLC
Rickels[a]	111	PAR > PLC
Claghorn[a]	72	PAR > PLC
Smith[a]	77	PAR = PLC
Kiev[a]	81	PAR > PLC
Naylor	47	PAR = PLC
Placebo + Imipramine[b]		
Feighner	120	PAR > PLC
Cohn	120	PAR > PLC
Mendels	125	PAR = PLC
Shrivastava	120	PAR > PLC
Fieve	121	PAR > PLC
Fabre	120	PAR > PLC

PAR, paroxetine; PLC, placebo.
[a] These studies were cited in ref. 13.
[b] These studies were cited in ref. 22.

TABLE 6. *Placebo-controlled studies of sertraline*

Study	N	Result
Placebo		
Fabre (24)	369	SER > PLC
Placebo + Amitriptyline		
Reimherr et al. (55)	448	SER = AMI > PLC

protocols compared paroxetine with placebo in 273 patients and three were positive (13). Six studies compared paroxetine with placebo and an active control, imipramine, in 726 patients and five of these were positive (22).

In the direct comparison with placebo in the merged four-study analysis a significantly better response was found in the group treated with paroxetine at 2 weeks. In the larger six-study comparison this apparently early onset of effect was also seen at 1 week. The response in the imipramine and paroxetine groups was seen to be very similar, and a quantitative difference large enough to be considered clinically important did not emerge until 3 to 4 weeks.

Sertraline

Sertraline has been shown to be effective as an antidepressant in two large multicenter placebo- or placebo- and reference-controlled studies (24,55) (Table 6). In the large placebo-controlled study (24), which included 369 patients, sertraline showed unequivocal efficacy. This study compared three fixed doses of sertraline between 50 mg and 150 mg. All these doses were seen to be effective, although there was some indication of a better response with the higher dose. In the reference- and placebo-controlled study, which included 448 patients, sertraline and amitriptyline were both shown to be significantly better than placebo with rather similar antidepressant response on the active drugs.

RELATIVE EFFICACY OF SELECTIVE SEROTONIN REUPTAKE INHIBITORS

The SSRIs have been extensively compared with reference antidepressants, both in the placebo-controlled studies that included a reference comparator and in standalone active comparator studies of varying size. Comparator antidepressants have included amitriptyline, imipramine, clomipramine, maprotiline, oxaprotiline, mianserin, and dothiepin; these studies have generally found no significant differences between treatment groups.

Relatively small active control studies can only provide support for the concept of equivalent efficacy because a very large number of patients is needed to indicate similar efficacy. In general, these studies have reported similar efficacy with occasional studies reporting either increased efficacy with the SSRI (26,52) or less efficacy (3). However the multicenter studies that have been conducted with the SSRIs during the clinical development program have been large enough to demonstrate that the SSRIs are of the same order of efficacy as the reference TCAs.

Another way of assessing the relative efficacy of antidepressants is to carry out metaanalyses of the databases. This has been done for some of the SSRIs; for example, fluoxetine (54) and paroxetine (22) appear to have very similar efficacy to the TCAs. This judgment is supported by the metaanalysis of the published literature on all of the SSRIs taken together (47). In this analysis, the SSRIs and TCAs were associated with the same rate of drop outs because of lack of efficacy, but there were significantly fewer dropouts because of side effects with the SSRIs.

Direct comparisons between SSRIs are generally lacking, so that we cannot state categorically that one is more effective than another. The results of the efficacy studies and the similar size of therapeutic effect indicate that there are unlikely to be clinically significant differences between them in efficacy.

DOSAGE

The selection of the correct dose for antidepressants has often been based on a combination of guess work, following observation of the effects of drugs in animals, and dose titration studies. Neither provide an adequate basis for selecting the optimum therapeutic dose. In dose titration studies, it is customary to increase the dose to the maximum tolerated at which a response is observed. Because of the delay in antidepressant response, this approach can lead to the dose being raised beyond necessary; the response to a low dose may be attributed to the later higher dose. Patients may thus be exposed unnecessarily to high doses of antidepressants, which are often accompanied by increased side effects, without any advantage in therapeutic efficacy. The more reliable way of establishing the optimum dose is via fixed dose studies that directly compare response to a range of doses given in a fixed dosage regimen. Without this type of study to establish the minimum effective dose, a drug may be introduced at too high a dose.

Fixed-dose studies with several of the SSRIs have shown that the earlier studies in the development program were carried out using too high a dose. The initial studies of fluoxetine, for example, were carried out using an 80-mg/day maximum dose. Later fixed-dose studies showed that 20 mg and 40 mg were significantly better than placebo and that the 60 mg dose although effective was associated with increased side effects and an increased number of withdrawals because of side effects (68). In a later fixed-dose study, 5 mg, 20 mg, and 40 mg of fluoxetine were found to be significantly better than placebo

although a larger treatment effect was seen with the 20 mg and 40 mg dose (67). The minimum effective dose of fluoxetine has not therefore been established, and the dose of 20 mg may be more than is necessary in some patients.

It is possible that fluvoxamine was introduced at too high a dose and that the side effect of nausea could have been reduced without a loss of efficacy if a lower dose had been recommended. It has become more routine in recent years to carry out fixed-dose studies of new antidepressants, and as a result data are available for most of the SSRIs to indicate the minimum effective dose. Thus the minimum effective dose of paroxetine was established in fixed dose studies as 20 mg (32). There is some suggestion that a higher dose may be more effective in patients with melancholia. The minimum effective dose of citalopram is thought to lie between 20 mg and 40 mg. The 20-mg dose has been found to be effective in a general practice population, but in a hospital-based population 40 mg was found to be more effective (50).

Some patients may need higher doses than the generally optimum therapeutic dose, and here the SSRIs, which are safer and more tolerable than the TCAs, offer an advantage. A study in which the dose was raised from 20 mg to 60 mg of fluoxetine in nonresponders at 3 weeks showed no advantage compared to patients continued on 20 mg. The evidence with paroxetine and citalopram, however, does suggest that raising the dose may be helpful for nonresponders, particularly those with melancholia symptoms or severe depression. Higher doses may also benefit patients with both depression and concomitant obsessive–compulsive disorder.

The SSRIs have been studied in both acute and long-term treatment; the long-term treatment studies have found that full antidepressant doses are needed for prophylaxis or maintenance treatment. Fluoxetine has been found to be effective in reducing the risk of new episodes of depression in doses of 20 mg (57) and 40 mg (45). The dose shown to be effective in both the continuation and prophylactic phase of treatment was approximately 100 mg of sertraline (21) and 20 to 30 mg of paroxetine (46). Citalopram was found to be effective at doses of both 20 and 40 mg in a 6-month continuation treatment study (51).

SELECTIVE EFFICACY OF ANTIDEPRESSANTS

The overview of the efficacy of SSRIs is that they are as effective as the TCAs with which they have been compared. Their speed of onset of action of general antidepressant effect also appears for the most part to be similar. There are however certain aspects of efficacy that seem to differentiate the SSRIs from the TCAs.

It is a difficult task to establish efficacy in subgroups

of depression, as the clinical trials are often too small in size to permit a legitimate analysis. However the databases with the new SSRIs are sufficiently large to enable metaanalyses to be carried out to investigate differential effects in different subgroups.

Severe Depression

Efficacy in severe depression is an important aspect of treatment, and when new drugs are introduced their efficacy in this respect is often challenged. Because severe depression is not usually studied separately, a metaanalysis of the database can provide answers. Several of these have been carried out to see if the SSRIs are as effective as the reference TCAs in severe depression. The approach has been to stratify patients included in studies into moderate and severe depression, defined by a cutoff score on a severity rating scale at the start of treatment. The answer provided by this type of metaanalysis has been that the SSRIs are as effective as the reference comparator in both moderate and severe depression; for example, such a metaanalysis has been carried out for fluoxetine (41).

There is also evidence to suggest that in some cases the SSRIs are more effective in severe depression than the comparator TCA. An example is the analysis of the placebo- and reference-TCA-controlled studies with paroxetine, which divided patients into severe [baseline Hamilton Depression (HAMD) score ≥ 28] and moderate depression (baseline HAMD score < 28). In the moderate depression group, there was little difference between the responses on par oxetine and imipramine, both of which appeared to have rather similar levels of efficacy in moderate depression. In the severe depression group, however, patients responded significantly better to paroxetine than imipramine, which was not significantly different from placebo (42).

Although the results of metaanalyses must be viewed with caution, this was not an isolated result. A similar metaanalysis of the fluvoxamine database also found an advantage for the SSRI compared with imipramine in severe depression (40).

Anxiety in Depression

A characteristic side effect of the SSRIs as a class is a transitory increase in nervousness or anxiety early in treatment in some patients. This quality might be expected to be prejudicial in treating depressed patients with prominent anxiety symptoms. Furthermore, it has often been thought that a sedative antidepressant was necessary for the treatment of anxiety in depression, and SSRIs, which lack the sedative effects of the TCAs, might therefore appear to be at a disadvantage. The metaanalyses that have been carried out indicate that, on the contrary, the

SSRIs have a differential advantage in treating anxiety within depression.

An advantage compared with a reference TCA in treating the anxiety component of depression was reported in the early small comparator study of zimelidine (48), an early SSRI briefly available in Europe. This could have been a chance finding because of the small size of the study. However metaanalyses of the databases of three SSRIs (fluvoxamine, fluoxetine, and paroxetine) have all reported an advantage for the SSRI. The advantage is reflected in an earlier response of the anxiety symptoms measured on the Hamilton Rating Scale for depression (23,41,43,66) and the Covi anxiety scale (43).

The response to SSRIs has also been investigated in metaanalyses of the databases in the subgroup of patients with more severe anxiety symptoms at the start of treatment. For example, a significant advantage was reported for fluoxetine compared with the comparator TCA in 786 patients identified as suffering from moderate or severe levels of agitation at entry to the study (41).

These results are all from retrospective analyses and have to be treated with caution. Nevertheless efficacy on anxiety symptoms accords with the positive results seen in the treatment of anxiety disorders such as panic disorder with SSRIs. The differential effects are interesting because they suggest that sedative antidepressants are not the automatic treatment of choice for the amelioration of anxiety symptoms in depression.

Suicidal Thoughts in Depression

Suicidal thoughts are present in a very high proportion of depressed patients. In studies of clinical efficacy the frequency of suicidal thoughts is high in spite of the attempts that are made to exclude these patients. It has been hypothesized that serotonin reuptake inhibitors might have a beneficial effect on suicidality and small early studies reported a differential advantage for SSRIs compared with comparator antidepressants early in treatment (48,52). Both paroxetine and fluvoxamine were found to reduce the number of suicidal thoughts more than comparator antidepressants in the metaanalyses of the databases (42,43). The response of patients with frequent suicidal thoughts at the start of treatment was also reported to be less frequent during treatment with fluvoxamine than with imipramine (66).

There have been a small number of anecdotal reports of a provocation or worsening of suicidal thoughts attributed by the authors to treatment with the SSRI fluoxetine (18,38,63). These were open observations in patients in whom suicidal thoughts did not occur de novo, many of whom were receiving concomitant medication; therefore, attribution to a particular treatment is hazardous. Suicidal thoughts are integral to depressive illness and fluctuate during the course of an episode. There is a natural increase associated with the illness, so that, if the depression worsens, so may the suicidal thoughts. This increase has been reported during treatment with placebo in the metaanalysis of the database of fluvoxamine and of paroxetine (42,43).

The metaanalyses of the databases of the SSRIs have been scrutinized for the possibility that these drugs might provoke suicidal thoughts and the evidence clearly suggests that, rather than provoking, the SSRIs protect against the emergence of suicidal thoughts. The number of patients who at the start of the study had zero or very low scores on suicidal thoughts items of rating scales and who subsequently developed high suicidal thoughts scores is seen to be significantly higher on placebo than on the active antidepressants in these metaanalyses (8,42,43).

PHARMACOKINETICS AND DRUG INTERACTIONS

Pharmacokinetics

Clinically the SSRIs discussed here behave in very similar ways and are effective in the same range of patients. They do, however, vary to some extent both in their selectivity for 5-HT receptors and in their potency. There are also some differences in the pharmacokinetics and pharmacodynamics between compounds, and these may have a bearing on clinical practice. In any discussion of relative selectivity, potency, or pharmacokinetics the metabolites of the drugs have also to be taken into account. For example clomipramine, which is a potent 5-HT reuptake inhibitor, is not included with the SSRIs because it has an active desmethyl metabolite that is a potent norepinephrine reuptake inhibitor.

Citalopram, fluoxetine, and sertraline are converted to their active metabolites which are potent and selective for serotonin. Paroxetine and fluvoxamine are transformed to inactive metabolites. The activity of the active metabolites of SSRIs on neurotransmitter reuptake varies from little in therapeutic doses, and probably not clinically relevant in the case of sertraline, to being more selective and potent than the parent drug, for example fluoxetine. Norfluoxetine is three times more selective than fluoxetine and is probably more important than fluoxetine for clinical efficacy.

The drugs discussed here are rapidly absorbed and distributed with a time-to-peak plasma concentration of 2 to 8 hr. Clearance times vary widely. The plasma half-life of citalopram is approximately 36 hr, fluvoxamine 15 hr, paroxetine 20 hr, and sertraline and norsertraline 25 hr and 66 hr, respectively. The longest is with fluoxetine, which, although the parent drug has a half-life of approximately 1 to 3 days, remains in the blood for very long periods because of the long 7- to 15-day half-life of the active metabolite, norfluoxetine. The long half-life of

fluoxetine and its metabolite imposes cautious management when treatment is to be changed, because the drug lingers in the blood for some time after the treatment has been discontinued, thereby increasing the risk of drug interactions. The persistence of the drug has some advantages for patients with irregular compliance.

There is a wide interindividual variation in steady-state plasma levels achieved with SSRIs. These drugs do not appear to be associated with a narrow therapeutic window, although there have been reports of poorer response associated with high plasma concentrations with some drugs (1,48).

Interactions

Combinations of antidepressants are sometimes used, although the benefit to be derived from polypharmacy has not been demonstrated in blinded studies and is in any case likely to be outweighed by the increased risks of the combined side effects. Drug interactions have been reported for a variety of drugs. For example, a large variety of commonly used antiarhythmics, beta blockers, neuroleptics, and TCAs, such as amitriptyline, imipramine, clomipramine, desipramine, and nortriptyline, are metabolized by the same cytochrome P450-P2-D6 system. Interactions are therefore expected and caution is needed with concomitant therapy. The SSRIs fluoxetine, citalopram, paroxetine, and sertraline are also metabolized by the same system and the same need for caution applies in varying degrees. It is not surprising therefore that interactions have been reported between TCAs and SSRIs leading to increased drug plasma levels (4,7,65). This matters less with the SSRIs, which have a wider safety margin, but may be important for the TCAs, which are often used at doses close to their toxic limit. The situation is complicated by the genetic polymorphism that exists for these enzyme systems and allows some 7% of Caucasians, for example, to be poor metabolizers of these drugs. Inhibition of their own enzyme system by some neuroleptics, antiarythmics, and SSRIs suggests that clinicians should become more cautious in the concomitant use of a wide variety of drugs and more circumspect in the use of drugs with a narrow therapeutic range or a poor safety margin. The potency of the SSRIs as inhibitors of the metabolism of the P450-P2-D6 varies and is reported in descending order of potency as paroxetine, fluoxetine, sertraline, citalopram, and fluvoxamine (17).

The combination of SSRIs with MAO inhibitors can lead to the appearance of the serotonin syndrome, which is potentially lethal. Rapid death from hyperthermia following combination of SSRI and irreversible MAO inhibitors have been reported (14) and the newer reversible MAO inhibitors may not be entirely free of risk (61). There should be an interval between treatments with an MAO inhibitor and SSRIs, which should be of a length to take the pharmacokinetics of the SSRI into account.

SAFETY AND TOLERABILITY

The SSRIs have been shown to have significantly less anticholinergic side effects compared with the TCAs and this is considered to be an important explanation for their improved tolerability. They are associated with characteristic side effects expected from their pharmacological actions.

The main side effects, which are generally mild and short-lived, are gastrointestinal symptoms and male sexual difficulties. The gastrointestinal symptoms are generally found to be mild and to reduce with continued treatment. It is important to base any assessment of the relative level of side effects on blinded comparisons with placebo in order to obtain an unbiased estimate. For example, 4% of those given paroxetine and 3% given a placebo withdrew because of nausea, which is the most common side effect (32). The gastrointestinal symptoms appear to be dose related, so that too high a dose is likely to cause nausea. Significant weight loss, mainly in those who are overweight, is seen, especially with higher doses of SSRIs. Sexual difficulties in men seems to be a consistent effect, with some two to three times more men reporting abnormal ejaculation than with active controls.

Although the SSRIs as a group are seen to improve the anxiety symptoms of depression somewhat more than comparator TCAs, a few patients experience an increase in anxiety symptoms or agitation early in treatment. These appear to have been reported more frequently with fluoxetine, which may relate to the 5-HT$_{1C}$ agonist properties of fluoxetine (69).

There are also reports of movement disorders with the SSRIs, which is perhaps not surprising in view of the close role that serotonin plays in dopamine autoregulation. Extrapyramidal symptoms are a class effect, rather than relating to one or other SSRI in particular. There have been a number of reports of movement disorders with fluoxetine, although a causal relationship has not been established (6,10,11,35,62). The number of spontaneous reports to the Committee on Safety of Medicines in the United Kingdom of this type of reaction appeared to be higher with paroxetine (15), but prescription-event monitoring studies suggest that the rate is low and that paroxetine does not cause a greater frequency of extrapyramidal reactions than other SSRIs (30).

The level of convulsions reported with the TCAs is high; a figure of 0.5% is frequently cited for the doses of TCAs used in the comparator trials. At higher doses, convulsion rates increase substantially and rates between 1% and 2% have been reported (19,27). The convulsion rate seen at doses over 200 mg of TCAs is of concern. The SSRIs as a group appear to have fewer reports of convulsions. Paroxetine, fluvoxamine, and sertraline have been reported to have significantly fewer reports of convulsions than the TCAs.

The potential for antidepressants to precipitate manic episodes in bipolar patients is widely accepted, and the use of TCAs, where the risk is elevated, is contraindicated. It has been postulated that manic switches may be associated with altered levels of 3-methoxy-4-hydroxyphenylglycol (MHPG), the metabolite of norepinephrine, it seems possible that SSRIs might have a safer profile. There is a suggestion from the controlled studies that some of the SSRIs may be associated with fewer cases of switches to mania in bipolar patients. For example, the database on paroxetine reveals that the rate of switches on paroxetine was 2.2% compared with 11.6% with comparator antidepressants (44). However this type of comparison has to be based on relatively small numbers, as bipolar patients are generally excluded from the early stages of a clinical trial program. This type of effect needs closer examination and needs to be confirmed in prospective studies.

The TCAs are associated with a high level of completed suicides attributed to overdose with the drug per million prescriptions (12). This has been attributed to the cardiotoxicity due to the ionotrophic effect of the TCAs on the myocardium. By contrast, there have been very few reports of suicide with SSRIs. In the United Kingdom, for example, the rates of suicides per million prescriptions is 34 with the TCAs compared with 1.7 with the SSRIs (Henry, *personal communication*). The SSRIs appear therefore to be relatively safe in overdose.

The level of side effects reported in placebo-controlled studies is consistently low with the SSRIs at the lower effective dose with few effects occurring with greater frequency than placebo. This contributes to the tolerability of these antidepressants and results in fewer side-effect–attributed discontinuations than is usual with the TCAs (47).

CONCLUSIONS

The SSRIs have now established themselves as a welcome new class of antidepressants. They are clearly effective with a somewhat wider spectrum of action and selective efficacy in obsessive–compulsive disorder and its concomitant depression, where the traditional TCAs are apparently ineffective. The major clinical advantage of the SSRIs lies in their improved side-effect profile and better tolerance, which is reflected in the better compliance seen even in the controlled studies. They appear safer than the TCAs on cardiotoxic measures and are associated with fewer deaths from overdosage. Increasingly clinicians are recognizing the importance of using these safer well-tolerated antidepressants as first line treatment.

REFERENCES

1. Altamura AC, Montgomery SA. Fluoxetine dose, pharmacokinetics and clinical efficacy. *Rev Contemp Pharmacother* 1990;1:75–81.

2. Amin MM, Anath JV, Coleman BS, et al. Fluvoxamine: antidepressant effect confirmed in a placebo controlled international study. *Clin Neuropharmacol* 1984;7(Suppl 1):317–318.

3. Andersen J, Bech P, Benjaminsen S, et al. Citalopram: clinical effect profiles in comparison with clomipramine. A controlled multicentre study. *Psychopharmacologia* 1986;90:131–138.

4. Aranow RB, Hudson JI, Pope HG, et al. Elevated antidepressant levels after addition of fluoxetine. *Am J Psychiatry* 1989;146:911–913.

5. Asberg M, Traskman L, Thoren P, Bertilsson L, Ringberger V-A. "Serotonin depression": A biochemical subgroup within the affective disorders? *Science* 1976;191:478–480.

6. Baldwin D, Fineberg NA, Montgomery SA. Fluoxetine, fluvoxamine and extrapyramidal tract disorders. *Int Clin Psychopharmacol* 1991;6(Suppl 1):51–58.

7. Baumann P, Bertschy G. Pharmacodynamic and pharmacokinetic interactions of selective serotonin re-uptake inhibiting antidepressants (SSRIs) with other psychotropic drugs. *Nord J Psychiatry* 1993;47(Suppl 30):13–19.

8. Beasley CM, Dornseif BE, Bosomworth JC. Fluoxetine and suicidality: absence of association in controlled depression trials. *Br Med J* 1991;303:685–692.

9. Bech P, Cialdella P. Citalopram in depression: meta-analysis of intended and unintended effects. *Int Clin Psychopharmacol* 1992;6(5):45–54.

10. Bouchard RH, Pourcher E, Vincent P. Fluoxetine and extrapyramidal side effects. *Am J Psychiatry* 1989;146:1352–1353.

11. Brod TM: Fluoxetine and extrapyramidal side effects. *Am J Psychiatry* 1989;146:1353.

12. Cassidy S, Henry J. Fatal toxicity of antidepressant drugs in overdose. *Br Med J* 1987;295:1021–1024.

13. Claghorn J. A double-blind comparison of paroxetine and placebo in the treatment of depressed outpatients. *Int Clin Psychopharmacol* 1992;6(Suppl 4):25–41.

14. Committee on Safety of Medicines. Fluvoxamine and fluoxetine—interaction with monoamine oxidase inhibitors, lithium and tryptophan. *Curr Prob* 1989;26.

15. Committee on Safety of Medicines. Dystonia and withdrawal symptoms with paroxetine (Seroxat). *Curr Prob* 1993;19:1.

16. Conti L, Dell'Osso LRF, Mussetti L, Cassano GB. Fluvoxamine maleate: double-blind clinical trial vs placebo in hospitalized depressed patients. *Curr Ther Res* 1988;43:468–480.

17. Crewe HK, Lennard MS, Tucker GT, Woods FR, Haddock RE. The effect of selective serotonin reuptake inhibitors on cytochrome P4502D6 (CYP2D6) activity in human liver microsomes. *Br J Clin Pharmacol* 1992;34:262–265.

18. Dasgupta K. Additional case of suicidal ideation associated with fluoxetine. *Am J Psychiatry* 1990;147:1570.

19. Dillier N. Worldwide clinical experience with Ludiomil. *Activ Nerv Sup* 1982;24:40–52.

20. Dominguez RA, Goldstein BJ, Jacobson AF, et al. A double-blind placebo-controlled study of fluvoxamine and imipramine in depression. *J Clin Psychiatry* 1985;46:84–87.

21. Doogan DP, Caillard V. Sertraline in the prevention of depression. *Br J Psychiatry* 1992;160:217–222.

22. Dunbar GC, Cohn JB, Fabre LF, et al. A comparison of paroxetine, imipramine and placebo in depressed out-patients. *Br J Psychiatry* 1991;159:394–398.

23. Dunbar GC, Fuell DL. The anti-anxiety and anti-agitation effects of paroxetine in depressed patients. *Int Clin Psychopharmacol* 1992;6(Suppl 4):81–90.

24. Fabre LF. A double-blind multicenter study comparing the safety and efficacy of sertraline with placebo in major depression. *Biol Psychiatry* 1991;29:353S.

25. Fabre LF, Crismon L. Efficacy of fluoxetine in outpatients with major depression. *Curr Ther Res* 1985;37:115–123.

26. Feighner J, Boyer WF, Meredith CH, Hendrickson GG. A placebo-controlled inpatients comparison of fluvoxamine maleate and imipramine in major depression. *Int Clin Psychopharmacol* 1989;4:239–244.

27. Geltzer J. Limits to chemotherapy of depression. *Psychopathology* 1986;19:108–117.

28. Glassman AH, Bigger JT. Cardovascular effects of therapeutic doses of tricyclic antidepressants. A review. *Arch Gen Psychiatry* 1981;38:815–820.

29. Heiligenstein JH, Tollefson GD, Faries DE. A double-blind trial of fluoxetine, 20 mg, and placebo in out-patients with DM-III-R major depression and melancholia. *Int Clin Psychopharmacol* 1993;8:247–251.

30. Inman WH. Paroxetine and dystonia. *Pharmaceut J* 1993;303.

31. Itil TM, Shrivastava RK, Mukherjee S, Coleman BS, Michael ST: A double-blind placebo-controlled study of fluvoxamine and imipramine in out-patients with primary depression. *Br J Clin Pharmacol* 1983;15(Suppl 3):433–438.

32. Jenner PN. Paroxetine: an overview of dosage, tolerability, and safety. *Int Clin Psychopharmacol* 1992;6(Suppl 4):69–80.

33. Johnson DAW. Depression: treatment compliance in general practice. *Acta Psychiatr Scand* 1981;63(Suppl 290):447–453.

34. Lapierre YD, Browne M, Horn E, et al. Treatment of major affective disorder with fluvoxamine. *J Clin Psychiatry* 1987;48:65–68.

35. Levinson ML, Lipsky RJ, Fuller DK. Adverse effects and drug interactions associated with fluoxetine therapy. *Ann Pharmacother* 1991;25:657–661.

36. Lydiard RB, Laird LK, Morton WA, et al. Fluvoxamine, imipramine and placebo in the treatment of depressed outpatients: effects on depression. *Psychopharmacol Bull* 1989;25:68–70.

37. March JS, Kobak KA, Jefferson JW. A double-blind, placebo-controlled trial of fluvoxamine versus imipramine in outpatients with major depression. *J Clin Psychiatry* 1990;51:200–202.

38. Masand P, Gupta S, Dewan M. Suicidal ideation related to fluoxetine treatment. *New Engl J Med* 1991;324:420.

39. Mendels J, Fabre L, Kiev A. A double blind placebo controlled study of citalopram in major depressive disorder. *NCDEU (Florida)* 1990; (abst).

40. Mendlewicz J. Efficacy of fluvoxamine in severe depression. *Drugs* 1992;43(Suppl 2):32–39.

41. Montgomery SA. The efficacy of fluoxetine as an antidepressant in the short and long term. *Int Clin Psychopharmacol* 1989;4(Suppl 1):113–119.

42. Montgomery SA. Suicide and antidepressants. *Drugs* 1992;43 (Supp 2):24–31.

43. Montgomery SA: The advantages of paroxetine in different subgroups of depression. *Int Clin Psychopharmacol* 1992;6(Suppl 4):91–100.

44. Montgomery SA. A review of the safety of paroxetine. *Eur Psychiatry* 1993;8(Suppl 1):25–30.

45. Montgomery SA, Dufour H, Brion S, et al. The prophylactic efficacy of fluoxetine in unipolar depression. *Br J Psychiatry* 1988;153 (Suppl 3):69–76.

46. Montgomery SA, Dunbar GC. Paroxetine is better than placebo in relapse prevention and the prophylaxis of recurrent depression. *Int Clin Psychopharmacol* 1993;8:189–195.

47. Montgomery SA, Henry J, McDonald G, et al. Selective serotonin reuptake inhibitors: meta-analysis of discontinuation rates. *Int Clin Psychopharmacol* 1994;9:47–53.

48. Montgomery SA, McAulay R, Rani SJ, Roy D, Montgomery DB. A double blind comparison of zimelidine and amitriptyline in endogenous depression. *Acta Psychiatr Scand* 1981;63(Suppl 290):314–327.

49. Montgomery SA, Pinder RM. Do some antidepressants promote suicide. *Psychopharmacologia* 1987;92:265–266.

50. Montgomery SA, Rasmussen JGC, Lyby K, Connor P, Tanghoj P. Dose response relationship of citalopram 20 mg, citalopram 40 mg, and placebo in the treatment of moderate and severe depression. *Int Clin Psychopharmacol* 1992;6(Suppl 5):65–70.

51. Montgomery SA, Rasmussen JGC, Tanghoj P. A 24 week study of 20 mg citalopram, 40 mg citalopram and placebo in the prevention of relapse of major depression. *Int Clin Psychopharmacol* 1993;8:181–188.

52. Muijen M, Roy D, Silverstone T, Mehmet A, Christie M. A comparative clinical trial of fluoxetine, mianserin and placebo with depressed outpatients. *Acta Psychiatr Scand* 1988;78:384–390.

53. Norton KRW, Sireling LI, Bhat AV, Rao B, Paykel ES. A double-blind comparison of fluvoxamine, imipramine and placebo in depressed patients. *J Affect Dis* 1984;7:297–308.

54. Pande AC, Sayler ME. Severity of depression and response to fluoxetine. *Int Clin Psychopharmacol* 1993;8:243–245.

55. Reimherr FW, Chouinard G, Cohn CK, et al. Antidepressant efficacy of sertraline: a double-blind placebo- and amitriptyline-controlled, multicenter comparison study in outpatients with major depression. *J Clin Psychiatry* 1990;51:18–27.

56. Rickels K, Amsterdam JD, Avallone MF. Fluoxetine in major depression—a controlled study. *Curr Ther Res* 1986;39:559–563.

57. Rosenbaum JF, Quitkin FM, Fava M, et al. Fluoxetine vs placebo: long-term treatment of MDD. *Proceedings of the American College of Neuropsychopharmacology Annual Meeting. Hawaii* 1993;32 (*abst*).

58. Roth D, Mattes J, Sheenan KH, Sheenan DV. A double blind comparison of fuvoxamine, desipramine and placebo in out-patients with depression. *Prog Neuropsychopharm Biol Psychiat* 1990;14:929–939.

59. Shaw DM, Harris B, Lloyd AT, et al. A comparison of the antidepressant action of citalopram and amitriptyline. *Br J Psychiatry* 1986;149:515–517.

60. Stark P, Hardison CD. A review of multicenter controlled studies of fluoxetine vs imipramine and placebo in outpatients with major depressive disorder. *J Clin Psychiatry* 1985;46:53–58.

61. Sternbach H. The serotonin syndrome. *Am J Psychiatry* 1991;148:705–713.

62. Tate JL. Extrapyramidal symptoms in a patient taking haloperidol and fluoxetine. *Am J Psychiatry* 1989;146:399–400.

63. Teicher MH, Glod C, Cole JO. The emergence of intense suicidal preoccupation during fluoxetine treatment. *Am J Psychiatry* 1990;147:207–210.

64. van Praag HM, Korf J. Endogenous depressions with and without disturbances of 5-hydroxytryptamine metabolism: a biochemical classification? *Psychopharmacologia* 1971;19:148–152.

65. Vandel S, Bertschy G, Bonin B, et al. Tricyclic antidepressant plasma levels after fluoxetine addition. *Neuropsychobiology* 1992;25:202–207.

66. Wakelin JS. The role of serotonin in depression and suicide: do serotonin reuptake inhibitors provide a key? *Adv Biol Psychiatry* 1988;17:70–83.

67. Wernicke JF, Dunlop SR, Dornseif BE, Bosomworth JC, Humbert M. Low dose fluoxetine therapy for depression. *Psychopharmacol Bull* 1988;24:183–188.

68. Wernicke JF, Dunlop SR, Dornseif BE, Zerbe RL. Fixed-dose fluoxetine therapy for depression. *Psychopharmacol Bull* 1987;23:164–168.

69. Zhang X, Peng L, Chen Y, Hertz L. Stimulation of glycogenolysis in astrocytes by fluoxetine, and antidepressant acting like 5-HT. *NeuroRep* 1993;4:1235–1238.

Psychopharmacology: The Fourth Generation of Progress, edited by Floyd E. Bloom and David J. Kupfer. Raven Press, Ltd., New York © 1995.

CHAPTER 90

Short-Term Treatment of Mood Disorders with Standard Antidepressants

Michael J. Burke and Sheldon H. Preskorn

This chapter surveys and synthesizes our current knowledge of the standard pharmacological treatment of acute depression and points out areas requiring further research. The information presented is based on a literature review of clinical trials, postmarketing studies, and meta-analyses since the last volume of this text. We have restricted our scope to antidepressant drugs marketed or soon to be marketed in the United States.

The treatment of mood disorders has been and continues to be in a state of dynamic evolution. In the last volume of this text, tricyclic antidepressants (TCAs) and irreversible monoamine oxidase inhibitors (MAOIs) were considered the standard antidepressant pharmacotherapy. All other antidepressant drugs were designated as ''new.'' Since that time, multiple antidepressant drugs have been approved in the United States, enjoy widespread use, and have become part of the standard pharmacopoeia for the acute treatment of major depressive disorder.

There are several different ways to classify these antidepressant drugs. One approach is by structure. Another is by the mechanism of action presumed to be responsible for the antidepressant effects (Table 1). Although the connection between these mechanisms of action and antidepressant response is hypothetical, this classification has the advantage of being based on the established pharmacology of the drugs. Such pharmacology clearly mediates some of the actions of the drugs, even if it is eventually proven that it is not responsible for their antidepressant effects. A classification based on presumed mechanism(s) of action also is more consistent with how these medications are being developed.

The focus of this chapter is to conceptualize and differentiate these major classes of antidepressant drugs in terms of efficacy, safety, and tolerability, because it is in fact the interaction of these three parameters that ultimately determines treatment effectiveness. An examination of antidepressant pharmacotherapy in terms of these three parameters generates a number of issues and questions germane to the research-oriented psychiatrist.

From the standpoint of antidepressant efficacy, important questions include, but are not limited to, dose– and concentration–response relationships, predicting response in depressive subtypes and special populations of patients, time to onset of antidepressant effect, and determining when a drug treatment trial is a failure. Important issues relative to antidepressant drug safety and tolerability include the relative adverse-effect profiles of the different antidepressant drugs and their significance with regards to special populations of depressed patients, relationship of dose and plasma concentration to adverse effects, and the potential significance of drug interactions.

One major class of standard antidepressant drugs, the selective serotonin reuptake inhibitors (SSRIs), is discussed in Chapter 89, which is devoted exclusively to this class of compounds. Only general principles of the drugs from the SSRI class or specific drug interactions will be referred to in this chapter. At present, data suggest possible antidepressant efficacy of benzodiazepines, psychostimulants, and azaspirones (e.g., buspirone) in some patients. However, drugs from these classes cannot be considered standard antidepressants at this time. Hence, they are not included in this chapter.

For more practical guidelines on the selection and usage of the currently marketed antidepressant drugs, the reader is referred to a recent how-to publication (42). This how-to approach is reasonable now that there are multiple pharmacotherapy options for treating depression, and it

M. J. Burke: Department of Psychiatry, University of Kansas School of Medicine—Wichita, Wichita, Kansas 67214.
S. H. Preskorn: Department of Psychiatry, University of Kansas School of Medicine—Wichita, and Psychiatric Research Institute, Wichita, Kansas 67214.

TABLE 1. *Classification of antidepressant pharmacotherapy by presumed mechanism of action*

Classification	Examples
Mixed NE/5-HT reuptake inhibitors	TCAs, venlafaxine
Serotonin selective reuptake inhibitors	fluoxetine, sertraline, paroxetine
Mixed serotonin effects−5 HT$_2$ receptor antagonism	phenylpiperazines like trazodone, nefazodone
Mixed NE/DA reuptake inhibitors	aminoketones like bupropion
Monamine oxidase inhibitors	
Irreversible	phenelzine, tranylcypromine
Reversible	moclobemide

NE, norepinephrine; 5-HT, serotonin; DA, dopamine; TCA, tricyclic antidepressants.

offers several advantages, not the least of which is consistency of treatment practices and improved quality of clinical data. In a sense, depression has become to psychiatry what hypertension is to internal medicine. Although the pathophysiology of depression remains elusive, the clinician can now choose from multiple drug therapies with different mechanisms of action. Failure to respond to a drug from one antidepressant class does not predict a failed response to a drug from another major class.

EVOLUTION OF ANTIDEPRESSANT PHARMACOTHERAPY

Over the last decade, drug discovery and development in psychiatry has gone from a process based almost exclusively on serendipity to a process of rational drug design by molecular targeting. Antidepressant pharmacotherapy is the first area in psychopharmacology to have benefitted significantly from such targeted development. Figure 1 illustrates the evolution of antidepressants over the past three decades. Tricyclic antidepressants and monoamine oxidase inhibitors (MAOIs) were the first successful antidepressants but their antidepressant properties were discovered by chance. Originally, TCAs were developed to be better neuroleptics. The antidepressant properties of MAOIs were found while searching for antitubercular drugs.

Such chance discoveries proved to be of seminal importance. First, they demonstrated that major depression was amenable to medical intervention just like other medical conditions, such as hypertension and diabetes. Second, they served as roadmaps to improve our understanding of the mechanisms of action mediating both their desired antidepressant effects and their undesired effects. The latter was critical to the rational drug development that followed.

The problem with drugs discovered by chance is that they frequently have multiple mechanisms of action, as is the case with TCAs, or they have such a basic mechanism of action that they impact on a wide variety of systems, such as MAOIs. Chance discovery is usually dependent on the drug having a large signal-to-noise ratio. The signal, or effect, must be larger than the background or random noise. Unfortunately, multiple mechanisms of

action also means that the drug will produce a number of undesired as well as desired effects and will also have a narrower therapeutic index than a drug rationally developed to affect only the mechanism(s) of action mediating the desired effect.

This issue can be better understood by examining the pharmacology of TCAs, which served as the cornerstone of antidepressant pharmacotherapy for almost 30 years. The TCAs have multiple mechanisms of action that occur over a relatively narrow concentration range, such that patients are likely to experience multiple effects while taking these medications (see Fig. 2 on page 1059). Some of these effects, such as the inhibition of Na+:K+ ATPase mediate potentially serious effects on cardiac conduction and occur at a concentration less than an order of magnitude above the concentration needed to inhibit the neuronal pumps for norepinephrine (NE) and serotonin (5-HT), the mechanisms of action that appear to mediate their antidepressant effects (45). This is the reason that an overdose of these drugs of only 10 times their therapeutic dose can have serious cardiotoxic effects.

From this discussion, one of the obvious goals of rational drug development is to produce agents with improved tolerability and safety. A potential downside to this strategy, given our limited understanding of the pathophysiology underlying major depression, is that a drug or class of drugs having a highly specific and hence limited range of actions might have a narrower spectrum of clinical activity in a syndromic illness like major depression. The history of medicine repeatedly shows that syndromic illnesses are usually composed of groups of heterogenously distinct conditions with different underlying pathophysiology and pathogenesis.

The dilemma then is to develop new medications with the optimal balance between the number of mechanisms of action needed for wide spectrum antidepressant activity and maximum safety and tolerability. Narrowing the pharmacological profile of new antidepressant agents offers potential advantages in terms of safety and tolerability. However, when coupled with the heterogenous nature of syndromal major depression, this may reduce our ability to detect efficacy and lead to false-negative results. With increasingly precise mechanisms of action, at what point will similar efficacy results shift from representing the

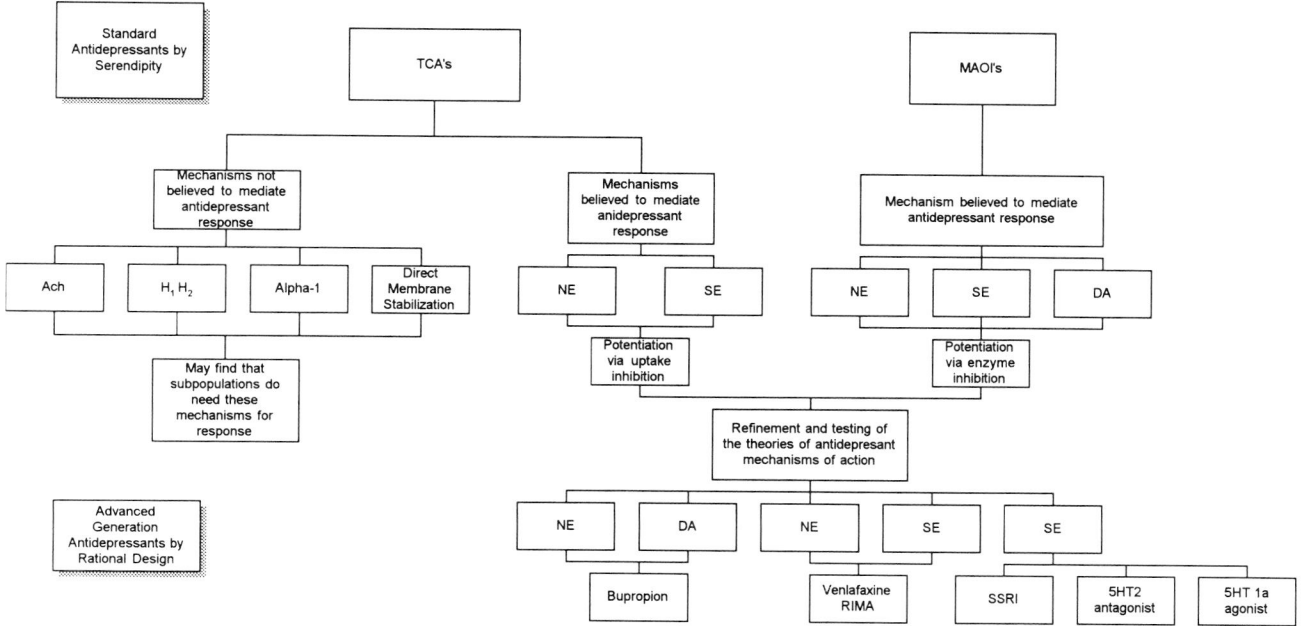

FIG. 1. The evolution of antidepressant pharmacotherapy from classes discovered by chance observation, tricyclic antidepressants (TCAs) and monoamine oxidase inhibitors (MAOIs), to those that were rationally designed to have specific mechanism(s) of action while also avoiding other effects. *NE*, norepinephrine; *SE*, serotonin; *DA*, dopamine; *Ach,* acetylcholine receptor antagonism; H_1H_2, histamine receptor antagonism; *Alpha 1,* alpha adrenergic receptor antagonism; *RIMA,* reversible inhibitor of MAO-A; *5HT1a,* serotonin$_{1a}$ receptor agonist (buspirone); *5HT2,* serotonin$_2$ receptor antagonist (nefazodone, trazodone); *SSRI,* serotonin selective reuptake inhibitor (sertraline, fluoxetine, paroxetine).

agents being studied to primarily reflecting the heterogenous patient population? How to conduct clinical trials to avoid this situation is a critical research issue.

CLINICAL TRIALS

Our ability to determine the merits of one drug over another is quite limited. To understand those limitations, one must understand the clinicals trials research done as part of the drug development process. The first thing to understand is that it is an expensive process. The cost is estimated at over 250 million dollars to bring a new antidepressant to market. For that reason, the focus of this development process is to successfully support the new drug application, which is what the Food and Drug Administration (FDA) evaluates to determine whether the drug is sufficiently safe and effective to warrant approval for marketing.

Typically, in the total clinical trials 2,500 or fewer people are treated with the new drug. Of these, only a few hundred are treated for more than a few months and even fewer patients are exposed to medications for over a year (Table 2). Hence, the cumulative human exposure to the active agent is relatively small during typical investigational drug development. As such, there are substan-

tial limits to drawing conclusions about long-term adverse effects and the cumulative safety risk of a new compound. The vast majority of data comes from trials in which the goal was to establish an optimal dose. As a result, it is not uncommon that over 90% of patients are treated with doses other than what will be commonly used in clinical practice. Also, the databases are frequently limited to at most a couple of comparator agents. Almost invariably most of the comparisons are done with a tertiary amine TCA (e.g., amitriptyline or imipramine).

The entry criteria for clinical trials in drug development is such that the population studied is a narrow subset of the population that the clinician treats. In fact, the population studied is more representative of the patients treated by primary care physicians rather than those treated by psychiatrists. The reason for limiting the scope of the patients treated goes back to the concern that if widely divergent groups are included in the trial, it will compromise the ability to determine the effects of the drug versus the natural variability of the sample being studied.

The typical clinical trial participant suffers from mild to moderate depression. All participants are screened and generally excluded if they have concomitant psychiatric illness such as psychosis, specific types of personality disorders (e.g., antisocial personality disorder), substance abuse, suicide risk, unstable medical conditions, and con-

TABLE 2. *Percent of all patients according to duration of therapy in phase II and III studies for three recently FDA-approved antidepressants*

Duration (days)	537-18-8548 (n = 1173)	534-30-9348 (n = 2171)	537-19-9348 (n = 2256)
<14	100	90	91
14–30	86	82	86
31–90	66	77	71
91–182	34	38	23
183–365	19	31	12
>365	6	17	2
>720	<1	<2	<1

Each antidepressant is identified by a nine digit number used during the premarketing research. n = total number of patients who received the investigational drug during premarketing trials.

comitant medications. There are also age (i.e., less than 18 and greater than 65 years old) and frequently gender (i.e., females of childbearing potential) exclusion criteria. The matter of restricting women of childbearing potential from the early stages of clinical trials is currently undergoing review given recent attempts to encourage research on the treatment of illnesses affecting women. An interesting area for future research would be to characterize the subpopulation of depressed patients who participate in clinical trials research. Why these patients answer advertisements for clinical trials, enter cumbersome treatment programs that disrupt their daily schedules, and agree to accept a chance of receiving a placebo is not known. Readers are referred to a specific review for further discussion of clinical trials (58).

Much of the information that clinicians would like to know will not be available for years after the medication has been released. For a new drug, the extent, duration, and diversity of human exposure expands exponentially in the first several years after marketing. However, the studies that follow marketing often suffer from significant design limitations from a research standpoint. The most frequent limitation is the absence of a placebo control group and inadequate power to separate the efficacy of one drug from another except in the most obvious ways. Properly controlled studies require funding by agencies such as the National Institute of Mental Health (NIMH). Such funding is quite limited. Hence, there are still many unanswered questions about TCAs, despite the fact that these drugs were the gold standard of treatment for major depression for nearly 30 years. The remainder of this chapter reviews the issues of efficacy, tolerability, and safety as they relate to the currently marketed antidepressants to the extent that existing data permit.

EFFICACY AND UNIQUE SPECTRA OF ACTIVITY

Efficacy is a fundamental criteria in the selection of an antidepressant agent. It would seem likely that antidepres-

sants with different mechanisms of action would have differences in either their spectrum of activity (i.e., subtypes of the disorder in which they work preferentially) or in terms of their overall efficacy (i.e., antidepressants with certain mechanisms of action would work in a larger percentage of patients). Despite this logic, there is no compelling evidence that any one antidepressant has greater efficacy than another.

There are now hundreds of antidepressant efficacy studies comparing a single drug to placebo or in the case of the newer antidepressants, the test drug may have also been compared to a TCA. Many of these studies have been well controlled, others have been partially controlled, and still others are open-label trials. Despite the size of the clinical trial literature, the ability to compare efficacy among the different classes of antidepressants has been limited in part because the average efficacy study compares only one or two agents to a placebo. More recently, the metaanalysis approach has been used to integrate the results of these separate studies into an evaluation of the relative efficacy of multiple antidepressant drugs. Meta-analysis is a well-established research method for making quantitative comparisons using the data from multiple sources (59).

Restricting the data sources to double-blind, placebo-controlled studies, the general finding from metaanalyses by independent research groups has been that (a) marketed drugs from the five major classes of antidepressants are effective when compared to placebo; (b) the overall response rate for these antidepressant drugs, in nonpsychotic depressed patients, was approximately 65% with an average placebo response of 35%; and (c) there was no evidence that the efficacy of a specific drug or drug from a specific antidepressant class was superior (4, 25,64).

When a comparator agent is used in an antidepressant clinical trial, a tertiary amine TCA, (e.g., amitriptyline or imipramine) is invariably used as the classic antidepressant. An underlying and unresolved question in this regard is what defines a "good" study when using TCAs? Comparison studies with tertiary amine TCAs are technically difficult to do because of the narrow therapeutic and tolerability ranges of these drugs. The investigator almost invariably finds himself in a no-win situation. If the study permits gradual titration of the dose, most patients on TCAs will finish on doses that many psychiatrists consider inadequate to test the efficacy of these drugs. The reason is that many patients simply cannot or will not tolerate such doses. If the study calls for aggressive dosing of the tertiary amine TCA, then there will be a large dropout rate. In that instance, the study can again be faulted for being an inadequate test of the efficacy of the TCA. In fact, both of these outcomes correctly reflect the difficulty with using tertiary amine TCAs in clinical practice.

With a 30-fold interindividual variability in plasma

drug concentration at a given dose, what is an adequate TCA dose to use for efficacy comparisons? There is compelling data to suggest that response rate to TCAs can be markedly increased by adjusting drug dose based on plasma level determinations (44). Does this mean that TCA dosing in clinical trials should be based on therapeutic drug monitoring (TDM)? If so, how should results be interpreted from studies failing to use TDM? The vast majority of clinical trials use tertiary amine TCAs. Is this the most appropriate comparison or should a secondary amine, like desipramine, which is better tolerated, be used? There are no ready answers to these questions. However, secondary amine TCAs are more potent as antidepressants than tertiary amine TCAs, and, as a result, lower concentrations of these drugs are needed for treatment. Secondary amine TCAs are also better tolerated, and there is an increased likelihood that the patient will complete a therapeutic treatment trial. These features of secondary amine TCAs suggest they would be a better comparator in efficacy studies of new agents.

For these and other reasons, we are often left to conclude that there is no difference in the overall efficacy of different types of antidepressants. The response rate (i.e., percentage of patients who experience at least a 50% reduction in the severity of their depressive episode) will be between 55% and 70%. Although remission rates (i.e., the percentage of patients who experience a complete resolution of their depressive episode) are usually not reported, these rates are approximately 10% to 20% less than response rates. Neither measure convincingly separates the existing classes of drugs.

Mixed Norepinephrine–Serotonin Reuptake Inhibitors

Among the tricyclic antidepressants (TCAs), amitriptyline and imipramine have been by far the most frequently studied, either directly or as a control for another active agent. In the vast majority of these studies, the TCA has been more effective than or equally effective to the placebo (25). In general, there was a 30% drug–placebo difference. Studies failing to demonstrate a definite superiority of TCA over placebo typically suffered from methodological inadequacies (e.g., insufficient dose, inappropriate rating scales, and small nonhomogeneous patient populations). In studies comparing amitriptyline, another tertiary amine TCA, with imipramine, the two drugs were found to be equally effective. Likewise studies comparing the secondary amine TCAs, desipramine and nortriptyline, to tertiary amine TCAs found no difference in efficacy, although secondary amines were more potent (e.g., lower doses and lower TCA plasma levels necessary for antidepressant response) (44).

The TCAs are broad acting and have been shown effective in treating all depressive subtypes. There has developed a general belief among psychiatrists that TCAs are the most effective treatment for the severe melancholic subtype of major depressive disorder, also referred to as endogenous depression and mood-nonreactive depression. In fact, the most striking response to TCAs [e.g., change on the Hamilton Depression Rating Scale (HDRS)] has been seen in severely depressed patients. This observation is consistent with work showing that higher HDRS scores and a full neurovegetative syndrome predict the greatest drug–placebo response difference (26,34).

The belief that TCAs are a more effective treatment for severely depressed inpatients is supported by the Danish University Antidepressant Group (DUAG) studies (10,11). In these controlled, multicenter trials, severely depressed inpatients had a superior response to chlorimipramine in comparison to treatment with the serotonin selective reuptake inhibitors (SSRIs) citalopram and paroxetine.

One can speculate as to why TCAs may be more effective than SSRIs in severely depressed patients. Is there an advantage to targeting more than one biogenic amine system (e.g., 5-HT and NE)? Do the other, presumed nonantidepressant effects of TCAs (e.g., antihistaminic sedation) give them an advantage in treating the severely depressed population? The former explanation is supported by a recent study with venlafaxine, also a mixed 5-HT and NE reuptake inhibitor. This drug was found to be more effective than fluoxetine, another SSRI, in treating severely depressed inpatients (62a). Like TCAs, venlafaxine is selective for NE and 5-HT systems but unlike TCAs is devoid of nonantidepressant effects on the histamine, acetylcholine, and adrenergic receptors.

Why there may be a differential response between inpatients and outpatients to antidepressants from different classes is unclear. How do depressed inpatients actually differ from outpatients? Is it only a function of severity of illness? Is it a function of comorbidity? What are the variables leading to a patient's admission for depression? Suicidality? Psychosis? Substance abuse? Once in the hospital, what factors may affect treatment response? Does inpatient status allow for more rapid titration to higher drug doses, particularly of more poorly tolerated drugs like chlorimipramine, because the patient can go to their room and lie down? Since the severely depressed patients requiring hospitalization and those with concomitant illness have been excluded from most clinical trials, the differential treatment response of these populations has yet to be clearly determined.

Serotonin Selective Reuptake Inhibitors

There is a substantial body of data to indicate that SSRIs (e.g., fluoxetine, sertraline, paroxetine) are superior to placebo and equal in efficacy to the TCAs. Like the

TCAs, the SSRIs are a broad-acting class of antidepressants. Patients who fail to respond to TCAs can still respond to SSRIs and vice versa. In double-blind crossover studies (1,16,32), 60% to 65% of patients who fail to respond to single-drug therapy with an SSRI responded when switched without breaking the blind to a secondary amine TCA such as nortriptyline or desipramine. The same percentage held true when switching TCA nonresponders to an SSRI. From a research perspective, this data is provocative, suggesting possible depressive subgroups based on pathophysiology (e.g., NE-mediated versus 5-HT-mediated). Characterizing these populations of drug-specific responders is an important direction for further study.

Phenylpiperazines

Trazodone, is currently the only marketed antidepressant from the phenylpiperazine class. In all likelihood, a second drug from this class, nefazodone, will be marketed in the United States in 1994. At one time, trazodone was the most widely prescribed antidepressant drug. Reviews of the randomized, controlled trials show that the average response rate achieved with trazodone is comparable to that seen with either TCAs or SSRIs and superior to placebo (17,28). Similar to TCAs and SSRIs, the phenylpiperazines (i.e., trazodone and nefazodone) are broadly effective with no substantial evidence to support a unique spectrum of activity. Despite this data, trazodone is considered by many psychiatrists to be a weaker antidepressant and has been criticized as being less effective in severely depressed patients. At this time, there is not ample data to resolve this issue.

One possible explanation is the dose-limiting problems of sedation and cognitive slowing or a drugged feeling on trazodone. These adverse effects may limit the number of patients who can reach therapeutic doses for antidepressant response. The problem is compounded by the short half-life of trazodone (i.e., 3 to 9 hr), which requires dosing to be divided into equal amounts given at least three times per day (36). These features of the drug may contribute to noncompliance and subtherapeutic treatment and in that way adversely affect remission rates in clinical practice. A review of trazodone efficacy studies found that those studies reporting a relatively poor response rate were characterized by use of a rapid dose escalation paradigm and a higher dropout rate (53). The conclusion was that a slower dose titration and overall lower doses (150 to 300 mg/day) maximized response.

Aminoketones

Bupropion, the only marketed aminoketone antidepressant, has been found to be an effective antidepressant in a number of double-blind studies (31,67). It is unique in both its apparent mechanism of action and its spectrum of antidepressant efficacy. It has no appreciable effect on the uptake of serotonin and its most potent action is blockade of dopamine uptake. Nonetheless, its antidepressant mechanism is unclear. Interestingly, in vitro studies using rat brain synaptosomes, found bupropion to be an order of magnitude less potent than sertraline (an SSRI) at blocking dopamine uptake (Fig. 2) (7).

There is evidence that bupropion is effective in patients who are TCA nonresponders. In double-blind, placebo-controlled trials of this agent, the largest difference between bupropion and placebo occurred in patients who had historically failed to respond to TCAs (55). In a parallel study, bupropion was compared to amitriptyline in patients with either primary or secondary major depressive disorder (MDD). In this study, secondary referred to an MDD that became apparent after the onset of another axis I diagnosis, almost invariably an anxiety disorder. Although amitriptyline was equally effective in both groups of patients, bupropion was substantially more effective in primary as opposed to secondary MDD (33). Consistent with this finding, bupropion in contrast to TCAs has been found to be ineffective in treating panic disorder patients (54). Taken together, this data supports a distinction between the clinical psychopharmacological activity of bupropion and that of TCAs.

There is limited data from uncontrolled, open trials suggesting that bupropion may have particular application in the treatment of the bipolar subtype of depression (i.e., depressed phase of bipolar disorder). In these studies, bupropion was effective in treating the depressed phase of bipolar disorder and unlike TCAs did not appear to induce rapid cycling or an affective shift to mania (24,65). Based on this data and an increasing number of anecdotal case reports, psychiatrists perceive this agent as more effective or at least less risky to use in the bipolar population. This conclusion is premature. There is clearly a need for controlled studies examining antidepressant therapy in patients with this complex mood disorder. The reader is referred to a recent review for a more detailed discussion of the somatic treatment of depression in bipolar disorder (66).

Monoamine Oxidase Inhibitors

In a recent metaanalysis of controlled efficacy studies, the response rate to MAOIs was comparable to the cyclic antidepressants (25). At one time, the TCAs were considered to be more effective than the MAOIs. A review of earlier studies showing a poorer response to MAOIs as compared to TCAs, suggested this conclusion was the result of subtherapeutic doses of MAOIs administered to treatment-resistant populations (e.g., psychotic depression). Several large, double-blind studies, which established the efficacy of phenelzine and tranylcypromine as

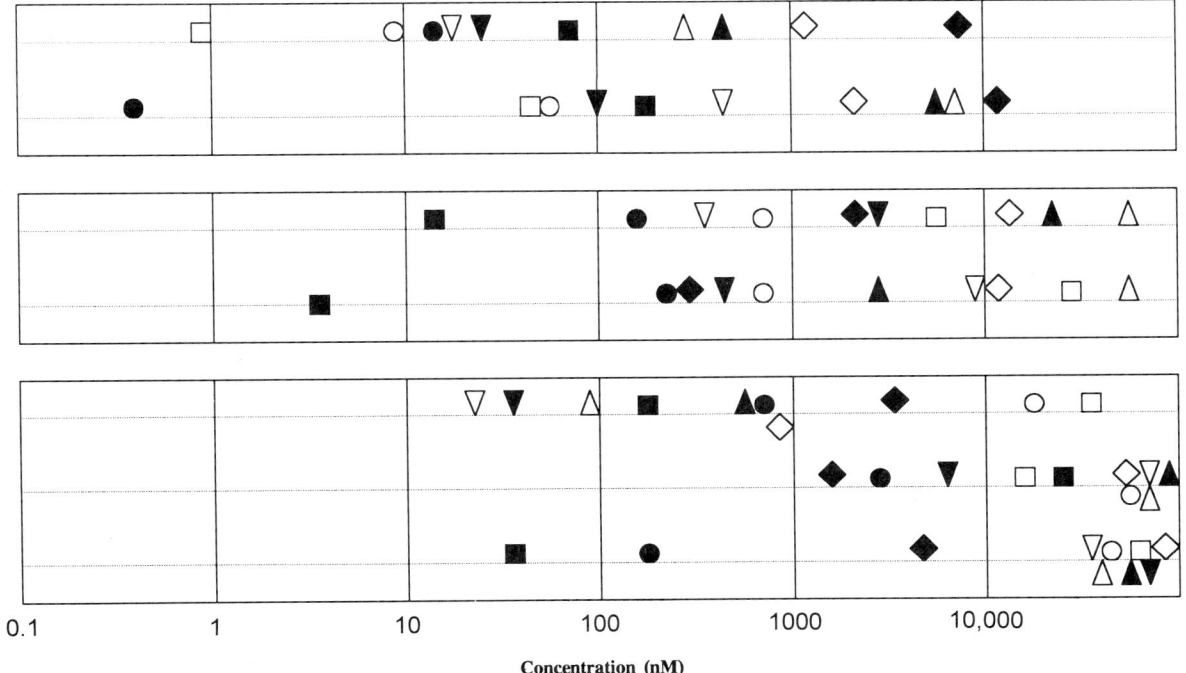

FIG. 2. Relative potencies of different antidepressants for neurotransmitter uptake inhibition and binding affinity for various types of receptors. K_i is the inhibition constant for the inhibition of neurotransmitter uptake as determined using rat brain synapatosomes and K_d is the equilibrium disassociation constant as determined using human brain receptors. Both are in nanomolar concentrations. ● NE uptake, ■ 5-HT uptake, ◆ DA uptake, △ 5-HT$_2$, ▽ 5-HT$_{1a}$, ▼ alpha^{NE}1, ▲ alpha^{NE}2, ○ Ach (musc.), □ H$_1$, ◇ D$_2$. The values are geometric mean based on results from Bolden-Watson and Richelson (7) and Cusak et al. (9).

equal to TCAs and superior to placebo, have recently been reviewed (56).

The spectrum of activity for MAOIs differs somewhat from that of TCAs (29). Whereas phenomenological predictors of response have not been identified for TCAs, SSRIs, phenylpiperazines, and bupropion, there are some clinical features that predict preferential response to MAOIs. These features include mood reactivity, irritability, hypersensitivity to rejection, hypersomnia, hyperphagia, and psychomotor agitation. They are collectively referred to as "reverse vegetative symptoms" and are thought to define an atypical subtype of depressive disorder. This subtype of depression has also been referred to as hysteroid dysphoria and mood-reactive depression. Repeated studies have found a preferential response to MAOIs in this selected population (30,56).

Uncontrolled studies and anecdotal reports have led to a belief among many psychiatrists that there is significant risk of inducing mania in depressed bipolar patients treated with an MAOI or TCA. However, a double-blind comparison with imipramine suggests that anergic, bipolar patients respond particularly well to MAOIs (60). As is the case for bupropion, further controlled studies are needed to determine the best treatment of depressive episodes in bipolar disorder. These gaps in our knowledge of treatment response in complicated depression (e.g., bipolar disorder, hospitalized patients) reflect the practice

of excluding several populations of patients important to psychiatrists from clinical trials research.

The MAOIs currently marketed in the United States are irreversible and nonselective inhibitors of monoamine oxidase. Phenelzine, tranylcypromine, and isocarboxazid inhibit both forms of monoamine oxidase (e.g., A and B). Moclobemide, marketed in 1993 in Europe, is the first selective and reversible inhibitor of monoamine oxidase-A (RIMA). Clinical trials of moclobemide in Europe have found them equal in efficacy to TCAs and superior to placebo (6). A unique spectrum of activity has not been defined for this compound.

Time To Onset of Action

The rate of onset of antidepressant action is important. The faster the illness can be brought into remission, the less the patient suffers, and the less the likelihood of suicide. Many, if not all antidepressants, have aspired to the throne of fastest onset of action; as of yet, none have convincingly claimed it (4).

In the case of TCAs, their antihistamine-mediated effects may offer the possibility of a faster drop in the total HDRS score due to sedation. Trazodone has been reported to provide early anxiolysis, but this claim has not been demonstrated under controlled conditions (51). The SSRIs have been reported to show both early activation and alternately anxiolysis. Bupropion and MAOIs have frequently been reported to have activating effects on anergic patients. Although these reported features may contribute to a psychiatrist's antidepressant selection for a given patient, there is no data to support a superior rate of onset of clinically meaningful antidepressant activity.

Part of the problem is the pharmacology of the drugs, but another part is the way onset of antidepressant action has been measured. Onset of action is usually defined as the time when the difference (on average) between a group of patients treated with the antidepressant can be separated from a group of patients treated with placebo or in rarer instances from a group treated with a comparator agent. This approach obscures and confuses the issue. It is based on the ability to detect an average difference between drug and placebo efficacy as opposed to determining the true onset of antidepressant action. The problem is further complicated by the fact that the most reproducible phenomenon in psychiatric research is the first 2-week drop in the average depression severity score in patients with major depression entered into a double-blind, placebo-controlled study.

There is also the question of what the phrase, "onset of antidepressant action" means. Some have suggested that the phrase can be defined as a drop of at least a specified minimum in the severity of the patient's depressive syndrome assessed by a standardized rating scale [e.g., Montgomery-Asberg Depression Rating Scale (MADRS) or the Hamilton Depression Rating Scale (HDRS)]. This suggestion raises many questions including what size drop would be clinically significant. Some have proposed four points on such a scale. However, these changes are not equivalent; a four-point drop at one place on the scale does not equal a four-point drop somewhere else: a drop from 8 to 4 or a drop from 34 to 30 on the HDRS may not have the same clinical impact as a drop from 20 to 16. A score of 8 on the HDRS is generally considered remission, whereas the patient with a score of 30 or 34 is severely ill. In contrast, a score of 20 is often the minimum severity score needed to enter a clinical trials treatment program, whereas a patient with a score of 16 could not. A further question concerns which four points change? If the patient has prominent insomnia, which can account for six points on the HDRS, a tertiary amine TCA can produce a four-point drop quickly due to antihistamine mediated sedation, but this is not onset of antidepressant action.

Despite these problems, the issue of rapid onset of antidepressant action is important and will continue to demand attention. It has been suggested that patients who begin to exhibit some improvement within the first week of treatment will go on to be treatment responders (18). Other researchers have suggested that the patient with an early, robust response is likely to be a placebo responder. At the other end of the spectrum, a subpopulation of slow responders has been identified (14,19). These patients were observed to require more than 8 weeks before significant improvement was observed. Because of the variance in rate of response, it has been suggested that a likely drug responder should begin to demonstrate some significant symptom reduction within the first three weeks of treatment (26). Based on this belief, clinical guidelines suggest a minimum 4- to 6-week treatment trial duration (25,42).

Therapeutic Drug Monitoring

Therapeutic drug monitoring (TDM) can serve several purposes including checking compliance and increasing the safe and efficacious use of drugs with well-defined concentration–response relationships. The underlying principles and goals of TDM of psychotropic drugs have recently been reviewed (43). General features of psychotropic drugs that make TDM useful include a small therapeutic index, large interindividual variability in the relationship between dose and plasma level, difficult detection of early toxicity, long delay in onset of action, and well-defined concentration–response relationships.

Among all classes of antidepressants, the use of TDM has been only well established for TCAs (43). The application of TDM is particularly suited to the TCAs because, as a class (a) there can be as much as a 30-fold variability in plasma TCA levels despite administration of the same dose of the same TCA to physically healthy individuals (36,41); (b) the drugs exhibit a narrow therapeutic index; and (c) plasma concentration–therapeutic response relationships have been determined (43).

The strongest of these plasma concentration–response relationships have been demonstrated for nortriptyline, desipramine, amitriptyline, and imipramine (Table 3) (44). In terms of likelihood of response, TCAs, when used based on clinically determined dose titration alone, will generally produce a response rate (i.e., at least a 50% drop in depressive symptom severity) of 60% to 70% and a remission rate of 30% to 40% (44). When the dose is adjusted based on plasma drug level monitoring, TCA remission rates increase, for example, from 30% to 42% for imipramine and from 45% to 70% for nortriptyline (35,44).

Unlike the TCAs, the SSRIs do not fit the profile of drugs that require TDM for their safe and effective use. They have a wide therapeutic index and flat dose–response curves (2,15,43). As would be predicted based on a flat dose-antidepressant response curve, attempts to determine a fluoxetine plasma concentration–response relationship have been unsuccessful (27,47). The utility of TDM with fluoxetine is even limited as a means of checking compliance due to the long half-lives of the parent compound and its metabolite. There would have to be gross noncompliance for TDM to detect it with a drug

TABLE 3. *Therapeutic drug monitoring guidelines*

Class	Concentration–efficacy	Concentration–toxicity	Recommendation

Tricyclic antidepresants (TCAs)
Tertiary amines:
  amitriptyline
  doxepin
  imipramine
  trimipramiine
Secondary amines:
  desipramine
  nortriptyline
  protriptyline
	Established ranges for 4 TCAs for efficacy in major depressive disorder:
	  nortriptyline: 50–150 ng/ml
	  desipraniine: 100–160 ng/ml
	  amitriptyline: 75–175 ng/ml
	  imipramine: 200–300 ng/ml
	Remission rates of 42%–70% in range versus 15%–29% outside range. Thus, the likelihood of full antidepressant response is 2- to 3-fold greater inside versus outside these optimal ranges.
		For all TCAs (tertiary amine > secondary amine), incidence and severity of toxicity (delirium, seizures, cardiac arrhythmias) increase as the plasma TCA level exceeds the antidepressant therapeutic range. For example, the increase in relative risk for delirium above 300 and 450 ng/ml was 13.7- and 37-fold, respectively.	Measurement of a TCA plasma level at least once during a course of treatment with these drugs at antidepressant doses. No need for repeat measurenient unless a change in clinical status of the patient, a compliance concern, or a suspected change in ability to metabolize and eliminate TCAs.

Adapted from Preskorn et al. (42).

like fluoxetine (36). The flat dose–response curves for SSRIs is compatible with their presumed mechanism of action, serotonin uptake inhibition, since the minimum effective doses of all SSRIs produce approximately 80% inhibition of platelet serotonin uptake in patients (29,36).

There is good reason to believe that TDM might be advantageous in guiding the dose adjustment of bupropion (36,43). A number of concentration–response studies have produced surprisingly consistent findings (21,23,39). These studies suggest that the highest antidepressant response rate occurs at plasma levels of bupropion in a range of 20 to 75 ng/ml. Only one of these studies measured the metabolite levels in addition to the parent compound (21). This fact is unfortunate because bupropion has a complex metabolism with three active metabolites that circulate in concentrations in excess of the parent compound (39). This issue is of more than academic interest, because in the study by Golden et al. (21) high plasma levels of these metabolites were associated with poorer antidepressant response and may be in part responsible for the seizure risk on this drug (39).

There is no substantial database to suggest utility of TDM with the use of trazodone. The metabolite of trazodone, m-chlorphenylpiperazine (m-CPP), can achieve higher plasma levels than the parent compound (36). However, the activity and function of this metabolite have not been clearly determined and plasma level–response studies on trazodone have not reported on the mCPP metabolite.

Conventional TDM is not applicable to MAOIs. However, the degree of platelet MAO inhibition appears to be a useful bioassay to guide dose adjustment. Studies support that maximum antidepressant response to the three irreversible MAOIs requires over 80% inhibition of platelet MAO (13).

Antidepressant Metabolites

The ratio of metabolites to parent compound can be highly variable based on interindividual differences in rates of biotransformation and elimination. Clinical response may at times be primarily a function of the metabolite. Therefore we need to know the pharmacology of antidepressant metabolites to properly interpret the clinical response observed in patients. We know surprisingly little about the metabolites of antidepressant drugs. Even for drug classes like the TCAs and MAOIs, after 30 years of marketing, the significance of their metabolites is unclear. The hydroxylated metabolites of TCAs inhibit biogenic amine uptake, but their potency and significance relative to the tertiary and secondary amine parent compounds is unknown. We do know that, in the elderly persons and patients with decreased renal function, the polar metabolites can accumulate several times in excess of the parent compound (37). However the clinical significance of increased levels of circulating hydroxylated metabolites, both in terms of antidepressant response and adverse effects is obscure.

In the case of clomipramine, the most potent TCA in terms of serotonin uptake inhibition, its metabolite, desmethylclomipramine, like other secondary amine TCAs, is actually a more potent norepinephrine uptake inhibitor. In some patients receiving clomipramine, more than 70% of their circulating drug concentration will be the demethylated metabolite (36). Without knowledge of the metabolite's activity and relative plasma concentration, the clinician might conclude incorrectly that a patient who fails to respond to clomipramine is not responsive to serotonin uptake inhibition and hence not use an SSRI. Further study of antidepressant drug metabolites is critical to understanding how these drugs work and how best to use them in clinical practice.

TOLERABILITY

Antidepressant tolerability is critical in the short-term treatment of mood disorders and is a critical factor in antidepressant treatment selection. Patients are already experiencing considerable morbidity secondary to their illness. Additional burden associated with the adverse effects of antidepressant treatment can lead to poor compliance and treatment failure.

Tolerability is assessed in several ways during the clinical trials development program for a new drug. One way is to note any adverse event that occurs to the patient during the treatment interval, whether or not it is believed to be related to the treatment. At the conclusion of the study, all reports of treatment-emergent adverse effects are tallied and summarized by major categories (e.g., complaints of lightheadedness, vertigo, woozy sensation, or unsteadiness may be combined into the category, "lightheadedness"). The incidence of a given adverse event category can then be compared across treatments in the same double-blind controlled studies (e.g., the incidence on the investigational drug versus the incidence on placebo versus the incidence on another marketed antidepressant).

This approach is limited by the fact that all reports of adverse effects are given the same weight whether the adverse effect occurred once during treatment or was persistent throughout the treatment period. Nonetheless, the same is also true for the placebo condition, so that the difference should be meaningful. Of clinical importance is the rate-limiting quality of a given adverse effect. This quality can be determined by whether the patient discontinues treatment as a result of an adverse effect. Such information is also recorded during the treatment trial.

It is worth emphasizing that after a drug is marketed there is never again the large-scale studies needed to address the important questions concerning tolerability and safety. Despite this importance, clinical trials have a number of limitations in determining the tolerability and safety profiles of antidepressant drugs. In a 6 to 8 week clinical trial, the development of tolerance to acute adverse effects and the occurrence of late-emergent adverse effects will likely be missed. The case of rare adverse effects (i.e., effects with a frequency of less than 1%) is particularly problematic. There may only be a chance to study 4 or 5 patients who develop the effect out of the 2,000 to 3,000 trial participants, which limits efforts to characterize rare adverse effects and determine their significance. Once the drug is marketed, the detection of adverse effects is generally dependent on spontaneous reporting by clinicians.

In terms of study design, a confounding issue is how to best assess the participants for adverse effects. This debate varies from fear of overendorsement of adverse effects by using a laundry check list approach to fear of missing important drug effects by relying completely on spontaneous reports by the trial participant. The significance of the assessment approach becomes particularly important with regard to adverse effects the patient may be hesitant to report (e.g., sexual dysfunction).

An equally important limitation in clinical trials is the focus on pharmacodynamic-mediated adverse effects at the near exclusion of those that are pharmacokinetically mediated. This is due in large part to the fact that participants are screened for medical illness and the use of other medications. As a result, significant pharmacokinetic drug interactions may not be determined until years after marketing (e.g., inhibition of P450 hepatic enzymes by fluoxetine) (36).

The problems with the tolerability of TCAs is that a number of the mechanisms of action responsible for producing adverse effects (e.g., those mediated by histamine or muscarinic receptor blockade, etc.) occur at concentrations lower than or the same as those needed to block the neuronal uptake for NE and 5-HT (Fig. 2) (7,50). As a result, rational dose adjustment based on therapeutic drug monitoring does not substantially improve the tolerability of the TCAs. The patient has to experience a large number of effects to receive the benefit of the mechanism that mediates antidepressant response.

In repeated studies, a number of adverse effects of TCAs occur in excess of placebo controls. These include anticholinergic effects (e.g., dry mouth, constipation, urinary retention, blurred vision), antihistaminic effects (e.g., sedation, weight gain), and anti-α_1-adrenergic effects (e.g., orthostatic hypotension). This adverse effect profile becomes increasingly problematic as a function of the age of the patient, because (a) elderly patients develop higher TCA plasma levels on a given dose (8); (b) older patients are more sensitive to the adverse effects (e.g., they develop TCA-induced delirium at lower plasma drug levels) (40); and (c) the multiple pharmacodynamic actions of TCAs increase the potential for additive or synergistic interaction with other drugs the elderly are likely to be taking.

There is a belief among psychiatrists that as a group the newer antidepressants have substantially fewer adverse effects. In fact, as a group the newer antidepressants have less anticholinergic and antihistaminic effects than tertiary amine tricyclics (42). As a class, the SSRIs are considerably more selective than TCAs in terms of their presumed antidepressant mechanism of action (7,50). Not surprisingly in comparison studies with tertiary amine TCAs, the average adverse effect burden and discontinuation rate secondary to adverse effects has been generally less for SSRIs (38,49,57).

However, non-TCA antidepressants are not without adverse effects. The SSRIs potentiate the effect of serotonin at all presynaptic terminals and affect a number of different regional systems in the CNS. Their adverse effect profile is consistent with this broad serotonin agonism and includes agitation, somnolence or insomnia, tremor, anorexia, sexual dysfunction, and dizziness (25,38). The incidence of nausea, diarrhea, and sexual dysfunction occur in excess of that seen in active control patients receiving tertiary amine TCAs (49).

Similar to the SSRIs, trazodone and bupropion are essentially devoid of anticholinergic and antihistaminic effects but are not without significant adverse effects. In the case of bupropion, the principal adverse effects include restlessness, activation, tremors, insomnia, and nausea (46). Although these adverse effects rarely require discontinuation, aggravation of psychosis, which has been reported, and seizures do (22).

In the case of trazodone, sedation, cognitive slowing and orthostasis are dose-limiting adverse effects (3). However, it is possible that these effects will not generalize to all drugs in this class. Results from the clinical trial development program for nefazodone (i.e., a new phenylpiperazine) suggest that these effects may be less of an issue than for trazodone (38).

The MAOIs are generally well tolerated if the patient observes the tyramine-restricted diet and avoids medications containing sympathomimetic amines. The most common and treatment-limiting adverse effect is hypotension (25,48). Although changes in blood pressure are most often orthostatic in nature, a general reduction in blood pressure can be seen in some patients. This adverse effect may present as fatigue or decreased motivation which emphasizes the importance of routine blood pressure monitoring in patients treated with a drug from this class.

SAFETY

There is perhaps no other area where rational drug development has proven more successful than in widening the therapeutic index of new antidepressant drugs and increasing their safety. This need has long been recognized, because patients with depressive episodes are at risk for taking overdoses of their medication either intentionally or through inattentiveness. Some patients who are slow metabolizers of a drug may also achieve toxic plasma concentrations on conventional doses. The latter is the case with TCAs whether the patient is a slow metabolizer due to a genetic deficiency or drug-induced (e.g., fluoxetine) deficiency in the hepatic isoenzyme 2D6 (36).

Acute Therapeutic Index

Bupropion and TCAs are the classes of antidepressants with a narrow therapeutic index. The difference between a therapeutic dose of TCA and a dose with the likelihood of causing serious toxicity can be as little as 5-fold (e.g., 150 mg/day versus 750 mg/day). The toxicity of TCAs affect the brain producing delirium and seizures and the heart producing various types of conduction disturbances and even sudden death.

There is an even narrower therapeutic index with the immediate release formulation of bupropion than with TCAs although the consequences are generally much less serious. Doses of bupropion above 450 mg/day are associated with a substantial increase in the risk of grand mal seizures (12). Seizures are themselves typically nonlethal and death is a rare possibility in overdoses of bupropion alone due to the absence of adverse effects on the cardiovascular or respiratory systems (46).

Phenylpiperazines (e.g., trazodone, nefazodone) and SSRIs have wide therapeutic indices and are nonlethal in overdose (42). However, MAOIs are somewhere between TCAs and SSRIs in terms of safety in acute overingestion.

Neurotoxicity

The CNS toxicity of TCAs is plasma concentration-dependent, often exhibiting the sequential clinical stages of agitation, delirium, seizures, coma, and death. The relative risk for delirium on a tertiary amine TCA increases 14- and 38-fold above plasma levels of 300 ng/ml and 450 ng/ml respectively (44).

The CNS toxicity of bupropion leading to seizures is dose-dependent. The seizure incidence is >0.4% at doses of 450 mg/day or less; approximately 1% at doses of 451 to 600 mg/day; and over 2% at doses of 601 to 900 mg/day (12). The pathogenesis of bupropion-induced seizures is likely to be in part pharmacokinetically mediated (36,39). This conclusion is based upon several observations: (a) the incidence of seizures is dose-dependent; (b) seizures generally occur within days of a dose increase; (c) seizures generally occur within the first few hours after the dose; and (d) bulimic patients with increased lean body mass may have a higher risk for seizures than do other patients.

Cardiotoxicity

As a class, the fundamental feature of TCAs responsible for their toxicity, in contrast to the other major classes of antidepressant drugs, is the ability to stabilize electrically excitable membranes through the inhibition of Na+:K+ ATPase. This action is responsible for their cardiotoxicity and lethality in overdose (45). The most characteristic and serious sequelae of this mechanism of action involves slowing of cardiac conduction manifested as prolongation of the QT interval, intraventricular conduction defects, and atrioventricular block leading to malignant arrhythmias (20).

The cardiotoxicity of TCAs is directly related to plasma concentration of the drug (36). The slowing of cardiac conduction by TCAs occurs even at therapeutic plasma concentrations. As TCA levels increase above the recommended therapeutic range, the incidence and severity of the cardiotoxicity increases. Above plasma levels of 350 ng/ml, 70% of physically healthy young depressed patients will develop a first-degree heart block versus less than 3% below 350 ng/ml (44).

The cardiac effects of TCAs are similar to the electrophysiological properties of the Type 1A antiarrhythmic compounds (e.g., quinidine, procainamide, disopyramide). This slowing of cardiac conduction by TCAs was believed to be of possible benefit in some patients with preexisting ventricular arrhythmias, causing reduction in premature ventricular contractions (20). Recently, this belief has been upset by findings from the Cardiac Arrythmia Suppression Trial (CAST) which demonstrated an increased mortality in cardiac patients treated with antiarrhythmic drugs. In this long-term follow up study, patients with cardiac arrhythmias and those suffering an acute myocardial infarction were more likely to have a fatal outcome if they were being treated with an antiarrhythmic drug of the type 1A class (61,62).

Since TCAs are indistinguishable from type 1A antiarrhythmic drugs, in terms of their effects on intracardiac conduction, this CAST data must now be included in the risk/benefit consideration when prescribing TCAs. Although the full interpretation is yet unclear, TCAs may become a second-line treatment for any patients suffering from cardiovascular disease or at risk for an acute myocardial infarction (e.g., age over 45, positive family history) (52).

Among the newer antidepressant drugs, SSRIs (5) and bupropion (46) have no direct effects on cardiac conduction. Trazodone had little direct action on the heart in preclinical and clinical trials. However, since its release there have been reports that trazodone aggravated arrhythmias in patients with preexisting ventricular conduction disease (63).

An important point is that TCAs were available for over 30 years before we have fully understood some of their risks. What do we actually know about the safety of newer antidepressant drugs? As discussed in the earlier section on clinical trials, results from clinical trial development programs have real limitations in terms of number of patients exposed to a new drug, the duration of that exposure, and the doses used (Table 2). Given the widespread use of antidepressants and the increasing emphasis on long-term treatment of depression, there is a pressing need for ongoing controlled studies of cumulative drug safety.

SUMMARY

Great strides have been made in the treatment of depression over the past decade due to the ability to rationally develop medications with targeted mechanisms of action. The major benefits of the new generation antidepressants have been in the areas of drug tolerability, safety, and ease of administration. The major disappointment is that remission rates have not improved. As a result, a substantial portion of patients fail to respond to single-drug therapy. This means that either there are forms of the illness that do not respond to pharmacother-

apy or that there are different forms of the illness requiring different pharmacological mechanisms of action for treatment. If the latter is the case, the challenge is to identify subpopulations of patients responding to specific pharmacological interventions rather than having to continue the trial-and-error approach with the sequential use of different agents. An alternative possibility is to develop drugs with multiple mechanisms of action that will treat a broad spectrum of patients but yet retain the tolerability and safety of the new generation of antidepressants.

REFERENCES

1. Aberg-Wistedt A. Comparison between zimelidine and desipramine in endogenous depression: a crossover study. *Acta Psychiatry Scand* 1982;66:129–138.
2. Altamura A, Montgomery S, Wernicke J. The evidence for 20 mg a day fluoxetine as the optimal in the treatment of depression. *Br J Psychiatry* 1988;153(Suppl 3):109–112.
3. Beasley C, Dornseif B, Pultz J. Fluoxetine versus trazodone: efficacy and activating–sedating effects. *J Clin Psychiatry* 1990;52:294–299.
4. Bech P. Acute therapy of depression. *J Clin Psychiatry* 1993;54(8, Suppl):18–27.
5. Benfield P, Heel R, Lewis S. Fluoxetine: a review of its pharmacodynamic and pharmacokinetic properties and therapeutic efficacy in depressive illness. *Drugs* 1986;32:481–508.
6. Berwish N, Amsterdam J. An overview of investigational antidepressants. *Psychosomatics* 1989;30:1–17.
7. Bolden-Watson C, Richelson E. Blockade by newly developed antidepressants of biogenic amine uptake into rat brain synaptosomes. *Life Sci* 1993;52:1023–1029.
8. Bupp S, Preskorn S. The effect of age on plasma levels of nortriptyline. *Ann Clin Psychiatry* 1991;3:61–65.
9. Cusack B, Nelson A, Richelson E. Binding of antidepressants to human brain receptors: focus on newer generation compounds. *Psychopharmacology* [in press].
10. Danish University Antidepressant Group. Citalopram: clinical effect profile in comparison with clomipramine. A controlled multicenter study. *Psychopharmacology* 1986;90:131–138.
11. Danish University Antidepressant Group. Paroxetine: a selective serotonin reuptake inhibitor showing better tolerance, but weaker antidepressant effect than clomipramine in a controlled multicenter study. *J Affect Dis* 1990;18:289–299.
12. Davidson J. Seizures and bupropion: a review. *J Clin Psychiatry* 1989;50:256–261.
13. Davidson J, McCleod M, Blum M. Acetylation phenotype, platelet monoamine oxidase inhibition, and effectiveness of phenelzine in depression. *Am J Psychiatry* 1978;135:467–469.
14. Dornseif B, Dunlop S, Potrin J, et al. Effect of dose escalation after low dose fluoxetine therapy. *Psychopharmacol Bull* 1989;25:71–79.
15. Dunner D, Dunbar G. Optimal dose regiment for paroxetine. *J Clin Psychiatry* 1992;53(2, Suppl):21–26.
16. Emrich H, Berger M, Riemann D, et al. Serotonin reuptake inhibition versus norepinephrine reuptake inhibition: a double-blind differential therapeutic study with fluvoxamine and oxaprotiline in endogenous and neurotic depressives. *Pharmacopsychiatrica* 1987;20:60–63.
17. Feighner J, Boyer W. Overview of USA controlled trials of trazodone in clinical depression. *Psychopharmacology* 1988;95:S50–S53.
18. Gelenberg A, Schoonover S. In: Gelenberg A, Bassuk E, Schoonover S, eds. *The practitioner's guide to psychoactive drugs.* New York: Plenum; 1991:77.
19. Georgotas A, McCue R, Cooper T, et al. Factors effecting the delay of antidepressant effect in responders to nortriptyline and phenelzine. *Psychiatry Res* 1989;28:1–9.
20. Glassman A, Preud'homme X. Review of the cardiovascular effects

of heterocyclic antidepressants. *J Clin Psychiatry* 1993;54(2, Suppl):16–22.

21. Golden R, DeVane C, Laizure S, et al. Bupropion in depression: the role of metabolites in clinical outcome. *Arch Gen Psychiatry* 1985;45:145–149.

22. Golden R, James S, Sherer M. Psychosis associated with bupropion treatment. *Am J Psychiatry* 1985;142:1459–1462.

23. Goodnick P, Sandoval R. Blood levels and acute response to bupropion. *Am J Psychiatry* 1992;149:399–400.

24. Haykal R, Akiskal H. Bupropion as a promising approach to rapid cycling bipolar II patients. *J Clin Psychiatry* 1990;51:450–455.

25. Janicak P, Davis J, Preskorn S, Ayd F. *Principles and practice of psychopharmacotherapy.* Baltimore: Williams and Wilkens; 1993: 223–240.

26. Katz M, Koslow S, Maas J, et al. The timing, specificity and clinical prediction of tricyclic drug effects in depression. *Psychol Med* 1987;17:297–309.

27. Kelly M, Perry P, Holstad S, et al. Serum fluoxetine and norfluoxetine concentrations and antidepressant response. *Ther Drug Monit* 1989;11:165–170.

28. Kerr T, McClelland H, Stephens D, et al. Trazodone: a comparative clinical and predictive study. *Acta Psychiatry Scand* 1984;70: 573–577.

29. Lemberger L, Bergstrom R, Wolen R, et al. Fluoxetine: clinical pharmacology and physiologic disposition. *J Clin Psychiatry* 1985;46(3, sec 2):14–19.

30. McGrath P, Stewart J, Harrison W, et al. Predictive value of symptoms of atypical depression for differential drug outcome. *J Clin Psychopharmacol* 1992;12:197–202.

31. Meredith C, Feighner J. The use of bupropion in hospitalized depressed patients. *J Clin Psychiatry* 1983;44(5, sec. 2):85–87.

32. Nystrom C, Ross S, Hallstrom T, et al. Comparison between serotonin and norepinephrine reuptake blocker in the treatment of depressed outpatients: a crossover study. *Acta Psychiatry Scand* 1987;75:377–382.

33. Othmer S, Othmer E, Preskorn S, et al. Differential effect of amitriptyline and bupropion on primary and secondary depression: a pilot study. *J Clin Psychiatry* 1988;49:310–312.

34. Paykel E, Hollyman J, Freeling P, et al. Predictor for therapeutic benefit from amitriptyline in mild depression: a general practice placebo controlled trial. *J Affect Dis* 1988;145:83–95.

35. Perry P, Browne J, Alexander B, et al. Relationships of free nortriptyline levels to therapeutic response. *Acta Psychiatry Scand* 1985;72:120–125.

36. Preskorn S. Pharmacokinetics of antidepressants: why and how are they relevant to treatment. *J Clin Psychiatry* 1993;54(9, suppl): 14–34.

37. Preskorn S. Recent pharmacologic advances in antidepressant therapy for the elderly. *Am J Medicine* 1993;94(suppl 5A):2S–12S.

38. Preskorn S. Safety and tolerability of antidepressants. *J Clin Psychiatry* [in press].

39. Preskorn S. Should bupropion dose be adjusted based upon therapeutic drug monitoring? *Psychopharmacol Bull* 1991;27:637–643.

40. Preskorn S. Tricyclic antidepressants: the whys and hows of therapeutic drug monitoring. *J Clin Psychiatry* 1989;50(Suppl):34–42.

41. Preskorn S, Bupp S, Weller E, et al. Plasma levels of imipramine and metabolites in 68 hospitalized children. *J Am Acad Child Adolesc Psychiatry* 1989;3:373–375.

42. Preskorn S, Burke M. Somatic therapy for major depressive disorder: selection of an antidepressant. *J Clin Psychiatry* 1992;53(9, Suppl):5–18.

43. Preskorn S, Burke M, Fast G. Therapeutic drug monitoring: principles and practice. *Psychiatr Clin N Am* 1993;16(3):611–645.

44. Preskorn S, Fast G. Therapeutic drug monitoring for antidepressants: efficacy, safety, and cost effectiveness. *J Clin Psychiatry* 1991;52(6, Suppl):23–33.

45. Preskorn S, Irwin H. Toxicity of tricyclic antidepressants: kinetics,

mechanism, intervention: a review. *J Clin Psychiatry* 1982;43: 151–156.

46. Preskorn S, Othmer S. Evaluation of bupropion hydrochloride: the first of a new class of atypical antidepressants. *Pharmacotherapy* 1984;4:20–34.

47. Preskorn S, Silkey B, Beber J, et al. Antidepressant response and plasma concentration of fluoxetine. *Ann Clin Psychiatry* 1991;3: 147–151.

48. Rabkin J, Quitkin F, Harrison W, et al. Adverse reactions to monoamine oxidase inhibitors, part I: a comparative study. *J Clin Psychopharmacol* 1984;4:270–278.

49. Reimherr F, Chouinard G, Cohn C, et al. Antidepressant efficacy of sertraline: a double-blind, placebo- and amitriptyline-controlled, multicenter comparison study in outpatients with major depression. *J Clin Psychiatry* 1990;51(12, Suppl B):18–27.

50. Richelson E. Biological basis of depression and therapeutic relevance. *J Clin Psychiatry* 1991;52(6, Suppl):4–10.

51. Rickels K, Downing R, Schweizer E, Hassman H. Antidepressants for the treatment of anxiety disorders. *Arch Gen Psychiatry* 1993;50:884–895.

52. Roose S. What is the role of concomitant cardiovascular disease in the selection of an antidepressant? *J Clin Psychiatry* [in press].

53. Schatzberg A. Dosing strategies for antidepressant agents. *J Clin Psychiatry* 1991;52(5, Suppl):14–20.

54. Sheehan D, Davidson J, Manschreck T, et al. Lack of efficacy of a new antidepressant (bupropion) in the treatment of panic disorder with phobias. *J Clin Pharmacol* 1983;3:28–31.

55. Stern W, Harto-Truax N, Bauer N. Efficacy of bupropion in tricyclic resistant or intolerant patients. *J Clin Psychiatry* 1983;44(5, sec 2):148–152.

56. Stewart J, McGrath P, Rabkin J, Quitkin F. Atypical depression: a valid clinical entity? *Psychiatr Clin N Am* 1993;16(3):479–495.

57. Stokes P. Fluoxetine: a five year review. *Clin Ther* 1993;15 (2):216–243.

58. Stokes P. The changing horizon in the treatment of depression: scientific/clinical publication overview. *J Clin Psychiatry* 1991;52 (5, Suppl):35–43.

59. Thacker S. Meta-analysis: a quantitative approach to research integration. *JAMA* 1988;259:1685–1689.

60. Thase M, Mallinger A, McKnight D, Himmelhoch J. Treatment of imipramine-resistant recurrent depression. IV: a double blind crossover study of tranylcypromine for anergic bipolar depression. *Am J Psychiatry* 1992;149:195–198.

61. The Cardiac Arrythmia Suppression Trial (CAST) Investigators. Preliminary report: effect of encainide and felcainide on mortality in a randomized trial of arrythmia suppression after myocardial infarction. *N Engl J Med* 1989;321:406–412.

62. The Cardiac Arrythmia Supression Trial II Investigators. Effect on the antiarrythmic agent moricizine on survival after a myocardial infarction. *N Engl J Med* 1992;327:227–233.

62a. The Venlafaxine Inpatient Study Group. A double-blind comparison of venlafaxine and fluoxetine in patients hospitalized for major depression and melancholia. *Int J Clin Psychopharmacol* [in press].

63. Vitullo R, Wharton J, Allen N, et al. Trazodone-related exercise-induced nonsustained ventricular tachycardia. *Chest* 1990;98: 247–248.

64. Workman E, Short D. Atypical antidepressants versus imipramine in the treatment of major depression: a meta-analysis. *J Clin Psychiatry* 1993;54:5–12.

65. Wright G, Galloway L, Kim J, et al. Bupropion in the long-term treatment of cyclic mood disorders: mood stabilizing effects. *J Clin Psychiatry* 1985;46:22–25.

66. Zornberg G, Pope H. Treatment of depression in bipolar disorder: new directions for research. *J Clin Psychopharmacol* 1993;13: 397–408.

67. Zung W. Review of placebo controlled trials with bupropion. *J Clin Psychiatry* 1983;44(5, sec 2):104–114.

Psychopharmacology: The Fourth Generation of Progress, edited by Floyd E. Bloom and David J. Kupfer. Raven Press, Ltd., New York 1995.

CHAPTER 91

Long-Term Treatment of Mood Disorders

Robert F. Prien and James H. Kocsis

This chapter deals with research findings, issues, and strategies relating to the long-term treatment of unipolar and bipolar mood disorders (see Chapter 73, *this volume*). There is increasing recognition of the importance of looking beyond the acute episode in treatment planning. This is evidenced by recent clinical practice guidelines developed by the U.S. Agency for Health Care Policy and Research (AHCPR) and the American Psychiatric Association (APA) that provide information on continuation and maintenance treatment of depression and encourage strategic planning to meet the long-term treatment needs of the patient (6,17). A set of APA guidelines for bipolar disorder also emphasize the need for long-term therapy (5).

For the purpose of this chapter, the term *unipolar depression* refers to a depressive disorder with no history of a manic or unequivocal hypomanic episode. *Bipolar disorder* refers to a mood disorder with a history of at least one manic episode, sometimes labeled as bipolar I to distinguish it from bipolar II that requires at least one episode of major depression and a history of hypomania but not mania.

COURSE OF ILLNESS AND NEED FOR LONG-TERM TREATMENT

A significant proportion of individuals with major depressive disorder have a course of illness characterized by recurrence and/or chronicity. Longitudinal naturalistic studies and placebo-controlled therapeutic trials indicate that over 50% of individuals who have an initial episode

R. F. Prien: Clinical Treatment Research Branch, Division of Clinical and Treatment Research, National Institute of Mental Health, Rockville, Maryland 20857.
J. H. Kocsis: Department of Psychiatry, Cornell University Medical College–New York Hospital, New York, New York 10021.

of major depression will have one or more recurrences (17). Bipolar disorder presents an even higher risk of recurrence. Patients with an initial episode of mania have an 80% to 90% probability of a recurrence (29). Recurrences for both unipolar and bipolar disorder tend to occur more frequently with each successive episode (8). These recurring episodes not only cause significant disruption in social, familial, and occupational functioning but may be fatal. Approximately 15% of individuals with a mood disorder commit suicide.

Although the prevention of recurrence is a priority objective for treatment research and practice, it should not divert attention from the disruption that can occur during the intervals between major episodes. The classical portrayal of recurrent mood disorders as a series of discrete episodes with minimal or no symptoms between episodes has been modified by studies showing that many patients with major mood disorder have a course characterized by insidious onset of episodes with incomplete symptom recovery and impaired functioning between episodes (38,78). An estimated 20% to 35% fail to recover fully from any given episode (6,38). The incomplete recovery may be from inadequate treatment of the episode, a preexisting chronic disorder, or the progressive deteriorative effects of recurring episodes.

PHASES OF TREATMENT

The treatment of mood disorders can be categorized into three interlocking phases: acute, continuation, and maintenance. Figure 1 illustrates these phases in a schematized episode of unipolar depression. This figure was developed to conceptually frame the sequence of significant change points in the course of a depressive disorder rather than to set standard practice guidelines (43). The relationship of the phases and possible outcomes represented in the figure are discussed below.

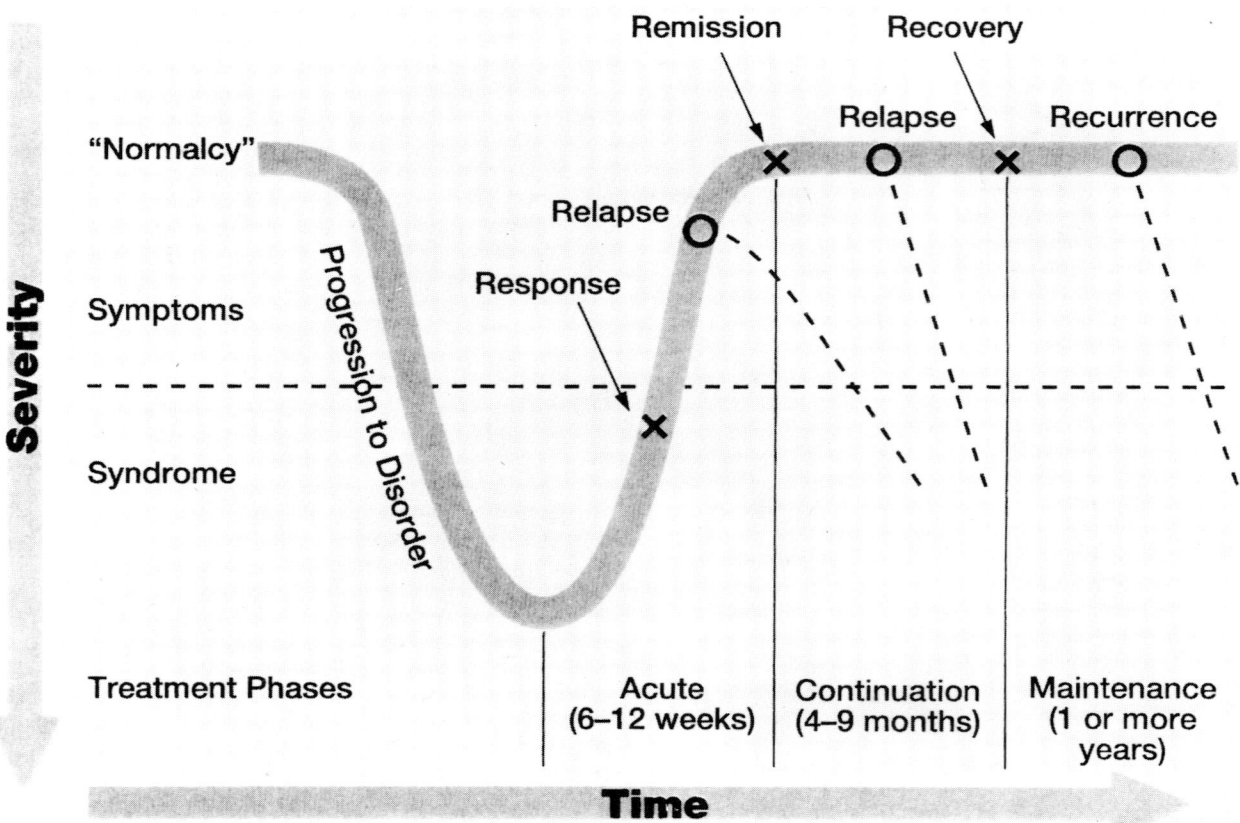

FIG. 1. Phases of unipolar depression. Adapted with permission from ref. 43 and reprinted from *Depression in Primary Care: Detection, Diagnosis, and Treatment. Quick Reference Guide for Clinicians, Number 5,* Agency for Health Care Policy and Research, AHCPR Publication No. 93-0552, 1993.

Acute Treatment

The acute phase of treatment aims at achieving remission of the acute symptoms of the episode. Remission may be defined as the return to the individual's premorbid or well self (72). In research, a remission often is declared when the individual no longer meets diagnostic criteria for the syndrome and has no more than minimal symptoms (25). When a treated patient shows significant improvement (with or without a remission), a treatment response is declared. In the research literature, a treatment response often is defined in terms of reduction in the severity of the syndrome. Usually, a clinically significant response requires at least a 40% to 50% reduction in the baseline level of severity. Failure to achieve a treatment response within 6 to 8 weeks with an adequate dose of an antidepressant or within 12 to 16 weeks with a psychotherapy targeted for symptom relief should cause one to consider an alternative treatment.

Continuation Treatment

Continuation treatment will be discussed more fully in the next section. Briefly, the purpose of this phase of treatment is to stabilize the remission and prevent a return of the symptoms of the acute phase, that is, a relapse. The pharmacotherapy that led to remission is usually maintained during the continuation phase. It is recommended that continuation therapy be maintained for at least 4 months if there is no reappearance of acute symptoms (17,61). Typically, however, there are symptomatic breakthroughs that prolong the continuation phase, sometimes for as long as 9 to 12 months.

Maintenance Treatment

The declaration of a recovery designates that the episode is over and presents the option of either discontinuing treatment or continuing it as a maintenance therapy with the aim of preventing a new episode. Following recovery, a subsequent episode traditionally is labeled a "recurrence" rather than a "relapse" to signify that it represents a new episode rather than a continuation or reemergence of the original episode.

CONTINUATION TREATMENT

Need for Continuation Treatment

Continuation treatment is based upon the assumption that episodes of depression or mania do not necessarily end with the treatment-induced remission of acute symptoms. One theory is that antidepressant and antimanic drugs may suppress symptoms without immediately correcting the postulated biological process or pathophysiology underlying the episode (33,61). As a result, even with successful treatment there may be a gap of months between the disappearance of overt symptoms and the end of the episode.

There is evidence from over a dozen placebo-controlled studies to support the need for continuation of pharmacotherapy following remission of symptoms for both unipolar and bipolar disorders (58,61,72). All of the studies used a double-blind discontinuation design in which an antidepressant or lithium was used to achieve remission, after which approximately half of the sample received a placebo and the other half continued to receive the medication. All provide relapse rates for the 6 months following randomization to continuation treatment. Overall, approximately 50% of the patients treated with placebo relapsed, compared to only 20% receiving medication. Most of the relapses occurred within 3 months.

Discontinuation studies for electroconvulsive therapy (ECT) show a rate of relapse similar to that occurring after withdrawal of antidepressants or lithium (4,58,68). A standard practice is to initiate continuation treatment with an antidepressant following the ECT-induced remission of acute symptoms. However, patients do not appear to benefit from continuation treatments that were ineffective in treating prior acute episodes. Sackeim et al. (68) suggested that one alternative is to continue ECT on an intermittent basis following symptomatic response. Recent retrospective reports tend to find continuation ECT helpful. Continuation ECT is endorsed by an APA report (4).

Duration

The most critical decision with continuation treatment is how long treatment should be maintained to ensure that the episode is over. The decision is not a problem if the patient is to be maintained on the same treatment for prevention of new episodes. However, if the intention is to discontinue the medication after recovery from the episode, uncertainty as to when the episode is over may result in premature withdrawal of treatment, resulting in relapse or unnecessary prolongation of treatment.

When a medication is successful in suppressing manifest symptoms, it is difficult to determine when the episode is over and continuation treatment is no longer required. A further complication is raised by Hollen et al. (33) who suggested that there may be two types of continuation treatment: (1) suppressive and (2) curative. Suppressive treatment blocks manifest symptoms without alleviating the underlying episode, whereas curative treatment alters the episode by shortening the time period that the episode would have run if left untreated. Although these categories have heuristic significance, they require further research to differentiate one from the other in making treatment decisions.

With major depression, a frequent practice is to continue medication for 4 to 12 months following remission of symptoms and then gradually reduce dosage while carefully monitoring the patient for signs of an emerging episode (6,17). The recommendation for continuing medication for at least 4 months is based upon findings indicating that risk of relapse is significantly reduced after the patient has remained in remission for at least 16 to 20 weeks (23,49,61,64). A recent review of both controlled and naturalistic data indicates that a continuation treatment period of 4 to 5 months reduces relapse rates to approximately 20% (45). This finding is used sometimes to define the boundary between remission of symptoms and recovery from the episode. For some patients, however, 4 to 5 months is not enough. The presence of residual (subsyndromal) symptoms is a sign that the patient may still require continuation treatment. Reports from three multicenter collaborative studies and several other trials suggest that even mild or moderate symptoms signal that the patient is at high risk for relapse if treatment is withdrawn (40,48,61,73).

In making decisions about withdrawal of continuation therapy, the clinician should be wary about relying solely upon clinical symptoms. A study on maintenance drug therapy coordinated by the National Institute of Mental Health (NIMH) found that the Global Assessment Scale (19) which evaluates both clinical symptoms and impairment of functioning was a more sensitive predictor of relapse than assessment instruments that focus exclusively on clinical symptoms. This finding and data from other studies (78) tend to support the need for instruments that can be used to evaluate both clinical state and functional status in predicting outcome for the continuation and maintenance phases of treatment. There should also be increased attention to the numerous other risk factors for relapse, including chronicity that does not respond to appropriate therapies, patient noncompliance, comorbid medical illnesses, and psychiatric disorders, especially personality disorders, and ongoing or renewed psychosocial stressors (10,45).

Biological Markers

During the past decade, there has been increased effort to identify a biological marker of recovery from a depressive episode (a state-dependent marker). A valid state marker would not only aid in determining when continuation treatment can be safely withdrawn but also might be useful in detecting an emerging episode before the appearance of overt symptoms. Some progress has been made with rapid eye movement (REM) dysregulation, slow-wave sleep (SWS) alterations, and dysregulations in the hypothalamic–pituitary–adrenal axis and hypothalamic–pituitary–thyroid axis (10,44,74). Kupfer (44) has proposed an innovative biological model of recurrent depression that attempts to differentiate biological measures associated with persistent features of depressive disorder (type 1) from episodic features (type 2). Type 2 episodic changes appear to be strongly correlated with REM sleep dysregulation and level of acute stress whereas type 1 alterations seem more associated with SWS alterations and growth hormone regulation. Data suggest that the model may allow predictions for acute and long-term treatment and provide a better understanding of the pathophysiology of depressive disorder. However, currently this and related research is not at a stage where it can be applied in clinical practice. This concurs with the conclusion from a European Consensus Conference (8) that no single biological marker could be recommended for determination of the endpoint of a depressive episode or the evaluation of treatment outcome.

Dose

There are three basic dosage strategies for continuation treatment: (a) maintaining the dose at the level that effectively treated acute symptoms; (b) reducing the dose to a fixed level, for example, to half of the acute therapeutic level or to the equivalent of 150 mg/day of imipramine; and (c) reducing the dose in graduated steps, with a rapid buildup at the signs of an emerging relapse. This has been a controversial issue. However, recent research with recurrent depression suggests that patients should continue to receive the full therapeutic dose used to attain remission of acute symptoms, providing that there are no significant adverse reactions or dose-related negative effects on patient compliance (6,17,24). A similar finding has been reported for treatment of dysthymia (41).

Withdrawal of Continuation Medication

Care should be taken in withdrawing continuation medication following completion of the episode. Rapid discontinuation of heterocyclic antidepressants, particularly tertiary amine tricyclics, can produce withdrawal effects such as sleep disturbance, gastrointestinal symptoms, behavioral activation, agitation, and irritability (66). Many of these withdrawal symptoms are indistinguishable from an emerging relapse and may lead the clinician to misinterpret the need for continued medication. Also, there is

evidence suggesting that rapid withdrawal of an antidepressant may produce an increased risk of early mania in susceptible patients (29). Current convention is that the dose of heterocyclic agents be tapered over a period of a month or more. It is not clear if a similar tapering schedule is needed for newer antidepressants. Fluoxetine with its long life does not appear to require a slow taper. In any case, the patient should be monitored during and after withdrawal to ensure that recovery from the episode is complete. Similar care should be applied to the management of bipolar disorder with lithium.

Continuation Psychotherapy

The need for continuation treatment following standardized short-term psychotherapies (cognitive therapy, interpersonal therapy, and behavioral treatment approaches) has not been as well studied as continuation therapy for medication. Published data from naturalistic follow-up studies suggest that the relapse rate following successful acute-phase cognitive therapy is on the order of 40% to 60%, similar to that for medication (17). Two studies that extended cognitive therapy for 8 months following successful acute treatment of major depression report low relapse rates of 19% (35) and 23% (12).

A recent study of cognitive therapy reports that patients who show only partial remission during acute treatment are at higher risk for relapse than patients who achieve a full remission (73). The relapse rate during the 6 months following a 20-week program of cognitive therapy was 52% for patients with partial remission and only 9% for patients with a full remission. The investigators strongly recommend that models of longer term psychotherapy be developed for depressed patients who do not show full remission during time-limited cognitive therapy. The need for longer term models for short-term psychotherapies is further emphasized by a follow-up study of patients from the NIMH Treatment of Depression Collaborative Research Program who had been successfully treated with cognitive behavior therapy, interpersonal therapy, or imipramine over a 16-week period (70). The major finding is that 16 weeks of these specific treatments is insufficient for most patients to sustain remission and achieve full recovery from the episode.

There is only one study of continuation interpersonal therapy. It found that patients who received continuation interpersonal therapy had better social, vocational, and marital adjustment after a 1-year follow-up than patients who had no continuation therapy (77). This study, conducted in the 1970s, has not been replicated.

Continuation Treatment For Bipolar Disorder

Continuation treatment for bipolar illness may pose a different set of problems than exist for unipolar disorder.

Because of the high risk of recurrence, patients with bipolar disorder are likely to be maintained on medication following recovery from an episode. Thus, there may be no need for the clinician to judge when the episode is over and when continuation medication can be safely withdrawn. However, there may be a need for adjustment of treatment during or after the continuation phase. Lithium, the treatment of choice for pure mania, often is supplemented by neuroleptics for more rapid onset of action or by anticonvulsants or benzodiazepines if the patient fails to respond adequately to lithium alone (63). With the waning of acute symptoms, consideration should be given to discontinuing the neuroleptic before it becomes a routine adjunct to lithium for long-term maintenance and exposes the patient to risk of tardive dyskinesia or other adverse reactions. Other combinations also may warrant dismantling to determine whether the patient needs more than one medication to sustain improvement. Other problems arise with patients who have dysphoric mania, bipolar major depression, or acute rapid cycling. There is only limited information on the appropriate long-term treatment for these subtypes of bipolar disorder (see the section on maintenance treatment).

MAINTENANCE TREATMENT

There is ample evidence supporting the efficacy of antidepressants and mood stabilizers for the maintenance treatment of mood disorders. The major issues are (a) who should receive treatment; (b) what treatments should be used; and (c) how long treatment should continue.

Who To Treat

A critical factor in deciding whether or not to initiate maintenance treatment is the likelihood of a recurrence in the near future and the impact it might have on the patient's career, family relations, and overall functioning. Most investigators who have published an opinion on the use of maintenance therapy recommend that patients with major depression should have two or three well-defined episodes before receiving maintenance treatment. The AHCRP Clinical Practice Guideline (17) strongly recommends maintenance treatment for individuals who have three or more episodes. The Guideline also recommends maintenance medication for individuals with two episodes who have one or more of the following characteristics: (1) a family history of bipolar disorder or recurrent depression; (2) early onset of the first episode (before age 20); and (3) both episodes occurred during the past 3 years and were sudden and severe or life-threatening. The World Health Organization (WHO) consensus statement on the pharmacotherapy of depressive disorders also recommends that maintenance therapy be initiated after three episodes, particularly if there have been two episodes in

the last 5 years (79). There is general agreement that patients who have only a single episode of major depression, mild episodes, or a lengthy interval between episodes (e.g., 5 years) probably should not be started on maintenance treatment. The exception is the patient for whom a second episode would have severely disruptive or life-threatening consequences.

Naturalistic studies tend to support the aforementioned recommendations, confirming that patients with a history of three or more episodes are at high risk for an early recurrence or unremitting chronic course (40). A study by Maj et al. (47) assessing the pattern of recurrence after recovery from an episode of major depression found that a history of three or more episodes was the most powerful predictor of an early recurrence. In a study of over 400 patients followed for 20 years, Angst (7) reports that patients who have two major episodes within 5 years have a 70% probability of developing two or more episodes during the following 5 years.

In general, bipolar disorder generates more urgency for early intervention than unipolar disorder. The WHO consensus statement recommends that patients with bipolar illness receive maintenance treatment after two episodes (79). Goodwin and Jamison (29) suggest more stringent guidelines. They recommend that maintenance treatment be considered after the initial manic episode if the episode has a sudden onset, is highly disruptive or life-threatening, or occurs in an adolescent, especially if there is substantial genetic loading.

There are factors other than the frequency and severity of prior episodes that should be considered in decisions about maintenance treatment. These include the rapidity of onset of prior episodes, contraindications to treatment, extenuating circumstances that may have contributed to prior episodes, and, perhaps most important, the patient's willingness to commit himself or herself to the treatment program.

Choice of Treatment: Unipolar Disorder

Evidence From Maintenance Studies

There have been numerous placebo-controlled trials evaluating long-term pharmacotherapy in unipolar disorder. Table 1 lists studies that used a placebo control and had a duration of at least 1 year. The 15 listed studies evaluated 11 medications, 10 of which were found to be superior to placebo in at least one study. Ideally, a design for determining the efficacy of an antidepressant in preventing recurrence should have four components: (1) a sample at high risk for recurrence; (2) a placebo control; (3) a minimum 4-month period of remission or symptom-free interval preceding randomization to maintenance treatment; and (4) at least a 2-year maintenance phase. Three of the studies listed in Table 1 satisfied all four

TABLE 1. *Maintenance treatment studies for unipolar disorder*

Study	Symptom-free interval	Length of study (yr)	Treatment	Total N	Outcome[a]
Bjork et al. (11)	4 months	1	Zimelidine	38	Z > P
			Placebo		
Coppen et al. (15)	6 weeks	1	Amitriptyline	29	A > P
			Placebo		
Coppen et al. (16)	Undefined[b]	2	Lithium	26	L > P
			Placebo		
Doogan et al. (18)	Undefined	1	Sertraline	295	S > P
			Placebo		
Eric et al. (20)	Undefined	1	Paroxetine	125	Pa > P
			Placebo		
Frank et al. (23)	17 weeks	3	Imipramine	51	I > P
			Placebo		
Georgotis et al. (27)	4 months	1	Phenelzine	51	Ph > P
			Nortriptyline		Ph > N
			Placebo		N = P
Glen et al. (28)	Undefined	3	Lithium	28	L = A = P
			Amitriptyline		
			Placebo		
Kane et al. (37)	6 months	2	Lithium	19	L > P
			Imipramine		L > I
			Placebo		I = P
Montgomery et al. (49)	18 weeks	1	Fluoxetine	220	F > P
			Placebo		
OADIG (53)	8 weeks	2	Diothepin	69	D > P
			Placebo		
Prien et al. (60)	Undefined[b]	2	Lithium	88	L > P
			Imipramine		I > P
			Placebo		L = I
Prien et al. (62)	2 months	2	Lithium	110	L > P
			Imipramine		I > P
			Placebo		L > I
Robinson et al. (65)	16 weeks	2	Phenelzine	47	Ph > P
			Placebo		
Rouillan et al. (67)	Undefined	1	Maprotiline	1141	M > P
			Placebo		

[a] Based on *p* = 0.05 level of significance.
[b] Maintenance treatment initiated at discharge from hospital.

components (23,37,65). Eight met all but one requirement (11,16,27,28,49,53,60). The remaining four failed to satisfy two or more requirements (15,18,20,67). Six studies did not include a defined symptom-free interval (16,18, 20,28,60,67). All six were multisite trials in which patients who showed a satisfactory response during acute treatment were randomly assigned to maintenance treatment without an intervening stabilization of remission or a symptom-free period. Two of these studies made no distinction between a relapse and a recurrence (28,67).

Despite the variation in design of the maintenance trials, the significant difference between drug and placebo in the large majority of studies provides evidence that antidepressants and mood stabilizers such as lithium can reduce the occurrence of new episodes in unipolar disorder. In most studies, the recurrence rate for placebo was more than twice that for active medication. The findings also show that none of the medications is a panacea. Even the most favorable results indicate failure in at least one-fourth of patients. Overall, there is no solid evidence that any one treatment is superior to another in preventing recurrences. Success with a given medication may vary from one study to another, often due to differences in study design and application of treatment. The classic example is imipramine which was evaluated in four of the studies. The recurrence rates were 22% (23), 46% (62), 48% (60), and 83% (37). Corresponding rates of recurrence for placebo were 78%, 71%, 92%, and 100%. The best results with imipramine were obtained by Frank et al. (23) who, paradoxically, used the patient sample at highest risk for recurrence among the four studies. Patients had to have at least three prior episodes (including the current episode) to enter the study. The low incidence of recurrence (22%) in this study may have been due, in part, to the use of the full therapeutic dose of imipramine throughout the maintenance phase. The mean dose at the start of the maintenance treatment was 200 mg/day. By contrast, the mean dose for the other three studies ranged from 135 to 138 mg/day, with doses seldom exceeding 150 mg/day.

Selecting a Maintenance Medication

In contemporary practice, the medication that induces remission of the acute episode generally is used for maintenance therapy. Unless the original medication presents special risks when used on a long-term basis, the advantages of continuing the medication for maintenance therapy clearly outweigh the disadvantages. Replacing a medication that is producing a good response can create logistical, compliance, and ethical problems. Also, there may be a loss of control over symptoms during and after replacement, particularly if the episode has not run its course.

It is important that the clinician carefully consider the side-effect profile of medication to be used for maintenance treatment and the effect it may have on patient compliance. Reactions that may be viewed by the clinician as being relatively mild may be troublesome enough for the patient to stop treatment. Examples include weight gain, dry mouth, and sexual dysfunction with antidepressants, and weight gain, hand tremor, and polyuria with lithium. An average of 4% of the patients receiving long-term treatment with an antidepressant discontinue medication because of unwanted effects (66). These unwanted effects are not significantly different from those occurring during treatment of the acute episode. The newer antidepressants, particularly the serotonin-selective reuptake inhibitors, appear to have an advantage over the standard tricyclic antidepressants (TCAs) in terms of attrition from side effects.

Side effects are not the only factor contributing to noncompliance. Other factors are dislike of having one's mood controlled by a drug, feeling well and seeing no need for medication, and the inconvenience in taking daily medication. The clinician and patient should discuss these and other problems that might interfere with the treatment program and come to an agreement as to how they may best be handled.

Role of Lithium in Treating Unipolar Disorder

Lithium has long been the cornerstone for the maintenance treatment of bipolar disorder but has generated conflicting findings as a long-term treatment for unipolar disorder (58). A NIMH consensus development conference on maintenance therapy for mood disorders (51) concluded that both lithium and TCAs are effective maintenance treatments for unipolar recurrent depression, each with advantages for certain patients. Lithium has potent antimanic properties, whereas TCAs and other antidepressants are ineffective in preventing manic episodes and may even precipitate hypomania, mania, or rapid cycling

in vulnerable patients (76). Because of the devastating effects of a manic episode, lithium may be the preferred treatment when there is suspicion of a previously unrecognized bipolar disorder or higher than usual risk of a subsequent manic episode. A major risk factor is a prior hypomanic episode that may have been missed in evaluating the patient. Other factors increasing the risk of a manic episode are a family history of mania, a high frequency of depressive recurrences, and early age of onset of the mood disorder (55). Overall, 10% to 15% of patients originally diagnosed as unipolar eventually develop a manic episode (51).

The advantages of TCAs and other antidepressants is that they are used far more frequently than lithium in treating acute unipolar depression and, thus, are a more logical choice for maintenance treatment. Also, there is evidence that lithium may not be as effective as an antidepressant in preventing severe depression (28,62). Adding lithium to an antidepressant regimen for the long-term treatment of unipolar disorder has demonstrated no significant advantages over an antidepressant alone (62).

Maintenance Psychotherapy

Psychotherapies designed for the treatment of depressed patients (cognitive and interpersonal) and certain behavioral, marital, brief dynamic, and group therapies have demonstrated efficacy in alleviating acute depressive symptoms. However, there has been only one randomized controlled trial evaluating the efficacy of psychotherapy as a maintenance treatment. The 3-year study by Frank et al. (23) found that monthly maintenance interpersonal therapy (IPT) delayed, but did not ultimately prevent, a new episode. Interpersonal therapy was found to be significantly less effective than maintenance imipramine. Furthermore, the combination of IPT and imipramine was no more effective than imipramine alone. The investigators emphasize that the delay in onset of a new episode with IPT may be of value to patients who cannot tolerate medication or wish to interrupt medication for selected clinical conditions such as pregnancy. They also question whether more frequent IPT sessions (e.g., twice monthly) would produce better results. Another 3-year study using a similar design to evaluate the combination of IPT and nortriptyline with elderly depressed patients is underway and should provide further information on the use of maintenance psychotherapy alone and in combination with medication (64).

From a clinical standpoint, maintenance psychotherapy is not recommended as the sole treatment for preventing recurrences unless the patient needs to avoid pharmacotherapy. The value of combining psychotherapy and pharmacotherapy for long-term maintenance has not been established in controlled trials. Nonetheless, many practitioners believe that psychotherapy may aid in preventing recurrence by improving social and occupational functioning and the capability to cope with life events that may precipitate a new episode. Psychosocial programs may also improve compliance with medication.

Choice of Treatment: Bipolar Disorder

Efficacy of Lithium

Lithium is the medication of choice for the maintenance treatment of bipolar disorder and is the only therapy to be compared to placebo for this indication. Several studies conducted in the 1970s found that lithium was significantly more effective than placebo in preventing both manic and depressive episodes (9,16,22,60). The pooled mean failure rate for lithium was 33% compared to 81% for placebo. More recent studies of lithium therapy report a less positive outcome. A multicenter study sponsored by the NIMH found that only one-third of patients receiving maintenance lithium treatment remained episode-free over a 18- to 24-month period (62). Similar results were reported for a multisite study conducted by the Medical Research Council in England (28). One explanation for the poorer outcome with lithium compared to earlier years is the change in patient selection for clinical studies. Many of the earlier studies were initiated when lithium was still an investigational drug and study centers were among the few places where lithium was available. These early trials included a high proportion of patients with classic manic-depressive disorder characterized by clear-cut onset and recovery and good interepisode functioning. In the current era, many of the classic cases are treated satisfactorily in the community and are not referred to the university medical centers or receiving hospitals that conduct most of the maintenance treatment studies. Thus, patient samples available for maintenance trials tend to include a larger proportion of difficult-to-treat patients who have failed to respond to traditional therapies in the community and may be unresponsive to lithium.

Recent follow-up studies and reviews of the literature on the long-term use of lithium across the entire spectrum of bipolar disorder suggest that lithium may be an inadequate treatment for as many as 50% or more of bipolar patients (26,52,75). However, these newer estimates of lithium's efficacy should be interpreted with caution. Partial or unsatisfactory response to lithium can have many causes that need to be addressed before labeling the medication a failure. These include misdiagnosis, poor compliance unrelated to adverse reactions, inadequate dose, hypothyroidism, and failure to allow sufficient time for lithium to exert full prophylactic effect.

Predictors of Maintenance Response to Lithium

Numerous studies and reviews have identified clinical features associated with lithium response (29,46,59,63).

Maintenance lithium appears to be most effective with patients who have an uncomplicated manic episode, good functioning between episodes, and a family history of bipolar disorder. Negative predictors of response to lithium include a history of dysphoric mania or rapid/continuous cycling, severe or chronic depression, mood-incongruent psychotic features, alcohol or drug abuse not associated with mood change, and co-occurring personality disorder. A pattern of course of illness characterized by a cycle starting with depression followed by mania and euthymia tends to respond poorly to lithium whereas a sequence of mania-depression-well interval tends to respond positively (21,42). Reports also suggest that patients who have three or four prior episodes are less likely to respond to lithium therapy than patients with fewer episodes (26,56).

Alternatives to Lithium

The anticonvulsants carbamazepine and valproate have emerged as the leading alternatives to lithium. The results from nearly a dozen maintenance studies of carbamazepine have reported positive results, suggesting that the compound may be beneficial with patients who fail to respond adequately to lithium (54,63). However, studies comparing carbamazepine to either lithium or placebo have significant methodological flaws that confound interpretation of data (59). The strongest evidence for the maintenance efficacy of carbamazepine comes from longitudinal studies in which carbamazepine is periodically replaced by a placebo and from mirror image studies in which the course of illness during treatment with carbamazepine is compared to the course of illness during an equivalent period preceding carbamazepine (59). Most of these studies suffer from small sample size. Valproate provides the same difficulties, although a recent 3-week study comparing valproate to lithium and placebo in patients with classic mania indicate that valproate is as effective as lithium and superior to placebo (13). Several open studies and naturalistic trials have evaluated valproate as a maintenance treatment (14,63) but, to date, there is no published study that systematically compares valproate with lithium, carbamazepine, or other treatments for bipolar disorder.

In the absence of clinical predictors for identifying patients who will respond to one anticonvulsant and not the other, the choice depends upon the clinician's preference and the side-effect profile. Usually, the anticonvulsant is used as an adjunct to lithium, thus avoiding the problem of sequential discontinuation of lithium and initiation of the anticonvulsant. An unresolved issue is whether an anticonvulsant alone or in combination with lithium is an appropriate first line maintenance treatment for certain subgroups of patients (e.g., rapid cyclers) or should be limited to patients who are resistant to lithium.

The most frequently used medications other than lithium for long-term treatment of bipolar disorder are the neuroleptics. They often are added to lithium for rapid control of manic episodes that occur during lithium maintenance treatment. Although neuroleptics are not routinely recommended for long-term use in bipolar disorder, they may be helpful for patients who suffer repeated breakthrough manias while receiving lithium. In such cases, the risk of tardive dyskinesia and other adverse effects of neuroleptic treatment must be balanced against the highly disruptive and life-threatening consequences of repeated manic attacks. Evidence suggesting that patients with major mood disorders are at higher risk for tardive dyskinesia than patients with schizophrenia makes this decision all the more difficult (36). Several case studies suggest that clozapine may be useful in the treatment of refractory bipolar disorder, including rapid cycling. The availability of newer atypical neuroleptics such as risperidone may provide protection against manic recurrence without the risks associated with clozapine and the traditional compounds, but this is yet to be determined.

Breakthrough depression occurring during maintenance treatment with lithium poses special problems. Initial steps include a reevaluation of the patient's lithium plasma level, thyroid function, and physical condition. The possibility of noncompliance in taking medication should be carefully explored. There should also be a reevaluation of life situations or psychosocial stressors that may be contributing to the depression state. Although some breakthrough depressions can be treated successfully by enhancing thyroid function or increasing the dose of lithium to levels of 1.2 mEq/L or higher (63), the standard practice is to add an antidepressant to the lithium regimen. This practice has been criticized by some investigators who claim that antidepressants may precipitate rapid or continuous cycling or mania in susceptible patients (42,76). This risk, however, must be balanced against the suffering, occupational and social impairment, and risk of suicide of a persisting severe depression. The efficacy of newer antidepressants for breakthrough depression has not been established; bupropion appears to be the most promising (31). Although anticonvulsants may be useful in preventing the development of rapid cycling, their efficacy in combating primary bipolar depression has not been demonstrated. Electroconvulsive therapy may be required for severe depression but should be used with caution if the patient remains on lithium. Administered with lithium, ECT has been reported to cause memory loss and neurological abnormalities (71).

Breakthrough rapid cycling or dysphoric (mixed) mania during lithium treatment is also a problem. As with breakthrough depression, there should be medical evaluation with particular attention to thyroid status. Carbamazepine or valproate may be useful in attenuating rapid cycling and mixed states (5). Other strategies reported to aid in stabilization of mixed or rapid cycling states are withdrawal of antidepressants, neuroleptics, or other potential cycle-inducing medications, the use of adjunct clorgyline, thyroid treatment, and repetitive sleep deprivation (5,29, 63). None of these strategies have been well studied and should be carefully monitored. In particular, the withdrawal of an antidepressant may raise ethical concerns about allowing a patient to endure severe depression. Substance abuse may pose an additional complication in patients with rapid cycling or mixed states and needs to be dealt with aggressively.

Psychosocial Treatment

It is clear that pharmacotherapy alone does not meet the needs of many bipolar patients. Even with adequate medication treatment, many patients fail to show full recovery from acute episodes and display symptomatic, interpersonal, and social deficits during interepisode periods. There are several reports citing the value of combined pharmacological–psychosocial treatment following remission or recovery from a bipolar episode (5,34,63). Most involve family or marital-based therapeutic intervention and psychoeducational programs. Research has not yet provided a standardized therapy tailored to maintenance treatment that has demonstrated definitive efficacy in a controlled trial. The slow progress in developing and evaluating adjunct psychosocial maintenance therapies may be due, in part, to the earlier misconception that most bipolar patients have a "clear" recovery between episodes and do not benefit from nonbiological treatments. As a result, the development of long-term psychotherapeutic treatments for bipolar disorder lags far behind similar efforts for schizophrenia as well as unipolar depression. It is noteworthy that despite the popularity of cognitive therapy for the treatment of depression, there have been few efforts to apply this treatment following an episode of mania. This may be a fertile ground for cognitive-behavioral therapeutic approaches.

One innovative maintenance treatment under study is Interpersonal and Social Rhythm Therapy developed by Frank et al. (personal communication). Its basic goal is to attenuate or prevent recurrences by stabilizing the social rhythms of bipolar patients. The primary focus of this intervention is on sleep rhythms, exercise rhythms, patterns of social interaction, and patterns of interpersonal, intellectual and emotional stimulation. It is being evaluated as an adjunct to lithium in a 2-year controlled maintenance study.

Dose

An important decision facing the clinician is what dose to use for maintenance treatment. With the exception of lithium, there are few dose–response studies for long-term therapy. A standard practice with antidepressants is to maintain the patient on a dose equivalent to 75 to 150 mg/day of imipramine. This level often represents a 40% to 60% reduction in the dose that was used to treat the acute episode. The study on maintenance treatment of recurrent depression by Frank et al. (23) suggests that the common practice of reducing dosage following recovery from the episode warrants reconsideration. Full-dose treatment tended to be more successful that half-dose treatment in a 3-year subset of the trial (24). Other maintenance studies suggest a difference in outcome relating to dose. Rouillon et al. (67) found that a 75-mg dose of maprotiline was superior to a 37.5 mg dose. However, 75 mg is only a half-standard therapeutic dose. It is possible that even better results may have been obtained with the standard dose of 150 mg. A study of long-term use of phenelzine (65) favored the use of a 60-mg dose over a 45-mg dose, although there was not a statistically significant difference. Montgomery et al. (49) achieved highly successful results with a 40-mg maintenance dose of fluoxetine, twice the dose level eventually approved for marketing. The aforementioned studies emphasize the need for dose–response trials that extend beyond the treatment of acute symptoms to the prevention of relapse and recurrence.

The maintenance dose range for lithium has been studied more carefully than that for the antidepressants. The dose generally is targeted at 0.6 to 0.8 mEq/L with a level of 0.5 not uncommon for elderly patients (51,63). Some patients may benefit from higher levels. A controlled trial by Gelenberg et al. (26) found that the risk of recurrence was 2.6 times greater for patients assigned a low dose (0.4–0.6 mEq/L) than a standard dose (0.6–0.8 mEq/L). However, there were two other critical findings. First, patients with three or more prior episodes did poorly at both levels, suggesting that even higher doses may be required for this subgroup. The finding may also mean that patients with a history of frequent recurrences are not responsive to lithium at any dose level. Second, the standard dose produced more side effects than the low dose, a factor that can adversely affect compliance. There are no studies evaluating the maintenance dose for other treatments used for bipolar disorder. Because of the difficulty in conducting these studies. it is questionable whether such trials will be undertaken. The most likely candidates are valproate and carbamazepine, both of which are being evaluated by pharmaceutical companies in the United States as a treatment for acute mania.

Duration

The decision of how long to continue maintenance treatment is not easy to determine from existing data. There is evidence that some patients with a long duration of illness who have not suffered a recurrence for several years may not require maintenance treatment. Angst et

al. (7) suggest that approximately one of three patients with bipolar disorder and one of eight with unipolar disorder who are over age 65 with a long history of illness appear to stop having recurrences. However, there are no valid predictors for identifying patients who no longer require maintenance treatment. Overall, existing data indicates that recurrent major depression and bipolar disorder can be a lifelong illness requiring treatment. The only way to determine whether the patient still needs medication is to gradually withdraw medication and carefully monitor the patient for signs of a recurrence. Schou (69) suggests that after the patient has remained well for 3 or 4 years, the clinician and patient should discuss whether the medication should be continued, taking into account the course of illness before and during treatment, the risk and consequences of a subsequent episode, and the patient's tolerance to the medication. Special precautions should be taken with patients having a history of episodes characterized by suicide attempts, need for hospitalization, or severe disruption of familial or career functioning, particularly if the episodes had a rapid onset.

Even with the most careful review of course of illness, discontinuation of medication can provide unanticipated difficulties. For example, Post (55) reports that some patients who have maintained long-term stability on lithium and discontinue treatment have a recurrence and then fail to respond to reinstated lithium, even when administered at higher doses. This phenomenon is labeled *discontinuation-induced refractoriness*. Post conceptualizes that the occurrence of new episodes despite renewal of previously effective lithium treatment is a manifestation of the kindling model. Adding one or more episodes to the cumulative load may impact the neurobiological mechanisms mediating mood dysregulation such that the disorder is no longer responsive to lithium. Although others have also observed this disturbing development, it is by no means clear that it is common. Its application to decisions regarding clinical treatment awaits further research.

TREATMENT OF DYSTHYMIC DISORDER

The diagnostic category of dysthymic disorder was developed by the American Psychiatry Association DSM-III (3). By definition, the disorder is long standing (at least 2 years duration in adults) and is characterized by a persistent or intermittent depressive syndrome of insufficient severity to satisfy the criteria for major depression. It soon became apparent that many patients with dysthymic disorder subsequently develop a major depressive episode, a condition commonly referred to as "double depression" (39). A naturalistic follow-up study by Keller et al. (39) found that a high proportion of patients with double depression had a remission of the superimposed episode of major depression during a 2-year period. However, overall, the outcome was relatively poor. A high percentage failed to remit from the underlying dysthymia and there was a high recurrence rate for episodes of major depression. It is noted, however, that treatment, particularly pharmacotherapy, was less than optimal for most of the patients. Subsequent placebo-controlled studies suggest that antidepressants are efficacious in treating both double depression and pure dysthymia (dysthymia without a super-imposed major depression) (32,41,50). All have been short-term studies, mostly of 6-week duration.

Overall, there has been relatively little research on the long-term treatment of dysthymic disorder. In a continuation treatment study, patients with double depression who responded to short-term phenelzine treatment were randomly assigned to continue phenelzine or receive a placebo for 6 months (30). Four of five patients assigned to placebo relapsed compared to none of seven who continued to receive active medication. An ongoing large-scale study by Kocsis and coworkers is evaluating the use of desipramine as a maintenance treatment for dysthymic disorder. The sample consists of patients who require acute treatment for either double depression or pure dysthymic disorder. Patients who respond to desipramine and remain in remission for 16 weeks are randomly assigned to continue desipramine or receive a placebo for 2 years. Preliminary results show that only 3 of 23 desipramine-treated patients (13%) have had a recurrence compared to 11 of 21 patients receiving placebo (52%). There is no significant difference in rate of recurrence between the double depression and pure dysthymic subgroups, suggesting the need for long-term treatment for both subgroups of chronic depression.

OBSTACLES TO LONG-TERM THERAPEUTIC STUDIES

Despite the increased attention to the long-term treatment of mood disorders during the past few years, the development and evaluation of maintenance treatments has progressed at only a moderate pace. One problem is that the pharmaceutical industry, which fuels much of the therapeutic drug development for mood disorders, is required for regulatory purposes only to demonstrate the efficacy of an investigational drug during the acute episode. Efficacy trials for antidepressants and mood stabilizers average 6 to 8 weeks in duration, despite the fact that most episodes of major depression and bipolar disorder extend for much longer periods. Also, partial remission of symptoms often is accepted as confirmatory evidence of the therapeutic efficacy of a new compound if the compound shows a statistically significant superiority over a placebo. Unfortunately, it cannot be assumed that partial remission will convert into a full remission with continued treatment. Nor can it be assumed that the efficacy of a drug in treating an acute episode necessarily

translates into long-term efficacy in preventing relapse or recurrence.

Efficacy studies of psychotherapy also tend to focus on the acute episode. Many of the studies use follow-up evaluations after discontinuation of treatment to determine whether the therapy has an enduring effect on the course of the disorder. These follow-up trials are difficult to interpret. In most cases, the researcher has no control over the patient's treatment and evaluations are conducted at infrequent intervals under nonblind conditions.

In general, longitudinal studies of therapeutic strategies are limited by the considerable expense, sample size requirements, and staffing resources needed to conduct well-controlled long-term trials. Sample attrition is a particularly pressing problem. Most studies of maintenance treatment enter patients during an acute episode and randomize them to long-term treatment groups following recovery from the episode. The attrition from the time of admission into the acute phase to entrance into the maintenance phase averages about 50% in reported studies. This heavy loss of patients often creates samples that are not representative of the population defined by study intake criteria and confounds generalization of results.

RECOMMENDATIONS AND AREAS REQUIRING RESEARCH

The chapter on long-term treatment of mood disorders in *Psychopharmacology: the third generation of progress* (57) identified several research needs, many of which are still relevant. The needs identified in the earlier chapter included (a) evaluation of the maintenance efficacy of drugs other than lithium for bipolar disorder and the TCAs and lithium for unipolar disorder; (b) long-term studies to identify treatment-responsive subgroups and areas of functioning that benefit from psychotherapy alone and in combination with medication; (c) determination of the efficacy of long-term treatments in attenuating the psychopathology and impairment in functioning that often is present during interepisode periods; (d) treatment strategies for alleviating or managing dysthymic disorder; (e) identification of biological markers for determining when continuation treatment can be safely withdrawn and for detecting an emerging recurrence before the appearance of clinical symptoms; (f) the effective dose range of lithium and antidepressants for maintenance treatment; (g) the use of maintenance ECT for patients who are refractory to medication and responsive to ECT; (h) the appropriate treatment for rapid-cycling and breakthrough depression during lithium maintenance therapy; and (i) development and evaluation of programs to reduce the high rate of attrition from noncompliance.

There have been significant advances with some of the aforementioned needs. There has been progress in evaluating alternatives to lithium and the TCAs, particularly with the anticonvulsants and serotonin reuptake inhibitors. There are also increased efforts to extend the clinical evaluation of investigational and newly marketed drugs beyond the acute episode. Traditional antidepressants are also being reevaluated in long-term trials. Other areas that have received attention are dosing strategies for long-term treatment, biological markers, treatment of rapid cycling, and treatment for dysthymia. Research on the extended use of combined pharmacotherapeutic–psychosocial treatments also has progressed, but is still more than a decade behind multimodality research for schizophrenia. A promising sign is the development of extended models of short-term psychotherapies for use as continuation or maintenance treatments.

A continuing under-served area of research is the study of the effect of maintenance treatments on interepisode functioning and subsyndromal psychopathology. Too often, the interepisode period is viewed as a well interval not requiring extensive study. Clinical instruments used in controlled clinical trials continue to be selected primarily for their capacity to identify and describe major episodes. As a result, the treatment of interepisode functioning and subthreshold symptoms often is neglected in the study design or in the report of results, omitting what could be useful information for judging the efficacy of individual treatments. This omission assumes particular importance in light of findings that subthreshold depressive symptoms and poor functional status can have a significant impact on a subsequent course of illness. The degree to which maintenance treatments effect the overall course of unipolar and bipolar disorder in domains extending beyond relapse and recurrence will be a challenge for the next generation of research.

REFERENCES

1. Abou-Saleh MT. Lithium and bipolar illness. In: Montgomery S, Rouillon F, eds. *Long-term treatment of depression.* New York: John Wiley; 1992:113–138.
2. Akiskal HS, Haykal RF. Dysthymic and chronic depressive conditions. In: Georgotis A, Cancro R, eds. *Depression and mania: comprehensive textbook.* New York: Elsevier; 1988.
3. American Psychiatric Association. *Diagnostic and statistical manual of mental disorders.* 3rd ed. Washington, DC: American Psychiatric Association; 1980.
4. American Psychiatric Association. *The practice of electroconvulsive therapy: recommendation for treatment, training and privileging.* Washington, DC: American Psychiatric Association Press; 1990.
5. American Psychiatric Association. Practice Guidelines for Bipolar Disorder. *Am J Psychiatry* (in press).
6. American Psychiatric Association. Practice Guideline for Major Depressive Disorder in Adults. *Am J Psychiatry* 1993;150(suppl):1–26.
7. Angst J. Clinical course of affective disorders. In: Mendlewicz J, Coppen A, van Pragg HM, eds. Depressive illness—biological psychopharmacological issues. *Adv Biol Psychiatry.* Vol 7. Basal: Karger; 1981:218–219.
8. Angst J, Bech P, Boyer P, Bruinvels R. Consensus conference on the methodology of clinical trials of antidepressants. Reports of the consensus committee. *Pharmacopsychiatry* 1988;22:3–7.
9. Baastrup PC, Paulsen JC, Schou M, Thomsen K, Amidsen A. Pro-

10. phylactic lithium: double-blind discontinuation in manic-depressive and recurrent depressive disorders. *Lancet* 1970;2:326–330.
10. Belsher G, Costello CG. Relapse after recovery from unipolar depression: a critical review. *Psychol Bull* 1988;104:84–96.
11. Bjork K. The efficacy of zimelidine in preventing depressive episodes in recurrent major depressive disorders—a double-blind placebo-controlled study. *Acta Psychiol Scand* 1983;68(Suppl):182–189.
12. Blackburn IM, Eunson KM, Bishop S. A two-year naturalistic follow-up of depressed patients treated with cognitive therapy, pharmacotherapy and a combination of both. *Affect Disord* 1986;10:67–75.
13. Bowden CL. What new data are available on lithium and anticonvulsants? Presented at the American Psychiatric Association Annual Meeting, San Francisco, May 1992.
14. Calabrese JR, Woyshville MJ, Kimmel SE, Rapport DJ. Mixed states and bipolar rapid cycling and their treatment with divalproex sodium. *Psychiatric Ann* 1993;23:70–78.
15. Coppen A, Ghose K, Montgomery S, Rao V, Bailey J, Jorgensen A. Continuation therapy with amitriptyline in depression. *Br J Psychiatry* 1978;133:28–33.
16. Coppen A, Noguera R, Bailey J, et al. Prophylactic lithium in affective disorders: controlled trial. *Lancet* 1971;2:326–330.
17. Depression Guideline Panel. *Depression in primary care: Vol. 1. Treatment of major depression. Clinical practice guideline.* Rockville, MD: U.S. Department of Health and Human Services, Public Health Service, Agency for Health Care Policy and Research; 1993. AHCPR Publication No. 93-0551.
18. Doogan DP, Caillard V. Sertraline in the prevention of depression. *Br J Psychiatry* 1993;160:217–222.
19. Endicott J, Spitzer RL, Fleiss JL. The global assessment scale. A procedure for measuring overall severity of psychiatric disturbance. *Arch Gen Psychiatry* 1976;33:766–771.
20. Eric L. A prospective double-blind comparative multicentre study of paroxetine and placebo in preventing recurrent major depressive episodes. *Biol Psychiatry* 1991;29:2545.
21. Faedda GL, Baldessarini RJ, Tohen M, Strakowski SM, Waternaux C. Episode sequence in bipolar disorder and response to lithium treatment. *Am J Psychiatry* 1991;148:1237–1239.
22. Fieve RR, Kumbaraci T, Dunner DL. Lithium prophylaxis of depression in bipolar I, bipolar II, and unipolar patients. *Am J Psychiatry* 1976;133:925–930.
23. Frank E, Kupfer DJ, Perel JM, et al. Three-year outcomes for maintenance therapies in recurrent depression. *Arch Gen Psychiatry* 1990;47:1093–1099.
24. Frank E, Kupfer DJ, Perel JM, et al. Comparison of full-dose versus half-dose pharmacotherapy in the maintenance treatment of recurrent depression. *J Affect Dis* 1993;27:139–145.
25. Frank E, Prien R, Jarrett RB, et al. Conceptualization and rationale for consensus definitions of terms in major depressive disorder. *Arch Gen Psychiatry* 1991;48:851–855.
26. Gelenberg AJ, Kane JM, Keller MB. Comparison of standard and low serum levels of lithium for maintenance treatment of bipolar disorder. *N Engl J Med* 1989;321:1489–1493.
27. Georgotis A, McCue RE, Cooper TB. A placebo-controlled comparison of nortriptyline and phenelzine in maintenance therapy of elderly depressed patients. *Arch Gen Psychiatry* 1989;46:783–786.
28. Glen AIM, Johnson AL, Shepherd M. Continuation therapy with lithium and amitriptyline in unipolar depressive illness: a randomized double-blind controlled trial. *Psychol Med* 1984;14:37–50.
29. Goodwin FK, Jamison KR. *Manic-depressive illness.* New York: Oxford University Press; 1990.
30. Harrison W, Rabkin J, Stewart JW, et al. Phenelzine for chronic depression: a study of continuation treatment. *J Clin Psychiatry* 1986;47:346–349.
31. Haykal RF, Akiskal HS. Bupropion as a promising approach to rapid cycling bipolar II patients. *J Clin Psychiatry* 1990;51:450–455.
32. Hellerstein DJ, Yanowitch P, Rosenthal J, et al. A randomized double-blind study of fluoxetine versus placebo in treatment of dysthymia. *Am J Psychiatry* 1993;150:1169–1175.
33. Hollen SD, Evans MD, DeRubein RJ. Cognitive medication of relapse prevention following treatment for depression: implications

of differential risk. In: Ingram RE, ed. *Psychological aspects of depression.* New York: Plenum Press; 1990:117–136.

34. Jamison KR. Psychotherapy. In: Goodwin FK, Jamison KR, eds. *Manic-depressive illness.* New York: Oxford University Press; 1990:725–745.

35. Jarrett RB, Ramanan J, Eaves GG, Kobes R, Basco MR, Rush AJ. How prophylactic is cognitive therapy in treating depressed outpatients? Paper presented at The World Congress of Cognitive Therapy. Toronto; 1992.

36. Kane JM. The role of neuroleptics in manic-depressive illness. *J Clin Psychiatry* 1988;49(Suppl):12–14.

37. Kane JM, Quitkin FM, Rifkin A, Ramos-Lorenzo JR, Novak DD, Howard A. Lithium carbonate and imipramine in the prophylaxis of unipolar and bipolar II illness. A prospective placebo-controlled comparison. *Arch Gen Psychiatry* 1982;39:1065–1069.

38. Keller MB. Diagnostic issues and clinical course of unipolar illness. In: Francis AJ, Hales RE, eds. *Review of psychiatry.* Vol. 7. Washington DC: American Psychiatry Press; 1988:188–212.

39. Keller MB, Lavori PW, Endicott J, Coryell W, Klerman GL. "Double-depression:" two-year follow-up. *Am J Psychiatry* 1983; 140:689–694.

40. Keller MB, Shapiro RW, Lavori PW, Wolfe N. Relapse in major affective disorders. *Arch Gen Psychiatry* 1982;39:911–915.

41. Kocsis JH, Francis AJ, Voss C, et al. Imipramine treatment for chronic depression. *Arch Gen Psychiatry* 1988;45:253–257.

42. Kukopulos A, Reginaldi D, Laddomada P, Floris G, Serra G, Tondo L. Course of manic-depressive cycle and changes caused by treatments. *Pharmakopsychiatr Neuropsychopharmakol* 1980;13:156–167.

43. Kupfer DJ. Long-term treatment of depression. *J Clin Psychiatry* 1991;52(Suppl):28–34.

44. Kupfer DJ. Maintenance treatment in recurrent depression: current and future directions. The first William Sargant Lecture. *Br J Psychiatry* 1992;161:309–316.

45. Kupfer DJ, Frank E. The minimum length of treatment for recovery. In: Montgomery S, Rouillon F, eds. *Long-term treatment of depression.* New York: John Wiley; 1992:33–52.

46. Maj M. Clinical prediction of response to lithium prophylaxis in bipolar patients: a critical update. *Lithium* 1992;3:15–21.

47. Maj M, Veltro F, Pirozzi S, Lobrace S, Magliano L. Pattern of recurrence of illness after recovery from an episode of major depression: a prospective study. *Am J Psychiatry* 1992;149:795–800.

48. Mindham RHS, Howland C, Shepperd M. An evaluation of continuation therapy with tricyclic antidepressants in depressive illness. *Psychol Med* 1973;3:5–17.

49. Montgomery SA, Dufour H, Brion S, et al. Prophylactic efficacy of fluoxetine in unipolar depression. *Br J Psychiatry* 1988;153 (Suppl):69–76.

50. Nardi E, Capponi R, Costa DA, Magistris W, Ucha R, Versiani M. Moclobamide compared with imipramine in the treatment of chronic depression (Dysthymia DSM-III-R). A double-blind placebo controlled trial. *Clin Neuropharmacol* 1992;15(Suppl):148.

51. NIMH/NIH Consensus Development Conference. Mood disorders: prevention of recurrences. *Am J Psychiatry* 1985;142:469–472.

52. O'Connell RA, Mayo JA, Flatow L, Cuthbertson B, O'Brien BE. Outcome of bipolar disorder on long-term treatment with lithium. *Br J Psychiatry* 1991;159:123–129.

53. Old Age Depression Interest Group (OADIG). How long should the elderly take antidepressants? A double-blind placebo-controlled study of continuation/prophylaxis therapy with diothepin. *Br J Psychiatry* 1993;162:175–182.

54. Post RM. Anticonvulsants and novel drugs. In: Paykel ES, ed. *Handbook of affective disorders.* London: Churchill Livingstone; 1992:387–417.

55. Post RM. Issues in the long-term management of bipolar affective illness. *Psychiatric Ann* 1993;23:86–92.

56. Post RM, Kramlinger KG, Altshuler IL, Ketter TA, Denicoff K. Treatment of rapid cycling bipolar illness. *Psychopharmacol Bull* 1990;26:37–47.

57. Prien RF. Long-term treatment of affective disorders. In: Meltzer

HY, ed. *Psychopharmacology: the third generation of progress.* New York: Raven Press; 1987:1051–1058.

58. Prien RF. Maintenance therapy. In: Paykel E, ed. *Handbook of affective disorders.* London: Churchill Livingston; 1992:419–435.

59. Prien RF, Gelenberg AJ. Alternatives to lithium for preventive treatment of bipolar disorder. *Am J Psychiatry* 1989;840–848.

60. Prien RF, Klett J, Caffey EM. Lithium carbonate and imipramine in prevention of affective episodes. A comparison in recurrent affective illness. Report of the Veterans Administration and National Institute of Mental Health Collaborative Study. *Arch Gen Psychiatry* 1973;29:420–425.

61. Prien RF, Kupfer DJ. Continuation drug therapy for major depressive episodes: how long should it be maintained? *Am J Psychiatry* 1986;143:18–23.

62. Prien RF, Kupfer DJ, Mansky PA, et al. Drug therapy in the prevention of recurrences in unipolar and bipolar affective disorders. Report of the NIMH Collaborative Study Group. *Arch Gen Psychiatry* 1984;41:1096–1104.

63. Prien RF, Potter WZ. NIMH workshop on treatment of bipolar disorder. *Psychopharm Bull* 1990;26:409–427.

64. Reynolds CF, Frank E, Perel J, et al. Combined pharmacotherapy and psychotherapy in the acute and continuation treatment of elderly patients with recurrent major depression: a preliminary report. *Am J Psychiatry* 1992;149:1687–1691.

65. Robinson DS, Lerfald SC, Bennett B, et al. Continuation and maintenance treatment of major depression with the monoamine oxidase inhibitor phenelzine: a double-blind placebo-controlled discussion study. *Psychopharm Bull* 1991;27:31–39.

66. Rouillon F. Unwanted effects of long-term treatment. In: Montgomery S, Rouillon F, eds. *Long-term treatment of depression.* New York: John Wiley; 1992:81–112.

67. Rouillon F, Serrurier D, Miller H, Gerard M. Prophylactic efficacy of maprotiline on unipolar depression relapse. *J Clin Psychiatry* 1991;52:423–431.

68. Sackeim H, Prudic J, Devanand DP, Decina P, Kerr B, Malitz S. The impact of medication resistance and continuation pharmacotherapy on relapse following responses to electroconvulsive therapy in major depression. *J Clin Psychopharm* 1990;10:96–104.

69. Schou M. *Lithium treatment of manic-depressive illness. A practical guide.* Basal: Karger; 1989.

70. Shea MT, Elkin I, Imber SM, et al. Course of depressive symptoms over follow-up: findings from the National Institute of Mental Health Treatment of Depression Collaborative Research Program. *Arch Gen Psychiatry* 1992;49:782–787.

71. Small JG, Milstein V, Klapper MH, Kellams JJ, Sharply PH. Electroconvulsive treatment compared with lithium in the management of manic states. *Arch Gen Psychiatry* 1988;45:727–732.

72. Thase ME. Long-term treatments of recurrent depressive disorders. *J Clin Psychiatry* 1992;53(Suppl):32–44.

73. Thase ME, Simons AD, McGeary J, et al. Relapse after cognitive therapy of depression: potential implication for longer courses of treatment. *Am J Psychiatry* 1992;149:1046–1052.

74. Van Bardeleben U, Holsboer F. Effect of age on the cortisol response to human corticotropin-releasing hormone in depressed patients pretreated with dexamethasone. *Biol Psychiatry* 1991;29: 1042–1050.

75. Vestergaard P. Treatment and prevention of mania: a Scandinavian perspective. *Neuropsychopharmacology* 1992;7:249–259.

76. Wehr TA, Goodwin FK. Can antidepressants cause mania and worsen the course of affective illness? *Am J Psychiatry* 1987; 144:1403–1411.

77. Weissman MM, Klerman GL, Paykel ES, Prusoff BA, Hanson B. Treatment effects on the social adjustment of depressed patients. *Arch Gen Psychiatry* 1974;30:771–778.

78. Wells KB, Burnam A, Rogers W, Hays R, Camp P. The course of depression in adult outpatients. Results from the Medical Outcomes study. *Arch Gen Psychiatry* 1992;49:788–801.

79. World Health Organization Mental Health Collaborating Centres. Pharmacotherapy of depressive disorders: a consensus statement. *J Affect Dis* 1989;17:197–198.

Psychopharmacology: The Fourth
Generation of Progress, edited by
Floyd E. Bloom and David J. Kupfer.
Raven Press, Ltd., New York © 1995.

CHAPTER 92

Treatment-Resistant Depression

Michael E. Thase and A. John Rush

An essential characteristic of mood disorders is their relatively favorable prognosis. Nevertheless, only 60% to 70% of patients who can tolerate an antidepressant medication will respond to the drug of first choice, and 5% to 10% remain depressed despite multiple interventions (66,104). The poorly responsive group has been variously described as resistant, refractory, or intractable. This chapter reviews the literature on the definition, assessment, and treatment of treatment-resistant depressions (TRD).

DEFINITIONS

Table 1 summarizes common definitions relevant to the concept of treatment resistance. The definition of an adequate treatment trial of antidepressant medication has varied widely over the years, as have the corresponding definitions of treatment resistance. In actuality, TRD patients present with histories of varying degrees of treatment adequacy. A high proportion of cases referred to university settings specifically for evaluation and treatment of "refractory" depressions have not received even a single adequate antidepressant trial (9,91).

An Adequate Treatment Trial

There is no absolutely correct dosage for a specific antidepressant, since dosage requirements vary depending on factors such as age, weight, general health, concomitant medication usage, and tolerance of a particular medication. Confirmation of treatment adequacy by more objective means (e.g., serial plasma drug levels) is not the rule in clinical practice, and valid plasma level–response

relationships are limited to only a subgroup of the tricyclic antidepressants (TCAs) and lithium salts. With respect to psychotherapy, adequacy of treatment may depend on the number of sessions, the expertise of the practitioner, the therapist's adherence to a particular form of therapy, and/or the interaction of the patient–therapist dyad. Electroconvulsive therapy (ECT) may be gauged by the total number of treatments, the use of bilateral electrode placement, and the verification of seizure time by electroencephalographic monitoring. Therefore, the terms "relative" and "absolute" treatment resistance may best describe lesser and greater degrees of certainty about the adequacy of a specific treatment trial (104).

Treatment Response

Similarly substantial variability exists as to the definition of an acceptable treatment response (109). The most common response criteria in clinical trials are a rating of at least "much improved" on the Clinical Global Impressions (CGI) scale, a prespecified level of improvement on a depression symptom rating scale (e.g., >50% reduction in Hamilton Depression Rating Scale scores), a final absolute score on a symptom measure (e.g., a Beck Depression inventory score of ≤9), or some combination of the above. Both the use of composite outcome criteria and documentation of persistent improvement (e.g., for 2 weeks or longer) may improve reliability and validity of classification (109).

At least a 50% reduction in depressive symptom severity generally corresponds to the clinician's global clinical impression of a moderate level of improvement (104). However, some patients meeting this commonly used response definition continue to have considerable residual symptomatology. Residual symptoms convey a higher risk of relapse during continuation treatment and likely contribute to suboptimal restoration of vocational or interpersonal functioning (104). Therefore, complete symptom

M. E. Thase: Department of Psychiatry, University of Pittsburgh School of Medicine, Pittsburgh, Pennsylvania 15213.
A. J. Rush: Department of Psychiatry, University of Texas Southwestern Medical Center, Dallas, Texas 75235.

TABLE 1. *Suggested terminology for treatment-resistance depressions*

Treatment nonresponse (e.g., significant residual depressive symptoms). A response that is poor enough that a change in the treatment plan is called for (e.g., failure to evidence at least a 50% reduction in the HRS-D score (or equivalent scale).

Treatment response. A response that is good enough that a change in the treatment plan is not usually called for (e.g., at least a 50% reduction in HRS-D score).

Remission. Attainment of a virtually asymptomatic status (e.g., HRS-D ≤ 7) for at least 2 consecutive weeks.

Recovery. Remission for ≥6 consecutive months.

Relative treatment resistance. Nonresponse to an adequate dose of a potentially effective medication for an adequate length of time.

Absolute treatment resistance. Failure to respond to a maximal trial of a single treatment for an extended period of time (e.g., IMI at 300 mg/d for 6 weeks).

Treatment refractory depression (TRD). Treatment nonresponse (i.e., persistence of significant depressive symptoms) despite at least two treatment trials with drugs from different pharmacological classes, each used in an adequate dose for an adequate time period.

Adequate dose. An oral dose that is close to the manufacturer's recommended maximal dose. Adequate dose may be smaller for elderly patients.

Adequate length of treatment. At least 4 consecutive weeks of treatment, during which the patient has had an adequate dose for at least 3 weeks.

Medication intolerance. Inability to achieve or maintain an adequate therapeutic dose of an antidepressant drug due to idiosyncratic reactions or side effects.

Adapted from Thase et al. (109).

remission is the desired outcome of acute treatment. The term *remission* describes a response in which a formerly depressed person's level of residual symptomatology is essentially indistinguishable from someone who has never been depressed. With respect to standardized scales, a score of 6 or less on the 17-item Hamilton Rating Scale for Depression is often used to define a remission (109).

Relative and Absolute Treatment Resistance

The concept of *relative treatment resistance* (104) refers to a patient who has received at least an average dose of a specific class of antidepressant for a minimally adequate period of time. For example, a relative TCA resistant depression would describe a patient who failed to respond to a typically adequate dose of imipramine, such as 200 mg/day or its equivalent, for at least 4 weeks (66,104). Similarly, relative resistance to a selective serotonin reuptake inhibitor (SRI) could be described as failure to benefit from a comparable trial of fluoxetine (20 mg/day).

Relative resistance recognizes that some patients would respond if they were treated with higher dosages and/or longer treatment periods. By contrast, *absolute resistance* refers to a patient failing to respond to a maximal, nontoxic dose of a given antidepressant, with confirmed compliance over an extended treatment period (e.g., an 8-week trial of imipramine at 300 mg per day and therapeutic blood levels or an 8-week trial of sertraline at 200 mg per day). Unfortunately, drug plasma levels are only of value for imipramine, desipramine, and nortriptyline (23).

The words resistance, refractory, and intractable are sometimes used interchangeably in the literature (66,104). Such definitional imprecision probably does the field little good. A more narrow application of the term treatment-resistant depression (as it pertains to failure to respond to an adequate trial of a specific antidepressant treatment) allows for a more precise description of each patient's past treatment history. For example, patients can be staged according to the number and classes of antidepressants that have failed to produce a response. Staging typically moves from more common (e.g., TCAs and SRIs) to less common [e.g., monoamine oxidase inhibitors (MAOIs) or ECT] treatments (see, for example, Table 2).

Staging of the treatment responsiveness of patients previously treated by other practitioners can be difficult, since both patient recollection and medical records often provide insufficient documentation of previous treatment trials. Several investigators have developed interviews or standardized rating scales to try to improve this process (29,64,89). However, the reliability of such measures has not been documented, and the major obstacle continues to be the source of the information not the means to elicit and record the data.

CORRELATES OF TREATMENT RESISTANCE

The psychobiological heterogeneity of major depressive disorder is well recognized and may be mirrored

TABLE 2. *Proposed staging of depression based on prior treatment response*

Stage	Treatment response
0	Has not had a single adequate trial of medication
1	Nonresponse to an adequate trial of one medication (monotherapy)
2	Failure to respond to two different adequate monotherapy trials of medications with different pharmacological profiles (e.g., a TCA and an SRI)
3	Stage 2 plus failure to response to one augmentation strategy (e.g., Li or thyroid augmentation) of one of the monotherapies
4	Stage 3 plus a failure on a second augmentation strategy
5	Stage 4 plus failure to respond to ECT

by heterogeneity of antidepressant response. To some extent, such heterogeneity can be attributed to sociodemographic factors, such as patient age and gender (104). Elderly patients, for example, may be somewhat less treatment responsive than those at midlife. Conversely, younger women may benefit less from TCAs than men or women treated with MAOIs (17,104). Individuals with fewer interpersonal or economic resources also may be less responsive to treatment (104). Perhaps these poorer outcomes reflect a higher level of objective stress, poorer social supports, and/or a greater risk of noncompliance.

Other correlates of response include symptomatic and diagnostic variables. One of the best studied symptomatic correlates is global severity (10,104). For example, the probability of placebo response appears to decrease as initial symptom severity increases. Although pharmacotherapy response rates may also decline in relation to more marked levels of severity, a significant drug-placebo difference remains even in the most markedly severe cases (104).

The broad grouping of major depressive disorders includes a number of clinical subtypes that show greater or lesser degrees of responsivity to different classes of antidepressants. For example, optimum response (particularly with respect to the drug-placebo difference) to TCAs appears to occur in unipolar (nonbipolar, nonpsychotic) major depressions of moderate severity (31,104). Although less well established, the proportional difference between active drug and placebo (PBO) may be highest when patients manifest classic melancholic features (i.e., psychomotor retardation or early morning awakening) (104). Some evidence exists indicating poorer response to TCAs in the following subforms of major depressive disorder: atypical depressions (including patients manifesting reversed vegetative signs and/or anxiety features such as phobia, panic attacks, or obsessions), bipolar depressions, psychotic depressions, and depressions associated with significant Axis I, Axis II, or Axis III comorbidity (104). In fact, patients with severe, concomitant Axis I, Axis II, or Axis III illnesses are typically excluded from contemporary efficacy trials, which greatly limits the generalizability of their findings to clinical practice. We believe that PBO-controlled trials of more complicated patients should be included within phase III and phase IV efficacy studies, as should trials of patients with a confirmed history of nonresponse to a standard TCA or SRI.

RESEARCH STRATEGIES FOR TREATMENT RESISTANT DEPRESSIONS

Controlled studies of the efficacy of alternative therapies for TRD are difficult to conduct for both pragmatic and ethical reasons. Consequently, controlled studies of TRD account for less than 1% of publications on the treatment of depression since 1959 (109).

Efforts to identify and sustain a large enrollment of patients in a study of treatment(s) for TRD are administratively and financially daunting. If, for example, cell sizes of 30 patients per condition are necessary to detect a clinically meaningful difference between two types of treatment for TRD, the investigator must recruit and treat as many as 300 patients in order to obtain 60 with a documented failure on the initial treatment (e.g., assuming an 80% completion rate and a 40% treatment nonresponse rate). Formation of multicenter collaborative study groups or the creation of regional data bases to pool the experience of a number of clinical investigators might help to remedy these logistical problems.

Other difficulties in designing studies of TRD result from the need to include either a standard comparator treatment and a placebo-expectancy control group. Although ECT may be thought of as the standard of efficacy for TRD (40), its use is largely limited to inpatients, and biased sampling may result if too many TRD patients decline to be in a randomized clinical trial utilizing ECT as one option. As discussed in subsequent sections of this review, augmentation of an ineffective agent with either lithium or thyroid or alternate treatment with an MAOI could be considered as possible comparators for outpatient studies of TRD.

Unlike uncomplicated new cases of depression, which typically have a 25% to 40% placebo response rate (23), most patients with TRD are relatively unresponsive to placebo (i.e., rates of 0% to 10%) (109). Thus, placebo control may be considered unnecessary in comparative studies of TRD, particularly if treatment resistance is established prospectively. The elimination of the placebo treatment condition might enhance the desirability of a study to eligible patients, facilitating research recruitment, and, as a result, improving generalizability of results. However, because response rates to active treatments may be as low as 25% to 35% in randomized controlled trials (RCT) of TRD (66,109), use of a placebo control provides the best opportunity to determine the statistical significance of a novel treatment in the context of such modest outcomes.

Alternatives to this dilemma include randomization strategies such as "play the winner" or the use of high-versus-low doses of a novel treatment (109). Another option is for patients to be randomly assigned to either the novel strategy or continued treatment with the ineffective agent currently received. The latter design, which provides a more ethically acceptable variation of the waiting list control design for TRD (109), controls for the passage of time and does not deprive patients of receiving some form of ongoing treatment. Staged criteria for level of treatment resistance afford another possibility to obviate placebo control. For example, for patients with a confirmed history of nonresponse to a TCA or SRI, the novel treatment strategy may be contrasted against a new trial of an alternate member of a previously ineffective drug class (66,109).

TREATMENT STRATEGIES FOR TRD

Maximizing Initial Treatment

Extending the Initial Medication Trial

The simplest strategy for nonresponse is to extend the initially ineffective treatment trial for another 2 to 4 weeks (109). Advantages of longer medication trials have been summarized by Quitkin et al. (53). This strategy capitalizes on the natural history of episodic depressions to remit over time and counteracts the tendency of some to discontinue the antidepressant prematurely. It also helps distinguish an enduring ''true'' antidepressant response from a more transient placebo response. Specifically, placebo responders have a greater likelihood of relapse between weeks 6 and 12 than patients who have responded to an active antidepressants (53).

The value of extending an ineffective, yet optimized, antidepressant beyond the sixth week of treatment has not been established for most agents. Indeed, in controlled trials comparing standard TCAs with various forms of psychotherapy, most of the variance associated with antidepressant response occurs during the first 4 to 6 weeks of treatment (23). In the Pittsburgh group's study of recurrent depression, a group of slower responders was identified who typically required 10 to 16 weeks of treatment to remit (33). This group, about one-third of the sample, was characterized by partial response between weeks 4 and 8 with a considerable degree of symptomatic fluctuations. These patients were characterized by higher levels of personality pathology and life stress, and somewhat lower levels of neurobiologic disturbance (33).

In sum, empirical evidence supports an extension of an optimized medication trial from the previous standard of 4 weeks up to 6 weeks. Past week 6, however, there is little empirical basis for this strategy, *unless* patients have shown at least a partial response or are receiving concomitant psychotherapy. An exception to this suggestion may be treatment with fluoxetine, which has been associated with continued evolution of treatment response for at least 8 weeks of treatment (94).

Adjusting the Dosage

Underdosage of the antidepressant is a common cause of treatment failure, although psychiatrists may be less likely to underdose than 10 or 20 years ago. An older literature suggests that routine prescription of maximal dosages of TCAs or MAOIs is associated with a greater likelihood of response than more modest dosages. Case reports similarly suggest response to megadosages of TCAs, SRIs, or MAOIs in some individuals unresponsive to typical maximum dosages (109). It is likely that the strategy to use higher dosages of antidepressants will prove more fruitful for agents with linear dose–response

pharmacokinetics. For example, approximately 5% to 10% of patients will have subtherapeutic TCA plasma levels despite compliance with conventionally maximal dosages (e.g., 300 mg/day of imipramine or 200 mg/day of nortriptyline) (109). In such cases, a supranormal dosage is necessary to achieve a blood level within the therapeutic range.

Treatment with nortriptyline has an apparent therapeutic window for blood levels. Although not as extensively documented as may be desired, the therapeutic-window phenomenon has been illustrated in several patients who, while nonresponsive at higher blood levels (e.g., >200 mg/ml), responded when blood levels were reduced to within the proposed therapeutic range (i.e., 50 to 150 ng/ml) (53). A therapeutic window has not yet been clearly shown for the SRIs, though anecdotal reports suggest such a possibility (12). The SRIs pose additional challenges to pharmacotherapists trying to implement rational treatment plans based on the dose–response behavior of this class of drugs. For example, initial randomization to either low dosages (e.g., 20 mg/day of fluoxetine or paroxetine or 50 mg/day of sertraline) or high dosages (e.g., 60 mg/day of fluoxetine, 50 mg/day of paroxetine, or 200 mg/day of sertraline) appear to yield comparable responses over 4 to 6 weeks of pharmacotherapy (1,26,116). In a study of patients not responsive to fluoxetine at 20 mg per day for 3 weeks (94), patients were randomly assigned to either an additional 8 weeks of continued therapy at 20 mg/day or an increased dosage of fluoxetine (60 mg/day). Both groups had similar outcomes at week 8, failing to identify any advantage for the higher dose. Further research on the efficacy of higher dosages of SRIs (after failure to respond to lower doses) is essential.

The dose–response relationships for trazodone and bupropion also are not well established. Both agents were initially tested in relatively high dosages (i.e., up to 600 mg/day) when compared to the dosages now typically prescribed. Much evidence of the efficacy of these drugs in severe depressive states was derived from studies at higher doses. However, concern about dose-dependent side effects now largely limits their prescription to dosages in the 200–450 mg/day range. Evidence of the relationship of plasma level to clinical response has not been established for either drug. In the absence of controlled data, a case for an 8-week, two-phase trial can be made for both trazodone and bupropion, in which 4 weeks of treatment at low-to-moderate doses is followed, when necessary, by 4 weeks of treatment at higher-to-maximal dosages.

SWITCHING STRATEGIES

A time-honored dictum in medicine is that a combination of two drugs should not be used if one drug will suffice. Accordingly, the most common pharmacological approach to TRD over the past 30 years has been to discontinue the ineffective agent and substitute an alternate antidepressant (109). Prior to 1980, clinicians in the United States were limited to substitutions within the first generation of antidepressants. Given the unfortunate reluctance to prescribe MAOIs that characterized the era, most psychiatrists would first opt to switch from one TCA to another. For example, a secondary amine TCA, such as desipramine, often would be prescribed when a relatively dissimilar tertiary amine TCA, such as amitriptyline, was ineffective. The introduction of a large number of novel antidepressant compounds over the past 15 years has broadened therapeutic options substantially.

The evidence tables used in the following sections were originally prepared for use by the Agency for Health Care Policy and Research (AHCPR) for development of guidelines for treatment of depression in primary care (23).

Switching from One Tricyclic Antidepressant to Another

Despite the apparent frequency of substitution of one TCA for another in clinical practice, only two controlled studies of this strategy have been published (see Table 3). Both studies document TCA response rates of only 10% to 30% in patients with a past history of TCA nonresponse. Preliminary evidence from an ongoing trial employing a plasma level-guided course of nortriptyline similarly suggests a 30% response in patients with a prior history of TCA failure (Nierenberg, *personal communication*).

Such low response rates are particularly unimpressive when compared to the outcomes reported in studies of patients treated by switching to alternate drug classes (see below). Moreover, the theoretical rationale that originally guided this practice, namely, that depressions might be subdivided on the basis of the primacy of noradrenergic or serotonergic dysfunction and matched to an appropriate TCA (e.g., amitriptyline for serotonergic depressions and desipramine for noradrenergic depressions), has not been supported by the available data. This is perhaps in part because the more serotonergic tertiary amine TCAs, amitriptyline and imipramine, are readily converted in vivo to noradrenergically active metabolites, nortriptyline and desipramine.

The tertiary amine TCA, clomipramine (CMI) is the most potent reuptake inhibitor of serotonin among this class of antidepressants, and CMI's active metabolite, desmethylclomipramine, is also a potent noradrenergic reuptake blocker. Generally, CMI is not widely used as an antidepressant in the United States, in part because of the decision of its manufacturer to obtain approval from the Food and Drug Administration (FDA) as an antiobsessional agent, but not as an antidepressant. Nevertheless, CMI is an effective primary antidepressant and, in addition to antiobsessional and antidepressant effects, CMI has broad anxiolytic and antipanic coverage. Also, CMI

is a potent suppressor of REM sleep and it can be safely administered parenterally (110). Thus, CMI might represent a logical first choice in a study or treatment sequence in which TCA nonresponse is confirmed prospectively. However, it has not been established that the CMI response rate in patients with tricyclic TRD would exceed the 30% ceiling observed in controlled studies utilizing other TCAs.

Switching from a Tricyclic Antidepressant to a Second-Generation Heterocyclic

The first generation TCAs and the second-generation heterocyclic antidepressants (HCAs) (e.g., trazodone, maprotiline, amoxapine, nomifensine, and bupropion) differ in both chemical structures and side-effect profiles. Therefore, it is reasonable to expect that a second-generation antidepressant may prove effective in some patients who either do not respond to or cannot tolerate adequate or maximal doses of TCA. The psychiatric literature from the early 1980s is replete with case reports of patients who responded to newer antidepressants after failure to respond to one or more TCAs (109).

As summarized in Table 3, the efficacy of bupropion treatment of tricyclic TRD has been examined by Stern et al. (100) in a report including both a double-blind, placebo-controlled inpatient study (n = 30) and an open-label outpatient trial of 56 patients intolerant or nonresponsive to TCAs. The findings of both controlled and open-label protocols indicate that bupropion is an effective treatment of tricyclic TRD, although response rates were not reported. A 56% response rate to trazodone was observed by Cole et al. (14) in an open-label study of a diverse group of 25 TCA nonresponders. However, only about half of these patients had clearly robust responses. Nomifensine, an approved HCA withdrawn from the market nearly 10 years ago because of toxicity concerns, has been studied by two groups. Nolen et al. (69) found only a 10% response rate in TRD patients resistant to both TCAs and SRIs. Schmauss et al. (92) similarly found intravenous infusions of nomifensine to be relatively ineffective in TRD (10%), although a slightly higher response rate (30%) was observed with oral administration. Although fondly remembered by some, the absence of nomifensine does not appear to be a marked loss for most TRD patients.

No controlled data have examined amoxapine or maprotiline in TCA failures. Alprazolam, a potent triazolobenzodiazepine anxiolytic with provisional efficacy in anxious depressed patients, also has not been studied in TCA failures. With respect to other HCAs not available in the United States, Nolen et al. (68) found that the relatively selective noradrenergic reuptake inhibitor oxaprotiline had statistically significant symptomatic effects in 33 TRD patients. However, the response rate to oxaprotiline was only 27% (9/33), placing its effectiveness in tricyclic TRD in a range comparable to currently available TCAs.

TABLE 3. *Alternate treatment of TCA nonresponders with TCAs or HCAs*

Antidepressant	Ref.	Sample and Dosage	Prior Medication and Design	Results
Tricyclics (TCAs)				
Desipramine	Charney et al. (13)	11 UP inpatients (DMI; 2.5 mg/kg)	TCAs (by history), open label	1 of 11 (9%) responders
Imipramine	Reimherr et al. (86)	27 UP outpatients (IMI; 150–300 mg)	TCAs (by history), double blind	8 of 27 (30%) responders
Imipramine	Peselow et al. (74)	15 UP outpatients (IMI; 150–300 mg)	Paroxetine, double blind crossover	11 of 15 (73%) responders
Imipramine	McGrath et al. (58)	UP outpatients, n = 22 atypical depression (IMI: 150–300 mg/day)	Phenelzine (60–90), double blind crossover	9 of 22 (41%) responders
Approved Heterocyclics (HCAs)				
Bupropion	Stern et al. (100)	30 UP inpatients (BUP, 675 mg/d; n = 19; PBO, n = 11); 4 weeks	TCAs (by history), placebo controlled	BUP significantly better than PBO on CGI and HRSD (response rate not reported)
		55 UP outpatients, >2 wks of BUP, 350 mg	IMI, double blind 4 week controlled trial, followed by open label BUP	Significant improvement in both intolerant (n = 18) and resistant (n = 38) patients on CGI and HRSD (response rate not reported)
Nomifensine	Nolen et al. (69)	10 UP inpatients	TCAs (by history), double blind crossover vs. TCP	1 of 10 (10%)
	Schmauss et al. (92)	20 Recurrent UP and BP inpatients	TCAs (by history), open label	4 of 20 (20%) (pooled; po, 30%, n = 10; iv, 10%, n = 10)
Trazodone	Cole et al. (14)	25 outpatients (mixed UP, BP) TRAZ: 264 mg.	TCAs (by history), open label	14 of 25 (56%) responders
Oxaprotiline	Nolen et al. (68)	Initial drug: n = 33, UP inpatients (260 mg); crossover: n = 31, UP inpatients (267 mg)	TCAs (by history), double blind; TCAs (by history) + FLV, double blind crossover	9 of 33 (27%) } pooled: 33% responders; 12 of 31 (38%) }
SRIs				
Fluoxetine	Reimherr et al. (86)	40 UP outpatients FLU: 60–80 mg/d	TCAs (by history), double blind	17 of 40 (43%) responders
	Beasley et al. (7)	35 UP outpatients FLU: 60–80 mg/d	Confirmed TCA nonresponse, double blind	18 of 35 (51%) responders
Fluvoxamine	Nolen et al. (69)	Initial drug: n = 35, UP inpatients (288 mg); crossover: n = 21, UP inpatients (286 mg)	TCAs (by history), double blind TCAs (by history) + OXAP, double blind	0 of 35 (0%) } pooled: 2 of 56 (4%) responders; 2 of 21 (10%) }
	Delgado et al. (20)	28 UP; inpatients (n = 21), outpatients (n = 7)	TCAs (by history), open label	Pooled: 8 of 28 (28%) responders Inpatients: 14% (3/21) Outpatients: 71% (5/7)
	White et al. (117)	12 UP outpatients FLV: 50–300 md/d	DMI 150–300 mg/d, 6 weeks; double blind crossover	9 or 12 (75%) responders
Paroxetine	Peselow et al. (74)	10 UP outpatients PAR:30–50 mg/d	IMI 150–250 mg/d, 6 weeks; double blind crossover	5 of 10 (50%) responders
	Gagiano et al. (34)	28 UP outpatients; PAR: 30 mg/d	TCAs (13 by history, 15 AMI), open label	18 of 28 (64%) responders
Viqualine	Faravelli et al. (28)	20 UP outpatients	TCA ≥ 150 mg > 4 weeks, double blind crossover	5 of 10 (50%) VIQ 0 of 10 (0%) PBO VIQ > PBO

In summary, the studies grouped on Table 3 indicate that a 20% to 50% response rate may be expected when a TCA nonresponder is crossed-over to a second generation HCA. However, this conclusion rests on only a modest number of studies, of which the largest effects were found with bupropion and trazodone.

Switching from Tricyclic or Heterocyclic Antidepressants to Serotonin Reuptake Inhibitors

Several small ($n_s \leq 10$) double-blind, crossover studies of the prototypic SRI, zimelidine, showed some degree of efficacy (i.e., 25% to 75% response rates) in patients who had failed to respond to trials of desipramine or maprotiline (109). Following the introduction of fluoxetine to the United States in 1988, a spate of published case reports emerged attesting to this SRI's effectiveness for TCA nonresponders (109). Studies of SRI treatment of TCA failures are summarized on Table 3. The utility of fluoxetine in patients with a history of TCA nonresponse subsequently has been confirmed in two outpatient studies, with response rates of 43% and 51% observed in these trials. Peselow et al. (74) similarly reported that paroxetine was significantly more effective than placebo in IMI nonresponders, with a 50% response rate to the SRI. Most recently, Gagiano et al. (34) conducted a 6-week, open-label study of paroxetine in 28 patients with a history of TCA nonresponse, including 15 patients who had failed to respond to amitriptyline (150 mg/day) in a controlled clinical trial. Eighteen patients (64%) responded to paroxetine treatment. No controlled data are yet available for sertraline or nefazodone treatment of tricyclic TRD.

Fluvoxamine, like clomipramine, has been approved by the FDA for treatment of obsessive–compulsive disorder; its manufacturer apparently will not seek an indication for major depression even though this drug is widely used for this purpose in Canada and Europe. Three inpatient studies of fluvoxamine in tricyclic TRD have yielded disappointing results. Fluvoxamine had response rates of 17% (1 of 6) and 14% (3 of 21) in two small inpatient studies of patients with a history of TCA nonresponse. Moreover, Nolen et al. (69) found almost no evidence of efficacy in a larger study of TRD inpatients: only 2 of 56 patients (4%) responded to a 4 week trial. Outpatient trials of fluvoxamine have yielded substantially more promising results. Delgado et al. (20) reported a 71% (5 of 7) response rate in an open-label study of outpatient desipramine nonresponders. White et al. (117) reported a 75% response rate (9 of 12) in a double-blind, crossover study of desipramine failures. The pooled outpatient response rate to fluvoxamine across outpatient studies (74%; 14 of 19) is both clinically and significantly greater than observed in inpatients (7%; 6 of 83) ($p < 0.0001$). Given the magnitude of this difference, it is important to note that all of the evidence pertaining to the effectiveness of other SRIs are crossover treatments derived from outpatient studies. With respect to investigational SRIs, Faravelli et al. (28) reported that viqualine was superior to placebo (5/10 versus 0/10) in a small study of outpatients with TRD.

In summary, the studies listed on Table 3 indicate that SRI treatment of tricyclic TRD typically yields 30% to 70% outpatient response rates, with fluvoxamine appearing to be an ineffective strategy for hospitalized TRD cases.

Switching from a Serotonin Reuptake Inhibitor to a Tricyclic Antidepressant

American psychiatrists are now much more likely to initiate outpatient treatment with an SRI than a TCA. Therefore, it is important to establish the efficacy of TCA in SRI-treated TRD. No studies were identified of TCA treatment of fluoxetine, sertraline, fluvoxamine, or citalopram nonresponders. Several small crossover studies of desipramine or maprotiline in patients resistant to zimelidine suggest a TCA response rate of approximately 50%. Peselow et al. (74) studied imipramine in a double-blind

trial of 15 paroxetine nonresponders, in which 11 (73%) responded to 6 weeks of IMI therapy. Although not yet extensively studied, it seems reasonable to anticipate that the TCAs will prove to be a strategy of first choice for SRI nonresponders. Comparable data for bupropion and venlafaxine treatment of SRI failures are needed.

Substituting One Serotonin Reuptake Inhibitor for Another

The proliferation of different SRIs begs the question of their interchangeability. Should patients nonresponsive to one SRI receive a trial of another or should they be routinely switched to another class of agents? As of yet, there are no controlled studies to address this important question. Clinical experience suggests that intolerance to one SRI does not necessarily convey intolerance to the whole class. A large prospective study by Brown and Harrison (11) found that 91% (85 of 93) patients intolerant to fluoxetine were able to complete an adequate trial of sertraline (50 to 200 mg/day), of which 69 (76%) responded. There are, as of yet, no controlled data to address the equally important question about the effectiveness of an alternate SRI when another member of this class is not effective.

AUGMENTATION STRATEGIES

Augmenting a Tricyclic Antidepressant with a Serotonin Reuptake Inhibitor

Two uncontrolled studies on the addition of fluoxetine (20 to 40 mg/day) to an adequate, but ineffective, dose of a TCA reported improvement rates on the order of 80% (39,72). Although the failure of fluoxetine monotherapy was not established in these open-label studies prior to the use of the combined strategy, the magnitude of response reported certainly surpasses those observed in the crossover studies of the SRIs reviewed earlier. Studies of the effectiveness of sertraline or paroxetine in combination with a TCA have yet to be published. Controlled studies are needed to confirm the effectiveness of this now-popular strategy.

It is not clear if the apparently robust effects of SRI–TCA cotherapy represent pharmacodynamic synergy or, more simply, a pharmacokinetic interaction. A study contrasting TCA cotherapy with sertraline, which has a lesser effect on TCA metabolism, versus fluoxetine or paroxetine might help to elucidate the mechanism as pharmacodynamic or pharmacokinetic, especially if TCA blood levels are carefully monitored.

Price et al. (50) studied the efficacy of an alternate serotonergic cotherapy strategy by adding the direct agonist fenfluramine (40 to 120 mg/day) to ongoing desipramine therapy in 15 patients with tricyclic TRD. In contrast to the positive reports regarding the use of the fluoxetine–

TCA combination, fenfluramine cotherapy was virtually useless in this small study (1/15; 8% response).

Thyroid Augmentation

One of the oldest augmentation strategies is the addition of small doses of thyroid hormone [e.g., 25 to 50 μg of L-triiodothyronine (T_3)] to the ineffective antidepressant agent. The theoretical underpinnings for this practice have been reviewed extensively (78,96). Thyroid augmentation can be traced to several early reports in which simultaneous initiation of TCA treatment and concomitant thyroid hormone was found to reduce the time to response in depressed women (see ref. 96). Of note, thyroid supplementation has not been demonstrated convincingly to speed response in depressed men (78). Suggested mechanisms include potentiation of effects on noradrenergic receptor sensitivity, increased efficiency of nonadrenergic neurotransmission, and correction of subtle thyroid abnormalities (78,96).

Studies of thyroid augmentation in TRD are summarized in Table 4. Early uncontrolled clinical series reported efficacy rates approaching 80% (5,27,71,111). The value of T_3 (25 to 50 μg/day) subsequently was documented by Goodwin et al. (39) in a placebo-controlled, within-subject study of 12 severely depressed inpatients, and by Joffe and Singer (46) in a study comparing T_3 and T_4 augmentation in outpatient TCA nonresponders. In the latter study, response to T_3 (53%; 9/17) was significantly greater than T_4 (19%; 4/21).

Interpretation of the studies of Goodwin et al. (39) and Joffe and Singer (46) is limited by the lack of a randomized, *parallel* control group receiving continued antidepressant treatment but not thyroid supplementation. Several contemporaneous studies were not generally supportive of the utility of the thyroid augmentation strategy. Targum et al. (101), for example, found that the effectiveness of thyroid augmentation (either T_3 or T_4) was limited to a small subgroup of patients with exaggerated thyroid-stimulating-hormone responses to thyrotropin-releasing hormone, an indicator of early thyroid dysfunction. Two other groups found T_3 augmentation to be no more effective than continued TCA treatment (37,105). Although none of these negative reports can be considered definitive (e.g., two were open-label and the third had relatively small cell sizes), they do raise questions about the generalizability of the effectiveness of thyroid augmentation across clinical settings and/or patient populations. Most recently, Joffe et al. (47) published a randomized, placebo-controlled, parallel groups study contrasting T_3 and lithium (Li) augmentation. Thyroid augmentation was significantly more effective than placebo and was comparable to lithium augmentation in this study.

Despite some variability (and, possibly, regionality) in outcomes, the studies summarized in Table 4 indicate that augmentation of TCA antidepressants with T_3 in doses of 25 to 50 μg/day appears to be effective in 25% to 60% of TCA-treated TRD cases, with very little risk of associated toxicity. The effectiveness of T_3 augmentation in SRI, venlafaxine, and bupropion nonresponders remains to be established. Of note, Stern et al. (63) recently found T_3 treatment (50 μg per day) to have a significant accelerative effect on speed of ECT response in a small, but well-controlled trial. Although it is not clear what proportion of these cases suffered from TRD, this promising finding warrants further attention.

Lithium Augmentation

The use of lithium salts in dosages of 600 to 1200 mg/day (or blood levels of 0.4 to 0.8 mmol) to augment antidepressant response has also been extensively reviewed (52,79). As summarized in Table 5, lithium augmentation is the best-studied outpatient treatment strategy for TRD.

The utility of the lithium augmentation was heralded by a number of reports in the 1970s, suggesting that the concomitant use of lithium and antidepressants or antipsychotic agents resulted in responses in patients who had otherwise been resistant to treatment (109). In 1981, de Montigny and associates (21) reported a rapid and dramatic response to lithium augmentation in eight TRD patients. These patients had not benefitted from at least 3 weeks of treatment with a variety of antidepressants, yet all eight responded within 48 hr of beginning lithium treatment. The effectiveness of lithium augmentation was subsequently supported by a large number of enthusiastic case reports and small series (see ref. 109). The efficacy of lithium augmentation has been further underscored by the results of six placebo-controlled trials of TRD and four open-label series (see Table 5). Several small series and case reports have suggested that the utility of lithium augmentation extends to combined TCA–neuroleptic treatment of psychotic forms of TRD (see ref. 109). Of note, both Garbutt et al. (30) and Thase et al. (106) have described small groups of tricyclic TRD patients who responded to lithium augmentation after an initial unsuccessful trial of T_3 augmentation.

Most investigators have not observed a large number of the dramatic 48-hr responses initially reported by de Montigny and colleagues (21). Thase et al. (106) reported a bimodal distribution of lithium augmentation responses in their 6-week study. One subgroup of patients responded within the first 2 weeks of therapy, whereas a second subgroup required 4 to 6 weeks of treatment. This observation could suggest two modes of action: an acute synergistic effect (such as that described by DeMontigny and associates) and a more slowly emerging primary antidepressant effect.

Variable results have been reported when lithium is used in combination with the more serotonergic TCA clomipramine (109). In one of the more positive reports,

TABLE 4. Triiodothyronine (T₃) potentiation in patients resistant to TCAs

Ref.	Sample	Medications and Design	Results
Earle (27)	25 retarded UP/BP outpatient females	IMI 150 mg + thyroid hormone, open label, trial length not reported	14 of 25 (56%) responders
Ogura et al. (71)	44 UP/BP males and females	TCA + T₃; open label, trial length not reported	29 of 44 (66%) responders
Banki (5)	49 UP/BP females (33 T₃; 16 controls)	AMI 75–200 mg or AMI 75–200 mg + 20–40 μg of T₃, open label, trial length not reported	T₃: 23 of 33 (70%) responders Controls: 4 of 16 (25%) responders T₃ > control
Tsutsui et al. (111)	11 males	TCA + 5–25 μg of T₃, open label, trial length not reported	10 of 11 (91%) responders
Goodwin et al. (39)	6 males, 6 females; 3 UP/9 BP	IMI or AMI 150–300 mg + 25 or 50 μg of T₃, 3 wks, double blind (within-subject-design)	8 of 12 (67%) responders 4 of 12 (33%) remitted
Targum et al. (101)	7 males, 14 females; all UP	TCA + 25 μg of T₃ or 100 mg of thyroxine, 3 wks, open label	7 of 21 (33%) responders Subclinically hypothyroid: 5 of 6 (83%) Euthyroid patients: 2 of 15 (13%)
Gitlin et al. (37)	9 males, 7 females; all UP	IMI, mean dose 206 mg, 4 wks, ±25 μg of T₃ or placebo, 2 wks, double blind/crossover	T₃ = PBO. Patients in both groups improved significantly. Response rates not reported.
Thase et al. (105)	4 males, 16 female; all UP	IMI, mean dose 240 mg, ≥12 wks + 25 μg T₃, 4 wks; 20 controls received continued IMI without T₃	T₃: 5 of 20 (25%) responders Controls: 4 of 20 (20%) responders
Joffe and Singer (46)	14 males, 24 females; all UP	Desipramine (n = 35) or IMI (n = 5); dose 2.5–3.0 mg/kg. T₃ (37.5 μg; n = 17) vs. T₄ (150 μg; n = 21), 3 wks	T₃: 10 of 17 (59%) responders T₄: 4 of 21 (19%) responders T₃ > T₄
Joffe et al. (47)	20 males, 31 females; all UP outpatients	Desipramine (n = 46) or IMI (n = 5); T₃ (37.5 μg) vs. Li₂CO₃ (900 mg) vs PBO; randomized, double-blind	T₃: 10 of 17 (59%) responders LI: 9 of 17 (53%) responders PBO: 3 of 16 (19%) responders T₃ = Li > PBO

the combination of clomipramine, lithium carbonate, and L-tryptophan (i.e., the "New Castle Cocktail") was particularly effective in seven markedly resistant cases (42). At present, the evidence pertaining to the effectiveness of lithium augmentation of other second generation HCAs and SRIs is largely limited to a number of case reports (109). Delgado et al. (20) found a 50% response to lithium augmentation in an open-label study of 18 fluvoxamine nonresponders. In a more recent study, Fontaine et al. (32) found that lithium augmentation of fluoxetine or desipramine was equally effective. However, lithium augmentation of fluoxetine was associated with both significantly more side effects and a greater number of transient responses or relapses than lithium augmentation of desipramine. Controlled trials evaluating the efficacy and side-effects of lithium augmentation of the SRIs should be considered a priority.

Only two randomized prospective trials have compared lithium augmentation against an alternate active treatment. Dinan and Barry (25) reported that a group of 15 TRD patients treated with lithium augmentation responded significantly more rapidly than 15 patients who were randomly assigned to treatment with ECT. By the end of the 3-week trial, however, the lithium augmentation and ECT groups had comparable levels of improve-

ment. As noted previously, Joffe et al. (47) found lithium and T₃ augmentation strategies to be equally effective in their placebo-controlled study.

In summary, the studies included on Table 5 indicate that lithium augmentation of an ineffective TCA or HCA yields variable responses, ranging from as low as 20% up to 100% in reported series. A response rate of 50% to 65% is suggested by published data drawn from studies permitting dosage adjustments and at least 4 weeks of augmentation treatment.

Neuroleptic Augmentation

Reviews of older data suggest that antipsychotic medications have a modest efficacy (i.e., 20% to 30%) in TRD (61,87). It is likely that neuroleptics help in the treatment of severe nonpsychotic depression with respect to anxiolytic and sedative effects, as well as more specific control of psychomotor agitation. Some phenothiazine neuroleptics, such as perphenazine, also may potentiate TCA response via competitive inhibition of the antidepressant's metabolism. Although many clinicians continue to use neuroleptic augmentation in severe, nonpsychotic TRD syndromes, empirical data to specifically support this

TABLE 5. *Lithium augmentation in major depression patients resistant to TCAs or HCAs*

Ref.	Sample UP + BP (UP only)	Medications and design	Results	Latency of response (days)
de Montigny et al. (22)	42 (42) depressed inpatients	AMI, IMI, doxepin, iprindole, or trimipramine + Li; mixed open label and placebo controlled	31 of 42 (74%) responders Li > PBO	2
Heninger et al. (43)	15 (14) depressed inpatients	Desipramine, AMI, or mianserin + Li or placebo; double blind, 3 wks.	12 of 15 (80%) responders Li > PBO	6–18
Nelson and Mazure (62)	21 (12) psychotically depressed inpatients	Desipramine + (neuroleptic) + Li; open label, 3 wks.	12 of 21 (57%) responders BP: 8 of 9 (89%) UP: 3 of 12 (25%)	6–14
Price et al. (81)	84 (73) depressed, mixture of inpatients and outpatients	Desipramine, AMI, adinazolam, bupropion, fluvoxamine, mianserin, or trazodone + Li; Open label, 3 wks.	40 of 84 (48%) responders Marked: 26 of 84 (31%) Partial: 21 of 84 (25%)	up to 21 days
Delgado et al. (20)	18 (16) depressed, mixture of inpatients and outpatients	Fluvoxamine, open label	9 of 18 (50%) responders UP: 9 of 16 (56%) BP: 0 of 2	up to 21 days
Thase et al. (106)	40 (40) outpatients with recurrent major depression	IMI (256 mg/d) + Li ($n = 20$) vs. IMI only (266 mg/d), Historical controls ($n = 20$), open label, 6 wks	Li 13 of 20 (65%) Controls: 5 of 20 (25%) Li > controls	up to 42 days
Dinan and Barry (25)	30 (24) inpatients	AMI (175 mg or equivalent) + Li ($n = 15$) versus 6 bilat. ECT ($n = 15$); 3 weeks, randomized, nonblind	Li: 10 of 15 (67%) responders ECT: 11 of 15 (73%) responders Li = ECT	up to 21 days
van Marwijk et al. (112)	51 (42) elderly inpatients with major depression	AMI ($n = 39$), maprotiline ($n = 5$) mianserin ($n = 3$), imipramine ($n = 2$), chlorimipramine ($n = 1$), dothiepin ($n = 1$) + Li; open, uncontrolled, 3 wks	33 of 51 (65%) responders 35% marked 30% partial	up to 42 days
Joffee et al. (47))	50 outpatients with major depression	Desipramine ($n = 46$), IMI ($n = 5$). Random assignment to Li (900 mg; $n = 17$), T_3 (37.5 mcg; $n = 17$), or PBO ($n = 16$).	Li 0 of 17 (53%) responders T_3: 10 of 17 (59%) responders PBO: 3 of 16 (19%) responders Li = T_3 > PBO	up to 14 days
Schopf et al. (93)	27 (25 inpatients and 2 outpatients with endogenous depression	TCA, HCA, and SRI antidepressants; random assignments to 1 wk of PBO ($n = 13$) or Li (600–800 mg/d); All patients received 14 days of Li treatment	Li > PBO 48% Li response after 14 days	up to 14 days
Fontaine et al. (32)	60 outpatients with major depression with melancholia	Desipramine ($n = 30$), fluoxetine ($n = 30$), open, uncontrolled, 6 wks plus 8 weeks further follow-up; Li (300–1,200 mg)	DMI: 17 of 30 (57%) responders FXT: 18 of 30 (60%) responders Relapse rates: DMI (0%), FXT (25%)	up to 42 days up to 14 weeks
Stein & Bernadt (97)	34 outpatients with major depression	Multiple tricyclics: Group 1 ($n = 16$): Li 250 mg/d × 3 wks, 750 mg/d × 6 wks Group 2: PBO × 3 wks, Li: 250 mg × 3 wks, Li: 750 mg × 6 wks	PBO = Li 250 mg < Li 750 mg Li (750 mg): 44% (15/34)	up to 21 days

Adapted from Katona (52).

practice are sparse. Furthermore, both significant short-term extrapyramidal side effects and the long-term risk of tardive dyskinesia associated with these agents certainly dampens enthusiasm for their systematic application. By contrast, the concomitant use of neuroleptics with TCAs is clearly indicated in delusional (psychotic) forms of TRD (61), yielding response rates that approach those for ECT.

Augmenting an Serotonin Reuptake Inhibitor with Another Agent

Beyond augmentation of a failed SRI trial with a TCA, lithium, or T_3, some anecdotal experience using postsynaptic serotonergic antagonists, such a buspirone (45), or mixed agents like trazodone (65), is accumulating. These strategies have not yet been subjected to randomized, placebo controlled investigation in TRD.

OTHER LESS-COMMON AUGMENTATION STRATEGIES FOR HCAS

Psychostimulant Treatment

The use of stimulant agents, such as dextroamphetamine and methylphenidate, in TRD has a long history but little empirical support (4). Some patients refractory to MAOI and tricyclic combinations may be treated successfully with the addition of methylphenidate or D-amphetamine (30,32). Safety concerns often dictate that patients treated with this rather heroic combination be started as inpatients. Unfortunately, no controlled studies of stimulant augmentation therapy have been conducted. Moreover, the abuse potential of these substances certainly places their role in TRD at a lower priority level.

Reserpine Pretreatment and Augmentation

The use of reserpine in TRD has been reviewed by Zohar et al. (119). This strategy has been hypothesized to induce changes in postsynaptic receptor sensitivity in response to a reserpine-induced depletion of brain monoamines. It should also be recalled that reserpine has modest antipsychotic potency, providing a second possible mechanism of action. Several poorly controlled early studies reported outcomes on the order of 70% to 90% in patients treated with repeated intramuscular injections of 5 to 10 mg of reserpine (see ref. 119). Given such dramatic findings, it is curious that reserpine strategies have received so little subsequent attention. Perhaps this is because two recent controlled clinical trials have failed to support the value of this approach for TRD patients (3,83).

Estrogen Treatment and Augmentation

Oppenheim et al. (72) have reviewed the use of estrogen supplementation strategies in women suffering from TRD. However, the value of estrogen supplementation in TRD has not been confirmed in a single double-blind, placebo-controlled trial.

Monoamine Agonists, Antagonists, and Precursors

The rationale for use of β-adrenergic agonists in TRD has been reviewed by Zohar et al. (118) and Charney et al. (13) have discussed the rationale for use of the α_2 antagonist yohimbine as an augmentation treatment. Both strategies are intended to speed down-regulation of cortical β-receptors, although no convincing evidence exists to support their effectiveness in TRD.

The use of various of monoamine precursors has received considerably more study in TRD (see ref. 109). The literature is rather mixed with respect to whether two common serotonin precursors, L-tryptophan (5-HT) and 5-hydroxytryptamine (5-HTP), are useful as either primary antidepressants or as augmentors (18,48). Walinder et al. (113) found no evidence of 5-HT enhancement of the efficacy of the relatively specific SRI zimelidine. Furthermore, Steiner and Fontaine (98) reported severe idiosyncratic reactions in a series of five patients receiving fluoxetine combined with 5-HT.

Sleep Alterations and Sleep Deprivation

The potential use of alterations in the sleep–wake cycle and sleep deprivation in TRD has been reviewed by several groups (e.g., refs. 51 and 114). Case vignettes and results in small series of patients suggest the utility of these methods in TRD, though randomized controlled trials are typically not available.

MONOAMINE OXIDASE INHIBITORS

Alternate Treatment with Monoamine Oxidase Inhibitors

The MAOIs have been used as a second- or third-line strategy for TRD for over 30 years. A number of reviews of the use of MAOIs in TRD have been published (e.g., ref. 24).

A number of open-label reports of MAOI treatment of TRD have been published (see Table 6). In a series of comparative studies, Nolen et al. (67,69,70) found tranylcypromine (TCP) to be significantly more effective than sleep deprivation, 5-HPT, and nomifensine; 50% of their highly refractory patients responded to TCP. In an open-label, crossover study of 42 recurrent unipolar depressives who had been vigorously treated with both IMI (mean dose 257 mg/day) and interpersonal psychotherapy, Thase et al. (107) found MAOI response to be both statistically and clinically significant (57% response rate). Moreover, MAOI treatment outcome was comparable to that observed in an earlier cohort treated with lithium augmentation and superior to thyroid augmentation. Most recently, Nolen et al. (70) compared responses to tranylcypromine (n = 17) with the novel MAO-type A selective agent brofaromine (n = 22) in hospitalized TRD patients. Response rates to the two MAOIs were identical (59%), although the novel MAOI was significantly better tolerated.

Several groups have conducted comparative studies of MAOI efficacy in TRD using double-blind, crossover methodology (see Table 6). As noted above, Nolen et al. (67,69,70) found both tranylcypromine (TCP) and brofaromine to be effective in patients resistant to either nortriptyline or maprotiline. Thase et al. (107) found TCP to

TABLE 6. *Studies of MAOIs in major depression patients resistant to TCAs*

Ref.	Sample	Medication and design[a]	Medication resistant to[a]	Results
Himmelhoch et al. (44)	21 depressed patients (13 BP, 11 UP)	Tranylcypromine (30 mg) added to lithium; open trial; ? duration	Recent (11) or past (8) trials TCA	16 of 21 (76%) responders
Price et al. (82)	12 depressed inpatients (6 psychotic UP, 2 BP)	Tranylcypromine (30–60 mg) added to Li; open crossover with blinded rater; 4 or more weeks	Lithium added to desipramine or adinazolam or bupropion	8 of 12 (67%) responders
Georgotas et al. (36)	20 depressed, UP elderly patients	Phenelzine (15–75 mg); open crossover, 2–7 weeks	Imipramine 150–300 mg or equivalent for 1–8 months	11 of 20 (55%) responders
Nolen et al. (69)	26 depressed, UP patients	Tranylcypromine (82 mg) or L-5HTP; open randomized crossover, 4 weeks	Imipramine >150 mg or equivalent followed by trials oxaprotiline, fluvoxamine, and sleep deprivation	TRP: 7 of 14 (50%) responders (L-5HTP: 0 of 12 responders) TRP > L-5HTP
Nolen et al. (67)	13 depressed, UP patients	Tranylcypromine (71 mg) or nomifensine; double blind randomized crossover, 4 weeks	Imipramine >150 mg. followed by trials of oxaprotiline, fluvoxamine, and sleep deprivation	TRP: 4/8 (50%) responders nomifensine: 0/5 responders TRP > NOM
Nolen et al. (70)	39 major depression inpatients (31 UP, 8 BP)	Brofaramine (218 mg; n = 22), tranylcypromine (85 mg; n = 17)	Prospective trial of nortriptyline or maprotiline	TRP 10/17 (59%) BRO: 13/22 (59%) BRO better tolerated than TRP.
Ryan et al. (88)	23 major depression adolescent outpatients, ages 11–18	Phenelzine (n = 1 alone; + TCA, n = 7); tranylcypromine (n = 3) alone; + TCA, n = 12); open trial; ? duration	Adequate doses of TCAs for ≥ 6 weeks weeks	12 of 23 (56%) responders
McGrath et al. (58)	46 depressed outpatients, UP (atypical) depression	Phenelzine (60–90 mg); double blind randomized crossover, 6 weeks	Imipramine (200–300 mg) for 6 weeks	31 of 46 (67%) responders PHZ > IMI
Thase et al. (107)	42 patients recurrent UP depression	Phenelzine (n = 4; 60 mg) or tranylcypromine (38.5 mg); open crossover, 6 weeks	Imipramine (257 mg) and interpersonal psychotherapy	17 of 26 (65%) responders
Thase et al. (108)	12 patients with anergic BP depression	Tranylcypromine (30–60 mg), double blind, randomized crossover, 6 weeks	Imipramine (242 mg/day)	9 of 12 (75%) responders TRP > IMI

Adapted from Devlin and Walsh (24).
[a] Dosage refers to mean prescribed dosage, where provided, or to dosage range.

be an effective treatment of anergic bipolar depressions resistant to IMI. Similarly, McGrath et al. (58) found phenelzine to be significantly effective in IMI-resistant nonbipolar patients with atypical depression (as defined by Columbia criteria).

As summarized in Table 6, the spectrum of MAOI efficacy in TRD appears to extend from adolescent to elderly patients. Unconventionally high doses of MAOIs also may be effective in carefully selected, side-effect-free patients who fail to respond to conventional doses of these agents (2,40).

It is unclear if the MAOIs are particularly useful in TRD because the structural dissimilarity between MAOIs and TCAs reflects distinctly different mechanisms of action or, more simply, because the two families of antidepressants have substantially different side-effect profiles.

This interesting line of research requires verification. As reviewed earlier, subgroups of TRD patients more responsive to MAOIs may include atypical, anergic bipolar, and comorbid anxious/phobic subgroups (17,104). For example, Thase et al. (102) found a MAOI response in TRD of only 33% in patients with typical major depressions, whereas nearly 80% of patients with reversed vegetative features responded to MAOI therapy.

Given such apparent selectivity for synergic or atypical syndromal presentations, it remains to be seen if other nonsedating compounds such as the SRIs, venlafaxine, or bupropion can be used in a similar fashion (38,86). The finding of Nolen et al. (69) that nomifensine apparently lacks efficacy would suggest that the relative efficacy of MAOIs in TRD goes beyond a nonsedating clinical pharmacology. Conversely, the effectiveness of the

MAOIs, which have potent effects on serotonergic neurotransmission, has not yet been confirmed in patients who have failed therapy with a SRI. Nevertheless, the MAOIs are probably the treatments of choice for Stage 3 TRD (i.e., patients resistant to both SRIs and TCAs, as well as their augmentation).

Augmentation of Monoamine Oxidase Inhibitors

A number of open-label case reports in small groups have described positive responses to lithium or T_3 augmentation when patients had not benefitted from treatment with an MAOI alone (see ref. 109). These strategies have not, however, been tested prospectively. Among other possible augmentation strategies for use with MAOIs, an older literature indicates that response to MAOIs may be enhanced by the addition of L-tryptophan (5-HT) (109). However, some individuals have developed serotonin syndrome when these agents are used in tandem (75). Similarly, SRIs are not to be used in combination with MAOIs because of several deaths reported with this combination suggestive of malignant hyperthermia (5).

Tricyclic Antidepressant and Monoamine Oxidase Inhibitor

The combined use of TCAs and MAOIs violates an explicit prohibition against their concurrent use in the *Physician's Desk Reference*. Nevertheless, a number of case reports and open-label studies dating to the 1960s, suggest that these agents may be synergistically effective in TRD (109). The general safety of combined TCA and MAOI treatment has been demonstrated in several controlled trials of nonresistant depressed patients. Combined therapy appears well-tolerated when moderate-to-low doses of both agents are used and the MAOI is added to an established dose of a TCA. However, these studies did not find evidence that the MAOI–TCA combination was more effective than either agent used alone in adequate dosages. Only one clinical trial has specifically dealt with the efficacy of combined MAOI and TCA treatment of TRD (16). In this trial, the combination of amitriptyline and phenelzine was clearly less effective than ECT. The combination of a TCA and MAOI thus is probably best reserved for after failure to respond to monotherapies, augmentation trials, and ECT.

ANTICONVULSANTS

The literature on the use of anticonvulsants in TRD has been reviewed by Kahn (50) and Post and Uhde (76). The value of anticonvulsants, such as carbamazepine and valproate as treatments of bipolar affective disorder has been recently established. Several series and case studies suggest that a subset of unipolar TRD patients, ranging from 20% to 40%, may respond to acute antidepressant treatment with carbamazepine (15,50,76). Kramlinger and Post (54) found additional improvement in 8 of 15 patients when lithium augmentation was added to an ineffective course of carbamazepine. Pending further study, the anticonvulsants seem particularly indicated for use in bipolar TRD syndromes or in clinically labile variants of unipolar disorder.

ELECTROCONVULSIVE THERAPY

The oldest available treatment of TRD is still the most consistently effective (89,109), and response rates of 50% to 70% are consistently observed (see Table 7). Although the ECT response rate in TRD is significantly lower than typically seen in nonresistant cases (84), at the worst the response rate reported for ECT is equivalent to response rates to MAOI treatment or lithium augmentation, and superior to all other therapeutic options for TRD (109). Electroconvulsive therapy response also may be enhanced by switching from unilateral to bilateral treatment modes and monitoring duration of seizure time to prevent missed treatments (89). Thus, ECT remains the treatment of choice for the most severe, incapacitating forms of TRD.

Although ECT is clearly an effective treatment of TRD, it has also recently been shown that relapse rates are significantly higher in TRD patients after a successful course of therapy (90). Research is necessary to establish the efficacy of alternate methods to prevent relapse following successful ECT, including maintenance ECT and combination pharmacotherapy strategies.

Patients who fail to respond to ECT (proposed Stage 5 TRD), represent some of the most challenging cases of TRD. Assuming that the course of ECT has been optimized (i.e., at least 12 total treatments, including at least 6 bilateral treatments with confirmation of the adequacy of seizure duration), it would seem prudent to allow a brief medication-free washout and proceed with one of the major strategies that have not yet been tried. Anecdotal clinical experience suggests that some patients are more responsive to antidepressant agents after an unsuccessful course of ECT, perhaps because of treatment-induced changes in postsynaptic receptor sensitivity (95). Thus, failure on ECT does not forbode nonresponsiveness to all somatic therapies.

PSYCHOTHERAPY

The value of various forms of psychotherapy in the management of patients with TRD has been reviewed elsewhere (see ref. 103). Traditionally, psychotherapy has been considered useful in the management of TRD primarily as an adjunct to help patients maintain morale and optimism. However, data to support these suggested indications are sparse, and those studies that are available are limited to the newer forms of psychotherapy, such as

TABLE 7. *ECT in patients resistant to HCAs*

Ref.	Sample	Resistant to[a]	Results
DeCarolis et al. (19)	190 mixed (UP & BP) depressed inpatients (109 psychotic)	Imipramine (200–350 mg/day) for 30 days; crossover, ECT (8–10 treatments), open trial	72% ECT response rate (proportions not reported)
Medical Research Council (59)	250 depressed inpatients	Medication failures (IMI or phenelzine), crossover ECT (4–8 treatments), open trial	50% response in TRD versus 71% in nonresistant patients (proportions not reported)
Mandel et al. (57)	76 TCA-resistant or TCA-intolerant depressed inpatients	Retrospective review of 100 charts yielded 76 TCA resistant cases (IMI @ 150 mg/day × 3 weeks); open trial	54 of 76 (71%) ECT responders
Paul et al. (73)	9 medication-resistant inpatients	Adequate pharmacotherapy; open trial	8 of 9 (89%) ECT responders
Hamilton (41)	146 melancholic inpatients	Medication failure or intolerant to either IMI or phenelzine; open trial	82 of 146 (68%) responders
Magni et al. (56)	28 medication-resistant patients	Adequate pharmacotherapy; Open trial	17 of 28 (61%) responders
Prudic et al. (84)	24 depressed inpatients (6 psychotic)	IMI (or equivalent) ≥ 200 mg × 4 wks, Open trial	TRD 12 of 24 (50%) ECT responders nonTRD: 24 of 29 (86%) ECT responders
Dinan and Barry (25)	15 depressed inpatients	AMI (or equivalent) 175 mg; Randomized trial (versus Li augmentation, *n* = 15); 6 bilat. ECT	ECT: 11 of 15 (73%) responders Li: 10 of 15 (67%) responders

[a] Dosages refer to mean prescribed dosage, where provided, or dosage range.

cognitive behavior therapy (CBT). Among several small groups of TRD patients, CBT response rates of 25% to 40% have been reported (see ref. 103). Cognitive behavior therapy thus may have about the same probability of response in TRD outpatients as retreatment with a similar antidepressant agent. The magnitude of this estimated effect is likely to be smaller than those observed for lithium augmentation, MAOIs, and ECT. Some evidence suggests that TRD patients benefit from more intensive models of therapy, for example, those offering frequent sessions and an admixture of individual, group, and milieu modalities. Such regimens are most practicable in partial-hospital or inpatient settings. Inpatient treatment with intensive CBT (in lieu of alternate somatic modalities) would appear to be best suited for patients who are poor candidates for further medication trials or for those who refuse ECT (103). A preliminary study by Miller et al. (60) suggests that CBT also might may be usefully combined with pharmacotherapy in TRD. In this regard, provision of psychotherapy may reduce attrition rates from pharmacological treatment and strengthen therapeutic alliances during the long-term management of chronic mood disorders (103).

PSYCHOSURGERY

The use of psychosurgery in TRD has been reviewed by Bridges (8). Although a number of early reports described dramatic success following stereotactic leukotomy (i.e., sustained improvement rates of 50% to 80%), more recent studies suggest that sustained remission rates of only about 25% to 50% can be expected (55,77). Complications include epilepsy and irreversible personality changes (8). Psychosurgery, therefore, remains the last line of somatic treatment for patients with TRD.

CONCLUSIONS

Whereas mood disorders have generally been viewed as episodic and of good prognosis, a large subset of this population (45% to 50%) can be expected to either be intolerant to or fail to respond to an initial medication trial (27,104). Evidence to date indicates that a second monotherapy will effectively treat about 40% to 50% of those who have failed with the initial treatment, especially if the second drug has a pharmacological profile distinct from the initial medication. The remaining 25% of mood-disordered patients are candidates for one or more augmentation strategies, followed by treatment with a MAOI. Electroconvulsive therapy has a place in the treatment plan for patients failing multiple monotherapies or augmented treatment packages. The need for randomized controlled studies utilizing innovative designs to identify the preferred therapies for those patients with varying degrees of treatment resistance is clear. Even now, however, present evidence argues for carefully conducted sequenced medication trials in patients who do not respond satisfactorily to the initial treatment.

ACKNOWLEDGMENTS

The review was supported in part by NIMH grants MH-41115 (to A. J. Rush), MH-30915 (University of Pittsburgh Mental Health Clinical Research Center), and MH-41884 (to M. E. Thase). The authors appreciate the secretarial support of Fast Word, Inc. of Dallas, Lisa Stupar, and David Savage, and the administrative support of Kenneth Z. Altshuler, Stanton Sharp Professor and Chairman of the Department of Psychiatry of the University of Texas Southwestern Medical Center, and David J. Kupfer, Chairman of the Department of Psychiatry of the University of Pittsburgh Medical Center.

REFERENCES

1. Amin M, Lehmann H, Mirmiran J. A double-blind, placebo-controlled dose-finding study with sertraline. *Psychopharm Bull* 1989;25:164–167.
2. Amsterdam JD, Berwish NJ. High dose tranylcypromine therapy for resistant depression. *Pharmacopsychiatry* 1989;22:21–25.
3. Amsterdam JD, Berwish NJ. Treatment of refractory depression with combination reserpine and tricyclic antidepressant therapy. *J Clin Psychopharmacol* 1987;7:238–242.
4. Ayd FJ, Zohar J. Psychostimulant (amphetamine or methylphenidate) therapy for chronic and treatment-resistant depression. In: Zohar J, Belmaker RH, eds. *Treating resistant depression.* New York: PMA Publishing; 1987:343–355.
5. Banki CM. Cerebrospinal fluid amine metabolites after combined amitriptylinetriiodothyronine treatment of depressed women. *Eur J Clin Pharmacol* 1977;11:311–315.
6. Beasley CM, Masica DN, Heiligenstein JH, Wheadon DE, Zerbe RL. Possible monoamine oxidase inhibitor-serotonin uptake inhibitor interaction: fluoxetine clinical data and preclinical findings. *J Clin Psychopharm* 1993;13:312–320.
7. Beasley CM, Sayler ME, Cunningham GE. Weiss AM, Masica DN. Fluoxetine in tricyclic refractory major depressive disorder. *J Affect Disord* 1990;20:193–200.
8. Bridges P. Psychosurgery for resistant depression. In: Zohar J, Belmaker RH, eds. *Treating resistant depression.* New York: PMA Publishing; 1987:397–411.
9. Bridges PK. ". . . and a small dose of an antidepressant might help." *Br J Psychiatry* 1983;142:626–628.
10. Brown RP, Sweeney J, Frances A, Kocsis JH, Loutsche E. Age as a predictor of treatment response in endogenous depression. *J Clin Psychopharmacol* 1983;3:176–178.
11. Brown WA, Harrison W. Are patients who are intolerant to one SSRI intolerant to another. *Psychopharm Bull* 1992;28:253–256.
12. Cain JW. Poor response to fluoxetine: underlying depression, serotonergic overstimulation, or a "therapeutic window." *J Clin Psychiatry* 1992;53:272–277.
13. Charney DS, Price LH, Heninger GR. Desipramine–yohimbine combination treatment of refractory depression. *Arch Gen Psychiatry* 1986;43:1155–1161.
14. Cole JO, Schatzberg AF, Sniffin C, Zolner J, Cole JP. Trazodone in treatment-resistant depression: An open study. *J Clin Psychopharmacol* 1981;1(Suppl.):49–54.
15. Cullen M, Mitchell P, Brodaty H, Boyce P, Parker G, Hickie I, Wilhelm K. Carbamazepine for treatment-resistant melancholia. *J Clin Psychiatry* 1991;52:472–476.
16. Davidson J, McLeod M, Law-Yone B, Linnoila M. A comparison of electroconvulsive therapy and combined phenelzine-amitriptyline in refractory depression. *Arch Gen Psychiatry* 1978;35:639–642.
17. Davidson J, Pelton S. Forms of atypical depression and their response to antidepressant drugs. *Psychiatry Res* 1986;17:87–95.
18. d'Elia G, Hanson L, Raotma H. L-Tryptophan and 5-hydroxytryptophan in the treatment of depression. A review. *Acta Psychiatr Scand* 1978;57:239–252.
19. DeCarolis V, Gilberti F, Roccatagliata G, et al. Imipramine and electroshock in the treatment of depression: A clinical statistical analysis of 437 cases. *Dis Nerv Syst* 1964;16:29–42.
20. Delgado PL, Price LH, Charney DS, Heninger GR. Efficacy of fluvoxamine in treatment-refractory depression. *J Affect Disord* 1988;15:55–60.
21. deMontigny C, Grunberg F, Mayer A, Deschenes JP. Lithium induces rapid relief of depression in tricyclic antidepressant drug non-responders. *Br J Psychiatry* 1981;138:252–256.
22. deMontigny C, Cournoyer G, Morissette R, Langlois R, Caille G. Lithium carbonate addition in tricyclic antidepressant-resistant unipolar depression. *Arch Gen Psychiatry* 1983;40:1327–1334.
23. Depression Guideline Panel. *Clinical practice guideline. Depression in primary care: Vol. 2. Treatment of major depression.* Rockville, MD: U.S. Dept. of Health and Human Services, Agency for Health Care Policy and Research; 1993:AHCPR publication no. 93-0551.
24. Devlin MJ, Walsh BT. Use of monoamine oxidase inhibitors in refractory depression. In: Tasman A, Goldfinger SM, Kaufman CA, eds. *American psychiatric press review of psychiatry,* Vol. 9. Washington, DC: American Psychiatric Press; 1990:74–90.
25. Dinan TG, Barry S. A comparison of electroconvulsive therapy with a combined lithium and tricyclic combination among depressed tricyclic nonresponders. *Acta Psychiatr Scand* 1989; 80:97–100.
26. Dunner DL, Dunbar GC. Optimal dose regimen for paroxetine. *J Clin Psychiatry* 1992;53:21–26.
27. Earle BV. Thyroid hormone and tricyclic antidepressants in resistant depressions. *Am J Psychiatry* 1970;126:143–145.
28. Faravelli C, Albanesi G, Sessarego A. Viqualine in resistant depression: A double-blind, placebo-controlled trial. *Neuropsychobiology* 1988;20:78–81.
29. Fawcett J, Kravitz HM. Treatment refractory depression. In: Schatzberg AE, ed. *Common treatment problems in depression.* Washington, DC: American Psychiatric Press; 1985.
30. Fawcett J, Kravitz HM, Zajecka JM, Schaff MR. CNS stimulant potentiation of monoamine oxidase inhibitors in treatment-refractory depression. *J Clin Psychopharmacology* 1991;11:127–132.
31. Feighner JP, Herbstein J, Damlouji N. Combined MAOI, TCA, and direct stimulant therapy of treatment-resistant depression. *J Clin Psychiatry* 1985;46:206–209.
32. Fontaine R, Ontiveros A, Elie R, Vézina M. Lithium carbonate augmentation of desipramine and fluoxetine in refractory depression. *Biol Psychiatry* 1991;29:946–948.
33. Frank E, Kupfer DJ. Axis II personality disorders and personality features in treatment-resistant and refractory depression. In: Roose SP, Glassman AH, eds. *Treatment strategies for refractory depression.* Washington, DC: American Psychiatric Press; 1990:205–221.
34. Gagiano CA, Muller PGM, Gourie J, LeRoux JF. The therapeutic efficacy of paroxetine: (a) an open study in patients with major depression not responding to antidepressants; (b) a double blind comparison with amitriptyline in depressed outpatients. *Acta Psychiatr Scand* 1993;80:130–131.
35. Garbutt JC, Mayo JP, Gillette GM, Little KY, Mason GA. Lithium potentiation of tricyclic antidepressants following lack of T_3 potentiation. *Am J Psychiatry* 1986;143:1038–1039.
36. Georgotas A, Friedman E, McCarthy M, Mann J, Krakowski M, Siegel R, Ferris S. Resistant geriatric depressions and therapeutic response to monoamine oxidase inhibitors. *Biol Psychiatry* 1983; 18:195–205.
37. Gitlin MJ, Weiner H, Fairbanks L, Hershman JM, Friedfeld N. Failure to T3 to potentiate tricyclic antidepressant response. *J Affect Dis* 1987;13:267–272.
38. Goodnick PJ, Extein IL. Bupropion and fluoxetine in depressive subtypes. *Ann Clin Psychiatry* 1989;1:119–122.
39. Goodwin FK, Prange AJ, Post RM, Muscettola F, Lipton MA.

Potentiation of antidepressant effects by L-triiodothyronine in tricyclic nonresponders. *Am J Psychiatry* 1982;139:34–38.

40. Guze BH, Baxter LR, Rego J. Refractory depression treated with high doses of a monoamine oxidase inhibitor. *J Clin Psychiatry* 1987;48:31–32.

41. Hamilton M. The effect of treatment on the melancholias (depressions). *Br J Psychiatry* 1982;40:223–230.

42. Hale AS, Procter AW, Bridges PK. Clomipramine, tryptophan and lithium in combination for resistant endogenous depression: seven case studies. *Br J Psychiatry* 1987;151:231–217.

43. Heninger GR, Charney DS, Sternberg DE. Lithium carbonate augmentation of antidepressant treatment. *Arch Gen Psychiatry* 1983;40:1335–1342.

44. Himmelhoch JM, Detre T, Kupfer DJ, Swartzburg M, Byck R. Treatment of previously intractable depressions with tranylcypromine and lithium. *J Nerv Mental Dis* 1972;155:216–220.

45. Joffe RT, Schuller DR. An open study of buspirone augmentation of serotonin reuptake inhibitors in refractory depression. *J Clin Psychiatry* 1993;54:269–271.

46. Joffe RT, Singer W. A comparison of triiodothyronine and thyroxine in the potentiation of tricyclic antidepressants. *Psychiatry Res* 1990;32:241–251.

47. Joffe RT, Singer W, Levitt AJ, MacDonald C. A placebo-controlled comparison of lithium and triiodothyronine augmentation of tricyclic antidepressants in unipolar refractory depression. *Arch Gen Psychiatry* 1993;50:387–393.

48. Jones JS, Stanley M. Serotonergic agents in the treatment of refractory depression. In: Roose SP, Glassman AH, eds. *Treatment strategies for refractory depression.* Washington, DC: American Psychiatric Press; 1990:143–167.

49. Joyce PR, Paykel ES. Predictors of drug response in depression. *Arch Gen Psychiatry* 1989;46:89–99.

50. Kahn D. Carbamazepine and other antiepileptic drugs in refractory depression. In: Roose SP, Glassman AH, eds. *Treatment strategies for refractory depression.* Washington, DC: American Psychiatric Press; 1990:75–107.

51. Kasper S, Ruhrmann S, van den Hoofdaker RH. Therapeutic sleep derivation in patients resistant to antidepressants. In: Maecher JP, Crocq MA, eds. *The bioclinical interface. Proceedings from the IXth conference.* Rouffach, France, Sept. 23–26 1992. Amsterdam: Elsevier (in press).

52. Katona CLE. Lithium augmentation in refractory depression. *Psychiatr Devel* 1988;2:153–171.

53. Kragh-Sorensen P, Hansen CE, Baastrup PC, Hvidberg FF. Self-inhibiting action of nortriptyline's antidepressive effect at high plasma levels. *Psychopharmacologia* 1976;45:305–312.

54. Kramlinger KG, Post RM. The addition of lithium to carbamazepine: antidepressant efficacy in treatment-resistant depression. *Arch Gen Psychiatry* 1989;46:794–800.

55. Lovett LM, Crimmins R, Shaw DM. Outcome in unipolar affective disorders after stereotactic tractotomy. *Br J Psychiatry* 1989;155:547–550.

56. Magni G, Fisman M, Helmes E. Clinical correlates of ECT-resistant depression in the elderly. *J Clin Psychiatry* 1988;49:405–407.

57. Mandel MR, Welch CA, Mieskie M, McCormick M. Prediction of response to ECT in tricyclic intolerant or tricyclic-resistant depressed patients. *McLean Hosp J* 1977;2:203–209.

58. McGrath PJ, Stewart JW, Nunes EV, Ocepek-Welikson K, Rabkin JG, Quitkin FM, Klein DF. A double-blind crossover trial of imipramine and phenelzine for outpatients with treatment-refractory depression. *Am J Psychiatry* 1993;250:118–123.

59. Medical Research Council. Clinical trial of the treatment of depressive illness. *Br Med J* 1965;5439:881–886.

60. Miller IW, Bishop SB, Norman WH, Keitner GI. Cognitive/behavioural therapy and pharmacotherapy with chronic, drug-refractory depressed inpatients: a note of optimism. *Behav Psychother* 1985;13:320–327.

61. Nelson JC. The use of antipsychotic drugs in the treatment of depression. In: Zohar J, Belmaker RH, eds. *Treating resistant depression.* New York: PMA Publishing, 1987;131–146.

62. Nelson JC, Mazure CM. Lithium augmentation in psychotic depression refractory to combined drug treatment. *Am J Psychiatry* 1986;143:363–366.

63. Nelson JC, Mazure CM, Bowers MB, Jatlow P. A preliminary, open study of the combination of fluoxetine and desipramine for

64. Nierenberg AA. Methodological problems in treatment resistant depression research. *Psychopharm Bull* 1990;26:461–464.

65. Nierenberg AA, Cole JO, Glass L. Possible-trazodone potentiation of fluoxetine: a case series. *J Clin Psychiatry* 1992;53:83–85.

66. Nierenberg AA, White K. What next? A review of pharmacologic strategies for treatment resistant depression. *Psychopharm Bull* 1990;26:429–460.

67. Nolen WA, Van De Putte JJ, Dijken WA, Kamp JS. L-5HTP in depression resistant to reuptake inhibitors: an open comparative study with tranylcypromine. *Br J Psychiatry* 1985;147:16–22.

68. Nolen WA, Van de Putte JJ, Dijken WA, Kamp JS, Blansjaar BA, Kramer HJ, Haffmans J. Treatment strategy in depression: I. Nontricyclic and selective reuptake inhibitors in resistant depression: A double-blind partial crossover study on the effects of oxaprotiline and fluvoxamine. *Acta Psychiatr Scand* 1988;78:668–675.

69. Nolen WA, Van De Putte JJ, Dijken WA, Kamp JS, Blansjaar BA, Kramer HJ, Haffmans J. Treatment strategy in depression: II. MAO inhibitors in depression resistant to cyclic antidepressants: Two controlled crossover studies with tranylcypromine versus L-5-hydroxytryptophan and nomifensine. *Acta Psychiatr Scand* 1988;78:676–683.

70. Nolen WA, Haffmans PMJ, Bouvy PF, Duivenvoorden HJ. Monoamine oxidase inhibitors in resistant major depression. A double-blind comparison of brofaromine and tranylcypromine in patients resistant to tricyclic antidepressants. *J Affect Disord* 1993;28:189–197.

71. Ogura C, Okuma T, Uchida Y, Imai S, Yogi H, Sumami Y. Combined thyroid (triiodothyronine)-tricyclic antidepressant treatment in depressive states. *Folia Psychiatr Neurol Jpn* 1974;28:179–186.

72. Oppenheim G, Zohar J, Shapiro B, Belmaker RH. The role of estrogen in treating resistant depression. In: Zohar J, Belmaker RH, eds. *Treating resistant depression.* New York: PMA Publishing; 1987:357–366.

73. Paul SM, Extein I, Calil HM, et al. Use of ECT with treatment resistant depressed patients at the National Institute of Mental Health. *Am J Psychiatry* 1981;138:486–489.

74. Peselow ED, Filippi AM, Goodnick P, Barouche F, Fieve RR. The short-and long-term efficacy of paroxetine HCl: B. Data from a double-blind crossover study and from a year-long trial vs. imipramine and placebo. *Psychopharmacol Bull* 1989;25:272–276.

75. Pope HW, Jonas JM, Hudson JI, Kafka MP. Toxic reactions to the combination of monoamine oxidase inhibitors and tryptophan. *Am J Psychiatry* 1985;142:491–492.

76. Post RM, Uhde TW. Carbamazepine as a treatment for refractory depressive illness and rapidly cycling manic-depressive illness. In: Zohar J, Belmaker RH, eds. *Treating resistant depression.* New York: PMA Publishing; 1987:175–235.

77. Poynton A, Bridges PK, Bartlett JR. Resistant bipolar affective disorder treated by stereotactic subcaudate tractotomy. *Br J Psychiatry* 1988;152:354–358.

78. Prange AJ. L-Triiodothyronine (T₃): its place in the treatment of TCA-resistant depressed patients. In: Zohar J, Belmaker RH, eds. *Treating resistant depression.* New York: PMA Publishing; 1987:269–278.

79. Price LH. Lithium augmentation in tricyclic-resistant depression. In: Extein IL, ed. *Treatment of tricyclic-resistant depression.* Washington, DC: American Psychiatric Press; 1989:49–79.

80. Price LH, Charney DS, Delgado PL, Heninger GR. Fenfluramine augmentation in tricyclic-refractory depression. *J Clin Psychopharmacol* 1990;10:312–317.

81. Price LH, Conwell Y, Nelson JC. Lithium augmentation of combined neuroleptic-tricyclic treatment in delusional depression. *Am J Psychiatry* 1983;140:318–322.

82. Price LH, Charney DS, Heninger GR. Efficacy of lithium-tranylcypromine treatment in refractory depression. *Am J Psychiatry* 1985;142:619–623.

83. Price LH, Charney DS, Heninger GR. Reserpine augmentation of desipramine in refractory depression: clinical and neurobiological effects. *Psychopharmacology [Berlin]* 1987;92:431–437.

84. Prudic J, Sackheim HA, Devanand DP. Medication resistance and clinical response to electroconvulsive therapy. *Psychiatry Res* 1990;31:287–296.

85. Quitkin FM. The importance of dosing in prescribing antidepressants. *Br J Psychiatry* 1985;247:593–597.

86. Reimherr FW, Woods DR, Byerley B, Brainard J, Grosser BI. Characteristics of responders to fluoxetine. *Psychopharm Bull* 1984;20:70–72.

87. Robertson MM, Trimble MR. Major tranquilizers used as antidepressants. A review. *J Affect Disorders* 1982;4:173–193.

88. Ryan ND, Puig-Antich J, Rabinovich H, Fried J, Ambrosini P, Meyer V, Torres D, Dachille S, Mazzie D. MAOIs in adolescent major depression unresponsive to tricyclic antidepressants. *J Am Acad Child Adolesc Psychiatry* 1988;27(6):755–758.

89. Sackheim HA, Prudic J, Devanand DP. Treatment of medication resistant depression with electroconvulsive therapy. In: Tasman A, Goldfinger S, Kaufman CA, eds. *American psychiatry press review of psychiatry,* Vol. 9. Washington, DC: American Psychiatric Press; 1990:91–115.

90. Sackheim HA, Prudic J, Devanand DP, Decina P, Kerr B, Malitz S. The impact of medication resistance and continuation pharmacotherapy on relapse following response to electroconvulsive therapy in major depression. *J Clin Psychopharmacol* 1990;10:96–104.

91. Schatzberg AF, Cole JO, Cohen BM, Altesman RJ, Sniffin CM. Survey of depressed patients who have failed to respond to treatment. In: Davis JM, Maas J, eds. *The affective disorders.* Washington, DC: American Psychiatric Press; 1983:73–85.

92. Schmauss M, Laakmann G, Dieterle D. Nomifensine: A double-blind comparison of intravenous versus oral administration in therapy-resistant depressed patients. *Pharmacopsychiatry* 1985; 18:88–90.

93. Schopf J, Baumann P, Lemarchand T, Rey M. Treatment of endogenous depressions resistant to tricyclic antidepressants or related drugs by lithium addition: Results of a placebo-controlled double-blind study. *Pharmacopsychiatry* 1989;22:183–187.

94. Schweizer E, Rickels K, Amsterdam JD, Fox I, Puzzuoli G, Weise C. What constitutes an adequate antidepressant trial for fluoxetine? *J Clin Psychiatry* 1990;51:8–11.

95. Shapira B, Kindler S, Lerer B. Medication outcome in ECT-resistant depression. *Convulsive Therapy* 1988;4:192–198.

96. Stein D, Avni J. Thyroid hormones in the treatment of affective disorders. *Acta Psychiatr Scand* 1988;77:623–636.

97. Stein G, Bernadt M. Lithium augmentation therapy in tricyclic-resistant depression. A controlled trial using lithium in low and normal doses. *Br J Psychiatry* 1993;162:634–640.

98. Steiner W, Fontaine R. Toxic reaction following the combined administration of fluoxetine and L-tryptophan: five case reports. *Biol Psychiatry* 1986;21:1067–1071.

99. Stern RA, Nevels CT, Shelhorse ME, Prohaska ML, Mason GA, Prange AJ. Antidepressant and memory effects of combined thyroid hormone treatment and electroconvulsive therapy: Preliminary findings. *Biol Psychiatry* 1991;30:623–627.

100. Stern WC, Harto-Truax N, Bauer N. Efficacy of bupropion in tricyclic-resistant or intolerant patients. *J Clin Psychiatry* 1983; 44:148–152.

101. Targum SD, Greenberg RD, Harmon RL, Kessler K, Salerian AJ, Fram DH. Thyroid hormone and the TRH stimulation in refractory depression. *J Clin Psychiatry* 1984;45:345–346.

102. Thase ME, Frank E, Mallinger AG, Hammer T, Kupfer DJ. Treat-

103. Thase ME, Howland RH. Refractory depression: relevance of psychosocial factors and therapies. *Psychiatr Ann* [*in press*].

104. Thase ME, Kupfer DJ. Characteristics of treatment-resistant depression. In: Zohar J, Belmaker RH, eds. *Treating resistant depression.* New York: PMA Publishing; 1987:23–45.

105. Thase ME, Kupfer DJ, Jarrett DB. Treatment of imipramine-resistant recurrent depression: I. An open clinical trial of adjunctive L-triiodothyronine. *J Clin Psychiatry* 1989;50:385–388.

106. Thase ME, Kupfer DJ, Frank E, Jarrett DB. Treatment of imipramine-resistant recurrent depression: II. An open clinical trial of lithium augmentation. *J Clin Psychiatry* 1989;50:413–417.

107. Thase ME, Frank E, Mallinger AG, Hammer T, Kupfer DJ. Treatment of imipramine-resistant recurrent depression: III. Efficacy of monoamine oxidase inhibitors. *J Clin Psychiatry* 1992;53:5–11.

108. Thase ME, Mallinger AG, McKnight D, Himmelhoch JM. Treatment of imipramine-resistant recurrent depression: IV. A double-blind, cross-over study of tranylcypromine in anergic bipolar depression. *Am J Psychiatry* 1992;149:195–198.

109. Thase ME, Rush AJ, Kasper S, Nemeroff C. Tricyclics and newer antidepressant medications: treatment options for treatment resistant depressions. *Depression* [*in press*].

110. Thase ME, Shipley JE. Tricyclic antidepressants. In: Last CG, Hersen M, eds. *Handbook of anxiety disorders.* New York: Pergamon Press; 1988:460–477.

111. Tsutsui S, Yamazaki Y, Namba T, Tsushima M. Combined therapy of T_3 and antidepressants in depression. *J Int Med Res* 1979; 7:138–146.

112. van Marwijk HWJ, Bekker FM, Nolen WA, Jansen PAF, van Nieuwkerk, Hop WCJ. Lithium augmentation in geriatric depression. *J Affect Disord* 1990;20:217–223.

113. Walinder J, Carlsson A, Persson R. 5-HT reuptake inhibitors plus tryptophan in endogenous depression. *Acta Psychiatr Scand* 1981;290(Suppl):179–190.

114. Wehr TA, Rosenthal NE. Sleep deprivation, phototherapy, and other nonpharmacological treatments of affective illness. In: Extein IL, ed. *Treatment of tricyclic-resistant depression.* Washington, DC: American Psychiatric Press; 1989:153–167.

115. Weilburg JB, Rosenbaum JF, Biederman J, Sachs GS, Pollack MH, Kelly K. Fluoxetine added to non-MAOI antidepressants converts nonresponders to responders: a preliminary report. *J Clin Psychiatry* 1989;50:447–449.

116. Wernicke JF, Dunlop SR, Dornseif BE, Zerbe RL. Fixed-dose fluoxetine therapy for depression. *Psychopharm Bull* 1987;23: 164–168.

117. White K, Wykoff W, Tynes LL, Schneider L, Zemansky M. Fluvoxamine in the treatment of tricyclic-resistant depression. *Psychiatr J Univ Ottawa* 1990;15:156–158.

118. Zohar J, Lerer B, Belmaker RH. Beta-2 adrenergic agonists for depression as a potential treatment. In: Zohar J, Belmaker RH, eds. *Treating resistant depression.* New York: PMA Publishing; 1987:375–380.

119. Zohar J, Moscovich D, Mester R. Addition of reserpine to tricyclic antidepressants in resistant depression. In: Zohar J, Belmaker RH, eds. *Treating resistant depression.* New York: PMA Publishing; 1987:367–374.

Psychopharmacology: The Fourth Generation of Progress, edited by Floyd E. Bloom and David J. Kupfer. Raven Press, Ltd., New York © 1995.

CHAPTER 93

Lithium and the Anticonvulsants in the Treatment of Bipolar Disorder

Joseph R. Calabrese, Charles Bowden, and Mark J. Woyshville

Although lithium remains the treatment of choice for bipolar disorder, only 60% to 80% of classic bipolar patients have a satisfactory clinical response. Fewer than half of all bipolar patients have classical, elated syndromes. When the response rate of lithium is considered across the wide spectrum of bipolar disorders, it probably only approaches 50%. Among mixed manics who account for 16% to 67% of all bipolar patients, only 30% to 40% respond to lithium (11). Rapidly cycling patients who constitute 13% to 20% of all bipolar disorders also have low (20% to 30%) response rates to lithium (5,16,34). Although there are numerous other predictors of lithium nonresponse, these two variants (mixed manics and rapid cycling) appear to account for the largest proportion of those who exhibit poor response to lithium. Serendipitously, emerging data suggest that these two predictors of lithium nonresponse may be putative predictors of positive response to both carbamazepine (57) and valproate (10,21).

Although controlled trials have demonstrated the efficacy of carbamazepine in the acute treatment of mania, initial responsiveness is often lost over time (59). Recent data also suggest that only one-third of acutely manic patients have moderate to marked improvement during the first 2 months of treatment with either lithium or carbamazepine as monotherapy (63). In addition, more severe mania was noted to predict nonresponse to carbamazepine. Such findings suggest that large numbers of bipolar patients are not responsive to lithium and that substantial numbers of both classic and rapid-cycling bi-

polar patients eventually become resistant to carbamazepine. Recent multicenter controlled data suggest valproate has efficacy equal to lithium in the acute management of mania (6). A large valproate maintenance study is currently underway. This chapter critically reviews recent information regarding the efficacy of lithium and its use in the treatment of bipolar disorder and the rapidly developing data regarding the evolving role of carbamazepine and valproate.

Extrapolation of results generated from controlled, blinded clinical trials to clinical practice is difficult. It is plausible that results from the better-designed trials emphasized here may actually underestimate patient outcome. For example, the enrollment of refractory patients in trials with monotherapy arms that allow only for the limited use of adjunctive medications depart substantially from the practice of psychiatry in the community (see Chapter 73 and 91, *this volume*).

LITHIUM

Acute Mania

Recent studies have indicated that 30% to 66% of acutely manic patients do not respond well to lithium (34,62,63). Furthermore, the benefits of response appear to be more compromised by adverse effects than earlier thought (24,72). Such reports have led to reassessment of the data on which approval of lithium was based and new studies to clarify these issues, utilizing improved research methodologies and patient samples that reflect the diagnostic spectrum of bipolar disorder in the 1990s. The evidence for the efficacy of lithium in acute mania largely came from three double-blind, placebo controlled crossover studies of a total of 78 patients (23). Outcome criteria

J. R. Calabrese and M. J. Woyshville: Department of Psychiatry, Case Western Reserve School of Medicine, University Hospitals of Cleveland, Cleveland, Ohio 44106.

C. Bowden: Division of Biological Psychiatry, Department of Psychiatry, University of Texas Health Science Center, San Antonio, Texas 78284-7792.

differed across the studies and diagnostic criteria were not consistently specified. In one study, patients with any degree of improvement on a nurse-rated seven-point global scale were reported as responders. In two of the studies, initial assignment to study medication was not randomized. No placebo-controlled study of using lithium in acute mania was published between 1971 and 1993.

A recently completed study provides the first parallel group, randomized, double-blind data on lithium-treated acutely manic patients. Of the 36 patients treated with lithium, 49% had moderate or better improvement in manic symptoms during the 3-week trial, a rate of response significantly greater than the 28% seen in patients treated with placebo (6). The efficacy of lithium did not differ from that of valproate. Of the patients treated with lithium, 31% had some degree of worsening manic symptoms at the end of the trial. The percentage of patients discontinuing because of medication intolerance was not significantly higher among lithium-treated than valproate-treated patients (11% vs. 6%). No neuroleptics were used during the study, and the only other psychotropic medication allowed was lorazepam during the first week of study medication. These results generally conform to recent impressionistic data, and indicate that although lithium is clearly effective, substantial numbers of patients remain unresponsive during monotherapy of an acute episode.

Clinical improvement with lithium is relatively slow, with an initial response generally occurring 7 to 14 days after initiation of lithium treatment. Initial improvement may not occur sooner than the 4th week for some patients. Because of aggressive, disruptive behavior of the acutely manic patient, adjunct medications are often required during this lag period. Lithium plasma concentrations required for acutely manic patients are often higher than needed for maintenance therapy. Although a loading dose strategy is ineffective, dosage should be increased as rapidly as tolerated until response occurs or a plasma level of approximately 1.2 mEq/L is reached. The side effects of lithium are generally less apparent during acute treatment than maintenance therapy.

Acute Bipolar Depression

Six of seven placebo-controlled studies have reported significant antidepressant effects of lithium (23). However, methodological problems limit generalizability. Most included unipolar as well as bipolar depressed patients. Most studies comparing tricyclic antidepressants with lithium lacked placebo controls. The single study that compared lithium, imipramine, and placebo in bipolar depressed patients found imipramine more effective than lithium (20). The protective effect of lithium against subsequent episodes appears to be lower for depressive episodes than from manic episodes (14,16,46). Additionally, most depressive episodes in bipolar patients will occur

in patients already taking lithium or alternative mood-stabilizing agents. Therefore, early use of other antidepressant agents is important if the patient does not respond to an increase in lithium dosage.

Prophylaxis

Maintenance phase studies of lithium are more extensive, better designed, and more conclusive than acute treatment studies regarding lithium's efficacy in preventing relapses (1,14). However, no placebo-controlled maintenance treatment study of lithium's efficacy in bipolar disorder has been conducted in over 20 years. Several recent naturalistic studies suggest that at present a substantial number of bipolar patients have inadequate responses to lithium. Harrow and colleagues reported that 40% of lithium-treated patients had a manic relapse during a mean 1.7-year period of treatment, a result similar to that of patients on no medication (26). Maj and colleagues found that among a group of patients selected for lithium responsiveness (successful acute response and no episodes over the first 2 years of follow-up), only half remained episode free over the ensuing 5 years (41). Tohen and colleagues also reported that 46% of patients remained stable for 4 years after their first episode, with outcome being unrelated to treatment (72).

Issues of dosage and approach to discontinuation of lithium have been clarified by recent studies. Discontinuation of lithium therapy in bipolar patients is followed by a high rate of relapse, with most episodes being manic rather than depressed (70). This study by Suppes et al., as well as other withdrawal study data, strongly suggest that lithium's prophylactic effect is principally in reducing the frequency of manic rather than depressive episodes (46). Furthermore, abrupt discontinuation is followed early on by a much higher rate of relapse than is gradual discontinuation (18).

Relapse rates following discontinuation were 50% higher among bipolar I than bipolar II patients. In addition, Post and colleagues have presented anecdotal evidence to suggest that some patients who had experienced long-term benefit from lithium and have it discontinued will, following relapse, be unresponsive to reintroduction of the lithium. Among patients with two or fewer prior episodes, maintenance lithium levels of 0.8 to 1.0 mEq/L were associated with lower rates of relapse than were levels of 0.4 to 0.6 mEq/L. Relapse rates into depression did not differ between the two groups. The severity of adverse effects was greater in the higher plasma level group (22).

Predictors of Response to Lithium

As evidence has developed that a substantial percentage fail to do well with acute or maintenance treatment with lithium, and as alternative treatments for bipolar disorder have developed, it has become important to know which illness characteristics are associated with a favorable or unfavorable response to lithium and alternative treatments. Acutely, patients with elated, less severe episodes without psychotic features, also referred to as classical mania, appear to have the best response to lithium during an acute manic episode (23). Patients who move from a depressive episode into a period of euthymia and then mania do better than those who move directly from a depressive episode into a manic episode (24). It is not well established that these differences hold equally during maintenance treatment.

Several syndromal variants of bipolar disorder are associated with relatively low response rates to lithium. The best studied is mixed mania, with more than half a dozen studies consistently indicating lower acute and chronic response rates to lithium treatment (23). Rapidly cycling patients also do not respond as well to lithium (16,34). This illness course of bipolar disorder will be defined in the DSM-IV as four or more depressions, hypomanias, or manias in the prior 12 months, with episodes being demarcated by a switch to an episode of opposite polarity or by a period of remission. This phenomenon appears to be late in onset, occurs most commonly in bipolar type II females, and is not usually associated with antidepressant use (5,16,34). Rapid cycling, and possibly mixed states, appear to be nonfamilial modifiers of state and course that transiently come and go during the natural history of bipolar disorder and its treatment (12). When these variants are present during treatment with lithium therapy, prognosis worsens and the morbidity and mortality associated with the illness increases (11,19).

As evidence has emerged that antidepressant medications increase the likelihood of rapid cycling, it is prudent to be cautious in interpreting the data about rapid cycling, because a component of the poor response may have been secondary to recent heterocyclic antidepressant therapy. Patients with bipolar disorder that appears to be secondary to other medical disorders respond poorly to lithium. Patients with comorbid substance abuse respond relatively poorly to lithium therapy, although this may be simply because of the conservative management of their substance abuse.

During maintenance therapy with lithium, the development of hypomania is strongly predictive of a subsequent full manic episode, with 65% having a subsequent major manic relapse. By contrast, minor depressive episodes were not usefully predictive of either subsequent manic or depressive episodes, as 61% of the minor depressive episodes were not followed by any major relapse (30).

Pharmacokinetics and Adverse Effects

The clearance of lithium is delayed by most nonsteroidal antiinflammatory drugs (NSAID). Sulindac appears not to alter lithium clearance. Several nonsteroidal antiinflammatory agents have been marketed in recent years, but effects on lithium clearance has not been assessed. A conservative approach is to monitor plasma lithium levels closely for several months following introduction of NSAID.

Lithium consistently impairs urinary concentrating ability. The ensuing frequent day- and nighttime urinations are often functionally impairing to the patient. Therefore, if such symptoms are prominent, one should consider discontinuing lithium and utilizing valproate or carbamazepine, or possibly, adding a diuretic that reduces the concentration impairment. Both loop diuretics and thiazides are effective. Although thiazides usually increase the plasma concentration of lithium, this can be managed by dosage adjustment. It is plausible, although it has not been studied, that the reduction in distal tubule exposure to lithium associated with thiazide use could reduce long-term risk of renal impairment.

Although several recent reviews have drawn sanguine conclusions regarding the effect of long-term lithium treatment on renal function, several other studies have reported a small number of cases of renal insufficiency, probably at incident rates no higher than 1% (60,65). Duration of lithium use, dosage, plasma level, and prior experiencing of polydipsia are possible, but not clearly established, risk factors in cases of renal insufficiency. Regular monitoring of creatinine levels in plasma is warranted indefinitely, and consultation indicated if creatinine levels rise to and remain above 1.6 mg/100 ml.

Long-term lithium use is also associated with a significant increase in subclinical hypothyroidism, a risk that may be greater in women. The duration of lithium use was positively correlated to antithyroid antibody titer. It thus seems advisable to check thyroid function regularly in patients treated with lithium, perhaps semiannually for the first 2 years of treatment. Some authorities recommend addition of T_4 to the regimen of any lithium-treated bipolar patient if indices of thyroid function are in the low-normal range, such as a TSH greater than 5 μIU. This may be particularly important if the patient exhibits signs of poor control of illness, such as subsyndromal depression.

The risks of using lithium during pregnancy remain unresolved. Earlier studies suggested that lithium increased the risk of the cardiovascular anomaly Ebstein's atresia. The low base rate of Ebstein's atresia of approximately 1 in 20,000 live births makes conclusive study of this risk difficult. A recent study suggested no increased risk, but was of such a small number of subjects that its ability to recognize two- to threefold increases in risk was negligible (74). Another recent study of 148 prospectively studied women using lithium during the first trimester of pregnancy indicated rates of major congenital malformations did not differ between the lithium (2.8%) and control (2.4%) group and concluded that lithium is not an important human teratogen (29). Since neuroleptics may control some aspects of manic symptoms, it may be advisable to try discontinuing lithium as soon as pregnancy is recognized and, if any manic symptoms emerge during the first trimester, first try neuroleptics and secondly use electroconvulsive therapy.

The most frequently reported subjective side effects of lithium have been long known (excessive thirst, polyuria, memory problems, tremor, and weight gain); however, the implications of lithium's adverse effects, especially their role in contributing to noncompliance, have more recently been reconsidered (23). It seems likely that the absence of alternatives to lithium inclined psychiatrists to try to manage adverse effects that seriously interfered with function rather than discontinue use. As evidence for the efficacy of alternative mood stabilizers emerged, earlier consideration of alternative regimens has become prudent. Recent studies underscore the frequency and degree to which lithium impairs cognitive functions and the contribution of such adverse effects to poor compliance (23).

CARBAMAZEPINE

The clinical efficacy of carbamazepine (or oxcarbamazepine) in bipolar disorder has been documented under controlled conditions in 288 acutely manic patients, 31 acutely depressed patients, and 116 patients for prophylaxis. Additionally, another 581 bipolar patients were treated with carbamazepine in open studies. Carbamazepine has been established as having marked acute and prophylactic antimanic and anti-mixed-states properties with poor to moderate antidepressant responses. Predictors of response data suggest this drug's profile may complement that of lithium and have particular application in the management of mixed states and rapid cycling.

Acute Mania

In 16 controlled studies, acute antimanic efficacy data was generated for 571 predominately bipolar manic patients (of whom at least 288 were treated with carbamazepine) and indicated that carbamazepine is superior to placebo and at least equal in efficacy to lithium and neuroleptics. Six comparisons each between carbamazepine and placebo, neuroleptics, and lithium were made.

Although reports of carbamazepine's efficacy appear in the literature as early as 1971 (70), the first placebo-controlled study of this drug's acute antimanic efficacy was published by Post and colleagues in 1978 (3). Reporting their results to date in 1980 (4), they found that better than 50% of manic patients experienced a moderate-to-marked improvement relative to their placebo baseline, and, again in 1987 (56), aggregate experience with 19 acutely manic patients (nine previously reported in ref.

4) indicated that 12 had a moderate-to-robust response. Although these findings are in support of carbamazepine's acute antimanic efficacy, Post and colleagues observed that, as a group, the responders remained symptomatic and that response in this study represented clinical improvement and not necessarily remission (56). Other placebo-controlled studies (15,17,31,43,44) demonstrated the superiority of carbamazepine over placebo, but frequently used adjunctive therapy with neuroleptics (31,43,44) or lithium (15).

Because, in part, of the morbidity normally associated with the acutely manic patient, the majority of controlled studies in this population compare carbamazepine with an active treatment, such as lithium or a neuroleptic. Post and colleagues reported a comparison between carbamazepine, lithium, and neuroleptics in which equal efficacy was demonstrated (57). Following a placebo lead-in, 19 patients received carbamazepine, 19 received lithium, and 17 received neuroleptics. By 3 weeks, all three groups showed substantial improvement over the placebo phase and the same degree of symptomatic severity despite higher degrees of baseline mania in the carbamazepine and neuroleptic groups. Other neuroleptic-controlled studies found that carbamazepine is at least as effective (25,43,44,47), or more effective (8,66) than neuroleptics. Okuma and colleagues carried out the largest double-blind comparison of carbamazepine and a neuroleptic in their study of 55 patients randomized to either carbamazepine or chlorpromazine. Rescue medications, such as benzodiazepines, were permitted in most of these studies (25,43,44,47).

Controlled studies of carbamazepine versus lithium in the management of acute mania give results paralleling the findings of the carbamazepine versus neuroleptic literature. Specifically, carbamazepine was found to be at least as efficacious as lithium in five studies (37,38,50,57,63). Small and colleagues carried out the largest ($n = 48$) and best designed double-blind parallel group comparison of carbamazepine to lithium. Although they found that carbamazepine was equal in efficacy to lithium, only one-third of patients in each cohort were described as responders. There is additional evidence that carbamazepine is at least as effective acutely as lithium from a maintenance study (52), which had an acute phase in which 20 of 29 bipolar patients treated with carbamazepine continued the trial past 2 months, as opposed to 16 of 27 lithium-treated patients. Three studies permitted neuroleptics as rescue medication (37,50,52) and one permitted antidepressants (56). These studies support the conclusion that carbamazepine and lithium have comparable antimanic efficacy; however, it should be noted that a substantial number of lithium nonresponders are among the participants in such studies. Thus, interpretation of the above results might be skewed by the presence of patients with inherently more severe illness. For example, the study of Small and colleagues (63), which contains a high proportion of lithium and other treatment nonresponders, only demonstrated response in one-third of patients treated with either carbamazepine or lithium as monotherapy. There is some evidence, however, that lithium and carbamazepine may possess a synergistic action that converts some failures of each drug as monotherapy into responders when used in combination. Kramlinger and Post added lithium in a blinded fashion to seven patients responding poorly to carbamazepine, of whom six were previous lithium failures, the remaining patient responding to lithium and neuroleptics in combination (33). Complete remission was seen in five (one of whom also required haloperidol), marked improvement in one, and no response in one (who was one of four rapid cyclers).

Acute Bipolar Depression

There is much less controlled data addressing the acute efficacy of carbamazepine in the treatment of bipolar depression than there is for mania. In placebo-controlled studies, Post and colleagues reported acute antidepressant efficacy in bipolar depression, but the response was less robust than seen in acute mania. Specifically, in their 1980 study (4), three of seven bipolar depressed patients had a good response to carbamazepine; in their 1986 update of their experience treating bipolar depression (55), they report on 24 patients with bipolar depression, of which 16 were bipolar I and eight were bipolar II. Fifteen of the 24 patients exhibited moderate improvement.

Prophylaxis

Seven controlled studies produced prophylactic data on 217 bipolar patients, of whom 116 were treated with carbamazepine. Carbamazepine was compared to placebo in two studies, and to lithium in five. Although carbamazepine is superior to placebo, the lithium results suggest equal efficacy overall; however, some evidence suggested that carbamazepine-treated patients relapsed earlier in the course of prophylaxis than their lithium-treated counterparts.

In 1978, Post and colleagues published the first placebo-controlled prophylactic study of carbamazepine using a crossover design in 10 patients (3). Several years later, Okuma and colleagues replicated these findings, noting moderate to marked responses in six of 10 patients treated with carbamazepine as opposed to two of nine patients treated with placebo followed for 1 year (48). Both studies permitted rescue medication to manage breakthrough episodes.

Although still arguing for the efficacy of carbamazepine, prophylactic studies comparing this agent to lithium have been less impressive than the acute studies. Two studies found that the two treatments were equally efficacious (40,52), but other studies (13,63,73) demonstrate superior prophylactic efficacy of lithium. Patients given carbamazepine appeared to relapse earlier. Placidi and colleagues (52) found that although both drugs were effective in two-thirds of patients, a higher dropout rate for patients with mood incongruent psychotic features was observed in the lithium cohort. Watkins and colleagues observed that ''[Lithium] significantly lengthens the time in remission'' (73). Small and colleagues (63) reported that all carbamazepine-treated patients dropped out during the first 24 weeks of prophylaxis, whereas lithium group dropouts occurred over the first year of follow-up. Coxhead and colleagues (13) stated that nearly all carbamazepine dropouts occurred in the first month of follow-up, but may have been due to precipitous withdrawal of lithium (as all patients entering prophylaxis were initially stabilized on lithium). As in the placebo studies, rescue medications were permitted and included neuroleptics (40,52) and antidepressants (40,52,73).

In addition to the above controlled studies, there are many open studies which in the main support the conclusions drawn from the controlled studies. By and large, over the broad spectrum of bipolar disorder, the literature suggests that carbamazepine is a safe and effective alternative and adjunct to lithium in the acute and prophylactic management of both classic bipolar disorder and atypical lithium nonresponsive variants. Carbamazepine appears to have its greatest clinical impact on the manic phase of the illness as opposed to the depressed phase but may lose some prophylactic efficacy over time (69).

Predictors of Response

Findings in the controlled literature bearing on predictors of response have been uneven. Initially, it seemed that predictors of lithium nonresponse, particularly dysphoria complicating mania and rapid cycling, predicted a differential response to carbamazepine relative to lithium (4,54,57). Summarizing predictors of response in mania, Ballenger (2) noted that rapid and circular continuously cycling patients respond much better to carbamazepine than to lithium; in fact, their response rate rivals that of patients without rapid cycling who are treated with lithium. He indicated that the predictors of response of bipolar illness to carbamazepine include mania complicated by dysphoria/anxiety (a subset of mixed states), rapid cycling, and greater severity of illness. Indeed, for mixed states, the work of Post and colleagues (57,58) supports the use of carbamazepine in this lithium-resistant population. For rapid cycling, a focused review of the literature reveals 19 open studies and 3 controlled studies yielding 119 and 6 rapid cyclers, respectively, in whom acute response rates were 32% for depression and 51% for mania. Prophylactically, responses were 60% for the depressed and 64% for mania. It should be noted that the great majority of these patients required acute and prophylactic adjunctive medications including neuroleptics, antidepressants, and lithium. Accordingly, these combination therapy predictors of response data may not extend to the drug's use in monotherapy.

Findings at variance with the prevailing view of predictors of response include acute work by Klein and colleagues which suggests that carbamazepine does not have a unique response profile (31). Stromgren and Boller's comprehensive review of carbamazepine treatment of bipolar illness (67) reported that scrutiny of the case histories of the literature reviewed gave no impression of pretreatment clinical differences between responders and nonresponders to carbamazepine. Lovett and colleagues (39) evaluated age of illness onset, predominant affective typology, and sequential pattern; they found no correlation with response. In contrast to Post's prior data, Small and colleagues (63) found that decreasing severity of mania predicted positive response to not only lithium, but carbamazepine as well. Coxhead and colleagues (13) found that previous morbidity predicted future morbidity, regardless of assignment to carbamazepine or lithium treatment groups. This is consistent with recent data suggesting that patients without rapid cycling respond better to carbamazepine than those with rapid cycling (50). These findings indicate that the initial optimism regarding the efficacy of carbamazepine in the management of the traditionally lithium refractory patient may need to be tempered somewhat, particularly in the case of rapid cycling.

VALPROATE

There now are over 1,042 psychiatric patients that have undergone various trials of valproate.[1] Of these, 256 acute manic patients underwent controlled trials, 528 open longitudinal trials for bipolar or schizoaffective disorder–bipolar subtype patients, and 258 open longitudinal trials for miscellaneous diagnoses including schizophrenia, unipolar depression, and personality disorders.

Acute Mania

Well-designed studies have demonstrated the efficacy of valproate in comparatively large samples of acutely manic patients (6,53). These studies are consistent with the findings of an extensive open longitudinal literature dating back to the mid-1960s. Prospective studies have documented poor to moderate acute and prophylactic efficacy in the management of the depressed phase of the bipolar disorder, but these were not controlled and await replication (10).

---

[1] In this chapter we refer to all similarly active preparations of the compound as valproate, including divalproex sodium, sodium valproate, valproic acid, valpromide, and dipropylacetamide.

Six controlled studies have evaluated the antimanic efficacy of valproate in 256 acutely manic patients in randomized double-blind trials. All of the placebo-controlled studies found valproate superior (6,7,17,53). Most (6,7,17,53), but not all (21), lithium-controlled studies found valproate to be equal in efficacy. Of the six, five had placebo arms and two had lithium arms. Emrich first documented the efficacy of valproate in a controlled study. When valproate and placebo was administered to five acutely manic patients in a double-blind ABA crossover study, four of five showed marked responses (17). Brennan et al. replicated these initial findings in 1984 by documenting marked efficacy in six of eight acutely manic patients that received valproate and placebo in a double-blind ABA crossover study (7). In a case study, Post et al. then showed valproate and phenytoin nonresponse in one patient who responded to carbamazepine in a double-blind crossover fashion. They concluded that nonresponse to one anticonvulsant did not predict nonresponse to others in bipolar disorder (56).

The first well-designed double-blind placebo-controlled study of valproate was published in 1991 by Pope and colleagues (52). Patients ($n = 36$) were randomly assigned to treatment for 7 to 21 days with no other medications permitted after day 10. Valproate was significantly superior to placebo. The 17 patients randomized to valproate treatment demonstrated a 54% decrease in scores on the Young Mania Rating Scale as compared with a median 5.0% decrease among the 19 patients receiving placebo. Significant differences also emerged on the Global Assessment Scale and the Brief Psychiatric Rating Scale. Substantial antimanic effects appeared within 1 to 4 days of achieving therapeutic valproate concentration. No adverse effects occurred more frequently with valproate than with the placebo. Although responders had an older age of onset, shorter duration of illness, and higher valproate levels, rapid cycling and dysphoric mania did not predict response during this short trial (54). Until Pope et al. (52) published their data, there were no studies available in the literature comparing the efficacy of valproate to a placebo. Although this study only randomized 36 patients, its sample size compared favorably to the three double-blind placebo-controlled crossover studies of lithium that used a total of 78 patients and was superior in design in that it employed random assignment to parallel groups. Freeman studied 27 acute manics who were randomized into a double-blind parallel-group trial comparing lithium to valproate (21). Favorable response to valproate was associated with high pretreatment depression scores. The coexistence of high pretreatment depression scores was found to be a predictor of response to valproate. They determined that valproate and lithium were both effective in improving manic symptoms, although lithium was slightly more effective overall, and they found valproate to be superior to lithium in the management of acute episodes of mania accompanied by co-

TABLE 1. *Degree of improvement at final evaluation of 179 patients*

	% Patients			Fisher p Values	
% Improvement	Valproate	Lithium	Placebo	Placebo vs Valproate	PLB vs LI
30	66	49	35	<0.001	0.022
40	54	49	28	<0.001	0.005
50	48	49	25	0.004	0.025

existing depression, i.e., mixed states or dysphoric mania. This study's unusually high response rate to lithium (90%) suggested the need for a placebo.

The completion of the Abbott-sponsored multicenter acute double-blind comparison of valproate to lithium and placebo (n = 179) increased the number of acutely manic patients studied in a double-blind fashion from a total of 77 to 256 (6). Patients were randomly assigned to parallel groups (valproate 40%, placebo 40%, lithium 20%) and studied over a 21-day experimental period. Rescue medications (up to 4 g/day chloral hydrate and/or 2 mg/day lorazepam) were permitted up the 10th day. The Mania Rating Scale, composed of the Manic Syndrome Scale and the Behavior and Ideation Scale from the Schedule for Affective Disorders and Schizophrenia, constituted the primary efficacy variable. Results were similar for the intent-to-treat sample, composed of all patients who received at least one dose of study drug or placebo, and the evaluable sample, composed of patients who received the study medication for at least 8 days and had adequate serum levels. Valproate-treated patients had significantly greater improvement than placebo-treated patients on the Manic Syndrome Scale from day 5 through the end of the 21-day trial. From day 10 on, the Mania Rating Scale and the Behavior and Ideation Scale indicated significantly greater improvement for valproate-treated patients than those treated with placebo. Lithium-treated patients had profiles of response similar to those of the valproate-treated patients on every efficacy variable throughout the entire study. Categorical outcome among the three groups was also analyzed. Mild, moderate, and marked improvements were defined as 30%, 40%, and 50% improvement from baseline to the final evaluation on efficacy measures (see Table 1). Thus, at all levels, the response to the two active medications was approximately twice that of response to placebo and was highly clinically significant. Analysis of individual behavioral items indicated that manic mood, reduced sleep, increased activity, generalized motor hyperactivity, elation/grandiosity, and psychosis improved significantly more in valproate- than placebo-treated patients and that manic mood improved significantly more in lithium- than in placebo-treated patients. During the 21-day trial, both drugs were relatively well tolerated. However, there was a trend toward more lithium-treated patients dropping out prematurely for intolerance to treatment than in the placebo group. Forty-eight percent of the valproate-treated group, 61% of the lithium-treated group, and 64% of the placebo-treated

group failed to complete all 21 days of treatment. The completion of the Abbott-sponsored multicenter acute mania study earmarked the advent of the beginning, and hopefully not the end, of a new era in bipolar disorder research. For the first time, resources were made available to carry out a large well-designed trial that employed random assignment to parallel groups that included a placebo arm. However, most patients at the end of its 21-day experimental period were still significantly impaired, suggesting that additional definition could have been obtained if patients were studied for a longer period of time and that alternative agents with more rapid onset of effects are still needed.

Prophylaxis

Although there are no published double-blind controlled studies comparing the prophylactic efficacy of valproate to any psychotropic agent, such a trial is ongoing. This study began in spring of 1993, and its principal objective is to evaluate the safety and efficacy of valproate compared to a placebo in the prevention of mania. In addition, it is comparing the efficacy and safety of lithium to that of a placebo in the prevention of mania to gauge study reliability. Three hundred patients are being randomly assigned to parallel groups of valproate, lithium, and placebo in ratios of 2:1:1. The duration of the maintenance phase is up to 12 months or the time to the first manic relapse.

Eleven open longitudinal studies investigated the prophylactic use of valproate in a total of 786 psychiatric patients have been published (7,10,17,27,35,36,59,61, 64,71,75). Of these 786 patients, there were 528 with bipolar disorder or the bipolar subtype of schizoaffective disorder with enough detail to allow for conclusions (see Table 2). Those of particular importance are described. The French investigator, Lambert, first began using valproate in 1966. He administered the drug to 393 psychiatric patients: 244 affective disorders (141 bipolar), 27 schizophrenics, and 122 character disorders (35). In open trials, 141 bipolar patients received an average of 900 to 1800 mg of valproate monotherapy for 6 to 163 months. Although his studies were methodologically compromised, he noted marked acute and prophylactic antimanic effects with poor to moderate antidepressant effects. Unfortunately, he did not comment on the degree to which rapid cycling and mixed states predicted response to valproate.

TABLE 2. *Open maintenance valproate studies in bipolar/schizoaffective disorders*

Study	No.[a]	Duration (mos)	Results
Lambert (35)	141 BP	6–163	Marked acute and prophylactic antimanic effects, moderate antidepressant effects
Semadeni (61)	32 BP 50% LI resistant	6–48	Recurrence in 50%
Puzynski and Klosiewicz (59)	10 BP 5 SA 80% LI resistant	26–51	Episodes decreased 46% efficacy in mania greater than depression
Brennan et al. (7)	4 BP 100% LI resistant	9–33	No recurrence in 100%
Emrich et al. (17)	12 SA 100% LI resistant	18–78	No recurrence in 83%
Vencovsky et al. (71)	60 BP	varied	Fewer side effects than LI
Zapletalek et al. (75)	14 BP	7.7	Fewer side effects than LI
Hayes (27)	12 BP 16 SA	14	Improvement in 88%
Sovner (64)	5 BP	2–6	No recurrence in 2 patients
Lambert and Venaud (36)	121 BP	24	Equal efficacy to lithium 15% fewer valproate dropouts
Calabrese et al. (11)	101 BP	9–46	Marked acute and prophylactic antimanic effects, moderate antidepressant effects

[a] BP, bipolar; SA, schizoaffective-bipolar subtype; LI, lithium.

Recently, Lambert and Venaud conducted a novel open prospective longitudinal study by randomly assigning patients for 2 years to either lithium or valproate (36). Of 150 patients studied, 121 were bipolar and 29 unipolar. Rapid cyclers, circular continuous cyclers, and patients with mood-incongruent psychotic symptoms were excluded. The frequency of episodes was compared between groups and then within groups (the 2 years prior to study was compared to the 2-year experimental period). When outcome or tolerance of the treatment was judged poor by the investigator, a switch to the alternative experimental agent was permitted. The main outcome measure was the number of episodes of mania or depression occurring during the follow-up. The number of episodes was 39 (0.51 per patient) in the valproate group and 42 (0.61 per patient) in the lithium group. The number of episodes for patients receiving valproate decreased from 4.12 during the 2 years prior to study to 0.51 during the experimental period, and the number of episodes for those receiving lithium decreased from 3.92 to 0.61. Therefore, efficacy rated by the number of episodes was similar between groups. For both drugs, efficacy was slightly higher in preventing mania than depression. Although valproate was equal in efficacy to lithium, at the end of the study there were fewer dropouts in the group treated with valproate (10%) than in the group treated with lithium (25%). The dropout rates were comparable for first year, but a disparity showed up during the second year of study, particularly toward the end of the study. Patients leaving the study for inefficacy were the same for the two treatments. Four subjects initially treated with valproate changed treatment because of lack of efficacy. Ten subjects initially treated with lithium changed treatment; of the ten, four changed because of lack of efficacy and

six because of poor tolerance. Poor tolerance rates were evaluated by combining the important and very important side effects: 4% for valproate and 10% for lithium. This lower incidence of important or very important side effects in the valproate group was evident at three months and led to valproate never being replaced by lithium, whereas lithium was replaced by valproate six times. Further information regarding side-effect profiles was not reported. The above literature suggests valproate is superior to placebo, equal in efficacy to lithium, and preliminarily better tolerated than lithium.

The published literature on the safety and efficacy of valproate is compromised by its open, and sometimes retrospective, designs but is distinguished by the large sample sizes evaluated by Lambert and his colleagues. Lambert's more recent use of open naturalistic designs with random assignment to parallel groups was a major advance and will probably usher in their more widespread use. There remains a need for studies that compare one of the anticonvulsants to lithium in the acute and prophylactic treatment of homogeneous cohorts of rapid cyclers and those patients with mixed states (dysphoric mania or hypomania). Until such studies are conducted, the treatment of choice for such variants of illness will remain controversial.

Valproate in Rapid Cycling and Mixed States

In addition to studies evaluating outcome in classic bipolar patients, there are now data from six published open trials that have assessed the efficacy of valproate in the management of a total 147 rapid-cycling bipolar patients (10,17,28,32,42,59). A combination therapy was used to treat 71 rapid cyclers and valproate monotherapy in 76 rapid cyclers. Marked acute and prophylactic antimanic effects, marked anti-mixed-state effects, and poor to moderate acute and prophylactic antidepressant effects were observed. Of the 147 patients, only 101 comprised a homogeneous patient population and were evaluated prospectively. The results from prospective studies of the acute and prophylactic efficacy of valproate in the management of bipolar rapid cycling (9) have recently been updated (10) with samples adequate in size to allow for predictors of response. A trial of valproate was given to 101 bipolar patients in a prospective, longitudinal, naturalistic design. Predictors of good antimanic response included decreasing or stable episode frequencies and nonpsychotic mania. Predictors of good antidepressant response included nonpsychotic mania worsening over the years of the illness and absence of borderline personality disorder comorbidity. Episode frequency did not predict response. Although there appeared to be a minimum therapeutic concentration of 50 to 80 μg/ml, there was no correlation between dose, level, and response at the upper limits of the therapeutic range. The data suggested that although comorbidity with borderline personality negatively impacted on the management of depression, it did not do so with hypomania or mania and mixed states (10). These predictors are consistent with recent data indicating that both decreasing or stable episode frequencies (59) and decreasing mania severity predict good outcome to carbamazepine (63). Calabrese's initial report of valproate's acute and prophylactic anti-mixed-state efficacy was replicated by Freeman and colleagues with a double-blind parallel group comparison of lithium to valproate (21).

PHARMACOKINETICS OF CARBAMAZEPINE AND VALPROATE

Carbamazepine and valproate possess pharmacokinetics different from lithium, and as a result, unique drug–drug interactions occur that affect clinical course and outcome. Three features of the pharmacology of carbamazepine and valproate incur particular clinical relevance: absorption, protein binding, and metabolism. Because lithium is not protein bound and excreted by the kidney unchanged, the last two of these concerns are not relevant to its use. In contrast, the pharmacology of anticonvulsants is somewhat more complicated, and these three pharmacological concerns frequently have clinical consequence.

Absorption

The general pharmacokinetic features of orally administered carbamazepine and valproate are clinically rele-

vant (Table 3). Normally, the side effects associated with anticonvulsants are either related to peak serum levels (i.e., tremors) or the speed and location of absorption (i.e., nausea and stomach cramps). Anticonvulsants are absorbed quickly, completely, and primarily in the stomach and are more likely to cause nausea and stomach cramps. Anticonvulsants like carbamazepine and either sodium valproate or valproic acid, but not divalproex sodium, have steep absorption curves and are more likely to cause such side effects at the upper limits of the therapeutic range. In contrast to valproate, there is only one preparation of carbamazepine readily available, so one is unable to change preparations in response to toxicity.

The absorption profiles of the different preparations of valproate vary substantially, provide flexibility, and influence the likelihood of such side effects as nausea, stomach cramps, or tremors. For example, the enteric coated preparation of valproate (divalproex sodium) causes nausea or stomach cramping much less frequently than the older preparations, valproic acid or sodium valproate. Divalproex sodium, which is actually the dimer of sodium valproate and valproic acid, reaches peak serum levels in 4 to 6 hrs and is better tolerated than valproic acid, which is absorbed rapidly (1 to 3 hr). The gastric absorption of valproic acid and sodium valproate is rapid and complete. Divalproex sodium is enterically coated and dissolves at the more basic pHs associated with the small intestine, thereby delaying its release and absorption. Occasionally, patients are unable to take valproate because of difficulty swallowing the capsules (valproic acid) or tablets (divalproex sodium); others cannot tolerate the aftertaste associated with the elixir (sodium valproate). The more recently released preparation of divalproex sprinkle is a hard gelatin, pull-apart capsule containing divalproex sodium-coated particles designed to be administered intact or opened to sprinkle on soft foods. Whereas valproate absorption with enteric-coated divalproex is delayed, the sprinkle preparation is a smooth release formulation since particles are released over an extended period of time. This minimizes fluctuation in levels between doses and makes it possible to be administered once daily in some patients. This preparation also offers additional flexibility for children and older adults, because it can be sprinkled on food for consumption. In addition to these currently available preparations, an intravenous preparation that reaches peak serum level in 10 to 20 min is currently under study.

Protein Binding

Most anticonvulsants are protein bound. Protein binding occurs predominantly on serum albumin and is proportional to the albumin concentration. The proportion of unbound, free, or bioactive drug is increased in patients with low levels of circulating albumin (caused by severe

TABLE 3. *Pharmacokinetic profiles*

	Peak absorption (hr)[a]	Elimination half-life (hr)		Time to steady state (days)	Protein binding (%)	Therapeutic range
		Children	Adults			
LI	1.5–4.5	24–36	24–72	5–15	0	0.6–1.2 mEq/L
CBZ	4–5	6–15	10–25	2–4	70–80	4–12 μg/ml
VPA	1–6	4–8	10–12	2–4	80–95	50–120 μg/ml

[a] Peak serum levels vary substantially due to preparations available: lithium carbonate and citrate (1.5–2 hr), controlled released lithium (4–4.5 hr); valproic acid and sodium valproate (1–3 hr), divalproex sodium (4–6 hr), and divalproex sprinkle (greater than 4 hr).

malnutrition, liver or renal failure, etc.) Unbound drug is important because it affects drug clearance. When using drugs that have concentration-dependent kinetics, such as valproate, it is important to note that an increase in the amount of unbound drug increases the rate of metabolism and ultimately lowers the blood concentration through what appears to be accelerated metabolism. For this reason, valproate does not have a truly linear relationship between total blood level and dose. The relationship between increasing dose and blood levels breaks down at the upper limits of the therapeutic range. Although blood levels are of critical importance in the dosing of valproate at the lower limits of the therapeutic range, at higher doses total blood levels provide only a rough guide. In the absence of toxicity, higher doses of valproate should be titrated against side effects rather than levels. This is in notable contrast to lithium, in which the upper limit of the therapeutic range is well defined. In other cases, competition for binding sites becomes important when two anticonvulsants with significant protein-binding properties are coadministered. The more highly protein-bound drug (valproate) increases the free or unbound fraction of the less highly protein-bound drug (carbamazepine), leading to occult carbamazepine toxicity.

Metabolism

Carbamazepine is metabolized by a liver microsomal P450 cytochrome oxidase to carbamazepine-10,11-epoxide. This metabolite is active, stable, and can produce toxic symptoms when significant levels accumulate. Carbamazepine is also metabolized through conjugation with glucuronides and sulfates. The ability of carbamazepine to autoinduce and heteroinduce drug metabolism complicates its routine clinical use. During the continuation phase of treatment, carbamazepine autoinduces its single dose $T_{\frac{1}{2}}$ of 20 to 30 hr down to a maintenance dose $T_{\frac{1}{2}}$ of 10 to 15 hr at some poorly defined interval between 3 weeks and 6 months. Not infrequently, this results in a return to subtherapeutic blood levels and cycling. Patients appear to have relapsed from a previously remitted state, and at this time some clinicians incorrectly consider the phenomenon of tolerance. Carbamazepine may also exhibit enzyme induction with many other psychiatric

medications, including haloperidol, valproate, and clonazepam, as well as oral contraceptives and most medications that employ P450 cytochrome oxidase as their main route of metabolism. For these reasons, before carbamazepine is prescribed to a woman currently taking oral contraceptives, routinely administered low-dose contraceptives should be changed to higher doses. A variety of other drugs, including fluoxetine, erythromycin, calcium channel blockers, cimetidine, and propoxyphene, cause clinically significant increases in carbamazepine levels and occasionally produce a picture similar to tricyclic antidepressant toxicity.

The metabolism of valproate is unusually complex and many active metabolites are produced. There are two major routes for metabolism of valproate: the P450 microsomal enzyme system and the mitochondrial β oxidation system. Metabolites are formed through both pathways, and it is currently believed that the 2-en-valproate metabolite has antiepileptic properties and that 4-en-valproate is a toxin. The more toxic metabolites are produced through the P450 pathway, and it is this pathway that tends to be enhanced by the coadministration of carbamazepine. Therefore, significantly higher doses of valproate are needed to produce effective drug levels when the drug is prescribed in combination therapy. Conversely, valproate is known to inhibit the metabolism of 10,11-epoxide carbamazepine. This metabolite is active, not usually included in blood monitoring, and may cause occult toxicity. With the exception of the coadministration of carbamazepine, valproate's drug–drug interactions rarely result in clinically significant problems in the management of bipolar patients.

The coadministration of carbamazepine and valproate in the treatment of patients with bipolar disorder occasionally leads to a series of drug–drug interactions that include the heteroinduction of valproate metabolism by carbamazepine, the displacement of protein-bound carbamazepine by valproate, and the inhibition of the metabolism of the primary metabolite of carbamazepine (10,11-epoxide carbamazepine) by valproate. When valproate is added to carbamazepine, anticipate an increased carbamazepine effect, as well as the eventual reduction in $T_{\frac{1}{2}}$ of valproate. When carbamazepine is added to valproate, anticipate decreasing valproate levels.

Side Effects

The side-effect profile of carbamazepine and most other anticonvulsants can be loosely categorized as dose related, not related to dose, and idiosyncratic. However, one occasionally sees dose-related side effects that do not subside until the dose is substantially decreased or the drug is discontinued, for example, carbamazepine-related fatigue and valproate-related hair thinning or stomach cramping.

The dose-related side effects of carbamazepine are benign and include leukopenia (15%), lethargy, double vision, cognitive changes, elevated liver functions tests, and hyponatremia. The non-dose-related side effects include nausea and vomiting and fluid retention. The idiosyncratic side effects include aplastic anemia (seen in less than 1 in 125,000), hepatic failure, Stevens-Johnson syndrome, rash (15%), and fetal drug effects. Nausea, benign leukopenia, fatigue, tremors, weight gain, and cognitive changes can be ameliorated by a decrease in dose, but occasionally beta blockers are required for treatment of tremors. Fetal drug effects can be minimized by use of folic acid supplements during pregnancy.

The dose-related side effects of valproate are benign and include nausea, vomiting, stomach cramps, increased liver functions tests, lethargy, hair thinning, and benign thrombocytopenia. Non-dose-related side effects include weight gain. Idiosyncratic side effects include hepatic failure (seen in less than 1 in 118,000), pancreatitis, agranulocytosis, and fetal drug effects. Nausea, vomiting, or stomach cramps can be managed by decreased dose, using divalproex sodium rather than valproic acid or sodium valproate, histamine type-2 blockers, or if necessary switching to the sprinkle preparation. Tremors can be managed by decreasing dose or use of beta blockers. Fatigue can be managed by decreasing dose. Hair thinning can be managed by decreasing the dose or zinc and selenium supplements. The benign thrombocytopenia and the benign increase in liver function tests can be managed by decreasing dose. Fetal drug effects of valproate can also be minimized by use of folic acid supplements during pregnancy.

METHODOLOGIC ISSUES

Although one can work toward treatment with bimodal monotherapy, it is clear that many patients require combination therapy during acute episodes of mania or depression. In fact, during the course of the illness most patients will eventually require adjunctive or augmentation pharmacotherapy with either other bimodal mood stabilizers or benzodiazepines, antidepressants, and/or antipsychotic agents. Informed combination therapy (polypharmacy) is routine and the state of the art in longitudinal management of this illness. Despite the above and the preexisting litera-

ture, the Food and Drug Administration requires that studies be designed to evaluate monotherapies against placebo so as to gauge study reliability. Accordingly, the design and completion of studies comparing different acute combination therapy paradigms is normally preceded by acute monotherapy designs with placebo arms. This practice has slowed the development of pharmacotherapy for bipolar disorder.

In addition, it has become increasingly clear that major mood disorders should be viewed longitudinally rather than solely in terms of the acute episode. Unfortunately, the rigor of the scientific literature evaluating the prophylactic pharmacotherapy of bipolar disorder is seriously encumbered by the three mood states that accompany this illness and multiple patterns of presentation. Because of the illness's inherent complexity, no method is available that allows controlled acute and prophylaxis studies to simultaneously focus on antidepressant, antimanic, and antimixed prophylactic efficacy with similar degrees of rigor. Naturalistic longitudinal studies more adequately address this need. Optimally, these prospective naturalistic studies, such as the one recently published by Lambert and Venaud, might openly randomize patients to different treatment groups and then allow for either crossovers or augmentation for nonresponders. If these designs are not employed, the patient population remaining at the end of maintenance studies will be so small and atypical that it will not have general relevance to the pool of patients normally treated. Studies involving rapid cycling and mixed states (dysphoric mania and hypomania, mixed mania) are particularly challenging because these phenomena appears to migrate unpredictably throughout the natural course of the illness.

Study designs employing placebo arms are feasible for research subjects who are hospitalized for acute studies, but not practical for evaluations of maintenance therapies. A survey of response rates in early double-blind placebo-controlled lithium studies in classic bipolar patients has been conducted. Whereas 55% to 100% of patients given placebo relapse over 5 months to 2 years, 0% to 49% of those given lithium relapse (14). The data of Schou suggest the average time of the untreated patient in remission is approximately 4.5 months. More recently, and consistent with this finding, a metaanalysis of 14 studies involving 257 patients with bipolar type I illness reported a 50% mania relapse rate after 5 months when lithium was rapidly discontinued (68). Given the remarkably high relapse rate for classic bipolar patients given placebo and the human cost in suicide attempts documented in the early studies, it is not clear that the additional methodological rigor obtained from a placebo arm merits the additional risk. On the other hand, current study designs employing random assignment to double-blind parallel treatment groups appear superior to older designs in which patients were crossed over to either other active arms or to placebo. The periodic recurrent nature of bipolar disorder makes these crossover designs vulnerable to false positives from the likelihood of spontaneous remissions. Accordingly, bipolar disorders research has been viewed as labor-intensive, expensive, not practical, and generally not funded by the National Institute of Mental Health or the pharmaceutical industry.

REFERENCES

1. Baastrup PC, Poulsen JC, Schou M, et al. Prophylactic lithium: double-blind discontinuation in manic-depressive and recurrent-depressive disorders. *Lancet* 1970;2:326–330.
2. Ballenger JC. The use of anticonvulsants in manic-depressive illness. *J Clin Psychiatry* 1988;49[11, Suppl]:21–24.
3. Ballenger JC, Post RM. Therapeutic effects of carbamazepine in affective illness: a preliminary report. *Commun Psychopharmacol* 1978;2:159–175.
4. Ballenger JC, Post RM. Carbamazepine in manic-depressive illness: a new treatment. *Am J Psychiatry* 1980;137:782–790.
5. Bauer MS, Calabrese JR, Dunner DL, et al. Multi-site data reanalysis: validity of rapid cycling as a course modifier for bipolar disorder in DSM-IV. *Am J Psychiatry* 1994;151:506–515.
6. Bowden CL, Brugger AM, Swann AC, et al. Efficacy of divalproex sodium vs. lithium and placebo in the treatment of mania. *JAMA* [*in press*].
7. Brennan MJW, Sandyk R, Borsook D. Use of sodium VPA in the management of affective disorders: basic and clinical aspects. In: Emrich HM, Okuma T, Muller AA, eds. *Anticonvulsants in affective disorders.* Amersterdam: Excerpta Medica; 1984.
8. Brown D, Silverstone T, Cookson J. Carbamazepine compared to haloperidol in acute mania. *Int Clin Psychoparmacol* 1989;4:229–238.
9. Calabrese JR, Delucchi GA. Spectrum of efficacy of VPA in 55 rapid-cycling manic depressives. *Am J Psychiatry* 1990;147:431–434.
10. Calabrese JR, Woyshville MJ, Kimmel SE, Rapport DJ. Predictors of valproate response in bipolar rapid cycling. *J Clin Psychopharmacology* 1993;13:280–283.
11. Calabrese JR, Woyshville MJ, Kimmel SE, Rapport DJ. Mixed states and bipolar rapid cycling and their treatment with VPA. *Psychiatr Ann* 1993;23:70–78.
12. Coryell W, Endicott J, Keller M. Rapid cycling affective disorder: demographics, diagnosis, family, and course. *Arch Gen Psychiatry* 1992;49:126–131.
13. Coxhead N, Silverstone T, Cookson J. Carbamazepine versus lithium in the prophylaxis of bipolar affective disorder. *Acta Psychiatry Scand* 1992;85:114–118.
14. Davis JM. Overview of maintenance therapy in psychiatry II: affective disorders. *Am J Psychiatry* 1976;133:1–13.
15. Desai NG, Gangadhas BN, Channabasavanna SM, et al. Carbamazepine hastens therapeutic action of lithium in mania. In: *Proceedings of the International Conference on New Directions in Affective Disorders.* Jerusalem, April 5–9, 1987:97 (*abst.*).
16. Dunner DL, Fieve RR. Clinical factors in LI carbonate prophylaxis failure. *Arch Gen Psychiatry* 1974;30:229–233.
17. Emrich HM, Dose M, von Serssen D. The use of sodium VPA and oxyCBZ in patients with affective disorders. *J Affect Dis* 1985;8:243–250.
18. Faedda GL, Tondo L, Baldessarini RJ, Suppes T, Tohen M. Outcome after rapid vs gradual discontinuation of lithium treatment in bipolar disorders. *Arch Gen Psychiatry* 1992;50:448–456.
19. Fawcett J, Scheftner A, Clark D, Hedeker D, Gibbons R, Coryell W. Clinical predictors of suicide in patients with major affective disorders: a controlled prospective study. *Am J Psychiatry* 1987;144:35–40.
20. Fieve RR, Platman SR, Plutchik RR. The use of lithium in affective disorders I: Acute endogenous depression. *Am J Psychiatry* 1968;125:487–491.
21. Freeman TW, Clothier JL, Passaglia P, Lesem MD, Swann AC. A double blind comparison of VPA and LI in the treatment of acute mania. *Am J Psychiatry* 1992;149:108–111.
22. Gelenberg AJ, Kane JN, Keller MB, et al. Comparison of the standard and low serum levels of lithium for maintenance treatment of bipolar disorders. *N Engl J Med* 1989;321:1489–1493.
23. Goodwin FK, Jamison KR. *Manic-depressive illness.* New York: Oxford University Press; 1990.
24. Grof E, Haag M, Grof P, et al. Lithium response and the sequence of episode polarities: preliminary report on a Hamilton sample. *Prog Neuropsychopharmacol Biol Psychiatry* 1987;11:199–203.
25. Grossi E, Sacchetti E, Vita A, et al. Carbamazepine vs. chlorpromazine in mania: a double blind trial. In: Emrich HM, Okuma T, Muller AA, eds. *Anticonvulsants in affective disorders.* Amsterdam: Excerpta Medica; 1984:177–187.
26. Harrow M, Goldberg JF, Grossman LS, et al. Outcome in manic disorders: a naturalistic follow-up study. *Arch Gen Psychiatry* 1990;47:665–671.
27. Hayes SG. Longterm use of VPA in primary psychiatric disorders. *J Clin Psychiatry* 1989;50(3):35–39.
28. Herridge PL, Pope HG. Treatment of bulimia and rapid cycling bipolar disorder with sodium VPA: a case report. *J Clin Psychopharmacol* 1985;5:229–230.
29. Jacobson SJ, Jones K, Johnson K, et al. Prospective multicentre study of pregnancy outcome after lithium exposure during first trimester. *Lancet* 1992;339:530–533.
30. Keller MB, Lavori PW, Kane JM, et al. Subsyndromal symptoms in bipolar disorder: a comparison of standard and low serum levels of lithium. *Arch Gen Psychiatry* 1992;49:371–376.
31. Klein E, Bental E, Lerer B, Belmaker RH. Carbamazepine and haloperidol v placebo and haloperidol in excited psychoses. *Arch Gen Psychiatry* 1984;41:165–170.
32. Klosiewicz L. The prophylactic influence of valproic acid amide in affective illness. *Psychiatr Pol* 1985;1:23–29.
33. Kramlinger KG, Post RM. Adding lithium carbonate to carbamazepine: antimanic efficacy in treatment-resistant mania. *Acta Psychiatr Scand* 1989;79:378–385.
34. Kukopulos A, Reginaldi D, Laddomada P, Floric G, Serra G, Tondo L. Course of the manic depressive cycle and changes caused by treatment. *Pharmacopsychiatry* 1980;13:156–167.
35. Lambert PA. Acute and prophylactic therapies of patients with affective disorders using valpromide (Dipropylacetamide). In: Emrich HM, Okuma T, Muller AA, eds. *Anticonvulsants in affective disorders.* Amsterdam: Excerpta Medica; 1984:33–44.
36. Lambert PA, Venaud G. Comparative study of valpromide versus LI in treatment of affective disorders. *Nervure* 1992;5(2):57–65.
37. Lenzi A, Lazzerine F, Grossi E, Massimetti G, Placidi GF. Use of carbamazepine in acute psychosis: a controlled study. *J Int Med Res* 1986;14:78–84.
38. Lerer B, Moore N, Meyendorff E, Cho S-R, Gershon S. Carbamazepine versus lithium in mania: a double-blind study. *J Clin Psychiatry* 1987;48:89–93.
39. Lovett L, Watkins SE, Shaw DM. The use of alternative drug therapy in nine patients with recurrent affective disorder resistant to conventional prophylaxis. *Biol Psychiatry* 1986;21:1344–1347.
40. Lusznat RM, Murphy DP, Nunn CMH. Carbamazepine vs lithium in the treatment and prophylaxis of mania. *Brit J Psychiatry* 1988;153:198–204.
41. Maj M, Priozzi R, Kemali D. Long-term outcome of lithium prophylaxis in patients initially classified as complete responders. *Psychopharmacology* 1989;98:535–538.
42. McElroy SL, Keck PE, Pope HG, Hudson JI. Valproate in the treatment of rapid cycling bipolar disorder. *J Clin Psychopharmacol* 1988;8:275–278.
43. Moller H-J, Kissling W, Riehl T, Bauml J, Binz U, Wendt G. Double-blind evaluation of the antimanic properties of carbamazepine as a comedication to haloperidol. *Prog NeuroPsychopharmacol Biol Psychiatry* 1989;13:127–136.
44. Muller AA, Stoll K-D. Carbamazepine and oxcarbazepine in the treatment of manic syndromes—studies in Germany. In: Emrich HM, Okuma T, Muller AA, eds. *Anticonvulsants in affective disorders.* Amsterdam: Excerpta Medica; 1984:139–147.
45. Nilsson A, Axelsson R. Lithium discontinuation. I. Clinical characteristics and outcome. *Acta Psychiatr Scand* 1990;82(6):433–438.
46. Okuma T, Inanaga K, Otsuki S, et al. Comparison of the antimanic

efficacy of carbamazepine and chlorpromazine: a double-blind controlled study. *Psychopharmacology* 1979;66:211–217.

47. Okuma T, Inanaga K, Otsuki S, et al. A preliminary double-blind study on the efficacy of carbamazepine in prophylaxis of manic-depressive illness. *Psychopharmacology* 1981;73:95–96.

48. Okuma T. Therapeutic and prophylactic effects of carbamazepine in bipolar disorders. *Psychiatr Clin North Am* 1983;6:147–174.

49. Okuma T, Yamashita I, Takahashi R, et al. Comparison of the antimanic efficacy of carbamazepine and lithium carbonate by double-blind controlled study. *Pharmacopsychiatry* 1990;23:143–150.

50. Okuma T. Effects of carbamazepine and other antiepileptic drugs on affective disorders. Presented at the symposium on Antiepileptic Drugs in Psychiatry, Freiburg, Germany; January 29–30, 1993.

51. Placidi GF, Lenzi A, Lazzerini F, Cassano GB, Akiskal HS. The comparative efficacy and safety of carbamazepine versus lithium: a randomized, double-blind 3-year trial in 83 patients. *J Clin Psychiatry* 1986;47:490–494.

52. Pope HG, McElroy SL, Keck P, Brown S. Valproate in the treatment of acute mania: a placebo controlled study. *Arch Gen Psychiatry* 1991;48:62–68.

53. Post RM, Uhde TW, Ballenger JC, Squillace KM. Prophylactic efficacy of carbamazepine in manic-depressive illness. *Am J Psychiatry* 1983;140:1602–1604.

54. Post RM, Berrettini W, Uhde T, Kellner C. Selective response to the anticonvulsant CBZ in manic depressive illness: a case study. *J Clin Psychopharmacol* 1984;4:178–185.

55. Post RM, Uhde TW, Roy-Byrne PP, Joffe RT. Antidepressant effects of carbamazepine. *Am J Psychiatry* 1986;143:29–34.

56. Post RM, Uhde TW, Roy-Byrne PP, Joffe RT. Correlates of antimanic response to carbamazepine. *Psychiatr Res* 1987;21:71–83.

57. Post RM, Rubinow DR, Uhde TW, et al. Dysphoric mania: clinical and biological correlates. *Arch Gen Psychiatry* 1989;46:353–358.

58. Post RM, Leverich GS, Rosoff AS, Altshuler LL. Carbamazepine prophylaxis in refractory affective disorders: a focus on long term follow-up. *J Clin Psychopharmacol* 1990;10:318–327.

59. Puzynski S, Klosiewicz L. Valproic acid amide in the treatment of affective and schizoaffective disorders. *J Affect Dis* 1984;6:115–121.

60. Schou M. Effects of long-term lithium treatment on kidney function: an overview. *J Psychiatr Res* 1988;22:287–296.

61. Semadeni GW. Study of the clinical efficacy of dipropylacetamide in mood disorders. *Acta Psychiatr Belg* 1967;76:458–466.

62. Small JG, Klapper MH, Kellams JJ, et al. Electroconvulsive treatment compared with lithium in management of manic states. *Arch Gen Psychiatry* 1988;45:727.

63. Small JG, Klapper MH, Milstein V, et al. Carbamazepine compared with LI in the treatment of mania. *Arch Gen Psychiatry* 1991;48:915–921.

64. Sovner R. The use of VPA in the treatment of mentally retarded persons with typical and atypical bipolar disorders. *J Clin Psychiatry* 1989;50(3):40–43.

65. Stancer HC, Forbath N. Hyperparathyroidism, hypothyroidism and impaired renal function after 10 to 20 years of lithium treatment. *Arch Intern Med* 1989;149:1042–1045.

66. Stoll KD, Bisson HE, Fischer E, et al. Carbamazepine versus haloperidol in manic syndromes—first report of a multicentric study in Germany. In: Shagass C, Josiassen RC, Bridger WH, et al., eds. *Biological psychiatry 1985: proceedings of the IVth World Congress of Biological Psychiatry.* Sept. 8–13, 1985; Philadelphia, PA. New York: Elsevier; 1986:332–334.

67. Stromgren LS, Boller S. Carbamazepine in treatment and prophylaxis of manic-depressive disorder. *Psychiatr Devel* 1985;4:349–367.

68. Suppes T, Baldessarini RJ, Faedda GL, Tohen M. Risk of recurrence following discontinuation of LI treatment in bipolar disorder. *Arch Gen Psychiatry* 1991;48:1082–1088.

69. Tohen M, Waternaux CM, Tsuang MT, Hunt AT. Four year follow-up of twenty four first-episode manic patients. *J Affect Dis* 1990;19:79–86.

70. Takezaki H, Hanaoka M. The use of carbamazepine (Tegretol) in the control of manic-depressive psychosis and other manic, depressive states. *Seishin-igaku (Clin Psychiatr)* 1971;13:173–183.

71. Vencovsky E, Peteriva E, Kabes J. Preventive effect of dipropylacetamide in bipolar manic depressive psychoses. *Psychiatr-Neurol-MedPsychol (Leipz)* 1987;39(6):362–364.

72. Vestergaard P, Aagaard J. Five-year mortality in lithium-treated manic-depressive patients. *J Affect Dis* 1991;21:33–38.

73. Watkins SE, Callender K, Thomas DR, Tidmarsh SF, Shaw DM. The effect of carbamazepine and lithium on remission from affective illness. *Br J Psychiatry* 1987;150:180–182.

74. Zalzstein E, Koren G, Einarson T, Freedom RM. A case-control study on the association between first trimester exposure to lithium and Ebstein's anomaly. *Am J Cardiol* 1990;65:817–818.

75. Zapletalek M, Hanus H, Kindernayova H. Experiences with the prophylactic action of dipropylacetaminde. *Cesk Psychiatrie* 1988;84:7–10.

Psychopharmacology: The Fourth Generation of Progress, edited by Floyd E. Bloom and David J. Kupfer. Raven Press, Ltd., New York © 1995.

CHAPTER 94

Psychosocial Predictors of Outcome in Depression

Robert M. A. Hirschfeld

Identification of predictors of outcome is useful because they provide clues to the etiology of depression and its pathogenesis. They are also useful clinically because they enable the physician to formulate a more accurate prognosis. Predictors of response to specific medications are especially helpful in selecting treatments.

The focus of this chapter is on psychosocial predictors of outcome in depression. Also included are general demographic predictors and a few prevalent clinical predictors, such as comorbid anxiety symptoms. The chapter is organized by type of predictor. For each predictor, the general relationship between the particular variables and depression is briefly presented, followed by research findings relevant to the variable's general utility as a predictor of general outcome and data available on the response to treatment, specifically pharmacotherapy.

After these presentations on predictors of outcome is a discussion of psychosocial outcomes. The issue of psychosocial outcomes, as contrasted with symptomatic outcomes, is of growing importance in medicine, as quality-of-life concerns are becoming part of investigations of all treatments. Fortunately, quality of life and other psychosocial measures have been of interest in psychiatry for a long time.

To be included in this review, the study had to use an objective measure of the particular variable, and the clinical sample had to be systematically ascertained and carefully evaluated, usually with a semistructured diagnostic interview (such as the SCID.)

SOCIODEMOGRAPHIC AND PSYCHOSOCIAL PREDICTORS OF RESPONSE

Age

Major depression and dysthymia are distributed across adulthood with a modest peak in early adulthood. How-

R. M. A. Hirschfeld: Department of Psychiatry and Behavioral Sciences, University of Texas Medical Branch, Galveston, Texas 77555-0429.

ever, there has been a trend over the last 50 years for the age of onset to decrease and the prevalence of depression to increase among young adults (39). Twice over a 6-year period, Coryell and his associates looked at major depression in a nonclinical sample of 965 relatives, controls, and spouses of affectively ill probands who had never been mentally ill when first examined. They found that subjects younger than 40 years were three times more likely to develop depression than were older subjects (17).

Robinson and Starkstein found that the older age of onset for a first major depressive episode was associated with greater likelihood of an undiagnosed neurological (or other general medical) disorder (64). Also, an older age of onset lessened the probability of atypical personality or a family history of depression (8).

With regard to recovery, the findings are mixed. In several studies, age was found to be positively associated with speed of recovery (36). However, Akiskal (3), Keller et al. (35,37), and Lewinsohn et al. (41), along with several others, did not find a relationship between age and recovery. Also, in a naturalistic study of 248 outpatients with bipolar disorder, O'Connell et al. found that neither current age nor age of onset was predictive of outcome (53).

In a community study of 119 married respondents with depression, McLeod and her colleagues found that age at episode onset was the only significant predictor of recovery in the total sample among other demographic variables, such as education, sex, and income. Specifically, persons who were older than 30 years at onset experienced longer episodes than did persons who were younger. Additionally, age was found to be more strongly predictive of recovery during early stages of an episode of depression, but not so much from later stages. Once an episode had lasted six or more weeks, age was no longer a predictive factor for the probability of recovery (47). With regard to medication, Brown and his coworkers found that older age predicted poorer response to tricyclic antidepressants in nonpsychotic, endogenously depressed patients (9).

In summary, age is clearly related to the prevalence of depression. With regard to recovery and other outcome variables, though, the relationship between age and depression is not clear.

Gender

With the exception of bipolar disorders, mood disorders occur twice as frequently in women as in men (12,76). This well-established finding suggests that gender plays an important role in the etiology and/or pathogenesis of depression.

Gender does not appear to be a predictor of recovery or relapse when treatment is uncontrolled, as in longitudinal studies (37,38). In the Zurich study of a community sample of young adults first interviewed at age 21, Vollrath and Angst found that gender did not predict recovery rates or response to medication (70).

The literature on differential sex response to antidepressant medications is rather limited. Hamilton and her colleagues reported a modest differential response to clorgyline by sex (24). In a study of 82 depressed subjects, Croughan et al. found that the clinical differences between male and female patients were minimal with regard to response to imipramine or amitriptyline. The women had equally good response to treatment, but that response tended not to be as strongly correlated with the clinical predictors as it was for men (19). In a study of atypical depression with 151 inpatients and outpatients, Davidson and Pelton found a gender difference when comparing responses to TCAs and monoamine oxidase inhibitors. Atypically depressed women responded better to MAOIs than to TCAs; and atypically depressed men showed a greater response to TCAs than to MAOIs (21).

In an examination of patients used for two multihospital collaborative studies of drug treatment in depression, Raskin found that younger women (i.e., those under the age of 40 years) responded less well to imipramine than did older women and men. Men under 40 years of age were seen to have responded better to chlorpromazine, but to have responded than younger women to phenelzine (60). However, O'Connell and his coworkers did not find any significant differences in outcome between the sexes in response to long-term treatment with lithium (53).

The findings with regard to the sex differences in pharmacokinetics of antidepressants, particularly amitriptyline and nortriptyline, have been inconsistent. Zeigler and Biggs (78) found no significant gender differences in plasma levels, but Preskorn and Mac (73) found higher plasma levels of either imipramine or amitriptyline in women. These differences may have occurred because of the coadministration of medications, including oral contraceptives, which could affect tricyclic antidepressant plasma levels (1). In their review of gender differences in pharmacokinetics and pharmacodynamics of psychotropic medication, Yonkers and colleagues concluded that there is little evidence to support claims of sex differential metabolism or actions of tricyclic antidepressants.

However, some differences have been reported for lithium. There appears to be a relationship between menstrual physiology and lithium pharmacology (77). Some studies have shown that adverse reactions to lithium may occur more frequently in women (7). This may be because lithium-induced hypothyroidism is more common in women (54). In addition, rapid-cycling bipolar illness is more prevalent in women (72); and this has been associated with thyroid abnormalities (54).

In summary, although there are a few scattered reports of modest or minimal gender effects predicting response to medication, the great majority of clinical studies did not find any evidence of gender relating to either outcome or medication response.

Marital Status

Depression has been found to be much higher among the nonmarried than among the married population. In the Epidemiology Catchment Area Study (ECA) studies, rates of major depression were lowest among the married, particularly those who were never divorced; whereas those who were divorced or cohabiting had the highest rates (67). This was also true of bipolar disorder in which married people had lower rates than did the divorced and never married.

Onset of depression is also more likely among the unmarried. In the Psychobiology of Depression Collaborative Study, Coryell and colleagues reported that onset of depression was most likely among single women. Divorce or separation increased the likelihood of a first-depressive episode (17). Coryell and associates (18), also found that both unipolar and bipolar patients were half as likely to marry as the comparison group. Bipolar patients with a predominance of manic episodes were also more likely not to be married, as reported by Romans and McPherson (65) in their study of 58 bipolar patients.

In their study of 101 patients with major depressive disorder in the Psychobiology Collaborative Study, Keller et al. (36) found a nonsignificant trend toward lower recovery rate in divorced or separated patients compared to married and single patients (45%, 63%, and 61%, respectively).

In the overwhelming majority of pharmacotherapy clinical trials in depression, marital status did not predict response to treatment (37,38,52,68). However, in one study, O'Connell and colleagues found that unmarried status was associated with poor outcome in 248 bipolar patients enrolled in an outpatient lithium program (53).

In summary, marital status is greatly associated with onset and prevalence of depression. As with gender, the majority of studies found that marital status is not a significant predictor of outcome. However, one study did find that an unmarried status was associated with poor outcome to medication response.

Quality of Marriage and Family Relationships

The quality of marital and family relationships and their effect on outcome in depressed patients has long been of interest. However, methodological problems have limited the utility and generalizability of these reports. For example, many studies have confounded individual characteristics that influence outcome (e.g., personality features, severity, and duration of symptoms) with familial factors.

An emotional atmosphere of calm and control at the time of discharge from the hospital was predictive of steady improvement in patients (48). If the environment lacked these positive features, it would predispose the patient to dangerous or undesirable activities, such as alcohol or drug abuse (4).

Expressed emotion is a key measure of intimate relationships within the family. The presence of expressed emotion has been noted to result in closeness and better functioning within the family setting (56). O'Connell and colleagues found that patients whose families showed high expressed emotion were overrepresented in the poorer outcome groups (53). Hooley and Teasdale reported that along with high expressed emotion, marital distress and the depressed person's perception of the amount of criticism of his or her spouse was predictive of relapse (30).

Similarly, Hooley and her associates (29) reported that depressed patients with relatives with high levels of expressed emotion had a poor course of illness. Those depressed patients from dysfunctional families whose relatives had high expressed emotion were three times more likely to relapse within the first 9 months following depression than were those patients whose relatives had low levels.

Miklowitz and his partners (48) found that the emotional atmosphere of the family during the postdischarge period was an important predictor of the clinical course of bipolar disorder. In their sample of 23 manic patients recruited from two inpatient wards, the risk of relapse for patients from high-expressed-emotion homes was 5.5 times that of patients from low-expressed emotion homes. The risk of relapse for patients from negative affective style homes was 5.9 times that of similar patients from benign affective-style homes. Thus, if either high rates of expressed emotion or negative affective style were present in a patient's home, relapse was highly likely (94%); whereas patients whose families demonstrated low stress had low relapse rates (17%).

In a study of 68 inpatients with major depression who had been categorized as belonging to functional or dysfunctional families at index, Miller et al. (49) found that impaired family functioning was an important predictor of the course of depressive illness. At the 12-month follow-up, depressed patients with dysfunctional families had a significantly poorer course of illness, as was apparent by higher levels of depression, lower levels of overall adjustment, and a lower proportion of recovered patients (34.9% with dysfunctional families and 69.6% rate with functional families). Keitner and his colleagues found that better family functioning was one of the five most important factors related to recovery in major depression (34).

In general, supportive and positive response to a patient's depression predicts a more rapid recovery than nonsupport. In a community study of 119 married men and women in which one partner had experienced a depressive episode, McLeod and her colleagues (47) found that recovery was more rapid in those relationships where the nondepressed spouse was perceived as being compassionate and warm toward the depressed individual. Positive feedback seemed to be especially important for predicting recovery, especially during the early stages of an episode.

In the same study, when McLeod and her affiliates (47) examined the impact of six indicators of social support on recovery, the only ones that reached significance in the total sample were conflict with friends and spouse warmth. Even though conflict with a spouse did not consistently predict speed of recovery as did conflictual relations with friends (i.e., less rapid recovery), spouses' reports of their reactions to the respondents' depression did. Patients whose spouse reported feeling positively toward them (i.e., feeling warmth and compassion) were much more likely to recover in any given time period than were patients whose spouse did not report those feelings.

Impaired family functioning (i.e., negative affective style) predicted poor outcome from treatment with lithium (53). For patients to be able to have a good outcome, their family relationships and home environment needed to be benign as opposed to critical and overinvolved (53).

In summary, in spite of many methodological concerns, three studies reported that an atmosphere of calm and control (expressed emotion) and spousal acceptance was predictive of steady improvement, closeness, and better family functioning within a depressed patient's family. This led to a greater possibility that the patient would recover and with a more rapid recovery. Six other studies consistently reported that high levels of expressed emotion and impaired family functioning was predictive of poorer outcome (i.e., more likely to relapse and lower proportion of recovered patients). Within those six studies, one study showed that impaired family functioning was predictive of poorer response to medication treatment with lithium.

Social Support

Similar to marital and familial support, social support has been of interest as a predictor of outcome in depressed patients. Several studies have examined the link of social support to depression. Clayton and her colleagues (15) have reported that a close, confiding relationship and physical proximity (i.e., social support) offers protection against the development of depression in persons in stressful situations. Warheit (71) provided evidence that individuals with low social support are at much greater risk of developing depressive symptoms. In their study of 44 outpatients with unipolar depression, Flaherty and colleagues found that patients with high social support had significantly better depression rating scores than did patients with low social support (22).

In general, the presence of social support has predicted successful outcome. In their study of 60 bipolar patients treated with lithium for one year, O'Connell and associates found positive social support, among other demographic measures such as sex, marital status, race, age, or education, to be most strongly correlated with a good outcome (52). Brugha and colleagues found that social support predicted clinical improvement in depressed patients in psychiatric hospitals, even when other potential risk factors such as age, sex, diagnosis, and severity of depression were controlled (11). In their more recent study of 248 bipolar outpatients, O'Connell et al. found that persons who had poor outcome to lithium treatment had less adequate social support than did those with better response to lithium (53).

Level of function in depressed subjects influences outcome (16,68). In depressed individuals, low social dysfunction was predictive of good response to interpersonal psychotherapy; high work dysfunction was predictive of good response to imipramine; and high impairment of function was predictive of good response to combined treatment (68).

In summary, social support has a strong connection to depression. Quality social support reduces the likelihood of developing depression. Furthermore, the presence of positive social support predicts successful outcome, and its absence has been associated in one study to poor outcome to lithium treatment.

Socioeconomic Status

Whether socioeconomic status is a predictor of outcome from pharmacotherapy is unresolved. With regard to prevalence, persons meeting poverty level criteria had higher rates for major depression than those persons who were not in poverty (10). People of low socioeconomic status were more likely to have chronic or recurrent depression than others in higher socioeconomic strata (50).

In a study of bipolar disorder, O'Connell found that lower socioeconomic status was associated with poor outcome for treatment with lithium (53). On the other hand, in the Biological Psychobiology Collaborative Study, those with lower annual income were more likely to recover (19). This latter study was of very severely ill inpatients.

In summary, depression is slightly more prevalent in individuals of lower socioeconomic status. The findings with regard to socioeconomic status as a predictor of outcome are mixed.

Race, Ethnicity, and Cultural Differences

In general, racial and cultural variables have not been reported as predictors of outcome in clinical trials and other studies, although one study did address this issue.

In a study of 159 black and 555 white depressed patients looking at the differential effects of chlorpromazine, imipramine, and a placebo, Raskin and Crook reported some differences in response between racial groups. They found that black patients evidenced a higher improvement rate at one week, irrespective of treatment, than did the white patients (61).

Personality Traits and Disorders

The relationship between personality and depression has received much attention in the literature (26). Four models have been described regarding the relationship between personality and depression: (a) predisposition, (b) complication, (c) spectrum, and (d) pathoplasty. The predisposition model proposes that certain personality characteristics render an individual vulnerable to depression and, in specific situations, can lead to depression. The complication model proposes that the experience of depression itself can cause personality change in an individual following recovery. The spectrum model proposes that certain personality characteristics may be genetically related to forms of depression. The pathoplasty model suggests that certain personality types may be associated with specific symptoms in a depressive episode (e.g., a histrionic personality may be associated with hostility, anger, and complaining during a depressive episode) (28).

To assess the connection between premorbid personality characteristics and onset of depression, Hirschfeld and his associates (27) looked at a sample of first-degree relatives, spouses, and controls of patients with mood disorders. Overall, differences were not found on measures of interpersonal dependency or extraversion. However, younger age (17 to 30 years old) predicted first onsets, both alone and in interaction with personality measures. With the younger subjects, personality variables did not significantly discriminate between the groups. Older subjects (31 to 41 years old), however, had decreased emotional strength, increased interpersonal dependency, and increased thoughtfulness. In another study, Maier et al. found that individuals with high levels of rigidity (men and women) and neuroticism (men only) were at risk for onset of depression (44).

Several studies of personality traits have been reported to predict response to antidepressant medication. For example, depressed individuals with assertive, independent, and competitive personality features were more likely to respond to medication treatment than were others who lacked these traits (33). High neuroticism in depressed persons predicted poor response to tricyclic antidepressants (33) and to lithium (45). In contrast, Davidson and his colleagues found that high neuroticism did not predict a poorer response to antidepressants (20).

Other personality traits that predicted outcome include sociotropy and autonomy. Sociotropy, a quality similar to interpersonal dependency, is a personality trait in which the individual seeks to have needs fulfilled by other people. An individual high in sociotropy is concerned about rejection from others and frequently acts in ways to please them to secure a strong interpersonal attachment. Autonomy refers to 14 qualities directed toward self-sufficiency. A highly autonomous individual is one who is concerned about personal failure and who strives to maximize control over his or her environment. Subjects with high autonomous and low sociotropic traits were more likely to show a greater response to antidepressants than were those subjects who displayed low autonomous and high sociotropic traits (58).

Depressed individuals with an associated personality disorder did not respond as well to antidepressants as those without personality disorders (33). In contrast, Davidson and his colleagues found that the presence of a personality disorder did not predict a poorer response to antidepressants (20).

In summary, personality traits and disorders have been found to be highly predictive of response to antidepressant medication. High neuroticism predicts a poor response to medication. Positive predictors of response to pharmacotherapy include high autonomy–low sociotropy, assertiveness, independence, and competitiveness.

The findings with respect to personality disorders are not as clear. One study reported that in depressed individuals with associated personality disorders, response to antidepressants was reduced. Another study did not find this.

Life Events

Life events have been associated with the onset of depression for many years. Paykel and his colleagues found that depressed patients, when compared with matched general population controls, had three times the number of life events in the 6-month period preceding the onset of depression (57). Other studies conducted more recently have been reasonably consistent in supporting this association (6,43).

In their longitudinal study of 65 depressed college students, Needles and Abramson found that individuals who displayed a reduction in hopelessness and experienced positive events were more likely to have a remission of depressive symptoms and subsequent recovery (51). In corroboration, Paykel and Cooper reported that, when

events occurred during treatment, negative events were more predictive of poorer outcome and neutral events were more predictive of better outcome (56).

Other studies have examined the relationship between life events and relapse. Hunt and his associates found that in approximately one-third of their 62 bipolar patients, a large number of severe life events had occurred during the month immediately preceding relapse. However, the actual number of manic and depressive relapses were not different (31).

O'Connell et al. found a trend for the poorer outcome groups to have experienced more life events in the year before a depressive episode (53).

Some specific drug and life event interactions have been reported. In a study of 116 patients suffering from major depression with melancholia, those individuals treated with imipramine who had an absence of life events during a 6-month follow-up had a better outcome at 6 months. For individuals treated with phenelzine, however, an absence of life events prior to the onset of an episode predicted a poorer outcome at 6 months (69).

In summary, life events are associated with depression, with relapse, and with prediction of response to medication. The more negative a life event, the more possibility of a relapse into a depressive episode.

Bereavement

The prevalence of depression is increased among the bereaved, especially among those who have lost a spouse or a child. Widows and widowers were found to be at an increased risk for developing major depression compared with married women and men (79). In their study of widowhood, Clayton et al. found that 35% of individuals had enough symptoms to meet criteria for major depression 1 month after the death of a spouse. At 4 months, 25% met the criteria, and at 1 year, 17% met the criteria (15).

In an analysis of 350 widows and widowers at 2 and 7 months following the death of their spouses, Zisook and Shuchter found that subjects who were most susceptible to depression were those with a history of major depression and who were younger (79).

In treating depression associated with bereavement, two studies have shown that the depressive symptoms improve with antidepressant treatment (32,55). However, even though the depressive symptoms do improve substantially, there is little, if any, improvement in the manifestation of bereavement (e.g., the intensity of grief). These differential responses to treatment suggest that major depression and bereavement are separate and distinguishable phenomena (55) and that treatment of depression may foster the process of grieving, not block it or "cover it over."

Whether depressions associated with bereavement respond better to pharmacotherapy or to psychotherapy is not known.

CLINICAL PREDICTORS OF RESPONSE

The chapter, thus far, has addressed demographic and psychosocial predictors of outcome. This section will address two important *clinical* predictors of response to pharmacotherapy—anxiety and substance abuse. These two clinical factors were selected because of their high comorbidity with depression.

Anxiety

Anxiety disorders are the second most common psychiatric disorders in the United States and often cooccur with depression. Between 15% and 33% of depressed patients have frank panic attacks (14).

The presence of anxiety symptoms in patients with major depression predicts more intense severity and greater likelihood of chronicity of depressive episodes, a decreased ability to respond to treatment, an increase in family prevalence of anxiety and/or depression, and increased impairment in social and vocational functioning (42). Outpatients with unipolar depressive disorder with higher ratings for anxiety recovered more slowly than those with lower levels of anxiety (14).

McLeod and colleagues found that a lifetime history of anxiety disorders significantly predicted a slower rate of recovery in their sample of outpatients with depression. They also found that a lifetime history of substance abuse predicted a slower rate of recovery (47).

In summary, anxiety disorders frequently cooccur with depression. Their cooccurrence predicts a slower recovery rate.

Alcohol and Drug Abuse

According to the ECA, the lifetime prevalence rate of alcoholism is 13.8% in the total population (25), and 6.2% had a history of drug abuse/dependence (5). The prevalence rates for major depressive disorder for alcohol abuse, drug abuse, and other mental disorders was 2.3% at 1 month, 3.0% at 6 months, and 5.9% for lifetime (62).

A history of alcohol or substance abuse in patients with depression increases the likelihood of hospitalization, committing suicide, and not complying with treatment (4).

Current alcohol and drug abuse in depressed individuals is known to hamper active treatment and is predictive of poor outcome in response to antidepressant treatment (3,53). In the O'Connell et al. study of bipolar disorder, 36% of the people in the poor outcome group were found to have substance abuse problems but only 7% of the people in the good outcome group (53). Akiskal found that concurrent sedative or alcohol abuse with depression was more likely to be associated with a poorer response to antidepressants (3).

In summary, the cooccurrence of substance abuse with depression is very common. Alcohol and drug abuse, in combination with depression, are predictors of poor outcome to medication treatment.

PSYCHOSOCIAL OUTCOMES

Earlier attention in this chapter has been on psychosocial variables at index, their relation to depression, and their value as predictors of treatment response. Now, the focus is on these variables as outcome measures in depressed individuals.

Social Functioning

In several follow-up studies, patients with major depression were found to be at higher risk of impairment in physical, social, and role functioning which resulted in lower levels of overall functioning (46,75).

Wells and colleagues demonstrated that outpatients with major depression had poorer physical functioning and feelings of well being than did patients with chronic medical conditions, including arthritis, hypertension, diabetes, and back pain. The only patients who scored lower than depressive patients on these measures were those with current heart conditions (75).

Work Functioning

Antidepressant therapy resulted in a significant improvement in functioning, generally, and a significant improvement in work and house functioning, specifically (2). Improved social and vocational functioning was seen in responders following treatment with imipramine (40).

When compared with symptom improvement, work functioning appeared to have a delayed reaction. After taking medication for approximately 6 weeks, symptoms in depressed patients began to lessen; but the bulk of improvement in work functioning did not occur until the patient had been taking medication for 6 to 24 weeks (23).

In summary, work functioning improves with successful treatment of depression, particularly antidepressants; but there appears to be a delay in improvement in work functioning compared with symptomatic improvement.

Marital and Family Functioning

Persons with major depression were found to have more marital and family problems than those without the disorders. In a study by Rounsaville et al. (66) of 76 moderately depressed married women who received outpatient maintenance treatment for depression, approximately 25% of those with marital disputes at treatment onset had a substantial improvement in their marriage over the course of 8 months of treatment. Those whose marriages did not improve were more symptomatic than those whose marriages improved. The married women in the dispute group at index were found to be more socially impaired (in terms of adjustment) than the married women in the nondispute group. Despite the poor prognosis for depressed women with marital disputes, those who did show improvement in their marital relationships were more likely to experience an improvement in depressive symptoms and overall social functioning by the end of their treatment.

In a follow-up study, persons with major depression were at an increased risk for not getting along with their partners and for not being able to confide in their partners (46). In support of this, Weissman showed that there was an approximate sixfold increase in the likelihood that persons with major depression would have trouble functioning in their marriage or within their families (73).

CONCLUSIONS

Sociodemographic and psychosocial variables clearly are related to depression and may be important in its etiology. There has been a trend in the last 50 years for the age of onset of depression to become younger. Nearly all types of depression are two times more prevalent in women than in men. Depression is more prevalent among the unmarried, and the onset of depression is more likely among the unmarried. There is some increase in prevalence of mood disorders (i.e., depression) in the lowest socioeconomic classes. However, these same variables have not been found to predict outcome generally or to influence the response to pharmacotherapy. There have been scattered findings reported in the literature, but no consistent pattern has emerged, that would suggest that these variables are helpful in predicting response to pharmacotherapy.

Although marital status per se does not predict outcome, the *quality* of marital, familial, and social relationships does seem to be an important predictor of outcome and response. A number of studies have found that calm, positive, steady support is associated with and predictive of a better outcome, a better response to medication, and often a speedier recovery. On the other hand, high criticism, distress, less support, and high expressed emotion is predictive of a poorer outcome in general and a poorer response to specific treatment. In addition, these same variables are predictive of relapses.

Other important predictors are personality features and disorders. High neuroticism, low autonomy, high sociotropy, are predictive of a poor response to tricyclic antidepressants. The presence of personality disorders also has an adverse affect on response to treatment. Comorbid anxiety disorders and substance abuse complicates the course of depression and reduces positive outcomes.

Depression rarely produces nonsymptomatic outcomes. Patients with depression appear to suffer from impairments in physical, social, and role functioning and a variety of other problems, including many common general medical illnesses. Successful treatment is associated with an improvement of psychosocial outcomes, but improvement in these outcomes tends to temporally lag behind symptomatic outcomes. This makes sense intuitively in that interpersonal relationships in role functioning often take time to improve.

Whether patients achieve nonclinical outcomes and what the effects of depression are on quality of life over time are very important questions, and should receive more attention in the future.

ACKNOWLEDGMENT

The author would like to express his thanks and appreciation to Ms. Victoria Trimm whose assistance in the preparation of this chapter was invaluable.

REFERENCES

1. Abernethy DR, Greenblatt DJ, Shader RI. Imipramine disposition in users of oral contraceptive steroids. *Clin Pharmacol Ther* 1984;35(6):792–797.
2. Agosti V, Stewart JW, Quitkin FM. Life satisfaction and psychosocial functioning in chronic depression: effect of acute treatment with antidepressants. *J Affect Dis* 1991;23:35–41.
3. Akiskal HS. Factors associated with incomplete recovery in primary depressive illness. *J Clin Psychiatry* 1982;43:266–271.
4. American Psychiatric Association. Practice guideline for major depressive disorder in adults. *Am J Psychiatry* 1993;150(4, Suppl):4–26.
5. Anthony JC, Helzer JE. Syndromes of drug abuse and dependence. In: Robins LN, Regier DA, eds. *Psychiatric disorders in America.* New York: The Free Press; 1991:116–154.
6. Billings A, Moos R. Psychosocial theory and research on depression: an integrative framework and review. *Clin Psychol Rev* 1982;2:213–237.
7. Bottiger LE, Furhoff AK, Holmberg L. Fatal reactions to drugs. *Acta Med Scand* 1979;205:451–456.
8. Brodaty H, Peters K, Boyce P, et al. Age and depression. *J Affect Dis* 1991;23(3):137–149.
9. Brown RP, Sweeney J, Frances A, Kocsis JH, Loutsch E. Age as a predictor of treatment response in endogenous depression. *J Clin Psychopharmacol* 1983;3:176–178.
10. Bruce ML, Takeuchi DT, Leaf PJ. Poverty and psychiatric status. *Arch Gen Psychiatry* 1991;48:470–474.
11. Brugha TS, Bebbington PE, MacCarthy B, Sturt E, Wykes T, Potter J. Gender, social support and recovery from depressive disorders: a prospective clinical study. *Psychol Med* 1990;20:147–156.
12. Clayton PJ. Gender and depression. In: Angst J, ed. *The origins of depression: current concepts and approaches.* New York: Springer-Verlag; 1983:77–89.
13. Clayton PJ. The comorbidity factor: establishing the primary diagnosis in patients with mixed symptoms of anxiety and depression. *J Clin Psychiatry* 1990;51(11, Suppl):35–39.
14. Clayton PJ, Grove WM, Coryell W, Keller M, Hirschfeld RMA, Fawcett J. Follow-up and family study of anxious depression. *Am J Psychiatry* 1991;148(11):1512–1517.
15. Clayton P, Halikes J, Mauvie W. The bereavement of the widow. *Dis Nerv Syst* 1974;32:597–604.
16. Coryell W, Endicott J, Keller M. Outcome of patients with chronic affective disorder: a five-year follow-up. *Am J Psychiatry* 1990;147:1627–1633.
17. Coryell W, Endicott J, Keller M. Major depression in a nonclinical sample. Demographic and clinical risk factors for first onset. *Arch Gen Psychiatry* 1992;49:117–125.
18. Coryell W, Scheftner W, Keller M, Endicott J, Maser J, Klerman

GL. The enduring psychosocial consequences of mania and depression. *Am J Psychiatry* 1993;150(5):720–727.

19. Croughan JL, Secunda SK, Katz MM, et al. Sociodemographic and prior clinical course characteristics associated with treatment response in depressed patients. *J Psychiatr Res* 1988;22(3):227–237.

20. Davidson J, Miller R, Strickland R. Neuroticism and personality disorder in depression. *J Affect Dis* 1985;8:177–182.

21. Davidson J, Pelton S. Forms of atypical depression and their response to antidepressant drugs. *Psychiatry Res* 1986;17:87–95.

22. Flaherty JA, Gaviria FM, Black EM, Altman E, Mitchell T. The role of social support in the functioning of patients with unipolar depression. *Am J Psychiatry* 1983;140(4):473–476.

23. Giller E Jr, Bialos D, Riddle MA, Waldo MC. MAOI treatment response: multiaxial assessment. *J Affect Dis* 1988;14:171–175.

24. Hamilton JA, Alagna SW, Pinkel S. Gender differences in antidepressant and activating drug effects on self-perceptions. *J Affect Dis* 1984;7:235–243.

25. Helzer JE, Burnam A, McEvoy LT. Alcohol abuse and dependence. In: Robins LN, Regier DA, eds. *Psychiatric disorders in America.* New York: The Free Press; 1991:81–115.

26. Hirschfeld RMA, Klerman GL, Clayton PJ, Keller MB. Personality and depression. *Arch Gen Psychiatry* 1983;40:993–998.

27. Hirschfeld RMA, Klerman GL, Lavori P, Keller MB, Griffith P, Coryell W. Premorbid personality assessments of first onset of major depression. *Arch Gen Psychiatry* 1989;46:345–350.

28. Hirschfeld RMA, Shea MT. Personality. In: Paykel ES, ed. *Handbook of affective disorders.* New York: Churchill-Livingstone; 1992:185–194.

29. Hooley JM, Orley J, Teasdale JD. Levels of expressed emotion and relapse in depressed patients. *Br J Psychiatry* 1986;148:642–647.

30. Hooley JM, Teasdale JD. Predictors of relapse in unipolar depressives: expressed emotion, marital distress, and perceived criticism. *J Abnorm Psychol* 1989;98:229–235.

31. Hunt N, Bruce-Jones W, Silverstone T. Life events and relapse in bipolar affective disorder. *J Affect Dis* 1992;25(1):13–20.

32. Jacobs SC, Nelson JC, Zisook S. Treating depressions of bereavement with antidepressants. *Psychiatr Clin North Am* 1987;10(3):501–510.

33. Joyce PR. Prediction of treatment response. In: Paykel ES, ed. *Handbook of affective disorders.* New York: Churchill-Livingstone; 1992:453–462.

34. Keitner GI, Ryan CE, Miller IW, Norman WH. Recovery and major depression: factors associated with twelve-month outcome. *Am J Psychiatry* 1992;149(1):93–99.

35. Keller MB, Klerman GL, Lavori PW, Coryell W, Endicott J, Taylor J. Long-term outcome of episodes of major depression: clinical and public health significance. *JAMA* 1984;252:788–792.

36. Keller MB, Lavori PW, Rice J, Coryell·W, Hirschfeld RMA. The persistent risk of chronicity in recurrent episodes of nonbipolar major depressive disorder: a prospective follow-up. *Am J Psychiatry* 1986;143(1):24–28.

37. Keller MB, Shapiro RW, Lavori PW, Wolfe N. Recovery in major depressive disorder. *Arch Gen Psychiatry* 1982;39:905–910.

38. Keller MB, Shapiro RW, Lavori PW, Wolfe N. Relapse in major depressive disorder. *Arch Gen Psychiatry* 1982;39:911–915.

39. Klerman GL, Lavori PW, Rick J, et al. Birth-cohort trends in rates of major depressive disorder among relatives of patients with affective disorder. *Arch Gen Psychiatry* 1985;42:689–693.

40. Kocsis JH, Sutton BM, Frances AJ. Long-term follow-up of chronic depression treated with imipramine. *J Clin Psychiatry* 1991;52(2):56–59.

41. Lewinsohn PM, Fenn DS, Stanton AK, Franklin J. Relation of age at onset to duration of episode in unipolar depression. *Psychol Aging* 1986;1:63–68.

42. Liebowitz MR. Depression with anxiety and atypical depression. *J Clin Psychiatry* 1993;54(2, Suppl):10–14.

43. Lloyd C. Life events and depressive disorders reviewed. 2. Events as precipitating factors. *Arch Gen Psychiatry* 1980;37:541–548.

44. Maier W, Lichtermann D, Minges J, Heun R. Personality traits in subjects at risk for unipolar major depression: a family study perspective. *J Affect Dis* 1992;24(3):153–163.

45. Maj M, Del-Vecchio M, Starace F, Pirozzi R, Kemali D. Prediction of affective psychoses responses to lithium prophylaxis: the role of sociodemographic, clinical, psychological and biological variables. *Acta Psychiatr Scand* 1984;69:37–44.

46. Markowitz JS, Weissman MM, Ouellette R, Lish JD, Klerman GL. Quality of life in panic disorder. *Arch Gen Psychiatry* 1989;46:984–992.

47. McLeod JD, Kessler RC, Landis KR. Speed of recovery from major depressive episodes in a community sample of married men and women. *J Abnorm Psychol* 1992;101(2):277–286.

48. Miklowitz DJ, Goldstein MJ, Nuechterlein KH, Snyder KS, Mintz J. Family factors and the course of bipolar affective disorder. *Arch Gen Psychiatry* 1988;45:225–231.

49. Miller IW, Keitner GI, Whisman MA, Ryan CE, Epstein NB, Bishop DS. Depressed patients with dysfunctional families: description and course of illness. *J Abnorm Psychol* 1992;101(4):637–646.

50. Murphy JM, Oliver DC, Monson RR, Sobol AM, Federman EB, Leighton AH. Depression and anxiety in relation to social status. *Arch Gen Psychiatry* 1991;48:223–229.

51. Needles DJ, Abramson LY. Positive life events, attributional style and hopefulness: testing a model of recovery from depression. *J Abnorm Psychol* 1990;99(2):156–165.

52. O'Connell RA, Mayo JA, Eng LK, Jones JS, Gabel RH. Social support and long-term lithium outcome. *Br J Psychiatry* 1985;147:272–275.

53. O'Connell RA, Mayo JA, Flatow L, Cuthbertson B, O'Brien BE. Outcome of bipolar disorder on long-term treatment with lithium. *Br J Psychiatry* 1991;159:123–129.

54. Parry BL. Reproductive factors affecting the course of affective illness in women. *Psychiatr Clin North Am* 1989;12(1):207–220.

55. Pasternak RE, Reynolds CF, Schlernitzauer M, et al. Acute open-trial nortriptyline therapy of bereavement-related depression in late life. *J Clin Psychiatry* 1991;52(7):307–310.

56. Paykel ES, Cooper Z. Life events and social stress. In: Paykel ES, ed. *Handbook of affective disorders.* New York: Churchill-Livingstone; 1992:149–170.

57. Paykel ES, Myers JK, Dienelt MN, et al. Life events and depression: a controlled study. *Arch Gen Psychiatry* 1969;21:753–760.

58. Peselow ED, Robins CJ, Sanfilipo MP, Block P, Fieve RR. Sociotropy and autonomy: relationship to antidepressant drug treatment response and endogenous-nonendogenous dichotomy. *J Abnorm Psychol* 1992;101(3):479–486.

59. Preskorn SH, Mac DS. Plasma levels of amitriptyline: effect of age and sex. *J Clin Psychiatry* 1985;46(7):276–277.

60. Raskin A. Age-sex differences in response to antidepressant drugs. *J Nerv Ment Dis* 1974;159(2):120–130.

61. Raskin A, Crook TH. Antidepressants in black and white inpatients. *Arch Gen Psychiatry* 1975;32:643–649.

62. Regier DA, Farmer ME, Rae DS, et al. Comorbidity of mental disorders with alcohol and other drug abuse. *JAMA* 1990;264(19):2511–2518.

63. Robins CJ. Congruence of personality and life events in depression. *J Abnorm Psychol* 1990;99(4):393–397.

64. Robinson RG, Starkstein SE. Current research in affective disorders following stroke. *J Neuropsychiatry Clin Neurosci* 1990;2:1–14.

65. Romans SW, McPherson HM. The social networks of bipolar affective disorder patients. *J Affect Dis* 1992;25(4):221–228.

66. Rounsaville BJ, Weissman MM, Prusoff BA, Herceg-Baron RL. Marital disputes and treatment outcome in depressed women. *Compr Psychiatry* 1979;20(5):483–490.

67. Smith AL, Weissman MM. Epidemiology. In: Paykel ES, ed. *Handbook of affective disorders.* New York: Churchill-Livingstone; 1992:111–129.

68. Sotsky SM, Glass DR, Shea T, et al. Patient predictors of response to psychotherapy and pharmacotherapy: findings in the NIMH treatment of depression collaborative research program. *Am J Psychiatry* 1991;148:997–1008.

69. Vallejo J, Gaston C, Catalan R, Bulbena A, Menchon JM. Predictors of antidepressant treatment outcome in melancholia: psychosocial, clinical and biological indicators. *J Affect Dis* 1991;21:151–162.

70. Vollrath M, Angst J. Outcome of panic and depression in a seven-year follow-up: results of the Zurich study. *Acta Psychiatr Scand* 1989;80:591–596.

71. Warheit GJ. Life events, coping, stress, and depressive symptomatology. *Am J Psychiatry* 1979;136:502–507.

72. Wehr TA, Sack DA, Rosenthal NE, Cowdry RW. Rapid cycling affective disorder: contributing factors and treatment responses in 51 patients. *Am J Psychiatry* 1988;145(2):179–184.

73. Weissman MM. Panic disorder: impact on quality of life. *J Clin Psychiatry Suppl* 1991;52(2):6–8.

74. Weissman MM, Klerman GL, Prusoff BA, Sholomskas D, Padian N. Depressed outpatients. *Arch Gen Psychiatry* 1981;38:51–55.
75. Wells KB, Stewart A, Hays RD, et al. The functioning and well-being of depressed patients. *JAMA* 1989;262(7):914–918.
76. Wittchen H, Essau CA, von Zerssen D, Krieg J, Zaudig M. Lifetime and six-month prevalence of mental disorders in the Munich follow-up study. *Eur Arch Psychiatry Clin Neurosci* 1992;241:247–258.
77. Yonkers KA, Kando JC, Cole JO, Blumenthal S. Gender differences in pharmacokinetics and pharmacodynamics of psychotropic medication. *Am J Psychiatry* 1992;149(5):587–595.
78. Ziegler VE, Biggs JT. Tricyclic plasma levels. Effect of age, race, sex and smoking. *JAMA* 1977;238:2167–2169.
79. Zisook S, Shuchter SR. Depression through the first year after the death of a spouse. *Am J Psychiatry* 1991;148(10):1346–1352.

Psychopharmacology: The Fourth Generation of Progress, edited by Floyd E. Bloom and David J. Kupfer. Raven Press, Ltd., New York © 1995.

CHAPTER 95

Electroconvulsive Therapy

Harold A. Sackeim, D. P. Devanand, and Mitchell S. Nobler

Convulsive therapy was introduced in 1934 by Meduna. He produced chemically induced generalized seizures in schizophrenic patients, based on the mistaken belief that schizophrenia and epilepsy were mutually incompatible (1). Despite a false rationale, it was soon evident that convulsive therapy often resulted in dramatic clinical improvement in psychiatric patients. At the time of the near simultaneous introduction of convulsive therapy and other physical treatments, such as insulin coma therapy and psychosurgery, the predominant view in biological psychiatry was that the major forms of mental illness were due to degenerative brain diseases, unyielding to therapeutic intervention. The early experience with convulsive therapy challenged this therapeutic nihilism and presaged the introduction of psychopharmacological agents.

Electrical induction of the generalized seizure soon became the preferred method, and electroconvulsive therapy (ECT) was the mainstay of biological treatment in psychiatry through the 1940s and 1950s. It was widely applied and central facts about the treatment emerged, such as its impressive efficacy in mood disorders (24). Nonetheless, most of the information regarding ECT was anecdotal, as modern standards for clinical trial methodology only emerged with the introduction of psychopharmacological agents. While initially ECT was the ''gold standard'' used to test the efficacy of the new psychotropics (29,51), research in therapeutics soon focused almost exclusively on the medications. At the same time, particularly in the United States, the clinical use of ECT diminished (65), because it was apparent that pharmacological strategies often were efficacious and free of the cognitive side effects associated with ECT. In addition, with ECT perceived as the most invasive of the commonly used treatments in psychiatry, it became the bell weather for ideological debate about the biological bases of mental

illness and the role of biological interventions. This in turn led to a virtual abandonment of ECT in some countries and a sharp reduction in its availability in public sector hospitals within the United States.

Spurred by growing awareness of the limitations of pharmacological approaches, as reflected in medication resistance, medication intolerance, safety concerns, and persistent side effects (e.g., tardive dyskinesia), a new era of research in ECT began in the late 1970s. This work incorporated more exacting methodological standards and led to new information about indications, treatment technique, side effects, and mechanisms of action. The role of ECT in therapeutics was the subject of a National Institutes of Health Consensus Conference (37) and its use was supported by a variety of national psychiatric and medical organizations (2,48). In 1990, the American Psychiatric Association Task Force on ECT issued a report that represents a particularly comprehensive statement of standards of care (2).

PATTERNS OF UTILIZATION

Within the United States, there was a sharp decline in the use of ECT from the 1960s to 1980s (65). After 1980, rates of utilization stabilized and may have increased in recent years (66). ECT is administered to a far greater extent in private hospitals and academic centers than in public sector facilities. Indeed, a NIMH survey found that in 1980 not a single, non-white patient received ECT in a state facility in the United States (65). In contrast to the claims by opponents that the treatment is a method of behavior control inflicted on the destitute, the evidence indicates that, in general, the treatment is more readily available among the affluent.

Recent surveys indicate that within the United States approximately 80% of patients who receive ECT present with major depression (65,66). Schizophrenia and mania are the next most common indications. Because of its use

H. A. Sackeim, D. P. Devanand, and M. S. Nobler: Department of Biological Psychiatry, Columbia University College of Physicians and Surgeons, New York State Psychiatric Institute, New York, New York 10032.

in major depression, females are more likely to receive ECT than males. The elderly also represent a high percentage of ECT recipients, presumably because ECT has a superior medical safety profile compared to some pharmacological alternatives and because rates of medication resistance and intolerance are elevated among the elderly (53).

EFFICACY

Major Depression

The short-term efficacy of ECT in major depression is well established. Current recommendations suggest that ECT is an effective treatment for all subtypes of unipolar and bipolar major depression (2). In the absence of major depression, its use in the treatment of dysthymia has not been investigated and is generally discouraged. Electroconvulsive therapy is recommended as a treatment of first choice when medical or psychiatric considerations dictate a particular need for a rapid or definitive clinical response, when the risks of other treatments outweigh those of ECT, when there is a clear history of medication resistance and/or a history of favorable ECT response, or when patients indicate a preference for this modality. Increasingly, patients with major depression receive ECT after failing one or more adequate antidepressant medication trials during the index episode (45). There is considerable variability in practice about when the use of ECT is considered during the course of somatic treatment. Relevant issues here include the benefit of identifying a successful pharmacological approach that may then also be used as continuation therapy to prevent relapse, compared to the risk of unsuccessful pharmacological treatment prolonging the index episode (see Chapter 92, *this volume*).

Uncontrolled Trials

Within a few years of the introduction of ECT, it was recognized that therapeutic results in depressive illness were striking and often superior to those in schizophrenia (24). In the prepharmacological era, a large number of uncontrolled studies of depressed patients reported response rates of between 80% and 100% (2,14). Post (43) suggested that prior to the introduction of ECT, the elderly depressed often manifested a chronic course or died of intercurrent medical illnesses in psychiatric institutions. A number of studies have contrasted the clinical outcome of depressed patients who received inadequate or no biological treatment to that of patients who received ECT. Although none of this work involved prospective, random assignment designs, the findings have been largely uniform. Electroconvulsive therapy resulted in decreased chronicity, decreased morbidity, and possibly decreased rates of mortality (53). In much of this work, the advan-

tages of ECT were particularly pronounced in elderly populations.

Sham Controlled Trials

Electroconvulsive therapy is a highly ritualized treatment, involving a complex, repeatedly administered procedure that is accompanied by high expectations of therapeutic success. Such conditions could augment placebo effects. Given this concern, a set of double-blind, random assignment trials were conducted in England during the late 1970s and 1980s that contrasted real ECT with that of the repeated administration of anesthesia alone—sham ECT. With one exception, real ECT was found consistently to be more efficacious than sham treatment (see ref. 51 for a review). The exceptional study (31) used a form of real ECT now known to have limited efficacy (54). Overall, these studies demonstrated that the passage of an electrical stimulus and/or the elicitation of a generalized seizure was necessary for ECT to exert antidepressant effects. Furthermore, the use of a repeated administration of anesthesia as a sham or active placebo condition may have underestimated therapeutic effects. There is some concern that repeated administration of anesthesia, by itself, may have mild antidepressant properties (51).

Comparative Trials with Antidepressant Medications

Following the introduction of tricyclic antidepressants (TCAs) and monoamine oxidase inhibitors (MAOIs), ECT was often used as the gold standard by which to calibrate the efficacy of the newer treatments (23,51). Janicak et al. (53), in a meta-analysis of this work, reported that the average response rate to ECT was 20% higher when compared to TCAs and 45% higher when compared to MAOIs. No study has ever found a pharmacological agent to be superior in antidepressant effects when compared to ECT. Rather, ECT has been found to have either equal or superior efficacy. At the same time, this literature was characterized by major methodological limitations. Most critically, the era in which the bulk of these trials were conducted had different standards regarding the dose and duration of adequate pharmacological treatment. By modern standards, the pharmacological treatments used were often suboptimal (45,57). In addition, given that patients must recognize whether they are receiving a medication or ECT, such comparisons could not be double blind.

Other issues intrinsic to the comparison of ECT with other biological treatments concern the speed and quality of clinical response. Since ECT is most often administered to inpatients, with severe and often psychotic depressive illness, rapid and definitive response is a fundamental concern. In the United States, the average course of ECT involves approximately eight to nine treatments, administered thrice weekly. This 3-week period to achieve full response indirectly supports the belief that symptomatic improvement is often more rapid with ECT compared to standard pharmacological treatments. However, only one recent study has tested this view (10). Patients who had failed an adequate TCA trial were randomized to treatment with ECT or lithium augmentation of the TCA. While both treatment conditions had equivalent efficacy, speed of improvement was more rapid with the TCA-lithium combination. Similarly, the extent of residual symptomatology following pharmacological treatment and ECT has rarely been compared. Hamilton (21), in a naturalistic, open study, reported that a higher percentage of depressed patients became asymptomatic after ECT compared to a similar group who received TCAs.

Comparisons of Treatment Technique

In recent years, the bulk of clinical trials involving ECT have focused on how variations in treatment technique impact on efficacy and side effects (58,69). Historically, such work has provided critical information that has constrained theories of mechanisms of action and, recently such research has provided compelling controlled data regarding the overall efficacy of ECT.

The real–sham studies of the 1980s demonstrated that the passage of an electrical stimulus and/or the elicitation of a seizure were fundamental to antidepressant effects. Earlier research had underscored the importance of seizure elicitation. One set of studies found inferior clinical outcome when patients were administered subconvulsive electrical stimuli, as opposed to electrical stimuli of sufficient intensity to elicit generalized seizures (67). Another set of comparisons suggested that seizures elicited by chemical induction (e.g., flurothyl) were equivalent, if not superior, in therapeutic properties to those elicited with an electrical stimulus (50,51). Furthermore, chemically induced seizures appeared to produce fewer cognitive side effects. This work further tied antidepressant effects to seizure induction, whereas adverse cognitive effects were related to the passage of an electrical stimulus. In line with this, Ottosson (41) performed a critical experiment, comparing three groups of patients. One group received standard suprathreshold electrical stimulation. Another group received the same electrical dosage, but with simultaneous administration of lidocaine, which, in addition to its antiarrhythmic properties, is an anticonvulsant and markedly reduced both the duration and amplitude of ictal activity. The third group received standard ECT, but with a substantially higher electrical intensity. The use of lidocaine to suppress expression of the seizure discharge resulted in diminished efficacy, whereas the high electrical intensity condition was associated with aggravated acute cognitive side effects. Consequently, this body of work lead to the view that, regardless of method, the elicitation of generalized seizures of adequate

duration provides the necessary and sufficient conditions for antidepressant effects (14,37). In contrast, the intensity of the electrical stimulus does not impact on efficacy, but contributes to the magnitude of cognitive side effects.

In recent years, these basic tenets have been substantially revised. The Columbia University group demonstrated that at low electrical intensity, generalized seizures of adequate duration are reliably produced with right unilateral ECT, but with remarkably weak therapeutic properties (54). In contrast, at low electrical dosage, bilateral ECT remained an efficacious treatment. Robin and de Tissera (47), using bilateral ECT, compared three different electrical waveforms that differed in overall stimulus intensity. They found that speed of clinical response was slower with less intense stimulation. Conjointly these findings led to the hypotheses that electrical dosage determines the efficacy of right unilateral ECT and influences speed of response, regardless of electrode placement. Both of these hypotheses were confirmed in a recent, random assignment, double-blind study by the Columbia University group (58). Crossing the factors of stimulus dosage (low or high) and electrode placement (right unilateral or bilateral), they found that short-term response rates to ECT varied between 17% and 65%. In addition, this work suggested that the effects of stimulus intensity on efficacy and efficiency (speed of response) were not related to the absolute electrical dose administered, but to the degree that the absolute dose exceeded the individual patient's seizure threshold (55,58).

These new studies contradicted the fundamental tenets on mechanisms of action and offered a new perspective. Generalized seizures of adequate duration can be reliably produced that lack therapeutic properties. Therefore, the generalized seizure may be a necessary, but insufficient, condition for efficacy. Furthermore, there are electrical dose–response relationships in ECT, indicating that technical aspects in how the treatment is performed can have a major impact on efficacy. The interactions of electrode placement and electrical dosage in determining efficacy also suggest that antidepressant effects are dependent on current paths, implicating anatomic specificity in the functional systems therapeutically altered by ECT. With regard to broader considerations of efficacy, the new studies went beyond the real–sham ECT trials. Using double-blind methods in which each patient not only underwent repeated anesthetic administration but had generalized seizures of adequate duration, this work demonstrated that technical factors in treatment delivery (stimulus dosage and electrode placement) can have a dramatic effect on response rates (54,58). Consequently, the neurobiological consequences of manipulating these parameters should be fundamental in accounting for antidepressant effects.

Prediction of Outcome

In the 1950s and 1960s, a series of studies showed impressive power to predict clinical outcome in depressed patients on the basis of pre-ECT symptomatological features and histories (see refs. 2 and 38 for reviews). This work is largely of historical interest, because the changes in nosology have resulted in more diagnosticly homogeneous samples being referred for ECT. Indeed, whereas the early research had emphasized the importance of vegetative or melancholic features as prognostic of positive outcome, recent studies restricted to patients with major depression suggest that subtyping as endogenous or melancholic has little predictive value (1,2,38). It appears that the early positive associations derived from the inclusion of neurotic depressives or dysthymics in the sampling.

In recent research, a few clinical features have been related to short-term ECT outcome. Several studies have noted that patients with a long duration of their current episode are less likely to respond (38). The majority of studies that have examined the distinction between psychotic and nonpsychotic depression found superior response rates among the psychotic subtype (38). This is of particular note given the established inferior response rate of this subtype to monotherapy with antidepressant or neuroleptic medications. In addition, in a relatively large number of studies patient age was positively associated with superior ECT outcome (53).

Although the predictive relationships between ECT outcome and episode duration, psychosis, and age are of theoretical interest, they are of insufficient strength to guide treatment recommendations. Recently, an alternative approach has been suggested: Electroconvulsive therapy was introduced in the prepharmacological era and was commonly used as a treatment of first choice. Increasingly, however, depressed patients now referred for ECT have frequently failed adequate trials of antidepressant medications. Despite this major shift in the nature of patient populations, there has been little research examining whether expectations about ECT response rates require recalibration. Prudic et al. (45) reported that patients who failed one or more adequate TCA trials prior to ECT had a 50% rate of response to bilateral ECT compared to an 86% rate in patients not found to be medication resistant during the index episode. Furthermore, medication resistance was particularly common in patients whose current episode was of long duration and particularly uncommon in psychotic depression, with the findings suggesting that the predictive power of these clinical features may be due to their relations with medication history. There is a need to replicate and extend this approach to prediction of ECT outcome. For example, it is unknown whether failure to respond to adequate treatment with a serotonin reuptake inhibitor (SSRI) has the same predictive power as TCA failure, an issue of both clinical and theoretical importance.

There have also been a variety of attempts to examine biological measures as predictors of short-term ECT outcome, including levels of neurotransmitter metabolites, neuroendocrine measures, and electroencephalographic

(EEG) and other brain-imaging parameters. To date, none of these approaches has yielded consistent findings (1,38). In the past, it was believed that as long as generalized seizures were of sufficient duration, maximal therapeutic effects would be obtained. It is now recognized, however, that seizure duration bears little relation to efficacy (55) and that generalized seizures of adequate duration can be consistently produced that lack therapeutic properties. Therefore, the field lacks a marker to indicate that therapeutically optimal treatment is being delivered. Because ECT results in acute changes in the levels of a variety of transmitters and peptides, the predictive power of these acute changes have been examined with regard to clinical outcome. Most of this work has documented null results. An exception, however, are reports by Scott and colleagues (46) that the acute release of oxytocin-associated neurophysin following the first ECT is associated with ultimate clinical outcome. Recently, this group suggested that this effect may pertain more to the adequacy of treatment methods than to patient characteristics. They found that the release of oxytocin acutely following ECT was sensitive to stimulus intensity and presumed that this sensitivity accounted for the relationship with clinical outcome. Other recent research avenues have concentrated on providing electrophysiological markers of treatment adequacy. There are consistent findings that forms of ECT that differ in efficacy also differ in the EEG parameters during and immediately following the seizure (39). Ongoing work is examining the sensitivity and specificity of such effects relative to clinical outcome.

Mania

As in major depression, ECT has been used to treat acute manic episodes for more than five decades. A recent review compiling this experience indicated that approximately 80% of 589 manic patients achieved remission following ECT (36). In contrast, surveys of utilization indicate that the use of ECT in the treatment of acute mania is often unappreciated. Particularly when patients manifest manic delirium, ECT may be life saving.

Uncontrolled Trials

The bulk of the literature on the use of ECT in mania involves uncontrolled case series. In addition, pharmacological intervention, particularly with lithium, is typically the first-choice treatment and there are limited data on the efficacy of ECT in medication-resistant manic patients. Further complicating the use of ECT in mania was the belief expressed in early reports that manic patients required particularly intense forms of ECT (more than one treatment per day) or prolonged ECT courses to achieve remission (15,24). A related view was that ECT did not exert a primary antimanic effect but that apparent clinical improvement was due to the masking effects of a treatment-induced organic mental syndrome.

Controlled Trials

Some of the limitations of the uncontrolled case series were addressed in a group of retrospective and prospective controlled comparisons of ECT and pharmacological treatments. In retrospective comparisons of ECT with lithium and chlorpromazine, the short-term efficacy of ECT was found in one study to be equivalent to both lithium and chlorpromazine and in another study to be superior to chlorpromazine (36). There have been only two prospective studies of ECT in acute mania, and both involved relatively small samples. In one study, patients were randomly assigned to treatment with ECT or lithium, with a neuroleptic used adjunctively in both treatment groups (61). At the end of this 8-week trial, the ECT and lithium groups had equivalent response rates, but the differences observed during the trial in discrete aspects of psychopathology all favored the ECT group. The second prospective study selected only patients who had failed to respond to robust treatment with lithium or neuroleptics (36). Patients were randomized to various forms of ECT or to pharmacological treatment with combined lithium and haloperidol. Among these medication-resistant patients, there was an impressive rate of response to ECT, but none of the small group of patients in the combined pharmacology condition met response criteria.

The findings of the retrospective and prospective studies were consonant with those of the uncontrolled reports in indicating that ECT is effective in acute mania and may be of particular value in manic patients who do not benefit from traditional pharmacotherapy. It is noteworthy, however, that there has yet to be a comparison of the efficacy of ECT and anticonvulsant medications. There is also limited information on the efficacy of ECT in rapid cycling patients. The recent prospective studies suggested that manic patients with poor premorbid functioning or those with symptoms of anger and irritability may be less likely to respond to ECT (36). This work and the recent retrospective studies also contradicted the view that particularly intensive forms of ECT are required in acute mania. In these studies, ECT was administered at twice- or thrice-a-week schedules and the average number of treatments ranged from 5.4 to 11. Indeed, recent evidence suggests that speed of improvement is often more rapid in acute mania than in major depression. The prospective studies have also rejected the view that improvement with ECT in acute mania is secondary to the induction of persistent confusion. Shortly following the ECT course, manic patients who responded generally manifested improved cognitive functioning without evidence of an organic mental syndrome (36).

Schizophrenia

There is considerable controversy about the role of ECT in the treatment of schizophrenia. Surveys of utilization indicate marked disparity in rates of use between and within countries. Likewise, recommendations of expert groups and professional organizations have been contradictory. For example, an National Institutes of Health consensus panel stated that evidence regarding the efficacy of ECT in schizophrenia was not compelling (37). The American Psychiatric Association Task Force on ECT recommended that ECT be considered particularly for schizophrenic patients who manifest prominent affective features or catatonia during exacerbations (2). In contrast, the Royal College of Psychiatrists expressed skepticism that any symptomatological features were predictive of response to ECT in schizophrenia (48).

Uncontrolled Trials

Many of the earlier reports on this use of ECT consisted of uncontrolled case material (29). Diagnostic practice preceded the introduction of operationalized criteria for schizophrenia and patient samples and outcome criteria were often poorly specified. International differences in the rate of diagnosis of schizophrenia have been described previously. In particular, earlier American studies describing samples of schizophrenic patients may have contained substantial representation of mood disorder patients, who may be particularly likely to respond to ECT.

Overall, the earlier reports were enthusiastic about the use of ECT for schizophrenic patients with relatively recent onset of illness, with recovery or marked improvement noted in a large proportion of cases, typically on the order of 75% (1,14,29). Historical comparisons and comparisons to psychotherapy or milieu therapy suggested that the introduction of ECT resulted in both superior short-term clinical outcome and more sustained remissions (29). However, in this early era, the view was also frequently expressed that ECT was considerably less effective in schizophrenic patients with insidious onset and long duration of illness (24). In addition, it was suggested that schizophrenic patients often required intensive courses of ECT, involving more frequent and closely spaced treatments (14,24).

Comparison of Real and Sham ECT

A surprising number of prospective, controlled studies have addressed the efficacy of ECT in schizophrenia. As in major depression, ECT was initially used as the gold standard by which to establish the efficacy of pharmacological agents, in this case, neuroleptics. This work included comparisons of real and sham ECT, monotherapy with ECT or neuroleptic medications, and the combined use of ECT and neuroleptics.

Using real–sham designs, four studies were conducted in the 1950s and 1960s, and three recent studies in the 1980s (29). With the possible exception of Ulett et al. (67), the early studies failed to demonstrate a therapeutic advantage for real ECT compared to repeated administration of anesthesia alone. In contrast, at least in the short-term, the three recent studies each found clinically significant therapeutic advantages for real over sham ECT (29). The source of this discrepancy is unknown. The recent studies have had small sample sizes, but this should have limited the possibility of obtaining statistically significant findings. It is noteworthy that Taylor and Fleminger (64) explicitly focused on a middle-prognostic group, and excluded patients with chronic conditions. The high representation of patients with chronic schizophrenia in the early studies may have mitigated against a real ECT advantage (29). Another possibility is that in each of the recent studies, patients were maintained on neuroleptic medications during the clinical trial. There is evidence that the combination of ECT and neuroleptics is a more effective treatment than either form of monotherapy (29).

In the recent work the advantages of real relative to sham ECT only pertained to the period of time during and immediately following the acute treatment course. Within months of trial termination, symptomatic differences between the groups were not evident. The importance of these negative findings is questionable. In each case, the treatment received following the randomized trial was uncontrolled. Indeed, in some cases, patients assigned to the sham condition went on to receive ECT.

Monotherapy with Neuroleptics or ECT

Ten prospective, controlled trials compared the efficacy of ECT with that of monotherapy with neuroleptics and/or other somatic treatments (e.g., insulin coma, reserpine). Since 1980, only one such study has been reported. The limitations of this literature in fundamental aspects of clinical trial methodology, particularly the reliability and validity of diagnosis, the nature of assignment to treatment groups, treatment adequacy, and the blindness and reliability of clinical evaluations, underscore the need for caution in interpretation (29). With these caveats, it appears that short-term ECT outcome was generally inferior or equivalent to antipsychotic medication (29,33), although there were exceptions (12). There is little indication from this literature about the clinical or treatment history features that might distinguish schizophrenics who preferentially respond to antipsychotic medications or ECT. In contrast, a seemingly consistent and surprising theme in this literature was the suggestion that patients who were administered ECT had superior long-term outcome compared to medication groups (12,33). This pattern emerged in other retrospective studies (29), as well as in the most rigorous of the prospective controlled investigations, the work conducted by May and colleagues (33). This type of effect is unexpected, given the predominant perspective that virtually all the behavioral and physiological effects of ECT are relatively short-lived (50). Furthermore, most of these studies were conducted in an era when the importance of continuation and maintenance treatment was not appreciated and no study controlled the treatment received following resolution of the schizophrenic episode. Nonetheless, the possibility that ECT may have beneficial long-term effects merits attention.

Neuroleptics and ECT in Monotherapy or in Combination

There have been three prospective clinical trials comparing the efficacy of combination treatment with ECT and neuroleptics with that of ECT alone, and seven such trials compare the combination treatment to monotherapy with a neuroleptic (29). This literature is also characterized by a host of methodological problems. Relatively few of these studies involved random assignment, and fewer still involved fully blind assessment of treatment outcome. Nonetheless, it is noteworthy that in each of the three studies in which ECT alone was compared to ECT combined with antipsychotic medication there were indications that the combination was more effective (29). With one exception, in each of seven comparisons, the combination of ECT with antipsychotic medication was more effective than treatment with an antipsychotic medication alone. In some cases, a superior outcome was obtained despite lower average neuroleptic dose in the combination condition. This pattern is particularly impressive when one considers that monotherapy with neuroleptics has established efficacy and the resultant constraints on statistical power in establishing superior response to a combination condition. At the least, these studies suggest that neuroleptic medication should not be discontinued when schizophrenic patients are referred for ECT. Few of these studies followed patients beyond the acute treatment period, and in none was there standardization of continuation or maintenance treatments. Therefore, the relative persistence of any advantage for combination treatment is unknown. Nonetheless, the findings in some of these studies suggested a lower relapse rate in patients treated acutely with neuroleptics and ECT relative to neuroleptics alone. When considered with the follow-up results of May et al. (33), there is added reason to explore whether ECT, particularly in combination with antipsychotic medication, exerts a long-term beneficial effect in schizophrenia.

Medication Resistance and Prediction of Outcome

Antipsychotic medication is the first-choice treatment in schizophrenia, and ECT is typically reserved for medication-resistant patients. There have been eight, largely impressionistic reports on the use of ECT in such patients. We have yet to have a double-blind, random assignment study contrasting the efficacy of combined ECT and neuroleptic treatment with continued neuroleptic treatment alone in medication-resistant schizophrenic patients. Nonetheless, starting in the early 1960s there have been a series of reports that some medication-resistant schizophrenic patients benefit substantially by the addition of ECT (29). In some cases these positive reports contradict the clinical tenet that ECT is of limited value in chronic schizophrenic patients, with long durations of illness (1,24), and there are a variety of unanswered questions. It could be that the recent set of positive case series contained samples with high representation of patients with prominent affective symptomatology (29). It could be that, in the absence of affective symptoms, the combination of ECT and neuroleptic treatment is particularly valuable for medication-resistant patients who have relatively short duration of illness. Regardless, it is clear that better information is needed, particularly about the clinical and historical features of those medication-resistant patients who may benefit from combination treatment. The patient that fails neuroleptic treatment and clozapine presents a serious treatment dilemma. It is noteworthy that the literature on the combined use of clozapine and ECT is confined to small case series (29).

Early studies of ECT suggested that the features associated with positive short-term clinical outcome in schizophrenia included being married, having at least a skilled or clerical occupation, an absence of premorbid personality disturbance and poor premorbid functioning, manifestation of catatonic symptoms, affective symptoms, and, most commonly, acute onset and short illness duration (29). It is noteworthy that many of these features have been found to predict outcome with pharmacological treatment and may be more general markers of prognosis. Nonetheless, the validity of these findings is questionable given that the early studies often used assessment techniques of doubtful reliability and lacked standardized diagnostic criteria. Although more recent research has replicated relationships between chronicity and outcome, predictive relationships were not observed for the presence of affective or catatonic symptoms (11,29).

Movement Disorders

The potential for acute extrapyramidal syndromes, particularly neuroleptic-induced parkinsonism (NIP), and for persistent tardive dyskinesia are major drawbacks of traditional neuroleptic treatment. Although extrapyramidal symptoms are generally considered to be reversible, prospective studies have suggested that neuroleptic-induced parkinsonism may predict the subsequent development of tardive dyskinesia.

Because ECT is unique in having both antipsychotic and antiparkinsonian properties, it may exert ameliorative effects on neuroleptic-induced parkinsonism (1,2,19). For

example, Goswami et al. (19) studied nine schizophrenic inpatients with a longitudinal triphasic design, first using neuroleptics, then neuroleptics and ECT, and then neuroleptics. Neuroleptic-induced parkinsonism was significantly reduced in stepwise fashion when patients were treated with ECT. Recently, Mukherjee and Debsikdar (35) introduced the notion that ECT may protect against the later development of neuroleptic-induced parkinsonism and tardive dyskinesia. They examined 35 DSM-IIIR schizophrenic patients who were on neuroleptics for at least 2 weeks, all of whom were receiving ($n = 15$) or had received ($n = 20$) a course of unmodified bilateral ECT during the index episode. None of the patients had bradykinesia, rigidity, or postural instability and only one patient met the research diagnostic criteria for probable tardive dyskinesia. Mukherjee and Debsikdar (35) speculated that if neuroleptic-induced parkinsonism is a risk factor in the development of tardive dyskinesia, ECT may ultimately protect against tardive dyskinesia by preventing initial neuroleptic-induced parkinsonism. At the neurophysiological level, there is evidence in rodents that electroconvulsive shock (ECS) prevents the development of dopamine receptor supersensitivity with exposure to dopamine antagonists (29) and results in increased D_1 receptor density without impact on the D_2 receptor density (16).

There are also suggestions that a history of ECT may be associated with a low prevalence or delayed development of tardive dyskinesia. Gardos et al. (18) evaluated 122 schizophrenic outpatients in Hungary and reported a striking absence of severe tardive dyskinesia. They suggested that the low prevalence was due to the use of ECT to treat exacerbations and the avoidance of high dosage neuroleptic treatment. In an American sample, Cole et al. (3) recently reported that a history of ECT was associated with a lower risk and delayed appearance of tardive dyskinesia. As noted, Mukherjee and Debsikdar (35) found virtually no tardive dyskinesia in an Indian sample, which they attributed to the use of ECT. Schwartz et al. (59), in an Israeli sample, reported a reduced incidence of tardive dyskinesia among male schizophrenic patients with a history of ECT. If, in fact, ECT does offer long-term protection against the iatrogenic effects of concurrent or later exposure to neuroleptics, this would also contradict the general impression that the behavioral and physiological effects of ECT are uniformly transient (50).

Less Common Indications

Psychiatric Disorders

There is limited information on the use of ECT in other psychiatric disorders. Among the anxiety disorders, traditionally it has been felt that ECT lacks efficacy in obsessive–compulsive disorder (OCD) and generalized anxiety disorder (14). Aside from clinical implications, the putative lack of efficacy of ECT in OCD is of theoretical interest, given the established efficacy of antidepressant medication, particularly those with strong serotonergic effects. Only one recent study examined this issue. Khanna et al. (26) reported on a small, prospective series of nondepressed OCD patients who had failed trials of antidepressant medications and behavior therapy. Shortly following ECT, marked improvement was documented, but patients were not given continuation treatment and quickly relapsed. Antidepressant medications are also efficacious in panic disorder. Surprisingly, there is virtually no information on the effects of ECT on panic disorder, even in patients with comorbid major depression.

Catatonia may be manifested in a variety of psychiatric disorders or as a consequence of medical illness. Impressionistic data support the use of ECT in catatonia, particularly following poor response to treatment with benzodiazepines (42). The syndrome of lethal catatonia is a life-threatening condition, characterized by stupor or excitement, hyperthermia, clouded consciousness, and autonomic dysregulation (32). Mann et al. (32) identified 292 cases in the world literature, with deaths in 176 (60%) of these cases. The literature on this syndrome, which consists solely of case series, suggests that neuroleptic treatment is of limited efficacy. Given the difficulty in distinguishing lethal catatonia from neuroleptic malignant syndrome (NMS), escalation of neuroleptic dosage may be counterproductive. Particularly when instituted prior to a comatose stage, ECT appears to be effective (29). In a recent study of schizophrenic and schizoaffective patients, perplexity was a clinical sign associated with positive ECT outcome (11). Confusion or perplexity is a common feature of the European categorization of cycloid psychoses, which may be a variant of schizoaffective disorder, that traditionally has been thought to be exquisitely responsive to ECT.

Neurological and Medical Conditions

A variety of organic affective and psychotic states, as well as certain states of delirium, have shown rapid and favorable response to ECT. These include delirium associated with alcohol withdrawal, toxic delirium or psychosis associated with use of phencyclidine, and mental syndromes associated with lupus erythematosus and enteric fevers (2). However, because of the availability of alternative treatments, ECT is rarely used in such cases.

In both open and sham-controlled trials, ECT has been found to improve clinical symptoms in idiopathic Parkinson's disease, at least on a short-term basis (1,2,29). Typically, L-dopa requirements are sharply reduced when parkinsonian patients receive ECT. The persistence of the beneficial effects are unpredictable and highly variable. The utility of ECT as a long-term treatment for medication-resistant Parkinson's disease has yet to be tested, as use of maintenance ECT has not been evaluated.

NMS shares clinical features with lethal catatonia and has been considered to be an iatrogenic form of lethal catatonia induced by neuroleptics (32). When the clinical community became cognizant of NMS, there was reluctance to treat these patients with ECT, based on the fact that NMS has similar symptoms to malignant hyperthermia, a familial syndrome provoked by exposure to general anesthesia and depolarizing muscle relaxants, such as succinylcholine. However, NMS and malignant hyperthermia have been shown to be unrelated syndromes and several reviews have documented that ECT is an effective treatment for NMS (e.g., see ref. 6). Davis et al. (6) found that mortality rates in NMS patients were equivalent with ECT compared to bromocriptine, dantrolene, L-dopa, or amantadine, and averaged approximately half that of untreated patients. The complications and deaths that have been observed with use of ECT have been tied to continued administration of neuroleptic medication and to cardiac dysregulation. Given the marked hemodynamic alterations associated with ECT in the NMS patient, it is advisable to first use medication strategies to stabilize autonomic function before starting ECT. These patients must often be discontinued from antipsychotic medication; therefore, ECT may have the advantage of treating both the NMS and the underlying psychotic condition.

In a variety of animal models and in humans, ECT exerts pronounced anticonvulsant effects (44,55). There is a case literature suggesting efficacy in some patients with medication-resistant epilepsy and instances of prolonged status epilepticus (2). The possible utility of ECT in status epilepticus may be of clinical relevance, because the mortality rate with standard pharmacological protocols remains high.

Relapse

Pharmacological Strategies Following ECT

Electroconvulsive therapy is most commonly used as a short-term treatment for acute episodes or exacerbations of psychiatric illness. In major depression, it is established that relapse rates during the first 6 months following response to ECT will be high if continuation treatment is not provided (57). A similar pattern is expected in mania and schizophrenia. For depressed patients, it has long been thought that relapse rates can be markedly reduced by the use of classical antidepressant medications, specifically TCAs or MAOIs, as continuation treatment following response to ECT. This view was based on the results of three double-blind, placebo controlled, randomized trials conducting in England during the 1960s (57). This work focused on patients receiving ECT as a first-choice treatment. Since then, ECT samples increasingly contain patients who fail to respond to these medications during the acute episode. Theoretically, if an agent that proved ineffective in treating the acute episode was effective as a continuation or maintenance therapy following ECT, then either of two hypotheses would be supported. From a neurobiological perspective, this might suggest that what needs to be accomplished to prevent relapse differs in degree or kind from what is required to treat the acute episode. Alternatively, ECT may change the neurobiology so that a medication can exert an action as a continuation treatment that it could not exert during pre-ECT acute-phase treatment. However, recent studies document high relapse rates following response to ECT in major depression in patients receiving traditional continuation pharmacotherapy (57). Furthermore, there is preliminary evidence that patients with established resistance to adequate trials of antidepressant medications during the acute episode have particularly elevated relapse rates and that adequate continuation therapy with a TCA may only benefit those who did not fail this class of medication during the acute episode (57). Consequently, there is considerable uncertainty about optimal continuation pharmacotherapy following ECT and a clear need for controlled research to reevaluate traditional and alternative strategies. Such efforts are in progress.

Continuation or Maintenance ECT

The problem of relapse is likely related to the fact that ECT is the only somatic treatment in psychiatry that is typically discontinued once it has been shown to be effective. An alternative is to use ECT as a form of continuation or maintenance treatment (2). There is a long history of such a use of ECT in both mood disorders and schizophrenia. On the one hand, this impressionistic literature suggests that, continuation ECT may be broadly effective; however there are also problems with its acceptability to patients and with compliance. Furthermore, no prospective, controlled study has compared the efficacy of continuation ECT with that of continuation pharmacotherapy. Research of this type is also indicated.

SIDE EFFECTS

Medical Adverse Effects

The mortality rate associated with ECT is comparable to that of general anesthesia in minor surgery and estimated to be approximately one death per 10,000 patients treated (1,2). Patients believed to have increased risk of morbidity are those with space-occupying cerebral lesions or other conditions that increase intracranial pressure, recent myocardial infarction associated with unstable cardiac function, recent intracerebral hemorrhage, unstable vascular aneurysm or malformation, retinal detachment, pheochromocytoma, or any patient rated at ASA level 4 or 5. The prevalence of these conditions increases with aging (53). There is strong consistency in the literature documenting that ECT-related medical complications are

more likely in the elderly, particularly the oldest age groups, in those with preexisting medical conditions, particularly cardiac illness, and in those receiving concurrent medication for medical conditions (53). Electroconvulsive therapy is often described as safer than classical antidepressant medications, particularly among the frail elderly. There are few controlled comparisons that have tested this claim (70), and naturalistic data are compromised by the fact that high-risk patients are preferentially referred for ECT.

Cardiovascular Effects

The application of an electrical stimulus results in immediate vagal stimulation, parasympathetic outflow, and bradycardia. With the elicitation of a generalized seizure, there is outpouring of catecholamines, markedly enhanced sympathetic tone, and resultant tachycardia and hypertension. The magnitude of the hemodynamic changes is often great, but short-lived, with a return to baseline levels within minutes of seizure termination. Benign arrhythmias are common in the immediate postictal period (2,70).

Mortality or significant morbidity during a course of ECT typically occurs immediately following the seizure or during the postictal recovery period. Cardiovascular complications are the leading cause of such events (2,34). Controlled investigation has shown that the likelihood of cardiovascular complications is substantially increased in patients with preexisting cardiac illness and that the type of preexisting illness strongly predicts the nature of the complication, that is, ischemic disease or ventricular arrhythmia (70). In recent years, there has been considerable variability among practitioners in the prophylactic use of β-adrenergic blocking agents, such as labetalol or esmolol, to reduce the hypertensive effects of seizure induction (34). Whether this strategy is effective in limiting cardiovascular morbidity has not been documented, and there is a theoretical concern that this approach may be counterproductive. The increased cardiac output and peripheral hypertension associated with the seizure may contribute to the profound ictal increase in cerebral blood flow (CBF). In turn, enhanced CBF provides for the transport of the oxygen and carbohydrate supplies that are necessary to sustain the large ictal increase in cerebral metabolic rate (22). Indeed, it is established that some of the β-adrenergic blocking agents, and newer anesthetics, like propofol, that reduce ictal hypertension, are also associated with shortened seizure duration (34,55). Prospective investigation is needed of the efficacy and safety of pharmacological strategies that limit the cardiovascular morbidity of ECT.

Neurological Effects

Despite increased CBF and intracranial pressure, cerebrovascular events are extremely rare among patients receiving ECT. Other sources of morbidity are prolonged and tardive seizures. The risk of prolonged seizures or status epilepticus is increased by some concomitant pharmacological treatments. These include use of adenosine antagonists, such as theophylline, high dosage of some neuroleptics, and lithium (2,55). This risk may also be increased among patients with a preexisting electrolyte imbalance and when more than one seizure is induced in the same treatment session (2).

When the phenomenon of kindled seizures in animals was first demonstrated, concern was expressed that ECT may result in kindling, producing a persistent decrease of seizure threshold and creating a vulnerability for the later development of seizure disorder (28). However, ECS in animals exerts an anticonvulsant effect, blocking the development or expression of kindling (44,55). For the most part, epidemiological studies of the frequency of spontaneous seizures and related EEG phenomena in former ECT patients have also not supported this concern (28). Recently, no relation with history of ECT was found in quantitative studies of human seizure threshold (28).

Adverse Cognitive Effects

The cognitive effects of ECT are the major factor limiting its use. These effects are stereotyped, are expected to be independent of psychiatric diagnosis, and are well modeled in animal studies (52). Central facts to be kept in mind when considering the cognitive consequences of ECT concern the slope of recovery functions, the impact of technical factors in treatment administration, and individual differences among patients.

In most cognitive domains, there is rapid recovery of function shortly following ECT (52). Consequently, the type and magnitude of cognitive deficits are heavily determined by when they are observed (4,58). When additive, progressive deficits occur during the ECT course, this is partly attributable to the spacing of treatments, with incomplete recovery before the imposition of further treatment (4).

How ECT is performed strongly impacts on the breadth and severity of short-term cognitive deficits. These factors include the anatomic positioning of electrodes, the type of electrical waveform used, the intensity of the electrical stimulus, and the spacing of treatments (52,58,69). Compared to application of electrodes over the right hemisphere (right unilateral ECT), the traditional bifrontotemporal placement of electrodes (bilateral ECT) results in prolonged recovery of orientation during the postictal period, a greater probability of developing an organic mental syndrome, and more extensive and severe amnesic effects. The fact that left and right unilateral ECT differ in the extent of amnesia they produce for verbal rather than nonverbal material clearly indicates lateralized neurophysiological effects (52). Electrical waveforms that are inefficient in seizure-eliciting properties (e.g., sine wave)

produce greater cognitive disturbance than more efficient waveforms (brief and ultrabrief pulse) (52,69). Similarly, there is evidence that, within a waveform, the extent to which electrical dosage exceeds seizure threshold contributes to the magnitude of short-term cognitive side effects (55,58).

Patients also vary considerably in the extent and severity of cognitive side effects. There are limited data on the individual factors that predict this vulnerability. A set of mainly retrospective studies has suggested that advanced age heightens the probability of prolonged confusion and that this effect is most pronounced among the very old (53). In addition, receiving psychotropic medication during ECT or experiencing major medical illnesses prior to ECT appear to be additional risk factors, particularly among the elderly. However, in much of this work, the manner in which ECT was conducted was not optimal. This problem is fundamental, because, depending on ECT technique, at some centers more than 50% of elderly patients have been found to develop an organic mental syndrome and elsewhere virtually no patient develops this adverse effect (58). It is commonly suggested that preexisting cognitive deficit is also a risk factor for more pronounced ECT-induced cognitive effects (2). Here as well, the data are extremely limited. Retrospective studies of patients with poststroke depression, depression and dementia, and depression and Parkinsonism, and other neurological disorders have generally reported favorable clinical outcome, with only a suggestion of increased tendency for prolonged postictal confusion (53). This issue is complicated by the fact that depressed patients with pseudodementia typically show progressive improvement in cognitive function during the ECT course. Recently, it has been suggested that manifestation of T_2-weighted MRI signal abnormalities in the basal ganglia is associated with post-ECT delirium (13).

Objective Cognitive Side Effects

In the immediate postictal period, patients may manifest, as they do with spontaneous seizures, transient neurological abnormalities, alterations of consciousness [e.g., disorientation or attentional dysfunction], sensorimotor abnormalities, and disturbance in higher cognitive functions, particularly learning and memory (52). The severity and persistence of these acute effects show marked sensitivity to technical factors in ECT administration. These factors determine, for instance, whether patients require a few minutes to achieve full reorientation following seizure elicitation or several hours (4,52,58).

Recovery of cognitive function following a single treatment is rapid. However, with forms of ECT that exert more severe acute cognitive effects, recovery may be incomplete by the time of the next treatment. In such cases, repeated acute assessment at the same time points relative to seizure induction demonstrates deterioration over the treatment course (4,52). In some cases, patients may develop an organic mental syndrome with marked disorientation during the ECT course (13,52). Milder forms of ECT have been developed in which cumulative deterioration in cognitive functions does not occur. Indeed, with specific alterations of ECT technique, cumulative improvement in some acute cognitive measures has been demonstrated (52).

Associations between the magnitude of cognitive effects and ECT treatment parameters rapidly diminish as time from ECT progresses. More than a week or two following the end of the ECT course, differences between electrode placements are difficult to establish (52,58,69). Within days of the end of the ECT course, depressed patients manifest performance superior to their pretreatment baseline in most cognitive domains. For example, patients typically show superior IQ scores on tests of intelligence shortly following ECT relative to those in the untreated depressed state (52). Similarly, prior to treatment, depressed patients often manifest deficits in the acquisition of information, as revealed by tests of immediate recall or recognition of item lists. Within several days following the ECT course, patients are typically unchanged or improved in the immediate memory measures, with the change in clinical state being the critical predictor of the magnitude of improvement. In contrast, patients often manifest a marked disturbance in their ability to retain information over a delay. This reflects a double dissociation between the effects of depression and ECT on anterograde learning and memory (52). Depression is associated with an acquisition deficit, most likely related to disturbances in attention and concentration, which frequently recedes following treatment with ECT. In contrast, ECT introduces a new deficit in consolidation or retention, so that information that is newly learned is rapidly forgotten.

During and shortly following a course of ECT, patients also display retrograde amnesia. Deficits in the recall or recognition of both personal and public information are usually evident, and there is evidence that these deficits are greatest for events that occurred temporally closest to the treatment (63). Therefore, memory for more remote events is usually intact, but patients may have difficulty recalling events that transpired during and several months to years prior to the ECT course. The retrograde amnesia is rarely dense, as patients typically show spottiness in memory for recent events. As time from treatment increases, there is typically improved retrograde functioning, with a return of more distant memories. This temporally graded pattern indicating greatest vulnerability for more recent events is compatible with similar findings of the effects of repeated ECS in animals (52). Both the anterograde and retrograde amnesia are most marked for explicit or declarative memory, whereas there should be no effect on implicit or procedural memory (52,63).

Within a few weeks following the end of ECT, objective evidence of persistent cognitive deficit is difficult to document (52). The anterograde amnesia typically resolves within a few weeks of ECT termination (58). The retrograde amnesia often shows a more gradual reduction, with substantial return of memory for events that were seemingly forgotten immediately following the treatment course. However, persistent effects of ECT have been identified (69). Most likely because of a combination of retrograde and anterograde effects, patients may manifest, even when tested at substantial time periods after treatment, persistent amnesia for some events that transpired in the interval of several months prior to and following the ECT course (52,69).

Patient Attitudes

There has been concerted investigation of the perceptions of former patients regarding the effects of ECT on their cognitive functioning. Using a variety of instruments to elicit self-reports and to assess memory, investigators have not observed significant relations between changes in subjective and objective measures of memory functioning at any testing interval (52,58,69). With noted consistency, symptomatic severity has been found to strongly correlate with patients' evaluations of their memory functioning, both before and after ECT (52,58,69). Early studies by Squire (63), suggested that there was no change in the level of memory complaints shortly following right unilateral ECT, but that there was an increase in memory complaints and a redistribution in the nature of perceived deficits with bilateral ECT. When patients were tested several months after bilateral ECT, they showed a reduction of memory complaints, reaching the global level that was observed in patients after unilateral ECT; nonetheless, they showed a persistent redistribution in the nature of complaints. However, since this work, a series of studies has found that the great majority of depressed patients report fewer memory difficulties within a week of the ECT course than they had prior to the course. This improvement in subjective reports has been observed both for groups treated with right unilateral and bilateral ECT (52,58,69).

A small minority of former patients report profound and long-lasting cognitive impairment, which they attribute to this treatment modality. The validity of this phenomenon has not been established with objective testing (17) and the reasons for this discrepancy are not clear. Complicating this issue are the effects of current psychopathology on cognitive functions (17), the natural progression of some forms of psychiatric illness, the effects of current and past treatments other than ECT, and the methodological difficulties intrinsic in isolating a rare phenomenon. In addition, because of the public and scientific attention that has been given to the cognitive side effects of ECT, patients who receive this modality may be primed to attribute perceived changes in cognitive functioning to this treatment relative to other causes (63).

MECHANISMS OF THERAPEUTIC ACTION

It is astonishing that repeated seizures in humans can exert such profound therapeutic effects. From a practical viewpoint, investigations of the mechanisms of action of ECT have the advantage of typically studying the most severely depressed patients who subsequently show marked improvement in clinical state. Furthermore, unlike pharmacological treatments, ECT is administered in a punctate manner, and the course of biological changes can be examined relative to the timing of the intervention. Because ECT is essentially a nonpharmacological physical treatment, patients can be studied while medication-free both prior to and following the intervention, removing a major complication in many human studies of the mode of action of psychotropics. Finally, it is evident that the anatomic positioning of electrodes (bilateral or unilateral ECT) has marked impact on neurophysiological and cognitive sequelae, and, in some circumstances, on efficacy. This potential to restrict the anatomy of the sites involved in seizure initiation and propagation is presently limited by the use of an electrical stimulus and the intrinsic geometry and impedance properties of the scalp and skull (56). The development of new focal methods of brain stimulation and seizure induction will likely involve the use of time-varying, focused magnetic fields and may afford new opportunities to isolate the functional neural systems involved in antidepressant and other therapeutic effects (56).

Over a hundred theories have been offered to account for the efficacy of ECT, and skepticism has often been expressed about the possibility of uncovering its mode of action, in part because ECT produces a wide variety of effects on neurophysiological, neurotransmitter, and neuroendocrine systems. The provocation of generalized seizures results in so many systemic changes that isolating those critical to efficacy from epiphenomena was believed to be relatively hopeless (50). The demonstrations that generalized seizures can be reliably produced that lack therapeutic properties has engendered greater optimism. Using subtraction methods, preclinical and clinical research has begun to isolate neurobiological changes that accompany therapeutically effective forms of stimulation from nonspecific changes intrinsic to seizure induction (e.g., see ref. 39).

Comparison to Pharmacological Treatments

Hundreds of preclinical studies have compared the neurochemical effects of ECS and antidepressant medications. Some investigators have argued that a unitary mode of action underlies the efficacy of ECT and antidepressant medications, highlighting the common changes in noradrenergic and serotonergic transmission. Others have reached the opposite conclusion, emphasizing the disparities (15). Failing a firmer understanding of the pathophysi-

ology of depressive illness or the bases of therapeutic response, information from preclinical investigation alone is unlikely to resolve this controversy.

At the clinical level, it is evident that ECT and antidepressant medications have different spectra of therapeutic action. The breadth of conditions that are posited as responsive to ECT from a single mode of action will strongly influence the search for mechanisms. For example, Post and colleagues (44) emphasized the efficacy of ECT in both depression and mania, and suggested parallels to lithium, carbamazepine, and valproate, supporting anticonvulsant theories of the mode of action of ECT (55). However, although it is clear that antidepressant medications (TCAs, MAOIs, and SSRIs) may aggravate mania, there is no assurance that the mode of action of ECT is uniform across major depression and mania.

An alternative strategy is to investigate the relationship between the response to a class of medications and to ECT (45,57). It had long been assumed that among depressed patients, clinical outcome with ECT was independent of history of response to antidepressant medications (15). Were this the case, it would suggest at least partial independence in modes of action. For example, high rates of ECT response in patients clearly resistant to TCAs would suggest that ECT differs from TCAs in the degree or kind of therapeutic neurobiological changes induced. However, although it is evident that many TCA-resistant patients respond to ECT, the preliminary evidence suggests that their response rate is reduced compared to that of patients without established medication resistance (45). This, in turn, is compatible with some overlap in mechanisms of action.

Psychological Effects

One group of theories focuses on psychological factors as largely accounting for the antidepressant effects of ECT. Various theories have emphasized psychodynamic themes, viewing ECT is as a punitive intervention, the high expectations of recovery with ECT, focusing on the induction of placebo effects, or the adverse cognitive consequences of ECT, implicating amnesia or gross cognitive as the basis for perceived therapeutic response (50). The findings of the double-blind, random-assignment studies using real vs. sham designs rule out the psychodynamic and placebo explanations (51). Furthermore, the findings that, independent of seizure elicitation, the efficacy of ECT is contingent on technical factors in its administration, such as the anatomic positioning of electrodes and the intensity of electrical dosage, substantially contradict this kind of explanation (58). A large number of studies have sought relationships between cognitive and therapeutic changes. When significant relationships have been observed, invariably they have indicated better cognitive functioning in those patients with greatest improvement in symptomatic status (52).

Neurophysiological Effects

Brain Imaging and EEG Studies

The generalized seizures produced during ECT reflect the hypersynchronous discharge of large neuronal populations. They are hypermetabolic states, involving pronounced increases in CBF, oxygen consumption, and glucose metabolism. Typically, the magnitude of the CBF increase outstrips metabolic demands, and, with modified ECT changes are not expected in cerebral arterial-venous pO_2, pCO_2, or lactate gradients (22).

There is a refractory period immediately following electrically induced seizure in which seizure threshold is markedly elevated and repeated seizure induction is difficult (55). Spontaneous cortical electrical activity may also be suppressed immediately following seizure termination. Manifestation of this isoelectric electroencephalogram (EEG) pattern is more common with bilateral than with unilateral electrode placement and with high- than with low-intensity electrical stimulation; it also may be predictive of superior clinical outcome (39). During the postictal period, the isoelectric pattern is typically replaced by high-amplitude slow-wave (delta) activity. Likewise, pronounced cortical reductions in CBF and glucose metabolism have been demonstrated (Nobler et al., *unpublished data*). The increase in EEG slow-wave activity and the decrease in CBF and glucose metabolism are greatest in anterior cortical regions and when unilateral ECT is administered, in the hemisphere ipsilateral to electrode placement (68, Nobler et al., *unpublished data*).

These neurophysiological effects have been interpreted as reflecting the recruitment of endogenous inhibitory processes to terminate the seizure (55). Several of these anticonvulsant effects are progressive during the ECT course. Seizure threshold typically shows a cumulative increase, and there is a decrease in seizure duration (55). These two effects are at least partially independent, and pharmacological agents have been shown to have distinct impact on seizure threshold and duration (28,55). Slow-wave EEG activity also shows progressive enhancement during the ECT course. There are preliminary data suggesting that the change in seizure threshold is related to efficacy in both major depression and mania (55). In particular, forms of ECT administration that exert weak antidepressant effects produce smaller increases in seizure threshold (58). However, a relationship between clinical outcome and changes in seizure duration has not been observed. A large number of studies have also sought to establish a relationship between changes in EEG slow-wave activity and clinical outcome (1,68). These findings were inconclusive and largely limited by the fact that few investigations examined topographic effects. Furthermore, this work was largely conducted with high intensity forms of bilateral ECT, producing ceiling effects by inducing large increases in slow-wave activity across patients, possibly masking a relationship with treatment out-

come. New findings suggest that greater CBF reductions in bilateral anterior cortical regions, as observed following both a single treatment and a complete course, are associated with superior antidepressant response (Nobler et al., *unpublished data*). To date, brain imaging studies of ECT have focused on cortical effects. The positive findings support the use of high-resolution technologies to outline the anatomy of the cortical–subcortical functional systems that subserve therapeutic response.

Protein Synthesis

In man and other animals, electrical induction of generalized seizures results in a short-lasting reversible inhibition of protein synthesis (60). No comprehensive theory has related this effect to efficacy. However, there is a substantial body of evidence that suggests that medications that inhibit protein synthesis interfere with long-term memory (5). This may be relevant to the cognitive effects of ECT, suggesting disruption of the neuronal plasticity mechanisms necessary for memory consolidation. Alternatively, recent evidence suggests that unmodified ECS in rodents activates astrocytes, as measured by increased staining for glial fibrillary acid protein, and also leads to an increase in the ratio of a marker of newly formed synapses relative to a marker of mature synapses (27). This has been interpreted as suggesting that ECS results in increased synaptic remodeling, an effect that may be relevant to a variety of biochemical theories of mode of action.

Blood–Brain Barrier Disruption

There is evidence that in man and animals electrically induced seizures also result in transient disruption of the blood–brain barrier. This disruption is dependent on transient systemic hypertension and cerebral vasodilatation, with the presumed mechanism being increased vesicular transport by pinocytosis (22,60). This effect is short lasting, and no increase in cerebrovascular permeability to serum proteins can be demonstrated by 24 hours after the last ECS in a series. Findings with repeat MRI in ECT patients of transient increases in T_1 relaxation times, an index of water content in the brain, have been interpreted as reflecting this transient disruption.

In turn, ECT results in an acute, and typically transient, increase in the plasma of a variety of transmitters and peptides including epinephrine, norepinephrine, prolactin, β-endorphin immunoreactivity, vasopressin, oxytocin, adrenocorticotropin (ACTH), cortisol, insulin, follicle-stimulating hormone, and luteinizing hormone (50). Increased brain permeability to endogenous, circulating molecules with putative antidepressant effects has been raised frequently as a process related to efficacy (15). Furthermore, in schizophrenia, the seeming superiority of ECT combined with a neuroleptic to either treatment alone has been attributed to the enhanced permeability, which produces higher brain concentration of the neuroleptic. In contrast, with the exception of oxytocin-related neurophysin (46), findings relating the antidepressant effects of ECT to the magnitude of acute surges of endogenous substances in plasma have been negative.

The magnitude of the systemic hypertensive changes, a factor contributing to increased blood–brain barrier permeability, is also unrelated to clinical outcome. During the postictal period in schizophrenic patients, plasma and red blood cell levels of haloperidol have been shown to increase transiently, indicating a redistribution phenomenon. However, recent work has demonstrated a similar effect in rats but did not find any changes in cerebral concentrations of haloperidol (29).

Biochemical Effects

Electroconvulsive shock has many consistent effects on transmitter and peptide concentrations, receptor density, and signal transduction mechanisms (see ref. 40 for a review). This evidence comes mainly from studies of physiologically normal rodents, and generalizability to human clinical context is uncertain. Criteria have been offered to screen ECS biochemical alterations for relevance to the mechanisms of action of ECT (40). For example, a single ECT treatment rarely results in clinical remission, and candidate neurochemical changes induced by ECS are expected to evolve with repeated application. However, critical aspects of methodology remain uncertain. Early work in which ECS was massed, with repeated application in the same day, was criticized as failing to mimic the schedule used in the human context, usually twice or thrice weekly. In turn, it is well known that there are fundamental differences between humans and rodents in the onset, peak, and recovery functions for a variety of biological processes. For example, following a single ECT treatment, seizure threshold in the human remains elevated at least for a matter of days. The elevation in the rat appears to last for about 1 hr (20). Studies of the neurochemistry subserving this anticonvulsant effect would have to take this difference in time course into account. Using such behavioral end points to guide parameter selection is largely unavailable in ECS studies aimed at accounting for the therapeutic effects of electrical induction of seizures.

In the human, in addition to neuroendocrine strategies, biochemical studies of ECT have concentrated on alterations in monoamine concentrations and turnover and receptor physiology in peripheral body fluids and tissue (49; see ref. 25 for a review). Here the relations to brain neurochemistry are often uncertain, in part due to concerns about the specificity of neuroendocrine probes or the strength of association between peripheral measures and central transmitter or peptide function. The development of in vivo brain imaging techniques to selectively probe central neurochemical systems may substantially advance knowledge in this area.

Norepinephrine

There are a number of effects that ECS has in common with chronic administration of TCAs in altering noradrenergic function. Repeated ECS results in a decrease in the density of β-adrenergic receptors (25,40). This change appears to be an adaptive down-regulation, as microdialysis and other studies have shown prominent acute and basal increases in brain norepinephrine and tyrosine hydroxylase activity. The β-receptor reduction also appears to be functional, as it is associated with reduced receptor-mediated cyclic adenosine monophosphate production and behavioral response to β agonists are attenuated after ECS. The changes in norepinephrine (NE) concentration and β-receptor density appear to show regional specificity, being most marked in cortex and hippocampus, but not in striatum, cerebellum, or hypothalamus. In general, the evidence is less consistent with regard to α_1- and α_2-adrenergic receptors. There are discrepant reports regarding decreased α_2-adrenergic receptor density, but behavioral data suggest presynaptic subsensitivity, perhaps accounting for increased basal NE concentrations. In the human, there is a surge in the levels of plasma catecholamines, particularly epinephrine, with seizure induction. These changes are transient and may be more relevant to ECT effects on cardiac function than to efficacy. With the possible exception of cerebrospinal fluid (CSF) homovanillic acid (HVA), studies of more chronic changes in peripheral or CSF measures of catecholamines and their metabolites have been negative or inconsistent (49). In general, the evidence is consistent with the view that repeated ECS enhances noradrenergic function.

Serotonin

The comparison of TCAs or MAOIs and ECS in altering serotonergic function is intriguing, since they have opposite effects on 5-HT$_2$ receptor density (25,40). Chronic ECS results in an increase, whereas antidepressant medications produce a decrease. Acutely following a single ECS, there is also increased serotonin (5-HT) concentrations, but no consistent effect has been observed on basal levels. However, as with some antidepressant medications, chronic ECS enhances electrophysiological and behavioral serotonergic responses mediated by the 5-HT$_2$ receptor subtype. The effects of chronic ECS on 5-HT$_2$ density and responsivity require intact serotonergic and noradrenergic innervation and can be blocked by inhibiting serotonin or NE synthesis. Studies of 5-HT$_1$ receptor density and function have not reported theoretically consistent effects, but much of this work predated identification of specific 5-HT$_1$ receptor subtypes. In humans, most studies have reported small or unchanged levels of plasma, urinary, and CSF 5-hydroxyindoleacetic acid (5-HIAA) following ECT, but a recent study with medication-free depressed patients suggests that CSF 5-HIAA may increase (49). Tritiated imipramine binding (^{3}H-IMI) on platelet membranes has been used to assess 5-HT transporter mechanisms (25). There are suggestions that ECT may normalize decreased ^{3}H-IMI platelet binding, but time course and a relationship with clinical outcome are uncertain. Recently, tritiated paroxetine binding has been shown to provide a more specific measure of the high-affinity 5-HT transporter site on platelet membrane, but effects with ECT have yet to be reported. Prolactin response to thyrotropin-releasing hormone (TRH) and to fenfluramine are believed to be serotonergicly mediated. In both cases, there is some evidence that these responses are enhanced following ECT. Overall, this work suggests that ECT enhances serotonergic throughput and function (25,40,49). The fact that antidepressant medications and ECS have distinct effects on the 5-HT$_2$ receptor may be relevant to the utility of ECT in medication-resistant patients and its superior efficacy in psychotic depression relative to monotherapy with antidepressant medications.

Dopamine

Antipsychotic effects are exerted by ECT across a range of diagnostic categories (e.g., psychotic depression, mania, schizophrenia), and yet ECT also has antiparkinsonian properties. This would suggest a distinct profile on alterations of dopaminergic function relative to classic antipsychotic medications. Recent microdialysis studies suggest that the concentration of dopamine and its metabolites are markedly increased acutely following a single ECS and that there appear to be increases in basal levels with chronic administration (40). This work also suggests that there is regional specificity in these changes in dopamine levels. A highly consistent finding is that there is increased behavioral responsivity to dopamine agonists following single or chronic ECS. This potentiation of dopamine-mediated behavior is contingent on intact noradrenergic, but not serotonergic, innervation. Effects on the D$_2$ receptor have not been observed. Rather, there is evidence for increased D$_1$ receptor density and increased second-messenger potentiation at this receptor (16). In addition, there is preliminary evidence that behavioral responsivity is enhanced with D$_1$ receptor agonists but not with D$_2$ receptor agonists. In man, growth hormone or prolactin response to apomorphine has been used as a neuroendocrine probe of dopaminergic function. Although there are reports that these responses are enhanced following ECT, there are also negative findings (25). Plasma HVA appears to be unaltered following a course of ECT and CSF HVA has been found to increase shortly following a single treatment. Most reports indicate no persistent effect of ECT on CSF HVA; however, a recent study in medication-free patients reported a marked in-

crease (49). In general, the findings in humans are less consistent than in animals, but similarly suggest enhanced dopaminergic function. This effect appears tied to regionally specific alterations of D$_1$-receptor physiology. Furthermore, there is evidence that the acute release of dopamine and its metabolites is sensitive to the dosage of electrical stimulation and is not contingent on seizure induction. Enhanced dopamine concentrations are not observed with chemically induced seizures, but are unaltered when the seizure discharge with electrical stimulation is blocked by concurrent administration of a barbiturate. If these effects are relevant to the antiparkinsonian properties of ECT, they suggest examination of electrical stimulation and pharmacological combinations that block the production of generalized seizures.

Acetylcholine

Chronic ECS results in significant but small reductions in muscarinic cholinergic receptor density in cortex and hippocampus and a functional decrease in second messenger response in the hippocampus (40). This is coupled with acute reductions in brain acetylcholine levels and acute increases in choline acetyltransferase and acetylcholinesterase activities shortly following ECS. In humans, there is evidence for increased CSF acetylcholine levels following ECT and spontaneous seizures (25). These findings are compatible with a reduction in central cholinergic function following ECT. Supporting this, chronic ECS has been shown to produce reduced behavioral responsivity to the muscarinic agonists pilocarpine and arecoline. These effects are compatible with a view that ECT exerts antidepressant effects through a reduction of cholinergic supersensitivity. However, reduction of cholinergic tone theoretically should be counterproductive in the treatment of mania and ECT has marked antimanic properties (36). Cholinergic mechanisms are strongly implicated in various aspects of learning and memory. Regionally specific reduction in cholinergic function may be relevant to the cognitive side effects of ECT (30).

Gamma Aminobutyric Acid

In animals and humans electrical induction of seizures results in a subsequent increase in seizure threshold (55). ECS raises the threshold of a variety of convulsant agents that produce seizures through antagonism of γ-aminobutyric acid (GABA). Pharmacological specificity obtains, since ECS will not raise the threshold for seizures evoked with a glycine antagonist or a serotonergic agonist (20). This suggests that ECS results in a functional increase in GABAergic activity. Indeed, single and repeated ECS raises GABA concentrations in specific brain regions. Furthermore, ECS, like most antidepressant medications, results in increased density of the GABA$_B$ receptor (40). Behavioral response to the GABA$_B$ agonist, baclofen, appears to be enhanced following ECS. In turn GABA_B receptors modulate the release of other neurotransmitters. For example, chronic administration of the GABA-mimetic agent, progabide, produces many of the same changes in monoamine biochemistry as ECS, including up-regulation of $5-HT_2$ receptors (25). There is preliminary data that some GABA-mimetics may have antidepressant properties. Complicating interpretation is evidence that GABA synthesis and release are reduced acutely following ECS (40). Several studies have reported reduced plasma and CSF levels of GABA in depressed patients. The one study to examine plasma GABA levels during ECT found acute reductions immediately following seizure elicitation. This effect was unusual in that virtually every other substance in plasma showed no change or an acute surge immediately following ECT.

Endogenous Opioids

Chronic ECS increases met-enkephalin and β-endorphin concentrations and synthesis in several brain regions (40). Like models of morphine tolerance, chronic ECS also results in changes in binding to a number of opioid ligands, with suggestions that the δ-opioid receptor may be the most affected. Consistent with these data is behavioral evidence that ECS exhibits cross sensitization to acute morphine challenge. In addition, a variety of postictal behavioral phenomena (e.g., antinociception, hyperthermia, hypoventilation, EEG slowing) have been modulated by selective opioid antagonists. There is strong evidence that immediately following ECS one or more endogenous anticonvulsant substances are released in CSF. Antagonist and ultrafiltration studies implicate a large-molecular-weight opioid peptide. Similarly opioid antagonists can block the progressive decrease in the severity and duration of seizures elicited by ECS. Antagonist studies have also modulated the extent of retrograde amnesia following ECS (30). In humans, there are marked acute increases in plasma β-endorphin immunoreactivity immediately following ECT (25). Although it seems likely that ECT results in enhanced function in some aspects of opioid systems, there has been limited research with humans using selective subtype antagonists to determine the involvement of these systems in anticonvulsant, amnesic, or therapeutic effects.

Adenosine

Adenosine has been implicated in the regulation of cerebral excitability. In addition to the increase in seizure threshold, seizure duration shortens during the course of ECT (55). Adenosine antagonists, such as caffeine or theophylline, increase the duration of seizures elicited with ECT. In humans, there is evidence that the effects of caffeine on seizure duration are not associated with a change in seizure threshold, again indicating at least par-

tial independence of these phenomena. Chronic ECS results in a persistent increase in the density of A_1 adenosine receptors, whereas effects on A_2 adenosine receptors have been inconsistent (40).

Gene Expression

The development of in situ hybridization techniques has led to extensive research on ECS effects on gene expression. Electroconvulsive shock results acutely in induction of a variety of protooncogene products, including c-fos, c-jun, jun-B, and zif/268. The regional distribution of these effects and their time course differ qualitatively from the changes associated with stress manipulations and other methods of seizure induction (e.g., caffeine) (40). This approach may offer a novel method for identifying the common anatomic systems activated by seizure induction methods which possess therapeutic properties (ECT, flurothyl, metrazol). Since oncogenes, like c-fos, are regulatory, it would be expected that ECS changes the expression of many proteins. Indeed, there are preliminary findings that ECS results in altered messenger ribonucleic acid (mRNA) levels in a variety of enzymatic, peptidergic, and transmitter systems. These include mRNA coding for the α_1- and γ_2-GABA_A receptor subunits in hippocampus and cerebellum, β_1-adrenergic receptor in frontal cortex, $5-HT_2$ receptor in frontal cortex, tyrosine hydroxylase and neuropeptide Y in the locus coeruleus, cerebral ornithine decarboxylase in cortex, somatostatin in the hippocampus, preproenkephalin in hypothalamus and entorhinal cortex, prodynorphin in hypothalamus and hippocampus, peptidylglycine α-amidating monooxygenase in the hippocampus, and preprocholecystokinin, preprotachykinin-A, corticotropin-releasing factor, arginine vasopressin, and heat shock cognate protein. Initial findings with this approach suggest notable differences in how ECS and antidepressant medications modulate the same transmitter system. For example, chronic ECS and imipramine both result in down-regulation of the β_1-adrenergic receptor in the frontal cortex. Electroconvulsive shock produces decreased β_1-mRNA levels in a time-dependent fashion, parallel to the receptor changes. In contrast, imipramine appears to produce an initial increase in β_1 mRNA levels, and decreases are seen only after approximately 3 weeks of treatment.

Other Systems

One class of theories regarding the mechanisms of action of ECT has concentrated on the neuromodulatory functions exerted by endocrine hormones. In general, these theories have emphasized the effectiveness of ECT in treating vegetative or endogenous symptoms, presumed to reflect hypothalamic dysregulation (15). In addition, there has been a view that the generalized seizure in ECT, a fundamental constituent of efficacy, emanates from a centroencephalic pacemaker. Finally, it is evident that a variety of peptides are elevated in plasma immediately following seizure induction in humans (50).

There are limited data supporting these conjectures. Electroconvulsive shock appears to have complex effects on brain concentrations of TRH and on TRH-receptor function, although some have reported consistent increases of TRH concentration following ECS in specific brain regions (40). Early studies suggested that following ECT most depressed patients showed decreased blunting in thyrotropin stimulating hormone (TSH) response to TRH and that manifestation of this change was predictive of long-term remission. More recent work failed to replicate this observation and, if anything, observed increased blunting following ECT (7). A recent preliminary study suggests that L-triiodothyronine (T₃) supplementation of ECT may improve clinical response and reduce cognitive side effects (30).

Investigations of the hypothalamic-pituitary-adrenal axis have proved inconsistent. There is preliminary evidence that the CSF level of corticotropin-releasing hormone is increased following ECT. The dexamethasone suppression test (DST) has not been useful in predicting ECT outcome, and it appears that ECT may have opposite short-term effects on the DST (9). Most patients show decreased postdexamethasone cortisol levels following ECT, but an effect of ECT producing abnormal DST responses has also been detected (9). In any case, changes in DST response appear to be independent of clinical outcome. Surprisingly, it was recently observed that plasma levels of exogenously administered dexamethasone typically increase during and following ECT, and this effect was associated with the degree of symptomatic improvement (9).

MECHANISMS OF ADVERSE COGNITIVE EFFECTS

Neuropathological Effects

Some have interpreted the adverse cognitive side effects of ECT as reflecting irreversible structural brain damage (50). The transient nature of most cognitive changes is incompatible with this position, although the permanent gaps in memory for events surrounding the treatment course hypothetically could reflect either functional or structural effects. The evidence from neuropathological investigations has been recently reviewed (8). Human postmortem studies have not linked neuronal cell loss to current ECT practice. Prospective structural brain imaging studies in cohorts of ECT patients have not observed any changes (8). The most critical work in this area involves animal investigation in which more intensive treatment paradigms can be used with more sensitive pathological techniques. Controlled studies using perfusion fixation techniques have failed to observe pathological changes following ECS. Indeed, cell counts in hippocampal fields in animals receiving intensive and chronic ECS have shown no difference from controls, despite the same technique demonstrating cell loss in epilepsy patients with frequent seizures (8). Furthermore, considerable information has accrued about the metabolic and molecular conditions required for cellular death following seizures (22,60). Conservatively, under conditions of oxygenation, seizures must be continuous for at least 25 to 30 min to result in cell death. This effect is thought to depend on mismatches between metabolic demand and supply in vulnerable neurons and agonist-receptor interactions that trigger dissipative fluxes of sodium and calcium ions across postsynaptic membranes (22,60). In any case, there is agreement that the minimum conditions for cellular necrosis do not apply to ECT.

Neurophysiological Theories

The adverse cognitive effects of ECT are stereotyped and pertain largely to discrete aspects of the retention of new information and the recall or recognition of recent events (52,63). This pattern suggests that ECT has particularly important effects on medial temporal structures long implicated as subserving long-term memory function (50,63). A large number of theories have been offered to account for the selective amnesic effects of ECT. Among the most attractive is the view that the anterograde and retrograde memory disturbances reflect dysfunctions of consolidation. Months to years after encoding, information may be vulnerable to loss, because the process of consolidation is not complete. Memories that are more remote in time may be least vulnerable, whereas interference with consolidation may result in permanent loss of recently acquired information. We have noted that ECT transiently inhibits protein synthesis and may disrupt the plasticity mechanisms needed for consolidation or maintenance of long-term memories (27,60).

Relatively little research has been conducted on the neurophysiological correlates of these cognitive effects. As indicated, ECT results in postictal reductions of cortical CBF and cerebral glucose metabolism. Little is known about the persistence of such effects, although reductions have been observed a week following the ECT course (Nobler et al., *unpublished data*). Regional reductions in CBF and metabolism in many neurological conditions are associated with particular profiles of cognitive deficit. Such correlations have not been examined following ECT. This is particularly important, because the ECT cognitive pattern is suggestive of medial temporal lobe dysfunction; yet the most prominent effects reported in brain-imaging studies have been in the anterior frontal cortex. In contrast, it has been established that the induction of slow-wave EEG activity may persist for weeks following ECT. Several studies have shown significant correlations between the magnitude of this effect and that of amnesic deficits (1,68). However, this work rarely involved examination of topographic EEG changes.

Pharmacological Treatment of ECT Amnesic Effects

In animals, ECS is a standard screening procedure for pharmacological compounds that may have beneficial effects on memory. A large variety of agents have been shown to diminish or block ECS amnesic effects, including opioid antagonists, calcium-channel blockers, cholinesterase inhibitors, acetylcholine precursors, corticosteroids, thyroid hormone, vasopressin analogs, somatostatin, melanocyte-stimulating hormone, atrial natriuretic peptide, substance P, nootropics, ergoloid mesylates, and psychostimulants (30). Typically, when the efficacy of such agents has been evaluated in humans, it has been in the context of clinical trials targeting various forms of dementia, often with disappointing results. There have been few attempts to use pharmacological strategies to reduce the cognitive side effects of ECT, despite the wealth of candidate agents and similarities in the cognitive effects of ECS and ECT (30). This approach holds considerable promise for improving this form of treatment. It is evident that distinct pathophysiologies underlie the cognitive disturbance in most dementia conditions and that associated with ECT. Efficacy of pharmacological strategies in one context and not the other would underscore this distinction. On the other hand, repeated failure to discern protective effects in human ECT for compounds that reduce the amnesic effects of ECS in rodents and nonhuman primates would introduce uncertainty about the relevance of particular animal models of amnesia.

CONCLUSIONS

Electroconvulsive therapy is a highly effective treatment for episodes of major depression and mania. Its role in the treatment of exacerbations of schizophrenia requires reconsideration. Considerable progress has been made in optimizing ECT technique. This work indicates that technical factors in ECT administration have pronounced impact on both efficacy and cognitive side effects and has contradicted the original view that the generalized seizure provides both the necessary and sufficient conditions for antidepressant effects. The central clinical issue in the use of ECT is the problem of rapid relapse. Research is needed into the efficacy of traditional and alternative continuation medication strategies, as well as the use of continuation ECT, particularly in relation to history of medication resistance. Brain-imaging studies are beginning to outline the functional anatomy of the neural systems associated with antidepressant effects. This work needs to be extended to adverse cognitive consequences. In addition, animal studies have identified a plethora of chronic ECS effects on neurochemical systems. Extension of this work to humans using in vivo imaging techniques and distinguishing between the nonspecific changes associated with seizure induction and those unique to seizures with therapeutic properties offer new approaches to investigation of mechanisms of action.

ACKNOWLEDGMENT

Preparation of this chapter was supported in part by grants MH35636 and MH47739 from the National Institute of Mental Health.

REFERENCES

1. Abrams R. *Electroconvulsive therapy.* New York: Oxford University Press, 1992.
2. American Psychiatric Association. Weiner RD, Fink M, Hammersley D, Moench L, Sackeim HA, Small I, eds. *The practice of ECT: recommendations for treatment, training and privileging.* Washington, DC: American Psychiatric Press, 1990.
3. Cole JO, Gardos G, Boling LA, Marby D, Haskell D, Moore P. Early dyskinesia—vulnerability. *Psychopharmacology (Berl)* 1992; 107:503–510.
4. Daniel WF, Crovitz HF. Acute memory impairment following electroconvulsive therapy. 1. Effects of electrical stimulus waveform and number of treatments. *Acta Psychiatr Scand* 1983;67:1–7.
5. Davis H, Squire L. Protein synthesis and memory. *Psychol Bull* 1984;96:518–559.
6. Davis JM, Janicak PG, Sakkas P, Gilmore C, Wang Z. Electroconvulsive therapy in the treatment of the neuroleptic malignant syndrome. *Convulsive Ther* 1991;7:111–120.
7. Decina P, Sackeim HA, Kahn DA, Pierson D, Hopkins N, Malitz S. Effects of ECT on the TRH stimulation test. *Psychoneuroendocrinology* 1987;12:29–34.
8. Devanand DP, Dwork AJ, Hutchinson ER, Bolwig TG, Sackeim HA. Does electroconvulsive therapy alter brain structure? *Am J Psychiatry* 1994;151:957–970.
9. Devanand DP, Sackeim HA, Lo ES, Cooper T, Huttinot G, Prudic J. Serial dexamethasone suppression tests and plasma dexamethasone levels. Effects of clinical response to electroconvulsive therapy in major depression. *Arch Gen Psychiatry* 1991;48:525–533.
10. Dinan TG, Barry S. A comparison of electroconvulsive therapy with a combined lithium and tricyclic combination among depressed tricyclic nonresponders. *Acta Psychiatr Scand* 1989;80:97–100.
11. Dodwell D, Goldberg D. A study of factors associated with response to electroconvulsive therapy in patients with schizophrenic symptoms. *Br J Psychiatry* 1989;154:635–639.
12. Exner JE Jr, Murillo LG. A long term follow-up of schizophrenics treated with regressive ECT. *Dis Nerv Syst* 1977;38:162–168.
13. Figiel GS, Coffey CE, Djang WT, Hoffman GJ, Doraiswamy PM. Brain magnetic resonance imaging findings in ECT-induced delirium. *J Neuropsychiatry Clin Neurosci* 1990;2:53–58.
14. Fink M. *Convulsive therapy: theory and practice.* New York: Raven Press; 1979.
15. Fink M. How does ECT work? *Neuropsychopharmacology* 1990; 3:77–82.
16. Fochtmann LJ, Cruciani R, Aiso M, Potter WZ. Chronic electroconvulsive shock increases D-1 receptor binding in rat substantia nigra. *Eur J Pharmacol* 1989;167:305–306.
17. Freeman CP, Weeks D, Kendell RE. ECT: II: patients who complain. *Br J Psychiatry* 1980;137:17–25.
18. Gardos G, Samu I, Kallos M, Cole JO. Absence of severe tardive dyskinesia in Hungarian schizophrenic out-patients. *Psychopharmacology (Berl)* 1980;71:29–34.
19. Goswami U, Dutta S, Kuruvilla K, Papp E, Perenyi A. Electroconvulsive therapy in neuroleptic-induced parkinsonism. *Biol Psychiatry* 1989;26:234–8.
20. Green A, Nutt D, Cowen P. Increased seizure threshold following

convulsion. In: Sandler M, ed. *Psychopharmacology of anticonvulsants.* Oxford: Oxford University Press, 1982;16–26.

21. Hamilton M. The effect of treatment on the melancholias (depressions). *Br J Psychiatry* 1982;140:223–30.
22. Ingvar M. Cerebral blood flow and metabolic rate during seizures: relationship to epileptic brain damage. *Ann NY Acad Sci* 1986;462:194–206.
23. Janicak PG, Davis JM, Gibbons RD, Ericksen S, Chang S, Gallagher P. Efficacy of ECT: a meta-analysis. *Am J Psychiatry* 1985; 142:297–302.
24. Kalinowsky LB, Hoch PH. *Shock treatments and other somatic procedures in psychiatry.* New York: Grune & Stratton, 1946.
25. Kapur S, Mann JJ. Antidepressant action and the neurobiologic effects of ECT: human studies. In: Coffey CE, ed. *The clinical science of electroconvulsive therapy.* Washington, DC: American Psychiatric Press; 1993:235–250.
26. Khanna S, Gangadhar BN, Sinha V, Rajendra PN, Channabasavanna SM. Electroconvulsive therapy in obsessive-compulsive disorder. *Convulsive Ther* 1988;4:314–320.
27. Kragh J, Bolwig TG, Woldbye DP, Jørgensen OS. Electroconvulsive shock and lidocaine-induced seizures in the rat activate astrocytes as measured by glial fibrillary acidic protein. *Biol Psychiatry* 1993;33:794–800.
28. Krueger RB, Fama JM, Devanand DP, Prudic J, Sackeim HA. Does ECT permanently alter seizure threshold? *Biol Psychiatry* 1993;33: 272–276.
29. Krueger RB, Sackeim HA. Electroconvulsive therapy and schizophrenia. In: Hirsch SR, Weinberger DR, eds. *Schizophrenia.* Oxford: Blackwell [*in press*].
30. Krueger RB, Sackeim HA, Gamzu ER. Pharmacological treatment of the cognitive side effects of ECT: a review. *Psychopharmacol Bull* 1992;28:409–424.
31. Lambourn J, Gill D. A controlled comparison of simulated and real ECT. *Br J Psychiatry* 1978;133:514–519.
32. Mann SC, Caroff SN, Bleier HR, Welz WK, Kling MA, Hayashida M. Lethal catatonia. *Am J Psychiatry* 1986;143:1374–1381.
33. May PR, Tuma AH, Dixon WJ, Yale C, Thiele DA, Kraude WH. Schizophrenia. A follow-up study of the results of five forms of treatment. *Arch Gen Psychiatry* 1981;38:776–784.
34. McCall WV. Antihypertensive medications and ECT. *Convulsive Ther* 1993;9:317–325.
35. Mukherjee S, Debsikdar V. Absence of neuroleptic-induced parkinsonism in psychotic patients receiving adjunctive electroconvulsive therapy. *Convulsive Ther* [*in press*].
36. Mukherjee S, Sackeim HA, Schnur DB. Electroconvulsive therapy of acute manic episodes: a review of 50 years of experience. *Am J Psychiatry* [*in press*].
37. National Institute of Health Consensus Conference. Electroconvulsive therapy. *JAMA* 1985;254:2103–2108.
38. Nobler MS, Sackeim HA. Prediction of response to electroconvulsive therapy. In: Goodnick P, ed. *Prediction of response to antidepressant treatments.* Washington, DC: American Psychiatric Press [*in press*].
39. Nobler MS, Sackeim HA, Solomou M, Luber B, Devanand DP, Prudic J. EEG manifestations during ECT: effects of electrode placement and stimulus intensity. *Biol Psychiatry* 1993;34:321–330.
40. Nutt DJ, Glue P. The neurobiology of ECT: animal studies. In: Coffey CE, ed. *The clinical science of electroconvulsive therapy.* Washington, DC: American Psychiatric Press; 1993:213–234.
41. Ottosson J-O. Experimental studies of the mode of action of electroconvulsive therapy. *Acta Psychiatr Scand* [*Suppl.*] 1960;145:1–141.
42. Pataki J, Zervas IM, Jandorf L. Catatonia in a university inpatient service (1985–1990). *Convulsive Ther* 1992;8:163–173.
43. Post F. The management and nature of depressive illness in late life: a follow-through study. *Br J Psychiatry* 1972;121:393–404.
44. Post RM, Putnam F, Uhde TW, Weiss SR. Electroconvulsive therapy as an anticonvulsant. Implications for its mechanism of action in affective illness. *Ann NY Acad Sci* 1986;462:376–388.
45. Prudic J, Sackeim HA, Devanand DP. Medication resistance and clinical response to electroconvulsive therapy. *Psychiatry Res* 1990;31:287–296.
46. Riddle WJ, Scott AI, Bennie J, Carroll S, Fink G. Current intensity and oxytocin release after electroconvulsive therapy. *Biol Psychiatry* 1993;33:839–841.

47. Robin A, de Tissera S. A double-blind controlled comparison of the therapeutic effects of low and high energy electroconvulsive therapies. *Br J Psychiatry* 1982;141:357–366.
48. Royal College of Psychiatrists. Freeman CP, Crammer JL, Deakin JFW, McClelland R, Mann SA, Pippard J, eds. *The practical administration of electroconvulsive therapy (ECT).* London: Gaskell; 1989.
49. Rudorfer MV, Manji HK, Osman TO, Risby ED, Potter WZ. The biochemical effects of electroconvulsive therapy in depressed patients. I. Changes in cerebrospinal fluid monoamine metabolite concentrations. *Arch Gen Psychiatry* [*in press*].
50. Sackeim HA. Mechanisms of action of electroconvulsive therapy. In: Hales RE, Frances J, eds. *Annual review of psychiatry.* Vol. 7. Washington, DC: American Psychiatric Press; 1988:436–457.
51. Sackeim HA. The efficacy of electroconvulsive therapy in treatment of major depressive disorder. In: Fisher S, Greenberg RP, eds. *The limits of biological treatments for psychological distress: comparisons with psychotherapy and placebo.* Hillsdale, NJ: Erlbaum; 1989:275–307.
52. Sackeim HA. The cognitive effects of electroconvulsive therapy. In: Moos WH, Gamzu ER, Thal LJ, eds. *Cognitive disorders: pathophysiology and treatment.* New York: Marcel Dekker; 1992:183–228.
53. Sackeim HA. Use of electroconvulsive therapy in late life depression. In: Schneider LS, Reynolds III CF, Liebowitz BD, Friedhoff AJ, eds. *Diagnosis and treatment of depression in late life.* Washington, DC: American Psychiatric Press; 1993:259–277.
54. Sackeim HA, Decina P, Kanzler M, Kerr B, Malitz S. Effects of electrode placement on the efficacy of titrated, low-dose ECT. *Am J Psychiatry* 1987;144:1449–1455.
55. Sackeim HA, Devanand DP, Prudic J. Stimulus intensity, seizure threshold, and seizure duration: impact on the efficacy and safety of electroconvulsive therapy. *Psychiatr Clin North Am* 1991; 14:803–843.
56. Sackeim HA, Long J, Luber B, Prohovnik I, Devanand DP, Nobler MS. Physical properties and quantification of the ECT stimulus: I. Basic principles. *Convulsive Ther* [*in press*].
57. Sackeim HA, Prudic J, Devanand DP, Decina P, Kerr B, Malitz S. The impact of medication resistance and continuation pharmacotherapy on relapse following response to electroconvulsive therapy in major depression. *J Clin Psychopharmacol* 1990;10:96–104.
58. Sackeim HA, Prudic J, Devanand DP, et al. Effects of stimulus intensity and electrode placement on the efficacy and cognitive effects of electroconvulsive therapy. *N Engl J Med* 1993;328:839–846.
59. Schwartz M, Silver H, Tal I, Sharf B. Tardive dyskinesia in northern Israel: preliminary study. *Eur Neurol* 1993;33:264–266.
60. Siesjö BK, Ingvar M, Wieloch T. Cellular and molecular events underlying epileptic brain damage. *Ann NY Acad Sci* 1986; 462:207–223.
61. Small JG, Klapper MH, Kellams JJ, et al. Electroconvulsive treatment compared with lithium in the management of manic states. *Arch Gen Psychiatry* 1988;45:727–732.
62. Smith K, Surphlis WR, Gynther MD, Shimkunas AM. ECT-chlorpromazine and chlorpromazine compared in the treatment of schizophrenia. *J Nerv Ment Dis* 1967;144:284–290.
63. Squire LR. Memory functions as affected by electroconvulsive therapy. *Ann New York Acad Sci* 1986;462:307–314.
64. Taylor P, Fleminger JJ. ECT for schizophrenia. *Lancet* 1980; 1:1380–1382.
65. Thompson JW, Blaine JD. Use of ECT in the United States in 1975 and 1980. *Am J Psychiatry* 1987;144:557–562.
66. Thompson JW, Weiner RD. An update on the use of ECT in the United States. *Am J Psychiatry* [*in press*].
67. Ulett G, Smith K, Gleser G. Evaluation of convulsive and subconvulsive shock therapies utilizing a control group. *Am J Psychiatry* 1956;112:795–802.
68. Weiner RD, Rogers HJ, Davidson JR, Kahn EM. Effects of electroconvulsive therapy upon brain electrical activity. *Ann NY Acad Sci* 1986;462:270–281.
69. Weiner RD, Rogers HJ, Davidson JR, Squire LR. Effects of stimulus parameters on cognitive side effects. *Ann NY Acad Sci* 1986; 462:315–325.
70. Zielinski RJ, Roose SP, Devanand DP, Woodring S, Sackeim HA. Cardiovascular complications of ECT in depressed patients with cardiac disease. *Am J Psychiatry* 1993;150:904–909.

Psychopharmacology: The Fourth Generation of Progress, edited by Floyd E. Bloom and David J. Kupfer. Raven Press, Ltd., New York 1995.

CHAPTER 96

Novel Pharmacological Approaches to the Treatment of Depression

Dennis L. Murphy, Philip B. Mitchell, and William Z. Potter

The search to find safer, more effective and more rapidly acting antidepressants that might also benefit currently treatment-resistant patients continues unabated in the mid 1990s. This review summarizes recent trends in antidepressant drug development. It focuses on agents with relatively novel suggested mechanisms of action, and only briefly surveys other antidepressants under development that are not yet available in the United States whose mechanisms are thought to resemble those of already marketed drugs (36,69). Chemical structures of many of these novel agents are depicted in Fig. 1 and 2. Only an abbreviated reference list, citing reviews or more recent publications is provided, because of space limitations (see Chapter 89, *this volume*).

Major progress in new antidepressant development has been slow, with the notable exception of a group of serotonin selective reuptake inhibitors (SSRIs) introduced in the last 5 years. Although the SSRI's therapeutic effects are accompanied by fewer serious side effects and overdosage hazards than the first- and second-generation antidepressants, their principal mechanism of action, neurotransmitter uptake inhibition, is certainly not a novel one.

Before considering specific drug classes, several criteria need to be considered. Discussion of the pharmacological treatment of depression depends on what patients are subsumed under this broad diagnostic category and what assessment measures and criteria are accepted as indicating a meaningful antidepressant effect. Diagnostic criteria employed in many recent outpatient studies yield popula-

tions that sometimes show a high (>50%) 6-week placebo response rate, requiring large numbers of subjects (over 100) to demonstrate significant therapeutic advantage over placebo for a new, active antidepressant. In these populations, even such established antidepressants as imipramine sometimes do not emerge as clearly superior to placebo. European and some U.S. studies of potential antidepressants that are based on comparisons with standard tricyclics alone often may reveal no difference, suggesting equal efficacy for the new drug. However, judgment may need to be reserved as to claims of efficacy when adequate comparisons with a placebo group are unavailable. Possible differences in the clinical characteristics of patients studied in U.S. versus European settings must also be taken into account in assessing response data.

In addition, some psychotherapeutic agents such as alprazolam and trazodone have sometimes uncritically been referred to as antidepressants in the broad sense, that is, they have been reported to be equivalent to first-generation tricyclic or other antidepressants in some studies and thus, by implication, considered equally effective in severely depressed, nonpsychotic hospitalized patients. It is doubtful whether most experienced clinicians would consider using alprazolam or trazodone as the mainstay treatment for a patient so dysfunctional with depression as to require hospitalization. On the other hand, recent comparisons provide difficult-to-ignore evidence that certain agents [e.g., the irreversible monoamine oxidase (MAO) inhibitors] may be superior to tricyclic antidepressants in subgroups of depression such as bipolar or atypical depression (66). All of this highlights a level of uncertainty about selecting and evaluating novel pharmacological approaches for treating patients with depression and allied disorders.

One possible organizing principle to survey potential novel antidepressants would be to select compounds on

D. L. Murphy: Laboratory of Clinical Science, National Institute of Mental Health, Bethesda, Maryland 20892.

P. B. Mitchell: School of Psychiatry, University of New South Wales, Prince Henry Hospital, Little Bay, N.S.W. 2036, Australia.

W. Z. Potter: Section on Clinical Pharmacology, Experimental Therapeutics Branch, National Institute of Mental Health, Bethesda, Maryland 20892.

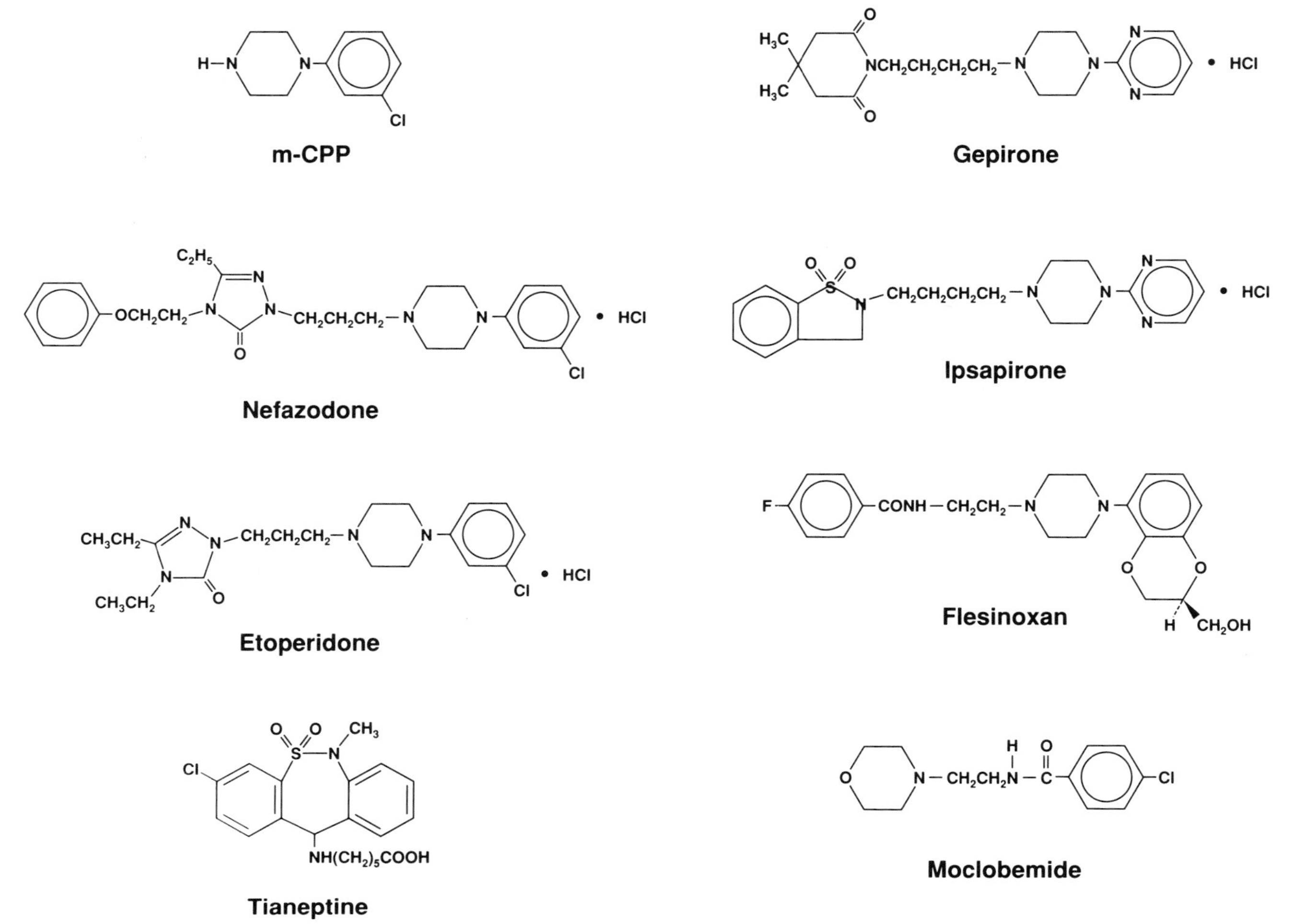

FIG. 1. Chemical structures of some putative novel antidepressant compounds.

the basis of their activity in animal models sensitive to antidepressant drug effects. However, this approach does not answer the question, because many animal models have multiple limitations for identifying novel antidepressants, ranging from circularity (e.g., the test merely reflects a biochemical property of standard drugs) to failure to detect any activity of certain established agents (e.g., inability of the MAO inhibitors to reverse passive-avoidance deficits) (78,84). Although some widely used behavioral paradigms (for example, the learned helplessness paradigm, the forced swim test, and the restraint stress-induced reduction of locomotor activity) yield positive results for most currently used antidepressant drugs, false positives and false negatives have been found for some novel compounds. Only clinical testing can definitively establish the utility of a new compound in the treatment of depression, whether narrowly or broadly defined, and a strong case can be made for clinical serendipity being involved in the discovery of most effective antidepressant agents thus far identified. Ultimately, we must depend on the observations of skilled clinicians employing well-targeted populations to find truly novel antidepressants with distinct efficacy in areas of need, rather

than on drug–placebo differences established solely in large trials with relatively fewer impaired outpatients.

NOVEL SEROTONERGIC ANTIDEPRESSANTS

The single largest class of new antidepressants, in the last decade is the SSRIs, but because several of these agents, namely fluoxetine, sertraline, and paroxetine, have recently been approved for use in the United States, only a few features of these agents specifically relevant to the development of new drugs affecting serotonin transport will be noted in this chapter. These agents, however, have drawn special attention to the potential involvement of brain serotonin subsystems in the modulation of mood, anxiety, sleep, and other physiological functions relevant to depressive symptoms (18).

The inhibition of serotonin (5-HT) uptake is by far the most established initial mechanism of action of serotonergic antidepressants; other non-uptake-inhibiting serotonergic drugs are active in animal models sensitive to antidepressant drugs, and have at least a modicum of clinical evidence supportive of antidepressant effects, including

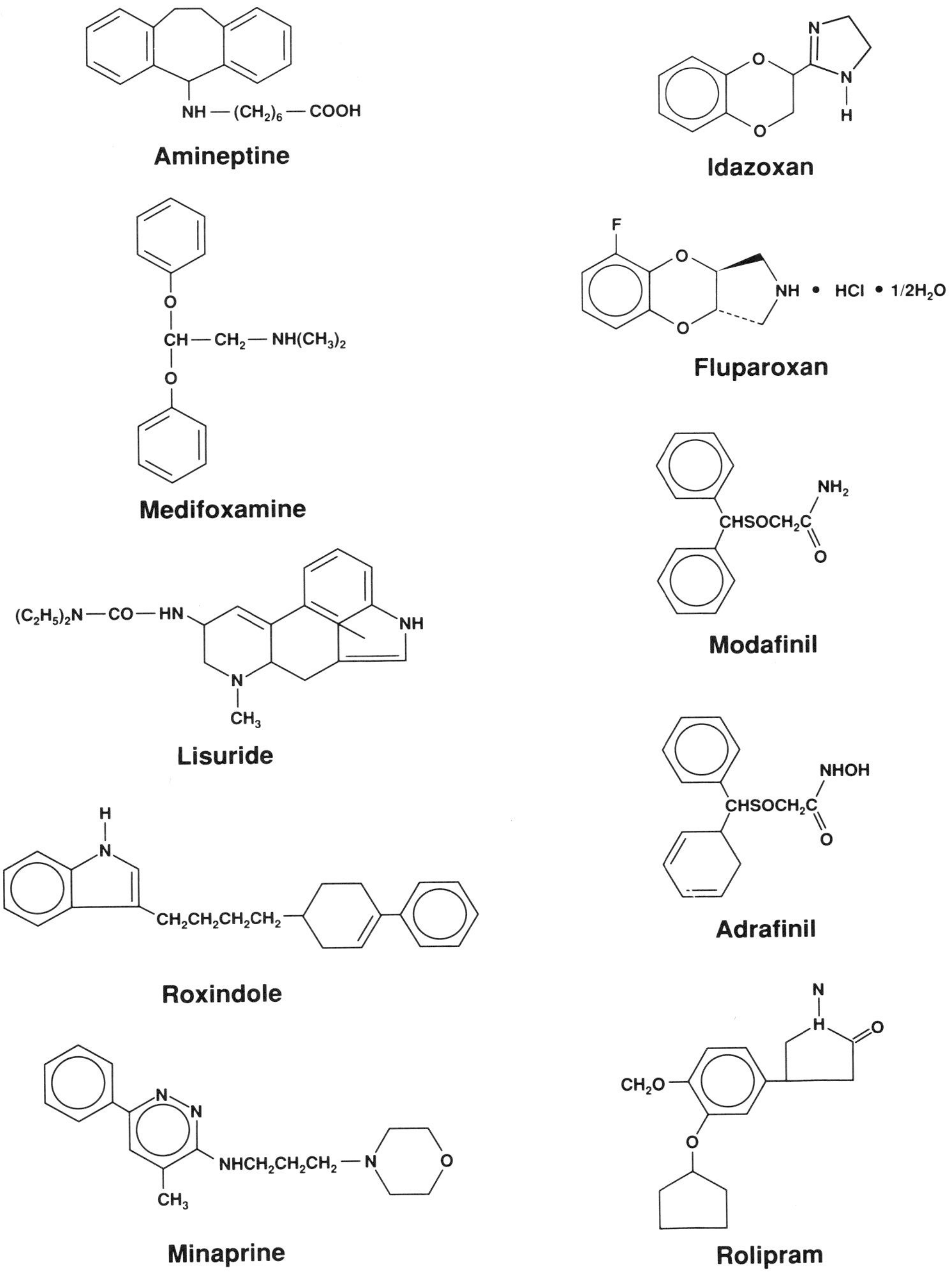

FIG. 2. Chemical structures of additional putative novel antidepressant compounds.

the following: (a) several 5-HT$_{1A}$ partial agonists, including buspirone, gepirone, ipsapirone, and flesinoxan (39); (b) a 5-HT$_{2C}$ partial agonist, m-chlorophenylpiperazine, with additional antagonist effects at 5-HT$_{2A}$ and 5-HT$_3$ sites (58); (c) other 5-HT$_{2A/2C}$ antagonists such as ritanserin, etoperidone and nefazodone (3,26,37); and (d) an enhancer of 5-HT uptake, tianeptine (44). Inhibitors of serotonin metabolism by MAO type A (MAO-A) inhibition, for which enzyme serotonin is a highly selective substrate, such as moclobemide, brofaromine, and clorgyline, are also effective antidepressants but are not available in the United States (15,47,83).

Reconciliation of the diverse serotonin receptor and related neurochemical mechanisms of action for the antidepressant effects of these agents is not immediately apparent. When consideration is given to adaptational events that follow repeated administration of these agents (as chronic administration is required for clinical therapeutic efficacy), even more complex schema are required. In the case of the SSRI's, a case for a net change leading to enhanced serotonergic neurotransmission responsible for antidepressant efficacy has been postulated, based upon drug-induced changes in electrophysiological events at serotonergic synapses and changes in releasable serotonin measured in microdialysis studies (28). However, because the more than 13 molecularly identified serotonin receptors may have opposing rather than potentiating effects measured on even one target cell, to say nothing of the multiple other neurotransmitter systems (dopamine, γ-aminobutyric acid, norepinephrine, and peptide systems) that are modulated by the widespread serotonin subsystems (45), adequate interpretations of mechanisms of action of these drugs would seem some distance in the future.

5-HT$_{1A}$ Receptor Agonists as Potential Antidepressants

Buspirone is the one representative of this drug class available in the United States; it is approved as an anxiolytic but not yet as an antidepressant. Studies of buspirone and related azapirones including gepirone and ipsapirone, as well as the prototypical 5-HT$_{1A}$ agonist, 8-hydroxy-2-(di-n-propylamino)tetralin(8-OHDPAT), revealed potential antidepressant effects in such animals models as the forced swim test and other stress-induced behavioral deficit tests (71).

Buspirone and gepirone both had significantly greater effects than placebo in patients with major depression in a series of studies that included over a hundred patients, each studied under double-blind conditions (39). Melancholic patients improved to an equal extent as nonmelancholic patients, which was interpreted as evidence that the moderate overall degree of improvement was unlikely to represent only a reduction in anxiety symptoms associated with depression. A smaller study that compared ipsapirone and a placebo in neurotic depressed patients demonstrated significantly greater antidepressant effects for ipsapirone (35). However, the lack of additional, more recent major reports on antidepressant efficacy of the azapirones is of concern.

Studies of the preclinical neuropharmacology of buspirone and related azapirones went through several phases, because the initial focus of the investigations was on antianxiety models. Additionally, buspirone elicited dopamine system effects not found with gepirone or ipsapirone that were puzzling to interpret. It has since become increasingly clear that the activity of these agents in animal models of anxiety and depression fits best with their 5-HT$_{1A}$ partial agonist effects (89).

The predominant initial effect of these drugs in rodents is a slowing of the firing rate of dorsal raphe neurons and, to a considerably lesser extent, medial raphe neurons, a consequence of a direct full agonist effect of these agents on autoreceptor 5-HT$_{1A}$ sites located in the midbrain raphe areas (9). In addition, these drugs act as partial agonists at postsynaptic 5-HT$_{1A}$ sites in the hippocampus and other forebrain areas, although drug concentrations required are up to tenfold higher at these sites, and, among both the azapirones and some newer 5-HT$_{1A}$ agonists with different chemical structures, partial agonist and antagonist properties differ (9,74). With sustained administration

for 10 days or more, some desensitization of the raphe response occurs when measured electrophysiologically (9). However, microdialysis studies indicate sustained reductions in hippocampal 5-HT release during chronic treatment (74). Lesion studies have suggested that the actions of these drugs in animal models of anxiolytic drug effects fit best with a primarily presynaptic mode of action. In contrast, the action of these drugs in animal antidepressant models is blocked by 5-HT$_{1A}$ antagonists but is essentially unaffected by lesions or by drugs that decrease presynaptic function such as the tryptophan hydroxylase inhibitor, p-chlorophenylalanine, which suggests that postsynaptic 5-HT$_{1A}$ partial agonist effects are more important for their antidepressant effects (8,51,71). An additional mechanism that might contribute is the metabolism of the azapirones to 1-(2-pyramidal)-piperazine (1-PP), which achieves brain concentrations tenfold higher than the parent component (13); 1-PP is an α_2-adrenergic antagonist, a drug class that has been hypothesized to have antidepressant properties (see below). In one clinical study, 1-PP plasma levels were significantly correlated with improvement in depressive symptoms in patients treated with buspirone (79).

5-HT$_{2A}$/5-HT$_{2C}$ Antagonists as Antidepressants

The moderate efficacy of the selective 5-HT$_{2A}$/5-HT$_{2C}$ antagonist ritanserin in several double-blind controlled trials in depressed, dysthymic, and anxiety disorder patients suggested the possibility of a different profile of therapeutic action than that found with earlier, less serotonin receptor subtype-selective 5-HT$_{1/2}$ antagonists such as methysergide, cyproheptidine, or metergoline. Only one study using ritanserin was placebo controlled; in others, ritanserin's effects equaled those of amitriptyline or flupenthixol, and were superior to trazodone (3). Another related agent, nefazodone, like trazodone, has prominent 5-HT$_{2A}$ and probably 5-HT$_{2C}$ antagonist effects; these effects may contribute more to the clinical effects of nefazodone and trazodone than the relatively weak uptake inhibitory effects of these agents on 5-HT (both) or 5-HT and norepinephrine (nefazodone) (26,37). Of note, mianserin, an earlier antidepressant in wide use in Europe and other regions, but not available in the United States, also has prominent 5-HT$_{2A,2C}$ antagonist properties (12,37).

Serotonin Transport Modulators Including Tianeptine

The recently available SSRIs are more selective than the tricyclics and other earlier antidepressants in their lack of effects at cholinergic, adrenergic and other neurotransmitter receptors, which improves their side-effect profile and reduces the risk of overdosage. Other SSRIs, such as citalopram, fluvoxamine, and Ro-15-8081 are also under development, along with some novel compounds that combine serotonin uptake-inhibiting actions with 5-HT$_{1A}$

agonist effects (LY 233708) or 5-HT$_3$ antagonist effects (litoxetine) (69). With advancing knowledge of serotonin receptors, it is of note that (−)-norfluoxetine, an active fluoxetine metabolite with a longer half-life than the parent compound, has only slightly lower affinity for the 5-HT$_{2C}$ receptor than for the 5-HT transporter in rat brain (87). Other examples of more complicated molecular interactions are the newly discovered 5-HT$_6$ and 5-HT$_7$ receptors, which have very high affinities for a number of tricyclic and other psychotropic drugs, including clomipramine, amitriptyline, ritanserin, mianserin, and clozapine, suggesting additional sites of action for these drugs (50,57).

Another interesting focus has been on drugs with combined 5-HT and norepinephrine uptake-inhibiting effects, but lacking tricycliclike interactions with neurotransmitter receptors, a therapeutic strategy that reflects recent evidence that 5-HT selective and norepinephrine selective uptake inhibitors act through separate serotonergic or noradrenergic mechanisms to yield equivalent antidepressant effects (55); the dual action uptake inhibitors might affect patient subgroups insensitive to 5-HT or norepinephrine changes alone. Venlafaxine and duloxetine (formerly LY 248686) are two examples of such agents; a substantial number of controlled clinical trials have demonstrated definite antidepressant efficacy for venlafaxine, which has a side-effect profile similar to that of the SSRIs (36,86).

A novel 5-HT uptake modulatory agent is tianeptine, which appears to enhance 5-HT uptake in vivo—in contrast to the 5-HT uptake-inhibiting action of the SSRIs and earlier tricyclics. Only limited clinical data is available for tianeptine. One double-blind study in 265 patients with dysthymic disorder and anxiety found tianeptine to be equipotent with amitriptyline (32). A similar result was found for tianeptine and amitriptyline in depressed alcoholics (49). In general, tianeptine appears to be well tolerated, with no anticholinergic or cardiovascular effects. Adverse effects leading to treatment discontinuation in these clinical trials included insomnia, anxiety, irritability, dizziness, nausea, and vomiting.

In a number of animal models sensitive to antidepressant drugs, tianeptine's profile was indicative of antidepressant activity: Tianeptine decreased aggressive behavior in the isolated mouse, decreased reserpine-induced ptosis and hypothermia, suppressed behavioral despair in the forced swim test, and also blocked pontogeniculooccipital waves induced by Ro 4-1284 in the cat (44). Tianeptine also antagonized deficits in open-field activity after a two-hour restraint, as well as deficits induced by immobilization stress; it also was active in the learned-helplessness paradigm (21,78).

Tianeptine is an atypical tricyclic molecule with a substituted dibenzothiadiazepine nucleus containing two heteroatoms, and a long amino-heptanoic chain with a terminal acidic group. It is similar in structure to the older antidepressant, amineptine (discussed below) (44). Enhanced 5-HT uptake was first reported in brain synapto-

somes from rats treated either acutely or chronically with tianeptine; it did not result from a reduction in 5-HT release, and was not found upon in vitro addition of the drug to synaptosomal preparations. In some studies, tianeptine led to an enhanced depletion of 5-HT, increased brain 5-hydroxyindoleacetic acid brain (5-HIAA) concentrations, and an attenuation of the potassium-induced rise in hippocampal extracellular 5-HT (44).

In an electrophysiological study that examined the effect of both tianeptine and clomipramine on the 5-HT-induced reduction of firing rates of rat hippocampal CA1 pyramidal cells, tianeptine accelerated the recovery of firing rates after 5-HT iontophoresis, in contrast to the delay in recovery found after clomipramine—a result consistent with tianeptine reducing intrasynaptic 5-HT concentrations (25). A similar study demonstrated a reduction in the time required for recovery of neuronal firing activity following microiontophoretic application of 5-HT in rats treated chronically, but not acutely, with tianeptine. Further studies indicated that the enhancement of 5-HT uptake by chronic tianeptine did not appear to be from an adaptive alteration of the 5-HT transporter (65), a finding consistent with earlier studies which found that tianeptine did not affect ^{3}H-imipramine binding. Thus, the mechanism of this 5-HT uptake-enhancing action of tianeptine remains elusive.

Enhancement of 5-HT uptake by tianeptine also occurs in humans, as demonstrated by a study of platelet 5-HT uptake in depressed patients that found an increase in apparent V_{max} which persisted after chronic treatment (16). Tianeptine has no effect on either 5-HT receptors (5-HT$_{1A/1B/2}$) or β-adrenergic receptors. It reduced acetylcholine release, an effect apparently mediated by an action on serotonergic neurons (6). Tianeptine also increased concentrations of dopamine and its metabolites in rat striatum, nucleus accumbens, brainstem and cerebral cortex (38). There is some uncertainty as to whether these dopaminergic effects are primary effects of tianeptine or secondary to the serotonergic actions of this agent.

NOVEL DOPAMINERGIC ANTIDEPRESSANTS

Drugs that directly or indirectly facilitate dopamine function have often been used as either primary agents or adjuncts in the treatment of depression, especially for patients not responding to standard noradrenergic or serotonergic uptake inhibitors. Such compounds have included the psychostimulants amphetamine and methylphenidate, the antiparkinsonian bromocriptine, the MAO inhibitors, and, while it was available, the dopamine uptake inhibitor, nomifensine. Nomifensine gained a reputation for being particularly effective in treatment-resistant patients with chronic depression. Preclinical investigations have demonstrated that most antidepressants, whatever their other actions, affect dopamine function. Facilitation of dopamine function is striking after repeated electroconvulsive therapy. Whether antidepressant effects on dopamine are primary or secondary (e.g., to primary facilitation of 5-HT, see above) is unknown (for reviews see refs. 67 and 73). Nonetheless, it has been hypothesized that some depressed patients require compounds with more potent and direct dopaminergic effects to achieve a therapeutic outcome.

Novel Drugs Affecting Dopamine Uptake and Release, Including Amineptine

Amineptine was originally marketed as an antidepressant in France and is now available in some other European, African, and South American countries. In 11 controlled studies, amineptine has generally been found to be of equivalent therapeutic efficacy to established antidepressants, although only two of these studies exceeded 50 patients per treatment group, many used relatively low doses of standard drugs, and the only study that included a placebo group was of depressed inpatients with psychomotor retardation, who showed greater improvement with amineptine compared to placebo, clomipramine, or minaprine (68). This result may be pertinent to the fact that amineptine has stimulant effects and associated abuse potential.

Amineptine is an atypical tricyclic, differing from the typical compounds in its 7-aminoheptanoic acid side chain. In animal screening models, amineptine antagonized reserpine-induced ptosis and hypothermia, decreased immobility in a behavioral despair test, and ameliorated impaired social behavior in monkeys; it also antagonized apomorphine-induced hypothermia and behavioral responses and had direct locomotor stimulatory effects in mice (14,30). Amineptine selectively inhibited the uptake of dopamine into rat striatal synaptosomes, and, at higher concentrations, also caused a release of dopamine, norepinephrine, and serotonin. A microdialysis study found dose-dependent elevations of dopamine in the striatum, nucleus accumbens, and frontal cortex, without changes in dopamine metabolites (38). Chronic administration of amineptine reduced the number of striatal dopamine binding sites (14).

Among other dopamine uptake inhibitors, medifoxamine is a monoamine reuptake inhibitor that preferentially inhibits dopamine uptake (70). Although in clinical use in France, there has been only one report of antidepressant efficacy (23), and there are few studies of its neurochemistry. GBR12909, GBR12783 and GBR13069 are piperazine compounds with potent, highly selective dopamine uptake blocking effects and locomotor stimulatory effects; GBR12909 is active in animal models for antidepressant drug effects, but apparently has not yet been evaluated in humans (2).

Dopamine Receptor Agonists and Antagonists

Several direct dopamine agonists were evaluated for antidepressant effects in the 1980s, including bromocrip-

tine and piribedil (40). The lack of recent studies may be because of both a high incidence of adverse effects and a rapid loss of efficacy with continued administration. A recent animal study found no effect of bromocriptine in the forced swim test (60). Lisuride is a centrally acting dopamine and serotonin agonist of the ergot type, which is marketed in Europe as an antidepressant (81). Animal screening studies indicate that lisuride may have clinical antidepressant properties. Unfortunately, there are no published controlled clinical studies to confirm its possible antidepressant activity. Lisuride also has very high affinity for the 5-HT$_6$ and 5-HT$_7$ receptor sites, which also exhibit high affinity for a number of other agents with antidepressant and antipsychotic efficacy (57). Roxindole is a potent dopamine autoreceptor agonist, which also inhibits 5-HT uptake and has 5-HT$_{1A}$ agonistic actions. It was originally developed for the treatment of schizophrenia and has been found to be particularly effective in the treatment of the negative features of schizophrenia. A recent open trial of roxindole in patients with major depression indicated that it may also possess antidepressant properties (31).

Somewhat paradoxically, certain drugs that block D$_2$ and/or D$_1$ receptors and are marketed as atypical antipsychotics, sulpiride (in Europe) and clozapine, are also reported to have antidepressant properties. Sulpiride has been reported to have equivalent antidepressant properties to amitriptyline in a double-blind comparison (76) and clozapine's combination of properties has been suggested to be particularly beneficial in schizoaffective disorder. Antidepressant properties of clozapine could be related either to its 5-HT$_2$ or α_2-adrenergic antagonistic properties, the latter suggested by the finding that in a controlled study the addition of the α_2-antagonist idazoxan (see below) to a standard neuroleptic produced improvement similar to that seen with clozapine in refractory schizophrenic patients (48). No controlled trials, however, of clozapine in any form of depression, even psychotic depression, have yet been reported.

NOVEL NORADRENERGIC ANTIDEPRESSANTS

Classification of putative antidepressants as primarily noradrenergic agents rests on preclinical demonstrations of selective norepinephrine (NE) uptake inhibition, α_2-adrenergic antagonism, and/or agonistic effects at α_1- or β-adrenergic receptors. It is noteworthy that, to date, among drugs with these actions, only NE uptake inhibition has been consistently associated with antidepressant responses in double-blind, placebo-controlled trials. Perhaps because alterations of noradrenergic function are so often found in depressed patients and often follow chronic treatment with any type of antidepressant, the search for drugs selectively facilitating NE throughput continues.

α_2-Adrenergic Antagonists

For many years, it has been hypothesized that inhibitors of α_2 receptors would functionally have a sufficient effect on central nervous system (CNS) α_2-adrenergic autoreceptors to increase intrasynaptic NE and therefore reproduce the consequences of NE reuptake-inhibiting antidepressants (64). The clinical efficacy of mianserin, which has some α_2-blocking properties in the absence of other effects on NE sites, has been invoked as supporting this notion (24), although it is now appreciated that mianserin more potently antagonizes 5-HT$_{2A}$ and 5-HT$_{2C}$ receptors (see above).

Preclinical studies showing that the addition of an α_2 antagonist to a tricyclic accelerated the rate of β-adrenergic receptor down-regulation in rat cortex led to a trial in which yohimbine, the most selective α_2 antagonist available for clinical use at the time, was added in patients who had failed to respond to monotherapy with desipramine. In this group, the addition of yohimbine did not produce significant improvement (17).

More recently, both the imidazoline, idazoxan, and the benzodioxinopyrrole, fluparoxan, which show favorable α_2/α_1 potency ratios have been available for clinical studies (34). Although controlled trials of both are said to have been carried out in several hundred depressed patients, no reports have emerged. Thus, it is uncertain whether monotherapy with selective α_2 antagonists is effective in unipolar depression. A preliminary report suggests that idazoxan may be an antidepressant in bipolar depression alone or in combination with lithium (Osman O. T., et al., *personal communication*). Furthermore, it is possible that the compounds available to date do not show the effects that would be achieved with a truly selective, full α_2 antagonist without partial agonist activity and without the binding at imidazoline sites shown by idazoxan. A Belgium compound, R47,243, may be such a potent full antagonist (20) but it does not appear to have been developed for clinical trials.

Other Novel Noradrenergic Antidepressants

Three selective NE uptake inhibitors have been recently reported, two of which are nontricyclics: tomoxetine, a benzenepropanamine; viloxazine, a morpholine; and the newer tricyclic, lofepramine. Since these do not involve a novel mechanism, they are not discussed further.

Modafanil is an interesting compound; it is structurally unrelated to any known antidepressant. It has been used in France for a number of indications including depression, although there have as yet been no published studies establishing clinical antidepressant efficacy. Most of the published investigations have examined its psychostimulant properties in humans and animals (10). It has been tentatively classified as an α_1-adrenergic agonist based on the ability of α_1 antagonists to block its behavioral activity in animals. Another French compound, adrafinil, is also classified as a central α_1 agonist and is said to be helpful for depression and other symptomatology in cognitively impaired subjects (22).

There continues to be an interest in indirect noradrenergic agonists, although salbutamol and clenbuterol, the latter almost exclusively a β_2 agonist, show at best mixed evidence of antidepressant efficacy (reviewed in ref. 67). Because those established antidepressants shown to down-regulate β-adrenergic receptors consistently reduce the β_1 subtype and clenbuterol reduces only β_2 receptors, there remains the possibility that a different type of β agonist without limiting peripheral effects would possess antidepressant potency. SR58611A may be such an agent and is being proposed for clinical studies based on its novel identity as a selective atypical β agonist (75).

OTHER MONOAMINERGIC AGENTS

Subtype-selective Inhibitors of Monoamine Oxidase

The first true antidepressants were nonselective, irreversible inhibitors of both MAO-A and MAO-B (e.g., phenelzine and tranylcypromine). The discoveries that antidepressant efficacy required only MAO-A and not MAO-B inhibition (47) and that the hazardous potentiation of pressor responses to dietary tyramine that accompanied MAO-A inhibition could be markedly attenuated by reversible inhibitors of MAO-A led to the current situation where there are at least ten new MAO-A inhibitors under development; unfortunately, none are yet available in the United States (15). A similar number of selective MAO-B inhibitors are also under development, primarily because neuroprotective and moderate treatment effects were reported for the MAO-B inhibitor selegiline (formerly named (−)deprenyl) in Parkinson's disease and dementia (15,59), although it is noteworthy that when given in higher non-MAO-B selective doses, selegiline is an effective antidepressant in treatment-resistant elderly depressed patients as well as younger patients (77).

Moclobemide is probably the most well-studied reversible, selective MAO-A–inhibiting antidepressant now available in Europe, Canada, and much of the world, except the United States. Efficacy has been demonstrated in multiple comparisons with placebo and conventional antidepressants of all types, including irreversible MAO inhibitors (27). A metaanalysis of over 2000 patients yielded evidence of equivalent efficacy for unipolar and bipolar patients, endogenous and nonendogenous, melancholic and nonmelancholic patients and younger and older patients. The drug is generally well tolerated with no anticholinergic or cardiovascular side effects; only nausea appeared more frequently as a side effect after moclobemide versus placebo treatment (27).

Dietary restrictions for moclobemide have been minimized to include only avoidance of very large servings of possibly tyramine-rich cheeses; the drug is taken after meals to lessen potential interactions with foods containing tyramine. Moclobemide is a weak MAO inhibitor in vitro, but apparently is rapidly and extensively biotransformed to a yet unknown predominantly MAO-A selective metabolite(s). Its effects on rapid-eye-movement sleep suppression and on catecholamine metabolite changes are somewhat less than those found with irreversible MAO-A selective inhibitors; as with earlier MAO-inhibitors, whether moclobemide's clinical effects result from delayed consequences of the enhanced synaptic availability of neurotransmitter amines like serotonin and norepinephrine or from adaptive responses at autoreceptors and other receptors and their signal transducing systems remains conjectural (15).

Another example of a reversible selective MAO-A inhibitor is brofaromine. Its MAO-A selectivity (100-fold) and relative reversibility over 48 hr depend upon in vivo kinetics, as brofaromine in vitro manifests only slight selectively for MAO-A versus MAO-B and only slowly dissociates from the enzyme (15,83). Brofaromine has a second property at higher doses—serotonin uptake inhibition in vitro and in vivo—which has been suggested to contribute to its clinical efficacy, because MAO-A inhibition becomes maximum at 50 mg/day doses, although clinical studies indicate increasing antidepressant efficacy with increasing doses up to at least 150 mg/day (83).

Minaprine

Minaprine is a nontricyclic compound that appears to enhance dopaminergic, serotonergic, and cholinergic transmission. Of the nine double-blind studies of minaprine published, eight compared minaprine with standard antidepressants and reported equivalent efficacy, although no study had 50 or more subjects per treatment group and doses of the comparison agents were often low. The single placebo-controlled study is worthy of note, because it compared four doses of minaprine (100 to 400 mg/day) with placebo, and found a significant difference from placebo only at 400 mg/day, a finding of particular concern as the usual dose range employed in other studies was ≤300 mg/day (1). In general, minaprine was well tolerated. Animal studies indicated no potential for abuse despite its enhancement of dopamine function. There have been no clinical reports of stimulant effects or abuse, and the most common side effects are nausea, anxiety, and insomnia.

Minaprine, which is a 3-amino-6-phenylpyridazine derivative, has an atypical molecular structure. In animal models for antidepressant drugs, minaprine antagonized reserpine-induced ptosis in mice, decreased immobility in a behavioral despair test, and antagonized muricidal behavior in rats (7). Minaprine has been suggested to enhance dopaminergic, serotonergic, and cholinergic neurotransmission, although there are relatively few basic

pharmacological studies of this compound. Minaprine given to rats reduced striatal homovanillic acid (HVA) and dihydroxyphenylacetic acid (DOPAC) concentrations, while concomitantly increasing levels of 3-methoxytyramine in a dose-dependent fashion; such findings are consistent with increased dopaminergic transmission, although the mechanism of this enhancement is unclear. A weak reversible inhibition of MAO-A might best explain these neurochemical changes (41). Minaprine has no effect on dopamine release or uptake; it also has no affinity for dopamine D_1 or D_2 receptors. Low doses of minaprine antagonized haloperidol-induced catalepsy, and higher doses induced stereotypic behavior in rats, consistent with enhancement of dopamine activity (7).

Additionally, minaprine has been shown to increase 5-HT and decrease 5-HIAA concentrations in rat cortex, striatum, brainstem, and hypothalamus (7). As with its dopaminergic actions, these effects would be consistent with MAO inhibition. Minaprine affected neither the release nor uptake of 5-HT. Similarly, it had no affinity for either $5-HT_1$ or $5-HT_2$ receptors. Minaprine also produced an increase in acetylcholine concentrations in rat striatal, hippocampal, and cortical regions (29). Minaprine displaced the M_1-muscarinic antagonist pirenzapine from cortical and hippocampal binding sites and antagonized intrastriatal pirenzapine-induced rotations in rats. These findings suggested the possibility that the cholinomimetic action of minaprine may be mediated by affinity for the M_1 receptor. However, other studies have suggested that the cholinomimetic action may be primarily mediated by effects on a serotonergic subsystem by $5-HT_{1B}$ or $5-HT_2$ receptors (11). Whatever the specific mechanism, minaprine has aroused interest as a potential agent for patients with cognitive impairment, particularly because there is some evidence that it may improve memory in animal models (88).

ADDITIONAL AGENTS WITH TRULY NOVEL BIOCHEMICAL ACTIONS

Phosphodiesterase Inhibitors and Inositol

Rolipram (a dialkoxyphenyl-2-pyrrolidone) is one of a series of isoenzyme-selective phosphodiesterase inhibitors that have been developed for the treatment of a broad range of medical disorders (33). It increases the availability of cyclic adenosine monophosphate (cAMP) by inhibiting cAMP phosphodiesterase and enhances the availability of NE by stimulating tyrosine hydroxylase and NE release. Despite marked optimism in the 1980s that this agent appeared to be a unique antidepressant, recent controlled trials have thrown considerable doubt upon the clinical efficacy of this compound. Although early controlled trials indicated clinical antidepressant efficacy, more recent studies have found rolipram to be less effective than either imipramine or amitriptyline (72). For example, in the latter study of 50 patients with DSM-III major depression, only 8% recovered with rolipram compared to 44% with amitriptyline. These two negative studies have clouded the future investigation of this compound as a potential antidepressant. Rolipram's action in animal screening models indicated its potential as a clinical antidepressant. It reversed the effects of reserpine on body temperature and locomotor activity and reduced muricidal behavior in olfactory bulbectomized rats (56,82). There is some uncertainty, however, about the mechanism of these effects. Because they were not prevented by depletion of monoamines or blockade of central β-adrenergic or dopamine receptors, rolipram appeared to be acting by a postreceptor mechanism (82). However, forskolin activation of adenyl cyclase did not replicate the behavioral effects of rolipram, suggesting that rolipram might not act by increasing cAMP (63).

Inositol is essential for the synthesis of phosphatidyl inositol, the precursor of the important second messenger for many neurotransmitter receptors, phosphatidyl inositol triphosphate. Although inositol crosses the blood–brain barrier with difficulty, large inositol doses (12 g) increased inositol concentrations in human cerebrospinal fluid (CSF) by 70% and led to improvement in depression ratings in an open trial (46). A recent double-blind controlled trial demonstrated improvement in depressed patients treated with 12 g/day inositol compared to placebo (46). Although inositol apparently has not been studied in any animal models sensitive to antidepressant drug effects, antidepressants from several classes increase cellular concentrations of inositol triphosphates.

Angiotensin-converting Enzyme Inhibitor

Captopril, one of the angiotensin-converting enzyme (ACE) inhibitors, has been reported to have mood elevating properties in some patients (19). This is consistent with the observation that animal screening models indicate putative antidepressant activity for this compound (54), although there has been one negative study (5). Formal clinical trials in depressed patients have not been reported.

Calcium Channel Modulators

Investigations of patients with bipolar disorder who demonstrated increased CSF calcium levels in the depressed phase have suggested a possible role for this cation in mood disorders, and a potential role of calcium channel modulators in their treatment. Most studies have focused on nifedipine. Animal studies indicate that nifedipine blocks immobility in behavioral despair tests, suggesting a potential for antidepressant action (42). The only clinical trial of nifedipine, however, found no antidepressant efficacy (43). This finding would appear to have been emphatically confirmed by other reports that nifedipine may, in fact, induce depression (52).

Glucocorticoid Antagonists

As elevated corticotropin-releasing hormone (CRH)/adrenocorticotropic hormone (ACTH)/cortisol activity is frequently associated with depression, consideration has been given to treatments that reduce glucocorticoid function. Positive open clinical trials have been reported for amino glutethamide, ketoconazole, and metapyrone in treatment-resistant depressed patients (58) and ketoconazole in hypercortisolemic depressed patients (85). Animal model studies using either normocortisolemic animals or the hypercortisolemic Fawn-hooded rat strain that manifests depressionlike behavior (4) have not yet been completed.

N-Methyl-D-aspartic Acid Receptor Partial Agonists and Antagonists

In two models for antidepressant drug effects, the forced swim test in mice and rats and tail suspension-induced immobility in mice, a noncompetitive N-methyl-D-aspartic acid (NMDA) antagonist, dizolcipine (MK-801) and a partial agonist at the glycine regulatory site of the NMDA receptor, 2-amino-7-phosphoheptanoic acid (AP-7), produced antidepressant-like effects (53,80). Although apparently no clinical antidepressant trial data with tolerated agents that have comparable effects on the NMDA receptor are available, these results have engendered considerable interest, as imipramine, AP-7, and 17 representatives of almost all major classes of antidepressant drugs given chronically, but not acutely, led to common, possibly adaptive changes in ligand binding at the cortex glycine binding receptor site of the NMDA receptor (61,62) and to associated changes in NMDA receptor mRNA (K.-P. Lesch, et al., *personal communication*).

CONCLUSIONS

In the present search for novel pharmacological approaches to the treatment of depression and allied disorders, we have taken a broad inclusive perspective of depression. Given that drugs principally classified as antidepressants are also effective in other disorders (e.g., obsessive–compulsive disorder, panic disorder, social phobia) and in some other neuropsychiatric patient populations, this strategy seemed justified. Thus, any compound that has shown some significant therapeutic benefit in any form of depression has been considered to be a possible candidate, as long as it also appeared biochemically distinct from currently available antidepressants. In many instances, considerable additional clinical-trials data in appropriate patient populations and subpopulations employing placebo groups will be needed to clearly establish efficacy. Regrettably, there exists at present an almost universal inverse relationship between novelty of action and convincing clinical evidence of efficacy for the new agents under development considered in this review. Nonetheless, there is some basis for cautious enthusiasm in the small hints from both clinical investigations and animal model studies that at least a few of the novel agents considered in this review may eventually contribute to our therapeutic armamentarium.

REFERENCES

1. Amsterdam JD, Dunner DL, Fabre LF, Kiev A, Rush AJ, Goodman LI. Double-blind, placebo-controlled, fixed dose trial of minaprine in patients with major depression. *Pharmacopsychiatry* 1989; 22:137–143.
2. Andersen PH. The dopamine uptake inhibitor GBR 12909: selectivity and molecular mechanism of action. *Eur J Pharmacol* 1989;166:493–504.
3. Anonymous. Ritanserin. *Drugs Fut* 1992;17:431–433.
4. Aulakh CS, Hill JL, Murphy DL. Attenuation of hypercortisolemia in Fawn-hooded rats by antidepressant drugs. *Eur J Pharmacol* 1993;240:85–88.
5. Baran L, Siwanowicz J, Nowak G, Przegalinski E. Captopril lacks the antidepressant-like activity in animal models. *Pol J Pharmacol Pharm* 1991;43:265–270.
6. Bertorelli R, Amoroso D, Girotti P, Consolo S. Effect of tianeptine on the central cholinergic system: involvement of serotonin. *Naunyn Schmiedebergs Arch Pharmacol* 1992;345:276–281.
7. Biziere K, Worms P, Kan JP, Mandel P, Garattini S, Roncucci R. Minaprine, a new drug with antidepressant properties. *Drugs Exp Clin Res* 1985;11:831–840.
8. Blier P, de Montigny C. Differential effect of gepirone on presynaptic and postsynaptic serotonin receptors: single-cell recording studies. *J Clin Psychopharmacol* 1990;10:13S–20S.
9. Blier P, Serrano A, Scatton B. Differential responsiveness of the rat dorsal and median raphe 5-HT systems to 5-HT$_1$ receptor agonists and p-chloroamphetamine. *Synapse* 1990;5:120–133.
10. Boivin DB, Montplaisir J, Petit D, Lambert C, Lubin S. Effects of modafinil on symptomatology of human narcolepsy. *Clin Neuropharmacol* 1993;16:46–53.
11. Bolanos F, Fillion G. Minaprine antagonizes the serotonergic inhibitory effect of trifluoromethylphenylpiperazine (TFMPP) on acetylcholine release. *Eur J Pharmacol* 1989;168:87–92.
12. Brogden RM, Heel RC, Speight TM, Avery GS. Mianserin: a review of its pharmacologic properties and therapeutic efficacy in patients with depressive illness. *Drugs* 1978;16:273–301.
13. Caccia S, Conti I, Vigano G, Garattini S. 1-(2-Pyrimidinyl)-piperazine an active metabolite of buspirone in man and rat. *Pharmacology* 1986;33:46–51.
14. Ceci A, Garattini S, Gobbi M, Mennini T. Effect of long term amineptine treatment on pre- and postsynaptic mechanisms in rat brain. *Br J Pharmacol* 1986;88:269–275.
15. Cesura AM, Pletscher A. The new generation of monoamine oxidase inhibitors. *Prog Drug Res* 1992;38:171–297.
16. Chamba G, Lemoine P, Flachaire E, et al. Increased serotonin platelet uptake after tianeptine administration in depressed patients. *Biol Psychiatry* 1991;30:609–617.
17. Charney DS, Price LH, Heninger GR. Desipramine–yohimbine combination treatment for refractory depression. *Arch Gen Psychiatry* 1986;45:1155–1161.
18. Coccaro EF, Murphy DL. *Serotonin in major psychiatric disorders.* Washington, DC: American Psychiatric Press; 1990:255–258.
19. Cohen BM, Zubenko GS. Captopril in the treatment of recurrent major depression. *J Clin Psychopharmacol* 1988;8:143–144.
20. Colpaert FC, Raymaekers L. In vivo pharmacological activity of R 47 243 in rat: a comparison with putative α_2-adrenoceptor antagonists. *Drug Dev Res* 1986;8:361–371.
21. Curzon G, Kennett GA, Sarna GS, Whitton PS. The effects of

22. tianeptine and other antidepressants on a rat model of depression. *Br J Psychiatry* 1992;15:51–55.
22. Defrance D, Raharison S, Herve MA, Fondarai J, Betrancourt JC, Lubin S. Malades ages institutionnalises et Olmifon® (adrfinil$^{(1)}$: Determination d'un profil de "respondeurs" a loccasion d'un "effet centre" lors d'un essai controle versus placebo. *Acta Med Int—Psychiatrie* 1991;8:1815–1823.
23. Delaunay J, Meynard J, Elie JC. Medifoxamine 50, an antidepressant drug without atropine-like side effects. *Ann Med Psychol* 1982;140:148–156.
24. Dickinson SL. Alpha$_2$-adrenoceptor antagonism and depression. *Drug News Perspect* 1990;4:197–203.
25. Dresse A, Scuvee-Moreau J. Electrophysiological effects of tianeptine on rat locus coeruleus, raphe dorsalis, and hippocampus activity. *Clin Neuropharmacol* 1988;11:S51–58.
26. Eison AS, Eison MS, Torrente JR, Wright RN, Yocca FD. Nefazodone: preclinical pharmacology of a new antidepressant. *Psychopharmacol Bull* 1990;26:311–315.
27. Fitton A, Faulds D, Goa KL. Moclobemide: a review of its pharmacological properties and therapeutic use in depressive illness. *Drugs* 1992;43:561–596.
28. Fuller RW. Basic advances in serotonin pharmacology. *J Clin Psychiatry* 1992;53:36–45.
29. Garattini S, Forloni GL, Tirelli S, Ladinsky H, Consolo S. Neurochemical effects of minaprine, a novel psychotropic drug, on the central cholinergic system of the rat. *Psychopharmacology* 1984;82:210–214.
30. Garattini S, Mennini T. Pharmacology of amineptine: synthesis and updating. *Clin Neuropharmacol* 1989;12:S13–18.
31. Gruender G, Wetzel H, Hammes E, Benkert O. Roxindole, a dopamine autoreceptor agonist, in the treatment of major depression. *Psychopharmacology* 1993;111:123–126.
32. Guelfi JD, Pichot P, Dreyfus JF. Efficacy of tianeptine in anxious-depressed patients: results of a controlled multicenter trial versus amitriptyline. *Neuropsychobiology* 1989;22:41–48.
33. Hall IP. Isoenzyme selective phosphodiesterase inhibitors: potential clinical uses. *Br J Clin Pharmacol* 1993;35:1–7.
34. Halliday CA, Jones BJ, Skingle M, Walsh DM, Wise H, Tyers MB. The pharmacology of fluparoxan: a selective α_2-adrenoceptor antagonist. *Br J Pharmacol* 1991;102:887–895.
35. Heller AH, Beneke M, Kuemmel B, Spencer D, Kurtz NM. Ipsapirone: evidence for efficacy in depression. *Drug Lit* 1990;26:219–222.
36. Hollister LE, Claghorn JL. New antidepressants. *Annu Rev Pharmacol Toxicol* 1993;32:165–177.
37. Hoyer D. 5-Hydroxytryptamine receptors and effector coupling mechanisms in peripheral tissues. In: Fozard JR, ed. *The peripheral actions of 5-hydroxytryptamine.* Oxford: Oxford University Press; 1990:72–99.
38. Invernizzi R, Pozzi L, Garattini S, Samanin R. Tianeptine increases the extracellular concentrations of dopamine in the nucleus accumbens by a serotonin-independent mechanism. *Neuropharmacology* 1992;31:221–227.
39. Jenkins SW, Robinson DS, Fabre LF, Andary JJ, Messina MD, Reisch LN. Gepirone in the treatment of depression. *J Clin Psychopharmacol* 1990;10:77S–85S.
40. Jimerson DC, Post RM. Psychomotor stimulants and dopamine agonists in depression. In: Post RM, Ballenger JD. eds. *Neurobiology of mood disorders. Frontiers of clinical neuroscience.* Baltimore: Williams and Wilkins; 1984:619–628.
41. Kan JP, Mouget-Goniot C, Worms P, Biziere K. Effect of the antidepressant minaprine on both forms of monoamine oxidase in the rat. *Biochem Pharmacol* 1986;35:973–978.
42. Kostowski W, Dyr W, Pucilowski O. Activity of diltiazem and nifedipine in some animal models of depression. *Pol J Pharmacol Pharm* 1990;42:121–127.
43. Kramer MS, Caputo K, De Johnson C, et al. Negative trial of nifedipine in depression. *Biol Psychiatry* 1988;24:958–959.
44. Labrid C, Mocaer E, Kamoun A. Neurochemical and pharmacological properties of tianeptine, a novel antidepressant. *Br J Psychiatry* 1992;160:56–60.
45. Lesch K-P, Aulakh CS, Wolozin BL, Murphy DL. Serotonin (5-HT) receptor, 5-HT transporter and G protein-effector expression: implications for depression. *Pharmacol Toxicol* 1992;71:49–60.
46. Levine J, Barak Y, Gonzalves M, Szor H, Elizur A. A double-blind

controlled trial of inositol treatment of depression. *Am J Psychiatry* [*in press*].

47. Lipper S, Murphy DL, Slater S, Buchsbaum MS. Comparative behavioral effects of clorgyline and pargyline in man: a preliminary evaluation. *Psychopharmacology* 1979;62:123–128.

48. Litman RE, Hong WW, Weissman EM, Su T-P, Potter WZ, Pickar D. Idazoxan, an α_2 antagonist, augments fluphenazine in schizophrenic patients: a pilot study. *J Clin Psychopharmacol* 1993;13: 264–267.

49. Loo H, Deniker P. Position of tianeptine among antidepressive chemotherapy's. *Clin Neuropharmacol* 1988;11:S97–102.

50. Lovenberg TW, Baron BM, de Lecea L, et al. A novel adenylyl cyclase-activating serotonin receptor (5-HT$_7$) implicated in the regulation of mammalian circadian rhythms. *Neuron* 1993;11:449–458.

51. Luscombe GP, Martin KF, Hutchins LJ, Grosen J, Heal DJ. Mediation of the antidepressant-like effect of 8-OH-DPAT in mice by postsynaptic 5-HT$_{1A}$ receptors. *Br J Pharmacol* 1993;108:669–677.

52. Lyndon RW, Johnson G, McKeough G. Nifedipine-induced depression. *Br J Psychiatry* 1991;159:447–448.

53. Maj J, Rogoz Z, Skusa G, Sowinska H. Effects of MK-801 and antidepressant drugs in the forced swimming test in rats. *Eur Neuropsychopharmacol* 1992;2:37–41.

54. Martin P, Massol J, Peuch AJ. Captopril as an antidepressant? Effects on the learned helplessness paradigm in rats. *Biol Psychiatry* 1990;27:968–974.

55. Miller HL, Delgado PL, Salomon RM, Licinio J, Barr LC, Charney DS. Acute tryptophan depletion: a method of studying antidepressant action. *J Clin Psychiatry* 1992;53:28–35.

56. Mizokawa T, Kimura K, Ikoma Y, et al. The effect of a selective phosphodiesterase inhibitor, rolipram, on muricide in olfactory bulbectomized rats. *Jap J Pharmacol* 1988;48:357–364.

57. Monsma FJ Jr, Shen Y, Ward RP, Hamblin MW, Sibley DR. Cloning and expression of a novel serotonin receptor with high affinity for tricyclic psychotropic drugs. *Mol Pharmacol* 1993;43:320–327.

58. Murphy BEP, Dhar V, Ghadirian AM, Chouinard G, Keller R. Response to steroid suppression in major depression resistant to antidepressant therapy. *J Clin Psychopharmacol* 1991;11:121–126.

59. Murphy DL, Sunderland T. MAOIs in the neurodegenerative disorders. In: Kennedy SH, eds. *Clinical advances in monoamine oxidase inhibitor therapies.* Washington, DC: American Psychiatric Press; 1993:293–305.

60. Nikulina EM, Skrinskaya JA, Popova NK. Role of genotype and dopamine receptors in behaviour of inbred mice in a forced swimming test. *Psychopharmacology* 1991;105:525–529.

61. Nowak G, Layer RT, Skolnick P, Paul IA. Adaptation of the *N*-methyl-D-aspartate receptor following chronic antidepressants. *J Neurochem* 1993;61:S51.

62. Nowak G, Trullas R, Layer RT, Skolnick P, Paul IA. Adaptive changes in the *N*-methyl-D-aspartate receptor complex after chronic treatment with imipramine and 1-aminocyclopropanecarboxylic acid. *J Pharmacol Exp Ther* 1993;265:1380–1386.

63. O'Donnell JM. Antidepressant-like effects of rolipram and other inhibitors of cyclic adenosine monophosphate phosphodiesterase on behaviour maintained by differential reinforcement of low response rate. *J Pharmacol Exp Ther* 1993;264:1168–1178.

64. Pinder RM. α_2-Adrenoceptor antagonists as antidepressants. *Drugs Fut* 1985;10:841–857.

65. Pineyro G, Blier P, Dennis T, de Montigny C. Effect of the tricyclic drug tianeptine on 5-HT reuptake: electrophysiological and biochemical studies in the rat brain. *Proceedings of the Canadian College of Neuropsychopharmacology 16th Annual Meeting.* 1993:T20.

66. Potter WZ, Rudorfer MV, Manji H. The pharmacologic treatment of depression. *Drug Ther* 1991;325:633–642.

67. Potter WZ, Rudorfer MV, Manji HK. Potential new pharmacotherapies for refractory depression. In: Hales RE, eds. *Psychiatry update: annual review.* Washington, DC: American Psychiatric Press; 1990:145–169.

68. Rampello L, Nicoletti G, Raffaele R. Dopaminergic hypothesis for

69. Robertson DW, Fuller RW. Progress in antidepressant drugs. *Annu Rep Med Chem* 1991;3:23–32.

70. Saleh S, Johnston A, Turner P. Absolute bioavailability and pharmacokinetics of medifoxamine in healthy humans. *Br J Clin Pharmacol* 1990;30:621–624.

71. Schreiber R, de Vry J. 5-HT$_{1A}$ receptor ligands in animal models of anxiety impulsivity and depression: multiple mechanisms of action? *Prog. NeuroPsychopharmacol Biol Psychiatry* 1993;17:87–104.

72. Scott AIF, Perini AF, Shering PA, Whalley F. In-patient major depression: is rolipram as effective as amitriptyline? *Eur J Clin Pharmacol* 1991;40:127–129.

73. Serra G, Collu M, D'Aquila PS, Gessa GL. Role of the mesolimbic dopamine system in the mechanism of action of antidepressants. *Pharmacol Toxicol* 1992;71:72–85.

74. Sharp T, McQuade R, Bramwell S, Hjorth S. Effect of acute and repeated administration of 5-HT$_{1A}$ receptor agonists on 5-HT release in rat brain in vivo. *Naunyn-Schmiedeberg's Arch Pharmacol* 1993;348:339–346.

75. Simiand J, Keane PE, Guitard J, et al. Antidepressant profile in rodents of SR 58611A, a new selective agonist for atypical beta-adrenoceptors. *Eur J Pharmacol* 1992;219:193–201.

76. Standish-Barry HM, Bouras N, Bridges PK, Watson JP. A randomized double blind group comparative study of sulpiride and amitriptyline in affective disorder. *Psychopharmacology (Berl)* 1983;81: 258–260.

77. Sunderland T, Cohen RM, Molchan S, et al. High dose selegiline in treatment-resistant older depressives. *Arch Gen Psychiatry* [*in press*].

78. Thiebot MH, Martin P, Puech AJ. Animal behavioral studies in the evaluation of antidepressant drugs. *Br J Psychiatry* 1992;15:44–50.

79. Tollefson GD, Lancaster SP, Montague-Clouse J. The association of buspirone and its metabolite 1-pyrimidinylpiperazine in the remission of comorbid anxiety with depressive features and alcohol dependency. *Psychopharmacol Bull* 1991;27:163–170.

80. Trullas R, Skolnick P. Functional antagonists at the NMDA receptor complex exhibit antidepressant actions. *Eur J Pharmacol* 1990; 185:1–10.

81. Vinar O, Klein DF, Potter WZ, Gause EM. A survey of psychotropic medications not available in the United States. *Neuropsychopharmacology* 1991;5:201–217.

82. Wachtel H, Schneider HH. Rolipram, a novel antidepressant drug, reverses the hypothermia and hypokinesia of monoamine-depleted mice by an action beyond postsynaptic monoamine receptors. *Neuropharmacology* 1986;25:1119–1126.

83. Waldmeier PC. Newer aspects of the reversible inhibitor of MAO-A and serotonin reuptake, brofaromine. *Prog NeuroPsychopharmacol Biol Psychiatry* 1993;17:183–198.

84. Willner P. Animal models of depression. In: Willner P, ed. *Behavioral models in psychopharmacology.* Cambridge: Cambridge University Press; 1991:91.

85. Wolkowitz OM, Reus VI, Manfredi F, Ingbar J, Brizendine L, Weingartner H. Ketoconazole administration in hypercortisolemic depression. *Am J Psychiatry* 1993;150:810–812.

86. Wong DT, Bymaster FP, Mayle DA, Reid LR, Krushinski JH, Robertson DW. LY248686, a new inhibitor of serotonin and norepinephrine uptake. *Neuropsychopharmacology* 1993;8:22–33.

87. Wong DT, Threlkeld PG, Robertson DW. Affinities of fluoxetine, its enantiomers, and other inhibitors of serotonin uptake for subtypes of serotonin receptors. *Neuropsychopharmacology* 1991;5:43–47.

88. Yamamoto T, Yatsugi S-I, Ohno M, Furuya Y, Kitajima I, Ueki S. Minaprine improves impairment of working memory induced by scopolamine and cerebral ischemia in rats. *Psychopharmacology* 1990;100:316–322.

89. Yocca FD. Neurochemistry and neurophysiology of buspirone and gepirone: interactions at presynaptic and postsynaptic 5-HT$_{1A}$ receptors. *J Clin Psychopharmacol* 1990;10:6S–12S.

retarded depression: a symptom profile for predicting therapeutical responses. *Acta Psychiatr Scand* 1991;84:552–554.

Psychopharmacology: The Fourth Generation of Progress, edited by Floyd E. Bloom and David J. Kupfer. Raven Press, Ltd., New York 1995.

CHAPTER 97

The Neurobiology of Treatment-Resistant Mood Disorders

Robert M. Post and Susan R. B. Weiss

In 1921, Kraepelin (30) not only differentiated manic–depressive illness from schizophrenia, but he crystallized the critical observations on the longitudinal development of the illness based on his systematic patient records and life-chart methodology. He described the pleomorphic aspects of its clinical presentation and the tremendous variability in its clinical course. At the same time, he abstracted the general principle that patients often undergo a pattern of cycle acceleration with longer intervals occurring between the first and second episodes than those occurring later in the illness. He also noted a progression from precipitated to autonomous episodes, such that psychosocial stresses (particularly loss or the threat of loss) appeared to be implicated in initial episodes but not in subsequent episodes, which occur more spontaneously, that is, without apparent external precipitating factors. It is against this backdrop of a potentially progressive and evolving illness that issues of treatment resistance should be considered.

In the ensuing decades, these initial clinical observations have been documented and redocumented in more formal clinical studies (46). In systematic studies examining the issue of cycle acceleration, the general pattern of decreasing duration of well intervals as a function of successive episodes has been supported in virtually every study (for reviews, see refs. 46 and 51). Many of these studies occurred in the prepsychopharmacological era or before systematic prophylactic treatments were utilized. Even in the current era of long-term treatments, if one examines patients with treatment-refractory illness a pattern of cycle acceleration is often apparent (51). The impact of psychopharmacological treatment on the course of illness is obviously a major confounding variable, par-

ticularly since some agents, such as the heterocyclic antidepressants, have been implicated in illness exacerbations, that is, either in the precipitation of manias or in cycle acceleration (70). Rouillon (62) has reviewed the controlled literature and suggests that in prospectively followed bipolar patients, the switch rate is approximately 25% on placebo (or with lithium and an antidepressant) but approximately 50% in bipolar patients treated with tricyclic antidepressants alone. In our National Institute of Mental Health (NIMH) cohort of treatment-refractory patients, we have observed a high incidence of switches during treatment with tricyclic antidepressants based on retrospective life-chart methodology. Approximately 35% of switches appear to be related to the antidepressant treatment and not typical of the patient's prior course of illness (2). Additionally, Wehr and Goodwin (70) have highlighted the earlier suggestions of Kukopulos and others that antidepressants might also be associated with increasing cycle acceleration and conversion from intermittent to continuous cycling patterns. Kukopulos et al. (32) have argued that this pharmacological impact is associated with lithium treatment resistance. In the study by Wehr and associates, the impact of tricyclics on cycle length was found to be a deceleration upon drug discontinuation, and reacceleration once antidepressant treatment was reinstituted. In our series, approximately 26% of patients showed cycle acceleration during treatment with antidepressants, with 35% of patients showing definite or likely patterns attributed to the antidepressant and not the course of illness (2). In each of the instances of cycle acceleration, antidepressant discontinuation confirmed the association because it slowed the cycles.

Patients who either begin their illness with a pattern of rapid cycling (four or more episodes in a given year) or who progressively evolve to this faster pattern also tend to be resistant to treatment with lithium (see ref. 47 for a review). It is of interest that many patients with initial

R. M. Post and S. R. B. Weiss: Biological Psychiatry Branch, National Institutes of Health, National Institute of Mental Health, Bethesda, Maryland 20892.

episodes of depression appear to go on to more rapid cycling forms of the illness and that the pattern of illness associated with biphasic episodes of depression, followed by mania, and then a well interval (D-M-I) is less responsive to lithium than the pattern of illness in patients who show an initial mania, followed by a depression, and then a well interval (M-D-I) (44). Recent data of Okuma and associates (40) also indicate that carbamazepine is less effective in patients with rapid cycling and the D-M-I pattern of illness.

It had previously been assumed that patients with 48-hr cycles represented the limit of cycle acceleration in manic-depressive illness. However, more recently, faster patterns of mood oscillation have been identified and are associated with relative treatment resistance (31). In these instances, patients not only show ultrarapid cycling, where episode durations are approximately one week or less, but ultra-ultra rapid (ultradian) cycling, where marked fluctuations in mood occur faster than once every 24 hrs. In these latter instances, mood fluctuations are distinct, dysrhythmic, or chaotic. George et al. (18) have modified the equations used by May and Gottschalk to model this chaotic pattern. In this model, systematic variation of a single constant can be associated with progressively more marked alterations in rhythmicity of the illness. This or related mathematical models may be of assistance in defining and classifying different phases of illness ranging from (a) isolated, intermittent episodes, to (b) more rapid, rhythmic, and continuous patterns, and, (c) to ultrafast frequencies associated with chaotic mood oscillations. These course-of-illness observations are of interest for several reasons. The chaotic patterns of mood oscillations often tend to occur late in the course of illness and may represent not only an evolving neural substrate but also one that tends to be lithium and, in many instances, carbamazepine-refractory (31). In some instances, combination treatment appears to be required to treat this phase of the illness, and, as noted below, preliminary observations suggest the potential utility of the calcium-channel blocker nimodipine in this phase of illness as well (42,49). Such a progression could represent either the increasing dysregulation of a single biochemical variable or a much more complex series of evolving biological processes, similar to those described in the evolution of behavioral sensitization and kindling. Sensitization and kindling are related in that they provide a conceptual framework for considering evolving processes that may be pertinent to treatment resistance.

COCAINE INDUCED BEHAVIORAL SENSITIZATION AND ITS CROSS-SENSITIZATION TO STRESS

Chronic cocaine administration is a pertinent model for consideration of refractory mood illness from three different perspectives. First, acute low-dose cocaine ad-

ministration produces an important model for the euphoric and psychomotor components of hypomania (55). However, with repeated administration, particularly involving higher doses, chronic cocaine administration also models the dysphoric and psychotic components of mania. As such, it represents a model for mania in evolution. Understanding the neurobiological mechanisms underlying the progressive increases in behavioral responsivity to the same dose of cocaine, which is the hallmark of behavioral sensitization, may thus provide a useful paradigm for elucidating progressive alterations in manic symptomatology and their differential response or lack of response to pharmacotherapeutic interventions.

Second, cocaine itself is an interesting model of a stressor, with many of its effects on neurotransmitters and peptide hormones mimicking the stress response, including increases in corticotropin-releasing hormone (CRH), adrenocorticotropic hormone (ACTH), and cortisol. In addition, behavioral sensitization to the psychomotor stimulants cocaine and amphetamine in many instances shows cross-sensitization to stress (4,27). That is, stimulant-induced behavioral sensitization results in increased reactivity to stress, and pretreatment of animals with acute or repeated stressors of appropriate frequencies, intensities, and modalities (such as tail pinch and mild foot shock) results in increased reactivity to psychomotor stimulant administration. Thus, consideration of the mechanisms underlying repeated cocaine administration may provide insights into those underlying long-term changes in responsivity to stressors as well as to maniclike syndromes of hyperactivity.

Third, there is a very high incidence of comorbidity in primary affective disorders, particularly bipolar illness with substance abuse disorders, where cocaine is often the substance abused (see the review in ref. 56). There is some evidence supporting the conclusion that substance abuse impacts negatively on treatment and provides one route to treatment resistance, perhaps through such mechanisms as increased incidence of noncompliance with therapeutic regimes, particularly lithium (48) and other agents, as highlighted in the studies of Aangaard and Vestergaard (1). Treatment resistance could also emerge because of lack of responsivity of patients with comorbid substance abuse to otherwise therapeutic regimes. For example, it has been widely reported that those patients with substance abuse are less responsive to lithium carbonate than those without such a variable (22). It is possible that neurobiological alterations accompanying chronic cocaine administration may interact with the primary pathophysiology of mood disorders in such a fashion that pharmacological responsivity is altered.

Our understanding of the mechanisms underlying cocaine-induced behavioral sensitization is, in itself, in the process of evolution; however, a preliminary blueprint of the critical processes involved is now available. The quality, magnitude, and duration of sensitization varies as a function of dose, frequency of repetition, intervals between drug administration, and a variety of other factors, including the environment (51,54,55,76). For example, in some paradigms, all of the behavioral sensitization appears attributable to conditioning variables; animals repeatedly pretreated and tested in the same environment show increased reactivity, whereas animals with equal exposures to cocaine but in different environments do not show sensitization (i.e., their behavior is like that of saline-pretreated controls). However, with higher doses of cocaine and more chronic administration, some components of behavioral sensitization can be demonstrated to be independent of the environmental context.

As such, dissection of the neurobiological mechanisms involved must necessarily distinguish between these two components of behavioral sensitization—conditioned and unconditioned. For example, in a 1-day cocaine sensitization paradigm with a low-dose challenge on the second day, Fontana and associates (15) found evidence of increased dopamine overflow in the nucleus accumbens measured by in vivo dialysis in animals pretreated with cocaine in the context of the test cage but not in those pretreated in a different environment or in controls treated with saline. Following repeated cocaine challenge paradigms, Brown et al. (10) failed to see significant evidence of conditioned sensitization when a saline challenge was utilized, however. This difference may have been attributable to either the difference in the pretreatment regimen, the greater pharmacological or interoceptive cueing associated with a cocaine compared to a saline challenge, and/or the presence of cocaine as a dopamine reuptake blocker in the test dialysate. Kalivas and Duffy (25,26) and Kalivas and Stewart (27) have elucidated a time course of unconditioned increases in dopamine overflow in terminal field areas (nucleus accumbens) or in dendritic autoreceptor fields (ventral tegmental area) following repeated cocaine administration compared with saline in an unconditioned paradigm as well. In these and other studies, behavioral sensitization to cocaine outlasted the regional alterations in dopamine overflow, suggesting that other mechanisms, over time, subserved behavioral sensitization. In this regard, White et al. (78) reported an increased responsivity of dopamine D_1 receptors in the accumbens, as revealed by direct iontophoretic application studies. These effects were longer lasting but, in some instances, behavioral sensitization can last for months, exceeding the period of time of increased dopamine receptor responsivity.

Cocaine has been reported to increase the immediate early gene (IEG) transcription factors c-*fos* (and *zif*-268) through a D_1 receptor mechanism (20,36,81). These substances acting through leucine zipper and zinc finger motifs, respectively, are thought to alter subsequent transcription of late effector genes and regulate levels of peptides, receptors, and enzymes. For example, chronic cocaine administration is associated with increases in dynorphin, substance P, and neurotensin, as well as decreases in neuropeptide Y (NPY), somatostatin, and, in some areas of brain, thyrotropin-releasing hormone (TRH) (56). Receptor binding is increased for μ-opiate and central- and peripheral-type benzodiazepine receptors and decreased for quinuclidinyl benzylate (QNB) and corticotropin-releasing factor (CRF) receptor binding. Although none of these neuropeptide or receptor changes has been specifically linked to alterations in immediate early gene regulation, it is thought that induction of c-fos and fos-related antigens (FRAS), zif-268, and a variety of other transcription factors and their interactions, initiate a sequence for transcription of these late effector adaptations that could help convey the altered neurobiochemical and behavioral responsivity to cocaine in a long-lasting fashion. Thus, prior experience with cocaine changes the brain not only in a short-term fashion at the level of neurotransmitters and receptors and their nongenomic adaptations, but also in a much more long-lasting fashion through alterations in genomic expression, which may affect not only biochemistry but neural structure in much longer-lasting temporal domains. Evolving processes in different neural systems may similarly occur with the experience of repeated stressors and episodes of mood illness; that is, stress and episode sensitization could ultimately affect treatment response.

KINDLING AS A MODEL FOR ILLNESS EVOLUTION AND TRANSITION TO AUTONOMY

In contrast to the behavioral sensitization described above, which directly models many aspects of mood illness (particularly euphoric and dysphoric manias), kindling is a nonhomologous model for mood illness evolution. Increased behavioral reactivity is measured with a seizure endpoint and none of the behaviors in kindling evolution are similar to those observed in patients with bipolar illness. Thus, although we might consider how various aspects of bipolar illness undergo kindlinglike transitions, it must be restated that kindling is only a conceptual bridge that might help describe the kinds of neurobiological processes and their spatial and temporal evolution in the brain that could be associated with the progression of a disorder.

Given these caveats, which violate most of the traditional principles of animal modeling of mood disorders, why discuss kindling as a potentially useful model in this context at all? In kindling, there is (a) increased behavioral responsivity to the same stimulation over time and (b) a progression to spontaneity following sufficient numbers of triggered kindled seizures. These syndrome characteristics are paralleled in vastly different time domains in some patients with mood disorders. We can then ask whether any of the neurobiological principles underlying kindling evolution at the level of gene expression and neuronal microstructure uncovered in seizure kindling provide a conceptual framework for making predictions about illness evolution and pharmacological responsivity in mood disorders. Finally, seizures are easily observable and measurable, thus making the quantification of kindling evolution relatively precise. Given the fact that there are few well-accepted or validated models for mood disorders that are easy to induce, reliably manifest, and long-lasting in terms of their memory characteristics, kindled seizure evolution and its robustness offers certain practical and logistical advantages.

In kindling, repeated and necessarily intermittent stimulation of the brain eventually results in a lowering of the threshold for afterdischarges (enhanced excitability); increases in the duration, spread, and complexity of the afterdischarges (the development phase); and finally, the reliable appearance of full-blown seizures in response to the previously subthreshold stimulation (completed phase of kindling) (19,57). In arriving at this completed phase of kindling, animals go through successive behavioral seizure-stage transitions from immobility and behavioral arrest (stage 1) to head nodding (stage 2), unilateral forepaw twitching (stage 3), and, finally, full-blown bilateral tonic/clonic seizures involving head, trunk, and forepaws (stage 4) with rearing and falling (stage 5). Following sufficient numbers of seizures (for example, several hundred kindled from the amygdala with once-a-day stimulation for one second at 200 to 800 μA), animals may be observed to undergo spontaneous seizures without any exogenous electrophysiological triggering.

Similar to what is observed in behavioral sensitization, it is now apparent that kindling induces an intricate cascade of neurobiological events at the level of gene expression that help code for the spatiotemporal evolution of neurobiological changes that accompany and may underlie kindling. For example, Clark et al. (12) have mapped the spread of the kindled seizure or memory trace during the developmental stages of kindling utilizing radiolabeled c-fos as the marker of what cellular pathways are being activated. This technique of in situ hybridization allows one to assess what cells are turning on their messenger ribonucleic acid (mRNA) for a transcription factor such as c-fos following activation or depolarization (Fig. 1). These effects at the level of the nucleus are similar to those observed while mapping metabolic pathways with deoxyglucose, although in the latter instance, it is the terminal areas of the neuron that are thought to be involved. With this in situ hybridization technique, Clark and associates have observed that initial phases of amygdala kindling are associated with unilateral activation of either the piriform cortex or the dentate gyrus of the hippocampus. With successive brain stimulations and seizure stage evolution, the piriform cortex and dentate gyrus become activated bilaterally. With completion of full-blown kindled seizures, there is increasingly widespread cortical involvement. Thus, in situ hybridization mapping of c-fos mRNA demonstrates the progressively more widespread activation of neural pathways associated with the evolution and development of amygdala kindling.

Most recently, Clark et al. (unpublished observation) have observed that a spontaneous kindled seizure induced unilateral c-fos activation in the dentate gyrus on the side opposite to that originally kindled, further suggesting that as the seizure process evolves, so does its neuroanatomy, in this case, to the contralateral side of the brain.

Alterations in IEGs appear to be only the initial phase of impact on gene expression, as c-fos and FRAS are rapidly induced, returning to baseline over a period of minutes to hours. Their transient induction, as noted above, may be associated with longer-lasting events and transcription of late effector genes (Fig. 2). For example, Rosen and associates (61) have found that following c-fos induction, the mRNA for TRH is induced in similar areas of brain (piriform cortex and dentate gyrus) first unilaterally and then bilaterally, and it remains elevated for longer durations of time (hours to days) than c-fos. Rosen et al. (60) have also found that c-fos and TRH coexist in the same cells, further suggesting the likelihood that the two events may be related. In addition, the gene for TRH has an AP-1-like binding site at which fos and FRAS may affect transcription of this neuropeptide. In different cells in the dentate hilar region of the hippocampus, kindling is associated with induction of the mRNA for CRH in cells that previously did not manifest CRH (67). Thus, kindling is associated with the activation of presumably novel neuropeptide synthesis in cells that ordinarily did not express this substance. This finding is of potential interest not only in its own right, in relationship to kindling, but as it might relate to the repeated observations of neuropeptide receptor mismatches in the central nervous system (CNS) where peptide receptors often appear to exist in areas of brain not associated with the neuropeptide itself (21). It is possible that these receptors are there to receive neuropeptides that some day may be turned on in a cellular program related to a variety of neural functions induced by the environment.

As with TRH or CRH, a variety of alterations in enzymes, receptors, and protein kinases have been reported to be altered during kindling in a subacute to long-lasting fashion (Fig. 2). These are not detailed further other than to indicate that a multitude of adaptations may occur in different spatiotemporal sequences and the IEG c-fos induction and some of its associated neuropeptide correlates may be only two examples in that vastly more complicated process. In this regard, it is important to emphasize that not only are neurobiological alterations induced in kindling but micro- and macroneuroanatomical changes occur as well. For example, Geinisman et al. (16) have observed alterations in synapse formation in pathways thought to be intimately involved in kindling evolution and Sutula et al. (69) have demonstrated neuronal sprouting in the dentate granule cells of the hippocampus. Sutula and his group have also demonstrated that some cells in the dentate and hilar areas are dying in a fashion that is in proportion to the number of kindled seizures.

Thus, an active process of synaptic and neural remodel-

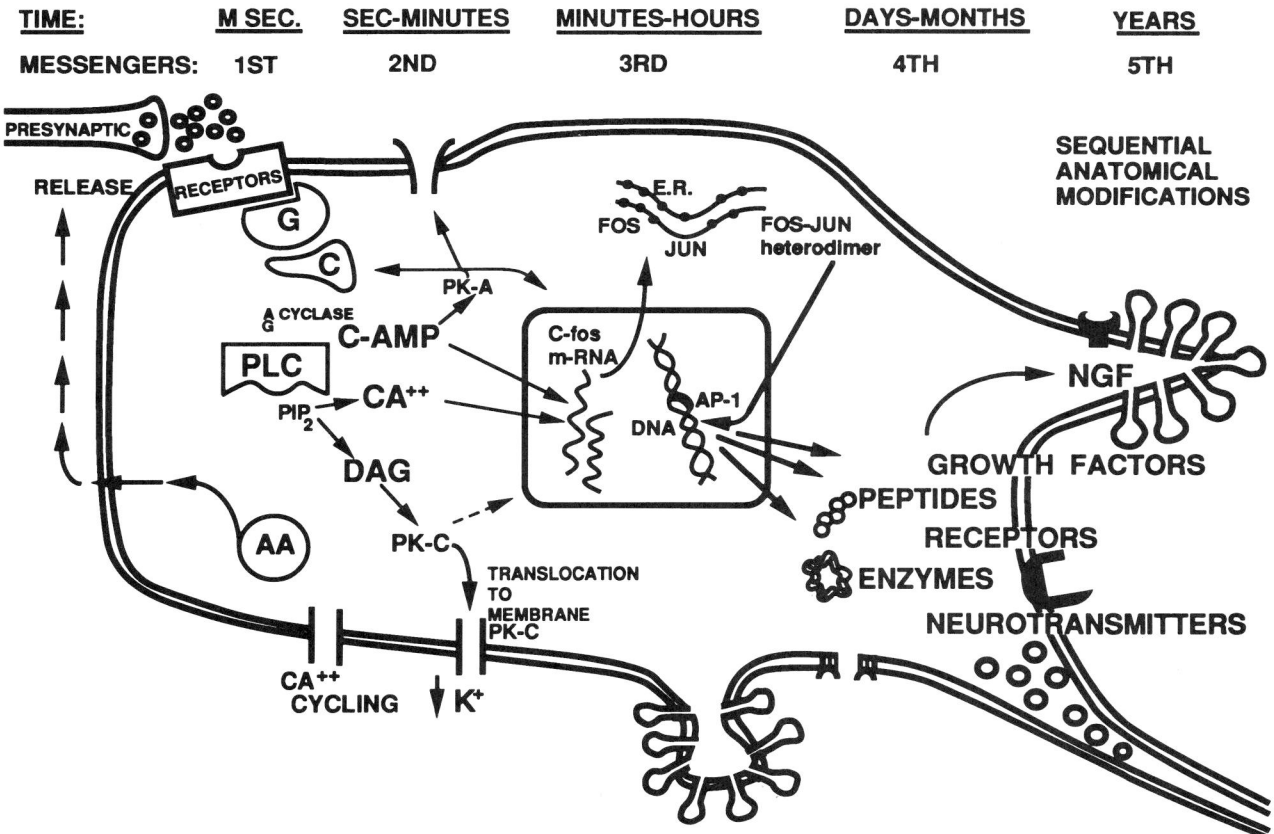

FIG. 1. The schematic illustrates how transient synaptic events induced by external stimuli can exert longer-lasting effects on neuronal excitability and the microstructure of the brain via a cascade of effects involving alterations in gene transcription. Neurotransmitters activate receptors and second messenger systems, which then induce immediate early genes (IEGs) such as c-*fos* and c-*jun*. Fos and Jun proteins are synthesized on the endoplasmic reticulum and then bind to DNA to further alter transcription of late effector genes (LEGs) and other regulatory factors, the effects of which could last for months or years.

ing may occur during kindling evolution and may account for some of the permanent alterations in neural and behavioral excitability that accompany kindling evolution. Because kindling is associated with the induction of nerve growth factors as well as neuropeptides which may exert tropic effects, there is a potential link between the intermediate neuropeptide inductions and the longer-lasting if not permanent alterations in synaptic microstructure and neuronal macrostructure and circuitry (Fig. 1). Although the process of preprogrammed cell death or apoptosis (35) is not definitively documented in the process of kindling, it is likely that cell death occurs by this process rather than by more classic toxic or degenerative forms of cell death, which are associated with obvious lesions, scarring, and glial proliferation. In the process of apoptosis, it is generally thought that a cell engages active cellular machinery, requiring ongoing protein synthesis, to activate an inherent cell death program and commit suicide. It is likely that there is a continuum of processes involved in cell death from those occurring in the absence of appropriate trophic factors to those occurring by more traditional excitotoxic processes. Similar processes of sculpt-

ing the CNS are thought to underlie not only critical stages of neural embryogenesis, but also the formation of the basic wiring diagram of the brain during development. The kindling data raise the possibility that related phases of neuroplasticity, synaptic reorganization, and neuronal tract sculpting could be occurring throughout adult life in relationship to processes of adaptation in response to environmental impact. Similar processes underlying memory-like events may be revealed by the kindling paradigm, which has been considered as a model of neuronal learning and memory (3).

STRESS AND EPISODE SENSITIZATION IN THE RECURRENT MOOD DISORDERS

Utilizing the principles derived from the sensitization and kindling models discussed above, one is now in a position to formulate a template for how stressors and episodes of mood illness could impact on the long-term course of recurrent mood disorders. The postulate is that, as in sensitization and kindling, appropriate psychosocial

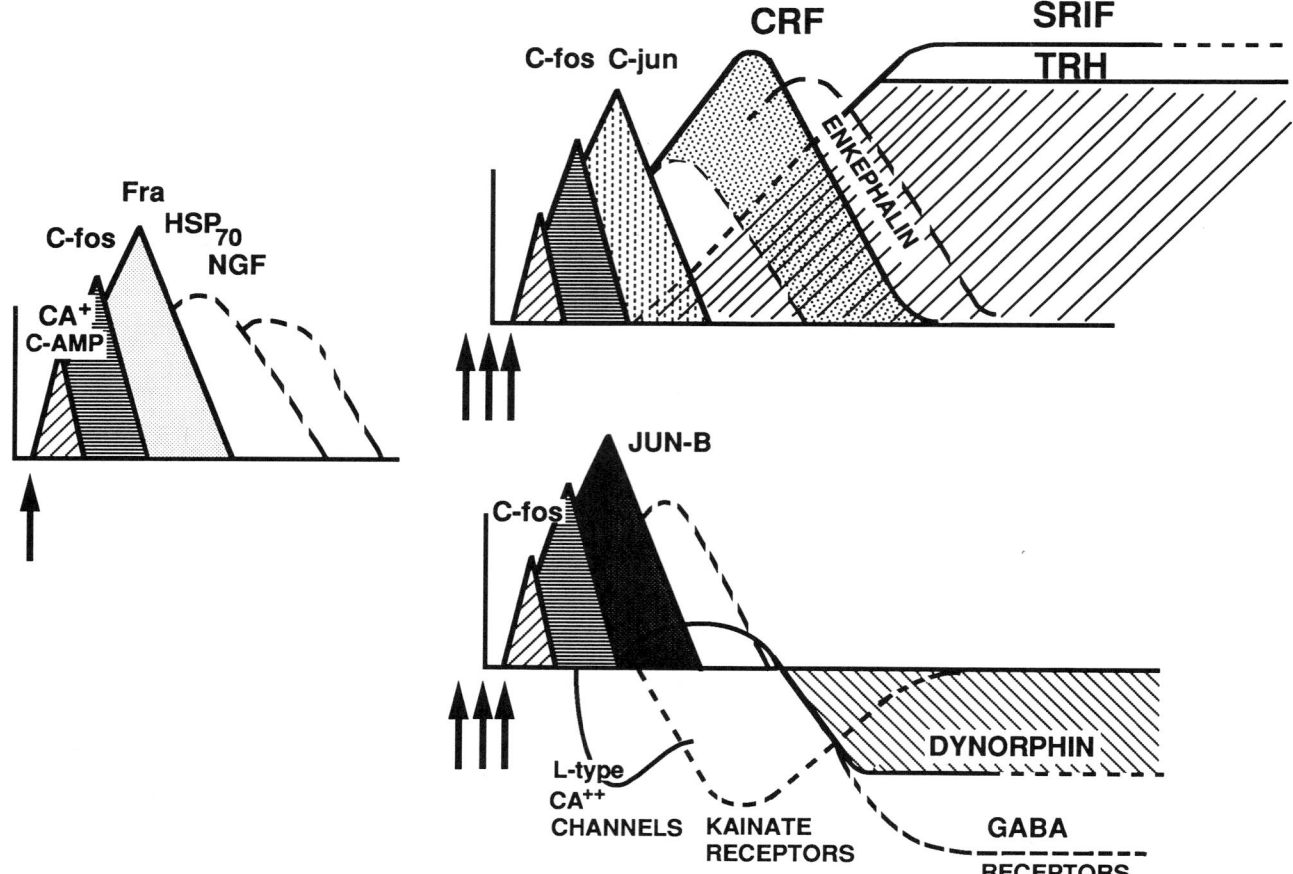

FIG. 2. In kindling, a single stimulation (*arrow*) affects receptors and second-messenger systems (calcium and cyclic-AMP) and activates a variety of transcription factors including c-*fos* and *fos*-related antigens (FRAS), as well as heat-shock proteins (HSP70) and growth factors (NGF). However, multiple stimulations (*triple arrows*) also result in the induction of longer-lasting changes in peptides or other late effector genes and regulatory factors that are either increased (**top right**) or decreased (**bottom right**) by the appropriate mix of transcription factors.

stressors may, through their impact on IEGs and late effector genes, reach a threshold for inducing full-blown episodes of affective illness. As in the kindling model, initial stressors may be insufficient to precipitate full-blown episodes, but with sufficient genetic vulnerability, repetition of stressor, or magnitude of stimulation, they become capable of inducing the neurobiological alterations associated with full-blown episodes. This formulation is consistent with the data that stresses not only induce IEGs (37), but also have a longer-lasting impact on neuropeptides and other transmitter and receptor alterations thought to be intimately involved in mood disorders. For example, increases in CRF and TRH have been reported in some studies of the CSF of depressed patients (6,38), whereas state-dependent decreases in somatostatin have also been observed in multiple studies of depressed patients (64). As illustrated in Fig. 3, it is possible that repeated occurrences of stressors become capable of triggering the appropriate combination of transcription factors that then result in the longer lasting regulation of mRNAs for CRH, TRH, and somatostatin in the appropriate direction with levels of respective neuropeptides remaining altered for much of the duration of the depressive episode. The long-term vulnerability to the stressor induction of episodes may be manifest in the observation that lesser degree or incidence of stress induction is required to induce subsequent episodes (46).

These observations also imply that another phenomenon is occurring simultaneously—that of episode sensitization. That is, it is the recurrence of sufficient numbers of triggered affective episodes themselves (similar to that observed with amygdala-kindled seizures) that not only leaves the organism progressively more vulnerable to subsequent episodes, but eventually results in the occurrence of episodes in the absence of exogenous triggers. The nature of the long-lasting memory traces left behind by episodes of mood illness remain to be adequately described, but the conditioned and unconditioned components of stimulant-induced behavioral sensitization discussed above suggest that a vast array of mechanisms induced by episodes of affective illness may be capable themselves of impacting on gene transcription, both of

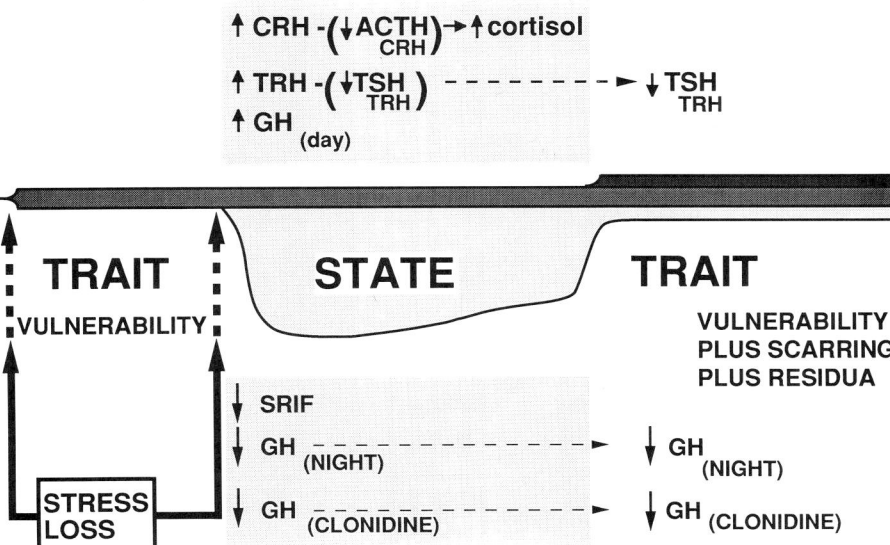

FIG. 3. As indicated in Fig. 2 for electrical stimulation, initial stressors might not be sufficient to trigger the full neurobiological concomitants of a depressive episode (*STATE*), but may nonetheless leave behind biological (*TRAIT*) vulnerabilities (shaded center line) to further alterations. The state of depression with its associated putative peptide and hormonal increases (**top**) and decreases (**bottom**) may then leave behind further trait vulnerabilities and residua, propelling the illness to further episode recurrence and automaticity.

the immediate early and late effector variety. This formulation would not be inconsistent with the existing data which show that a variety of the neurotransmitter and neuropeptide alterations postulated to occur during episodes of mood illness (such as increases in dopamine and norepinephrine during mania, increases in acetylcholine during depression, and increases in CRH and associated peptide abnormalities) have all been reported to impact on IEGs. The manic and depressive behaviors associated with these and a multiplicity of other biological abnormalities may thus become sensitized with recurring episodes.

Preliminary endocrinological data are also compatible with this; patients who fail to normalize their pathological escape from dexamethasone suppression during their well interval are at risk for increased incidence of relapse into another depressive episode (5). Similar observations have also been made for failure to normalize the blunted TSH response to TRH (putatively linked to TRH hypersecretion). Banki and colleagues (7) have observed that patients who do not decrease their high CSF levels of CRH during a depressive episode are also at higher risk for relapse when they are restudied during a euthymic episode. These data suggest the possibility that some of the neurobiological abnormalities associated with acute affective episodes may persist in some fashion into the euthymic or apparently clinically well interval. Even those patients demonstrating a full recovery based on clinical characteristics and neurobiological assessment, may still be at increased risk for episode recurrence compared with patients whose episodes have been prevented with adequate long-term prophylaxis. This postulate of episode sensitization requires direct clinical demonstration in appropriate clinical trials to ascertain whether patients undergoing long-term prophylaxis with episode prevention become less vulnerable to episode recurrence than patients who only receive acute and intermittent treatment

of their recurrent mood disorder. Other indirect evidence does exist, however, that suggests that episodes may change pharmacological responsivity, if not the course of untreated illness.

DISCONTINUATION AND REFRACTORINESS

We have observed a series of patients who have been well maintained on lithium prophylaxis, discontinue their medication, experience a relapse, and then fail to respond to the reinstitution of lithium at the same or higher dosages (48,49). In some instances, patients have been capable of re-responding after the first period of lithium discontinuation, but not after the second. The duration of time on lithium with the patients maintained in a relatively euthymic state does not appear to preclude the phenomenon of discontinuation-induced refractoriness as it has been observed after patients have been well for as long as 10 to 15 years.

These data are subject to a variety of interpretations, but one possibility is that the reemergence of an additional episode itself is sufficient to alter the neurobiology of the illness in such a fashion that it is no longer responsive to initially effective treatment. It is possible that this phenomenon is not unique to lithium. The Hillside Hospital group have observed that schizophrenic patients undergoing neuroleptic discontinuation and suffering relapses become more refractory to antipsychotic treatment with neuroleptics following each relapse (33). Thus, as in neuroleptic refractoriness in the late (expression) phase of cocaine sensitization (76), it may be the emergence of new behavioral pathology and its associated biochemical alterations that impacts on the degree of pharmacological response. Consistent with this perspective are the data of Gelenberg et al. (17) and O'Connell et al. (39), who observed that patients with greater numbers of prior episodes of mood illness before instituting lithium prophylaxis were at higher risk for lithium nonresponsiveness than patients who had had only three or four prior episodes.

It is noteworthy that neuroleptics are able to block the development, if not the expression, of cocaine-induced behavioral sensitization (76). This implies that the sensitizing effect of repeated cocaine-induced behavioral alterations or their associated biochemical changes are capable of conveying neuroleptic nonresponsiveness. In a similar fashion, new episodes engendered following lithium or neuroleptic discontinuation could alter the neurobiological substrate in such a fashion that patients become less responsive.

The kindling paradigm offers an additional perspective for treatment resistance. During kindling evolution, not only does the neuroanatomy and biochemistry appear to evolve, as discussed below, but the pharmacology does as well. That is, the three major phases of kindling evolution, a, development; b, completed; c, spontaneous, each show a differential pharmacology (51). Some drugs that are effective in one phase are not effective in another. For example, carbamazepine is ineffective in blocking the

development of amygdala-kindled seizures, but it is highly effective on the completed variety. Classical N-methyl-D-aspartate (NMDA) antagonists appear to show the opposite pattern. Diazepam is effective in the first two phases of kindling, but does not appear to be useful in blocking spontaneous seizures, whereas phenytoin shows the opposite pattern (43). These data suggest the possibility that as recurrent affective syndromes evolve, they too might change their pharmacological responsivity, as outlined in Figs. 4 and 5 and discussed in the last section.

TOLERANCE EMERGENCE DURING LONG-TERM PROPHYLAXIS

Another route to treatment resistance is the development of tolerance to a previously effective prophylactic agent. We have noted a substantial incidence of loss of efficacy during long-term treatment with carbamazepine, either alone or adjunctively with lithium (45). During long-term prophylaxis with lithium, some loss of efficacy is being reported with this agent as well (34,49). In assessing the possible routes of loss of responsivity to lithium in a group of 66 lithium-refractory patients referred to our clinical research unit because of treatment resistance, we observed that 45% had originally shown a good response to lithium but developed tolerance. Fourteen percent of the patients in this cohort of lithium-resistant patients developed lithium-discontinuation-induced refractoriness; that is, responsiveness was not lost during lithium treatment but following its discontinuation.

In our patients observed to show eventual loss of efficacy to carbamazepine prophylaxis, those with a more rapid progression of their illness in the 4 years prior to institution of treatment appeared to be at greatest risk (45,50). This may be consistent with observations in the preclinical model that animals kindled at higher currents (greater pathological drive) develop tolerance faster than those kindled at threshold currents (Weiss et al., *unpublished data*). As discussed below, tolerance may be conceptualized as either a loss of drug efficacy or the possibility that an underlying pathological process is remanifesting itself through an otherwise effective treatment modality.

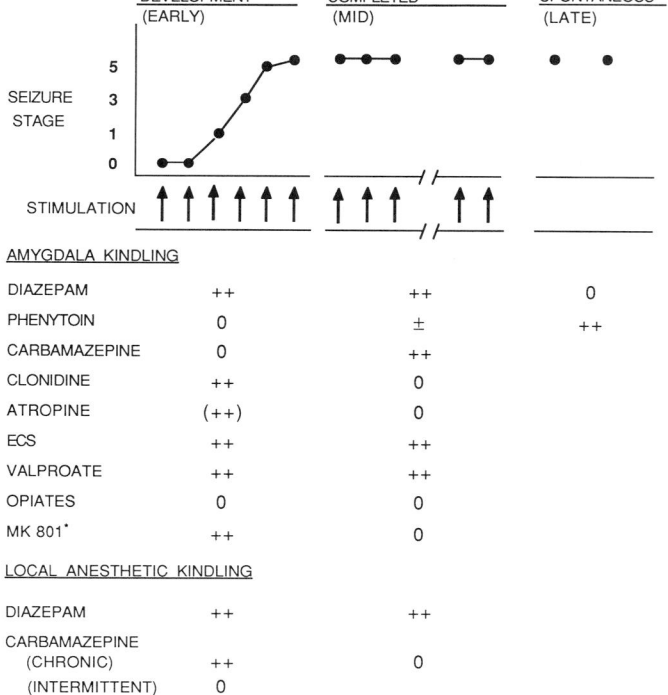

	DEVELOPMENT (EARLY)	COMPLETED (MID)	SPONTANEOUS (LATE)
AMYGDALA KINDLING			
DIAZEPAM	++	++	0
PHENYTOIN	0	±	++
CARBAMAZEPINE	0	++	
CLONIDINE	++	0	
ATROPINE	(++)	0	
ECS	++	++	
VALPROATE	++	++	
OPIATES	0	0	
MK 801*	++	0	
LOCAL ANESTHETIC KINDLING			
DIAZEPAM	++	++	
CARBAMAZEPINE			
(CHRONIC)	++	0	
(INTERMITTENT)	0		

FIG. 4. Early (developmental), mid (completed), and late (spontaneous) phases of amygdala (**top**) or pharmacological (**bottom**) kindling evolution show differences in pharmacological responsivity (++ = very effective, 0 = not effective). The double dissociation in response to diazepam and phenytoin in the early versus the late phases, as described by Pinel, are particularly striking. Note also that carbamazepine is effective in inhibiting the development phase of local anesthetic but not amygdala kindling, whereas the converse is true for the mid (completed) phase.

CONTINGENT TOLERANCE

Loss of efficacy to the anticonvulsant effects of carbamazepine can also occur in some patients with seizure disorders, and tolerance to the antinociceptive effects of carbamazepine is a well-recognized problem in the long-term treatment of patients with trigeminal neuralgia. In this latter instance, carbamazepine shows an initial 80% to 90% response rate, but as many as 50% of patients will demonstrate some degree of loss of efficacy over time. A better understanding of the neurobiological aspects of tolerance development may allow for the genera-

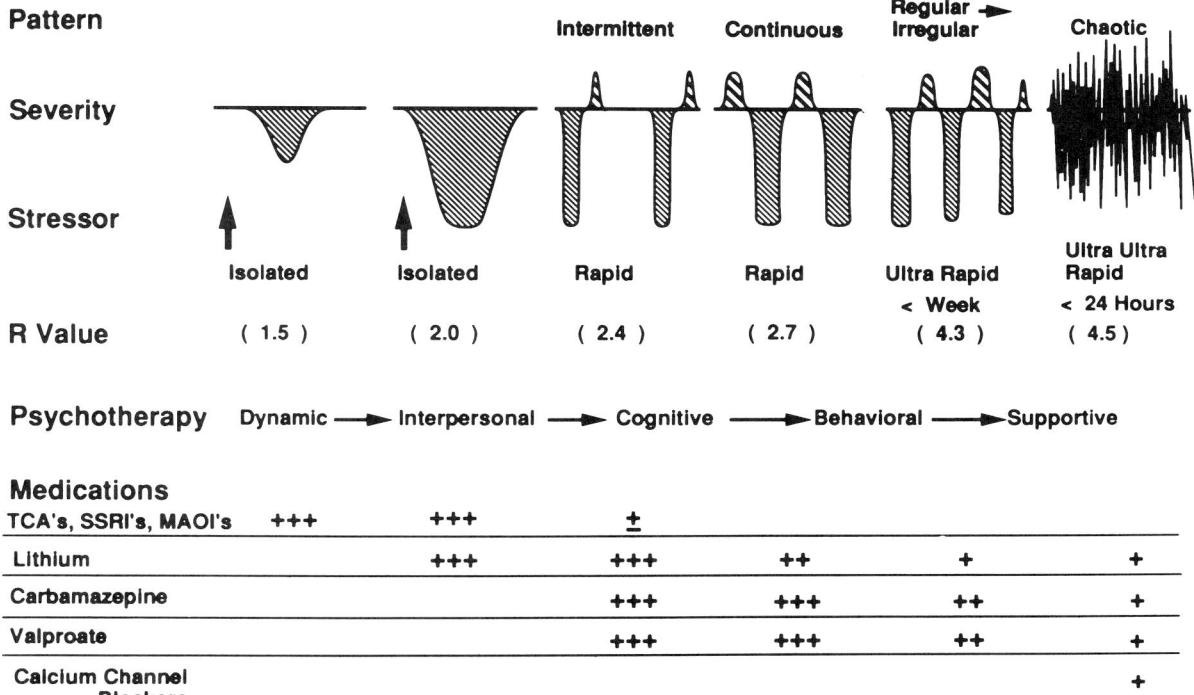

FIG. 5. In an analogous fashion to kindling, episodes of mood illness may progress from triggered (*arrows*) to spontaneous and show different patterns and frequencies (**top row**) as a function of stage of syndrome evolution. Just as different neural substrates are involved in different phases of kindling evolution, a similar principle is postulated in mood illness; these phases might also be responsive to different types of pharmacotherapies or psychotherapies. Although systematic and controlled studies have not examined the relationship of the illness phase to treatment response, anecdotal observations provide suggestive data that some treatments may be differentially highly effective (+++), moderately effective (++), or possibly effective (+) as a function of course of illness. Note that the pharmacological dissociations in the nonhomologous model of kindling (Fig. 4) are different from those postulated in mood illness; nonetheless, the principle of differential response as a function of stage may be useful and deserves to be specifically examined and tested. The use of multiple agents in combination as a function of late or severe illness stage is standard in many medical illnesses and also should be studied systematically in the refractory mood disorders.

tion and testing of new clinical approaches to both its prevention and reversal once it has become manifest.

To this end, Weiss and associates have begun to study development of tolerance to the anticonvulsant effects of carbamazepine on amygdala-kindled seizures as a paradigm that may help unravel different components of tolerance phenomenology, pharmacology, physiology, and biochemistry. Weiss et al. (71,72,74,77) have elucidated a type of tolerance related to a unique type of pharmacodynamic mechanism rather than pharmacokinetic ones. In this instance, tolerance is not related to the mere presence of the drug in the organism, but is dependent upon its being present during the episode being treated; that is, it is contingent tolerance.

Once the animal has been made tolerant to the anticonvulsant effects of carbamazepine with repeated administration of the drug before seizures have occurred, kindling the animal with no drug (or even continuing to give daily drug, but after the seizure has occurred) is sufficient to reverse the tolerance and reinstate anticonvulsant efficacy when the drug is then given before the kindling stimula-

tion. Following further drug exposure, the animal will again become tolerant at approximately the same rate as initially observed. These data demonstrate that drug efficacy in this model can be manipulated at will, depending on whether the drug is given before or after the seizure has occurred.

Animals made tolerant to the anticonvulsant effects of carbamazepine compared with those receiving equal drug treatment but that were not tolerant (i.e., those given carbamazepine after seizures have occurred) show a differential seizure susceptibility when tested in the drug-free condition. That is, tolerant animals have a lower seizure ... (increased convulsive responsivity) compared with nontolerant animals. When tolerance is reversed by a period of kindling with no drug (or with drug after kindling), the threshold returns to the baseline kindled state (72,77). These data suggest that endogenous biochemical and physiological processes occur during tolerance development that render the animals more seizure prone in a long-lasting fashion.

Dr. Weiss and colleagues have begun to examine the

possible neural substrates mediating this altered responsivity during carbamazepine tolerance. During the generation of amygdala-kindled seizures, a variety of biochemical effects in the hippocampus have been observed in our laboratory, as summarized below. When animals have become tolerant to the anticonvulsant effects of carbamazepine, some of these biochemical adaptations normally associated with kindled seizures are inhibited or fail to occur altogether. These biochemical changes are intimately associated with contingent tolerance as they are observed only when animals are treated with carbamazepine before kindled seizures occur, but do not occur in animals treated with equal doses of carbamazepine after the seizure has occurred; that is, a situation not associated with tolerance development. In these studies, animals were matched for number of seizures, as well.

Following amygdala-kindled seizures, increases in c-fos are observed in the granule cells of the dentate gyrus as well as increases in the neuropeptide TRH, benzodiazepine and GABA receptors, mineralocorticoid, and glucocorticoid receptors. Kindled seizures also increase CRH and CRH-binding protein in the dentate hilar region (66). In animals that have been rendered contingently tolerant to the anticonvulsant effects of carbamazepine by repeated pretreatment, the seizures are no longer associated with the same degree of increase in c-fos, $GABA_A$ receptors, or mRNA for TRH (Weiss et al. and Clark et al., unpublished observations) (Fig. 6). Again, these biochemical alterations are selective to the contingently tolerant rats as nontreated animals exposed to equal numbers of kindled seizures and drug doses (but after the seizures have occurred) do not show this failure to increase these indices.

To the extent that some of the changes following kindled seizures are endogenous compensatory adaptive processes (attempting to prevent or terminate the seizure process; i.e., endogenous anticonvulsant mechanisms), a failure to increase these substances during carbamazepine treatment could account for the loss of efficacy. As a major inhibitory neurotransmitter in brain, GABA is thought to exert its endogenous anticonvulsant effects through the $GABA_A$ receptor. Thus, failure to increase $GABA_A$ receptors during carbamazepine-induced contingent tolerance could be associated with the drug's loss of efficacy. Similarly, the neuropeptide TRH is thought to exert anticonvulsant effects when administered intrathecally (80).

Post and Weiss have observed, paradoxically, that animals given a period of time off from seizures for 4 days or more lose their ability to respond to carbamazepine (52). It is of interest that seizure-induced increases in TRH occur over a period of approximately 4 days. Thus, increases in TRH induction as well as other intermediately lasting changes in neurotransmitters or receptors (such as the increase in $GABA_A$ and benzodiazepine receptors) remain candidates for the time-off-from seizure effect.

Whatever turns out to be the precise mechanism of this effect, it is clear that endogenous processes, which have occurred in response to seizures, enable the anticonvulsant effects of carbamazepine.

These data become all the more intriguing in relationship to mechanisms underlying loss of efficacy to carbamazepine during contingent-tolerance development as this process, too, is associated with a failure to increase $GABA_A$ receptors, TRH mRNA, as well as other variables. Thus, contingent tolerance may, in part, resemble an animal in the time-off effect where increases in TRH, $GABA_A$ receptors, or some other endogenous mechanism are no longer apparent, and this loss or failure of adaptive response is associated with a loss of anticonvulsant effects of carbamazepine on amygdala-kindled seizures. The time-off data are consistent with the formulation that some of the neurobiological changes associated with amygdala-kindled seizures represent secondary or compensatory adaptations (i.e., they are good guys attempting to provide an endogenous anticonvulsant mechanism), whereas others are a more primary part of the pathophysiological process of kindling (i.e., the bad guys, relating to kindling persistence or progression). Differentiating between the two may be of considerable import as one would want to facilitate the good effects but inhibit the bad effects to maximize anticonvulsant efficacy.

This perspective raises the possibility that some of the biochemical alterations associated with the evolution of mood disorders could similarly be divided into those representing a part of the primary pathophysiological process (bad guys) and those representing secondary compensatory attempts at endogenous psychotropic effects (good guys) (52). For example, it is likely that sleep loss in depression represents a secondary adaptive response, as one night's sleep deprivation results in substantial amelioration of depression in 50% to 60% of severely depressed patients (63,79). If it were part of the primary pathophysiology of the illness it would be expected that further deprivation of sleep would exacerbate rather than ameliorate the depressive process. In a similar fashion, one would postulate that other neurobiological alterations in the illness may similarly be dichotomized. This raises the question of whether the postulated increases in TRH during depression based on increases in CSF levels of TRH (7) and blunted TSH responses to intravenous TRH are pathological or compensatory and adaptive. Obviously such a distinction is of considerable importance in developing better therapeutics.

One prediction of the contingent tolerance model is that a period of time off medication may be associated with the renewal of therapeutic efficacy. Preliminary data in epilepsy (14), trigeminal neuralgia, and mood illness (41) based on small case series are consistent with this hypothesis but remain to be directly tested in prospective clinical trials.

It should be noted from the outset, however, that oppo-

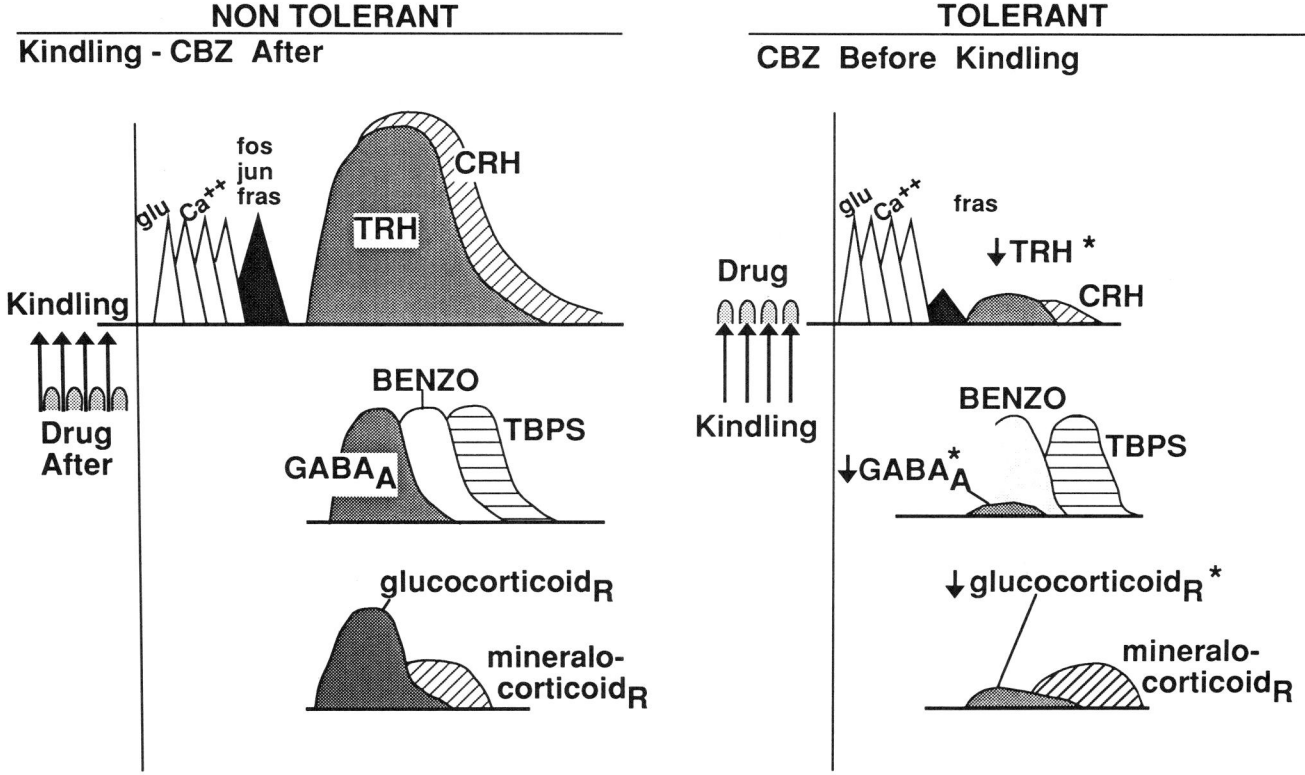

FIG. 6. Schematic illustration of seizure-induced changes in nontolerant animals (*left*) who receive carbamazepine (CBZ) after the seizure has occurred. (These effects are also similar to those observed in medication-free kindled animals.) When CBZ-tolerant animals (*right*) experience the same number of seizures and drug administrations, they fail to show the typical seizure-induced changes in TRH, CRH, GABA_A, and glucocorticoid receptors. * indicates the putative endogenous anticonvulsant adaptations that may be lost with contingent tolerance.

site predictions of the utility of a period of time off medications are derived from the two phenomena described in this manuscript: discontinuation-induced refractoriness and contingent tolerance. In the case of a patient who is continuing to show adequate response, a period of time off medication may be deleterious (48). In contrast, for a patient who has already lost responsiveness to a given treatment, as in the contingent-tolerance paradigm, the current model holds the possibility that renewed responsivity could occur (41). These formulations highlight the possibility that the history of drug responsivity (rather than mere presence of the drug in an organism) could differentially affect treatment strategies in the treatment-resistant mood disorders. In the case of the well-maintained patient, drug discontinuation could not only result in relapse (68) but also in treatment resistance (48,49), whereas the opposite could hypothetically occur in the patient who has already become tolerant (72). In addition, because there is some mechanistic specificity to contingent-tolerance development, at least on amygdala-kindled seizures (71), using a new drug with a different mechanism of action may not be associated with cross-tolerance. However, unexpectedly, when animals demonstrated tolerance to the anticonvulsant effects of carba-

mazepine, they were also tolerant to the anticonvulsant effects of valproate (77). Because carbamazepine causes a failure of kindled seizures to up-regulate GABA_A receptors during tolerance development, as discussed above, this relative loss of GABA_A-receptor tone might provide a basis for the cross-tolerance to valproate.

It is also hoped that understanding the mechanisms underlying development of the contingent tolerance to carbamazepine's anticonvulsant effects might provide additional clues toward its prevention or reversal as well as in pertinent clinical syndromes. In the contingent-tolerance paradigm described, all of the loss of efficacy to the anticonvulsant effects of carbamazepine are related to contingent administration of the drug, and noncontingent drug administration (i.e., drug that administered after each seizure has occurred) is not associated with any loss of efficacy compared with vehicle-treated controls. These data suggest that even in clinical situations with chronic drug administration, a contingent component of tolerance development may account for a greater degree of loss of efficacy than had previously been surmised. Moreover, if this proves to be the case, it would provide for additional predictions regarding vulnerability to drug discontinuation effects. Chronic treatment with a given drug may be associated with long-lasting adaptations that change polarity during the drug discontinuation phase, leaving the patient more prone to illness emergence in this withdrawal period.

In addition to the classic drug withdrawal effects, the current analysis raises the possibility that an additional vulnerability could occur during the withdrawal period in patients who are contingently tolerant to the effects of a drug. That is, they have not only lost the primary effects of the drug, but they have also lost the illness-induced endogenous adaptations associated with tolerance development. These two liabilities may then combine to make the patient who has lost drug responsivity via contingent tolerance more vulnerable to withdrawal phenomena than a patient similarly treated with a drug, but who has not shown loss of efficacy or never responded in the first place; in other words, this patient would only be vulnerable on the basis of classic withdrawal effects. This proposition could be directly tested in patients with refractory seizure, mood, or anxiety disorders, where the prediction would be that patients who had lost efficacy through tolerance would be more seizure prone during the discontinuation phase compared with patients who had never shown response to the drug.

FURTHER PREDICTIONS OF THE SENSITIZATION AND KINDLING MODELS

As illustrated in Table 1, the sensitization and kindling paradigms as they apply to the long-term course of mood disorders have specific predictions that have long-term treatment implications. To the extent that the experience of episodes of mood illness impacts on gene expression and other mechanisms conveying a long-lasting vulnerability to recurrence, early institution of long-term maintenance treatment should have an impact on not only the course of illness but also, potentially, drug response. A dual role for long-term prophylaxis is postulated. Patients undergoing prophylaxis would gain the benefit of amelioration and prevention of affective episodes, and, if the current formulation proves correct, upon drug discontinuation, say after a decade of treatment, they would be less vulnerable to recurrences than other patients who received only intermittent acute treatment of multiple recurrent episodes as they emerged. Although such a study is technically feasible, it would be extremely difficult to perform in an ideal or systematic fashion at this time. Not only would the study be extremely expensive because of its duration, but even the initial randomization of patients to intermittent versus prophylactic treatment would raise ethical dilemmas, as would the period of drug discontinuation after a given number of years of successful prophylaxis.

Thus, less ideal designs are required to assess the possibility of a dual impact of prophylaxis in prevention of episodes and prevention of sensitization (i.e., increased vulnerability to subsequent recurrences). Clearly, the initial data of Gelenberg et al. (17) and O'Connell et al. (39) are consistent with the notion that a greater number of prior episodes before instituting a prophylaxis is associ-

TABLE 1. *Phenomena in the course of mood disorders modeled by kindling and behavioral sensitization*

Descriptors	Kindling	Sensitization	Phenomenon[a]
Stressor vulnerability	++	++	Initial stressors early in development may be without effect but predispose to greater reactivity upon rechallenge
Stressor precipitation	++	++	Later stress may precipitate full-blown episode
Conditioning may be involved	—	++	Stressors may become more symbolic
Episode autonomy	++	—	Initially-precipitated episodes may occur spontaneously
Cross-sensitization with stimulants	—	++	Comorbidity with drug abuse may work in both directions (affective illness ⇌ drug abuse)
Vulnerability to relapse	++	++	S and K demonstrate long-term increases in responsivity
Episodes may:			
a. become more severe	++	++	S and K both show behavioral evolution in severity or stages
b. show more rapid onsets		++	Hyperactivity and stereotypy show more rapid onsets
Anatomical and biochemical substrates evolve	++	++	K memory-trace evolves from unilateral to bilateral
IEGs involved	++	++	IEGs, such as c-*fos* induced
Alterations in gene expression occur	++	++	IEGs may change gene expression, especially of peptides over long time domains
Change in synaptic microstructure occurs	++	—	Neuronal sprouting and cell loss indicate structural changes
Pharmacology differs as a function or stage of evolution	++	++	K differs as a function of stage; S differs as a function of development versus expression

[a] S, sensitization; K, kindling.

ated with a lesser degree of lithium response; however, a variety of other interpretations are possible, including that these patients were preselected for a more refractory illness to begin with. Nonetheless, one could make the conservative argument that even if earlier institution of treatment did not affect the long-term course of illness and its drug responsiveness, one is still better off for having successfully prevented the episodes with effective prophylaxis, and such a single benefit is worthwhile, even in the absence of a convincing demonstration of a dual benefit (i.e., the additional prevention of episode sensitization). Nonetheless, the current data regarding the impact of lithium, carbamazepine, and valproate on the illness and the recent metaanalysis of Suppes et al. (68) showing that 80% to 90% of patients relapse following lithium discontinuation provide a very strong empirical basis for the institution and maintenance of long-term prophylaxis, even in the absence of the demonstration of the sensitization factor. Alas, it is highly likely that both the clinician and the patient will be left to struggle with these risk–benefit formulations for a long time to come in the absence of highly convincing data about the long-term impact of prophylaxis on course of illness and treatment response.

EFFICACY OF NIMODIPINE IN ULTRAFAST MOOD OSCILLATIONS: IMPLICATIONS FOR CALCIUM-BASED MECHANISMS

In an ongoing double-blind, controlled trial, Pazzaglia and collaborators (42) found preliminary evidence of the efficacy of the L-type calcium channel antagonist nimodipine in ameliorating the amplitude and frequency of mood swings in patients with ultrafast mood oscillations. This included some patients with ultra-ultra-rapid (ultradian) cycling and one patient with recurrent brief depression where responses to treatment were confirmed in a B-A-B-A design. Patients with more traditional and slower cycle frequencies did not appear to respond as often. Should these observations be confirmed in a larger patient sample, they suggest the possibility that alterations in calcium flux through L-type channels could play a pathophysiological role in these ultrafast cycle frequencies.

In one patient whose significant but partial response to nimodipine was confirmed and reconfirmed in a B-A-B-A design, the addition of carbamazepine yielded further clinical improvement and attenuation in the frequency and amplitude of this patient's ultradian oscillations. Thus, this patient, who was inadequately responsive to either carbamazepine or nimodipine alone, showed an additive effect when the two drugs were used in combination, achieving the first clinical remission (absence of nurses' blind ratings of functional incapacity) for the first time in more than 4 years.

The efficacy of nimodipine in patients with ultradian mood fluctuations suggests that erratic fluxes in calcium

channel regulation could underlie this type of chaotic mood dysregulation. The additive effects of carbamazepine and nimodipine, should they occur in a larger series of patients, also raise the possibility that blockaded L-type calcium channels, in addition to the concurrent effects of carbamazepine on other neurotransmitter or ion channel systems, could provide the basis for the efficacy of these two agents in combination therapy. Of particular interest among the panoply of neurotransmitter second-messenger and ion-channel effects of carbamazepine (53) is the recent recognition that carbamazepine can block calcium flux through NMDA receptors, at least in cerebellar granule cells (Hough, Ragowski, and Chuang, *unpublished observations*). If this were the mechanism of carbamazepine-induced potentiation of nimodipine, similar clinical effects should be achievable by more traditional glutamate antagonists. It is also possible that effects of carbamazepine on entirely different mechanisms unrelated to calcium could be important to its potentiative effects with nimodipine.

Nevertheless, the efficacy of nimodipine alone, and possibly in combination with carbamazepine in patients with ultradian and chaotic mood fluctuations, does raise the possibility of important alterations in calcium dysregulation in these patients with ultrafast frequencies of mood disorder. Calcium oscillations appear to be fundamental aspects of neurobiology at various spatial and temporal domains ranging from molecular fluctuations in intracellular calcium and membrane-bound calcium involved in neurosecretion and various aspects of neuroplasticity to more global aspects of neuronal function (9,58,59). Clarifying the role for L-type and other types of calcium channel blockers in mood dysregulation may not only provide a new class of compounds for the therapeutic armamentarium (13,23), but may also provide clues to some of the pathophysiological mechanisms involved in the neurobiology of treatment-refractory bipolar illness.

CONCLUSIONS

The kindling and sensitization formulations suggest the possibility that alterations in a series of transcriptional activating and suppressor factors could also occur, not by somatic mutation as in carcinogenesis, but by environmental and experiential impact (Figs. 1, 2, and 3) in addition to the more typically considered inherited genetic vulnerability. In the course of affective evolution, we have postulated that, based on alterations in experience-induced gene expression, there is sensitization both to stressors and to episodes themselves. In the kindling process, each apparently similar and behaviorally stereotyped occurrence of a seizure episode appears, nonetheless, to propel the process gradually toward autonomy (i.e., the spontaneous occurrence of seizures with their differential anatomy and pharmacology). If a similar phenomenon were found to occur in the different neural systems implicated in the mood disorders, then one would postulate not only that repeated episodes may propel the illness toward autonomy, but that a differential pharmacology may also exist as a function of stage-of-illness evolution (Fig. 4).

Preliminary data that are available to date are consistent with such a formulation (Fig. 5). For example, multiple studies have documented that lithium is less effective in rapid-cycling compared with non-rapid-cycling patients (47). Although some patients begin to show rapid cycling from the onset of their illness, this phase is often a late manifestation of the illness. Moreover, initially, all of the patients we have seen with ultradian cycling illness have been inadequately responsive to lithium (18,31). In rapid, ultrarapid, and ultradian cycling, the anticonvulsants carbamazepine and valproate have shown some success (44). Whether these agents are selectively more effective in this phase of the illness is unclear from the current data. A recent study of Okuma (40) suggests that carbamazepine, like lithium, is more effective in less rapid cycling patients. Nonetheless, in the late rapid cycling and ultrarapid cycling phases of the illness, these newer mood stabilizing drugs (carbamazepine and valproate), either alone or in combination with lithium, may prove to be effective. In addition, Ketter et al. (29) and Keck et al. (28) have demonstrated that, in some instances, patients will respond to carbamazepine and valproate in combination when they have been inadequately responsive to either agent alone. In addition, some patients appear to respond to one anticonvulsant but not the other (44).

These data on differential responsivity among the anticonvulsants and their use in combination with or without lithium augmentation, raise the possibility that, as in cancer chemotherapy, patients in late phases of their illness with severe manifestations of symptomatology and rapid cycling, may require complex treatment regimens to target multiple mechanisms of action. It is of interest that each of the drugs used in long-term prophylaxis (lithium, carbamazepine, and valproate) has been postulated to have multiple targets of drug action and are putative dirty drugs. When these agents are used in combination, perhaps their multiple targets of action converge or diverge on multiple neurobiological processes that are increasingly disordered in the most severely cycling patients. In this fashion, cleaner drugs might not necessarily be more effective treatments in late phases of the illness unless they were more precisely and multiply targeted to block the ''bad guys'' and assist the ''good guys'', as discussed above. However, it is also possible that endogenous antidepressant adaptations that are the good guys for a depressive episode could (like tricyclic antidepressants) help precipitate the next manic episodes and contribute to cycle induction. Mood stabilizers may then be unique in their ability to dampen or prevent both manic and depressive episodes by targeting both types of endogenous adaptations.

To the extent that the development of clinical loss of

efficacy in long-term prophylaxis is mediated by processes parallel to those seen in contingent tolerance in the kindling model, there may be an associated failure of positive, illness-related endogenous adaptations to occur. In the case of such tolerance development, a sufficient period of time off medications could lead to renewed efficacy because of the reinduction of these illness-driven putative good guys. Conversely, in lithium-discontinuation refractoriness, it is postulated that the primary pathological process of the illness is predominately facilitated by the occurrence of a new episode, propelling the illness to a new stage (like metastases in malignancy), which is now no longer responsive to the previously effective medication. That is, in this instance of the ongoing battle of the pathophysiological illness process versus endogenous, adaptive compensations, the bad guys win. This battle may be taking place at multiple levels of the neuroaxis from ion channels in the membrane and effects on gene expression in the nucleus to more global changes in the balance within and between nuclei (amygdala versus hippocampal) or whole regions of brain and its lateralized function.

The kindling and sensitization models suggest that this balance process between pathological and compensatory mechanisms may be constantly evolving in a complex spatiotemporal pattern, providing multiple targets for conceptualizing new treatment interventions and for systematically testing some of the preliminary formulation offered based on these indirect preclinical models. In this fashion, it is hoped that a more detailed understanding of the primary and adaptive neurobiological processes involved in the recurrent mood disorders will rapidly advance therapeutics. In addition, these formulations add a growing theoretical foundation for the already substantial empirical data base indicating the importance of early institution and long-term maintenance of pharmacoprophylaxis in the recurrent unipolar and bipolar mood disorders. In addition to preventing the considerable morbidity and potential mortality of the illness, appropriate prophylaxis may prevent the bad guys from engaging the long-term biochemistry and microstructure of the brain and propelling the illness to cycle acceleration, autonomy, and treatment resistance.

REFERENCES

1. Aagaard J, Vestergaard P. Predictors of outcome in prophylactic lithium treatment: a 2-year prospective study. *J Affect Dis* 1990;18:259–266.
2. Altshuler LL, Post RM, Leverich GS, Mikalauskas K, Rosoff A, Ackerman L. Antidepressant-induced mania and cycle acceleration: a controversy revisited. 1994;[*submitted*].
3. Anokhin KV, Mileusnic R, Shamakina IY, Rose SP. Effects of early experience on c-*fos* gene expression in the chick forebrain. *Brain Res* 1991;544:101–107.
4. Antelman SM, Eichler AJ, Black CA, Kocan D. Interchangeability of stress and amphetamine in sensitization. *Science* 1980;207:329–331.
5. Arana GW, Baldessarini RJ, Ornsteen M. The dexamethasone sup-

pression test for diagnosis and prognosis in psychiatry. Commentary and review. *Arch Gen Psychiatry* 1985;42:1193–1204.

6. Banki CM, Bissette G, Arato M, Nemeroff CB. Elevation of immunoreactive CSF TRH in depressed patients. *Am J Psychiatry* 1988;145:1526–1531.

7. Banki C, Karmacsi L, Bissette G, Nemeroff CB. CSF corticotropin-releasing hormone and somatostatin in major depression: response to antidepressant treatment and relapse. *Eur Neuropsychopharmacol* 1992;2:107–113.

8. Bauer MS, Whybrow PC. Rapid cycling bipolar affective disorder. II. Treatment of refractory rapid cycling with high-dose levothyroxine: a preliminary study. *Arch Gen Psychiatry* 1990;47:435–440.

9. Berridge MJ. The Albert Lasker Medical Awards. Inositol trisphosphate, calcium, lithium, and cell signaling. *JAMA* 1989;262:1834–1841.

10. Brown EE, Fibiger HC. Cocaine-induced conditioned locomotion: absence of associated increases in dopamine release. *Neuroscience* 1992;48:621–629.

11. Brown EE, Robertson GS, Fibiger HC. Evidence for conditional neuronal activation following exposure to a cocaine-paired environment: role of forebrain limbic structures. *J Neurosci* 1992;12:4112–4121.

12. Clark M, Post RM, Weiss SRB, Cain CJ, Nakajima T. Regional expression of c-*fos* mRNA in rat brain during the evolution of amygdala-kindled seizures. *Mol Brain Res* 1991;11:55–64.

13. Dubovsky SL, Murphy J, Thomas M, Rademacher J. Abnormal intracellular calcium ion concentration in platelets and lymphocytes of bipolar patients. *Am J Psychiatry* 1992;149:118–120.

14. Engel J Jr. *Molecular neurobiology of epilepsy.* New York: Elsevier, 1992.

15. Fontana DJ, Post RM, Pert A. Conditioned increase in mesolimbic dopamine overflow by stimuli associated with cocaine. *Brain Res* 1993;629:31–39.

16. Geinisman Y, de Toledo-Morrell L, Morrell F. The brain's record of experience: kindling-induced enlargement of the active zone in hippocampal perforated synapses. *Brain Res* 1990;513:175–179.

17. Gelenberg AJ, Kane JM, Keller MB, et al. Comparison of standard and low serum levels of lithium for maintenance treatment of bipolar disorder. *N Engl J Med* 1989;321:1489–1493.

18. George MS, Jones M, Post RM, Mikalauskas K, Leverich GS. The longitudinal course of affective illness: mathematical models involving chaos theory. *World Congr Biol Psychiatry Abstracts* 1992;31:86–87A(abst 58).

19. Goddard GV, McIntyre DC, Leech CK. A permanent change in brain function resulting from daily electrical stimulation. *Exp Neurol* 1969;25:295–330.

20. Graybiel AM, Moratalla R, Robertson HA. Amphetamine and cocaine induce drug-specific activation of the c-*fos* gene in striosome-matrix compartments and limbic subdivisions of the striatum. *Proc Natl Acad Sci USA* 1990;87:6912–6916.

21. Herkenham M. Mismatches between neurotransmitter and receptor localizations in brain: observations and implications. *Neuroscience* 1987;23:1–38.

22. Himmelhoch JM, Garfinkel ME. Sources of lithium resistance in mixed mania. *Psychopharmacol Bull* 1986;22:613–620.

23. Hoschl C. Do calcium antagonists have a place in the treatment of mood disorders. *Drugs* 1991;42:721–729.

24. Joffe RT, Singer W. A comparison of triiodothyronine and thyroxine in the potentiation of tricyclic antidepressants. *Psychiatry Res* 1990;32:241–251.

25. Kalivas PW, Duffy P. Effect of acute and daily cocaine treatment on extracellular dopamine in the nucleus accumbens. *Synapse* 1990;5:45–58.

26. Kalivas PW, Duffy P. Time course of extracellular dopamine and behavioral sensitization to cocaine. I. dopamine axon terminals. *J Neurosci* 1993;13:266–275.

27. Kalivas PW, Stewart J. Dopamine transmission in the initiation and expression of drug- and stress-induced sensitization of motor activity. *Brain Res Rev* 1991;16:223–244.

28. Keck PE Jr, McElroy SL, Vuckovic A, Friedman LM. Combined valproate and carbamazepine treatment of bipolar disorder. *J Neuropsychiatry Clin Neurosci* 1992;4:319–322.

29. Ketter TA, Pazzaglia PJ, Post RM. Synergy of carbamazepine and valproic acid in affective illness: case report and review of literature. *J Clin Psychopharmacol* 1992;12:276–281.

30. Kraepelin E. *Manic-depressive insanity and paranoia.* Edinburgh: Livingstone; 1921. Barclay RM, Robertson GM, translators.

31. Kramlinger KG, Post RM. Ultra-rapid and ultradian cycling in bipolar affective illness. 1994;[*submitted*].

32. Kukopulos A, Reginaldi D, Laddomada P, Floris G, Serra G, Tondo L. Course of the manic–depressive cycle and changes caused by treatment. *Pharmakopsychiatria Neuropsychopharmakol* 1980;13:156–167.

33. Lieberman JA, Mayerhoff DI, Loebel A, Geisler S, Alvir J. Evidence for sensitization in early stage of schizophrenia. *Clin Neuropharmacol* 1992;15(Suppl):54B.

34. Maj M, Pirozzi R, Kemali D. Long-term outcome of lithium prophylaxis in patients initially classified as complete responders. *Psychopharmacology (Berl)* 1989;98:535–538.

35. Margolis RL, Chuang D-M, Post RM. Programmed cell death: implications for neuropsychiatric disorders. *Biol Psychiatry* 1994;[*in press*].

36. Moratalla R, Robertson HA, Graybiel AM. Dynamic regulation of NGFI-A (zif268, egr1) gene expression in the striatum. *J Neurosci* 1992;12:2609–2622.

37. Nakajima T, Daval JL, Gleiter CH, Deckert J, Post RM, Marangos PJ. c-*Fos* mRNA expression following electrical-induced seizure and acute nociceptive stress in mouse brain. *Epilepsy Res* 1989;4:156–159.

38. Nemeroff CB, Widerlov E, Bissette G. Elevated concentrations of CSF corticotropin-releasing factor-like immunoreactivity in depressed patients. *Science* 1984;226:1342–1344.

39. O'Connell RA, Mayo JA, Flatow L, Cuthbertson B, O'Brien BE. Outcome of bipolar disorder on long-term treatment with lithium. *Br J Psychiatry* 1991;159:123–129.

40. Okuma T. Effects of carbamazepine and other anticonvulsant drugs on affective disorders. *Neuropsychobiology* 1993;27:138–145.

41. Pazzaglia PJ, Post RM. Contingent tolerance and reresponse to carbamazepine: a case study in a patient with trigeminal neuralgia and bipolar disorder. *J Neuropsychiatry Clin Neurosci* 1992;4:76–81.

42. Pazzaglia PJ, Post RM, Ketter TA, George MS, Marangell LB. Preliminary controlled trial of nimodipine in ultra-rapid cycling affective dysregulation. *Psychiatry Res* [*in press*].

43. Pinel JPJ. Effects of diazepam and diphenylhydantoin on elicited and spontaneous seizures in kindled rats: a double dissociation. *Pharmacol Biochem Behav* 1983;18:61–63.

44. Post RM. Alternatives to lithium for bipolar affective illness. In: Tasman A, Goldfinger SM, Kaufmann CA, eds. *Review of psychiatry,* vol. 9. Washington DC: American Psychiatric Press; 1990:170–202.

45. Post RM. Prophylaxis of bipolar affective disorders. *Int Rev Psychol* 1990;2:277–320.

46. Post RM. Transduction of psychosocial stress into the neurobiology of recurrent affective disorder. *Am J Psychiatry* 1992;149:999–1010.

47. Post RM, Kramlinger KG, Altshuler LL, Ketter TA, Denicoff K. Treatment of rapid cycling bipolar illness. *Psychopharmacol Bull* 1990;26:37–47.

48. Post RM, Leverich GS, Altshuler L, Mikalauskas K. Lithium discontinuation-induced refractoriness: Preliminary observations. *Am J Psychiatry* 1992;149:1727–1729.

49. Post RM, Leverich GS, Pazzaglia PJ, Mikalauskas K, Denicoff K. Lithium tolerance and discontinuation as pathways to refractoriness. In: Birch NJ, Padgham C, Hughes MS, eds. *Lithium in medicine and biology.* Lancashire, UK: Marius Press; 1993:71–84.

50. Post RM, Leverich GS, Rosoff AS, Altshuler LL. Carbamazepine prophylaxis in refractory affective disorders. A focus on long-term followup. *J Clin Psychopharmacol* 1990;10:318–327.

51. Post RM, Rubinow DR, Ballenger JC. Conditioning and sensitization in the longitudinal course of affective illness. *Br J Psychiatry* 1986;149:191–201.

52. Post RM, Weiss SRB. Endogenous biochemical abnormalities in affective illness: therapeutic vs. pathogenic. *Biol Psychiatry* 1992;32:469–484.

53. Post RM, Weiss SRB, Chuang D-M. Mechanisms of action of anticonvulsants in affective disorders: comparisons with lithium. *J Clin Psychopharmacol* 1992;12:23S–35S.

54. Post RM, Weiss SRB, Fontana D, Pert A. Conditioned sensitization to the psychomotor stimulant cocaine. *Ann NY Acad Sci* 1992;654:386–399.

55. Post RM, Weiss SRB, Pert A. Animal models of mania. In: Willner P, Scheel-Kruger J, eds. *The mesolimbic dopamine system: from motivation to action.* Chichester: John Wiley; 1991:443–472.

56. Post RM, Weiss SRB, Rosen J, Smith M, Thomas N, Pert A. Comorbidity of cocaine abuse and affective disorders. *Am J Psychiatry* [*submitted*].

57. Racine RJ. Modification of seizure activity by electrical stimulation. I. After-discharge threshold. *Electroencephalogr Clin Neurophysiol* 1972;32:269–279.

58. Rasmussen H. The cycling of calcium as an intracellular messenger. *Sci Am* 1989;261:66–73.

59. Rawlings SR, Hoyland J, Mason WT. Calcium homeostasis in bovine somatotrophs: calcium oscillations and calcium regulation by growth hormone-releasing hormone and somatostatin. *Cell Calcium* 1991;12:403–414.

60. Rosen JB, Abramowitz J, Post RM. Co-localization of TRH mRNA and Fos-like immunoreactivity in limbic structures following amygdala kindling. *Mol Cell Neurosci* 1993;4:335–342.

61. Rosen JB, Cain CJ, Weiss SRB, Post RM. Alterations in mRNA of enkephalin, dynorphin and thyrotropin releasing hormone during amygdala kindling: an in situ hybridization study. *Mol Brain Res* 1992;15:247–255.

62. Rouillon F. Adverse drug reaction in long term antidepressant treatment. *Eur Neuropsychopharmacol* 1991;1:216–218.

63. Roy-Byrne PP, Uhde TW, Post RM. Antidepressant effects of one night's sleep deprivation: clinical and theoretical implications. In: Post RM, Ballenger JC, eds. *Neurobiology of mood disorders.* Baltimore: Williams & Wilkins; 1984:817–835.

64. Rubinow DR, Post RM, Davis CL. Somatostatin. In: Nemeroff CB, ed. *Neuropeptides and psychiatric disorders.* Washington, DC: American Psychiatric Press; 1991:30–49.

65. Sakai S, Baba H, Sato M, Wada JA. Effect of DN-1417 on photosensitivity and cortically kindled seizure in Senegalese baboons, *Papio papio. Epilepsia* 1991;32:16–21.

66. Smith M, Weiss SRB, Abedin T, Post RM, Gold P. Effects of amygdala-kindling and electroconvulsive seizures on the expression of corticotropin releasing hormone (CRH) mRNA in the rat brain. *Mol Cell Neurosci* 1991;2:103–116.

67. Smith MA, Banerjee S, Gold PW, Glowa J. Induction of c-*fos* mRNA in rat brain by conditioned and unconditioned stressors. *Brain Res* 1992;578:135–141.

68. Suppes T, Baldessarini RJ, Faedda GL, Tohen M. Risk of recurrence following discontinuation of lithium treatment in bipolar disorder. *Arch Gen Psychiatry* 1991;48:1082–1088.

69. Sutula TP, Golarai G, Cavazos J. Assessing the functional significance of mossy fiber sprouting. *Epilepsy Res Suppl* 1992;7:251–259.

70. Wehr TA, Goodwin FK. Do antidepressants cause mania? *Psychopharmacol Bull* 1987;23:61–65.

71. Weiss SRB, Post RM. Contingent tolerance to carbamazepine: a peripheral-type benzodiazepine mechanism. *Eur J Pharmacol* 1991;193:159–163.

72. Weiss SRB, Post RM. Development and reversal of conditioned inefficacy and tolerance to the anticonvulsant effects of carbamazepine. *Epilepsia* 1991;32:140–145.

73. Weiss SRB, Post RM. Sensitization and kindling: the hidden liabilities of cocaine. *Scientific Am* [*in press*].

74. Weiss SRB, Post RM, Anthony P, Ferrer J. Contingent tolerance to carbamazepine is not affected by calcium-channel or NMDA-receptor blockers. *Pharmacol Biochem Behav* 1993;45:439–443.

75. Weiss SRB, Post RM, Costello M, Nutt DJ, Tandeciarz S. Carbamazepine retards the development of cocaine-kindled seizures but not sensitization to cocaine's effects on hyperactivity and stereotypy. *Neuropsychopharmacology* 1990;3:273–281.

76. Weiss SRB, Post RM, Pert A, Woodward R, Murman D. Context-dependent cocaine sensitization: differential effect of haloperidol on development versus expression. *Pharmacol Biochem Behav* 1989;34:655–661.

77. Weiss SRB, Post RM, Sohn E, Berger A, Lewis R. Cross tolerance between carbamazepine and valproate on amygdala-kindled seizures. *Epilepsy Res* [*in press*].

78. White FJ, Henry DJ, Hu X-T, Jeziorski M, Ackerman JM. Electrophysiological effects of cocaine in the mesoaccumbens dopamine system. In: Lakoski JM, Galloway MP, White FJ, eds. *Cocaine: pharmacology, physiology and clinical strategies.* West Caldwell, NJ: Telford Press, 1992:261–293.

79. Wu JC, Bunney WE. The biological basis of an antidepressant response to sleep deprivation and relapse: review and hypothesis. *Am J Psychiatry* 1990;147:14–21.

80. Yatsugi S, Yamamoto M. Anticonvulsive properties of YM-14673, a new TRH analogue, in amygdaloid-kindled rats. *Pharmacol Biochem Behav* 1991;38:669–672.

81. Young ST, Porrino LJ, Iadarola MJ. Cocaine induces striatal c-*fos* immunoreactive proteins via dopaminergic D1 receptors. *Proc Natl Acad Sci USA* 1991;88:1291–1295.

Psychopharmacology: The Fourth Generation of Progress, edited by Floyd E. Bloom and David J. Kupfer. Raven Press, Ltd., New York 1995.

CHAPTER 98

Neurodevelopmental Perspectives on Schizophrenia

Daniel R. Weinberger

A dramatic conceptual shift in thinking about the neurobiology of schizophrenia has taken place since the previous volume in this series. After many decades of speculation that schizophrenia occurs because of cerebral pathological events that happen or are expressed around early adult life, it has recently become *de rigeur* to refer to schizophrenia as a neurodevelopmental disorder in which the primary cerebral insult or pathological process occurs during brain development long before the illness is clinically manifest (14,20,52,71).

The reasons for this shift are primarily threefold: scientific data confirming adult onset pathological cerebral changes have remained elusive; replicable evidence implicating cortical maldevelopment has emerged; and neurobiological models that may explain the relationship between such maldevelopment and the clinical features of the illness exist. This chapter reviews several issues underlying this conceptual reorientation of schizophrenia (see Chapters 59 and 60, *this volume* for background).

DEVELOPMENTAL NEUROPATHOLOGY

An association between putative abnormalities in intrauterine development and schizophrenia has been reported throughout this century. The evidence ranges from highly circumstantial and weak (e.g., slight overrepresentation of minor physical anomalies) to compelling (e.g., replicated cytoarchitectural anomalies). When viewed in total, the evidence might be interpreted to weave a coherent story of developmental abnormalities; however, individual findings show many inconsistencies and methodological

problems. The most important research questions at present are whether evidence of cytoarchitectural deviations can be more widely replicated and whether lingering methodological uncertainties can be resolved. If these questions are answered positively, most of the research controversies and theoretical speculation considered below (e.g., obstetrical complications, pruning defects) will be irrelevant, because a "smoking gun" will have been found.

Minor Physical Anomalies

Because abnormal intrauterine events might be expected to affect the development of extracerebral tissues, reports of somatic morphological variations are of potential relevance. The spectrum of potential minor physical anomalies (MPA) and their relationship to abnormal brain development is not clearly defined. In the schizophrenia literature, there is no consistent pattern of associations, and often the samples have to be broken down post hoc into putative subgroups for any associations to be found (68). Many different anomalies have been reported, including high palate, low set ears, webbed digits, and variations in limb length and angle, finger print patterns and ridge counts. Proponents of the relevance of MPAs have stressed that many of these abnormalities are seen as a result of second-trimester insults, timing that is consistent with a putative defect in neuronal migration. They also stress that MPAs are seen in other neurodevelopmental disorders such as intrauterine viral encephalopathies and in other psychiatric disorders of presumed developmental origin (e.g., autism) (68).

However, the circumstantial nature of these arguments does not obscure problems with the fundamental data base. The true frequency of MPAs in patients with schizo-

D. R. Weinberger: Clinical Brain Disorders Branch, Intramural Research Program, National Institute of Mental Health, National Institutes of Health, Washington, DC 20032.

phrenia is not known, as large unselected samples of patients and well-matched controls have not been studied. Whether all the morphological characteristics reported are actually pathological is also uncertain. Moreover, few of the studies have used the same methods of assessment, and it is uncertain if any of the studies were truly blind comparisons. The studies that report increases in MPAs tend to lump them all together as if each signified the same thing, when, in fact, their relative frequencies seem not to correlate with each other (68). Because the search for MPAs has not been a centerpiece of schizophrenia research, it is doubtful that investigators who failed to find MPAs in their samples reported the negative results. Another uncertainty is that the timing of events that cause MPAs is not well established, and considerable variability exists. In light of these questions and other contradictory data [e.g., no difference in MPAs within pairs of discordant monozygotic twins (68), no consistent abnormalities in birth weights of schizophrenic births compared with healthy sibling births (48), and no relationship of MPAs to birth weight or other clinical signs of intrauterine adversity (48,68)], the relevance of MPAs to understanding potential cerebral maldevelopment in schizophrenia is weak.

Premorbid Neurological Abnormalities

If the brains of patients with schizophrenia have not developed normally, it might be expected that some evidence of subtle abnormalities of neural function would be apparent during their childhood before they become clinically ill. Several lines of circumstantial data support this possibility. Studies of premorbid neuropsychological test performance and school achievement have tended to report that individuals who later manifest schizophrenia did worse than their healthy siblings. Reports of no difference have also appeared (68). Four series of reports of high-risk subjects, that is children with at least one schizophrenic parent, have found various abnormalities of motor function (31,51), autonomic responsivity (51), and attention (6,27). The abnormalities vary somewhat from one study to another and are not linked with schizophrenia per se. Fish et al. (31) have provided a detailed description of what they refer to as a *pandysmaturational defect* in high-risk children, consisting of gross abnormalities of gait, posture, muscle tone, and reflexes in early childhood. It is uncertain how representative these relatively dramatic findings are of most children who subsequently manifest the illness. Moreover, the findings disappear to some degree over time, further complicating their interpretation. Finally, Walker and colleagues (70) recently reported a novel study of home movies of families having a child who later developed schizophrenia. In a blind comparison of affected and unaffected siblings in four sibships, they reported clear differences in bimanual dexterity, in gait,

and in other gross motor functions that allowed them to invariably identify the affected family member even in the first few years of life. To clinicians, the severity of the observations of Fish and the severity and consistency of the observations of Walker et al. may seem surprising. Clearly, further replication is needed. Nevertheless, the results of these studies, although open to other interpretations, are consistent with the possibility of brain-maldevelopment.

Cerebral Morphometric Abnormalities

In Vivo Studies

Beginning in 1976 with an in vivo study of cerebral ventricular size using computerized axial tomography (CAT) scanning (63), literally hundreds of reports have appeared of subtle variations in cerebral anatomy associated with schizophrenia. The CAT data base established that as a group patients with schizophrenia have slightly enlarged ventricles and wider cortical fissures and sulci (63). These findings suggested a nonfocal reduction in cerebral and probably cortical volume. Moreover, the data did not support the widely expressed assumption that morphological abnormalities characterized only a subgroup of patients. Instead, they seemed to describe a continuum of pathological change (22,63) that characterized the majority of the patient population. Recently, using magnetic resonance imaging (MRI), which produces images of much greater contrast and resolution, the CAT data have been confirmed and refined. Evidence of cortical volume loss, most frequently replicated in but not confined to mesial temporal cortex in the area of the rostral hippocampus, has been a relatively consistent finding (74). Again, the data do not implicate only a subgroup of patients (66,74).

In some studies, evidence of pathological changes appears to favor the left side of the brain. This has been especially true for the size of the ventricles (20) and for the volume of the superior temporal gyrus (64). Reports of relatively greater reductions in other regions of the left temporal cortex have also appeared (66). Indeed, when asymmetric findings have been reported, they usually involve the left hemisphere. This has prompted some to suggest that this lateralization tendency is consistent with a putative delay in the development of the left hemisphere during the second trimester, leaving it more vulnerable to adverse events that might otherwise affect the brain diffusely (20). This is an interesting hypothesis, but it depends on a number of assumptions and probably overinterprets the morphometric literature. Whether the slight delay in the appearance of surface gyri means that the left hemisphere is developing slower or that it is more vulnerable to injury or vulnerable for a longer period is unknown. Moreover, most of the morphometric studies, even those that report unilateral findings (20,64,66), have observed bilateral changes as well.

Although in vivo evidence of subtle morphometric deviations might implicate a neuropathological process as being related to schizophrenia, it does not by itself implicate a neurodevelopmental one. However, beginning with the results of the second CAT study of schizophrenia, the correlative data have not been consistent with what would be expected of a degenerative condition of adult onset and have been consistent with what would be expected of a neurodevelopmental one. In particular, in the majority of cross-sectional studies, ventricular size has been found not to correlate with duration of illness (63), as would have been expected if the neuropathological process responsible for ventricular enlargement advanced as the illness progressed. More recently, lack of progression has been confirmed by prospective studies that have followed the same individuals for up to 10 years from the first psychotic episode (38). Thus, it appears that, for most patients, the pathological process responsible for the in vivo morphometric changes associated with schizophrenia has arrested at least by the time their clinical illness is diagnosed.

Circumstantial and correlational evidence that the pathological process might have arrested early in life if not during early development also emerged from in vivo imaging studies. Ventricular enlargement has been found in most studies of patients at the onset of the clinical illness in early adulthood (15,24,63) and reduced hippocampal volume has been observed in at least one first-break study (15). This suggests that these findings do not develop during the early phases of illness and probably predate the onset of the illness. Several, although not all, studies have found an unexpected correlation between ventricular enlargement in patients with schizophrenia and poor premorbid social and educational adjustment during early childhood (26,40,63). This finding further suggests the possibility that the morbid pathology had occurred early in life and manifested itself in different ways at different times of life.

Postmortem Studies

Data from postmortem morphometric studies of brains of patients who died with schizophrenia are generally consistent with the conclusions from the in vivo studies (63). In general, volumetric assessments of cerebral ventricular size (20,55), of various cortical regions, the hippocampal formation (including the parahippocampal cortex), and of various periventricular subcortical nucleii have found differences between patients and normals (3,39,55,63). Likewise, neuronal counts have been reported to be reduced in patients in selected cortical and periventricular regions (12,20,29). These studies, like the in vivo studies, implicate a fairly widespread neuropatho-

logical process. It should be noted, however, that there have also been negative reports (35), and the reasons for the inconsistencies are unclear.

One observation that has been consistent is lack of gliosis. In fact, it was the absence of gliosis that prompted many classical neuropathologists during the first half of the twentieth century to dismiss reports of neuropathological changes in schizophrenic brain specimens. Recent studies, whether in neocortex (60,63), hippocampus (60), or parahippocampal cortex (29), have not found evidence of either acute or chronic gliosis. Because proliferation of glial cells is seen in most degenerative brain conditions and encephalopathies that arise after birth, this negative result would seem more consistent with neuropathological events that predate the responsivity of glial cells to injury, which is before the third trimester of gestation.

It is also interesting to note that, as in the in vivo morphometry data, correlational results are not consistent with a neuropathological process that progresses once the illness has manifested. Ventricular size and cortical volume have not been correlated with duration of illness (20,55). Pakkenberg (55) reported, moreover, that ventricular size did not correlate with cognitive deficits noted in the hospital records at the time of death, but instead, correlated with those noted at the time of onset of the illness. This curious finding is more consistent with an underlying pathological defect that set the neurobiological stage for an illness rather than one that evolved over the course of the illness.

Anomalous Lateralization

The possibility that normally lateralized aspects of the brain might be anomalous in patients with schizophrenia has come from several experimental directions. Studies of lateralized cerebral function, such as handedness, dichotic listening asymmetries, and lateralized cognitive tasks, have suggested that patients with schizophrenia may be less completely lateralized than normal individuals (20). If these functional asymmetries are related to mechanisms of the development of normal anatomical asymmetries, the findings may have implications for abnormal cerebral development in schizophrenia. Since the times when many of the well-characterized normal anatomical asymmetries originate are known; the time of developmental disruption might be inferred.

Although some in vivo imaging studies have reported diminished asymmetry of the widths of the occipital lobes, at least as many have failed to replicate this finding (63). Such inconsistency appears to characterize the majority of the other literature on cerebral anatomical asymmetries in schizophrenia. For example, some groups have reported less asymmetry of normally asymmetric perisylvian structures, such as the sylvian fissure (28) and the planum temporale (61), but other groups have failed to replicate these findings (8,44). Based on a finding of asymmetry of the ventricles seen in two-dimensional x-ray films of postmortem brain specimens, Crow et al. (20) went so far as to hypothesize that schizophrenia is caused by a gene that controls the normal development of temporal lobe asymmetries. A test of this hypothesis in a sample of discordant monozygotic twins, where the abnormalities of asymmetry would be expected in the unaffected twin as well as in the affected twin, has been negative (8).

In summary, notwithstanding the uncertainties about lateralization, the data from morphometric studies, in general, have a considerable degree of internal consistency and lead to the interpretation of neurodevelopmental deviance, most likely occurring before the end of the second trimester. The strongest feature of the morphometric data is its replicability. Moreover, the weight of the evidence does not fit into the model of adult-onset brain disorders. Unfortunately, measurements of the size of various cerebral structures and counts of cell numbers are not conclusive evidence of any neuropathological condition, developmental or otherwise, and could conceivably be accounted for by other explanations (e.g., nonpathological volume changes on in vivo scanning due to dehydration or coincidental neuronal loss or other artifacts unrelated to illness in postmortem studies, which usually involve elderly subjects). The possibility that the development of normal anatomical asymmetries is disrupted in patients with schizophrenia also is inconclusive and does not necessarily implicate a neuropathological condition. The most conceptually unimpeachable evidence comes from qualitative studies of cytoarchitecture.

Cytoarchitectural Abnormalities

The laminar patterns of neurons in cortex, the orientation of neurons, and their internal relationships are fixed during the second trimester of birth. It is generally assumed that such relationships and patterns do not change during life, even if cells are lost or if secondary pathological conditions arise. If this assumption is correct, and this is not certain, then abnormalities of cytoarchitecture would strongly implicate pathological development.

Kovelman and Sheibel reported in 1984 (43) that the orientation of hippocampal pyramidal cells in nissl stained sections of left hemispheres from ten patients with chronic schizophrenia was abnormal in most of the specimens as compared with eight normal controls. Conrad et al. (19) subsequently reported the identical finding in the right hemispheres of mostly the same subjects. They interpreted their findings as consistent with a defect in neural migration, arguing that disorientation reflected a fault of neuronal settling into their target sites. This finding has not been independently replicated, and negative studies have been reported (4,18).

In contrast to the data on pyramidal cell orientation,

the data on laminar organization in neocortex and limbic cortex are more consistent, although still far from ideal. Jakob and Beckman (37) made a potentially landmark observation in the entorhinal cortex. In nissl stained sections of the brains of 64 patients with the diagnosis of schizophrenia and 10 controls, they reported that in the majority of ill cases there were cytoarchitectural anomalies of laminar organization. Specifically, they described attenuation of cellularity in superficial layers I and II, incomplete clustering of neurons into normal glomerular structures in layer II, and the inclusion of such clusters in deeper layers where they are not normally found. They studied the rostral entorhinal cortex in the region of the amygdala and pes hippocampus. Interestingly, this is similar to the area of mesial temporal cortex where the most consistent morphometric abnormalities have been found both in vivo and postmortem (3,15,29,39,66). They interpreted their findings as the result of a failure of cortical development, probably an arrest of migration, whereby relatively recent generation neurons destined for the superficial cortical lamina were held up in deeper layers. Perhaps the most compelling aspect of their observations is that these findings are difficult if not impossible to attribute to an insult that occurred to an already developed brain. The three major uncertainties about their findings are as follows: (a) Are they artifacts of localization within the entorhinal cortex? (b) Are they related to schizophrenia per se? (c) Are they replicable? Other problems with the study included that it was not blind, that the controls were neurologically impaired in nine of the cases, and that the patient population was probably atypical (e.g., mean age of illness onset was 36).

Normal entorhinal cortex anatomy is characterized by remarkable regional variability. In fact, as one moves caudal in the entorhinal cortex, the normal appearance looks increasingly like what Jakob and Beckman reported in schizophrenia. Therefore, it is critical that patients and controls be very carefully examined in the same cytoarchitectonic areas. The possibility that what Jakob and Beckman observed may not be related to schizophrenia per se also must be considered. They subsequently reported the identical abnormalities in four patients with bipolar disorder, although two of these patients had originally been diagnosed with schizophrenia (10).

In spite of these questions, the basic findings of Jakob and Beckman have been independently replicated using the same methods and further supported by other recent data from different approaches to cortical cytoarchitecture. Arnold et al. (5) studied nissl-stained sections of six brains of patients with schizophrenia from the Yakovlev Collection and 16 controls. They observed essentially the same abnormalities as described by Jakob and Beckman and in addition reported anomalous mesial temporal sulci in their specimens. They felt that all six cases were abnormal, but in five the abnormalities were dramatic and unequivocal. None of their controls had similar findings. The authors acknowledged the importance of location within entorhinal cortex and attempted to control for this. Moreover, they reported that as they moved caudally, the differences between patients and controls disappeared, an observation that again corresponds to reports from the morphometric literature. The authors believed that their findings indicated an abnormality of entorhinal cortex development, probably a migration failure, that would render normal neocortical-hippocampal communication impossible. In addition to its small sample size, this study suffered from one other obvious problem. The entire patient sample had undergone prefrontal leukotomies. To control for the possible effect of this, they had included three controls who underwent leukotomy for nonpsychiatric indications (e.g., chronic pain). Although the potential confound of leukotomy cannot be conclusively ruled out by this control group, it is difficult to imagine how the pattern of changes could be explained by this procedure.

Akbarian and colleagues (1) took a different approach to studying cytoarchitecture, but their results suggest the same defect as do those of Jakob and Beckman and Arnold et al. Using a histochemical stain for cortical neurons that express the enzyme, nicotinamide adenine dinucleotide diaphorase (NADPH-diaphorase), a neuronal population said to be remnants of the embryological subplate zone, they studied the superior frontal gyrus region of the dorsolateral prefrontal cortex in the brains of five patients with schizophrenia and five controls matched for age, gender, and postmortem interval before fixation. They found reduced numbers of these neurons in superficial cortical layers I, II, and III and increased numbers in deep layers, especially in subcortical white matter, the putative vestigial subplate neurons. In essence, they observed a qualitative shift in the representation of NADPH-diaphorase positive neurons, as if the younger neurons destined to migrate last from the subplate zone got held up and never made it to their superficial cortical targets. The interpretations of the findings are remarkably similar to those of Jakob and Beckman and Arnold et al.

It is also possible that the underlying defect reflected in the findings of Akbarian and colleagues is the same as that of yet another recent report, a study of nissl sections of frontal cortex by Benes et al. (12). They found decreased numbers of small presumably γ-aminobutyric acid-ergic (GABA-ergic) neurons in prefrontal cortex of patients with schizophrenia and larger numbers of pyramidal cells in deeper layers. This finding also might suggest a failure of completion of the normal inside-out migratory gradient. The potential coherence of these two studies may be underscored by the fact that NADPH-diaphorase positive neurons appear to be GABA-ergic. Unfortunately, there are some inconsistencies. Subsequent cell counts of small presumably GABA-ergic neurons in nissl-stained sections of the samples of Akbarian et al. could not directly confirm the finding of Benes et al. of a reduction in the small neuron population (16).

In a subsequent study of the NADPH-diaphorase neurons of the temporal lobe, including the lateral temporal neocortex and the mesial limbic cortex, Akbarian and colleagues (2) extended their abnormal findings to this region, suggesting a more widespread cortical developmental defect. This also would be consistent with the morphometric data. However, this second study presented some new inconsistencies. Although they did find gradient abnormalities in the hippocampus and lateral temporal neocortex, the entorhinal cortex was normal. It is conceivable that the abnormalities of the entorhinal cortex observed by Jakob and Beckman and by Arnold et al. did not involve the subset of neurons that express NADPH-diaphorase. This might be consistent with the latter neurons being primarily GABA-ergic and the layer II entorhinal cortex neurons being primarily glutamatergic. On the other hand, the involvement of NADPH-diaphorase neurons in each of the other cortical areas examined by Akbarian et al. make this explanation seem a bit strained. It also should be noted that the small sample size of the Akbarian et al. studies necessitated a matched-pair statistical analysis. It is unclear whether the findings would have held up if the matching had been done differently. Clearly, further studies of this type are needed before these uncertainties can be resolved.

In summary, if one looks at the research data base about brain abnormalities in schizophrenia as a whole, the most coherent impression is of subtle multifocal or diffuse anatomical deviations that predate the onset of the illness and are static, that are most consistent with the notion of a developmental defect, and that may implicate a failure of second-trimester neuronal migration leading to cortical maldevelopment. The most potentially incriminating evidence comes from studies of cortical cytoarchitecture. The possibility of cortical maldevelopment in the second trimester is also critical to a discussion of the additional speculation about neurodevelopmental factors and models that follows.

ETIOLOGICAL CONSIDERATIONS

Obstetrical Abnormalities

The possibility that obstetrical complications (OC) could contribute to or even cause schizophrenia has been the subject of a surprisingly large number of investigations over the past three decades. The literature on this issue is difficult to interpret, as the same methods are rarely used, the same findings are rarely reported, and the implications of the data are rarely critically addressed (68). Nevertheless, the weight of the evidence suggests that there is a statistical association between OCs and schizophrenia (68). An overview of the recent literature in which obstetrical histories of patients were compared with that of their unaffected siblings is shown in Tables

TABLE 1. *Obstetrical complications in adult schizophrenics and sibling controls*

Study	Samples	Recall/records	Findings[a]
Pollack et al. (57)	33 patients 33 sibs	recall	n.s. differences
Woerner et al. (73)	52 patients 54 sibs	both	↑ OCs in schizophrenia and other abnormal sibs
McCreadie et al. (47)	54 patients 114 sibs	recall	no differences
DeLisi et al. (23)	123 patients 148 sibs	recall	↑ OCs
Eagles et al. (25)	27 patients 27 sibs	records	↑ OCs

[a] n.s., not significant; OCs, obstetrical complications; ↑, increase.

1 and 2. Sibship studies are particularly important because uncertainty about the validity of maternal recall is less problematic. Although the twin studies tend to be less conclusive, perhaps because twin pregnancies are often complicated, the sibling data suggest an association.

The controversial aspects of the OC literature concern the specific nature of the complications themselves [e.g., prenatal or delivery, (48)], their neuropathological correlations, and their overall significance. The neuropathological implications that have been attributed to OCs are difficult to reconcile with the neuropathological findings associated with schizophrenia. Murray et al. (52) and Mednick et al. (49) have suggested that OCs result in periventricular hemorrhages, hypoxic-ischemic injury, and ultimately abnormalities of pruning, cell death, and developmental connectivity. McNeil (48) also suggests that delivery complications result in brain damage by virtue of hypoxic-ischemic injury. Such injuries are typically characterized by gliosis and could not account for the cytoarchitectural changes described above, which presumably occur at least 3 months before delivery. If cytoarchitectural abnormalities and lack of gliosis are a neuropathological signature of schizophrenia, it is virtually certain that these occur independent of delivery events. Other inconsistencies in the OC literature have to do with the overall pathogenic significance of the findings. Mednick and colleagues have proposed that OCs are related to genetic risk for schizophrenia and that somehow the gene for schizophrenic liability increases the neuropathological effects of OCs, including of anesthesia used during delivery (17,49). This complex hypothesis emerged as a result of correlational data from arbitrarily defined patient subgroups, when in fact, these investigators did not find an absolute increase of OCs in their entire sample of patients with schizophrenia (56) or in their entire high-risk population (17). Moreover, the interpretation of OCs being related to increased genetic risk is exactly the opposite interpretation of Murray et al. (52), who argued from their data that OCs are especially relevant to nongenetic forms of schizophrenia.

A sober perspective on the OC literature and the pathogenic implications of OCs was offered by Goodman (34) in an enlightening critique of the subject. He pointed out that even if one accepts the frequency data, OCs increase the risk of schizophrenia by, at most, 1%. Moreover, OCs are much more common in certain environments, but the frequency of schizophrenia does not parallel this geographical and cultural distribution. Thus, OCs appear to be poor predictors of schizophrenia. Finally, he suggested that a more likely scenario for a relationship between OCs and schizophrenia was that the latter caused the former, and not the other way around. It has become increasingly apparent, as first proposed by Freud in reference to cerebral palsy, that preexisting fetal abnormalities predispose to OCs. This synthesis of the OC literature also would be more compatible with the neuropathological data.

Prenatal Viral Exposure

Another potential cause of developmental injury that has occasionally been considered as a pathogenic factor

TABLE 2. *Obstetrical complications in twins with schizoprenia*

Study	Samples	Recall/records	Findings
Torrey et al. (68)	26 discordant pairs	recall	no differences between affected and unaffected
Pollin and Stabeneau (58)	100 discordant pairs	both	↑ OCs[b] in affected twin
Reveley et al. (59)	21 schizophrenic MZ[a] pairs 18 normal MZ pairs	recall	Complex interactions with family history
Onstad et al. (54)	16 discordant pairs 8 concordant pairs	recall	no differences

[a] MZ, monozygotic.
[b] OCs, obstetrical complications.

in schizophrenia is prenatal viral exposure. Recently, interest in this potential etiology has mushroomed as a result of a remarkable result reported by Mednick and colleagues (50) in 1988. They examined the hospital admission records of 1781 adult individuals in Finland, some of whom were born around the time of the Helsinki influenza A-2 epidemic of 1957 (the index cases) and others who were born before the epidemic (control cases). They found that both males and females who had been in their second trimester of gestation during the height of the epidemic had a significantly higher percentage of subsequent admission diagnoses of schizophrenia than either the control cases or the index cases exposed during other trimesters. The implications were that influenza itself or a related phenomena (e.g., fever) interfered with second-trimester brain development and that such interference was an etiological risk factor for schizophrenia. This study has spawned at least six other studies (summarized in Table 3), opening a new area of research controversy. While there have been positive reports supporting the findings of Mednick and colleagues, negative reports are virtually as frequent, and methodological uncertainties cloud the interpretation of the results.

Kendell and Kemp (42) compared hospital admission records throughout Scotland of individuals who had been in utero during the influenza A epidemics of 1918–1919 and 1957. Although they did find an increased risk of schizophrenia for those in the second trimester in 1957 in a sample from Edinburgh, the overall Scottish admission data revealed no such effect. These authors tended to dismiss the Edinburgh data and emphasized their negative findings. Moreover, they have argued that a reanalysis of the data of Mednick et al. using absolute numbers of patients with schizophrenia rather than proportions of such patients relative to other diagnoses is also negative (41).

Subsequent studies have only added to the controversy. Torrey et al. (66) looked at a large birth cohort in the United States and found no association of increased risk with the U.S. influenza A-2 epidemic of 1957. Barr et al. (7) attempted to replicate the study of Mednick et al. (50) in a Danish sample. Regrettably, they chose a different approach to data collection and analysis. They collected hospital admission data about all patients in Denmark with a diagnosis of schizophrenia born between 1911 and 1951, divided them into three groups based on the relative frequency of influenza infections in the general population during their birth month as recorded in public health infectious disease records, and analyzed the birth-rate data as a deviation score from the expected schizophrenia birth rate for a particular month. This complex analysis was justified as an attempt to control for spurious associations that might result from seasonal variations in influenza exposure and in schizophrenia birth rates. The authors reported that in the high seasonal influenza exposure subgroup, those exposed during the sixth month of gestation had the highest rates of schizophrenia. Unfortunately, the data also appear to show that the other two groups have lower than expected schizophrenia birthrates during the same month (i.e., the sixth) of gestation. Moreover, it appears, although this analysis is not reported, that unless the tripartite approach to subgrouping is used, there is no overall association between schizophrenia birth rate and exposure to influenza A-2. Indeed, the authors acknowledge that even in their positive subgroup, the association between schizophrenia and influenza is weak, accounting for at most 4% of the variance.

Another example of the confusing nature of this litera-

TABLE 3. Prenatal influenza and adult schizophrenia

Study	Sample	Findings[a]
Mednick et al. (50)	pregnancies coincident with Helsinki 1957 A-2 epidemic	↑ in schizophrenia in second-trimester cohort, especially at 6th months' gestation
Kendell and Kemp (42)	pregnancies coincident with Scottish 1918, 1991, and 1957 A-2 epidemics	↑ in Edinburgh samples for 1957, second trimester. No ↑ association in entire sample
Torrey et al. (65)	43,814 schizophrenic births between 1950–1959 in USA	No ↑ in association with 1957 A-2
Barr et al. (7)	Danish schizophrenic samples born between 1911 and 1950 (N = 7239)	↑ in schizophrenia in 6 to 7-month gestational group coincident with high incidence of influenza compared with group coincident with low incidence
O'Callaghan et al. (53)	339 schizophrenic patients born around English 1957 A-2 epidemic	abnormal distribution of schizophrenia births in index year in women only, *appearance* of ↑ in risk in 5th gestational month
Sham et al. (59)	British Hospital First Admission between 1970–1979 with schizophrenia, N not specified	weak statistical association between frequency pattern of influenza deaths between 1939 and 1960 and second trimester of schizophrenic births
Crow and Done (21)	1620 pregnancies with history of 1957 A-2 influenza infection in Great Britain	no increased risk of schizophrenia

[a] ↑, increase.

ture is the study by O'Callaghan et al. (53). These investigators compared admission diagnoses in eight health regions of England and Wales with birth records around the time of the 1957 influenza epidemic. They reported that for patients in utero during the second trimester (especially the fifth month) "the number of births of individuals who later developed schizophrenia was 88% higher" than expected. In fact, what they actually found was that the overall monthly distribution of affected births (i.e., subsequent schizophrenia) was different in the exposure and the control years. Because they did not perform post hoc tests on individual months, they did not statistically determine which month(s) accounted for the overall distribution differences. Indeed, their data also show a peak at around 3 months and a trough at around 8 months, both of which may have been important factors in the overall distribution analysis. In a related study, Sham et al. (62) examined the numbers of first-time admissions with a diagnosis of schizophrenia throughout England and Wales from 1970 to 1979 and compared them to the number of deaths from influenza during the period 1930 to 1969. Arguing that the latter was a relative index of likelihood of influenza exposure in utero for the former, they found a statistical relationship using a complex model-fitting paradigm of the two frequency distributions, with greatest correspondence during the third and seventh months of gestation. The data suggested, however, that at most 1% to 2% of schizophrenic births could be explained by this relationship.

An important limitation of each of the perinatal exposure studies is that none of them documented actual maternal, let alone, intrauterine infection. In the only study to attempt this, Crow and Done (21) investigated psychiatric admissions of individuals born around the 1957 epidemic who had been enrolled in a perinatal injury and child development research project in England. They identified 945 individuals whose mothers had been diagnosed during their second trimester of pregnancy as having influenza. They did not find an increased risk of subsequent schizophrenia in the offspring of these mothers.

In summary, the perinatal viral exposure literature is provocative but inconclusive. The reasons for the inconsistencies are uncertain, and it is doubtful that they will be resolved in the near future. Even if the inconsistencies can be resolved and the positive results prevail, exposure to influenza will account for at most a small minority of cases. Moreover, although the positive results may add circumstantially to the notion that second-trimester maldevelopment increases the risk of schizophrenia, the mechanisms by which this happens will be difficult to establish from epidemiological studies of potential viral exposure.

Other Etiological Factors

Because of the possibility that neural development may be disrupted by a number of adverse environmental events

in addition to viral exposure, other causes have been considered. For example, in a recent study of the potential impact of maternal malnutrition, Susser and Lin (67) studied the effects of starvation in occupied Holland during World War II and found that first- but not second-trimester starvation was associated with increased risk of schizophrenic births. Because the implications of this finding for the neuropathological changes associated with schizophrenia are unclear, if not contradictory, this study is difficult to integrate with the rest of the neurodevelopmental data base. Also, this study did not control for the implications of social class both on access to food and on risk for schizophrenia.

In light of the widely accepted data that genetic factors convey susceptibility to schizophrenia, it is not surprising that there has been speculation about genetic factors that may affect brain development in schizophrenia. Approximately 30% of the genome is expressed in brain, and many genes are turned on and off during discrete phases of brain development; therefore, there are many potential candidates. No existing data link schizophrenia with a defect in any known gene related to brain development. Nevertheless, Murray et al. (52) have hypothesized that the fundamental neuropathological deviations in the schizophrenic brain arise because of a primary genetic defect in at least a substantial subgroup of patients. Mednick et al. (49) have hypothesized that a genetic defect predisposes the schizophrenic brain to being adversely affected by intrauterine or perinatal environmental events. These hypotheses and undoubtedly many others that will be advanced must await the discovery and practicability of scientific methods to test them.

MECHANISMS OF DELAYED ONSET

The possibility that schizophrenia is related to an abnormality of early brain development poses yet another interesting challenge, for the clinical expression of the illness is delayed typically for about two decades after birth. If the neurological abnormality is present at birth, why is the illness itself not manifested earlier in life and what accounts for its predictable clinical expression in early adulthood? Speculation about the answers to these questions has come primarily from two perspectives: (a) the possibility of an additional pathological process occurring around the time of onset of the clinical illness; and (b) an interaction between a static developmental defect and normal developmental programs or events that occur in early adult life.

As the foremost proponent of the first perspective, Feinberg (30) focused on the age of onset of schizophrenia as a clue to neurodevelopmental abnormalities that might explain the illness. He posited that schizophrenia is caused by a defect in adolescent synaptic reorganization, because either "too many, too few, or the wrong synapses are eliminated.'' In effect, he argues for a second pathological process, a specific pathology of synaptic elimination not necessarily related to possible maldevelopment in utero. His hypothesis does not take into account the replicable neuropathological data base (most of which did not exist at the time of his original proposal), and he does not address the biological mechanisms that might be responsible for this putative disorder of synaptic elimination. In light of the neuropathological data base that implicates maldevelopment in utero, this hypothesis would require the unlikely scenario of a second primary pathology. Another problem with this hypothesis is that it is unclear how one could directly test it, especially because it accommodates all potential variations (i.e., too much, too little, or the "wrong" pruning).

An alternative scenario that might be considered is that maldevelopment in utero sets the stage for secondary synaptic disorganization that has its greatest neurobiological and clinical impact in adolescence. This integration of the neuropathological data with the Feinberg hypothesis would tend to regard irregularities of synaptic pruning as epiphenomena. It would be consistent with the notion that neuronal circuitry that is anomalous from early in development may have particularly profound implications for eventual connectivity. In other words, perhaps primary migratory or other developmental defects lead to the creation of abnormal circuits that compete successfully for survival, whereas certain normal circuits either do not form or are structurally disadvantaged, so that they cannot avoid elimination.

Other mechanisms for delayed onset that emphasize a new process going wrong around the time of clinical onset have been proposed. These include abnormalities of myelination (11), of neuronal sprouting (65), and of adverse effects of stress-related neural transmission (14). Each of these involves a variation on the theme of another abnormality taking place in early adult life. In essence, they are dual pathology hypotheses, either positing that maldevelopment in utero is not sufficient pathology, or is coincidental, or that it is only one of two relatively independent pathologies that characterize the illness.

The second perspective maintains that it might be possible to accommodate both maldevelopment in utero and delayed clinical onset without positing an additional abnormal process in adolescence. This perspective involves an interaction between cortical maldevelopment in utero and normal developmental events that occur much later (71). This view rests on several assumptions: that the clinical implications of a developmental defect vary with the maturational state of the brain; that the neural systems disrupted by the defect in early brain development in schizophrenia are normally late-maturing neural systems; and that a defect in the function of these neural systems will not be reliably apparent until their normal time of functional maturation. In other words, it is posited that certain neural systems are destined from early development to malfunction in a manner that accounts for the illness, but until a certain state of postnatal brain development they either do not malfunction to a clinically significant degree, or their malfunctioning can be compensated for by other systems. The first of these assumptions has been repeatedly validated in developmental neurobiology. Indeed, a fundamental principle of the clinical impact of developmental neuropathology is that in general early brain damage is apparent early and tends to become less so over time. The young brain has a greater capacity for functional compensation than does the old brain. It is also a fundamental principle of pediatric neurology that, in some cases, congenital brain damage can have delayed or varying clinical effects if the neural systems involved are neurologically immature at birth (71).

In the case of schizophrenia, these fundamental principles appear to be violated, in that the impact of putative early damage is less apparent early and more apparent late. In this respect, the other two assumptions of this perspective are much more speculative. It is not known whether the principle of clinical effects being delayed until the affected neural systems reach functional maturity applies to those neural systems implicated in schizophrenia. More data are needed about the neural systems that develop abnormally in schizophrenia and about their normal course of functional maturation. Nevertheless, in the absence of such data, the following speculation seems appropriate. The neuropathological data base about schizophrenia has highlighted subtle maldevelopment of the cerebral cortex. Correlative data from studies of cortical function in patients with schizophrenia, including neuropsychological testing results (32) and studies of cortical physiology using functional brain-imaging techniques (13), indicate that cortical dysfunction is a prominent characteristic of the illness and that prefrontal–temporal functional connectivity is especially impaired. Even if cortical maldevelopment is widespread, the functional neural systems that appear to be particularly relevant to the clinical characteristics of schizophrenia are those involved in prefrontal–temporal connectivity (13,72). This pattern is consistent with the developmental neuropathology reviewed above. If the function of systems that subserve such connectivity matures late, as a number of lines of evidence suggest, then this would fit the model of this perspective about delayed onset. The molecular events that account for the functional maturation of these systems are probably complex and may involve stabilization of synapses, leveling off of the growth of dendritic arbors, and other processes related to the refinement of cortical connectivity, all of which seem to plateau in early adult life.

These alternative perspectives on mechanisms of delayed onset, although differing on the question of whether neurodevelopmental processes of adolescence are abnormal, share an emphasis on cortical connectivity being abnormal, as do the in vivo imaging, neuropsychological, and postmortem data. This raises an additional problem for the explanatory power of neurodevelopmental models of schizophrenia, in that the diagnostic symptoms of the illness, that is, hallucinations and delusions, have not been classically imputed to cortical dysfunction. Moreover, it is unclear how this apparent inconsistency could be resolved by the added complexity of the neurodevelopmental frame of reference. Potential insights into these issues have come from studies of neurological illnesses associated with developmental neuropathology and psychosis and from animal models of delayed effects of perinatal injury.

NEUROBIOLOGICAL MODELS

Neurological Analogies

Hallucinations and delusions are not unique to schizophrenia. They are encountered in a number of neurological conditions, involving many areas of the brain. It has been pointed out that one of the better predictors of whether a neurological condition presents with psychosis is the age at which it presents (72). Of those disorders that may have psychopathology as a prominent symptom, psychosis is much more likely to be manifest in late adolescence and early adulthood than at other times of life. This is true even if the neuropathological changes do not vary with age. In other words, simply disrupting the neural systems related to psychosis is not necessarily sufficient to cause the syndrome. The brain needs to be at a certain state of development for the maximum likelihood of psychosis.

Metachromatic leukodystrophy (MLD) is an informative example of this age association and also of the potential importance of functional "dysconnection" of cortical regions. Hyde and colleagues (36) have demonstrated that when MLD presents between the ages of 13 and 30, it presents in the majority of cases as a schizophrenialike illness. Moreover, the clinical presentation is probably more similar to schizophrenia than is seen in any other neurological disease. Patients have disorganized thinking, act bizarrely, have complex delusions, and when hallucinated, invariably have complex, Schneiderian-type auditory hallucinations. The condition is often misdiagnosed as schizophrenia, sometimes for years, before neurological symptoms appear. Interestingly, MLD is not a disease of mesial temporal cortex or of frontal cortex. It is a pure connectivity disorder in that the neuropathological changes involve white matter connections. In its early neuropathological stages, when it is most likely to present with psychosis, the changes are especially prominent in subprefrontal white matter. This suggests that a neural dysfunction with a high valence for producing psychotic symptoms is failure of some aspects of prefrontal connec-

tivity, analogous functionally to what has been implicated in schizophrenia.

In the case of MLD, however, this functional "dysconnection" does not appear to be enough. When MLD presents outside of this critical age range, it almost never presents with psychosis, even though the location of the neuropathology is not age dependent. In other words, the involvement of critical neural systems is not by itself sufficient for the expression of psychosis. An age-related factor that appears to be independent of the illness is also required. Because this age factor transends specific illness boundaries, it is probably a function of normal postnatal brain maturation. Thus, the example of MLD supports the theoretical perspective that psychosis may reflect a cortical defect that interacts with developmental programs normally linked to a late adolescent brain.

Animal Models

The analogy of MLD suggests that a putative defect in intracortical connectivity occurring at a critical period in postnatal brain maturation may clinically manifest as psychosis. It does not, however, suggest that a defect in such connectivity existing at birth could remain clinically silent until late adolescence. Studies in animals have supported this possibility.

Goldman (33) showed that a perinatal ablation of the dorsolateral prefrontal cortex did not impair performance on delayed response tasks in animals before adolescence as a similar lesion placed in adult animals did. However, when animals with perinatal lesions of this cortical region reached adolescence, their performance on these tests actually became impaired. She suggested that prior to puberty other brain regions (e.g., the caudate) took responsibility for this behavior, but by adolescence, the brain was developmentally committed to use the cortex for this activity. In other words, the other neural strategies or systems were no longer available or were incapable of performing normally in the context of a more developed brain. She also showed that this delay in presentation of the cognitive deficit was a characteristic of some neural systems and not others. In animals with ablations of orbital frontal cortex, a phylogenetically older cortical region, deficits were manifest early in life, and if anything, they improved as the animals grew older.

Recently, Beauregard et al. (9) reported preliminary data suggesting that an analogous delay in the appearance of certain cognitive deficits can be seen after perinatal hippocampal ablations. In rhesus monkeys with selective ablations of the rostral hippocampus, performance on delayed nonmatching to sample tests, tests that are sensitive to hippocampal dysfunction in adult monkeys, are only mildly impaired until after puberty when they become more profoundly so.

These studies indicate that perinatal injury to prefrontal

and limbic cortices, two regions that are strongly implicated in schizophrenia, can have minimal impact on cognitive function before puberty and clinically significant impact afterward. This suggests that the apparent deterioration in cognitive function seen in patients with schizophrenia around the time of onset of their illness (32) could conceivably be the result of early developmental brain injury by itself. However, these studies do not suggest that psychotic symptoms, symptoms that tend to respond to antipsychotic drugs presumably through the blockade of dopamine receptors, also could suddenly emerge during early adulthood as a result of early developmental brain injury by itself. Recent studies in the rat, however, have made it possible to conceive of this as well.

In a series of studies, Lipska and colleagues (45,46) have shown that perinatal excitotoxic damage of the ventral hippocampus of the rat represents an interesting model of delayed emergence of hyperdopaminergic behaviors. These animals show no evidence of abnormalities of mesolimbic or nigrostriatally mediated behaviors until after puberty, whereupon they become hyperresponsive to dopaminergic drugs and to a variety of experiential stresses. They also manifest the delayed emergence of other abnormalities associated with schizophrenia, such as abnormal prepulse inhibition of startle. Moreover, in some respects they grow up to look like animals with adult prefrontal lesions, suggesting that the neonatal hippocampal lesion has affected prefrontal development as well. Their abnormal dopaminergic behaviors are ameliorated by antipsychotic drugs.

This provocative animal model illustrates that early developmental damage to cortical systems that have been implicated in schizophrenia may also have delayed effects on the regulation of brain dopamine systems. These delayed effects may have something to do with the maturation of these dopamine systems. They might also reflect the maturation of experience-based cortical systems which are programmed to take responsibility in early adulthood for regulating subcortical dopamine systems when they are needed. It seems theoretically possible that if these cortical systems developed abnormally, they may be unable to appropriately regulate subcortical dopamine systems when it is their time to do so.

OVERVIEW

The research summarized in this chapter tends, on the whole, toward the interpretation that individuals who manifest schizophrenia in early adult life have suffered some form of subtle cerebral maldevelopment in utero. This assumption is based on imperfect studies and inconclusive data. Nevertheless, there are a number of converging lines of evidence. The morphometric anatomical data from in vivo and postmortem investigations are difficult to attribute to a neuropathological process of adult life.

The static nature of the structural findings, the correlations with early life adaptation, and the absence of gliosis are much more consistent with the possibility of a developmental anomaly. By far, the most important anatomical data concerns the evidence of cytoarchitectural disorganization of the cortex. These findings are virtually pathognomonic of a defect in cortical development occurring during the second trimester of gestation. If these data can be replicated in methodologically unimpeachable studies, a "smoking gun" will have been identified. Further efforts in this regard should be at the top of the list of priorities in schizophrenia research.

The other issues in thinking about schizophrenia as a neurodevelopmental disorder pivot on the validity of the cytoarchitectural findings. If these postmortem results are valid, then the etiology is one that affects brain development during this critical period. The etiology would clearly not be birth complications. Moreover, the question of why the clinical manifestations of such congenital damage are not present in recognizable form until early adulthood also becomes increasingly important, because answering this question may hold clues to the mechanisms of clinical compensation and decompensation. The scenario stressed in this chapter involves an interaction of cortical maldevelopment with normal programs of postnatal functional development of critical intracortical neural systems. The systems that appear to be especially relevant to the cortical functional impairments of schizophrenia involve prefrontal and limbic cortices and their connectivity. Such highly evolved, late maturing systems may be especially important in coping with the vicissitudes of independent psychosocial functioning and may be critical as well for the stress-related management of subcortical dopamine activity. As recently demonstrated in a new wave of heuristically meaningful animal models, it is conceivable that a congenital defect in such systems would remain submerged until early adult life and then fail to properly regulate critical secondary systems (e.g., subcortical dopamine activity) in the context of environmental stress. It is further conceivable that genetically determined variations in intracortical connectivity or in responsivity of the limbic dopamine system, which would not be clinically significant by themselves, could become clinically devastating when combined with the manner of cortical maldevelopment implicated above.

REFERENCES

1. Akbarian S, Bunney WE Jr, Potkin SG, et al. Altered distribution of nicotinamide-adenine dinucleotide phosphate-diaphorase cells in frontal lobe of schizophrenics implies disturbances of cortical development. *Arch Gen Psychiatry* 1993;50:169–177.
2. Akbarian S, Viñuela A, Kim JJ, Potkin SG, Bunney WE Jr, Jones EG. Distorted distribution of nicotinamide-adenine dinucleotide phosphate-diaphorase neurons in temporal lobe of schizophrenics implies anomalous cortical development. *Arch Gen Psychiatry* 1993;50:178–187.

3. Altshuler LL, Casanova MF, Goldberg TE, Kleinman JE. The hippocampus and parahippocampus in schizophrenic, suicide, and control brains. *Arch Gen Psychiatry* 1990;47:1029–1034.
4. Altshuler LL, Conrad A, Kovelman JA, Scheibel A. Hippocampal pyramidal cell orientation in schizophrenia. A controlled neurohistologic study of the Yakovlev collection. *Arch Gen Psychiatry* 1987;44:1094–1098.
5. Arnold SE, Hyman BT, van Hoesen GW, Damasio AR. Some cytoarchitectural abnormalities of the entorhinal cortex in schizophrenia. *Arch Gen Psychiatry* 1991;48:625–632.
6. Asarnow JR. Children at risk for schizophrenia: converging lines of evidence. *Schizophr Bull* 1988;14:613–631.
7. Barr CE, Mednick SA, Munk-Jorgensen P. Exposure to influenza epidemics during gestation and adult schizophrenia. A 40-year study. *Arch Gen Psychiatry* 1990;47:869–874.
8. Bartley AJ, Jones DW, Torrey EF, Zigun JR, Weinberger DR. Sylvian fissure asymmetries in monozygotic twins: a test of laterality in schizophrenia. *Biol Psychiatry* 1993;34:853–863.
9. Beauregard M, Malkova L, Bachevalier J. Is schizophrenia a result of early damage to the hippocampal formation? A behavioral study in primates. *Soc Neurosci Abst* 1992;18:872.
10. Beckmann H, Jakob H. Prenatal disturbances of nerve cell migration in the entorhinal region: a common vulnerability factor in functional psychoses? *J Neural Transm* 1991;84:155–164.
11. Benes FM. Myelination of cortical-hippocampal relays during late adolescence. *Schizophr Bull* 1989;15:585–593.
12. Benes FM, McSparren J, Bird ED, SanGiovanni JP, Vincent SL. Deficits in small interneurons in prefrontal and cingulate cortices of schizophrenic and schizoaffective patients. *Arch Gen Psychiatry* 1991;48:996–1001.
13. Berman KF, Weinberger DR. Functional localization in the brain in schizophrenia. In: Tasman A, Goldfinger SM, ed. *American Psychiatric Press review of psychiatry*. Vol 10. Washington, DC: American Psychiatric Press; 1991:5–6, 136–137.
14. Bogerts B. Limbic and paralimbic pathology in schizophrenia: interaction with age- and stress-related factors. In: Schulz SC, Tamminga CA, eds. *Schizophrenia: scientific progress*. New York: Oxford University Press; 1989:216–226.
15. Bogerts B, Ashtari M, Degreef G, Alvir JMJ, Bilder RM, Lieberman JA. Reduced temporal limbic structure volumes on magnetic resonance images in first episode schizophrenia. *Psychiatry Res Neuroimag* 1990;35:1–13.
16. Bunney WE Jr, Akbarian S, Kim JJ, Hagman JO, Potkin SG, Jones EG. Gene expression for glutamic acid decarboxylase is reduced in prefrontal cortex of schizophrenics. *Neurosci Abst* 1993;19:199.
17. Cannon TD, Mednick SA, Parnas J, Schulsinger F, Praestholm J, Vestergaard A. Developmental brain abnormalities in the offspring of schizophrenic mothers. I. Contributions of genetic and perinatal factors. *Arch Gen Psychiatry* 1993;50:551–564.
18. Christison GW, Casanova MF, Weinberger DR, Rawlings R, Kleinman JE. A quantitative investigation of hippocampal pyramidal cell size, shape, and variability of orientation in schizophrenia. *Arch Gen Psychiatry* 1989;46:1027–1032.
19. Conrad AJ, Abebe T, Austin R, Forsythe S, Scheibel AB. Hippocampal pyramidal cell disarray in schizophrenia as a bilateral phenomenon. *Arch Gen Psychiatry* 1991;48:413–417.
20. Crow TJ, Ball J, Bloom SR, et al. Schizophrenia as an anomaly of development of cerebral asymmetry. A postmortem study and a proposal concerning the genetic basis of the disease. *Arch Gen Psychiatry* 1989;46:1145–1150.
21. Crow TJ, Done DJ. Prenatal exposure to influenza does not cause schizophrenia. *Br J Psychiatry* 1992;161:390–393.
22. Daniel DG, Goldberg TE, Weinberger DR. Lack of a bimodal distribution of ventricular size in patients with schizophrenia. *Biol Psychiatry* 1991;30:887–903.
23. DeLisi LE, Dauphinais ID, Gershon ES. Perinatal complications and reduced size of brain limbic structures in familial schizophrenia. *Schizophr Bull* 1988;14:185–191.
24. DeLisi LE, Hoff AL, Schwartz JE, Shields GW, et al. Brain morphology in first-episode schizophrenic-like psychotic patients: a quantitative magnetic resonance imaging study. *Biol Psychiatry* 1991;29:159–175.
25. Eagles JM, Gibson I, Bremner MH, Clunie F, Ebmeier KP, Smith NC. Obstetric complications in DSM-III schizophrenics and their siblings. *Lancet* 1990;335:1139–1141.
26. Erel O, Cannon TD, Hollister JM, Mednick SA, Parnas J. Ventricular enlargement and premorbid deficits in school-occupational attainment in a high risk sample. *Schizophr Res* 1991;4:49–52.
27. Erlenmeyer-Kimling L. High risk research in schizophrenia: a summary of what has been learned. *J Psychiatr Res* 1987;21:401–411.
28. Falkai P, Bogerts B, Greve B, et al. Loss of sylvian fissure asymmetry in schizophrenia. A quantitative postmortem study. *Schizophr Res* 1992;7:23–32.
29. Falkai P, Bogerts B, Rozumek M. Limbic pathology in schizophrenia: the entorhinal region—a morphometric study. *Biol Psychiatry* 1988;24:515–521.
30. Feinberg I. Schizophrenia: caused by a fault in programmed synaptic elimination during adolescence? *J Psychiat Res* 1982;17:319–334.
31. Fish B, Marcus J, Hans SL, Auerbach JG, Perdue S. Infants at risk for schizophrenia: sequelae of a genetic neurointegrative defect. A review and replication analysis of pandysmaturation in the Jerusalem infant development study. *Arch Gen Psychiatry* 1992;49:221–235.
32. Goldberg TE, Gold JM, Braff DL. Neuropsychological functioning and time-linked information processing in schizophrenia. In: Tasman A, Goldfinger SM, eds. *American Psychiatric Press: review of psychiatry*. Vol 10. Washington, DC: American Psychiatric Press; 1991:60–78.
33. Goldman PS. Functional development of the prefrontal cortex in early life and the problem of neuronal plasticity. *Exp Neurol* 1971;32:366–387.
34. Goodman R. Are complications of pregnancy and birth causes of schizophrenia? *Devel Med Child Neurol* 1988;30:391–395.
35. Heckers S, Heinsen H, Heinsen YC, Beckmann H. Limbic structures and lateral ventricle in schizophrenia. *Arch Gen Psychiatry* 1990;47:1016–1022.
36. Hyde TM, Ziegler JC, Weinberger DR. Psychiatric disturbances in metachromatic leukodystrophy: insight into the neurobiology of psychosis. *Arch Neurology* 1992;49:401–406.
37. Jakob H, Beckmann H. Prenatal developmental disturbances in the limbic allocortex in schizophrenics. *J Neural Transm* 1986;65:303–326.
38. Jaskiw GE, Juliano DM, Goldberg TE, Hertzman M, Urow-Hamell E, Weinberger DR. Cerebral ventricular enlargement in schizophreniform disorder does not progress—a seven year follow-up study. *Schizophr Res* [in press].
39. Jeste DV, Lohr JB. Hippocampal pathologic findings in schizophrenia. *Arch Gen Psychiatry* 1989;46:1019–1024.
40. Keefe RSE, Mohs RC, Losonczy MF, et al. Premorbid sociosexual functioning and long-term outcome in schizophrenia. *Am J Psychiatry* 1989;146:206–211.
41. Kendell RE, Kemp IW. Influenza and schizophrenia: Helsinki vs Edinburgh. *Arch Gen Psychiatry* 1990;47:877–878.
42. Kendell RE, Kemp IW. Maternal influenza in the etiology of schizophrenia. *Arch Gen Psychiatry* 1989;46:878–882.
43. Kovelman JA, Scheibel AB. A neurohistological correlate of schizophrenia. *Biol Psychiatry* 1984;19:1601–1621.
44. Kulynych JJ, Vladar K, Fantie BD, Jones DW, Weinberger DR. Normal asymmetry of the planum temporale in patients with schizophrenia: three-dimensional cortical morphometry with MRI. *Br J Psychiatry* [in press].
45. Lipska BK, Jaskiw GE, Weinberger DR. Postpubertal emergence of augmented exploration and amphetamine supersensitivity after neonatal deeferentation of the rat ventral hippocampus: a potential animal model of schizophrenia. *Neuropsychopharmacol* 1993;9:67–75.
46. Lipska BK, Weinberger DR. Cortical regulation of the mesolimbic dopamine system: implications for schizophrenia. In: Kalivas PW, ed. *The mesolimbic motor circuit and its role in neuropsychiatric disorders*. Boca Raton, FL: CRC Press; 1993:329–349.
47. McCreadie RG, Hall DJ, Berry IJ, Robertson LJ, Ewing JI, Geals MF. The Nithsdale schizophrenia surveys. X: obstetric complications, family history and abnormal movements. *Br J Psychiatry* 1992;161:799–805.
48. McNeil TF. Obstetric factors and perinatal injuries. In: Tsuang MT, Simpson JC, eds. *Nosology, Epidemiology and Genetics*. New York:

Elsevier Science Publishers; 1988:319–344. (*Handbook of Schizophrenia,* vol. 3).

49. Mednick SA, Cannon TD, Barr CE, Lyon M, eds. *Fetal neural development and adult schizophrenia.* Cambridge: Cambridge University Press; 1991.

50. Mednick SA, Machon RA, Huttunen MO, Bonett D. Adult schizophrenia following prenatal exposure to an influenza epidemic. *Arch Gen Psychiatry* 1988;45:189–192.

51. Mednick SA, Silverton L. High risk studies of the etiology of schizophrenia. In: Tsuang MT, Simpson JC, eds. *Nosology, Epidemiology and Genetics of Schizophrenia.* New York: Elsevier Science Publishers, 1988:543–562. (*Handbook of Schizophrenia,* vol. 3).

52. Murray RM, O'Callaghan E, Castle DJ, Lewis SW. A neurodevelopmental approach to the classification of schizophrenia. *Schizophr Bull* 1992;18:319–332.

53. O'Callaghan E, Sham P, Takei N, Glover G, Murray RM. Schizophrenia after prenatal exposure to 1957 A2 influenza epidemic. *Lancet* 1991;337:1248–1250.

54. Onstad S, Skre I, Torgersen S, Kringlen E. Birthweight and obstetric complications in schizophrenic twins. *Acta Psychiatr Scand* 1992;85:70–73.

55. Pakkenberg B. Post-mortem study of chronic schizophrenic brains. *Br J Psychiatry* 1987;151:744–752.

56. Parnas J, Schulsinger F, Teasdale TW, Schulsinger H, Feldman PM, Mednick SA. Perinatal complications and clinical outcome within the schizophrenia spectrum. *Br J Psychiatry* 1982;140:416–420.

57. Pollack M, Woerner MG, Goodman W, Greenberg IM. Childhood development patterns of hospitalized adult schizophrenic and nonschizophrenic patients and their siblings. *Am J Orthopsychiatry* 1966;36:510–517.

58. Pollin W, Stabeneau JR. Biological, psychological and historical differences in a series of monozygotic twins discordant for schizophrenia. In: Rosenthal D, Kety S, eds. *The Transmission of Schizophrenia.* New York: Pergamon Press; 1968:317–322.

59. Reveley AM, Reveley MA, Murray RM. Cerebral ventricular enlargement of non-genetic schizophrenia: A controlled twin study. *Br J Psychiatry* 1984;144:89–93.

60. Roberts GW, Colter N, Lofthouse R, Bogerts B, Zech M, Crow TJ. Gliosis in schizophrenia: a survey. *Biol Psychiatry* 1986;21:1043–1050.

61. Rossi A, Stratta P, Mattei P, et al. Planum temporale in schizophrenia: a magnetic resonance study. *Schizophr Res* 1992;7:19–22.

62. Sham PC, O'Callaghan E, Takei N, Murray GK, Hare EH, Murray RM. Schizophrenia following prenatal exposure to influenza epidemics between 1939 and 1960. *Br J Psychiatry* 1992;160:461–466.

63. Shelton R, Weinberger DR. Brain morphology in schizophrenia. In: Meltzer H, Bunney W, Coyle J, David K, Schuster R, Shader R, Simpson G, eds. *Psychopharmacology: the third generation of progress.* New York: Raven Press; 1987:773–781.

64. Shenton ME, Kirkinis R, Jolesz FA, et al. Abnormalities of the left temporal lobe and thought disorder in schizophrenia. A quantitative magnetic resonance imaging study. *N Engl J Med* 1992;327:604–612.

65. Stevens JR. Abnormal reinnervation as a basis for schizophrenia: a hypothesis. *Arch Gen Psychiatry* 1992;49:238–243.

66. Suddath RL, Christison GW, Torrey EF, Weinberger DR. Cerebral anatomical abnormalities in monozygotic twins discordant for schizophrenia. *N Engl J Med* 1990;322:789–794.

67. Susser ES, Lin SP. Schizophrenia after prenatal exposure to the Dutch hunger winter of 1944–1945. *Arch Gen Psychiatry* 1992;49:983–988.

68. Torrey EF, Bowler AE, Taylor EH, Gottesman II. *Schizophrenia and manic depression disorders: the biological roots of mental illness as revealed by a landmark study of identical twins.* New York: Basic Books [*in press*]

69. Torrey EF, Rawlings R, Waldman IN. Schizophrenic births and viral diseases in two states. *Schizophr Res* 1988;1:73–77.

70. Walker E, Lewine RJ. Prediction of adult-onset schizophrenia from childhood home movies of the patients. *Am J Psychiatry* 1990;147:1052–1056.

71. Weinberger DR. Implications of normal brain development for the pathogenesis of schizophrenia. *Arch Gen Psychiatry* 1987;44:660–669.

72. Weinberger DR, Berman KF, Suddath R, Torrey EF. Evidence for dysfunction of a prefrontal-limbic network in schizophrenia: an MRI and rCBF study of discordant monozygotic twins. *Am J Psychiatry* 1992;149:890–897.

73. Woerner MG, Pollack M, Klein DF. Pregnancy and birth complications in psychiatric patients: A comparison of schizophrenic and personality disorder patients with their siblings. *Acta Psychiatr Scand* 1973;49:712–721.

74. Zigun J, Weinberger DR. In vivo studies of brain morphology in patients with schizophrenia. In: Lindenmayer J-P, Kay SR, eds. *New biological vistas on schizophrenia.* New York: Brunner Mazel; 1992:57–81.

Psychopharmacology: The Fourth Generation of Progress, edited by Floyd E. Bloom and David J. Kupfer. Raven Press, Ltd., New York © 1995.

CHAPTER **99**

Functional Brain-Imaging Studies in Schizophrenia

Raquel E. Gur

Functional brain-imaging methods have been applied to the study of schizophrenia, aiming at elucidating the neurobiology of this heterogeneous and complex disorder. These methods have included the [133]xenon technique for measuring cerebral blood flow (CBF); positron emission tomography (PET) for assessing metabolism, CBF, and neuroreceptor functioning; and single photon emission computerized tomography (SPECT) for studying CBF and neuroreceptors. This chapter reviews the application of this technology in schizophrenia research. Studies are summarized and integrated with our current understanding of brain function in schizophrenia.

Links between clinical features of schizophrenia and brain function have been guided by hypotheses relating behavior to specific brain regions and systems that have been implicated in schizophrenia. These links are based on preclinical research and the emergence of symptoms, commonly seen in schizophrenia, which also occur following brain lesions. Persistent negative, deficit symptoms have been related to frontal lobe dysfunction also evident in neurobehavioral sequelae of frontal lobe damage, such as impairment in abstraction, verbal fluency, mental flexibility, and concept formation. Positive, productive symptoms of hallucinations and delusions have been related to the temporal–limbic system with evidence of impaired learning and memory. Subcortical regions, with special emphasis on the basal ganglia, have been examined in the context of the dopamine hypothesis. Across these dimensions, laterality measures of the relation between left and right hemispheric parameters have been compared in patients and normal controls. Although necessarily simplistic and not reflecting on other brain

systems that modulate normal and pathological psychotic behavior, these dimensions have generated hypotheses that can be examined with functional brain imaging.

CEREBRAL METABOLISM AND BLOOD FLOW STUDIES

Studies of cerebral metabolism and blood flow can be divided into those measuring the physiological parameters at a resting state and those that introduced a perturbation, or challenge, in the form of a neurobehavioral probe or a pharmacological intervention. Initially, investigators have aimed at assessing whether resting blood flow and glucose metabolism differ between patients with schizophrenia and healthy controls. The topography of physiological activity was examined along the dimensions stated above. This research is summarized in special issues of the *Schizophrenia Bulletin* (12,32).

The frontal lobes were implicated in early physiological studies of CBF, reporting that patients with schizophrenia did not show the normal pattern of increased anterior relative to posterior CBF (38). This hypofrontal disturbance in the anterior–posterior gradient has been supported in some (e.g., 12,47,70), but not all (e.g., 14,30,33,35) studies of resting CBF, with the [133]xenon method and glucose metabolism with PET.

The relationship between this pattern of metabolic activity and clinical variables has also been examined (62). Decreased frontal metabolic activity is associated with duration of illness; longer duration is associated with lower anteroposterior gradient (69) and negative symptoms (63). Liddle et al. (43) found that patients with poor performance on the Stroop test, which measures attention, have abnormal CBF in the anterior cingulate cortex.

Differences in resting values between patients and con-

R. E. Gur: Neuropsychiatry Section, Department of Psychiatry, University of Pennsylvania, Philadelphia, Pennsylvania 19104.

trols were also found in laterality indices, suggesting relatively higher left hemispheric values in severely disturbed patients (34,58). Furthermore, improvement in clinical status correlated with a shift toward lower left hemispheric rather than right hemispheric metabolism (35). This supports hypotheses derived from behavioral data concerning lateralized abnormalities in schizophrenia (16), and perhaps the more specific form of the hypothesis which proposes that schizophrenia is associated both with left hemispheric dysfunction and overactivation of the dysfunctional left hemisphere (37).

These reports varied in the technology applied and definition of regional parameters. Most studies used regional ratios, such as region-to-whole brain or anterior–posterior ratios, rather than absolute values of activity. Some of the inconsistencies in findings may be related to sample heterogeneity, analytical approaches, and the individual techniques. Another potentially important source of variability in results is the definition of resting state. Investigators have been reluctant to include an unstructured resting state because of concern that such measures will be uncontrolled and therefore produce unreliable results. Some studies used partial sensory deprivation (eyes and ears occluded), and other used sensory stimulation in the form of electrical shock to the forearm to standardize this condition. However, several studies have examined the reproducibility of resting baseline measures with relatively unstructured conditions (i.e., eyes open, ears unoccluded, with ambient noise kept to a minimum). These studies found very high reproducibility among healthy subjects (35,65) and patients with schizophrenia (4).

Given the demonstrated reliability of the standardized resting baseline condition, we believe it is important to include such a condition in physiological neuroimaging studies. This serves three main purposes. First, it permits comparison across studies within a center, as technology evolves and patient characteristics change. Without a common resting baseline condition, it would be impossible to determine the source of differences in results. Second, it permits comparability across centers. Imagine the need to explain why two centers using the same or similar tasks find evidence for different regional abnormalities in schizophrenia. If resting baseline values are available and are comparable in the two samples, different task effects could be legitimately attributed to theoretically meaningful sources, such as task condition or symptomatic variability. A third advantage of standardized resting baseline is the provision of a reference point for evaluating whether a given task or condition has increased neural activity. In studies that have included such a condition, cognitive activation was consistently shown to increase cortical activity both in patients and controls (e.g., 28,30,36). Using a resting baseline condition enables the investigator to make much stronger statements in the interpretation of regional effects. Rather than being restricted to statements that a given region has changed in its activation relative to the remainder of the brain, resting baseline availability permits stating whether the task has induced increased neural activity.

Regardless of one's position in the debate over the value of obtaining resting baseline measures, it is apparent that measures of CBF and metabolism during the performance of cognitive tasks tend to accentuate differences between patients and controls. Perhaps even more importantly, such measures are critical for establishing the link between behavioral deficits and the ability of brain regions to become activated in response to task demand. This expectation has been supported in studies which employed neurobehavioral probes (26). This approach begins with hypotheses, derived from neurobehavioral data, which associate behavioral measures with regional brain function. Task selection can be made to include a target task, where patients are expected to have differential deficit, and control tasks. Patients are then compared to healthy controls in the pattern of task-induced changes in regional brain activity.

This can be illustrated in several investigations using CBF measures. In the first study in which medicated patients with schizophrenia were compared to sociodemographically balanced healthy controls, no differences were found in overall or hemispheric CBF using the [133]xenon clearance technique. However, distinct abnormalities were seen in the pattern of hemispheric changes induced by verbal (analogies) and spatial (line orientation) tasks. Healthy controls showed the expected greater left hemispheric increase for the verbal and greater right hemispheric increase for the spatial task. However, patients with schizophrenia had a bilaterally symmetric activation for the verbal task and greater left hemispheric activation for the spatial task. Thus, patients failed to show the normal left hemispheric dominance for the verbal task, and instead showed left hemispheric overactivation for the spatial task (Fig. 1).

Similarly, Weinberger et al. (68) found no regional abnormalities in resting CBF of patients with schizophrenia. However, distinct abnormalities were reported in the dorsolateral prefrontal region during activation with the Wisconsin Card Sorting Test of abstraction and mental flexibility, which is sensitive to frontal lobe damage (66). The application of this paradigm to the study of monozygotic twins discordant for schizophrenia (67), revealed that all affected twins had reduced dorsolateral prefrontal cortex CBF response compared to discordant co-twins. These results have been corroborated by other investigators (39,53). Furthermore, negative symptoms, which have been related to frontal lobe dysfunction, showed a negative correlation with frontal CBF during performance of executive but not control tasks (61). Measuring CBF with SPECT during the application of another task sensitive to frontal lobe function, Andreasen et al. (3) also

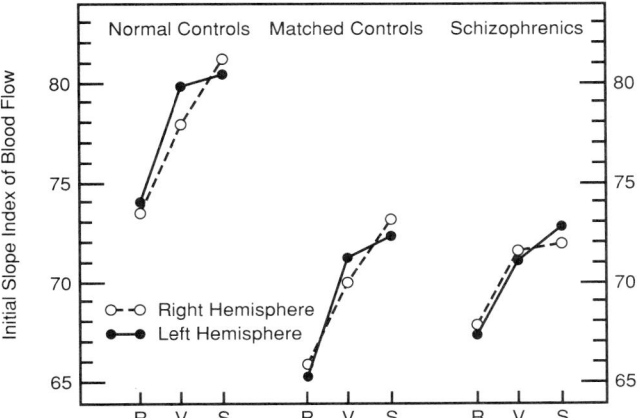

FIG. 1. Regional cerebral blood flow in two hemispheres of schizophrenics and matched controls when resting (*R*), solving verbal analogies (*V*), and performing spatial task (*S*). Normal control values are from earlier study for comparison with latest matched sample. From Gur et al. (36).

reported failure in patients with schizophrenia to show the expected increase in blood flow to the frontal region.

Subsequent to assessing global, anterior–posterior, and laterality dimensions, investigators have begun the study of functional changes in temporal lobe regions. Dysfunction in temporal–limbic structures, including the hippocampus and the temporal cortex, is supported by recent neuroanatomical and neuropsychological studies (7,54). Lateralized abnormalities in these regions, with greater left than right hemispheric dysfunction, are implicated by characteristic clinical features of schizophrenia, such as thought disorder, auditory hallucinations, and language disturbances. Positron emission topography studies of temporal lobe metabolism include findings of both increased (e.g., ref. 18) and decreased glucose utilization. Decreased metabolism was also noted in the hippocampus and the anterior cingulate cortex (60). Studies in this region have been limited in part by instrument resolution.

Metabolism and flow pattern in temporal–limbic regions have also been related to symptoms. Liddle et al. (43) used ^{15}oxygen-labeled water with PET, and described abnormal CBF in parahippocampal gyrus associated with positive symptoms. Musalek et al. (50) found hallucinations to be associated with SPECT flow changes in the hippocampus, parahippocampus, and amygdala. There are conflicting reports of superior temporal gyrus functional changes in schizophrenia during active auditory hallucinations. Cleghorn et al. (15) suggested that patients with hallucinations have significantly lower relative metabolism in Wernicke's region. Anderson et al. (1) showed asymmetric temporal lobe perfusion, lower in the left than the right, in schizophrenic patients with auditory hallucinations. Delisi et al. (18) found greater metabolic activity in the left anterior temporal lobe, which was related to the severity of symptoms. This is consistent with Gur's (34,35) reported association between severity of symptoms and relative increase in left hemispheric metabolism measured with PET.

Further research is needed to elucidate the nature and extent of temporal lobe changes in schizophrenia. Given that this region is linked to memory functions, an appropriate neurobehavioral probe would be aimed at memory (29,75). We have applied verbal and facial memory tasks in schizophrenia with the ^{133}xenon clearance method (29) and the results are presented in Fig. 2.

As can be seen, patients had normal resting CBF values and topography, but showed abnormalities in activation-induced changes. These abnormalities were both in degree of activation and in lateralized changes as a function of whether the memory task required processing of words or faces. In healthy controls the midtemporal region was the only cortical area showing hemispherically appropriate changes (left more than right for words, right more than left for faces). By contrast, patients did not show a significantly lateralized response in this region and instead showed such responses in other regions.

Functional changes in the basal ganglia have been examined with PET and SPECT. Several PET studies implicate basal ganglia dysfunction in schizophrenia (9,19,33,35,41). The withdrawal-retardation factor (emotional withdrawal, blunted affect, and motor retardation) of the Brief Psychiatric Rating Scale, has been negatively correlated with PET basal ganglia metabolic activity (72). Neuroleptic-naive schizophrenic patients were reported to have relatively increased blood flow in the left globus pallidus (20). Other PET studies report decreased basal ganglia metabolism in schizophrenia (9,12). Some studies found increased basal ganglia metabolic rates following administration of neuroleptic medication (e.g., see ref. 9).

Thus, although the contribution of PET metabolic and blood flow studies so far has added to the growing evidence implicating basal ganglia involvement in schizophrenia, the exact nature of the dysfunction remains unclear. In particular, the relationship between basal ganglia and frontal lobe activity in schizophrenia needs further scrutiny. There is emerging evidence of interrelationships between the various key regions, revealed by structural and functional imaging. Rubin et al. (52) showed that patients with schizophrenia not only fail to activate the dorsolateral prefrontal cortex in response to the Wisconsin Card Sorting Test, but they also fail to inhibit caudate activation. Hence, in schizophrenia, basal ganglia continue to show relatively increased blood flow in the caudate during performance of the task, as opposed to normal controls who seem to demonstrate a reciprocal relationship in which decreasing blood flow in basal ganglia is associated with increasing perfusion to the frontal region.

The pharmacological status of patients undergoing metabolic and blood flow studies has varied. Research has ranged from investigations in which neuroleptics were considered a variable that needed controls to those in which pharmacological intervention was introduced in a

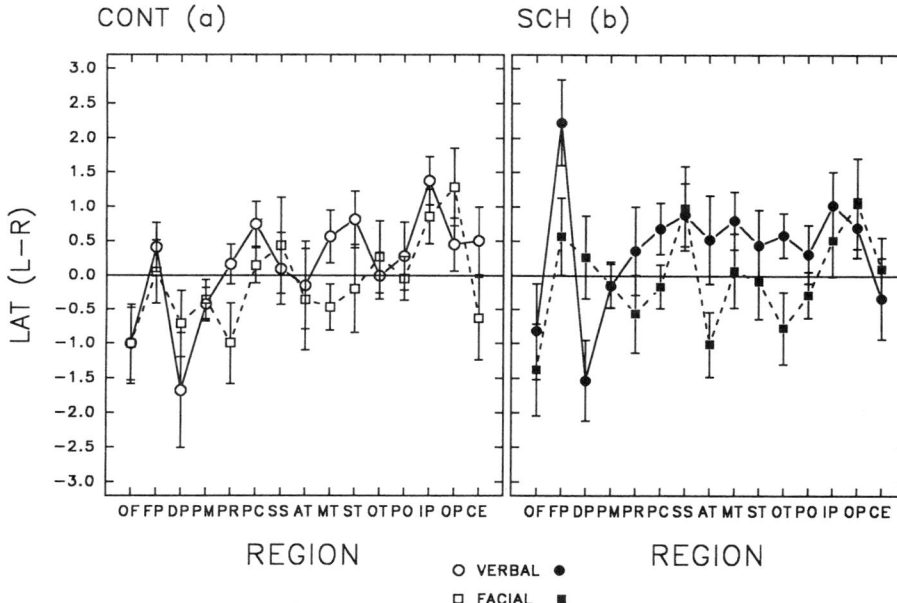

FIG. 2. Means and SEMs regional laterality (L−R) for the verbal and facial tasks in controls (*empty*) and patients (*filled symbols*). From Gur RE et al. Cerebral blood flow in schizophrenia: effects of memory processing on regional activation. *Biol Psychiatry* 1994; 35:3−15.

standardized fashion to examine treatment effects on the regional metabolic landscape. The washout period in studies that controlled for the effects of neuroleptics on CBF and metabolism has been commonly short, ranging from 2 to 4 weeks. This period is a compromise from what is feasible and desirable. Siegel et al. (59) examined glucose activity in cortical–striatal–thalamic circuits in a large sample of unmedicated schizophrenic males; they found low metabolic activity in medial–frontal–cortical regions and basal ganglia and impaired lateralization in the frontal and temporal regions. A strategy applied more recently in schizophrenia research, which is especially important in functional neuroimaging, is the study of neuroleptic-naive first-episode patients. This population is particularly informative when studying the effects of pharmacological intervention. The study of neuroleptic-naive patients before pharmacological intervention permits evaluation of the disease state separate from its treatment. However, progress can be made in metabolic studies using complementary methods when the integration of pharmacological probes in metabolic studies has been restricted.

A repeated-measures design has been applied in a limited number of PET studies. In addition to examining symptom severity over time (33,35), this paradigm is especially useful when pharmacological intervention is standardized. Bartlett et al. (5) compared the effects of thiothixene and haloperidol in chronic patients who were scanned off and after 4 to 6 weeks on medication. A different pattern of global and regional glucose metabolism was seen in the two groups. In 25 patients with schizophrenia, PET scans were obtained at weeks 5 and 10 of a double-blind cross-over trial of haloperidol and placebo (11). Lower metabolism in the striatum on placebo was associated with improved symptomatology. Responders had higher metabolism in the striatum after treat-

ment. Nonresponders failed to show such a change and had more marked hypofrontality on medication. In a subsequent study, 12 patients were scanned before and 4 to 6 weeks after treatment with clozapine or thiothixene (10). The drugs had a differential effect, with clozapine increasing and thiothixene decreasing metabolism in the basal ganglia, right more than left. Larger scale studies relating subcortical to cortical networks are needed and can contribute to the understanding of the neurobiology of schizophrenia (59,60). The study of neuroreceptors provides an important window to assessing the nature of subcortical abnormalities in schizophrenia.

NEURORECEPTOR STUDIES

Since advances in elucidating the pathophysiology of schizophrenia require understanding of neurotransmitter function, the application of PET and SPECT to the study of receptor occupancy is an important research domain. These efforts have been guided both by an extensive psychopharmacological literature and by advances in basic neuroscience on neuroreceptor subtyping. Functional neuroimaging is the meeting ground of preclinical and clinical neuropharmacology. Human neuroreceptor PET studies have built on progress with in vitro binding measurements of receptor density and affinity and neuroreceptor autoradiography (56,74). Psychotic symptoms seen in schizophrenia have been associated with dysfunction of dopamine, and the dopamine hypothesis has undergone revisions (17,44).

The development of radioligands for PET studies first focused on the D_2 receptor because of its clinical significance. The study of neuroleptic-naive patients could potentially differentiate effects of the psychotic state, before

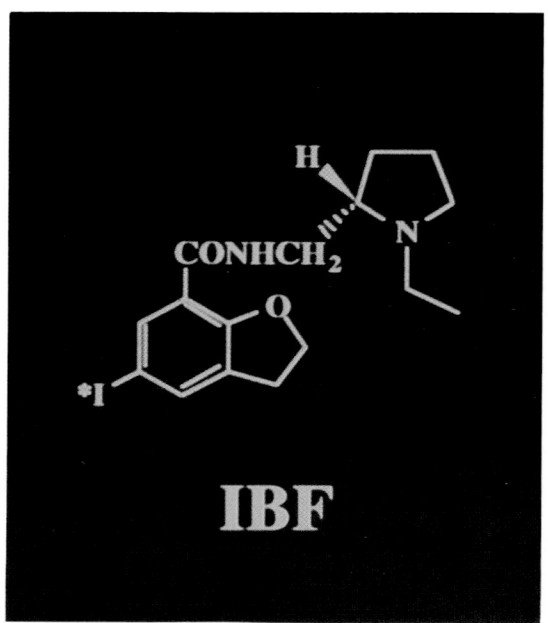 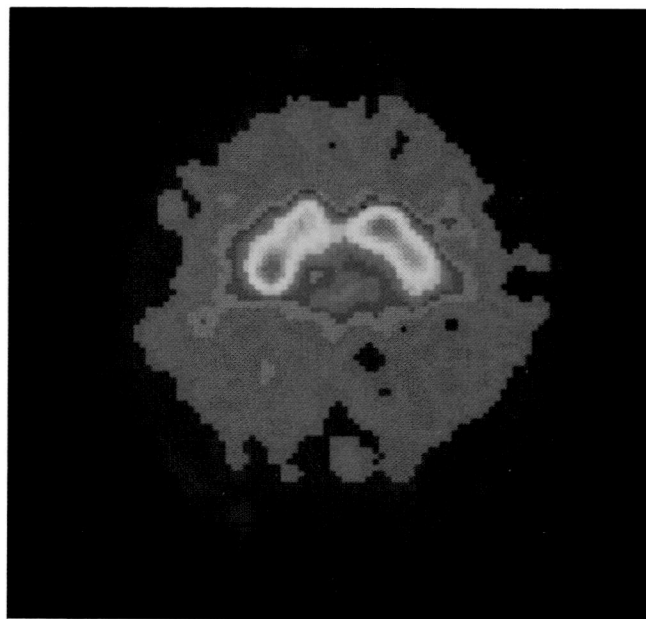

FIG. 3. Transaxial sections of SPECT imaging of D_2 dopamine receptors in normal brain after an intravenous injection of 5 mCi of [^{123}I]-IBF. High accumulation was observed in the basal ganglia area of the brain where D_2 dopamine receptors are concentrated.

neuroleptic intervention. Two major methodologies for quantitative measurement were developed and applied in the study of schizophrenia. Investigators at Johns Hopkins University applied ^{11}C-N-methylspiperone (NMSP) (64) and reported that patients have higher D_2 B_{max} values than controls (74). Studies at the Karolinska Institute using ^{11}C-raclopride, reported similar B_{max} and K_d values in patients and controls (23,24).

These apparent differences have been discussed and summarized extensively, and are likely related to multiple factors including patient variables, ligand properties, and PET modeling methods (2,32). Because the ligands differ in binding properties and sensitivity to endogenous dopamine, studies permitting a more direct comparison will be particularly helpful. Furthermore, it is not clear whether the results are specific to schizophrenia or other psychotic disorders might be implicated (32).

Martinot et al. (46) measured D_2 striatal dopamine receptors using [76]Br-bromospiperone in a PET study of 12 untreated schizophrenics and found similar amounts in patients and controls. In a subsequent study (45), [76]Br-bromolisuride was applied to the measurement of striatal D_2 receptors in 19 untreated patients and 14 controls. Again, no differences in striatum–cerebellum ratios emerged. In both studies, no relationship to symptoms or subtypes was evident. Recently, investigators at John Hopkins (32) replicated the initial report in a new sample of drug-naive schizophrenic patients. Other data reveal D_2 density increases in psychotic but not in nonpsychotic bipolar patients. The degree of increase is comparable to that reported in schizophrenia (73). This raises questions regarding the specificity of the dopamine hypothesis to schizophrenia versus other psychotic syndromes.

The study of neuroreceptors can also address issues about the relationship between receptor function and signs, such as akathisia, which are commonly seen in patients treated with neuroleptics. Farde (25) found central ^{11}C-SCH 23390, a selective D_1 dopamine receptor antagonist, in four control subjects. Two PET studies, at low and high dose of the radioligand, were conducted per subject. Transient akathisia occurred only when binding in the basal ganglia was at a high level with 45% to 59% occupancy. The D_2-dopamine receptor antagonist ^{11}C-raclopride was measured in 20 controls and 13 patients. Akathesia was associated in patients and controls with maximal ligand binding in the basal ganglia. Wolkin et al. (71), found that neuroleptic-resistant schizophrenics did not differ from neuroleptic responders in degree of D_2 receptor occupancy by the neuroleptics. The regional distribution and kinetics of haloperidol binding were studied with ^{18}F-haloperidol in a PET study of nine controls and five schizophrenics examined while on haloperidol and after a drug washout (55). Wide regional distribution of the ligand was evident in the cerebellum, basal ganglia, and thalamus, in contrast to the specific binding to the basal ganglia of ^{18}F-N-methylspiroperidol. Thus, small structural differences among butyrophenones are associated with changes in kinetics and distribution.

Positron emission tomography neuroreceptor methods have also been applied in comparing typical to atypical antipsychotic drugs. The properties of clozapine binding to D_1 and D_2 dopamine receptors was examined in an open study of five patients, relative to 22 patients treated with typical neuroleptics (21,22). Clozapine induced lower D_2 occupancy (38% to 63%), whereas D_2 receptor occupancy with typical neuroleptics at conventional doses was 70% to 89%. Neuroleptic-induced extrapyramidal syndromes were associated with higher D_2 occupancy. In a followup study, Nordstrom et al. (51) examined the relationship between D_2 receptor occupancy and antipsychotic drug effect in a double-blind PET study using ^{11}C-raclopride. Seventeen patients with schizophrenia were randomly assigned to three groups treated with a varied dose of raclopride. A PET study was conducted at steady-state on 13 patients during the third to fourth week of treatment. A curvilinear relation between plasma concentration of raclopride and D_2 receptor occupancy was obtained. A significant relationship was noted between D_2 receptor occupancy and Brief Psychiatric Rating Scale percent change as a measure of outcome. The D_2 receptor occupancy in patients who had extrapyramidal side effects (EPS) was higher than in patients with no EPS.

These research paradigms illustrate the integration of functional neuroimaging with pharmacological research. Clearly, incorporation of these research strategies to psychopharmacological studies of schizophrenia with available therapeutic agents can advance the field and guide treatment intervention. Other advances are on the way as new ligands become available.

The ligand 3-iodobenzamide (IBZM) has become available (8) and is being used in SPECT studies of dopamine D_2 receptors in patients with schizophrenia (42). Kessler (40) has used epidepride, a D_2 receptor antagonist, to explore extrastriatal D_2 receptors in autoradiographic and in vivo neuroimaging studies. Iodine-labeled epidepride may be a useful agent for exploration of D_2 sites, because it labels receptors in the prefrontal and cingulate cortex as well as in the striatum. Subsequent developments have introduced IBF, which has more specific affinity for D_2 receptors with SPECT (48), as well as TISCH and fluorinated and iodinated dopamine agents (FIDA) (13,49). Figure 3 illustrates the application of such ligands in human studies.

CONCLUSIONS

Functional neuroimaging research in schizophrenia has made progress in two areas: regional brain energy metabolism and blood flow and neuroreceptor studies. In a recent review of this field Sedvall (57) concluded that the major future contribution for understanding the pathophysiology of schizophrenia will be achieved through advanced resolution and development of new ligands for neurotransmitter systems. Although we agree on the potential of these developments, we believe metabolic studies can make unique contributions that will prove essential for finding the neural basis of schizophrenia and ultimately for improved treatment (31). Functional neuroimaging studies in the context of the overall effort in neurobiological research in schizophrenia, have contributed and will continue to advance the understanding of brain dysfunction as it relates to neurobehavior and neuropharmacology. The field has reached some maturity in developing appropriate paradigms, and there is now a need for adequate sample size in patient and normal populations with attention to clinical heterogeneity and variability in brain function in relation to gender and age.

Two complementary types of probes can enhance our understanding of brain function in schizophrenia: The first is the study of neuroreceptors as described by Sedvall (57). The second is neurobehavioral probes (26), which provide a useful paradigm for metabolic studies. Although there are a number of reports in which glucose studies were undertaken during cognitive activation procedures (see refs. 12 and 32 for review), a better ligand for such studies is ^{15}O-labeled water for measuring cerebral blood flow. The short half-life of the ligand permits repeated measures under different task conditions. This strengthens the design by eliminating sampling error and enabling the demonstration of task–region interactions. Studies with other physiological neuroimaging methods, such as the ^{133}xenon clearance technique, have used this approach profitably in the study of schizophrenia (6,30,68). This study is now underway with PET and requires consideration of several factors: task appropriateness for the PET environment, task difficulty, validity and reliability of tasks in relation to the concepts they measure, specificity of effect for task and population, and availability of performance data that can be correlated with metabolism (27,29).

One of the major challenges in this research is the integration of neuroimaging data, across anatomical and functional measures, with clinical and neurobehavioral variables. A potential strength of functional neuroimaging is the integration of neuroreceptor and metabolic studies. Ultimately, dysfunctional neurotransmitter systems translate into aberrant metabolism. Because CBF and metabolism reflect neuronal activity, relating these domains is a prerequisite for understanding the neurobiology of schizophrenia. As new receptor subtypes are cloned and as radioligands are developed and become available for human studies, it will be necessary to know which neuroreceptor measures result in increased neuronal activity and how regional activation relates to behavior.

Thus, although new receptor ligands and improved resolution are welcome and exciting (and now add the development of methods for magnetic resonance spectroscopy and flow measures), it is unlikely that finding the neural basis of schizophrenia will come simply as a product of applying the right method with sufficient resolution. Rather, it seems that we will have to undertake the harder and longer route of understanding the interaction between regional brain activity and neuroreceptors as they affect the clinical and neurobehavioral manifestations of schizophrenia. On the positive side, in the process of this examination, we will be in a position to find partial answers of immediate benefit for treatment, and, in the evolution of this work, we will systematically improve our ability to articulate a neuropsychiatric perspective of this devastating disorder.

ACKNOWLEDGMENTS

This work was supported by U.S. Public Health Service grants MH-00586, MHCRC-43880, and MH40391, from the National Institute of Mental Health. The author thanks Ruben C. Gur, Ph.D., for input, Hank Kung, Ph.D., and P. David Mozley, M.D., for providing Fig. 3, and Helen Mitchell-Sears for assistance in preparation of the manuscript.

REFERENCES

1. Anderson J, Fawdry R, Gordon E, Coyle S, Gruenewald S, Meares RA. SPECT asymmetry of left temporal lobe in hallucinated schizophrenics. Biol Psychiatry 1991;29:291.
2. Andreasen NC, Carson R, Diksic M, et al. PET and dopamine D$_2$ receptors in the human neostriatum. Schiz Bull 1988;14:471–484.
3. Andreasen NC, Rezai K, Alliger R, et al. Hypofrontality in neuroleptic-naive patients and in patients with chronic schizophrenia: assessment with Xenon 133 single-photon emission computed tomography and the tower of London. Arch Gen Psychiatry 1992;49(12):943–958.
4. Bartlett EJ, Barouche F, Brodie JD, et al. Stability of resting deoxyglucose metabolic values in PET studies of schizophrenia. Psychiatry Res 1991;40:11–20.
5. Bartlett EJ, Woklin A, Brodie JD, Laska EM, Wolf AP, Sanfilipo M. Importance of pharmacologic control in PET studies: effects of thiothixene and haloperidol on cerebral glucose utilization in chronic schizophrenia. Psychiatry Res 1991;40:115–124.
6. Berman KF, Weinberger DR. Lateralization of cortical function during cognitive tasks: regional cerebral blood flow studies of normal individuals and patients with schizophrenia. J Neurol Neurosurg Psychiatry 1990;53:150–160.
7. Bogerts B, Falkai P, Greve B. Evidence of reduced temporolimbic structure volumes in schizophrenia letter. Arch Gen Psychiatry 1991;48:956–958.
8. Brucke T, Tsai YF, McLellan CA, et al. In vitro binding properties and autoradiographic imaging of 3-iodobenzamide ([125I]-IBZM): a potential imaging ligand for D$_2$ dopamine receptors in SPECT. Life Sci 1988;42:2097–2104.
9. Buchsbaum MS, Ingvar DH, Kessler R, et al. Cerebral glucography with positron tomography. Arch Gen Psychiatry 1987;39:251–259.
10. Buchsbaum MS, Potkin SG, Marshall JF, et al. Effects of clozapine and thiothixene on glucose metabolic rate in schizophrenia. Neuropsychopharmacology 1992;6:155–163.
11. Buchsbaum MS, Potkin SG, Siegel BV Jr, et al. Striatal metabolic rate and clinical response to neuroleptics in schizophrenia. Arch Gen Psychiatry 1992;49:966–974.
12. Buchsbaum MS. The frontal lobes, basal ganglia, and temporal lobes as sites for schizophrenia. Schiz Bull 1990;16:377–387.

13. Chumpradit S, Kung M-P, Billings J, Mach R, Kung HF. Fluorinated and iodinated dopamine agents (FIDA): D_2 imaging agents for PET and SPECT. *J Med Chem* 1993;36:221–228.

14. Cleghorn JM, Garnett ES, Nahmias C, et al. Increased frontal and reduced parietal glucose metabolism in acute untreated schizophrenia. *Psychiatry Res* 1989;28:119–133.

15. Cleghorn JM. Regional brain metabolism during auditory hallucinations in chronic schizophrenia. *Br J Psychiatry* 1990;157:562–570.

16. Crow TJ. Temporal lobe asymmetries as the key to the etiology of schizophrenia. *Schiz Bull* 1990;16:433–443.

17. Davis KL, Kah RS, Ko G, Davidson M. Dopamine in schizophrenia: a review and reconceptualization. *Am J Psychiatry* 1991;148:1474–1486.

18. DeLisi LE, Buchsbaum MS, Holcomb HH, et al. Increased temporal lobe glucose use in chronic schizophrenic patients. *Biol Psychiatry* 1989;25(7):835–851.

19. DeLisi LE, Holcomb HH, Cohen RM, et al. Positron emission tomography in schizophrenic patients with and without neuroleptic medication. *J Cerebr Blood Flow Metab* 1985;5:201–206.

20. Early TS, Reiman EM, Raichle ME, Spitznagel EL. Left globus pallidus abnormality in never-mediated patients with schizophrenia. *Proc Nat Acad Sci USA* 1989;84:561–563.

21. Farde L, Nordstrom AL. PET analysis indicates atypical central dopamine receptor occupancy in clozapine-treated patients. *Br J Psychiatry* 1992;160:30–33.

22. Farde L, Nordstrom AL, Wiesel FA, Pauli S, Halldin C, Sedvall G. PET analysis of central D_1 and D_2 dopamine receptor occupancy in patients treated with chemical neuroleptics and clozapine: relation to extra-pyramidal side effects. *Arch Gen Psychiatry* 1992;49:538–544.

23. Farde L, Wiesel FA, Stone-Elander S, et al. D_2 dopamine receptors in neuroleptic-naive schizophrenic patients: a positron emission tomography study with ^{11}C raclopride. *Arch Gen Psychiatry* 1990;47:213–219.

24. Farde L, Wiesel FA, Halldin C, Sedvall G. Central D_2-dopamine receptor occupancy in schizophrenic patients treated with antipsychotic drugs. *Arch Gen Psychiatry* 1988;45:71–76.

25. Farde L. Selective D_1- and D_2-dopamine receptor blockade both induces akathisia in humans—a PET study with $[^{11}C]SCH$ 23390 and $[^{11}C]$raclopride. *Psychopharmacology* 1992;107:23–29.

26. Gur RC, Erwin RJ, Gur RE. Neurobehavioral probes for physiologic neuroimaging studies. *Arch Gen Psychiatry* 1992;49:409–414.

27. Gur RC, Gur RE, Skolnick BE, et al. Effects of task difficulty on regional cerebral blood flow: relationships with anxiety and performance. *Psychophysiology* 1988;25:392–399.

28. Gur RC, Gur RE, Obrist WD, et al. Sex and handedness differences in cerebral blood flow during rest and cognitive activity. *Science* 1982;217:659–661.

29. Gur RC, Jaggi JL, Ragland JD, et al. Effects of memory processing on regional brain activation: cerebral blood flow in normal subjects. *Int J Neurosci* 1993;72:31–44.

30. Gur RE, Gur RC, Skolnick BE, et al. Brain function in psychiatric disorders: III. Regional cerebral blood flow in unmedicated schizophrenics. *Arch Gen Psychiatry* 1985;42:329–334.

31. Gur RE, Gur RC. Neurotransmitters are important, but so is metabolism. *Neuropsychopharmacology* 1992;7:63–65.

32. Gur RE, Pearlson GD. Neuroimaging in schizophrenia research. *Schiz Bull* 1993;19:337–353.

33. Gur RE, Resnick SM, Alavi A, et al. Regional brain function in schizophrenia. I. A positron emission tomography study. *Arch Gen Psychiatry* 1987;44:119–125.

34. Gur RE, Resnick SM, Gur RC. Laterality and frontality of cerebral blood flow and metabolism in schizophrenia: relationship to symptom specificity. *Psychiatry Res* 1989;27:325–334.

35. Gur RE, Resnick SM, Gur RC, et al. Regional brain function in schizophrenia. II. Repeated evaluation with positron emission tomography. *Arch Gen Psychiatry* 1987;44:126–129.

36. Gur RE, Skolnick BE, Gur RC, et al. Brain function in psychiatric disorders: I. Regional cerebral blood flow in medicated schizophrenics. *Arch Gen Psychiatry* 1983;40:1250–1254.

37. Gur RE. Left hemisphere dysfunction and left hemisphere overactivation in schizophrenia. *J Abnorm Psychol* 1978;87:226–238.

38. Ingvar DH, Franzen G. Abnormalities of cerebral blood flow distribution in patients with chronic schizophrenia. *Acta Psychiatr Scand* 1974;50:425–462.

39. Kawasaki Y, Maeda Y, Suzuki M, et al. SPECT analysis of rCBF changes during Wisconsin Card Sorting Test. *Biol Psychiatry* 1991;29:333S–701S.

40. Kessler RM, Ansari MS, Schmidt DE, et al. High affinity dopamine D_2 receptor radioligands. 2.[125I]epipride, a potent and specific radioligand for the characterization of striatal and extrastriatal dopamine D_2 receptors. *Life Sci* 1991;49:617–628.

41. Kling AS, Metter EJ, Riege WH, Kuhl DE. Comparison of PET measurement of local brain glucose metabolism and CAT measurement of brain atrophy in chronic schizophrenia and depression. *Am J Psychiatry* 1986;143:175–180.

42. Konig P, Benzer MK, Fritzsche H. SPECT technique for visualization of cerebral dopamine D_2 receptors. *Am J Psychiatry* 1991;148:1607–1608.

43. Liddle PF, Friston KJ, Frith CD, Hirsch SR, Jones T, Frackowiak RSJ. Patterns of cerebral blood flow in schizophrenia. *Br J Psychiatry* 1992;160:179–186.

44. Lieberman JA, Koreen AR. Neurochemistry and neuroendocrinology of schizophrenia: a selective review. Special report. *Schizophrenia* 1993;19:197–255.

45. Martinot JL, Paillere-Martinot ML, Loc'h C, et al. The estimated density of D_2 striatal receptors in schizophrenia: a study with positron emission tomography and ^{76}Br-bromolisuride. *Br J Psychiatry* 1991;158:346–350.

46. Martinot JL, Peron-Magnan P, Huret JD, et al. Striatal D_2 dopaminergic receptors assessed with positron emission tomography and $[^{76}Br]$bromospiperone in untreated schizophrenic patients. *Am J Psychiatry* 1990;147:44–50.

47. Mathew RJ, Wilson WH, Tant SR, Robinson L, Prakash R. Abnormal resting regional cerebral blood flow patterns and their correlates in schizophrenia. *Arch Gen Psychiatry* 1988;45:542–549.

48. Mozley PD, Stubbs JB, Kung HF, Selikson MH, Stabin MG, Alavi A. The dosimetry of I-123 IBF: a reversible SPECT ligand with a high affinity for the D_2 dopamine receptor. *J Nucl Med* 1993;34:1910–1917.

49. Mozley PD, Zhu X, Kung HF, et al. The dosimetry of I-123 labeled TISCH: a SPECT imaging agent for the D_1 dopamine receptor. *J Nucl Med* 1993;34:208–213.

50. Musalek M, Podreka I, Walter H, et al. Regional brain function in hallucinations: a study of regional cerebral blood flow with 99m-Tc-HMPAO-SPECT in patients with auditory hallucinations, tactile hallucinations, and normal controls. *Comprehens Psychiatry* 1989;30:99–108.

51. Nordstrom AL, Farde L, Wiesel FA, et al. Central D_2-dopamine receptor occupancy in relation to antipsychotic drug effects: a double-blind PET study of schizophrenic patients. *Biol Psychiatry* 1993;33:227–235.

52. Rubin P, Holm S, Friberg L, et al. Altered modulation of prefrontal and subcortical brain activity in newly diagnosed schizophrenia and schizophreniform disorder: a regional cerebral blood flow study. *Arch Gen Psychiatry* 1991;48:987–995.

53. Rubin P, Holm S, Friberg L, et al. rCBF (SPECT) and CT measurements during first episode schizophrenia and schizophreniform psychosis. *Biol Psychiatry* 1991;29:270.

54. Saykin AJ, Gur RC, Gur RE, et al. Neuropsychological function in schizophrenia: selective impairment in memory and learning. *Arch Gen Psychiatry* 1991;48:618–624.

55. Schlyer DJ, Voklow ND, Fowler JD, et al. Regional distribution and kinetics of haloperidol binding in human brain: a PET study with $[^{18}F]$haloperidol. *Synapse* 1992;11:10–19.

56. Sedvall G, Farde L, Persson A, Weisel FA. Imaging of neurotransmitter receptors in the living human brain. *Arch Gen Psychiatry* 1986;3:995–1005.

57. Sedvall GC. The current status of PET scanning with respect to schizophrenia. *Neuropsychopharmacology* 1992;7:41–54.

58. Sheppard G, Gruzelier J, Manchanda R, et al. 15-O positron emission tomographic scanning in predominantly never-treated acute schizophrenic patients. *Lancet* 1983;2:1448–1452.

59. Siegel BV, Buchsbaum MS, Bunney WE Jr, et al. Cortical–striatal–thalamic circuits and brain glucose metabolic activity in 70 unmedicated male schizophrenic patients. *Am J Psychiatry* 1993;150:1325–1336.

60. Tamminga CA, Thaker GK, Buchanan R, et al. Limbic system abnormalities identified in schizophrenia using positron emission tomography with fluorodeoxyglucose and neocortical alterations with deficit syndrome. *Arch Gen Psychiatry* 1992;49:522–530.

61. Vita A, Giobbo GM, Dieci M, Garbarini M, Castignoli G, Invernizzi G. Frontal lobe dysfunction in schizophrenia: Evident from neuropsychological testing and brain imaging techniques. *Biol Psychiatry* 1991;29:647S.

62. Volkow ND, Wolf AP, Van Gelder P, et al. Phenomenological correlates of metabolic activity in 18 patients with chronic schizophrenia. *Am J Psychiatry* 1987;144:151–158.

63. Volkow ND, Wolf AP, Brodie JD, et al. Brain interactions in chronic schizophrenics under resting and activation conditions. *Schiz Res* 1988;1:47–53.

64. Wagner HN, Burns HD, Dannals RF, et al. Imaging dopamine receptors in the human brain by positron emission tomography. *Science,* 1983;221:1264–1266.

65. Warach S, Gur RC, Gur RE, Skolnick BE, Obrist WD, Reivich M. The reproducibility of the Xe-133 inhalation technique in resting studies: task order and sex related effects in healthy young adults. *J Cerebr Blood Flow Metab* 1987;7:702–708.

66. Weinberger DR, Berman KF, Illowsky B. Physiological dysfunction of dorsolateral prefrontal cortex in schizophrenia III. A new cohort and evidence for a monoaminergic mechanism. *Arch Gen Psychiatry* 1988;45:609–615.

67. Weinberger DR, Berman KF, Suddath R, Torrey EF. Evidence of dysfunction of a prefrontal-limbic network in schizophrenia: a magnetic resonance imaging and regional cerebral blood flow study of discordant monozygotic twins. *Am J Psychiatry* 1992;149:890–897.

68. Weinberger DR, Berman KF, Zec RF. Physiologic dysfunction of dorsolateral prefrontal cortex in schizophrenia: I. Regional cerebral blood flow evidence. *Arch Gen Psychiatry* 1986;43:114–125.

69. Wiesel FA, Wiik G, Sjogren I, Blomqvist G, Greitz T, Stone-Elander S. Regional brain glucose metabolism in drug free schizophrenic patients and clinical correlates. *Acta Psychiatr Scand* 1987;76:628–641.

70. Wolkin A, Angrist B, Wolf A, et al. Low frontal glucose utilization in chronic schizophrenia: a replication study. *Am J Psychiatry* 1988;145:251–253.

71. Wolkin A, Barouche F, Wolf AP, et al. Dopamine blockade and clinical response: evidence for two biological subgroups of schizophrenia. *Am J Psychiatry* 1989;146:905–908.

72. Wolkin A, Jaeger J, Brodie JD, et al. Persistence of cerebral metabolic abnormalities in chronic schizophrenia as determined by positron emission tomography. *Am J Psychiatry* 1985;142:564–571.

73. Wong DF, Wagner HN, Pearlson G, et al. Dopamine receptor binding of C-11-3-*N*-methylspiperone in the caudate in schizophrenia and bipolar disorder: a preliminary report. *Psychopharmacol Bull* 1985;21:595–598.

74. Wong DF, Wagner HN, Tune LE, et al. Positron emission tomography reveals elevated D_2 receptors in drug-naive schizophrenics. *Science* 1986a;239:1473–1624.

75. Wood F, Flowers DL. Hypofrontal vs. hypo-sylvian blood flow in schizophrenia. *Schiz Bull* 1990;16:413–424.

Psychopharmacology: The Fourth Generation of Progress, edited by Floyd E. Bloom and David J. Kupfer. Raven Press, Ltd., New York © 1995.

CHAPTER **100**

New Developments in Dopamine and Schizophrenia

René S. Kahn and Kenneth L. Davis

The last 10 years have witnessed far-reaching changes in the understanding of dopamine (DA) and its possible role in the pathogenesis of schizophrenia. Although the original hypothesis that has so stimulated the study of DA in schizophrenia has proven to be untenable, a role for DA in schizophrenia appears even more likely than it did 10 years ago.

The original DA hypothesis of schizophrenia postulated that schizophrenia was characterized by increased DA function (1). This hypothesis was based primarily on the correlation between the ability of neuroleptics to displace DA antagonists in vitro and their clinical potency (2). However, in the last decade it has become increasingly evident that this hypothesis was in need of revision. One of the principal reasons driving the demand for reconceptualizing the original DA hypothesis was the appreciation that some core symptoms of schizophrenia are negative symptoms and cognitive deficits. These symptoms, though amenable to some extent to neuroleptic treatment, are far less responsive to treatment with DA antagonists than are psychotic, positive symptoms. This, in turn, suggests that some of the core symptoms of schizophrenia may be unrelated to increased DA activity. Additionally, knowledge about the DA system has expanded considerably over the last decade and, combined with the above questions, has stimulated further studies into DA and schizophrenia, leading to an increased and refined understanding of its role in that illness. (See Chapters 25 and 26, *this volume,* for related discussion.)

IDENTIFICATION OF MULTIPLE DA RECEPTOR SUBTYPES

The discovery of multiple DA receptors serves as a good illustration of the progress made over the last decade

in understanding the DA system. Ten years ago, D_2 and D_1 were the only DA receptors known, but now D_3, D_4, and D_5 receptors have also been identified. D_1 receptors are coupled to adenylate cyclase, have a low binding affinity to [^{3}H]spiperone, and are found predominantly in the cortex of humans (3). D_5 receptors resemble D_1 (4), but they have a higher affinity for DA than do D_1 receptors (5). D_2 receptors are negatively coupled to adenylate cyclase, display high binding affinity to [^{3}H]spiperone (6), and are most prominent in the striatal and limbic structures in humans; and their presence, if at all, in the human cortex, is limited (3). The D_2 receptor has also been cloned and two D_2 isoforms, labeled D_2a and D_2b, have been identified (7). The D_3 receptor has been cloned and is primarily present in the nucleus accumbens with very low levels in the caudate and putamen (8). It also exists in two isoforms (9). [In one study, no linkage was found in four Icelandic pedigrees between schizophrenia and the D_3 receptor gene (10).] It bears no resemblance to either the D_1 or the D_2 system (11). Finally, D_4 receptors have been identified displaying a higher affinity for the atypical neuroleptic, clozapine (12). The identification of these various DA receptors has important implications. The high affinity of clozapine to the DA_4 receptor, for instance, raises the issue of whether atypical neuroleptics are effective by blocking D_4 receptors more effectively than they block D_2 receptors. Indeed, it has been argued that blockade of D_4 receptors is related to the efficacy of neuroleptics, whereas blockade of D_2 receptors is related to their extrapyramidal side-effect profile (13). The anatomical localization of D_3 receptors to limbic regions has intriguing possibilities for the development of antipsychotic compounds.

MODULATION OF THE DA SYSTEM

Another discovery of importance in understanding the role of dopaminergic transmission in schizophrenia has

R. S. Kahn: Department of Psychiatry, University Hospital Utrecht, 3508 GA Utrecht, The Netherlands.
K. L. Davis: Department of Psychiatry, Mount Sinai School of Medicine, New York, New York 10029.

been the elucidation of an interaction between cortical and striatal DA systems: An inhibitory regulation of cortical DA systems on striatal DA neurons has been found. When DA neurons are lesioned in the prefrontal cortex (PFC) in rats, increased levels of DA and its metabolites as well as increased D_2 receptor binding sites and D_2 receptor responsivity are found in striatum (14–18). Conversely, injection of the DA agonist, apomorphine, in the PFC of rats reduced the DA metabolites, homovallic acid (HVA) and dihydroxyphenylacetic acid (DOPAC), by about 20% in the striatum (19).

In a modification to the model proposed by Pycock et al. (14), Deutch (20) proposed that the effect of DA depletion in the PFC on striatal DA activity is particularly revealed after the animal has been stressed. Specifically, when animals were stressed, larger increases in striatal DA activity were found in animals whose mesocortical DA neurons had been lesioned than in animals with intact PFC DA systems (20). This suggests that the sensitivity of striatal (mesolimbic) DA neurons to physiological (i.e., stress) challenge is enhanced when DA function in the PFC is decreased. These studies therefore indicate that decreasing prefrontal cortical DA activity increases striatal DA turnover, D_2 receptor sensitivity, and D_2 receptor function, whereas increased DA function in the PFC decreases striatal DA activity particularly in response to stress. Thus, it appears that DA systems in the PFC display an inhibitory modulatory effect on subcortical, striatal DA systems. Decreased activity in the PFC may render the subject particularly sensitive to stress-induced increases in subcortical DA activity.

Others suggest an additional link between (diminished) DA activity in the PFC and stress-sensitive changes in subcortical DA activity. It has been hypothesized that the release of DA in subcortical sites is under the control of two independent mechanisms: phasic and tonic DA release (21). Phasic DA release appears associated with behavioral stimuli (stress, for instance), whereas the degree of tonic DA activity determines the magnitude of the phasic response to environmental stimuli. Decreased prefrontal DA activity in schizophrenic patients is hypothesized to reduce tonic DA release, leading to compensatory increases in (for instance) receptor sensitivity, resulting in exaggerated responses to phasic release of DA in response to stress (21).

In summary, findings suggesting a regulatory effect for PFC DA systems on subcortical DA function have changed the focus from solely subcortical DA systems to the interaction between the subcortical and cortical DA systems as one of the primary regions of interest in schizophrenia. These findings have far-reaching and important implications for the role of DA in schizophrenia: Not only do they suggest the usefulness of increasing DA activity (in the PFC), but even more importantly, increasing DA function in the PFC may be used as an intervention to prevent (stress-induced) increases in subcortical DA activity (i.e., psychosis) and thus may be considered as maintenance treatment in schizophrenia (see also Chapter 103, *this volume*).

METHODOLOGICAL ADVANCE

Understanding of the DA system in humans has also been enhanced by the development of peripheral measures that reflect central DA function. Measurement of the DA metabolite, homovanillic acid (HVA), in plasma has proven to be such a tool, appearing particularly useful when DA function is putatively manipulated, as during administration of neuroleptics. The HVA found in plasma is produced primarily by brain DA neurons and peripheral noradrenergic (NA) neurons. Secondary sources of HVA

TABLE 1. *Plasma homovanillic acid studies in schizophrenia: treatment studies[a]*

Reference	Subjects (N)	Duration	Dose/day	Result
Bowers et al. (48)	PSYCHOT* (29)	10 days	HAL 0.2–0.4 mg/kg	pHVA ↑ in responders
Pickar et al. (56)	SCZ (16)	5 weeks	FLU 30 mg	pHVA ↓, week 3–5
Davila et al. (45)	SCZ (14)	4 weeks	HAL 10 mg	pHVA ↑, day 4
Wolkowitz et al. (51)	SCZ (12)	10 weeks	FLU 27 mg + ALP 2.9 mg	pHVA ↓ in responders
Bowers et al. (95)	PSYCHOT** (37) SCZ (11)	9 days	PER 0.5 mg/kg + HAL 0.2 mg/kg	pHVA ↓, day 7–9 ΔpHVA: responders > nonresponders, pHVA =, week 4
Sharma et al. (47)	PSYCHOT (6)	4 weeks	TFP 40 mg	
Chang et al. (49)	SCZ (33)	6 weeks	HAL 20 mg	pHVA ↓ in responders
Davidson et al. (23)	SCZ (30)	6 weeks	HAL 20 mg	pHVA ↑, day 1
Davidson et al. (57)	SCZ (20)	5 weeks	HAL 20 mg	pHVA ↓ in responders
Pickar et al. (60)	SCZ[b] (21)	12 weeks	CLZ 300–900 mg	pHVA ↓ responders > nonresponders

[a] Abbreviations in Tables 1–4. SCZ, schizophrenic patients; NC, normal controls; PSYCHOT, patients suffering from different psychotic disorders; pHVA, plasma homovanillic acid concentration; HAL, haloperidol; PER, perphenazine; TFP, trifluoperazine; r, correlation coefficient; ns, not significant; *, only two patients were schizophrenic; **, only four patients were schizophrenic; =, no change; ↑, increase; ↓, decrease.
[b] Three patients were schizoaffective (DSM IIIR).

TABLE 2. *Plasma homovanillic acid studies in schizophrenia: baseline pHVA as prediction of treatment response*[a]

Reference	Subjects (N)	Drug-free	Duration	Result
Bowers et al. (52)	Psychosis (85)	7	10 days	Baseline pHVA correlated with outcome at day 10
Davila et al. (45)	SCZ (14)	37	4 weeks	Baseline pHVA similar in responders and nonresponders
Bowers et al. (95)	Psychosis (47)	7	10 days	Baseline pHVA higher in responders
Van Putten et al. (53)	SCZ (22)	28	6 weeks	Baseline pHVA higher in responders
Javaid et al. (55)	SCZ (25)	—	4 weeks	Baseline pHVA similar in responders and nonresponders
Chang et al. (49)	SCZ (33)	28	6 weeks	Baseline pHVA higher in responders
Davidson et al. (50,51)	SCZ (20)	14	5 weeks	Baseline pHVA higher in responders
Mazure et al. (54)	Psychosis (37)	7	10 days	Baseline pHVA higher in responders

[a] Abbreviations are defined in footnote *a* of Table 1.

are peripheral DA and brain NA neurons. Animal and human studies suggest that brain DA turnover can be reflected by plasma HVA (pHVA) concentrations (22,23). Although the precise proportion of pHVA deriving from brain HVA has not been fully elucidated (24), measurement of this DA metabolite in plasma of schizophrenic patients appears to be a valid method to investigate DA in this disorder provided certain conditions are met.

For example, highly consistent findings have been produced when HVA is measured in plasma prior to and during neuroleptic treatment in schizophrenic patients. All studies found chronic neuroleptic treatment to lower pHVA, and all found this decrement to relate to treatment outcome (Table 1). Moreover, six out of eight studies found higher pretreatment pHVA concentrations to be related to good neuroleptic treatment response (Table 2). When HVA is measured during the steady state, however, less consistent results have been generated: pHVA differentiates patients from controls only in some studies, and results of studies trying to link pHVA concentrations to specific schizophrenic symptoms, or even to severity of illness, have been inconsistent (Table 3).

Thus, while the results when HVA is used as an indication of baseline DA function are conflicting, when HVA is used as an index of *change* in DA function the results are quite consistent. This may be the result of the relatively large changes in HVA production when DA activity is manipulated as compared to the steady state. For instance, when striatal HVA is reduced (after administration of apomorphine) by about a third, pHVA decreases by about 25% in rodents (22); when HVA increases fourfold (after administration of haloperidol) in striatum, it almost doubles in plasma of rats (25). A single administration of haloperidol roughly doubles pHVA concentrations in human subjects (26). Thus, the changes induced by perturbation of DA function lead to large changes in both central and peripheral HVA concentrations. Possibly, when DA function is manipulated, the changes that occur are profound enough to be detected in metabolite concentrations in plasma. In contrast, when steady-state DA function is assessed, DA metabolite concentrations may be much more prone to multiple confounding factors (27).

MODULATION OF DA SYSTEMS IN ANIMALS

The distribution and development of the DA system in primates have recently been elucidated. This may indirectly help to understand the role of DA in schizophrenia (see ref. 28). In contrast to those in rodents, DA fibers in adult monkeys are widespread in every cortical region, although they are most pronounced in layers I and III (28). Neonatal monkeys, however, display a more uneven distribution of DA fibers—that is, fewer DA axons in layers III–VI. Axonal growth in these layers takes place during the first 2–3 months of life, so that in early adult life the distribution of DA fibers resembles that in adult monkeys. Interestingly, in monkeys that have been socially isolated since birth, the neuronal growth in layers III–VI appears to have been stunted (29), suggesting that

TABLE 3. *Plasma homovanillic acid studies in schizophrenia: baseline studies*[a]

Reference	Subjects (N)	Weeks off drug	Result
Pickar et al. (46)	SCZ (8)	2	$r = 0.82$
Davis et al. (61)	SCZ (18)	4	$r = 0.66$
Pickar et al. (56)	SCZ (11)	5	$r = 0.81$
Davidson and Davis (62)	SCZ (14), NC (14)	3	pHVA SCZ < NC
Kirch et al. (63)	SCZ (22)	6	ns
Maas et al. (96)	SCZ (23)	2	$r = 0.38$
Sharma et al. (47)	SCZ (11) PSYCHOT (6)	2.5	$r = -0.08$
Van Putten et al. (53)	SCZ (22)	4	ns
Markianos et al. (97)	SCZ (0)	Neuroleptic-naive ns	ns

[a] Abbreviations are defined in footnote *a* of Table 1.

early age is critical for the normal development of DA neuronal networks.

MODULATIONS OF DA SYSTEMS IN HUMANS

Evidence for Cortical Hypofunction

Anatomical Imaging Studies

Multiple studies using computerized tomography (CT) have found evidence of enlarged ventricles in schizophrenic patients as compared to healthy controls (for a review see ref. 30). These studies provide only nonspecific evidence of diminished brain tissue. With the advent of magnetic resonance imaging (MRI), evidence of more localized abnormalities have materialized. Decreased volume of the frontal and temporal cortex have been found as well as decreased volume of the hippocampus, although the findings have not been consistent (see ref. 30). Differences in results may depend on imaging techniques (resolution of MRI scanners) including the slice thickness of the images. The potential significance of these findings can best be viewed in relation to functional imaging studies.

Functional Imaging Studies

Decreased function of the frontal lobes has been repeatedly demonstrated with both measurements of cerebral blood flow as measured by single photon emission computerized tomography (SPECT) and positron emission tomography (PET) (for a review see ref. 31). In a cognitive task linked to frontal lobe function, the Wisconsin Card Sort Task (WCST), schizophrenic patients failed to show an increase in cerebral blood flow to the same degree as normal controls (32). Facility at this task has been associated with the dorsolateral prefrontal lobe. Similarly, schizophrenic patients showed decreased blood flow and activation of the left mesial frontal cortex on performing the "Tower of London" task (31). This lack of activation and decreased blood flow was similar in drug-naive and medicated patients, but occurred only in patients with high negative symptoms scores (31). Indeed, negative symptomatology has been associated with prefrontal hypometabolism (33). Furthermore, decreased frontal blood flow is not related to medication effects (34). Hence, frontal hypofunction seems a key feature of schizophrenia, particularly to patients with prominent negative or deficit symptoms. However, a critical question is whether the findings of decreased volume and function of the prefrontal cortex in schizophrenia have any relationship to the role of DA in schizophrenia. Obviously, atrophy of the frontal cortex could affect various neurotransmitter systems. Similarly, decreased function of the PFC may be the result of hypofunction of multiple neurotransmitters.

However, several lines of evidence suggest that decreased function of the PFC may be related to decreased activity of mesocortical DA neurons.

Relationship Between Cerebrospinal Fluid HVA (CSF HVA) and Function of the PFC

Indirect evidence has suggested that cortical hypofunctionality is associated with diminished cortical DA activity. For example, a strong positive correlation was found between the ability to activate the PFC (on the Wisconsin Card Sort Test) and CSF HVA concentrations (32). Indeed, cognitive deficits attributed to activity of the frontal cortex, such as WCST performance, were associated with lowered CSF HVA concentrations, suggesting a relationship between decreased DA function and impaired frontally mediated cognitive function (35). Moreover, blood flow in the prefrontal cortex increases in schizophrenic patients after administration of the DA agonists amphetamine (36) and apomorphine (37), suggesting that the hypofrontality found in schizophrenic patients can be redressed by increasing DA activity in the PFC. The increase in prefrontal blood flow after amphetamine also correlated significantly with improved performance on the WCST (36), indicating that increasing DA activity improves a cognitive deficit linked to diminished prefrontal cortical activity.

Effect of DA Agonists on Negative Symptoms

If negative symptoms were related to decreased function of the mesocortical DA system, one would expect treatment with DA agonists to improve negative symptoms of schizophrenia. Various studies have attempted to improve schizophrenic symptoms by increasing DA activity. Most have failed to find clinically meaningful effects (see ref. 38). However, recently the DA reuptake inhibitor, mazindole (2 mg/day), improved negative symptoms as compared to placebo (39). In that study, mazindole or placebo were added to neuroleptic treatment after patients had been stabilized on neuroleptic for 4 weeks. However, well-controlled large studies are needed to explore the efficacy of increasing DA activity in the negative symptoms of schizophrenia, although the data reviewed here certainly encourage such an approach.

Conclusion

In summary, evidence suggests that the negative symptoms and some of the cognitive deficits of schizophrenia may be related to decreased PFC function which, in turn, based on indirect evidence, may be associated with decreased mesocortical DA activity.

Evidence for Subcortical Hyperfunction

Increased DA activity of the subcortical, striatal DA neurons has been the basis of the original DA hypothesis. Although unlikely to be the only, or even the main, dopaminergic abnormality in schizophrenia, some evidence does suggest that increased striatal or mesolimbic DA activity is related to some schizophrenic symptoms. Increased activity in those areas is suggested by anatomical and functional imaging studies and more indirectly by measurement of pHVA.

Anatomical Imaging Studies

Only very recently have imaging studies been able to focus on volumetric measurement of the subcortical structures with the availability of high-resolution MRI scanners with section thickness of 3 mm. Increased volume of the left caudate nucleus has been described in a study comparing 44 schizophrenic patients with 29 healthy controls (40). This effect may be medication-related, because it was not found in neuroleptic-naive patients but, instead, appeared only after patients had been receiving neuroleptic treatment.

Functional Imaging Studies

In vivo measurement of D_2 receptor affinity in humans, using PET, has provided conflicting results. An increase in D_2 receptor numbers in striatum of 10 neuroleptic-naive schizophrenic patients has been reported, using [^{11}C]methylspiperone as a D_2 ligand (41). In contrast, D_2 receptor density was not different in 15 (42) and 18 (43) similarly drug-naive schizophrenic patients as compared to normal controls when studied with [^{11}C]raclopride. Similarly, when [^{76}Br]bromospiperone was used to compare D_2 receptor density in 12 schizophrenic patients (who were either drug-naive or at least 1 year drug-free) with 12 controls, no group differences in D_2 receptor density were found (44). Interestingly, the more acutely ill patients had higher D_2 receptor density in the striatum than did the more chronically ill patients and higher than the control subjects, suggesting that DA_2 receptor density may be state-dependent. Part of these conflicting data may be due to the ligand used. For instance, methylspiperone, but not raclopride, binds potently to $5HT_2$ receptors. Moreover, the methods with which PET data were analyzed varied across studies. In addition, as the study using [^{76}Br]bromospiperone suggests, differences in patient population may partly explain the different D_2 receptor densities found in schizophrenic patients. Finally, the ligands used occupied different populations of DA receptors, and they may therefore point toward an increase in number in only the receptors occupied by methylspiperone but not raclopride.

pHVA and the Mechanism of Action of Neuroleptics

The relationship between pHVA concentrations and neuroleptic treatment response suggests an association between the effects of neuroleptics on DA activity and treatment outcome (Table 1). Neuroleptics initially increase (45) and subsequently decrease pHVA concentrations (49–53). Both the initial increase and the subsequent decrease by neuroleptics are associated with clinical response. Interestingly, increased pretreatment pHVA concentrations (49,50,52–54 but also see refs. 45 and 55) are predictive of good treatment response to neuroleptics. Conversely, clinical decompensation after discontinuation of neuroleptic is associated with increases in pHVA levels (56–58). Thus, pHVA studies suggest that neuroleptics initially increase and subsequently decrease DA activity. This is consistent with studies in rodents where, in the nigrostriatal (A9) and mesolimbic (A10) DA systems, a single dose of a neuroleptic increases DA neuron firing (59) while chronic (3–4 weeks) neuroleptic administration decreases DA neuron firing in A9 and A10 below pretreatment levels. Interestingly, atypical neuroleptics— that is, antipsychotics that do not induce extrapyramidal side effects, such as, for instance, clozapine—are anatomically more selective in their effect on DA neuronal firing than typical neuroleptics in that they decrease DA activity in A-10 only (59). On the basis of these data, it has been proposed that decreased activity in A9 is responsible for induction of extrapyramidal side effects, while in A10 it leads to the antipsychotic effects of neuroleptics (59).

The effects of clozapine on pHVA are less clear-cut than those of typical neuroleptics. Clozapine treatment decreased pHVA concentrations with larger decrements associated with good treatment response (60). However, in another study the effect of clozapine on pHVA was less robust, although treatment responders tended to show a decrement in pHVA while nonresponders did not (57). A complicating factor in examining clozapine's effect on pHVA concentrations is the fact that, unlike typical neuroleptics such as haloperidol (Davidson, *unpublished results*) and fluphenazine (60), it increases plasma norepinephrine (NE) concentrations. Because about one-third of NE is metabolized into HVA in the peripheral nervous system (24), the clozapine-induced increase in plasma NE (pNE), may partially overshadow a possible lowering effect of clozapine on pHVA. Consequently, measurement of pHVA as a reflection of clozapine's effect on (central) DA turnover may be compromised by its concomitant opposite effect on NE metabolism. Therefore, a relationship between symptom improvement on clozapine and its effects on pHVA could be obscured by this potent effect of clozapine on pNE.

pHVA and Positive Symptoms

Studies examining a relationship between steady-state pHVA and schizophrenic symptoms have been less consistent than studies examining the effect of neuroleptic treatment on pHVA (Table 3). Four studies have found a positive correlation between pHVA levels and clinical severity (27,46,61,62), while three studies did not (47,53,63). The most likely explanation for the different results across studies is the number of pHVA samples taken as a basis for the correlational studies. The studies employing more than one sampling of pHVA found significant positive correlations between pHVA and severity of symptoms, whereas studies using one single measurement of pHVA did not. The studies producing significant correlations between pHVA and severity of schizophrenic symptoms averaged two (27), three (46), four (61), or thirteen (62) pHVA samples, whereas the studies that produced negative findings assessed pHVA only once (47,53,63). Repeated pHVA measurements in the same individual therefore appears to increase the signal/noise ratio for pHVA by reducing the intra-individual variance in pHVA concentrations (see also Chapter 103, *this volume*).

Postmortem Studies

Although HVA and DA concentrations in postmortem brains of schizophrenic patients consistently show patient–control differences, the localization of these differences are not consistent. Increased HVA concentrations in schizophrenic patients have been found in caudate and nucleus accumbens (64) and cortex as compared to normal brains. The difference in caudate was attributable to prior medication history, while the finding in accumbens only applied in the medication-free patients. Similarly, although DA was found to be increased in nucleus accumbens in schizophrenic patients compared to controls (65), another study found increased DA in the caudate of schizophrenic patients, but not in nucleus accumbens (66). Finally, increased DA has been found in the amygdala of schizophrenic patients, mostly in the left hemisphere (67). These inconsistencies may be due to differences in medication status of the patients studied, varying analytical and statistical methods used, and, finally, genuine variability in the location of DA abnormalities in schizophrenia.

Receptor affinity studies have found increases in D_2, but not D_1, receptors in the striatum of schizophrenics (68–72; see Table 4). Although these results could have been a result of prior medication use, most studies show that those patients who were neuroleptic-free for at least 1 year prior to study or were drug-naive still have increased striatal D_2 receptors. Moreover, a bimodal distribution of D_2 receptor numbers in brains of schizophrenic patients indicates that neuroleptics do not uniformly increase D_2 receptor numbers (68). That neuroleptic treatment alone cannot explain the increased D_2 receptor affinity in schizophrenia is also suggested by postmortem studies in other patient groups treated with neuroleptics: Patients

with Alzheimer's disease and Huntington's disease who had been treated with neuroleptics prior to death showed increases in striatal DA receptors of only 25% as compared to controls, whereas schizophrenics had greater than 100% increases (68). Thus, the available data indicate that D_2 (but not D_1) receptor density is increased in schizophrenia, and that this finding cannot be accounted for by medication history alone.

D_4 receptors have also been reported to be elevated in postmortem schizophrenic brain in subcortical regions (73). Because a selective D_4 ligand was not used in this study, subtraction of two different ligands was used to infer the D_4 receptor number. The differences found between schizophrenic and controls was quite robust, but awaits confirmation (see all Chapter 75, *this volume*).

Conclusion

Increased striatal DA activity has not been demonstrated directly in schizophrenia. Postmortem and in vivo receptor binding studies provide some, but not consistent, evidence that striatal DA function is increased, while studies examining pHVA prior to and after neuroleptic treatment only provide an indirect suggestion that modulatory DA activity in schizophrenia can alter symptomatology. pHVA appears to be a useful indicator of central DA activity, and studies examining pHVA justify the following conclusions: (a) Increased DA turnover is related to good response to neuroleptic treatment, and (b) neuroleptic treatment decreases DA turnover, and this effect is related to treatment response.

Temporal Lobe Function and Dopamine

An increasing number of MRI studies indicate abnormalities in the temporal lobes (more pronounced on the left side) in schizophrenic patients. Decreases of 10% in total temporal lobe volume (74) or 20% of temporal lobe gray matter have been found, present at first episode (75). Interestingly, the abnormalities of the temporal cortex in schizophrenia appears to be associated with specific positive symptoms, such as auditory hallucinations (76) and thought disorder (77). Additional, indirect evidence that the temporal lobes are associated with (positive) schizophrenic symptoms is the discovery that stimulation of the superior temporal gyrus (left and right) elicits auditory experiences (78) and that psychotic symptoms in temporal lobe epilepsy patients appear related to anatomical abnormalities in the medial temporal lobe (established at postmortem examination) (79). Although speculative, since increased D_2 receptor binding has been found in the temporal cortex of brains of schizophrenic patients (80), the abnormalities found in the temporal cortices of schizophrenic patients and its association with some of the schizophrenic symptoms may be related to dysfunctional DA systems in those areas. These findings are particularly

TABLE 4. *Postmortem studies in schizophrenia: DA receptors[a]*

Reference	Subjects (N)	Site	Ligand used	Results
Crow et al. (69)	SCZ (19) NC (19)	Caudate	[^{3}H]Spiroperidol	D2: SCZ > NC
Seeman et al. (68)	SCZ (92) NC (242)	Striatum	[^{3}H]Spiperone	D2: SCZ > NC D1: SCZ = NC
Cross et al. (70)	SCZ (15) NC (8)	Caudate	[^{3}H]Flupethixol	D2: SCZ > NC D1: SCZ = NC
Mackay et al. (65)	SCZ (12) NC (17)	Caudate	[^{3}H]Spiperone	D2: SCZ > NC
Mita et al. (71)	SCZ (11) NC (9)	Caudate	[^{3}H]Spiperone	D2: SCZ > NC
Hess et al. (72)	SCZ (8) NC (8)	Caudate	[^{3}H]Spiperone	D2: SCZ > NC D1: SCZ < NC
Toru et al. (64)	SCZ (10) NC (10)	Putamen	[^{3}H]Spiperone	D2: SCZ > NC

[a] Abbreviations are defined in footnote *a* of Table 1.

provocative in light of the fact that hippocampal lesions to rat pups produces subcortical hyperdopaminergia and an enhanced stress response at adulthood (81).

Frontal Cortical DA Function and Negative Symptoms

Negative Symptoms and Cortical Function

The negative or deficit symptoms—that is, decreased social interaction, apathy and avolition—are considered to be core symptoms of schizophrenia. Indeed, Bleuler proposed that deficit state symptoms represent pathognomonic signs of schizophrenia and are at the root of the poor social and work function that characterize people with chronic schizophrenia. Primate studies suggest that insufficient frontal cortical functioning is responsible for poor social skills: Monkeys with frontal lobe ablations not only have an inability to suppress irrelevant stimuli, poor concentration, and impaired delayed response testing, but also exhibit the poor social function that is reminiscent of deficit state symptoms which characterize schizophrenia (82).

Only a handful of studies have directly attempted to link decreased activity of the PFC in schizophrenia with negative symptoms. Decreased activation of the PFC as measured by SPECT was only found in schizophrenic patients with predominantly negative symptoms (31). Furthermore, negative symptoms were associated with decreased frontal blood flow as assessed by PET (33). Although preliminary, these data do suggest a link between negative symptoms and impaired cortical function in schizophrenia.

There are data indicating that frontal lobe dysfunction can be associated with psychotic symptoms. Evidence of frontal lobe damage leading to abnormal behaviors strikingly similar to some of the more persistent symptoms observed in schizophrenia can be found in anecdotal and case series describing (a) patients with frontal lobe

injury and (b) primates with frontal lobe ablations (e.g., see ref. 83). Although there is great individual variation in the severity and constancy of the symptoms that emerge in patients even with severely damaged frontal lobes, some of these bear a remarkable resemblance to the deficit state symptoms in schizophrenia. For example, orbito-frontal and anteromedial lesions can produce flattened affect.

That negative symptoms are associated with decreased DA function (in the mesocortical DA system) is suggested indirectly. pHVA concentrations levels were lower in chronic, treatment refractory schizophrenic patients than in normal subjects (62). Treatment with the DA reuptake blocker, mazindole (35), or with the DA agonist, SKF393939 (84), appears to ameliorate negative symptoms in some schizophrenic patients. Although indirect, these data imply that decreased DA activity can modulate negative symptoms in schizophrenia.

Negative Symptoms and Decreased Frontally Mediated Cognitive Function

Schizophrenic patients perform poorly on cognitive tests that are thought to depend on activation of the PFC, such as the WCST (e.g., see ref. 32) and the "Tower of London" (31). Animal studies suggest that some of these cognitive deficits may be due to decreased mesocortical DA activity: (a) Surgical ablation of the PFC or selective destruction of mesocortical DA neurons in monkeys impaired performance of the spatial delayed-response task, a test thought to depend on activation of the frontal cortical areas in monkeys (85); (b) iontophoretically applied DA in area 46 [corresponding to the dorsolateral aspects of the PFC (DLPFC) in humans] improved performance in the delayed-response task in monkeys (86); and (c) administration of D_1 antagonists dose-dependently produced deficits in performance during the delayed response task, while the selective D_2 antagonist raclopride did not (86). Because the terminals of the mesocortical DA system consists of the D_1 (and likely D_5) receptor subtype (87), these findings suggest that the mesocortical DA system is important for memory and retrieval functions in high-order primates, and by inference in humans as well. These data are consistent with the notion that the decreased cognitive performance on frontally mediated tasks in schizophrenia may be the result of decreased activity of the mesocortical ($D_{1/5}$) system. Indeed, single-dose administration of DA agonists, such as apomorphine and amphetamine, ameliorate cognitive performance on frontally mediated tasks (36). Studies examining the effect of selective $D_{1/5}$ agonists on cognitive function in schizophrenia have yet to be conducted.

Andreasen et al. (31) and Wolkin et al. (33) demonstrated that these cognitive deficits occur predominantly in negative-symptom schizophrenics. By inference, the cognitive deficits and negative symptoms in schizophrenia may both be related to decreased mesocortical DA function.

Therapeutic Implications

DA_1 Agonists: Increasing DA Function in Cortex?

The persistent symptoms of schizophrenia appear to be the deficit state symptoms rather than the positive symptoms and appear to be related to decreased DA function in the cortex rather than being related to increased DA activity in the subcortical regions. Thus, it is not surprising that these symptoms are resistant to treatment with DA antagonists. Indeed, one would expect these symptoms to be amenable to treatment with DA agonists with cortical selectivity. Because mesocortical DA neurons are primarily of the D_1 and D_5 type, it can be hypothesized that selective D_1 or D_5 agonists would be particularly helpful for these symptoms. Moreover, consistent with the finding by Jaskiw et al. (88) that increasing prefrontal cortical DA activity reduces striatal DA activity, D_1 or D_5 agonists would be expected to decrease the hypothesized increased DA activity in subcortical DA neurons and thus be useful (in combination with traditional D_2 antagonists) in the treatment of acute psychoses as well. Preliminary data from treatment of nonresponsive patients treated with mazindole or SKF39393 are consistent with this notion (39,84).

To treat both positive and negative symptoms of schizophrenia, a balance between increasing DA activity at $D_{1/5}$ receptors and decreasing it at D_2, D_3, or D_4 receptors may be needed. Studies examining such combination treatments, using selective D_1 agonists and D_2, D_3, or D_4 antagonists, have yet to be conducted, but promise to be scientifically and possibly practically fruitful.

$5HT_2$ and $5HT_3$ Antagonists: Roles in Regulating DA Function

It would be overly simplistic to hypothesize that the pathophysiology of schizophrenia is only dopaminergic in nature. Several authors have suggested that it may be abnormalities in the interaction between monoaminergic systems in general and between serotonin (5HT) and DA systems in particular (38), rather than abnormalities in any one system, that is relevant to the pathophysiology of schizophrenia. Indeed, it is particularly difficult to discuss DA without mentioning its interactions with 5HT. Both neurotransmitter systems are highly intertwined, anatomically and functionally, with 5HT having an inhibitory modulation on DA function (89). Moreover, human studies consistently find high correlations in CSF between the DA and 5HT metabolites HVA and 5-hydroxyindolic acid (5HIAA), respectively (see ref. 90). This appears to be the result of a functional interaction, with 5HIAA "controlling" HVA (90), and is not due to a shared transport mechanism (91).

Blockade of 5HT receptors diminishes extrapyramidal side effects induced by DA antagonists. Indeed, ritanserin, a selective $5HT_{1c/2}$ antagonist, significantly reduced extrapyramidal side effects when added to neuroleptic treatment in schizophrenic patients in several placebo-controlled, double-blind studies (92). Thus the addition of $5HT_2$ antagonism to DA_2 receptor blockade may lead to decreased extrapyramidal side-effect potential of DA receptor blockade. Although more speculative, it has also been suggested that blockade of $5HT_2$ (38) or 5HT1c (89) receptors mediates, in part, the superior clinical efficacy of clozapine.

Another interesting relationship is the one between $5HT_3$ systems and DA function. For instance, $5HT_3$ antagonists fail to alter basal DA activity, but they reverse the increase in DA release that results from behavioral and biological stressors (93,94). This may have important implications for the treatment of schizophrenia and schizophrenia spectrum disorders. If $5HT_3$ antagonists prevent stress-induced increases in DA activity, these drugs would be particularly useful in the prevention of relapse in schizophrenic patients and may also have a role in patients that are prone to display psychotic decompensations, such as borderline personality disorders.

FUTURE DIRECTIONS

The explosion in knowledge concerning DA in general, and its possible role in modulating the symptoms of schizophrenia in particular, offers rich ground for drug development and for further elucidating the biology of schizophrenia and its symptomatology. The following seem to be particularly exciting directions.

1. The development of drugs with selectivity for frontal cortical regions could be a viable approach to the treatment of the negative or deficit symptoms of schizophrenia. Dopamine D_1 or D_5 receptors would be most appropriate targets.

2. The development of specific D_4 antagonists will be an important test of the centrality of this DA receptor

subtype in alleviating the positive symptoms of schizophrenia, and it will further our understanding of the relatively unique properties of clozapine.

3. The role of the corticostriatal glutamatergic pathway and its likely role in mediating the reciprocal relationship between cortical and subcortical dopaminergic activity needs to become a target for investigation both in antemortem and postmortem protocols. With the generation of new antibodies for the glutamatergic receptors, the latter may be a particularly worthwhile pursuit.

4. The importance of stress in precipitating subcortical hyperdopaminergia following lesions to the cortex has obvious implications for understanding the initiation of schizophrenic symptoms. Studies in schizophrenic patients that attempt to rigorously document stressful events in a longitudinal context, and correlate them with changes in dopaminergic parameters as well as with symptom fluctuation, would be particularly informative.

5. Some link must be sought between the morphometric abnormalities that have been found in postmortem examination of schizophrenic tissue and the bidirectionality of dopaminergic systems.

With the inevitable conduct of the above investigations, real advances in testing the validity of current conceptualizations regarding DA and schizophrenia will finally be made.

ACKNOWLEDGMENTS

This work was supported, in part, by the Schizophrenia Biological Research Center Grant from the Veterans Administration (4175-020) and by RO1-MH3792206.

REFERENCES

1. Matthyse S. Antipsychotic drug actions: a clue to the neuropathology of schizophrenia? *Fed Proc* 1973;32:200–205.
2. Creese I, Burt DR, Snyder SH. DA receptor binding predicts clinical and pharmacological potencies of antischizophrenic drugs. *Science* 1976;192:481–483.
3. Bunzow JR, Van Tol HHM, Grandy DK, et al. Cloning and expression of a rat D2 DA receptor cDNA. *Nature* 1988;336:783–787.
4. Sanshara RK, Hong Chang G, O'Dowd BF, et al. Cloning of the gene for a human dopamine D$_5$ receptor with higher affinity for dopamine than D$_1$. *Nature* 1991;350:614–619.
5. Sunahara RK, Guan HC, O'Dowd BF, et al. Cloning of the gene for a human dopamine D$_5$ receptor with higher affinity for dopamine than D$_1$. *Nature* 1991;18:350(6319), 614–619.
6. Robakis NK, Mohamadi M, Fu DY, Sambamurti K, Refolo LM. Human retina D2 receptor cDNA's have multiple polyadenylation sites and differ from a pituitary cloae at the 5' non-coding region. *Nucleic Acids Res* 1990;18:1299.
7. Todd RD, Khurana TS, Sajovic P, Stone KR, O'Malley KL. Cloning of ligand-specific cell lines via gene transfer: identification of a D2 dopamine receptor subtype. *Proc Natl Acad Sci USA* 1989;86: 10134–10138.
8. Landwehrmeyer-B, Mengod G, Palacios JM. Dopamine D$_3$ receptor mRNA and binding sites in human brain. *Brain Res Mol Brain Res* 1993;18:(1–2)187–192.
9. Schmauss C, Haroutunian V, Davis KL, Davidson M. Selective loss of dopamine D$_3$-type receptor mRNA expression in parietal and

10. motor cortices of patients with chronic schizophrenia. *Proc Natl Acad Sci USA* 1993;90:8942–8946.
10. Wiese C, Lannfelt L, Kristbjarnarson H, et al. No evidence of linkage between schizophrenia and D$_3$ dopamine receptor gene locus in Icelandic pedigrees. *Psychiatry Res* 1993;46(1),69–78.
11. Sokoloff P, Giros B, Martres MP, et al. Molecular cloning and characterization of a novel dopamine receptor (D3) as a target for neuroleptics. *Nature* 1990;347:146–151.
12. Van Tol HHM, Bunzow IJ, Hong-Chang G, et al. Cloning of the gene for a human dopamine D$_4$ receptor with high affinity for the antipsychotic clozapine. *Nature* 1991;350:610–614.
13. Seeman P. Dopamine receptor sequences. Therapeutic levels of neuroleptics occupy D$_2$ receptors, clozapine occupies D$_4$. *Neuropsychopharmacology* 1992;7:4,261–284.
14. Pycock CJ, Kerwin RW, Carter CJ. Effect of lesion of cortical DA terminals on subcortical DA receptors in rats. *Nature* 1980;286:74–77.
15. Haroutunian V, Knott P, Davis KL. Effects of mesocortical DAergic lesions upon subcortical DAergic function. *Psychopharmacol Bull* 1988;24(3):341–344.
16. Roskin DL, Deutch AY, Roth RH. Alterations in subcortical dopaminergic function following dopamine depletion in the medial prefrontal cortex. *Soc Neurosci Abstr* 1987;13:560.
17. Leccesse AP, Lyness WH. Lesions of dopamine neurons in the medial prefrontal cortex: effects on self-administration of amphetamine and dopamine synthesis in the brain of the rat. *Neuropharmacology* 1987;26:1303–1308.
18. Glowinski J, Tassin JP, Thierru AM. The mesocortical–prefrontal DAergic neurons. *Trends Neurosci* 1984;7:415–418.
19. Jaskiw GE, Karoum F, Freed WJ, et al. Effect of medial prefrontal cortex lesions on dopamine turnover and dopamine agonism. *Soc Neurosci Abstr* 1987;13:599.
20. Deutch AY. The regulation of subcortical dopamine systems by the prefrontal cortex: interactions of central dopamine systems and the pathogenesis of schizophrenia. *J Neural Trans* 1992;36(Suppl):61–89.
21. Grace AA. Commentary. Phasis versus tonic dopamine release and the modulation of dopamine system responsivity: a hypothesis for the etiology of schizophrenia. *Neuroscience* 1991;41:1, 1–24.
22. Kendler KS, Heninger GR, Roth RH. Influence of dopamine agonists on plasma and brain levels of homovanillic acid. *Life Sci* 1982;30:2063–2069.
23. Davidson M, Miklos F, Losonczy F, et al. Effects of debrisoquin and haloperidol on plasma homovanillic acid concentration in schizophrenic patients. *Neuropsychopharmacology* 1987;1:17–23.
24. Kopin I, Bankiewicz KS, Harvey-White J. Assessment of brain dopamine metabolism from plasma HVA and MHPG during debrisoquin treatment: validation in monkeys treated with MPTP. *Neuropsychopharmacology* 1988;1:119–126.
25. Kendler KS, Heninger GR, Roth RH. Brain contribution to the haloperidol-induced increase in plasma homovanillic acid. *Eur J Pharmacol* 1981;71:321–326.
26. Davila R, Zumarraga M, Perea K, Andia I. Elevation of plasma homovanillic acid level can be detected within four hours after initiation of haloperidol treatment. *Arch Gen Psychiatry* 1987; 44:837–838.
27. Maas JW, Contreras SA, Miller AL, et al. Studies of catecholamine metabolism in schizophrenia/psychosis—I. *Neuropsychopharmacology* 1993;8(2):97–109.
28. Lewis DA. The catecholaminergic innervation of primate prefrontal cortex. *J Neural Transm* 1992;36:179–200.
29. Morrison JH, Hof PR, Janssen W. Quantitive neuroanatomic analyses of cerebral cortex in rhesus monkeys from different rearing conditions. *Soc Neurosci Abstr* 1990;16:789.
30. Gur RE, Pearlson GD. Neuroimaging in schizophrenia research. *Schizophr Bull* 1993;19:337–353.
31. Andreason NC, Rezai K, Alliger R, et al. Hypofrontality in neuroleptic-naive patients and in patients with chronic schizophrenia: assessment with xenon 133 single-photon emission computed tomography and the tower of London. *Arch Gen Psychiatry* 1992;12:943–958.
32. Weinberger DR, Berman KF, Illowsky BP. Physiological dysfunction of dorsolateral prefrontal cortex in schizophrenia. III. A new cohort and evidence for a monoaminergic mechanism. *Arch Gen Psychiatry* 1988;45(7):609–615.
33. Wolkin A, Sanfilipo M, Wolf AP, Angrist B, Brodle JD, Rotrosen

J. Negative symptoms and hypofrontality in chronic schizophrenia. *Arch Gen Psychiatry* 1992;49:959–965.

34. Buchsbaum MS, Haier RJ, Potkin SG, et al. Frontostriatal disorder of cerebral metabolism in never-medicated schizophrenics. *Arch Gen Psychiatry* 1992;12:935–942.

35. Kahn RS, Davidson M, Siever L, Gabriel S, Apter S, Davis KL. Serotonin function and treatment response to clozapine in schizophrenic patients. *Am J Psychiatry* 1993;150:1337–1342.

36. Daniel DG, Weinberger DR, Jones DW, et al. The effect of amphetamine on regional cerebral blood flow during cognitive activation in schizophrenia. *J Neurosci* 1991;11(7):1907–1917.

37. Daniel DG, Berman KF, Weinberger DR. The effect of apomorphine on regional cerebral blood flow in schizophrenia. *J Neuropsychiatry* 1989;1:377–384.

38. Meltzer HY. Clinical studies on the mechanism of action of clozapine: the dopamine–serotonin hypothesis of schizophrenia. *Psychopharmacology* 1989;99:S18–S27.

39. Krystal JH, Seibyl JP, Erdos J, et al. Neuroleptic augmentation with medications enhancing dopaminergic function: focus on mazindol. In: *ACNP proceedings, 1992;*17.

40. Breier A, Buchanan RW, Elkashef A, Munson RC, Kirkpatrick B, Gellad F. Brain morphology and schizophrenia. *Arch Gen Psychiatry* 1992;49:921–926.

41. Wong DF, Wagner HN, Tune LE, et al. Positron emission tomography reveals elevated D2 DA receptors in drug-naive schizophrenics. *Science* 1986;234:1558–1563.

42. Farde L, Halldin C, Stone-Elander S, Sedvall G. PET analysis of human dopamine receptors using 11C-SCH23390 and 11C-raclopride. *Psychopharmacology* 1987;92:278–284.

43. Farde L, Wiesel FA, Stone-Elander S, et al. D2 dopamine receptors in neuroleptic-naive schizophrenic patients: a positron emission tomography study with [11c]raclopride. *Arch Gen Psychiatry* 1990;47:213–219.

44. Martinot JL, Peron-Magnan P, Huret JD, et al. Striatal D2 dopaminergic receptors with positron emission tomography and 76Br-bromospiperone in untreated schizophrenic patients. *Am J Psychiatry* 1989;147:44–50.

45. Davila R, Manero E, Zumarraga-Andia I, Andia I, Schweitzer JW, Friedhoff AJ. Plasma homovanillic acid as a predictor of response to neuroleptics. *Arch Gen Psychiatry* 1988;45:564–567.

46. Pickar D, Labarca R, Linnoila M, et al. Neuroleptic induced decrease in plasma homovanillic acid and antipsychotic activity in schizophrenic patients. *Science* 1984;225:954–956.

47. Sharma R, Javaid JI, Janicak P, Faull K, Comaty J, Davis JM. Plasma and CSF HVA before and after pharmacological treatment. *Psychiatry Res* 1989;28:97–104.

48. Bowers MB, Swigar ME, Jatlow PI, et al. Plasma catecholamine metabolism and early response to haloperidol. *J Clin Psychiatry* 1984;45:284–251.

49. Chang WH, Chen TY, Lin SK, et al. Plasma catecholamine metabolites in schizophrenics: evidence for the two-subtype concept. *Biol Psychiatry* 1990;27:510–518.

50. Davidson M, Kahn RS, Knott P, et al. The effect of neuroleptic treatment on plasma homovanillic acid concentrations and schizophrenic symptoms, *Arch Gen Psychiatry* 1991;48:910–913.

51. Wolkowitz OM, Breier A, Doran A, et al. Alprazolam augmentation of the antipsychotic effect of flophenazine in schizophrenic patients. *Arch Gen Psychiatry* 1988;45:664–672.

52. Bowers M, Swiger ME, Jatlow PI, et al. Early neuroleptic response. Clinical profiles and catecholamine metabolites. *J Clin Psychopharmacol* 1987;7:83–86.

53. Van Putten T, Marder S, Aravagiri M, Chabert N, Mintz J. Plasma homovanillic acid as a predictor of response to flephenazine treatment. *Psychopharmacol Bull* 1989;89–91.

54. Mazure CM, Nelson G, Jatlow PI, Bowers MB. Plasma free homovanillic acid (HVA) as a predictor of clinical response in acute psychosis. *Biol Psychiatry* 1991;30:475–482.

55. Javaid JI, Sharma RP, et al. Plasma HVA in psychiatric patients; Longitudinal studies. *Psychopharmacol Bull* 1990;26:361–365.

56. Pickar D, Labarca R, Doran A, et al. Longitudinal measurement of plasma homovanillic acid levels in schizophrenic patients. *Arch Gen Psychiatry* 1986;43:669–676.

57. Davidson M, Kahn RS, Warne P, et al. Changes in plasma homovanillic acid concentrations in schizophrenic patients following neuroleptic discontinuation. *Arch Gen Psychiatry* 1991;48:73–76.

58. Glazer WM, Bowers MB, Charney DS, et al. The effect of neuroleptic discontinuation on psychopathology, involuntary movements, and biochemical measures in patients with persistent tardive dyskenesia. *Biol Psychiatry* 1989;26:224–233.

59. Chiodo LA, Bunney BS. Possible mechanisms by which repeated clozapine administration differentially affects the activity of two subpopulations of midbrain dopamine neurons. *J Neurosci* 1985; 5:2539–2544.

60. Pickar D, Owen RR, Litman RE, Konicki PE, Gutierrez R, Rapaport MH. Clinical and biological response to clozapine in patients with schizophrenia: crossover comparison with fluphenazine. *Arch Gen Psychiatry* 1992;49:345–353.

61. Davis KL, Davidson M, Mohs RC, et al. Plasma homovanillic acid concentration and the severity of schizophrenic illness. *Science* 1985;227:1601–1602.

62. Davidson M, Davis KL. A comparison of plasma homovanillic acid concentrations in schizophrenics and normal controls. *Arch Gen Psychiatry* 1988;45:561–563.

63. Kirch DG, Jaskiw G, Linnoila M, Weinberger DR, Wyatt RJ. Plasma amine metabolites before and after withdrawal from neuroleptic treatment in chronic schizophrenic inpatients. *Psychiatry Res* 1988;25:233–242.

64. Toru M, Watanabe S, Shibuya H, et al. Neurotransmitters, receptors and neuropeptides in post-mortem brains of chronic schizophrenic patients. *Acta Psychiatr Scand* 1988;78:121–137.

65. Mackay AVP, Iversen LL, Rossor M, et al. Increased brain DA and DA receptors in schizophrenia. *Arch Gen Psychiatry* 1982;39:991–997.

66. Owen F, Crow TJ, Poulter M, et al. Increased DA-receptor sensitivity in schizophrenia. *Lancet* 1978;29:223–225.

67. Reynolds GP. Increased concentrations and lateral asymmetry of amygdala DA in schizophrenia. *Nature* 1983;305:527–529.

68. Seeman P, Bzowej NH, Guan HC, et al. Human brain D1 and D2 DA receptors in schizophrenia, Alzheimer's, Parkinson's, and Huntington's diseases. *Neuropsychopharmacology* 1987;1:5–15.

69. Crow TJ, Johnstone EC, Longden AJ, et al. Dopaminergic mechanisms in schizophrenia: the antipsychotic effect and the disease process. *Life Sci* 1978;23:563–568.

70. Cross AJ, Corw TJ, Owen F. 3H-flupenthixol binding in postmortem brains of schizophrenics: evidence for a selective increase in dopamine D2 receptors. *Psychopharmacology* 1981;74:122–124.

71. Mita T, Hanada S, Nishino N. Decreased serotonin S2 and increased dopamine D2 receptors in chronic schizophrenics. *Biol Psychiatry* 1986;21:1407–1414.

72. Hess EJ, Bracha S, Kleinman JE, Creese I. Dopamine receptor subtype imbalance in schizophrenia. *Life Sci* 1987;40:1487–1497.

73. Seeman P, Guan H-C, Van Tol HHM. Dopamine D4 receptors elevated in schizophrenia. *Nature* 1993;365:441–445.

74. Dauphinais D, DeLisi LE, Crow TJ, et al. Reduction in temporal lobe size in siblings with schizophrenia: a magnetic resonance imaging study. *Psychiatry Res Neuroimaging* 1990;35:137–147.

75. Bogerts B, Ashtari M, Degreef G, Alvir Jose Ma J, Bilder RM, Lieberman JA. Reduced temporal limbic structure volumes on magnetic resonance images in first episode schizophrenia. *Psychiatry Res Neuroimaging* 1990;35:1–13.

76. Barta PE, Pearlson GD, Powers RE, Richards SS, Tune LE. Auditory hallucinations and smaller superior temporal gyral volume in schizophrenia. *Am J Psychiatry* 1990;147;11:1457–1462.

77. Shenton ME, Kikinis R, Jolesz FA, et al. Abnormalities of the left temporal lobe and thought disorder in schizophrenia. *N Engl J Med* 1992;327:604–612.

78. Penfield W, Perot P. The brain's record of auditory and visual experience. A final summary and discussion. *Brain* 1963;86,4:596–697.

79. Roberts GW, et al. A ''mock up'' of schizophrenia: temporal lobe epilepsy and schizophrenia-like psychosis. *Biol Psychiatry* 1990; 28:127–143.

80. Joyce JN. The dopamine hypothesis of schizophrenia: limbic interactions with serotonin and norepinephrine. *Psychopharmacology* 1993;112:16–34.

81. Lipska BK, Jaskin GE, Chrapusta S, Karoum F, Weinberger DR. Ibotenic acid lesion of the ventral hippocampus differentially affects dopamine and its metabolites in the nucleus accumbens and prefrontal cortex in the rat. *Brain Res* 1992;585:1–6.

82. Myers RE, Swett C, Miller M. Loss of social group affinity following prefrontal lesions in free-ranging macaques. *Brain Res* 1973;64:257–269.

83. Mesulam M-M. Frontal cortex and behavior [Editorial]. *Ann Neurol* 1986;19:320–325.
84. Davidson M, Harvey PD, Bergman PL, et al. Effects of the D1 agonist SKF 38393 combined with haloperidol in schizophrenic patients. *Arch Gen Psychiatry* 1990;47:190–191.
85. Brozoski TJ, Brown RM, Rosvold HE, Goldman PS. Cognitive deficit caused by regional depletion of dopamine in prefrontal cortex of rhesus monkey. *Science* 1979;205:929–931.
86. Sawaguchi T, Goldman-Rakic PS. D$_1$ dopamine receptors in prefrontal cortex: involvement in working memory. *Science* 1991; 251:947–950.
87. Bannon ML, Roth RH. Pharmacology of mesocortical dopamine neurons. *Pharmacol Rev* 1983;35:53–68.
88. Jaskiw GE, Weinberger DR, Crawley JN. Microinjection of apomorphine into the prefrontal cortex of the rat reduces dopamine metabolite concentrations in microdialysate from the caudate nucleus. *Biol Psychiatry* 1991;29:703–706.
89. Kahn RS, Davidson M. Serotonin dopamine and their interaction in schizophrenia: an editorial. *Psychopharmacology* 1993;112: 1–4.
90. Agren H, Mefford IN, Rudorfer MV, Linnoila M, Potter WZ. Interacting neurotransmitter systems. A non-experimental approach to the 5HIAA–HVA correlation in human CSF. *J Psychiatry Res* 1986;20:175–193.
91. Jibson M, Faull KF, Csernansky JG. Intercorrelations among monoamine metabolite concentrations in human lumbar CSF are not due to a shared acid transport system. *Biol Psychiatry* 1990;28:595–602.
92. Gelders Y, Bussche GV, Reyntjens A, Janssen JAP. Serotonin S2 receptor blockers in the treatment of chronic schizophrenia. *Clin Neuropharmacol* 1986;9:325–327.
93. Hagan RM, Kilpatrick GL, Tyers MB. Interactions between 5HT3 receptors and cerebral dopamine function: implications for the treatment of schizophrenia and psychoactive substance abuse. *Psychopharmacology* 1993;112:68–75.
94. Palfreyman MG, Schmidt CJ, Sorensen SM. Electrophysiological, biochemical and behavioral evidence for 5HT2 and 5HT3 mediated control of dopaminergic function. *Psychopharmacology* 1993;112: 60–67.
95. Bowers MB, Swigar ME, Jatlow PI, Hoffman J. Plasma catecholamine metabolites and treatment response at neuroleptic steady state. *Biol Psychiatry* 1989;25:734–738.
96. Maas JW, Contreras SA, Miller AL, et al. Dopamine metabolism and disposition in schizophrenic patients. *Arch Gen Psychiatry* 1988;45:553–560.
97. Markianos M, Botsis A, Arvanitis Y. Biogenic amine metabolites in plasma of drug-naive schizophrenic patients: associations with symptomatology. *Biol Psychiatry* 1992;32:288–292.

Psychopharmacology: The Fourth Generation of Progress, edited by Floyd E. Bloom and David J. Kupfer. Raven Press, Ltd., New York © 1995.

CHAPTER 101

Schizophrenia and Glutamate

Blynn Garland Bunney, William E. Bunney, Jr., and Arvid Carlsson

Innovative approaches to the study of schizophrenia have provided compelling evidence suggesting a role for glutamate in schizophrenic illness (5,6,7,10). Although the neurotransmitters dopamine, appears to play an important role in the illness, dopamine models of schizophrenia fall short of providing the optimal model for clinical symptoms. For example, in nonpsychiatric controls, dopamine agonists such as amphetamine and amphetamine-like compounds produce positive symptoms of schizophrenia such as hallucinations. However, they fail to produce some of the formal thought disorders usually associated with schizophrenia (27).

An alternative model of schizophrenia has been proposed that involves the amino acid, glutamate. Two divergent clinical observations led to the glutamate hypothesis. One observation was that compounds that blocked the glutamate receptor, such as phencyclidine (PCP) and PCP-like compounds, produced both negative and positive schizophrenic-like symptoms in normals. Luby et al. (41) administered PCP (0.1 mg/kg iv) to normals and reported changes in behavior that progressed from loss of body boundaries and estrangement to profound disorganization of thought. These investigators subsequently administered PCP to four chronic schizophrenics who were ill for an average of 8 to 10 years. In the chronic patients, there was an intensification of thought disorder and as Domino and Luby (17) observed, "it was as though the acute, agitated phase of the illness had been reinstated." The chronic patients became more assertive, hostile, and unmanageable. They noted that all four chronic schizophrenics had behavioral changes that lasted from 4 to 6 weeks.

In normals, the effects of PCP-induced changes in behavior usually last from 1 to 4 hours (21). Because of the dramatic PCP-induced exacerbation of symptoms in schizophrenics and the chronicity of its effects as compared to normals, Luby et al. (41) concluded that PCP touched upon "some fundamental aspect of the disease," which almost 35 years ago was thought to involve a disturbance in the proprioceptive feedback system.

A second line of controversial evidence involved observations of abnormal glutamatergic activity in schizophrenics. Kim et al. (32) measured cerebrospinal fluid levels of (CSF) glutamate in a group of 20 schizophrenics and compared them with 44 controls. All of the schizophrenics had a paranoid psychosis with hallucinations. Of the 20 schizophrenics, 16 were treated with neuroleptic drugs. Results indicated that CSF levels in schizophrenics were reduced by as much as 50% as compared to controls. Comparisons between neuroleptic-treated patients and drug-free patients were not significant, although the lack of significance could be attributed to the small number of unmedicated patients ($N = 4$). Based on these findings, Kim et al. (32) proposed a glutamatergic hypothesis of schizophrenia, which postulated a deficiency in glutamatergic function and/or an increase in dopaminergic function associated with schizophrenia. A corollary to the hypothesis suggested an interaction of dopamine and glutamate in which dopamine inhibits glutamatergic actions. The antipsychotic efficacy of neuroleptics, therefore, could be justified in that neuroleptics decrease dopamine function.

However, other laboratories failed to replicate Kim's et al. results (32). Based on suggestions of a dysfunction of glutamatergic neurons in schizophrenics, it was hypothesized that a degeneration of glutamatergic neurons or a failure to release glutamate would be associated with a decrease in CSF levels of glutamate. Gattaz et al. (20) measured CSF glutamate in 28 paranoid schizophrenics (15 taking medication) and 15 healthy controls. The overall findings of the group reported no difference in CSF

B. Garland Bunney and W. E. Bunney, Jr.: Department of Psychiatry, University of California, Irvine, College of Medicine, Irvine, California 92717.

A. Carlsson: Department of Pharmacology, University of Göteborg, S-413 90 Göteborg, Sweden.

levels. Further analyses of the data revealed increases in CSF levels in patients taking neuroleptics as compared to controls. In addition, significant increases in CSF glutamate were reported in neuroleptic-treated patients compared to medication-free schizophrenics. The investigators hypothesized a relationship between the efficacy of neuroleptics and what appeared to be the resultant increases in cerebral glutamate. A study by Perry (50) compared CSF glutamate in 100 neurological controls requiring a lumbar puncture with 33 patients with Huntington's Disease and 13 patients with schizophrenia (medications were not specified). No significant differences in CSF levels of glutamate were reported in any of the groups. These same investigators also measured glutamate content in six autopsied brain regions in controls (32 nonpsychiatric and non-neurological control adults) and in 21 schizophrenics and reported no differences between schizophrenics and controls (50). Korpi et al. (36) measured CSF levels of glutamate in 23 drug-free chronic schizophrenics and 12 inpatients with neurological diagnoses. An additional six drug-free patients were treated with haloperidol (0.4 mg/kg day) for an average of 60 days and CSF glutamate was measured before and after haloperidol treatment. Results indicated no difference between schizophrenics and controls and no difference in CSF glutamate levels pre- and post-treatment with haloperidol in the six schizophrenic patients. A possible difference in assay techniques between the studies by Kim et al. (32) and Korpi et al. (36) may be a factor in the observed discrepancies.

Animal studies addressed the relationship between drugs and alterations in CSF and brain glutamate. Kim et al. (33) administered chronic amphetamine, a dopamine agonist, to rats and measured brain and CSF levels of glutamate. Results indicated a significant increase in brain glutamate levels and a significant decrease in CSF glutamate levels. A study by Kornhuber et al. (34) showed that chronic treatment with the dopamine blocker, haloperidol, did not produce significant changes in CSF glutamate levels in rats. Finally, Perry et al. (49) injected rats daily for 100 days with large doses of the dopamine blockers, chlorpromazine or haloperidol, and reported no changes in glutamate levels in mesolimbic brain regions.

A number of postmortem studies measuring glutamate activity provide additional data of glutamatergic function. In general, postmortem studies of glutamate receptors labeled with the neuroexcitatory agonists [³H]-aspartate and [³H]-kainate suggest an increase in cortical glutamate–N-methyl-D-aspartate (NMDA) receptors. A number of studies documented increased binding in the frontal cortex of schizophrenics than in controls. These included increased [³H]-aspartate (15) and [³H]-kainate binding (15,56) in the orbital frontal cortex (15) and increased [³H]-kainate binding in the medial frontal cortex (64).

Data from postmortem studies of temporal lobe areas including the hippocampus did not show significant differences in glutamate receptor binding between schizophrenics and controls (15,35), although Kerwin et al. (31) reported decreased [³H]-kainate binding in these areas. Simpson et al. (57) measured [³H]-aspartate receptor binding in basal ganglia regions and reported significant reductions in binding in the lateral pallidum and putamen.

Increased binding in the cortex was also reported in studies using noncompetitive NMDA antagonists (PCP-like) ligands in schizophrenia. Postmortem measurements of [³H]-MK-801 receptor sites in schizophrenic brains suggest an overall increase in [³H]-MK-801 receptor sites in the brain regions studied including the frontal cortex, amygdala, entorhinal cortex, hippocampus, and putamen. However, only the putamen, which was previously described as having a moderate number of [³H]-MK-801 receptors (36), reached statistical significance (there was a 44% increase in [³H]-MK-801 binding in schizophrenics as compared to controls) (35). Studies of [³H]-TCP, another PCP-like ligand, revealed increases in NMDA receptors in the orbital frontal cortex of schizophrenics as compared to controls (56). However, a negative study by Weissman et al. (73) reported no difference in [³H]-TCP binding in the frontal cortex and a decrease in [³H]-TCP binding in the occipital cortex of schizophrenics, although the controls in this study consisted of a mixture of nonpsychiatric subjects and nonschizophrenic suicide victims.

Other technologies assessing glutamatergic activity in schizophrenics include measurements of messenger ribonucleic acid (mRNA). Collinge and Curtis (13) describe a dramatic loss of mRNA that encodes for non-NMDA receptors in the hippocampus of schizophrenics as compared to controls. In a study that measured glutamate release in response to amino acid stimulation, a significant decrease was reported in brain synaptosomes derived from schizophrenics as compared to normals. In addition, the amount of L-glutamate-induced release of γ-aminobutyric acid (GABA) was also significantly reduced in the schizophrenic-derived synaptosomes (54).

Taken together, clinical studies provide preliminary evidence for a disturbance in glutamate activity in schizophrenics. The relationship between decreases in glutamatergic function and increases in glutamatergic receptors remains to be defined, although some evidence supports a negative relationship between receptor density and glutamate function (64). Nishikawa et al. (43) speculate that the proliferation of subtypes of glutamate receptors may reflect a glutamate supersensitivity in response to a decrease in glutamatergic activity at the synapse. A study by Weihmuller et al. (70) investigated postmortem striata from Parkinson's patients and age-matched controls and reported a reduction in dopamine transporter receptors (labeled with [³H]-mazindol) by approximately 70% to 80% in caudate and putamen regions in the parkinsonian patients. In contrast, L-[³H]-glutamate binding increased by 20% to 40% in the same parkinsonian patient group. The data from the Weihmuller et al. (70) study suggest the development of a glutamatergic supersensitivity (increased number of $[^3H]$-glutamate receptors) in regions where dopamine transporter sites are reduced. However, the relationship between dopamine and glutamate activity is unclear and further studies may evaluate such factors as the effects of the antipsychotic agents (dopamine receptor antagonists and the role of the schizophrenic process upon the alteration of glutamate receptors).

POSSIBLE ROLE OF DOPAMINE AND GLUTAMATE IN THE PRODUCTION OF SCHIZOPHRENIC SYMPTOMS

Although the focus of this review is on glutamate, the involvement of dopamine in the schizophrenic process should not be underestimated. Of all the compounds producing schizophrenic-like symptoms only two classes of drugs closely mimic schizophrenia. These are PCP and PCP-like compounds and amphetamine and amphetamine-like compounds (27). Briefly, PCP is a noncompetitive NMDA antagonist that binds inside the glutamatergic–NMDA receptor ion channel and decreases glutamate release. Amphetamine and similar compounds are indirect dopamine agonists that increase the release of presynaptic dopamine and block dopamine reuptake. It is hypothesized that the net changes in the neurotransmitter activity of glutamate and dopamine, respectively, are associated with the production of negative symptoms (e.g., poor work history, poor self-care, poor social interactions, and flat affect) and positive symptoms (e.g., hallucinations, incoherence, loose associations, paranoia, catatonia, and formal thought disorder) of schizophrenia. However, unlike PCP, acute amphetamine does not induce formal thought disorder symptoms, which has led some investigators to suggest that the PCP model is better than the amphetamine model for schizophrenia (27).

It is generally agreed that all the PCP-like compounds administered to man have the capability of producing psychoses. Drug-associated psychoses have been reported with ketamine (37; Wu et al., *unpublished*), dexoxadrol (38) and MK-801 (Zukin, *personal communication*). One question to be addressed is whether PCP and PCP-like compounds exacerbate preexisting schizophrenic symptoms or whether PCP induces novel psychotic symptoms in schizophrenic patients.

THE NMDA RECEPTOR SITE

Glutamate is an excitatory neurotransmitter whose pre- and postsynaptic actions are characterized by its receptor binding properties. The glutamate receptors have been divided into classes, which include postsynaptic sites (ionotropic receptors) and a presynaptic metabotropic receptor. Ionotropic receptors are excitatory, contain glutamate-gated cation channels and have distinct agonist binding sites including NMDA, AMPA and kainate receptor sites. Activation of the presynaptic metabotropic site via a G-protein decreases release of glutamate, decreases N-type Ca^{2+} release, and decreases GABA. The NMDA receptor is thought to be comprised of a recognition site and an ion channel. Competitive NMDA antagonists bind outside the ion channel, whereas noncompetitive antagonists such as PCP bind inside the ion channel at a PCP receptor site (there is also a Mg^+ site within the ion channel). Binding inside the channel is dependent on the state of the ion channel (open or closed), and noncompetitive antagonists such as PCP and PCP-like compounds appear to bind only when the channel is open. In the presence of NMDA agonists, binding of PCP and PCP-like compounds is enhanced. According to MacDonald et al. (58), an open ion channel allows molecules such as PCP to enter and bind. However, binding of PCP inside the ion channel results in closing the ion channel, which traps the molecules inside. When the molecules are trapped, they cannot escape until the ion channel reopens. The potency of molecules such as PCP and ketamine is calculated at the relative rate at which they can escape from the open channels, with PCP having a potency greater than ten times that of ketamine because its rate of escape is ten times slower (58). However, it should be noted that PCP and PCP-like compounds do not bind exclusively to the PCP receptor and may affect other ionotropic receptor sites and the metabotropic site. In addition (as reviewed below), PCP also binds to brain sigma receptor sites.

Information about the NMDA receptor complex can be applied to develop new drugs that can alter PCP-associated receptor effects. In addition, the NMDA receptor contains allosteric receptor binding sites outside the ion channel and substances that bind to these sites such as glycine have been shown to potentiate the binding of NMDA agonists. Similarly, a polyamine recognition site exists on the NMDA receptor, and spermidine and spermine (polyamines) have been reported to increase NMDA responses. If PCP-like compounds are trapped, the effect of increased agonist binding would be to more efficiently open the NMDA ion channels, allowing the PCP molecules to escape.

Recent studies suggest that the opening of the NMDA ion channel is facilitated by NMDA, glycine, and the polyamines, whereas it is negatively modulated by Mg^{2+}, Zn^{2+}, H^+ and noncompetitive antagonists. Therapeutic approaches in the treatment of schizophrenia, for example, could address these multiple sites of activity for the development of novel compounds.

EFFECT OF PCP ON SIGMA RECEPTORS

Although it appears that the major action of PCP is to block glutamate transmission by noncompetitively binding inside the NMDA ion channel, another activity of PCP is to bind to the sigma receptor. The relevance of PCP binding to the sigma site is currently unknown and the potency is only one-tenth of its activity at the PCP receptor. However, the sigma site is of interest in that one of the compounds that binds most tightly to this site is the antipsychotic, haloperidol. In addition, the benzomorphan class of opioids, such as the mixed agonist–antagonists pentazocine and cyclazocine, which are known to produce hallucinations in man, also bind to the sigma receptor (58).

Postmortem studies of sigma receptors in the brains of schizophrenics show discrete but not consistent regional changes. Weissman et al. (73) reported a decrease in sigma ([³H]-haloperidol binding) in the temporal cortex and cerebellar dentate nucleus as compared to controls. Shibuya et al. (55) reported an increase in sigma receptors in the superior parietal cortex of 12 schizophrenics as compared to 10 controls. No other significant changes in sigma receptors were seen in the 17 areas of the cerebral cortex examined. Simpson et al. (56) using [³H](+)-PPP to label sigma sites, reported reductions in neuroleptic-treated schizophrenics but not in drug-free schizophrenics in the amygdala and hippocampus.

Evidence from basic research suggests that administration of antipsychotic compounds may alter binding to the sigma receptor. Chronic haloperidol was shown to down-regulate sigma sites (labeled with [³H]-haloperidol) in mice although no change was reported in PCP sites (29).

Can chronic PCP alter brain sigma or PCP sites? A clinical study of postmortem brain tissue from PCP-abusers and suicide victims (controls) showed no difference between PCP addicts and controls in sigma or PCP binding sites providing preliminary evidence that repeated exposure to PCP does not alter these receptor sites (74).

EFFECT OF PCP AND PCP-LIKE COMPOUNDS ON BRAIN METABOLISM

Data from receptor binding studies in animals show that the limbic regions (especially the hippocampus) contain high concentrations of NMDA receptors (35). A review of the acute effects in animals of the administration of PCP and PCP-like compounds show that these non-competitive glutamate antagonists (e.g., [³H]-MK-801) increase regional glucose metabolism in the brain, specifically in the hippocampal regions (62,72). Ketamine, a PCP-like compound, was similarly shown to increase glucose metabolism in hippocampal regions in animals (14,68). In a rat study, Gao et al. (21) reported that PCP had a delayed effect, decreasing glucose metabolism in limbic regions. A number of review studies of regional changes in brain metabolism are compatible with this suggestion (4,63).

INTERACTIONS BETWEEN GLUTAMATE AND DOPAMINE

Several investigators have documented the behavioral interactive effects of glutamate antagonists and dopamine agonists. In a series of experiments, Carlsson and Carlsson (8,9) showed that, in monoamine-depleted mice, neither low-dose MK-801 (which has a high affinity for the PCP receptor) nor low-dose apomorphine (a dopamine agonist) administration produce significant effects on motor behavior. However, administration of the combination of apomorphine and MK-801 produced a marked increase in locomotor activity, suggesting a synergistic effect of these two compounds.

PCP-like drugs have also been reported to alter behavioral effects of dopamine agonists. For example, MK-801 blocked stimulatory locomotor effects induced by a single injection of amphetamine within the first 30 min of exposure to amphetamine (53). However, 30 min after the injection of amphetamine, MK-801 had the opposite effects on behavior and potentiated the amphetamine-induced locomotor responses. Another study by Weihmuller et al. (69) using in vivo microdialysis techniques similarly demonstrated interactive effects of dopamine and glutamate. A single methamphetamine injection in rats was shown to produce prolonged increases in extracellular dopamine and to increase locomotor behavior. Pretreatment with MK-801 significantly decreased methamphetamine-induced dopamine and increased methamphetamine-induced locomotor effects; this result suggests a dual interactive effect of MK-801 on dopamine release and dopamine-related locomotor activity.

However, MK-801 did not significantly alter methamphetamine-induced increases in stereotypy. In another set of studies, Ujike et al. (66) studied the acute effects of MK-801 and methamphetamine administration and found that at the higher doses of methamphetamine (6 mg/kg), MK-801 attenuated stereotypy and rearing but enhanced locomotor activity. Repeated administration of the combined treatment of MK-801 (0.5 mg/kg) and methamphetamine (6 mg/kg) for 7 and 10 days, respectively, revealed that MK-801 significantly abolished methamphetamine-induced stereotypy but did not reduce locomotor activity. Following a 7-day withdrawal period, rats pretreated with methamphetamine alone or the combination of methamphetamine and MK-801 (or the glutamate antagonist, PCP) were challenged with methamphetamine (2 mg/kg). Results indicated that the rats pretreated with methamphetamine had significantly higher stereotypy scores than those rats pretreated with saline. Furthermore, neither pretreatment with methamphetamine nor the combination of methamphetamine and MK-801 significantly altered the methamphetamine-induced increases in stereotypy. These results suggest that pretreatment with glutamatergic antagonists can modulate acute methamphetamine-induced behaviors but do not have long-lasting chronic effects, which is compatible with data from Weihmuller et al. (71), which illustrates the need for repeated MK-801 pretreatments to block methamphetamine-induced effects.

It should be noted that glutamate antagonists can induce motility even in the seemingly complete absence of dopamine in mouse brain (8–10).

GLUTAMATE INTERACTIONS WITH DOPAMINE RECEPTOR SUBTYPES

Current investigations on the interaction between dopamine and glutamate suggest that glutamate acts differentially on subtypes of dopamine receptors. NMDA receptor antagonists enhance the actions of D_1 and mixed D_1/D_2 agonists. In monoamine-depleted mice, MK-801 was observed to potentiate the effects of SKF-39393 (D_1 agonist) and the mixed D_1/D_2 agonist, apomorphine (8,10).

However, NMDA receptor antagonists can also serve an inhibitory role when combined with D_2 agonists. Svensson et al. (60) experimentally demonstrated the inhibitory effects of MK-801 on the locomotor stimulation induced by D_2 agonists. Similar findings were reported by other investigators using different methodologies (23). Thus, the inhibitory and excitatory actions of glutamate appear to be dependent on the specific interactions with the dopamine subtypes D_1 and D_2.

There is some evidence suggesting that the actions of glutamate antagonists may be dependent on the level of NMDA receptor sensitization. A study by Svensson et al. (61) demonstrated that MK-801 given to animals exposed to low doses of apomorphine (i.e., apomorphine-induced low levels of locomotor activity) produced a stimulatory effect on locomotor behavior. However, if animals were administered high doses of apomorphine, resulting in increased levels of locomotor activity, the effect of MK-801 was shown to inhibit the apomorphine-induced locomotor response.

A more complex model illustrating the interactions of dopamine and glutamate are based on observations by Svensson et al. (59). In their model, they injected the competitive NMDA antagonist, AP-5, into the nucleus accumbens of the mouse, which produced a unilateral loss of glutamatergic tone. In monoamine-depleted mice, AP-5 induces behavioral activation and contralateral turning. In non-monoamine-depleted mice, AP-5 induces ipsilateral turning. Based on these data, one could assume that increasing dopamine would produce the same behavioral effects observed with AP-5 in non-monoamine-depleted mice (i.e., ipsilateral turning). The data support this hypothesis. The systematic administration of the D_2 receptor agonist, quinpirole, in monoamine-depleted mice treated with AP-5, produced a switch in rotation from contralateral to ipsilateral. The same results were observed when apomorphine (a mixed D_1/D_2 agonist) was substituted for quinpirole. However, the combination of AP-5 and the

D_1 agonist, SKF 38393, increased contralateral turning in monoamine-depleted mice. These experiments strongly support a differential interaction of glutamate with dopamine in the nucleus accumbens depending on the involvement of D_1 or D_2 receptors.

HYPOTHESIZED NEURONAL MECHANISMS FOR THE INTERACTION OF DOPAMINE AND GLUTAMATE

The striatum is a possible site for the interaction of dopamine and glutamate neurons. Two major inputs to the striatum include the corticostriatal glutamatergic pathway and the nigrostriatal dopaminergic pathway, which converge on medium spiny GABA-ergic cells. The GABA-ergic cells are inhibitory and project to the pallidum and substantia nigra pars reticulata (24). The relatively recent discoveries of neuronal phosphoproteins, specifically DARPP-32 and its localization in the striatum, provide a mechanism for interaction between dopamine and glutamate. Briefly, the administration of dopamine stimulates cyclic adenosine monophosphate (cAMP)-dependent phosphorylation of DARPP-32 via the activation of the D_1 receptor. This process converts DARPP-32 from an inactive state into a potent inhibitor of protein phosphatase. Activation of the NMDA receptor reverses the cAMP-stimulation of DARPP-32 through an NMDA-induced dephosphorylation of DARPP-32. Thus, activation of this cycle by either glutamate or dopamine can result in different neuronal responses depending on the activity level of the neuronal phosphoprotein DARPP-32 (25).

A number of biochemical investigations have suggested that glutamate increases dopamine release. However, more recent investigations suggest that these effects are complex and may depend on such factors as axonic impulse flow and the dose of glutamate (77).

An electrophysiological study of NMDA-induced dopamine release used a technique called terminal excitability to measure glutamate/dopamine interactions in rats (46). Terminal excitability of nigrostriatal dopamine cells was measured before and after NMDA administration and before and after AP-7 (a competitive NMDA antagonist) administration. AP-7 did not have a significant effect on dopamine terminal excitability. However, NMDA administration was associated with a dose-dependent increase in dopamine terminal excitability. This in vivo technique provides preliminary evidence that glutamate enhances striatal dopamine release via the NMDA receptor. This same group (46) measured firing rates of selected nigrostriatal neurons following the direct, intrastriatal administration of the glutamate agonist NMDA and reported that NMDA produced a short latency increase in dopamine cell firing rates, which was often accompanied by increases in dopamine terminal excitability. These studies provide further electrophysiological evidence for the interaction of dopamine and glutamate in the striatum.

CIRCUITRY

A hypothesized circuitry is proposed to integrate substrates for both potentiating and antagonizing effects of NMDA antagonists on dopaminergic stimulation. It has been thought that a direct route from the striatum to the thalamus, encompassing two GABA-ergic neurons via the medial globus pallidus (in rodents, the entopeduncular nucleus) or substantia nigra pars reticulata is under the excitatory influence of the nigrostriatal dopamine system (2,48), thus cooperating with the corticostriatal glutamatergic system. The indirect route, on the other hand, encompassing three GABA-ergic neurons between the striatum and the thalamus is under the inhibitory control of striatal dopamine, thus opposing the corticostriatal glutamatergic system.

Corticostriatal glutamatergic neurons impinging on the direct pathways could act as a driving force with respect to psychomotor functions; they would mediate the excitatory glutamatergic input from the cortex to the striatum and further on to the thalamus, and the loops involved in this case would mediate positive feedback. Conversely, the corticostriatal glutamatergic system impinging on the indirect pathway would inhibit the thalamus and act as a break with respect to psychomotor functions. The loops in this case should mediate negative feedback. Dopamine would be behaviorally stimulating via both pathways.

Based on the results reported by Svensson et al. (61), it might be hypothesized that D_2 receptors are primarily involved in the direct and D_1 receptors in the indirect route, although there is neuroanatomical evidence for the opposite organization (22).

POSSIBLE IMPLICATION OF NEUROTOXIC EFFECTS

In an extensive review, Wyatt (76) presents evidence that untreated psychoses may be toxic. He reviews data from 22 studies, 19 of which consisted of a majority of first-break patients, and showed that patients treated with long-term neuroleptics have a better long-term outlook than those left untreated. Thus, neuroleptics may be neuroprotective, but more importantly, the process of psychosis itself may be biologically toxic. These findings are consistent with those of Lieberman et al. (40) who reported that prompt and efficient treatment of acute psychotic episodes and the prevention of relapses limit the morbidity associated with schizophrenia and that those patients having increases in dopaminergic activity (possibly associated with the psychotic process) will have the worst outcomes.

A study by Weihmuller et al. (71) demonstrates in ani-

mals acute toxic effects of methamphetamine. Repeated administration of methamphetamine produced dramatic increases in extracellular levels of dopamine, which can result in dopamine terminal damage. In these experiments, rats were injected with either the glutamate antagonist MK-801 (0.5 mg/kg ip) or saline. Each animal was injected with methamphetamine (4 mg/kg sc) 15 min later. The injection sequence was repeated at 2-hr intervals for a total of four sets of injections. One week after drug treatment, striata from these animals were analyzed to determine tissue catecholamine levels. Treatment with saline plus methamphetamine produced a 40% decrease in striatal dopamine tissue as compared to controls. Pretreatment with MK-801 prior to methamphetamine completely blocked the methamphetamine-induced striatal dopamine decrease. Interestingly, results showed that MK-801 was most effective if administered at each of the four 2-hr intervals prior to methamphetamine administration. Data from conditions in which MK-801 was administered either once or twice prior to the four methamphetamine injections revealed less MK-801-associated protective effects.

Using microdialysis techniques and the same drug treatment paradigm as described above, Weihmuller et al. (71) showed that four injections of methamphetamine produced a significant increase in striatal dopamine overflow as compared to saline or MK-801 (given alone). Although the first three methamphetamine injections produced increases in striatal dopamine overflow, the fourth injection of m-amphetamine produced a striking increase in dopamine overflow which was significantly greater than the dopamine increases produced after the first three methamphetamine injections. If MK-801 was administered 15 min prior to the methamphetamine treatment, striatal dopamine overflow induced by methamphetamine was significantly reduced. MK-801 was most effective in preventing methamphetamine-induced dopamine overflow if it was administered prior to each of the four injections of methamphetamine. O'Dell et al. (45) similarly demonstrated that MK-801 prevents methamphetamine-induced striatal dopamine damage and reduces extracellular dopamine overflow.

The data from these experiments suggest a possible neurotoxic effect following surges in dopamine activity in striatal tissue, associated with damage of dopamine terminals. A dramatic rise in striatal dopamine overflow after the fourth treatment of methamphetamine suggests the development of a sensitized response to dopamine. Hypothetically, in man, dramatic changes in dopaminergic function might similarly produce a neurotoxic response. One could speculate that psychosis is a disease process associated with surges in dopamine activity and left untreated, the episodic psychoses become neurotoxic. The neuroprotective properties of the glutamate antagonist, MK-801, has interesting implications for a possible treatment strategy. Compatible with these findings, chronic MK-801 was shown to block the development of dopamine supersensitivity in another animal model of dopamine supersensitivity. Following chronic imipramine treatment, a challenge with the dopamine receptor agonist (D_2/D_3 agonist) quinpirole was shown to increase locomotor behavior, demonstrating dopaminergic supersensitivity. Chronic treatment with MK-801 (0.3 mg/kg i.p.) in the imipramine treated rats blocked the quinpirole response (42).

Glutamatergic excitotoxicity, which is apparently involved in the methamphetamine-induced neurotoxicity, seems to act preferentially on cell bodies rather than on axons. It thus seems reasonable to hypothesize that the excessive glutamate release leading to neurotoxicity is, in this case, mediated via glutamatergic fibers impinging directly on mesencephalic dopaminergic neurons. These fibers may be corticofugal (26). One could thus envisage a positive-feedback system, driven by excessive dopamine release in the basal ganglia and stimulating cortical glutamatergic neurons via striatothalamocortical pathways (11). A similar mechanism may operate in acute psychosis with fulminant positive symptomatology, and this would be compatible with the irreversible deterioration apparently induced by psychotic episodes.

FILTERING DEFICITS IN SCHIZOPHRENIA

As has been documented by a number of investigators over the years, a subgroup of schizophrenics have a sensory-gating deficit, which is represented by a general lack of an ability to efficiently filter incoming external sensory information. Distortions have been reported to affect the five sensory modalities resulting in perceptual disturbances.

Drugs that affect the PCP receptor, including PCP and ketamine, have been reported to produce alterations in external sensory perception. Oye et al. (47) administered ketamine to six normal volunteers and observed changes in perception that were strikingly similar to those observed in schizophrenia. Luby et al. (41), in a series of studies, similarly reported that the effects of PCP produced changes in external sensory perception which at times were almost indistinguishable from similar changes seen in schizophrenia.

One of the most reliable and generalizable models for the study of sensory filtering deficits in schizophrenics is the acoustic startle response. Briefly, a small auditory stimulus is presented 80 to 120 msec prior to a larger stimulus pulse. Eyeblink responses are recorded in response to the stimulus. In normals, there is an inhibition in eyeblink response following the second intensified pulse of sound. The inhibition observed in normals is usually diminished in schizophrenics. In addition, schizophrenics have demonstrated a failure to habituate to auditory stimuli. These findings were reported by Braff et al. (3) and then later confirmed by Wu et al. (75).

Basic studies in animals have demonstrated that drugs that antagonize glutamate produce startle deficits in animals (59). These drugs include MK-801, PCP, and ketamine. (A number of other neurotransmitters may also play a role in disrupting startle responses including serotonin and GABA.)

Electrophysiological (EEG) recordings of evoked potentials (P50) following stimuli presentation have been used to measure sensory gating. Similarly, the administration of drugs known to disrupt the glutamatergic and dopaminergic circuitries produced abnormalities in sensory gating in animals (1) that were similar to the changes seen in schizophrenics (19,30).

POSSIBLE THERAPEUTIC AGENTS

Glycine

An innovative approach to the treatment of psychoses in schizophrenics involves the administration of glycine (for review, see ref. 16) or proglycine (e.g., milacemide) (52) with the goal of potentiating NMDA receptor agonist effects. An encouraging study in mice demonstrated that glycine was able to antagonize behavioral effects of PCP in certain strains of mice (65). However, more studies are needed in this area.

One study on the measurement of glycine receptors in schizophrenic brains reported an increased number of [^{3}H]-glycine receptors in discrete brain regions in schizophrenics as compared to controls. Ishimaru et al. (28) reported increased [^{3}H]-glycine binding in the brains of 13 chronic schizophrenics (seven of whom had not been treated with neuroleptics) in the sensory cortex (supramarginal cortex, angular gyrus, somesthetic cortex, visual area 1, visual area 2) and in the premotor cortex. Whether this reflects a glycine receptor supersensitivity remains to be determined. Waziri et al. (68) reported increases in glycine levels in mesial but not lateral temporal lobe regions in schizophrenic brains as compared to controls. However, the integration of these results with Ishimaru's (28) findings of increased glycine sites is preliminary.

A number of clinical studies have been completed measuring the response of schizophrenics to glycine. In open clinical studies, Waziri et al. (67) administered high doses of glycine (5 to 25 g/day) to 11 schizophrenic patients and reported improvement in 4 of the 11 patients. The majority of the responders to glycine were refractory to treatment with neuroleptics. However, in another open study using similarly high doses of glycine, Potkin et al. (51) was unable to replicate the Waziri et al. (67) study and reported improvement in only one of eight schizophrenics. In an open study, treatment in schizophrenics with low dose milacemide, a proglycine drug, produced no significant changes in behavior (52).

Interestingly, the combination of neuroleptics and glycine appeared to be more efficacious than treatment with glycine alone. Two open studies reported overall improvement in a subgroup of schizophrenics with glycine and neuroleptic administration. Two double-blind studies (44,51) reported improvement in schizophrenics treated with the combination of glycine and neuroleptics. Zukin et al. (78) noted specific improvement in negative symptoms, and a trend toward improvement on a cognitive task (Wisconsin Card Sort Task) when glycine was coadministered with neuroleptics.

Polyamines

An alternative therapeutic class of agents might involve polyamines. Data from a series of studies as reviewed by Enomoto et al. (18) showed that several natural polyamines such as spermidine and spermine augment neuronal responses mediated by NMDA receptors. A detailed study of spermidine suggested that spermidine significantly increased the binding of [^{3}H]-MK-801 in the presence of glycine and glutamate in hippocampal and cortical but not cerebellar membranes. As is known, some noncompetitive NMDA antagonists can displace [^{3}H]-MK-801 from the receptor. However, when spermidine was added to glutamate and glycine, the potency of these noncompetitive antagonists was significantly increased. The authors conclude that the polyamine spermidine promotes the transition of sites responsible for mediating NMDA responses within the channel to a higher affinity for the noncompetitive NMDA antagonists. It is noteworthy that compounds having high affinity for the [^{3}H]-MK-801 receptor including MK-801, TCP, and PCP were affected by spermidine. However, several compounds from another class of drugs, benzomorphans, which bind to both [^{3}H]-MK-801 and sigma receptors, were shown to be potentiated by spermidine. These compounds are cyclazocine and pentazocine and have psychotomimetic properties. Although cyclazocine has slightly less potency at the [^{3}H]-MK-801 receptor than PCP, other compounds having much greater affinity for the [^{3}H]-MK-801 receptor than pentazocine, were not significantly affected by spermidine.

Preliminary data in rats suggest that polyamine antagonists inhibit [^{3}H]-MK-801 binding. Lehmann et al. (39) measured [^{3}H]-MK-801 binding to rat cortical membranes and reported that the polyamine antagonist arcaine dramatically blocked [^{3}H]-MK-801 binding. However, the investigators argue that, in spite of the data, the polyamine site is only modulatory and binding at this site is not necessary for NMDA channel opening. Therefore, they question the selectivity of arcaine for the polyamine site.

D-Cycloserine

Another compound acting as an agonist at the NMDA receptor is D-cycloserine which binds at the strychnine-

insensitive glycine recognition site on the NMDA receptor-ionophore complex. In a postmortem study of Alzheimer's patients, binding of [^{3}H]-MK-801 was measured in membranes from the inferior parietal cortex. D-Cycloserine in the presence of fixed concentrations of glycine was shown to increase [^{3}H-MK-801] binding. These data are compatible with findings that D-cycloserine is a partial agonist at the glycine site (12).

SUMMARY

In summary, evidence from a number of clinical and basic scientific investigations suggest the involvement of the neurotransmitter glutamate in schizophrenia. Specific brain circuitries and relevant interactions with receptor subtypes support the involvement of glutamate. Future studies may elucidate the mechanisms of glutamate in the brain and its genetic modulation in the production of schizophrenic symptoms.

REFERENCES

1. Adler LE, Rose G, Freedman R. Neurophysiological studies of sensory gating in rats: effects of amphetamine, phencyclidine, and haloperidol. *Biol Psychiatry* 1986;21:787–798.
2. Alexander GE, Crutcher MD. Functional architecture of basal ganglia circuits: neural substrates of parallel processing. *Trends Neurosci* 1990;13:266–271.
3. Braff D, Stone C, Callaway E, Geyer M, Glick I, Bali L. Prestimulus effects on human startle reflex in normals and schizophrenics. *Psychophysiology* 1978;15:339–343.
4. Buchsbaum MS, Haier RJ, Potkin SG, et al. Frontostriatal disorder of cerebral metabolism in never-medicated schizophrenics. *Arch Gen Psychiatry* 1992;49:935–942.
5. Bunney WE Jr. PCP receptor ionophore complex: basic mechanisms and possible relevance to schizophrenia. *21st Annual Winter Conference on Brain Research,* Steamboat Springs, Colorado, 1988, No. 20 (abst.).
6. Bunney WE Jr., Bunney BG. New hypotheses in schizophrenia. In: Stefanis CN, Soldatos CR, Rabavilas AD, eds. *Psychiatry: a world perspective.* Vol. 2. Amsterdam: Elsevier; 1990:37–44.
7. Carlsson A. The current status of the dopamine hypothesis of schizophrenia, *Neuropsychopharmacology* 1988;1:179–186.
8. Carlsson M, Carlsson A. The NMDA antagonist MK-801 causes marked locomotor stimulation in monoamine-depleted mice. *J Neural Transm* 1989;75:221–226.
9. Carlsson M, Carlsson A. Dramatic synergism between MK-801 and clonidine with respect to locomotor stimulatory effect in monoamine-depleted mice. *J Neural Transm* 1989;77:65–71.
10. Carlsson M, Carlsson A. Schizophrenia: a subcortical neurotransmitter imbalance syndrome? *Schizophrenia Bull* 1990;16:425–432.
11. Carlsson A. Search for the neuronal circuitries and neurotransmitters involved in "positive" and "negative" schizophrenic symptomatology. *Fidia Research Foundation neuroscience award lectures.* Vol. 5. New York: Raven Press, 1991.
12. Chessell IP, Proctor AW, Francis PT, Bowen DM. D-Cycloserine, a putative cognitive enhancer, facilitates activation of the *N*-methyl-D-aspartate receptor-ionophore complex in Alzheimer brain. *Brain Res* 1991;565:345–348.
13. Collinge J, Curtis D. Decreased hippocampal expression of a glutamate receptor gene in schizophrenia. *Br J Psychiatry* 1991;159:857–859.
14. Davis DW, Mans AM, Biebuyck JF, Phil D, Hawkins RA. The influence of ketamine on regional brain glucose use. *Anesthesiology* 1988;69:199–205.

15. Deakin JF, Slater P, Simpson MD, et al. Frontal cortical and left temporal glutamatergic dysfunction in schizophrenia. *J Neurochemistry* 1989;52:1781–1786.

16. Deutsch SI, Mastraopaolo Y, Schwartz BL, Rosse RB, Morihisa JM. A "glutamatergic hypothesis" of schizophrenia; rationale for pharmacotherapy with glycine. *Clin Neuropharmacol* 1989;12:1–13.

17. Domino EF, Luby E. Abnormal mental states induced by phencyclidine as a model of schizophrenia. In: Domino EF, ed. *PCP (Phencyclidine): historical and current perspectives.* Michigan: NPP Books;1981:401–418.

18. Enomoto R, Ogita K, Han D, Yoneda Y. Differential potentiation by spermidine of abilities of a variety of displacers for 3H-MK-801 binding in hippocampal synaptic membranes. *Neuro Sci Res* 1993;16:217–224.

19. Freedman R, Adler LE, Waldo MC, Pachtman E, Franks RD. Neurophysiological evidence for a defect in inhibitory pathways in schizophrenia: comparison of medicated and drug-free patients. *Biol Psychiatry* 1983;18:537–551.

20. Gattaz WF, Gattaz D, Beckmann H. Glutamate in schizophrenics and healthy controls. *Arch Psychiatr Nervenkr* 1982;231:221–225.

21. Gao XM, Shirikawa O, Tamminga CA. Delayed phencyclidine-induced alterations in local cerebral glucose utilization in rat brain. *Neuro Sci Abst* 1991;575:1473.

22. Gerfen CR, Engber TM, Mahan LC, et al. D_1 and D_2 dopamine receptor-regulated gene expression of striatonigral and striatopallidal neurons. *Science* 1990;250:1429–1432.

23. Goodwin P, Starr BS, Starr MS. Motor responses to dopamine D_1 and D_2 agonists in the reserpine-treated mouse are affected differentially by the NMDA receptor antagonist MK-801. *J Neural Trans* 1992;4:15–26.

24. Graybiel AM. Neurotransmitters and neuromodulators in the basal ganglia. *Trends Neurosci* 1990;13:244–253.

25. Halpain S, Girault JA, Greengard P. Activation of NMDA receptors induces dephosphorylation of DARPP-32 in rat striatal slices. *Nature* 1990;343:369–372.

26. Heimer L, Alheid GF, Zaborszky L. "Perestroika" in the basal forebrain: Opening the border between neurology and psychiatry. *Prog Brain Res* 1991;87:109–165.

27. Heresco-Levy U, Javitt DC, Zukin SR. The phencyclidine/N-methyl-D-aspartate (PCP/NMDA) model of schizophrenia: theoretical and clinical implications. *Psychiatr Ann* 1993;23:135–143.

28. Ishimaru M, Kurumaji A, Toru M. NMDA-associated glycine binding site increases in schizophrenic brains. *Biol Psychiatry* 1992;32:379–381.

29. Itzhak Y, Alerhand S. Differential regulation of sigma and PCP receptors after chronic administration of haloperidol and phencyclidine in mice. *FASEB J* 1989;3:1868–1873.

30. Judd LL, McAdams L, Budnick B, Braff DL. Sensory gating deficits in schizophrenia: New results. *Am J Psychiatry* 1992;149:488–493.

31. Kerwin R, Patel S, Meldrum B. Quantitative autoradiographic analysis of glutamate receptor binding sites in the hippocampal formation in normal and schizophrenic postmortem brain. *Neuroscience* 1990;39:25–32.

32. Kim JS, Kornhuber HH, Schmid-Burgk, Holzmuller B. Low cerebrospinal fluid glutamate in schizophrenic patients and a new hypothesis of schizophrenia. *Neurosci Lett* 1980;20:379–382.

33. Kim JS, Kornhuber HH, Brand U, Menge HG. Effects of chronic amphetamine treatment on the glutamate concentration in cerebrospinal fluid and brain: implications for a theory of schizophrenia. *Neurosci Lett* 1981;24:93–96.

34. Kornhuber J, Kim JS, Kornhuber ME, Kornhuber HH. Chronic haloperidol administration enhances the gamma-aminobutyric acid level in the rat striatum without altering the glutamate level. *Eur Neurol* 1984;23:269–273.

35. Kornhuber J, Mack-Burkhardt F, Hebenstreit GF, Reynolds GP, Andrews HB, Beckmann H. 3H-MK-801 binding sites in postmortem brain regions of schizophrenic patients. *J Neural Trans* 1989;77:231–236.

36. Korpi ER, Kaufmann CA, Marnela KM, Weinberger DR. Cerebrospinal fluid amino acid concentrations in chronic schizophrenia. *Psychiatry Res* 1987;20:337–345.

37. Lahti AC, Gao XM, Cascella NG, Mokriski B, LaPorte D, Lahti

38. RA, Tamminga CA. Can NMDA antagonists help us understand the psychosis mechanisms in schizophrenia? *Schiz Res* 1993;9:241.

38. Lasagna L, Pearson JW. Analgesic and psychotomimetic properties of dexoxadrol. *Proc Soc Exp Biol Med* 1965;118:352–354.

39. Lehmann J, Colpaert F, Karbon EW. Glutamate and glycine coactivate while polyamines merely modulate the NMDA receptor complex. *Neurosci Lett* 1991;132:146–150.

40. Lieberman JA. Prediction of outcome in first-episode schizophrenia. *J Clin Psychiatry* 1993;54(suppl):13–17.

41. Luby ED, Cohen BD, Rosenbaum F, Gottlieb J, Kelley R. Study of a new schizophrenomimetic drug, Sernyl. *Arch Neurol Psychiatry* 1959;81:363–369.

42. Marshall JF, O'Dell SJ, Weihmuller FB. Dopamine-glutamate interactions in methamphetamine-induced neurotoxicity. *J Neural Trans* 1993;91:241–254.

43. Nishikawa T, Takashima M, Toru M. Increased [3H]kainic acid binding in the prefrontal cortex of schizophrenics. *Neurosci Lett* 1983;40:245–250.

44. Nussenzweig IZ, Javitt DC, Silipo GS, et al. High-dose glycine in the treatment of schizophrenia. Presented at the 145th annual meeting American Psychiatric Association. Washington, DC, 1992.

45. O'Dell SJ, Weihmuller FB, Marshall JF. MK-801 prevents methamphetamine-induced striatal dopamine damage and reduces extracellular dopamine overflow. *Ann NY Acad Sci* 1992;648:317–319.

46. Overton P, Clark D. Electrophysiological evidence that intrastriatally administered N-methyl-D-aspartate augments striatal dopamine tone in the rat. *J Neurosci Transmission* 1992;4:1–14.

47. Oye I, Paulsen O, Maurset A. Effects of ketamine on sensory perception: evidence for a role of N-methyl-D-aspartate receptors. *J Pharm Exp Ther* 1992;260:1209–1213.

48. Pan HS, Penney JB, Young AB. GABA and benzodiazepine receptor changes induced by unilateral 6-hydroxydopamine lesions of the medial forebrain bundle. *J Neurochem* 1985;45:1396–1404.

49. Perry TL, Hansen S, Kish SJ. Effects of chronic administration of antipsychotic drugs on GABA and other amino acids in the mesolimbic area of rat brain. *Life Sci* 1979;24:460–466.

50. Perry TL. Normal cerebrospinal fluid and brain glutamate levels in schizophrenia do not support the hypothesis of glutamatergic neuronal dysfunction. *Neurosci Lett* 1982;28:81–85.

51. Potkin S, Costa J, Roy S, Sramek J, Jin Y, Gulasekaram B. Glycine in the treatment of schizophrenia: theory and preliminary results. In: Meltzer HY, ed. *Novel antipsychotic drugs.* New York: Raven Press; 1992:179–188.

52. Rosse RB, Schwartz BL, Davis RE, Deutsch SI. An NMDA intervention strategy in schizophrenia with "low-dose" milacemide. *Clin Neuropharmacol* 1991;14:268–272.

53. Schenk S, Valadez A, McNmara C, Horger BA. Blockade of sensitizing effects of amphetamine pre-exposure on cocaine self-administration by the NMDA antagonist MK-801. 22nd Annual Meeting of the Society of Neuroscience, Anaheim, CA, October 25–30, 1992:1237 (abst.).

54. Sherman AD, Hegwood TS, Baruah S, Waziri R. Deficient NMDA-mediated glutamate release from synaptosomes of schizophrenics. *Biol Psychiatry* 1991;30:1191–1198.

55. Shibuya H, Mori H, Toru M. Sigma receptors in schizophrenic cerebral cortices. *Neurochem Res* 1992;17:983–990.

56. Simpson MDC, Slater P, Royston MC, Deakin JFW. Alterations in phencyclidine and sigma binding sites in schizophrenic brains: effects of disease process and neuroleptic medication. *Schiz Res* 1992;6:41–48.

57. Simpson MD, Slater P, Royston MC, Deakin JF. Regionally selective deficits in uptake sites for glutamate and gamma-aminobutyric acid in the basal ganglia of schizophrenics. *Psychiatry Res* 1992;42:273–282.

58. Snyder SH, Largent BL. Receptor mechanisms in antipsychotic drug action: focus on sigma receptors. *J Neuropsychiatry* 1989;1:7–15.

59. Svensson A, Carlsson M. Injection of the competitive NMDA receptor antagonist AP-5 into the nucleus accumbens of monoamine-depleted mice induces pronounced locomotor stimulation. *Neuropharmacology* 1992;31:513–518.

60. Svensson A, Carlsson M, Carlsson A. Differential locomotor interactions between the dopamine D_1 and D_2 receptor agonists and

NMDA antagonist dizolcipine in monoamine-depleted mice. *J Neural Transm* 1992;90:199–212.

61. Svensson A, Carlsson ML, Carlsson A. Interaction between glutamatergic and dopaminergic tone in the nucleus accumbens of mice. Evidence for a dual glutamatergic function with respect to psychomotor control. *J Neural Trans* 1992;88:235–240.

62. Tamminga CA, Tanimoto K, Kuo S, et al. PCP-induced alterations in cerebral glucose metabolism in rat brain: blockade by metaphit, a PCP receptor acylating agent. *Synapse* 1987;1:497–504.

63. Tamminga CA, Thanker GK, Buchanan R, et al. Limbic system abnormalities identified in schizophrenia using positron emission tomography with fluorodeoxyglucose and neocortical alterations with deficit syndromes. *Arch Gen Psychiatry* 1992;49:522–530.

64. Toru M, Watanabe S, Shibuya H, et al. Neurotransmitters, receptors and neuropeptides in postmortem brains of chronic schizophrenic patients. *Acta Psychiatr Scand* 1988;78:121–137.

65. Toth E, Lajtha A. Antagonism of phencyclidine-induced hyperactivity by glycine in mice. *Neurochem Res* 1986;11:393–400.

66. Ujike H, Tsuchida H, Kanzaki A, Akiyama K, Otsuki S. Competitive and noncompetitive N-methyl-D-aspartate antagonists fail to prevent the induction of methamphetamine-induced sensitization. *Life Sci* 1992;50:1673–1681.

67. Waziri R. Glycine therapy of schizophrenia. *Biol Psychiatry* 1988;23:210.

68. Waziri R, Baruah S, Sherman AD. Abnormal serine-glycine metabolism in the brains of schizophrenics. *Neurosci Lett* 1990;120:237–240.

69. Weihmuller FB, O'Dell SJ, Cole BN, Marshall JF. MK-801 attenuates the dopamine-releasing but not the behavioral effects of methamphetamine: an in vivo microdialysis study. *Brain Res* 1991;549:230–235.

70. Weihmuller FB, Ulas J, Nguyen L, Cotman CW, Marshall JF. Elevated NMDA receptors in parkinsonian striatum. *Neuroreport* 1992;3:977–980.

71. Weihmuller FB, O'Dell SJ, Marshall JF. MK-801 protection against methamphetamine-induced striatal dopamine terminal injury is associated with attenuated dopamine overflow. *Synapse* 1992; 11:155–163.

72. Weissman AD, Dam M, London ED. Alterations in local cerebral glucose utilization induced by phencyclidine. *Brain Res* 1987; 435:29–40.

73. Weissman AD, Casanova MF, Kleinman E, London ED, DeSouza EB. Selective loss of cerebral sigma, but not PCP binding sites in schizophrenia. *Biol Psychiatry* 1991;29:41–54.

74. Weissman AD, Casanova MF, Kleinman JE, DeSouza EB. PCP and sigma receptors in brain are not altered after repeated exposure to PCP in humans. *Neuropsychopharmacology* 1991;4:95–102.

75. Wu J. Acoustic startle response in schizophrenics. Presented at West Coast College of Biological Psychiatry, San Diego, 1990.

76. Wyatt RJ. Neuroleptics and the natural course of schizophrenia. *Schiz Bull* 1991;17:325–351.

77. Youngren KD, Daly DA, Moghaddam B. Distinct actions of excitatory amino acids on the outflow of dopamine in the nucleus accumbens. *J Pharm Exp Ther* 1993;264:289–293.

78. Zukin R, Nussenveig IZ, Javitt DC, Heresco-Levy U, Sircar R, Lindenmayer J-P. NMDA receptor stimulation schizophrenia: candidate mechanisms and effect of oral glycine. 31st meeting of the American College of Neuropsychopharmacology, San Juan, Puerto Rico, December 14–18, 1992:21 (abst.).

Psychopharmacology: The Fourth Generation of Progress, edited by Floyd E. Bloom and David J. Kupfer. Raven Press, Ltd., New York © 1995.

CHAPTER 102

The Role of Serotonin in Schizophrenia

Bryan L. Roth and Herbert Y. Meltzer

Schizophrenia is generally considered to be a syndrome comprised of a number of different disorders that produce overlapping but not identical disturbances in reality testing, cognition, mood, social function, interpersonal relations, and so on. The evidence that schizophrenia is characterized by structural brain damage appears incontrovertible, although it is far from clear if there is a specific group of structural abnormalities that are crucial to the disorder. For decades, the biochemical basis of schizophrenia and the mechanism of action of antipsychotic drugs was overly concentrated on the role of dopamine (DA) (see Chapter 100, *this volume*). However, in recent years, the possible importance of the role of other neurotransmitters acting in conjunction with DA for the etiology of schizophrenia and the mechanism of action of psychotropic drugs has been intensively studied.

This chapter reviews the evidence for the role of serotonin (5-hydroxytryptamine; 5-HT) in the etiology and pathophysiology of schizophrenia and, to a limited extent, the mechanism of action of antipsychotic drugs. We critically review current methods to study the 5-HT system in schizophrenia. Additionally, the potential of serotonergic agents to treat or exacerbate schizophrenia is scrutinized. The evidence for 5-HT/DA interactions in vivo, which could be the basis for the role of 5-HT in schizophrenia, is also examined. Finally, we synthesize these findings and present them in the form of a wiring diagram of the brain serotonergic system.

EARLY HYPOTHESES LINKING HALLUCINOGENS AND SCHIZOPHRENIA

The first hypotheses of an involvement of 5-HT in schizophrenia were provided by Wooley and Shaw (87)

and Gaddum (17) based on the attribution of the psychotomimetic effects of lysergic acid diethylamide (LSD), which is structurally related to 5-HT, to its antagonist action at brain 5-HT receptors. Accordingly, Gaddum (17) and Wooley and Shaw (87) proposed that serotonergic activity might be decreased in schizophrenia. One of the major problems with this hypothesis was the recognition that LSD-induced primarily visual hallucinations, which are relatively rare in schizophrenia, whereas auditory hallucinations are characteristic of schizophrenia. Additionally, paranoid delusions, conceptual disorganization, and certain types of cognitive impairment characteristic of schizophrenia are generally absent during LSD intoxication (79). An additional problem with the LSD hypothesis of schizophrenia is the recognition that LSD is a full or partial agonist (not antagonist) at many 5-HT receptors (19).

The hypothesis of Wooley and Shaw (87) was followed by the proposal that the production of endogenous methylated indoleamines with psychotomimetic properties might be important to the etiopathology of schizophrenia (discussed in ref. 7). However, no differences in the amounts of the methyltransferase enzyme or the levels of methylated indoleamines excreted in plasma or urine of schizophrenic patients and normal controls have been consistently reported (reviewed in ref. 7).

SEROTONIN HYPOTHESIS OF SCHIZOPHRENIA

It is beyond the scope of this chapter to review the many normal and abnormal behaviors linked to 5-HT. This was previously discussed in the context of the role of 5-HT in the etiology of depression (see Chapter 81, *this volume*), one of the many psychiatric disorders in which 5-HT has been implicated. Serotonin has been implicated in a variety of behaviors and somatic functions

B. L. Roth and H. Y. Meltzer: Department of Psychiatry, Laboratory of Biological Psychiatry, Case Western Reserve University School of Medicine, Cleveland, Ohio 44106.

that are disturbed in schizophrenia (e.g., perception, attention, mood, aggression, sexual drive, appetite, motor behavior, and sleep). Given the complexity of the serotonergic system (see Chapter 36, *this volume*) and its interactions with multiple neurotransmitters, it seems likely that a variety of disturbances of the 5-HT system might play a role in specific aspects of schizophrenia. In 1988, Bleich et al. (7) reviewed the role of 5-HT in schizophrenia and concluded that alterations in brain 5-HT metabolism could be related to Crow's concept of Type II (deficit) schizophrenia. In particular, these authors proposed that the 5-HT abnormality in schizophrenia "might involve 5-HT postsynaptic receptor hypersensitivity" (7).

Meltzer (48) suggested that there might be enhanced serotonergic neurotransmission in schizophrenia, leading to a secondary down-regulation of some 5-HT_{2A} receptors. Specifically, a serotonin–dopamine hypothesis, was proposed; abnormalities in the serotonergic modulation of dopaminergic activity (e.g., decreased inhibition by 5-HT of the release of DA in the mesencephalon and cortex) might be contributory to schizophrenia (48). It was also proposed that the enhanced antipsychotic effect of clozapine and related drugs such as risperidone to improve schizophrenic psychopathology might be due to normalization of the various interactions between 5-HT and DA in relevant brain regions. A more general statement of the 5-HT hypothesis of schizophrenia, however, is that functional alterations in the serotonergic neuronal system (including pre- and postsynaptic elements) occur in schizophrenia, that these affect multiple neurotransmitter systems (e.g., glutamate, norepinephrine, and acetylcholine, as well as DA), and that pharmacological manipulation of the serotonergic system can either reduce or exacerbate positive, negative, or disorganization symptoms and cognitive function, as well as modulate extrapyramidal function [e.g., extrapyramidal symptoms (EPS) and tardive dyskinesia or dystonia (TD)].

CRITICAL TESTS OF THE SEROTONIN HYPOTHESIS OF SCHIZOPHRENIA

The DA hypothesis of schizophrenia has been supported by three types of findings: first, that neuroleptics (in general) are D_2 receptor antagonists; second, that functional alterations in brain dopaminergic function have been reported in schizophrenia; and third, that drugs that increase brain dopaminergic activity can either induce psychosis in normal individuals or exacerbate symptoms in schizophrenies (see Chapter 100, *this volume*). The extent to which comparable data are available with regard to 5-HT and schizophrenia will now be reviewed.

Fundamental to testing the 5-HT hypothesis of schizophrenia is the determination of whether serotonergic drugs can affect the core psychopathology of schizophrenia

(both to exacerbate or ameliorate these symptoms) as do drugs that act on the dopaminergic system, (e.g., amphetamine and neuroleptics). Additionally, alterations in serotonergic neurotransmission should be demonstrable. In the 5 years since Bleich reviewed this topic (7), a large number of potential antipsychotic agents that block 5-HT receptors have been evaluated in patients with schizophrenia. Additionally, a number of serotonergic agonists [fenfluramine, (5-HTP), m-chlorophenylpiperazine (mCPP), and tryptophan] have been shown to sometimes exacerbate symptoms of schizophrenia (36,46,57). Finally, as we summarize below, many studies have demonstrated consistent alteration of serotonergic neurotransmission (measured by receptor binding, 5-HT metabolism, or hormone response to serotonergic drugs) in schizophrenia.

Complicating the study of the role of 5-HT in schizophrenia has been the discovery of a multiplicity of 5-HT receptors. To date, 14 distinct 5-HT receptors have been identified using molecular biology and pharmacological techniques (see Chapters 36–38, and 40, *this volume*). Additional evidence in favor of a 5-HT hypothesis of schizophrenia comes from the observation that many typical and atypical antipsychotics have relatively high affinities for multiple cloned 5-HT receptors (68,69).

Clozapine, for instance, has a high affinity for at least five of the 5-HT receptors (5-HT_{2A}, 5-HT_{2C}, 5-HT_3, 5-HT_6, and 5-HT_7) (68,69) and has been shown (26) to be more effective than typical neuroleptic drugs in treatment-resistant schizophrenia. Additionally, a number of other atypical antipsychotic agents have been shown to have greater affinity for 5-HT_{2A} (formerly 5-HT_2 receptors) (54,68) than 5-HT_{2C} (formerly 5-HT_{1C}) (68) receptors in vitro. Reports that risperidone (a drug with high 5-HT_{2A} receptor-blocking activity relative to its D_2 affinity, see ref. 51) has greater efficacy for treating negative symptoms of schizophrenia than haloperidol (11) supports the hypothesis that 5-HT_{2A} receptor antagonism is of value in an antipsychotic drug. It has been suggested that the strong 5-HT_{2A} relative to D_2 affinity is the key factor, not merely the absolute affinity for the 5-HT_{2A} receptor (48,51).

The fact that the 5-HT_{2A} receptor appears to be an important site of action of atypical antipsychotic agents is interesting in light of the fact that hallucinogens primarily utilize the 5-HT_{2A} or 5-HT_{2C} receptors to achieve their functional effects (19). However, many atypical antipsychotic drugs also bind to 5-HT_6 and 5-HT_7 receptors (69). Importantly, 5-HT_6 and 5-HT_7 receptors are present in the striatal and corticolimbic areas, respectively, which are major sites of action of antipsychotic drugs (54,73). Antagonism of these receptors could also contribute to the action of atypical antipsychotics, but it does not seem likely that potent 5-HT_6 or 5-HT_7 receptor affinities or 5-HT_6 to D_2 ratios *alone* are essential features of atypical antipsychotic drugs (22).

A comparison of the effect of the D_2 blocker raclopride

or the D_1 blocker SCH 23390 with the 5-HT$_{1A}$ agonist 8-OH-DPAT or the 5-HT$_{2A/2C}$ antagonist ritanserin on catalepsy and conditioned avoidance behavior also suggested actions on D_2 and 5-HT$_{1A}$ receptors might be the basis for at least some of clozapine's spectrum of advantages (83). Thus, although there is compelling evidence for an involvement of 5-HT in the special efficacy and low-side-effect profile of atypical antipsychotic drugs (see Chapters 39 and 40, *this volume*), it is likely that effects on other neurotransmitter systems (e.g., DA, norepinephrine, glutamate, acetylcholine, neurotensin) contribute importantly to its efficacy (see Chapter 108, *this volume*).

CRITICAL TECHNIQUES FOR INVESTIGATING BRAIN SEROTONERGIC SYSTEMS IN SCHIZOPHRENIA

Cerebrospinal Fluid

There have been many studies measuring the concentration of 5-HT and its major metabolite, 5-hydroxyindoleacetic acid (5-HIAA), in the cerebrospinal fluid (CSF) of schizophrenic patients. Pretreatment with probenecid to inhibit the active transport of 5-HIAA was employed in many of those studies. The assumption of these studies is that CSF levels of 5-HIAA reflect neuronal release and/or metabolism of 5-HT and provide an estimate of 5-HT turnover in the CNS. Studies by Stanley et al. (reviewed in ref. 7) suggest that CSF levels of 5-HIAA positively correlate with frontal cortex and hindbrain levels of 5-HT.

As reviewed by Bleich et al. (7), no clear consensus has emerged from studies prior to 1988 concerning the levels of 5-HIAA in the CSF of patients with schizophrenia. Most investigators found no gross differences in CSF levels of 5-HIAA comparing schizophrenic patients and controls, although Ashcroft (4) and Bowers (8) reported decreased CSF concentrations of 5-HIAA in schizophrenia. Some studies have found a significant inverse relationship between CSF concentrations of 5-HIAA and brain atrophy as determined by computerized tomography (CT) in schizophrenia (64). Studies by Van Praag (82) Cooper et al. (12) and Roy et al. (72) reported that suicidal schizophrenic patients have low CSF levels of 5-HIAA, whereas two other studies did not replicate these results (see ref. 12). A prospective study by Cooper et al. (12) found an inverse correlation between CSF levels of 5-HIAA and suicidal behavior in schizophrenic patients. One strength of this particular study is that CSF levels of 5-HIAA were measured prospectively and a 10-year follow-up was performed.

More recent studies have attempted to correlate CSF levels of 5-HIAA with other biological and psychological measures. Thus, Csernansky et al. (15) reported a positive correlation between CSF 5-HIAA, and various deficit symptoms of schizophrenia (Brief Psychiatric Rating Scale negative symptom score, work history, and results of the WAIS-R), which were incorporated into a combined deficit syndrome score. They suggested that increased serotonergic activity could play a role in the pathogenesis of deficit schizophrenic symptoms.

Weinberger et al. (84) found CSF levels of 5-HIAA and homovanillic acid (HVA) correlated positively with prefrontal regional cerebral blood flow (rCBF) on one neuropsychologic test (Wisconsin Card Sort) which has been shown to be dependent, in part, upon frontal lobe function. The authors suggested that the primarily relationship might be with HVA, that is, DA not 5-HIAA or 5-HT. Interestingly, CSF concentrations of 5-HIAA did not correlate with resting cerebral blood flow (rCBF) under two other conditions in which frontal lobe activity was not predominant (resting state and a number matching test), suggesting a close relationship between CSF levels of 5-HIAA and prefrontal cortical activity.

Lindström et al. (43) found a significant negative relationship between CSF concentrations of 5-HIAA and abnormal brainstem, which produced auditory evoked potentials in never-treated first-episode schizophrenics. These authors suggested brainstem dysfunction might be related to decreased serotonergic activity in schizophrenia. In a subsequent study, these authors noted that schizophrenic patients who showed reduced skin conductance responsiveness had low CSF concentrations of 5-HIAA and HVA (61). The significance of these findings is unknown.

There is evidence that the ratio of dopaminergic to serotonergic activity may be relevant to schizophrenia. Lewine et al. (42) reported that, although neither CSF levels of HVA or 5-HIAA alone correlated with ventricular brain ratio (VBR) in 45 patients with schizophrenia, the ratio of HVA to 5-HIAA was negatively correlated with VBR ($r = 0.45$, $p < 0.005$). This suggests that structural brain abnormalities in schizophrenia might be related to a relatively increased serotonergic or decreased dopaminergic activity. Hsiao et al. (26) reported that typical neuroleptics produced a greater increase in CSF levels of HVA and 5-HIAA than did clozapine, but they did not separate out responders and nonresponders. These authors also noted an increased correlation between CSF levels of HVA and 5-HIAA after neuroleptic treatment and proposed that one effect of neuroleptic drug treatment may be to alter the relative activities of 5-HT and DA systems in concert.

Pickar et al. (63) found that low CSF ratios of HVA to 5-HIAA predicted a positive response to clozapine in 21 neuroleptic-resistant patients; neither metabolite alone predicted a good clozapine response. They suggested that these findings were consistent both with the hypothesis that the efficacy of clozapine depended on a combined effect on 5-HT and DA neurotransmission and with the notion of a combined 5-HT/DA malfunction in schizophrenia.

Taken together, these findings support, in a general way, the role of brain 5-HT in schizophrenia. The Csernansky et al. (15) and Weinberger et al. (84) findings lend general support to the notion that alterations in serotonergic activity might be related to the deficit symptoms of schizophrenia. However, CSF levels of 5-HIAA, at best, provide an integrated measure of serotonergic activity in multiple brain regions. They cannot distinguish between selective changes in different regions or provide any index of the necessary integration between serotonergic activity and that of other neurotransmitters. Additionally, because of the correlational nature of these studies, cause and effect relationships cannot be established.

NEUROENDOCRINE CHALLENGE STUDIES

The rationale and background for the use of neuroendocrine challenge studies to clarify pathophysiology and study psychotropic drug action in psychiatric disorders has been previously summarized (56). Briefly, it has been proposed that alterations in brain 5-HT receptor sensitivities may be inferred from altered neuroendocrine responses to serotonergic agonists. Thus, for instance, a blunted prolactin (PRL), cortisol, or temperature response to MK-212 (a direct-acting $5\text{-HT}_{2A}/5\text{-HT}_{2C}$ agonist) could be attributed to a diminished number of 5-HT_{2A} or 5-HT_{2C} receptors and/or coupling to second-messenger systems. Limitations to these types of studies include (a) the lack of specificity of the challenge agents; (b) the lack of suitable receptor subtype-specific antagonists; and (c) the paucity of full dose–response studies.

The 5-HT hypothesis of schizophrenia predicts that patients with schizophrenia should have abnormal responses to serotonergic challenge studies, if the hypothalamic neurons that transduce 5-HT responses are also abnormal. Among the serotonergic drugs that have been studied in schizophrenia are fenfluramine (which induces the release of 5-HT), mCPP (a full or partial agonist at multiple 5-HT receptors as discussed below; see Tables 1 and 2), L-tryptophan (a precursor of 5-HT, and thus, a potential agonist at all 5-HT receptors), and MK-212 (a potent 5-HT_{2A} and 5-HT_{2C} agonist, and a weak agonist at 5-HT_{1A} receptors). Previous investigators have suggested that mCPP has the highest affinities for 5-HT_{2C} receptors and, hence, should be considered a selective 5-HT_{2C} agonist (28). However, a careful study of more recent data obtained with cloned 5-HT receptors has clearly shown that mCPP has a high affinity (and efficacy) for at least seven 5-HT receptors subtypes: $5\text{-HT}_{1D\alpha}$, $5\text{-HT}_{1D\beta}$, 5-HT_{2A}, 5-HT_{2B}, 5-HT_{2C}, 5-HT_6, 5-HT_7 (Table 2). Additionally, mCPP is a partial agonist at cloned 5-HT_{2A} receptors stably expressed in NIH3T3 cells (Roth, *unpublished observation*). These results all suggest that caution should

be used when interpreting results obtained from the use of serotonergic agonists in neuroendocrine challenge tests. Tables 1 and 2 summarize the pharmacology of agents used in challenge studies.

Kolakowska et al. (34) found the growth hormone (GH) response to L-tryptophan was reduced, whereas the PRL responses to L-trytophan were enhanced. Because the Kolakowska studies were performed in medicated schizophrenics, the interpretation of the results are not straightforward. Price et al. (65) found that the PRL response to L-tryptophan was normal in nonmedicated schizophrenic patients. Lee et al. (38) reported that the temperature response to MK-212 was blunted in unmedicated schizophrenic patients. The PRL and cortisol responses to MK-212 were also blunted in unmedicated schizophrenic patients compared to normal controls (Meltzer, *unpublished data*). These results are consistent with the hypothesis that $5\text{-HT}_{2A/2C}$ responsivity is diminished in schizophrenia. The mCPP-induced elevations in serum PRL and cortisol levels were also reported to be blunted in schizophrenic patients (31). Lerer et al. (41) found a blunted PRL response to fenfluramine in schizophrenia and that fenfluramine exacerbated positive symptoms. The increase in cortisol and decrease in body temperature due to ipsapirone, a 5-HT_{1A} partial agonist, however, are normal in unmedicated male schizophrenic patients (Meltzer, *unpublished data*), suggesting that there is no abnormality in the function of those postsynaptic 5-HT_{1A} receptors that mediate the cortisol response following 5-HT_{1A} stimulation. Meltzer et al. (50) recently found that the cimetidine-induced increase in PRL levels was blunted in male but not in female patients with schizophrenia. This finding is of particular interest because of the well-known gender difference in age of onset and severity of illness in schizophrenics. If the blunted response is from a compensatory down-regulation of the serotonergic system, further blockade would be predicted to relieve psychotic symptoms.

When patients are treated with atypical antipsychotic agents like clozapine, it is clear that significant attenuation of 5-HT receptor-mediated responses is attained. Thus, Lemus et al. (39) found that the fenfluramine induced PRL response was blunted by clozapine treatment. Meltzer et al. (50) reported blockade of the PRL, cortisol, and temperature responses to MK-212 by clozapine. Kahn et al. (31) found absent nocturnal GH responses in clozapine-treated schizophrenic patients. Additionally, Kahn et al. (31) found that clozapine but not haloperidol, blocked the mCPP-induced ACTH and PRL response in schizophrenia (50). Treatment with clozapine totally abolished the cimetidine-induced prolactin response in schizophrenia. Based on previous studies suggesting that the cimetidine response is indirectly mediated via 5-HT_{2A} receptors (perhaps via induction of 5-HT release; see ref. 53), Meltzer et al. (50) concluded that these findings were further evidence of a complex serotonergic abnormality in schizo-

TABLE 1. *Serotonergic agents used in neuroendocrine studies in schizophrenia*

Test agent	Receptor occupied (agonist/antagonist)	Result
mCPP	5-HT$_{1C}$, 5-HT$_{1D}$, 5-HT$_2$ (weak agonist), 5-HT$_6$, 5-HT$_7$	Diminished PRL response compared to controls
mCPP	5-HT$_{1C}$, 5-HT$_{1D}$, 5-HT$_2$ (weak agonist), 5-HT$_6$, 5-HT$_7$	Diminished cortisol response compared to controls
L-Tryptophan	All 5-HT receptors activated	No difference in PRL response compared to controls
Fenfluramine	All 5-HT receptors activated	Diminished PRL response compared to controls
MK-212	5-HT$_{2C}$, 5-HT$_{2A}$, 5-HT$_{1A}$(?)	Diminished temperature response compared to controls
MK-212 + clozapine	5-HT$_2$, 5-HT$_{1C}$ activated; 5-HT$_2$, 5-HT$_{1C}$, 5-HT$_6$, 5-HT$_7$ blocked	Blocked PRL and cortisol response to MK-212
Fenfluramine + clozapine	All 5-HT receptors activated; 5-HT$_2$, 5-HT$_{1C}$, 5-HT$_6$, 5-HT$_7$ blocked	Blocked PRL response to fenfluramine
L-Tryptophan + typical neuroleptics	All 5-HT receptors activated; D$_2$ receptors blocked	Augmented PRL response to L-tryptophan; Diminished GH response
Cimetidine	5-HT$_2$ activated (indirect)	Diminished PRL response in schizophrenia compared to control
Cimetidine + clozapine	5-HT$_2$ activated (indirect); 5-HT$_2$, 5-HT$_{1C}$, 5-HT$_6$, 5-HT$_7$ blocked)	Clozapine abolishes the PRL response induced by cimetidine

phrenia. A direct effect of cimetidine on several 5-HT receptors (5-HT$_{1C}$, 5-HT$_2$, 5-HT$_6$, 5-HT$_7$) was ruled out by radioligand binding studies with cloned receptors (see Table 2).

Taken together, these results generally also support the 5-HT hypothesis of schizophrenia because (a) most investigators have found blunted responses to indirect-acting 5-HT agonists (e.g., fenfluramine) or 5-HT$_{2A/2C}$ agonists, and (b) atypical but not typical antipsychotic agents block the neuroendocrine responses to serotonergic agonists. Future studies with more selective agonists and antagonists should help to clarify the 5-HT receptor subtype involved in these alterations. The fact that these responses are blocked by clozapine favors the idea that 5-HT$_{2A}$ or 5-HT$_{2C}$ receptors are responsible; however the recent discovery that clozapine and other neuroendocrine challenge agents bind to multiple 5-HT receptors (5-HT$_6$; 5-HT$_7$) suggests caution is necessary at this point.

POSITRON EMISSION TOMOGRAPHY SCANNING

In theory, positron emission tomography (PET) studies should permit measurement of 5-HT receptor density in the brains of schizophrenic patients, both on and off medication. To date, there are no reliable PET data on the density of any 5-HT receptor subtype in unmedicated patients with schizophrenia. Using [^{11}C]-N-methylspiperone as a ligand, our laboratory compared occupancy of cortical 5-HT$_2$ and striatal D$_2$ receptors in six clozapine-treated and five typical neuroleptic-treated patients (21). The occupancy of the 5-HT$_2$ receptors in cortex and the ratio of 5-HT$_2$ to D$_2$ occupancy was significantly greater in the clozapine-treated patients ($p < 0.01$). These results are consistent with expected differences between clozapine and typical neuroleptics. Nyberg et al. (60) have shown, however, using [^{11}C]-N-methylspiperone, that the putative atypical antipsychotic drug risperidone binds to both cortical 5-HT$_2$ and striatal D$_2$ receptors in normal volunteers. Risperidone occupied approximately 60% of the 5-HT$_2$ receptors and 50% of the D$_2$ receptors after a single 1-mg oral dose. Because the recommended dose of risperidone in schizophrenia is 6 mg (11), high occupancy of both 5-HT$_{2A}$ and D$_2$ receptors would be expected during treatment (21).

Studies in rats (78) indicate that, as a group, atypical antipsychotic agents have a higher ratio of 5-HT$_{2A}$/D$_2$ receptor occupancy in vivo compared with typical anti-

TABLE 2. *Affinity of mCPP, TFMPP, 5-HT, and MK-212 for various cloned 5-HT receptors (in nM)[a]*

	5-HT	mCPP	TFMPP	MK-212	Cimetidine
5-HT$_{1D\beta}$	0.59	90	28	N.D.	N.D.
5-HT$_{2A}$	1,320	231	256	8,532	>10,000
5-HT$_{2B}$	10	26.8	84.8	408	N.D.
5-HT$_{2C}$	22	204	150	332	>10,000
5-HT$_6$	56	2300	682	71,000	>10,000
5-HT$_7$	1.84	352	532	N.D.	>10,000

[a] N.D. = not determined.

TABLE 3. *Alterations of 5-HT receptors in schizophrenia*

Receptor	Ligand	Direction of change	Brain regions	Ref.
5-HT$_{1A}$	[^{3}H]-8-OH-DPAT	Increase	Crotex (Brodmann areas 10 and 11)	Hashimoto et al. (24)
5-HT$_{1A}$	[^{3}H]-8-OH-DPAT	Increase	Prefrontal cortex	Hashimoto et al. (24)
5-HT$_1$	[^{3}H]-5-HT	No change	Prefrontal cortex	Bennett et al. (6)
5-HT$_2$	[^{3}H]-spiperone	No change	Nucleus accumbens	MacKay (47)
5-HT$_2$	[^{3}H]-LSD	Decrease	Brodmann areas 6, 8, 11, 44, 47	Bennett et al. (6)
5-HT$_2$	[^{3}H]-LSD	No change	Caudate nucleus	Owen (62)
5-HT$_2$	[^{3}H]-LSD	No change	Brodmann areas 4, 10, 11	Whitaker et al. (85)
5-HT$_2$	[^{3}H]-LSD	Increase (drug free)	Brodmann areas 4, 10, 11	Whitaker et al. (85)
5-HT$_2$	[^{3}H]-ketanserin	No change	Brodmann area 10	Reynolds et al. (66)
5-HT$_2$	[^{3}H]-ketanserin	Decrease (on and off drugs)	Brodmann area 9	Mita et al. (52)
5-HT$_2$	[^{3}H]-spiperone	Decrease	Brodmann areas 8 and 9	Arora and Meltzer (2)
5-HT$_2$	[^{125}I]-LSD	Increase	Postcingulate cortex, ventral putamen, n. accumbens, hippocampus	Joyce et al. (30)
5-HT$_{1A}$	[^{3}H]-8-OH-DPAT	Increase	Hippocampus, postcingulate cortex, motor and temporal cortex	Joyce et al. (30)
5-HT uptake sites	[^{3}H]-cyanoimipramine	Decrease	Anterior cingulate, postcingulate, prefrontal and temporal cortex	Joyce et al. (30)
5-HT uptake sites	[^{3}H]-cyanoimipramine	Increase	Dorsal caudate, dorsal putamen, ventral putamen, n. accumbens, motor cortex	Joyce et al. (30)

psychotic agents. Taken together, these results suggest that atypical antipsychotic agents exert profound effects on 5-HT$_{2A}$ receptors in vivo at clinically effective doses.

POSTMORTEM STUDIES

A number of authors have measured 5-HT receptor density in postmortem brain tissue from patients with schizophrenia (Table 3). Bennett et al. (6) found a decrease in [^{3}H]-LSD binding in Brodmann areas 6, 8, 11, 44, and 47, whereas Whitaker et al. (85) found increased [^{3}H]-LSD binding in unmedicated schizophrenics in cortical regions 4, 10, and 11 (discussed in ref. 7). By contrast, using the 5-HT$_{2A}$ antagonist [^{3}H]-ketanserin as a ligand, Mita et al. (53) found a decrease in binding in cortical area 9, but Reynolds et al. (see ref. 66) found no change in cortical area 10. One potential problem with [^{3}H]-ketanserin as a ligand is that, although it has little affinity for other types of 5-HT$_2$ receptors, it does have high affinity for both α_1-adrenergic receptors (25) and tetrabenazine-sensitive sites (see refs. 69 and 70). Importantly, Mita et al. (53) found a decrease in 5-HT$_{2A}$ receptor number in cortical area 9 in unmedicated schizophrenics, whereas Arora and Meltzer (2), using [^{3}H]-spiperone found a similar decrease in cortical areas 8 and 9. Laruelle et al. (37) also found a decrease in cortical 5-HT$_{2A}$ receptor density in schizophrenia. However, Joyce et al. (30), using quantitative receptor autoradiography, recently reported an increase of [^{125}I]-LSD- and [^{3}H]-ketanserine-labeled 5-HT$_2$ receptors in the temporal and posterior cingulate, frontal and parietal cortices, and in the ventral putamen, nucleus accumbens, and hippocampus, but not in the caudate nucleus, motor, prefrontal, entorhinal, or

anterior cingulate cortices. It is difficult to draw any firm conclusions from these studies for any region of the brain because of the inherent difficulties with postmortem receptor binding research, as will be discussed below. There is no data on 5-HT$_6$ or 5-HT$_7$ receptors.

There are some data on other brain 5-HT receptors in schizophrenia. Bennett et al. (6) found no change in 5-HT$_1$ receptor number using [^{3}H]-5-HT in the prefrontal cortex. Hashimoto et al. (24) using [^{3}H]-8-OH-DPAT found an increase in 5-HT$_{1A}$ receptors in cortical areas 10 and 22 and in the prefrontal cortex. The difference in these two studies could simply be because [^{3}H]-5-HT binds to many distinct 5-HT receptors (5-HT$_{1A}$, 5-HT$_{1D\alpha/\beta}$, 5-HT$_{1E\alpha/\beta}$, 5-HT$_{2C}$, 5-HT$_5$, 5-HT$_7$). Finally, Joyce et al. (30), using quantitative autoradiographic techniques, reported that 5-HT$_{1A}$ receptors were increased in several brain regions of schizophrenic patients (hippocampus, posterior cingulate cortex, motor and temporal cortex). There are no data on other types of the 5-HT$_1$ family of receptors.

Several methodological issues make it impossible to come to a firm conclusion regarding possible changes in 5-HT receptor density in schizophrenia. [^{3}H]-LSD binds to at least six distinct 5-HT receptors with high affinity (5-HT$_{2C}$, 5-HT$_{1E}$, 5-HT$_{2A}$, 5-HT$_5$, 5-HT$_6$, 5-HT$_7$); so even when changes are found, it is not possible to determine which type of receptor is responsible. Similarly, [^{3}H]-ketanserin is not specific for 5-HT$_{2A}$ sites either. Results may be influenced by agonal changes, prolonged neuroleptic treatment in most cases, possible effects of substance abuse, and so on. Because any abnormalities may be confined to specific regions, it is not possible to directly compare studies that did not examine the same cortical region since 5-HT receptor binding in the cortex is highly laminar, whereas it is highly regional in areas such as the hippocampus and striatum. Also, studies of binding in homogenates may obtain results different from those using autoradiographic methods. Finally, all the studies cited above were of small size ($N < 15$/group); further large-scale autoradiographic studies with highly specific ligands with appropriate controls and extensive clinical information are desperately needed.

Joyce et al. (30) reported a large increase in the number of 5-HT uptake sites in all striatal regions in schizophrenia. They also noted a marked increase in the density of 5-HT uptake sites in the ventral striatum and patches of dense binding in the dorsal striatum of schizophrenic patients but not in controls. They suggested that this is evidence for hyperserotonergic innervation of the striatum in schizophrenia. This needs to be verified in independent studies, but is interesting in light of data (see below) suggesting that marked denervation of DA terminals leads to a serotonergic hyperinnervation of the striatum.

PERIPHERAL MEASURES

The platelet has been proposed as a model of 5-HT neurons, and a number of similarities do exist between 5-HT physiology in platelets and neurons. It has also been suggested that platelet 5-HT function might parallel changes that occur in the brain. Bleich et al. (7) reviewed the data prior to 1988 on levels of 5-HT in platelets and whole blood. They concluded that platelet or whole blood concentrations of 5-HT did not differ in schizophrenic patients and in controls. By contrast, significant positive correlations between platelet and/or blood 5-HT levels and cortical atrophy as well as auditory hallucinations have been reported (7). Braunig et al. (9) reported decreased blood concentrations of 5-HT only in female schizophrenic patients who were suicidal. Increased platelet 5-HT concentrations was found in schizophrenic patients with paranoid features, but a decrease was found in patients with nonparanoid features (55).

Many studies of platelet–5-HT uptake performed prior to 1988 gave inconsistent results (19). Arora and Meltzer (3) reported that platelet 5-HT$_2$ receptor density (B_{max}) was increased in nine schizophrenic patients with a recent history of suicidal ideation or attempts compared to 24 nonsuicidal schizophrenic patients and 42 normal controls. Grahame-Smith et al. (22) found that chronic treatment with phenothiazines or thioxanthines (which have a high affinity for 5-HT$_2$ receptors) caused an up-regulation of platelet 5-HT$_2$ receptors. Arora and Meltzer found that chronic clozapine treatment also increased the number of platelet 5-HT$_2$ receptors. It should be noted that these effects of antipsychotic drugs on the platelet 5-HT$_2$ receptors are opposite to those found on brain 5-HT$_2$ sites (reviewed in ref. 70). The fact that the effects of antipsychotic drugs on peripheral and central 5-HT$_2$ receptors differ so markedly suggests that the platelet is not an ideal model to study brain 5-HT$_2$ receptor regulation.

There have been two studies of plasma 5-HIAA concentrations in schizophrenia. Alfredsson and Weisel (1) reported an inverse relationship between depressive and autistic symptoms in 24 schizophrenic patients as well as response to sulpiride, a selective D$_2$ antagonist. Markianos et al. (45) reported a positive association between plasma 5-HIAA and paranoia. The origin of most of plasma 5-HIAA is not likely to be brain, so these associations may be fortuitous.

ROLE OF SEROTONERGIC DRUGS IN THE TREATMENT OF SCHIZOPHRENIA

One potentially powerful technique for evaluating the role of 5-HT in schizophrenia is to show that drugs that act on serotonergic receptors or serotonergic systems either exacerbate or ameliorate the symptoms of schizophrenia. Precursors of 5-HT such as 5-HTP and tryptophan (plus monoamine oxidase inhibitor) have generally been found to exacerbate schizophrenia (reviewed in ref. 7). Paradoxically, L-5-HTP administration significantly antagonized amphetamine-induced increases in thought disturbance, activation, and hallucinations in five neuroleptic-treated schizophrenic patients (28). This is unexpected, because 5-HT agonists have been found to enhance amphetamine-induced DA release in rat striatum (Meltzer, *unpublished data*).

Fenfluramine

Fenfluramine is an anorectic agent that acutely induces 5-HT release and chronically depletes 5-HT, at least in rodents. Two recent studies have suggested that chronic fenfluramine administration causes a worsening of psychotic symptoms in schizophrenics. Soper et al. (75) found that fenfluramine worsened performance on a neuropsychological battery and impaired communication. Marshall et al. (46) found fenfluramine worsened psychotic symptoms, and that the degree of worsening inversely correlated with the fenfluramine-induced decline in blood 5-HT levels. Kolakowska et al. (34) found that some patients worsened and others improved on fenfluramine. It is unclear whether 5-HT release is increased, decreased, or unchanged in man during chronic fenfluramine treatment. Therefore, the apparent worsening with fenfluramine cannot be used to infer a particular relationship between 5-HT and psychosis.

Fluoxetine

Chronic administration of a selective serotonin reuptake inhibitor would be expected to increase serotonergic activity by inhibiting 5-HT uptake and also by desensitizing the 5-HT autoreceptor, leading to increased 5-HT release. Chronic fluoxetine may also alter postsynaptic receptor responsivity (e.g., increasing responsivity to 5-HT_{1A} agonists). In an open 6-week clinical trial, augmentation of typical neuroleptic drugs with fluoxetine has been reported to ameliorate positive and negative symptoms in nine neuroleptic-resistant schizophrenic patients (20).

Buspirone

Buspirone, a partial 5-HT_{1A} agonist, has been reported to either exacerbate, improve, or have no effect on positive and negative symptoms in schizophrenic patients receiving typical neuroleptics (10). It appeared that the major effect was positive.

m-Chlorophenylpiperazine

m-Chlorophenylpiperazine is a 5-HT agonist/partial agonist for a number of different 5-HT receptor subtypes (5-HT_{1D}, 5-HT_{1C}, 5-HT_2, 5-HT_{2F}, 5-HT_6) (Table 2). It may also have α-adrenergic and 5-HT uptake-inhibiting effects. Two studies have recently reported that iv infusions of mCPP induce an exacerbation of positive symptoms of schizophrenia (31,36). Krystal et al. (36) showed that pretreatment with ritanserin (a 5-HT_{2A}/5-HT_{2C} receptor antagonist) decreased the mCPP-induced psychotic symptoms in four out of six patients. This same group also demonstrated that clozapine, but not haloperidol, blocked the behavioral and neuroendocrine effects of mCPP (33). However, oral mCPP at a dose of 0.5 mg/kg only rarely causes significant changes in positive symptoms (Meltzer, *unpublished observations*). Taken together, these results lend some support to the hypothesis of Meltzer that overactive 5-$HT_{2A/2C}$ receptors may contribute to the positive symptoms of schizophrenia. In light of this idea, though, it is important to remember that mCPP and clozapine both occupy 5-HT_{2A}, 5-HT_{2C}, 5-HT_6, and 5-HT_7 receptors, so that a multiplicity of receptors might be involved in mCPP and clozapine responses.

Methysergide

Methysergide is a 5-HT antagonist that has partial agonist activity at certain DA receptors. Methysergide binds potently to many 5-HT receptors, including the 5-HT_1, 5-HT_2, and 5-HT_6 families of receptors (Roth, *unpublished observation*). Skorzewska and Lal (74) reported that methysergide induced psychosis in a single individual with a family history of schizophrenia, whereas Mendels et al. (52) found some schizophrenic patients had a worsening of their psychotic symptoms following methyser-

gide administration. These data with methysergide are difficult to interpret as its adverse effects could be due to its dopamine agonist or serotonergic effects.

THE 5-HT_2 FAMILY OF ANTAGONISTS

Clozapine

In the last few years, a large number of clinical studies have been performed with 5-HT_{2A}/5-HT_{2C} antagonists. Clinical studies with clozapine are summarized elsewhere (Chapter 108, *this volume*). Clozapine has potent antagonist effects at many subtypes of 5-HT receptors, for example, 5-HT_{2A}, 5-HT_{2C}, 5-HT_3, 5-HT_6, and 5-HT_7 (see Table 3). It has a much lower affinity for the 5-HT_{1A} receptor, but this action could be relevant to its antipsychotic effect. Meltzer et al. (51) have demonstrated that a large number of atypical antipsychotic drugs are characterized by a higher ratio of 5-HT_2/D_2 receptor binding compared to typical antipsychotics in vitro and of receptor occupancy in vivo (78). Since the discovery of the unique efficacy and low EPS profile of clozapine, many drugs with high 5-HT_2/D_2 affinity ratios have been identified and are in clinical testing. Preliminary results have been favorable enough to warrant wide-scale clinical testing of many of these drugs.

Ritanserin

Initial studies using ritanserin (which binds with high affinity to 5-HT_{2C} and 5-HT_{2A} receptors reported that it decreased EPS induced by haloperidol. However, one recent study of seven patients reported that chronic ritanserin treatment increased psychotic symptoms in four of the patients (reviewed in ref. 49). Mianserin, a 5-$HT_{2A/2C}$ antagonist, has also been reported to improve positive and negative symptoms when used to augment typical neuroleptic drugs (67). Further controlled trials of mixed 5-$HT_{2A/2C}$ antagonists, selective 5-HT_{2A}, or selective 5-HT_{2C} are needed.

Other Agents

Table 4 lists the dissociation constants for a number of typical and atypical antipsychotic agents for several cloned 5-HT receptors (5-HT_{1C}, 5-HT_2, 5-HT_6, and 5-HT_7). It is clear that clozapine, the protypical atypical antipsychotic agent, has a high affinity for several of these receptors (5-HT_{2A}, 5-HT_{2C}, 5-HT_6, and 5-HT_7). By comparison, as a group, the atypical antipsychotic agents bind with high affinity only to 5-HT_{2A} receptors. This spectrum of receptor binding lends further support to the idea that the 5-HT_{2A} receptor binding affinity is essential for the atypical nature of many antipsychotic drugs. 5-HT_6 and

TABLE 4. *Affinities of representative typical and atypical antipsychotic drugs for cloned 5-HT receptors*

Drugs	$5\text{-HT}_{2A}K_i$ (nM)	$5\text{-HT}_{2C}K_i$ (nM)	5-HT_6K_i (nM)	5-HT_7K_i (nM)
Spiperone	0.33	1595	1095	9.9
Loxapine	0.82	9.4	14.9	43
Chlorpromazine	2.3	27	4.1	21
Clozapine	4	7.2	4.5	6.3
Fluperlapine	6.7	18.2	16.5	13.9
Haloperidol	41.6	2320	>5000	262
MDL 100907	0.2	18	>5000	ND

5-HT_7 binding could be important for some of the unique actions of clozapine.

OTHER 5-HT RECEPTORS

Monsma et al. (54) recently reported that the 5-HT_6 serotonin receptor possessed high affinity for clozapine ($IC_{50} = 12$ nM), whereas loxapine and amoxapine had relatively weak affinities. This group has also presented data for the 5-HT_7 receptor, finding that it also had high affinity for clozapine (73). The 5-HT_7 receptor is highly enriched in the striatum, but the greatest concentrations of the 5-HT_7 receptor are found in the hypothalamus. When microinjected into the hypothalamus, 5-HT_7 active agents appear to regulate sleep. A potential action of atypical antipsychotic agents at 5-HT_7 receptors is interesting in light of reports of altered sleep activity in schizophrenia which may be normalized by clozapine (Lee and Meltzer, *unpublished data*). Table 4 presents the calculated K_d values using the 5-HT_6, 5-HT_7, 5-HT_{2A}, and 5-HT_{2C} receptors stably expressed in cell lines. As can be seen, clozapine had high affinities for all four 5-HT receptors. Methysergide and LSD, two compounds with psychotomimetic potential, also have high affinities for these four receptors (data not shown); LSD is a full or partial agonist at these receptors. Further studies will be required to determine the physiological relevance of these receptors for the treatment and/or etiopathology of schizophrenia.

GENETIC STUDIES OF SEROTONIN RECEPTORS IN SCHIZOPHRENIA

Linkage of a particular 5-HT receptor and/or metabolic enzyme to schizophrenia would be compelling evidence in favor of the idea of a link between 5-HT and schizophrenia. One published finding (23) could find no evidence in favor of a relationship between the 5-HT_{2A} receptor gene and schizophrenia using linage analysis.

SEROTONIN-DOPAMINE INTERACTIONS: RELEVANCE TO SCHIZOPHRENIA?

One additional manner in which 5-HT could be involved in schizophrenia is via a modulatory role on DA neuronal and/or receptor function in vivo. Over the past several years, a number of studies have emerged that suggest that 5-HT receptors may modulate DA neuronal function in vivo. This has been reviewed in detail elsewhere (48).

Studies by Costall et al. (14) have shown that chronic administration of 5-HT_3 antagonists block the effect of DA agonists in the mesolimbic area. Additionally, certain relatively potent $5\text{-HT}_{2A}/D_2$ antagonists (e.g., clozapine, sertindole, olanzepine) can induce depolarization blockade in mesolimbic but not nigrostriatal DA cell bodies in rats following chronic administration (reviewed in ref. 76). Also, recent studies with MDL 100,907 (76) (the most selective 5-HT_{2A} drug currently available; see Table 4) showed that chronic administration induced selective depolarization blockade of mesolimbic DA cell bodies. These results convincingly demonstrate that 5-HT_{2A} receptors modulate dopaminergic tone.

There is also a wealth of information suggesting that 5-HT may regulate DA release from strionigral systems. However, this effect is complex: 5-HT may have both inhibitory and excitatory actions on dopaminergic activity. Thus, 5-HT may induce local release of dendritic nigral DA (81). Others have suggested that 5-HT_{1A} receptors may exert subtle inhibitory effects on DA cell bodies in the substantia nigra (33,58). Additionally, there is evidence that 5-HT_2 receptors may reduce KCl-stimulated DA release in the caudate nucleus in vitro. Microdialysis studies of the ability of direct-acting 5-HT agonists into the striatum, with and without pretreatment with specific antagonists, suggests that 5-HT_{1B} and 5-HT_3 receptors, but not 5-HT_2 receptors, modulated striatal DA release (5). These results suggest important effects of 5-HT on the DA presynaptic terminals mediated via heteroreceptors.

Recent anatomical studies of 5-HT_2 receptor protein suggests that $DA-5\text{-HT}$ interactions could occur on postsynaptic elements as well. Garlow et al. (18) have demonstrated that 5-HT_{2A} receptors are found in interneurons in caudate nucleus and in certain cortical areas. Since at least some D_2 receptors are found on similar neuronal populations, it is conceivable that direct $5\text{-HT}_{2A}/D_2$ interactions occur on interneurons in the caudate nucleus and other regions. A diagram listing the wiring of $5\text{-HT}-DA$ interactions is found in Fig. 1. Taken together, all of these

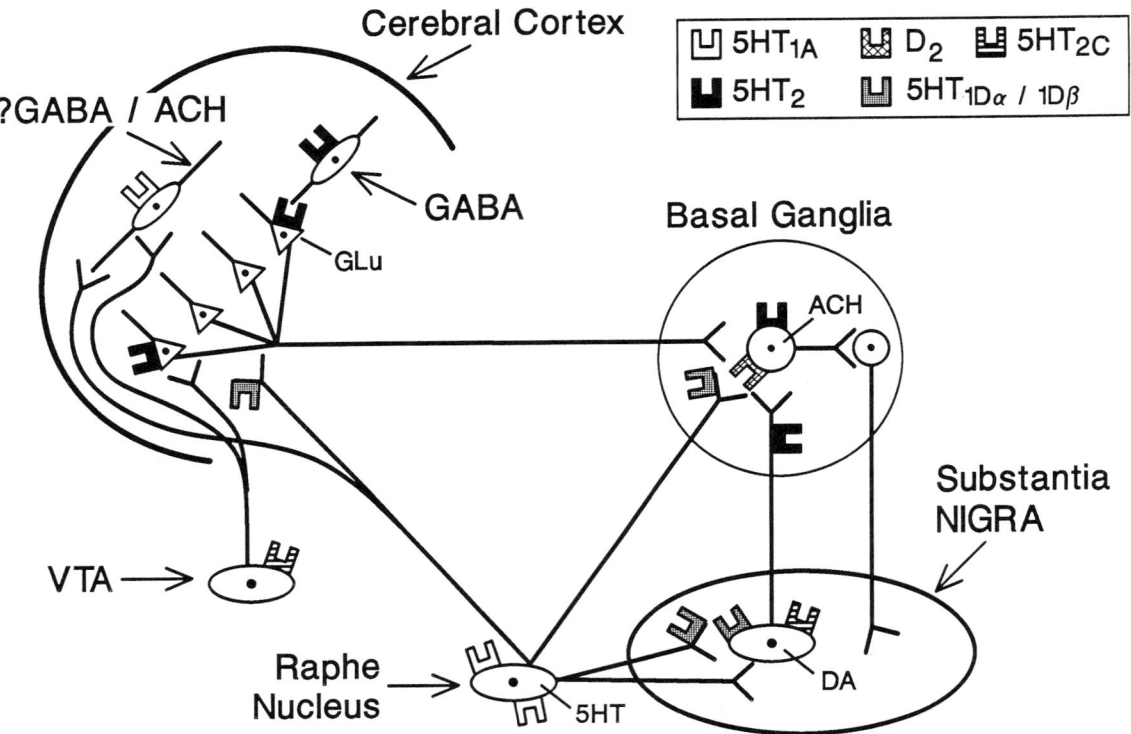

FIG. 1. Potential DA–5-HT interaction in schizophrenia. Shown is a diagram of potential DA–5-HT interactions and the specific 5-HT receptor subtypes that could be involved. In general, 5-HT exerts an inhibitory effect on neurotransmitter release. ACH, cholinergic neuron; DA, dopaminergic neuron; GABA, gaba-ergic neuron; GLu, glutamatergic neuron; VTA, ventral tegmental area; 5HT, serotonergic neuron.

results suggest that serotonergic systems physiologically modulate dopaminergic tone and/or receptors in vivo via interests with pre- and/or postsynaptic elements.

As is seen in Fig. 1, a large number of sites exist for the modulation of DA receptor/dopaminergic neuronal firing by serotonergic agents. The raphé nucleus sends dense projections to the caudate nucleus, cortex, nucleus accumbens, and substantia nigra. In the substantia nigra and caudate nucleus, there is evidence that 5-HT can modulate DA release by interactions with dendritic, somatic, and terminal 5-HT receptors. Additionally, 5-HT receptors in the substantia nigra appear to affect DA neuronal activity by affecting GABA release (16). These results indicate that $5\text{-HT}_{1D\beta}$ (5-HT_{1B}) receptors decrease dopaminergic tone and $5\text{-HT}_{2A/2C}$ receptors increase dopamine release.

As suggested by Meltzer, given the probable heterogeneity of schizophrenia and the complexity of the serotonergic system, no single type of abnormality of the serotonergic (or other neurotransmitter system) is likely to emerge as characteristic of all patients who meet current criteria for this syndrome. It seems more likely that specific symptoms and signs of schizophrenia, ranging from cognitive dysfunction, disorganization, negative and positive symptoms, motoric abnormalities, decreased sexual development, insomnia, and compulsive behaviors may be related to specific individual or combinatorial serotonergic abnormalities. A comprehensive examination of pre- and postsynaptic serotonergic function in a wide range of schizophrenic patients at various stages of the evolution of the syndrome will be needed to assess this hypothesis.

A NEURODEVELOPMENTAL PERSPECTIVE

Many investigators have speculated that schizophrenia may be a neurodevelopmental disease, perhaps involving the dopaminergic neuronal system. In this regard, it is interesting to note that serotonergic terminals have been shown to sprout after neonatal lesions of dopaminergic terminals (reviewed in ref. 20). Most recently, Jackson and Abercrombie (29) demonstrated that rats depleted of DA at birth showed enhanced release of 5-HT when evaluated as adults and that ketanserin blocked the hypermotility of neonatally dopamine-lesioned rats. These results suggest that a functional deficit of DA release during the perinatal period can lead to a functional supersensitivity of the $5\text{-HT}_{2A}/5\text{-HT}_{2C}$ receptors and enhanced release of 5-HT at adulthood.

Roth et al. (70,71) previously demonstrated that 5-HT_{2A} and 5-HT_{2C} receptors developed in a precisely regulated fashion. The principal increases in 5-HT_{2A} and 5-HT_{2C} receptors occurred postnatally, between postnatal days 7 and 14 with a subsequent decrease in 5-HT_{2A} receptor and mRNA levels after this time. After postnatal day 21, little change in 5-HT_{2A} or 5-HT_{2C} receptor and mRNA levels were measured. 5-HT_{2A} receptor gene expression and receptor levels appeared to be unregulated by brain 5-HT levels, because neonatal 5,7-dihydroxytryptamine lesions did not alter adult levels of 5-HT_2 mRNA or receptors. Additionally, perinatal treatment of rats with mianserin (a $5\text{-HT}_{2A/2C}$ antagonist) did not alter levels of 5-HT_{2A} mRNA or receptors (Roth and Ciaranello, *unpublished observations*).

Taken together, these results suggest that the immediate perinatal period of the rat (which corresponds to the third trimester in humans) might represent a stage of vulnerability of the $5\text{-HT}_{2A}/5\text{-HT}_{2C}$ receptor system, and that dopaminergic, but not serotonergic, inputs could be important for regulating 5-HT_{2A} receptor activity. It is conceivable, then, that the alterations of 5-HT_{2A} receptors and receptor activity measured in schizophrenic patients could be due to abnormalities of dopaminergic neurotransmission, which occur during early brain development. Future studies aimed at examining the effects of dopaminergic lesions on 5-HT receptor subtypes will be important for verifying this hypothesis.

CONCLUSIONS

From the foregoing, it is clear that a role for 5-HT in the pathogenesis and treatment of schizophrenia is compelling. Thus, (a) alterations of 5-HT receptors have been found in schizophrenia by many (but not all) investigators; (b) neuroendocrine challenge studies are consistent with a subsensitivity of postsynaptic alteration of some types of serotonin receptors; (c) many typical and atypical antipsychotic agents bind with high affinity to 5-HT (particularly 5-HT_{2A}) receptors; (d) alterations in serotonergic systems have been correlated with key deficit symptoms of schizophrenia; (e) novel antipsychotic agents which function as 5-HT_{2A} antagonists appear superior to neuroleptics for treating negative symptoms and treatment-resistant schizophrenia; (f) functional blockade of 5-HT_{2A} receptors occurs in vivo in patients treated with atypical antipsychotic agents; and (g) animal pharmacological studies are consistent with the notion that the 5-HT system may serve as one of the regulators of dopaminergic tone in vivo. Clearly, then, there is a large amount of internally consistent information to suggest a role for 5-HT in the etiology and/or treatment of schizophrenia. Future studies examining the role of multiple serotonin receptors in the etiopathology and/or treatment of schizophrenia are likely to yield productive results.

REFERENCES

1. Alfredsson G, Wiesel FA. Relationship between clinical effects and monoamine metabolites and amino acids in sulpiride-treated schizophrenic patients. *Psychopharmacol (Berl)* 1990;101: 324–331.
2. Arora RC, Meltzer HY. Serotonin$_2$ (5-HT$_2$) receptor binding in the frontal cortex of schizophrenic patients. *J Neurotransm* 1991; 85:19–29.
3. Arora RC, Meltzer HY. Serotonin$_2$ receptor binding in blood platelets of schizophrenic patients. *Psychiatry Res* 1993;47:111–119.
4. Ashcroft GW, Crawford TBB, Eccleston D, Sharman DF, MacDougall EG, Stanton JB, Binns JK. 5-hydroxyindole compounds in the cerebrospinal fluid of patients with psychiatric or neurologic disease. *Lancet* 1966;11:1049–1052.
5. Benloucif S, Keegan MJ, Galloway MP. Serotonin-facilitated dopamine release in vivo: pharmacological characterization. *J Pharmacol Exp Ther* 1993;265:373–377.
6. Bennett JP, Enna SJ, Bylund DB, Gillin JC, Wyatt RC, Snyder SH. Neurotransmitter receptors in the frontal cortex of schizophrenics. *Arch Gen Psych* 1979;36:927–934.
7. Bleich A, Brown SL, Kahn R, van Praag HM. The role of serotonin in schizophrenia. *Schizophr Bull* 1988;14:297–315.
8. Bowers MB, Serotonin (5HT) systems in psychotic states. *Psychopharmacol Commun* 1975;1:655–662.
9. Braunig P, Rao ML, Flimmers R. Blood serotonin levels in suicidal schizophrenic patients. *Acta Psychiatr Scand* 1989;79:186–189.
10. Brody D, Adler LA, Kuo T, Aubust B, Rotrosen J. Effects of buspirone in seven schizophrenic subjects. *J Clin Psychopharmacol* 1990;10:68–69.
11. Chouinard G, Jones B, Ronnington G, et al. A Canadian multicenter placebo-controlled study of fixed doses of risperidone and haloperidol in the treatment of chronic schizophrenic patients. *J Clin Psychopharmacol* 1993;13:25–40.
12. Cooper SJ, Kelly CB, King DJ. 5-Hydroxyindoleacetic acid in cerebrospinal fluid and prediction of suicidal behaviour in schizophrenia. *Lancet* 1992;340:940–941.
13. Corbett R, Hartman H, Klerman LL, et al. Effects of atypical antipsychotic agents on social behavior in rodents. *Pharmacol Biochem Behav* 1993;45:9–17.
14. Costall B, Naylor RJ, Tyers MB. The psychopharmacology of 5-HT$_3$ receptors. *Pharmacol Ther* 1990;47:181–202.
15. Csernansky JG, King RJ, Faustman WO, Moses JA, Poscher ME, Faull KF. 5-HIAA in cerebrospinal fluid and deficit schizophrenic characteristics. *Br J Psychiatr* 1990;156:501–507.
16. Ennis C, Kemp JD, Cox B. Characterisation of inhibitory 5-hydroxytryptamine receptors that modulate dopamine release in the striatum. *J Neurochem* 1981;36:1515–1520.
17. Gaddum JH, Hameed KA. Drugs which antagonize 5-hydroxytryptamine. *Br J Pharmacol* 1954;9:240–248.
18. Garlow S, Morilak D, Dean RS, Roth BL, Ciaranello RD. Production and characterization of an antibody for the 5-HT$_2$ receptor which labels a subpopulation of rat forebrain neurons. *Brain Res* 1993;615:113–120.
19. Glennon RA. Do classical hallucinogens act as 5-HT$_2$ agonists or antagonists? *Neuropsychopharmacology* 1990;3:509–517.
20. Goff DC, Brotrian AW, Aiates M, McCormack S. Trial of fluoxetine added to neuroleptics for treatment resistant schizophrenic patients. *Am J Psychiatry* 1990;14:492–493.
21. Goyer PF, Berridge MS, Semple WE, et al. Dopamine-2 and serotonin-2 receptor indices in clozapine treated schizophrenic patients. *Schiz Res* 1993;9:199.
22. Grahame-Smith DG, Geaney DP, Schachter M, Elliott JM. Human platelet 5-hydroxytryptamine receptors: binding of [^{3}H]-LSD. Effects of chronic neuroleptic and antidepressant drug administration. *Experentia* 1988;44:142–145.
23. Hallmayer J, Kennedy JL, Wetterberg L, et al. Exclusion of linkage between the serotonin$_2$ receptor and schizophrenia in a large Swedish kindred. *Arch Gen Psychiatry* 1992;45:9–17.
24. Hashimoto T, Nishino N, Nakai H, Tanaka C. Increase in serotonin 5-HT$_{1A}$ receptors in prefrontal and temporal cortices of brains from patients with chronic schizophrenia. *Life Sci* 1991;48:355–363.
25. Hoyer D. Functional correlates to 5-HT$_1$ recognition sites. *J Recept Res* 1988;8:59–81.

26. Hsiao JK, Potter WZ, Agren H, Owen RR, Pickar D. Clinical investigation of monoamine neurotransmitter interactions. *Psychopharmacology* 1993;112:S76–S84.

27. Iqbal N, Asnis GM, Kahn RS, Kay SR, van Praag HM. The mCPP challenge test in schizophrenia: hormonal and behavioral responses. *Biol Psychiatry* 1991;30:770–778.

28. Irwin MR, Marder SR, Fuentenebro F, Yuwiler A. 1-5-hydroxytryptophan attenuates positive psychotic symptoms induced by D-amphetamine. *Psychiatr Res* 1987;22:283–289.

29. Jackson D, Abercrombie O. In vivo neurochemical evaluation of striatal serotonergic hyperinnervation in rats depleted of dopamine at infancy. *J Neurochem* 1992;58:890–897.

30. Joyce JN, Shane A, Lexow N, Winokur A, Casanova MF, Kleinman JE. Serotonin uptake sites and serotonin receptors are altered in the limbic system of schizophrenics. *Neuropsychopharmacology* 1993;8:315–336.

31. Kahn RS, Siever L, Davidson M, Greenwald C, Moore C. Haloperidol and clozapine treatment and their effect on *m*-chlorophenylpiperazine-mediated responses in schizophrenia: implications for the mechanism of action of clozapine. *Psychopharmacology* 1993;112:S90–S94.

32. Kane J, Honigfield G, Singer J, Meltzer HY, Clozaril Collaborative Study Group. Clozapine for the treatment-resistant schizophrenic. *Arch Gen Psychiatry* 1988;45:789–796.

33. Kelland MD, Freeman AS, Chiodo LA. Serotonergic afferent regulation of the basic physiology and pharmacological responsiveness of nigrostriatal dopamine neurons. *J Pharmacol Exp Ther* 1990;253:803–811.

34. Kolakowska T, Cowen PJ, Murdock P. Endocrine responses to tryptophan infusion in schizophrenic patients treated with neuroleptics. *Psychoneuroendocrinology* 1987;12:193–202.

35. Kolakowska T, Gadhvi H, Molyneux S. An open clinical trial of fenfluramine in chronic schizophrenia: a pilot study. *Int Clin Psychopharmacol* 1987;2:83–88.

36. Krystal JH, Seibyl JP, Price LH, et al. *m*-Chlorophenylpiperazine (MCPP) effects in neuroleptic-free schizophrenic patients. *Arch Gen Psychiatr* 1993;50:624–635.

37. Laruelle M, Abi-Dargham A, Casanova MF, Toti R, Weinberger DR, Kleinman JE. Selective abnormalities of prefrontal serotonergic receptors in schizophrenia. A postmortem study. *Arch Gen Psych* 1993;50:810–818.

38. Lee HS, Bastani B, Friedman L, Ramirez L, Meltzer HY. Effect of the serotonin agonist, MK-212, on body temperature in schizophrenia. *Biol Psychiatry* 1992;31:460–470.

39. Lemus CZ, Lieberman JA, Johns CA, et al. CSF 5-hydroxyindoleacetic acid levels and suicide attempts in schizophrenia. *Biol Psychiatry* 1990;27:923–926.

40. Lemus CZ, Lieberman JA, Johns CA, et al. Hormonal response to fenfluramine challenges in clozapine-treated schizophrenic patients. *Biol Psychiatry* 1991;29:691–694.

41. Lerer B, Ran A, Blacker M, et al. Neuroendocrine responses in chronic schizophrenia. Evidence for a serotonergic dysfunction. *Schiz Res* 1988;1:405–410.

42. Lewine RR, Risch SC, Risby E, et al. Lateral ventricle-brain ratio and balance between CSF HVA and 5-HIAA in schizophrenia. *Am J Psychiatry* 1991;148:1189–1194.

43. Lindström LH, Wieselgren IM, Klockhoff I, Svedberg A. Relationship between abnormal brainstem auditory-evoked potentials and subnormal CSF levels of HVA and 5-HIAA in first-episode schizophrenic patients. *Biol Psychiatry* 1990;28:435–442.

44. Losonczy MF, Song IS, Mohs RS, et al. Correlates of lateral ventricular size in chronic schizophrenia II: biological measures. *Am J Psychiatry* 1986;143:1113–1118.

45. Markianos M, Botsis A, Ananitis Y. Biogenic amine metabolites in plasma of drug-naive schizophrenic patients: associations with symptomatology. *Biol Psychiatry* 1992;32:288–292.

46. Marshall BD, Glynn SM, Midha KK, et al. Adverse effects of fenfluramine in treatment refractory schizophrenia. *J Clin Psychopharmacol* 1989;9:110–115.

47. MacKay AV. New antipsychotic agents and the future. *J Clin Psych* 1985;46:51–53.

48. Meltzer HY. Clinical studies on the mechanism of action of clozapine: the dopamine-serotonin hypothesis of schizophrenia. *Psychopharmacology* 1989;99:S18–S27.

49. Meltzer HY. Clozapine: clinical advantages and biological mechanisms. In: Schulz SC, Tamminga C, eds. *Schizophrenia: a scientific focus*. New York: Oxford University Press; 1989:302–309.

50. Meltzer HY, Maes M, Lee MA. The cimetidine-induced increase in prolactin secretion in schizophrenia: effect of clozapine. *Psychopharmacology* 1993;112:S95–S104.

51. Meltzer HY, Matsubara S, Lee J-C. Classification of typical and atypical antipsychotic drugs on the basis of dopamine D-1, D-2 and serotonin$_2$ pKi values. *J Pharmacol Exp Ther* 1989;251:238–246.

52. Mendels J. The effect of methysergide (a serotonine agent) on schizophrenia: a preliminary report. *Br J Psychiatry* 1967;124:157–160.

53. Mita T, Hanada S, Nishino N, et al. Decreased serotonin S$_2$ and increased dopamine D$_2$ receptors in chronic schizophrenics. *Biol Psychiatry* 1986;21:1407–1414.

54. Monsma FJ, Shen Y, Ward RP, Hamblin MW, Sibley DR. Cloning and expression of a novel serotonin receptor with high affinity for tricyclic psychotropic drugs. *Mol Pharmacol* 1993;43:320–327.

55. Muck-Seler D, Jakavljevic M, Deanovic Z. Platelet serotonin in subtypes of schizophrenia and unipolar depression. *Psychiatry Res* 1991;38:105–131.

56. Nash JF, Meltzer HY. Neuroendocrine studies in psychiatric disorders: the role of serotonin. In: Brown S-L, van Praag HM, eds. *The role of serotonin in psychiatric disorders*. New York: Brunner/Mazel 1991;57–90.

57. Nasrallah HA, Smith RE, Dunner FJ, McCalley-Whitter M. Serotonin precursor effect in tardive dyskinesia. *Psychopharmacology* 1982;11:234–235.

58. Nedergaard S, Bolam JP, Greenfield SA. Facilitation of dendritic calcium conductance by 5-hydroxytryptamine in the substantia nigra. *Nature* 1988;333:174–177.

59. Nisstriandt H, Waters N, Hyarth S. The influence of serotonergic drugs on dopaminergic neurotransmission in rat substantia nigra, striatum and limbic forebrain in vivo. *N-S Arch Pharmacol* 1992;346:12–19.

60. Nyberg S, Farde L, Eriksson L, Halldin C. 5-HT$_2$ and D$_2$ dopamine receptor occupancy in the living human brain. A PET study with risperidone. *Psychopharmacology* [in press].

61. Ohlund LS, Lindstrom LH, Ohman A. Electrodermal orienting response and central nervous system dopamine and serotonin activity in schizophrenia. *J Nerv Mental Dis* 1992;180:304–313.

62. Owen F, Cross AJ, Crow TJ, Lofthouse R, Poulter M. Neurotransmitter receptors in brain in schizophrenia. *ACTA Psych Scand Suppl* 1991;291:20–28.

63. Pickar D, Owen RR, Litman RE, Konicki E, Gutierrez R, Rapaport MH. Clinical and biologic response to clozapine in patients with schizophrenia. Crossover comparison with fluphenazine. *Arch Gen Psych* 1992;49:345–353.

64. Potkin SG, Weinberger DR, Linoila M, Wyatt RJ. Low CSF 5-hydroxyindoleacetic acid in schizophrenic patients with enlarged cerebral ventricles. *Am J Psychiatry* 1983;140:21–25.

65. Price LH, Charney DS, Delgado PL, et al. Clinical studies of 5-HT function using i.v. L-tryptophan. *Prog Neuropsychopharmacol Biol Psychiatry* 1990;14:459–472.

66. Reynolds GP, Rossor M, Iversen LL. Preliminary studies of human cortical 5-HT2 receptors and their involvement in schizophrenia and neuroleptic drug action. *J Neural Trans* 1983;18[Suppl]:273–277.

67. Rogue A, Rogue P. Mianserin in the management of schizophrenia. In: *Schizophrenia 1992: an international conference.* 1992:135.

68. Roth BL, Ciaranello RD, Meltzer HY. Binding of typical and atypical antipsychotic agents with transiently expressed 5-HT$_{1C}$ receptors. *J Pharmacol Exp Ther* 1992;260:1361–1365.

69. Roth BL, Craigo SC, Choudhary MS, et al. Binding of typical and atypical antipsychotic agents to 5-hydroxytryptamine$_6$ (5-HT$_6$) and 5-hydroxytryptamine$_7$ (5-HT$_7$) receptors. *J Pharmacol Exp Ther* 1994;268:1403–1410.

70. Roth BL, Hamblin MW, Ciaranello RD. Regulation of 5-HT$_2$ and 5-HT$_{1C}$ serotonin receptor levels: methodology and mechanisms. *Neuropsychopharmacology* 1990;3:427–433.

71. Roth BL, Hamblin MW, Ciarnello RD. Developmental regulation of 5-HT$_2$ and 5-HT$_{1C}$ mRNA and receptor levels. *Develop Brain Res* 1991;58:51–58.

72. Roy A, Ninan P, Mazonson A, et al. CSF monoamine metabolites

in chronic schizophrenic patients who attempt suicide. *Psychol Med* 1985;15:335–340.

73. Shen Y, Monsma FJ, Metcalf MA, Jose PA, Hamblin MW, Sibley DR. Molecular cloning and expression of a 5-HT$_7$ serotonin receptor subtype. *J Biol Clin* 1993;268:18200–18204.

74. Skorzewsak A, Lal S. Methysergide-induced psychosis: case report with long-term follow-up. *Neuropsychobiology* 1989;22:125–127.

75. Soper HV, Elliott RO, Rejzer AA, Marshall BD. Effects of fenfluramine on neuropsychological and communicative functioning in treatment-refractory schizophrenic patients. *J Clin Psychopharmacol* 1990;10:168–175.

76. Sorensen SM, Kehne JH, Fadayl EM, et al. Characterization of the 5-HT$_2$ antagonist MDL 100907 as a putative atypical antipsychotic: behavioral, electrophysiological and neurochemical studies. *J Pharmacol Exp Ther* 1993;266:684–691.

77. Stanley M, Mann JJ. Increased serotonin-2 binding sites in frontal cortex of suicide victims. *Lancet* 1983;1:214–216.

78. Stockmeier CA, DiCarlo JJ, Zhang Y, Thompson P, Meltzer HY. Characterization of typical and atypical antipsychotic drugs based on in vivo occupancy of serotonin$_2$ and dopamine$_2$ receptors. *J Pharmacol Exp Ther* 1993;266:1374–1384.

79. Szara S. *Hallucinogenic amines and schizophrenia.* New York: Pergamon Press; 1967.

80. Szymanski S, Lieberman J, Pollack S, et al. The dopamine-serotonin relationship in clozapine response. *Psychopharmacology* 1993; 112,S85–S89.

81. Trent F, Tepper JM. Dosal raphe stimulation modifies striatal-evoked antidromic invasion of nigral dopaminergic neurons in vivo. *Exp Brain Res* 1991;84:620–630.

82. Van Praag HM. CSF 5HIAA and suicide in non-depressed schizophrenics. *Lancet* II:1983;977–978.

83. Wadenberg ML. Antagonism by 8-OH-DPAT, but not ritanserin, of catalepsy induced by SCH 23390 in the rat. *J Neural Transm* 1992;89:49–59.

84. Weinberger DR, Berman KF, Illowsky BP. Physiological dysfunction of dorsolateral prefrontal cortex in schizophrenia. III. A new cohort and evidence for a monoaminergic mechanism. *Arch Gen Psychiatry* 1988;45:609–615.

85. Whitaker PM, Crow TJ, Ferrer IN. Tritiated LSD binding in frontal cortex in schizophrenia. *Arch Gen Psych* 1981;38:278–280.

86. Williams J, Davies JA. The involvement of 5-hydroxytryptamine in the release of dendritic dopamine from slices of rat substantia nigra. *J Pharm Pharmacol* 1983;35:734–737.

87. Wooley DW, Shaw E. A biochemical and pharmacological suggestion about certain mental disorders. *Proc Natl Acad Sci USA* 1954;40:228–231.

Psychopharmacology: The Fourth Generation of Progress, edited by Floyd E. Bloom and David J. Kupfer. Raven Press, Ltd., New York © 1995.

CHAPTER 103

The Effects of Neuroleptics on Plasma Homovanillic Acid

Arnold J. Friedhoff and Raul R. Silva

One of the most dramatic observations in psychopharmacology is that various changes in plasma homovanillic acid (pHVA) are highly correlated with the therapeutic response to neuroleptic drugs. In an early study, Bowers' group (4) showed that patients with schizophrenia who responded to a neuroleptic had a decline in pHVA over several weeks of treatment, whereas nonresponders showed little change from baseline. Subsequently Pickar et al. (19) found an impressively high correlation (0.82) between improvement in symptoms of schizophrenia and decline in pHVA. More recently Davila and colleagues (11) found that the extent of the increase in pHVA that occurs early in treatment (4 days after initiation of treatment in this study) was also predictive of therapeutic outcome. A vigorous increase in initial response was predictive of a good therapeutic outcome as was a later decline. The ability to predict outcome after only a few days of treatment could be useful in making decisions about whether to continue treatment with a given drug.

Davis et al. (12), looking at pHVA from a different perspective, reported that the severity of symptoms as schizophrenia and basal pHVA levels were correlated. In the interim, many other investigations have confirmed all or part of these early observations. Green et al. (15) confirmed the previous findings of Davila et al. (11) showing that an early increase in pHVA followed by a subsequent decrease in pHVA, was a good predictor of a favorable clinical response. Chang et al. (6) also found pretreatment pHVA levels higher in patients who turned out to be good responders to haloperidol when compared with a poor responder group. The good outcome group also showed a significant decline in pHVA over time.

Interestingly, Green and coworkers (15) found similar changes in plasma dopamine during haloperidol treatment, although no early surge was detected as there was with pHVA. Although Meltzer (20) found no significant difference when comparing pHVA levels between unmedicated schizophrenic patients and normal controls, clozapine treatment in this study also was associated with a resulting decrease in pHVA. Bowers et al. (5) established a significant relationship between pretreatment pHVA levels and early neuroleptic treatment response in psychotic patients. Likewise Mazure et al. (19) determined that in a group of patients treated with perphenazine, pretreatment pHVA was significantly correlated with posttreatment outcome. In that study, as in the study by Chang et al. (6), good responders had higher mean levels of pHVA than did nonresponders. Additionally, Davidson et al. (8) also showed that patients who have neuroleptics discontinued and develop symptom exacerbation, experience an increase in pHVA. Davila and Friedhoff (10), determining both pHVA and prolactin, reported that the ratio of prolactin to pHVA had stronger correlations with clinical outcome than pHVA alone. Considering all of the studies, most of which are concordant in major detail, there is little question that one or more aspects of the pHVA response to neuroleptics is a predictor of the therapeutic response. The mechanism of this effect, however, remains a matter for speculation, debate, and disagreement.

It is now generally agreed that the response of pHVA to the initiation of neuroleptic treatment follows a typical pattern. Neuroleptics are potent D2 antagonists, blocking signal transduction to postsynaptic D2 receptors, and interfering with the sensing function of presynaptic D2 receptors (for review, see ref. 13). The presynaptic neurons, not sensing excess dopamine in the synaptic cleft, release massive amounts of this transmitter into the synaptic

A. J. Friedhoff and R. R. Silva: Department of Psychiatry, Millhauser Laboratories, New York University Medical Center, New York, New York 10016.

space. The high concentration of dopamine impinging on the blocked postsynaptic receptors competes with the neuroleptic for the binding site; however, the neuroleptic antagonist has a much higher affinity than dopamine for the postsynaptic D2 receptor and thus is probably only minimally displaced. Signal transduction, therefore, remains largely disrupted at early stages of treatment.

Continued interference with neurotransmission invokes another compensatory response—the appearance of new D2 receptors on the postsynaptic neuron (for review, see ref. 14). The density of these receptors can increase by as much as 25% or 30%; however the density in the postsynaptic region of the neuron could be substantially higher. If treatment is continued and blockade is maintained, ultimately the increased release of dopamine from presynaptic terminals returns to baseline levels or below through a process called depolarization blockade (22). The mechanism for this phenomenon is not well understood; however, it is accompanied by a reduction in the activity of the rate-limiting enzyme in dopamine synthesis, tyrosine hydroxylase (17), just as the initial increase in dopamine release was accompanied by an increase in tyrosine hydroxylase activity.

This sequence of events, which has been shown to occur at dopaminergic synapses in the brain, is paralleled almost exactly by changes in pHVA: (a) the initial increase in pHVA that follows initiation of neuroleptic treatment parallels the initial increase in dopamine release from presynaptic terminals, (b) the return of pHVA to baseline levels or below parallels the increase in the number of postsynaptic receptors and the reduction in dopamine release and synthesis as a result of depolarization blockade. Nonetheless serious questions remain as to whether these central events are responsible for the changes in the HVA found in plasma.

A major problem in understanding the mechanism of the pHVA response is the fact that most pHVA does not come from the central nervous system (CNS). It is almost certain, however, that neuroleptics work via their effects on central dopaminergic neurons. Dopamine has several roles in the body. It acts as a neurotransmitter in a network of dopaminergic neurons in the prefrontal cortex and in a number of interacting subcortical nuclei. It also acts on peripheral dopamine receptors principally in the vascular system and kidneys. Dopamine has another important role as a precursor of norepinephrine. To meet kinetic requirements for the synthesis of norepinephrine, dopamine must be produced in excess from its precursor L-dopa. An additional factor to be taken into consideration is that dopamine cannot cross the blood–brain barrier in either direction. Thus all dopamine in the brain is made from L-dopa, which can cross the barrier, and all dopamine found in the periphery originates in the periphery.

The HVA found in circulating plasma thus, comes from (a) dopamine released from central dopaminergic neurons and subjected to the action of monamine oxidase and catechol-O-methyltransferase, (b) dopamine acting as a precursor in the biosynthesis of norepinephrine in noradrenergic neurons in the brain, (c) dopamine released from peripheral dopaminergic neurons, (d) dopamine acting as a precursor in peripheral noradrenergic neurons, or (e) dopamine originating as a metabolite of L-dopa in any tissue in which 1-amino acid decarboxylase, the enzyme converting L-dopa to dopamine can be found. Finally the level of HVA in plasma is determined not only by its rate of synthesis but also by its rate of excretion, primarily in urine (16). The net result of all of this is that most pHVA does not originate in the brain or even from dopamine acting as a neurotransmitter.

These observations led us to ask the question, How can changes in a metabolite that comes mainly from sources other than from dopamine acting as a transmitter so successfully predict the outcome of a treatment that acts by modifying dopaminergic transmission? To attempt to understand this, we reviewed an experiment we carried out in 1978 (2). In this study, we used therapeutic response to haloperidol and resting finger tremor as outcome measures. Resting finger tremor reflects the continuous microoscillation of the fingers. This oscillation probably increases finger dexterity by making it possible to initiate a finger movement with a running start. The tremor is under strong dopaminergic control. Neuroleptic drugs, which are D2 antagonists, increase tremor amplitude and slow its frequency. Parkinsonism, a hypodopaminergic syndrome, also has this effect. Dopaminergic agonists, on the other hand, decrease amplitude and increase frequency. This tremor is largely under the control of spinal, not brain, neurons.

In our experiment, carried out years before pHVA could be assayed by high-performance liquid chromatography (HPLC), we measured baseline finger tremor in patients with schizophrenia, then began treatment with haloperidol. We proposed that subjects in whom neuroleptic administration had little effect on tremor released large amounts of dopamine which overcame the blockade. Four days after haloperidol treatment was begun we again measured tremor. Those subjects who best overcame the neuroleptic blockade, presumably by a large compensatory release of dopamine, had the least increase in amplitude and slowing of frequency. We then continued haloperidol treatment for 28 days and measured improvement in mental status. The subjects showing the least change in either tremor amplitude or frequency on the 4th day of the haloperidol treatment had the best therapeutic response to the haloperidol. Subjects with the most vigorous release of dopamine on the 4th day of haloperidol treatment would tend to overcome the haloperidol blockade of D2 receptors and not suffer a change in tremor. Those with a sluggish release, on the other hand, would have slowing of tremor frequency and increased amplitude.

Somewhat to our surprise those subjects with evidence of preexisting low dopaminergic activity did not do well therapeutically, whereas those with evidence of an active dopaminergic system did. This seeming paradox is addressed later in this chapter. It should be noted that haloperidol treatment tends to reduce dopaminergic activity in responders (as reflected by pHVA) to the point it was before treatment in nonresponders.

Despite the fact that plasma HVA is a peripheral dopaminergic measure, it is at least as good a predictor as HVA found in cerebrospinal fluid. Van Kammen (24) reviewed the literature and theorized that dopaminergic turnover in certain regions of the brain (such as cortical areas) are greater than in other brain regions. As a result, measurements of CSF HVA may predominantly represent dopaminergic turnover in cortical areas, rather than reflecting what transpires in specific striatal dopaminergic regions. Interestingly, Davidson and colleagues reported that the results of a study utilizing debrisoquin provided preliminary evidence correlating the relationship between pHVA and central HVA. Thus measuring pHVA may represent a practical approach to estimating dopamine turnover in the human brain.

One plausible explanation as to why pHVA changes, in response to neuroleptic treatment, is that neuroleptics have a correlated effect on the diverse sources of pHVA. If a number of different pools of origin of HVA contribute to the plasma pool in a correlated manner, changes in pHVA could be highly predictive of therapeutic response, even though it does not reflect only that fraction of pHVA that originates in presynaptic terminals of relevant brain neurons.

Surprisingly little has been reported about the relationship of pHVA changes during neuroleptic treatment and the emergence of side effects, in particular extrapyramidal side effects. Early in the use of neuroleptics it was proposed that the emergence of Parkinsonianlike tremor and rigidity was a good therapeutic indicator (1). Inasmuch as extrapyramidal side effects (EPS) result from low dopaminergic activity, and neuroleptics reduce dopaminergic activity, it was felt that EPS reflected the fact that hypodopaminergia was achieved. However, EPS has not turned out to be a good predictor of therapeutic outcome, perhaps because it occurs, initially, at relatively low levels of neuroleptic blockade, often before effective doses are achieved.

One complication in studying predictors of therapeutic response is the definition of a responder. As more data have been accumulated, a more specific definition of responders and nonresponders has begun to emerge. From clinical studies, it has been found that two types of manifestations of schizophrenia cluster together. These have been variously named but are now generally called positive and negative symptom types of schizophrenia. Positive symptoms are those generally found in more acute patients or in those having an acute recurrence and include delusions, labile affect, auditory hallucinations, and disturbances in associative processing. Negative symptoms include social withdrawal, flat affect, and anhedonia (for a complete list of negative symptoms see ref. 3). Few patients have a pure distillate of one type of symptom or the other; thus the characterization of a patient as positive or negative generally refers to the dominant symptom type. There are a number of studies showing that positive-symptom patients respond better to treatment with typical neuroleptics than negative symptom types, but pHVA has been measured in only a few of these studies (7,11,21). In a study by Davila et al. (11), it has been found that negative symptom patients do not have the initial increase in pHVA associated with the beginning of neuroleptic treatment, nor do they have the later decline in pHVA. Also there have been several reports that nonresponders have lower baseline pHVA, although these have not been rated for positive or negative symptoms (4,6,19,23,25).

Flat affect has been considered to be the *sine qua non* of the negative subtype. This is of interest because of the flat affectual responses of Parkinson's patients who have a central hypodopaminergic syndrome, and because neuroleptics, which reduce dopaminergic activity pharmacologically, produce blunted or flat affect in many cases. There is, therefore, reason to believe that affect is under strong dopaminergic regulation. This conclusion can also be supported by data obtained from observations of patients with extreme affective lability, as seen in hypomania, for example. In these patients, treatment with neuroleptic drugs frequently reduces affectivity. Thus we have proposed that a reduction of central dopaminergic activity may produce blunting of affective responses and that affect is under dopaminergic control. If this is the case, then one could conclude that negative-symptom patients have low central dopaminergic activity.

Affect may also play a central role in regulating thinking processes. There may be an association between flat affect and concrete thinking and between labile affect and looseness of associations. In mania, for instance, associations are made between thoughts that are related in nonsubstantive ways, because they sound alike, for example, or rhyme with each other. At one end of the affect spectrum, flatness is associated with concrete thinking in which a conceptual or symbolic dimension is missing. On the other end in a highly labile affective state, relationships are seen between thoughts, based on trivial connections, characterized as flight of ideas. Creative thinking, which involves making new associations, may lie somewhere between these two extremes and be dependent on more modest affectivity.

This chapter is not about thinking or affect, thus only scant attention can be given to those subjects. A consideration of these topics is necessary, however, to begin to address questions concerning the mechanism of the pHVA response. If overactivity of the dopaminergic system were the primary etiology of schizophrenia, as was proposed in the early dopamine hypothesis (18) then it would not be possible to understand patients with negative symptoms who have clinical evidence of low dopaminergic activity (flat affect) confirmed by generally low pHVA in these subjects. On the other hand if dopamine plays a role in the pHVA response only as a mediator of the treatment response, then it may be possible to reconcile pHVA changes with clinical response.

A new element has been introduced by the widespread use of clozapine, and the experimental use of many so-called atypical drugs. It is reported that these compounds can be used to effectively treat many patients with negative symptoms (low pHVA). These patients frequently have low baseline pHVA, which is not affected by treatment with typical neuroleptics, nor does their clinical state improve significantly. What is perplexing is the fact that responders (generally positive-symptom type) have a decrease in pHVA only to the baseline level of poor outcome patients (4). Do atypical drugs, more particularly clozapine, reduce pHVA further in negative-symptom patients than typical neuroleptics? This question is being pursued by several groups but cannot yet be answered definitively.

We have formulated a hypothesis in which we attempt to reconcile observations of the pHVA response with well-established clinical observations of patients with schizophrenia and their response to treatment. The proposal that best fits the existing facts is that the dopaminergic system in the brain is a restitutive or compensatory system. In the face of inescapable stress of either internal or external origin, of such nature as to threaten the integrity of the thinking function, the dopaminergic system turns itself down, resulting in affectual blunting, an increase in concrete thinking, and through a poorly understood mechanism, a decrease in pHVA. Patients with positive- or negative-type schizophrenia would carry a schizophrenia gene, but not necessarily the same one. In negative-symptom patients, a compensatory decrease in dopaminergic activity would have taken place resulting in affectual blunting and an increase in concrete thinking, but that did not overcome the deficit produced by the schizophrenia gene. Thus these patients would remain incapacitated but with the addition of flat affect and concrete thinking as manifestations of the invocation of a decrease in dopaminergic activity resulting from the action of the compensatory system. Flat affect and concrete thinking, in this proposal, are not manifestations of schizophrenia, but result from the turning down of the dopaminergic compensatory system. It should be noted that normal subjects, in response to intractable stress, also often manifest blunted affect.

We have proposed that positive patients have two defects: (a) In one a schizophrenia gene or a defect in a gene is involved in regulating activity of the dopaminergic compensatory system. The dopaminergic system in these patients cannot turn itself down but can be turned down pharmacologically by neuroleptics. (b) Negative-symptom patients, by contrast, get little benefit from neuroleptics, because their dopaminergic system has reduced itself spontaneously; thus typical neuroleptics have little additional effect. One important challenge of this hypothesis will be to see if clozapine can reduce pHVA more than typical neuroleptics do in those patients who respond to this drug.

Measurement of pHVA over only a few days of neuroleptic treatment makes it possible to predict the therapeutic outcome of the treatment. It is not clear why this works as a predictor because much of the HVA in plasma does not originate in the brain or even from dopamine released during neurotransmission. Further understanding of this mechanism may clarify the physiological role of the dopaminergic system in maintaining mental stability.

ACKNOWLEDGMENTS

This work was supported in part by Grant MH 35976 and Research Scientist Award MH 14024, both from the National Institute of Mental Health.

REFERENCES

1. Alpert M, Diamond F, Kesselman M. Correlation between extrapyramidal and therapeutic effects of neuroleptics. *Comp Psychiatry* 1977;18(4):333–338.
2. Alpert M, Diamond F, Weisenfreund J, Taleporos E, Friedhoff AJ. The neuroleptic hypothesis: study of covariation of extrapyramidal and therapeutic drug effects. *Br J Psychiatry* 1978;133:169–175.
3. Andreasen N. *Modified scale for the assessment of negative symptoms (SANS).* Iowa City: University of Iowa, 1984.
4. Bowers MB, Swigar ME, Jatlow PI, Giocoechea N. Plasma catecholamine metabolites and early response to haloperidol. *J Clin Psychiatry* 1984;45:248–251.
5. Bowers MB, Swigar ME, Jatlow PI, Hoffman FJ, Goicoecha N. Early neuroleptic response: clinical profiles and plasma catecholamine metabolites. *J Clin Psychopharmacol* 1987;7:83–86.
6. Chang WH, Chen TY, Lee CF, Hung JC, Hu WH, Yeh EK. Plasma homovanillic acid levels and subtyping of schizophrenia. *Psychiatry Res* 1988;23:239–244.
7. Davidson M, Davis KL. A comparison of plasma homovanillic acid concentrations in schizophrenic patients and normal controls. *Arch Gen Psychiatry* 1988;45(6):561–563.
8. Davidson M, Kahn RS, Warne P, et al. Changes in plasma homovanillic acid concentrations in schizophrenic patients following neuroleptic discontinuation. *Arch Gen Psychiatry* 1991;48:73–76.
9. Davidson M, Losonczy MF, Mohs RC, et al. Effects of debrisoquin and haloperidol on plasma homovanillic acid concentration in schizophrenic patients. *Neuropsychopharmacology* 1987;1:17–23.
10. Davila R, Gonzales-Torres M, Zumarraga M, Andia I, Guimon J, Friedhoff AJ. The ratio of plasma prolactin to homovanillic acid: a good predictor of clinical response in schizophrenia. [*Submitted.*]
11. Davila R, Manero E, Zumarraga M. Plasma homovanillic acid as a predictor of response to neuroleptics. *Arch Gen Psychiatry* 1988;45:564–567.
12. Davis KL, Davidson M, Mohs RC, et al. Plasma homovanillic acid concentration and the severity of schizophrenic illness. *Science* 1985;227:1601–1692.
13. Davis KL, Kahn RS, Ko G, et al. Dopamine in schizophrenia. *Am J Psychiatry* 1991;148:1474–1486.
14. Friedhoff AJ. Catecholamines and behavior. In: Ramachandran VS, ed. *Encyclopedia of human biology.* San Diego: Academic Press; 1991:217–224.
15. Green AI, Alam MY, Boshes RA, et al. Haloperidol response and plasma catecholamines and their metabolites. *Schizophr Res* 1993; 10:33–37.

16. Grodsky GM. Chemistry and functions of the hormones: in thyroid, pancreas, adrenal and gastrointestinal tract. In: Harper HA, Rodwell VW, Mayers PA, eds. *Review of physiological chemistry.* California: Lang Medical; 1979:511–555.

17. Landsberg L, Young JB. Physiology and pharmacology of the autonomic nervous system. In: Wilson JD, Braunwald E, Isselbacher KF, et al. eds. *Principles of internal medicine.* New York: McGraw-Hill; 1991:380–389.

18. Matthysse S. Antipsychotic drug actions: a clue to neuropathology of schizophrenia? *Fed Proc* 1973;32:200–205.

19. Mazure CM, Nelson JC, Jatlow PI, Bowers MB. Plasma free homovanillic acid (HVA) as a predictor of clinical response in acute psychosis. *Soc Biol Psychiatry* 1991;30:475–482.

20. Meltzer H. Duration of a clozapine trial in neuroleptic-resistant schizophrenia. *Arch Gen Psychiatry* 1989;46:672.

21. Pickar D, Labarca R, Linnoila M, et al. Neuroleptic-induced decrease in plasma homovanillic acid and antipsychotic activity in schizophrenic patients. *Science* 1984;225:954–957.

22. Pickar D, Labarca R, Doran AR. Longitudinal measurement of plasma homovanillic acid levels in schizophrenic patients. *Arch Gen Psychiatry* 1986;43:669–676.

23. Steinberg JL, Garver DL, Moeller FG, Raese JD, Orsulak PL. Serum homovanillic acid levels in schizophrenic patients and normal control subjects. *Psychiatry Res* 1993;48:93–106.

24. Van Kammen DP. The biochemical basis of relapse and drug response in schizophrenia: review and hypothesis. *Psychol Med* 1991;21:881–895.

25. Van Putten T, Marder SR, Aravagiri M, Chabert N, Mintz J. Plasma homovanillic acid as a predictor of response to fluphenazine treatment. *Psychopharm Bull* 1989;1:89–91.

Psychopharmacology: The Fourth
Generation of Progress, edited by
Floyd E. Bloom and David J. Kupfer.
Raven Press, Ltd., New York © 1995.

CHAPTER 104

Neurophysiological and Psychophysiological Approaches to Schizophrenia

Keith H. Nuechterlein and Michael E. Dawson

Schizophrenia is characterized by psychotic states in which there are striking abnormalities of perception, thinking, and speech, suggesting that alterations in the normal neural control of information processing play a critical role (12,42,55). In addition, negative symptoms such as flat affect, apathy, and poverty of speech (3) seem to entail decreased integration of emotional and motivational functions with perceptual and cognitive functioning. Thus, it is fitting that a substantial body of research has attempted to delineate neurophysiological and psychophysiological abnormalities that are characteristic of this disorder or group of disorders. We will describe several of the more prominent methods and a sampling of relevant results and provide sources for further information.

One prominent psychophysiological dysfunction in schizophrenia that is not reviewed here is eye-tracking dysfunction, which is among the most promising indicators of genetic vulnerability to schizophrenia. Fortunately, excellent recent reviews of the extensive literature on eye-tracking abnormalities offer easy access to this important topic (e.g., see refs. 43, 44, and 50).

ELECTROENCEPHALOGRAM AND EVENT-RELATED POTENTIAL MEASURES

Basic Concepts and Measures

Studies of the electrical activity of the brain can be divided into those that examine the *electroencephalogram*

K. H. Nuechterlein: Department of Psychiatry and Biobehavioral Sciences, University of California, Los Angeles, Los Angeles, California 90024.
M. E. Dawson: Department of Psychology, University of Southern California, Los Angeles, California 90089.

(*EEG*) and those that focus on *event-related potentials* (*ERPs*). The EEG is a measure of a combination of excitatory and inhibitory postsynaptic electrical potentials as recorded between pairs of electrodes on the scalp. The brain regions that give rise to these potentials involve the neocortex that lies near the electrodes, but the potentials also appear to involve influences from ascending pathways from limbic, thalamic, and reticular nuclei. The EEG is fundamentally a physiological measure of the momentary *functional state* of the underlying cerebral structures, although it may be affected by any neuroanatomical abnormalities. In a recent extensive review, Shagass (63) has noted that the critical advantages of the EEG for psychiatric research are that it is (a) noninvasive and radiation-free, (b) repeatable as often as needed, (c) closer to brain effects for pharmacological studies than blood levels, (d) multidimensional (frequency, amplitude, wave symmetry, and the temporal and spatial aspects of each), and (e) extremely sensitive to changes in alertness and cognitive activity. Accompanying these advantages are the limitations that (a) the usual scalp recordings index primarily surface cortical activity, (b) scalp electrodes pick up potentials that include attenuation by tissue conduction, (c) recordings at any given site involve some overlap between potentials that originate at different locations, (d) care must be taken to eliminate artifacts from electrical potentials from noncerebral sources, and (e) the subject's state of alertness and cognitive activity need to be considered and possibly controlled when a psychopathological characteristic is the object of study (63). The typical EEG scoring procedure involves power spectral analyses, which provides an indication of the amount of electrical activity in delta (<4 Hz), theta ($5-7$ Hz), alpha ($8-13$ Hz), and beta ($14-30$ Hz) frequency bands. Fourier analysis also allows estimation of coherence, which involves the correlation between EEG waveforms at two recording sites. EEG applications also now often include topographic mapping of the power or amplitude values across the surface of the head.

In contrast to EEG, ERP methods involve examination of the electrical activity of the brain that is time-locked to presentation of various stimulus events. By averaging the electrical activity recorded in the first few hundred milliseconds following a number of discrete presentations of a stimulus, the background EEG can be removed and the electrical potentials that are related to the stimulus can be examined (40). Figure 1 is a schematic diagram of this process and the resulting waveform for an auditory stimulus. The temporal resolution allowed by this technique is excellent, as seen in the number of distinct positive and negative deflections within 1000 msec in Fig. 1. This temporal resolution is a distinct advantage for studies of information processing in schizophrenia, because a large literature suggests that schizophrenic patients often show abnormalities in processing information in the period immediately following stimulus presentation (5,12,55). Topographic mapping of ERPs is also increasingly popular, and better methods for location of generator sources are being developed. In comparison to other current methods of examining the physiological processes of the brain in response to stimuli, such as positron emission tomography (PET) or regional cerebral blood flow, ERP methods at present have better temporal resolution but less spatial resolution.

The ERP temporal components can be used to detect successive aspects of registration and processing of a stimulus. Auditory ERP components are often divided into brainstem components (first 10 msec), middle-latency components (10 to about 90 msec), and long-latency components (100 msec and later) (28,30). Starting with the positive-polarity response at about 50 msec, the components are labeled by positive or negative polarity (P or N) and by either their latency in milliseconds or their order (e.g., P50 or P1, N100 or N2). The ERP components through 200 msec have usually been called *exogenous* or *stimulus-driven,* because they mainly reflect particular physical properties of the stimulus. The components after 200 msec are referred to as *endogenous, concept-driven,* or *context-dependent,* because they are strongly influenced by internal stimulus representations and the role or significance of the stimulus as defined by the task and the subject (28,30,45).

EEG Findings in Schizophrenia

The EEGs of schizophrenic patients have been found to differ from those of normal subjects in a variety of ways, some of which may be dependent on the level and type of psychiatric symptoms that the patient is experiencing at the time of assessment. Medication effects have sometimes been difficult to separate from effects of

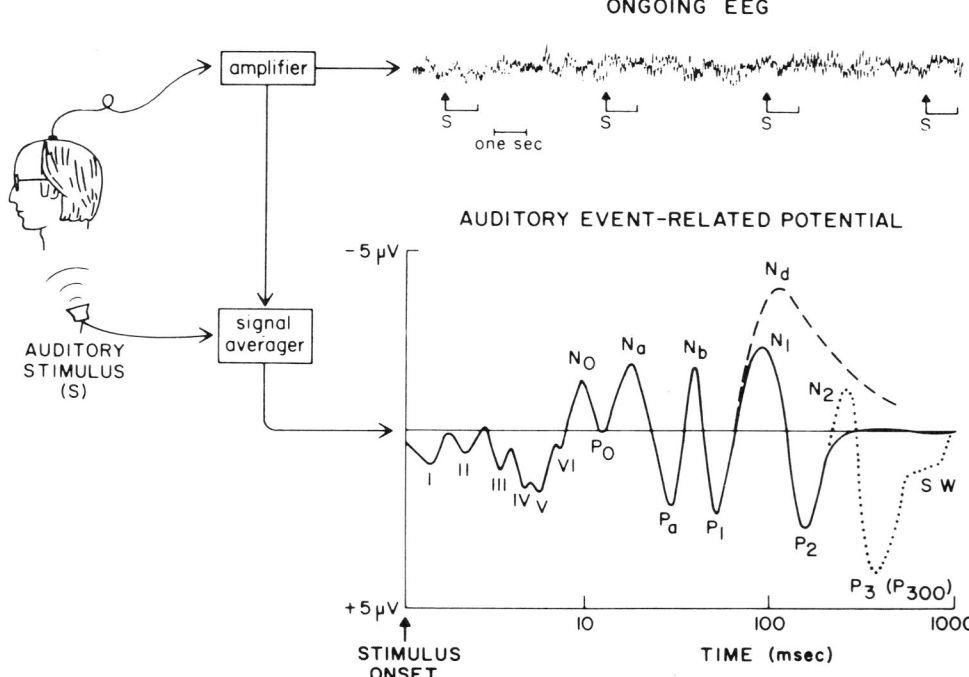

FIG. 1. Idealized form of the averaged event-related potential to a sequence of auditory stimuli (S). Component numbers represent approximate latency ×100 msec. Other labels are early brainstem responses (I to VI), midlatent component (N$_O$, P$_O$, N$_a$, P$_a$, N$_b$), and slow wave (SW). Note log units on time axis. (From ref. 40, with permission.)

schizophrenia, although some EEG differences were reported even before the introduction of neuroleptic drugs. One prominent finding is an increased frequency of EEG records reflecting high activation levels, as judged by reactivity of the EEG upon opening the eyes, among schizophrenic patients in an unmedicated state (63). Consistent with hyperactivation are quantitative results showing that EEGs of schizophrenic subjects have lower alpha power, increased variability of frequency, and higher wave symmetry than comparison subjects (63). Given that excesses in both slow and fast EEG activity have been reported, however, Shagass (63) suggests that dysregulation of brain activity in schizophrenia might be a more basic problem than hyperactivation per se.

Koukkou and her colleagues have emphasized an information-processing approach to EEG research and have addressed more directly than most investigators the issue of whether EEG abnormalities represent trait-like vulnerability to schizophrenia or are characteristics of a schizophrenic psychotic state. Koukkou and Manske (48) selected schizophrenic subjects who were either in an unmedicated state with a recent onset of positive symptoms or who had shown a full symptomatic remission after a first episode and had been medication-free for 3 months. Abnormal power in low-frequency bands (2–8 Hz) in reaction to auditory stimuli was found to be present only in the symptomatic schizophrenic patients and therefore is apparently a reflection of clinical state. Possible indicators of a vulnerability trait were also suggested, but they need evaluation in longitudinal studies across clinical states before any clear conclusions can be drawn.

Several topographic EEG studies have found evidence of excessive slow activity (delta) in frontal areas (e.g., see refs. 38 and 53). This EEG evidence is conceptually consistent with PET and regional cerebral blood flow evidence of reduced frontal activity in at least some schizophrenic patients, and increased frontal delta activity has been shown to be correlated within schizophrenic samples with PET hypofrontal metabolic patterns (38).

Prominent ERP Findings in Schizophrenia

The most common ERP paradigm has examined P300 (P3) amplitude and latency in a situation in which an occasional, unpredictable physical change in a stimulus occurs within a series of identical stimulus presentations (the "oddball" paradigm). The oddball stimulus may, for example, differ from the repeated standard stimulus in pitch or duration. The P300 response in this situation is an index of cortical response related to processing the significance of the novel stimulus. Schizophrenic patients were first found to show reduced P300 amplitude in this paradigm a little more than 20 years ago, and this characteristic has been among the most robust of ERP results for schizophrenia (32,45). Because P300 is believed to be

an index of consciously controlled aspects of information processing, this P300 abnormality contributed to the view that controlled information processing is impaired in schizophrenia but more automatic information processing is intact (16). More recently, a specific aspect of P300 amplitude reduction—that is, smaller amplitude over left as compared to right lateral sites—has been linked to thought disorder levels and reductions in the volume of the left posterior superior temporal gyrus among schizophrenic patients (51).

Decreased auditory P300 amplitude or increased P300 latency has also been found in some recent studies of first-degree relatives of schizophrenic patients (9,47), suggesting the possibility that P300 latency or amplitude might be an indicator of a genetic vulnerability factor for schizophrenia. However, Friedman and Squires-Wheeler (32) argue that these findings might reflect the older age of the first-degree relatives of schizophrenic probands relative to control subjects. P300 findings in children at increased genetic risk by virtue of having a schizophrenic parent have been mixed. Friedman et al. (31) found no evidence of P300 abnormalities among the complete initial sample from the New York High Risk Project, and Squires-Wheeler et al. (66) found that P300 amplitude recorded in adolescent offspring of schizophrenic probands did not predict later young adult clinical assessments. On the other hand, Schreiber et al. (62) found that children of schizophrenic patients had prolonged P300 latencies (although not reduced amplitude) when compared to control children matched for age, sex, and educational level. The interested reader should consult the excellent recent review by Friedman and Squires-Wheeler (32) for discussion of additional methodological issues that need to be faced in order to determine whether P300 latency or amplitude may serve as a useful vulnerability indicator for schizophrenia.

An earlier positive ERP component, P50, has been the focus of substantial recent research as a possible vulnerability indicator for schizophrenia, particularly as an index of the initial processing of sensory stimuli that occur in close succession. The concept of a sensory or sensorimotor gating process has been central to this work with the P50 component and to work with a paradigm that we discuss in the next section, namely, prepulse inhibition of the startle blink response. As we navigate through the world, we are constantly bombarded with a multitude of external and internal stimuli. The stimuli include a variety of visual, auditory, tactile, and olfactory stimuli, as well as interoceptive sensations and thoughts. For the most part, we are able to select and consciously process those specific stimuli most relevant to our current activities and goals and somehow screen out, or gate, irrelevant stimuli, often to the point that we are not even consciously aware of them.

Acute schizophrenic patients in the early stage of their psychosis frequently vividly describe disturbances suggestive of an impaired ability to gate irrelevant stimuli and focus on the relevant stimuli (52). For example, one patient reported that "I am attending to everything at once and as a result I do not really attend to anything." Another stated that "I am speaking to you now but I can hear noises going on next door and in the corridor. I find it difficult to shut these out and it makes it more difficult for me to concentrate on what I am saying to you." McGhie and Chapman (52) hypothesized that a breakdown in the selective-inhibitory function of attention occurs in schizophrenia, leading to a sense of being flooded with incoming sensory data.

The notion of an impaired sensory filter, or sensory gate, in schizophrenia remains a popular one today (12,13,29). In the P50 conditioning-testing paradigm, two brief auditory stimuli (usually clicks) are presented in rapid succession, typically 500 msec apart. Series of these paired stimuli are presented, usually at 10-sec intervals. Freedman, Adler, Waldo, and their colleagues have shown that the P50 response to the first stimulus in normal subjects is typically reasonably large, but the P50 response to the second stimulus is attenuated by inhibitory effects associated with the first stimulus (29). This temporary inhibitory effect presumably serves to protect processing of the initial stimulus from the potentially disruptive effects of the second stimulus. Schizophrenic subjects, in contrast, often do not show this decreased P50 response to the second stimulus (1). While about 90% of control subjects without a family history of schizophrenia show a reduction of more than 50% in the amplitude of the second stimulus relative to the first, about 85% of schizophrenic patients show less than a 50% reduction (29). This inhibitory deficit is seen in both unmedicated and medicated patients (27). Two other independent groups have now been able to replicate this basic P50 inhibitory deficit in schizophrenia (11,46). Of at least equal interest is the finding that the abnormality in P50 gating is also present in a disproportionate number of the first-degree relatives of schizophrenic patients (64,73). In addition, the P50 gating deficit has been associated within biological relatives with increased Sc scores on the Minnesota Multiphasic Personality Inventory. Thus, it shows promise as an indicator of an extended phenotype that may be associated with vulnerability to schizophrenia.

Freedman et al. (27) have demonstrated that the P50 gating phenomenon may involve cholinergic mechanisms at the level of the hippocampus and temporal lobes and have emphasized hippocampal mediation of the gating deficit. The P50 inhibitory deficit in unaffected biological relatives of schizophrenic patients appears to be normalized by nicotine, consistent with animal studies which indicate that administration of nicotinic antagonists can induce temporary gating deficits (2). Additional work is needed to determine the degree to which the neural mechanisms that account for the P50 gating phenomenon overlap with those involved in another popular procedure for examining sensory gating—namely, prepulse inhibition of the startle reflex response.

PREPULSE INHIBITION OF THE STARTLE REFLEX

The Prepulse Inhibition Paradigm

The so-called "prepulse inhibition" (PPI) paradigm for study of sensorimotor gating also involves the presentation of two stimuli in close succession, but examines the inhibition of the amplitude of the startle reflex rather than the attenuation of the P50 response. Operationally, it consists of presenting a startle-eliciting stimulus pulse (e.g., a brief burst of loud noise) sometimes alone and sometimes shortly following a nonstartling stimulus (e.g., a mild tone). As shown in Fig. 2, when the nonstartling "prepulse" precedes the startling "pulse" by an interval ranging from approximately 30 to 300 msec, the startle reflex amplitude is markedly inhibited compared to when the startle pulse is presented alone. On average, the startle reflex amplitude is inhibited by 50% or more, and in some individuals it is completely inhibited. The PPI phenomenon has been demonstrated to occur reliably in lower animals using measures of whole-body startle (41), as well as in humans using the eye-blink component of the startle reflex (4). The optimal interval between onset of the prepulse and onset of the startle pulse for producing PPI in both humans and animals is approximately 100 msec. The general working model is that the first nonstartling stimulus initiates a brief inhibitory process that attenuates responses to the second startling stimulus.

In human research, PPI is usually measured as a change in eye-blink amplitude (and/or change in blink latency) because the eye blink is one of the most reliable components of the startle reflex and is relatively easy to measure with electromyographic techniques. The startle-eliciting pulse is usually a brief burst of loud noise (95–105 dB) with a rapid rise time, although tactile stimuli (airpuffs) and visual stimuli (bright flashes) also have been used effectively. The nonstartling prepulse is usually a brief mild innocuous tone, although it too can be in other modalities. The prepulse may be discrete (onset and offset before the startle pulse is presented) or it may be continuous (sustained until or beyond the presentation of the startle pulse).

Graham (35) suggested that the PPI may reflect an automatic sensory gating mechanism initiated by the prepulse that serves to protect initial processing of the prepulse from the distractive effects of other sensory events, such as startle stimuli. Moreover, it has recently been demonstrated that directing attention to the prepulse enhances the PPI effect (e.g., ref. 25). The latter finding is important in the present context for at least two reasons. First, it indicates that PPI is not solely an automatic effect in all situations because it can be modulated by conscious attentional strategies. Thus, PPI offers the opportunity to evaluate both automatic and controlled information processing. Second, because controlled attentional deficit has long been recognized in schizophrenia, it may be that the attentional modulation of the PPI effect would be a sensitive index of schizophrenia impairments. We therefore turn next to an examination of PPI in schizophrenic patients.

PPI Findings with Schizophrenic Patients

Three studies have examined the basic PPI effect in schizophrenic patients to date. Braff et al. (15), Braff et al. (14), and Grillon et al. (36) measured PPI in heterogeneous groups of hospitalized chronic and acute medicated schizophrenic patients. Braff et al. (15) employed a continuous innocuous tone as the prepulse and a burst of loud white noise as the startle pulse, Braff et al. (14) employed a discrete mild white noise as the prepulse and either a burst of loud white noise or a tactile stimulus as the startle pulse, and Grillon et al. (36) employed a discrete white noise as the prepulse and a burst of loud white noise as the startle pulse. In each study, schizophrenic patients exhibited impaired PPI compared to normal control subjects when the prepulse preceded the startle stimulus by between 60 and 120 msec. Impaired PPI was documented across different modalities of the startling stimulus (14) and across different intensities of the prepulse (36). These findings have been interpreted as reflecting an impairment in automatic, preattentive central nervous system inhibition (sensorimotor gating) in schizophrenia (13).

Dawson et al. (19) extended this line of research by studying attentional modulation of PPI in relatively asymptomatic schizophrenic outpatients. In the basic PPI paradigm, subjects are not given specific instructions to attend to the stimuli, but Dawson et al. (19) instructed subjects to attend to one auditory prepulse and simply ignore another auditory prepulse. A group of normal controls demographically matched to the schizophrenic patients exhibited greater PPI following the attended prepulse than it exhibited following the ignored prepulse, whereas the patients exhibited similar PPI following the attended and ignored prepulses. This finding illustrates defective attentional modulation of PPI by schizophrenic outpatients and suggests that the patients have a deficit in controlled cognitive processes. The fact that the outpatients were relatively asymptomatic at the time of testing suggests that the failure to attentionally modulate PPI may be a trait-like index related to ongoing vulnerability to schizophrenia rather than a secondary effect of psychotic symptoms.

Neuropsychopharmacological Models of PPI

One of the methodological advantages of studying the PPI phenomenon is that it can be examined in lower animals (e.g., see ref. 70). These studies add significantly to our understanding of the neurobiological mechanisms underlying PPI and its impairments. For example, a neural circuit for the primary acoustic startle reflex has been established in rats by Davis et al. (17). This circuit consists of the auditory nerve, ventral cochlear nucleus, nuclei of the lateral lemniscus, nucleus reticular pontis caudalis, spinal neuron, and muscle.

More relevant to the present discussion of PPI, neural circuits are being established for the modification of the startle reflex. Leitner and co-workers have proposed a basic midbrain circuit for PPI by auditory prepulses based on brain lesion findings in rats (e.g., see ref. 49). This hypothesized circuit for auditory prepulse input parallels that proposed by Davis et al. (17) for the acoustic startle

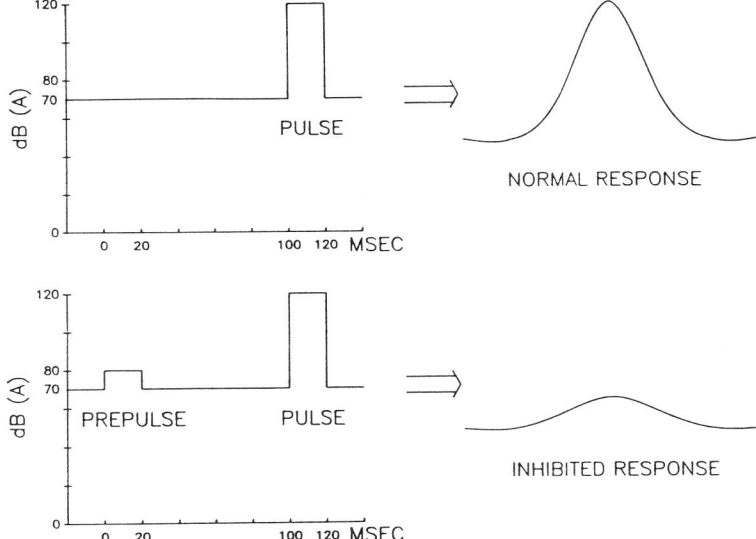

FIG. 2. Diagrammatic representation of prepulse inhibition. The **top figure** illustrates the pulse-alone trial in which startle is elicited by a loud noise burst presented for 20–40 msec. The **bottom figure** illustrates the prepulse + pulse trial in which startle is inhibited by a weak prepulse given shortly (in this case 100 msec) before the same startle eliciting pulse used in the pulse-alone trial. (From ref. 34, with permission.)

stimulus up to the level of the lateral lemniscus (i.e., it consists of the auditory nerve, ventral cochlear nucleus, nuclei of lateral lemniscus), but then it continues to ascend to the inferior colliculus and lateral tegmentum, from where it then descends to a hindbrain area such as the reticularis pontis caudalis. Leitner and Cohen (49) also suggest that the lateral tegmentum area serves as a convergence point for descending information from prepulses in other sensory modalities.

Although the primary startle reflex circuit is located in the hindbrain and the basic PPI circuit appears to be located in the midbrain, there is considerable evidence that forebrain structures can modulate PPI (34,70,72). This, of course, would be expected given that higher-order attention can modulate PPI. Evidence indicates that PPI can be modulated by a complex cortical–striatal–pallidal–thalamic circuit. This proposed circuit includes glutamate innervation from the limbic area to the nucleus accumbens, dopamine innervation from the mesolimbic area to the nucleus accumbens, and GABAergic efferents from the nucleus accumbens to the ventral pallidum (71). Both lesion and biochemical manipulations at various points of this circuitry cause impaired PPI. For example, infusion of dopamine into the nucleus accumbens disrupts normal PPI in rats, and this disruption can be reversed or prevented by D2-receptor-blocking antipsychotics. Data such as these support the suggestion that impaired PPI in rats may be a valid animal model of deficient sensorimotor gating in schizophrenic patients (70).

Unresolved Issues and Directions for Future Research

There is currently an upsurge of interest in the plasticity of the startle reflex in general, and of PPI in particular, among both human and animal investigators. We believe that we are on the threshold of a period of heightened research activity dealing with this phenomenon that will focus on a number of clinical and preclinical issues in the next few years. Some of the more prominent clinical issues include whether the PPI deficits are specific to schizophrenia, and whether they are state-related episode indicators or trait-related vulnerability indicators in schizophrenia and other disorders. The relation of the deficits to subtypes, course, and prognosis of schizophrenia is another area in need of research. Some of the more important preclinical issues include (a) the better definition of the neural substrates of PPI and its modulation and (b) their relationships to psychobiological deficits in schizophrenia. Functional brain imaging technology will no doubt be used in conjunction with the PPI paradigm to productively address these issues.

The significance of PPI within an information processing theoretical framework also will be a focus of future research. In this regard, the distinction between the automatic PPI phenomenon and its attentional modulation may be a critical issue. The time course of PPI may be revealing here because basic PPI can occur at very short lead intervals (30–60 msec), but attentional modulation is evident only with longer lead intervals (120 msec). The differential time course suggests different underlying mechanisms, and it will be interesting to determine whether both mechanisms have the same relationship to schizophrenia. All in all, we believe that PPI provides a unique opportunity to meaningfully integrate cognitive science, neuroscience, and clinical science approaches to schizophrenia (18).

ELECTRODERMAL ACTIVITY

Measures of Electrodermal Activity

Electrodermal activity (*EDA*) refers to a variety of electrical phenomena measured from the skin, particularly changes in the electrical conductivity of the skin. EDA is usually measured by passing a small and imperceptible electric current through a pair of electrodes placed on the surface of the skin, typically on the volar surfaces of the fingertips or on palmar sites. In this way one can measure the electrical conductivity of the skin and changes in that conductivity that occur under different stimulus conditions. The principal peripheral effectors mediating skin conductance are the eccrine sweat glands, which are quite dense on the palmar surfaces of the hands. Increases in sweat gland activity, which lead to increases in skin conductance, are under the neural control of the sympathetic branch of the autonomic nervous system.

The empirical study of EDA began over 100 years ago, and it continues to be one of the most popular measures in contemporary human psychophysiology. The popularity of EDA is due to its apparent sensitivity to psychological states and processes, combined with its relative easy of measurement and quantification. The reader is referred to (a) Boucsein (10) and Roy et al. (61) for thorough book-length treatments of EDA and (b) Dawson et al. (24) and Fowles (26) for shorter chapter-length reviews. A brief overview of EDA also is available in Dawson and Nuechterlein (20, pp. 205–208).

Electrodermal phenomena can be divided into *tonic* and *phasic* measures. A *phasic measure* is a relatively fast-changing aspect of EDA that is stimulus-elicited. For example, presentation of a novel, unexpected, significant, or aversive stimulus will very likely elicit a momentary increase in skin conductance beginning within 1–3 sec following stimulus onset, known as a *skin conductance response* (*SCR*). If the eliciting stimulus is innocuous, the SCR is considered to be a component of the "orienting response." When the stimulus is repeated several times, the elicited SCR amplitude usually becomes smaller and eventually completely habituates. The phasic SCR can be quantified as the mean magnitude of the elicited SCR (in microsiemen), the proportion of stimulus presentations that elicited SCRs, or the number of stimulus presentations required to reach complete habituation. The SCR orienting response is generally thought to reflect the subject's attention to, and cognitive processing of, the eliciting stimulus.

Tonic measures are relatively stable or slowly changing aspects of EDA. One common measure of tonic EDA is *skin conductance level* (*SCL*). In normal subjects, SCL usually begins relatively high in the novel laboratory environment, decreases gradually while at rest, and then sharply increases when stimulation is introduced or some task is required. A second measure of tonic EDA is the frequency of ''nonspecific skin conductance responses'' (NS-SCRs). NS-SCRs appear similar to stimulus-elicited SCRs described above but are called ''nonspecific'' because they occur in the absence of identifiable eliciting stimuli, and they are considered a tonic measure rather than phasic measure because their rate of occurrence is fairly stable over time. In addition, both SCL and NS-SCRs are considered to be useful indices of sympathetic arousal.

Phasic and Tonic EDA in Schizophrenia Research

Since the research of Gruzelier and Venables (37), EDA research with schizophrenic patients has focused primarily on phasic responding to innocuous stimuli (e.g., soft tones without task significance). As indicated in several extensive reviews (7,20,42,57,74), approximately 40–50% of schizophrenic patients fail to exhibit any SCR orienting responses to innocuous tones, compared to only 5–10% in the normal population. In contrast to the ''nonresponders,'' the remaining 50–60% of the patients do respond with SCRs to innocuous tones and also show abnormally high tonic arousal.

The responder/nonresponder distinction generally has been treated as a dichotomy. However, we believe that it may be more useful to treat it as a continuous variable. The continuous approach allows one to use correlational analyses and take advantage of the full range of variability in electrodermal responsivity. That is, the continuous approach distinguishes between subjects with one versus many SCRs, whereas the dichotomous approach lumps these subjects together as ''responders.'' We (23) found significant correlations of SCRs and symptoms using the continuous approach, whereas the effects were less frequently significant when one simply dichotomized patients into ''responder'' and ''nonresponder'' subgroups. Thus, the degree of responding within the ''responder'' subgroup appears to contain important information, and this argues for analyzing electrodermal responding as a continuous measure rather than as a dichotomous variable.

A key question in current research concerns the meaning of the individual differences among schizophrenic patients in electrodermal responsivity and arousal. This general question has been addressed by relating electrodermal measures to current symptomatology and prognosis, and by determining whether electrodermal activity changes with changes in symptomatic state when both are assessed longitudinally.

Regarding EDA relationships with current symptoms, several early studies suggested that EDA nonresponding tends to be related to presence of negative symptoms (e.g., see refs. 8 and 67). Others, however, have suggested that the relationship may not be this simple. For example, Bernstein (6) later suggested that SCR nonresponding may be related specifically to a subgroup that is conceptually disorganized and emotionally withdrawn, thereby displaying both positive and negative symptom features. Dawson et al. (23) suggested that SCR responding might be related ''to a dimension of behavioral and emotional activation rather than to the dimension of positive and negative symptoms.''

Regarding relationships between EDA and prognosis, several studies have reported that high electrodermal responsivity or activation measured during the inpatient phase is associated with poor short-term symptomatic outcome (23,33,68,75). However, Öhman et al. (58) reported that SCR nonresponding, rather than hyperactivation, was associated with poor social and employment outcome. These studies appear inconsistent, but it must be remembered that studies reporting that poor outcome was associated with EDA hyperresponsivity used measures of symptomatic outcome rather than social or employment outcome measures. Social and employment outcome are often only mildly correlated with symptomatic outcome in schizophrenia (69) and likely involve mechanisms that only partially overlap with those determining symptomatic outcome.

Finally, longitudinal studies of EDA and symptomatic changes are just beginning to appear. Dawson et al. (21), for example, summarized EDA findings recorded from schizophrenic patients and matched normal controls on two occasions, one while the patients were in a symptomatic remitted state and the other while the same patients were in a psychotic state. The primary result was that tonic EDA became abnormally high during the psychotic period. These findings suggest that schizophrenic psychotic states are accompanied by high sympathetic nervous system activation. Moreover, longitudinal study of three remitted schizophrenic patients has suggested that increased EDA activity may occur in the week or two before a psychotic exacerbation (21). These results are consistent with a theoretical model that sympathetic activation is a ''transient intermediate state'' that precedes psychotic episodes in vulnerable individuals (54,56). Thus, tonic electrodermal measures may be more useful than previously thought in understanding the nature of the process by which psychotic symptoms return and in obtaining objective early warning signs of that process.

Recent analyses suggest that phasic SCR findings are more complicated than tonic electrodermal data in their relationship to clinical state, but of no less theoretical interest (22). Phasic hyporesponsiveness to innocuous external stimuli relative to levels of electrodermal activation is apparently present in both remitted and psychotic states, but is significantly greater in the psychotic state. Thus, phasic SCOR hyporesponsiveness appears to be a mediating vulnerability factor that might be related to attentional deficits. Indices of phasic skin conductance responses that control statistically for tonic electrodermal activation level look promising and need additional consideration in this context.

In contrast to the longitudinal results described above, some other studies have reported both phasic and tonic electrodermal activity to be relatively stable across different symptomatic states (59,65,75). The previous studies differed in several ways from that of Dawson et al. (21,22), and it is clear that more longitudinal research is needed to fully test the state versus trait role of EDA in schizophrenia.

Neuropsychopharmacological Models of EDA

The central neurophysiological and pharmacological mechanisms mediating EDA appear to be multiple and complex. Boucsein (10, p. 34) describes at least two and possibly three independent cerebral pathways for EDA. The first involves hypothalamic and limbic structures, with excitatory influences stemming primarily from the amygdala and inhibitory influences stemming mainly from the hippocampus. The second involves the basal ganglia together with the premotor cortex. The third involves the reticular system, which may have eliciting as well as a modulating influences on EDA.

The use of brain imaging techniques promises to greatly increase the understanding of the central origins of EDA, and both structural and functional brain imaging studies are now beginning to be reported (60). For example, the first preliminary PET study of SCR responder and nonresponder schizophrenic patients has recently been reported (39). In comparison to both normal controls and responder patients, the nonresponders showed about a 20% reduction in metabolic rate across the entire brain. More specifically, nonresponders also had significantly lower glucose metabolic rates relative to that of the whole brain in medial frontal and hippocampal areas as well as in the right amygdala as compared to responders. More studies are needed, with larger samples of schizophrenic patients and also samples of SCR responders and nonresponders from the normal population, to determine the reliability and specificity of these preliminary PET/EDA relationships.

Unresolved Issues and Directions for Future Research

The electrodermal measures continue to make important contributions to our understanding of the nature of schizophrenia. Of particular promise are the individual differences in electrodermal measures that are typically found within schizophrenic samples. That is, most studies do not find that a single electrodermal abnormality characterizes the entire group of schizophrenic patients; instead, there is usually one subgroup of *tonic hyperaroused* patients and another subgroup of *phasic hyporesponsive* patients. A major task of future research is to probe the clinical, psychological, and physiological meaning of this individual difference. The electrodermal measures will have more to contribute when the various levels of meaning of the individual differences in tonic and phasic activity are better understood.

REFERENCES

1. Adler LE, Pachtman E, Franks RD, Pecevich M, Waldo MC, Freedman R. Neurophysiological evidence for a defect in neuronal mechanisms involved in sensory gating in schizophrenia. *Biol Psychiatry* 1982;17:639–654.
2. Adler LE, Hoffer LJ, Griffith J, Waldo M, Freedman R. Normalization of deficient auditory sensory gating in the relatives of schizophrenics by nicotine. *Biol Psychiatry* 1992;32:607–616.
3. Andreasen NC. Negative symptoms in schizophrenia: definition and reliability. *Arch Gen Psychiatry* 1982;39:784–788.
4. Anthony BJ. In the blink of an eye: implications of reflex modification for information processing. In: Ackles PK, Jennings JR, Coles MGH, eds. *Advances in Psychophysiology*, vol 4. Greenwich, CT: JAI Press, 1985;167–218.
5. Asarnow RF, Granholm E, Sherman T. Span of apprehension in schizophrenia. In: Steinhauer SR, Gruzelier JH, Zubin J, eds. *Neuropsychology, psychophysiology, and information processing. Handbook of schizophrenia*, vol 5. Amsterdam: Elsevier, 1991;335–370.
6. Bernstein AS. Orienting response research in schizophrenia: where we have come and where we might go. *Schizophr Bull* 1987; 13:623–641.
7. Bernstein AS, Frith CD, Gruzelier JH, et al. An analysis of the skin conductance orienting response in samples of American, British, and German schizophrenics. *Biol Psychol* 1982;14:155–211.
8. Bernstein A, Taylor KW, Starkey P, Juni S, Lubowsky J, Paley, H. Bilateral skin conductance, finger pulse volume, and EEG orienting response to tones of differing intensities in chronic schizophrenics and controls. *J Nerv Ment Dis* 1981;169:513–528.
9. Blackwood DHR, St. Clair DM, Muir WJ, Duffy JC. Auditory P300 and eye tracking dysfunction in schizophrenic pedigrees. *Arch Gen Psychiatry* 1991;48:899–909.
10. Boucsein W. *Electrodermal activity*. New York: Plenum Press, 1992.
11. Boutros NN, Zouridakis G, Overall J. Replication and extension of P50 findings in schizophrenia. *Clin Electroencephalogr* 1991; 22:40–45.
12. Braff DL. Information processing and attention dysfunctions in schizophrenia. *Schizophr Bull* 1993;19:233–259.
13. Braff DL, Geyer MA. Sensorimotor gating and schizophrenia: human and animal model studies. *Arch Gen Psychiatry* 1990;47:181–188.
14. Braff DL, Grillon C, Geyer MA. Gating and habituation of the startle reflex in schizophrenic patients. *Arch Gen Psychiatry* 1992;49:206–215.
15. Braff D, Stone C, Callaway E, Geyer M, Glick I, Bali L. Prestimulus

effects on human startle reflex in normals and schizophrenics. *Psychophysiology* 1978;15:339–343.

16. Callaway E, Naghdi S. An information processing model for schizophrenia. *Arch Gen Psychiatry* 1982;39:339–347.

17. Davis M, Gendelman DS, Tischler MD, Gendelman PM. A primary acoustic startle circuit: lesion and stimulation studies. *J Neurosci* 1982;2:791–805.

18. Dawson, ME. Psychophysiology at the interface of clinical science, cognitive science, and neuroscience. *Psychophysiology* 1990; 27:243–255.

19. Dawson ME, Hazlett EA, Filion DL, Nuechterlein KH, Schell AM. Attention and schizophrenia: impaired modulation of the startle reflex. *J Abnorm Psychol* 1993;102:633–641.

20. Dawson ME, Nuechterlein KH. Psychophysiological dysfunctions in the developmental course of schizophrenic disorders. *Schizophr Bull* 1984;10:204–232.

21. Dawson ME, Nuechterlein KH, Schell AM. Electrodermal abnormalities in recent-onset schizophrenia: relationships to symptoms and prognosis. *Schizophr Bull* 1992;18:295–311.

22. Dawson ME, Nuechterlein KH, Schell AM, Gitlin M, Ventura J. Autonomic abnormalities in schizophrenia: state or trait indicators? *Arch Gen Psychiatry* [in press].

23. Dawson ME, Nuechterlein KH, Schell AM, Mintz J. Concurrent and predictive electrodermal correlates of symptomatology in recent-onset schizophrenia patients. *J Abnorm Psychol* 1992; 101:153–164.

24. Dawson ME, Schell AM, Filion DL. The electrodermal system. In: Cacioppo JT, Tassinary LG, eds. *Principles of psychophysiology.* Cambridge: Cambridge University Press, 1990;295–324.

25. Filion DL, Dawson ME, Schell AM. Modification of the acoustic startle-reflex eyeblink: a tool for investigating early and late attentional processes. *Biol Psychology* 1993;35:185–200.

26. Fowles DC. The eccrine system and electrodermal activity. In: Coles MGH, Donchin E, Porges SW, eds. *Psychophysiology: systems, processes, and applications.* New York: Guilford Press, 1989;51–96.

27. Freedman R, Adler LE, Waldo MC, Pachtman E, Franks RD. Neurophysiological evidence for a defect in inhibitory pathways in schizophrenia: comparison of medicated and drug-free patients. *Biol Psychiatry* 1983;18:537–551.

28. Freedman R, Mirsky AF. Event-related potentials: exogenous components. In: Steinhauer SR, Gruzelier JH, Zubin J, eds. *Neuropsychology, psychophysiology, and information processing. Handbook of schizophrenia,* vol 5. Amsterdam: Elsevier, 1991;71–90.

29. Freedman R, Adler LE, Gerhardt GA, Waldo M, Baker N, Rose GM, Drebing C, Nagamoto H, Bickford-Wimer P, Franks R. Neurobiological studies of sensory gating in schizophrenia. *Schizophr Bull* 1987;13:669–678.

30. Friedman D. Endogenous scalp-recorded brain potentials in schizophrenia: a methodological review. In: Steinhauer SR, Gruzelier JH, Zubin J, eds. *Handbook of schizophrenia, vol 5. Neuropsychology, psychophysiology, and information processing.* Amsterdam: Elsevier, 1991;91–127.

31. Friedman D, Cornblatt B, Vaughan HG Jr, Erlenmeyer-Kimling L. Auditory event-related potentials in children at risk for schizophrenia: the complete initial sample. *Psychiatr Res* 1988;26:203–221.

32. Friedman D, Squires-Wheeler E. Event-related potentials (ERPs) as indicators of risk for schizophrenia. *Schizophr Bull* 1994;20:63–74.

33. Frith CD, Stevens M, Johnstone EC, Crow TJ. Skin conductance responsivity during acute episodes of schizophrenia as a predictor of symptomatic improvement. *Psychol Med* 1979;9:101–106.

34. Geyer MA, Swerdlow NR, Mansbach RS, Braff D. Startle response models of sensorimotor gating and habituation deficits in schizophrenia. *Brain Res Bull* 1990;25:485–498.

35. Graham FK. The more or less startling effects of weak prestimulation. *Psychophysiology* 1975;12:238–248.

36. Grillon C, Ameli R, Charney DS, Krystal J, Braff DL. Startle gating deficits occur across prepulse intensities in schizophrenic patients. *Biol Psychiatry* 1992;32:939–943.

37. Gruzelier JH, Venables PH. Skin conductance orienting activity in a heterogeneous sample of schizophrenics: possible evidence of limbic dysfunction. *J Nerv Ment Dis* 1972;155:277–287.

38. Guich SM, Buchsbaum MS, Burgwald L, Wu J, Haier R, Asarnow

R, Nuechterlein K, Potkin S. Effect of attention on frontal distribution of delta activity and cerebral metabolic rate in schizophrenia. *Schizophr Res* 1989;2:439–448.

39. Hazlett EA, Dawson ME, Buchsbaum MS, Nuechterlein KH. Reduced regional brain glucose metabolism assessed by PET in electrodermal nonresponder schizophrenics: A pilot study. *J Abnorm Psychol* 1993;102:39–46.

40. Hillyard SA, Kutas M. Electrophysiology of cognitive processing. *Ann Rev Psychol* 1983;34:33–61.

41. Hoffman HS, Ison JR. Reflex modification in the domain of startle. 1. Some empirical findings and their implications for how the nervous system processes sensory input. *Psychol Rev* 1980;87:175–189.

42. Holzman PS. Recent studies of psychophysiology in schizophrenia. *Schizophr Bull* 1987;13:49–75.

43. Holzman PS. Eye movement dysfunctions in schizophrenia. In: Steinhauer SR, Gruzelier JH, Zubin J, eds. *Neuropsychology, psychophysiology, and information processing. Handbook of schizophrenia,* vol 5. Amsterdam: Elsevier, 1991;129–145.

44. Iacono WG, Clementz BA. A strategy for elucidating genetic influences on complex psychopathological syndromes (with special reference to ocular motor functioning and schizophrenia). *Prog Exp Pers Res* 1993;16:11–65.

45. Javitt DC. Neurophysiological approaches to analyzing brain dysfunction in schizophrenia. *Psychiatric Ann* 1993;23:144–150.

46. Judd LL, McAdams LA, Budnick B, Braff DL. Sensory gating deficits in schizophrenia: new results. *Am J Psychiatry* 1992; 149:488–493.

47. Kigogami Y, Yoneda H, Asaba H, Sakai T. P300 in first degree relatives of schizophrenics. *Schizophr Res* 1992;6:9–13.

48. Koukkou M, Manske W. Functional states of the brain and schizophrenic states of behavior. In: Shagass C, Josiassen RC, Roemer RA, eds. *Brain electrical potentials and psychopathology.* New York: Elsevier, 1986;91–114.

49. Leitner DS, Cohen ME. Role of the inferior colliculus in the inhibition of acoustic startle in the rat. *Physiol Behav* 1985;34:65–70.

50. Levy DL, Holzman PS, Matthysse S, Mendell NR. Eye tracking dysfunction and schizophrenia: a critical perspective. *Schizophr Bull* 1993;19:461–536.

51. McCarley RW, Shenton ME, O'Donnell BF, et al. Auditory P300 abnormalities and left posterior superior temporal gyrus volume reduction in schizophrenia. *Arch Gen Psychiatry* 1993;50:190–197.

52. McGhie A, Chapman J. Disorders of attention and perception in early schizophrenia. *Br J Med Psychol* 1961;34:103–116.

53. Morihisa JM, Duffy FH, Wyatt RJ. Brain electrical activity mapping (BEAM) in schizophrenic patients. *Arch Gen Psychiatry* 1983; 40:719–728.

54. Nuechterlein KH, Dawson ME. A heuristic vulnerability/stress model of schizophrenic episodes. *Schizophr Bull* 1984;10:300–312.

55. Nuechterlein KH, Dawson ME. Information processing and attentional functioning in the developmental course of schizophrenic disorders. *Schizophr Bull* 1984;10:160–203.

56. Nuechterlein KH, Dawson ME, Gitlin M, et al. Developmental Processes in Schizophrenic Disorders: longitudinal studies of vulnerability and stress. *Schizophr Bull* 1992;18:387–425.

57. Öhman A. Electrodermal activity and vulnerability to schizophrenia: a review. *Biol Psychol* 1981;12:87–145.

58. Öhman A, Ohlund LS, Alm T, Wieselgren I-M, Istm K, Lindstrom LH. Electrodermal nonresponding, premorbid adjustment, and symptomatology as predictors of long-term functioning in schizophrenics. *J Abnorm Psychol* 1989;98:426–435.

59. Olbrich R. The contributions of psychophysiology to vulnerability models. In: Häfner H, Gattaz WF, eds. *Search for the causes of schizophrenia,* vol II. Berlin: Springer-Verlag, 1991;192–204.

60. Raine A, Lencz T. Brain imaging research on electrodermal activity in humans. In: Roy JC, Boucsein W, Fowles DC, Gruzelier JH, eds. *Progress in electrodermal research.* New York: Plenum Press, 1993;115–130.

61. Roy JC, Boucsein W, Fowles DC, Gruzelier JH. *Progress in electrodermal research.* New York: Plenum Press, 1993.

62. Schreiber H, Stolz-Born G, Kornhuber A, Kornhuber HH, Born J. Endogenous event-related potentials and psychometric performance in children at risk for schizophrenia. *Biol Psychiatry* 1991;30:177–189.

63. Shagass C. EEG studies of schizophrenia. In: Steinhauer SR, Gruzelier JH, Zubin J, eds. *Neuropsychology, psychophysiology, and information processing. Handbook of schizophrenia,* vol 5. Amsterdam: Elsevier, 1991;39–69.

64. Siegel C, Waldo M, Mizner G, Adler LE, Freedman R. Deficits in sensory gating in schizophrenic patients and their relatives. *Arch Gen Psychiatry* 1984;41:607–612.

65. Spohn HE, Coyne L, Wilson JK, Hayes K. Skin-conductance orienting response in chronic schizophrenics: The role of neuroleptics. *J Abnorm Psychol* 1989;98:478–486.

66. Squires-Wheeler E, Friedman D, Erlenmeyer-Kimling L. A longitudinal study relating P3 amplitude to schizophrenia spectrum disorders and to global personality functioning. *Biol Psychiatry* 1993;33:774–785.

67. Straube ER. On the meaning of electrodermal nonresponding in schizophrenia. *J Nerv Ment Dis* 1979;167:601–611.

68. Straube ER, Wagner W, Forerster K, Heimann H. Findings significant with respect to short- and medium-term outcome in schizophrenia—a preliminary report. *Prog Neuropsychopharmacol Biol Psychiatry* 1989;13:185–197.

69. Strauss JS, Carpenter WT. Prediction of outcome in schizophrenia. III. Five year outcome and its predictors. *Arch Gen Psychiatry* 1977;34:159–163.

70. Swerdlow NR, Braff DL, Taaid N, Geyer MA. Assessing the validity of an animal model of deficient sensorimotor gating in schizophrenic patients. *Arch Gen Psychiatry* 1994;51:139–154.

71. Swerdlow NR, Caine SB, Braff DL, Geyer MA. The neural substrates of sensorimotor gating of the startle reflex: a review of recent findings and their implications. *J Psychopharmacol* 1992;6:132–146.

72. Swerdlow NR, Koob GF. Dopamine, schizophrenia, mania, and depression: toward a unified hypothesis of cortico-striato-pallido-thalamic function. *Behav Brain Sci* 1987;197–245.

73. Waldo M, Carey G, Myles-Worsley M, Cawthra E, Adler LE, Nagamoto HT, Wender P, Byerley W, Plaetke R, Freedman R. Codistribution of a sensory gating deficit and schizophrenia in multi-affected families. *Psychiatr Res* 1991;39:257–268.

74. Zahn TP. Psychophysiological approaches to psychopathology. In: Coles MGH, Donchin E, Porges SW, eds. *Psychophysiology: systems, processes, and applications.* New York: Guilford Press, 1986;508–610.

75. Zahn TP, Carpenter WT, McGlashan TH. Autonomic nervous system activity in acute schizophrenia. II. Relationship to short-term prognosis and clinical state. *Arch Gen Psychiatry* 1981;38:260–266.

Psychopharmacology: The Fourth
Generation of Progress, edited by
Floyd E. Bloom and David J. Kupfer.
Raven Press, Ltd., New York 1995.

CHAPTER 105

Neurocognitive Functioning in Patients with Schizophrenia

An Overview

Terry E. Goldberg and James M. Gold

Increasingly, neurocognitive paradigms have been used to study patients with schizophrenia. Such paradigms use experimental and clinical tests to better characterize the cognitive abnormalities in schizophrenia. This approach differs from earlier psychological research, in that neurocognitive tests have been validated, often in a principled manner, in brain-damaged populations or by functional neuroimaging studies in normal controls, such that inferences can be made about the cerebral regions or neural systems that subserve them. Use of these techniques has also indicated that some types of cognitive impairment are central and enduring features of schizophrenia and are reliably present. Moreover, impairments may account for a significant proportion of the social and vocational morbidity in schizophrenia. The remainder of this chapter marshalls evidence that bears on this view.

Cognitive abnormalities were noted by early investigators of schizophrenia. In the original clinical descriptions of schizophrenia made by Kraepelin (45), he commented "Mental efficiency is always diminished to a considerable degree. The patients are distracted, inattentive . . . , they 'cannot keep the thought in mind.' " Some years later, Shakow (66) began a series of studies in which he examined abnormalities in patients' readiness to respond to different types of imperative stimuli. Hunt and Cofer (38) noted that schizophrenic patients' intellectual quotient

was lower than that of normal controls. However, the increasing influence of psychodynamic theory tended to minimize the significance of cognitive deficits of schizophrenia. It was thought that the deficits displayed on formal psychological testing were secondary to impaired motivation, gross breakdowns in reality testing, or disordered thought processes. Early application of neuropsychological testing in the assessment of schizophrenia was therefore to "rule out" an organic basis for psychiatric symptomatology that was thought somehow to be instantiated in mind, but not brain. It was within this context that a series of studies using broad neuropsychological test batteries found that chronic schizophrenic patients could not be reliably discriminated from heterogeneous brain-damaged populations on the basis of discriminant scores (48). The possibility that these results indicated that schizophrenia was, in fact, a brain disease was considered, but rejected by many researchers, who continued to emphasize the role of motivation, institutionalization, medication, and psychiatric symptomatology in cognitive impairment.

This view changed rapidly with the advent of in vivo brain imaging techniques. First, it became evident that patients with schizophrenia had larger lateral cerebral ventricles than did controls on computed tomography (CT) scans (68). Second, functional brain imaging suggested that schizophrenic patients had decreased frontal lobe blood flow and/or metabolism. Moreover, one type of cognitive impairment, namely, poor performance on the Wisconsin Card Sorting Test (WCST) was directly linked to impaired activation of the prefrontal cortex in regional cerebral blood flow (rCBF) (77). These findings

T. E. Goldberg: Clinical Brain Disorders Branch, National Institute of Mental Health, Neurosciences Center at St. Elizabeths, Washington, DC 20032.
J. M. Gold: Clinical Research Services Branch, National Institute of Mental Health, Neurosciences Center at St. Elizabeths, Washington, DC 20032.

led to a reinterpretation of the original neuropsychological studies. There was growing realization that patients with schizophrenia performed in the range typically found in brain-damaged populations, because schizophrenia involved structural and functional abnormalities of the brain that were, in some sense, primary.

Despite the consistency of the neurocognitive findings and the relevance they have to the interpretation of old findings, the relationship between symptomatology and cognitive impairment has been a continuing subtext in the scientific literature on schizophrenia. The distraction of hallucinations, lack of cooperation, distortions in interpersonal relationships caused by paranoid delusions, and neuroleptic medication have been thought to have an adverse effect on cognitive functions. Further complicating interpretation of the significance of these results is the heterogeneity in the clinical presentation of schizophrenia. A number of different subtyping schemes have been devised to account for this and include distinctions between patients with primarily positive symptoms (hallucinations, delusions, thought disorder) and those with negative symptoms (flat affect, impoverished speech), patients with family histories of schizophrenia and those without, male patients and female patients, and paranoid and nonparanoid patients.

We examine these crucial conceptual issues in turn: Are the deficits restricted to various subgroups given the clinical variability of the disorder within and across patients or are they present in nearly every patient? Are the cognitive deficits in some way real or are they artifactual? What are the core neurocognitive impairments in schizophrenia? What is the course of cognitive impairment in schizophrenia? What is the specificity of cognitive impairment both in terms of profile and severity level to schizophrenia as compared to other neuropsychiatric disorders? We conclude this chapter by noting that neurocognitive impairments may have prognostic significance in schizophrenia because of the importance of such functions in orienting to relevant environmental information, remembering new information, propitiously retrieving old information, and working on-line with old and new information to make responses or decisions. In this account, cognitive impairments in schizophrenia should be considered a target symptom that requires amelioration.

FREQUENCY OF NEUROCOGNITIVE IMPAIRMENT

The frequency of cognitive impairment in schizophrenia has often been examined by using binary cut-offs. In these studies, less than 40% of cases are generally considered to be abnormal (6). Variations of this approach have been used when various subgroups of schizophrenic patients are compared. In particular, the paranoid–nonparanoid distinction has been examined. When differences were found, they usually favored the paranoid group; that is, the paranoid group was less severely impaired. Classification schemes have also distinguished between patients with primarily positive symptoms and those with primarily negative symptoms. Patients with negative symptoms often have been considered to exhibit more cognitive impairment. Factor analytical studies of symptomatology have led to refinements in classification between positive and negative symptoms with the addition of a third factor involving disorganized behavior and thought. Liddle (47) found evidence for differences in profile and frequency of cognitive impairment between the three symptom-driven syndromes.

However, using a paradigm that involved monozygotic twins discordant for schizophrenia, it is possible to arrive at different conclusions (28). In this paradigm, each affected individual is yoked to an ideal control, namely, his or her unaffected cotwin. Thus age, sex, and genetic factors are completely controlled, and educational opportunity, socioeconomic status, and family emotional climate are well controlled. Goldberg et al. found that the affected twins performed consistently worse than their unaffected cotwins on many of the tests from a large neuropsychological battery. Crucially, even when affected twins were ostensibly performing within the normal range, their cotwins performed at still higher levels. Thus, cognitive impairment was apparent throughout the whole range of the distribution and was not restricted to a subgroup of outliers. Hit ratios (the proportion of affected twins that performed below unaffected cotwins) for tests involving memory (Wechsler Memory Scale), attention and vigilance, verbal fluency, lexical access and response speed (Stroop), psychomotor speed and scanning (trailmaking), intelligence quotient or IQ [Wechsler Adult Intelligence Scale-Revised (WAIS-R)], and set shifting and abstraction (WCST) were very high, that is, greater than 85%. These differences occurred irrespective of patients' diagnosis (paranoid, undifferentiated, schizoaffective) or symptom profile. Moreover, these data suggest that it is important to note not only patients' current level of functioning, but the magnitude of decline relative to their potential. The finding is important because it suggests that while the level of a cognitive score may be an admixture of insult and endowment, the magnitude of decline may reflect more accurately the severity of insult.

In summary, a variety of findings suggest that a simple model in which patients with schizophrenia vary along a severity dimension on cognitive impairment cannot easily be rejected and, for parsimony's sake, can even be favored. Moreover, recent neurobiological studies support a view of homogeneity in schizophrenia. Daniel et al. (11) could not discern a bimodal distribution of ventricular brain ratios using mixture distribution analysis of over 1,000 published data points. Furthermore, Suddath et al. (71) using magnetic resonance imaging (MRI) data obtained from monozygotic twins discordant for schizophrenia, demonstrated consistent enlargement in various components in the ventricular system and diminution of the left anterior hippocampus. Similarly, Berman et al. (72) found that prefrontal cerebral blood flow measured while twins were being administered the WCST was lower in the affected than unaffected twin in all pairs discordant for schizophrenia. Thus, one of the more interesting features of schizophrenia may be that beyond the phenomenological level, which is exceptionally heterogeneous, patients may display unexpected homogeneity at the neuropsychological, neuroanatomical, and neurophysiological levels of analysis.

SYMPTOMS, COGNITION, AND MEDICATION

Impact of Medication on Cognition

The clinical efficacy of a variety of antipsychotic medications in the reduction of positive psychotic symptoms in many patients with schizophrenia is beyond dispute. However, the cognitive effects of antipsychotic medications remain more poorly understood. Indeed, most of the literature examining this issue comes from the 1950s and 1960s when these medications were first widely utilized and the paucity of positive findings using cognitive outcome measures may well have led to their abandonment as a means of assessing the impact of medications whose clinical, symptomatic benefits were frequently obvious and dramatic. This abandonment was particularly unfortunate given the recent prominence of cognitive and neuropsychological research in the illness. Not unexpectedly, this older literature has a number of serious methodological limitations. Despite these limitations, several reviews of literature over the past decade have come to similar conclusions on the limited cognitive impact of chronic treatment with antipsychotic agents (36,52).

Clearly, the most important question for neuropsychological research in schizophrenia is whether the impairments observed in patients might not be, in fact, the results of treatment. There are three major lines of evidence that argue strongly against this view. First, there is clear evidence of cognitive impairment noted in the literature from the preneuroleptic era. For example, Rapaport et al. (59) noted impairments of judgment, concentration, and planning ability and anticipation, and described memory and concept formation deficits. The work of Shakow and colleagues (66), documenting impairments in motor speed and reaction time, preceded the introduction of neuroleptic medications, as did the observation that the general intellectual function of patients appeared to have declined from premorbid levels. Thus, the basic cognitive "profile" of schizophrenic patients has been observed for nearly half a century, long before the introduction of antipsychotic medications. Recently, Saykin et al. (61) reported striking cognitive impairments in a sample of unmedicated patients. Thus, unmedicated patients meeting current diagnostic criteria for schizophrenia as well as older samples (which may have been heterogeneous) demonstrate deficits. Second, as noted (see below) many of the impairments observed in patients treated with neuroleptics have also been observed, albeit typically to a lesser degree, in unmedicated first-degree relatives of patients, in the premorbid histories of ill patients, and in populations of children at genetic risk for the illness. Thus, it appears that at least some deficits are related to vulnerability or risk for the illness rather than the treated full clinical syndrome. Third, and most directly addressing the issue, is the fact that there is simply very little evidence that chronic neuroleptic treatment impairs neuropsychological performance in ill patients. The data base supporting this conclusion involves multiple studies examining variables ranging from intelligence test performance, the Halstead Reitan Battery, reaction time, and graphomotor speed. Recent studies are generally in agreement with this older literature. For example, Seidman et al. (64) found that a marked reduction in neuroleptic dosage in patients who did not relapse had virtually no effect on performances in a wide variety of neurocognitive tests.

Several reviewers (see above) have pointed out two potentially important exceptions to this overall conclusion. First, timed measures of motor dexterity, such as the Purdue Pegboard, may be particularly vulnerable to the impact of neuroleptic dopamine blockade, a finding which is expected given the prominent role of dopaminergic neural transmission in the motor system. The extent to which this is a persistent deficit or a more temporary effect of treatment initiation remains unclear. Indeed, what is most remarkable is that simpler speed measures such as finger tapping, reaction time, and complex graphomotor tasks such as digit symbol coding, rarely demonstrate drug-related performance decrements.

A second area in which drug-related performance decrements have been reported involves memory functions. These appear to be sensitive to the impact of anticholinergic activity inherent in neuroleptics or in the medications used as adjunctive treatment of extrapyramidal side effects, such as rigidity and tremor, a negative effect fully expectable given the effect of anticholinergics in normal subjects (70). Although this adverse effect has been demonstrated in a number of study designs, its size generally appears to be small, and there is little reason to believe that the recent work documenting memory impairment in schizophrenic patients is the result of negative treatment effects: such effects were noted prior to neuroleptics and in unmedicated groups.

Neuroleptics do appear to offer certain limited cognitive benefits. It is clear that neuroleptics reduce formal thought disorder. Insofar as thought disorder interferes with performance (19), particularly on tasks requiring open-ended and coherent verbal responses, such as certain measures of verbal conceptualization and proverb interpretation, improvement has been noted following neuroleptic treatment. Perhaps the clearest evidence of neuroleptic-related performance enhancement has come on several measures of attention. The most consistent results have been observed on visual and auditory versions of the Continuous Performance Test (CPT), which generally span several minutes and require the subject to selectively respond to a specified target, such as a letter or sequential combination of letters (70). It should be noted that there is evidence that CPT deficits are also observed in high-risk populations and in subjects in states of relative symptomatic remission, suggesting that there are both stable trait- and clinical state-related dimensions of impairment (55). In addition to this evidence for improvements in sustained attention, there are several reports of improvement in measures of distractibility: patients are less stimulus bound while on active treatment (56). Mixed, but largely positive findings, have also emerged from studies using span of apprehension type tasks to assess selective attention during time-dependent visual information processing (1).

Although positive cognitive effects have typically coincided with symptomatic improvements, these may not be related in a simple causal fashion. Serper et al. (65) recently reported that patients on neuroleptics were able to benefit from extended practice on a dual task paradigm, whereas unmedicated patients at the same level of symptom severity were not. This suggests a direct pharmacological cognitive effect of antipsychotic treatment, independent of symptomatic status. It is intriguing that these enhancements appear to be somewhat selective, as many other measures of attention such as reaction time or digit symbol do not appear overly sensitive to neuroleptic effects.

Admittedly, the literature addressing the cognitive effects of neuroleptics has many shortcomings and several investigators have recently again raised the issue of negative effects on the basis of finding a correlation of impaired performance and drug dose or by comparing patients on and off neuroleptics when treatment status was not randomly assigned. Although the results of such studies are of interest, they remain difficult to interpret as the issue of clinical state, compliance, and dose are inevitably confounded. Furthermore, there may be large individual differences in the relationship between oral neuroleptic dose and actual central nervous system bioavailability. Thus, the possibility of specific adverse effects remains an open issue, which will require a new generation of studies to answer. Indeed, the comparison of the newer atypical antipsychotics with current standard treatments will offer another opportunity to examine the relationship of symptomatic status and cognitive functions. Initial results suggest that atypical neuroleptics do not offer cognitive benefits concomitant with more effective treatment of psychotic symptoms, and in this way very much resem-

ble the lack of cognitive benefits associated with conventional treatments (see below).

Dissociating Symptoms from Cognition

The prototypical atypical neuroleptic clozapine has been used to dissociate symptoms from cognition (27). The design of the study was straightforward: Patients were first neuropsychologically examined while receiving a variety of typical neuroleptic medications. Symptoms were rated on the Brief Psychiatric Rating Scale (BPRS). Patients then received clozapine for an average of 15 months and were reassessed. Psychiatric symptoms improved significantly; symptom scores declined by 35% as had been shown previously (41). However, no cognitive measure improved. Thus, no significant changes were observed in WAIS-R; trailmaking; the WCST; the Category Test; tests of visual processing, namely, facial recognition and judgment line orientation; and measures of verbal memory from the Wechsler Memory Scale. Visual memory for designs declined. Moreover, the subgroup of patients that improved the most psychiatrically did not differ from the subgroup that improved least on tests of cognitive function (as measured by change in scores). These results suggested that symptoms and cognitive function in this sample of patients with schizophrenia were dissociable, in that despite remarkable improvement in symptom status due to clozapine, no change in cognitive function was noted. Thus, it appeared that the data were consistent with the conclusion that neuropsychological deficits might be fundamental manifestations of the illness, and that the cognitive and symptomatic effects of neuroleptic treatment are independent.

A second study found that clozapine improved tasks requiring speeded motor output including verbal fluency, mazes, and digit symbol coding, but not executive set shifting on the WCST (35). These results may have been attributable to reductions in extrapyramidal toxicity associated with clozapine. Moreover, performances generally remained in the impaired range and had tenuous relations to changes in symptomatology.

Another approach that is useful in assessing the strength of the association between psychiatric symptoms and cognitive function in schizophrenia involves correlational statistics. Faustman et al. (14) found no relation between Luria Nebraska Battery neurocognitive performance and symptoms in unmedicated patients. These results are consistent with those found in a study that directly compared the relationship between symptoms and cognition in patients with schizophrenia and mood disorder (25). In unipolar depressed and bipolar groups, redundancy analysis (derived from canonical correlations) indicated that symptom factors of the BPRS accounted for 15% to 30% of the variance in cognition. However, in the schizophrenic group, analysis suggested that symptoms accounted for less than 5% of variance in cognition.

Based on an extensive review of original and variegated studies, Gold et al. (19) concluded that overall symptom severity had little impact on the cognitive level of neuropsychological tests or indices. Moreover, the association of positive symptoms and cognition has been found to be limited. This is surprising, as on the face of it such symptoms might be thought to interfere with information processing. The relation between cognitive failures and negative symptoms is somewhat stronger. However, it is often the case that negative symptoms improve with treatment, whereas cognition does not. Thus, neurocognitive testing may be a more reliable and more precise way of measuring deficiencies in volition, planning, and productivity that have a chronic, adverse effect on a patient's adjustment.

COURSE

There are two sharply contrasting views of the course of cognitive function in schizophrenia. One view suggests that cognitive deficits become progressively worse throughout the long duration of the illness. After an insidious onset, patients intellectual functions become weaker and social skills become coarser (53). A second view suggests that cognitive deficits, once they arise, are relatively stable. It is thus consistent with the notion of a static encephalopathy. There is much longitudinal, cross-sectional, and correlational evidence that supports the latter view.

A number of different research designs have been utilized to study cognitive performance in schizophrenia prior to overt onset of the disorder. In the high-risk approach, consistent deficits have been found on various measures of vigilance, including the degraded version of the CPT and selective attention in tachistoscopically presented span of apprehension task in children (10,55). Comparison of unaffected and affected members of monozygotic twin pairs discordant for schizophrenia and comparisons of the unaffected group and normal monozygotic twins have also yielded information on premorbid neurocognitive function. Given that prior to the onset of illness in the affected twin, members of these discordant pairs were similar cognitively (31) on measures of putative premorbid IQ and school grades, the functioning of the unaffected twin may be an accurate representation of the premorbid performance of the affected twin. Observations of subtle attenuations (i.e., performance was at the low end of average) on some aspects of visual and verbal memory, psychomotor speed and scanning, speed of access to the lexicon on automatized naming, and abstraction and set shifting were found in the unaffected group in comparisons with the normal twins and suggest a premorbid "forme fruste" profile of dysfunction.

Once the clinical manifestations of the illness become overt, there is evidence to suggest that a sharp decline in cognitive ability occurs. In longitudinal studies spanning the premorbid and morbid periods, Schwartzman and Douglass (63) found that schizophrenic patients who were tested on an army intelligence examination displayed a significant decrement (of nearly 0.5 standard deviations) in performance, whereas controls improved their score. (The patients were similar to controls in the premorbid period.)

Recent studies of patients during their first episode of schizophrenia substantiate the view that marked cognitive abnormalities are present at the very onset of the illness. Goldberg et al. (26) found that adolescents with diagnoses of schizophreniform disorder or schizophrenia demonstrated patterns in IQ similar to those of patients with chronic schizophrenia (i.e., lower performance IQ than verbal IQ), but dissimilar to psychiatric controls with adjustment and conduct disorders (who had lower verbal IQ than performance IQ.) Both groups had similar premorbid abilities as measured by a reading test. Hoff et al. (37) found that the neuropsychological profile of first-episode schizophrenic patients was remarkably similar to that of patients with chronic schizophrenia. Both groups performed poorly on a wide range of tests that included those assessing memory, executive functioning, and attentional abilities. Bilder et al. (4) examined a large group of first-break patients and found neuropsychological deficits in language, motor, attention, executive, and memory ability. Deficits were as frequent, though not as severe, as those found in a group of chronic patients.

During the chronic phase of the illness, a number of longitudinal studies have suggested that there is no progressive deterioration. For example, Klonoff et al. (43) studied a large group of patients with chronic schizophrenia over an 8-year period and observed that no deterioration was evident in Wechsler IQ.

A number of cross-sectional studies also examined decline during the chronic phase of the illness. Davidson et al. (12) found that large cohorts of patients lost approximately one to two points on the Mini Mental State Examination per decade of life. This rate is greater than that which occurs in normal groups. It is, however, much slower than that found in patients with a progressive cortical dementia such as Alzheimer's disease. Goldstein and Zubin (33) found no differences on the complex cognitive tasks of the Halstead Reitan Battery between large samples of younger and older chronic schizophrenic patients. Hyde et al. (39) also used a cross-sectional approach, in which successive cohorts of schizophrenic patients were assessed. Although a cross-sectional paradigm has obvious shortcomings, including increased variability, as comparisons are made between groups rather than within subjects and decreased power, the study design also had strengths in that it allowed comparison over an extremely wide range of duration of illness (patients ranged in age from 18 to 70 years) and it minimized attrition. In addition, each cohort was matched on a measure of premorbid intellectual ability, and patients with confounding neurological or systemic diseases were excluded. No significant age cohort differences were noted on tests known to be sensitive to progressive dementias: the Mini Mental State Examination, Dementia Rating Scale, verbal list learning, and semantic fluency. A cohort effect was found for the Boston Naming Test, but this appeared to be due to age rather than duration of illness. Thus, over five decades of illness, there was no indication of relentless cognitive decline.

This view of the natural history of schizophrenia is consistent with a neurodevelopmental perspective (76) in that a prenatal lesion remains silent for years before manifesting itself in overt symptomatology and cognitive impairment. There is much evidence that the markers of such a lesion are static. Thus, serial CT scan studies have indicated that there is no progression in enlargement of the ventricular system, nor are gliotic changes indicative of atrophy (26). Contrary to recent interpretations, Kraepelin (45) held to this account, stating, "As a rule, if no essential improvement intervenes in at most two of three years after the appearance of the more striking morbid phenomena, a state of weak mindedness will be developed which usually changes slowly and insignificantly."

COGNITIVE FUNCTIONS

Attention

Early description of the clinical phenomenology of schizophrenia emphasized the impairment of volitional attention. This clinical observation has been amply supported by many years of experimental study using a wide variety of tasks. Recent neuropsychological research has suggested that attention is not a unitary construct and is likely to involve several different component operations mediated by multiple brain areas (54). However, even these more specific frameworks do not appear to provide a useful heuristic for understanding the impairment in schizophrenia as available data would suggest that most, if not all, attentional processes (such as alerting, sustaining attention, rapid encoding, shifting) are impaired to some degree. This conclusion is similar to that voiced earlier in a review of work inspired by information-processing models, which were the focus of intense research interest a decade ago. The promise of these models was to isolate a particular stage of processing that was particularly impaired in schizophrenia. However, impairment limited to a specific stage could not be identified, leading to the notion that schizophrenia involves a general limitation of attentional processing resources, a limitation likely to effect a wide range of tasks. Although these results may be disappointing from the point of view of anatomical specificity, there is little doubt that impairments of attention are among the most frequently ob-

served cognitive deficits in schizophrenia, and further developments in the understanding of normal attentional processes may allow for a reinterpretation of this rich experimental literature.

Several experimental paradigms have played a central role in this research tradition. The study of various reaction-time paradigms has produced reliable evidence that patients are typically slow and variable in initiating volitional responses. Such slowing may also be a characteristic of perceptual processes as patients often require longer stimulus exposures in backward masking paradigms before they are able to identify various target stimuli (7).

The CPT has played a central role in the study of sustained attention. Typically patients make an excessive number of errors, both failing to respond to targets and responding incorrectly to nontarget stimuli. Although the CPT is typically regarded as a test of the ability to sustain attention, it appears that patients make errors throughout the test, suggesting that the deficit is one in selective attention and maintaining a readiness to respond.

Such a readiness deficit has also been demonstrated in the reaction time literature where patients fail to benefit normally from a regular predictable series of preparatory intervals between warning cues and imperative stimuli (66). This type of inability to benefit from warning cues has been elaborated in studies of the startle reflex and electrophysiological studies of the P_{50}, an evoked potential that is elicited when pairs of stimuli are presented and the initial stimulus serves to prepare the subject for the forthcoming stimulus resulting in a lessened response to the second stimulus (7). Thus, across paradigms, it appears that patients often fail to benefit from a variety of cues to facilitate either overt responses or perceptual processes.

Studies with span-of-apprehension type tasks demonstrate that patients are unable to quickly process large amounts of data. In this task, subjects view very brief presentations of up to 12 letters and have to identify the presence of a specific target. Patients can perform such discriminations fairly well with small arrays. However, their performance declines rapidly with large arrays. This type of paradigm suggests a failure in the amount of selective information that can be processed (1). In addition, several studies have demonstrated that patients are unusually sensitive to the presence of distraction, with their already diminished processing capabilities deteriorating even further when the additional demand is made to ignore irrelevant stimuli (56).

The literature documenting attentional impairment is voluminous, and we have only discussed some of the more prominent themes. As noted above, the cognitive-anatomical interpretation of these results remains highly ambiguous. On a more practical level, the relationship between attentional deficits and the compromise of more complex cognitive processes in schizophrenia remains unclear. Certainly, other patient populations with attentional disorders such as children with Attention Deficit Hyperactivity Disorder, do not typically present with severe generalized deficits. Furthermore, it appears that treatment with antipsychotic medications often improves (but fails to fully normalize) attentional functions in patients with schizophrenia, but has little benefit for more complex cognitive functions (see above). Thus, impairment of attention does not necessarily predict impairment in other cognitive domains, and change in attentional performance may not be predictive of broader cognitive changes.

Memory

Memory functions have been frequently assayed in schizophrenia. Recall of verbal paired associates, stories, recurring digits, and geometric designs has been reported to be deficient (61). These deficits are often prominent even against a background of general intellectual impairment. For example, Gold et al. (22) found that schizophrenic patients frequently displayed large discrepancies between IQ and the Wechsler Memory Scale-Revised General Memory Index, with the latter test being lower, and that these deficits were not attributable to attentional dysfunction.

Various stages in the processing of declarative memory (material encoded in distinct, event-related, spatiotemporal contexts) have been implicated. A number of investigators have suggested that schizophrenic patients use inefficient encoding strategies and thus do not take advantage of semantic regularities (21). Inefficient retrieval strategies or poor effortful recall have also been noted. When memory for materials after delays of 20 min or more is assessed, schizophrenic patients demonstrate only mildly accelerated rates of forgetting (22,30), in contradistinction to amnesic patients, whose rate of forgetting is markedly accelerated. The rate of learning for item-based lists of words has also been studied. Schizophrenic patients display the capacity to learn lists, but do so at rates slower than that of normal subjects. Reduced memory for the initial portions of verbal lists (the primacy effect) has also been found (51). These three pieces of information (slowed rate of learning, mildly increased rate of forgetting, and lack of a primacy effect) may indicate that patients have difficulty consolidating material in a long-term store.

Recognition paradigms, which involve less elaborate search strategies (subjects simply state whether a target is more familiar or has been presented more recently than a foil) and thus may measure consolidation, have elicited conflicting results. Patients sometimes display relatively better, although not necessarily normal, performance on these tasks compared to recall memory. However, it is possible that these results are an artifact of differences in the difficulty between recall and recognition tests (8).

Moreover, in some studies, recall and recognition have been highly correlated (21).

Another type of memory system that is theoretically dissociable from the explicit or declarative memory system is the implicit system. In implicit paradigms, subjects are not called upon to consciously recall material, but demonstrate item-specific learning when required to perform certain tasks in which stimuli have in some way been encountered previously. In a systematic study, Schwartz et al. (62) found that schizophrenic patients exhibited normal implicit memory on tasks involving the identification of perceptually degraded material and on semantic category production tasks, whereas explicit cued recall was impaired.

Motor skill or procedural learning has also been tested. In paradigms that involved pursuing a rotating target with a stylus, schizophrenic patients appear to be able to increase their ability to track as well as controls (30).

Language

Perhaps the widest discrepancy between clinical observations and formal assessment occurs in the language domain. While the conversation of schizophrenia is often marked by lack of pronominal referents, illogicality, and derailment, patients may perform unexpectedly well on tests of language. Rausch et al. (60) found that schizophrenic patients performed similarly to normal controls and significantly better than aphasic patients on tests of the ability to apply linguistic rules. Core verbal tests from the WAIS-R that include expressive vocabulary, knowledge of commonplace information, abstraction of similarities, and expression of comprehension of social situations may be near normal (20).

The basis for patients' disordered use of language might theoretically lie in abnormalities in the semantic organization. Semantic priming studies (50) have indicated that patients with schizophrenia demonstrate greater facilitation of reaction time to a semantically primed target word than do normal subject (i.e., a response to cat is faster if preceded by dog rather than stone). Furthermore, Gourovitch et al. (34) also found that semantic fluency performances were more impaired than phonological fluency. This also implicates the organization of the semantic system. However, the relationship between these types of semantic system abnormalities and disordered speech has not been empirically tested.

Visual Perception

The performance of patients with schizophrenia on various tests of visual processing has often been found to be intact. Two distinct cognitive systems are thought to play a role in this type of processing. An object location system determines the orientation of objects in space and the relationship between one object and another in space, or where something is; an object recognition system determines an object's identity based on a critical set of perceptual attributes, or what something is. Tests of location, involving spatial analysis including block design and object assembly from the WAIS-R test and judgment of line orientation, generally elicit normal performance in patients with schizophrenia (28,44). Tests of the object recognition system, which includes facial perceptual matching have elicited somewhat more equivocal data as group differences or effect sizes are often larger than those on object location tests, but are not often significant. These findings imply that some posterior cortical zones may be relatively uncompromised in schizophrenia.

Executive Processes

Patients with schizophrenia often seem unable to maintain some form of volitional control over information processing. They appear to have difficulty formulating plans, initiating them, and recovering from errors once a plan has begun (i.e., using feedback efficiently). Moreover, patients sometimes have problems when their behavior is interrupted: They appear to forget what they had been formerly doing even after short delays.

Such behavior can be elicited by formal tests. Several investigators demonstrated that schizophrenic patients have deficits on the WCST of set shifting, response to feedback, and abstraction (15). Patients seem to have both difficulty abstracting concepts and make perseverate responses to incorrect responses. Shallice et al. (67) stressed the consistency of frontal deficits in their detailed analyses of single cases, as most patients in their series displayed difficulties generating rules to the WCST or solving Tower of Hanoi type puzzles.

Patients with schizophrenia have difficulty on the Brown-Petersen test in which words have to be remembered over short delays during which overt rehearsal is prevented (i.e., behavior is interrupted). Interference conditions that imposed even moderate processing loads caused a sharp decline in Brown Petersen performance in schizophrenic patients, suggesting that coordination or allocation of resources is deficient or that resource capacity itself is limited (17). Interestingly, Brown-Petersen performance has been correlated to a test of executive function as well as short-term memory and anterograde memory. As such, it might be a test that demands working with information in various memory stores. In an elegant study that also emphasized the role of delay in information control in schizophrenia, Cohen and Servan-Schreiber (9) found that patients had difficulty understanding sentences in which they (the patients) had to retain information over short periods to resolve ambiguity (by comprehending semantic context). The authors went on to note that patients may have difficulty maintaining

or using the internal representation of context to control action.

One construct that attempts to capture this type of processing involves notions of working memory. Because working memory theoretically involves the simultaneous storage and processing of information, it is presumed that a central executive component partitions or allocates limited resources during complex, novel, or dual tasks and deploys additional cognitive resources to aid in maintenance of material in some short-term store or computational workspace.

There is evidence that the Wisconsin Card Sort might involve the working memory system. For instance, Sullivan et al. (72) found that WCST perseveration was strongly associated with other tests that are thought to require working memory including self-ordered pointing (in which a subject monitors his or her own series of responses). A second line of evidence comes from attempts to teach patients with chronic schizophrenia how to do the WCST. In one such study, Goldberg et al. (32) provided incremental instructions about categorization and set shifting, followed by intensive card-by-card teaching in an effort to ensure that patients maintained an optimal test taking set. Goldberg et al. found that incremental information did not aid patients (the performance was poor), but, when card-by-card teaching was withdrawn and normal testing procedures were resumed, patients' performance returned to baseline. These results suggested that psychological factors were not the primary explanation of the patients' difficulties, but rather failures were manifestations of unique task-specific computational systems. In particular, it appeared that patients could not maintain information in some working memory store to control responses. A number of other studies have also demonstrated that it is exceedingly difficult to normalize patients performance on the WCST, although not necessarily to improve it (32).

Another study also argues for a deficit in working memory's visual scratchpad. Using an ocular motor-delayed response paradigm that was developed by Goldman-Rakic and colleagues for use in primates, Park and Holzman (57) found that patients with schizophrenia had grave difficulties maintaining information for location over a brief delay in which they had to perform an interference task. Although interpretation of results in this particular study was complicated because patients also had difficulty on a control task that did not involve a delay, the corpus of the work suggests that schizophrenic patients have difficulty maintaining and transforming information over short delays in the service of a response.

Motor Function

Abnormal voluntary and involuntary movements have long been recognized as common in schizophrenic patients. With the introduction of neuroleptic medications and the apparent link between such medications and the development of tardive dyskinesia, motor abnormalities have not been widely studied (with the exception of eye movements), perhaps out of concern that such symptoms are treatment-induced rather than inherent features of the illness. However, this being said, there is a large, consistent literature suggesting abnormal motor function in schizophrenia. Patients with schizophrenia tend to be slow in initiating movements as demonstrated in prolonged reaction time. Repetitive movements are carried out slowly (as in finger tapping) and this slowing is often exaggerated by the complexity of the required motor act. The abnormality is not simply one of the psychomotor retardation. When patients perform a simple motor act, such as button pressing, their physical effort has been characterized as abnormally discontinuous and irregular (75). There is direct electrophysiological evidence that the voluntary preparation processing typically seen in normal subjects prior to the initiation of a motor act is delayed in onset in patients (69).

Unsurprisingly, more complex forms of motor performance that involve continuous adjustment to feedback are also impaired in patients. Thus patients have been reported to have remarkable difficulties monitoring their own actions and often fail to correct errors (49). It has been suggested that this failure to monitor action execution represents a fundamental deficit in schizophrenia and may be one of the mechanisms implicated in the genesis of psychotic symptoms (18). The motor abnormalities extend beyond slowing and lack of normal refinement of action sequences; there are reports of gross perseverative behavior in patients with schizophrenia when performing graphomotor tasks (3). Thus, many of the themes that are well developed in the literature on more complex cognitive functions in schizophrenia can be traced to the purely motor domain. Indeed, this may suggest that many of the abnormalities in schizophrenia are primarily located at the stage of response preparation, execution, and monitoring, abnormalities that are evident in any modality and at any level of processing complexity where responses are not fully specified by the imperative stimulus involved in task presentation.

The motor abnormality most thoroughly documented in schizophrenia has involved the oculomotor system. More than 80 years ago, Difendorf and Dodge reported impaired eye tracking in schizophrenic patients. This observation has been replicated numerous times in recent years and has been comprehensively reviewed by Levy et al. (46). When engaged in pursuit of an object, patients with schizophrenia demonstrate several abnormalities including impaired gain. That is, they fail to match the velocity of the target. They also demonstrate the intrusion of saccadic movements into what should be smooth tracking. Abnormal tracking has been observed in both chronically ill and first-episode samples. It is a matter of dispute

whether there is any effect of illness chronicity or severity on tracking performance. Neuroleptic medications do not appear to have a significant effect on eye tracking, although other psychotropic medications, such as lithium, may impair tracking. Several independent groups have reported an increased frequency of abnormal tracking in the first-degree relatives of patients, suggesting that eye movement abnormalities may be a marker of vulnerability to schizophrenia. Poor smooth pursuit, and poor performance in an antisaccade task has been associated with poor performance on neuropsychological tests of frontal cortical function by several investigators, suggesting that the eye movement deficits of patients may be another manifestation of frontal pathology (46).

MAPPING COGNITION ONTO THE BRAIN

Mapping cognitive performance onto neuroanatomical measures has met with mixed results. It is an important endeavor because positive associations suggest that cognitive impairments do not arise de novo, but may have a specific or circumscribed neurobiological substrate. Inconsistent findings may have been due in part to difficulties in ascertaining precisely to what degree each measure deviates from its genetically and environmentally determined potential level. Goldberg et al. (29) attempted to surmount this problem by examining difference scores derived from the unaffected member and affected member of a twin pair, reasoning that such scores should represent the degree of pathological involvement irrespective of actual level. In correlating intrapair difference scores of anatomical structures measured from MRI with cognitive abilities (after partialling IQ), they found strong associations between the left hippocampus and a parameter of verbal memory.

Despite the theoretical power of this technique, there was a general paucity of significant correlations. In contrast, Goldberg et al. found a wider array of significant association between some cognitive performances and a neurophysiological measure, prefrontal rCBF, assayed during administration of the Wisconsin Card Sorting Test. In particular, correlations between perseveration and a prefrontal rCBF were robust (>0.60). These results suggest that (a) physiological measures may be better measures of the functional integrity of a neural system than anatomical volumes and (b) the restriction of range inherent in both cognitive and anatomical measures compared to a neurodegenerative disease like Alzheimer's, may limit positive findings. These results, although limited, do support other research implicating medial temporal and prefrontal regions as important in the symptomatic expression and cognitive failures of schizophrenia.

SPECIFICITY OF NEUROCOGNITIVE IMPAIRMENT

Delineating the characteristic neurocognitive profile and global level in schizophrenia has implications for (a) weighing the fundamental validity of accumulated neuropsychological findings, (b) inferring neuroanatomical and neurophysiological dysfunction, (c) identifying measures to be used in high-risk or linkage studies, and (d) providing targets for rehabilitative efforts. Recent evidence suggests that relative neuropsychological specificity may be present in schizophrenia. This has not always been viewed as the case, as cluster analytical techniques delineated groups of psychiatric patients with unique profiles of cognitive impairments that were independent of diagnosis (74). However, these studies did not always use DSM-III diagnoses and did not include key neurocognitive measures that tapped memory and set shifting.

Two obvious groups of patients to contrast with schizophrenic patients are those with unipolar and bipolar mood disorders. Differences in neuropsychological performance between patients with schizophrenia and patients with mood disorder might account for some of the differences in outcome between these disorders. Schizophrenia is characterized by a chronic course with much associated morbidity, whereas mood disorder is thought to be more episodic and less disabling. If cognitive impairment is frequent in schizophrenia and accounts for some proportion of social and vocational disability, it would be expected at the very least that patients with schizophrenia should have more severe deficits on neuropsychological tests. In a recent study, Goldberg et al. (25) found that patients with schizophrenia performed significantly and consistently below unipolar and bipolar affective patients on test of attention, psychomotor speed, verbal and visual memory, and problem solving and abstraction. Also, IQ was lower in the schizophrenic group and appeared to have deteriorated from normal premorbid levels. Such a decline was not apparent in the mood-disordered groups. When IQ was controlled, differences in problem solving on the WCST and visual memory for design remained. These results were consistent with outcome data and also suggested prominent executive and mnemonic deficits in the schizophrenic group against a background of more generalized impairment.

Various neurological groups have been considered to be ''mock-ups'' of schizophrenia. Temporal lobe epilepsy, for instance, is thought to have neurodevelopmental origins, and left temporal lobe epilepsy is thought to be associated with an increased incidence of psychosis. When directly compared to patients with left temporal lobe epilepsy and right temporal lobe epilepsy, Gold et al. (20) found that patients with schizophrenia exhibited superior semantic memory relative to the left temporal group and more severe attentional and problem-solving deficits relative to both the right and left epilepsy groups.

Memory performance, especially in the verbal domain and including immediate and delayed recall appeared to fall between the two epilepsy groups. Thus a unilateral (left) temporal lobe model of schizophrenia does not appear to be consonant with the neurocognitive data.

Subcortical dementias also share certain clinical features, including bradyphrenia and motor abnormalities, with schizophrenia. A group with subcortical dementia comprised of patients with Huntington's disease was compared to patients with schizophrenia (23). In this study, the groups were matched on WCST perseveration. Both groups also had equivalent full scale IQs. Patients with schizophrenia exhibited better perceptual organization on the WAIS-R than did patients with Huntington's, while concomitantly exhibiting slightly better verbal and poorer attentional abilities. A double dissociation at the neurophysiological level was also observed. Patients with schizophrenia exhibited reduced prefrontal and augmented parietal flow, whereas patients with Huntington's disease exhibited the reverse of this pattern upon rCBF testing with WCST cognitive activation.

CONCURRENT AND PREDICTIVE VALIDITY OF NEUROPSYCHOLOGICAL IMPAIRMENT

There is increasing evidence that neuropsychological impairment is associated with deficits in social and vocational functioning and with long-term outcome. For instance, Goldberg et al. (31) found that intrapair differences between neuropsychological test scores of the unaffected and affected monozygotic twins discordant for schizophrenia correlated with intrapair differences in social and vocational functioning on the Global Assessment Scale. In particular, IQ, memory for stories, fluency, and WCST perseveration were significantly associated with global level of functioning. These results suggests that patients' deficits in learning new information, purposefully recalling old information, and generating novel plans or hypotheses may have an impact on their capacity to efficiently perform a job, take part in social transactions, and make decisions. Moreover, using intrapair differences in twins concordant for schizophrenia, Goldberg et al. (31) observed that nearly all of the variance on the Global Assessment Scale could be accounted for by differences in the performance of four neuropsychological variables. In this design, the experience of illness, institutionalization, medication, psychotic symptomatology, and, of course, genome are shared.

Although in one sense the design ''stacks the deck'' because of its artificiality, it does illustrate the often underappreciated importance of neurocognition in predicting level of functioning. The aforementioned study of schizophrenic patients' response to clozapine (27) also is relevant. The investigators found that patients' living arrangement and job status did not change significantly with clozapine treatment, although patients' symptoms were much reduced. Because neuropsychological impairments remained substantial and constant, they may have been rate limiting in the rehabilitation on this group of patients. In another study long-term inpatients could be discriminated from patients who lived outside the hospital on the basis of memory, attention, and motor tests (58). This is not to say that symptoms do not have an impact on social and vocational outcome; they do, at least in the short term. What is important to note is that cognitive impairment may also contribute in a unique manner to outcome as well.

PHARMACOLOGICAL ENHANCEMENT OF COGNITION

Based on the preceding arguments that cognitive impairment is an enduring and frequent aspect of schizophrenia, it would appear reasonable to target these deficits for treatment. This being said, few pharmacological studies have set out to directly improve cognition in schizophrenia (as opposed to improving it by ameliorating symptoms). In the first study, Fields et al. (16) used clonidine, an α2-adrenergic agonist, to increase memory performance in schizophrenia. Clonidine had been previously shown to improve memory in amnesics. After approximately 3 weeks of treatment with the drug, patients, who were otherwise unmedicated, scored higher on memory quotients and delayed recall scores than they had while receiving placebo. This change occurred independently of changes in severity of psychosis. However, the exact mechanisms responsible for the improvement were obscure, as clonidine may act as a direct postsynaptic agonist or exert presynaptic inhibition. In another study, Goldberg et al. (24) used dextroamphetamine as a cognitive enhancer. The rationale was as follows. Cognitive failure and psychiatric symptoms might be the result of an imbalance between dopamine systems, the latter the result of dopamine overactivity in limbic regions, the former the result of dopamine underactivity in prefrontal cortical regions. With this in mind and capitalizing on differences in distribution of dopamine type I and type II receptors, patients were maintained on chronic haloperidol treatment to blockade dopamine type II receptors in subcortical regions and administered an oral dose of amphetamine (at 0.25 mg/kg) to stimulate cortical type I receptors. On cognitive measures, patients demonstrated significant improvement in psychomotor speed and a near-significant improvement on concept formation on the WCST. The latter finding was consistent with changes in regional cerebral blood flow in dorsolateral prefrontal cortex as detected by SPECT (12). In fact, increases in prefrontal flow were correlated with improvements in the Card Sort.

The complexity of cognitive enhancement in schizophrenia was recently demonstrated by Bilder et al. (4) who found that verbal fluency was reduced by neuroleptic treatment relative to placebo, but that the impact of methylphenidate infusion differed as a function of treatment status. Performance was enhanced in patients on neuroleptic and decreased in neuroleptic-free patients to whom it was administered. Bilder et al. suggested that there is an optimal level of dopamine tone for cognitive function; both too little and too much dopaminergic activity have deleterious effects.

CONCLUSIONS

In the lay imagination, schizophrenic patients experience problems in living because they are divided against themselves, out of touch with reality, and disorganized. The view of scientists, once not altogether different, has begun to change. Not only have the symptoms been defined and codified, but the neurobiological underpinnings of the disorder have begun to be described. Emerging also is a view in which cognitive impairments may be a relatively central feature of the disorder. Why central? First, they seem enduring in that they are dissociable from psychiatric symptomatology. Second, they are very frequent: most patients exhibit cognitive impairments to a greater or lesser degree. Third, cognitive impairments also may have a relatively well-delineated profile in which executive, memory, and attentional deficits are prominent and are associated with social and vocational disability. This account carries with it implications for treatment in that cognitive impairments should also be considered target symptoms in the way that hallucinations, delusions, and anergia are. That is, drugs or a combination of drugs in conjunction with various cognitive rehabilitational techniques should be marshalled against the impairments, because certain cognitive functions are necessary for even rudimentary successes in modern life.

REFERENCES

1. Asarnow RF, Granholm E, Sherman T. Span of apprehension in schizophrenia. In: Steinhauer SR, Gruzelier JH, Zubin J, eds. *Handbook of schizophrenia, Vol. 5, Neuropsychology, psychophysiology and information processing.* New York: Elsevier; 1991.
2. Berman KF, Torrey EF, Daniel DG, Weinberger DR. Regional cortical blood flow in monozygotic twins discordant and concordant for schizophrenia. *Arch Gen Psychiatry* 1992;49:927–934.
3. Bilder RM, Goldberg E. Motor perseveration in schizophrenia. *Arch Clin Neuropsychol* 1987;2:195–214.
4. Bilder RM, Lieberman JA, Kim Y, Alvir JA, Reiter G. Methylphenidate and neuroleptic effects on oral word production in schizophrenia. *Neuropsychiatry Neuropsychol Behav Neurol* 1992;5:262–271.
5. Bilder RM, Lipschutz-Broch L, Reiter G, Geisler S, Mayerhoff D, Lieberman JA. Intellectual deficits in first episode and chronic schizophrenia: evidence for progressive deterioration? *Schiz Bull* [in press].
6. Braff DL, Heaton R, Kuck J, et al. The generalized pattern of neuropsychological deficits in outpatients with chronic schizophrenia with heterogeneous Wisconsin Card Sorting Test results. *Arch Gen Psychiatry* 1991;48:891–898.
7. Braff DL, Saccuzzo DP, Geyer MA. Information processing dys-

functions in schizophrenia: studies of visual backward masking, sensorimotor gating, and habituation. In: Steinhauer SR, Gruzelier JH, Zubin J, eds. *Neuropsychology, Psychophysiology and Information Processing*. New York: Elsevier; 1991:303–334. (*Handbook of schizophrenia*, vol. 5).

8. Calev A. Recall and recognition in mildly disturbed schizophrenics: the use of matched tasks. *Psychol Med* 1984;14:425–429.

9. Cohen JD, Servan-Schreiber D. Context, cortex and dopamine: a connectionistic approach to behavior and biology in schizophrenia. *Psychol Rev* 1992;99:45–77.

10. Cornblatt RA, Erlenmeyer-Kimling L. Global attentional deviance as a marker of risk for schizophrenia: specificity and predictive validity. *J Abnorm Psychol* 1985;96:470–486.

11. Daniel DG, Goldberg TE, Gibbon R, Weinberger DR. Lack of a bimodal distribution of ventricular size in schizophrenia: a Gaussian mixture analysis of 1056 cases and controls. *Biol Psychiatry* 1991;30:887–903.

12. Daniel DG, Weinberger DR, Jones DW, et al. The effect of amphetamine on regional cerebral blood flow during cognitive activation in schizophrenia. *J Neurosci* 1991;11:1907–1917.

13. Davidson M, Powchik P, Losonczy MF, et al. Dementia in elderly schizophrenic patients clinical and neuropathological correlates. *Biol Psychiatry* 1991;29:91A.

14. Faustman WO, Moses JA Jr, Csernansky JB. Neuropsychological performance and symptomatology: Correlations in medicated and unmedicated schizophrenic patients. *Psychiatry Res* [in press].

15. Fey ET. The performance of young schizophrenics and young normals on the Wisconsin Card Sorting Test. *J Consult Psychol* 1951;15:311–319.

16. Fields RB, Van Kammen DP, Peters JL, et al. Clonidine improves memory function in schizophrenia independently from change in psychosis: Preliminary findings. *Schizophr Res* 1988;1:417–423.

17. Fleming K, Goldberg TE, Gold JM, Weinberger DR. Brown Peterson performance in patients with schizophrenia. *Psychiatr Res* [in press].

18. Frith C. *The cognitive neuropsychology of schizophrenia*. Hove, UK: Lawrence Erlbaum Associates, Publishers; 1993.

19. Gold JM, Goldberg TE, Kleinman JE, Weinberger DR. The impact of symptomatic state and pharmacological treatment on cognitive functioning of patients with schizophrenia and mood disorders. In: Mohr E, Brouwers P eds. *Handbook of clinical trials. The neurobehavioral and injury*. Amsterdam: Swets and Zeitlinger; 1991:185–214.

20. Gold JM, Hermann BP, Wyler A, Randolph C, Goldberg TE, Weinberger DR. Schizophrenia and temporal lobe epilepsy: a neuropsychological study. *Arch Gen Psychiatry* 1994;51:265–272.

21. Gold JM, Randolph C, Carpenter CJ, Goldberg TE, Weinberger DR. Forms of memory failure in schizophrenia. *J Abnorm Psychol* 1992;101:487–494.

22. Gold JM, Randolph C, Carpenter CJ, Goldberg TE, Weinberger DR. The performance of patients with schizophrenia on the Wechsler Memory Scale-Revised. *Clin Neuropsychol* 1992;6:367–373.

23. Goldberg TE, Berman KF, Mohr E, Weinberger DR. Regional cerebral blood flow and cognitive function in Huntington's disease and schizophrenia. *Arch Neurol* 1990;47:418–422.

24. Goldberg TE, Bigelow LB, Kleinman JE, Daniel DG, Weinberger DR. Effects of the coadministration of amphetamine and haloperidol on the affect, motor behavior, and cognition of patients with schizophrenia. *Am J Psychiatry* 1991;148:78–84.

25. Goldberg TE, Gold JM, Greenberg R, et al. Contrasts between patients with affective disorder and patients with schizophrenia on a neuropsychological screening battery. *Am J Psychiatry* 1993;150:1355–1362.

26. Goldberg TE, Hyde TM, Kleinman JE, Weinberger DR. Course of schizophrenia: neuropsychological evidence for a static encephalopathy. *Schiz Bull* 1993;19:797–804.

27. Goldberg TE, Greenberg R, Griffin S, et al. The impact of clozapine on cognition and psychiatric symptoms in patients with schizophrenia. *Br J Psychiatry* 1993;162:43–48.

28. Goldberg TE, Ragland DR, Gold J, Bigelow LB, Torrey EF, Weinberger DR. Neuropsychological assessment of monozygotic twins discordant for schizophrenia. *Arch Gen Psychiatry* 1990;47:1066–1072.

29. Goldberg TE, Torrey EF, Berman KB, Weinberger DR. Relations between neuropsychological performance and brain morphological and physiological measures in monozygotic twins discordant for schizophrenia: use of an intrapair difference method. *Psychiatry Res Neuroimag* 1994;55:51–61.

30. Goldberg TE, Torrey EF, Gold JM, Ragland JD, Bigelow LB, Weinberger DR. Learning and memory in monozygotic twins discordant for schizophrenia. *Psychol Med* 1993;23:71–85.

31. Goldberg TE, Torrey EF, Gold JM, Ragland JD, Taylor E, Weinberger DR. Risk of cognitive impairment in monozygotic twins concordant and discordant for schizophrenia. *Schiz Res* [in press].

32. Goldberg TE, Weinberger DR. Schizophrenia, training paradigms, and the Wisconsin Card Sorting Test redux. *Schiz Res* 1994;11:291–296.

33. Goldstein G, Zubin J. Neuropsychological differences between young and old schizophrenics with and without associated neurological dysfunction. *Schiz Res* 1990;3:117–126.

34. Gourovitch M, Goldberg TE, Weinberger DR. Differential verbal fluency deficits in schizophrenic patients as compared to normal controls. *Schiz Res* 1993;9:175–176.

35. Hagger C, Buckley P, Kenny JT, et al. Improvement in cognitive functions and psychiatric symptoms in treatment-refractory schizophrenic patients receiving clozapine. *Biol Psychiatry* 1993;34:702–712.

36. Heaton RK, Crowley TJ. Effects of psychiatric disorders and their somatic treatment on neuropsychological test results. In: Filskov SB, Boll TJ, eds. *Handbook of clinical neuropsychology*. New York: John Wiley; 1981:481–525.

37. Hoff AL, Riordan H, O'Donnell DW, Morris L, DeLisi LE. Neuropsychological functioning of first-episode schizophreniform patients. *Am J Psychiatry* 1992;149:898–903.

38. Hunt JMcV, Cofer CN. Psychological deficit. In: Hunt JMcV (ed.) *Personality and the behavior disorders*. New York: Ronald Press; 1944.

39. Hurt SW, Holzman PS, Davis JM. Thought disorder: the measurement of its changes. *Arch Gen Psychiatry* 1983;40:1281–1285.

40. Hyde TM, Nawroz S, Goldberg TE, et al. Is there cognitive decline in schizophrenia? Results from a cross-sectional study. *Br J Psychiatry* [in press].

41. Kane J, Honigfeld G, Singer J, et al. Clozapine for the treatment-resistant schizophrenic: a double-blind comparison with chlorpromazine. *Arch Gen Psychiatry* 1988;45:789–796.

42. Kay S, Lindenmayer J-P. Stability of psychopathology dimensions in chronic schizophrenia: Response to clozapine treatment. *Compr Psychiatry* 1991;32:28–35.

43. Klonoff H, Hutton GH, Fibiger CH. Neuropsychological patterns in chronic schizophrenia. *J Nerv Ment Dis* 1970;150:291–300.

44. Kolb B, Whishaw IQ. Performance of schizophrenic patients on tests sensitive to left or right frontal temporal, and parietal function in neurologic patients. *J Nerv Ment Dis* 1983;171:435–443.

45. Kraepelin E. *Dementia praecox and paraphrenia*. Melbourne, FL: Robert E. Krieger, 1971. Robertson GM, ed. (original published in 1919).

46. Levy DL, Holzman PS, Matthysse S, Mendell NR. Eye tracking dysfunction and schizophrenia: a critical perspective. *Schiz Bull* 1993;19:461–536.

47. Liddle PF. Schizophrenic syndromes, cognitive performance and neurological dysfunction. *Psychol Med* 1987;17:49–57.

48. Malec J. Neuropsychological assessment of schizophrenia versus brain damage: a review. *J Nerv Ment Dis* 1978;166:507.

49. Malenka RC, Angel RW, Thiemann S, Weitz CJ, Berger PA. Central error-correcting behavior in schizophrenia and depression. *Biol Psychiatry* 1986;21:263–273.

50. Manschreck TC, Maher BA, Milavetz JJ, Ames D, Weisstein CC, Schneyer ML. Semantic priming in thought disordered schizophrenic patients. *Schiz Res* 1988;1:61–66.

51. Manschreck TC, Maher BA, Rosenthal JE, Berner J. Reduced primacy and related features in schizophrenia. *Schiz Res* 1991;5:35–41.

52. Medalia A, Gold JM, Merriam A. The effects of neuroleptics on neuropsychological test results of schizophrenics. *Arch Clin Neuropsychol* 1988;3:249–271.

53. Miller R. Schizophrenia as a progressive disorder relations to EEG, CT, neuropathological and other evidence. *Progress Neurobiol* 1989;33:17–44.

54. Mirsky AF. Research on schizophrenia in the NIMH Laboratory of Psychology and Psychopathology, 1954–1987. *Schiz Bull* 1988; 14:151–156.

55. Nuechterlein KH. Converging evidence for vigilance deficit as a vulnerability indicator for schizophrenic disorders. In: Alpert M, ed. *Controversies in schizophrenia.* New York: Guilford Press; 1985:175–198.

56. Oltmanns TF, Ohayon J, Nezle JM. The effect of medication and diagnostic criteria on distractibility in schizophrenia. *J Psychiatric Res* 1979;14:81–91.

57. Park S, Holzman PS. Schizophrenics show spatial working memory deficits. *Arch Gen Psychiatry* 1992;49:975–982.

58. Perlick D, Mattis S, Stasny P, Teresi J. Neuropsychological discriminators of long-term inpatient or outpatient status in chronic schizophrenia. *J Neuropsychiatry Clin Neurosci* 1992;4:428–434.

59. Rapaport D, Gill M, Schafer R. *Diagnostic psychological testing.* Chicago: Year Book Publishers, 1945/46.

60. Rausch MA, Prescott TE, DeWolfe AS. Schizophrenic and aphasic language: discriminable or not? *J Consult Clin Psychol* 1980; 48:63–70.

61. Saykin JA, Gur RC, Gur RE, et al. Neuropsychological function in schizophrenia: selective impairment in memory and learning. *Arch Gen Psychiatry* 1991;48:618–624.

62. Schwartz BL, Rosse RB, Deutsch SI. Limits of the processing view in accounting for dissociations among memory measures in a clinical population. *Memory Cognition* 1993;21:63–72.

63. Schwartzman AE, Douglas VI. Intellectual loss in schizophrenia part II. *Can J Psychol* 1962;16:161–168.

64. Seidman LJ, Pepple JR, Faraone SV, et al. Neuropsychological performance in chronic schizophrenia in response to neuroleptic dose reduction. *Biol Psychiatry* 1993;33:575–584.

65. Serper MR, Bergman RL, Harvey PD. Medication may be required for the development of automatic information processing in schizophrenia. *Psychiatry Res* 1990;32:281–288.

66. Shakow D. Adaptation in schizophrenia: the theory of segmental set. New York: John Wiley; 1979.

67. Shallice T, Burgess PW, Frith CD. Can the neuropsychological case-study approach be applied to schizophrenia? *Psychol Med* 1991;21:661–673.

68. Shelton RC, Weinberger DR. X-ray computerized tomography studies in schizophrenia: a review and synthesis. In: Nasrallah HA, Weinberger DR, eds. *Handbook of schizophrenia.* Amsterdam: Elsevier; 1986:207–250.

69. Singh J, Knight RT, Rosenlicht N, Kotun JM, Beckley DJ, Woods DL. Abnormal premovement brain potentials in schizophrenia. *Schiz Res* 1992;8:31–41.

70. Spohn HE, Strauss ME. Relation of neuroleptic and anticholinergic medication to cognitive function in schizophrenia. *J Abnorm Psychol* 1989;98:367–380.

71. Suddath RL, Christison GW, Torrey EF, Casanova MF, Weinberger DR. Anatomical abnormalities in the brains of monozygotic twins discordant for schizophrenia. *New Engl J Med* 1990;22:789–794.

72. Sullivan EV, Mathalon DH, Zipursky RB, Kersteen-Tucker Z, Knight RT, Pfefferbaum A. Factors of the Wisconsin Card Sorting Test as measures of frontal-lobe function in schizophrenia and in chronic alcoholism. *Psychiatry Res* 1992;46:175–199.

73. Torrey EF, Bowler AE, Taylor EH, Gottesman II. *Schizophrenia and manic-depressive disorder.* New York: Basic Books; 1994.

74. Townes BD, Martin DC, Nelson D, Prosser R, Pepping M, Maxwell J. Neurobehavioral approach to classification of psychiatric patients using a competency model. *J Consult Clin Psychol* 1985;53:33–42.

75. Vrtunski PB, Simpson DM, Weiss KM, Davis GC. Abnormalities of fine motor control in schizophrenia. *Psychiatry Res* 1986; 18:275–284.

76. Weinberger DR. Implications of normal brain development for the pathogenesis of schizophrenia. *Arch Gen Psychiatry* 1987;44:660–669.

77. Weinberger DR, Berman KF, Zec RF. Psychologic dysfunction of dorsolateral prefrontal cortex in schizophrenia: I. Regional cerebral blood flow evidence. *Arch Gen Psychiatry* 1986;43:114–124.

Psychopharmacology: The Fourth
Generation of Progress, edited by
Floyd E. Bloom and David J. Kupfer.
Raven Press, Ltd., New York 1995.

CHAPTER 106

Acute Treatment of Schizophrenia

William C. Wirshing, Stephen R. Marder, Theodore Van Putten,
and Donna Ames

The illness schizophrenia is, for many so afflicted, a chronic relapsing and remitting condition. Although a person rarely returns to full psychosocial functioning during the periods of remission, the oftentimes dramatic worsenings that punctuate the typical clinical course have been the focus of much of the pharmacological treatment research. These deteriorations, also called relapses and exacerbations, define the target symptoms of acute treatment studies. Their prevention is the goal of the various maintenance strategies (see Chapter 107, *this volume*).

The acute pharmacological phase of schizophrenia treatment concerns the introduction or reintroduction of medication to alleviate (or at least palliate) an exacerbation of psychosis. These episodes are usually marked by an increase in positive symptoms, such as delusions, hallucinations, thought disorder, and agitation; however, an increase in negative symptoms, such as extreme withdrawal or mutism, can also occur. An episode may be rapid or insidious in onset, and the form and content of the symptoms may change from one exacerbation to the next. Since the most important aspects of schizophrenic psychopathology involve subjective experiences (e.g., delusions and hallucinations), the ability or willingness of the individual to describe these phenomena reliably may also vary over time. Thus, the symptomatic target of acute pharmacotherapy is clinically elusive and at times simply unquantifiable.

Conventional neuroleptic agents have, since the mid-1950s, proven to be the most consistently effective compounds in the treatment of acute and chronic schizophrenic patients. This efficacy, though, has come at the cost of a number of untoward neurological side effects.

Prominent among these are disturbances of the extrapyramidal system including dystonia, tremor, akinesia, bradykinesia, rigidity, akathisia, and a variety of tardive dyskinetic (TD) syndromes. These side effects have been linked to notorious patient noncompliance and iatrogenic morbidity (11,14,29,30,41,56,61,62). Additionally, conventional neuroleptics have been shown to be only partially effective at ameliorating the psychosis which contributes to persistent disability, subjective distress, and family burden. Finally, a substantial minority of patients derive little if any benefit from drug treatment (9).

This chapter reviews the efficacy of conventional antipsychotic agents, the utility of plasma level monitoring, and the use of adjunctive agents in treating unresponsive cases. See Chapter 108 (*this volume*) for a discussion of the unconventional compounds.

EFFICACY

The major considerations in acute pharmacological treatment (once appropriate diagnostic, neuromedical, and psychosocial evaluations have taken place) are the choice of drug, drug dosage, and dosage escalation schedule. Subsequently, the pharmacological treatment plan should involve the assessment of therapeutic efficacy and adverse effects, the need for further dosage adjustment, and adjunctive or alternative treatments in those patients who fail to respond.

Several different classes of antipsychotic drugs have been introduced over the last 35 years. With the exception of clozapine (27), there are no convincing data that any one drug or drug class is more effective than any other. It is possible that differences do exist, but studies with appropriate methodology have not been conducted to demonstrate these differences. Most comparisons involve random assignment and parallel group designs (see

W. C. Wirshing, S. R. Marder, T. Van Putten (*deceased*),
and D. Ames: University of California at Los Angeles School
of Medicine and West Los Angeles Veterans Affairs Medical
Center, Los Angeles, California 90073.

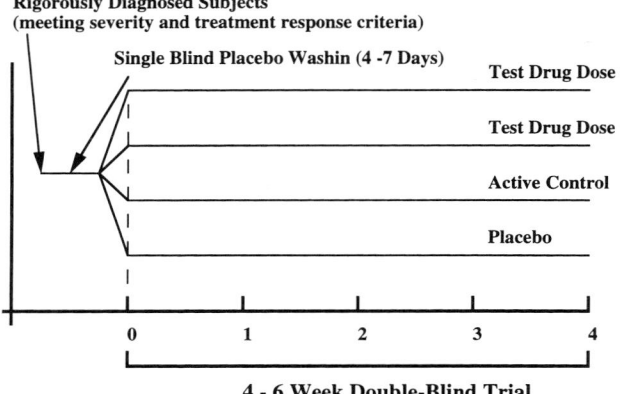

FIG. 1. Schematic flow of a typical pharmacological study in acute schizophrenia. The placebo arm is frequently omitted after a compound has previously been shown to have clear efficacy over placebo.

Fig. 1) that contrast one drug with another and demonstrate a lack of significant difference in overall response rate. These results do not necessarily mean that a given individual would respond equally well to either drug. As such designs typically exclude subjects with historical neuroleptic unresponsiveness and placebo response, they also greatly limit the generalizability of the results to a standard clinical population.

The equal efficacy data across classes of neuroleptics apply to the primary effects of these agents but not to the secondary or side effects. Generally, when compared to the low-potency neuroleptics, the high-potency compounds like fluphenazine, haloperidol, and droperidol have less sedation, fewer anticholinergic effects, and fewer cardiovascular effects (e.g., orthostatic hypotension) but at a cost of producing more acute extrapyramidal side effects (e.g., akathisia, drug-induced parkinsonism, and dystonia). The choice then of which neuroleptic to use is generally made by considering which particular constellation of side effects would be least harmful or most beneficial to a given patient. Although no consensus is available, many feel that the side-effect profile of the high-potency agents is easier to manage for the clinician and better tolerated by the patient.

This clinical impression may account for the fact that the high-potency agents are prescribed at two to seven times the dose (in chlorpromazine equivalents) as the low-potency agents (4). However, because the high-potency agents carry with them a higher extrapyramidal liability, adjunctive medication (anticholinergic, dopaminergic, antiadrenergic) is frequently required. One notion that continues to be widespread is that sedating drugs, such as chlorpromazine, are more effective for agitated or highly excited patients than nonsedating drugs, such as fluphenazine or haloperidol. The latter, in turn, are supposedly more appropriate for withdrawn or psychomotorically retarded patients. This relationship has never been established, and numerous studies suggest that high- and low-potency drugs are equally effective in both types of patients.

Drug Dosage

Despite years of clinical and research experience, we do not have definitive dose–response curves for antipsychotic drugs. However, recent research provides much guidance to clinicians. In the early stages of antipsychotic drug development, it became apparent that chlorpromazine doses below 400 to 600 mg/day were much less likely to prove superior to placebo than doses above that range. Subsequently, particularly in the 1970s, there was considerable interest in exploring the upper ranges of tolerated doses to determine if such doses might produce any added benefit, either in terms of rapidity of therapeutic effect or the ultimate degree of improvement. Studies comparing high-dose (defined as >2,000 mg chlorpromazine equivalents) to standard-dose treatment showed no statistically significant advantage for the high dose (12,13,15,44,50,52,67). These findings do not exclude the possibility that some patients may benefit from higher than usual dosages, but such patients appear to be in the minority and better means are needed to identify those individuals who might be appropriate candidates for high-dose treatment.

As Reardon et al. (51) have shown, there had been an increase in the use of high dosages of high-potency neuroleptics during the late 1970s and 1980s despite the lack of clinical research data supporting such use. The use of these high-dose regimens may have resulted from increasing pressure to treat patients rapidly, the increasing acuity and severity of those being hospitalized, the belief by many clinicians that high doses of high-potency drugs are well tolerated, and the profound lack of treatment options for the neuroleptic unresponsive patient. As a result of these trends, several studies in recent years have focused on clarifying the benefit-to-risk ratios of different neuroleptic dosages.

Levinson et al. (36) studied 53 patients with acute exacerbations of schizophrenic, schizoaffective (mainly schizophrenic), and other nonaffective psychoses. Patients were randomly assigned to fixed-dose, double-blind treatment with either 10, 20, or 30 mg/day of oral fluphenazine. After 24 to 28 days of treatment, improvement in the sample as a whole was not related to dosage. However, among patients who showed a 40% or greater improvement in positive symptoms, dosages of 0.3 mg/kg/per day were associated with the most clinical improvement, but also with a higher incidence of extrapyramidal side effects (EPS). They suggested that a linear relationship between fluphenazine dosage and clinical response exists among patients who respond to a certain degree, and that the nonresponder group may include many patients in whom dose is not a factor because they would be unresponsive to any of the dosages studied. The authors concluded that although the best clinical response was seen at dosages of 0.3 mg/kg/per day, the increase in adverse effects was such that they would recommend daily dosages in the lower end of the 0.2 to 0.3 mg/kg range. The authors also found that the presence of akathisia during the study (regardless of whether or not it was treated) also predicted poor response during the 4-week trial. Antiparkinsonian drugs were given as needed, not prophylactically.

Van Putten et al. (64) reported on the treatment of 80 newly admitted men with schizophrenia who were assigned openly by cohort to receive 5, 10, or 20 mg/day of haloperidol for 4 weeks. Patients with a history of nonresponse to neuroleptic drugs were excluded, and patients with a history of severe dystonic reactions (28%) were given prophylactic benztropine mesylate 2 mg b.i.d. After 7 days of treatment, the proportion of patients who remained in the study and were described as ''much improved'' for the 5-, 10-, and 20-mg doses were 6%, 33%, and 47%, respectively. Although the 20-mg dose appeared superior in efficacy during the first 2 weeks, the highest dosage group subsequently experienced a worsening in emotional withdrawal and psychomotor retardation as well as a higher incidence of akinesia and akathisia. In addition, the 20 mg/day group had a 35% dropout rate (leaving hospital against medical advice) in comparison to only 5 percent for the 5- and 10-mg dose groups. These investigators concluded that 20 mg may be more effective for controlling psychoses in the first week or two, but a higher incidence of adverse effects subsequently undermines this initial benefit. It is important to note that this was an open study (investigators were not blind to dosage), and it is possible that the prophylactic or early use of antiparkinsonian agents or propranolol to treat akathisia could improve the therapeutic index.

Rifkin et al. (52) randomly assigned 87 newly admitted patients meeting Research Diagnostic Criteria (RDC) for schizophrenia (59) to receive 10, 30, or 80 mg/day of oral haloperidol on a double-blind basis for 6 weeks. All subjects were given benztropine mesylate 2 mg t.i.d. (Among these patients, 93% received DSM-III diagnoses of schizophrenia and 7% schizophreniform disorder.) Although 22% of the subjects dropped out, there was no difference in dropout rate between the treatment groups. Nor were there any significant differences between the treatment groups either in terms of clinical response or the occurrence of EPS. Thus, these investigators found no advantage to treating patients with haloperidol dosages >10 mg/day, but they also did not find a significant increase in EPS among patients treated with higher dosages and prophylactic antiparkinsonian medication.

There is a considerable degree of consistency in these studies despite differences in patient populations and methodology. It would appear that there are no significant advantages to using dosages of haloperidol or fluphenazine >10–20 mg/day for acute treatment and that even dosages of 20 mg may be associated with a substantial number of neurologic adverse effects if prophylactic antiparkinsonian medication is not used.

McEvoy et al. (42) used the neuroleptic threshold to determine optimal dosages for neuroleptic treatment of patients with acute schizophrenia. This involves a hypothesis first proposed by Haase (22) suggesting that the lowest neuroleptic dosages on which patients develop slight increases in rigidity are also the lowest dosages at which the patients will attain maximum therapeutic benefit. Of the 106 patients who participated, 25 had schizoaffective disorder and 32 had no prior exposure to neuroleptics. On day 1 of the protocol, 2 mg of oral haloperidol was given and the daily dosage was subsequently increased by 2 mg every other day until the neuroleptic threshold was crossed (i.e., rigidity increased from baseline) or a dosage of 10 mg/day was reached. Once the neuroleptic threshold was reached within the first 10 to 12 days (very few patients failed to show an increase in rigidity on 10 mg/day), the dosage was fixed and the patient was treated openly for 14 days. After 24 days, patients were randomly assigned, double-blind, to either continue at their neuroleptic threshold dosage or to have the dosage increased by 2 to 10 times. The average high dosage between days 24 and 38 was 11.6 ± 4.7 mg/day versus 3.4 ± 2.3 mg/day for those continuing at their neuroleptic threshold dosage. Neuroleptic-naive patients crossed the threshold at a significantly lower average (2.1 mg/day) dosage than those who had been previously treated (4.3 mg/day). After 24 days (14 at the neuroleptic threshold dosage), 54% were considered responders. After the double-blind comparison was completed at day 38, 42% of those who hadn't responded at day 24 had become responders, but there was no difference between those remaining on the neuroleptic threshold dosage and those randomized to a higher dosage. The only therapeutic measures on which the higher dosage was superior, were ratings of hostility and suspiciousness. Unlike the study by Rifkin et al. (52) described above, higher dosages were associated with more EPS. In addition, the authors reported a significantly poorer response rate in those patients who had been actively psychotic for more than 6 months before treatment was initiated compared to those with shorter periods of psychoses.

The McEvoy et al. findings (42) differ from those of Levinson et al. (36) and Van Putten et al. (63), who found clear therapeutic advantages for the 10-mg dose in comparison to lower doses. It may be that the inclusion of more first-episode and drug-naive patients in the McEvoy et al. (42) study could account for this if one assumes that such patients are initially more sensitive to both the therapeutic and neurotoxic side effects of haloperidol. The monitoring for such subtle signs of neurotoxicity requires careful scrutiny and much clinical experience. Thus, the extent to which these findings are generalizable to routine clinical practice remains to be established.

Taken together, these results build a strong case that dosages above 15 to 20 mg/day of haloperidol or fluphenazine should not be the first-line treatment in patients who are judged to be capable of responding (i.e., those without an established history of neuroleptic refractoriness). It is also clear that neuroleptic side effects such as akathisia and akinesia are serious clinical problems even with dosages in this range, and efforts to prevent and treat them should be a high priority for clinicians.

Plasma Level Monitoring

Plasma level monitoring of the antipsychotic agents has been of decidedly limited utility in both clinical and research settings, in part, because the dose–to–plasma-level correlations are generally low (with intersubject variability high) and clinical effect typically lags behind steady-state plasma levels by days or even weeks. Some recent studies focusing on the relationship between plasma level and clinical response have, however, helped to characterize the potential usefulness and underscore the limitations of plasma-level measurement of antipsychotics. Early studies focused on drugs, such as chlorpromazine, that have a complex metabolism. Measurement of plasma levels does not give a true picture, because some of the antipsychotic activity may result from metabolites of the drug in the plasma. Thus, drug selection and methodological errors may explain why early studies failed to find a reliable relationship.

More recent studies have focused on drugs other than chlorpromazine and have had more promising results. Recent studies have also employed improved methodology, including the use of fixed dosages, particularly for haloperidol. This is partially because this drug has only a single important metabolite (reduced haloperidol), which may not have significant antipsychotic activity. Five studies have found a therapeutic-window relationship between plasma levels and clinical response, and five other studies have not. In most cases, failure to find a relationship may be explained by methodological shortcomings, such as the use of patients with a history of poor drug responses or the use of doses that were either too high or too low. At the same time, those studies reporting poor response at higher blood levels may reflect an increase in adverse effects rather than a true decrease in efficacy.

The findings of Van Putten et al. (63) indicated a curvilinear relationship between plasma haloperidol levels that were averaged during a fixed-dose treatment period and change in psychosis on the Brief Psychiatric Rating Scale (BPRS) (46,68). Patients demonstrated the most improvement when their levels were between 5 and 12 ng/ml. Patients with levels above 12 ng/ml also improved as a group, suggesting that some patients tolerate these higher

levels. However, when poor responders had levels above 12 ng/ml, they failed to improve, and some actually worsened. Volavka et al. (66) randomized 176 acutely ill schizophrenic patients to one of three plasma ranges of haloperidol: low (2 to 13 ng/ml), medium (13.1 to 24), and high (24.1 to 35). This is an innovative design that permits clinicians to evaluate the usefulness of targeting a particular plasma concentration. Overall, the three groups had approximately the same rate of response, although there was a suggestion that higher levels were associated with less improvement. However, the low plasma-level range overlapped with what others consider the optimal range (i.e., 2 to 12 ng/ml) (65). The findings of this study seem to indicate that there is no advantage to raising haloperidol levels above this low plasma range.

Given the array of studies in this area and their varying results, it is understandable that there is no consensus as to whether plasma levels of antipsychotics should be monitored by clinicians. However, some conclusions may reasonably be drawn from an evaluation of the most recent generation of studies. There is probably little to be gained by monitoring plasma concentrations on a routine basis, because a high proportion of patients will respond when they are prescribed moderate doses of antipsychotics. On the other hand, a plasma level may provide useful information in the following circumstances: (a) when patients fail to respond to what is usually an adequate dose; (b) when it is difficult for the clinician to discriminate drug side effects, particularly akathisia or akinesia, from symptoms of schizophrenia such as agitation or negative impairments (a high blood level might be associated with increased adverse effects); (c) when antipsychotic drugs are combined with other drugs that may affect their pharmacokinetics, such as fluoxetine, beta blockers, cimetidine, barbiturates, and carbamazepine; (d) in the very young, the elderly, and the medically compromised, in whom the pharmacokinetics of neuroleptics may be significantly altered; (e) if noncompliance or poor compliance is suspected; (f) when compliance is compelled by the legal system.

ADJUNCTIVE TREATMENTS

The majority of controlled clinical trials have reported that 10% to 20% of schizophrenics derive little benefit from typical neuroleptic drug therapy (10). Although the near future holds the promise of providing clinicians and researchers with the pharmacological tools to effectively and safely treat this recalcitrant population (see Chapter 108, *this volume*), the present state of the art is largely empirical trial and error.

High-dose Treatment

Arguably the most common clinical choice for the treatment-resistant patient is high-dose neuroleptic therapy.

The literature has a number of anecdotal (17,48,53) and controlled (25) reports that support the use of very large doses (up to 60,000 mg/day of chlorpromazine equivalents) in a treatment-resistant population. However, the study by Quitkin et al. (50) blindly compared two fixed doses of fluphenazine (1,200 and 30 mg/day) in a nonchronic but treatment-resistant group. The results favored the standard dose above the megadose. Thus, although experience would support a high-dose trial for the treatment-resistant patient, it would also predict little benefit of such an approach.

Lithium

Lithium has been used for over two decades to effectively treat the symptoms of bipolar illness. When combined with neuroleptics it has also been reported to benefit patients with excited schizoaffective illness (5) and schizophreniform illness (23). Small et al. (58) showed that combining lithium and neuroleptics in a chronically hospitalized and relatively treatment-refractory population somewhat reduced symptomatology. Therefore, it is reasonable to try lithium in the neuroleptic-refractory patient but, as with the high dose, little optimism is warranted.

Propranolol

After Atsmon and colleagues (3) anecdotally reported that adjunctive high dose propranolol positively influenced acute schizophrenia, a number of controlled studies have addressed its utility as an adjunctive agent in treatment-refractory patients. Most (38,49,69), but not all (43), have reported improvement with the addition of propranolol (400 to 2,000 mg/day) to standard neuroleptic regimens. Taken together, these results hint that high-dose propranolol might be a useful adjunctive agent, but they do little to guide the clinician in the choice of a target dose. A dose of 1,000 mg is probably a reasonable (54) middle-ground choice, but support for even higher doses (up to 2,000 mg) can be found (38). As propranolol, like the antidepressants, elevates neuroleptic (and metabolite) levels (47), care should be exercised in monitoring for an increase in neuroleptic-induced neurotoxic or endocrinological side effects.

Carbamazepine

When used alone, carbamazepine has little to recommend it for stable but refractory schizophrenics. There is even some suggestion that it may destabilize some of these patients (60). However, some controlled-study evidence indicates that, when combined with neuroleptics, it may have benefit over neuroleptic alone in excited psy-

choses, including schizophrenia (35). Additional anecdotal reports and uncontrolled studies have indicated that it may be of adjunctive utility in schizophrenics with evidence of temporal lobe EEG abnormalities (21,45) or violence (39).

Others, though, have found no benefit or even some worsening in nonexcited but refractory schizophrenics (33). Kidron and colleagues (33) hypothesized that the measured reduction in neuroleptic plasma levels caused by the addition of carbamazepine (presumably through induction of hepatic metabolic enzymes) caused this clinical worsening.

So where does all this leave the clinician considering adjunctive carbamazepine for the treatment-refractory patient? It is probably reasonable to try it (at typical anticonvulsant levels) in refractory subjects with either known EEG abnormalities or with violent clinical manifestations. In addition to the usual hematological, hepatic, and dermatological concerns one has when using carbamazepine, the clinician must also be alert to the possibility that it may necessitate increasing the neuroleptic above the baseline.

Benzodiazepines

The literature on the use of benzodiazepines in schizophrenia is divided, but it is somewhat skewed to negative or null effects. Some investigators have been mildly encouraging (26,31,37) but others have been frankly negative (20,24,28). Karson and colleagues (28) not only reported a lack of efficacy for adjunctive clonazepam, but described the new development of violent behaviors in 4 of 13 patients during treatment. Thus, benzodiazepines should probably be reserved for those cases that fail all other adjunctive modalities or in whom clear anxious symptoms predominate.

Opiates

There have been some investigators who have reasoned that opiate agonists may have antipsychotic efficacy (19,32). Brizer et al. (7) used this reasoning to conduct a double-blind, single crossover, controlled study that compared methadone (25 to 40 mg/day) to a nonactive placebo as adjunctive compounds with neuroleptics in a group of seven treatment-refractory schizophrenics. The results indicated that methadone resulted in clinically modest but statistically significant improvement. The authors also stated that there were no difficulties getting these subjects off the methadone. Although encouraging, such limited results cannot be extrapolated to routine clinical practice. Except in the most desperate and wretched of treatment-resistant cases the use of adjunctive opiates cannot be justified.

Antidepressants

Siris (57) continued his excellent clinical investigations into the etiology and treatment of postpsychotic depression and negative schizophrenic symptoms. His group reported on the effects of adjunctive imipramine in neuroleptic-stabilized schizophrenics who met criteria for both postpsychotic depression and negative symptoms. Importantly, the protocol excluded any subjects whose symptom complex responded to a week's trial of adjunctive anticholinergics. This was an attempt to reduce the contribution and confound of a neuroleptic-induced "akinetic" syndrome to the measured outcome. Even though the groups were small (17 placebo and 10 imipramine), the results showed that both the depressive and negative symptoms improved together in the imipramine treated group. This study is somewhat important from a clinical perspective, because it provides the clinician with some medication options in this traditionally resistant group of schizophrenics. From the research point of view, it demonstrates that it is only through methodical pharmacological probing at the junction of depression, negative symptoms, and neuroleptic toxicity that we will be able to understand and treat each component.

Adjunctive specific serotonin reuptake inhibitors (SSRIs) can be beneficial to schizophrenic patients (2,18). Also, the addition of the $5HT_{1A}$ agonist, buspirone has been shown to be of some benefit to small samples of patients (2,8). Considering that serotonergic antagonism is among the explanations posited for clozapine's enhanced efficacy (see Chapter 108, *this volume*), it is theoretically curious that adjunctive putative serotonergic enhancing agents would improve some schizophrenic symptoms. Fluoxetine (or other SSRIs) may result in down-regulation of postsynaptic serotonin receptors, thus causing the overall effect of the medication to be similar to serotonin blockade. Alternatively (or perhaps additionally), it may work by increasing the plasma level of the neuroleptic through competitive metabolism (2,18). Higher levels of haloperidol, however, are not clearly correlated with good clinical response, and indeed may be associated with poorer response (64). The fact that some patients respond to drugs that have opposite effects on serotonin function underscores the need to develop better ways to select patients for one type of drug treatment or another. It may, for example, be that patients with schizophrenia who have obsessive–compulsive and depressive tendencies may benefit more from a trial of combined therapy with a conventional neuroleptic and an SSRI. Further research, particularly double-blind studies with SSRIs, is needed to substantiate the efficacy of these agents in schizophrenia treatment.

Electroconvulsive Therapy

Although electroconvulsive therapy (ECT) is not as effective as medication across the range of schizophrenia patients, it has been shown to be of some value (55), and its relative merits in refractory patients deserves further study. Those patients with illness duration greater than 6 months, significant affective symptoms, or catatonia are most likely to benefit from ECT.

Newer Neuroleptics

The two main contenders vying for a position alongside of clozapine on the atypical shelf are remoxipride and risperidone. The former, like the already widely used agent sulpiride, is a substituted benzamide that is a highly selective D_2 (but not D_4) blocker. It also possesses even greater affinity for the sigma site, but this is of unclear clinical significance. It was approved for clinical use in Sweden in January, 1991 and is generally thought to possess antipsychotic activity that is comparable to conventional neuroleptics but with less EPS liability and less mental dulling. The results of a placebo-controlled study in stabilized chronic schizophrenics revealed that remoxipride is effective (compared to placebo) at preventing relapse (34). In another study (16), normal volunteers were administered several doses of remoxipride (30, 60, and 120 mg) and its effects on psychomotor performance were measured. The upper dose was abandoned when two of the first three subjects developed moderately severe akathisia. In addition to possibly demonstrating akathisic liability, the data indicated that remoxipride did have a mild negative effect on attention and arousal. Because there was no conventional agent comparison arm, it is difficult to know whether remoxipride has a milder impact on psychomotor performance. These results, when combined with the previous clinical data on remoxipride, seem to confirm that this agent is an effective antipsychotic that is relatively nonsedating and generally well tolerated. Unfortunately, after a cumulative world wide experience exceeding 25,000 patients, eight developed fatal aplastic anemia. This agent will, therefore, never be used again in a general clinical population. However, its chemical successors will predictably be developed and used.

Risperidone is a benzisoxizole derivative that is pharmacologically characterized by potent central antagonism of both serotonin (type 2 subclass; S_2) and D_2 receptors. It has also demonstrated substantial antagonism of α_1, α_2, and histamine receptors. Preclinical animal experimentation has indicated that although it is slightly less potent than haloperidol at D_2 antagonism (canine emesis model), it is several times less potent than haloperidol at inducing catalepsy. Taken together, these data would predict risperidone would have antipsychotic efficacy and reduced EPS liability in humans. The potent S_2 antagonism might theoretically be of utility in ameliorating the negative symptoms of schizophrenia, mirroring clozapine's enhanced efficacy in this spectrum of symptoms (see Chapter 108, *this volume*).

The initial clinical reports released in 1993 (6,40) hint that the most effective dose of risperidone (6 mg) may be more effective than 20 mg of haloperidol in controlling acute psychotic symptoms and has an EPS liability that is not significantly greater than placebo. The data from the multicenter North American study further hint that it has dose-related extrapyramidal liability that begins to develop at a daily dose of approximately 10 mg. Even more interesting, its antipsychotic efficacy begins to wane at and above that same dose. This inverted U-shaped dose–response curve has been described by some investigators of conventional compounds, but this is the first report of such an occurrence in the newer agents. This molecule is currently available for general clinical use in many countries. Extrapolating from the premarketing results, it will almost surely replace some of the high-potency oral neuroleptics.

CONCLUSIONS

The last few years have seen an incremental advance in our clinical experience with some of the new generation of antipsychotics and a fine tuning of our understanding of the safest ways to treat acutely psychotic patients with conventional agents. The increasing clinical availability of new and different antipsychotic molecules will undoubtedly fuel even greater advances along these fronts in the near future. The experience gained from designing and enacting experimental clinical protocols with conventional compounds will clearly be carried over to the newer agents in the future.

ACKNOWLEDGMENTS

The authors thank the National Alliance for Research on Schizophrenia and Depression (NARSAD), the Department of Veterans Affairs, and the National Institute of Mental Health for supporting this research work and Andrew Berisford for his assistance with the manuscript.

REFERENCES

1. American Psychiatric Association. *DSM-III: diagnostic and statistical manual of mental disorders,* 3rd ed. Washington, DC: American Psychiatric Association; 1980.
2. Ames D, Wirshing WC, Marder SM, Yuwiler A, Brammer GL. Fluoxetine and haloperidol stabilized schizophrenics. *New research programs and abstracts.* APA 146th Annual Meeting, San Francisco, May 1993, NR 66,76.
3. Atsmon A, Blum I, Wijsenbeek H, Maoz B, Steiner M, Ziegelman G. Short-term effects of adrenergic-blocking agents in a small group of psychotic patients: preliminary clinical observations. *Psychiatr Neurol Neurochir* 1971;74:251–258.
4. Baldessarini RJ, Katz B, Cotton P. Dissimilar dosing with high-potency and low-potency neuroleptics. *Am J Psychiatry* 1984; 141:748–752.
5. Biederman J, Lerner Y, Belmaker RH. Combination of lithium carbonate and haloperidol in schizo-affective disorder: a controlled study. *Arch Gen Psychiatry* 1979;36:327–333.
6. Bollen CA, DeCuyper H, Eneman M, Malfroid M, Peuskens J, Heylen S. Risperidone versus haloperidol in the treatment of chronic schizophrenic inpatients: a multicentre double-blind comparative study. *Acta Psychiatr Scand* 1992;85:295–305.
7. Brizer DA, Hartman N, Sweeney J, Millman RB. Effect of methadone plus neuroleptics on treatment-resistant chronic paranoid schizophrenia. *Am J Psychiatry* 1985;142(9):1106–1107.
8. Brody D, Adler LA, Kim T, et al. Effects of buspirone in seven schizophrenic subjects. *J Clin Psychopharmacol* 1990;10:68–69.
9. Davis JM, Casper R. Antipsychotic drugs: clinical pharmacology and therapeutic use. *Drugs* 1977;14:260–282.
10. Davis JM, Schaffer CB, Killian GA, Kinard C, Cahn C. Important issues in the drug treatment of schizophrenia. *Schiz Bull* 1980;6:70–87.
11. Diamond R. Drugs and the quality of life: the patient's point of view. *J Clin Psychiatry* 1985;42:636–637.
12. Donlon PT, Hopkin JT, Tupin JP, Wicks JJ, Wahba M, Meadow A. Haloperidol for acute schizophrenic patients: an evaluation of three oral regimens. *Arch Gen Psychiatry* 1980;37:691–695.
13. Donlon PT, Meadow A, Tupin JP, Wahba M. High versus standard dosage fluphenazine HCl in acute schizophrenia. *J Clin Psychiatry* 1978;39:800–804.
14. Drake RE, Ehrich J. Suicide attempts associated with akathisia. *Am J Psychiatry* 1985;142:499–501.
15. Ericksen SE, Hurt SW, Chang S, Davis JM. Haloperidol dose, plasma levels, and clinical response: a double-blind study. *Psychopharmacol Bull* 1978;14:15–16.
16. Fagan D, Scott DB, Mitchell M, Tiplady B. Effects of remoxipride on measures of psychological performance in healthy volunteers. *Psychopharmacology* 1991;105:225–229.
17. Fouks L. Originalite et specificite de la fluphenazine. In: *Proceedings of the fifth International Congress of Neuropsychopharmacology,* Washington, DC. Amsterdam: Exerpta Medica, 1967:1128–1134 (International Congress Series No. 192).
18. Goff DG, Brotman AW, Waites M, McCormick S. Trial of fluoxetine added to neuroleptics for treatment resistant schizophrenic patients. *Am J Psychiatry* 1990;147:492–494.
19. Gold MS, Donabedian RK, Dillard M Jr, Slobetz FW, Riordan CE, Kleber HD. Antipsychotic effect of opiate agonists [Letter]. *Lancet* 1977;2:398–399.
20. Gundlach R, Engelhardt DM, Hankoff L, Paley H, Rudorfer L, Bird E. A double-blind outpatient study of diazepam (Valium) and placebo. *Psychopharmacology (Berl)* 1966;9:81–92.
21. Hakola HPA, Laulumaa VA. Carbamazepine in treatment of violent schizophrenics [Letter]. *Lancet* 1982;2:1358.
22. Haase HJ. Extrapyramidal modification of fine movements—a "conditio sine qua non" of the fundamental therapeutic action of neuroleptic drugs. In: Bordeleau JM, ed. *Systeme extrapyramidal et neuroleptiques.* Montreal: Editions Psychiatriques; 1961:329–353.
23. Hirschowitz J, Casper R, Garver DL. Lithium response in good prognosis schizophrenia. *Am J Psychiatry* 1980;137(8):916–920.
24. Hollister LE, Bennett JL, Kimbell I Jr, Savage C, Overall JE. Diazepam in newly admitted schizophrenics. *Dis Nerv Syst* 1963;12:746–750.
25. Ital T, Keskiner A, Heinemann L, et al. Treatment of resistant schizophrenics with extreme high dosage fluphenazine. *Psychosomatics* 1970;11:496–499.
26. Jimerson DC, Van Kammen DP, Post RM, Docherty JP, Bunney WE Jr. Diazepam in schizophrenia: preliminary double-blind trial. *Am J Psychiatry* 1982;139(4):489–491.
27. Kane JM, Honigfeld G, Singer J, Meltzer HY. Clozapine for the treatment-resistant schizophrenic: a double-blind comparison with chlorpromazine. *Arch Gen Psychiatry* 1988;45:789–796.
28. Karson CN, Weinberger DR, Bigelow L, Wyatt RJ. Clonazepam treatment of chronic schizophrenia: negative results in a double-blind, placebo-controlled trial. *Am J Psychiatry* 1982;139(12):1627–1628.
29. Keckish WA. Neuroleptics. Violence as a manifestation of akathisia. *JAMA* 1978;240:2185.
30. Keepers GA, Clappison VJ, Casey DE. Initial anticholinergic pro-

phylaxis for neuroleptic-induced extrapyramidal syndromes. *Arch Gen Psychiatry* 1983;40:1113–1117.

31. Kellner R, Wilson RM, Muldawer MD, Pathak D. Anxiety in schizophrenia: responses to chlordiazepoxide in an intensive design study. *Arch Gen Psychiatry* 1975;32:1246–1254.

32. Khantzian EJ, Mack JE, Schatzberg AF. Heroin use as an attempt to cope: clinical observations. *Am J Psychiatry* 1974;131(2):160–164.

33. Kidron R, Auerbuch I, Klein E, Belmaker RH. Carbamazepine-induced reduction of blood levels of haloperidol in chronic schizophrenia [Brief Report]. *Biol Psychiatry* 1985;20:219–222.

34. King DJ, Blomqvist M, Cooper SJ, Doherty MM, Mitchell MJ, Montgomery RC. Placebo controlled trial of remoxipride in the prevention of relapse in chronic schizophrenia. *Psychopharmacology* 1992;107:175–179.

35. Klein E, Bental E, Lerer B, Belmaker RH. Carbamazepine and haloperidol v placebo and haloperidol in excited psychoses. *Arch Gen Psychiatry* 1984;41:165–170.

36. Levinson DF, Simpson GM, Singh H, et al. Fluphenazine dose, clinical response, and extrapyramidal symptoms during acute treatment. *Arch Gen Psychiatry* 1990;47:761–768.

37. Lingjaerde O. Effect of the benzodiazepine derivative estazolam in patients with auditory hallucinations: a multicentre double-blind, cross-over study. *Acta Psychiatr Scand* 1982;65:339–354.

38. Lindstrom LH, Persson E. Propranolol in chronic schizophrenia: controlled study in neuroleptic-treated patients. *Br J Psychiatry* 1980;137:126–130.

39. Luchins DL. Carbamazepine in violent non-epileptic schizophrenics. *Psychopharmacol Bull* 1984;20(3):569–571.

40. Marder SR. Risperidone: clinical development: North American results. *Clin Neuropharm* 1992;15(suppl 1):92A–93A.

41. Marder SR, Van Putten T, Mintz J, et al. Costs and benefits of two doses of fluphenazine. *Arch Gen Psychiatry* 1984;41:1025–1029.

42. McEvoy JP, Hogarty G, Steingard S. Optimal dose of neuroleptic in acute schizophrenia: a controlled study of the neuroleptic threshold and higher haloperidol dose. *Arch Gen Psychiatry* 1991;48:739–745.

43. Myers DH, Campbell PL, Cocks NM, Flowerdew JA, Muir A. A trial of propranolol in chronic schizophrenia. *Br J Psychiatry* 1981;139:118–121.

44. Neborsky R, Janowsky D, Munson E, Depry D. Rapid treatment of acute psychotic symptoms with high and low dose haloperidol. *Arch Gen Psychiatry* 1981;38:195–199.

45. Neppe VM. Carbamazepine in nonresponsive psychosis. *J Clin Psychiatry* 1988;49(4, Suppl):22–28.

46. Overall JE, Gorham DR. The Brief Psychiatric Rating Sale. *Psychol Rep* 1962;10:799–812.

47. Peet M, Middlemiss DN, Yates RA. Pharmacokinetic interaction between propranolol and chlorpromazine in schizophrenic patients, *Lancet* 1980;2:978.

48. Povan N, Yagcioglu V, Itil M, et al: High and very high dose fluphenazine in the treatment of chronic psychosis. In: Cerletti A, Bore FD, eds. *The present status of psychotropic drugs, pharmacological and clinical aspects* (*Proceedings of the Sixth International Congress of the Collegium Internationale Neuropsychopharmacologicum,* Tarrangona, Spain, April 1968). Amsterdam: Exerpta Medica; 1969:495–497 (International Congress Series, No. 180).

49. Pugh CR, Steinert J, Priest RG. Propranolol in schizophrenia: a double blind, placebo controlled trial of propranolol as an adjunct to neuroleptic medication. *Br J Psychiatry* 1983;143:151–155.

50. Quitkin F, Rifkin A, Klein DF. Very high dosage versus standard dosage fluphenazine in schizophrenia: a double-blind study of nonchronic treatment refractory patients. *Arch Gen Psychiatry* 1975;32:1276–1281.

51. Reardon GT, Riflkin A, Schwartz A, Myerson A, Siris SH. Changing pattern of neuroleptic dosage over a decade. *Am J Psychiatry* 1989;146:726–729.

52. Rifkin A, Doddi S, Karagi B, Borenstein M, Wachpress M. Dosage of haloperidol for schizophrenia. *Arch Gen Psychiatry* 1991;48:166–170.

53. Rifkin A, Quitkin F, Carrillo C, et al. Very high dose fluphenazine for nonchronic treatment-refractory patients. *Arch Gen Psychiatry* 1971;25:398–403.

54. Rifkin A, Siris S. Drug treatment of acute schizophrenia In: Meltzer HY, ed. *Psychopharmacology: the third generation of progress.* New York: Raven Press; 1987;1095–1101.

55. Salzman C. The use of ECT in the treatment of schizophrenia. *Am J Psychiatry* 1980;137:1032–1041.

56. Simpson GM, Varga E, Haber EJ. Psychotic exacerbations produced by neuroleptics. *Dis Nerv Syst* 1976;37:367–369.

57. Siris SG, Bermanzohn PC, Gonzalez A, Mason SE, White CV, Shuwall MA. Use of antidepressants for negative symptoms in a subset of schizophrenic patients. *Psychopharmacol Bull* 1991;27:331–335.

58. Small JG, Kellams JJ, Milstein V, Moore J. Placebo-controlled study of lithium combined with neuroleptics in chronic schizophrenic patients. *Am J Psychiatry* 1975;132(12):1315–1317.

59. Spitzer RL, Endicott J, Robbins E. Research diagnostic criteria: rationale and reliability. *Arch Gen Psychiatry* 1978;35:773–782.

60. Sramek J, Herrera J, Costa J, Heh C, Tran-Johnson T, Simpson G. A carbamazepine trial in chronic, treatment-refractory schizophrenia. *Am J Psychiatry* 1988;145(6):748–750.

61. Teicher MH, Baldessanni RJ. Selection of neuroleptic dosage. *Arch Gen Psychiatry* 1985;42:636–637.

62. Van Putten T. Why do schizophrenic patients refuse to take their drugs? *Arch Gen Psychiatry* 1974;31:67–72.

63. Van Putten T, Marder SR, Mintz J. A controlled dose comparison of haloperidol in newly admitted schizophrenic patients. *Arch Gen Psychiatry* 1990;47:754–758.

64. Van Putten T, Marder SR, Mintz J, Poland RE. Haloperidol plasma levels and clinical response: a therapeutic window relationship. *Am J Psychiatry* 1992;49:500–505.

65. Van Putten T, Marder SR, Wirshing WC, Aravagiri M, Chabert N. Neuroleptic plasma levels. *Schiz Bull* 1991;17:197–216.

66. Volavka J, Cooper T, Czobor P, et al. Haloperidol blood levels and clinical effects. *Arch Gen Psychiatry* 1992;49:354–361.

67. Wijsenbeck H, Steiner M, Goldberg SC. Trifluoperazine: a comparison between regular and high doses. *Psychopharmacologia* 1974;36:147–150.

68. Woerner MG, Mannuza S, Kane JM. Anchoring the BPRS: an aid to improved reliability. *Psychopharmacol Bull* 1988;24:112–117.

69. Yorkston NJ, Zaki SA, Pitcher DR, Gruzelier JH, Hollander D, Sergeant HGS. Propranolol as an adjunct to the treatment of schizophrenia. *Lancet* 1977;2:575–578.

Psychopharmacology: The Fourth Generation of Progress, edited by Floyd E. Bloom and David J. Kupfer. Raven Press, Ltd., New York © 1995.

CHAPTER 107

Maintenance Drug Treatment for Schizophrenia

John G. Csernansky and John G. Newcomer

Pharmacological treatment is required in most patients who suffer from schizophrenia for an indefinite period of time, because schizophrenia is a life-time disorder and prevention of psychotic episodes is preferable to reversing them. Therefore, increasing emphasis should be placed on evaluating the risks and benefits of maintenance drug treatment for patients with schizophrenia. The major goal of this chapter is to review current knowledge about maintenance pharmacological treatment for schizophrenia, in the hope that such a review will be instructive for clinicians and stimulate new research.

In the case of acute pharmacological treatments for schizophrenia, the goals of treatment have been relatively well defined by the literature and emphasize the reduction of the key elements of psychosis (i.e., hallucinations, delusions, bizarre behavior, positive formal thought disorder). However, in the case of maintenance pharmacological treatments, therapeutic goals have been less clearly delineated (see Chapter 73, *this volume*). This chapter will be oriented around a discussion of three appropriate goals for maintenance pharmacological treatment in schizophrenic patients. They are (a) prevention of relapse, (b) improvement of quality of life (including the treatment of negative symptoms), and (c) minimization of chronic side-effects. The first of these goals is obvious and has been well studied in the literature, the latter two perhaps less so. Little emphasis will be placed on the prevention and treatment of tardive dyskinesia, as this is covered in detail in another chapter. Also, recent research indicates that minimization of other chronic side-effects, such as

J. G. Csernansky and J. G. Newcomer: Department of Psychiatry, Washington University School of Medicine, and the Schizophrenia Research Program, Malcolm Bliss Mental Health Center, St. Louis, Missouri 63110.

akathisia, may be closely related to achieving the first and second goals.

PREVENTION OF PSYCHOTIC RELAPSE

Dose–Response Studies

The efficacy of antipsychotic medications for the prevention of psychotic relapses in schizophrenic patients has been well established for many years (19). Although individual variations in the course of schizophrenia suggest that some patients might not need continuous prophylactic treatment with an antipsychotic medication, no clinically feasible means of predicting who will or will not relapse after treatment discontinuation is currently available (see below). Overall, 50% of patients treated with placebo relapse within 4 to 6 months, in contrast to 20% of patients treated with neuroleptic medications (19). Kane and Lieberman (40) in their review of this issue noted that the average rate of psychotic relapse in placebo-treated patients in remission or partial remission appears to be approximately 60% to 80% within 1 year.

Relapse prevention with neuroleptic medications can only be accomplished when the medications are taken correctly. Poor compliance with prescribed medication occurs in large numbers of schizophrenic patients and seriously undermines treatment efficacy. Although poor compliance of schizophrenic patients with their medications can, in part, be ascribed to poor insight and judgement (61), many patients are also reluctant to take their medications because of unpleasant neurological side effects, such as pseudoparkinsonism and akathisia (67). Although long-acting depot neuroleptics may effectively address some compliance issues, recognition and treatment of neurological side effects remains a critical consideration in maintaining a cooperative relationship with the patient. Such side effects also represent a strong motivation to use the lowest effective doses of neuroleptics for maintenance treatment.

Several groups of investigators have studied the use of lower maintenance doses of neuroleptics (57). These studies suggest that minimum effective doses for commonly used depot antipsychotics are between 5 and 10 mg every 2 weeks for fluphenazine decanoate (32,41,46) and 50 mg every 4 weeks for haloperidol decanoate (39). Controlled trials of lower doses compared with higher neuroleptic doses have demonstrated equivalent efficacy for the prevention of relapse in most patients, with additional benefits in the reduction of neurological side effects and patient reports of an improved sense of well-being (41,46). However, at least some patients treated with lower maintenance doses of neuroleptics may be at higher risk for psychotic relapse. Kane et al. (39) have recently reported the results of a multicenter, double-blind evaluation of haloperidol decanoate, with patients randomly assigned to one of four fixed monthly doses for 48 weeks: 25 mg, 50 mg, 100 mg, or 200 mg. The relapse rates for the four treatment groups were 63%, 25%, 23%, and 15%, suggesting comparable efficacy for the 50 mg and 100 mg doses, and only a small increase in relapse protection for patients treated with the 200 mg dose.

These studies suggest that the use of lower doses of maintenance antipsychotics will benefit most patients with schizophrenia. However, attempts to reduce the dose of maintenance antipsychotic doses may result in the reappearance of psychotic symptoms in some patients. Careful clinical management, with particular attention paid to prodromal signs and symptoms of relapse, should be followed whenever dose adjustments are made. Although prompt treatment of prodromal symptoms may avert a psychotic relapse, it remains uncertain whether assessments of prodromal symptoms are sensitive or accurate enough in most patients with schizophrenia to be reliable (28,34).

Constant or Intermittent Treatment

The average rate of psychotic relapse over a 1-year period in placebo-treated patients, as cited above, suggests that 20% to 40% of patients might avoid relapse for up to a year without receiving any neuroleptic medications. Such data also suggest that neuroleptic treatment could be instituted on an intermittent basis, when prodromal symptoms appear. This strategy of identifying the earliest signs of psychotic exacerbation for targeted, time-limited treatment with neuroleptics was first suggested by Herz and Melville (29). The feasibility of this approach, at least when special expertise is available, has been demonstrated by more than one group (11,30).

Controlled, prospective studies of intermittent dosing strategies of antipsychotic drugs have generally demonstrated higher rates of relapse or rehospitalization, lower total neuroleptic doses over the period of study, a lower incidence of side-effects, and either no differences or modest disadvantages for the intermittent dosing group with regard to other measures of psychopathology and social functioning (9,36,50). However, there are substantial differences in the methods of these studies, with regard to the nondrug treatments used as adjuncts, and in the rating scales used to measure psychopathology and social functioning. Furthermore, a concern has been noted that repeated interruptions of neuroleptic treatment might be associated with a higher risk for a persistent form of tardive dyskinesia (33). Overall, an intermittent-dosing strategy may still offer advantages for some carefully selected patients, particularly those for whom a lower total cumulative dose of neuroleptics is indicated.

A comparison of lower dose treatment (2.5 to 10 mg fluphenazine decanoate every 2 weeks), standard dose treatment (12.5 to 50 mg fluphenazine decanoate every 2 weeks), and intermittent dosing treatment has recently been accomplished in a pivotal multicenter study, entitled the "Treatment Strategies in Schizophrenia Study." Schooler and colleagues (55,56) have recently reported preliminary results of this study, which compares the three medication treatment conditions described above in combination with either applied (monthly group meetings and home sessions) or supportive family management (monthly group meetings alone) therapies. Following successful completion of a psychoeducational workshop for family members, subjects were randomly assigned to either applied or supportive ongoing family management. Subjects entering the double-blind, randomized medication treatment phase of the study were first stabilized on neuroleptic medication over a period of 16 to 26 weeks. Five sites participated in this study and a total of 313 patients were randomized to both family management and medication treatment.

The preliminary analysis of the data revealed a significant advantage of standard dose treatment over lower dose treatment, and of lower dose treatment over intermittent dosing treatment with regard to the rate of psychotic relapse. However, the standard dose treatment group did not significantly differ from the lower dose treatment group in the amount of time prior to their first rehospitalization or the likelihood of rehospitalization during the 2-year study period. However, both treatments were significantly better than the intermittent dosing treatment on these measures. Negative symptoms seemed to be best treated by intermittent dosing and lower dose treatment compared to standard dose treatment. In summary, this study appears to provide definitive support for the findings of earlier comparisons of low-dose and intermittent-dosing treatments with regular dose treatments.

Nondrug Predictors of Relapse during Maintenance Treatment

There is substantial interest in determining nondrug predictors of relapse in schizophrenic patients undergoing maintenance treatment. Because of the limitations of both lower dose and intermittent dosing treatments, it would be clinically useful to be able to identify those individuals most vulnerable to relapse under such conditions (i.e., when treatment is interrupted or the dose is reduced below an effective level). This topic has recently been reviewed in detail by van Kammen (68) and will only be briefly summarized here. A variety of clinical variables (e.g., age of onset, number of hospitalizations, brain atrophy) have not been found to consistently predict relapse. Buchanan et al. (8) have recently reported that neuroleptic dose prior to treatment discontinuation is predictive of subsequent relapse (i.e., higher doses are related to a higher rate of relapse). Lieberman et al. (45), but not Buchanan et al. (8), have found that the presence of tardive dyskinesia prior to drug discontinuation was predictive of early relapse. Lieberman et al. (45) have also reported that behavioral responses, blink rate, and pulse rate during a challenge with methylphenidate infusion may be predictive of increased rates of relapse after drug discontinuation.

Plasma concentrations of prolactin (pPRL) may reflect ambient levels of dopamine in the vicinity of the anterior pituitary lactotrophs. However, pPRL have only been variably related to early relapse (23,26). Calculating the ratio of pPRL to plasma neuroleptic concentrations may improve the ability of this neuroendocrine measure to predict relapse using pPRL. Csernansky et al. (16) found an inverse relationship between the ratio of pPRL to plasma neuroleptic activity and both residual paranoid symptoms and tardive dyskinesia during maintenance treatment of younger, but not older, schizophrenic patients.

Plasma homovanillic acid concentrations (pHVA) have also been investigated as a peripheral marker of central nervous system (CNS) dopamine activity in schizophrenic patients during and after discontinuation of maintenance neuroleptic treatment. Lower values for pHVA during maintenance antipsychotic drug treatment have been suggested to predict early relapse during subsequent neuroleptic discontinuation (26) and increases in pHVA following discontinuation have been associated with clinical decompensation (18). Newcomer et al. (53) performed a parallel assessment of pPRL and pHVA as markers of central dopamine activity during maintenance neuroleptic treatment and following an abrupt 50% dose decrease. However, in this study, no relationship was found between pPRL or pHVA prior to the dose decrease and relapse following the dose decrease. Further research is needed to establish the sensitivity and specificity of pPRL, pHVA, and responses to provocative challenge paradigms, such as methylphenidate infusions, as predictors of the vulnerability for relapse in schizophrenic patients.

Limitations of Current Work and Needs for Future Research

The last decade has seen a tremendous amount of work aimed at establishing optimal drug treatments for the prevention of relapse. Yet, the drugs available for use in the treatment of schizophrenia are now changing (see Chapter 108, *this volume*). The introduction of atypical antipsychotic drugs, such as clozapine and risperidone will present the field with new opportunities and challenges. A recent report, indicating that clozapine has superior benefits compared to haloperidol for both short-term improvements in psychopathology and for the prevention of relapse (7), suggests that atypical antipsychotic drugs may be the drugs of choice during the maintenance phase of treatment. Few data have been reported concerning optimal doses of clozapine for the prevention of relapse and comparisons of clozapine treatment with optimal strategies of using typical neuroleptics. In addition, further work needs to be accomplished to discover predictors of relapse and exacerbation that are reliable and readily obtainable.

TREATMENT FOR NEGATIVE SYMPTOMS AND IMPROVED QUALITY OF LIFE

Varying Doses of Typical Drugs

Efficacy for the treatment of negative symptoms during the maintenance phase of treatment may be highly related to the relative absence of neurological side effects. Recently, Van Putten et al. have shown that greater severity of pseudoparkinsonism, dysphoria, and depression and poor efficacy for the treatment of negative symptoms occur together with the use of greater than optimal doses and plasma concentrations of conventional antipsychotic drugs during acute treatment (62,63). In these studies, Van Putten and colleagues suggest that haloperidol doses of 20 mg/day or more and plasma concentrations above 12 ng/ml are associated with increased pseudoparkinsonism, greater dysphoria, the loss of efficacy for negative symptom treatment, and with no substantial additional antipsychotic benefits compared to lower doses (5 to 10 mg/day) and blood levels (5 to 12 ng/ml) after 4 weeks of treatment. Such relationships between the ability to assess a drug's efficacy for negative symptoms and the severity of confounding side effects in all likelihood also persist into the maintenance phase of treatment (see below).

Typical and Atypical Drug Selection

There are few available studies that have addressed the question of the efficacy of typical neuroleptics for the treatment of negative symptoms during maintenance treatment. With regard to acute treatment studies of inpatients, there remains considerable controversy regarding the effects of typical neuroleptics on negative symptoms. Some early studies indicate that the negative symptoms of schizophrenia respond poorly to typical neuroleptic drugs (3,35). However, Meltzer (49) has criticized these studies because of inadequate sample size, the use of rating instruments that may be insensitive to negative symptom assessment, and the fact that the patients had not been chosen to have a minimum level of negative symptoms. Meltzer (49) and Goldberg (27) have conducted comprehensive reviews of the relevant literature and suggested that typical neuroleptic drugs are efficacious for the treatment of negative symptoms, although the magnitude of the effect is small compared to their efficacy for positive symptoms. In addition, Van Putten's work suggests that efficacy of typical neuroleptics for the treatment of negative symptoms may be masked by pseudoparkinsonism in those patients who are prescribed higher than optimal doses (63).

It should be remembered, however, that there are few data to determine whether typical neuroleptic drugs have efficacy for the treatment of negative symptoms that develop or persist in the absence of positive symptoms. In all of the studies reported above, both positive and negative, the negative symptoms in question were concurrent with positive symptoms. Negative symptoms that are enduring and occur independently of positive symptoms (i.e., primary negative symptoms) have been used to identify patients with the so-called deficit syndrome (10). Increasing efforts have been made in recent years to distinguish primary negative symptoms from secondary negative schizophrenic symptoms, that may derive from positive symptoms, depression, or social isolation (10). The responsiveness of primary negative symptoms versus secondary negative symptoms to typical neuroleptics in acute or maintenance treatment settings has not yet been adequately studied to permit meaningful conclusions.

In studies of schizophrenic patients who are resistant to the antipsychotic effects of typical neuroleptics, these drugs have also failed to demonstrate efficacy for negative symptoms (38). It should be noted, however, that most such studies are of only 4- to 6-weeks duration. The possibility of a delayed effect of these drugs on negative symptoms in neuroleptic-resistant patients has not been fully investigated.

There is growing evidence that atypical neuroleptics have substantial efficacy for the treatment of negative symptoms, at least in the acute setting. Clozapine, the prototypical drug in this category, has been shown to be effective for the treatment of negative symptoms in both neuroleptic-responsive (13) and neuroleptic-resistant schizophrenic patients (38). However, Breier et al. (7) showed that clozapine only had a modest advantage over haloperidol for the treatment of negative symptoms in outpatients with schizophrenia. Clozapine's efficacy for the treatment of negative symptoms in neuroleptic-refractory patients may be associated with long-term benefits for the patients' quality of life. In an open study of refractory schizophrenic patients followed for 6 months in the community, Meltzer and colleagues showed that clozapine treatment was able to improve deficits in social functioning in a variety of areas, including work ability and interpersonal relationships (48). However, the question of whether clozapine is effective for the treatment of primary negative symptoms has yet to be answered.

Hopefully, other new antipsychotics may be more effective than typical neuroleptics for the treatment of negative symptoms. For example, risperidone, has been shown to improve negative symptoms in a manner superior to haloperidol, but perhaps only at certain intermediate doses (i.e., 6 mg/day) (12,14).

Adjunctive Drugs for the Treatment of Negative Symptoms

Given the similarity of negative symptoms and depression (see below), it is not surprising that antidepressants have been tried for the treatment of negative symptoms in schizophrenic patients. In a study of schizophrenic patients with negative symptoms who also met criteria for postpsychotic depression, the addition of imipramine to ongoing fluphenazine treatment produced a modest improvement in the patients' negative symptoms (59). Some (15,70), but not all (1), investigators have suggested that alprazolam, a triazolobenzodiazepine with antidepressant properties, may also be of some benefit for negative symptoms when added to typical neuroleptics (15,70), but tolerance may develop to these effects (17). Taken together, these studies suggest that drug treatments that have shown efficacy for the treatment of depression may also have limited efficacy for the treatment of negative schizophrenic symptoms.

Limitations of Current Work and Needs for Future Research

No firm conclusions can be drawn from the available research studies as to the efficacy of drug treatments for the maintenance treatment of negative symptoms in schizophrenic patients. Nonetheless, negative symptoms adversely affect quality of life and need to be emphasized as a target of drug therapy. Atypical neuroleptics, such as clozapine, and risperidone, have tentatively been shown to be more effective than typical neuroleptics for the treatment of negative symptoms in the acute setting, but further studies are needed to determine whether these drugs will have similar efficacy for the treatment of negative symptoms in outpatients, in particular those who have the most primary, enduring negative symptoms. Adjunctive drugs with antidepressant activity, such as tricyclics and alprazolam, may be useful in some patients, but overlaps between negative symptoms and other syndromes (e.g., postpsychotic depression) confound current research results.

MINIMIZATION OF DRUG SIDE EFFECTS

Pseudoparkinsonism and Akathisia

Maintenance treatment with neuroleptics is often complicated by persistent neurological side effects, similar to those that develop during acute treatment (e.g., pseudoparkinsonism and akathisia). Pseudoparkinsonism is a well-described side effect of neuroleptic treatment, occurring with a frequency and severity determined by neuroleptic dose (see below). Akathisia, defined as a subjective restlessness with or without objective motor signs, is also a frequent side effect of neuroleptic treatment (2), occurring in approximately 20% of patients (6). Both pseudoparkinsonism and akathisia can compromise patients' quality of life either directly or through decreased medication compliance leading to subsequent relapses (67). Investigations with both schizophrenic inpatients and outpatients have supported the finding that overall neuroleptic treatment outcome may be worse in patients who develop akathisia (43,52,63).

Both pseudoparkinsonism and akathisia appear to be dose-related side effects, with a threshold for onset. Farde et al. (24) recently reported that clinical efficacy with typical neuroleptics is associated with approximately 70% striatal D_2 receptor occupancy, whereas pseudoparkinsonism is associated with approximately 80% or greater occupancy. These results suggest that effective antipsychotic treatment without pseudoparkinsonism might be achieved by using careful dose titration. In this regard, McEvoy et al. (47) have reported on the use of a threshold neuroleptic dosing strategy, in which an effective antipsychotic dose was achieved by gradually titrating the dose to a level just below the threshold of pseudoparkinsonism. However, neuroleptic-naive subjects were overrepresented in this sample, and the generalizability of these results to more chronically ill patients remains to be established.

Neuroleptic-induced akathisia is also associated with higher neuroleptic doses and higher plasma neuroleptic concentrations. Following a metaanalysis of several investigations, Baldessarini et al. (4) suggested that the diminishing clinical benefits of higher neuroleptic doses

may be due, at least in part, to worsening side effects, such as akathisia. However, other investigations have failed to find a relationship between either haloperidol dose or plasma concentration and the severity of akathisia (43,52). The results of these latter studies suggest a threshold model for akathisia, with no further increases in severity following dose increases beyond the onset threshold. Overall, these findings provide support for the idea that careful selection of lower neuroleptic doses during acute and maintenance treatment can minimize the severity of pseudoparkinsonism and akathisia and enhance therapeutic efficacy.

While the primary approach to minimizing neuroleptic side effects is to use the lowest effective drug doses, this approach may not be advisable or attainable in all patients, due to individual risks of relapse, suicide, or other complications. In some patients, pseudoparkinsonism can be readily treated with anticholinergic medications, such as benztropine mesylate or trihexyphenidyl. Akathisia may also respond to anticholinergic medication, especially when it appears in concert with pseudoparkinsonism. However, some groups of patients or variants of akathisia appear to be refractory to treatment with anticholinergic drugs (6,25,64). Other proposed treatments for akathisia include amantadine, benzodiazepines, clonidine, and the beta blockers (2). Beta blockers appear to act rapidly through a central mechanism, are effective at relatively low doses (e.g., 20 to 80 mg of propranolol/day), and their use does not appear to be limited by the development of tolerance during extended treatment. Finally, atypical antipsychotics, such as clozapine (38) and risperidone (12,14), may offer a lower incidence and severity of neurological side effects, such as pseudoparkinsonism and akathisia.

Overlap between Schizophrenic Symptom Groupings, Depression, and Side Effects

There are important relationships between groupings of schizophrenic symptoms, especially negative symptoms,

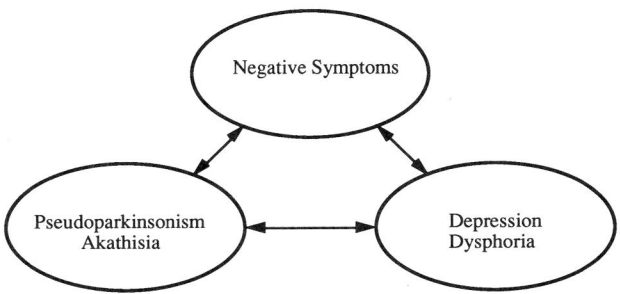

FIG. 1. Interrelationships among negative schizophrenic symptoms, antipsychotic drug side-effects, and disturbances of mood.

and neurological side effects in schizophrenic patients receiving maintenance treatment (see Fig. 1). Thus, any attempt to minimize neurological side effects during maintenance treatment may have important additional benefits in enhancing the apparent efficacy of treatment. Neuroleptic-induced pseudoparkinsonism, sedation, and dysphoria can confound the assessment of negative symptoms (10,67). Over the last several years, there have been substantial improvements in our understanding of negative symptoms, and the overlap between negative symptoms and neuroleptic-induced pseudoparkinsonism (54) and some forms of depressive symptomatology (51,54).

Prosser et al. (54) evaluated the relationship between negative symptoms, depression, and pseudoparkinsonism in outpatients with schizophrenia undergoing maintenance treatment with neuroleptics. A significant correlation was found between the severity of negative symptoms and pseudoparkinsonism. Negative symptoms were unrelated to subjective feelings of depression in this group of patients, but they were significantly correlated with some specific behavioral and vegetative features of depression, such as decreased work and activities, motor retardation, and decreased libido. While these results suggest a substantial overlap between negative symptoms and both neuroleptic-induced pseudoparkinsonism and some features of depression, the apparent relationship between depression and negative symptoms may have been neuroleptic-induced, at least in part. To address this issue, Newcomer et al. (51) examined a large sample of inpatients with schizophrenia, following the withdrawal of neuroleptics. Again, the severity of negative symptoms was not found to be correlated with the severity of subjective feelings of depression. However, several specific features of depression, such as motor retardation and loss of initiative for work and other activities were significantly correlated with the severity of negative symptoms. Overall, these studies suggest that although the subjective features of depressed mood and thought content can be distinguished from the flattened affect associated with negative symptoms, some features related to motor activity and behavior appear to be common to depression and negative symptoms.

Several recent investigations of both inpatient and outpatient schizophrenic patients also suggest a substantial relationship between neuroleptic-induced akathisia and poorer efficacy for the treatment of positive symptoms (43,52). For example, Levinson et al. (43) found that development of akathisia during treatment of schizophrenic inpatients with fluphenazine was associated with a poor antipsychotic response. However, Van Putten et al. (63) failed to find a relationship between akathisia and higher levels of psychotic symptoms during the acute treatment of inpatients with schizophrenia.

Neuroleptic-induced akathisia has also been linked to higher levels of anxiety and depression (64), suicide (20), and violence (42) in schizophrenic patients undergoing maintenance treatment. Given the fragile limitations of most outpatient treatment settings, these complications of maintenance neuroleptic treatment are particularly of concern. The nature of these interrelationships has been recently clarified in a combined study of both acute inpatients and clinically stabilized schizophrenic outpatients, both receiving haloperidol treatment (52). The acute inpatients participated in a fixed-dose (20 mg/day), 2-week, haloperidol treatment protocol. The stabilized outpatients had previously received at least 2 years of neuroleptic treatment, were on a stable dose of haloperidol for at least 3 weeks, and were without current evidence of clinical instability. In both the acute inpatients and in the stabilized outpatients, the severity of akathisia was strongly correlated with the overall level of psychopathology. Furthermore, a stepwise regression revealed that symptoms of depression and dysphoria best explained this correlation. Notably, neither the acute nor the stabilized outpatient treatment sample met syndromal criteria for a mood disorder.

These results are consistent with the previous proposal by Van Putten et al. (63) that neuroleptic-induced dysphoria may largely explain the relationship between residual psychopathology and akathisia during both acute and maintenance neuroleptic treatment. This is also consistent with an early observation that the clinical presentation of akathisia can be mistaken for agitated depression (37). The hypothesis that a common brain mechanism underlies both akathisia and poor treatment response (43) may be seen as a variant of the earlier suggestion of Van Putten and May (65) and Singh (58) that neuroleptic-induced dysphoria predicts a poor treatment response.

Limitations of Current Work and Needs for Future Research

Although atypical antipsychotic drugs, such as clozapine, appear to have a lower incidence of neurological side effects, additional research will be required to establish optimal relapse prevention doses. Although low-dose versus high-dose studies have been conducted with typical neuroleptics, this work is just beginning with atypical neuroleptics drugs. For example, the risperidone study of Chouinard et al. (12) suggests that 6 mg/day may be an optimal dose, yielding both fewer side effects and greater efficacy for the treatment of both psychosis and negative symptoms.

Much attention has been given to the overlap between neuroleptic-induced pseudoparkinsonism and negative symptoms, but the overlap of akathisia-associated dysphoria with negative symptoms deserves further study. Prospective studies would be of value in clarifying the direction of cause-and-effect relationships among akathisia, dysphoria, and residual symptoms. In the studies cited above, no relationships were found between the severity of symptoms prior to treatment and the subsequent severity of akathisia, which suggests that neuroleptic treatment produced the relationships among these variables. However, a stronger case for this hypothesis could be made by altering neuroleptic dose or treating the akathisia and then evaluating effects on dysphoria and selected symptom groupings.

COMBINED PHARMACOLOGICAL AND PSYCHOSOCIAL TREATMENTS

Although the efficacy of psychosocial treatments for schizophrenia is not the central topic of this chapter, there is little doubt that the optimization of maintenance treatment paradigms for schizophrenic patients must involve attention to important psychosocial variables. Psychosocial treatments can alter environmental features related to relapse, offer opportunities and training to improve quality of life, and enhance compliance with drug treatments. Furthermore, combinations of drug treatments and psychosocial interventions are carried out on an everyday basis in most outpatient clinics, although there are few studies to adequately guide practice.

Efficacy of Psychosocial Treatments for Relapse Prevention and Negative Symptoms

The relationship between environmental stressors and a poor outcome in schizophrenia has been discussed for many years (69). In particular, high levels of interpersonal stress within the patient's family, sometimes referred to as high expressed emotion, have been linked to higher rates of relapse in remitted patients. Psychosocial treatments aimed at educating family members about important management issues and diminishing interpersonal criticism have been found to be effective in diminishing rates of relapse while patients are receiving maintenance neuroleptics (22). This benefit appears to have some specificity, since behavioral interventions related to decreasing high levels of expressed emotion have been found to be superior to a general educational program involving patients and their families (60). Long-term follow-up studies of the efficacy of such psychosocial interventions suggest that the benefits of this intervention can be relatively long-lasting (31).

Psychosocial approaches to treatment may also decrease negative symptoms and enhance quality of life in schizophrenic patients. In a controlled study of schizophrenic outpatients, Liberman and colleagues demonstrated that the application of specific social skills training techniques improved social adjustment and decreased rates of relapse and rehospitalization (44). Furthermore,

Bellack and colleagues have shown that a specific social skills training program could lead to ongoing improvements in symptomatology and functioning, even after treatment has been completed (5).

Combining Drug Treatments and Psychosocial Treatment

There have been relatively few studies where the interaction of psychosocial treatments and drug treatments has been specifically studied. In general, such studies are complex and expensive, requiring a variety of control conditions. Hogarty et al. (32) examined the efficacy of a psychosocial treatment program in patients treated with either a standard or low dose of fluphenazine decanoate. In this study, patients who came from a high expressed-emotion environment showed higher rates of relapse in particular when treated with the lower neuroleptic dose. This study suggests that when attempting to minimize the dose of maintenance neuroleptic, special attention should be given to the patient's psychosocial environment. In addition, psychosocial treatment may also be used to enhance compliance with drug treatments. For example, Eckman et al. (21) recently demonstrated that the implementation of a behaviorally oriented program for teaching medication compliance was feasible in a large urban care–delivery system and was effective in improving the intended skills.

Needs for Future Research

Further research is needed to determine the optimal ways of combining drug treatments and psychosocial interventions. In particular, the combination of psychosocial treatment with atypical antipsychotic drugs, that have fewer side effects and greater benefits for negative symptoms would appear to be an attractive approach to minimizing relapse rates and maximizing quality of life in schizophrenic patients.

REFERENCES

1. Adan F, Siris SG. Trials of adjunctive alprazolam in "negative symptom" patients. *Can J Psychiatry* 1989;34:326–328.
2. Adler LA, Angrist B, Reiter S, Rotrosen J. Neuroleptic-induced akathisia: a review. *Psychopharmacology* 1989;97:1–11.
3. Angrist B, Rotrosen J, Gershon S. Differential effects of amphetamine and neuroleptics on negative vs. positive symptoms in schizophrenia. *Psychopharmacology* 1980;72:17–19.
4. Baldessarini RJ, Cohen BM, Teicher MH. Significance of neuroleptic dose and plasma level in the pharmacological treatment of psychoses. *Arch Gen Psychiatry* 1988;45:79–91.
5. Bellack AS, Turner SM, Hersen M, Luber RF. An examination of the efficacy of social skills training for chronic schizophrenic patients. *Hosp Community Psychiatry* 1984;35:1023–1028.
6. Braude WM, Barnes TRE, Gore SM. Clinical characteristics of akathisia. *Br J Psychiatry* 1983;143:134–150.

7. Breier A, Buchanan RW, Kirkpatrick B, et al. Clozapine in schizophrenic outpatients: efficacy, long-term outcome, and relationship to prefrontal cortex. *Schiz Res* 1993;9:257–258.

8. Buchanan RW, Kirkpatrick B, Summerfelt A, Hanlon TE, Levine J, Carpenter WT Jr. Clinical predictors of relapse following neuroleptic withdrawal. *Biol Psychiatry* 1992;32:72–78.

9. Carpenter WT Jr, Hanlon TE, Heinrichs DW, et al. Continuous versus targeted medication in schizophrenic outpatients: outcome results. *Am J Psychiatry* 1990;147:1138–1148.

10. Carpenter WT Jr, Heinrichs DW, Wagman AM. Deficit and non-deficit forms of schizophrenia: the concept. *Am J Psychiatry* 1988;145:578–583.

11. Carpenter WT Jr, Heinrichs DW, Hanlon TE. A comparative trial of pharmacologic strategies in schizophrenia. *Am J Psychiatry* 1987;144:1466–1470.

12. Chouinard G, Jones B, Remington G, et al. A Canadian multicenter placebo-controlled study of fixed doses of risperidone and haloperidol in the treatment of chronic schizophrenic patients. *J Clin Psychopharmacol* 1993;13:25–40.

13. Claghorn J, Honigfeld G, Abuzzahab F, et al. The risks and benefits of clozapine versus chlorpromazine. *J Clin Psychopharmacol* 1987;7:377–384.

14. Claus A, Bollen J, De Cuyper H, et al. Risperidone versus haloperidol in the treatment of chronic schizophrenic inpatients: a multicenter double-blind comparative study. *Acta Psychiatr Scand* 1992;85:295–305.

15. Csernansky JG, Lombrozo L, Gulevich GD, Hollister LE. Treatment of negative schizophrenic symptoms with alprazolam: a preliminary open-label study. *J Clin Psychopharmacol* 1984;4:349–352.

16. Csernansky JG, Prosser E, Kaplan J, Mahler E, Berger PA, Hollister LE. Possible associations among plasma prolactin levels, tardive dyskinesia, and paranoia in treated male schizophrenics. *Biol Psychiatry* 1986;21:632–642.

17. Csernansky JG, Riney SJ, Lombrozo L, Overall JE, Hollister LE. Double-blind comparison of alprazolam, diazepam and placebo for the treatment of negative schizophrenic symptoms. *Arch Gen Psychiatry* 1988;45:655–659.

18. Davidson M, Kahn RS, Powchik P, et al. Changes in plasma homovanillic acid concentrations in schizophrenic patients following neuroleptic discontinuation. *Arch Gen Psychiatry* 1991;48:73–76.

19. Davis JM. Maintenance therapy and the natural course of schizophrenia. *J Clin Psychiatry* 1985;11:18–21.

20. Drake RE, Ehrlich J. Suicide attempts associated with akathisia. *Am J Psychiatry* 1985;142:499–501.

21. Eckman TA, Liberman RP, Phipps CC, Blair KE. Teaching medication management skills to schizophrenic patients. *J Clin Psychopharmacol* 1990;10:33–38.

22. Falloon IRH, Boyd JL, McGill CW, et al. Family management in the prevention of morbidity of schizophrenia. Clinical outcome of a two-year longitudinal study. *Arch Gen Psychiatry* 1985;42:887–896.

23. Faraone SV, Brown WA, Laughren TP. Serum neuroleptic levels, prolactin levels, and relapse: a two-year study of schizophrenic outpatients. *J Clin Psychiatry* 1987;48:151–154.

24. Farde L, Nordstrom A-L, Wiesel F-A, Pauli S, Halldin C, Sedvall G. Positron emission tomographic analysis of central dopamine receptor occupancy in patients treated with classical neuroleptics and clozapine: relation to extrapyramidal side effects. *Arch Gen Psychiatry* 1992;49:538–544.

25. Friis T, Christensen TR, Gerlach J. Sodium valproate and biperiden in neuroleptic-induced akathisia, parkinsonism and hyperkinesia: a double-blind cross-over study with placebo. *Acta Psychiatr Scand* 1982;67:178–187.

26. Glazer WM, Bowers MB Jr, Charney DS, Heninger GR. The effect of neuroleptic discontinuation on psychopathology, involuntary movements, and biochemical measures in patients with persistent tardive dyskinesia. *Biol Psychiatry* 1989;26:224–233.

27. Goldberg SC. Negative and deficit symptoms in schizophrenia do respond to neuroleptics. *Schiz Bull* 1985;11:453–456.

28. Herz MI, Lamberti JS, Schwarzkopf SB, Crilly JF. Prodromal symptoms in schizophrenia: a prospective study and review. *Schiz Res* 1993;9:266.

29. Herz MI, Melville C. Relapse in schizophrenia. *Am J Psychiatry* 1980;137:801–805.

30. Herz MI, Szymanski HV, Simon JC. Intermittent medication for stable schizophrenic outpatients: an alternative to maintenance medication. *Am J Psychiatry* 1982;139:918–922.

31. Hogarty GE, Anderson CM, Reiss DJ, et al. Family psychoeducation, social skills training, and maintenance chemotherapy in the aftercare treatment of schizophrenia. II. Two-year effects of a controlled study on relapse and adjustment. *Arch Gen Psychiatry* 1991;48:340–347.

32. Hogarty GE, McEvoy JP, Munetz M, et al. Dose of fluphenazine, familial expressed emotion, and outcome in schizophrenia. *Arch Gen Psychiatry* 1988;45:797–805.

33. Jeste DV, Potkin SG, Sinha S, et al. Tardive dyskinesia—reversible and persistent. *Arch Gen Psychiatry* 1979;36:585–590.

34. Johnston-Cronk K, Marder SR, Wirshing WC, et al. Prediction of schizophrenic relapse using prodromal symptoms. *Schiz Res* 1993;9:259.

35. Johnstone EC, Frith CD, Gold A, Crow TJ. The outcome of severe acute schizophrenic illnesses after one year. *Br J Psychiatry* 1979;134:28–33.

36. Jolley AG, Hirsch SR, Morrison E, McRink A, Wilson L. Trial of brief intermittent neuroleptic prophylaxis for selected schizophrenic outpatients: clinical and social outcome at two years. *Br Med J* 1990;301:837–842.

37. Kalinowsky LB. Appraisal of the "tranquilizers" and their influence on other somatic treatments in psychiatry. *Am J Psychiatry* 1958;115:294–300.

38. Kane J, Honigfeld G, Singer J, Meltzer H. Clozapine for the treatment-resistant schizophrenic. A double-blind comparison with chlorpromazine. *Arch Gen Psychiatry* 1988;45:789–796.

39. Kane JM, Davis JM, Schooler NR, Marder SR, Brauzer B, Casey DE. A one-year comparison of four dosages of haloperidol decanoate. *Schiz Res* 1993;9:239–240.

40. Kane JM, Lieberman JA: Maintenance pharmacotherapy in schizophrenia. In: Meltzer HY, ed. *Psychopharmacology: the third generation of progress. The emergence of molecular biology and biological psychiatry.* New York: Raven Press; 1987:1103–1109.

41. Kane JM, Rifkin A, Woerner M, et al. Low-dose neuroleptic treatment of outpatient schizophrenics: I. Preliminary results for relapse rates. *Arch Gen Psychiatry* 1983;40:893–896.

42. Keckica WA. Violence as a manifestation of akathisia. *JAMA* 1978;240:2185.

43. Levinson DF, Simpson GM, Singh H, et al. Fluphenazine dose, clinical response, and extrapyramidal symptoms during acute treatment. *Arch Gen Psychiatry* 1990;47:761–768.

44. Liberman RP, Mueser RP, Mueser KT, Wallace CJ. Social skills training for schizophrenic individuals at risk for relapse. *Am J Psychiatry* 1986;143:523–526.

45. Lieberman JA, Kane JM, Sarantakos S, et al. Prediction of relapse in schizophrenia. *Arch Gen Psychiatry* 1987;44:597–603.

46. Marder SR, Van Putten T, Mintz J, Lebell M, McKenzie J, May PRA. Low- and conventional-dose maintenance therapy with fluphenazine decanoate: two-year outcome. *Arch Gen Psychiatry* 1987;44:518–521.

47. McEvoy JP, Hogarty GE, Steingard S. Optimal dose of neuroleptic in acute schizophrenia. *Arch Gen Psychiatry* 1991;48:739–745.

48. Meltzer HY, Burnett S, Bastani B, Ramirez LF. Effects of six months of clozapine treatment on the quality of life of chronic schizophrenic patients. *Hosp Community Psychiatry* 1990;41:892–897.

49. Meltzer HY. Dopamine and negative symptoms in schizophrenics: critique of the type I-type II hypothesis. In: M. Alpert, ed. *Controversies in schizophrenia: changes and constancies.* New York: Guilford Press; 1985:10–136.

50. Müller P, Bandelow B, Gaebel W, et al. Intermittent medication, coping and psychotherapy interactions in relapse prevention and course modification. *Br J Psychiatry* 1992;161(Suppl 18):140–144.

51. Newcomer JW, Faustman WO, Yeh W, Csernansky JG. Distinguishing depression and negative symptoms in unmedicated patients with schizophrenia. *Psychiatry Res* 1990;243–250.

52. Newcomer JW, Miller LS, Faustman WO, Wetzel MW, Vogler GP, Csernansky JG. Correlations between akathisia and residual

psychopathology: a by-product of neuroleptic-induced dysphoria. *Br J Psychiatry* [*in press*].

53. Newcomer JW, Riney SJ, Vinogradov S, Csernansky JG. Plasma prolactin and homovanillic acid as markers for psychopathology and abnormal movements after neuroleptic dose decrease. *Psychopharmacol Bull* 1992;28:101–107.

54. Prosser ES, Csernansky JG, Kaplan J, Thiemann S, Becker TJ, Hollister LE. Depression, parkinsonian symptoms, and negative symptoms in schizophrenics treated with neuroleptics. *J Nerv Ment Dis* 1987;175:100–105.

55. Schooler NR, Keith SJ, Severe JB, et al. Acute treatment response and short term outcome in schizophrenia: first results of the NIMH treatment strategies in schizophrenia study, Treatment Strategies in Schizophrenia Collaborative Study Group. *Psychopharmacol Bull* 1989;25:331–335.

56. Schooler NR, Keith SJ, Severe JB, Matthews SM. Treatment strategies in schizophrenia: effects of dosage reduction and family management on outcome. *Schiz Res* 1993;9:260.

57. Schooler NR. Maintenance medication for schizophrenia: strategies for dose reduction. *Schizophrenia Bull* 1991;17:311–324.

58. Singh MM. Dysphoric response to neuroleptic treatment in schizophrenia and its prognostic significance. *Dis Nerv Syst* 1976;37:191–196.

59. Siris SG, Adan F, Cohen M, Mandeli J, Aronson A, Casey E. Postpsychotic depression and negative symptoms: an investigation of syndromal overlap. *Am J Psychiatry* 1988;145:1532–1537.

60. Tarrier N, Barrowclough C, Vaughn C, Bamrah JS, Porceddu K, Watts S, Freeman H. The community management of schizophrenia.

61. Van Putten T, Crumpton E, Yale C. Drug refusal in schizophrenia and the wish to be crazy. *Arch Gen Psychiatry* 1976;33:1443–1446.

62. Van Putten T, Marder SR, Mintz J, Poland RE. Haloperidol plasma levels and clinical response: a therapeutic window relationship. *Am J Psychiatry* 1992;149:500–505.

63. Van Putten T, Marder SR, Mintz J. A controlled dose comparison of haloperidol in newly admitted schizophrenic patients. *Arch Gen Psychiatry* 1990;47:754–758.

64. Van Putten T, May PRA, Marder SR. Akathisia with haloperidol and thiothixene. *Arch Gen Psychiatry* 1984;41:1036–1039.

65. Van Putten T, May PRA. Subjective response as a predictor of outcome in pharmacotherapy. *Arch Gen Psychiatry* 1978;35:477–480.

66. Van Putten T. The many faces of akathisia. *Compr Psychiatry* 1975;16:43–47.

67. Van Putten T. Why do schizophrenic patients refuse to take their drugs? *Arch Gen Psychiatry* 1974;31:67–72.

68. van Kammen DP. The biochemical basis of relapse and drug response in schizophrenia: review and hypothesis. *Psychol Med* 1991;21:881–895.

69. Vaughn CE, Leff JP. The influence of family and social factors on the course of psychiatric illness: a comparison of schizophrenic and depressed neurotic patients. *Br J Psychiatry* 1976;129:125–137.

70. Wolkowitz OM, Pickar D, Doran AR, Breier A, Tarell J, Paul SM. Combination alprazolam-neuroleptic treatment of the positive and negative symptoms of schizophrenia. *Am J Psychiatry* 1986;143:85–87.

The controlled trial of a behavioral intervention with families to reduce relapse. *Br J Psychiatry* 1988;153:532–542.

Psychopharmacology: The Fourth Generation of Progress, edited by Floyd E. Bloom and David J. Kupfer. Raven Press, Ltd., New York © 1995.

CHAPTER **108**

Atypical Antipsychotic Drugs

Herbert Y. Meltzer

The distinction between typical and atypical antipsychotic drugs has attained considerable importance since the last edition of this book, because of evidence, reviewed below, that a new generation of antipsychotic drugs with important advantages over the first generation of antipsychotic drugs (i.e., the "typical" antipsychotics, usually referred to as neuroleptics) has been introduced into clinical practice or is in an advanced stage of development (44). Ironically, the best-studied atypical antipsychotic drug is not a new drug at all but an old one, clozapine. Although first synthesized in 1959, the scope and importance of the differences between clozapine and atypical neuroleptics was not appreciated until 1988, following the demonstration of its greater efficacy in at least 30% of schizophrenic patients who had failed to respond to at least three trials of neuroleptic drugs of different classes (27). Other atypical antipsychotic drugs have not been as well studied as clozapine, but there is enough evidence of their relationship to clozapine and of clinically important differences between them and neuroleptics to warrant the new designation.

It should be noted that not all investigators approve of the designation of a group of atypical antipsychotic drugs, preferring to describe all antipsychotic agents in terms of their currently perceived key pharmacological properties (22). This is, in part, because of a lack of agreement on what is the essential definition of atypicality in an antipsychotic drug (42). Common to all definitions of atypical antipsychotic drugs of which I am aware is the ability to produce an antipsychotic action in most patients at doses that do not cause significant acute or subacute extrapyramidal side effects (EPS), such as parkinsonism and akathisia. By this definition, remoxipride, a substituted benzamide, is atypical (32), as is risperidone, a benzisoxazole, although the latter drug's low EPS profile is

evident only at lower doses (e.g., 6–8 mg/day) (9,14). At higher doses, risperidone may be indistinguishable from haloperidol with regard to EPS, indicating that the distinction between typical and atypical antipsychotics requires careful study of dose–response relationships for both EPS and efficacy. Other characteristics that have been included in some definitions of atypicality include (a) failure to increase serum prolactin (PRL) levels; (b) superior efficacy for positive, negative, and disorganization symptoms; and (c) no evidence of tardive dyskinesia or dystonia following chronic administration. This second cluster of properties has been shown to be characteristic of clozapine (43), which is why they are considered by some to be criteria for atypicality. There is evidence that some antipsychotic drugs that satisfy the low acute EPS criterion meet some, but not all of these criteria (e.g., both risperidone and remoxipride elevate serum PRL levels) (72,78). The lower rate and intensity of acute and subacute EPS produced by different atypical antipsychotics may be the result of a variety of biological properties, which they may not share. The differences in clinical profile among atypical antipsychotics identified solely on the basis of low EPS suggests that multiple biological mechanisms may be responsible for the diverse differences between clozapine and typical antipsychotic drugs.

This chapter reviews the recent studies of efficacy, side effects, and indications for clozapine, risperidone, and remoxipride, the other atypical antipsychotic drugs that have been approved for use in a number of countries. Other strategies for developing atypical antipsychotic drugs are also briefly discussed (see also Chapters 106 and 107, *this volume*).

CLOZAPINE

H. Y. Meltzer: Departments of Biological Psychiatry and Psychiatry, Case Western Reserve University, School of Medicine, Cleveland, Ohio 44106.

Clozapine, a dibenzazepine tricyclic that is chemically related to loxapine, which is a neuroleptic, was first clinically tested in the 1960s in Europe. The preclinical profile of clozapine is consistent with a drug that would be an effective antipsychotic with few EPS (i.e., it does not produce catalepsy but does block amphetamine-induced locomotor activity) (42). Its effectiveness as an antipsychotic without producing EPS was confirmed in early clinical trials (3). However, it was observed to produce agranulocytosis at a rate much higher than that usually found with standard neuroleptic drugs (29), approximately 1 in 2,000. This led to the withdrawal of clozapine from clinical use in Europe and the cessation of widespread testing in the United States. However, when many of the schizophrenic patients withdrawn from clozapine at that time did not respond as well to typical neuroleptic drugs or expressed strong preference for clozapine because of its low EPS profile, they were permitted to continue receiving clozapine for prolonged periods. This led to a body of clinical information unparalleled in the history of psychotropic drugs which lack formal approval for general use in a developed society. Clinical experience with clozapine suggested that it differed from typical neuroleptic drugs in causing fewer EPS, had a greatly diminished liability to cause tardive dyskinesia, and that it possibly had superior efficacy for some patients with schizophrenia. Definitive evidence that it did not cause elevations of serum PRL concentrations in man was also noted (42).

A double-blind six-week trial comparing clozapine with chlorpromazine in hospitalized neuroleptic-resistant patients established that is was superior to chlorpromazine for alleviating both positive and negative symptoms as well as improving ward behavior (27). This study also showed that clozapine was well-tolerated in a small group of neuroleptic-intolerant patients. On the basis of this study, clozapine was approved for use in the United States and subsequently in other countries.

Because of its ability to cause granulocytopenia or agranulocytosis in 1% to 2% of patients (29), clozapine has usually not been considered to be a first line drug for the initial treatment of schizophrenia or for those chronic patients whose positive symptoms respond to typical antipsychotic drugs (see below). Rather, the chief indication for clozapine is considered to be neuroleptic-resistant schizophrenic patients (i.e., those patients with schizophrenia who have an unsatisfactory response to at least two trials of typical neuroleptic drugs of adequate dosage and duration) (27,43). There appears to be no need for three trials if two are unsuccessful. These patients are characterized by persistent moderate positive, negative, or disorganization symptoms, along with impaired cognitive and social function. Conservatively, at least 30% of schizophrenic patients are neuroleptic-resistant. Some schizophrenic patients are resistant to neuroleptics from the first episode, whereas other patients become resistant at a later phase of their illness (38). Pharmacokinetic factors do not account for the poor response to neuroleptic drugs as positron emission studies using D_2 ligands such as ^{11}C-N-methylspiperone demonstrate adequate occupancy of central D_2 receptors in neuroleptic-resistant patients.

The minimum standard for an unsatisfactory response to neuroleptic drugs has not been established. If even moderate social impairment, persistent negative symptoms, and mild-to-moderate positive symptoms are present despite treatment with neuroleptics, it would be reasonable to consider clozapine, because clozapine should produce clinically significant benefits in the majority of such patients.

Patients that are neuroleptic intolerant (i.e., patients with tardive dyskinesia of at least moderate severity despite optimal adjustment of neuroleptic dosage) and patients who cannot tolerate therapeutic doses of even low EPS-producing antipsychotic drugs, such as thioridazine, and are frequently noncompliant because of it, should also be considered candidates for clozapine (43).

The criteria for use of clozapine will change when other drugs are approved that possess some or all of clozapine's advantages. Trials of these agents may be expected to precede trials with clozapine if the risk–benefit ratio of these newer drugs for specific indications is superior. This may be the case for risperidone in neuroleptic-intolerant patients. The risk–benefit ratio for clozapine treatment of neuroleptic-responsive schizophrenic patients must be developed in controlled trials that evaluate multiple dimensions of outcome, including psychopathology, cognition, social function, work function, hospitalization, and cost effectiveness.

There is limited clinical evidence that clozapine is effective in neuroleptic-resistant psychotic children and young adolescents, as well as in elderly, neuroleptic-resistant, or intolerant schizophrenic patients (43). Clozapine is also useful in alleviating psychotic symptoms in demented psychogeriatric patients.

Twelve studies have compared the efficacy of clozapine with standard neuroleptic drugs in non-treatment-resistant schizophrenia (see ref. 3 for a review of these studies). Clozapine was reported to be superior to typical neuroleptic drugs with regard to global psychopathology or specific positive symptoms in seven of these studies whereas five studies failed to show a difference between clozapine and typical drugs. Differences in dosage, duration of study, sample size, and patient composition may account for these differences.

Other Indications

There is limited evidence from case reports that clozapine may be at least as, or more, effective than other antipsychotics in a variety of conditions, such as treatment-resistant mood disorders, including: (a) rapid cycling and dysphoric mania (13); (b) psychotic depression (59); (c) organic psychoses, such as cases of Huntington's chorea refractory to neuroleptic drugs; and (d) refractory psychoses due to severe head injury (51). Clozapine has also proven useful to treat polydypsia in schizophrenic patients (31). Clozapine, at low doses, is extremely useful in treating L-dopa-induced psychoses (19). It seems reasonable that clozapine should be evaluated for use in refractory patients with a variety of neuropsychiatric disorders in which neuroleptic drugs have been shown to be therapeutic.

Administration

Initiation of clozapine treatment should ordinarily be done in patients free of other psychotropic drugs to minimize side effects such as hypotension, sedation, and anticholinergic effects and to avoid interference with those benefits of clozapine that are dependent upon weak D_2-receptor blockade (e.g., low EPS and possibly increased efficacy and cognitive improvement) (43). If typical neuroleptic drugs are coadministered with clozapine to initiate treatment, they should be stopped within the first 2 to 3 weeks. However, controlled trials of the combination of clozapine and neuroleptic drugs versus clozapine alone, are needed to establish whether the use of a neuroleptic does, in fact, delay or impair response to clozapine.

The recommended starting dose of clozapine is 12.5 mg to test for possible hypotensive reactions. Slow titration is recommended until doses of 300 to 450 mg/day are reached, generally by 2 to 3 weeks. This may be done on an outpatient basis. Optimal doses usually range between 450 and 600 mg/day in younger adults, but doses up to 900 mg/day may be needed. Twice-a-day dosage is recommended because the half-life of clozapine is 12 to 16 hr (27). Elderly patients usually respond to 200 to 300 mg/day or even lower doses. There is no data available as to whether lower doses of clozapine may be effective for maintenance treatment.

There are, as yet, no fixed-dose studies to determine optimal dosage. In Europe, clinical practice has been to use doses of 200 to 300 mg/day or even lower (55), whereas in the United States and England, doses of 400 to 600 mg/day are most common (43). The reasons for this discrepancy require further study. It is possible that lower doses are required for neuroleptic-responsive or neuroleptic-intolerant patients than for neuroleptic-resistant cases.

Clozapine improves the three main syndromes of psychopathology in schizophrenia: positive symptoms, negative symptoms, and disorganization (27,45). Improvement is greatest in disorganization followed by positive and then negative symptoms. Although the change in negative symptoms may be slight (10), it can be shown to be independent of the change in positive symptoms, EPS, and depression (52). Affective symptoms in schizoaffective patients improve concurrently. Clozapine appears to be effective in treating aggression and hostility in schizophrenic patients (76). Improvement in social functioning during clozapine treatment has been reported (46). Even

some previously regressed patients with marked defect symptoms have been able to return to work after clozapine (36,46). The marked reduction in rehospitalization that usually results from clozapine treatment also contributes to improvement in social function (42). Psychosocial treatments have been advocated as necessary to facilitate recovery during clozapine treatment (43).

One of the major advantages of clozapine is the ability to improve some aspects of cognitive dysfunction in schizophrenia (23) Cognitive dysfunction is characteristic of schizophrenia from the first episode and may not differ between neuroleptic-resistant and intolerant cases. Typical antipsychotics have rarely been found to produce significant improvement in any aspect of cognitive function. Clozapine has been found to have modest effects to improve attention, verbal fluency, recall memory, and executive function (23) It does not improve performance on the Wisconsin Card Sort Test (23). It remains to be determined if other atypical antipsychotic drugs can also improve cognitive function.

Response to clozapine in neuroleptic-resistant patients may not be evident until after 6 months or after even longer treatment periods (41). Approximately 30% respond by 6 weeks and another 30% respond more slowly. The reasons for such a delayed response to clozapine are unknown. Because of the frequent delay in the onset of its effect and its potential for clinical superiority to standard drugs, clozapine should probably not be discontinued for lack of apparent efficacy before less than six months of treatment have elapsed.

Clozapine may be no more effective than standard neuroleptics in treating positive symptoms in up to 25% of neuroleptic-resistant schizophrenic patients, despite a trial of adequate dose (up to 900 mg/day) or duration (up to 6 months or longer) (46–48). Addition of typical neuroleptic drugs or electroconvulsive therapy (ECT) has been reported to be helpful in some cases, but controlled data is lacking. Selective serotonin uptake inhibitors such as fluoxetine and paroxetine have proven useful to alleviate persistent or emergent depression or obsessive–compulsive symptomatology that is sometimes increased by clozapine (2).

Abrupt withdrawal of clozapine may sometimes be associated with a rapid, severe, and sometimes prolonged exacerbation of psychotic symptoms (58), but this is relatively rare. When clozapine treatment is terminated because of noncompliance or for some other reason and then reinstituted, the response is usually similar but some cases of greatly diminished responsivity have been reported. The reason for this is unknown.

Clinical Pharmacology and Plasma Levels

Peak clozapine plasma levels following the oral administration of clozapine are achieved in 1 to 4 hr (26). The half-life after twice-a-day dosing at the steady state is approximately 14 hr (range 6 to 33 hr). Thus, steady-state levels should be achieved approximately 1 week after constant dose twice-daily administration. The major metabolites of clozapine are desmethylclozapine and clozapine-N-oxide; but they appear to be inactive.

Optimal plasma levels of clozapine in treatment-resistant schizophrenia have been reported to be ≥ 350 ng/ml, range 60 to 1000 ng/ml (24,60), but some patients respond at lower levels. There is no evidence for a therapeutic window. It may be prudent in very carefully selected cases to exceed the recommended limit of 900 mg/day if plasma levels of clozapine are less than 350 ng/ml, and there are no major cardiovascular or other side effects (24). Clozapine metabolism may be blocked by cimetidine, phenytoin, valproic acid, and fluoxetine (see 43 for a review).

Prefrontal sulcal prominence as measured by CT has been reported to be inversely related to response to clozapine, but ventricular brain ratio (VBR) does not predict clinical response (19). Shorter duration of illness, female gender, and younger age are significant predictors of a more favorable response to clozapine.

Drug Interactions

There has been considerable concern about combining clozapine and benzodiazepines because of possible respiratory arrest. However, reliable evidence for a negative interaction between clozapine and benzodiazepines is very slight. Benzodiazepines are sometimes useful in diminishing anxiety when initiating clozapine treatment in neuroleptic-free schizophrenic patients (34).

The combination of clozapine and lithium has been implicated in several cases of neuroleptic malignant syndrome (61) as well as in other types of neurotoxicity (8). These reports suggest lithium should be used with clozapine only if hypomanic symptoms are not adequately controlled with clozapine. Valproic acid may be the safest agent to combine with lithium carbonate therapy if supplemental mood stabilization is required. However, valproic acid may also increase clozapine plasma levels.

Side Effects

Granulocytopenia and Agranulocytosis

The major side effect of clozapine, which limits its use, is its significant risk of granulocytopenia or agranulocytosis (1,29). In the United States, indefinite weekly total white blood cell (WBC) or neutrophil counts are required to permit rapid detection of this potentially fatal side effect. Some countries require only monthly monitoring after the first 4 to 6 months of treatment, because approximately 50% to 80% of cases of neutropenia or agranulocytosis occur within the first 18 weeks of treatment.

The fall in WBC count due to clozapine may be abrupt or gradual. Steadily falling total WBC or neutrophil counts should increase concern, even if none are below 3000/mm^3. An abrupt drop of 3000/mm^3 or more in a single week may signal impending agranulocytosis. When the total WBC count falls below 3000/mm^3 or the neutrophil count below 1500/mm^3, clozapine must be discontinued and the white count with differential must be followed for 4 weeks. Patients who are withdrawn from clozapine during a neutropenic phase (WBC count between 2500 and 3500/mm^3), may be rechallenged, but more intensive and differential monitoring is indicated.

The etiology of clozapine-induced agranulocytosis is unknown. Clozapine itself or its metabolite desmethylclozapine have been implicated in the etiology of agranulocytosis or granulocytopenia (21). Because the duration of agranulocytosis may be longer than for other drug-induced blood dyscrasias, neutropenia fever, should it develop, is often a challenging management problem. Upon withdrawal of clozapine, the hematological status usually returns to normal within 2 to 3 weeks. The successful use of granulocyte colony stimulating factor (G-CSF) to promote more rapid recovery from agranulocytosis has recently been reported (4).

Patients who have developed agranulocytosis on clozapine will experience it again, after only 1 to 4 weeks of treatment (29). Thus, rechallenge with clozapine after clear granulocytopenia or agranulocytosis should not be tried.

Extrapyramidal Reactions

The absence, or very low incidence, of EPS is a major clinical advantage associated with clozapine therapy (43) and contributes significantly to patient acceptance and compliance. There have been no reported cases of dystonic reactions in patients receiving clozapine monotherapy. Compared to typical neuroleptic drugs, clozapine produces much less akathisia. It does not worsen parkinsonian symptoms in Parkinson's disease and may even produce some improvement in bradykinesia, tremor, and rigidity (19). There have been no definite reported cases of tardive dyskinesia linked to clozapine treatment alone. At the same time, clozapine appears effective in blocking this syndrome in up to 67% of patients (12,35). Here again response may be delayed. Approximately 30% of cases with tardive dyskinesia (TD) treated with clozapine will have a remission of TD and another 30% will have a reduction in severity. However, symptoms recur when clozapine is stopped. Clozapine can cause neuroleptic malignant syndrome, which should be managed in the same manner as when the etiology is a typical neuroleptic.

Other Side Effects

Clozapine decreases the seizure threshold, sometimes causing a dose-related increase in major motor seizures or myoclonus (18). Major motor seizures are induced in 1% to 2% of patients at doses below 300 mg/day, 2% to 4% at doses greater than 300 mg/day, and 4% to 6% risk at doses greater than 600 mg/day. Management of these seizures is usually possible, so that discontinuation because of seizures is rarely necessary. Decreasing the dose and pharmacological management of seizures (e.g., addition of valproic acid) is usually able to control the seizures. The electroencephalogram (EEG) is usually abnormal in clozapine-treated patients and is, therefore, of little clinical value (37).

There have been numerous reports of clozapine-induced exacerbations of obsessive–compulsive symptoms (2). This may be due to serotonin$_2$ (5-HT$_2$) receptor blockade and usually responds to treatment with selective serotonin reuptake inhibitors (SSRIs).

The main cardiovascular side effects of clozapine are orthostatic hypotension, tachycardia, and some conduction abnormalities (34). Tachycardia, in patients receiving clozapine, is predominantly the result of the anticholinergic effects of clozapine. Mean heart rate can increase 20 to 25 beats per minute and can persist for over a year in some patients. Similar to orthostatic hypotension, this effect is also dose dependent. Tolerance to the tachycardia develops slowly. β-Adrenergic blockers have been successfully used to decrease clozapine-induced tachycardia. Hypertension may also be observed, most frequently in the first 2 weeks of treatment.

Hypersalivation occurs in about 30% of clozapine-treated patients. Reduction in the dosage of clozapine or treatment with an anticholinergic medication such as benztropine can prove beneficial (34). The α_2-adrenergic agonist clonidine, which causes dry mouth by suppressing sympathomimetic sialagogic mechanisms, may also be helpful in treating hypersalivation due to clozapine.

Weight gain is common with clozapine. In a recent study, the mean clozapine-induced weight gain was 6 kg or 8.9% of body weight (30). The magnitude of weight gain has been reported to be positively correlated with clinical response.

Clozapine does not elevate serum PRL levels (43).

Cost Effectiveness

Two studies have examined the cost effectiveness of clozapine in treatment-resistant schizophrenia. Revicki et al. (63) reported that by the second year of treatment, total costs had decreased more than $24,000 per year in 86 treatment-resistant schizophrenic patients. In a prospective study, Meltzer et al. (47) compared the total costs of treatment for 2 years before and 2 years after clozapine treatment in 37 treatment-resistant schizophrenic patients. The median total cost for 2 years decreased from $42,934 (1987 dollars) to $23,772, a decrease of $19,162. These studies suggest that large savings are possible with clozapine treatment for treatment-resistant schizophrenic patients who have had frequent hospitalizations.

Conclusions

Clozapine provides the possibility of significant help for at least 60% of patients with schizophrenia who fail to respond adequately to typical neuroleptics, as well as a reduced potential to cause EPS, including TD. On the other hand, because of its side-effect profile and the need for blood monitoring, the use of clozapine has been relatively limited. As of April, 1994, it has been tried on 65,000 of the approximately 2,000,000 schizophrenic patients in the United States. Its fate will depend upon the ability of other novel antipsychotic agents, described below, to have similar advantages in efficacy, EPS, and TD, without other serious adverse effects.

RISPERIDONE

Risperidone is a benzisoxazole derivative, chemically unrelated to any other currently available antipsychotic drug. Risperidone, like clozapine, is a potent 5-HT$_{2A}$, 5-HT$_7$, α_1-, α_2-adrenergic and histamine H$_1$ and a relatively weak (in comparison with its affinity for the 5-HT$_2$ receptor) D$_2$ dopamine (DA) receptor antagonist (34). However, its absolute affinity for the D$_2$ receptor is similar to that of haloperidol (1 to 5 nM). It has low potency as an antagonist at D$_1$ and D$_4$ receptors. In vivo, risperidone blocks DA agonist-induced locomotor activity at doses that cause weak catalepsy, a profile that suggests it should produce less EPS at effective antipsychotic doses than typical neuroleptics (40). Risperidone, unlike clozapine, stimulates prolactin secretion in man (6,73), suggesting that at clinically effective doses, it produces a net decrease in dopaminergic activity at the pituitary lactotrophs and should cause galactorrhea in some females.

Clinical Pharmacology

Risperidone is rapidly and completed absorbed following oral administration and reaches peak plasma levels within 2 hr (73). It is extensively metabolized in the liver; 9-hydroxyrisperidone, the major metabolite, has a half-life of 17 to 22 hr compared to 2 to 4 hr (mean 2 to 8 hr) for risperidone. Thus, the pharmacologically active moiety is the sum of risperidone and 9-hydroxyrisperidone. Poor metabolizers of debrisoquine (8% of the Caucasian population) will also be unable to metabolize risperidone because the 9-hydroxylation of risperidone is catalyzed by CYP2 D6. Poor metabolizers of risperidone have half the active moiety of good metabolizers because risperidone levels will be much higher in the poor metabolizers. Elimination of the active moiety is independent of metabolic phenotype with a half-life of 20 hr. For this reason, poor metabolizers of risperidone require the same daily dosage as good metabolizers. There is no data about a relationship between plasma levels of the active moiety and clinical response. No parenteral formulation, either short- or long-acting, is currently available.

Efficacy

Risperidone, in doses of 4 to 10 mg/day, appears to be at least equivalent and possible superior to haloperidol, 10 to 20 mg/day, in decreasing positive and negative symptoms (6,9,13,14,16,50). For some patients, slightly lower or higher doses may be needed. Some studies have reported risperidone to be superior to haloperidol in treating positive and negative symptoms in schizophrenia and to possibly have a faster onset of action (14,16). Risperidone was found to be superior to placebo as add-on therapy to reduce behavioral disturbances in mentally retarded patients (72). There is no evidence yet as to its effect on cognition. The long-term benefits of risperidone and its cost-effectiveness has not yet been studied. The proportion of patients for whom risperidone have superior efficacy to standard treatment is not entirely clear and needs further study. Two of the above studies (14,16) included some apparently neuroleptic-resistant schizophrenic patients, raising the possibility that risperidone might be effective in some, if not all, the patients for whom clozapine is effective. However, no double-blind comparison of risperidone and clozapine has been conducted to date, and, until definitive evidence is available, it would be premature to broaden the indication for risperidone to this class of patients, except for experimental purposes or for patients who fail or cannot tolerate clozapine.

There is some evidence that risperidone can partially mask TD symptoms (14). It has been suggested that risperidone has a lower potential to cause TD or dystonia than typical neuroleptic drugs because it produces fewer EPS, but this is not necessarily the case, as indicated by thioridazine.

Side Effects

Risperidone has been reliably reported to produce fewer EPS than haloperidol at doses of 4 to 6 mg/day (9). Consistent with this, antiparkinsonian agents are needed less frequently with risperidone than with haloperidol but may be required by approximately 20% of patients (14,16). There is clear evidence that the incidence of EPS with risperidone is dose-related, and it should be comparable to haloperidol at higher doses ($\geq$12 mg/day). In clinical practice, it is important to keep the dose of risperidone in the 4 to 8 mg/day range wherever possible. This may require lowering the dose after the acute phase of psychosis is over.

The most common adverse effects of risperidone are insomnia, anxiety, agitation, sedation, dizziness, rhinitis, hypotension, weight gain, and menstrual disturbances (9). Risperidone does not produce granulocytopenia or agranulocytosis, so no weekly monitoring is required, as is

the case with clozapine. For this reason, it may be more acceptable to patients, all other aspects being equal. It may be expected to cause neuroleptic-malignant syndrome and galactorrhea.

Usage

The usual starting dose of risperidone is 1 mg twice daily, increasing to 2 mg twice daily and 3 mg twice daily over the next 2 days. Thus, it can be titrated to optimal therapeutic dose more rapidly than clozapine. The mean optimal dose appears to be 6 mg/day but higher doses may be needed to control positive symptoms in some patients. Since higher doses would increase the risk of EPS and presumably TD, lower dosages should be tried for adequate periods of time. If higher doses are needed acutely, lower doses should be substituted for maintenance treatment. Risperidone, like clozapine, should usually be given without concomitant typical neuroleptic drugs to avoid EPS. However, in a recent study, risperidone was superior to placebo as add-on-therapy to typical neuroleptic drugs in mentally retarded patients with persistent behavioral disturbances (72). This may reflect the value of 5-HT$_2$ antagonism as a supplement to D$_2$ receptor blockade.

Conclusions

Risperidone should prove to be useful as a first line antipsychotic agent. It could prove useful in a myriad of indications where typical neuroleptic drugs have been used: manic–depressive illness, psychotic depression, organic psychoses, especially in the elderly, L-dopa–induced psychoses, schizotypal and borderline psychoses, childhood psychoses, and so on. Its place in the armamentarium of antipsychotic drugs may well depend upon the ability of prescribers to obtain good control over psychopathology using doses of 4 to 6 and possibly 8 mg/day. If higher doses are frequently needed, the risk of clinically significant EPS, including TD, will be increased. The tendency of clinicians to keep increasing doses to achieve rapid response or to use typical neuroleptics concomitantly, will have to be altered for risperidone, if it is to fulfill its full potential as the first atypical first-line antipsychotic drug.

REMOXIPRIDE

Remoxipride, a substituted benzamide, is a selective D$_2$ receptor antagonist. Substituted benzamides such as sulpiride and amisulpride have been very widely used in Europe and Asia. Remoxipride is the first of this interesting class of drugs to be developed for use in North America. This class of compounds has been considered to have advantages with regard to treating negative symptoms and EPS, although the clinical trials to support this have not had the rigor to unequivocally establish these claims. A detailed review of the pharmacodynamic, pharmacokinetic, and early clinical literature is available (78). Animal studies indicate that doses required to block amphetamine-induced locomotor activity are significantly lower than those that produce catalepsy, indicating a potentially atypical profile. It may be expected to reduce mesolimbic dopaminergic activity while sparing the striatum (56). Because of its lack of effect on muscarinic, adrenergic, and histaminergic receptors (56), it produces few side effects. Patients often feel they are not taking any antipsychotic drug. It has a potent affinity for the sigma receptor, but it is unclear whether it is a sigma agonist or antagonist. The contribution of this property to its clinical profile is unknown (28).

Pharmacokinetics

The pharmacokinetics of remoxipride have been summarized (77). It is rapidly absorbed and has good bioavailability, with a plasma half-life of 4 to 7 hr. It has no active metabolites and is approximately 80% bound to plasma proteins. There are, as yet, no known drug interactions, but further study is required.

Clinical Studies

Remoxipride has been extensively studied in large double-blind, multicenter trials in comparison with haloperidol. Lewander et al. (32) provided a combined analysis of nine trials, involving 667 remoxipride- and 437 haloperidol-treated patients. After 4 to 6 weeks of treatment, 55% to 60% of patients in both groups were rated as much or very much improved. Haloperidol and remoxipride produced similar effects on positive and negative symptoms, with approximately 60% and 30% improvement in each class of symptoms, using an intention to treat analysis (32).

There is limited data on the usefulness of remoxipride in neuroleptic-resistant patients. In an open long-term trial of remoxipride in 45 chronic, neuroleptic-resistant schizophrenic patients, there was an 80% drop-out rate despite the absence of EPS. Ten patients (22%) showed a 30% or greater decrease in their total BPRS scores. These patients had relatively low mean BPRS scores at baseline: 18.4. Only 5 out of the 45 patients were considered very much improved (75). The clinically effective dose of remoxipride appears to be between 120 and 600 mg/day (32).

Side Effects

In the composite summary of side effect data from nine multicenter trials, remoxipride appeared to have clear advantages over haloperidol with regard to EPS (32). This was especially true for interference with gait, elbow rigidity, fixation of position, head dropping, tremor, and salivation. However, 20% of remoxipride-treated patients required anticholinergic drugs, indicating that it does have significant EPS liability for vulnerable individuals. There is no evidence to suggest that remoxipride would not induce TD if given for prolonged periods. Of remoxipride-treated patients, 10% to 30% report drowsiness, tiredness, and difficulty concentrating, significantly less than haloperidol but not dramatically so.

Following the introduction of remoxipride in Europe, a significant number of cases of aplastic anemia were reported. The rate may be as high as 1 in 10,000. For this reason, the further use of remoxipride has been halted until the incidence, cause, and possible prevention of this side effect can be further studied. It is not clear if it will ever again be available without major restrictions and monitoring.

Conclusion

Remoxipride appears to be an effective antipsychotic drug that should be particularly useful in treating patients who experience significant EPS and sedation with standard neuroleptic drugs. Because of its ability to cause aplastic anemia, it may not be available for general use. Other substituted benzamides such as amisulpride, should be studied as possible substitutes.

FUTURE DEVELOPMENTS IN ATYPICAL ANTIPSYCHOTIC DRUGS

There are now numerous drugs in advanced stages of clinical testing as potential atypical antipsychotic drugs. These are listed in Table 1 and briefly commented on here. The major focus of drugs in development is on 5-HT_{2A} antagonists, based on the hypothesis that this prop-

TABLE 1. *Novel atypical antipsychotic drugs*

5-HT_2/D_2 antagonists	D_1 antagonist
HP 873	NO-01-0687
Melperone	SCH-39166
Olanzapine	DA autoreceptor agonists
Org 5222	BHT-920
Sertindole	CGS 15873A
Seroquel	DD 118717E
SM-9018	Pramipexole
Zaprisidone	3-PPP
5-HT_{2A} antagonists	SND919
Amperozide	U-66444B
MDL 100,907	Partial DA Agonists
Ritanserin	MER-327
5-HT_3 antagonist	SDZ-208-911
GR 68755C	SD-208-912
Sigma Antagonist	
DUP 734	

erty is a critical facet of the pharmacology of clozapine and risperidone. Melperone, a butyrophenone, which has been used in Europe for two decades, produces low EPS and has a definitely reduced liability to cause TD (48). It has also been found to be a relatively potent $5\text{-}HT_{2A}$ antagonist compared to its D_2 antagonist effects. Its absolute affinity for the $5\text{-}HT_{2A}$ receptor is 30 nM (49). A large number of other antipsychotic drugs with a similar $5\text{-}HT_2/D_2$ profile have been identified. These include Zaprisidone (65), olanzepine (53), Organon 5222 (66), seroquel (64), sertindole (67), and SM-9018 (25). In general, these compounds produce low catalepsy at doses that block amphetamine- or apomorphine-induced locomotor activity and the conditioned-avoidance response, and they have selective effects on the mesolimbic DA neurons, sparing the nigrostriatal system. Because they differ in relative potency as antagonists of a variety of other key receptors (e.g., D_1, D_3, D_4, $5\text{-}HT_{1A}$, $5\text{-}HT_{2C}$, $5\text{-}HT_3$, $5\text{-}HT_6$, $5\text{-}HT_7$, M_1, α_1- and α_2-adrenergic receptors), it is likely that these drugs will have significantly different side effect and efficacy profiles. Some may be effective in treating negative symptoms and improving cognitive dysfunction, others may not, and so on. Meticulous clinical research will be required to delineate the spectrum of action of these compounds. Olanzapine has recently been shown to produce significantly fewer EPS and to produce significantly greater decreases in positive and negative symptoms than haloperidol in schizophrenic patients in an acute exacerbation.

Two drugs related to this class are of special interest: amperozide (7,15) and MDL 100,937 (70). Both are potent $5\text{-}HT_{2A}$ antagonists but have no apparent D_2-receptor blocking effects in vivo and yet have the preclinical or clinical profile, or both, of atypical antipsychotic drugs. Another drug that is a specific $5\text{-}HT_{2A}$ blocker, ritanserin, has also been reported to be effective in treating positive and negative symptoms in schizophrenia. These results suggest that $5\text{-}HT_{2A}$ antagonism *by itself,* may be a sufficient means of treating the full spectrum of symptoms in some types of schizophrenia.

There is considerable behavioral, biochemical, and electrophysiological evidence that $5\text{-}HT_3$ antagonists may be effective antipsychotic drugs (57), but clinical evidence is lacking to support this strategy (17). Blockade of $5\text{-}HT_3$ would be expected to decrease the release of DA, so this strategy is another variation on the theme of decreasing dopaminergic activity to alleviate psychosis. Whether $5\text{-}HT_6$ or $5\text{-}HT_7$ antagonists will be useful to treat psychosis or ameliorate EPS is unknown (see Chapters 37 and 42, *this volume*). There is also some interest in the hypothesis that $5\text{-}HT_{1A}$ agonist properties, in conjunction with D_2-receptor antagonism, may increase the effectiveness and decrease the EPS liability of an antipsychotic drug.

The D_1 receptor has long been known to modulate D_2 receptor function in complex ways (see Chapter 26, *this volume*). D_1-receptor blockade has been thought to be a

potential way to achieve an antipsychotic effect with low EPS (39). There are various D_1 antagonists in clinical development (e.g., SCH 39166, NO-01-0687, DOD 647). Early clinical results with SCH 39166 have been unimpressive. However, this compound may be a partial D_1 agonist. Trials with full D_1 antagonists are underway. Since the cloning of the D_3 and D_4 receptors, which are localized in the mesolimbic, cortical, or striatal areas (see Chapters 14, 25, and 26, *this volume*), the possibility of developing antipsychotic drugs based upon antagonists of these receptors has excited great interest (68,74). There is as yet no preclinical evidence or clinical trials to suggest that drugs that are specific antagonists of the D_3 or D_4 receptors would be advantageous. Partial DA agonists (i.e., drugs that can possibly enhance mesocortical dopaminergic activity by a direct agonist effect while blocking DA-induced stimulation of the mesolimbic system) are being developed. To date, none of the D_2 partial agonists (e.g., SDZ 208-911, SDZ 208-912 and terguride) have been systematically studied in schizophrenia (70).

The strategy of administering DA autoreceptor agonists to suppress the synthesis and release of DA is being studied. Several such compounds have now been developed, including BHT-920, 3-PPP, CGS 15873A, pramipexole, PD 118717, SND 919, WAY-124866 (see ref. 62 for a review of these compounds). The initial clinical studies with these drugs suggest a weak effect on negative symptoms (5).

Finally, the sigma receptor has been implicated in psychosis, but this has been disputed (54). There have been several attempts to test sigma receptor antagonists as antipsychotics (e.g., BMY 14802) without success. A new sigma antagonist with $5\text{-}HT_2$–receptor blocking properties DUP 734 appears to be of particular interest based upon its ability to block the behavioral effects of phencyclidine (71).

Conclusions

It seems clear that antipsychotic drugs that produce fewer EPS than typical neuroleptic drugs may do so via a variety of pharmacological strategies. The key to clozapine's advantages for positive, negative, and cognitive symptoms and signs in schizophrenia is not yet fully known. New antipsychotics that can be shown to share these advantages of clozapine will help identify its key pharmacological properties. It is likely that a multiplicity of effects contribute to the end result.

ACKNOWLEDGMENT

The research reported was supported in part by a U.S. Public Health Service grant MH 41684, and grants from the Elisabeth Severance Prentiss, Milton Maltz, and John Pascal Sawyer Foundations. The author is the recipient of a U.S. Public Health Service Research Career Scientist

Award MH 47808. The secretarial assistance of Ms. Lee Mason is greatly appreciated.

REFERENCES

1. Alvir JMJ, Lieberman JA, Safferman AZ, Schwimmer JL, Schaaf JA. Clozapine-induced agranulocytosis incidence and risk factors in the United States. *New Engl J Med* 1993;329:162–167.
2. Baker RW, Chengappa KN, Baird JW, Steengard S, Christ MA, Schooler NR. Emergence of obsessive-compulsive symptoms during treatment with clozapine. *J Clin Psychiatry* 1992;53:439–442.
3. Baldessarini R, Frankenburg FR. Clozapine: a novel antipsychotic agent. *New Engl J Med* 1991;324:746–754.
4. Barnas C, Swierzina H, Hummer M, Sperner-Unterweger B, Stern A, Fleishchacker WW. Granulocyte-macrophase colony-stimulating factor (GM-CSF) treatment of clozapine-induced agranulocytosis: a case report. *J Clin Psychiatry* 1992;53:245–247.
5. Bankert O, Grüner G, Wetzel H. Dopamine autoreceptor agonists in the treatment of schizophrenia and major depression. *Pharmacopsychiatry* 1992;25:254–260.
6. Bersani G, Bressa GM, Meco G, Pozzi F. Mixed D_2 and S_2 antagonism in a preliminary study with risperidone (R64766). *Hum Psychopharmacol* 1990;5:225–231.
7. Björk A, Bergman I, Gustavsson G. Amperozide in the treatment of schiozprenic patients: a preliminary report. In: Meltzer HY, ed. *Novel atypical antipsychotic drugs*. New York: Raven Press; 1992:47–58.
8. Blake LM, Marks RC, Luchins DJ. Reversible neuroleptic symptoms with clozapine. *J Clin Psychopharmacol* 1992;12:297–298.
9. Borison RL, Diamond BI, Pathiragja A, Meibach RC. Clinical overview of risperidone. In: Meltzer HY, ed. *Novel atypical antipsychotic drugs*. New York: Raven Press; 1992:223–239.
10. Brier A, Buchanan RW, Kirkpatrick B, Davis OR, Irish D, Sumnerfelt, Carpenter WT. Effects of clozapine on positive and negative symptoms in outpatients with schizophrenia. *Am J Psychiatry* 1994;151:20–26.
11. Calabrese JR, Meltzer HY, Markovitz PJ. Clozapine prophylaxis in rapid cycling: bipolar disorder. *J Clin Psychopharmacol* 1991;11:396–397.
12. Casey DE. Clozapine: neuroleptic-induced EPS and tardive dyskinesia. *Psychopharmacol Suppl* 1989;99:S47–S53.
13. Castelao JF, Ferrerira L, Gelders YG, Heylen SLE. The efficacy of the D_2 and 5-HT_2 antagonist risperidone (R64766) in the treatment of chronic psychoses. An open dose finding study. *Schiz Res* 1989;2:411–415.
14. Chouinard G, Jones B, Remington G, et al. A Canadian multicenter placebo-controlled study of fixed doses of risperidone and haloperidol in the treatment of chronic schizophrenic patients. *J Clin Psychopharmacol* 1993;13:35–40.
15. Christensson EG. Amperozide and some other atypical compounds with antipsychotic effect. In: Meltzer HY, ed. *Novel atypical antipsychotic drugs*. New York: Raven Press; 1992:19–32.
16. Claus A, Bollen J, de Cuyper H, et al. Risperidone versus haloperidol in the treatment of chronic schizophrenic inpatients: a multicentre double-blind comparative study. *Acta Psychiatr Scand* 1992;85:295–305.
17. DeVeaugh-Geiss J, McBain S, Gooksey PG, Bell JM. The effects of a novel 5-HT_3 antagonist, ondansetron, in schizophrenia: results from uncontrolled trials. In: Meltzer HY, ed. *Novel atypical antipsychotic drugs*. New York: Raven Press; 1992:225–232.
18. Devinsky O, Honigfeld G, Patin J. Clozapine-related seizures. *Neurology* 1991;41:369–371.
19. Friedman JH, Lannon MC. Clozapine in the treatment of psychosis in Parkinson's disease. *Neurology* 1989;39:1219–1221.
20. Friedman L, Knutson L, Shurell M, Meltzer HY. Prefrontal sulcal prominence is inversely related to response to clozapine in schizophrenic patients. *Biol Psychiatry* 1991;29:865–877.
21. Gerson SL, Meltzer HY. Mechanisms of clozapine-induced agranulocytosis. *Drug Safety* 1992;7:17–25.
22. Gerlach J, Casey DE. Drug treatment of schizophrenia: myths and realities. *Curr Opin Psychiatry* 1994;7:65–70.
23. Hagger C, Buckley P, Kenny JT, Friedman L, Ubogy D, Meltzer HY. Improvement in cognitive function and psychiatric symptoms in treatment-refractory schizophrenic patients receiving clozapine. *Biol Psychiatry* 1993;34:702–712.
24. Hasegawa M, Gutierrez-Esteinou R, Way L, Meltzer HY. Relationship between clinical efficacy and clozapine plasma concentrations in schizophrenia: effect of smoking. *J Clin Psychopharmacol* 1993;13:383–390.
25. Hirose A, Kato T, Ohno Y, et al. Pharmacological actions of SM-9018, a new neuroleptic drug with both potent 5-hydroxy-tryptamine$_2$ and dopamine$_2$ antagonistic actions. *Jap J Pharmacol* 1990;53:321–329.
26. Jann MW, Grimstey SR, Gray EC, Change W-H. Pharmacokinetics and pharmacodynamics of clozapine. *Clin Pharmacokinet* 1993;24:161–176.
27. Kane J, Honigfeld G, Singer J, Meltzer HY, the Clozaril Collaborative Study Group. Clozapine for the treatment-resistant schizophrenic: a double-blind comparison with chlorpromazine. *Arch Genl Psychiatry* 1988;45:789–796.
28. Köhler C, Hall H, Magnusson O, Lewander T, Gustaffson K. Biochemical pharmacology of the atypical neuroleptic remoxipride. *Acta Psychiatr Scand* 1990;82(Suppl 358):27–36.
29. Krupp P, Barnes P. Leponex®-associated granulocytopenia: a review of the situation. *Psychopharmacol Suppl* 1989;99:S118–S121.
30. Leadbetter R, Schulty M, Pavalonis D, Vieweg V, Hippius P, Downs P. Clozapine-induced weight gain: prevalence and clinical relevance. *Am J Psychiatry* 1992;149:68–72.
31. Lee HS, Kwon KY, Alphs LD, Meltzer HY. Buspirone does not produce a 5-HT_{1A}-mediated decrease in temperature in man. *J Clin Psychopharmacol* 1991;11:222–223.
32. Lewander T, Westerberg S-E, Morrison D. Clinical of remoxipride—a combined analysis of a comparative double-blind, multi-centre trial programme. *Acta Psychiatr Scand* 1990;82(Suppl 358):92–98.
33. Leysen JC, Gommeren W, Eens A, de Chaffoy de Courcelles D, Stoff JC. Janssen PAJ. Biochemical profile of risperidone, a new antipsychotic. *J Pharmacol Exp Ther* 1988;247:661–670.
34. Lieberman JA, Kane JM, Johns CA. Clozapine: guidelines for clinical management. *J Clin Psychiatry* 1989;50:329–338.
35. Lieberman JA, Saltz BL, Johns CA, Pollack S, Borenstein M, Kane J. The effect of clozapine on tardive dyskinesia. *Br J Psychiatry* 1991;158:503–510.
36. Lindström LH, The effect of long-term treatment with clozapine in schizophrenia: a retrospective study in 96 patients treated with clozapine for up to 13 years. *Acta Psychiatr Scand* 1988;77:524–529.
37. Luikkonen J, Kopenen HJ, Nousiainen J. Clinical picture and long-term course of epileptic seizures that occur during clozapine treatment. *Psychiatry Res* 1992;44:107–112.
38. McGlashan TH. A selective review of recent North American long-term follow-up studies of schizophrenia. *Schiz Bull* 1988;14:515–542.
39. McHugh D, Coffin V. The reversal of extrapyramidal side effects with SCh 39166, a dopamine D_1 receptor antagonist. *Eur J Pharmacol* 1991;202:133–134.
40. Megens AA, Awouters FH, Niemegeers CJ. Differential effects of the new antipsychotic risperidone on large and small motor movements in rats: a comparison with haloperidol. *Psychopharmacology* 1988;95:493–496.
41. Meltzer HY. Duration of a clozapine trial in neuroleptic-resistant schizophrenia. *Arch Gen Psychiatry* 1989;46:672.
42. Meltzer HY. The mechanism of action of novel antipsychotic drugs. *Schiz Bull* 1991;17:263–287.
43. Meltzer HY. Treatment of the neuroleptic non-responsive schizophrenic patient. *Schiz Bull* 1992;18:515–542.
44. Meltzer HY. The concept of atypical antipsychotics. In: den Boer JA, Westenberg HGM, van Praag HM, eds. *Advances in the Neurobiology of Schizophrenia*, London: Wiley (*in press*).
45. Meltzer HY, Bastani B, Kwon KY, Ramirez LF, Burnett S, Sharpe J. A prospective study of clozapine in treatment-resistant patients: I: preliminary report. *Psychopharmacol Suppl* 1989;99:S68–S72.
46. Meltzer HY, Burnett S, Bastani B, Ramirez LF. Effect of six months of clozapine treatment on the quality of life of chronic schizophrenic patients. *Hosp Commun Psychiatry* 1990;41:892–897.
47. Meltzer HY, Cola P, Way L, et al. Cost effectiveness of clozapine in neuroleptic-resistant schizophrenia. *Am J Psychiatry* 1993;150:1630–1638.

48. Meltzer HY, Koenig JI, Nash JF, Gudelsky GA. *Acta Psychiatrica Scand* 1989;80(Suppl 352):24–26 (Sedval G, Suppl ed.).
49. Meltzer HY, Matsubara S, Lee J-C. Classification of typical and atypical antipsychotic drugs on the basis of dopamine D-1, D-2 and serotonin$_2$ pKi values. *J Pharmacol Exp Ther* 1989;251:238–246.
50. Mesotten F, Suy E, Pictquin M, Burton P, Heylen S, Gelders Y. Therapeutic effect and safety of increasing doses of risperidone (R 64 766) in psychotic patients. *Psychopharmacology* 1989;99:445–449.
51. Michaels ML, Crimson ML, Robert S, Childs A. Clozapine response and adverse effects in nine brain-injured patients. *J Clin Psychopharmacology* 1993;13:192–203.
52. Miller DD, Perry PJ, Cadoret RJ, Andreasen NC. Clozapine's effects on negative symptoms in treatment-refractory schizophrenics. *Comprehen Psychiatry* 1994;35:8–15.
53. Moore NA, Tye NC, Axton MS, Risius RC. The behavioral pharmacology of olanzepine, a novel "atypical" antipsychotic agent. *J Pharmacol Exp Ther* 1992;262:545–551.
54. Musacchio JM. The psychotomimetic effects of opiates and the α receptor. *Neuropsychopharmacology* 1990;3:191–200.
55. Naber D, Leppig M, Grohmann R, Hippius H. Efficacy and adverse effects of clozapine in the treatment of schizophrenia and tardive dyskinesia—a retrospective study of 387 patients. *Psychopharmacol Supple* 1989;99:S73–S76.
56. Ögren S-O, Florvall L, Hall H, Magnusson O, Ängeby-Möller K. Neuropharmacological and behavioral properties of remoxipride in the rat. *Acta Psychiatr Scand* 1990;82(Suppl 358):21–26.
57. Palfreyman MG, Sorensen SM, Baron BM, Humphreys TM, Moser PC, Dudley MW. Antipsychotic potential of 5-HT$_3$ antagonists: preclinical data. In: Meltzer HY, ed. *Novel atypical antipsychotic drugs.* New York: Raven Press; 1992:211–224.
58. Parsa M, Al-Lanhram Y, Ramirez LF, Meltzer HY. Prolonged psychotic relapse after abrupt clozapine withdrawal. *J Clin Psychopharmacol* 1993;13:154–155.
59. Parsa MA, Ramirez LF, Loula EC, Meltzer HY. Effect of clozapine on psychotic depression and Parkinsonism. *J Clin Psychopharmacol* 1991;11:330–331.
60. Perry PJ, Miller DD, Arndt SV, Cadoret RJ. Clozapine and norclozapine plasma concentrations and clinical response of treatment-refractory schizophrenic patients. *Am J Psychiatry* 1991;148:231–235.
61. Pope HG Jr, McElroy SL, Keek PE, Hudson JI. Valproate in the treatment of acute mania. *Arch Genl Psychiatry* 1991;44:113–118.
62. Pugsley TA, Christofferson CM, Corbin A, et al. Pharmacological characterization of PD 118717, a putative piperazinyl benzopyranone dopamine autoreceptor agonist. *J Pharmacol Exp Ther* 1992;263:1147–1158.
63. Revicki DA, Luce BR, Wechsler JM, Brown RE, Adler MA. Cost-effectiveness of clozapine for treatment-resistant schizophrenic patients. *Hosp Commun Psychiatry* 1990;41:850–855.
64. Saller CF, Salama AI. Seroquel: biochemical profile of a potential atypical antipsychotic. *Psychopharmacology* 1993;112:285–292.
65. Seymour PA, Seegar TF, Guanowsky V, Robinson GL, Howard H, Heym J. Behavioral pharmacology of CP-88,059, a new antipsychotic with both 5-HT$_2$ and D$_2$ antagonist properties. *Neurosci Abstr* 1993;19:599.
66. Sitsen JMA, Vrijmoed-de Vries MC. Org 5222: preliminary clinical results. In: Meltzer HY, ed. *Novel Atypical Antipsychotic drugs.* New York: Raven Press; 1992:15–28.
67. Skarsfeldt T, Perregaard J. Sertindole, a new neuroleptic with extreme selectivity on A10 versus A9 dopamine neurons in the rat. *Eur J Pharmacol* 1990;182:613–614.
68. Sokoloff P, Martres M-P, Giros B, Bouthenet M-L, Schwartz J-C. The third dopamine receptor (D$_3$) as a novel target for antipsychotics. *Biochem Pharmacol* 1992;43:659–666.
69. Sorensen SM, Kehne JH, Fadayel GM, et al. Characterization of the 5-HT$_2$ receptor antagonist MDL 100907 as a putative atypical antipsychotic: behavioral, electrophysiological and neurochemical studies. *J Pharmacol Exp Ther* 1993;266:684–691.
70. Svensson K, Ekman A, Piercey MF, Hoffmann WE, Lum JT, Carlsson A. Effects of the partial dopamine receptor agonists SDZ 208-911, SDZ 208-912 and terguride on central monoamine receptors. *Naunyn-Schmiedeberg's Arch Pharmacol* 1991;344:263–274.
71. Tam SW, Steinfels GF, Gilligan PJ, Schmidt WK, Cook L. DuP 734 [1-(cyclopropylmethyl)-4-(2′(4″-fluorophenyl)-2-oxoethyl)-piperidine HBR], a sigma and 5-hydroxytryptamine$_2$ receptor antagonist: receptor binding, electrophysiological and neuropharmacological profiles. *J Pharmacol Exp Ther* 1992;263:1167–1174.
72. Van den Borre R, Vermite R, Buttiens M, et al. Risperidone as add on therapy in behavioral disturbances in mental retardation: a double-blind placebo-controlled cross-over study. *Acta Psychiatr Scand* 1993;87:167–171.
73. Van den Bussche G, Heykants J, De Coster R. Pharmacokinetic profile and neuroendocrine effects of the new antipsychotic risperidone. *Psychopharmacology* 1988;96(Suppl):334.
74. Van Tol HHM, Bunzow JR, Guan HC, et al. Cloning of the gene for a human dopamine D$_4$ receptor with high affinity for the antipsychotic clozapine. *Nature* 1991;350:610–614.
75. Vartiainen H, Leinonen E, Putkonen A, Lang S, Hagert U, Tolvanen U. A long-term study of remoxipride in chronic schizophrenic patients. *Acta Psychiatr Scand* 1993;87:114–117.
76. Volavka J, Zito JM, Vitrai J, Czobar P. Clozapine affects on hostility of aggression in schizophrenia. *J Clin Psychopharmacol* 1993;13:287–289.
77. von Bahr C, Movin G, Yisak W-A, Jostell KG, Widman M. Clinical pharmacokinetics of remoxipride. *Acta Psychiatr Scand* 1992;82(Suppl 358):41–44.
78. Wadworth AM, Heel RC. Remoxipride. A review of its pharmacodynamic and pharmacokinetic properties, and therapeutic potential in schizophrenia. *Drugs* 1990;40:863–879.

Psychopharmacology: The Fourth Generation of Progress, edited by Floyd E. Bloom and David J. Kupfer. Raven Press, Ltd., New York © 1995.

CHAPTER 109

Neuroimaging Studies of Human Anxiety Disorders

Cutting Paths of Knowledge through the Field of Neurotic Phenomena

Lewis R. Baxter, Jr.

We may look forward to a day when paths of knowledge and, let us hope, of influence will be opened up, leading from organic biology and chemistry to the field of neurotic phenomena, . . .

—*Sigmund Freud, 1926 (25)*

Freud's remark, actually concluded: ". . . That day still seems a distant one." Were he alive today, however, Freud might not be so pessimistic about the distance in time to an understanding of brain mechanisms mediating these psychological disorders (26,72). Present day instruments for studing the chemistry and physiology of the living human brain are helping to bring to psychiatry the scientific analysis about which Freud could only dream.

In the past 5 years, there has been significant progress in in vivo brain-imaging studies of some of the anxiety disorders that interested Freud, especially obsessive–compulsive disorder (OCD), sufficient to warrant this fresh optimism. The purpose of this chapter is to aquaint the reader with relevant human brain-imaging studies that shed light on how the central nervous system (CNS) may mediate the symptomatic expression of anxiety disorders.

L. R. Baxter, Jr.: Department of Psychiatry and Biobehavioral Sciences, The Laboratory of Nuclear Medicine, Laboratory of Structural Biology and Molecular Medicine, The Crump Institute for Biological Imaging, The Brain Research Institute, University of California at Los Angeles School of Medicine, Los Angeles, California 90024.

The author does not believe that all the DSM-IV designated anxiety disorders are intrinsicly any more closely related to each other than some of them are to other psychiatric problems, like depression or Gilles de la Tourette's syndrome, in the case of OCD (12,16,56), but this is the conventional lumping, and all these maladies do share anxiety (or dread) as a major symptom.

Of the official nonorganic anxiety disorders, social phobia and posttraumatic stress disorder have not been investigated sufficiently to merit review at this time. In this chapter, discussion of the other anxiety disorders are frequently interwoven, because this seems most efficient and the only large body of brain-imaging work to date is on OCD. In this vein, studies of induced anxiety states in normals are discussed, where appropriate, as they are often relevant. Review of studies in normals are limited, however, to those works judged directly relevant to understanding psychiatric disorders. Likewise, studies on the pharmacological effects of antianxiety agents in normals or animals, of which there are many, or anxiety states induced by structural brain lesions or drugs, are omitted. Brain-imaging studies of medication effects in the primary anxiety disorders themselves are reviewed when they illuminate possible brain mechanisms of symptom mediation.

The technical modalities covered are the present tomographic brain-imaging techniques—X-ray computed tomography (CT), magnetic resonance imaging (MRI) for structural anatomy (there are no published functional MRI studies of anxiety disorders to date, although several are in progress), single photon computed tomography (SPECT), and positron emission tomography (PET). The first two give information on brain structure, the latter two probe biochemical and physiological functions. The nontomographic brain-mapping techniques, such as various electroencephalographic (EEG) methods, are not surveyed. Although some relevant technical information on the functional imaging techniques will be given in passing in the context of critical review, readers are referred to other chapters of this volume, and other references (2,3,57,58) for discussion of the methods for each form of brain imaging.

GENERALIZED ANXIETY, SIMPLE PHOBIA AND INDUCED ANXIETY STATES IN NORMALS

A search of the literature uncovered no structural brain-imaging studies of a series of patients with these disorders. Wu and colleagues (75) have studied 18 patients diagnosed with primary generalized anxiety disorder (GAD) with PET and the fluorodeoxyglucose (FDG) method to determine local cerebral metabolic rates for glucose (lCMR-Glc). Patients were studied during a passive viewing task off medication, and then in an active visual vigilence task after oral clorazepate (7.5 mg; $n = 8$) or placebo ($n = 10$); there were 15 normal controls. Significant findings included lower basal ganglia lCMR-Glc in patients compared to normal controls during passive visualization, but increased lCMR-Glc in the left inferior primary visual cortex, right posterior temporal cortex, and right precentral frontal gyrus. Active vigilance resulted in basal ganglia activation in GAD compared to controls, although the benzodiazepine decreased metabolic rates in the whole cortex, basal ganglia, and some limbic structures. Interpretation of this study is difficult because of the extreme number of post hoc analyses and summaries reporting of lCMR-Glc for various brain regions, but it is significant in noting that basal ganglia were significantly lower in anxious patients in the passive state—different than in FDG-PET studies of OCD (see below).

Two studies have looked at regional cerebral blood flow (CBF) in patients with small animal phobias. Mountz and colleagues (50) examined seven such phobics in a test–retest manner with PET for regional CBF. Studies were done as an intrasubject cross-over at baseline and when exposed to the animal. Eight normal controls studied under similar conditions. Although global absolute CBF was lower in the phobics when stimulated than at baseline and compared to results in the controls, when the method was corrected for hypocapnia, no global or regional differences were significant for either group. Wik and coworkers (73), on the other hand, studied six women with snake phobia in three states: (a) at baseline viewing

a neutral stimulus, (b) viewing a video tape of snakes, and (c) viewing a tape of other adverse scenes not involving snakes. They observed significant increases in secondary visual cortex CBF, and reduced CBF in the hippocampus, orbitofrontal, prefrontal, temporal poles, and posterior cingulate cortex with snake exposure, compared to the neutral stimulation. The nonsnake adverse stimulus showed similar, but less intense patterns as those seen with snake viewing.

Two studies of normals are relevant to the phenomona of generic situational anxiety. In one (28), 43 normal volunteers were administered the State-Trait Anxiety Inventory before and after FDG-PET scanning with no specific stimuli. No relationship was observed between measured anxiety level and lCMR-Glc findings, and the authors concluded that the effects of simple situational anxiety at the levels experienced under these study conditions, if they exist, are obscured by the normal variance inherent in the FDG-PET method used. Reiman and colleagues (63) studied anticipatory anxiety (threatened painful electrical shock) and measured CBF changes compared to baseline in normal volunteers ($n = 8$). They observed significant increases in CBF in the region of the lateral temporal poles, bilaterally, and attributed these to anxiety-related brain activation. Unfortunately, subsequent work by the same and other groups suggest that the temporal pole findings may have been generated by an artifact resulting from jaw clenching and consequent increased glucose metabolism in maseter and temporalis muscles. The data reduction methods employed, whereby brain regions are identified by idealized stereotactic coordinates, may have resulted in misidentification of muscle activity as being inside rather than outside the skull (22). Whether there are any specific patterns of functional brain activation in normals with situational anxiety is unclear at this time.

PANIC DISORDER

Structural Imaging Studies

Panic disorder patients ($n = 30$) were studied with X-ray CT by Lepola and colleagues (39). Despite the fact that this patient group had a high baseline suspicion of organic lesions, only six had any identifiable structural abnormality, and these did not fit any recognizable patterns. On the other hand, Ontiveros and collaborators (54) when studying 30 lactate-sensitive panic disorder subjects with MRI did find 43% of the panic subjects with right temporal lobe dysmorphias, whereas only 10% of normals ($n = 20$) could be so classified. Furthermore, panic disorder patients with these temporal abnormalities were significantly younger and had more panic attacks than those with normal MRI scans. These results are in line with a single CT report of a patient developing panic disorder after right parahippocampal infarction (42) and with functional brain-imaging studies (below).

Studies of In Vivo Brain Physiology and Biochemistry

Reiman and collegues have published two PET studies of panic disorder subjects. In the first (61), 16 patients with lactate-induced panic attacks were compared with 11 controls in the resting state; the panic disorder patients had L < R asymmetry of blood flow, blood volume, and metabolic rates for oxygen in the parahippocampal gyrus. In a follow-up report of these subjects and others (24 patients with panic disorder, 18 normals), subjects were studied before and during lactate infusion to induce a panic attack (62). Patients who did not experience panic, as well as normal controls, showed no significant change in CBF on lactate infusion, but patients who panicked with this challenge showed increased CBF in temporal poles, insular cortex, claustrum, lateral putamen, and superior colliculus—all bilaterally—and near the left anterior cerebellar vermis. This study, however, is subject to the same questions concerning neuroanatomical localization as the study of induced anxiety in normals (22,63) above.

Two studies using very different functional imaging methods do tend to support the general finding of parahippocampal abnormalities in panic disorder subjects at baseline. Nordhal and coworkers (53) studied 12 panic disorder patients and 30 normal controls with FDG-PET tracer uptake during an auditory discrimination task. This investigation also found a left–right (L < R) hippocampal region asymmetry compared to normal controls, this time in lCMR-Glc. They also reported decreased left inferior parietal and anterior cingulate lCMR-Glc and trend-level increases in medial orbital frontal cortex. Teresa et al. (71), used CT and ^{99m}Tc-hexamethyl-propyleneamine oxime (HMPAO) SPECT, an indirect index of blood flow, to study seven lactate-sensitive panic disorder patients compared to five controls. No CT abnormalities were noted in the patients, but they did report a decrease in hippocampal perfusion (relative to the rest of the brain) bilaterally and in the left occipital cortex in patients compared to control subjects.

Thus, there are several functional and even structural brain-imaging studies that suggest abnormality in brain regions around the hippocampus in panic disorder. This should be noted in comparison to results in OCD.

OBSESSIVE–COMPULSIVE DISORDER

My colleagues and I have published several reviews of brain-imaging studies of obsessive–compulsive disorder and related conditions (4,5,11,12,13,16). Although many new and significant studies are reviewed here that have not been reviewed before, of necessity much will be but a repetition of those previous reviews.

Structural Imaging Studies

Insel and associates (32) studied 18 patients with DSM-III OCD, using neuropsychological testing (Wechsler Adult Intelligence Scale and Halstead-Reitan Battery) and EEG recordings. As part of this work they also studied a subgroup of 10 patients with CT. Two subjects with EEG abnormalities, four with neuropsychological testing abnormalities, and four others chosen at random underwent CT scanning. Controls were age- and gender-matched subjects without evidence of psychiatric or known CNS illness, although seven had other known "peripheral illnesses." The findings in this study were unremarkable. There were no significant differences between OCD subjects and controls.

Another CT study, this time of childhood-onset OCD by Behar and colleagues (17), did find significant differences in the ventricle-to-brain ratios (VBRs) between OCD and normal subjects. The 17 OCD subjects could have had secondary depression, the severity of which was not reported. The 16 control subjects, had CT scans that were not "questionable clinically" (it is not clear whether they were truly "normal") and were not from individuals with altered consciousness, psychiatric symptoms, or hard neurological signs. All controls were suspected of having CNS pathology, however; this was the clinical reason for the CT study. Here, VBRs were judged significantly greater in OCD subjects than in controls. The ventricular measures did not show a significant correlation with demographic, disease severity, or prior treatment variables, but it was noted that those with compulsions without obsessions tended to have higher VBRs than those who had obsessions.

This second research group also reported results of another CT study in late adolescents with childhood-onset OCD (40). In addition to examining VBRs, the investigators also examined caudate nuclei volumes. Subjects were ten young males. Control subjects were ten males in good health. In this study, volumes of the caudate nuclei were found to be significantly smaller in OCD subjects than in controls. All other structures and ventricles were remarkably similar in volume across the two groups, and there were no significant left–right asymmetries.

To date only two studies of OCD patients studied with MRI have been published, although several are reported in progress. Garber and colleagues (27) studied 32 patients with OCD during a double-blind treatment study while on either clomipramine ($n = 19$) or placebo ($n = 13$). These patients were compared with normal controls. There were no distinct structural abnormalities noted in the OCD patients by inspection. Neuroanatomic structure volumes or other morphological measurements were not calculated. In both patients and controls, a variety of non-specific T_2 hyperintensity lesions were seen in the white matter. The authors also used the controversial approach of T_1 mapping in comparing OCD subjects to control subjects. Subjects with OCD with a positive family history had more negative mean and right–left (R > L) hemisphere asymmetry T_1 differences in the anterior cingulate than other patients or controls. Right–left T_1 differences for the orbital cortex gave significant correlations with symptom severity in unmedicated patients and patients with a family history positive for OCD. Although the exact meaning of such findings is not clear, the authors did feel that the findings were consistent with frontal–limbic–striatal pathology.

Kellner et al. (37) studied with MRI 12 OCD subjects and 12 age- and sex-matched healthy controls. Patients were five females and seven males, average age 40. They had Yale-Brown OCD scale scores above 16. Scanning was for T_1- and T_2-weighted images. Measures were made of the caudate, cingulate gyrus thickness, intracaudate/frontal horn ratio, and the corpus callosum. No significant differences were found between the OCD patients and the normal control subjects.

Studies of In Vivo Brain Physiology and Biochemistry with Functional Brain Imaging

Cerebral Blood Flow

Two HMPAO studies of pretreatment OCD have been published at the time of this review, although several others are known to be in progress. In the first study (41), ten nondepressed, medication-free OCD subjects were compared to eight Johns Hopkins employees or students, matched by age, race, and sex (three females in each group). Studies were done on the Toshiba GCA-90B single-rotating Anger camera (resolution, 16 mm; slice thickness, 11 mm). Patients had higher medial frontal perfusion than controls (109.7% ± 3.7% of cortical mean vs. 102.9% ± 3.6), but this gave a significant correlation with anxiety ($r = -0.84$, $p = 0.002$), not OCD severity ($p > 0.50$). Orbital metabolic rates were not significantly different between the two groups. Besides the difficulty with the significant finding correlating only with anxiety and not OCD symptoms, and there being no other pathological comparison group to control for anxiety, there are inherent technical problems with this study. The SPECT camera used is of low resolution. It is doubtful that the orbital region, which is not trivial to localize even with higher resolution PET technology, could be reliably identified. Furthermore partial volume effects (58), would likely lead to serious overestimation of activity in midline structures, given the present resolution limitations of this technology.

The much higher resolution (8 to 9.6 mm) Shimadzu Headtome, Model SET/031 SPECT system was used for both ^{133}Xe- and HMPAO-measured blood flow by Rubin et al. (64). They studied 10 nondepressed, drug-free males with OCD and 10 matched controls. Although there were no significant differences between the two groups with ^{133}Xe (although blood flow did give a significant correlation with OCD symptom severity), on HMPAO scanning the OCD patients had significantly increased uptake in the bilateral orbital frontal cortex, normalized to either cerebellum or whole brain, and in the left posterofrontal cortex and bilaterally in the high dorsal parietal cortex. They also had decreased HMPAO uptake in the caudate nuclei, bilaterally. Although the most likely reason for detecting differences with HMPAO and not ^{133}Xe is the resolution difference between the two methods, the authors also thought an HMPAO-sensitive difference in blood–brain barrier permeability or a difference in HMPAO trapping through hydrophilic conversion between the experimental groups might be responsible for the effects observed (see below).

Fluorodeoxyglucose Positron Emission Tomography for Cerebral Glucose Metabolic Rates

Our group at UCLA examined a sample of OCD patients ($n = 14$), compared to both normal controls ($n = 14$) and patients with unipolar-type major depression ($n = 14$) (7). All subjects were matched for age, and OCD and depressed subjects had similar Hamilton Depression Rating Scale and Brief Psychiatric Rating Scale tension and anxiety item scores. Nine of the OCD subjects were in a clear-cut secondary major depression at the time of study. Nine of the OCD subjects were drug-free for at least two weeks, but the other five were on a variety of antidepressants, benzodiazepines, and neuroleptics. The normal and depressed subjects were all drug-free. The normal control group had equal numbers of males and females, whereas the male–female ratio in the depressed group was 5:9, but was 9:5 for OCD.

Scanning by FDG-PET was done with the Neuro ECAT (in-plane resolution = 11 mm, axial = 12.5 mm) in the eyes and ears open state, without specific stimuli. Arteriolized venous blood was used for the calculation of absolute metabolic rates, and an idealized, calculated (rather than measured), attenuation correction was employed. Absolute glucose metabolic rates were determined for the whole cerebral hemispheres, hippocampal–parahippocampal complexes, anterior cingulate gyri, heads of the caudate nuclei, putamen nuclei, and thalamic nuclei, as well as various gyri in the prefrontal and temporal cortex. A one-way ANOVA was run among the subject groups for each structure, using the first seven subjects only. For those structures yielding significant results, a second, prospective analysis was run using the second group of seven. A separate analysis was also done excluding OCD subjects on drugs. Neuroanatomical regions of interest had to pass all tests to be considered significant. This approach was chosen to decrease the likelihood of type I (false-positive) statistical error, but greatly increased the likelihood of type II (false-negative) error.

Absolute glucose metabolic rates for the whole cerebral hemispheres, caudate nuclei, and orbital gyri were found to be significantly elevated in OCD, compared to the control groups, by these criteria. Furthermore, metabolic rates in the left orbital gyrus, divided by those of the ipsilateral hemisphere (normalized metabolic rates) were significantly higher than those found in normals on the left. There was only a trend for this to be the case in the right hemisphere. However, there was no statistically significant left–right asymmetry on this measure, and values on the right were higher in OCD than in normal controls. Normalized caudate metabolic rates in OCD were not different from normal control values.

The subject groups in this first FDG-PET study had several characteristics that were not optimal: (a) There was an unequal number of male and female subjects across the experimental groups (8); (b) most of the OCD subjects also had concomitant major depression; (c) some of the OCD subjects were on medications; and (d) handedness was not equal across the groups. Therefore, a second FDG-PET study was undertaken to compare a new group of drug-free, nondepressed, right-handed OCD patients to normal control subjects of similar age, scanned under the same conditions as before (9).

Glucose metabolic rates in the cerebral hemispheres, heads of the caudate nuclei, and orbital gyri were examined, using an a priori design in an attempt to confirm or refute previous findings. The results obtained in this study were similar to those of the previous study. The OCD subjects had significantly higher glucose metabolic rates for the whole cerebral hemispheres, heads of the caudate nuclei, and orbital gyri than those found in normal control subjects. The orbital gyrus–hemisphere ratio (the normalized rate) was also elevated in OCD when compared to normal controls, but in this second study this finding was bilateral. In the previous study, where significant results had obtained only on the left, there was a higher percentage of males in the OCD group than in the normal control group (male–female OCD = 9:5; controls = 7:7). The data in this second study, when analyzed with a repeated measures ANOVA for variance and covariance, showed that there was a significant effect of sex by hemisphere on this measure (with males showing higher values on the left and females showing higher values on the right). The unbalanced sex ratios between the diagnostic groups that obtained in the first study probably accounted for the observation of statistical significance between OCD and normals for the left orbital gyrus–hemisphere ratio, whereas there was only a trend toward significance in the right hemisphere. We now believe that there are significant elevations in both left and right orbital gyrus–

hemisphere ratios in OCD, compared to normals. (Why both OCD and normal control females should have a higher orbital gyrus–hemisphere ratio on the right than the left, whereas males of both groups show the opposite pattern, is a mystery at this time.)

At the same time that the second UCLA study was being undertaken, two separate groups at the National Institute of Mental Health were performing similar studies independently. Nordahl et al. (52) studied eight nondepressed OCD subjects. These subjects were compared with 30 normal volunteers with no personal or family history of psychiatric problems. Scanning by FDG-PET was done with tracer uptake taking place during an auditory continuous-performance task with eyes closed. Arterial blood was used, and attenuation was measured with a transmission scan. Neuroanatomical regions of interest were determined by two independent raters. Sixty regions of interest were examined, with those found significant in the previous UCLA studies examined a priori with one-tailed Student's t test. Calculations of global brain metabolic rates, which were also used to normalize rates, were done with gray matter structures only, rather than all supratentorial brain regions, as in the UCLA work. Absolute metabolic rates for whole-brain gray matter were calculated, but only normalized values for individual regions of interest were examined.

This group also found normalized regional brain metabolic rates higher in OCD than in normals in both orbital gyri and normalized OCD caudate rates similar to normals. This group did not find elevated absolute global brain glucose metabolic rates, however. Two-tailed Student's t tests, with $p < 0.05$ considered significant, were done for other regions of interest in an exploratory analysis, with no corrections for the number of tests done. Normalized values in the right parietal and left occipital-parietal regions were higher in normals than in OCD subjects by this criterion. This group interpreted their findings in the orbital cortex as consistent with those of the UCLA group.

The other NIMH group (69) examined nine men and nine women with childhood-onset OCD but no concurrent major depression or other anxiety disorders. All were drug-free for at least 2 weeks and physically healthy. These subjects were compared to age- and sex-matched, physically and mentally healthy control subjects. Scanning by FDG-PET was done in the eyes- and ears-closed condition, with arterial blood sampling and measured attenuation correction. The global metabolic rate was calculated based on the simple mean of cortical gray matter only. This measure was used also for normalizing other regions of interest.

The OCD patient group showed increased absolute glucose metabolism in left orbital and right sensorimotor regions and, bilaterally, in the anterior cingulate gyri and lateral prefrontal areas. Normalized values were significantly increased in right lateral prefrontal and left anterior cingulate regions only. These authors, however, did observe a significant correlation between absolute and normalized right orbital glucose metabolic activity and a measure of OCD severity. Furthermore, six of these patients, who failed to respond to a subsequent trial of clomipramine had significantly higher right anterior cingulate and right orbital metabolism than 11 patients who did respond. This research group interpreted their findings in light of other work on OCD to suggest a dysfunction of a frontal cortex–basal ganglia loop (67,69). This team, along with other collaborators, subsequently reported a complicated correlational analysis of data from these patients (31), but the methods are hard to follow, and the conclusions to be drawn are unclear at this time.

Another FDG-PET study (43) found results at odds with those of the other PET studies reviewed above. Sixteen OCD patients were compared to eight normal controls in the resting state. Both absolute rates and rates normalized to whole brain were analysed. All brain regions examined were reported to show lower absolute rates in the OCD subjects than in the controls. For normalized values, however, the lateral prefrontal cortex had significantly lower rates in the OCD subjects than in normal controls. They could not confirm orbital abnormalities. Given the similarity between these results and our data on depressed OCD subjects (see below), it is particularly important to note that the authors assure us that no subjects were depressed at the time of PET scanning and results of drug-free subjects were similar to those scanned while on medication. However, it is possible that a different threshold of depression severity for a diagnosis of major depression was applied in this study than in those done in the United States. In a PET study of depression by this same group, recovered patients had a mean score of 32 on the 26-item Hamilton Depression Rating Scale (44).

Thus, four separate FDG-PET studies have found evidence for inferior prefrontal cortex abnormalities in OCD, and one has not.

An FDG-PET Study of Depression in OCD

Yet another FDG-PET study provides information relevant to the phenomenon of secondary, major depression in OCD. In this study (10), drug-free, age- and sex-matched, right-handed patients with unipolar depression ($n = 10$), bipolar depression ($n = 10$), OCD with secondary major depression ($n = 10$), OCD without depression ($n = 14$), and normal controls ($n = 12$) were evaluated under the same conditions and with the same machinery as in the other UCLA studies. Six non-sex-matched manic subjects (four males) were also evaluated under conditions that were otherwise the same. Depressed patients in all three groups had similar levels of depression on the Hamilton Depression Rating Scale (HDRS) and OCD patients with

and without depression were of similar severity of OCD symptoms, measured on the NIMH OCD scale.

As predicted a priori, ipsilateral-hemisphere-normalized glucose metabolic rates for the left dorsal anterolateral prefrontal cortex were similar in the unipolar and bipolar subjects and significantly lower than values obtained for both normals and OCD subjects without depression. Bipolar depressed patients were significantly lower than manics on this measure. Likewise, OCD with major depression showed significantly decreased glucose metabolic values in this brain region, compared to OCD without depression. Furthermore, there was a significant negative correlation ($r = -0.5$; $p = 0.0002$) between this brain metabolism measure and scores on the HDRS.

With antidepressant medication, normalized left dorsal anterolateral prefrontal cortex activity increased significantly, and the percentage change in HDRS scores gave a significant ($r = -0.5$; $p = 0.045$) negative correlation with percentage change on the metabolic variable. It was concluded that, despite being different on other measures of cerebral glucose metabolic rates, OCD with major depression, like the other two primary major depressions, is distinguished from the nondepressed (OCD) state by a decrease in normalized left dorsal anterolateral prefrontal glucose metabolic rates.

Brain Function Studies of Obsessive–Compulsive Symptom Treatment and Provocation

Zohar et al. (76) studied ten subjects using SPECT and ^{133}Xe, a low resolution but direct method for determining CBF. All the subjects had washing compulsions and reports of focal stimuli for their obsessions concerning contamination. The design was complicated. There were six women and four men, and all were drug-free for at least 3 weeks. Subjects underwent two single-blind "placebo Xe" test runs in an attempt to diminish test-situation anxiety. All studies were done with eyes closed for 16 min, with 30-min intervals in between. The subjects underwent, in sequence, Xe–flow studies (a) in a relaxation state, (b) during imaginal flooding, and (c) during in vivo exposure to stimuli that, in the past, had tended to induce contamination obsessions and washing rituals. All three stimulus state studies were done during a 4-hr time period on the same day. The relaxation stimulus was done with an audiotape of a relaxation scene (the same for all subjects), and the flooding was done with an audiotape of a situation specific to the subject's individual contamination fears. Exposure in vivo was done with the flooding tape, accompanied by placing the contaminating object in contact with the dorsum of the right hand. In an attempt to gain information as to whether results were biased by the fixed sequence of presentation, three subjects returned, 5 to 10 days later, for testing in which exposure was given before flooding.

Both symptom-rating-scale scores and physiological measures gave highest values during in vivo exposure and were lowest during relaxation. In contrast, CBF was significantly increased in the imaginal flooding over the relaxation state, but only in the temporal cortex, and was significantly decreased in virtually all cortical regions (specifically temporal, parietal, posterior, and in the cortex as a whole) during exposure in vivo. In all three conditions, flow in the left hemisphere was greater than on the right, and the left prefrontal cortex appeared slightly more reactive than the right in the directions cited above. There did not appear to be an effect of order of presentation in the three subjects in whom this was evaluated.

The authors found the results of this study puzzling. They had predicted that the peripheral physiological measures of anxiety would increase going from relaxation to imaginal flooding to in vivo stimulation, which they did. However, they predicted the same direction of effect on CBF as well. Instead, blood flow *decreased* in in vivo stimulation.

A number of speculations were offered that might have accounted for the results. Differences in the sensory modalities of the stimuli (i.e., auditory versus touch) could have been important. Imaginal flooding might require more active cortical involvement than the passive touch situation, but this explanation was not favored, due to patient reports of the degree of conscious activity in the various situations. Another possible explanation was that, in the highly anxiety provoking in vivo exposure situation, blood was being shunted away from the cortical areas of the brain to other areas, such as the caudate nucleus or orbital gyri (see PET studies, below), which cannot be visualized with the ^{133}Xe-flow method.

One group has used ^{11}C-glucose and PET to measure cerebral glucose metabolism in five patients with OCD refactory to conventional treatment who were studied 10 days before and 1 year after surgical capsulotomy (47–49). Drug status is not clear. These patients' scans were compared to scans of ten healthy males. The PET scanning and blood sampling were done over a 15-min period and the model for calculating metabolic rates used estimates of ^{11}C—CO_2 loss from brain based on other experiments in anesthetized monkeys where the arteriovenous difference across the brain is measured after an iv bolus and the Fick Principle applied. We are told that orbital and caudate metabolic rates in patients were significantly higher before than after surgery, but it is not clear whether these are absolute or normalized metabolic rates. We are told further that although the orbital region was not determined in normals, that Brodmann area 11 was higher in the five normal controls where it could be located than was the orbital cortex in OCD patient pretreatment. The investigators also correlated measured lCMR-Glc changes with various personality measures on the Karolinska Scales of Personality. They observed significant positive correlations of the left caudate nucleus lCMR-Glc with decreases in somatic anxiety, psychic anxiety, psychasthenia, and guilt, and in the right orbital gyri with decreases in psychic anxiety, psychasthenia, suspicion, and guilt. Although this report finds similar pre- to posttreatment changes in orbital and caudate metabolic rates as reported with other methods (below), besides the multiple questions about patient status and the small subject numbers, there are the problems with the ^{11}C-glucose method itself. If the orbital region of the brain is in fact overstimulated in OCD, as supported by most FDG studies and theories advanced about brain function in OCD (see below), then the ^{11}C-glucose method would underestimate the glucose metabolic rate in OCD patients versus normals.

The Johns Hopkins group examined six of the OCD subjects of their HMPAO-SPECT study after 3 to 4 months of 80 to 100 mg/day of fluoxetine (29). Obsessive–compulsive symptoms showed significant decreases with treatment, as did ratios of medial-frontal cortex to mean cortex. No Pearson correlations with clinical symptoms were significant, but this method of correlation is decidedly not valid with subject numbers this low. The orbital region of the brain did not change pre- to posttreatment. It should be noted that, although the exact localization of the medial-frontal region is not clear in these reports, it is said to include the anterior cingulate cortex (29,41).

Benkelfat et al. (18) restudied eight of their initial FDG-PET study OCD subjects after an average of 16 weeks of drug treatment with clomipramine. For the group as a whole, whether responders to treatment or not, metabolic rates normalized to whole brain decreased in some regions of the medial and right orbital cortex. Left caudate rates also decreased significantly, but right anterior putamen values increased. When poor responders were compared to those showing good clinical response, good responders showed a significantly greater decrease in left caudate values than poor responders (10.9% ± 5%, mean ± sd, vs 2.1% ± 3.6%). There was a similar directional change between these groups for the right caudate (7.4% ± 18.6% vs −0.07% ± 8.7%), but there was not a significant difference due to the higher variance in the data than on the left.

Swedo et al. (67) restudied 13 of their OCD patients, eight on clomipramine, two on fluoxetine, and three off drug, after at least 1 year of treatment (mean 20 months). Seven patients were treatment responders and six had not changed significantly. Normalized glucose metabolic rates were examined in orbital (lateral), prefrontal, and cingulate cortical regions and in the caudate nuclei. In responders, the orbital cortex decreased 9.0% ± 9.7%, whereas in nonresponders only 0.4% ± 6.1% ($p = 0.04$). (It should be noted, however, that orbital metabolic rates showed highly significant, positive correlations with levels of clomipramine and its metabolite desmethylclomipramine.) No other brain regions tested showed significant changes. Interestingly, both normalized orbital and caudate metabolic rates were higher in nonresponders before treatment than in responders.

Baxter et al. (15) have studied patients pre- and posttreatment either with fluoxetine alone ($n = 9$) or behavior treatment using exposure and response-prevention without medication ($n = 9$). Both treatment groups were well matched on OCD severity, anxiety, age, and sex. All were drug-free on initial scan. They were rescanned after 10 weeks of treatment. In both groups, normalized right caudate metabolic rates decreased significantly in treatment responders ($-5.2\% \pm 2.3\%$ for drug treatment and $-8.0\% \pm 4.8\%$ for behavior treatment), not in nonresponders ($0.3\% \pm 1.0\%$ and $2.6 \pm 3.2\%$, respectively) and the differences between responders and nonresponders were significant for both treatment groups. They were also significant compared to normalized right caudate changes in a small group of normals ($0.4\% \pm 2.0\%$) rescanned after a similar interval. Percentage change in normalized right caudate rates gave a significant correlation with percentage change on the Yale-Brown Obsessive–Compulsive Disorder Scale for drug treatment, although there was a trend in behavior-treated subjects. The left caudate decreased in responders to each treatment, but not significantly. The right anterior cingulate (cf., SPECT study, above) and left thalamus decreased with fluoxetine, but not with behavior modification.

We also found in this study (15) and by subsequent analysis (5) that, before treatment, eventual positive treatment responders had significant, positive, pathological correlations between glucose metabolic rates in the orbital cortex and the caudate nucleus, bilaterally, and between the orbital cortex and the thalamus, bilaterally. After effective treatment, however, these correlations were abolished, and the change in correlation strength pre- and posttreatment was significant. Although numbers were too small to establish significance, it did not appear that treatment nonresponders had such positive correlations among these structures before treatment (Baxter et al., *unpublished data*). Both normal controls and patients with unipolar depression do not show these significant correlations of glucose metabolic rates among the orbit, caudate, and thalamus (11). See Table 1.

Rauch and colleagues at Harvard (60) have used PET measures of CBF before and while acutely exposing subjects ($n = 8$) with OCD to stimuli that acutely increase their OCD symptoms (see Fig. 1). They demonstrated significant and striking increases in CBF in the right head of the caudate nucleus and orbital gyri, and lesser increases in thalamus, anterior cingulate, and dorsolateral cortex. Caudate laterality comes up again, this time consistent with our report (15), rather than with Benkelfat et al. (18). Because regional brain blood flow and glucose metabolism are usually tightly correlated (58), many of these PET findings by Rausch and collaborators on augmentation of OCD symptoms can be viewed as the

TABLE 1. *Metabolic rate correlation coefficients (Kendall's tau)*

Location[a]	Normal controls ($n = 12$)	Unipolar depressives ($n = 10$)	Obsessive–compulsives ($n = 13$)	
			preTx	postTx[b]
L Cd to orb	−0.09	−0.20	0.49[a]	0.00
R Cd to orb	0.05	−0.20	0.44[c]	−0.03
L orb to thal	0.09	−0.24	0.33	−0.21
R orb to thal	0.13	−0.11	0.41[c]	−0.21

[a] Cd, caudate head; orb, orbital gyri; thal, thalamus.
[b] All pre- to posttreatment (Tx) changes $p < 0.05$. Significant changes occurred pre- to posttreatment.
[c] $p < 0.05$.

reciprocal of changes we and others have noted with FDG-PET after effective treatment of OCD, and quite compatible with most FDG studies of OCD at rest. This is a remarkable validation that these brain regions are involved in the mediation of OCD symptoms. (Other regions, for example, the cingulate, may be for nonspecific distress; the same Harvard group has now studied six humans with small animal phobia in a similar manner, and found a different activation pattern than in OCD, namely cingulate and medial temporal blood flow increases (Jenike and Rausch, *personal communication*).

Rubin and colleagues have recently repeated the SPECT procedure on eight of the subjects of their initial [133]Xe- and HMPAO-SPECT study (above) while still on clomipramine, after a mean treatment interval of 7 months (range 2 to 10 months) (Rubin, *personal communication*, and ref. 65). On clomipramine the previous increases in HMPAO uptake in the orbital, posterofrontal, and high dorsal parietal cortex showed significant reductions compared to the range of normal controls. Significantly reduced caudate HMPAO uptake in OCD patients compared to controls before treatment did not change with clomipramine.

Specific Critiques of Methods in Obsessive–Compulsive Disorder Treatment Studies

We must note the conflicts in the functional brain-imaging reports of treatment effects on the brains of OCD patients. These could relate to specific differences in the treatment chosen for each study (e.g., clomipramine vs. fluoxetine), different stimulus conditions at the time of scanning, the scanning technique used, or other factors.

Specifically, although FDG and ^{11}C-glucose PET both measure a form of cerebral glucose metabolic rates, they are not at all equivalent. Unfortunately, this is not always recognized, leading to needless confusion. For this reason a few lines are necessary about each technique. Fluorodeoxyglucose is phosphorylated and transported into cells proportionally to glucose transport and equated to glucose

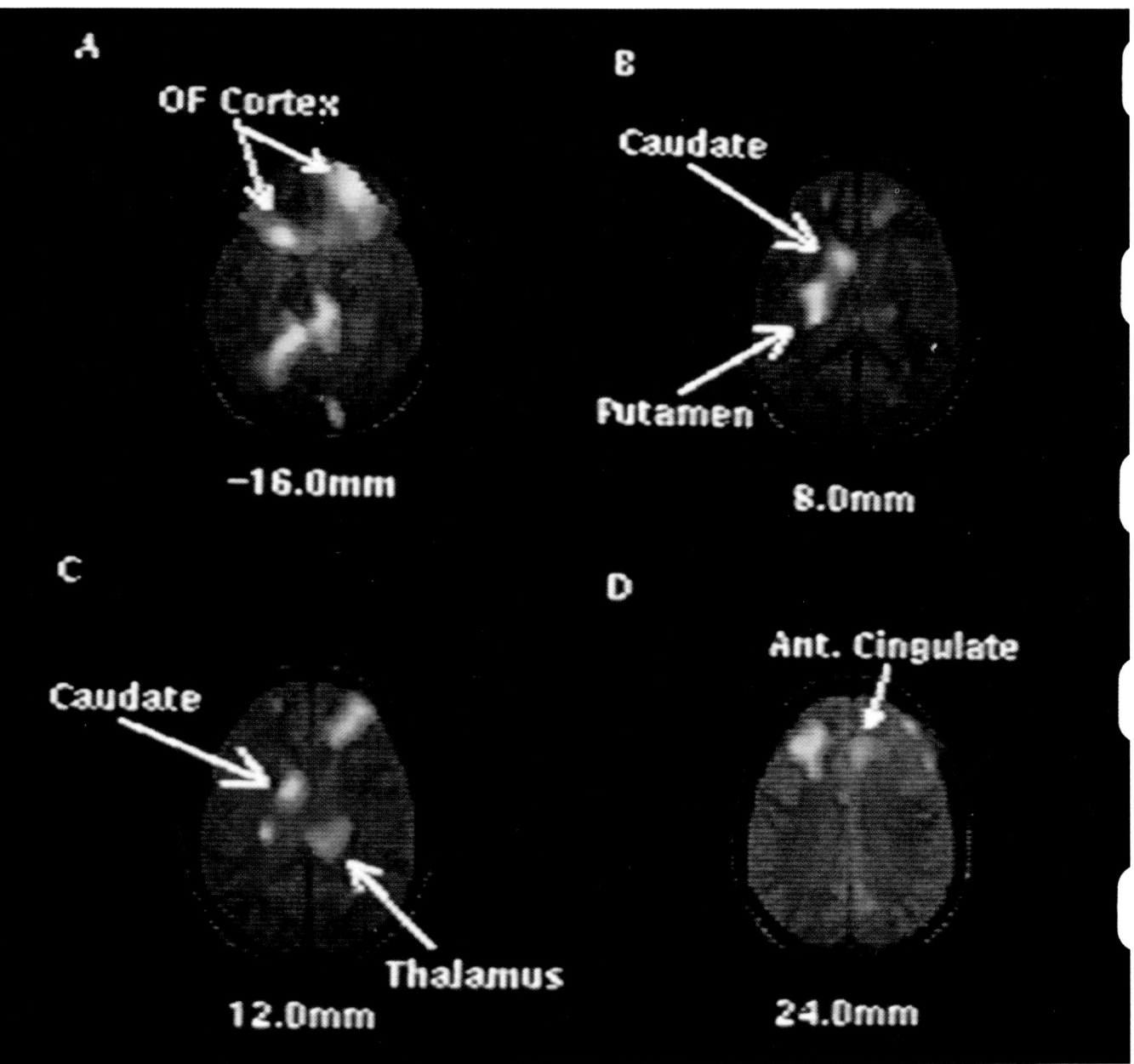

FIG. 1. PET study measuring cerebral blood flow rates in eight OCD subjects exposed to a neutral stimulus, then with one designed to provoke obsessive thoughts and anxiety. Shown are omnibus subtraction images (summed for all subjects) with the provoked state minus the resting condition, displayed with a hot-iron scale in units of z scores, superimposed over a normal magnetic resonance image transformed to a standard brain, for the purpose of anatomic reference. Increasing z score indicates activity in the provoked state that is increased to levels above that in the resting state.

Orbital cortex, bilaterally, and right head of caudate nucleus were a priori brain regions of interest, which showed significant ($p < 0.01$) changes (increases); other regions were significant at the trend level ($p < 0.10$). From Rausch et al. (60).

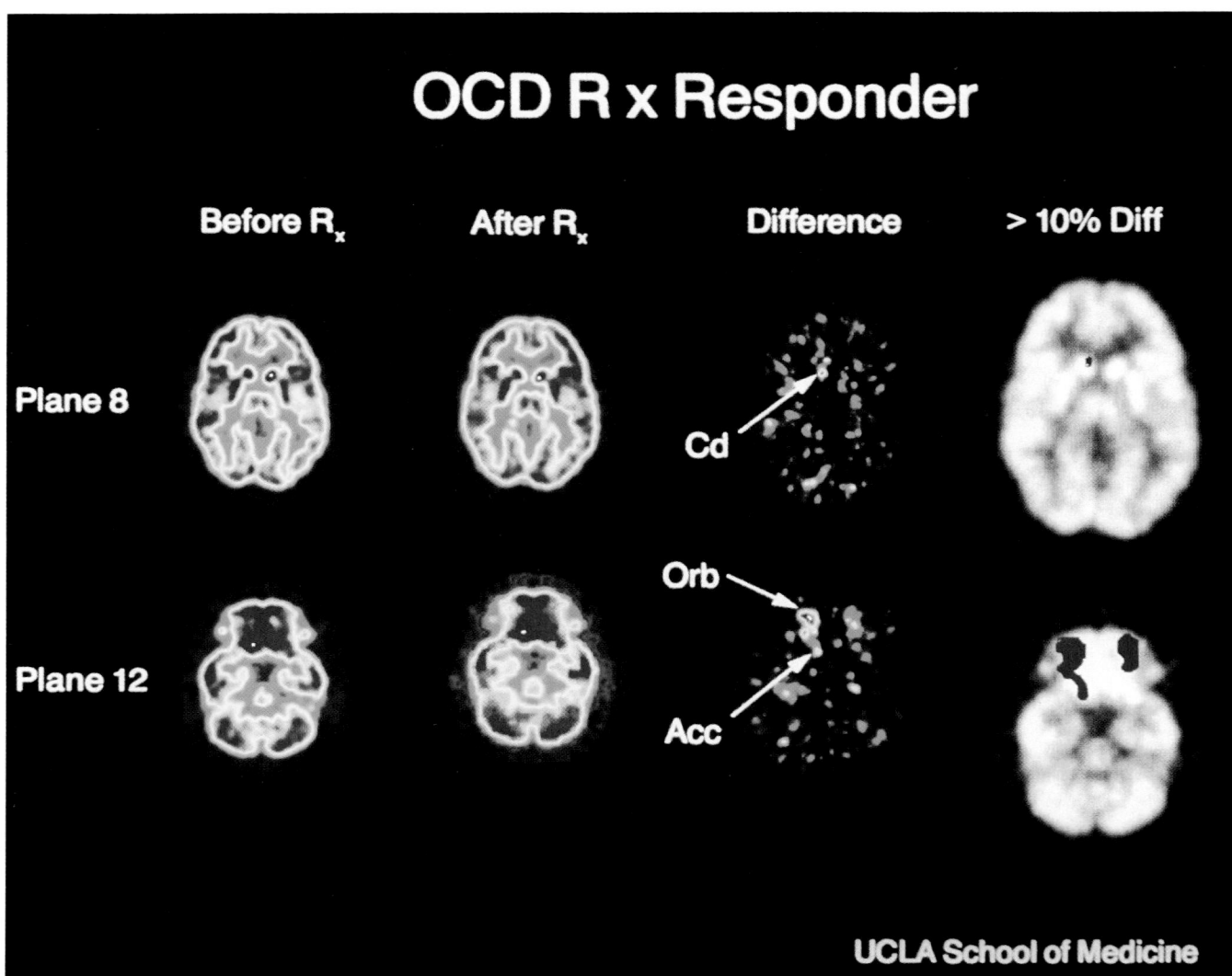

FIG. 2. Subject with severe OCD studied with FDG-PET for glucose metabolic rates before and after effective treatment with paroxetine hydrochloride. PET image plane 8 is at the level of the head of the caudate nucleus, whereas plane 12 is at the level of the orbital gyri and nucleus accumbens. The *first two columns (left to right)* show normalized glucose metabolic rate images before and after 6 weeks of paroxetine treatment. *Difference column* shows subtraction of posttreatment from pretreatment image to show *decreases* in glucose metabolic rates. The *last column* shows difference data windowed to show regions of significant (>10%) decreases in glucose metabolic rate, *in red,* and superimposed on image of underlying neuroanatomy in the same patient. These PET results seen after decreasing OCD symptoms with drug treatment can be viewed as the inverse of those seen in Fig. 1, where OCD symptoms were increased with provocation.

via the lumped constant in the modified Sokoloff equation (58), but once in the cell FDG undergoes no further metabolism and is trapped. Thus, not only is FDG-PET scanning done after uptake is complete, but it also reflects total glucose uptake, whether that glucose is being used for aerobic or anaerobic processes.

^{11}C-glucose, on the other hand, undergoes metabolism rapidly and the ^{11}C label is lost. How rapidly depends on the position of the ^{11}C in the glucose molecule. Under complete aerobic conditions, the carbon skeletons of glucose are largely retained in the amino acid pools of the Krebs cycle during the time period of dynamic PET scanning used for this tracer. Glucose metabolism in nonstimulated (baseline condition) brain regions is thought to be mainly aerobic. However, even in the baseline condition, although glucose labeled with ^{11}C in the 1- or 6-position gives metabolic rates comparable to deoxyglucose in rats sacrificed quickly (6 min), labeling in the other four possible positions of the glucose molecule gives severe underestimations of glucose metabolic rates. This problem is worse in brain regions undergoing physiological stimulation where the underestimation even with ^{11}C-glucose labeled at the 6-position can be as high as 10% in rats just 6 min after administration of the tracer. The error is even higher with ^{11}C-glucose labeled at other positions.

Although the exact reason for this underestimation of brain glucose metabolic rates in stimulated regions with glucose versus deoxyglucose is still somewhat controversial, it is probably accounted for by the fact that, under physiological stimulation, a significant amount of cerebral glucose is metabolized anaerobically. Here, the tracer is quickly converted into lactate, which is quickly carried off and not available for counting in PET. (Remember that deoxyglucose does not undergo metabolism after initial phosphorylation, and is trapped in the cell.) This results in a serious underestimation of total glucose metabolism with ^{11}C-glucose, which only accurately reflects oxidative metabolism. Fluorodeoxyglucose measures total glucose metabolism in stimulated or unstimulated brain regions. Readers interested in more detail are referred elsewhere (38,58).

The studies by Zohar et al. (76), Rubin et al. (64), and Hoehn-Saric et al. (29) used SPECT techniques, which is itself of special concern. Using ^{133}Xe is a very low-resolution technique that only measures summed activity across the brain surface and provides no information on deep structures. On the other hand, HMPAO SPECT with a high-resolution camera, as that used by Rubin et al. (64) does provide data on deep structures. How HMPAO is used to derive an index of blood flow must be kept in mind, however.

^{99m}Tc-hexamethyl-propyleneamine oxidase is a highly lipophililc compound that crosses the blood–brain barrier quickly, but once in cells is metabolically converted to a hydrophilic form that is trapped in the brain at concentrations roughly proportional to the blood flow through the region. Any HMPAO not so metabolized is in equilibrium across the blood–brain barrier, and is therefore subject to redistribution kinetics, that is, it can be carried off by the blood to other lipid sinks in the body. Thus, although HMPAO uptake is usually interpreted as a valid method of measuring the blood flow of one brain structure relative to that of another, there may be circumstances when the rate of the metabolic conversion from the lipophilic to the hydrophilic form in the brain may be a more important confound than usually admitted in the SPECT literature. Although the most likely reason for Rubin and coworkers detecting differences in brain function between OCD patients and normals with HMPAO and not with ^{133}Xe is the resolution difference between the two methods, the authors also thought an HMPAO-sensitive difference between patients and controls in blood–brain barrier permeability, or even a difference in the rate of HMPAO trapping through hydrophilic conversion, might be responsible. Such possibilities must also be borne in mind when considering these studies compared to those using PET glucose and blood flow techniques (the later is a direct measure of blood flow). Rubin and coworker's finding of continued HMPAO abnormality in the head of the caudate nucleus after effective treatment might point to an important abnormality related to an OCD trait dysfunction that is partially compensated by other elements in the system after effective treatment, as measured with FDG-PET. In fact, it fits well with the model proposed by Swedo et al. (67) for a possible cause of one subtype of OCD in which autoantibodies selectively bind in the striatum, where they would be expected to disrupt the blood–brain barrier coating the microvasculature.

The reports of both Benkelfat et al. (18) and of Baxter et al. (15) found decreases in normalized caudate metabolic rates bilaterally; they differed only on which side made statistical significance. Rausch et al. (60) found that stimulating OCD thoughts increased blood flow in the right striatum. Although there is no proven explanation, we note that Rauch et al. (60) stimulated patients on the left side of the body; we performed blood sampling (often an intense focus of patient attention) on the left, whereas Benkelfat et al. sampled blood on the right. In all these studies, many of the subjects had doubting and checking; a lateralized focus of concern may have led to lateralized brain findings, clearly in need of control in further experiments.

Besides laterality, there are differences in the brain region of interest that are reported to change in the three PET reports of treatment effects in the brains of OCD patients. Our group has noted (15) that the report of both Benkelfat et al. and Baxter et al. found decreases in normalized caudate metabolic rates bilaterally but differed on which side made statistical significance. Swedo et al. (67) found only changes in orbital glucose metabolic rates after treatment, whereas Baxter et al. reported only changes in the striatum, although correlations among orbital cortex and other brain regions were broken up after effective treatment. Time-interval differences between pre- and posttreatment scans among these three studies may have been a critical factor. Our group defined the orbital cortex as involving all orbital gyri, whereas Swedo et al. looked at subregions of the orbital cortex. In addition, other PET work done at UCLA (44) has shown that as a person learns to execute a task more efficiently, the brain region mediating the behavior shows a decrease in both the extent and degree of activation on PET scanning, compared to when the task was new. With time the caudate might become more efficient in limiting OCD symptoms, and its change in a critical function might no longer be detectable with present FDG-PET methods (12).

Recent data from our laboratory may help to resolve these apparent conflicts. We have studied seven OCD subjects with FDG-PET pre- and posttreatment with paroxetine hydrocholoride. New image-subtraction techniques have been employed in data analysis that allow unbiased assessment of small brain regions that change from one scanning session to another. With this treatment and these techniques we observed significant (>10%) reductions of glucose metabolic rates in the medial orbital gyri, bilaterally, when there is treatment response. There are also glucose metabolic decreases localized to the anterior medial inferior region of the head of the caudate nucleus and nucleus accumbens [precisely that striatal region to which the medial orbital gyri project (13)] with effective treatment (Colgan et al. *unpublished data*) (see Fig. 2).

We believe we missed detecting a significant change in orbital gyri glucose metabolic rates with effective OCD treatment in previous studies because we lumped the whole orbital gyri, rather than evaluating the medial gyrus separately. Similarly, in studies by other groups, changes in the head of the caudate nucleus may have been missed because only that subregion of the striatum that receives limbic cortex projections is affected. These specific orbital and striatal subregions are the ones that theory would predict are the points of OCD symptom mediation (13).

A Theory of the Functional Neuroanatomy Mediating the Symptoms of Obsessive-Compulsive Disorder and Certain Other Psychiatric Disorders

Many of the brain-imaging studies reviewed here provide evidence for symptom-related functional activity in the orbital prefrontal cortex and caudate nucleus in OCD. This pattern of orbital-striatal dysfunction is different from that reported in panic (above), depression (4), and schizophrenia (3).

Based on these functional-imaging results reviewed above, the results of neurosurgeries for OCD that interrupt tracts coursing among these brain elements (48), and studies in animals (36,76), we have proposed (15) a model

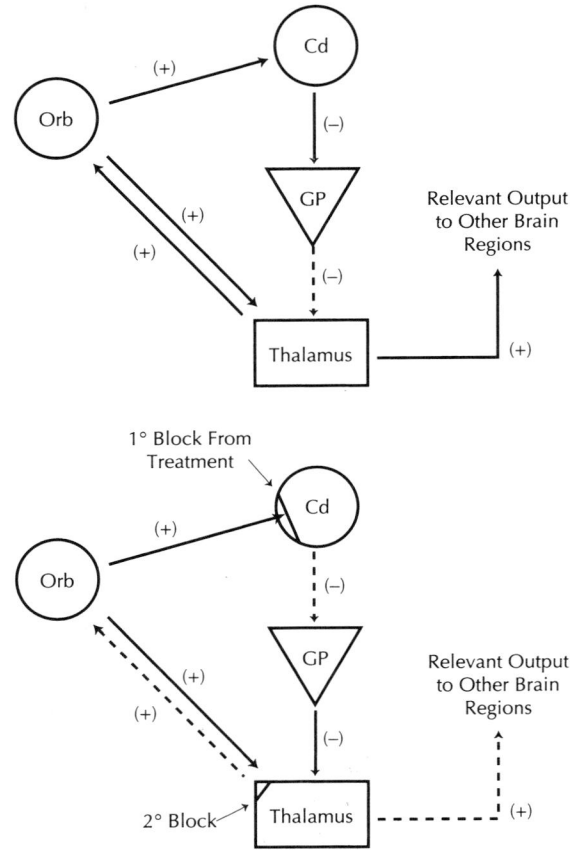

FIG. 3. Proposed model of brain system dysregulation that may mediate the symptom expression of OCD. In the symptomatic state (**top**) worry output from the medial orbital region (*Orb*), largely glutimate, may be driving OCD-relevant circuits in the anterior medial ventral regions of the head of the caudate nucleus (*Cd*), and thus increase inhibitory GABA output to relevant regions of the globus pallidus (*GP*). This would reduce inhibition of the thalamus by GABA, making it vulnerable to being driven (glutimate) by the orbit as well. The excitatory connections between thalamus and orbit make this a potentially self-sustaining circuit, and thus difficult to break (fixation). With effective treatment (**bottom**), however, increases in filtering functions in the Cd may reduce its inhibitory output to the GP, which in turn would increase inhibitory output to the thalamus. This would result in an uncoupling of this fixed worry circuit and allow the patient to more easily terminate OCD behaviors. *Arrows* indicate the effect of stimulating one brain region on the rate of neuronal firing in the other; +, excitatory output; −, inhibitory output; and − − −, reduced effect. From Baxter et al. (15).

for the mediation of symptoms in treatment-responsive OCD (see Fig. 3). These ideas grew from theories first put forward by others (20,33,35,49,60; see ref. 15 for review) of a dysfunctional ''[cortico/limbic]-basal ganglia-thalamic circuit'' in OCD.

In the present formulation of this theory, inadequate sensory information gating (66), sieving, or, to use Freud's term, ''repressive'' functions in the basal ganglia might allow cortical (in this case orbital) inputs to capture and drive a self-sustaining loop (see Fig. 3). In turn, this loop drives behavioral routines (adaptive in other circumstances) that are difficult to interrupt, even when maladaptive. It should be considered that sources of such context-specific behavioral interference (referant to survival needs) may consist not only of irrelevant sensory stimuli (external interference or distractors) but may also consist of well-established but currently irrelevant sensory or motor representations (internal interference) that assert themselves regardless of new, significant environmental inputs that, if they could get through, would alter behavior.

In this regard, we have argued (see ref. 15 for further discussion and literature review) that one function of the orbital cortex, in conjunction with the neostriatum and thalamus as an interactive system, is to help the animal **rivet** critical, prepackaged response behavior (macros) to specific stimuli that are judged significant, to the exclusion of less important signals clamoring for other actions. Such a system may have evolved to allow significant threats to capture and direct attention for needed action to the exclusion of other distractors and to rivit behavior to such concerns until the danger is judged passed. To function optimally, however, such a system would have to be adjusted so that goal-directed behavior would continue to implementation, despite insignificant external distractors that may intervene to redirect behavior, yet could still be suppressed if more significant new information intervenes that requires a change in behavior. Thus, we have postulated that if orbital cortex function is set too high in relationship to the rest of this critical circuitry (i.e., in relationship to the strength of the gate closure in the basal ganglia), such internal inputs might capture behavior to the exclusion of significant new information (resulting in preoccupation), whereas if the orbital region is hypofunctional, less important external inputs may prevail, resulting in distractability.

With successful OCD treatment, however, we believe that the gating functions of the caudate are adequately restored, and this driving circuit broken up.

What is not at all clear at this time is what neurotransmitter system(s) might mediate the proposed critical changes in caudate function that might facilitate treatment response. Studies by PET and SPECT with more specific chemical tracers, especially probes for specific neurotransmitter systems, are clearly needed. Since such radioligand development is difficult and expensive, precluding a shot gun approach, the selection of likely candidates might best be persued with autoradiographic studies of many possibilities in animal models.

Circuits involving limbic- and prefrontal–striatal–thalamic systems have been postulated to mediate the symptomatic expression of several psychiatric disorders (21), including schizophrenia (70) and depression (6,22,70), as well as OCD and Gilles de la Tourette's syndrome (16). Indeed, the sensory gating functions of the striatum (70) seem to fit the metaphor of successful vs. unsuccessful repression, classically invoked by Freud

in many mood and anxiety disorders (72). We propose that specific, different patterns of abnormal neural function in subcircuits of these general cortical- and limbic–basal ganglia–thalamic systems (1,12,13,16,51) may mediate the symptomatic expression of many of the neurotic phenomana of whose neurological basis Freud could only dream.

ACKNOWLEDGMENTS

This work was supported, in part, by a Research Scientist Development Award (KO1-MH00752), and ROI MH37916 from the National Institute of Mental Health, an Established Investigator Award from the National Alliance for Research on Schizophrenia and Affective Disorders, contract AM03-76 SF00012 from the Department of Energy, the Jennifer Jones Simon Foundation, Los Angeles, and the Judson Braun Chair in Psychiatry at UCLA.

I am indebted to many collaborators, but especially would like to acknowledge here the late Daniel X. Freedman, M.D., a psychiatrist who had a life-long interest in both the workings of the brain and the observations of the classical psychoanalysis, and without whose encouragement and support this work would not have progressed.

REFERENCES

1. Alexander GE, DeLong MR, Strick PL. Parallel organization of functionally segregated circuits linking basal ganglia and cortex. *Ann Rev Neurosci* 1986;9:357–381.
2. Andreasen NC: Brain imaging: applications in psychiatry. *Science* 1988;239:1381–1388.
3. Andreasen NC: *Brain imaging: applications in psychiatry.* Washington, DC: American Psychiatric Press; 1989.
4. Baxter LR. PET studies of cerebral function in major depression and obsessive-compulsive disorder: the emerging prefrontal cortex consensus. *Ann Clin Psychiatry* 1991;3:103–109.
5. Baxter LR. Neuroimaging studies of obsessive-compulsive disorder. *Psychiatr Clin No Am* 1992;15:871–884.
6. Baxter LR, Phelps ME, Mazziotta JC, et al. Cerebral metabolic rates for glucose in mood disorders. *Arch Gen Psychiatry* 1985;42:441–447.
7. Baxter LR, Phelps ME, Mazziotta JC, Guze BH, Schwartz JM, Selin CE. Local cerebral glucose metabolic rates in obsessive-compulsive disorder—a comparison with rates in unipolar depression and in normal controls. *Arch Gen Psychiatry* 1987;44:211–218.
8. Baxter LR, Mazziotta JC, Phelps ME, Selin CE, Guze BH, Fairbanks L. Cerebral glucose metabolic rates in normal human females vs. normal males. *Psychiatry Res* 1987;21:237–245.
9. Baxter LR, Schwartz JM, Mazziotta JC, et al. Cerebral glucose metabolic rates in nondepressed obsessive–compulsives. *Am J Psychiatry* 1988;145:1560–1563.
10. Baxter LR, Schwartz JM, Phelps ME, et al. Reduction of prefrontal cortex glucose metabolism common to three types of depression. *Arch Gen Psychiatry* 1989;46:243–250.
11. Baxter LR, Schwartz JM, Guze BH, Bergman K, Szuba MP. PET imaging in obsessive–compulsive disorder with and without depression. *J Clin Psychiatry* 1990;51(s):61–69.
12. Baxter LR, Schwartz JM, Guze BH, Bergman K, Szuba MP. Neuroimaging in obsessive–compulsive disorder: seeking the mediating

neuroanatomy. In: Jenike MA, Baer L, Minichiello WE, eds. *Obsessive–compulsive disorders: theory and management,* 2nd ed. Chicago: Year Book Medical Publishers; 1990:167–188.

13. Baxter LR, Schwartz JM, Guze BH. Brain Imaging: toward a neuro-anatomy of OCD. In Zohar Y, Insel TR, Rasmussen S, eds. *The psychobiology of obsessive–compulsive disorder.* New York: Springer-Verlag; 1991:101–125.

14. Baxter LR, Mazziotta JC, Pahl JJ, et al. Psychiatric, genetic, and positron emission tomographic evaluation of persons at risk for Huntington's disease. *Arch Gen Psychiatry* 1992;49:148–154.

15. Baxter LR, Schwartz JM, Bergman KS, et al. Caudate glucose metabolic rate changes with both drug and behavior therapy for obsessive–compulsive disorder. *Arch Gen Psychiatry,* 1992; 49:681–689.

16. Baxter LR, Guze BH. Neuroimaging in Tourette's and related disorders. In: Kurland R, ed. *Handbook of Tourette's syndrome and related tic and behavioral disorders.* Paris: Marcel Dekker; 1993:289–304.

17. Behar D, Rapoport JL, Berg CJ, Computerized tomography and neuropsychological test measures in adolescents with obsessive–compulsive disorder. *Am J Psychiatry* 1984;141:363–369.

18. Benkelfat C, Nordhal TE, Semple WE, King AC, Murphy DL, Cohen RM. Local cerebral glucose metabolic rates in obsessive–compulsive disorder: patients treated with clomipramine. *Arch Gen Psychiatry* 1990;47:840–848.

19. Blomqvist G, Bergstrom K, Bergstrom M, et al. Models for ^{11}C-glucose. In: Greitz T, Ingvar DH, Widen L, eds. *The metabolism of the human brain studied with positron emission tomography.* New York: Raven Press; 1985.

20. Cummings JL, Frankel M. Gilles de la Tourette's syndrome and the neurological basis of obsessions and compulsions. *Biol Psychiatry* 1985;20:1117–1126.

21. Cummings JL. Frontal-subcortical circuits and human behavior. *Arch Neurol* 1993;50:873–880.

22. Drevets WC, Videen TO, MacLeod AK, Haller JW, Raichle ME. PET images of blood flow changes during anxiety: correction. *Science* 1992;256:1696.

23. Drevets WC, Videen TO, Price JL, Preskorn SH, Carmichael T, Raichle ME. A functional anatomical study of unipolar depression. *J Neurosci* 1992;12:3628–3641.

24. DeCristofaro MTR, Sessarego A, Pupi A, Biondi F, Faravelli C. Brain perfusion abnormalities in drug-naive, lactate-sensitive panic patients: a SPECT study. *Biol Psychiatry* 1993;33:505–512.

25. Freud S. The question of lay analysis (1926). In: Strachey J, ed. *The standard edition of the complete psychological works of Sigmund Freud.* Vol. 20. London: Hogarth Press; 1964:231.

26. Freud S. Project for a scientific psychology. In: Strachey J, ed. *The standard edition of the complete psychological works of sigmund freud.* Vol. 1. London: Hogarth Press; 1964:283–294.

27. Garber HJ, Ananth JV, Chiu LC, Griswold VJ, Oldendorf WH. Nuclear magnetic resonance study of obsessive–compulsive disorder. *Am J Psychiatry* 1989;146:1001–1005.

28. Giodani B, Boivin MJ, Berent S, Anxiety and cerebral cortical metabolism in normal persons. *Psychiatry Res Neuroimag* 1990;35:49–60.

29. Hoehn-Saric R, Pearlson GD, Harris GJ, Machlin SR, Camargo EE. Effects of fluoxetine on regional cerebral blood flow in obsessive–compulsive patients. *Am J Psychiatry* 1991;148:1243–1245.

30. Horwitz B, Swedo SE, Grady CL, et al. Cerebral metabolic pattern in obsessive–compulsive disorder: altered intercorrelations between regional rates of glucose utilization. *Psychiatry Res Neuroimag* 1991;40:221–237.

31. Husby G, van de Rijn I, Zabriskie JB, Abdin ZH, Williams RC. Antibodies reacting with cytoplasm of subthalamic and caudate nuclei neurons in chorea and acute rheumatic fever. *J Exp Med* 1976;144:1094–1110.

32. Insel TR, Donnelly EF, Lalakea ML, Alterman IS, Murphy DL. Neurological and neuropsychological studies of patients with obsessive–compulsive disorder. *Biol Psychiatry* 1983;18:741–751.

33. Insel TR. Obsessive–compulsive disorder: a neuroethological perspective. *Psychopharmacol Bull* 1988;24:365–369.

34. Insel TR, Winslow JT. Neurobiology of obsessive–compulsive disorder. In: Jenike MA, Baer L, Minichiello WE, eds. *Obsessive–*

compulsive disorders: theory and management, 2nd ed. Chicago: Year Book Medical Publishers; 1990:116–131.

35. Insel TR. Toward a neuroanatomy of obsessive–compulsive disorder. *Arch Gen Psychiatry* 1992;49:739–744.

36. Iversen SD. Behavioral aspects of cortico–subcortical interaction with special reference to frontostriatal relations. In: Reinoso-Suarez G, Ajmone-Marsan C, eds. *Cortical integration.* New York: Raven Press; 1984.

37. Kellner CH, Jolley RR, Holgate RC, et al. Brain MRI in obsessive–compulsive disorder. *Psychiatry Res* 1991;36:45–49.

38. Lear JL, Ackermann RF. Autoradiographic comparison of FDG-based and GLU-based measurements of cerebral glucose transport and metabolism: normal and activated conditions. In: Lassen NA, Ingvar DH, Raichle ME, Friberg L, eds. *Brain work and mental activity: quantitative studies with radioactive tracers.* Copenhagen: Munksgaard; 1991:142–157. (31st Alfred Benson Symposium).

39. Lepola U, Nousiainen U, Puranen M, Riekkinen P, Rimon R. EEG and CT findings in patients with panic disorder. *Biol Psychiatry* 1990;28:721–727.

40. Luxenberg JS, Swedo SE, Flament MF, Friedland RP, Rapoport J, Rapoport SI. Neuroanatomical abnormalities in obsessive–compulsive disorder determined with quantitative x-ray computed tomography. *Am J Psychiatry* 1988;145:1089–1093.

41. Machlin SR, Harris GJ, Pearlson GD, Hoehn-Saric R, Jeffery P, Camargo EE. Elevated medial-frontal cerebral blood flow in obsessive–compulsive patients: a SPECT study. *Am J Psychiatry* 1991;148:1240–1242.

42. Maricle RA, Sennhauser S, Burry M. Panic disorder associated with right parahippocampal infarction. *J Nerv Ment Dis* 1991;179:374–375.

43. Martinot JL, Allilaire JF, Mazoyer BM, et al. Obsessive–compulsive disorder: a clinical, neuropsychological and positron emission tomography study. *Acta Psychiatr Scand* 1990;82:233–242.

44. Martinot JL, Hardy P, Feline A, et al. Left prefrontal glucose hypo-metabolism in the depressed state: a confirmation. *Am J Psychiatry* 1990;147:1313–1317.

45. Mazziotta JC, Grafton ST, Woods RC. The human motor system studied with PET measurements of cerebral blood flow: topography and motor learning. In: Lassen NA, Ingvar DH, Raichle ME, Friberg L, eds. *Brain work and mental activity: quantitative studies with radioactive tracers.* Copenhagen: Munksgaard; 1991:280–293. (31st Alfred Benson Symposium).

46. Mindus P, Nyman H, Mogard J, Meyerson BA, Ericson K. Orbital and caudate glucose metabolism studied by positron emission tomography (PET) in patients undergoing capsulotomy for obsessive–compulsive disorder. In: Jenike MA, Asberg M, eds. *Understanding obsessive–compulsive disorder (OCD).* Toronto: Hogrefe & Huber Publishers; 1991:52–57.

47. Mindus P, Nyman HL. Normalization of personality characteristics in patients with incapacitating anxiety disorders after capsulotomy. *Acta Psychiatr Scand* 1991;83:283–291.

48. Mindus P. *Capsulotomy in anxiety disorders: a multidisciplinary study.* Stockholm: Karolinska Institute; 1991.

49. Modell JG, Mountx JM, Curtis GC, Greden JF. Neurophysiological dysfunction in basal ganglia/limbic striatal and thalamocortical circuits as a pathogenetic mechanism of obsessive–compulsive disorder. *J Neuropsychiatry* 1989;1:27–36.

50. Mountz JM, Modelll JG, Wilson MW, et al. Positron emission tomographic evaluation of cerebral blood flow during state anxiety in simple phobia. *Arch Gen Psychiatry* 1989;46:501–504.

51. Nauta WJH, Domesick VB. Afferent and efferent relationships of the basal ganglia. *Functions of the basal ganglia.* London: Pitman; 1984:3–29. (CIBA foundation Symposium #107).

52. Nordahl TE, Benkelfat C, Semple WE, Gross M, King AC, Cohen RM. Cerebral glucose metabolic rates in obsessive–compulsive disorder. *Neuropsychopharmacology* 1989;2:23–28.

53. Nordahl TE, Semple WE, Gross M, et al. Cerebral glucose metabolic differences in patients with panic disorder. *Neuropshchopharmacology* 1990;3:261–272.

54. Ontiveros A, Fontaine R, Breton G, Elie R, Fontaine S, Dery R. Correlation of severity of panic disorder and neuroanatomical changes on magnetic resonance imaging. *J Neuropsychiatry Clin Neurosci* 1989;1:404–408.

55. Parent A. *Comparative Neurobiology of the Basal Ganglia.* New York: John Wiley; 1986.

56. Pauls DL, Leckman JF. The inheritance of Gilles de la Tourette's syndrome and associated behaviors—evidence for autosomal dominant transmission. *N Engl J Med* 1986;315:993–997.

57. Phelps ME, Mazziotta JC. Positron emission tomography: human brain function and biochemistry. *Science* 1985;228:799–809.

58. Phelps ME, Mazziotta JC, Shelbert HR, eds. *Positron emission tomography and autoradiography.* New York: Raven Press; 1986.

59. Rapaport JL, Wise SP. Obsessive–compulsive disorder: is it a basal ganglia dysfunction? *Psychopharm Bull* 1988;24:380–384.

60. Rauch SL, Jenike MJ, Alpert NA. Regional cerebral blood flow measured during symptom provocation in obsessive-compulsive disorder using ^{15}O-labeled CO_2 and positron emission tomography. *Arch Gen Psychiatry* 1994;51:62–70.

61. Reiman EM, Raichle ME, Butler FK, Herscovitch P, Robins E. A focal brain abnormality in panic disorder, a severe form of anxiety. *Nature* 1984;310:683–685.

62. Reiman EM, Raichle ME, Robins E, et al. Neuroanatomical correlates of a lactate-induced anxiety attack. *Arch Gen Psychiatry* 1989;46:493–500.

63. Reiman EM, Fusselman MJ, Fox PT, Raichle ME. Neuroanatomical correlates of anticipatory anxiety. *Science* 1989;243:1071–1074.

64. Rubin RT, Villanueva-Meyer J, Ananth J, Trajmar PG, Mena I. Regional ^{133}Xe cerebral blood flow and cerebral ^{99m}HMPAO uptake in unmedicated obsessive–compulsive disorder patients and matched normal control subjects: determination by high-resolution single-photon emission computed tomography. *Arch Gen Psychiatry,* 1992;49:695–702.

65. Rubin RT, Ananth J, Villanueva-Meyer J, Trajmar PG, Mena I. Regional xenon 133 cerebral blood flow and cerebral technetium 99m HMPAO uptake in patients with obsessive–compulsive disorder before and during treatment. *Arch Gen Psychiatry* [submitted].

66. Schneider JS. Review: basal ganglia role in behavior: importance of sensory gating and its relevance to psychiatry. *Biol Psychiatry* 1984;19:1693–1710.

67. Swedo SE, Rapoport JL, Cheslow DL, et al. High prevalence of obsessive–compulsive symptoms in patients with Sydenham's chorea. *Am J Psychiatry* 1989;146:246–249.

68. Swedo SE, Pietrini P, Leonard HL, et al. Cerebral glucose metabolism in childhood-onset obsessive–compulsive disorder: revisualization during pharmacotherapy. *Arch Gen Psychiatry* 1992;49:690–694.

69. Swedo SE, Schapiro MB, Grady CL, et al. Cerebral glucose metabolism in childhood-onset obsessive–compulsive disorder. *Arch Gen Psychiatry* 1989;46:518–523.

70. Swerdlow NR, Koob GF. Dopamine, schizophrenia, mania and depression: toward a unified hypothesis of cortico-striato-pallido-thalamic function. *Behav Brain Sci* 1987;10:197–245.

71. Teresa M, De Cristofaro DER, Sessarego A, Pupi A, Biondi F, Faravelli C. Brain perfusion abnormalities in drug-naive, lactate-sensitive panic patients: a SPECT study. *Biol Psychiatry* 1993;33:505–512.

72. Thompson JM, Baxter LR, Schwartz JM. Freud, obsessive–compulsive disorder and neurobiology. *Psychoanal Contemp Thought* 1992;15:483–505.

73. Wik G, Fredrikson M, Ericson K, Driksson L, Stone-Elander S, Greitz T. A functional cerebral response to frightening visual stimulation. *Psychiatry Res Neuroimag* 1993;50:15–24.

74. Winslow JT, Insel T. Neuroethological models of obsessive–compulsive disorder. In: Zohar J, Insel T, Rasmussen S, eds. *The psychobiology of obsessive–compulsive disorder* New York: Springer-Verlag; 1991.

75. Wu JC, Buchsbaum MS, Hershey TG, Hazlett E, Sicotte N, Johnson JC. PET in generalized anxiety disorder. *Biol Psychiatry* 1991;29:1181–1199.

76. Zohar J, Insel TR, Berman KF, Foa EB, Hill JL, Weinberger DR. Anxiety and cerebral blood flow during behavioral challenge: dissociation of central from peripheral and subjective measures. *Arch Gen Psychiatry* 1989;46:505–510.

77. Zohar J, Insel TR. Obsessive-compulsive disorder: psychobiological approaches to diagnosis, treatment, and pathophysiology. *Biol Psychiatry* 1987;22:667–687.

Psychopharmacology: The Fourth Generation of Progress, edited by Floyd E. Bloom and David J. Kupfer. Raven Press, Ltd., New York © 1995.

CHAPTER 110

Anxiety and the Serotonin$_{1A}$ Receptor

Jeremy D. Coplan, Susan I. Wolk, and Donald F. Klein

The serotonin (5-HT) receptor was first described in 1957 (25). Since then, there has been an explosion of knowledge regarding this ubiquitous neurotransmitter system. Despite extensive documentation of a role for the central 5-HT system in regulation of mood, anxiety, feeding, sleep, sexual activity, body temperature, and nociception (for review, see ref. 5), the mechanisms by which disorders of these functions are mediated remain unclear. At least eight receptor subtypes with specific neuroanatomical location and multiple intracellular effects following receptor activation have been identified (for review, see ref. 30 and Chapter 39, *this volume*). Such diversification of function implies an exceedingly complex system. Rheostat models of neural dysfunction propose that reductions or increases of a single neurotransmitter system are responsible for clinical psychopathology and are inadequate in understanding 5-HT receptor-related abnormalities. These authors (16,37) have previously proposed a cybernetic model describing the inability of the system to maintain or regain homeostatic control of its neurotransmitters to facilitate understanding of 5-HT–related abnormalities in panic–anxiety. The neural substrate for cybernetic dysfunction is unclear, although the observation that certain psychotherapeutic drugs may act, in part, through regulatory 5-HT$_{1A}$ autoreceptors is of interest.

The 5-HT$_{1A}$ receptor was first described in 1981 (49), and is probably the best characterized of the 5-HT receptors. The recognition of anxiolytic effects of nonbenzodiazepine azapirones agents, which act as 5-HT$_{1A}$ partial agonists, such as buspirone, gepirone, and ipsapirone and their therapeutic role in clinical anxiety and mood disorders has further focused attention on the 5-HT$_{1A}$ receptor. Although the azapirones interact with other neurotransmitter systems, such as the dopaminergic (56) and norad-

renergic (60), the azapirones display nanomolar affinity for 5-HT$_{1A}$ receptor sites (66). Interestingly, the anxiolytic effects of azapirones follow a time course observed with antidepressants where therapeutic effects are delayed for 3 to 4 weeks, which is unlike the rapid effects observed with benzodiazepine anxiolytics. The putative mechanism of therapeutic effects of these piperazine derivatives are complex and involve both pre- and postsynaptic receptor sites of action. We first review the preclinical studies followed by the available clinical data (see Chapter 37, *this volume*).

PRECLINICAL CONSIDERATIONS

Basic science and animal studies have facilitated identification of the 5-HT$_{1A}$ partial agonists, as well as delineated a role of the 5-HT$_{1A}$ receptor in the regulation of animal models of anxiety. From a preclinical perspective, the 5-HT$_{1A}$ receptor is discussed regarding its neuroanatomical location, its pharmacological properties, molecular biological structure, and intracellular signal transduction. The effects of the azapirones on behavioral responses reflective of anxiety in rodents are divided according to Lucki and Wieland (42) into three categories: (a) unconditioned behaviors elicited by 5-HT$_{1A}$ agonists (b) drug discrimination studies, and (c) conditioned behaviors. Studies suggesting an effect of 5-HT$_{1A}$ ligands on rodent distress vocalizations elicited by mother–infant separation are reviewed. Despite the recent extensive elaboration of the 5-HT system in preclinical studies, the emerging complexity of its function has only complicated clarification of its role in clinical anxiety.

NEUROANATOMICAL CONSIDERATIONS

Serotonergic pathways may be divided into ascending and descending pathways that project to the spinal cord

J. D. Coplan, S. I. Wolk, and D. F. Klein: Department of Psychiatry, Columbia University College of Physicians and Surgeons, and New York State Psychiatric Institute, New York, New York 10032.

and brainstem and to cortical and subcortical structures, respectively. There is good evidence that 5-HT modulates both motor and sensory processing at the level of the brainstem and spinal cord. Certain serotonergic nuclei are closely associated and modulate other brainstem structures implicated in anxiety, such as the nucleus locus coeruleus (47) and the nucleus paragigantocellularis (4). Serotonin-related dysfunction of sensory and motor modulatory processes may have consequences for nociceptive and cardiorespiratory psychophysiology.

Dense ascending serotonergic pathways project to the monkey amygdala (especially the entorhinal and dentate gyrus), the rectus gyrus of the frontal lobe, and the inferior and superior gyri of the temporal lobe. The lowest levels in primates are seen in the occipital lobe and the precentral motor cortex of the frontal lobe (for review, see ref. 5). In man, rat, and guinea pig, 5-HT$_{1A}$ receptors are found in high concentration in the dorsal raphe nuclei, the hippocampal pyramidal cell layer, the lateral septum, the frontal cortex, and the dorsal horn of the spinal cord (19,72). Neurotoxicity studies using 5,7-DHT (dihydroxytryptamine) indicate that the 5-HT$_{1A}$ receptors of the dorsal raphe are generally presynaptic, whereas hippocampal 5-HT$_{1A}$ receptors are largely postsynaptic (72).

PHARMACOLOGICAL PROPERTIES

Specific ligand studies with high affinity for the 5-HT$_{1A}$ receptor have facilitated characterization of the functional consequences of receptor activation. 8-OH-DPAT [8-hydroxy-2-(di-*n*-propylamino)-tetralin] possesses an almost 1000-fold selectivity for the 5-HT$_{1A}$ binding site (45). Many other ligands have been developed (30), although 8-OH-DPAT possesses the greatest specificity and has been most studied. In contrast to 5-HT$_{1A}$ agonists, ligands that are not strong 5-HT$_{1A}$ agonists (e.g., 1-3-fluoromethyl)phenyl]-piperazine (TFMPP) which is predominantly a 5-HT$_{1B}$ agonist) (65) and 1-(3-chlorophenyl)piperazine (*m*CPP, a functional 5-HT$_2$ and 5-HT$_{1C}$ agonist) (29) are weak dorsal raphe autoreceptor agonists (1). β-Adrenoceptor antagonists including (−)-propranolol, spiperone, and pindolol may possess 5-HT$_{1A}$ antagonistic properties (1), but also show affinity for 5-HT$_{1C}$ receptors. Intracellular recordings from hippocampal pyramidal cells (CA1) in rat-brain slices have shown that direct application of 5-HT produces a membrane hyperpolarization and reduction in the input resistance from an opening of potassium channels (3). Buspirone and ipsapirone, which displace 5-HT binding in hippocampal preparations (26), produce only small hyperpolarizations, which is in accordance with their partial agonistic action at postsynaptic sites (2) but also reduces in a dose-dependent fashion certain firing patterns of the pyramidal cell layer (CA1) of the hippocampus (7). Low-dose microiontophoretic applications of ipsapirone, which do not affect spon-

taneous firing rates, attenuate excitation of pyramidal cells induced by the excitatory amino acid, glutamate (1).

MOLECULAR BIOLOGY

The 5-HT$_{1A}$ receptor has been cloned and sequenced (see ref. 30, for review). The receptor structure is similar to that of the G-protein–coupled superfamily of neurotransmitter receptors. In the presence of guanosine triphosphate (GTP), the receptor complex dissociates into two components. The smaller 60-kd component is the actual receptor, whereas the larger 90-kd component is the associated G protein.

The human receptor is approximately 420 amino acids long and has seven putative transmembrane regions with four intervening peptide sequences facing the extracellular space, whereas four others face the cytoplasm. Like other receptors that inhibit adenylate cyclase, the 5-HT$_{1A}$ receptor has a relatively long third cytoplasmic peptide loop (C3), portions of which have been used to generate antibodies. In transmembrane regions 3, 6, and 7, the 5-HT$_{1A}$ receptor shares significant levels of amino acid sequences with the α$_2$-, β$_1$- and β$_2$-adrenergic receptors. Interestingly, single-point mutations in the seventh transmembrane loop of the 5-HT$_{1A}$ receptor reduces receptor affinity by 100-fold for the β-antagonist, pindolol, but not for 5-HT and 8-OH-DPAT (see ref. 30, for review). Such data suggest that point mutations of receptor peptide sequences may have profound consequences for 5-HT receptor sensitivity.

INTRACELLULAR SIGNAL TRANSDUCTION

The second messenger effects of the 5-HT$_{1A}$ receptor are diverse. Activation of the 5-HT$_{1A}$ receptor in rat hippocampal membranes was noted to inhibit forskolin-induced increases in adenylate cyclase. This 5-HT$_{1A}$-mediated effect was abolished by pertussis toxin, suggesting involvement of the pertussis-sensitive Gi-protein. The Gi protein is negatively coupled to adenylate cyclase and thereby reduces cyclic adenosine monophosphate (cAMP) dependent protein kinase activity. Cloning studies using human 5-HT$_{1A}$ receptors transfected in cell cultures support the view that 5-HT$_{1A}$ receptor activation mediates inhibition of adenylate cyclase via the pertussis-sensitive Gi protein and also stimulates phosphoinositide turnover. The clinical relevance of abnormal intracellular signal transduction following 5-HT receptor activation is relatively unexplored (for review, see ref. 30).

PUTATIVE MECHANISMS OF ACTION

Based on in vivo electrophysiological experiments, Blier et al. (8) have postulated that 5HT$_{1A}$ partial agonists mediate antidepressant effects through a net increase in serotonergic neurotransmission following adaptive receptor changes. The firing activity of 5-HT neurons of the dorsal raphe nucleus during the course of gepirone administration was studied. The responsiveness of 5-HT neurons to autoreceptor stimulation by lysergic acid diethylamide given intravenously (LSD) and microiontophoretic dorsal raphe applications of 5-HT, LSD, 8-OH-DPAT, and gepirone was decreased after 14 days of 15 mg/kg per day of gepirone treatment. Gepirone applied microiontophoretically to postsynaptic sites of the hippocampal pyramidal neurons decreased firing rates, as does 5-HT application, although the responsiveness of hippocampal neurons did not diminish after 14 days of gepirone administration. Thus, gepirone activates postsynaptic 5-HT receptors without inducing a desensitization upon long-term administration. The recovery of presynaptic release of 5-HT in combination with pharmacological activation of unaltered postsynaptic 5-HT receptors putatively results in an enhancement of 5-HT neurotransmission. The usefulness of the Blier et al. (8) model is limited by the extent to which single dorsal raphe neuron studies are representative of 5-HT neurons in general. In addition, the postsynaptic effects described are localized and may not generalize to other projection sites. For instance, in radioligand studies, chronic antidepressants down-regulate 5-HT$_2$ binding in the rat cortex, which would tend to reduce 5-HT neurotransmission (51).

Schreiber and DeVry (62) hypothesized that the anxiolytic effects of 5-HT$_{1A}$ partial agonists result predominantly from an interaction with presynaptic 5-HT$_{1A}$ receptors, resulting in a decrease of hyperactive serotonergic neurotransmission. The same authors report that reduction of serotonergic function by the neurotoxin 5,7-dihydroxytryptamine (5,7-DHT) and depletion of 5-HT by the competitive antagonist, parachlorphenylalanine (PCPA), diminishes conditioned inhibition in rat studies. The observation that PCPA and 5,7-DHT also induce muricidal behavior in rodents calls into question the specificity of conditioned inhibition as a model of anxiety. Rats in an elevated maze (an anxiety paradigm) have increased 5-HT levels in the ventral hippocampus (74). Nevertheless, the lack of anxiolytic (or anxiogenic) effect in panic disorder patients following depletion of central 5-HT using a tryptophan-free amino acid preparation (27) contradicts the view that anxiety is consistently due to an increase of 5-HT neurotransmission. Moreover, based on the Blier et al. studies (8), 5-HT$_{1A}$ partial agonists would be predicted to exert immediate clinical anxiolytic effects that would dissipate following desensitization of raphe autoreceptors. The limitations of extrapolating animal models directly to clinical psychopathology are evident.

The antidepressant effects of the 5-HT$_{1A}$ partial agonists are postulated to result from an enhancement of serotonergic neurotransmission through their interaction with postsynaptic 5-HT$_{1A}$ sites (62). However, evidence

for low 5-HT function in clinical depression is conflicting. Although cerebrospinal fluid (CSF) concentrations of 5-hydroxyinositolacetic acid (5-HIAA) is found to be reduced in depressed subjects, its strong association with impulsive–aggressive behaviors implies a secondary rather than central role in depression (12). Supporting the view of hypoactive 5-HT neurotransmission in depression is that the prolactin response to intravenous tryptophan is reduced in patients with the disorder (31), although similar reduced prolactin responses in response to fenfluramine have been reported in impulsive-aggressives (12). Augmentation of prolactin response to intravenous tryptophan by a range of antidepressant medications occurs irrespective of clinical response (54), suggesting that simple augmentation of 5-HT activity is desirable but not always sufficient for therapeutic response. Further casting doubt on the rheostat model of the association of low 5-HT with depression is the finding by Delgado et al. (20) that rapid 5-HT depletion using an oral tryptophan-free amino-acid preparation causes relapse in 73% of selective serotonin reuptake inhibitor (SSRI)-treated subjects, but only 15% of desipramine (DMI) treated subjects, and does not acutely worsen depression in untreated subjects. These conflicting data suggest a complex interaction between 5-HT and other unknown target systems, which produces manifestations of clinical anxiety and mood disorders and their therapeutic response.

With respect to receptor function, Schreiber and DeVry (62) have postulated a preliminary distinction between receptors that mediate anxiolytic and antidepressants effects and those that produce opposing effects. For instance, in vivo rat studies demonstrate that acute administration of 5-HT$_{1A}$ agonists lead to hyperpolarization of the neuron (8) whereas down-regulation of 5-HT$_2$ receptors by many antidepressant treatments may contribute to reductions of anxiety, although it should be noted that many antidepressants also down-regulate 5-HT$_{1A}$ receptors (50).

RODENT BEHAVIORAL STUDIES OF THE SEROTONIN$_{1A}$ RECEPTOR

Unconditioned Behaviors Elicited by Serotonin$_{1A}$ Agonists

The 5-HT syndrome is most studied in rats and can be produced by administering a direct or indirect 5-HT agonist (70). In addition to the standard features of the rodent serotonin syndrome, other behaviors include low outstretched posture, hyperreactivity, hyperactivity, intense salivation, backward walking, and piloerection. Serotonin agonists that do not have high affinity for the 5-HT$_{1A}$ receptor do not produce the syndrome as strongly. In contrast to β-receptor antagonists with high 5-HT$_{1A}$ affinity, 5-HT2 antagonists do not block the syndrome. Acute depletion of 5-HT does not affect the syndrome, suggesting postsynaptic mediation. Destruction of 5-HT neurons may in fact enhance susceptibility to the 5-HT syndrome by the 5-HT$_{1A}$ agonist 8-OH-DPAT (70). Recent data suggest that the 5-HT syndrome may be mediated by descending pathways of the nucleus raphe obscurus. Such 5-HT$_{1A}$ partial agonists as buspirone induce the syndrome weakly and antagonize the effects of more potent 5-HT$_{1A}$ agonists, such as 8-OH-DPAT (for review, see ref. 42).

In humans, excessive increase of synaptic 5-HT may lead to a clinical 5-HT syndrome, which may respond to nonspecific 5-HT antagonists, such as cyproheptadine (see ref. 16, for review). A more frequently encountered observation (34) regarding the use of SSRIs and the 5-HT precursor, 5-hydroxytryptophan in panic disorder patients was that there appeared to be a biphasic treatment response. Patients initially experienced a worsening of generalized anxiety accompanied by a cluster of stimulation symptoms, including jitteriness, insomnia, diarrhea, and a sensation of jumping out one's skin. Of note, panic frequency appeared unchanged despite an overall increase in anxiety symptoms. If patients were able to tolerate these symptoms for several weeks, an ensuing reduction in panic attacks and anxiety was evident. Such stimulation reactions have also been noted with imipramine and desipramine (75) suggesting that they are not specific to the SSRIs or 5-HT. However, the syndrome itself is most frequently encountered in patients with panic attacks in contrast to subjects with other SSRI, clomipramine (CMI), and/or tricyclic-antidepressant (TCA) responsive psychiatric disorders (16). Of note, partial 5-HT$_{1A}$ agonists do not, to our knowledge, consistently produce the jitteriness syndrome, suggesting a necessity for full 5-HT agonism at postsynaptic sites. The relationship of the jitteriness syndrome to the rodent 5-HT syndrome remains unclarified. Reports of subsensitivity of the 5-HT$_{1A}$ receptor in panic disorder as reflected by hypothermic and corticoid response (41) suggests that 5-HT$_{1A}$ receptors are not likely to be associated with the jitteriness syndrome. Nevertheless, a parallel pattern is shown with the rodent 5-HT syndrome—induction by full but not partial agonism (42)—suggesting some similarity to the human jitteriness syndrome.

Drug Discrimination Studies

Rats trained to discriminate the stimulus properties of 8-OH-DPAT generalized this stimulus to the 5-HT$_{1A}$ partial agonists. Benzodiazepines, on the other hand, do not generalize to the stimulus properties of the 5-HT$_{1A}$ partial agonists, suggesting that the stimulus properties of these two classes of anxiolytics are mediated by distinct mechanisms. Interestingly, fenfluramine, which acts as a nonspecific 5-HT agonist through enhancement of presynap-

tic release and reuptake blockade and sertraline, a 5-HT reuptake inhibitor, fail to substitute for the 5-HT$_{1A}$ agonist 8-OH-DPAT, but do generalize to non-5-HT$_{1A}$ agonists such as TFMPP (largely a 5-HT$_{1B}$ agonist) and [+/−)-1-(2,5-dimethoxy-4-iodophenyl)-2-aminopropane (DOI), a 5-HT$_2$ agonist. These data suggest preferential stimulation of non-5-HT$_{1A}$ receptors (particularly 5-HT$_{1B}$ and 5-HT$_2$) by nonspecific indirect agonists, whereas the stimulus properties of 8-OH-DPAT are probably mediated by the inhibition of 5-HT release by 5-HT$_{1A}$ autoreceptor activation. This view is supported by the observation that PCPA-induced 5-HT depletion generalizes to 8-OH-DPAT but not TFMPP (for review, see ref. 42).

Conditioned Behaviors

Drugs with therapeutic effects in humans exert effects on various animal models of anxiety. These models facilitate the prediction of the effects of novel compounds. The 5-HT$_{1A}$ agonist (8-OH-DPAT) and 5-HT$_{1A}$ partial agonists increase punished responding in rats (18), similar to the effects of the benzodiazepines (71). However, it should be noted that the magnitude of buspirone's effects on punished responding is weak relative to the benzodiazepine anxiolytics. In addition, benzodiazepines enhance punished responding in certain paradigms where azapirones fail to exert such effects. Further evidence for the distinction between benzodiazepine versus azapirone effects on punished responding is the observation that flumazenil antagonizes benzodiazepine-induced suppression of scheduled behavior but has no effect on azapirone-induced effects (6). Again, the enhanced punished responding effects of the 5-HT$_{1A}$ partial agonists appear to be mediated by presynaptic receptors as PCPA-induced depletion, neurotoxic destruction of 5-HT neurons, and direct raphe injection of 5-HT$_{1A}$ agonists antagonize the effects of the azapirones. In accordance with their clinical effects, the azapirones, in contrast to benzodiazepines, exert behavioral effects in rodent task tests that are analogous to antidepressant drugs, but these effects appear to be postsynaptically mediated (for review, see ref. 42). These rodent studies suggest that benzodiazepines may exert a more generalized anxiolytic effect than the azapirones, but the latter class of drugs possess the advantage of antidepressant properties.

RODENT DISTRESS VOCALIZATION STUDIES

A modulatory role for 5-HT has been described for the development and expression of the ultrasonic call of infant rat pups during brief maternal separations. Serotonin reuptake inhibitors reduce the rate of calling following acute administration to 9- to 11-day-old pups, and a 5-HT neurotoxin [3,4-methylenedioxymethamphetamine (MDMA)] systematically disrupted the development of ultrasonic vocalizations but not other measures of motor development (73). Consistent with their clinical effects, acute administration of the 5-HT$_{1A}$ agonists buspirone and 8-OH-DPAT (73) and ipsapirone (62) reduces the rate of calling at doses that did not affect motor activity or core body temperature. In the same study, administration of the purported 5-HT$_{1B}$ receptor agonist, CGS12066B {7-trifluoromethyl-4(4-methyl-1-piperazinyl)-pyrro lo[1,2-a] quinoxaline} and the 5-HT$_{1B}$ agonist TFMPP increased the rate of calling. D,L-Propranolol, a 5-HT$_1$ receptor antagonist, blocked the effects of both 8-OH-DPAT and TFMPP. Calling was decreased by both m-CPP (an agonist at 5-HT$_{1C}$ and 5-HT$_2$ receptor sites) and DOI (a drug with putative agonistic action at 5-HT$_2$ sites). Ritanserin, a 5-HT$_2$ and 5-HT$_{1C}$ antagonist, produced a dose-related increase in call rate. These data suggest that in certain models of anxiety, 5-HT$_2$ receptor activation may exert an anxiolytic and not anxiogenic effect. The possibility is raised that ontogenetic or species factors may influence the function of specific 5-HT receptor subtypes.

THERAPEUTIC EFFECTS OF SEROTONIN$_{1A}$ PARTIAL AGONISTS IN ANXIETY

Bearing the preclinical correlates in mind, we review below the therapeutic effects of the 5-HT$_{1A}$ partial agonists in the DSM-IIIR anxiety disorder categories.

Generalized Anxiety Disorder

The azapirones, such as buspirone, are the first modern pharmacotherapeutic alternative to benzodiazepines for the treatment of generalized anxiety disorder (GAD). The 3- to 4-week delay in onset of anxiolytic effects of the azapirones closely resembles that of imipramine treatment of GAD (33), but benzodiazepine effects are more rapid. Several well-controlled studies have shown that buspirone is superior to placebo and are equivalent to a range of benzodiazepines in the treatment of GAD. Goldberg and Finnerty (28) first reported anxiolytic properties of buspirone. Rickels et al. (57) subsequently reported in a placebo-controlled study that buspirone (20 to 25 mg/day) was as effective as diazepam (20 to 25 mg/day) over a 4-week period in the treatment of 212 anxious outpatients, although diazepam appeared slightly better than buspirone for somatic anxiety symptoms, whereas the opposite was observed for interpersonal difficulties. Subsequent controlled studies indicate similar efficacy for buspirone as compared to diazepam (22) and clorazepate (13), lorazepam, and alprazolam (14). Subsequent studies by Petracca et al. indicate similar efficacy for buspirone and lorazepam, although abrupt termination of treatment at 8 weeks resulted in discontinuation symptoms only in the lorazepam group (52). Strand et al. (67) have reported on the similar efficacy of buspirone and oxazepam treat-

ment of GAD in a primary care setting, where anxiety disorders are the most frequently encountered psychiatric disorders. Rickels (58) has suggested that buspirone, the only azapirone approved by the U.S. Food and Drug Administration, may be particularly appropriate in those with chronic variants of GAD, the anxious elderly, and possibly those with mixed anxiety and depression. Buspirone, according to the authors, appears most helpful in GAD patients who do not insist on the immediate relief provided by the benzodiazepines. If GAD patients are able to wait for a more gradual onset of anxiolytic effects, they avoid the dependency-producing effects of benzodiazepines.

Anxiety with Comorbid Depression

Anxious patients frequently present with complicating depressive symptomatology. Early clinical observation of buspirone-treated patients suggested antidepressant properties in addition to anxiolytic effects. Robinson and colleagues (59) report on five placebo-controlled studies involving 382 patients with DSM-III major depression and significant associated anxiety symptoms (i.e., Hamilton Anxiety Rating Scales (HARS) greater than or equal to 18). Buspirone, initiated at 15 mg/day, and increased to a maximal dose of 90 mg/day was effective for both depressive and anxiety symptoms. In general patients with higher HARS and HDRS scores responded better to buspirone than did less severely ill patients. A limitation of this analysis was the absence of separate evaluation of depressive symptoms, raising the possibility that improvement of HDRS scores were primarily related to improvement of overlapping anxiety-related items. Other depression studies using azapirones are remarkable for their high drop-out rates. Fabre (23) reports a 64% drop-out rate from a buspirone-treated group for various reasons. Jenkins et al. (32) reports a 71% drop-out rate from a group treated with high doses of gepirone, whereas a 57% drop-out rate was observed for the low-dose group. Other controlled studies have confirmed gepirone's antidepressant properties (55). The high drop-out rates observed with azapirone treatment combined with the lack of confirmatory data supporting primary antidepressant efficacy suggests a limited role where a range of other effective antidepressant treatments are available.

Generalized Anxiety Disorder and Alcohol Abuse

Tollefson treated recently detoxified patients who met criteria for DSM-III-R GAD criteria (69). In a placebo-controlled double-blind trial involving 51 dually diagnosed subjects, buspirone was superior to placebo in reducing measures of anxiety and number of days craving alcohol with increases in clinical global improvement scores observed. At the final study dose, blood levels of the buspirone metabolite 1-pyrimidinyl-piperazine (1-PP) were correlated to improvement in anxiety, global depressive symptoms, and number of days not using alcohol. Because this was not a fixed-dose study, this result is ambiguous. Also, the lack of a significant relationship between the parent compound and metabolite concentrations needs explanation. Nevertheless, buspirone may be a useful anxiolytic agent in alcoholic patients when the use of conventional anxiolytics such as the benzodiazepines are to be avoided. However, the specificity of these therapeutic effects to the 5-HT$_{1A}$ receptor is unclear, as the 1-PP derivative lacks 5-HT$_{1A}$ affinity and may function as an α_2 antagonist (24).

Panic disorder

Buspirone does not appear to be effective in panic disorder in several controlled studies. The role of other 5-HT$_{1A}$ partial agonists such as gepirone and ipsapirone in panic disorder have not, to our knowledge, been formally studied.

Sheehan et al. (64) compared the relative efficacy of buspirone, imipramine, and placebo in a double-blind controlled study of 52 randomly assigned patients with panic disorder. Imipramine was superior to placebo on many outcome measures. Although sample differences favored buspirone, these differences were not statistically significant. Of note, buspirone, like its 1-PP metabolite, may increases locus coeruleus firing modestly (60). That patients did not worsen on buspirone is therefore of interest, since an increase of noradrenergic locus coeruleus activity has been associated with worsening anxiety (10).

Pohl and associates (53) tested the efficacy of buspirone in 60 panic disorder patients in a placebo-controlled imipramine comparison design. There were no significant differences between treatments on outcome measures, although 25% of the buspirone patients were panic free as compared to 7% on imipramine and 14% on placebo. At the end of the study, mean doses of imipramine were 140 mg/day and of buspirone 29.5 mg/day. The authors attribute the lack of a treatment effect to the relatively small number of patients in each group and the robust placebo response observed in the study sample. The lack of imipramine–placebo difference raises questions about the nature of this sample and the measures used. Since a type II error is likely, one cannot evaluate buspirone effects. Further confirmation of the lack of buspirone efficacy in panic disorder is reported in a small controlled study by Schweizer and Rickels (57).

Investigators have speculated that activation of 5-HT$_{1A}$ and 5-HT$_2$ receptors may produce opposing effects (62). Such 5-HT$_2$ antagonists as ritanserin may therefore facilitate preferential 5-HT$_{1A}$ receptor activation with putative anxiolytic effects. Den Boer and Westenberg (21) administered ritanserin and the SSRI, fluvoxamine in a double-blind placebo-controlled design. Fluvoxamine treatment significantly reduced panic attacks, whereas ritanserin was indistinguishable from placebo. Ritanserin has been reported as effective as lorazepam in the treatment of GAD (9). The study suggests that the previously proposed relationship (62) between 5-HT$_{1A}$ (anxiolytic) and 5-HT$_2$ (anxiogenic) receptors does not apply to therapeutic effects in panic disorder but may be of relevance in GAD.

To explore the sensitivity of the 5-HT$_{1A}$ receptor in panic disorder, Lesch and colleagues (38,41) investigated the hypothermic, neuroendocrine, and behavioral responses in 14 patients and matched controls to a single oral dose of 0.3 mg/kg of ipsapirone and placebo. Ipsapirone produced hypothermia and corticotropin (ACTH)/cortisol release but had only minimal effects on behavior. The panic disorder patients showed reduced hypothermic and corticoid responses to ipsapirone when compared to controls. Hypothermia is postulated to reflect presynaptic 5-HT$_{1A}$ receptor activation, whereas corticoid responses reflect activation of postsynaptic 5-HT$_{1A}$. Although the prototype 5-HT$_{1A}$ agonist, 8-OH-DPAT, produces hypothermic and corticoid responses in rodents and these responses are blocked by selective 5-HT$_{1A}$ antagonists (spiperone and (−)-pindolol) (46), evidence for this functional distinction is lacking in humans. Nevertheless, these data are of interest as Targum (68) reports greater corticoid responses in panic-disorder patients to oral fenfluramine (a nonspecific indirect 5-HT agonist) challenge than in healthy controls. Although fenfluramine induces anxiety, it is described by the authors as not resembling panic but rather waves of generalized anxiety. In rodent studies, mCPP does not functionally interact with 5-HT$_{1A}$ receptor sites but acts as a 5-HT$_{1C}$ and 5-HT$_2$ agonist (73). Also, mCPP produces enhanced anxiety responses and exaggerated corticoid responses when administered orally in panic-disorder subjects (34) but produces equivalent anxiety and corticoid responses when administered intravenously (11). As dyspnea is not evident during mCPP-induced anxiety, a question is posed as to its validity in producing panic attacks. Taken together, these data raise the possibility of normosensitive, supersensitive, and subsensitive 5-HT receptors in panic disorder, suggesting a mosaic of receptor abnormalities. The effects of treatment on challenge response to the various 5-HT ligands may further facilitate characterization of 5-HT receptor abnormality in panic disorder.

Obsessive–Compulsive Disorder

In an open trial, Markovitz et al. (43) reported modest benefits in 9 out of 11 patients with obsessive–compulsive disorder (OCD) when buspirone was added to fluoxetine treatment, suggesting a potential ancillary role for 5-HT$_{1A}$ partial agonists in OCD. McDougle et al. (44) subsequently performed a placebo-controlled double-blind study to test the augmenting efficacy of buspirone in OCD patients treated with standard medications for OCD. Buspirone was not different from placebo as an augmenting agent. The role of buspirone in OCD, therefore, appears limited, particularly since 5-HT reuptake blockers and clomipramine are generally effective in this population. Its role as an augmenting agent in specific refractory cases is of interest.

Challenge studies using the 5-HT$_{1A}$ partial agonist, buspirone, in ten OCD patients and ten controls did not show differences in prolactin responses. Lesch and colleagues (39) examined hypothermic, neuroendocrine, and behavioral responses to the selective 5-HT$_{1A}$ receptor ligand ipsapirone in patients with OCD and healthy controls. A single dose of ipsapirone (0.3 mg/kg) or placebo was administered to 12 patients and 22 controls under double-blind, random-assignment conditions. Ipsapirone induced hypothermia (presynaptic effect) and release of corticotropin and cortisol (postsynaptic effect) but had no effect on behavior, including obsessive or compulsive symptoms. Thermoregulatory and neuroendocrine responses to ipsapirone were not consistently different between healthy controls and patients with OCD. In a double-blind random-assignment study of 10 OCD patients, Lesch and colleagues (40) challenged subjects with ipsapirone and placebo before and during open fluoxetine treatment. The authors report ipsapirone-induced hypothermia and ACTH/cortisol release was significantly attenuated following chronic fluoxetine when compared to the pretreatment ipsapirone challenge. Although fluoxetine was effective in reducing the severity of obsessive–compulsive symptoms, no significant correlation between attenuation of ipsapirone-induced responses and fluoxetine improvement in OCD symptoms was detected. Thus, it remains unclear whether the ability of fluoxetine to down-regulate pre- and/or postsynaptic 5-HT$_{1A}$ receptors is specific to its antiobsessional effects. Moreover, the absence of repeat ipsapirone challenges in a healthy control group limits evaluation of the possibility of a nonspecific reduction in ipsapirone response.

Social Phobia

Of an original 21 social phobia patients, Schneier et al. (61) reported modest improvement in 8 of 17 (47%) patients who tolerated at least 2 weeks in an open 12-week trial of buspirone. Of the 12 patients who were able to tolerate a dose of 45 mg/day or greater, 9 (67%) were at least much improved on the clinical global improvement scale. Of note, one patient was unable to tolerate the drug because of panic-like side effects. Other side effects included gastrointestinal upset, dizziness, and increased anxiety. The authors noted that response status related to the ability to tolerate high doses of the drug. Similar results have been reported by Munjack et al. (48) in open

buspirone treatment of SP. The drug may provide a non-monoamine-oxidase-inhibitor alternative to the treatment of social phobia with a substance abuse history, although systematic controlled studies are required.

To our knowledge, 5-HT$_{1A}$ receptors have not been systematically studied for the treatment of posttraumatic stress disorder or simple phobia.

SUMMARY

That the azapirones are effective in GAD but not in panic-anxiety supports the tenet of pharmacological dissection proposed by Klein. Moreover, azapirones appear effective as antidepressants and therefore are included in the group of antidepressants that do not block panic attacks—buproprion, trazodone, deprenyl, and maprotiline (see ref. 16 for review). The differing therapeutic responses to the azapirones support the nosological distinction between GAD and panic disorder. Specific potential for the azapirones in the treatment of GAD patients with comorbid alcoholism requires replication. Use of the azapirones in social phobia requires systematic study, whereas the initial open observations in OCD have not been replicated under double-blind placebo controlled conditions. Considered in the context of the advent of the 5-HT reuptake inhibitors, effective agents in non-GAD anxiety disorders with a favorable side effects profile, the therapeutic role of the azapirones is greatly restricted. Moreover, the high doses of azapirone that are often required for adequate therapeutic effects are often associated with significant side effects, such as gastrointestinal upset, dizziness, and anxiety. Of note, SSRIs have not been systematically studied in GAD. The development of compounds with selective 5-HT receptor binding profiles is nevertheless an important psychopharmacological advance and expands the clinician's armamentarium, particularly for atypical cases.

Dysfunction of putatively reciprocal and interdependent 5-HT pathways, possibly as a result of pathological receptor sensitivities may account for disparate clinical disorders and effects of 5-HT related compounds. We have previously proposed homeostatic failure along cybernetic lines, that is, an inability of the neural system to buffer pertubations in either direction. We hypothesize a neural substrate for 5-HT dysfunction in anxiety disorders whereby a distinction is made between raphe pathways that mediate inhibitory effects, particularly to brainstem and limbic sites, and raphe projections that mediate stimulatory effects, such as hypothalamic activation and the elicitation of a corticoid response. Loss of 5-HT tone in the inhibitory systems is hypothesized to be associated with depression and panic. Panic-anxiety may preferentially involve descending inhibitory pathways to medullary respiratory centers, and disruption of such activity may contribute to the misevaluation of the threat for suf-

1308 / THE 5-HT$_{1A}$ RECEPTOR IN ANXIETY

TABLE 1. *Serotonin function in psychiatric disorders*

	Azapirone	SSRI	Inhibitory pathways	Stimulatory pathways	Orbitofrontal cortex	GH response to clonidine
GAD	+	?	−	↑	—	↓
Panic disorder	—	+	↓ brainstm	↑	—	↓
OCD	+?	+	−	↓	↑	—
Depression	+	+	↓ limbic	↑	—	↓

GAD, generalized anxiety disorder; OCD, obsessive-compulsive disorder.

focation. The available data suggest that either partial 5-HT$_{1A}$ agonism is not sufficient to suppress ventilatory overdrive or other inhibitory 5-HT receptors are involved. In panic disorder, an exaggerated reciprocal relationship between inhibitory and stimulatory 5-HT pathways may exist. Recent data by our group (15) suggest that 5-HT–modulated functions, such as ventilation (pCO$_2$) and corticoid response are negatively correlated during the pre-lactate period in patients who panic when challenged with lactate. Depressive symptoms may relate to a loss of 5-HT tone in the ascending projections to limbic (and cortical) structures which may be corrected by an enhancement of serotonergic neurotransmission produced by most antidepressants (8).

Overactivity of stimulatory pathways is hypothesized to generate generalized or anticipatory anxiety. In this instance, azapirones may act as antagonists, attenuating raphe hyperactivity. Of note, SSRIs and 5-hydroxytryptophan transiently worsen generalized anxiety, conceivably due to increased synaptic cleft 5-HT, until adaptive receptor changes have taken place. OCD is characterized by overactivity of stimulatory projections to the caudate nuclei and orbitofrontal cortex and blunted corticoid responses to 5-HT agonists (see Table 1).

In conclusion, despite an unprecedented increase in knowledge of the 5-HT receptors and their role in anxiety, the study of the relationship between serotonin and clinical pathophysiology is in its infancy. Future studies are required to delineate functional and neuroanatomical correlations and receptor sensitivity profile status of the multiple raphe nuclei and their projections.

ACKNOWLEDGMENTS

This work has been supported in part by a National Institute of Mental Health Scientist Development Award for Clinicians (1-K20-MH01039-01A1 to JDC and a Mental Health Clinical Research grant (NIMH P50-MH-30906.

REFERENCES

1. Aghajanian GK, Sprouse JS, Rasmussen K. Physiology of the midbrain serotonin system. In: Meltzer HY, ed. *Psychopharmacology: the third generation of progress.* New York: Raven Press, 1987:141–149.
2. Andrade R, Nicoll RA. *Soc Neurosci Abstr* 1985:11:597.
3. Andrade R, Nicoll RA. Pharmacologically distinct actions of serotonin on single pyramidal neurons of the rat hippocampus recorded in vitro. *J Physiol Lond* 1987;394:99–124.
4. Aston-Jones G, Ennis M, Pieribone VA, Nickell WT, Shipley MT. The brain nucleus locus coeruleus: restricted afferent control of a broad efferent network. *Science* 1986;234:734–737.
5. Azmitia EC, Whitaker-Azmitia PM. Awakening the sleeping giant: anatomy and plasticity of the brain serotonergic system. *J Clin Psychiatry* 1991;52(12,Suppl):4–16.
6. Barrett JE, Witkin JM, Mansbach RS, Skolnick P, Weissman BA. Behavioral studies with anxiolytic drugs. III. Antipunishment actions of buspirone in the pigeon do not involve benzodiazepine receptor mechanisms. *J Pharmacol Exp Ther* 1986;238:1009–1013.
7. Beck SG, Clarke WP, Goldfarb J. Spiperone differentiates multiple 5-hydroxytryptamine responses in rat hippocampal slices in vitro. *Eur J Pharmacol* 1985;116:195–197.
8. Blier P, De Montigny C, Chaput Y. Modifications of the serotonin system by antidepressant treatments: Implications for the therapeutic response in major depression. *J Clin Psychopharmacol* 1987;7(6,Suppl):24S–35S.
9. Bressa GM, Marini S, Gregori S. Serotonin S2 receptors blockade and generalized anxiety disorders. A double-blind study on ritanserin and lorazepam. *Int J Clin Pharmacol Res* 1987;7(2):111–119.
10. Charney DS, Redmond DE. Neurobiological mechanisms in human anxiety: evidence supporting central noradrenergic hyperactivity. *Neuropharmacology* 1983;22:1531–1536.
11. Charney DS, Woods SW, Goodman WK, Heninger GR. Serotonin function in anxiety. II. Effects of the serotonin agonist mCPP in panic disorder patients and healthy subjects. *Psychopharmacology* 1987;92(1):14–24.
12. Coccaro EF, Siever LJ, Klar HM, Maurer G, et al. Serotonergic studies in patients with affective and personality disorders: correlates with suicidal and impulsive aggressive behavior. *Arch Gen Psychiatry* 1989;46(7):587–599.
13. Cohn JB, Bowden CL, Fisher JG, Rodos JJ. Double-blind comparison of buspirone and clorazepate in anxious outpatients. *Am J Med* 1986;80(3B):10–16.
14. Cohn JB, Wilcox CS. Low-sedation potential of buspirone compared with alprazolam and lorazepam in the treatment of anxious patients: a double blind study. *J Clin Psychiatry* 1986;47(8):409–412.
15. Coplan JD, Goetz R, Klein DF, Gorman JM, Papp LA. Determinants of lactate-induced panic: an extended sample review. Presented at the American Psychiatric Association, 1992, New Orleans, Louisiana.
16. Coplan JD, Gorman JM, Klein DF. Serotonin related functions in panic-anxiety: a critical overview. *Neuropsychopharmacology* 1992a;6(3):189–200.
17. Coplan JD, Gorman JM. Detectable levels of fluoxetine metabolites after discontinuation; an unexpected serotonin syndrome. *Am J Psychiatry* 1993;150(5):837.
18. Cunningham KA, Callahan PM, Appel JB. Discriminative stimulus properties of 8-hydroxy-2-(di-n-propylamino)tetralin (8-OH-DPAT): implications for understanding the actions of novel anxiolytics. *Eur J Pharmacol* 1987;138:29–36.
19. Daval G, Verge D, Basbaum AI, et al. Autoradiographic evidence of serotonin I binding sites on primary afferent fibres in the dorsal horn of the rat spinal cord. *Neurosci Lett* 1987;83:71–76.
20. Delgado PL, Price LH, Miller HL, et al. Rapid serotonin depletion as a provocative challenge test for patients with major depression:

relevance to antidepressant action and the neurobiology of depression. *Psychopharmacol Bull* 1991;27:321–330.

21. Den Boer JA, Westenberg HGM. Serotonin function in panic disorder: a double blind placebo controlled study with fluvoxamine and ritanserin. *Psychopharmacology* 1990;102(1):85–94.

22. Fabre LF. Double-blind comparison of buspirone with diazepam in anxious patients. *Curr Ther Res* 1987;41(5):751–759.

23. Fabre LF. Buspirone in the management of major depression: a placebo-controlled comparison. *J Clin Psychiatry* 1990;51(Suppl): 55–61.

24. Fuller RW, Perry KW. Effects of buspirone and its metabolite, 1-(2-pyrimidinyl)piperazine, on brain monoamines and their metabolites in rats. *J Pharmacol Exp Ther* 1989;248(1):50–6.

25. Gaddum JH, Picarelli ZP. Two kinds of tryptamine receptor. *Br J Pharmacol Chemother* 1957;12:323–328.

26. Glaser T, Traber J. Buspirone: action on serotonin receptors in calf hippocampus. *Eur J Pharmacol* 1983;88:137–138.

27. Goddard AW, Goodman WK, Woods SW, Heninger GR, Charney DS, Price LH. Effects of tryptophan depletion on panic anxiety. American College of Neuropsychopharmacology, 1992, San Juan, Puerto Rico. (abst).

28. Goldberg HL, Finnerty RJ. The comparative efficacy of buspirone and diazepam in the treatment of anxiety. *Am J Psychiatry* 1979;136(9):1184–1187.

29. Hamik A, Peroutka SJ. 1-(*m*-Chlorophenyl) piperazine (mCPP) interactions with neurotransmitter receptors in the human brain. *Biol Psychiatry* 1989;25:569–575.

30. Harrington MA, Zhong P, Garlow SJ, Ciaranello RD. Molecular biology of serotonin receptors. *J Clin Psychiatry* 1992; 53(10,Suppl):8–27.

31. Heninger GR, Charney DS, Sternberg DE. Serotonergic function in depression. Prolactin response to intravenous tryptophan in depressed patients and healthy subjects. *Arch Gen Psychiatry* 1984;41:398–402.

32. Jenkins SW, Robinson DS, Fabre LF Jr, Andary JJ, Messina ME, Reich LA. Gepirone in the treatment of major depression. *J Clin Psychopharmacol* 1990;10(3,Suppl):77S–85S.

33. Kahn RJ, McNair DM, Frankenthaler LM. Tricyclic treatment of generalized anxiety disorder. Special issue: drug treatment of anxiety disorders. *J Affective Disord* 1987;13(2):145–151.

34. Kahn RS, Asnis GM, Wetzler S, Van Praag HM. Neuroendocrine evidence for serotonin receptor hypersensitivity in panic disorder. *Psychopharmacology* 1988;96(3):360–364.

35. Kendall DA, Nahorski SR. 5-Hydroxytryptamine stimulated inositol phospholipid hydrolysis in rat cerebral cortex slices: pharmacological characterization and effects of antidepressants. *J Pharmacol Exp Ther* 1985;233:473–479.

36. Klein DF, Coplan JD, Gorman JM. Theoretical and empirical basis for serotonergic drug use in panic avoidance behavior. In: Cassano GB, Akiskal HS, eds. *Serotonin-related psychiatric syndromes: clinical and therapeutic links.* London: Royal Society of Medicine Services Limited; 1991:93–97.

37. Klein DF, Gittelman R, Quitkin F, Rifkin A. *Diagnosis and drug treatment.* 2nd ed. Baltimore: Williams & Wilkins; 1980.

38. Lesch KP. 5-HT$_{1A}$ receptor responsivity in anxiety disorders and depression. *Prog Neuropsychopharmacol Biol Psychiatry* 1991; 15(6):723–733.

39. Lesch KP, Hoh A, Disselkamp-Tietze J, Wiesmann M, Osterheider M, Schulte HM. 5-Hydroxytryptamine$_{1A}$ receptor responsivity in obsessive-compulsive disorder. Comparison of patients and controls. *Arch Gen Psychiatry* 1991;48(6):540–547.

40. Lesch KP, Hoh A, Schulte HM, Osterheider M, Muller T. Long term fluoxetine treatment decreases 5-HT$_{1A}$ receptor responsivity in obsessive-compulsive disorder. *Psychopharmacology* 1991; 105(3):415–420.

41. Lesch KP, Wiesmann M, Hoh A, et al. 5-HT$_{1A}$ receptor-effector system responsivity in panic disorder. *Psychopharmacology* 1992;106(1):111–117.

42. Lucki I, Wieland S. 5-Hydroxytryptamine$_{1A}$ receptors and behavioral responses. *Neuropsychopharmacology* 1990;3:481–493.

43. Markovitz PJ, Stagno SJ, Calabrese JR. Buspirone augmentation of fluoxetine in obsessive–compulsive disorder. *Am J Psychiatry* 1990;147(6):798–800.

44. McDougle CJ, Goodman WK, Leckman JF, et al. Limited therapeutic effect of addition of buspirone in fluvoxamine-refractory obsessive-compulsive disorder. *Am J Psychiatry* 1993;150(4): 647–649.

45. Middlemiss DN, Fozard JR. 8-Hydroxy-2(di-*n*-propylamino)tetralin dicriminates between subtypes of the 5-HT$_1$ recognition site. *Eur J Pharmacol* 1983;90:151–153.

46. Millan MJ, Rivet JM, Canton H, LeMarouille-Girardon S, Gobert A. Induction of hypothermia as a model of 5-hydroxytryptamine$_{1A}$ receptor-mediated activity in the rat: a pharmacological characterization of the actions of novel agonists and antagonists. *J Pharmacol Exp Ther* 1993;264(3):1364–1376.

47. Morgane PJ, Jacobs MS. Raphe projections to the locus coeruleus in the rat. *Brain Res Bull* 1979;4(4):519–534.

48. Munjack DJ, Brun SJ, Baltazar PL, et al. A pilot study of buspirone in the treatment of social phobia. *J Anxiety Disord* 1991;5:87–98.

49. Pedigo NW, Yamamura HI, Nelson DL. Discrimination of multiple [^{3}H]-5-hydroxytryptamine binding sites by the neuroleptic spiperone in rat brain. *J Neurochem* 1981;36:220–226.

50. Peroutka SJ, Sleight AJ, McCarthy BG, Pierce PA, Schmidt AW, Hekmatpanah CR. The clinical utility of pharmacological agents that act at serotonin receptors. *J Neuropsychiatry Clin Neurosci* 1989;1:253–262.

51. Peroutka SJ, Snyder SH. Long term antidepressant treatment lowers spiroperidol-labeled serotonin receptor binding. *Science* 1980;210: 88–90.

52. Petracca A, Nisita C, McNair D, Melis G, Guerani G, Cassano GB. Treatment of generalized anxiety disorder: preliminary clinical experience with buspirone. *J Clin Psychiatry* 1990;51(Suppl):31–39.

53. Pohl R, Balon R, Yeragani VK, Gershon S. Serotonergic anxiolytics in the treatment of panic disorder: a controlled study with buspirone. *Psychopathology* 1989;22(Suppl 1):60–67.

54. Price LH, Charney DS, Delgado PL, et al. Effects of desipramine and fluvoxamine treatment on the prolactin response to tryptophan: serotonergic function and the mechanism of antidepressant action. *Arch Gen Psychiatry* 1989;46(7):625–631.

55. Rausch JL, Ruegg R, Moeller FG. Gepirone as a 5-HT$_{1A}$ agonist in the treatment of major depression. *Psychopharmacol Bull* 1990;26(2):169–171.

56. Riblet LA, Taylor DP, Eison MS, Stanton HC. Pharmacology and neurochemistry of buspirone. *J Clin Psychiatry* 1982;43:11–16.

57. Rickels K. Antianxiety therapy: potential value of long-term treatment. *J Clin Psychiatry* 1987;48(Suppl):7–11.

58. Rickels K, Weisman K, Norstad N, et al. Buspirone and diazepam in anxiety: a controlled study. *J Clin Psychiatry* 1982; 43(12,Sect.2):81–86.

59. Robinson DS, Rickels K, Feighner J, et al. Clinical effects of the 5-HT$_{1A}$ partial agonists in depression: a composite analysis of buspirone in the treatment of depression. *J Clin Psychopharmacol* 1990;10(3,Suppl):67S–76S.

60. Sanghera MK, McMillen BA, German DC. Buspirone, a non-benzodiazepine anxiolytic, increases locus coeruleus noradrenergic neuronal activity. *Eur J Pharmacol* 1982;86(1):107–110.

61. Schneier F, Campeas R, Fallon B, et al. Buspirone in social phobia. Presented at the 17th Congress of Collegium Internationale Neuro-Psychopharmacologicum, Sept. 1991; Kyoto, Japan (abst).

62. Schreiber R, DeVry J. 5-HT$_{1A}$ receptor ligands in animal models of anxiety, impulsivity, and depression: multiple mechanisms of action? *Prog Neuro-Psychopharmacol Biol Psychiatry* 1993; 17(1):87–104.

63. Schweizer E, Rickels K. Buspirone in the treatment of panic disorder: a controlled pilot comparison with clorazepate. *J Clin Psychopharmacol* 1988;8(4):303.

64. Sheehan DV, Raj AB, Sheehan KH, Soto S. Is buspirone effective for panic disorder? *J Clin Psychopharmacol* 1990;10(1):3–11.

65. Sills MA, Wolfe BB, Frazer A. Determination of selective and nonselective compounds for the 5-HT1a and 5-HT$_{1B}$ receptor subtypes in rat frontal cortex. *J Pharmacol Exp Ther* 1984;231:480–487.

66. Sprouse JS, Aghajanian GK. Electrophysiological responses of serotoninergic dorsal raphe neurons to 5-HT$_{1A}$ and 5-HT$_{1B}$ agonists. *Synapse* 1987;1:3–9.

67. Strand M, Hetta J, Rosen A, et al. A double-blind, controlled trial in primary care patients with generalized anxiety: a comparison

between buspirone and oxazepam. *J Clin Psychiatry* 1990;51 (Suppl):40–45.

68. Targum SD. Differential responses to anxiogenic challenge studies in patients with major depressive disorder and panic disorder. *Biol Psychiatry* 1990;28(1):21–34.

69. Tollefson GD, Montague-Clouse J, Tollefson SL. Treatment of comorbid generalized anxiety in a recently detoxified alcoholic population with a selective serotonergic drug (buspirone). *J Clin Psychopharmacol* 1992;12(1):19–26.

70. Trulson ME, Eubanks EE, Jacobs BL. Behavioral evidence for supersensitivity following destruction of central serotonergic nerve terminals by 5,7-dihydroxytryptamine. *J Pharmacol Exp Ther* 1976;198:23–32.

71. Tye NC, Iversen SD, Green AR. The effects of benzodiazepines and serotonergic manipulations on punished responding. *Neuropharmacology* 1979;18:689–695.

72. Verge D, Daval G, Marcinkiewicz M, et al. Quantitative autoradiography of multiple 5-HT$_1$ receptor subtypes in the brain of control or 5,7-dihydroxytryptamine-treated rats. *J Neurosci* 1986;6:3474–3482.

73. Winslow JT, Insel TR. Serotonergic modulation of the rat pup ultrasonic isolation call: studies with 5-HT$_1$ and 5-HT$_2$ receptor subtype-selective agonists and antagonists. *Psychopharmacology* 1991;105(4):513–520.

74. Wright IK, Upton N, Marsden CA. Effect of potential anxiolytics on extracellular 5-HT in the ventral hippocampus of rats observed on the elevated X-maze using in vivo microdialysis. In: Rollema H, Westerink B, Drijfhout WJ, eds. *Monitoring molecules in neuroscience. Proceedings of the 5th International Conference on in vivo methods,* Krips Repro, Meppel; 1991:208–211.

75. Zitrin CM, Klein DF, Woerner MG, Ross DC. Treatment of phobias. I. Comparison of imipramine hydrochloride and placebo. *Arch Gen Psychiatry* 1983;40:125–138.

Psychopharmacology: The Fourth Generation of Progress, edited by Floyd E. Bloom and David J. Kupfer. Raven Press, Ltd., New York © 1995.

CHAPTER **111**

Pharmacological Challenges in Anxiety Disorders

Lawrence H. Price, Andrew W. Goddard, Linda C. Barr, and Wayne K. Goodman

The pharmacological challenge strategy involves administering a test agent under controlled conditions to elucidate some aspect of biological or behavioral function in the organism being studied. It is based on the assumption that true functional abnormalities may not be evident in the basal state because of the action of compensatory mechanisms. Under such circumstances, pharmacological perturbation of a specific target system may reveal information about the functional integrity of both that system and systems that modulate it. Uses of this approach include (a) generation and testing of hypotheses regarding the pathophysiology of a disorder, (b) delineation of the effects and mechanisms of action of treatments, (c) identification of pathophysiologically distinct diagnostic subtypes, and (d) clinical applications (as a diagnostic test, as a predictor of treatment response, as a means of assessing treatment adequacy, and as a predictor of relapse).

In studies of neuropsychiatric disorders, the ideal challenge probe should have a mechanism of action that is well-characterized at the preclinical level, be pharmacologically selective for the system under investigation, have no active metabolites, and induce responses that are sensitive, reliable, accessible to clinical measurement, and reflective of brain function. Safety and convenience are desirable qualities. Drug dosage, route and rate of administration, environmental conditions of the testing situation, and rater–observer characteristics are additional factors that should be standardized, because they may contribute to unwanted response variance.

L. H. Price, A. W. Goddard, and L. C. Barr: Clinical Neuroscience Research Unit, Abraham Ribicoff Research Facilities, Connecticut Mental Health Center, Department of Psychiatry, Yale University School of Medicine, New Haven, Connecticut 06519.
W. K. Goodman: Department of Psychiatry, University of Florida College of Medicine, Gainesville, Florida 32610.

In practice, few challenge probes meet all of the ideal criteria. Despite this, the pharmacological challenge paradigm continues to enjoy popularity among investigators. Clinically relevant neurobiological processes are otherwise difficult to study in vivo in patients, and the promise of the paradigm for clarifying pathophysiology still seems great. In some instances, that promise has been at least partially realized [e.g., probes of serotonin (5-HT) function in depression], whereas other lines of investigation have foundered [e.g., prolactin (PRL) responses to dopamine (DA) agonists and antagonists in schizophrenia].

In light of these factors, this chapter reviews the use of the pharmacological challenge strategy in patients with anxiety disorders. The chapter is divided into two major sections: panic and related anxiety disorders and obsessive–compulsive disorders (OCD). Within each major section, the use of specific probes is considered according to the major neurotransmitter systems they engage. Doses and routes of administration are specified to underscore the dependence of response sensitivity and specificity on these parameters. This chapter updates the detailed review of Gorman et al. (34) on the pharmacological provocation of panic attacks and additionally considers other response measures to pharmacological challenges.

PANIC AND RELATED ANXIETY DISORDERS

The use of pharmacological challenges in panic disorder is unique in that the clinical phenomenon of central interest (i.e., the panic attack) can be readily provoked and assessed in the clinical laboratory setting (34). This has proved far more difficult in other disorders (e.g., depression and schizophrenia). The primary focus of this section on panic disorder reflects the extensive study of this condition by means of the pharmacological challenge strategy. Consideration of related anxiety disorders, such as social phobia, generalized anxiety disorder (GAD), and posttraumatic stress disorder (PTSD), is included where appropriate.

Noradrenergic Probes

Historically, the noradrenergic system has dominated preclinical theoretical and empirical approaches to anxiogenesis (79). The extensive clinical literature on the involvement of norepinephrine (NE) in panic has been made possible through the long-standing availability of several relatively selective probes of this system.

Yohimbine

Yohimbine is an indole alkaloid with α_2-adrenoceptor antagonist properties. It increases NE function by blocking inhibitory α_2-adrenoceptors located presynaptically on NE neurons in the locus coeruleus (LC), resulting in activation of those neurons (79). Although generally considered selective for α_2-adrenoceptor blockade, yohimbine also has effects on the DA and 5-HT systems.

In a 1984 study, Charney et al. (14) gave yohimbine (20 mg po) to 39 drug-free patients with panic disorder or agoraphobia and 20 healthy controls. Ratings of anxiety and nervousness, physical symptoms, and blood pressure responses were greater in the patients. Yohimbine-induced increases in plasma levels of the NE metabolite 3-methoxy-4 hydroxyphenylglycol (MHPG) correlated with increases in anxiety in patients but not in controls. Patients with frequent panic attacks had greater MHPG responses than controls. In a subsequent study in 1987 using yohimbine (20 mg po), panic attacks were provoked in 37 out of 68 (54%) panic patients and 1 out of 20 (5%) controls (19). Patients reporting yohimbine-induced panic attacks had greater increases in plasma MHPG, cortisol, blood pressure, and heart rate than controls. More recently, Charney et al. (20) reported that yohimbine (0.4 mg/kg iv) provoked panic attacks in 24 out of 38 (63%) panic patients and 1 out of 15 (7%) controls, again finding that MHPG responses were greater in patients who panicked. Gurguis and Uhde in 1990 replicated the relationship between anxiety and MHPG responses to yohimbine (20 mg po) in 11 panic patients and 7 controls. Albus et al. (3) administered yohimbine (20 mg po) to panic patients treated with placebo ($n = 8$) or alprazolam ($n = 7$) and 12 healthy controls. Patients had greater anxiety responses than controls, but none experienced panic attacks, apparently because instructions during the test were designed to minimize the likelihood of an attack. The central effects of yohimbine (0.4 mg/kg iv) in six drug-free panic patients and six controls were studied by Woods et al. (95) using single-photon emission computed tomography (SPECT) imaging with ^{99m}Tc-HMPAO. Decreased fronto-cortical cerebral blood flow occurred in patients compared to controls, with six out of six patients and one out of six controls experiencing increased anxiety following yohimbine.

These studies strongly suggest involvement of the NE system in some panic patients. However, there are limitations to yohimbine as a panicogen. Over one-third of panic patients are insensitive to its panicogenic effects. Moreover, such effects are not specific to panic disorder: in a study of 20 drug-free PTSD patients and 18 controls utilizing yohimbine (0.4 mg/kg iv), Southwick et al. (83) observed panic attacks in 14 out of 20 (70%) and flashbacks in 8 out of 20 (40%) patients, with none in controls. Contrary to expectation, Charney and Heninger found in 1985 (17) that long-term treatment with the antipanic agent imipramine, which significantly affects NE function, did not block yohimbine-induced panic in 11 patients. However, the behavioral response to yohimbine is attenuated by long-term treatment with other antipanic drugs, such as the benzodiazepine alprazolam ($n = 14$) (17) and the selective serotonin reuptake inhibitor (SSRI) fluvoxamine ($n = 16$) (31). Effects of yohimbine on 5-HT and DA function could account for the lack of reversal of yohimbine's behavioral effects by imipramine.

Phenomenologically, yohimbine does not produce a panic attack that is identical to naturally occurring episodes. Patients and controls describe euphoria, lacrimation, and rhinnorhea, which are not typical of naturalistic panic. Finally, Albus et al. (4) have noted the influence of expectancy and cognitive set on behavioral responses to yohimbine (20 mg po). While this may be viewed as a limitation of the challenge paradigm in general, it also reflects the real modulation of anxiety by such factors in the natural environment.

Clonidine

Clonidine, an imidazoline derivative, is an α_2-adrenoceptor agonist with some anxiolytic properties. It decreases neuronal activity in the LC by stimulating presynaptic autoreceptors, consequently reducing sympathetic outflow (78). Sedation and hypotension limit its clinical use as an anxiolytic.

Charney and Heninger found in 1986 (18) that clonidine (0.15 mg iv) caused greater hypotension, greater decreases in plasma MHPG, and less sedation in 26 drug-free panic patients than in 21 controls. In 1989 Nutt (see ref. 66) replicated these observations in 16 panic patients and 16 controls using clonidine (1.5 μg/kg iv). Recently, these finding were also replicated with clonidine (2 μg/kg iv) in a subgroup of panic patients who had manifested yohimbine-induced panic (20). These data suggest that presynaptic α_2-adrenoceptor sensitivity is increased in panic disorder, although it is unclear whether this reflects changes in receptor affinity (K_d), receptor binding (B_{max}), or second-messenger function. Uhde et al. (90), in a study of 11 drug-free panic patients, 11 depressed patients, and 11 controls, first reported a blunted growth hormone (GH) response to clonidine (2 μg/kg iv) in panic disorder, suggesting subsensitivity of central postsynaptic α_2-adrenoceptors. This finding, already well established in depression, was confirmed by other investigators (18,66). A recent study has found blunted GH responses to both clonidine (2 μg/kg iv) and GH-releasing factor (GHRF; 1 μg/kg iv) in 13 panic patients compared to 20 controls (86), suggesting that intrinsic hypothalamic–pituitary dysfunction may be present in panic disorder. Other anxiety disorders may also manifest a blunted GH response to clonidine. Abelson et al. (1) observed this phenomenon in a study of 11 drug-free GAD patients and 14 controls given clonidine (2 μg/kg iv). However, normal GH responses to clonidine (5 μg/kg po) were found in a study of 21 social phobia patients and 22 controls (85).

In summary, panic patients consistently manifest altered responses to α_2-adrenoceptor agonists and antagonists. Whether this reflects some primary defect in the α_2-adrenoceptor itself is unclear. The large number of non-NE neurotransmitter systems with significant input to the LC leaves open the possibility that dysregulation of one or more of these systems could lead to abnormalities of LC function manifested as panic attacks (79).

β-Adrenoceptor Agonist and Antagonists

Isoproterenol, a synthetic sympathomimetic amine, is a peripherally acting agent with selectivity for the β-adrenoceptor. Early studies suggested that patients predisposed to anxiety-related symptoms experienced exacerbation of such symptoms when given isoproterenol, and that this could be reversed with the β-adrenoceptor antagonist propranolol (34).

Extending their own earlier findings, Pohl et al. (70) reported that 57/86 (66%) panic patients and 4/45 (9%) controls developed panic after isoproterenol 1 μg/min iv. These findings support the hypothesis of increased β-adrenoceptor sensitivity in panic disorder. In contrast, Nesse et al. in 1984 (64) observed no differences between 14 drug-free panic patients and 6 controls in behavioral responses to isoproterenol 0.06–4.0 mg iv. The discrepancy could be explained by differing methods of isoproterenol administration (i.e., continuous infusion (70) vs multiple boluses (64)). Differences in panic attack criteria may also have contributed to conflicting results. Nesse et al. (64) additionally found smaller heart rate responses in patients than controls, which suggests decreased β-adrenoceptor sensitivity and a generalized increase in NE function in the nonpanic state. In another study casting doubt on the necessity of β-adrenoceptor supersensitivity for the occurrence of panic, Gorman et al. observed in 1983 (34) that pretreatment with propranolol (0.2 mg/kg iv) failed to block lactate-induced panic in all six panic patients studied.

The reliability and mechanism of isoproterenol-induced panic remain to be clarified. A singular limitation of isoproterenol is its inability to cross the blood–brain barrier. In addition, it is not differentially selective between β_1- and β_2-adrenoceptor subtypes. Finally, the fact that it is metabolized by monoamine oxidase, which could be altered in panic disorder, constitutes a disadvantage relative to some other β-adrenoceptor agonists.

Epinephrine and Norepinephrine

Epinephrine and NE are endogenous amines that are secreted in response to stress; they do not cross the blood–brain barrier. Epinephrine is a more potent agonist of β- than α-adrenoceptors, whereas NE is primarily an α-adrenoceptor agonist with some β activity. This lack of specificity compromises their use as pharmacological challenge agents.

The effects of these substances in anxiety disorders are not established, as they have rarely been studied in well-diagnosed patients. Early studies suggested that epinephrine tended to induce social withdrawal rather than panic, whereas NE was seen as weakly anxiogenic (34). In 1986, Pyke and Greenberg (73) evaluated the response of six panic patients to a NE infusion starting at 0.25 mg/min and increasing up to 16 mg/min. All six patients experienced panic attacks, but the study included neither a placebo infusion nor healthy subjects as controls.

Serotonergic Probes

Preclinical interest in the role of 5-HT in the pathogenesis of anxiety has been building over the past decade, but clinical studies have begun to appear in number only in the past several years.

m-Chlorophenylpiperazine

Often described as a 5-HT partial agonist, m-CPP has complex effects on brain 5-HT systems. It binds equipotently and with greatest affinity to 5-HT$_{1C}$ and 5-HT$_3$ receptors, and less potently to 5-HT$_2$ and 5-HT$_{1A}$ receptors (52). m-Chlorophenylpiperazine appears to act as an agonist at the 5-HT$_{1C}$ receptor, and perhaps at the 5-HT$_{1A}$ receptor as well. Effects at the 5-HT$_3$ receptor seem primarily antagonistic, whereas mixed agonist and antagonist activity has been found at the 5-HT$_2$ site. Serotonin releasing properties have been reported. Although m-CPP has little affinity for most non-5-HT receptors, it does bind to α_2-adrenergic sites, the functional significance of which is unknown.

Kahn et al. found in 1988 (52) that m-CPP (0.25 mg/kg po) caused panic attacks in six out of ten drug-free panic patients but not in 10 depressed patients or 11 healthy controls. Cortisol responses to m-CPP were also greater in panic patients (52). These investigators posited 5-HT receptor supersensitivity in panic disorder. However, no differences were found in the behavioral and neuroendocrine responses of 23 drug-free panic patients and 19 controls to *m*-CPP (0.1 mg/kg iv) (19,52), or of 27 panic patients and 22 controls to *m*-CPP (0.05 mg/kg iv) (27). A possible explanation for these discrepant findings is that intravenous administration at these doses leads to receptor overstimulation in both patients and controls, with loss of resolution of the behavioral and neuroendocrine signal demonstrated with the oral route.

Germine et al. (27) administered *m*-CPP (0.1 mg/kg iv) to ten drug-free GAD patients and 19 controls. Patients showed greater increases in anxiety symptoms, subjective anger, and GH, consistent with supersensitivity of postsynaptic 5-HT receptors. Similarly, Krystal et al. (54) found that 14 drug-free PTSD patients experienced more panic and dissociative symptoms (including flashbacks) following *m*-CPP (0.1 mg/kg iv) than placebo.

These findings are consistent with other evidence that *m*-CPP may exacerbate psychopathology across several disorders (52). However, *m*-CPP's complex neuropharmacology makes it difficult to draw conclusions about specific abnormalities within the 5-HT system. Moreover, the drugged feeling reported by many panic patients following *m*-CPP administration suggests an important dissimilarity between *m*-CPP-induced and naturalistic panic. Nonetheless, *m*-CPP may prove useful in evaluating interactions between 5-HT and other neurotransmitter systems. For example, Asnis et al. (6) recently tested 22 drug-free panic patients, 17 depressed patients, and 10 healthy controls with *m*-CPP (0.25 mg/kg po) and desipramine (75 mg im). Cortisol responses to each challenge were negatively correlated in the total sample, but particularly in the patient groups, suggesting some dysregulation of 5-HT/NE interactions in these disorders.

Fenfluramine

Fenfluramine is a phenylethylamine derivative with marked effects on brain 5-HT function. Upon acute administration, it potently releases presynaptic 5-HT and inhibits 5-HT reuptake, with weaker action as a postsynaptic 5-HT agonist. Long-lasting reductions in brain levels of 5-HT and its principal metabolite, 5-hydroxyindoleacetic acid (5-HIAA), have been observed following a single dose. Although structurally similar to amphetamine and classified as a sympathomimetic, fenfluramine causes little activation or euphoria.

Targum and Marshall in 1989 (87) administered DL-fenfluramine (60 mg po) to nine drug-free panic patients, nine depressed patients, and nine healthy controls. Panic patients exhibited greater anxiety, prolactin, and cortisol responses than the other groups, with six (67%) experiencing a panic attack. No depressed patients had an anxiety reaction, and two healthy controls experienced a mild

increase in anxiety. In a subsequent study by Targum in 1991 (88), 26 drug-free panic patients and 12 controls were given 0.5-M sodium DL-lactate (10 ml/kg iv) followed one day later by fenfluramine (60 mg po). Nine out of twelve patients (75%) with frequent panic attacks had prominent anxiety responses to both challenges, compared with none of the 14 patients with infrequent panic attacks. The investigator concluded that these responses reflected an elevated level of anticipatory anxiety due to frequent recent attacks, rather than some trait of panic patients. More recently, Targum (88) reported cortisol responses to lactate and fenfluramine in 12 drug-free panic patients with known anxiety responses to both agents and eight nonresponsive healthy controls. Patients had greater cortisol responses to fenfluramine than controls, but were similar to controls in showing no cortisol response to lactate. Some authors have remarked that the quality of the fenfluramine-provoked anxiety in panic patients is more suggestive of anticipatory or generalized anxiety than true panic (44). Targum's 1991 finding is consistent with this view. Fenfluramine might be conceptualized as a probe of one facet of panic disorder, that is, anticipatory fear, whereas lactate might be a better probe of true panic. The differential cortisol response of panic patients to these challenges is consistent with this view.

Tancer and Golden (85) gave fenfluramine (60 mg po) to 21 social phobia patients and 22 controls, observing an elevated cortisol response in the patients. This preliminary evidence suggests that social phobia patients exhibit dysregulated 5-HT neurotransmission, consistent with the clinical efficacy of the MAO inhibitor phenelzine in this population.

Serotonin Precursors

L-tryptophan is the initial dietary precursor of 5-HT. After competing with other large neutral amino acids for uptake into the brain, it is converted by the rate-limiting enzyme tryptophan hydroxylase into 5-hydroxytryptophan (5-HTP), which is then decarboxylated to 5-HT. Neuroendocrine effects of intravenous L-tryptophan are believed to result from the central synthesis and release of 5-HT, although there is debate as to whether other mechanisms (e.g., decreased availability of tyrosine for DA synthesis, activation of kynurenine metabolism) might be involved.

Serotonin-precursor loading is not anxiogenic. Charney and Heninger (18) gave L-tryptophan (7 g iv) to 23 drug-free panic patients and 21 controls, observing no difference in behavioral or prolactin responses between the groups. Westenberg and Den Boer in 1989 (91) administered 5-HTP (60 mg iv) to seven drug-free panic patients and seven controls, also finding little behavioral or neuroendocrine difference between groups. The discrepancy of these data with the *m*-CPP findings could be due to differential 5-HT receptor subtype activation by these agents or to the presynaptic effects of the precursors.

Tryptophan Depletion

Administration of a tryptophan-free amino acid mixture lowers plasma tryptophan, brain tryptophan, and 5-HT in laboratory animals, with behavioral effects consistent with a state of 5-HT depletion (24). Similar effects on plasma tryptophan have been demonstrated in humans by giving a tryptophan-free amino acid mixture preceded by a 24-hour low tryptophan diet (24).

Double-blind sham-controlled tryptophan depletion in six drug-free panic patients demonstrated no effects on anxiety symptoms (30). In a related study evaluating the role of 5-HT/NE interactions in anxiogenesis, a combination challenge of tryptophan depletion followed by yohimbine (0.4 mg/kg iv) caused greater nervousness in 11 healthy subjects than did either challenge condition alone (29). The NE metabolite MHPG and cortisol responses to the combination test were not augmented above those in the yohimbine alone condition. Investigation of panic patients with this paradigm should further clarify recent evidence of dysregulated 5-HT/NE interactions in panic disorder (6).

Ipsapirone

Ipsapirone is an azapirone derivative that acts selectively as a full agonist at presynaptic 5-HT$_{1A}$ autoreceptors and as a partial agonist at postsynaptic 5-HT$_{1A}$ sites. Lesch et al. (57) gave ipsapirone (0.3 mg/kg po) to 14 drug-free panic patients and 14 controls. Corticotropin (ACTH), cortisol, and hypothermic responses were blunted in the patients, but anxiety responses did not differ from controls. These findings support some role, perhaps modulatory in nature, of 5-HT$_{1A}$ receptors in the pathogenesis of panic disorder.

Metabolic and Respiratory Probes

This area, constituting the largest single body of pharmacological challenge research into the anxiety disorders, has recently been reviewed (34,53,66). Although the findings are impressively robust and reproducible, their theoretical impact has been limited by a paucity of relevant preclinical data regarding mechanism(s) of action.

Sodium Lactate and Bicarbonate

Lactic acid plays a key role in carbohydrate and energy metabolism. Pitts and McClure first showed in 1967 (69) that infusing sodium lactate caused panic attacks in anxious patients but not controls. This finding has been replicated often, with few contradictions. The challenge probe generally consists of 0.5-M sodium DL-lactate (10 ml/kg) given iv over 20 min. Lactate-induced anxiety appears specific to panic disorder (23) and is antagonized by treatment with antipanic agents (34).

Early investigators suggested that lactate might provoke panic by causing hypocalcemia, but this has not been substantiated. Carr and Sheehan hypothesized in 1984 (13) that panic patients have enhanced sensitivity of ventral medullary chemoreceptors to fluctuations in pH. They argued that lactate infusion could lower the pH in these cells by increasing the local lactate:pyruvate ratio, a consequence of passive diffusion of lactate into these areas and of hypoxemia secondary to cerebrovascular vasoconstriction caused by lactate-induced metabolic alkalosis. Panic attacks would result from the chemoreceptors' "misperception" of life-threatening central hypoxia and acidosis. To date, the assumptions underlying this model are unproven.

In an alternative model, Gorman et al. speculated in 1989 (37) that as lactate is metabolized to bicarbonate, resulting in a metabolic alkalosis, bicarbonate is in turn metabolized to CO_2, which stimulates both medullary chemoreceptors and the LC, causing panic in vulnerable individuals. Consistent with this is evidence that clonidine partially attenuates lactate-induced panic (20). Against this theory is the finding by Gorman et al. in 1990 (38) that D-lactate is also panicogenic, although it is not metabolized to CO_2. The lactate–CO_2 hypothesis has nonetheless been of great value in considering the relationship between respiration and panic (53).

Hyperventilation and CO_2

Voluntary hyperventilation, causing hypocapnia, can precipitate panic in panic patients, although some authorities suggest that this is only weakly panicogenic. Panic may also be induced by hypercapnia. Gorman et al. found in 1988 (36) that CO_2 inhalation (5% in air) precipitated panic in 12 out of 31 (39%) drug-free panic patients, one out of 13 (8%) healthy controls, and none of 12 patients with other anxiety disorders. Woods et al. in 1986 (93) provoked panic attacks in 8 out of 14 (57%) drug-free panic patients rebreathing 5% CO_2 in air; anxiety responses were similar in 8 controls given 7.5% CO_2, but less in 11 controls given 5% CO_2, suggesting greater sensitivity in the patients. These investigators also observed marked attenuation of the anxiety response to 5% CO_2 in seven panic patients treated with alprazolam. Griez et al. in 1987 (39) reported that one or two deep breaths of a 35% CO_2/65% O_2 mixture could induce panic in panic patients ($n = 12$) but not healthy controls ($n = 11$).

The ability of both hypo- and hypercapnia to trigger panic remains an enigma. Carr and Sheehan (13) suggested that both states may lead to a fall in brainstem pH, either directly (hypercapnia leading to respiratory acidosis) or indirectly (hypocapnia leading to respiratory alkalosis leading to cerebrovascular vasoconstriction leading to hypoxia). Related to this is the theory of enhanced chemoreceptor or LC sensitivity to CO_2 in panic patients (37), although this does not address the issue of hypocapnia. A less specific, but more encompassing, psychological explanation is that both states produce internal somatic cues that are misinterpreted as "dangerous" and therefore evoke panic (77). Nutt and Lawson (66) have enumerated the flaws in this explanation, which might be advanced to account for all pharmacological panicogens. Among these flaws is the failure to explain why panic patients are prone to such misinterpretations in the first place. Moreover, Goetz et al. (32) have shown that cardiorespiratory activation occurs even in panic attacks during placebo pharmacological challenges, suggesting that these changes are a manifestation, rather than a cause, of panic. Most recently, Klein (53) has advanced a comprehensive theory suggesting that both CO_2 and lactate induce panic by triggering a suffocation false-alarm in individuals with a hypersensitive suffocation detector. An attractive feature of this theory is its attempt to differentiate the neurobiological and phenomenological underpinnings of fear, acute and chronic anxiety, and panic.

Benzodiazepine Agonist and Antagonist Probes

The major behavioral effects of benzodiazepine (BZ) agonists and antagonists are mediated through saturable high-affinity BZ receptor sites located on a subunit of the γ-aminobutyric acid$_A$ (GABA$_A$) receptor (45). In this location, BZ receptors allosterically modulate GABA$_A$ receptor function to increase conductance through the associated chloride channel. Benzodiazepine receptor agonists (e.g., diazepam) have marked anxiolytic effects. Inverse agonists (e.g., the β-carboline FG 7142) are proconvulsant and anxiogenic. Antagonists (e.g., flumazenil) have little intrinsic activity, but block the effects of agonists and inverse agonists.

Roy-Byrne et al. (80) administered iv diazepam in dosages of 25, 25, 50, and 100 μg/kg 15 minutes apart to nine drug-free panic patients and ten controls, measuring saccadic eye movement velocity as an index of brainstem BZ receptor function. Patients had less diazepam-induced slowing of saccadic eye movement than controls, suggesting subsensitivity of BZ receptors.

Nutt et al. (65) gave flumazenil (2.0 mg iv) to ten drug-free panic patients and ten controls. Panic attacks occurred in 80% of patients but not in the controls. Studying oral flumazenil in 11 drug-free panic patients, however, Woods et al. (94) obtained panic attack rates of four out of ten at 200 mg, none of 11 at 600 mg, and none of eight with placebo. Nutt and Lawson (66) speculated that BZ receptor functioning is shifted in panic patients so that antagonists are recognized as partial inverse agonists. This is consistent with evidence of BZ receptor subsensitivity in panic disorder (80). An alternative interpretation is that flumazenil exacerbates a functional deficiency of some endogenous anxiolytic in the patients. The data do

not support the hypothesis that panic patients have increased levels of some endogenous inverse agonist, since this would predict anxiolytic effects of the antagonist. In a recent study of flumazenil given in doses of 2.0 mg iv to seven drug-free panic patients and seven controls, Wilson et al. (92) found that flumazenil decreased saccadic eye movements in both groups, suggesting a slight partial agonist effect.

Two novel compounds acting at the GABA$_A$/BZ receptor deserve mention. The partial inverse agonist Ro-16-0154 is being evaluated for behavioral effects in humans, and the partial agonist abecarnil (ZK 112–119) may have clinical efficacy as an anxiolytic. These new agents, together with the developments that have recently occurred in this area, will significantly advance understanding of BZ receptor pathophysiology in anxiety disorders.

Peptidergic Probes

Cholecystokinin

Cholecystokinin (CCK) is an octapeptide found regionally in the gastrointestinal tract and brain, where it acts as a neurotransmitter and neuromodulator. In some neurons, it is colocalized with other neurotransmitters, particularly DA and GABA, and GABA seems to be involved in the regulation of CCK release. Interest in CCK's role in anxiogenesis arose from evidence that it stimulates rat cortical and hippocampal neurons, effects that are blocked by benzodiazepine agonists (25).

DeMontigny (25) reported that seven out of ten healthy subjects experienced panic anxiety after receiving 20 to 100 mg iv of CCK-4, a selective CCK-B receptor agonist that crosses the blood–brain barrier. Bradwejn et al. found in 1991 (12) that CCK-4 (50 μg iv) induced panic in all eleven drug-free panic patients; patients rated these attacks as very similar to their naturalistic panics. Bradwejn et al. (12) subsequently observed that 50 μg iv of CCK-4 provoked panic in all 12 drug-free panic patients and 7 out of 15 (47%) controls, whereas 25 μg iv of CCK-4 induced panic in 10 out of 11 (91%) patients and 2 out of 12 (17%) controls. These investigators concluded that panic patients were more sensitive than controls to the anxiogenic effects of CCK-4. Abelson and Nesse (2) have also found that the CCK-B agonist pentagastrin (0.6 μg/kg iv) provokes panic symptoms in four out of five drug-free panic patients and one out of four controls.

Cholecystokinin-4 is an attractive new probe of anxiety. Its anxiogenic effects are reliable and dose-dependent, with 25 μg iv of CCK-4 producing panic responses similar to 35% CO_2 inhalation in patients and controls (11). Its ease of administration and similarity of effect to naturalistic panic are also strengths. Studies of CCK-4's interactions with non-CCK neurotransmitter systems have already begun. DeMontigny (25) reported that lorazepam prevented CCK-4–induced anxiety in four healthy sub-

55. Parent A. *Comparative Neurobiology of the Basal Ganglia.* New York: John Wiley; 1986.

56. Pauls DL, Leckman JF. The inheritance of Gilles de la Tourette's syndrome and associated behaviors—evidence for autosomal dominant transmission. *N Engl J Med* 1986;315:993–997.

57. Phelps ME, Mazziotta JC. Positron emission tomography: human brain function and biochemistry. *Science* 1985;228:799–809.

58. Phelps ME, Mazziotta JC, Shelbert HR, eds. *Positron emission tomography and autoradiography.* New York: Raven Press; 1986.

59. Rapaport JL, Wise SP. Obsessive–compulsive disorder: is it a basal ganglia dysfunction? *Psychopharm Bull* 1988;24:380–384.

60. Rauch SL, Jenike MJ, Alpert NA, Regional cerebral blood flow measured during symptom provocation in obsessive-compulsive disorder using ^{15}O-labeled CO_2 and positron emission tomography. *Arch Gen Psychiatry* 1994;51:62–70.

61. Reiman EM, Raichle ME, Butler FK, Herscovitch P, Robins E. A focal brain abnormality in panic disorder, a severe form of anxiety. *Nature* 1984;310:683–685.

62. Reiman EM, Raichle ME, Robins E, et al. Neuroanatomical correlates of a lactate-induced anxiety attack. *Arch Gen Psychiatry* 1989;46:493–500.

63. Reiman EM, Fusselman MJ, Fox PT, Raichle ME. Neuroanatomical correlates of anticipatory anxiety. *Science* 1989;243:1071–1074.

64. Rubin RT, Villanueva-Meyer J, Ananth J, Trajmar PG, Mena I. Regional ^{133}Xe cerebral blood flow and cerebral ^{99m}HMPAO uptake in unmedicated obsessive–compulsive disorder patients and matched normal control subjects: determination by high-resolution single-photon emission computed tomography. *Arch Gen Psychiatry,* 1992;49:695–702.

65. Rubin RT, Ananth J, Villanueva-Meyer J, Trajmar PG, Mena I. Regional xenon 133 cerebral blood flow and cerebral technetium 99m HMPAO uptake in patients with obsessive–compulsive disorder before and during treatment. *Arch Gen Psychiatry* [*submitted*].

66. Schneider JS. Review: basal ganglia role in behavior: importance of sensory gating and its relevance to psychiatry. *Biol Psychiatry* 1984;19:1693–1710.

67. Swedo SE, Rapoport JL, Cheslow DL, et al. High prevalence of obsessive–compulsive symptoms in patients with Sydenham's chorea. *Am J Psychiatry* 1989;146:246–249.

68. Swedo SE, Pietrini P, Leonard HL, et al. Cerebral glucose metabolism in childhood-onset obsessive–compulsive disorder: revisualization during pharmacotherapy. *Arch Gen Psychiatry* 1992; 49:690–694.

69. Swedo SE, Schapiro MB, Grady CL, et al. Cerebral glucose metabolism in childhood-onset obsessive–compulsive disorder. *Arch Gen Psychiatry* 1989;46:518–523.

70. Swerdlow NR, Koob GF. Dopamine, schizophrenia, mania and depression: toward a unified hypothesis of cortico-striato-pallido-thalamic function. *Behav Brain Sci* 1987;10:197–245.

71. Teresa M, De Cristofaro DER, Sessarego A, Pupi A, Biondi F, Faravelli C. Brain perfusion abnormalities in drug-naive, lactate-sensitive panic patients: a SPECT study. *Biol Psychiatry* 1993; 33:505–512.

72. Thompson JM, Baxter LR, Schwartz JM. Freud, obsessive–compulsive disorder and neurobiology. *Psychoanal Contemp Thought* 1992;15:483–505.

73. Wik G, Fredrikson M, Ericson K, Driksson L, Stone-Elander S, Greitz T. A functional cerebral response to frightening visual stimulation. *Psychiatry Res Neuroimag* 1993;50:15–24.

74. Winslow JT, Insel T. Neuroethological models of obsessive–compulsive disorder. In: Zohar J, Insel T, Rasmussen S, eds. *The psychobiology of obsessive–compulsive disorder* New York: Springer-Verlag; 1991.

75. Wu JC, Buchsbaum MS, Hershey TG, Hazlett E, Sicotte N, Johnson JC. PET in generalized anxiety disorder. *Biol Psychiatry* 1991;29:1181–1199.

76. Zohar J, Insel TR, Berman KF, Foa EB, Hill JL, Weinberger DR. Anxiety and cerebral blood flow during behavioral challenge: dissociation of central from peripheral and subjective measures. *Arch Gen Psychiatry* 1989;46:505–510.

77. Zohar J, Insel TR. Obsessive-compulsive disorder: psychobiological approaches to diagnosis, treatment, and pathophysiology. *Biol Psychiatry* 1987;22:667–687.

jects. However, Couetoux-Dutertre et al. (22) recently found that flumazenil (2.0 mg iv) did not block the anxiogenic effects of CCK-4 (50 μg i.v) in 30 healthy subjects, indicating that CCK-4 is not acting as an inverse agonist at the GABA$_A$/BZ receptor. Studies with selective antagonists (e.g., the CCK-B antagonists CI-988, L-365,260, and LY-262691) will help clarify the mechanism of CCK-4's anxiogenic effects. The clinical efficacy of CCK-B antagonists is currently under investigation.

Corticotropin-releasing Hormone

Preclinical evidence strongly implicates corticotropin-releasing hormone (CRH) in the mediation of stress responses in animals (26). Roy-Byrne et al. in 1986 (80) first reported blunted ACTH and cortisol responses to CRH (1 μg/kg) in eight drug-free panic patients compared with 30 controls, a finding that was replicated by Holsboer et al. in 1987 (45). These data are consistent with a chronic hypercortisolemic state in panic disorder. However, Rapaport et al. (75) observed no difference between eight drug-free panic patients and 11 controls in response to ovine CRH (0.03 μg/kg iv). Reconciliation and extension of these findings awaits further clinical studies.

Growth Hormone-releasing Factor

Rapaport et al. reported in 1989 (76) that the GH response to 1 μg/kg iv of growth hormone-releasing factor (GHRF) was markedly blunted in 11 drug-free panic patients compared with 11 controls. This finding, recently replicated by Tancer et al. (86) (cf. above), suggests that hypothalamic–pituitary dysfunction merits further scrutiny as a possible factor in the pathophysiology of panic disorder.

Thyrotropin-releasing Hormone

In addition to the voluminous literature documenting thyroid axis abnormalities in affective disorders, reports with small samples have suggested that the thyrotropin response to thyrotropin-releasing hormone (TRH) is blunted in panic disorder. Stein and Uhde (84) recently conducted a careful investigation of the effects of TRH (500 μg iv) in 26 drug-free panic patients and 22 controls. Prolactin, thyrotropin, blood pressure, and heart rate responses were similar between groups. Despite robust increases in heart rate and blood pressure following TRH, only one patient experienced a panic attack. This finding contradicts the theory that cognitive elaboration of interoceptive cues is sufficient to trigger panic attacks in these patients.

Caffeine

Caffeine is a methylxanthine with central effects as an adenosine receptor antagonist. It is a mild psychostimulant, well-known for its dose-dependent anxiogenic properties in healthy subjects and psychiatric patients.

In a 1985 study utilizing caffeine (10 mg/kg po), Charney et al. (15) provoked panic attacks in 15 out of 21 (71%) drug-free panic patients and none of the 17 controls. Uhde et al. (89) observed panic in 9 out of 24 (54) panic patients and none of the 14 controls after 480 mg po of caffeine.

Caffeine-induced anxiety could be from blockade of central adenosine receptors followed by activation of the LC, resulting in increased release of brain NE. Other possible mechanisms include inhibition of phosphodiesterase and BZ receptor antagonism. Unfortunately, the pharmacological and behavioral effects of caffeine are neither selective nor potent, which limits its utility as a probe for anxiety disorders. Major advances in this area await the availability of adenosine receptor ligands with more selectivity than the xanthines or purines.

Miscellaneous Probes

Hypoglycemia

Neuroglycopenia has many symptoms in common with panic, but Schweizer et al. (81) found that insulin (0.1 units/kg) did not precipitate panic attacks in ten drug-free panic patients, even though prominent symptoms of hypoglycemia were evident. This study argues against the hypothesis that nonspecific sympathetic activation is sufficient to cause panic in predisposed individuals via cognitive elaboration of interoceptive cues.

Cholinergic Probes

Early reports suggested that cholinergic agonists such as the central cholinesterase inhibitor physostigmine had anxiogenic properties in healthy subjects. Following pretreatment with propantheline (45 mg po) to block peripheral effects, Rapaport et al. (74) administered physostigmine (0.022 mg/kg iv) to nine drug-free panic patients and nine controls. Behavioral, cortisol, and cardiovascular responses did not differ between groups, and no subjects experienced panic attacks. These data do not support a role for the central cholinergic system in the pathogenesis of anxiety disorders.

Dopaminergic Probes

Pitchot et al. (68) observed a greater GH response to the DA agonist apomorphine (0.5 mg sc) in nine drug-free panic patients compared with nine major depressive and nine minor depressive patients. These investigators concluded that DA function was increased in panic disorder compared with depression, but the lack of healthy controls limits the interpretation of this study. In their study of 21 social phobia patients and 22 controls, Tancer and Golden (85) found no difference between groups in the prolactin response to oral L-dopa (500 mg). Abnormal neuroendocrine responses to fenfluramine, but not clonidine, were observed, suggesting that social phobia patients manifest dysregulated 5-HT neurotransmission in the face of normal DA and NE function.

OBSESSIVE–COMPULSIVE DISORDERS

Use of the pharmacological challenge strategy in OCD is a relatively recent development, and the high context dependency of OC symptoms has made studies of behavioral responses more problematic than in panic disorder. Despite these limitations, a significant literature has begun to emerge.

Serotonergic Probes

Potent SRIs are superior to other agents in the treatment of OCD. This, rather than theoretical considerations, accounts for the fact that studies of 5-HT function have dominated research into the clinical neurobiology of OCD over the past decade (7).

m-Chlorophenylpiperazine

m-Chlorophenylpiperazine has been the most frequently used probe in studies of OCD, appearing in six reports involving drug-free patients. Zohar et al. in 1987 (96) gave m-CPP (0.5 mg/kg po) to 12 OCD patients and 20 controls. Patients manifested a greater anxiety response than controls and specific exacerbation of their obsessive–compulsive (OC) symptoms. Cortisol responses were blunted in patients, whereas increased prolactin and hyperthermia occurred equally in both groups. Charney et al. in 1988 (16) administered m-CPP 0.1 mg/kg iv to 21 OCD patients and 21 controls. Basal prolactin levels were lower and prolactin responses were blunted in female, but not male, patients. There were no differences between patients and controls in cortisol, GH, or anxiety responses, and OC symptoms were unchanged. Hollander et al. (43) studied m-CPP (0.5 mg/kg po) in 20 OCD patients and 10 controls. Obsessive–compulsive symptoms were exacerbated and prolactin responses attenuated in patients, with no difference between groups in anxiety or cortisol responses. To clarify the mechanism of oral m-CPP's behavioral effects, Pigott et al. in 1991 (67) administered m-CPP (0.5 mg/kg po) to 12 OCD patients following acute pretreatment with the 5-HT antagonist metergoline (4 mg po). Metergoline blocked the worsen-

ing of OC symptoms and the prolactin increase caused by m-CPP. However, in a subsequent study designed to reconcile conflicting behavioral findings with oral and intravenous m-CPP, Pigott et al. (67) administered m-CPP (0.5 mg/kg po) to 17 OCD patients and m-CPP (0.1 mg/kg iv) to a separate group of 10 OCD patients. Oral m-CPP did not increase OC or anxiety symptoms, but intravenous m-CPP increased both. Exacerbation of OC and anxiety symptoms caused by intravenous m-CPP was blocked by metergoline (4 mg po). Recently, Goodman et al. in 1991 (33) gave 0.1-mg/kg iv and 0.5-mg/kg po doses of m-CPP to the same 12 OCD patients on two different occasions. Neither route of administration resulted in worsening OC symptoms.

Two studies have described the effects of long-term treatment with SRIs on responses to m-CPP in OCD patients. Zohar et al. (96), using a 0.5-mg/kg po dose of m-CPP found that clomipramine treatment abolished the m-CPP–induced exacerbation of OC and anxiety symptoms and the hyperthymic response observed pretreatment in nine patients; prolactin and cortisol responses were unaffected. Using the same m-CPP dosage and route of administration, Hollander et al. in 1991 (43) reported that fluoxetine treatment also abolished pretreatment m-CPP–induced exacerbation of OC symptoms in six patients, although no anxiety response was detected pre- or posttreatment. In this study, prolactin and cortisol responses were increased during fluoxetine treatment, but this may have reflected increased m-CPP plasma levels.

To summarize, the most controversial finding with m-CPP is its putative ability to exacerbate OC symptoms, as reported by two groups (43,96) but contested by a third (16). Differences in dosage and route of administration have been adduced to explain the discrepancy, but this argument has recently been weakened by evidence that oral and intravenous routes have comparable effects (7). Additionally, one group (67) has failed to replicate its own finding of symptom exacerbation with oral m-CPP, but now observes this effect with the intravenous route, in contrast to the other group which has studied intravenous m-CPP (16). Behavioral and neurobiological variability across patients, interacting with the multiplicity of m-CPP's pharmacological effects, could account for these disparate findings, which are reminiscent of the inconsistencies in the m-CPP–panic literature. In contrast, attenuated neuroendocrine responses to m-CPP is a consistent finding, although not all studies report blunting of the same hormone.

Fenfluramine

Three studies have utilized DL-fenfluramine as a probe in drug-free OCD patients. Hollander et al. (43) gave fenfluramine (60 mg po) to 20 OCD patients and 10 controls. Prolactin and cortisol responses did not differ between groups. In a study of 21 OCD patients and 27 controls, McBride et al. (63) also found no difference in prolactin responses to fenfluramine (60 mg po). In neither study did fenfluramine significantly affect OC symptoms. However, Hewlett et al. (41) reported that fenfluramine (60 mg po) caused a blunted prolactin response in 26 OCD patients compared with 20 controls, a finding significant in females only.

Lucey et al. (62) studied D-fenfluramine (30 mg po) in 10 OCD patients, 10 depressed patients, and 10 controls, all drug-free. Preference for the D-isomer over the racemate has been advocated based on its greater potency and specificity for 5-HT (as opposed to DA) systems. Both OCD and depressed patients had blunted prolactin and cortisol responses compared with controls, with no differences between the patient groups.

These four studies provide some support for the hypothesis that net 5-HT neurotransmission is impaired in OCD. Fenfluramine studies have yielded similarly equivocal evidence of blunted 5-HT function in depression. Fenfluramine's ability to provoke panic attacks in panic patients (88) contrasts with its lack of behavioral effects in OCD.

L-Tryptophan

In the only study using this agent in OCD, Charney et al. (16) gave L-tryptophan (7 g iv) to 21 drug-free OCD patients and 21 controls. The prolactin response to L-tryptophan was slightly but significantly greater in patients than controls, with no difference in GH response and no exacerbation of OC symptoms. The enhanced prolactin response in OCD contrasts with findings in panic disorder patients, who do not differ from controls (18), and depressed patients, who manifest blunted responses in some subtypes (72). However, Price et al. (72) found that melancholic depressed patients show an enhanced prolactin response. This disappeared when baseline plasma tryptophan levels, which were nonsignificantly lower in melancholic patients than controls, were used as covariates. Baseline plasma tryptophan levels were not measured by Charney et al. (16), but this factor might also account for the finding in OCD patients.

Ipsapirone

Lesch et al. (56) administered ipsapirone (0.3 mg/kg po) to 12 drug-free OCD patients and 22 controls. Cortisol, ACTH, hypothermic, and behavioral responses did not differ between groups. Lesch et al. (57) found that long-term treatment with fluoxetine in 10 OCD patients attenuated the cortisol, ACTH, and hypothermic responses to ipsapirone. This suggests that SRI treatment down-regulates 5-HT$_{1A}$ receptor sensitivity, although the lack of 5-HT$_{1A}$−mediated differences between drug-free patients and controls raises doubts regarding the mediation of antiobsessional effects through this mechanism. Cortisol, ACTH, and hypothermic responses to ipsapirone

are blunted in panic disorder (58) and depression relative to controls.

Buspirone

Like ipsapirone, buspirone is also an azapirone derivative with high affinity for the 5-HT$_{1A}$ receptor. However, mediation of its neuroendocrine effects through the 5-HT$_{1A}$ site is questionable, since it also antagonizes DA receptors.

Lucey et al. (60) studied buspirone (30 mg po) in 10 drug-free OCD patients and 10 controls. There was no difference in prolactin responses between groups, and OCD patients showed no worsening of symptoms. Acknowledging the lack of pharmacological selectivity of buspirone, these findings are nonetheless consistent with the ipsapirone findings (56) in arguing against 5-HT$_{1A}$ involvement in the pathogenesis of OCD.

MK-212

MK-212 [6-chloro-2-(1-piperazinyl)-pyrazine] is a 5-HT agonist that binds to 5-HT$_{1A}$, 5-HT$_{1B}$, 5-HT$_{1C}$, and 5-HT$_2$ receptors (9). Bastani et al. (9) gave MK-212 (20 mg po) to 17 drug-free OCD patients and 9 controls. Compared with controls, patients had blunted cortisol responses to the probe, but prolactin and behavioral responses did not differ. Since selective 5-HT$_2$ antagonists block the cortisol response to MK-212 in laboratory animals, this study suggests that 5-HT$_2$ receptors may be subsensitive in OCD.

Metergoline

Metergoline is a nonselective 5-HT$_1$/5-HT$_2$ antagonist that blocks neuroendocrine and hyperthermic responses to m-CPP in humans. Three studies have examined responses to metergoline (4 mg po) in drug-free OCD patients. Zohar et al. in 1987 (96) observed no behavioral changes in 12 patients. In subsequent efforts to assess the effects of metergoline on m-CPP-induced responses in OCD (cf. above), Pigott et al. (67) found no behavioral effects of metergoline alone in 12 patients in a 1991 study or in 10 patients in a later study.

Benkelfat et al. in 1989 (10) administered metergoline (4 mg/day) or placebo for 4 days to 10 OCD patients whose symptoms had responded to long-term clomipramine treatment. Patients experienced worse OC symptoms during metergoline administration than during placebo, but this reflected a slight improvement from baseline in symptoms during placebo treatment; worsening of symptoms from baseline during metergoline treatment was even smaller and nonsignificant.

These studies indicate that nonspecific antagonism of 5-HT receptors has no unique effects on the neurobiology or phenomenolgy of OCD. Although such antagonism may interfere with the antiobsessional action of SRIs, relevant data are equivocal.

Tryptophan Depletion

Barr et al. (8) administered double-blind sham-controlled tryptophan-depletion tests to 15 OCD patients who had responded to long-term SRI treatment. Tryptophan depletion had no effect on OC symptoms, but depressive symptoms increased compared with the sham test. A similar worsening of depressive symptoms has been reported in remitted depressed patients being treated with antidepressants (24). These findings suggest that the vulnerability unmasked by tryptophan depletion is more central to the regulation of mood than of core OC symptoms.

Noradrenergic Probes

Theoretical and pharmacotherapeutic considerations have traditionally generated interest in NE mechanisms of depression and panic disorder. Phenomenological similarities of these conditions to OCD have stimulated some studies of NE function in OCD.

Clonidine

Clonidine has been used as a pharmacological probe in three studies of drug-free OCD patients. Siever et al. in 1983 (82) gave clonidine (2 μg/kg iv) to nine OCD patients and nine controls and found the GH response blunted in patients. Lee et al. in 1990 (55) administered clonidine (2 μg/kg iv) to 10 OCD patients and 13 controls. They observed no differences between groups in GH or behavioral responses. Hollander et al. in 1991 (42) gave clonidine (2 μg/kg iv) to 18 OCD patients and 10 controls. Cortisol, GH, MHPG, and blood pressure responses did not differ between groups, but patients manifested transient improvement in OC symptoms.

These studies do not support major involvement of α_2-adrenoceptors in the pathogenesis of OCD. Independent replication of the improvement in OC symptoms noted by Hollander et al. (42) would be important, but it will be difficult to establish that this does not reflect nonspecific sedation. These findings contrast with the blunted GH response to clonidine seen in depression and panic disorder (90).

Yohimbine

Rasmussen et al. in 1987 (78) administered yohimbine (20 mg po) to 12 drug-free OCD patients and 12 controls. Groups did not differ in behavioral or MHPG responses to yohimbine, but patients had an increased cortisol re-

sponse. This recalls the increased cortisol responses to yohimbine in depression and panic disorder (20). In panic disorder, however, yohimbine also induces panic attacks associated with an enhanced MHPG response (20).

Desipramine

Desipramine is a selective inhibitor of presynaptic NE reuptake. Given acutely, it increases GH secretion, apparently reflecting α_2-adrenoceptor stimulation. Lucey et al. (59) gave desipramine (1 mg/kg po) to 10 drug-free OCD patients and 10 controls. Growth hormone and behavioral responses did not differ between groups. This contrasts with studies showing blunted GH responses to desipramine in depression.

Mixed Monoamine Probes

Psychostimulants were among the first agents used in challenge studies of mood disorders. Although specific mechanisms vary, the principal effect of these drugs is to increase synaptic availability of monoamines via enhanced presynaptic release and/or reuptake inhibition. Their action as euphoriants is often attributed to their effects on DA function, although they have comparable effects on NE and 5-HT.

Three studies have examined the effects of psychostimulants in drug-free OCD patients. Insel et al. in 1983 (48) administered D-amphetamine (30 mg po) or placebo to 12 OCD patients; a significant improvement in OC symptoms was observed after active drug administration only. Joffe and Swinson in 1987 (50) found no change in OC symptoms in 13 OCD patients given open methylphenidate (40 mg po). In a subsequent placebo-controlled study of 11 OCD patients, Joffe et al. (51) again found that D-amphetamine (30 mg po) improved OC symptoms, whereas methylphenidate (40 mg po) had no effect.

Miscellaneous Probes

Naloxone

Insel and Pickar reported in 1983 (49) that administration of the nonselective opiate antagonist naloxone (0.3 mg/kg iv) to two drug-free OCD patients in a placebo-controlled study caused worsening of OC symptoms. This contrasts with reports that high-dose naloxone infusions transiently decrease psychotic symptoms in schizophrenia.

Sodium Lactate

Gorman et al. (35) gave 0.5-M sodium DL-lactate (10 ml/kg iv) to seven drug-free OCD patients and 48 drug-free panic disorder patients. Only one of the 7 (14%)

OCD patients developed panic attacks, whereas 26 of the 48 (56%) panic disorder patients did so. These findings are consistent with other studies showing that known panicogens have little behavioral effect in OCD (7,41,43,63).

Hypertonic Saline

In laboratory animals, arginine vasopressin (AVP) is associated with abnormal persistence of behaviors acquired under aversive conditioning and expression of stereotypic grooming behaviors. To examine the role of AVP in OCD, Altemus et al. (5) administered 3% hypertonic saline (0.1 mg/kg) over 2 hr to 12 drug-free OCD patients and 24 controls. Patients showed greater secretion of plasma AVP than controls, and, in many patients, the normal linear relationship between AVP and serum osmolality was disrupted. Additional findings of elevated cerebrospinal fluid levels of AVP and CRH in OCD patients in this study suggest that the effect of these synergistic arousal-producing hormones may be increased in OCD.

Cholinergic Probes

Lucey et al. (61) recently reported that the cholinesterase inhibitor pyridostigmine (120 mg po) caused greater GH responses in nine drug-free OCD patients than in nine controls. This evidence suggesting cholinergic supersensitivity in OCD is tempered by knowledge of pyridostigmine's poor entry into the brain.

SUMMARY

The pharmacological challenge strategy has proven remarkably productive in the study of anxiety disorders. Unfortunately, some of the best-replicated findings (e.g., the panicogenic effects of lactate and CO_2) remain most resistant to simple explanations of mechanism. However, this may accurately reflect the complexity of the etiopathologic factors underlying these disorders.

Particularly encouraging are emerging data suggesting real differences in responses to the same challenge agents in different anxiety disorders. Panic disorder differentiates clearly from OCD, with recent evidence suggesting that social phobia and PTSD may also manifest distinctive response profiles. These observations underscore the lack of specificity inhering in the concept of anxiety that serves as the purported common factor linking these conditions to each other. Although it is disappointing that these findings so far have had relatively little clinical application, they could ultimately serve as the basis for a diagnostic nosology based on neurobiology as well as phenomenology. This process will be greatly facilitated if progress in understanding the neuroanatomy of anxiety as a phenomenon (71), as well as that of the discrete disorders

(37,47), can be married to pharmacological challenge findings.

Equally exciting are recent developments in which clinical treatments have led to preclinical advances (e.g., BZ receptor studies) and preclinical findings have suggested new treatments (e.g., CCK antagonists). The reciprocal nature of these interactions epitomizes an ideal in the relationship between preclinical and clinical neuroscience that is rarely realized. In the anxiety disorders, the pharmacological challenge strategy continues to serve this ideal well.

ACKNOWLEDGMENTS

This work was supported in part by grants MH-25642, MH-30929, MH-45802, and MH-50641 from the U.S. Public Health Service and by grant DA-04060 from the State of Connecticut Department of Mental Health. Elizabeth Kyle prepared the manuscript.

REFERENCES

1. Abelson JL, Glitz D, Cameron OG, Lee MA, Bronzo M, Curtis GC. Blunted growth hormone response to clonidine in patients with generalized anxiety disorder. *Arch Gen Psychiatry* 1991;48:157–162.
2. Abelson J, Nesse R. Cholecystokinin-4 and panic. *Arch Gen Psychiatry* 1990;47:395.
3. Albus M, Zahn TP, Breier A. Anxiogenic properties of yohimbine. I. Behavioral, physiological and biochemical measures. *Eur Arch Psychiatry Clin Neurosci* 1992;241:337–344.
4. Albus M, Zahn TP, Breier A. Anxiogenic properties of yohimbine. II. Influence of experimental set and setting. *Eur Arch Psychiatry Clin Neurosci* 1992;241:345–351.
5. Altemus M, Pigott T, Kalogeras KT, et al. Abnormalities in the regulation of vasopressin and corticotropin factor secretion in obsessive-compulsive disorder. *Arch Gen Psychiatry* 1992;49:9–20.
6. Asnis GM, Wetzler S, Sanderson WC, Kahn RS, van Praag HM. Functional interrelationship of serotonin and norepinephrine: cortisol response to MCPP and DMI in patients with panic disorder, patients with depression, and normal control subjects. *Psychiatry Res* 1992;43:65–76.
7. Barr LC, Goodman WK, Price LH, McDougle CJ, Charney DS. The serotonin hypothesis of obsessive compulsive disorder: implications of pharmacologic challenge studies. *J Clin Psychiatry* 1992;53[4, Suppl]:17–28.
8. Barr LC, Goodman WK, McDougle CJ, et al. Tryptophan depletion in patients with obsessive-compulsive disorder who respond to serotonin reuptake inhibitors. *Arch Gen Psychiatry* 1994;51:309–317.
9. Bastani B, Nash JF, Meltzer HY. Prolactin and cortisol responses to MK-212, a serotonin agonist, in obsessive-compulsive disorder. *Arch Gen Psychiatry* 1990;47:833–839.
10. Benkelfat C, Murphy DL, Zohar J, et al. Clomipramine in obsessive-compulsive disorder: further evidence for a serotonergic mechanism of action. *Arch Gen Psychiatry* 1989;46:23–28.
11. Bradwejn J. CCK agonists and antagonists in clinical studies of panic and anxiety. *Clin Neuropharm* 1992;15(Suppl 1):481–482A.
12. Bradwejn J, Koszycki D, Shriqui C. Enhanced sensitivity to cholecystokinin tetrapeptide in panic disorder. Clinical and behavioral findings. *Arch Gen Psychiatry* 1991;48:603–610.
13. Carr DB, Sheehan DV. Panic anxiety: a new biological model. *J Clin Psychiatry* 1984;45:323–330.
14. Charney DS, Heninger GR, Breier A. Noradrenergic function in panic anxiety: effects of yohimbine in healthy subjects and patients with agoraphobia and panic disorder. *Arch Gen Psychiatry* 1984;41:751–763.

15. Charney DS, Heninger GR, Jatlow PI. Increased anxiogenic effects of caffeine in panic disorders. *Arch Gen Psychiatry* 1985;42:233–243.

16. Charney DS, Goodman WK, Price LH, Woods SW, Rasmussen SA, Heninger GR. Serotonin function in obsessive compulsive disorder: a comparison of the effects of tryptophan and MCPP in patients and healthy subjects. *Arch Gen Psychiatry* 1988;45:177–185.

17. Charney DS, Heninger GR. Noradrenergic function and the mechanism of action of antianxiety treatment: I. The effect of long-term alprazolam treatment. *Arch Gen Psychiatry* 1985;42:458–467.

18. Charney DS, Heninger GR. Serotonin function in panic disorders: the effect of intravenous tryptophan in healthy subjects and patients with panic disorders before and during alprazolam treatment. *Arch Gen Psychiatry* 1986;43:1059–1065.

19. Charney DS, Woods SW, Goodman WK, Heninger GR. Neurobiological mechanisms of panic anxiety: biochemical and behavioral correlates of yohimbine-induced panic attacks. *Am J Psychiatry* 1987;144:1030–1036.

20. Charney DS, Woods SW, Krystal JH, Nagy LM, Heninger GR. Noradrenergic neuronal dysregulation in panic disorder: the effects of intravenous yohimbine and clonidine in panic disorder patients. *Acta Psychiatr Scand* 1992;86:273–282.

21. Coplan JD, Liebowitz MR, Gorman JM, et al. Noradrenergic function in panic disorder. Effects of intravenous clonidine pretreatment on lactate induced panic. *Biol Psychiatry* 1992;31:135–146.

22. Couetoux-Dutertre A, Bradwejn J, Koszycki D, Paradis M, Bourin M. Lack of effect of flumazenil on CCK-4-panic. *1992 New Research Program and Abstracts* 145th Annual Meeting, Washington, DC: American Psychiatric Association; 1992:NR138.

23. Cowley DS, Arana GW. The diagnostic utility of lactate sensitivity in panic disorder. *Arch Gen Psychiatry* 1990;47:277–284.

24. Delgado PL, Charney DS, Price LH, Aghajanian GK, Landis H, Heninger GR. Serotonin function and the mechanism of antidepressant action: reversal of antidepressant induced remission by rapid depletion of plasma tryptophan. *Arch Gen Psychiatry* 1990;47:411–418.

25. De Montigny C. Cholecystokinin tetrapeptide induces panic like attacks in healthy volunteers. *Arch Gen Psychiatry* 1989;46:511–517.

26. Dunn AJ, Berridge CW. Physiological and behavioral responses in corticotropin-releasing factor administration: is CRF a mediator of anxiety or stress responses? *Brain Res Rev* 1990;15:71–100.

27. Germine M, Goddard AW, Woods SW, Charney DS, Heninger GR. Anger and anxiety responses to *m*-chlorophenylpiperazine in generalized anxiety disorder. *Biol Psychiatry* 1992;32:457–461.

28. Goddard AW, Charney DS, Germine M, Heninger GR, Woods SW. Anxiety responses to IV MCPP in healthy subjects and patients with panic disorder. *Soc Neurosci Abstr* 1991;17:1456.

29. Goddard AW, Germine M, Woods SW, Delgado PL, Heninger GR, Charney DS. Effects of tryptophan depletion on anxiety responses to yohimbine in humans. Presented at the Annual Meeting of the American College of Neuropsychopharmacology, San Juan, Puerto Rico, 1991.

30. Goddard AW, Goodman WK, Woods SW, Heninger GR, Charney DS, Price LH. Effects of tryptophan depletion on panic anxiety. Presented at the Annual Meeting of the American College of Neuropsychopharmacology, San Juan, Puerto Rico, 1992.

31. Goddard AW, Woods SW, Sholomskas DE, Goodman WK, Charney DS, Heninger GR. Effects of the serotonin reuptake inhibitor fluvoxamine on noradrenergic function in panic disorder. *Psychiatry Res* 1993;48:119–133.

32. Goetz RR, Klein DF, Gully R, et al. Panic attacks during placebo procedures in the laboratory. Physiology and symptomatology. *Arch Gen Psychiatry* 1993;50:280–285.

33. Goodman WK, McDougle CJ, Price LH, et al. M-chlorophenylpiperazine in patients with obsessive-compulsive disorder: absence of symptom exacerbation. *Biol Psychiatry* 1994;[in press].

34. Gorman JM, Fyer MR, Liebowitz MR, Klein DF. Pharmacologic provocation of panic attacks. In: Meltzer HY, ed. *Psychopharmacology: the third generation of progress*. New York: Raven Press; 1987:985–993.

35. Gorman JM, Liebowitz MR, Fyer AJ, et al. Lactate infusions in obsessive–compulsive disorder. *Am J Psychiatry* 1985;142:864–866.

36. Gorman JM, Fyer MR, Goetz R, et al. Ventilatory physiology of patients with panic disorder. *Arch Gen Psychiatry* 1988;45:31–39.

37. Gorman JM, Liebowitz MR, Fyer AJ, Stein J. A neuroanatomical hypothesis for panic disorder. *Am J Psychiatry* 1989;146:148–161.

38. Gorman JM, Goetz RR, Dillon D, et al. Sodium D-lactate infusion in panic disorder patients. *Neuropsychopharmacology* 1990;3:181–189.

39. Griez E, Lousberg H, Van den Hout MA, et al. Carbon dioxide vulnerability in panic disorder. *Psychiatry Res* 1987;20:87–95.

40. Gurguis GNM, Uhde TW. Plasma 3-methoxy-4-hydroxyphenylethylene glycol (MHPG) and growth hormone responses to yohimbine in panic disorder patients and normal controls. *Psychoneuroendocrinology* 1990;15:217–224.

41. Hewlett WA, Vinogradov S, Martin K, Berman S, Csernansky JG. Fenfluramine stimulation of prolactin in obsessive–compulsive disorder. *Psychiatry Res* 1992;42:81–92.

42. Hollander E, DeCaria C, Gully R, et al. Effects of chronic fluoxetine treatment on behavioral and neuroendocrine responses to metachlorophenylpiperazine in obsessive compulsive disorder. *Psychiatry Res* 1991;36:1–17.

43. Hollander E, DeCaria CM, Nitescu A, et al. Serotonergic function in obsessive–compulsive disorder: behavioral and neuroendocrine responses to oral *m*-chlorophenylpiperazine and fenfluramine in patients and healthy volunteers. *Arch Gen Psychiatry* 1992;49:21–28.

44. Hollander E, Liebowitz MR, DeCaria C, Klein DF. Fenfluramine, cortisol, and anxiety. *Psychiatry Res* 1990;31:211–213.

45. Holsboer F, von Bardeleben U, Buller R, Heuser I, Steiger A. Stimulation response to corticotropin-releasing hormone (CRH) in patients with depression, alcoholism, and panic disorder. *Horm Metab Res* 1987;16(suppl):80–88.

46. Hommer DW, Skolnick P, Paul SM. The benzodiazepine/GABA receptor complex and anxiety. In: Meltzer HY, ed *Psychopharmacology: the third generation of progress*. New York: Raven Press; 1987:977–983.

47. Insel TR. Toward a neuroanatomy of obsessive-compulsive disorder. *Arch Gen Psychiatry* 1992;49:739–744.

48. Insel TR, Hamilton JA, Guttmacher LB, Murphy DL. D-amphetamine in obsessive-compulsive disorder. *Psychopharmacology* 1983;80:231–235.

49. Insel TR, Pickar D. Naloxone administration in obsessive-compulsive disorder: report of two cases. *Am J Psychiatry* 1983;140:1219–1220.

50. Joffe RT, Swinson RP. Methylphenidate in primary obsessive-compulsive disorder. *J Clin Psychopharmacol* 1987;7:420–422.

51. Joffe RT, Swinson RP, Levitt AJ. Acute psychostimulant challenge in primary obsessive-compulsive disorder. *J Clin Psychopharmacol* 1991;11:237–241.

52. Kahn RS, Wetzler S. *m*-Chlorophenylpiperazine as a probe of serotonin function. *Biol Psychiatry* 1991;30:1139–1166.

53. Klein DF. False suffocation alarms, spontaneous panics, and related conditions. An integrative hypothesis. *Arch Gen Psychiatry* 1993;50:306–317.

54. Krystal JH, Southwick SM, Morgan CA, et al. Noradrenergic and serotonergic mechanisms in PTSD. Presented at the Annual Meeting of the American College of Neuropsychopharmacology, San Juan, Puerto Rico, 1991.

55. Lee MA, Cameron OG, Gurguis GNM, et al. Alpha₂-adrenoreceptor status in obsessive-compulsive disorder. *Biol Psychiatry* 1990;27:1083–1093.

56. Lesch KP, Hoh A, Disselkamp-Tietze J, et al. 5-hydroxytryptamine$_{1A}$ receptor responsivity in obsessive-compulsive disorder: comparison of patients and controls. *Arch Gen Psychiatry* 1991;48:540–547.

57. Lesch KP, Hoh A, Schulte HM, et al. Long-term fluoxetine treatment decreases 5-HT$_{1A}$ receptor responsivity in obsessive compulsive disorder. *Psychopharmacology* 1991;105:415–420.

58. Lesch KP, Wiesmann M, Hoh A, et al. 5-HT$_{1A}$ receptor-effector system responsivity in panic disorder. *Psychopharmacology* 1992;106:111–117.

59. Lucey JV, Barry S, Webb MGT, Dinan TG. The desipramine-induced growth hormone response and the dexamethasone suppression test in obsessive–compulsive disorder. *Acta Psychiatr Scand* 1992;86:367–370.

60. Lucey JV, Butcher G, Clare AW, Dinan TG. Buspirone induced prolactin responses in obsessive–compulsive disorder (OCD): is

OCD a 5-HT$_2$ receptor disorder? *Int Clin Psychopharmacol* 1992;7:45–49.

61. Lucey JV, Butcher G, Clare AW, Dinan TG. Elevated growth hormone responses to pyridostigmine in obsessive–compulsive disorder: evidence of cholinergic supersensitivity. *Am J Psychiatry* 1993;150:961–962.

62. Lucey JV, O'Keane V, Butcher G, Clare AW, Dinan TG. Cortisol and prolactin responses to D-fenfluramine in non-depressed patients with obsessive–compulsive disorder: a comparison with depressed and healthy controls. *Br J Psychiatry* 1992;161:517–521.

63. McBride PA, DeMeo MD, Sweeney JA, et al. Neuroendocrine and behavioral responses to challenge with the indirect serotonin agonist DL-fenfluramine in adults with obsessive–compulsive disorder. *Biol Psychiatry* 1992;31:19–34.

64. Nesse RM, Cameron OG, Curtis GC, McCann DS, Huber-Smith MJ. Adrenergic function in patients with panic anxiety. *Arch Gen Psychiatry* 1984;41:771–776.

65. Nutt DJ, Glue P, Lawson CW, Wilson S. Flumazenil provocation of panic attacks: evidence for altered benzodiazepine receptor sensitivity in panic disorder. *Arch Gen Psychiatry* 1990;47:917–925.

66. Nutt D, Lawson C. Panic attacks. A neurochemical overview of models and mechanisms. *Br J Psychiatry* 1992;160:165–178.

67. Pigott TA, Hill JL, Grady TA, et al. A comparison of the behavioral effects of oral versus intravenous mCPP administration in OCD patients and the effect of metergoline prior to IV mCPP. *Biol Psychiatry* 1993;33:3–14.

68. Pitchot W, Ansseau M, Moreno AG, Hansenne M, von Frenckell R. Dopaminergic function in panic disorder: comparison with major and minor depression. *Biol Psychiatry* 1992;32:1004–1011.

69. Pitts FM, McClure JN. Lactate metabolism in anxiety neurosis. *N Engl J Med* 1967;277:1329–1336.

70. Pohl R, Yeragani VK, Balon R, et al. Isoproterenol-induced panic attacks. *Biol Psychiatry* 1988;24:891–902.

71. Pratt JA. The neuroanatomical basis of anxiety. *Pharmacol Ther* 1992;55:149–181.

72. Price LH, Charney DS, Delgado PL, Heninger GR. Serotonin function and depression: neuroendocrine and mood responses to intravenous L-tryptophan in DSM-III-R depressive subtypes and healthy controls. *Am J Psychiatry* 1991;148:1518–1525.

73. Pyke RE, Greenberg HS. Norepinephrine challenges in panic patients. *Psychopharmacol* 1986;6:279–285.

74. Rapaport MH, Risch SC, Gillin JC, Golshan S, Janowsky D. The effects of physostigmine infusion on patients with panic disorder. *Biol Psychiatry* 1991;29:658–664.

75. Rapaport MH, Risch SC, Golsham S, Gillin JC. Neuroendocrine effects of ovine corticotropin-releasing hormone in panic disorder patients. *Psychiatry* 1989;26:344–348.

76. Rapaport MH, Risch SC, Gillin JC, Golshan S, Janowsky DS. Blunted growth hormone response to peripheral infusion of human growth hormone-releasing factor in patients with panic disorder. *Am J Psychiatry* 1989;146:92–95.

77. Rapee RM, Ancis JR, Barlow DH. Emotional reactions to physiological sensations: panic disorder patients and non-clinical Ss. *Behav Res Ther* 1988;26:265–269.

78. Rasmussen SA, Goodman WK, Woods SW, Heninger GR, Charney DS. Effects of yohimbine in obsessive compulsive disorder. *Psychopharmacology* 1987;93:308–313.

79. Redmond DE. Studies of the nucleus locus coeruleus in monkeys and hypotheses for neuropsychopharmacology. In: Meltzer HY, ed. *Psychopharmacology: the third generation of progress.* New York: Raven Press; 1987:967–975.

80. Roy-Byrne PP, Cowley DS, Greenblatt DJ, Shader RI, Hommer D. Reduced benzodiazepine sensitivity in panic disorder. *Arch Gen Psychiatry* 1990;47:534–538.

81. Schweizer E, Winokur A, Rickels K. Insulin-induced hypoglycemia and panic attacks. *Am J Psychiatry* 1986;143:654–655.

82. Siever LJ, Insel TR, Jimerson DC, et al. Growth hormone response to clonidine in obsessive-compulsive patients. *Br J Psychiatry* 1983;142:187–187.

83. Southwick SM, Krystal JH, Morgan CA, et al. Abnormal noradrenergic function in posttraumatic stress disorder. *Arch Gen Psychiatry* 1993;50:266–274.

84. Stein MB, Uhde TW. Endocrine, cardiovascular, and behavioral effects of intravenous protirelin in patients with panic disorder. *Arch Gen Psychiatry* 1991;48:148–156.

85. Tancer ME, Golden RN. Monoamine neurotransmitter function in social phobia. Presented at the Annual Meeting of the American College of Neuropsychopharmacology, San Juan, Puerto Rico, 1992.

86. Tancer ME, Stein MB, Black B, Uhde TW. Blunted growth hormone responses to growth hormone-releasing factor and to clonidine in panic disorder. *Am J Psychiatry* 1993;150:336–337.

87. Targum SD, Marshall LE. Fenfluramine provocation of anxiety in patients with panic disorder. *Psychiatry Research* 1989;28:295–306.

88. Targum SD. Cortisol response during different anxiogenic challenges in panic disorder patients. *Psychoneuroendocrinology* 1992;17:453–458.

89. Uhde TW. Caffeine provocation of panic: a focus on biological mechanisms. In: Ballenger JC, ed. *Neurobiology of panic disorder.* New York: Wiley-Liss; 1990:219–242.

90. Uhde TW, Vittone BJ, Siever LJ, Kaye WH, Post RM. Blunted growth hormone response to clonidine in panic disorder patients. *Biol Psychiatry* 1986;21:1077–1081.

91. Westenberg HGM, Den Boer JA. Serotonin function in panic disorder: effect of L-5-hydroxytryptophan in patients and controls. *Psychopharmacology* 1989;98:283–285.

92. Wilson S, Glue P, Nutt D. Flumazenil and saccadic eye movements in patients with panic disorder and normal controls. *Hum Psychopharmacol* 1992;7:45–50.

93. Woods SW, Charney DS, Lake J, Goodman WK, Redmond DE, Heninger DR. Carbon dioxide sensitivity in panic anxiety: Ventilatory and anxiogenic response to carbon dioxide in healthy subjects and panic anxiety patients before and after alprazolam treatment. *Arch Gen Psychiatry* 1986;43:900–909.

94. Woods SW, Charney DS, Silver JM, Krystal JH, Heninger GR. Behavioral, biochemical, and cardiovascular responses to the benzodiazepine receptor antagonist flumazenil in panic disorder. *Psychiatry Res* 1991;36:115–127.

95. Woods SW, Koster K, Krystal JK, et al. Yohimbine alters regional cerebral blood flow in panic disorder. *Lancet* 1988;2:678.

96. Zohar J, Insel TR, Zohar-Kadouch RC, Hill JL, Murphy DL. Serotonergic responsivity in obsessive–compulsive disorder: effects of chronic clomipramine treatment. *Arch Gen Psychiatry* 1988;45:167–172.

Psychopharmacology: The Fourth Generation of Progress, edited by Floyd E. Bloom and David J. Kupfer. Raven Press, Ltd., New York 1995.

CHAPTER 112

Environmental Factors in the Etiology of Anxiety[1]

Karrie J. Craig, Kelly J. Brown, and Andrew Baum

Anxiety is a common human emotional state, and anxiety disorders represent a major class of clinical problems that occur throughout the lifespan. The construct has become intertwined with concepts such as stress and uncertainty, and anxiety disorders have been extended to include syndromes that do not feature anxiety as a primary presenting symptom. Regardless, anxiety remains a central concept in psychopharmacology. This chapter considers the etiology and maintenance of anxiety, with emphasis on exogenous factors such as stress. Research on environmental influences in the development of anxiety and anxiety disorders is described and major models of anxiety, emphasizing exogenous factors in the etiology and maintenance of these affective states, are considered. Distinctions between anxiety and fear and among the different anxiety disorders, as well as an evaluation of research linking these two constructs, provide a useful perspective on the origins of anxiety.

ANXIETY AND ANXIETY DISORDERS

Anxiety is a complicated concept, in part because it represents different things in different contexts. Most think of it either as a mood state or a mood disorder, some view it as a proxy for stress, and still others discuss its cognitive aspects with little reference to mood. As a mood state or feeling state, anxiety usually refers to the experience of fear, apprehensiveness, nervousness, panic, restlessness, tension, and agitation (69). Manifest symptoms include trembling, fainting, headaches, and sweat-

ing, possibly elevated blood pressure, and changes in other psychophysiological indices such as heart rate, muscle tone, and skin conductance. Anxiety disorders are also associated with these physical and emotional symptoms, but are several magnitudes more severe, debilitating, and/ or intrusive. The defining features of anxiety disorders in DSM III-R are symptoms of anxiety and avoidance behavior (2). Hyperarousal is also a frequent symptom of these syndromes. Representative of these disorders are (a) panic disorder and generalized anxiety disorder, in which anxiety is usually the primary symptom, and (b) phobic disorders, in which anxiety is experienced as if one is confronted by the feared stimulus and avoidance is very common.

Researchers have adopted a range of outcomes used to measure anxiety. Self-report of mental state, mood, behavior, and symptom experience has been used extensively, as in the State-Trait Anxiety Inventory (65). Other scales also measure anxious symptoms, and consensus has identified primary and secondary symptoms of anxiety: nervousness and fear, fears of fainting and losing control, and avoidance (69). Adequate understanding and study of anxiety requires additional attention to several complicating factors.

Anxiety and Fear

One of the primary reasons for confusion about anxiety is its similarity to fear. Both of these mood states involve some sense of dread or apprehensiveness, and fear may be experienced as ''part'' of anxiety. Because they share

K. J. Craig and K. J. Brown: Uniformed Services University of the Health Sciences, Bethesda, Maryland 20814.
A. Baum: Pittsburgh Cancer Institute, University of Pittsburgh, Pittsburgh, Pennsylvania 15213.

[1]The opinions or assertions contained herein are the private ones of the authors and are not to be construed as official or reflecting the views of the Department of Defense or the Uniformed Services University of the Health Sciences.

a number of characteristics, it is often difficult to distinguish between them; some researchers have suggested that they are indistinguishable (53). Others believe that fear and anxiety are clearly distinct and separate phenomena (4).

Initial distinctions between anxiety and fear appear to have arisen accidently by early translations of Freud, mistaking "Angst," the German word for fear, to mean anxiety (35, p. 389). Freud did not make the distinctions between fear and anxiety that are made by some modern psychotherapists—namely, that anxiety is associated with a repressed unconscious object and fear is linked with a known external stimulus. In other words, an approaching storm would cause fear, and unresolved conflict might cause anxiety. Although intuitively attractive, this distinction does not always hold because fear may be manifested by the displacement of a repressed internal thought to an external object. In addition, a specific external threat can cause anxiety and fear as correlates of the primary threat.

Other distinctions between fear and anxiety focus on (a) the presence or absence of a "consensually determined" threat, (b) the degree to which responses to the threat are in line with its dangerousness, and (c) the potential adaptive value of these responses (4). In these instances, *fear* refers to realistic or adaptive responses, whereas *anxiety* refers to less realistic or more inappropriate reactions. Distinctions based on these features are based on self-report of similar phenomena, making them less useful and sometimes arbitrary. However, they provide some additional context for defining anxiety in spite of the difficulty inherent in operationalizing the constructs.

Both fear and anxiety function as alerting signals to warn of danger. Fear involves sympathetic arousal, readying the body and preparing it for action against immediate danger. Miller (45) described two general responses to fear: (i) the excitatory fight or flight response initially postulated by Cannon (14) and (ii) an inhibitory, presumably parasympathetic-based response. As sympathetic arousal, the fight or flight response includes increased heart rate, increased cardiac output, antidiuresis, dilation of skeletal blood muscles, constriction of gut blood vessels, and a surge of catecholamine release. This excitatory reaction can be contrasted with the inhibitory pattern, involving tonic immobility and freezing or feigning death in extreme cases (45). This behavior appears to help conceal or protect the body from harm. The physiological correlates of this inhibitory response include inhibition of skeletal movement, increased peripheral resistance, and little or no change in diuresis or heart rate. The nature of the stimulus, intensity of the fear, previous experience, and genetic factors appear to influence these general patterns and determine which will be elicited.

Anxiety is also composed of two components. Unlike fear, however, the responses are temporally linked such that one follows the other. The first response to anxiety is the initiation of physiological arousal and recognition of impending danger (35). Coincident with the elicitation of sympathetic arousal, as this arousal and activity are unfolding, one becomes aware of a range of bodily changes. This second aspect of anxiety is primarily cognitive, serves to differentiate anxiety from fear, and may influence the extent to which one suffers from anxiety disorders.

Because anxiety and fear are among the body's first defenses against harm, they may share redundant mechanisms; in general, psychometric and physiological data suggest that they share considerable overlap. Based on a review of studies that manipulated anxiety and fear through brain lesions, electrical stimulation, and pharmacological manipulations, it appears that both fear and anxiety operate through activation of the noradrenergic pathway originating in the locus coeruleus (30). In contrast to fear, which triggers the fight or flight response through this mechanism, anxiety appears to activate the noradrenergic system in conjunction with serotonergic pathways originating in the raphe nuclei (30). The result is a priming of the fight or flight response, which is simultaneously suppressed through serotonergic inhibitory pathways.

Different etiologies, response patterns, time courses, and intensities of anxiety and fear make distinctions between them justifiable. Although both anxiety and fear are alerting signals, they appear to prepare the body for different actions. Anxiety implies that danger may be near and that the fight or flight response may be necessary—hence the priming effect described by Gray (30). Anxiety is a generalized response to an unknown threat or internal conflict, whereas fear is focused on known or unknown external danger. Anxiety is usually long-lived (there is no obvious stimulus to escape or avoid), but fear is usually event-limited. Where fear represents response to finite potential harm that can be avoided if something is done, anxiety is characterized by less well-defined threats that are not readily addressed. Fear also differs from anxiety in that it is usually unanticipated, is dependent upon the termination of the feared object, is often very intense, and occurs in self-limiting single episodes.

Anxiety Disorders

Both anxiety and fear are usually experienced well within the range of normal emotional experience. To some extent, anxiety is a routine emotional state experienced as part of everyday life. The ability to anticipate and prepare is associated with the ability to experience fear and anxiety as we continually strive to adapt to a changing world. When anxiety becomes abnormally intense and/or prolonged, it ceases to play a role in this continual adaptation. Pathological anxiety occurs when normal daily functioning is disrupted by inappropriate responses to internal conflicts or anticipation of some unknown threat. These exaggerated responses can be qualified in terms of duration or intensity. Characteristics of pathological anxiety can include repressed thoughts, negative conditioned responses, counterproductive thought patterns, poor coping strategies, and increased sympathetic tone of the autonomic system (35).

Pathological anxiety is reflected in symptoms of organic anxiety syndrome, adjustment disorder with anxious mood, or an anxiety disorder. The DSM-III R (2) lists six separate categories of anxiety disorders: generalized anxiety, panic disorders, obsessive–compulsive disorder, post-traumatic stress disorder, and phobias (e.g., simple, social, and agoraphobia). Disorders that characteristically involve prominent anxiety or phobic avoidance but do not meet the diagnostic criteria for a particular anxiety or adjustment disorder with anxious mood are classified as anxiety disorders not otherwise specified (NOS). The DSM-III R (2) also includes a subclass of anxiety disorders found in children and adolescents, including separation anxiety, avoidant disorder, and overanxious disorder. Although the anxiety disorders are grouped together because the fundamental symptom in all these syndromes is thought to be anxiety, these disorders represent a heterogeneous group of dysfunctional states, each with its own etiology and responses to treatment (35).

Generalized Anxiety Disorder

This syndrome is characterized by unrealistic and excessive apprehension about unspecified future events. It has been classified as a chronic disorder lasting longer than 6 months and encompassing at least two or more life circumstances (2). Specific symptoms include motor tension (e.g., trembling, twitching, restlessness), autonomic hyperactivity (e.g., shortness of breath, tachycardia, sweating, nausea, abdominal distress), vigilance, and scanning (e.g., exaggerated startle, difficulty concentrating, irritability). At least six of these symptoms must be persistent and bothersome and not just experienced during an acute episode.

Panic Disorder

Panic disorders are defined as conditions in which anxiety manifests itself as recurrent panic attacks characterized by discrete periods of intense fear and discomfort (2). They typically begin with the sudden onset of extreme apprehension or terror and are often accompanied by feelings of impending doom. The attacks are unpredictable and do not occur immediately before or during exposure to specific situations. However, some circumstances can increase the likelihood of an attack at some time during exposure. In these situations, panic attacks can lead to the avoidance of specific events, and the disorder is said to be accompanied by agoraphobia.

Panic attacks are accompanied by a shortness of breath,

the sensation of smothering, dizziness, faintness, tachycardia, shaking, abdominal distress, depersonalization, numbness or tingling, chills, chest pains, and a fear of dying or going crazy. During an attack, some of these symptoms develop suddenly and increase in intensity within 10 min of the beginning of the first noticed symptom (2). To be diagnosed as having a panic disorder, four such attacks must occur within a 4-week period or one or more attacks must have been followed by a prolonged period of persistent fear of having another.

Obsessive–Compulsive Disorder

The essential features of obsessive–compulsive disorder are recurrent obsessions or compulsions that are strong or persistent enough to cause distress (2). Obsessions are defined as persistent ideas, thoughts, or images about some object or action. Attempts to ignore or suppress these intrusive and often senseless obsessions with other thoughts or actions are usually time-consuming and can interfere with normal daily functioning. Compulsions are repetitive, purposeful, and intentional behaviors that may accompany obsessive thoughts. These behaviors are performed in a stereotypic manner, are ordinarily excessive, and usually follow rules that are not clearly tied to the thoughts or ideas they are trying to neutralize. These acts are initially performed as a function of a conflict between wanting to perform the behavior and wanting to resist it. This conflict may end with repeated failure and mounting tension. The person may recognize that the behavior is unreasonable and may find it unpleasurable, but compulsive behaviors typically provide a release of tension.

Post-traumatic Stress Disorder (PTSD)

Unlike most of the anxiety disorders, PTSD does not feature anxiety as a primary presenting symptom. It typically follows a psychologically distressing event that is outside the realm of normal human experience, events that often involve a threat to life (2). These events may be experienced alone (as in assault or rape) or in groups (e.g., combat, disasters) and include natural and accidental or deliberate human-made emergencies. Symptoms characteristic of PTSD are often intensified or precipitated when cues or reminders of the event are present. The disorder is characterized by victims' reexperiencing the traumatic event in a variety of ways. The event can be relived through recurrent, intrusive thoughts, vivid and distressing dreams, and flashbacks accompanied by intense feelings of reliving the trauma in a dissociative state. Cues or symbols that resemble the event can cause intense psychological distress and are persistently avoided in controllable thoughts and actions.

''Psychic numbing'' is another common symptom of

PTSD and is characterized by diminished responsiveness to everyday events, feelings of detachment and estrangement to loved ones, loss of interest in previously enjoyed activities, and difficulty in experiencing emotions. In addition, PTSD victims have a persistent elevated level of arousal, manifested in sleep problems, irritability, difficulty concentrating, hypervigilance, an exaggerated startle response, aggression, and increased sympathetic arousal and reactivity. Diagnostic criteria require that all categories of symptoms (reexperiences, emotional numbness, and increased arousal) be met during the same period of at least a month. A delayed-onset diagnosis is applied if the symptoms appear more than 6 months after the event has passed (2).

Phobias

The DSM-III R (2) divides phobias into three specific types: agoraphobia, social phobias, and simple phobias. Agoraphobia is a fear of being in places or situations from which escape may not be immediately available (fear may be generated by the desire to avoid embarrassment if a limited symptom attack should occur). Symptoms often include dizziness, depersonalization, falling, loss of bladder or bowel control, vomiting, and cardiac distress. These symptoms need not have been experienced before.

Social phobias are reflected in the persistent fear that one or more situations may expose a person to unusual or unacceptable scrutiny by others, causing the person to act inappropriately. Exposure to these stimuli usually leads to immediate symptoms of anxiety, including panic, tachycardia, sweating, and breathing difficulty. Anticipation of encountering a social situation usually leads to avoidance, and this often interferes with normal functioning. The afflicted individual recognizes that the fear is excessive and unreasonable; this may, in turn, increase distress associated with the situation.

Simple phobias are characterized by persistent fear of a circumscribed object or situation other than having a panic attack or being socially embarrassed. Sometimes referred to as *specific phobias,* these disorders are initiated by exposure to the stimulus which invariably evokes an immediate anxiety response which will predictably increase or decrease in intensity as the location or nature of the stimulus changes. Anticipatory anxiety is common and these stimuli are avoided, which can lead to a disruption in daily living. As with other phobias, individuals are normally aware of the extent of experienced fear and this adds to the anxiety evoked by the stimulus.

Childhood Disorders

Anxiety disorders found in children include separation anxiety disorder, avoidant disorder, and overanxious disorder (2). In separation anxiety and avoidant disorder, anxiety is focused on a specific situation. Overanxious disorder is generalized to a variety of situations. Separation anxiety manifests itself as excessive anxiety over separation from someone to whom the child is attached. The reaction can be so strong that the victim experiences panic. The child may display clinging behavior and be unable to stay alone in a room for fear that something will happen to the person they are attached to or to them.

Children may also fear animals, monsters, and situations that are perceived as a threat to the integrity of the family. Some children may experience anticipatory anxiety when separation is imminent, and this anticipation is commonly accompanied by physical complaints such as gastric distress, headaches, nausea, and vomiting. Behavioral problems such as trouble sleeping alone, recurrent nightmares, social withdrawal, apathy, sadness, temper tantrums, difficulty concentrating, and aggressive behavior can occur during times of separation. Similarly, avoidant disorders are characterized by the excessive avoidance of contact with unfamiliar people and a desire for involvement with family members and friends who the child finds warm and satisfying. Social functioning with peers is hampered and the child appears socially withdrawn, embarrassed, and timid when around strangers.

Unlike separation and avoidant disorders, overanxious disorder is a generalized excessive or unrealistic anxiety or worry. A child with this disorder has the tendency to be self-conscious and worried about future events and past behaviors. The disorder is accompanied by feelings of inadequacies, constantly being judged by authority figures or peers and an excessive need of reassurance. Somatic symptoms such as gastrointestinal distress, headaches, a lump in the throat, shortness of breath, and nausea are manifest in some cases. Difficulties sleeping are also common. In general, the child appears nervous and tense, and symptoms persist for at least 6 months.

MODELS OF ANXIETY

A number of human models of anxiety have been proposed, and several are linked to different approaches to nonpharmacologic treatment of anxiety disorders. In this section, two major developments in the evolution of these models are described. Animal models of anxiety are also of considerable interest to those interested in the biological bases of anxiety and in psychopharmacologic treatments for anxiety disorders. Because of the ethical problems inherent in studying extreme or disturbing human emotions, animals are frequently used to study conditions or emotions such as fear, phobias, and anxiety. Comparisons are usually made between a proposed animal model and the human disorder in terms of underlying mechanisms, treatment responsiveness, and etiology. There is no single comprehensive animal model of anxiety, but there are a number of models that meet specific criteria necessary for meaningful comparisons to at least one aspect of the human experience. Models discussed in this section will include the subset of animal models designed to study environmental factors that contribute to the development of anxiety or anxiety disorders.

Animal Models of Anxiety

Animal models used to test etiologic theories of anxiety are typically designed to produce fear and "anxious behaviors." Both can be adaptive if they inhibit potentially harmful behaviors or, conversely, cause the animal to act in such a way to allow it to escape an aversive situation. As noted earlier, anxiety and fear are not readily separable behaviorally or physiologically, but are differentiated by their distinct etiology. Causes of anxiety are usually associated with nonspecific events or stimuli such as being in a novel environment. Consequently, anxiety is usually defined as a generalized, unfocused response. Fear normally results from an experienced or known danger in the immediate environment. A rat that has been shocked in a particular setting might vocalize or try to escape when placed in the same setting. Thus, fear is usually used to describe a focused response to a known object or experience.

Animal models of anxiety and fear are often based on the assumption that the cause of the emotional response in the animal would be sufficient to cause a similar emotional response in a human. Situations involving the unknown, reminders of negative experiences, conflict, unpredictability, and uncontrollability are commonly used as anxiety-evoking agents in both human and animal studies. Using animals to approximate human conditions involves operationalizing these environmental factors in order to evaluate potential anxiety-inducing effects. The goal is to develop models that closely parallel theories based on clinical observations, including the conditioned emotional response, fear-potentiated startle, punishment–conflict, and separation and abandonment models of anxiety.

Conditioned Emotional Response

Conditioned emotional responses are readily produced in animals through a series of pairings and nonpairings of an unconditioned stimulus (US) (such as shock) with a conditioned stimulus (CS) (such as a tone). The US–CS contingency is important in determining whether emotional conditioning is developed, inhibited, or retarded (54). In time, shock-tone pairings come to elicit a conditioned emotional response that is characterized by a decrease in baseline behavior, usually measured in number of lever responses. This specific phenomenon is referred to as *conditioned emotional response* (CER). Conversely,

when a shock and a tone are explicitly not paired, the tone represents a period of safety and becomes a conditioned inhibitor of fear or anxiety (59). The result is a suppression of lever pressing only in the absence of the tone.

The situations that are produced by this conditioning procedure are thought to closely approximate the human fear experience, but they are not readily generalizable to feelings of anxiety. In the CER paradigm the unpleasant affect or absence thereof is predictable and expected. In contrast, anxiety is often triggered by uncertainty and anticipation of unknown events. This type of environment is produced in animal models by designing conditions where the tone and shock are neither paired nor unpaired (58). In this situation, the tone provides no information about the likelihood or actual occurrence of the impending negative event, producing a general state of suppressed activity at all times. Unpredictable and uncontrollable shocks or experiences in environments appear to produce a negative emotional state and leave animals susceptible to the development of ulcers and unrestricted tumor growth (e.g., see ref. 71).

Fear-Potentiated Startle

The acoustic startle reflex in the rat can be exaggerated by presenting an eliciting auditory startle stimulus in the presence of a conditioned stimulus that has previously been paired with shock (12). This is referred to as the *fear-potentiated startle paradigm,* in which fear or anxiety is operationally defined as an elevated startle response. Under normal conditions, the acoustic startle response occurs naturally in mammals as a defensive reaction to external auditory stimulation, characterized by a series of rapid movements beginning at the head and moving towards the tail, causing the contraction and extension of major muscle groups (19). In the fear-potentiated startle paradigm the conditioned stimulus itself does not elicit a response and the startle-eliciting stimulus is never paired with shock. Fear-potentiated startle is said to occur only when the startle-eliciting stimulus creates a greater response in the presence of the conditioned stimulus compared to when it is presented alone (19).

Potentiated startle only occurs following paired presentations of the conditioned stimulus and the stressor. Unlike other animal models of fear and anxiety that use the suppression of ongoing behaviors as an indicator of an emotional state, the potentiated startle paradigm equates enhanced response output with the desired affect (19). Because emotionality in the potentiated startle paradigm is manifested as increased responding, it provides a distinct measurable symptom of anxiety separate from other animal models of affective disorders characterized by behavioral inhibition such as depression or learned helplessness. In addition, the fear-potentiated startle response provides a parallel to increased arousal seen in humans in many cases of PTSD. Symptoms of PTSD include elevated sympathetic arousal and an exaggerated startle response (2). Furthermore, drugs such as yohimbine, which induce anxiety in normal people and enhance it in anxious people, increase the potentiated startle reflex in rats (19). Drugs that reduce anxiety in people also decrease the fear-potentiated startle response in rats (43). Again, these drug effects are of particular value because they cannot be attributed to a decrease in general performance as with animal models that measure anxiety through marked changes in making or withholding required learned responses.

Punishment–Conflict

In general, punishment–conflict tasks involve the use of operant techniques to elicit well-established behaviors and then use aversive stimuli to suppress them by punishing the behaviors when they occur. This suppression of responding is thought to mimic the passive–avoidant component of anxiety, manifested in many animals and humans in anxious or fearful situations. It is characterized by the expending of energy to extinguish specific behaviors to avoid contact with feared objects and situations.

The development of this model of anxiety was initially based on Estes and Skinner's (21) discovery that a conditioned stimulus such as shock will suppress the performance of appetitive instrumental responding. In contrast to conditioned emotional response paradigms, punishment procedures do not use explicit conditioned stimuli to signal the impending aversive unconditioned stimuli. Instead the environment provides the necessary cues that signal that repeated exposure is paired with punishment. These environmental cues come to elicit conditioned emotional responses which are incompatible with the punished behavior. Animals are left in a state of conflict by having to balance the positive features of the reward (i.e., food, water) against the negative aspects of receiving shock (26). The punished behavior is eventually suppressed, presumably by inhibiting motivation to respond to the positive reinforcement (50).

Suppressed behavior is based on the predictability and objectivity of the presentation of an aversive stimulus, and the resulting conditioned responses are quite different from generalized anxiety, which is often unpredictable and uncontrollable and often involves some aspect of uncertainty. Although these variables are manipulated in animal models of depression, they have generally been overlooked in models of anxiety. Animal models of depression assume that uncontrollability leads to escape and avoidance deficits, whereas anxiety models characterize anxiety as the use of excessive avoidant behaviors. This discrepancy is somewhat resolved by distinguishing between active and passive avoidance. It is suggested that while uncontrollability may lead to impaired active avoidance, it can facilitate the use of passive avoidance (55).

Animal models have shown that uncontrollable and/or unpredictable aversive events produce a wide range of emotional disturbances in animals, compared to controllable and predictable events of the same duration and intensity. These emotions include intense and persistent fear and physiological arousal (46,47). It has been suggested that these models produce generalized fear and arousal accompanied by discrete fear, analgesia, and avoidant behaviors and may parallel the symptom cluster of post-traumatic stress disorder consisting of hyperarousal, reexperiencing, numbing, and avoidance (24).

Separation and Abandonment

Animal models of anxiety also have been based on the manipulation of social interactions. One such model involves the separation of an animal from an object of attachment. Rhesus monkeys that have been forcibly separated from an attached object during rearing have been shown to exhibit fear behaviors in the absence of any immediate danger (67). During maternal or peer separation, nonhuman infant primates become hyperactive and show a marked increase in adrenal–pituitary activity (10). Behaviors following this initial reactive stage have been linked to a panic attack. Like anxiety, the intensity and frequency with which these behaviors are induced are dependent upon the type and amount of stress encountered (67).

Human Models of Anxiety

One of the major developments in the study of human anxiety was the distinction between state and trait anxiety. Initially differentiated by Cattell and Scheier (15) in 1958, state and trait anxiety have been used to indicate different constructs. Spielberger (65) has proposed a conceptual definition of state anxiety (S-anxiety), suggesting that it consists of subjective, consciously perceived feelings of tension, apprehension, nervousness, and worry, accompanied by or associated with activation and arousal of the autonomic nervous system. It has become essential in the study of anxiety and stress to differentiate between (a) S-anxiety as a transitory emotional state and (b) relatively stable individual differences in anxiety as a personality or dispositional trait (T-anxiety).

There are several paper and pencil instruments that can be used to measure fluctuations in S-anxiety as various events (stressors) occur. These self-report scales include the Affect Adjective Check List (75) and the S-anxiety scale of the State-Trait Anxiety Inventory [STAI (65)]. The STAI has been used to measure anxiety in thousands of studies since it was published in 1970, using a set of questions referencing feelings of anxiety currently experienced (S-anxiety) as well as items that are directed toward typical patterns of feelings (T-anxiety). The STAI has undergone several translations and adaptations and is available in many languages. There are also versions that have been created for use across the lifespan, such as the STAI for children (STAIC), and versions for use with more elderly subjects (48).

Salzman (56) measured state anxiety using a different method in an elderly sample by using a 100-mm line with anchoring adjectives. He and his colleagues used 13 such items, each with an adjective in the center (e.g., calm, nervous, jittery) and anchored with "absent" and "severe." Participants were asked to make a mark on the line indicating the degree to which they were currently experiencing the feeling. Physiological indices, including heart rate, blood pressure, and muscle action potential, can also be measured to tap activation of the autonomic nervous system due to the experience of anxiety, although differentiating anxiety (from distress or other affective states) can be difficult using only these physiological indices.

There are differences among individuals in the frequency and duration of S-anxiety. However, everyone experiences S-anxiety occasionally. Experience of S-anxiety over long periods of time and the general tendency to view the world as threatening and dangerous is used as a marker of T-anxiety (65). People who are high in T-anxiety do not constantly exhibit elevated levels of anxiety but are predisposed to exhibit anxiety when activated by a specific danger situation. For example, research has shown that people who are high in T-anxiety are more prone to perceive danger in their personal relationships and respond to these threats with greater elevations in S-anxiety than are persons who are lower in T-anxiety (65). In general, people high in T-anxiety are more vulnerable to situations that require evaluation by others because they tend to have poor self-esteem and lack confidence in themselves. High trait anxiety is associated with a lower threshold for experiencing threat or anxious affect. An inverse relationship has been found between pain sensitivity and state anxiety; the more anxious a person was (S-anxiety), the poorer the ability to discriminate varying intensities of painful stimuli (68).

The initiation and maintenance of trait anxiety have generated research suggesting that childhood relationships may contribute to the development of high levels of T-anxiety. Withdrawal of love by parental figures and negative evaluations by parents, teachers, or peers in the past may all contribute to general trait anxiety (65). However, these influences are not immutable, and T-anxiety can change. Davidson (18) investigated the effects of meditation on trait anxiety by using four groups that differed by the extent to which they were practicing meditation and found that T-anxiety was progressively lowered by extent of meditation. This was an important finding because it showed that meditation could be used to reduce the experience of trait anxiety and also because it pro-

vided evidence that trait anxiety levels can change over time.

Self-Efficacy and Anxiety

Another model of anxiety that has received increasing attention posits self-efficacy as a key construct in anxiety. Self-efficacy theory is based on the notion that a sense of personal mastery or ability to control the environment and/or what happens to people is a primary determinant of mood and behavior (3). Self-efficacy refers to one's beliefs and expectations regarding achievement of goals; it is related to control, personal agency beliefs, and other constructs that focus on contingencies and perceived success. Changes in self-efficacy should affect mood and behavior, and evaluation of an individual's expectations provide a window on his or her motivation and likelihood of success.

Evaluations of self-efficacy are derived from several sources, including a review of one's accomplishments (taking into consideration such attributional properties as task difficulty, help received, effort, and external circumstances) and vicarious experiences such as observational learning and modeling (3). State variables, including arousal, appraisal, and social influence, may also affect evaluation of self-efficacy.

In some ways, self-efficacy is similar to self-esteem or what theorists have referred to as "self-concept." In fact, efficacy is related to both self-esteem and one's self-concept, contributing to positive esteem and overall self-perception when one's sense of efficacy is high and relatively strong. Anxiety is associated with low self-efficacy or other problems that interfere with one's perceived ability to cope with fear or with anxiety-arousing events. Avoiding feared objects may not be controlled by the fearful stimulus but rather by evaluations of self-efficacy as suggested by studies that show strong relationships between perceived efficacy and anxious behavior (e.g., see ref. 74). In these studies, covarying for self-efficacy reduced the relationship between fear and avoidance of feared stimuli, suggesting that fear and self-efficacy are distinct predictors of anxious affect and behavior.

Davison et al. (20), for example, have shown that the ratio of positive to negative self-efficacy was related to anxiety in a stressful situation, based on articulated thoughts elicited by the situation. Similarly, a study of undergraduates considering treatment alternatives for test anxiety yielded significant relationships between self-efficacy and test anxiety, though the relationship was stronger for women than for men (63).

Application of self-efficacy theory to anxiety treatment has also proven useful. Here the assumption is that anxiety reduction will be facilitated when self-efficacy is reinforced and that treating anxiety will be more difficult when evaluations of efficacy yield poor self-assessments. Behavioral achievements, verbal persuasion, information about self-efficacy, and beneficial changes in arousal detected by monitoring of symptoms of arousal are useful in increasing self-efficacy, and all of these have been used in efforts to reduce anxiety (e.g., see ref. 3). Like perceived control, self-efficacy appears to bolster one's expectations regarding success and, in doing so, increases the likelihood that one can accomplish desired goals.

SOURCES OF ANXIETY

Anxiety has its origins in a complex interaction of environmental, psychological, and biological events and processes. Perhaps the most critical are (a) stress and life events requiring adaptation or change and (b) early familial and school experiences.

Stress and Anxiety

Stress may be defined as a process linking external events, perception and appraisal of them, and responses directed at changing the event or one's relationship to it (e.g., see ref. 39). It can also be viewed as an emotional state characteristic of perception and evaluation of stressor events (e.g., see ref. 7). Stress has been defined as a nonspecific general adaptation syndrome through which we struggle to rebuff the wear and tear of life (60), whereas Cannon (14) and Mason (44) have proposed models of stress that define it as an integrated neuroendocrine response that supports our ability to cope—to fight or flee. Common to these perspectives are a shared emphasis on interactive aspects of the process or state and the purposive nature of the syndrome. Regardless of whether stress was as adaptive as Cannon (14) believed or whether it remains adaptive today, it is clear that the demands of daily life require continuous adjustment to changing surroundings and that stress characterizes some of these adjustments.

If one thinks of stress as a process, its constituents include stressors, or initiating events, and appraisal and interpretation of these stressors. Recognition of a dangerous event or situation demanding more than routine adjustment initiates an appraisal of the relevant events, the person's assets and experience, and other factors that might affect whether the event seems to be stressful. When these appraisals are benign, stress responses do not occur. However, when appraisal is not benign (i.e., when excessive demand or threat is likely), stress responses occur. These stress responses include emotional and psychological changes accompanying and following appraisal, behavioral changes, coping, and bodily responses characterized by sympathetic and pituitary–adrenal cortical arousal. Consequences of these responses, such as

health changes or performance deficits, may accrue if responses are unusually intense or prolonged.

As was suggested at the beginning of this section, stress has been defined as a stimulus, a response, and a process linking them. A close listen to modern lay discussions of stress or of scientists discussing it in a research context will quickly reveal this confusing use of the word. The process view is clearly more inclusive than the others and focuses on the emotional and motivational state associated with appraised threat, harm, loss, or excessive demand. For this reason, we define stress here as the emotional experience resulting from appraisal of information about a stressor and one's ability to deal with it. This emotional state is ordinarily accompanied by physiological arousal, either as a direct co-effect of the appraisal of danger or as a part of the emotional state itself. Together these changes support one's ability to cope and motivate people to change the stressor and reduce its effects or to insulate themselves from its effects.

Viewed this way, stress is characterized by aversive emotional experience and a highly aroused state. The former is conative; if the emotional experience of stress is negative, people will be motivated to reduce or relieve it. Thus, the experience of stress motivates coping by creating tension that is aversive to the subject. This coping is, in turn, facilitated by heightened sympathetic activity, by increased circulating levels of glucose, and by other aspects of the catabolic physiological responses that occur during stress. In this way, the experience resulting from evaluation of the situation leads to a motivational and supportive arousal state that initiates further appraisal and coping (39).

Anxiety, in this context, may be seen as a component of the emotional state associated with stress and is a major part of the motivational strength of the construct. Definitions of anxiety that focus on its role as an alerting signal or indication of danger that cues mobilization of energy and resources suggest that anxiety may be an immediate affective component of stressful appraisals (6). The extent to which anxious affect becomes prolonged or intense enough to create enduring problems will depend on the nature of other aspects of the stress process. In this way, anxiety is also a sign of disorganization and dysfunction (6). Before focusing on this and other issues, the general relationship between stress and mental or physical pathology needs to be addressed.

We have portrayed stress as an adaptive process, and this is consistent with most modern models of stress. However, it is also becoming clearer that stress is an important pathological process in the development and progression of mental health problems and organic disease states. Some have suggested that modern stressors defy the "hard-wired" or biologically determined stress response because they are not readily addressed in the same ways as were stressors common as the stress process was evolving. While adaptive in many situations, stress responses include features that may not be as suitable for more "sedentary" stressors of modern life. The hyper-arousal associated with stress may interfere with some coping options and may contribute to disease processes. In addition, it is possible that as stressors become more chronic, the persistence of a hyperaroused negative state may cause organic damage as well as emotional distress.

Krantz, Grunberg, and Baum (37) described three general pathways by which stress may contribute to ill health. Direct effects include physiological changes that occur as part of stress and that have specific disease-relevant consequences (e.g., increased blood pressure, reduced immunosurveillance, altered corticosteroid release). Behaviorally mediated effects are less direct: Stress may alter behaviors or motivation to perform behaviors that are healthy and/or protective against illness, resulting in possible changes in health (e.g., increased smoking or drug use, poor diet, and abnormal sleep). Finally, stress can affect the behavior of patients or people who are already ill, by increasing delay for seeking help, by causing self-medication or masking of symptoms, or by reducing adherence with medical treatment. In general, stress should not be viewed as a problem unless it becomes sufficiently intense or cumulatively burdensome to disrupt ongoing behavior. Abnormally intense or abnormally persistent stress is most likely to cause problems.

This same logic holds for the various aspects of the stress response. Psychological changes including heightened anxiety and arousal need not be viewed as a problem. Under "normal" conditions, arousal and affect are unpleasant and aversive enough to be motivating, but are not debilitating. Similarly, arousal, particularly if it is of brief duration, need not be experienced aversively. These affective changes are instrumental in increasing motivation to respond and reflect on the nature of the appraisals that are made. Resulting coping responses may be generally directed at the source of distress in attempts to reduce or eliminate its effects. Alternatively, coping may be directed inward in attempts to regulate distress and reduce unpleasant feelings.

When anxiety or any affective component of stress becomes severe, it may suppress problem-focused coping so that all effort can be focused on reducing negative affect (40). One could argue, for example, that an approaching stressor, one which we can anticipate but not predict, would be most likely to evoke apprehensiveness and anxiety. This state is then seen as contributing to the unique mixture of coping efforts that is optimal for each situation. If a stressor will be better met if one prepares for it, anxiety or apprehensiveness will be functional to the extent that it motivates anticipatory activity. However, an unusually intense anxiety response might freeze efforts at coping and focus all attention on reducing distress and fear, thereby ignoring the danger and failing to resist it. Similarly, abnormally prolonged episodes of anxious affect can predispose appraisals of subsequent stressors,

limit the effectiveness of one's coping, and shape the essential experience of even routine events. Recent research suggests that individual factors, including memory, perceived control, and other variables, play important roles in maintaining stressful appraisals or responses across long periods of time (e.g., see ref. 7). Prior psychopathology or dysfunction could also increase the likelihood of prolonged distress and/or exacerbate the consequences of anxiety by intensifying the magnitude of experienced anxiety or triggering symptoms and consequences more quickly.

This theme is also present in Sarason's (57) description of an anxious person's reactions to stress, a response that includes catastrophizing, self-blame, and feelings of helplessness. To a large extent, anxiety may reflect a perceived inadequacy of resources or ability when required to act: Anxiety does not appear to obscure ability to see solutions but does increase the likelihood of perseveration, rumination, and nonproductive worrying in the face of task-related demands (57). This is also consistent with Leventhal's (40) parallel process model of emotion and predictions about overwhelming threat and responses channeled into reducing fear.

Another way of distinguishing anxiety from stress focuses on its selective and pathological aspects. Anxiety can be defined as a sense of apprehension due to perception of threat. Anticipatory responses can help prepare one for dealing with threat but carries a price in terms of distress during the pre-event period. Consistent with Lazarus and Folkman (39), nearly any and all stimuli or events are capable of posing threat or causing one to perceive the possibility of danger. The entire universe of potential threats can be broken down into those that are more likely to be viewed as a threat (e.g., tornadoes, assault, illness) and events that are less likely to evoke such an appraisal (e.g., a picnic, visiting family and friends, going to work). Those events that are likely to elicit threat appraisals can be thought of as stressors, whereas those that are less likely to cause apprehension can be viewed as anxiety stimuli when a given person reacts to them (6). While this distinction may not be as appealing as those based on other dimensions, it may provide insight into the relationships between stress and anxiety disorders.

Life Events

The link between stress and anxiety is suggested by several studies of life events that show that the experience of change and the magnitude of adaptation required are related to a range of mental and physical illnesses or symptoms of illness (e.g., see ref. 32). More specifically, Johnson and McCutcheon (34) found evidence of a relationship between negative life events and trait anxiety (measured on the STAI). Adolescents were asked to indicate life events they had experienced the previous year, and rate whether each was negative or positive. Those who had experienced more life change reported more anxiety. These data are correlational, and compelling arguments can be made for all possible causal orders. However, these findings provide reason to believe that stress causes or includes anxious affect.

Uncertainty

Anxiety can also be seen as a product of uncertainty. Life events, especially transitions, are often stressful, and the uncertainty surrounding these transitions contributes to distress and anxiety. Ambiguous situations, particularly ambiguous stressors, are associated with both uncertainty and anxiety. These situations, lacking in clear indications of situational contingencies or likely outcomes, are associated with considerable stress. The uncertainty regarding these situations highlights a lack of control that contributes to feelings of anxiety and makes coping more difficult. For example, Coelho (16) studied adolescents experiencing anxiety about the future, a stressor marked by uncertainty, finding that anxiety experienced by adolescent subjects was expressed by attempts to reduce anxiety and alter mood, much like coping with stress. These motives were often reflected in drug-taking and impulsive behavior, palliative behaviors that can lead to impaired physical health. Uncertainty regarding the future was linked with anxiety, which in turn was associated with dangerous behavior and eventual illness.

Uncertainty about an upcoming event or situation is frequently marked by anxiety. When a person is unsure about what course an event will take, they may also be uncertain as to what type of coping response will be required in order to meet the demands of the impending situation. If the event itself is unclear, there are no effective means of assessing available coping supports and identifying coping options that will be effective. This inability to "diagnose" the situation and appraise it for coping-relevant information can leave one uncertain not only about the stressful event but also about one's coping abilities.

Stress and Anxiety Disorders

Research on the relationship between stress and anxiety disorders is not extensive, due in part to changing diagnostic criteria and shifts in the way in which anxiety has been conceptualized. These data appear to suggest a relationship between stress and anxiety disorders but do not specify a causal path nor go beyond simple demonstration that stress and anxiety disorders co-occur. Evidence of stress as a trigger of phobic disorders, for example, is not limited to clinical reports. Several reports indicate that up to two-thirds of people experiencing pho-

bic episodes could identify a stressful, precipitating incident. Other studies find far fewer being able to identify a trigger, and the relative role of stressor and personality factors in precipitating anxiety disorders are not clearly quantified or understood.

Post-traumatic Stress Disorder

In some cases an individual will experience a life event that is out of the realm of normal human experience. These are referred to as *traumatic events* and can have substantial impact on the development and experience of anxiety. One of the most extreme reactions to a traumatic experience is seen in the anxiety disorder known as *post-traumatic stress disorder* (PTSD). This syndrome is marked by intrusive thoughts and reliving of the trauma, psychic numbing, hyperarousal, and sleep disturbances (2). The triggering events themselves vary and may include assault, rape, combat, disasters, and major injuries or mishaps such as motor vehicle accidents. Reactions to traumatic events vary, and most people experiencing them recover with a reasonable degree of speed and efficacy. However, some do not, and it is estimated that the lifetime prevalence of PTSD is about 1% in the general population, about 3.5% among civilians exposed to physical attack (including rape) and among Vietnam veterans who were not wounded, and up to 20% among veterans wounded in Vietnam (31). It is also estimated that as many as 55,000 individuals experience an acute PTSD response precipitated by a motor vehicle accident each year (31). Prevalence of PTSD among victims of natural disasters and technological accidents has been difficult to pin down, and its estimated range is from 2.3% to 53% (64).

Despite the fact that external stressors or traumatic events typically begin and end suddenly, the internalized event or the response to it does not subside quickly. Traumatic events usually involve several stimuli, including sights, sounds, and smells. As we know from the literature regarding conditioning, the pairing of these stimuli with the trauma lends power to the environmental stimuli that were present at the time of the event. These sounds, odors, and sights become cues for re-experiencing the traumatic event. Encountering a trigger for the traumatic event can lead to a reexperiencing or reliving of the psychological and physiological reactions that were initially elicited.

This conditioned responding is suggested by studies that have found elevated heart rates among Vietnam veteran PTSD patients when listening to combat sounds in the laboratory (e.g., see refs. 9 and 42). The intrusive thoughts and memories caused by these cues may be responsible for continued responding to the event after it occurs (7). Intrusive thoughts can be regarded as positive in the sense that a reworking and reexperiencing of the traumatic event can help a survivor to come to terms with and understand the experience. Through the intrusions and forced reconsideration of his or her circumstances, a victim can confront the actual images of the experience as well as the anxiety associated with these thoughts. These intrusive recollections may have a curative effect because through repeated exposure the anxiety may be gradually diminished (52).

Exposure to a traumatic event can lead to increased anxiety after the event and can also have long-term effects that surface with future exposure to traumatic events. This idea was noted by Freud (25) when he suggested that once a person has experienced a traumatic event and a panic state associated with the event, he/she will be more vulnerable to developing another panic state if exposed to a similar trauma; this is not unlike Horowitz' (33) notion of intrusive and avoidant phases of post-stressor distress. Once an individual has experienced a trauma-induced panic state, the occurrence of a new event that threatens injury or loss is likely to lead to a state similar to or greater than that in the past. All things being equal, this person is more likely to experience panic or distress when minimally or moderately exposed to threat than a person who had not had that previous traumatic experience.

Many studies support the association of traumatic events and anxiety. The Buffalo Creek dam collapse and flood in 1972 has been extensively examined in longitudinal field studies of responses to this sudden traumatic event (e.g., see ref. 28). Buffalo Creek survivors reported more anxiety 14 years post-disaster on both the Symptom Checklist 90 and the Psychiatric Evaluation Form (29). These survivors also had significantly more diagnoses based on the Structured Clinical Interview for DSM-IIIR than did a control population, with 18% of the sample diagnosed as having generalized anxiety disorder, 2% with panic disorder, 4% social phobia, 15% simple phobia, 23% current PTSD, and 63% PTSD-lifetime. Both the generalized anxiety disorder and PTSD diagnoses were significantly greater in the Buffalo Creek sample compared to the control group (29).

The accident at the Three Mile Island (TMI) nuclear power station in 1979 allowed for the study of responses and reactions to a technological disaster of traumatic proportion over a fairly long period of time. For 5 years after the accident, TMI-area residents reported more anxiety and exhibited greater stress-related arousal than did residents of control areas (8). Bromet (11) reported that young mothers living near TMI had an increased risk of anxiety disorders compared to those living near an undamaged plant up to 9 months post-accident. These studies provide some evidence that traumatic events, natural and human-caused, are associated with anxiety.

Mediating Variables

Not everyone who experiences a traumatic event develops PTSD or other chronic problems. A number of factors

appear to be important in defining vulnerability to stress and the likelihood that it will become unusually intense or prolonged. Many of these variables have been investigated in relationship to PTSD, including coping strategies, social support, and previous psychopathology. It is important to understand what role, if any, these factors play in the development of or protection from PTSD.

As suggested earlier, stress is an emotional state resulting from appraisal of information about a stressor or one's ability to deal with it. What Lazarus (39) call "secondary appraisal" of personal coping capacity is an important component in the reaction to an experience. If an event is perceived as being outside of one's coping repertoire, the implicit inability to cope effectively can lead to a state of anxiety. In some instances a person may find that they do not have adequate coping skills to deal with a stressor, so they may turn to an alternative method of coping in order to protect their self-esteem. Coehlo (16) found that students blaming others or luck, the personality of teacher, or background to explain test results managed to conserve their self-esteem and to tolerate anxiety.

Other variables of interest in the study of anxiety disorders and PTSD include social support and the concordance of previous psychopathology with current PTSD. Research has found a positive correlation between prior psychopathology and PTSD as well as negative relationships with social support. For example, the Epidemiologic Catchment Area Survey found that nearly 80% of those people with PTSD had previously had another psychiatric disorder, but that only a third of people reporting no PTSD symptoms had ever had some other psychiatric disorder (31).

Developmental Factors in Anxiety

The roles of developmental or age-related changes on mood and behavior are the subjects of entire disciplines, so that one's approach to understanding lifespan influences on anxiety should be one of specifying effects and differences over the life course. The childhood environment, including one's interactions with parents and family, child-rearing practices applied, and early reactions to separation, may have long-term effects on anxiety levels. The school environment is also an important shaper of adult life, and anxieties related to academic performance, social acceptance, and one's self-concept become more important in adolescence. Adults cope with the sequelae of these previous experiences and cope with stressors and additional sources of anxiety related to career, family, security, and realization of one's dreams and goals. As one enters middle age or older adulthood, concerns may become more associated with physical health issues, and there is some evidence that fear of aging can be an important determinant of mental health.

Child-Rearing Practices

The belief that child-rearing practices or early experience affects later behavior and personality is neither new or surprising. However, evidence of such a relationship, particularly from studies examining anxiety-related outcomes, is surprisingly lacking. Studies of repression and sensitization, for example, have not yielded evidence of a relationship between child-rearing and anxiety proneness (e.g., see ref. 13). Child-rearing antecedent conditions associated with anxiety during adolescence have been identified and include environmental factors (e.g., broken home, family conflict) as well as specific attitudes and child-rearing practices (49). Lack of clear family rules, a strong concern for a family's reputation, a poor relationship with the father, and frequent criticism and disagreement all were associated with anxiety. However, parents of children who were low or high in manifest anxiety were not different from one another on this dimension, suggesting that experiencing particular environmental and social conditions rather than having an anxious parent led to development of anxiety during early adolescence (49).

Research on child rearing and later behavior and affect is difficult for several reasons. Partly as a result, the literature on the relationship between parent–child interactions and anxiety has been inconsistent. However, some variables have begun to emerge as reliable predictors of anxiety. Parental support, child-rearing style, authoritarian personality of the mother, teachers' authoritarian attitudes, and maternal punitiveness have all been linked to anxiety in adolescence or adulthood (e.g., see ref. 38), but the only clear conclusion that can be drawn from these studies is that there are links between child rearing and anxiety that require additional investigation. Inconsistency, harsh and unyielding attitudes, ambiguity, and family conflict appear to be among the primary predictors of the development of anxiety.

School

Consistent with the magnitude of its impact on children, school experiences have received a good deal of attention as potential sources of anxiety. Some attention has been focused on the role of anxiety in school phobias, but most studies have considered its causes and effects on school performance (e.g., see ref. 51). Low self-concept appears to be associated with concurrent anxiety, and it may be a product of how others perceive one's academic performance (23). Other studies suggest that anxiety and self-concept have separable effects on school performance, and evidence of links between emergent anxiety and self-concept or image in social as well as academic settings in school has also been reported (22).

As one would expect, the causes and consequences of anxiety in school settings vary with age. At younger ages, when influences from parents are still stronger than those from peers, academic doubts and fears, separation from parents, and similar concerns appear to be related to anxiety (36). As they grow older, children become increasingly aware of peer influences as well, and the influence of these sources of anxiety increase (1). Anxiety in this context may be viewed as a complex of experiences including how parents react to early achievement motivation, children's ability to interpret their performance and compare it to others, and their reactions to evaluative practices applied in school (73).

It should be noted that anxiety due to particular aspects of school performance have been examined in some detail. For example, math anxiety, related specifically to performance at mathematics, does not necessarily generalize to other aspects of school (66). Similarly, test-taking anxiety, which clearly has very broad implications for students, and computer anxiety, of increasing concern during the past decade, have received attention (57). Review of the literatures on these topics is beyond the scope of this chapter, but these and other specific sources of anxiety in school settings have been considered as targets for interventions to improve school performance.

Aging

Anxiety and anxiety disorders are common in the elderly, in part due to concerns and worries about bodily symptoms and changes in health (41). Fear of aging is one antecedent condition of anxiety in some, though worries about aging may occur across the entire adult life cycle. Some of this is related to the fear of death and dying, as suggested by Vickio and Cavanaugh (70), who studied 133 nursing home employees across a range of ages and jobs. Results indicated that increasing fear of death was associated with more anxiety toward aging. For the most part, however, most attention in this area has been on treatment rather than etiology, with concerns about drug interactions and synergistic effects of drugs and declining cognitive resiliency (61). It seems likely that in a population marked by increasing concerns about one's health, changes in bodily sensations would evoke more worry and apprehensiveness, and this alone could yield higher rates of anxiety and dysfunction among older people than among younger ones (decreases in other causes could offset these increases). Etiological changes in anxiety disorders over the lifespan would suggest more targeted pharmacologic and nonpharmacologic interventions.

Familial Influences

The distribution of anxiety disorders in populations, as revealed by epidemiological and twin studies over the past 25 years, suggests strong familial patterns and genetic–

environmental interactions in the etiology of these disorders (e.g., see refs. 17 and 72). In general, this is consistent with broader findings for affective disorders, indicating that close relatives of patients are more likely to share disorders and that nearly two-thirds of monozygotic twins are concordant for particular disorders (27). Though limited by the nature of the variables assessed in these epidemiological studies, there now appears to be considerable evidence for genetic determination of some aspects of anxiety. Investigation of 215 probands (including 82 controls, 52 patients with major depression, 51 patients with major depression and anxiety disorders, and 30 patients with anxiety disorders only) and more than 1500 adult and child first-degree relatives has provided further evidence of familial influence (72). First-degree relatives of the 51 probands with both depression and anxiety were generally more likely to show major depression and anxiety disorders than were relatives of patients with major depression alone. Similarly, relatives of patients with anxiety disorders that were not associated with major depression showed higher rates of anxiety disorders than did relatives of patients with major depression or with no diagnosis. It is important to note, however, that the rates of dysfunction among these relatives were relatively low: For anxiety disorders, relatives of normals showed a rate of 5 in 100, relatives of patients with major depression were somewhat more likely to experience anxiety disorders (9/100), and among patients with anxiety disorders with or without depression, 14 or 15 of 100 relatives exhibited anxiety problems (72). Though these rates suggest that most relatives of patients with these disorders did not exhibit symptoms of anxiety or depression, they suggest that relatives of patients with anxiety disorders were more likely to show symptoms of similar dysfunction (72).

The causes of such familial patterns are unclear. Genetic predispositions are indicated as potential mechanisms, either as direct tendencies to develop symptoms of anxiety or as physiological or biochemical predispositions to respond to environmental events in particular ways. Examination of shared patterns of response to drugs, to external events, and to other stimuli may provide important information about the underlying bases of inherited risk for anxiety disorders. Differences in cardiovascular or sympathetic reactivity, implicated in the development of hypertension and sociopathy, may be one such mechanism. Research has not systematically addressed these possibilities, and future investigations could include response by gamma-aminobutyric acid (GABA) and responses to benzodiazepines as well as interaction of genetic and behavioral history factors as described by Barrett (5). Similarly, activity of endogenous opioid peptides as well as exogenously applied opiates may vary across individuals. The point here is not to catalog the various systems and neurotransmitters involved in anxiety so much as to suggest points at which inherited predispositions may make a difference in the development of anxiety. Experimental induction of anxiety, by administration of drugs or by enforcing withdrawal from them, may offer one way of identifying genetic–environmental interactions.

CONCLUSIONS

Sheehan and Soto (62) have suggested that research and treatment of anxiety disorders will be facilitated by conceptualization of anxiety and associated dysfunction as either exogenous or endogenous. This distinction rests on the notion that some anxiety and anxiety disorders are caused by, or are sensitive to, environmental changes and stimuli outside the organism. Others, related to internal causes and events, are endogenous and more resistant to behavioral treatment (62).

Our focus in this chapter has been on exogenous anxiety with emphasis on the environmental factors responsible for the etiology and course of anxiety and anxiety disorders. Exogenous anxiety may be manifest in simple phobias, where responsiveness is limited to a single stimulus, and in adjustment disorders accompanied by anxiety (62). Exogenous anxiety is also involved in the development of PTSD, where anxiety and distress are linked to profound stressors and to stimuli reminiscent of these stressors. Stress, whether early in development or during adulthood, appears to be an important process in the experience and expression of anxiety, and though more work is needed to address the role of stress in dysfunctional anxiety, it also appears to be an important factor in anxiety disorders. Under benign conditions, anxiety appears to serve an alerting function, keying an alarm reaction and letting the organism know that something is wrong. Also under these conditions, anxiety may be a principal component of the stress experience and may play a major role in motivating the organism to act to decrease or eliminate distress. However, when stress is unusually intense or prolonged the functional nature of anxiety may diminish and, because it no longer motivates effective coping and tension reduction, may become abnormally intense or persistent. When this occurs, and when anxious affect begins to cause dysfunction and interference with daily life, anxiety disorders develop and require effective management and treatment.

REFERENCES

1. Allsopp M, Williams T. Self-report measures of obsessionality, depression, and social anxiety in a school population of adolescents. *J Adolesc* 1991;14:149–156.
2. American Psychiatric Association. *Diagnostic and statistical manual of mental disorders*, 3rd ed. (revised). Washington, DC: American Psychiatric Association, 1987;235–253.
3. Bandura A. *Social foundations of thought and action: a social cognitive theory*. Englewood Cliffs, NJ: Prentice–Hall, 1986.

4. Barlow DH. *Anxiety and its disorders: the nature and treatment of anxiety and panic.* New York: Guilford, 1988.
5. Barrett JE. Non-pharmacological factors determining the behavioral effects of drugs. In: Meltzer, HY, ed. *Psychopharmacology: the third generation of progress.* New York: Raven Press, 1987;1493–1501.
6. Basowitz H, Persky H, Korchlin S, Grinker R. *Anxiety and stress.* New York: McGraw–Hill, 1955.
7. Baum A, Cohen L, Hall M. Control and intrusive memories as possible determinants of chronic stress. *Psychosom Med* 1993;55:274–286.
8. Baum A, Gatchel RJ, Schaeffer MA. Emotional, behavioral, and physiological effects of chronic stress at Three Mile Island. *J Consult Clin Psychol* 1983;51:565–572.
9. Blanchard EB, Kolb LC, Pallmeyer TP, Gerardi RJ. The development of a psychological assessment procedure for post-traumatic stress disorder in Vietnam veterans. *Psychiatr Q* 1982;54:220–229.
10. Breese GR, Smith RD, Mueller RA, et al. Induction of adrenal catecholamine synthesizing enzymes following mother–infant separation. *Nature New Biol* 1973;246:94–96.
11. Bromet E. *Three Mile Island: Mental health findings.* Pittsburgh: University of Pittsburgh, Western Psychiatric Institute and Clinic, 1980.
12. Brown JS, Kalish HI, Farber IE. Conditioned fear as revealed by magnitude of startle response to auditory stimulus. *J Exp Psychol* 1951;41:317–328.
13. Byrne D. Childrearing antecedents of repression-sensitization. *Child Dev* 1964;35:1033–1039.
14. Cannon WB. The James–Lange theory of emotions: a critical examination and an alternative. *Am J Psychol* 1927;39:106–124.
15. Cattell RB, Scheier IH. The nature of anxiety: a review of thirteen multi-variate analyses comprising 814 variables. *Psychol Rep* 1958;4:351–388.
16. Coehlo GV. Environmental stress and adolescent coping behavior: key ecologial factors in college student adaptation. In: Sarason IG, Spielberger CD, eds. *Stress and anxiety,* vol 7. Washington, DC: Hemisphere Publishing Corporation, 1980;247–263.
17. Crowe RR, Noyes R Jr, Pauls DL, Slyman D. A family study of panic disorder. *Arch Gen Psychiatry* 1983;40:1065–1069.
18. Davidson JM. The physiology of meditation and mystical states of consciousness. *Perspect Biol Med* 1976;19:345–379.
19. Davis M. The role of the amygdala in fear-potentiated startle: Implications for animal models of anxiety. *Trends Pharmacol Sci* 1992;13:35–41.
20. Davison GC, Haaga DA, Rosenbaum J, et al. Assessment of self-efficacy in articulated thoughts: "states of mind" analysis and association with speech-anxious behavior. *J Cognitive Psychother* 1991;5:83–92.
21. Estes WK, Skinner BF. Some quantitative properties of anxiety. *J Exp Psychol* 1941;29:390–400.
22. Fisher M, Schneider M, Pegler C, Napolitano B. Eating attitudes, health-risk behaviors, self-esteem, and anxiety among adolescent females in a suburban high school. *J Adolesc Health* 1991;12:377–384.
23. Fite K, Howard S, Garlington NK, Zinkgraf S. Self-concept, anxiety, and attitude toward school: a correlational study. *TACD J* 1992;20:21–28.
24. Foa EB, Zinbarg R, Rothbaum BO. Uncontrollability and unpredictability in post-traumatic stress disorder: an animal model. *Psychol Bull* 1992;112:218–238.
25. Freud S. Inhibition, symptoms, and anxiety (1926). In: *Standard edition of the complete psychological works of Sigmund Freud,* vol 20. London: Hogarth Press, 1959.
26. Geller I, Seifter J. The effects of meprobamate, barbiturates, diamphetamines and promazine on experimentally, induced conflict in the rat. *Psychopharmacologica* 1960;1:482–492.
27. Gershon ES, Targum SD, Kessler LR, Mazure CM, Bunney WE Jr. Genetic studies and biologic strategies in the affective disorders. *Prog Med Genet* 1977;2:101–164.
28. Gleser GC, Green BL, Winget CW. *Prolonged psychosocial effects of disaster: a study of Buffalo Creek.* New York: Academic Press, 1981.
29. Grace MC, Green BL, Lindy JD, Leonard AC. The Buffalo Creek disaster; a 14-year follow-up. In: Wilson JP, Raphael B, eds. *International handbook of traumatic stress syndromes.* New York: Plenum Press, 1993;441–449.
30. Gray JA. *The neuropsychology of anxiety: an enquiry into the functions of the septo-hippocampal system.* New York: Oxford University Press, 1982.
31. Helzer JE, Robins LN, McEvoy L. Post-traumatic stress disorder in the general population. *N Engl J Med* 1987;317:1630–1634.
32. Holmes TH, Rahe RH. The social readjustment rating scale. *J Psychosom Res* 1967;11:213–218.
33. Horowitz MJ. Anxious states of mind induced by stress. In: Tuma AH, Maser JD, eds. *Anxiety and the anxiety disorders.* Hillsdale, NJ: Lawrence Erlbaum Associates, 1985;619–631.
34. Johnson JH, McCutcheon S. Assessing life stress in older children and adolescents: preliminary findings with the life events checklist. In: Sarason IG, Spielberger CD, eds. *Stress and anxiety,* vol 7. Washington, DC: Hemisphere Publishing Corporation, 1980;111–125.
35. Kaplan HI, Sadock BJ. *Synopsis of psychiatry: behavioral sciences clinical psychiatry,* 6th ed. Baltimore: Williams & Wilkins, 1991;389–415.
36. King NJ, Ollendick TH. Children's anxiety and phobic disorders in school settings: classification, assessment, and intervention issues. *Rev Educ Res* 1989;59:431–470.
37. Krantz DS, Grunberg NE, Baum A. Health psychology. *Annu Rev Psychol* 1985;36:349–383.
38. Krohne HW, Rogner J. Parental child-rearing styles and the development of anxiety and competencies in the child. *Arch Psychol* 1982;134:117–136.
39. Lazarus RS, Folkman S. *Stress, appraisal and coping.* New York: Springer, 1984.
40. Leventhal H. Toward a comprehensive theory of emotion. In: Berkowitz, L. *Advances in experimental social psychology,* vol 13. New York: Academic Press, 1980;140–207.
41. Malauzat D, Noel F, Clement J, Bourlot D. Anxiety and aging. *Psychol Med* 1989;21:1181–1186.
42. Malloy PF, Fairbank JA, Keane TM. Validation of a multimethod assessment of post-traumatic stress disorders in Vietnam veterans. *J Consult Clin Psychol* 1983;51:488–494.
43. Mansbach RS, Geyer MA. *Eur J Pharmacol* 1988;156:375–383.
44. Mason JW. A historical view of the stress field. *J hum stress* 1975;1:22–36.
45. Miller N. Theoretical models relating animal experiments on fear to clinical phenomena. In: Tuma AH, Maser JD, eds. *Anxiety and the anxiety disorders.* Hillsdale, NJ: Lawrence Erlbaum Associates, 1985;261–272.
46. Mineka S, Henderson R. Controllability and predictability in acquired motivation. *Annu Rev Psychol* 1985;87:256–271.
47. Mineka S, Cook M, Miller S. Fear conditioned with escape and inescapable shock: effects of a feedback stimulus. *J Exp Psychol* 1984;10:307–323.
48. Patterson RL, O'Sullivan MJ, Spielberger CD. Measurement of state and trait anxiety in elderly mental health clients. *J Behav Assess* 1980;2:89–97.
49. Perry NW, Millimet CR. Child-rearing antecedents of low and high anxiety eighth-grade children. In: Spielberger CD, Sarason IG, eds. *Stress and anxiety,* vol 4. Washington, DC: Hemisphere Publishing Corporation, 1977;189–204.
50. Pich EM, Samanin R. Disinhibitory effect of buspirone and low doses of sulpiride and haloperidol in two experimental anxiety models in rats: possible role of dopamine. *Psychopharmacology* 1986;89:125–130.
51. Pilkington CL, Piersel WC. School phobia: a critical analysis of the separation anxiety theory and an alternative conceptualization. *Psychol Schools* 1991;28:290–303.
52. Rachman S. Emotional processing. *Behav Res Ther* 1979;18:1–60.
53. Rachman SJ. Disorders of emotion: causes and consequences. *Psychol Inquiry* 1991;2:86–87.
54. Rescorla RA. Conditioned inhibition of fear resulting from negative CS–US contingencies. *J Comp Physiol Psychol* 1969;67:504–509.
55. Rush DK, Mineka S, Suomi SJ. The effects of control and lack of control on active and passive avoidance in rhesus monkeys. *Behav Res Ther* 1982;20:135–152.
56. Salzman C. Psychometric rating of anxiety in the elderly. In: *Diag-*

nosis and treatment of anxiety in the aged, part II: measurement of anxiety. Nutley, NJ: Hoffman–LaRoche, 1977;5–21.

57. Sarason IG. Life stress, self-preoccupation, and social supports. In: Sarason IG, Spielberger CD, eds. *Stress and anxiety,* vol 7. Washington, DC: Hemisphere Publishing Corporation, 1980;73–92.

58. Schwartz B. *Psychology of learning and behavior,* 2nd ed. New York: WW. Norton and Company, 1984;91–138.

59. Seligman MEP, Binik YM. The safety signal hypothesis. In: Davis H, Hurwitz H, eds. *Pavlovian operant interaction.* Hillsdale, NJ: Lawrence Erlbaum Associates, 1977.

60. Selye H. *The stress of life,* revised edition. New York: McGraw–Hill, 1976.

61. Shader RI, Kennedy JS, Greenblatt DJ. Treatment of anxiety in the elderly. In: Meltzer HY, ed. *Psychopharmacology: the third generation of progress.* New York: Raven Press, 1987;1141–1147.

62. Sheehan DV, Soto S. Diagnosis and treatment of pathological anxiety. *Stress Med* 1987;3:21–32.

63. Shelton DM, Mallinckrodt B. Test anxiety, locus of control, and self-efficacy as predictors of treatment preference. *College Student J* 1991;25:544–551.

64. Smith EM, North CS. Posttraumatic stress disorder in natural disasters and technological accidents. In: Wilson JP, Raphael B, eds. *International handbook of traumatic stress syndromes.* New York: Plenum Press, 1993;405–419.

65. Spielberger CD. *Understanding stress and anxiety.* New York: Harper & Row, 1979.

66. Suinn RM, Taylor S, Edwards RW. Suinn mathematics anxiety rating scale for elementary school students (MARS-E): psychometric and normative data. *Educ Psychol Meas* 1988;48:979–986.

67. Suomi SJ, Kraemer GW, Baysinger CM, DeLizio RD. Inherited and experiential factors associated with individual differences in anxious behavior displayed by rhesus monkeys. In: Klein DF, Rabkin J, eds. *Anxiety: new research and changing concepts.* New York: Raven Press, 1981;179–200.

68. Uhde TW, Bowlenger JP, Siever LJ, DuPont RL, Post RM. Animal models of anxiety: implications for research in humans. *Psychopharmacol Bull* 1982;18:47–52.

69. Van Riezen H, Segal M. Introduction to the evaluation of anxiety and related disorders. In: *Comparative evaluation of rating scales for clinical psychopharmacology.* New York: Elsevier, 1988;225–228.

70. Vickio CJ, Cavanaugh JC. Relationships among death anxiety, attitudes toward aging, and experience with death in nursing home employees. *J Gerontol* 1985;40:347–349.

71. Visintainer M, Volpicelli JR, Seligman MEP. Tumor rejection in rats after inescapable or escapable shock. *Science* 1982;216:437–439.

72. Weissman MM. The epidemiology of anxiety disorders: rates, risks, and familial patterns. In: Tuma AH, Maser JD, eds. *Anxiety and the anxiety disorders.* Hillsdale, NJ: Lawrence Erlbaum Associates, 1985;275–296.

73. Wigfield A, Eccles JS. Test anxiety in elementary and secondary school students. *Educ Psychol* 1989;24:159–183.

74. Williams SL, Dooseman G, Kleifeld E. Comparative effectiveness of guided mastery and exposure treatments for intractable outcomes. *J Consult Clin Psychol* 1984;52:505–518.

75. Zuckerman M. The development of an affect adjective check list for the measurement of anxiety. *J Consult Psychol* 1960;24:462–475.

Psychopharmacology: The Fourth
Generation of Progress, edited by
Floyd E. Bloom and David J. Kupfer.
Raven Press, Ltd., New York © 1995.

CHAPTER 113

The Pharmacotherapy of Acute Anxiety

A Mini-Update

Richard I. Shader and David J. Greenblatt

Panic attacks are a prototypical presentation for acute anxiety. Rapid in onset, they quickly build to a crescendo of symptoms of sympathetic overactivity and typically last from a few minutes to a few hours. Experientially, panic attacks differ from other attack-like episodes of intense anxiety mostly because of their rapidly mounting pattern of symptoms and because patients usually feel they must flee from their current location or fear they will suffocate, ''go crazy,'' or even die during the height of the attack. Panic attacks can occur without obvious triggers and are not simply acute bouts of fear or intense worry. Approximately 10% of the adult population reports having experienced at least one panic attack. Fewer have had recurrent attacks, and estimates of the lifetime prevalence for those meeting criteria for panic disorder range from 0.1% to 2.3%. Panic attacks can occur in conjunction with other disorders or as a component of the symptomatology of other disorders. When seen with other disorders, their response to treatment may differ. For example, patients with schizophrenia may worsen rather than improve when tricyclic antidepressants are used for their anti-panic effects (5). About one-half of patients who present with panic disorder will eventually develop depressive symptoms, and about 20% of patients with recurrent major depressive episodes report having panic attacks. Some data suggest that when panic attacks accompany depression, treatment response may be less favorable (22). This observation, however, may be confounded by the duration of untreated panic disorder prior to the initiation of effective therapy or by the type of pharmacotherapy chosen (61).

R. I. Shader and D. J. Greenblatt: Department of Pharmacology and Experimental Therapeutics, Tufts University School of Medicine, Boston, Massachusetts 02111.

Generalized anxiety disorder (GAD) is another prominent anxiety disorder. It appears to be about three to four times more common than panic disorder. GAD is a somewhat confusing disorder; its diagnostic criteria have shifted considerably over the last 10–15 years (79). When codified in 1980, the time-course criterion required 1 month of continuous or persistent symptoms. In DSM-IIIR this was lengthened to 6 months, and a greater emphasis was placed on the presence of unrealistic worry as a key symptom. In DSM-IV, the 6-month time frame has been maintained, and excessive worry is now the cardinal feature. Because of these changes, studies done in the 1980s may not be comparable to those of agents evaluated in the early 1990s. Patients seen in primary care settings often do not meet full GAD diagnostic criteria. This is particularly important because marketing data suggest that about 75–80% of prescribing of anxiolytic agents is by primary care physicians; benzodiazepines account for the vast majority of these prescriptions.

Additional aspects of panic disorder and other forms of anxiety disorders are considered in more detail elsewhere in this volume (see Chapters 109 and 110, *this volume*). In this chapter, we discuss selected aspects of the understanding and pharmacotherapy of acute anxiety and briefly explore future directions for treatment. Because the benzodiazepines are still the major class of compounds used in anxiety, considerable attention will be devoted to their molecular pharmacology, current patent status including new agents, regulatory issues, drug interactions, and receptor partial agonists (benzodiazepines and 5-HT$_{1A}$). The remaining sections of the chapter deal with other drugs, namely, SSRI and tricyclic antidepressants, cholecystokinin antagonists, and 5-HT$_3$ receptor antagonists.

BENZODIAZEPINES

Benzodiazepines remain the mainstay of our treatment armamentarium for acute anxiety. They have been extensively utilized and studied, and their efficacy and relative safety compared to other antianxiety agents currently marketed in the United States are well established; the interested reader is urged to consult recent comprehensive reviews that have appeared elsewhere (47,78,94). Although thousands of benzodiazepine-like drugs have been synthesized, no new benzodiazepines have been introduced into clinical practice in the United States as antianxiety agents since the last volume in this series.

MOLECULAR PHARMACOLOGY

Central nervous system (CNS)-active benzodiazepines bind at complex, membrane-spanning, heteromeric protein structures that comprise the GABA-A receptors in gray matter. The current assumption is that these structures are pentameric. The highest receptor densities are found in synaptosomal fractions from cortex, followed by hypothalamus, cerebellum, hippocampus, and striatum. Receptor populations are also found in midbrain, medulla oblongata-pons, and spinal cord. Benzodiazepines allosterically modify GABA-mediated opening of a chloride ion channel in the center of the GABA-A receptor. Other modifiers acting at different binding sites include barbiturates, ethanol, and neurosteroids. Benzodiazepine-induced conformational changes increase GABA's receptor affinity, and thus increase the frequency of ion channel openings. Chloride ion influx hyperpolarizes GABA neurons and produces GABA's inhibitory interneuronal effects, including actions on dopaminergic, serotonergic, and noradrenergic neurons. For example, inhibition by GABA-ergic neurons decreases locus coeruleus noradrenergic neuron firing.

The noncovalently associated protein subunits surrounding the chloride channel by convention are labeled alpha (α), beta (β), and gamma (γ). Other polypeptide subunits have been identified (e.g., δ, ρ), but their functional significance is not established. Various GABA-A receptor isoforms are assembled from gene family products that yield six, three, and three different subtypes of α, β, and γ subunits, respectively. In vitro transfection data and other studies suggest that there is considerable regional heterogeneity in the subunit composition of GABA-A receptors, but most are comprised of an $\alpha1\beta2\gamma2$ pattern. In this type of receptor complex, sometimes called the *type I benzodiazepine subtype*, GABA per se binds to β subunits, while photoaffinity labeling studies suggest that benzodiazepines bind to a site on the α subunit ($\alpha1$) (85). So-called type II imidazopyridine-sensitive (e.g., alpidem, zolpidem) subunits contain $\alpha2/\alpha3$ subunits, while an imidazopyridine-insensitive type II receptor subtype contains the $\alpha5$ subunit. Receptors containing $\alpha4$ or $\alpha6$ subunits have low affinity for benzodiazepines and are sometimes called *diazepam-insensitive receptors*. Receptors containing γ subunits have increased affinity for benzodiazepines (89). Unfortunately, in vivo strategies are not available to establish the accuracy or clinical significance of these in vitro observations. Also, it is not known what subunits or combinations are expressed in vivo in single neurons; it is surely possible that a single cell could carry multiple receptor subtypes. GABA-A receptors have a clear homology with glycine and nicotinic acetylcholine receptors.

PATENT STATUS AND NEW AGENTS

All eight benzodiazepines currently indicated for GAD have exceeded their patent protection; nevertheless, alprazolam, diazepam, and lorazepam remain among the top 100 drugs in sales in the United States. Alprazolam recently received approval (but without a patent extension) as the only benzodiazepine specifically for use in panic disorder (50,68,86). Other benzodiazepines, however, have also been used successfully in panic disorder (32,47,77,78). A slow-release formulation of alprazolam has been developed and is being reviewed by the FDA. Clonazepam's sole approved indication is as an anticonvulsant even though it is frequently prescribed for its anti-panic (47,78,87) and anti-manic effects. Adinazolam, with its active metabolite [mono-N-desmethyladinazolam (NDMAD)], is a potent triazolobenzodiazepine which, in a slow-release formulation, appears to have efficacy in patients with panic disorder (35,37,70,82). There is some suggestion that use of the slow-release preparation may be associated with less interdose (therapeutic tolerance) and discontinuation-associated (rebound) intensification of symptoms than occurs with some rapidly eliminated, shorter half-life benzodiazepines (e.g., alprazolam). As with other triazolobenzodiazepines, the biotransformation of adinazolam to NDMAD appears to involve the cytochrome P-450 3A subfamily pathway. NDMAD, which is more potent than its parent compound, is renally eliminated (34). It seems likely that caution will be required in the use of adinazolam in patients with renal impairment. (N.B., A recent review by an FDA advisory panel did not recommend approval of adinazolam for use in panic disorder.)

REGULATORY ISSUES

Perhaps in part because of their extensive use and cost impact, benzodiazepine use has been subjected to increasingly close scrutiny and monitoring. In New York State, for example, the promulgation of triplicate prescription procedures since 1989 has significantly reduced their use. Ostensibly, such programs are initiated to reduce alleged inappropriate prescribing practices and illicit diversion. Unfortunately, however, what has mainly been accomplished is a decrement in state (e.g., Medicaid) and third-party (e.g., Blue Cross and Blue Shield) outlays for benzodiazepines. Other anxiolytic agents and alcohol-containing products are routinely substituted by some physicians or patients; these substituted therapies generally are less safe or less effective. There have been negative impacts not only in patients with anxiety disorders, but also in elderly patients in nursing homes and patients with epilepsy. An increase in deaths due to overdosages with meprobamate has been reported. Adequate impact data have not been collected and analyzed, and the larger community of concerned clinicians and scientists has not become adequately involved with this increasingly problematic issue (4,10,72,74–76,80,91,96). Other regulatory actions have been under consideration, including class labeling for benzodiazepines used as hypnotics and unit-of-use packaging (57).

Underlying many of these actions is an unsubstantiated belief that benzodiazepine misuse and abuse are widespread and a significant public health problem. In this regard, a survey conducted by the late Mitchell B. Balter and colleagues is of interest (8). A peer selection process using primary nominators from 44 countries generated a panel of international experts on the pharmacotherapy of anxiety. Sixty-six members of this clinician–researcher cohort overwhelmingly concluded that strict and differential restrictions on the use of benzodiazepines are not warranted. This conclusion reflected the opinion of the expert panel that the relative abuse liability of benzodiazepines is low and that qualitative differences in abuse liability among the benzodiazepines are minimal.

DRUG INTERACTIONS

Pharmacodynamic drug interactions (e.g., CNS depression and its consequences) between benzodiazepines and other CNS agents, including ethanol, are well-recognized. However, during their initial years of use, one of the ''virtues'' of benzodiazepines was thought to be their relative lack of clinically significant pharmacokinetic interactions. This property was a clear advantage, for example, over the barbiturates and meprobamate which are known inducers of hepatic oxidative metabolism. This conclusion reflected the fact that a few benzodiazepines are metabolized mainly by conjugation (e.g., oxazepam, lorazepam), whereas others such as diazepam, with its active metabolite desmethyldiazepam, may have alternative pathways via different cytochrome P-450 isozymes (e.g., 2C3, 2D6, 3A4) that could mitigate the clinical significance of any pharmacokinetic interactions. Triazolobenzodiazepines (e.g., alprazolam, midazolam, triazolam), however, present different concerns: They are metabolized preferentially by 3A subfamily isozymes, and

both in vitro and in vivo data suggest that clinically significant increments in sedation and its consequences may occur when triazolobenzodiazepines are coadministered with other agents that inhibit this pathway either competitively (e.g., fluoxetine) or through complex formation (e.g., erythromycin and other macrolides, cimetidine) (36,40,55,58,88,90,95). Benzodiazepines do not appear to have significant effects on the metabolism of other agents (i.e., when they are viewed not as substrates but as potential competitive inhibitors).

RECEPTOR PARTIAL AGONISTS

A partial agonist by commonly accepted classical definition has less intrinsic activity than a full agonist for the same receptor. Potency is not the differentiating variable, because potency comparisons are made from the dose at which a given drug attains 50% of a target pharmacodynamic effect (i.e., its ED_{50}). Two drugs (e.g., a full agonist and a partial agonist) could differ according to their intrinsic activities and yet have the same ED_{50} or potency. Another view of partial agonists presumes that they have reduced intrinsic activity and require a greater degree of receptor occupancy as compared to full agonists to achieve the same effect. However, it is also possible for the same drug to be a partial agonist at one receptor site and a full agonist at another. For ligand-gated ion channels, full and partial agonists modulate their allosteric transition from their inactive (closed) to active (open) states to varying degrees, perhaps because of different affinities for specific protein subunits in the receptor complex. This understanding of full and partial agonists fits well with drug actions at ligand-gated chloride ion channels (e.g., GABA-A receptors) where no second messengers are involved. It is possible that more frequent contact with the benzodiazepine receptor is required for partial agonists than for full agonists to maintain the GABA receptor in the active (open) conformation.

When G proteins and second messengers are involved (e.g., 5-HT$_{1A}$ receptors), the same drug acting at the same receptor type can produce effects ranging from antagonism to almost full agonism (48). Drug action may depend on the state of the coupling in the G-protein–receptor complex which may vary from precoupling to dissociation. Receptor coupling to different combinations of G-protein subunits can also influence second messenger effects. Some of this variation may also be a function of the degree of receptor reserve (i.e., spare receptors). For the medications in the following two subsections, there is still limited understanding about the specifics of their actions as partial agonists.

BENZODIAZEPINE RECEPTOR PARTIAL AGONISTS

The search for benzodiazepine receptor partial agonists derives from the desire to find agents that will have comparable or better efficacy, tolerability, and safety when compared to currently available benzodiazepines, and yet cause fewer of the unwanted properties attributed to benzodiazepines (e.g., sedation, physical dependence, tolerance) (41). It should be kept in mind that GABA-A receptors in contrast to GABA-B receptors do not couple to second messengers.

A variety of structurally distinct compounds have been studied that have partial agonist properties at GABA-A receptors. Some act as full agonists at certain GABA-A receptor subtypes while acting as partial agonists at others; some appear to act as partial agonists at all GABA-A receptor subtypes. Among the agents that have received the most attention are abecarnil (84), alpidem (66), bretazenil (54,62), and suriclone (53). All have been investigated for their effectiveness in animal models and in patients with anxiety. Bretazenil, for example, has reasonable effectiveness in animal models and yet in comparison to benzodiazepines (e.g., diazepam) produces less sedation, anticonvulsant tolerance, muscle incoordination, self-administration, and discontinuation-related behaviors (62). Alpidem (an imidazopyridine) (66,67), abecarnil (a β-carboline) (7), and suriclone (a cyclopyrrolone) (3) appear to be the most extensively studied of these agents in humans.

Alpidem is a high-affinity full agonist comparable to benzodiazepines at $\alpha2\beta1\gamma2S$ recombinant receptors, but it is a low-potency partial agonist at $\alpha2\beta1\gamma1$ recombinant receptors at which benzodiazepines act as higher-potency partial agonists (89). Abecarnil, by contrast, is a partial agonist at both of these recombinant receptors (89). Although not studied in this same way, suriclone binds to membranes that have been fully and irreversibly photolabeled with flunitrazepam, which suggests some binding at a locus that is not identical to the $\alpha1\beta2\gamma2$ subtype (97). In standard models, however, suriclone has high affinity for both type I and type II benzodiazepine receptors. Curiously, some cyclopyrrolones do not potentiate the sedative effects of ethanol (31).

Despite their presumed advantages, no benzodiazepine partial agonists have been approved for anxiolytic use in the United States. Abecarnil's development program is currently quiescent, although anxiolytic research in Europe is quite active. Suriclone is no longer under study, and alpidem was recently withdrawn from clinical use in Europe because of hepatotoxicity (note that hepatotoxicity does not appear to be a problem with zolpidem, a structurally and pharmacologically similar agent recently marketed in the United States as a hypnotic). Although it seems likely that other benzodiazepine partial agonists will be developed, it remains unclear whether their putative selectivity based on in vitro binding data will translate into any demonstrable clinical advantages (e.g., reduced sedation, tolerance development, or dependence liability).

5-HT$_{1A}$ RECEPTOR PARTIAL AGONISTS

Understanding the role of serotonergic agents in anxiety disorders is not straightforward. The CNS actions of serotonin are mediated by multiple receptor subtypes and subfamilies that can be present on the same neuron and involve different intracellular signaling systems (42). Azapirones such as buspirone and ipsapirone (13) are generally classified as 5-HT$_{1A}$ receptor partial agonists. The role of the 5-HT$_{1A}$ receptor in the pathogenesis of anxiety disorders is discussed in detail elsewhere in this volume (see chapter by Coplan et al.). In vitro studies suggest that these compounds are full agonists at presynaptic autoreceptors and partial agonists at postsynaptic receptors. Presynaptic 5-HT$_{1A}$ receptors also appear to have a large receptor reserve, whereas postsynaptic receptors do not. A given agonist acting at the same receptor in a specific cell line can show differences in intrinsic activity depending on receptor density. Receptor–effector coupling also can vary as a function of the second messenger system involved (e.g., adenylyl cyclase versus phospholipase C) (48). It is unclear how such putative differences translate into the effectiveness of these agents in GAD. Agonist effects at presynaptic autoreceptors could temporarily reduce serotonin concentrations and have anxiolytic effects, but desensitization should occur with chronic administration. Postsynaptic partial agonist effects could lead to reduced postsynaptic agonist effects from serotonin per se. This overly simplified explanation based on in vitro findings does not adequately take into account the increasingly complex information accumulating about serotonin receptors and their varied nature and second messenger systems. Some non-azapirone 5-HT$_{1A}$ receptor full agonists are in the early stages of development. Their availability may help to clarify the role of this receptor in anxiety. The slow onset of action of the azapirones is consistent with the idea that second messenger systems set into motion a cascade of downstream events that takes more time to effect change than drugs that work directly on ligand-gated ion channels.

Azapirones are not as consistently effective as benzodiazepines in patients with GAD. Some evidence suggests that these agents have a better chance of helping patients not previously benefited by or exposed to benzodiazepines. In such a population, 60–80% of patients could be expected to benefit. (45). Compared to benzodiazepines, they cause less sedation, motor impairment, and memory loss. They also do not appear to cause clinically significant discontinuation syndromes. Unfortunately, they do not seem to stop panic attacks (50,81). However, when they are effective at reducing overall levels of anxiety they may decrease the frequency of panic attacks in some patients.

SPECIFIC SEROTONIN REUPTAKE INHIBITORS AND TRICYCLIC ANTIDEPRESSANTS

Tricyclic antidepressants (TCAs) and specific serotonin reuptake inhibitors (SSRIs) appear to be beneficial in some patients with GAD, mixed anxiety and depression, or panic disorder. The numbers of such patients in placebo-controlled trials are growing, but none of these drugs has received FDA approval for any of these indications. Among the TCAs, imipramine (6,20,25,45,49, 63,93) and clomipramine (21,30,51) have been the most extensively studied. Among the SSRIs, fluoxetine and fluvoxamine have been the most extensively studied, especially for their role in panic disorder (6,11,20,25,28–30,38,39,45,46,59,63,73,83,92,93). Relative to benzodiazepines, onset of action in any of these anxiety disorders for any of these agents is slow, ranging from 2 to 6 weeks. Patients with panic disorder have received the most attention in controlled trials with SSRIs, and their ability to reduce the frequency of panic attacks appears to be independent of concomitant depressive symptomatology. Because of their relative lack of unwanted anticholinergic and cardiovascular effects and weight gain, SSRIs are favored over TCAs by many clinicians. In panic-disorder patients treated with TCAs and SSRIs, there may be an initial increase in jitteriness that decreases treatment acceptance (tolerability) (65,69). Prior warning through patient education or the temporary use of β-adrenergic receptor antagonists or a benzodiazepine may be beneficial. Sexual dysfunction (e.g., anorgasmia, retarded ejaculation) associated with SSRI use can also affect patient acceptance and compliance. In clinical practice, it is increasingly common for patients with panic disorder to be started on a benzodiazepine (e.g., alprazolam, clonazepam) while an antidepressant (e.g., imipramine, fluoxetine) is being phased in. Such combination regimens need to take into account potential drug interactions (see above).

CHOLECYSTOKININ ANTAGONISTS

Cholecystokinin (CCK), in addition to its peripheral role as a regulator of gastrointestinal functions (e.g., inhibition of gastric emptying), is also a centrally acting neuropeptide with high-affinity binding sites in cortex, hippocampus, and amygdala (9,71). Its predominant form in brain is a sulfated octapeptide (CCK-8). Data suggest that some forms of CCK may be mediators of anxiety symptomatology; benzodiazepine receptor agonists (both full and partial) have been shown to antagonize CCK-induced excitation of hippocampal neurons in the rat (15,16), and long-term benzodiazepine use in the rat has also been shown to lower CCK-induced CNS activation (14). Animal models also support the anxiogenic effects of a naturally occurring metabolite of CCK-8 [i.e., the COOH-terminal tetrapeptide (CCK-4)] (26). This anxiogenic effect is likely mediated by both CCK-A and CCK-B receptors in brain, and it may explain the anxiolytic properties of devazepide, a non-benzodiazepine CCK-A receptor antagonist (43). Devazepide also causes a dose-dependent inhibition of CCK-8-stimulated increases in levels of ACTH and β-endorphin in rat brain (64). In small-cohort studies, the anxiogenic properties of CCK-4 have been observed in normal volunteers (an effect that could be blocked by lorazepam) (27) and in patients with panic disorder (17–19). In two patients studied by the latter group, CCK-4-induced panic attacks were blocked by pretreatment with imipramine (17,18), an observation that curiously is not reported in Ref. 19. Others have noted the anxiogenic effects (in a small series of panic disorder patients and controls) of the homologous CCK pentapeptide fragment, pentagastrin (1). In one study, patients with panic disorder had lower CCK-8 CSF levels than did normal controls (60). Possible explanations for this finding include (a) altered metabolism of CCK-8 or conversion into CCK-4, (b) reduced CCK-A or CCK-B receptor density, or (c) increased CCK-A or CCK-B receptor sensitivity in panic disorder patients as compared to controls. Taken together, these studies support a possible role for CCK in the pathogenesis of anxiety, the use of CCK-4 as a diagnostic challenge test for panic disorder, and a potential role for specific CCK-A or CCK-B receptor antagonists in the acute treatment of anxiety.

5-HT₃ RECEPTOR ANTAGONISTS

The 5-HT₃ receptor antagonist and antiemetic agent, ondansetron, is currently being investigated as a potential treatment for GAD, panic disorder, and social phobia. Because the 5-HT₃ receptor is a ligand-gated ion channel for cations, it is possible that drug actions at this receptor subtype may be more rapid than for drugs acting at other serotonin receptor subtypes. Some data also suggest that 5-HT₃ receptors may mediate CCK release. From microinjection studies in rats, the amygdala has been postulated to be a key site for the anxiolytic activity of 5-HT₃ antagonists (44). Some rodent models that quantify social interaction or time spent in dark versus light test boxes and primate (marmoset) responses to a confrontational human threat test have supported the further testing of ondansetron as an antianxiety agent (23,24,52,56). Data available from human trials are limited but supportive at the present time. Four hundred and two patients with GAD were treated in the United Kingdom in a multicenter (58 general practitioners), 4-week, fixed-dose, double-blind trial comparing ondansetron at 1.0 mg t.i.d. and 4.0 mg t.i.d. to diazepam 2.0 mg t.i.d. and placebo (16,17). Using HAM-A total scores, both the higher-dose ondansetron patients and the diazepam patients were significantly more improved by 3 weeks than those on placebo. At trial completion (i.e., 4 weeks), the lower-dose ondansetron and diazepam patients were more improved than those on placebo. This study, which slightly favored the 1.0 mg t.i.d. ondansetron group, was complicated by a high placebo response (45% met improvement criteria on the

HAM-A). On the Global Improvement Scale, the improvement rates were 50%, 43%, 48%, and 38%, respectively, for patients on ondansetron 1.0 mg t.i.d., ondansetron 4.0 mg t.i.d., diazepam 2.0 mg t.i.d., and placebo. The study author also claims an absence of abrupt discontinuation-related rebound anxiety for both ondansetron groups yet "significant rebound" for the diazepam patients (i.e., a 1-week later HAM-A increment of 2.3 points) (56).

Further discussion and understanding of ondansetron is not possible at this time because the trial just noted is published only in summary form, and no other data, including trials in the United States, appear to be published. Limited data have also been published for other 5-HT₃ receptor antagonists (e.g., zacopride [its enantiomers may have differential activity] (2,12), tropisetron, zatosetron) but not for granisetron or bemesetron.

Hepatic metabolism data have recently been published for both ondansetron and tropisetron (33). In studies using human liver microsomes, the oxidative metabolism of tropisetron was reduced to a greater degree by 1.0 μM quinidine than was the case for ondansetron (67% and 18%, respectively), suggesting that both drugs are substrates for cytochrome P-450 2D6. By contrast, ondansetron hydroxylation was modestly reduced (27%) by the 3A subfamily inhibitors, cyclosporin and triacetyloleandomycin, and this was even less the case for tropisetron (<10%). Coadministration of drugs that are known inhibitors of these isozymes (e.g., specific serotonin reuptake inhibitors) could have both pharmacokinetic and pharmacodynamic consequences. In addition to being substrates to varying degrees for these isozymes, both 5-HT₃ antagonists appear to be weak competitive inhibitors of the 2D6 pathway; however, the inhibitory constants for both drugs are well above their likely therapeutic concentrations. Ondansetron ($K_i = 31$ μM) appears to have comparable effects as a weak competitive inhibitor for the 3A subfamily pathway (e.g., cyclosporin metabolism), while tropisetron's inhibiting effects would seem to be inconsequential ($K_i = 2.1$ mM).

COMMENT

Benzodiazepines continue to be consistently effective agents for acute anxiety in patients with GAD and panic disorder. Although not totally free from unwanted problems, their benefit-to-risk ratio is extremely favorable. Unfortunately, no benzodiazepine receptor partial agonist has emerged as a viable alternative. Azapirone 5-HT₁A receptor partial agonists are somewhat less predictably effective than benzodiazepines in patients with GAD and are relatively ineffective in the acute treatment of panic attacks; nevertheless, they offer some advantages over benzodiazepines in patients for whom they prove to be effective (e.g., less sedation or memory impairment). A

major limitation in the use of azapirones is their slow onset of action. Tricyclic antidepressants and SSRIs also have a slow onset of action. For patients who tolerate the side effects that are characteristic of either class, agents from both classes may reduce symptomatology in GAD or significantly lower the frequency of panic attacks in patients with panic disorder. Cholecystokinin antagonists and 5-HT₃ receptor antagonists have the potential for a more rapid onset of anxiety reduction; unfortunately, further research will be essential to clarify their place in the treatment of acute anxiety.

ACKNOWLEDGMENT

This work was supported, in part, by a grant (MH-34223) from the Department of Health and Human Services.

REFERENCES

1. Abelson JL, Nesse RM. Cholecystokinin-4 and panic. *Arch Gen Psychiatry* 1990;47:395.
2. Andrews N, File SE. Are there changes in sensitivity to 5-HT₃ receptor ligands following chronic diazepam treatment? *Psychopharmacology* 1992;108:333–337.
3. Ansseau M, Olie JP, von Frenckell R, et al. Controlled comparisons of the efficacy and safety of four doses of suriclone, diazepam and placebo in generalized anxiety disorder. *Psychopharmacology* 1991;104:439–443.
4. Applebaum PS. Controlling prescriptions of benzodiazepines. *Hosp Community Psychiatry* 1992;43:12–13.
5. Argyle N. Panic attacks in chronic schizophrenia. *Br J Psychiatry* 1990;157:430–433.
6. Aronson TA. A naturalistic study of imipramine in panic disorder and agoraphobia. *Am J Psychiatry* 1987;144:1014–1019.
7. Ballenger JC, McDonald S, Noyes R, et al. The first double-blind, placebo-controlled trial of a partial benzodiazepine agonist abecarnil (ZK 112–119) in generalized anxiety disorder. *Psychopharmacol Bull* 1991;27:171–179.
8. Balter MB, Ban TA, Uhlenhuth EH. International study of expert judgment on the therapeutic use of benzodiazepines and other psychotherapeutic medications. I. Current concerns. *Hum Psychopharmacol* 1993;8:253–261.
9. Beinfeld MC. Cholecystokinin in the central nervous system: a mini review. *Neuropeptide* 1983;3:411–427.
10. Berner R. The patient's perspective. *N Y State J Med* 1991; 91(11)(suppl):37S–39S.
11. Black DW, Wesner R, Bowers W, et al. A comparison of fluvoxamine, cognitive therapy and placebo in the treatment of panic disorder. *Arch Gen Psychiatry* 1993;50:44–50.
12. Blackburn TP. 5-HT receptors and anxiolytic drugs. In: Marsden CA, Heal DJ, eds. *Central serotonin receptors and psychotropic drugs.* London: Blackwell Scientific Publishers, 1992;175–197.
13. Borison RL, Albrecht JW, Diamond BI. Efficacy and safety of a putative anxiolytic agent: ipsapirone. *Psychopharmacol Bull* 1990;26:207–210.
14. Bouthillier A, de Montigny C. Long-term benzodiazepine treatment reduces neuronal responsiveness to cholecystokinin: an electrophysiological study in the rat. *Eur J Pharmacol* 1988;151:135–138.
15. Bradwejn J, de Montigny C. Benzodiazepines antagonize cholecystokinin-induced activation of rat hippocampal neurons. *Nature* 1984;313:363–364.
16. Bradwejn J, de Montigny C. Antagonism of cholecystokinin-induced activation by benzodiazepine receptor agonists. *Ann NY Acad Sci* 1985;448:575–580.
17. Bradwejn J, Koszycki J, Payeur R, et al. Replication of action

of cholecystokinin tetrapeptide in panic disorder patients. In: *New research program and abstracts of the 144th meeting of the American Psychiatric Association,* May 11–16, 1991, New Orleans, LA, Abstract NR367.

18. Bradwejn J, Koszycki D, Shriqui C. Enhanced sensitivity to cholecystokinin tetrapeptide in panic disorder. *Arch Gen Psychiatry* 1991;48:603–610.

19. Bradwejn J, Koszycki D, Payeur R, et al. Replication of action of cholecystokinin tetrapeptide in panic disorder: clinical and behavioral findings. *Am J Psychiatry* 1992;149:962–964.

20. Brady K, Zarzar M, Lydiard RB. Fluoxetine in panic disorder patients with imipramine-associated weight gain. *J Clin Psychopharmacol* 1989;9:66–67.

21. Cassano GB, Petracca A, Perugi G, et al. Clomipramine for panic disorders. I. the first 10 weeks of a long-term comparison with imipramine. *J Affect Dis* 1988;14:123–127.

22. Clayton PJ, Grove WM, Coryell W, et al. Follow-up and family study of anxious depression. *Am J Psychiatry* 1991;148:1512–1517.

23. Costall B. The breadth of action of the 5-HT₃ receptor antagonists. *Int Clin Psychopharmacol* 1993;8(suppl 2):3–9.

24. Costall B, Naylor RJ. Anxiolytic potential of 5-HT₃ receptor antagonists. *Pharmacol Toxicol* 1992;70:157–162.

25. Cross-national collaborative panic study second phase investigators. Drug treatment of panic disorder: comparative efficacy of alprazolam, imipramine and placebo. *Br J Psychiatry* 1992;160:191–202.

26. Csonka E, Fekete M, Nagy G, et al. Anxiogenic effect of cholecystokinin in rats. In: Penke B, Torok A, eds. *Peptides.* New York: Walter de Gruyter & Co, 1988;249–252.

27. de Montigny C. Cholecystokinin tetrapeptide induces panic-like attacks in healthy volunteers: preliminary findings. *Arch Gen Psychiatry* 1989;46:511–517.

28. den Boer JA, Westenberg HGM. Effect of serotonin and noradrenaline uptake inhibitors in panic disorder; a double blind comparative study with fluvoxamine and maprotiline. *Int J Clin Pharmacol* 1988;3:59–74.

29. den Boer JA, Westenberg HGM. Serotonin function in panic disorder: a double blind placebo controlled study with fluvoxamine and ritanserin. *Psychopharmacology* 1990;102:85–94.

30. den Boer JA, Westenberg HGM, Kamerbeek WDJ, et al. Effect of serotonin uptake inhibitors in anxiety disorders; a double blind comparison of clomipramine and fluvoxamine. *Int J Psychopharmacol* 1987;2:21–32.

31. Doble A, Canton T, Dreisler S, et al. RP 59037 and RP 60503: anxiolytic cyclopyrrolone derivatives with low sedative potential. interaction with the γ-aminobutyric acid_A/benzodiazepine receptor complex and behavioral effects in the rodent. *J Pharmacol Exp Ther* 1993;266:1213–1226.

32. Dunner DL, Ishiki D, Avery DH, et al. Effect of alprazolam and diazepam on anxiety and panic attacks in panic disorder: a controlled study. *J Clin Psychiatry* 1986;47:458–460.

33. Fischer V, Vickers AEM, Heitz F, et al. The polymorphic cytochrome P-4502D6 is involved in the metabolism of both 5-hydroxytryptamine antagonists, tropisetron and ondansetron. *Drug Metab Dispos Biol Fate Chem* 1994;22:269–274.

34. Fleishaker JC, Friedman H, Pollock SR, et al. Clinical pharmacology of adinazolam and N-desmethyladinazolam mesylate after single oral doses of each compound in healthy volunteers. *Clin Pharmacol Ther* 1990;48:652–664.

35. Fleishaker JC, Smith TC, Friedman H, et al. N-Desmethyladinazolam pharmacokinetics and behavioral effects following administration of 10–50 mg oral doses in healthy volunteers. *Psychopharmacol* 1991;105:181–185.

36. Fleishaker JC, Hulst LK. Effect of fluvoxamine on the pharmacokinetics and pharmacodynamics of alprazolam in healthy volunteers. *Pharmacol Res* 1992;9:294.

37. Fleishaker JC, Greist JH, Jefferson JW, et al. Relationship between concentrations of adinazolam and its primary metabolite in plasma and therapeutic/untoward effects in the treatment of panic disorder. *J Clin Psychopharmacol* 1994;14:28–35.

38. Goddard AW, Woods SW, Scholomskas DE, et al. Effect of the serotonin uptake inhibitor fluvoxamine on yohimbine-induced anxiety in panic disorder. *Psychiatry Res* 1993;8:119–133.

39. Gorman JM, Liebowitz MR, Fyer AJ. An open trial of fluoxetine

40. Greenblatt DJ, Preskorn SH, Cotreau MM, et al. Fluoxetine impairs the clearance of alprazolam but not of clonazepam. *Clin Pharmacol Ther* 1992;52:479–486.

41. Haefely W, Martin JR, Schoch P: Novel anxiolytics that act as partial agonists at benzodiazepine receptors. *Trends Pharmacol Sci* 1990;11:452–456.

42. Harrington MA, Zhong P, Garlow SJ, et al. Molecular biology of serotonin receptors. *J Clin Psychiatry* 1992;53(suppl 10):8–27.

43. Hendrie CA, Dourish CT. Anxiolytic profile of the cholecystokinin antagonist devazepide in mice. *Br J Pharmacol* 1990;99(suppl):138.

44. Higgins GA, Jones BJ, Oakley NR, et al. Evidence that the amygdala is involved in the disinhibitory effects of 5-HT₃ receptor antagonists. *Psychopharmacology* 1991;104:545–551.

45. Hoehn-Saric R, McLeod DR, Zimmerli WD. Differential effects of alprazolam and imipramine in generalized anxiety disorder: somatic vs psychic symptoms. *J Clin Psychiatry* 1988;49:293–301.

46. Hoehn-Saric R, McLeod DR, Hipsley PA. Effects of fluvoxamine on panic disorder. *J Clin Psychopharmacol* 1993;13:321–326.

47. Hollister LE, Müller-Oerlinghausen B, Rickels K, et al. Clinical uses of benzodiazepines. *J Clin Psychopharmacol* 1993;13(suppl 1):1S–169S.

48. Hoyer D, Boddeke HWGM. Partial agonists, full agonists, antagonists: dilemmas of definition. *Trends Pharmacol Sci* 1993;14:270–275.

49. Jann MW, Kurtz NM. Treatment of panic and phobic disorders. *Clin Pharmacol* 1987;6:947–962.

50. Jann MW. Buspirone: an update on a unique anxiolytic agent. *Pharmacotherapy* 1988;8:100–116.

51. Johnston DG, Troyer IE, Whitsett SF. Clomipramine treatment of agoraphobic women. *Arch Gen Psychiatry* 1988;45:453–459.

52. Jones BJ, Costall B, Domeney AM, et al. The potential anxiolytic activity of GR38032F, a 5-HT₃ receptor antagonist. *Br J Pharmacol* 1988;93:985–993.

53. Julou L, Blanchard JC, Dreyfus JF. Pharmacological and clinical studies of cyclopyrrolones: zopiclone and suriclone. *Pharmacol Biochem Behav* 1985;23:653–659.

54. Katshnig H. Attack-related treatment of panic disorder with bretazenil. *Biol Psychiatry* 1991;29:59S.

55. Kronbach T, Mathys D, Umeno M, et al. Oxidation of midazolam and triazolam by human liver cytochromes P450 IIIA4. *Mol Pharmacol* 1989;36:89–96.

56. Lader MH. Ondansetron in the treatment of anxiety. From a satellite symposium at the 5th World Congress of Biological Psychiatry, Florence, Italy, June 9, 1991, pp. 16–19.

57. Lasagna L, Shader RI. A white paper on the appropriateness of proposals by the FDA to modify the labeling of benzodiazepine sedative-hypnotics. *J Clin Pharmacol* 1994;34:812–815.

58. Lasher TA, Fleishaker JC, Steenwyk RC, et al. Pharmacokinetic pharmacodynamic evaluation of the combined administration of alprazolam and fluoxetine. *Psychopharmacology* 1991;104:323–327.

59. Laws D, Ashford JJ, Anstee JA. A multicentre double-blind comparative trial of fluvoxamine versus lorazepam in mixed anxiety and depression treated in general practice. *Acta Psychiatr Scand* 1990;81:185–189.

60. Lydiard RB, Ballenger JC, Laraia MT, et al. CSF cholecystokinin concentrations in patients with panic disorder and in normal comparison subjects. *Am J Psychiatry* 1992;149:691–693.

61. Maddock RJ, Carter CS, Blacker KH, et al. Relationship of past depressive episodes to symptom severity and treatment response in panic disorder with agoraphobia. *J Clin Psychiatry* 1993;54:88–95.

62. Martin JR, Pieri L, Bonetti EP, et al. Ro16-608: a novel anxiolytic acting as a partial agonist at the benzodiazepine receptor. *Pharmacopsychiatry* 1988;21:360–362.

63. Mavissakalian MR, Perel JM. Imipramine dose–response relationship in panic disorder with agoraphobia: preliminary findings. *Arch Gen Psychiatry* 1989;46:127–131.

64. Millington WR, Mueller GP, Lavigne GJ. Cholecystokinin type A and type B receptor antagonists produced opposing effects on cholecystokinin-stimulated β-endorphin secretion from the rat pituitary. *J Pharmacol Exp Ther* 1992;261:454–461.

in the treatment of panic attacks. *J Clin Psychopharmacol* 1987;7:329–332.

65. Modigh K. Antidepressants in anxiety disorders. *Acta Psychiatr Scand* 1987;76(suppl 335):57–71.

66. Morselli PL. On the therapeutic action of alpidem in anxiety disorders: an overview of European data. *Pharmacopsychiatry* 190;23(suppl 2):129–135.

67. Morton S, Lader M. Alpidem and lorazepam in the treatment of patients with anxiety disorders: comparison of physiological and psychological effects. *Pharmacopsychiatry* 1992;25:177–181.

68. Munjack DJ, Crocker B, Cabe D, et al. Alprazolam, propranolol, and placebo in the treatment of panic disorder and agoraphobia with panic attacks. *J Clin Psychopharmacol* 1989;9:22–27.

69. Pohl R, Yeragani VK, Balon R, et al. The jitteriness syndrome in panic disorder patients treated with antidepressants. *J Clin Psychiatry* 1988;49:100–104.

70. Pyke RE, Greenberg HS. Double-blind comparison of alprazolam and adinazolam for panic and phobic disorders. *J Clin Psychopharmacol* 1989;9:15–21.

71. Ravard S, Dourish CT. Cholecystokinin and anxiety. *Trends Pharmacol Sci* 1990;11:271–273.

72. Reidenberg MM. Effect of the requirement for triplicate prescriptions for benzodiazepines in New York State. *Clin Pharmacol Ther* 1991;50:129–131.

73. Schneier FR, Liebowitz MR, Davies SO, et al. Fluoxetine in panic disorder. *J Clin Psychopharmacology* 1990;10:119–121.

74. Schwartz HI. Negative clinical consequences of triplicate prescription regulation of benzodiazepines. *New York State J Med* 1991;91(11)(suppl 11):9S–12S.

75. Schwartz HI. An empirical review of the impact of triplicate prescription of benzodiazepines. *Hosp Community Psychiatry* 1992;43:382–385.

76. Schwartz HI, Blank K. Regulation of benzodiazepine prescribing practices: clinical implications. *Gen Hosp Psychiatry* 1991;13:219–224.

77. Schweizer E, Fox I, Case G, et al. Lorazepam versus alprazolam in the treatment of panic disorder. *Psychopharmacol Bull* 1988;24:224–227.

78. Shader RI, Greenblatt DJ. Use of benzodiazepines in anxiety disorders. *N Engl J Med* 1993;328:1398–1405.

79. Shader RI, Greenblatt DJ. Approaches to the treatment of anxiety. In: Shader RI, ed. *Manual of psychiatric therapeutics*. Boston: Little, Brown and Co, 1994;275–298.

80. Shader RI, Greenblatt DJ, Balter MB. Appropriate use and regulatory control of benzodiazepines. *J Clin Pharmacol* 1991;31:781–784.

81. Sheehan DV, Raj AB, Harnett Sheehan K, et al. The relative efficacy of buspirone, imipramine and placebo in panic disorder: a preliminary report. *Pharmacol Biochem Behav* 1988;29:815–817.

82. Sheehan DV, Raj AB, Harnett-Sheehan K, et al. Adinazolam sustained release formulation in the treatment of panic disorder. *Ir J Psychol Med* 1990;7:124–128.

83. Solyom L, Solyom C, Ledwidge B. Fluoxetine in panic disorder. *Can J Psychiatry* 1991;36:378–379.

84. Stephens DN, Schneider HH, Kehr W, et al. Abecarnil, a metabolically stable anxioselective β-carboline acting at benzodiazepine receptors. *J Pharmacol Exp Ther* 1990;253:334–343.

85. Stephenson FA, Duggan MJ, Pollard S: The $\gamma 2$ subunit is an integral component of the γ-aminobutyric acid$_A$ receptor but the $\alpha 1$ polypeptide is the principal site of the agonist benzodiazepine photoaffinity labeling reaction. *J Biol Chem* 1990;265:21160–21165.

86. Taylor CB, Hayward C, King R, et al. Cardiovascular and symptomatic reduction effects of alprazolam and imipramine in patients with panic disorder: results of a double-blind, placebo-controlled trial. *J Clin Psychopharmacol* 1990;10:112–118.

87. Tesar GE, Rosenbaum JF, Pollack MH, et al. Clonazepam versus alprazolam in the treatment of panic disorder: interim analysis of data from a prospective, double-blind, placebo-controlled trial. *J Clin Psychiatry* 1987;48(suppl):S16–S19.

88. von Moltke LL, Greenblatt DJ, Harmatz JS, et al. Alprazolam metabolism in vitro: studies of human, monkey, mouse, and rat liver microsomes. *Pharmacology* 1993;47:268–276.

89. Wafford KA, Bain CJ, Whiting PJ, et al. Functional comparison of the role of γ subunits in recombinant human γ-aminobutyric acid$_A$/benzodiazepine receptors. *Mol Pharmacol* 1993;44:437–442.

90. Warot D, Bergougnan L, Lamiable D, et al. Troleandomycin–triazolam interaction in healthy volunteers: pharmacokinetic and psychometric evaluation. *Eur J Clin Pharmacol* 1987;32:389–393.

91. Weintraub M, Singh S, Byrne L, et al. Consequences of the 1989 New York State triplicate benzodiazepine prescription regulations. *JAMA* 1991;266:2392–2397.

92. Westenberg HGM, den Boer JA. Selective monoamine uptake inhibitors and a serotonin antagonist in the treatment of panic disorder. *Psychopharmacol Bull* 1989;25:119–123.

93. Wilkinson G, Balestrieri M, Ruggeri M, et al: Meta-analysis of double-blind placebo-controlled trials of antidepressants and benzodiazepines for patients with panic disorders. *Psychol Med* 1991;21:991–998.

94. Woods JH, Katz JL, Winger G. Benzodiazepines: use, abuse, and consequences. *Pharmacol Rev* 1992;44:151–347.

95. Wright CE, Lasher-Sisson TA, Steenwyk RC, et al. A pharmacokinetic evaluation of the combined administration of triazolam and fluoxetine. *Pharmacotherapy* 1992;12:103–106.

96. Zullich SG, Grasela TH, Fiedler-Kelly JB, et al: Impact of triplicate prescription programs on psychotropic prescribing patterns in long-term care facilities. *Ann Pharmacother* 1992;26:539–546.

97. Zundel JL, Blanchard JC, Julou L. Partial chemical characterization of cyclopyrrolones ([^{3}H]-suriclone) and benzodiazepines ([^{3}H]-flunitrazepam) binding site: differences. *Life Sci* 1985;36:2247–2255.

Psychopharmacology: The Fourth Generation of Progress, edited by Floyd E. Bloom and David J. Kupfer. Raven Press, Ltd., New York © 1995.

CHAPTER 114

Issues in the Long-Term Treatment of Anxiety Disorders

Edward Schweizer, Karl Rickels, and Eberhard H. Uhlenhuth

The goal of this chapter is to review issues relating to the long-term treatment of anxiety disorders. The review does not pretend to be exhaustive, but it has been written with the intention of critically addressing clinically important aspects of long-term anxiolytic therapy. The scope of the review is limited to panic disorder with or without agoraphobia, generalized anxiety disorder (GAD), and social phobia. Most of the emphasis is placed on drug therapy. Space limitations, and the limitations of the authors themselves, have dictated that results from psychotherapy studies could only be highlighted. It was felt, though, that the rapidly expanding literature of controlled psychotherapy research simply could not be ignored, because their preliminary results stake a claim to the achievement of sustained efficacy *post treatment.*

The review will first undertake to establish whether there is any need for long-term or maintenance anxiolytic therapy. Long-term therapy can only be justified if there is evidence that the course of illness of panic/agoraphobia, GAD, and social phobia are frequently chronic. The longitudinal nature of these disorders will be evaluated in terms of retrospective reports, prospective studies of community samples (ideal but not generally available), and follow-up studies of treated samples. Acute (short-term) treatment studies will also be reviewed: High rates of relapse or recurrence in the months and years following acute treatment suggest that such treatment is inadequate, and that continuation or maintenance treatment may be beneficial. Establishing how beneficial leads us to a brief review of recent research on the degree of disability and impairment

in quality of life caused by the anxiety disorders. The justification section will conclude with a brief review of the extent to which the natural history of the three anxiety disorders is complicated by Axis I and Axis II comorbidity. Long-term treatment planning cannot be undertaken without considering these high rates of comorbidity.

Next will come a brief review of published evidence for the efficacy of long-term treatment of each of the three anxiety disorders. Evidence for long-term efficacy will be reviewed for the various classes of antidepressants, as well as for the benzodiazepines and buspirone. Long-term treatment will be conceptualized, in keeping with the terminology employed in the affective disorders literature, as either "continuation" treatment or "maintenance" treatment. Continuation treatment consists of the extension of drug therapy for 6 months beyond the acute phase in an attempt to prevent relapse, defined as a return of the *current* episode of anxiety. Maintenance treatment consists of the long-term use of drugs whose goal is to prevent a recurrence of a subsequent episode of anxiety in a patient who has demonstrated high chronicity, a high rate of recurrence, and/or significant levels of severity or disability associated with previous episodes.

The putative benefits of long-term (continuation or maintenance) therapy, insofar as they have been established, will be contrasted with the potential risks attendant upon such therapy. The abuse liability, dependence, and withdrawal risks associated with the benzodiazepines will be especially emphasized. Miscellaneous issues relating to long-term therapy, such as predictors of chronicity, safety and benefits of combination therapy (drug–drug or drug–psychotherapy), compliance, and intermittent medication strategies, will be reviewed next. The chapter will conclude with a review of methodologic issues in studying long-term treatment, suggest some promising research designs, and identify areas for future research.

E. Schweizer and K. Rickels: Psychopharmacology Research and Treatment Unit, Department of Psychiatry, University Science Center, University of Pennsylvania, Philadelphia, Pennsylvania 19104.
E. H. Uhlenhuth: Department of Psychiatry, University of New Mexico, Albuquerque, New Mexico 87131.

THE EVIDENCE FOR CHRONICITY

Only belatedly has it been recognized that the anxiety disorders tend to be chronic and/or recurrent conditions. This recognition has not yet reshaped our basic treatment approach, which still focuses almost exclusively on the acute control of symptoms and only secondarily acknowledges that treatment may need to be either continued or reinitiated. Treatment planning for bipolar disorder, for schizophrenia, and, recently, for unipolar depression is premised on the chronicity of each illness, whether a maintenance or an intermittent drug treatment strategy is ultimately utilized.

But what is the evidence for chronicity for panic disorder (with or without agoraphobia), GAD, and social phobia? The evidence comes mostly from cross-sectional and retrospective assessments of duration of illness and, much less frequently, from prospective studies. These latter prospective studies are not long-term, but generally consist of patient samples followed naturalistically post treatment, in which case they provide evidence not only for the chronicity of the disorder, but also for the insufficiency of acute therapy alone.

Panic Disorder

In the ECA community survey (51), the median age of onset was 23, and the mean duration of panic disorder was 7.1 years for the subset of patients whose panic was in remission. The duration of panic in the majority (81%) who continued to report panic was apparently not computed, because the illness was still ongoing. Treatment studies find a similar mean duration of illness (ongoing at the time of evaluation) in the range of 5–12 years (4,56,59). The retrospectively assessed age of panic onset in these treatment studies was in the mid-twenties, comparable to the results obtained in the ECA community survey, suggesting that the reported duration of illness was long not simply due to a sampling bias with respect to the type of patient applying for treatment in a drug study. Overall, the course of illness of panic disorder appears to be chronic in the majority of patients, but with many reporting periods of remission lasting 6 months or longer.

Generalized Anxiety Disorder

For GAD, the ECA community survey reported a median age of onset in the early twenties (51). For the good outcome cases that had remitted, mean duration was 4.5 years, with 40% reporting durations of illness of longer than 5 years. For currently active cases of GAD, the mean duration of illness to date was reported as 8.5 years. Duration of illness for still-active cases of GAD entering both drug and psychotherapy treatment studies (45,47) ranges from 5 to 15 years, confirming that GAD has high chronicity. Several researchers (5,29) have noted that the clinical course of GAD is both more chronic and more unremitting than panic disorder. Noyes et al. (35), in one of the few prospective studies (of anxiety neurosis), reported that 48% of patients continued to have moderate-to-marked symptoms at the 4- to 9-year follow-up.

Social Phobia

Much less information is available about the course of illness of social phobia, but available data from both community (23,54) and patient samples (19,24) suggest an age of onset in the mid to late teens, with a chronicity that is equal to or greater than that of panic disorder, with mean duration of illness exceeding 5 years.

AGE OF ONSET: EVIDENCE FROM ADOLESCENT POPULATIONS

As has been mentioned, panic/agoraphobia appears to have a mean age of onset, estimated retrospectively, to be in the early to mid twenties, GAD in the early twenties, and social phobia in the mid teens. Because retrospective recollection is prone to bias, in the direction of either over- or underestimation, it would be a useful corrective to study anxiety directly in its early incarnations. This is especially true in light of the lack of reliable course of illness data from prospective community samples followed over time. Fortunately, recent research provides data on the onset of panic, social phobia, and GAD in contemporaneous child and adolescent populations. Structured, prospectively conducted DSM-III-R assessments of a random community sample of 1710 adolescents found a lifetime prevalence rate, to date, of 1.2% for panic disorder, 0.6% for agoraphobia, 1.5% for social phobia, 4.3% for separation anxiety disorder, and 1.2% for overanxious disorder (23). A similar community survey of adolescents (70) found prevalence rates of 0.6% for panic disorder and 3.7% for GAD. Other community prevalence estimates place the rate of panic attacks post puberty as high as 12–13%. The panic/agoraphobia, GAD, and social phobia prevalence rates for adolescents are in the range of rates reported for adults, suggesting that the age of onset and duration of illness estimates gleaned from retrospective reports in adults are, if anything, an underestimate.

THE ADEQUACY OF SHORT-TERM (ACUTE) TREATMENT

Panic Disorder

Accumulated evidence across multiple controlled trials suggests that the high-potency *benzodiazepines* (the most studied is alprazolam) are effective drugs for the short-term treatment of panic disorder, either with or without agoraphobia (e.g., see refs. 4, 12, and 58). Similar short-term treatment efficacy has been reported for the tricyclic antidepressants (12,58), the MAOI antidepressants (59), and, in pilot studies, the SSRI antidepressants (8).

Only a few studies, though, have examined clinical and drug treatment status after naturalistic follow-up 1–3 years post acute study treatment. Studies reporting outcome after short-term benzodiazepine therapy find that many patients experience transient rebound anxiety symptoms to a level above their pretreatment baseline (38,56). By 1–3 years, approximately 50% or more of acutely treated patients have had a recurrence (34), and at least 50% have resumed treatment, either with a benzodiazepine or with an antidepressant.

Acute treatment with *antidepressants* appears to have a similar clinical and drug treatment outcome at follow-up, with reports of relapse ranging from 25% to 70% (30,36). Less data are available at follow-up for the MAOI antidepressants, but here again clinical experience suggests that relapse rates are comparable. The similar relapse rates after both antidepressant and benzodiazepine therapy suggest the need for continuation therapy. They also suggest that relapse is not simply an iatrogenic by-product of benzodiazepine therapy.

Generalized Anxiety Disorder

We are not aware of any published research that reports reliable relapse/recurrence rates for GAD patients treated with *antidepressants*. With *azapirones*, however, Rickels and Schweizer (48) found GAD patients treated with buspirone for 6 months to have a lower relapse at 3 years post treatment than did patients treated with clorazepate.

A few studies have examined relapse/recurrence rates after acute benzodiazepine therapy. Rickels et al. (42) reported an 81% anxiety recurrence rate at 1 year for patients who had received 4 weeks of benzodiazepine therapy. In another study, Rickels et al. (44) treated 138 GAD patients for a minimum of 6 weeks with diazepam. A recurrence rate of 63% was reported at 1 year, with 50% of the patients sustaining improvement for at least 3 months. Overall, it appears that 60–80% of GAD patients (at least the ones applying for drug therapy) require additional treatment by 1 year.

Another index of the inadequacy of acute benzodiazepine treatment is the percent of patients who relapse in the week or two immediately after discontinuation of acute treatment. In a 4-week treatment study utilizing both a long-and a short-half-life benzodiazepine, 30% of patients had relapsed by 2 weeks (46). In fact, approximately 20% achieved HAM-A scores that were equal to or higher than their pretreatment baseline, indicating a rebound anxiety that, it has been speculated, might be an early precursor of the benzodiazepine withdrawal syndrome. Other studies have reported similar rates of rebound anxiety after short-term benzodiazepine therapy, ranging from 25% to 44% (17). It is unclear what percent of patients experience rebound anxiety as a transient and self-limited phenomenon, and in what percent it serves to trigger a recrudescence of the underlying generalized anxiety.

Relapse/Recurrence Rates After Psychotherapy

The published outcome research for the psychotherapy of GAD is hampered by small sample sizes and low-power, frequently inadequate inclusion/exclusion criteria and characterization of the study populations, as well as a variety of other methodological problems. Therapies that appear to have the most well-established efficacy are cognitive therapy (with various degrees of behavior therapy added in) and anxiety management therapies. Despite poor power, the tentative evidence to date consistently suggests some degree of acute efficacy for the psychotherapies (6,9,16,40). Of special interest is that 3- to 12-month follow-up suggests that GAD treated by cognitive or anxiety management therapy may be unusually effective in sustaining improvement, with less than one-third of patients relapsing in the immediate 6- to 12-month follow-up period. If these results are confirmed, especially in drug versus psychotherapy trials, it would be a significant advance in the long-term management of GAD.

Social Phobia

Much less treatment research has been conducted on social phobia. Treatment experience with MAOI antidepressants consists of at least two open-label studies (63,64) and three controlled studies (19,24), all of which suggest efficacy over 8–16 weeks of acute treatment. Only one of these studies (69) examined efficacy during continuation therapy for up to 1 year. This latter study found efficacy to be sustained. None of the studies examined rates of relapse or recurrence after MAOI discontinuation.

Clonazepam has also shown pilot evidence of efficacy, but only in open-label studies (13). Fluoxetine and buspirone have both also been used successfully in short-term pilot studies (55). Again, no data were reported for post-drug relapse or recurrence rates, so no conclusions can be drawn concerning whether there is a role for continuation therapy. Anecdotal experience, though, with all its shortcomings, does suggest, at least for the MAOIs and clonazepam, that relapse frequently occurs within 3–6 months of discontinuing short-term treatment.

LEVEL OF DISTRESS, DISABILITY, AND QUALITY OF LIFE IMPAIRMENT ASSOCIATED WITH ANXIETY DISORDERS

It can be concluded with some degree of confidence (albeit with methodological caveats) that the evidence is fairly strong and very consistent and that the three anxiety disorders all have substantial chronicity. But to what extent is this chronicity associated with significant distress, disability, and impairment in functioning and quality of life? In the end, judgments about the benefits and risks of long-term anxiolytic therapy must be placed in this broader context.

The evidence regarding disability and quality of life is not substantial, but appears to be fairly consistent as far as it goes. For *panic disorder,* significant psychosocial impairment appears to be a common feature of the disorder. In the 1979 National Survey of Psychotherapeutic Drug Use, significant proportions of respondents with anxiety syndromes reported impaired role performance due to psychological and other factors: for panic/agoraphobia, 41% and 25%; for other phobias, 33% and 23%; for general anxiety, 22% and 45% (66). The rates for panic/agoraphobia were comparable to those for major depression in the same study: 47% and 31%. Substantial proportions of respondents with anxiety syndromes utilized treatment during the year prior to the survey: panic/agoraphobia, 62%; other phobias, 32%; general anxiety, 50%; compared to 26% of the general population (67).

The ECA survey reported that approximately 58% of their community sample of persons with *panic disorder* had some degree of financial disability, whether welfare, disability, or social security payments (28,51). Massion et al. (29), reporting on 234 panic patients in an outpatient setting, found approximately 50% to be employed full time and found 27% to be receiving some form of public assistance. In the ECA community survey, 86% had sought medical outpatient evaluation and treatment in the previous 6 months (compared to 8% of persons without panic), and 51% had sought mental health evaluation and treatment. In keeping with these figures, 35% of the community ECA sample rated their physical health as fair to poor, and 38% rated their emotional health as fair to poor (28). In the ECA survey, 7% of panic patients without comorbid depression reported a history of suicide attempts, while Massion and colleagues (29) found a rate of 3%. In a large group of high utilizers of medical outpatient care, Katon et al. (20) found a 12% rate of current panic disorder and a 30% rate of lifetime panic. This overrepresentation of panic disorder is especially high in medical subspecialty clinics, where rates of panic range from 20% to 50% for medically unexplained episodes of chest pain, tinnitus, dizziness, irritable bowel, and chronic fatigue (7,27).

For *GAD,* the best information currently available probably comes from the ECA community survey (51) and

from a multisite survey of psychiatric outpatients (29). The overall picture for GAD is one of significant psychosocial impairment (albeit somewhat less severe than is observed with panic disorder), with 38% of ECA subjects and 71% of outpatients characterizing their emotional health as fair to poor; 27% and 25%, respectively, were receiving disability payments, and only about one-half worked full time. Of those who were working, 38% of the patient population had missed at least 1 week of work in the past year due to their anxiety. The ECA survey found a strong correlation between occupational status/income and GAD, with presence of GAD being associated with (a) a threefold greater likelihood of working at a low occupational level and (b) a more than twofold greater likelihood of earning less than $10,000 per year. Medically, 35% of the ECA sample with GAD, and 23% of the patient population of Massion et al. (29), reported that their physical health was fair to poor. This latter finding is corroborated in an outpatient medical setting by Katon et al. (20), who found that 24% of all high utilizers of medical outpatient care had a diagnosis of GAD.

The early onset and the high degree of chronicity, disability, and medical and psychiatric morbidity associated with GAD have led some researchers to speculate that GAD might not be an independent diagnosis, but instead a trait or vulnerability factor that predisposes to later problems. Whatever its status, the chronicity and disability associated with GAD make it an unlikely candidate for a cure or sustained remission after short-term drug therapy.

Quality-of-life issues and the degree of disability associated with *social phobia* have been much less well studied. Unfortunately, social phobia was not analyzed as a separate part of the ECA survey, so good community-based information is not available.

As can be seen, the anxiety disorders are not only chronic in nature, but are often accompanied by a wide range of moderate impairments in both psychosocial functioning and quality of life. The impairment and early onset of these disorders raise questions about what developmental distortions they may produce and what benefits early treatment may provide.

THE DEVELOPMENT OF COMORBIDITY DURING THE LONGITUDINAL COURSE OF ANXIETY DISORDERS

One of the most important issues in the long-term treatment of the anxiety disorders is the presence of comorbidity. Any long-term anxiolytic treatment strategy must take account of the high rates of comorbidity that appear to develop during the longitudinal course of panic, GAD, and social phobia—and that complicate these disorders, in fact, from their very inception. Comorbidity rates for adolescent anxiety disorders have been reported to range from approximately 20% to 60%, with higher rates recorded for patient samples that are under treatment (21).

It is well-established that comorbidity is significantly higher for patients seeking treatment than for persons not in treatment in the community. Nonetheless, even community surveys suggest a high rate of comorbidity, especially for GAD. In the ECA survey (51), 1-year prevalence estimates, reflecting *current* comorbidity, showed that approximately 25% of patients with a diagnosis of GAD also suffered from either panic or major depression, while an additional 30% (approximately) suffered from another Axis I diagnosis, leaving only about 40–45% of patients with "pure" GAD (at least from an Axis I standpoint, though the extent to which social phobia might have been an undetected source of comorbidity is unclear). This figure reports only 1-year prevalence rates for comorbidity, and as such is a likely underestimate because anxiety has been shown frequently to evolve into either depression or panic (10) over time.

Patient surveys show even higher rates of comorbidity, though the samples studied are obviously much smaller. Massion et al. (29) found that of 123 psychiatric outpatients diagnosed with GAD, 51% had a history of comorbid panic disorder. When these patients were edited out, 46% of the remaining patients had a history of comorbid major depression and 27% had social phobia. Overall, only 1.6% (2 of 123 patients in a psychiatric treatment setting) were felt to have "pure" GAD, with no history of comorbid depressive or anxiety disorders. Similarly, Brown and Barlow (10) have reported high comorbidity rates for outpatients with a principal diagnosis of GAD. Thirty-six percent suffered from concurrent panic disorder with or without agoraphobia, 29% suffered from concurrent social phobia, and 29% suffered from concurrent major depression or dysthymic disorder. In another study (37) of outpatients who had been recruited through the media, 34% had a history of major depression and 17% had a history of social phobia (a panic disorder diagnosis was a reason for exclusion).

The ECA community survey (51), as well as the Zurich cohort of Angst (2), found that 73% of patients with *panic disorder* had other comorbid conditions. Massion et al. (29), in their outpatient sample of 294, reported the following rates of comorbidity, depending on whether the patient was diagnosed with panic alone versus panic with agoraphobia: social phobia, 6% versus 15%; major depression, 27% versus 22%; OCD, 10% versus 7%. Twenty percent of panic patients suffered from comorbid GAD, but these patients were excluded from the previously reported comorbidity rates. Brown and Barlow (10), in a sample of 232 outpatients with a panic disorder diagnosis (both with and without agoraphobia), reported comorbid social phobia ranging from 6% to 36%, comorbid GAD ranging from 20% to 36%, and comorbid major depression ranging from 7% to 36%, largely depending on the presence and severity of the associated agoraphobia. In a sample of patients with panic disorder alone versus panic with agoraphobia who were recruited for a trial of psychotherapeutic medication, substantially higher rates of comorbidity were found; for example, social phobia, 26% versus 64%; GAD, 32% versus 68%; major depression, 26% versus 68% (61).

Comorbidity patterns for *social phobia* are less well-studied. The ECA community survey offers no data on social phobia. Brown and Barlow (10) reported the following comorbidity rates among 76 outpatients with a principal diagnosis of social phobia: panic disorder, 9%; GAD, 17%; major depression, 11%; and dysthymic disorder, 13%.

Substance abuse and Axis II personality disorders constitute two other important, but often neglected, categories of comorbidity which may complicate the natural history of the anxiety disorders and which must be taken into account when planning treatment interventions over time (39,62). Studies of *alcoholic patients* suggest a range of 25–45% for comorbid anxiety disorders, with social phobia and panic/agoraphobia being the most prevalent (60). Conversely, prevalence rates of alcoholism in anxiety disorder populations range from 15% to 40% (29,37,61,63). The ECA community survey found, not surprisingly, much lower rates of alcohol dependence/abuse. Van Ameringen et al. (68) have reported a 28% rate of alcoholism in a group of outpatient social phobics.

Comorbidity rates for *substance abuse* are lower for all three anxiety disorders, ranging from about 10% to 36% in patient samples (29,37,61). Again, these rates are much lower in the ECA community survey (51).

Multiple studies have reported rates of comorbidity for the anxiety disorders and *Axis II disorders,* most commonly the anxious "Cluster C" type. Axis II comorbidity rates for panic/agoraphobia generally range from about 30% to 60% (18,37), with more severe agoraphobia being associated with increased rates (18). Axis II comorbidity rates for GAD have been reported in the same 30–60% range (37,53).

As can be seen from the above review, comorbidity is the rule and not the exception in the clinical picture of the anxiety disorders. Long-term treatment planning cannot be undertaken except on the assumption that the majority of patients suffering from a principal anxiety disorder diagnosis also suffer from another disorder, or will suffer from one in the near future. This clinical reality makes it important to maintain an index of suspicion concerning the development of other disorders, and to carefully reevaluate the patient at intervals. This is especially true if patients fail to respond fully to a course of drug therapy or if an initial good response is lost. In both instances, unsuspected comorbidity is frequently the culprit.

The high rates of comorbidity among anxiety and depressive disorders also raise serious questions about the true independence of these disorders. An alternative way of conceptualizing comorbidity, with depression for example, is to view the two disorders as varying manifestations of one underlying diathesis—that is, two phenotypic expressions of a common underlying "genotype." Such a view has been proposed by Tyrer et al. (65), who speak of a "general neurotic syndrome." Recent genetic analyses of women suffering from major depression and GAD (22) provide some confirmation for this perspective, with results suggesting that the genetic vulnerability for *both* disorders is largely shared.

EVIDENCE FOR SUSTAINED EFFICACY (PREVENTION OF RELAPSE AND RECURRENCE) DURING CONTINUATION AND MAINTENANCE THERAPY

Previous sections of this chapter have established that the anxiety disorders are frequently chronic conditions associated with (a) a high degree of comorbidity and (b) impairment in both psychosocial functioning and quality of life. Furthermore, evidence has been presented that acute (4–12 weeks) drug therapy frequently results in early return of symptoms (relapse) or subsequent episodes (recurrence) when treatment is discontinued. What is the evidence, though, that continuation therapy is effective in preventing relapse, or that maintenance therapy is effective in preventing recurrences?

Unfortunately, there is little controlled research addressing these issues for panic/agoraphobia or GAD, and none for social phobia. The evidence for the efficacy of continuation and/or maintenance therapy of *panic disorder* is currently being studied in an NIMH-funded multicenter trial that compares imipramine to a form of cognitive-behavioral therapy.

Schweizer et al. (58) have conducted an 8-month, placebo-controlled study of continuation therapy for *panic disorder* with alprazolam and imipramine that found sustained efficacy for both compounds with no dose escalation, suggesting an absence of tolerance to the therapeutic effect. When drug was discontinued after 8 months of maintenance therapy, at 3 weeks post discontinuation, approximately 25% of patients had experienced a return of their panic attacks. At 1 year follow-up, 30% of patients had a recurrence of their panic, and 49% had restarted or never stopped their medication (50). Of course, the selection bias that was likely operating in the choice of patients for the initial study, as well as the naturalistic nature of the follow-up, makes this only a suggestive pilot study.

Preliminary evidence for the efficacy of continuation therapy of *GAD* comes from two studies (43,47). In both studies the benzodiazepine therapy achieved sustained remission of anxious symptomatology with no tolerance and no dose escalation over a 6-month period. In the second study, buspirone also achieved a comparable sustained remission of anxious symptoms, though the significantly higher attrition rate by patients treated with buspirone complicates the interpretation of results. In both studies, about 25% of the patients experienced a return of their initial anxiety within 4 weeks of drug discontinuation.

There is no good published evidence for the sustained efficacy of either antidepressants or the benzodiazepines in the continuation or maintenance treatment of *social phobia*. The only published reports found both tranylcypromine (69) and clonazepam (13) to sustain efficacy over an 11- to 12-month period of treatment.

The 1979 National Survey of Psychotherapeutic Drug Use (67) indicates that a small fraction of patients with anxiety syndromes take psychotherapeutic medications for a year or more (panic/agoraphobia, 25%; other phobias, 6%; general anxiety, 6%). On the other hand, experts in the pharmacotherapy of these disorders, aware that they are chronic, severe, and disabling, generally recommend vigorous, long-term treatment. Here, as is so often the case, clinicians have had to use their best judgment in addressing clinical problems that lie beyond the scope of existing empirical evidence. Whether long-term drug treatment represents effective continuation or maintenance therapy, or patients continue to take medication because it elicits only a partial response, is uncertain. Two of the present authors have reported HAM-A scores of 16 in anxious patients with a mean of 6 years of benzodiazepine therapy, suggesting that long-term drug therapy, at least in this population, may have been continued even though (and perhaps because!) it was less than effective. The public health interest urgently requires clinical research to address these long-term issues of efficacy.

RISKS OF LONG-TERM MEDICATION TREATMENT

The efficacy obtained from drug therapy must always be weighed carefully against the potential adverse effects of the drug. This is especially true when it comes to long-term or maintenance drug therapy. What is considered tolerable, and even safe, during acute treatment may be neither of the above during chronic administration. This section will focus most intensively on the safety of long-term administration of the benzodiazepines. Not only have they been the object of intense scrutiny and concern, both publicly and scientifically, over the past 10–15 years (see ref. 71 for an excellent review), but they continue to be widely prescribed, sometimes for long-term therapy. The most recent survey data indicate that 1.6% of the adult population in 1980 took benzodiazepine for 12 months or longer in the previous reporting year (32). Some decline in long-term usage appears to have occurred since then, but it is still estimated that approximately 1% of the adult population has currently or recently received long-term benzodiazepine therapy.

Benzodiazepines

Discussion of the safety of the benzodiazepines during chronic use can be usefully reviewed under two headings: (i) the psychological and behavioral effects and (ii) the medical or physiological effects.

A variety of psychological and behavioral effects have been attributed to the benzodiazepines when chronically administered. These include: persistent attentional, psychomotor, cognitive, and memory-impairing effects; abuse liability; physical dependence and withdrawal; post-withdrawal craving; and effects on coping and stress response capabilities. A brief review of each of these potential safety concerns is necessary in order to obtain a more complete picture of the benefit–risk equation regarding long-term therapy.

Attentional, Psychomotor, Cognitive, and Memory Effects

Substantial tolerance appears to develop to the attentional and psychomotor effects of benzodiazepines, beginning after the first few weeks of acute administration. The actual clinical significance (e.g., effects on driving ability) of subtle residual impairments, or the potentiation of these impairments by low levels of alcohol consumption that otherwise would pose no problem, is uncertain. Results of laboratory assessments, including driving simulation, have had very variable and contradictory results (see refs. 1 and 71 for reviews). But there appears to be some persistent attentional and psychomotor impairment that may be relevant to the execution of complex real-world tasks.

Preliminary research suggests that cognitive tasks and (especially) short-term memory tasks continue to be impaired even after long-term (5–10 years) daily administration of benzodiazepines (25), apparently exhibiting less tolerance than psychomotor function. The existence of differential rates of tolerance development is an intriguing phenomenon, and may depend on subtle regional differences in the monomeric constituents of the benzodiazepine receptor. The amnestic effect of benzodiazepines, which appears to be relatively resistant to tolerance in humans, probably has a hippocampal substrate. It should be cautioned that statistically "significant" amnestic findings ascertained, for example, using meaningless word lists may have little generalizability to life situations. Furthermore, since moderate-to-severe anxiety frequently has been noted to impair performance, the net effect of benzodiazepine treatment may be an enhancement of performance. Nonetheless, the subtle effects on learning and motivation of chronic, mild benzodiazepine-induced amnesia have not been well-studied.

A final behavioral effect for which there is no good evidence that tolerance does, or does not, develop with long-term benzodiazepine administration is irritability and hostility.

Abuse Liability

Benzodiazepines have a *potential* for recreational abuse (1,71). But *actual* recreational abuse appears to occur principally in persons who abuse other drugs (see ref. 71 for review).

The abuse liability of the benzodiazepines in drug and alcohol abusers appears to stem in large part from marked individual differences in the euphoriant effects of benzodiazepines. Drug addicts, alcoholics, and even the nonalcoholic sons of alcoholics appear to be much more susceptible to the euphorogenic properties of the benzodiazepines (11). In most other populations, even among anxious persons (14), benzodiazepines do not appear to have much of a euphoric effect. In fact, the reinforcing properties of the benzodiazepines appear to be relatively low compared to every other drug of abuse (71). The reinforcing property of a drug appears to be an important behavioral correlate of abuse liability that tends to be fairly consistent across primate species. Even when one corrects for availability, diazepam and alprazolam are more widely abused in at-risk populations. It is unknown whether this reported effect is due to methodological problems with the adjustment for availability or to the rapidity of onset of action (lipophilicity, etc), or to differences in the intrinsic efficacy of the benzodiazepine at the receptor.

Another indicator of abuse liability that has been identified is drug liking or preference in normal human subjects. Here, again, the benzodiazepines appear to elicit much less drug liking than do traditional drugs of abuse (14,31).

Physical Dependence and Withdrawal

An ineluctable consequence of chronic benzodiazepine therapy is physical dependence, along with the likelihood of developing a withdrawal syndrome upon drug discontinuation. The clinical picture of benzodiazepine withdrawal is not always easy to distinguish from anxiety, though the temporal pattern of onset is of some help. Further confounding the clinical picture is that the experience of benzodiazepine withdrawal may serve, in turn, to trigger a recrudescence of the patient's underlying anxiety. Common symptoms of the benzodiazepine withdrawal syndrome consist of increased anxious mood and nervousness, insomnia, restlessness, tension, irritability, lethargy, nausea, depression, hyperacusis, and tinnitus. There appear to be no pathognomonic symptoms that are unique to the withdrawal syndrome and that do not commonly occur in anxiety disorders. After abrupt discontinuation of a short half-life benzodiazepine (e.g., alprazolam or lorazepam), withdrawal symptoms begin to appear within 6–12 hr, with a peak severity generally at 2–4 days. Symptoms usually subside within 1–3 weeks. After abrupt discontinuation of a long half-life benzodiazepine (e.g., diazepam or clorazepate), withdrawal symptoms begin to appear within 24–36 hr, peak at 4–7 days, and subside within 2–4 weeks. The benzodiazepine withdrawal syndrome, unless complicated by other medical or psychiatric illness or by other drug or alcohol problems, can be managed in an outpatient setting.

Several factors have been identified that appear to contribute to the development of benzodiazepine withdrawal and that add to its severity. The first of these is *duration* of therapy. Rebound anxiety (to a level above pretreatment baseline) has been observed after as little as 4 weeks of benzodiazepine treatment (46). Such transient rebound reactions are thought to be the prodromal signs of a developing pattern of dependence and withdrawal. By 3–4 months, physical dependence is likely to have been established, and a withdrawal syndrome upon benzodiazepine discontinuation can clearly be observed in a significant number of patients. There is no good evidence that longer durations of maintenance therapy beyond 12 months contributes to greater dependence and withdrawal liability (49,57).

A second factor that contributes to dependence and withdrawal is the *daily dose* of the drug. It is important to note, though, that dependence and withdrawal do not require aggressive dosing. Patients treated with as low as 5–10 mg of diazepam or its equivalent have been noted to experience withdrawal reactions upon drug discontinuation. The clinical implications of the dose and duration of treatment factors is that only the most short-term treatment is without risk of physical dependence and withdrawal. The medical–legal implication of this situation is that information on dependence and withdrawal effects should probably be a routine part of the educational introduction of all patients to the benefits and risks of benzodiazepine therapy.

Several other factors contribute to the severity of benzodiazepine withdrawal. These include the *rate of taper* (obviously abrupt discontinuation poses a greater problem than a gradual taper over 4–8 weeks) and the presence of Axis I and II disorders. *Residual anxiety, panic,* and *depressive symptoms* also predict greater difficulty with withdrawal.

One unresolved issue is whether the benzodiazepine withdrawal syndrome may persist, in some form and in some patients, for many months, or even years. A subset of patients subjectively reported ongoing symptoms and complaints (3), and a "post-withdrawal syndrome" has even been proposed (64). The pharmacologic mechanism of this proposed state of persistent withdrawal is unclear, though a putative "receptor shift" has been suggested. It is, of course, difficult to disentangle persistent symptoms of withdrawal from a recrudescence of anxiety. The fact that the symptoms differ from a patient's previous experience of anxiety is no guarantee that an iatrogenic state has been triggered, because symptoms of anxiety can change over time. It is also of interest that two of the authors (Rickels and Schweizer) have noted an absence of any reports of persistent withdrawal states in abstinent patients with a history of benzodiazepine dependence, but in whom benzodiazepines were not prescribed for anxiety. In most cases, such post-benzodiazepine discontinuation symptoms are most likely related to the patient's Axis I and Axis II disorders. Still, it is a topic of concern, and deserves further research, whether chronic administration of benzodiazepines may in some way permanently alter the benzodiazepine-GABAergic system.

Post-withdrawal Craving of Drug and Restarting Benzodiazepine

It is an almost universal feature of drugs of abuse that they intermittently evoke craving in the user long after the withdrawal syndrome has subsided. Alcohol, tobacco, cocaine, amphetamines, opiates, and even coffee engender cravings in the months and years after drug discontinuation. Preliminary research (26) suggests that there is little or no craving associated with long-term dependence on benzodiazepines. Certainly former benzodiazepine-dependent patients do restart their benzodiazepine, but resumption of benzodiazepine use is almost exclusively caused by a recurrence of symptoms of anxiety. Naturalistic follow-up studies of chronic benzodiazepine users find a clear trend over time toward lower daily doses, and eventual discontinuation. The pharmacoepidemiological data (32) also indicate that the vast majority of regular daily benzodiazepine use continues less than a year (85%) and usually less than a month (67%).

Long-Term Medical/Physiological Effects

The risk of adverse medical or physiological effects from chronic benzodiazepine therapy has not been systematically studied. Medical evaluations of over 400 benzodiazepine-dependent patients (mean duration of use: >5 years), which included blood chemistries, complete blood count with differential, urinalysis, and electrocardiogram, have yielded no obvious abnormalities (Rickels et al., *personal communication*). A question has been raised concerning whether chronic benzodiazepine treatment might be associated with increased ventricular–brain ratios on computerized tomography scans. Several studies have yielded conflicting results on this subject, but because a variety of other comorbid medical factors, particularly alcohol use, were not excluded, the issue remains unresolved (1).

Several other physiological effects appear to result from chronic benzodiazepine treatment. Preliminary data suggest that chronic treatment alters the functional status of one or more components of the benzodiazepine–GABAergic receptor complex (33). One of the hypothesized mechanisms for benzodiazepine withdrawal suggests that the symptoms can be explained by the "overdrive" of downstream noradrenergic, serotonergic, and cholinergic receptors that have been released from inhibitory control (that had been previously augmented by the exogenously administered benzodiazepine agonists).

Parenthetically, clinical anxiety may be due to a subsensitivity of the benzodiazepine receptors (52). If additional data establish that a functional deficit in benzodiazepine receptors is one of the pathological substrates of anxiety, then the rationale for maintenance therapy with benzodiazepines would be greatly strengthened.

Antidepressants and Azapirones

Long-term safety assessments of the tricyclic antidepressants, and of the newer SSRI antidepressants, has long been a routine part of the drug development and FDA approval process. Most safety research on antidepressants has been conducted on depressed populations, but from a behavioral and medical standpoint one might tentatively extrapolate to a population of patients suffering from anxiety disorders. Safety and benefit–risk issues relating to antidepressants as a class are discussed elsewhere in this volume (see Chapters 89, 90, and 91). Noyes et al. (36) have reported safety data on long-term use of tricyclic antidepressants in a population of panic patients followed-up naturalistically for 1–4 years. They found that 35% of these patients were unable to tolerate tricyclic antidepressants (TCAs) and discontinued them. Early discontinuations (in the first 6 weeks) were most commonly for overstimulation, orthostatic reactions, and allergic reactions. Late discontinuations were most commonly for weight gain and persistent anticholinergic effects. Forty percent of long-term patients reported weight gain, with the mean weight gained being 22 pounds.

Abrupt discontinuation of long-term antidepressants (TCAs, MAOIs, and short half-life SSRIs) has also been reported to result in a withdrawal reaction (15). The exact prevalence, or consequences, of such withdrawal reactions has not been systematically studied for panic disorder patients, though it appears to be correlated with the rapidity of the taper schedule. For TCAs, the withdrawal reaction may be related to cholinergic rebound, with common symptoms consisting of insomnia, nausea, headache, and tremor. For the MAOIs, vivid dreams associated with rapid eye movement (REM) rebound are also observed. The extent to which these withdrawal reactions trigger a recrudescence of panic is uncertain.

Buspirone appears to be safe in maintenance therapy (41,47). Unlike the TCAs, no significant side effects were found to emerge with long-term therapy. In general, buspirone was well-tolerated during maintenance treatment. No withdrawal reaction has been reported to occur upon discontinuation.

BENEFITS AND RISKS OF COMBINED TREATMENTS

Combined Drug Therapies

Surveys of prescribing practices suggest that perhaps one-quarter to one-third of anxiolytic drug therapy consists of treatment with combinations of drugs. The addition of a second or third drug may be clinically indicated because of the presence of a comorbid condition—most commonly either another anxiety disorder or an affective illness. But virtually no controlled research exists concerning the effectiveness of long-term drug treatment for comorbid conditions with one, not to mention two, drugs.

Combined Drug and Psychotherapy

Again, it is common clinical practice to combine anxiolytic drug therapy with some form of psychotherapy. Yet there are virtually no controlled studies that establish the clinical indications or additive efficacy of such treatment. Nor can it be confidently predicted that the addition of psychotherapy to a drug regimen, or vice versa, will result in enhanced efficacy. In fact, experienced cognitive therapy researchers (A. T. Beck, *personal communication*, May 1993) believe that the efficacy of cognitive therapy in panic disorder is *reduced* by the concomitant administration of benzodiazepines. The reason for this, if it is confirmed, is uncertain. Perhaps the cognitive effects of benzodiazepines hamper psychotherapy, or perhaps learning under the influence of a benzodiazepine does not carry over to the drug-free state (state-dependent learning).

NEED FOR FUTURE RESEARCH ON MAINTENANCE TREATMENT

The high chronicity and/or recurrence rate of the major anxiety disorders suggest that studies of the safety and efficacy of maintenance therapy should be integral to the assessment of any drug or psychotherapy. Acute symptom reduction is important to achieve, but is a hollow victory over the distress and disability associated with clinical anxiety if it cannot be sustained.

Research questions, largely unanswered, concerning maintenance treatment of GAD, social phobia, and panic disorder are legion and include the following: What constitutes an adequate course of maintenance drug therapy? What are the predictors (e.g., duration, severity, rate of recurrence, comorbidity) that suggest the need for further continuation therapy? What are optimal doses for both maintenance and continuation therapy? When, if ever, are intermittent medication strategies indicated as opposed to maintenance or continuation therapy? Does any further clinical improvement accrue from maintenance therapy compared to what is achieved by acute therapy? Is there any prophylactic benefit, in terms of long-term outcome, from continuation therapy? What is the safety of continuation drug therapy—including withdrawal, rebound, and other behavioral effects? Does tolerance develop during the course of maintenance or continuation drug therapy, or is efficacy maintained? What is the optimal way to discontinue maintenance or continuation drug therapy? How should emergent comorbidity be optimally managed? When are combination drug therapies indicated, and what are the safety and efficacy of such combination therapies? What is the comparative safety and long-term efficacy of drug versus psychotherapy? Can response predictors be identified for choosing drug versus psychotherapy? What are the clinical indications, safety, and efficacy of combined drug and psychotherapy?

All of these questions can, and should, be asked, not only for each anxiety diagnosis, but for each treatment modality: benzodiazepine, TCA, MAOI, SSRI, azapirones, cognitive therapy, dynamic therapy, and so on. The investigation of the long-term treatment and outcome of the anxiety disorders is a difficult area of research. It is afflicted with its own methodological problems that daunt even the most seasoned researcher who dares to enter this largely uncharted domain. These problems include: issues of sample size; patient retention over time; the influence of retention strategies on outcome; how to handle a host of potentially significant intervening variables (e.g., nonstudy medication usage, life events, etc.) that cannot be simply excluded as they can in acute treatment studies; how and when to randomize for maintenance therapy; how to handle emergent comorbidity; how to handle taper and discontinuation of study medication; how to undertake long-term follow-up post study; and how to determine appropriate outcome measures.

ACKNOWLEDGMENTS

Preparation of this chapter was supported, in part, by USPHS Research Grant MHO-8957.

REFERENCES

1. American Psychiatric Association. *Benzodiazepine dependence, toxicity, and abuse.* A Task Force Report of the American Psychiatric Association, 1990.
2. Angst J, Vollrath M, Merikangas KR, Ernst C. Comorbidity of anxiety and depression in the Zurich cohort study of young adults. In: Maser and Cloninger, eds. *Comorbidity of mood and anxiety disorders.* Washington, DC: American Psychiatric Press, 1990; 123–137.
3. Ashton H. Benzodiazepine withdrawal: an unfinished story. *Br Med J* 1984;288:1135–1140.
4. Ballenger JC, Burrows GD, DuPont RL Jr, Lesser IM, Noyes R Jr,

Pecknold JC, Rifkin A, Swinson RP. Alprazolam in panic disorder and agoraphobia: results from a multicenter trial. I. Efficacy in short-term treatment. *Arch Gen Psychiatry* 1988;45:413–422.
5. Barlow DH, Blanchard EB, Vermilyea JA, Vermilyea BB, DiNardo PA. Generalized anxiety and generalized anxiety disorder: description and reconceptualization. *Am J Psychiatry* 1986;143:40–44.
6. Barlow DH, Cohen AS, Waddell MT, Vermilyea BB, Klosko JS, Blanchard EB, Di Nardo PA. Panic and generalized anxiety disorders: nature and treatment. *Behav Ther* 1984;15:431–449.
7. Beitman BD, Mukerji V, Lamberti JW, Schmid L, De Rosear L, Kushner M, Flaker G, Basha I. Panic disorder in patients with chest pain and angiographically normal coronary arteries. *Am J Cardiol* 1989;63:1399–1403.
8. Black DW, Wesner R, Bowers W, Gabel J. A comparison of fluvoxamine, cognitive therapy, and placebo in the treatment of panic disorder. *Arch Gen Psychiatry* 1993;50:44–50.
9. Borkovec TD, Mathews AM. Treatment of nonphobic anxiety disorders: a comparison of nondirective, cognitive, and coping desensitization therapy. *J Consult Clin Psychol* 1988;56:877–884.
10. Brown TA, Barlow DH. Comorbidity among anxiety disorders: implications for treatment and DSM-IV. *J Consult Clin Psychol* 1992;60:835–844.
11. Ciraulo DA, Sands BF, Shader RI. Critical review of liability for benzodiazepine abuse among alcoholics. *Am J Psychiatry* 1988;145:1501–1506.
12. Cross-National Collaborative Panic Study, Second Phase Investigators. Drug treatment of panic disorder. Comparative efficacy of alprazolam, imipramine, and placebo. *Br J Psychiatry* 1992;160: 191–202.
13. Davidson JR, Ford SM, Smith RD, Potts NL. Long-term treatment of social phobia with clonazepam. *J Clin Psychiatry* 1991;52 (Suppl):16–20.
14. de Wit H, McCracken SM, Uhlenhuth EH, Johanson CE. Diazepam preference in subjects seeking treatment for anxiety. *NIDA Res Monogr* 1987;76:248–254.
15. Dilsaver SC. Antidepressant withdrawal syndromes: phenomenology and pathophysiology. *Acta Psychiatr Scand* 1989;79:113–117.
16. Durham RC, Turvey AA. Cognitive therapy vs behavior therapy in the treatment of chronic general anxiety. *Behav Res Ther* 1987;25:229–234.
17. Fontaine R, Chouinard G, Annable A. Rebound anxiety in anxious patients after abrupt withdrawal of benzodiazepine treatment. *Am J Psychiatry* 1984;141:848–852.
18. Friedman CJ, Shear MK, Frances AJ. DSM-III personality disorders in panic patients. *J Personal Dis* 1987;1:132–135.
19. Gelernter CS, Stein MB, Tancer ME, Uhde TW. An examination of syndromal validity and diagnostic subtypes in social phobia and panic disorder. *J Clin Psychiatry* 1992;53:23–27.
20. Katon W, Von Korff M, Lin E, Lipscomb P, Russo J, Wagner E, Polk E. Distressed high utilizers of medical care: DSM-III-R diagnoses and treatment needs. *Gen Hosp Psychiatry* 1990;12:355–362.
21. Kendall PC, Kortlander E, Chansky TE, Brady EU. Comorbidity of anxiety and depression in youth: treatment implications. *J Consult Clin Psychol* 1992;60:869–880.
22. Kendler KS, Neale MC, Kessler RC, Heath AC, Eaves LJ. Major depression and generalized anxiety disorder. Same genes, (partly) different environments? *Arch Gen Psychiatry* 1992;49:716–722.
23. Lewinsohn PM, Hops H, Roberts RE, Seeley JR, Andrews JA. Adolescent psychopathology. I. Prevalence and incidence of depression and other DSM-III-R disorders in high school students. *J Abnorm Psychol* 1993;102:133–144.
24. Liebowitz MR, Schneier F, Campeas R, Hollander E, Hatterer J, Fyer A, Gorman J, Papp L, Davies S, Gully R. Phenelzine vs atenolol in social phobia. A placebo-controlled comparison. *Arch Gen Psychiatry* 1992;49:290–300.
25. Lucki I, Rickels K. The effect of anxiolytic drugs on memory in anxious subjects. In: Hindmarch I, Ott H, eds. *Benzodiazepine receptor ligands, memory and information processing.* Berlin: Springer-Verlag, 1988;128–139.
26. Lucki I, Volpicelli JR, Schweizer E. Differential craving between recovering abstinent alcoholic-dependent subjects and therapeutic users of benzodiazepines. *NIDA Res Monogr* 1991;105:322–323.
27. Lydiard RB, Fossey MD, Ballenger JC. Irritable bowel syndrome

in patients with panic disorder [Letter]. *Am J Psychiatry* 1991;148:1614.

28. Markovitz JS, Weissman MM, Ouellette R, Lish JD, Klerman GL. Quality of life in panic disorder. *Arch Gen Psychiatry* 1989;46:984–992.

29. Massion AO, Warshaw MG, Keller MB. Quality of life and psychiatric morbidity in panic disorder and generalized anxiety disorder. *Am J Psychiatry* 1993;150:600–607.

30. Mavissakalian M, Michelson I. Two-year follow-up of exposure and imipramine treatment of agoraphobia. *Am J Psychiatry* 1986;143:1106–1112.

31. McCracken SG, de Wit H, Uhlenhuth EH, Johanson CE. Preference for diazepam in anxious adults. *J Clin Psychopharmacol* 1990;10:190–196.

32. Mellinger GD, Balter MB, Uhlenhuth EH. Prevalence and correlates of the long-term regular use of anxiolytics. *JAMA* 1984;251:375–379.

33. Miller LG, Woolverton S, Greenblatt DJ, Lopez F, Roy RB, Shader RI. Chronic benzodiazepine administration. IV. Rapid development of tolerance and receptor downregulation associated with alprazolam administration. *Biochem Pharmacol* 1989;38:3773–3777.

34. Nagy LM, Krystal JH, Woods SW, Charney DS. Clinical and medication outcome after short-term alprazolam and behavioral group treatment in panic disorder: 2.5 year naturalistic follow-up study. *Arch Gen Psychiatry* 1989;46:993–999.

35. Noyes R, Clancy J, Hoenk PR, Slymen DJ. The prognosis of anxiety disorders. *Arch Gen Psychiatry* 1980;37:173–178.

36. Noyes R, Garvey MJ, Cook BL. Follow-up study of patients with panic disorder and agoraphobia with panic attacks treated with tricyclic antidepressants. *J Affective Disord* 1989;16:249–256.

37. Noyes R Jr, Woodman C, Garvey MJ, Cook BL, Suelzer M, Anderson DJ. Generalized anxiety disorder versus panic disorder: distinguishing characteristics and patterns of comorbidity. *J Nerv Ment Dis* 1992;180:369–379.

38. Pecknold JC, Swinson RP, Kuch K, Lewis CP. Alprazolam in panic disorder and agoraphobia: results from a multicenter trial. III. Discontinuation effects. *Arch Gen Psychiatry* 1988;45:429–436.

39. Pollack MH, Otto MW, Rosenbaum JF, Sachs GS. Personality disorders in patients with panic disorder: association with childhood anxiety disorders, early trauma, comorbidity, and chronicity. *Compr Psychiatry* 1992;33:78–83.

40. Power KG, Simpson RJ, Swanson V, Wallace LA, Feistner ATC, Sharp D. A controlled comparison of cognitive-behavior therapy, diazepam, and placebo, alone and in combination, for the treatment of generalized anxiety disorder. *J Anx Disorders* 1990;4:267–292.

41. Rakel RE. Long-term buspirone therapy for chronic anxiety: a multicenter international study to determine safety. *South Med J* 1990;83:194–198.

42. Rickels K, Case WG, Diamond L. Relapse after short-term drug therapy in neurotic outpatients. *Int Pharmacopsychiatry* 1980;15:186–192.

43. Rickels K, Case WG, Downing RW, Winokur A. Long-term diazepam therapy and clinical outcome. *JAMA* 1983;250:767–771.

44. Rickels K, Case WG, Downing RW, Fridman R. One-year follow-up of anxious patients treated with diazepam. *J Clin Psychopharmacol* 1986;6:32–36.

45. Rickels K, Downing R, Schweizer E, Hassman H. Antidepressants for the treatment of generalized anxiety disorder: a placebo-controlled comparison of imipramine, trazodone and diazepam. *Arch Gen Psychiatry* 1993;50:884–895.

46. Rickels K, Fox IL, Greenblatt DJ. Clorazepate and lorazepam: clinical improvement and rebound anxiety. *Am J Psychiatry* 1988;145:312–317.

47. Rickels K, Schweizer E, Csanalosi I, Case WG, Chung H. Long-term treatment of anxiety and risk of withdrawal. Prospective comparison of clorazepate and buspirone. *Arch Gen Psychiatry* 1988;45:444–450.

48. Rickels K, Schweizer E. The clinical course and long-term management of generalized anxiety disorder. *J Clin Psychopharmacol* 1990;10:101S–110S.

49. Rickels K, Schweizer E, Case WG, Greenblatt DJ. Long-term therapeutic use of benzodiazepines. I. Effects of abrupt discontinuation. *Arch Gen Psychiatry* 1990;47:899–907.

50. Rickels K, Schweizer E, Weiss S, Zavodnick S. Maintenance drug treatment for panic disorder. II. Short and long-term outcome after drug taper. *Arch Gen Psychiatry* 1993;50:61–68.

51. Robins L, Regier DA, eds. *Psychiatric disorder in America.* New York: Free Press, 1991.

52. Roy-Byrne PP, Cowley DL, Greenblatt DJ, Shader RI, Hommer D. Reduced benzodiazepine sensitivity in panic disorder. *Arch Gen Psychiatry* 1990;47:534–538.

53. Sanderson WC, Wetzler S. Chronic anxiety and generalized anxiety disorder: issues in comorbidity. In: Rapee RM, Barlow DH, eds. *Chronic anxiety, generalized anxiety disorder, and mixed anxiety depression.* New York: Guilford Press, 1991;119–135.

54. Schneier FR, Johnson J, Hornig CD, Liebowitz MR, Weissman MM. Social phobia. Comorbidity and morbidity in an epidemiologic sample. *Arch Gen Psychiatry* 1992;49:282–288.

55. Schneier FR, Saoud JB, Campeas R, Fallon BA, Hollander E, Coplan J, Liebowitz MR. Buspirone in social phobia. *J Clin Psychopharmacol* 1993;13:251–256.

56. Schweizer E, Patterson W, Rickels K, Rosenthal M. Double-blind, placebo-controlled study of a once-a-day, sustained-release preparation of alprazolam for the treatment of panic disorder. *Am J Psychiatry* 1993;150:1210–1215.

57. Schweizer E, Rickels K, Case WG, Greenblatt DJ. Long-term therapeutic use of benzodiazepines. II. Effects of gradual taper. *Arch Gen Psychiatry* 1990;47:908–915.

58. Schweizer E, Rickels K, Weiss S, Zavodnick S. Maintenance drug treatment for panic disorder. I. Results of a prospective, placebo-controlled comparison of alprazolam and imipramine. *Arch Gen Psychiatry* 1993;50:51–60.

59. Sheehan DV, Ballenger J, Jacobsen G. Treatment of endogenous anxiety with phobic, hysterical, and hypochondriacal symptoms. *Arch Gen Psychiatry* 1980;37:51–59.

60. Smail P, Stockwell T, Canter S, Hodgson R. Alcohol dependence and phobic anxiety states. I. A prevalence study. *Br J Psychiatry* 1984;144:53–57.

61. Starcevic V, Uhlenhuth EH, Kellner R, Pathak D. Patterns of comorbidity in panic disorder and agoraphobia. *Psychiatry Res* 1992;42:171–183.

62. Starcevic V, Uhlenhuth EH, Kellner R, Pathak D. Comparison of primary and secondary panic disorder: a preliminary report. *J Affective Disord* 1993;27:81–86.

63. Thyer BA, Parrish RT, Himle J, Cameron OG, Curtis GC, Nesse RM. Alcohol abuse among clinically anxious patients. *Behavior Res Ther* 1986;24:357–359.

64. Tyrer P. The benzodiazepine post-withdrawal syndrome [Guest editorial]. *Stress Med* 1991;7:1–2.

65. Tyrer P, Seivewright N, Ferguson B, Tyrer J. The general neurotic syndrome: a coaxial diagnosis of anxiety, depression and personality disorder. *Acta Psychiatr Scand* 1992;85:201–206.

66. Uhlenhuth EH, Balter MB, Mellinger GD, Cisin IH, Clinthorne J. Symptom checklist syndromes in the general population: correlations with psychotherapeutic drug use. *Arch Gen Psychiatry* 1983;40:1167–1173.

67. Uhlenhuth EH, Balter MB, Mellinger GD, Cisin IH, Clinthorne J. Anxiety disorders: prevalence and treatment. *Curr Med Res Opin* 1984;8(Suppl 4):37–47.

68. Van Ameringen M, Mancini C, Styan G, Donison D. Relationship of social phobia with other psychiatric illness. *J Affective Disord* 1991;21:93–99.

69. Versiani M, Mundim FD, Nardi AE, Liebowitz MR. Tranylcypromine in social phobia. *J Clin Psychopharmacol* 1988;8:279–283.

70. Whitaker A, Johnson J, Shaffer D, Rapoport JL, Kalikow K, Walsh T, Davies M, Braiman S, Dolinsky A. Uncommon troubles in young people: prevalence estimates of selected psychiatric disorders in a nonreferred adolescent population. *Arch Gen Psychiatry* 1990;47:487–496.

71. Woods JH, Katz JL, Winger G. Benzodiazepines: use, abuse, and consequences. *Pharmacol Rev* 1992;44:155–186.

*Psychopharmacology: The Fourth
Generation of Progress,* edited by
Floyd E. Bloom and David J. Kupfer.
Raven Press, Ltd., New York © 1995.

CHAPTER 115

Towards an Understanding of the Genetics of Alzheimer's Disease

Corinne L. Lendon and Alison M. Goate

THE CLINICAL AND PATHOLOGICAL FEATURES OF ALZHEIMER'S DISEASE

Alzheimer's disease (AD) is the most common dementia in the elderly. It affects around 5% of the population over 65 years of age, and this figure rises rapidly with increasing age, to approximately 10–20% of those over 80 years old (29). Although the majority of those suffering from AD are elderly, the age of onset can be much younger: some cases as young as 35 have been documented. Clinically, AD is an insidious fatal dementia. The first symptom is usually a loss of short-term memory followed progressively by worsening memory loss, deterioration of mental ability, impairment of visuospatial skills, impairment of the perception and association of language, and progressive physical disability. Death occurs about 10 years after the onset of symptoms, mainly as a result of opportunistic infections. The latter years of a patient's life invariably require constant care, and in many cases they are spent institutionalized. As a result of its profound debilitating nature and the large number of individuals affected (4 million in the United States alone), AD constitutes a major health problem in aging populations.

AD is associated with a characteristic neuropathology: extracellular neuritic plaques and intraneuronal neurofibrillary tangles mainly within the temporal cortex. Histological detection of neuritic plaques and neurofibrillary tangles is used to diagnose "definite" AD when accompanied by a clinical history of "probable" AD dementia (29). The major proteinaceous component of the plaque core is β-A4, an aggregated form of a 39- to 43-amino-acid fragment of the β-amyloid precursor protein (β-APP)

(17). β-A4 deposits occur diffusely and/or as dense cores surrounded by dystrophic neurites that comprise the extracellular neuritic plaques. Neurofibrillary tangles (NFTs) are largely composed of paired helical filaments containing an abnormally phosphorylated form of the microtubule associated protein, tau. The greatest numbers of these inclusions are found in the temporal cortex and hippocampus.

DEPOSITION OF β-A4 IN OTHER DISORDERS

β-A4 deposition is a feature of "normal" aging. However, the number of plaque cores observed are fewer than in AD. Premature β-A4 deposition occurs in several other disorders; for example, AD-like neuropathology occurs in Down's syndrome (DS) subjects who live beyond their third or fourth decade (37). Studies of the brains of subjects with DS over a range of ages indicate that β-A4 deposition is an early event and that NFTs form decades after the first signs of β-A4 deposition. Cognitive decline has also been reported in aging DS individuals, suggesting that they may also dement. NFTs and diffuse deposits of β-A4 are also found in the brains of victims with *dementia pugilistica,* a rare disorder seen in boxers and battered wives where sufferers had received repeated head trauma (32). β-A4 deposition also occurs in the cerebral vasculature and as diffuse plaques in the brain parenchyma of individuals with the rare disorder *hereditary cerebral hemorrhage with amyloidosis—Dutch type* (HCHWA-D) (27). Cerebral hemorrhage occurs at an average age of 52 in these apparently healthy, normotensive subjects who do not normally develop symptoms of dementia (27).

The amyloid deposited in AD brains was isolated from cerebral vascular plaques (17) and shown to be a 4.2-kb polypeptide with a partial β-pleated sheet structure. Oligonucleotides corresponding to part of the peptide se-

C. L. Lendon and A. M. Goate: Department of Psychiatry, Washington University Medical School, St. Louis, Missouri 63110.

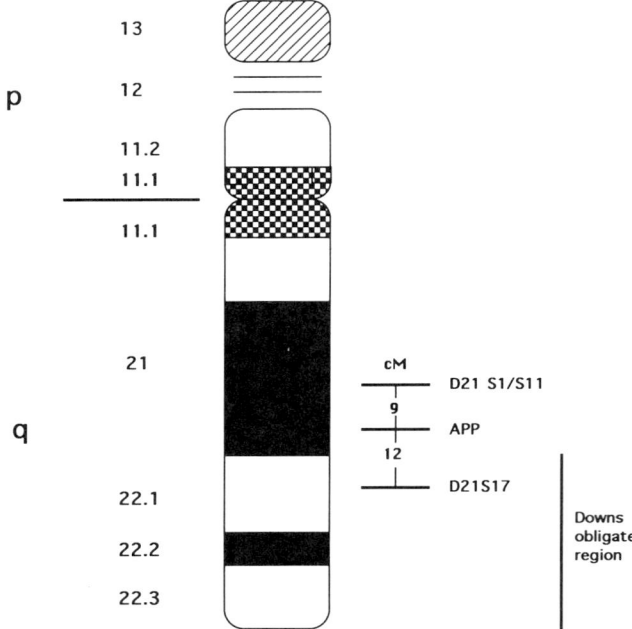

FIG. 1. Ideogram of human chromosome 21 showing the position of the APP gene and two polymorphic DNA markers used in the linkage studies (D21S1/S11 and D21S17). The numbers (9 and 12) indicate the genetic distance in centimorgans between these loci.

quence were used to screen cDNA libraries. The cDNAs isolated were much larger than expected and appeared to code for an amyloid precursor protein (APP). Mapping in a somatic cell hybrid panel revealed that the APP gene mapped to a single locus in the middle of the long arm of chromosome 21 (Ch 21) between 21q11.2 and 21q22.1 (see Fig. 1) (24). The human APP gene contains 19 exons and covers 400 kb of genomic DNA (45).

ALZHEIMER'S DISEASE IS A GENETIC DISORDER

AD was first described by Alois Alzheimer in 1907. The disorder was later reported to occur at high frequency in some families, suggesting a genetic component (30). In these families, AD was shown to follow an autosomal dominant pattern of inheritance with apparent 100% penetrance. The age of onset differs markedly between pedigrees but is quite consistent between affected members of the same family (66). Many epidemiological studies have shown that a positive family history is a consistent risk factor for AD (22). However, the vast majority of cases of AD do not show a clear pattern of inheritance. It is difficult to determine what proportion of cases are genetic in etiology for two reasons. Firstly, among late-onset cases some family members die of other causes before the age of onset of AD, which may lead to a failure to recognize a case as genetic. Secondly, the high frequency of AD in the elderly means that familial cluster-

ing could occur by chance quite often even when genetic factors are not involved.

Other risk factors that have been suggested to be involved in AD include head trauma, thyroid disease, and aluminum intake. Only in the case of head trauma, however, does there appear to be any significant correlation with disease (65). It has been suggested that a combination of genetic and environmental factors must predispose to AD because about a third of AD patients have affected first-degree relatives (see Chapters 2, 69, and 155 for related topics and background).

FACTORS LEADING TO THE SEARCH FOR AN AD LOCUS ON CHROMOSOME 21

One of the aims of the geneticist is to find the defective genes causing hereditary disorders. Two factors directed workers to search for an AD locus on Ch 21: (i) β-A4, the principal proteinaceous material of the senile plaque core, is a product of the much larger APP which is encoded by a gene which maps to Ch 21 and (ii) DS subjects, who invariably develop AD-like neuropathology, are trisomic for all or part of Ch 21. It is thought that an extra copy of a normal APP gene on Ch 21 in these individuals leads to overexpression of APP and the premature deposition of β-A4 (47). This is supported by findings of overexpression of APP in mouse trisomy 16, the mouse homologue to human Ch 21 (3).

These observations led to the suggestion that the APP gene on Ch 21 was a good candidate gene for the AD locus in the inherited forms of the disease. Support for this hypothesis could be drawn from the analogous situation of the prion dementias where prion protein is found in plaque deposits. Six mutations which co-segregate with the various forms of the prion dementias have been found in the human prion protein gene (PrP), which encodes the prion peptide deposited in Creutzfeldt–Jakob disease (CJD) and Gerstmann–Sträussler–Scheinker syndrome (GSS) (43).

GENETIC LINKAGE TO CHROMOSOME 21 OR NOT

The first indication of linkage to Ch 21 was reported by St. George-Hyslop et al. (60) in 1987. They described linkage to Ch 21 in four large AD pedigrees with histologically confirmed familial Alzheimer's disease (FAD). Each family had affected members over 6–8 generations, with a mean age of onset between 39.9 and 52 years. The putative location of a defective gene was deduced to be near two markers on the long arm of Ch 21. This was not in the 21q22 region, the so-called "Down's obligate region," but was closer to the centromere between 21q11.2 and 21q21, in the region of the APP gene. The highest lod scores, 4.25 and 4.06, occurred as two peaks on either side of markers D21S1 and D21S11. The story seemed well on its way to a tidy conclusion, especially when duplication of the APP gene was described in two cases of sporadic AD and not in seven controls (13). However, not only did other sporadic cases fail to reveal a gene duplication, but recombinants were reported between the APP gene and the disease in several large pedigrees (64). These findings appeared to rule out the APP gene as the disease locus. Subsequent reports appeared to exclude other areas of the long arm of Ch 21 and shed doubt on the original report (41,51). Only one report confirmed a linkage to the proximal region of the long arm of Ch 21 in early-onset families (EOAD) (19).

The situation became clearer as a result of a large multicenter collaboration. In this study, 48 pedigrees were genotyped with five polymorphic DNA markers mapping to the proximal region of the long arm and two independent methods of statistical analysis were used: relative likelihood and affected pedigree member methods. Both methods indicated significant evidence for linkage on Ch 21 around four of the five markers. However, the majority of pedigrees did not contribute to the positive lod scores at these loci. When divided on the basis of age of onset, late-onset families showed no evidence for linkage to Ch 21, whereas the early-onset group gave significant evidence of linkage to this region. However, the observation of two peak lod scores on either side of the marker map even in early-onset families suggested the possibility of genetic heterogeneity even within this group. These results clearly indicated that despite the general uniformity of the AD phenotype, FAD was not a single homogeneous disorder. It now became clear that failure to detect and localize the disease locus on Ch 21 had been due, at least in part, to genetic heterogeneity. Indeed, each candidate gene would need to be excluded in each family (see Chapters 116 and 118 for related topics).

MUTATIONS IN THE APP GENE

Although it was recognized that most cases of AD were not due to a gene defect on Ch 21, interest in the APP gene as a candidate disease locus was revived for some EOAD cases. Researchers were fortunate that a single large family existed with Ch 21-linked EOAD. This family (F23) provided a large part of the positive lod score in the collaborative study (60) and in our own study (19). Typing all individuals in the family for markers along the entire length of Ch 21 led to the identification of two recombination events which delineated a region between D21S1 and D21S17 in which the disease locus must lie. Approximately 20–30 megabases lying between these DNA markers, including the APP gene, was inherited in all affected family members (18).

At this time a mutation in exon 17 of the APP gene was reported in association with HCHWA-D. A G-to-C mutation resulting in a glutamic acid to glutamine substitution was discovered at position 693 of the full-length

APP770 transcript (25) (see Fig. 2). These workers had found the mutation by sequencing the two exons which encode the deposited β-A4 peptide. This strategy was employed for F23 and led to the discovery of the first mutation that co-segregates with AD: a G-to-A transition at codon 717 in exon 17, causing a valine-to-isoleucine substitution (18). The mutation was detected in all affected family members but not in unaffected individuals over the age of onset nor in 100 unrelated controls; this provided evidence that the mutation could be pathogenic. Since then the mutation has been reported in an additional five Japanese families, one family from the United States, one Canadian family, two Italian families, and one British family (9,16,18). Further support for the probable pathogenicity of this mutation is the failure to reveal other mutations in the other 17 exons or a 330-bp regulatory region of the APP promoter in either of the two British families exhibiting this mutation (16). Soon after this, two other mutations were reported in codon 717: (i) a valine-to-glycine substitution in a British family (7) and (ii) a valine-to-phenylalanine substitution in a US family (35) both multiply affected by AD.

A double point mutation was found in two large Swedish families with EOAD (probably related) (33). Here a G-to-T and an A-to-C transversion result in amino acid changes: lysine to asparagine and methionine to leucine, respectively. These mutations were found in exon 16 at codons 670 and 671 of the APP770 transcript. A family was described with an unusual mixed phenotype that associates with a single base change in codon 692 of exon 17. One patient exhibited presenile dementia (onset 49.3 years), and four others had cerebral hemorrhage at a mean age of 39.5 years. The biopsies from one hemorrhaging patient showed extensive β-A4 immunological reactivity. The mutation is a C-to-G transversion resulting in an alanine-to-glycine substitution and has been detected in the histologically confirmed AD case in the absence of the HCHWA-D or other known AD mutations (21). This mutation was found in four other patients with cerebral hemorrhage and in seven who developed dementia, with a mean age of onset of 49 years and from the same family. The mutation did not occur in unaffected individuals ranging in age from 64 to 76; however, the pathogenicity of this mutation is in some doubt because of the absence of the mutation in a single elderly dementing patient (onset 61 years). The age of onset in this individual was significantly higher than in the individuals with mutations and may represent a nongenetic case of AD (a phenocopy). In addition, two other individuals of expected onset age had the 692 mutation and were healthy at the time of reporting. A C-to-T base change has also been reported in codon 713 of exon 17 (23). The resulting alanine-to-valine substitution was described in a single patient with schizophrenia who had a family history of the disorder. However, no other living relatives were available for study, and the mutation was not found in 86 unrelated schizophrenics or 156 controls (10). An alanine-to-

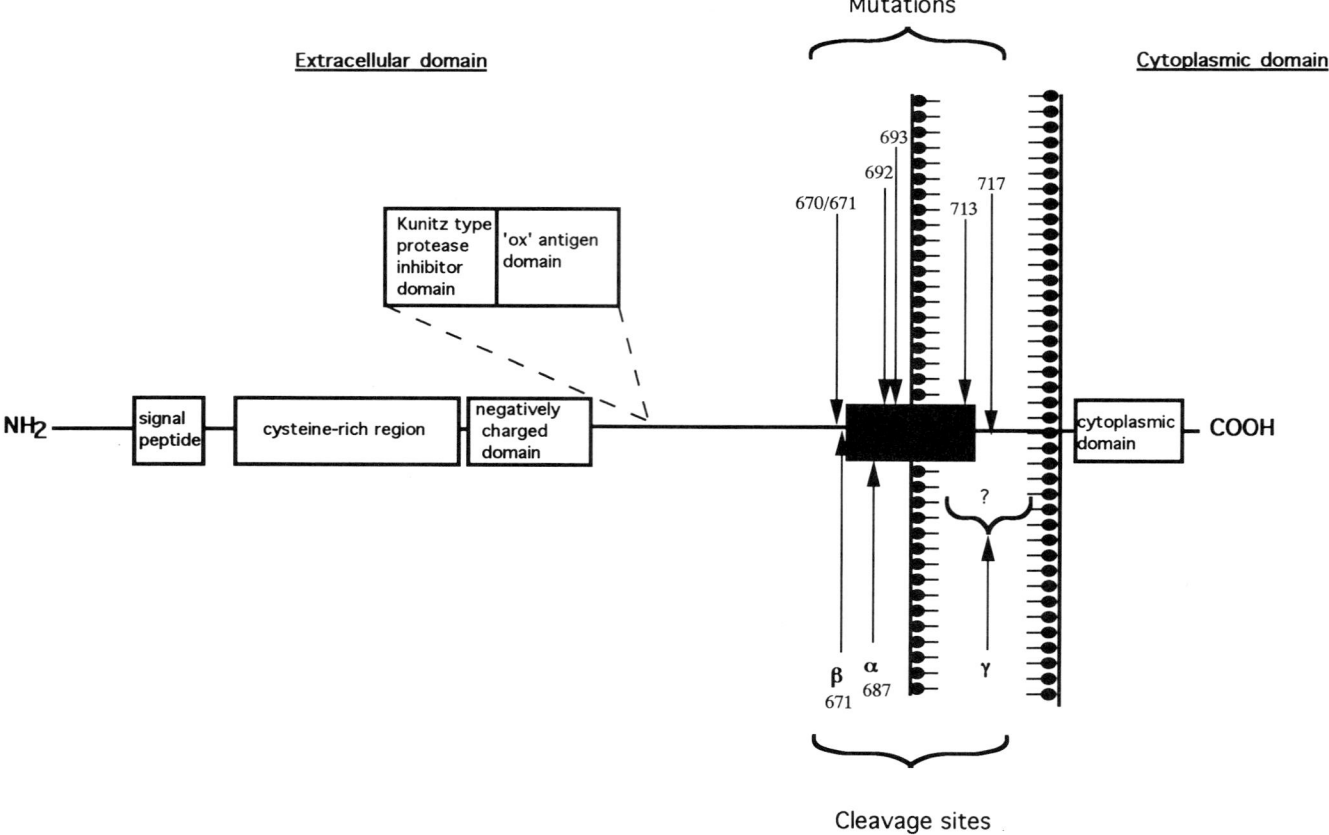

FIG. 2. Diagram showing the structural domains of APP and the position of disease causing mutations with respect to the sites of cleavage by proteolytic processing enzymes (α, β, and γ secretase). The *black box* represents β-A4, and |●—   —●| represents the plasma membrane.

threonine mutation also in codon 713 was described in a sporadic case of AD (onset 59 years) but not in five unaffected elderly relatives (6). Caution should be exercised with such findings because they may simply be rare polymorphisms. Alternatively, the observation of mutations in elderly unaffected relatives may reflect incomplete penetrance.

In summary, four mutations have been found in a total of 15 families with EOAD. This only represents a small proportion of familial EOAD [estimates range from 5% to 25% (65)] and an even smaller proportion of the total number of cases of AD (50).

THE PATHOGENICITY OF THE MUTATIONS IN THE APP GENE

Although mutations have been found in the APP gene in several AD families, it has not yet been demonstrated definitively that the mutations are sufficient to cause the disease. It is possible that they merely predispose to AD. However, a primary causal role is supported by the detection of mutations only in affected family members. Further supporting evidence comes from the fact that families with the 717 valine-to-isoleucine mutation are from dif-

ferent racial origins and that none of the Japanese or Caucasian families share APP haplotypes, indicating independent mutational events.

There are several possibilities as to how mutations in the APP gene might cause disease. The presence of an extra copy of a normal APP gene in trisomy 21 suggests that overexpression of normal APP may be sufficient to cause premature β-A4 deposition. These mutations could theoretically have their effect at one of several different levels: They could influence the rate of transcription or mRNA stability; they could affect the rate of translation of the mRNA or the post-translational modification of the protein; they could alter the proteolytic processing of APP; or for those mutations within the β-A4 sequence they may alter the physicochemical properties of the peptide. The mutations in the APP gene which are associated with the AD phenotype (i.e., mutations at codons 670/671 and 717) do not lie within the sequence encoding the β-A4 peptide, whereas mutations associated with HCHWA-D at codons 692 and 693 lie within this sequence (see Fig. 2). The 717 mutations lie 3 amino acid residues from the predicted carboxyl terminal end of β-A4. However, to-date, β-A4 has not been sequenced from the brain of an individual with an APP717 mutation, and these mutations may or may not be within the deposited sequence in such individuals. It has been suggested that these mutations affect proteolytic processing of APP because all four seem to occur in sequences flanking β-A4.

APP proteolytic processing is complicated and, as yet, not completely understood, although evidence suggests that the proportion of APP processed by different routes varies in different cell types. The detection of extracellular amino-terminal fragments in cultured mammalian cells transfected with full-length APP cDNA and a variety of hybrid and modified APPs indicated that specific cleavage occurs within the extracellular domain of β-A4 (57) (see Fig. 2). This was corroborated by results from non-transfected neuronal PC12 cells (1). The enzyme, termed "α-secretase," cleaves at lysine 16 of β-A4 (encoded by codon 687) but appears to have a broad sequence specificity (67). α-Secretase cleaves cell-surface-membrane-bound APP to produce a soluble "secreted" amino-terminal derivative extracellularly and a short C-terminal fragment that is degraded within the endosomal/lysosomal compartment of the cell. The cleavage occurs within the β-A4 fragment and therefore cannot lead to deposition of intact fragments. The 692 mutations for mixed AD/HCHWA-D and 693 HCHWA-D mutation occur only about 6 amino acid residues away from the α-secretase cleavage site, but as yet there is no evidence that these mutations have any effect on cleavage.

Cellular studies have revealed that there are alternative pathways of APP processing. A lysosomal route of APP degradation is indicated by the finding of C-terminal fragments within lysosomes. These fragments are both (a) the C-terminal fragment derived from the α-secretase cleavage and (b) a larger fragment which contains an intact β-A4 sequence (probably derived from the "β-secretase" cleavage. The "β-secretase" activity was detected by studying APP processing in mixed brain cell cultures. This activity cleaves APP between the methionine residue of APP770 at codon 671 and the aspartic acid residue at APP672 (55). Cleavage at this site produces fragments containing intact β-A4. The Swedish mutation (33) occurs in the two amino acids preceding this cleavage site. It is likely that this cleavage site is crucial to the production of soluble β-A4, a normal processing product detectable in body fluids (20,56). Indeed, transient transfection of human kidney 293 cells with DNA constructs encoding APP containing the base substitutions at 670 and/or 671 of the Swedish double mutation leads to a six- to eightfold increase in soluble β-A4 production. The 670 mutation is largely responsible for this increase in soluble β-A4 detectable in the media compared to wild-type control (8). It would appear that the production of soluble β-A4 is distinct from the endosomal/lysosomal pathway of C-terminal degradation because truncation of the cytoplasmic tail of APP does not prevent enhanced generation of soluble β-A4 in these cells. Recently, similar increases in the production of β-A4 derivatives were produced in human neuroblastoma cells transfected with constructs

containing the mutation at codon 670 (4). No effect on soluble β-A4 levels was observed upon transfection of constructs containing APP717 mutations. Similar transfection of human neuroglioma cells with constructs containing the HCHWA-D mutation do not cause any detectable changes (15).

Preliminary evidence suggests that the mutation causing HCHWA-D may cause premature β-A4 deposition by altering the secondary structure of the peptide rather than altering APP processing (14).

In summary, there are several possible processing pathways involving membrane-bound APP, all of which could be perturbed by the known mutations to accelerate β-A4 deposition. However, as already noted, the known mutations only account for a very small number of FAD cases. If β-A4 deposition is central to the disease process, then defects in any of the enzymes, precursors, cofactors, activators, and inhibitors that are involved in the processing of APP could lead indirectly to premature β-A4 deposition. Because potentially amyloidogenic fragments of APP occur in normal brain and cerebrospinal fluid (CSF), AD could result from abnormal polymerization of normal degradation products. It is possible that the APP mutations merely predispose to AD and other amyloidopathies, perhaps simply by bringing forward the age of onset. Other genetic and environmental factors may be involved, particularly because most cases of AD are sporadic.

EVIDENCE FOR OTHER DISEASE LOCI

Chromosome 19

The search for other disease loci gathered pace following the recognition of the genetic heterogeneity of AD. One of the early genetic investigations of FAD that failed to show linkage to Ch 21 (40) used a mixture of families, but the majority were of late onset (mean age: >60 years). When this group was reexamined using the affected pedigree member method of linkage analysis which excludes unaffected members, two chromosomal regions gave significant results: proximal 19q (see Fig. 3a) and the FAD-linked region of Ch 21 (40). Division of the families by age of onset revealed that the associations were between LOAD and Ch 19 and between EOAD and Ch 21. Indeed one of the EOAD families was later found to have a mutation in the APP gene (18). Independently, several groups have presented supporting evidence for linkage to Ch 19 (46). Two association studies have provided further support for this region of the genome.

Recently, several independent lines of evidence have provided support for the hypothesis that the disease locus on Ch 19 is the apolipoprotein E (ApoE) gene. ApoE is one of the many different proteins found to associate with β-A4 amyloid fibrils (5,36,58). Immunohistochemical studies show that ApoE accumulates extracellularly in

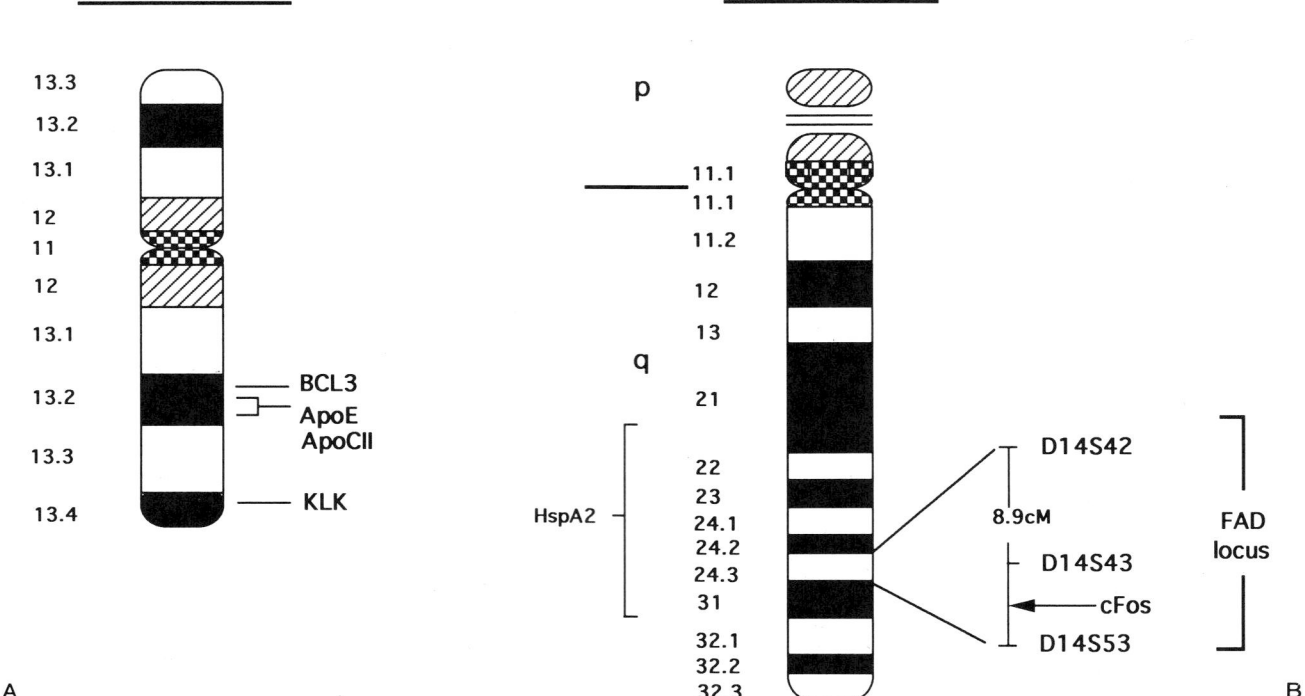

FIG. 3. (a) An ideogram of chromosome 19 showing the position of genes which have been linked to late-onset AD or used in association studies (not to scale). (b) An ideogram of chromosome 14 showing the position of markers linked to the early-onset FAD locus and the approximate location of two candidate genes *c-fos* and *HspA2* (not to scale).

senile plaques and intracellularly in NFT in both autopsy and biopsy samples (36,70). This ApoE seems to bind tightly to β-A4 because ApoE immunoreactivity is enhanced when sections are pretreated with formic acid, which is thought to denature amyloid polymers (36). ApoE staining colocalizes with Congo red stain as evidenced by ultrastructural studies of autopsy tissue. However, local ApoE production, as well as leakage and neuronal uptake of serum protein occurring in the aged brain, could contribute to ApoE immunoreactivity in the brain (70). In vitro binding studies have also shown tight binding of ApoE to β-A4 (61,62). ApoE and a related protein apolipoprotein CII (Apo CII) map to the region of Ch 19 originally implicated in the linkage studies. Association studies have recently been carried out using polymorphisms within both of these genes. The frequency of the "F" allele of Apo CII was found to be increased in family members affected by AD compared to unrelated controls in one study (53) but was not reproduced in a second study (49). However, association studies using polymorphism within the ApoE gene has demonstrated a robust and reproducible increase of the ApoE4 allele within familial and sporadic cases of late onset AD (11,48,49,62). This is perhaps somewhat surprising when one considers that the ApoCII locus is less than 50 kb from the ApoE locus.

There are three common isoforms of ApoE encoded by the alleles E2, E3, and E4. The variants differ at residues

112 and 158: ε3 cysteine 112, cysteine 158; ε4 arginine 112, cysteine 158; ε2 cysteine 112, arginine 158. A study of 2000 chromosomes estimates the frequency of the E3 and E4 alleles in the normal population to be 0.78 and 0.14, respectively (31). The ε2 variant is defective in binding to the low-density-lipoprotein receptor (LDL-R). Individuals with abnormal lipoprotein metabolism and E2/E2 homozygosity are at increased risk for developing type III hyperlipoproteinemia. The ε4 variant has a greater affinity for lipoprotein particles than does ε3, resulting in more efficient lipid clearance, leading to down-regulation of hepatic LDL-R and enhanced plasma levels of cholesterol and triglycerides (28).

In an initial study of 30 AD families with mixed age of onset, the E4 allele frequency was 0.52 ± 0.06 compared to that of age-matched unrelated controls, 0.16 ± 0.03 (62). When restricted to affected and unaffected family members from 42 LOAD onset families, AD occurred in 91% of individuals homozygous for the E4 allele and in 47% of those with the E3/E4 allele, whereas only 20% had AD with allele combinations E3/E3, E3/E2, and E2/E4 (11). Similar trends have since been described (39). Enrichment for the E4 allele has also been observed in cases of sporadic AD (42,44,48). Immunocytochemistry of autopsy material from LOAD patients has revealed that the β-A4 burden (plaque numbers and amount of congophilic angiopathy) shows a positive correlation with the number of E4 alleles (44,54).

ApoE is one of the several glycosylated proteins associated with plasma lipids (28). It plays a major role in regulation of lipid transport by acting as a ligand for binding ApoE-containing lipoproteins to the low-density lipoprotein receptor (LDL-R) and for binding chylomicron remnants to the LDL-R-related protein (LRP) (2). The ApoE gene is located on the proximal long arm of Ch 19q13.2 and consists of 4 exons and 3 introns covering 3597 bp. The gene encodes a 299-amino-acid protein, a third of which is rich in the basic residues arginine and lysine and is involved in receptor binding. The remaining 976-bp C-terminal region is the amphipathic α-helical lipid-binding domain (12,38). ApoE is synthesized in many organs, and the highest levels are produced in the liver and the brain. It is the main lipoprotein in the CSF, where it is brain-derived from glia and astrocytes but not from neurons. LRP is the major receptor that binds ApoE in the brain and is particularly abundant in astrocytes (44). The lipid transport function of ApoE is thought to extend to the delivery of lipid to regenerating nerves and is postulated to be involved in response to neuronal injury. The levels of ApoE in the CSF rise significantly with several central nervous system disorders (5).

The genetic data reviewed here strongly support the hypothesis that possession of an Apo E4 allele is an important risk factor for the development of LOAD and sporadic AD but not for EOAD. It has been proposed that ApoE4 acts as a "pathological molecular chaperone" that binds to soluble β-A4 and enhances β-pleated sheet formation and amyloid fibril stability (70). Investigation of possible differences in the binding characteristics of ApoE alleles to synthetic β-A4 are underway (61).

The genetic evidence for the E4 allele as a risk factor above is compelling, yet many cases of LOAD sporadic AD (29% and 38%, respectively) have no E4 allele (11,44). However, the precise risk associated with the ApoE4 allele requires use of an epidemiologically based sample. Unpublished data, presented at the 1993 Society for Neuroscience meeting by Schellenberg and colleagues, showed that in an epidemiologically based sample of 11,000 individuals there was a much smaller enrichment of the E4 allele with AD (0.26 compared to 0.19 nondementing individuals) than observed in previous studies. The presence of an E4 allele is therefore not diagnostic for AD. The allelic association between AD and ApoE could arise from linkage disequilibrium with a nearby predisposing locus on Ch 19. One possible candidate for such a role is an APP-like protein which has recently been mapped to the proximal portion of the long arm of human Ch 19 (68). The dosage effects of the ApoE4 allele (11), if confirmed by other groups, would strongly support the notion that ApoE is the disease locus rather than being linked to the real disease locus. Whatever the role of ApoE, the pronounced allelic association in many cases of LOAD and sporadics has served to bring the hitherto little supported disease locus on Ch 19 back into hot contention.

Chromosome 14

Convincing evidence of an alternative locus for FAD was reported by four independent groups in 1992. Linkage was reported to the marker D14S43 on Ch 14 at q24.3 in a collection of EOAD families (52) (see Fig. 3b). Schellenberg's findings were quickly followed by others reporting an AD locus on Ch 14 in unrelated families. The strongest evidence for linkage to Ch 14 was found in two large EOAD Belgian pedigrees. Linkage to D14S43 was found with a maximum lod score of +13.25 at zero recombination (63). St. George-Hyslop (59) reported linkage to Ch 14 near markers D14S43 and D14S53 with a maximum multipoint lod score of +23.4. The pedigrees were a combination of 21 families of mixed origin, with a mean family age of onset ranging from 42 to 84 years. These workers report that significant linkage to Ch 14 was found in the four EOAD families used in the original linkage report to Ch 21 (60). The lod scores for each family are much higher with the Ch 14 markers, suggesting that the small positive lod scores on Ch 21 were a chance event and did not represent true linkage. A peak lod score of +7.8 at no recombination was generated from nine EOAD families, indicating tight linkage to D14S43 (34). Subsequent to these original reports, genetic linkage maps for Ch 14 have been published using additional polymorphic markers in q24.3 (69). Use of these markers in the linked AD families has identified D14S63/S57 and D14S61 as the centromeric and telomeric flanking markers, respectively. Four markers show no recombination with the disease (D14S43, D14S76, D14S71, and D14S77). The distance between the flanking markers is approximately 12 cM, but the majority of this distance is between D14S63/S57 and D14S77. It is therefore a high priority to identify additional polymorphic markers in this region of the chromosome. Two candidate genes map to this portion of the long arm of Ch 14: c-fos and heat-shock protein 70. So far, no defects in these genes have been reported.

The Volga Germans, a group of families originating from the Volga region of Russia, do not show linkage to markers on Ch 21, 14, or 19, indicating further genetic heterogeneity in AD (52).

Other Loci

A mutation has been reported in codon 331 of mitochondrial NADH dehydrogenase subunit 2 (ND2) (26). The mutation occurred in 10 of 19 AD patients and in two of six patients with amyotrophic lateral sclerosis (ALS). Mutations within the mitochondrial genome are known to accumulate with aging although their pathological significance is unclear, particularly because the mitochondrial genome is highly polymorphic. The 331 mutation could be a common polymorphism or the discovery of a mutation that increases the risk of AD. If AD-causing mutations enhance susceptibility of neurons to damage, then defects in a host of metabolically sensitive cellular processes, which might otherwise be below a threshold for damage or be compensated for, may be sufficient to initiate a pathway leading to AD and AD-like pathology.

SUMMARY

A small proportion of EOAD appears to be caused by mutations in the APP gene encoding β-A4, a major component in diffuse and aggregated plaques. One of the mutations appears to initiate a pathogenic process by overproduction of soluble β-A4. A second disease locus causing EOAD has been localized to the long arm of Ch 14 in band q24.3. Linkage and molecular genetic studies are underway to both narrow down the candidate region and to clone the region in yeast artificial chromosomes: a prelude to gene isolation and characterization. A third locus on the long arm of Ch 19 has been implicated in predisposition to late-onset AD. Evidence from association studies supports the notion that this locus is the apolipoprotein E gene or another gene very close by. It is clear that the number of genetic defects causing AD will not be confined to the loci on chromosomes 14, 19, and 21 because linkage cannot be demonstrated in families of Volga German origin. The determination of whether APP or β-A4 plays a major role in the pathogenesis of all cases of AD awaits the isolation of these other genes. As more gene defects are discovered, and a knowledge of the role and properties of their products are accumulated, the potential for drug design of many-fold greater phenotypic specificity and efficacy increases.

REFERENCES

1. Anderson JP, Esch FS, Keim PS, Sambamurti K, Lieberburg I, Robakis NK. Exact cleavage site of Alzheimer amyloid precursor in neuronal PC-12 cells. Neurosci Lett 1991;128:126–128.
2. Beisiegel U, Weber W, Ihrke G, Herz J, Stanley K. The LDL-receptor-related protein, LRP, is an apolipoprotein E-binding protein. Nature 1989;341:162–164.
3. Bendotti C, Forloni G, Morgan R, et al. Neuroanatomical localisation and quantification of amyloid precursor protein mRNA by in situ hybridisation in the brains of normal, aneuploid and lesioned mice. Proc Natl Acad Sci USA 1988;85:3628–3632.
4. Cai X-D, Golde TE, Younkin SG. Release of excess amyloid β protein from a mutant amyloid β protein precursor. Science 1993;259:514–516.
5. Carlsson J, Armstrong V, Reiber H, Felgenhauer K, Seidel D. Clinical relevance of the quantification of apolipoprotein E in cerebrospinal fluid. Clin Chim Acta 1991;196:167–176.
6. Carter DA, Desmarais E, Bellis M, et al. More missense in amyloid gene. Nature Genet 1992;2:255–256.
7. Chartier Harlin MC, Crawford F, Houlden H, et al. Early onset Alzheimer's disease caused by mutations at codon 717 of the β-amyloid precursor protein gene. Nature 1991;353:844–846.
8. Citron M, Oltersdorf T, Haass C, et al. Mutation of the β-amyloid precursor protein in familial Alzheimer's disease increases β-protein production. Nature 1992;360:672–674.
9. Clark R, Goate A. Molecular genetics of Alzheimer's disease. Arch Neurol 1993;50:1164–1172.
10. Coon H, Hoff M, Holik J, et al. C to T nucleotide substitution in codon 713 of amyloid precursor protein gene not found in 86 unrelated schizophrenics from multiplex families. Am J Med Gen (Neuropsychiatr Genet) 1993;48:36–39.
11. Corder E, Saunders A, Strittmatter W, et al. Gene dose of apolipoprotein E type 4 allele and the risk of Alzheimer's disease in late onset families. Science 1993;261:921–923.
12. Das H, McPherson J, Bruns G, Karathanasis S, Breslow J. Isolation, characterization and mapping to chromosome 19 of the human apolipoprotein E gene. J Biol Chem 1985;260:6240–6247.
13. Delabar JM, Goldgaber D, Lamour Y, et al. Beta amyloid gene duplication in Alzheimer's disease and karyotypically normal Down syndrome. Science 1987;235:1390–1392.
14. Fabian H, Szendrei G, Mantsch H, Otvos L Jr. Comparative analysis of human and Dutch-type Alzheimer beta-amyloid peptides by infrared spectroscopy and circular dichroism. Biochem Biophys Res Commun 1993;191(1):232–239.
15. Felenstein K, Lewis-Higgins L. Processing of the β-amyloid precursor protein carrying the familial, Dutch-type, and a novel recombinant C-terminal mutation. Neurosci Lett 1993;152:185–189.
16. Fidani L, Rooke K, Chartier-Harlin MC, et al. Screening for mutations in the open reading frame and promoter of the β-amyloid precursor protein gene in familial Alzheimer's disease: identification of a further family with APP717 Val→Ile. Hum Mol Genet 1992;1:165–168.
17. Glenner GG, Wong CW. Alzheimer's disease: initial report of the purification and characterization of a novel cerebrovascular amyloid protein. Biochem Biophys Res Commun 1984;120:885–890.
18. Goate A, Chartier Harlin MC, Mullan M, et al. Segregation of a missense mutation in the amyloid precursor protein gene with familial Alzheimer's disease. Nature 1991;349:704–706.
19. Goate AM, Haynes AR, Owen MJ, et al. Predisposing locus for Alzheimer's disease on chromosome 21. Lancet 1989;1:352–355.
20. Haass C, Schlossmacher M, Hung A, et al. Amyloid β-peptide is produced by cultured cells during normal metabolism. Nature 1992;359:322–325.
21. Hendriks L, van Duijn C, Cras P, et al. Presenile dementia and cerebral haemorrhage linked to a mutation at codon 692 of the β-amyloid precursor protein gene. Nature Genet 1992;1(3):218–221.
22. Heyman A, Wilkinson WE, Stafford JA, Helms MJ, Sigmon AH, Weinberg T. Alzheimer's disease: a study of epidemiological aspects. Ann Neurol 1984;15:335–341.
23. Jones LM, Knowler JT. Role of ribonuclease and ribonuclease inhibitor activities in Alzheimer's disease. J Neurochem 1989;53:1341–1344.
24. Kang J, Lemaire HG, Unterbeck A, et al. The precursor of Alzheimer's disease amyloid A4 protein resembles a cell-surface receptor. Nature 1987;325:733–736.
25. Levy E, Carman MD, Fernandez Madrid IJ, et al. Mutation of the Alzheimer's disease amyloid gene in hereditary cerebral hemorrhage, Dutch type. Science 1990;248:1124–1126.
26. Lin F-H, Lin R, Wisniewski H, et al. Detection of point mutations in codon 331 of mitochondrial NADH dehydrogenase subunit 2 in Alzheimer's disease. Biochem Biophys Res Commun 1992;182:238–246.
27. Luyendijk W, Bots GT, Vegter Van der Vlis M, Went LN, Frangione B. Hereditary cerebral haemorrhage caused by cortical amyloid angiopathy. J Neurol Sci 1988;85:267–280.
28. Mahley RW. Apolipoprotein E: cholesterol transport protein with expanding role in cell biology. Science 1988;240:622–630.
29. McKhann G, Drachman D, Folstein M, Katzman R, Price D, Stadlan EM. Clinical diagnosis of Alzheimer's disease: report of the NINCDS-ADRDA Work Group under the auspices of Department of Health and Human Services Task Force on Alzheimer's disease. Neurology 1984;34:939–944.
30. Meggendorfer F. Uber familiengeschichtliche Untersuchungen bei arteriosklerotischer und seniler Demenz. Zentralbl Neurol Psychiatr 1925;40:359.
31. Menzel H, Kladetzky R, Assmann G. Apolipoprotein E polymorphism and coronary artery disease. Arteriosclerosis 1983;3:310–315.
32. Mortimer JA, van Duijn CM, Chandra V, et al. Head trauma as a risk factor for Alzheimer's disease: a collaborative re-analysis of case-control studies. Int J Epidemiol 1991;20(Suppl 2):S28–S35.
33. Mullan M, Crawford F, Axelman K, et al. A pathogenic mutation for probable Alzheimer's disease in the APP gene at the N-terminus of β-amyloid. Nature Genet 1992;1(4):345–347.

34. Mullan M, Houlden H, Windelspecht M, et al. A locus for familial early-onset Alzheimer's disease on the long arm of chromosome 14, proximal to the α1-antichymotrypsin gene. *Nature Genet* 1992;2:340–342.

35. Murrell J, Farlow M, Ghetti B, Benson M. A mutation in the amyloid precursor protein associated with hereditary Alzheimer's disease. *Science* 1991;254:97–99.

36. Namba Y, Tomonaga M, Kawasaki H, Otomo E, Ikeda K. Apolipoprotein E immunoreactivity in cerebral amyloid deposits and neurofibrillary tangles in Alzheimer's disease and kuru plaque amyloid in Creutzfeldt–Jakob disease. *Brain Res* 1991;541:163–166.

37. Oliver C, Holland AJ. Down's syndrome and Alzheimer's disease: a review. *Psychol Med* 1986;16:307–322.

38. Paik Y-K, Chang D, Reardon C, Davies G, Mahley R, Taylor J. Nucleotide sequence and structure of the human apolipoprotein E gene. *Proc Natl Acad Sci USA* 1985;82:3445–3449.

39. Payami H, Kaye J, Heston L, Bird T, Schellenberg G. Apolipoprotein E genotype and Alzheimer's disease. *Lancet* 1993;342:738.

40. Pericak-Vance MA, Bebout JL, Gaskell PC Jr, et al. Linkage studies in familial Alzheimer disease: evidence for chromosome 19 linkage. *Am J Hum Genet* 1991;48:1034–1050.

41. Pericak-Vance MA, Yamaoka LH, Haynes CS, et al. Genetic linkage studies in familial Alzheimer's disease. *Exp Neurol* 1988;102:271–279.

42. Poirier J, Davignon J, Kogan S, Bertrand P, Gauthier S. Apolipoprotein E polymorphism and Alzheimer's disease. *Lancet* 1993;342:697–699.

43. Prusiner SB. Molecular biology of prion diseases. *Science* 1991;252:1515–1522.

44. Rebeck G, Reiter J, Strickland D, Hyman B. Apolipoprotein E in sporadic Alzheimer's disease: allelic variation and receptor interactions. *Neuron* 1993;11:575–580.

45. Rooke K, Talbot C, James L, Anand R, Hardy J, Goate A. A physical map of the human APP gene in YACs. *Mammalian Genome* 1993;4:662–669.

46. Ropers HH, Pericak-Vance MA, Siciliano MJ, Mohrenweiser HW. Report of the second international workshop on human chromosome 19 mapping. *Cytogenet Cell Genet* 1992;60:87–95.

47. Rumble B, Retallack R, Hilbich C, et al. Amyloid A4 protein and its precursor in Down's syndrome and Alzheimer's disease. *N Engl J Med* 1989;320:1446–1452.

48. Saunders A, Schmader K, Breitner J, et al. Apolipoprotein E e4 allele distributions in late onset Alzheimer's disease and in other amyloid forming diseases. *Lancet* 1993;342:710–711.

49. Saunders A, Strittmatter W, Schmechel D, et al. Association of apolipoprotein E allele e4 with late-onset familial and sporadic Alzheimer's disease. *Neurology* 1993;43:1467–1472.

50. Schellenberg GD, Anderson L, O'Dahl S, et al. APP717, APP693, and PRIP gene mutations are rare in Alzheimer's disease. *Am J Hum Genet* 1991;49:511–517.

51. Schellenberg GD, Bird TD, Wijsman EM, et al. Absence of linkage of chromosome 21q21 markers to familial Alzheimer's disease. *Science* 1988;241:1507–1510.

52. Schellenberg GD, Bird TD, Wijsman EM, et al. Genetic linkage evidence for a familial Alzheimer's disease locus on chromosome 14. *Science* 1992;258:668–671.

53. Schellenberg GD, Boehnke M, Wijsman EM, Moore DK, Martin GM, Bird TD. Genetic association and linkage analysis of the apolipoprotein C11 locus and familial Alzheimer's disease. *Ann Neurol* 1992;31:223–227.

54. Schmechel D, Saunders A, Strittmatter W, et al. Increased amyloid beta-peptide deposition in cerebral cortex as a consequence of apolipoprotein E genotype in late-onset Alzheimer disease. *Proc Natl Acad Sci USA* 1993;90:9649–9653.

55. Seubert P, Oltersdorf T, Lee MG, et al. Secretion of β-amyloid precursor protein cleaved at the amino terminus of the β-amyloid peptide. *Nature* 1993;361:260–263.

56. Seubert P, Vigo-Pelfrey C, Esch F, et al. Isolation and quantification of soluble Alzheimer's β-peptide from biological fluids. *Nature* 1992;359:325–327.

57. Sisodia S, Koo E, Beyreuther K, Unterbeck A, Price D. Evidence that beta-amyloid protein in Alzheimer's disease is not derived by normal processing. *Science* 1990;248:492–494.

58. Snow AD, Mar H, Nochlin D, et al. The presence of heparan sulfate proteoglycans in the neuritic plaques and congophilic angiopathy in Alzheimer's disease. *Am J Pathol* 1988;133:456–463.

59. St. George-Hyslop P, Haines J, Rogaev E, et al. Genetic evidence for a novel familial Alzheimer's disease locus on chromosome 14. *Nature Genet* 1992;2:330–334.

60. St. George-Hyslop PH, Tanzi RE, Polinsky RJ, et al. The genetic defect causing familial Alzheimer's disease maps on chromosome 21. *Science* 1987;235:885–890.

61. Strittmatter W, Weisgraber K, Huang D, et al. Binding of human apolipoprotein E to synthetic amyloid beta-peptide: isoform-specific effects and implications for late-onset Alzheimer disease. *Proc Natl Acad Sci USA* 1993;90:8098–8102.

62. Strittmatter WJ, Saunders AM, Schmechel D, et al. Apolipoprotein E: high-avidity binding to β-amyloid and increased frequency of type 4 allele in late-onset familial Alzheimer's disease. *Proc Natl Acad Sci USA* 1993;90:1977–1981.

63. Van Broeckhoven C, Backhovens H, Cruts M, et al. Mapping of a gene predisposing to early-onset Alzheimer's disease to chromosome 14q24.3. *Nature Genet* 1992;2:335–339.

64. Van Broeckhoven C, Genthe AM, Vandenberghe A, et al. Failure of familial Alzheimer's disease to segregate with the A4-amyloid gene in several European families. *Nature* 1987;329:153–155.

65. van Duijn CM, Stijnen T, Hofman A. Risk factors for Alzheimer's disease: overview of the EURODEM collaborative re-analysis of case–control studies. *Int J Epidemiol* 1991;20(Suppl 2):S4–S12.

66. van Duijn CM, Van Broechhoven C, Hardy JA, et al. Evidence for allelic heterogeneity in familial early onset Alzheimer's disease. *Br J Psychiatry* 1991;158:471–474.

67. Wang R, Meschai J, Cotter R, Sisodia S. Secretion of the β/A4 amyloid precursor protein. *J Biol Chem* 1991;266(25):16960–16964.

68. Wasco W, Brook JD, Tanzi RE. The amyloid precursor-like protein (aplp) gene maps to the long arm of human chromosome-19. *Genomics* 1993;15(1):237–239.

69. Weissenbach J, Gynapay G, Dib C, et al. A second-generation linkage map of the human genome. *Nature* 1992;359:794–801.

70. Wisniewski T, Frangione B. Apolipoprotein E: a pathological chaperone protein in patients with cerebral and systemic amyloid. *Neurosci Lett* 1992;135:235–238.

Psychopharmacology: The Fourth Generation of Progress, edited by Floyd E. Bloom and David J. Kupfer. Raven Press, Ltd., New York © 1995.

CHAPTER 116

Amyloidogenesis in Alzheimer's Disease and Animal Models

Sangram S. Sisodia and Donald L. Price

Alzheimer's disease (AD) is the most common type of dementia in adults (13,41). The major risk factors for AD are age (13) and, in families with early-onset disease, genetic loci on chromosomes 21 and 14 (16,23,42,50,57). The disease involves a variety of neuronal circuits in several regions of the brain, including nerve cell populations within the brainstem, basal forebrain, thalamus, amygdala, hippocampus, and neocortex. The consequence of these lesions is deafferentation of targets, particularly in the hippocampus and neocortex (5,24,30,62,70). Affected neurons develop neurofibrillary tangles (NFTs), neuropil threads, and neurites, all of which reflect abnormalities of the neuronal cytoskeleton (6,17,37). A characteristic feature of AD is the presence of deposits of the β-amyloid protein ($A\beta$) in the hippocampus and neocortex. Derived from the amyloid precursor proteins (APPs), $A\beta$ is a 4-kD peptide comprised of 11–15 amino acids of the transmembrane domain and 28 amino acids of the extracellular domain of APP (15,28,39).

This review, which complements other chapters dealing with aspects of AD, describes the current status of our understanding of (a) the biology of APP, (b) mechanisms that lead to the formation of deposits of $A\beta$, (c) the pathogenesis of amyloidogenesis in the brains of aged nonhuman primates, and (d) the results of attempts to develop transgenic animal models that show AD-type abnormalities (see also Chapters 115 and 118, *this volume*).

BIOLOGY OF APP

Located on the midportion of the long arm of human chromosome 21 (28), the APP gene, encompassing ~400 kb of DNA (B. Lamb and J. Gearhart, *personal communication*), gives rise by alternative splicing of APP pre-mRNA to at least four transcripts that encode $A\beta$ containing proteins of 695, 714, 751, and 770 amino acids (18,28,31,46). APP-751 and -770 contain a domain that shares homology with the Kunitz class of serine protease inhibitors (31,46). In cultured mammalian cells, full-length APP isoforms are modified by the addition of both N- and O-linked carbohydrates and terminal sulfation events (68). Dependent on cell type, levels of newly synthesized APP molecules appear at the cell surface (21), and some of these proteins are cleaved by an enzyme, designated APP secretase, within the $A\beta$ sequence (2,12,54,65) to release the ectodomain of APP, including residues 1–16 of $A\beta$, into the medium. Thus, APP cleavage within the $A\beta$ domain precludes the formation of $A\beta$. The presence of secreted APP isoforms that contain $A\beta$ epitopes in cerebrospinal fluid suggests that similar processing events occur in vivo (44,68). A fraction of cell-surface APP is also internalized and degraded via endosomal–lysosomal pathways (19,21). It appears that the sequence NPXY in the cytoplasmic domain of APP is required for internalization by a clathrin-coated-pit-mediated pathway (S. Sisodia, *personal observations*). Processing via the endosomal–lysosomal pathway results in the production of potentially amyloidogenic C-terminal-containing fragments (19,21). Moreover, recent reports indicate that peptides similar to $A\beta$ (4 kD) and truncated forms of $A\beta$ (~3 kD) are secreted to the media of primary cell cultures and various tissue culture cell lines. $A\beta$-related peptides have also been detected in cerebrospinal fluid (52,53). Although these studies suggest

S. S. Sisodia: Department of Pathology and the Neuropathology Laboratory, The Johns Hopkins University School of Medicine, Baltimore, Maryland 21205.

D. L. Price: Departments of Pathology, Neurology, and Neuroscience and the Neuropathology Laboratory, The Johns Hopkins University School of Medicine, Baltimore, Maryland 21205.

that Aβ may be produced and released in vitro and in vivo, it is not clear whether these Aβ-related fragments of variable lengths are the source of cerebral Aβ (which is principally 42–43 amino acids) found in cases of AD. In any event, the observation that APP mutations in early-onset familial AD invariably flank the Aβ sequence indirectly suggests that altered processing of APP is central to the formation of amyloid in these individuals (see below).

Despite advances in our understanding of APP metabolism in cultured cells and the description of APP mutations in early-onset familial AD, little is known regarding the biological function of APP in the brain and its metabolism in in vivo settings. In the central nervous system, APP transcripts and proteins are expressed in most neurons. In many regions of the nervous system, including the neocortex, APPs are present in cell bodies, proximal dendrites, and axons (10,38). In the rat peripheral nervous system, neuronal APPs are delivered to axons and terminals via the fast anterograde axonal transport system (34), and holo-APP-695 is the predominant transported isoform (55). It has been suggested that APPs may play roles in synaptic adhesion, interactions, and plasticity. Recent studies indicate that a sequence in the APP cytoplasmic domain catalyzes GTP exchange with the trimeric G protein, G$_o$. These results suggest a role of APP as a G$_o$-coupled receptor (43). Additional studies (56,66) have documented the expression of APP homologues in vertebrates. Unfortunately, relatively little is known about the subcellular distributions, targeting, processing, or functions of APP or the amyloid-precursor-like proteins (APLPs) at pre- or postsynaptic sites. The distribution and fates of transported APP isoforms in the central nervous system can be examined in vivo by labeling APP synthesized by specific populations of neurons followed by examination of APP processing in defined target fields. In transgenic mice, this approach will be invaluable in assessing the processing of overexpressed or mutated APP isoforms in transgenic animals.

MECHANISMS OF Aβ AMYLOIDOGENESIS

Senile plaques, comprised of amyloid deposits in proximity to neurites, are common in amygdala, hippocampus, and neocortex (30) and are a histological hallmark of AD (41). Amyloid, visualized by staining with thioflavin S or Congo red and consisting of 8-nm straight extracellular filaments, typically appears as diffuse parenchymal deposits in the cores of plaque and around blood vessels. The presence of amyloid has also been documented in the brains of aged primates (38,51,59,72) and in the brains of older patients with Down's syndrome (48), as well as in cases of hereditary cerebral hemorrhage with amyloidosis, Dutch type (HCHWA-D).

Several mutations have been described in the APP gene that are linked to early-onset AD (22). Mutations at codon 717 (of APP-770) and 693 (of APP-770) are linked genetically to early-onset familial AD and HCHWA-D, respectively (8,16,23,42). In nine families of early-onset autosomal dominant AD, the valine residue at position 717 is replaced by either isoleucine, phenylalanine, or glycine; mutations occur within the transmembrane domain of APP, two amino acids downstream from the C-terminus of Aβ (16). Although the conservative substitution of isoleucine for valine at position 717 does not appear to alter APP processing in transfected cells (7), the effects of isoleucine and other 717 substitutions on APP metabolism in vivo remain to be established. In addition, a mutation in APP that leads to a Glu-Gln substitution at position 693, corresponding to amino acid 22 of Aβ, is associated with HCHWA-D, a disease in which Aβ is deposited around blood vessels. As with the 717 mutation, the maturation of APP harboring this substitution is indistinguishable from wild-type APP (S. Sisodia, *unpublished observations*). More recently, a double mutation at codons 670 and 671 has been demonstrated in two large, related, early-onset AD families from Sweden (42). This double mutation results in substitution of the normal Lys-Met dipeptide for Asn-Leu. As yet, the pathology has not been fully documented. Remarkably, Aβ-related peptides are secreted at elevated levels from cells transfected with cDNA encoding APPs that harbor this double amino acid distribution (7,9). Finally, recent studies have shown that the majority (~80%) of early-onset non-Volga German kindreds exhibit linkage to markers localized to 14q24.3 on the distal part of chromosome 14 (50,57). The gene involved in these early-onset cases is presently unknown, although candidate loci mapping to 14q24 includes genes encoding c-*fos* and HSP-70. Future research should clarify the relationship of the product encoded by this locus to amyloidogenesis.

The cellular origins of APP that give rise to Aβ are beginning to be clarified. Neurons are one likely source (10,38), and morphological evidence suggests that APP-immunoreactive neurites, often decorated or capped by Aβ deposits (10,38), are one source of parenchymal amyloid. However, others cells, including astroglia, microglia, and vascular cells, may contribute to the formation of Aβ and may produce other constituents that colocalize with Aβ (1,35,58,67,73).

Aβ AMYLOIDOGENESIS IN AGED NONHUMAN PRIMATES

With a lifespan of 25–30 years (61), *Macaca mulatta* develop age-associated impairments in performance on cognitive and memory tasks early in the third decade of life (3). It is likely that these impairments in performance of specific behavioral tasks are associated, in individual animals, with the formation of neurites (32,38), the deposition of amyloid (51,59), and alterations in neurotransmitter markers (4,20,69). In many old animals, Aβ appears as diffuse deposits, as the cores of senile plaques, and as congophilic angiopathy (i.e., Aβ within the walls of blood vessels) (1,51,59,63,64). In neural parenchyma, Aβ is readily demonstrable in proximity to swollen APP-enriched neurites filled with lysosomes and abnormal membranes (38). It has been speculated that, normally, APP may play an important role in synaptic interactions, and alterations in the biology of APP at synapses could lead to changes in synaptic functions, including synaptic disjunction (a potentially reversible process) followed by irreversible synaptic disconnection. Loss of synapses has been well documented in AD (11,49,60). Disconnected axons may then "die back," and retrograde abnormalities, similar to those that occur following axotomy, appear in cell bodies. Subsequently, the organization of cytoskeletal elements in perikarya becomes perturbed, leading to the formation of NFT, a pathology eventually associated with death of neurons. Research during the next few years will identify the influences of other cells (i.e., astroglia, astrocytes, and vascular cells), colocalized proteins [i.e., apolipoprotein E (58)], and constituents of the complement cascade (40) on Aβ amyloidogenesis.

ATTEMPTS TO PRODUCE Aβ AMYLOIDOGENESIS IN TRANSGENIC MICE

Transgenic strategies have been used to test some of the hypothetical mechanisms of amyloidogenesis. Although initial studies designed to examine age- or disease-associated alterations in ratios of different APP transcripts and isoforms did not disclose consistent patterns in these measures (25,33,45), one in situ hybridization study suggested that levels of APP-751 mRNA (relative to APP-695 mRNA) were increased in subsets of affected neurons in AD (25). The hypothesis that the overexpression of APP-751 could facilitate the formation of Aβ was tested in transgenic mice that expressed a human APP-751 cDNA under the control of a neuron-specific enolase promoter (47). Immunocytochemistry of the brains of transgenic animals was interpreted to suggest a relative increase in APP in neurons and the presence of some extracellular Aβ deposits in hippocampus and cortex. Although the present report suggests that increased neuronal expression of APP-751 may promote amyloidogenesis, absolute levels of transgene-derived products or the prevalence of deposits in aged animals are presently unknown.

Transgenic animals were also generated by introduction of a transgene that encodes the 4-kD Aβ peptide under the transcriptional control of ~1.8 kb of the human APP promoter (71). Although initial immunocytochemical analyses were interpreted to show small clusters of Aβ immunoreactivity in the hippocampus of older mice, it soon became apparent that C57BL/6J mice, a contributor

to the Aβ transgenic mouse line, develop nonspecifically stained age-related clusters of intracytoplasmic inclusions within astrocytic processes (26).

On the basis of several lines of evidence suggesting that Aβ-containing C-terminal APP fragments may exhibit potential neurotoxicity, Gordon and colleagues (29) produced transgenic mice that utilized the human Thy-1 promoter to drive the expression of the C-terminal 100 amino acids of APP. Animals were reported to show neuritic plaques, NFT, and neuronal degeneration in silver-stained preparations similar to those seen in cases of AD (29). However, discrepancies were noted in the original report, and subsequent studies of additional littermates failed to replicate the initial observations.

Neve and colleagues (27) generated transgenic animals that express the C-terminal 100 amino acids of APP under the control of a brain dystrophin promoter. The authors documented (a) accumulations of Aβ-immunoreactive deposits in cell bodies and neuropil of the brains of 4- and 6-month-old transgenic animals and (b) the presence of abnormal aggregates of C-terminal epitopes in vesicular structures in the cytoplasm and in abnormal-appearing neurites in hippocampal CA2/3 regions. However, because polypeptide expression has not been documented by these investigators, the relationship between transgene expression and the observed phenotypes is unclear.

In related experiments, Fukuchi and colleagues (14) created transgenes that encode the APP signal peptide fused to APP C-terminal 100 amino acids driven by a cytomegalovirus (CMV) promoter. Cells transfected with this gene showed evidence of cytotoxicity (14). In transgenic mice, the CMV-driven transgene expressed substantial levels of the transgene-derived APP C-terminal 100 amino acids. However, these animals have not shown clinical signs or histopathological abnormalities in any tissues (G. M. Martin, *personal communication*).

Thus, at the present time, none of the transgenic models reproduce the features of AD-type pathology. It is uncertain whether the relative lack of success is caused by differences between species in their ability to form Aβ, the inappropriate selection of transgenes, or insufficient levels of transgenic product expression in cells that have the capacity to generate Aβ.

Because it has been difficult to overexpress APP by using conventional transgenic technologies, Lamb et al. (36) have recently used yeast artificial chromosome(s)/embryonic stem cell (YAC-ES) technologies to create a dosage imbalance and overexpression of APP in mice. A 650-kb YAC that contained the entire unrearranged 400-kb APP gene was transferred into ES cells by lipid-mediated transfection; ES cells that expressed human APP were introduced into mouse blastocytes to generate a number of chimeric mice. Subsequent breeding efforts resulted in mice that harbor human sequences in the germline. Levels of expression of the human transgene-encoded mRNA and protein in brain and peripheral tissues are approximately equivalent to endogenous levels, and, remarkably, the splicing pattern of human APP transcripts mirrors the stoichiometry spliced products derived from the endogenous mouse APP gene. This approach, which allows the introduction and expression of large DNA fragments, represents a technology that should prove useful in generating animal models of disorders that involve large genes, such as APP, and that has proven intractable for manipulation and expression by standard transgenic technologies.

CONCLUSION

Over the past 5 years, cellular and molecular biological approaches have significantly advanced our understanding of Aβ amyloidogenesis. Research in the area of trafficking and processing of APP in specific cell types, along with in vivo paradigms, will provide additional insights into APP biology. Moreover, the descriptions of mutations in the APP gene in some early-onset familial AD provide compelling reasons to pursue transgenic approaches in which the effects of these mutations on Aβ amyloidogenesis can be evaluated.

ACKNOWLEDGMENTS

The authors thank Drs. Lary Walker, Lee Martin, Linda Cork, Cheryl Kitt, Bruce Lamb, David Borchelt, and John Gearhart for helpful discussions.

This work was supported by grants from the U.S. Public Health Service (NS AG 05146, NS 20471) as well as from the American Health Assistance Foundation, the Metropolitan Life Foundation, and the Claster Family Fund. Dr. Price is the recipient of a Leadership and Excellence in Alzheimer's Disease (LEAD) award (AG 07914) and a Javits Neuroscience Investigator Award (NS 10580).

REFERENCES

1. Abraham CR, Selkoe DJ, Potter H, Price DL, Cork LC. α_1-Antichymotrypsin is present together with the β-protein in monkey brain amyloid deposits. *Neuroscience* 1989;32:715–720.
2. Anderson JP, Esch FS, Keim PS, Sambamurti K, Lieberburg I, Robakis NK. Exact cleavage site of Alzheimer amyloid precursor in neuronal PC-12 cells. *Neurosci Lett* 1991;128:126–128.
3. Bachevalier J, Landis LS, Walker LC, et al. Aged monkeys exhibit behavioral deficits indicative of widespread cerebral dysfunction. *Neurobiol Aging* 1991;12:99–111.
4. Beal MF, Walker LC, Storey E, Segar L, Price DL, Cork LC. Neurotransmitters in neocortex of aged rhesus monkeys. *Neurobiol Aging* 1991;12:407–412.
5. Braak H, Braak E. Alzheimer's disease affects limbic nuclei of the thalamus. *Acta Neuropathol* 1991;81:261–268.
6. Brion J-P. Molecular pathology of Alzheimer amyloid and neurofibrillary tangles. *Semin Neurosci* 1990;2:89–100.
7. Cai X-D, Golde TE, Younkin SG. Release of excess amyloid β protein from a mutant amyloid β protein precursor. *Science* 1993;259:514–516.
8. Chartier-Harlin M-C, Crawford F, Houlden H, et al. Early-onset Alzheimer's disease caused by mutations at codon 717 of the β-amyloid precursor protein gene. *Nature* 1991;353:844–846.
9. Citron M, Oltersdorf T, Haass C, et al. Mutation of the β-amyloid precursor protein in familial Alzheimer's disease increases β-protein production. *Nature* 1992;360:672–674.
10. Cras P, Kawai M, Lowery D, Gonzalez-DeWhitt P, Greenberg B, Perry G. Senile plaque neurites in Alzheimer disease accumulate amyloid precursor protein. *Proc Natl Acad Sci USA* 1991;88:7552–7556.
11. Davies CA, Mann DMA, Sumpter PQ, Yates PO. A quantitative morphometric analysis of the neuronal and synaptic content of the frontal and temporal cortex in patients with Alzheimer's disease. *J Neurol Sci* 1987;78:151–164.
12. Esch FS, Keim PS, Beattie EC, et al. Cleavage of amyloid β peptide during constitutive processing of its precursor. *Science* 1990;248:1122–1124.
13. Evans DA, Funkenstein HH, Albert MS, et al. Prevalence of Alzheimer's disease in a community population of older persons. Higher than previously reported. *JAMA* 1989;262:2551–2556.
14. Fukuchi K-i, Kamino K, Deeb SS, Smith AC, Dang T, Martin GM. Overexpression of amyloid precursor protein alters its normal processing and is associated with neurotoxicity. *Biochem Biophys Res Commun* 1992;182:165–173.
15. Glenner GG, Wong CW. Alzheimer's disease: initial report of the purification and characterization of a novel cerebrovascular amyloid protein. *Biochem Biophys Res Commun* 1984;120:885–890.
16. Goate A, Chartier-Harlin M-C, Mullan M, et al. Segregation of a missense mutation in the amyloid precursor protein gene with familial Alzheimer's disease. *Nature* 1991;349:704–706.
17. Goedert M, Sisodia SS, Price DL. Neurofibrillary tangles and β-amyloid deposits in Alzheimer's disease. *Curr Opin Neurobiol* 1991;1:441–447.
18. Golde TE, Estus S, Usiak M, Younkin LH, Younkin SG. Expression of β amyloid protein precursor mRNAs: recognition of a novel alternatively spliced form and quantitation in Alzheimer's disease using PCR. *Neuron* 1990;4:253–267.
19. Golde TE, Estus S, Younkin LH, Selkoe DJ, Younkin SG. Processing of the amyloid protein precursor to potentially amyloidogenic derivatives. *Science* 1992;255:728–730.
20. Goldman-Rakic PS, Brown RM. Regional changes of monoamines in cerebral cortex and subcortical structures of aging rhesus monkeys. *Neuroscience* 1981;6:177–187.
21. Haass C, Koo EH, Mellon A, Hung AY, Selkoe DJ. Targeting of cell-surface β-amyloid precursor protein to lysosomes: alternative processing into amyloid-bearing fragments. *Nature* 1992;357:500–503.
22. Hardy J, Mullan M. In search of the soluble. *Nature* 1992;359:268–269.
23. Hendriks L, van Duijn CM, Cras P, et al. Presenile dementia and cerebral haemorrhage linked to a mutation at codon 692 of the β-amyloid precursor protein gene. *Nature Genet* 1992;1:218–221.´
24. Hyman BT, Van Hoesen GW, Kromer LJ, Damasio AR. Perforant pathway changes and the memory impairment of Alzheimer's disease. *Ann Neurol* 1986;20:472–481.
25. Johnson SA, McNeill T, Cordell B, Finch CE. Relation of neuronal APP-751/APP-695 mRNA ratio and neuritic plaque density in Alzheimer's disease. *Science* 1990;248:854–857.
26. Jucker M, Walker LC, Martin LJ, Kitt CA, Kleinman HK, Ingram DK, Price DL. Age-associated inclusions in normal and transgenic mouse brain. *Science* 1992;255:1443–1445.
27. Kammesheidt A, Boyce FM, Spanoyannis AF, et al. Deposition of β/A4 immunoreactivity and neuronal pathology in transgenic mice expressing the carboxyterminal fragment of the Alzheimer amyloid precursor in the brain. *Proc Natl Acad Sci USA* 1992;89:10857–10861.
28. Kang J, Lemaire H-G, Unterbeck A, et al. The precursor of Alzheimer's disease amyloid A4 protein resembles a cell-surface receptor. *Nature* 1987;325:733–736.
29. Kawabata S, Higgins GA, Gordon JW. Amyloid plaques, neurofibrillary tangles and neuronal loss in brains of transgenic mice over-

expressing a C-terminal fragment of human amyloid precursor protein. *Nature* 1991;354:476–478.

30. Kemper T. Neuroanatomical and neuropathological changes in normal aging and in dementia. In: Albert ML, ed. *Clinical neurology of aging.* New York: Oxford University Press, 1984;9–52.

31. Kitaguchi N, Takahashi Y, Tokushima Y, Shiojiri S, Ito H. Novel precursor of Alzheimer's disease amyloid protein shows protease inhibitory activity. *Nature* 1988;331:530–532.

32. Kitt CA, Price DL, Struble RG, et al. Evidence for cholinergic neurites in senile plaques. *Science* 1984;226:1443–1445.

33. König G, Salbaum JM, Wiestler O, et al. Alternative splicing of the β/A4 amyloid gene of Alzheimer's disease in cortex of control and Alzheimer's disease patients. *Mol Brain Res* 1991;9:259–262.

34. Koo EH, Abraham CR, Potter H, Cork LC, Price DL. Developmental expression of α_1-antichymotrypsin in brain may be related to astrogliosis. *Neurobiol Aging* 1991;12:495–501.

35. Koo EH, Sisodia SS, Archer DR, et al. Precursor of amyloid protein in Alzheimer disease undergoes fast anterograde axonal transport. *Proc Natl Acad Sci USA* 1990;87:1561–1565.

36. Lamb BT, Sisodia SS, Lawler AM, et al. Introduction and expression of the 400 kilobase *precursor amyloid protein* gene in transgenic mice. *Nature Genetics* 1993;5:22–30.

37. Lee VM-Y, Balin BJ, Otvos L Jr, Trojanowski JQ. A68: a major subunit of paired helical filaments and derivatized forms of normal tau. *Science* 1991;251:675–678.

38. Martin LJ, Sisodia SS, Koo EH, et al. Amyloid precursor protein in aged nonhuman primates. *Proc Natl Acad Sci USA* 1991;88:1461–1465.

39. Masters CL, Simms G, Weinman NA, Multhaup G, McDonald BL, Beyreuther K. Amyloid plaque core protein in Alzheimer disease and Down syndrome. *Proc Natl Acad Sci USA* 1985;82:4245–4249.

40. McGeer PL, Akiyama H, Itagaki S, McGeer EG. Activation of the classical complement pathway in brain tissue of Alzheimer patients. *Neurosci Lett* 1989;107:341–346.

41. McKhann G, Drachman D, Folstein M, Katzman R, Price D, Stadlan EM. Clinical diagnosis of Alzheimer's disease: report of the NINCDS-ADRDA Work Group under the auspices of Department of Health and Human Services Task Force on Alzheimer's Disease. *Neurology* 1984;34:939–944.

42. Mullan M, Crawford F, Axelman K, et al. A pathogenic mutation for probable Alzheimer's disease in the APP gene at the N-terminus of β-amyloid. *Nature Genet* 1992;1:345–347.

43. Nishimoto I, Okamoto T, Matsuura Y, et al. Alzheimer amyloid protein precursor complexes with brain GTP-binding protein G_o. *Nature* 1993;362:75–79.

44. Palmert MR, Golde TE, Cohen ML, et al. Amyloid protein precursor messenger RNAs: differential expression in Alzheimer's disease. *Science* 1988;241:1080–1084.

45. Palmert MR, Podlisny MB, Witker DS, et al. The β-amyloid protein precursor of Alzheimer disease has soluble derivatives found in human brain and cerebrospinal fluid. *Proc Natl Acad Sci USA* 1989;86:6338–6342.

46. Ponte P, Gonzalez-DeWhitt P, Schilling J, et al. A new A4 amyloid mRNA contains a domain homologous to serine proteinase inhibitors. *Nature* 1988;331:525–532.

47. Quon D, Wang Y, Catalano R, Scardina JM, Murakami K, Cordell B. Formation of β-amyloid protein deposits in brains of transgenic mice. *Nature* 1991;352:239–241.

48. Rumble B, Retallack R, Hilbich C, et al. Amyloid A4 protein and its precursor in Down's syndrome and Alzheimer's disease. *N Engl J Med* 1989;320:1446–1452.

49. Scheff SW, Price DA. Synapse loss in the temporal lobe in Alzheimer's disease. *Ann Neurol* 1993;33:190–199.

50. Schellenberg GD, Bird TD, Wijsman EM, et al. Genetic linkage evidence for a familial Alzheimer's disease locus on chromosome 14. *Science* 1992;258:668–671.

51. Selkoe DJ, Bell DS, Podlisny MB, Price DL, Cork LC. Conservation of brain amyloid proteins in aged mammals and humans with Alzheimer's disease. *Science* 1987;235:873–877.

52. Seubert P, Oltersdorf T, Lee MG, et al. Secretion of β-amyloid precursor protein cleaved at the amino terminus of the β-amyloid peptide. *Nature* 1993;361:260–263.

53. Shoji M, Golde TE, Ghiso J, et al. Production of the Alzheimer amyloid β protein by normal proteolytic processing. *Science* 1992;258:126–129.

54. Sisodia SS, Koo EH, Beyreuther K, Unterbeck A, Price DL. Evidence that β-amyloid protein in Alzheimer's disease is not derived by normal processing. *Science* 1990;248:492–495.

55. Sisodia SS, Koo EH, Hoffman PN, Perry G, Price DL. Identification and transport of full-length amyloid precursor proteins in rat peripheral nervous system. *J Neurosci* 1993;13:3136–3142.

56. Slunt HH, Thinakaran G, Von Koch C, Lo ACY, Tanzi RE, Sisodia SS. Expression of a ubiquitous, cross-reactive homologue of the mouse β-amyloid precursor protein (APP). *J Biol Chem* 1994;269:2637–2644.

57. St George-Hyslop P, Haines J, Rogaev E, et al. Genetic evidence for a novel familial Alzheimer's disease locus on chromosome 14. *Nature Genet* 1992;2:330–334.

58. Strittmatter WJ, Saunders AM, Schmechel D, et al. Apolipoprotein E: high-avidity binding to β-amyloid and increased frequency of type 4 allele in late-onset familial Alzheimer disease. *Proc Natl Acad Sci USA* 1993;90:1977–1981.

59. Struble RG, Price DL Jr, Cork LC, Price DL. Senile plaques in cortex of aged normal monkeys. *Brain Res* 1985;361:267–275.

60. Terry RD, Masliah E, Salmon DP, et al. Physical basis of cognitive alterations in Alzheimer's disease: synapse loss is the major correlate of cognitive impairment. *Ann Neurol* 1991;30:572–580.

61. Tigges J, Gordon TP, McClure HM, Hall EC, Peters A. Survival rate and life span of rhesus monkeys at the Yerkes Regional Primate Research Center. *Am J Primatol* 1988;15:263–273.

62. Vogels OJM, Broere CAJ, Ter Laak HJ, Ten Donkelaar HJ, Nieuwenhuys R, Schultz BPM. Cell loss and shrinkage in the nucleus basalis Meynert complex in Alzheimer's disease. *Neurobiol Aging* 1990;11:3–13.

63. Walker LC, Kitt CA, Cork LC, Struble RG, Dellovade TL, Price DL. Multiple transmitter systems contribute neurites to individual senile plaques. *J Neuropathol Exp Neurol* 1988;47:138–144.

64. Walker LC, Masters C, Beyreuther K, Price DL. Amyloid in the brains of aged squirrel monkeys. *Acta Neuropathol* 1990;80:381–387.

65. Wang R, Meschia JF, Cotter RJ, Sisodia SS. Secretion of the β/A4 amyloid precursor protein. Identification of a cleavage site in cultured mammalian cells. *J Biol Chem* 1991;266:16960–16964.

66. Wasco W, Gurubhagavatula S, Paradis MD, et al. Isolation and characterization of *APLP2* encoding a homologue of the Alzheimer's associated amyloid β protein precursor. *Nature Genet* 1993;5:95–99.

67. Wegiel J, Wisniewski HM. The complex of microglial cells and amyloid star in three-dimensional reconstruction. *Acta Neuropathol* 1990;81:116–124.

68. Weidemann A, König G, Bunke D, et al. Identification, biogenesis, and localization of precursors of Alzheimer's disease A4 amyloid protein. *Cell* 1989;57:115–126.

69. Wenk GL, Pierce DJ, Struble RG, Price DL, Cork LC. Age-related changes in multiple neurotransmitter systems in the monkey brain. *Neurobiol Aging* 1989;10:11–19.

70. Whitehouse PJ, Price DL, Struble RG, Clark AW, Coyle JT, DeLong MR. Alzheimer's disease and senile dementia: loss of neurons in the basal forebrain. *Science* 1982;215:1237–1239.

71. Wirak DO, Bayney R, Ramabhadran TV, et al. Deposits of amyloid β protein in the central nervous system of transgenic mice. *Science* 1991;253:323–325.

72. Wisniewski HM, Terry RD. Morphology of the aging brain, human and animal. *Prog Brain Res* 1973;40:167–186.

73. Wisniewski HM, Wegiel J, Wang KC, Lach B. Ultrastructural studies of the cells forming amyloid in the cortical vessel wall in Alzheimer's disease. *Acta Neuropathol* 1992;84:117–127.

Psychopharmacology: The Fourth
Generation of Progress, edited by
Floyd E. Bloom and David J. Kupfer.
Raven Press, Ltd., New York © 1995.

CHAPTER 117

Neuropsychological Assessment of Patients with Alzheimer's Disease

Richard C. Mohs

The aims of this chapter are to review the cognitive and behavioral abnormalities associated with Alzheimer's disease (AD), to review instruments used to measure those impairments, and to describe how those instruments can be used to evaluate treatments. During the past 20 years and especially during the past 10 years a great deal has been learned about the pathophysiology of AD and related dementias, and this knowledge has led to the development of many potential treatments for the cognitive impairments which are the hallmarks of AD (see Chapter 110, *this volume*). In addition, there is substantial interest in the use of drugs which are already available but designed for other indications (such as psychosis, depression, or anxiety) as therapeutic agents for the management of AD patients (see Chapter 121, *this volume*). The efficacy of all of these agents is determined, in large part, by their effects on the behavior of AD patients, and many different instruments have been used to assess behavior of AD patients in clinical trials. The present review starts with a brief overview of the abnormal behaviors associated with AD and distinguishes the core cognitive abnormalities of AD such as memory loss, dysphasia, and dyspraxia from other symptoms such as agitation, depression, and anxiety, which are not invariably present. The roles of different assessment methods (including neuropsychologic tests, psychiatric rating scales, global clinical scales, and functional scales) in evaluating treatments for AD are discussed with emphasis on the need for neuropsychologic assessment in trials of drugs designed to treat cognitive symptoms. Desirable characteristics of instruments for evaluating AD treatments are then introduced, fol-

lowed by a discussion of specific neuropsychologic and other assessment instruments along with data on the extent to which they have the desirable reliability and validity characteristics. The review indicates that existing instruments for evaluating cognitive symptoms of AD are adequate to evaluate most drugs proposed for the treatment of AD's cognitive symptoms, but areas of continuing controversy remain. Available instruments for evaluating psychiatric symptoms, functional capacity, and global clinical utility are less well developed, and considerable work needs to be done before these aspects of AD can be evaluated with confidence in clinical trials.

CLINICAL SYMPTOMS OF ALZHEIMER'S DISEASE

Cognitive Symptoms

Alzheimer's is a disease characterized by a progressive loss of cognitive functions including memory, language, praxis, judgment, and orientation (50). Modern diagnostic criteria for AD require that a patient be given a diagnosis of AD only if they have a progressive loss of memory and at least one other cognitive function sufficient to interfere with social or occupational functioning (2,37). The terminology used to describe the cognitive functions lost in AD varies among clinical investigators, but there is general agreement on two points. The first is that the disorder is progressive (50), and the second is that, if a patient lives long enough after disease onset, all of the cognitive functions dependent upon the neocortex—particularly memory, language, praxis, and orientation—will be impaired (26,32,50). These defining deficits are referred to in this review as the core cognitive deficits of

R. C. Mohs: Department of Psychiatry, Mount Sinai School of Medicine, New York, New York 10029; and Psychiatry Service, Veterans Affairs Medical Center, Bronx, New York 10468.

TABLE 1. *Prevalence of symptoms by etiology of dementia upon presentation*[a]

Symptom or difficulty	SDAT[b] (N = 264)		Vascular (N = 18)		Mixed (N = 34)	
	N	Percent	N	Percent	N	Percent
Memory loss	252	95.5	15	83.3	33	97.1
Disorientation	95	36.0	4	22.2	11	32.4
Personality change	82	31.1	7	38.9	14	41.2
Language difficulty	74	28.0	2	11.1	11	32.4
Poor calculations	62	23.5	5	27.8	7	20.6
Psychotic behavior	45	17.0	2	11.1	6	17.6
Depression	39	14.8	4	22.2	4	11.8
Agnosia	32	12.1	0	0.0	5	14.7
Apraxia	18	6.8	0	0.0	0	0.0
Uncleanliness	17	6.4	1	5.6	4	11.8
Weight loss	16	6.1	0	0.0	1	2.9
Incontinence	14	6.1	4	22.2	1	2.9
Gait difficulty	6	2.3	8	44.4	1	2.9
Transient neurologic symptom	3	1.1	5	27.8	2	5.9
Seizures	3	1.1	0	0.0	0	0.0
Focal weakness	1	0.4	0	0.0	3	8.8

[a] Adapted from ref. 61, with permission.
[b] Senile dementia of the Alzheimer type.
From Thal et al. (61).

AD. Drugs that are designed to treat these core cognitive deficits are referred to as *antidementia drugs.*

Psychiatric Symptoms

Along with these cognitive abnormalities, however, AD patients have a variety of other symptoms and behaviors. Table 1, reproduced from Thal et al. (61), lists the symptoms and abnormal behaviors observed in a large group of AD patients, patients with vascular dementia, and patients with mixed AD and vascular dementia when they were first evaluated in a research clinic. As expected, virtually all patients with AD or vascular dementia had a prominent memory impairment, and many had clinically evident deficits in other cognitive areas. Many patients also had significant psychiatric symptoms such as depression, psychosis, agitation, and personality change. There is considerable controversy over the extent to which these symptoms are typical of AD and the way in which these symptoms change during the course of AD (26). What is evident, however, is that these symptoms, when present, are troublesome and produce excess disability in AD patients (60). In current clinical practice a variety of available psychotropic agents are used to treat these symptoms (see Chapter 121, *this volume*). However, drugs that alleviate such symptoms but do not improve cognition are not antidementia drugs. They are used very differently from antidementia drugs in clinical practice, and new agents to treat psychiatric symptoms must be evaluated with different procedures than are antidementia drugs.

Functional Impairments

Both the cognitive and the psychiatric symptoms of AD lead to functional impairment manifested by poor performance in everyday activities of daily living (ADLs) such as feeding, dressing, holding a job, doing household chores, and managing money. These functional impairments rather than symptoms, per se, are often the most troubling aspects of AD because they result in loss of autonomy for the patient, increased need for care by family members or professional caregivers, and economic hardship (60). Consequently, it is important both in studies of antidementia drugs and in studies of drugs for the psychiatric symptoms of AD to consider the effects of those treatments on patient functioning. As indicated below, functional measures often serve as a useful adjunct to measures of symptom severity in trials of drug treatments for AD.

Approaches to Assessment

Given the wide variety of symptoms and behavioral abnormalities associated with AD, it is not surprising that many different types of assessments are used in clinical trials. Roughly, these assessments can be grouped into two categories, each with its own rationale and historical development. The two categories are illustrated in Table 2, adapted from a review by Yesavage et al. (67) of the clinical trials of vasodilators done prior to 1979. Although the vasodilators are no longer considered viable treatments for AD, the table indicates one of the major prob-

TABLE 2. *Outcome measures used in two or more clinical treatment trials of vasodilators in senile dementias conducted prior to 1979*[a]

Measure	Times used
Psychological tests	
Wechsler Adult Intelligence Scale	10
Raven's Progressive Matrices	5
Bender–Gestalt	4
Babcock Sentence Completion	2
Critical Flicker Fusion	2
Behavioral ratings	
Sandoz Clinical Assessment—Geriatric	5
Mental Status Check List	5
Brief Psychiatric Rating Scale	3
Crichton Royal Behavior Rating Scale	2
Nurses' Observation Scale for Inpatient Evaluation	2

[a] Adapted from ref. 67, with permission.

lems encountered in trying to evaluate studies of antidementia drugs conducted prior to 1979—namely, the fact that there was little agreement about how to assess the efficacy of such drugs. The table presents all of the outcome measures used in two or more clinical trials. No instrument was used consistently enough to allow comparisons across studies, and most of the commonly used instruments (e.g., the WAIS) were not designed to evaluate symptoms or behaviors associated with AD. Almost none of the instruments listed in Table 2 are still used in trials of treatments for AD, but the grouping of these assessments into those involving psychological tests and those involving psychiatric ratings illustrates the two general approaches to assessment still followed today. Performance-based neuropsychological tests in which the patient is actually required to perform specific tasks are generally used to assess drug effects on the core cognitive symptoms of AD. Clinician ratings based on interviews of the patients, caregivers, or others are used to assess drug effects on psychiatric symptoms and ADLs and to provide global clinical assessments. As indicated below, both of these approaches have important, but complementary, roles to play in the evaluation of treatments for AD.

NEUROPSYCHOLOGICAL ASSESSMENT IN DIAGNOSIS

Part of the diagnostic process for patients with AD or other dementia is to document that the patient has a cognitive impairment. Several neuropsychologic batteries have been shown to be useful for screening persons at risk for AD and for evaluating patients during a diagnostic work-up. However, neuropsychologic tests do not, by themselves, permit a diagnosis of AD or other dementia. Furthermore, the characteristics of a good screening test or diagnostic aid for dementia do not necessarily make it a

good instrument for use in clinical trials. Most current diagnostic criteria for AD (37) require that a patient be evaluated with some standard mental status examination before a diagnosis of AD is made. Community screening studies (27) indicate that poor performance on a standard cognitive screening instrument may be the best single predictor of who is likely to develop a dementing illness in the near future. Clinical studies (64) indicate that specific neuropsychologic measures can distinguish even mildly demented persons from matched normal controls very reliably. The tests most sensitive to early AD are delayed recall memory measures (64), while tests of speeded psychomotor performance and tests of verbal ability also show decrements very early (57,65). Many different kinds of dementia produce similar cognitive impairments, however, and therefore neuropsychologic tests are relatively poor at distinguishing different types of dementia in the absence of a complete clinical examination. The difficulty is exemplified by the data in Table 1 which indicate that vascular dementia and AD share most of the same cognitive abnormalities. Performance on neuropsychologic tests is also very much affected by education (24), age (16), cultural background (16,24), illnesses other than AD (16), and situational factors, so that a poor score on a test must be examined in light of all these clinical variables before a diagnosis of dementia is made.

Thus for a dementia screening test it is important to have information about how these factors affect performance so that they can be factored into clinical decision-making. For outcome measures in clinical trials, this information is often less crucial because performance is compared between groups of patients (rather than between individuals) who are randomized to different treatment conditions. Other factors, including the availability of longitudinal data and the availability of alternate forms, are more important for determining the utility of treatment assessment instruments.

NEUROPSYCHOLOGICAL TESTS IN CLINICAL TRIALS

Clinical and Regulatory Issues

Neuropsychological tests are an essential part of the evaluation of antidementia drugs but are of secondary importance in evaluating drugs designed to treat the psychiatric manifestations of AD. In ordinary clinical practice the severity of cognitive impairment in AD or other dementia is best evaluated with neuropsychological tests. A formal assessment of cognitive functioning with some performance-based test is used both as part of a standard diagnostic evaluation (37) and to monitor progression of illness (18). Recently developed regulatory guidelines for the development of antidementia drugs mandate that an

1380 / Assessment of Alzheimer's Disease

antidementia drug be superior to placebo on two types of measures: (i) a performance-based measure of cognitive function and (ii) an independent clinician-rated measure of global severity (10,34). Originally developed in the United States following extensive discussion among many clinicians involved in clinical trials of antidementia drugs (1), this "dual outcome" strategy was adopted to ensure that any approved antidementia drug would improve the core cognitive symptoms of AD and that the magnitude of improvement would be large enough to be clinically significant (34). The pivotal studies used to demonstrate the efficacy of tacrine, the only drug yet approved as an antidementia drug in the United States, utilized outcome measures designed to satisfy this requirement (11,14). Guidelines for the Community of European Nations (10) which are currently under review have adopted this dual outcome strategy with some modifications, particularly in that they permit a wider variety of measures to be used to assess the clinical impact of a drug.

At present there are no formal regulatory guidelines either in the United States or in Europe for the development of drugs to treat the psychiatric symptoms associated with dementia. Presumably, neuropsychologic tests would play a lesser role in the evaluation of such drugs because their primary target symptoms would be agitation, depression, psychosis, and anxiety, all of which are traditionally evaluated with rating scales completed by a clinician following an interview (see Chapter 121, *this volume*). It is reasonable, however, to expect that cognitive assessments would be included in trials of such agents to determine whether the drug improved, worsened, or had no effect on cognition.

Criteria for Neuropsychological Tests

To be used successfully in clinical trials of drugs for the treatment of dementia, a neuropsychologic test battery must meet certain criteria. In many respects, these criteria are similar to those which must be met by instruments used satisfactorily to evaluate other psychoactive agents such as neuroleptics, antidepressants, or drugs for movement disorders. One difference between the antidementia field and other areas of psychopharmacology, however, is that in many other areas, effective drugs were developed before the most commonly used assessment tools were accepted as valid measures of efficacy. This enabled instruments such as the Hamilton Depression Rating Scale (23) and the Brief Psychiatric Rating Scale (43) to be validated in studies with treatments for depression or psychosis, respectively, that were already accepted as effective. The first drug approved as effective in the treatment of AD was only approved in 1993, and this drug has relatively modest beneficial effects (11,14). Conse-

quently, another measure of validity had to be used to assess potential instruments. Virtually all clinicians and clinical follow-up studies agree that AD is a progressive condition, and any instrument that is a valid measure of clinical severity must reflect this change over time. As a result, longitudinal studies have played an important role in establishing the utility of instruments for evaluating patients with AD.

Following is a list of some properties that any instrument used to evaluate treatments for AD should have. The list expands upon the criteria originally proposed by Mohs et al. (40). Although the criteria are specifically designed for performance-based cognitive assessments, they are, with minor modifications, applicable to other types of assessments for AD as well. There are two reliability criteria:

1. The instrument should have high inter-rater reliability.
2. The instrument should have high retest reliability. In studies of cognitive instruments the interval for evaluating retest reliability is usually 1–4 weeks because a patient's cognitive status is not likely to change substantially in that period. However, the appropriate retest interval for psychiatric assessment instruments is probably shorter because these symptoms may fluctuate more quickly.

There are two practicality criteria:

3. The instrument should be brief enough to be completed in 1 hr or less.
4. Alternate, but equivalent, forms should be available so that patients can be tested repeatedly. This criteria applies only to cognitive tests.

There are three validity criteria:

5. The instrument should measure all of the major symptoms judged to be clinically important; and if instruments are to be used in pivotal trials, they should yield a single overall symptom severity score.
6. The instrument should be suitable for use in AD patients with a broad range of dementia severity because patients enter clinical trials with different baseline levels of dementia.
7. The instrument should measure increases in symptom severity known to occur as patients progress longitudinally. This criterion does not apply to instruments for psychiatric symptoms because the symptoms do not invariably worsen as the disease progresses.

Comparison of Available Instruments and Batteries

Table 3 presents a list of some of the neuropsychological test batteries commonly used to assess cognition in clinical trials of drugs for AD. The table also lists the

TABLE 3. *Comparison of neuropsychologic tests as tools for the assessment of antidementia drugs*[a]

Instrument	Reference	Reliable		Practical		Valid		
		1	2	3	4	4	5	6
MMSE[b]	17	+++	+++	+++	0	+	++	+++
BIMC[c]	4	+++	++	+++	0	+	+	+++
ADAS-Cog[d]	49	+++	+++	++	+++	+++	+++	+++
SKT[e]	13	+++	+	++	+++	++	+	++
Mattis Dementia Scale	8	++	++	+	0	+++	++	++
CERAD Battery[f]	42	+++	+++	++	+	+++	+++	+++
NYU Battery	15	+++	++	+	+++	+++	+	+
Everyday Memory	31	++	++	+	+++	++	+	+
WAIS-R[g]	63	+++	+++	0	0	0	0	+

[a] Degree to which each criterion has been met based on available data; 0 = does not meet; +, ++, +++ = satisfied to slight, moderate, or high degree, respectively.
[b] Mini Mental State Exam.
[c] Blessed Test of Information, Memory, and Concentration.
[d] Alzheimer's Disease Assessment Scale, Cognitive Subscale.
[e] Syndrome Kurtztest.
[f] Consortium to Establish a Registry for Alzheimer's Disease.
[g] Wechsler Adult Intelligence Scale, Revised.

seven criteria for such tests mentioned above and gives a rating of the extent to which each test satisfies the criteria. While it is hardly exhaustive, this list includes all of the tests used very frequently and also includes a variety of different types of tests so that the strengths and weaknesses of various approaches can be discussed.

1. *The Mini Mental State Exam (MMSE; see ref. 17).* This is an 11-item test with a total score of 0 (severe impairment) to 30 (no impairment). It is probably the most widely used screening instrument for dementia in the world (18), and it has been used in clinical trials. It includes very brief assessments of memory, language, praxis, and orientation. Major strengths of the MMSE are its coverage of a variety of relevant cognitive areas in a very brief test and the fact that a large amount of cross-sectional and longitudinal data are available. Weaknesses are that it is probably too brief, particularly in its assessment of memory, to be very sensitive, and, because there are no alternate forms, nonspecific carry-over effects make it difficult to use in trials where patients are assessed many times.

2. *Blessed Test of Information, Memory, and Concentration (BIMC; see ref. 4).* This is a short test which assesses primarily orientation and memory. Originally developed in Great Britain as a 37-point scale, most American investigators use adaptations with 27 items and a total score ranging from 0 (no impairment) to 33 (severe impairment). Strengths of this instrument are that it is very brief, that scores on the Blessed test have been correlated with both the neuropathologic (4) and neurochemical (45) abnormalities of AD, and that extensive longitudinal data are available (53). Principal weaknesses of the scale are that it does not cover all of the cognitive symptoms evident in AD patients, that it is so brief that it is

relatively insensitive (54), and that there are no alternate forms to enable repeated administration in clinical trials.

3. *Alzheimer's Disease Assessment Scale—Cognitive Portion (ADAS-Cog; see ref. 49).* This is probably the most widely used cognitive assessment instrument in clinical trials of antidementia drugs done in the United States (11,14) and has been recognized by the U.S. Food and Drug Administration (34). Although less well known outside the United States, this scale has been used extensively in Europe (7,66), where it has been recognized as acceptable by the Commission of the European Communities (10), and in Japan (39). Table 4 presents a list of the items included in both the cognitive and noncognitive portions of this scale. The cognitive portion includes seven performance items and four clinician-rated items assessing memory, language, praxis, and orientation, with a total score ranging from 0 (no impairment) to 70 (severe impairment). The noncognitive portion includes 10 clinician-rated items assessing psychosis, agitation, depression, and other abnormalities. Strengths of the scale are its broad coverage of relevant cognitive domains, its widespread use, the availability of alternate forms for the memory tests, and the availability of extensive longitudinal data (54). Weaknesses are that it is somewhat long (approximately 45 min per administration) and that severely demented patients cannot be assessed with this instrument.

4. *Syndrome Kurtztest (SKT; see ref. 13).* This is a timed test with 60 sec allowed for each of nine subtests. The tests are designed to assess memory, attention, naming, and object arrangement. The test was originally developed in Germany, where it has been administered to hundreds of persons (13). Recently, an English-language version was developed and used in a large clinical trial

TABLE 4. *Contents of the Alzheimer's Disease Assessment Scale (ADAS)*

Subscale Symptom area Item	Points (range)
Cognitive	0–70
Memory	0–25
Word recall	0–10
Word recognition	0–12
Remembering test instructions[a]	0–5
Orientation	0–8
Language	0–25
Naming	0–5
Following commands	0–5
Spoken language ability[a]	0–5
Word-finding difficulty[a]	0–5
Comprehension of spoken language[a]	0–5
Praxis	0–10
Copying drawings	0–5
Ideational praxis	0–5
Noncognitive	0–50
Agitation	0–20
Excess motor activity[a]	0–5
Pacing[a]	0–5
Uncooperative to testing[a]	0–5
Tremors[a]	0–5
Depressed mood	0–10
Depressed mood[a]	0–5
Tearfulness[a]	0–5
Psychosis	0–10
Delusions[a]	0–5
Hallucinations[a]	0–5
Miscellaneous	0–10
Attention/concentration[a,b]	0–5
Weight change[a,c]	0–5
Total score	0–120

[a] Clinician rated item.
[b] May be included as a cognitive item.
[c] May be associated with depression or cognitive impairment.

with AD patients (29). Strengths of the test are its brevity and inclusion of items specifically designed to measure attention. The principal weakness of the SKT is that the scale is suitable only for patients with very mild symptoms. There are few longitudinal data on the SKT and the fact that it is a timed test suggests that performance on many items may be difficult to interpret.

5. *Mattis Dementia Rating Scale (see ref. 8).* This is an instrument with five subscales measuring attention, initiation and perseveration, conceptualization, construction, and memory. The items are administered in a stepwise fashion such that patients who make errors on simple items do not receive more complex ones. The usual time for administration is about 45 min, and the total scale is from 0 (no impairment) to 144 (severe impairment). Strengths of the scale are its broad coverage of relevant cognitive domains and its inclusion of items to assess attention. The instrument has no alternate forms for repeated testing. Although the instrument has been used to

assess severity of demented patients in clinical studies (8) and in some longitudinal studies (51), the scale has not been widely used in treatment trials.

6. *Neuropsychological Battery of the Consortium to Establish a Registry for Alzheimer's Disease (CERAD).* The CERAD project was funded by the U.S. National Institute on Aging (NIA) with the aim of developing standardized methods for the clinical (42), neuropsychological (64,65), neuropathological (38), and neuroradiological (12) evaluation of patients with AD. The CERAD neuropsychological battery consists of seven subtests including the MMSE and three others which are adapted from the ADAS-Cog. These tests assess memory, language, praxis, and orientation. Because the tests were designed to characterize patients along different dimensions, there is no established algorithm for calculating a single dementia severity score. Advantages of the CERAD battery are its broad coverage of cognitive domains, applicability to a broad range of dementia severity, the availability of extensive longitudinal data (41), and the utility of the battery for measuring symptoms in early AD (64,65). Disadvantages are that alternate forms are not readily available, the lack of an obvious summary measure, and its extensive overlap with other instruments.

7. *New York University Computerized Test Battery (NYU Battery; see ref. 15).* This is a collection of 12 tests that have been adapted for administration by computer. The battery is quite long and measures memory, language, concept formation, psychomotor speed, and attention. The tests in this battery are primarily adaptations of tests used to measure the effects of aging and, as a result, are suitable for nondemented aged and mildly demented persons but not for moderate or severe AD patients. Some of the tests are designed to simulate real-world memory tasks such as telephone number recall, and others were designed as human analogs of tests used to evaluate drug effects in nonhuman primates. There is no standard method for calculating an overall dementia score, and few longitudinal data have been published (15). The primary value of the battery may be as a tool for assessment early in drug development when there is a need to investigate possible drug effects on a broad array of cognitive functions and where statistical concerns about multiple outcome measures are not critical.

8. *Everyday Memory Battery (see ref. 31).* This is a collection of 14 memory and attention tests which are administered by computer. The tests were selected to mimic real-world activities such as telephone dialing and remembering of faces. Like the NYU Battery, this battery is suitable for nondemented elderly and mildly impaired patients but not for moderate or severe AD. There is no summary dementia score, and the battery does not cover all of the domains impaired in AD. This battery may also have some utility in the early phases of drug development

when highly selected patients with mild dementia can be assessed on a broad array of measures.

9. *Wechsler Adult Intelligence Scale (WAIS; see ref. 63).* Until recently, this test was often used to assess deficits in patients with AD (67). It consists of five verbal subtests including vocabulary and general information and four nonverbal subtests including block design and digit symbol substitution. The test is very widely used as a general measure of intelligence, so extensive population data are available. The test has almost none of the features desirable in an assessment instrument for AD. It does not cover the major cognitive symptoms of AD (particularly memory), it is not suitable for a broad range of demented patients, there are no alternate forms, and few longitudinal data are available in AD patients. Fortunately, few recent clinical studies have used tests such as this.

Longitudinal Data and Their Implications

Extensive longitudinal data have been collected on several of the tests listed above, particularly the MMSE (18,41), the BIMC test (18,53,61), the ADAS-Cog (30,54), and the CERAD battery (41). All of these tests have been shown to measure deterioration in AD patients followed over time and to be relatively insensitive to age-related cognitive changes in nondemented elderly persons. Several studies have attempted to identify demographic or clinical factors that might predict rate of cognitive decline. With a few exceptions (36), most studies have not found any relationship between rate of deterioration and gender, age of onset, or presence of family history of dementia (28,51,53). While there may be some tendency for early-onset patients to have a more severe language and praxis impairment relative to memory impairment (6), these differences at initial presentation do not alter the longitudinal course. An implication is that we have, at present, no rationale for stratifying patients at entry into clinical trials on the basis of demographic factors. While there is some evidence that psychosis early in the disease may be predictive of more rapid deterioration (56), most studies of antidementia drugs do not include psychotic patients.

With all of these instruments, the reliability of measured change increases with longer follow-up. This has implications for the design of clinical trials, particularly those in which the aim is not to determine the acute effects of a drug, but to determine the ability of the drug to alter the course of the illness. Relevant data from Stern et al. (53) for the BIMC illustrate this point very clearly. Their data were obtained in a study of 111 patients assessed every 6 months. Over a 12-month follow-up the mean change on the BIMC test was 4.1 points with a standard deviation of 4.1 points. Over a 6-month follow-up period the mean change was 2.2 points, with a standard deviation

of 3.2 points (53). Power calculations were done to determine the sample sizes needed to detect the effect of a drug which slows the rate of deterioration by one-half relative to placebo. Regardless of other parameters, the sample size needed for such a study was over twice as large when drug and placebo patients were compared for 6 months than when they were compared for 12 months. This results from the fact that the mean change relative to the standard deviation of change increases dramatically the longer patients are followed. Similar points have been made using MMSE (41), CERAD (41), and ADAS-Cog (54) data. For clinical investigators this implies that they can perform shorter studies with larger sample sizes or longer studies with smaller sample sizes.

Annual rates of progression have been published for several of the commonly used instruments. Table 5 presents a summary of some of the rates along with measures of variability. This table is not an exhaustive list but does include nearly all of the studies with large enough samples to yield stable estimates. Because the CERAD battery does not have an obvious summary score, annual rates of change for three selected subtests are presented. In most instances the standard deviation of the annual change is equal to or greater than the mean annual change. For the ADAS-Cog the standard deviation is slightly less, possibly indicating greater sensitivity of this instrument. However, the instruments do not all cover the same range of symptom severity, with the BIMC and MMSE probably covering the smallest severity range. One direct comparison of the range of two instruments compared the ADAS-Cog and the BIMC. This study found that the ADAS-Cog was more sensitive both to mild dementia and to change in severe dementia than was the BIMC (54). One study found that in clinically demented persons with MMSE scores above 24, portions of the CERAD battery were still able to detect marked impairment (64). The greater length of the ADAS-Cog and the CERAD battery relative to the MMSE and the BIMC test enable them to have items covering a greater range of dementia severity.

Rate of change for these tests is not independent of baseline dementia severity. For the BIMC test the rate of change is linear over most of the scale's range (53), but the rate of change slows for severely demented persons who are reaching the limit of the scale. For the other tests there is evidence that rate of change is slower both for mild dementia and for severe dementia than for moderate dementia. This phenomenon is illustrated by the graph in Fig. 1 [adapted from Stern et al. (54)], which shows annual change in the ADAS-Cog as a function of baseline. Annual change was a curvilinear function of baseline such that expected annual change went from less than 5 points for mild patients to a maximum of nearly 13 points for baselines of 35–40 and again decreased to 5 for baselines of over 60. A similar phenomenon was observed in the CERAD study when MMSE scores were plotted as a

TABLE 5. *Annual rates of change for instruments used to assess cognitive function in Alzheimer's disease*

Instrument	Range	Reference	N	Annual change	S.D.
		62	120	2.2	5.0
MMSE	0–30	59	106	2.8	4.6
		41	430	3.9	3.7
BIMC	0–33	53	213	4.1	4.1
		28	161	4.4	3.6
ADAS-Cog	0–70	54	253	9.6	8.2
Mattis Scale	0–144	51	55	11.4	11.1
CERAD Battery		41			
Word list	0–30		430	2.0	2.4
Naming	0–15		430	2.0	2.2
Drawings	0–11		428	1.3	1.9

function of overall dementia severity during the follow-up period (41). Expected annual MMSE change was approximately 2 points for patients whose mean MMSE level during follow-up was over 20, annual change was nearly 5 for patients whose overall level was 10, and annual change was approximately 2 for patients whose level was 5. What this means is that the expected amount of deterioration for patients in a clinical trial will depend heavily upon dementia severity at entry. Consequently, stratification by severity will be wise, and these scales may be most sensitive to change, not in the most mild patients but in moderately demented patients.

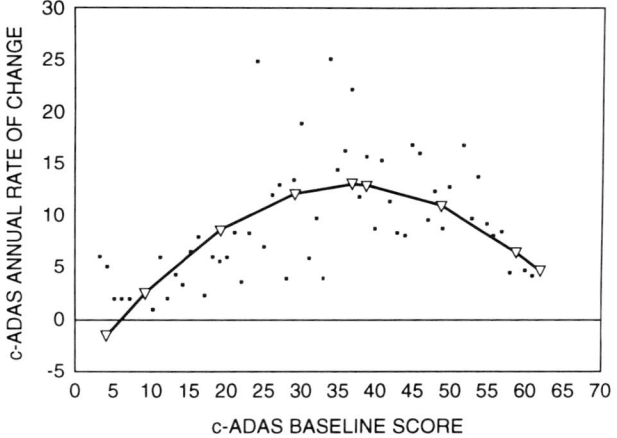

FIG. 1. Annual rate of cognitive change (ARCC) scores obtained from Alzheimer patients in a longitudinal study. *Squares* representing mean change scores on the cognitive portion of the Alzheimer's Disease Assessment Scale (c-ADAS) are shown as a function of the baseline score (base). *Triangles* represent predicted values calculated from the quadratic equation fit by the method of least squares to the original 253 annual change scores: ARCC = −6.357 + 1.022 × base − 0.01339 × base^2 ($R = 0.42$, $F = 27.46$, df = 2250, $p < .001$). *Straight lines* connecting the estimated points approximate the actual quadratic equation. (From ref. 54, with permission. Copyright 1994, American Psychiatric Association.)

RELATIONSHIP TO OTHER OUTCOME MEASURES

Global Change and Staging Instruments

These are instruments which provide an assessment not only of the patient's cognitive status, but of the patient's overall clinical condition as well. Staging instruments such as the Clinical Dementia Rating Scale (CDR; see refs. 3 and 5) and the Global Deterioration Scale (GDS; see ref. 47) evaluate patient's according to fixed external standards, whereas change instruments such as the Clinical Global Impression of Change (CGIC; see ref. 22) rate the patient relative to their own previous condition. In the evaluation of antidementia drugs, these instruments provide one way of assessing the clinical impact of proposed treatments that have been shown to improve cognitive symptoms as measured by neuropsychological tests (10,34). In and of themselves, global instruments cannot be used to demonstrate that a drug has antidementia effects, because a variety of treatments that do not improve cognition might have globally beneficial effects in demented patients; this would include (a) neuroleptic drugs for agitated patients and (b) antidepressants for AD patients with depressive symptoms. There is considerable debate about whether staging instruments or change measures are best for this purpose and about the kinds of information that should be considered in assigning a global score. There is agreement that the global measure should be done independently of the neuropsychological test measure (10,34).

When administered according to specified procedures, global scales can be highly reliable (5), although procedures for administering most are not well-specified. Scores on staging instruments correlate highly with performance-based cognitive measures (42) in AD patients, and they also can be used to document longitudinal change (3,41). Few studies have been done to evaluate the reliability and sensitivity of global change measures such as the CGIC in AD. In theory, change measures might be more sensitive than global staging instruments because they are, by definition, adjusted for baseline. Some trials of antidementia drugs last a year or more, however, so that elaborate procedures for completing global change measures might be necessary to remind the rating clinician of the patient's baseline condition and to minimize the effect of intervening patients. Clearly, additional work needs to be done to evaluate the factors which make these instruments more or less reliable and more or less valid. Recent clinical trials have shown that even modestly effective cholinergic drugs (see Chapter 120, *this volume*) can be shown to have beneficial effects measured with unstructured global change instruments.

Functional Measures

These are scales designed to measure the patient's ability to perform everyday activities of daily living (ADLs). The primary use of such measures in clinical trials of drugs for AD is to document the functional or clinical impact of either antidementia drugs or drugs used to manage psychiatric symptoms. The fact that ADLs are impaired in AD is well known, but at present no ADL instrument has been accepted as a valid measure of clinical significance for antidementia or other drugs (10,34). This probably results from the fact that no ADL instrument has been shown both to capture all of the major functional impairments in AD patients and to measure progression of those impairments over a broad range of severity.

Most ADL instruments are derived, at least in part, from the work of Katz et al. (25), who identified and developed a scale to measure six basic ADLs (feeding, toileting, dressing, physical ambulation, bathing, and grooming) which represent biologically necessary activities common to all persons. Later functional assessment instruments designed for older persons include many of these basic ADLs, but also contain clinician ratings of cognitive symptoms such as memory impairment or language loss (21,35), ratings of psychiatric symptoms such as personality change (4), or ratings of higher-level ADLs such as managing money, driving, and shopping (52). If a functional assessment instrument is to be used to provide independent validation of the effects of a drug designed to treat cognitive or psychiatric symptoms, then it would not be desirable to include items that also evaluate cognitive or psychiatric symptoms in the functional scale. While they may have some utility as global measures in some situations, functional scales with cognitive or psychiatric symptom items are not useful validators for clinical trials.

The distinction between universal, biologically necessary ADLs such as feeding and dressing and higher-level

ADLs performed by most (but not all) individuals was formalized by Lawton and Brodie (33). They developed two scales: (i) the Physical and Self-Maintenance Scale (PSMS), which evaluates basic ADLs, and (ii) the Instrumental Activities of Daily Living Scale (IADLS), which evaluates higher-level activities that tend to be more specific for certain groups of individuals. The PSMS is similar to the original ADL scale of Katz et al. (25), whereas the IADLS includes items such as "shopping," "doing laundry," and "handling finances." Several studies have shown that these higher-level, instrumental activities are impaired in patients with AD (18,52). A recent study of 104 patients followed for up to 8 years demonstrated the strengths and weaknesses of these two scales (19). While all of the PSMS items had high reliability, raters had substantial difficulty in rating many of the IADLS items, particularly for men, because they tended not to perform these activities even prior to onset of dementia (33). Thus, more universally applicable IADLS items would be desirable. The difficulty with using the PSMS alone is illustrated by the longitudinal data in Fig. 2, which presents the 12-month change scores plotted against the BIMC test scores obtained at the start of each follow-up interval. For follow-up intervals beginning when patients were mild to moderately demented (i.e., BIMC scores < 25) there was usually little change on the PSMS, indicating that the PSMS would be relatively insensitive to change in most clinical trials. Scores on the IADLS began to change substantially even for follow-up intervals beginning when patients had mild dementia, but tended to change very little in moderate-to-severe patients largely because of a ceiling on the scale. Thus, to be sensitive over a broad range of disease severity, an ADL scale for use in clinical trials would have to include items to assess both basic and instrumental ADLs, with items designed to be less gender-specific than those of the IADLS.

Psychiatric Rating Scales

These are scales designed to assess symptoms such as depression, agitation, psychosis, anxiety, and personality change in patients with AD. While there is general agreement that such symptoms are of clinical significance in patients with AD, it is not yet clear how prevalent these symptoms are, how best to assess them, or how they are related to other aspects of AD. Because the different types of psychiatric symptoms are likely to be treated with different drugs, it will probably be necessary to have different items or instruments for each type of symptom. It is not possible to review all of the issues involved in evaluating these symptoms here, but a few general principles involved in selecting instruments for evaluating these symptoms should be mentioned. First is that AD patients are, by definition, demented, so that traditional

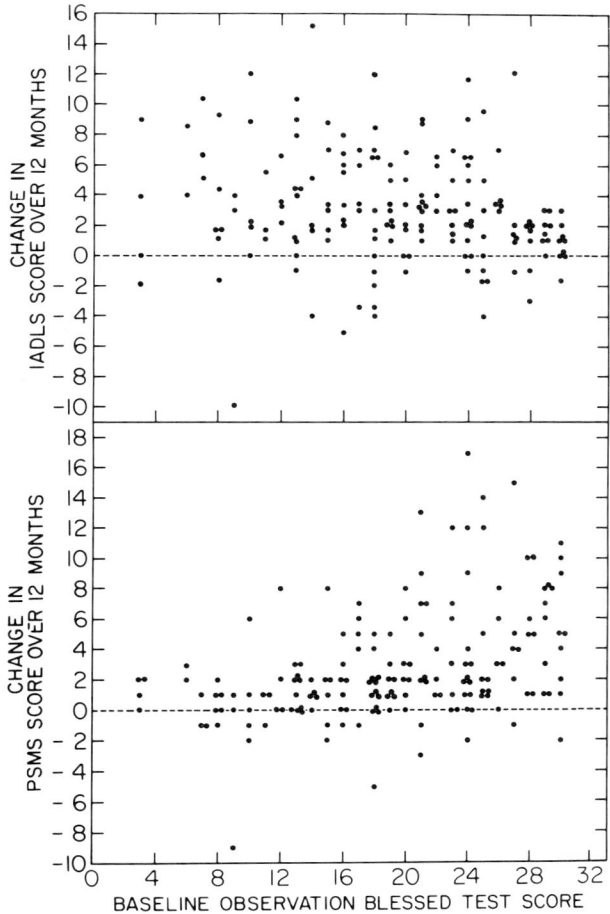

FIG. 2. Annual change scores on the Instrumental Activities of Daily Living Scale (IADLS) and the Physical and Self-Maintenance Scale (PSMS) for Alzheimer patients in a longitudinal study. Change scores on both scales are shown for 172 annual follow-up periods with baseline scores on the Blessed Test of Information, Memory, and Concentration of less than 31. Where points overlap, approximate values have been graphed so that all points are visible. (From ref. 19, with permission. Copyright 1992, American Geriatrics Society.)

rating scales which rely upon information from the patients themselves are generally not appropriate for AD patients. Secondly, because these symptoms may be different in AD patients than in other diagnostic groups, the assessments used for AD patients should be shown to measure symptoms in AD patients.

Depressive symptoms are common in AD patients (46), but the prevalence of major depressive disorder is probably quite low (20,48). Some (44), but not all (55), studies find a relationship of depression to functional impairment in AD. Depressive symptoms are usually found to be more common in the early stages of AD (44), but they can appear in severe cases (20). Newer instruments for evaluating depression in demented patients, such as the NIMH Scale for Depression in Dementia (58), will proba-

bly enhance the validity of clinical trials of antidepressant drugs in demented patients, but additional data are needed to document the prevalence, natural history, and consequences of depression in AD patients.

Agitation is clearly a clinically significant problem in AD, and many demented patients are treated at least temporarily with psychotropic drugs in an effort to manage agitation (60). In general, agitation is more of a problem in advanced dementia (9), but the degree of agitation varies among patients and does not necessarily show the inexorable progression characteristic of cognitive impairment (68). Recently, some scales [such as the Cohen-Mansfield scale (9)] that are specifically designed to measure agitation or behavioral disturbance in AD have been developed. Only limited longitudinal data are available on these scales, so it is not certain that they are adequate measures for patients at all levels of severity or in all settings.

FUTURE DIRECTIONS

Present standards for evaluating the efficacy of antidementia drugs are likely to remain useful with only minor modifications for the forseeable future. These standards require that an antidementia drug be shown to be superior to placebo on a performance-based assessment of cognitive function as well as on an independent measure of clinical efficacy. The available performance-based cognitive instruments, such as the ADAS-Cog and the MMSE, are adequate but not optimal for evaluating potential antidementia drugs. Modified versions of these instruments might be necessary for special populations such as very mild or very severe patients or for drugs that have effects primarily on attention, which is not assessed directly by these scales. More work needs to be done to determine the best procedures for administering global staging and change instruments and to determine how these instruments behave when used in longitudinal studies. Functional measures could ultimately be very useful for evaluating the "real world" impact of proposed treatments, but more research is needed to identify reliable and valid ways of measuring the key functional capacities lost in AD patients. Instrumentation for evaluating psychiatric symptoms, particularly agitation, needs to be developed further. Such instrumentation will facilitate the evaluation of drugs currently used to manage behavioral symptoms and will help speed the development of new, more effective agents.

REFERENCES

1. Ad Hoc FDA Dementia Assessment Task Force. Meeting report: Antidementia drug assessment symposium. *Neurobiol Aging* 1991;12:379–382.

2. American Psychiatric Association. *Diagnostic and statistical manual of mental disorders*, 3rd ed. (revised). Washington, DC: American Psychiatric Association, 1987.

3. Berg L, Miller JP, Bary J, Rubin EH, Morris JC, Figiel G. Mild senile dementia of the Alzheimer type. 4. Evaluation of intervention. *Ann Neurol* 1992;31:242–249.

4. Blessed G, Tomlinson BE, Roth M. The association between quantitative measures of dementia and of senile change in the cerebral grey matter of elderly subjects. *Br J Psychiatry* 1968;114:797–811.

5. Burke WJ, Miller JP, Rubin EH, Morris JC, Coben LA, Duchek J, Wittels IG, Berg L. Reliability of the Washington University clinical dementia rating. *Arch Neurol* 1988;45:31–32.

6. Chui HC, Teng EL, Henderson VW, Moy AC. Clinical subtypes of dementia of the Alzheimer type. *Neurology* 1985;35:1544–1550.

7. Clinical Research Working Group from the Pharmaceutical Industry on Dementia. Recommendations for clinical drug trials in dementia. *Dementia* 1990;1:292–295.

8. Coblentz JM, Mattis S, Zingesser LH, Kasoff SS, Wisniewski HM, Katzman R. Presenile dementia: clinical aspects and evaluation of cerebrospinal fluid dynamics. *Arch Neurol* 1973;29:299–308.

9. Cohen-Mansfield J. Agitated behaviors in the elderly. II. Preliminary results in the cognitively deteriorated. *J Am Geriatr Soc* 1986;34:722–727.

10. CPMP Working Party on Efficacy of Medicinal Products. Antidementia medicinal products. Commission of the European Communities, Brussels, November 1992.

11. Davis KL, Thal LJ, Gamzu ER, et al. A double-blind, placebo-controlled multicenter study of tacrine for Alzheimer's disease. *N Engl J Med* 1992;327:1253–1259.

12. Davis PC, Gray L, Albert M, et al. The Consortium to Establish a Registry for Alzheimer's Disease (CERAD). Part III. Reliability of a standardized MRI evaluation of Alzheimer's disease. *Neurology* 1992;42:1676–1680.

13. Erzigkeit H. The SKT—a short cognitive performance test as an instrument for the assessment of clinical efficacy of cognitive enhancers. In: Bergner W, Reisberg B, eds. *Diagnosis and treatment of senile dementia.* Heidelberg: Springer, 1989;164–174.

14. Farlow M, Gracon SI, Hershey LA, et al. A controlled trial of tacrine in Alzheimer's disease. *JAMA* 1992;268:2523–2529.

15. Ferris SH, Flicker C, Riesberg B. NYU computerized test battery for assessing cognition in aging and dementia. *Psychopharmacol Bull* 1988;24:699–702.

16. Folstein M, Anthony JC, Parhad I, Duffy B, Gruenberg EM. The meaning of cognitive impairment in the elderly. *J Am Geriatr Soc* 1985;33:228–235.

17. Folstein MF, Folstein SE, McHugh PR. ''Mini-Mental-State.'' A practical method for grading the cognitive state of patients for the clinician. *J Psychiatr Res* 1975;12:189–198.

18. Galasko D, Corey-Bloom J, Thal LJ. Monitoring progression in Alzheimer's disease. *J Am Geriatr Soc* 1991;39:932–941.

19. Green CR, Mohs RC, Schmeidler J, Aryan M, Davis KL. Functional decline in Alzheimer's disease: a longitudinal study. *J Am Geriatr Soc* 1993;41:654–661.

20. Greenwald BS, Kramer-Ginzberg E, Marin DB, Laitman LB, Herman CK, Mohs RC, Davis KL. Dementia with coexistent depression. *Am J Psychiatry* 1989;146:1472–1478.

21. Gurel L, Linn MW, Linn BS. Physical and mental impairment-of-function evaluation in the aged: the PAMIE scale. *J Gerontol* 1972;27:83–90.

22. Guy W, ed. *ECDEU assessment manual.* Rockville, MD: U.S. Department of Health Education and Welfare Publication No. (ADM) 76-338, 1976.

23. Hamilton M. A rating scale for depression. *J Neurol Neurosurg Psychiatry* 1960;23:56–62.

24. Inouye SK, Albert MS, Mohs RC, Sun K, Berkman L. Cognitive performance in a high-functioning community-dwelling elderly population. *J Gerontol: Med Sci* 1993;48:M146–M151.

25. Katz S, Ford AB, Moskowitz RW, Jackson BA, Jaffe MW. Studies of illness in the aged. *JAMA* 1963;185:914–919.

26. Katzman R. Alzheimer's disease. *N Engl J Med* 1986;314:964–973.

27. Katzman R, Aronson M, Fild P, Kawas C, Brown T, Morgenstern H, Frishman W, Gidez L, Eder H, Ooi WL. Development of dementing illnesses in an 80-year-old volunteer cohort. *Ann Neurol* 1989;25:317–324.

28. Katzman R, Brown T, Thal LJ, et al. Comparison of rate of annual change of mental status score in four independent studies of patients with Alzheimer's disease. *Ann Neurol* 1988;24:384–389.

29. Kim YS, Nibbelink DW, Overall JE. Factor structure and scoring of the SKT test battery. *J Clin Psychol* 1993;49:61–71.

30. Kramer-Ginzberg E, Mohs RC, Aryan M, Lobel D, Silverman JM, Davidson M, Davis KL. Predictors of course for Alzheimer patients in a longitudinal study. *Psychopharmacol Bull* 1988;24:458–462.

31. Larrabee GJ, Crook T. A computerized everyday memory battery for assessing treatment effects. *Psychopharmacol Bull* 1988;24:695–697.

32. Larsson T, Sjogren T, Jacobson G. Senile dementia. *Acta Psychiatr Scand* 1963;39(Suppl 167):3–259.

33. Lawton MP, Brodie EM. Assessment of older people: Self-maintaining and instrumental activities of daily living. *Gerontologist* 1969;23:349–357.

34. Leber P. Guidelines for the clinical evaluation of antidementia drugs, first draft. Rockville, MD: U.S. Food and Drug Administration, 1990.

35. Loewenstein DA, Amigo E, Duara R, et al. A new scale for the assessment of functional status in Alzheimer's disease and related disorders. *J Gerontol Psychol Sci* 1989;44:P114–P121.

36. Luchins DJ, Cohen D, Hanrahan P, et al. Are there clinical differences between familial and nonfamilial Alzheimer's disease? *Am J Psychiatry* 1992;149:1023–1027.

37. McKhann G, Drachman D, Folstein M, Katzman R, Price D, Stadlan EM. Clinical diagnosis of Alzheimer's disease: Report of the NINCDS-ADRDA Work Group under the auspices of Department of Health and Human Services Task Force on Alzheimer's Disease. *Neurology* 1984;34:939–944.

38. Mirra SS, Heyman A, McKeel D, et al. The Consortium to Establish a Registry for Alzheimer's Disease (CERAD). Part II. Standardization of the neuropathologic assessment of Alzheimer's disease. *Neurology* 1991;41:479–486.

39. Mohs RC. Assessment of cognitive symptoms in clinical studies of antidementia drugs (Homma A, trans.). *Jpn J Geriatr Psychiatry* 1991;2:1195–1201.

40. Mohs RC, Rosen WG, Davis KL. Defining treatment efficacy in patients with Alzheimer's disease. In: Corkin S, Davis KL, Growden JH, Usdin E, Wurtman RJ, eds. *Alzheimer's disease: a report of progress in research.* New York: Raven Press, 1982;351–356.

41. Morris JC, Edland S, Clark C, et al. Consortium to Establish a Registry for Alzheimer's Disease (CERAD). Part IV. Rates of cognitive change in the longitudinal assessment of probable Alzheimer's disease. *Neurology* 1993;43:2457–2465.

42. Morris JC, Heyman A, Mohs RC, et al. The Consortium to Establish a Registry for Alzheimer's Disease (CERAD). Part I. Clinical and neuropsychological assessment of Alzheimer's disease. *Neurology* 1989;39:1159–1165.

43. Overall JE, Gorham DR. The Brief Psychiatric Rating Scale. *Psychol Rep* 1962;10:799–812.

44. Pearson JL, Teri L, Reifler BV, Raskind MA. Functional status and cognitive impairment in Alzheimer's patients with and without depression. *J Am Geriatr Soc* 1989;37:1117–1121.

45. Perry EK, Tomlinson BE, Blessed G, Bergman K, Gibson PH, Perry RH. Correlation of cholinergic abnormalities with senile plaques and mental test scores in senile dementia. *Br Med J* 1978;2:1457–1459.

46. Reifler BV, Larson E, Hanley R. Coexistence of cognitive impairment and depression in geriatric outpatients. *Am J Psychiatry* 1982;139:623–626.

47. Reisberg B, Ferris SH, de Leon MJ, Crook T. The Global Deterioration Scale for assessment of primary degenerative dementia. *Am J Psychiatry* 1982;139:1136–1139.

48. Rosen J, Zubenko GS. Emergence of psychosis and depression in the longitudinal evaluation of Alzheimer's disease. *Biol Psychiatry* 1991;29:224–232.

49. Rosen WG, Mohs RC, Davis KL. A new rating scale for Alzheimer's disease. *Am J Psychiatry* 1984;141:1356–1364.

50. Roth M. The natural history of mental disorder in old age. *J Mental Sci* 1955;101:281–301.

51. Salmon DP, Thal LJ, Butters N, Heindel WC. Longitudinal evaluation of dementia of the Alzheimer type. *Neurology* 1990;40:1225–1230.

52. Spiegel R, Brunner C, Ermini-Funfschilling D, Monsch A, Notter M, Puxty J, Tremmel L. A new behavioral assessment scale for geriatric out- and in-patients: the NOSGER (Nurses Observation Scale for Geriatric Patients). *J Am Geriatr Soc* 1991;39:339–347.

53. Stern RG, Mohs RC, Bierer LM, Silverman JM, Schmeidler J, Davidson M, Davis KL. Deterioration on the Blessed Test in Alzheimer's disease: longitudinal data and their implications for clinical trials and identification of subtypes. *Psychiatry Res* 1992;42:101–110.

54. Stern RG, Mohs RC, Davidson M, Schmeidler J, Silverman JM, Kramer-Ginzberg E, Searcey T, Bierer LM, Davis KL. A longitudinal study of Alzheimer's disease: measurement, rate and predictors of cognitive deterioration. *Am J Psychiatry* 1994;151:390–396.

55. Stern Y, Hesdorffer D, Sano M, Mayeux R. Measurement and prediction of functional capacity in Alzheimer's disease. *Neurology* 1990;40:8–14.

56. Stern Y, Mayeux R, Sano M, Hauser WA, Brush T. Predictors of disease course in patients with probable Alzheimer's disease. *Neurology* 1987;37:1649–1653.

57. Storandt M, Hill RD. Very mild senile dementia of the Alzheimer type. *Arch Neurol* 1989;46:383–386.

58. Sunderland T, Alterman I, Young D, Hill JL, Tariot PN, Newhouse PA, Murphy DL, Cohen RM. A new scale for the assessment of depressed mood in dementia subjects. *Am J Psychiatry* 1988;145:955–959.

59. Teri L, Hughes JP, Larson EB. Cognitive deterioration in Alzheimer's disease: behavioral and health factors. *J Gerontol* 1990;45:P58–P63.

60. Teri L, Rabins P, Whitehouse P, Berg L, Riesberg B, Sunderland T, Eichelman B, Phelps C. Management of behavior disturbance in Alzheimer disease: Current knowledge and future directions. *Alzheimer's Dis Assoc Disord* 1992;6:77–88.

61. Thal LJ, Grundman M, Klauber MR. Dementia: characteristics of a referral population and factors associated with progression. *Neurology* 1988;38:1083–1090.

62. Uhlman RF, Larson EB, Koepsell TD. Hearing impairment and cognitive decline in senile dementia of the Alzheimer's type. *J Am Geriatr Soc* 1986;34:207–210.

63. Wechsler D. *The measurement and appraisal of adult intelligence,* 4th ed. Baltimore: Williams & Wilkins, 1958.

64. Welsh KA, Butters N, Hughes J, Mohs RC, Heyman A. Detection of abnormal memory decline in mild cases of Alzheimer's disease using CERAD neuropsychological measures. *Arch Neurol* 1991;48:278–281.

65. Welsh KA, Butters N, Hughes J, Mohs RC, Heyman A. Detection and staging of dementia in Alzheimer's disease: use of the neuropsychological measures developed for the Consortium to Establish a Registry for Alzheimer's Disease (CERAD). *Arch Neurol* 1992;49:448–452.

66. Weyer G, Ihl R, Mohs RC, Schambach M, Denkel A, Kaiser-Kehl H. Validierungsuntersuchungen zu einer deutschen version der Alzheimer's Disease Assessment Scale (ADAS). *Z Gerontopsychol Psychiatr* 1993;6:67–81.

67. Yesavage JA, Tinklenberg JR, Hollister LE, Berger PA. Vasodilators in senile dementia: a review of the literature. *Arch Gen Psychiatry* 1979;36:220–223.

68. Zec RF, Landreth ES, Vicari SK, Belman J, Feldman E, Andrise A, Robbs R, Becker R, Kumar V. Alzheimer's Disease Assessment Scale: a subtest analysis. *Alzheimer's Dis Assoc Disord* 1992;6:164–181.

Psychopharmacology: The Fourth
Generation of Progress, edited by
Floyd E. Bloom and David J. Kupfer.
Raven Press, Ltd., New York 1995.

CHAPTER 118

Biological Markers in Alzheimer's Disease

Trey Sunderland, Susan E. Molchan, and George S. Zubenko

Biological markers in medicine are usually considered diagnostic or prognostic tools in the treatment of serious illness. However, Alzheimer's disease (AD) remains largely a clinical diagnosis of exclusion. While elegant neuropathologic procedures allow final diagnoses at autopsy, the current consensus histopathological criteria have not been validated. Because patients rarely undergo a diagnostic brain biopsy because of the general lack of subsequent therapeutic options, discovering a readily accessible biological marker in AD which is firmly associated with the diagnostic neuropathology would be a major scientific major step forward.

In this chapter, several approaches in the study of biological markers will be reviewed:

1. Cerebrospinal fluid (CSF)
2. Peripheral tissue markers
3. Pharmacologic and neuroendocrine probes
4. Behavioral and biochemical correlates

Because the expanding study of biologic markers in AD is such a vast topic, not all approaches can be included. These areas each represent a fertile research field, and many of the major studies will be highlighted. Although the underlying neurobiology of AD is still elusive, these biologic probes offer a way to study potential etiologic mechanisms in affected and at-risk subjects, for both diagnostic and prognostic purposes. They may also provide a mechanism to follow treatment response once more effective therapies are available.

CSF MARKERS IN ALZHEIMER'S DISEASE

Given the physiologic proximity of the CSF to the brain and the usual lack of biopsy confirmation of AD, CSF

T. Sunderland and S. E. Molchan: Section on Geriatric Psychiatry, Laboratory of Clinical Science, National Institute of Mental Health, Bethesda, Maryland 20892.
G. S. Zubenko: Department of Psychiatry, Western Psychiatric Institute and Clinic, University of Pittsburgh, Pittsburgh, Pennsylvania 15213.

studies have long held promise for the antemortem diagnosis of the illness. Unfortunately, that promise has mostly been unfulfilled, because conflicting results have been the rule rather than the exception. There are multiple reasons for these conflicting results, not the least of which is the diagnostic uncertainty in any clinical study of AD. Other obvious clinical sources of variance include the severity of dementia, concomitant medical and neuropsychiatric variables, status of the subject at the time of the lumbar puncture (i.e., inpatient or outpatient), concurrent medications, and recent dietary history. There are also technical factors which may play a role in the final results, including the delay between sampling and assays, aliquot sampling, possible freezer thaw effects, and, of course, differing assay techniques across laboratories. Despite these multiple issues, enthusiasm runs high in the scientific community regarding CSF studies, and the search continues to discover the aberrant CSF marker that might better distinguish AD from control populations or other neuropsychiatric conditions.

Cholinergic System

An obvious starting point for any investigation with CSF in AD would be with markers of the cholinergic system. Postmortem studies uniformly reveal decreases in cholinergic indices, including choline acetyl transferase (CAT), acetylcholinesterase (AChE), and the number of cholinergic neurons (see Chapters 11–13, and 121, *this volume*). Furthermore, these changes have long been correlated with clinical measures of cognitive decline (11). However, the results of numerous studies of cholinergic markers in the CSF have been disappointing. In an early study, Johnson and Domino (34) reported no differences between demented subjects and healthy young controls in CSF CAT. Subsequently, the results have been mixed (35), perhaps due to methodologic differences among groups and the fact that CAT is known to be highly variable across CSF samples.

Similarly, measures of AChE have been found to be normal (61) or reduced (41). At best, the overlap between normals and Alzheimer patients is considerable, obviating the diagnostic utility of this measurement. In what is perhaps a more important measure of dynamic cholinergic change with AD, there is a report of a continuous decline in specific activity of the AChE enzyme with progression of the disease process over a 2-year period (22). Interestingly, this group had previously reported no significant changes after the first year of their study (22). When studying familial versus nonfamilial AD patients, Kumar and Giacobini (37) showed a significant decrease in CSF choline in the familial patients but no differences between the groups in CSF AChE. Butylcholinesterase (BuChE) activity has also been measured in AD and controls. As with the other cholinergic markers, there are reports of decreases (2), but most of the studies show no significant changes (4,34). When studying the ratio of AChE to BuChE, there is still mixed opinion as to whether there is increased separation between the patient group and controls.

CSF Monoamine Metabolites

The CSF monoamine metabolites are the most studied substances in the CSF of AD, but the picture is still confusing. Despite the fact that there are marked decreases in total brain norepinephrine, serotonin, and dopamine at autopsy, the in vivo measures of the metabolites do not reveal consistent decreases. Most studies reveal the levels to be within normal limits, some show reductions, and one even reports an increase in norepinephrine metabolites (see Table 1). For example, Hartikainen et al. (29) showed no significant differences in CSF measures of MHPG, 5HIAA, or HVA between 27 Alzheimer patients and 34 elderly controls. On the other hand, Parnetti et al. (53) revealed lower CSF HVA in a subgroup of Alzheimer patients with a later onset of illness. Interestingly, this later-onset group also showed a significant correlation between their CSF HVA levels and several neuropsychological measures. Within the serotonergic system, Gottfries (26) has consistently reported a reduction in 5-HIAA. Concerning the noradrenergic system, Raskind et al. (59) have previously reported increases of CSF MHPG in a group of advanced AD patients ($N = 9$) compared to age-matched controls or more mildly affected AD patients ($N = 7$). However, in a separate study of histologically verified AD, the CSF MHPG was normal in spinal fluid compared to that of normal controls, but the CSF HVA and 5HIAA levels were indeed lower in patients than in controls (51) (see also Chapter 103 for related discussion).

CSF Somatostatin

CSF somatostatin levels represent a special case in AD studies, because there is remarkable consistency in the world literature. Following the initial report of a decrease in brain somatostatin in AD brains, Oram and colleagues (50a) were the first to report a substantial decrease in CSF somatostatin-like immunoreactivity (SLI) in AD patients versus neurologic controls. Since then, there have been multiple other reports of lowered CSF somatostatin levels in AD patients versus normal controls; interestingly, the CSF SLI deficit is not limited to AD, because several other neuropsychiatric conditions have been found to show reduced levels (29,65). Such diagnostic overlap may be important, because when biopsy-proven AD patients have been compared to normal controls, only the presenile and not the senile patients have been shown to have the SLI reduction (24). Nonetheless, there appears to be a significant relationship between lumbar CSF SLI and frontal lobe SLI, at least as measured in cortical biopsies of a limited number of patients (25). In the only long-term study of CSF SLI in AD thus far published, there was no evidence of significant reductions with progression of the illness over 18 months of follow-up (3). However, when CSF SLI was measured during tetrahydroaminoacridine (THA) treatment, positive responders were noted to have increased levels post treatment, and that change was significantly correlated with neuropsychological improvement following a 4-week trial (1) (see also Chapter 48, *this volume*).

CSF Amyloid Markers

One of the more interesting recent developments in the antemortem study of AD has been the detection of altered absolute and relative amounts of amyloid derivatives in the CSF of AD patients versus older normal controls using antisera to amino acids 45–62 in the beta-amyloid precursor protein (52). Significant decreases in the larger forms (125 and 105 kD) and increases in relative amount of the smaller form (25 kD) of these derivatives have also been found in elderly controls compared to younger controls, although to a lesser extent than the changes found in AD (52). Significant decreases in the larger APP fragment thought to include the Kunitz inhibitor domain (PN-2) were also reported using a monoclonal mouse antibody which recognizes the amino-terminal epitope of all three major isoforms of APP (76); however, this method has also led to reports of quantitative increases in APP with the Kunitz-type inhibitor domain in the CSF of AD patients (75). Using a double-sandwich ELISA procedure with densitometric analysis of Western blots, a reduction of total APP, APP 695, and APP 751/770 has been reported in cases of sporadic AD (57). In a study of a family affected by presenile AD, clinical symptoms in one

TABLE 1. *Baseline monoamine metabolite levels in Alzheimer patients and controls*[a]

Study	N	Group	Age	MHPG	HIAA	HVA	Units
Hartikainen et al. (29)	27	AD	72.1 ± 7.5	35.0 ± 7.5	145 ± 44	222 ± 77	nmol/liter
	34	NC	49.3 ± 16.7	33.8 ± 4.7	135 ± 44	209 ± 73	
Molchan et al. (44)	60	AD	66.2 ± 8.7	51.3 ± 16	93 ± 31	188 ± 74	nmol/liter
	12	NC	65.8 ± 10.7	51.1 ± 15	95 ± 34	202 ± 66	
Parnetti et al. (53)	15	AD	65.9 ± 2.5	46.0 ± 8.3	85 ± 30*	168 ± 51**	nmol/liter
	30	SDAT	79.8 ± 4.9	47.0 ± 8.7	100 ± 30	193 ± 80**	
	14	NC	76.8 ± 8.8	47.3 ± 13.4	101 ± 11	281 ± 42	
Tohgi et al. (72)	11	AD	70.8 ± 8.2	11.6 ± 4.1*	29.3 ± 11.2	29.5 ± 16.4	ng/ml
	15	NC	69.1 ± 9.5	8.2 ± 2.3	29.6 ± 11.0	29.0 ± 17.4	
Blennow et al. (10)	123	AD	72.0 ± 7.2	48 ± 14	116 ± 49**	203 ± 101	nmol/liter
	57	NC	72.2 ± 10.8	50 ± 11	159 ± 63	301 ± 121**	
Malm et al. (41)	14	AD	71.2 ± 4.0	36.3 ± 8.9	153 ± 63	247 ± 104	nmol/liter
	21	NC	73.8 ± 8.2	46.4 ± 33.4	157 ± 191	243 ± 102	
Kawakatsu et al. (35)	22	AD	55.6	7.3 ± 2.5	6.7 ± 3.5**	15.8 ± 11.2*	ng/ml
	21	NC		6.3 ± 1.0	10.2 ± 2.5	21.6 ± 5.6	
Kaye et al. (35a)	27	AD	69.4 ± 1.7	40.3 ± 2.5	113 ± 9.1	161 ± 15	nmol/liter†
	14	NC	68.0 ± 2.9	39.8 ± 3.4	91 ± 13.7	202 ± 27	
Sunderland et al. (65)	13	AD	57.8 ± 5.1	51.9 ± 4.5	109 ± 10	229 ± 22	nmol/liter†
	7	NC	61.6 ± 3.2	54.3 ± 4.8	109 ± 11	228 ± 21	
Raskind et al. (59)	9 S	AD	68 ± 8	10.8 ± 1.8*	n/a	n/a	ng/ml
	7 M	AD	61 ± 6	7.6 ± 1.0			
	6	NC	67 ± 10	7.6 ± 2.4			
Palmer et al. (51)	21	AD	69 ± 12	8.3 ± 2.4	15.3 ± 5.7*	28.1 ± 13.4*	ng/ml
	38	NC	60 ± 6	7.2 ± 2.3	21.4 ± 8.4	42.3 ± 17.1	

[a] Data expressed in means ± standard deviation except where noted in the units column (dagger denotes mean ± standard error). * $p < 0.05$, ** $p < 0.01$ compared to control value; n/a, not available; S, severe; M, moderate; AD, Alzheimer's disease; NC, normal control.

subject were associated with low levels of APP similar to those with sporadic disease, whereas two symptom-free family members had normal levels (23).

Other CSF Markers in Alzheimer's Disease

Another major strategy in studying CSF has been to examine the fluid for evidence of increased breakdown or "wear and tear" substances that would be likely byproducts of a degenerative process like AD. Glycosphingolipids are present in all human cells, particularly plasma membranes, and are produced during normal cell turnover; however, they have been found in higher quantities or different ratios in the CSF of AD patients (9). Examining the neuroimmune system has also led to interesting discoveries with evidence of (a) higher CSF levels of interleukin-1β in AD patients when compared to other neurological controls, including multiple sclerosis patients (13), and (b) higher SP-40,40 levels, a modulatory protein of the complement system, in the CSF of AD patients versus that of normal controls (15).

Using other approaches, the reactivity of ubiquitin, a small (8.5 kD) protein found in most cells, has been shown to be significantly higher in AD over control CSF, perhaps reflecting the extensive ubiquitinylation of paired helical filaments (PHFs) in the brains of AD patients (78). Neuronal thread protein, a 20-kD protein of unknown function which nonetheless accumulates in the brains of

AD patients, has also been found in larger quantities in the CSF of AD patients than in that of both normal and other neurologic controls (17). On the other hand, levels of biopterin, peptidyl-glycine-alpha-amidating monooxygenase (PAM), and superoxidase dismutase have all been reported to be lower in the CSF of AD patients than in that of controls (12). When looking at metals and trace elements, Basun et al. (5) showed reduced levels of cadmium and calcium but increased levels of copper in the CSF of AD patients when compared to that of normal controls. Aluminum, lead, manganese, and mercury levels were measured and were not found to be statistically different amongst groups. One study reported significant increases in CSF xanthines, uric acid, and creatinine in AD patients, but the controls were younger patients with psychiatric problems and not age-matched controls (18). Finally, cyclic GMP, but not cyclic AMP, has previously been reported to be elevated in AD patients versus normal controls (74).

ALTERATIONS OF PERIPHERAL TISSUES IN AD

While AD is generally considered a central nervous system disorder, numerous biological alterations in tissues outside of the cerebral nervous system have been reported to show associations with AD. These peripheral abnormalities have been found in platelets, blood cells, skin fibroblasts, and peripheral vessels, just to name a few, and they present researchers with readily accessible tissue for further study of potential biological markers of AD. Rather than present a comprehensive review of this literature, this section serves to revisit associations that have been replicated and those for which plausible connections to the pathophysiology of AD could be formulated. A more complete review of this literature can be found elsewhere (68).

Cell Membranes

Increased platelet membrane fluidity (PMF) in AD, as reflected by decreased fluorescence anisotropy of 1,6-diphenyl-1,3,5-hexatriene in labeled membranes, was initially reported by Zubenko et al. (84,85) and has since been replicated by most (21,28,30,56,77), but not all, investigators (36). Using a threshold value for DPH anisotropy of 0.1920 at 37°C (the 90th percentile for neurologically intact elderly controls), increased PMF identifies a subgroup of patients with AD who have distinct clinical features. Increased PMF (DPH anisotropy less than 0.1920) appears to be associated with a group of AD patients with an earlier age of onset, more rapid progression of illness, less frequent focal abnormalities on electroencephalogram, decreased prevalence factors, and an earlier age of onset of AD in family members (for review see ref. 82).

Among demented patients, increased PMF is relatively specific for AD. This membrane abnormality is not shared by elderly patients with major depression (85), patients with multi-infarct dementia (MID) (30), or cognitively intact patients with Parkinson's disease (82). Moreover, increased PMF has been shown to be a stable characteristic over a 1-year follow-up period and to be a familial trait (92). The last finding provides strong evidence against unidentified medication exposure or a nonspecific effect of chronic illness as the source of the platelet membrane alteration. Finally, segregation analysis of 14 pedigrees revealed that at least 80% of the variance of PMF within families could be explained by the inheritance of a single major locus which has yet to be identified (14). It should be noted that while PMF appears to be under genetic control, increased PMF is not specifically associated with familial AD (21,86). This finding suggests that the PMF locus may influence the likelihood of developing AD and may modify its clinical expression without being sufficient to cause AD.

Increased PMF does not seem to be a manifestation of a generalized cell membrane defect in AD. Instead, several lines of evidence converge to suggest that increased PMF in AD results, at least in part, from a selective abnormality of internal platelet membranes. Intact platelets exposed to DPH for a short time so that external membranes are preferentially labeled do not exhibit the increase in membrane fluidity associated with AD (92). Furthermore, ultrastructural studies have revealed an increased frequency of platelets bearing accumulations of trabeculated cisternae bounded by smooth membranes resembling smooth endoplasmic reticulum (SER) (28,87).

Biochemical markers of SER function in platelets with increased membrane fluidity are also altered in AD. Activity of the SER marker, antimycin-A-insensitive NADH-cytochrome reductase, is decreased in platelets from AD patients (28), specifically those with increased PMF (83). Furthermore, there is evidence of disturbance in SER-mediated calcium homeostasis in AD. The percentage increase in cellular calcium following thrombin stimulation is significantly higher in platelets from AD patients than in those from matched controls. Both calcium/magnesium ATPase and calcium ATPase, SER-associated enzymes that regulate free calcium, show decreased specific activity in platelets from patients with AD (28). Overall, these results provide evidence that increased PMF in patients with AD is associated with a structural and functional impairment of internal platelet membranes that may affect protein maturation, localization, and calcium homeostasis.

Skin Fibroblasts

Alterations in calcium homeostasis have been reported in several cell types in patients with AD, though most work has been done in cultured skin fibroblasts. Peterson and Goldman (54) reported increases in total bound calcium and intracellular calcium in fibroblasts derived from both AD and normal elderly groups, when compared to younger controls. Both findings, however, were more marked in the AD group. Cytosolic free calcium, by contrast, was decreased in fibroblasts from the AD group when compared with young controls, again with intermediate results in the normal elderly (55). These results suggest an impairment of calcium homeostasis in AD, though the observed changes may represent an exaggeration of those seen in normal aging. Caution must be used in interpreting these studies, because the actual number of AD patients involved was small.

Changes in calcium homeostasis appear to be associated with impairments in mitochondrial function and cytoskeletal organization. Mitochondrial processes such as the oxidation of glucose and glutamine and their incorporation into proteins and lipids were decreased in a fashion parallel to that of cytosolic free calcium, with cells from the AD group affected most. By comparison, markers of cytosolic and nuclear processes, such as incorporation of leucine into protein and thymidine into DNA, were depressed more by aging than by AD (54). There was decreased spreading (a measure of cytoskeletal function) of fibroblasts from AD patients which improved when these cells were treated with calcium ionophores (55).

An alternative model of pathogenesis hypothesizes the presence of impaired mitochondrial function in AD, with resulting impairments of calcium homeostasis (8). Changes in mitochondrial oxidative functions have been reported in cultured skin fibroblasts; Blass et al. (8) have postulated that uncoupling of mitochondrial oxidative phosphorylation may lead to the accumulation of the abnormal cytoskeletal elements seen in AD. The mechanism linking mitochondrial uncoupling to the development of abnormal cytoskeletal elements, however, remains speculative and may be related to the effects of mitochondrial function on calcium homeostasis (8).

Olfactory Neuroblasts

Mammalian olfactory receptor cells are located in the epithelium of the upper nasal cavity beneath the cribriform plate. Each of these neuronal cells extends a dendritic process that terminates in a ciliated olfactory vesicle at the mucosal surface of the nasal epithelium, while projecting an axonal process that terminates on the olfactory bulb. Because of their intimate connection to the central nervous system, olfactory neurons are a promising model that may provide insights into the molecular pathology of neuropsychiatric disorders including AD. Indeed, pathological changes in morphology, distribution, and immunoreactivity of olfactory neurons have been reported in biopsy samples of olfactory epithelium obtained at autopsy from patients with AD (69).

Olfactory neurons are continuously generated from stem cells located within the epithelial layer and appear to be unique among neurons in their ability to regenerate throughout life. Recent success has been reported in the establishment of primary cultures of olfactory epithelium from adult human cadavers and living subjects (80). Cells from cloned cell lines have been reported to exhibit neuronal properties including neuron-specific enolase, olfactory marker protein, neurofilaments, and growth-associated protein 43. In addition, the cells express non-neuronal molecules, suggesting properties of neuroblasts or stem cells. The clonal cultures have been reported to contain 5–10% of cells sufficiently differentiated to manifest odorant-dependent biochemical responses to submicromolar concentrations of odorants.

Olfactory neuroblasts, as well as several other cell lines associated with the central nervous system, have been reported to contain detectable levels of carboxyl terminal degradation products (CTDs) of the amyloid precursor protein. The levels of these potentially amyloidogenic peptides are significantly elevated by incubation of cells in the presence of low concentrations of chloroquine, an inhibitor of lysomal function, and leupeptin, a protease inhibitor (81). In contrast, incubation in the presence of monensin, an endosomal specific inhibitor, was not accompanied by a significant change in the baseline level of these degradation products (81). Overall, these results suggest that lysosomes or some closely related internal membrane compartment play an important role in the degradation of APP CTDs.

Wolozin et al. (81) also reported considerable variation in the basal levels of APP CTDs across cell lines. Cell types associated with the pathology of AD, such as olfactory neuroblasts and cortical vascular endothelial cells, had higher levels of CTDs than did lymphoblasts and melanoma cells. These differences became even greater after incubation in the presence of inhibitors of lysosomal function. Consistent with previous evidence, this observation suggests that the degradation of APP may be highly tissue-specific. This finding has obvious significance for studies of amyloidogenesis and may have important implications for the pathophysiology of AD.

PHARMACOLOGIC AND NEUROENDOCRINE PROBES IN ALZHEIMER'S DISEASE

Alterations in neurotransmitter and neurohormone function are thought to be involved in the physiology, if not the etiology, of neuropsychiatric illnesses such as AD. Because of these changes, and the modulatory effects that neurochemicals have on each other, it has been hypothesized that studies of peripherally obtained neuroendocrine measures will give clues about neurochemical alterations in the brain. Besides neuroendocrine measures, cognitive, behavioral, and physiologic responses can also be studied in response to drug challenges in an attempt to characterize patient subgroups and allow for better diagnostic or prognostic accuracy during subsequent clinical treatment.

Cholinergic System

Because of the central importance of the cholinergic deficit in AD, there has been a significant emphasis on probes of the cholinergic system. Table 2 lists studies published since 1985, in which a cholinergic agent has been used acutely in AD patients to assess effects on cognition, behavior, physiologic, and/or neuroendocrine measures. While a number of studies have shown a positive effect on memory function or activation level in these patients, many others were negative. Few studies have compared neuroendocrine responses after cholinergic stimulation between AD and age-matched normal control subjects. Challenges with the cholinesterase inhibitor, physostigmine, showed that AD subjects had blunted plasma arginine vasopressin, β-endorphin, and epinephrine responses as compared with controls (60). These data suggested that deterioration in AD results in decreased responsiveness of neuroendocrine systems regulated by central cholinergic systems.

The cholinergic system deficits in AD led to the hypothesis that patients with AD should be more sensitive than

TABLE 2. *Cholinergic pharmacologic challenge studies in Alzheimer's disease patients and controls*

Pharmacologic agent	N	Group	Dose/route	Results	References
Scopolamine	10	AD	0.1, 0.25, 0.5 mg i.v.	↑ Cognitive and behavioral sensitivity	66
	10	NC			
	10	AD	0.1–0.5 mg i.m.	↑ Cognitive sensitivity in AD	32a
	6	NC			
Arecoline	12	AD	1, 2, 4 mg/liter i.v.	No cognitive improvement	70
	15	AD	5 mg i.v.	No cognitive improvement	58
	6	AD	4 mg i.v.	↑ CSF HVA in AD versus controls	56a
	4	NC			
Physostigmine	12	AD	0.75 mg i.v.	↑ Picture recognition	7
	11	Dementia	0.004–0.013 mg/kg i.m.	↑ Selective reminding, ↓ intrusions	63
	10	AD	0.50 mg i.v. + variable infusion	↑ Reaction time, no memory ↑	27
	10	AD	60 mg/kg p.o.	↑ Plasma cortisol & ↓ cholinesterase	37
	12	AD	0.0125 mg/kg i.v.	↓ Plasma vasopressin, endorphin, epinephrine versus controls	60
	12	NC			
Edrophonium	14	AD	0.13/kg i.v.	↓ GH response versus control	71
	8	NC			
	12	AD	0.15 mg/kg i.v.	No difference versus controls	16
	8	NC			
Nicotine	6	AD	0.125, 0.25, 0.5 mg/kg/min	↓ Intrusion errors	50
	11	AD	0.125, 0.25, 0.5 mg/kg/min i.v.	↑ Prolactin in AD, no difference from controls for ACTH, cortisol	48

normal controls to the memory-impairing and other central effects of the muscarinic antagonist scopolamine. A centrally mediated "functional hypersensitivity" was indeed documented in AD patients as compared with normals, on a number of behavioral and cognitive measures (66). Similar increases in sensitivity have also been noted in other elderly neuropsychiatric populations including Parkinson's patients and Korsakoff's patients but not elderly depressives (64). At least five muscarinic receptor subtypes have been subsequently identified by molecular genetic studies. It is hoped that more receptor-subtype selective agonist and antagonists will become available for use as probes to help discern their physiologic roles.

Serotoninergic System

The serotonin (5-HT) agonist *m*-chlorophenylpiperazine (*m*-CPP) is thought to be relatively selective for 5-HT$_1$ receptors (38). One study examined the effects of *m*-CPP in AD patients, and it found that they had increased behavioral responsivity and cognitive sensitivity to intravenous infusion of the drug as compared with elderly control subjects (38). AD patients became anxious and restless, experienced psychomotor activation and perceptual abnormalities, and had a greater performance decrement on some measures of memory as compared with controls. Neuroendocrine responses (plasma levels of cortisol and prolactin) did not differ between the two groups (38). The increased behavioral sensitivity to *m*-CPP in AD patients was hypothesized to be secondary to decreased

inhibition on 5-HT$_1$ receptors from the loss of 5-HT$_2$ receptors, or possibly from decreased inhibition from damaged cholinergic neurons on 5-HT systems. This hyperresponsiveness has been postulated to reflect a contribution of 5-HT systems to some of the behavioral disturbances (anxiety, depression, agitation, sleeplessness) which occur in AD (38) (see also Chapters 41 and 42, *this volume*).

GABAergic System

The benzodiazepine class of drugs interacts with the benzodiazepine–gamma-aminobutyric acid (GABA) receptor complex to enhance GABA activity, which is thought to lead to their anxiolytic action. Few studies of this neurotransmitter system have been done in AD. In one utilizing lorazepam as a probe, AD patients experienced more attentional impairment as compared with controls after drug administration (67). It was hypothesized that one possible reason for the difference between the groups was altered benzodiazepine sensitivity in the AD patients, secondary to decreased benzodiazepine receptor numbers.

Dexamethasone Suppression Test and Corticotropin-Releasing Hormone (CRH) Stimulation Test

AD and major depression can have overlapping clinical symptoms (e.g., depressed mood, sleep disturbance, psychomotor retardation, anxiety, agitation, and cognitive impairment). There also have been reports of overlapping biological markers, including nonsuppression of serum cortisol after a dose of dexamethasone (usually 1.0 mg, taken orally). The dexamethasone suppression test (DST) has been widely studied in samples of patients with AD, both with and without symptoms of major depression (see ref. 43 for review). The consensus has been that the rate of nonsuppression of cortisol during the test in nondepressed patients with AD is similar to that found in patients with major depressive disorder (about 50%) (43). Therefore, the DST is not useful in distinguishing dementia from depression. Positive relationships between post-dexamethasone cortisol levels and measures of dementia severity have been reported in some, though not all, studies (43).

Serum adrenocorticotropic hormone (ACTH) levels following administration of dexamethasone were reported to be elevated in two studies of AD patients (39). This change may be an indication of less effective feedback inhibition of cortisol, which could be caused by down-regulation of glucocorticoid receptors in the brain. Two studies have reported that, like patients with major depression, AD patients had a blunted ACTH response and a normal cortisol response to CRH infusion; this would be consistent with hypersecretion of CRH, and it implies a pathological process at the level of the hypothalamus or above. Two other studies found no difference in response to CRH between AD patients and controls (31) (see Chapter 84, *this volume*).

TRH Stimulation Test

Many studies have reported associations between thyroid dysfunction and psychiatric symptoms, especially depressed mood. Clinically, patients with AD and major depression often have overlapping clinical syndromes, so it was hypothesized that a blunted TSH response to TRH may occur in some AD patients as it does in depressed patients. Most studies report no significant difference in the TSH response in AD patients as compared with normals, although two report blunted responses (45,73). Some studies have reported that patients with a blunted TSH response tended to have higher levels of free T4, indicating normal feedback inhibition at the pituitary (45). Hypothalamic neuropathology has been documented in AD, but most studies have not found a significant change in TRH concentration in AD brain. It is therefore unknown why some of these patients have increased levels of T4; the mechanism may involve decreased feedback or increased stimulation of thyroid hormones by some other substance, such as norepinephrine. A few studies have examined the relationship between degree of dementia severity and TSH response; results have generally been negative (6,20,45). Measures of depression and TSH response do not appear to be significantly correlated (45).

The prolactin response in AD patients, usually to TRH, has been studied by a number of investigators. Dopamine has a strong inhibitory effect on prolactin, and serotonin and TRH stimulate its release. Deficits in the dopaminergic and serotoninergic systems have been reported in AD, so alterations in prolactin response may be expected. Over half the studies of prolactin response in AD found no significant difference from controls, one reported a blunted response, and two reported an enhanced response as compared with controls (20,73). Two studies looked for correlations in response to measures of dementia severity but found none (6,20) (see Chapter 44, *this volume*).

Growth Hormone Stimulation Tests

Acetylcholine has a stimulatory effect on growth hormone (GH), so alterations in it have been hypothesized in AD given the cholinergic deficit. Also, decreased levels of the peptide somatostatin, a major inhibitory modulator of GH, in both CSF and brain of AD patients is well-documented (44). The adrenergic and GABAergic systems also have regulatory actions on GH secretion, and alterations have been reported in those systems in AD. GH responses to a number of substances, including GH-releasing hormone, TRH, and cholinergic agents, have been explored in AD patients. Over half of them show no difference between AD patients and controls, a few reported a blunted response, and one an enhanced response as compared with controls (16,73).

Second Messenger Systems

The understanding of mechanisms of actions of drugs and hormones has recently moved beyond receptors, to the level of second messengers and genes. Evidence has also accumulated that AD is a systemic disorder, because many abnormalities have been identified in tissues other than brain (68). Some of these abnormalities therefore should be amenable to exploration with pharmacologic probes. In the brain, as well as in fibroblasts of patients with AD, alterations in the phosphoinositide second messenger system, including the enzyme protein kinase C (PKC), have been reported (62). There is evidence that PKC is involved in memory mechanisms, and increasing evidence suggests that lithium affects PKC function. In AD, chronic lithium resulted in significantly less membrane-associated (activated) PKC when compared to controls in three of the four isoenzymes examined (46), suggesting possible differential regulation in the platelets of AD subjects. Such aberrations in peripheral cells indicate that PKC may be involved early in the pathophysiology of the illness, and is not simply a secondary response to neuronal loss (62). Studies pursuing other possible alterations in phosphoinositide system components such as guanine-nucleotide-binding (G) proteins and membrane phospholipids in this paradigm are underway. In fact, future pharmacologic challenges may even link examinations of second messenger systems with dynamic brain imaging techniques.

BEHAVIORAL CORRELATIONS WITH BIOCHEMICAL AND NEUROPATHOLOGIC CHANGES IN AD

Depression and psychosis often complicate the course of primary dementia, exaggerating the functional impairment suffered by patients and increasing the burden experienced by their caregivers (91). These behavioral abnormalities appear to occur independently in demented patients and, once they emerge, to be chronic or recurrent. Available evidence suggests that these syndromes of major depression and psychosis are less responsive to treatment when they occur in the context of primary dementia than when they develop in cognitively intact elders (91). Both syndromes are associated with poorer outcomes among demented patients who develop them. The emergence of major depression appears to be associated with an increased mortality rate (88,93), but has no effect on the rate of cognitive decline (40). Conversely, psychosis appears to be associated with a faster rate of cognitive decline (19) without affecting mortality (19).

Autopsy studies of the neuropathologic and neurochemical correlates of major depression and psychosis in primary dementia have been guided by preexisting studies suggesting anatomic substrates for the idiopathic forms of these behavioral syndromes. The catecholamine hypothesis of affective disorders was attractive in this regard, because the cell bodies of the majority of the catecholaminergic neurons in the brain are localized in relatively discrete brainstem nuclei. In contrast, chronic idiopathic psychotic disorders are associated with decreases in blood flow glucose metabolism, cell loss, and cytoarchitectural changes in the neocortex and allocortex (see ref. 82 for review).

In a study of 37 demented patients who had participated in a longitudinal clinical study prior to death, Zubenko and Moossy (88) found that the emergence of major depression was associated with degeneration of the locus coeruleus and substantia nigra. However, patients who developed major depression did not differ from those who did not with respect to other clinical features or neuropathologic indices of global severity including cortical dementia of senile plaques (SPs) or neurofibrillary tangles (NFTs), reflecting the specificity of the brainstem findings. A logistic regression model that included the degenerative features of both the locus coeruleus and substantia nigra predicted the emergence of major depression with significantly greater accuracy than models employing the characteristics of either nucleus alone. This observation suggests an interaction of both noradrenergic and dopa-

minergic systems in the pathogenesis of major depression in primary dementia. Zweig et al. (93) have also reported an association of major depression with degeneration of the locus coeruleus and dorsal raphe nuclei in AD.

In a neurochemical analysis of the same 37 cases, Zubenko et al. (89) reported that the demented patients with major depression exhibited a 10-fold or greater reduction in the concentration of norepinephrine in the cortex, along with the relative preservation of choline acetyltransferase (ChAT) activity in subcortical regions, compared to demented patients without depression. The level of serotonin and its metabolite 5-HIAA showed a trend toward reduction in all cortical and subcortical regions examined. A paradoxical elevation in dopamine levels was observed in one region of the hippocampus in the depressed patients, but no consistent pattern emerged across brain regions. These findings did not appear to be related to medication exposure.

Zubenko et al. (90) reported an analogous study of 27 autopsy-confirmed cases of AD, with or without psychosis. In contrast to major depression, psychosis was associated with (a) increased cortical densities of SPs and NFTs and (b) a relative preservation of norepinephrine in the substantia nigra with trends in this direction for the remaining brain regions examined. Like major depression, psychosis was associated with a significant reduction of serotonin in the hippocampus that was accompanied by trends toward reduction of this amine and its metabolite 5-HIAA in the remaining regions. In their morphometric study of brainstem aminergic nuclei, Zweig et al. (93) did not observe a significant change in the numbers of neurons in either the locus coeruleus or dorsal raphe nuclei in AD patients who developed hallucinations or delusions.

The significance of these findings is manifold. Overall, these results provide the first direct evidence addressing the neurochemical and anatomic substrates of major depression and are largely consistent with the aminergic hypotheses of depression (42). Whether the relative preservation of ChAT activity in depressed, demented patients implicates cholinergic hyperactivity specifically in the pathogenesis of major depression (33) or, instead, reflects the inability to express or detect major depression in severely demented patients cannot be determined from these studies. It is noteworthy that the neuropathologic and neurochemical correlates of major depression and psychosis in dementia differ qualitatively from each other and from those associated with primary dementia alone. This observation reflects the specificity of the findings and may be related to the clinical observation that depression and psychosis appear to emerge independently of each other. The diffuse, but modest, reduction in the brain levels of serotonin and its metabolite 5-HIAA in both behavioral complications may be related to the apparent nonspecific therapeutic effect of trazodone in the management of agitated patients with dementia (32). Moreover, the degenerative nature of these changes may explain the clinical observation that major depression and psychosis are less responsive to treatment in the context of dementia than when they emerge in cognitively intact patients (91).

It is tempting to speculate that the biological correlates of major depression and psychosis in dementia may explain the negative prognoses associated with each of these complications of dementia (91). If the brainstem degenerative changes in depressed, demented patients extend beyond the resident aminergic nuclei, it may not be surprising that this behavioral complication is associated with a higher mortality rate. Moreover, greater cognitive impairment would seem a predictable consequence of the exaggerated cortical degeneration in demented patients with delusions or hallucinations. In summary, continued clinicopathologic and neurochemical studies of the behavioral complications of dementia may provide additional insights into the nature of AD as a multifocal brain disorder, may better define the relationship of depression to cognitive impairment in late life, and may suggest novel pharmacologic interventions. This area has been reviewed in detail elsewhere (47,91).

REFERENCES

1. Alhainen K, Sirvio J, Helkala E-L, Reinikainen K, Riekkinen P Sr. Somatostatin and cognitive functions in Alzheimer's disease—the relationship of cerebrospinal fluid somatostatin increase with clinical response to tetrahydroaminoacridine. *Neurosci Lett* 1991; 130:46–48.
2. Appleyard ME, Smith AD, Berman P, et al. Cholinesterase activities in cerebrospinal fluid of patients with senile dementia of Alzheimer type. *Brain* 1987;110:1309–1322.
3. Atack JR, Beal MF, May C, et al. Cerebrospinal fluid somatostatin and neuropeptide Y. *Arch Neurol* 1988;45:269–274.
4. Atack JR, May C, Kaye JA, Kay AD, Rapoport SI. Cerebrospinal fluid cholinesterases in aging and in dementia of the Alzheimer type. *Ann Neurol* 1988;23:161–167.
5. Basun H, Forssell LG, Wetterberg L, Winblad B. Metals and trace elements in plasma and cerebrospinal fluid in normal ageing and Alzheimer's disease. *J Neural Transm* 1991;4:231–258.
6. Bille A, Olafsson K, Jensen HV, Andersen J. Prolactin responses to thyrotropin-releasing hormone in multi-infarct dementia and senile dementia of the Alzheimer type. *Acta Psychiatr Scand* 1991; 83:321–323.
7. Blackwood DHR, Christie JE. The effects of physostigmine on memory and auditory P300 in Alzheimer-type dementia. *Biol Psychiatry* 1986;21:557–560.
8. Blass JP, Baker AC, Ko L. Induction of Alzheimer antigens by an uncoupler of oxidative phosphorylation. *Arch Neurol* 1990;47:864–869.
9. Blennow K, Davidsson P, Wallin A, et al. Differences in cerebrospinal fluid gangliosides between ''probable Alzheimer's disease'' and normal aging. *Aging Clin Exp Res* 1992;4:301–306.
10. Blennow K, Wallin A, Gottfries CG, et al. Significance of decreased lumbar CSF levels of HVA and a5-HIAA in Alzheimer's disease. *Neurobiol Aging* 1991;13:107–113.
11. Blessed G, Tomlinson BE, Roth M. The association between quantitative measures of dementia and of senile change in the cerebral grey matter of elderly subjects. *Br J Psychiatry* 1968;114:797–811.
12. Bracco F, Scarpa M, Rigo A, Battistin L. Determination of superoxide dismutase activity by the polarographic method of catalytic currents in the cerebrospinal fluid of aging brain and neurologic degenerative diseases. *Proc Soc Exp Biol Med* 1991;196:36–41.
13. Cacabelos R, Barquero M, Garcia P, Alvarez XA, Varela de Seijas

E. Cerebrospinal fluid interleukin-1β (IL-1β) in Alzheimer's disease and neurological disorders. *Methods Find Exp Clin Pharmacol* 1991;13:455–458.
14. Chakravarti A, Slaugenhaput S, Zubenko GS. Inheritance pattern of platelet membrane fluidity in Alzheimer's disease. *Am J Hum Genet* 1989;44:799–805.
15. Choi-Miura N-H, Ihara Y, Fukuchi K, et al. SP-40,40 is a constituent of Alzheimer's amyloid. *Acta Neuropathol* 1992;83:260–264.
16. Davidson M, Davis BM, Bastiaens L, et al. Growth hormone response to edrophonium in patients with Alzheimer's disease and normal control subjects. *Am J Psychiatry* 1988;145:1007–1009.
17. de la Monte SM, Volicer L, Hauser SL, Wands JR. Increased levels of neuronal thread protein in cerebrospinal fluid of patients with Alzheimer's disease. *Ann Neurol* 1992;32:733–742.
18. Degrell I, Niklasson F. Purine metabolites in the CSF in presenile and senile dementia of Alzheimer type, and in multi infarct dementia. *Arch Gerontol Geriatr* 1988;7:173–178.
19. Drevets WC, Rubin EH. Psychotic symptoms and the longitudinal course of senile dementia of the Alzheimer type. *Biol Psychiatry* 1989;25:39–48.
20. Dysken MW, Falk A, Pew B, Kuskowski M, Krahn DD. Gender differences in TRH-stimulated TSH and prolactin in primary degenerative dementia and elderly controls. *Biol Psychiatry* 1990; 28:144–150.
21. Eagger S, Hajimohammadreza I, Fletcher K. Platelet membrane fluidity, family history, severity and age on onset in Alzheimer's disease. *Int J Geriatr Psychiatry* 1990;5:395–400.
22. Elble R, Giacobini E, Scarsella GF. Clolinesterases in cerebrospinal fluid. *Arch Neurol* 1987;44:403–407.
23. Farlow M, Ghetti B, Benson MD, Farrow JS, van Nostrand WE, Wagner SL. Low cerebrospinal-fluid concentrations of soluble amyloid β-protein precursor in hereditary Alzheimer's disease. *Lancet* 1992;340:453–454.
24. Francis PT, Bowen DM, Neary D, Palo J, Wikstrom J, Olney J. Somatostatin-like immunoreactivity in lumbar cerebrospinal fluid from neurohistologically examined demented patients. *Neurobiol Aging* 1984;5:183–186.
25. Gomez S, Puymirat J, Valade P, Davous P, Rondot P, Cohen P. Patients with Alzheimer's disease show an increased content of 15K dalton somatostatin precursor and a lowered level of tetradecapeptide in their cerebrospinal fluid. *Life Sci* 1986;39:623–627.
26. Gottfries CG. Disturbance of the 5-hydroxytryptamine metabolism in brains from patients with Alzheimer's dementia. *J Neural Transm* 1990;30:33–43.
27. Gustafson L, Edvinsson L, Dahlgren N, et al. Intravenous physostigmine treatment of Alzheimer's disease evaluated by psychometric testing, regional cerebral blood flow (rCBF) measurement, and EEG. *Psychopharmacology* 1987;93:31–35.
28. Hajimohammadreza I, Brammer MJ, Eagger S. Platelet and erythrocyte membrane changes in Alzheimer's disease. *Biochim Biophys Acta* 1990;1025:208–214.
29. Hartikainen P, Reinikainen KJ, Soinien H, Sirvio J, Soikkeli R, Rickkinen PJ. Neurochemical markers in the cerebrospinal fluid of patients with Alzheimer's disease, Parkinson's disease and amyotrophic lateral sclerosis and normal controls. *J Neural Transm* 1992;4:53–68.
30. Hicks N, Brammer MJ, Hyumas N. Platelet membrane properties in Alzheimer and multi-infarct dementias. *J Alzheimer's Dis Relat Disord* 1987;1:90.
31. Holsboer F, Spengler D, Heuse RI. The role of corticotropin-releasing hormone in the pathogenesis of Cushing's disease, anorexia nervosa, alcoholism, affective disorders and dementia. *Prog Brain Res* 1992;93:385–417.
32. Houlihan DJ, Mulsant BH, Sweet RA, et al. A naturalistic study of trazodone in the treatment of behavioral complications of dementia. *Am J Geriatr Psychiatry* 1994;2:78–85.
32a.Huff FJ, Mickel SF, Corkin S, Growdon JH. Cognitive functions affected by scopolamine in Alzheimer's disease and normal aging. *Drug Dev Res* 1988;12:271–278.
33. Janowsky DS, Risch SC. Role of acetylcholine mechanisms in the affective disorders. In: Meltzer HY, ed. *Psychopharmacology: the third generation of progress.* New York: Raven Press, 1987;527–533.
34. Johnson S, Domino EF. Cholinergic enzymatic activity of cerebro-

spinal fluid of patients with various neurologic diseases. *Clin Chim Acta* 1971;35:421–428.

35. Kawakatsu S, Morinobu S, Shinohara M, Totsuka S, Kobashi K. Acetylcholinesterase activities and monoamine metabolite levels in the Cerebrospinal fluid of patients with Alzheimer's disease. *Biol Psychiatry* 1990;28:387–400.

35a.Kaye JA, May C, Daly E, Atack JR, Sweeney DJ, Luxenberg JS, Kay AD, Kaufman S, Milstien S, Friedland RP, Rapoport SI. Cerebrospinal fluid monoamine markers are decreased in dementia of the Alzheimer type with extrapyramidal features. *Neurology* 1988;38:554–557.

36. Kukull WA, Hinds TR, Schellenberg GD. Increased platelet membrane fluidity as a diagnostic marker for Alzheimer's disease. *Neurology* 1992;42:607–614.

37. Kumar V, Giacobini E. Cerebrospinal fluid choline, and acetylcholinesterase activity in familial vs. non-familial Alzheimer's disease patients. *Arch Gerontol Geriatr* 1988;7:111–117.

38. Lawlor BA, Sunderland T, Mellow AM, Hill JL, Molchan SE, Murphy DL. Hyperresponsivity to the serotonin agonist m-chlorophenylpiperazine in Alzheimer's disease: a controlled study. *Arch Gen Psychiatry* 1989;46:542–549.

39. Leake A, Charlton BG, Lowry PJ, Jackson S, Fairbairn A, Ferrier IN. Plasma N-POMC, ACTH and cortisol concentrations in a psychogeriatric population. *Br J Psychiatry* 1990;156:676–679.

40. Lopez OL, Boller F, Becker JT. Alzheimer's disease and depression: neuropsychological impairment and progression of the illness. *Am J Psychiatry* 1990;147:855–860.

41. Malm J, Kristensen B, Ekstedt J, Adolfsson R, Wester P. CSF Monoamine metabolites, cholinesterases and lactate in the adult hydrocephalus syndrome (normal pressure hydrocephalus) related to CSF hydrodynamic parameters. *J Neurol Neurosurg Psychiatry* 1991;54:252–259.

42. Meltzer HY, Lowy MT. The serotonin hypothesis of depression. In: Meltzer HY, ed. *Psychopharmacology: the third generation of progress.* New York: Raven Press, 1987;513–526.

43. Molchan SE, Hill JL, Mellow AM, Lawlor BA, Martinez R, Sunderland T. The dexamethasone suppression test in Alzheimer's disease and major depression: relationship to dementia severity, depression, and CSF monoamines. *Int Psychogeriatr* 1990;2:99–122.

44. Molchan SE, Lawlor BA, Hill JL, et al. CSF monoamine metabolites and somatostatin in Alzheimer's disease and major depression. *Biol Psychiatry* 1991;29:1110–1118.

45. Molchan SE, Lawlor BA, Hill JL, et al. The TRH stimulation test in Alzheimer's disease and major depression: relationship to clinical and CSF measures. *Biol Psychiatry* 1991;30:567–576.

46. Molchan SE, Manji H, Chen G, et al. Effects of chronic lithium treatment on platelet PKC isozymes in Alzheimer's and elderly control subjects. *Neurosci Lett* 1993;162:187–191.

47. Mulsant BH, Zubenko GS. Clinical, neuropathological, and neurochemical correlates of depression and psychosis in primary dementia. In: Emery VOB, Oxmanan TE, eds. *Dementia: presentations, differential diagnosis, and nosology.* Baltimore: Johns Hopkins University Press, 1994;336–352.

48. Newhouse PA, Sunderland T, Narang PK, et al. Neuroendocrine, physiologic, and behavioral responses following intravenous nicotine in nonsmoking healthy volunteers and in patients with Alzheimer's disease. *Psychoneuroendocrinology* 1990;15:471–484.

49. Newhouse PA, Sunderland T, Tariot PN, Mueller EA, Murphy DL, Cohen RM. Prolactin response to TRH in Alzheimer's disease and elderly controls. *Biol Psychiatry* 1986;21:963–967.

50. Newhouse PA, Sunderland T, Tariot PN, et al. The effects of acute scopolamine in geriatric depression. *Arch Gen Psychiatry* 1988;45:906–912.

50a.Oram JJ, Edwardson J, Millard PH. Investigation of cerebrospinal fluid neuropeptides in idiopathic senile dementia. *Gerontology* 1981;27:216–223.

51. Palmer AM, Sims NR, Bowen DM, et al. Monoamine metabolite concentrations in lumbar cerebrospinal fluid of patients with histologically verified Alzheimer's dementia. *J Neurol Neurosurg Psychiatry* 1984;47:481–484.

52. Palmert MR, Usiak M, Mayeux R, Raskind M, Tourtellote WW, Younkin SF. Soluble derivatives of the b amyloid protein precursor in cerebrospinal fluid: alterations in normal aging and in Alzheimer's disease. *Neurology* 1990;40:1028–1034.

53. Parnetti L, Gaiti A, Reboldi GP, et al. CSF Monoamine metabolites in old age dementias. *Mol Chem Neuropathol* 1992;16:143–157.

54. Peterson C, Goldman JE. Alterations in calcium content and biochemical processes in cultured skin fibroblasts from aged and Alzheimer donors. *Proc Natl Acad Sci USA* 1986;83:2758–2762.

55. Peterson C, Ratan RR, Shelanski ML. Cytosolic free calcium and cell spreading decrease in fibroblasts from aged and Alzheimer donors. *Neurobiology* 1986;83:7999–8001.

56. Piletz JE, Sarasua M, Whitehouse P. Intracellular membranes are more fluid in platelets of Alzheimer's disease patients. *Neurobiol Aging* 1991;12:401–406.

56a.Pomara N, Stanley M, LeWitt PA, Galloway M, Singh R, Deptula D. Increased CSF HVA response to arecoline challenge in Alzheimer's disease. *J Neural Transm* 1992;90:53–65.

57. Prior R, Monning U, Schreiter-Gasser U, et al. Quantitative changes in the amyloid βA4 precursor protein in Alzheimer cerebrospinal fluid. *Neurosci Lett* 1991;124:69–73.

58. Raffaele KC, Berardi A, Morris PP, et al. Effects of acute infusion of the muscarinic cholinergic agonist arecoline on verbal memory and visuo-spatial function in dementia of the Alzheimer type. *Prog Neuropsychopharmacol Biol Psychiatry* 1991;15:643–648.

59. Raskind MA, Peskind ER, Halter JB, Jimerson DC. Norepinephrine and MHPG levels in CSF and plasma in Alzheimer's disease. *Arch Gen Psychiatry* 1984;41:343–346.

60. Raskind MA, Peskind ER, Veith RC, et al. Neuroendocrine responses to physostigmine in Alzheimer's disease. *Arch Gen Psychiatry* 1989;46:535–540.

61. Ruberg M, Villageois A, Bonnet A-M, Pillon B, Rieger F, Agid Y. Acetylcholinesterase and butyrylcholinesterase activity in the cerebrospinal fluid of patients with neurodegenerative diseases involving cholinergic systems. *J Neurol Neurosurg Psychiatry* 1987;50:538–543.

62. Saitoh T, Masliah E, Jin L-W, Cole GM, Wieloch T, Shapiro IP. Biology of disease: protein kinases and phosphorylation in neurologic disorders and cell death. *Lab Invest* 1991;65:596–616.

63. Schwartz AS, Kohlstaedt EV. Physostigmine effects in Alzheimer's disease: Relationship to dementia severity. *Life Sci* 1986;38:1021–1028.

64. Sunderland T, Molchan SE, Martinez RA, Vitiello B, Martin P. Drug challenge strategies in Alzheimer's disease: a focus on the scopolamine model. In: Becker RE, Giacobini E, eds. *Alzheimer's disease: current research in early diagnosis.* New York: Taylor & Francis, 1990;173–181.

65. Sunderland T, Rubinow DR, Tariot PN, et al. CSF somatostatin in patients with Alzheimer's disease, older depressed patients, and age-matched control subjects. *Am J Psychiatry* 1987;144:1313–1316.

66. Sunderland T, Tariot PN, Cohen RM, Weingartner H, Mueller EA, Murphy DL. Anticholinergic sensitivity in patients with dementia of the Alzheimer type and age-matched controls: a dose–response study. *Arch Gen Psychiatry* 1987;44:418–426.

67. Sunderland T, Weingartner H, Cohen RM, et al. Low-dose oral lorazepam administration in Alzheimer subjects and age-matched controls. *Psychopharmacology* 1989;99:129–133.

68. Sweet RA, Zubenko GS. Peripheral markers in Alzheimer's disease. In: Burns A, Levy R, eds. *Dementia.* London: Chapman & Hall, 1994;387–403.

69. Talamo BR, Rudel R, Kosik KS. Pathological changes in olfactory neurons in patients with Alzheimer's disease. *Nature* 1989;337:736–739.

70. Tariot PN, Cohen RM, Welkowitz JA, et al. Multiple-dose arecoline infusions in Alzheimer's disease. *Arch Gen Psychiatry* 1988;45:901–905.

71. Thienhaus OJ, Zemlan FP, Bienenfeld D. Growth hormone response to edrophonium in Alzheimer's disease. *Am J Psychiatry* 1987;144:1049–1052.

72. Tohgi H, Ueno M, Abe T, Takahashi S, Nozaki Y. Concentrations of monoamines and their metabolites in the cerebrospinal fluid from patients with senile dementia of the Alzheimer type and vascular dementia of the Binswanger type. *J Neural Transm* 1992;4:69–77.

73. Tsuboyama GK, Gabriel SS, Davis BM, et al. Neuroendocrine dysfunction in Alzheimer's disease: results following TRH stimulation. *Biol Psychiatry* 1992;32:195–198.

74. Tsuji M, Takahashi S, Akazawa S. CSF Vasopressin and cyclic

nucleotide concentrations in senile dementia. *Psychoneuroendocrinology* 1981;6:171–176.

75. Urakami K, Takahashi K, Saito H, et al. Amyloid b protein precursors with kunitz-type inhibitor domains and acetylcholinesterase in cerebrospinal fluid from patients with dementia of the Alzheimer type. *Acta Neurol Scand* 1992;85:343–346.

76. Van Nostrand WE, Wagner SL, Shankle WR, et al. Decreased levels of soluble amyloid β-protein precursor in cerebrospinal fluid of live Alzheimer disease patients. *Proc Natl Acad Sci USA* 1992;80:2551–2555.

77. van Rensburg SJ, Carsten ME, Potocnik FCV. Membrane fluidity of platelets and erythrocytes in patients with Alzheimer's disease and the effect of small amounts of aluminum on platelet and erythrocyte membranes. *Neurochem Res* 1982;1:825–829.

78. Wang GP, Iqbal K, Bucht G, Winblad B, Wisniewski HM, Grundke-Iqbal I. Alzheimer's disease: paired helical filament immunoreactivity in cerebrospinal fluid. *Acta Neuropathol* 1991;82:6–12.

79. Winderlov E, Brane G, Ekman R, Kihlgren M, Norberg A, Karlsson I. Elevated CSF somatostatin concentrations in demented patients parallel improved psychomotor functions induced by integrity-promoting care. *Acta Psychiatr Scand* 1989;79:41–47.

80. Wolozin B, Bacic M, Merrill MJ. Differential expression of carboxyl-terminal derivatives of amyloid precursor protein among call lines. *J Neurosci Res* 1992;33:163–169.

81. Wolozin B, Sunderland T, Zheng B, et al. Continuous culture of neuronal cells from adult human olfactory epithelium. *J Mol Neurosci* 1992;3:137–146.

82. Zubenko GS. Biological correlates of clinical heterogeneity in primary dementia. *Neuropsychopharmacology* 1992;6:77–93.

83. Zubenko GS. Endoplasmic reticulum abnormality in Alzheimer's disease: selective alteration in platelet NADH-cytochrome C reductase activity. *J Geriatr Psychiatry* 1989;2:3–10.

84. Zubenko GS, Cohen BM, Growdon J. Cell membrane abnormality in Alzheimer's disease. *Lancet* 1984;2:235.

85. Zubenko GS, Cohen BM, Reynolds CF. Platelet membrane fluidity in Alzheimer's disease and major depression. *Am J Psychiatry* 1987;238:539–542.

86. Zubenko GS, Huff FJ, Beyer J. Familial risk of dementia associated with a biologic subtype of Alzheimer's disease. *Arch Gen Psychiatry* 1988;45:889–893.

87. Zubenko GS, Malinakova I, Chojnacki B. Proliferation of internal membranes in platelets from patients with Alzheimer's disease. *J Neuropathol Exp Neurol* 1987;46:407–418.

88. Zubenko GS, Moossy J. Major depression in primary dementia: clinical and neuropathologic correlates. *Arch Neurol* 1988;45:1182–1186.

89. Zubenko GS, Moossy J, Kopp U. Neurochemical correlates of major depression in primary dementia. *Arch Neurol* 1990;47:209–214.

90. Zubenko GS, Moossy J, Martinez J, et al. Neuropathologic and neurochemical correlates of psychosis in primary dementia. *Arch Neurol* 1991;48:619–624.

91. Zubenko GS, Rosen J, Sweet RA, Mulsant BH, Rifai AH. Impact of psychiatric hospitalization on behavioral complications of Alzheimer's disease. *Am J Psychiatry* 1992;149:1484–1491.

92. Zubenko GS, Wusylko M, Cohen BM. Family study of platelet membrane fluidity in Alzheimer's disease. *Science* 1987;238:539–542.

93. Zweig RM, Ross CA, Hedreen JC, et al. The neuropathology of aminergic nuclei in Alzheimer's disease. *Ann Neurol* 1988;24:233–242.

Psychopharmacology: The Fourth Generation of Progress, edited by Floyd E. Bloom and David J. Kupfer. Raven Press, Ltd., New York 1995.

CHAPTER 119

Anatomic and Functional Brain Imaging in Alzheimer's Disease

Stanley I. Rapoport

Currently, there is no certain biological marker for Alzheimer's disease (AD), and the pathophysiological mechanisms of neurodegeneration in AD are not understood. Furthermore, diagnosis is not absolutely certain and depends in large part on excluding other causes of dementia. In life, therefore, AD is diagnosed as "possible" [progressive decline in single cognitive sphere (usually memory), or atypical course of presentation of dementia, or other illness sufficient to cause dementia but not considered the cause of dementia] or "probable" (progressive memory deficit plus additional cognitive defect), according to NINCDS-ADRDA criteria (54). "Definite" AD is diagnosed with a history of dementia and postmortem evidence of critical densities of senile (neuritic) plaques and of neurofibrillary tangles with paired helical filaments within the brain. Possible or probable AD are considered "dementia of the Alzheimer type" (16).

Before the introduction of in vivo brain imaging, information was limited about the brain metabolic and anatomic abnormalities that underlay the signs and symptoms of AD in a given individual. Furthermore, until brain imaging was employed, AD could not be readily diagnosed in life nor readily distinguished from other causes of dementia, which include vascular dementia, normal pressure hydrocephalus, stroke, hemorrhage, neoplasm, frontal lobe atrophy of Pick's disease, caudate nucleus atrophy of Huntington's disease, Wernicke–Korsakoff disease, and some cases Parkinson's disease (4,17).

Structural imaging in the form of computer-assisted x-ray tomography (CT) was introduced just 20 years ago (39), after which diagnostic accuracy for AD rose from 43% to greater than 70% (4). CT replaced invasive methods of pneumoencephalography and cerebral angiogra-phy, which had been used sparingly in the elderly because of associated morbidity. More recently, magnetic resonance imaging (MRI) has been introduced to examine brain structure. In the future, magnetic resonance spectroscopy (MRS) looks promising for measuring brain metabolites and metabolite fluxes through brain compartments (72).

With regard to functional imaging, the low-resolution ^{133}Xe clearance technique provided initial evidence for a relation between reduced regional cerebral blood flow (rCBF) in the cerebral cortex and dementia severity in AD (30). This technique was replaced in the early 1980s by the more quantitative positron emission tomography (PET), which provided numerical values for (a) regional cerebral metabolic rates for glucose (rCMR$_{glc}$) and for O$_2$ (rCMRo$_2$) and (b) the regional oxygen extraction fraction (rOEF) (19,22; also see Chapters 76 and 77, *this volume*), in deep brain structures as well as in the neocortex. PET also has elucidated blood–brain barrier integrity, dopamine metabolism, and specific receptors in brains of AD patients (56,59,71,74). More recently, single photon emission computed tomography (SPECT) has been introduced as a cheaper and more available imaging tool than PET, for clinical measurements of rCBF in AD, and to distinguish AD from vascular dementia (37; see also Chapter 130, *this volume*). Dynamic MRI also promises to allow measurements of rCBF in AD patients, with temporal resolutions in seconds and anatomic resolutions in millimeters, free of radiation exposure (47). In this chapter, we consider each of these in vivo imaging techniques with regard to the nature and diagnosis of AD, and we show how the cognitive deficits of AD in individual patients are related to the local functional and structural changes in the brains of these patients.

Because AD is a heterogeneous disease with regard to severity of dementia and cognitive profile (33,53), our consideration of brain imaging in AD will be most infor-

S. I. Rapoport: Laboratory of Neurosciences, National Institute on Aging, National Institutes of Health, Bethesda, Maryland 20892.

TABLE 1. *Cognitive profiles for AD patients with mild or moderate dementia*[a,b]

Neuropsychological test	Controls (N = 21–29)		Mild AD (N = 11)		Moderate AD (N = 13)	
Omnibus Tests						
Wechsler intelligence scale						
Full-scale IQ	126	± 10	117	± 8	92	± 17**
Deviation quotients						
Verbal comprehension	129	± 10	123	± 9	102	± 17**
Memory and distractibility	116	± 13	113	± 8	90	± 15**
Perceptual organization	119	± 13	109	± 13	84	± 26**
Memory						
Wechsler memory scale						
Immediate story recall	22	± 15	11	± 15**	5	± 3**
Immediate figure recall	10	± 3	7	± 4*	1	± 2**
Delayed story recall	17	± 5	2	± 4**	1	± 1**
Delayed figure recall	7	± 3	1	± 1**	0	± 1**
Attention, planning and abstract reasoning						
Trailmaking (Trail A) (sec)	40	± 17	54	± 30	153	± 98**
Trailmaking (Trail B) (sec)	82	± 40	192	± 155*	428	± 139**
Stroop color–word inference, no/45s	37	± 8	24	± 8*	12	± 8**
Porteus mazes (age in years)	15.4	± 1.6	12.8	± 3.9	7.7	± 3.8**
Language						
Syntax comprehension	24	± 2	23	± 2	17	± 5**
Controlled word association (FAS)	42	± 2	34	± 13	25	± 12**
Boston naming	37	± 4	35	± 7	25	± 8**
Visuospatial Function						
Extended range drawing	21	± 2	19	± 4	13	± 5**
Hiskey–Nebraska block patterns	15	± 4	11	± 5	4	± 3**
Benton facial recognition	44	± 4	42	± 5	39	± 5*

[a] Neuropsychological tests classified by cognitive sphere that they are considered to evaluate. Data from ref. 31.
[b] Mean ± SD differs from control mean, * $p < 0.05$; ** $p < 0.001$.

mative if the results are correlated explicitly with cognitive status. Dementia severity can be defined by scores on the Mini Mental State Examination (MMSE): mild, 22–30; moderate, 11–21; and severe, 0–10 (20). Cognitive profiles are summarized with regard to dementia severity in Table 1, for a group of AD patients as compared with healthy controls, as mean scores on tests of different spheres of cognitive function: memory; attention, planning, and abstract reasoning; language; and visuospatial function. The details of these tests and why they were chosen are described elsewhere (31). Moderately demented patients had significantly reduced means scores on all the cognitive tests that were administered. In contrast, mildly demented patients had significantly reduced mean scores only on measures of verbal and visual recent memory (Wechsler Memory Scale), attention to a complex set (Trailmaking B and Stroop Color Interference Task), and planning (Porteus Mazes), but performance on most tests of ''focal'' neuropsychological functions was not significantly impaired. These findings confirm that a memory deficit usually is the first prominent complaint in AD and show that attention, planning and abstract reasoning are also affected. Indeed, with an appropriate history and neurologic examination and laboratory testing, a memory deficit is sufficient to make a diagnosis of ''possible'' AD (16,54).

Cognitive profiles even for patients of equivalent dementia severity are heterogeneous, and their rates of change, which iikely are biphasic, can differ markedly among individual patients (33,53). When the Wechsler Adult Intelligence Scale (WAIS) and the Dementia Rating Scale were repeated over periods of 2.7–6.8 years in 16 AD patients, an initial plateau phase, during which language and cognitive functions did not change for 9–35 months, was observed in five patients who presented with an isolated memory impairment (33). Once nonmemory functions began to decline in the second phase in these patients, the rate of decline was remarkably steady in each patient but varied two- to threefold among patients.

IMAGING IN ALZHEIMER'S DISEASE WITH COMPUTER-ASSISTED X-RAY TOMOGRAPHY AND MAGNETIC RESONANCE

Quantitative Volumetric Imaging

Computer-Assisted X-Ray Tomography

Computer-assisted x-ray tomography (CT), whether analyzed qualitatively or quantitatively, cannot easily distinguish mildly or moderately demented AD patients from healthy age-matched controls, when causes of dementia other than AD are excluded (12,50). This lack of sensitivity is due largely to a marked overlap in brain atrophy between AD patients and healthy elderly (9,17,42).

Measures of ''cortical atrophy'' which have been used to try to discriminate individual AD patients from normals include the width of the largest sulci and the outlined perimeter of the brain, standardized to cranial size (12,50). In an attempt to overcome limitations of irregular ventricular shape, net ventricular volumes have been calculated by summing ventricular area on serial CT slices, and then multiplying the sum by interslice distance. However, volumetric measurements also have proven of limited use (12,24).

CT-derived estimates of volume demonstrated statistically significant reductions in mean gray matter volume and in the mean gray/white matter volume ratio, and significant increases in mean cerebrospinal fluid (CSF) and lateral ventricular volumes, in relation to dementia severity in a cross-sectional study (9). When brain atrophy then was examined in a longitudinal design, that the mean rate of enlargement of linear indices of ventricular size over 1 year was significantly larger in mildly demented AD patients than in controls (24). In another longitudinal study, rates of change of lateral ventricle volume on CT (cm^3/year) completely separated a group of 12 male AD patients (including 8 with mild dementia), examined during a mean interval of 1.4 years, from controls who were examined during a mean interval of 3.3 years (51). Furthermore, rates of ventricular enlargement in individual AD patients were correlated significantly with rates of decline on a composite neuropsychological test battery.

A more extensive longitudinal CT study was conducted on 11 men and 9 women with presumed AD (6 of whom had an isolated memory impairment), who were followed for 9 months to 7 years, and on 9 male and 8 female controls (11). The rate of total lateral ventricle enlargement (cm^3/year) differed significantly between patients and controls, with a 94% specificity (the ability to make a correct positive diagnosis) and 90% sensitivity (the ability to correctly exclude AD) (one control and two patients were misdiagnosed). For six initially ''possible'' AD patients, the rate of ventricular enlargement during the period of isolated memory impairment was significantly less than that after the appearance of focal neuropsychological deficits, suggesting a biphasic atrophic process. The diagnostic power of the volumetric measurements from two CT scans taken 1 year apart was only 0.33 in the mildly demented patients (11).

In summary, single CT scans, whether analyzed qualitatively or quantitatively, cannot distinguish AD patients from normals because of overlap of brain atrophy in the two groups. Serial quantitative CT of lateral ventricular volume has demonstrated a distinct difference in rate of dilatation between AD and normal subjects, and it deserves to be evaluated further for identifying AD patients.

Magnetic Resonance Imaging

Limitations of CT include its low spatial resolution and low tissue contrast differences, as well as an artifactual elevation of brain CT density adjacent to the skull (''bone hardening artifact'') which renders CT unreliable for measuring subarachnoid CSF and cortical atrophy. MRI can overcome some of these limitations, because MRI requires no ionizing radiation, repeated measures are without known risk, and images are free of a bone hardening artifact (although MRI scans do contain spectral inhomogeneities) (17,58). A thorough description of MRI methodology, and of the limitations and advantages of MRI, is presented elsewhere in this volume (Chapter 76). Thus MRI, but not CT, can be used to quantitate lobar and cortical atrophy as well as volumes of subarachnoid CSF. MRI is more costly than CT ($1200–$1800 as compared to $450 for contrast studies of the head), and it should be used clinically when CT is considered inadequate for diagnosis.

Whereas a cross-sectional volumetric CT study of the brain demonstrated no mean difference between mildly demented AD patients and controls (see above) (9), a comparable MRI study did show statistically significant group differences. Mildly demented AD patients had significantly smaller mean cerebral brain matter and temporal lobe volumes and significantly larger volumes of the lateral ventricles and of temporal lobe CSF than did controls (58). Severity of dementia correlated significantly with reduced brain matter volume and increased lateral ventricular volume, confirming progression of brain atrophy. Sparing of caudate, lenticular, and thalamic nuclear groups was evident, consistent with their lesser neuropathology post mortem (64) and their lesser PET-derived metabolic reductions in life (see below).

Discriminant analysis is a statistical procedure that constructs a linear combination of observed variables that best describes group differences, and it can classify group membership of any individual. When applied to MRI volumetric data, a discriminant analysis distinguished each of 31 mildly demented AD patients from sex- and age-matched controls (13). Age and brain volume were the most significant discriminators for men, whereas temporal lobe and CSF volumes were best for women. Because 10 of the patients had a diagnosis of ''possible'' AD, with impaired memory as the only apparent cognitive deficit (54), it appears that discriminant analysis using volumetric MRI variables can add diagnostic certainty in mildly demented, ''possible'' AD patients and should be explored further in this regard.

CT and MRI Densities to Distinguish Alzheimer's Disease from Vascular Dementia

Of 2143 demented patients reported as of 1988 with a diagnosis of AD and/or vascular dementia, having 15%

pathological confirmation, 51% had a diagnosis of AD alone, 23% had a diagnosis of vascular dementia alone, and 15% were considered to have AD plus cerebrovascular disease (4). Thus, vascular disease contributes to 38% of reported dementias, and its distinction from AD is a major clinical problem. This is particularly important because many of the cardiovascular risk factors for vascular dementia can be prevented or treated (29). There are a number of different causes of vascular dementia, including arteriosclerotic encephalopathy (lacunar state, multiple small infarcts, large cerebral infarcts), hypertensive arteriosclerosis (including mixed cortical and subcortical leukoencephalopathy of Binswanger), and congophilic angiopathy (7,40). In subcortical disease (leukoencephopathy), CT and T_2-weighted MRI images demonstrate periventricular and deep white matter changes, referred to as *leukoaraiosis*.

To date, diagnostic criteria to distinguish vascular dementia from AD have not formally incorporated neuroimaging, which published data nevertheless demonstrate can be very helpful (7,54,69). DSM-III-R identifies the following diagnostic criteria for AD: dementia, insidious onset with a generally progressive deteriorating course, and exclusion of other specific causes. Diagnostic criteria for multi-infarct (vascular dementia), as listed by DSM-III-R, are as follows: dementia; stepwise deteriorating course with "patchy" distribution of deficits, focal neurological signs and symptoms, and evidence of significant cerebrovascular disease judged to be etiologically related to the disturbance (16). A Hachinski Ischemia Scale Score exceeding 6, with emphasis on focal neurological signs, points to vascular dementia (7,69).

The relation between white matter hyperintensities on CT or MRI and cognitive and metabolic function is not entirely evident. Studies indicate that 30–80% of elderly individuals without neurologic signs have focal density abnormalities in cerebral white matter, and that the frequency of these abnormalities increases with hypertension (7). Abnormalities can be small focal or confluent areas of increased signal intensity on T_2-weighted MRI, which demonstrates them more frequently than does CT (17). Abnormalities often are scattered throughout deep white matter and basal ganglia, and they cap lateral ventricular margins and are thought to indicate increased tissue water due to vascular disease (17). However, cognitive testing has failed to demonstrate differences between healthy aged adults with and without white-matter hyperintensities (1).

In the absence of hypertension, AD patients do not demonstrate a higher frequency of grade 2–3 white-matter abnormalities (17%) than do elderly nonhypertensive healthy controls (27%) (44). Nevertheless, in demented AD and vascular disease patients, severity of cognitive impairment, particularly in tests of subcortical function, has been related to the grade of white-matter hyperintensities by MRI (1). This suggests that in the absence of hypertension, white-matter hyperintensities

can represent brain changes that are clinically subthreshold, but that the subcortical pathology they represent in the presence of hypertension is more severe and can add to cognitive impairment in vascular dementia as well as AD patients.

In this regard, 14 AD patients with severe leukoencephalopathy on MRI, 9 of whom were hypertensive, were compared by cognitive testing and PET (see below) with 13 age- and severity-matched nonhypertensive AD patients free of leukoencephalopathy (10). No significant difference was found on any psychological test score or grade of leukoencephalopathy between the groups, but a ratio analysis of PET data indicated lesser $rCMR_{glc}$ in the caudate nucleus and thalamus of the patients with white-matter changes than of the patients without these changes, consistent with subcortical dysfunction.

In the above study, three of the leukoencephalopathic patients who were not hypertensive have come to autopsy (10). Each demonstrated the senile plaques and tangles of AD, as well as extensive myelin pallor in white matter in the area of distribution of the white matter hyperintensities during life. Furthermore, in each, Congo-red staining revealed striking amyloid deposition (amyloid angiopathy) in meningeal and cerebral perforating arteries, but normal-appearing arteries in white matter and in the lenticulo-striate vasculature. There was no evidence of hypertensive lipohyalinosis or atherosclerosis in these vessels. Thus, white-matter changes in nonhypertensive AD patients may reflect the amyloid angiography that is found frequently in the AD brain (severe in 30% of cases).

Grading of white-matter lesions on MRI to distinguish AD from vascular dementia has been of limited success. In one study, scores of periventricular lesions could not distinguish the two groups; scores of subcortical lesions, although somewhat better, showed too much overlap to be useful (5). Forty percent of the AD patients did not have subcortical white-matter changes, whereas such changes were present in all the vascular dementia patients. In another study, vascular dementia patients had higher mean frequencies of infarcts and lacunae ($p < 0.001$) and of focal signal hyperintensities ($p < 0.05$) in the basal ganglia and thalamus than did AD patients (48).

In summary, MRI or CT evidence of infarcts or lacunae, particularly in the basal ganglia and thalamus, points to a clinical diagnosis of cerebrovascular disease plus AD, or of vascular dementia alone. Whereas significant leukoencephalopathy on CT likely reflects cerebrovascular disease, on the more sensitive MRI the pathological significance is less certain. In the absence of hypertension and a high Hachinski Ischemic Score to point to vascular dementia rather than AD, white-matter lesions on MRI alone are of questionable clinical import. In nonhypertensive AD patients, they may represent amyloid angiopathy.

Magnetic Resonance Spectroscopy

In vivo magnetic resonance spectroscopy (MRS) produces spectra of relatively weak magnetic signals from nuclei of phosphorus, carbon, or non-water hydrogen (the signals are weak due to the small concentrations of these nuclei). These spectra provide information about chemical compounds and the energy state within the brain, and they can be localized to specific brain regions (72).

Phosphomonoesters (e.g., phosphoethanolamine and phosphocholine) are considered anabolic precursors of membrane phospholipids, whereas phosphodiesters (e.g., glycerol-3-phosphoethanolamine and glycerol-3-phospho-choline) are thought to represent catabolic products from the breakdown of phospholipids (61). Using in vivo ^{31}P MRS, AD patients were reported to have a larger-than-normal concentration of phosphomonoesters in the temporo-parietal cortex (6). This observation, as well as evidence that phosphomonoesters and phosphodiesters are abnormal in the postmortem AD brain (61), suggested that regenerative processes involving phospholipids occur early in AD, whereas degenerative process occur later on. The phosphocreatinine-to-inorganic phosphorus ratio with ^{31}P MRS was reported to distinguish AD from vascular dementia patients (6).

Disturbed phospholipid metabolism in AD also is suggested by ^{1}H MRS evidence of an increased ratio (by 11–22%) of myoinositol to creatine in the parietal and occipital cortices of AD patients compared to controls, when the ratio of the neuronal marker N-acetylaspartate to creatine was reduced by 5–11% (55). Because myo-inositol is part of the phosphatidylinositol molecule, its increased brain concentration in AD could reflect accelerated breakdown of phosphatidylinositol and other phospholipids.

Despite these reports, a careful study which used ^{1}H MRS to localize and calculate dimensions of a brain volume of interest, and ^{31}P MRS to quantitate phosphorus metabolites in this volume of interest when employing internal standards (57), found no significant difference between AD patients and controls in absolute concentrations of adenosine triphosphate, phosphocreatine, inorganic phosphate, phosphomonoesters, or phosphodiesters. Nor was any absolute concentration or concentration ratio in AD related to dementia severity, or to rCMR$_{glc}$ as measured with PET, in the volume of interest. It was concluded that reduced rCMR$_{glc}$ in AD (see below) is unrelated to rate-limited delivery of glucose or oxygen to brain, and that normal levels of high-energy phosphorus metabolites are maintained even with severe dementia. However, because the volume of interest studied with MRS was large and included primary as well as association brain regions, localized changes in association areas may have been obscured. A quantitative MRS study of association cortex in severely demented patients is needed to confirm the conclusions (57).

In the future, in vivo MRS combined with anatomic localization should help to clarify whether there is an energy deficit in AD, and whether abnormalities of phospholipid turnover or of phospholipids in second messenger systems are part of the AD process. In vivo MRS also

could be used to determine the actual flux of ^{13}C-glucose moieties into brain glutamate, glutamine and aspartate compartments, in relation to rCMR$_{glc}$ (72).

FUNCTIONAL IMAGING: POSITRON EMISSION TOMOGRAPHY

PET Methods

Measurements of rCMR$_{glc}$, rCMRO$_2$, rOER, and rCBF with PET have contributed to our understanding of brain functional activity and oxidative metabolism in AD. As described in detail elsewhere in this volume (Chapters 76 and 77), with PET, a positron-emitting compound that is administered systemically is taken up by brain, where it releases positrons (positively charged electrons). These collide with electrons and are annihilated, to release two gamma rays at 180° to each other. A ring or sphere of radiation detectors surrounding the head identifies, by coincidence counting with appropriate reconstruction and attenuation algorithms, the quantities and locations of radioactivity within the brain. ^{18}F-2-fluoro-2-deoxy-D-glucose (^{18}F-FDG; radioactive half-life of ^{18}F is 110 min) or ^{11}C-DG (radioactive half-life of ^{11}C is 20 min) has been used to measure rCMR$_{glc}$ with PET, whereas H$_2$^{15}O and ^{15}O$_2$ or ^{15}O-CO$_2$ (radioactive half-life of ^{15}O is 2.03 min) have been used to generate rCMRO$_2$ and rCBF images, respectively.

PET can be performed during specific cognitive or pharmacologic activation, or in the absence of direct activation when the subject is in a "resting state" (eyes covered, ears plugged to reduce sensory input) or otherwise at rest with visual and auditory inputs uncontrolled. In the absence of activation, rCBF is proportional (coupled) to both rCMR$_{glc}$ and rCMRO$_2$ in normal subjects and in patients with chronic stable brain disease, including AD (63). During focal stimulation, however, coupling is maintained between rCBF and rCMR$_{glc}$, but can be disrupted between each of these measures and rCMRO$_2$ (21), implying glycolytic at the expense of oxidative metabolism. Thus, rCBF or rCMR$_{glc}$, but not rCMRO$_2$, can be employed to quantify focal activation.

Resting Cerebral Metabolism in Alzheimer's Disease

More than 20 cross-sectional PET studies of brain functional activity have been reported for AD patients who were diagnosed by DSM-III and/or NINCDS-ADRDA criteria (16,54). Individual publications and supporting references are summarized elsewhere (66). These data were obtained with scanners differing with regard to anatomic resolution [full width at half-maximum (FWHM) of line spread function], sensitivity, and attenuation correction. Patients studied differed with regard to dementia severity and scanning conditions, whereas controls differed with regard to quality of medical screening. Despite

TABLE 2. *Glucose metabolism in AD patients of different dementia severity, in relation to metabolism in age-matched healthy controls[a]*

	rCMR$_{glc}$(mg/100 g/min)			
Region	Controls (N = 30)	Mild AD (N = 17)	Moderate AD (N = 19)	Severe AD (N = 11)
Association neocortex				
Prefrontal	7.96 ± 1.09	6.59 ± 1.34 (83)[b,c]	6.22 ± 1.40 (78)[c]	4.69 ± 1.64 (59)[c]
Premotor	8.69 ± 1.16	6.90 ± 1.46 (79)[c]	6.26 ± 1.43 (72)[c]	4.70 ± 1.74 (54)[c]
Parietal	8.27 ± 1.13	6.09 ± 1.37 (74)[c]	5.36 ± 1.28 (65)[c]	3.83 ± 1.46 (46)[c]
Temporal	7.53 ± 0.79	5.98 ± 0.91 (79)[c]	5.63 ± 1.23 (75)[c]	3.97 ± 1.28 (52)[c]
Occipital	7.72 ± 0.94	6.65 ± 1.28 (86)[c]	6.13 ± 1.23 (79)[c]	5.00 ± 1.83 (65)[c]
Primary neocortex				
Sensorimotor	8.31 ± 1.00	7.27 ± 1.03 (87)[c]	6.75 ± 1.14 (82)[c]	5.61 ± 1.71 (68)[c]
Calcarine	8.06 ± 1.12	7.02 ± 1.09 (87)[c]	7.09 ± 1.02 (88)[c]	6.52 ± 1.89 (81)[c]
Subcortical nuclei				
Caudate	9.24 ± 1.64	8.35 ± 1.26 (90)	7.72 ± 1.87 (84)[c]	5.45 ± 1.21 (70)[c]
Lenticular	9.41 ± 1.37	8.76 ± 1.45 (93)[c]	8.71 ± 1.85 (93)[c]	6.87 ± 1.48 (73)[c]
Thalamus	8.99 ± 1.37	8.27 ± 1.46 (92)[c]	8.15 ± 0.94 (91)[c]	6.42 ± 2.05 (71)[c]

[a] From ref. 45.
[b] Mean ± SD (percent of control mean).
[c] Differs significantly from control mean ($p < 0.05$), corrected for six comparisons.

these differences, the overall picture is remarkably consistent. Metabolic reductions were reported throughout the neocortex, more so in association than in primary areas, in AD patients of equivalent dementia severity. Reductions were more severe in relation to dementia severity, ranging from −17% in the prefrontal association cortex of mildly demented patients to −54% in the parietal association cortex of severely demented patients.

The most extensive study with a high-resolution multislice PET scanner [Scanditronix PC 1024-7B, 6-mm in-plane and 10-mm axial resolution] was performed by Kumar et al. (45) on 47 carefully screened AD patients of differing dementia severity, as well as on 30 controls, in the "resting state." Table 2 illustrates rCMR$_{glc}$ values from this study for representative right-sided regions. With the exception of the caudate nucleus, mean metabolic rates even in mildly demented AD patients were significantly less than control means. At each dementia severity in AD, rCMR$_{glc}$ generally was lower in association than in primary neocortices or subcortical nuclei. For example, whereas percent (of control) association cortex metabolism in mildly demented subjects ranged from 74% to 86%, the percent equaled 87% for the primary cortices and 90–93% for the subcortical nuclei. Figure 1 illustrates such selectivity in PET scans from a severely demented patient with a disease of 8 years' duration.

When high-resolution Scanditronix data were subjected to discriminant analysis (see above), a discriminant function of rCMR$_{glc}$ values in frontal and parietal association areas was derived which correctly identified 87% of mildly to moderately demented AD patients and controls (2). This function thus could be used to convert a "possible" to a "probable" AD diagnosis in mildly demented patients. In this regard, this discriminant function later identified as "AD" an individual with an isolated mem-

ory impairment and a family history for autosomal dominant AD, whose PET scan had normal absolute and ratio values of rCMR$_{glc}$ (62). The patient subsequently developed severe dementia and a reduced parietal rCMR$_{glc}$.

Can PET Distinguish AD from Vascular Dementia?

Independently of clinical history and evaluation and of CT or MRI, PET (like SPECT, see below) cannot easily distinguish AD from vascular dementia. Both syndromes demonstrate global reductions in brain metabolism and flow in relation to dementia severity (22), as well as heterogeneity of cognitive and local metabolic deficits. Large asymmetric metabolic or flow reductions that correspond to CT or MRI abnormalities, or reductions in the basal ganglia or thalamus, suggest vascular dementia, whereas sparing of primary as compared with association cortical areas suggests AD (3). Neither AD nor vascular dementia is accompanied by an elevated rOER (22). However, prior to the appearance of dementia in some subjects with leukoaraiosis and hypertension (a major risk factor for vascular dementia), rOER can be elevated (77). Recently, PET demonstrated that the rCBF response to hypercapnia is normal in AD but defective in vascular dementia of the Binswanger type (46).

COGNITIVE AND METABOLIC CORRELATIONS IN ALZHEIMER'S DISEASE

Metabolic and Cognitive Groups

Mean PET measures of brain metabolism and blood flow (Table 2) mask distinct but heterogeneous metabolic patterns that are found in different AD patients. Four

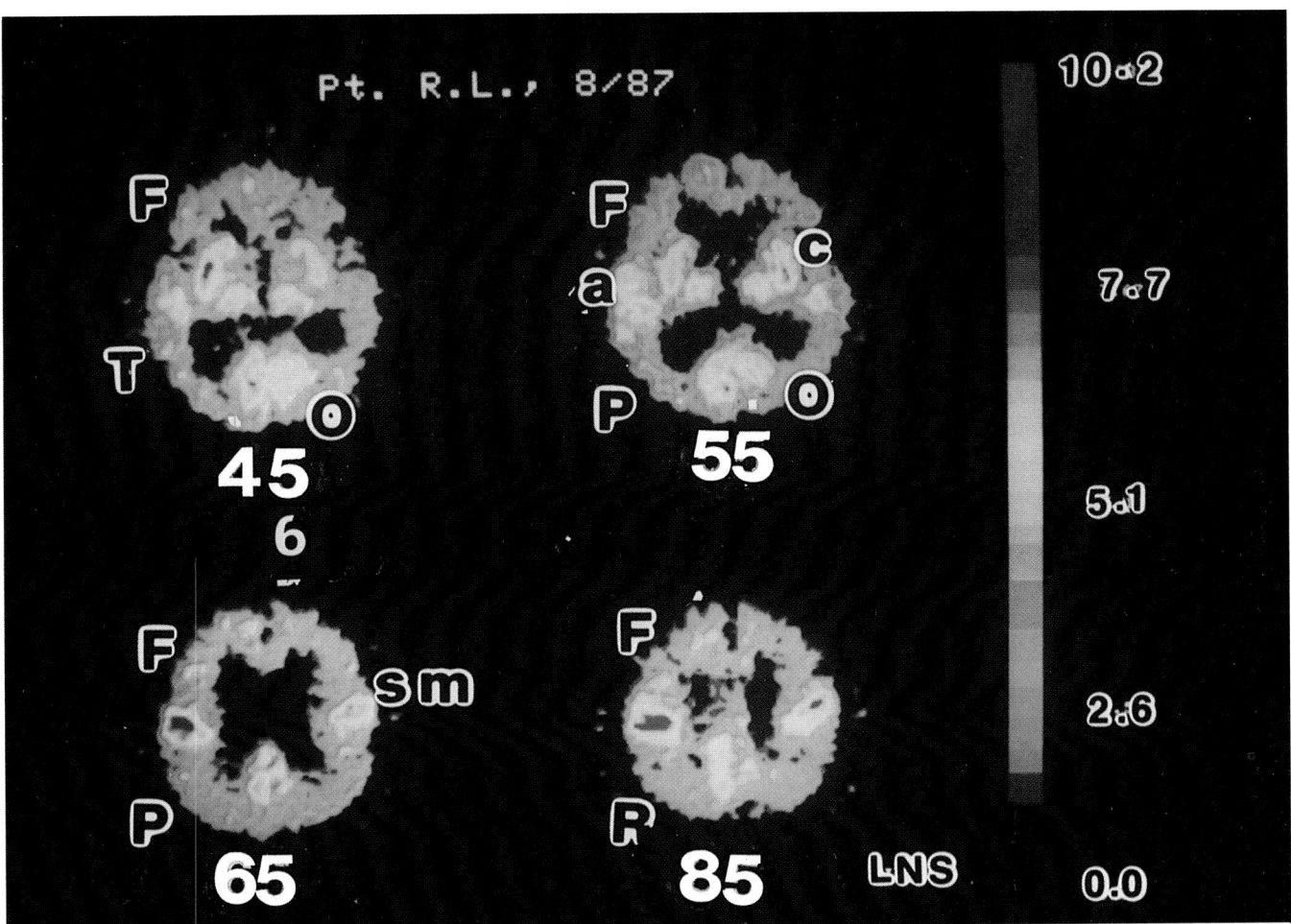

FIG. 1. PET scans of a severely demented AD patient. rCMR$_{glc}$, derived with Scanditronix PC 1024-7B tomograph, in units of mg/100 g brain/min. Higher metabolic rates are retained in the primary sensorimotor cortex (sm), primary visual cortex (o), primary auditory cortex (a), and caudate and lenticular nuclei (c), but are reduced in association neocortices. P, parietal lobe; F, frontal cortex; T, temporal cortex; O, occipital cortex. Numbers represent millimeters above inferior orbitomeatal line. (Courtesy of Laboratory of Neurosciences, National Institute on Aging.)

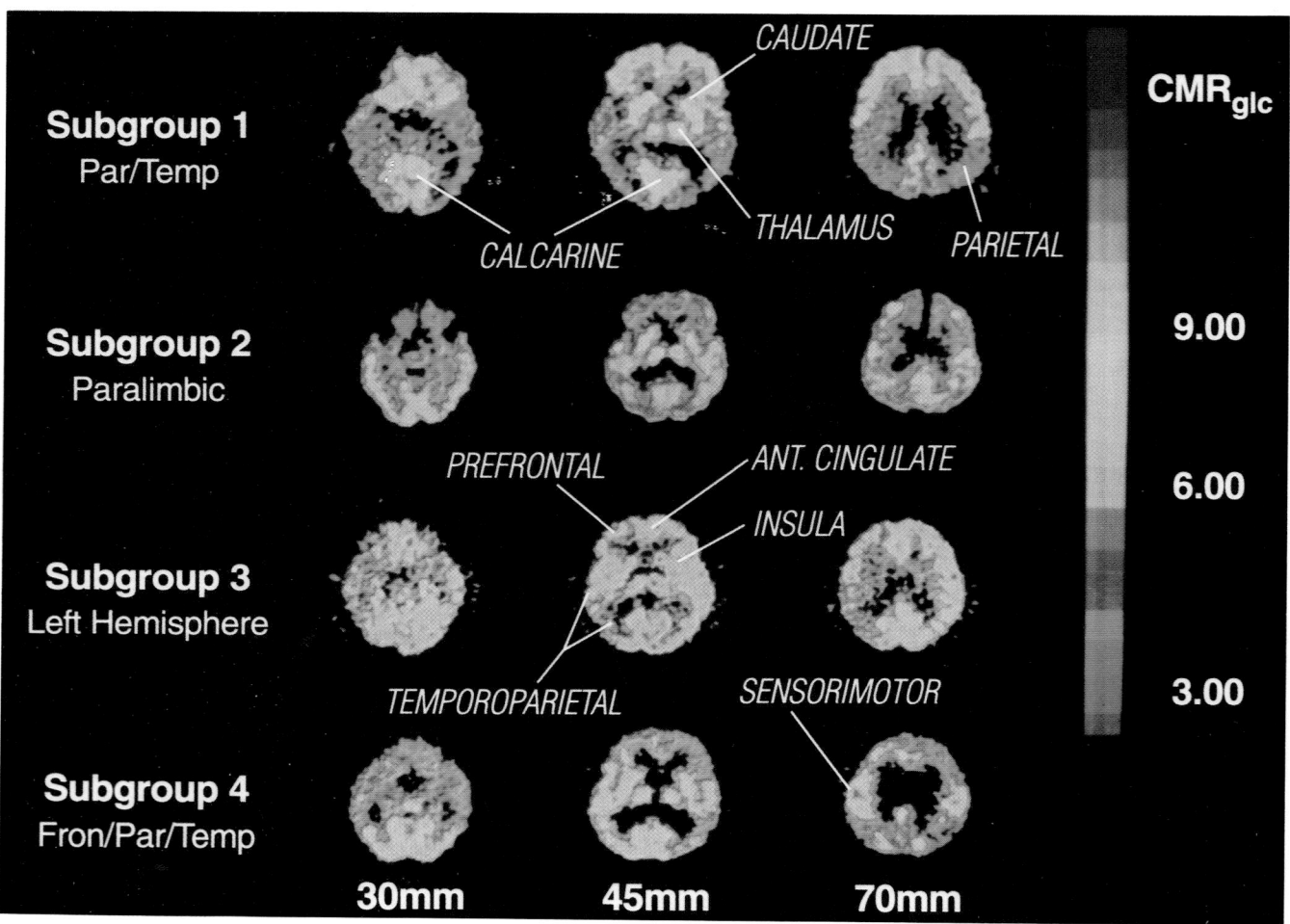

FIG. 2. PET scan images from four AD patients that best characterize four independent subgroups of metabolic patterns. Three planes are shown for each subject: *left*, at level of orbitofrontal cortex 30 mm above inferior orbitomeatal (IOM) line; *middle*, at level of basal ganglia 45 mm above IOM line; *right*, at level of centrum ovale 70 mm above IOM line. rCMR$_{glc}$ scale in mg/100 g/min. (From ref. 28.)

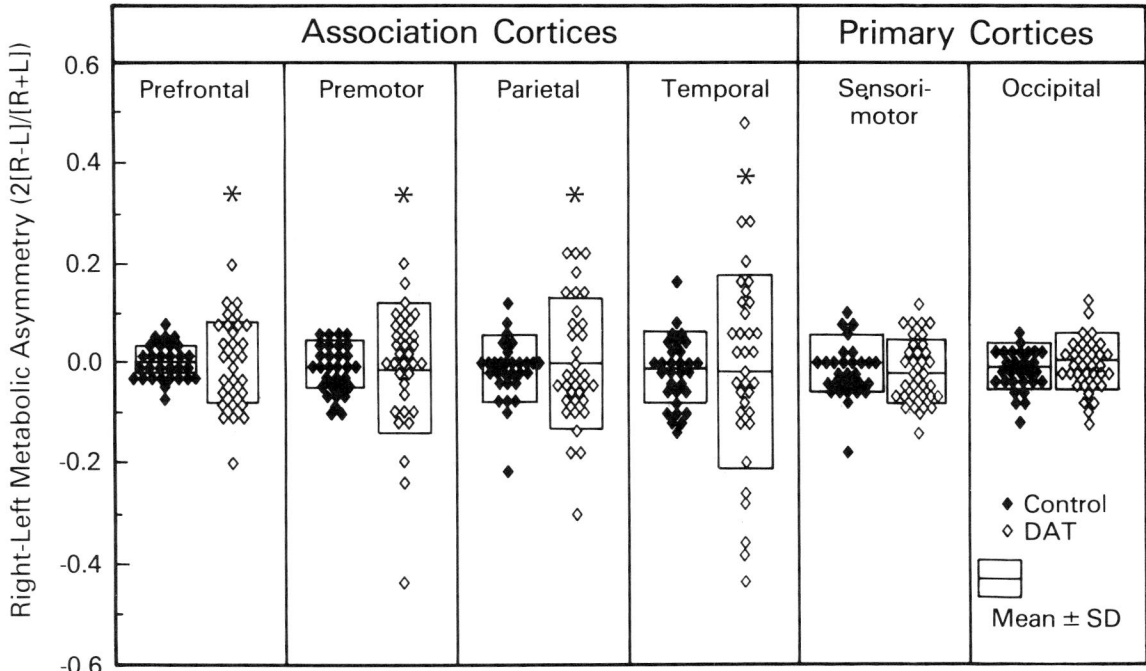

FIG. 3. Right–left metabolic asymmetries [Eq. (1)] in association and primary cortical regions in mildly to severely demented AD patients and control subjects. R, $rCMR_{glc}$, right; L, $rCMR_{glc}$, left; asterisk denotes that coefficient of variation differs from control value ($p < 0.05$). (High-resolution Scanditronix PC 1024-7B data from ref. 31.)

statistically significant patterns have been identified by a principal components analysis of high-resolution $rCMR_{glc}$ data, normalized via Z scores, from 16 regions of 36 mildly to severely demented AD patients (28). The group patterns are illustrated in Fig. 2. The most common pattern (Group 1, 17 patients) had $rCMR_{glc}$ reduced in superior and inferior parietal lobules and posterior medial temporal lobe. Group 2 (paralimbic) patients (8 of 36) had reduced metabolism in orbitofrontal and anterior cingulate gyri, whereas parietal regions were relatively spared. Group 3 (5 of 36) patients showed reduced left hemisphere metabolism, whereas Group 4 (6 of 36) patients had reductions in frontal, parietal, and temporal cortices.

Each patient group had a characteristic neuropsychological–behavioral profile. Group 2 patients had poorer verbal performance and fluency than did Group 1 (parietal/temporal) patients, but better visuospatial performance and spatial memory. Group 3 patients (left hemisphere) had worse verbal memory, verbal fluency, and calculating ability than did Group 1 patients, but better visuoperceptual performance and drawing. Group 1 patients were likely to be depressed, whereas Group 4 patients tended to show inappropriate behavior and psychotic symptoms. Group 2 patients demonstrated agitation, inappropriate behavior, and personality change, whereas those in Group 3 frequently had depressive symptoms (28).

Different PET metabolic patterns do not appear to be related to etiology in AD. No relation exists between metabolic asymmetry and early- or late-onset AD (27),

nor can PET distinguish familial from sporadic AD (35). Another etiologic subgroup is Down's syndrome, in which AD neuropathology and dementia become evident after 35 years of age (70). In nondemented Down's syndrome adults, patterns and absolute values of $rCMR_{glc}$ are the same as in age-matched controls, whereas in demented Down's syndrome adults, PET abnormalities appear which cannot be distinguished from abnormalities in AD.

Metabolic–Cognitive Correlations in Individual Patients

We have seen that reductions in mean PET measures of regional brain metabolism are more severe in more demented AD patients, that they are more profound in association than primary neocortical areas at each level of dementia severity, and that they fall into at least four statistically independent patterns. PET also has been used to show that cognitive deficits in individual AD patients correspond to specific metabolic deficits. Thus, PET has extended our understanding of brain networks that subserve specific cognitive processes, conceived of from lesion and stimulation studies in humans and higher primates (49). In this section, we discuss right/left asymmetries and parietal/frontal gradients of metabolism in individual AD patients, in relation to test scores of cognitive functions thought to be mediated by the right and left hemispheres or by the parietal and frontal lobes, respectively.

TABLE 3. *Right–left metabolic asymmetries [Eq. (1)] in control subjects and in AD patients of differing dementia severity[a,b]*

Brain regions	Right–left metabolic asymmetries			
	Controls (31)	Mild AD (11)	Moderate AD (13)	Severe AD (8)
Association cortex				
Prefrontal	0.01 ± 0.03	−0.01 ± 0.07*	−0.01 ± 0.08***	0.05 ± 0.10***
Premotor	0.01 ± 0.05	−0.01 ± 0.10**	−0.02 ± 0.16***	0.05 ± 0.11**
Orbitofrontal	−0.01 ± 0.06	−0.03 ± 0.08	−0.03 ± 0.11**	0.00 ± 0.11*
Parietal	−0.01 ± 0.06	−0.01 ± 0.11*	−0.03 ± 0.13*	0.08 ± 0.13*
Lateral temporal	−0.01 ± 0.07	−0.05 ± 0.17**	−0.03 ± 0.18***	0.08 ± 0.23***
Primary cortex				
Sensorimotor	−0.02 ± 0.05	−0.01 ± 0.07	0.00 ± 0.06	0.01 ± 0.08
Occipital[c]	−0.01 ± 0.04	0.00 ± 0.05	−0.01 ± 0.03	0.03 ± 0.08*

[a] Values are means ± SD (number of subjects). Scanditronix PC 1024-7B data from ref. 31.
[b] Variance greater than in controls: * $p < 0.05$; ** $p < 0.01$; *** $p < 0.001$.
[c] Primary and unimodal association cortex.

Based on evidence that Extended Range Drawing and Visual Recall tests reflect right neocortical function, and that Syntax Comprehension and Verbal Recall Tests reflect left neocortical function, AD patients and controls were ranked separately on these test scores and differences between ranks were quantified as a "drawing/comprehension discrepancy" or a "visual recall/verbal recall discrepancy" to reflect hemispheric functional asymmetry (31). These discrepancies then were correlated with a metabolic asymmetry index derived with high-resolution PET data, where $rCMR_{glc,right}$ is metabolic rate in a right hemisphere region and where $rCMR_{glc,left}$ is the rate in the homologous left hemisphere region:

Metabolic asymmetry index (%)

$$= \frac{rCMR_{glc,\ right} - rCMR_{glc,\ left}}{(rCMR_{glc,\ right} + rCMR_{glc,left})/2} \times 100 \quad (1)$$

Asymmetry indices for four association and two primary cortical areas are illustrated in Fig. 3 for mildly to severely demented AD patients and controls. As shown by asterisks, patients had significantly greater variances

(SD^2) than did controls in association but not in primary cortices. Distinct metabolic asymmetries were visually evident in PET scans of individual patients (Fig. 2, Group 3). Abnormal variances of metabolic asymmetry were found at each dementia severity (Table 3). They were correlated significantly and in expected directions with cognitive discrepancies in moderately but not in mildly demented patients (Table 4). In the moderately demented patients, relatively lower right-sided metabolism corresponded to worse drawing and visual recall test scores, compared with syntax comprehension and verbal recall test scores, respectively. The opposite was true for relative left-sided hypometabolism (31).

PET scans of AD patients also can display gradients in metabolism between the parietal and frontal lobes (Fig. 2, Groups 1 and 3). Accordingly, cognitive tests of parietal lobe function—Arithmetic Subtest of the WAIS, Syntax Comprehension Test, Extended Range Drawing Test, Block Tapping Span test—were compared in terms of rank ordering and cognitive discrepancies (see above) with tests of prefrontal integrity—Controlled Word Association (FAS) and Trailmaking (Trail A) tests. The cogni-

TABLE 4. *Spearman rank-sum correlations between right–left metabolic asymmetries [Eq. (1)] and drawing/syntax comprehension or visual recall/verbal recall discrepancies in AD patients of varying dementia severity[a,b]*

Neuropsychological discrepancy	Right–left metabolic asymmetry			
	Prefrontal	Premotor	Parietal	Lat temporal
Controls (N = 15–16)				
Drawing versus comprehension	−0.10	−0.33	0.00	0.12
Visual versus verbal recall	−0.30	−0.39	−0.30	−0.17
Mildly demented AD (N = 10)				
Drawing versus comprehension	0.04	−0.15	0.04	−0.24
Visual versus verbal recall	−0.22	−0.21	−0.16	−0.18
Moderately demented AD (N = 13)				
Drawing versus comprehension	0.76**	0.76**	0.79**	0.53
Visual versus verbal recall	0.49	0.55*	0.69**	0.48

[a] Positive correlation indicates that better drawing capacity or better visual recall is associated with relative high right-sided metabolism. Scanditronix PC 1024-7B data from ref. 31.
[b] Spearman rank-sum correlation differs from zero: * $p < 0.05$; ** $p < 0.01$.

TABLE 5. *Spearman correlations between parietal/prefrontal rCMR$_{glc}$ ratios and parietal/prefrontal neuropsychological test score discrepancies in AD patients*[a,b]

Neuropsychological discrepancy	Parietal/prefrontal metabolic ratio					
	Controls (14–17)[c]		Mild AD (10)[c]		Moderate AD (14)[c]	
	Right	Left	Right	Left	Right	Left
Arithmetic versus						
Verbal fluency	−0.02	0.00	−0.14	0.04	0.63*	0.57*
Attention (Trail A)	−0.34	−0.08	−0.02	−0.21	0.43	0.46
Verbal comprehension versus						
Verbal fluency	0.00	0.03	−0.30	−0.06	0.66*	0.67*
Attention (Trail A)	−0.12	0.11	0.04	−0.01	0.51	0.56*
Drawing versus						
Verbal fluency	−0.02	0.11	−0.02	0.22	0.66*	0.57
Attention (Trail A)	−0.21	0.21	0.42	0.32	0.44	0.43
Immediate memory span for visuospatial location (block tapping) versus						
Verbal fluency	0.16	0.05	−0.25	−0.11	0.62*	0.54
Attention (Trail A)	0.14	0.32	0.26	0.11	0.73**	0.72**

[a] Neuropsychological discrepancy is rank on a test of arithmetic, syntax comprehension, and extended range drawing minus rank on controlled word association or attentional trailmaking (Trail A) test score. Scanditronix PC 1024-7B data from ref. 32.

[b] Spearman correlation coefficient in AD differs from control: * $p < 0.05$; ** $p < 0.01$.

[c] Number of subjects are in parentheses.

tive discrepancies then were correlated with parietal/frontal metabolic ratios in AD patients of differing dementia severity (32). As noted in Table 5, statistically significant correlations in the expected directions were evident between cognitive discrepancies and the metabolic ratios in moderately but not in mildly demented patients.

Longitudinal studies of individual AD patients with PET demonstrated frequent retention of initial directions of right/left metabolic asymmetry and parietal/frontal metabolic ratios over many years. The initial direction of metabolic asymmetry in each of 11 mildly demented AD patients was shown not to change for up to 4 years (Fig. 4) (27). Likewise, Spearman correlations between initial and follow-up metabolic ratios at least 1.5 years later

ranged from 0.67 to 0.86 ($p < 0.01$) (32). These results indicate that the AD process leading to regional hypometabolism may start in one hemisphere before the other [there is no predilection for either hemisphere because mean asymmetries do not differ from unity (Table 3)], or in the parietal before the frontal lobe, and that subsequently rates of decline in both lobes or hemispheres are sufficiently consistent in a given patient to prevent crossover in direction.

This consistency likely explains why metabolic asymmetries in initially mildly demented AD patients were significant predictors of expected cognitive discrepancies that appeared 1–3 years later (language worse with initial left-sided hypometabolism, visuospatial function worse

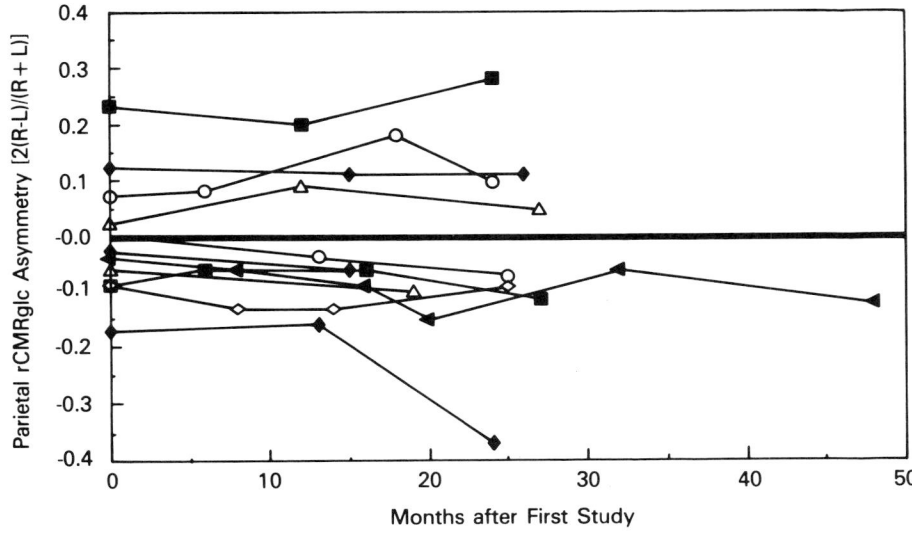

FIG. 4. Stability over time of right–left metabolic asymmetries in parietal association cortex of 11 initially mildly demented AD patients. (From ref. 31.)

TABLE 6. *Spearman rank-sum correlations between visuospatial–verbal neuropsychological discrepancies and right–left metabolic asymmetries in AD patients when initially mildly demented and at last evaluation[a–c]*

Neuropsychological discrepancy	Cerebral metabolic asymmetry			
	Prefrontal	Premotor	Parietal	Lat temporal
Controls				
WAIS PDQ minus MDQ				
(N = 29)	−0.07	−0.06	0.02	0.03
Visual minus verbal recall				
(N = 15)	−0.30	−0.39	−0.40	−0.17
Mild AD (N = 10)				
Initial evaluation				
WAIS PDQ minus MDQ	0.04	−0.09	−0.16	0.04
Visual minus verbal recall	−0.22	−0.21	−0.16	−0.18
Last evaluation				
WAIS PDQ minus MDQ	0.78**	0.67*	0.50	0.59
Visual minus verbal recall	0.44	0.41	0.68*	0.71*

[a] From ref. 31.
[b] WAIS, Wechsler Adult Intelligence Scale; PDQ, perceptual organization deviation quotient; MDQ, memory and freedom from distractibility quotient.
[c] Statistically significant: ** $p < 0.01$; * $p < 0.05$.

with initial right-sided hypometabolism), and why parietal as compared with frontal hypometabolism in mildly demented patients accurately predicted worst scores on cognitive tests of parietal than of frontal integrity (27,31). Thus, in initially mildly demented AD patients in whom the direction of metabolic asymmetry was maintained (Fig. 4), Spearman rank-sum correlations between asymmetries and appropriate neuropsychological discrepancies were significant at the last but not at the first evaluation (Table 6) (31).

In summary, PET is a more sensitive marker of early AD than are neuropsychological measures of cognitive functions mediated by the neocortex. Metabolic reductions, asymmetries, and parietal/frontal gradients can be found in mildly demented patients, where they indicate very early dysfunction within neocortical association areas. The directions of asymmetries and gradients are retained over many years in individual patients, in whom they predict either (a) deficits in language as compared with visuospatial function that later appear or (b) discrepancies of parietal compared to prefrontal cognitive test scores, which appear in the later stages of disease. Thus, metabolic asymmetry or an abnormal prefrontal/parietal metabolic ratio in a patient with a diagnosis of "possible" AD patient and only a memory deficit implies a diagnosis of "probable" AD.

Causes of Reduced rCMR$_{glc}$ in Alzheimer's Disease

If rCMR$_{glc}$ largely represents functional activity of terminal synapses and their postsynaptic dendritic connections (see Chapters 56, 76, and 77, *this volume*) a reduced rCMR$_{glc}$ in early AD could be due to synaptic pathology and reduced synaptic efficacy (67). Indeed, synaptic markers are down in the AD brain, and presynaptic ele-

ments have been shown by biopsy to drop out very early in disease (15). Reduced synaptic functioning is evidenced in life by fewer significant positive correlations between pairs of PET-derived rCMR$_{glc}$ values in AD as compared with control subjects (38). Fewer correlations imply, furthermore, that rCMR$_{glc}$ in regions without marked pathology (e.g., basal ganglia or thalamus; see Table 2) may decline because of disrupted connections with pathological regions elsewhere in the brain. The fact that uptake of ^{18}F-fluoro-DOPA into the basal ganglia was not altered in AD patients even with extrapyramidal signs, whereas uptake into the putamen was reduced in Parkinson's disease, further indicates that basal-ganglia–substantia-nigra circuitry is not directly affected in AD (74).

In demented patients proven on autopsy to have AD, neurofibrillary tangle densities were common in cortical association areas which had the most reductions in rCMR$_{glc}$ prior to death, but were much less common in primary cortical areas (14). This correlation is consistent with other reports on gradients of tangle distribution and atrophy in the neocortex in AD (64,66). Because focal atrophy in AD may artificially reduce PET metabolic values due to partial voluming, anatomic registration will be needed in future PET studies to obtain true estimates of metabolism or of flow per gram tissue (see Chapters 76 and 77, *this volume*).

Metabolic deficits and neuropathology in association as compared with primary neocortex represent a more general AD neurodegeneration in regions closely connected with the association neocortex—the hippocampal formation, amygdaloid complex, entorhinal cortex, nucleus basalis of Meynert, and catecholaminergic projecting neurons from the brainstem and pons. These regions constitute a telencephalic "association system" that evolved coherently and preferentially in higher primates,

TABLE 7. *rCBF in occipitotemporal visual association areas in AD patients and normals performing control or face-matching tasks[a]*

Parameter	Normals	Alzheimer patients
Control task		
rCBF ratio[b]	0.81 ± 0.02	0.74 ± 0.02[c]
rCBF (ml/100 g/min)	52.5 ± 3.0	45.0 ± 4.1
Face-matching task		
rCBF (ml/100 g/min)	59.0 ± 3.2	50.7 ± 4.2
Difference, face matching − control task		
rCBF (ml/100 g/min)	6.52 ± 0.82	5.63 ± 1.43

[a] From ref. 67.
[b] Ratio of rCBF in occipitotemporal visual association areas (Brodmann 19 and part of 37) to rCBF in primary occipital area (Brodmann 17).
[c] Mean ± SE differs significantly from normal mean, $p < 0.05$.

particularly in hominids, leading to the hypothesis that AD is a human phylogenic, or evolution-related, neurodegenerative disease (64,65).

Reduced brain metabolism in AD is unlikely to result from blood–brain barrier damage or ischemia. PET with ^{68}Ga-EDTA demonstrates normal blood–brain barrier permeability in AD (71). Furthermore, a ^{31}P MRS study indicates normal brain concentrations of phosphocreatine, adenosine triphosphate, and inorganic phosphate in AD (58), and PET shows that the rOER is not reduced (22). PET also indicates that transfer coefficients for glucose between blood and brain are not abnormal in AD (23), although capillary density of the glucose carrier is reduced in affected brain regions (41).

PET STUDIES DURING BRAIN ACTIVATION IN ALZHEIMER'S DISEASE

Cognitive Stimulation

By localizing and quantifying focal activation, PET promises to provide a new order of information about neural networks that are defective in AD, about the basis and possible reversibility of these defects, and about how these defects might be altered by appropriate drugs. Thus, Grady et al. (26) used $H_2^{15}O$ and a high-resolution Scanditronix multislice scanner to examine rCBF in occipitotemporal visual association regions while AD patients or normals performed a control or face-matching task. rCBF during the control task (a button was pressed alternately with right and left thumbs in response to a neutral visual stimulus) was subtracted from rCBF during the face-matching task (the button was pressed with the appropriate thumb after deciding whether the right or left face was to be matched) to produce a ''difference'' image. Mildly to moderately demented AD patients were chosen who were capable of performing the face-matching task as accurately [85 ± 8 (SD)% correct choices] as the normals (92 ± 5%, respectively).

As illustrated in Table 7, a reduced rCBF ratio during the control task, between association occipitotemporal (Brodmann areas 19 and 37) and primary occipital (Brodmann areas 17) regions, indicated impaired functional activity in a visual association area of the AD patients. However, during face matching, the mean increment in absolute rCBF (ml/100 g/min) did not differ between patients and controls (26,67). Thus, reduced unstimulated functional activity in visual association areas in some mildly demented AD patients is not accompanied by a reduced capacity of these areas to respond fully during face recognition, suggesting a degree of reversibility of functional failure, possibly through recovery of synaptic efficacy (67). It also was noted that frontal lobe regions were activated in the AD patients but not in the normals during face matching (26). This was ascribed to greater effort by the patients, whose reaction times during the task were more variable than in normals; 3.34 ± 1.46 (SD) sec as compared with 2.07 ± 0.54 sec.

Another study measured $rCMR_{glc}$ twice during the same PET session, in AD patients and normal subjects who first performed a control and then a reading memory task (18). Patients and normals had equivalent global activation [11% ± 13 (SD)% compared to 15 ± 15% (as percent control task)] and equivalent regional activations.

Pharmacologic Stimulation

Limited useful data are available with regard to PET and drug effects. In one study, AD patients who were scanned before and during physostigmine infusion demonstrated increments as well as decrements of normalized $rCMR_{glc}$ (73). The one patient who improved clinically had the maximum elevation of $rCMR_{glc}$. With regard to efficacy of cholinergic therapy, three mildly to moderately demented AD patients, treated orally with the cholinesterase inhibitor tetrahydroaminoacridine for several months, were shown by PET to have increased uptake of (S)(−) ^{11}C-nicotine in the frontal and temporal cortices, suggesting restoration of nicotinic cholinergic receptors and improved $rCMR_{glc}$ as well as neuropsychological performance (59). In another study, when phosphatidylserine was administered to AD patients over a 6-month period, both resting and visual stimulation $rCMR_{glc}$ values were higher after treatment than before, whereas decreases were observed after 6 months in AD patients not given phosphatidylserine (34). Cognitive performance was not markedly changed in drug and nondrug groups.

A large number of positron-emitting ligands for receptors have been developed for use with PET, but few have as yet been applied to AD. These include ^{11}C-nicotine (see above). ^{11}C-Carfentanil has been used to demonstrate early loss of mu opiate receptors in the amygdaloid complex of AD patients, even after correction for atrophy (56).

SINGLE PHOTON EMISSION COMPUTED TOMOGRAPHY (SPECT) IN ALZHEIMER'S DISEASE: COMPARISON WITH PET AND UTILITY FOR CLINICAL DIAGNOSIS

Its high cost (approximately $4000) and its requirements for extensive cyclotron and technical support limit PET as a routine clinical tool for the diagnosis and characterization of AD. In response, SPECT has been introduced into clinical settings to estimate rCBF and receptor densities. SPECT is cheaper than PET ($500–$700) and requires less personnel and technical support. As described elsewhere in this volume (Chapter 77), high-sensitivity special-purpose gamma cameras can be used with ^{133}Xe gas to image single slices during 4–7.5 min with a resolution (FWHM) approaching 8 mm. Alternatively, low-sensitivity rotating gamma cameras can provide volumetric information, using commercially available long-lived ^{123}I- or ^{99m}Tc-labeled radiopharmaceuticals (36,37). The use of long-lived isotopes with a need for long signal acquisition times extends scanning time to 30–60 min and allows only 1 scan per day. SPECT is not truly quantitative because photon scatter and attenuation compensation have not been adequately addressed in its reconstruction paradigms. Ratios of radioactivity between one brain region and another usually are determined, and arterial input functions for absolute flow or density calculations usually are not obtained.

Estimates of specificity in diagnosing AD, based on studies using ^{123}I-N-isopropyl-p-iodoamphetamine SPECT, range from 50% to 100%, whereas estimates of sensitivity range from 97% to 100% (43). Because most of these reports lacked pathological confirmation and used moderately to severely demented patients, their relevance to the early diagnosis of AD is limited.

Whereas four statistically distinct PET patterns of $rCMR_{glc}$ have been reported in AD (see above) (28), seven qualitative rCBF patterns have been identified using ^{99m}Tc-HMPAO SPECT from a prospective study of 132 consecutive demented patients of varying dementia severity (36). Probability of AD was 82% for bilateral temporoparietal defects, 72% for bilateral temporoparietal plus additional defects, 57% for unilateral temporoparietal defects, 43% for frontal defects, 18% for large focal defects, and 0% for multiple small cortical defects. In another study of mildly to moderately demented AD patients, ^{99m}Tc-HMPAO SPECT demonstrated depressed rCBF ratios of frontal, anterior, posterior temporoparietal, and occipital regions to cerebellum (60). However, a normal SPECT pattern has been reported in 45% of mildly demented patients (68). Another study concluded that ^{99m}Tc-HMPAO SPECT has minimal diagnostic utility in mildly demented AD patients unless considerable doubt about the diagnosis exists on clinical ground (8).

A rule of thumb derived from SPECT studies of moderately to severely demented patients is that a temporoparietal reduction in rCBF is more likely with AD, whereas a patchy whole brain reduction is more likely with vascular dementia (48). But this rule is not always followed, because normal SPECT images occur in mildly demented AD and vascular dementia patients, and an asymmetric presentation in AD may be indistinguishable from pattern of cerebral infarction in another patient (37). A parietal deficit may favor the diagnosis of AD, whereas involvement of the motor cortex may favor vascular dementia, but some patients may have a mixture of both diseases. In a study of AD and vascular dementia patients matched for dementia severity (rarely done), with controls, ^{99m}Tc-HMPAO ratios of temporo-parietal cortex, parietal cortex, or frontal cortex to cerebellar radioactivity did not distinguish between the two dementia groups (76).

With regard to neuropharmacology, 0.5 mg intravenous physostigmine was shown by SPECT to increase rCBF in the left posterior parietotemporal region of AD patients whose baseline rCBF was reduced, but not of normals, suggesting up-regulation of postsynaptic cholinergic sensitivity (25). The muscarinic M_2-receptor subtype is selectively lost in AD (52), but currently no M_2-selective ligand which can penetrate the blood–brain barrier is available for use with SPECT. However, the radioligand ^{123}I-QNB has different pharmacokinetic properties for the M_1 as compared with the M_2 receptors. These properties may allow SPECT imaging with ^{123}I-QNB to quantitate loss of the M_2 subtype in the AD brain, if the regional M_2/M_1 receptor ratio normally is 1/1 or higher (78). This is unlikely in the parietal cortex, however, where M_1 = 88 nM and M_2 = 12 nM in normal brain (78). Focal reductions of ^{123}I-QNB binding by SPECT, in excess of reductions in $rCMR_{glc}$ by PET, have been reported in the thalamus and frontal cortex of AD patients, and they suggest selective loss of M_2 receptors in these regions (75).

In summary, SPECT measures of rCBF are of limited application for identifying mildly demented AD patients, except those with an atypical disease presentation, and of limited value for distinguishing moderately to severely demented patients with AD or vascular dementia. If a diagnosis of probable AD has been made by clinical history and examination, by evaluation of the Hachinski Ischemic Scale, and by anatomical imaging, the addition of SPECT usually is not necessary. Further use of SPECT for exploring receptor changes in AD would be of interest.

DISCUSSION

Prior to the introduction of functional brain imaging, AD was considered a progressive global dementia whose neuropsychological defects were an expression of overall damage and not dependent on the localization of more severe tissue changes. It was argued that there are homogeneous stages of deterioration, involving simultaneous worsening of aphasic, apraxic, and agnosic symptoms (66). Consistent with staging is evidence that mean metabolic reductions within the neocortex are proportional on average to dementia severity in AD patients (Table 2), and that memory and attention test scores are defective in mildly demented AD patients, whereas moderately to severely demented changes have more global defects (Table 1). Furthermore, volumetric CT demonstrates progressive dilatation of the lateral ventricles in relation to overall dementia severity (9).

Nevertheless, quantitative MRI now indicates more atrophy in the neocortex than in the basal ganglia and thalamus (58), in agreement with in vivo PET measurements and postmortem observations that AD is a disease of a phylogenically distinct, telencephalic association system which does not include these subcortical regions (64). With regard to the neocortex, PET-derived right–left metabolic asymmetries, posterior/anterior metabolic ratios, and metabolic group patterns defined by a principal-component analysis (28) have demonstrated marked metabolic heterogeneity in AD, and that staging of metabolic reductions as homogeneous is an oversimplification. Metabolic heterogeneities are not related to disease etiology, but they correlate with appropriate patterns of cognitive dysfunction and clinical profiles in individual patients and probably have underlying heterogeneous neuropathological profiles as their basis (14).

The consensus from cross-sectional and longitudinal studies of AD patients, using PET and cognitive testing, is that the disease has an initial and maintained predilection for the frontal, parietal, temporal, and occipital association neocortices compared with primary sensory and motor regions. Right–left metabolic asymmetries and abnormal posterior/anterior metabolic ratios appear in mildly demented patients, are maintained over years, and predict and correspond to neuropsychological discrepancies between language and visuospatial test scores, and between parietal and frontal lobe test scores, that appear with progressing dementia. Vulnerability of the association cortex early and throughout the disease course reflects an overall vulnerability, confirmed by neuropathol-

ogy, for a telencephalic association system that evolved disproportionately during higher primate evolution (64,65).

Initial PET studies suggest that some brain regions with low resting rCBF can be fully activated during cognitive stimulation (18,26). Such stimulation studies deserve to be extended, because they suggest that early functional failure in AD might be reversed by administering drugs which increase synaptic efficacy (67). Dynamic MRI should be of help in this regard, because it can provide signals proportional to rCBF with a spatial resolution of a few millimeters and a temporal resolution of a few seconds, in the absence of ionizing radiation (47).

Future advances in anatomic and functional imaging technology and in tracer development promise to provide further insights into AD, and additional diagnostic applications. High-resolution, high-sensitivity PET scanners, combined with better localization and atrophy correction through MRI–PET superimposition (see Chapters 76 and 77, *this volume*), should afford critical information about functional activation of the amygdaloid formation and hippocampal complex, regions known to be pathological in AD, and perhaps help to identify mildly demented patients with only a memory deficit, or even subjects at risk for AD.

REFERENCES

1. Almkvist O, Wahlund L-O, Andersson-Lundman G, Basun H, Bäckman L. White-matter hyperintensity and neuropsychological functions in dementia and healthy aging. *Arch Neurol* 1992;49:626–632.
2. Azari NP, Pettigrew KD, Schapiro MB, et al. Early detection of Alzheimer's disease: a statistical approach using positron emission tomographic data. *J Cereb Blood Flow Metab* 1993;13:438–447.
3. Benson DF, Kuhl DE, Hawkins RA, Phelps ME, Cummings JL, Tsai SY. The fluorodeoxyglucose ^{18}F scan in Alzheimer's disease and multi-infarct dementia. *Arch Neurol* 1983;40:711–714.
4. Boller F, Lopez OL, Moossy J. Diagnosis of dementia: clinicopathologic correlations. *Neurology* 1989;39:76–79.
5. Bowen BC, Barker WW, Loewenstein DA, Sheldon J, Duara R. MR signal abnormalities in memory disorder and dementia. *AJR* 1990;154:1285–1292.
6. Brown GG, Levine SR, Gorell JM, et al. In vivo ^{31}P NMR profiles of Alzheimer's disease and multiple subcortical infarct dementia. *Neurology* 1989;39:1423–1427.
7. Chui HC, Victoroff JI, Margolin D, Jagust W, Shankle R, Katzman R. Criteria for the diagnosis of ischemic vascular dementia proposed by the State of California Alzheimer's disease diagnostic and treatment centers. *Neurology* 1992;42:473–480.
8. Claus JJ, Hasan D, van Harskamp FH, et al. SPECT with ^{99m}Tc-HMPAO is of limited diagnostic value in mild Alzheimer's disease: a population-based study. *Neurology* 1993;43(Suppl 2):A406.
9. Creasey H, Schwartz M, Frederickson H, Haxby JV, Rapoport SI. Quantitative computed tomography in dementia of the Alzheimer type. *Neurology* 1986;36:1563–1568.
10. DeCarli C, Grady CL, Clark CM, et al. Leukoencephalopathy in dementia of the Alzheimer type. Submitted for publication.
11. DeCarli C, Haxby JV, Gillette JA, Teichberg D, Rapoport SI, Schapiro MB. Longitudinal changes in lateral ventricular volume in patients with dementia of the Alzheimer type. *Neurology* 1992;42:2029–2036.
12. DeCarli C, Kaye JA, Horwitz B, Rapoport SI. Critical analysis of the use of computer-assisted transverse axial tomography to study

human brain in aging and dementia of the Alzheimer type. *Neurology* 1990;40:872–883.

13. DeCarli C, Murphy DGM, McIntosh AR, Teichberg D, Schapiro MB, Horwitz B. Discriminate analysis of MRI measures determines the presence of dementia of the Alzheimer type in males and females. [*Submitted.*]

14. DeCarli CS, Atack JR, Ball MJ, et al. Post-mortem regional neurofibrillary tangle densities but not senile plaque densities are related to regional cerebral metabolic rates for glucose during life in Alzheimer's disease patients. *Neurodegeneration* 1992;1:113–121.

15. DeKosky ST, Scheff SW. Synapse loss in frontal cortex biopsies in Alzheimer's disease: correlation with cognitive severity. *Ann Neurol* 1990;27:457–464.

16. Spitzer RL, ed. *Diagnostic and statistical manual of mental disorders*, 3rd ed. (revised) (DSM-III-R). Washington, DC: American Psychiatric Association, 1987;567.

17. Drayer BP. Imaging of the aging brain. Part II. Pathologic conditions. *Radiology* 1988;166:797–806.

18. Duara R, Barker WW, Chang J, Yoshii F, Loewenstein DA, Pascal S. Viability of neocortical function shown in behavioral activation state PET studies in Alzheimer disease. *J Cereb Blood Flow Metab* 1992;12:927–934.

19. Duara R, Grady C, Haxby J, et al. Positron emission tomography in Alzheimer's disease. *Neurology* 1986;36:879–887.

20. Folstein MF, Folstein SE, McHugh PR. "Mini Mental State"—a practical method for grading the cognitive state of patients for the clinician. *J Psychiatr Res* 1975;12:189–198.

21. Fox PT, Raichle ME, Mintun MA, Dence C. Nonoxidative glucose consumption during focal physiologic neural activity. *Science* 1988;241:462–464.

22. Frackowiak RSJ, Pozzilli C, Legg NJ, Du Boulay GH, Marshall J, Lenzi GL, Jones T. Regional cerebral oxygen supply and utilization in dementia. A clinical and physiological study with oxygen-15 and positron tomography. *Brain* 1981;104:753–778.

23. Friedland RP, Jagust WJ, Huesman RH. Regional cerebral glucose transport and utilization in Alzheimer's disease. *Neurology* 1989;39:1427–1434.

24. Gado M, Hugh CP, Danziger W, Chi D. Aging, dementia, and brain atrophy: a longitudinal computed tomographic study. *AJNR* 1983;4:699–702.

25. Geaney DP, Soper N, Shepstone BJ, Cowen PJ. Effect of central cholinergic stimulation on regional cerebral blood flow in Alzheimer's disease. *Lancet* 1990;335:1484–1487.

26. Grady CL, Haxby JV, Horwitz B, et al. Activation of cerebral blood flow during a visuoperceptual task in patients with Alzheimer-type dementia. *Neurobiol Aging* 1993;14:35–44.

27. Grady CL, Haxby JV, Horwitz B, et al. Longitudinal study of the early neuropsychological and cerebral metabolic changes in dementia of the Alzheimer type. *J Clin Exp Neuropsychol* 1988;10:576–596.

28. Grady CL, Haxby JV, Schapiro MB, et al. Subgroups in dementia of the Alzheimer type identified using positron emission tomography. *J Neuropsychol Clin Neurosci* 1990;2:373–384.

29. Hachinski V. Preventable senility: a call for action against the vascular dementias. *Lancet* 1992;340:645–648.

30. Hagberg BO, Ingvar DH. Cognitive reduction in presenile dementia related to regional abnormalities of cerebral blood flow. *Br J Psychiatry* 1976;128:209–222.

31. Haxby JV, Grady CL, Koss E, et al. Longitudinal study of cerebral metabolic asymmetries and associated neuropsychological patterns in early dementia of the Alzheimer type. *Arch Neurol* 1990;47:753–760.

32. Haxby JV, Grady CL, Koss E, Horwitz B, Schapiro M, Friedland RP, Rapoport SI. Heterogeneous anterior–posterior metabolic patterns in dementia of the Alzheimer type. *Neurology* 1988;38:1853–1863.

33. Haxby JV, Raffaele K, Gillette J, Schapiro MB, Rapoport SI. Individual trajectories of cognitive decline in patients with dementia of the Alzheimer type. *J Clin Exp Neuropsychol* 1992;14:575–592.

34. Heiss W-D, Kessler J, Slansky I, Mielke R, Szelies B, Herholz K. Metabolic activation by a visual recognition task for assessment of therapeutic efficacy in Alzheimer's disease. *Ann Nucl Med [Suppl]* 1993;7:S124–S125.

35. Hoffman JM, Guze BH, Baxter L, et al. Metabolic homogeneity in familial and sporadic Alzheimer's disease: an FDG-PET study. *Neurology* 1989;39(Suppl 1):167.

36. Holman BL, Johnson KA, Gerada B, Carvalho PA, Satlin A. The scintigraphic appearance of Alzheimer's disease: a prospective study using technetium-99m-HMPAO SPECT. *J Nucl Med* 1992;33:181–185.

37. Holman BL, Nagel JS, Johnson KA, Hill TC. Imaging dementia with SPECT. *Ann NY Acad Sci* 1991;620:165–174.

38. Horwitz B, Grady CL, Schlageter NL, Duara R, Rapoport SI. Intercorrelations of regional cerebral glucose metabolic rates in Alzheimer's disease. *Brain Res* 1987;407:294–306.

39. Hounsfield GN. Computerized transverse axial scanning (tomography), part I: description of system. *Br J Radiol* 1973;46:1016–1022.

40. Jellinger K. Neuropathological aspects of dementias resulting from abnormal blood and cerebrospinal fluid dynamics. *Acta Neurol Belg* 1976;76:83–102.

41. Kalaria RN, Harik SI. Reduced glucose transporter at the blood–brain barrier and in cerebral cortex in Alzheimer disease. *J Neurochem* 1989;53:1083–1088.

42. Kaye JA, DeCarli C, Luxenberg JS, Rapoport SI. The significance of age-related enlargement of the cerebral ventricles in healthy men and women measured by quantitative computed X-ray tomography. *J Am Geriatr Soc* 1992;40:225–231.

43. Killen AR, Oster G, Colditz GA. An assessment of the role of ^{123}I-N-isopropyl-p-iodoamphetamine with single-photon emission computed tomography in the diagnosis of stroke and Alzheimer's disease. *Nucl Med Commun* 1989;10:271–284.

44. Kozachuk WE, DeCarli C, Schapiro MB, Wagner EE, Rapoport SI, Horwitz B. White matter hyperintensities in dementia of Alzheimer's type and in healthy subjects without cerebrovascular risk factors. A magnetic resonance imaging study. *Arch Neurol* 1990;47:1306–1310.

45. Kumar A, Schapiro MB, Grady C, et al. High-resolution PET studies in Alzheimer's disease. *Neuropsychopharmacology* 1991;4:35–46.

46. Kuwabara Y, Ichiya Y, Otsuka M, Masuda K, Ichimiya A, Fujishima M. Cerebrovascular responsiveness to hypercapnia in Alzheimer's dementia and vascular dementia of the Binswanger type. *Stroke* 1992;23:594–598.

47. Kwong KK, Belliveau JW, Chesler DA, et al. Dynamic magnetic resonance imaging of human brain activity during primary sensory stimulation. *Proc Natl Acad Sci USA* 1992;89:5675–5679.

48. Lechner H, Bertha G. Multiinfarct dementia. *J Neural Transm [Suppl.]* 1991;33:49–52.

49. Luria AR. *Higher cortical functions in man.* New York: Basic Books, 1966;513.

50. Luxenberg JS, Friedland RP, Rapoport SI. Quantitative X-ray computed tomography (CT) in dementia of the Alzheimer type (DAT). *Can J Neurol Sci* 1986;13:570–572.

51. Luxenberg JS, Haxby JV, Creasey H, Sundaram M, Rapoport SI. Rate of ventricular enlargement in dementia of the Alzheimer type correlates with rate of neuropsychological deterioration. *Neurology* 1987;37:1135–1140.

52. Mash DC, Flynn DD, Potter LT. Loss of M_2 muscarine receptors in the cerebral cortex in Alzheimer's disease and experimental cholinergic denervation. *Science* 1985;31:1115–1117.

53. Mayeux R, Stern Y, Spanton S. Heterogeneity in dementia of the Alzheimer type: evidence of subgroups. *Neurology* 1985;35:453–461.

54. McKhann G, Drachman D, Folstein M, Katzman R, Price D, Stadlan EM. Clinical diagnosis of Alzheimer's disease: Report of the NINCDS-ADRDA work group under the auspices of Department of Health and Human Services task force on Alzheimer's disease. *Neurology* 1984;34:939–944.

55. Miller BL, Moats RA, Shonk T, Ernst T, Woolley S, Ross BD. Alzheimer disease: depiction of increased cerebral *myo*-inositol with proton MR spectroscopy. *Radiology* 1993;187:433–437.

56. Mueller-Gaertner HW, Mayberg HS, Tune L, et al. Mu opiate receptor binding in amygdala in Alzheimer's disease: in vivo quantification by 11C carfentanil and PET. *J Cereb Blood Flow Metab* 1991;11(Suppl 2):S20.

57. Murphy DGM, Bottomley PA, Salerno J, et al. An in vivo study of glucose and phosphorus metabolism in Alzheimer's disease using magnetic resonance spectroscopy and PET. *Arch Gen Psychiatry* 1993;50:341–349.

58. Murphy DGM, DeCarli C, Daly E, et al. Volumetric magnetic resonance imaging in men with dementia of the Alzheimer type: correlations with disease severity. *Biol Psychiatry* 1993;34:612–621.

59. Nordberg A, Lilja A, Lundqvist H, et al. Tacrine restores cholinergic

nicotinic receptors and glucose metabolism in Alzheimer patients as visualized by positron emission tomography. *Neurobiol Aging* 1992;13:747–758.

60. Parani D, Di Piero V, Vallar G, et al. Technetium-99m HM-PAO-SPECT study of regional cerebral perfusion in early Alzheimer's disease. *J Nucl Med* 1988;29:1507–1514.

61. Pettegrew JW, Moossy J, Withers G, McKeag D, Panchalingam K. [31]P nuclear magnetic resonance study of the brain in Alzheimer's disease. *J Neuropathol Exp Neurol* 1988;47:235–248.

62. Pietrini P, Azari NP, Grady CL, et al. Pattern of cerebral metabolic interactions in a subject with isolated amnesia at risk for Alzheimer's disease: a longitudinal evaluation. *Dementia* 1993;4:94–101.

63. Raichle ME, Grubb RL Jr, Gado MH, Eichling JO, Ter-Pogossian MM. Correlation between regional cerebral blood flow and oxidative metabolism. *Arch Neurol* 1976;33:523–526.

64. Rapoport SI. Brain evolution and Alzheimer's disease. *Rev Neurol (Paris)* 1988;144:79–90.

65. Rapoport SI. Integrated phylogeny of the primate brain, with special reference to humans and their diseases. *Brain Res Rev* 1990; 15:267–294.

66. Rapoport SI. Positron emission tomography in Alzheimer's disease in relation to disease pathogenesis: a critical review. *Cerebrovasc Brain Metab Rev* 1991;3:297–335.

67. Rapoport SI, Grady CL. Parametric in vivo brain imaging during activation to examine pathological mechanisms of functional failure in Alzheimer disease. *Int J Neurosci* 1993;70:39–56.

68. Reed BR, Jagust WJ, Seab JP, Ober BA. Memory and regional cerebral blood flow in mildly symptomatic Alzheimer's disease. *Neurology* 1989;39:1537–1539.

69. Rosen WG, Terry RD, Fuld PA, Katzman R, Peck A. Pathological verification of ischemic score in differentiation of dementias. *Ann Neurol* 1980;7:486–488.

70. Schapiro MB, Haxby JV, Grady CL, et al. Decline in cerebral glucose utilization and cognitive function with aging in Down's syndrome. *J Neurol Neurosurg Psychiatry* 1987;50:766–774.

71. Schlageter NL, Carson RE, Rapoport SI. Examination of blood–brain barrier permeability in dementia of the Alzheimer type with [68-Ga]EDTA and positron emission tomography. *J Cereb Blood Flow Metab* 1987;71:1–8.

72. Shulman RG, Blamire AM, Rothman DL, McCarthy G. Nuclear magnetic resonance imaging and spectroscopy of human brain function. *Proc Natl Acad Sci USA* 1993;90:3127–3133.

73. Tune L, Brandt J, Frost JJ, et al. Physostigmine in Alzheimer's disease: effects on cognitive functioning, cerebral glucose metabolism analyzed by positron emission tomography and cerebral blood flow analyzed by single photon emission tomography. *Acta Psychiatr Scand [Suppl]* 1991;366:61–65.

74. Tyrrell PJ, Sawle GV, Ibanez V, Gloomfield PM, Leenders KL, Frackowiak RS, Rossor MN. Clinical and positron emission tomography studies in the "extrapyramidal syndrome" of dementia of the Alzheimer type. *Arch Neurol* 1990;47:1318–1323.

75. Weinberger DR, Jones D, Reba RC, et al. A comparison of FDG PET and IQNB SPECT in normal subjects and in patients with dementia. *J Neuropsychiatry Clin Neurosci* 1992;4:239–248.

76. Weinstein HC, Haan J, van Royen EO, et al. SPECT in the diagnosis of Alzheimer's disease and multi-infarct-dementia. *Clin Neurol Neurosurg* 1991;93:39–43.

77. Yao H, Sadoshima S, Ibayashi S, Kuwabara Y, Ichiya Y, Fujishima M. Leukoaraiosis and dementia in hypertensive patients. *Stroke* 1992;23:1673–1677.

78. Zeeberg BR, Kim H-J, Reba RC. Pharmacokinetic simulations of SPECT quantitation of the M_2 muscarinic neuroreceptor subtype in disease states using radioiodinated (R,R)-4IQNB. *Life Sci* 1992; 51:661–670.

Psychopharmacology: The Fourth
Generation of Progress, edited by
Floyd E. Bloom and David J. Kupfer.
Raven Press, Ltd., New York © 1995.

CHAPTER 120

Experimental Therapeutics

Deborah B. Marin and Kenneth L. Davis

Several pharmacologic strategies have been used in attempts to treat the cognitive deficits in Alzheimer's disease. Trials with nootropics that presumptively alleviate the symptoms of mental aging and cerebral insufficiency exemplify nonspecific empirical treatments. In distinction, the neurotransmitter replacement strategies that have been explored are based on specific neurotransmitter deficits demonstrated in the brains of Alzheimer's disease patients. The consistently reported central cholinergic depletion in Alzheimer's disease in conjunction with the cholinergic system's involvement in learning have generated many studies that have focused on cholinergic enhancement. Although the cholinergic strategy has yielded some promising findings, including the approval of the first drug indicated for Alzheimer's disease, the results have not yet demonstrated robustness and universality. The results observed with cholinergic replacement may in part be due to the fact that other neurotransmitter systems are affected in Alzheimer's disease. It can therefore be argued that multiple neurotransmitter replacements may be more efficacious than a purely cholinergic approach.

An alternative to these palliative treatments of Alzheimer's disease is the development of approaches that interfere with the neurodegenerative process of the illness. This chapter will review the cholinergic and combined neurotransmitter approaches and will then discuss strategies designed to modify the course of Alzheimer's disease because of their presumed alteration of the fundamental pathophysiological processes in the disease.

THE CHOLINERGIC SYSTEM

There is a convergence of evidence supporting the critical role of the cholinergic system in Alzheimer's disease:

D. B. Marin and K. L. Davis: Department of Psychiatry, Mount Sinai Medical Center, New York, New York 10029.

(a) Centrally active anticholinergic agents produce attention and memory deficits; (b) cholinergic neurotransmission modulates memory and learning; (c) lesions of the central cholinergic system create learning and memory impairments which are attenuated with cholinergic agents; and (d) postmortem studies of Alzheimer's patients consistently document cholinergic abnormalities with the degree of cognitive impairment (45,47).

Both muscarinic and nicotinic receptors have been implicated in cognition and in Alzheimer's disease. Five muscarinic receptor subtypes, known as m1–m5, have been demonstrated and localized in the central nervous system (CNS) (71). Studies with pharmacological antagonists have identified four classes of muscarinic receptors that are known as M1, M2, M3, and M4. The subtypes identified by antisera (m1–m5) show substantial overlap with the receptor types identified pharmacologically (M1–M4) (71). The postsynaptic M1 receptors, whose main subtype is found in the cerebral cortex, have been implicated in memory processes (42). Activation of the m1, m3, and m5 receptors causes cellular excitation, whereas activation of the m2 and m4 subtypes produces inhibitory effects. The excitatory role of the m1 and m3 receptors, combined with their location in the cortex and hippocampus, makes these sites potential targets for pharmacologic treatment of the cognitive deficits in Alzheimer's disease.

There exist at least three different subtypes of nicotinic receptors in the human frontal cortex. The nicotinic receptors can be divided into three types, termed super-high, high, and low affinity (42). Brains of patients with Alzheimer's disease demonstrate decrements in the high-affinity nicotinic sites (42). In animal studies, nicotinic antagonists produce a dose-dependent impairment of memory comparable to what is observed with scopolamine (17). The nicotinic and muscarinic systems appear to jointly modulate performance in learning and memory (51). Animal data suggest that presynaptic nicotinic receptors mediate a positive feedback mechanism that modulates cholinergic activity (17). The development and implementation of safe and effective pharmacologic treatments have not yet fully utilized the above basic science findings (see also Chapters 11–13, and 125, *this volume*).

Cholinergic Agonists

The use of muscarinic agonists for the treatment of Alzheimer's disease is supported by their beneficial effects on memory and learning in animals in hypocholinergic states (25) and by the observed relative preservation of postsynaptic M1 sites in Alzheimer's disease (69).

RS86

RS-86 (2-ethyl-8-methyl-2,8-diazospiro-4,5-decan-1,3-dianhydrobromide) is a muscarinic receptor agonist that has a relatively higher affinity for M1 sites than for M2 sites. Oral administration of RS-86 has been shown to produce minimal or no effects in patients with Alzheimer's disease (26).

Bethanecol

Bethanecol is a synthetic β-methyl analogue of acetylcholine that acts on both M1 and M2 receptors. Studies conducted on small samples of patients have demonstrated modest improvement with this agent (50). Variable dose responses may contribute to this agent's heterogeneous efficacy (50). Bethanecol must be administered by an intracerebroventricular (ICV) route because of its poor blood–brain barrier permeability. ICV administration carries substantial risks, including perioperative complications, pneumocephalus, seizures, and chronic subdural hematoma. Thus, ICV bethanecol treatment is not likely to be a viable option for cholinergic enhancement in Alzheimer's disease.

Arecoline

Arecoline is a natural alkaloid with both muscarinic and nicotinic agonist properties. Modest improvement in picture recognition, verbal memory, and visuospatial construction after arecoline infusion have been observed in patients with Alzheimer's disease (49).

Oxotremorine

Oxotremorine is a synthetic nonselective muscarinic agonist with a half-life lasting several hours. Oxotremorine administration to Alzheimer's disease patients did not have cognitive enhancing effects and was associated

with significant side effects, including panic and depression (14).

Other Agonists

AF102B [$\pm cis$-2-methyl-spiro(1,3-oxathiolane-5,3') quinuclidine] is a structurally rigid analogue of acetylcholine. Unlike most of the cholinergic agents described above, AF102B is a selective M1 agonist (21). This characteristic is desirable because activation of the M2 autoreceptors can result in decreased acetylcholine release. AF102B, like other cholinergic agonists, reverses the cognitive impairments observed in hypocholinergic animals (21). Azaspirodecanes (2-methyl-1,3-dioxaazaspiro[4,5]-decanes) are a group of muscarinic compounds that are analogues of the tertiary amine AF-30. Some of these analogues are potent muscarinic agonists that have yet to be clinically tested.

Nicotine

Intravenous nicotine administration to Alzheimer's disease patients has been shown to improve performance in recall (40). Unfortunately, the anxiety and depressive symptoms associated with nicotine administration represent toxic effects that lessen the clinical utility of this compound.

None of the cholinergic agonists have yielded robust clinical benefit. Yet, it may very well be that the potential benefits of cholinergic agonists have not been adequately tested. The diverse physiologic effects of muscarinic and nicotinic activation limit the clinical usefulness of the agents currently employed. Arecoline, RS-86, and bethanecol probably do not have much effect on the m1 and m3 receptor sites in the cortex. The importance of targeting the appropriate site is exemplified by the compound oxotremorine, which actually decreases acetylcholine release through its action on the presynaptic m2 receptor. Targeting the appropriate receptor subtype in order to enhance cognition may be true for nicotinic receptors as well because there exist at least three different subtypes of these receptors. Optimal pharmacological manipulation of cholinergic subtypes has yet to be attempted.

Future directions in cholinergic agonist development may include manipulation of the subtypes of muscarinic and nicotinic receptors that are most likely to enhance cognitive function without adverse side effects. Such agents may be used in conjunction with other cholinergic strategies to treat the cognitive deficits in Alzheimer's disease. Postsynaptic therapy, however, is limited by the fact that agonist administration provides a nonphysiologic tonic stimulation, whereas the physiologic state is characterized by phasic mechanisms.

Cholinesterase Inhibitors

Acetylcholinesterase inhibitor treatment for Alzheimer's disease is based on the rationale that cholinergic neurotransmission is enhanced through preventing the breakdown of acetylcholine. The agents to be reviewed are physostigmine, tetrahydroaminoacridine, HP 029, and galanthamine.

Physostigmine

Physostigmine is a natural alkaloid that is absorbed in the gastrointestinal tract, subcutaneous tissue, and mucous membranes. Most studies using parenteral administration of physostigmine have documented transient cognitive improvement in at least a subgroup of patients with Alzheimer's disease (34). Oral administration of the compound has been shown to have some efficacy as well. It has been suggested that long-term treatment with physostigmine may delay deterioration in Alzheimer's disease (28). Obviously, these intriguing reports will stimulate further investigation. The limited efficacy of physostigmine may be due to several factors. The unpredictable blood, and therefore CNS, concentrations achieved with a given dose necessitate individual titration of medication. This agent's peripheral-to-brain partitioning also lessens its clinical utility. Blood levels required to achieve CNS concentrations necessary for cognitive enhancement may be associated with significant adverse effects. Physostigmine's short half-life is also problematic because this characteristic causes continuous fluctuations in blood levels and the need for frequent administration. The compound's inverted U-shape dose–response curve can lead to nonoptimal blood levels which also limit beneficial effects.

HP 029

HP 029 (velnacrine maleate) is a tetrahydroaminoacridine derivative that inhibits true cholinesterase and pseudocholinesterase. The drug reverses scopolamine- or lesion-induced memory impairment in rodents (20). There is marked intersubject variability in tolerance to the drug within the therapeutic dose range. A double-blind, placebo-controlled, enriched population design consisting of a 7-week dose-ranging phase followed by a 6-week dose replication phase demonstrated modest clinical improvement in a subset of the 195 patients with Alzheimer's disease (39). Unfortunately, a high incidence of liver toxicity is observed with this agent.

Galanthamine

Galanthamine is a tertiary amine of the phenthrene group. Administration of this medication results in cere-bral concentrations that are three times higher than its plasma level. Galanthamine's half-life of 7 hr is longer than that observed with tetrahydroaminoacridine or physostigmine (65). Some studies have suggested the efficacy of galanthamine in AD (65), whereas others have not (12).

THA

9-Amino-1,2,3,4-tetrahydroaminoacridine (THA) is a synthetic acetylcholinesterase inhibitor. THA has been shown to increase presynaptic acetylcholine release through blocking slow K channels and to increase postsynaptic monoaminergic stimulation by interfering with norepinephrine and serotonin uptake. These latter characteristics of THA occur at concentrations higher than those required to achieve acetylcholinesterase inhibition and therefore probably do not contribute to the drug's clinical effects.

Double-blind, placebo-controlled studies have assessed the efficacy of THA in large samples of Alzheimer's disease patients (7,15–17,19,23). THA and lecithin administration produced statistically significant improvement in the Mini Mental State score in two investigations (16,23) and minimal cognitive improvement in another study of Alzheimer's patients (17). A 6-week crossover trial using an enriched-population design with 215 patients (15) demonstrated that patients treated with THA showed significantly less decline in cognitive function than did the placebo-treated group, as assessed by the Alzheimer's Disease Assessment Scale cognitive subscale. A 12-week parallel group design that included 273 patients demonstrated a significant cognitive improvement with THA (19). Side effects with THA are nausea, abdominal distress, tachycardia, and liver toxicity. The liver damage noted with this agent is dose-dependent and reversible upon its discontinuation. The THA data indicate that anticholinesterase therapy is likely to benefit a subgroup of patients with Alzheimer's disease. The lack of efficacy in some patients in these investigations may be due to underdosing. Improvement with THA appears to be dose-dependent, with over 50% of patients improving at the highest doses (19). The results from these large-scale studies contributed to THA being the first FDA-approved drug for the treatment of Alzheimer's disease. Nonetheless, the ideal cholinesterase has not yet been tested. This agent would have (a) a long enough half-life that permits one dose per day, (b) minimal peripheral side effects and toxicity, and (c) good absorption and CNS penetration.

Cholinergic Releasing Agents

The use of acetylcholine releasers is based on their enhancement of stimulus-induced acetylcholine delivery into the synapse. Such an action would improve the signal-to-noise ratio during neuronal transmission without the toxicity associated with cholinesterase inhibitors or the distorted temporal pattern of neurotransmission observed with cholinergic agonists.

DuP 996

Linopirdine [DuP 996; 3,3-bis(4-pyrindinylmethyl)-1-phenylindolin-2-one] enhances potassium-stimulated release of acetylcholine, dopamine, and serotonin without affecting basal neurotransmitter release. DuP 996 has been shown to protect against hypoxia-induced passive avoidance deficits in rodents. In humans, DuP 996 administration induces electroencephalographic changes consistent with vigilance-improving properties (56).

HP 749

HP 749 [N-(n-propyl)-N-(4-pyridinyl)-1H-indol-1-amine] is an indole-substituted analogue of 4-aminopyridine which is well-absorbed after oral administration. Preclinical studies demonstrate that HP 749 reverses the passive avoidance deficit produced by nucleus basalis and dual lesions in rodents (10). Clinical trials to determine the efficacy of HP 749 in humans have yet to be performed.

Combined Treatment Approaches

Several lines of evidence demonstrate that multiple neurotransmitter systems are involved in cognition and in Alzheimer's disease, thereby suggesting that combined treatment approaches are likely to be more efficacious than cholinergic monotherapy. Animal studies demonstrate that noradrenergic brain lesions negate cholinomimetic enhancement of memory in hypocholinergic animals (25). Administration of the alpha-adrenergic agonist clonidine will, in turn, restore the efficacy of cholinomimetic treatment in animals with noradrenergic and cholinergic lesions (25). Furthermore, postmortem studies demonstrate major neurotransmitter losses of the noradrenergic system in Alzheimer's disease patients. All these findings support the use of a combination of cholinergic and noradrenergic agents to treat Alzheimer's disease. This combined approach has been shown to be safe in humans. A pilot study with clonidine and physostigmine treatment in nine patients demonstrated the feasibility and safety of combining these agents in Alzheimer's disease (13).

Studies evaluating the efficacy of combination treatment have primarily been performed with cholinesterase inhibitors and the monoamine oxidase B inhibitor 1-deprenyl. Double-blind, placebo-controlled trials with small patient samples suggest that subchronic treatment

with 1-deprenyl (10 mg/day) improves performance on attention, memory, and learning tasks (32).

A double-blind, placebo-controlled 4 week crossover study demonstrated that 1-deprenyl augmentation of either THA or physostigmine treatment significantly improved performance on the cognitive subscale scores of the Alzheimer's Disease Assessment Scale (59), suggesting possible additive effects of 1-deprenyl and cholinesterase inhibitors. However, another study of 16 Alzheimer's disease patients found no significant improvement with the combination of physostigmine and deprenyl (63). Inadequate physostigmine levels achieved in this latter trial might have led to spuriously poor results.

Future studies are needed to determine the potential efficacy of combination treatments. The 1-deprenyl results need to be replicated with larger patient samples and longer treatment trials to determine if this agent alone or in combination with other agents have clinically significant effects on cognition in patients with Alzheimer's disease.

APPROACHES TO SLOW PROGRESSION

The approaches described above generally offer palliative treatment to augment the functioning of deficient neurotransmitter systems in Alzheimer's disease. However, the suggestion that restoring either cholinergic transmission or some other property of cholinesterase inhibitors may slow the course of the illness needs to be pursued. Advances in the understanding of the biology of Alzheimer's disease permit the development of strategies that interfere with the underlying pathophysiology of the illness. The rationale for, and description of, potential neuroprotective strategies will be discussed.

Glutamatergic Approaches

Glutamate is the major excitatory neurotransmitter of the pyramidal neurons. The postsynaptic effects of glutamate are mediated via several different receptor subtypes that can be classified according to their prototypic agonists, namely, N-methyl-D-aspartate (NMDA), quisqualate (QUIS), and kainate (KAIN). Extensive loss of NMDA sites has been demonstrated in some, but not all, studies of brains of Alzheimer's disease patients (61). These findings suggest that development of glutamatergic treatment strategies must consider whether there is a glutamate deficiency to treat in Alzheimer's disease.

The glutamatergic system has been implicated in learning and memory (30). NMDA receptor blockade with aminophosphonopentanoic acid disrupts spatial learning and prevents long-term potentiation, which is considered a physiological model for memory. In addition to its beneficial properties, glutamate is neurotoxic and implicated in the pathogenesis of several CNS neurodegenerative disorders. The neurotoxic effects of glutamate can occur via both NMDA and non-NMDA receptors.

Given that glutamate can enhance learning as well as produce neurotoxicity, determination of the optimal glutamatergic strategy has to consider the complex functions of glutamate and the various glutamatergic receptors. Both NMDA and non-NMDA sites could be potential targets for therapeutic approaches. A strategy that enhances glutamatergic transmission is supported by the presynaptic glutamatergic losses observed in Alzheimer's disease. However, augmentation of glutamatergic functioning could increase neuronal damage. Glutamatergic blockade could protect against neurotoxic effects, yet potentially interfere with memory processing.

Antagonism of the glycine modulatory site of the NMDA receptor could decrease neurotoxicity mediated by glutamate. 1-Hydroxy-3-amino-2-pyrrolidone (HA-966) and 1-aminocyclobutane (ACBC) appear to inhibit NMDA-specific binding and block NMDA responses (27,68). An optimal antagonist at the glycine site would interfere with glutamate's neurotoxicity without causing cognitive impairment.

Non-NMDA antagonism may provide a potential therapeutic strategy to interfere with glutamatergic functioning and neurotoxicity. Antagonists of the non-NMDA receptors include 2,3-dihydroxy-6-nitro-7-sulfamoyl-benzo (F)quinoxaline (NBQX), 6,7-dinitroquinoxaline-2,3-dione (DNQX), and 6-cyano-7-nitroquinoxaline-2,3-dione (CNQX) (60). These agents have been shown to protect against the effects of ischemia (60). Clinical trials are necessary to determine whether these agents can alter the course of Alzheimer's disease.

Given the complex sequelae of glutamatergic activation, a partial agonist approach is rational. The glycine agonist milacemide enhances learning in normal and amnestic rodents. One clinical trial of this drug, however, did not enhance cognition and was accompanied by significant liver toxicity (48). As with other glutamatergic modulating agents, further clinical studies are necessary to test their potential efficacy (also see Chapter 7, *this volume,* for related topic).

Antioxidants

Several studies demonstrate increased free radical production in aging and Alzheimer's disease. Metal ions, increased superoxide-dismutase-derived hydrogen peroxide fluxes, and damaged mitochondria can contribute to cell damage mediated by free radicals. Free radical production in Alzheimer's disease might also be caused by amyloid beta protein, glutamate, increased levels of monoamine oxidase, or another toxic event (3). All these findings suggest the use of antioxidants to treat Alzheimer's disease.

L-Deprenyl's inhibition of monoamine oxidase B support its use as a free radical scavenger for the treatment of Alzheimer's disease. Vitamin E and idebenone are also potential antioxidant treatments for Alzheimer's disease. Alpha tocopherol, a biologically active constituent of vitamin E, interferes with the effects of lipid peroxidation by trapping free radicals (70). Vitamin E and idebenone have been shown to prevent cell death caused by glutamate and amyloid beta protein (3,43). Because of their antioxidant properties, L-deprenyl and vitamin E have been investigated as therapies to slow the progression of Parkinson's disease. A multicenter double-blind, placebo-controlled trial has demonstrated that deprenyl given at 10 mg/day delays the onset of disability associated with early Parkinson's disease (46). A multicenter double-blind, placebo-controlled trial is now underway to determine the ability of L-deprenyl and vitamin E, administered alone or in combination, to slow the progression of Alzheimer's disease.

Immunological Approaches

Several lines of evidence demonstrate the involvement of the immune system and inflammation in Alzheimer's disease. Histochemical studies demonstrate the presence of several markers of inflammation in Alzheimer's disease brains. Furthermore, components of the immune response have been localized in senile plaques, suggesting a role for the immune response in the pathophysiology of Alzheimer's disease. The implication of the presence of an immune response in the brain is that host cells can be inadvertently attacked and destroyed by these molecules.

Increased numbers of reactive glia and microglia (believed to be related to macrophages) have been observed in postmortem brain tissue (24). Of particular relevance is that complement proteins, including the membrane attack components C5–C9, have also been identified in senile plaques, tangles, and dystrophic neurites (36). These findings suggest that the complement system could be involved in the tissue destruction in Alzheimer's disease. Although the stimulus for complement activation in Alzheimer's disease brains is unclear, it has been shown that a beta protein can activate the classical complement pathway (54).

Elevated concentrations of cytokines, agents which signal cell proliferation and the production of mediators of the inflammatory response, exist in Alzheimer's disease patients. Because interleukins can enhance amyloid precursor protein (APP) production, their presence in the Alzheimer's disease brain may have substantial import (1). Acute-phase proteins, inflammatory response molecules that are induced by cytokines, are elevated in Alzheimer's disease. Alpha-2 macroglobulin and alpha-1 antichymotrypsin (ACT) have been demonstrated in amyloid deposits in Alzheimer's disease (2). Increased ACT concentrations is particularly intriguing because it is a proteinase inhibitor.

Clinical data derived from other illnesses support the

use of antiinflammatory agents to treat Alzheimer's disease. The prevalence of Alzheimer's disease in rheumatoid arthritis clinic patients, a population who was very likely to have received chronic anti-inflammatory therapy, was significantly less than that observed in the general population over age 64 (37). Thus, therapies for autoimmune diseases can serve as models for the choice of anti-inflammatory treatment strategies in Alzheimer's disease.

Given the host of immunological reactions noted in AD and their implication in cell death, immunomodulatory therapies might offer treatments to slow the course of the illness. A 6-month double-blind study with the nonsteroidal anti-inflammatory agent indomethacin demonstrated that Alzheimer's disease patients who received active drug declined significantly less than did patients who received placebo (53). Steroids offer a logical anti-inflammatory therapy for Alzheimer's disease, because these agents are widely used and efficacious for several inflammatory diseases in the CNS, including lupus cerebritis and multiple sclerosis. Unfortunately, the systemic toxicity of steroids limits the use of high doses or long-term treatments with these agents. Animal studies suggest that prolonged exposure to high doses of glucocorticoids is toxic to hippocampal neurons (57). Low-dose steroid therapy (e.g., 10 mg/day of prednisone) may be the safest strategy because this dose is well-tolerated and effective in patients with rheumatoid arthritis.

Colchicine is another possible candidate for the treatment of Alzheimer's disease. This drug effectively treats familial Mediterranean fever, a condition in which recurrent inflammation and renal amyloidosis occur. Although the amyloid constituents in familial Mediterranean fever and Alzheimer's disease differ, both illnesses involve chronic inflammation, elevated acute-phase proteins, and abnormal processing of a precursor protein leading to deposition of insoluble amyloid fragments. These similarities suggest the potential therapeutic efficacy of colchicine for patients with Alzheimer's disease.

Hydroxychloroquine has been used as an antimalarial agent, but it has been adopted as a safe and effective second-line agent for the treatment of rheumatoid arthritis and lupus erythematosus. This agent suppresses cytokine and acute-phase reactant levels in these illnesses. The efficacy of hydroxychloroquine is thought to be related to its effects on the immune response and lysosomal functioning. Hydroxychloroquine is a lysomotropic agent that interferes with lysosomal enzymatic activity by increasing the pH in these organelles and by stabilizing lysosomal membranes. Hydroxychloroquine's safe clinical profile as a chronic treatment for rheumatoid arthritis support it as a possible candidate for the treatment of Alzheimer's disease.

Antiamyloid Agents

Alzheimer's disease is characterized by neurofibrillary tangles and extracellular deposits of amyloid beta protein

($A\beta$). $A\beta$ is derived from processing of APP (52). The presence of $A\beta$ in Alzheimer's disease may result from several causes. APP can undergo secretory processing that occurs within the domain of $A\beta$, thereby precluding amyloidogenesis (64). In contrast, lysosomal processing of amyloid precursor protein can produce amyloidogenic fragments (18). Increased synthesis of APP could, in turn, overwhelm the capacity of the cell to degrade its substrate through the regular pathway. A disrupted balance between protease and protease inhibitors in the brain could lead to abnormal degradation of APP and increased production of $A\beta$ (52). Two forms of APP contain a Kunitz-type protease inhibitor (KPI) insert that may provide protease inhibitor activity to APP. Protease inhibitors have been shown to modulate cell growth and might be involved in the neuronal sprouting activity associated with plaques (35). The presence of ACT in plaques further supports a role of plasma proteinase inhibitors in amyloidogenesis.

Agents that interfere with $A\beta$'s production or deposition offer potential therapeutic strategies to alter the course of Alzheimer's disease. The lysomotropic properties of colchicine and hydroxychloroquine suggest these agents as candidates to interfere with $A\beta$ production. Although colchicine is used as a neurotoxin in laboratory studies, no significant CNS toxicity has been reported with clinical use of this agent. A study using cell cultures suggests that a lysosomal inhibitor may shunt APP to the secretase pathway, thereby leading to the release of nonamyloidogenic fragments (5). Numerous pharmaceutical companies have active drug discovery programs directed at inhibiting amyloidogenesis through specific protease inhibitors. The findings that apolipoprotein type 4 allele is a risk factor for the development of Alzheimer's disease and is localized in senile plaques suggest that modulation of this chaperone may prevent amyloid deposition (62) (see also Chapter 116, *this volume*).

Neurotrophic Factors

The cell loss in Alzheimer's disease and in other neurodegenerative illnesses suggests a role of neurotrophic factors in their pathophysiology and treatment. Several neurotrophic factors (i.e., proteins capable of altering neuronal survival, innervation, and function) have been identified (67). Nerve growth factor (NGF) represents one of these neurotrophins and has been most studied in relation to AD. NGF is primarily located in the basal forebrain, hippocampus, and cortex and acts selectively on cholinergic neurons (67). The basal forebrain cholinergic neurons possess the NGF receptor and express increased choline acetyltransferase activity in response to NGF. NGF administration has been shown to attenuate degenerative changes in cholinergic cells caused by transections of the septohippocampal pathway. NGF treatment also elevates choline acetyltransferase activity, acetylcholine synthesis, and release following partial lesions of the fimbria.

The basic and preclinical findings support the utility of NGF for the treatment of Alzheimer's disease. A case report of a patient treated subchronically with NGF demonstrates that one month of treatment was associated with improvement in verbal episodic memory, increased nicotine binding in frontal and temporal cortices, and increased cerebral blood flow (44). Limitations of NGF treatment, however, include the morbidity associated with the required intraventricular dosing, and the unknown neuronal and behavioral sequelae of its long term administration (see Chapter 55 for related topic).

Chelating Agents

There is evidence to suggest an association between aluminum and neurodegenerative diseases, including Alzheimer's disease. Aluminum administration has been shown to be neurotoxic to the cholinergic system (9). These data suggest the use of chelating agents for the treatment of Alzheimer's disease.

Desferrioxamine mesylate has been investigated as a chelating agent to treat Alzheimer's disease. This compound has a high stability constant for aluminum and has been extensively used to treat iron and aluminum overload (6). In a study of 48 Alzheimer's patients, intramuscular administration of desferrioxamine was compared to placebo or no treatment over a 2-year period (38). Patients who received desferrioxamine treatment evidenced a significant reduction in the rate of decline of daily living skills when compared to the placebo group, suggesting that this agent may slow the clinical progression of Alzheimer's disease. The therapeutic effects observed with this agent, however, may not necessarily be due to its chelating action because it has been shown to inhibit free radical formation and inflammation (38). In addition, it was hard to keep the blind in that investigation because patients receiving active treatment received injections, whereas the controls did not. The required intramuscular administration and toxic side effects of this compound do limit its clinical utility. In addition, the role of aluminum in Alzheimer's disease has been questioned (29).

Calcium Channel Blockers

Neurotransmitter synthesis and release, neuron action potentials, receptor affinity, and memory storage are calcium-dependent functions. Therefore, the age-related deficits in calcium homeostasis have been implicated in the pathophysiology of neurodegenerative conditions, including Alzheimer's disease. It has been suggested that excessive calcium influx represents the final common pathway of neuronal death after a variety of insults, including hypoglycemia, excitotoxin release, and hypoxia

(8). Calcium influx has also been associated with neurofibrillary tangle-like changes in tau (8).

Calcium channel antagonists are logical choices to prevent excessive calcium influx into neurons. Alzheimer's patients treated with nimodipine at 30 mg t.i.d. have been shown to experience a prophylactic benefit from the agent (66). Higher doses of nimodipine were not as efficacious. NGF administration also is protective of cell death associated with excessive calcium influx (8). These findings suggest further investigation of calcium antagonists for the treatment of Alzheimer's disease.

METHODOLOGICAL PROBLEMS IN DRUG DEVELOPMENT

Animal Models

Animal models have been very useful in determining the cognitive results of disruption of neurotransmitter systems in the CNS. These studies have supported the role of the cholinergic, noradrenergic, and glutamatergic systems in memory and learning and have been used for drug development for the treatment of Alzheimer's disease. However, there are limitations inherent in these models. Lesion experiments provide only an approximation of the neurodegenerative process in Alzheimer's disease. In addition, the tasks used to assess learning and memory in animals do not necessarily represent the complex cognitive processes disrupted in Alzheimer's disease. The discrepancy between animal study findings and clinical trials can be understood in light of these limitations. The development of an animal model that has the pathophysiology observed in Alzheimer's disease will undoubtedly enhance development of new strategies to treat the illness. It is hoped that transgenic animals will offer such a model, although thus far these efforts have been disappointing (see also Chapter 116, *this volume*).

Outcome Measures

The nature of the assessments used to determine medication response needs to be considered when reviewing the efficacy of pharmacotherapies for Alzheimer's disease. Neuropsychological tests that require the patient to perform specific tasks are often used to assess drug effects on cognitive symptoms. Clinician ratings that rely on interviews with patients and caregivers are usually used to determine psychiatric symptoms, activities of daily living, and global impressions of clinical improvement. These approaches are useful and complement each other. However, the use of different measures to evaluate drug efficacy can contribute to variable treatment outcomes. A "dual outcome" strategy that measures both improvement on core cognitive symptoms and the overall magnitude of clinical improvement has been suggested as the most comprehensive assessment of the efficacy of antidementia drugs (31).

Neuropsychological Tests

The severity of cognitive compromise in Alzheimer's disease is best evaluated with neuropsychological assessments. An instrument that measures outcome of drug trials should provide a valid measurement of cognitive impairment across several stages of the illness, have alternate forms to avoid practice effects, and have high inter-rater and retest reliability. The instruments discussed below are those that have been most often used in clinical trials.

The Mini Mental State and Blessed test (4,22) are easy to administer, measure relevant areas of cognition, are available in multiple languages, and have available longitudinal data. However, both instruments do not comprehensively cover all domains of cognitive functioning and don't offer enough sensitivity to detect subtle changes in cognition. They also do not have alternate forms, leading to nonspecific carry-over effects that are problematic in clinical trials with multiple assessments.

The Alzheimer's Disease Assessment Scale (ADAS; see ref. 55) provides broad coverage of cognitive functioning and has alternate forms for the memory tests. The greater length of the ADAS relative to the Blessed and the Mini Mental State enables this instrument to assess in more depth a range of cognitive domains. Because of its greater sensitivity to cognitive change over a broad range of severity, the ADAS has been accepted as a standard outcome measure for treatment and longitudinal studies. Longitudinal studies that have been conducted with the ADAS provide data on the expected rate of cognitive decline in Alzheimer's patients. This information permits investigators to estimate the sample size required to determine the presence of a desired drug effect over varying time intervals. For example, power calculations can be done to determine the sample size needed to detect the effect of a drug which slows the rate of deterioration by one-half relative to placebo. The sample size needed for such a study is over twice as large when drug and placebo patients are compared for 6 months than when they are compared for 12 months.

The rate of change in cognition observed with these tests is not independent of the baseline severity of dementia. For the ADAS, the rate of change is slower for both mild and severe dementia than for moderate dementia (33). The implication for clinical trial development is that the expected amount of deterioration for patients in a study will depend substantially upon the dementia severity at entry, suggesting stratifying patients by their severity at entry (33). Modifications of these instruments might be required for special populations, such as very mildly or severely impaired patients.

Global Change and Staging Instruments

These instruments assess both the cognitive status and the overall clinical condition of a patient. Used alone, these instruments cannot determine the cognitive efficacy of a drug because improvement on these measures may reflect noncognitive outcomes (15,19). In addition, use of such global measures hampers quantification of the magnitude of drug effect. Global scales can be highly reliable when administered with specified procedures. However, there are few studies that evaluate the reliability and sensitivity of global change measures.

Functional Measures

These assessments measure the patient's ability to perform everyday activities of daily living (ADLs). In clinical trials, these instruments are used to document the functional or clinical impact of therapeutic agents. The ADL instruments are not very sensitive for documenting subtle deficits in the very mildly impaired patients and usually show little change in clinical trials with this subgroup. Instruments which evaluate higher level activities [e.g., the Instrumental Activities of Daily Living Scale (IADLS)] tend to be more specific for less impaired individuals. Scores on the IADLS change substantially at follow-up with mildly impaired patients, but then change very little in moderate-to-severe patients because of a ceiling effect. Although ADL impairment is well-documented in Alzheimer's disease, no specific instrument is accepted as a valid measurement of clinical efficacy of agents that treat the cognitive deficits in Alzheimer's disease (31). An ADL scale that would be optimal for clinical trials would be sensitive over a broad range of disease severity and include items to assess both basic and instrumental ADLs.

Patient Populations

While rigorous efforts are made to document the presence of Alzheimer's disease in all subjects entered into treatment trials, patients diagnosed with this illness are a heterogeneous population because of the following factors. The criteria used to determine the presence of the illness do not have 100% concordance with neuropathological findings at autopsy. The cognitive deficits in the illness have variable presentations and course. The severity of cognitive compromise in patients at entry is not uniform. All these issues introduce heterogeneity into the patient population that can increase variability into the results of clinical trials.

Study Designs

The study designs used to assess drug efficacy also introduce methodological problems. The crossover designs which are usually employed for drug studies may create carry-over effects that lessen the drug's effect in comparison to placebo. The repeated assessments used in trials lead to learning effects that can erroneously inflate a patient's response to medication. Practice effects can be avoided by administration of the key outcome measures at longer time intervals and by the use of parallel design studies. Finally, another problem is the shifting baseline due to the progression of the severity of Alzheimer's disease. The longer the study, the more this becomes a factor that needs to be addressed.

CONCLUSIONS

Several strategies for cognitive enhancement have been attempted with Alzheimer's disease patients. An adequate acetylcholinesterase inhibitor has not yet been tested with all the necessary parameters. Combined neurotransmitter therapies have also not been adequately tested to determine the level of efficacy that could be achieved with this approach. Strategies to delay progression of the illness are beginning to be explored and may provide the most effective means to treat the cognitive deterioration observed in Alzheimer's disease. It is essential to choose the appropriate measures and optimal study designs in order to determine drug efficacy.

REFERENCES

1. Altstiel L, Sperber K. Cytokines in Alzheimer's disease. *Prog Neuropsychopharmacol Biol Psychiatry* 1991;15:481–495.
2. Bauer J, Strauss S, Schreiter-Gasser U, et al. Interleukin-6 and alpha-2-macroglobulin indicate an acute phase response in Alzheimer's disease cortices. *FEBS Lett* 1991;285:111–114.
3. Behl C, Davis J, Cole GM, et al. Vitamin E protects nerve cells from amyloid B protein toxicity. *Biochem Biophys Res Commun* 1992;186:944–950.
4. Blessed G, Tomlinson BE, Roth M. The association between quantitative measures of dementia and of senile change in the cerebral grey matter of elderly subjects. *Br J Psychiatry* 1968;114:797–811.
5. Caporaso GL, Gancy SE, Buxbaum JD, et al. Chloroquine inhibits intracellular degradation but not secretion of Alzheimer B/A4 amyloid precursor protein. *Proc Natl Acad Sci USA* 1992;89:2252–2256.
6. Chang TMS, Barre P. Effect of desferrioxamine on removal of aluminum and iron by coated charcoal haemoperfusion and haemodialysis. *Lancet* 1983;1051–1053.
7. Chatellier G, Lacomblez L on behalf of Groupe Francais d'Etude de la Tetraaminoacridine. Tacrine (tetrahydroaminoacridine; THA) and lecithin in senile dementia of the Alzheimer's type: a multi-center trial. *Br Med J* 1990;495–499.
8. Cheng B, Mattson MP. Glucose deprivation elicits neurofibrillary tangle-like antigenic changes in hippocampal neurons: prevention by NGF and bFGF. *Exp Neurol* 1992;117:114–123.
9. Clayton RM, Sedowofia SKA, Rankin JM, Manning A. A long term effect of aluminum in the fetal mouse brain. *Life Sci* 1992;51:1921–1928.
10. Cornfeldt M, Wirtz-Burgger, Szewczak M, Blitzer R, Haroutunian V, Effland RC, Klein JT, Smith C. *Abstr Soc Neurosci* 1990;16:612.
11. Crutcher KA, Scott SA, Liang S, et al. Detection of NGF-like activity in human brain tissue: increased levels in Alzheimer's disease. *J Neurosci* 1993;13:2540–2550.
12. Dal-Bianco P, Maly J, Wober C, et al. Galanthamine treatment in Alzheimer's disease. *J Neural Transm [Suppl]* 1991;59–63.
13. Davidson M, Bierer LM, Kaminsky R, et al. Combined administration of physostigmine and clonidine to patients with dementia of the Alzheimer type: a pilot safety study. *Alzheimer's Dis Assoc Disord* 1989;4:1–4.
14. Davis KL, Hollander E, Davidson M, et al. Induction of depression with oxotremorine in Alzheimer's disease patients. *Am J Psychiatry* 1987;144:4.
15. Davis KL, Thal LJ, Gamzu E, et al. Tacrine in patients with Alzheimer's disease: a double blind placebo controlled multicenter study. *N Engl J Med* 1992;327:1374–1379.
16. Eagger S, Morant N, Levy R, Sahakian B. Tacrine in Alzheimer's disease time course of changes in cognitive function and practice effects. *Br J Psychiatry* 1992;160:36–40.
17. Elrod K, Buccafusco JJ. Correlation of the amnestic effects of nicotinic antagonists with inhibition of regional brain acetylcholine synthesis in rats. *J Pharmacol Exp Ther* 1991;403–409.
18. Estus S, Golde T, Kunishita T, et al. Potentially amyloidogenic, carboxyl-terminal derivatives of the amyloid protein precursor. *Science* 1992;255:726–730.
19. Farlow M, Gracon SI, Hershey LA, Lewis KW, Sadowsky CH, Dolan-Ureno J. A controlled trial of tacrine in Alzheimer's disease. *JAMA* 1992;2523–2529.
20. Fielding S, Cornfeldt ML, Szewczak MR, et al. HP-029, a new drug for the treatment of Alzheimer's disease: its pharmacological profile. Presented at fourth world conference on clinical pharmacology and therapeutics, Berlin (West), July 28–30, 1989.
21. Fisher A, Brandeis R, Karton I, et al. (±)-*cis*-2-Methyl-spiro(1,3-oxathiolane-5,3')quinuclidine, an M1 selective cholinergic agonist, attenuates cognitive dysfunctions in an animal model of Alzheimer's disease. *J Pharmacol Exp Ther* 1991;392–403.
22. Folstein MF, Folstein SE, McHugh PR. "Mini-Mental-State". A practical method for rating the cognitive state of patients for the clinician. *J Psychiatry Res* 1975;12:189–198.
23. Gauthier S, Bouchard R, Lamontagne A, et al. Tetrahydroaminoacridine–lecithin combination treatment in patients with intermediate-stage Alzheimer's disease. *N Engl J Med* 1990;322:1272–1276.
24. Haga S, Akai K, Ishii T. Demonstration of microglial cells in and around senile (neuritic) plaques in the Alzheimer brain: an immunohistochemical study using a novel monoclonal antibody. *Acta Neuropathol* 1989;77:569–575.
25. Haratounian V, Kanof PD, Tsuboyama G, et al. Restoration of cholinomimetic activity by clonidine in cholinergic plus adrenergic lesioned rats. *Brain Res* 1990;507:261–266.
26. Hollander E, Davidson M, Mohs RC, et al. RS 86 in the treatment of Alzheimer's disease: cognitive and biological effects. *Biol Psychiatry* 1987;22:1067–1078.
27. Hood WF, Sun ET, Compton RP, et al. 1-Aminocyclo-butane 1-carboxylate (ACBC): a specific antagonist of the *N*-methyl-D-asoartate receptor coupled glycine receptor. *Eur J Pharmacol* 1989;161:281–282.
28. Jenike MA, Albert MS, Baer L. Oral physostigmine as treatment for Alzheimer's disease: a long term outpatient trial. *Alzheimer's Dis Assoc Dis* 1990;4(4):226–231.
29. Kruck TPA. Aluminum in Alzheimer's disease. Is there a link? *Nature* 1993;363(6425):119.
30. Lawlor BA, Davis KL. Does modulation of glutamatergic function represent a viable therapeutic strategy in Alzheimer's disease? *Biol Psychiatry* 1992;31:337–350.
31. Leber P. Guidelines for the clinical evaluation of antidementia drugs, first draft. Rockville, MD: US Food and Drug Administration, 1990.
32. Mangoni A, Grassi MP, Frattola L, et al. Effects of a MAO-B inhibitor in the treatment of Alzheimer's disease. *Eur Neurol* 1991;31(2):100–107.
33. Mohs RC. Neuropsychologic assessment of patients with Alzheimer's disease. In: Bloom FE, Kupfer DJ, eds. *Psychopharmacology The Fourth Generation of Progress*. New York: Raven Press, 1994:1377–1388.
34. Mohs RC, Davis BM, Johns CA, et al. Oral physostigmine treatment of patients with Alzheimer's disease. *Am J Psychiatry* 1985;142:28–33.

35. Monard D. Role of protease inhibition in cellular migration and neuritic growth. *Biochem Pharmacol* 1987;36:1389–92.
36. McGeer PL, McGeer EG. Complement proteins and complement inhibitors in Alzheimer's disease. *Res Immunol* 1992;143:621–624.
37. McGeer PL, McGeer EG, Rogers J, et al. Does anti-inflammatory treatment protect against Alzheimer's disease? In: Khachaturian ZS, Blass JP, eds. *Alzheimer's disease: new treatment strategies.* New York: Marcel Dekker, 1992;165–171.
38. McLachlan Crapper DR, Dalton AJ, Kruck TPA, Bell MY, Smith WL, Kalow W, Andrews DF. Intramuscular desferrioxamine in patients with Alzheimer's disease. *Lancet* 1991;337:1304–1308.
39. Murphy MF, Hardiman ST, Nash RJ, et al. Evaluation of HP 029 (velnacrine maleate) in Alzheimer's disease. *Ann NY Acad Sci* 1991;253–262.
40. Newhouse PA, Sunderland T, Tariot PN, et al. Intravenous nicotine in Alzheimer's disease: a pilot study. *Psychopharmacology* 1988;95:171–175.
41. Nicholson VJ, Tam SW, Myers MJ, et al. DuP996 (3,3-bis(4-pyrindinylmethyl)-1-phenylindolin-2-one) enhances the stimulus-induced release of acetylcholine from rat brain in vitro and in vivo. *Drug Rev Res* 1990;19:285–300.
42. Nordberg A, Alafuzoff I, Winblad B. Nicotinic and muscarinic subtypes in the human brain: changes with aging and dementia. *J Neurosci Res* 1992;103–111.
43. Oka A, Belliveau MF, Rosenberg PA, et al. Vulnerability of oligodendroglia to glutamate. Pharmacology, mechanisms, and prevention. *J Neurosci* 1993;13:1441–153.
44. Olson L, Nordberg A, von Holst H, et al. Nerve growth factor affects C-nicotine binding, blood flow, EEG, and verbal episodic memory in an Alzheimer patient. *J Neural Transm* 1992;4:79–95.
45. Olton DS, Wenk GL. Dementia: animal models of the cognitive impairments produced by degeneration of the basal forebrain cholinergic system. In: Meltzer HY, ed. *Psychopharmacology: the third generation of progress.* New York: Raven Press, 1987;941–953.
46. The Parkinson Study Group. Effect of deprenyl on the progression of disability in early Parkinson's disease. *N Engl J Med* 1989;321:1364–1371.
47. Perry EK, Tomlinson BE, Blessed G, et al. Correlation of cholinergic abnormalities with senile plaques and mental test scores in senile dementia. *Br Med J* 1978;2:1457–1459.
48. Pomara N, Mendels J, Lewitt PA, et al. Multicenter trial of milacemide in the treatment of Alzheimer's disease. *Biol Psychiatry [Suppl]* 1991;29:718.
49. Raffaele KC, Berardi A, Morris P, et al. Effects of acute infusion of the muscarinic cholinergic agonist arecoline on verbal and visuospatial function in dementia of the Alzheimer's type. *Prog Neuropsychopharmacol Biol Psychiatry* 1991;15:643–648.
50. Read SL, Frazee J, Shapira J, et al. Intracerebroventricular bethanechol for Alzheimer's disease. Variable dose-related responses. *Arch Neurol* 1990;47:1025–1030.
51. Riekkinen P Jr, Sirvio J, Aaltonen M, et al. Effects of concurrent manipulations of nicotinic and muscarinic receptors on spatial and passive avoidance learning. *Pharmacol Biochem Behav* 1990;405–410.
52. Robakis NK, Anderson JP, Lawrence MR, et al. Expression of the Alzheimer amyloid precursor in brain tissue and effects of NGF and EGF on its metabolism. *Clin Neuropharmacol* 1991;14(Suppl):15–23.
53. Rogers J, Kirby LC, Hempelman SR, et al. Clinical trial of indomethacin in Alzheimer's disease. *Neurology* 1993;43:1609–1611.
54. Rogers J, Schultz J, Brachova L, et al. Complement activation and B-amyloid-mediated neurotoxicity in Alzheimer's disease. *Res Immunol* 1992;143:624–630.
55. Rosen WG, Mohs RC, Davis KL. A new rating scale for Alzheimer's disease. *Am J Psychiatry* 1984;141(11):1356–1364.
56. Saletu B, Darragh A, Salmon P, et al. EEG brain mapping in evaluating the time course of the central action of DuP 996: a new acetylcholine release drug. *Br J Pharmacol* 1989;28:1–16.
57. Sapolsky RM, Krey LM, McEwen BS. Prolonged glucocorticoid exposure reduces hippocampal neuron number: implications for aging. *J Neurosci* 1985;5:1222–1227.
58. Sara SJ, Debaugesw B. Idazoxam, an alpha 2 agonist, facilitates memory retrieval in the rat. *Behav Neurol Biol* 1989;51:401–411.
59. Schneider LS, Olin JT, Pawluczyk S. A double-blind crossover pilot study of L-deprenyl (selegeline) combined with cholinesterase inhibitors in Alzheimer's disease. *Am J Psychiatry* 1993;150:21–23.
60. Sheardon MJ, Nielsoen EO, Hansen AJ, et al. 2,3-Dihydroxy-6-nitro-7-sulfamoyl-benzo(F)quinoxaline: a neuroprotectant for cerebral ischemia. *Science* 1990;247:571–574.
61. Simpson MDC, Royston MC, Deakin JFW, et al. Regional changes in [H]D-aspartate and [H] TCP binding sites in Alzheimer's disease brains. *Brain Res* 1988;462:850–852.
62. Strittmatter WJ, Saunders AM, Schmechel D, et al. Apolipoprotein E: high-avidity binding to B-amyloid and increased frequency of type 4 allele in late-onset familial Alzheimer's disease. *Proc Natl Acad Sci USA* 1993;90:1977–1981.
63. Sunderland T, Molchan S, Lawlor B, et al. A strategy of "combination chemotherapy" in Alzheimer's disease: rationale and preliminary results with physostigmine plus deprenyl. *Int Psychogeriatr* 1992;4(Suppl 2):291–309.
64. Suzuki T, Nairn AC, Gandy SE, Greengard P. *Neuroscience* 1992;48:755–761.
65. Thomsen T, Bickel U, Fischer JP, et al. Galanthamine hydrobromide in a long-term treatment of Alzheimer's disease. *Dementia* 1990;1:46–51.
66. Tollefson GD. Short-term effects of the calcium channel blocker nimodipine (Bay-e-9736) in the management of primary degenerative dementia. *Biol Psychiatry* 1990;27:1133–1142.
67. Vantini G. The pharmacological potential of neurotrophins: a perspective. *Psychoneuroendocrinology* 1992;17:401–410.
68. Watson GB, Bolanowski MA, Baganoff MP, et al. Glycine antagonist action of 1-aminocyclobutane-1-carboxylate (ACBC) in *Xenopus* oocytes injected with rat brain mRNA. *Eur J Pharmacol* 1989;167:291–294.
69. Whitehouse PJ. Neuronal loss and neurotransmitter receptor alterations in Alzheimer's disease. In: Fisher JA, Hanin I, Lachman C, eds. *Alzheimer's and Parkinson's diseases: strategies for research and development.* New York: Plenum Press, 1986;85–94.
70. Willson RL. Free radical protection: why vitamin E, not vitamin C, B-carotene or glutathione? In: Porter R, Whelan J, eds. *Biology of vitamin E.* Ciba Foundation Symposium 101. London: Pitman, 1983;19–44.
71. Yasuda RP, Ciesla W, Flores LR, et al. Development of antisera selective for m4 and m5 muscarinic cholinergic receptors: distribution of m4 and m5 receptors in rat brain. *Mol Pharmacol* 43:149–157.

Psychopharmacology: The Fourth
Generation of Progress, edited by
Floyd E. Bloom and David J. Kupfer.
Raven Press, Ltd., New York © 1995.

CHAPTER 121

Alzheimer's Disease

Treatment of Noncognitive Behavioral Abnormalities

Murray A. Raskind

The original patient described by Dr. Alois Alzheimer in 1907 (3) was remarkable both for her progressive cognitive impairment and for her prominent noncognitive behavioral abnormalities. Clinical interest in these noncognitive abnormalities in Alzheimer's disease (AD) has been substantial because of their high prevalence (70) and because noncognitive behavioral problems complicate patient management and often precipitate institutionalization (64). The real or apparent resemblance of delusions, hallucinations, depressed mood, agitation, hostility, and other noncognitive behavioral abnormalities of AD to the signs and symptoms expressed in such classic psychiatric disorders as depression, schizophrenia, and anxiety disorders has prompted the widespread use of psychotropic drugs in the management of AD (29). However, widespread use does not imply established efficacy. In fact, data establishing efficacy of psychotropic drugs for noncognitive behavioral problems in AD and other dementing disorders are limited. Carefully designed treatment outcome studies incorporating reliable and valid outcome measures, well-defined patient samples, and randomization to an adequate trial of active medication or placebo are few. This chapter will review informative studies of psychopharmacologic management of noncognitive behavioral problems in AD. These include depression (or depressive signs and symptoms), psychotic symptoms (delusions and hallucinations), and nonpsychotic disruptive behaviors (such as physical and verbal aggression, motoric hyperactivity, and uncooperativeness with activities necessary for personal hygiene and safety). Placebo-

controlled studies will be emphasized, but results of other studies and reports will be discussed when they suggest directions for future investigation.

DEPRESSION

The diagnosis and treatment of depression complicating the course of AD has received considerable attention. Because depression per se can impair cognitive function (14), it is reasonable to hypothesize that effective treatment of depression in the AD patient may maximize potential cognitive capacity. Furthermore, there is consensus that reduction of depressive signs and symptoms improves quality of life (16). Unfortunately, the apparently straightforward goal of treating depression complicating AD becomes complex when the problems involved in the diagnosis of depression in the context of AD or other dementing illnesses are considered. A fundamental problem is the substantial overlap of signs and symptoms between depression and AD. Common to both disorders are apathy and loss of interest, impaired ability to think and concentrate, psychomotor changes (both retardation and agitation), and sleep disturbance. The ability to diagnose depression in AD is further compromised by the patient's lack of insight and poor recollection of symptoms.

Even if investigators agreed on uniform diagnostic criteria for syndromal depression in AD and used uniform assessment instruments and interviews, discrepant prevalence rates would likely arise from the differential characteristics of the samples of AD patients studied. Prevalence rates of AD with concurrent depression derived from clinical populations are higher than those derived from re-

M. A. Raskind: Department of Psychiatry and Behavioral Sciences, Seattle VA Medical Center, University of Washington School of Medicine, Seattle, Washington 98195.

search registries that select "pure" AD subjects without a history of major depressive disorder. For example, in an outpatient geriatric clinic, Reifler et al. (48) found that 20% of AD patients met DSM-III criteria for major depressive episode. In contrast, Burke et al. (11) found no incident case of major depression patients in an AD research registry population followed longitudinally through the course of illness. This latter study included a longitudinally followed normal control group matched for age, sex, race, and social position. Signs and symptoms of depression occurred in both AD patients and controls, but major depression could not be diagnosed. A similarly low prevalence of major depression in a sample of AD subjects screened to exclude those with past histories of major psychiatric disorders was reported by Kumar et al. (37). Although depressed mood was more frequent in AD subjects than in age-matched normal controls, depressed mood in AD subjects was unaccompanied by classic vegetative signs and symptoms of depression. These investigators, therefore, interpreted depressed mood as reflecting "demoralization" rather than major depressive disorder. Given these problems, it is not surprising that estimates of the prevalence of depression in AD are widely disparate, ranging from 0% to more than 80% (70).

Perhaps the true prevalence of concurrent depression in AD lies somewhere in between these disparate estimates. As early as 1955, Sir Martin Roth (54) addressed the issue of differentiating the common "affective coloring" seen in dementia patients from the relatively uncommon "sustained depressive symptom complex." He found that the latter syndrome, which can probably be equated with DSM-III-R major depressive episode, occurred in only 3% of dementia patients. In a recent carefully performed study of AD patients admitted to an inpatient geropsychiatry service, Greenwald et al. (25) reported that 8% of patients with AD met DSM-III criteria for major depressive episode. Application of DSM-III-R as opposed to DSM-III criteria may reduce even further the rate of diagnosable major depressive episode in patients with AD (39). Regardless of the true prevalence of major depressive episode complicating AD, when such an episode occurs it produces excessive functional disability (44).

It is disappointing that the extensive interest in defining the prevalence of depression complicating AD has not generated many interpretable studies evaluating the outcome of antidepressant treatment in such patients. The database consists primarily of anecdotal case reports and non-placebo-controlled outcome studies. Although some of these reports appear useful, the only placebo-controlled treatment trial in the literature (50) raises concerns about the interpretability of uncontrolled studies.

Anecdotal reports have suggested that depression complicating AD may respond to tricyclic antidepressants (49), monoamine oxidase (MAO) inhibitor antidepressants (34), or electroconvulsive therapy (ECT) (18,63). In a carefully performed open trial of nortriptyline, given in doses sufficient to achieve therapeutic plasma concentrations, or ECT in eight inpatients with AD complicated by depression, Reynolds et al. (52) reported significant reduction of mean Hamilton Depression Rating scores from 17 prior to treatment to 9 following treatment. Although the reduction in depressive signs and symptoms was substantial in AD patients with concurrent depression, it was less robust than in a similarly treated group of elderly nondemented depressed patients. Another open trial of "naturalistic" somatic antidepressant treatment of inpatients with dementia and concurrent depression was reported by Greenwald et al. (25). This study carefully documented the presence of major depressive episode in six patients with AD and four with multi-infarct dementia (MID) (see Chapter 130). Patients were treated for a mean duration of 11 weeks with a variety of conventional somatic antidepressants (doses not reported) and/or ECT. Hamilton scores significantly and substantially decreased from a mean of 19 on admission to a mean of 5 at discharge. This degree of improvement did not differ significantly from an elderly nondemented depressed inpatient group treated in a similar naturalistic manner. However, the mean length of stay to achieve comparable improvement in the elderly nondemented/depressed group was substantially shorter than in the demented/depressed group. Possible differential treatment responses between AD subjects with major depression and MID subjects with major depression were not reported. Both Reynolds et al. (52) and Greenwald et al. (25) interpreted their results as suggesting that major depression complicating dementia is responsive to standard somatic antidepressant treatments, but both investigators acknowledged that standardized, double-blind placebo-controlled studies of dementia patients with major depression are needed.

In the only placebo-controlled study of treatment of major depressive episode complicating AD reported in the literature, Reifler et al. (50) randomly assigned either the tricyclic imipramine ($n = 13$) or placebo ($n = 12$) to subjects who met DSM-III criteria for both primary degenerative dementia of the Alzheimer's type and major depressive episode. AD outpatients (mean age = 72 years) had a mean Mini Mental State Exam (MMSE) score of 17 [very comparable to the mean MMSE scores of the demented/depressed patients studied by Greenwald et al. (25) and Reynolds et al. (52)] and were suffering from a similarly moderate degree of depression (mean Hamilton score = 19). Imipramine (mean dose = 83 mg/day; mean plasma level of imipramine plus desmethylimipramine = 116 ng/ml) or placebo were prescribed for 8 weeks. Substantial, highly significant, and almost identical improvements occurred in mean Hamilton scores in both the imipramine subjects (19.3 prior to treatment compared to 11.5 following treatment) and placebo subjects (18.6 prior to treatment compared to 10.8 following treatment). The improvement of Hamilton scores was similar to those achieved in the open inpatient studies reported by Greenwald et al. (25) and Reynolds et al. (52). This outpatient study demonstrated that depressive signs and symptoms can be reduced in outpatients with AD, but the mechanism of treatment efficacy did not appear to be a specific antidepressant effect of imipramine. It is possible that more aggressive antidepressant medication treatment or a different type of somatic antidepressant treatment may have revealed a difference between an active treatment and placebo in this study. However, the substantial placebo response and the low likelihood that mean Hamilton scores much below 5 are achievable in patients with AD [mean Hamilton scores of 6 or 7 have been reported in samples of AD subjects in whom concurrent depression has been specifically excluded (25,68)] make this possibility unlikely. At the least, this study (50) makes it mandatory that future antidepressant trials in AD patients with concurrent depression be placebo-controlled.

PSYCHOTIC SYMPTOMS AND NONPSYCHOTIC DISRUPTIVE BEHAVIORS

Prevalence of Psychotic Symptoms

Prevalence rates of psychotic symptoms (delusions and hallucinations) complicating AD cluster between 30% and 40% in carefully performed cross-sectional studies (17,70). Because psychotic symptoms can emerge at any time during the course of AD and probably are more prevalent in the later stages of the illness, longitudinal studies reveal even higher prevalence rates. Drevets and Rubin (22) longitudinally followed subjects with AD from the early through the later stages of illness and documented the occurrence of psychotic symptoms both cross-sectionally and cumulatively. This study was strengthened by the inclusion of a longitudinally followed age-matched normal control population (none of whom developed psychotic symptoms during the course of the study). Slightly more than 50% of AD subjects manifested psychotic symptoms at some point during the course of their illness. Subjects were not considered positive if psychotic symptoms occurred only rarely or if they occurred only in the context of a possible delirium. As in other studies of psychotic symptoms in AD (51,70), delusions were usually simple and persecutory, most commonly involving theft. Systematized delusions were uncommon. Hallucinations were most frequently visual, although auditory hallucinations were also common.

Nonpsychotic Disruptive Behaviors

Verbal and physical aggression, motor agitation, uncooperativeness with essential care, persistent irritability, and other disruptive or potentially disruptive behaviors are common in moderately to markedly demented patients with AD (15). In one well-conducted nursing home study, Rovner et al. (55) documented the occurrence of problematic disruptive behaviors in the majority of a random sample of 50 demented residents. Most frequently reported were restlessness, noisiness, and aggressive behaviors. Less demented AD patients still able to reside in the community also manifest disruptive behaviors. Ryden (56) surveyed caregivers of outpatients with AD and found a prevalence of aggressive behavior occurring at least once a week in 31% of subjects and daily in 16% of subjects.

Although psychotic symptoms and "nonpsychotic" disruptive behaviors may not always reflect the same underlying pathophysiologic process or processes, these two classes of noncognitive behavioral problems appear associated. Lopez et al. (38) evaluated the presence of belligerence, uncooperativeness, and physical and verbal aggression in AD patients with ($n = 17$) and without ($n = 17$) delusions and hallucinations. A greater proportion of psychotic AD patients (11 of 17) than of nonpsychotic AD patients (1 of 17) manifested these behavioral disturbances. A study addressing the relationship between psychotic symptoms and physical aggression in AD patients was reported by Deutsch et al. (19). Delusions (most commonly persecutory) and misidentifications (such as the patient believing his or her house was not their home or that strangers were living in the house) frequently preceded and were significantly associated with episodes of physical aggression. However, the presence of delusions could account for episodes of physical aggression in only a minority of cases. Therefore, other factors not clearly apparent were involved in the precipitation of physically aggressive behavior.

PSYCHOTIC SYMPTOMS AND DISEASE COURSE

A number of studies consistently suggest that the presence of psychotic symptoms in AD is associated with more rapid deterioration of cognitive function. Stern et al. (66) were the first to report this phenomenon, and the association between psychotic symptoms and more rapid decline has since been confirmed by other groups. Lopez et al. (38) reported that AD patients with delusions and hallucinations had a more rapid decline in MMSE scores over a 1-year follow-up than did nonpsychotic AD patients and appeared to manifest a specific defect in receptive language. Drevets and Rubin (22) reported that the presence of psychotic symptoms predicted increased rate of cognitive deterioration. Recently, Jeste et al. (35) compared the performance of delusional and nondelusional AD patients on a neuropsychological test battery. Patients with delusions had a more rapid rate of dementia progression than did nondelusional AD patients. The explanation for this apparent association between psychotic symptoms and more rapid cognitive deterioration in AD is unclear.

ANTIPSYCHOTIC DRUG USE FOR PSYCHOTIC AND DISRUPTIVE BEHAVIORS

Psychotropic drugs are widely prescribed to AD patients in long-term care facilities (29). In fact, the repeated documentation of widespread and often chronic prescription of antipsychotic and other psychotropic drugs in the long-term care setting has prompted Federal regulations designed to limit this practice to short-term treatment regimens with clear indications (30). Although the goals of such regulations are laudable, their application in the absence of empirically and soundly derived treatment guidelines continues to be problematic. Typical of studies documenting a high use rate for psychotropic medications in elderly long-term care recipients is a study of intermediate care facility residents in the state of Massachusetts (8). To ensure that the institutions surveyed represented typical geriatric facilities rather than those caring for deinstitutionalized patients with such long-term illnesses as chronic schizophrenia, facilities were not studied if they had greater than 20% of their residents admitted from inpatient psychiatric hospitals. More than half of all elderly residents surveyed were prescribed a psychotropic medication. Twenty-six percent were receiving an antipsychotic medication, and 28% were receiving a sedative-hypnotic medication (primarily benzodiazepines) or a sedating antihistamine. In a survey of nursing homes in Illinois (10), 60% of residents received at least one psychotropic medication during a 1-year period. The antipsychotics haloperidol and thioridizine and the benzodiazepine flurazepam were most frequently prescribed. Similarly, a random sample of 55 long-term care facilities in Massachusetts (5) found that over half of the residents were prescribed at least one psychoactive medication. In this study, antipsychotic medications were being administered to 39% of patients.

ANTIPSYCHOTIC DRUGS

The rationale for the use of antipsychotic drugs in AD is partially attributable to the phenomenologic similarities of delusions and hallucinations and other disruptive behaviors occurring in AD to the symptoms occurring in schizophrenia. Unfortunately, this analogy to psychotic and other behavioral signs and symptoms in schizophrenia is imperfect. For example, delusions in AD are usually unelaborated persecutory beliefs often involving theft. Systematized, complex, and grandiose delusions are uncommon (70). In addition, the memory deficits basic to AD often appear to play a role in the development of delusional beliefs. For example, an AD patient who has forgotten where an item has been placed and who lacks insight as to his or her cognitive deficits might assume that it has been stolen. Or, an AD patient can stubbornly insist in a delusional manner that long-deceased persons who still remain alive in available memory traces are, in fact, alive. Although such beliefs of theft, of decreased persons continuing to exist, or of a spouse being an impostor may meet formal criteria for delusions, they are in some ways phenomenologically dissimilar to the delusions of schizophrenia for which the antipsychotic drugs have been demonstrated to be so effective. In fact, a meta-analysis of studies evaluating antipsychotic drugs in behaviorally disturbed dementia patients (60) concluded that although these drugs are more effective than placebo in patients with AD, the effect size is relatively small. The phenomenologic differences between psychotic features of AD and psychotic features of schizophrenia as well as the inclusion of nonpsychotic disruptive behaviors as target symptoms in outcome studies of antipsychotic drugs in AD may explain why the overall efficacy of antipsychotic drugs in AD is modest.

EARLY CLINICAL TRIALS OF ANTIPSYCHOTIC DRUGS

Interpretation of antipsychotic drug outcome studies in dementia patients performed prior to the introduction of DSM-III are often hampered by the use of unclear diagnostic nomenclature. For example, the term ''senile psychosis'' connoted severe dementia rather than the presence of delusions and hallucinations. In addition, early studies were usually performed in state hospital populations which included patients with degenerative neurologic dementing disorders (the majority of whom presumably were suffering from AD) and patients with chronic schizophrenia who had grown old in the institutional setting. In one of these early studies (61), 29 patients with the diagnosis of dementia complicated by disturbed behaviors were treated with either chlorpromazine or placebo in a double-blind crossover trial. Global ratings favored chlorpromazine, but serious adverse effects such as excessive sedation and falls also were more common in the active drug group. In a small study of dementia patients who manifested ''hyperactive behaviors'' such as assaultiveness, irritability, and hyperexcitability, acetophenazine was more effective than a placebo (26). Again, excessive sedation was a major adverse effect of active medication. In another small placebo-controlled study (67), haloperidol was more effective than placebo for the control of agitation, overactivity, and hostility in a group of elderly demented patients. The haloperidol group had more subjects who developed unsteady gait and/or extrapyramidal symptoms than did the placebo group. In this study, the best responders to haloperidol were those patients with the most severe agitated behaviors prior to study entry. All three of the above small placebo-controlled positive studies are notable for having included only dementia patients with disruptive behaviors.

Other early studies of antipsychotic drugs in dementia patients which did not include psychotic or nonpsychotic disruptive behaviors as target symptoms and signs found antipsychotic drugs no more effective than placebo. A comparison of trifluoperazine and placebo on target symptoms of apathy, withdrawal, and cognitive and behavioral deterioration (loss of ambulation, disorientation, and incontinence) demonstrated no therapeutic effect of the active medication and was most remarkable for a high prevalence of trifluoperazine-induced sedation and extrapyramidal signs and symptoms (27). In a comparison of thiothixene and placebo for the amelioration of cognitive deficits in a group of demented patients, therapeutic response to active drug again did not differ from placebo (47). Thirteen of 22 patients receiving thiothixene were rated as globally improved, and 11 of 20 patients in the placebo group were rated as globally improved. The presence of an apparent placebo response in this study confirmed an earlier report (1) which documented a positive placebo response in elderly demented patients.

RECENT ANTIPSYCHOTIC DRUG OUTCOME STUDIES

Since the introduction of DSM-III, a small number of placebo-controlled studies have evaluated the efficacy of antipsychotic drugs in dementia patients. Diagnostic criteria for AD and MID increase confidence that elderly patients with chronic psychiatric disorders beginning in early life, such as schizophrenia, have been excluded. In addition, these latter studies have targeted psychotic and disruptive nonpsychotic behaviors as outcome measures. Perhaps the study which best supports the efficacy of an antipsychotic drug in the treatment of psychotic signs and symptoms complicating AD is a small but carefully performed outpatient study by Devanand et al. (20). Nine outpatients with predominantly early-onset AD (mean age = 67) were treated with either haloperidol (mean dose = 3 mg/day) or placebo in a crossover design. All nine AD subjects had clear delusions and/or hallucinations, and eight of the nine had other nonpsychotic disruptive behaviors. Although haloperidol was superior to placebo for psychotic symptoms, cognitive function worsened during active drug treatment and extrapyramidal adverse effects limited the improvement in quality of life achieved by subjects in the haloperidol condition.

Petrie et al. (45) compared low-dose haloperidol and loxapine to placebo in 64 inpatients of a state psychiatric hospital (mean age = 73 years). The sample included subjects who met diagnostic criteria for either AD or MID. Both antipsychotic medications were more effective

than placebo for improvement of hallucinations, suspiciousness, hostility, excitement, and uncooperativeness. Global improvement ratings, however, only modestly favored the active medications. Thirty-five percent of haloperidol subjects and 32% of loxapine subjects as compared to 9% of placebo subjects were rated as moderately or markedly improved. Not only were therapeutic responses to active drugs in these elderly demented patients lower than would have been predicted from outcome studies in younger subjects with schizophrenia, adverse drug effects including sedation and extrapyramidal signs and symptoms were frequent. In the only placebo-controlled study of antipsychotic drugs in a typical community nursing home sample of elderly demented patients, Barnes et al. (7) randomized 60 behaviorally disturbed dementia patients (mean age = 83 years) to thioridazine, loxapine, or placebo. All subjects met diagnostic criteria for either AD or MID. Both active antipsychotic drugs were more effective than placebo for ratings of excitement and uncooperativeness. Although suspiciousness and hostility tended to improve more with active drugs than with placebo, substantial improvements in these two factors also were documented in subjects receiving placebo. Therefore, differences between active drugs and placebo for improvement in suspiciousness and hostility were not statistically significant. As in the Petrie study (45), Barnes et al. (7) found that only approximately one-third of patients in the active medication conditions achieved global ratings of either moderate or marked improvement. In both of these studies, classic delusions and hallucinations were present only in a minority of patients, and the heterogeneous target symptoms may have limited the ability to detect antipsychotic drug efficacy in specific subgroups of subjects with more schizophreniform delusions and hallucinations. Taken together, these three studies suggest that antipsychotic drugs are modestly effective for psychotic and nonpsychotic disruptive behaviors in AD. They also suggest that adverse effects limit their utility in these elderly subjects.

The high frequency of adverse effects in elderly dementia patients receiving low doses of antipsychotic drugs also raises the possibility that pharmacokinetic factors may be clinically important in elderly patients. Several recent studies of haloperidol pharmacokinetics in human aging suggest that pharmacodynamic factors may be more important than pharmacokinetic factors in the differential responsivity with aging to low-dose antipsychotics. Aoba et al. (4) failed to demonstrate an age effect on plasma haloperidol neuroleptic levels. Dysken et al. (23) measured haloperidol and reduced haloperidol concentrations in plasma and red blood cells in 29 inpatients with AD assigned to fixed doses of haloperidol (1, 2, or 4 mg/day for 3 weeks) to treat noncognitive behavioral problems. Although plasma concentrations achieved at these low doses were substantially below the haloperidol therapeutic window (5–12 ng/ml) postulated by Van Putten et al.

(69), substantial behavioral improvement was noted in the majority of subjects. Similarly low plasma haloperidol concentrations measured by radioimmunoassay were reported by Devanand et al. (21) in 19 patients with AD treated with low dose haloperidol. These subjects included the smaller group previously reported (20) who showed substantial therapeutic (compared to placebo) as well as substantial adverse effects at these doses of haloperidol and the plasma concentrations achieved. In a recent study more directly addressing pharmacokinetic and pharmacodynamic effects of aging on response to haloperidol, Kelly et al. (36) administered intravenous haloperidol (0.014 mg/kg) in a double-blind, placebo-controlled crossover study to 13 young subjects (mean age = 27 years) and 10 older subjects (mean age = 72 years). There were no statistically significant age differences in plasma haloperidol pharmacokinetics. However, older subjects showed significantly greater decreases in cognitive function following drug administration. These data suggest important pharmacodynamic mechanisms for the increased sensitivity to haloperidol with aging. In contrast, pharmacokinetic factors with aging may be important for some other antipsychotic drugs. Movin et al. (42) found that both total and unbound remoxipride following fixed oral doses increased with age. They demonstrated a twofold increase in area under the curve of both total and unbound remoxipride concentrations in elderly subjects compared to young subjects.

MAINTENANCE ANTIPSYCHOTIC DRUG THERAPY IN DEMENTIA

When a satisfactory response to antipsychotic drugs is achieved during an acute treatment trial, the clinician must next decide how long to maintain patients on these drugs. This question recently was addressed by Risse et al. (53) in a small but informative antipsychotic drug discontinuation study in behaviorally disturbed elderly dementia patients who appeared to have benefited from an acute course of antipsychotic medications and who had then been maintained on these medications chronically. Placebo was substituted for maintenance antipsychotic medication in nine male dementia patients (mean age = 65 years) who had shown clear improvement in noncognitive behavioral problems following treatment with antipsychotic medication and who subsequently had been maintained on antipsychotic medication for at least 90 days. At the end of the 6-week placebo substitution period, only one patient had developed disruptive behaviors severe enough to warrant reinstitution of antipsychotic medication. Of the remaining eight patients, five actually were less agitated, two were unchanged, and only one was determined to be more agitated than when receiving maintenance antipsychotic medication. This small but important study supports the wisdom of periodic discontinu-

ation of chronic antipsychotic medication to evaluate the need for long-term maintenance.

OTHER PHARMACOLOGICAL APPROACHES TO MANAGEMENT OF DISRUPTIVE BEHAVIORS IN AD

Given the limited efficacy and the frequent adverse effects of antipsychotic drugs in the elderly patient with AD, attempts to demonstrate efficacy for other types of psychotropic drugs with more benign adverse effect profiles are both reasonable and important. Unfortunately, the database derived from well-designed clinical trials of non-antipsychotic drugs for the management of disruptive behaviors in AD is even less robust than for the antipsychotic drugs. The following review, therefore, will rely heavily on anecdotal reports and non-placebo-controlled studies.

BENZODIAZEPINES

The use of benzodiazepines in patients with AD and other dementing disorders recently has been reviewed (65). In a group of "emotionally disturbed" elderly patients (mean age = 81), Sanders (59) evaluated the efficacy of oxazepam compared to placebo in an 8-week treatment trial. Oxazepam was superior to placebo, particularly for reduction of agitation and anxiety. Interpretation of this study is hampered by the vagueness of the diagnoses and the likelihood that many subjects were not demented. Coccaro et al. (13) compared oxazepam, haloperidol, and the sedating antihistamine diphenhydramine in elderly institutionalized patients. The mean age of these subjects was 75 years, most met criteria for AD, and target signs and symptoms included tension, excitement, aggressiveness, pacing, and increased motor activity. Ratings of target signs and symptoms improved over an 8-week period in all treatment groups. Although statistically significant differences among groups did not emerge, there was a trend for greater improvement with diphenhydramine and haloperidol than with oxazepam. The lack of a placebo group in this study complicates interpretation of the modest improvements in objective ratings of disruptive behaviors. A recent study (32) which used an "n of 1" design methodology (6) compared oxazepam, diphenhydramine, and the antipsychotic thiothixene in resistive dementia patients. Results were interpreted as supporting efficacy for the antipsychotic, and benzodiazepines had little to offer to behaviorally disruptive dementia patients. Salzman et al. (58) tapered and then discontinued benzodiazepines in 13 elderly nursing home residents and compared memory function and ratings of depression, anxiety, irritability, and sleep to 12 nursing home residents who continued their benzodiazepine therapy. The drug discontinuation group showed greater improvements in memory than did the drug maintenance group, and there were no differences between groups in measures of depression, anxiety, irritability, or sleep. This study suggests that at least a subgroup of patients maintained chronically on short-acting benzodiazepines may benefit from a trial of drug discontinuation. In addition to adverse effects on cognitive function, benzodiazepines have been associated with falls in geropsychiatric inpatients (2). Taken together, these studies of benzodiazepine use in behaviorally disturbed dementia patients suggest that the widespread prescription of these drugs noted in several epidemiologic studies (8,10) needs stronger justification.

BUSPIRONE

Buspirone is a partial 5-HT$_{1A}$ agonist which has antianxiety activity and a benign adverse effect profile. Two recent uncontrolled studies of buspirone in dementia patients with agitated behavior have been reported. Sakauye et al. (57) prescribed buspirone to 10 patients with AD complicated by agitated behaviors in an open-label study. A modest but statistically significant overall reduction of agitated behaviors was noted. There was substantial variability in response, with 4 of the 10 patients demonstrating marked declines in disruptive behaviors. In a similar study, Hermann et al. (31) prescribed buspirone to a group of elderly nursing home residents who exhibited heterogeneous types of dementia (AD, MID, and alcoholic dementia). All subjects had demonstrated severe behavioral disturbances including agitation and aggression, and all had failed to improve with previous trials of other types of psychotropic medications, principally antipsychotic drugs. Six of 16 patients were rated as much or very much improved in terms of agitation and aggressive behavior. In both of these studies, adverse effects were unusual. Although neither of these studies was placebo-controlled, they suggest that a subgroup of dementia patients with disruptive behaviors may benefit from buspirone. Given the low toxicity of this drug, further placebo-controlled investigations appear warranted.

SEROTONIN DRUGS

Because of the clear serotonergic deficit demonstrated in AD postmortem brain tissue (28) and cerebrospinal fluid (9), studies addressing the behavioral efficacy of drugs which purport to enhance central serotonergic activity in AD would be of interest. Simpson and Foster (62) treated four dementia patients who manifested disruptive behaviors with trazodone after antipsychotic drug treatment had proved ineffective. In this anecdotal report, trazodone in doses of 200–500 mg daily was associated with decreased agitation and aggressive behavior. Pinner and Rich (46) treated seven dementia patients with trazo-

done for symptomatic aggressive behavior. Again, all subjects had failed to improve with antipsychotic drug therapy. Three of the seven patients demonstrated an apparent marked decrease in aggressive behavior following 4–6 weeks of trazodone at doses ranging from 200 to 350 mg/day. Olafsson (43) reported a placebo-controlled trial of fluvoxamine in a mixed group of nondepressed demented patients with MID and AD. There was a trend ($p = 0.08$) for greater improvement with fluvoxamine than with placebo for noncognitive symptoms (irritability, anxiety, mood level, and restlessness).

ANTIMANIC AND ANTICONVULSIVE DRUGS

Because the hyperactive and aggressive behaviors encountered in the manic phase of bipolar disorder at least superficially can resemble agitated behaviors in AD and other dementias, drugs effective in the treatment of mania have been used in open trials in behaviorally disturbed dementia patients. Marin and Greenwald (40) treated two AD patients and one MID patient with carbamazepine in an attempt to reduce combative agitated behaviors. Within 2 weeks of carbamazepine treatment at doses ranging from 100 to 300 mg/day, behavioral improvement was noted in all subjects. In a larger open study in AD patients who had failed to respond to antipsychotic drugs (24), reduction in hostility, agitation, and uncooperativeness was noted in five of nine patients. In this study, two patients whose agitated behaviors decreased manifested ataxia and confusion which resolved with carbamazepine dose reduction. The mean dose of carbamazepine in this study was 480 mg/day. In contrast to these enthusiastic open studies, Chambers et al. (12) noted no overall benefit from carbamazepine in 19 elderly dementia patients who were prescribed carbamazepine at 100–300 mg/day. Target symptoms in this study were wandering, overactivity, and restlessness.

Sodium valproate is another anticonvulsant drug with demonstrated antimanic activity. Mellow et al. (41) treated four AD patients who manifested disruptive and agitated behaviors for 1–3 months at doses of valproate ranging from 500 mg/b.i.d. to 500 mg/t.i.d. Substantial behavioral improvement was noted in two of the four patients, and adverse effects did not appear. The classic antimanic drug lithium was evaluated by Holton and George (33) in an open study of 10 dementia patients who manifested disruptive behaviors. Although no improvement in disruptive behaviors was observed, the low dose of lithium (250 mg/day) administered may have been inadequate.

CONCLUSION

It is remarkable how little is really known about specific pharmacologic management of noncognitive behavioral abnormalities in AD despite the prevalence of these problems and their impact on patient management. Extrapolating from psychotherapeutic drug outcome studies in younger patients with such diseases as depression and schizophrenia is not a satisfactory way to develop a meaningful database for the pharmacologic management of noncognitive behavioral disturbances in elderly patients with dementia. The clear placebo responses noted in several carefully performed pharmacologic trials in AD patients with noncognitive behavioral problems emphasize the necessity for inclusion of a placebo condition if a study is to be interpretable. These placebo responses also suggest that nonpharmacologic behavioral and environmental strategies deserve careful evaluation in the management of behaviorally disturbed dementia patients. Critical needs in all further studies are careful phenomenologic descriptions of target behavioral abnormalities and blind randomization to active treatment and placebo conditions.

REFERENCES

1. Abse DW, Dahlstrom WG. The value of chemotherapy in senile mental disturbances. *JAMA* 1960;174:2036–2042.
2. Aisen PS, DeLuca T, Lawton BA. Falls among geropsychiatry inpatients are associated with PRN medications for agitation. *Int J Geriatr Psychiatry* 1992;7:709–712.
3. Alzheimer A. About a peculiar disease of the cerebral cortex (1907 article translated by L Jarvik and H Greenson). *Alzheimer's Dis Assoc Disord* 1987;1:7–8.
4. Aoba A, Kakita Y, Yamaguchi N, et al. Absence of age effect on plasma haloperidol neuroleptic levels in psychiatric patients. *J Gerontol* 1985;40:303–308.
5. Avorn J, Dreyer P, Connelly MA, Soumerai SB. Use of psychoactive medication and the quality of care in rest homes. *N Engl J Med* 1989;320:227–232.
6. Barlow D, Kersen M. *Single case experimental designs.* New York: Pergamon Press, 1984.
7. Barnes R, Veith R, Okimoto J, et al. Efficacy of antipsychotic medications in behaviorally disturbed dementia patients. *Am J Psychiatry* 1982;139:1170–1174.
8. Beers M, Avorn J, Soumerai SB, Everitt DE, Sherman DS, Salem S. Psychoactive medication use in intermediate-care facility residents. *JAMA* 1988;260:3016–3020.
9. Blenow KAH, Wallin A, Gottfries CG, Lekman A, Karlsson I, Skoog I, Svennerholm L. Significance of decreased lumbar CSF levels of HVA and 5-HIAA in Alzheimer's disease. *Neurobiol Aging* 1991;13:107–113.
10. Buck JA. Psychotropic drug practice in nursing homes. *J Am Geriatr Sci* 1988;36:409–418.
11. Burke WJ, Rubin EH, Morris JC, Berg L. Symptoms of "depression" in dementia of the Alzheimer type. *Alzheimer's Dis Assoc Disord* 1988;2:356–362.
12. Chambers CA, Bain J, Rosbottom R, et al. Carbamazepine in senile dementia and overactivity—a placebo controlled double blind trial. *IRCS Med Sci* 1982;10:505–506.
13. Coccaro EF, Zembishlany Z, Thorne A, et al. Pharmacologic treatment of noncognitive behavioral disturbances in elderly demented patients. *Am J Psychiatry* 1990;147:1640–1645.
14. Cohen RM, Weingartner HW, Smallberg A, Pickar D, Murphy DL. Effort and cognition in depression. *Arch Gen Psychiatry* 1982;39:593–597.
15. Cohen-Mansfield J, Billig N. Agitated behavior in the elderly. *J Am Geriatr Soc.* 1986;34:711–727.
16. Consensus Development Panel. Diagnosis and Treatment of Depression in late life: the NIH Consensus Development Conference Statement. *Psychopharmacol Bull* 1993;29:87–100.
17. Cummings JL, Miller B, Hill MA, et al. Neuropsychiatric aspects of multi-infarct dementia and dementia of the Alzheimer type. *Arch Neurol* 1987;44:389–393.
18. Demuth GW, Rand GH. Atypical major depression in a patient with severe primary degenerative dementia. *Am J Psychiatry* 1980;137:1609–1610.
19. Deutsch LH, Bylsma FW, Rovner BW, Steele C, Folstein MF. Psychosis and physical aggression in probable Alzheimer's disease. *Am J Psychiatry* 1991;148:1159–1163.
20. Devanand DP, Sackeim HA, Brown RP, Mayeux R. A pilot study of haloperidol treatment of psychosis and behavioral disturbance in Alzheimer's disease. *Arch Neurol* 1989;46:854–857.
21. Devanand DP, Cooper T, Sackeim HA, Taurke E, Mayeux R. Low dose oral haloperidol and blood levels in Alzheimer's disease: a preliminary study. *Psychopharmacol Bull* 1992;28:169–173.
22. Drevets WC, Rubin EH. Psychotic symptoms and the longitudinal course of senile dementia of the Alzheimer type. *Biol Psychiatry* 1989;25:39–48.
23. Dysken MW, Johnson SB, Holden L, et al. Haloperidol concentrations in patients with Alzheimer's disease. *Am J Geriatr Psychiatry* 1994;2:124–133.
24. Gleason RP, Schneider LS. Carbamazepine treatment of agitation in Alzheimer's outpatients refractory to neuroleptics. *J Clin Psychiatry* 1990;51:115–118.
25. Greenwald BS, Kramer-Ginsberg E, Marin DB, et al. Dementia with coexistent major depression. *Am J Psychiatry* 1989;146:11:1472–1478.
26. Hamilton LD, Bennett JL. Acetophenazine for hyperactive geriatric patients. *Geriatrics* 1962;17:596–601.
27. Hamilton LD, Bennett JL. The use of trifluoperazine in geriatric patients with chronic brain syndrome. *Am Geriatr Soc* 1962;10:140–147.
28. Hardy J, Adolfsson R, Alafuzoff I, et al. Review: transmitter deficits in Alzheimer's disease. *Neurochem Int* 1985;7:545–563.
29. Harrington C, Tompkins C, Curtis M, Grant L. Psychotropic drug use in long-term care facilities: a review of the literature. *Gerontologist* 1992;32:822–833.
30. Health Care Financing Administration. Medicare and Medicaid: requirements for long-term care facilities. Final rule with request for comments. *Fed Regist* 1989;5316–5336.
31. Hermann N, Eryavec G. Buspirone in the management of agitation and aggression associated with dementia. *Am J Geriatr Psychiatry* 1993;1:249–253.
32. Herz LR, Volicer L, Ross V, Rheaume Y. Pharmacotherapy of agitation in dementia. *Am J Psychiatry* 1992;149:1757–1758.
33. Holton A, George K. The use of lithium in severely demented patients with behavioral disturbance. *Br J Psychiatry* 1985;146:99–100.
34. Jenike MA. Monoamine oxidase inhibitors as treatment for depressed patients with primary degenerative dementia (Alzheimer's disease). *Am J Psychiatry* 1985;162:6:763–764.
35. Jeste DV, Wragg RE, Salmon DP, Harris MJ, Thal LJ. Cognitive deficits of patients with Alzheimer's disease with and without dementia. *Am J Psychiatry* 1992;149:184–189.
36. Kelly JF, Berardki A, Raffaele K, Szcepanick J, Haxby JV, Soncrant TT. Intravenous haloperidol causes greater memory impairment in old compared to young healthy subjects. Presented at American Geriatrics Society Annual Meeting, New Orleans, LA, November 1993.
37. Kumar A, Koss E, Metzler D, Moore A, Friedland RP. Behavioral symptomatology in dementia of the Alzheimer type. *Alzheimer's Dis Assoc Disord* 1988;2:363–365.
38. Lopez OL, Becker JT, Brenner RP, Rosen J, Bajulaiye OI, Reynolds CF, III. Alzheimer's disease with delusions and hallucinations: neuropsychological and electroencephalographic correlates. *Neurology* 1991;41:906–912.
39. Mackenzie TB, Robiner WN, Knopman DS. Differences between patient and family assessments of depression in Alzheimer's disease. *Am J Psychiatry* 1989;46:9:1174–1178.
40. Marin DB, Greenwald BS. Carbamazepine for aggressive agitation in demented patients. *Am J Psychiatry* 1989;46:805.
41. Mellow AM, Solano-Lopez C, Davis S. Sodium valproate in the

treatment of behavioral disturbance in dementia. *J Geriatr Psychiatry Neurol* 1993;6:28–32.

42. Movin G, Gustafson L, Franzen G, et al. Pharmacokinetics of remoxipride in elderly psychotic patients. *Acta Psychiatr Scand* 1990;82(Suppl 358):176–180.
43. Olafsson K, Jorgensen S, Jensen HV, Bille A, Arup P, Anderson J. Fluvoxamine in the treatment of demented elderly patients: a double-blind, placebo-controlled study. *Acta Psychiatr Scand* 1992;85:453–456.
44. Pearson JL, Teri L, Reifler BV, Raskind MA. Functional status and cognitive impairment in Alzheimer's patients with and without depression. *J Am Geriatr Soc* 1989;37:1117–1121.
45. Petrie WM, Ban TA, Berney S, et al. Loxapine in psychogeriatrics: a placebo- and standard-controlled clinical investigation. *J Clin Psychopharmacol* 1982;2:122–126.
46. Pinner E, Rich CL. Effects of trazodone on aggressive behavior in seven patients with organic mental disorders. *Am J Psychiatry* 1988;145:1295–1296.
47. Rada RT, Kellner R. Thiothixene in the treatment of geriatric patients with chronic organic brain syndrome. *J Am Geriatr Soc* 1976;24:105–107.
48. Reifler BV, Larson E, Hanley R. Coexistence of cognitive impairment and depression in geriatric outpatients. *Am J Psychiatry* 1982;139:623–626.
49. Reifler BV, Larson E, Teri L, Poulsen M. Alzheimer's disease and depression. *J Am Geriatr Soc* 1986;14:855–859.
50. Reifler BV, Teri L, Raskind M, Veith R, et al. Double-blind trial of imipramine in Alzheimer's disease patients with and without depression. *Am J Psychiatry* 1989;146:45–49.
51. Reisberg B, Borenstein J, Salob SP, et al. Behavioral symptoms in Alzheimer's disease: phenomenology and treatment. *J Clin Psychiatry* 1987;48(5, Suppl):9–15.
52. Reynolds CF, III, Perel JM, Kupfer DJ, Zimmer B, Stack JA, Hoch CC. Open-trial response to antidepressant treatment in elderly patients with mixed depression and cognitive impairment. *Psychiatry Res* 1987;21:111–122.
53. Risse SC, Cubberly L, Lampe TH, et al. Acute effects of neuroleptic withdrawal in elderly dementia patients. *J Geriatr Drug Ther* 1987;2:65–67.
54. Roth M. The natural history of mental disorders in old age. *J Ment Sci* 1955;101:281–301.
55. Rovner BW, Kafonek S, Filipp L, Lucas MJ, Folstein MF. Prevalence of mental illness in a community nursing home. *Am J Psychiatry* 1986;143:1446–1449.
56. Ryden MB. Aggressive behavior in persons with dementia who live in the community. *Alzheimer's Dis Assoc Disord* 1988;2:342–355.
57. Sakauye KM, Camp CJ, Ford PA. Effects of buspirone on agitation associated with dementia. *Am J Geriatr Psychiatry* 1993;1:82–84.
58. Salzman C, Fisher J, Nobel K, et al. Cognitive improvement following benzodiazepine discontinuation in elderly nursing home residents. *Intl J Geriatr Psychiatry* 1992;7:89–93.
59. Sanders JF. Evaluation of oxazepam and placebo in emotionally disturbed aged patients. *Geriatrics* 1965;20:739–746.
60. Schneider LS, Pollock VE, Lyness SA. A metaanalysis of controlled trials of neuroleptic treatment in dementia. *J Am Geriatr Soc* 1990;38:553–563.
61. Seager CP. Chlorpromazine in treatment of elderly psychotic women. *Br Med J* 1955;1:882–885.
62. Simpson DM, Foster D. Improvement in organically disturbed behavior with trazodone treatment. *J Clin Psychiatry* 1986;47:191–193.
63. Snow SS, Wells CE. Case studies in neuropsychiatry: diagnosis and treatment of coexistent dementia and depression. *J Clin Psychiatry* 1981;42:11:439–441.
64. Steele C, Rovner B, Chase GA, Folstein M. Psychiatric symptoms and nursing home placement of patients with Alzheimer's disease. *Am J Psychiatry* 1990;147:1049–1051.
65. Stern RG, Duffelmeyer ME, Zemishlani Z, Davidson M. The use of benzodiazepines in the management of behavioral symptoms in dementia patients. *Psychiatr Clin North Am* 1991;14:375–384.
66. Stern Y, Mayeux R, Sano M, Hauser WA, Bush T. Predictors of disease course in patients with probable Alzheimer's disease. *Neurology* 1987;37:1649–1653.
67. Sugarman AA, Williams BH, Adlerstein AM. Haloperidol in the psychiatric disorders of old age. *Am J Psychiatry* 1964;120:1190–1192.
68. Teri L, Reifler BV, Veith RC, Barnes R, White E, McLean P, Raskind M. Imipramine in the treatment of depressed Alzheimer's patients: impact on cognition. *J Gerontol* 1991;46:P373–377.
69. Van Putten T, Marder SR, Mintz J, Poland RE. Haloperidol plasma levels and clinical response: a therapeutic window relationship. *Am J Psychiatry* 1992;149:4:500–505.
70. Wragg RE, Jeste DV. Overview of depression and psychosis in Alzheimer's disease. *Am J Psychiatry* 1989;146:577–587.

Psychopharmacology: The Fourth Generation of Progress, edited by Floyd E. Bloom and David J. Kupfer. Raven Press, Ltd., New York © 1995.

CHAPTER **122**

Late-Onset Schizophrenia and Other Related Psychoses

Dilip V. Jeste, Jane S. Paulsen, and M. Jackuelyn Harris

The goal of this chapter is to discuss (a) the nomenclature of late-onset schizophrenia (LOS) and related psychoses, (b) diagnostic boundaries among these conditions, (c) neurobiologic findings in late-life schizophrenia, (d) the relationship of LOS to early-onset schizophrenia (EOS), and (e) therapeutic considerations in the treatment of late-life schizophrenia. In general, much less attention has been given to late-onset psychoses than to psychoses with onset during adolescence and early adulthood. One of the first steps toward meaningful research in this area is defining and distinguishing among different psychoses with late onset, especially schizophrenia, delusional disorder, psychotic mood disorder, and so-called "organic" psychoses. Furthermore, LOS needs to be contrasted with EOS in terms of clinical characteristics, course, treatment, and pathogenesis.

Most theories of the pathophysiology of schizophrenia are based upon its onset being restricted to adolescence or early adulthood. Yet it should be apparent that comprehensive theories of schizophrenia need to address LOS. We will discuss the available literature on LOS and related psychoses and consider the implications for improving our understanding of the neurobiology of schizophrenia (and other psychoses) in general (see Chapter 98, *this volume*).

NOMENCLATURE

Historical Background

At the turn of the century, Kraepelin (35) used the term "dementia praecox" to refer to a disorder we now know

as schizophrenia. "Praecox" suggested the onset of the disorder in youth, and "dementia" referred to a deterioration of function in the "emotional and volitional spheres of mental life." Kraepelin (37) himself later questioned the appropriateness of the term "dementia" because the disorder was not always accompanied by a permanent deterioration; remissions did occur in some cases. In addition, he noted that not all of the patients first presented in youth. There was a subset of patients with onset of symptoms well into the fifth, sixth, or seventh decade of life. Kraepelin used the term "paraphrenia" to describe those patients with a relatively late onset of delusions and hallucinations, characterized by a predominance of paranoid symptoms and relatively preserved personality (36). Follow-up studies of Kraepelin's paraphrenic patients, however, indicated that a substantial proportion of them had clinical features (including course) similar to those of dementia praecox (44). Mayer (44) concluded that paraphrenia and dementia praecox were more similar than dissimilar. Subsequently, the label "paraphrenia" fell out of use in favor of the broader category of "schizophrenic syndrome" introduced by Bleuler (4). Later the term "paraphrenia" resurfaced (59), but its definitions were often inconsistent.

Variations in Terminology

Although the literature on LOS and related psychoses dates back to the early 1900s, there are several confounding problems with its interpretation. The most confusing feature of the controversy has been the bewildering array of terms and definitions used to refer to psychotic symptoms beginning in late life. Variously referred to as paraphrenia, late paraphrenia, paranoia, and involutional paranoid disorder, there has been no consensus about the

D. V. Jeste, J. S. Paulsen, and M. J. Harris: Department of Psychiatry, University of California, San Diego, and San Diego VA Medical Center, San Diego, California 92161.

terminology. Although most investigators agree that patients do present with schizophrenia-like psychosis in late life, consensus regarding the grouping and labeling of such patients has been less forthcoming. The term "paraphrenia" has been popular in the European literature, whereas LOS has gained acceptance in the recent American literature. One problem with the term "paraphrenia" has been the wide variation in the diagnostic criteria used for paraphrenia (18). Some investigators have used that term synonymously with paranoid schizophrenia, some refer to it as a combination of all "nonorganic" paranoid psychoses in late life, while still others even include patients with obvious metabolic or other organic etiology of late-onset paranoid psychoses under the category of paraphrenia.

It is notable that the term "paraphrenia" is rarely used for early-onset paranoid psychoses. When a young patient develops a paranoid psychosis, considerable attention is paid to distinguishing among schizophrenia, mood disorder with psychotic features, delusional disorder, and so on. Yet, there is sometimes a tendency to lump different types of late-onset paranoid psychoses under the broad, ill-defined category of paraphrenia. We believe that the diagnostic rigor used for differentiating among various late-onset paranoid psychoses should be no less than that used in younger patients. The term "paraphrenia" is not included in the ICD-10 (66), the DSM-III, the DSM-III-R, or the DSM-IV Draft Criteria. Some authors avoid the problem of nomenclature altogether by the cautious description of such patient groups under "persistent persecutory states of the elderly" (55).

Age of Onset

There has been no general agreement on the definition of late onset. Some studies chose 40 years of age as the cutoff, whereas others defined late onset as onset after 45, 60, or 65 years of age (18). Furthermore, it is often difficult to determine the age of onset of schizophrenia, especially in older subjects. Elderly patients may not remember and significant others may have died, making corroboration of the patient's history difficult. The presence of premorbid paranoid or schizoid personality traits may further confuse the issue, and older patients with psychotic symptoms may be thought to have organic mental syndromes, mood disorders, or simple sensory deficits (17). The earlier versions of the Diagnostic and Statistical Manuals (DSMs) did not have an upper age limit for the diagnosis of schizophrenia. It was not until the DSM-III (1) that it was stipulated that the onset of symptoms for schizophrenia had to be before age 45. Subsequently, the DSM-III-R (2) allowed an onset of schizophrenic symptoms after age 45, and it used the term LOS for these individuals. The DSM-IV Draft Criteria (3) do not specify an upper age limit, nor do they include a separate categorization of LOS.

Diagnostic Criteria for LOS

To diagnose LOS, the patient should meet the DSM-III-R (2) criteria for schizophrenia (including duration of at least 6 months), with the additional requirement that the onset of symptoms (including the prodrome) be at or after age 45. The prototypical patient is a middle-aged or elderly person who functioned moderately well through early adulthood (despite some premorbid schizoid or paranoid personality traits) and who exhibits persecutory delusions and auditory hallucinations and shows some improvement in positive symptoms with low-dose neuroleptic therapy, yet has a chronic course.

Diagnostic Validity

Although debate regarding the utility of diagnosis without etiologic distinction has been present for years, the current atheoretical system (namely, DSM) is usually considered to be reasonably valid for clinical and research purposes. Spitzer and Williams (61) have discussed certain methods for assessing the validity of a classification of mental disorders and its component categories. Face validity requires expert consensus regarding the description of a diagnostic group. Studies of LOS using DSM-III-R criteria support the face validity of LOS (29). Descriptive validity is present when the characteristics of a particular disorder are unique to that condition. Although the diagnostic specificity of psychiatric symptoms, in themselves, is poor, the DSM-III-R criteria for LOS adequately describe (a) its similarity with EOS and (b) its differences from delusional and mood disorders. Predictive validity requires that course, complications, and treatment response be homogeneous in diagnostically similar patients. From the available data the treatment response, course, and complications of LOS are generally similar to those of EOS, although there is heterogeneity among both groups. Construct validity is the extent to which evidence supports a hypothesis that is helpful in understanding the etiology or pathophysiology of the disorder. At the present time, we can address the face validity, descriptive validity, and predictive validity of LOS. We still do not know enough about the etiopathology of schizophrenia in general to assess the construct validity of LOS.

CLINICAL CHARACTERISTICS

Psychopathology of LOS

Late-onset schizophrenia is often characterized by bizarre delusions, which have a predominantly persecutory flavor. Auditory hallucinations are the second most prominent psychotic symptom. Systematized delusions of physical or mental influence are seen in many of the patients. Grandiose, erotic, or somatic delusions may occur in some cases. Schneiderian first-rank symptoms, such as thought broadcasting or two voices arguing with each other, are less common but are not rare. Depressive symptoms are reported by a number of these patients. In contrast, looseness of association and inappropriateness of affect are less common than in younger schizophrenic patients (29).

Clinical Evaluation

Whenever an older patient presents with psychotic symptoms, organic pathology must first be ruled out. A complete history, followed by a careful neurologic evaluation, other physical examinations, and appropriate laboratory tests (including tests of thyroid function, toxicology screening, and serologic tests for syphilis), is usually part of the assessment. Computed tomography (CT) or magnetic resonance imaging (MRI) may be needed to identify cases where structural brain abnormalities are suspected (48).

Differential Diagnosis

In a recent study of 367 geriatric inpatients in four different hospitals, 50% of patients had paranoid symptoms (16). Given the relatively high incidence of paranoia in geriatric patients, diagnostic specificity becomes imperative. Two important conditions in the differential diagnosis of LOS (other than the ''organic mental syndromes'') are mood disorders with psychotic features and delusional disorder. These diagnoses are more likely to have onset during middle age or old age than during early adulthood. Mood disorders with psychotic features may present for the first time after age 45, and they can be confused with LOS. The predominance of affective symptoms and periodicity of the illness should make the clinician consider a mood disorder. A diagnosis of schizophrenia is made when the total duration of all mood symptoms has been brief relative to that of the primary psychotic symptoms. Delusional disorder may mimic LOS, but the latter diagnosis is more likely in the presence of bizarre delusions or prominent auditory hallucinations, Schneiderian first-rank symptoms, deteriorated functioning, and flattening of affect (67). Delusional disorder is distinguished from LOS by the presence of nonbizarre delusions and the absence of prominent auditory or visual hallucinations, disorganized speech, negative symptoms, and functional impairment outside the area of delusions (2).

Differentiation from EOS

Similar to EOS, there is an insidious deterioration of personal and social adjustment. A sizable proportion of LOS patients have abnormal premorbid personality traits of a paranoid or schizoid nature (23,33). Some patients have never been married and have been previously considered by acquaintances to be eccentric, reserved, and suspicious. In our recent study of clinical characteristics in LOS, the LOS and EOS groups were both impaired (compared to normal controls) in childhood adjustment. These findings suggest that the LOS patients might have had a perinatal predisposition similar to that in the EOS group. Nevertheless, when compared to EOS subjects, patients with LOS were more likely to have been married, to have held a job, and to have had better adjustment during adolescence and early adulthood (28).

Caution is required in determining the age of onset of schizophrenia strictly on the basis of a first psychiatric hospitalization for psychosis. It is prudent to obtain a detailed history of the disease from both the patient and his or her family or friends because some patients might have had the prodromal symptoms for some time prior to the first hospitalization. In patients with suspected LOS, it is important to establish an absence of prodromal symptoms before age 45 to exclude the diagnosis of EOS. Prodrome is characterized by a clear deterioration in functioning before the active phase of psychosis, and it includes symptoms such as the following: marked social isolation; marked impairment in role functioning; peculiar behavior; marked impairment in personal hygiene; blunted or inappropriate affect; digressive, vague, overelaborate, or circumstantial speech; odd beliefs or magical thinking influencing behavior and inconsistent with cultural norms; unusual perceptual experience; and marked lack of initiative (2). The prodrome differs from premorbid personality disorder in that it requires a clear deterioration in a previous level of functioning. Also, some patients with an apparently late onset of psychosis may have had a more benign illness which never required hospitalization until age 45.

LOS patients show a female predominance not found among EOS cases (8,18,54). Most studies of LOS show a 2–10 times higher proportion of women than men. In a review by Pearlson and Rabins (52), the authors concluded that there seemed to be an age-related fall in the number of dopamine D2 receptors but men lost them at a faster rate with increasing age, leaving older women with a relative excess. It has also been suggested that estrogen in premenopausal women might have a protective role. The contribution of these and other factors to the later onset of schizophrenia in women is unclear.

Course of LOS

Many schizophrenic patients survive into old age, yet comparatively little is known about the long-term course of LOS. A review of the literature on the course of schizophrenia in general suggests that a majority of patients either undergo remission or are left with mild symptoms over the long term (45). The more positive, dramatic symptoms of schizophrenia seem to lessen in severity with the passage of time. In a recent study of a 3-year follow-up of older schizophrenic patients, negative symptoms were prevalent, moderately severe, and quite stable over time (24). Studies of the course of LOS have generally found it to be chronic (23,33,67). Hafner et al. (32) found a higher frequency of negative symptoms and a more extended course of negative symptoms in women over the age of 35 with a diagnosis of schizophrenia, again supporting a tendency towards chronicity.

Epidemiology

Studies have reported the frequency of LOS among consecutive admissions to inpatient psychiatric facilities to range from 3–4% (13,67) to as high as 8–10% (41,59). These studies have utilized varying diagnostic criteria, however. A review by Harris and Jeste (18) estimated that 13% of the hospitalized schizophrenic patients were reported to have had onset of psychosis in their forties, 7% had onset in their fifties, and only 3% first presented after age 60. These percentages cannot be considered definitive, however, given the methodological issues in terms of diagnosis of schizophrenia and determination of age of onset, as well as policies and practices for hospitalizing patients.

NEUROBIOLOGY

The following discussion of neurobiology is limited by the problems in clinical methodology considered above. Nonetheless, the more recent studies in this area have had considerably greater diagnostic rigor than the older ones.

Imaging Studies

Ventricular Brain Ratio

A structural brain finding in LOS reported by several groups of investigators in younger schizophrenic adults has been increased ventricle-to-brain ratio (VBR) seen on CT or MRI. Rabins (57) reported that 25 of 29 LOS patients had VBRs that were higher than the mean for an age-matched cohort; however, the mean VBR was smaller than that in an age-matched group of patients with probable Alzheimer's disease who had concurrent psychotic symptoms. In a more recent study of patients with LOS ($N = 11$), Alzheimer's disease ($N = 12$), and age- and gender-matched normal controls ($N = 18$), only one of three VBR measures was found to be increased in LOS (40). There were significant increases in third ventricular volume, lateral VBR, and total percentage CSF in Alzhei-

mer's disease; by comparison, only third ventricular volume was significantly increased compared to controls in LOS. In one report directly comparing EOS and LOS patients on visual analog measures of atrophy, Pearlson et al. (53) showed similar ratings of atrophy in these two patient groups. In one of the few longitudinal studies to date, Naguib and Levy (49) reported that VBR was not associated with clinical course or outcome (26).

White-Matter Hyperintensities

In addition to the quantification of ventricular and sulcal size, several reports have documented large areas of white-matter hyperintensities in patients with LOS and related psychoses compared to age-matched normal comparison subjects (6,10,38,39,47,48). In addition, some reports have noted an increased number of vascular lesions in such patients (6,14).

Functional Brain Imaging

Only a few studies of functional brain imaging have been done in LOS patients. Single photon emission computed tomography (SPECT) studies by Miller et al. (48) revealed evidence of blood flow changes suggestive of cerebrovascular disease in some late-onset psychotic patients. Eighty-three percent of their late-life psychotic subjects and 27% of normals had one or more small temporal or frontal areas of hyperfusion (40). Similarly, Dupont et al. (12) found lower global cortical uptake (particularly in the left posterior frontal region and bilateral inferior temporal regions) in late-life schizophrenic patients ($N = 11$) than in normal comparison subjects ($N = 11$). The uptake did not correlate with age of onset, duration of illness, current daily neuroleptic dose, severity of psychopathology, or global cognitive impairment. In the only available published study of positron emission tomography (PET) in LOS, Pearlson et al. (53) reported elevated B_{max} (receptor density) values for dopamine D2 receptors in 13 neuroleptic-naive LOS patients compared to age and gender norms. An important question arises as to whether brain abnormalities associated with LOS are of pathogenetic significance, and how they compare with those in EOS.

Neuropsychological Investigations

Neuropsychology of Schizophrenia

There is presently a considerable amount of published research on neuropsychological functioning in schizophrenia. Despite notable heterogeneity in the behavioral presentation of schizophrenia, there is general agreement regarding the presence of neuropsychological impairments that accompany the disorder. Relatively little is known, however, about the potential interaction between the cognitive deficits associated with schizophrenia and aging (19,22).

Outcome Studies in Schizophrenia

A number of long-term follow-up studies of schizophrenia patients have shown that the clinical prognosis of schizophrenia is better than that implied in Kraepelin's use of the term "dementia praecox." Bleuler, Huber, and Ciompi all came to the same conclusion—that is, that schizophrenia was in no sense a "basically" or even "predominantly" unfavorable disease process that ran an inexorably deteriorating course (9). The proportion of patients with favorable outcome (either recovery or mild end state) was 53% in Bleuler's study, 57% in the study by Huber et al., and 59% in that by Ciompi (9). Only 18% of Ciompi's patients had "severe" end stage. These findings were corroborated in the 10 North American long-term follow-up studies of schizophrenia reviewed by McGlashan (46), who concluded that the schizophrenia process appeared to plateau after 5–10 years of manifest illness. Neuropsychological abilities were not addressed in these studies, however, so the nature and degree of cognitive impairment in late-life schizophrenia remain unclear.

In a review addressing this issue, Heaton and Drexler (22) examined 100 cross-sectional studies and 10 longitudinal studies of neuropsychological functioning in schizophrenia. The results generally argued against the possibility of a progressive neuropsychological impairment, and in particular suggested that schizophrenia patients probably did not have more rapid neuropsychological decline associated with the aging process. Heaton and Drexler (22) noted numerous methodological limitations of the available literature, however, qualifying the conclusions made. Despite an obvious need, there have been very few neuropsychological studies of LOS.

Heaton et al. (20) recently investigated neuropsychological performance in patients with EOS, LOS, and Alzheimer's disease and in normal comparison subjects. All the schizophrenia groups were worse than the normal comparison group on all the ability areas except for memory; no schizophrenia group showed impairment on the memory deficit score. By contrast, the Alzheimer's disease group was worse than the normal comparison group on memory as well as on all the other areas. Discriminant function analyses further indicated that the neuropsychological discriminant functions rarely misclassified a schizophrenia subject as having Alzheimer's disease, or vice versa; moreover, there was no tendency for this type of error to be made more often with LOS subjects than with EOS patients.

Effects of Medication on Cognition

It can be argued that some of the neuropsychological deficits in schizophrenic patients may be due to the effects of medication. There is evidence that anticholinergic drugs can interfere with cognitive functioning, especially learning and attention (21,62). Typically, learning impairment is associated with higher anticholinergic dosage or acute change in anticholinergic medication regimen. In terms of the reported effects of neuroleptic drugs on cognitive and psychomotor functions in patients and normal controls, there has been some variability and inconsistency in the literature (34). In general, sedative phenothiazines have been found to depress psychomotor function and sustained attention, but higher cognitive functions are relatively unaffected. In the majority of studies of schizophrenic patients, both cognitive function and attention improved with neuroleptic treatment, in parallel with clinical recovery. In general, the studies of neuropsychological effects of neuroleptic therapy have not been addressed specifically in older schizophrenic patients.

Neuropsychology of Tardive Dyskinesia

An additional concern with regard to cognitive functions associated with late-life psychosis is whether tardive dyskinesia (TD) affects neuropsychological performance. It is well known that the risk of TD increases with age (27,31). Thus, neuroleptic-treated patients with psychosis in late life are more likely to develop persistent TD than their younger counterparts. Less is known, however, about the interaction of cognition and TD. In a review of 31 studies we found that TD was generally associated with greater cognitive impairment (51). In a recent study of neuropsychological abilities in older schizophrenia patients we showed that severity of TD was highly associated with severity of neuropsychological impairment. Findings demonstrated that schizophrenia patients with TD had greater global cognitive deficits and greater deficits in learning than did age-, education- and subtype-matched schizophrenia patients without TD. These results suggest that research on neuropsychological abilities in schizophrenia needs to address the presence and severity of TD.

Neuropsychology Summary

This brief summary of the neuropsychology of schizophrenia and aging emphasizes the need for further longitudinal research of cognitive functioning over the course of the schizophrenic illness. There are a number of methodological issues raised by the current research in this area which limit the conclusions made (22,42,62). Some of the methodological limitations include: (a) the methods for identification and selection of schizophrenic subjects;

(b) the variable course of schizophrenic illness such that clinical state must be considered to determine which cognitive deficits are state- or trait-related requiring repeated assessments over time; (c) the issue of treatment effects (i.e., medication) and the cognitive pattern of patients with tardive dyskinesia; and (d) the evaluation of generalized and specific neuropsychological deficits. Future research in this area needs to control for these clinical and treatment factors as well as consider more specific analyses of cognition in addition to traditional global indices of performance.

Neurochemical Correlates of LOS and Related Psychoses

Neurochemical investigation has played a major role in the search for the pathophysiology of schizophrenia. Historically, there has been an emphasis on the dopamine neurotransmitter system and its role in the etiology of schizophrenia. More recently, increased evidence for the role of other neurotransmitters, coupled with limitations in the dopamine hypothesis of schizophrenia, has extended the scope of clinical neurochemical studies. The neurotransmitters that have come under increasing scrutiny include serotonin, norepinephrine, glutamate, and related excitatory amino acids, as well as the neuropeptides cholecystokinin and neurotensin. To our knowledge, no large-scale systematic study has specifically evaluated the plasma or cerebrospinal fluid of patients with LOS or related psychoses for neurochemical or neuroendocrine abnormalities. The ability to predict neuroleptic responsiveness and psychotic relapse in older schizophrenic patients using neuropeptide, neurohormone, and neurochemical parameters may provide insight into the role of limbic/mesolimbic pathogenic mechanisms in the schizophrenic disease process.

Genetic and Other Risk Factors

Studies to evaluate the prevalence of schizophrenia in families of LOS patients have been hindered by methodologic problems. For example, not all family members have been followed into old age to ensure that every case of LOS is detected. Physical illness, geographic relocation, and untimely death of relatives make it difficult to conduct such studies. The published studies suggest that the prevalence of schizophrenia (whether early or late in onset) is approximately 7% in siblings and 3% in parents of all probands with LOS. Rokhlina (58) reported that the overall prevalence of schizophrenia in the first-degree relatives of LOS patients was lower than that in the families of EOS patients.

Funding (15) and some other authors conclude that the mode of inheritance of LOS, similar to that of EOS, is probably polygenic, with many nongenetic factors being

influential. In a more recent study of HLA antigens, however, Naguib and McGuffin (50) postulated that the syndrome of LOS might be genetically distinct from EOS. Despite the previously reported association between HLA-A9 and paranoid schizophrenia, the investigators were unable to replicate this finding when 31 LOS patients were HLA-typed. Although their sample size was too small to refute confidently an association with A9, they did not even detect a trend in this direction. The authors concluded that the possibility of LOS being genetically distinct from EOS required further study.

Sensory Deficits

Several studies have reported an association between hearing impairment and late-life schizophrenia. Cooper and Porter (11) noted an increased incidence of cataracts in a population of paranoid patients compared to affective controls and also noted an association between bilateral conductive hearing loss and paranoid illness. Prager and Jeste (56) recently reviewed 27 published studies of a possible association between sensory (visual or hearing) impairment and late-life psychosis with paranoid features. A majority of these investigations supported the postulated association between hearing impairment and LOS/paranoid disorder. Many of the published studies, however, had important methodologic limitations. Also, a causal relationship between sensory deficits and LOS remains to be established. In a case–control study, Prager and Jeste (56) assessed visual and hearing impairments in 87 middle-aged and elderly subjects, including 16 with LOS, 25 with EOS, 20 with mood disorder, and 26 normal comparison subjects. Uncorrected and corrected (with eyeglasses and hearing aids) visual and hearing impairments were assessed in a "blind" manner, using standardized quantitative assessments. The two schizophrenia groups as well as the mood disorder group had greater impairments in most variables of corrected visual acuity and in self-reported hearing deficit, but not in uncorrected (constitutional) visual acuity or in pure-tone audiometry, compared to normal subjects. This suggests that schizophrenia (LOS and EOS) and mood disorder patients may have equivalent sensory deficits but inadequate correction of their sensory impairments compared to normal comparison subjects. Hence a specific contribution of sensory deficits to the etiopathology of LOS remains uncertain.

Summary of Neurobiology

Late-onset psychotic disorders may be fundamentally similar to their early-onset counterparts in the underlying neurobiologic predisposition. Certain specific protective factors may, however, prevent an earlier breakdown, whereas other aging-related precipitants may be responsible for onset of symptoms during later life. Specificity of neurobiologic substrates for different types of late-onset psychoses is yet to be established.

Integration of Findings

Attempts at an integration of neuroimaging, neuropsychology, neurochemical, and genetic research in schizophrenia have recently begun. Similar efforts must now be made to link clinical and basic research in late-onset psychoses with those findings already established in younger cohorts. Only with unified nomenclature, hypotheses, and research can the study of late-onset psychosis progress further.

According to the neurodevelopmental model, which is primarily based on studies of schizophrenia with onset during adolescence or early adulthood, the brain lesions putatively related to the pathogenesis of schizophrenia are of developmental origin (65). Furthermore, long-term treatment with neuroleptics and other environmental factors are not the principal causes of cognitive deficits and brain abnormalities reported in chronic schizophrenic patients (20,65).

At the present state of our knowledge, we may hypothesize that the neurodevelopmental model applies to LOS too. Differences in severity and specific locations or nature of these ''lesions'' may be at least partly responsible for a delay in the onset of schizophrenia (e.g., lesser severity of the nonprogressive brain lesions that presumably occurred during the developmental period may explain the relatively better social, heterosexual, and occupational functioning during early adulthood in the LOS group). Another possibility is that the peak in dopaminergic activity related to the schizophrenic breakdown, as per the neurodevelopmental theory (65), may be delayed until later in life in the patients with LOS. For obvious reasons, this discussion must be considered speculative. Nonetheless, our suggestions may offer some interesting leads to pursue in this relatively unstudied entity.

THERAPEUTIC CONSIDERATIONS

Pharmacological Management of LOS

Neuroleptic Efficacy

Neuroleptics have been shown to be the most effective treatment modality for schizophrenia, although pharmacotherapy in the older patient is complicated by alterations in both the pharmacokinetic and pharmacodynamic responses. Unfortunately, the published literature on neuroleptic treatment of late-life psychosis is extremely sparse, although the available studies suggest that a significant number of late-life schizophrenic patients improve symptomatically with neuroleptic treatment (30). Most of the

published reports do not, however, distinguish between LOS patients and elderly subjects with EOS.

In a 24-week, double-blind, placebo-controlled study involving 13 hospitals and 308 schizophrenic men aged 54–74 years, acetophenazine and trifluoperazine were both more effective than placebo in motor disturbances, conceptual disorganization, manifest psychosis, and a lack of personal neatness (25). In another study of 50 psychogeriatric (mostly chronic schizophrenic) patients, Tsuang et al. (64) reported a significant decrease in psychopathology for both haloperidol and thioridazine treatments in a 12-week double-blind study. Finally, Branchey et al. (5) demonstrated efficacy of orally administered fluphenazine and thioridazine in chronic schizophrenic patients (mean age 67 years) in a double-blind, crossover study.

With the possible exception of clozapine, the available data suggest that the commonly prescribed antipsychotic medications are equally efficacious. Therefore, selection of an antipsychotic for use in the elderly should be based primarily on the following: (a) the side effect profile of the particular drug; (b) the potential adverse consequences of the additional antipsychotic to preexisting medication regimen or a concomitant physical illness; and (c) a history of a patient's previous therapeutic response to a specific neuroleptic.

Side Effects

An important consideration is the higher incidence of side effects seen in elderly patients, as compared to younger patients, upon administration of a given amount of neuroleptic. Some studies have shown positive correlations between age and serum level of neuroleptic when equivalent doses of neuroleptic are administered (63). Usually, small doses of neuroleptics are sufficient for improvement in older patients. The side effect profiles of individual neuroleptics differ considerably, and such differences may be important in prescribing a particular medication to a patient for whom the occurrence of a particular side effect might prove dangerous (43). For example, in patients with preexisting parkinsonian symptoms, high-potency antipsychotics (e.g., haloperidol) may worsen tremor and rigidity. On the other hand, high-potency neuroleptics (especially haloperidol) are reported to have lower cardiovascular toxicity than low-potency neuroleptics. Hence, haloperidol may be a better choice than low-potency neuroleptics among patients with preexisting cardiovascular disorders. Low-potency neuroleptics (e.g., thioridazine) have marked anticholinergic activity and should be avoided in patients with prostatic hypertrophy or in those who are already on other anticholinergics. Finally, an agent that previously produced a positive response in that patient or in a blood relative may be tried first, whereas an agent that led to an unfavorable reaction may be avoided.

Tardive Dyskinesia

A number of cross-sectional investigations have found a significantly greater prevalence of neuroleptic-induced tardive dyskinesia (TD) in older patients than in younger ones (27). Saltz et al. (60) reported a 31% incidence of TD after 43 weeks of cumulative treatment with neuroleptics in a group of 160 elderly subjects (mean age 77 years), predominantly female, with a sizable proportion being institutionalized.

In a recent prospective, longitudinal study of TD in older persons, Jeste et al. (28) evaluated the overall cumulative incidence of TD (i.e., the total number of new cases of TD) over a 1-year period in a sample of 236 middle-aged and elderly outpatients with a mean age of 66 years. The annual incidence was 29.87% for schizophrenia patients ($N = 48$), 30.73% for the patients with Alzheimer's disease ($N = 55$), 33.34% for patients with mood disorders ($N = 33$), and 33.96% for patients with miscellaneous organic diagnoses ($N = 100$). These data suggest that the risk of TD over a 1-year period is no different in schizophrenic outpatients than in other diagnostic groups among middle-aged and elderly subjects. The notably high incidence of TD among all the patient groups over age 45 years points to a need for caution in prescribing neuroleptics in this population. There have been few, if any, systematic studies of the incidence of TD with "atypical" neuroleptics such as clozapine and risperidone in elderly schizophrenic patients.

Neuroleptic Dosage in LOS

Although there have been a number of studies of neuroleptic dosage in young adults with schizophrenia, little is known about the neuroleptic dose requirement in older schizophrenic patients. We recently reported the results of cross-sectional data on associations of neuroleptic dose with selected demographic, clinical, and neuropsychological variables in a group of 64 schizophrenic outpatients over the age of 45 (30). The neuroleptic dose correlated significantly with current age, age at onset of illness, severity of negative symptoms, and impairment on a variety of neuropsychological test measures such as the Halstead Reitan Average Impairment Rating, Story and Figure Learning, and psychomotor speed. An inverse correlation between age and neuroleptic dose is consistent with studies reporting pharmacokinetic (high blood levels) and pharmacodynamic (increased sensitivity to drug response) changes associated with aging (63). Age-related pharmacokinetic alterations in drug disposition may produce higher plasma concentrations of specific neuroleptic medications in older patients than in younger ones. Age-related pharmacodynamic alterations at the receptor or neurotransmitter level may increase the intensity of drug response in the elderly. The association of later age at onset of schizophrenia with lower dosages may also be consistent with the suggestion that LOS has a better prognosis than EOS (7,18). Well-controlled, prospective studies are required before one can interpret the correlation that we observed between neuroleptic dose and either the severity of negative symptoms or that of the neuropsychological impairment.

Nonpharmacologic Treatment

The results of controlled research on psychological treatment suggest that intervention may improve the outcome of schizophrenia, although many patients require long-term treatment due to the chronic nature of the illness. A widely studied psychological intervention for schizophrenia is social skills training, although cognitive retraining and didactic family counseling have also shown positive effects. However, despite more than two decades of psychological treatment research in young schizophrenic patients, no published study to our knowledge has evaluated the efficacy of these treatment strategies in older schizophrenic patients or in those with late-onset psychosis. Given the numerous psychological issues that become paramount in later life (e.g., retirement, grief over losses, financial limitations), future research needs to evaluate the efficacy of various psychological treatment strategies in patients with LOS and other late-onset psychoses.

CONCLUSIONS

In the past, most of the research interest in schizophrenia focused on younger adults. With the aging of the general population, there is now an increase in the attention being given to older schizophrenic patients, including those with a late onset of the disorder. Other late-onset psychotic disorders are also beginning to be studied more comprehensively. The literature in this area is still very limited, however, and is also fraught with a number of methodologic problems. Nonetheless, the following "conclusions" can be made with at least some degree of certainty at this time:

1. There is clinical evidence to support the face validity, descriptive validity, and predictive validity of LOS.
2. Schizophrenia can have onset after the age of 45, although such late onset of schizophrenia is much less common than onset prior to age 45.
3. Delusional disorder and psychotic (delusional) depression are more likely to have onset during middle age and old age than during early adulthood.
4. Late-onset psychotic disorders may be fundamentally similar to their early-onset counterparts in the underlying neurobiologic predisposition. Certain specific protective factors may, however, prevent an earlier break-

down, whereas other aging-related precipitants may be responsible for the onset of symptoms during later life.

5. Specificity of neurobiologic substrates for different types of late-onset psychoses is yet to be established.

6. Late-onset psychosis patients have neuroleptic responsiveness that is qualitatively similar to that of younger patients. The late-onset patients, however, need and tolerate much lower dosages than do the early-onset patients.

7. Late-onset schizophrenia and other related psychoses must be considered in any comprehensive theories of psychosis, especially schizophrenia.

FUTURE DIRECTIONS

There is a need for longitudinal, multicenter, collaborative studies of late-onset psychosis using well-defined diagnostic criteria and reliable, validated instruments for assessment. Apart from clinical characteristics (including course and treatment-response), the other aspects that should be investigated include: neuropsychological performance, structural and functional brain imaging, neurochemical and neuroendocrine parameters, and neuropathological variables.

Comparisons of early-onset and late-onset psychosis patients using age-corrected measures are warranted. Also, the utility of the current diagnostic differentiation of late-onset psychosis (i.e., schizophrenia, delusional disorder, psychotic depression, etc.) needs to be established from both clinical and neurobiologic perspectives.

ACKNOWLEDGMENTS

This work was supported, in part, by NIMH grants MH45131, MH43693, and MH49671-01 and by the Department of Veterans Affairs.

REFERENCES

1. American Psychiatric Association. *Diagnostic and statistical manual of mental disorders*, 3rd ed. Washington, DC: American Psychiatric Association, 1980.
2. American Psychiatric Association. *Diagnostic and statistical manual of mental disorders*, 3rd edition (revised). Washington, DC: American Psychiatric Association, 1987.
3. Andreasen NC, Carpenter WT. Diagnosis and classification of schizophrenia. *Schizophr Bull* 1993;19(2):199–214.
4. Bleuler E. *Dementia praecox, or the group of schizophrenias* (translated by J Zinkin, 1950). New York: International Universities Press, 1911.
5. Branchey MH, Lee JH, Ramesh A. High- and low-potency neuroleptics in elderly psychiatric patients. *JAMA* 1978;239:1860–1862.
6. Breitner J, Husain M, Figiel G, Krishnan K, Boyko O. Cerebral white matter disease in late-onset psychosis. *Biol Psychiatry* 1990;28:266–274.
7. Castle DJ, Murray RM. The neurodevelopmental basis of sex differences in schizophrenia. *Psychol Med* 1991;21:565–575.
8. Castle DJ, Sham PC, Wessely S, Murray RM. Sex and the subtyping of schizophrenia. Paper presented at International Conference

"Schizophrenia: Poised for Change," Vancouver, Canada, July, 1992.
9. Ciompi L. Catamnestic long-term study on the course of life and aging of schizophrenics. *Schizophr Bull* 1980;6:606–618.
10. Coffey CE, Figiel GS, Djang WT, Weiner RD. Subcortical hyperintensity on magnetic resonance imaging: a comparison of normal and depressed elderly subjects. *Am J Psychiatry* 1990;47:187–189.
11. Cooper AF, Porter R. Visual acuity and ocular pathology in the paranoid and affective psychoses of later life. *J Psychosom Res* 1976;20:107–114.
12. Dupont RM, Lehr P, Lamoureaux G, Halpern S, Harris MJ, Jeste DV. Preliminary report: cerebral blood flow abnormalities in late-life schizophrenia. *Psychiatry Res* 1994;[in press].
13. Fish F. Senile schizophrenia. *J Ment Sci* 1960;106:938–946.
14. Flint AJ, Rifat SI, Eastwood MR. Late-onset paranoia: distinct from paraphrenia? *Int J Geriatr Psychiatry* 1991;6:103–109.
15. Funding T. Genetics of paranoid psychosis of later life. *Acta Psychiatr Scand* 1961;37:267–282.
16. Grief C, Eastwood RM. Paranoid disorders in the elderly. *Int J Geriatr Psychiatry* 1993;8:681–684.
17. Harris MJ, Cullum CM, Jeste DV. Clinical presentation of late-onset schizophrenia. *J Clin Psychiatry* 1988;49:356–360.
18. Harris MJ, Jeste DV. Late-onset schizophrenia: an overview. *Schizophr Bull* 1988;14:39–55.
19. Harrow M, Marengo J, Pogue-Geile M, Pawelski TJ. Schizophrenic deficits in intelligence and abstract thinking: influence of aging and long-term institutionalization. In: Miller D, Cohen G, eds. *Schizophrenia, paranoia, schizophreniform disorders in later life*. New Haven: Yale University Press, 1986;133–144.
20. Heaton R, Paulsen J, McAdams LA, et al. Neuropsychological deficits in schizophrenia: relationship to age, chronicity and dementia. *Arch Gen Psychiatry* 1994;[in press].
21. Heaton RK, Crowley TJ. Effects of psychiatric disorders and their somatic treatments on neuropsychological results. In: Filskov SB, Ball TJ, eds. *Handbook of clinical neuropsychology*. New York: Wiley–Interscience, 1981;481–525.
22. Heaton RK, Drexler M. Clinical neuropsychological findings in schizophrenia and aging. In: Miller NE, Cohen GD, eds. *Schizophrenia and aging*. New York: The Guilford Press, 1987;145–161.
23. Herbert ME, Jacobson S. Late paraphrenia. *Br J Psychiatry* 1967;113:461–469.
24. Hoffman WF, Ballard L, Turner EH, Casey DE. Three-year follow-up of older schizophrenics: extrapyramidal syndromes, psychiatric symptoms, and ventricular brain ratio. *Biol Psychiatry* 1991;30:913–926.
25. Honigfeld G, Rosebaum MP, Blumenthal IJ, Lambert HL, Roberts AJ. Behavioral improvement in the older schizophrenic patient: drug and social therapies. *J Am Geriatric Soc* 1965;13:57–71.
26. Hymas N, Naguib M, Levy R. Late paraphrenia—a follow-up study. *Int J Geriatr Psychiatry* 1989;4:23–29.
27. Jeste DV, Caligiuri MP. Tardive dyskinesia. *Schizophr Bull* 1993;19:303–315.
28. Jeste DV, Harris MJ, Krull A, Kuck J, McAdams LA, Heaton R. Late onset schizophrenia: clinical and neuropsychological characteristics. [*Submitted*.]
29. Jeste DV, Harris MJ, Pearlson GD, et al. Late-onset schizophrenia: studying clinical validity. *Psychiatr Clin North Am* 1988;11:1–14.
30. Jeste DV, Lacro JP, Gilbert PL, Kline J, Kline N. Treatment of late-life schizophrenia with neuroleptics. *Schizophr Bull* 1993;19(4):817–830.
31. Kane JM, Jeste DV, Barnes TRE, et al. *Tardive dyskinesia: a task force report of the American Psychiatric Association*. Washington, DC: American Psychiatric Association, 1992.
32. Kaplan E, Goodglass H, Weintraub S. *The Boston naming test*. Philadelphia: Lea & Febiger, 1983.
33. Kay DWK, Roth M. Environmental and hereditary factors in the schizophrenias of old age ("late paraphrenia") and their bearing on the general problem of causation in schizophrenia. *J Ment Sci* 1961;107:649–686.
34. King DJ. The effect of neuroleptics on cognitive and psychomotor function. *Br J Psychiatry* 1990;157:799–811.
35. Kraepelin E. *Psychiatrie, Ein Lehrbuch fur Studierende und Artzte*, 6th ed. Leipzig: Barth, 1899.

36. Kraepelin E. *Psychiatrie ein Lehrbuch fur Studierende und Aertzte*, 8th ed. Leipzig: Barth, 1909.
37. Kraepelin E. *Dementia praecox and paraphrenia* (translated by RM Barclay). Chicago: Chicago Medical Book, 1919.
38. Lesser IM, Jeste DV, Boone KB, et al. Late-onset psychotic disorder, not otherwise specified: clinical and neuroimaging findings. *Biol Psychiatry* 1992;31:419–423.
39. Lesser IM, Miller BL, Boone KB, Hill-Gutierrez E, Mena II. Brain injury and cognitive function in late-onset psychotic depression. *J Neuropsychiatry Clin Neurosci* 1991;3:33–40.
40. Lesser IM, Miller BL, Swartz JR, Boone KB, Mehringer CM, Mena I. Brain imaging in late-life schizophrenia and related psychosis. *Schizophr Bull* 1993;19:773–782.
41. Leuchter AF, Spar JE. The late-onset psychoses. *J Nerv Ment Dis* 1985;173:488–494.
42. Levin S, Yurgelun-Todd D, Craft S. Contributions of clinical neuropsychology to the study of schizophrenia. *J Abnorm Psychol* 1989;98:341–356.
43. Lohr JB, Jeste DV, Harris MJ, Salzman C. Treatment of disordered behavior. In: Salzman C, ed. *Clinical geriatric psychopharmacology*. Baltimore: Williams & Wilkins, 1992;79–113.
44. Mayer W. On paraphrenic psychoses (in German). *Z Gesamte Neurol Psychiatr* 1921;71:187–206.
45. McGlashan TH. Predictors of shorter-, medium-, and longer-term outcome in schizophrenia. *Am J Psychiatry* 1986;143:50–55.
46. McGlashan TH. A selective review of recent North American long-term follow-up studies of schizophrenia. *Schizophr Bull* 1988;14:515–542.
47. Miller BL, Lesser IM. Late-life psychosis and modern neuroimaging. In: Jeste DV, Zisook S, eds. *The psychiatric clinics of North America: psychosis and depression in the elderly*, Philadelphia: WB Saunders, 1988;33–46.
48. Miller BL, Lesser IM, Boone KB, Hill E, Mehringer CM, Wong K. Brain lesions and cognitive function in late-life psychosis. *Br J Psychiatry* 1991;158:76–82.
49. Naguib M, Levy R. Late paraphrenia: neuropsychological impairment and structural brain abnormalities on computed tomography. *Int J Geriatr Psychiatry* 1987;2:83–90.
50. Naguib M, McGuffin P. Genetic Markers in late paraphrenia: a study of HLA antigens. *Br J Psychiatry* 1987;150:124–127.
51. Paulsen JS, Heaton R, Jeste DV. Neuropsychological impairment in tardive dyskinesia. *Neuropsychology* 1993;in press.
52. Pearlson G, Rabins P. The Late-onset psychoses: possible risk factors. In: Jeste DV, Zisook S, eds. *The psychiatric clinics of North America: psychosis and depression in the elderly*. Philadelphia: WB Saunders, 1988;15–32.
53. Pearlson GD, Tune LE, Wong DF, et al. Quantitative D2 dopamine receptor PET and structural MRI changes in late onset schizophrenia. *Schizophr Bull* 1993;19:783–795.
54. Pilowsky L, Kerwin R, Murray RM. Neurodevelopment and schizophrenia. In: Kringham E, et al., eds. *Etiology of mental disorder*. London: University of Soho Press, 1991;169–181.
55. Post F. *Persistent persecutory states of the elderly*. London: Pergamon Press, 1966.
56. Prager S, Jeste DV. Sensory impairment in late-life schizophrenia. *Schizophr Bull* 1993;19(4):755–772.
57. Rabins P. Coexisting depression and dementia. *J Geriatr Psychiatry* 1989;22:17–24.
58. Rokhlina ML. A comparative clinico-genetic study of attack-like schizophrenia with late and early manifestations with regard to age [in Russian]. *Zh Nevropatol Psikhiatr* 1975;75:417–424.
59. Roth M. The natural history of mental disorder in old age. *J Ment Sci* 1955;101:281–301.
60. Saltz BL, Woerner MG, Kane JM, et al. Prospective study of tardive dyskinesia incidence in the elderly. *JAMA* 1991;266:2402–2406.
61. Spitzer RL, Williams JBW. Classification of mental disorders. In: Kaplan HI, Sadock BH, eds. *Comprehensive textbook of psychiatry*, vol 1. Baltimore: Williams & Wilkins, 1985;591–613.
62. Spohn HE, Strauss ME. Relation of neuroleptic and anticholinergic medication to cognitive functions in schizophrenia. *J Abnorm Psychol* 1989;98:367–380.
63. Tran-Johnson TK, Krull AJ, Jeste DV. Late life schizophrenia and its treatment: the pharmacologic issues in older schizophrenic patients. In: Alexopoulos GS, ed. *Clinics in geriatric medicine*. Philadelphia: WB Saunders, 1992;401–410.
64. Tsuang MM, Lu LM, Stotsky BA, Cole JO. Haloperidol versus thioridazine for hospitalized psychogeriatric patients: double-blind study. *J Am Geriatr Soc* 1971;19:593–600.
65. Weinberger DR. Implications of normal brain development for the pathogenesis of schizophrenia. *Arch Gen Psychiatry* 1987;44:660–669.
66. World Health Organization. *The International Pilot Study of Schizophrenia*, vol 1. Geneva, Switzerland: World Health Organization, 1993.
67. Yassa R, Dastoor D, Nastase C, Camille Y, Belzile L. The prevalence of late-onset schizophrenia in a psychogeriatric population. *J Geriatr Psychiatry Neurol* 1993;6:120–125.

Psychopharmacology: The Fourth Generation of Progress, edited by Floyd E. Bloom and David J. Kupfer. Raven Press, Ltd., New York © 1995.

CHAPTER 123

Cognitive Impairment in Geriatric Schizophrenic Patients

Clinical and Postmortem Characterization

Michael Davidson and Vahram Haroutunian

The outcome of schizophrenia in old age remains among the most debated topics in schizophrenia research. The debate between the Kraepelinian pronouncement that the outcome is invariably bleak and the view that the outcome of schizophrenia in old age is variable (20,33) focuses on the schizophrenic cognitive capacities in old age and not on the psychosis, which for many (but not all) patients ameliorates. There is consensus among investigators that nearly all young and middle-aged schizophrenic patients suffer from moderate cognitive impairment (see Chapter 105, *this volume*), and that a certain proportion of geriatric patients suffer from a very severe form of cognitive impairment (20,36). There is, however, no consensus on the proportion of geriatric schizophrenic patients who suffer from the severe form of cognitive impairment, on the specific manifestations of the cognitive impairment in old age, or on how moderate impairment of specific cognitive aspects progresses, if at all, into severe and possibly global cognitive impairment.

The debate on the outcome of schizophrenia in general, and on the cognitive impairment in particular, is complicated by the fact that the criteria used to define good or poor outcome are influenced by (a) the level of care needed by the patients and (b) the type of health facility where this care is delivered. For example, good outcome is associated with patients discharged from psychiatric hospitals into the community, and with care delivered by outpatient clinics, whereas poor outcome is associated

with continued inpatient status. Early in the schizophrenic illness the need for inpatient psychiatric care is determined by the severity of psychotic symptoms and cognitive impairment (13). However, as psychotic symptoms ameliorate with age, cognitive impairment may become the major determinant of the type of care necessary and of the facility where this care will be provided. For example, of the 300,000 geriatric schizophrenic patients in the United States, approximately 200,000 live in nursing homes, while only 15,000 live in psychiatric hospitals (32,61,63,71). It is plausible to assume that, among many other factors, amelioration of psychotic symptoms has enabled the discharge of geriatric schizophrenics from psychiatric hospitals. It is also plausible to assume that cognitive impairment has required that these patients continue to live in protected environments such as nursing homes. Therefore, if living in a protected environment is used as a criteria for outcome, cognitive impairment may be a major determinant of outcome.

The paucity of investigations on the cognitive impairment in geriatric schizophrenics can be understood in light of the methodological difficulties inherent in studying the long-term outcome of schizophrenia in general (33) and those inherent in studying cognition in the context of a chronic illness and aging in particular. Cohort attrition, diagnostic uncertainty and heterogeneity, and changes in the social and treatment environment not accounted for in the original study design are a few of the difficulties common to schizophrenia outcome studies. Interactions of cognitive functioning with positive and negative symptoms, other schizophrenic symptoms, poor cooperation, depression, poor education, somatic treatment, length of

M. Davidson and V. Haroutunian: Department of Psychiatry, Mount Sinai School of Medicine/Bronx Veterans Affairs Medical Center, Bronx, New York 10468.

hospitalization, and concomitant neurological illnesses are some of the specific methodological difficulties which can confound or affect cognitive performance.

Furthermore, in young and middle-aged schizophrenic patients, findings that executive and memory functions, believed to be subserved by the frontal and temporal lobes respectively, are disproportionately impaired (29,65) have been invoked in directing neuroradiological and neuropathological research to these areas (7,76). However, as chronic schizophrenia and aging interact, separating the domains of cognition which are disproportionately affected from those which are not may not be feasible, and the question of generalized versus specific cognitive impairment, which is still debated in young patients, becomes even more difficult to resolve in geriatric schizophrenics. Thus, the already tenuous inferences made about brain dysfunction and structural lesions based on neuropsychological test results become even more speculative in geriatric patients.

Despite methodological difficulties, investigating the cognitive impairment in geriatric schizophrenic patients is essential to elucidate the pathophysiology of this illness and improve the care given to this population. For example, investigating the lifelong course of cognitive impairment may add support to either the developmental or the degenerative hypothesis of schizophrenia. An abrupt decline in cognitive performance in late adolescence or early adulthood without additional progression, or with very slow progression over the rest of the lifespan, would lend support to the evolution of an early static lesion in the context of a chronic disease and aging (see Chapter 98, *this volume*). Conversely, periods of rapid and progressive cognitive decline, or the appearance in geriatric patients of novel aspects of cognitive impairment not found in young patients, in conjunction with a characteristic neurohistological signature, would lend support to an active, possibly degenerative type of disorder.

Equally relevant to schizophrenia research is the fact that most schizophrenic patients who come to autopsy die at a very advanced age and are cognitively impaired, making it plausible that some of the plethora of neuroanatomical and neurochemical findings which are attributed to schizophrenia are in fact causally related to the cognitive impairment of schizophrenia. It would not be implausible to suspect that not accounting for the presence and severity of the cognitive impairment and for the age-related changes in schizophrenia symptomatology in general has contributed to the inconsistencies reported in neuropathological and neurochemical studies of this illness. Comparing cognitively impaired and cognitively nonimpaired schizophrenic patients in terms of demographic correlates, associated symptoms, and course in conjunction with postmortem studies might resolve these inconsistencies and help delineate a subtype of schizophrenia with a biologically distinct substrate.

Finally, in terms of the contribution to the care of geriatric schizophrenics, characterizing the cognitive impairment and knowing its course might predict the degree and type of support needed (13,80) and thus assist in a rational planning of care delivery. Furthermore, in order to evaluate the efficacy of the treatments currently available for geriatric schizophrenic patients and to conceptualize treatments specifically targeted at ameliorating the cognitive impairment or delaying its onset, it is essential to know its course and manifestations.

This chapter will review the course and severity of cognitive impairment, the factors associated with it (i.e., other schizophrenic symptoms, demographic variables, and somatic treatment), and the potential biological substrates which may be responsible for this condition in geriatric schizophrenic patients whose illness started before age 45 (for a review of late onset schizophrenia, see Chapters 98 and 122, *this volume*). For the purposes of this review, cognitive impairment will refer to impairment in more than one area of cognition which is sufficiently severe to affect daily social functioning.

CLINICAL STUDIES

Cognitive Impairment Through the Lifespan of Chronic Schizophrenic Patients

Despite the shortcomings of long-term follow-up studies, they remain the preferred method to investigate the course of cognitive impairment and to place it in the overall context of the outcome of schizophrenia. The ideal study would administer psychometric tests to a cohort of first-episode, very young schizophrenic patients drawn from a catchment area and would then repeat the testing periodically until very old age or death. Unfortunately, published long-term studies either are (a) limited to narrative descriptions of cognitive decay without formal cognitive assessments of the entire cohort (20) or (b) cover a restricted range of patients' lives (e.g., early life or middle age; see refs. 27 and 36 for reviews). A number of "first-episode" psychosis catamnestic studies which periodically administer psychometric tests were initiated in the late 1980s (14), but their long-term results will not be available in the near future.

A more feasible approach to estimate the progression of the cognitive impairment in geriatric schizophrenics is to compare cognitive performance between geriatric (>65 years of age) and nongeriatric schizophrenic patients in cross-sectional studies. However, results of cross-sectional studies are vulnerable to "sample biases," because geriatric schizophrenic patients who participate in cross-sectional studies are recruited mostly, but not exclusively, from psychiatric inpatient facilities (27,36). In contrast, patients who require no psychiatric care, and for whom old age is associated with independent living in the community, are difficult to locate and are rarely included in cross-sectional studies. Because the ability to live independently in the community is associated with better cognitive functioning (13), results of cross sectional studies may overestimate the prevalence of cognitive impairment in geriatric schizophrenia.

Cross-sectional studies are also subject to "birth cohort effects." If younger patients have a less severe form of illness than older patients [due, for example, to treatment early in their illness with neuroleptics (79)] or if the younger patients were more educated (a factor associated with better cognitive performance), this "birth cohort effect" could be misinterpreted as age-related deterioration in individual patients (66). Similarly, comorbid neurological conditions which affect cognitive performance and whose prevalences increase with age (such as Alzheimer's disease, multi-infarct dementia, and Parkinson's dementia) could likewise be misinterpreted as age-related deterioration in individual patients (see below for a discussion of this topic). In contrast, cross-sectional studies have the advantage of covering large age ranges and including large numbers of patients so that potential differences in cognitive functioning between age groups are not underestimated.

With the aforementioned limitations in mind, reviews of cross-sectional comparison studies have found that young schizophrenic patients performed better than geriatric patients on some (but not the majority of) psychometric tests, and they concluded that the differences between the younger and older patients were not sufficient to support a progressively deteriorating course of the already existing cognitive impairment (27,36). However, a most comprehensive review of over 100 studies (36) and the only very long-term catamnestic study (20) agree that a progressively deteriorating course of cognitive function may occur in a subgroup of schizophrenic patients whose illness is characterized by (a) very severe and persistent symptoms throughout life and (b) lengthy or uninterrupted hospitalization.

In order to investigate if such a subgroup exists and to overcome the limitations related to too narrow an age-range comparison, we divided the entire inpatient population of chronic schizophrenics residing at a long-term psychiatric hospital into seven age groups ranging from 25+ to 85+ years of age (25–34, 35–44, 45–54, etc.) and compared their cognitive performance (22). After excluding the patients who on medical screening were found to suffer from neurological or medical conditions which could affect cognitive performance, 393 subjects remained, 308 of whom were geriatric (>65 years of age or older). All 393 patients had been admitted to this chronic care psychiatric hospital after they had failed several treatment trials, and the majority of them are very chronic and severely ill patients. A battery of tests sensitive to progressive, cognitive deterioration used by the Consortium to Establish a Registry for Alzheimer's Disease (CERAD) (51) was administered. Analyses of vari-

TABLE 1. Cognitive performance in schizophrenic patients by age group[a]

Age	Boston naming	Praxis	Word list learning	Word list recall
25+	13.3	6.6	6.5	5.0
	(1.4)	(0.5)	(1.9)	(2.6)
35+	13.0	6.7	5.4	4.2
	(1.9)	(0.8)	(2.9)	(3.0)
45+	11.4	5.9	5.2	3.0
	(4.7)	(1.6)	(3.3)	(2.5)
55+	9.1	5.1	4.8	2.9
	(4.8)	(1.1)	(2.8)	(2.3)
65+	8.5	4.4	3.2	1.5
	(3.6)	(2.9)	(2.5)	(2.0)
75+	8.0	4.5	3.2	1.4
	(4.6)	(3.7)	(3.3)	(2.7)
85+	5.6	3.3	2.2	0.5
	(4.5)	(3.2)	(2.4)	(1.6)

[a] Values are means per age group. Standard deviations in parentheses.

ance examining the effect of age group (i.e., decade) on the performance of each of the five tests found statistically significant effects of age group for each measure (see Table 1).

The results indicated that all chronic schizophrenic patients have poor learning, memory, recognition, and praxis abilities; however, young schizophrenic patients have better cognitive functioning than do geriatric schizophrenic patients. Despite the fact that every age group obtained a better mean score than the following (older) age group on virtually every measure, in order for the age-associated differences to reach statistical significance it was necessary to compare age groups separated by at least 20 years and to include in the comparison patients older than 65 years of age. Thus, the differences between age groups would have been overlooked if the age range was not broad enough or if the older groups were left out of the comparison, suggesting that if the differences in performance between age groups reflect cognitive decline in individual patients the decline is very slow.

Despite the relatively small differences in scores between each age group of schizophrenics, these differences are much larger than the differences between the same age groups of equivalently educated normal control individuals. Furthermore, in a multiple regression analysis, the contribution of age to the variance of psychometric scores in the population of geriatric schizophrenic patients was approximately 5%, which is much lower than the contribution of age to the variance in cognitive performance in a group of geriatric normal controls (57). Together, this and other data (67) suggest that for severely ill schizophrenic patients, the age-related differences in cognitive performance are larger than differences associated with normal aging. On the other hand, the differences are significantly smaller than the decline observed in individuals suffering from a typical degenerative dementia such as Alzheimer's disease (51).

In summary, these data are consistent with a very slow decline in cognitive performance over the lifespan of severely ill, chronically hospitalized schizophrenic patients, and they are inconsistent with either normal aging or a typical degenerative disease. These results are not in conflict with three reviews of this topic (27,36), which concluded that because the differences between younger and older schizophrenic patients are not very large, the data are not consistent with a progressive deterioration of a degenerative type. The study presented here found larger differences between age groups perhaps because it compared cognitive function over a much broader age range in larger age groups and in a more severely ill patient population. In fact, the population presented here consists of (a) young and middle-aged patients who have repeatedly failed several consecutive treatment trials and (b) geriatric patients, the overwhelming majority of whom have been in the same institution for over 20 years. The question of whether the young and middle-aged patients included in this cross-sectional study will eventually develop the same kind of severe cognitive impairment as the geriatric patients, and if they all belong to a phenomenologically and biologically distinct subtype of schizophrenia, can only be conclusively answered with a long-term follow-up study. However, the chronicity and the already impaired cognitive functioning of the young and middle-aged patients evidenced by the scores presented in Table 1 suggest an affirmative answer to this question.

Cognitive Impairment and Institutionalization

Of the geriatric schizophrenic patients who reside in chronic psychiatric hospitals, over 50% suffered from severe impairment in more than one area of cognition which affected social functioning (46,53), thus meeting DSM-III-R criteria A to D for dementia. Despite persistent suggestions that the unstimulating institutional social environment contributes to the cognitive impairment (78), and despite this suggestion's face validity, a cause–effect relationship has not been established (1,31,40).

To investigate the role of institutionalization in the cognitive impairment of geriatric schizophrenic patients, several strategies can be employed, all of which have serious methodological flaws. For example, a case–control study could compare cognitive performance in pairs of schizophrenic patients admitted at the same time, preferably in the same institution, and match them on most demographic and illness related variables, with the exception that one patient has been continuously institutionalized for most of his/her life and the other immediately discharged and never or only briefly readmitted. While no such study has been reported, an observation (40), though not confirmed (47), suggested that patients discharged

from an institution had slightly better cognitive functioning than did patients who remained institutionalized, and it could be interpreted as evidence that institutionalization is causally related to cognitive impairment. However, this conclusion is flawed because the assignment of patients to remain in an institution or to be discharged cannot be randomized. Patients who have better cognitive performance are more likely to be discharged and to stay in the community (13); thus, it may very well be that cognitive impairment serves as a selection factor for long-term institutionalization, rather than long-term institutionalization being the cause of cognitive impairment (1).

An alternative approach to separate the contributions of institutionalization and the schizophrenic illness to cognitive impairment is to compare the cognitive performance of the geriatric schizophrenics to the performance of another diagnostic group of chronically institutionalized patients such as geriatric patients suffering from mood disorder. Of the 50 mood disorder inpatients identified by our study, most of whom have been institutionalized for more than 20 years, only 30% met DSM-III-R criteria A to D for dementia, which is significantly less than the proportion (50%) of geriatric schizophrenic patients who met the criteria and reside in the same institution. Furthermore, the average Mini Mental State Examination (MMSE) scores of the mood disorder patients were significantly higher (better) than the scores of the schizophrenic patients, and there was no correlation between years of institutionalization and MMSE scores in mood disorder patients, while there was a correlation, albeit weak, between these variables in the geriatric schizophrenic patients. Taken together, the data indicate that institutionalized geriatric patients suffering from mood disorder have better cognitive functioning than do institutionalized geriatric schizophrenic patients; however, the differences between the two diagnostic groups were not clinically substantial. Thus, while the comparison between the two diagnostic groups implicates the specific schizophrenic illness rather than a generalized institutionalization effect, it does not rule out that institutionalization contributes to the cognitive impairment of both geriatric schizophrenic and mood disorder patients. On the other hand, it could be hypothesized that cognitive impairment is a point of convergence for very severe forms of schizophrenia and mood disorder, possibly mediated by a biological abnormality shared by the two disorders (77).

In summary, evidence can be accumulated to suggest that cognitive impairment is a selection factor for long-term institutionalization and is responsible for patients' continued hospitalization, rather than supporting the notion that cognitive impairment is the inevitable result of long-term institutionalization (1,31,40). In fact, at least one study investigating the long-term effects of deinstitutionalization has suggested an association between deinstitutionalization and worsening in cognitive functions and positive symptoms (80). Symptom aggravation even after a long period of deinstitutionalization was observed in patients who suffered from mild-to-moderate cognitive impairment before deinstitutionalization, suggesting that these patients did not benefit from community care and supporting the notion that cognitive function is predictive of independent living (13) and level of care required.

Cognitive Impairment and Other Schizophrenic Symptoms

Correlational analyses in samples of young and middle-aged schizophrenic patients have consistently revealed associations between severity of cognitive impairment and negative symptoms (5,48). Similarly, our study of 393 schizophrenic patients between the ages 25 and 85 revealed strong correlations between cognitive impairment and negative symptoms. The correlations remained significant, and their magnitude did not change throughout the entire lifespan. These correlations between cognitive impairment and negative symptoms led to the hypothesis that the two symptoms share a common biological substrate. Components of cognitive dysfunction and of negative symptoms have both been attributed to structural and functional abnormalities of the dorsolateral prefrontal cortex and its connectivities to the medial temporal lobe (65; also see Chapter 98, *this volume*).

Common schizophrenic symptoms such as preoccupation with delusions and hallucinations, as well as poor cooperation with the testing process, have been invoked to explain the poor performance of the geriatric schizophrenic patients on cognitive testing. However, in our study of geriatric schizophrenic patients and in most other studies of schizophrenics of all ages, severity of delusions and hallucinations did not correlate with severity of cognitive impairment. Furthermore, investigations have demonstrated that the cognitive impairment in schizophrenia is not a result of poor cooperation but is, instead, a result of the inability to perform the task (29).

The severity of cognitive impairment was also found to correlate with the number of years of formal education in our sample of geriatric schizophrenics. Similar findings have emerged for younger schizophrenics (31) and for normal geriatric individuals (74). In the schizophrenic patients, these associations may reflect a shared biological substrate for (a) poor educational achievement at younger age and (b) an enhanced risk for cognitive impairment in old age. However, confounding factors such as cohort effects or anxiety with test taking in the less educated individuals cannot be ruled out.

In summary, of all schizophrenic symptoms and factors associated with them, negative symptoms seem to show the strongest association with cognitive impairment, an association which remains constant throughout all age ranges. The immutable association throughout life between cognitive impairment and negative symptoms could be the phenomenological signature of a biological lesion which mediates both cognitive impairment and negative symptoms.

Cognitive Impairment and Somatic Treatment

The generation of schizophrenic patients who are currently in their seventh or eighth decade of life have been exposed to leukotomy, insulin coma, electroconvulsive therapy (ECT), and at least 30 years of treatment with neuroleptic and anticholinergic drugs. Furthermore, many of them are still being treated with neuroleptics and few with anticholinergic drugs. Depending on the specific aspect of cognitive functioning tested, somatic treatments have been found to have therapeutic, deleterious, or negligible effects on the cognitive performance of geriatric schizophrenic patients (36,69; see also Chapter 122, *this volume*).

Our own review of the treatments given to geriatric schizophrenic patients showed no significant effects on current MMSE scores of past treatment with leukotomy, insulin coma, or ECT or of cumulative lifetime exposure to neuroleptics. At the time of the assessment, the majority of the geriatric schizophrenic patients were still treated with neuroleptics, and their mean MMSE scores were higher (better) than the scores of the patients not currently treated with neuroleptics. However, there were no differences in the MMSE scores associated with a particular class of neuroleptics despite the fact that they differed in their anticholinergic potencies or other pharmacological properties (atypical neuroleptics were not included in the comparison because none of the geriatric patients were receiving this treatment).

These data, consistent with previous reports, suggested that past or current somatic treatment (including treatment with anticholinergic drugs) has no obvious deleterious effects on cognitive functioning (42,68). Despite the fact that patients currently being treated with neuroleptics had better MMSE scores than the nontreated patients, and that neuroleptic medication has been demonstrated to improve attention (68), better cognitive functioning cannot easily be attributed to current neuroleptic treatment. Until a prospective study of administration or discontinuation of typical neuroleptics to geriatric schizophrenics is conducted, typical neuroleptics cannot be unequivocally "absolved" of deleterious effects nor can cognitive enhancing effects be attributed to this class of drugs.

In summary, studies suggest that chronic treatment with neuroleptics or other somatic treatments are not responsible for the cognitive impairment in geriatric schizophrenics. However, while most of the studies compared different degrees of exposure to somatic treatments, they did not compare patients exposed and not exposed to the treatments.

Cognitive Impairment and Concomitant Neurological and Medical Disorders

Presence of concomitant neurological disorders (such as seizures) or a history of severe head trauma has been suggested to contribute to the schizophrenic cognitive impairment in young and geriatric patients (30). These disorders, along with medical disorders associated with increased risk for vascular dementia such as hypertension or diabetes, have constituted exclusion criteria from samples of schizophrenic patients in whom cognitive performance was evaluated in some (27), but not all, studies (see ref. 36 for a review). Furthermore, although each of these neurological and medical conditions have been invoked as a risk factor for dementia, their actual contribution to cognitive impairment is far from established. On the other hand, if presence of a risk factor was used to account for poor cognitive performance (i.e., patients who had poor cognitive performance and diabetes or hypertension were excluded from studies assessing cognitive performance), then the true prevalence of cognitive impairment associated with schizophrenia could have been underestimated because these variables' contribution in an individual patient's cognitive impairment cannot be ascertained.

Other neurological disorders such as Alzheimer's disease, multi-infarct dementia, and Parkinson's dementia could account for the cognitive impairment in schizophrenics. Because the disorders are more prevalent in geriatric individuals in general, they could enhance the differences in cognitive performance between young and geriatric schizophrenic patients. However, our own clinicopathological studies (see following sections) and those of others indicate that degenerative or vascular disorders known to cause dementia in nonschizophrenic individuals are not responsible for the cognitive impairment in geriatric schizophrenics.

Tardive dyskinesia (TD), and particularly orofacial TD, was found to be associated with cognitive impairment in schizophrenic patients in 24 of 37 studies reviewed (56). However, because establishing the presence, severity, and characteristics of schizophrenia, cognitive impairment, and TD is not an unambiguous task, the controversy surrounding the nature of the association among the three is not surprising (see Chapter 127, *this volume*). Elucidating this association is further complicated by the fact that TD and cognitive impairment share common risk factors such as advanced age, and maybe exposure to neuroleptic treatment (45,56). Although some animal studies and observations in humans have led to the speculation that a striatal abnormality may mediate both the cognitive impairment and the limbotruncal TD (45), there is no support for a causal relationship between cognitive impairment and TD (42).

Finally, abuse of illicit drugs could theoretically contribute to the schizophrenic cognitive impairment; however, no direct evidence for this assertion exists. Furthermore, even if illicit drug abuse contributed to cognitive impairment, it could not be responsible for cognitive impairment in geriatric schizophrenics because illicit drug abuse is not common in this generation of patients.

In summary, similar to nonschizophrenic patients, cognitive impairment in schizophrenics could be associated with medical and neurological disorders; however, there is no evidence that the prevalence of medical or neurological disorders which induce cognitive impairment or dementias is increased in schizophrenics, nor is there evidence that these disorders can account for the high prevalence of cognitive impairment among geriatric institutionalized schizophrenic patients (also see following sections).

Cognitive Impairment: Treatment Options

Available anti-schizophrenia drugs target positive and some negative symptoms, and occasionally agitation. There is, however, no specific pharmacological strategy for the treatment of the cognitive impairment in schizophrenia. The realization that cognitive impairment is a major contributor to the social disability in schizophrenia (8) has prompted investigators to evaluate what effects, if any, neuroleptics have on cognitive performance, and, more importantly, to include cognitive testing in efficacy trials of new anti-schizophrenia drugs. For example, despite its marked anticholinergic activity, clozapine was shown to benefit cognitive performance (49). Clozapine has been shown to release dopamine (DA) by in vivo microdialysis studies (18), and DA deficiency in the frontal cortex has produced cognitive impairment in primates (64). Thus, clozapine might benefit cognitive performance by enhancing DA neurotransmission. However, a second study which examined the effects of clozapine treatment on cognition reported no improvement in performance of chronic schizophrenic patients (28). Furthermore, because of clozapine's propensity to produce blood dyscrasia and occasionally hypotension and tachycardia, its large-scale use in geriatric schizophrenics is unlikely; therefore, other options to improve cognitive performance should be considered.

Because preliminary data regarding the pathophysiology of the cognitive impairment in schizophrenia are barely available, it is difficult to design rational therapies for this condition. In Alzheimer's disease, for example, finding a cholinergic deficiency led to the idea that cholinomimetic drugs might ameliorate Alzheimer's symptoms (see Chapter 120, *this volume*). It would not be implausible, however, to hypothesize that despite the fact that cognitively impaired schizophrenic patients do not show cortical cholinergic deficiencies (34) (also see following sections), cholinomimetic drugs might, nevertheless, benefit these patients. Cholinomimetics have been shown to improve learning behavior and attention in cholinergically intact rodents, and they have been shown to improve attention in normal volunteers (52). Furthermore, schizophrenic patients have an auditory gating deficit which in experimental animals is reversed by a nicotinic agonist (62). Moreover, in a brain region responsible for vigilance and attention, the levels of choline acetyltransferase were found to be decreased in schizophrenic patients (41). Together these data lead to the hypothesis that increasing cholinergic neurotransmission and maybe dopaminergic and noradrenergic neurotransmission (26) may improve attention, and hence cognitive functions, in schizophrenic patients.

Cognitive Impairment in Schizophrenia Versus Alzheimer's Disease

Alzheimer's disease (AD) is among the best characterized types of dementia in terms of specific areas of neuropsychological impairments and neurohistological abnormalities. By contrasting the cognitive profile of geriatric schizophrenics to that of AD patients (22), it is hoped that insight into the neural basis of dementing illnesses will be achieved. An overlap of specific cognitive deficits would suggest that clinically similar types of dementias could be associated with different neurohistological and neurochemical abnormalities. Partial dissimilarities in neuropsychological performance, together with the neurohistological investigation (see below), would support the view that these conditions involve different neural substrates.

In a comparison between the neuropsychological performance of geriatric schizophrenics and AD patients matched on level of global cognitive impairment, age, sex, and Z score education, we found that the schizophrenic patients performed worse than the AD patients on the Boston Naming test and the Praxis test. In contrast, the schizophrenic patients performed better than the AD patients on Delayed Recall, retaining 38% of the information presented relative to 23% retained by the AD patients. On the learning task, both groups performed poorly but not differently. This pattern of performance was present at all levels of global dementia severity. In spite of very close matching on measures known to affect psychometric performance (i.e., global dementia, severity, MMSE scores, age, and education), the schizophrenics and the AD patients could still be discriminated from one another on the basis of their neuropsychological test profiles. This pattern of double dissociation of neuropsychological performance indicated that despite equivalent levels of global dementia, schizophrenic and AD patients presented divergent profiles of cognitive dysfunction consistent with the notion that each dementia is associated with different neural abnormalities which in turn affect specific cognitive functions. It could be hypothesized that the cognitive impairments of geriatric schizophrenic patients are related to abnormalities of a mesial frontal–temporal neural circuit, whereas the impairments of AD are related to a disturbed temporal–parietal circuit, linking structures in the mesial temporal lobe (hippocampus, entorhinal cortex) to associational cortices in temporal and parietal lobes (see also Chapters 117 and 119, *this volume*).

POSTMORTEM STUDIES

Alzheimer's Disease-like Neuropathology in Schizophrenia

The most widely accepted neurochemical and neuropathological lesions believed to be associated with dementia in the elderly are those attributable to AD. The best correlates of dementia in AD have been deficits in cortical cholinergic markers, lesions of the basal forebrain cholinergic system, cortical neuritic plaques and neurofibrillary tangles, and deficits in cortical synaptic vesicular marker proteins, such as synaptophysin. In general (but note exceptions below), when these variables have been studied in schizophrenia they have not been found to be severely abnormal or to account for the cognitive impairment in those patients. For example, Burton et al. (16) examined the brains of 48 schizophrenic cases ranging in age between 22 and 99 years of age and found no significant differences from age-matched controls in neuritic plaques and neurofibrillary tangles. In a similar study, the brains of 12 schizophrenic cases (mean age 77, range 54–100) with evidence of cognitive impairment were compared to the brains of age- and sex-matched AD cases (60). No evidence of AD-like neuropathology in the schizophrenic group was observed in this study, nor in another study which extended these findings and demonstrated a lack of significant AD-like neuropathology even when severely cognitively impaired schizophrenics were contrasted to cases of non-cognitively impaired schizophrenics (6).

Sixty-two schizophrenic cases were compared to 116 AD cases using the CERAD neuropathology diagnostic battery. Brain specimens from each case were assessed for over 73 separate neuropathological categories, including neuritic plaques, neuritic plaques with amyloid cores, neurofibrillary tangles, neuronal cell loss, and gliosis in the cortex (midfrontal gyrus, middle and superior temporal gyrus, inferior parietal gyrus, entorhinal cortex) and in the hippocampus, amygdala, and nucleus basalis. Both cognitively impaired and cognitively nonimpaired schizophrenic groups differed significantly from the AD group on every neuropathological category assessed. Importantly, the significant differences between schizophrenics and AD cases were maintained even when 34 schizophrenic and AD pairs were matched on the basis of the severity of their cognitive impairment. Cognitively impaired and nonimpaired schizophrenic groups did not differ in any of the neuropathological categories assessed—with the exception of neurofibrillary tangles in the entorhinal cortex, which showed higher densities in the cognitively impaired patients. These results indicate that cognitive impairment in geriatric schizophrenic patients cannot be explained by an association with AD-like neuropathological variables such as the density of neuritic plaques or the density of neurofibrillary tangles in cortical and subcortical structures.

In sharp contrast to these conclusions are the results of a large study reported by Prohovnik et al. (59). The prevalence of AD-like neuropathology was found to be significantly increased in patients dying at state institutions with a chart diagnosis of schizophrenia relative to expected rates of AD in the general population. As pointed out by the authors, the diagnoses of schizophrenia obtained from clinical reports after death may not have been accurate in all 1046 cases reviewed. Furthermore, a selection bias for the demented cases remaining institutionalized may have been operating in this population. Moreover, the neuropathology criteria applied to diagnose AD differed from the CERAD diagnostic criteria. Nevertheless, the marked increase in the prevalence of AD-like neuropathology in schizophrenia reported in this study cannot be easily dismissed. The use of prospectively diagnosed cases of schizophrenia—and, more importantly, the use of modern diagnostic criteria for AD neuropathology (50) and of antibodies which recognize AD brain pathology, such as ALZ-50—may help clarify this apparent discrepancy.

In fact, immunoreactivity with the AD-related protein antibody, ALZ-50, has been studied in a small sample of schizophrenics. Cortical specimens from geriatric cognitively impaired schizophrenic cases were compared to specimens derived from geriatric controls and AD cases (58). Despite significant cognitive impairment, the ALZ-50 immunoreactivity of the cortical specimens derived from the schizophrenic cases was significantly different from the AD cases and indistinguishable from that of normal controls. There was no overlap of values between the AD group and the schizophrenic group. Similar results have been reported when ALZ-50 immunoreactivity has been examined in the nucleus accumbens, caudate nucleus, amygdala, temporal cortex, and cingulate cortex (39).

Cortical cholinergic marker deficits and the loss of cholinergic neurons in the basal forebrain are also characteristic of AD and have been shown to be causally related to compromised cognitive functioning in animals (35). Recently, cholinergic marker activity in six different cortical regions derived from geriatric controls, chronically institutionalized geriatric schizophrenic patients, and AD patients were compared (34). Cholinergic marker activity (choline acetyltransferase and acetylcholinesterase) was significantly diminished relative to controls in the AD cohort but not in the schizophrenic cohort. Additionally, cortical choline acetyltransferase activity was significantly and negatively correlated with the severity of cognitive impairment in the AD cohort, whereas no such correlations were evident in the schizophrenic cohort, suggesting that cognitive impairment in geriatric schizophrenics is not due to diminished cortical cholinergic activity.

Additionally, cognitively impaired geriatric schizophrenics did not differ from geriatric controls with respect to the number of large neurons (>30 μm) in the nucleus basalis of Meynert (23), suggesting that the basal forebrain neurons providing cholinergic afferents to the cortex are not affected in schizophrenia. Support for these findings was recently provided by another neuroanatomical study (38) which quantitatively assessed the density of acetylcholinesterase-positive fibers in five different cortical areas in schizophrenic and schizoaffective patients. A normal, age-appropriate pattern of cortical acetylcholinesterase staining was found in the study cohort.

On the other hand, some evidence in favor of brain cholinergic system involvement in schizophrenia does exist. The numbers of cholinergic interneurons in the striatum have been reported to be diminished in schizophrenic cases (38). In some studies, choline acetyltransferase activity is reported to be diminished in the nucleus accumbens and hippocampus by approximately 20% relative to controls, still a substantially smaller deficit than that which is normally noted in AD cases. The levels of choline acetyltransferase are also reported to be significantly reduced in the pedunculopontine nucleus of schizophrenic patients (41), but the relevance of this finding to dementia is not entirely clear.

In AD patients, decreased cortical immunoreactivity with antibodies against synaptic vesicular marker proteins such as synaptophysin has been found and interpreted as evidence consistent with synaptic loss (72). Synaptophysin-like immunoreactivity was found to be selectively decreased in the prefrontal cortex of schizophrenics in one study (25), whereas in another study (39) using an enzyme-linked immunosorbent assay (ELISA) technique and a different antibody for synaptophysin (EP10), the levels of synaptophysin-like immunoreactivity were found to be increased in the nucleus accumbens and temporal cortex of schizophrenics. Differences in technique (ELISA using tissue homogenates versus photodensitometry and immunocytochemistry), brain regions, age of subjects, and small sample sizes may well account for these disparate results. These observations, especially the correlations between synaptophysin-like immunoreactivity and severity of dementia in AD (72), argue in favor of a more intensive study of synaptic marker proteins in multiple brain regions of well-characterized schizophrenic populations with and without evidence of cognitive impairment.

In summary, the majority of the evidence suggests that

the dementia-like cognitive impairment of geriatric schizophrenics is *not* related to (a) the neuropathological features associated with dementia in AD (e.g., neuritic plaques, neurofibrillary tangles, neuronal loss in the basal forebrain), (b) diminished cortical cholinergic marker activity, or (c) increased immunoreactivity with antibodies to the AD-related protein ALZ-50. The most parsimonious conclusion which can be derived from the studies reviewed above is that the biological substrates of dementia-like cognitive impairment in schizophrenia are not similar to those of AD. This conclusion is consistent with clinical studies demonstrating (a) differences in specific areas of cognitive impairment between the two diseases and (b) the marked differences in rates of cognitive deterioration (see previous sections). The failure of the aforementioned class of central nervous system (CNS) lesions to account for the severe cognitive impairment of schizophrenia serves to direct research toward other variables which may more adequately explain the cognitive impairment of geriatric schizophrenic patients such as catecholamines, synaptophysin, and other markers of neuroanatomical lesions.

Other Non-Alzheimer's Disease-Related Histopathology in Schizophrenia

There is considerable cumulative evidence from the past century of postmortem research to suggest that there is significant, albeit inconsistent, neuropathology associated with the antemortem diagnosis of schizophrenia. This evidence could be interpreted to suggest that in schizophrenia there is an increased susceptibility to a wide range of neuropathological lesions, and that many of these lesions could lead to a general syndrome of dementia-like cognitive impairment in old age. A related "threshold" hypothesis would suggest that the presence of several concomitant lesions is necessary to produce the dementia-like clinical picture. These hypotheses, for which there is some support (see below), while partially accounting for the inconsistencies reported in neuropathological studies of schizophrenia, are unsatisfying because they fail to attribute the schizophrenic trait and the cognitive impairment associated with schizophrenia to any specific cause.

A number of findings of structural abnormalities appear to be replicable, but the specific nature of the abnormalities and of the precise anatomical locations differ from study to study (70). Other less vague abnormalities, including changes in cortical (cingulate and prefrontal) and hippocampal cytoarchitecture (9,10,21), await replication by independent laboratories using independent autopsy samples. However, these cytoarchitectural abnormalities are relevant because they elegantly demonstrate alterations in the fine structure of the frontal and cingulate cortices. Although the centrality of these cytoarchitectural abnormalities to the cognitive impairment of schizophre-

nia has not been determined, they do occur in (a) cortical regions (prefrontal cortex and cingulate cortex) known to be involved in the processes which subserve learning and memory in nonhuman primates (64) and (b) regions implicated by functional imaging studies of schizophrenia (76). As such, these cytoarchitectural abnormalities must be considered to be potential contributors to the cognitive deficits of geriatric schizophrenics.

The evidence suggests that reductions in the size or volume of the brain or certain cortical or subcortical regions and increases in ventricular volume are among the most readily replicable findings in the neuropathology of schizophrenia (37), but their relevance to the specific cognitive impairment is unclear. Typical of this class of findings are data reported from a cohort of 41 schizophrenic cases (15) showing significant ventricular enlargements, diminished overall brain weight, and thinner parahippocampal cortices relative to specimens derived from patients bearing diagnoses of affective disorder. Similar results, especially with respect to ventricular volume, have been reported when schizophrenic cases have been compared to age- and sex-matched controls without histopathological evidence of CNS disease (16,55). It is also interesting to note that when the study samples have included a relatively large age range, significant correlations between age of death and the severity of the neuropathologic lesions have not been reported (15). These findings are clearly supported by (a) the wealth of imaging studies of schizophrenic patients who often show clear evidence of enlarged ventricles and (b) some studies that report evidence of diminished cortical mantle width and length. Whether these nonspecific structural abnormalities contribute to the development of cognitive impairment in geriatric schizophrenics must still be determined.

Neurochemical Studies

There is little question that innumerable neurochemical abnormalities have been identified in the schizophrenic brain, and that at least some of these abnormalities, such as those associated with the dopaminergic system and some of the peptidergic systems, have been replicated in a number of different studies (11,54). Like the neuropathological and cytoarchitectural studies mentioned above, however, neurochemical investigations have not focused on age-related changes in schizophrenia and, with a few exceptions, have not related their findings to the cognitive impairment of geriatric schizophrenics. Once again, most specimens studied neurochemically have been derived from geriatric cases, a significant proportion of whom would be expected to suffer from severe cognitive impairment. Thus, it is possible that some of the neurochemical deficits noted in these patients and attributed to the schizophrenic illness provide, instead, a biological basis for cognitive impairment.

Different from the cholinergic system of the forebrain, which is not severely affected in geriatric schizophrenics, there is reason to believe that the catecholaminergic system of the forebrain, especially of the prefrontal and cingulate cortices, is affected and may contribute to the cognitive impairment of geriatric schizophrenics. The normal functioning of the mesocortical dopaminergic system has been found to be essential for normal cognitive functioning in nonhuman primates, and to be severely affected by the aging process (64). Given the hypothesized involvement of the mesocortical dopaminergic system in schizophrenia (11; see also Chapters 100 and 103, *this volume*), it is possible that poor cognitive functioning is among the consequences of the dopaminergic or other catecholaminergic deficits in schizophrenia. At least one study (12) reports deficits of norepinephrine in the hypothalamus and nucleus accumbens in cognitively impaired schizophrenics. Furthermore, nucleus accumbens DA and 3-methoxy-4-hydroxyphenylglyde (MHPG) were found to relate inversely to the degree of cognitive impairments, supporting a role for catecholaminergic modulation of cognitive functioning in geriatric schizophrenics. Unfortunately, this intriguing finding has not been confirmed or disconfirmed by follow-up independent studies.

Abnormalities in peptidergic systems have also been observed in schizophrenic patients (43), but their association with the cognitive impairment has not been addressed. In contrast, the involvement of peptidergic systems in dementing illnesses such as AD is not questioned (24). In a recent study, we investigated the concentrations of five neuropeptides [somatostatin (SLI), cholecystokinin (CCK), vasoactive intestinal polypeptide (VIP), corticotropin-releasing hormone (CRH), and neuropeptide Y (NPY)] in six different cortical regions representing the frontal, temporal, parietal, and occipital lobes was investigated. The specimens were derived from a cohort of cognitively impaired schizophrenics. The concentrations of these peptides in the schizophrenic group were compared to the concentration of the same neuropeptides in the same brain regions of normal geriatric controls and AD cases. Relative to geriatric controls, the concentrations of SLI, NPY, VIP, and CCK were significantly reduced in the schizophrenic cohort. Furthermore, a discriminant function analysis using NPY and SLI concentrations in the frontal and temporal lobes correctly identified 100% of the schizophrenic patients. Of particular relevance to the current discussion were the similarities and differences in the pattern of neuropeptide deficits in the cortices of the cognitively impaired schizophrenic group relative to patients suffering from AD dementia. First, although significant somatostatinergic deficits were present in the schizophrenic and AD cohorts, the SLI deficits were significantly more pronounced in the temporal cortex of the schizophrenic group than in the same cortical regions of the AD cohort, underscoring the role of the temporal lobe abnormalities in schizophrenia

(7,69). In addition, significant deficits were observed in the concentrations of VIP and CCK in the cortices of the schizophrenic cases, whereas deficits in these peptides were absent in the AD cohort. On the other hand, the concentrations of CRH were reduced in the cortices of the AD cases, but not in the cortices of the schizophrenics, indicating that the reported findings in schizophrenia were not reflective of generalized peptidergic deficits, but of deficits specific to schizophrenia. The profound reductions in the concentrations of SLI in the cortices of the schizophrenic group may be of relevance to the cognitive impairment observed in these cases because in AD the cortical concentrations of SLI have been found to correlate with the degree of cognitive impairment (4).

These results demonstrate that the pattern of neuropeptide deficits observed in cognitively impaired schizophrenics is markedly different from that in normal controls and from the pattern of neuropeptide deficits observed in AD, but that reduced SLI concentrations could be a marker for cognitive impairment shared by the two diseases. The findings further demonstrate that it is possible to isolate deficits in neurochemical variables which are relatively specific to schizophrenia and to begin to distinguish between those neurochemical deficits which can be directly attributed to known neurodegenerative processes and those which may be nondegenerative and static in nature (see Chapters 51 and 84 for related issues).

A speculative but intriguing aspect of the neuropeptide deficits observed in the schizophrenic cohort is that the decrements in the cortical concentrations of NPY and SLI in the schizophrenic cohort may be manifestations of the potential neurodevelopmental lesions hypothesized in schizophrenia (see Chapter 98, *this volume*). NPY and SLI have been shown to be colocalized in human cortical neurons exhibiting nicotinamide-adenine dinucleotide phosphate (NADPH)-diaphorase activity (44,75). Recent evidence suggests that neurodevelopmental abnormalities may lead to the aberrant dislocation of NADPH-positive neurons to the cortical white matter in schizophrenics (2,3). It is possible that the NPY and SLI deficits noted above are manifestations of the same neurodevelopmental "lesions" which cause the dislocation of NADPH-positive neurons in schizophrenia.

In summary, because very few studies have directly addressed the question of the neurochemical correlates of the cognitive impairment of schizophrenia, it is difficult to associate the cognitive impairments of geriatric schizophrenics with any specific neurochemical abnormalities. The available results do suggest, however, that abnormalities in neuropeptide-containing neurons (such as those associated with SLI and NPY) and possible alterations in cortical catecholaminergic functioning may contribute to the cognitive impairment.

An emerging awareness of factors which contribute to variability in postmortem studies, combined with increasingly sophisticated neurochemical and neuropathoanatomical techniques, promises a bright future in the next generation of studies. Critically important to the potential for future research is (a) the accumulation of normative neurochemical and neuropathoanatomical data from prospectively studied cognitively intact populations and (b) prospective atheoretical characterization of the symptoms and histories of the cases used in the neurochemical and neuropathoanatomical studies of schizophrenia. The historical characterization of the cases studied is important because the principal goal of research in the years to come must be the elucidation and discrimination of the neurochemical and neuropathoanatomical substrates of the schizophrenic trait, independent of the prevailing state of the patients shortly prior to, or at the time of, death. There is every reason to believe that studies currently underway using brain specimens derived from schizophrenic patients with varying degrees of cognitive impairment will help us to address the question of the neurochemical and neuroanatomical substrates of cognitive impairment in geriatric schizophrenics.

CONCLUSIONS

Investigations reviewed in this chapter indicate that a subtype of the schizophrenic illness exists in which severe cognitive impairment in old age is a predominant and incapacitating symptom. Indirect evidence suggests that this subtype of illness is characterized by (a) moderate cognitive impairment and persistent negative symptoms early in the course of the illness, (b) age-associated worsening of cognitive impairment with persistent negative symptoms for most of the lifespan, and (c) dementia-like cognitive impairment in old age. Illness severity and chronicity in general, and cognitive impairment and negative symptoms in particular, seem to be the cause, not the result, of lengthy or uninterrupted hospitalization and of intensive somatic treatment.

Without a 60-year catamnestic follow-up study it is not possible to estimate what proportion of all individuals who in late adolescence or early adulthood receive a diagnosis of schizophrenia suffer in senescence from cognitive impairment which is severe enough to distinguish it from normal aging and to significantly affect social functioning. Because this is impractical, the only other solution to address this question is to conduct an epidemiological study of the geriatric schizophrenic patients who reside in nursing homes. The study, which would verify if indeed the estimate that the majority (200,000) of all (300,000) geriatric schizophrenic patients in the United States reside in nursing homes is accurate, would determine what proportion of these patients suffer from cognitive impairment and whether the outcome of the geriatric schizophrenic patients who have remained in long-term psychiatric hospitals is not representative of the outcome of schizophrenia in general. Investigating the proportion of cognitively impaired geriatric schizophrenic patients would help elucidate the role of cognitive impairment in determining the long-term outcome of schizophrenia in general and the need to live in protected environments such as nursing homes in particular.

When differences between age groups are not very large, this observation in conjunction with the postmortem data are not supportive of a rapid degenerative process occurring across the lifespan or during the latter decades of life of the schizophrenic patients. A number of studies have reported a slow decrease in some CNS structural and functional parameters with advancing age in "cognitively intact," normal populations (17,73). Of particular interest to schizophrenia are (a) age-related changes reported in normals in neuronal numbers of the dopaminergic and noradrenergic systems and (b) reports that aging primates are hyporeactive to pharmacological dopaminergic challenges (17,19; Arnsten, 1994, *personal communication*). Age-associated reduction in DA activity superimposed on static dopaminergic abnormalities in areas relevant to cognitive functioning could produce the appearance of slow progression of cognitive impairment and alteration of symptom clusters in schizophrenic patients. This superimposition is probably most apparent and damaging in the most severely ill schizophrenic patients with the greatest preexisting cognitive impairment and possibly dopaminergic hypoactivity. Thus, the extent to which current neuropathological studies contribute to the debate concerning the static versus degenerative nature of the disease process is to suggest that clinical evidence of age-related differences in cognitive functioning in a subgroup of patients with early, preexisting cognitive impairment is not sufficient to warrant a conclusion of progressive neuropathology. The data are rather consistent with an interaction between preexisting lesion(s) and aging in the context of chronic illness. The available data suggest that it is unlikely that the cognitive impairment in schizophrenia can be attributed to neuropathological conditions with known degenerative etiology. On the other hand, it must be kept in mind that the numbers of studies directly addressing this question are so few that this conclusion is tenuous, and far from one which comes after having taken into account all possible alternatives and problems associated with testing the null hypothesis.

ACKNOWLEDGMENTS

This work was supported by the following: National Institute of Mental Health (NIMH) grant 46436-05, awarded to Michael Davidson, M.D.; NIMH grant 45212-02, awarded to Kenneth L. Davis, M.D.; and a Veterans Affairs Merit Review grant, 5118-011, awarded to Vahram Haroutunian, Ph.D., and Michael Davidson, M.D. The authors wish to acknowledge Paul Hartel for his assistance in the preparation of this manuscript.

REFERENCES

1. Abrahamson D. Institutionalization and the long-term course of schizophrenia. *Br J Psychiatry* 1993;162:533–538.
2. Akbarian S, Bunney WE, Potkin SG, et al. Altered distribution of nicotinamide-adenine dinucleotide phosphate-diaphorase cells in frontal lobe of schizophrenics implies disturbances of cortical development. *Arch Gen Psychiatry* 1993;50:169–177.
3. Akbarian S, Vinuela A, Kim JJ, Potkin SG, Bunney WE, Jones EG. Distorted distribution of nicotinamide-adenine dinucleotide phosphate-diaphorase neurons in temporal lobe of schizophrenics implies anomalous cortical development. *Arch Gen Psychiatry* 1993;50:178–187.
4. Alhainen K, Sirviö J, Helkala EL, Reinikainen K, Riekkinen P. Somatostatin and cognitive functions in Alzheimer's disease—the relationship of cerebrospinal fluid somatostatin increase with clinical response to tetrahydroaminoacridine. *Neurosci Lett* 1991;130:46–48.
5. Andreason NC, Olsen S. Negative vs. positive schizophrenia. *Arch Gen Psychiatry* 1982;39:789–794.
6. Arnold SE, Franz BR, Trojanowski JQ. Lack of neuropathological findings in elderly patients with schizophrenia and dementia. *Neurosci Abstr* 1993;18:340–350.
7. Arnold SE, Hyman BT, Van Hoesen GW, Damasio AR. Some cytoarchitectural abnormalities of the entorhinal cortex in schizophrenia. *Arch Gen Psychiatry* 1991;48:625–632.
8. Bellack AS, Mueser KT. Psychosocial treatment for schizophrenia. *Schizophr Bull* 1993;19(2):199–448.
9. Benes FM, Majocha R, Bird ED, Marotta CA. Increased vertical axon counts in cingulate cortex of schizophrenics. *Arch Gen Psychiatry* 1987;44:1017–1021.
10. Benes F, McSparren J, Bird E, SanGiovanni J, Vincent S. Deficits in small interneurons in prefrontal and cingulate cortices of schizophrenic and schizoaffective patients. *Arch Gen Psychiatry* 1991;48:996–1001.
11. Bird E, Barnes J, Iversen L, Spokes E, Mackay A, Shepherd M. Increased brain dopamine and reduced glutamic acid decarboxylase and choline acetyl transferase activity in schizophrenia and related psychoses. *Lancet* 1977;3:1157–1159.
12. Bridge TP, Kleinman JE, Karoum F, Wyatt RJ. Postmortem central catecholamines and antemortem cognitive impairment in elderly schizophrenics and controls. *Neuropsychobiology* 1985;14:57–61.
13. Brier A, Schreiber JL, Dyer J, Pickar D. National Institute of Mental Health longitudinal study of schizophrenia: prognosis and predictors of outcome. *Arch Gen Psychiatry* 1991;48:239–246.
14. Bromet EJ, Schwartz JE, Fennig S, et al. The epidemiology of psychosis: the Suffolk County Mental Health Project. *Schizophr Bull* 1992;18(2):243–255.
15. Brown R, Colter N, Corsellis N, et al. Postmortem evidence of structural brain changes in schizophrenia. *Arch Gen Psychiatry* 1986;43:36–42.
16. Burton C, Crow T, Frith C, Johnstone E, Owens D, Roberts G. Schizophrenia and the brain: a prospective clinico-neuropathological study. *Psychol Med* 1990;20:285–304.
17. Calne D, Peppard R. Aging of the nigrostriatal pathway in humans. *Can J Neurol Sci* 1987;14:424–427.
18. Chai B, Meltzer HY. The effect of chronic clozapine on basal dopamine release and apomorphine-induced DA release in the striatum and nucleus accumbens as measured by in vivo brain microdialysis. *Neurosci Lett* 1992;140(1):47–50.
19. Chan-Palay V, Asan E. Quantitation of catecholamine neurons in the locus coeruleus in human brains of normal young and older adults and in depression. *J Comp Neurol* 1989;287:357–372.
20. Ciompi L. The natural history of schizophrenia in the long-term. *Br J Psychiatry* 1980;136:413–420.
21. Conrad A, Scheibel A. Schizophrenia and the hippocampus: the embryological hypothesis extended. *Schizophr Bull* 1987;3(4):577–587.
22. Davidson M, Haroutunian V, Gabriel SM, et al. Cognitive impairment in elderly schizophrenic patients. *Schizophr Res* 1994;11(2):162.
23. El-Mallakh RS, Kirch DG, Shelton R, et al. The nucleus basalis of Meynert, senile plaques, and intellectual impairment in schizophrenia. *J Neuropsychiatry Clin Neurosci* 1991;3:383–386.
24. Gabriel SM, Bierer LM, Haroutunian V, Purohit DP, Perl DP, Davis KL. Widespread deficits in somatostatin but not neuropeptide-Y concentrations in Alzheimer's disease cerebral cortex. *Neurosci Lett* 1993;155:116–120.
25. Glantz LA, Lewis DA. Synaptophysin immunoreactivity is selectively decreased in the prefrontal cortex of schizophrenic subjects. *Neurosci Abstr* 1993;18:84–90.
26. Goldberg TE, Bigelow LB, Weinberger DR, et al. Cognitive and behavioral effects of the coadministration of dextroamphetamine and haloperidol in schizophrenia. *Am J Psychiatry* 1991;148:78–84.
27. Goldberg TE, Hyde TM, Lleinman JE, Weinberger DR. Course of schizophrenia: neuropsychological evidence for a static encephalopathy. *Schizophr Bull* 1993;19(4):797–804.
28. Goldberg TE, Greenberg R, Griffin S, et al. Impact of clozapine on cognitive impairment and clinical symptoms in patients with schizophrenia. *Br J Psychiatry* 1993;162:43–38.
29. Goldberg TE, Weinberger DR, Berman KF, Pliskin NH, Podd MH. Further evidence for dementia of the pre-frontal type in schizophrenia. *Arch Gen Psychiatry* 1987;44:1008–1014.
30. Goldstein G, Zubin J. Neuropsychological differences between young and old schizophrenics with and without associated neurological dysfunction. *Schizophr Res* 1990;3:117–126.
31. Goldstein G, Zubin J, Pogue-Geile MF. Hospitalization and the cognitive deficits of schizophrenia: the influences of age and education. *J Nerv Ment Dis* 1991;179(4):202–205.
32. Gurland BJ, Cross PS. Epidemiology of psychopathology in old age. *Psychiatr Clin North Am* 1982;98(4):478–486.
33. Harding CM, Zubin J, Strauss JS. Chronicity in schizophrenia revisited. *Br J Psychiatry* 1992;161(Suppl 18):27–37.
34. Haroutunian V, Davidson M, Kanof PD, et al. Cortical cholinergic markers in schizophrenia. *Schizophr Res* 1994;12:137–144.
35. Haroutunian V, Santucci AC, Davis KL. Neurotransmitter interactions and responsivity to cholinomimetic agents. In: Levin ED, Decker MW, Butcher LL, eds. *Neurotransmitter interactions and cognitive function.* Boston: Birkhauser, 1992;118–143.
36. Heaton RK, Drexler M. Clinical neuropsychological findings in schizophrenia and aging. In: Miller NE, Cohen GD, eds. *Schizophrenia and aging.* New York: Guilford Press, 1987.
37. Heckers S, Heinsen H, Heinsen Y, Beckmann H. Limbic structures and lateral ventricle in schizophrenia. *Arch Gen Psychiatry* 1990;47:1016–1022.
38. Heckers S, Mash D, Geula C, Mesulam MM. Basal forebrain and striatal cholinergic neurons in schizophrenia. *Neurosci Abstr* 1993;18:340.6.
39. Honer WG, Kaufmann CA, Kleinman JE, Casanova MF, Davies P. Monoclonal antibodies to study the brain in schizophrenia. *Brain Res* 1989;500:379–383.
40. Johnstone EC, Owens DGC, Gold A, Crow TJ, Macmillan JF. Institutionalization and the defects of schizophrenia. *Br J Psychiatry* 1981;139:195–203.
41. Karson CN, Casanova MR, Kleinman JE, Griffin WST. Choline acetyltransferase in schizophrenia. *Am J Psychiatry* 1993;150(3):454–459.
42. Karson CN, Lyon N, Bracha HS, Guggenheim FG. The profile of cognitive impairment in elderly dyskinetic subjects. *J Neuropsychiatry Clin Neurosci* 1993;5:61–65.
43. Kerwin R, Robinson P, Stephenson J. Distribution of CCK binding sites in the human hippocampal formation and their alteration in schizophrenia: a post-mortem autoradiographic study. *Psychol Med* 1992;22:37–43.
44. Kowall NW, Beal MF. Cortical somatostatin, neuropeptide Y, and NADPH diaphorase neurons: normal anatomy and alterations in Alzheimer's disease. *Ann Neurol* 1988;23:105–114.
45. Lohr J, Wisniewski A, Jeste DV. Neurological aspects of tardive dyskinesia. In: Nasrallah HA, Weinberger DR, eds. *The neurology of schizophrenia.* Amsterdam: Elsevier Science Publishers, 1986;97–119.
46. Lyon N, Lawson W, Amick R, Karson C. The profile of cognitive impairment in elderly schizophrenic subjects. *Biol Psychiatry* 1992;31:193(A).
47. Mathai PJ, Gopinath PS. Deficits of chronic schizophrenia in relation to long-term hospitalization. *Br J Psychiatry* 1985;148:509–516.

48. McKenna PJ, Lund CE, Mortimer AM. Negative symptoms: relationship to other schizophrenic symptom classes. *Br J Psychiatry* 1989;155(Suppl 7):104–107.
49. Meltzer HY. Dimensions of outcome with clozapine. *Br J Psychiatry [Suppl]* 1992;17:46–53.
50. Mirra SS, Heyman A, McKeel D, et al. The Consortium to Establish a Registry for Alzheimer's Disease (CERAD). Part II. Standardization of the neuropathologic assessment of Alzheimer's disease. *Neurology* 1991;41:479–486.
51. Morris JC, Edland S, Clark C, et al. The Consortium to Establish a Registry for Alzheimer's Disease (CERAD). Part IV. Rates of cognitive change in the longitudinal assessment of probable Alzheimer's disease. *Neurology* 1993;43:2457–2465.
52. Muir JL, Dunnett SB, Robins TW, Everitt BJ. Attentional functions of the forebrain cholinergic systems: effects of intraventricular hemicholinium, physostigmine, basal forebrain lesions and intracortical grafts on a multiple-choice serial reaction time task. *Exp Brain Res* 1992;89:611–622.
53. Mukherjee P, Decina P, Scapicchio PL. Temporal course of cognitive impairment in elderly, chronic schizophrenic patients: a prospective longitudinal study. *Schizophr Res* 1993;9(2):105–106.
54. Nemeroff CB, Bissette G. Neuropeptides, dopamine, and schizophrenia. *Ann NY Acad Sci* 1988;537:273–291.
55. Pakkenberg B. Post-mortem study of chronic schizophrenic brains. *Br J Psychiatry* 1987;151:744–752.
56. Paulsen JS, Heaton R, Jeste DV. Neuropsychological impairment in tardive dyskinesia. *Neuropsychology* 1994;8(2):227–241.
57. Peterson RC, Smith E, Kokmen E, Ivnik RJ, Tangalos EG. Memory function in normal aging. *Neurology* 1992;42:396–401.
58. Powchik P, Davidson M, Nemeroff CB, et al. Alzheimer's disease related protein in geriatric schizophrenic patients with cognitive impairment. *Am J Psychiatry* 1994;150:1726–1727.
59. Prohovnik I, Dwork AJ, Kaufman MA, Willson N. Alzheimer-type neuropathology in elderly schizophrenia patients. *Schizophr Bull* 1993;19:805–816.
60. Purohit DP, Davidson M, Perl DP, et al. Severe cognitive impairment in elderly schizophrenic patients: a clinicopathological study. *Biol Psychiatry* 1993;33:255–260.
61. Regier DA, Boyd JH, Burke JD, et al. One-month prevalence of mental disorders in the United States. *Arch Gen Psychiatry* 1988;45(11):977–986.
62. Rollins LY, Logel J, Drebing C, et al. Evidence for association of the α7 neuronal nicotinic cholinergic receptor with auditory evoked potential deficits in schizophrenia [Abstract 340.4]. *Soc Neurosci Abstr* 1993;19:837.
63. Rosenstein MJ, Milazzo-Sayre LJ, Manderscheid RW. Characteristics of persons using specialty inpatient, outpatient, and partial care programs in 1986. In: Manderscheid RW, Sonnenschein MA, eds. National Institute of Mental Health. *Mental Health, United States, 1990.* DHHS publication no. (ADM)90-1708. Washington, DC: Superintendent of Documents, US Government Printing Office, 1990;139–172.
64. Sawaguchi T, Goldman-Rakic PS. D1 dopamine receptors in prefrontal corex: involvement in working memory. *Science* 1991;251:947–950.
65. Saykin AJ, Gur RC, Gur RE, et al. Neuropsychological function in schizophrenia. *Arch Gen Psychiatry* 1991;48:618–632.
66. Schaie KW. The impact of methodological changes in gerontology. *Int J Aging Hum Dev* 1992;35(1):19–29.
67. Schwartzman AE, Douglas VI. Intellectual loss in schizophrenia, Part I. *Can J Psychol* 1962;16:1–10.
68. Serper MR, Bergman RL, Harvey PD. Medication may be required for the development of automatic information processing in schizophrenia. *Psychiatr Res* 1990;32(3):281–288.
69. Shenton ME, Kikinis R, Ferenc A, et al. Abnormalities of the left temporal lobe and thought disorder in schizophrenia: a quantitative magnetic resonance imaging study. *N Engl J Med* 1992;327(9):604–612.
70. Stevens J. Neuropathology of schizophrenia. *Arch Gen Psychiatry* 1982;39:1131–1139.
71. Strahan GW. Prevalence of selected mental disorders in nursing and related care homes. In: Manderscheid RW, Sonnenschein MA, eds. National Institute of Mental Health. *Mental Health, United States, 1990.* DHHS publication no. (ADM)90-1708. Washington, DC: Superintendent of Documents, U.S. Government Printing Office, 1990;227–240.
72. Terry RD, Masliah E, Salmon DP, et al. Physical basis of cognitive alterations in Alzheimer's disease: synapse loss is the major correlate of cognitive impairment. *Ann Neurol* 1991;30:572–580.
73. Terry R, DeTeresa R, Hansen L. Neocortical cell counts in normal human adult aging. *Ann Neurol* 1987;21(6):530–539.
74. Uhlmann RF, Larson EB. Effect of education on the Mini-Mental State Examination as a screening test for dementia. *J Am Geriatr Soc* 1991;39(9):876–880.
75. Unger JW, Lange W. NADPH-diaphorase-positive cell populations in the human amygdala and temporal cortex: neuroanatomy, peptidergic characteristics and aspects of aging and Alzheimer's disease. *Acta Neuropathol (Berl)* 1992;83:636–646.
76. Weinberger DR, Berman KF, Suddath R, Torrey EF. Evidence of dysfunction of a prefrontal-limbic network in schizophrenia: a magnetic resonance imaging and regional cerebral blood flow study of discordant monozygotic twins. *Am J Psychiatry* 1992;149:890–897.
77. Wexler BE. Beyond the Kraepelinian dichotomy. *Biol Psychiatry* 1992;31:539–541.
78. Wing JK, Brown J. *Institutionalism and Schizophrenia* London: Cambridge University Press, 1970.
79. Wyatt RJ. Neuroleptics and the natural course of schizophrenia. *Schizophr Bull* 1991;17:325–351.
80. Wykes T. The prediction of outcome in community care. *Schizophr Res* 1994;11(2):174–175.

Psychopharmacology: The Fourth Generation of Progress, edited by Floyd E. Bloom and David J. Kupfer. Raven Press, Ltd., New York © 1995.

CHAPTER 124

Psychotropic Drug Metabolism in Old Age

Principles and Problems of Assessment

Lisa L. von Moltke, David J. Greenblatt, Jerold S. Harmatz, and Richard I. Shader

As our capacity to understand and treat medical problems of the elderly becomes more refined, the proportion of the American population that is over the age of 65 is increasing. Emotional and psychiatric disorders are commonplace in the elderly population and are disproportionately prevalent in geriatric populations when compared to groups of younger age (9,53,66). As such, the appropriate use of psychotropic drugs in the elderly assumes major importance in clinical medicine (11,46,47, 61,64,77). Elderly individuals may respond uniquely to psychotropic drug treatment as a consequence of alterations in disease characteristics associated with old age or because of intrinsic age-related changes in drug sensitivity occurring at the neuroreceptor site mediating drug action (6). Pharmacologic response may also change in the elderly due to alterations in pharmacokinetics associated with the aging process.

Changes in drug absorption, distribution, elimination, and clearance in elderly populations have been the subject of many studies over the past two decades or more (13,20,26,30,33,34,45,47,58,64,65,69,70). Although many of these studies focus on psychotropic drugs, the quality of the data base is variable, often because the elderly present special problems and constraints. Previous reports have extensively reviewed the status of understanding of age-related changes in psychotropic drug disposition, and we will not present the entire data

base again in this chapter. Instead we will focus on theoretical and practical methodological considerations in the design and interpretation of studies of altered psychotropic drug disposition in old age. The first section deals with fundamental pharmacokinetic principles, including the concepts of clearance, distribution, elimination, absorption, and protein-binding. Emphasis is placed on the biologic bases of these concepts, methods of measurement, their relation to physiologic changes in the elderly, and implications for psychotropic drug use in the aging population. The second section outlines options available for the design and implementation of studies of drug disposition in old age, including their benefits and limitations, and implications for the quality of the current data base.

PHARMACOKINETIC PRINCIPLES

Clearance

The concept of clearance is a cornerstone of the understanding of the discipline of pharmacokinetics (22,24,25,28,72,73). Clearance is a mathematical construct having units of volume divided by time (i.e., ml/min or liters/hr). It refers to the total amount of blood, serum, or plasma from which a substance is completely removed per unit time. Alternatively, clearance may be viewed as the rate of drug removal per unit of plasma concentration. Physicians usually first encounter the concept of clearance in the context of renal function, whereby creatinine clearance is used as an indirect index of renal function. Under the assumption that the endogenous sub-

L. L. von Moltke, D. J. Greenblatt, J. S. Harmatz, and R. I. Shader: Department of Pharmacology and Experimental Therapeutics, Tufts University School of Medicine, Boston, Massachusetts 02111; and Division of Clinical Pharmacology, New England Medical Center, Boston, Massachusetts 02111.

stance, creatinine, is completely cleared by the kidney, renal clearance of creatinine can be used as an indicator of glomerular filtration rate.

Clearance also applies to the removal of drugs and other foreign chemicals. Clearance is the single most reliable index of the capacity of a given patient to remove a given drug. For most drugs used in clinical practice, the major mechanisms of drug clearance are hepatic biotransformation or renal excretion. For drugs cleared by the kidney, a significant fraction of the administered drug is recovered unchanged in the urine (Fig. 1). For hepatically metabolized drugs, products of biotransformation may ultimately be recovered in the urine, although this does not imply that the intact drug undergoes renal clearance.

Of the drugs encountered in psychopharmacology, lithium is cleared primarily by renal clearance (36,39), as are the hydroxylated metabolites of the cyclic antidepressants (78). Essentially all other psychotropic drugs are cleared by hepatic biotransformation. The effect of age on renal clearance of drugs excreted intact by the kidney is relatively straightforward to understand and predict, since renal function, as measured by glomerular filtration rate or other functional indexes, on the average declines with age (12,18,43,44,51,55). As such, an age-related decline in clearance of lithium can be anticipated (36,39). The problem is not so straightforward in the case of hepatic biotransformation. Liver metabolism of drugs is mediated by a variety of groups of enzymes and enzyme systems whose activities are not uniformly influenced by age (10,35,50,71,76).

Hepatic blood flow constitutes an upper limit of clearance for drugs that are metabolized by the liver, since clearance cannot exceed the rate of drug delivery to the clearing organ. In healthy individuals, hepatic blood flow

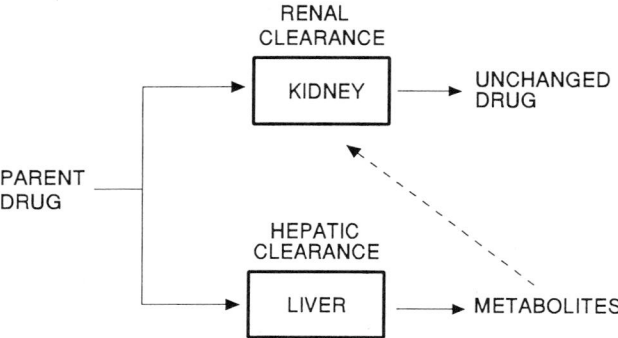

FIG. 1. Renal clearance and hepatic biotransformation are two possible mechanisms of drug clearance. When a drug undergoes renal clearance, a significant fraction of the dose is recovered in the urine in unchanged form. When a drug undergoes hepatic clearance, liver enzyme systems change the molecular structure of the parent compound. The metabolites produced by hepatic biotransformation often appear in the systemic circulation and are excreted by the kidney (*dashed line*), but this does not imply renal clearance of the parent drug.

usually falls in the range of 1500–1800 ml/min, although there is considerable individual variation. Some studies suggest a decline in hepatic blood flow with age. Unfortunately, there is no straightforward noninvasive clinical test that can be used routinely to quantitate this parameter.

The numeric value of a drug's clearance relative to hepatic blood flow has important clinical implications (24,52,72,73). Many of the benzodiazepine anxiolytics have low values of hepatic clearance (less than 10% of hepatic blood flow). For such drugs, first-pass metabolism (presystemic extraction) after oral dosage is minimal, and absolute bioavailability after oral dosage is generally greater than 80%. That is, more than 80% of an orally administered dose ultimately reaches the systemic circulation. For these low-clearance drugs, a reduction in hepatic clearance associated with old age will have the effect of prolonging elimination half-life rather than changing the peak plasma concentration after oral dosage. In contrast, many of the cyclic antidepressants and antipsychotic agents have values of hepatic clearance exceeding 50% of hepatic blood flow (4,8,14,19,57,68,70). These drugs undergo substantial presystemic extraction after oral administration, such that a relatively small fraction of an oral dose actually reaches the systemic circulation. Oral doses needed to produce a particular therapeutic endpoint generally will be higher than parenteral doses of the same drug needed for the same endpoint. For these drugs, a reduction in hepatic clearance may lead to a prolongation of half-life but will also be associated with an increase in the peak plasma concentration after oral dosage (24,52,72,73).

For any drug metabolized by the liver, the predicted hepatic extraction ratio (ER) can be calculated as the ratio of clearance after intravenous dosage divided by hepatic blood flow. The maximum systemic availability of an orally administered dose (F) can then be calculated as:

$$F \leq 1 - \text{ER} \quad [1]$$

Thus, the greater a drug's intravenous clearance relative to hepatic blood flow, the lower the maximum systemic availability after oral dosage (Fig. 2).

Clearance is the major biologic determinant of steady-state plasma concentration (C_{ss}) during chronic administration. Assuming that a drug has been administered long enough for the steady state to be reached, C_{ss} can be calculated as:

$$C_{ss} = \frac{\text{Dosing rate}}{\text{Clearance}} \quad [2]$$

Dosing rate, presumably determined by the health care professional, can be viewed as the "input" determinant: It is the rate at which the drug is given to the patient. If clearance is constant, C_{ss} will increase in proportion to dosing rate in any given patient. It is important to remember that *actual* dosing rate is influenced by patient compli-

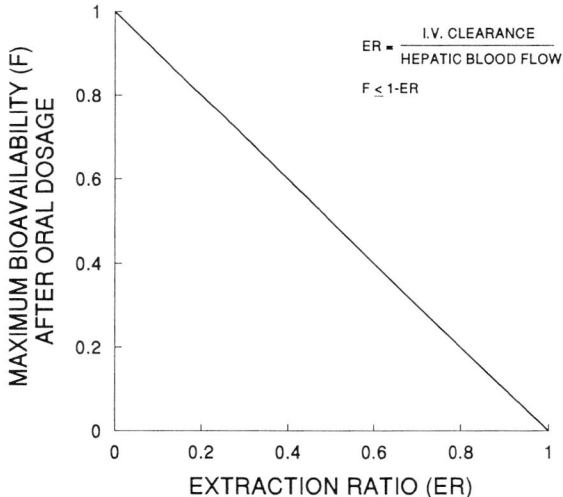

FIG. 2. The relation of hepatic extraction ratio (*x* axis) to maximum bioavailability of a drug after oral dosage (*y* axis) for a drug whose clearance is due entirely to hepatic biotransformation. Extraction ratio (ER) is calculated as the ratio of clearance after intravenous dosage divided by hepatic blood flow. Oral bioavailability (*F*) cannot exceed the quantity 1 − ER.

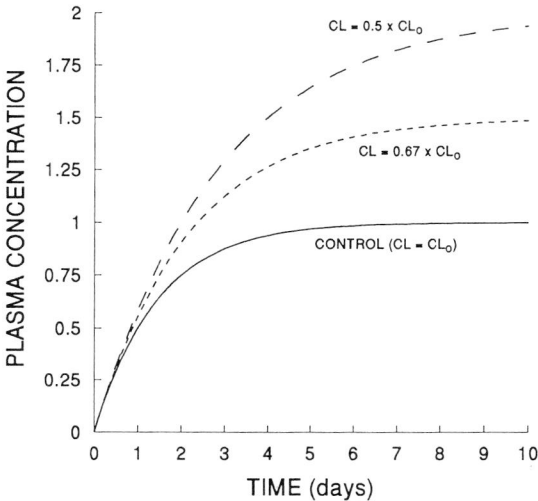

FIG. 3. Effect of a change in clearance on the extent of drug accumulation during chronic dosage, and on the rate of attainment of steady state. In the control condition, clearance = CL_0, and elimination half-life = 1.0 days. After initiation of a constant dosage regimen at time = 0 (*solid line*), the steady-state plasma concentration is 1.0 units, and approximately 4 days (4 × $t_{1/2}$) are required for steady state to be more than 90% attained. Assuming the same volume of distribution and dosing rate, reduction of clearance relative to the control value (*dashed lines*) increases the steady-state plasma concentration and prolongs the time necessary to attain steady state. When CL = 0.5 × CL_0, the steady-state plasma concentration is 2.0 units, half-life is 2.0 days, and 8 days (4 × $t_{1/2}$) are necessary for 90% attainment of steady state.

ance and therefore does not necessarily correspond to the *intended* dosing rate as decided upon by the health care professional. The denominator of this equation is clearance, which represents the capacity of that particular patient to eliminate that particular drug.

Clearance then is a biologic variable that cannot be directly measured or predicted without actually giving that particular patient a test dose of the drug in question. Because clearance appears in the denominator, its importance is evident. If drug clearance declines with old age, C_{ss} will correspondingly increase unless dosing rate is appropriately reduced (Fig. 3). Increases in C_{ss} may be associated with a greater likelihood of drug toxicity. For this reason, clearance is almost always a major focus of studies of altered drug disposition and old age.

Distribution

Drug distribution is not a measure of drug clearance or removal and is completely independent of clearance. Drug distribution is determined by physicochemical properties: the drug's relative solubility in lipid as opposed to water (lipophilicity), its affinity for various body tissues, the blood flow to each of these tissues, and the drug's binding to plasma protein. Only a small fraction of the total amount of a psychotropic drug present in the body interacts with the specific neuroreceptor recognition site in the brain. Uptake of drug by peripheral sites will accordingly influence the amount that is available to the brain.

Body habitus typically changes with age, even if total body weight does not change significantly (5,16,28,60,62). The amount of adipose tissue relative to total body weight generally will increase as a person ages, while the fraction of lean body mass correspondingly decreases. The same pattern of age-related change will occur in both men and women, but at any age, women have a higher fraction of body weight comprised of adipose tissue than do men. Thus both age and gender influence body habitus, and gender is therefore a potential confounding factor in pharmacokinetic studies in the elderly.

The extent of drug distribution can be quantitated using the pharmacokinetic concept of volume of distribution (V_d). This is a hypothetical quantity having units of volume (liters) that is defined as follows:

$$V_d = \frac{\text{Amount of drug in the body}}{\text{Concentration in reference compartment}} \quad [3]$$

The "reference compartment" in this equation usually refers to blood, serum, or plasma, and therefore V_d represents the amount of drug in the body divided by the blood or plasma concentration. Lipophilic drugs, including most psychotropic agents, have large values of V_d, indicating that the plasma concentration is small relative to the amount of drug in the body. For cyclic antidepressants, for example, the pharmacokinetic V_d may be 10 times the size of the body, or even more. On the other hand, relatively nonlipophilic drugs such as lithium will have smaller V_d, indicating that a larger fraction of what is present in the body is found in blood, serum, or plasma. It must be emphasized that pharmacokinetic V_d is hypothetical, and does not refer to any specific anatomic entity.

Because of age-related changes in body habitus, pharmacokinetic V_d for many drugs will change with increasing age (28,33). V_d for lipophilic drugs typically will be larger in elderly subjects when compared to young individuals of the same gender, even when total body weight does not differ between groups. This is explained by the greater fraction of total body weight comprised of adipose tissue in the elderly. Conversely, V_d of nonlipophilic drugs may be reduced in the elderly relative to young controls.

V_d itself, and changes in V_d with age, are of importance for two reasons. First, elimination half-life depends on both V_d and clearance, as described below. Second, the duration of action of many lipophilic psychotropic drugs following single doses is dependent mainly on distribution rather than elimination or clearance. This phenomenon is described in detail elsewhere in this volume (see Chapter 74, *this volume*). The duration of action of some psychotropic drugs may be expected to change in the elderly as a consequence of a change in distribution, but this theoretical possibility has not been tested in controlled studies.

Elimination

The rate of drug disappearance in the post-distributive phase after a single dose, or after termination of multiple dose treatment, is quantitated as an elimination half-life. The same half-life applies to the rate of attainment of steady-state after initiation of multiple dose therapy (without a loading dose), or the rate of attainment of a new steady-state condition if the maintenance dose is increased or decreased. Elimination half-life is currently recognized as potentially misleading as a pharmacokinetic variable, because it is a dependent quantity related to V_d and clearance as follows:

$$\text{Elimination half-life} = \frac{0.693 \cdot V_d}{\text{Clearance}} \qquad [4]$$

We ordinarily think of elimination half-life as being inversely related to clearance. That is, low clearance (inefficient drug removal) implies long elimination half-life, and the reverse. This intuitive relationship is correct only in situations when V_d is relatively constant, an untenable assumption when pharmacokinetic properties are being evaluated in relation to age. For any given drug, V_d may increase or decrease as a function of age, depending on lipophilicity and body habitus. V_d also will be influenced

by gender. Since either or both V_d and clearance may be affected by aging, elimination half-life should not be used as the sole index of the capacity for drug removal. The relationship of half-life to V_d is most evident in pharmacokinetic studies of lipophilic drugs in obese individuals (1,2,29). In such studies, clearance may not be significantly different between obese subjects and normal-weight controls matched for age and sex. Elimination half-life, however, greatly increases in obese individuals only because of their increased V_d.

Absorption

Studies of the pharmacokinetics of drug absorption commonly address questions on the rate and the extent of drug absorption from the gastrointestinal tract. That is, how fast the drug is absorbed, and how much of what is administered actually reaches the systemic circulation. Structural and functional changes in the aging gastrointestinal tract are well-documented (15,21,40,41,48). Cytochrome P450-3A4 is present in human gastrointestinal tract mucosa and may contribute to presystemic extraction of some drugs, such as cyclosporine (38,75). It is possible that the apparent activity of gastrointestinal as well as hepatic Cytochrome P450-3A4 may change with age. Observations such as these have led to speculation that absorption of orally administered medications may be reduced and/or delayed in old age. However, systematic studies of drug absorption in the elderly fail to validate this presumption. The rate and extent of absorption of several orally administered psychotropic medications are not importantly changed in elderly subjects when compared to young controls (Table 1).

Protein Binding

Many psychotropic drugs are extensively though reversibly bound to plasma protein. For some drugs, such as diazepam, the extent of binding is very high, with only 1–2% of the total concentration in plasma being in the unbound state (49). Albumin and alpha-1 acid glycoprotein (AAG) are the two plasma proteins usually responsible for drug binding (32,42,54,56,63,67,74).

Old age may be associated with a reduced extent of

TABLE 1. *Psychotropic drugs for which the rate and extent of absorption after oral dosage is uninfluenced by age*

Chlordiazepoxide
Diazepam
Lorazepam
Midazolam
Trazodone
Flumazenil

drug binding to plasma protein (26,33). This is best documented for drugs bound to plasma albumin. Because albumin concentrations tend to decline with age (23), the extent of drug binding may also be reduced, leaving higher fractions of unbound drug in plasma. The effect of age on plasma binding for drugs bound to AAG is not clearly established (3).

A widely disseminated but incorrect dictum in the medical literature states that reduced plasma binding of psychotropic drugs in the elderly yields increased amounts of unbound drug available for pharmacologic action, and therefore a greater intensity of drug action. The free fraction (FF) of drug in plasma can be calculated as the ratio of free (unbound) concentration divided by total (free plus bound) concentration. This relationship is arithmetically correct but biologically wrong (32). The form of the equation which correctly delineates the dependent and independent biological variables is as follows:

$$\text{Total concentration} = \frac{\text{Free concentration}}{\text{Free fraction}} \quad [5]$$

The independent variables are on the right-hand side of the equation. FF is a physicochemical variable determined by the concentration of the binding protein, the concentration of the drug, and the drug's affinity for the binding protein. In the numerator is free concentration, which is completely independent of FF. Free concentration depends on the dosing rate and the liver's capacity to remove the free drug ("free clearance"), as described in Equation 2. The dependent variable, on the left side of the equation, is total concentration. Assume a physiologic situation in which dosing rate and free clearance are constant; therefore, free concentration is constant. If drug protein binding decreases (FF increases), the result will be a reduction in total concentration (32). Thus FF influences total drug concentration, but by itself has no effect on either free concentration or the drug's pharmacologic action (Fig. 4) Since most drug assays measure total rather than free concentration, interpretation of total concentrations may be influenced by changes in FF (17,32). In studies of clinical situations (such as old age) in which drug binding to plasma protein may be altered, FF must be measured to assure correct interpretation of pharmacokinetic data based on total drug concentrations in plasma.

APPLICATION OF THE PRINCIPLES: OPTIONS FOR STUDY DESIGN

The design and execution of experimental protocols evaluating age-related changes in psychotropic drug disposition requires investigators to integrate an understanding of the principles described above together with the practical and ethical limits of various design options. Two broad categories of design can be applied. Each has benefits and drawbacks, but neither by itself will provide the

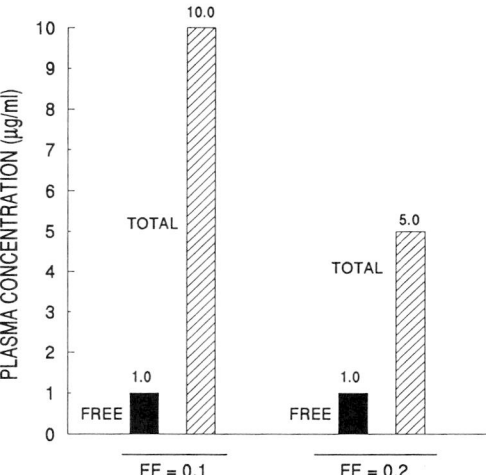

FIG. 4. Effect of a change in protein binding (free fraction, FF) on steady-state plasma concentrations of free (unbound) drug and total (free plus bound) drug. It is assumed that dosing rate and free clearance are constant. **Left:** Free fraction is 0.1; that is, the drug is 90% bound to plasma protein. The free concentration is 1.0 μg/ml, and the total concentration is 10.0 μg/ml. **Right:** An intervening factor reduces the extent of plasma protein binding. The free fraction is now 0.2; the drug is 80% bound to protein. Since dosing rate and free clearance are not changed, steady-state free concentration remains at 1.0 μg/ml. However, the total concentration falls to 5.0 μg/ml.

complete answer. This section considers the two major design options, along with an example of how each can be applied to the same research question.

Controlled Pharmacokinetic Studies

Important data on psychotropic drug disposition in the elderly have been generated through well-controlled clinical pharmacokinetic studies. These studies generally involve healthy volunteers who can be screened to exclude potentially confounding factors such as medical disease, concurrent medications, or extremes of body habitus. The interacting effects of age and gender on pharmacokinetics can be separated by study of separate cohorts of young male, young female, elderly male, and elderly female volunteers.

The study design typically involves administration of a single dose of the medication in question to subjects in all cohorts. Plasma concentrations of the drug are measured at multiple points in time after the dose, and pharmacokinetic methods are used to determine pertinent variables such as clearance, V_d, and elimination half-life. Multiple dosing schemes may be used to verify the relation between the single-dose kinetic profile and plasma concentrations during multiple dosage.

Well-controlled intensive-design studies provide the most complete and accurate description of the pharmacokinetic properties of a given drug in volunteer cohorts. Important confounding factors can be controlled for or eliminated, and the influence of age by itself on drug disposition can be isolated. This approach also has drawbacks. Sample sizes within each cohort generally are limited by the time, patience, and financial resources of the investigators. The representativeness of the study cohorts to the general population can never be determined. If variability within groups is large, the statistical power of comparisons will be reduced, with an increased possibility of failing to detect an important difference that would be demonstrable with a larger sample size. Finally, not all categories of psychotropic drugs are equally suitable for study in healthy volunteers. With proper subject selection and monitoring, and appropriate choice of dosage size, young and elderly volunteers can participate in single-dose kinetic studies of anxiolytics, hypnotics, and most antidepressants. Many such studies are reported in the medical literature (30,34,70). Controlled pharmacokinetic studies of neuroleptics, on the other hand, are few in number, owing to the potential hazards and discomfort associated with these agents, particularly in the elderly (14,19). A further complication is that analytic techniques for quantitation of neuroleptics in plasma following single doses are technically difficult and not widely available.

Population Studies

A second important methodological approach involves the study of plasma concentrations of psychotropic drugs during actual clinical use by larger groups of patients taking the medications for clinical purposes. The prinicpal advantages of this approach are that large numbers of patients can be studied at relatively low cost with essentially no unwarranted risk to the participants. A further benefit is that the study population is "real"; that is, it is precisely the group of patients that actually needs and takes the medication. The population study design also has drawbacks. At most only a few steady-state plasma concentrations are available for any given patient. The only pharmacokinetic variable that can be calculated is clearance. This requires an accurate record of dosing rate, which still can be influenced to an unknown degree by compliance. The time of sampling relative to dosage usually is not controlled and may not even be known. Therefore, steady-state concentrations may be influenced by interdose fluctuation as well as by dosing rate and clearance. Additional confounding factors must be suspected, since real patient populations may have concurrent medical disease, and be taking other medications which could alter plasma concentrations of the drug in question. Finally, drug doses in clinical populations generally are titrated to optimize response, and variations in plasma concentrations will reflect differences in dosage as well as possible effects of age. The statistical analysis must incorporate the effect of dosage when evaluating the influence of age on steady-state plasma concentration.

Application of the Methods

To illustrate the nature of these two approaches, two studies on the benzodiazepine derivative alprazolam are described. An intensive design study evaluated the pharmacokinetics of single 1-mg oral doses of alprazolam in healthy young and elderly male volunteers (27). Age-related differences in alprazolam clearance are shown in Fig. 5. The effect of age was highly significant, with alprazolam clearance reduced an average of 50% in the elderly men compared to the young male controls. A second study evaluated steady-state plasma concentrations of alprazolam in male patients receiving the drug for the treatment of panic disorder in a controlled clinical trial (31). A plasma alprazolam concentration was measured at week 10 of treatment. Daily dosage of alprazolam varied widely among patients, ranging from 1 to 10 mg/day. Because dose was a major determinant of steady-state plasma level, the effect of age could be evaluated only after normalization for dosage. This dose-normalized plasma concentration is shown on the y-axis of fig. 6, while patient age is shown on the x-axis. Dose-normalized plasma level increased significantly with age ($r = 0.24$, $p < 0.05$), but the size of the squared correlation coefficient ($r^2 = 0.06$) indicates that age explains only a small fraction of the variance.

Thus the intensive design pharmacokinetic study in a small group of carefully screened normal volunteers does not yield identical findings as a study of steady-state alprazolam concentrations during actual treatment of panic

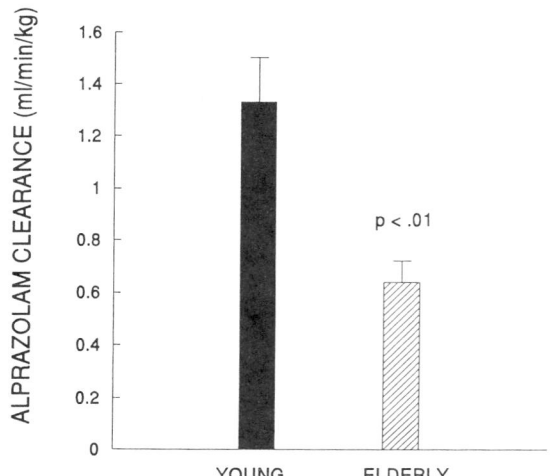

FIG. 5. Mean ($\pm$SE) values of alprazolam clearance in a series of healthy young and elderly male volunteers ($N = 8$ in each group) who ingested a single 1.0-mg oral dose of alprazolam. The difference is highly significant. (Adapted from ref. 27, with permission.)

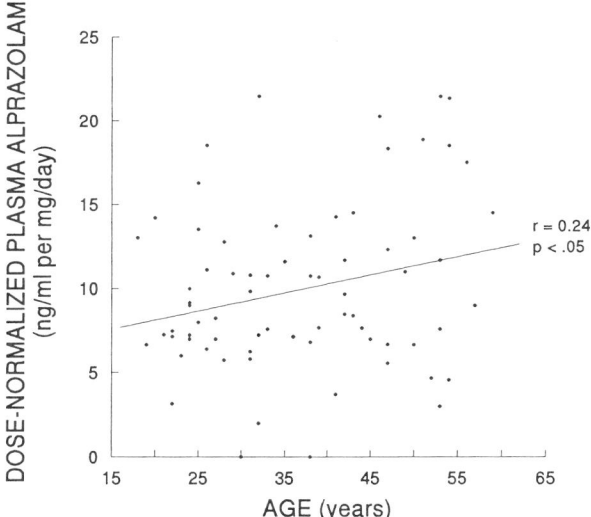

FIG. 6 Relation of age (*x* axis) to dose-normalized steady-state plasma alprazolam concentration (ng/ml per mg/day, *y* axis) in a series of 74 male patients receiving alprazolam for the treatment of panic disorder in a multicenter clinical trial (31). Dose-normalized plasma concentration increases significantly with age ($r = 0.24$, $p < 0.05$), but the size of the squared correlation coefficient ($r^2 = 0.06$) indicates that age accounts for only a small proportion of variance.

TABLE 2. *Psychotropic drugs whose hepatic clearance is impaired in healthy elderly subjects*

Chlordiazepoxide
Diazepam[a]
Desmethyldiazepam
Alprazolam[a]
Triazolam[a]
Midazolam[a]
Bromazepam
Desalkylflurazepam
Clobazam
Loprazolam
Imipramine[a]
Trazodone

[a] Established as probable substrates for the Cytochrome P450-3A4 subfamily.

disorder in a clinical trial. However, the possibility cannot be excluded that confounding factors masked an actual effect of age in the population study. Furthermore, the maximum age in the population study was 59 years, whereas the mean age in the intensive-design study was 70 years (range: 62–77 years).

QUALITY OF THE DATA BASE

The effects of age on the pharmacokinetics of psychotropic drugs have been extensively reviewed elsewhere. The quality of the data base is highly variable. It is most solid in the case of benzodiazepine derivaties (30,34). Reasonable data are also available for a number of cyclic antidepressants and for trazodone, although the antidepressant data base is not nearly as reliable as that for benzodiazepines (70). Some data are available for the serotonin-reuptake-inhibitor antidepressants, although the information has been slow to reach the peer-reviewed medical literature (68). Data on the neuroleptic agents are relatively weak, largely due to ethical problems with studies in volunteers, and difficulties with analytical methodology (14,19).

Most benzodiazepines are metabolized by microsomal oxidation, with Cytochrome P450-3A4 identified as a major responsible cytochrome (Table 2). The weight of the data indicate impairment of clearance of these drugs in old age, particularly among men (30,34). For benzodiazepines metabolized by glucuronide conjugation, the weight of

the data indicates that age has only a small effect on clearance. A similar conclusion can be drawn for nitrazepam, which is biotransformed by nitroreduction (30). Since clonazepam is metabolized by the same pathway, it can be expected that age would not greatly influence its clearance, but this has not been studied.

Among cyclic antidepressants, clearance of imipramine (also mediated in part by P450-3A4) appears impaired in old age (4,8,20,70). Some data suggest that amitriptyline clearance may also be reduced in the elderly, but this is not a consistent observation (59,70). Clearance of trazodone appears to be impaired in old age, particularly among men (7,29). For other antidepressants, study findings of age effects on clearance either are conflicting, or are affected by methodologic drawbacks that preclude definitive interpretation (37,70).

THE FUTURE OF GERIATRIC PHARMACOKINETICS

The pharmacokinetic profile of a new psychotropic medication usually is elucidated in the pre-marketing phase of drug development by studies of healthy young normal male volunteers. Yet the target population of afflicted individuals who ultimately are treated with the drug may consist largely of women and the elderly, about whom little or no pharmacokinetic data are available before the drug reaches the market. This is changing, as women and the elderly are becoming priorities for pre-marketing studies of drug disposition. Understanding age-related alterations in pharmacokinetics is critical to the decision-making by clinicians who must estimate modifications in dosage needed for treatment of elderly patients.

ACKNOWLEDGMENTS

This work was supported by Grant MH-34223 from the Department of Health and Human Services. Dr. von

Moltke is the recipient of an Abbott Laboratories Fellowship in Clinical Pharmacology.

REFERENCES

1. Abernethy DR, Greenblatt DJ. Pharmacokinetics of drugs in obesity. *Clin Pharmacokinet* 1982;7:108–124.
2. Abernethy DR, Greenblatt DJ. Drug disposition in obese humans: an update. *Clin Pharmacokinet* 1986;11:199–213.
3. Abernethy DR, Kerzner L. Age effects on alpha-1-acid glycoprotein concentration and imipramine plasma protein binding. *J Am Geriatr Soc* 1984;32:705–708.
4. Abernethy DR, Greenblatt DJ, Shader RI. Imipramine and desipramine disposition in the elderly. *J Pharmacol Exp Ther* 1985;232:183–188.
5. Barlett HL, Puhl SM, Hodgson JL, Buskirk ER. Fat-free mass in relation to stature: ratios of fat-free mass to height in children, adults, and elderly subjects. *Am J Clin Nutr* 1991;53:1112–1116.
6. Barnhill JG, Greenblatt DJ, Miller LG, Gaver A, Harmatz JS, Shader RI. Kinetic and dynamic components of increased benzodiazepine sensitivity in aging animals. *J Pharmacol Exp Ther* 1990;253:1153–1161.
7. Bayer AJ, Pathy MSJ, Ankier SI. Pharmacokinetic and pharmacodynamic characteristics of trazodone in the elderly. *Br J Clin Pharmacol* 1983;16:371–376.
8. Benetello P, Furlanut M, Zara G, Baraldo M. Imipramine pharmacokinetics in depressed geriatric patients. *Int J Clin Pharmacol Res* 1990;10:191–195.
9. Blazer D. Depression in the elderly. *N Engl J Med* 1989;320:164–166.
10. Cholerton S, Daly AK, Idle JR. The role of individual human cytochromes P450 in drug metabolism and clinical response. *Trends Pharmacol Sci* 1992;13:434–439.
11. Chrischilles EA, Foley DJ, Wallace RB, Lemke JH, Semla TP, Hanlon JT, Glynn RJ, Ostfeld AM, Guralnik JM. Use of medications by persons 65 and over: data from the established populations for epidemiologic studies of the elderly. *J Gerontol* 1992;47:M137–M144.
12. Cockcroft DW, Gault MH. Prediction of creatinine clearance from serum creatinine. *Nephron* 1976;16:31–41.
13. Durnas C, Loi C-M, Cusack BJ. Hepatic drug metabolism and aging. *Clin Pharmacokinet* 1990;19:359–389.
14. Ellenbroek BA. Treatment of schizophrenia: a clinical and preclinical evaluation of neuroleptic drugs. *Pharmacol Ther* 1993;57:1–78.
15. Evans MA, Triggs EJ, Cheung M, Broe GA, Creasey H. Gastric emptying rate in the elderly: implications for drug therapy. *J Am Geriatr Soc* 1981;29:201–205.
16. Forbes GB, Reina JC. Adult lean body mass declines with age: some longitudinal observations. *Metabolism* 1970;19:653–663.
17. Friedman H, Greenblatt DJ. Rational therapeutic drug monitoring. *JAMA* 1986;256:2227–2233.
18. Friedman JR, Norman DC, Yoshikawa TT. Correlation of estimated renal function parameters versus 24-hour creatinine clearance in ambulatory elderly. *J Am Geriatr Soc* 1989;37:145–149.
19. Froemming JS, Lam YWF, Jann MW, Davis CM. Pharmacokinetics of haloperidol. *Clin Pharmacokinet* 1989;17:396–423.
20. Furlanut M, Benetello P. The pharmacokinetics of tricyclic antidepressant drugs in the elderly. *Pharmacol Res* 1990;22:15–25.
21. Geokas MC, Haverback BJ. The aging gastrointestinal tract. *Am J Surg* 1969;117:881–892.
22. Greenblatt DJ. Pharmacokinetic principles in clinical practice (Clinical Therapeutic Conference). *J Clin Pharmacol* 1992;32:118–123.
23. Greenblatt DJ. Reduced serum albumin concentration in the elderly: a report from the Boston Collaborative Drug Surveillance Program. *J Am Geriatr Soc* 1979;27:20–22.
24. Greenblatt DJ. Presystemic extraction: mechanisms and consequences. *J Clin Pharmacol* 1993;33:650–656.
25. Greenblatt DJ, Koch-Weser J. Clinical pharmacokinetics. *N Engl J Med* 1975;293:702–705, 964–970.
26. Greenblatt DJ, Abernethy DR, Shader RI. Pharmacokinetic aspects of drug therapy in the elderly. *Ther Drug Monit* 1986;8:249–255.
27. Greenblatt DJ, Divoll M, Abernethy DR, Moschitto LJ, Smith RB, Shader RI. Alprazolam kinetics in the elderly: relation to antipyrine disposition. *Arch Gen Psychiatry* 1983;40:287–290.
28. Greenblatt DJ, Divoll M, Abernethy DR, Shader RI. Physiologic changes in old age: relation to altered drug disposition. *J Am Geriatr Soc* 1982;30(suppl):s6–s10.
29. Greenblatt DJ, Friedman H, Burstein ES, Scavone JM, Blyden GT, et al. Trazodone kinetics: effect of age, gender, and obesity. *Clin Pharmacol Ther* 1987;42:193–200.
30. Greenblatt DJ, Harmatz JS, Shader RI. Clinical pharmacokinetics of anxiolytics and hypnotics in the elderly: therapeutic considerations. *Clin Pharmacokinet* 1991;21:165–177, 262–273.
31. Greenblatt DJ, Harmatz JS, Shader RI. Plasma alprazolam concentrations: relation to efficacy and side effects in the treatment of panic disorder. *Arch Gen Psychiatry* 1993;50:715–722.
32. Greenblatt DJ, Sellers EM, Koch-Weser J. Importance of protein binding for the interpretation of serum or plasma drug concentrations. *J Clin Pharmacol* 1982;22:259–263.
33. Greenblatt DJ, Sellers EM, Shader RI. Drug disposition in old age. *N Engl J Med* 1982;306:1081–1088.
34. Greenblatt DJ, Shader RI, Harmatz JS. Implications of altered drug disposition in the elderly: studies of benzodiazepines. *J Clin Pharmacol* 1989;29:866–872.
35. Guengerich FP. Human cytochrome P-450 enzymes. *Life Sci* 1992;50:1471–1478.
36. Hardy BG, Shulman KI, MacKenzie SE, Kutcher SP, Silverberg JD. Pharmacokinetics of lithium in the elderly. *J Clin Psychopharmacol* 1987;7:153–158.
37. Harmatz JS, Greenblatt DJ. Falling off the straight line: some hazards of correlation and regression. *J Clin Psychopharmacol* 1992;12:75–78.
38. Hebert MF, Roberts JP, Prueksaritanont T, Benet LZ. Bioavailability of cyclosporine with concomitant rifampin administration is markedly less than predicted by hepatic enzyme induction. *Clin Pharmacol Ther* 1992;52:453–457.
39. Hewick DS, Newbury P, Hopwood S, Naylor G, Moody J. Age as a factor affecting lithium therapy. *Br J Clin Pharmacol* 1977;4:201–205.
40. Holt PR, Balint JA. Effects of aging on intestinal lipid absorption. *Am J Physiol* 1993;264:G1–G6.
41. Horowitz M, Maddern GJ, Chatterton BE, Collins PJ, Harding PE, Shearman DJC. Changes in gastric emptying rates with age. *Clin Sci* 1984;67:213–218.
42. Koch-Weser J, Sellers EM. Binding of drugs to serum albumin. *N Engl J Med* 1976;294:311–316, 526–531.
43. Levi M, Rowe JW. Aging and the kidney. In: Schrier RW, Gottschalk W, eds. *Diseases of the kidney*. Boston: Little Brown and Co, 1988;2657–2679.
44. Lindeman RD. Changes in renal function with aging: implications for treatment. *Drugs Aging* 1992;2:423–431.
45. Loi C-M, Vestal RE. Drug metabolism in the elderly. *Pharmacol Ther* 1988;36:131–149.
46. Mellinger GD, Balter MB, Uhlenhuth EH. Prevalence and correlates of the long-term regular use of anxiolytics. *JAMA* 1984;251:375–379.
47. Montamat SC, Cusack BJ, Vestal RE. Management of drug therapy in the elderly. *N Engl J Med* 1989;321:303–309.
48. Moore JG, Tweedy C, Christian PE, Datz FL. Effect of age on gastric emptying of liquid–solid meals in man. *Dig Dis Sci* 1983;28:340–344.
49. Moschitto LJ, Greenblatt DJ. Concentration-independent plasma protein binding of benzodiazepines. *J Pharm Pharmacol* 1983;35:179–180.
50. Murray M. P450 enzymes: inhibition mechanisms, genetic regulation and effects of liver disease. *Clin Pharmacokinet* 1992;23:132–146.
51. Nicoll SR, Sainsbury R, Bailey RR, King A, Frampton C, Elliot JR, Turner JG. Assessment of creatinine clearance in healthy subjects over 65 years of age. *Nephron* 1991;59:621–625.
52. Pond SM, Tozer TN. First-pass elimination: basic concepts and clinical consequences. *Clin Pharmacokinet* 1984;9:1–25.
53. Regier DA, Boyd JH, Burke JD, Rae DS, Myers JK, Kramer M, Robins LN, George LK, Karno M, Locke BZ. One-month preva-

lence of mental disorders in the United States. *Arch Gen Psychiatry* 1988;45:977–986.

54. Rothschild MA, Oratz M, Schreiber SS. Serum albumin. *Hepatology* 1988;8:385–401.

55. Rowe JW, Andres R, Tobin JD, Norris AH, Shock NW. Age-adjusted standards for creatinine clearance. *Ann Intern Med* 1976;84:567–568.

56. Salive ME, Cornoni-Huntley J, Phillips CL, Guralnik JM, Cohen HJ, Ostfeld AM, Wallace RB. Serum albumin in older persons: relationship with age and health status. *J Clin Epidemiol* 1992;45:213–221.

57. Sallee FR, Pollock BG. Clinical pharmacokinetics of imipramine and desipramine. *Clin Pharmacokinet* 1990;18:346–364.

58. Schmucker DL. Aging and drug disposition: an update. *Pharmacol Rev* 1985;37:133–148.

59. Schultz P, Turner-Tamiyasu K, Smith G, Giacomini KM, Blaschke TF. Amitriptyline disposition in young and elderly normal men. *Clin Pharmacol Ther* 1983;33:360–366.

60. Schwartz RS, Shuman WP, Bradbury VL, Cain KC, Fellingham GW, Beard JC, Kahn SE, Stratton JR, Cerqueira MD, Abrass IB. Body fat distribution in healthy young and older men. *J Gerontol* 1990;45:M181–M185.

61. Shader RI, Greenblatt DJ. Use of benzodiazepines in anxiety disorders. *N Engl J Med* 1993;328:1398–1405.

62. Shimokata H, Tobin JD, Muller DC, Elahi D, Coon PJ, Andres R. Studies in the distribution of body fat. I. Effects of age, sex, and obesity. *J Gerontol* 1989;44:M66–M73.

63. du Souich P, Verges J, Erill S. Plasma protein binding and pharmacological response. *Clin Pharmacokinet* 1993;24:435–440.

64. Thompson TL, Moran MG, Nies AS. Psychotropic drug use in the elderly. *N Engl J Med* 1983;308:134–138, 194–199.

65. Tumer N, Scarpace PJ, Lowenthal DT. Geriatric pharmacology: basic and clinical considerations. *Annu Rev Pharmacol Toxicol* 1992;32:271–302.

66. Uhlenhuth EH, Balter MB, Mellinger GD, Cisin IH, Clinthorne J. Symptom checklist syndromes in the general population: correlations with psychotherapeutic drug use. *Arch Gen Psychiatry* 1983;40:1167–1173.

67. Vallner JJ. Binding of drugs by albumin and plasma protein. *J Pharm Sci* 1977;66:447–465.

68. van Harten J. Clinical pharmacokinetics of selective serotonin reuptake inhibitors. *Clin Pharmacokinet* 1993;24:203–220.

69. Vestal RE. Pharmacology and aging. *J Am Geriatr Soc* 1982;30:191–200.

70. von Moltke LL, Greenblatt DJ, Shader RI. Clinical pharmacokinetics of antidepressants in the elderly: therapeutic implications. *Clin Pharmacokinet* 1993;24:141–160.

71. von Moltke LL, Greenblatt DJ, Harmatz JS, Shader RI. Cytochromes in psychopharmacology. *J Clin Psychopharmacol* 1994;14:1–4.

72. Wilkinson GR. Clearance approaches in pharmacology. *Pharmacol Rev* 1987;39:1–47.

73. Wilkinson GR, Shand DG. A physiological approach to hepatic drug clearance. *Clin Pharmacol Ther* 1975;18:377–390.

74. Wood M. Plasma drug binding: implications for anesthesiologists. *Anesth Analg* 1986;65:786–804.

75. Watkins PB. Drug metabolism by cytochromes P450 in the liver and small bowel. *Gastrointest Clin North Am* 1992;21:511–526.

76. Wrighton SA, Stevens JC. The human hepatic cytochromes P450 involved in drug metabolism. *Crit Rev Toxicol* 1992;22:1–21.

77. Wysowski DK, Baum C. Outpatient use of prescription sedative–hypnotic drugs in the United States, 1970 through 1989. *Arch Intern Med* 1991;151:1779–1783.

78. Young RC. Hydroxylated metabolites of antidepressants. *Psychopharmacol Bull* 1991;27:521–532.

Psychopharmacology: The Fourth Generation of Progress, edited by Floyd E. Bloom and David J. Kupfer. Raven Press, Ltd., New York © 1995.

CHAPTER 125

Pharmacological Treatment of Depression in Late Life

Carl Salzman, Lon S. Schneider, and George S. Alexopoulos

Major depression is a serious disorder in late life. Although common, it is less frequent in elderly adults than in younger adults. The 1-year prevalence of major depression among community-dwelling persons aged 65 years or older is approximately 1%, with an approximately 2% prevalence of dysthymic disorder (5,40).* The prevalence is greater in women than in men. Significant depressive symptoms without a major depression diagnosis occur in approximately 8–15% of community residents over 65 years of age (6). Elderly patients hospitalized for a medical illness have an even higher prevalence of depression, with a rate of 40% for combined major and minor depression (38) (see Chapters 89–90, *this volume*).

In nursing home residents, major depression has been estimated at approximately 12%, while lesser but clinically significant depression occurs in an additional 30–35% (19). The rates of new cases of depression in nursing homes are striking, with a 14% incidence of major depression over a 6-month period. Those at highest risk for major depression are the cognitively intact nursing home patients who are sickest, most disabled, and most dependent, compared to cognitively impaired residents (24% versus 10%, respectively). Patients with major depression show increased mortality, with death rates between 1.5 and 3 times those of other residents (33).

Compared to early-onset geriatric depressives, patients with late-onset depression appear to have less frequent family histories of mood disorders, higher prevalence of dementing disorders, more impairment in neuropsycho-logical tests, higher rate of dementia follow-up, and more neurosensory hearing impairment.

As in younger people, the course of depression in the elderly is characterized by exacerbations and remissions, as well as chronicity. Sixty percent of elderly patients who recover from an index episode have at least another subsequent one; relapse and chronicity occur in up to 40% of depressed patients (3). Mortality is significant, with an annual death rate of about 10%; delusional depression is associated with greater morbidity and mortality than in patients without delusions (29). The rate of completed suicides for older people is over twice as high as that of the general population (26.5/100,000 in 80- to 84-year-olds compared to 12.4/100,000 overall) (8).

Despite progress in treatment with antidepressant drugs, longitudinal studies indicate significant chronicity (42). Although about 60% of elderly depressed patients remain well at 1–6 years follow-up, the other 40% show relapse, only partial improvement, chronicity, or death (29). Chronicity of depression in the elderly may be predicted by coexisting medical illness, high severity of depression, nonmelancholic presentation, and delusions.

Although depression in the elderly may symptomatically resemble younger life depression, there is considerable diagnostic heterogeneity. Consequently, the search for diagnostic biological markers of depression has been particularly important in the elderly. In addition to symptomatic variability from patient to patient (7,60), there is diagnostic overlap with dementia, as well as the presence of medical illnesses which may obscure the diagnosis (2). Data summarizing attempts to identify a biological marker are presented in Table 1. As with young persons, no spe-

C. Salzman: Department of Psychiatry, Harvard Medical School, Boston, Massachusetts 02115.

L. S. Schneider: Department of Psychiatry, University of Southern California School of Medicine, Los Angeles, California 90033.

G. S. Alexopoulos: Department of Psychiatry, Cornell University Medical College, White Plains, New York 10605.

NOTE: Owing to space limitation, complete references have not been provided for this chapter. When multiple citations were possible, the authors have chosen to select the single most recent citation. Complete references are available from the first author on request.

TABLE 1. *Biological markers for depression in the elderly*[a]

Marker	Comment
MHPG	Poorly correlated with depression. Effect of age uncertain. May correlate with late age of onset.
Increased α_2 binding	Poorly correlated with depression. May correlate with late age of onset.
Platelet MAO	Higher in elderly hospitalized females. Associated with presence of medical illness in elderly depressives. Reported in elderly depressives with "reversible dementia."
[3]IMI	Decrease in geriatric depression in all but one study. Also decrease more in primary depression as compared with depression secondary to medical illness. Associated with poor response to AD treatment. Normal in Alzheimer's dementia.
DST	More frequent in geriatric as compared with younger depressed patients. Low specificity; also occurs in one-third of demented patients.
TRH–TSH	Low specificity: reported in geriatric depressives and in Alzheimer's disease.
CT	Decreased lateral brain ventricle size in geriatric depression. More pronounced in late-onset compared to early-onset patients. Associated with poor AD response.
MRI	White-matter hypersensitivity in elderly as well as young depressives. More pronounced in late- compared to early-onset depression. Associated with poor AD response.
REM latency	Found in elderly as well as young depressives. High specificity; not found in Alzheimer's disease.
CSF somatostatin	Not affected by age. Not specific: decreased in depression and Alzheimer's disease.
CSF CRF	Possible increase with age. Increased in major depression. Decreased in dementia.
CSF arginine vasopressin	Not specific: decreased in unipolar depression and in dementia.

[a] Owing to space limitations, references are not included; complete table and chapter references are available from the first author on request.

MHPG, 3-methoxy-4-hydroxyphenylglycol; MAO, monoamine oxidase; [3]IMI, tritiated imipramine binding; DST, Dexamethasone Suppression Test; TRH-TSH, Thyrotropin-Releasing Hormone Test; CT, computed axial tomography; MRI, magnetic resonance imaging; REM, rapid eye movement; CSF, cerebrospinal fluid; CRF, corticotropin-releasing factor.

cific diagnostic test for late-life depression has yet been developed.

TREATMENT OF DEPRESSION

Appreciation of the age-associated changes in the bioavailability of antidepressants is important when treating older patients. The aging process is associated with changes in the pharmacokinetic characteristics of antidepressant drugs, including altered absorption, distribution, metabolism, and excretion of medications. The most clinically significant changes, however, occur in hepatic and renal clearance.

Hepatic clearance of antidepressants is, in general, decreased in the elderly due to reduced hepatic blood flow and enzyme activity. Renal clearance is reduced by the aging process as well as by disease. Although there is great individual variability (12,61), these changes are reflected in higher plasma levels and prolonged elimination half-lives (Table 2).

Studies of tricyclic antidepressant hydroxymetabolites have been of particular relevance to the elderly. It was initially assumed that these metabolites, produced by hepatic aromatic hydroxylation, were inactive; current evidence suggests that they are active and potentially cardiotoxic (see section entitled "Side Effects," below). Because these hydroxymetabolites are water-soluble, their clearance depends on renal function which is likely to be reduced by age, disease, or medications. Significant elevations of hydroxymetabolites have been reported in elderly patients with nortriptyline (28,50,63) and desipramine (21).

The relationship between antidepressant blood levels and therapeutic response in the elderly is also characterized by a large degree of interindividual variation (61). For nortriptyline and desipramine, elderly patients have been shown to require approximately the same therapeutic plasma levels as young adults, although lower doses may produce these levels (9,10,18,23,25,31). Blood levels of imipramine and amitriptyline tend to be higher in the elderly than in young adults (1,32), but these levels have

TABLE 2. *Elimination half-life of antidepressants in the elderly[a]*

Drug	Half-life (hr)
Imipramine	23–26
	27–32
Desipramine (from imipramine)	75–92
Desipramine	26
	21
Amitriptyline	37
	21.7
	27
Nortriptyline	37–45
Maprotiline	32
Trazodone	5–8
	6.0–16.2
Fluoxetine	72
Paroxetine	10–25
	8–65

[a] Owing to space limitations, references are not included; complete table and chapter references are available from the first author on request.

not clearly been correlated with therapeutic response. Plasma levels of doxepin and trazodone similarly have not been correlated with clinical response, although higher levels in the elderly are associated with greater side effects (55). Plasma levels of selective serotonin reuptake inhibitors (SSRIs) have not been correlated with therapeutic response in the elderly.

In elderly patients, it has been possible to predict therapeutic daily doses of nortriptyline by measuring the plasma level 24 hr after the administration of a single 50-mg dose of nortriptyline (9,10,52). The usefulness of this technique in clinical treatment settings, however, is not clear.

The efficacy of antidepressants for the treatment of late-life depression has been frequently described in the literature (e.g., 20,35,37,39–41,43–49,54,56). Most recently, a National Institute of Mental Health (NIMH)-sponsored consensus conference on depression in the elderly (53) included a comprehensive review of all efficacy studies; conclusions regarding the efficacy of heterocyclics, SSRIs,* and monoamine oxidase inhibitors (MAOIs) are presented in Tables 3 and 4 (49). There are no double-blind, controlled trials of bupropion in patients exclusively above the age of 65; one trial in a mixed older-age population demonstrated its efficacy and safety (15). In the only study of delusional elderly patients (4), antidepressants were found to be effective in only about 50% of delusional patients, and residual symptoms were common.

Several meta-analyses of antidepressant treatment in the elderly have also been performed confirming short-term efficacy (22,54). These indicate that drug–placebo

differences are only modest (in terms of Hamilton scale points), and significant residual symptomatology remains in the drug-treated group.

Morning presystolic orthostatic blood pressure has been shown to correlate inversely with response to nortriptyline in some elderly patients (14,51,57). The applicability of this finding in clinical treatment settings, however, is not clear.

There are no clinical or research data to suggest that one MAOI is therapeutically superior to any other in the elderly. Starting and treatment doses are substantially lower for elderly patients than for younger depressed adults. Adequate therapeutic ranges for MAOIs have never been carefully established for older patients, and it is possible that some elderly patients may require full therapeutic doses. Monitoring platelet MAO inhibition activity as a guide to dosing is of uncertain value.

Stimulants are sometimes used to treat anergia and apathy in nondepressed elderly patients (36). No controlled or methodologically acceptable studies have been conducted to date.

Six reports suggest a modest effect of lithium in augmenting tricyclic antidepressant response in the elderly (16,24,26,59,64,65). Not all who receive lithium respond with enhanced therapeutic effect, however, and in those who did improve, the necessary lithium dose was one-third to one-half that of younger adults. Augmentation with carbamazepine or thyroid medication has not been systematically studied in geriatric patients.

SIDE EFFECTS

Common heterocyclic antidepressant side effects that are particularly hazardous in the elderly include orthostatic hypotension, sedation, cardiac toxicity, and anticholinergic reactions. Side effects of selective serotonin reuptake inhibitors do not differ between young and elderly populations; agitation, anxiety, insomnia, sedation, gastrointestinal difficulties, and sexual dysfunction have been reported with all currently available SSRIs. Based on the available data, it is not possible to state whether or not the elderly are more sensitive to these side effects than younger patients at therapeutic doses.

Side effects of MAOIs, especially orthostatic hypotension, are common in the elderly. Other side effects include agitation, insomnia, sedation, hypertensive crisis, weight gain, peripheral neuropathy, exacerbation of cognitive dysfunction, and inhibition of orgasm.

The most serious side effect of heterocyclic antidepressant treatment in older patients is cardiotoxicity. Patients with preexisting conduction defects present the highest risk. The quinidine-like effects produce sinus tachycardia and stabilization of abnormal cardiac rhythms at low plasma drug levels. However, at higher plasma levels, these effects interfere with cardiac conduction. Serious

---

*Fluvoxamine (62) was not yet released for clinical use in the United States when this chapter was prepared.

TABLE 3. *Summary of acute treatments for major depression in the elderly*[a]

Treatment	Efficacy	Comments
Antidepressant medications	Numerous (25–30) randomized, placebo-controlled trials of several tricyclics, bupropion, trazodone, and others. Currently no placebo-controlled, published information in the elderly on the newer antidepressants fluoxetine, sertraline, paroxetine. Trial results are for acute treatment responses.	Adequate doses, plasma levels, and treatment duration are essential in order to maximize response. Response may take 6–12 weeks, somewhat longer than in younger patients. Side effects may limit use.
Psychostimulants	Evidence for efficacy over the short term; onset of action is rapid; randomized trials results are limited; responders are usually converted to a standard antidepressant.	Particularly in medically ill, hospitalized patients; when there is an increased risk from other antidepressants; and when rapid response may be needed.
Combined antidepressants and neuroleptic (antipsychotic) medications	More effective than either medication alone for depression with delusions or severe agitation. However, convulsive therapy is more effective than the combination.	Need controlled studies in the elderly.
Augmentation of antidepressants with lithium, thyroid, carbamazepine	Patients nonresponsive to several weeks of treatment with standard antidepressant medications may respond rapidly after lithium is added. Evidence is based on case series and reports.	May be useful in patients who are not responding or only partially responding to standard antidepressant medications.
Electroconvulsive therapy	Clearly effective in severe depression, depression with melancholia, and depression with delusions, as well as when antidepressants are not fully effective; sometimes combined with antidepressants.	In medication-resistant patients, acute response rate is approximately 50%. Relapse rate is high, requiring attention to maintenance treatments. Favorable effect of increasing age.
Psychotherapy	More effective than waiting list, no treatment, or pill-placebo; equivalent to antidepressant medications in geriatric outpatient populations studied, but distribution of responses may be different from the response to medication.	All studies have been in elderly depressed outpatients who were not suicidal and for whom hospitalization was not indicated. No evidence for efficacy in severe depression.
Combined antidepressant medication and psychotherapy	Effective in outpatients using manual-based therapies; the relative contributions of each component is not well understood.	Combined therapy has not been explicitly studied in the elder.

[a] Owing to space limitations, references are not included; complete table and chapter references are available from the first author on request.

Adapted from LS Schneider: Efficacy of treatment for geropsychiatric patients with severe mental disorder. *Psychopharmacology Bulletin* 1993;29(4):497–519.

conduction alterations (including right and left bundle branch block or partial or complete atrioventricular (AV) block occur at very high or toxic plasma levels and are reflected in the electrocardiogram (ECG) as prolonged PR, QRS, and QT intervals and T-wave flattening or inversion (11,13,34,58). These effects have not been reported with trazodone (13). High plasma levels of 10-hydroxynortriptyline (27) and 2-hydroxydesipramine (30) are also associated with cardiac conduction defects in older patients and are reflected in the ECG.

Several comprehensive reviews (49) have concluded that amitriptyline and imipramine cause significant orthostatic hypotension and probably should be avoided in

the elderly. Anticholinergic effects also limit the use of tertiary amine tricyclic antidepressants in the elderly.

PROBLEMS IN RESEARCH METHODOLOGY USED TO STUDY ANTIDEPRESSANT EFFECTS IN THE ELDERLY

Several methodological problems face the clinician who wishes to study the pharmacologic treatment of depression in the elderly.

Age. Although age 65 is conventionally considered to be the onset of "old age," most published reports in-

TABLE 4. *Summary of antidepressant efficacy in the elderly[a]*

Drug	Number of reports	Approximate number of subjects	Conclusions
Amitriptyline	12	678	Effective AD. More anticholinergic SEs than fluoxetine. More SEs than trazodone. Effect not predicted by methylphenidate challenge.
Doxepin	4	124	Partially effective at low dose. One-third nonresponsive; efficacious maintenance AD. More SEs than fluoxetine.
Imipramine	10	311	Effective AD; ECT better. One-third significant improvement; one-third no improvement. Significant agitation and anticholinergic SEs.
Nortriptyline	12	447	Effective AD. Effective maintenance AD. One-quarter to one-half have significant residual Sx. Association between high E-10-OH-NT and poor response. Significant anticholinergic and orthostatic SEs.
Desipramine	4	46	Effective AD. As effective as NT, AMI, IMI; ECT better. Response predicted by methylphenidate challenge. Response associated with plasma level but not to 2-OH-DMI level.
Trazodone	9	561	Partially effective. Significant residual Sx. High dropout due to SEs. Fewer SEs than amitriptyline and imipramine.
Maprotiline	4	77	More effective than doxepin. No correlation between blood level and response.
Fluoxetine	8	331	Effective AD. Fewer SEs than TCAs and trazodone. Bipolar patients become manic. Effective maintenance AD. Increases blood levels of other antidepressants.
Paroxetine	8	1079	Effective AD. Fewer anticholinergic SEs than amitriptyline. Low doses may be effective in elderly. SE's include nausea and headache.
Sertraline	3	253	Effective AD. One-quarter drop out because of SEs. SEs include sedation, GI Sx.
Bupropion	1	21	Effective AD. Dose range 150–450 mg/day. No cardiovascular SEs.
Monoamine oxidase inhibitors	6	158	Superior to PBO. Equally efficacious to nortriptyline. Response correlates with 80% platelet MAO inhibitor.

[a] Owing to space limitations, references are not included; complete table and chapter references are available from the first author on request.

AD, antidepressant; SE, side effect; ECT, electroconvulsive therapy; D-10-OH-NT, hydroxynortriptyline; NT, nortriptyline; AMI, amitriptyline; IMI, imipramine; DMI, desipramine; TCA, tricyclic antidepressants; GI, gastrointestinal; PBO, placebo; MAO, monoamine oxidase.

cludes subjects who are under 65, and the greatest majority of patients are between the ages of 55 and 65. There are only five studies of depressed patients exclusively 75 and older, and there is only one study (17) of patients all 80 or older (47).

Medical illness. Elderly patients in randomized clinical trials are usually outpatients who do not have concomitant physical illness and who are not taking medication for concomitant physical disorders. Thus, they represent an atypical sample of depressed elderly patients, most of whom may be suffering from a variety of disorders as well as taking several medications simultaneously.

Criteria for depression. Virtually all depressed patients in research studies suffer from moderately severe depression as suggested by Hamilton depression rating scores ranging between 18 and 22. There are no studies of elderly patients with Hamilton scores higher than 30, and there is only one study of delusional (psychotic) depressed elderly patients.

Criteria for therapeutic response. In nearly all studies,

therapeutic response consists of a percentage decline of baseline rating-scale scores (e.g., 50% from the original score). In elderly subjects, final Hamilton scores are often greater than 10. Consequently, patients who were initially the most depressed prior to treatment are still likely to be depressed at the end of the treatment course (albeit somewhat less so than placebo-treated patients). In most studies, patients are left with significant residual depressive symptoms. No study has asked patients about their quality of life or the degree to which they felt they had returned to their normal baseline affective status, and only a few studies consider the final depression rating scale to be an outcome criterion.

CONCLUSIONS

It is becoming apparent that many of the conclusions regarding antidepressant pharmacology and therapeutic efficacy in the elderly are based on (a) information that has not adequately reflected the heterogeneity of the elderly patient sample, (b) problems in patient selection, (c) wide range of interindividual variability, (d) concomitant medication, and (e) definition of both depression and treatment response. The NIMH Consensus Conference called for further research on the effect of antidepressants in the elderly, especially in the over-80 age-group range.

Considering the numerous methodologic problems of available studies with this population, the following tentative conclusions can be offered:

1. No individual antidepressant is best for elderly patients.
2. Among the tricyclic antidepressants, secondary amines are usually recommended.
3. Therapeutic blood levels of tricyclics in the elderly are similar to levels required for response in younger patients; lower doses may achieve these levels. Elimination half-life of parent compounds, desmethylated metabolites, and hydroxymetabolites tend to be prolonged.
4. Tricyclic antidepressants produce water-soluble hydroxymetabolites whose excretion is dependent of renal function. These metabolites may produce clinically relevant cardiotoxicity.
5. Selective serotonin reuptake inhibitors may be effective, well-tolerated antidepressants in the elderly, but more data are needed. No data suggest a therapeutic superiority for one SSRI.
6. Augmentation of tricyclic antidepressant effect may be helpful for some elderly patients, but this effect is neither reliable nor predictable. Further data are required to form definitive conclusions.
7. Monoamine oxidase inhibitors may be therapeutic, but most of the data come from studies employing a heterogeneous patient population. The clinical use of these compounds in the elderly may be complicated by numerous problems.

REFERENCES

1. Abernethy DR, Greenblatt DJ, Shader RI. Imipramine and desipramine disposition in the elderly. *J Pharmacol Exp Ther* 1985;232:183–188.
2. Alexopoulos G. Biological correlates of late-life depression. In: Schneider LS, Reynolds CF, Lebowitz BD, Friedhoff A, eds. *Diagnosis and treatment of depression in late life: results of the NIH consensus development conference.* Washington, DC: American Psychiatric Press, 1994;99–116.
3. Alexopoulos GS, Chester JG. Outcomes of geriatric depression. *Clin Geriatr Med* 1992;8:363–376.
4. Baldwin RC. Delusional and non-delusional depression in late life. Evidence for distinct subtypes. *Br J Psychiatry* 1988;152:39–44.
5. Blazer D, Burchett B, Service C, et al. The association of age in depression among the elderly: an epidemiologic exploration. *J Gerontol* 1991;46:M210–M215.
6. Branconnier RJ, Cole JO, Ghazvinian S, Spera KF, Oxenkrug GF, Bass JL. Clinical pharmacology of bupropion and imipramine in elderly depressives. *J Clin Psychiatry* 1983;44(5, section 2):130–133.
7. Caine E, Lyness JM, King DA, Connor L. Clinical and diagnostic heterogeneity in depression in late life. In: Schneider LS, Reynolds CF, Lebowitz BD, Friedhoff A, eds. *Diagnosis and treatment of depression in late life: results of the NIH consensus development conference.* Washington, DC: American Psychiatric Press, 1994; 21–54.
8. Conwell Y. Suicide in elderly patients. In: Schneider LS, Reynolds CF, Lebowitz BD, Friedhoff A, eds. *Diagnosis and treatment of depression in late life: results of the NIH consensus development conference.* Washington, DC: American Psychiatric Press, 1994;397–418.
9. Dawling S. Pharmacokinetics of single oral doses of nortriptyline in depressed elderly hospital patients and young healthy volunteers. *Clin Pharmacokinet* 1980;5:394–401.
10. Dawling S, Crome P, Heyer EJ. Nortriptyline therapy in elderly patients: dosage prediction from plasma concentration at 24 hours after a single 50 mg dose. *Br J Psychiatry* 1981;139:413–416.
11. Dietch JT. The effect of nortriptyline in elderly patients with cardiac conduction disease. *J Clin Psychiatry* 1990;51:65–67.
12. Furlanut M, and Benetello P. The pharmacokinetics of tricyclic antidepressant drugs in the elderly. *Pharmacol Res* 1990;22:15–25.
13. Hayes RL. ECG findings in geriatric depressives given trazodone, placebo or imipramine. *J Clin Psychiatry* 1983;44:180–183.
14. Jarvik LF, Read SL, Mintz J, Neshkes RE. Pretreatment orthostatic hypotension in geriatric depression: predictor of response to imipramine and doxepin. *J Clin Psychopharmacol* 1983;3:368–372.
15. Kane JM, Cole K, Sarantakos S, Howard A, Borenstein M. Safety and efficacy of bupropion in elderly patients: preliminary observations. *J Clin Psychiatry* 1983;44(5, section 2):134–136.
16. Katona CLE, Finch EJL. Lithium augmentation for refractory depression in old age. *Adv Neuropsychiatry Psychopharmacol* 1991;2:177–184.
17. Katz IR, Simpson GM, Curlik SM, Parmelee PA, Muhly C. Pharmacologic treatment of major depression for elderly patients in residential care settings. *J Clin Psychiatry* 1990;51(Suppl):41–47.
18. Katz IR, Simpson GM, Jethanandani V, et al. Steady state pharmacokinetics of nortriptyline in the frail elderly. *Neuropsychopharmacology* 1989;2:229–236.
19. Katz IR, Parmelee PA. Depression in elderly patients residential care settings. In: Schneider LS, Reynolds CF, Lebowitz BD, Friedhoff A, eds. *Diagnosis and treatment of depression in late life: results of the NIH consensus development conference.* Washington, DC: American Psychiatric Press, 1994;437–462.
20. Kim KY. Diagnosis and treatment of depression in the elderly. *Int J Psychiatry Med* 1988;18:211–221.
21. Kitanaka I, Ross RJ, Cutler NR, et al. Altered hydroxydesipramine

concentrations in elderly depressed patients. *Clin Pharmacol Ther* 1992;31:51–55.

22. Klawansky S. Meta-analysis on the treatment of depression in late life. In: Schneider LS, Reynolds CF, Lebowitz BD, Friedhoff A, eds. *Diagnosis and treatment of depression in late life: results of the NIH consensus development conference.* Washington, DC: American Psychiatric Press, 1994;331–352.
23. Kumar V. Plasma levels and effects of nortriptyline in geriatric depressed patients. *Acta Psychiatr Scand* 1987;75:20–28.
24. Kushnir SL. Lithium—antidepressant combinations in the treatment of depressed, physically ill geriatric patients. *Am J Psychiatry* 1986;143:378–379.
25. Kutcher SP, Shulman KI, Reed K. Desipramine plasma concentration and therapeutic response in elderly depressives: a naturalistic pilot study. *Can J Psychiatry* 1986;31(8):752–754.
26. Lafferman J, Solomon K, Ruskin P. Lithium augmentation for treatment-resistant depression in the elderly. *J Geriatr Psychiatry Neurol* 1988;1:49–52.
27. McCue RE. Plasma levels of nortriptyline and 10-hydroxynortriptyline and treatment-related electrocardiographic changes in the elderly depressed. *J Psychiatry Res* 1989;23:73–79.
28. McCue RE. 10-Hydroxynortriptyline and treatment effects in elderly depressed patients. *J Neuropsychiatry Clin Neurosci* 1989;1:176–180.
29. Murphy E. The course and outcome of depression in late life. In: Schneider LS, Reynolds CF, Lebowitz BD, Friedhoff A, eds. *Diagnosis and treatment of depression in late life: results of the NIH consensus development conference.* Washington, DC: American Psychiatric Press, 1994;81–98.
30. Nelson JC, Atillasoy E, Mazure C, et al. Hydroxydesipramine in the elderly. *J Clin Psychopharmacol* 1988;8:428–433.
31. Nelson JC, Jatlow PI, Mazure C. Desipramine plasma levels and response in elderly melancholic patients. *J Clin Psychopharmacol* 1985;5(4):217–220.
32. Nies A, Robinson DS, Friedman MJ. Relationship between age and tricyclic antidepressant plasma levels. *Am J Psychiatry* 1977;134:790–793.
33. Parmelee PA, Katz IR, Lawton MP. Depression and mortality among institutionalized aged. *J Gerontol Psychol Sci* 1992;47:P3–P10.
34. Pascualy M, Murburg MM, Veith RC. Cardiac risks of antidepressants in the elderly. In: Shamoian CA, ed. *Psychopharmacological treatment complications in the elderly.* Washington, DC: American Psychiatric Press, 1992;17–44.
35. Peabody CA, Whiteford HA, Hollister LE. Antidepressants and the elderly. *J Am Geriatr Soc* 1986;34:869–874.
36. Pickett P, Masand P, Murray GB. Psychostimulant treatment of geriatric depressive disorders secondary to medical illness. *J Geriatr Psychiatry Neurol* 1990;3(3):146–151.
37. Plotkin DA, Gerson SG, Jarvik LF. Antidepressant drug treatment in the elderly. In: Meltzer HY, ed. *Psychopharmacology: the third generation of progress.* New York: Raven Press, 1987;1149–1158.
38. Rapp SR, Parisi SA, Walsh DA. Psychological dysfunction and physical health among elderly medical inpatients. *J Consult Clin Psychol* 1988;56:851–855.
39. Reynolds CF, Schneider LS, Lebowitz BD, Kupfer DJ. Treatment of depression in the elderly: guidelines for primary care. In: Schneider LS, Reynolds CF, Lebowitz BD, Friedhoff A, eds. *Diagnosis and treatment of depression in late life: results of the NIH consensus development conference.* Washington, DC: American Psychiatric Press, 1994;463–490.
40. Reynolds CF. Treatment of depression in special populations. *J Clin Psychiatry* 1992;53:9(Suppl):45–53.
41. Reynolds CF, Frank E, Perel JM, et al. Combined pharmacotherapy and psychotherapy in the acute and continuation treatment of elderly patients with recurrent major depression: a preliminary report. *Am J Psychiatry* 1992;149:1687–1692.
42. Reynolds CF, Perel JM, Frank E, et al. Open-trial maintenance

pharmacotherapy in late-life depression: survival analysis. *Psychiatry Res* 1989;27:225–231.
43. Rockwell E, Lam RW, Zisook S. Antidepressant drug studies in the elderly. *Psychiatr Clin North Am* 1988;11:215–233.
44. Salzman C, ed. *Clinical geriatric psychopharmacology,* 2nd ed. Baltimore: Williams & Wilkins, 1992.
45. Salzman C. Monoamine oxidase inhibitors and atypical antidepressants. *Clin in Geriatr Med* 1992;8:335–348.
46. Salzman C. Antidepressants. In: PF Lamy, ed. *Clinics in geriatric medicine.* Philadelphia: WB Saunders, 1990;399–410.
47. Salzman C, Schneider L, Lebowitz B. Antidepressant treatment of very old patients. *Am J Geriatr Psychiatry* 1993;1:21–29.
48. Salzman C. Pharmacologic treatment of depression in the elderly. *J Clin Psychiatry* 1993;54(Suppl):23–28.
49. Salzman C. Pharmacological treatment of depression in the elderly. In: Schneider LS, Reynolds CF, Lebowitz BD, Friedhoff A, eds. *Diagnosis and treatment of depression in late life: results of the NIH consensus development conference.* Washington, DC: American Psychiatric Press, 1994;181–244.
50. Schneider LS, Cooper TB, Severson JA. Electrocardiographic changes with nortriptyline and 10-hydroxynortriptyline in elderly depressed outpatients. *J Clin Psychopharmacol* 1988;8:402–408.
51. Schneider LS, Sloane RB, Staples FR, Bender M. Pretreatment orthostatic hypotension as a predictor of response to nortriptyline in geriatric depression. *J Clin Psychopharmacol* 1986;6(3):172–176.
52. Schneider LS, Cooper TB, Staples FR, et al. Prediction of individual dosage of nortriptyline in depressed elderly outpatients. *J Clin Psychopharmacol* 1987;7:311–314.
53. Schneider LS, Reynolds CF, Lebowitz B, Friedhoff A, eds. *Diagnosis and treatment of depression in late life: proceedings of the NIH consensus development conference.* Washington, DC: American Psychiatric Press, 1994.
54. Schneider LS. Metaanalysis from a clinician's perspective. In: Schneider LS, Reynolds CF, Lebowitz B, Friedhoff A, eds. *Diagnosis and treatment of depression in late life: proceedings of the NIH consensus development conference.* Washington, DC: American Psychiatric Press, 1994;361–374.
55. Schneider LS. Decreased platelet ^{3}H-imipramine binding in primary major depression compared with depression secondary to medical illness in elderly outpatients. *J Affective Disord* 1988;15:195–200.
56. Shamoian CA, ed. *Psychopharmacological treatment complications in the elderly.* Washington DC: American Psychiatric Press, 1992.
57. Stack JA. Pretreatment systolic orthostatic blood pressure (PSOP) and treatment response in elderly depressed inpatients. *J Clin Psychopharmacol* 1988;8:116–120.
58. Thayssen P. Cardiovascular effects of imipramine and nortriptyline in elderly patients. *Psychopharmacology* 1981;74:360–364.
59. van Marwijk HW, Bekker FM, Nolen WA, Jansen PA, van Nieuwkerk JF, Hop WC. Lithium augmentation in geriatric depression. *J Affective Disord* 1990;20(4):217–223.
60. Veith RC, Raskind MA. The neurobiology of aging: does it predispose to depression? *Neurobiol Aging* 1988;9:101–117.
61. von Moltke L, Greenblatt DJ, Shader RI. Clinical pharmacokinetics of antidepressants in the elderly. *Clin Pharmacokinet* 1993;24:141–160.
62. Wakelin JS. Fluvoxamine in the treatment of the older depressed patient, double-blind, placebo-controlled data. *Int Clin Psychopharmacol* 1986;1:221–230.
63. Wilkins JN. Desipramine increased circulating growth hormone in elderly depressed patients: a pilot study. *Psychoneuroendocrinology* 1989;14:195–202.
64. Zimmer B, Rosen J, Thorton JE, Perel JM, Reynolds CF. Adjunctive lithium carbonate in nortriptyline-resistant elderly depressed patients. *J Clin Psychopharmacol* 1991;11:254–256.
65. Zusky PM. Adjunct low dose lithium carbonate in treatment-resistant depression: a placebo-controlled study. *J Clin Psychopharmacol* 1988;8:120–124.

Psychopharmacology: The Fourth
Generation of Progress, edited by
Floyd E. Bloom and David J. Kupfer.
Raven Press, Ltd., New York © 1995.

CHAPTER 126

Parkinson's Disease

Amos D. Korczyn

Parkinson's disease (PD) is one of the common chronic diseases of old age. It is a prototypical disease in the sense that the understanding of its pathophysiology and treatment have advanced hand in hand at a very impressive rate during the past two or three decades. In this review, these developments will be discussed.

CLINICAL FEATURES

PD is primarily a disease of the motor system. It has a gradual onset, slowly progressing to eventual severe disability. The motor symptoms include tremor at rest, poverty or slowness of movement, rigidity, and loss of postural reflexes. None of these four primary manifestations are specific to PD, and therefore the clinical diagnosis can only be tentative. The slow evolution and the lack of other features (e.g., pyramidal, sensory, or marked autonomic disturbances) support the diagnosis although some vegetative symptoms, and particularly constipation, are common (26). As will be discussed below, the clinical diagnosis is also supported by a positive response to levodopa.

Several other brain diseases can mimic PD. The assumption that vascular brain disease can result in similar manifestations was favored several years ago, leading to the clinical designation of *arteriosclerotic parkinsonism*. This nosologic entity has been disfavored but has recently re-emerged. Its eventual destiny is unclear. Historically, the encephalitis pandemic of the 1920s resulted in a multitude of cases with postencephalitic parkinsonism. Six decades after the disappearance of new cases of lethargic encephalitis, patients with recent-onset PD are highly unlikely to be due to encephalitis.

Other disorders with extrapyramidal features resem-

bling PD include progressive supranuclear palsy, olivopontocerebellar atrophy, and Shy–Drager syndrome, all of which can frequently be identified by specific clinical features. However, several reports indicate that the accuracy of the clinical diagnosis is limited and that as many as one-quarter or one-third of patients will be found at autopsy to have alternative diagnoses (24).

In addition to the motor abnormalities, patients with PD frequently have cognitive and affective disturbances. Depression is common in PD and in many patients predates the extrapyramidal features. The nosologic entity of the association of the motor and affective features is still unclear, but for reasons discussed below it is quite likely that depression should be regarded as one of the features of PD rather than one of its complications.

Dementia also commonly occurs in PD patients; prevalence data suggest that about 50% of PD cases have significant cognitive impairment. This too seems to be an integral part of the spectrum of clinical manifestations of PD.

NEUROPATHOLOGY

The pathological hallmark of PD is intracellular inclusions called *Lewy bodies*. These occur inside neurons in the substantia nigra, presumably dopamine (DA)-containing cells. These inclusions probably accumulate in neurons undergoing degeneration. The number of DA neurons progressively diminishes in PD. It is important to note that only DA neurons in the substantia nigra whose axons are destined to go to the putamen (less so to the caudate) in the nigrostriatal tract are affected. Chemical analysis shows progressive loss of DA in the striatum; clinical symptoms first appear when DA content in the striatum is reduced by about 70%. This may imply that a long preclinical stage, of 20 years or more, occur (19,38,46).

A. D. Korczyn: Sackler Faculty of Medicine, Tel Aviv University, Ramat Aviv 69978, Israel.

Other neurotransmitter systems are also affected in PD. These include norepinephrine (NE) loss in the cell bodies of the locus coeruleus, serotonin [5-hydroxytryptamine (5-HT)] loss in the raphe nuclei, and cholinergic cell loss in the nucleus basalis of Meynert. These deficiencies probably contribute to the affective and cognitive changes in PD but may also be involved in motor dysfunction. However, it is clear that the motor disturbances are primarily related to DA deficits, because replacement of endogenous DA can miraculously alleviate the motor disability.

Until recently, it was impossible to demonstrate the DA deficiencies during life. However, this was changed by the use of positron emission tomography (PET). Using radioactive tracer techniques it can be demonstrated that DA markers accumulation is reduced in the corpus striatum in PD, presumably because of the loss of DA terminals which take up these markers. At the present state, the PET is not sensitive enough to detect the progression of the disease (5), but easily correlates with the side of the clinical abnormalities in unilateral parkinsonism.

PATHOPHYSIOLOGY

The pathophysiology of PD is still rather clouded (33). The dopaminergic denervation of the basal ganglia (and particularly the striatum) is obviously central in the basic movement abnormalities. The existence of "motor loops" involving the basal ganglia, subthalamic nucleus, thalamus and cortex was recently established. However, their function is poorly understood (2,4). How the loss of dopamine causes tremor at rest, enhanced tone both at rest and during action, and bradykinesia or hypokinesia still needs to be explained. The pathophysiology of the fourth cardinal feature of PD, loss of postural reflexes, is totally unclear. Some gains were made through the use of kinematic studies, such as of arm trajectories. These quantify the defects and demonstrate some unexpected findings (e.g., regarding the importance of visual feedback), demonstrating how the "motor loops" incorporate sensory information (12).

The nigrostriatal pathway activates, in the corpus striatum, dopaminergic receptors. Four subtypes have been identified and while the most important seem to be of the D_2 type, the role of the others, and particularly D_1, in normal activity is unclear and it is therfore not completely established what is the functional correlate of activation of these receptors. In particular it is not clear whether activation of D_1 receptors is important for the elicitation of dyskinesias or other motor complications occurring in advanced cases who are treated by levodopa.

PATHOGENESIS OF PD

There is no consensus on the pathogenesis of the disease. The fact that only a selected population of neurons die off may suggest the involvement of a toxin affecting DA cells. Drugs are known which can selectively damage catecholaminergic neurons—for example, 6-hydroxydopamine (6-OHDA). This substance is uptaken by the DA transporter (vide infra), and it is concentrated in DA cells and causes their degeneration. Because 6-OHDA does not cross the blood–brain barrier, it cannot account for human PD. But recently another chemical, MPTP, was identified as causing in humans a disorder quite similar to PD in most characteristics. The mechanisms of MPTP toxicity have been explored in depth and although there is no doubt that this chemical only accounts for very few cases of PD, the possible existence of MPTP-ioids has been explored (50). While epidemiological and toxicological studies have generally failed to support the theory of an environmental toxin, the possibility of endogenous production of a substance similar to MPTP in its mechanism of action is still actively explored (48).

If such endogenous substances account for PD, occurrence of the disease in only a minority of elderly humans may suggest a genetic abnormality responsible for the production of this MPTP-ioid. Preliminary data have strongly suggested that there is no genetic contribution, but there has recently been a reappraisal of these conclusions. Some families have been described in which genetic transmission may well account for the high frequency. These families constitute a small minority, but it is possible that in others, multigenic transmission (or perhaps mitochondrial mutations), may contribute to the occurrence of PD.

Excessive concentrations of excitatory amino acids, particularly glutamate, may be involved in causing irreversible neuronal damage (47). This is particularly relevant for PD because of the existence of strong glutamatergic innervation of the corpus striatum. The neurotoxicity is produced by activation of N-methyl-D-aspartate (NMDA) receptors, and competitive antagonists can limit this damage. Although the assumption that the development of PD is preceded, or accompanied, by excessive excitatory amino acid bombardment is presently speculative, preliminary data suggest that NMDA antagonists, like memantine, may slow the process (40).

It is quite likely that several factors may contribute to the occurrence of PD, and an important question focuses on whether some or all of them operate through one common pathway that leads to DA cell loss. Along these lines, several authors have suggested that a selective increase exists in lipid peroxidation in the substantia nigra in PD, which may lead to excessive production of free radicals; these may in turn result in cellular damage and death (3). Of particular relevance is that DA degradation, like that of 6-OHDA, may cause free radical formation. As will be discussed later, these hypotheses have important immediate therapeutic implications.

The substantia nigra and globus pallidum are rich in iron, and the iron concentration increases with age and particularly in PD. This may suggest involvement of this metal in the process of lipid peroxidation (3). (See Chapters 7, 24, and 26, *this volume,* for related topics.)

TREATMENT OF PD

The basic treatment of PD is by DA replacement using levodopa. Levodopa is absorbed from the gastrointestinal tract and transported through the blood–brain barrier by active amino acid transport mechanisms. In the brain, as well as in the periphery, levodopa is metabolized to DA by an enzyme, 1-amino acid decarboxylase. This enzyme can be blocked by the substances benserazide and carbidopa. Employing either of these inhibitors can prevent the peripheral conversion of levodopa to DA. Most patients today are treated by a combination of levodopa and one of those enzyme inhibitors. The aim of using this fixed dose drug combination is to prevent the peripheral conversion to DA, because otherwise DA may act in the periphery to produce undesirable side effects such as orthostatic hypotension and nausea (6,7).

Levodopa replacement is extremely effective in controlling much of the disability in PD. It is most efficacious against rigidity and hypokinesia, but tremor also responds. However, postural instability does not respond well to dopaminergic therapy. Because the progressive loss of DA neurons continues despite levodopa treatment, patients gradually require higher doses of the drug. These increments may cause significant problems, particularly *peak-dose dyskinesias.* Basically these reactions are to be expected because when brain DA concentrations are very high, the patient is in a state opposite to the baseline DA deficiency. The requirement to increase the dose will be obvious to the patient who becomes less and less mobile as time elapses since the last dose was ingested, manifested as *end-of-dose hypokinesia.*

Treating this stage is usually done by dividing the dose into several daily administrations. While initially three daily doses are sufficient, as the disease progresses six or more doses may be required. Additional mechanisms may be relevant. In normal subjects, levodopa will not produce dyskinesias (at least by doses used in PD). Presumably this is because presynaptic terminals in the corpus striatum take up any excessive DA and either store or degrade it to inactive metabolites. This mechanism will necessarily fail in PD because of the progressive loss of DA neurons and terminals (25).

The loss of this buffering capacity may be responsible also for the eventual and most problematic complication of therapy, the so-called *"on–off"* phenomenon. Patients fluctuate from being normal in their function, or even dyskinetic as a manifestation of excessive DA stimulation (''on''), to severe parkinsonian hypokinesia and rigidity (''off''). These fluctuations may initially be regular but later come on unexpectedly (''random on–off''). In addi-

tion to the loss of buffering capacity, pharmacokinetic factors (e.g., changes of levodopa serum concentration) may contribute to the occurrence of this disabling state (27,35,36). These fluctuations could be due to erratic absorption (possibly related partly to competition by amino acids derived from dietary proteins), distribution factors, or transportation across the blood–brain barrier. Attempts to reduce such fluctuations, which are of some benefit, include low-protein diet (23), gastric administration of levodopa at a constant rate (45), or by duodenal infusion (44), addition of vitamin C to facilitate absorption, controlled-release levodopa preparations (30), and administration of direct-acting water-soluble DA agonists (e.g., lisuride and apomorphine) subcutaneously, rectally, or intranasally (14,20,29,53).

The revolutionary introduction of levodopa into the therapeutics of PD was so dramatic that its impact is unlikely to be superseded by another drug any time soon (56). However, as has been discussed above, this treatment does not solve all the problems (49).

One critical question relates to the time at which levodopa therapy should be initiated. The basic aim of levodopa therapy is to replace endogenous DA; it is thus a symptomatic therapy which, however, also masks to some extent the relentless progression of neuron cell loss. However, it is still unclear whether levodopa treatment itself accelerates or retards this loss. There are views suggesting that levodopa reduces the oxidative stress which results from the excessive burden on the remaining neurons. Alternatively, it is possible that the pharmacological concentrations of extrinsic levodopa will contribute to the formation of toxic free radicals inside neurons. Therefore, diverging views exist on whether levodopa should be started immediately upon diagnosing PD, or delayed as much as possible, with the aid of nondopaminergic therapy (9).

Monoamine oxidase (MAO), the enzyme which metabolizes several catecholamine and indole amines, exists in two forms. MAO-A metabolizes not only dopamine but also NE and 5-HT, whereas MAO-B does not metabolize either NE or 5HT. Selective inhibitors of MAO-B, and particularly deprenyl, are effective against MPTP toxicity. In PD patients, deprenyl provides symptomatic benefit (10,18). This may be related to an amphetamine-like action in releasing DA from terminals or preventing DA reuptake or metabolism. Interestingly, a large study has shown that newly diagnosed PD patients can be maintained on deprenyl alone for a long period (51,52).

There is significant controversy about the interpretation of this study, specifically whether the benefit results from a transient symptomatic effect of deprenyl or whether the drug actually slows down the progress of the disease (28,37,43). At present, many patients are being treated with deprenyl in addition to levodopa. The usefulness of this combination in retarding the progression of the disease has not been convincingly demonstrated.

Direct-acting DA agonists are important in the treatment of PD. These include apomorphine (14,20,29), bromocriptine, pergolide, and lisuride, but newer agents such as ropinirole and cabergoline are being introduced (39,41). Theoretically, the use of such agents could be advantageous. In initial stages, they relieve the excessive burden of remaining neurons without being subject to metabolism into toxic free radicals inside DA neurons as has been hypothesized for levodopa (42,54). In later stages, it is easier to maintain constant levels at receptor sites because these drugs do not depend on active transport in the gut and through blood–brain barrier. Particularly cabergoline, which has a very long biological half-life, may be advantageous in PD patients who develop motor fluctuations.

However, these drugs have significant drawbacks and side effects.Their potency is lower than that of levodopa and they can rarely be used as monotherapy, except in the initial stages of the disease. As ergoline derivatives, they are not very specific and interact with several subtypes of DA receptors as well as with 5-HT receptors. D_1 stimulation may contribute to the occurrence of dyskinesias, while 5-HT and D_4 stimulation may result in hallucinations and other psychiatric manifestations. Ropinirole, a novel synthetic non-ergoline derivative, is specific to DA (particularly D_2) receptors and may therefore be advantageous. In addition, DA agonists act also at the periphery, and this may contribute to significant side effects such as orthostatic hypotension and nausea.

The inactivation of DA after its release into the synaptic cleft involves both reuptake by DA terminals and metabolism by catechol O-methyl transferase (COMT). The reuptake is performed by specialized DA transporter molecules in the membrane. Inhibitors of this transporter, as well as those of COMT, may prolong the action of DA and thus potentially could affect the response fluctuations (32).

Surgical interventions of PD include ablative and transplanting approaches. Targets for functional stereotactic neurosurgical lesions, which reduce tremor, are the ventrolateral thalamus and the posteroventral pallidum. There has been extensive interest in transplanting DA tissue into the caudate or putamen in PD. Originally, autologous adrenal tissue was used, but the benefits, if any, were less than the risks (13). This approach was discarded, and more recently dopaminergic transplants were used where the tissue was removed from aborted fetal midbrains. It is difficult to assess the success of this approach, because frequently the patients who were recruited had a poor prognosis to start with and also because this intervention is associated with a high placebo factor (55).

COGNITIVE CHANGES IN PD

The prevalence of frank dementia in PD is far greater than that in the general population. PD dementia may be preceded by mild memory loss, transient confusional episodes, or hallucinosis. The progression of the cognitive decline is unrelated to that of the motor disability, and the only robust predictor for the development of dementia is the patient's age. Clinically, the dementia of PD differs from that of Alzheimer's disease (AD). PD patients rarely develop dysfunctions of the isocortical association areas, such as dysphasia or agnosia, and resemble a "frontal" type of dementia. But while the differentiation between cortical and subcortical dementia is of theoretical importance, it cannot be applied to individual PD patients who may develop a clinical AD-like picture. Cell loss in PD is not limited to DA neurons. The degeneration of cholinergic neurons in the nucleus basalis of Meynert, as well as 5-HT, NE, and somatostatin damage, was documented. These deficiencies are similar to those observed in AD and therefore suggest similarities in pathogenesis and treatment, as well as a clinical overlap.

During the past decade it became obvious that Lewy bodies are not limited to the substantia nigra in PD, but may occur in a widespread distribution in the cortex. Diffuse Lewy body disease is a pathological entity whose clinical correlates have not yet been defined. Patients commonly have cognitive decline and Parkinsonian features, and either one may dominate the picture.

Treatment of the cognitive changes of PD is unsatisfactory. The cholinergic defect suggests that drugs with antimuscarinic action may be detrimental, and these include of course not only specific antiparkinsonian agents such as benzhexol or trihexyphenidyl but also antidepressants such as amitryptiline. Contrariwise, cholinomimetic agents such as tacrine, presently used in AD, may increase the motor disability. Treatment of hallucinations and delusions similarly poses difficult problems because the use of D_2 blockers may well cause exacerbation of the motor symptomatology. Recently the use of clozapine, a specific D_4 blocker, was suggested as an efficacious treatment of this condition (16). In addition, if the cognitive decline and the motor deterioration both result from similar processes of neurotoxicity, it is possible that deprenyl may retard both. (See Chapters 105 and 107, *this volume,* for related topics.)

DEPRESSION IN PD

Exactly how frequently depression occurs in PD is a question that is extremely difficult to answer. There is quite a spectrum of answers, which diverge depending on (a) the criteria used to diagnose depression, (b) possible inclusion or exclusion of demented patients or those with parkinsonism due to causes other than PD (e.g., vascular etiology and progressive supranuclear palsy), and (c) the severity of their neurological impairment. In addition, referral bias to specialized centers may result in excessive numbers of depressed patients. However, and regardless of these factors, it is safe to conclude that depression is rather common in PD. Because depression is potentially treatable, this conclusion is of significant importance (8).

Several tests are available for diagnosing depression. These include neuropsychological evaluations, self-reports, projection tests, and others. However, while all these tests have important roles in research, none is superior to the clinical assessment by a competent clinician. Nor is such a test likely to ever be developed, because the manifestations of PD are quite varied.

The clinical evaluation of the affective state of PD patients may be difficult because the motionless face, the slowness of movement, and the bradyphrenia may create an erroneous impression of depression. The distinction from depressive motor retardation is obviously very important.

Decisions about the therapeutic approaches should be based not solely, perhaps not even primarily, on an objective measure but rather on the context and repercussions of the affective state of the patient.

Based on the above, every patient with PD *must* be assessed for possible depressive symptomatology, and adequate consideration should be given to the therapeutic implications.

The therapeutic considerations regarding the depression in PD may be quite unlike those for major depression. In the latter situation, massive treatment with tricyclic antidepressants is recommended, with the expected benefits occurring only several weeks later. If not efficacious, other treatment options exist, eventually leading to the employment of electroconvulsive therapy (ECT) (1,11). However, in the parkinsonian patient who is depressed, less aggressive therapy is usually sufficient, and high doses may in fact cause intolerable side effects.

The present knowledge of therapeutic options for parkinsonian depression is limited because of the scarcity of drug evaluations in this condition, let alone of comparative studies of different agents.

Tricyclic antidepressants (TCAs) have marked antimuscarinic effects. These are potentially advantageous for the PD patient because they reduce the motor symptoms, particularly the tremor. Another feature of TCAs is their anxiolytic action, and of course this is helpful in those patients manifesting anxiety symptomatology. The third relevant feature is the soporific effect of TCAs which is of significant value in those suffering from insomnia (although some patients respond to TCAs with increased alertness and restlessness) (17).

Because of their supposed mechanism of action—namely, blockade of the reuptake of 5-HT and NE by nerve terminals—these drugs are of potential value in the depression of PD (31,35). Previous attempts to differentiate depressive symptomatology related to 5-HT as opposed to NE dysfunction have been largely unrewarding. In addition, most drugs block the reuptake of both neurotransmitters. For example, while amitriptyline

mainly blocks 5-HT reuptake, its active metabolite, nortriptyline, preferentially blocks NE reuptake.

The antimuscarinic action of TCAs, already alluded to, may well lead to disorientation and confusion. This is particularly true when patients with more limited cognitive reserves are being treated (i.e., those with imminent or actual dementia), when relatively high doses are prescribed, or when employed together with antiparkinsonian drugs with antimuscarinic actions (18). Although these newer drugs do have specific actions, it remains to be demonstrated that this is of practical significance.

Selective 5-HT reuptake blockers include clomipramine, fluvoxamine, and fluoxetine. Clomiprimine is a tricyclic derivative, while the others have novel structures. Fluoxetine and fluvoxamine lack antimuscarinic actions and thus may be particularly useful in those patients for whom the use of anticholinergic drugs is contraindicated.

The use of monoamine oxidase inhibitors (MAOIs) is of course well established for the treatment of depression; although they have a bad reputation regarding safety, they continue to be used. Ever since it was realized that DA deficiency is responsible for PD, attempts were made to treat it by MAOIs, but the response was limited. It is probably true that MAOIs can successfully be used in PD patients who are depressed, with expected mild benefits also in the motor function.

The use of ECT is reserved to patients with severe depression. Although previous reluctance to use this treatment in the elderly seems to have been excessive, there is only anecdotal information on its use in PD. Some case reports suggested improvement in both affective and motor symptomatology (1,11).

Meager data exist suggesting an independent antidepressant action of levodopa. Bromocriptine is also reputed to have some antidepressant activity, although, again, this depends on unconfirmed, uncontrolled observations (21). Lastly, some anticholinergic drugs used in the treatment of PD have mood-elevating actions. This is particularly true for orphenadrine.

REFERENCES

1. Abrams R, Douvon R, Serby M, Klutchoko B, Rotrosen J. ECT and Parkinson's disease. *Am J Psychiatry* 1989;146:451–455.
2. Alexander GE, DeLong, MR, Strick, PL. Parallel organization of functionally segregated circuits linking basal ganglia and cortex. *Ann Rev Neurosci* 1986;9:357–381.
3. Ben Shachar D, Riederer P, Youdim MBH. Iron melanin interaction and lipid peroxidation: implication for Parkinson's disease. *J Neurochem* 1991;57:1609–1614.
4. Bergman H, Wichmann T, DeLong MR. Reversal of experimental parkinsonism by lesions of the subthalamic nucleus. *Science* 1990;249:1436–1438.
5. Bhatt MH, Snow BJ, Martin WRW, Pate BD, Calne DB. Positron emission tomography suggests that the rate of progression of idiopathic parkinsonism is slow. *Ann Neurol* 1991;29:673–677.
6. Cederbaum JM, Gardy SE, McDowell FH. "Early" initiation of levodopa treatment does not promote the development of motor response fluctuations, dyskinesias or dementia in Parkinson's disease. *Neurology* 1991;41:622–629.

7. Clough CG. Parkinson's disease: management. *Lancet* 1991; 337:1324–1327.

8. Cummings JL. Depression and Parkinson's disease: review. *Am J Psychiatry* 1992;149:443–454.

9. Diamond SG, Markham CH, Hoehn MM, McDowell FH, Muenter MD. Multicenter study of Parkinson mortality with early versus later dopa treatment. *Ann Neurol* 1987;22:8–12.

10. Elizan TS, Moros DA, Yahr MD. Early combination of selegiline and low-dose levodopa as initial symptomatic therapy in Parkinson's disease. *Arch Neurol* 1991;48:31–34.

11. Faber R, Trimble MR. Electroconclusive therapy in Parkinson's disease and other movement disorders. *Mov Disord* 1991;6:293–303.

12. Flash T, Inzelberg R, Schechtman E, Korczyn AD. Kinematic analysis of upper limb trajectories in Parkinson's disease. *Exper Neurol* 1992;118:215–226.

13. Forno LS, Langston JW. Unfavourable outcome of adrenal medullary transplant for Parkinson's disease. *Acta Neuropathol* 1991; 81:691–694.

14. Frankel JP, Lees AJ, Kempster PA, Stern GM. Subcutaneous apomorphine in the treatment of Parkinson's disease. *J Neurol Neurosurg Psychiat* 1990;53:96.

15. Freed WJ, Wyatt RJ. In: Meltzer HY, ed: *Psychopharmacology: the third generation of progress.* New York: Raven Press, 1987;471–479.

16. Friedman JH, Lannon MC. Clozapine in the treatment of psychosis in Parkinson's disease. *Neurology* 1989;39:1219–1221.

17. Goetz CG, De Long MR, Penn RD, Bakay AE. Neurosurgical horizons in Parkinson's disease. *Neurology* 1993;43:1–7.

18. Golbe JI. Deprenyl as symptomatic therapy in Parkinson's disease. *Clin Neuropharmacol* 1988;11:387–400.

19. Hornykiewicz O. Neurochemical pathology and the etiology of Parkinson's disease: basic facts and hypothetical possibilities. *Mt Sinai J Med* 1988;55:11–20.

20. Hughes AJ, Bishop S, Lees A, Stern GM, Webster R, Bovingdon M. Rectal apomorphine in Parkinson's disease. *Lancet* 1991;337:118.

21. Inzelberg R, Bornstein NM, Reider I, Korczyn AD. Basal ganglia lacunes and parkinsonism. *Neuroepidemiol* 1994;13:108–112.

22. Jouvent R, Abensour P, Bonnet AM, et al. Antiparkinsonian and antidepressant effects of high doses of bromocriptine. *J Affect Disord* 1983;5:141–145.

23. Karstaedt PJ, Pincus JH. Protein redistribution diet remains effective in patients with fluctuating parkinsonism. *Arch Neurol* 1992;49: 149–151.

24. Koller WC. How accurately can Parkinson's disease be diagnosed? *Neurology* 1992;42(Suppl 1):6–16.

25. Korczyn AD. Pathophysiology of drug-induced dyskinesias. *Neuropharmacol* 1973;11:601–607.

26. Korczyn AD. Autonomic nervous system dysfunction in Parkinson's disease. In: Calne DB, ed. *Parkinsonism and aging.* New York: Raven Press, 1989;211–219.

27. Kostic V, Przedborski S, Flaster E, Sternic N. Early development of levodopa-induced dyskinesias and response fluctuations in young onset Parkinson's disease. *Neurology* 1991;41:202–205.

28. Landau WM. Pyramid sale in the bucket shop: datatop bottoms out. *Neurology* 1990;40:1337–1339.

29. Lees AJ, Montastruc JL, Turjanski N, Rascol O, Kleedorfer B. Sublingual apomorphine and Parkinson's disease. *J Neurol Neurosurg Psychiatry* 1989;52:1440.

30. LeWitt P. Controlled-release carbidopa/levodopa (Sinemet 50/200 CR4): Clinical and pharmacokinetic studies. *Neurology* 1989;39 (Suppl 2):45.

31. McCance-Katz E, Marek KL, Price LH. Serotonergic dysfunction in depression associated with Parkinson's disease. *Neurology* 1992;42:1813–1814.

32. Mannisto PT, Kaakola S. Rationale for selective COMT inhibitors as adjuncts in the drug treatment of Parkinson's disease. *Pharmacol Toxicol* 1993;66:317–323.

33. Marsden CD. The mysterious motor function of the basal ganglia. *Neurology* 1982;32:514–539.

34. Mayeux R, Stern Y, Sano M, Williams JBW, Cote LJ. The relationship of serotonin to depression in Parkinson's disease. *Mov Disord* 1988;3:237–244.

35. Nutt JG, William R, Woodward WR, Hammerstad JP, Carter JH, Anderson JL. The ''on-off'' phenomenon in Parkinson's disease. Relation to levodopa absorption and transport. *New Engl J Med* 1984;310:483–488.

36. Nutt JG, Woodward WR, Carter JH, Gancher ST. Effect of long term therapy on the pharmacodynamics of levodopa. *Arch Neurol* 1992;49:1123–1130.

37. Olanow CW, Calne DB. Does selegiline monotherapy in Parkinson's disease act by symptomatic or protective mechanisms? *Neurology* 1992;42(Suppl 4):13–26.

38. Paulus W, Jellinger K. The neuropathological basis of different clinical subgroups of Parkinson's disease. *J Neuropathol Exp Neurol* 1991;50:743–755.

39. Rabey JM, Nissipeanu P, Inzelberg R, Korczyn AD. Beneficial effect of cabergoline, a new long-lasting D_2 agonist in the treatment of Parkinson's disease. *Clin Neuropharmacol* 1994;17:286–293.

40. Rabey JM, Nisipeanu P, Korczyn AD. Efficacy of memantine, an NMDA receptor antagonist, in the treatment of Parkinson's disease. *J Neural Transm* 1992;4:277–282.

41. Rabey JM, Streiffler M, Treves T, Korczyn AD. The beneficial effect of chronic lisuride administration compared with levodopa in Parkinson's disease. In: Streifler MB, Korczyn AD, Melamed E, Youdim MBH, eds, *Advances in Neurology, vol. 53: Parkinson's disease: anatomy, pathology and therapy.* New York: Raven Press, 1990;451–455.

42. Rinne UK. Early dopamine agonist therapy in Parkinson's disease. *Mov Disord* 1989;4:86–94.

43. Rinne JO, Ryotta M, Paljarvi L, Rummukainen J, Rinne U. Selgiline (deprenyl) treatment and death of nigral neurons in Parkinson's disease. *Neurology* 1991;41:859–861.

44. Sage JI. Long term duodenal infusion of levodopa for motor fluctuations in parkinsonism. *Ann Neurol* 1988;24:87–89.

45. Sage JI, McHale DM, Sonsalla P, Vitagliano D, Heikkila RE. Continuous levodopa infusions to treat complex dystonia in Parkinson's disease. *Neurology* 1989;39:888–891.

46. Scherman D, Desnos C, Darchem F, Pollack P, Javoy-Agid F, Agid Y. Striatal dopamine deficiency in Parkinson's disease: role of aging. *Ann Neurol* 1989;26:551–557.

47. Sonsalla PK, Nicklas J, Heikkila RE. Role for excitatory amino acids in methamphetamine induced nigrostriatal dopaminergic toxicity. *Science* 1989;247:398–400.

48. Stevenson GB, Heafield MTE, Waring RH, Williams AC. Xenobiotic metabolism in Parkinson's disease. *Neurology* 1989;39:883–887.

49. Stroessl AJ. The prevention and management of late stage complications in Parkinson's disease. *Can J Neurol Sci* 1992;19:113–116.

50. Tanner CM, Langston JW. Do environmental toxins cause Parkinson's disease? A critical review. *Neurology* 1990;40(Suppl 3):17–30.

51. The Parkinson Study Group. Effect of deprenyl on the progression of disability in early Parkinson's disease. *New Engl J Med* 1989;321:1364–1371.

52. The Parkinson Study Group. Effects of tocopherol and deprenyl on the progression of disability in early Parkinson's disease. *New Engl J Med* 1993;328:176–183.

53. Vaamonde J, Luquin MR, Obeso JA. Subcutaneous lisuride infusions in Parkinson's disease. Response to chronic administration in 34 patients. *Brain* 1991;114:601–614.

54. Weiner WJ, Factor SA, Sanchez-Ramos, JR. Early combination therapy (bromocriptine and levodopa) does not prevent motor fluctuations in Parkinson's disease. *Neurology* 1993;43:21–27.

55. Widner H, Rechcronal S. Transplantation and surgical treatment of Parkinsonian syndromes. *Curr Opin Neurol Neurosurg* 1993;6: 344–349.

56. Yahr MD, Duvoisin RS, Schear MK, Barre HRE, Hoehn MM. Treatment of parkinsonism and levodopa. *Arch Neurol* 1969; 21:343–354.

Psychopharmacology: The Fourth Generation of Progress, edited by Floyd E. Bloom and David J. Kupfer. Raven Press, Ltd., New York © 1995.

CHAPTER 127

Tardive Dyskinesia:

Epidemiological and Clinical Presentation

John M. Kane

Tardive dyskinesia continues to be an important concern in the long-term use of antipsychotic (neuroleptic) medication. Considerable research has been conducted on the clinical presentation, epidemiology, and risk factors associated with the development of tardive dyskinesia. There is certainly increased awareness of the difference of ways in which this condition can manifest itself and the extent to which it can produce a variety of disabilities either directly or indirectly (see Chapters 128 and 129, *this volume*).

DIFFERENTIAL DIAGNOSIS

It is critical to emphasize that any and all abnormal involuntary movements experienced by neuroleptic-treated patients should not necessarily be considered to be tardive dyskinesia. There are numerous clinical conditions which may produce abnormal involuntary movements that may be mistaken for tardive dyskinesia.

The word *dyskinesia* refers to a broad range of abnormal involuntary movements including chorea, athetosis, and dystonia. There are a variety of abnormal movements which would not be considered dyskinesias, including akathisia, compulsive movements, mannerisms, stereotypic movements, tics, or tremors.

Neuroleptic drugs can produce dyskinetic movements which are not tardive (late-occurring), but rather acute. Ayd (3) reported dyskinesias in 2.3% of patients early in the course of neuroleptic treatment. Dystonic reactions

may be part of acute dyskinesia. These intermittent or sustained muscle contractions can involve the eyes, neck, diaphragmatic muscles, jaw, larynx, or truncal musculature. This reaction responds well to acute treatment with anticholinergic or antihistaminic agents. (A phenomenon known as *tardive dystonia* may be identical phenomenologically, but is late-occurring and is considered to be a subtype of tardive dyskinesia. This will be discussed subsequently.)

Dyskinesia may be produced or precipitated by a variety of other drugs besides neuroleptics. Caffeine, phenytoin, estrogens, and other drugs can produce reactions which are rapidly reversed when the drug is discontinued. Movements which mimic tardive dyskinesia can frequently be seen with L-dopa treatment of Parkinson's disease and have been reported in isolated cases with an array of other drugs such as tricyclic antidepressants and antihistamines.

Disorders of the basal ganglia can produce an array of abnormal involuntary movements including chorea, athetosis, and dystonia. Examples would include Huntington's disease, Wilson disease, Sydenham's chorea, and Fahr's syndrome. In most cases an appropriate evaluation can succeed in identifying such causes of abnormal movements. Because patients with Huntington's disease and Wilson's disease may have psychotic symptomatology, the differential diagnosis is particularly critical in the context of the present discussion. Since patients with Huntington's disease may receive neuroleptic drugs, the possibility of having concurrent abnormal movements with different etiologies exists. Patients with Huntington's disease may have marked postural instability and/or atrophy of the caudate nucleus on brain imaging, both of which would not be likely in true dyskinesia. Wilson's disease can be diagnosed if suspected with a serum ceruloplasmin.

J. M. Kane: Department of Psychiatry, Hillside Hospital, A Division of Long Island Jewish Medical Center, Glen Oaks, New York 11004; and Department of Psychiatry, Albert Einstein College of Medicine, Bronx, New York 10467.

Hyperthyroidism, hypoparathyroidism, and systemic lupus erythematosus are also capable of producing dyskinesias. Tourette's disorder, torsion dystonia, and spasmodic torticollis are all movement disorders which should be differentiated from tardive dyskinesia based on history and clinical presentation. Meige syndrome is an idiopathic condition which can produce dystonic facial movements and blepharospasm. When these phenomena are seen subsequent to neuroleptic treatment, it is suggested that the term *tardive facial dystonia* be employed.

Critical in any assessment of abnormal involuntary movement disorder in a patient receiving neuroleptics is a good history as to whether or not movements were present prior to the initiation of antipsychotic medication. Dyskinesia can occur which are not attributable to known causes. Some may occur in patients with psychiatric illnesses who have not been treated with neuroleptics or may be a manifestation of a conversion reaction. In addition, some elderly individuals may have so-called spontaneous dyskinesias with no obvious cause, and some individuals with ill-fitting or absent dentures may have abnormal movements of the tongue or lips.

Abnormal Movements in Schizophrenia

Prior to the introduction of neuroleptic drugs, there were a number of descriptions of abnormal involuntary movements occurring in patients with apparent schizophrenia (14,36). These descriptions included tic-like movements, grimacing, and stereotypic movements, as well as occasional choreiform movements and orofacial dyskinesias. However, choreiform or choreoathetoid movements were felt to be fairly rare in chronic psychiatric patients prior to the neuroleptic era (40).

Given problems in diagnostic reliability and validity of the diagnoses in both the psychosis and the movement disorder in historical reports, attempts have been made to identify special populations which might help shed some light on this issue. Owens et al. (41) reported a prevalence of dyskinesia (defined as a rating of 2 or more on one or more AIMS items) of 53% among a group of patients with chronic schizophrenia who had apparently never been treated with neuroleptic drugs. This cohort of 47 individuals satisfied Feighner criteria for schizophrenia and had an average age of 67. In comparison, these investigators found a 67% prevalence of dyskinesia among a somewhat younger (mean age 57) group of chronic patients who had received neuroleptic drugs.

Chorfi and Moussaoui (12) did not find any dyskinesias in never-medicated schizophrenic patients. Fenton et al. (15) reviewed detailed medical records on 100 lifetime neuroleptic-naive schizophrenic patients treated at Chestnut Lodge. Descriptions of abnormal movements were reviewed and rated by investigators blind to the treatment history of the patient. Fifteen percent of the records documented oral/facial dyskinesias with sufficient detail to be considered definite. If less stringent criteria are employed, 28% of the patient records documented some form of movement disorder.

Fenton et al. (15) reported that patients with spontaneous dyskinesia received significantly greater ratings on negative symptoms and conceptual disorganization than those with no movement disorders. Owens et al. (41) have suggested that in some patients a syndrome of abnormal involuntary movements reflects the cerebral pathology underlying severe chronic schizophrenia. Lidsky et al. (38) have postulated that some repetitive motor acts exhibited by patients with schizophrenia could be a manifestation of an underlying dysfunction of the basal ganglia associated with the condition.

Yarden and Discipio (60) described a sample of young, drug-free schizophrenic patients who exhibited a variety of abnormal involuntary movements (choreiform, athetoid, tics, stereotypies, and mannerisms). After following-up these patients 2.5 to 3.5 years later, those investigations concluded that these patients constituted a group with early onset and a steadily progressive course. In addition, they showed marked thought disorder and poor response to pharmacologic treatment. In studying disturbances in voluntary motor activity apparently unrelated to drug effects, Manschrek et al. (39) also reported an association between movement disorders, cognitive impairment, affective blunting, and formal thought disorder.

These findings complicate suggestions that patients with negative symptoms, cognitive dysfunction, and possibly relative abnormalities on neuroimaging are at increased risk for developing tardive dyskinesia because some of the movements attributed to neuroleptic treatment may in fact be spontaneous dyskinesias associated with the schizophrenic illness itself. Waddington (53) has suggested that neuroleptic drug treatment may precipitate or hasten the appearance of dyskinesias in those people who may have ultimately developed the movements "spontaneously."

DIAGNOSTIC CRITERIA FOR TARDIVE DYSKINESIA

As suggested by the report of the American Psychiatric Association Task Force on Tardive Dyskinesia (28), the diagnosis of tardive dyskinesia should not be solely one of exclusion, but it should also be based on satisfying some criteria. The following were suggested by the Task Force.

Phenomenology

1. *Nature of abnormal movements.* Choreiform, athetoid, or rhythmic abnormal involuntary movements are reduced by voluntary movements of the affected parts

and increased by voluntary movements of the unaffected parts.

2. *Other characteristics.* The abnormal movements increase with emotional arousal and decrease with relaxation and volitional effort. The movements are absent during sleep.

3. *Specific localization of neuroleptic-induced tardive dyskinesia.* The tongue, jaw, or extremities are involved in most cases.

4. *Severity.* At least "moderate" abnormal, involuntary movements in one or more body areas or "mild" movements in two or more body areas (face, lips, jaw, tongue, upper extremities, lower extremities, and trunk) are present. Because of the variability in the manifestation of movements associated with tardive dyskinesia, if the examination reveals movements that are only "minimal" or "mild" in only one body area, the examination should be repeated within 1 week to confirm their presence. Determination of the presence of these movements should be made using a standardized examination procedure and rating scale (e.g., the AIMS or the Rockland/Simpson Tardive Dyskinesia Rating Scale).

History

1. *Duration of dyskinesia.* The abnormal movements should be present continually for at least 4 weeks.

2. *Neuroleptic treatment.* There should be a history of at least 3 months of total cumulative neuroleptic exposure. Exposure may be continuous or discontinuous. Patients who fail to meet the criterion for duration of neuroleptic exposure should receive the appropriate diagnosis with the qualification "less than 3 months of neuroleptic exposure."

3. *Onset of dyskinesia.* The onset of the dyskinesia should be either while the patient is on neuroleptics or within a few weeks of discontinuing neuroleptics.

Treatment Response

1. *Antiparkinsonian agents.* Antiparkinsonian agents usually have no effect or may even aggravate tardive dyskinesia (although they may improve tardive dystonia).

2. *Changes in neuroleptic doses.* Increasing the dose of neuroleptics usually suppresses dyskinesia. Reduction or discontinuation of neuroleptics may worsen the symptoms temporarily (but are likely to result in improvement over the long-term).

Tardive Dystonia

Tardive dystonia is viewed sometimes as a subtype of tardive dyskinesia and sometimes as a distinct entity. Burke and Kang (6) have suggested that tardive dystonia

is distinguished from the classic oral–buccal–lingual choreiform movements of tardive dyskinesia not only by the dystonic nature of the movement, but also by the frequency with which it causes significant neurologic disability. The movements seen in tardive dystonia are not dissimilar to those presenting in primary torsion dystonia. The face and neck are the most frequently involved body regions. Some patients may exhibit aspects of both tardive dystonia and tardive dyskinesia either concurrently or sequentially. Because the dystonic disorder is in many cases more disabling, the rationale for neuroleptic discontinuation may be even greater. Tardive dystonia usually benefits from anticholinergic medications, whereas tardive dyskinesia generally does not (6).

Acute dystonia reactions usually occur in the first 24–48 hr of treatment with a dopamine D2 antagonist, whereas tardive dystonia tends to occur much later. In a series of 67 patients, Kang et al. (34) reported that tardive dystonia occurred after a median of 5 years of drug exposure.

ASSESSMENT OF TARDIVE DYSKINESIA: RATING METHODS

There are several factors specific to tardive dyskinesia that make accurate assessment a particular problem. Although diagnostic criteria have been developed, investigators may differ in the threshold they set for defining a case. On a cross-sectional assessment, it is obviously difficult to rule out other conditions discussed previously and rating instruments or assessment measures cannot be utilized to make a diagnosis, though they may be useful as a screening tool.

There is considerable variability (even within patients) in the severity and presentation of abnormal movements over time. Some changes in severity may also be apparent in relation to changes in level of arousal or focus. Anxiety may aggravate the dyskinesias, whereas relaxation may improve them; however, these influences are not consistent across patients.

A critical source of variability in the presentation of tardive dyskinesia is the role of medication, because changes in antipsychotic drug dosage may influence the severity of the movements. In addition, the administration of anticholinergic medication can influence the presentation of tardive dyskinesia.

The most frequently employed methods of assessment are: instrumentation, frequency counts, and multi-item rating scales.

Instrumentation (e.g., electromyography, accelerometry, force procedures, or ultrasound) has been employed in an attempt to provide objective and automated assessments. Some studies have found quantitative instrumental methods to correlate with traditional rating scales. These techniques may also prove useful in helping to identify the early or subclinical case and to help differentiate tardive dyskinesia from other movement disorders.

Frequency counts of abnormal movements provide the number of movements occurring within a certain time frame. This method can be difficult to employ when multiple movements are present, and there are inherent problems in comparing patients who may have different types of movements. In addition, a frequency count may not be an accurate reflection of the overall severity of the condition in terms of body areas involved and the magnitude of the movements themselves.

Multi-item scales remain the mainstay in clinical research. A variety of scales are available (for listing see ref. 28, page 42). Many instruments have also been developed with a standard examination format for increased standardization. Brief multi-item scales can be employed in the context of routine clinical care to monitor patients for the development of abnormal involuntary movements. As emphasized previously, these instruments are not diagnostic though they can be used to screen patients, and threshold criteria can be developed for defining the severity of movements necessary to be identified as a definite case.

There remain a variety of problems in utilizing rating scales. It is not always clear where one draws the line between normal and abnormal movements (e.g., occasional tongue protrusion or movements of the lips may not constitute tardive dyskinesia). The perceived severity of movements could be based on quality, frequency, duration, or amplitude of the movement, and it is far from clear how to integrate these different aspects.

Satisfactory levels of interrater reliability have been demonstrated for several widely used scales. Attempts to validate scales have not been extensive, particularly because there are no established criteria for the condition which could be used to demonstrate concurrent validity.

There are special populations which present particular challenges in assessing abnormal involuntary movements. As previously discussed among patients with schizophrenia, some proportion of abnormal involuntary movements may be spontaneous. This also applies to elderly populations where a relatively high prevalence of a variety of neuromedical conditions may also contribute to the presence of abnormal movements.

Antipsychotic medications are frequently employed in those with developmental disabilities. In this population of patients, a variety of abnormal movements (stereotypies, mannerisms, adventitious movements) may be seen unrelated to exposure to medication. Clearly, the training of raters in the assessment of abnormal movements takes on added importance when special populations are involved.

EPIDEMIOLOGY

Although as discussed previously there remains some debate as to what extent neuroleptic treatment is either necessary or sufficient to produce abnormal involuntary movements, the consensus at present remains that antipsychotic drugs do play an important role in producing or evoking abnormal involuntary movements. Studies of the epidemiology of tardive dyskinesia have had to confront a variety of methodologic problems including: differential diagnosis, fluctuations in symptomatology, the potential masking effect of antipsychotic drug treatment, and the absence of validating criteria.

Numerous prevalence surveys of tardive dyskinesia have been conducted and extensively reviewed (7,31). Prevalence estimates have been useful in helping to identify populations at particular risk and helping to provide some sense of the overall scope of the problem. Clearly, prevalence estimates will vary depending upon the population studied (e.g., age, sex, length of neuroleptic treatment), the assessment strategy utilized, and the criteria employed to define caseness.

Yassa and Jeste (61) reviewed 76 published studies on the prevalence of tardive dyskinesia representing a total of 39,187 patients. The reported prevalence ranged from 3% to 62%, with a mean of 24%.

Woerner et al. (57) completed a large-scale prevalence survey designed to address a variety of methodologic concerns by including a wide range of clinical populations, while employing the same raters, assessment techniques, and definition of caseness throughout. The prevalence of presumptive tardive dyskinesia varied enormously across the different populations; 13% in a voluntary hospital with a relatively young patient population, 23% in a Veterans Administration Hospital, and 36% in a state hospital. The proportion of apparent cases of tardive dyskinesia that could be attributed to other neuromedical conditions following clinical laboratory evaluation and examination by a neurologist experienced in the assessment of movement disorders was surprisingly low (0.1%). A somewhat larger group (3.7%) had abnormal movements in the context of a variety of neuromedical conditions that might have played an etiologic role. As a result, the most conservative estimate of overall prevalence among the 1441 patients examined was 19.6%.

In order to estimate the rate of false-negative cases due to masking by the neuroleptic, a subgroup of patients with no evidence of tardive dyskinesia was withdrawn from neuroleptic drugs and examined weekly for 3 weeks. Seventy subjects were discontinued; of these, 24 (34%) showed emergent dyskinesias. The rate of emergent dyskinesia at the state facility was strikingly higher (67%) than at the voluntary hospital (18%) or the Veterans Administration facility (17%).

Patients discontinued from fluphenazine decanoate (a minimum of 5 weeks from the last injection) were less likely to show covert dyskinesia than were patients discontinued from oral medication, confirming a previous finding by Levine et al. (37). The dose of antipsychotic medication prior to drug discontinuation was not related to the emergence of tardive dyskinesia; however, a history of treatment with very high doses (3000 mg/day in chlorpromazine equivalents) was negatively correlated with covert dyskinesia. Age and total months of antipsychotic drug treatment were found to be positively correlated with emergent tardive dyskinesia.

Interpretation of the results of prevalence surveys especially with regard to analysis of potential risk factors is complicated by the fact that prevalence estimates are influenced by the persistence of the condition within a given population. Because many cases of tardive dyskinesia will remit over time, particularly with drug discontinuation or dosage reduction, while others may persist, any analysis of risk factors in a prevalence survey will be complicated by those factors that influence course. If, for example, advanced age is a risk factor for the development of tardive dyskinesia and a risk factor for the relative persistence of tardive dyskinesia, then the prevalence would be particularly high in an elderly population.

The approach involved in the prevalence survey has definite limitations, and further progress in understanding and preventing tardive dyskinesia will require more sophisticated methodology.

Incidence

Several prospective studies have been conducted in the past decade, and this strategy overcomes many, but not all, of the methodologic problems inherent in cross-sectional prevalence surveys.

Kane et al. (32,33) have reported interim results from a long-term prospective study of tardive dyskinesia involving more than 850 patients. The design of the study allows for reassessment every 3 months, and patients are selected without regard to their psychiatric diagnosis or history of antipsychotic drug treatment. A subgroup of approximately 100 patients recruited into the study have never received antipsychotic drugs. The average age of the cohort at entry was 29, and 43% were female. Of those individuals who did have a history of antipsychotic treatment at study entry, the median length of lifetime exposure was 12 months; therefore, patients are followed from a relatively early stage in their drug treatment experience. The findings regarding incidence thus far indicate that the cumulative incidence of tardive dyskinesia is 5% at 1 year, 10% at 2 years, 15% at 3 years, and 19% after 4 years of antipsychotic drug exposure. For the fifth and sixth years the figures have continued to increase; 23% and 26%, respectively. These results certainly support the notion that increasing duration of antipsychotic drug exposure is associated with an increasing cumulative incidence of tardive dyskinesia (at least for the first several years of such exposure). It remains to be seen whether or not the risk decreases after some point in time.

Yassa et al. (63,64) have carried out a prospective study involving 108 patients (55 men and 53 women) who were assessed over a 2-year period. Sixty-five percent of the patients had a diagnosis of schizophrenia. In eight patients the tardive dyskinesia persisted through at least two separate examinations at some time during the 2 years. The condition was considered to be of a moderate severity in one case and mild in the remainder. An incidence of 7.4% for persistent tardive dyskinesia is reported by the investigators, but this figure is not based on a life-table analysis or a cumulative proportion remaining free of tardive dyskinesia, which would allow inclusion of the dropouts in the incidence calculation.

Glazer et al. (21) have reported prospective data on a cohort of 362 chronic psychiatric outpatients who were free of tardive dyskinesia at baseline and who were maintained on neuroleptic medication. Many of these patients had lengthy neuroleptic treatment prior to baseline (mean 8 year); however, the investigators made every attempt to rule out prior evidence of tardive dyskinesia.

This study demonstrated an average incidence rate of 5% per year during the 5-year follow-up, with a cumulative incidence of 20% at the end of the 5 years. By combining data from patients with different durations of neuroleptic exposure at baseline, the investigators also estimated the risk of developing tardive dyskinesia for exposure periods that exceeded the observed follow-up duration of 5 years. Using this strategy, they estimated the 10-year risk to be 49% and the 25-year risk to be 68%.

Saltz et al. (46) have reported on a prospective study of tardive dyskinesia development in a large cohort of elderly subjects whose mean age was 77 and who exhibited no evidence of abnormal involuntary movements prior to antipsychotic drug treatment. Fifty-eight percent of this sample received a diagnosis of organic mental syndrome, and 42% had a primary psychiatric diagnosis. The incidence of tardive dyskinesia observed after 43 weeks of cumulative antipsychotic drug exposure was 31%.

Jeste et al. (23) have presented preliminary data on 236 elderly patients followed prospectively. Forty-eight patients received a diagnosis of schizophrenia, 55 Alzheimer's disease, 33 affective disorders, and 100 patients received miscellaneous diagnoses. The mean age of this cohort is 66, and patients were enrolled early in the course of their neuroleptic treatment, many with less than 90 days of total lifetime exposure.

The overall cumulative incidence of tardive dyskinesia by the end of 1 year is 26%. The investigators found no significant difference among the four diagnostic groups in terms of tardive dyskinesia incidence.

Risk Factors

The elucidation of factors that might contribute to individual vulnerability to tardive dyskinesia should be of help in the development of preventive strategies; however, there is a paucity of data resulting from long-term prospective studies which could test the predictive value of potentially relevant risk factors.

Age

Age is one of the most consistently replicated risk factors, particularly in prevalence surveys. Extensive reviews of the topic have concluded that increasing age remains the most consistently implicated factor for the risk of tardive dyskinesia development. In addition, advanced age is associated with the development of more severe and persistent types of the disorder. Data from the Saltz et al. (46) and Jeste and Caligiuri (23) prospective studies confirm a strikingly high incidence of tardive dyskinesia within the first year of neuroleptic treatment.

Clearly the elderly are also at risk for the development of spontaneous dyskinesias or abnormal involuntary movements associated with a variety of neuromedical conditions independent of their exposure to antipsychotic drugs. At the same time, prevalence surveys of healthy elderly volunteers suggest that spontaneous dyskinesias are not that common in the absence of some form of brain disease or dysfunction, even in late life (31,57).

The potential mechanism producing the effect of age on risk for tardive dyskinesia remains speculative. It is possible that neuronal damage, degeneration, age-related changes in receptor number, sensitivity, or plasticity and the reduced efficiency of restorative processes may be relevant.

Studies of neuroleptic effects in children indicate that they are also vulnerable to tardive dyskinesia and even persistent dyskinesias (7).

Gender

Sex differences in the prevalence of tardive dyskinesia have been reported by a number of investigators. Yassa and Jeste (61) conducted a meta-analysis of published reports providing prevalence data in men and women. The mean prevalence rate was found to be 26.6% in women and 21.6% in men. In addition, women were found to have more severe tardive dyskinesia and a higher prevalence of spontaneous dyskinesia in comparison to men. They also found an interaction between age and gender as suggested by numerous individual prevalence surveys. The prevalence of tardive dyskinesia appeared to reach its peak in the sixth and seventh decades among men, whereas it continued to rise after the seventh decade in women. It remains unclear as to what extent these sex differences are a result of biological variables or how much they are due to external risk factors such as differences in neuroleptic treatment, dosage, or duration.

Psychiatric Diagnosis

As previously discussed, a variety of abnormal involuntary movements have been described in psychiatric patients, particularly those with schizophrenia, long before the introduction of antipsychotic medication.

Another line of evidence supporting the possibility that schizophrenia includes motor disturbance is the occurrence of abnormal movements in amphetamine-induced psychosis. Chronic use of amphetamines can produce a paranoid state almost indistinguishable from schizophrenia and which may be accompanied by patterns of perseverative, stereotyped behavior and impulsive fidgety movements, as well as grimacing, chewing, and twisting of the trunk and limbs (47).

As previously discussed, tardive dyskinesia may be more common in patients with predominant negative features (4,26,51). There are a variety of caveats that should be kept in mind in drawing firm conclusions regarding this association. It is particularly important to recognize the inherent difficulty in differentiating negative symptoms from depression or drug-induced parkinsonism, especially on a cross-sectional basis. It may be particularly complicated if affective symptoms and/or vulnerability to drug-induced parkinsonian symptoms convey a higher risk for the development of tardive dyskinesia among neuroleptic-treated patients.

Affective Disorder

Several investigators (8,44,45) have suggested that patients with affective disorder may be at increased risk for the development of tardive dyskinesia. This may be particularly true among patients with recurrent unipolar depressions. It is important to keep in mind that a diagnosis of depression may also be associated with intermittent antipsychotic drug administration, the concurrent use of tricyclic antidepressants, or alcohol abuse, all of which may be more common in depressed patients and potentially increase the vulnerability to tardive dyskinesia.

Even within the population of patients with schizophrenia there has been some evidence that the presence of a familial history positive for affective disorders may increase the risk of tardive dyskinesia (43,56).

In the prospective study of elderly neuroleptic-treated patients, Saltz et al. (46) found a higher incidence of tardive dyskinesia developing in elderly individuals with psychiatric diagnoses as compared to elderly individuals with organic brain syndromes. This finding runs counter to the notion that "organicity" increases the risk for tardive dyskinesia, but it supports the notion that some psychiatric disorders may predispose to the development of abnormal involuntary movements following neuroleptic treatment. The dichotomy is outmoded in that schizophrenia is also now considered to be a largely "organic" disorder.

DRUG TREATMENT VARIABLES

Drug Type

Enormous attention has been directed towards whether or not any specific antipsychotic drug or drug class differs from others in their propensity to produce tardive dyskinesia. Unfortunately a great deal of this attention has focused on the implications of animal models and preclinical studies that may not be entirely relevant to the clinical condition. At the present time, there are no compelling data from prospective clinical studies that any currently available antipsychotic drug has a lower risk for tardive dyskinesia, with the possible exception of clozapine. Studies which are retrospective in nature are difficult to interpret because such factors as polypharmacy, noncompliance, co-administration of other drugs, and so on, remain a problem. Some reports have suggested that depot injectable forms of fluphenazine may carry an increased risk of tardive dyskinesia (19,48); however, this could be a result of increased antipsychotic drug exposure due to guaranteed medication delivery overcoming noncompliance. There are a variety of other difficulties in arriving at meaningful conclusions regarding relative risk with a specific drug. The ideal design for such studies would involve random assignment of patients to treatment groups, systematic evaluation, and control of such variables as length of drug exposure, dose equivalents and age. Pharmaceutical companies have tended to shy away from conducting prospective studies involving the risk of tardive dyskinesia development because the assumption has been that hundreds of patients would be required and a very lengthy follow-up would be necessary. Based on previously discussed results from prospective studies, it would appear that relatively high risk groups (e.g., elderly individuals with early signs of drug-induced parkinsonism) could be recruited and might allow the development of a relatively rapid comparison between an experimental and a standard medication.

The best evidence for a reduced liability in producing tardive dyskinesia has been found for sulpiride and clozapine, and for both compounds a variety of theories have been put forward to explain this potential advantage. The best claims for low propensity to produce tardive dyskinesia have been made for clozapine. Recent data in the United States indicate that more than 60,000 patients have been treated with clozapine and that approximately 40,000 are currently receiving the medication (H. Sykes-Gomez, July 1993, *personal communication*). To date, there have been no confirmed cases of definite tardive dyskinesia occurring amongst these patients attributable to treatment with clozapine.

Casey (8) also concluded that this compound has a very low incidence of parkinsonism and there are virtually no reports of dystonia. Clozapine is associated with a relatively high rate of agranulocytosis. Experience in the United States reveals a cumulative incidence of 0.8% for this reaction after 1 year of treatment (2).

Drug Dosage

Although it must be true that at some level there is a significant relationship between neuroleptic dosage, duration of treatment, and the risk of tardive dyskinesia, this has been a very difficult relationship to establish. Because most patients do not develop tardive dyskinesia, it may be difficult to establish such a relationship which would only be apparent in those individuals who are in fact vulnerable to the disorder.

The overwhelming majority of cross-sectional studies and follow-up studies that have addressed this issue have not been able to identify a clear association between the risk of tardive dyskinesia development and drug variables such as duration, total amount of drug administered, type of drug, or current dosage. Although one study (30) did suggest the possibility of a reduced incidence of tardive dyskinesia among patients receiving very low doses of neuroleptic maintenance treatment, this finding has not been consistently borne out in other studies of dosage reduction or intermittent treatment.

Kane and Smith (31) have pointed out that most studies reporting a significant relationship between tardive dyskinesia and medication dosage or duration have included samples of patients in the relatively early years of their drug treatment history. It is possible that the relationship between these variables and tardive dyskinesia risk is more apparent or more of a risk factor in the relatively early development of tardive dyskinesia as opposed to those cases which occur after 5–10 years of cumulative neuroleptic exposure.

Several recent studies have employed an intermittent or targeted strategy to attempt to reduce cumulative neuroleptic exposure. One important outcome measure in these studies is the potential impact on tardive dyskinesia. To date, none of these studies have demonstrated significant advantages for intermittent treatment in reducing the risk of tardive dyskinesia (29).

Antipsychotic Drug Blood Levels

In exploring the relationship between dosage, duration, and tardive dyskinesia, risk analyses are also complicated by the fact that there are enormous individual differences in the absorption and metabolism of antipsychotic drugs. Therefore, patients receiving similar oral doses of a specific drug may develop very different levels of active drug in relevant brain areas. To date, results are not consistent across studies to suggest that patients with tardive dyskinesia experience higher blood levels following equivalent doses of antipsychotic drugs; therefore, the results are inconclusive. Most of the studies have not found a significant correlation (13,24). Some other investigators, however, have reported that patients with tardive dyskinesia had higher drug serum levels (25,65). A comparison between prescribed dosage regimens in oral form is a far cry from an accurate reflection of the drug exposure at a specific receptor. It is not surprising, therefore, that relationships between drug treatment variables and tardive dyskinesia have been difficult to demonstrate. It remains unclear as to whether or not drug blood levels are a critical predictive factor, but as indicated in the previous discussion of dosage and duration, it may be that we have not applied adequate methodology to establish the point in time and for which patients such a relationship might exist.

Concomitant Medication—Anticholinergic Drugs

Many observers have noted that the addition of anticholinergic medication can exacerbate existing tardive dyskinesia and that discontinuing anticholinergic drugs may improve the condition. The observation has led to the hypothesis that these compounds might also contribute to the development of tardive dyskinesia; however, there is no clear-cut evidence that an increased incidence or prevalence of tardive dyskinesia is seen among patients chronically treated with antiparkinsonian drugs (17). It may also be possible that any association seen between vulnerability to tardive dyskinesia and anticholinergic administration is really an epiphenomenon because those individuals who are vulnerable to drug-induced extrapyramidal side effects may also have an increased risk of developing tardive dyskinesia. Because such patients are probably more likely to receive anticholinergic medication, this relationship may suggest anticholinergic drugs as a risk factor when in fact it is the extrapyramidal side effects that are increasing relative risk (31).

In the case of tardive dyskinesia, it is clearly difficult to make inferences regarding etiology based on the effects of a particular manipulation on preexisting tardive dyskinesia. The ability of antipsychotic drugs to mask the condition is an example because we assume that antipsychotic drugs play a critical role in etiology. The chronic administration of cholinergic receptor antagonists has been shown in animal models to increase antagonist-induced supersensitivity of dopamine receptors. It is also apparent that there is considerable difference among commonly used anticholinergic drugs in their relative affinities for different subtypes of muscarinic receptors.

Lithium

Some animal studies have explored the effect of concomitantly administered lithium in models of tardive dys-

kinesia (42). The results from these studies have been somewhat mixed, however, and it is difficult to draw conclusions. There are very few clinical data available, but Kane et al. (32) did find an effect of concomitant lithium administration in reducing the incidence of tardive dyskinesia among a group of patients receiving neuroleptic treatment.

Smoking

Some investigators have found that among neuroleptic-treated patients, smoking was associated with an increased of prevalence of tardive dyskinesia. It is possible that nicotine stimulates dopamine release from nigrostriatal neurons (62).

Diabetes Mellitus

Several investigators have suggested that diabetes may increase the risk of tardive dyskinesia (16,58). The possible mechanism underlying this apparent increased susceptibility remains unclear.

Structural Brain Pathology

Several investigators have studied the relationship between abnormalities on brain imaging and the prevalence of tardive dyskinesia (1,35,50). Overall, the findings are rather mixed and a variety of methodologic problems complicate the drawing of firm conclusions. Waddington (52) had suggested the possibility that associations between structural brain abnormalities and measures of abnormal involuntary movements may be more robust for orofacial dyskinesia than for limb and truncal dyskinesias.

Neuropsychological Deficits

The relationship between a variety of measures of cognitive functioning and tardive dyskinesia has been subject of several investigations. This area is obviously complicated by the fact that some degree of cognitive dysfunction is found in a substantial proportion of patients with schizophrenia. The question as to whether or not such dysfunction is more common in those patients who are most vulnerable to the development of tardive dyskinesia has been difficult to pursue. It is also possible, as discussed previously, that those schizophrenic patients with cognitive dysfunction (and negative symptoms, etc.) are overall more vulnerable to developing tardive dyskinesia and that cognitive dysfunction represents one aspect of a particular schizophrenia subtype.

Waddington (51) reviewed 11 studies in which patients with schizophrenia underwent neuropsychological testing, and contrasts were made between those with and those without tardive dyskinesia. These investigations involved a variety of test measures and very heterogeneous patient populations; however, in eight of these reports there was evidence supporting an association between cognitive dysfunction and the prevalence of tardive dyskinesia. In many of these studies, the investigators failed to control for such potentially important variables as age and psychiatric diagnosis. Waddington et al. (54,55) also reported a significant relationship between tardive dyskinesia and cognitive dysfunction in neuroleptic-treated bipolar patients.

Most of those studies that have included a wide range of cognitive functions in their assessment methodology failed to detect significant differences between individuals with and without tardive dyskinesia (5,49).

At the present time, it is difficult to draw firm conclusions on the relationship between cognitive dysfunction and drug-induced movement disorders.

NATURAL HISTORY

The outcome of tardive dyskinesia appears to be very heterogeneous. Many patients, particularly younger individuals, will experience considerable improvement over time (10,59). In general, follow-up studies suggest that tardive dyskinesia does not commonly progress, but tends to follow a fluctuating course with an overall trend towards improvement (18). Time may be the most important factor in outcome. The length of follow-up in most studies is positively correlated with increasing improvement or remission of tardive dyskinesia. Therefore, studies examining outcome after more than 5 years provide results that are more favorable than those obtained from shorter follow-up assessments. If drug treatment is stopped or if medication dosage is reduced, the tardive dyskinesia has a more favorable outcome (11).

Kane et al. (*unpublished data*) have assessed the outcome of tardive dyskinesia developing among patients followed in the prospective study previously alluded to by Kane et al. (32). In this study, 144 patients whose mean age is 29 were followed for an average of 4.3 years after the development of tardive dyskinesia. Approximately 60% showed remission in tardive dyskinesia at some point during the follow-up period. However, because tardive dyskinesia can have a fluctuating course, it is possible that some patients who experience a remission will be at risk for subsequent reemergence of tardive dyskinesia. Examining only those patients in whom tardive dyskinesia remitted and never recurred, Kane et al. found that approximately 40% were so characterized after 5 years of follow-up. These investigators found that age, gender, diagnosis, and length of neuroleptic treatment prior to the diagnosis of tardive dyskinesia bore no relationship to the outcome. On the other hand, the proportion of time on medication following the development of tar-

dive dyskinesia, as well as modal dose of neuroleptic following the diagnosis of tardive dyskinesia, did appear to be associated with outcome. Interestingly, it appeared that those patients who were either on neuroleptics all of the time or less than 50% of the time had a significantly better outcome than those patients who were on neuroleptics between 51% and 99% of the time. This might suggest that intermittent treatment or on/off medication manipulations are associated with a worse outcome than either continuous treatment or relatively long-term drug withdrawal. This association will require further study, but has important implications for clinical management of tardive dyskinesia, particularly in the context of those patients who are likely to benefit from or require continued neuroleptic treatment.

Glazer et al. (20,22) reported the results of a retrospective follow-up study of 192 patients seen two or more times during a 3- to 55-month period while continuing to receive neuroleptics. One hundred twelve subjects (58% of the sample) demonstrated a "chronic persistent" pattern in contrast to an intermittent pattern in the remainder of the patients. These investigators found that the most important predictors of chronic persistent tardive dyskinesia included increased age and the presence of nonorofacial dyskinesia at baseline. Glazer et al. (20,22) reported results on a separate cadre of tardive dyskinesia patients who were withdrawn from neuroleptic and who were reexamined monthly for a mean of 10 months. These investigators reported complete and persistent reversibility of tardive dyskinesia in only 2% of these patients; however, many patients showed substantial improvement without complete remission.

The fact that tardive dyskinesia is most often not severe and may improve or remit over time is important clinically in establishing the benefit-to-risk ratio of continued neuroleptic treatment in those patients who clearly require continued medication.

RESEARCH IMPLICATIONS AND FUTURE DIRECTIONS

Given the promise offered by clozapine and other potentially atypical medications, it will be essential to conduct adequately designed and controlled tests to establish the relative merits of new compounds in this regard.

As new compounds with more specific effects on particular receptors become available, it is hoped that new knowledge with regard to mechanisms of drug action will be forthcoming. It may also be particularly valuable to study those patients who appear invulnerable to tardive dyskinesia despite years of neuroleptic treatment in terms of providing clues to pathophysiology and risk factors.

Given the fact that at present there are no proven safe and effective treatments for tardive dyskinesia, identification of risk factors and the development of preventive strategies remains an important goal.

ACKNOWLEDGMENTS

This work was supported by NIMH grants MH-32369, MH-40015, and MH-41960.

REFERENCES

1. Albus M, Naber D, Muller-Spahn E, et al. Tardive dyskinesia: relation to computer tomographic, endocrine and psychopathological variables. *Biol Psychiatry* 1985;20:1082–1089.
2. Alvir JMAJ, Lieberman JA, Safferman AZ, et al. Clozapine-induced agranulocytosis: incidence and risk factors in the United States. *N Engl J Med* 1993;329:162–167.
3. Ayd FJ. A survey of drug-induced extrapyramidal reactions. *JAMA* 1961;175:1054–1060.
4. Barnes TRE, Liddle PF. Tardive dyskinesia: implications for schizophrenia? In: Schiff AA, Roth M, Freeman HL, eds. *Schizophrenia: new pharmacological and clinical development.* London: Royal Society of Medicine Services, 1985;81–87.
5. Barr WB, Mukherjee M, Caracci G, et al. Neuropsychological studies in tardive dyskinesia: a possible relationship with anomalous dominance. Society of Biological Psychiatry, 42nd Annual Convention and Scientific Program, 295, 1987.
6. Burke RE, Kang UJ. Tardive dystonia: clinical aspects and treatment. In: Jankovic J, Tolosa E, eds. *Facial dyskinesias.* New York: Raven Press, 1988;199–210.
7. Campbell M, Grega DM, Green WH, et al. Review: neuroleptic-induced dyskinesias in children. *Clin Neuropharmacol* 1983;6:207–222.
8. Casey DE. Affective disorders and tardive dyskinesia. *Enephale* 1988;14:221–226.
9. Casey DE. Clozapine: neuroleptic-induced EPS and tardive dyskinesia. *Psychopharmacology* 1989;99:S47–S53.
10. Casey DE, Gardos G. Tardive dyskinesia: outcome at 10 years. *Schizophr Res* 1990;3:11.
11. Casey DE, Gerlach J. Tardive dyskinesia: What is the long-term outcome. In: Casey DE, Gardos G, eds. *Tardive dyskinesia and neuroleptics: from dogma to reason.* Washington, DC: American Psychiatric Press, 1986;75–97.
12. Chorfi M, Moussaoui D. Lack of dyskinesias in unmedicated schizophrenics. *Psychopharmacology* 1989;97:423.
13. Fairbairn AF, Rowell FJ, Hui SM, et al. Serum concentration of depot neuroleptics in tardive dyskinesia. *Br J Psychiatry* 1983;142:579–583.
14. Farran-Ridge C. Some syndromes referrable to the basal ganglia occurring in dementia praecox and epidemic encephalitis. *J Ment Sci* 1926;72:513–523.
15. Fenton WS, Wyatt RJ, McGlashan TH. Risk factors for spontaneous dyskinesia in schizophrenia. Paper presented at the American Psychiatric Association meeting, May 1993.
16. Ganzini L, Heintz RT, Hoffman WF, Casey DE. The prevalence of tardive dyskinesia in neuroleptic-treated diabetics. *Arch Gen Psychiatry* 1991;48:259–263.
17. Gardos G, Cole JO. Tardive dyskinesia and anticholinergic drugs. *Am J Psychiatry* 1993;140:200–202.
18. Gardos G, Cole JO, Haskell D, et al. The natural history of tardive dyskinesia. *J Clin Psychopharmacol* 1988;8(suppl 4):31–33.
19. Gardos G, Cole JO, La Brie RA. Drug variables in the etiology of tardive dyskinesia: application of discriminant function analysis. *Prog Neuropsychopharmacol* 1977;1:147–154.
20. Glazer WM, Morgenstern H, Doucette JT. The prediction of chronic persistent versus intermittent tardive dyskinesia: a retrospective follow-up study. *Br J Psychiatry* 1991;158:822–828.
21. Glazer WM, Morgenstern H, Doucette JT. Predicting the long-term risk of tardive dyskinesia in outpatients maintained on neuroleptic medication. *J Clin Psychiatry* 1993;54:133–139.
22. Glazer WM, Morgenstern H, Schooler N, et al. Predictors of improvement in tardive dyskinesia following discontinuation of neuroleptic medication. *Br J Psychiatry* 1990;157:585–592.
23. Jeste DV, Caligiuri MP. Tardive dyskinesia. *Schizophr Bull* 1993;19:303–315.
24. Jeste DV, DeLisi LE, Zaleman S, et al. A biochemical study of tardive dyskinesia in young male patients. *Psychiatry Res* 1981;4:327–331.
25. Jeste DV, Linnoila M, Wagner RL, et al. Serum neuroleptic concentrations and tardive dyskinesia. *Psychopharmacology* 1982;76:377–386.
26. Jeste DV, Karson CM, Iager AC, et al. Association of abnormal involuntary movements and negative symptoms. *Psychopharmacol Bull* 1984;20:380–381.
27. Jeste DV, Wyatt RJ. Changing epidemiology of tardive dyskinesia: an overview. *Am J Psychiatry* 1981;138:297–309.
28. Kane JM, Jeste DV, Barnes TRE, et al. Tardive dyskinesia: a Task force report of the American Psychiatric Association. Washington, DC: American Psychiatric Association, 1992.
29. Kane JM, Marder SR. Pharmacologic treatment of schizophrenia. *Schizophr Bull* 1993;19:287–302.
30. Kane JM, Rifkin A, Woerner M, et al. Low-dose neuroleptic treatment of outpatient schizophrenics. *Arch Gen Psychiatry* 1983;40:893–896.
31. Kane JM, Smith JM. Tardive dyskinesia: prevalence and risk factors, 1959–1979. *Arch Gen Psychiatry* 1982;39:473–481.
32. Kane J, Woerner M, Borenstein M. Integrating incidence and prevalence of tardive dyskinesia. *Psychopharmacol Bull* 1986;22:254–258.
33. Kane JM, Woerner M, Lieberman J. Tardive dyskinesia: prevalence, incidence and risk factors. *J Clin Psychopharmacol* 1988;8:52S–56S.
34. Kang UJ, Burke RE, Fahn S. Natural history and treatment of tardive dystonia. *Mov Disord* 1986;1:193–208.
35. Kaufmann CA, Jeste DV, Shelton RC, et al. Noradrenergic and neuroradiologic abnormalities in tardive dyskinesia. *Biol Psychiatry* 1986;21:799–812.
36. Kraepelin EP. *Dementia praecox and paraphrenia.* Translated by Barclay RM and edited by Robertson GM. Edinburgh: E & S Livingstone, 1919.
37. Levine J, Schooler N, Severe J, et al. Discontinuation of oral and depot fluphenazine in schizophrenic patients after one year of continuous medication: a controlled study. *Psychopharmacology* 1980;24:483–493.
38. Lidsky TI, Weinhold PM, Levine FM. Implications of basal ganglionic dysfunction for schizophrenia. *Biol Psychiatry* 1979;14:3–12.
39. Manschrek TC, Maher BA, Rucklos ME, et al. Disturbed voluntary motor activity in schizophrenic disorder. *Psychol Med* 1982;12:73–84.
40. Mettler FA, Crandell A. Neurologic disorders in psychiatric institutions. *J Nerv Ment Dis* 1959;128:148–159.
41. Owens DGC, Johnstone EC, Frith CD. Spontaneous involuntary disorders of movement: their prevalence, severity and distribution in chronic schizophrenics with and without treatment with neuroleptics. *Arch Gen Psychiatry* 1982;39:452–461.
42. Pert A, Rosenblatt JE, Sivit C, et al. Long-term treatment with lithium prevents the development of dopamine receptor supersensitivity. *Science* 1978;201:171–173.
43. Richardson MA, Pass R, Bregman Z, et al. Tardive dyskinesia and depressive symptoms in schizophrenics. *Psychopharmacol Bull* 1985;21:130–135.
44. Rosenbaum AH, Niven RG, Hanson HP, et al. Tardive dyskinesia: relationship with primary affective disorder. *Dis Nerv Syst* 1977;38:423–426.
45. Rush M, Diamond F, Alpert M. Depression as a risk factor in tardive dyskinesia. *Biol Psychiatry* 1982;17:387–392.
46. Saltz BL, Woerner MG, Kane JM, et al. Prospective study of tardive dyskinesia incidence in the elderly. *JAMA* 1991;266:2402–2406.
47. Segal DS, Janowsky DS. Psychostimulant-induced behavioral effects: Possible models of schizophrenia. In: Lipton MA, DiMascio AD, Killam KF, eds. *Psychopharmacology: a generation of progress.* New York: Raven Press, 1978;1113–1123.
48. Smith RC, Strizich M, Klass D. Drug history and tardive dyskinesia. *Am J Psychiatry* 1978;135:1402–1403.
49. Soni SD, Neill D. Tardive dyskinesia and cognitive functions in schizophrenia. *Schizophr Res* 1990;3:78.
50. Sorokin JE, Giordani B, Mohs RC, et al. Memory impairment in schizophrenic patients with tardive dyskinesia. *Biol Psychiatry* 1988;23:129–135.

51. Waddington JL. Tardive dyskinesia in schizophrenia and other disorders: association with aging, cognitive dysfunction and structural brain pathology in relation to neuroleptic exposure. *Hum Psychopharmacol* 1987;2:11–22.
52. Waddington JL. Schizophrenia, affective psychoses and other disorders treated with neuroleptic drugs: the enigma of tardive dyskinesia, its neurobiological determinants and the conflict of paradigms. *Int Rev Neurobiol* 1989;31:297–353.
53. Waddington JL. Spontaneous orofacial movements induced in rodents by very long-term neuroleptic drug administration: phenomenology, pathophysiology and putative relationship to tardive dyskinesia. *Psychopharmacology* 1990;101:431–447.
54. Waddington JL, Brown K, O'Neill J. Cognitive impairment, clinical course and treatment history in outpatients with bipolar affective disorder: relationship to tardive dyskinesia. *Psychol Med* 1989;19:897–902.
55. Waddington JL, Youssef HA, Dolphin C, et al. Cognitive dysfunction, negative symptoms and tardive dyskinesia in schizophrenia: their association in relation to topography of involuntary movements and criterion of their abnormality. *Arch Gen Psychiatry* 1987;44:907–912.
56. Wegner JT, Catalano F, Gibralter J, et al. Schizophrenics with

tardive dyskinesia: neuropsychological deficit and family psychopathology. *Arch Gen Psychiatry* 1985;42:860–865.
57. Woerner M, Kane JM, Lieberman JA, et al. The prevalence of tardive dyskinesia. *J Clin Psychopharmacol* 1991;11:34–42.
58. Woerner M, Saltz BL, Kane JM, Lieberman JA, Alvir JMJ. Diabetes and development of tardive dyskinesia. *Am J Psychiatry* 1993;150:966–968.
59. Yagi G, Itoh H. Follow-up study of 11 patients with potentially reversible tardive dyskinesia. *Am J Psychiatry* 1987;144:1496–1498.
60. Yarden PE, Discipio WJ. Abnormal movements and prognosis in schizophrenia. *Am J Psychiatry* 1971;128:317–323.
61. Yassa R, Jeste DV. Gender differences in tardive dyskinesia: a critical review of the literature. *Schizophr Bull* 1992;18:701–715.
62. Yassa R, Lal S, Korpassy A, Ally J. Nicotine exposure and tardive dyskinesia. *Biol Psychiatry* 1987;22:67–72.
63. Yassa R, Nair V, Schwartz G. Tardive dyskinesia and the primary psychiatric diagnosis. *Psychosomatics* 1984;25:135–138.
64. Yassa R, Nair V, Schwartz G. Tardive dyskinesia: a two-year follow-up study. *Psychosomatics* 1984;25:852–855.
65. Yesavage JA, Tauke ED, Sheikh. Tardive dyskinesia and steady-state serum levels of thiothixene. *Arch Gen Psychiatry* 1987;44:913–915.

Psychopharmacology: The Fourth Generation of Progress, edited by Floyd E. Bloom and David J. Kupfer. Raven Press, Ltd., New York © 1995.

CHAPTER 128

Tardive Dyskinesia

Pathophysiology

Daniel E. Casey

Tardive dyskinesia (TD), a syndrome of potentially irreversible, involuntary hyperkinetic dyskinesias that occurs during long-term neuroleptic treatment, is a major limitation of chronic antipsychotic drug therapy. This has stimulated substantial research to identify the underlying pathophysiological mechanisms of TD, with the hope that these results will lead to new drugs that maintain antipsychotic efficacy but are free of TD risk. Data from multiple lines of investigation in both the preclinical and clinical realms have been brought to bear on the topic, but have not yet produced a parsimonious explanation. Hypotheses span a wide range of concepts that incorporate neurochemical and/or structural abnormalities associated with the underlying psychoses as well as the drug therapies for these disorders. Each hypothesis utilizes multiple models to marshal data relevant to specific issues. The aim of this chapter is to review and critique the results that are in support of, or in conflict with, the major hypotheses about the pathophysiology of TD (see Chapter 127, *this volume*).

DOPAMINE HYPERSENSITIVITY

The hypothesis of dopamine hypersensitivity has dominated the conceptual approaches to studying TD. It proposes that the nigrostriatal dopamine system develops increased sensitivity to dopamine as a consequence of chronic dopamine receptor blockade induced by neuroleptic drugs (45,68). This derives from the classic studies of denervation-induced hypersensitivity seen in peripheral muscles. The very large database generated by investigating this hypothesis can be interpreted as limited support for, or ample evidence against, the dopamine hypersensitivity hypothesis (12).

Behavioral evidence of dopamine hypersensitivity following neuroleptic treatment is seen in many different models in several species. The most common is exaggerated oral stereotyped behavior in response to acute dopamine agonist challenges after discontinuing neuroleptic drugs. Such increased behavior can be seen after a single dose, a few days, several weeks, or 1 year of neuroleptics in rodents (18,20,45,64,68) and nonhuman primates (10). Biochemical changes of increased numbers of dopamine D2 receptors are also usually found after repeated neuroleptic treatment (8), but this is not the case in all studies (73).

Though this model has served as the bedrock of the dopamine D2 receptor hypersensitivity hypothesis of TD, there are several fundamental flaws. The principal problems center around the incompatibility between features of the model and the clinical TD syndrome. In patients, the symptoms gradually develop over many months or years of treatment and continue to be present without the requirement of dopamine agonist provocation. In contrast, all animals rapidly develop behavioral and biochemical measures of hypersensitivity, which quickly resolve following neuroleptic discontinuation, whereas only a subgroup of patients develop TD, and it persists for long periods of time (14), except in the case of withdrawal dyskinesias (3). Perhaps these behavioral and biochemical models in rodents are better conceptualized as characterizing the acute and subacute effects of neuroleptics in extrapyramidal syndromes (EPS) or antipsychotic actions (12).

D.E. Casey: Psychiatric Research and Psychopharmacology, VA Medical Center, Portland, Oregon 97207; Department of Psychiatry and Neurology, Oregon Health Sciences University, Portland, Oregon 97207; and Oregon Regional Primate Research Center, Beaverton, Oregon 97006.

The model of spontaneous vacuous chewing movements (VCMs) that increase with chronic neuroleptic treatment has been proposed as a closer fit to the time course of clinical TD (24). In this setting, traditional neuroleptics show a wide range of inducing VCMs that correspond to the milligram potency continuum (i.e., haloperidol produces more and chlorpromazine produces fewer movements) (33). However, this is not a clinical feature of TD, because all neuroleptics used in the clinic appear to have similar TD liability, with the exception of clozapine (13,42). These VCMs increase with age and neuroleptic treatment (60,73) but may or may not correlate with changes in dopamine receptor numbers (73). Reversibility of VCMs is also unclear, because one study noted prompt resolution when discontinuing neuroleptics or giving anticholinergics (60), but another observed persistence for at least 2.5 months (73). Perhaps this VCM model also reflects more of the neuroleptic effects in acute EPS than in TD. Alternatively, it may be modeling both early and late aspects of neuroleptics in rodents, but those differ in some important features from the clinical findings. It is also possible that the chewing movements, which are variously described by different investigators, are actually different phenomena seen in these different studies.

The model of TD in nonhuman primates much more closely fits the clinical features (10,11,34) but provides only limited support for the dopamine hypersensitivity hypothesis. Dopamine turnover was significantly decreased in the caudate and substantia nigra in monkeys with TD 2 months after neuroleptics were discontinued (35), though no receptor quantification was done to compare and contrast findings with other species.

A modification of the D2-receptor hypersensitivity hypothesis incorporates a role for D1 dopamine receptors. The core of this hypothesis is that clozapine has a unique biochemical profile at D1 and D2 receptors that may be associated with atypical behavioral and clinical features. Clozapine in rodents does not produce biochemical or behavioral indications of basal ganglia-related D2 hypersensitivity (21). Similarly, clozapine produces very little EPS and TD in patients (13) and has relatively high D1 and moderate D2 occupancy rates, as measured by positron emission tomography (PET) (25). These observations have led to the proposal that TD develops from an imbalance between D1- and D2-mediated effects in the basal ganglia (29,30). This possibility is supported by the wealth of data documenting the functional interactions of D1 and D2 receptors (72), but it is too soon to know if there is a critical role for D1–D2 interactions in TD.

Data from the clinic are also difficult to fully reconcile with the dopamine-receptor hypersensitivity hypothesis. Efforts at finding direct evidence of support for this proposal have been unsuccessful. Receptor binding studies of human postmortem brain tissue comparing schizophrenic patients with and without TD found no significant differences in either D1 or D2 receptors (22,23). However, these data must be considered in the context of concern about (a) the time of, and conditions at, death and (b) current and past drug treatment that may obscure the role of dopamine in TD. Neuroimaging with PET to assess functional evidence of dopamine-receptor hypersensitivity has not been systematically applied to the question.

Biochemical data from the clinic also fail to support dopamine dysfunction as the explanation of TD. When comparing TD patients with non-TD patients, there were no consistent differences in (a) dopamine-mediated endocrine measures of prolactin or growth hormone or (b) cerebrospinal fluid (CSF), plasma, or urinary homovanillic acid assessments (40,44,66).

Clinical pharmacological observations suggest an important role for dopamine in TD. There is an increased incidence and prevalence of involuntary hyperkinetic dyskinesias in patients receiving dopamine antagonists in most (42,43,62), but not all, reports (71,74). Additionally, dopamine antagonists suppress TD, whereas dopamine agonists usually aggravate TD symptoms (14). However, even in these findings, observations are conflicting, because potent direct dopamine agonists such as bromocriptine fail to markedly worsen TD (37), and neuroleptics may paradoxically increase TD in a few patients (16,31). These clinical data, which in part seem to support the dopamine hypersensitivity hypothesis, may best be incorporated into an understanding of TD if dopamine plays a secondary or modulatory role. If the primary pathophysiology lies outside the dopamine system but is indirectly influenced by dopaminergic mechanisms, the clinical pharmacological impact of perturbations from dopamine agonists and antagonists could be parsimoniously combined (12,14,71), with the absence of any direct evidence of dopamine hypersensitivity.

NEUROTOXICITY

An alternate hypothesis recently receiving considerable interest is the proposal that TD is due to neurotoxic effects of free radical byproducts from catecholamine metabolism. The basal ganglia, by virtue of their high oxidative metabolism, would be particularly vulnerable to membrane lipid peroxidation as a result of the increased catecholamine turnover induced by neuroleptic drugs (9,50,51). This concept has also been proposed as an explanation for several dyskinetic syndromes referable to the basal ganglia (50). While this hypothesis is speculative, there are data to support the proposal.

Animal studies in rodents receiving acute or subacute neuroleptic treatment show a mitigating effect of vitamin E (α-tocopherol) on behavioral measures of dyskinesias (50). This benefit is purportedly on the basis of vitamin E serving as a free radical scavenger, thus reducing the potentially cytotoxic effects of free radicals.

Clinical studies have produced conflicting data in this area. Some studies have found increased levels of lipid peroxidation byproducts in blood or CSF of TD compared to non-TD patients (52,58). In clinical trials with TD, the majority of patients with TD did not show major (>50%) improvement (1,51,65). However, there was a more favorable outcome in those patients who were younger and had shorter durations of TD (1,51,65)—both of which are factors associated with a greater likelihood of spontaneous recovery from, or improvement in, TD (15). Other possible explanations for these findings that are yet to be explored include alterations in neuroleptic metabolism or brain drug levels from vitamin E, which could have the effect of raising the amount of neuroleptic antagonism at dopamine receptors and thus mask or suppress TD.

GABA INSUFFICIENCY

Another competing hypothesis involves gamma-aminobutyric acid (GABA) insufficiency in the neuroanatomical loop controlling movement (26,27,63). Again the data are conflicting. In rodent models there may (27,63) or may not (55,61) be consistent alterations in GABA function associated with acute and chronic neuroleptic treatment. Studies in nonhuman primates indicate a GABA association with TD because decreased glutamic acid decarboxylase (GAD), the GABA synthesizing enzyme, was noted in the substantia nigra, medial globus pallidus, and subthalamic nuclei in dyskinetic monkeys compared to similarly neuroleptic treated non-TD monkeys (35,36). These were the same animals that also have abnormalities in dopamine parameters listed above (35).

Clinical biochemical data suggest that GABA may play a role, whereas clinical treatment trials are not as supportive. A small postmortem study found a trend toward decreased GAD in the medial globus pallidus, but normal levels in the nigra in TD in patients (2), and a separate study reported decreased CSF levels in TD patients (70). However, treatment trials with drugs that enhance GABA have been disappointing. Single doses of muscimol partially decreased TD but produced unacceptable toxicity and sedation (67), and trials with other agonists produced negative (17,46,47) or mixed results (69). Thus, it has not been possible to effectively treat TD with GABA acting agents, which raises important questions about a primary role for GABA in this disorder.

OTHER NEUROCHEMICAL HYPOTHESES

Because most neuroleptics also antagonize many other receptor types besides dopamine, it is possible that these play an important role in the pathophysiology of TD. A noradrenergic dysfunction theory derives some support from findings of greater dopamine β-hydroxylase activity in TD patients compared to non-TD patients (40) and a positive CSF norepinephrine correlation with TD severity (44). However, noradrenergic agents have not been successful treatments for TD (32,41).

Serotonin may modulate dopamine activity and thus be involved with TD. However, efforts to find consistent abnormalities of serotonin parameters or effective serotonin treatments for TD (41) offer little support for this hypothesis.

There is some evidence that nutritional or metabolic issues may play a role in TD, but these concepts are currently more heuristic than well-developed. Meals which alter the phenylalanine/large amino acid ratio temporarily decrease TD movements (59). Another interesting observation is the increased risk of TD in diabetics (28,56,76), suggesting that alterations in glucose and/or insulin parameters may interact with neuroleptics.

Cholinergic hypofunction has been proposed as a cause of TD, but this is not adequately supported. Several other possible avenues of exploration include (a) roles for neuropeptides, such as cholecystokinin, substance P, neurotensin, and somatostatin (71), and (b) disorders of mineral metabolism, such as iron (4).

Electrophysiological measures of decreased activity in the nigrostriatal dopamine system (depolarization inactivation) following chronic treatment in rodents with traditional neuroleptics but not with clozapine (7) indicate this mechanism may be involved with TD. In contrast, some drugs known to produce TD, such as thioridazine, do not cause striatal depolarization block (75), and adding anticholinergics to traditional neuroleptics in rodents makes them appear atypical in this model (7), when this is not the case in patients. Thus, the role of depolarization inactivation in TD is unknown.

STRUCTURAL ABNORMALITIES

Attempts to identify a structural basis for TD have involved animals and patients. Electron-microscopic studies have recently shown that treatment for 2 weeks or more with traditional neuroleptics such as haloperidol increases perforated postsynaptic densities in the head of the caudate nucleus, but this is not seen with clozapine (54). The D1 antagonist SCH 23390 also produces this effect, but when combined with haloperidol to make D1 and D2 antagonism similar to clozapine, the combination does not alter structure (53). Thus, there are selective drug-induced neuroanatomical alterations that are site-specific and may be related to TD, but require much more investigation. Whether long-term neuroleptic treatment causes cell loss is unclear. Brains from rodents receiving several months of neuroleptics show either cell loss or no change (57) or cytoarchitectural alterations (5).

Postmortem studies in humans have also produced conflicting results. One light-microscopic study noted higher rates of nigral degeneration and gliosis in patients with

TD (19), but another suggested that these findings may be nonspecific age-related changes (39). Neuroimaging investigations have similarly found variable results. Computerized tomography studies often find abnormalities, but the wide range of different methodologies makes it impossible to conclude if there are consistent structural defects associated with TD (38). The few reports of magnetic resonance imaging in TD also find several different questionable lesions that do not yet lead to a conclusion (4).

SPONTANEOUS DYSKINESIAS

Up to this point in the search for the underlying pathophysiology of TD, considering neuroleptics as the sole etiological agent has not been fruitful. Expanding the issue to incorporate important patient parameters (e.g., disease, age) in addition to drug factors seems prudent (11).

Kraepelin (48) and Bleuler (6) observed abnormal movements of the orofacial and limb regions when they were describing the fundamental aspects of schizophrenia. Unfortunately, it is not possible to know the true prevalence of these phenomena or whether the movements described were the same as, or fundamentally distinct from, TD. A more recent report found that the type and severity of dyskinesias were similar in treated and untreated patients, but the prevalence was significantly higher in the neuroleptic group when age was controlled (23). Additionally, several studies indicate that TD patients often have greater cognitive dysfunction, negative symptoms, poor premorbid function, and poor prognosis (71).

Age may make a similarly important contribution to the expression of TD. Spontaneously occurring orofacial dyskinesias occur more often in aging humans and monkeys (11) and in patients with more neuromedical illnesses (49). The long observed positive correlation between age and neuroleptic-associated TD risk further emphasizes the role of age.

Thus, an important coalescence of critical factors may best explain TD. The underlying syndromes of psychosis, particularly schizophrenia, advancing age, and some unknown component of neuroleptic action, may combine to convert a covert vulnerability to dyskinesias to overt symptomology in the clinical constellation of TD (11). The central challenge which has not yet been fully overcome is to accurately attribute the relative contribution of each of these factors to the pathogenesis and pathophysiology of TD.

CONCLUSION

The pathophysiology of TD has been actively pursued, but remains elusive. Human studies and animal models have been a rich but incomplete source of data about the effects of neuroleptic treatment. A major limitation is that most of the animal models utilize short-term paradigms, which may more accurately assess the effects of acute or subacute treatment. To date, no direct evidence of any pathophysiological process has been identified, though indirect evidence suggests that dopamine, and perhaps other neurotransmitters, play a modulating or secondary role. A cogent argument can be made for a critical interaction between patient and drug parameters, but the specific contribution of these factors is unknown. In the current state of conflicting findings, it is best to keep an open mind about the pathogenesis and pathophysiology of the complex syndrome known as TD.

ACKNOWLEDGMENT

This work was supported, in part, by funds from the Veterans Administration Research Program and by NIMH grant 36657.

REFERENCES

1. Adler LA, Peselow E, Rotrosen J, et al. Vitamin E treatment of tardive dyskinesia. *Am J Psychiatry* 1993;150(9):1405–1407.
2. Andersson U, Häggström JE, Levi ED, Bondessan U, Valverius M, Gunne LM. Reduced glutamate decarboxylase activity in the subthalamic nucleus in patients with tardive dyskinesia. *Movement Disord* 1989;4:37–46.
3. Baldessarini RJ, Cole JO, Davis JM, Gardos G, Preskorn SH, Simpson GM, Tarsy D. *Tardive dyskinesia: a task force report.* Washington, DC: American Psychiatric Press, 1980.
4. Bartzokis G, Garber HJ, Marder SR, Olendorf WH. MRI in tardive dyskinesia. Shortened left caudate T2. *Biol Psychiatry* 1990;28:1027–1036.
5. Benes FM, Pashevich PA, Davidson J, Domesick VB. The effects of haloperidol on synaptic patterns in the rat striatum. *Brain Res* 1985;329:265–273.
6. Bleuler E. *Dementia praecox or the group of schizophrenias.* New York: International Universities Press, 1950.
7. Bunney BS, Sesack SR, Silva N. Midbrain dopaminergic systems: neurophysiology and electrophysiological pharmacology. In: Meltzer HY, ed. *Psychopharmacology: the third generation of progress.* New York: Raven Press, 1987;113–126.
8. Burt DR, Creese I, Synder SH. Antischizophrenic drugs: chronic treatment elevates dopamine receptor binding in the brain. *Science* 1977;196:326–328.
9. Cadet JL, Lohr JB, Jeste DV. Free radicals and tardive dyskinesia. *Trends Neurosci* 1986;9:107–108.
10. Casey DE. Tardive dyskinesia—animal models. *Psychopharmacol Bull* 1984;20:376–379.
11. Casey DE. Spontaneous and tardive dyskinesias: clinical and laboratory studies. *J Clin Psychiatry* 1985;46:42–47.
12. Casey DE. Tardive dyskinesia. In: Meltzer HY, ed. *Psychopharmacology: the third generation of progress.* New York: Raven, 1987;1411–1419.
13. Casey DE. Clozapine: neuroleptic-induced EPS and tardive dyskinesia. *Psychopharmacology* 1989;99:S47–S53.
14. Casey DE. Tardive dyskinesia. *West J Med* 1990;153:535–541.
15. Casey DE. Neuroleptic-induced acute extrapyramidal syndromes and tardive dyskinesia. In: Dunner DL, ed. *The psychiatric clinics of North America. Psychopharmacology I,* vol 16, part 3. Philadelphia: WB Saunders, 1993;589–610.
16. Casey DE, Denney D. Pharmacological characterization of tardive dyskinesia. *Psychopharmacology* 1977;54:1–8.
17. Casey DE, Gerlach J, Magelund G, Rosted Christensen T. The effect of gamma-acetylenic GABA in tardive dyskinesia. *Arch Gen Psychiatry* 1980;37:1376–1379.

18. Christensen AV, Fjalland B, Moller Nielsen I. On the supersensitivity of dopamine receptors induced by neuroleptics. *Psychopharmacology* 1976;48:1–6.

19. Christensen E, Moller JE, Faurbye A. Neuropathological investigation of 28 brains from patients with dyskinesia. *Acta Psychiatr Scand* 1970;46:14–23.

20. Clow A, Jenner P, Marsden CD. Changes in dopamine-mediated behaviour during one year's neuroleptic administration. *Eur J Pharmacol* 1979;57:365–375.

21. Coward DM, Imperato A, Urwyler S, White TG. Biochemical and behavioural properties of clozapine. *Psychopharmacology* 1989; 99:S6–S12.

22. Cross AJ, Crow TJ, Ferrier IN, Johnson JA, Johnstone EC, Owen F, Owens DGC, Poulter M. Chemical and structural changes in the brain in patients with movement disorder. In: Casey DE, Chase TN, Christensen AV, Gerlach J, eds. *Dyskinesia: research and treatment.* Berlin: Springer-Verlag, 1985;104–110.

23. Crow TJ, Cross AJ, Johnstone EC, Owens DG, Waddington JL. Abnormal involuntary movements in schizophrenia: are they related to the disease process or its treatment? Are they associated with changes in dopamine receptors? *J Clin Psychopharmacol* 1982;2:336–340.

24. Ellison G, See RE. Rats administered chronic neuroleptics develop oral movements which are similar in form to those in humans with tardive dyskinesia. *Psychopharmacology* 1989;98:564.

25. Farde L, Nordström A-L, Wiesel F-A, Pauli S, Halldin C, Sedvall G. Positron emission tomographic analysis of central D1 and D2 dopamine receptor occupancy in patients treated with classical neuroleptics and clozapine—relation to extrapyramidal side effects. *Arch Gen Psychiatry* 1992;49:538–544.

26. Fibiger HC, Lloyd KG. Neurobiological substrates of tardive dyskinesia: the GABA hypothesis. *Trends Neurol Sci* 1984;7:462–464.

27. Gale K. Chronic blockade of dopamine receptors by antischizophrenic drugs enhances GABA binding in substantia nigra. *Nature* 1980;283:569–570.

28. Ganzini L, Heintz R, Hoffman W, Casey DE. Prevalence of tardive dyskinesia in neuroleptic treated diabetics. *Arch Gen Psychiatry* 1991;48:259–263.

29. Gerfen CR, Engber TM, Mahan LC, et al. D1 and D2 dopamine receptor-regulated gene expression of striatonigral and striatopallidal neurons. *Science* 1990;250:1429–1432.

30. Gerlach J, Casey DE. Tardive dyskinesia. *Acta Psychiatr Scand* 1988;77:369–378.

31. Gerlach J, Reisby N, Randrup A. Dopaminergic hypersensitivity and cholinergic hypofunction in the pathophysiology of tardive dyskinesia. *Psychopharmacology* 1974;34:21–35.

32. Glazer WM. Noradrenergic function and tardive dyskinesia. *Psychiatr Ann* 1989;19(6):297–301.

33. Gunne LM, Andersson U, Bondesson U, Johansson P. Spontaneous chewing movements in rats during acute and chronic antipsychotic drug administration. *Pharmacol Biochem Behav* 1986;25:897–901.

34. Gunne LM, Barany S. Haloperidol-induced tardive dyskinesia in monkeys. *Psychopharmacology* 1976;50:237–240.

35. Gunne LM, Häggström JE. Pathophysiology of tardive dyskinesia. In: Casey DE, Chase T, Christensen AV, Gerlach J, eds. *Dyskinesia: research and treatment.* Berlin: Springer, 1985;191–193.

36. Gunne LM, Häggström JE, Sjöquist B. Association with persistent neuroleptic-induced dyskinesia of regional changes in brain GABA synthesis. *Nature* 1984;309:347–349.

37. Häggström JE. Bromocriptine in the treatment of tardive dyskinesia—an update. *Integr Psychiatry* 1989;6:171–179.

38. Hoffman WF, Casey DE. Computed tomographic evaluation of patients with tardive dyskinesia. *Schizophr Res* 1991;5:1–12.

39. Hunter R, Blackwood W, Smith MC. Neuropathological findings in three cases of persistent dyskinesia following phenothiazine medication. *J Neurol Sci* 1968;7:263–273.

40. Jeste DV, Lohr JB, Kaufmann CA, Wyatt RJ. Pathophysiology of tardive dyskinesia: evaluation of supersensitivity theory and alternative hypotheses. In: Casey DE, Gardos G, eds. *Tardive dyskinesia and neuroleptics: from dogma to reason.* Washington, DC: American Psychiatric Press, 1986;15–32.

41. Jeste DV, Wyatt RJ. Therapeutic strategies against tardive dyskinesia. *Arch Gen Psychiatry* 1982;39:803–816.

42. Kane JM, Jeste DV, Barnes TRE, Casey DE, Cole JO, Davis JM, Gualtieri CT, Schooler NR, Sprague RL, Wettstein RM. *Tardive dyskinesia: a task force report of the American Psychiatric Association.* Washington, DC: American Psychiatric Association, 1992.

43. Kane JM, Woerner M, Weinhold P, Wegner J, Kinon B, Borenstein M. Incidence of tardive dyskinesia: five year data from a prospective study. *Psychopharmacol Bull* 1984;20:39–40.

44. Kaufmann CA, Jeste DV, Shelton RC. Noradrenergic and neuroradiologic abnormalities in tardive dyskinesia. *Biol Psychiatry* 1986;21:799–812.

45. Klawans HL, Rubovits R. An experimental model of tardive dyskinesia. *J Neural Transm* 1972;33:235–246.

46. Korsgaard S, Casey DE, Gerlach J. Effect of gamma-vinyl-GABA in tardive dyskinesia. *Psychiatry Res* 1983;8:261–269.

47. Korsgaard S, Casey DE, Gerlach J, Hetmar O, Kaldan B, Mikkelsen LB. The effect of tetrahyroisoxazolopyridinol (THIP) in tardive dyskinesia. *Arch Gen Psychiatry* 1982;39:1017–1021.

48. Kraepelin E. *Dementia praecox and paraphrenia.* Edinburgh: E and S Livingstone, 1919.

49. Lieberman J, Kane JM, Woerner M. Prevalence of tardive dyskinesia in elderly samples. *Psychopharmacol Bull* 1984;20:22–26.

50. Lohr JB. Oxygen radicals and neuropsychiatric illness. Some speculations. *Arch Gen Psychiatry* 1991;48:1097–1106.

51. Lohr JB, Cadet JL, Lohr MA, et al. Vitamin E in the treatment of tardive dyskinesia: the possible involvement of free radical mechanisms. *Schizophr Bull* 1988;14:291–296.

52. Lohr JB, Kuczenski R, Bracha HS, Moir M, Jeste DV. Increased indices of free radical activity in the cerebrospinal fluid of patients with tardive dyskinesia. *Biological Psychiatry* 1990;28:535–539.

53. Meshul CK, Janowsky A, Casey DE, Stallbaumer RK, Taylor B. Coadministration of haloperidol and SCH-23390 prevents the increase in "perforated" synapses due to either drug alone. *Neuropsychopharmacology* 1992;7(4):285–293.

54. Meshul CK, Janowsky A, Casey DE, Stallbaumer RK, Taylor B. Effect of haloperidol and clozapine on the density of "perforated" synapses in caudate, nucleus accumbens, and medial prefrontal cortex. *Psychopharmacology* 1992;106:45–52.

55. Mithani S, Atymadja A, Bainbridge KG, Fibiger HC. Neuroleptic-induced oral dyskinesias: effects of progabide and lack of correlation with regional changes in glutamic acid decarboxylase and choline acetyltransferase activities. *Psychopharmacology* 1987;93:94–100.

56. Mukherjee S, Roth SD, Sandyk R, Schnur DB. Persistent tardive dyskinesia and neuroleptic effects on glucose tolerance. *Psychiatry Res* 1989;29:17–27.

57. Nielsen EB, Lyon M. Evidence for cell loss in corpus striatum after long-term treatment with a neuroleptic drug (Flupenthixol) in rats. *Psychopharmacology* 1978;59:85–89.

58. Peet M, Laugharne J, Rangarajan N, Reynolds GP, Watson REB, Cutts AJ. Tardive dyskinesia, lipid peroxidation and vitamin E. *Schizophr Res* 1993;9(2,3):279.

59. Richardson MA, Suckow R, Whittaker R, et al. The plasma phenylalanine/large neutral amino acid ratio: a risk factor for tardive dyskinesia. *Psychopharmacol Bull* 1989;25:47–51.

60. Rupniak NMJ, Jenner P, Marsden CD. Cholinergic manipulation of perioral behavior induced by chronic neuroleptic administration to rats. *Psychopharmacology* 1983;79:226–230.

61. Rupniak NMJ, Prestwick SA, Horton RW, Jenner P, Marsden CD. Alterations in cerebral glutamic acid decarboxylase and [³H]-flunitrazepam binding during continuous treatment of rats for one year with haloperidol, sulpiride, or clozapine. *J Neurol Transm* 1987;68:113–125.

62. Saltz BL, Woerner M, Kane JM, et al. Prospective study of tardive dyskinesia incidence in the elderly. *JAMA* 1991;266:2402–2406.

63. Scheel-Kruger J, Arnt J. New aspects on the role of dopamine, acetylcholine and GABA in the development of tardive dyskinesia. In: Casey DE, Chase T, Christensen AV, Gerlach J, eds. *Dyskinesia: research and treatment.* Berlin: Springer-Verlag, 1985;19–30.

64. Schelkunov EL. Adrenergic effect of chronic administration of neuroleptics. *Nature* 1967;214:1210–1212.

65. Shriqui CL, Bradwejn J, Annable L, et al. Vitamin E in the treatment of tardive dyskinesia: a double-blind placebo-controlled study. *Am J Psychiatry* 1992;149:391–393.

66. Stahl SM, Faull KF, Barchas JD, Berger PA. CSF monoamine metabolites in movement disorders and normal aging. *Arch Neurol* 1985;42:166–169.

67. Tamminga CA, Crayton JW, Chase TN. Improvement in tardive dyskinesia after muscimol therapy. *Arch Gen Psychiatry* 1979;36:595–598.
68. Tarsy D, Baldessarini RJ. Pharmacologically induced behavioral supersensitivity to apomorphine. *Nature* 1973;245:262–263.
69. Thaker GK, Nguyen JA, Strauss ME, Jacobson R, Kaup BA, Tamminga CA. Clonazepam treatment of tardive dyskinesia: a practical GABAmimetic strategy. *Am J Psychiatry* 1990;147:445–451.
70. Thaker GK, Tamminga CA, Alphs LA, Lafferman J, Ferraro TN, Hare TA. Brain gamma-aminobutyric acid abnormality in tardive dyskinesia. *Arch Gen Psychiatry* 1987;44:522–529.
71. Waddington JL. Schizophrenia, affective psychoses, and other disorders treated with neuroleptic drugs: the enigma of tardive dyskinesia, its neurobiological determinants, and the conflict of paradigms. *Int Rev Neurobiol* 1989;31:297–353.
72. Waddington JL. Implications of recent research on dopamine D1 and D2 receptor subtypes in relation to schizophrenia and neuroleptic drug action. *Neurosci Neuropsychiatry* 1989;2:89–92.
73. Waddington JL, Cross AJ, Gamble SJ, Bourne RC. Spontaneous orofacial dyskinesia and dopaminergic function in rats after 6 months of neuroleptic treatment. *Science* 1983;220:530–532.
74. Waddington JL, Youssef HA. The lifetime outcome and involuntary movements of schizophrenia never treated with neuroleptic drugs. *Br J Psychiatry* 1990;156:106–108.
75. White FJ, Wang RY. Differential effects of classical and atypical antipsychotic drugs on A9 and A10 dopamine cells. *Science* 1983;221:1054–1057.
76. Woerner MG, Saltz BL, Kane JM, Lieberman JA, Alvir JMJ. Diabetes and development of tardive dyskinesia. *Am J Psychiatry* 1993;150(6):966–968.

Psychopharmacology: The Fourth Generation of Progress, edited by Floyd E. Bloom and David J. Kupfer. Raven Press, Ltd., New York © 1995.

CHAPTER 129

The Treatment of Tardive Dyskinesias

George Gardos and Jonathan O. Cole

The treatment of tardive dyskinesia (TD) poses unusual problems. This iatrogenic condition is at the interface of psychiatry and neurology insofar as psychiatric patients are most likely to develop TD, while, by being a movement disorder, TD is in the province of neurology. A second difficulty is that TD is a heterogeneous entity with respect to its clinical features, topography, and pathophysiology. A third anomaly is that most cases of TD also involve an underlying psychiatric disorder with major impact on the development, course, and therapy of TD (see Chapters 127 and 128, *this volume*).

MANAGEMENT OF TARDIVE DYSKINESIA

The coexistence of TD and a psychiatric disorder, frequently but not invariably a chronic psychosis, raises complex risk–benefit issues in treatment planning.

The prevalent strategy is to arrest the progression of TD by minimizing neuroleptic (NL) exposure while simultaneously providing appropriate pharmacotherapy. Implied in this paradigm, although seldom stated explicitly, is the notion that the psychiatric disorder, most often schizophrenia, is the more disabling condition while the movement disorder is usually less severe and does not cause functional impairment.

Neuroleptic drug discontinuation is the method which appears straightforward and conforms to the principle that removal of a causative agent may result in cure. In this instance, clinical thinking is partly supported by research data. Jeste and Wyatt (38) reviewed 23 studies in which NL were withdrawn for the purpose of treating TD for periods varying from 1–2 weeks to 3 years. Of the 631 patients, 37% had remission of symptoms defined as a 50% or greater decrease in rating scale scores. A more

recent review by the same group (36) cited three additional NL withdrawal studies where the averaged remission rate of TD was 55%. The clinical feasibility of neuroleptic withdrawal is severely limited by the high risk of psychotic relapse in chronic psychotic patients. The risk of relapse appears to be higher in TD patients (48).

Long-term studies have shown that TD can be successfully managed within the context of appropriate NL treatment of coexistent severe mental illness (17). Follow-up studies of TD for 5 years or longer have tended to confirm that TD typically stays stable or improves even with continued neuroleptic treatment (27), although neuroleptic dose reduction may offer benefit for both TD and clinical status (40). Alternatives to NL treatment, including mood stabilizers (lithium carbonate, carbamazepine, divalproex sodium, benzodiazepines, or antidepressants) (43), are sometimes effective clinically and may lead to amelioration of TD in the absence of NL.

Specific step-by-step recommendations for the clinical management of patients with TD, including algorithms, have been offered (6,14). The doctor–patient relationship and the provision of adequate information to patient and family are also key aspects of the appropriate clinical management of TD.

THERAPEUTIC AGENTS FOR TARDIVE DYSKINESIA

Methodological Issues

Studies often distinguish between reversible and irreversible TD, but no agreement exists as to whether reversible TD implies a complete disappearance of all TD symptoms. Similarly, whether the definition of irreversible TD allows for improvement of TD, but with continued TD symptoms, is unresolved (14). Persistent versus remitting TD is a more flexible dichotomy, and, when coupled with

---

G. Gardos and J. O. Cole: Department of Psychopharmacology, McLean Hospital, Belmont, Massachusetts 02178.

operational criteria such as Schooler and Kane's research diagnoses for TD (65), a better description of TD outcome may result. However, to assess treatment response a criterion for improvement is also needed. A statistically significant treatment effect does not always reflect clinically significant improvement in particular patients (37). The criterion of at least 50% improvement was chosen as the indicator of positive drug response in the treatment studies to be cited.

Placebo Response

Sizable placebo response was found in double-blind studies: Groups of placebo patients showed mean improvement in TD of as much as 50% (69), and the proportion of placebo patients improving by ≥50% could reach as high as one-third (36). The placebo effect makes interpretation of uncontrolled positive studies problematic.

Shifting Baseline

Tardive dyskinesia severity is often subject to diurnal variations as well as to apparently spontaneous fluctuations over days or weeks (47) which inflate the variance in treatment studies and may lead to Type II errors. A different problem causing Type I errors may arise when, as is often the case, patients enter a treatment study at or near their worst level of TD. Such patients sometimes improve spontaneously no matter what the treatment and will inflate both the drug and placebo response rate although not the drug–placebo differences.

Other methodological issues which are not specific to TD treatment studies are carry-over effects which may confound cross-over studies as well as problems handling dropouts.

Criteria for an Adequate Trial

Compounds which may be effective in treating TD should prove their therapeutic efficacy in well-designed studies. Based on Mackay and Sheppard's (55) recommendations, the following criteria for a methodologically sound therapeutic trial in TD are suggested: double-blind design, adequate number of cooperative patients, clear diagnostic and descriptive definitions, valid and reliable rating scales, attention to the timing of ratings, and holding nonresearch medications constant. While few studies in the literature measure up to these standards, studies will be judged on how far they approximate the ideal study design.

Agents Used for Treating Tardive Dyskinesia

The assertion by Casey (15) in the previous volume of this series remains true: (a) No drugs are both safe and effective over extended periods, and (b) the long list of agents attests to their general ineffectiveness.

Dopamine Antagonists

The earliest class of compounds to have been employed in the treatment of TD were drugs which reduce DA activity.

Classical Neuroleptics

Neuroleptics are the most effective drugs available to reduce TD. Jeste and Wyatt (38) reviewed 50 studies with 501 patients and found an improvement rate of TD of 66.9% in NL-treated patients, which was higher than that obtained with any other class of therapeutic agents. The APA Task Force Report (40) similarly found that NL treatment produced a ≥50% improvement in 60% of TD patients. The rate of 63% improvement in the 19 double-blind studies was not significantly different from the 69% rate of improvement in open and single-blind studies (38).

Jeste and Wyatt (38) summarized studies with different NL and found haloperidol (7 studies with an average of 79% improvement), thiopropazate (10 studies, 62% improvement), and other NLs (13 studies, 84% improvement) to have been essentially equipotent in antidyskinetic action. Suppression or masking are terms often used to refer to the antidyskinetic action of NLs on TD. The use of NLs in treating TD is considered paradoxical and controversial (38) because NL therapy is the presumed cause of the condition. The amelioration of TD by NL is tempered by concerns that the improvement in TD occurs at the expense of increased parkinsonian symptoms and that the antidyskinetic effect may be temporary (42). The potentially harmful effects of TD suppression are also suggested by the rebound increase in TD after NL withdrawal, with the amount of rebound aggravation of TD proportional to the degree of TD suppression (30). There is little compelling evidence to differentiate NL suppression or masking from antidyskinetic effect since the mechanism of action for most antidyskinetic drugs has not been clarified.

Catecholamine Depleters

These compounds deplete catecholamines from nerve terminals and have been employed as antipsychotic as well as antidyskinetic drugs for several decades. Reserpine, tetrabenazine, and oxypertine have been the drugs most extensively studied in the treatment of TD.

In a double-blind, placebo-controlled study, Huang et al. (33) obtained a statistically significant improvement by reserpine 0.75–1.5 mg daily; 5 of 10 reserpine patients showed >50% improvement. More recently, Fahn (25) used reserpine in doses up to 8 mg/day and found marked and long-lasting improvement in 8 of 17 patients. Reserpine appears more effective as an antidyskinetic drug without concurrent NL therapy (25). Side effects such as hypotension, sedation, parkinsonism, and depression limit the clinical usefulness of this compound.

Tetrabenazine, a nonindole benzoquinolizine, is a presynaptic monoamine-depleting agent as well as a postsynaptic dopamine receptor blocker (56). It is not marketed in the United States. Tetrabenazine in typical doses of 150–200 mg daily produced positive results in both open and controlled studies, but side effects of parkinsonism, depression, drowsiness, and akathisia restrict the drug's therapeutic potential (56). Oxypertine is a potent depleter of norepinephrine, while its dopamine-depleting activity is less than that of reserpine or tetrabenazine (40). Despite its apparent efficacy both as an antipsychotic and as an antidyskinetic agent, and the lack of major side effects (69), oxypertine is rarely used today.

Although little recent research has been carried out with these compounds, they remain potentially useful. Reserpine and tetrabenazine are still frequently employed by neurologists (43).

Atypical Neuroleptics

Recently introduced antipsychotic drugs are credited with lesser propensity to cause extrapyramidal symptoms and TD and are potential antidyskinetic agents as well. Clozapine, a dibenzodiazepine compound, rarely causes extrapyramidal symptoms and practically never causes TD (47). Numerous studies have addressed the drug's therapeutic potential in TD. Jeste and Wyatt's comprehensive early review of TD treatment (38) found clozapine the least effective NL for suppressing TD: Of eight studies involving 75 patients, 51% improved by 50% or more, while classical NL showed an improvement rate between 62% and 84%. In one of the important early studies, Gerbino et al. (29) demonstrated that after at least 1 year on an average dose of 650 mg/day clozapine, 14 of 17 patients reached at least 90% improvement. No breakthrough of TD was noted even when dosage was tapered by 40–50%. The greater efficacy of higher doses of clozapine was confirmed by Lieberman et al. (50), who treated 30 TD patients for an average of 27.8 months and obtained >50% improvement in 16 (53%) patients. The average daily doses at week 6 and endpoint were 653 and 483 mg, respectively. Lieberman et al. (50) concluded that clozapine exerts a specific antidyskinetic effect rather than simple TD suppression mainly because of the absence of rebound of TD after drug withdrawal, and because the drug seemed to have greater efficacy in severe TD and in cases of tardive dystonia as well. The long-term outcome of TD in clozapine-treated patients and the lack of rebound of TD after clozapine discontinuation, however, need to be confirmed by controlled studies.

The benzamides are selective D_2-receptor antagonists without significant actions on receptors of other brain neurotransmitter systems (19). Sulpiride in doses of 400–1200 mg/day was found to reduce TD significantly ($p < 0.01$) without affecting parkinsonism in a placebo-controlled trial with 11 elderly patients; however, there was reemergence of TD symptoms after sulpiride withdrawal (16). Haggstrom (31) found a dose-dependent reduction in TD and psychosis by sulpiride 200–1200 mg/day in six patients with marked TD. Tiapride, another substituted benzamide, showed an antidyskinetic effect in two controlled trials with 12 (12) and 5 (16) patients, respectively.

Risperidone is a novel benzisoxazole derivative characterized by potent central 5-HT$_2$ antagonism at low doses and potent dopamine D_2-receptor antagonism at higher doses (18). In a double-blind multicenter study of 135 schizophrenic inpatients at doses of 6–16 mg daily, risperidone significantly lowered dyskinesia scores compared to placebo. TD patients treated with the optimal dose of 6 mg/day risperidone showed a significantly greater decrease in dyskinesia scores than did haloperidol-treated patients. The greatest improvement was observed in patients with severe TD treated with 6 and 10 mg/day of risperidone. Risperidone is a potentially important antidyskinetic agent as well as an effective antipsychotic.

Other Catecholamine Antagonists

Based on prevailing theories that striatal dopamine and/or norepinephrine overactivity may be associated with TD, a host of dopamine and norepinephrine antagonists in addition to those already discussed above have been tested for potential antidyskinetic effects. Most of them are of theoretical or research interest only.

Alpha-methyl-paratyrosine (AMPT) inhibits tyrosine hydroxylase, the rate-limiting enzyme in the synthesis of dopamine. Modest improvement in TD by AMPT was seen in several studies, but the samples were small and the period of observations varied between a few days and 4 weeks (38,40). Other putative dopamine antagonists—alpha-methyldopa, papaverine, metoclopramide, droperidol, and oxiperomide—have shown unimpressive antidyskinetic effects in small and/or uncontrolled studies.

Noradrenergic antagonists, primarily the beta-adrenergic blocker propranolol and the alpha-2 agonist clonidine, have been tested in several treatment studies. Propranolol produced mixed results in doses of 20–40 mg/day in open studies. A double-blind study with intensive case design using up to 800 mg/day of propranolol in four TD patients suggested that therapeutic effects may appear slowly: Two of the four subjects showed a substantial therapeutic response during weeks 20–50 of observation (66). In a double-blind study of eight TD patients, clonidine 0.2–0.9 mg/day produced a mean improvement of 63% (26), whereas in another double-blind, placebo-controlled study all seven patients improved on 0.4 mg/day (9). Significant side effects, especially hypotension, restrict the clinical usefulness of clonidine for TD. Disulfiram and the dopamine beta-hydroxylase inhibitor fusaric acid are of theoretical interest, but appropriate treatment studies have not been conducted.

Catecholamine Agonists

Apomorphine, hydergine, piribedil, methylphenidate, amphetamine, and amantadine have been tried for TD without notable success. Bromocriptine, an ergotalkaloid derivative, possesses both dopamine agonist and antagonist activities. In doses of 0.75–7.5 mg daily, it failed to show satisfactory improvement in TD in small open (36) and double-blind (46) studies. In a placebo-controlled study of 11 TD patients, Lieberman et al. (49) added increasing doses of bromocriptine (15–60 mg/day) to NL for 10 weeks, followed by 8 weeks of observation off bromocriptine. No significant therapeutic effects were found. The Receptor Sensitivity Modification Hypothesis (4) postulates that dopamine agonists in relatively high doses may counteract postsynaptic dopamine-receptor hypersensitivity. Positive results with L-DOPA treatment (54) were not supported by several negative studies (15,36,68). The potential for increased psychotic symptoms further limits the clinical applicability of L-DOPA therapy.

L-Deprenyl has recently attracted interest for neurological conditions, including TD (73), but controlled studies are needed. The dopamine autoreceptor agonist 3-PPP, which decreases the release of dopamine, has been shown in monkeys to improve TD (44), but human studies are yet to be completed.

Catecholamine agonists appear to be more useful as tools to elucidate the pathophysiology of TD than as reliable treatment for patients.

Cholinergic Treatments

The application of centrally acting cholinergic compounds is based on the hypothesis that the pathophysiology of TD is linked to a relative imbalance between cholinergic and dopaminergic activity within the striatum (5).

Most of the relevant research was carried out in the 1970s and has been reviewed by Alphs and Davis (5). Intravenous physostigmine in doses of 0.5–3 mg with methscopolamine was given in 11 studies: Results ranged from marked improvement (>50%) to no change or worsening, with no clear differences between double-blind, single-blind, and open studies (5). Because the drug is short-acting and toxic, its main clinical application appears to be as a pharmacological probe and as a potential predictor of response to cholinergic therapy (5). Deanol,

an orally administered putative cholinergic drug, enjoyed intense but brief popularity. Alphs and Davis (5) reviewed no fewer than 14 double-blind studies involving 199 patients, as well as numerous single-blind and open studies. The prolific research on deanol is astonishing when considering that only one of the double-blind studies showed it to be significantly superior to placebo; furthermore, serious doubt exists as to whether and how deanol increases central acetylcholine content (5).

Choline chloride (3–18 g/day) demonstrated therapeutic efficacy in one double-blind and four other trials, but distressing side effects severely limit the drug's clinical applicability (5). Lecithin is much better tolerated than choline. Open treatment trials tended to produce positive findings, whereas three double-blind studies reported mixed results (5). The clinical use of lecithin is hampered by the fact that phosphatidylcholine content varies greatly between different manufacturers; therefore, accurate dosing is difficult to achieve. Another problem is the need to prescribe large doses (sometimes >50 g daily), which represent a large caloric intake. In a double-blind crossover study, Gelenberg et al. (28) gave 20 g lecithin daily to 21 patients for 8 weeks and obtained statistically significant drug–placebo differences. Clinically, however, the lecithin effect was negligible. The newer cholinergic agents—meclofenoxate (34) and RS86, a specific muscarinic agonist (62)—yielded disappointing results in clinical trials.

Overall, the early encouraging results with cholinergic compounds have not been sustained.

Anticholinergics

The same rationale which led to the enthusiastic trials of cholinergics for TD would predict worsening by anticholinergics. Although this expectation is generally borne out, there are reports of TD improving in a minority of affected patients. Jeste and Wyatt (38) reviewed 14 studies involving 177 patients in which anticholinergic drugs were given systematically for TD and found that 7.3% of patients improved. The anticholinergics included benztropine (2 mg IV and 1–5 mg PO), trihexyphenidyl (2–27 mg/day), biperiden (6–18 mg/day), and procyclidine (30 mg/day); the duration ranged from single-dose studies to 2 months of observation. One explanation for the improvement in TD is that antimuscarinic antiparkinsonian agents such as benztropine have potent dopaminergic and noradrenergic agonist activities in the central nervous system (57).

GABAergic Drugs

The inhibiting effect of gamma-aminobutyric acid (GABA) on dopamine neurons provides the rationale for treating TD with drugs which increase GABA influences

(15). Thaker et al. (71) traced the evolution of GABAergic treatments in TD. Muscimol, the first specific GABA$_A$ agonist to be tried for TD, produced a 48% decrease in TD symptoms in doses up to 9 mg/day in a placebo-controlled trial of seven NL-free schizophrenics. Another GABA$_A$ agonist THIP was, at best, slightly beneficial in two small studies (71). Progabide, which is active at GABA$_A$ and GABA$_B$ receptors, yielded 40–60% improvement in TD in one open and two double-blind clinical trials (71). The GABA transaminase inhibitors GABA-acetylenic GABA and gamma-vinyl GABA were tested in small-scale trials and resulted in modest improvement which in some patients was clinically significant (71). Distressing side effects of dizziness, sedation, confusion, myoclonic jerks, and increases in parkinsonian and psychotic symptoms impose limitations on the therapeutic potential of these specific GABAergic drugs.

Sodium valproate may increase brain GABA via GABA-transaminase inhibition, although it is unclear whether in usual clinical doses this does in fact occur. Double-blind studies in which 900–2500 mg sodium valproate was added to ongoing NL treatment failed to improve TD in the majority of patients (51,60). Baclofen, a structural analogue of GABA, has shown variable effects on TD in a few double-blind studies (15).

Benzodiazepines may enhance GABA function (15). These widely used and generally safe compounds have been extensively used in patients with TD, although most often unsystematically. In open studies an average of 58% patients improved, while in double-blind studies the improvement rate was 43% (13,15,38).

Despite the high rate of improvement, benzodiazepines have not been established as specific treatments in TD. The mechanism of action and the influence of nonspecific factors such as sedation or antianxiety effect remain unclear (13). Nonetheless, benzodiazepines enjoy widespread use in the clinical management of TD of all types and severity.

Serotonergic Drugs

The rationale for using serotonergic drugs in TD is based on clinical and biochemical data suggesting that 5-HT inhibits dopamine functioning. No clear therapeutic effects have been demonstrated clinically with the 5-HT precursors L-tryptophan or 5-HTP or with cyproheptadine (64). Sandyk and Fisher (64) pioneered a dietary approach of L-tryptophan (8 g/day) combined with nicotinic acid (25 mg/day) to slow hepatic degradation of L-tryptophan, and they devised a high-carbohydrate–low-protein diet to further promote brain levels of serotonin. Improvement in TD was obtained in three patients (64). The dietary manipulation of neurotransmitter precursors is a novel approach which awaits experimental and clinical confirmation.

Lithium Carbonate

A series of case reports and small uncontrolled studies suggested that lithium carbonate benefited TD as well as Huntington's chorea, tics, and dystonias (20). Systematic open and double-blind studies, however, revealed modest (at best) benefit resulting from lithium carbonate, whether used as the sole therapeutic agent or when added to NL (20). There was an apparent trend in these studies for serum lithium levels of ≤0.8 mEq/liter to be more likely to reduce TD than lithium levels of over 0.8 mEq/liter. Some investigators reported worsening of existing TD or development of new TD on lithium carbonate, especially at toxic lithium levels (20). The lack of clear therapeutic efficacy still leaves open the question of whether lithium carbonate may prevent TD development (20).

Calcium-Channel Antagonists

Case reports of unexpected benefit in TD patients stimulated clinical trials. A rationale was provided by data from animal experiments which demonstrated that calcium-channel blockers possess dopamine antagonist properties (8,53). Borison et al. (8) stressed the pharmacological differences among the calcium-channel antagonists. Verapamil, for instance, crosses the blood–brain barrier more readily than diltiazem or nifedipine and was also found to exhibit dopamine-antagonist properties. Clinical studies tend to bear out these differential effects. Adler et al. (1) added up to 80 mg q.i.d. of verapamil or up to 60 mg q.i.d. of diltiazem to ongoing antipsychotic drug treatment in 21 patients with TD. AIMS rating were done blindly. There was a 19% decrease in AIMS ($p < 0.05$) in the verapamil patients, whereas the 11% decrease in AIMS in the 12 diltiazem patients was not statistically significant. Borison et al. (8) treated 13 treatment-refractory male schizophrenics with verapamil 80 mg t.i.d. and chlorpromazine 600 mg daily. Average AIMS scores decreased by over 50% ($p < 0.001$) after 3 weeks and rebounded after verapamil discontinuation. By contrast, a double-blind, placebo-controlled crossover study found diltiazem ineffective (53). Studies with nifedipine have likewise been disappointing.

Adequately controlled longer-term studies are yet to be done. All these drugs, however, have serious limitations: hypotension, increase in anxiety, hostility and depression, and the dissipation of antidyskinetic effect after 1–3 months.

Vitamin E (Alpha-tocopherol)

Vitamin E (alpha-tocopherol) is a lipid-soluble antioxidant located on cell membranes near enzymes that produce free radicals (70). Neuroleptics increase catecholamine turnover and may increase free radical formation which in turn may cause neurotoxicity and may induce TD. Szymanski et al. (70) recently reviewed treatment studies of vitamin E in TD, which were all double-blind and placebo-controlled. Lohr et al. (52) treated 15 patients with persistent TD with 1200 I.U. of vitamin E daily and found an average of 43% decrease in AIMS scores. The seven patients who showed a >50% response had a shorter duration of TD than did the eight patients with ≤50% improvement. Elkashef et al. (23) treated eight schizophrenics with TD with 1200 I.U. for 4 weeks, in addition to their regular psychotropics; despite a significant drug–placebo difference, only one patient showed >50% reduction of AIMS scores. Egan et al. (22) gave 1600 I.U./day of vitamin E to 21 TD patients. Data from the 18 patients with high blood levels of vitamin E showed no significant drug–placebo differences except in the subgroup of 9 patients who had had TD for 5 years or less, where an 18.5% average decrease in AIMS scores was obtained. Adler et al. (3) administered 1600 I.U. of vitamin E daily; during the initial 8-week trial, 2 of 16 patients showed >50% improvement. When the trial was extended to 36 weeks, 4 of 8 patients on vitamin E and 0 of 9 placebo patients improved by >33% (2). Junker et al. (39) used 1200 I.U./day of vitamin E in 16 TD patients and found significant improvement only in patients over age 40. A double-blind crossover study with 6-week treatment periods of vitamin E 1200 I.U./day or placebo was carried out on 27 outpatients with TD by Shriqui et al. (67); no significant drug placebo differences were obtained in AIMS scores.

The impression gained from these studies is that while vitamin E is safe and well-tolerated, it confers only modest benefits. Those with shorter duration of TD improve more, but the usual response criterion of 50% improvement is infrequently reached. Longer-term trials may yield better results.

Electroconvulsive Therapy

Hay et al. (32) reviewed 22 published cases of electroconvulsive therapy (ECT) in patients with TD; these authors noted five cases of disappearance of TD and reported improvement in another six patients. Nine of these 11 patients received a diagnosis of depression; the age range was 49–92 years, and 10 of the 11 patients were NL-free during ECT treatment.

Miscellaneous Compounds

Neuropeptides have received attention because of the connection of endogenous opiates with brain dopamine systems and with motor behavior. An acute study with eight TD patients showed weak antidyskinetic effects by morphine (10 mg SC) and by the synthetic encephalon

FK 33-824 (3 mg IM), but showed no effect by naloxone (0.8 mg IM) (7).

Ceruletide [a cholecystokinin octapeptide (CCK-8) analogue], in doses of 0.8 mg/kg, was found to reduce TD in a small number of patients (61).

Estrogens in clinical trials in TD have produced negative results.

Prostaglandin precursor *essential fatty acids* (EFAs) were tested in 16 TD patients in a double-blind, placebo-controlled, 6-week trial. Six hundred milligrams of γ-linolenic acid produced no significant effects on TD (75).

Insulin (10 units SC) was tested in a double-blind, placebo-controlled study in 20 DSM-III schizophrenics with persistent severe TD (mean AIMS at baseline: 13.7). Daily injections for 15 days were followed by injections every other week for a total of 90 days. At day 7 the insulin group ($N = 10$) showed a significant decrease in TD scores in comparison with the placebo group ($N = 10$); the significant drug–placebo differences persisted throughout the study ($p < 0.001$) (59). The authors believe that decreased glucose availability may have reversed receptor hypersensitivity and led to improvement in TD.

Carbamazepine was found to be ineffective in reducing TD in small uncontrolled trials.

Inadequate stores of *manganese* found through analysis of hair samples have been suggested to be involved in TD development (45). Open studies reported improvement in TD from the administration of manganese, but these studies have not been confirmed.

Pyridoxine (vitamin B_6) has been considered for treatment of TD because of its role in the metabolic breakdown of L-DOPA. High doses of pyridoxine (1000–1400 mg daily) have been advocated as both therapy and prophylaxis for TD (21). However, controlled studies are lacking.

Buspirone, an azopirone antianxiety agent, exerts a partial agonist effect at the serotonin 5-HT$_{1A}$ receptor and exerts mixed agonist and antagonist effects at the dopamine D$_2$ receptor. An open trial of increasing doses of buspirone in eight TD patients found the highest dose of 180 mg/day to have been most effective: There was a mean improvement of 4.4 on the AIMS ($p < 0.01$), and three of the eight patients showed ≥50% improvement (58).

TARDIVE DYSKINESIA VARIANTS

Several distinct forms of NL-induced involuntary movements have been recognized which may coexist with choreo-athetoid dyskinesia or may occur separately. Although much less prevalent than typical TD, they may become severe and disabling. The pathophysiology and treatment of these TD variants show important differences from typical TD.

Tardive dystonia is a syndrome of sustained muscle

contractions, frequently causing either (a) twisting and repetitive movements or (b) abnormal postures (10). Blepharospasm, grimacing, torticollis, retrocollis, and the Pisa syndrome are characteristic movements of tardive dystonia.

Methodologically adequate treatment studies of tardive dystonia are conspicuously absent, probably because of the lack of a sufficiently large cohort of suitable patients at any site. The best information available on the treatment of tardive dystonia comes from series of patients treated at centers specializing in movement disorders (10,41). The general principles of therapy are similar to those for treating TD. Because tardive dystonia is an NL-induced condition, NL discontinuation is considered whenever feasible, but the results have been disappointing: In Burke's series (10), only five of 42 (12%) NL-withdrawn patients remitted, which was defined as prolonged cessation of dystonic movements. Specific therapy often employs either dopamine-depleting or anticholinergic drugs. Reserpine is typically started at a low dose of 0.25 mg daily and raised gradually to an average of 5 mg/day and occasionally to as high as 9 mg/day (10). Tetrabenazine has also been employed with some benefit.

Anticholinergic treatment of tardive dystonia has yielded mixed results. Trihexyphenidyl, the anticholinergic studied most, is usually started at around 5 mg daily, and the dose is raised gradually until adequate benefit occurs or until distressing side effects are met (24). Doses of as high as 120 mg/day have been used, but the average dose of trihexyphenidyl for treating tardive dystonia is 20 mg/day (24). Ethopropazine, a phenothiazine derivative with antimuscarinic anticholinergic effects, has also been used with some success in doses of 50–350 mg daily (24,63). Drawbacks of high-dose anticholinergic treatment are as follows: relapse after transient therapeutic effects, distressing anticholinergic side effects, and exacerbation of choreo-athetoid dyskinesia (74).

Benzodiazepines such as diazepam, clonazepam, and lorazepam have been sometimes helpful (10). Occasional patients have benefited from baclofen, propranolol, bromocriptine, clonidine, carbamazepine, or ECT. Botulinum A toxin injections into affected muscles was found effective in a placebo-controlled trial in focal cranial dystonias such as blepharospasm and torticollis (35).

Burke (10) advocates dopamine antagonist treatment ("suppression") for either (a) severe generalized tardive dystonia causing muscle pain or muscle damage (with elevated CPK) or (b) instances where other drugs have failed. Clozapine may be a suitable alternative. Lieberman et al. (50) found that clozapine was particularly effective for TD patients showing dystonia.

Tardive akathisia, consisting of both motor restlessness and subjective discomfort, is considered a subtype of TD (11). Treatment strategy is similar to those of TD and tardive dystonia. Neuroleptic discontinuation resulted in remission in a minority of patients only (8% in Burke's

series) (10). Dopamine-depleting drugs reserpine and tetrabenazine in place of, or added to, NL were found beneficial: of 15 patients treated with reserpine, three had full remission and eight showed marked improvement; tetrabenazine was effective in 7 of 12 (58%) patients (10). Beta-adrenergic blockers (such as propranolol), which show clear therapeutic efficacy in acute NL-induced akathisia, have produced mixed results in tardive akathisia. Occasional patients may improve on benzodiazepines, antiparkinsonian drugs, L-deprenyl, or clozapine.

Tardive myoclonus refers to NL-induced myoclonus manifested by sudden, brief, shock-like jerks (10). Clonazepam may be effective for this condition (10,72). *Tardive tics and Tardive Tourette's syndrome* may be observed after chronic NL treatment. Burke (10), however, points to the difficulty of ascribing tics to NL therapy, because tics often occur and disappear spontaneously. No effective treatment has been identified.

The TD variants discussed above often coexist with typical TD, and, like typical TD, they do not have effective therapies. Research into the treatment of TD variants may be particularly rewarding by elucidating pathophysiological mechanisms of NL-induced movement disorders.

ACKNOWLEDGMENT

Partial support was obtained from NIMH grant #TDA-2 2 RO1 MH32675-12.

REFERENCES

1. Adler L, Duncan E, Reiter S, Angrist B, Peselow E, Rotrosen J. Effects of calcium-channel antagonists on tardive dyskinesia and psychosis. *Psychopharmacol Bull* 1988;24:421–425.
2. Adler L, Peselow E, Angrist B, et al. Vitamin E in tardive dyskinesia: effects of longer term treatment. Poster at 31st Annual Meeting of ACNP, San Juan, Puerto Rico, December 16, 1992.
3. Adler LA, Peselow E, Rosenthal M, et al. Vitamin E treatment of tardive dyskinesia. *Biol Psychiatry* 1992;31:160A.
4. Alpert M, Diamond F, Friedhoff AJ. Receptor sensitivity modification in the treatment of tardive dyskinesia. *Psychopharmacol Bull* 1982;18:90–92.
5. Alphs LD, Davis JM. Cholinergic treatments for tardive dyskinesia. In: Bannet J, Belmaker RH, eds. *New directions in tardive dyskinesia research. Modern problems in pharmacopsychiatry,* vol 21, Basel: Karger, 1983;168–186.
6. Baldessarini RJ, Cole JO, Davis JM, et al. *Tardive dyskinesia.* Task Force Report 18. Washington, DC: American Psychiatric Association, 1980.
7. Bjørndal N, Casey DE, Gerlach J. Enkephalin, morphine, and naloxone in tardive dyskinesia. *Psychopharmacology* 1980;69:133–136.
8. Borison RL, McLarnon MC, DeMartines N, Diamond B. Calcium channel antagonists: interaction with dopamine, schizophrenia and tardive dyskinesia. In: Wolf ME, Mosnaim AD, eds. *Tardive dyskinesia: biological mechanisms and clinical aspects.* Washington, DC: American Psychiatric Press, 1988;217–231.
9. Browne J, Silver H, Martin R, et al. The use of clonidine in the treatment of neuroleptic-induced tardive dyskinesia. *J Clin Psychopharmacol* 1986;6:88–92.
10. Burke RE. Neuroleptic-induced tardive dyskinesia variants. In: Lang AE, Weiner WJ, eds. *Drug-induced movement disorders.* New York: Futura, 1992;167–198.

11. Burke RE, Kang UK, Jankovic J, Miller LG, Fahn S. Tardive akathisia: an analysis of clinical features and response to open therapeutic trials. *Movement Disord* 1989;4:157–175.

12. Buruma OJS, Roos RAC, Bruyn GW, Kemp B, Van Der Velde FA. Tiapride in the treatment of tardive dyskinesia. *Acta Neurol Scand* 1982;65:81–88.

13. Casey DE. Tardive dyskinesia: nondopaminergic treatment approaches. In: Casey DE, Chase TN, Christensen AV, Gerlach J, eds. *Dyskinesia—research and treatment. Psychopharmacology,* supplement 2. Berlin: Springer-Verlag, 1985;137–144.

14. Casey DE. Tardive dyskinesia: reversible and irreversible. In: Casey DE, Chase TN, Christensen AV, Gerlach J, eds. *Dyskinesia—research and treatment. Psychopharmacology,* supplement 2. Berlin: Springer-Verlag, 1985;88–97.

15. Casey DE. Tardive dyskinesia: In: Meltzer HY, ed. *Psychopharmacology: The third generation of progress.* New York: Raven Press, 1987;1411–1419.

16. Casey DE, Gerlach J, Simmelgaard H. Sulpiride in tardive dyskinesia. *Psychopharmacology* 1974;66:73–77.

17. Casey DE, Toenniessen LM. Neuroleptic treatment in tardive dyskinesia: can it be developed into a clinical strategy for long-term treatment? In: Bannet J, Belmaker RH, eds. *New directions in tardive dyskinesia research.* Basel: Karger, 1983;65–79.

18. Chouinard G, Jones B, Remington G, et al. A Canadian multicenter placebo-controlled study of fixed doses of risperidone and haloperidol in the treatment of chronic schizophrenic patients. *J Clin Psychopharmacol* 1993;13:25–40.

19. Chouza C, Caamano JL, Romero S, Lorenzo J, Feres S. Extrapyramidal effects of benzamides. In: Kemali D, Racagni G, eds. *Chronic treatments in neuropsychiatry.* New York: Raven Press, 1985;43–59.

20. Cole JO, Gardos G, Rapkin RM. Lithium carbonate in tardive dyskinesia and schizophrenia. In: Gardos G, Casey DE, eds. *Dyskinesia and affective disorder.* Washington, DC: American Psychiatric Press, 1984;49–73.

21. Devaux A. Dyskinesies tardives: rôle de la pyridoxine dans la prevention. *Semin Hôp Paris* 1987;63:1476–1480.

22. Egan MF, Hyde TM, Albers GW, et al. Treatment of tardive dyskinesia with vitamin E. *Am J Psychiatry* 1992;149:773–777.

23. Elkashef AM, Ruskin PE, Bacher N, Barrett D. Vitamin E in the treatment of tardive dyskinesia. *Am J Psychiatry* 1990;147:505–509.

24. Fahn S. High dosage anticholinergic therapy in dystonia. *Neurology* 1983;33:1255–1261.

25. Fahn S. A therapeutic approach to tardive dyskinesia. *J Clin Psychiatry* 1985;464:195–245.

26. Freedman R, Bell J, Kirch D. Clonidine therapy for coexisting psychosis and tardive dyskinesia. *Am J Psychiatry* 1980;137:629–630.

27. Gardos G, Casey D, Cole JO, Perenyi A, Kocsis E, Arato M, Samson JA, Conley C. Ten year outcome of tardive dyskinesia. *Am J Psychiatry* 1994;151:836–841.

28. Gelenberg AJ, Dorer DJ, Wojcik JD, Falk WE, Brotman AW, Leahy L. A crossover study of lecithin treatment of tardive dyskinesia. *J Clin Psychiatry* 1990;51:149–153.

29. Gerbino L, Shopsin B, Collora M. Clozapine in the treatment of tardive dyskinesia: an interim report. In: Fann WF, Smith RC, Davis JM, Domino EF, eds. *Tardive dyskinesia.* New York: Spectrum, 1980;475–489.

30. Gerlach J, Simmelsgaard H. Tardive dyskinesia during and following treatment with haloperidol, haloperidol plus biperiden, thioridazine, and clozapine. *Psychopharmacology* 1978;59:105–112.

31. Haggstrom JE. Sulpiride in tardive dyskinesia. *Curr Ther Res* 1980;27:164–169.

32. Hay DP, Hay L, Blackwell B, Spiro HR. ECT and tardive dyskinesia. *J Geriatric Psychiatr Neurol* 1990;3:106–109.

33. Huang CC, Wang RH, Hasegawa A, Alverno L. Reserpine and alpha-methyldopa in the treatment of tardive dyskinesia. *Psychopharmacology* 181;73:359–362.

34. Izumi K, Tominaga H, Koja T, et al. Meclofenoxate therapy in tardive dyskinesia: a preliminary report. *Biol Psychiatry* 1986;21:151–160.

35. Jankovic J, Arman J. Botulinum A toxin for cranial-cevical dystonia: a double-blind placebo controlled study. *Neurology* 1987;37:616–623.

36. Jeste DV, Lohr JB, Clark K, Wyatt RJ. Pharmacological treatments of tardive dyskinesia in the 1980s. *J Clin Psychopharmacol* 1988;8:385–485.

37. Jeste DV, Wyatt RJ. In search of treatment for tardive dyskinesia: review of the literature. *Schizophr Bull* 1979;5:251–295.

38. Jeste DV, Wyatt RJ. *Understanding and treating tardive dyskinesia.* New York: Guildford Press, 1982.

39. Junker D, Steigleider P, Gattaz WF. Alpha-tocopherol in the treatment of tardive dyskinesia. *Schizophr Res* 1992;6:122–123.

40. Kane JM, Jeste DV, Barnes JRE, et al, eds. *Tardive dyskinesia: a task force report of the American Psychiatric Association.* Washington, DC: American Psychiatric Association, 1992.

41. Kang UJ, Burke RE, Fahn S. Tardive dystonia. *Adv Neurol* 1988;50:415–429.

42. Kazamatsuri H, Chien C, Cole J. Therapeutic approaches to tardive dyskinesia. *Arch Gen Psychiatry* 1972;27:491–499.

43. Khot V, Egan MF, Hyde TM, Wyatt RJ. Neuroleptics and classic tardive dyskinesia. In: Lang AE, Weiner WJ, eds. *Drug-induced movement disorders.* Mt. Kisco, NY: Futura, 1992;121–166.

44. Kovacic B, LeWitt P, Clark D. Suppression of neuroleptic-induced persistent abnormal movements in *Cebus apella* monkeys by enantiomers of 3-PPP. *J Neurol Transm* 1988;74:97–107.

45. Kunin RA. Manganese in dyskinesias. *Am J Psychiatry* 1976;133:105.

46. Lenox RH, Weaver LA, Saran BM. Tardive dyskinesia: clinical and neuroendocrine response to low dose bromocriptine. *J Clin Psychopharmacol* 1985;5:286–292.

47. Lieberman JA. Neuroleptic-induced movement disorders and experience with clozapine in tardive dyskinesia. *J Clin Psychiatry* 1990;8:3–8.

48. Lieberman JA. Prediction of outcome in first-episode schizophrenics. *J Clin Psychiatry* 1993;54(Suppl):13–17.

49. Lieberman JA, Alvir J, Mukherjee S, Kane JM. Treatment of tardive dyskinesia with bromocriptine. *Arch Gen Psychiatry* 1989;46:908–913.

50. Lieberman JA, Saltz BL, Johns CA, Pollack S, Borenstein M, Kane J. The effects of clozapine on tardive dyskinesia. *Br J Psychiatry* 1991;158:503–510.

51. Linnoila M, Viukari M, Hietala O. Effect of sodium valproate on tardive dyskinesia. *Br J Psychiatry* 1976;129:114–119.

52. Lohr JB, Cadet JL, Lohr MA, Jeste DV, Wyatt RJ. Alpha-tocopherol in tardive dyskinesia [Letter]. *Lancet* 1987;1:913–914.

53. Loonen AJM, Verwey HA, Roels PR, vanBavel LP, Doorschot CH. Is diltiazem effective in treating the symptoms of (tardive) dyskinesia in chronic psychiatric inpatients? A negative double-blind, placebo-controlled trial. *J Clin Psychopharmacol* 1992;12:39–42.

54. Ludatscher JI. Stable remission of tardive dyskinesia by L-Dopa. *J Clin Psychopharmacol* 1989;9:39–41.

55. Mackay AVP, Sheppard GP. Pharmacotherapeutic trials in tardive dyskinesia. *Br J Psychiatry* 1979;135:489–499.

56. Miller LG, Jankovic J. Drug-induced movement disorders: an overview. In: Joseph AB, Young RR, eds. *Movement disorders in neurology and neuropsychiatry.* Boston: Blackwell Scientific, 1992;5–32.

57. Modell JG, Tandon R, Beresford TP. Dopaminergic activity of the antimuscarinic antiparkinsonian agents. *J Clin Psychopharmacol* 1989;9:347–351.

58. Moss LE, Neppe VM, Drevets WC. Buspirone in the treatment of tardive dyskinesia. *J Clin Psychopharmacol* 1993;13:204–209.

59. Mouret J, Khomais M, Lemoine P. Low doses of insulin as a treatment of tardive dyskinesia: a double-blind, placebo-controlled study. *17th CINP Meeting, Kyoto, Japan* 1990;1:155A.

60. Nasrallah HA, Dunner FJ, McCalley-Whitters M, et al. Pharmacologic probes of neurotransmitter systems in tardive dyskinesia: implications for clinical management. *J Clin Psychiatry* 1986;47:56–59.

61. Nishikawa T, Tanaka M, Tsuda A, Kuwahara H, Koga I, Uchida Y. Effect of ceruletide on tardive dyskinesia: a pilot study of quantitative computer analyses on electromyogram and microvibration. *Psychopharmacology* 1986;90:5–8.

62. Noring U, Poulsen UJ, Casey DE, et al. Effect of a cholinomimetic drug (RS 86) in tardive dyskinesia and drug related parkinsonism. *Psychopharmacology* 1984;84:569–571.

63. Pakkenberg H, Pedersen B. Medical treatment of dystonia. In: Casey DE, Chase TN, Christensen AV, Gerlach J, eds. *Dyskinesia—research and treatment. Psychopharmacology,* supplement 2. Berlin: Springer-Verlag, 1985;111–117.

64. Sandyk R, Fisher H. Serotonin in involuntary movement disorders. *Int J Neurosci* 1988;42:185–205.

65. Schooler NR, Kane JM. Research diagnoses for tardive dyskinesia. *Arch Gen Psychiatry* 1982;39:486–487.

66. Schrodt GR, Wright JH, Simpson R, Moore DP, Chase S. Treatment of tardive dyskinesia with propranolol. *J Clin Psychiatry* 1982;43:328–331.

67. Shriqui CL, Bradwejn J, Annable L, Jones BD. Vitamin E in the treatment of tardive dyskinesia: a double-blind placebo-controlled study. *Am J Psychiatry* 1992;149:391–393.

68. Simpson GM, Yadalam KG, Stephanos MJ. Double-blind carbidopa/levodopa and placebo study in tardive dyskinesia. *J Clin Psychopharmacol* 1988;8:49s–51s.

69. Soni SD, Freeman HL, Hussein EM. Oxypertine in tardive dyskinesia: an 8-week controlled study. *Br J Psychiatry* 1984;144:48–52.

70. Szymanski S, Maune R, Gordon MF, Lieberman J. A selective review of recent advances in the management of tardive dyskinesia. *Psychiatr Ann* 1993;23:209–215.

71. Thaker GK, Ferraro TN, Hare TA, Tamminga CA. Pathophysiology and therapy of tardive dyskinesia: the GABA connection. In: Wolf ME, Mosnaim AD, eds. *Tardive dyskinesia—biological mechanisms and clinical aspects.* Washington, DC: American Psychiatric Press, 1988;199–215.

72. Tominaga H, Fukuzako H, Izumi K, et al. Tardive myoclonus [Letter]. *Lancet* 1987;1:322.

73. Wirshing W, Ames D, Cummings JL, vanPutten T, Marder SR, Bartzokis G, Lee MA. Selegiline and akathisia, tardive dyskinesia and negative symptoms. *18th CINP Meeting, Nice, France* 1992;3:17–65.

74. Wolf ME, Koller WC. Tardive dystonia: treatment with trihexyphenidyl. *J Clin Psychopharmacol* 1985;5:247–248.

75. Wolkin A, Jordan B, Peselow E, Rubinstein M, Rotrosen J. Essential fatty acid supplementation in tardive dyskinesia. *Am J Psychiatry* 1986;143:912–914.

Psychopharmacology: The Fourth Generation of Progress, edited by Floyd E. Bloom and David J. Kupfer. Raven Press, Ltd., New York © 1995.

CHAPTER 130

Multi-Infarct Dementia

David S. Geldmacher and Peter J. Whitehouse

Cerebrovascular disease is a leading contributor to dementia worldwide. In most populations which have been studied, only Alzheimer's disease (AD) is a more common cause of dementia (8). In 1974, Hachinski et al. (24) popularized the phrase "multi-infarct dementia" (MID) to represent the syndrome of dementia accompanied by focal neurologic signs or symptoms, characterized by stepwise deterioration, and frequently associated with hypertension. In some populations with a high prevalence of hypertension (such as African American men and the Japanese), MID is more common than AD (26,56). The nomenclature of MID is complicated by several overlapping terms. Though criteria for the diagnosis of MID were published in DSM-III-R in 1987 (2) and have been widely adopted, their reliability has been questioned and nonstandard alternatives have arisen (14). Furthermore, "vascular dementia" (VaD) has emerged as a diagnostic category that includes not only the multiple discrete infarcts of MID, but other dementing syndromes attributed to cerebrovascular origins. Among these is a dementia associated with diffuse subcortical white-matter disease putatively attributed to chronic subcortical ischemia. This state is commonly, but controversially, known as "Binswanger's disease" or "subcortical arteriosclerotic encephalopathy." In contrast, "Leuko-araiosis" was proposed by Hachinski et al. (25) as a description of radiologic and pathologic subcortical white-matter abnormalities such as those encountered in Binswanger's disease, but these changes are not obligately associated with dementia. Other less common causes of dementia, such as vasculitides, are also considered under the rubric of VaD.

MID has been considered a "subcortical dementia" (10). The term "subcortical dementia" provides a clinical

shorthand for dementia with prominent motor effects and relative rarity of the "cortical syndromes" of aphasia, agnosia, and apraxia. Erkinjuntti (13) reported, however, that 65 of 79 MID patients in his series had sustained a cortical stroke and that 56% of the subjects had evidence of cortical strokes alone. Mahler and Cummings (41) have subsequently considered large-vessel and small-vessel behavioral subtypes of vascular dementia. This distinction further clouds the concept of MID as a subcortical syndrome because the behavioral neurology of large-vessel infarctions typically involves "cortical" signs. The theoretical problems inherent in a cortical–subcortical dichotomy for the description of dementia have also been previously addressed (61). The interpretation of what constitutes MID is further complicated by a lack of specificity and uniform application of proposed criteria for diagnosis. Given the high prevalence of cerebrovascular disease, strokes frequently contribute to the cognitive morbidity of individuals with dementia of all types, including AD. Although antemortem clinical evaluations and imaging may confirm the presence of multiple strokes, those techniques cannot exclude the presence of AD pathology contributing to the overall condition. For instance, the presence of cerebral infarctions may allow the clinical expression of Alzheimer-type dementia even though the pathologic criteria for AD are not met. Consequently, the frequency of pure MID in autopsy studies is 10–23%, comparable to that of "mixed dementia" with changes of both MID and AD (35) (see Chapters 118 and 119, *this volume,* for related issues).

CLINICAL FEATURES

Recurrent cerebral infarctions are, by definition, the pathophysiologic basis of MID. The risk factors for MID are, not surprisingly, those for cerebrovascular disease, especially age and hypertension. There appear to be no

D. S. Geldmacher and P. J. Whitehouse: Department of Neurology, Case Western Reserve University, Cleveland, Ohio 44106; and Alzheimer Center and Division of Behavioral and Geriatric Neurology, University Hospitals of Cleveland, Cleveland, Ohio 44106.

TABLE 1. *Hachinski ischemia score*

Abrupt onset	2
Stepwise progression	1
Fluctuating course	2
Nocturnal confusion	1
Relative preservation of personality	1
Depression	1
Somatic complaints	1
Emotional incontinence	1
History of hypertension	1
History of strokes	2
History of associated atherosclerosis	1
Focal neurologic symptoms	2
Focal neurologic signs	2

From ref. 9, with permission.

risks specific for the development of MID within the context of cerebrovascular disease. In about 90% of pathologically verified cases of MID there is a history of acute unilateral motor or sensory dysfunction consistent with stroke (14). There may also be a history of acute impairment of "cortical" functions manifest as aphasia, apraxia, or agnosia. Urinary dysfunction and gait disturbance have been suggested as early markers for the development of MID (38). With accumulation of ischemic brain lesions there is typically incremental impairment of memory and behavioral initiation, along with extrapyramidal features such as facial masking and rigidity.

An "ischemic score" (IS) was proposed by Hachinski et al. (23) as a means of distinguishing MID from primary degenerative dementia. A number of variants have been employed since the introduction of the original IS; a typical example is shown in Table 1. These scales share the common weaknesses that they are sensitive but not specific indicators of MID and do not address the presence or absence of AD pathology (8). In the clinical setting, an IS is most useful as an instrument for suggesting the presence of cerebrovascular contributors to a dementia syndrome.

The diagnosis of MID depends on the establishment of dementia—that is, a sustained decrement from previously attained levels of cognitive ability, sufficient to interfere with everyday activities, without an associated impairment of consciousness. Dementia may be stable or progressive. If strokes are the cause of a dementia, it is conceivable that there might be an improvement in cognitive status as the deficits from an acute stroke resolve without returning to baseline. When dementia is accompanied by a history of strokes temporally linked to stepwise deterioration in intellectual abilities, the clinical diagnosis of MID is obvious, though mixed dementia is also a possibility. A more difficult diagnostic situation is the patient with a history of strokes not temporally associated with onset of worsening of cognitive impairment. Recently, Chui et al. (9) proposed criteria for the diagnosis of "ischemic vascular dementia," based on the model for diagnosis of AD (44). These criteria are summarized in Table

2. An even more broadly defined set of international diagnostic criteria for research studies of VaD has been proposed (52), but these have been criticized for being overly inclusive and failing to address the importance of temporal association of vascular events with onset of intellectual impairment (12). Of particular note is the inability of any criteria, short of autopsy examination, to differentiate mixed dementia from MID. These factors have led to considerable controversy over the clinical usefulness of the "vascular dementia" concept (7,49). Hachinski (22) has further argued that diagnostic criteria for vascular dementia fail to account for the fact that it is a syndromic diagnosis of multiple origins and outcomes.

NEUROPSYCHOLOGICAL FEATURES

Because they are sensitive to site of dysfunction as opposed to the mechanism causing it, neuropsychological tests have been incapable of consistently distinguishing between MID, AD, and mixed dementias (41). Gainotti et al. (19) reported that AD patients were more likely than those with MID to make "globalistic" or "odd" type errors on Raven's Colored Progressive Matrices task, and on a design copy task were more likely to demonstrate the "closing-in" phenomenon—that is, copying figures such that they overlap the model. Mendez and Ashla-Mendez (45) suggested that unstructured neuropsychological tasks, such as the Tinker Toy test, may be able to distinguish between AD and MID, because of prominent aspontaneity in the latter. As with other neuropsychological measures, the ranges of performance of AD and MID patients overlap, which limits the diagnostic specificity in any individual patient. Furthermore, how well these results generalize to a populations not selected for the "classic" clinical courses of the syndromes is unknown. Rothlind and Brandt (53) have proposed the use of a Frontal/Subcortical Assessment Battery as a supplement to common bedside cognitive examinations for differentiating dementia types characterized by prominent subcortical pathology from AD.

IMAGING

As with most central nervous system diseases, imaging studies have an important role in the diagnosis of MID. In contrast to the diagnosis of AD, in which cerebral images are used to "rule out" structural changes contributing to the dementia, the images in MID can clearly identify significant pathology. In the neuropathologically verified series of Erkinjuntti's group (14), 74% of MID patients had cortical infarcts and 13% had deep infarcts on x-ray computed tomography (CT). Magnetic resonance imaging (MRI) is more sensitive to lesions in the brain than CT, but this is not necessarily an advantage in the diagnosis of MID. Cavities present on T1-weighted im-

TABLE 2. *Criteria for the diagnosis of ischemic vascular dementia (IVD)*

I. Dementia

Dementia is a deterioration from a known or estimated prior level of intellectual function sufficient to interfere broadly with the conduct of the patient's customary affairs of life, which is not isolated to a single narrow category of intellectual performance and which is independent of level of consciousness.

This deterioration should be supported by historical evidence and documented either by bedside mental status testing or, ideally, by more detailed neuropsychological examination, using tests that are quantifiable and reproducible and for which normative data are available.

II. Probable IVD

A. The criteria for the clinical diagnosis of **probable ivd** include *all* of the following:
  1. Dementia
  2. Evidence of two or more ischemic strokes by history, neurologic signs, and/or neuroimaging studies (CT of T1-weighted MRI

B. The diagnosis of **probable ivd** is supported by:
  1. Evidence of multiple infrared in brain regions known to affect cognition
  2. A history of multiple transient ischemic attacks
  3. History of vascular risk factors (e.g., hypertension, heart disease, diabetes mellitus)
  4. Elevated Hachinski Ischemia Scale (original or modified version)

C. Clinical features that are thought to be associated with IVD but await further research include:
  1. Relatively early appearance of gait disturbance
  2. Periventricular and deep white-matter changes on T2-weighted MRI that are excessive for age
  3. Focal changes in electrophysiologic studies (e.g., EEG, evoked potentials) or physiologic neuroimaging studies (e.g., SPECT-ET-NMR spectroscopy)

D. Other clinical features that do not constitute strong evidence either for or against a diagnosis of **probable ivd** include:
  1. Periods of slowly progressive symptoms
  2. Illusions, psychosis, hallucinations, delusions
  3. Seizures

E. Clinical features that cast doubt on a diagnosis of **probable ivd** include:
  1. Transcortical sensory aphasia in the absence of corresponding focal lesions on neuroimaging studies
  2. Absence of central neurologic symptoms/signs, other than cognitive disturbance

III. Possible IVD

A clinical diagnosis of **possible ivd** may be made when there is:
  1. Dementia
      and one or more of the following:
  2a. A history or evidence of a single stroke (but not multiple strokes) without a clearly documented temporal relationship to the onset of dementia or
  2b. Binswanger's syndrome (without multiple strokes) which includes all of the following:
      i. Early-onset urinary incontinence not explained by urologic disease, or gait disturbance (e.g., parkinsonian, magnetic, apraxic, or "senile" gait) not explained by peripheral cause
      ii. Vascular risk factors
      iii. Extensive white-matter changes on neuroimaging

IV. Definite IVD

Diagnosis of **definite ivd** requires histopathologic examination of the brain, as well as:
A. Chemical evidence of dementia
B. Pathologic confirmation of multiple infarcts, some outside of the cerebellum

V. Mixed dementia

A diagnosis of **mixed** dementia should be made in the presence of one or more other systemic or brain disorders that are thought to be *causally* related to the dementia.

The degree of confidence in the diagnosis of IVD should be specified as possible, probably, or definite, and the other disorder(s) contributing to the dementia should be listed. For example: mixed dementia due to probable IVD and possible Alzheimer's disease, or mixed dementia due to definite IVD and hypothyroidism.

Note: If there is evidence of Alzheimer's disease or some other pathologic disorder that is thought to have contributed to the dementia, a diagnosis of **mixed dementia** should be made.
From ref. 9, with permission.

ages are consistent with cerebral infarction, but many of the changes observed on MRI may represent the effects of healthy aging, such as dilated perivascular spaces. The typical changes include small, focal areas of increased signal as well as patchy or confluent periventricular white-matter hyperintensity on T2-weighted images. These nonspecific changes are the basis of the term "leuko-araiosis" (LA). It is important to recognize that a large volume of diffuse signal change may be present on CT or MRI without meaningful impairment of cognition. Nonetheless, LA is a frequent correlate of MID. In Erkinjuntti et al.'s (15) clinical series, 72% of MID patients had LA, as opposed to 19% of AD patients.

For many years, "cerebral arteriosclerosis" was considered an important component of most senile dementia—hence the popular use of the phrase "hardening of the arteries" as a synonym for dementia. This perception understandably led to extensive study of cerebral blood flow and metabolism, but with little concern over clinical differentiation of dementia types. The earliest studies employed inert gas measures of global cerebral metabolic rate for O_2 ($CMRO_2$). Such studies demonstrated diminished cerebral metabolism in demented subjects, both with and without known cerebrovascular disease (39).

Developing technology subsequently allowed regional cerebral blood flow (CBF) measurements using the gamma-emitter ^{133}Xe and multiple extracranial radiation detectors for planar or tomographic imaging. Simultaneously, a greater understanding of dementia subtypes improved the discriminative abilities of the techniques. Patients with vascular dementia, including MID, demonstrate patchy, irregular areas of decreased CBF consistent with areas of infarction or ischemia, whereas AD patients have more uniform frontal, parietal, and temporal decreases in CBF (36,62). There is no general agreement that diminished CBF by ^{133}Xe methods correlates with dementia severity. Some studies have found good correlation in MID only (23), and others have reported it in AD only (62); however most studies have found it in both (6).

Positron emission tomography (PET) using ^{15}O allows detailed mapping of O_2 metabolism. Neither AD nor MID patients typically demonstrate chronic ischemia by this method (18). Despite early enthusiasm for [^{18}F]-fluorodeoxyglucose (FDG) PET as a useful technique for the differentiation of MID and AD (4), subsequent investigations have not been as conclusive (6).

Single photon emission computed tomography (SPECT) is more widely available than PET and has been used clinically to differentiate MID from AD, though the validity of SPECT for this purpose is not known. Neither of the two isotopes in general use, ^{123}I-labeled amphetamine (IMP) and ^{99m}Tc-labeled hexamethylpropylene amine oxime (HMPAO), has been shown to be superior in the differential diagnosis of dementia (20). As with other imaging modalities, MID patients tend to show patchy or multifocal hypoperfusion whereas AD patients show more diffuse changes, but there is sufficient overlap to prevent diagnostic surety in any individual patient (55).

EPIDEMIOLOGY

The reported frequency of MID in demented populations ranges from 4.5% to 39% (34). Karasawa and Homma (33) have suggested that the prevalence of MID, at least in Japan, has decreased since 1980 as the result of fewer strokes affecting the elderly.

Jorm et al.'s (29) extensive review of previous studies provides the basis for much of the current understanding of the demographics of MID. They calculated the prevalence of MID as doubling with every 5.3 years of age, which is in contrast to a popular perception that the prevalence of MID declines after age 75 because of mortality associated with recurrent strokes (43). Men are affected with MID more frequently—as opposed to AD, which is more common among women (29). In Europe, there is also a trend toward higher rates of MID in rural populations than in urban ones (34).

Meta-studies of the epidemiology of MID have been complicated by the lack of clear-cut and uniform diagnostic criteria. Another problem in the interpretation of MID epidemiology is that the illness is often defined on the basis of its risk factors regardless of temporal course. As pointed out by Kase (34), in the presence of dementia, the IS items of (a) history of hypertension, (b) history of stroke, (c) evidence of associated atherosclerosis, and (d) focal findings on neurologic exam are considered sufficient to diagnose MID. Prospective studies, using uniform diagnostic criteria and paying careful attention to the timing and character of stroke and dementia, will be required to more fully understand the epidemiology and natural history of MID.

PATHOLOGY

Tomlinson, Blessed, and Roth's landmark article (59) on the neuropathology of demented older individuals clarified the importance of AD pathology in senile dementia. It also reported a 20% frequency of multiple, discrete infarcts. These findings, along with Hachinski et al.'s (24) popularization of the term MID, defined the role of focal infarctions as a cause of dementia. Lacunar infarctions, also known as *lacunes,* are commonly implicated as a major contributor to MID because of the "subcortical" features often prominent in the clinical presentation of the illness. Lacunes are small cavitary lesions attributed to the occlusion of deep penetrating arteries. There is no uniform definition based on size, but most lacunes are less than 2 cm in diameter.

Lacunar infarctions are strongly associated with a history of hypertension. In Fisher's (16) report, 97% of 114 autopsy cases of lacunar infarction had a diagnosis of hypertension, though more recent studies with stricter criteria for hypertension suggest rates ranging from 60% to 75% (47). The importance of lacunes per se as contributors to the dementia has been questioned. Both Tomlinson et al. (59) and Fisher (17) minimized the role of these lesions in cognitive deficits. Cases of MID with lacunes also typically show myelin-stain evidence for extensive white-matter degeneration (27,48). Whether an accumulation of lacunes themselves is able to produce dementia in the absence of associated noncavitary white-matter damage is unknown. Though frequently referred to as *demyelination,* electron microscopy (EM) indicates that axons within the myelin-stain lesions are lost as well (63). Because the diffuse white-matter changes and the cavitary lesions almost always co-occur and share a common pathophysiology, it is unlikely that their differential effects will be elucidated from human clinical material. The problem in differentiating "pure" MID pathologically is one factor contributing to the evolution of the more inclusive concept of ischemic vascular dementia.

Two other types of discrete infarctions contribute to many cases of MID. Large-vessel infarctions are usually identifiable by history with features of hemiparesis, hemianopia, aphasia, and so on. These are also unequivocally evident on CT or MRI. The volume of tissue loss from such lesions is an important factor in the development of dementia. Tomlinson et al. (59) reported that all their autopsy subjects with greater than 100 ml of tissue loss were demented. However, it is clear that dementia can follow much smaller losses of brain tissue if these are strategically located (11). The second type of cortical lesion contributing to MID is the micro-infarct. These have been reported as the sole basis of dementia (32,59) and consist of 0.5- to 2-mm-diameter lesions within the cortical ribbon. They are associated with a history of transient ischemic attacks (48).

Other factors which predispose to the development of multiple cerebral infarctions are associated with MID or VaD. Conditions leading to thromboembolic showers, such as endocarditis or atrial myxoma, can lead to the rapid development of a demented state often after a period of acute encephalopathy or coma. Autoimmune vasculitides, such as in systemic lupus erythematosus or granulomatous angiitis of the central nervous system, contribute to areas of cerebral ischemia and infarction. They can be associated with long-term cognitive impairments. Tertiary Lyme disease and syphilis can also cause dementia on the basis of vasculitic thromboses. Cerebral amyloid angiopathy, though often linked to AD, may lead to multiple intracerebral hemorrhages and play a significant role in the development of VaD (28). One other lesion of vascular origin which can present as dementia is chronic subdural hematoma. These intracranial fluid collections can mimic the fluctuating, stepwise cognitive deterioration and prominent motor symptoms characteristic of MID, and they are largely reversible with surgical drainage of fluid and relief of mass effect.

PATHOGENESIS

To date, there remains no concise explanation for the pathogenesis of MID except for infarctions causing loss of brain volume or loss of strategic, localized, areas integral to normal cognition, or a combination of these two factors.

Although CBF is diminished in MID, this is a feature common to most dementia and probably represents a response to reduced cerebral metabolism, rather than the cause of the cognitive impairment. Some MID patients show foci of elevated regional oxygen extraction fraction (rOEF) suggestive of areas of chronic compensated ischemia (21). Rogers et al. argued (51) that a state of insufficient blood flow to the brain precedes the onset of dementia in MID patients by up to 2 years. Brown and Frackowiak (6) have cautioned, however, that such rOEF changes are not common among MID patients and therefore cannot be the major factor in the development of most MID. Two conditions associated with global diminution in CBF—cardiac disease (58) and hypertension (3)—have nonetheless been long recognized as contributors to impairment on neuropsychological testing. Meyer et al. (46), for example, reported that careful control of blood pressure improved cognition in some in MID patients, but overcontrol (with presumed diminution of CBF) worsened cognitive performance.

MID and, more inclusively, VaD are associated with changes in the blood–brain barrier (BBB). Elevated cerebrospinal fluid (CSF) concentrations of albumin and immunoglobulin G (IgG) have been reported for MID patients (40), though other studies have found no difference for albumin (1) or IgG (5). Interestingly, Blennow et al. (5) also reported increased CSF/serum ratios for albumin in AD patients with white-matter lesions or vascular risk factors. This indicates that BBB dysfunction in VaD may result from risk factors for cerebrovascular disease rather than represent a unique contributor to MID. Wallin and Blennow (60) have argued that, because myelin lipids are significantly reduced in vascular dementia, the myelin sheath is a primary lesion site. They further hypothesize that the high metabolic demands of the oligodendrocytes render them prone to ischemic damage. These views are at odds with (a) the PET data, which suggest that chronic ischemia is not a contributor to MID (6), and (b) the EM studies, which show axonal loss in areas of noncavitary demyelination (63). Although myelin loss and BBB dysfunction may contribute to some vascular dementia syndromes, their causative role in MID is questionable. One of the difficulties in assessing the pathophysiology of VaD is the considerable frequency of dementia with findings of both vascular disease and AD. Although this may simply represent the co-occurrence of two common illnesses, there is evidence that links cerebrovascular disease and AD pathology. Kalaria et al. (31), for instance, found that cerebral ischemia promotes deposition of potentially neurotoxic amyloid in the brain. Sofroniew et al. (57) reported that focal cerebral damage causes neuronal loss in the nucleus basalis of Meynert similar to that observed in AD. Furthermore, such changes in the basal forebrain, when associated with AD, have been linked to alterations of cerebral vascular regulation and diminution of CBF (54). The synthetic sites for the biogenic amines are also affected in AD (42,50). Degeneration in these sites, the locus coeruleus and dorsal raphe nuclei, may adversely affect cerebrovascular function, because norepinephrine and serotonin also influence vascular autoregulation (53). The distinction between causes of vascular and "primary degenerative" dementias may therefore be more difficult than is commonly accepted.

ANIMAL MODELS

Although a number of animal models for the development of MID have been employed, none have been satisfactory. Rodents tend not to have profound long-lasting behavioral effects from cerebral infarctions, and the multiple or diffuse, gradually acquired lesions characteristic of MID in humans have not been reproduced. The promising technique of inducing embolic ischemia in rats by injecting $35\text{-}\mu\text{m}$-diameter microspheres into rat carotid arteries produced effects on memory, but these were not sustained (37).

TREATMENT

Drugs of many classes and presumed mechanisms of action have been tried in the treatment of the cognitive symptoms in MID, but none have consistently been demonstrated to be effective. No agent has been approved for such use in the United States. There are, however, potential means of symptomatic treatment. Improvement among selected MID patients on a screening instrument for cognition, the Cognitive Capacity Screening Exam (CCSE), was reported with treatment of vascular risk factors such as hypertension and smoking. Similar treatments did not affect the cognition of AD patients in the same paradigm (46). In systemic conditions that decrease CBF, such as valvular heart disease and hypertension, neuropsychological test performance can improve with treatment of the causative factor(s) (30).

Alteration of the course of the illness may also be accomplished. Reduction of blood pressure is a primary goal of treatment in order to diminish the risk for recurrent stroke (43). Other risk factors, such as smoking and diabetes mellitus, can be addressed to reverse or slow the progression of vascular pathology. Any treatment approach that reduces the likelihood of stroke, such as carotid endarterectomy in moderate stenoses or the use of aspirin or ticlopidine in primary and secondary prevention, is likely to alter the course of MID, but no definitive analyses have been reported. It is important, however, to emphasize that many of the vascular changes contributing to strokes are the result of long-term pathologic processes which are not reversed with treatment. As Meyer et al. (46) found, overreduction in blood pressure can actually worsen cognition. That risk factor modification can affect the course of MID after diagnosis has not been conclusively demonstrated, but a reduction in VaD prevalence has been attributed to attention to risk factors (26).

CONCLUSIONS

Multi-infarct dementia is a syndrome which varies according to the site, size, nature, number, and timing of the lesions. Although criteria for the diagnosis of vascular dementia as a whole have been proposed, the long-term utility of such criteria has been questioned (22). No specific risk factors beyond those for cerebral ischemia have been identified, but it is likely that with control of the risk factors, progression of the illness, and perhaps current function, can be affected. The challenge lies in the early identification of those at risk for subsequent development of cognitive impairments and intervention. Prevention of vascular dementia through risk factor management may have further impact because of potential interactions between cerebral ischemia and the expression of AD.

FUTURE DIRECTIONS

Hachinski (22) has claimed that "Few areas in medicine are as ripe for action as the vascular dementias." The success of further efforts to understand VaD depends on several factors. Included among them are (a) a commonly accepted definition of what constitutes VaD and (b) the recognition that multiple, potentially treatable causes contribute to a final common clinical state of dementia. Early recognition of risk, and subsequent intervention, are then possible before the evolution of the dementia. The development of more useful animal models and new techniques of functional imaging to understand the pathogenesis of dementia in the face of vascular compromise will be vital in settling many of the controversies surrounding the field today. Despite those controversies, and the impediments to progress engendered by them, it is apparent that prevention and treatment of VaD is an achievable goal.

ACKNOWLEDGMENT

This work was supported by NIA Alzheimer's Disease Research Center grant AG08012.

REFERENCES

1. Alafuzoff I, Adolfsson R, Bucht G, Winblad B. Albumin and immunoglobulin in plasma and cerebrospinal fluid, and blood-cerebrospinal fluid barrier in patients with dementia of Alzheimer type and multi-infarct dementia. *J Neurol Sci* 1983;60:465–472.
2. American Psychiatric Association Committee on Nomenclature and Statistics. *Diagnostic and statistical manual of mental disorders (DSM-III-R)*, 3rd ed. (revised). Washington, DC: American Psychiatric Association, 1987.
3. Apter NS, Halstead WC, Heimburger RF. Impaired cerebral functions in essential hypertension. *Am J Psychiatry* 1951;107:808–813.
4. Benson DF, Kuhl DE, Hawkins RA, Phelps ME, Cummings JL,

Tsai SY. The fluorodeoxyglucose ^{18}F scan in Alzheimer's disease and multi-infarct dementia. *Arch Neurol* 1983;40:711–714.

5. Blennow K, Wallin A, Fredman P, Karlsson I, Gottfries CG, Sverrholm L. Blood–brain barrier disturbance in Alzheimer's disease is related to vascular factors. *Acta Neurol Scand* 1990;81:323–326.

6. Brown WD, Frackowiak RSJ. Cerebral blood flow and metabolism studies in multi-infarct dementia. *Alzheimer's Dis Assoc Disord* 1991;5:131–143.

7. Brust JCM. Vascular dementia is overdiagnosed. *Arch Neurol* 1988;45:799.

8. Chui HC. Dementia: a review emphasizing clinicopathologic correlation and brain-behavior relationships. *Arch Neurol* 1989;46:806–814.

9. Chui HC, Victoroff JI, Margolin D, Jagust W, Shankle R, Katzman R. Criteria for the diagnosis of ischemic vascular dementia proposed by the State of California Alzheimer's Disease Diagnostic and Treatment Centers. *Neurology* 1992;42:473–480.

10. Cummings JL, Benson DF. *Dementia: a clinical approach.* Boston: Butterworth, 1983.

11. del Ser T, Bermejo F, Portera A, Arredondo JM Bouras C, Constantinidis J. Vascular dementia: a clinicopathological study. *J Neurol Sci* 1990;96:1–17.

12. Drachman DA. New criteria for the diagnosis of vascular dementia: do we know enough yet? *Neurology* 1993;43:243–245.

13. Erkinjuntti T. Types of multi-infarct dementia. *Acta Neurol Scand* 1987;75:391–399.

14. Erkinjuntti T, Haltia M, Palo J, Sulkava R, Paetau A. Accuracy of the clinical diagnosis of vascular dementia: a prospective clinical and post-mortem pathological study. *J Neurol Neurosurg Psychiatry* 1988;51:1037–1044.

15. Erkinjuntti T, Ketonen L, Sulkava R, Vuorialho M, Palo J. CT in the differential diagnosis between Alzheimer's disease and vascular dementia. *Acta Neurol Scand* 1987;75:262–270.

16. Fisher CM. Lacunes: small, deep, cerebral infarcts. *Neurology* 1965;15:774–784.

17. Fisher CM. Lacunar strokes and infarcts: a review. *Neurology* 1982;32:871–876.

18. Frackowiak RSJ, Pozzilli C, Legg NJ, et al. Regional cerebral oxygen supply and utilization in dementia: a clinical and physiological study with oxygen-15 and positron tomography. *Brain* 1981;104:753–778.

19. Gainotti G, Parlato V, Monteleone D, Carlomagno S. Neuropsychological markers of dementia on visuospatial tasks: a comparison between Alzheimer's type and vascular forms of dementia. *J Clin Exp Neuropsychol* 1992;14:239–252.

20. Gemmell HG, Sharp PF, Besson JAO, Ebmeier KP, Smith FW. A comparison of Tc-99m HM-PAO and I-123 IMP cerebral SPECT images in Alzheimer's disease and multi-infarct dementia. *Eur J Nucl Med* 1988;14:463–466.

21. Gibbs JM, Frackowiak RSJ, Legg NJ. Regional cerebral blood flow and oxygen metabolism in dementia due to vascular disease. *Gerontology* 1986;32(Suppl):84–88.

22. Hachinski V. Preventable senility: a call for action against the vascular dementias. *Lancet* 1992;340:645–648.

23. Hachinski VC, Iliff LD, Zilhka E, et al. Cerebral blood flow in dementia. *Arch Neurol* 1975;32:632–637.

24. Hachinski VC, Lassen NA, Marshall J. Multi-infarct dementia: a cause of mental deterioration in the elderly. *Lancet* 1974;2:207–210.

25. Hachinski VC, Potter P, Merskey H. Leuko-araiosis. *Arch Neurol* 1987;44:21–23.

26. Homma A, Hasegawa K. Recent developments in gerontopsychiatric research on age associated dementia in Japan. *Int Psychogeriatr* 1989;1:31–49.

27. Ishii N, Nichihara Y, Imamura T. Why do frontal lobe symptoms predominate in vascular dementia with lacunes? *Neurology* 1986;36:340–345.

28. Jellinger K. Cerebrovascular amyloidosis with cerebral hemorrhage. *J Neurol* 1977;214:195–206.

29. Jorm AF, Korten AE, Henderson AS. The prevalence of dementia: a quantitative integration of the literature. *Acta Psychiatr Scand* 1987;76:465–479.

30. Juolasmaa A, Outakoski J, Hirvenoja R, Tienari P, Sotaniemi K,

Takunen J. Effect of open heart surgery on intellectual performance. *J Clin Neuropsychol* 1981;3:181–197.

31. Kalaria RN, Bhatti SU, Palatinsky EA, et al. Accumulation of the beta amyloid precursor protein at sites of ischemic injury in rat brain. *Neuroreport* 1993;4:211–214.

32. Kaplan JG, Katzman R, Horoupin DS, Field PA, Mayeux R, Mays AP. Progressive dementia, visual deficits, amyotrophy and microinfarcts. *Neurology* 1985;35:789–796.

33. Karasawa A, Homma A. Recent changes in the prevalence of dementia in the Tokyo metropolis. In: Hasegawa K, Homma A, eds. *Psychogeriatrics: biomedical and social advances.* Tokyo: Excerpta Medica, 1990;24–29.

34. Kase CS. The epidemiology of multi-infarct dementia. *Alzheimer's Dis Assoc Disord* 1991;5:71–76.

35. Katzman R, Lasker B, Bernstein N. Advances in the diagnosis of dementia: accuracy of diagnosis and consequence of misdiagnosis of disorders causing dementia. In: Terry RD, ed. *Aging and the brain.* New York: Raven Press, 1988;17–62.

36. Kitigawa Y, Meyer JS, Tachibana H, Mortel KF, Rogers RL. CT-CBF correlations of cognitive deficits in multi-infarct dementia. *Stroke* 1984;15:1000–1009.

37. Kiyoto Y, Miyamoto M, Nagayoka A, Nagawa Y. Cerebral embolization leads to memory impairment of several learning tasks in rats. *Pharmacol Biochem Behav* 1986;24:687–692.

38. Kotsoris H, Barclay LL, Kheyfets S, Hulyalkar A, Dougherty J. Urinary and gait disturbances as markers for early multi-infarct dementia. *Stroke* 1987;18:138–141.

39. Lassen NA, Munck O, Tottey ER. Mental function and cerebral oxygen consumption in organic dementia. *Arch Neurol Psychiatry* 1957;77:126–133.

40. Leonardi A, Gandolfo C, Caponetto C, Arata L, Vecchia R. The integrity of the blood-brain barrier in Alzheimer's type and multi-infarct dementia evaluated by the study of albumin and IgG in serum and cerebrospinal fluid. *J Neurol Sci* 1985;67:253–261.

41. Mahler ME, Cummings JL. The behavioral neurology of multi-infarct dementia. *Alzheimer's Dis Assoc Disord* 1991;5:122–130.

42. Mann DMA, Yates PO, Hawkes J. The noradrenergic system in Alzheimer and multi-infarct dementias. *J Neurol Neurosurg Psychiatry* 1982;45:113–119.

43. Marshall J. Vascular dementias. In: Whitehouse PJ, ed. *Dementia.* Philadelphia: FA Davis, 1993;215–236.

44. McKhann G, Drachman D, Folstein M, Katzman R, Price D, Stadlan EM. Clinical iagnosis of Alzheimer's disease: report of the NINCDS-ADRDA work group under the auspices of the Department of Health and Human Services Task Force on Alzheimer's Disease. *Neurology* 1984;34:939–944.

45. Mendez MF, Ashla-Mendez M. Differences between multi-infarct dementia and Alzheimer's disease on unstructured neuropsychological tasks. *J Clin Exp Neuropsychol* 1991;13:923–932.

46. Meyer JS, Judd BW, Tawaklna T, Rogers RL, Mortel KF. Improved cognition after control of risk factors for multi-infarct dementia. *JAMA* 1986;256:2203–2209.

47. Miller VT. Lacunar stroke: a reassessment. *Arch Neurol* 1983;40:129–134.

48. Munoz DG. The pathological basis of multi-infarct dementia. *Alzheimer's Dis Assoc Disord* 1991;5:77–90.

49. O'Brien M. Vascular dementia is underdiagnosed. *Arch Neurol* 1988;45:799.

50. Reinikainen KJ, Paljarvi L, Huuskonen M, et al. A post mortem study of noradrergic, serotonergic and GABAergic neurons in Alzheimer's disease. *J Neurol Sci* 1988;84:101–116.

51. Rogers RL, Meyer JS, Mortel KF, Mahurin RK, Judd BW. Decreased cerebral blood flow precedes multi-infarct dementia, but follows senile dementia of the Alzheimer type. *Neurology* 1986;36:1–6.

52. Roman GC, Tatemichi TK, Erkinjuntti T, et al. Vascular dementia: diagnostic criteria for research studies; report of the NINDS-AIREN International Workshop. *Neurology* 1993;43:250–260.

53. Rothlind JC, Brandt J. A brief assessment of frontal and subcortical functions in dementia. *J Neuropsychiatry Clin Neurosci* 1993;5:73–77.

54. Sato A, Sato Y. Regulation of regional cerebral blood flow by cholinergic fibers originating in the basal forebrain. *Neurosci Res* 1992:242–274.

55. Sharp PF, Gemmell HG, Besson JAO, Smith FW. Perfusion patterns in dementia. *J Nucl Med* 1986;27:1939–1940.

56. Smyth K, Whitehouse PJ, Rust M, Kahana J. Epidemiology, diagnosis, and management of Alzheimer's disease and related disorders: implications for minority populations. *Health Matrix* 1988;4:28–32.

57. Sofroniew MV, Pearson RCA, Eckenstein F, Cuello AC, Powell TPS. Retrograde changes in cholinergic neurons in the basal forebrain of the rat following cortical damage. *Brain Res* 1983;289:370–374.

58. Spieth W. Cardiovascular health status, age and psychological performance. *J Gerontol* 1964;19:277–284.

59. Tomlinson BE, Blessed G, Roth M. Observations on the brains of demented old people. *J Neurol Sci* 1970;11:205–242.

60. Wallin A, Blennow K. Pathogenetic basis of vascular dementia. *Alzheimer's Dis Assoc Disord* 1991;5:91–102.

61. Whitehouse PJ. The concept of subcortical and cortical dementia: another look. *Ann Neurol* 1986;19:1–6.

62. Yamaguchi F, Meyer JS, Yamamoto M, Sakai F, Shaw T. Noninvasive regional blood flow measurements in dementia. *Arch Neurol* 1980;37:410–418.

63. Yamanoucki H, Suguira S, Tomonage M. Decrease in nerve fibers in cerebral white matter in progressive vascular encephalopathy of Binswanger type: an electron microscopy study. *J Neurol* 1989;236:382–387.

Psychopharmacology: The Fourth Generation of Progress, edited by Floyd E. Bloom and David J. Kupfer. Raven Press, Ltd., New York © 1995.

CHAPTER 131

Prion Diseases

Stephen J. DeArmond and Stanley B. Prusiner

The prion diseases, sometimes referred to as the "transmissible spongiform encephalopathies," include kuru, Creutzfeldt–Jakob disease (CJD), and Gerstmann–Sträussler–Scheinker disease (GSS) of humans as well as scrapie and bovine spongiform encephalopathy (BSE) of animals (Tables 1 and 2). For many years, prion diseases were thought to be caused by viruses despite intriguing evidence to the contrary (1). The unique characteristic common to all of these disorders whether sporadic, dominantly inherited, or acquired by infection is that they involve the aberrant metabolism of the prion protein (PrP) (59). In many cases, the normal cellular prion protein, PrP^C, is converted into an abnormal, protease-resistant isoform, PrP^{CJD} in humans and PrP^{Sc} in animals, by a post-translational process which involves a conformational change. The particle (prion) which transmits scrapie appears to be composed largely, if not exclusively, of PrP^{Sc} (58). In the case of human prion diseases, many sporadic and familial cases have been transmitted to experimental animals (30,34,50).

TERMINOLOGY

Because of the complexity of prion diseases, the nomenclature to designate the wild-type and mutant prion protein genes, the pathogenic prion protein synthesized by humans and animals, the prion protein associated with the infectious prion and different prion isolates, and the normal and artificial prion proteins expressed in transgenic mice are currently evolving. A provisional, simplified nomenclature is used here. PrP^C designates the normal cellular isoform synthesized constitutively by hu-

mans and animals. PrP^{Sc} designates pathogenic PrP synthesized in any animal whether its synthesis is initiated by inoculation with human or animal prions or by expression of a mutated PrP gene. PrP^{CJD} designates pathogenic PrP synthesized in humans irrespective of whether the human prion disorder is sporadic, familial, or acquired by prion infection. The human PrP gene maps to the short arm of chromosome 20 and is designated PRNP. The mouse PrP gene maps to the homologous region of chromosome 2 and is designated *Prn-p* (67). Transgenic (Tg) mice expressing foreign or mutant PrP genes are labeled with the transgene in parentheses. For example, transgenic mice harboring a mouse (Mo) PrP gene which mimics the codon 102 mutation of human GSS, which causes a leucine for proline substitution, is designated Tg(MoPrP-P102L) (see Chapter 2, *this volume*, for background).

PRNP GENE MUTATIONS IN HUMAN NEURODEGENERATIVE SYNDROMES

Until recently, only two familial forms of human prion disease were recognized based on dominant inheritance, transmissibility to animals, and the type of amyloid plaques: familial CJD (50,52) and Gerstmann–Sträussler–Scheinker syndrome (GSS) (50). By definition, the diagnosis of GSS requires multicentric PrP amyloid plaques. GSS cases in which ataxia predominates have been linked to a mutation in PRNP gene codon 102 which leads to a proline-to-leucine substitution (41). The cause–effect relationship between the codon 102 mutation and prion disease was verified in Tg mice expressing a mouse (Mo) PrP transgene mimicking the human codon 102 mutation, Tg(MoPrP-P102L) mice (45). The founder and its offspring expressing the transgene developed a spontaneous neurodegenerative disorder with spongiform degeneration and multicentric amyloid plaques similar to

S. J. DeArmond: Departments of Pathology and Neurology, University of California, San Francisco, California 94143.

S. B. Prusiner: Departments of Neurology and of Biochemistry and Biophysics, University of California, San Francisco, California 94143.

TABLE 1. *Human prion diseases*

Etiologic categories	Traditional name[a]
Infectious prion diseases	Kuru
	Iatrogenic CJD
Inherited prion diseases	
Inherited prion disease (P102L)	GSS[b]
Inherited prion disease (A117V)	GSS[c]
Inherited prion disease (D178N)	Familial CJD[d], FFI[e]
Inherited prion disease (F198S)	GSS-nft[f]
Inherited prion disease (E200K)	Familial CJD[g]
Inherited prion disease (Q217R)	GSS-nft[h]
Inherited prion disease (4 octarepeat insert)	Familial CJD[i]
Inherited prion disease (5 octarepeat insert)	Familial CJD[i]
Inherited prion disease (6 octarepeat insert)	Familial CJD[i]
Inherited prion disease (7 octarepeat insert)	Familial CJD[i]
Inherited prion disease (8 octarepeat insert)	Familial CJD[i]
Inherited prion disease (9 octarepeat insert)	Familial CJD[i]
Sporadic prion disease	CJD

[a] CJD, Creutzfeldt–Jakob disease; GSS, Gerstmann–Sträussler–Scheinker syndrome; GSS-nft, GSS with neurofibrillary tangles; FFI, fatal familial insomnia.
[b] Ref. 41.
[c] Refs. 22 and 44.
[d] Refs. 6 and 37.
[e] Refs. 37 and 51.
[f] Ref. 21.
[g] Refs. 28,29,35, and 39.
[h] Ref. 42.
[i] Refs. 38,54, and 57.

the neuropathology in human GSS. The primarily dementing form of GSS has been linked to a PRNP gene codon 117 mutation (22,44). A PRNP gene codon 200 mutation has been identified in some familial CJD pedigrees (28, 35,39,43). This mutation among Libyan Jews represents the largest focus of CJD in the world, with an incidence about 100 times greater than in the worldwide population (52). To date, this mutation has been found in 51 Libyan Jews with CJD and except for one homozygous patient, all were heterozygous for the mutation (29). In addition to point mutations in the PRNP gene, octapeptide-repeat insertions at codon 53 have been identified in other families with CJD (38,54). Molecular genetics has led to the discovery of new prion disorders. PRNP gene codon 198 and 217 mutations (21,42) have been found in a unique form of GSS in which Alzheimer's disease-like neuropathological changes, including neuritic plaques and neurofibrillary tangles, are associated with deposition of PrP amyloid plaques and not the βA4 peptide (31,32,68).

These unique pedigrees raise questions about the relationship of the βA4 peptide deposition and senile plaques in Alzheimer's disease and suggest that there is an overlap of pathogenic mechanisms in Alzheimer's disease and prion diseases. A codon 178 mutation (51) has been found in families with fatal familial insomnia; however, the same codon 178 mutation has also been described in some familial CJD pedigrees without features of insomnia (37). Although the mutation at codon 178 causes an Asn-for-Asp substitution in both FFI and 178-CJD, the two diseases differ in clinical presentation and distribution of neuropathology. In FFI, neuropathological changes were confined largely to the mediodorsal and anterior ventral nuclei of the thalamus whereas they were widespread in 178-CJD. Subsequently, in a collaborative molecular genetic effort, it was discovered that the 178 mutation in FFI is also associated with a methionine (Met) polymorphism at codon 129 (37). Furthermore, it was reported that methionine homozygosity at codon 129 in FFI results in a more severe form of FFI, and valine (Val) homozygosity results in a more severe form of 178-CJD.

Therefore, molecular genetic studies indicate that both CJD and GSS are not single, discrete disorders, but instead are both syndromes with multiple molecular, clinical, and neuropathological characteristics. While we only know of familial forms of GSS, those disorders we classify as CJD because of common clinical and neuropathological features are clearly more complicated because they can have familial, infectious, or sporadic etiologies.

THE MOLECULAR PATHOGENESIS OF PRION DISEASES

Much has been assumed about the pathogenesis of infectious, genetic, and sporadic human prion diseases from studies of infectious forms of scrapie in experimental animals and, more recently, by creating genetic forms of prion disease in Tg mice. As a result of these studies, it appears that abnormal forms of the prion protein play the predominant role in both the etiology and pathogenesis of all forms of prion disorders. The data argue that a protease-resistant form of the prion protein, PrP^{Sc}, is the

TABLE 2. *Animal prion diseases*

Infectious prion diseases
  Bovine spongiform encephalopathy
  Feline spongiform encephalopathy
  Transmissible mink encephalopathy
  Chronic wasting disease
  Exotic ungulate encephalopathy
  Experimental scrapie
Inherited prion disease
  Transgenic mice expressing GSSMoPrP
  Natural scrapie?
Sporadic prion disease
  Natural scrapie?

sole functional component of the infectious particle, termed a *prion*, which transmits scrapie (58). Multiple studies have verified that PrP^{Sc} purifies with scrapie infectivity and have shown that procedures which hydrolyze or modify proteins inactivate prions (26,27,58). In contrast, those procedures that alter nucleic acids do not affect infectivity (1,3,58). Physicochemical analysis of nucleic acids in highly purified prion preparations have failed to reveal viral-like polynucleotides; however, small nucleic acid fragments were found, the vast majority of which were between 40 and 80 nucleotides in length (48). Whether these nucleic acids are contaminants or a functional component of the prion is unknown. It has been proposed that an accessory cellular RNA, designated a "co-prion," can modify the properties of PrP^{Sc} to account for strain-like differences among different prion isolates; however, the failure of ultraviolet (UV) radiation to modify the properties of prions argues against the nucleic acid co-prion hypothesis.

PrP^C is synthesized by a single copy cellular gene in which the entire open reading frame is in a single exon (2,53). PrP^C is distinguished from PrP^{Sc} in several ways. PrP^C is completely digested by limited hydrolysis with proteinase K, whereas it only removes the N-terminal 67 amino acids from PrP^{Sc} to yield PrP 27-30 without loss of infectivity. PrP^{Sc} accumulates in the brain during scrapie infection and attains concentrations locally 10–100 times greater than that of PrP^C (17,46). PrP 27-30 forms into rod-like particles in vitro, whereas PrP^C does not. These rods resemble the structures purified from amyloids and, like them, bind Congo red dye, which displays green birefringence in polarized light. Immunogold studies for electron microscopy verify that the rods are composed of PrP (16). PrP-specific antibodies indicate that the amyloid plaques which form in scrapie-infected brains (16), as well as those found in cases of CJD, GSS, and kuru (60,64,66), are composed of protease-resistant PrP.

Whether mutated PrP in inherited forms of human prion disease is protease-resistant or must act on PrP^C to transform it into protease-resistant PrP^{CJD} is not known. Transgenic mice which express PrP containing the P102L mutation mimicking the PRNP mutation of ataxic human GSS spontaneously develop a neurodegenerative disorder with neuropathological characteristics of scrapie (45). Subsequently we found that about 30% of these mice form PrP-immunopositive amyloid plaques spontaneously (Fig. 1).

PRION ISOLATES ("STRAINS")

A single host animal species can synthesize multiple types of scrapie prions each capable of faithfully transmitting a different clinical–pathological syndrome (18,40). We have chosen to avoid using the term "strain" to describe distinct prion inocula which differ in their indi-

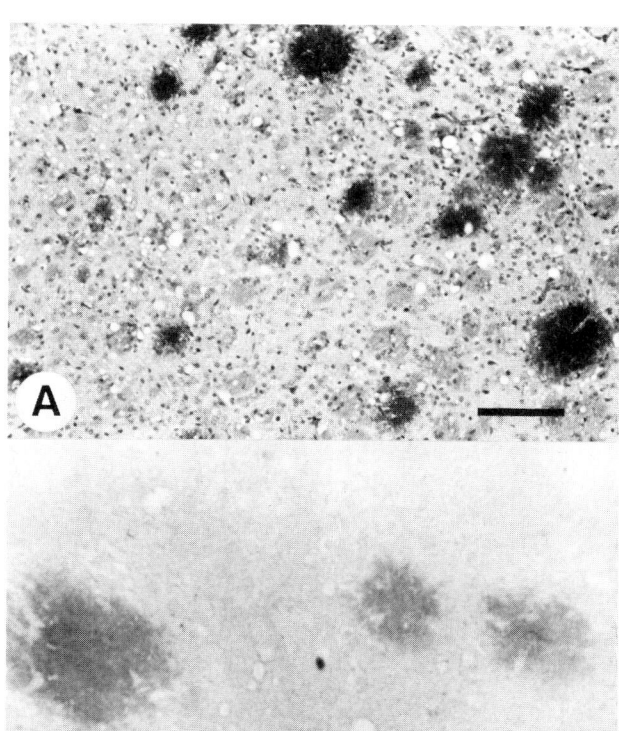

FIG. 1. PrP cerebral amyloid plaques develop in the spontaneous neurodegenerative disease of transgenic mice which express a mouse PrP gene mimicking the codon 102 mutation genetically linked to human ataxic GSS, Tg (MoPrP-P102L)-174 mice (Hsiao et al., *in preparation*). Most of the amyloid plaques were located in the caudate nucleus but also occurred in the hippocampus and cerebellar cortex. **A:** Multiple amyloid plaques in the caudate nucleus. Bar represents 100 μm. Periodic acid–Schiff stain. **B:** Amyloid plaques in the caudate nucleus react specifically with PrP antibodies (R073). Peroxidase immunohistochemistry following proteinase K digestion. Bar represents 50 μm.

vidual passage history among animals and which produce distinct clinical–neuropathological syndromes because of the implication from strains of bacteria, viruses, and viroids that diversity resides in the sequence of their nucleic acid genomes. We currently prefer to use the term "isolate" for prions to avoid prejudging the molecular mechanisms which determine reproducible clinical and neuropathological features.

The existence of distinct prion isolates was first discovered during laboratory transmission studies of sheep scrapie to sheep and goats (56). Subsequently, more than 15 scrapie prion isolates were identified in rodents (8) which could be distinguished by scrapie incubation time, the distribution and intensity of spongiform degeneration, and whether or not cerebral amyloid plaques formed. These characteristics were preserved during multiple sequential passages of a given prion isolate within a single mouse or hamster strain but varied markedly or even failed to appear when transferred to a different animal species (host species barrier). Classic genetic studies in different mouse strains which exhibited short (100–180 days) or long (greater than 280 days) incubation times with different prion isolates indicated that scrapie incubation time was determined largely by a single autosomal gene (20). Following the discovery of PrP, molecular genetic studies showed that the scrapie incubation time gene is tightly linked to, or identical to, the *Prn-p* gene (11).

ORIGIN OF PrP^{Sc}

There is considerable evidence from studies of PrP turnover in scrapie-infected cell lines that PrP^{Sc} is derived from preexisting PrP^{C} (5,12,69). It is believed that exogenous PrP^{Sc} in the form of inoculated prions, as well as nascent PrP^{Sc} produced endogenously, form a transient complex (a heterodimer) with PrP^{C} molecules and that this interaction leads to the conversion of PrP^{C} into nascent PrP^{Sc}. The fact that each animal species can synthesize multiple prion isolates with strain-like characteristics implies that specific information is transferred from PrP^{Sc} to PrP^{C} during its conversion to nascent PrP^{Sc}. It is further assumed that the information must be "coded" by specific stable structural configurations of PrP^{Sc}.

There are three possible mechanisms to explain how PrP^{Sc} can attain multiple stable structural states. First, it has been proposed that an accessory cellular RNA called a "co-prion" can modify the properties of PrP^{Sc}; however, there is no physical or chemical evidence to support the existence of a co-prion. The alternative hypothesis is that transferable information is stored exclusively in prion protein molecules. Thus, a second mechanism may be that each cell in an animal synthesizes a single isoform of PrP^{C} with the same amino acid sequence and same secondary and tertiary structures. In this case, one would have to postulate that specific structural information coding for individual prion isolate behavior in PrP^{Sc} of the infecting prion is transferred stably to PrP^{C}. A third mechanism has been suggested by studies with transgenic mice which express both Syrian hamster (SHa) PrP^{C} and mouse (Mo) PrP^{C} (62,65), as well as by our recent studies of the patterns of PrP^{Sc} deposition in the brain as a function of prion isolate (18,19,40). The former study indicates that prion isolates selectively bind to homologous PrP^{C} molecules and convert them into specific kinds of PrP^{Sc} molecules. Syrian-hamster-adapted Sc237 scrapie prions which contain SHaPrP^{Sc} selectively interacted with SHaPrP^{C} in these Tg(SHaPrP) mice to form nascent Sc237 prions, and mouse-adapted RML scrapie prions which contain MoPrP^{Sc} selectively interacted with MoPrP^{C} to form nascent RML prions. In the second set of studies, the histoblot technique revealed that the neuro-

anatomical location of PrP^{Sc} deposition was different and characteristic for each prion isolate (Fig. 2). When combined, these findings argue for the possibility that each subset of neurons synthesizes a different PrP^{C} isoform with the same amino acid sequence but with perhaps different secondary or tertiary structures. Prion-stimulated conversion of PrP^{C} into nascent PrP^{Sc} would occur only in those neurons which synthesize an isoform of PrP^{C} which is compatible with PrP^{Sc} of the infecting prion.

There is ample evidence for variation in the glycosylation patterns of PrP^{Sc} isolated from SHa brain. Multiple charge isomers due to variations in sialylation have been demonstrated by 2-D electrophoresis (4). The diversity of PrP^{Sc} glycoforms is sufficient to account for a large number of prion isolates. Furthermore, cells potentially possess distinct repertoires of glycosyltransferases which could synthesize PrP^{C} molecules with diverse carbohydrate structures. Presumably, the interaction between PrP^{Sc} and PrP^{C} would be fostered by receptors on the surface of cells which recognize PrP^{Sc} carbohydrates homologous to those which are attached to PrP^{C} synthesized within the cells. This hypothesis not only is supported by a number of experimental observations, but also might explain how each prion isolate exhibits a specific scrapie incubation time, neuropathologic lesion profile, and pattern of PrP^{Sc} accumulation. The postulate set forth here does not preclude PrP^{Sc} interacting with receptor proteins on the surface of cells which might restrict its entry into the cell or its binding to PrP^{C}.

Although the diversity of structures found among Asn-linked sugar chains is attractive as a possible source of the biological diversity manifest by prion isolates, the large array of complex-type oligosaccharides found linked to PrP 27-30 isolated from Syrian hamster brains inoculated with the Sc237 isolate is also at odds with this hypothesis. Bi-, tri-, and tetraternary structures were found, some of which contained branched fucoses (24). Some of the sugar chains were also sialylated. The extreme diversity of Asn-linked oligosaccharides found in one isolate makes it difficult to envision entirely distinct populations of Asn-linked sugar chains for each of five additional isolates or "strains." However, these PrP27-30 preparations were made from whole hamster brains and not from specific brain regions, and therefore the hypothesis has not yet been rigorously tested. It is also possible that many different PrP^{Sc} molecules are formed in the brain, but that only a subset will determine clinical behavior.

Although the differences in location of PrP^{Sc} accumulation raise the possibility of the neuronal origin of prion isolates, the fact that there are also regions common to each of the prion isolates in which PrP^{Sc} accumulated (19) requires comment. One possibility is that these regions contain subpopulations of neurons, each with differential susceptibility to prion infection. Another possibility is that they represent neurons which nonspecifically accumulate

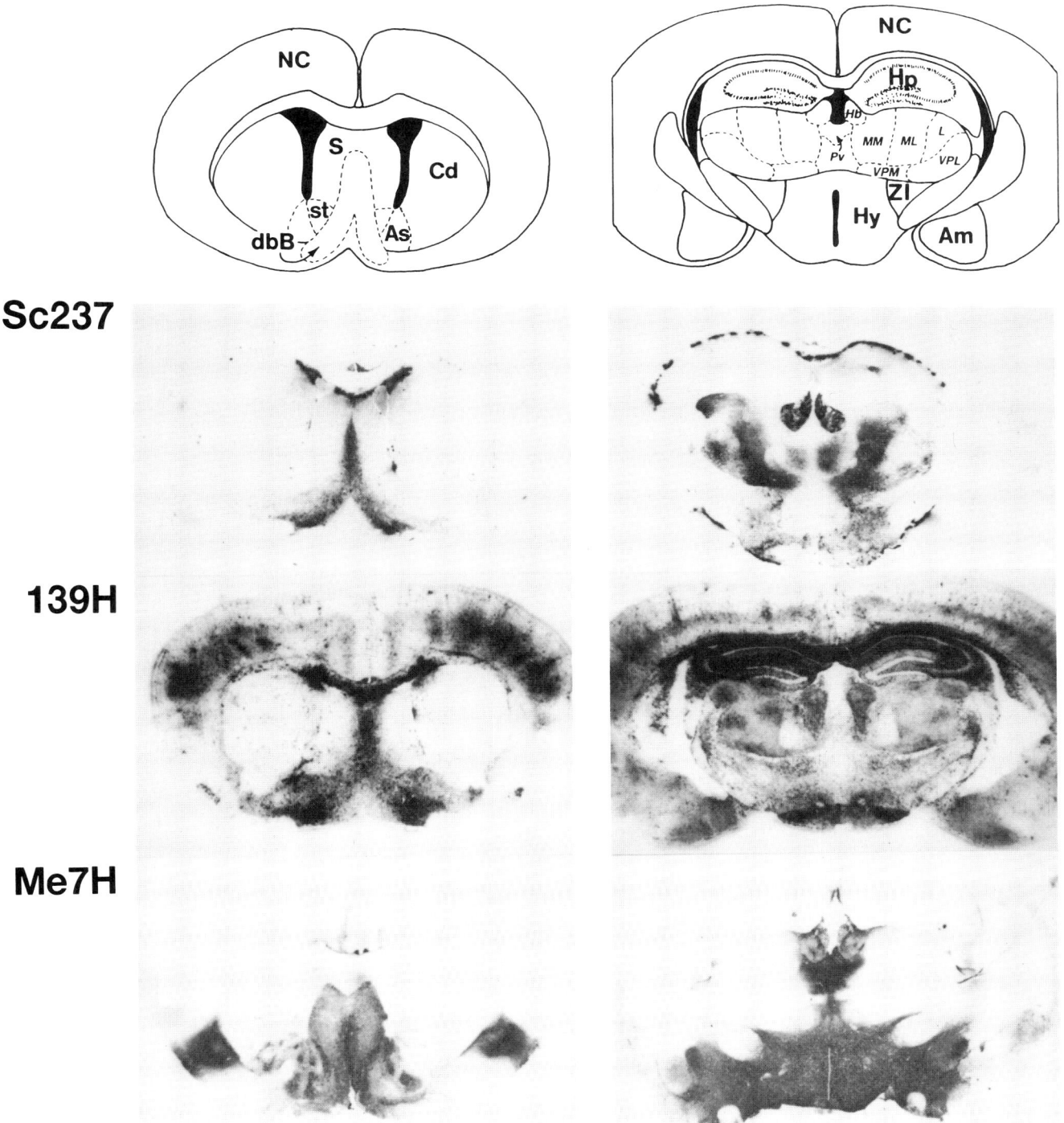

FIG. 2. The distribution of PrP^{Sc} in the brain of Tg(SHaPrP)-7 mice which express high levels of Syrian hamster PrP^{C} is unique for the Sc237, 139H, and Me7H prion isolates (19). Histoblots from two levels of the brain are compared for each prion isolate. The location of PrP^{Sc} was obtained by pressing 10-μm cryostat sections to nitrocellulose paper, digesting the resulting histoblot with proteinase K to eliminate PrP^{C}, and denaturing the remaining protease resistant PrP^{Sc} with quanidinium to enhance antibody binding followed by immunohistological localization with PrP-specific antibodies.

PrP^{Sc} of any form perhaps through a retrograde transport mechanism. Similarly, it is possible that PrP^{Sc} is transported by anterograde axonal transport from multiple neurons, each with their own selective vulnerability to prion infection.

THE DISTRIBUTION OF PrP^{Sc} IS THE MOST FUNDAMENTAL DIFFERENTIATING CHARACTERISTIC OF PRION ISOLATES

Our recent finding that the pattern of PrP^{Sc} deposition is different for each prion isolate argues that it is another fundamental characteristic (18,19,40). The neuropathological feature common to all forms of human and animal prion disorders is spongiform (vacuolar) degeneration of synaptic regions of the grey matter. This is accompanied by varying degrees of nerve cell loss and reactive astrocytic gliosis. Immunohistochemical and neurochemical localization of PrP^{Sc} during scrapie have revealed a precise topographical correlation between PrP^{Sc}, spongiform degeneration, and reactive astrocytic gliosis (17). This correlation has been found with both Sc237 and 139H isolates of the scrapie agent (40) and more recently with the Me7H isolate (19). There is also a temporal correlation between the accumulation of PrP^{Sc} and the development of neuropathology (46). However, the most convincing argument that abnormal PrP causes pathology comes from the molecular genetic studies which link dominantly inherited human prion diseases with mutations in the PRNP gene described above.

Thus a wealth of the experimental data argues that PrP^{Sc} is a necessary component of the scrapie infectious agent and that its accumulation in the brain causes the clinically relevant neuropathology. Furthermore, the rate and pattern of PrP^{Sc} accumulation—and, therefore, the rate of formation of neuropathology—determine scrapie incubation time (15,40). For these reasons, it appears that the rate and pattern of PrP^{Sc} deposition may be the most relevant characteristics of each prion isolate.

SPORADIC CJD

A major unresolved issue concerns the etiology and pathogenesis of sporadic forms of CJD which account for the great majority, about 85%, of human prion diseases. Because neither an infectious nor familial etiology has been found for these cases and because molecular genetic studies of familial prion disorders indicate that multiple mutations of the PRNP gene are pathogenic, the possibility of an age-related acquired mutation of the PRNP gene must be considered. In this regard, sporadic CJD is an age-related disorder with a peak onset at about 60 years of age. It is likely that the PRNP genes in neurons or other cell types occasionally experience mutations. Some of these may be repaired and some may not be pathogenic;

however, some may be pathogenic mutations and not repaired. If a mutation leads to the formation of PrP^{CJD} even in a single neuron, the experience from infectious scrapie argues that a chain reaction could result which leads to the spread of disease to other susceptible neurons. During the process of spreading, the neuron in which the mutated PrP was synthesized might degenerate, leaving no objective evidence of a somatic mutation. Because prions do not stimulate neoplastic growth of cells to produce a tumor in which the putative mutation leads to the production of PrP^{CJD}, this hypothesis will be difficult to verify. The incidence of CJD in populations throughout the world is about 1 case per 10^6. This may represent the combined probabilities that a mutation occurs in the PRNP gene, the probability that the mutation leads to the synthesis of PrP^{CJD}, and the probability that the resultant PrP^{CJD} targets other neurons for the synthesis of more PrP^{CJD} at a rate fast enough to cause clinical disease in the patient's lifetime.

The somatic mutation hypothesis predicts that any neuron could be the source of PrP^{CJD}. In the context of the hypothesis that neurons determine prion isolates through an inherent control of PrP structure, one would predict that sporadic CJD consists of multiple distinct clinical–neuropathological syndromes. Consistent with this postulate, multiple clinical–neuropathological subtypes of CJD have been described, including primarily cortical, corticostriatal with visual impairment, corticostriatal without visual impairment, corticostriatocerebellar, corticospinal, and corticonigral types. That there are "strains" of CJD prions is also suggested by transmission experiments. Transmission of CJD and kuru from many patients into a variety of subhuman primates, cats, and rodents revealed that the susceptible host range, incubation times, duration of illness, and type of clinical disease varied significantly among human prion isolates (33). Once a CJD isolate was transmitted to one rodent species or strain, other rodent strains which had previously been resistant to primary infection with that particular prion isolate could be infected with it. In terms of the prion protein hypothesis, the explanation for this form of species barrier breach is that human CJD prions, composed of PrP^{CJD}, when passaged in a mouse, become composed of rodent PrP^{Sc}.

While the somatic mutation hypothesis may account for some cases of CJD, equally plausible is the notion that sporadic CJD results from the spontaneous conversion of PrP^C into PrP^{Sc} in one or a limited subpopulation of cells. Most of the features of sporadic CJD described above are equally plausible with this model. A third possible mechanism of sporadic CJD is suggested by its association with homozygousity at PRNP codon 129 (see below).

IATROGENIC CJD

Molecular studies of iatrogenic CJD, particularly those related to human growth hormone treatment, suggest that normal polymorphisms of the PRNP gene may cause a predisposition to prion infection.

It is believed that kuru, which is virtually indistinguishable from CJD, was transmitted among the Fore people of New Guinea by ritualistic cannibalism. It is conjectured that this infectious form of human prion disease was initiated in the Fore as the result of spontaneous development of a case of sporadic CJD in one of its members. The only proven cases of infectious CJD in the "civilized" world have resulted from medical procedures (7). Cases of CJD thought to be transmitted by medical procedures include the following: (a) Depth-recording electroencephalographic electrodes sterilized with 70% ethanol and formaldehyde vapor (two cases); electrodes were used previously in a patient with known CJD. While this sterilization procedure was effective for viruses, it was not effective for prions which requires 1 N NaOH denaturation of PrP^{CJD}. (b) Corneal transplant; brain extracts from the donor transmitted CJD to chimpanzee. (c) Cadaveric dura homografts have been implicated in seven cases of iatrogenic CJD. Five of the seven dura specimens came from a single manufacturer where they had been treated with 10% hydrogen peroxide and ionizing radiation. They are now treated for 1 hr with 1 N NaOH. (d) A pericardial homograft replacement for a tympanic membrane has been implicated in one case. (e) The most devastating in terms of numbers has been the transmission of CJD via human growth hormone (hGH) therapy (47). In the past, hGH was prepared from pools containing as many as 20,000 pituitaries obtained at necropsy. The first case of growth-hormone-associated CJD was described almost 10 years ago (49). Today, more than 43 cases are known. Most of these have occurred before the age of 40. The risk among those who have been treated with hGH is estimated to be about 1 per 200 currently, whereas the risk of CJD in the general population under 40 years of age is about 1 per 20×10^6 (25). (f) Human gonadotropin therapy has been associated with CJD in two Australian women (13,23).

DOES A GENETIC PREDISPOSITION TO INFECTIOUS AND SPORADIC CJD EXIST?

Seventeen patients who developed CJD following hGH inoculations did not have any known pathogenic mutations of the PRNP gene (14). However, Collinge et al. (14) found that four of seven patients in the United Kingdom with iatrogenic CJD were homozygous for Val at PRNP codon 129. Brown et al. (7) found that four of nine patients from the United States and France were homozygous for Val, while four others were homozygous for Met. One of the nine was heterozygous for this polymorphism. The normal distribution of the codon 129 polymorphism in the general Caucasian population of the United States, France, and United Kingdom was found to be virtually identical: Val/Val = 11–12%, Met/Met = 37–38%, and Met/Val = 51% (7,14). These findings indicate that homozygosity at codon 129 is not necessary for the development of infectious CJD, but they do suggest that it is associated with increased susceptibility. Interestingly, two of three kuru patients were reported to be homozygous for Val at codon 129 (36).

Because of this association, Palmer et al. (55) tested the possibility that there is a significant homozygosity at codon 129 among cases of sporadic CJD. Twenty-two sporadic CJD cases and 23 suspected sporadic CJD cases in the United Kingdom were examined. Ninety-five percent of the sporadic CJD cases were homozygous (16 Met/Met, 5 Val/Val, and 1 Met/Val). Whether the one heterozygous patient was truly a sporadic case came into question when it was learned that his father died of dementia, raising the possibility that it was familial CJD. Eighty-two percent of the suspected sporadic CJD cases were also homozygous (11 Met/Met, 6 Val/Val, and 4 Met/Val).

Other examples of the apparent importance of homozygosity at codon 129 was its association with more severe forms of fatal familial insomnia and 178-CJD mentioned above. It has also been reported that individuals with CJD associated with a heterozygous 144-base-pair insert between codons 51 and 91 in the PRNP gene and homozygous for Met at codon 129 died at a significantly earlier age than those heterozygous at codon 129 (mean age 42.7 years versus 56.9 years) (57). The PRNP allele containing the insert always coded for methionine at codon 129.

One implication of these findings concerns the etiology of sporadic CJD. They present an alternative to the acquired mutation hypothesis by raising the possibility that some cases of "sporadic" CJD are due to a codon-129-determined susceptibility to environmental prions. That it is possible to acquire a prion disease from the environment is attested to by the experience with kuru and its association with ritualistic cannibalism and by the recent bovine spongiform encephalopathy (BSE) epidemic (70). With regard to the latter, cattle developed BSE, a spongiform encephalopathy with accumulation of protease-resistant PrP^{Sc} primarily in the brainstem (61), after they were given sheep-scrapie-contaminated feed.

The influence of codon 129 homozygosity on the severity and rapidity of prion diseases may shed some light on the mechanism of PrP^C transformation to PrP^{Sc} in which a PrP^C–PrP^{Sc} complex is believed to be an essential step. It raises the possibility that the interaction of PrP^{Sc} with PrP^C requires the formation of a heterodimer composed of a dimer of PrP^{Sc} and a dimer of PrP^C. Putative PrP^C dimer formation would be favored when the amino acids at codon 129 are the same.

The Met and Val polymorphism at codon 129 appears to be the most common and generally nonpathogenic polymorphism among human PrP alleles in the general population. An uncommon polymorphism has been identified in some kindreds with the D178N mutation which consists of 24-base-pair deletion of the PRNP gene in the octapeptide repeat portion of the prion protein (6).

PrP NULL MICE AND THE TREATMENT AND PREVENTION OF PRION DISEASES

PrP gene knockout mice appear to live a normal lifespan with no morphological or behavioral abnormalities (10). These animals do not develop scrapie following inoculation with a spectrum of prion isolates (9,63). The negative results with the PrP null mice are consistent with the preeminence of the prion protein in prion disorders. They also argue that scrapie and CJD are not due to the loss of the normal isoform, PrP^C. PrP null mice are now being used to express a broad variety of PrP genes in the absence of normal mouse PrP gene expression.

The apparent normal mouse phenotype in PrP null mice suggests possible methods for treatment and/or prevention of prion diseases. In the case of the economically devastating animal diseases related to the prion protein, scrapie in sheep and BSE in beef and dairy cattle, it may be possible to breed animals without PrP genes to produce prion-disease-resistant animal strains which are safe for humans. It is interesting to conjecture whether elimination of prion diseases in domestic animals would have an impact on the incidence of ''sporadic'' CJD. The results with null mice also raise the possibility of gene therapy for human prion diseases. Human prion diseases are universally fatal with a relatively rapid, unrelenting course to death once signs and symptoms present. One can hope that someday with antisense PrP gene therapy, it will be possible to diminish synthesis of PrP^C and therefore prevent or slow the formation of PrP^CJD as well as prevent the synthesis of mutated forms of PrP. The experience with PrP null mice suggests that attenuating PrP^C synthesis may not be detrimental; however, we do not yet know the normal function of PrP^C or whether critical cell functions become dependent on it when it is expressed normally throughout life. These as well as multiple other questions remain to be answered about the etiology, pathogenesis, and treatment of this set of neurodegenerative diseases which are uniquely manifest as genetic and infectious disorders.

ACKNOWLEDGMENTS

The authors wish to thank Dr. Shu-Lian Yang and Audrey Lee for preparing histoblots, Mrs. Juliana Cayetano-Canlas for neurohistology, and Mrs. Jo Nelson for help in manuscript preparation. This work was supported by research grants AG02132, NS14069, AG08967, and NS22786 from the National Institutes of Health as well as by gifts from the Sherman Fairchild Foundation and National Medical Enterprises.

REFERENCES

1. Alper T, Haig DA, Clarke MC. The scrapie agent: evidence against its dependence for replication on intrinsic nucleic acid. *J Gen Virol* 1978;41:503–516.
2. Basler K, Oesch B, Scott M, Westaway D, Wälchli M, Groth DF, McKinley MP, Prusiner SB, Weissmann C. Scrapie and cellular PrP isoforms are encoded by the same chromosomal gene. *Cell* 1986;46:417–428.
3. Bellinger-Kawahara C, Diener TO, McKinley MP, Groth DF, Smith DR, Prusiner SB. Purified scrapie prions resist inactivation by procedures that hydrolyze, modify, or shear nucleic acids. *Virology* 1987;160:271–274.
4. Bolton DC, Meyer RK, Prusiner SB. Scrapie PrP 27-30 is a sialoglycoprotein. *J Virol* 1985;53:596–606.
5. Borchelt DR, Taraboulos A, Prusiner SB. Evidence for synthesis of scrapie prion proteins in the endocytic pathway. *J Biol Chem* 1992;267:6188–6199.
6. Bosque PJ, Vnencak-Jones CL, Johnson MD, Whitlock JA, McLean MJ. A PrP gene codon 178 base substitution and a 24-bp interstitial deletion in familial Creutzfeldt–Jakob disease. *Neurology* 1992;42:1864–1870.
7. Brown P, Preece MA, Will RG. ''Friendly fire'' in medicine: hormones, homografts, and Creutzfeldt–Jakob disease. *Lancet* 1992;340:24–27.
8. Bruce ME, Fraser H. Scrapie strain variation and its implications. *Curr Top Microbiol Immunol* 1991;172:125–138.
9. Büeler H, Aguzzi A, Sailer A, Greiner R, Autenried P, Aguet M, Weissmann C. Mice devoid of PrP are resistant to scrapie. *Cell* 1993;73:1339–1347.
10. Büeler H, Fischer M, Lang Y, Blüthmann H, Lipp H-L, DeArmond SJ, Prusiner SB, Aguet M, Weissmann C. The neuronal cell surface protein PrP is not essential for normal development and behavior of the mouse. *Nature* 1992;356:577–582.
11. Carlson GA, Lovett M, Epstein CJ, Westaway D, Goodman PA, Marshall ST, Prusiner SB. The prion gene complex: polymorphism of *Prn-p* and its linkage with agouti. In: *Fourteenth molecular and biochemical genetics workshop,* Bar Harbor, Maine, 1986.
12. Caughey B, Raymond GJ. The scrapie-associated form of PrP is made from a cell surface precursor that is both protease- and phospholipase-sensitive. *J Biol Chem* 1991;266:18217–18223.
13. Cochius JI, Hyman N, Esiri MM. Creutzfeldt–Jakob disease in a recipient of human pituitary-derived gonadotrophin: a second case. *J Neurol Neurosurg Psychiatry* 1992;55:1094–1095.
14. Collinge J, Palmer M, Dryden A, Campbell T. Molecular genetics of inherited, sporadic and iatrogenic prion disease. In: *Prion diseases in humans and animals conference,* London, UK, 1991.
15. DeArmond SJ, Jendroska K, Yang S-L, Taraboulos A, Hecker R, Hsiao K, Stowring L, Scott M, Prusiner SB. Scrapie prion protein accumulation correlates with neuropathology and incubation times in hamsters and transgenic mice. In: Prusiner SB, Collinge J, Powell J, Anderton B, eds. *Prion diseases of humans and animals.* London: Ellis Horwood, 1992;483–496.
16. DeArmond SJ, McKinley MP, Barry RA, Braunfeld MB, McColloch JR, Prusiner SB. Identification of prion amyloid filaments in scrapie-infected brain. *Cell* 1985;41:221–235.
17. DeArmond SJ, Mobley WC, DeMott DL, Barry RA, Beckstead JH, Prusiner SB. Changes in the localization of brain prion proteins during scrapie infection. *Neurology* 1987;37:1271–1280.
18. DeArmond SJ, Prusiner SB. The neurochemistry of prion diseases. *J Neurochem* 1993;61:1589–1601.
19. DeArmond SJ, Yang S-L, Lee A, Bowler R, Taraboulos A, Groth D, Prusiner SB. Three distinct scrapie prion isolates exhibit different patterns of PrP^Sc accumulation. *Proc Natl Acad Sci USA* 1993;90:6449–6453.
20. Dickinson AG, Meikle VMH, Fraser H. Identification of a gene which controls the incubation period of some strains of scrapie agent in mice. *J Comp Pathol* 1968;78:293–299.
21. Dlouhy SR, Hsiao K, Farlow MR, Foroud T, Conneally PM, Johnson P, Prusiner SB, Hodes ME, Ghetti B. Linkage of the Indiana kindred of Gerstmann–Straussler–Scheinker disease to the prion protein gene. *Nature Genet* 1992;1:64–67.
22. Doh-ura K, Tateishi J, Sasaki H, Kitamoto T, Sakaki Y. Pro → Leu

change at position 102 of prion protein is the most common but not the sole mutation related to Gerstmann–Sträussler syndrome. *Biochem Biophys Res Commun* 1989;163:974–979.

23. Dumble LJ, Klein RD. Creutzfeldt-Jakob legacy for Australian women treated with human pituitary gonadotropins. *Lancet* 1992;340:847–848.

24. Endo T, Groth D, Prusiner SB, Kobata A. Diversity of oligosaccharide structures linked to asparagines of the scrapie prion protein. *Biochemistry* 1989;28:8380–8388.

25. Fradkin JE, Schonberger LB, Mills JL, Gunn WJ, Piper JM, Wysowski DK, Thomson R, Durako S, Brown P. Creutzfeldt–Jakob disease in pituitary growth hormone recipients in the United States. *JAMA* 1991;265:880–884.

26. Gabizon R, McKinley MP, Groth DF, Prusiner SB. Immunoaffinity purification and neutralization of scrapie prion infectivity. *Proc Natl Acad Sci USA* 1988;85:6617–6621.

27. Gabizon R, McKinley MP, Prusiner SB. Purified prion proteins and scrapie infectivity copartition into liposomes. *Proc Natl Acad Sci USA* 1987;84:4017–4021.

28. Gabizon R, Meiner Z, Cass C, Kahana E, Kahana I, Avrahami D, Abramsky O, Scarlato G, Prusiner SB, Hsiao KK. Prion protein gene mutation in Libyan Jews with Creutzfeldt–Jakob disease [Abstract]. *Neurology* 1991;41:160.

29. Gabizon R, Rosenman H, Meiner Z, Kahana I, Kahana E, Shugart Y, Ott J, Prusiner SB. Mutation and polymorphism of the prion protein gene in Libyan Jews with Cretuzfeldt–Jakob disease. *Am J Hum Genet* 1993;33:828–835.

30. Gajdusek DC, Gibbs CJ Jr, Alpers M. Experimental transmission of a kuru-like syndrome to chimpanzees. *Nature* 1966;209:794–796.

31. Ghetti B, Tagliavini F, Masters CL, Beyreuther K, Giaccone G, Verga L, Farlo MR, Dlouhy SR, Azzarelli B, Bugiani O. Gerstmann–Sträussler–Scheinker disease. II. Neurofibrillary tangles and plaques with PrP-amyloid coexist in an affected family. *Neurology* 1989;39:1453–1461.

32. Giaccone G, Tagliavini F, Verga L, Frangione B, Farlow MR, Bugiani O, Ghetti B. Neurofibrillary tangles of the Indiana kindred of Gerstmann–Sträussler–Scheinker disease share antigenic determinants with those of Alzheimer disease. *Brain Res* 1990;530:325–329.

33. Gibbs CJ Jr, Gajdusek DC, Amyx H. Strain variation in the viruses of Creutzfeldt–Jakob disease and kuru. In: Prusiner SB, Hadlow WJ, eds. *Slow transmissible diseases of the nervous system*, vol 2. New York: Academic Press, 1979;87–110.

34. Gibbs CJ Jr, Gajdusek DC, Asher DM, Alpers MP, Beck E, Daniel PM, Matthews WB. Creutzfeldt–Jakob disease (spongiform encephalopathy): transmission to the chimpanzee. *Science* 1968;161:388–389.

35. Goldfarb L, Korczyn A, Brown P, Chapman J, Gajdusek DC. Mutation in codon 200 of scrapie amyloid precursor gene linked to Creutzfeldt–Jakob disease in Sephardic Jews of Libyan and non-Libyan origin. *Lancet* 1990;336:637–638.

36. Goldfarb LG, Brown P, Goldgaber D, Asher DM, Strass N, Graupera G, Piccardo P, Brown WT, Rubenstein R, Boellaard JW, Gajdusek DC. Patients with Creutzfeldt–Jakob disease and kuru lack the mutation in the PRNP gene found in Gerstmann–Sträussler–Scheinker syndrome, but they show a different double-allele mutation in the same gene [Abstract]. *Am J Hum Genet [Suppl]* 1989;45:A189.

37. Goldfarb LG, Brown P, Haltia M, Cathala F, McCombie WR, Kovanen J, Cervenakova L, Goldin L, Nieto A, Godec MS, Asher DM, Gajdusek DC. Creutzfeldt–Jakob disease cosegregates with the codon 178^Asn PRNP mutation in families of European origin. *Annu Neurol* 1992;31:274–281.

38. Goldfarb LG, Brown P, McCombie WR, Goldgaber D, Swergold GD, Wills PR, Cervenakova L, Baron H, Gibbs CJJ, Gajdusek DC. Transmissible familial Creutzfeldt–Jakob disease associated with five, seven, and eight extra octapeptide coding repeats in the PRNP gene. *Proc Natl Acad Sci USA* 1991;88:10926–10930.

39. Goldfarb LG, Mitrova E, Brown P, Toh BH, Gajdusek DC. Mutation in codon 200 of scrapie amyloid protein gene in two clusters of Creutzfeldt–Jakob disease in Slovakia. *Lancet* 1990;336:514–515.

40. Hecker R, Taraboulos A, Scott M, Pan K-M, Torchia M, Jendroska K, DeArmond SJ, Prusiner SB. Replication of distinct prion isolates is region specific in brains of transgenic mice and hamsters. *Genes & Development* 1992;6:1213–1228.

41. Hsiao K, Baker HF, Crow TJ, Poulter M, Owen F, Terwilliger JD, Westaway D, Ott J, Prusiner SB. Linkage of a prion protein missense variant to Gerstmann–Sträussler syndrome. *Nature* 1989;338:342–345.

42. Hsiao K, Dlouhy S, Ghetti B, Farlow M, Cass C, Da Costa M, Conneally M, Hodes ME, Prusiner SB. Mutant prion proteins in Gerstmann–Straussler–Scheinker disease with neurofibrillary tangles. *Nature Genet* 1992;1:68–71.

43. Hsiao K, Meiner Z, Kahana E, Cass C, Kahana I, Avrahami D, Scarlato G, Abramsky O, Prusiner SB, Gabizon R. Mutation of the prion protein in Libyan Jews with Creutzfeldt–Jakob disease. *N Engl J Med* 1991;324:1091–1097.

44. Hsiao KK, Cass C, Schellenberg GD, Bird T, Devine-Gage E, Wisniewski H, Prusiner SB. A prion protein variant in a family with the telencephalic form of Gerstmann–Sträussler–Scheinker syndrome. *Neurology* 1991;41:681–684.

45. Hsiao KK, Scott M, Foster D, Growth DF, DeArmond SJ, Prusiner SB. Spontaneous neurodegeneration in transgenic mice with mutant prion protein of Gerstmann–Sträussler syndrome. *Science* 1990;250:1587–1590.

46. Jendroska K, Heinzel FP, Torchia M, Stowring L, Kretzschmar HA, Kon A, Stern A, Prusiner SB, DeArmond SJ. Proteinase-resistant prion protein accumulation in Syrian hamster brain correlates with regional pathology and scrapie infectivity. *Neurology* 1991;41:1482–1490.

47. Job JC, Maillard F, Goujard J. Epidemiologic survey of patients treated with growth hormone in France in the period 1959–1990: preliminary results. *Horm Res* 1992;38(Suppl 1):35–43.

48. Kellings K, Meyer N, Mirenda C, Prusiner SB, Riesner D. Further analysis of nucleic acids in purified scrapie prion preparations by improved return refocussing gel electrophoresis (RRGE). *J Gen Virol* 1992;73:1025–1029.

49. Koch TK, Berg BO, DeArmond SJ, Gravina RF. Creutzfeldt–Jakob disease in a young adult with idiopathic hypopituitarism. Possible relation to the administration of cadaveric human growth hormone. *N Engl J Med* 1985;313:731–733.

50. Masters CL, Gajdusek DC, Gibbs CJ Jr. Creutzfeldt–Jakob disease virus isolations from the Gerstmann–Sträussler syndrome. *Brain* 1981;104:559–588.

51. Medori R, Tritschler H-J, LeBlanc A, Villare F, Manetto V, Chen HY, Xue R, Leal S, Montagna P, Cortelli P, Tinuper P, Avoni P, Mochi M, Baruzzi A, Hauw JJ, Ott J, Lugaresi E, Autilio-Gambetti L, Gambetti P. Fatal familial insomnia, a prion disease with a mutation at codon 178 of the prion protein gene. *N Engl J Med* 1992;326:444–449.

52. Neugut RH, Neugut AI, Kahana E, Stein Z, Alter M. Creutzfeldt–Jakob disease: familial clustering among Libyan-born Israelis. *Neurology* 1979;29:225–231.

53. Oesch B, Westaway D, Wälchli M, McKinley MP, Kent SBH, Aebersold R, Barry RA, Tempst P, Teplow DB, Hood LE, Prusiner SB, Weissmann C. A cellular gene encodes scrapie PrP 27-30 protein. *Cell* 1985;40:735–746.

54. Owen F, Poulter M, Collinge J, Leach M, Shah T, Lofthouse R, Chen YF, Crow TJ, Harding AE, Hardy J. Insertions in the prion protein gene in atypical dementias. *Exp Neurol* 1991;112:240–242.

55. Palmer MS, Dryden AJ, Hughes JT, Collinge J. Homozygous prion protein genotype predisposes to sporadic Creutzfeldt–Jakob disease. *Nature* 1991;352:340–342.

56. Pattison IH, Millson GC. Scrapie produced experimentally in goats with special reference to the clinical syndrome. *J Comp Pathol* 1961;71:101–108.

57. Poulter M, Baker HF, Frith CD, Leach M, Lofthouse R, Ridley RM, Shah T, Owen F, Collinge J, Brown G, Hardy J, Mullan MJ, Harding AE, Bennett C, Doshi R, Crow TJ. Inherited prion disease with 144 base pair gene insertion. 1. Genealogical and molecular studies. *Brain* 1992;115:675–685.

58. Prusiner SB. Novel proteinaceous infectious particles cause scrapie. *Science* 1982;216:136–144.

59. Prusiner SB. Molecular biology of prion diseases. *Science* 1991;252:1515–1522.

60. Prusiner SB, DeArmond SJ. Biology of disease: prions causing nervous system degeneration. *Lab Invest* 1987;56:349–363.
61. Prusiner SB, Fuzi M, Scott M, Serban D, Serban H, Taraboulos A, Gabriel J-M, Wells G, Wilesmith J, Bradley R, DeArmond SJ, Kristensson K. Immunologic and molecular biological studies of prion proteins in bovine spongiform encephalopathy. *J Infect Dis* 1993;167:602–613.
62. Prusiner SB, Scott M, Foster D, Pan K-M, Groth D, Mirenda C, Torchia M, Yang S-L, Serban D, Carlson GA, Hoppe PC, Westaway D, DeArmond SJ. Transgenetic studies implicate interactions between homologous PrP isoforms in scrapie prion replication. *Cell* 1990;63:673–686.
63. Prusiner SB, Groth D, Serban A, Koehler R, Foster D, Torchia M, Burton D, Yang S-L, DeArmond SJ. Ablation of the prion protein (PrP) gene in mice prevents scrapie and facilitates production of anti-PrP antibodies. *Proc Natl Acad Sci USA* 1993;90:10608–10612.
64. Roberts GW, Lofthouse R, Allsop D, Landon M, Kidd M, Prusiner SB, Crow TJ. CNS amyloid proteins in neurodegenerative diseases. *Neurology* 1988;38:1534–1540.
65. Scott M, Foster D, Mirenda C, Serban D, Coufal F, Wälchli M, Torchia M, Groth D, Carlson G, DeArmond SJ, Westaway D, Prusiner SB. Transgenic mice expressing hamster prion protein produce species-specific scrapie infectivity and amyloid plaques. *Cell* 1989;59:847–857.
66. Snow AD, Kisilevsky R, Willmer J, Prusiner SB, DeArmond SJ. Sulfated glycosaminoglycans in amyloid plaques of prion diseases. *Acta Neuropathol (Berl)* 1989;77:337–342.
67. Sparkes RS, Simon M, Cohn VH, Fournier REK, Lem J, Klisak I, Heinzmann C, Blatt C, Lucero M, Mohandas T, DeArmond SJ, Westaway D, Prusiner SB, Weiner LP. Assignment of the human and mouse prion protein genes to homologous chromosomes. *Proc Natl Acad Sci USA* 1986;83:7358–7362.
68. Tagliavini F, Prelli F, Ghiso J, Bugiani O, Serban D, Prusiner SB, Farlow MR, Ghetti B, Frangione B. Amyloid protein of Gerstmann–Sträussler–Scheinker disease (Indiana kindred) is an 11-kd fragment of prion protein with an N-terminal glycine at codon 58. *EMBO J* 1991;10:513–519.
69. Taraboulos A, Raeber AJ, Borchelt DR, Serban D, Prusiner SB. Synthesis and trafficking of prion proteins in cultured cells. *Mol Biol Cell* 1992;3:851–863.
70. Wilesmith JW, Wells GAH, Cranwell MP, Ryan JBM. Bovine spongiform encephalopathy: epidemiological studies. *Vet Rec* 1988;123:638–644.

Psychopharmacology: The Fourth Generation of Progress, edited by Floyd E. Bloom and David J. Kupfer. Raven Press, Ltd., New York © 1995.

CHAPTER 132

Amyotrophic Lateral Sclerosis, Glutamate, and Oxidative Stress

Andreas Plaitakis and P. Shashidharan

Amyotrophic lateral sclerosis (ALS) is a devastating human disease affecting approximately one to two persons per 100,000 population each year—an incidence similar to multiple sclerosis. Clinically, ALS is manifested by muscle weakness, wasting, spasticity, and weight loss; pathologically, it is characterized by degeneration and loss of the motor neurons in the spinal cord, brainstem, and cerebral cortex. Death usually occurs within 2–5 years after onset of symptoms. While the overwhelming majority of cases are sporadic (primary or idiopathic ALS), about 5–10% of patients have a positive family history (familial ALS).

The cause of primary ALS is unknown, and no treatment is currently available. Recent studies, however, have shown that abnormal glutamate metabolism occurs in patients with sporadic ALS and is thought to cause motor neuron degeneration via neuroexcitotoxic mechanisms. Meanwhile, molecular genetic analyses have linked the familial form of ALS with mutations of Cu/Zn superoxide dismutase (SOD1), an enzyme that is part of the cellular antioxidant defense systems. Because there are indications that glutamate excitotoxicity is associated with increased oxidative stress, and that failure of the antioxidant defense systems can lead to excitotoxicity, these observations suggest common final pathways to motor neuron degeneration. Because glutamate is central to the main theme of this chapter, the role of this amino acid in the biology of nerve tissue in health and disease is discussed in detail (see also Chapters 4, 7, 54, and 58, *this volume*).

GLUTAMATE FUNCTION IN METABOLISM

Glutamate, a five-carbon skeleton dicarboxylic amino acid, is known to play a key role in mammalian intermedi-

ary metabolism. Glutamate is involved in the synthesis and/or catabolism of many compounds, including amino acids, ketoacids, and peptides. Gamma-aminobutyric acid (GABA), a major inhibitory neurotransmitter in mammalian central nervous system (CNS), is known to be formed from glutamate (Fig. 1) by decarboxylation. Glutamate can be reversibly transaminated via glutamate oxaloacetate transaminase (GOT) with oxaloacetate to form α-ketoglutarate and aspartate (Fig. 1). Also, it can be oxidatively deaminated to α-ketoglutarate and ammonia via glutamate dehydrogenase (GDH). As such, glutamate is associated directly with aerobic metabolism via the Krebs cycle.

Glutamate plays an essential role in ammonia homeostasis. In mammalian liver, oxidative deamination of glutamate (via GDH) provides ammonia for urea synthesis (12). However, in brain, as in other organs which lack an active urea cycle, formation of glutamate and glutamine via amination of α-ketoglutarate (GDH reaction) and glutamate (glutamine synthetase reaction), respectively, seems to be essential for ammonia detoxification (5). Glutamate is an important building block for polypeptides and accounts for over 10% of amino acid residues present in most proteins. It is also a constituent of many biologically active oligopeptides such as glutathione, a tripeptide present at high concentrations intracellularly and thought to be involved in cellular mechanisms dealing with oxidative stress (see below).

GLUTAMATE AS EXCITATORY TRANSMITTER

Curtis and Watkins (14) demonstrated in 1960 that glutamate and other acidic amino acids can produce potent excitation of spinal neurons. However, the possibility that

A. Plaitakis and P. Shashidharan: Department of Neurology, Mount Sinai School of Medicine, New York, New York 10029.

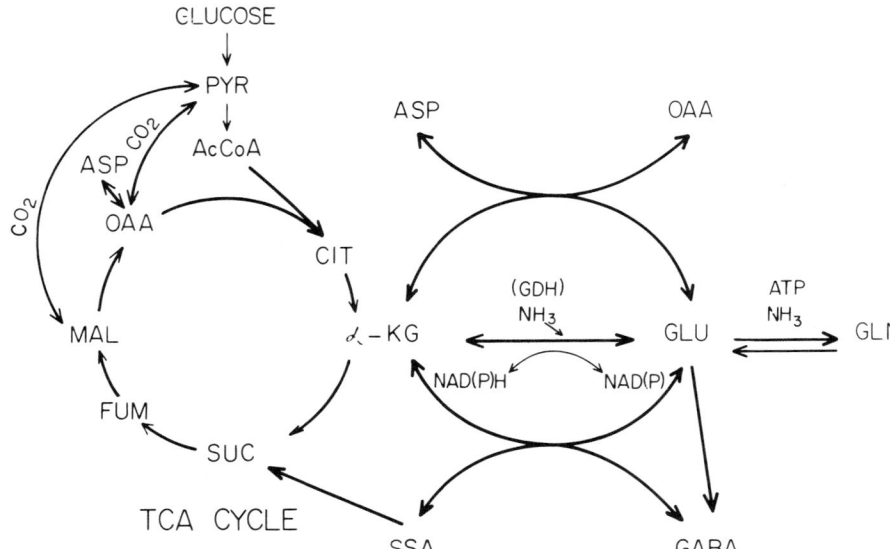

FIG. 1. Glutamate metabolism in brain and its relationship to the operation of the tricarboxylic acid (TCA) cycle. CO_2 indicates reactions in which CO_2 can be fixed to pyruvate to yield malate (MAL) or oxaloacetate (OAA) for replenishing α-ketoglutarate exported for de novo synthesis of glutamate (GLU) (anaplerotic reactions). AcCoA, acetyl CoA; ASP, aspartate; CIT, citrate; FUM, fumarate; GDH, glutamate dehydrogenase; GLN, glutamine; SSA, succinic semialdehyde; SUC, succinate.

excitatory amino acids serve as neurotransmitters in mammalian CNS was initially discounted for a number of reasons. Glutamate and other acidic amino acids are present at high concentrations in all cells. These compounds show little regional variation in their distribution in mammalian brain and are also known to be involved in many aspects of intermediary metabolism. These characteristics are in contrast to those of other biologically active compounds (i.e., dopamine, norepinephrine and acetylcholine) considered as classic neurotransmitters (13). In spite of these features, evidence has mounted over the past decade in favor of the neurotransmitter role. In fact, glutamate has been accepted as having satisfied the main criteria required for classification as an excitatory transmitter in mammalian CNS (13) (see Chapter 71, *this volume*).

Glutamate Compartmentation

A key feature which may permit glutamate to perform its many functions in nerve tissue is compartmentation of its distribution into distinct pools (6). The largest of these pools (about 50% of total) is related to the metabolism of neurons and is known as the *metabolic* pool (20). A smaller neuronal pool (20–30% of the total) is releasable from the nerve endings during neurotransmission and is thought to represent the glutamate *neurotransmitter* pool. A separate pool (10–30% of total) is contained in glial cells and is believed to serve the recycling of transmitter glutamate (*glial* pool). The smallest glutamate pool (5% of the total) is believed to be involved in the synthesis of GABA (GABA *precursor* pool).

Glutamate Transport

It appears that transmitter glutamate is stored presynaptically in specific nerve endings (glutamatergic) where it

can be released by a calcium-dependent mechanism (20). The synaptic action of the amino acid is believed to be terminated by rapid removal from the synaptic cleft via a high-affinity uptake system which is sodium-dependent and which does not discriminate between glutamate or aspartate. This uptake is present both in the surrounding astrocytes and in the nerve terminals, with the glial uptake thought to be particularly efficient. Recently, two sodium-dependent glutamate/aspartate transporters were cloned from cDNA libraries derived from rat brain mRNA and shown to be expressed specifically in brain (50,72). Both are thought to be glial-cell-specific. A third, sodium-dependent glutamate/aspartate transporter was recently isolated from a cDNA library derived from rabbit small bowel mRNA and found to be expressed in many tissues, including brain (25). In situ hybridization studies suggested the neuronal localization of this transporter (25). We have recently cloned a human glutamate transporter from a cDNA library derived from cerebellum (67) which shows a high degree of homology with the rat brain transporter described by Storck et al. (72). Similarly to the rat transporter, the human cDNA seems to be specific for brain (67).

Glutamate/Glutamine Cycle

Synaptic glutamate, removed by uptake into the surrounding glial cells, is believed to be recycled via the glutamine/glutamate cycle (20). The first step of this cycle is amination of glutamate to glutamine via the action of glutamine synthetase, an enzyme of exclusive glial localization. Glutamine, thus formed, readily crosses cell membranes and is transported back to the nerve terminals where it can be converted to transmitter glutamate via the action of the neuronal enzyme glutaminase. In addition, glutamate taken up by glial cells may be oxidatively deaminated by GDH (21) or transaminated by GOT to α-ketoglutarate, which can then enter the Krebs cycle and be oxidized to CO_2 and H_2O or be recycled, serving as a precursor of transmitter glutamate (66).

Recycling of glutamate at the glutamatergic synapses seems to be essential for preventing depletion of the transmitter because the brain seems to have a rather limited capacity to synthesize glutamate de novo from glucose. Synthesis of glutamate from glucose removes α-ketoglutarate from the Krebs cycle which, if not replenished, will eventually result in the failure of the cycle. On the other hand, replenishment of five-carbon skeleton substrates of the Krebs cycle requires fixation of CO_2 on pyruvate (Fig. 1) via either the pyruvate carboxylase or the malic enzyme reaction resulting in the formation of oxaloacetate and malate, respectively (anaplerotic reactions). These anaplerotic reactions are estimated to be only one-tenth as active in the brain as in the liver (78). However, enhanced CO_2 fixation has been found in brain under conditions of increased ammonia load (5) and attributed to de novo production of α-ketoglutarate, required for the synthesis of glutamate and glutamine as a means for ammonia detoxification.

Glutamate Receptors

Postsynaptic transduction of excitatory transmission is mediated by several classes of glutamate receptors (79). These include the NMDA (N-methyl-D-aspartate), the AMPA [amino-3-(3-hydroxy-5-methylisoxazol-4-yl)propionic acid]/kainate, and the metabotropic receptors. These receptors not only exhibit different ligand specificity, but they also differ in such features as duration and speed of postsynaptic transduction, desensitization, and other characteristics.

The NMDA receptor is coupled to an ion channel which is highly permeable to Ca^{2+} and which can be blocked by magnesium in a voltage-dependent manner. NMDA, quinolinic and ibotenic acid are selective agonists, whereas ketamide and phencyclidine are selective antagonists at this receptor (79). Glycine has been shown to potentiate excitatory transmission by acting on a strychnine-insensitive allosteric site of the NMDA receptor (31) (Fig. 2). Transduction through the NMDA receptor produces slow but sustained physiologic responses (79). Long-term potentiation is a long-lasting increase in synaptic sensitivity that can be induced by high-frequency stimulation and that has been implicated in memory and learning processes (79). Molecular biological techniques have led to the cloning of two main subunits of the NMDA receptor in the rat (39). Subunit NMDAR1 consists of seven isoforms generated by alternative mRNA splicing, whereas subunit NMDAR2 consists of four subtypes encoded by different genes (39).

The AMPA/kainate receptors seem to mediate predominantly fast excitatory synaptic transmission (79). Molecular cloning of these receptors has led to the realization that they exist physiologically at heteromeric combinations of multiple subunits (Glud1-Glud7; KA1-Ka2) with different ligand specificity (39). Depending on the particular subunit composition, the AMPA/kainate receptor may or may not be permeable to Ca^{2+} ions (39). CNQX is a nonselective antagonist at the AMPA/kainate receptor (79). Recently, the 2,3-benzodiazepine GYKI 52466 has been shown to be a highly selective antagonist at this receptor (18).

In contrast to the above receptors which are linked to ion channels, the metabotropic receptor mediates its action through G proteins (79). Activation of this receptor stimulates inositol 1,4,5-triphosphate (IP_3) metabolism and is associated with mobilization of Ca^{2+} from intracellular stores (79). At the molecular biological level, the metabotropic receptor consists of at least six subtypes (mGluR1 through mGluR6) (39). trans-(±)-ACPD [trans-(±)-1-amino-1,3-cyclopetanedicarboxylic acid] is shown to be a selective agonist, and quisqualate a nonselective agonist, at the glutamate metabotropic receptor (79) (see Chapter 7, this volume, for additional details).

GLUTAMATE NEUROTOXICITY

The Neuroexcitotoxicity Concept

Over three decades ago Lucas and Newhouse (28) observed that the systemic administration of monosodium glutamate to experimental animals resulted in degeneration of retinal ganglion cells. Olney et al. (43) subsequently showed that excitatory amino acids given systemically to immature animals can cause neuronal degeneration in areas of brain which lack an intact blood–brain barrier, such as the hypothalamus. They further noted that the neurotoxicity of acidic amino acids correlates with their ability to excite nerve cells and coined the term ''neuroexcitotoxicity.''

Neuroexcitotoxicity and Neurodegeneration

Following these early observations, additional studies (33) revealed that intracerebral injections of potent analogues of glutamate were capable of lesioning neuronal systems selectively. These data aroused considerable interest because the pattern of neuronal degeneration induced by the neuroexcitotoxic compounds was similar to that found in some disorders with system atrophy, such as in Huntington's disease (33). Additional studies showed marked losses in the NMDA subtype of glutamate receptor in affected brain regions of patients with Huntington's and Alzheimer's disease (30), thus providing further evidence for excitotoxic nerve cell death in these disorders. The recent cloning of the gene responsible for Hunting-

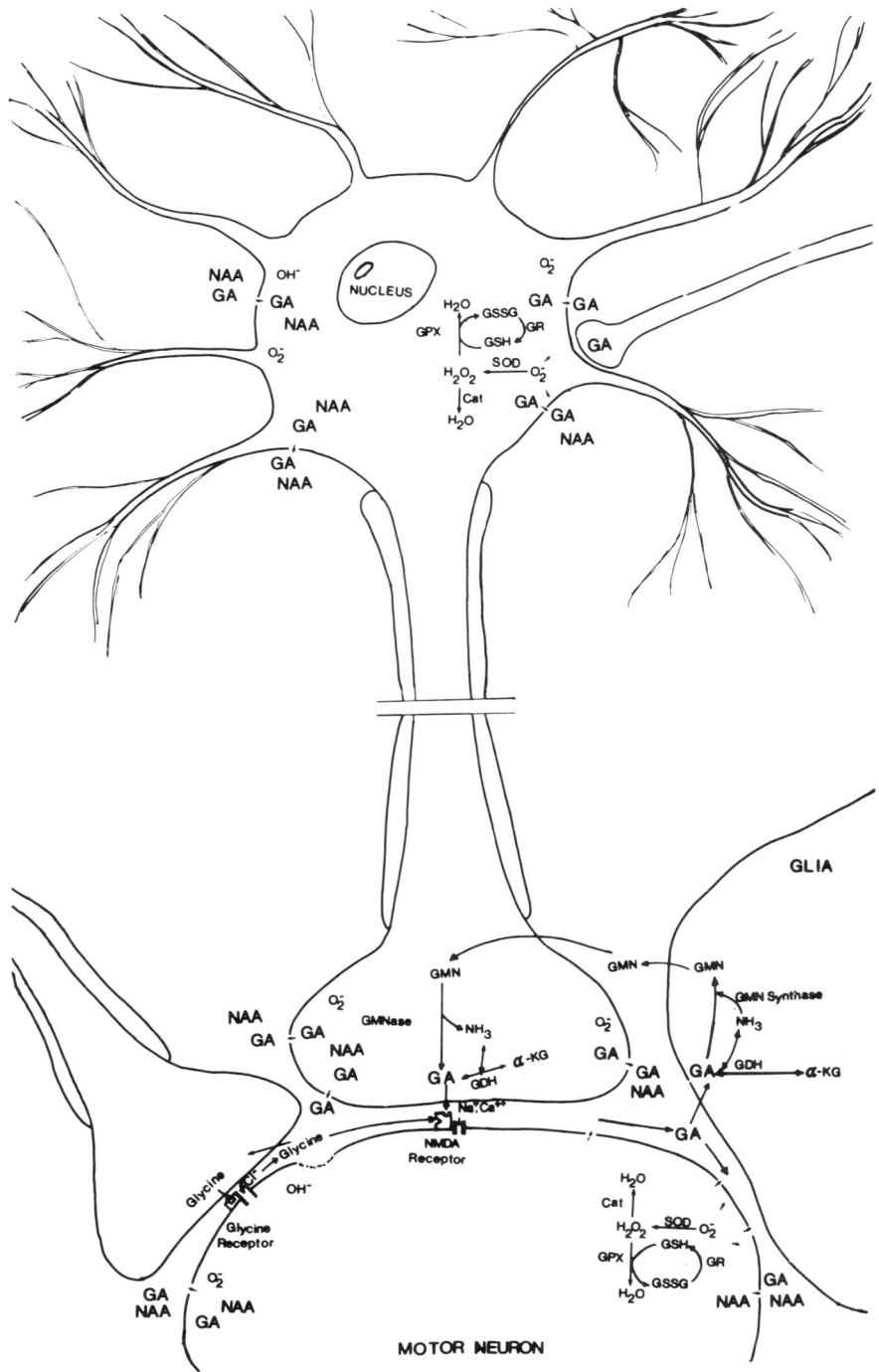

FIG. 2. Diagram showing a hypothetical glutamatergic corticospinal neuron forming a synapse with a hypothetical motor neuron. In primates, corticospinal fibers, originating from motor cortex areas, can form direct connections with spinal cord motor neurons, particularly with those innervating distal muscles of the extremities (26). Glutamate (GA) released from the glutamatergic terminal during neurotransmission is thought to bind to postsynaptic receptors, one of which, the *N*-methyl-D-aspartate (NMDA) receptor, is shown schematically. The NMDA receptor mediates excitatory transmission by activating the Na$^+$ channel, which is also highly permeable to Ca^{2+}. Synaptic glutamate is inactivated by uptake, primarily into the surrounding astrocytes (GLIA) where it can be converted to glutamine (GMN) via glutamine synthase or be metabolized to α-ketoglutarate (α-KG) via glutamate dehydrogenase (GDH) or via glutamate oxaloacetate transaminase. Astrocytes may then supply the nerve terminal by glutamine and/or α-KG, both of which can serve as precursors of transmitter glutamate (66). Glycinergic interneurons are also known to innervate motor neurons. Glycine, present at high concentrations in the vicinity of the NMDA receptor, is expected to potentiate glutamatergic transmission by acting on a strychine-insensitive allosteric site of the NMDA receptor. Glycine seems to

ton's disease (32) opens new avenues for testing this hypothesis and elucidating the primary pathogenetic process in this disease. Glutamate dysfunction has also been suggested in a variety of neuropsychiatric disorders, including schizophrenia (see Chapter 101, *this volume*).

Neuroexcitotoxicity in Metabolic Encephalopathies

Around the time when the potential role of excitotoxicity in neurodegeneration was first suggested, evidence implicating altered glutamatergic mechanisms in nerve cell death induced by various metabolic insults began to accumulate. Initial studies on experimental thiamine deficiency encephalopathy revealed altered glutamate metabolism in the brains of deficient animals (51). More recent observations have shown attenuation of brain lesions with the use of NMDA receptor antagonists (27). Also, metabolic alterations induced in the brain by the selective neurotoxin 3-acetylpyridine led to the finding (52) that the glutamate-metabolizing enzyme glutamate dehydrogenase is deficient in patients with neurodegenerative disorders affecting the cerebellum and its connections (see below). Glutamatergic excitotoxic mechanisms have also been implicated in the nerve cell death that occurs in hypoxia (4) and hypoglycemia (80).

A Defect of Glutamate Metabolism in Cerebellar Degeneration

As mentioned above, 3-acetylpyridine is a selective neurotoxin which, when administered to rats systemically, can lesion the inferior olives, olivocerebellar fibers, lower cranial nerve nuclei, and regions of pons and nigra. Because this pattern of neurodegeneration is similar to that which occurs in patients with olivopontocerebellar atrophy (OPCA), 3-acetylpyridine was suggested as a model for this human disorder (52). Acting as a nicotinamide antagonist, 3AP is incorporated into the NADP system;

this leads to formation of 3-APADP, a compound shown to be inhibitory to NADP-dependent oxidoreductases. Given these considerations, a search for abnormalities of these enzymes was undertaken in OPCA patients and led to the detection of GDH deficiency in patients with recessive or sporadic forms of this disease and other multisystem atrophies (52,53). In patients with decreased GDH activity, glutamate metabolism is abnormal (53) and is thought to be responsible for the selective degeneration of neuronal systems which receive glutamatergic innervation (22) and which are rich in GDH immunoreactivity (2) (inferior olive, pontine, and lower cranial nerve nuclei). Additional investigations (76) revealed decreased glutamate binding sites in the cerebellum of patients with decreased GDH activity. These data are consistent with the selective disappearance of postsynaptic neurons bearing glutamate receptors (76).

A similar strategy, based on the effect of 1-methyl-4-phenyl-1,2,5,6-tetrahydropyridine (another pyridine derivative capable of producing an animal model for Parkinson's disease) on mitochondrial oxidative systems (41), has been used to detect a defect in oxidative metabolism in patients with Parkinson's disease (44).

ABNORMAL GLUTAMATE METABOLISM IN SPORADIC ALS

Amyotrophic Lateral Sclerosis: Disease Types

The motor neuron diseases (MNDs) encompass a group of heterogeneous neurological disorders that are characterized by degeneration and atrophy of motor neurons. *Typical* ALS occurs sporadically and is the most common form of MND; it is often referred to as *primary* ALS. Patients affected by typical ALS exhibit a constellation of deficits that reflects involvement of both the lower motor neurons (progressive muscle weakness, wasting, and fasciculations) and the upper motor neurons (spas-

---

increase the frequency of the NMDA receptor channel openings by accelerating the recovery of the receptor from glutamate-induced desensitization. There are indications that in primary (sporadic) ALS, intracellular glutamate stores are depleted and extracellular levels are increased. A number of primary defects, capable of causing increased membrane permeability with resultant leakage of glutamate, NAA, and other compounds to the extracellular space, may be operational. Patients with familial ALS have mutations of Cu/Zn SOD, a cytosolic enzyme involved in the elimination of superoxide radicals (O^-) produced intracellularly during certain oxidation reactions. Non-detoxified O_2^- may cause lipid peroxidation with resultant increased membrane permeability. Leakage of glutamate to the extracellular space is expected to enhance excitatory transmission mediated by glutamate receptors. Under such conditions of increased synaptic glutamate, desensitization of the NMDA receptor may be essential for protecting postsynaptic neurons from excitotoxic damage. However, the presence of high levels of glycine in the spinal cord and brainstem may prevent these adaptive processes, leading to abnormal potentiation of excitatory transmission and selective degeneration of motor neurons. α-KG, α-ketoglutarate; Cat, catalase; GA, glutamate; GDH, glutamate dehydrogenase; GMN, glutamine; GMNase, glutaminase; GPX, glutathione peroxidase; GR, glutathione reductase; GSH, reduced glutathione; GSSG, oxidized glutathione; NAA, N-acetylaspartate; SOD, superoxide dismutase.

ticity and pathological reflexes). On the other hand, patients in whom the disease is limited to only the lower motor neurons are considered as suffering from *spinal muscular atrophy*. Conversely, when the disease affects the upper motor neurons only, it is referred to as *primary lateral sclerosis*. Lastly, the term *progressive bulbar palsy* is used to define the predominant involvement of bulbar muscles (causing dysarthria, dysphagia, tongue atrophy, and fasciculations) with or without corticospinal deficits. In addition to these clinicopathological characteristics, the natural history of these MND variants often differs from that of typical ALS, thus suggesting that distinct pathogenetic processes may be involved in these disorders.

About 5–10% of all MND cases are *familial,* with the majority of these showing a dominant pattern of inheritance. The features of most of these familial ALS cases, including age at onset, natural history, and clinical and pathological characteristics, are very similar to those of sporadic typical ALS. Thus, it is possible that both sporadic and familial ALS share common pathogenetic mechanisms. Should this prove to be the case, elucidation of the genetic defect(s) of the familial cases could help us to understand the etiopathogenesis of the most prevalent sporadic disease. Conversely, studies on the sporadic disease could provide clues for finding the defective gene(s) in the familial cases.

Plasma Glutamate Abnormalities

Studies on patients with decreased GDH activity have shown that signs of motor neuron involvement is commonly encountered in such patients (52). Innervation of anterior horn cells by the glutamatergic corticospinal fibers and interneurons is thought to render these cells susceptible to the neurodegenerative process (22). Moreover, these observations have raised the possibility that abnormalities of glutamate metabolism may also occur in patients with primary ALS and may be responsible for its neurodegeneration.

To test this possibility, Plaitakis and Caroscio (54) measured amino acid levels in the fasting plasma from 22 patients with MND (15 males, 7 females), 19 of whom had typical ALS (upper and lower motor neuron deficits). Results revealed that plasma concentrations of glutamate were selectively elevated (40.8 ± 12.7 μM; $p < 0.001$) in the ALS patients when compared to age-matched healthy controls (21.3 ± 7.9 μM) and to patients with other types of neurodegenerative or neuromuscular disorders (disease controls) (54). Oral loadings with monosodium glutamate produced excessive elevations in plasma glutamate associated with proportional increases in plasma aspartate levels (54). This abnormal glutamate clearance is thought to suggest defective glutamate transport across cellular or mitochondrial membranes, probably linked to the oxidative deamination of this amino acid (glutamate-OH trans-

locator). On the other hand, the rise in plasma aspartate levels after glutamate loading was interpreted as being consistent with an intact transamination pathway, including a normally functioning glutamate/aspartate translocator (54). These metabolic abnormalities were similar to those observed in OPCA patients with GDH deficiency, although activity of this enzyme was normal in leukocytes of ALS patients (54).

Plaitakis et al. (57) recently reported the results of plasma glutamate investigations involving 88 patients with MND; 62 had typical ALS, 23 had progressive bulbar palsy (PBP), and 3 had progressive muscular atrophy (PMA). As compared to control values, glutamate levels were increased by about 80% ($p < 0.0001$) in patients with typical ALS and by about 30% ($p < 0.005$) in those with PBP. No changes were found for PMA patients, although the small number of PMA patients studied makes it difficult to draw conclusions about this type of MND. Hence, these data indicate that dysregulation of glutamate metabolism occurs primarily in patients with typical ALS.

Several investigators also have reported altered glutamate levels in the plasma of ALS patients, but with varying interpretations. Perry et al. (47) studied 28 patients with various types of motor neuron disease. Of these, 16 had typical ALS, four suffered from disease limited to lower motor neurons (i.e., PMA) (C. Krieger, *personal communication*), seven had PBP, and one had familial ALS (47). Glutamate values in normal controls were 25 ± 12 μM ($N = 48$), and those in the mixed group of 28 MND patients were 33 ± 19 μM ($p < 0.05$). Perry et al. (47) attributed these differences to patients' older ages, although another study by Perry and Hansen (48), which was reported concurrently and evaluated 98 controls, showed no effect of aging on plasma glutamate levels. If the data of Perry et al. (47) are reanalyzed according to disease type, plasma glutamate values in patients with typical ALS were 38.2 ± 18.7 μM ($N = 16$). These values are close to those obtained in our laboratory in 52 patients with typical ALS (40.19 ± 17 μM) (65).

Recently, Blin et al. (7) studied 18 patients (12 males, 6 females) with primary ALS. They found significant glutamate elevations in the plasma of the ALS patients (168.3 ± 57.2 μM; $p < 0.01$) as compared to healthy controls (57.1 ± 31.7 μM; $N = 16$). Also, Iwasaki et al. (24) determined amino acid levels in the plasma of 10 ALS patients (6 males, 4 females) and compared them to 10 normal controls. Glutamate levels were significantly greater in the ALS (163.9 ± 117.3 μM; $p < 0.001$) than in the control group (34.1 ± 11.3 μM). Plasma aspartate and glycine levels showed lesser increases.

Hence, although plasma glutamate values have varied substantially among the different laboratories, these recent reports concur that glutamate levels are significantly higher in ALS patients than in controls. The reported glutamate variation seems to reflect differences in the methodology used. The methods used in our laboratory (54) and in Perry's laboratory (47) were very similar. Both techniques measured glutamate levels in fasting plasma that was free of platelets. Moreover, painstaking efforts were taken to eliminate to the extent possible any artifactual hydrolysis of glutamine to glutamate that can occur during processing or analysis of plasma samples. Control plasma glutamate values obtained in both laboratories were quite similar [our lab: 23.6 ± 9 μM, $N = 52$ (54); Perry's lab: 25 ± 12 μM, $N = 48$ (47) and 22 ± 10 μM, $N = 98$ (48)]. This is also true for patients with typical ALS as described above.

Glutamate in the Cerebrospinal Fluid

Recent studies evaluated amino acid levels in the cerebrospinal fluid (CSF) of ALS patients and produced seemingly conflicting results (47,62,63). It is now well established that levels of glutamate in the CSF are extremely low (~0.3 μM), whereas those of glutamine are as high as those present in plasma (~660 μM). Therefore, measurement of CSF glutamate is much more difficult than that of plasma. Because glial cells have a tremendous capacity to eliminate transmitter glutamate, it remains uncertain whether any glutamate measured in CSF reflects that present in the CNS extracellular space. It has been our experience (*unpublished data*) that, in controls, CSF glutamate is present at trace or nondetectable levels. Recently, Rothstein et al. (63) used a very sensitive analytical method to measure amino acids in the CSF and reported glutamate values which were about 10-fold lower than those previously reported by the same authors utilizing different methodology (62). Both of these studies (62,63) showed that glutamate and aspartate concentrations were significantly elevated in the CSF of ALS patients when compared to those of controls. Perry et al. (47), who have reported control CSF amino acid values similar to those of Rothstein et al. (63), did not find any differences in CSF glutamate levels between ALS patients and controls (47). However, Perry et al. (47) did not specify in their report the clinical syndromes of 17 ALS patients on whom CSF measurements were made. Hence, it is reasonable to conclude that the conflicting results on CSF glutamate in ALS relate to great technical difficulties involved in determining these levels and/or the selection of patients.

Glutamate in the Central Nervous System

Investigations which explored the free amino acid content of nerve tissue revealed that, in contrast to plasma, glutamate was decreased throughout the CNS of ALS patients (29,46,55,75). In absolute terms, the decrease in glutamate was the same in all brain areas studied (about 2 μM/gram wet tissue) (46,55). However, there were greater proportional decreases in the spinal cord due to its normally lower glutamate content. Changes in glutamate levels were selective because other amino acids were not significantly altered except for aspartate, which was reduced in the cervical and the lumbar spinal cord of ALS patients (29,55,75).

Reductions in glutamate levels did not correlate with regional degenerative changes occurring in ALS. Thus, decreased glutamate content was found not only in pathologically affected areas such as the spinal cord, brainstem, and motor cortex (29,46,55,75), but also in the basal ganglia, hippocampus, occipital cortex, and cerebellum (46,55)—regions which are spared in the degenerative process. Also within the spinal cord, glutamate and aspartate decreases were observed even in the dorsal horns (29), which are pathologically spared in ALS. Hence, it is unlikely that the decreased content of CNS glutamate relates simply to neuronal loss. Instead, it suggests a generalized abnormality in glutamate metabolism (55).

Based on these observations, Plaitakis et al. (55) first suggested in 1988 that the decreased nerve tissue content and the increased peripheral levels of glutamate are consistent with an altered distribution of the amino acid between its intracellular and extracellular pools. These authors further hypothesized (56–58) that defective transport, including impaired glial or neuronal glutamate uptake, could cause the presynaptic glutamate alterations (see below). Rothstein et al. (64) have accordingly measured the high-affinity glutamate uptake in nerve tissue of ALS patients obtained at autopsy. They found decreased accumulation of [^{14}C]glutamate by synaptosomes isolated from spinal cord, motor cortex, and somatosensory cortex (64). However, synaptosomes from visual cortex, hippocampus and striatum showed normal glutamate uptake. Kinetic analysis revealed decreased V_{max} but normal K_m. These findings are indicative of a decreased number of uptake sites but normal transport affinity (64).

Changes in *N*-Acetylaspartate and *N*-Acetylaspartylglutamate

In addition to glutamate, *N*-acetylaspartate (NAA) is also known to be present in high concentrations in the nerve tissue. In many regions of the mammalian CNS, NAA levels are second only to glutamate. As with glutamate, almost all NAA content is limited to the intracellular and, probably, neuronal compartment. *N*-acetylaspartylglutamate (NAAG), a dipeptide that can excite neurons, is also present at rather high concentrations intraneuronally. The contents of NAA and NAAG in human CNS exhibit a reciprocal distribution pattern consistent with rostrocaudal gradient of decreasing NAA and increasing NAAG concentrations (58). Because NAAG is thought to derive from NAA, this reciprocal distribution may reflect different regional turnover rates with the higher spinal cord NAAG, probably resulting from a high rate of conversion of NAA to NAAG (58).

Measurement of these compounds in postmortem brain and spinal cord tissue from ALS patients showed that both NAA and NAAG were significantly reduced in the cervical spinal cord of these patients by 40% and 48% ($p < 0.001$), respectively (11,58,75). In contrast, NAA and NAAG levels were not altered in postmortem frontal and cerebellar cortex of ALS patients (58). Pioro et al. (49) recently reported decreased NAA levels in the cerebrum of ALS patients, detected in vivo with [1]H-magnetic resonance spectroscopy.

Glutamate Receptors in ALS

We (54–58) and others (62–65) have hypothesized that the abnormality in glutamate metabolism is associated with altered presynaptic glutamatergic mechanisms leading to an abnormally enhanced excitatory transmission mediated by glutamate receptors and selective degeneration of postsynaptic motor neurons. Disappearance of neurons that bear glutamate receptors is expected to cause a decrease in the density of these receptors. Allaoua et al. (1) have accordingly measured the density of glutamate receptors in the spinal cord of ALS patients and reported that the NMDA receptor was decreased in these patients. In contrast, the non-NMDA receptors were not altered (1).

PATHOPHYSIOLOGY OF GLUTAMATE ALTERATIONS IN ALS

Altered Distribution of Intracellular/Extracellular Glutamate

Almost all glutamate measured in nerve tissue is intracellular (the extracellular levels are extremely small), whereas that present in the plasma and CSF may reflect the extracellular fluid content of the amino acid. As such, the findings of decreased nerve tissue glutamate content, taken together with the elevated concentrations in plasma and, perhaps, in the CSF, suggest that the distribution of glutamate is altered in the CNS with resultant depletion of intracellular pools and elevated extracellular concentrations (56). Plaitakis et al. (55,56) first suggested that the above changes may be a result of either (a) a defect in the transport of extraneuronal glutamate to intracellular stores or (b) an increased release of intracellular pools to extracellular space.

A Glutamate Transport Defect?

Given these considerations, the finding of decreased accumulation of [^{14}C]glutamate by spinal cord and brain synaptosomes of ALS patients is indeed consistent with a transport defect (64). Decreased glutamate transport is expected to disrupt the recycling of this transmitter with resultant depletion of its intracellular stores (decreased nerve tissue glutamate content). However, a correlation between regional changes in glutamate content and the high-affinity uptake, is lacking. Thus, in the striatum and visual cortex, areas which show decreased glutamate levels (46), synaptosomal glutamate uptake was normal (64). Hence, defective uptake cannot adequately account for the widespread depletion of CNS glutamate content in ALS.

Recent observations on the *Mnd* mouse, a genetic mutant used as a model for adult-onset MND disease (3), have provided some clues to the synaptosomal glutamate uptake changes. In these animals, decreased glutamate uptake was found in CNS regions analogous to those of ALS patients (spinal cord and motor cortex but not in the striatum) (3). These uptake changes did not precede the onset of the neurologic abnormalities, but, instead, they occurred after the development of the neuropathological changes. As with the human data, the high-affinity uptake of other neurotransmitters was not altered (3). Hence, a primary genetic defect affecting the glutamate/aspartate transport system seems to be unlikely in this mouse MND model.

Inhibition of the high-affinity glutamate uptake has been shown to cause neuronal degeneration in vitro systems (8,65,79). Studies utilizing organotypic cultures of rat spinal cord have shown that chronic treatment with glutamate uptake inhibitors leads to loss of motor neurons without concomitant damage to dorsal horn neurons (65). As discussed below, the dense glutamatergic innervation of ventral gray matter may render motor neurons susceptible to altered presynaptic glutamatergic mechanisms.

A Primary Membrane Abnormality?

An alternative possibility that could account for the altered glutamate distribution in nerve tissue is an increased release of glutamate from the nerve terminals and/or increased leakage of the amino acid through a defective cell membrane. This is expected to lead to depletion of the intracellular stores and to increased extracellular glutamate levels. The finding that, in addition to glutamate, other compounds with high intracellular/extracellular gradient, such as aspartate, NAA and NAAG, are also reduced in nerve tissue (11,58,75) and increased in the CSF (62) is consistent with this possibility. NAA is an anion that may contribute substantially to intraneuronal osmotic pressure. Hence, reduction in the nerve tissue levels of NAA is indicative of a diffuse membrane abnormality which may permit compounds with high intracellular concentrations to leak out of the cell (58). This is expected to increase the workload of the various membrane pumps responsible for transporting these substances against a concentration gradient. Ultimately, failure of these systems may lead to accumulation of toxic amounts of glutamate at the synapses and degeneration of the postsynaptic motor neurons. The recent detection of mutations affecting the Cu/Zn superoxide dismutase in familial ALS (61), a defect capable of affecting membrane permeability through lipid peroxidation (see below), is consistent with this possibility.

A Problem of Energy Metabolism?

Impaired energy metabolism or increased oxidative stress (see below) could render the nerve cells incapable of maintaining their high intracellular/extracellular gradients for many biologically important compounds. Decreased glucose utilization has been shown by the use of the PET technology in ALS patients (15). Defective glial uptake or metabolism could also lead to decreased detoxification of transmitter glutamate and impaired recycling of the amino acid at the nerve terminals.

DEFECTIVE HANDLING OF OXIDATIVE STRESS IN FAMILIAL ALS

Mutations of Cu/Zn Superoxide Dismutase in Familial ALS

The use of the "reverse genetic approach" has recently led to a major breakthrough in elucidating the primary genetic abnormality of a subgroup of familial ALS cases. The initial step was the linkage of dominant ALS to human chromosome 21 (69). Subsequent investigations, using highly polymorphic dinucleotide repeats, localized the disease locus to a narrow chromosomal region (21q22.1) containing the gene for the Cu/Zn superoxide dismutase (SOD1) (60). A tight linkage was found between the disease in several ALS families and the SOD1 gene, while direct sequencing of this gene revealed the presence of 11-point mutations in 13 families (61). Further investigations revealed additional single-point mutations in exons 2, 4, and 5 of SOD1 (16). Enzyme activity was reduced (by about 50%) in the red cells of patients with these mutations. Analysis of the crystal structure of human SOD suggested that all of the observed mutations affect subunit interactions critical to the tertiary form of this dimeric enzyme rather than its catalytic site(s) (16). Given the presence of SOD1 in almost all cellular systems, the selective degeneration of motor neurons is a remarkable phenomenon.

Implications for Understanding the Pathogenesis of ALS

Cu/Zn SOD is a cytosolic enzyme that is known to dismutate superoxide (O_2^-) generated intracellularly during oxidation of various compounds, such as hypoxanthine to xanthine via xanthine oxidase (10,70). This results in the formation of H_2O_2 which is then rapidly converted to H_2O and O_2 via the action of catalase, an enzyme present at high levels in most cells. Also, oxidation of glutathione via glutathione peroxidase is another way by which H_2O_2 can be converted to H_2O (10). Given the high intracellular levels of glutathione, this tripeptide may play an important role in cellular mechanisms against oxidative stress.

Malfunction of the cytosolic SOD is expected to impair the ability of the cell to eliminate O_2^- produced during certain oxidation reactions. The nondetoxified superoxide radical can oxidize a number of cellular systems, particularly lipids which are constituents of the many membrane systems present in each cell (70). Peroxidation of cell membrane lipids, in particular, is expected to alter the membrane properties. Membrane fluidity may be affected along with its permeability to various compounds. Because the cytoplasmic membrane is essential for the transport of many biologically important substances, these processes are expected to be impaired. Increased permeability to substances with high intracellular concentration will lead to an increased workload for the various membrane systems responsible for transporting these substances against a concentration gradient. This, in turn, is expected to enhance the metabolic demands of the cells and perhaps lead to increased superoxide formation. Peroxidation of membrane lipids may also occur in other membranous structures of the cell such as the endoplasmic reticulum (70), the Golgi apparatus, and the outer mitochondrial and nuclear membranes. In this regard, it may be relevant that fragmentation of the Golgi apparatus has been shown to occur in ALS (35). Also, oxidation of enzymes may impair energy metabolism or other metabolic processes (70). Given the limited ability of O_2^- to penetrate membranes (10), this oxidative damage may involve primarily cytosolic enzymes.

Although the SOD1 defect is limited to a small percentage of ALS patients (no mutations have been found in patients with sporadic ALS), its recognition is of paramount importance for the following reasons: (a) A motor neuron disease, similar in all respects to sporadic ALS, can result from a generalized metabolic abnormality, thus indicating that such defects are capable of damaging motor neurons selectively; (b) the consequences of SOD1 abnormalities on cellular functions are precisely those implicated in the pathogenesis of primary ALS that is associated with altered glutamate metabolism (increased membrane permeability, impaired transport, and/or energy metabolism); and (c) there are probably myriad abnormalities with pathophysiological consequences similar to those induced by SOD1 malfunction, and this is consistent with the proposed multifactorial origin of ALS.

THE PROBLEM OF SELECTIVE MOTOR NEURON VULNERABILITY

Although the defect in glutamate metabolism in primary ALS is generalized, motor neurons are the only targets of the degenerative process. The same is also true for the familial ALS that has been linked to Cu/Zn SOD mutations because this enzyme is expressed in many tissues with the brain showing rather low SOD1 activity (17). As such, there is no reason to believe that the above metabolic abnormalities are limited to the motor pathways. If this is so, why are only the motor neurons affected?

The Glycine-Potentiated Excitotoxic Hypothesis

Based on the pattern of neuronal connectivity and the characteristics of glutamate receptors, Plaitakis (56) advanced a hypothesis according to which glycinergic co-innervation renders motor neurons the selective targets of a glutamate-mediated neurodegenerative process. In motor neurons, unlike other neuronal systems, inhibition is in large part mediated through glycinergic interneurons. Glycine released from such glycinergic nerve terminals is known to inhibit motor neurons by binding to a Cl^--channel-linked glycinergic receptor which is strychnine-sensitive (13). In addition, glycine has been shown to potentiate glutamatergic transmission by acting on a strychnine-insensitive allosteric site of the NMDA subtype of glutamate receptor (31,79). Glycine increases the frequency of the NMDA receptor channel openings by shortening the desensitization period that follows glutamate action on this receptor (31,74). Some investigators (79) consider desensitization of glutamate receptors, rather than removal of the amino acid by uptake, as being the main mechanism by which the neurotransmitter action of glutamate is terminated.

There are indications that human motor neurons express NMDA receptors in high density (68), although the spinal cord as a whole is low in these receptors (81). [^{3}H]MK-801, a noncompetitive antagonist that binds to the NMDA channel, was recently used to study human spinal cord. Results revealed that, in addition to regions of dorsal horns, focal areas of high binding were found in the ventral gray matter that corresponded to motor neurons (68). Because both dorsal and ventral horn neurons express NMDA receptors in high density, the differential sensitivity of spinal cord neurons to ALS neurodegeneration cannot solely relate to the presence of NMDA receptors on these cells.

Studies on cultured chick motor neurons have shown that innervation by interneurons potentiates glutamate transmission (42). A substantial proportion of such interneurons are glycinergic, projecting to motor neurons with glycine levels known to be greater in the ventral than in the dorsal horns (13). There are also indications that motor neurons receive a dense glutamatergic innervation (36). Thus, an Na^+-dependent glutamate transporter, expected to be associated with glutamatergic synaptic elements, was found to be densely expressed in the ventral, but not the dorsal, horns of the cat (36). Hence, ventral and dorsal horns appear to differ in their presynaptic inputs.

Although the glycine allosteric site at the NMDA receptor is thought to be fully saturated by normal levels of nerve tissue glycine (81), Thomson et al. (73) obtained enhancement of excitatory postsynaptic potentials in cerebral cortex slices by applying increased concentrations of glycine. Similarly, Budai et al. (9) obtained enhancement of NMDA-evoked neuronal activity by glycine in the rat spinal cord in vivo and concluded that the glycine sites on NMDA receptors were not saturated. Also, neuronal toxicity induced by continuous intrathecal infusion of NMDA in rats was enhanced by coadministration of glycine (38).

Under conditions of enhanced synaptic glutamate, postsynaptic transduction seems to be mediated primarily by the NMDA receptor (79). As such, desensitization of this receptor may be of particular importance for protecting postsynaptic neurons from neurotoxicity. In the motor neurons, however, the presence of high glycine levels may lead to prolonged openings of the NMDA-linked channels with resultant excessive entrance of Ca^{2+} into these cells. This, in turn, is expected to activate intracellular proteases and lipases which can damage the cell by inducing a variety of secondary changes. Also, prolonged depolarization of postsynaptic neurons by glutamate analogues is shown to cause ATP depletion and accumulation of purine metabolites intracellularly (19,40). Depletion of ATP is thought to impair the function of ion-dependent ATPases and thus membrane fluxes (19). Studies on kainate toxicity in cerebellar slices showed that, in addition to ATP depletion, an increased leakage of glutamate and aspartate occurred into the medium (40).

The glycine hypothesis does not readily explain the degeneration of corticospinal neurons as well as the sparing of the oculomotor neurons (81) that occur in ALS. Cortical pyramidal neurons are thought to receive glutamatergic innervation (30), but the presence of glycinergic terminals on these neurons has not been established. With respect to neurotransmitter(s) involved in eye movements, recent studies have suggested glycine as the inhibitory transmitter of vestibular, reticular, and prepositus hypoglossi neurons that project to the abducens nucleus. In contrast, GABA seems to be the neurotransmitter of inhibitory vestibular neurons that project to oculomotor and trochlear motoneurons (71). Hence, the pattern of NMDAergic and glycinergic synapses in the motor cortex and oculomotor nuclei remains to be further studied.

Several investigators have been exploring whether neuroexcitotoxicity at the spinal cord level is mediated through the NMDA or the non-NMDA receptors. Studies on a limited number of patients dying of ALS showed significant reductions in the spinal cord NMDA receptors but not in the non-NMDA receptors (1). The NMDA-mediated toxicity has been supported by observations made on dissociated spinal cord neurons maintained in culture (59). Studies utilizing organotypic cultures of rat spinal cord that maintain intact synaptic connections, however, have shown that excitotoxicity induced by glutamate uptake inhibitors is mediated by the non-NMDA receptors (65). Intrathecal injection of kainic acid to rats is said to selectively damage motor neurons (23). Also, an outbreak of poisoning with domoic acid, an agonist at the kainate receptor, caused diffuse encephalopathy associated with motor neuron involvement (45).

In contrast to other potent glutamate analogues, kainate-induced neurodegeneration depends on the presence of intact presynaptic glutamatergic input and, thus, on the presence of the endogenous ligand(s). Because neurons can express several glutamate receptors, it is presently unclear whether neuroexcitotoxicity can be mediated exclusively by one type of these receptors. In fact, over a decade of experience with Huntington's disease models has established that striatal neurons, containing substance P and GABA, are sensitive to selective agonists that act at the kainate as well as at the NMDA receptor (77).

Glutamate or Oxidative Stress: Which Is Primary?

As already discussed, altered glutamate metabolism has been shown in patients with primary ALS which accounts for the overwhelming majority of patients with MND. These patients do not seem to have mutations of the SOD1 gene which are specifically associated with familial ALS (61). Because the glutamatergic abnormalities in primary ALS suggest a defect in membrane permeability and because SOD1 malfunction could also damage membranes via lipid peroxidation, it is possible that membrane abnormalities induced by diverse etiologies may cause altered presynaptic glutamatergic mechanisms and selective degeneration of motor neurons.

The question can be raised as to whether glycinergic co-innervation of motor neurons is a factor in the selective degeneration of these neurons in familial ALS. Because glutamate metabolism has not yet been studied in patients with familial ALS, a connection between glutamate and the SOD1 defect will be speculative. It seems, however, that even in the presence of normal synaptic glutamate, glycine-induced potentiation of NMDA function could increase the metabolic demands of motor neurons and/or make them bear, perhaps temporarily, increased Ca^{2+} loads. Both conditions may lead to an increased production of superoxide radicals (10,34). ATP breakdown is thought to generate increased amounts of hypoxanthine (10,34,40), oxidation of which may lead to superoxide

formation (10,70). Normal cells may compensate by enhancing their defenses against oxidative stress (10). However, motor neurons with SOD1 malfunction may be less well able to handle oxidative stress. Over the years, accumulation of superoxide radicals may damage cell membranes through lipid peroxidation, causing altered glutamate distribution and thus initiating a vicious cycle. Whether this explains the rapid downhill course patients often experience after remaining disease-free for decades remains to be established.

There is evidence that neuroexcitotoxicity is associated with increased oxidative stress which may contribute to nerve cell death (19,37). Kainate-induced degeneration of cultured cerebellar neurons was shown to be prevented by inhibiting xanthine oxidase or the formation of this enzyme from xanthine dehydrogenase (19). Also, addition of mannitol (a hydroxyl radical scavenger) or superoxide dismutase to these cultures attenuated kainate toxicity (19). Another mechanism by which glutamate toxicity may lead to increased oxidative stress is inhibition of cystine transport with a resultant reduction in intracellular glutathione levels (37). Conversely, failure of antioxidant mechanisms seems to potentiate neuroexcitotoxic cell damage. Nerve cell death, induced by agents capable of generating free radicals, is shown to be attenuated by glutamate receptor blockers (10). As such, multiple metabolic abnormalities capable of interfering with different aspects of glutamate transmission and/or cellular defenses against oxidative stress may underlie primary ALS. The primary abnormality(ies) remains to be defined, and therefore the questions raised by these observations are an important challenge to modern neurosciences.

ACKNOWLEDGMENTS

This work was supported by NIH grant NH-16871 and by Mount Sinai Research Center grant RR00071. We are indebted to Drs. D. D. Clarke and Pedro Pasik for reviewing the manuscript and for helpful suggestions.

REFERENCES

1. Allaoua H, Chaudieu I, Krieger C, et al. Alterations in spinal cord excitatory amino acid receptors in amyotrophic lateral sclerosis. *Brain Res* 1992;579:169–172.
2. Aoki C, Millner TA, Rex Sheu K-FR, et al. Regional distribution of astrocytes with intense immunoreactivity for glutamate dehydrogenase in rat brain: implications for neuron–glial interactions in glutamate transmission. *J Neurosci* 1987;7:2214–2231.
3. Battaglioli G, Martin DL, Plummer J, Messer A. Synaptosomal glutamate uptake declines progressively in the spinal cord of a mutant mouse with motor neuron disease. *J Neurochem* 1993;60:1567–1569.
4. Benevensite H, Drejer J, Schonsboe A, Diemer NH. Elevation of extracellular concentrations of glutamate and aspartate in rat hippocampus during transient cerebral ischemia monitored by intracerebral microdialysis. *J Neurochem* 1984;43:1369–1374.
5. Berl S. Cerebral amino acid metabolism in hepatic coma. *Exp Biol Med* 1971;4:78–84.

6. Berl S, Nicklas WJ, Clarke DD. Compartmentation of citric acid metabolism in brain: labeling of glutamate, glutamine, aspartate and GABA by several radioactive tracer metabolites. *J Neurochem* 1970;17:1009–1015.

7. Blin O, Desnuelle C, Guelton C, et al. Clinique des maladies du systeme nerveux et de l'appareil locomoteur. *Rev Neurol* 1991;147:292–294.

8. Brooks N. In vitro evidence for a role of glutamate in CNS toxicity of mercury. *Toxicology* 1992;76:245–256.

9. Budai D, Wilcox GL, Larsen AA. Enhancement of NMDA-evoked neuronal activity by glycine in the rat spinal cord in vivo. *Neurosci Lett* 1992;135:265–268.

10. Cohen G, Werner P. Free radicals, oxidative stress, and neurodegeneration. In: Calne DB, ed. *Neurodegenerative diseases.* WB Saunders, 1993;139–161.

11. Constantakakis E, Plaitakis A. *N*-acetyl-aspartate and *N*-acetyl-aspartyl-glutamate are altered in amyotrophic lateral sclerosis. *Ann Neurol* 1988;24:478.

12. Cooper AL, Nieves E, Rosenspire KC et al. Short term metabolic fate of L-(^{13}N)alanine, L-(^{13}N)glutamate, and L-(amide ^{13}N)glutamine in normal rat liver. *J Biol Chem* 1988;263:12268–73.

13. Cooper J, Bloom FE, Roth RH. *The biochemical basis of neuropharmacology,* 6th ed. New York: Oxford University Press, 1991.

14. Curtis DR, Watkins JC. The excitation and depression of spinal neurons by structurally related amino acids. *J Neurochem* 1960;6:117–141.

15. Dalakas MC, Harazawa J, Brooks RA, et al. Lowered cerebral glucose utilization in amyotrophic lateral sclerosis. *Ann Neurol* 1987;22:580–586.

16. Deng H-X, Hentati A, Tainer JA, et al. Amyotrophic lateral sclerosis and structural defects in Cu,Zn superoxide dismutase. *Science* 1993;261:1047–1051.

17. Dixon M, Webb EC, eds. *Enzymes,* 3rd ed. New York: Academic Press, 1979.

18. Donevan SD, Rogawski MA. GYKI 52466, a 2,3-benzodiazepine, is a highly selective, noncompetitive antagonist of AMPA/kainate receptor responses. *Neuron* 1993;10:51–59.

19. Dykens JA, Stern A, Trenkner E. Mechanism of kainate toxicity to cerebellar neurons in vitro is analogous to reperfusion tissue injury. *J Neurochem* 1987;49:1222–1228.

20. Fonnum F. Glutamate: a neurotransmitter in mammalian brain. *J Neurochem* 1984;42:1–11.

21. Hertz A, Schousboe A. In: Kvamme E, ed. *Glutamine and glutamate in mammals,* Vol. II. Boca Raton, FL: CRC Press, 1988;39–55.

22. Huang YP, Plaitakis A. Morphological changes of olivopontocerebellar atrophy in computed tomography and comments on its pathogenesis. In: Duvoisin RC, Plaitakis A, eds. *The olivopontocerebellar atrophies.* Adv Neurol 1984;41:39–81.

23. Hugon J, Vallat JM, Spencer PS, Leboutet MJ, Barthe D. Kainic acid induces early and delayed degenerative neuronal changes in rat spinal cord. *Neurosci Lett* 1989;104:258–262.

24. Iwasaki Y, Ikeda K, Kinoshita M. Plasma amino acid levels in patients with amyotrophic lateral sclerosis. *J Neurol Sci* 1992;107:219–222

25. Kanai Y, Hediger MA. Primary structure and functional characterization of a high-affinity glutamate transporter. *Nature* 1992;360:467–471.

26. Kuypers HGJM. Anatomy of the descending pathways. In: Brookhart JM, Mountcastle VB, Brooks VB, eds. *Handbook of physiology, section 1. The nervous system, vol II. Motor control.* Bethesda, MD: American Physiological Society, 1981;597–666.

27. Langlais PJ, Mair RG. Protective effects of the glutamate antagonist MK-801 on pyrithiamine-induced lesions and amino acid changes in brain. *J Neurosci* 1990;10:1664–1667.

28. Lucas DR, Newhouse JP. The toxic effect of sodium L-glutamate on the inner layer of the retina. *AMA Arch Ophthalmol* 1957;58:193–204.

29. Malessa S, Leigh PN, Bertel O, Sluga E, Hornykiewicz O. Amyotrophic lateral sclerosis, glutamate dehydrogenase and transmitter amino acids in the spinal cord. *J Neurol Neurosurg Psychiatry* 1991;54:984–988.

30. Maragos WF, Greenamyre T, Penny JB, Young AB. Glutamate dysfunction in Alzheimer's disease: an hypothesis. *Trends Neurosci* 1987;10:65–68.

31. Mayer ML, Ladislav V Jr, Clements J. Regulation of NMDA receptor desensitization in mouse hippocampal neurons by glycine. *Nature* 1989;338:425–427.

32. The Huntington's disease collaborative research group. A novel gene containing a trinucleotide repeat that is expended and unstable on Huntington's disease chromosomes. *Cell* 1993;72:971–983.

33. McGeer EG, McGeer PL. Duplication of biochemical changes of Huntington's chorea by intrastriatal injection of glutamic and kainic acid. *Nature* 1976;263:517–519.

34. McNamara J, Fridovich I. Did radicals strike Lou Gehrig? *Nature* 1993;362:20–21.

35. Mourelatos Z, Yachnis A, Rorke L, et al. The Golgi apparatus of motor neurons in amyotrophic lateral sclerosis. *Ann Neurol* 1993;33:608–615.

36. Mitchell JJ, Anderson KJ. Quantitative autoradiographic analysis of excitatory amino acid receptors in the cat spinal cord. *Neurosci Lett* 1991;124:269–272.

37. Murphy TH, Miyamoto M, Sastre A, et al. Glutamate toxicity in neuronal cell line involves inhibition of cystine transport leading to oxidative stress. *Neuron* 1989;2:1547–1558.

38. Nag S, Riopelle RJ. Spinal neuronal pathology associated with continuous intrathecal infusion of *N*-methyl-D-aspartate in the rat. *Acta Neuropathol* 1990;81:7–13.

39. Nakanishi S. Molecular diversity of glutamate receptors and implications for brain function. *Science* 1992;258:597–603.

40. Nicklas WJ, Krespan B, Berl S. Effect of kainate on ATP levels and glutamate metabolism in cerebellar slices. *Eur J Pharmacol* 62:209–215.

41. Nicklas WJ, Vyas I, Heikkila RE. Inhibition of NADH-linked oxidation in brain mitochondria by 1-methyl-4-phenyl-pyridine, a metabolite of the neurotoxin, 1-methyl-4-phenyl-1,2,5,6-tetrahydropyridine. *Life Sci* 1985;36:2503–2508.

42. O'Brien RJ, Fischbach GD. Modulation of embryonic chick motoneuron glutamate sensitivity by interneurons and agonists. *J Neurosci* 1986;6:3290–3296.

43. Olney JW, Ho OL, Rhee V. Cytotoxic effects of acidic and sulfur containing amino acids on the infant mouse central nervous system. *Exp Brain Res* 1971;14:61–76.

44. Parker WD, Boyson SJ, Parks JK. Abnormalities of the electron transport chain in idiopathic Parkinson's disease. *Ann Neurol* 1989;26:719–723.

45. Perl TM, Bedard L, Kosatsky T, et al. An outbreak of toxic encephalopathy caused by eating mussels contaminated with domoic acid. *N Engl J Med* 1990;322:1775–17780.

46. Perry TL, Hansen S, Jones K. Brain glutamate deficiency in amyotrophic lateral sclerosis. *Neurology* 1987;37:1845–1848.

47. Perry TL, Krieger C, Hansen S, Eisen A. Amyotrophic lateral sclerosis: amino acid levels in plasma and cerebrospinal fluid. *Ann Neurol* 1990;28:12–17.

48. Perry TL, Hansen S. What excitotoxin kills striatal neurons in Huntington's disease? Clues from biochemical studies. *Neurology* 1990;40:20–24.

49. Pioro EP, Preul MC, Antel JP, Arnold DL. ^{1}M-magnetic resonance spectroscopy demonstrates decreased *N*-acetyl-aspartate in the cerebrum of patients with amyotrophic lateral sclerosis. *Neurology* 1993;44(Suppl 2):405P.

50. Pines G, Danbolt NC, Bjoras M, et al. Cloning and expression of a rat brain L-glutamate transporter. *Nature* 1992;360:464–467.

51. Plaitakis A, Nicklas WJ, Berl S. Alterations in uptake and metabolism of aspartate and glutamate in brain of thiamine deficient animals. *Brain Res* 1979;171:489–502.

52. Plaitakis A, Nicklas WJ, Desnick RJ. Glutamate dehydrogenase deficiency in three patients with spinocerebellar syndrome. *Ann Neurol* 1980;7:297–303.

53. Plaitakis A, Berl S, Yahr MD. Abnormal glutamate metabolism in an adult-onset degenerative neurological disorder. *Science* 1982;216:193–196.

54. Plaitakis A, Caroscio JT. Abnormal glutamate metabolism in amyotrophic lateral sclerosis. *Ann Neurol* 1987;22:575–5759.

55. Plaitakis A, Constantakakis E, Smith J. The neuroexcitotoxic amino acids glutamate and aspartate are altered in the spinal cord and brain in amyotrophic lateral sclerosis. *Ann Neurol* 1988;24:446–449.

56. Plaitakis A. Glutamate dysfunction and selective motor neuron de-

generation in amyotrophic lateral sclerosis. A hypothesis. *Ann Neurol* 1990;28:3–8.

57. Plaitakis A, Mandeli J, Fesdjian CO, Smith J, Sivak M. Dysregulation of glutamate metabolism in ALS: correlation with gender and disease type. *Neurology* 1990;41(Suppl 1):392–393.

58. Plaitakis A, Constantakakis E. Altered metabolism of excitatory amino acids, N-acetyl-aspartate and N-acetyl-aspartyl-glutamate in amyotrophic lateral sclerosis. *Brain Res Bull* 1993;30:381–386.

59. Regan RF, Choi DW. Glutamate neurotoxicity in spinal cord cell culture. *Neuroscience* 1991;43:585–591.

60. Rosen DR, Sapp PC, Regan JO, et al. Dinucleotide repeat polymorphisms (D21S223 and D21S224) at 21q22.1. *Hum Mol Genet* 1992;1:547.

61. Rosen DR, Siddique T, Patterson D, et al. Mutations in CU/Zn superoxide dismutase gene are associated with familial amyotrophic lateral sclerosis. *Nature* 1993;362:59–62.

62. Rothstein JD, Tsai G, Kuncl RW, et al. Abnormal excitatory amino acid metabolism in amyotrophic lateral sclerosis. *Ann. Neurol* 1990;28:18–25.

63. Rothstein JD, Kuncl R, Chaudhry V, et al. Excitatory amino acids in amyotrophic lateral sclerosis: an update. *Ann Neurol* 1991;30:224–225.

64. Rothstein JD, Martin LJ, Kuncl RW. Decreased glutamate transport by the brain and spinal cord in amyotrophic lateral sclerosis. *N Engl J Med* 1992;326:1464–1468.

65. Rothstein JD, Jin L, Dykes-Hoberg M, Kuncl RW. Chronic inhibition of glutamate uptake produces a model of slow neurotoxicity. *Proc Natl Acad Sci USA* 1993;90:6591–6595.

66. Shank RP, Aprison MH. Glutamate as neurotransmitter. In: Kvamme E, ed. *Glutamine and glutamate in mammals,* Vol II. Boca Raton, FL: CRC Press, 1989; 3–19.

67. Shashidharan P, Plaitakis A. Cloning and characterization of a glutamate transporter cDNA from human cerebellum. *Biochim Biophys Acta* 1993;1216:161–164.

68. Shaw PJ, Ince PG, Johnson M, Perry EK, Candy J. The quantitative autoradiographic distribution of [^{3}H]MK-801 binding sites in the normal human spinal cord. *Brain Res* 1991;539:164–168.

69. Siddique T, Figlewicz D, Pericak-Vance M, et al. Linkage of a gene causing familial amyotrophic lateral sclerosis to chromosome 21 and evidence of genetic locus heterogeneity. *N Engl J Med* 1991;324:1381–1384.

70. Sies H, ed. *Oxidative stress* London: Academic Press, 1985;273–303.

71. Spencer RF, Whenthold RJ, Baker R. Evidence for glycine as an inhibitory neurotransmitter of vestibular, reticular, and prepositus hypoglossal neurons that project to the cat abducens nucleus. *J Neurosci* 1989;9:2718–2736.

72. Storck T, Shulte S, Hofmann K, Stoffel W. Structure, expression, and functional analysis of a Na$^+$-dependent glutamate/aspartate transporter from rat brain. *Proc Natl Acad Sci USA* 1992;89:10955–10959.

73. Thomson AM, Walker VE, Flynn DM. Glycine enhances NMDA-receptor mediated synaptic potentials in neocortical slices. *Nature* 1989;338:422–424.

74. Trussell LD, Thio LL, Zorumski CF, Fischbach GD. Rapid desensitization of glutamate receptors in vertebrate central neurons. *Proc Natl Acad Sci USA* 1988;85:2834–2838.

75. Tsai GC, Stauch-Sluser B, Sim L, et al. Reductions in acidic amino acids and N-acetylaspartylglutamate in amyotrophic lateral sclerosis. *Brain Res* 1991;556:151–156.

76. Tsiotos P, Plaitakis A, Mitsakos G, et al. L-Glutamate binding sites of normal and atrophic human cerebellum. *Brain Res* 1989;481:87–96.

77. Vecsei L, Beal MF. Comparative behavioral and neurochemical studies with striatal kainic or quinolinic acid-lesioned rats. *Pharmacol Biochem Behav* 1991;39:437–438.

78. Waelsch H, Berl S, Rossi CA, Clarke DD, Purpura DP. Quantitative aspects of CO$_2$ fixation in mammalian brain in vivo. *J Neurochem,* 1964;11:717–728.

79. Wheal HV, Thomson AM, eds. *Excitatory amino acids and synaptic transmission.* London: Academic Press, 1991.

80. Wieloch T. Hypoglycemia-induced damage prevented by N-methyl-D-aspartate antagonist. *Science* 1984;230:681–683.

81. Young AB. What's the excitement about excitatory amino acids in amyotrophic lateral sclerosis? *Ann Neurol* 1990;28:9–11.

Psychopharmacology: The Fourth
Generation of Progress, edited by
Floyd E. Bloom and David J. Kupfer.
Raven Press, Ltd., New York © 1995.

CHAPTER 133

Neuropsychiatric Manifestations of HIV-1 Infection and AIDS

Robert A. Stern, Diana O. Perkins, and Dwight L. Evans

By 1993, 172,000 individuals in the United States had died from acquired immunodeficiency syndrome (AIDS) and another 1,000,000 were estimated to be infected by human immunodeficiency virus type 1 (HIV-1), the retrovirus that causes AIDS. Currently, most individuals infected with HIV-1 develop AIDS after an estimated median latency period of 10 years. After developing AIDS, the average length of survival is approximately 11 months, and the maximum length of survival has been reported to be 9 years.

Until 1993, the Centers for Disease Control (CDC) defined AIDS as the development of at least one of 23 specific infectious, neoplastic, general systemic, or nervous system diseases that are rare in the absence of immunodeficiency. In 1993, the CDC case definition was modified to include individuals with CD4+ T-lymphocyte cell counts (CD4+) less than $200/\mu L$ or a CD4+ percentage of total lymphocytes of less than 14 (14). This expanded surveillance case definition for AIDS and classification system for HIV-1 infection also included additional clinical conditions seen in women, such as invasive cervical cancer.

Since the earliest descriptions of AIDS, neuropsychiatric and neurologic signs and symptoms have been reported in a subgroup of persons with this disease. The neuropsychiatric manifestations contained in these early reports include progressive dementia, depression with pronounced apathy and psychomotor slowing, and other psychiatric presentations including manic symptoms and atypical psychosis. Initially, these AIDS-related mental disturbances were attributed to psychological reactions to a systemic illness, the effects of psychosocial stressors associated with the disease, or the consequences of opportunistic infections or tumors within the central nervous system (CNS).

It is now estimated that 40–70% of patients with AIDS develop clinical neurologic abnormalities. Upon autopsy, 75% of AIDS patients exhibit neuropathologic changes, with 30% having multiple CNS lesions (37). In as many as 20% of HIV-1-infected individuals, neurologic or neuropsychiatric symptoms may be the presenting features, prior to other medical symptoms of AIDS (7). The most severe form of HIV-1-associated neuropsychiatric disorders, HIV-1 encephalopathy or HIV-1-associated dementia complex, affects at least 7% of persons with AIDS and is one of the most common causes of dementia in individuals age 20–59 in the United States (39).

CNS involvement in AIDS results from a variety of etiologies, including (a) the direct or primary effects of HIV-1 on nervous tissue, (b) the consequences of secondary viral and nonviral opportunistic infections, tumors, and cerebrovascular disease, and (c) the complications of systemic therapies for AIDS and associated disorders (Table 1).

HIV-1 AND NEUROPATHOLOGY

Direct CNS Effects of HIV-1

Early evidence for the neuropathogenicity of HIV-1 included (a) the presence of HIV-1 in the cerebrospinal

R. A. Stern: Department of Psychiatry and Human Behavior and Department of Clinical Neurosciences, Brown University School of Medicine, Providence, Rhode Island 02912; and Department of Psychiatry, Rhode Island Hospital, Providence, Rhode Island 02903.

D. O. Perkins: Department of Psychiatry, University of North Carolina School of Medicine, Chapel Hill, North Carolina 27599.

D. L. Evans: Departments of Psychiatry, Medicine, and Neuroscience, University of Florida College of Medicine, Gainesville, Florida 32610.

fluid (CSF) of patients with AIDS, (b) abnormal neuro-imaging findings in neurologically impaired AIDS patients, (c) the high frequency of peripheral neuropathies in AIDS patients, and (d) the presence of HIV-1 in tissue obtained by brain biopsy. It is now known that HIV-1 penetrates the blood–brain barrier early in the course of infection and is replicated in brain tissue using mono- and multinucleated macrophages as hosts (44). Once in the brain, the virus can have neurotoxic effects via direct or indirect mechanisms. For example, the HIV-1 envelope protein, gp120, elevates intracellular free calcium, leading to neuronal damage (17). In addition, patients with HIV-1 encephalitis have significantly higher levels of the excitatory amino acid and endogenous N-methyl-D-aspartate receptor agonist, quinolinic acid, in CSF and in brain tissue than do controls (1). Although these levels are not correlated with encephalitis severity, quinolinic acid may be an etiologic agent in HIV-1-related neuropathology. Chapter 134 (*this volume*) details the current knowledge of the neurotoxic process of HIV-1.

CNS Effects of Secondary Infections

In addition to the direct or primary effects of HIV-1 on the CNS, there are numerous and significant secondary effects of HIV-1 (Table 2). One of the most important with regard to CNS effects is the papovavirus, JC virus, because it leads to progressive multifocal leukoencephalopathy (PML), a severe demyelinating disease for which there is no proven treatment. Although PML is an infrequent complication of immunosuppressive therapy, it is highly prevalent among AIDS patients, with an incidence of at least 4–7% in this group (6). Among the nonviral secondary infections affecting the CNS, toxoplasmosis is by far the most significant and one of the most treatable, with up to 50% of HIV-1-infected patients experiencing this disorder (48).

Neuropathology

The neuropathological changes associated with HIV-1 infection are the result of both the primary effects of the virus on the CNS and the secondary effects of opportunistic infections, tumors, and cerebrovascular disease. The

TABLE 1. *Causes of CNS dysfunction in AIDS*

Primary effects of HIV-1
Secondary viral infections
Nonviral infections
Neoplasms/lymphoma
Cerebrovascular disease
Iatrogenic effects of systemic therapy

TABLE 2. *Secondary infections resulting in CNS dysfunction*

Viral infections
JC virus (leading to progressive multifocal leukoencephalopathy)
Human adenovirus
Cytomegalovirus
Herpes simplex I and II
Varicella zoster
Epstein–Barr
Nonviral infections
Toxoplasmosis
Cryptococcosis
Candidiasis
Histoplasmosis
Coccidioidomycosis
Aspergillus
Neurosyphilis

lesions are both focal and diffuse, with much variability across patients and within a single patient over time.

Primary neuropathological effects of the virus include (a) the presence of multinucleated giant cells, (b) the infiltration of both subcortical white and gray matter by macrophages, (c) myelin pallor, and (d) gliosis (12). HIV-1-specific neuropathological appearances that predominate in subcortical areas include: (a) HIV-1 encephalitis, characterized by perivascular, focal lesions with damage to axons and myelin, large, reactive astrocytes, focal vacuolization, and mono- and multinucleated macrophages; (b) HIV-1 leukoencephalopathy, a triad of myelin loss, infiltration by mono- and multinucleated macrophages/microglia, and reactive astrogliosis; and (c) vacuolar leukoencephalopathy, involving vacuolar myelin swellings in deep white matter. However, the neuropathology of HIV-1 is not restricted to subcortical regions; cortical gray matter changes have also been observed, including cell loss, synaptic loss, and gliosis.

Neuroimaging

Various neuroimaging techniques have been used for in vivo observations of HIV-1 neuropathology. Although computerized tomography (CT) has been employed to assess the structural lesions associated with HIV-1, magnetic resonance imaging (MRI) has proven to be the most revealing technique to date in identifying HIV-1 structural neuropathology. Common MRI findings in HIV-1-infected patients have involved the presence of cerebral atrophy, focal high signal intensities in subcortical white and gray matter (observed primarily using T_2-weighted images), confluent high-signal areas, and solitary high-signal areas (15,42). Abnormal MRI findings are mostly observed in patients with HIV-1 encephalopathy (Fig. 1) or in patients with focal neurologic lesions resulting from opportunistic infections such as toxoplasmosis (Fig. 2) or lymphoma. However, standard MRI interpretation is not as useful in depicting abnormalities in neurologically *asymptomatic* HIV-1-infected patients. If MRI abnormalities are detected in these patients, they tend to involve focal white-matter lesions only (76). More recently, quantitative morphometric analyses of MRIs have suggested that symptomatic HIV-1-infected individuals who do not have any neurologic signs do indeed exhibit cortical and central atrophy (41).

Functional neuroimaging techniques have also proven to be sensitive to the neuropathology associated with both asymptomatic and symptomatic HIV-1-infected patients. In fact, functional assessments of cerebral perfusion [using single photon emission computerized tomography (SPECT)], metabolism [using positron emission tomography (PET)], and biochemical abnormalities [using magnetic resonance spectroscopy (MRS)], appear to be more sensitive than structural techniques such as CT and MRI. For example, a SPECT study of HIV-1-infected men without AIDS or HIV-1-associated dementia revealed abnormal perfusion in approximately two-thirds of the asymptomatic and three-quarters of the symptomatic patients (88). The high prevalence of perfusion abnormalities in asymptomatic subjects have been reported by other

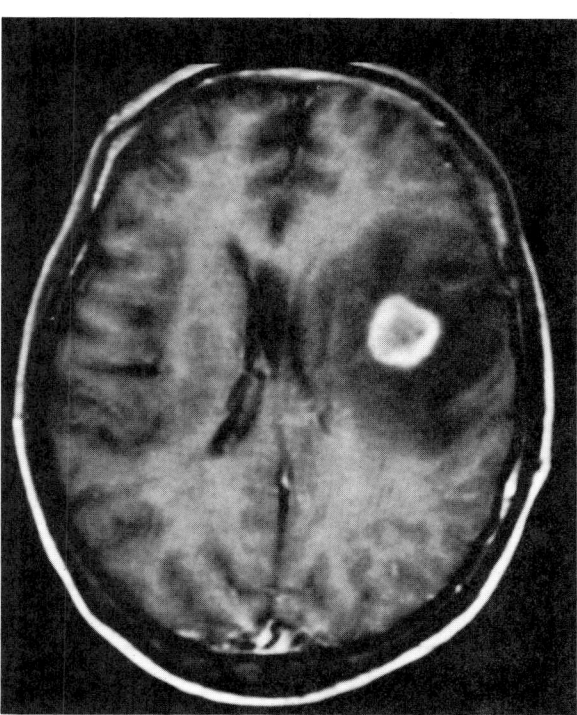

FIG. 2. T$_1$-weighted axial MRI of the brain with gadolinium enhancement of a patient with AIDS exhibiting a prototypic toxoplasmosis lesion, with a contrast-enhancing lesion with mass effect and ring enhancement.

investigators as well (95), providing further evidence that cerebral abnormalities can be detected early in the course of HIV-1 disease. In patients with AIDS and HIV-1-associated dementia, multifocal perfusion defects have been found (54). However, the relationship between SPECT findings and severity of neurocognitive impairment in either demented or nondemented patients is unclear.

Although not as widely employed, PET has been useful in detecting functional cerebral abnormalities throughout the course of HIV-1. For example, focal metabolic disturbance of the basal ganglia, thalamus, and temporal lobes has been reported (96). In this study, hypermetabolism of the basal ganglia and thalamus was observed in nondemented patients, with additional hypometabolism of the temporal lobes evidenced in demented patients. MRS has been the focus of several recent investigations (e.g., see ref. 40) and appears to be both sensitive and specific to the neurological and neuropsychiatric changes seen in both asymptomatic and symptomatic HIV-1-infected patients.

HIV-1-ASSOCIATED DEMENTIA COMPLEX

Early case reports suggested that patients with AIDS experience a variety of neuropsychiatric symptoms in-

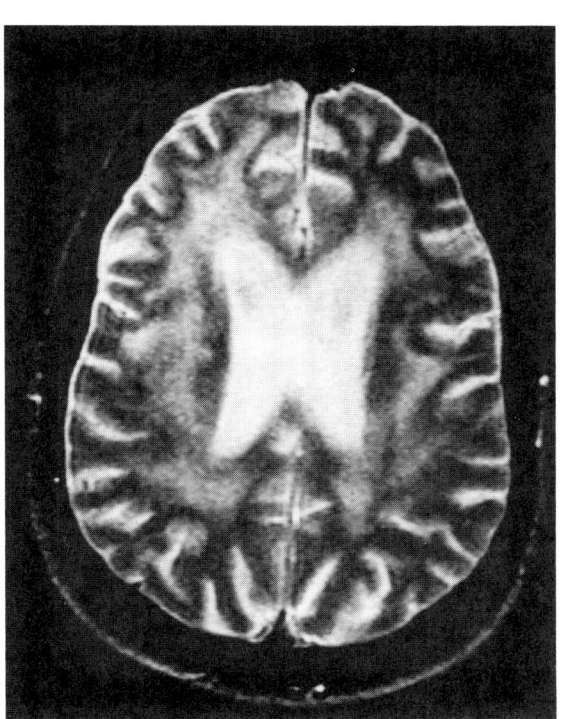

FIG. 1. T$_2$-weighted axial MRI of the brain of a patient with AIDS and HIV-1 encephalopathy exhibiting cortical and central atrophy as well as diffuse white-matter enhancement.

cluding mental slowing, lethargy, forgetfulness, apathy, and social withdrawal. The term, "AIDS dementia complex" (ADC) was coined, referring to the changes in cognition, motor function, and behavior associated with AIDS (61,77,78). However, the accuracy of this term has been heavily discussed and refined. Given that HIV-1 is the etiological agent responsible for the disorder, AIDS may not be an appropriate term. "Dementia" may also not be an adequate descriptor because early presentations of the disorder did not necessarily involve decline in intellectual functioning. Lastly, not all patients exhibit the full "complex" of cognitive, motor, and behavioral dysfunction, and may instead have only one or two of these disturbances.

In 1991, a working group of the American Academy of Neurology AIDS Task Force (38) developed consensus nomenclature and case definitions for HIV-1-associated neurological conditions to be used for research purposes. A major outcome of this working group was the replacement of the term "AIDS dementia complex" with the more descriptive term "HIV-1-associated cognitive/motor complex." The latter term was then divided into two categories: (i) a more severe form, "HIV-1-associated dementia complex" or "HIV-1-associated myelopathy" (the latter term reserved for patients whose myelopathic dysfunction is worse than their neurocognitive impairment), and (ii) a less severe form, "HIV-1-associated minor cognitive/motor disorder." The classification "HIV-1-associated dementia complex" can be further delineated based on the presence of behavioral and motor abnormalities. Therefore, a patient with cognitive and motor impairment but no behavioral dysfunction would be considered to have "HIV-1-associated dementia complex (motor)." A patient with cognitive and behavioral dysfunction but no motor involvement would have "HIV-1-associated dementia complex (behavior)."

The major difference between "HIV-1-associated dementia complex" and "HIV-1-associated minor cognitive/motor disorder" is the severity of impairment in activities of daily living. That is, by definition, dementia must have cognitive impairment severe enough to interfere with occupational or social functioning. In "HIV-1-associated minor cognitive/motor disorder," activities of daily living are generally intact with the possible exception of mild difficulties in the most demanding activities.

Differences in terminology aside, HIV-1-associated dementia arises in one-third of the AIDS patient population and is the most common neurological or neuropsychiatric disorder associated with HIV-1 infection (16). Although the dementia usually develops in patients who already show other AIDS manifestations, up to 25% of HIV-1-infected patients may develop it as their initial, AIDS-defining illness (62). An additional 15% develop dementia concurrent with other features of AIDS. HIV-1-associated

TABLE 3. *Clinical features of HIV-1-associated dementia complex*

Early features
Difficulty with concentration and memory
"Slowness" of thinking, losing track of conversation
Tasks take longer to complete
Cannot follow written material or television
Motor movement slowed and clumsy
Handwriting changes
Gait incoordination with tripping and ataxia
Apathy and indifference
Social withdrawal
Reduced spontaneity
Rarely dysphoric, but may be anxious or irritable
Neurologic signs
  Slowing of rapid movements of extremities and eyes
  Pathological ("frontal release") signs (e.g., snout)

Late features
Bowel and bladder incontinence
Myoclonus
Vegetative state

dementia is a rapidly progressing process, with the time of onset to severe dementia averaging only several months (11).

The initial features of HIV-1-associated dementia include an overall slowing in cognition (i.e., bradyphrenia) and movement (i.e., bradykinesia) as well as difficulties in motor dexterity and coordination, forgetfulness, poor concentration, and marked apathy (Table 3). Although dysphoric mood is not a common feature, the pronounced slowing and apathy may appear as if the patient is depressed. Furthermore, assessing other aspects of depression (e.g., weight loss, cognitive disturbance, insomnia) is difficult for patients with this disorder due to shared symptomatology that may be indistinguishable from the psychiatric symptoms.

Later in the course of HIV-1-associated dementia, the patient may exhibit myoclonus, bowel and bladder incontinence, and, eventually, mutism and a vegetative state. Once these advanced features are present, death is typically imminent.

Because the above initial symptoms are similar to those seen in other patient groups with subcortical impairment (e.g., Parkinson's disease, progressive supranuclear palsy, multiple sclerosis) and because of the neuroimaging findings of subcortical neuropathology, HIV-1-associated dementia was originally described as a subcortical dementia. However, in light of the more recent findings of cortical atrophy and higher cortical function deficits in AIDS patients, this characterization may not fully describe the spectrum of neuropsychiatric deficits associated with HIV-1 infection and AIDS.

EARLY HIV-1-ASSOCIATED COGNITIVE/MOTOR IMPAIRMENT

Although it is clear that neuropsychiatric symptoms and neuropathological changes are common in AIDS, the presence and severity of the neurocognitive changes during the early asymptomatic phase of HIV-1 infection remain unclear. In an early study addressing this issue, Grant et al. (28) reported that 44% of asymptomatic HIV-1-infected homosexual men exhibited abnormal neuropsychological performance, compared to only 9% of HIV-1-seronegative controls. This report received wide attention in the lay press, which, in turn, led to policy change in the military such that personnel infected with HIV-1 were removed from sensitive or stressful roles, such as aviation. Since that original report, scores of divergent studies have been published that have either supported the presence of early neurocognitive dysfunction or have argued against it (29). The most common deficits reported by the former studies include fine motor slowing, decreased dexterity, slowing of information processing, and memory difficulties mainly involving diminished free recall.

Confounding Variables

Between-study differences in sample composition may partially account for the discrepant findings described above. Subjects in these studies differed in terms of several factors that may have a major impact on neuropsychological test performance, such as past head trauma, alcohol and other substance abuse, premorbid psychiatric illness, learning or developmental disability, and previous CNS disorders. However, the actual impact of these possible confounds has also been the subject of debate. For example, Pakesch et al. (64) found that long-term drug abuse may account for the cognitive/motor deficits observed in HIV-1-infected subjects. Conversely, Bornstein et al. (8) found that alcohol use, despite its negative effect on neuropsychological performance, does not account for performance differences between HIV-1-seronegative and HIV-1-seropositive homosexual men (8).

Researchers have also focused on the impact of head injury on the neurocognitive status of HIV-1-infected asymptomatic individuals. In a study of homosexual and bisexual men, Bornstein et al. (9) found no difference in neuropsychological performance between asymptomatic HIV-1-infected subjects with a history of minor head injury and matched controls (HIV-1-seropositive and HIV-1-seronegative) without any history of head injury. In contrast, in a study of intravenous drug users, Marder et al. (51) found that previous head injury was associated with significantly worse neuropsychological performance in the HIV-1-infected group.

In a report addressing the effect of the above variables on the cognitive and motor functioning of HIV-1-infected patients, Wilkins et al. (98) found that confound severity was positively correlated with the degree of neurocognitive dysfunction. Although the impact of confounds on performance was the most striking for the asymptomatic group, this finding was also true for symptomatic individuals.

Cofactors

A variety of possible coexisting factors may account for the neurobehavioral impairment found in asymptomatic HIV-1-infected individuals. Beach et al. (5) have suggested that diminished vitamin B_{12} levels in some HIV-1-infected individuals may serve as one such potential cofactor because B_{12} deficiency has been associated with a variety of psychiatric, neurological, and neurocognitive dysfunction. However, the largest study of B_{12}–neuropsychological/neurological interactions to date in HIV-1 spectrum disease found no relationship between B_{12} levels and neuropsychological, psychiatric, neurophysiological, or neurological dysfunction at any stage of HIV-1 infection (85).

Depression has been proposed as another possible cofactor for early neuropsychological impairment (45). Almost all studies addressing this issue, however, have found that the presence and severity of depressive symptoms are not associated with the early neurocognitive disturbance in HIV-1 infection (e.g., see refs. 30 and 32).

In a recent study by Satz et al. (87), low education (i.e., less than 12 years) was associated with neuropsychological impairment in early HIV-1 infection. In this study, 38% of the subjects with low education exhibited cognitive abnormalities, compared to less than 17% of the high education group. These authors suggest that low education indirectly reflects a marker of lower "reserve capacity" that increases the risk of developing cognitive/motor impairment in neurological damage, such as that which may occur in early HIV-1 infection.

It has also been suggested that immunosuppression precedes neurobehavioral dysfunction (26). Other investigators, however, have found that neurocognitive and motor alterations in early HIV-1 infection are independent of degree of immunosuppression as measured by CD4+ count (97). More recently, Martin et al. (53) have suggested that typical markers of immunosuppression, such as CD4+ count, are not valid or reliable measures of CNS status. Rather, these authors indicated that increased levels of quinolinic acid may play a salient role in the development of early HIV-1-related cognitive/motor impairment. Additional promising work assessing the relationship between neurobehavioral functioning and quinolinic acid levels is ongoing.

Stern et al. (93) conducted a study of the presence and extent of neurocognitive impairment in early HIV-1 infection in subjects who met extensive inclusion criteria aimed at excluding individuals with the previously detailed confounding variables. In addition, several potential cofactors, such as vitamin B_{12} deficiency, depression, limited education, and immunocompromise (i.e., low CD4+ count), were controlled for statistically. Prior to controlling for the various potential cofactors, the seropositive group was found to have significantly worse performance in attention, information processing, and motor functioning than the group of HIV-1-seronegative homosexual men. However, once the influence of these cofactors was removed, the asymptomatic HIV-1-infected participants had significantly worse performance only on tasks sensitive to motor slowing and dexterity. These group differences were not *clinically* significant, however, because the asymptomatic group's performance was not in the impaired range compared to normative data. The results of this study suggest two important findings: (i) in a non-confounded group of asymptomatic HIV-1-infected homosexual men, neuropsychological dysfunction appears limited to mild, subclinical motor disturbance; and (ii) in order to assess the role of HIV-1 in the development of cognitive/motor disturbance during the asymptomatic stage, it is imperative to account for the possible impact of previously implicated cofactors.

Clinical Significance of Early Cognitive/Motor Disturbance and Its Relationship to Future Disease Course

Even with continued investigation of the impact of confounding variables and possible cofactors, two major questions remain to be addressed regarding early cognitive and motor disturbance in HIV-1: (i) Is the severity of the "impairment" clinically meaningful? That is, statistically significant between group differences on sensitive neuropsychological tests do not necessarily translate into noticeable impairments in occupational and/or daily living tasks. This issue of the "ecological validity" of early HIV-1 neuropsychological findings has yet to be addressed adequately. (ii) Is the presence of early cognitive/motor dysfunction indicative of either future presence or course of dementia, or of future disease course in general? With regard to the former, very little is known. With regard to prediction of disease course, an intriguing study by Mayeux et al. (55) suggests that the presence of impaired neuropsychological test performance in both asymptomatic and symptomatic HIV-1-infected individuals is associated with a significantly increased risk of mortality over a 36-month period.

Pharmacologic Treatment

Zidovudine (i.e., azidothymidine, AZT, Retrovir), an anti-retroviral, continues to be the mainstay in treatment of HIV-1 spectrum disease. It has been found to temporarily improve the prognosis in patients with AIDS and to reduce disease progression in asymptomatic HIV-1-infected individuals. However, neurotoxicity has been associated with chronic doses of zidovudine, including headache, seizures, Wernicke's encephalopathy, coma, and mania (83). In spite of these reports of neurotoxicity, there is also evidence that zidovudine significantly improves HIV-1-associated cognitive/motor abnormalities in symptomatic HIV-1-infected patients and in persons with AIDS (90). Recent data suggest that zidovudine may reverse, albeit transiently, the severity of HIV-1-associated dementia (94). However, the positive effects of zidovudine on neuropsychological function may be limited to patients with advanced HIV infection in light of a recent finding that the drug had no significant beneficial neuropsychological effects on HIV-1-infected individuals without AIDS (27).

Another anti-retroviral, 2',3'-dideoxyinosine (ddI), now used in the treatment of AIDS has also been shown to be effective in improving HIV-1-associated cognitive impairment in a small number of cases (100). However, controlled studies of the neurocognitive efficacy of ddI have yet to be completed.

Because of the bradyphrenia and attentional deficits exhibited by HIV-1-infected patients, the use of psychostimulants has been suggested. Results of anecdotal case reports and uncontrolled case series of methylphenidate and dextroamphetamine have indicated that these agents may be useful in diminishing the neurocognitive effects of HIV-1 (25). Once again, prospective, controlled investigations have not yet been conducted.

PSYCHIATRIC ASPECTS OF HIV-1 INFECTION

The psychiatric sequelae of HIV-1 infection and AIDS are numerous and have etiologies that involve neurobiological and psychosocial factors. These include the natural and expected grief response to being diagnosed with a terminal illness, later reactions to disability and illness, exacerbation of preexisting psychiatric illness, development of new primary psychiatric symptoms and syndromes, and the neuropsychiatric manifestations of HIV-1-associated neurological illness.

Psychiatric Sequelae of Notification of HIV Infection

Several investigators have examined the psychological impact of HIV testing. In a longitudinal study of individuals with a variety of HIV-1 risk factors, Perry and colleagues (36,74,75) found that all subjects reported moderate-to-high levels of depression and anxiety prior to receiving HIV test results. Subjects who received a negative HIV test result reported a significant reduction from pretest levels of depression and anxiety symptoms. This reduction was sustained at both 2- and 10-week follow-ups. Subjects who received a positive HIV test result reported no significant change from their pretest level of distress at 2-week follow-up. However, by the 10-week follow-up, these HIV-1-infected subjects also reported a significant reduction of depression and anxiety symptoms. Furthermore, by 1-year follow-up, both the HIV-1-infected and HIV-1-uninfected individuals reported similar levels of depression and anxiety. It is important to note that, compared to routine HIV counseling, counseling that included stress reduction techniques significantly reduced depression and anxiety symptoms in the HIV-1-infected individuals (72).

The findings by Perry and colleagues are supported by other studies. For example, Moulton et al. (59) found that 2 weeks after HIV test notification there were similar levels of negative mood, hopelessness, and anxiety in 66 individuals notified of positive results and in 41 notified of negative results. In this study most (78%) HIV-1-positive and about half (43%) HIV-1-negative subjects correctly anticipated their test result. Thus, similar levels of dysphoric mood may have reflected anticipatory adjustment of their presumed HIV-1 status.

It is understandable that individuals who receive notification of positive HIV test results will be emotionally distressed as they adjust to the knowledge of their HIV-1 serostatus. The severity of the acute distress will vary from individual to individual. Whereas some individuals may react with little distress, others may be at increased risk of suicide. Rundell et al. (86) found that 15 out of 826 (<2%) HIV-1-infected active duty members of the U.S. Air Force had attempted suicide, with 47% of the attempts occurring within 3 months of serostatus notification and 67% within 1 year. In contrast, Perry et al. (73) found that suicidal ideation remained at pretest levels among those who received notification of positive HIV test results. In addition, these levels dropped significantly by 2 months after positive test result notification, and, after comparing individuals who received a positive HIV test result with those who received a negative one, the authors found that the proportion of individuals with suicidal ideation was similar in both groups, suggesting little, if any, relationship between suicidal ideation and HIV test results. It is important to note, however, that the low level of suicidal ideation in Perry's HIV-1-infected subjects may have resulted from the extensive HIV counseling provided to participants in this study. Such counseling may serve to combat suicidal thoughts or intent that have been found to be associated

with greater levels of depression in both HIV-infected and HIV-uninfected individuals.

Psychiatric Symptoms in Asymptomatic HIV-1 Infection

Several controlled studies have shown that asymptomatic HIV-1 infection is not associated with increased depression or anxiety symptoms. For example, Perkins et al. (70) found similar levels of depression and anxiety symptoms in HIV-1-infected and HIV-1-uninfected homosexual men. Thus, it appears that although individuals are often distraught after receiving positive HIV-1 test results, after an adjustment period lasting weeks to a few months, most will cope well and will show a reduction in anxiety and depressive symptoms. Consequently, it appears that symptoms of depression and anxiety should not be considered ''normal'' in asymptomatic HIV-1 infection. Rather, significant symptoms should warrant careful clinical evaluation.

Controlled studies have shown that the prevalence of major depression and other mood disorders is higher in asymptomatic HIV-1-infected homosexual men than in the general population (82,84), but is similar to that in HIV-1-seronegative homosexual men (3,70,99). Several studies have shown that 4–9% of both HIV-1-infected and HIV-1-uninfected homosexual men report a major depression in the month prior to study evaluation. In one study, Perkins et al. (70) found that 6% of both HIV-1-infected and HIV-1-uninfected subjects developed a major depression during a 6-month follow-up period. There is also evidence that similar proportions (ranging from 0% to 5%) of HIV-1-infected and HIV-1-uninfected individuals meet DSM-III-R criteria for current anxiety disorders (70). Once again, these findings underscore the issue that mood disorders should not be considered a ''normal'' phenomenon in HIV-1-infected individuals. Rather, they should be assessed carefully and treated appropriately.

Differential diagnosis of major depression in HIV-1-infected patients is complicated because several symptoms of major depression (i.e., fatigue, sleep disturbance, and weight loss) are also common symptoms of HIV-1 disease progression (e.g., see refs. 58 and 63). Recent reports, however, have indicated that although complaints of fatigue and insomnia in asymptomatic HIV-1-infected homosexual men are significantly associated with severity of depressed mood and other symptoms of major depression, they are not associated with low CD4+ counts or decreased neuropsychological functioning (4,69). Thus, complaints of fatigue and insomnia in otherwise asymptomatic HIV-1-infected patients are highly suggestive of an underlying mood disorder and indicate that patients with such complaints should be assessed routinely for major depression.

Although factors that influence risk for development of mood symptoms in HIV-1-infected individuals have not yet been well-studied, a recent investigation found a relationship between major depression in asymptomatic HIV-1-infected homosexual men and a prior history of major depression (70). This study, however, found no relationship between major depression and neuropsychological functioning, suggesting that the depressive disorder is not related to the CNS effects of HIV-1. Therefore, in individuals infected by HIV-1, past history of a major depression may be a risk factor for subsequent development of major depression.

The strategies that an individual uses to cope with the threat of AIDS may be related to overall level of dysphoric mood (60). Leserman et al. (46) reported that asymptomatic HIV-1-infected men who used active coping strategies to deal with the threat of AIDS (e.g., fighting spirit, reframing stress to maximize personal growth, planning a course of action, seeking social support) had lower levels of depressed and anxious mood than those who used passive coping strategies (denial or feeling helpless). Importantly, there is also evidence that personality disorder is common in HIV-1-infected patients, and that these patients experience greater dysphoria and cope less well with the threat of AIDS (66). Therefore, the way in which an individual deals with his or her seropositive HIV status, vis-à-vis coping strategies, may influence the development of depression or anxiety.

Thus, the available data suggest that asymptomatic HIV-1-infected individuals have no greater dysphoric symptoms or clinical mood disorders than do uninfected control subjects. As has been reported of individuals with other life-threatening diseases, HIV-1-seropositive individuals are usually able to adjust successfully to their infection, and the majority are able to maintain hope over time. Furthermore, the available data suggest that by creating preventive intervention programs targeted at HIV-1-positive individuals at risk for developing depressive or anxious symptomatology (e.g., those with a history of clinical depression) and by fostering the development of active coping strategies in these individuals, the rates of depression and anxiety in this population may even be lowered.

Psychiatric Symptoms in Symptomatic HIV-1 Infection

The effects of HIV-1 on the CNS may result in a variety of psychiatric symptoms in the latter stages of the illness. In addition, individuals infected with HIV-1 may be at further risk for developing psychiatric symptoms due to diseases secondary to AIDS that also have CNS effects, as well as due to medications used to treat HIV-1. Furthermore, psychiatric symptoms in HIV-1-infected individu-

als in later stages of the illness may also represent new-onset psychiatric disorders. The direct CNS effects of HIV-1, HIV-1-related CNS disturbances, and CNS effects of medications used in the treatment of AIDS may each influence the development of mood disorders and psychosis. Several ongoing longitudinal cohort studies are currently examining psychiatric symptoms across the course of HIV-1 infection and should ultimately provide important data to address the relative contribution of each of these factors to the development of mood and related disorders.

There is some available evidence, however, that HIV-1 may cause organic mood disturbance. In a 17-month retrospective chart review of patients with AIDS, Lyketsos et al. (49) examined associated historical and clinical features in an attempt to separate organic and functional symptoms. They used family history of mood disorder as a ''marker'' for functional mood disorders. They further assumed that coexisting dementia and low CD4+ count were ''markers'' for HIV-1-related mood disorders. They found that none of the patients with a personal or family history of mood disorder had coexistent dementia, and that all but one of the patients without a personal or family history of mood disorder had coexistent dementia. In addition, among the 8% of the patients who experienced manic episodes, CD4+ count was significantly higher in those individuals without a personal history of mood disorder. Although these findings are not based on controlled studies, they do suggest that mania may be a consequence of the effect of HIV-1 on the brain.

Vitamin B_{12} deficiency may also place HIV-1-infected patients at risk for organic mood disturbance. Between 20% and 30% of patients with AIDS and 7% of asymptomatic HIV-1-infected patients have been reported to have a vitamin B_{12} deficiency. Furthermore, vitamin B_{12} deficiency has previously been shown to be associated with depression, and can occur in the absence of hematologic or neurologic signs (18). Although the relationship between vitamin B_{12} level and depressive symptomatology in HIV-1-infected individuals is not clear (85), it is prudent that the medical evaluation of depressive symptoms in HIV-1-infected individuals include assessment of serum B_{12} levels.

Psychosis may also result from CNS HIV-1 involvement. Numerous case studies of symptomatic HIV-1-infected individuals have reported psychotic symptoms, including delusions, bizarre behavior, and hallucinations. Mood disturbances, including euphoria, irritability, and labile or flat affect, have often accompanied psychotic symptoms in these patients. Similarly, anxiety and agitation were reported in almost half of the reported cases. In addition, there is some evidence that psychosis may be a symptom of the terminal stages of AIDS, because half of the patients described had a progressively worsening course, with dementia or death occurring within a few months after the onset of the psychotic symptoms.

Psychosis may be more frequently found in patients with significant AIDS-related neurocognitive impairment than in patients in earlier stages of the disease. In one retrospective chart review of 46 patients identified with HIV-1-associated dementia, Navia and Price (62) found that 15% had developed psychotic symptoms. Relatedly, data from an ongoing, prospective study suggests that HIV-1-infected patients with psychosis have greater neurocognitive impairment than do nonpsychotic HIV infected controls (Jeste, *personal communication*).

Other sequelae of HIV-1 infection may also result in psychiatric symptomatology. For example, CNS mass-occupying lesions and generalized metabolic disturbance may lead to depressive symptomatology. Furthermore, almost all of the medications used to treat HIV-1-related illnesses have psychiatric symptoms as potential side effects, and zidovudine has been reported to cause mania (20). Thus, a complete organic work-up should be considered for HIV-1-infected individuals with disturbance of mood or psychosis in order to determine if the etiology is CNS-based or idiopathic in nature.

Suicide and AIDS

Several epidemiological studies suggest that AIDS patients are at increased risk of death by suicide. The relative prevalence is estimated to range from 7 to 36 times the rate in demographically similar control populations. Other studies, however, have not found patients with AIDS to have higher suicidal ideation, especially when comparing persons with AIDS to other medically or neuropsychiatrically ill patients. For example, McKegney and O'Dowd (56) found that in hospitalized medical patients seen in psychiatric consultation, patients with AIDS were significantly less likely to have suicidal ideation than were asymptomatic HIV-1-infected patients and patients with unknown HIV-1.

Rather than finding a correlation between current suicidal ideation and AIDS, studies have found an association between past history of suicidal ideation or past psychiatric treatment and current level of suicidal ideation. Thus, the relationship between suicide risk and AIDS remains unclear. However, suicidal ideation in patients with AIDS should never be regarded as part of an "expected" or temporary grief reaction; rather, it should warrant careful evaluation for major depression and appropriate treatment (see also Chapter 85, *this volume*).

Treatment of Psychiatric Disorders in HIV-1 Infection

Treatment of Mood Symptoms

Available evidence suggests that mood symptoms and syndromes in the asymptomatic stage of HIV-1 infection are not secondary to the effects of HIV-1 on the brain, and should be evaluated and treated as in the general population. No controlled antidepressant clinical trials in patients with HIV-1 infection have been published, though several are currently underway and other open trials have been reported. Imipramine and fluoxetine have been shown to be effective in the treatment of major depression in asymptomatic HIV-1-infected patients (47,67,80). Fernandez and Levy (24) found that treatment with either bupropion or fluoxetine resulted in a moderate-to-marked improvement of major depressive symptoms in 81% of patients with AIDS and found that bupropion was superior to fluoxetine in activating anhedonic patients. Rabkin and Harrison (80) have found imipramine, fluoxetine, and sertraline to be as effective for the treatment of major depression in HIV-1-seropositive patients as for the treatment of depression in patients with no medical disease. They have also conducted the first double-blind, placebo-controlled trial of imipramine in HIV-1 and found a 74% response rate to imipramine. Although there is evidence that desipramine decreases natural immunity (natural killer cell activity) in vitro (57), Rabkin and Harrison (80) found no in vivo effects of imipramine on CD4+ cell counts. There is additional in vitro evidence that neither desipramine nor lithium enhances HIV-1 replication in cultured cells (21). Thus, there is no available evidence to suggest that antidepressants cause adverse immunological effects in the treatment of depression in HIV-1-infected individuals. In the selection of antidepressants, it appears that those with higher anticholinergic properties should be avoided; reports suggest that symptomatic HIV-1-infected patients may be more vulnerable to the anticholinergic side effects of tricyclic antidepressants than asymptomatic HIV-1-infected or HIV-1-uninfected patients (24).

Data on the treatment of mania in HIV-infected individuals have been limited to clinical anecdote and retrospective chart review. The few available findings suggest that while lithium may be effective, it is associated with significant adverse effects including neurotoxicity and gastrointestinal side effects; additional work suggests that anticonvulsants, including valproic acid, carbamazepine, and clonazepam, are effective alternatives.

Psychostimulants, such as methylphenidate and dextroamphetamine, have also been reported to improve depressive symptoms in symptomatic HIV-1-infected patients (33). Psychostimulant medication may be particularly effective in improving apathy and lethargy associated with the later stages of AIDS or with the more generalized HIV-1-associated dementia complex (79). In addition, there is also evidence from an open trial that testosterone is effective in treating low mood, anergy, and anhedonia in late-stage HIV-1 disease (Rabkin, *personal communication*).

To date, there have been no published studies of the

treatment of anxiety symptoms in HIV-1-infected individuals. However, clinical experience suggests that general treatment guidelines apply to this patient population. Benzodiazepines have been efficacious and safe in treating anxiety symptoms in HIV-1-infected patients. As with other medically ill populations, benzodiazepine dosage may need to be decreased in patients with AIDS in order to avoid CNS depressant effects. Furthermore, anecdotal clinical evidence suggests that the intermediate acting agent, lorazepam, is effective and well-tolerated in this population.

Treatment of Psychotic Symptoms

Although there have been no published controlled clinical trials of the treatment of psychosis in HIV-1-infected patients to date, several case studies have suggested that neuroleptics are generally effective (Perry, *personal communication*). Patients with psychosis who are in the symptomatic stages of HIV-1 infection, however, have consistently been reported to require very low doses of neuroleptics. Controlled studies are currently being conducted on the treatment of HIV-1-related delirium and HIV-1-associated psychosis. Brietbart (10) has found both haloperidol and chlorpromazine in low doses (40–80 mg chlorpromazine equivalents, mean daily dose) to be highly efficacious in the treatment of delirium. Lorazepam was ineffective as a single agent and was poorly tolerated. Both neuroleptics were well-tolerated at these low doses, and there was no evidence of significant extrapyramidal symptoms. Jeste and colleagues are conducting a controlled study of new onset psychosis in HIV-1-infected individuals. Results from this ongoing study suggest that mood symptoms, usually dysphoria, are extremely common, and there is evidence of greater neuropsychological impairment compared to nonpsychotic controls. Standard neuroleptics (haloperidol and thioridazine) are being compared for efficacy and adverse effects (Jeste, *personal communication*). Both neuroleptics are effective at low doses (124 mg chlorpromazine equivalents, mean daily dose). Thus, it appears that HIV-1-infected individuals are especially sensitive to neuroleptic side effects. Although a retrospective chart review demonstrated no significant increase in extrapyramidal symptoms in AIDS patients treated with dopamine antagonists as compared to non-HIV-1-infected control patients (34), the small sample size and the general methodology of this study would only allow for the detection of large differences in prevalence of extrapyramidal symptoms; moderate, but clinically relevant, differences could not be detected. Therefore, at this point, when treating psychotic symptoms in symptomatic HIV-1-infected patients it would appear clinically prudent to slowly titrate neuroleptic medications, minimize drug dose, and carefully monitor for side effects.

Nonpharmacologic Treatments

Although individuals with HIV-1 infection may exhibit psychiatric symptoms secondary to, or associated with, underlying CNS dysfunction, they also exhibit mood and anxiety symptoms as a result of psychosocial factors, such as loss of health, financial problems, social stigma, and other similar stressors associated with the progression of HIV-1 disease. Therefore, interventions that provide emotional support and enhance coping are important components of the treatment of functional mood symptoms in HIV-1-infected patients. Controlled studies are few, but stress prevention training has been associated with significantly lower depression and anxiety symptoms in individuals undergoing HIV testing (72). Interpersonal psychotherapy has also been found to be an effective treatment of major depression in patients with HIV-1 infection. Markowitz et al. (52) found that interpersonal psychotherapy resulted in significant improvement of symptoms in 20 out of 23 HIV-1-infected individuals. Collectively, these results suggest that individual and group psychotherapies as well as support groups may act to improve quality of life, including the ability to cope with AIDS, a factor that has been found to be associated with less depression and anxiety in HIV-1-infected individuals (46).

Psychoneuroimmunology of HIV-1 Infection

There is increasing evidence that the CNS influences the immune system, and there is considerable popular enthusiasm for the concept that stress and depression influence the course of physical diseases such as cancer and HIV-1 infection (31,68). Although there are many positive studies, there is still no consistent clinical evidence supporting this relationship. However, decreases in natural immunity as measured by reductions in the number and function of natural killer cells is the most consistent and reproducible finding to date (19,89,92). The potential clinical relevance of these findings are suggested by studies of cancer patients who have been reported to have increased natural killer cell number and function (23), as well as increased survival time, in association with a well-controlled psychoeducational group psychotherapy intervention (22,23,91). A number of studies have begun to address the question as to whether stress and depression are associated with immune suppression and disease progression in HIV-1 infection.

Rabkin et al. (81) found no relationship between psychosocial and psychiatric factors such as depressive disorders, distress, and stressors, on the one hand, and measures of HIV-1 disease progression, including CD4+ and CD8+ cell counts, on the other hand. However, they found a trend for depressive disorders, distress, and stressors to be associated with number of AIDS-related symptoms. Similarly, over a 12-month follow-up period, Perry et al. (71) did not find a relationship between social support, stressful life events, and a variety of psychological factors and CD4+ and CD8+ counts. They did find, however, that severity of physical symptoms was associated with greater levels of distress in HIV-1-infected subjects without AIDS.

There is evidence that the stress of HIV-1 testing is significant enough to alter both neuroendocrine and immune system function. In a group of individuals who ultimately were shown to be HIV-1-infected, Antoni et al. (2) found that abnormal elevations in serum cortisol decreased significantly after notification of a negative HIV test. Furthermore, higher-baseline cortisol was associated with lower lymphocyte functioning, suggesting that the stress of HIV testing impacted on immune system function. Lastly, use of denial as a coping mechanism was inversely associated with lymphocyte response to stimulation, suggesting that coping strategy may in part mediate the body's reaction to the stress of HIV testing in at-risk individuals.

In a negative study, Kertzner et al. (43) found no consistent evidence of stress-associated alterations of the hypothalamic–pituitary–adrenal axis in seropositive subjects and found no relationship between cortisol and CD4 cell counts. However, other measures of immune function may be more sensitive to the effects of emotional factors. Ironson et al. (35) have found alterations in mitogen stimulation of lymphocytes in subjects before and after HIV antibody testing. Extensive data from our laboratory also suggest that life event stress is greater in HIV-1-seropositive subjects than in HIV-1-seronegative controls and is associated with detriments in the number of natural killer cells and cytotoxic T cells (Evans et al., *submitted*). In a similar comprehensive assessment of stress and depression, Patterson et al. (65) have reported that stress and depressive symptoms predict a 6-month change in immunity as measured by percentage of CD4+ cells and serum β_2-microglobulin. These data suggest that stress and depression may accelerate the course of immunologic decline in HIV-1 infection, but are preliminary and require further longitudinal confirmation.

Recent data from population-based studies of HIV-1-infected individuals have yielded conflicting findings with respect to depression and immunity (13,50). In one investigation, Burack et al. (13) found depressive symptoms to predict a more rapid decline in CD4+ counts, while Lyketsos et al. (50) found no such relationship. Unfortunately, no available studies have followed cohorts through the course of HIV-1 infection using (a) comprehensive clinical examinations of stress and depression, (b) comprehensive endocrine and immune assessments, and (c) clinical measures of HIV-1 disease progression. Consequently, the relationship between psychological, psychiat-

ric, and psychosocial factors and course of disease in HIV-1 infection has not been resolved and warrants continued exploration (see Chapter 63, *this volume,* for more background).

CONCLUSION

Great strides have been made over the last decade in both describing the neuropsychiatric functioning associated with HIV-1 spectrum disease and increasing our understanding of the underlying neuropathological mechanisms. It is now clear that the virus enters the CNS early in the course of the disease and has both primary and secondary effects on neural tissue. Subtle abnormalities can be detected in pathology, neuroimaging, and neuropsychological studies prior to the onset of AIDS-defining illnesses, though the clinical significance of these findings remains unclear. In symptomatic AIDS, neuropsychiatric and neurological complications are highly prevalent and often can be the first manifestations of AIDS.

Although most individuals infected with HIV-1 cope well, major depression is highly prevalent in both HIV-1-seropositive and HIV-1-seronegative homosexual men, compared to epidemiologically based estimates of the general population. The interrelationship among the CNS, the endocrine system, and the immune system is only beginning to be understood in HIV-1 infection. Moreover, the effects of stress and depression on endocrine and immune function, as well as the potential effects on HIV-1 disease progression, will require comprehensive, longitudinal investigation. Future study is also necessary to understand the neuropsychiatric manifestations of HIV-1 infection in women, as well as the special effects on neurodevelopment. Cross-cultural comparisons are also needed.

Finally, early psychopharmacological treatment studies have yielded promising results for the alleviation of depression and psychotic symptoms, as well as for the improvement of neurocognitive impairment. Future neuropsychopharmacological approaches will certainly focus on both the direct and indirect effects of HIV-1 on the brain in order to develop interventions that could alter the course of disease, as well as focus on symptomatic treatments in order to improve clinical outcome and quality of life.

ACKNOWLEDGMENTS

This chapter was supported in part by a grant from the National Institute of Mental Health, MH R01 5-47486. The authors thank John R. Z. Abela and Isabell C. Leshko for editorial assistance.

REFERENCES

1. Achim CL, Heyes MP, Wiley CA. Quantitation of human immunodeficiency virus, immune activation factors, and quinolinic acid in AIDS brains. *J Clin Invest* 1993;91:2769–2775.
2. Antoni MH, August S, LaPerriere A, et al. Psychological and neuroendocrine measures related to functional immune changes in anticipation of HIV-1 serostatus notification. *Psychosom Med* 1990;52:496–510.
3. Atkinson JH, Grant I, Kennedy CJ, Richman DD, Spector SA, McCutchan A. Prevalence of psychiatric disorders among men infected with the human immunodeficiency virus. *Arch Gen Psychiatry* 1988;48:859–864.
4. Baum S, Perkins DO, Gray-Silva S, Stern RA, Golden RN, Evans DL. Asymptomatic HIV infection and insomnia. *Proceedings of the American Psychiatric Association*. New Research Program and Abstracts, 1993.
5. Beach RS, Morgan R, Wilkie F, et al. Plasma vitamin B_{12} level as a potential cofactor in studies of human immunodeficiency virus type-1-related cognitive changes. *Arch Neurol* 1992;49:501–506.
6. Berger JR, Laszovitz B, Post MJD, Dickinson G. Progressive multifocal leukoencephalopathy associated with human immunodeficiency virus infection. *Ann Intern Med* 1987;107:78–87.
7. Berger JR, Moskowitz L, Fischl M, Kelley RE. Neurologic disease as the presenting manifestation of acquired immunodeficiency syndrome. *South Med J* 1987;80:683–686.
8. Bornstein RA, Fama R, Rosenberger P, et al. Drug and alcohol use and neuropsychological performance in asymptomatic HIV infection. *J Neuropsychiatry Clin Neurosci* 1993;5:254–259.
9. Bornstein RA, Podraza AM, Para MF, et al. Effect of minor head injury on neuropsychological performance in asymptomatic HIV-1 infection. *Neuropsychology* 1993;7:228–234.
10. Breitbart W. HIV-1 and delirium. Abstract presented at Psychopharmacology of HIV-1 infection: Clinical Challenges and Research Directions. NIMH, Office of AIDS Programs, Washington, DC, April 1993.
11. Brew BJ, Rosenblum M, Price RW. Pathogenetic implications of neuropathological findings in the AIDS dementia complex. *Psychopharmacol Bull* 1988;24:307–310.
12. Budka H. Neuropathology of human immunodeficiency virus. *Brain Pathol* 1991;1:163–175.
13. Burack JH, Barrett DC, Stall RD, Chesney MA, Ekstrand ML, Coates TJ. Depressive symptoms and CD4 lymphocyte decline among HIV-infected men. *JAMA* 1993;270:2568–2573.
14. Chang SW, Katz MH, Hernadez S. The new AIDS case definition: implications for San Francisco. *JAMA* 1992;267:973–976.
15. Chrysikopoulos HS, Press GA, Grafe MR, Hesselink JR, Wiley CA. Encephalitis caused by human immunodeficiency virus: CT and MR imaging manifestations with clinical and pathologic correlation. *Radiology* 1990;175:185–191.
16. Day JJ, Grant I, Atkinson JH, et al. Incidence of AIDS dementia in a two-year follow-up of AIDS and ARC patients on an initial phase II AZT placebo-controlled study: San Diego cohort. *J Neuropsychiatry Clin Neurosci* 1992;4:15–20.
17. Dreyer EB, Kaiser PK, Offermann JT, Lipton SA. HIV-1 coat protein neurotoxicity prevented by calcium channel antagonists. *Science* 1990;248:364–367.
18. Evans DL, Edelsohn G, Golden R. Organic psychoses without anemia or spinal cord symptoms in vitamin B_{12} deficient patients. *Am J Psychiatry* 1983;140:218–221.
19. Evans DL, Folds JD, Petitto JM, et al. Circulating natural killer cell phenotypes in men and women with major depression. *Arch Gen Psychiatry* 1992;49:388–395.
20. Evans DL, Perkins DO. The clinical psychiatry of AIDS. *Curr Opin Psychiatry* 1990;3:96–102.
21. Evans DL, Smith MS, Golden RN. Antidepressants and HIV infection: effect of lithium chloride and desipramine and HIV replication. *Depression* 1993;1:205–209.
22. Fawzy FI, Fawzy NW, Hyun CS, et al. Malignant melanoma: effects of an early structured psychiatric intervention, coping, and affective state on recurrency and survival 6 years later. *Arch Gen Psychiatry* 1993;50:681–689.
23. Fawzy FI, Kemeny ME, Fawzy NW, et al. A structured psychiatric intervention for cancer patients. II. Changes over time in immunological measures. *Arch Gen Psychiatry* 1990;47:729–735.
24. Fernandez F, Levy JK. Psychopharmacotherapy of psychiatric syndromes in asymptomatic and symptomatic HIV infection. *Psychiatr Med* 1991;9:377–396.
25. Fernandez F, Levy JK, Ruiz P. The use of methylphenidate in HIV patients: a clinical perspective. In: Grant I, Martin A, eds. *Neuropsychology of HIV infection*. New York: Oxford University Press, 1994;295–309.
26. Gibbs A, Andrews DG, Szmukler G, Mulhall B, Bowden SC. Early HIV-related neuropsychological impairment: relationship to stage of viral infection. *J Clin Exp Neuropsychol* 1990;12:766–780.
27. Gorman JM, Mayeux R, Stern Y, et al. The effect of zidovudine on neuropsychiatric measures in HIV-infected men. *Am J Psychiatry* 1993;150:505–507.
28. Grant I, Atkinson JH, Hesselink JR, et al. Evidence for early central nervous system involvement in the acquired immunodeficiency syndrome (AIDS) and other human immunodeficiency virus (HIV) infections. *Ann Intern Med* 1987;107:828–836.
29. Grant I, Martin A, eds. *Neuropsychology of HIV infection*. New York: Oxford University Press, 1994.
30. Grant I, Olshen RA, Atkinson JH, et al. Depressed mood does not explain neuropsychological deficits in HIV-infected persons. *Neuropsychology* 1993;7:53–61.
31. Helsing KJ, Szklo M, Comstock GW. Factors associated with mortality after widowhood. *Am J Public Health* 1981;71:802–809.
32. Hinkin CH, van Gorp WG, Satz P, Weisman JD, Thommes J, Buckingham S. Depressed mood and its relationship to neuropsychological test performance in HIV-1 seropositive individuals. *J Clin Exp Neuropsychol* 1992;14:289–297.
33. Holmes VF, Fernandez F, Levy JK. Psychostimulant response in AIDS-related complex patients. *J Clin Psychiatry* 1989;50:5–8.
34. Hriso E, Kuhn T, Masdeu JC, Grundman M. Extrapyramidal symptoms due to dopamine-blocking agents in patients with AIDS encephalopathy. *Am Journal Psychiatry* 1991;148:1558–1561.
35. Ironson G, LaPerriere A, Antoni M, et al. Changes in immune and psychological measures as a function of anticipation and reaction to news of HIV-1 antibody status. *Psychosom Med* 1990;52:247–270.
36. Jacobsen PB, Perry SW, Hirsch DA. Behavioral and psychological effects of HIV antibody testing. *J Consult Clin Psychol* 1990;58:31–37.
37. Janssen RS. Epidemiology of human immunodeficiency virus infection and the neurological complications of the infection. *Semin Neurol* 1992;12:10–17.
38. Janssen RS, Cornblath DR, Epstein LG, et al. Nomenclature and research case definitions for neurologic manifestations of human immunodeficiency virus-type 1 (HIV-1) infection: report of a working group of the American Academy of Neurology AIDS Task Force. *Neurology* 1991;41:778–785.
39. Janssen RS, Nwanyanwu OC, Selik RM, Stehr-Green JK. Epidemiology of human immunodeficiency virus encephalopathy in the United States. *Neurology* 1992;42:1472–1476.
40. Jarvik JG, Lenkinski RE, Grossman RI, Gomori JM, Schnall MD, Frank I. Proton MR spectroscopy of HIV-infected patients: characterization of abnormalities with imaging and clinical correlation. *Radiology* 1993;186:739–744.
41. Jernigan TL, Archibald S, Hesselink JR, et al. Magnetic resonance imaging morphometric analysis of cerebral volume loss in human immunodeficiency virus infection. *Arch Neurol* 1993;50:250–255.
42. Keiburtz KD, Ketonen L, Zettelmaier AE, Kido D, Caine ED, Simon JH. Magnetic resonance imaging findings in HIV-1 cognitive impairment. *Arch Neurol* 1990;47:643–645.
43. Kertzner RM, Goetz R, Todak G, et al. Cortisol levels, immune status, and mood in homosexual men with and without HIV infection. *Am J Psychiatry* 1993;150:1674–1678.
44. Koenig S, Gendelman HE, Orenstein JM, et al. Detection of AIDS virus in macrophages in brain tissue from AIDS patients with encephalopathy. *Science* 1986;233:1089–1093.
45. Kovner R, Perecman E, Lazar W, et al. Relation of personality

and attentional factors to cognitive deficits in human immunodeficiency virus: infected subjects. *Arch Neurol* 1989;46:274–277.

46. Leserman J, Perkins DO, Evans DL. Coping with the threat of AIDS: the role of social support. *Am J Psychiatry* 1992;149:1514–1520.

47. Levine S, Anderson D, Bystritsky A. A report of eight HIV-seropositive patients with major depression responding to fluoxetine. *J AIDS* 1990;3:1074–1077.

48. Luft BJ, Remington JS. Toxoplasmic encephalitis in AIDS. *Clin Infect Dis* 1992;15:211–222.

49. Lyketsos CG, Hanson AL, Fishman M, Rosenblatt A, McHugh PR, Treisman GJ. Manic syndrome early and late in the course of HIV. *Am J Psychiatry* 1993;150:326–327.

50. Lyketsos CG, Hoover DR, Guccione M, et al. Depressive symptoms as predictors of medical outcomes in HIV infection. *JAMA* 1993;270:2563–2567.

51. Marder K, Stern Y, Malouf R, et al. Neurologic and neuropsychological manifestations of human immunodeficiency virus infection in intravenous drug users without acquired immunodeficiency syndrome: relationship to head injury. *Arch Neurol* 1992;49:1169–1175.

52. Markowitz JC, Klerman GL, Perry SW. Interpersonal psychotherapy of depressed HIV-seropositive patients. *Hosp Community Psychiatry* 1992;43:885–890.

53. Martin A, Heyes MP, Salazar AM, Law WA, Williams J. Impaired motor-skill learning, slowed reaction time, and elevated cerebrospinal-fluid quinolinic acid in a subgroup of HIV-infected individuals. *Neuropsychology* 1993;7:149–157.

54. Masdeu JC, Yudd A, VanHeertum RL. Single photon emission computerized tomography in small multifocal perfusion defects in human immunodeficiency virus encephalopathy: a preliminary report. *J Nucl Med* 1991;32:1471–1475.

55. Mayeux R, Stern Y, Tang M-X, et al. Mortality risks in gay men with human immunodeficiency virus infection and cognitive impairment. *Neurology* 1993;43:176–182.

56. McKegney FP, O'Dowd MA. Suicidality and HIV status. *Am J Psychiatry* 1992;149:396–398.

57. Miller AH, Asnis GM, van Praag HM, Norin AJ. Influence of desmethylimipramine on natural killer cell activity. *Psychiatry Res* 1986;19:9–15.

58. Moeller AA, Oechsner M, Backmund HC, Popescu M, Emminger C, Holsboer F. Self-reported sleep quality in HIV infection: correlation to the stage of infection and zidovudine therapy. *J AIDS* 1991;4:1000–1003.

59. Moulton JM, Stempel RR, Bacchetti P, Temoshok L, Moss AR. Results of a one year longitudinal study of HIV antibody test notification from the San Francisco General Hospital Cohort. *J AIDS* 1991;4:787–794.

60. Namir S, Wolcott DL, Fawzy FI, Alumbaugh MJ. Coping with AIDS: psychological and health implications. *J Appl Soc Psychol* 1987;17:309–328.

61. Navia BA, Jordon BD, Price RW. The AIDS dementia complex, 1: clinical features. *Ann Neurol* 1986;19:517–524.

62. Navia BA, Price RW. The acquired immunodeficiency syndrome dementia complex as the presenting or sole manifestation of human immunodeficiency virus infection. *Arch Neurol* 1987;44:65–69.

63. Norman SE, Chediak AD, Freeman C, Kiel M, Mendez A, Duncan R, Simoneau J, Nolan B. Sleep disturbances in men with asymptomatic human immunodeficiency (HIV) infection. *Sleep* 1992;15:150–155.

64. Pakesch G, Loimer N, Grunberger J, Pfersmann D, Linzmayer L, Mayerhofer S. Neuropsychological findings and psychiatric symptoms in HIV-1 infected and noninfected drug users. *Psychiatry Res* 1992;41:163–177.

65. Patterson TL, Semple S, Temoshok L, Atkinson JH, McCutchan JA, Grant I. Stress and depression predict immune change among HIV-infected men. Abstract presented at the 101st Annual Meeting of the American Psychological Association, Toronto, Canada, August 1993.

66. Perkins DO, Davidson EJ, Leserman J, Liao D, Evans DL. Personality disorder in men infected with HIV: a controlled study with implications for clinical care. *Am J Psychiatry* 1993;150:309–315.

67. Perkins DO, Evans DL. Fluoxetine treatment of depression in patients with HIV infection. *Am J Psychiatry* 1991;148:807–808.

68. Perkins DO, Leserman J, Gilmore JH, Petitto JM, Evans DL. Stress, depression, and immunity: research findings and clinical implications. In: N. Plotnikoff, A. Murgo, R. Faith, and J. Wybran, eds. *Stress and immunity*. London: CRC Press, 1991;167–188.

69. Perkins DO, Leserman J, Gray-Silva S, Baum SF, Stern RA, Evans DL. Fatigue and HIV infection: relationship to depressive symptoms and indicators of HIV disease. *Proceedings of the American Psychiatric Association*. New Research Program and Abstracts, 1993.

70. Perkins DO, Stern RA, Golden RN, Murphy C, Naftolowitz D, Evans DL. Mood disorders in HIV infection: prevalence and risk factors in a non-epicenter of the AIDS epidemic. *Am J Psychiatry* 1994;151:233–236.

71. Perry S, Fishman B, Jacobsberg L, Frances A. Relationship over 1 year between lymphocyte subsets and psychosocial variables among adults with infection by human immunodeficiency virus. *Arch Gen Psychiatry* 1992;49:396–401.

72. Perry S, Fishman B, Jacobsberg LB, Young J, Frances A. Effectiveness of psychoeducational interventions in reducing emotional distress after HIV antibody testing. *Arch Gen Psychiatry* 1991;48:143–147.

73. Perry S, Jacobsberg L, Fishman B. Suicidal ideation and HIV testing. *JAMA* 1990;263:679–682.

74. Perry S, Jacobsberg LB, Fishman B, Frances A, Bob J, Jacobsberg BK. Psychiatric diagnosis before serological testing for the human immunodeficiency virus. *Am J Psychiatry* 1990;147:89–93.

75. Perry SW, Jacobsberg LB, Fishman B, Weiler PH, Gold JWM, Frances AJ. Psychological responses to serological testing for HIV. *AIDS* 1990;4:145–152.

76. Post MJD, Berger JR, Quencer RM. Asymptomatic and neurologically symptomatic HIV-1-seropositive individuals: prospective evaluation with cranial MR imaging. *Radiology* 1991;178:131–139.

77. Price RW, Brew BJ. The AIDS dementia complex. *J Infect Dis* 1988;158:1079–1083.

78. Price RW, Sidtis J, Rosenblum M. The AIDS dementia complex: some current questions. *Ann Neurol* 1988;23:S27–S33.

79. Rabkin JG. Psychostimulant medication for depression and lethargy in HIV illness: a pilot study. *Newsletter Am Soc Clin Psychopharmacol* 1994;[in press].

80. Rabkin JG, Harrison WM. Effect of imipramine on depression and immune status in a sample of men with HIV infection. *Am J Psychiatry* 1990;147:495–497.

81. Rabkin JG, Williams JBW, Reimien RH, Goetz R, Kertzner R, Gorman J. Depression, distress, lymphocyte subsets, and human immunodeficiency virus symptoms on two occasions in HIV-positive homosexual men. *Arch Gen Psychiatry* 1991;48:111–119.

82. Reiger DA, Boyd JH, Rae DS, et al. One month prevalence of mental disorders in the United States. *Arch Gen Psychiatry* 1988;45:977–986.

83. Richman DD, Fischl MA, Grieco MH, et al. The toxicity of azidothymidine (AZT) in the treatment of patients with AIDS and AIDS-related complex: a double blind, placebo-controlled trial. *N Engl J Med* 1987;317:192–197.

84. Robins LN, Helzer JE, Weissman MM, et al. Lifetime prevalence of specific psychiatric disorders in three sites. *Arch Gen Psychiatry* 1984;41:949–958.

85. Robertson KR, Stern RA, Hall CD, et al. The relationship of vitamin B_{12} deficiency to nervous system disease in human immunodeficiency virus seropositive individuals. *Arch Neurol* 1993;50:807–811.

86. Rundell JR, Kyle KM, Brown GR, Thomason JL. Risk factors for suicide attempts in a human immunodeficiency virus screening program. *Psychosomatics* 1992;33:24–27.

87. Satz P, Morgenstern H, Miller EN, et al. Low education as a possible risk factor for cognitive abnormalities in HIV-1: findings from the Multicenter AIDS Cohort Study. *J AIDS* 1993;6:503–511.

88. Schielke E, Tatsch K, Pfister HW, et al. Reduced cerebral blood

flow in early stages of human immunodeficiency virus infection. *Arch Neurol* 1990;47:1342–1345.

89. Schliefer SJ, Keller SE, Meyerson AT, et al. Lymphocyte function in major depressive disorder. *Arch Gen Psychiatry* 1985;42:129–133.

90. Schmitt FA, Dickson LR, Brouwers P. Neuropsychological response to antiretroviral therapy in HIV infection. In: Grant I, Martin A, eds. *Neuropsychology of HIV infection.* New York: Oxford University Press, 1994;276–294.

91. Spiegel D, Bloom JR, Kraemer HC, Gottheil E. Effect of psychosocial treatment on survival of patients with metastatic breast cancer. *Lancet* 1989;2:888–891.

92. Stein M, Miller AH, Trestman RL. Depression, the immune system, and health and illness. *Arch Gen Psychiatry* 1991;48:171–177.

93. Stern RA, Singer NG, Silva SG, et al. Neurobehavioral functioning in a nonconfounded group of asymptomatic HIV-seropositive homosexual men. *Am J Psychiatry* 1992;149:1099–1102.

94. Tozzi V, Narciso P, Galgani S, et al. Effects of zidovudine in 30 patients with mild to end-stage AIDS dementia complex. *AIDS* 1993;7:683–692.

95. Tran Dinh YR, Mamo H, Cervoni J, Caulin C, Saimot AC. Disturbances in the cerebral perfusion of human immune deficiency virus-1 seropositive asymptomatic subjects: a quantitative tomography study of 18 cases. *J Nucl Med* 1990;31:1601–1607.

96. vanGorp WG, Mandelkern MA, Gee M, et al. Cerebral metabolic dysfunction in AIDS: findings in a sample with and without dementia. *J Neuropsychiatry Clin Neurosci* 1992;4:280–287.

97. Wilkie FL, Morgan R, Fletcher MA, et al. Cognition and immune function in HIV-1 infection. *AIDS* 1992;6:977–981.

98. Wilkins JW, Robertson KR, van der Horst C, Robertson WT, Fryer JG, Hall CD. The importance of confounding factors in the evaluation of neuropsychological changes in patients infected with human immunodeficiency virus. *J AIDS* 1990;3:938–942.

99. Williams JBW, Rabkin JG, Remien RH, Gorman JM, Ehrhardt AA. Multidisciplinary baseline assessment of homosexual men with and without human immunodeficiency virus infection: standardized clinical assessment of current and lifetime psychopathology. *Arch Gen Psychiatry* 1991;48:124–130.

100. Yarchoan R, Pluda JM, Thomas RV, et al. Long-term toxicity/activity profile of 2′,3′-dideoxyinosine in AIDS or AIDS-related complex. *Lancet* 1990;336:526–529.

Psychopharmacology: The Fourth Generation of Progress, edited by Floyd E. Bloom and David J. Kupfer. Raven Press, Ltd., New York 1995.

CHAPTER 134

Potential Mechanisms of Neurologic Disease in HIV Infection

Melvyn P. Heyes

Infection of humans with the human immunodeficiency virus (HIV) results in the eventual development of the acquired immune deficiency syndrome (AIDS). In the first month after infection, there is a phase of high virus replication in peripheral blood and entry of virus into lymphoid tissue and the brain (15,21,39). During seroconversion, flu-like symptoms and aseptic meningitis are experienced, and there is a transient phase of immunosuppression with a decrease in CD_4^+ cells. In subsequent years, viral load and replication rates in tissues where HIV is localized may be low, due to the effects of the hosts immune response (21). There is (a) chronic activation of the immune system, with increased levels of immune activation markers such as neopterin and β_2-microglobulin, and (b) gradual development of immune dysfunction, including loss of antibody production, increased production of cytokines that accelerate HIV replication, destruction of the microenvironment of lymphoid organs, and increased apoptosis of CD_4^+ and CD_8^+ cells (21). Patients usually develop a persistent lymphadenopathy and a gradual decline in the number of CD_4^+ cells, and some may also develop fever, weight loss, night sweats, and oral candidiasis. There is a marked secretion of cytokines during the course of disease. It has been hypothesized that increased activity of immunoprotective cytokines in the early phases of disease is beneficial [T_H-1 dominant phase; interleukin 2 (IL-2) and interferon γ (IFN-γ)], but is followed in the later phases of disease by secretion of proinflammatory cytokines (T_H-2 dominant phase; IL-4, IL-5, IL-6, and IL-10) (14,21,53). Secretion of tumor necrosis factor α (TNF-α) from B cells and macrophages has been linked to the wasting syndrome

associated with HIV infection (21). The secretion of cytokines is also important in the regulation of HIV expression; TNF-α, for example, promotes HIV replication (21,49). Eventually, immunosuppression and immune abnormalities increase in severity, and $CD4^+$ T lymphocytes become depleted. About 6–8 years after initial infection, patients suffer one or more opportunistic conditions of systemic tissues and brain (AIDS), including *Pneumocystis carinii* pneumonia, lymphoma, *Cryptococcus neoformans* meningitis, cytomegalovirus with encephalitis, and human papovavirus infection of brain, which causes progressive multifocal leukoencephalitis. Peripheral neuropathies and myopathies also occur. Death usually occurs within about 4 years of the onset of AIDS (21) (see Chapter 133, *this volume*).

HIV infection is also associated with the development of a broad spectrum of central nervous system (CNS) and neuropsychologic deficits, originally termed the "AIDS dementia complex" (55). More recently, the terms "HIV-associated dementia" and "HIV-associated motor cognitive and motor complex" have evolved (9). Meningitis may recur during throughout the course of disease (40). Motor slowing may begin early in HIV infection when patients are otherwise asymptomatic, and resemble those noted in basal-ganglia-related disorders, such as Huntington's disease (2,46). This has led to the notion that key components of HIV-related neurologic disease are a basal ganglia disorder or subcortical dementia (65). Nevertheless, it is clear that other brain regions are involved, particularly in the later stages of disease (52). Neuropsychologic symptoms that begin early in disease may be of constant severity. Once AIDS has developed, symptoms may rapidly increase in severity and can become an incapacitating dementia. These deficits are viewed as unrelated to opportunistic CNS conditions, although such conditions can cause additional neurologic problems. There

M. P. Heyes: Section on Analytical Biochemistry, Laboratory of Clinical Science, National Institute of Mental Health, Bethesda, Maryland 20892.

is evidence that CNS disease is associated with macrophage-tropic variants of virus rather than T-cell-tropic variants (18). About 30% of vertically transmitted HIV-infected children also show bilateral and symmetrical mineralization of the basal ganglia and periventricular frontal white matter (17). Postmortem studies have shown the presence of multinucleated giant cells, microglial nodules, perivascular monocyte infiltrates, astrogliosis, white-matter pallor, and neurodegeneration or neuronal injury with loss of dendritic spines (9,41,48,51,65,74,75, 81,82). The presence of multiple disseminated microglial nodules with macrophages and multinucleated giant cells, or the presence of HIV-infected cells within the CNS, is defined as HIV encephalitis (9). Vacuolar myelopathy occurs in about 20% of patients, particularly those with dementia (40).

The mechanisms responsible for neuropsychologic deficits has focused on the neuroanatomical lesions in the brain, i.e. HIV encephalitis. What is striking is that HIV is localized in macrophage infiltrates and microglia, rather than the "functional" elements of the brain, namely neurons, astrocytes and oligodendrocytes. These studies have led to the notion that neurologic deficits in HIV infection are mediated indirectly by either virus- or host-coded agents that produce neurologic symptoms by killing neurons, damaging neurons, disrupting neuronal electrical activity, or impairing neurotransmission. Neurologic dysfunction may also result from abnormalities in the functions of astrocytes or oligodendrocytes (20,22,57). Particular interest has focused on the macrophage, because of the distinct association between this cell type and the presence of HIV. Furthermore, although a direct cause-and-effect link between the presence of HIV encephalitis with neurologic deficits during life has not been firmly established, a large proportion of encephalitic patients are demented, which suggests that neurologic symptoms are linked to neuropathology, the presence of HIV, and inflammatory cell infiltrates. Nevertheless, there can be a disassociation between of HIV encephalitis and dementia (73).

Experimental investigations of these hypotheses have largely relied on studies of cells in vitro where neurons and other CNS cell types from various species and brain areas are incubated in the presence or absence of other cell types (macrophages, microglia, astrocytes, lymphocytes), or are treated from supernatants obtained from such cells. In some instances, the cell types other than neurons that are present in the cultures are not stated. Cells are then infected with HIV or stimulated by other HIV- or non-HIV-related agents, and the death of neurons is documented. A few studies have determined whether either systemic or intracerebral injections of putative neurotoxins produce functional or anatomical lesions in intact animals, usually rats.

Collectively, these studies have added significantly to the understanding of immune-mediated neurologic dis-

ease. Importantly, they have evolved new approaches to therapy. On the other hand, it has to be stated that the results and interpretations of some of these studies have been viewed as inconsistent, speculative, and perhaps difficult to accept. Some findings are unique or have not been reproduced between different laboratories, and consequently are difficult to evaluate (see also Chapters 7, 53, and 54, *this volume,* for related topics).

VIRUS-CODED TOXINS

gp120

Glycoprotein-160 (gp160) is a 160-kD glycoprotein on the surface of HIV, and it includes the gp120 viral envelope and the gp41 fusion protein. The gp120 envelope protein has a high affinity for binding to CD_4, a membrane receptor on the surface of several types of immune system cells. gp120 can be released from HIV-infected cells, a critical means by which HIV targets CD_4^+ cells (27). Brenneman et al. (7) were the first to report that gp120 was neurotoxic to mouse hippocampal neurons at concentrations of 100 aM to 10 pM (10^{-16} M to 10^{-10} M). Toxicity associated with gp120 was attenuated by monoclonal antibodies to CD_4 receptors. Both peptide T and vasoactive intestinal polypeptide, which share certain analogous sequences with gp120 from some HIV strains, appeared to block gp120 binding and reduce neurotoxicity (6,7,10). The neurotoxic effects of 20 to 200 pM (2×10^{-11} M to 2×10^{-10} M) gp120 on rat retinal ganglion cells have also been shown to be attenuated by either N-methyl-D-aspartate (NMDA) receptor antagonists or nimodipine, a calcium channel blocker (19,44). In this latter respect, gp120 resembles the classic excitotoxic response exemplified by NMDA itself, glutamate, kainate, ibotenate, and quinolinate. The receptors that mediate the neurotoxic effect of gp120, as well as its binding characteristics and specificity, are unclear, because rodent cells do not express CD_4, although receptors other than CD_4 have been implicated in HIV infection of neural cell lines (28).

There is other evidence that the neurotoxicity of gp120 may be indirect. Lipton et al. (44) have noted that the increase in intracellular calcium (19) and NMDA-receptor-mediated neurotoxicity of gp120 in rat retinal ganglion cells was attenuated by depletion of cell cultures of glutamate. Because gp120 alone had no discernible effect on ionic currents of ganglion cells, as determined by patch-clamp techniques, nor did gp120 enhance glutamate/NMDA-activated currents, a "synergistic" effect of gp120 on glutamate toxicity was postulated. Similarly, an increase in intracellular calcium levels and subsequent translocation of protein kinase C from the cytosol to the cell membrane of rat cortical neurons in response to gp120 was also blocked by removal of glutamate from the incubation medium (72). The mechanisms by which gp120 interacts with glutamate and NMDA receptors remains unclear. However, Sweetnam et al. (67) have reported that gp120 at a concentration of 10 nM to 100 nM (10^{-8} M to 10^{-7} M) inhibited the specific binding of NMDA receptor agonists, and blocked inward ion currents in *Xenopus* oocytes in response to NMDA and glycine (67). They also found that gp120 actually protected against neurotoxicity of rat cerebellar neurons in response to NMDA and glycine, and blocked calcium currents in response to NMDA (67). Peptide T had no effect on NMDA-induced calcium currents. Pulliam et al. (57) have noted no binding of biotinylated gp120 to human fetal neuronal cultures.

Piani et al. (54) showed that murine brain macrophages released glutamate, particularly after stimulation with either endotoxin or IFN-γ, and that such supernatants killed cerebellar granule cells via an NMDA-receptor-mediated mechanism. The effects of gp120 were not studied. In contrast, glutamate was eliminated as a neurotoxin involved in HIV-macrophage-mediated toxicity in other studies (24,56). Further evidence that gp120 can affect NMDA receptor function has been obtained in 7-day-old rats, where an injection of 100 ng of gp120 (but not 1 or 50 ng) into the hippocampus has been reported to produce focal pyramidal cell loss and to exacerbate the neurotoxic effects of NMDA (3). An intracerebroventricular injection of 5 μg of gp120, however, protected mice against an intraperitoneal injection of NMDA (67).

gp120 has also been shown to stimulate nitric oxide production from a human astrocyte cell line by 70% (50). Nitric oxide is an arginine-derived neuroactive free radical that has been implicated in NMDA-receptor-mediated neurotoxicity. Killing of cortical neurons in response to picomolar quantities of gp120 has also been linked to nitric oxide production (16). However, other studies of gp120 report neurotoxicity that is independent of nitric oxide (22,24,25,56).

While some studies suggest a direct effect of gp120 on neurons (64), it should be noted that other studies have reported no direct neurotoxic effects of gp120 on neurons obtained from chicken ciliary ganglion cells [100 pM to 10 nM (25)], fetal rat cerebral cortex [4 nM (4)], or rat cerebellar granule cells [10 nM to 100 nM (67)] or from cultures of neurons, astrocytes, and oligodendrocytes obtained from human fetus [1 pM to 1 nM (56,57)]. Giulian et al. (25) did, however, report that gp120-stimulated macrophages (but not lymphocytes or H9 cells) released neurotoxin(s) via binding of gp120 to monocytoid CD4 receptors. These toxin(s) co-purified with toxin(s) released from HIV-infected THP-1 cells, and could be blocked by antagonists to NMDA receptors (24,25). In contrast, Pulliam et al. (57) have reported that supernatant obtained from human macrophages that were stimulated with gp120 (1 pM to 1 nM) was not neurotoxic to human fetal brain cultures.

In intact rats, intracerebroventricular injections of 12

ng, but not 1.2 ng, of gp120 resulted in decreased spatial learning in rats (26). This effect of gp120 could be blocked by co-administration of vasoactive intestinal polypeptide, but was not replicated by injections of gp160. In subsequent studies, daily subcutaneous injections of 5 ng of gp120 for 28 days into newborn rats resulted in morphological damage of pyramidal neurons in the cerebral cortex consisting of reduced dendritic branching and length (38). A number of neurologic milestones were also delayed by gp120, although some were unaffected. Both peptide T and vasoactive intestinal polypeptide reduced the severity of neuroanatomical damage and behavioral abnormalities in response to gp120. To investigate whether a fragment of gp120 could be involved in neurotoxicity, 3.3 ng of ^{125}I-gp120 was injected subcutaneously into newborn rats, and gel-filtration chromatography was performed on brain extracts to isolate ^{125}I-labeled gp120 fragments (38). Several fragments were demonstrated and were shown to kill mouse spinal cord neurons. One fraction (#54) was diluted 1:400 (to an estimated concentration of 6×10^{-15} M) and was shown to kill neurons. Peptide T was able to block the toxic effects of fraction #54 (38). The metabolism of gp120 to these neuroactive fragments was not investigated. It is not known whether the production of fragments is essential for the neurotoxic effect of gp120, although filtration of gp120 to remove fragments of gp120 of <30 kD was associated with a 20% decrease in inward ion currents in *Xenopus* oocytes in response to NMDA and glycine (67). The composition of these molecules were not investigated, and it remains to be established whether they are derived from gp120 or not. Their presence in other preparations of gp120 has not been determined.

In a new approach, Toggas et al. (69) have created the expression of gp120 in the brains of mice by inserting the *env* sequence that codes for gp120, and placing it under the control of a modified glial fibrillary acidic protein gene promoter that is localized predominantly in astrocytes. Extensive vacuolization of dendrites, reductions in synaptodendritic complexity, astrogliosis, and increased numbers of F4/80-positive cells (microglia) were noted in these mice. Similarly, increased expression of IL-6, also under the regulation of the glial fibrillary acidic protein gene promoter in transgenic mice, was associated with tremors, ataxia, and seizures, as well as neurodegeneration, astrogliosis, angiogenesis, and induction of acute-phase protein production (11).

Tat, nef, rev, env, and gag

Tat, nef, rev, env, and *gag* are genes that code for structural, regulatory, and enzyme proteins (27). When HIV enters the hosts cells, viral RNA is converted to DNA by the action of the enzyme reverse transcriptase and is incorporated into the host cells' chromosomes (pro-virus) (27). Mistakes in the transcription of HIV nucleotide sequences occur during the reverse transcription step and contribute the high degree of virus mutation. Certain proteins from the host cell initiate transcription, and RNA molecules leave the nucleus to produce proteins via the hosts own translation system. The actual HIV genes code these different proteins. The long-term repeat is a binding site for host transcription factors (27). *Tat* is one of the first genes to be transcribed, and it binds to the enhancer element of the long-term repeat to enhance viral replication. *Nef* may suppress transcription or facilitate the manufacture of virus. *Rev* facilitates the export of intron containing HIV mRNA from the nucleus to the cytoplasm. *Tat, nef,* and *rev* are nonstructural regulatory proteins and are expressed early in HIV replication. *Env* codes for viral coat proteins that mediate CD4 binding and membrane fusion. Core proteins are coded for by *gag.* Other genes are also involved, including *pol,* which codes for reverse transcriptase, integrase, and ribonuclease (27). Release of these genes from HIV-infected cells have been reported or implicated.

Sabatier et al. (60) have studied the effects of *tat* protein and certain fragments of *tat.* ^{125}I-labeled *tat$_{38-68}$* was shown to bind to rat brain synaptosomes in a manner that could be blocked by very high concentrations of unlabeled *tat* derivatives with a 50% binding coefficient (K_0) of 3 μM. At 5 μM, *tat$_{2-86}$* caused a rapid depolarization of frog muscle fibers and cockroach giant interneuron synapses, via increases in non-ion-selective ion permeability. Murine neuroblastoma and rat neuroglioma were also damaged by *tat$_{2-86}$* at concentrations of 130 nM to 13 μM. Several *tat* derivatives and certain *rev* peptides were then shown to kill mice following intracerebroventricular injection in 10- to 180-μg quantities. The authors concluded that this was a ''neurotoxic'' effect, because muscular tremors, convulsions, wasting, and spastic paralysis were noted (45,60). No ''neurotoxicity'' was observed following systemic injection.

Other workers have reported that *tat* peptides derived from the maedi-visna virus or HIV produced excitotoxic-like lesions 7 days following direct injections into rat striata, consisting of neuronal loss, astrocytosis, microglial reactions, and macrophage infiltrates (29). Nanomoles of the toxin were injected, although the small volume of the injectate rendered the resultant solution in the milimolar range. These neurotoxic effects were attenuated by co-administration of N^G-nitro-L-arginine methyl ester, an inhibitor of the synthesis of nitric oxide, or systemic administration of MK-801, an antagonist of NMDA receptors. The authors also speculated that the large numbers of arginine residues in *tat* provided substrate for the synthesis of nitric oxide.

Nef protein has been reported to share sequence and structural similarities to neuroactive scorpion peptides and can reversibly increase total potassium currents in chick dorsal root ganglion cells (77). A recombinant fusion peptide, *env-gag,* has been reported to potentiate NMDA neurotoxicity in newborn rat hippocampus (3).

Giulian et al. (25) reported no neurotoxic effects of *gag* protein or *nef* protein in chicken cilliary ganglion cells.

HOST-CODED TOXINS

Cytokines

Cytokines are well-established mediators of immune function. Within the CNS, cytokines have many effects including toxicity to neurons and oligodendrocytes, stimuli to astrocyte proliferation, and mediators of fever (11,49). Although selective increases cytokine expression in brain have been shown to occur in HIV-1-infected patients, there is minimal correlation to the severity of encephalitis (1,70,78,80). The most consistent response has been an elevation in TNF-α, which is highest in patients with dementia (1,70,78,80). Cytokines are also important in protecting cells against intracellular parasites— including *Toxoplasma gondii,* an opportunistic infection in AIDS (13).

Quinolinic Acid

Quinolinic acid (QUIN) is a neurotoxic tryptophan–kynurenine pathway metabolite (see ref. 66) which increases neuronal activity and the entry of calcium and which can cause neurodegeneration and promote lipid peroxidation (59). QUIN is an agonist of NMDA receptors, and some brain regions and neuronal types are particularly sensitive to the neurotoxic effects of QUIN, including striatum, hippocampus, and spinal cord (66). Neurotoxicity has been reported in the nanomolar to micromolar range (23,24,42,79).

Immune activation in experimental animals was reported to result in an increase in QUIN levels in brain and blood (33). Elevated levels of QUIN were noted in patients with AIDS, thus implicating NMDA receptors in HIV-associated neurologic disease (34). Substantial increases in the concentrations of QUIN have also been observed in the brain and other tissues following immune activation unrelated to HIV infection (5,35,83). In the case of patients infected with HIV, the accumulations of QUIN in cerebrospinal fluid (CSF) begin soon after seroconversion (30,32), in association with the development of motor deficits (46,47). CSF QUIN levels are highest in the later stages of disease, particularly in those patients with neurologic deficits, inflammatory lesions in the brain, aseptic meningitis, or opportunistic CNS conditions (1,30,31,34,35,80). In brain tissue, QUIN levels were highest in the basal ganglia (1). Importantly, the concentrations of QUIN in CSF are also correlated with quantitative measures of neuropsychologic deficits in adults (30,47), children (8), and SIV-infected macaques (58). Treatment of HIV-infected patients with azidothymidine and antimicrobial therapies were associated with reductions in CSF QUIN levels (8,30). CSF QUIN concentrations are also correlated with measures of immune activation (neopterin, β_2-microglobulin), but not correlated with measures of blood–brain barrier abnormalities (31,35). In this context, QUIN may be a "marker" of immune activation and neurologic status. The mechanisms involved in increasing QUIN production involve increased activity of, and regulation by, indoleamine-2,3-dioxygenase and kynurenine-3-hydroxylase (35,36,63). Macrophages rather than astrocytes appear to be an important source of QUIN within the CNS (36,37,61). Cytokines released from activated lymphocytes, macrophages, and astrocytes are an important link between immune activation and QUIN production (36,61,62).

Reductions in CSF and blood L-tryptophan levels are associated with induction of indoleamine-2,3-dioxygenase. (31,76). L-Tryptophan is a precursor of indoleamines, such as serotonin. Evidence for reductions in serotonergic activity have been reported in the CSF of HIV-1-infected patients (43), which raises the possibility that such disturbances may have neuropsychologic consequences. Paradoxically, despite the long history of investigating neurotransmitter abnormalities in human neurodegenerative and psychiatric disorders, minimal studies of the neurochemistry of HIV-1-related CNS disease have been published. Interestingly, induction of indoleamine-2,3-dioxygenase and depletion of L-tryptophan has been implicated in the mechanisms by which interferon-γ exerts antiproliferative and antimicrobial effects (12). Depletion of L-tryptophan, an essential amino acid, may have a role in the wasting syndrome of AIDS and other inflammatory conditions.

While the micromolar concentrations of QUIN that are achieved in CSF and tissue QUIN of HIV-infected patients and simian immunodeficiency virus (SIV)-infected macaques (1,30,32,80) are neurotoxic and neuroactive to certain types of CNS neurons (23–25,42,66,79), there is currently no proof that QUIN is involved in the pathogenesis of HIV-associated neurologic disease.

UNIDENTIFIED TOXINS AND MECHANISMS

A number of independent studies with quite different paradigms have suggested the presence of additional factors related to HIV toxicity. Many of these factors have not been identified, and their presence in patients remains to be confirmed.

Giulian et al. (24) reported that chronic infection of either THP-1 cells or U-937 cells in vitro was associated with the release of a neurotoxin(s), as demonstrated by death of either rat spinal cord neurons or chick ciliary ganglion cells following application of monocyte super-

natants. In this study, neurons were kept separate from the HIV-infected cells. A number of potential toxins were eliminated as candidates for this toxic activity, including gp120, free radicals, nitric oxide, QUIN, glutamate, aspartate, cysteine, cytokines, and other peptides or molecules larger than 2000 daltons. A subsequent study suggested that toxin(s) are also released from gp120-stimulated monocytes (25). Pulliam et al. (56) have also reported neurotoxic activity of supernatants derived from HIV-infected macrophages, although this toxic activity was associated with high-molecular-weight molecules that were heat-labile. Toxicity was proportional to the levels of p24 expression, but unrelated to gp120 production (56).

Other studies have reported no neurotoxic activity in supernatants obtained from relatively acutely HIV-infected THP-1 cells when the fluids were applied to cultures of human neurons (68), SK-N-MC human neuroblastoma cells, or rat neurons (22). However, neurotoxicity associated with THP-1 infection was observed if PBMC or THP-1 cells had actually adhered to the neuron/astrocyte cultures ("cell-to-cell adhesion") (22,68). Free radicals were eliminated as mediating toxins, and neurotoxicity was not replicated by TNF-α, IL-1, or IFN-γ or by using fibroblasts instead of macrophages (68). Similarly, Genis et al. (22) noted no neurotoxic activity in supernatants obtained from HIV-infected monocytes when applied to cultures of SK-N-MC human neuroblastoma cells or rat brains. Neither TNF-α nor IL-1β was neurotoxic in their system.

Initially, Bernton et al. (4) reported that the neurotoxic effects of culture media obtained from HIV-infected monocyte cultures on rat cortical neurons could be explained by contamination of the HIV stock used with either *Mycoplasma arginini* or *M. hominis*. Both Pulliam et al. (56) and Giulian et al. (24), however, had already stated that such contamination was not present in their experimental systems. Bernton et al. (4) also showed that neurotoxicity could be replicated by exposure of neurons to mycloplasma, endotoxin, or TNF-α.

Pulliam et al. (57) have reported that gp120 in human fetal brain cultures or isolated human fetal brain astrocytes was toxic to astrocytes, resulting in decreased GFAP staining. Astrocytes have been reported to attenuate the neurotoxic effects of glutamate released from stimulated murine brain macrophages (54), and zymosan-activated astrocytes have been reported to release protein(s) that promote neuronal survival (23). In contrast, no astrocyte toxicity was found by Genis et al. (22) following exposure of rat cultures of supernatants from HIV-infected monocytes. However, cocultures of astrocytes and HIV-infected monocytes were reported to produce neurotoxic factor(s) (22). In association with toxicity, increased expression of TNF-α and IL-1β were demonstrated, although these cytokines were not toxic in and of themselves. Production of arachidonic acid metabolites were implicated in the production of TNF-α and

IL-1β. Platelet-activating factor, leukotrienes B$_4$ and D$_4$, and lipoxin A$_4$ were also shown to be produced. Neurotoxic activity in HIV-infected glial cultures was stated to be blocked by dexamethasone. Platelet-activating factor added to cocultures of uninfected monocytes, and astroglia produced neurotoxic activity (20). These results suggest that arachidonate metabolites, cytokine production, and neurodegenerative responses are linked in this particular system, and that "interactions" between HIV-infected monocytes and astrocytes were required for neurotoxicity.

Buzy et al. (10) have shown that CSF obtained from HIV-infected patients was not toxic when applied undiluted to mouse hippocampal neurons. However, neurotoxic activity appeared if the CSF was first diluted between 1:1000 to 1:1000000. Neurotoxicy was attenuated by peptide T and monoclonal antibodies to CD4. Neurotoxic activity was not found in CSF from non-HIV-related neurologic diseases.

Certain features of HIV encephalitis can be replicated in severe combined immunodeficiency mice by intracerebral injections with human peripheral blood mononuclear cells and HIV (71). Other models include macaques infected with SIV, mice infected with murine retroviruses, and cats infected with the feline immunodeficiency virus.

CONCLUSIONS

Neurotoxicity associated with HIV-1 infection has been described in a variety of experimental paradigms. Neurotoxic activity may be related to the presence of HIV and agents derived from the virus. Other toxins released from the host in response to the presence of HIV and/or immune activation are also candidates. The clinical manifestations of HIV-associated neurologic disease may result from the combined and separate effects of several of factors that operate to different degrees at different times in disease. NMDA receptors may be common mediators of toxicity in several experimental conditions.

The conflicting findings in the different experimental systems used indicate that caution should be exercised in the interpretation of results to generalized phenomenon in patients. It is clear that no one toxin can account for all neurotoxic activity described in vitro, and several remain to be identified or shown to be present in HIV-infected patients in significant and neuroactive amounts. Most studies that evaluate the "neurotoxin" hypothesis of HIV-associated neurologic disease use cell death as a measure of neurotoxic activity. More studies are required that evaluate subtle or noncytolytic neurologic dysfunction, particularly because there is no proof that HIV-associated neurologic disease in AIDS is dependent on nerve cell death per se. Alternative systems, such as transgenic mice, xenographs, and cells implanted into severe combined immunodeficiency mice, may prove useful

in modeling chronic mechanisms, rather than the acute systems currently available. The effects of anti-HIV drugs on neurotoxic activity also need to be studied. Certain mechanisms suggest generalized therapeutic strategies, including attenuation of HIV replication, reductions in the synthesis, or effects of key cytokines or antagonists to NMDA receptors. Other agents suggest highly specific approaches, such as drugs that attenuate the synthesis of quinolinate or attenuate the effects of gp120.

ACKNOWLEDGMENTS

I appreciate the useful comments made by Drs. A. Lackner, S. P. Markey, D. Rausch, K. Saito, and C. A. Wiley regarding this manuscript.

REFERENCES

1. Achim CL, Heyes MP, Wiley CA. Quantitation of human immunodeficiency virus, immune activation factors and quinolinic acid in AIDS brains. *J Clin Invest* 1993;91:2769–2775.
2. Arendt G, Hefter H, Elsing C, Strohmeyer G, Freund HJ. Motor dysfunction in HIV-infected patients without clinically detectable central-nervous deficit. *J Neurol* 1990;237:362–368.
3. Barks JD, Nair MPN, Schwartz SA, Silverstein FS Potentiation of *N*-methyl-D-aspartate-mediated brain injury by a human immunodeficiency virus-1-derived peptide in perinatal rodents. *Pediatr Res* 1993;34:192–198.
4. Bernton EW, Bryant HU, Decoster MA, Orenstein JM, Ribas JL, Meltzer MS, Gendelman HE. No direct neuronotoxicity by HIV-1 virions or culture fluids from HIV-1-infected T cells or monocytes. *AIDS Res Hum Retroviruses* 1992;8:495–503.
5. Blight AR, Saito K, Heyes MP. Increased levels of the excitotoxin quinolinic acid in spinal cord following contusion injury. *Brain Res* 1993;632:314–316.
6. Brenneman DE, Buzy JM, Ruff MR, Pert CB. Peptide T sequences prevent neuronal death produced by the envelope protein (gp120) of the human immunodeficiency virus. *Drug Dev Res* 1988;15:361–369.
7. Brenneman DE, Westbrook GL, Fitzgerald SP, Ennist DL, Elkins KL, Ruff MR, Pert CB. Neuronal cell killing by the envelope protein of HIV and its prevention by vasoactive intestinal peptide. *Nature* 1988;335:639–642.
8. Brouwers P, Heyes MP, Moss H, Wolters P, El-Amin D, Poplack D, Markey SP, et al. Quinolinic acid in the cerebrospinal fluid of children with symptomatic human immunodeficiency virus type-1 disease: relationships to clinical status and therapeutic response. *J Infect Dis* 1993;168:1380–1386.
9. Budka H, Wiley CA, Kleihues P, Artigas J, Asbury AK, Cho E-S, Cornblath DR, et al. Consensus report. HIV-associated disease of the nervous system: review of nomenclature and proposal for neuropathology-based terminology. *Brain Pathol* 1991;1:143–152.
10. Buzy J, Brenneman DE, Pert CB, Martin A, Salazar A, Ruff MR. Potent gp120-like neurotoxic activity in the cerebrospinal fluid of HIV-infected individuals is blocked by peptide T. *Brain Res* 1992;598:10–18.
11. Campbell IL, Abraham CR, Masliah E, Kemper P, Inglis JD, Oldstone MB, Mucke L. Neurologic disease induced in transgenic mice by cerebral overexpression of interleukin-6. *Proc Natl Acad Sci USA* 1993;90:10061–10065.
12. Carlin JM, Ozaki Y, Byrne GI, Brown RR, Borden EC. Interferons and indoleamine 2,3-dioxygenase: role in antimicrobial and antitumor effects. *Experientia* 1989;45:535–541.
13. Chao CC, Gekker G, Hu S, Peterson PK. Human microglial cell defense against *Toxoplasma gondii*: the role of cytokines. *J Immunol* 1994;152:1246–1252.

14. Clerici M, Shearer GM. A $T_H1\rightarrow T_H2$ switch is a critical step in the etiology of HIV infection. *Immunol Today* 1993;14:107–111.
15. Davis LE, Hjelle BL, Miller VE, Palmer DL, Llewellyn AL, Merlin TL, Young SA, et al. Early viral brain invasion in iatrogenic human immunodeficiency virus infection. *Neurology* 1992;42:1736–1739.
16. Dawson VL, Dawson TM, Uhl GR, Snyder SH. Human immunodeficiency virus type 1 coat protein neurotoxicity mediated by nitric oxide in primary cortical cultures. *Proc Natl Acad Sci USA* 1993;90:3256–3259.
17. DeCarli C, Civitello LA, Brouwers P, Pizzo PA. The prevalence of computed axial tomographic abnormalities of the cerebrum in 100 consecutive children symptomatic with the HIV. *Ann Neurol* 1993;34:189–205.
18. Desrosiers RC, Hansen-Moosa A, Mori K, Bouvier DP, King NW, Daniel MD, Ringler DJ Macrophage-tropic variants of SIV are associated with specific AIDS-related lesions that are not essential for the development of AIDS. *Am J Pathol* 1991;139:29–35.
19. Dreyer EB, Kaiser PK, Offermann JT, Lipton SA. HIV-1 coat protein neurotoxicity prevented by calcium channel antagonists. *Science* 1990;248:364–367.
20. Epstein LG, Gendelman HE. Human immunodeficiency virus type 1 infection of the nervous system: pathogenic mechanisms. *Ann Neurol* 1993;33:429–436.
21. Fauci AS. Multifactorial nature of human immunodeficiency virus disease: implications for therapy. *Science* 1993;262:1011–1018.
22. Genis P, Jett M, Bernton EW, Boyle T, Gelbard HA, Dzenko K, Keane RW, et al. Cytokines and arachidonic acid metabolites produced during human immunodeficiency virus (HIV)-infected macrophage–astrocyte interactions: implications for the neuropathogenesis of HIV disease. *J Exp Med* 1992;176:1703–1718.
23. Giulian D, Vaca K, Corpuz M. Brain glia release factors with opposing actions upon neuronal survival. *J Neurosci* 1993;13:29–37.
24. Giulian D, Vaca K, Noonan CA. Secretion of neurotoxins by mononuclear phagocytes infected with HIV-1. *Science* 1990;250:1593–1596.
25. Giulian D, Wendt E, Vaca K, Noonan CA. The envelope glycoprotein of human immunodeficiency virus type 1 stimulates the release of neurotoxins from monocytes. *Proc Natl Acad Sci USA* 1993;90:2769–2773.
26. Glowa JR, Panlilio LV, Brenneman DE, Gozes I, Fridkin M, Hill JM. Learning impairment following intracerebral administration of the HIV envelope protein gp120 or a VIP antagonist. *Brain Res* 1992;570:49–53.
27. Greene WC. AIDS and the immune system. *Sci Am* 1993;269:99–105.
28. Harouse JM, Bhat S, Spitalnik SL, Laughlin M, Stefano K, Silberberg DH, Gonzalez-Scarano F. Inhibition of entry of HIV-1 in neural cell lines by antibodies against galactosyl ceramide. *Science* 1991;253:320–323.
29. Hayman M, Arbuthnott G, Harkiss G, Brace H, Filippi P, Philippon V, Thomson D, et al. Neurotoxicity of peptide analogues of the transactivating protein tat from maedi-visna virus and human immunodeficiency virus. *Neuroscience* 1993;53:1–6.
30. Heyes MP, Brew BJ, Martin A, Price RW, Salazar AM, Sidtis JJ, Yergey JA, et al. Quinolinic acid in cerebrospinal fluid and serum in HIV-1 infection: relationship to clinical and neurologic status. *Ann Neurol* 1991;29:202–209.
31. Heyes MP, Brew BJ, Saito K, Quearry BJ, Price RW, Bhalla RB, Mouradian MM, et al. Inter-relationships between neuroactive kynurenines, neopterin and β_2-microglobulin in cerebrospinal fluid and serum of HIV-1 infected patients. *J Neuroimmunol* 1992;40:71–80.
32. Heyes MP, Jordan EK, Lee K, Saito K, Frank JA, Snoy PJ, Markey SP, et al. Relationship of neurologic status in macaques infected with the simian immunodeficiency virus to cerebrospinal fluid and serum quinolinic acid and kynurenic acid. *Brain Res* 1992;570:237–250.
33. Heyes MP, Kim P, Markey SP. Systemic lipopolysaccharide and pokeweed mitogen increase quinolinic acid content of mouse cerebral cortex. *J Neurochem* 1988;51:1946–1948.
34. Heyes MP, Rubinow D, Lane C, Markey SP. Cerebrospinal fluid quinolinic acid concentrations are increased in acquired immune deficiency syndrome. *Ann Neurol* 1989;26:275–277.
35. Heyes MP, Saito K, Crowley J, Davis LE, Demitrak MA, Der M,

Dilling L, et al. Quinolinic acid and kynurenine pathway metabolism in inflammatory and noninflammatory neurologic disease. *Brain* 1992;115:1249–1273.
36. Heyes MP, Saito K, Major EO, Milstein S, Markey SP, Vickers JH. A mechanism of quinolinic acid formation by brain in inflammatory neurologic disease: attenuation of synthesis from L-tryptophan by 6-chloro-tryptophan and 4-chloro-3-hydroxyanthranilate. *Brain* 1993;116:1425–1450.
37. Heyes MP, Saito K, Markey SP. Human macrophages convert L-tryptophan to the neurotoxin quinolinic acid. *Biochem J* 1992;283:633–635.
38. Hill JM, Mervis RF, Avidor R, Moody TW, Brenneman DE. HIV envelope protein-induced neuronal damage and retardation of behavioral development in rat neonates. *Brain Res* 1993;603:222–233.
39. Hurtrel B, Chakrabarti L, Hurtrel M, Maire MA, Dormont D, Montagnier L. Early SIV encephalopathy. *J Med Primatol* 1991;20:159–166.
40. Johnson RT, McArthur JC, Narayan O. The neurobiology of human immunodeficiency virus infections. *FASEB J* 1988;2:2970–2981.
41. Ketzler S, Weis S, Haug H, Budka H. Loss of neurons in the frontal cortex in AIDS brain. *Acta Neuropathol* 1990;80:92–94.
42. Kim JP, Choi DW. Quinolinate neurotoxicity in cortical cell culture. *Neuroscience* 1987;25:423–432.
43. Larsson M, Hagberg L, Norkrans G, Forsman A. Indole amine deficiency in blood and cerebrospinal fluid from patients with human immunodeficiency virus infection. *J Neurosci Res* 1989;23:441–446.
44. Lipton SA, Sucher NJ, Kaiser PK. Synergistic effects of HIV coat protein and NMDA-receptor mediated neurotoxicity. *Neuron* 1991;7:111–118.
45. Mabrouk K, Van RJ, Vives E, Darbon H, Rochat H, Sabatier JM. Lethal neurotoxicity in mice of the basic domains of HIV and SIV Rev proteins. Study of these regions by circular dichroism. *FEBS Lett* 1991;289:13–17.
46. Martin A, Heyes MP, Salazar AM, Kampen DL, Williams J, Law WA, Coates ME, et al. Progressive slowing of reaction time and increasing cerebrospinal fluid concentrations of quinolinic acid in HIV-infected individuals. *J Neuropsychiatr Clin Neurosci* 1992;4:270–279.
47. Martin A, Heyes MP, Salazar AM, Law WA, Williams J. Impaired motor-skill learning, slowed reaction time, and elevated cerebrospinal fluid quinolinic acid in a sub-group of HIV-infected individuals. *Neuropsychology* 1993;7:149–147.
48. Masliah E, Ge N, Morey M, DeTeresa R, Terry RD, Wiley CA. Cortical dendritic pathology in human immunodeficiency virus encephalitis. *Lab Invest* 1992;66:285–291.
49. Merrill JE, Chen ISY. HIV-1, macrophages, glial cells, and cytokines in AIDS nervous system disease. *FASEB J* 1991;5:2391–2397.
50. Mollace V, Colasanti M, Persichini T, Bagetta G, Lauro GM, Nistico G. HIV gp120 glycoprotein stimulates the inducible iso form of NO synthetase in human cultured astrocytoma cells. *Biochem Biophys Res Commun* 1993;194:439–445.
51. Navia BA, Cho E-S, Petito CK, Price RW. The AIDS dementia complex. II. Neuropathology. *Ann Neurol* 1986;19:525–535.
52. Neuen JE, Arendt G, Wendtland B, Jacob B, Schneeweis M, Wechsler W. Frequency and topographical distribution of CD68-positive macrophages and HIV-1 core proteins in HIV-associated brain lesions. *Clin Neuropathol* 1993;12:315–324.
53. Paul WE, Seder RA. Lymphocyte responses and cytokines. *Cell* 1994;76:241–251.
54. Piani D, Frei K, Do KQ, Cuenod M, Fontana A. Murine brain macrophages induce NMDA receptor mediated neurotoxicity in vitro by secreting glutamate. *Neurosci Lett* 1991;133:159–162.
55. Price RW, Brew B, Sidtis J, Rosenblum M, Scheck AC, Cleary P. The brain in AIDS: central nervous system HIV-1 infection and AIDS dementia complex. *Science* 1988;239:586–592.
56. Pulliam L, Herndier BG, Tang NM, McGrath MS. Human immunodeficiency virus-infected macrophages produce soluble factors that cause histological and neurochemical alterations in cultured human brains. *J Clin Invest* 1991;87:503–512.
57. Pulliam L, West D, Haigwood N, Swanson RA. HIV-1 envelope

gp120 alters astrocytes in human brain cultures. *AIDS Res Hum Retroviruses* 1993;9:439–444.

58. Rausch DM, Heyes MP, Murray EA, Lendvay J, Sharer LR, Ward JM, Rehm S, et al. Cytopathologic and neurochemical correlates to motor/cognitive impairments in SIV-infected rhesus monkeys. *J Neuropathol Exp Neurol* 1994;53:165–175.

59. Rios C, Santamaria A. Quinolinic acid is a potent lipid peroxidant in rat brain homogenates. *Neurochem Res* 1991;16:1139–1143.

60. Sabatier J-M, Vives E, Mabrouk K, Benjouad A, Rochat H, Duval A, Hue B, et al. Evidence for neurotoxic activity of *tat* from human immunodeficiency virus type-1. *J Virol* 1991;65:961–967.

61. Saito K, Chen CY, Masana M, Crowley J, Markey SP, Heyes MP. 4-Chloro-3-hydroxyanthranilic acid, 6-chlorotryptophan and norharmane attenuate quinolinic acid formation by interferon-γ stimulated monocytes (THP-1) cells. *Biochem. J.* 1993;291:11–14.

62. Saito K, Markey SP, Heyes MP. Effects of immune activation on quinolinic acid and kynurenine pathway metabolism in the mouse. *Neuroscience* 1992;51:25–39.

63. Saito K, Nowak TS Jr, Markey SP, Heyes MP. Mechanism of delayed increases in kynurenine pathway metabolism in damaged brain regions following transient cerebral ischemia. *J Neurochem* 1993;60:180–192.

64. Savio T, Levi G. Neurotoxicity of HIV coat protein gp120, NMDA receptors, and protein kinase C: a study with rat cerebellar granule cell cultures. *J Neurosci Res* 1993;34:265–272.

65. Spencer DC, Price RW. Human immunodeficiency virus and the central nervous system. *Annu Rev Microbiol.* 1993;46:655–693.

66. Stone TW. Neuropharmacology of quinolinic and kynurenic acids. *Pharmacol Rev* 1993;45:309–379.

67. Sweetnam PM, Saab OH, Wroblewski JT, Price CH, Karbon EW and Ferkany JW The envelope glycoprotein of HIV-1 alters NMDA receptor function. *Eur J Neurosci* 1993;5:275–283.

68. Tardieu M, H:ery C, Peudenier S, Boespflug O and Montagnier L. Human immunodeficiency virus type 1-infected monocytic cells can destroy human neural cells after cell-to-cell adhesion. *Ann Neurol* 1992;32:11–17.

69. Toggas SM, Masliah E, Rockenstein EM, Rall GF, Abraham CR, Mucke L. Central nervous system damage produced by expression of the HIV-1 coat protein gp120 in transgenic mice. *Nature* 1994;367:188–193.

70. Tyor WR, Glass JD, Griffin JW. Cytokine expression in the brain during AIDS. *Ann Neurol* 1992;31:249–360.

71. Tyor WR, Power C, Gendelman HE, Markham RB. A model of human immunodeficiency virus encephalitis in scid mice. *Proc Natl Acad Sci USA* 1993;90:8658–8662.

72. Ushijima H, Ando S, Kunisada T, Schroder HC, Klocking H-P, Kijoa A, Muller WEG. HIV-1 gp120 and NMDA induce protein kinase C translocation differentially in at primary neuronal cultures. *J AIDS* 1993;6:339–343.

73. Vazeux R, Lacroix CC, Blanche S, Cumont MC, Henin D, Gray F, Boccon GL, et al. Low levels of human immunodeficiency virus replication in the brain tissue of children with severe acquired immunodeficiency syndrome encephalopathy. *Am J Pathol* 1992;140:137–144.

74. Weis S, Haug H, Budka H. Astroglial changes in the cerebral cortex of AIDS brains: a morphometric and immunohistochemical investigation. *Neuropathol Appl Neurobiol* 1993;19:329–335.

75. Weis S, Haug H, Budka H. Neuronal damage in the cerebral cortex of AIDS brains: a morphometric study. *Acta Neuropathol (Berl)* 1993;85:185–189.

76. Werner ER, Fuchs D, Hausen A. Tryptophan degradation in patients infected by human immunodeficiency syndrome virus. *Biol Chem Hoppe Seyler* 1988;369:337–340.

77. Werner T, Ferroni S, Saermark T, Brack-Werner R, Banati RB, Mager R, Steinaa L, et al. HIV-1 Nef protein exhibits structural and functional similarity to scorpion peptides interacting with K^+ channels. *AIDS* 1991;5:1301–1308.

78. Wesselingh SL, Power C, Glass JD, Tyor WR, McArthur JC, Faber JM, Griffin JW, et al. Intracerebral cytokine messenger RNA expression in acquired immunodeficiency syndrome dementia. *Ann Neurol* 1993;33:576–582.

79. Whetsell WO, Schwarcz R. Prolonged exposure to submicromolar concentrations of quinolinic acid causes excitotoxic damage in organotypic cultures of rat corticostriatal system. *Neurosci Lett* 1989;97:271–275.

80. Wiley CA, Achim CL, Schrier RD, Heyes MP, McCutchan JA, Grant I. Relationship of cerebrospinal fluid immune activation associated factors to HIV encephalitis. *AIDS* 1992;6:1299–1307.

81. Wiley CA, Belman AL, Dickson DW, Rubenstein A, Nelson JA. Human immunodeficiency virus within the brains of children with AIDS. *Clin Neuropathol* 1990;9:1–6.

82. Wiley CA, Mesliah E, Morey M, Lemere C, DeTeresa R, Grafe M, Hansen L, et al. Neocortical damage during HIV infection. *Ann Neurol* 1991;29:651–657.

83. Yellon RF, Rose E, Kenna MA, W.J.D, Casselbrant M, Diven WF, Whiteside TL, et al. Sensorineural hearing loss from quinolinic acid: a neurotoxin present in middle ear effusions. *Laryngoscope* 1994;104:176–181.

Psychopharmacology: The Fourth Generation of Progress, edited by Floyd E. Bloom and David J. Kupfer. Raven Press, Ltd., New York © 1995.

CHAPTER 135

The Neuropsychopharmacology of Personality Disorders

Emil F. Coccaro and Larry J. Siever

The inclusion for the first time of a chapter on the neuropsychopharmacology of the personality disorders in the "ACNP Generation of Progress" series reflects the increasing appreciation of underlying neurobiologic substraits for these disorders and the value of targeted psychopharmacologic treatment. The personality disorders, located on Axis II in DSM-III-R and DSM-IV, consist of constellations of enduring or persistent maladaptive traits and/or symptoms that are characteristic of the way an individual experiences and interacts with his/her environment. In contrast with the Axis I disorders, which are primarily symptom-oriented and wax and wane in severity (often in episodic fashion), the Axis II personality disorders are conceived to be characteristic of an individual throughout his lifetime. This conceptual distinction between the Axis I and II disorders, while heuristically useful, is becoming increasingly blurred because studies into the neuropsychopharmacology of personality disorder suggest that enduring traits reflect underlying biologic variations that may be amenable to alteration with psychopharmacologic treatment. While some have argued that these considerations argue for the abolition of Axis II, the separation of these disorders on Axis II has highlighted the fact that traits considered to be part of an individual's stable personality can be substantially impacted by psychopharmacologic treatment.

While the DSM-III and III-R represented a significant advance over DSM-II in the identification of specific categories of personality disorder, many of these categories were found to be overlapping and have yet to be validated by external validators. By the advent of DSM-IV, validating antecedents and correlates in both biologic and psychosocial arenas have been found for some of the personality disorders, particularly schizotypal and borderline personality disorder. The total number of these disorders has been reduced from 11 to 10, and criteria have been sharpened with no major changes in the constructs (see Chapter 71, *this volume*).

Because the categories are highly overlapping and describe a range of interpersonal, attitudinal, and more fundamental psychologic traits, neurobiologic and psychopharmacologic approaches to the personality disorders can also be organized around "dimensional" or "cluster" approaches to the personality disorders that may cross categorical boundaries. DSM-III and DSM-III-R was organized for heuristic purposes into clusters: the "odd" cluster, the "dramatic" cluster, and the "anxious" cluster. These clusters also may be mapped into dimensions of *cognitive disorganization* for the "odd" cluster, *impulsivity and affective instability* for the "dramatic" cluster, and *anxiety* for the "anxious" cluster (53). *Cognitive organization* refers to the capacity of an individual to attend to and select relevant information from the environment, organize it in relation to past experience, and formulate appropriate strategies to interact with the environment. Impairment in this dimension ranges from the chronic psychosis of schizophrenia, where perception of reality is markedly distorted, to the psychotic-like symptoms of schizotypal personality disorder and perhaps even to more subtle deficits in interpretation of social cues. Impulsivity, which is characteristic of borderline, histrionic, and antisocial personality disorders, may be defined as a lowered threshold for motoric action, particularly aggressive behavior, in response to environmental stimuli. Individuals with a tendency toward impulsivity tend to externalize their problems and overreact

E. F. Coccaro: Department of Psychiatry, Medical College of Pennsylvania at Eastern Pennsylvania Psychiatric Institute, Philadelphia, Pennsylvania 19129.
L. J. Siever: Department of Psychiatry, Mt. Sinai School of Medicine, New York, New York 10029.

to environmental events. Affective-related symptoms are another dimension prominent in the "dramatic" cluster personality disorders. Affective instability is a criterion of borderline personality disorder and may be observed in histrionic and narcissistic personality disorders as well. Individuals with affective instability are characterized by rapidly occurring shifts in affect, changing from anger to disappointment to excitement in a matter of hours or minutes. These affective shifts are exquisitely sensitive to shifts in the environment, such as separation or frustration. Finally, anxiety thresholds vary between individuals. Individuals with high anxiety have a greater readiness to anticipate punishment or aversive consequences of their behavior and often show concomitant autonomic arousal associated with their fearfulness. They may inhibit a variety of behaviors they perceive as potentially assertive or competitive, fearing the consequences of their behavior. While a number of psychometric dimensional schema exist for the personality disorders, emerging evidence supports a biologic underpinning to these clinically based dimensions, which also may constitute target symptoms for psychopharmacologic intervention.

In this review, the available evidence regarding the biology of the personality disorders, particularly because they have implications for psychopharmacologic treatment, will be presented in relation to each of these target symptom dimensions, which may overlap with specific disorders. Most pharmacologic studies have focused on patients with specific personality disorders, such as borderline or schizotypal personality disorder, and have evaluated changes in target domains of psychosis, affect, anxiety, or impulsivity. Thus, both syndromal and dimensional considerations will be discussed. It should be noted, however, that there are few placebo-controlled pharmacologic trials in patients with well-characterized personality disorders. Therefore, the conclusions presented in this chapter must be considered tentative at this time. Accordingly, we will highlight trends in the data, both biologic and pharmacologic, and present possible future directions for research in the clinical psychopharmacologic management of patients with personality disorders.

PSYCHOBIOLOGY OF PSYCHOTIC-LIKE SYMPTOMS

The schizophrenia-related personality disorders of DSM-III and DSM-IV include schizotypal, paranoid, and schizoid personality disorders. Of these, schizotypal personality disorder is the best characterized and the most severe of the schizophrenia-related personality disorders, and it is the most closely related to schizophrenia biologically, phenomenologically, and genetically (53). In addition to psychotic-like symptoms, patients with schizotypal personality disorder also manifest social detachment and other deficit-related symptoms. Initial hypotheses cen-

tered around defining similarities between schizotypal personality disorder patients and schizophrenic patients in these domains, whereas more recent studies have pursued more specific correlates (particularly in the psychotic-like and deficit-like symptom complexes) of underlying psychopathologic processes in schizotypal personality disorder to better understand the fundamental pathophysiologic processes of the schizophrenia-related disorders (53).

Psychotic-like symptoms in these personality disorders include magical thinking, ideas of reference, and perceptual distortions and are some of the most discriminating criteria for clinically identified schizotypal personality disorder patients. Because psychotic symptoms in the schizophrenic disorders have been linked to excessive dopaminergic activity, most studies have explored this hypothesis in order to understand the biologic underpinnings of psychosis proneness in these individuals. The "dopamine hypothesis" of schizophrenia was stimulated by (a) the observation that antipsychotic medications had potent dopamine antagonist properties that correlate with their therapeutic efficacy (34) and (b) the observation of psychotogenic effects of dopamine-releasing agents such as amphetamine when administered over long periods of time. While studies measuring the dopamine metabolite homovanillic acid (HVA) in cerebrospinal fluid (CSF) in schizophrenic patients and comparing them with controls have been inconsistent (69), there are suggestions of increases in some paranoid subtypes and decreases associated with deficit-like symptoms (52). However, current hypotheses regarding the dopaminergic system in schizophrenia might suggest hypodopaminergia in frontal cortical areas and hyperdopaminergia in subcortical areas. However, indices of dopaminergic activity such as CSF and plasma HVA depend on contributions from multiple brain regions and the periphery, making interpretations of these measures problematic.

The study of schizotypal patients affords an opportunity to disentangle these two processes. Both CSF and plasma HVA levels are greater in clinically selected schizotypal patients than in normal and other personality disorder controls, specifically associated with the psychotic-like symptoms of schizotypal personality disorder (51,52). In schizotypal relatives of schizophrenic patients, characterized more by deficit-like symptoms, plasma HVA is reduced compared to relatives of nonschizotypal relatives (Amin et al., 1993, *unpublished data*).

PSYCHOPHARMACOLOGY OF PSYCHOTIC-LIKE SYMPTOMS

These considerations imply that the psychotic-like symptoms of the schizophrenia-related personality disorders may be ameliorated by neuroleptics and worsened by psychostimulants such as amphetamine. In one study of borderline/schizotypal patients, amphetamine induced psychotic-like symptoms, particularly in those patients with a schizotypal personality disorder diagnosis (48). In clinical psychopharmacologic trials, neuroleptic treatment has generally been associated with global improvement in patients with borderline and/or schizotypal personality disorder (7). In two relatively large placebo-controlled trials in patients with borderline and/or schizotypal personality disorder, psychotic-like symptoms (as well as symptoms of anxiety) were reduced by treatment with a neuroleptic (thiothixene in ref. 17, haloperidol in ref. 57). The generalizability of the data from one trial may be limited, however, to personality-disordered patients with histories of brief transient psychotic-like symptoms prior to the start of the trial. A smaller study involving only females with severe borderline personality disorder found only modest efficacy for the neuroleptic (trifluroperizine) over placebo. While these data are in general agreement with those of several other studies involving neuroleptic treatment in personality-disordered patients, the most recent study found no efficacy for the neuroleptic (haloperidol) on psychotic-like symptoms in borderline and/or schizotypal personality-disordered patients (56). The authors noted, however, that the patients in their previous study, where haloperidol had been efficacious in treating psychotic-like symptoms, had significantly higher ratings of "psychoticism," "schizotypal symptom severity," and "global impairment" than in the more recent study. In conjunction with the finding that "severity of schizotypal symptoms" was a favorable predictor of response to thiothixine (17), these results suggest that low-dose neuroleptic treatment may be best indicated for moderately to severely impaired patients with prominent histories of psychotic-like schizotypal symptoms.

PSYCHOBIOLOGY OF DEFICIT SYMPTOMS

The social detachment in interpersonal isolation of the schizophrenia spectrum personality disorders may be rooted in biologic processes impairing cortical processing of complex interpersonal cues as well as deficits in attachment behavior. Interpersonal relationships depend on selecting appropriate information and cues from other people and synchronizing one's responses in a reciprocal interaction. These interactional patterns might be set down in infancy and may be disrupted when there is neurologic immaturity on the part of the developing infant (53). Offspring of schizophrenic patients show pandevelopmental immaturities, raising the possibility that the diathesis to the schizophrenic disorders may impair the development of mutually satisfying interactions (53). A variety of studies implicate deficits in information processing, neuropsychological, and psychophysiologic tasks in the schizophrenia-related personality disorders, as in schizophrenia. These are often particularly associated

with the deficit-like symptoms of the schizophrenic spectrum personality disorders and have been hypothesized to be related to alterations in brain structure (53a). The cognitive impairment seems to be associated with decreased indices of dopaminergic activity, consistent with the notion that adequate dopaminergic tone, particularly at D_1 receptors in frontal cortical areas, may be necessary for the integrity of working memory and other executive cognitive functions. Preliminary evidence supporting this hypothesis comes from psychophysiologic, neuropsychologic, and imaging studies (53a).

Impaired eye movements tracking a smoothly moving target is one of the most consistent findings in the schizophrenia-related disorders. Abnormalities in smooth pursuit tracking are seen in schizophrenic patients and in schizotypal personality-disordered patients. Eye-tracking impairment is specifically associated with the "deficit-like" traits of schizotypal personality disorder (53).

In addition, patients with schizotypal personality disorder show abnormalities and other attentional tasks. These include the Continuous Performance Task (CPT) and the Backward Masking Task (BMT). The CPT is a test of sustained attention that involves identifying target stimuli from a continually presented array. Poor performance on the CPT has been observed in studies of schizotypal volunteers, patients, and offspring of schizophrenic patients (53a) and is correlated with social detachment in offspring of schizophrenic patients (12). The BMT is a visual information processing task which has also been reported to be abnormal in patients with schizotypal personality disorders as well as in volunteers selected because of their schizotypal traits (36). Abnormalities in electroencephalographic (EEG) responses to an unexpected stimuli provide a measure of brain responses to an attentional paradigm. Such evoked potential studies suggest alterations in a positive wave at 300 msec following a stimulus (P300) in schizotypal volunteers and patients similar to those demonstrated in schizophrenic patients. Abnormalities in galvanic skin orienting response and visual reaction time similar to that observed in schizophrenic patients also suggest altered information processing in schizotypal individuals (53a).

Imaging studies suggest that there may be increased ventricular size in the schizophrenia-related personality disorders (5). In one study, lateral ventricles were enlarged (particularly on the left side), and enlargement of the frontal horn and ventricle was associated with impaired performance on the Wisconsin Card Sort Test. In contrast, no such abnormalities have been found in patients with borderline personality disorder (53a). In exploratory analyses, increased ventricular size was associated with reduced concentrations of plasma HVA and deficit-like symptoms (53a), raising the possibilities that frontal cortical impairment may be associated with increased ventricular size and hypodopaminergia in this area. Also consistent with this possibility are magnetic resonance imaging (MRI) studies suggesting reduced frontal size correlated with schizotypal traits in volunteer subjects (44).

Schizotypal personality disorder patients or volunteers, like schizophrenic patients, also demonstrate impaired performance on tests sensitive to prefrontal function, including the Wisconsin Card Sort Test (WCST) (44,53a). On the other hand, performance on the verbal fluency test and Wechsler Adult Intelligence Scale (WAIS) vocabulary and block design that does not significantly differ from normal controls suggests that cortical impairment is not global and may be more selective for brain circuits including frontal and perhaps temporal regions.

Poor performance on the WCST as reflected in increased preseverative errors, as well as poor performance on the Trails B Test, tends to be associated with reduced concentrations of plasma HVA, the primary metabolite of dopamine in the brain (53a). Furthermore, increased ventricular size tends also to be associated with decreased concentrations of plasma HVA. In personality disorder patients, plasma HVA shows a trend to be negatively related to the deficit-like symptoms; that is, reduced concentrations of plasma HVA are related to increased social withdrawal and constricted affect (53a). A significant correlation between deficit-like symptoms and plasma HVA has been reported in relatives of schizophrenic patients with schizotypal traits (Amin et al., 1993, *unpublished data*). These results contrast with clinical studies suggesting that increases in plasma HVA are correlated with the psychotic-like symptoms of schizotypal personality disorder.

Together, these findings suggest that schizotypal personality-disordered patients, particularly those with deficit-like symptoms, are characterized by impairment on a variety of cortical processing tasks, increased ventricular size, and reduced indices of dopaminergic activity. Because the dopamine system is implicated in working memory via D1 receptors in frontal cortex, it is tempting to speculate that the cortical dysfunction (in areas such as prefrontal cortex) associated with reduced dopaminergic function may contribute to the "core" deficit-related psychopathology of the schizophrenia spectrum. Other factors must modify this core diathesis in the direction of chronic psychosis for true schizophrenia to emerge. Schizotypal patients with prominent deficit-like symptoms may, however, represent the most common expression of a genetic susceptibility to a neurodevelopmental lesion which results in cortical malfunction.

PSYCHOPHARMACOLOGY OF DEFICIT SYMPTOMS

If the theory discussed above is correct, deficits in cortical function and associated social deficits might be improved with administration of agents that enhance dopa-

minergic activity. Preliminary data from our laboratory suggests that amphetamine may improve cognitive performance on tests sensitive to prefrontal function (such as the WCST) in schizotypal patients (53a). Therapeutic trials with dopamine reuptake inhibitors such as mazindole, psychostimulants, L-DOPA, or monoamine oxidase (MAO) inhibitors might be warranted. Also intriguing is the possibility that selective D_1 agonists, when they become clinically available, might more selectively enhance cognitive function in such patients. If, as correlational analyses hint, social deficits are also related to these underlying cognitive impairments, these strategies may improve the interpersonal functioning of the withdrawn, schizophrenia spectrum personality-disordered patients.

PSYCHOBIOLOGY OF IMPULSIVE/ AGGRESSIVE BEHAVIORS

Impulsivity is a defining feature of borderline personality disorder and is prominent as well in antisocial personality disorder and, to a lesser degree, in histrionic and narcissistic personality disorders. Impulsive personality disorder patients are likely to act without reflecting, particularly when it comes to the expression of aggression. They are more easily irritated and are more likely to engage in assaultive behavior, substance abuse, self-damaging acts, and promiscuity. Their impulsive traits may account for the instability of relationships in these patients and their tendencies toward dramatic presentations of themselves. In this cluster of personality disorders, the impulsivity may be differently expressed in the various disorders. For example, in the borderline personality disordered patient, impulsivity is coupled with affective instability such that the patient often reacts with impulsive or aggressive action to the dysphoria engendered by a loss or separation. Such patients frequently present as depressed or feeling abandoned following the dissolution of a relationship. In contrast, antisocial personality disordered patients are much less likely to have affective instability, and their antisocial and aggressive behaviors are fairly persistent and more likely to result in their being seen in a forensic setting rather than in a psychiatric clinic.

Impulsivity as a personality trait appears to be partially heritable. Studies of twins reared apart suggest that impulsivity in healthy, nonpsychiatric populations may be heritable (8). Twin studies of patients with borderline personality disorder also suggest that impulsivity may be partially inherited, although the diagnosis of borderline personality disorder itself is not (66). While individuals with borderline personality disorder may aggregate in families, the core features of impulsivity and affective instability appear to independently aggregate in relatives of borderline patients and may thus combine to provide the susceptibility to borderline personality disorder (55).

The presence of a heritable substrate for impulsivity raises the possibility that biologic correlates of impulsivity might be identified.

Neuromodulators that play a role in stimulating and inhibiting external behavior are likely candidates for biologic systems that underlie impulsivity and/or aggression. The serotonergic system, which serves as a behavioral inhibitory system, has been increasingly implicated in the biology of these behavioral traits. In addition, impulsivity and/or aggression in personality-disordered patients may be associated with the presence of epileptiform disorders, attentional disorders, and elevated levels of circulating testosterone and/or endorphins.

Abnormalities of the serotonin are perhaps the most well-documented findings in relation to impulsive aggression and personality disorder patients. Studies in the rodent suggest that lesions of serotonergic neurons result in disinhibited aggression (6). Agents that enhance serotonergic activity can reverse this aggressive behavior as well as inhibit spontaneous or induced aggression. In primates, individual differences in serotonin activity as indexed by concentrations of CSF 5-hydroxyindoleacetic acid (5-HIAA) appear to be heritable and associated with aggressive, dominant behavior (20).

Reductions in indices of central 5-HT function are also seen in humans with impulsive aggression, whether directed towards the self (e.g., suicide attempt) or against others (3). Reduced indices of presynaptic serotonergic activity including CSF concentrations of 5-HIAA have been reported in depressed patients who have made suicide attempts or who have engaged in parasuicidal behavior (9). Furthermore, serotonin and its metabolites are decreased in postmortem studies of the brains of suicide victims regardless of diagnosis (9).

Neuroendocrine challenge studies also suggest that central serotonergic activity is reduced in personality disorder patients with impulsive aggression. Prolactin responses to fenfluramine (both d,l- and d-stereoisomer forms) are blunted in personality disorder patients, specifically borderline (11) and antisocial (39) personality disorder patients. In three studies, a negative correlation has been demonstrated between the prolactin response to d,l-fenfluramine (11), m-CPP (38), and buspirone (10) and inventories of irritability and aggression in patients with personality disorder. These studies provide support for the hypothesis that decreased serotonin activity is associated with aggression and impulsive behavior in patients with personality disorders. They raise the possibility, reviewed later, that selective serotonin reuptake inhibitors might ameliorate impulsive aggression in such patients.

In contrast to serotonin, the noradrenergic system may play a facilitatory role in promoting impulsivity and aggression. In preclinical studies, the noradrenergic system, with nerve cell bodies located in the locus coeruleus, plays a major role in the regulation of arousal and responsiveness to the environment. While increased activity of the locus coeruleus is associated with reactivity to novel and particularly threatening stimuli (2), decreased locus coeruleus activity has been documented during self-restitutive or vegetative activity such as eating, self-grooming, and sleeping. Heightened noradrenergic activity may be associated with increased irritable aggression (62), whereas a social withdrawal, such as is observed in separation of an infant primate from its mother, seems to be associated with decreased noradrenergic activity (35). Heightened noradrenergic activity may then be related to enhanced sensitivity or reactivity to stimuli in the environment, whereas reductions in noradrenergic activity appear to be more associated with withdrawal from the environment and restitutive functions.

These clinical observations are consistent with studies of noradrenergic abnormalities in the clinical arena. For example, reductions in the responsiveness of the noradrenergic system as indicated by responses to noradrenergic challenges such as clonidine are observed in patients with major depressive disorder, particularly those with endogenous depression (50). A hyporeactive noradrenergic system may thus be related to the disengagement from the environment observed in the patient with autonomous or endogenous depression, particularly with symptoms of withdrawal, psychomotor disturbance, and reduced concentration.

Conversely, increased engagement and reactivity to the environment seems to be associated with enhanced noradrenergic activity in clinical studies. For example, gamblers evidence increased arousal and enhanced noradrenergic activity associated with risk-taking, boredom, susceptibility, and sensation-seeking (47). Similarly, an augmented growth-hormone response to clonidine is positively correlated with scores on the irritability subscale of the Buss–Durkee Hostility Inventory (10). In a larger overlapping sample of personality-disordered patients, presynaptic measures of noradrenergic activity such as plasma norepinephrine were positively correlated with risk-taking and total scores on the Barratt Impulsivity Scale (BIS), and growth-hormone responses to clonidine were associated with irritability and verbal hostility on the BDHI (67). Thus, a heightened responsiveness of the noradrenergic system might contribute to the increased sensitivity and reactivity of personality-disordered patients with impulsivity and affective instability such as may be observed in those with "dramatic cluster" diagnoses. Agents that stabilize or reduce noradrenergic activity might be expected to partially improve irritability and reactivity in these patients.

An etiologic role for epileptiform activity in the limbic system in patients with personality disorder is suggested by some preliminary data related to (a) the presence of certain EEG abnormalities in patients with borderline personality disorder and (b) the response of dyscontrol behaviors to anticonvulsant medications (14; see below). Attention-deficit hyperactivity disorders (ADHDs) are associated with impulsivity and may persist into adulthood. The decrease in impulsivity and irritability in adults with ADHD in response to treatment with stimulants (70) suggests that some irritable impulsive patients may have an underlying adult ADHD syndrome. Finally, there are limited data which suggest that elevated testosterone (free, not total) and endorphin levels may play a contributing role in aggressive (1) and self-injurious behaviors (27), respectively.

PSYCHOPHARMACOLOGY OF IMPULSIVE AGGRESSIVE TRAITS AND BEHAVIORS

Our current understanding of these traits and behaviors suggests a number of potential treatment strategies. Evidence of a reduction in central 5-hydroxytryptamine (5-HT) neurotransmission suggests that impulsive aggressive behavior may be treated with agents which enhance 5-HT in the brain. Open-label clinical trials with fluoxetine in patients with a primary Axis II diagnosis of borderline personality disorder (7) provide evidence that these agents may be effective in reducing impulsive aggression. Effective doses in studies to date have ranged from 20 to 80 mg p.o. q.d., and positive effects have been reported to occur within the first week or within the first month of treatment (8) studies. Unfortunately, none of these studies were placebo-controlled, and the clinical presentations of the patients were varied. However, because impulsive aggressive behavior is intermittent and sensitive to environmental provocation, placebo-controlled trials of adequate duration and careful behavioral monitoring are required. Future studies need to assess the effect of 5-HT uptake inhibitors in patients who do not have comorbid disorders that are also responsive to these medications (e.g., major depression, obsessive–compulsive disorder). It is currently difficult to assess whether gains in impulsive aggressive behavior associated with treatment with fluoxetine have been due to a primary effect of the drug or occurred through a more primary effect on comorbid diagnoses such as depression or obsessive–compulsive disorder. Studies with some of the newer selective 5-HT uptake inhibitors have yet to be reported.

Other agents with putative antiaggressive properties include lithium, beta-adrenergic antagonists, carbamazepine (and other anticonvulsants), neuroleptics, stimulants, and opiate antagonists. While not all of these agents have been studied specifically in personality-disordered patients, specifically, all have demonstrated some efficacy in disorders associated with impulsive aggressive behavior.

As of this date, lithium carbonate is the only agent which has been shown in a blind placebo-controlled study to diminish the frequency of impulsive aggressive behaviors in individuals with probable antisocial personality disorder. In a landmark study, a 3-month treatment trial of lithium carbonate was associated with a cessation of

impulsive aggressive behavior in a group of prison inmates (49). Blind crossover to placebo, at the end of 3 months of treatment, resulted in a return to the baseline frequency of these behaviors. While these individuals would most likely be diagnosed with antisocial personality disorder, only acts of impulsive aggressive behavior were affected by the lithium treatment. These results suggest that other aspects of antisocial personality disorder related to "conning" or "disregard for the rights of others" may not be affected by lithium. The mechanism of lithium carbonate's antiaggressive action has been proposed to be secondary to its putative ability to increase 5-HT neurotransmission. However, lithium treatment enhanced prolactin responses to intravenous tryptophan, a measure of serotonin responsiveness, only at 1 week in normal controls and not at all in depressed patients, raising questions regarding serotonergic mechanisms (42). It is also possible that lithium's effect of dampening catecholaminergic function (4) plays a role in its antiaggressive properties observed in antisocial personality-disordered patients.

Beta-adrenergic antagonists (e.g., propranolol, pindolol) have also been shown to have antiaggressive properties in patients with a variety of diagnoses (although no studies have been reported in patients with primary diagnoses of personality disorder). In general, high doses of these agents are necessary to produce an antiaggressive effect. The mechanism of action for this effect is also unclear, although antagonism at beta-noradrenergic sites and possible agonism (especially at the higher doses usually employed) at 5-HT$_1$ receptors raise the possibility that these agents may work through both noradrenergic and serotonergic mechanisms. It is also possible, however, that these agents also work through a peripheral mechanism, either in concert with a central mechanism or exclusive of one. Consistent with this possibility, nadolol, a beta-adrenergic antagonist which does not cross the blood–brain barrier, has also been reported to have antiaggressive efficacy in violent individuals (73).

Carbamazepine treatment has been associated with a striking, and significant, reduction in the severity of episodic dyscontrol in a study of a small group of well-diagnosed female patients with DSM-III borderline personality disorder (14). In this sample, episodic dyscontrol (i.e., worst episode) was rated as moderate or severe in only 10% of cases, whereas placebo treatment was associated with episodic dyscontrol of moderate or severe intensity in 60% of cases. In addition to carbamazepine, diphenylhydantoin has been reported to decrease "anger," "irritability," "impatience," and "anxiety" in neurotic (DSM-II diagnosed) psychiatric outpatients (60). While it is not known how many of these patients would meet DSM-III criteria for a personality disorder, it is noteworthy that most patients entered into this trial were characterized by prominent histories of hostility and/or anxiety. The mechanism of action for the antiaggressive effect of these anticonvulsive agents is unknown, although it may involve stabilization of limbic neuronal discharges. Abnormal EEG patterns, similar to those seen in patients with partial complex seizures, have been reported for a small proportion of borderline personality-disordered patients in some, but not all (13), studies. It is possible that limbic excitability may underlie both the etiology and treatment responsiveness of some borderline personality-disordered patients to anticonvulsants. It is also possible that these anticonvulsive agents work partially through the central 5-HT system. Enhancement of the prolactin responses to intravenous tryptophan challenge during carbamazepine treatment has been reported, suggesting that carbamazepine may enhance 5-HT activity in humans (15).

The efficacy of neuroleptics in the treatment of impulsive aggressive behavior is likely to be associated with its effect on dopamine receptors. Low-dose high-potency neuroleptic agents have been shown to have modest efficacy in several placebo-controlled studies (17,57) involving the use of neuroleptics in the treatment of patients with personality disorder. In the most recent study of patients with borderline and/or schizotypal personality disorder, haloperidol's main effects were on observed measures of "hostile belligerence" and impulsive aggressive behaviors (56). In a placebo-controlled trial, treatment with the neuroleptic flupenthixol was associated with a significant reduction in suicidal behavior in personality-disordered patients with histories of recurrent suicidal behavior (37). While these patients were not formally diagnosed as personality-disordered, most of these patients would have met DSM-III criteria for borderline personality disorder.

Finally, there are some limited, but noteworthy, data regarding the effect of stimulants and opiate antagonists on impulsivity and aggression. In a placebo-controlled study of adult patients with attention deficit disorder (ADD), the stimulant pemoline was shown to significantly decrease ratings of both "impulsivity" and "hot or explosive temper" (70). Reductions in these symptoms occurred in the context of similar improvement in ratings of "attention difficulties" and "hyperactivity," but not of "affective lability." While patients with "borderline" or schizotypal personality disorders were excluded from study, at least 27% met Research Diagnostic Criteria for antisocial personality disorder (definite or probable). In addition, all patients had at least two or three of the following six symptoms (i.e., in addition to either motor hyperactivity or attentional deficits persisting from childhood): impulsivity, hot or explosive temper, affective lability, impaired interpersonal relationships, stress intolerance, and inability to complete tasks. It is noteworthy that the first four of these criteria are found in the DSM-III criteria for borderline personality disorder. Because patients with borderline personality disorder were excluded, this suggests that "impulsivity" and/or "hot or

explosive temper" may respond to stimulant medication in the absence of a full personality-disorder diagnosis. These findings were generally replicated in another sample with the stimulant methylphenidate (71). Hence, it is possible that stimulant medication may be beneficial in treating impulsivity and irritability/anger when it occurs in the context of adult ADD. Studies with opiate antagonists in the treatment of self-injurious behavior in a variety of psychiatric patients, mostly with mental retardation, have met with mixed success (27) but may offer another avenue for research for pharmacologic intervention in very difficult patients with borderline personality disorder who cut or otherwise mutilate themselves.

Exacerbation of aggressive behavior may represent an unwanted side effect at some psychopharmacologic agents in personality-disordered patients. The tricyclic antidepressants (e.g., amitriptyline), MAO inhibitors (e.g., tranylcypromine), and alprazolam, all of which may be presented to patients with personality disorder, may increase aggressive behavior. Evidence of potential enhancement of impulsive aggressive behavior during treatment with tricyclic antidepressants in personality-disordered patients was first reported by Soloff et al. (58). Soloff and colleagues noted that borderline personality-disordered patients who had no global improvement during treatment with amitriptyline (i.e., "nonresponders," defined as having a global assessment improvement score after medication below the average for the entire sample) demonstrated increases in ratings of impulsive and aggressive behavior compared to patients who similarly had no global improvement during placebo treatment. This increase in impulsive aggressive behavior occurred in spite of isolated improvements in measures of depression and psychoticism in the amitriptyline "nonresponders" compared to the placebo "nonresponders." These findings suggest a dissociation between antidepressant and antiaggressive responses to amitriptyline in a subset of patients with borderline personality disorder. Amitriptyline "nonresponders" in this study had significantly higher pretreatment ratings of hostility, psychoticism, and negativism than did amitriptyline "responders" (58), raising the possibility that personality-disordered patients with these characteristics may be at more risk for increased impulsive aggressive behavior during treatment with tricyclic antidepressants. Increases in impulsive and/or aggressive behaviors have previously been reported in depressives during treatment with tricyclic agents (43). While tricyclic antidepressants may enhance serotonergic actively, they can also enhance noradrenergic activity. Given indications of a positive relationship between noradrenergic system function and hostility and/or impulsive aggression, it is possible that tricyclic antidepressants may augment these behaviors by enhancing noradrenergic system function. Increased aggression in patients with borderline personality disorder has also been reported during treatment with MAO inhibitors (14), although this phenomenon is not well-characterized.

An increase in the severity of episodic dyscontrol in borderline personality-disordered patients treated with alprazolam was first noted by Cowdry and Gardner (14) in their placebo-controlled multiple-drug crossover study. The effect was so robust that the treatment arm involving alprazolam was discontinued after the entry of only 12 patients into the trial. This phenomenon is currently understood to represent another example of how benzodiazepine-like agents can disinhibit some individuals (18). Accordingly, caution should probably be taken in prescribing this agent to personality-disordered patients with prominent histories of impulsive aggression.

PSYCHOBIOLOGY OF AFFECTIVE-RELATED TRAITS

Depressive symptoms can appear in any patient with a personality disorder. However, affective-related traits are a common part of the diagnostic picture for several of the personality disorders in the dramatic and the anxious cluster. Affective instability characterizes one of the DSM-III criteria for borderline personality disorder, while exaggerated displays of emotion and rapidly shifting emotions characterize two of the DSM-III criteria for histrionic personality disorder. Rejection sensitivity, a trait often associated with depressive symptoms, characterizes two of the DSM-III criteria for dependent personality disorder and one for avoidant personality disorder. The clinical picture of a depressive syndrome in a patient with personality disorder offers a diagnostic challenge that is often difficult to resolve. Specifically, some personality-disordered patients presenting with depressive symptoms appear to have a type of "environmentally sensitive" affective disturbance that is part of their usual personality profile, whereas others appear to have a more sustained and discrete depressive syndrome indistinguishable from major depression.

Familial relationships have been noted between some personality-disordered patients (i.e., those with borderline personality disorder) and major mood disorder. However, recent data suggest that the relationship may be secondary to comorbid major depression in the personality-disordered probands. In recent studies (55) the familial relationship between borderline personality disorder and depression was attributed to the presence of major mood disorder in the proband itself. Family members of borderline personality-disordered patients without histories of depression had the same morbid risk of depression as did other personality-disordered patients without histories of depression. In contrast, family members of patients with borderline personality disorder had an elevated morbid risk of impulsive personality disorder traits and affective personality disorder traits (55). Individuals with impulsive personality disorder traits were characterized as having at least three of the following symptoms chronically: physical fighting with others, not associated with alcohol; nonpremeditated stealing (e.g., shoplifting); problems with drinking or drugs; binge eating; problems with gambling; sexual promiscuity; self-damaging acts (e.g., wrist-slashing etc.); and irrational angry outbursts, or overreaction to minor events, not associated with alcohol. Individuals with affective personality disorder traits were characterized as having either (a) a chronic dysphoria (e.g., depression, anxiety) or (b) fluctuations in mood not associated with highly severe mood disturbances, psychomotor agitation or retardation, psychotic features, or extreme guilt. In addition, these individuals had at least one of the following symptoms chronically: easily disappointed or self-pitying; low self-esteem; pessimistic attitude; and absence of satisfactory intimate relationships (55). These results suggest that a familial relationship exists between borderline personality disorder and personality disorder traits consistent more with the core features of borderline personality disorder (i.e., impulsivity, affective lability) than with major syndromal mood disorder.

Abnormally high rates of nonsuppression of plasma cortisol following dexamethasone has been reported in some, but not all, studies of patients with borderline personality disorder (28). Over all studies, rates of dexamethasone nonsuppression ranged from 9% to 73%. This difference in rates of dexamethasone nonsuppression appeared to be attributable to the presence of a comorbid diagnosis of major depression in most of these studies. In the studies where comorbidity of major depression is low, the rates of dexamethasone nonsuppression are correspondingly low. The same conclusion can be drawn from data from studies utilizing thyrotropin-releasing hormone (TRH) stimulation testing (33) in patients with borderline personality or other personality disorders (24). Two studies have reported elevated rates of blunted thyrotropin-stimulating hormone (TSH) in small samples of patients with DSM-III borderline personality disorder. Blunted TSH responses to TRH were 38–47% in borderline patients compared to 0–9% in healthy controls. The comorbidity of major depression or alcoholism (either of which can be associated with a blunted TSH response to TRH) in these samples, however, was between 80% and 100%, making a specific association between blunted TSH responses to TRH and borderline personality disorder unlikely. The most recent study investigating personality disorders of all types found no difference in the rate of TSH blunting or in the absolute magnitude of TSH responses to TRH in personality-disordered patients compared to healthy controls (24). These data suggest that abnormalities in TSH responses to TRH stimulation in patients with personality disorder are attributable to the presence of a comorbid diagnosis of depression or alcoholism and not to the personality disorder itself.

Other strategies designed to find biologic correlates of mood disorder in personality-disordered patients have met with mixed results. Growth-hormone responses to clonidine challenge, an index of central alpha-2 noradrenergic receptor sensitivity, in personality-disordered patients tend to be similar to those seen in healthy volunteers (10). This is in contrast to the reduction in growth-hormone responses to clonidine that are observed in depressed patients in either the acute-depressed or the remitted-euthymic state (54). Moreover, growth-hormone responses to clonidine in personality-disordered patients and healthy volunteers were correlated with irritability, not depression (10). Similarly, prolactin responses to d,l-fenfluramine challenge do not seem to discriminate personality-disordered patients with current (or past) history of depression from those who have never met criteria for depression (11); again, correlations between prolactin responses to fenfluramine challenge were seen with irritability and assaultiveness, but not with depression.

It is possible that mood dysregulation or instability is related to a dysfunction of more than one neurotransmitter system including both norepinephrine or serotonin (53). For example, amphetamine challenge is associated with an improvement in global function (including mood) in a subgroup of patients with borderline personality disorder (48). Moreover, behavioral responses to amphetamine challenge may correlate with trait indices of affective lability (23). Neurochemical events triggered by amphetamine stimulation may more accurately reflect the biologic substrate associated with affective lability and dysregulation than stimulation by more selective neurotransmitter agents. This hypothesis also may explain why treatment of mood dysfunction with tricyclic antidepressants is often not successful in patients with personality disorder.

Finally, it is possible that cholinergic sensitivity may play an important role in the mood dysregulation seen in many patients with personality disorder. An extensive body of evidence suggests that increased cholinergic receptor responsiveness may be associated with major depressive disorder (21). Physostigmine, an acetylcholinesterase inhibitor, and arecoline, a muscarinic agonist, both of which increase the signal at postsynaptic cholinergic receptors, induce a behavioral syndrome resembling depression in animals (21), acute and remitted depressed patients, and normal volunteers (21). Furthermore, these agents appear to have antimanic properties. These results raise the possibility that enhanced cholinergic receptor sensitivity may be associated with a broader sensitivity to dysphoria. In fact, in normal males, dysphoric responses to physostigmine correlate with traits of irritability and emotional lability (16).

Consistent with these studies, studies of rapid eye movement (REM) latency, partially modulated by cholinergic activity, suggest that borderline personality-disordered patients share disturbances in REM regulation with major depressive disorder. Borderline personality-disordered patients have been reported to have both decreased and more variable REM latency when compared to normal controls, and in a preliminary study they demonstrated exaggerated reduction in REM latency in response to a cholinomimetic agent. Preliminary studies suggest that personality-disordered patients with prominent affective instability, particularly borderline personality-disordered patients, have a significantly greater dysphoric response to the acetyl cholinesterase physostigmine than do patients with other personality disorder (59). The extent of the dysphoric response in this study as measured by the Profile of Mood States (POMS) was correlated with baseline affective instability. Therefore, it is possible that enhanced responsiveness of cholinergic receptors may play a role in the susceptibility to affective shifts observed in Cluster B personality disorders, such as borderline or histrionic personality disorder.

PSYCHOPHARMACOLOGY OF AFFECTIVE-RELATED TRAITS

Clinical trials designed to specifically treat depression in patients with personality disorders have tested the efficacy of standard psychotropic medications in patients with borderline and/or schizotypal personality disorder. In general, most medications which have been tested demonstrate some efficacy on measures related to state depression. These medications include chlorpromazine and loxapine (29), thiothixine (17), haloperidol (56,57), amitriptyline (57), imipramine (32), phenelzine (19,40), and tranylcypromine (14). In most studies, improvements in state depression in personality-disordered patients have been minimal to modest in studies involving neuroleptics and tricyclic antidepressants and modestly robust in some studies involving MAO inhibitors.

Of the MAO inhibitors, phenelzine has been the most extensively evaluated of the MAO inhibitors. In the pre-DSM-III era, phenelzine was reported to be globally efficacious in treating a subset of patients with pseudoneurotic schizophrenia (19). This diagnostic categorization describes patients characterized by the triad of pananxiety, panphobias, and chaotic sexuality but without psychosis or major depression. With regard to DSM-III Axis II disorders, this picture comes closest to that of patients falling into the Dramatic and/or Anxiety Cluster of personality disorders. A retrospective study comparing imipramine with phenelzine found that the response rate of atypical depressives with comorbid borderline personality disorder treated with phenelzine was nearly three times as great (89% versus 31%) as the response rate achieved with imipramine. In contrast, the efficacy of phenelzine in atypical depressives without borderline personality disorder was equal to that of imipramine (56% versus 57%;) (40). Despite this earlier literature, phenelzine was reported to be remarkably ineffective in treating state depression in the only prospective placebo-controlled study of phenelzine treatment in patients with borderline and/or schizotypal personality disorder (56). In this study, phenelzine was ineffective as an antidepressant in treating both the typical and atypical signs and symptoms of depression. Two reasons for the negative finding in the study of Soloff and colleagues may relate to differences in the patient selection and in the maximal phenelzine dose. First, patients in this study were inpatients with primary entry diagnoses of borderline or schizotypal personality disorder (less than half with a diagnosis of atypical depression), whereas patients in the previous studies were outpatients with a primary entry diagnosis of atypical depression. Second, the phenelzine dose administered in the Soloff study was probably lower than that administered in either of the previous studies. The average phenelzine dose in this study was 60 mg p.o. q.d., whereas that in the previous studies was higher (i.e., nonresponding patients received 90 mg p.o. q.d. of phenelzine after 4 weeks of treatment). In addition, treatment was 6 weeks or longer in the previous studies, and this may also have affected the response rates. The relatively high frequency of adverse events occurring in the personality-disordered patients prevented phenelzine doses from being raised much above 60 mg p.o. q.d.; only 18% of patients received doses as high as 75 mg p.o. q.d. In spite of the differences between the studies, the absence of efficacy for phenelzine in a well-defined sample of hospitalized personality-disordered patients suggests that phenelzine may not be an efficacious treatment in moderately to severely impaired patients with personality disorder.

Unlike phenelzine, tranylcypromine treatment was associated with a significant antidepressant/mood-enhancing effect in a small group of treatment-resistant females with borderline personality disorder (14). In this prospective comparison of tranylcypromine to carbamazepine, it was reported that trifluoperazine, alprazolam, and placebo treatment with tranylcypromine resulted in significantly greater improvement in self-rated assessments of mood (14). While this is yet to be replicated, it is possible that tranylcypromine's mood-enhancing effect was partly due to its amphetamine-like structure and pharmacologic effects. This hypothesis is supported by preliminary data demonstrating that some patients with borderline personality disorder have a marked mood-enhancing response to amphetamine challenge (48).

5-HT uptake inhibitors may also treat the depression seen in patients with personality disorder, specifically borderline personality disorder. However, all published data at this time are based on open-label trials (7). All three reports available suggest that fluoxetine is efficacious in treating state depression as well as other behavioral (e.g., obsessive–compulsive, impulsive) features which can respond to these agents.

Clinical trials designed to specifically treat affective lability have been few. The first placebo-controlled trial in this area compared chlorpromazine to imipramine in a group of patients with "emotionally unstable character disorder" (25). Affective lability in these patients was characterized as rapid autonomous (rather than reactive) shifts in mood. In addition, these patients displayed chronic personality traits such as difficulty with authority, job instability, and problems in interpersonal relations. Both chlorpromazine and imipramine were associated with positive outcomes compared to placebo, although there was clear superiority for chlorpromazine in these patients. Notably, the clinical responses of a subset of imipramine-treated patients was characterized by an increase in anger during the trial (see above discussion regarding tricyclic antidepressants and impulsive aggression). A second placebo-controlled trial with lithium as the experimental agent reported a decrease in the variability of mood in another group of emotionally unstable character-disordered patients (46). A more recent placebo-controlled study of lithium treatment in borderline personality disorder reported a trend for lithium over desipramine in terms of decreasing anger, but did not examine their data in terms of lithium's potential efficacy on mood instability. While limited, these data raise the possibility that other antimanic/anticonvulsant agents (e.g., carbamazepine) could be efficacious in reducing the affective instability of patients with borderline personality disorder, although one uncontrolled study of patients with emotionally unstable character disorder demonstrated no efficacy for the anticonvulsant, diphenylhydantoin (26). Finally, the efficacy of anticholinergic agents in treating affective instability remains to be tested.

PSYCHOBIOLOGY OF ANXIETY-RELATED TRAITS

The anxiety-related personality disorders include avoidant, dependent, obsessive–compulsive, and passive aggressive (now deleted from DSM-IV). All of these disorders share behavioral traits that may be related to a heightened susceptibility to anxiety and efforts to ward off potential anxiety. For example, patients with avoidant personality disorder have excessive anticipatory anxiety regarding the prospect of future rejection and thus avoid social interactions, while individuals with dependent personality disorder may submit to the wishes of others on whom they depend for fear of rejection or conflict. While there has been almost no systematic investigation into these specific personality disorders, there have been some studies of related or comorbid conditions such as social phobia. For example, the comorbidity of avoidant personality disorder and social phobia may be as high as 90% (72).

Family studies suggest familial transmission of "anxious" personality traits and disorders (45), while twin studies suggest significant heritability of social anxiety (65). Longitudinal studies of children suggest a stable dimension of fearfulness and inhibition (22). Thus, it is likely that at least social anxiety has a genetic basis with some longitudinal stability.

Otherwise, there is limited biologic data regarding social phobia/avoidant personality disorder. Clinical studies of hypothalamic–pituitary function suggest that neither the hypothalamic–adrenal (68) nor the hypothalamic–thyroid axis (63) of these patients differ from that of healthy volunteers. Preliminary results suggest enhanced responsiveness to serotonergic probes but not to adrenergic probes (64), suggesting potential increases of serotonin function associated with enhanced behavioral inhibition, but not noradrenergic system dysfunction. While lactate infusion is a potent stimulus of panic attacks in patients with panic disorder, it produces only inconsistent responses in patients with social phobia (31). One study has suggested decreased dopamine metabolism in social phobic patients (41), but this finding will require replication.

PSYCHOPHARMACOLOGY OF ANXIETY-RELATED PERSONALITY TRAITS

Little has been published which relates to the pharmacologic treatment of patients with anxiety-related personality disorders. Placebo-controlled, double-blind data are published documenting the efficacy of MAO inhibitors in the treatment of social phobia (30). Otherwise, there has been at least one open-label report suggesting that fluoxetine may be beneficial in the treatment of avoidant personality disorder/social phobia (61).

CONCLUSION

Research into the biologic and neuropsychopharmacologic correlates of behavioral and personality traits has produced many important insights which can aid the psychopharmacologist in the treatment of patients with personality disorders. First, there may be a heritable, biologic component to some selected personality and behavioral traits. Second, the efficacy of various psychotropic agents in treating the more extreme manifestations of these traits may be related to the specific psychopharmacologic properties of the agents (e.g., serotonin-enhancing, catecholamine-dampening properties of lithium) in question (7,56). Third, symptoms referable to different personality dimensions respond differentially to psychotropic agents within groups of patients with similar diagnoses (17,56,57) and within individuals (14). This latter phenomenon reflects the great biologic and clinical heterogeneity present in patients with DSM-III personality disorders.

These insights represent a clear advance in the psycho-

pharmacologic conceptualization of the personality disorders over the past few decades. Despite this, no definitive psychopharmacologic recommendations for specific groups of patients with personality disorders can be made at this time. Many more placebo-controlled clinical trials in well-defined (both clinically and biologically) patients with personality disorder will be required before such recommendations can be made in this area. A first step might be more placebo-controlled studies of agents which have already shown some promise in preliminary placebo-controlled trials (e.g., lithium, carbamazepine, tranylcypromine) of patients with personality disorder.

REFERENCES

1. Archer J. The influence of testosterone on human aggression. *Br J Psychology* 1991;82:1–28.
2. Aston-Jones G, Bloom FE. Norepinephrine-containing locus coeruleus neurons in behaving rats exhibit pronounced responses to nonnoxious environmental stimuli. *J Neurosci* 1981;1:887–890.
3. Brown GL, Ebert MH, Goyer PF, Jimerson DC, Klein WJ, Bunney WE, Goodwin FK. Aggression, suicide, and serotonin relationships to CSF metabolites. *Am J Psychiatry* 1982;139:741–745.
4. Bunney WE, Bunney-Garland BL. Mechanism of action of lithium in affective illness: basic and clinical implications. In: Meltzer NY, ed. *Psychopharmacology: third generation of progress.* New York: Raven Press, 1987;553–563.
5. Cazzullo CL, Vita A, Giobbio GM, Diecie M, Sacchetti E. Cerebral structured abnormalities in schizophreniform disorder in schizophrenia spectrum personality disorders. In: Tamminga CA, Schultz SC, eds. *Schizophrenia research. Advances in neuropsychiatry and psychopharmacology,* vol 1. New York: Raven Press, 1991;209–217.
6. Coccaro EF. Central serotonin in impulsive aggression. *Br J Psychiatry* 1989;155(S8):52–62.
7. Coccaro EF. Psychopharmacologic studies in patients with personality disorder: review and perspective. *J Pers Disord* 1993;7(Suppl):181–192.
8. Coccaro EF, Bergeman CS. Heritability of irritable impulsiveness: a study of twins reared together and apart. *Psychiatry Res* 1993;48:229–242.
9. Coccaro EF, Gabriel S, Siever LJ. Buspirone challenge: preliminary evidence for a role for 5-HT-la receptors in impulsive aggressive behavior in humans. *Psychopharmacol Bull* 1990;26:393–405.
10. Coccaro EF, Lawrence T, Trestman R, Gabriel S, Klar HM, Siever LJ. Growth hormone responses to intravenous clonidine challenge correlates with behavioral irritability in psychiatric patients and in healthy volunteers. *Psychiatry Res* 1991;39:129–139.
11. Coccaro EF, Siever LJ, Klar H et al. Serotonergic studies in patients with affective and personality disorders: correlates with suicidal and impulsive aggressive behavior. *Arch Gen Psychiatry* 1989;46:587–599.
12. Cornblatt BA, Lenzenweger MF, Dworkin RH, Erlenmeyer-Kimling L. Childhood attentional dysfunctions predict social deficits in unaffected adults at risk for schizophrenia. *Br J Psychiatry* 1992;161(Suppl 18):59–64.
13. Cornelius JR, Brenner RP, Soloff PH, Schulz SC, Tumuluru RV. EEG abnormalities in borderline personality disorder: specific or nonspecific. *Biol Psychiatry* 1986;21:977–980.
14. Cowdry RW, Gardner DL. Pharmacotherapy of borderline personality disorder: alprazolam, carbamazepine, trofluroperazine, and tranycypromine. *Arch Gen Psychiatry* 1988;45:111–119.
15. Elphick M, Yang JD, Cowen PJ. Effects of carbamazepine on dopamine- and serotonin-mediated neuroendocrine responses. *Arch Gen Psychiatry* 1990;47:135–140.
16. Fritze J, Sofic E, Muller T, Pfuller H, Lanczik M, Riederer P. Cholinergic–adrenergic balance, part 2: relationship between drug sensitivity and personality. *Psychiatry Res* 1990;34:271–279.

17. Goldberg SC, Schulz SC, Schulz PM, Resnick RJ, Hamer RM, Friedel RO. Borderline and schizotypal personality disorders treated with low-dose thiothixine versus placebo. *Arch Gen Psychiatry* 1986;43:680–686.

18. Hall RCW, Zisook S. Paradoxical reactions to benzodiazepines. *Br J Clin Pharmacol* 1981;11:99S–194S.

19. Hedberg DC, Hauch JH, Glueck BC. Tranylcypromine-trifluoperazine combination in the treatment of schizophrenia. *Am J Psychiatry* 1971;127:1141–1146.

20. Higley JD, Mehlman PT, Taub DM, Higley SB, Suomi SJ, Vickers JH, Linnoila M. Cerebrospinal fluid monoamine and adrenal correlates of aggression in free-ranging rhesus monkeys. *Arch Gen Psychiatry* 1992;49:436–441.

21. Janowsky DS, Risch CS. Role of acetylcholine mechanisms in the affective disorders. In: Meltzer HY, ed. *Psychopharmacology: the third generation of progress.* New York: Raven Press, 1987;527–534.

22. Kagan J, Reznick S, Snidman N, et al. Childhood derivatives of inhibition and lack of inhibition to the unfamiliar. *Child Dev* 1988;59:1580–1589.

23. Kavoussi RJ, Coccaro EF. The amphetamine challenge test correlates with affective lability in healthy volunteers. *Psychiatry Res* 1993;48:219–228.

24. Kavoussi RJ, Coccaro EF, Klar HM, Lesser J, Siever LJ. The TRH-stimulation test in DSM-III personality disorder. *Biol Psychiatry* 1993;34:234–239.

25. Klein DF. Psychiatric diagnosis and a typology of clinical drug effects. *Psychopharmacology* 1968;13:359–386.

26. Klein DF, Greenberg IM. Behavioral effects of diphenylhydantoin in severe psychiatric disorders. *Am J Psychiatry* 1967;124:847–849.

27. Konecki PE, Schulz SC. Rationale of clinical trials of opiate antagonists in treating patients with personality disorders and self-injurious behavior. *Psychopharmacol Bull* 1989;25:556–563.

28. Korzekwa M, Steiner M, Links P, Eppel A. The dexamethasone suppression test in borderlines: is it useful? *Can J Psychiatry* 1991;36:26–28.

29. Leone NF. Response of borderline patients to loxapine and chlorpromazine. *J Clin Psychiatry* 1982;43:148–150.

30. Liebowitz MR. Phenelzine versus atenolol in social phobia: a placebo controlled study. *J Clin Psychiatry* 1989;49:498–504.

31. Liebowitz MR, Fyer AJ, Gorman JM et al. Specificity of lactate infusions in social phobia versus panic disorder. *Am J Psychiatry* 1985;142:947–950.

32. Links PS, Steiner M, Boiago I, Irwin D. Lithium therapy for borderline patients: preliminary findings. *J Pers Dis* 1990;4:173–181.

33. Loosen PT, Prange AJ. Serum thyrotropin response to thyrotropin-releasing hormone in psychiatric patients. *Am J Psychiatry* 1982;139:405–415.

34. Losonczy MF, Song IS, Mohs RC, et al. Correlates of lateral ventricular size in chronic schizophrenia. II. Biological measures. *Am J Psychiatry* 1986;143:1113–1118.

35. McKinney WT, Moran EC, Kraemer GW. Separation in nonhuman primates as a model for human depression: neurobiological implications. In: Post RM, Ballenger JC, eds. *Neurobiology of mood disorders.* Baltimore: Williams & Wilkins, 1984;393–406.

36. Merritt RD, Balogh DW. Backward masking spatial frequency effects among hypothetically schizotypal individuals. *Schizophr Bull* 1989;15(4):573–583.

37. Montgomery SA, Montgomery D. Pharmacological prevention of suicidal behavior. *J Affective Dis* 1982;4:219–298.

38. Moss HB, Yao JK, Panzak GL. Serotonergic responsivity and behavioral dimensions in antisocial personality disorder with substance abuse. *Biol Psychiatry* 1990;28:325–338.

39. O'Keane V, Moloney E, O'Neill H, O'Connor A, Smith C, Dinan TG. Blunted prolactin responses to d-fenfluramine in sociopathy: evidence for subsensitivity of central serotonergic function. *Br J Psychiatry* 1992;160:643–646.

40. Parsons B, Quitkin FM, McGrath PJ. Phenelzine, imipramine, and placebo in borderline patients meeting criteria for atypical depression. *Psychopharmacol Bull* 1989;25:524–534.

41. Potts NLS, Davidson JRT. Social phobia: biological aspects and pharmacotherapy. *Prog Neuropsychopharmacol Biol Psychiatry* 1992;18:635–646.

42. Price LH, Charney DS, Delgado PL, Heninger GR. Lithium treatment and serotonergic function. Neuroendocrine and behavioral responses to intravenous tryptophan in affective disorders. *Arch Gen Psychiatry* 1989;46:13–19.

43. Rampling D. Aggression: a paradoxical response to tricyclic antidepressants. *Am J Psychiatry* 1978;135:117–118.

44. Raine A, Sheard C, Reynolds GP, Lencz T. Pre-frontal structural and functional deficits associated with individual differences in schizotypal personality. *Schizophr Res* 1992;7:237–247.

45. Reich JH. Avoidant and dependent personality traits in relatives of patients with panic disorder, patients with dependent personality disorder, and normal controls. *Psychiatry Res* 1991;39:89–98.

46. Rifkin A, Quitkin F, Curillo C, Blumberg AG, Klein DF. Lithium carbonate in emotionally unstable character disorders. *Arch Gen Psychiatry* 1972;27:519–523.

47. Roy A, DeJong J, Linnoila M. Extraversion in pathological gamblers: correlates with indices of noradrenergic function. *Arch Gen Psychiatry* 1989;46:679–681.

48. Schulz SC, Cornelius J, Schulz PM, Soloff PH. The amphetamine challenge test in patients with borderline personality disorder. *Am J Psychiatry* 1988;145:809–814.

49. Sheard M, Marini J, Bridges C, Wapner A. The effect of lithium on impulsive aggressive behavior in man. *Am J Psychiatry* 1976;133:1409–1413.

50. Siever LJ. The role of noradrenergic mechanisms in the etiology of the affective disorders. In: Meltzer HY, ed. *Psychopharmacology: the third generation of progress.* New York: Raven Press, 1987;493–504.

51. Siever LJ, Amin F, Coccaro EF, et al. Plasma homovanillic acid in schizotypal personality disorder. *Am J Psychiatry* 1991;148:1246–1248.

52. Siever LJ, Amin F, Coccaro EF, et al. Cerebrospinal fluid homovanillic acid in schizotypal personality disorder. *Am J Psychiatry* 1993;150:149–151.

53. Siever LJ, Davis KL. A psychobiological perspective on the personality disorders. *Am J Psychiatry* 1991;148:1647–1658.

53a. Siever LJ, Kalus OF, Keefe RS. The boundaries of schizophrenia. *Psychiatr Clin North Am* 1993;16:217–244.

54. Siever LJ, Trestman RL, Coccaro EF, et al. The growth hormone response to clonidine in acute and remitted depressed male patients. *Neuropsychopharmacology* 1992;6:165–177.

55. Silverman JM, Pinkhan L, Horvath TB, et al. Affective and impulsive personality disorder traits in the relatives of borderline personality disorder. *Am J Psychiatry* 1991;148:1378–1385.

56. Soloff PH, Cornelius JR, George A, Nathan RS, Schulz PM, Perel JM, Ulrich RF. Efficacy of phenelzine and haloperidol in borderline personality disorder. *Arch Gen Psychiatry* 1993;50:377–385.

57. Soloff PH, George A, Nathan RS, Schulz PM, Cornelius JR, Herring J, Perel JM. Amitriptyline versus haloperidol in borderlines: final outcomes and predictors of response. *J Clin Psychopharmacol* 1989;9:238–246.

58. Soloff PH, George A, Nathan RS, Schulz PM, Perel JM. Paradoxical effects of amitriptyline in borderline patients. *Am J Psychiatry* 1986;143:1603–1605.

59. Steinberg BJ, Trestman RL, Siever LJ. The cholinergic and noradrenergic neurotransmitter systems affective instability in borderline personality disorder. In: *Biological and neurobehavioral studies in borderline personality disorder.* American Psychiatric Press, in press.

60. Stephens JH, Schaffer JW. A controlled study of the effects of diphenylhydantoin on anxiety, irritability, and anger in neurotic outpatients. *Psychopharmacologia (Berlin)* 1970;17:169–181.

61. Sternbach HA. Fluoxetine treatment of social phobia. *J Clin Psychopharmacol* 1990;10:230.

62. Stolk JM, Conner RL, Levine S, Barchas JD. Brain norepinephrine metabolism and shock-induced fighting behavior in rats: differential effects of shock and fighting on the neurochemical response to a common footshock stimulus. *J Pharmacol Exp Ther* 1984;190:193–209.

63. Tancer ME, Stein MB, Gelernter CS, Uhde TW. The hypothalamic–pituitary–thyroid axis in social phobia. *Am J Psychiatry* 1990;147:929–933.

64. Tancer ME, Golden RN. A neuropharmacologic test of the tridimensional personality questionnaire in social phobia. *Biol Psychiatry* 1993;33:48A.

65. Torgerson AM, Kringlen E. Genetic aspects of temperamental differences in infants: a study of same-sexed twins. *J Am Acad Child Psychiatry* 1978;17:438–444.

66. Torgerson S. Genetic and nosological aspects of schizotypal and borderline personality disorders. *Arch Gen Psychiatry* 1984;41:546–554.

67. Trestman RL, Coccaro EF, Weston S, Mitropoulou V, Ramella F, Gabriel S, Siever LJ. Impulsivity, suicidal behavior, and major depression in the personality disorder: differential correlates with noradrenergic and serotonergic function. *Biol Psychiatry* 1992;31:68A.

68. Uhde TW, Tancer ME, Black B, Brown TM. Phenomenology and neurobiology of social phobia: comparison with panic disorder. *J Clin Psychiatry* 1991;52(11 Suppl):31–40.

69. van Kammen DP, Peters J, van Kammen WB. Cerebrospinal fluid studies of monoamine metabolism in schizophrenia. *Psychiatr Clin North Am* 1986;9:81–97.

70. Wender PH, Reimherr FW, Wood DR. Attention deficit disorder (minimal brain dysfunction) in adults. *Arch Gen Psychiatry* 1981;38:449–456.

71. Wender PH, Reimherr FW, Wood DR, Ward M. A controlled study of methylphenydate in the treatment of attention deficit disorder, residual type, in adults. *Am J Psychiatry* 1985;142:547–552.

72. Widiger TA. Generalized social phobia versus avoidant personality disorder: a commentary on three studies. *J Abnorm Psychol* 1992;101:340–343.

73. Yudofsky SC, Silver JM, Schneider SE. Pharmacologic treatment of aggression. *Psychiatr Ann* 1987;17:397–406.

Psychopharmacology: The Fourth Generation of Progress, edited by Floyd E. Bloom and David J. Kupfer. Raven Press, Ltd., New York © 1995.

CHAPTER 136

Psychopharmacology of Anorexia Nervosa, Bulimia Nervosa, and Binge Eating

B. Timothy Walsh and Michael J. Devlin

Disturbances of human eating behavior have been recognized as an appropriate focus of clinical intervention for centuries. Anorexia nervosa was clearly described as a syndrome in the late 19th century, and, in the over 100 years since, an impressive variety of behavioral and pharmacological interventions have been suggested, ranging from psychoanalysis to lobotomy, and including most of the pharmacological agents employed in psychiatry. In 1980, with the promulgation of DSM-III, an additional eating disorder—that of bulimia, now known as bulimia nervosa—was recognized. This recognition helped prepare the way for a number of important treatment studies, including trials of pharmacological interventions, in the last 15 years. With the advent of DSM-IV, another eating disorder, binge eating disorder, has been tentatively recognized and is likely to be a focus of psychological and pharmacological treatment research in the next decade.

This chapter will review our knowledge of the effectiveness of pharmacological interventions for these three disturbances of human eating behavior, and it will emphasize studies which have appeared since the publication of the *Psychopharmacology: Third Generation of Progress.* Much of the work in this time has focused on the treatment of bulimia nervosa and has clearly established the short-term efficacy of antidepressant medication in the treatment of this syndrome. Unfortunately, progress has not been as great in the treatment of anorexia nervosa. Work concerning binge eating disorder is just beginning.

PSYCHOPHARMACOLOGY OF ANOREXIA NERVOSA

In conceptualizing the psychopharmacological treatment of anorexia nervosa, it is useful to keep in mind the chronicity of its course in many patients (30). Treatment could theoretically include interventions at a number of different stages of the illness: preemptive treatment aimed at preventing disease onset in high-risk individuals, acute treatment emphasizing weight gain, treatment immediately following weight gain aimed at preventing relapse, and long-term maintenance treatment.

The *Third Generation of Progress* reviewed our knowledge of the efficacy of pharmacological interventions for anorexia nervosa in 1987 (40). At that time, virtually all published studies concerned treatment in the acute weight gain phase, usually given on an inpatient basis. While anecdotal case reports enthusiastically described impressive responses to a variety of pharmacological interventions, only a small number of controlled trials had been carried out, and these generally yielded negative or equivocal results. Unfortunately, in the ensuing 7 years, little additional information has become available. There are probably several reasons for the dearth of studies. First, over the last quarter century, a number of specialized eating disorder units have been established, and the experience of these units indicates that most patients with anorexia nervosa can achieve adequate weight gain during inpatient behavioral treatment. Most of the controlled trials reviewed in the *Third Generation of Progress* attempted to evaluate whether the addition of medication to structured inpatient treatment conferred any additional benefit. The fact that patients with anorexia nervosa can be, perhaps not easily, but nonetheless successfully, treated acutely on specialized units without the use of medication and the failure of controlled trials to suggest

B. T. Walsh and M. J. Devlin: Department of Clinical Psychiatry, Columbia University College of Physicians and Surgeons, New York, New York 10032; and Eating Disorders Unit, New York State Psychiatric Institute, New York, New York 10032.

impressive additional benefit from the use of medication have tended to focus the attention of investigators away from inpatient studies of acute weight gain treatment. Instead, interest is growing in the efficacy of psychopharmacological treatment in the prevention of relapse among weight-restored patients. There have as yet been no studies concerning the role of psychopharmacology in prevention of onset of the illness or in long-term maintenance of remission.

MEDICATION IN THE ACUTE WEIGHT GAIN PHASE

Studies of the use of antipsychotic medications in anorexia nervosa were based theoretically on evidence that feeding is, in part, mediated by dopaminergic neurons (5), and they were based clinically on the observation that these medications tend to produce weight gain. A series of early studies (11,13) reported that chlorpromazine, sometimes in combination with insulin to further stimulate hunger, produced more rapid weight gain and earlier hospital discharge. However, unwanted side effects included the onset of binge eating and seizures, and follow-up studies showed no benefit (14). Placebo-controlled studies of the higher-potency antipsychotics pimozide (55) and sulpiride (54) provided little evidence of clinical utility. Therefore, although particular patients may benefit from treatment with antipsychotic medications, existing studies do not support their routine use. As one might expect, long-term antipsychotic therapy in patients with anorexia nervosa, as in other patients, can lead to the development of tardive dyskinesia (10).

Studies of antidepressants were based on the observed comorbidity of eating and affective disorders and on the observation that semistarvation in previously healthy individuals produces depressive symptoms (23). Controlled trials of antidepressants, including clomipramine in low dosage (12,36) and amitriptyline (6,28), failed to provide compelling evidence for their clinical utility during the weight gain phase. Interestingly, weight gain even without pharmacological intervention produces an improvement in depressive symptoms (9,16), and animal work suggests that starvation may inhibit responsiveness to antidepressants (51). Earlier case reports, summarized in the *Third Generation of Progress,* suggest that individual patients may benefit from tricyclic antidepressants but tend to tolerate them poorly, and more recent case reports (20,27) suggest that the selective serotonin reuptake inhibitor fluoxetine may be useful. An open study of the antidepressant levoprotiline suggests improvement in various symptoms characteristic of anorexia nervosa (18). A small controlled study has suggested that lithium may enhance weight gain in inpatients with anorexia nervosa (26), but this has not been replicated.

Other clinical trials have utilized various agents that are thought to directly influence neurotransmitter systems involved in feeding behavior (see Chapter 138, *this volume*). The antihistaminic antiserotonergic orexigenic agent cyproheptadine has been studied in three controlled trials (25,28,56). The results suggest that although most inpatients do not benefit greatly from the addition of cyproheptadine, the drug may have some utility in more severely ill patients (25) and in nonbulimic anorectic patients, whereas in bulimic anorectic patients it may actually detract from clinical response (28). A small controlled crossover trial of the alpha-2 agonist clonidine, which is known to increase feeding behavior in several animal species including primates, showed no clinical benefit in patients with anorexia nervosa (8). Several case and small series reports summarized in the *Third Generation of Progress* (40) suggest that a variety of agents ranging from adrenocorticotropic hormone (ACTH) to zinc may enhance either the rate or the ease of weight gain, but there have been no controlled studies.

Medication in the Prevention of Relapse

The most innovative approach to the psychopharmacology of anorexia nervosa since the publication of the *Third Generation of Progress* has been the idea that psychotropic medications might be useful in the post-weight-gain phase—for example, for patients who have gained to their target weight, are about to leave the hospital, and are therefore at risk of relapse. Based on several lines of evidence suggesting the involvement of serotonergic systems in the pathophysiology of eating disorders, investigators, in particular the Pittsburgh group, have studied the selective serotonin reuptake inhibitor fluoxetine in weight-restored patients. Kaye et al. (33) have reported that of 31 anorexia nervosa patients who received fluoxetine for 11 ± 6 months following hospital discharge, 29 maintained their weight at or above 85 percent average body weight. Nonbulimic anorectics appeared to benefit more than bulimic anorectics. Although no data from placebo controlled double-blind trials have yet appeared, the open study data are encouraging and underscore the utility of further investigation of clinical interventions at times other than the acute weight gain phase.

Summary

The broadening of the sphere of inquiry to include the post-weight-gain phase of anorexia nervosa and continuing investigations of the biology of anorexia nervosa to provide a rational basis for identifying promising psychopharmacological interventions are encouraging developments. However, despite these new directions, the unfortunate fact is that little concrete progress has been made in the treatment of anorexia nervosa in the last decade. Follow-up studies indicate that for many patients hospitalized with anorexia nervosa, this illness has a chronic course with impressive morbidity and mortality. It would be surprising if biological interventions were eventually not found to be of use in the treatment of this syndrome, which is characterized by manifold biological disturbances. Additional effective interventions, perhaps at different points in the course of the illness, are sorely needed.

PSYCHOPHARMACOLOGY OF BULIMIA NERVOSA

Antidepressant Medication

Progress in establishing a scientific foundation for the treatment of bulimia nervosa has been much more rapid. In the early 1980s, as clinicians became more familiar with the features of this disorder, it was recognized that many individuals with bulimia nervosa were prone to mood disturbance. This observation led to open trials of antidepressant medication which were encouraging and which were promptly followed by placebo-controlled investigations. At the time of the publication of the *Third Generation of Progress,* the results of five double-blind, placebo-controlled trials of antidepressants in the treatment of bulimia nervosa were available. In the ensuing years, the results of an additional 13 trials have become available (see Table 1). Members of virtually all available

classes of antidepressants have been examined, including tricyclic antidepressants, monoamine oxidase (MAO) inhibitors, and selective serotonin reuptake inhibitors. The patients in these studies have, with few exceptions, been adult women of normal body weight who met DSM-IIIR criteria for bulimia nervosa, who regularly induced vomiting after binge eating, and who were treated on an outpatient basis. The controlled phase of these trials was generally of short duration, most commonly 8 weeks.

Several conclusions can be confidently reached on the basis of this work. First, antidepressant medication is more effective than placebo in the short-term treatment of bulimia nervosa. This finding is supported by virtually all the trials in Table 1. It is of note that most of the studies that failed to find a statistically significant difference between active medication and placebo were ones in which the response to placebo was considerable. In other words, the improvement on antidepressant medication was usually modest and, with the small number of subjects in many of the trials, was clearly distinguishable from improvement on placebo only when the latter was minimal.

Second, despite the number of agents that have been examined, there is no evidence that one antidepressant medication or one class of medication is dramatically more effective than another in the treatment of bulimia nervosa. This conclusion must be regarded with some

TABLE 1. *Summary of controlled outpatient trials of antidepressants in bulimia[a]*

Author	N	Design	Medication	Change in binge frequency (%)[b]		Remission (%)	
				Drug	Placebo	Drug	Placebo
Pope et al. (45)	19	Parallel	Imipramine[c]	−70.0	0.0	NR[d]	NR
Sabine et al. (50)	36	Parallel	Mianserin	NR	NR	NR	NR
Mitchell and Groat (42)	32	Parallel	Amitriptyline	−72.1	−51.8	NR	NR
Hughes et al. (32)	22	Parallel	Desipramine[c]	−91.0	19.0	NR	NR
Barlow et al. (4)	24	Crossover	Desipramine[c]	−46.8	−2.4	2.4	NR
Agras et al. (1)	20	Parallel	Imipramine[c]	−72.4	−43.1	30.0	10.0
Blouin et al. (7)	10	Crossover	Desipramine[c]	−40.0	NR	10.0	NR
Horne et al. (29)	81	Parallel	Bupropion[c]	−67.0	−1.9	29.7	NR
Walsh et al. (58)	50	Parallel	Phenelzine[c]	−64.2	−5.5	34.8	3.7
Kennedy et al. (35)	18	Crossover	Isocarboxazid[c]	−35.0	5.0	33.3	NR
Pope et al. (46)	42	Parallel	Trazodone[c]	−31.0	21.0	10.0	0.0
Mitchell et al. (43)	74[e]	Parallel	Imipramine[c]	−49.3	−2.5	16.0	NR
Fluoxetine Bulimia Nervosa Collaborative Study Group (22)	387	Parallel	Fluoxetine (60 mg)[c]	−67	−33	27[f]	14[f]
			Fluoxetine (20 mg)	−45		14[f]	
Freeman et al. (24)	40	Paralell	Fluoxetine[c]	−51.4	−16.8	NR	NR
Walsh et al. (59)	78	Parallel	Desipramine[c]	−47.0	7.0	12.5	7.9
Potvin et al. (47)	398	Parallel	Fluoxetine[c]	−50	−18	NR	NR
Alger et al. (3)	14	Parallel	Imipramine	−20	−30	NR	NR
Kennedy et al. (34)	36	Parallel	Brofaromine	−61.5	−50.0	19	13

[a] Adapted from ref. 57, with permission.
[b] Mean of individual subjects' percent reduction in binge frequency is given where available; otherwise percent reduction in group mean binge frequency is given.
[c] Statistically significant difference between active medication and placebo.
[d] NR, not reported.
[e] This study also examined the effects of group psychotherapy. These 74 patients received only imipramine or placebo.
[f] Approximate figures.

caution because it is based not on direct comparisons of one agent to another in a single study, but on comparisons between response rates in different studies. It is clear that factors other than which antidepressant agent was employed contribute importantly to response. For example, it can be noted from Table 1 that the change in frequency of binge eating on placebo ranges from 21% deterioration to 52% improvement. Similarly, the response to the same active agent varies substantially across the studies in which it has been used; for example, the improvement in binge frequency on desipramine ranges from 40% to 91%. These observations indicate that factors other than the choice of antidepressant have a major impact on the response of patients with bulimia nervosa. It is not clear what these other factors are, because the studies of antidepressant medication in bulimia nervosa, for the most part, have examined populations that appear comparable in terms of age, duration, and severity of illness.

Although these studies have established beyond question the superiority of antidepressant medication over placebo in the treatment of bulimia nervosa, concerns persist about the place of antidepressant medication in the therapeutic approach to this illness. One concern relates to the degree of improvement commonly achieved during antidepressant treatment. As indicated in Table 1, the average decline in binge frequency achieved during medication treatment was only about 50%, and the highest reported rate of remission was only 35%. Although improved, the average patient was significantly symptomatic at the conclusion of a course of antidepressant medication.

The long-term outcome of antidepressant treatment of bulimia nervosa also remains a significant concern. One of the earliest reports regarding the long-term response to medication was that of Pope et al. (44), who were instrumental in initiating studies of antidepressants in bulimia. In 1985, they described the follow-up of 20 patients an average of 18 months after they had been recruited to participate in a controlled trial of imipramine. Although a majority of patients reported being markedly or more improved, most had required multiple medication trials and most of those who were doing well remained on medication. Similar results were described by Fava et al. (19). In a retrospective follow-up study, they found that improvement in eating behavior symptomatology was generally maintained in 19 patients who had an initial favorable response to fluoxetine and who had been treated with fluoxetine for an average of 10 months. However, 13 of the 19 patients remained on fluoxetine, and all also received psychotherapy. These reports suggested that patients with bulimia nervosa who responded favorably to treatment with antidepressant medication often continued to do well if they remained on medication.

Two controlled studies attempted to determine how frequently bulimia nervosa could be successfully treated

with a time-limited course of antidepressant medication, and they were not as encouraging. Pyle et al. (48) examined the maintenance of change in nine patients who had improved during 3 months of treatment with imipramine by randomly assigning them to 4 months of continued treatment with either imipramine or placebo. Five of six patients randomized to placebo and two of three randomized to imipramine relapsed during the succeeding 4 months.

Our own group also attempted to address the issue of the long-term response to antidepressant treatment (59). We carried out a three-phase trial in which patients were initially randomized to either desipramine or placebo and treated for 8 weeks. Patients who responded to desipramine entered an open maintenance phase during which they continued active medication for an additional 4 months or until they relapsed. Patients who continued to do well were then randomly assigned to remain on desipramine for an additional 6 months or to switch to placebo in double-blind fashion. The results of this study were disappointing in that, of 21 patients who entered the maintenance phase, 29% relapsed despite continued desipramine, and only nine patients entered the discontinuation phase. Five were assigned to continue on desipramine, and only one of these patients relapsed during the succeeding 6 months. Two of the four patients assigned to placebo relapsed during maintenance. This study and that of Pyle et al. (48) are too small to permit definitive conclusions about the appropriate duration of antidepressant treatment for bulimia nervosa. However, both studies suggested that symptomatic relapse was frequent even after several months of significant improvement on medication. These studies provide a less optimistic impression of the long-term outcome of a single course of a single medication than do the reports of Pope et al. (44) and of Fava et al. (19), possibly because in the latter studies, patients received trials of additional medications or concurrent treatment with psychotherapy.

In summary, the work conducted to date suggests there are three major clinical problems with the use of antidepressant medication as a primary intervention for bulimia nervosa. First, although a single course of antidepressant medication is superior to treatment with placebo, the response commonly falls short of remission, the desired goal. Second, among patients who initially respond favorably to antidepressant medication, there is a substantial rate of relapse despite continuation of that medication. And, third, even patients who remain improved during long-term medication treatment appear prone to relapse when the medication is discontinued.

On a theoretical level, the studies of antidepressant medications in the treatment of bulimia nervosa leave open a major question about why these drugs are effective in this disorder. The earliest work in this area proceeded on the basis of the assumption that bulimia nervosa could be viewed as a variant of an affective illness and that the pharmacological treatment of bulimia nervosa could follow principles identical to those used in the treatment of mood disturbance. Two findings suggest that this simple model is deficient. First, it has been consistently noted that there is no relationship between the pretreatment level of depression in bulimia nervosa and the response to medication. Several studies have found that the response of patients without sufficient symptoms of mood disturbance to merit the diagnosis of depression respond as well as do patients with concurrent affective illness.

Second, the large study of the Fluoxetine Bulimia Nervosa Collaborative Study Group (22) found a different relationship between fluoxetine dose and clinical response than had been previously identified in studies of depression. In this trial, patients with bulimia nervosa were randomized to receive one of three treatments: placebo, fluoxetine at 20 mg/day, and fluoxetine at 60 mg/day. Only the group receiving 60 mg/day was found to have a consistently superior response to placebo. This contrasts with studies of major depressive disorder in which a dose of 20 mg/day of fluoxetine is consistently superior to placebo. Though only a single study, this work suggests that the pharmacological treatment of bulimia nervosa may not be identical to the pharmacological treatment of affective disorder.

Antidepressant Medication and Psychotherapy

As studies of the antidepressant treatment of bulimia nervosa were progressing, the utility of psychological interventions was also being examined. In the early and mid-1980s, most studies of psychotherapy for bulimia nervosa examined therapies that were based to a considerable degree on cognitive behavioral principles. Studies using waiting list controls convincingly demonstrated the superiority of such psychological treatment. In addition, a few studies suggested that the gains were enduring. Although not directly relevant to the focus of this chapter, it is of note that more recent studies have begun to challenge the notion that cognitive behavioral therapy is particularly advantageous in the treatment of this syndrome. There are now indications that other forms of therapy such as interpersonal psychotherapy and supportive expressive psychotherapy, which do not specifically focus on the cognitive and behavioral disturbances characteristic of bulimia nervosa, are capable of producing comparable degrees of improvement.

The development of effective forms of psychotherapy has led to questions about the relative efficacy of pharmacological and psychological intervention for bulimia nervosa and about the potential advantages of combined treatment. In the last few years, studies have begun to address these issues. Mitchell et al. (43) randomized patients with bulimia nervosa into one of four treatment groups. One group received placebo alone, and another received imipramine alone. The two other groups received an intensive form of group psychotherapy that involved instructional, cognitive-behavioral, and more traditional group psychotherapy elements. Half of the patients in the intensive group psychotherapy received imipramine and half received placebo. Consistent with other reports of the efficacy of medication, the reduction in binge frequency in the group receiving imipramine alone was significantly greater than that in the group receiving placebo alone. However, the reduction in binge frequency in the groups receiving intensive psychotherapy was significantly superior to the reduction in binge frequency in the group which received imipramine alone. The patients receiving psychotherapy attained an impressive degree of improvement, an average reduction in binge eating of 90%. Although there was no difference in the reduction in binge frequency for the patients who had received intensive group psychotherapy with imipramine compared to those who had received the same therapy with placebo, the investigators were able to detect a drug/placebo difference in the reduction in ratings of depression and of anxiety. Thus, even though the results of psychotherapy were substantially superior to those of medication alone, there were hints of a small additional benefit for patients who had received imipramine in combination with the psychotherapy.

A second study comparing the relative efficacy of medication and psychotherapy is that of Agras et al. (2). These investigators examined individual cognitive behavioral therapy (CBT) for 16 weeks, desipramine alone, given for 16 or 24 weeks, or a combination of CBT and desipramine, the latter again given for either 16 or 24 weeks. A clear result of this study, similar to that of the study of Mitchell et al. (43), was that patients treated with medication alone did not fare as well as did patients who received psychological therapy, either alone or in combination with medication. There were hints of a small advantage for the combination of medication and psychotherapy, but these were somewhat difficult to interpret. They were largely confined to the group that received CBT and 24 weeks of desipramine. Yet, the superior outcome of this group was achieved after 16 weeks of treatment when no suggestion of added benefit was seen in the other combined treatment group that received identical treatment up to 16 weeks.

A third trial comparing medication and cognitive behavioral therapy and its combination is that of Leitenberg et al. (37). This study attempted to compare individual CBT to desipramine alone, and to the combination of these two forms of treatment given for 4 months. The investigators terminated this study prematurely, with only seven patients in each treatment group, because of an unexpectedly high dropout rate largely due to side effects among patients receiving desipramine. In the results that were obtained, no evidence of an advantage for combined treatment was apparent.

Finally, Fichter et al. (21) compared the utility of flu-oxetine (60 mg/day) to placebo in the treatment of 40 patients with bulimia nervosa who were hospitalized on a specialized unit for the treatment of eating disorders and receiving an intensive course of psychological and behavioral treatment. Although both fluoxetine- and placebo-treated groups improved considerably over the 5-week trial, there was no indication of an advantage for fluoxetine over placebo.

In summary, there has been substantial progress in the treatment of bulimia nervosa in the last decade. Pharmacological treatments using antidepressant medication have been demonstrated to be efficacious, and this field has now turned to more challenging questions regarding the place of pharmacological treatment in the overall approach to this eating disorder. The available data suggest that, in general, structured psychotherapy is superior to a course of a single antidepressant medication. There are suggestions that the combination of antidepressant medication and psychotherapy may have some utility, but the advantages of a combined treatment approach over psychotherapy alone appear small and often offset by the occurrence of significant side effects, especially with tricyclic antidepressants. Our group is currently conducting a study that attempts to improve on previous designs by combining structured forms of psychotherapy with a sequential medication intervention in which patients are first treated with desipramine and, if this is ineffective or intolerable, are then treated with fluoxetine. This may enable us to determine whether a more complex but clinically realistic approach to pharmacological management is of significant benefit when provided in the context of psychotherapy.

Other Pharmacological Interventions

While antidepressant medication has received the most attention, other psychopharmacological interventions for bulimia nervosa have also been explored. Lithium was examined in a controlled trial, but was found to be no more effective than placebo (31).

Three studies have examined the potential utility of fenfluramine, which augments serotonergic activity in several ways, including the stimulation of presynaptic serotonin release and the blockade of reuptake. Because serotonergic activity appears to be involved in the development of satiety, fenfluramine is a theoretically appealing candidate for the treatment of bulimia nervosa. In a small ($N = 12$) controlled trial lasting 6 weeks, Blouin et al. (7) found that d,l-fenfluramine at a dose of 60 mg/day was superior to placebo. In a larger trial, Russell et al. (49) examined d-fenfluramine, the more active isomer, at a dose of 30 mg/day in 42 patients with bulimia nervosa, 21 of whom were assigned to active drug and 21 to placebo. The results of this study were ambiguous.

Using data from all 42 patients who were randomized, the investigators found d-fenfluramine to be superior to placebo in the effect on binge eating. However, 17 of the 42 patients withdrew prematurely, and there was no evidence of a significant drug effect compared to placebo when only data from patients who completed the 12-week trial were considered.

The same group carried out a second trial of d-fenfluramine with two important modifications (17). First, a higher dose (45 mg/day) was used. Second, all patients received an abbreviated 8-week course of CBT in addition to medication or placebo. This study was successful in reducing the dropout rate: Only 4 of 43 patients terminated the study prematurely. Both fenfluramine and placebo groups experienced a decline in binge frequency of about 50%, and there was no evidence that the addition of fenfluramine was of clinical benefit. The results of this study resemble those of studies of combined psychotherapy and antidepressant medication, which have had limited success in demonstrating that medication adds substantially to the effectiveness of psychotherapy.

Another theoretically based pharmacological intervention for bulimia nervosa is the use of opiate antagonists. There is substantial evidence that endogenous opiates are involved in the control of eating behavior (see Chapter 138, *this volume*), and, in a variety of paradigms, including some forms of stress-induced eating, opiate antagonists reduce food intake. Unfortunately, two placebo-controlled trials of the opiate antagonist naltrexone have failed to provide much support for the efficacy of this agent in bulimia nervosa (3,41).

PSYCHOPHARMACOLOGY OF BINGE EATING DISORDER

A significant development since the publication of *Third Generation of Progress* has been an increased interest in patients who report binge eating in the absence of attempted methods of compensation such as vomiting, laxative abuse, excessive exercise, or fasting. One formulation of this syndrome is that of Spitzer et al. (52,53), who have (a) referred to the syndrome as *binge eating disorder* (BED), (b) developed preliminary criteria, and (c) demonstrated that the syndrome exists in about one-third of obese patients presenting to weight control clinics and in 2–5% of individuals in the community. The challenges of characterizing and treating patients with BED have brought investigators of eating disorders together with obesity researchers, communities that have, until recently, remained surprisingly separate.

There have been four controlled studies of the use of medications, antidepressants for the most part, in the treatment of BED or related syndromes. The basic questions posed in these studies include the following: (a) Given the demonstrated efficacy of antidepressants in bulimia nervosa, do these medications produce a reduction in binge frequency in obese patients with BED? (b) Do antidepressant medications facilitate weight loss in obese BED patients? (c) Is there a differential efficacy of medications in obese patients with BED when compared to their efficacy in obese patients without binge eating?

McCann and Agras (39) studied desipramine at an average daily dose of 188 mg in the treatment of "nonpurging bulimics," many of whom would probably meet criteria for BED. Subjects ranged in weight from the upper limits of normal to morbidly obese. Reduction in binge frequency, measured as binge days per week, was substantially greater with desipramine than with placebo (63% decrease versus 16% increase). Neither group had a substantial weight change. Sixteen-week follow-up suggested that the decrease in binge frequency largely disappeared when medication was discontinued.

Marcus et al. (38) compared fluoxetine to placebo in obese binge eaters (many of whom would likely meet criteria for BED) who were receiving standard behavior modification treatment. Fluoxetine (60 mg/day) or placebo was given for 1 year. Patients receiving active medication lost significantly more weight than those who received placebo; however, there was no difference between obese binge eaters and obese non-bingers, suggesting that the drug did not specifically target binge eating. Follow-up data suggested that patients tended to regain weight following discontinuation of fluoxetine. Although binge frequency was not reported, the bulimia subscale of the Eating Disorders Inventory changed equally for both active medication and placebo groups; this suggested that although fluoxetine enhanced weight loss, it did not enhance binge suppression.

Alger et al. (3) studied the effect of imipramine up to 200 mg versus naltrexone up to 150 mg/day versus placebo in normal-weight bulimic patients (see above) and obese binge eaters, many of whom probably met criteria for BED. Both active medications were associated with a significant reduction in binge frequency, but the effect of the medications did not differ significantly from that of the placebo. Imipramine, but not naltrexone, was associated with a reduction in binge duration among obese binge eaters. Subjects were not placed on a reducing diet, and no group showed a substantial change in weight. Although this study did not provide compelling evidence for the utility of either medication, the authors speculate that, given the effect on binge duration, imipramine may enhance compliance in dietary treatment aimed at weight reduction.

De Zwaan et al. (15) conducted a two-by-two combined treatment study in which 22 overweight binge eaters and 42 non-binge eaters received either cognitive behavioral treatment (CBT) or dietary management (DM) and either fluvoxamine (100 mg/day) or placebo. All treatment groups responded similarly with a modest weight loss during treatment and regain at 1 year follow-up. There was a trend toward greater weight regain among binge eaters than among non-binge eaters. The only evidence of efficacy of fluvoxamine was among binge eaters, who showed a greater reduction in Hamilton depression scores with fluvoxamine than with placebo. There was no evidence of a specific effect of medication on binge eating. Limitations of this study included small sample size and possibly inadequate fluvoxamine dosage.

Clearly, the treatment of binge eating among the obese is an area that requires further study. However, the results, to date, are not particularly encouraging. In terms of the original questions, only one study (39) suggested a suppression of binge frequency with medication versus placebo, only one suggested an enhancement of weight loss with medication versus placebo (38), and both of these effects were lost when medication was discontinued. None of these studies provided evidence for a specific effect of medication among obese binge eaters. These results are somewhat surprising in view of the clearly established efficacy of antidepressant medications in reducing binge frequency among patients with bulimia nervosa. However, only two of the four studies reported binge frequency during treatment, and in one of these two studies there was a marked placebo response. Future studies will benefit from (a) more careful assessment of binge frequency along with weight and (b) increased attention to the long-term maintenance of change.

CONCLUSION

This chapter has reviewed developments in psychopharmacologic treatment of eating disorders since the publication of the *Third Generation of Progress*. In the case of anorexia nervosa, while the yield from acute treatment studies remains limited, there has been a potentially important refocusing of attention toward the use of medication in the prevention of relapse among weight-restored patients. Studies of antidepressants in the acute treatment of bulimia nervosa have continued to suggest that virtually all classes of antidepressants are more effective than placebo in the short term. However, the available data indicate that a single course of antidepressant medication is insufficient for most patients when they are followed over a longer term. The potential utility of combining antidepressant medication and psychotherapy remains to be clarified. In patients with the newly defined binge eating disorder, the role of medications in weight reduction and binge suppression are under active investigation, but given the preliminary nature of available data, a definitive statement concerning their efficacy must be deferred to the *Fifth Generation of Progress*.

ACKNOWLEDGMENT

This work was supported, in part, by grant MH-38355 from the National Institutes of Health.

REFERENCES

1. Agras WS, Dorian B, Kirkley BG, Arnow B, Bachman J. Imipramine in the treatment of bulimia: a double-blind controlled study. *Int J Eat Disord* 1987;6:29–38.
2. Agras WS, Rossiter EM, Arnow B, Schneider JA, Telch CF, Raeburn SD, Bruce B, Perl M, Koran LM. Pharmacologic and cognitive-behavioral treatment for bulimia nervosa: a controlled comparison. *Am J Psychiatry* 1992;49:82–87.
3. Alger SA, Schwalberg MD, Bigaouette JM, Michalek AV, Howard LJ. Effect of a tricyclic antidepressant and opiate antagonist on binge-eating in normoweight bulimic and obese, binge-eating subjects. *Am J Clin Nutr* 1991;53:865–871.
4. Barlow J, Blouin J, Blouin A, Perez E. Treatment of bulimia with desipramine: a double-blind crossover study. *Can J Psychiatry* 1988;330:129–133.
5. Barry VC, Klawans HL. On the role of dopamine in the pathophysiology of anorexia nervosa. *J Neural Transm* 1976;38:107–122.
6. Biederman J, Herzog DB, Rivinus TM, Harper GP, Ferber RA, Rosenbaum JF, Harmatz JS, Tondorf R, Orsulak PJ, Schildkraut JJ. Amitriptyline in the treatment of anorexia nervosa: a double-blind, placebo-controlled study. *J Clin Psychopharmacol* 1985;5:10–16.
7. Blouin AG, Blouin JH, Perez EL, Bushnik T, Zuro C, Mulder E. Treatment of bulimia with fenfluramine and desipramine. *J Clin Psychopharmacol* 1988;8:261–269.
8. Casper RC, Schlemmer RF, Javaid JI. A placebo-controlled crossover study of oral clonidine in acute anorexia nervosa. *Psychiatry Res* 1987;20:249–260.
9. Channon S, DeSilva WP. Psychological correlates of weight gain in patients with anorexia nervosa. *J Psychiatr Res* 1985;19:267–271.
10. Condon JT. Long-term neuroleptic therapy in chronic anorexia nervosa complicated by tardive dyskinesia. A case report. *Acta Psychiatr Scand* 1986;73:203–206.
11. Crisp AH. A treatment regime for anorexia nervosa. *Br J Psychiatry* 1966;112:505–512.
12. Crisp AH, Lacey JH, Crutchfield M. Clomipramine and 'drive' in people with anorexia nervosa: an in-patient study. *Br J Psychiatry* 1987;150:355–358.
13. Dally P, Sargant W. A new treatment of anorexia nervosa. *Br Med J* 1960;1:1770–1773.
14. Dally P, Sargant W. Treatment and outcome of anorexia nervosa. *Br Med J* 1966;2:793–795.
15. de Zwaan M, Nutzinger DO, Schoenbeck G. Binge eating in overweight women. *Compr Psychiatry* 1992;33:256–261.
16. Eckert ED, Goldberg SC, Halmi KA, Casper RC, Davis JM. Depression in anorexia nervosa. *Psychol Med* 1981;11:1–8.
17. Fahy TA, Eisler I, Russell GFM. A placebo-controlled trial of d-fenfluramine in bulimia nervosa. *Br J Psychiatry* 1993;162:597–603.
18. Faltus F, Janeckova E. Levoprotiline-function regulator of food and satiety centres? *Act Nerv Super (Praha)* 1989;31:282–283.
19. Fava M, Herzog DB, Hamburg P, Riess H, Anfang S, Rosenbaum JF. Long-term use of fluoxetine in bulimia nervosa: a retrospective study. *Ann Clin Psychiatry* 1990;2:53–56.
20. Ferguson JM. Treatment of an anorexia nervosa patient with fluoxetine [Letter]. *Am J Psychiatry* 1987;144:1239–1240.
21. Fichter MM, Leibl K, Rief W, Brunner E, Schmidt-Auberger S, Engel RR. Fluoxetine versus placebo: a double-blind study with bulimic inpatients undergoing intensive psychotherapy. *Pharmacopsychiatry* 1991;24:1–7.
22. Fluoxetine Bulimia Nervosa Collaborative Study Group. Fluoxetine in the treatment of bulimia nervosa: a multicenter, placebo-controlled, double-blind trial. *Arch Gen Psychiatry* 1992;49:139–147.
23. Franklin JC, Schiele BC, Brozek J, Keys A. Observations on human behavior in experimental semistarvation and rehabilitation. *J Clin Psychol* 1948;4:28–45.
24. Freeman CPL, Davies F, Morris J, Cheshire K, Hampson M. A double-blind controlled trial of fluoxetine versus placebo for bulimia nervosa. Unpublished report, 1989.
25. Goldberg SC, Halmi KA, Eckert ED, Casper RC, Davis JM. Cyproheptadine in anorexia nervosa. *Br J Psychiatry* 1979;134:67–70.
26. Gross HA, Ebert MH, Faden VB, Goldberg SC, Nee Le, Kaye WH. A double-blind controlled trial of lithium carbonate in primary anorexia nervosa. *J Clin Psychopharmacol* 1981;1:376–381.
27. Gwirtsman HE, Guze BH, Yager J, Gainsley B. Fluoxetine treatment of anorexia nervosa: an open clinical trial. *J Clin Psychiatry* 1990;51:378–382.
28. Halmi KA, Eckert ED, LaDu TJ, Cohen J. Anorexia nervosa: treatment efficacy of cyproheptadine and amitriptyline. *Arch Gen Psychiatry* 1986;43:177–181.
29. Horne RL, Ferguson JM, Pope HG, Hudson JI, Lineberry CG, Ascher J, Cato A. Treatment of bulimia with bupropion: a multicenter controlled trial. *J Clin Psychiatry* 1988;49:262–266.
30. Hsu LKG. *Eating disorders*. New York: The Guilford Press, 1990.
31. Hsu LKG, Clement L, Santhouse R, Ju ESY. Treatment of bulimia nervosa with lithium carbonate. A controlled study. *J Nerv Ment Dis* 1991;179:351–355.
32. Hughes PL, Wells LA, Cunningham CJ, Ilstrup DM. Treating bulimia with desipramine: a double-blind, placebo-controlled study. *Arch Gen Psychiatry* 1986;43:182–186.
33. Kaye WH, Weltzin TE, Hsu LKG, Bulik CM. An open trial of fluoxetine in patients with anorexia nervosa. *J Clin Psychiatry* 1991;52:464–471.
34. Kennedy SH, Goldbloom DS, Ralevski E, Davis C, D'Souza J, Lofchy J. Is there a role for selective MAO-inhibitor therapy in bulimia nervosa? A placebo-controlled trial of brofaromine. *J Clin Psychopharmacol* 1993;13:415–422.
35. Kennedy SH, Piran N, Warsh JJ, Prendergast P, Mainprize E, Whynot C, Garfinkel PE. A trial of isocarboxazid in the treatment of bulimia nervosa. *J Clin Psychopharmacol* 1988;8:391–396.
36. Lacey JH, Crisp AH. Hunger, food intake and weight: the impact of clomipramine on a refeeding anorexia nervosa population. *Postgrad Med J* 1980;56(Suppl 1):79–85.
37. Leitenberg H, Rosen JC, Wolf J, Vara LS, Detzer MJ, Srebnik D. Comparison of cognitive-behavior therapy and desipramine in the treatment of bulimia nervosa. *Behav Res Ther* 1994;32:37–45.
38. Marcus MD, Wing RR, Ewing L, Kern E, Gooding W, McDermott M. A double-blind, placebo-controlled trial of fluoxetine plus behavior modification in the treatment of obese binge eaters and nonbinge eaters. *Am J Psychiatry* 1990;147:876–881.
39. McCann UD, Agras WS. Successful treatment of nonpurging bulimia nervosa with desipramine: a double-blind, placebo-controlled study. *Am J Psychiatry* 1990;147:1509–1513.
40. Mitchell JE. Psychopharmacology of anorexia nervosa. In: Meltzer HY, ed. *Psychopharmacology: the third generation of progress*. New York: Raven Press, 1987;1273–1276.
41. Mitchell JE, Christenson G, Jennings J, Huber M, Thomas B, Pomeroy C, Morley J. A placebo-controlled, double-blind crossover study of naltrexone hydrochloride in outpatients with normal weight bulimia. *J Clin Psychopharmacol* 1989;9:94–97.
42. Mitchell JE, Groat R. A placebo-controlled, double-blind trial of amitriptyline in bulimia. *J Clin Psychopharmacol* 1984;4:186–193.
43. Mitchell JE, Pyle RL, Eckert ED, Hatsukami D, Pomeroy C, Zimmerman R. A comparison study of antidepressants and structured group psychotherapy in the treatment of bulimia nervosa. *Arch Gen Psychiatry* 1990;47:149–157.
44. Pope HG, Hudson JI, Jonas JM, Yurgelun-Todd D. Antidepressant treatment of bulimia: a two-year follow-up study. *J Clin Psychopharmacol* 1985;5:320–327.
45. Pope HG Jr, Hudson JI, Jonas JM, Yurgelun-Todd D. Bulimia treated with imipramine: a placebo-controlled, double-blind study. *Am J Psychiatry* 1983;140:554–558.
46. Pope HG Jr, Keck PE Jr, McElroy SL, Hudson JI. A placebo-controlled study of trazodone in bulimia nervosa. *J Clin Psychopharmacol* 1989;9:254–259.
47. Potvin JH, Rampey AH, Roberts AH, Wheadon VL, Wilson MG. Fluoxetine vs. placebo in long-term treatment of bulimia nervosa: parallel/double-blind. Unpublished report, 1990.
48. Pyle RL, Mitchell JE, Eckert ED, Hatsukami D, Pomeroy C, Zimmerman R. Maintenance treatment and 6-month outcome for bulimic patients who respond to initial treatment. *Am J Psychiatry* 1990;147:7:871–875.
49. Russell GFM, Checkley SA, Feldman J, Eisler I. A controlled trial of d-fenfluramine in bulimia nervosa. *Clin Neuropharmacol* 1988;11(Suppl 1):S146–S159.
50. Sabine EJ, Yonace A, Farrington AJ, Barratt KH, Wakeling A.

Bulimia nervosa: a placebo controlled double-blind therapeutic trial of mianserin. *Br J Clin Pharmacol* 1983;15:195S–202S.

51. Slaiman S. Restricted diets restrict antidepressant efficacy. *Practitioner* 1989;233:974–975.

52. Spitzer RL, Devlin MJ, Walsh BT, Hasin D, Wing RR, Marcus MD, Stunkard A, Wadden TA, Yanovski S, Agras WS, Mitchell J, Nonas C. Binge eating disorder: a multisite field trial for the diagnostic criteria. *Int J Eat Disord* 1992;11:191–203.

53. Spitzer RL, Yanovski S, Wadden T, Wing R, Marcus MD, Stunkard A, Devlin M, Mitchell J, Hasin D, Horne RL. Binge eating disorder: its further validation in a multisite study. *Int J Eat Disord* 1993;13:137–153.

54. Vandereycken W. Neuroleptics in the short-term treatment of anorexia nervosa: a double-blind placebo-controlled study with sulpiride. *Br J Psychiatry* 1984;144:288–292.

55. Vandereycken W, Pierloot R. Pimozide combined with behavior therapy in the short-term treatment of anorexia nervosa. *Acta Psychiatr Scand* 1982;66:445–450.

56. Vigersky RA, Loriaux DL. The effect of cyproheptadine in anorexia nervosa: a double-blind trial. In: Vigersky RA, ed. *Anorexia nervosa.* New York: Raven Press, 1977;349–356.

57. Walsh BT. Fluoxetine in the treatment of bulimia nervosa. *J Psychosom Res* 1991;35(Suppl 1):33–40.

58. Walsh BT, Gladis M, Roose SP, Stewart JW, Stetner F, Glassman AH. Phenelzine vs placebo in 50 patients with bulimia. *Arch Gen Psychiatry* 1988;45:471–475.

59. Walsh BT, Hadigan CM, Devlin MJ, Gladis M, Roose SP. Long-term outcome of antidepressant treatment for bulimia nervosa. *Am J Psychiatry* 1991;148:1206–1212.

Psychopharmacology: The Fourth Generation of Progress, edited by Floyd E. Bloom and David J. Kupfer. Raven Press, Ltd., New York © 1995.

CHAPTER 137

Obesity, Fat Intake, and Chronic Disease

George A. Bray

The life insurance industry has repeatedly pointed out the increased risks of mortality associated with being overweight. Their statistics have shown that the overweight individual has a greater risk of developing diabetes mellitus, heart disease, high blood pressure, and gallbladder disease (56). With this impetus, a large body of research on the mechanisms underlying the development of obesity and its risks has been assembled. This chapter will provide a perspective on several of the recent developments. First, the newer techniques for measuring fatness will be described, and we will discuss the way they can be used to quantitate total and regional body fat. Second, current ideas about prevalence will be presented. Third, the role of diet composition in regulation of fat stores will be discussed using a feedback model. Finally, the relative impact of total fatness versus regional fatness will be discussed.

DEFINITION, MEASUREMENT, AND CLASSIFICATION

Overweight is defined as an increase in body weight above a standard related to height. Obesity, on the other hand, is defined as an abnormally high percentage of body fat. Overweight and fat distribution are useful predictors of excess mortality and the risks of heart disease, hypertension, diabetes mellitus, and gallbladder disease, among others. In order to determine whether an individual is obese or simply overweight due to increased muscle mass, one needs techniques for measuring body fat and standards against which to compare these numbers. Table 1 shows a list of both the classic and newer methods which can be used for assessing body fat and its distribution. It

also provides an assessment of the relative ease, reliability, accuracy, and expense of these various methods.

Techniques for Measuring Body Fat

Anthropometric Methods

Measurements of height and weight as well as measurements of circumference of the chest, waist, hips, or extremities and skinfolds in the triceps, biceps, subscapular, abdominal, thigh, calf, and sometimes other regions are relatively inexpensive to perform, and they have been widely used in epidemiologic studies to assess total body fat, fat distribution, or the degree of overweight. Of these techniques, height and weight can be measured with the greatest accuracy (coefficient of variation < 1%). Circumferences can also be measured accurately (cv = 2.5%), but skinfolds have more variability in their measurement (cv = 11%). Interobserver variation and variability in precise site location for skinfolds limit their use to studies where trained investigators are involved. Because of the variability in skinfolds, they are of limited value in determining changes in body fat of individuals.

Anthropometric measurements provide several kinds of information. First they provide height and weight from which the degree of overweight can be calculated. Second, the ratio of the circumference of the waist divided by the circumference of the hips has provided a useful epidemiologic tool for estimating the health risk associated with central fat distribution. Finally, skinfold measurements with all their attendant limitations can be used to quantitate subcutaneous fat distribution and for determining the relative amount of truncal or peripheral fat (35).

G. A. Bray: Department of Medicine, Pennington Biomedical Research Center, Louisiana State University, Baton Rouge, Louisiana 70808.

TABLE 1. *Methods of estimating body fat and its distribution*

Method	Cost	Ease of use	Accuracy	Measures regional fat
Height and weight	Low	Easy	High	No
Skin folds	Low	Easy	Low	Yes
Circumferences	Low	Easy	Moderate	Yes
Density				
Immersion	Moderate	Moderate	High	No
Plethysmograph	High	Difficult	High	No
Heavy water				
Tritiated	Moderate	Moderate	High	No
Deuterium oxide, or heavy oxygen	Moderate	Moderate	High	No
Potassium isotope (^{40}K)	Very high	Difficult	High	No
Conductivity, total body electrical	High	Moderate	High	No
Bioelectric impedance	Moderate	Easy	High	No
Fat-soluble gas	Moderate	Difficult	High	No
Computed tomography	Very high	Difficult	High	Yes
Magnetic resonance	Very high	Difficult	High	Yes
Ultrasonography	High	Moderate	Moderate	Yes
Dual-energy x-ray or photon absorptiometry	High	Easy	High	±
Neutron activation	Prohibitive	Difficult	High	No

Quantitative Methods to Measure Body Compartments

Two Compartment Models

The data obtained from quantitative measurements of body composition can be used to partition the body into several compartments (64), some of which are summarized graphically in Fig. 1. There are several methods that provide two-compartment models where the first compartment is body fat and the second can be fat-free mass, lean body mass, body potassium, or body water.

Body density has generally been considered the gold standard for measuring body fat. It assumes a density for fat equal to 0.900 and a density for fat-free body mass equal to 1.100. These assumptions are satisfactory for normal individuals, but are frequently in error for children and adolescents, for athletes, for the markedly obese, and for the elderly. The simple technique of measuring body density provides data for a two-compartment model of body fat and fat-free mass. Whole-body plethysmographs are an alternative to body density, but are more expensive and have been more difficult to use although theoretically this method could provide information for a two-compartment model.

Determination of total body water is a second method for calculating body fat. Total body water may be mea-

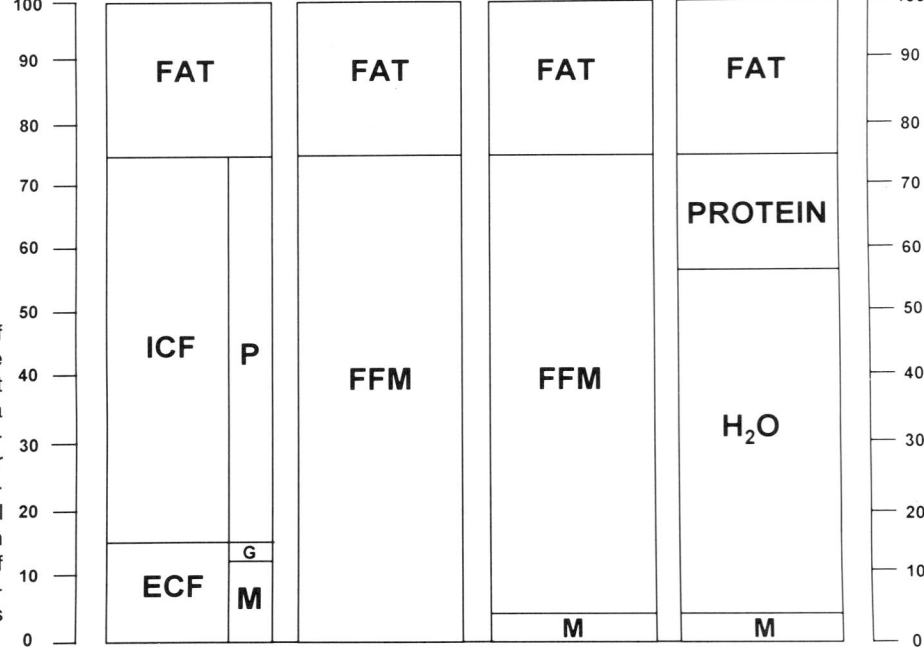

FIG. 1. Compartmental models of body composition. From left to right the columns represent a six-compartment model, a two-compartment model, a three-compartment model, and a four-compartment model. ICF, intracellular fluid; P, protein; G, glucose + glycogen; ECF, extracellular fluid; M, mineral mass; FFM, fat-free mass. For each model, fat is represented as 25% of weight. Mineral is 4% in the three-, four- and six-compartment model. Protein is 22%.

sured using tritiated water, deuterated water, ^{18}O-labeled water, or appropriate chemicals such as antipyrine, which dissolve in body water. The underlying assumption for this method is that water has a constant relation to fat free mass. This is assumed to be 73.2%. Body fat in kilograms and is obtained by subtracting lean body mass (body water/0.732) from total body weight.

A third two-compartment model is obtained by estimating total body potassium. The naturally occurring isotope of potassium, ^{40}K, can be estimated from its gamma emission using a whole-body scintillation counter. Assuming that lean body mass has 60 mEq/kg of K in females and 66 mEq/kg of K in males, one can calculate lean body mass, and by subtracting that from total body weight one can calculate fat mass. In a study by Heymsfield et al. (22), in a large group of males and females aged 52–58, the assumptions used in estimating total fat from total body water were shown to be highly reliable. Similarly, the density of fat-free mass was also shown to be very close to the assumed values. However, the potassium concentrations were lower for both males and females than the values used in most equations, indicating that calculating body fat from ^{40}K could produce considerably larger errors.

Two techniques providing two-compartment models of body fat use electrical conductivity. The first measures total body electrical conductivity using an expensive instrument called *total-body electrical conductivity* (TO-BEC). In contrast, determination of body electrical impedance using either a fixed- or variable-frequency electrical input at the wrist and ankle can provide a relatively inexpensive method for calculating body fat, provided that the degree of hydration is satisfactory. Using appropriate equations that include height, impedance, age, and sex can provide good estimates for body fat in all but the most obese individuals (53). Correlations between laboratories can provide interlaboratory coefficients of between $r = 0.95$ and $v = 0.99$. Because this method measures water, variation in hydration may bias the interpretation (15).

Multicompartment Models

The dual photon absorptiometer (DPA) and the dual-energy x-ray absorptiometer (DEXA) were originally developed for determination of bone mass for studies of osteoporosis. This technique provides body mineral, body fat, and fat-free mass (see Fig. 1). Comparison of the estimated three-compartment model obtained with these instruments to that obtained with neutron activation ^{40}K and body water determinations show a very high correlation (21). Thus, the accuracy for this method of fat mass estimated with DPA or DEXA is high, and it is probably the most appropriate ''gold standard'' for comparison of individuals who can be measured with this technique. Its

current limitation is the mass of the individual who can be fitted on the table of these instruments. This is approximately 150 kg.

The most expensive procedure for determination of total body mass and its components is neutron activation. At present, only the Brookhaven National Laboratory in New York is carrying out these highly expensive procedures (22). The neutron activation instruments can provide measurements of potassium, sodium, chloride, calcium, nitrogen, and carbon as well as a number of minor elements. The limitation of the method is its radiation dose, which is on the order of 500 mrem. With knowledge about the proportion of calcium in the hydroxyapatite of bone crystal and the fact that nitrogen represents 16% of protein mass, one can calculate a four- or six-compartment model based on neutron activation (Fig. 1).

Fat Distribution

Subcutaneous fat distribution can be determined by several methods. The first is the ratio of skinfolds measured on the trunk and on the limbs (35). A second technique is the use of ultrasound, that measures subcutaneous fat thickness at defined trunk and limb sites. The use of magnetic resonance imaging and computed tomography to assess the proportion of fat to muscle and bone in limbs or trunk provides the most quantitative data (27,54). The limitation of multiple CT scans is again radiation exposure, a problem that does not occur with magnetic resonance imaging.

Visceral fat is one of the most important fat depots, but is one of the most difficult depots to measure. The only reliable methods for measuring visceral fat at present are with computed tomography or magnetic resonance imaging. With either technique, a cut through the L-4, L-5 region provides a good estimate of the visceral to subcutaneous fat ratio.

Summary

DPA and DEXA

DPA and DEXA appear to have replaced density, total body water, and ^{40}K as the gold standard for body composition. For regional fat distribution, the ratio of trunk to peripheral skinfolds or ratio of waist circumference divided by hip circumference may be used. Visceral fat can only be adequately estimated at present by magnetic resonance imaging (MRI) or computed tomography (CT) scans.

Body Fat

Once measured, body fat can be divided into three main components. The first component is the total amount of body fat expressed as a percent of body weight. The second component is the regional distribution of subcutaneous fat into central fat—also called male, android, or upper body fatness—versus female, gynoid, or lower body fatness. This can best be done with CT scans, but one can also use either (a) subscapular fat fold, the ratio of truncal skinfolds to limb skinfolds, or (b) sex-specific measurements of waist circumference divided by hip circumference (waist-to-hip ratio). The third component of body fat is the amount of visceral fat located in the abdomen. This appears to be controlled differently than total fat or the regional distribution of subcutaneous fat and can only be accurately estimated with CT or MRI scans.

Body Weight for Epidemiologic Studies

For epidemiologic studies, two methods of relating body weight to height have been most widely used. These include relative weight and body mass index. Relative weight compares actual weight to the appropriate weight table for a given height obtained from life insurance or other tables. One problem with this approach is that many tables divide weight into "frame" sizes for which standards may be of dubious value:

$$\text{Percent overweight} = \frac{\text{Actual weight for height}}{\text{Table weight for height}} \times 100$$

The preferred method of relating height and weight is the body mass index that was developed by Quetelet more than 100 years ago. This relationship is expressed below and is usually called the body mass index (BMI), but might be more appropriately called the Quetelet index (QI):

$$\text{BMI or QI} = \frac{\text{Weight (kg)}}{[\text{Height (m)}]^2}$$

A nomogram for determining the body mass index is presented in Fig. 2.

Fat Distribution For Epidemiologic Studies

Measurement of either the subscapular skinfold or the ratio of the circumference of the abdomen at the minimal point between the ribs and iliac crest and the circumference of the gluteal region at the maximal gluteal protuberance expressed as the WHR (waist-to-hip circumference ratio) is most widely used. A nomogram for WHR is shown in Fig. 3. The ratio of trunk and peripheral skinfolds including biceps, triceps, subscapular abdominal, supra iliac, lateral calf, and lateral thigh can also be used. No satisfactory way exists to estimate visceral fat for epidemiologic studies.

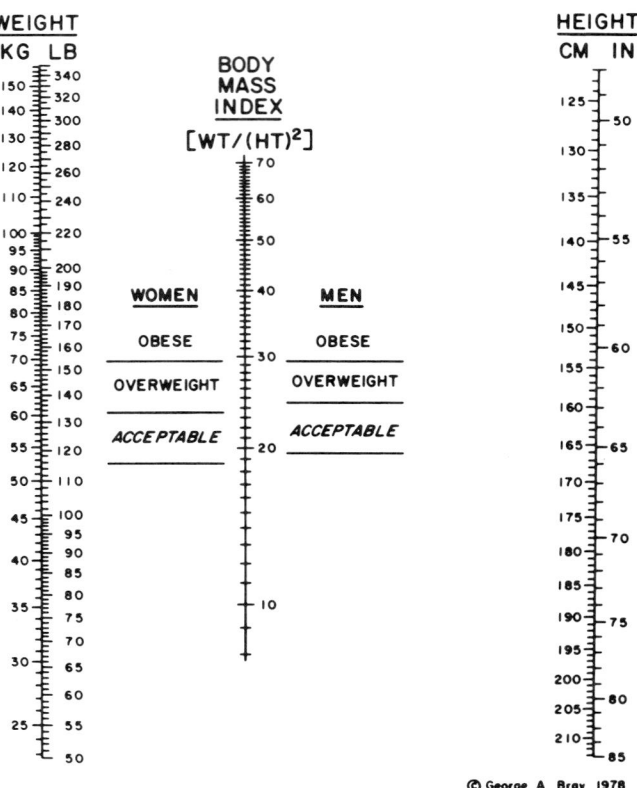

NOMOGRAM FOR BODY MASS INDEX

© George A Bray 1978

FIG. 2. Nomogram for determining body mass index. To use this nomogram, place a ruler or other straight edge between the body weight in kilograms or pounds (without clothes) located on the left-hand line and the height in centimeters or in inches (without shoes) located on the right-hand line. The body mass index is read from the middle of the scale and is in metric units. (Copyright 1978, George A. Bray. Reproduced with permission.)

Criteria for Determining Overweight and Obesity

Setting weight standards can be done in two ways. First, the normal distribution of body weight in relation to height can be measured in a large sample of the population and then arbitrarily divided into overweight and severely overweight categories. This approach has been used by the National Center for Health Statistics. They define overweight as individuals above the 85th percentile of weight for height, using as reference the weights of 20- to 29-year-old American males and females. With this technique, overweight is a BMI: $kg/m^2 > 27.8 \ kg/m^2$ for men and $27.3 \ kg/m^2$ for women. The top 5th percentile is considered severely overweight. There are four problems with this approach. First, the standards change as the weight distribution of the population changes. Second, the decimal values of BMI at the 85th percentile makes these numbers difficult to use or remember. Third, this approach defines 15% of the adult population as over-

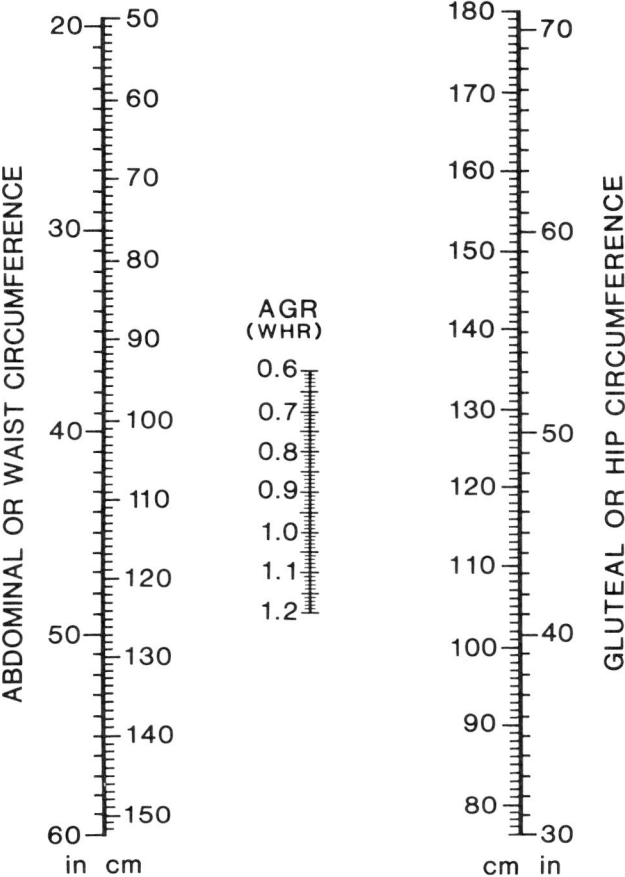

FIG. 3. Nomogram for determining waist-to-hips ratio. Place a straight edge between the column for waist circumference and the column for hip circumference and read the ratio from the point where this straight edge crosses the AGR or WHR line. The waist or abdominal circumference is the smallest circumference below the rib cage and above the umbilicus, and the hips or gluteal circumference is taken as the largest circumference at posterior extension of the buttocks. (Copyright 1987, George A. Bray. Reproduced with permission.)

TABLE 2. *Good body weights for adults*[a]

Height[b]	Age 19–34 years		Age 35 years and above	
	Target (pounds)[c]	Range (pounds)[c]	Target (pounds)[c]	Range (pounds)[c]
5'0"	112	97–128	123	108–138
5'1"	116	101–132	127	111–143
5'2"	120	104–137	131	115–148
5'3"	124	107–141	135	119–152
5'4"	128	111–146	140	122–157
5'5"	132	114–150	144	126–162
5'6"	136	118–155	148	130–167
5'7"	140	121–160	153	134–172
5'8"	144	125–164	158	138–178
5'9"	149	129–169	162	142–183
5'10"	153	132–174	167	146–188
5'11"	157	136–179	172	151–194
6'0"	162	140–184	177	155–199
6'1"	166	144–189	182	159–205
6'2"	171	148–195	187	164–210
6'3"	176	152–200	192	168–216
6'4"	180	156–205	197	173–222
6'5"	185	160–211	202	177–228
6'6"	190	164–216	208	182–234
BMI (kg/m^2)	22	19–25	24	21–27

[a] Derived from National Research Council, 1989.
[b] Without shoes.
[c] Weight without clothes.

weight, and by definition it is impossible to have less than 15% of the population overweight. Finally, the most serious problem with this approach is the underlying assumption that average weight is a healthy weight. There is little to support this idea.

An alternative approach to arriving at healthy weights is to use body weights associated with the lowest overall risk to health. The minimal death rate in several prospective studies is associated with a BMI between 22 and 25 kg/m^2. In an analysis of the data from the build study for 1979 (56), the population study from Norway (63), and the American Cancer Society study (32), Andres (*personal communication*) showed that the BMI associated with the lowest mortality for women increased with each decade of life. For men, on the other hand, the weight with the lowest mortality did not change with age in two of these three studies (Andres, *personal communication*).

Based on these data, the Dietary Guidelines of the U.S. Department of Agriculture and the U.S. Department of Health and Human Services (60) have adopted BMI standards of 19–25 kg/m^2 for men and women aged 19–35 and a BMI of 21–27 kg/m^2 for men and women over 35 years of age. These data are similar to standards adopted in Canada and in Europe, although they differ in some details. Tables 2 and 3 translate these numbers into weights and provides a middle target weight.

Because body fat increases with age and is substantially higher for any given height/weight relationship in women than in men, assigning standards in terms of percent body fat is more difficult and on less solid ground. Guidelines for defining obesity in terms of body fat for each sex are provided in Table 4.

Criteria for Regional Fat Distribution

Several approaches have been used to estimate body fat distribution. The simplest is the circumference of the waist divided by the circumference of the hips (WHR). A nomogram for determining this is presented in Fig. 3. The ratio of skin folds on the trunk to the skin folds on the extremities (T/E ratio) provides a second index of fat distribution. A third approach is the ratio of skinfold to circumference measurements on the upper arm and upper thigh as originally proposed by Vague (61).

At present, the only population-based criteria for the

TABLE 3. *Good body weights for adults*[a]

Height (cm)[b]	Age 19–34 years Target (kg)[c]	Age 19–34 years Range (kg)[c]	Age 35 years and above Target (kg)[c]	Age 35 years and above Range (kg)[c]
152	51	44–58	55	49–62
155	53	46–60	58	50–65
157	54	47–62	59	52–67
160	56	49–64	61	54–69
163	58	51–66	64	56–72
165	60	52–68	65	57–74
168	62	54–71	68	59–76
170	64	55–72	69	61–78
173	66	57–75	72	63–81
175	67	58–77	74	64–83
178	70	60–79	76	67–86
180	71	62–81	78	68–88
183	74	64–84	80	70–90
185	75	65–86	82	72–92
188	78	67–88	85	74–95
191	80	69–91	88	77–99
193	82	71–93	89	78–101
196	85	73–96	92	81–104
198	86	75–98	94	82–106
BMI (kg/m^2)	22	19–25	24	21–27

[a] Derived from National Research Council, 1989.
[b] Without shoes.
[c] Weight without clothes.

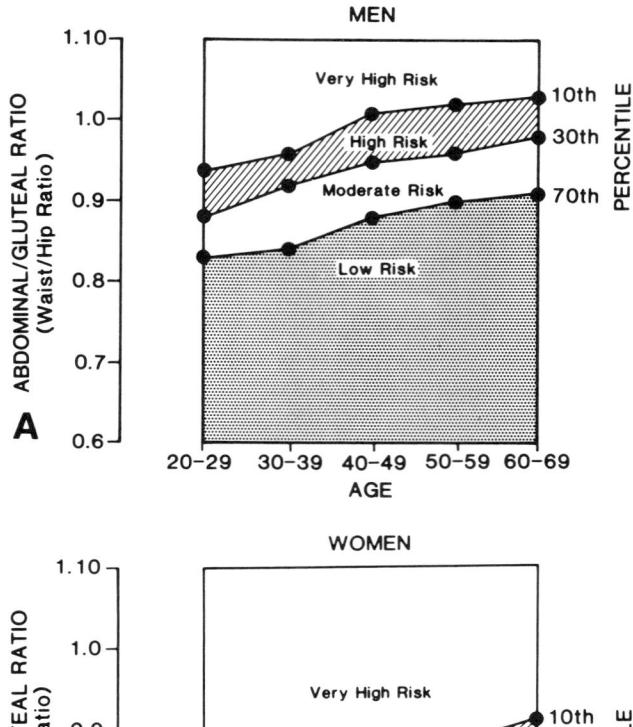

FIG. 4. Percentiles for fat distribution. The percentiles for the ratio of abdominal circumference to gluteal circumference (ratio of waist to hips) are depicted for men (4a) and women (4b) by age groups. The relative risk for these percentiles is indicated based on the available information. (Plotted from tabular data in the *Canadian Standardized Test of Fitness,* 3rd edition, 1986. Copyright 1987, George A. Bray.)

distribution of fat are the data from the Canadian National Survey in which waist and hip circumference were measured. These data are plotted in Fig. 4 for both sexes.

Visceral Fat

Visceral fat can be estimated reliably with CT or MRI scans taken at the fourth to fifth lumbar vertebrae (see Fig. 2). Other estimates of visceral fat remain to be validated. Visceral fat increases with age and changes pari passu with changes in body fat or fat distribution. At this writing, no standards are available.

Stability of Body Weight in Childhood, Adolescence, and Adult Life

Several epidemiological studies have examined the relationship between weight at two or more ages in the same population. The mean upward shift in body weight

TABLE 4. *Criteria for obesity in men and women*

Category	Body fat (%) 12–20	Body fat (%) Females
Normal	12–20	20–30
Borderline	21–25	31–33
Obesity	>25	>33

during adult life may well camouflage considerable individual and year-to-year fluctuations. In 1302 women from Gothenburg, Sweden, the mean weight gain over a 6-year period was 1.4 ± 5.1 kg (SD); 28 of the women lost more than 10 kg and 59 gained more than 10 kg (42). In the normative aging study from Boston, 168 of 1396 men increased their weight more than 10%, whereas 75 lost more than 10%. The baseline weight for those gaining weight was higher (84.1 kg) than for those losing weight (77.3 kg). Williamson et al. (68) at the National Center for Health Statistics have also reported on 10-year changes in body weight. As expected, younger people gained more weight than older ones. In men the gain was less than in women before age 55. After 55, men tended to lose less than women. Between the ages of 35 and 44, 14–16% became overweight. The 10-year incidence of gaining more than 10 kg (≥ 5 kg/m^2) peaks between ages 25–34 and is 3.9% in men and 8.4% in women. Thus, women are more than twice as likely as men to gain weight in middle life.

A number of studies have tracked childhood weight into adult life. Although many studies have examined this question, only a few of them have calculated the relative risk of being in the top weight category as an adult based on the weight status in childhood or adolescence. According to these reports, it is between 1.6 and 2.5 times more likely for the heaviest youngster to be overweight than the lightest youngster. In a 50-year follow-up of the Harvard Longitudinal Study of Child Health and Development, Casey et al. (10) found that the BMI of females in childhood had essentially no correlation with their BMI as adults. BMI of females in adolescence showed a better, but still low, correlation, with BMI at age 50 ($r = .25$ to .35). The low correlation of adolescent weight with later adult weights in women may account for the failure to show an effect of overweight in adolescent girls on mortality of adult women. In men, on the other hand, the correlation of BMI in childhood or adolescence with BMI at age 50 was better ($r +.44$ to $+.55$). Because the tracking of childhood and adolescent weight into adult life is of a low order, one must be careful in making public health recommendations to adolescents based on their adolescent weight status. A prospective follow-up over 36 years points to the variability of body weight with age (5). At age 36, 3,322 people born in 1946 were divided into weight categories according to BMI. In this cohort, 5.3% of the men and 8.4% of the women had a BMI greater than 30 kg/m^2, and 38% of the men and 24.2% of the women were overweight with a BMI between 25 and 29.9 kg/m^2. The correlation between BMI at ages 26 and 36 was $r = .64$ for men and $r = .66$ for women. The authors draw the following important conclusions about weight stability. First, that 25% of the obese cohort, men as well as women, were obese both as children and as adults. Second, the remaining 75% of this cohort became obese as adults, an event which could not be predicted from weights before age 20. Those who became obese between ages 11 and 36 were often not the heaviest during childhood. Only 50–60% of the men and women in the top decile at age 36 could be correctly predicted at age 26, using all socioeconomic, demographic, and other available weight data.

PREVALENCE

Prevalence data have been compiled from a number of countries around the world. Amongst these data are many comparisons of information on factors influencing the prevalence within countries. The following discussion will first focus on factors affecting prevalence estimates within countries and then examine the cross-country prevalence data.

Factors Affecting Weight Within Countries

Within any country there are a number of clear-cut differences in the frequency of obesity. These differences are related to age, sex, ethnic factors, and socioeconomic status. The ensuing discussion will illustrate these with data from the National Center for Health Statistics because this database provides two criteria with which to make assessments within a population.

Age

The prevalence of overweight (BMI 25–30 kg/m^2) as well as obesity (BMI > 30 kg/m^2) increases with age. The peak prevalence of overweight males occurs at age 50–59, whereas in females it occurs at age 70–74. For obesity, the peak is at age 40–49 in men and 50–59 in women.

Gender

In almost all populations, more women are overweight and obese than men.

Ethnic Factors

Among females in the United States there is a lower percentage of overweight white women than either African-American or Hispanic women. The nearly linear increase in prevalence with age is evident in all three groups, with peak values occurring between age 40 and 70. For males, the percentage of overweight is lower for African-Americans at all ages except the decade 40–49. Among males, the percentage of overweight becomes stable between the fourth and sixth decade of life.

White females are less obese at all ages than African-American or Hispanic females. The prevalence of obesity in the African-American and Hispanic groups rises to between 30% and 40% between the ages of 40 and 70. This contrasts with a figure of 20% for white females. In contrast to the large ethnic difference in obesity between women, the differences in obesity among males between ethnic groups is much smaller. White males have a smaller prevalence of obesity at all ages than do African-American or Hispanic males, but these differences are small: White males run close to 14% through most of their adult life, whereas African-American and Hispanic males run between 15% and 22%.

Socioeconomic Status

Socioeconomic status plays an important role in the prevalence of obesity. With the exception of the 20- to 29-year-old women, those defined as below the poverty level by the American government have a higher prevalence of obesity than those above the poverty level. This fact is clear for both white females and African-American females, but less so for Hispanic or Mexican/American females. These striking differences in the prevalence of obesity for white females are present but of much smaller values among the males.

Time Trends in Weight Status

Several studies suggest that there is a progressive increase in weight for height in the United States throughout the entire 20th century. Data on inductees into the military service show that for men 5'8" tall weights rose from 147 lbs in 1863 to 168 lbs in 1962. A similar increase has been observed in the Framingham cohort, with males showing steady increase throughout the early part of this century and females showing a slight downward average weight. Life insurance data and data from the National Center for Health Statistics also report a small increase in average weight for height. NCHS data from surveys conducted in 1960–1962, 1970–1974, and 1980–1981 (69) showed only a small change with time. Recent data from Denmark and the Netherlands also show a similar increase. Particularly striking is the Danish data in inductees into the military service showing a sudden sharp increase in the prevalence rates in the late 1970s.

NUTRIENT BALANCE AND FAT STORAGE

A nutrient balance model can be used to examine the role of dietary fat in the development of obesity. In the normal-weight adult, nearly 150,000 kcal of energy is available from the triacylglycerols stored in adipose tissue, 24,000 kcal is available in the peptide bonds and amino acids from protein, and barely 1000 kcal is available in glucose and glycogen. Obesity is a failure of nutrient balance that occurs when the intake of nutrients exceeds the daily need for nutrients to stoke the metabolic furnace.

The Nutrient Balance Model

A feedback model for nutrient balance consists of four components. The first is the controlled system comprising dietary intake, digestion, absorption, storage, and metabolism of the nutrients in food. The second component is the feedback signals that tell the controller about the state of the controlled system. The third component is a controller located in the brain. And finally, there are the efferent control mechanisms that modulate nutrient intake and energy expenditure.

The Controlled System

The 150,000 kcal of energy contained in body fat of the normal adult human being is some six times larger than what is stored as protein. By comparison, the quantity of carbohydrate is minute. An individual eating 2000 kcal, of which 40% is carbohydrate, will take in an amount of carbohydrate each day between 50% and 100% of their total body stores of carbohydrate. In contrast, average daily protein intake is a little over 1% of total stores, whereas fat intake is considerably less than 1%. This is depicted in Fig. 5. It should not be surprising that in studies of nutrient balance in experimental animals, changes in carbohydrate balance from day to day reciprocally affected carbohydrate intake on the subsequent day (14). That is, if carbohydrate balance is positive (i.e., the animal ate more carbohydrate than it oxidized), the animal would eat less carbohydrate tomorrow. Conversely, when carbohydrate balance is negative, the animal will eat more carbohydrate tomorrow. Although fat oxidation is related to body fat (52), the day-to-day relationship between fat balance and fat intake is very weak (14). Addition of fat to a meal does not acutely change energy expenditure (14). Access to a diet with more than 30% fat consistently produces obesity in most animals. Thus, it should not be surprising that there is a positive but weak correlation between fat intake and body weight in humans (49,70). As might be expected from this model, a low fat intake in women reduced body weight (33,55).

An analysis of this regulatory controlled system suggests the following concepts:

1. Each major nutrient may be regulated separately.
2. The time required to achieve balance for each nutrient varies as a function of the amount ingested each day in relation to the total body stores of that macronutrient. Thus, becoming obese by eating a high-carbohydrate diet would appear to be more difficult than when eating a high-fat diet because the body storage system for carbohydrate as glycogen is limited. Although excess carbohydrate can be converted to fatty acids, this is an energetically expensive transformation (12). Body fat stores, on the other hand, are many times larger than daily fat intake, implying a much greater capacity for fat storage and a much longer time constant to achieve balance.
3. Achievement of nutrient balance requires that the net oxidation of each macronutrient equals the average composition of the macronutrients in the diet (14,52). That is, ingestion of a high-fat diet requires greater oxidation of fat than when equilibrium is achieved eating a low-fat diet. For $\Delta E = 0$, the following conditions are required:

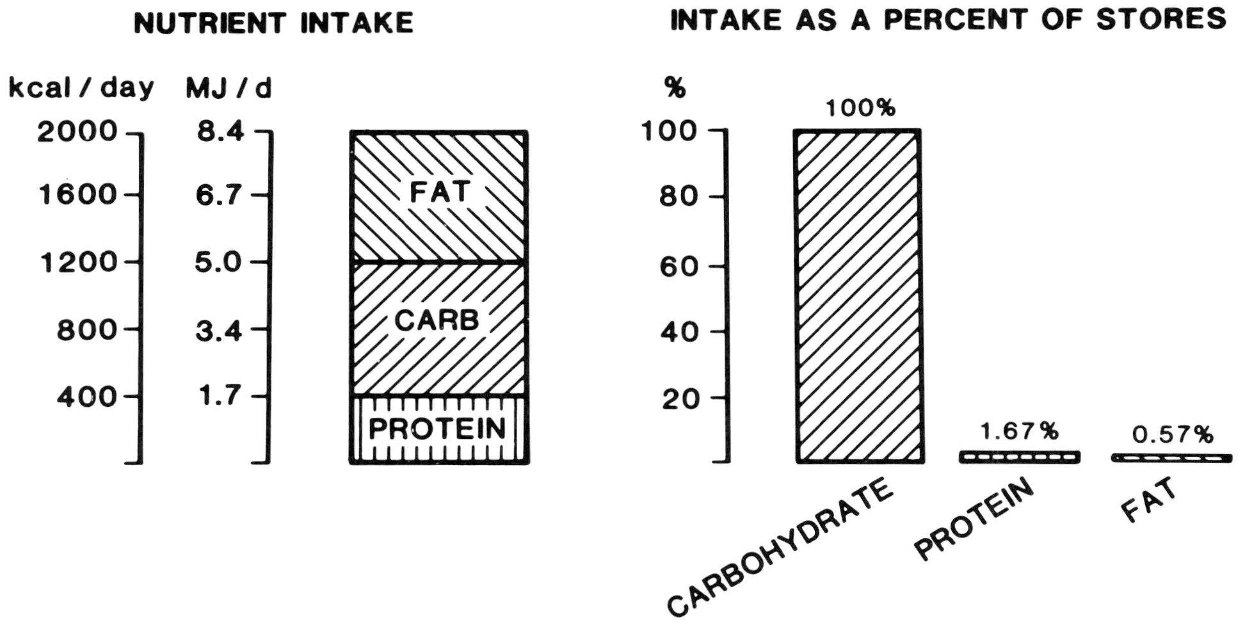

NUTRIENT INTAKE

INTAKE AS A PERCENT OF STORES

FIG. 5. Relationship of macronutrient intake to body stores of that macronutrient. A diet containing 40% fat, 40% carbohydrate, and 20% protein in terms of energy content is shown on the left. The relationship of each of these components to the body stores of the corresponding nutrient is shown on the left side as a percent of nutrient stores.

Fat intake = Fat oxidation

Carbohydrate intake = Carbohydrate oxidation

Protein intake = Protein oxidation

$$\Delta E = \text{Change in energy stores}$$

4. There are major differences between individuals in the incapacity to increase rapidly the oxidation of fat after beginning a high-fat diet (73). Much of this difference may be genetic (4).

5. Physical training can increase oxidation of fatty acids by muscle, and thus regular aerobic exercise might reduce the tendency to become obese or help maintain lower body weight after losing weight.

6. The regulation of nutrient stores is subject to positive and negative feedback signals that operate through the central controller.

Nutrient composition of the diet plays a variable role in the development of obesity in man and animals. At one extreme are the types of obesity due simply to excess food intake regardless of composition. In these cases, obesity may develop when the diet is composed primarily of carbohydrates (vegetables, fruits, and meat or vegetable protein) or fats. In these instances, genetic factors probably play an important role because experimental animals with a recessively inherited tendency develop obesity regardless of the composition of the diet. At the other extreme are those types of obesity where dietary composi-

tion is central to the development of obesity. These include a high-fat diet, access to beverages or solutions containing sucrose, or other soluble carbohydrates and diets with an abundance of highly palatable foods. Any of these types of dietary obesity can be controlled by changing diets or by restraint in the intake of food. In clinical studies, a low rate of fat oxidation (i.e., higher carbohydrate oxidation) in the basal state predicts an increase in body weight (73). The rate of fat oxidation is directly related to the degree of body fat (52). As weight is lost, fat oxidation declines. To keep from regaining weight that has been lost, the intake of fat must be reduced by approximately 20 g/day for each 10 kg of fat lost (52).

Afferent Feedback Signals

The brain receives information about the status of nutrient balance from several sources (6). Afferent signals can be transmitted over the somatic sensory nervous system via the autonomic nervous system or through blood-borne signals.

Sensory Signals

Sight and smell of food are important signals for identifying potential environmental sources of food and for initiating food intake. Along with the texture and taste of food in the mouth, the olfactory and sensory cues about the quality of the food can serve as positive feedback signals for initiating and sustaining food ingestion. Negative feedback signals that eventually slow down, terminate, or abort an eating incident also arise from olfactory or gustatory senses. The ability of most animals to avoid foods that have previously made them sick, a phenomenon known as bait-shyness, is an example of these afferent sensory signals integrated with a central learning system.

Gastrointestinal Signals

Information about the presence of food or nutrients in the gastrointestinal (GI) tract can be initiated by several mechanisms. The first is GI distension. The second is by the action of nutrients on the GI tract mucosa. For example, oleate, a long-chain fatty acid, decreases food intake when infused into the duodenum. The third is release of gastrointestinal hormones when nutrients act directly on the GI tract. The fourth is through the effects of absorbed nutrients. Apo-AIV, a protein component of the chylomicrons that is synthesized in the GI tract, decreases food intake (17).

Several gastrointestinal hormones, as well as other peptides, have been implicated in the inhibition of feeding. [This is also reviewed in relation to eating disorders by Halmi (Chapter 138, *this volume*).] The most prominent is cholecystokinin (CCK) (3). Intraperitoneal injections of CCK decrease food intake in hungry rats, sheep, and humans, and they inhibit sham feeding in rats and monkeys. The sequence of events associated with a response to CCK is similar to that of spontaneous postprandial satiety. CCK may terminate eating by acting on antral CCK receptors (CCK-A receptors) in the pylorus that constrict the pylorus and enhance gastric distension. This peripheral information generated in this way by CCK may be important in producing satiety because vagotomy and lesions to the central vagal connections of the vagus in the nucleus of the tractus solitarius will block the satiety effect of CCK.

Nutrient Signals

Nutrient signals may also act on the liver or brain to induce satiety. 2-Deoxy-D-glucose, a drug that inhibits cellular metabolism of glucose, increases food intake. Similarly, a drop in glucose precedes many meals in humans and animals (9,30). Manipulation of fatty acid oxidation also affects food intake. Blockade of fatty acid oxidation with either mercaptoacetate or methylpalmoxirate (etomoxir) increases food intake (8,16). Fatty acid metabolites, such as 3-hydroxybutyrate or acetoacetate, also reduce food intake (51). These observations point to a potential for nutrients as afferent feedback signals.

The Controller

Anatomy

Several anatomic regions of the mid- and hindbrain play an important role in the control of nutrient balance. Destruction of the ventromedial or paraventricular hypothalamus is associated with hyperphagia and obesity in most homeothermic species that have been studied. Lesions in the amygdala central nucleus also produce obesity. On the other hand, destruction of the lateral hypothalamus is associated with a decrease in food intake and a reduction in body fat.

Neurotransmitters

The neurotransmitters involved in regulation of nutrient intake can be divided into three groups:

1. The fast-acting amino acids, which modulate ion channels.
2. The monoamines, which act more slowly through second messengers.
3. The peptides, which may modulate monoamines and affect intake of specific nutrients (39).

Gamma-aminobutyric acid (GABA) is one of the fast-acting neurotransmitters that can increase or decrease food intake depending on where it is injected (45).

In addition to GABA, there are a number of slow-acting neurotransmitters that are involved in modulating feeding, including norepinephrine, serotonin, dopamine, and histamine. Serotonin [5-hydroxytryptamine (5-HT)] is derived from the dietary amino acid tryptophan. Increasing extraneuronal concentrations of serotonin by any one of several methods decreases food intake. Norepinephrine can either (a) decrease food intake by activating beta receptors in the perifornical area or (b) increase food intake by acting on alpha-2 adrenergic receptors in the paraventricular or ventromedial nucleus (23,31). Dopamine D1 receptors may be involved in decreasing food intake and in the hedonic effects of feeding. Activation of H3 receptors in the ventromedial hypothalamus also reduces food intake.

A number of peptides modulate global food intake or the intake of a single nutrient (7,39) (Table 5). Neuropeptide Y, beta-endorphin, dynorphin, growth-hormone-releasing hormone, somatostatin, and galanin all stimulate food intake when injected into the third ventricle or the medial hypothalamus. A variety of other peptides, including bombesin, cholecystokinin, enterostatin, anorectin, calcitonin (calcitonin gene-related peptide), neurotensin, corticotropin-releasing hormone, thyrotropin-releasing hormone, and vasopressin, inhibit feeding when injected into the medial hypothalamus or into the third ventricle (7).

TABLE 5. *Peptides that stimulate or suppress feeding*

Increase food intake	Decrease food intake
Dynorphin	Anorectin (CTPG)
β-Endorphin	Calcitonin (CRPG)
Galanin	Cholecystokinin (CCK)
Growth-hormone-releasing hormone (GHRH)	Corticotropin-releasing hormone (CRH)
Neuropeptide Y (NPY)	Cyclo-His-Pro
	Enterostatin (VPDPR)
	Glucagon
	Insulin
	Neurotensin
	Oxytocin
	Thyrotropin-releasing hormone (TRH)
	Vasopressin

One hypothesis to explain the role of neuropeptides in modulation of food intake is through their effects on specific types of eating (7). Neuropeptide Y injected into the paraventricular nucleus preferentially increases carbohydrate intake. Galanin injected into the same area increases fat intake. Enterostatin, an activation pentapeptide from pancreatic procolipase, specifically reduces fat intake, whether the peptide is injected peripherally or into the central nervous system (44). These examples suggest that the way in which some peptides may act is to modulate specific components of the homeostatic system dealing with individual nutrients and their "appetites." This hypothesis can be called the peptide-specific nutrient balance model of eating, and the peptides that have been identified as affecting specific measurements are listed in Table 6.

Sensory-specific satiety is a term that describes the fact that when given a choice of preferred foods including a food that had just been eaten, subjects will choose a new food that they have not eaten (48). The nutrient-specific effect of peptides could provide the molecular basis for this phenomenon of sensory-specific satiety.

Efferent Controls

The efferent controls include (a) the motor activities involved in identifying, obtaining, and ingesting food and

TABLE 6. *Peptides and monoamines affecting specific nutrient appetites*

Nutrient	Increase	Decrease
Fat	Galanin	Serotonin
		Enterostatin
	Opioids	Vasopressin
		Corticotropin-releasing hormone
		Cyclo-His-Pro
Carbohydrate	Norepinephrine	Cholecystokinin
	Neuropeptide Y	
Protein	Growth-hormone-releasing hormone	Glucagon
Sodium	Angiotensin	

(b) the efferent effects produced by the autonomic nervous system and several circulating hormones. The complex sequence of motor activities that leads to the initiation of food-seeking, the identification of food, and the killing and ingestion of this food is integrated in the lateral hypothalamus, because electrical stimulation in this area will lead to food-seeking and ingestive behavior. Further discussion of this system is beyond this paper.

Autonomic Nervous System

Both the sympathetic and parasympathetic nervous systems are involved in nutrient balance. In animals where obesity follows hypothalamic lesions, there is evidence for increased activity of the efferent parasympathetic nervous system (vagus nerve) (6). This may provide part of the explanation of the increase in insulin secretion which characterizes hypothalamic obesity.

Reduction in sympathetic activity is also characteristic of obesity and may participate in the enhanced insulin secretion (6). In the experimental animal there is an inverse relationship between the activity of the sympathetic nervous system and food intake (6). In spontaneously feeding rats there is a negative correlation throughout the 24 hr between basal activity of the sympathetic nervous system and spontaneous food intake. In addition, almost all of the experimental maneuvers that increase food intake, such as lesions in the ventromedial hypothalamus or genetic obesity, decrease the activity of the sympathetic nervous system. Conversely, those maneuvers that decrease food intake, such as lateral hypothalamic lesions or injections of fenfluramine, an appetite-suppressant drug, increase sympathetic activity (6).

Food intake is often initiated by a transient drop in circulating glucose levels (9,30). In anticipation of food intake, efferent vagal activity increases, producing an early phase of insulin release from the pancreas. As food enters the stomach and intestine, its digestion triggers vagal afferent signals producing a further rise in insulin secretion and an increase in peripheral efferent sympathetic activity that activates beta-3 adrenergic receptors and their thermogenic responses that may participate in mediating satiety. A rise in cholecystokinin, which slows gastric emptying and the release of other intestinal hormones, may also participate in the satiety sequence. In both animals and humans, ingestion of a meal enhances sympathetic efferent activity that may serve as one of the inhibitory factors in feeding and act as part of the satiety system.

Efferent Hormonal Mechanisms

Insulin

Increased levels of insulin are characteristic of obesity. Injections of insulin can increase food intake, especially glucose, probably by lowering glucose concentrations. The increased food intake following insulin injections also produces mild degrees of obesity. Chronic infusions of insulin, on the other hand, reduce food intake and body weight (62). Insulin has thus been proposed as a signal to the brain about the quantity of peripheral fat stores. One problem with this hypothesis is that most types of obesity have hyperphagia in the face of high concentrations of insulin. There are at least two other possible interpretations of the hyperinsulinemia of obesity. First, the rise in insulin may be a reflection of high levels of nutrient intake. Because insulin is essential for nutrient storage, increased flux of nutrients would be expected to increase insulin. Second, hyperinsulinemia may reflect actual or apparent hypothalamic resistance to the action of insulin. In this case, increased insulin secretion would be modulated by changes in the function of the autonomic nervous system resulting from resistance to the action of insulin in the central nervous system.

Adrenal Steroids

The development or progression of experimental obesity is either reversed or attenuated by adrenalectomy (6). In clinical medicine, Addison's disease with adrenal insufficiency is associated with leanness, whereas Cushing's syndrome, with high levels of adrenal steroid secretion, is associated with obesity. The fact that almost all defects in genetically obese animals are reversed by adrenalectomy and that clinical changes in adrenal status can produce leanness or obesity suggests that glucocorticoids play a key role in the development and maintenance of the obese state. In addition, steroids modulate intake of specific nutrients. In adrenalectomized animals, injections of aldosterone increases fat intake. Glucocorticoids such as corticosterone are essential for stimulation of carbohydrate intake following the injection of norepinephrine (58).

RISKS OF OBESITY AND ABDOMINAL FAT TO HEALTH

It is a cliche to say that "overweight is risking fate." However, the data presented below will argue that not only is an excess quantity of fat risky, but increased abdominal fat distribution may be an even more important external guide to health risks.

Epidemiologic data on the relationship between BMI and a given risk, such as overall mortality, heart disease, diabetes mellitus, or gallbladder disease, are curvilinear and often described as J- or U-shaped. This effect on overall mortality is shown in Fig. 6. Mortality or morbidity increases as BMI increases. There may also be an increase in excess mortality at weights below a lower limit of BMI of $18–19$ kg/m^2, but this may also be related largely to smoking.

Effects of Obesity and Fat Distribution on Overall Mortality

Retrospective Studies

Both retrospective and prospective studies have contributed to our understanding of the relationship between overweight, fat distribution, and mortality. The primary retrospective studies looking at the relationship between weight and obesity have come from the life insurance industry. Life insurance statistics published most recently in 1979 (56), as well as those assembled at intervals throughout this century, have shown that excess weight is associated with higher mortality rates. The minimal mortality for both men and women occurs among individuals 10% below average weight. Deviations in body weight above or below this figure are associated with an increase in mortality. Based on the 1979 data, a body weight that is 10% above average weight is accompanied by an 11% increase in excess mortality for men and a 7% increase for women. If body weight is 20% above average weight, the excess mortality rises to 20% for men and 10% for women.

A second major retrospective study has examined the relationship between body weight and mortality in Norwegian men and women (63). The same curvilinear relationship is observed in this study, with the minimum BMI observed between 23 and 27 kg/m^2. Individuals with lower body weights showed an increase, giving the U-shaped relationship described above.

Overweight generally increases the risk of death, especially sudden death, although in many studies it may not be an independent variable. Three major problems plague the interpretation of studies in this area (37). First, many studies fail to separate smokers from nonsmokers. Because smokers tend to have lower body weights and higher mortality, this influences the death rates and com-

ALL CAUSE MORTALITY

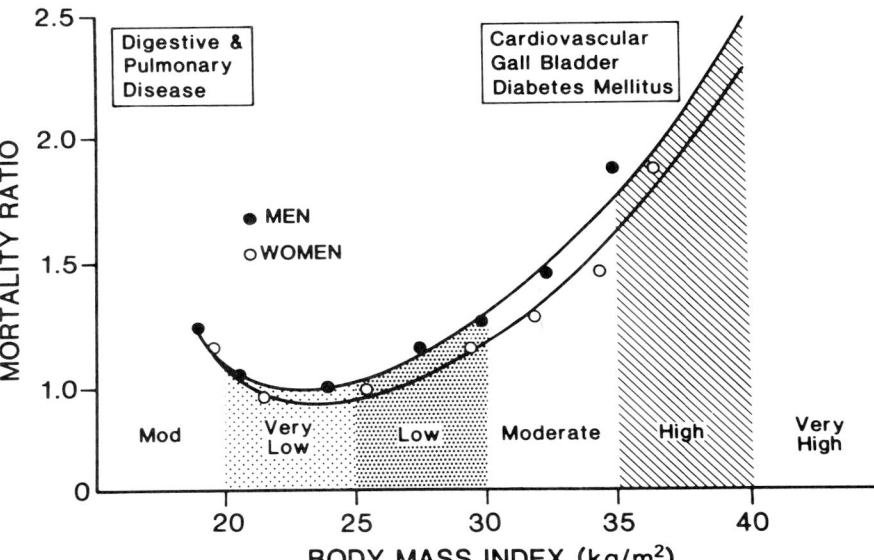

FIG. 6. Mortality ratio and body mass index. Data from the American Cancer Society study have been plotted for men and women to show relationship of body mass index to overall mortality. At a body mass index below 20 kg/m² and above 25 kg/m², there is an increase in relative mortality. The major causes for this increased mortality are listed along with division of body mass index groupings into various levels of risk. (Copyright 1987, George A. Bray. Used with permission.)

pounds the difficulty of assigning effects to body weight per se. Second, early mortality may bias the interpretation of weight status on life expectancy. Individuals who are losing weight at the time of initial survey may die early and thus overemphasize the effect of low body weights as a cause of higher mortality. The failure to identify obesity as an independent risk factor, therefore, has led many people to suggest that it is unimportant. This denies the important relationship that obesity has to diabetes, hypertension, and hyperlipidemia and through whose effects the increase in body weight is likely to cause the ill health. Because obesity must modify some intermediate mechanism, such as cardiac function or the metabolism of lipids or glucose to produce death or disease, overweight may serve as a useful identifier of risk factors.

Prospective Studies of Obesity and Mortality

A large number of prospective studies have now been published relating obesity and mortality. Interpretation of these data has varied because some studies found no relationship between weight and excess mortality, whereas others did. In a careful review of these data, Sjostrom plotted the relationship between the numbers of subjects studied, the duration of follow-up, and the mortality experience. As shown in Fig. 7, this clearly demonstrates that smaller studies of long duration or shorter studies with large numbers of subjects led to similar conclusions—that is, that there was a relationship between initial body weight and subsequent excess risk of mortality.

Effects of Change in Body Weight on Mortality

Weight gain in adults and children has been associated with an increase in blood pressure and blood lipids, as

well as an increase in glucose, uric acid, and risk of heart disease. From the data obtained in the Framingham study, it was concluded that a 10% reduction in relative weight for men was associated with a fall in serum glucose of 2.5 mg/dl, a fall in serum cholesterol of 11.3 mg/dl, a fall in systolic blood pressure of 6.6 mm Hg, and a fall in serum uric acid of 0.33 mm/dl (2). For each 10% reduction in body weight of men, these data predicted that there would be an anticipated 20% decrease in the incidence of coronary artery disease. "If everyone were at optimal weight, there would be 25% less coronary heart disease and 35% less congestive heart failure and brain infarction," based on the data collected in the Framingham study (24). A 10-kg increase in body weight in the Nurses Health Trial was associated with an increased frequency of cardiovascular events. Life insurance data also suggest that changes in body weight were associated with corresponding changes in relative risk of cardiovascular disease.

Losing and regaining weight, so-called weight cycling, may also be hazardous. Data from the Chicago Gas and Electric Company Study (20) showed that those who gained and lost weight had a significantly higher risk of death from cardiovascular disease than did the group of individuals with no change in weight. More recently, Lissner et al. (33), using data from the Framingham study, showed that significant changes in weight, whether in the obese or nonobese, were associated with higher likelihood of mortality. This is currently a controversial area.

Effects of Regional Fat Distribution

More than half a dozen studies have been published showing that central adiposity is positively correlated with

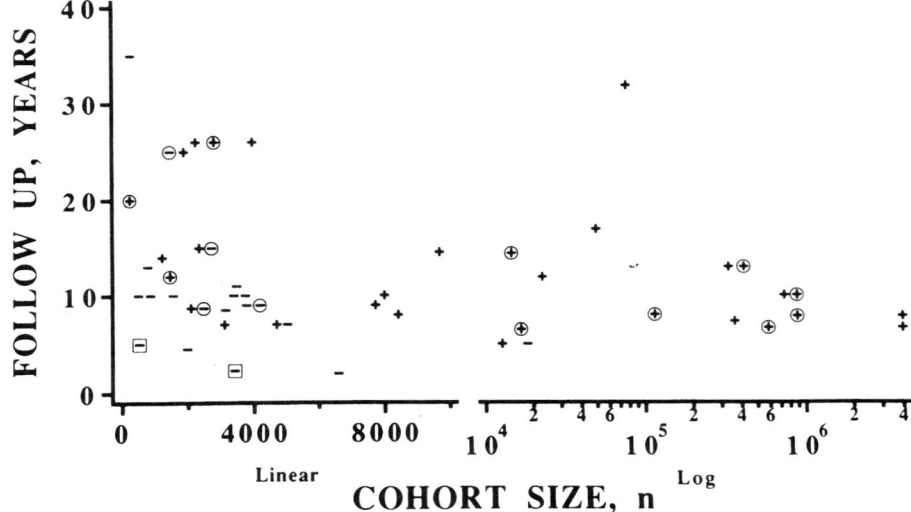

FIG. 7. Cohort size and follow-up period in relation to 40 employee, community, or random population studies finding (+) or not finding (−) a positive relationship between obesity and mortality. Encircled signs represent female cohorts, and signs inside squares indicate that men and women were analyzed together. For layout reasons, seven cohorts have been plotted in positions deviating as little as possible from the true values. Signs for cohort sizes increasing from 0 to 5000 in the follow-up interval 1–10 y correspond to refs. 11 (men plus women combined), 12–16 (men and women), 17–19 (men plus women combined, unpublished SOS mortality data), 20–22 (men and women), and 23 (urban and rural). Signs for cohort sizes increasing from 0 to 5000 in the follow-up interval 11–20 y correspond to refs. 24 (women), 25–27 (women), 28 (black men and women), and 29. Signs for cohort sizes increasing from 0 to 5000 in the follow-up interval 21–35 y correspond to refs. 30, 31 (women and men), 32 (men and women), and 33. Signs for cohort sizes increasing from 5000 to 10,000 correspond to refs. 34–38. Signs for cohort sizes increasing from 10,000 to 100,000 correspond to refs. 39, 38 (women), 40 (women), and 41–44. Signs for cohort sizes increasing from 100,000 to 4,000,000 correspond to refs. 45 (women), 46, 47 (women), 3 (women), 48 (men and women), and 2 (women and men). References without comments refer to studies in men. (Reprinted, with permission, from Sjostrom LV. Mortality of severely obese subjects. *Am J Clin Nutr* 1992;55(Suppl 2):516S–523S.)

increased mortality and increased risk for developing cardiovascular disease, diabetes mellitus, and stroke. Most of these studies have provided information about men. Only the Gothenburg cohort has also provided data on women (28). Among 14,462 women between 38 and 60 years of age, the 12-year age-specific incidence rates for myocardial infarction, stroke, and overall death rate were related to central adiposity. Among the highest quintile for central body fat, the relative risk of myocardial infarction was 8.2 times higher than that for the lowest quintile. For stroke and overall death rate, the relative risk was increased 3.8 and 2.8 times higher for those in the highest quintile compared to those in the lowest quintile. When women in the top 5% for central adiposity, measured as the ratio of the circumference of the waist divided by the circumference of the hips (WHR), were compared to women in the lowest quintile, the risk for myocardial infarction was increased 14.8 times, the risk of having a stroke was increased 11.0 times, and the risk of death from all causes was increased 4.8 times. The Swedish data allow a comparison of men and women in the same town. Larsson et al. (29) have suggested that differences in fat distribution between men and women may account for most of the sex differences in rates of myocardial infarction.

Morbidity Related to Individual Organ Systems

Cardiovascular Morbidity

Increased weight and central adiposity both produce a number of important changes in cardiovascular function. Heart mass increases, both on postmortem examination (1) and as assessed by echocardiographic measurements of posterior wall and interventricular septal thickness (71). The increased cardiac mass is associated with increased blood volume and an increase in both intra- and extracellular fluid volumes. Both cardiac output and cardiac stroke volume are elevated and positively correlated with body weight and with the degree of excess weight. Left and right ventricular end-diastolic pressures are also high, as are the pulmonary artery and pulmonary capillary wedge pressures. Studies using cardiac catheterization and echocardiography with pulsed Doppler techniques have revealed the presence of impaired left ventricular function in some obese patients (71), and a cardiomyopathy of obesity has been clearly identified (1). Abnormalities in both atrial and ventricular filling have been identified in 50% of morbidly obese patients. Heart rate, however, does not increase in obesity. Thus, the increased cardiac output occurs by increased stroke volume from an enlarged heart. Electrocardiographic alterations show a leftward shift in the mean QRS complex with increased fatness for both men and women. The PR interval, QRS duration, and QTc interval in voltage increase with increasing obesity. A prolonged QTc interval was present in 28.3% of those tested.

A number of lipoprotein abnormalities are associated with obesity (18). First, high-density lipoprotein (HDL) cholesterol decreases in obese males and females. Second, serum total cholesterol is usually normal or only slightly elevated, although the transport of low-density lipoprotein (LDL) cholesterol through the plasma compartment increases. This increased transport is consistent with the correlation between cholesterol production and obesity (41). As body fat accumulates, approximately 20 mg of additional cholesterol is synthesized for each extra kilogram of body fat. Third, the production of very-low-density lipoprotein triglyceride (VLDL) and the corresponding apoprotein B100 by liver tends to increase in relation to the degree of obesity in Caucasians and Pima Indians. The increased hepatic VLDL production in obesity is probably a reflection of the associated hyperinsulinemia. Fourth, the high rate of apoprotein-B synthesis in LDL is probably related to the high rate of synthesis apoprotein-B for incorporation into VLDL. Fifth, lipoprotein lipase, the enzyme that hydrolyzes triacylglycerols in VLDL and chylomicrons, increases in adipose tissue with obesity. In contrast to most abnormalities in obesity, LDL frequently rises with significant weight loss (25), whereas most other abnormalities return toward normal. Finally, free fatty acid concentrations frequently increase in obesity, reflecting their higher rate of turnover.

Hypertension

Increased blood pressure, like increased levels of insulin, is characteristic of obesity. Indeed, these two events may be related through the mechanism of insulin resistance (11,46). The use of indirect sphygmomanometric methods for indirect determination of blood pressure requires use of an appropriately sized blood pressure cuff. When the blood pressure cuff is too short, greater differences are observed between systolic and diastolic pressures measured by direct intra-arterial methods than those obtained by indirect measurements.

Hypertension has a striking correlation, not only with body weight but also with lateral body build, that is proportional to changes in both systolic and diastolic blood pressure. The cardiac response can include both concen-

tric hypertrophy and dilation (38). Both central body fat distribution and an increase in total body fat appear to be related to the appearance of hypertension. During periods of severe caloric deprivation, such as occurred in World War I and World War II, hypertension was almost nonexistent. In clinical studies correlating changes in blood pressure with weight reduction, approximately 50–70% of those who lose weight have a fall in blood pressure (36). One explanation might be reduced intake of salt, but careful studies have shown that blood pressure falls even if a fall in sodium intake is prevented by giving salt supplements (59). Weight reduction is more effective in lowering systolic blood pressure than in lowering diastolic blood pressure.

Pulmonary Function

A number of abnormalities in pulmonary function have been observed in obese subjects. At one extreme are patients with the Pickwickian syndrome, named after Joe the fat boy in Dickens' *Pickwick Papers*. This syndrome, called the obesity–hypoventilation syndrome (OHS), is characterized by somnolence, obesity, and alveolar hypoventilation. It is usually associated with obstructive sleep apnea and can represent a respiratory emergency. Weight loss will markedly reduce the detrimental effects of this syndrome, as will oxygenation of the patients airways by using nocturnal CPAP.

At the other extreme are the impairments in work capacity and pulmonary function due to obesity per se. There is a fairly uniform decrease in expiratory reserve function with obesity. Extensive alterations in pulmonary function are observed primarily in massively obese individuals or in obese individuals with some other underlying respiratory or cardiovascular problem. Thus, vital capacity, inspiratory capacity, residual volume, and diffusing capacity remain fairly constant over a wide range of body weights, except in subjects who are massively overweight—that is, those with a weight to height ratio greater than 1 cm/kg.

Diabetes Mellitus and Obesity

The U.S. Diabetes Commission reported that the chance of becoming diabetic more than doubles for every 20% of excess body weight. A curvilinear relationship between diabetes and obesity clearly exists. This has been demonstrated in the studies from Oslo, Norway (66), on the Pima Indians (26), and on members of a weight loss club (47). The curvilinear relationship with mortality is present in the data from the American Cancer Society Study (32). The excess mortality for individuals with a BMI of 35 kg/m^2 increased by nearly eightfold, compared to those of normal weight. All of the data cited above suggest a threshold effect for overweight and the development of Type II diabetes. When the BMI nears 20 kg/m², there is essentially no risk for developing Type II diabetes.

Central fat deposition increases the risk of diabetes. This was first suggested by Vague (61) and has been demonstrated repeatedly since that time (43). There was a greater risk for developing diabetes as WHR increased (i.e., abdominal fat increased). For those in the lowest tertile for central fat distribution, increasing total fat had no significant effect. Haffner et al. (19) in the San Antonio Heart Study have demonstrated that the presence of central adiposity in Mexican Americans was associated with high rates of Type II diabetes. In the women in this population, the BMI, a high WHR, and the ratio of subscapular to triceps skinfold measurements all made independent contributions to the risk of developing non-insulin-dependent diabetes mellitus.

Gallbladder Disease and Obesity

The association between obesity and gallbladder disease has been documented in several studies. In one study, 88% of the variation in frequency of gallbladder disease could be accounted for by weight, age, and parity, with weight being the most important variable. Within each age group, however, the frequency of gallbladder disease increases at higher body weights. Women with a BMI greater than 30 kg/m² had a yearly incidence of gallstones of 1%, and those with a BMI greater than 45 kg/m² had an annual rate of approximately 2% (57).

One mechanism for the increased risk of gallbladder disease is increased cholesterol production and secretion. As noted above, each kilogram of excess body fat increases cholesterol production by 20 mg/day (41). With weight loss, bile becomes more highly saturated with cholesterol and, if nidation factors are present, the risk of gallstone formation may increase sharply. Several recent studies have examined the formation of gallstones during the period of rapid weight loss. The incidence rates in these studies can be 15- to 25-fold higher than in the population of general obese subjects (65). The stones that form appear to produce symptoms in approximately one-third of the subjects, and a significant fraction in up to one-half of these may require surgery.

Cancer and Obesity

The American Cancer Society cohort study reported positive associations between excess weight and cancers of the gallbladder, biliary duct, endometrium, ovary, breast, and cervix among women, as well as positive relationships between excess weight and cancers of the colon and prostate among men (32). The finding of an increase in the risk for endometrial cancer with increasing weight has been a consistent finding in the majority of case–control studies. The relationship between obesity and

breast cancer has been primarily observed in postmenopausal women in studies in the Netherlands, Northern Italy, and Israel. Premenopausal women less frequently show an association between breast cancer and obesity. Indeed, Willett et al. (67), using data from the Nurses Health Trial, have found an inverse relationship between BMI and age-adjusted relative risk for breast cancer in premenopausal women. This discrepancy with other data might be explained by the recent finding that breast cancer risk is augmented in women with upper-body obesity (50).

Obesity and Joint Disease

Increasing body weight might be expected to add additional trauma to the weight-bearing joints and, thus, accelerate the development of osteoarthritis. The National Health and Nutrition Examination survey (NHANES I) examined the prevalence of osteoarthritis in the hands and ankles in relation to weight status race and physical demands. Within each age group, however, there was a clear increase in the prevalence of osteoarthritis in relation to body weight for all groups. The slope of increase with weight was sharpest below 90 kg, suggesting that body weight is only one factor. Weight loss was associated with a significant reduction in risk for osteoarthritis of the knee (13). In contrast with osteoarthritis, the risk of osteoporosis is reduced in the obese, possibly because of increased bone mass accrued during the early years of bone formation. Obesity is also associated with an increased risk of gout. In individuals whose weights were 15% of desirable, the frequency of gout was 3.0 times that of individuals who were less than 110% of desirable weight. There is also a significant correlation between uric acid levels and body weight (24).

Obstetrics and the Overweight Patient

Body weight before pregnancy and weight gain during pregnancy influence the course of labor and its outcome. Infants born to heavy women weigh more than those born to light women. There is also a direct relationship between placental weight and pre-pregnancy body weight. When these infants were compared with weight changes at age 7, 50% of the incremental weight gain could be accounted for by the differences in placental weight at birth. The remaining 50% of the difference was accounted for by the postnatal environment. Naeye (40) found that the fewest fetal and postnatal deaths occurred with mothers who were overweight at the beginning of pregnancy and who gained an average of 7.3 kg or less. The optimal weight gain during pregnancy was 9.1 kg for normal-weight women and 13.6 kg for those who were underweight.

Endocrine Function

Obesity produces a number of changes in endocrine function, but in almost all instances these appear to be secondary to the obesity rather than etiologic (72).

CONCLUDING REMARKS

This chapter has focused on some of the newer ideas about the definition and development of obesity, as well as the health risks associated with obesity and body fat distribution. Of these two, central or visceral fat has the highest relative risk for overall mortality, heart disease, stroke, hypertension, diabetes mellitus, and possibly cancer. Effective long-term treatment for the problem of obesity and excessive visceral fat, in particular, holds the promise of reducing national health budgets for a variety of chronic diseases.

REFERENCES

1. Alexander JK. The cardiomyopathy of obesity. *Prog Cardiovasc Dis* 1985;27(5):325-334.
2. Ashley FW, Kannel WB. Relation of weight change to changes in atherogenic traits: the Framingham study. *J Chronic Dis* 1974;27:103-114.
3. Boosalis MG, Gemayel N, Lee A, Bray GA, Laine L, Cohen H. Cholecystokinin and satiety: effect of hypothalamic obesity and gastric bubble insertion. *Am J Physiol* 1992;262[*Regul Integrative Comp Physiol* 31]:R241-R244.
4. Bouchard C, Despres J, Mauriege P. Genetic and nongenetic determinants of regional fat distribution [Review]. *Endocr Rev* 1993;14(1):72-93.
5. Bradden FE, Rodgers B, Wadsworth ME, Davies JM. Onset of obesity in the 36-year birth cohort study. *Br Med* 1986;293:299-303.
6. Bray GA. Obesity, a disorder of nutrient partitioning: the Mona Lisa hypothesis. *J Nutr* 1991;121:1146-1162.
7. Bray GA. Peptides affect the intake of specific nutrients and the sympathetic nervous system. *Am J Clin Nutr* 1992;55:265S-271S.
8. Calingasan NY, Ritter S. Hypothalamic paraventricular nucleus lesions do not abolish glucoprivic or lipoprivic feeding. *Brain Res* 1992;595(1):25-31.
9. Campfield LA, Brandon P, Smith FJ. On-line continuous measurement of blood glucose and meal pattern in free-feeding rats: the role of glucose in meal initiation. *Brain Res Bull* 1985;14(6):605-616.
10. Casey VA, Dwyer JT, Coleman KA, Valadian I. Body mass index from childhood to middle age: a 50-year follow-up. *Am J Clin Nutr* 1992;56:14-18.
11. DeFronzo RA, Ferranni E. Insulin resistance—a multifaceted syndrome responsible for NIDDM obesity, hypertension, dyslipidemia, and atherosclerotic cardiovascular disease. *Diabetes Care* 1991;14(3):173-194.
12. Donato K, Hegsted DM. Efficiency of utilization of various sources of energy for growth. *Proc Natl Acad Sci USA* 1985;82:4866-4870.
13. Felson DT, Zhang Y, Anthony JM, Naimark A, Anderson JJ. Weight loss reduces the risk for symptomatic knee osteoarthritis in women. *Ann Intern Med* 1992;116:535-539.
14. Flatt JP. Assessment of daily and cumulative carbohydrate and fat balances in mice [Technical note]. *J Nutr Biochem* 1991;2(4):193-202.
15. Forbes GB, Simon W, Amatruda JM. Is bioimpedance a good predictor of body-composition change? *Am J Clin Nutr* 1992;56:4-6.
16. Friedman MI. Body-fat and the metabolic control of food-intake. *Int J Obes* 1990;14(S3):53-67.
17. Fujimoto K, Machidori H, Iwakiri R, et al. Effect of intravenous administration of apolipoprotein A-IV on patterns of feeding, drinking and ambulatory activity of rats. *Brain Res* 1993;608:233-237.
18. Grundy SM, Barnett JP. Metabolic and health complications of obesity [Review]. *DM* 1990;36(12):641-696.
19. Haffner SM, Stern MP, Hazuda HP, Pugh J, Patterson JK. Do upper body and centralized adiposity measure different aspects of regional body-fat distribution? Relationship to non-insulin-dependent diabetes mellitus, lipids, and lipoproteins. *Diabetes* 1987;36:43-51.
20. Hamm P, Shekelle RB, Stamler J. Large fluctuations in body weight during young adulthood and twenty-five-year risk of coronary death in men. *Am J Epidemiol* 1989;129:312-318.
21. Heymsfield SB, Wang J, Heshka S, Kehayias JJ, Pierson RN. Dual-photon absorptiometry: comparison of bone mineral and soft tissue mass measurements in vivo with established methods. *Am J Clin Nutr* 1989;49(6):1283-1289.
22. Heymsfield SB, Waki M, Kehayias J, et al. Chemical and elemental analysis of humans in vivo using improved body composition models. *Am J Physiol* 1991;261(2 pt 1):E190-E198.
23. Jhanwar-Uniyal M, Roland CR, Leibowitz SF. Diurnal rhythm of alpha 2-noradrenergic receptors in the paraventricular nucleus and other brain areas: relation to circulating corticosterone and feeding behavior. *Life Sci* 1986;38(5):473-482.
24. Kannel WB, Gordon T. Physiological and medical concomitants of obesity: the Framingham study. In: Bray GA, ed. *Obesity in america,* Washington, DC: DHEW #79-249, 1979;125-153.
25. Kern PA, Ong JM, Saffari B, Carty J. The effects of weight loss on the activity and expression of adipose tissue lipoprotein lipase in very obese humans. *N Engl J Med* 1990;322(15):1053-1059.
26. Knowler WC, Pettitt DJ, Savage PJ, Bennett PH. Diabetes incidence in PIMA Indians: contributions of obesity and parental diabetes. *Am J Epidemiol* 1981;113:144-156.
27. Kvist H, Chowhury B, Grangard U, Tylen U, Sjostrom L. Total and visceral adipose-tissue volumes derived from measurements with computed tomography in adult men and women: predictive equations. *Am J Clin Nutr* 1988;48:1351-1361.
28. Lapidus L, Bengtsson C, Larsson B, Pennert K, Rybo E, Sjostrom L. Distribution of adipose tissue and risk of cardiovascular disease and death: a 12 year follow-up of participants in the population study of women in Gothenburg, Sweden. *Br Med J* 1984;289:1257-1261.
29. Larsson B, Bengtsson C, Bjorntorp P, et al. Is abdominal body fat distribution a major explanation for the sex difference in the incidence of myocardial infarction? The study of men born in 1913 and the study of women, Gothenburg, Sweden. *Am J Epidemiol* 1992;135(3):266-273.
30. LeMagnen J. *Hunger.* New York: Cambridge University Press, 1985.
31. Leibowitz SF. Reciprocal hunger-regulating circuits involving alpha- and beta-adrenergic receptors located, respectively, in the ventromedial and lateral hypothalamus. *Proc Natl Acad Sci USA* 1970;67(2):1063-1070.
32. Lew EA, Garfinkel L. Variations in mortality by weight among 750,000 men and women. *J Chronic Dis* 1979;32:563-576.
33. Lissner L, Levitsky DA, Strupp BJ, Kalkwark HJ, Roe DA. Dietary fat and the regulation of energy intake in human subjects. *Am J Clin Nutr* 1991;46(6):886-892.
34. Lissner L, Odell PM, D'Agostino RB, et al. Variability of body weight and health outcomes in the framingham population. *N Engl J Med* 1991;324:1839-1844.
35. Lohman TG. Skinfolds and body density and their relation to body fatness: a review. *Hum Biol* 1981;53:181-225.
36. MacMahon SW, Wilcken DE, MacDonald GJ. The effect of weight reduction on left ventricular mass. A randomized controlled trial in young, overweight hypertensive patients. *N Engl J Med* 1986;314:334-339.
37. Manson JE, Stampfer MJ, Hennekens CH, Willett WC. Body weight and longevity. A reassessment. *JAMA* 1987;257:353-358.
38. Messerli FH. Cardiovascular effects of obesity and hypertension. *Lancet* 1982;1:1165-1168.
39. Morley J. Neuropeptide regulation of appetite and weight. *Endocr Rev* 1987;8:256-287.

40. Naeye RL. Weight gain and the outcome of pregnancy. *Am J Obstet Gynecol* 1979;135:3–9.
41. Nestel PJ, Schreibman PH, Ahrens EH Jr. Cholesterol metabolism in human obesity. *J Clin Invest* 1973;52:2389–2397.
42. Noppa H, Hallstrom T. Weight gain in adulthood in relation to socioeconomic factors, mental illness and personality traits: a prospective study of middle-aged women. *J Psychosom Res* 1981;25:83–89.
43. Ohlson LO, Larsson B, Svardsudd K, et al. The influence of body fat distribution on the incidence of diabetes mellitus. 13.5 years of follow-up of the participants in the study of men born in 1913. *Diabetes* 1985;34:1055–1058.
44. Okada S, York DA, Bray GA, Erlanson-Albertsson C. Enterostatin (Val-Pro-Asp-Pro-Arg), the activation peptide of procolipase, selectively reduces fat intake. *Physiol Behav* 1991;49(6):1185–1189.
45. Paredes RG, Agmo A. GABA and behavior: the role of receptor subtypes. *Neurosci Biobehav Rev* 1992;16:145–170.
46. Reaven GM. Banting lecture 1988. Role of insulin resistance in human disease. *Diabetes* 1988;37(12):1596–1607.
47. Rimm AA, Werner LH, Yserloo BV, Bernstein RA. Relationship of obesity and disease in 73,532 weight-conscious women. *Public Health Rep* 1975;90:44–54.
48. Rolls BJ. Sensory-specific satiety. *Nutr Rev* 1986;44:93–101.
49. Romieu I, Willett WC, Stampfer MJ, et al. Energy intake and other determinants of relative weight. *Am J Clin Nutr* 1988;47:406–412.
50. Schapira DV, Kumar NB, Lyman GH, Cavanagh D, Roberts WS, LaPolla J. Upper-body fat distribution and endometrial cancer risk. *JAMA* 1991;266:1808–1811.
51. Scharrer E, Langhans W. Control of food intake by fatty acid oxidation. *Am J Physiol* 1986;250:R1003–R1006.
52. Schutz Y, Tremblay A, Weinsier RL, Nelson KM. Role of fat oxidation in the long-term stabilization of body weight in obese women. *Am J Clin Nutr* 1992;55:670–674.
53. Segal KR, Van Loan M, Fitzgerald PI, Hodgon JA, Van Itallie TB. Lean body mass estimation by bioelectrical impedance analysis: a four-site cross-validation study. *Am J Clin Nutr* 1988;47:7–14.
54. Seidell JC, Bakker CJ, van der Krooy K. Imaging techniques for measuring adipose-tissue distribution—a comparison between computed topography and 1.5-T magnetic resonance. *Am J Clin Nutr* 1990;51(6):953–957.
55. Sheppard L, Kristal AR, Kushi LH. Weight loss in women participating in a randomized trial of low-fat diets. *Am J Clin Nutr* 1991;54:821–828.
56. Society of Actuaries and Association of Life Insurance Medical Directors of America. *Society of Actuaries build study of 1979.* Chicago, 1980.
57. Stampfer MJ, Maclure KM, Colditz GA, Manson JE, Willet WC. Risk of symptomatic gallstones in women with severe obesity. *Am J Clin Nutr* 1992;55:652–658.
58. Tempel DL, McEwen BS, Leibowitz SF. Effects of adrenal steroid agonists on food intake and macronutrient selection. *Physiol Behav* 1992;52(6):1161–1166.
59. Tuck ML, Sowers J, Dornfeld L, Kledzik G, Maxwell M. The effect of weight reduction on blood pressure, plasma renin activity, and plasma aldosterone levels in obese patients. *N Engl J Med* 1981;304:930–933.
60. U.S. Dept of Agriculture. *Nutrition and your health: dietary guidelines for americans,* 3rd ed. Home and Garden Bulletin no. 232, 1990.
61. Vague J. Degree of masculine differentiation of obesities: factor determining predisposition to diabetes, atherosclerosis, gout, and uric calculous disease. *Am J Clin Nutr* 1956;4:20–34.
62. Van der Weele D. Insulin and satiety from feeding in pancreatic normal and diabetic rats. *Physiol Behav* 1993;54(3):in press.
63. Waaler HT. Height, weight and mortality: the Norwegian experience. *Acta Med Scand* 1984;679:1–56.
64. Wang ZM, Pierson RN, Heymsfield SB. The five-level model: a new approach to organizing body-composition. *Am J Clin Nutr* 1992;56(1):19–28.
65. Weinsier R, Ullmann DO. Gallstone formation and weight loss: a review. *Obes Res* 1993;1(1):51–56.
66. Westlund K, Nicolaysen JM. Ten-year mortality and morbidity related to serum cholesterol: a follow-up of 3,751 men aged 40–49. *Scand J Clin Lab Invest* 1972;30(Suppl 127):3–24.
67. Willett WC, Browne ML, Bain C, et al. Relative weight and risk of breast cancer among premenopausal women. *Am J Epidemiol* 1985;122:731–740.
68. Williamson DF, Kahn HS, Remington PL, et al. The 10-year incidence of overweight and major weight gain in US adults. *Arch Intern Med* 1990;150:665.
69. Wong FL, Trowbridge FL. Nutrition surveys and surveillance: their application to clinical practice. *Clin Nutr* 1984;36(3):94–99.
70. World Health Organization. Report of a WHO study group. *Diet, nutrition, and the prevention of chronic diseases.* Geneva: World Health Organization Technical Report Series 797, 1990.
71. Zarich SW, Kowalchuk GJ, McGuire MP, Benotti PN, Mascioli EA, Nesto RW. Left ventricular filling abnormalities in asymptomatic morbid obesity. *Am J Cardiol* 1991;68:377–381.
72. Zellisen PMJ. Neuroendocrine regulation in obesity. Thesis. University of Utrecht, 1991.
73. Zurlo F, Lillioja S, Esposito-Del Puente A, et al. Low ratio of fat to carbohydrate, oxidation as predictor of weight gain: study of 24-h RQ. *Am J Physiol* 1990;259(5 pt 1):E650–E657.

*Psychopharmacology: The Fourth
Generation of Progress*, edited by
Floyd E. Bloom and David J. Kupfer.
Raven Press, Ltd., New York © 1995.

CHAPTER 138

Basic Biological Overview of Eating Disorders

Katherine A. Halmi

The eating disorders anorexia nervosa and bulimia nervosa are complex syndromes that most likely result from, and are sustained by, environmental, psychological, and biological factors. Although they are disorders of eating, very little is known about psychobiological phenomena of hunger, satiety, taste, and eating behavior in these disorders. Both the chronicity and relapse rate of aberrant eating behavior is a serious problem (33). Many of the biological aberrations present in anorexia nervosa and bulimia nervosa reflect the nutritional state of the patient and revert to normal with weight gain, cessation of bingeing and purging, and eating a normal diet. Biological mechanisms that influence eating behavior, hunger, and satiety also affect mood, activity level, and cognitive states, which are disturbed in anorexia and bulimia nervosa (28). Thus, it seems reasonable to assume that studies of the basic biology of eating behavior will provide some insight into the aberrant eating behavior present in anorexia nervosa and bulimia nervosa. The first section of this chapter will provide a guide to the behavioral pharmacology of eating. Eating behavior hypotheses and experimental methods used to test those hypotheses are presented. The role of central neurotransmitters, neuropeptides, and peripheral physiology and metabolism in eating is discussed. The second section presents the actual neuroendocrine aberrations measured in anorexia and bulimia nervosa, and the third section integrates the psychological domain of eating behavior with basic physiological mechanisms of eating behavior (see also Chapters 47, 48, 52, 67, 68, 136, and 137, *this volume*).

BEHAVIORAL PHARMACOLOGY OF EATING

Eating behavior reflects an interaction between an organism's physiological state and environmental conditions. Blundell and Hill (4) proposed a model in which the salient physiological variables included the balance of various neuropeptides and neurotransmitters, metabolic state, metabolic rate, condition of the gastrointestinal tract, amount of storage tissue, and receptors for taste and smell. The environmental conditions included features of food such as taste, texture, novelty, accessibility, nutritional composition, and other external conditions such as ambient temperature, presence of other people, and stress. More succinctly, Blundell and Hill's formulation is that the capacity to control nutrient intake to meet bodily needs requires special mechanisms to harmonize physiological information in the internal milieu with nutritional information in the external environment. Hypothalamic eating centers are part of the broad complex of neuroregulator interactions that include a peripheral satiety system (gastrointestinal and pancreatic hormones released by food passing through the gastrointestinal tract) and a broad neural network affecting feeding within the brain. When an exogenous agent such as a drug or peptide is given to an animal or human, it not only activates a specific set of receptors that induce specific responses, but also intervenes in a complex transactional fabric (4). Perceptual capacities identify (a) the characteristics of food materials in the environment and (b) the mechanism to link the biochemical consequences of the ingested food with the consumed structured form. Thus, a control over selection of foods must involve both conditioned and unconditioned responses (5).

Booth (7) proposed a concept of nutritional hedonic conditioning that occurs from the integration of sensory characteristics of foods (including nutritional functioning), culturally derived attitudes, and satiation cues (gastrointestinal tract, peptide hormones, neurotransmitters). Thus, nutritional hedonic conditioning is the process whereby the nutritional functions of the food are related to its sensory characteristics and, thus, its conceptual identity. Immediate determinants of actual food intake in-

K. A. Halmi: Eating Disorders Program, Cornell Medical Center—Westchester Division, White Plains, New York 10605.

clude the influences of sensory input and somatic physiology (8).

Models developed to study feeding in animals have been successfully used with humans. Early test models in animals either (a) used food deprivation to induce eating or (b) observed the effects of hypothalamic lesions. Later, pharmacological agents, either agonists or antagonists to neurotransmitters present in the hypothalamus, were used to probe effects on eating behavior. A microstructural analysis of feeding behavior has been used that involves the simultaneous recording of many behaviors such as drinking, grooming, locomotor activity, resting, and the eating behavior of animals, within a short time frame. Blundell and Latham (6) used a microstructural analysis to obtain extensive data on serotonin manipulations and animal feeding behaviors.

The macroanalysis of feeding patterns is a measurement of long-term feeding patterns in free-feeding animals never subjected to food deprivation. This continuous monitoring procedure has improved the precision of measuring parameters of meal patterns such as meal size, meal duration, meal frequency, inter-meal intervals, and ratio of meal size to meal interval. It allows assessments to be made under normal physiological conditions.

The technique of using varied and palatable diets was used to produce experimental obesity in animals. This dietary self-selection model allows the study of pharmacological agents and exogenously administered hormones on macronutrient (fat, protein, and carbohydrate) consumption.

With a refined microstructural analysis technique, Rogers and Blundell (68) studied human eating behavior using videotaped records. This provided a means for studying intra-meal selection patterns. Using the microanalysis technique, amphetamine was found to inhibit the onset of eating and increase eating rate, whereas fenfluramine shortened the duration of the meal and markedly slowed the rate of eating. With the dietary self-selection method, Silverstone and Kyriakides (70) used an automated food dispenser to study the action of various anorectic drugs on eating profiles.

A sham feeding model has been used in animals (80) in order to determine whether satiety signals arise from oral, gastric, or intestinal sites. In this technique, cannulas are placed in the esophagus or stomach so that they can be temporarily opened during a test to allow drainage and recovery of an ingested food. During sham feeding (cannulas are open), all species overeat. This demonstrates that food stimuli in the mouth are not sufficient to exert a normal satiety reaction. Food infused directly into the intestine produces a dose-related suppression of sham feeding.

The effects of stress on eating has been studied on animals with a mild tail-pinching technique, immobilization, or exposure to a novel environment (64). Obviously,

these stress models and the sham feeding model are more difficult to adapt for studying human behavior.

The experimental models described above have been used to study the role of central neurotransmitters, neuropeptides, and peripheral physiology and metabolism in eating behavior.

Norepinephrine produces an appetite stimulant effect within the paraventricular nucleus (PVN), through α2-noradrenergic receptors (55). It appears to regulate feeding by inhibiting an inhibitor within the PVN. Tricyclic antidepressants stimulate food intake by activating the noradrenergic system in the PVN. During food deprivation there is a decrease of α-adrenergic receptor binding in the PVN and an increase in α-adrenergic receptor binding in the lateral hypothalamus (42). Norepinephrine, when injected in the PVN, causes preferential ingestion of carbohydrate-rich foods (55). Adrenergic β2 receptors in the perifornical hypothalamus (PFH) inhibit feeding when stimulated (54).

Hoebel (39) has used PVN injection studies to demonstrate the utility of serotonin, an indolamine, in the facilitation of satiety. Serotonin injected peripherally and centrally into the PVN suppresses deprivation-induced and norepinephrine-induced eating (53). The Wurtmans (79) demonstrated a feedback mechanism of carbohydrate intake and increased serotonin synthesis in the brains of rats. They demonstrated that increased carbohydrate intake increased the ratio of tryptophan to large neutral amino acids in the blood; this facilitated the entry of tryptophan across the blood–brain barrier, which, in turn, facilitated increased serotonin synthesis because tryptophan is a precursor of serotonin.

Dopaminergic systems are necessary for self-administration behaviors and could be a major link in the role of food as a reinforcer. Low doses of dopamine agonists stimulate feeding, whereas higher doses inhibit feeding (53). Glucose administration suppresses firing in the substantia nigra dopamine neurons. There is evidence of increased hypothalamic dopamine turnover during feeding (36). This finding suggests that central dopamine mechanisms mediate rewarding effects of food as they mediate rewarding effects of intracranial self-stimulation and self-administration of psychoactive drugs. Dopamine blockers, such as pimozide, can decrease intravenous self-injection, self-stimulation, or feeding (78). Self-administration behavior is stimulated by both opiates and nonopiate peptides (neurotensin), which activate dopamine neurons in the ventral tegmental area (VTA), and these cells project in the mesocortical pathway to limbic areas including the nucleus accumbens (24). (See also Chapters 22 and 66, this volume.)

The role of endogenous opioids in eating behavior is more complex. β-Endorphin, morphine, and long-acting enkephalin analogues all induce feeding when injected into the PVN (39). Opioid antagonism decreases feeding in many species, but has no effect in reducing food intake in other species. Under some physiological conditions, such as starving or insulin-induced hypoglycemia, naloxone fails to inhibit feeding. Stress-induced eating is probably driven by activation of the opioid system. Both the K-receptor agonist dynorphin and (to a lesser extent) the mu-opioid increase feeding. The major site of action for dynorphin appears to be the PVN (62). Endogenous opioids seem to influence the intake of foods with a high fat content (69). Morphine-treated rats tend to select fatty foods, whereas naloxone-treated rats tend to avoid fats (53).

Corticotropin-releasing factor (CRF) is a neuropeptide that acts within the PVN to inhibit feeding. Norepinephrine (NE) seems to inhibit the CRF inhibitory feeding affect (63). Continuous infusion of CRF produced weight loss associated with both decreased food intake and increased thermogenesis (2).

Two peptides stimulate eating behavior. The pancreatic polypeptide neuropeptide Y (NPY) increases both food and water intake when injected into the PVN. Another pancreatic polypeptide, peptide YY (PYY), is a more potent stimulator of feeding than NPY (62). Both of these peptides increase weight gain (14), and NPY specifically increases carbohydrate ingestion.

The peripheral satiety network is another important component in the regulation of eating behavior. Satiety may be produced by several gastrointestinal hormones released during the passage of food through the gut. These hormones—cholecystokinin (CCK), glucagon, somatostatin, and bombesin—all decrease food intake after pharmacologic administration. Some of these peptides inhibit feeding by activating ascending vagal fibers. CCK is the most extensively studied of these peptides. The effects of CCK, mediated by vagal fibers, have been traced to the PVN of the hypothalamus, where lesions abolish the CCK effect on feeding (15). Low doses of CCK infused into PVN attenuate feeding, and central infusion of CCK enhances feeding. There is variability of the potency of the satiety effects of CCK across various animal species, and it appears to have little satiety effect in females (71). It is of interest to note that tolerance to the appetite suppressant effects of CCK occurs with prolonged administration. Specifically, in an animal study, CCK continued to suppress meal size, but was ineffective in suppressing 24-hr intake because the animals ate more meals to maintain their food intake (77). Other peptides that appear to inhibit feeding via vagal fibers are glucagon, somatostatin, and thyroid-releasing hormone.

Bombesin is a gastric peptide that inhibits feeding independent of vagal fibers. Systemic injections of bombesin produced a potent and dose-related inhibition of normal feeding (23) and a similar effect on sham feeding (58).

A new glucostatic hypothesis postulates that a small decrease of blood glucose has informational value for the eating system that is not directly related to current metabolic need (57). This postulation is supported by the observation that a decrease in blood glucose occurs shortly before the initiation of a meal in rats with constant access to food. The decreases in glucose are small (approximately 10%), and presumably are not sufficient to decrease cellular glucose utilization in any tissue (12).

NEUROENDOCRINE ABERRATIONS IN ANOREXIA AND BULIMIA NERVOSA

Two studies of healthy men and women placed on diets showed that serotonin function, as measured by pharmacological challenge, was altered significantly in women but not in men (27), and the availability of circulating tryptophan, a precursor necessary for serotonin synthesis, was reduced in the dieting women but not in the dieting men (1). These findings suggest that women may have a biological vulnerability for developing eating disorders. Two studies in eating disorder patients give preliminary evidence that serotonin function may be disturbed in bulimic anorectics, and this may be related to the perception of satiety in those patients. Kaye et al. (47) showed a decreased serotonin turnover in bulimic anorectics compared with restricting anorectics by measuring 5-hydroxyindoleacetic acid (5-HIAA) in cerebrospinal fluid (CSF), after probenecid. Halmi et al. (32) showed that the serotonin antagonist drug, cyproheptadine, enhanced weight gain in restricting anorectics, but decreased weight gain in bulimic anorectics, compared with amitriptyline and placebo groups. Low concentrations of CSF 5-HIAA in low-weight restricting anorectic women, when compared to themselves after weight restoration and controls, suggest a starvation-dependent alteration in serotonin functioning (48). In another study, Kaye et al. (50) found elevated CSF 5-HIAA levels in long-term weight-restored anorectic women compared to controls. This finding suggests a trait contributing to pathological feeding behavior and weight loss. A popular speculation is that the proclivity in anorectic patients to be rigid, inhibited, ritualistic, and perfectionistic might also be associated with increased CSF 5-HIAA levels. Reduced prolactin responses to m-chlorphenylpiperazine (m-CPP), a direct serotonin agonist, and L-tryptophan, a serotonin precursor, in women with anorexia nervosa in both the emaciated state and at normal weight suggest that these anorectic patients have reduced postsynaptic serotonin receptor function in the hypothalamus (11). Serotonin agonists that are effective in reducing obsessive–compulsive behaviors and that are present in relation to food and weight in anorectic patients may be useful for the prevention of relapse in this disorder. At present, no definite conclusions can be drawn from studies of serotonin functioning in anorexia nervosa. Some studies suggest that alteration in the central serotonin system could develop as a result of weight loss, persisting long after weight restoration and contributing to the resistance to weight gain seen in patients with anorexia. Other studies suggest that people who develop anorexia nervosa have a preexisting dysfunction of the homeostatic mechanisms regulating the serotonin system, which then becomes easily destabilized by food restriction and weight loss.

Because serotonin facilitates satiety, it is reasonable to suspect reduced serotonin metabolism in bulimia. Jimerson et al. (43) found that bulimic patients who binge more than twice a day had a lower CSF 5-HIAA level than did controls and those who binge less often. This suggests that highly symptomatic, bulimic patients have a decreased presynaptic release of serotonin. However, studies by Kaye et al. (45) showed that bulimic patients had normal levels of CSF 5-HIAA.

Brewerton et al. (11) showed that bulimic patients given m-CPP had a blunted prolactin response compared with controls, suggesting an abnormality of postsynaptic serotonergic neurons. Only bulimic patients with major depression had a blunted prolactin response to L-tryptophan, suggesting an involvement with both pre- and postsynaptic serotonergic neurons in the depressed bulimics. McBride et al. (59) has shown that bulimic patients have a reduced prolactin response to the serotonin agonist fenfluramine.

In summary, there is a fair amount of evidence suggesting serotonergic dysfunction in anorexia nervosa and serotonergic hypofunction in bulimia nervosa.

There are few noteworthy findings of NE dysfunction in eating disorder patients. Kaye et al. (46) reported that long-term recovered anorexia nervosa patients have low CSF NE levels. In the same study, NE levels were similar in underweight anorexia nervosa patients and in normal controls.

This study needs to be replicated with a larger number of cases. Other studies have shown that plasma NE and urinary MHPG levels are reduced during the starvation state and are increased as anorectic patients gain weight (56).

Investigations using a variety of methodologies suggest that bulimic patients have decreased activity of the sympathetic nervous system. Plasma NE concentrations in bulimia nervosa have been found to be less than those in normal controls (47), as have CSF concentrations (45). Bingeing has been shown to increase plasma NE to higher-than-normal levels in bulimic patients, and abstinence from bingeing and vomiting appears to lower these levels. These findings suggest a state-dependent effect (47). In this same study, lower CSF levels of NE were associated with amenorrhea in bulimic women both when bingeing and abstinent. In another study of actively bingeing patients, CSF MHPG concentrations were normal (43). Kaplan et al. (44), using the $\alpha2$ agonist clonidine in challenge tests in depressed and nondepressed bulimics, found no evidence for adrenergic receptor abnormalities at the hypothalamic level in either group.

The changes in NE metabolism in both anorexia and bulimia nervosa are probably state-related changes associated with starvation and dieting effects.

The abnormal hedonic responses to food present in both anorexia and bulimia nervosa could be related to dopamine function. Halmi et al. (34) showed that anorexia nervosa patients have a decreased growth hormone response to L-DOPA during both the emaciated and the weight-recovered states. They also demonstrated that anorectic patients have a decreased prolactin response to chlorpromazine in both the emaciated and the weight-restored periods. This suggests that anorectic patients have an impairment at the postsynaptic dopamine receptor site. Bulimic patients without a history of anorexia nervosa appear to have lower CSF HVA levels and a less vigorous dopamine response to a clonidine challenge than do normal controls (43,44). These findings suggest that abnormalities in the dopaminergic pathways can lead to decreased satisfaction after eating, which in turn may facilitate binge-eating behavior.

Changes associated with opioid activity in anorexia nervosa are state-related. That is, both the increased levels of opioid activity in the CSF of severely underweight anorectic patients and the decreased CSF β-endorphin levels return to a normal range with nutritional rehabilitation (49,51). Brambilla et al. (9) found that anorectic patients had elevated plasma β-endorphin levels that did not correlate with the degree of weight loss, but rather with the depressive symptomatology.

CSF β-endorphin levels have been found to be lower in normal-weight bulimic women and correlate inversely with the degree of depression (10). In one study (75), plasma β-endorphin levels were found to be decreased in bulimics, and they correlated with the severity of eating disorder but not with the severity of depression. Conversely, another study found plasma β-endorphin levels to be increased in bulimic women when compared to controls (19). Bulimic women who binged but had not purged by vomiting for 1 month prior to this study were found to have normal plasma β-endorphin levels, whereas those actively bingeing and vomiting had elevated levels (20). At the present time, it is not clear that the changes present in the opioid system in bulimia are the result of active bingeing and vomiting, starvation, or a trait feature that might predispose a person to bulimia. The opioid antagonist naloxone decreased the size of binge-eating episodes in bulimic patients in one study (61). A double-blind study with nontoxic doses of the long-acting opioid antagonist naltrexone showed no response in diminishing the binge-eating episodes (60).

In the study of fasting and postprandial plasma CCK concentrations in anorectic women, normal levels were found both when they were underweight and following short-term weight restoration (22). These findings do not support a hypothetical role for the hypersecretion of CCK in the etiology of anorexia nervosa. Geracioti and Liddle (21) reported that, compared with normal control subjects, bulimia nervosa patients had a decreased CCK response to an experimental meal. After these patients were treated with tricyclic antidepressants and had a decrease in binge eating, an increase in the postprandial CCK response and an increase in the satiety response occurred. It remains to be answered whether CCK has a primary pathognomonic or physiological role in bulimia or whether it represents an epiphenomena reflecting chronic gastrointestinal overextension.

Underweight anorectic women have been found to have normal CSF PYY concentrations and elevated CSF NPY concentrations, which remain significantly elevated after short-term weight restoration (45). In long-term weight-restored anorectics the CSF NPY levels returned to normal in those women who regain regular menstruation and remained elevated in those who continued to be amenorrheic or oligomenorrheic. Elevations in NPY do not appear to stimulate eating in women with anorexia nervosa and may simply reflect the starvation condition.

In bulimic patients, CSF PYY concentrations were found to be normal when the bulimics were actively bingeing and purging. These levels became elevated after 30 days of abstinence from bingeing and purging. CSF NPY values remained normal before and after the bulimic patients' abstinent period (45). The elevation of PYY following abstinence from bingeing and vomiting in bulimic patients cannot be easily explained, and it needs to be replicated. It seems unlikely that the elevation of PYY is a trait in persons vulnerable to develop bulimia, and that bingeing and vomiting is an attempt to normalize some intrinsic aberration.

It was demonstrated almost 20 years ago that anorectic patients have an impaired ability to concentrate urine (74). Later studies showed that anorectic patients have abnormally high levels of plasma and CSF vasopressin that gradually return to normal with weight gain (25). Demitrack et al. (16) showed that an underweight anorectic patient also has reduced CSF oxytocin levels that return to normal with weight restoration. Demitrack et al. hypothesize that a low level of oxytocin and a high level of vasopressin could work in concert to enhance the retention of distorted thinking about food and contribute to the anorectic patient's obsessional concerns about it. Oxytocin appears to disrupt memory consolidation and retrieval, whereas vasopressin promotes the consolidation of learning. Oxytocin also inhibits vasopressin-induced adrenal corticotrophic hormone release from the anterior pituitary gland. Nishita et al. (66) showed that vasopressin secretion abnormalities with hypertonic saline infusion occur in both underweight and weight-restored anorectics, as well as in bulimic patients. Vasopressin abnormalities in the bulimic patients are probably an epiphenomena of the electrolyte changes associated with self-induced vomiting. Two studies have shown elevated levels of CRF in the CSF of patients with anorexia nervosa (41,49). These elevated CRF levels returned to a normal range with

weight gain. Central and peripheral adrenocorticotropic hormone (ACTH) and cortisol levels are elevated in underweight anorectic patients, and they returned to normal with weight restoration (29). Kaye et al. (49) did find a positive correlation between CSF corticotropin-releasing hormone (CRH) levels and depression in weight-restored but not underweight patients. CRF secretion may have a role in maintaining anorectic behaviors and initiating a relapse. There is a possibility that hypersecretion of CRH may pre-date the weight loss in some anorectic patients, particularly those where depression does exist.

Normal-weight bulimic women have been shown to have normal (76) and elevated 24-hr plasma cortisol levels (65). Nocturnal circadian patterns of cortisol production have been found to be both normal (18) and elevated (52). Also, cortisol and ACTH response to CRH administration has been shown to be normal (29) and blunted (65). Actively bingeing and vomiting bulimics have demonstrated both normal CSF and plasma ACTH and cortisol levels and decreased CSF and ACTH levels following a 30-day period of abstinence (29). These conflicting CRH findings need to be clarified and may be related to dieting behavior.

Casper et al. (13) studied menstruating, weight-recovered, anorectic patients and nonrecovered, amenorrheic, underweight patients. Recovered patients showed glucose tolerance curves and insulin responses similar to those of normal controls, whereas nonrecovered anorectic patients had persistently abnormal glucose tolerance and delayed insulin release. Glucose metabolism abnormalities appear to reverse with affective treatment in these patients.

Low fasting glucose levels have been found in bulimic women (17,67). Goldbloom et al. (26) showed that fasting glucose, alanine, pyruvic, fat-derived metabolites, insulin, and glucagon were similar in actively bingeing and purging bulimic women and normal controls. The C peptide (secreted by the pancreas in equal amounts with insulin) level in bulimic patients was 50% that of controls, indicating a decreased clearance of insulin in the patient group. Blouin et al. (3) found that after an intravenous glucose challenge, blood glucose level and insulin/glucagon ratio remained lower in bulimics than in controls for 45 min after injection. These observed physiological differences were accompanied by an increased subjective craving for sweets, an enhanced urge to binge, and less subjective control over food intake compared to controls.

INTEGRATING MECHANISMS OF THE PSYCHOLOGICAL AND PHYSIOLOGICAL ASPECTS OF EATING BEHAVIOR

In the section of this chapter entitled "Behavioral Pharmacology of Eating," Blundell and Hill's model of eating behavior was described (4). In summary, their formulation was that the capacity to control nutrient intake to meet bodily needs requires specialized mechanisms to harmonize the physiological information in the internal milieu with nutritional information in the external environment. Two essential features are perceptual capacities to identify the characteristics of food materials in the environment and a specialized mechanism to link the biochemical consequences of the ingested food with the consumed structured form (4). One of these integrating mechanisms is the perception of hunger and satiety (37). In this section, studies of hunger and satiety perceptions of eating disorders will be reviewed along with studies of macronutrient and taste influences on eating behavior in the eating disorders.

Using an experimental meal paradigm with a liquid formula, Halmi et al. (30,35) were able to demonstrate that eating-disorder patients have disturbances in the perception of hunger and satiety. The hunger and satiety curves before, during, and after the experimental meal demonstrated that anorexia nervosa and bulimia nervosa patients often have difficulty distinguishing between perceptions of hunger and satiety. Underweight anorectics had lower hunger levels, higher satiety levels, and less urge to eat than did normal-weight bulimics and normal-weight controls. Subjects who binged and purged were more preoccupied with thoughts of food, and normal-weight bulimics had more urge to eat after finishing a meal. Two patterns of responses emerged unaltered by treatment: (i) Those patients who were previously underweight (ANR and ANB) continued to have lower hunger ratings than did the other two groups, and (ii) ANR continued to have a higher level of satiety than did the other groups. After treatment, a difference emerged in those patients with a history of bingeing and purging. They had significantly higher palatability ratings than did ANR and controls. Urge to eat was positively correlated with monthly binge frequency for the bulimic subjects. Bulimic patients who binged the most were also the most depressed.

After establishing differences in hunger and satiety perceptions in eating-disorder patients with a standard liquid formula, Halmi et al. (31) studied the responses in anorectic and bulimic patients to meals differing in macronutrient content. In this preliminary report, there were distinct differences in the hunger and satiety responses in bulimia nervosa patients to meals that were high in carbohydrate and low in fat compared with meals that were low in carbohydrate and high in fat. In addition, the bulimic responses were different from both the unrestrained normal controls and the anorectic restrictors. It appears that the high-fat meals may indeed provoke a hunger stimulus in bulimic patients, but not in controls and not in anorectic restrictors.

The fullness or satiety ratings were consistently higher in the anorectic restrictors before both high-fat and high-carbohydrate meals; however, they remained higher compared with the other groups only after the high-fat meal. The bulimics had lower fullness or satiety ratings after the high-fat meal compared with the high-carbohydrate meal and compared with the anorectic restrictor ratings. Another interesting finding occurred with bulimics after the high-fat meal. After 8 min their ratings began to increase, and after 14 min their hunger ratings were only slightly below those they had at the beginning of the meal. This did not occur with the high-carbohydrate meal, after which the normal-weight bulimics had substantially lower hunger ratings compared with those before that meal. The hunger and satiety curve patterns before, during, and after the meal were markedly distorted in all of the eating-disorder patients.

There is ample evidence from the studies just described that the integrating processes for physiological information and perceptual capacities in the control of eating behavior is markedly disturbed in both anorexia and bulimia nervosa patients.

In a study of taste perceptions in eating-disorder patients (72), the anorectic restrictors and anorectic bulimics displayed a pronounced aversion to high-fat stimuli. The anorectic restrictors also showed a strong dislike for solutions that contained little or no sweetness. The negative responses to fat persisted following weight restoration, suggesting that this behavior may be a stable trait characteristic of anorexia nervosa. The bulimic patients did not differ in their hedonic ratings compared with control subjects. The results of the taste study match those of a cognitive preference study (73), in which all patients with a current or past history of anorexia nervosa significantly disliked high-fat, high-calorie foods compared with the control groups and the bulimic patients. After weight restoration, this intense dislike of high-fat and high-calorie foods persisted and, therefore, appears to be a stable trait characteristic in anorexia nervosa.

From the review presented here, it is obvious that there are aberrations or dysfunctions in many physiological systems in both anorexia and bulimia nervosa. Most of these physiological systems interact with each other, and most of the research conducted has studied individual isolated physiological mechanisms. Although it is a costly endeavor and difficult to accomplish, future research focusing on the interactions of these various systems would probably yield far more significant and helpful information for understanding the development of these disorders and providing clues for more affective treatment strategies.

What are some of the areas that warrant continued and more creative research? The studies of insulin secretion in anorexia and bulimia nervosa are contradictory, but there is enough evidence of changes present that warrant further investigation. CRH hypersecretion may have a role in maintaining anorectic behaviors and initiating a relapse and, therefore, deserves further study. There is considerable evidence for serotonin dysfunction in both anorexia and bulimia nervosa. Just how these aberrations interact and affect eating behavior in these disorders needs to be clarified. The persistent low CSF NE levels in long-term so-called weight-restored anorectics needs an explanation. Does this merely reflect continued aberrant eating behavior and dieting? If so, how does it affect and sustain abnormal eating behavior? Very little research has been conducted on the role of dopamine and eating behavior in the eating disorders. The abnormal hedonic food responses seen in both anorexia and bulimia nervosa could be related to dopamine function. There are only a few studies on neuropeptides in eating disorders. These studies indicate that aberrations in the neuropeptides affecting eating behavior are present in anorexia and bulimia nervosa. Creative studies in this area may show how changes in these neuropeptides and neurotransmitters affect the disturbed integrating mechanisms of hunger and satiety perceptions.

REFERENCES

1. Anderson IM, Perry-Billings SM, Newsholme EA, et al. Dieting reduces plasma tryptophan and alters brain 5-HT function in women. *Psychol Med* 1990;20:785–791.
2. Arase K, York DA, Chimizuh H. Effects of corticotropin releasing factor in food intake in brown adipose tissue thermogenesis in rats. *Am J Physiol* 1988;255:e255–e259.
3. Blouin AG, Blouin JH, Bratan JT, et al. Physiological and psychological responses to a glucose challenge in bulimia. *Int J Eating Disord* 1990;10:285–296.
4. Blundell JE, Hill AJ. Behavioral pharmacology of feeding: relevance of animal experiments in man. In: Carruba N, Blundell JE, eds. *Pharmacology of eating disorders.* New York: Raven Press, 1986; 51–70.
5. Blundell JE, Hill AJ. Nutrition, serotonin and appetite: case study in the evolution of a scientific idea. *Appetite* 1987;8:183–194.
6. Blundell JE, Latham M. Serotonergic influences on food intake: effect on 5-hydroxytryptophan on parameters of feeding behavior in deprived and free-feeding rats. *Pharmacol Biochem Behav* 1979;11:431–437.
7. Booth DA. How should questions about satiation be asked? *Appetite* 1981;2:237–244.
8. Booth DA. Food-conditioned eating preferences and aversions with interceptive elements: conditioned appetite and satieties. *Ann NY Acad Sci* 1985;443:22–41.
9. Brambilla F, Cavagnini F, Invitti C, et al. Neuroendocrine and psychopathological measures in anorexia nervosa: resemblances to primary affective disorders. *Psychiatry Res* 1985;16:165–176.
10. Brewerton TD, Lydiard RB, Laraia MT, et al. CSF beta-endorphins and dynorphin in bulimia nervosa. *Am J Psychiatry* 1992;149:1086–1090.
11. Brewerton TD, Mueller ED, Lesem MD. Neuroendocrine responses to *m*-chlorophenol piperazine and L-tryptophan in bulimia. *Arch Gen Psychiatr* 1992;49:852–861.
12. Campfield LA, Brandan B, Smith FJ. Reduction in blood sugar before initiation of meals. *Brain Res Bull* 1985;14:605–616.
13. Casper RC, Pandy G, Jaspen JB, et al. Eating attitudes and glucose tolerance in anorexia nervosa patients at 8-year follow-up compared to control subjects. *Psychiatry Res* 1988;25:283–299.
14. Clark JT, Crawley WR, Kalra SP. Neuropeptide-Y and human pancreatic polypeptide stimulate feeding behavior in rats. *Endocrinology* 1984;115:427–429.
15. Crawley JN, Kiss JZ. Central control of CCK. *Ann NY Acad Sci* 1985;488:586–588.
16. Demitrack MA, Lesem MD, Listwak SJ, et al. CSF oxytocin in anorexia nervosa and bulimia nervosa: clinical and pathophysiological considerations. *Am J Psychiatry* 1990;147:882–886.
17. Devlin MJ, Walsh T, Kral G, et al. Metabolic abnormalities in bulimia nervosa. *Arch Gen Psychiatry* 1990;47:144–148.
18. Fichter MM, Pirke KM, Pollinger J, et al. Disturbances in the hypothalamal–pituitary–adrenal and other neuroendocrine axes in bulimia. *Biol Psychiatry* 1990;27:1021–1037.
19. Fullerton DT, Swift WJ, Getto CJ, et al. Plasma immunoreactive β-endorphin in bulimics. *Psychol Med* 1986;16:59–63.
20. Fullerton DT, Swift WJ, Getto CJ, et al. Differences in the plasma β-endorphin levels of bulimics. *Int J Eating Disord* 1988;7:191–200.
21. Geracioti TD, Liddle RA. Impaired cholecystokinin secretion in bulimia nervosa. *N Engl J Med* 1988;319:683–688.
22. Geracioti TD, Liddle RA, Altemus M, et al. Regulation of appetite and cholecystokinin secretion in anorexia nervosa. *Am J Psychiatry* 1992;149:958–961.
23. Gibbs J, Madison SP, Rolles ET. Bombesin and eating. *J Comp Physiol Psychol* 1981;85:1003–1015.
24. Glimcher P, Margolin D. Dopamine pathways. *Brain Res* 1986;266:348–352.
25. Gold PW, Kaye WH, Robertson GL, et al. Abnormalities in plasma and cerebral spinal-fluid arginine vasopressin in patients with anorexia nervosa. *N Engl J Med* 1983;308:1117–1123.
26. Goldbloom DS, Zinman B, Hicks LK, et al. The baseline metabolic state in bulimia nervosa: abnormality and adaptation. *Int J Eating Disord* 1992;12:171–178.
27. Goodwin GM, Fairburn CG, Cowen PJ. Dieting changes serotonergic function in women but not men: implications for the etiology of anorexia nervosa? *Psychol Med* 1987;17:839–842.
28. Grossman SP. Eating behavior, the biology of motivation. *Annu Rev Psychol* 1979;30:209–242.
29. Gwirtsman HE, Kaye WH, George DT. Central and peripheral ACTH and cortisol levels in anorexia nervosa and bulimia. *Arch Gen Psychiatry* 1989;46:61–69.
30. Halmi KA, Sunday SR. Temporal patterns of hunger and fullness ratings and related cognitions in anorexia and bulimia. *Appetite* 1991;16:219–237.
31. Halmi KA, Sunday SR. Macronutrient effects on eating behavior in anorexia and bulimia nervosa. SSIB, June 24–28, 1992. Princeton University, Princeton, NJ.
32. Halmi KA, Eckert E, LaDu T, Cohen J. Anorexia nervosa: treatment efficacy of cyproheptadine and amitriptyline. *Arch Gen Psychiatry* 1986;43:177–181.
33. Halmi KA, Eckert E, Marchi PA, et al. Comorbidity of psychiatric diagnoses in anorexia nervosa. *Arch Gen Psychiatry* 1991;48:712–718.
34. Halmi KA, Owen WP, Lasley E, Stokes P. Dopaminergic regulation in anorexia nervosa. *Int J Eating Disord* 1983;21:192–233.
35. Halmi KA, Sunday SR, Puglisi A, Marchi PA. Hunger and satiety in anorexia and bulimia nervosa. In: Schnieder LH, Cooper SJ, Halmi KA, eds. *The psychobiology of human eating disorders.* New York: New York Academy of Sciences, 1989;431–445.
36. Heffner TG, Hartman JA, Seiden LS. Dopamine turnover in feeding. *Science* 1986;208:1168–1170.
37. Hill AJ, Magson LE, Blundell JE. Hunger and palatability: tracking ratings of selective experience before, during and after consumption of preferred and less preferred foods. *Appetite* 1984;8:361–371.
38. Hoebel BG. Pharmacological control with feeding. *Annu Rev Pharmacol Toxicol* 1977;17:605–621.
39. Hoebel BG. Hypothalamic self-stimulation and stimulation escape in relation to feeding and mating. *Fed Proc* 1979;30:2454–2461.
40. Hoebel BG. Neurotransmitters in the control of feeding and its rewards: monoamines, opiates, and brain–gut peptides. In: Stunkard AJ, Steller E, eds. *Eating and its disorders.* New York: Raven Press, 1984;15–38.
41. Hotta M, Chibasaki T, Masuda A, et al. The responses of plasma adrenal corticotropin and cortisol to corticotropin-releasing hormone and cerebral spinal fluid immunoreactive CRH in anorexia nervosa patients. *J Clin Endocrinol Metab* 1986;62:319–321.
42. Jhanvar-Uniyal M, Fleisher F, Levine BE. Alpha-adrenergic receptor binding in the lateral hypothalamus. *Abstr Soc Neurosci* 1982;8:711.
43. Jimerson DC, Lessem MD, Kaye WH, et al. Low serotonin and

dopamine metabolite concentrations in cerebral spinal fluid from bulimic patients with frequent binge episodes. *Arch Gen Psychiatry* 1992;49:132–138.

44. Kaplan AS, Garfinkel PE, Walsh FC, et al. Clonedine challenge test in bulimia nervosa. *Int J Eating Disord* 1989;8:425–435.

45. Kaye WH, Berrettini W, Gwirtsman HE, et al. Altered cerebral spinal fluid neuropeptide-Y and peptide-YY immunoactivity in anorexia and bulimia nervosa. *Arch Gen Psychiatry* 1990;47:548–556.

46. Kaye WH, Ebert N, Gwirtsman HE, et al. Serotonin metabolism in anorexia nervosa. *Am J Psychiatry* 1984;41:1598–1601.

47. Kaye WH, Ebert MH, Gwirtsman HE, et al. CSF monoamine levels in normal weight bulimia & evidence for abnormal noradrenergic activity. *Am J Psychiatry* 1990;147:225–229.

48. Kaye WH, Ebert N, Raleigh M, et al. Abnormalities in CNS monoamine metabolism in anorexia nervosa. *Arch Gen Psychiatry* 1984;41:350–355.

49. Kaye WH, Gwirtsman HE, George DT. Elevated cerebral spinal fluid levels of immunoreactive corticotropin-releasing hormones in anorexia nervosa: relation to state of nutrition adrenal function, and intensity of depression. *J Clin Endocrinol Metab* 1987;64:203–208.

50. Kaye WH, Gwirtsman HE, George DT, et al. Altered serotonin activity in anorexia nervosa after long-term weight restoration. *Arch Gen Psychiatry* 1991;48:556–562.

51. Kaye WH, Pickar D, Naber D, et al. Cerebral spinal fluid opioid activity in anorexia nervosa. *Am J Psychiatry* 1982;139:643–645.

52. Kennedy SH, Garfinkel PE, Parienti V, et al. Changes in mellatonin levels but not cortisol levels are associated with depression in patients with eating disorders. *Arch Gen Psychiatry* 1989;46:73–78.

53. Leibowitz SF. Opioids and food selection. In: Morgan PG, Pankse PP, eds. *Handbook of the hypothalamus,* vol 3. New York: Marcel Dekker, 1982;299–437.

54. Leibowitz SF. Neurochemical systems of the hypothalamus: control of feeding and drinking behavior and water electrolyte excretion. In: Morgan PJ, Panksepp J, eds. *Handbook of the Hypothalamus,* vol 3. New York: Raven Press, 1987;130–150.

55. Leibowitz SF, Brown O, Trettor JE Jr, et al. Norepinephrine, clonidine and tricyclic antidepressants selectively stimulate carbohydrate ingestion through noradrenergic system of the paraventricular nucleus. *Pharmacol Biochem Behav* 1985;23:541–550.

56. Lessem MD, George DT, Kaye WH. State-related changes in norepinephrine regulation in anorexia nervosa. *Biol Psychiatry* 1989;25:509–512.

57. Louis-Sylvester J, LeMagnen J. A new glucostatic hypothesis. *Neurosci Biobehav Rev* 1980;4:13–15.

58. Martin CF, Gibbs J. Bombesin effect on sham feeding. *Peptides* 1980;1:131–134.

59. McBride PA, Anderson GM, Khait V, Sunday SR, Halmi KA. Serotonergic responsivity in eating disorders. *Psychopharmacol Bull* 1991;27:365–372.

60. Mitchell JE, Christenson G, Jennings J, et al. A placebo-controlled, double-blind crossover study of naltrexone hydrochloride in outpatients with normal-weight bulimia. *J Clin Pharmacol* 1989;9:94–97.

61. Mitchell JE, Laine DE, Morley JE. Naloxone but not CCK-8 may attenuate binge eating in patients with bulimia syndrome. *Biol Psychiatry* 1986;21:1399–1406.

62. Morley JE, Levine AS, Grace M. Peptide-YY: a potent orexigenic agent. *Brain Res* 1985;340:200–203.

63. Morley JE, Levine AS. Corticotropin-releasing factor, grooming and ingestive behavior. *Life Sci* 1982;31:1459–1464.

64. Morley JE, Levine AS, Willenbirng NL. Stress induced feeding disorder. In: Carruba M, Blundell JE, eds. *Pharmacology of Eating disorders.* New York: Raven Press, 1986;71–100.

65. Mortola JF, Rasmussen BE, Yen SSC. Alterations of the adrenal corticotropin–cortisol axis in normal weight bulimic women: evidence for a central mechanism. *J Clin Endocrinol Metab* 1989;68:517–522.

66. Nishita JK, Ellinwood EH, Rockwell WJK, et al. Abnormalities in the response of plasma argenine vasopressin during hypertonic salene fusion in patients with eating disorders. *Biol Psychiatry* 1989;26:73–86.

67. Pirke KM, Pahl J, Schweiger U, et al. Metabolic and endocrine indices of starvation in bulimia: a comparison with anorexia nervosa. *Psychiatry Res* 1985;15:33–39.

68. Rogers PJ, Blundell JE. Effect of anorectic drugs on food intake, and the micro-structure of eating in human subjects. *Psychopharmacology* 1979;66:159–165.

69. Rosmos DR, Gosnell BA, Morley JE. Effects of kappa opiate agonist cholescystokinin and bombesin on intake of diets varying in carbohydrate to fat ratio in rats. *J Nutr* 1987;117:976–985.

70. Silverstone T, Kyriakides M. Clinical pharmacology of appetite. In: Silverstone T, eds. *Drugs and appetite,* New York: Academic Press, 1982;50–65.

71. Strohmeyer AJ, Smith G. A sex difference in the effect of CCK on food and water intake in obese and lean mice. *Peptides* 1987;8:845–848.

72. Sunday SR, Halmi KA. Taste perceptions and hedonics in eating disorders. *Physiol Behav* 1990;48:587–594.

73. Sunday SR, Einhorn A, Halmi KA. The relationship of perceived macronutrient and caloric content to affective cognitions about food. *Am J Clin Nutr* 1992;55:362–371.

74. Vigersky RA, Loriaux DL, Anderson AE, et al. Anorexia nervosa: behavioral and hypothalamic aspects. *Clin Endocrinol Metab* 1976;5:517–535.

75. Waller DS, Kiser RS, Hardy BW, et al. Eating behavior in plasma β-endorphin in bulimia. *Am Clin Nutr* 1986;44:20–23.

76. Walsh BT, Roose SP, Katz JL, et al. Hypothalamic–pituitary–adrenal cortical activity in anorexia nervosa and bulimia. *Psychoneuroendocrinology* 1987;12:131–140.

77. West BE, Fay ED, Woods CS. Cholescystokinin consistently suppresses meal sites but not food intake in free-feeding rats. *Am J Physiol* 1984;246:776–787.

78. Wise RA, Spindler J, DWit H, Gerber GJ. Sub-stimulation behaviors. *Science* 1978;201:262–264.

79. Wurtman JJ, Wurtman RJ. Drugs that enhance central serotonergic transmission diminish elective carbohydrate consumption by rats. *Life Sci* 1979;24:895–903.

80. Young RC, Gibbs J, Anton J, et al. Sham feeding. *J Comp Physiol Psychol* 1974;87:795–800.

Psychopharmacology: The Fourth Generation of Progress, edited by Floyd E. Bloom and David J. Kupfer. Raven Press, Ltd., New York © 1995.

CHAPTER 139

Disordered Sleep

Developmental and Biopsychosocial Perspectives on the Diagnosis and Treatment of Persistent Insomnia

Charles F. Reynolds III, Daniel J. Buysse, and David J. Kupfer

The maintenance of a robust circadian rhythm of sleep and waking is a vital component of successful adaptation across the life cycle, in that sleep and circadian rhythms help to regulate mood and govern the ability to perform cognitively. Changes in sleep, sleep quality, and daytime alertness have enormous impact on quality of life, level of functioning, and (particularly in late life) ability to remain independent (43,45,47,70). Hence, preserving the integrity of sleep across the life cycle is a major public health priority and is, we suggest, a critical correlate of "successful aging" (59).

In this chapter we will focus primarily on persistent insomnia as a prototypical sleep disorder because of its importance to psychiatry and neuropsychopharmacology. The symptom of persistent insomnia can result from numerous factors operating singly or in combination. The most important factors contributing to insomnia include psychiatric disorders, behavioral patterns destructive to sleep (e.g., worrying excessively about sleep, irregular sleep–wake schedule, spending excessive time in bed), medication and substance use, medical/neurological illness, circadian dyssynchrony, and intrinsic sleep pathologies (25) (see Chapter 86, *this volume*). However, considerable debate continues regarding the relative importance of these factors in the conceptualization and presumed etiology of persistent insomnia. Some investigators have argued that most insomnia complaints reflect psychiatric and psychological disturbances (32,64). Other investiga-

tors have emphasized the importance of other causes, often relying on polysomnographic information to make causal inferences (11,15,30).

Within this context, the goals of this chapter are as follows: (a) to review epidemiological data on the prevalence of sleep disturbance, particularly of persistent insomnia, in relation to psychiatric disorders; (b) to review medical correlates of persistent insomnia in clinical samples; (c) to review psychosocial correlates of persistent insomnia in clinical samples and in the general population; (d) to model the interrelationships of psychosocial, medical, and sleep-related factors in successful adaptation; (e) to review the major findings from the recent DSM-IV field trials on sleep disorders; and (f) to review promising leads which might help to elucidate the neurobiological significance of sleep physiological abnormalities in major psychiatric disorders, such as depression, schizophrenia, and Alzheimer's dementia. We will conclude by highlighting promising directions for intervention research and recent methodological developments pertinent to such research. Readers wishing to pursue specific conceptual and methodologic issues in relation to sleep and affective disorders are referred to Kupfer and Reynolds (38) and to Benca et al. (3). With respect to the Benca et al. (3) meta-analysis of electroencephalographic (EEG) sleep measures in psychiatric disorders, we underscored the importance of several issues: (a) the use of multivariate approaches in the ascertainment of sensitivity and specificity; (b) the use of quantitative automated measured of rapid eye movement (REM) and delta activity; and (c) the need to consider EEG sleep measures from remitted depressed patients, off medication (39).

C. F. Reynolds, D. J. Buysse, and D. J. Kupfer: Sleep and Chronobiology Center, Department of Psychiatry, Western Psychiatric Institute and Clinic, University of Pittsburgh School of Medicine, Pittsburgh, Pennsylvania 15213.

EPIDEMIOLOGICAL SIGNIFICANCE OF INSOMNIA: A DEVELOPMENTAL PERSPECTIVE

Epidemiological studies of insomnia have reported that between 10% and 20% of respondents characterize their sleep problems as severe or constant (4,33,41). Sleep maintenance insomnia is the most frequent problem, followed by difficulty falling asleep and then early morning awakening. Several important demographic trends also emerge: First, complaints of poor sleep or insomnia increase with age, apparently paralleling age-related changes in sleep-stage physiology (18,73). In addition, younger insomniacs more frequently complain of difficulty falling asleep, whereas older patients often complain of middle and terminal insomnia. Second, women of all ages have more sleep complaints than men. Third, complaints of poor sleep are more common in lower socioeconomic groups. However, despite the large number of people with insomnia complaints, only one-third seek medical help for this problem (71).

Epidemiological studies have also documented a robust association between insomnia and psychiatric disorders (particularly depression and anxiety) across the life cycle. For example, in the Zurich study, where the course of insomnia was examined over 7 years in a cohort of young adults, the authors reported the following: (a) specific associations between recurrent brief insomnia and recurrent brief depression; (b) an association between continued insomnia and major depression; and (c) an association between any form of insomnia and anxiety disorders (69). The authors also observed that insomnia tends to recur, regardless of subtype. Similarly, reporting on a study of a mixed-age clinical sample of 954 psychiatric patients with major affective disorders, Fawcett et al. (17) observed six clinical features which were associated with suicide within 1 year. They included global insomnia, which is potentially a modifiable suicide risk factor. Similarly, the prevalence of persistent sleep disturbance is quite high in community resident samples, particularly among the elderly, where a 12–15% 6-month prevalence rate of persistent sleep disturbance was noted in the epidemiological catchment area (ECA) survey by Ford and Kamerow (19).

Persistent sleep disturbance was identified in the ECA data set as a highly significant risk factor for the *subsequent* development of major depression, as well as a major factor in patient and family decisions to seek services from the primary care sector. Hence, Ford and Kamerow (19) suggested that early intervention to treat sleep disturbance might protect patients from developing major depression.

In the setting of sleep, psychiatric morbidity, and quality of life, a longitudinal study of depressed mood and sleep disturbances in the elderly by Rodin et al. (55) examined the association between frequency of depressed mood and self-reports of four sleep problems over a 3-year period in a randomly selected sample of 198 community residents (mean age of 72). A robust association between frequency of depressed mood and severity of sleep symptoms was noted, after controlling for health status, gender, and age. Longitudinal fluctuation in sleep complaints (particularly sleep continuity disturbance and early morning awakening) covaried strongly with intensity of depressive symptoms. This observation was confirmed and extended by Kennedy et al. (34), who studied the persistence or remission of depressive symptoms in late life in a sample of 1885 adults aged 65 or older from the NIMH ECA study. The authors observed that changes in health, sleep disturbance, and added formal support services distinguished the persistently depressed and remitted groups.

Taken together, these studies across the life cycle suggest that sleep disturbance is a consequence of depressive symptoms, a significant correlate of help-seeking behavior, and a major risk factor for the subsequent development of syndromal major depression. Other studies have shown that sleep-related behaviors often precipitate the decision of families to institutionalize an elderly dementing relative (45,48,60). Any understanding of how to attenuate the sleep changes and disturbances of usual and pathological aging that would reduce psychiatric morbidity, burden to families, and the rate of institutionalization would be of enormous public health significance. Thus, we believe that the challenge to researchers and clinicians is to understand how the successful functioning of the aging circadian time-keeping system can be preserved in the face of multiple medical and psychosocial challenges (12).

MEDICAL CORRELATES OF SLEEP DISTURBANCE

As recently reviewed by Bliwise (5), there is now considerable evidence underscoring the general effects, either direct or indirect, of medical illness burden in poor sleep. While such difficulties often reflect presumably nonspecific effects of pain, impaired mobility, poor nutrition, and poor physical conditioning, specific clinical symptoms or disorders have also been shown to have negative effects upon sleep quality, including nocturia (16,78), headache (13), gastrointestinal illness (40), bronchitis and asthma (40), cardiovascular symptoms (28), and Type II diabetes (28). Chronic pain from conditions like osteoarthritis also disrupts sleep in the elderly (74). In addition, elevated autonomic activity and a greater susceptibility to external arousal may be important predisposing factors to disturbed sleep, particularly in later life (46,58,76,77).

Medical and neurological illness and cognitive impairment may be related not only to sleep, but to mortality as well. We have reported increases in sleep-disordered breathing, as well as deterioration in sleep continuity and REM sleep, in patients with Alzheimer's dementia (54). These changes correlate with 2-year mortality (27). Furthermore, Kripke et al. (36), Ancoli-Israel et al. (2), and Bliwise (5) have observed (a) high prevalence of sleep-disordered breathing with aging and (b) attendant increases in morbidity and mortality. Other data—for example, those of He et al. (26)—suggest, however, that sleep-disordered breathing may have a stronger relationship to mortality in midlife (where it is often more severe) than in late life (where it is typically subsyndromal).

PSYCHOSOCIAL AND PSYCHIATRIC CORRELATES OF INSOMNIA

As we have recently reviewed (14), sleep problems are often reported to occur in the context of, or to be exacerbated by, other life stressors. By far the most extensive body of work has focused on sleep disturbances in treated psychiatric patient populations documenting the significant comorbidity between sleep abnormalities and psychiatric disorder, particularly in the area of mood disorders (38). The descriptive, primarily cross-sectional investigations in this domain have detailed a range of abnormalities in sleep continuity and architecture and have also considered the clinical and sociodemographic correlates of these abnormalities across the lifespan, both with respect to subjective self-report measures (7) and with respect to objective polysomnographic indices (23,27,54). The age of subjects in particular appears to be an important moderator of the sleep changes that accompany psychiatric disorders (35), and late-age sleep deterioration in general has been found to be influenced by a variety of psychosocial factors, including gender (53), major life events such as bereavement (51), and ongoing strains such as those arising from chronic medical illness (5).

These clinical sleep studies, recognizing the multifactorial nature of life stresses and their correlates, have begun to expand the breadth of their psychosocial assessments in order to yield a more accurate and detailed picture of the social circumstances in which subjects' lives and their sleep are embedded. As Dew et al. (14) have pointed out, an important limitation of most existing studies is that the generalizability of findings from selected patient groups to nonpatient-community samples, the majority of whom do not seek treatment, is questionable. In fact, Vitiello et al. (67) reported that polysomnographic sleep is undisturbed in depressed individuals who have not sought health care.

Several studies of nonpatient, community-based samples have carefully examined (a) the roles of multiple psychosocial factors in altered sleep patterns and (b) the impact of sleep and sleep quality on subsequent quality of life. These reports provide evidence that diverse variables such as life events, psychological state, age, and gender are robustly correlated with reduced sleep quality (9,55).

With few exceptions (9), however, studies employing nonpatient samples have relied on subjective reports of sleep problems, rather than objective polysomnographic data which is, by contrast, available in many clinical populations. Given this gap in the database, our group recently performed a study examining longitudinal data on psychosocial status and polysomnographic sleep collected annually from 57 healthy, community-residing elders aged 61–89 (14). Cluster analysis of variables reflecting sleep continuity and architecture at the baseline assessment identified three groups of elders: those whose sleep was either (a) superior to all remaining respondents across a variety of measures, (b) marred only by significantly reduced sleep efficiency relative to other respondents, or (c) poorer than all other respondents in multiple areas. Cross-validation procedures suggested that the three-group cluster solution was stable and replicable over persons and over time. Subsequent multivariate analyses indicated that recent life events, as well as psychosocial stability and support variables at baseline, distinguished the sleep-pattern groups. Moreover, sleep pattern group membership itself predicted subjects' subsequent sleep characteristics and psychosocial status at follow-up. Of special significance, the group of elderly subjects with poor sleep efficiency had more negative social circumstances at baseline, with an elevated number of major negative life events as well as less social stability and support (as reflected by reduced social rhythmicity, number of regular activities, and lower levels of perceived instrumental social support). This finding is consistent with the growing literature documenting the pathogenic role of life stress and the protective role of social stability and support with respect to mental health and well-being (for review focused on the elderly, see ref. 50).

These data led us to propose that specific psychosocial factors (e.g., major life events and social support) contribute to observed sleep variability. Furthermore, we hypothesize that EEG sleep disturbances will also themselves be likely to influence subsequent adaptation along physical, psychological, and psychosocial dimensions. These data clearly support the significance of considering a rich array of psychosocial variables in relation to sleep. Several points of intervention for improving sleep and waking life quality are also suggested: either by focusing on identified precursors of sleep disturbance (e.g., psychosocial stability and support) or by targeting elements of sleep which predict subsequent psychosocial changes.

Recent data on the sleep-disrupting effects of life events cast further light on these issues. Sleep, particularly dream sleep, may remain altered for prolonged periods of time after exceedingly negative or protracted stressors, as seen in the case of post-traumatic stress disorder (57). Indeed, a study of sleep in Holocaust survivors suggested that sleep disturbance with nightmares may persist for up to 50 years after extreme stressors (56).

We have suggested elsewhere that sleep may show

greater alteration when the experience of a life event and major transition leads to significant and persistent changes in mood, as seen in major depression or post-traumatic stress syndrome. Thus, for example, depressed divorcing women (9) and depressed bereaved elders (51) are more likely to show shorter REM sleep latency or greater disruption in sleep continuity (with early morning awakening) than subjects who negotiate these life events without becoming depressed. Furthermore, bereaved subjects with depression of subsyndromal intensity complain of disturbed sleep but appear to have generally normal EEG sleep, with the possible exception of diminished slow-wave sleep generation in the first non-REM sleep period (44). These data suggest, therefore, that the development of major depression may mediate sleep changes following major life events or transitions. In the absence of pre-event sleep measures, however, this inference must be regarded as tentative.

These observations give rise to another important question, namely, whether there are any stable EEG sleep correlates of life stresses not confounded by concurrent major depression. This is an important issue theoretically and clinically because major life changes require adaptation to new roles and often to a new view of self. For example, to adapt to the loss of a spouse without becoming depressed could be regarded as an example of successful adaptation, in the sense of showing resilience, or the ability to bounce back from a major negative life event. The question therefore becomes, Does sleep remain entirely normal under such circumstances? Could sleep be an important correlate, or even a mechanism, of the resilience of successful adaptation in the context of major life transitions? If so, what aspects of sleep, if any, change during successful adaption, and what inference about the functions of sleep might one draw from the presence or absence of such changes?

REM sleep is a theoretically appealing candidate for providing a psychobiological correlate of successful adaptation to major changes in life, such as bereavement (50). Although we still do not know the functions of REM sleep, it has been suggested by Cartwright (9) that REM sleep may be a state of the mind brain during which affective information processing and affect discharge take place. If so, the burden of affective information processing during adaptation to a major life change may well lead to changes in the timing or intensity of REM sleep.

To pursue these issues, we recently performed a comparison of EEG sleep in nondepressed, spousally bereaved elders and in a healthy control group, in order to search for possible psychobiological correlates of bereavement not confounded by concurrent major depression (52). Bereaved and control subjects showed consistent differences over 2 years of follow-up in the phasic measures of REM sleep (increased in bereaved subjects), but were similar on all other EEG sleep measures over the 2-year period of observation. The bereaved subjects showed a small

decline in the percentage of slow-wave sleep over the 2 years in which they were followed, but measures of sleep efficiency, REM latency, and delta sleep ratio were stable and did not differ from values seen in control subjects. Bereaved and control subjects were also similar on subjective sleep quality.

These data led us to conclude that during successful adaptation to the loss of a spouse, and in the absence of major depression, spousal bereavement is associated with elevation in the phasic measures of REM sleep, but does not appear to be associated with other physiological sleep changes typical of major depression when studied at 3–23 months after the spousal loss. This suggests that preservation of normal sleep following a major negative life event may be an important correlate, if not mechanism, of the resilience seen in successful adaptation to life events. Furthermore, the elevation in REM density may provide a psychobiological correlate of bereavement not confounded by concurrent major depression.

A CONCEPTUAL FRAMEWORK FOR UNDERSTANDING CHALLENGES TO SLEEP AND CIRCADIAN TIME-KEEPING

The perennial debate among sleep researchers about the relative importance of psychiatric and medical factors in insomnia led us to conceptualize a unified model of the multiple factors which challenge successful circadian time-keeping, including sleep, across the life cycle (50). This model provides a biopsychosocial framework in which to understand pathogenesis, assessment, and intervention for persistent insomnia. The model is based on the results of our own work, as well as on other data in the literature (reviewed above), and is shown in the Fig. 1.

The model explicitly shows important predictors of, as well as outcomes resulting from, the development of sleep and circadian function across the life cycle. Thus, changes in health and cognitive status and negative life events (particularly those associated with significant loss) are hypothesized to lead to decay in sleep and sleep quality. However, the model posits that much of the effect is not direct, but is instead mediated by two factors: changes in mood (negative shifts in affect balance) and worsening of sleep-disordered breathing. We also hypothesize that characteristics such as gender, stability of social rhythms, and social support serve as important moderators, helping to buffer the subject from the effects of medical burden, negative life events, and their mediators. It is also noteworthy that the model explicitly recognizes that sleep changes are also likely to influence subsequent adaptation to aging along physical and psychological dimensions. Thus, what appear as major predictors in the model may, over time, ultimately be influenced by the very outcomes that they have helped to produce. That is, the model also permits one to test empirically whether

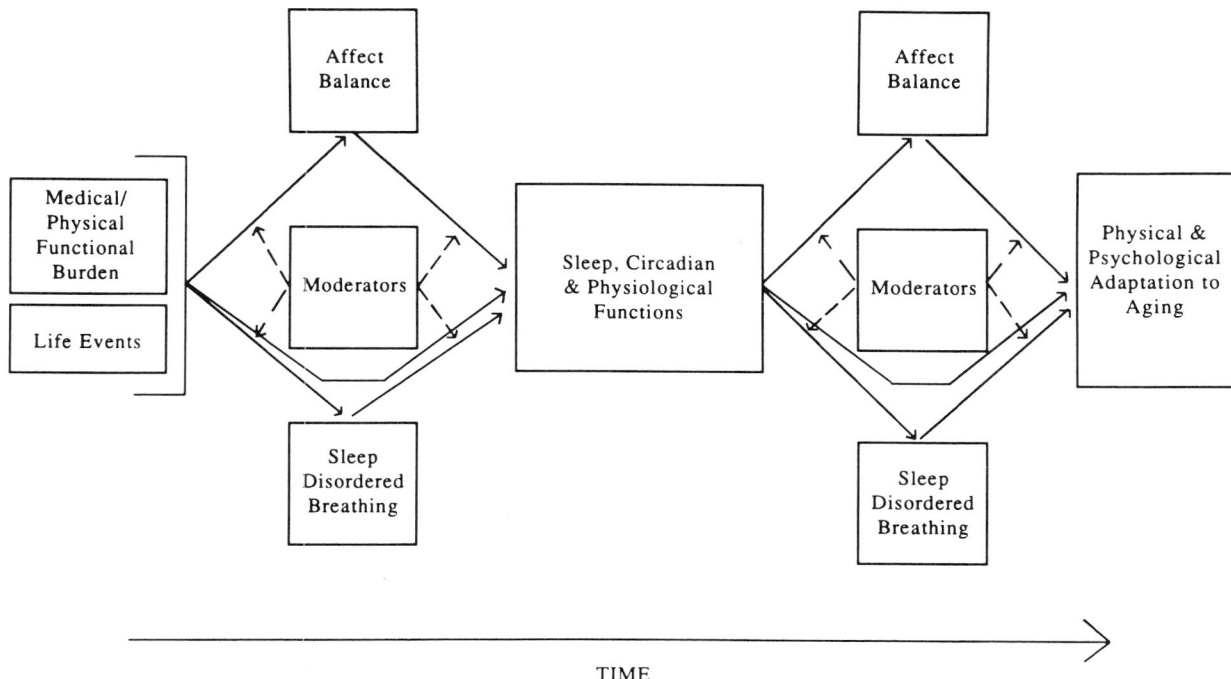

FIG. 1. Conceptual model of longitudinal relationships of sleep, circadian, and physiological parameters with other key variables. *Solid lines* denote direct effects; *dashed lines* denote moderating effects. (From ref. 50.)

sleep itself indicates changes or stability in psychosocial variables over time.

Medical burden and increasing physical functional limitations, together with other negative life events and ongoing difficulties (e.g., financial strain, family member illnesses and death), represent chronic stresses in the model and are among the vulnerability factors most frequently addressed in previous research on the precursors of psychiatric symptoms and disorders (for review, see ref. 50). More specifically, chronic stressors that have received the most empirical scrutiny in mixed age samples are job stress, chronic financial strain, and chronic physical illness; all three are related to increased risk of psychiatric morbidity, particularly depression, anxiety, and alcohol misuse. Similarly, the primary protective factor examined in previous research is social support, including the dimensions of social network, tangible support, and perceived social support. However, we do not know whether or not support exerts its effects directly upon such outcomes as sleep, or primarily serves to buffer the impact of other stressors.

Our own work on sleep in bereavement provides evidence linking negative affect balance (i.e., depression) and sleep outcomes. Among recently bereaved elders, sleep is disturbed among widows and widowers who present with a full depressive syndrome. Sleep efficiency is diminished, REM latency is short, and early slow-wave

sleep generation is reduced, compared to nondepressed recently bereaved subjects who are not depressed and compared to healthy elderly controls (51,52). Similar findings linking stress, depression, and EEG sleep disturbances, including decreased delta sleep and shortened REM latency, were reported by Cartwright et al. (10) in a study of middle-aged divorcing spouses.

An understanding of the proposed biopsychosocial model is not complete without also considering sleep in pathological aging. Given the theoretical interest in the impact of medical burden and cognitive impairment on sleep, we have published the observation that Alzheimer's dementia, in contrast to major depression, is associated with deficits in the production of phasic activity during sleep, including rapid eye movements, sleep spindles, and K complexes (54). Alzheimer's dementia is also associated with increased rates of sleep-disordered breathing (27). Furthermore, in studies in patients with depressive pseudodementia, the sleep physiological response to one night of sleep deprivation is characterized by robust REM sleep rebound (6). Such a rebound is absent in patients with Alzheimer's dementia. The relevance of this observation to the current model and to its prediction that sleep outcomes influence subsequent adaptation is that sleep measures predict survival status at 2 years in patients with mixed clinical presentations of depression and cognitive impairment (27). Nonsurvivors show impaired capacity to generate REM sleep and to maintain respiratory control during sleep.

NEUROBIOLOGICAL CORRELATES OF PERSISTENT SLEEP DISTURBANCE

The proposed model certainly does not preclude the possibility that some illnesses directly exert their effects on sleep, rather than being mediated by other factors. This becomes clear in considerations of the neurocircuitry and neurotransmitters involved in sleep. Several neurotransmitter systems have been extensively studied in sleep, including serotonin, dopamine, acetacholine, and noradrenergic systems. While the data in this area are not easily summarized, two particular observations appear relevant to the current discussion. First, as reviewed by Meltzer and Lowy (42), "Decreased serotonergic activity is consistent with many of the changes in mood and somatic function observed in depressed patients, for example, decreased mood, insomnia, decreased REM latency, and disturbed circadian rhythms." Secondly, as reviewed by Janowsky and Risch (31), "Cholinergic agonists generally cause a shortening of REM latency and an increase in REM density, particularly in patients with an affective disorder episode or a family history of affective disorder." These observations have led to the hypothesis that changes in sleep in depressed patients may reflect neurotransmitter abnormalities, particularly an increased ratio of cholinergic to aminergic neurotransmission. Conversely, the decreased capacity for REM sleep generation in Alzheimer's dementia may reflect impairment, loss, and underactivity in cholinergic systems.

The availability of positron emission tomography (PET) and its utilization in psychiatric sleep research may lead to a more direct testing of these hypotheses, as suggested by the Institute of Medicine Panel on Basic Sleep Research (29). In this context there are several promising approaches which might elucidate the neurobiological significance of sleep physiological abnormalities, in major depression and schizophrenia. These approaches include studies of (a) the effects of family history of psychiatric disorder on sleep abnormalities, (b) the clinical correlates of EEG sleep abnormalities, and (c) functional imaging correlates of EEG sleep changes.

The ongoing work of Giles et al. (22,23) illustrates the first approach, in which it is being asked whether EEG sleep is abnormal in persons at risk for major depression by virtue of family history. Data suggest that abnormal EEG sleep has shown an association within families, as well as a predictable relationship to lifetime development of depression (22) and an increased risk for new onset of depression (23).

Studies of clinical correlates of sleep abnormalities in schizophrenia have suggested that loss of slow-wave sleep (probably the most robust finding in schizophrenia) and

evidence of cerebral atrophy on computerized tomography (CT) scan are strongly correlated with severity of negative symptoms (21,65). Other studies in major depression have addressed EEG sleep correlates of long-term clinical response. For example, reduction in pretreatment REM latency was found by Giles et al. (24) to be associated with higher risk for recurrence of major depression. Kupfer and co-workers (37,38) reported that reductions in delta sleep ratio were associated with a significant increase in risk for recurrent major depression among midlife patients randomized to a maintenance psychotherapy condition.

Imaging correlates of EEG sleep changes in psychopathological states have now been conducted in patients with schizophrenia and major depression. These studies have led to several important observations: (a) increased cortical atrophy in relation to slow-wave sleep deficits in chronic schizophrenia (65) and (b) a finding of persistently increased limbic glucose metabolic rates in depressed patients who fail to show an antidepressant response to total sleep deprivation (75). In other words, total sleep deprivation appears to be associated with greater decreases in rates of glucose metabolism in limbic system among endogenously depressed patients who show an antidepressant response to this intervention.

Summary

By way of summarizing this discussion before proceeding to clinical issues, and attempting to tie together both neurobiological and psychosocial determinants of sleep changes, we are suggesting that successful adaptation across the life cycle is associated with preservation of sleep quality, ability to maintain daytime alertness, and physiological integrity of nocturnal EEG sleep (50). Failure to adapt is associated with loss of sleep continuity, alterations in the temporal distribution of delta wave activity, and either a relative increase of REM sleep (mood disorders) or a decrease in REM sleep (neurodegenerative disorders). As noted above, the increase in REM sleep which accompanies depression, whether endogenous or in the wake of negative life events, is also correlated with an attendant decrease in positive affect balance and diminished stability of social rhythms in the case of bereavement. By contrast, diminished capacity for REM sleep generation seems to accompany neurodegenerative disorders such as Alzheimer's dementia and is a correlate not only of cognitive impairment, but also of early mortality. The model we propose attempts to account for data at different points along the continuum of aging, from successful to pathological. Clearly, further longitudinal studies will be required to validate the hypothesized interrelationships among sleep, aging, neuromedical, and psychosocial variables.

In the next section of this chapter, we shall shift to

clinical considerations, such as issues of diagnostic classification, the utility of polysomnography in the evaluation of chronic insomnia, the impact of diagnosis and interviewer experience on treatment recommendations, and promising areas for intervention research.

TOWARD A RELIABLE AND VALID NOSOLOGY OF SLEEP DISORDERS

Because of long recognized links between certain types of sleep disorders (particularly insomnias) and psychiatric symptoms, psychiatry has played an integral role in the development of sleep disorders medicine over the past quarter century. Furthermore, given the clear association between sleep and psychiatric disorders, psychiatric clinicians and researchers need a comprehensible, reliable, and valid sleep disorders nosology. This need provided the impetus for the recently completed APA/NIMH/DSM-IV field trial on the diagnostic reliability of sleep disorders.

Several diagnostic classifications have been developed for sleep disorders in the past 15 years, including the *Diagnostic Classification of Sleep and Arousal Disorders,* 1st edition [DCSAD; American Sleep Disorders Association (62)], the *Diagnostic and Statistical Manual,* 3rd edition, revised [DSM-IIIR; American Psychiatric Association (1)], and the *International Classification of Sleep Disorders* [ICSD, 1991 (15)]. These systems differ with respect to (a) broad versus detailed diagnoses, (b) organizing categories by presenting symptom or presumed pathophysiology, and (c) intended users (general clinicians versus sleep specialists). Only DSM-IIIR and ICSD include specific diagnostic criteria, and only ICSD includes polysomnographic features among those criteria (although polysomnographic findings are not required to make a diagnosis). Recently, Schramm et al. (61) in Germany have completed a study showing excellent rates of interrater agreement (kappas in excess of .80) for DSM-IIIR sleep disorders, when sleep disorder specialists used a structured clinical interview to make diagnoses.

The sleep disorder section in the *Diagnostic and Statistical Manual,* 4th edition (DSM-IV) combines elements of previous diagnostic systems and takes into account controversies surrounding sleep disorders diagnosis, such as broad versus narrow diagnoses, the role of EEG sleep studies in diagnosis, and the intended users (see Table 1). DSM-IV includes a greater number of more specific categories than does DSM-IIIR (23 versus 15, including subtypes), but far fewer than the 84 total disorders enumerated in the ICSD. Like ICSD, DSM-IV includes major categories based on presumed pathophysiology, rather than on symptoms alone. Another proposed nosology, the *International Classification of Diseases,* 10th edition (ICD-10), is similar to DSM-IV in the number of specific diagnoses (17 total), but has only two general categories

compared to four for DSM-IV. Neither DSM-IV nor ICD-10 include specific polysomnographic criteria. (An outline of DSM-IV and ICSD is presented in Table 1).

The DSM-IV multisite field trial, sponsored by the American Psychiatric Association and the National Institute of Mental Health, was undertaken to determine rates of interrater agreement for sleep disorder diagnoses using the proposed classification systems, DSM-IV and ICD-10. The field trial focused on patients with insomnia complaints, because these are most relevant to psychiatric practice (Buysse et al., *in press*). Five sites interviewed a total of 257 patients (216 referred for insomnia complaints, and 41 control patients). One sleep specialist and one general clinician interviewed each patient, using a nonstructured clinical interview, and assigned DSM-IV and ICD-10 diagnoses.

We found that "insomnia due to another mental disorder" was the most frequent DSM-IV diagnosis, occurring in 76% of cases, as either a primary (43%) or secondary (33%) diagnosis. "Primary insomnia" was the next most frequent diagnosis, occurring in 48% of cases as either the primary (21%) or secondary (27%) diagnosis. "Insomnia due to emotional causes" was the most frequent ICD-10 diagnosis, occurring in 62% of cases. Interrater kappa value for multiple DSM-IV diagnoses was 0.47, with considerable range for individual diagnoses from 0 to 0.70. Individual sites varied considerably in the distribution of diagnoses, as well as in rates interrater agreement. Interviewers indicated greater confidence and better fit of diagnoses, as well as greater ease of use, for DSM-IV as compared to ICD-10.

The distribution of insomnia diagnoses in the DSM-IV field trial was similar, with some exceptions, to that reported by Coleman et al. (11), who used the *Diagnostic Classification of Sleep and Arousal Disorders* (ASDA) (62). These results confirm the importance of psychiatric and behavioral factors in clinicians' assessments of insomnia patients, and they suggest that ICSD and DSM-IV sleep disorder diagnoses have similar patterns of use by experienced clinicians. The results also suggested that rates of agreement were higher for more specific diagnostic categories and lower for less-well-defined diagnoses. Furthermore, site-related differences appeared to occur not only because of different patient populations but also because of different application of diagnostic criteria. In this context, the differentiation of primary from psychiatric forms of insomnia was frequently a source of disagreement between raters.

Although in both the DSM-IV field trial and the Coleman et al. (11) multisite trial psychiatric insomnia was the most prevalent, followed by psychophysiological (primary) insomnia, the DSM-IV field trial actually found a somewhat higher percentage of psychiatric insomnia (40% versus 35%) and a slightly lower percentage of psychophysiological (primary) insomnia (12.5% versus 15.3%). Other differences included in the DSM-IV field

TABLE 1. *Sleep disorder diagnoses*

DSM-IV sleep disorder diagnoses
Primary sleep disorders
  Dyssomnias
    Primary insomnia
    Primary hypersomnia
    Narcolepsy
    Breathing-related sleep disorder
    Dyssomnia not otherwise specified
  Circadian rhythm sleep disorders
    Delayed sleep phase syndrome
    Jet lag
    Shift work
    Unspecified
  Parasomnias
    Nightmare disorder
    Sleep terror disorder
    Sleep walking disorder
    Parasomnia not otherwise specified
Sleep disorders related to another mental disorder
  Insomnia related to another mental disorder
  Hypersomnia related to another mental disorder
Secondary sleep disorders due to an Axis III condition
  Insomnia type
  Hypersomnia type
  Parasomnia type
  Mixed type
Substance-induced sleep disorders
  Insomnia type
  Hypersomnia type
  Parasomnia type
  Other

International classification of sleep disorders (ICSD) sleep diagnoses
Dyssomnias
  Intrinsic sleep disorders
    Psychophysiological insomnia
    Sleep state misperception
    Idiopathic insomnia
    Narcolepsy
    Obstructive sleep apnea syndrome
    Central sleep apnea syndrome
    Central alveolar hypoventilation syndrome
    Periodic limb movement disorder
    Restless legs syndrome
    Intrinsic sleep disorder not otherwise specified
  Extrinsic sleep disorders
    Inadequate sleep hygiene
    Adjustment sleep disorder
    Nocturnal eating (drinking) syndrome
    Hypnotic-dependent sleep disorder
    Stimulant-dependent sleep disorder
    Extrinsic sleep disorder not otherwise specified
  Circadian rhythm sleep disorders
    Shift work sleep disorder
    Irregular sleep–wake pattern
    Delayed sleep phase syndrome
    Non-24-hour sleep–wake disorder
Parasomnias
  Arousal disorders
    Confusional arousals
    Sleepwalking
    Sleep terrors

International classification of sleep disorders (ICSD) sleep diagnoses (cont.)
Parasomnias (cont.)
  Sleep–wake transition disorders
    Rhythmic movement disorder
    Sleep starts
    Sleep talking
    Nocturnal leg cramps
  Parasomnias usually associated with REM sleep
    Nightmares
    Sleep paralysis
    Impaired sleep-related penile erections
    Sleep-related painful erections
    REM sleep-related sinus arrest
    REM sleep behavior disorder
  Other parasomnias
    Sleep bruxism
    Sleep enuresis
    Sleep-related abnormal swallowing syndrome
    Nocturnal paroxysmal dystonia
    Sudden unexplained nocturnal death syndrome
    Primary snoring
    Infant sleep apnea
    Congenital central hypoventilation syndrome
    Sudden infant death syndrome
    Benign neonatal sleep myoclonus
    Other parasomnia not otherwise specified
Sleep disorders associated with medical/psychiatric disorders
  Associated with mental disorders
    Psychoses
    Mood disorders
    Anxiety disorders
    Panic disorder
    Alcoholism
    Other mental disorder
  Associated with neurological disorders
    Cerebral degenerative disorders
    Dementia
    Parkinsonism
    Fatal familial insomnia
    Sleep-related epilepsy
    Electrical status epilepticus of sleep
    Sleep-related headaches
    Other neurological disorder
  Associated with other medical disorders
    Sleeping sickness
    Nocturnal cardiac ischemia
    Chronic obstructive pulmonary disease
    Sleep-related asthma
    Sleep-related gastroesophageal reflux
    Peptic ulcer disease
    Fibrositis syndrome
    Other medical disorder
Proposed sleep disorders

trial were lower percentages of substance-related insomnia (3.1% versus 12.4%) and periodic limb movements/restless legs (1.2% versus 12.2%), but a higher frequency of delayed sleep phase syndrome (7.0% versus approximately 3.6%) and a similar frequency of sleep apnea (5.4% versus 6.2%). In comparing these studies, it is important to note that Coleman et al. (14) collected diagnoses *after* polysomnography, while diagnoses in the DSM-IV field trial were assigned on purely clinical grounds after one initial interview.

An important conceptual difference between DSM-IV and ICSD consists of the greater subtyping of nonpsychiatric, nonmedical forms of insomnia in ICSD. Patients diagnosed with DSM-IV ''primary insomnia'' actually fall into three major ICSD categories: ''psychophysiological insomnia,'' ''inadequate sleep hygiene,'' and ''idiopathic (childhood-onset) insomnia.'' This type of difference relates to the conceptualization and presumed etiology of insomnia problems. Thus, in DSM-IV, ''primary insomnia'' is essentially atheoretical with regard to causation; ''psychophysiological insomnia'' in ICSD invokes conditioning and physiological factors; ''inadequate sleep hygiene'' attributes causation to voluntary behaviors; and ''idiopathic insomnia'' assumes a yet-to-be identified genetic or biological component. Whether the broader DSM-IV (and ICD-10) categories or the more specific ICSD categories have greater validity remains to be determined. Indications of validity may include differences in polysomnographic measure, longitudinal course, treatment response, and familial patterns. We have suggested elsewhere that such indicators of validity have not yet been demonstrated (53).

Although the overall rate of agreement for DSM-IV diagnoses was moderately good, it was lower than that usually reported for psychiatric disorders. We speculate that several factors probably contributed to the lower rate of agreement: (a) the absence of a structured interview; (b) the use of interviewers without specialized training in sleep disorders; and (c) relatively low base rates of certain disorders, which had the effect of lowering kappa values. These results provide a conservative estimate of diagnostic reliability—higher than that which may be seen in routine clinical practice where even more heterogeneous interviewers and lower rates of insomnias may occur, but lower than that which could be obtained using structured interviews and formal training (72). Finally, the higher kappa values seen for DSM-IV compared to ICD-10 diagnoses suggest that not only the total number of diagnostic categories, but also their familiarity and sensibility to interviewers, may relate to interrater agreement.

A PRACTICAL ALGORITHM FOR DSM-IV SLEEP DISORDERS

The findings of the DSM-IV field trial, together with the model proposed in this chapter, lend themselves to the formation of a practical algorithm for the diagnosis of DSM-IV sleep disorders. The intent of this algorithm, created by Nancy Vettorello and Harold Alan Pincus of the APA Office of Research (personal communication to Charles Reynolds and David Kupfer), is to translate into usable clinical form the results of the field trial and the findings reviewed from the literature and incorporated into our model of the medical and psychosocial correlates of sleep disturbance.

The clinician who is confronted by a complaint of sleep disturbance on the part of the patient or a family member must define the nature of the complaint, whether primarily of insomnia, excessive daytime sleepiness, disturbed mentation or behavior during sleep, or difficulties in the circadian placement of sleep. The first step in the diagnostic algorithm is to consider the patient's general medical condition, in order to determine whether the patient's complaint represents a secondary sleep disorder due to a general medical condition. Furthermore, if the patient is taking medication or using a substance, the clinician should consider the diagnostic possibility of a substance-induced sleep disorder (step 2 of the DSM-IV sleep disorders algorithm).

If sleep disturbance is suspected to be related to another mental disorder, the clinician should consider diagnoses such as major depression, anxiety disorders, or post-traumatic stress disorder as the etiology of the sleep complaint (step 3). If the sleep problem, particularly one of excessive daytime sleepiness, occurs in the context of a history of snoring or with obesity, the clinician should consider a breathing-related sleep disorder (step 4). If the patient frequently crosses time zones or is involved in shift work, or has a primary problem of sleep timing (rather than disturbance), a circadian rhythm sleep disorder or a sleep–wake schedule disorder should be considered (step 5).

If the patient's symptoms are predominantly behavioral or mental events during sleep (e.g., abrupt awakening, frightening dreams, or walking about while sleeping), the clinician should consider a diagnosis of nightmare disorder, sleep terror disorder, sleep walking disorder, or another type of parasomnia (step 6).

If the primary complaint is persistent insomnia and/or difficulty initiating or maintaining sleep, a diagnosis of primary insomnia is suggested if (a) symptoms have persisted for more than a month and (b) symptoms do not appear to be associated with another mental or physical disorder (step 7). Similarly, if the primary complaint is excessive sleepiness, the clinician should consider the differential diagnosis of a breathing-related sleep disorder, narcolepsy, or primary hypersomnia, in the absence of a mental or physical disorder which could explain the complaint (step 8).

Finally, if the criteria for previously described specific disorders are not met, a ''default'' diagnosis of dysomnia not otherwise specified should initiate a more complete evaluation (step 9).

For further reference, Table 1 summarizes the DSM-

IV sleep–wake disorders nosology and the International Classification of Sleep Disorders (ICSD).

THE USE OF POLYSOMNOGRAPHY IN THE EVALUATION OF INSOMNIA

The differential diagnosis of chronic insomnia inevitably leads to a review of the current controversies surrounding the use of polysomnography in the evaluation of insomnia, the subject of a recent task force report by the American Sleep Disorders Association (49). Two of the authors (Reynolds and Buysse) participated in the writing of this task force report. The central issue addressed in this report is whether polysomnographic findings are helpful clinically—that is, do they elucidate pathophysiology, establish a diagnosis, or guide treatment recommendations? The task force report concluded that "sleep studies are more likely to be helpful if there is a specific suspicion of an intrinsic sleep pathology (such as sleep apnea or periodic limb movements), or if the sleep complaints are not adequately explained by the type or degree of medical illness and medications. Examples would include a suspicion of periodic leg movements in a patient with chronic renal disease; a suspicion of apnea in a patient with neuromuscular or chronic pulmonary disease; or a suspicion of a seizure disorder in a patient who has suffered head trauma or stroke." Furthermore, as reviewed by Bliwise (5), older patients more frequently demonstrate unsuspected periodic leg movements and apnea. The incidence of secondary sleep disorders due to medical illness increases with age, suggesting that polysomnographic findings are more likely to be helpful in older patients. With respect to the goal of separating subtypes of insomnia, the task force report indicated that a more comprehensive assessment than is typically performed might be useful. Areas of potential interest include assessment of the circadian system (e.g., systematic temperature assessment) and use of computerized EEG analysis (e.g., period analysis and power spectral analysis).

The ASDA task force authors suggested that "far more important than polysomnography is a careful and thorough clinical evaluation of the patient with an insomnia complaint, and perhaps a therapeutic trial based upon the most probable cause(s), before polysomnography, in most cases." At the same time, however, the authors acknowledged that "there is no general agreement as to what constitutes an adequate therapeutic trial." Whatever approaches may be taken, we suggest that follow-up assessment is important in order to determine the stability of clinical response. With respect to the conduct of clinical trials, we also advocate the use of specific diagnostic criteria, such as those tested in the field trial, in order to constitute more homogeneous study groups. Finally, we advocate the use of both subjective and objective outcome measures in clinical trials of interventions in insomnia.

EFFECTS OF DIAGNOSIS AND INTERVIEW EXPERIENCE ON TREATMENT RECOMMENDATIONS IN CHRONIC INSOMNIA

The DSM-IV field trial was also designed to permit an examination of (a) whether different insomnia diagnoses are associated with different treatment recommendations and (b) whether sleep specialists and nonspecialists advise different treatments. The trial found that treatment and polysomnography recommendations differed significantly for different DSM-IV diagnoses (Buysse et al., *unpublished observations*). Sleep specialists recommended several behavioral strategies—including self-monitoring, sleep hygiene techniques, and stimulus control techniques—more highly than did nonspecialists. However, nonspecialists more strongly recommended relaxation training and medications for medical or neurological conditions. Nonspecialists also recommended polysomnography more strongly than did specialists.

Most treatment recommendations differed significantly for different diagnoses. For instance, position training, continuous positive airway pressure, and oxygen were all recommended more strongly for "breathing-related sleep disorder" than for the other diagnoses; psychiatric medications and interventions were more strongly recommended for "insomnia related to another mental disorder"; and behavioral intervention were more strongly recommended for "primary insomnia." Polysomnography was recommended for "breathing-related sleep disorders" more strongly than for other diagnoses.

Significant site-related differences also emerged in the treatment recommendations, even for the same diagnoses. Such site-related differences reflect the perennial debate in the sleep-disorders and research community about (a) the importance of nonpsychiatric factors in insomnia and (b) the proper method of subtyping insomnia diagnoses. On the one hand, numerous studies have shown elevations in MMPI scores and other measures of psychopathology in chronic insomnia patients, including categorical psychiatric diagnoses (30,32,64). These findings can lead to the conclusion that chronic insomnia is almost always associated with significant psychopathology, and that psychiatric treatment is indicated. On the other hand, other studies have shown that chronic insomnia not uncommonly results from either (a) more specific intrinsic disorders of sleep (e.g., periodic limb movements, sleep apnea), (b) concurrent medical or neurological illness, or (c) behavioral and conditioning factors (11,30). Such studies emphasize diversity in etiology—and presumably in the treatment—of chronic insomnia. Thus, site-related differences in the DSM-IV field trial suggest that some controversy remains in the conceptualization of sleep disorders, their evaluation, and their treatment. The array of contemporary treatment options for chronic insomnia is shown in

TABLE 2. *Treatment for chronic insomnia*

Psychiatric intervention (includes psychotherapy, hospitalization, etc.)
Medication for psychiatric disorder
Self-monitoring (e.g., completing sleep–wake log or diary)
Sleep hygiene techniques (e.g., establishing regular sleep–wake hours, limiting naps, limiting caffeine)
Relaxation training (included progressive muscular relaxation, biofeedback, guided imagery, etc.)
Stimulus control techniques (e.g., going to bed only when sleepy, using the bed only for sleep, getting out of bed in the event of prolonged awakenings)
Sleep restriction therapy (limiting time in bed to match actual sleep duration)
Medication for sleep disorder (included benzodiazepine hypnotics)
Chronotherapy (scheduling sleep to match endogenous circadian phase)
Continuous positive airway pressure
Supplemental oxygen
Position training (to prevent position-related apnea)
Medical intervention (includes diagnostic tests, procedures, surgery)
Neurological intervention (includes diagnostic tests, procedures)
Medication for medical/neurological disorder
Medication/substance discontinuation (includes prescribed and nonprescribed drugs, recreational substances)

Table 2, where they are grouped according to psychiatric, behavioral, and neuromedical interventions.

PROMISING LEADS FOR INTERVENTION RESEARCH

In concert with the 1990 NIH Consensus Development Conference on Sleep Disorders in Late Life, the authors believe that chronic primary insomnia, particularly sleep-maintenance insomnia, represents a significant public-health problem and an important opportunity for intervention research. The authors also suggest that, to be truly successful, intervention must be shown to be efficacious over long periods of time (because primary insomnia tends to be chronic and recurring). Based upon the work of Spielman et al. (63) and Friedman et al. (20), we suggest that therapy utilizing sleep-restricting techniques holds particular promise for short- and long-term efficacy in the management of primary, sleep maintenance insomnia, particularly in late life. Another promising lead, though less well researched to date, is the use of bright-light exposure in the evening (8). Properly timed bright-light exposure may help reduce sleep-maintenance difficulties and improve daytime alertness, possibly via internal phase realignments of circadian temperature and sleep–wake rhythms. Finally, based upon the work of Vitiello et al. (68), enhancing aerobic fitness may be associated with improved sleep quality.

Finally, although we endorse the need for further con-

trolled clinical trials to establish the short- and long-term efficacy of behavioral, psychotherapeutic, and naturalistic interventions for primary insomnia, we suggest that it would be premature to exclude a role for maintenance medication. Because significant progress has been made in the methodology of maintenance therapy trials, we endorse the application of such methodology to long-term intervention studies of chronic insomnia. We suggest that antidepressant medication or intermittent benzodiazepines could justifiably be investigated for chronic efficacy in sleep maintenance insomnia.

In conclusion, although the interventions which the authors regard as promising candidates for treatment research in chronic insomnia are quite diverse, such diversity attests to the heterogeneity of chronic insomnia. Conceptually, it is plausible to suggest that chronic primary insomnia is the behavioral expression of many different underlying factors. In some patients, diminished sleep drive will predominate; in others, misalignment of circadian rhythms will be etiologically important; and in still others, mood disorders, often of subsyndromal intensity, will lead to insomnia. Such heterogeneity provides, we suggest, a compelling theoretical rationale for different interventions and, possibly, a framework for understanding differential treatment response. It also underscores the need for the use of a more rigorous, structured approach to diagnosis for defining study groups. The possibility for more rigorous sample definition has been advanced, we feel, through the DSM-IV insomnia field study.

ACKNOWLEDGMENTS

This work was supported, in part, by NIMH grants MH30915, MH00295, MH37869, MH48891, MH47200.

REFERENCES

1. American Psychiatric Association. *Diagnostic and statistical manual of mental disorders,* 3rd ed. (revised). Washington, DC: American Psychiatric Association, 1987.
2. Ancoli-Israel S, Kripke DF, Klauber MR, Mason WJ, Fell R, Kaplan O. Sleep disordered breathing in community dwelling elderly. *Sleep* 1991;14:486–495.
3. Benca RM, Obermeyer WH, Thisted RA, Gillin JC. Sleep and psychiatric disorders: a meta-analysis. *Arch Gen Psychiatry* 1992; 49:651–668.
4. Bixler EO, Kales A, Soldatos CR, Kales JD, Healey S. Prevalence of sleep disorders in the Los Angeles metropolitan area. *Am J Psychiatry* 1979;136:1257–1262.
5. Bliwise D. Sleep in normal aging and dementia. *Sleep* 1993;16(1):40–81.
6. Buysse DJ, Reynolds CF, Kupfer DJ, et al. EEG sleep in depressive pseudodementia. *Arch Gen Psychiatry* 1988;45:568–576.
7. Buysse DJ, Reynolds CF, Hauri PJ, Roth T, Stepanski EJ, Thorpy MJ, Bixler ED, Kaks A, Manfredi RL, Vgontzas AN, Messiano DA, Houck PR, Kupfer DJ. Diagnostic concordance for sleep disorders using proposed DSM-IV categories: a report from the APA/NIMH/DSM-IV field trial. *Am J Psychiatry* (in press).

8. Campbell SS, Dawson D. Bright light treatment of sleep disturbance in older subjects. *Sleep Res* 1991;20:448.

9. Cartwright RD. REM sleep during and after mood-disturbing events. *Arch Gen Psychiatry* 1983;40:197–201.

10. Cartwright RD, Kravitz HM, Eastman CI, Wood E. REM latency and the recovery from depression. *Am J Psychiatry* 1991;148:1530–1535.

11. Coleman RM, Roffwarg HP, Kennedy SJ, et al. Sleep–wake disorders based on a polysomnographic diagnosis; a national cooperative study. *JAMA* 1982;247:997–1003.

12. Consensus Development Conference. *Diagnosis and treatment of sleep disorders in late life.* National Institutes of Health: Bethesda, MD, 1990.

13. Cook NR, Evans DA, Funkenstein H, et al. Correlates of headache in a population-based cohort of elderly. *Arch Neurol* 1989;46:1338–1344.

14. Dew MA, Reynolds CF, Monk TH, et al. Psychosocial correlates and sequelae of electroencephalographic sleep in healthy elders. *J Gerontol: Psychol Sci* 1994;49(1):P8–P18.

15. Diagnostic Classification Steering Committee, Thorpy MJ (Chairman). *International classification of sleep disorders: diagnostic and coding manual.* Rochester, MN: American Sleep Disorders Association, 1990.

16. Evans RW, Manninen DL, Garrison LP, et al. The quality of life of patients with end-stage renal disease. *N Engl J Med* 1985;312:553–559.

17. Fawcett J, Scheftner WA, Fogg L, et al. Time-related predictors of suicide in major affective disorder. *Am J Psychiatry* 1990;147(9):1189–1194.

18. Feinberg I, Koresko RL, Heller N. EEG sleep patterns as a function of normal and pathological aging in man. *J Psychiatr Res* 1967;5:107–144.

19. Ford DE, Kamerow DB. Epidemiologic study of sleep disturbances and psychiatric disorders. *JAMA* 1989;262:1479–1484.

20. Friedman L, Bliwise DL, Yesarage JA, Salom SR. A preliminary study comparing sleep restriction and relaxation treatments for insomnia in older adults. *J Gerontol: Psychol Sci* 1991;46:1–8.

21. Ganguli R, Reynolds CF, Kupfer DJ. EEG sleep in young, never-medicated, schizophrenic patients: a comparison with delusional and nondelusional depressives and with healthy controls. *Arch Gen Psychiatry* 1987;44:36–45.

22. Giles DE, Biggs MM, Rush AJ, Roffwarg HP. Risk factors in families of unipolar depression. I. Psychiatric illness and reduced REM latency. *J Affect Disord* 1988;14:51–59.

23. Giles DE, Etzel BA, Biggs MM. Risk factors in unipolar depression. II. Relation between proband REM latency and cognitions of relatives. *Psychiatry Res* 1990;33:39–49.

24. Giles DE, Jarrett RB, Roffwarg HP, Rush AJ. Reduced REM latency: a predictor of recurrence in depression. *Neuropsychopharmacology* 1987;1:33–39.

25. Gillin JC, Byerly WF. The diagnosis and management of insomnia. *N Engl J Med* 1990;322(4):239–248.

26. He J, Kryger MH, Zorick FJ, Conway W, Roth T. Mortality and apnea index in obstructive sleep apnea, experience in 385 male patients. *Chest* 1988;94(1):9–14.

27. Hoch CC, Reynolds CF, Houck PR, et al. Predicting mortality in mixed depression and dementia using EEG sleep variables. *J Neuropsychiatr Clin Neurosci* 1989;1:366–371.

28. Hyyppa MT, Kronholm E. Quality of sleep and chronic illness. *J Clin Epidemiol* 1989;42(7):633–638.

29. Institute of Medicine Panel on Basic Sleep Research. *Basic sleep research—research briefing.* Washington, DC: National Academy Press, 1990.

30. Jacobs EA, Reynolds CF, Kupfer DJ, Lovin PA, Ehrenpreis AB. The role of polysomnography in the differential diagnosis of chronic insomnia. *Am J Psychiatry* 1988;145:346–349.

31. Janowsky DS, Risch SD. Role of acetylcholine mechanisms in the affective disorders. In: Meltzer HY, ed. *Psychopharmacology: the third generation of progress.* New York: Raven Press, 1987;527–533.

32. Kales A, Caldwell A, Preston TA, Healey S, Kales JD. Personality patterns in insomnia: theoretical implications. *Arch Gen Psychiatry* 1976;33:1128–1134.

33. Karacan I, Thornby JI, Williams RL. Sleep disturbance: a community survey. In: Guilleminault C, Lugaresi E, eds. *Sleep/wake disorders: natural history, epidemiology, and long-term evolution.* New York: Raven Press, 1983;37–60.

34. Kennedy GJ, Kelman HR, Thomas C. Persistence and remission of depressive symptoms in late life. *Am J Psychiatry* 1991;148(2):174–178.

35. Knowles JB, MacLean AW. Age-related changes in sleep in depressed and healthy subjects. *Neuropsychopharmacology* 1990;3:251–259.

36. Kripke DF, Ancoli-Israel S, Mason WJ, Kaplan O. Sleep apnea: association with deviant sleep durations and increased mortality. In: Guilleminault C, Partinen M, eds. *Sleep apnea syndrome: clinical research and treatment.* New York: Raven Press, 1990;9–14.

37. Kupfer DJ, Frank E, McEachran AB, Grochocinski VJ. Delta sleep ratio: a biological correlate of early recurrence in unipolar affective disorder. *Arch Gen Psychiatry* 1990;47:1100–1105.

38. Kupfer DJ, Reynolds CF. Sleep and affective disorders. In: Paykel ES, ed. *Handbook of affective disorders*, 2nd ed. New York: Churchill Livingstone, 1992;311–323.

39. Kupfer DJ, Reynolds CF. Sleep and psychiatric disorders: a meta-analysis. Comment in *Arch Gen Psychiatry* 1992;49:669–670.

40. Mant A, Eyland EA. Sleep patterns and problems in elderly general practice attenders: an Australian survey. *Community Health Stud* 1988;12(2):192–199.

41. Mellinger GD, Balter MB, Uhlenhuth EH. Insomnia and its treatment: prevalence and correlates. *Arch Gen Psychiatry* 1985;42:225–232.

42. Meltzer HY, Lowy MT. The serotonin hypothesis of depression. In: Meltzer HY, ed. *Psychopharmacology: the third generation of progress.* New York: Raven Press, 1987;513–526.

43. Morin C, Gramling SE. Sleep patterns and coping: comparison of older adults with and without insomnia complaints. *Psychol Aging* 1989;4:290–294.

44. Pasternak RE, Reynolds CF, Hoch CC, et al. Sleep in spousally bereaved elders with subsyndromal depressive symptoms. *Psychiatry Res* 1992;43:43–53.

45. Pollak CP, Perlick D, Linsner JP, Wenston J, Hsieh F. Sleep problems in the community elderly as predictors of death and nursing home placement. *J Community Health* 1990;15:123–135.

46. Prinz PN, Halter J, Benedetti C, Raskind M. Circadian variation of plasma catecholamines in young and old men: relation to rapid eye movements and slow wave sleep. *J Clin Endocrinol Metab* 1979;49:300–304.

47. Prinz PN, Vitiello MV, Raskin MA, Thorpy MJ. Geriatrics: sleep disorders and aging. *N Engl J Med* 1990;323:520–526.

48. Rabins PV, Mace NL, Lucas MJ. The impact of dementia on the family. *JAMA* 1982;248:333–335.

49. Reite M, Buysse DJ, Reynolds CF, Mendelson WB. *The use of polysomnography in the evaluation of insomnia.* Prepared by the Standards of Practice Committee of The American Sleep Disorders Association, 1993.

50. Reynolds CF, Dew MA, Monk TH, Hoch CC. Sleep disorders in late life: a biopsychosocial model for understanding pathogenesis and intervention. In: Cummings J, Coffey CE, eds. *Textbook of geriatric neuropsychiatry.* Washington, DC: American Psychiatric Press, 1994;323–331.

51. Reynolds CF, Hoch CC, Buysse DJ, et al. EEG sleep in spousal bereavement and bereavement-related depression of late life. *Biol Psychiatry* 1992;31:69–82.

52. Reynolds CF, Hoch CC, Buysse DJ, et al. Sleep after spousal bereavement: a study of recovery from stress. *Biol Psychiatry* 1993;34:791–797.

53. Reynolds CF, Kupfer DJ, Buysse DJ, Coble PA, Yeager AL. Subtyping DSM-III-R ''primary'' insomnia: usefulness, reliability, and validity. *Am J Psychiatry* 1991;148(4):432–439.

54. Reynolds CF, Kupfer DJ, Houck PR, et al. Reliable discrimination of elderly depressed and demented patients by EEG sleep data. *Arch Gen Psychiatry* 1988;45:258–264.

55. Rodin J, McAvay G, Timko C. A longitudinal study of depressed mood and sleep disturbances in elderly adults. *J Gerontol* 1988;43:45–53.

56. Rosen J, Reynolds CF, Yeager AL, Houck PR, Hurwitz L. Sleep disturbance in survivors of the Nazi Holocaust. *Am J Psychiatry* 1991;148(1):62–66.

57. Ross RJ, Ball WA, Sullivan KA, Caroff SN. Sleep disturbance as the hallmark of post-traumatic stress disorder. *Am J Psychiatry* 1989;146(6):697–707.
58. Roth T, Kramer M, Trinder J. The effect of noise during sleep on the sleep patterns of different age groups. *Can Psychiatr Assoc J* 1972;17:197–201.
59. Rowe JW, Kahn RL. Human aging: usual and successful. *Science* 1987;237:143–149.
60. Sanford JRA. Tolerance of debility in elderly dependents by supports at home: significance for hospital practice. *Br Med J* 1975;3:471–473.
61. Schramm E, Hohagen F, Grasshoff U, et al. Test–retest reliability and validity of a structured interview for sleep disorders according to DSM-III-R (SIS-D). *Am J Psychiatry* 1993;150(6):857–858.
62. Sleep Disorders Classification Committee, Roffwarg HP (Chairman), Association of Sleep Disorders Centers. *Diagnostic classification of sleep and arousal disorders,* 1st ed. *Sleep* 1979;2:1–137.
63. Spielman AJ, Saskin P, Thorpy MJ. Treatment of chronic insomnia by restriction of time in bed. *Sleep* 1987;10:45–56.
64. Tan TL, Kales JD, Kales A, Soldatos CR, Bixler EO. Biopsychobehavioral correlates of insomnia, IV: Diagnosis based on DSM-III. *Am J Psychiatry* 1984;141:357–362.
65. van Kammen DP, van Kammen WB, Peters J, Goetz K, Neyland T. Decreased slow wave sleep and enlarged lateral ventricles in schizophrenia. *Neuropsychopharmacology* 1988;1:265–271.
66. Vettorello N, Pincus HA. *DSM-IV sleep algorithm.* Office of Research, American Psychiatric Association, 1993.
67. Vitiello MV, Prinz PN, Avery DH, et al. Sleep is undisturbed in elderly, depressed individuals who have not sought care. *Biol Psychiatry* 1990;27:431–440.
68. Vitiello MV, Schwartz RS, Bradbury VL, Abrass IB, Stratton JR, Prinz PN. Improved subjective sleep quality following fitness training in healthy elderly males. *Sleep Res* 1990;19:154.
69. Vollrath M, Wicki W, Angst J. The Zurich study. VIII. Insomnia: association with depression, anxiety, somatic syndromes, and course of insomnia. *Eur Arch Psychiatry Neurol Sci* 1989;239(2):113–124.
70. Wauquier A, Van Sweden B, Lagaay AM, Kamphuisen HAC. Ambulatory monitoring of sleep–wakefulness patterns in healthy elderly males and females. *J Am Geriatr Soc* 1992;40:109–114.
71. Welstein L, Dement WC, Redington D, Guilleminault C, Mitler MM. Insomnia in the San Francisco Bay area: a telephone survey. In: Guilleminault C, Lugaresi E, eds. *Sleep/wake disorders: natural history, epidemiology, and long-term evolution.* New York: Raven Press, 1983;73–85.
72. Williams JBW, Gibbon M, First MB, et al. The structured clinical interview for DSM-III-R (SCID). II. Multisite test–retest reliability. *Arch Gen Psychiatry* 1992;49:630–636.
73. Williams RL, Karacan I, Hursch CJ. *EEG of human sleep: clinical applications.* New York: John Wiley & Sons, 1974.
74. Wittig RM, Zorick FJ, Blumer D, Heilbronn M, Roth T. Disturbed sleep in patients complaining of chronic pain. *J Nerv Ment Dis* 1982;170:429–431.
75. Wu JC, Gillin JC, Buchsbaum MS, Hershey T, Johnson JC, Bunney WE. Effect of sleep deprivation on brain metabolism of depressed patients. *Am J Psychiatry* 1992;149(4):538–543.
76. Zepelin H, McDonald CS. Age differences in autonomic variables during sleep. *J Gerontol* 1987;42:142–146.
77. Zepelin H, McDonald CS, Zammit GK. Effects of age on auditory awakening thresholds. *J Gerontol* 1984;39:294–300.
78. Zepelin H, Morgan LE. Correlates of sleep disturbance in retirees. *Sleep Res* 1981;10:120.

Psychopharmacology: The Fourth
Generation of Progress, edited by
Floyd E. Bloom and David J. Kupfer.
Raven Press, Ltd., New York © 1995.

CHAPTER 140

Early-Onset Mood Disorder

David A. Brent, Neal Ryan, Ronald Dahl and Boris Birmaher

During the past decade, tremendous advances have been made in our knowledge of the natural history, risk factors, and psychobiology of early-onset affective illness. In this chapter, the epidemiology, natural history, and adult sequelae of early-onset affective illness are reviewed, followed by a discussion of family-genetic and high-risk studies of juvenile affective illness. The status of investigation into biological markers in prepubertal and adolescent depression is discussed, focusing on studies of secretory patterns of cortisol and growth hormone, provocative neuroendocrine challenge studies, and electroencephalographic (EEG) sleep studies. An emphasis is given to clinical and developmental variables that might explain differences between studies or apparent discontinuities from studies of adults with depression. The psychopharmacological treatment studies for prepubertal and adolescent depression are reviewed, and the possible reasons for negative findings in nearly all of them are discussed. Finally, areas of further investigations that may be particularly fruitful for the field are suggested (see Chapters 83 and 86, *this volume*).

EPIDEMIOLOGY

Affective illness is less common in prepubertal children than in adolescents. In prepuberty, the point prevalence of major depression has been estimated at 1.8–2.5%; "minor" forms of depression, including dysthymia, have been estimated at 2.5%; and bipolar illness has been estimated at 0.2–0.4% (23). For adolescents, the point prevalences of depression, dysthymic disorder, and bipolar disorder have been estimated at 2.9–4.7%, 1.6–8.0%, and

D. A. Brent, N. Ryan, R. Dahl, and B. Birmaher: Departments of Psychiatry (DB, RD, BB, NR), Epidemiology (DB), Pediatrics (DB, RD), Western Psychiatric Institute and Clinic, University of Pittsburgh School of Medicine, Pittsburgh, Pennsylvania 15213.

1%, respectively. Depressive illness is equally common in males and females prior to puberty, but is more common in females than in males postpubertally (23). On the other hand, bipolar disorder is of equal prevalence in both genders.

Early-onset affective illness appears to have become a much more significant public health problem in recent years. There is evidence of a secular trend for depression and suicide. Successive cohorts born after 1950 appear to have an increased risk for depression and suicide relative to earlier birth cohorts, based both on retrospectively and prospectively gathered data (34,46,90), with evidence of a secular trend for depression affecting even prepubertal and adolescent children (89).

NATURAL HISTORY

In clinically referred samples, major depression in childhood and adolescence is a chronic and recurrent condition. According to the results of one naturalistic study of depressed children aged 8–13 years, untreated major depression lasted an average of 7.2 months, whereas dysthymic disorder lasted an average of 45.9 months (48). Subsequent follow-up of these children revealed that a cumulative probability of a recurrence of depression could be expected of 40% within 2 years, and of 72% within 5 years (49). Earlier age of onset and underlying dysthymic disorder both increase the risk of depressive recurrence (49), but comorbidity with anxiety disorder or conduct disorder did not influence the course of depressive illness (50,51). Certain features of adolescent depression predictive of the development of bipolar illness include: (a) a symptom cluster consisting of rapid onset, psychomotor retardation, and mood-congruent psychotic features, (b) family history of bipolar disorder and three generations of family members with affective illness, and (c) pharmacologically induced hypomania (95).

SEQUELAE OF DEPRESSIVE DISORDERS

Both prepubertal and adolescent depressive disorders are associated with social impairment with peers, in school, and with parents (75,80). In a follow-up of remitted prepubertal depressives, some areas of functional impairment persist, particularly with respect to mother–child discord (76). There is evidence that, over time, early-onset depressives are likely to develop additional comorbid conditions—namely, conduct disorder, anxiety disorder, and substance abuse (41,50,51). However, anxiety disorders are more likely to antedate early-onset major depression than to develop secondary to depression (51).

Other studies have also supported the view that early-onset depression persists into adulthood. A 9-year follow-up of adolescents with prominent depressive symptomatology predicted (a) the persistence of depression and (b) functional impairment in school, work, and interpersonal relations with spouses and parents (41). Harrington et al. (36) found that child and adolescent-onset depressives were four times more likely than nonaffectively ill psychiatric controls to have had an affective disorder on follow-up; and of those with early-onset affective illness who had a second episode before age 17, 95% had a subsequent episode in adulthood. Earlier age of onset is associated with a very high risk of recurrence (49). Pure depression (e.g., no comorbid conduct disorder) tends to persist into adulthood, whereas those depressives with comorbid conduct disorder do not appear to be at increased risk for depression upon follow-up, but have a course more similar to those with "pure" conduct disorders (24,37).

Among the most significant sequelae of depression are suicidal behavior and completed suicide. Clinically significant suicidality (i.e., suicidal ideation with a plan or actual suicide attempt) is quite common among referred samples of affectively disordered youth and is associated with comorbid substance abuse and other nonaffective disorders, longer duration of disorder, family discord, and hopelessness (52,67,86). Furthermore, depression has been shown to be the single most significant clinical risk factor for completed suicide in adolescence in several case–control studies using a psychological autopsy approach (7,8,90,91), and some, but not all, studies also suggest that bipolar disorder, particularly in a mixed state, conveys significant risk for completed suicide (7,8). Longitudinal studies of youth with early-onset affective illness have also demonstrated a high risk for both attempted and completed suicide associated with affective illness upon follow-up (36,52,81), although the rate of re-attempt was heightened if the affective illness was associated with nonaffective comorbidity (52).

FAMILY-GENETIC STUDIES

Several family-genetic studies have demonstrated continuity between child and adult affective disorders. Puig-

Antich et al. (79) conducted a blind family history study comparing the morbid risk of disorders in the relatives of prepubertal major depressives, non-affectively ill "neurotic" psychiatric controls, and normal controls. The rates of depression were higher in the relatives of the depressive probands, particularly in male relatives. Looking within the major depressive group, familial loading for depression was greater in endogenous than in nonendogenous depressives, and the rate of mania in first-degree relatives was higher in psychotic than in nonpsychotic depressives. Major depression, when comorbid with conduct disorder, was associated with a *lower* familial morbid risk of depression than when depression occurred without conduct disorder (0.14 versus 0.39); the same was true when comparing the morbid risk of depression in the relatives of suicidal versus nonsuicidal prepubertal depressives (0.20 versus 0.46).

Strober et al. (96) reported on a family study of bipolar I disorder in children and adolescents, with schizophrenic probands as controls. Higher familial rates of bipolar disorder were found in the relatives of both prepubertal and adolescent-onset bipolars compared to schizophrenics. The morbid risk of bipolar disorder was 3.5-fold *higher* in the relatives of the prepubertal-onset bipolars than in the relatives of the adolescent-onset bipolars. Prepubertal onset was also associated with greater nonaffective comorbidity and resistance to the therapeutic effect of lithium.

Several high-risk studies have demonstrated that the offspring of affectively ill parents are at higher risk for affective illnesses than are psychiatric or normal controls (35,66), with evidence of both an increased risk and earlier onset of disorder. Orvaschel et al. (65) recently demonstrated that the greatest risk for the development of affective illness is in offspring who come from families with affectively ill parents and grandparents. On follow-up, at least half of the offspring of affectively ill parents will experience a depression by the time they reach late adolescence (35,99). Parent–child discord, low family cohesion, and affectionless control were associated with development of conduct disorder and substance abuse in offspring of parents with a history of depression, but these variables were not associated with the onset of depression or anxiety. However, in the offspring of parents without history of depression, these factors were associated with depression, as well as with conduct disorder and substance abuse (22). Greater functional impairment and more prolonged depressive episodes in high-risk children and adolescents has been associated with the degree of exposure to parental affective illness, early age of onset of affective illness in the parent, chronicity, severity, recurrence of the illness in the parent, psychopathology in the nonaffectively ill parent, and parental divorce (44,98).

Several high-risk studies of offspring of bipolar disordered parents also indicate familial transmission of bipolar disorder. Akiskal et al. (1), in an uncontrolled, high-risk study of the offspring and siblings of bipolar patients, found that fully 50% showed signs of bipolarity, often manifested by cyclothymic disorder. One controlled high-risk study found an association between parental bipolarity and affective and cyclothymic disorder (45), whereas another found a more nonspecific increase in a broad range of nonaffective disorders (33). The severity and chronicity of parental bipolar disorder, as well as psychopathology in the nonbipolar parent, were associated with psychopathology and functional impairment in offspring (33).

These family-genetic and longitudinal high-risk studies support a significant role for the familial transmission of affective illness, probably through both environmental and genetic mechanisms, and also support the view that depression is heterogeneous in etiology. Disorders that are both most recurrent and familial appear to be psychotic depression, endogenous depression, and bipolar disorder, whereas the least familial and recurrent disorders are depression comorbid with conduct disorder. It may be that the secular trend in affective illness is accounted for primarily by the latter type of early-onset depressives, who are genetically "phenocopies," presenting with comorbid conduct disorder, substance abuse, and suicidality.

Other life stressors may also be associated with risk for depression, including loss of a parent (100), loss of a sibling or friend to suicide (9), or physical or sexual abuse (42,43). With respect to loss, depression is much more likely to occur if a personal or family history of depression is present (9,100). Parent–child discord has also been associated with both prepubertal and adolescent depression, but it is hard to discern to what extent discord is a cause of depression or, alternatively, a byproduct of the irritability of depression in the child and its frequent co-occurrence in an affectively ill parent (75,76,80).

Chronic medical conditions have been associated with an increased risk of early-onset depression and depressive symptomatology, namely, juvenile-onset diabetes, inflammatory bowel disease, and epilepsy (6,10). The etiologies of depression in these diverse groups is likely to be heterogeneous relating to the general stress of chronic illness, neurobiological interplay between systemic, metabolic diseases and psychopathology, and the effect of medications such as steroids and phenobarbital on mood (6).

BIOLOGICAL MARKERS IN MAJOR DEPRESSION

The search for psychobiological markers is exceedingly important both for research in early-onset affective illness and for a better understanding of affective illness across the lifespan, for several reasons (84). First, such approaches have helped validate the diagnosis of major depression in prepubertal patients. Second, such markers

may shed light on the pathophysiology of depression by indicating which neurotransmitter systems may be most intimately involved with depression. Third, markers may be useful in predicting the course, symptomatology (e.g., mania, psychosis, suicidal behavior), risk of recurrence, and treatment response in patients with early-onset depression. Fourth, the identification of biological markers may make it possible to study more homogeneous populations for family-genetic and treatment studies. Fifth, the study of these markers in children at high risk for depression may identify trait markers, thereby enabling researchers and clinicians to identify who is vulnerable to depression before it occurs. This may lead to greater understanding of the etiology of depression and to the development of preventive strategies. Furthermore, the identification of trait markers may lead to more informative family-genetic studies which include children who have not yet passed through the age of risk. If such children are unaffected, but yet have a given marker, then they may be counted as informative family members, thereby increasing the power of genetic-linkage studies. Sixth, the study of psychobiological markers in prepubertal depression enables one to examine the biological correlates of affective illness unadulterated by substance abuse, personality disorder, psychopharmacologic exposure, or chronic medical illness. Furthermore, longitudinal studies of biological probes in early-onset depression can shed light on the interaction between normal development, environment, and intrinsic vulnerability to depression. In specific, the longitudinal study of prepubertal depressives (and those at high risk for depression) through pubescence is critical to an understanding of the relationship between puberty and the increased risk of depression. In studying the developmental sequence of the appearance of psychobiological markers, it may be that early-onset markers are more intrinsic to the pathophysiology of depression, whereas later-appearing markers may be more related to dysregulation that occurs with chronic stress (69,84). Among the studies to be reviewed are neuroendocrine and sleep studies of prepubertal children and adolescents with major depression.

BASELINE AND 24-HOUR CORTISOL

Cortisol hypersecretion is rare in prepubertal children with major depression, occurring in only about 10% of cases (78). This was true when 24-hr cortisol secretory patterns in prepubertal depressives were compared to themselves in episode and recovery, as well as in comparison to psychiatric and normal controls.

In a comparison of adolescent outpatients with depression to normal controls, there were also no group differences with respect to the 24-hr pattern of cortisol secretion (14,55). However, in a second sample of adolescents with both inpatients and outpatients, Dahl et al. (17) examined the 24-hr cortisol secretory pattern by symptomatic subgroup of adolescent depressives, and they found that inpatient and suicidal subgroups of patients did not have the usual nadir of cortisol secretion near sleep onset when compared to other adolescents with depression and to normal controls. It is uncertain if this subgroup was under greater stress, which led to both suicidality and inpatient status, whether inpatient status allowed for greater circadian entrainment and, thus, revealed this abnormality, or whether these findings represent an intrinsic biological difference between suicidal and nonsuicidal adolescents with major depression. These results suggest that cortisol hypersecretion associated with depression is developmentally mediated, is rarely seen in childhood, emerges inconsistently with adolescence, and is not observed commonly until adulthood. One study of the impact of maltreatment on children found that depression in maltreated children was associated with the loss of the expected diurnal pattern of cortisol secretion (43). While this study did not examine 24-hr cortisol secretion, it does point to the possibility that severe stress in a subgroup of children may lead to both depression and cortisol hypersecretion and that, in fact, the nature of the stress response may predict which children under severe stress will develop affective illness.

DEXAMETHASONE SUPPRESSION TEST (DST)

The early claims for the dexamethasone suppression test (DST) as a sensitive and specific test for endogenous major depression have been qualified considerably in more recent studies of adults (3). Overall, as reviewed by Dahl et al. (18), Casat et al. (11), and Ryan and Dahl (84), the sensitivity of the DST across studies was low in both children (58%) and adolescents (44%). Studies on inpatients yield much greater sensitivity than did studies on outpatients (61% versus 29%). Specificity was somewhat higher in adolescents than in children, compared to both normal controls (84% versus 74%) and psychiatric controls (solely inpatients, 85% versus 60%).

Other clinical and methodological variables have been reported to be associated with DST nonsuppression—most notably, concurrent suicidal behavior (68,82), subsequent suicidal lethality (82), and endogenous subtype (83). The findings associating suicidality with DST nonsuppression were among inpatients, and they are consistent with Dahl et al.'s (17) report of a loss of the usual decline in cortisol secretion at sleep onset in suicidal inpatient adolescents with major depression. The studies associating psychotic and endogenous subtype have not been replicated in DST studies which employed an indwelling catheter to obtain blood samples (4,5,18). This may be related to the fact that these studies were conducted in a relatively low-stress environment, on mostly outpatients. As in studies of 24-hr cortisol secretion, it is likely that

age, pubertal status, and degree of stress interact to yield abnormalities in cortisol secretion in depression, and that such abnormalities are less common in children and among outpatients than among adolescents and inpatients.

CRH STIMULATION TEST

Corticotropin-releasing hormone (CRH) infusion results in release of adrenocorticotropic hormone (ACTH) from the pituitary, followed by cortisol secretion from the adrenal. The CRH challenge has shown blunted ACTH response, despite normal-to-high cortisol levels in adults with depression (31). This has not been the case in studies of prepubertal children with major depression. Birmaher and colleagues (*unpublished data*) found no differences between prepubertal major depressives and normal controls on baseline cortisol or ACTH, or cortisol or ACTH response to CRH. However, subgroup analyses revealed that ten inpatient depressed children and four melancholic depressed subjects showed a significantly lower ACTH, but normal cortisol after CRH, consistent with findings in depressed adults. Another related subanalysis in this sample found that prior sexual abuse was associated with a blunted response of ACTH to CRH (Kaufman, *unpublished data*), a finding also reported by DeBellis et al. (20) in a different sample.

Taken together, the findings of 24-hr cortisol secretion, the DST, and the CRH challenge studies suggest that abnormalities of cortisol secretion are relatively rare in children and begin to emerge, albeit inconsistently, in adolescence. Children may be developmentally *protected* against manifesting these abnormalities associated with adult depression, and they may only consistently emerge after exposure to severe stress (e.g., sexual or physical abuse).

Several critical questions emerge from these results: (a) At what point in adolescence or adulthood do psychobiological abnormalities of cortisol homeostasis consistently emerge? (b) Why are children with depression ''protected'' from more commonly manifesting abnormalities in cortisol homeostasis? (c) What are the pathways from stress to perturbations in cortisol dynamics to the development of depression? Longitudinal studies of depressed and control samples with careful measures of both exogenous stress and the above-noted psychobiological probes will be critical to addressing these questions. On the basis of recent work, it is critical to take into account the presence of multiple feedback loops involving the hypothalamus, pituitary, and adrenals (13).

GROWTH HORMONE

There is consistent evidence for blunted growth hormone (GH) response to provocative pharmacologic challenges in prepubertal depressed patients. Puig-Antich et al. (73) showed blunted growth hormone response to insulin-induced hypoglycemia in prepubertal children with endogenous major depression, compared to a nondepressed neurotic psychiatric control group. This blunting in GH response to insulin persisted after a medication-free period of recovery (74). Furthermore, this abnormality has also been found in a subset of prepubertal children, who, by virtue of familial loading, were at high risk for depression, but were as yet unaffected (Ryan, *unpublished data*). These studies, taken together, support the view that this finding represents a trait marker for major depression. Jensen and Garfinkel (40) found blunted GH response to oral clonidine and to L-DOPA in prepubertal depressed versus normal subjects. Meyer et al. (63) found blunted growth hormone response to insulin-induced hypoglycemia, to arginine, and to oral clonidine, but *not* to L-DOPA or 5-hydroxytryptophan in comparing 7- to 13-year-old depressed boys and age-matched normal controls.

Ryan and colleagues (*unpublished data*) have replicated and extended the findings of Puig-Antich et al. (73,74) in a comparison of 38 prepubertal patients with major depression and 19 normal-aged and Tanner stage-matched controls. As in the above-noted studies, GH release was blunted after insulin-induced hypoglycemia in the depressed subjects, but the findings occurred *without* regard to endogenicity. There was a trend for GH release to be blunted at 1.3 μg/kg of intravenous clonidine, although the differences were not statistically significant. Of interest was that GH release was also significantly blunted after challenge with GH-releasing hormone (GHRH). This finding, which was initially unexpected, suggests that the abnormality in GH regulation is not solely at the level of the α_2-adrenergic system in the hypothalamus. Studies by Ryan and colleagues are ongoing to determine the origin of this abnormality, including the examination of somatostatin and of insulin-like growth factor (somatomedin C).

There has been less published on provocative GH challenges in adolescents with major depression, and what has been published is not as conclusive as the above-noted findings in prepubertal children. Ryan et al. (87) found blunted GH response to desmethylimipramine (DMI) in depressed adolescents compared to normal controls, but the difference between groups was entirely accounted for by blunting of GH in depressed, suicidal adolescents. Jensen and Garfinkel (40), in a small sample of adolescents (8 depressed and 5 normals), found no differences with respect to GH response to oral clonidine or L-DOPA. The variability in the findings in adolescents relative to prepubertal children may be attributable to the mediating effects of sex steroids on GH response to provocative challenges. For example, Matussek et al. (60) noted that GH response to clonidine was most consistently blunted in postmenopausal females. Studies have indicated that estrogen potentiates the effect of exercise and arginine on the release of GH (62), whereas others have

indicated that androgens, but not estrogens, potentiate the effect of GHRH on GH release (94).

The above-noted findings are consistent with work in adults. Adults with major depression have shown blunted GH response to clonidine (12,92), a finding that persists after recovery (92). More recently, studies have indicated that depressed adults show a blunted GH response to GHRH (58,64) and that this blunted response was related to a blunted GH response to clonidine (58) and to DMI (64), as well as to higher levels of circulating somatomedin (58).

GROWTH HORMONE: NOCTURNAL AND 24-HOUR PATTERNS

Puig-Antich et al. (71,72) found that prepubertal patients with major depression *hypersecreted* GH during sleep compared to nondepressed neurotic controls, both in episode and after a sustained medication-free recovery. Meyer et al. (63), in a comparison of the 24-hr patterns GH secretion in depressed and normal boys, found *decreased* GH secretion association with depression, both during the daytime and during nocturnal phases of GH secretion. More recently, Ryan and colleagues (*unpublished data*) have found *no difference* between prepubertal depressed children and normal controls in nocturnal GH secretion.

Studies of GH secretion in adolescent major depression are also inconsistent. Kutcher et al. (54), in a comparison of nine depressed adolescents and nine normal controls, found *increased* nocturnal secretion of GH, mostly in the first half of the night (midnight and 1:00 a.m.). This finding was replicated in a second study comparing 12 adolescent depressives and 12 normal adolescents (55). In both of these studies, nocturnal GH hypersecretion was unrelated to suicidality or endogenicity. In contrast, Dahl et al. (19) found *decreased* nocturnal GH in depressed, suicidal adolescents, compared to normal controls, but in contrast, nonsuicidal depressed adolescents were no different than normal controls. In a second adolescent sample, Dahl and colleagues (*unpublished data*) have found no difference in 24-hr GH secretion between depressed and control adolescents.

Results in adult depressives are similarly inconsistent. One study reported that adult male depressives *hypersecreted* GH during the day and had a normal nocturnal secretory pattern (61), whereas another found that adults with recurrent depression (males and females) *hyposecreted* GH during the time of sleep onset (39). In the latter study, this pattern of nocturnal GH hyposecretion persisted after sustained medication-free recovery.

SEROTONIN CHALLENGE STUDIES

In the only study reported to date of serotonergic functioning in early-onset depression, Ryan et al. (88)

compared 37 depressed children with 23 psychiatrically normal children using an intravenous challenge of L-5-hydroxytryptophan (L-5HTP), preceded by oral preloading with carbidopa, in order to prevent peripheral degradation of L-5HTP. In response to the L-5HTP challenge, the depressed children showed significantly greater prolactin response and a smaller rise in cortisol compared to controls. Cortisol response was unaffected by gender, but the difference in prolactin secretion between depressives and normals was only seen in females. There was no association between suicidality and either prolactin or cortisol response to L-5HTP, nor were there any correlates of either of these two markers with aggression, endogenicity, or melancholia.

These findings are consistent with studies in adults, insofar as several other studies have shown differences in neuroendocrine responses to serotonergic probes between adult depressives and controls. Similar to the findings of Ryan et al. (88), Maes et al. (59) found *enhanced* prolactin response to oral L-5HTP in melancholic women. In contrast to blunted cortisol response reported by Ryan et al. (88), *enhanced* cortisol response to L-5HTP has been reported associated with depression (59). While Ryan et al. (88) found gender differences for prolactin response, but not for cortisol, Maes et al. (59) reported that female, but not male, depressives differed from controls on *both* prolactin and cortisol response to L-5HTP.

The variability in responses reported in different studies may differ as a function of age, gender, the specificity of the serotonergic probes, and the balance of different subpopulations of serotonergic receptors in a given subject. The latter is likely to be the case because there is evidence that both prolactin and cortisol responses to serotonergic agonists are governed by both pre- and postsynaptic effects.

SLEEP

Sleep EEG changes are one of the most frequently found psychobiological markers associated with depression in adults (47). These findings include reduced rapid eye movement (REM) latency, decreased delta (stage 3 and 4) sleep, sleep continuity disturbances, increased REM density, and more even distribution of REM density across the entire night, as compared to the pattern of increased REM pressure during the second half of the night in normals. The above-noted sleep characteristics, while typically found in adult depressives, are much less consistently found in juvenile populations.

Puig-Antich et al. (69) compared 54 prepubertal depressives, 25 psychiatric controls with ''emotional'' disorders, and 11 normal controls, and they found no group differences with respect to any of the above-noted sleep parameters. In a follow-up study (70), 28 fully recovered prepubertal depressed children were studied in a

medication-free state. The recovered depressed subjects showed shorter REM latency upon follow-up compared to themselves while in episode, and to the two control groups upon follow-up. However, those followed up, compared to those who were not, had more normal sleep to begin with, so that the interpretation of these results is not straightforward; to our knowledge, a replication of this study has not been published. Emslie et al. (21), in contrast, compared 35 hospitalized depressed children and 20 age-matched controls, and they found evidence of decreased REM latency, increased REM time, and increased sleep latency in the depressed group. Dahl et al. (16) compared 36 prepubertal depressed children with 18 age- and Tanner stage-matched normal controls. Overall, there were no group differences, but one subgroup of eight depressed subjects was noted to have reduced REM latency, decreased stage 4 sleep, and increased REM time, and symptomatically these individuals were more severely depressed and more likely to be melancholic.

The picture in adolescent depression appears to be intermediate between that of prepuberty and adulthood. Lahmeyer et al. (57) compared 13 older adolescents with depression and 13 age-matched controls, finding evidence of decreased REM latency in the depressed group. Moreover, a negative correlation was found between REM latency and age, suggesting that this marker may not emerge until later in adolescence. Goetz et al. (30) studied 49 nonbipolar adolescents (mostly outpatients) with major depression and 40 normal adolescent controls. There was longer sleep latency in the adolescent depressive group, but no difference between depressives and controls with respect to REM latency, REM density, or delta sleep. Age was noted to be correlated with REM latency and delta sleep, more so in the depressives than in the controls, similar to the observation of Lahmeyer et al. (57). Dahl et al. (15) compared 27 adolescents with major depression and 30 normal controls. There were no age–diagnosis interactions for any of the relevant sleep parameters. There were no group differences when the depressed group was compared to the control group. However, the suicidal depressed adolescents showed increased sleep latency and decreased REM latency compared to both the nonsuicidal depressives and normal controls. There was substantial overlap between suicidality and inpatient status, such that it was uncertain if the findings could be attributed to suicidality or to inpatient status (15). Finally, Kutcher et al. (56) compared 23 endogenously depressed older adolescents with 23 normal controls. The depressed group showed decreased REM latency and increased sleep latency.

In summary, as reviewed by Ryan and Dahl (84), the ''classic'' sleep EEG findings associated with adult depression are found inconsistently in child and adolescent studies. Only three of the eight controlled studies reported decreased REM latency (21,56,57), and only one study found an increase in the total REM time (21). Decreases in sleep continuity were reported in two studies (2,30). An additional study found decreased REM latency and increased sleep latency *only* in depressed suicidal inpatients (15), and one study of prepubertal subjects found reduced REM latency, decreased stage 4 sleep, and increased REM time only in a subgroup of more severely depressed, prepubertal subjects who were more likely to be melancholic (16).

Therefore, consistent sleep EEG findings in depression do not emerge until late adolescence. When they appear earlier, the subjects are inpatients, suicidal or severely depressed, and possibly under considerable stress. Thus, similar to the discussion of cortisol HPA abnormalities, it may take an unusual amount of exogenous stress for children and adolescents to manifest sleep-EEG abnormalities. Moreover, as noted in the analyses of several of these studies (30,56,57), the REM and sleep continuity changes as a function of age with some evidence that the trend was *accelerated* in the depressive group. These findings are also consistent with the meta-analysis of Knowles and MacLean (47), which noted that the differences in the sleep findings between depressed and normal subjects seem to increase as a function of age.

TREATMENT

Several controlled studies have failed to find differences between antidepressant and placebo in depressed children and adolescents. There have not as yet been any controlled trials of treatment of bipolar disorder, although prepubertal-onset bipolar disease has been reported to be associated with lithium resistance (96).

The largest study of prepubertal depression examined 38 depressed children assigned to either imipramine or placebo (77). No difference in treatment response was found between imipramine (56% response) and placebo (68%). In a related study examining relationship of plasma level of imipramine and metabolites to clinical response, Puig-Antich et al. (77) noted that nonresponse was associated with lower plasma level of imipramine and desipramine, severe depression, and the presence of hallucinations.

Hughes et al. (38) reported on an inpatient treatment study using imipramine versus placebo in prepubertal depressed children. Children with "pure" depression, or depression complicated by anxiety, responded much better to imipramine than to placebo (57% versus 20%), whereas depression comorbid with conduct disorder responded better to placebo (33% versus 67%). Geller et al. (26), in a study of severely and chronically ill prepubertal depressed children, also found no difference between nortriptyline (NT) and placebo, with response rate. As defined by a score on the Child Depression Rating Scale (CDRS) of <20, 31% of those treated with NT versus 17% of those given placebo responded. Using Puig-

Antich et al.'s (77) criteria, the response rates were 46% versus 58% for medication versus placebo.

Two methodological issues were addressed in subsequent follow-up studies of Geller et al. (27,28). First, in a follow-up of subjects who had a response to placebo and hence "failed" the placebo washout phase, it was demonstrated that the subsequent risks of depression and mania were the same in the placebo responders and nonresponders. Moreover, these two groups were similar with respect to other clinical parameters, namely, severity, chronicity, age of onset, and comorbid psychopathology, and differed only insofar as placebo washout responders were more likely to be female. These results indicate that the placebo washout phase may not be necessary for clinical trials in this age group.

Second, Geller et al. (28) noted an association between the development of mania and tricyclic use, especially if the exposure to NT was greater than 25 weeks, whereupon the risk for mania was increased twofold. Bipolar I disorder developed *only* in subjects exposed to tricyclic antidepressants. However, there was no difference in the rate of bipolar I (or II) mania or hypomania between those who did and did not receive tricyclic antidepressants. A heavily loaded pedigree with affective illness in three generations conveyed a greatly increased risk for the development of mania, as was noted a decade earlier by Strober and Carlson (95). This may be a critical treatment and design issue in samples of clinically referred early-onset depressives, who often are enriched with those with a family history of bipolarity.

With respect to adolescents, there have been even fewer published studies. Ryan et al. (85), in an open-label study of adolescents, found only a 44% response rate to imipramine, with nonresponse associated with comorbid separation anxiety, endogenicity, and female gender. In one small controlled study of depressed adolescent inpatients, 80% responded to amitriptyline versus 60% of subjects receiving placebo (53). Two unpublished studies (Ryan, *personal communication;* Gittleman-Klein, *unpublished manuscript*) also note no difference between antidepressant and placebo. Geller et al. (25), in a study of chronically and severely ill adolescents with major depression, found only an 8% versus 21% response rate in NT-treated versus placebo-treated groups. Simeon et al. (93), in a comparison of adolescent depressives treated with fluoxetine versus placebo, also found no difference between the two treatment groups, with approximately two-thirds responding in both conditions.

This lack of difference in response between antidepressant and placebo in early-onset depression is a critical area for further research because of several reasons. First, no clinical intervention, either pharmacologic or psychosocial, has been demonstrated to be effective in clinically referred, affectively ill children or adolescents. Second, antidepressants continue to be used widely, and while most clinicians agree that on the basis of their clinical experience, treatment with antidepressants is warranted, there are no accepted guidelines as to which patients are most likely to respond, nor is there consensus with respect to optimal dosage or length of treatment. Finally, the apparent difference in the antidepressant placebo response in children and adolescents compared to adults raises questions as to possible developmentally mediated biological differences in depression across the lifespan. As reviewed in this chapter, there is strong evidence supporting a continuity between child-onset and adult depression, based on family-genetics, high-risk, longitudinal, and neuroendocrine challenge studies. Therefore, it is particularly puzzling why depressed children and adolescents do not show similar response to antidepressants as do depressed adults.

First, it should be noted that, in general, children and adolescents *do* respond well to antidepressants—it is just that the placebo-response rate is also high. The exception to this is the study of Geller et al. (25), where adolescents with depression responded to antidepressants only 8% of the time, and to placebo 21%. This particular sample was a very severely and chronically ill sample, enriched for family history of bipolar disorder, a population that in adults has been shown not to do well on tricyclic antidepressants (97). Puig-Antich et al. (77) also noted that those prepubertal, depressed patients with severe depression and/or hallucinations did not respond well to imipramine. It is possible that this subpopulation might respond better to a monamine oxidase inhibitor or to lithium.

A second possibility is developmental, and two possibilities have been advanced. From primate studies, it is known that the noradrenergic neurotransmitter system continues to mature and develop throughout puberty (32), so that it is possible that antidepressants do not exert the same impact on developing systems. However, neuroendocrine studies noted above—namely, the insulin tolerance and clonidine challenge studies of GH—are consistent with a noradrenergic deficit of neurotransmission, at least in endogenously depressed prepubertal children. Therefore, one could posit that noradrenergic agents should be effective in prepubertal endogenous depressives. A related issue is that perhaps the high level of circulating sex steroids in adolescents may explain their failure to respond to antidepressants. However, this would not explain a high placebo response that has been reported in some studies of adolescents (53,93).

A third possibility, as yet untested, is that younger populations of affectively ill patients are enriched for atypical depression, a group that has been demonstrated not to respond as well to tricyclic antidepressants as compared to monoamine oxidase inhibitors (97). With the availability of reversible monoamine oxidase inhibitors, studies using these much safer agents should be considered.

A fourth and related issue is that endogenomorphic features have been found to predict tricyclic antidepressant response in adults (97), yet endogenous features are relatively rare in clinical samples of early-onset affectively ill patients who participate in protocols. However, endogenicity did not predict response to imipramine in Puig-Antich et al.'s (77) study of prepubertal depressives, and it was associated with nonresponse in Ryan et al.'s (85) open-label study of depressed adolescents.

A fifth possibility is the observation that the psychosocial environment of depressed children and adolescents is sufficiently different from depressed adults enrolled in clinical trials such that the outcomes may differ by age. Specifically, family conflict, history of abuse, and parental depression are noted as potential risk factors for early-onset depression. It is possible that unless these potent factors are addressed in treatment, the sociotoxic impact of parent–child discord and parental depression may override any individually focused intervention, whether psychopharmacologic or psychosocial. This issue would not, however, explain the high placebo response rate seen in the reported studies.

At least one other untested possibility remains, as raised by Geller et al. (26): The failure to find differences in response to antidepressant versus placebo in more juvenile populations may be related to the recent secular trend in affective illness. It is likely that the secular trend has not occurred due to changes in the genetic make-up of the population, but rather that certain exogenous factors (e.g., social stressors) have contributed to the increased risk of depression in younger populations. Therefore, it is possible that, via the secular trend, the proportion of phenocopies with depressive symptoms has increased, and that most clinical samples are, in fact, enriched with them. One would predict that phenocopies might not show high familial loading for depression, would be more likely to be suicidal and to have comorbid symptoms of disruptive disorders and substance abuse, and might not show the core differences in neuroendocrine challenge studies (e.g., L-5HTP cortisol and prolactin, GH-GHRH). Among prepubertal children, there is some preliminary evidence to support this insofar as suicidal and conduct-disordered children show lower family loading for affective disorder (79). Also, certain neurobiological findings have been reported by some to be present only in endogenously depressed prepubertal children (found in refs. 73 and 74 but not found in refs. 84 and 88), and other biological changes (e.g., in blunted ACTH response to CRH) are found in association with maltreatment or sexual abuse (20,43). Additional evidence to support the role of family discord in ''phenocopies'' comes from the work of Fendrich et al. (22), in which family environmental factors such as ''affectionless control'' were associated with increased risk for depression in offspring of nondepressed parents only. Such familial risk factors were associated with comorbid substance abuse and conduct disturbance in *both* the high- and low-risk groups. Hence, the presence of comorbid disruptive disorder may signal the presence of a phenocopy with low familial loading. Longitudinal studies (24,37) also support the thesis that "pure" depression is much more likely to be continuous with adult depression than depression comorbid with conduct disorder. Additionally, Hughes et al. (38) found that the presence of conduct disorder predicted a lower response to antidepressant and a better response to placebo than in the "pure" depressive group, although these findings have not been replicated by others. The role of the exogenous stressors, family loading for affective illness, and the neuroendocrine profile of early-onset depressives may be helpful in delineating the subgroups of depressed patients who will respond more favorably to antidepressant than to placebo. From the extant literature, one might posit that children with strong familial loading for recurrent unipolar depression, who present with prominent endogenous features without extensive nonaffective comorbidity, would be the most likely to respond to antidepressants better than to placebo. Conversely, such studies may point the way to more precise ways of identifying those patient who might benefit from psychosocial interventions.

CONCLUSIONS

During the past decade, tremendous strides in our study of early-onset affective disorders have been achieved. The following are some of the "unsolved mysteries" in this fascinating field that should be addressed in the coming years:

1. *The etiology of the secular trend in early-onset depression.* As noted above, a better understanding of the secular trend has important implications for treatment and prevention. This could possibly be achieved by stratifying epidemiologic and clinical data sets on the basis of family history, psychobiologic markers, or antidepressant response, to learn if the secular trends are really influencing all subpopulations equally. For example, Giles et al. (29) found that the rate of unipolar depression was the same in siblings and in parents of unipolar depressed probands with reduced REM latency, whereas the rate was *higher* in siblings than in parents of depressed probands *without* reduced REM latency.

2. *The differential psychobiology of bipolar and unipolar depression.* This will perhaps be best achieved by following early-onset depressives studied psychobiologically to learn what are the predictors of the course of illness and of the onset of mania (84).

3. *Predictors of onset and course of affective illness.* This will probably best be understood by following populations at high risk for depression and studying them from family-genetic, family-environmental, and psychobiological points of view in order to learn what factors predict onset of depression and subsequent course. In this regard, the identification of trait markers that antedate the development of affective illness will be a critical step to prog-

ress in this area. Such studies may also lead to empirically based programs to prevent the onset of affective illness in those at risk.

4. *The genetics of early-onset affective illness.* If informative, trait psychobiological markers for depression can be identified, then they can be utilized to render unaffected members of pedigrees who are not yet through the age of risk much more informative, thereby increasing statistical power for linkage studies. For example, pedigrees now include many unaffected members who are not through the age of risk, and therefore do not contribute to estimates of linkage. If a reliable marker for vulnerability to affective illness could be identified, this would enable a greater proportion of family members in a pedigree to become informative. Use of animal, particularly primate, models for depression with subsequent linkage studies may also shed light on the genetic etiology of affective illness.

5. *The role of puberty in the increased risk for depression.* With the onset of puberty, the risk for depression increases dramatically, particularly in females, yet the role of puberty in the etiology of depression is poorly understood. Basic neurobiological studies of the effect of puberty on the development of neurotransmitter systems relevant to risk for affective disorder are critical, as are clinical psychobiological studies that follow normal, depressed, and high-risk children through puberty. Such studies are also likely to shed light on the gender difference in the rate of depression that occurs postpubertally.

6. *Predictor of suicidal behavior and suicide within the early-onset affectively ill.* Some psychobiological studies have indicated specific psychobiologic correlates of differential suicidality with depressed subjects (15,17,19, 82,87), although it has been difficult to disentangle the impact of inpatient status, depressive severity, and suicidality. Further cross-sectional and longitudinal studies of early-onset affectively ill subjects that assess in psychosocial, family-genetic, and psychobiological domains are likely to be the most informative in this regard.

7. *Integrating studies of individual variability in stress-responsivity with studies of risk for depression.* Animal models and follow-up studies of behaviorally inhibited infants suggest that individual differences in stress-responsivity may be related to subsequent risk for behavioral syndromes analogous to depression or anxiety. Such paradigms should also be applied to clinical populations, and particularly to children at risk for the development of depression, beginning with very young children.

8. *Better prediction of treatment response.* Up to this point, assessment and treatment studies of early-onset depression have not been well-integrated. In order to address the issues of heterogeneity, it is vital to integrate family-genetic, family-environmental, and psychobiological assessments with treatment studies in order to learn what characteristics from these different domains predict treat-

ment response to either psychosocial or psychopharmacologic agents.

ACKNOWLEDGMENTS

Preparation of this chapter was made possible, in part, by funding from the following grants: NIMH grant MH41712, "Psychobiology of Depression in Children and Adolescents" (Program Project) (Dr. Ryan); NIMH grant MH46510, "EEG Sleep Changes in Adolescent Depression" (Dr. Dahl); NIMH grant MH44711, "Youth Exposed to Suicide" (Dr. Brent); and NIMH grant MH30915, "Mental Health Clinical Research Center for the Study of Affective Disorders" (Dr. Kupfer, P.I.; seed award to Dr. Birmaher). The assistance of Ms. Susie Petrie in the preparation of this chapter is gratefully acknowledged.

REFERENCES

1. Akiskal HS, Downs J, Jordan P, Watson S, Daugherty D, Pruitt DB. Affective disorders in referred children and younger siblings of manic-depressives. Mode of onset and prospective course. *Arch Gen Psychiatry* 1985;42:996–1003.
2. Appleboom-Fondu J, Kerkhofs M, Mendlewicz J. Depression in adolescents and young adults—polysomnographic and neuroendocrine aspects. *J Affective Disord* 1988;14:35–40.
3. Arana GW, Baldessarini RJ, Ornsteen M. The dexamethasone suppression test for diagnosis and prognosis in psychiatry. *Arch Gen Psychiatry* 1985;42:1193–1204.
4. Birmaher B, Dahl RE, Ryan ND, et al. The dexamethasone suppression test in adolescent outpatients with major depressive disorder. *Am J Psychiatry* 1992;149:1040–1045.
5. Birmaher B, Ryan ND, Dahl RE, et al. Dexamethasone suppression test in children with major depressive disorder. *J Am Acad Child Adolesc Psychiatry* 1992;31:291–297.
6. Brent D, Crumrine P, Varma R, et al. Phenobarbital treatment and major depressive disorder in children with epilepsy. *Pediatrics* 1987;80:909–917.
7. Brent D, Perper J, Goldstein CE, et al. Risk factors for adolescent suicide: a comparison of adolescent suicide victims with suicidal inpatients. *Arch Gen Psychiatry* 1988;45:581–588.
8. Brent DA, Perper JA, Moritz G, et al. Psychiatric risk factors for adolescent suicide: a case–control study. *J Am Acad Child Adolesc Psychiatry* 1993;32:521–529.
9. Brent DA, Perper JA, Moritz G, et al. Psychiatric sequelae to the loss of an adolescent peer to suicide. *J Am Acad Child Adolesc Psychiatry* 1993;32:509–517.
10. Burke P, Meyer V, Kocoshis S, et al. Depression and anxiety in pediatric inflammatory bowel disease and cystic fibrosis. *J Am Acad Child Adolesc Psychiatry* 1989;28:948–951.
11. Casat CD, Arana GW, Powell K. The DST in children and adolescents with major depressive disorder. *Am J Psychiatry* 1989;146:503–507.
12. Checkley SA, Slade AP, Shyur E. Growth hormone and other responses to clonidine in patients with endogenous depression. *Br J Psychiatry* 1981;138:51–55.
13. Chrousos GP, Gold PW. The concepts of stress and stress system disorders. *JAMA* 1992;267:1244–1252.
14. Dahl R, Puig-Antich J, Ryan N, et al. Cortisol secretion in adolescents with major depressive disorder. *Acta Psychiatr Scand* 1989;80:18–26.
15. Dahl R, Ryan ND, Nelson B, Dachille S, Cunningham S, Trubnick L, Klepper T. EEG sleep in adolescents with major depression: the role of suicidality and inpatient status. *J Affect Disord* 1990;19:63–75.
16. Dahl RE, Ryan ND, Birmaher B, et al. Electroencephalographic sleep measures in prepubertal depression. *Psychiatry Res* 1991;38:201–214.
17. Dahl RE, Ryan ND, Puig-Antich J, et al. 24-hour cortisol measures in adolescents with major depression: a controlled study. *Biol Psychiatry* 1991;30:25–36.
18. Dahl RE, Kaufman J, Ryan ND, et al. The dexamethasone suppression test in children and adolescents: a review and a controlled study. *Biol Psychiatry* 1992;32:109–126.
19. Dahl R, Ryan ND, Williamson DE, et al. Regulation of sleep and growth hormone in adolescent depression. *J Am Acad Child Adolesc Psychiatry* 1992b;31:615–621.
20. DeBellis MD, Chrousos GP, Dorn L, et al. Hypothalamic-pituitary-adrenal axis dysregulation in sexually abused girls. *J Clin Endocrinol Metab* 1994;78(2):249–255.
21. Emslie GJ, Rush AJ, Weinberg WA, Rintelmann JW, Poffwarg HP. Children with major depression show reduced rapid eye movement latencies. *Arch Gen Psychiatry* 1990;47:119–124.
22. Fendrich M, Warner V, Weissman MM. Family risk factors, parental depression, and psychopathology in offspring. *Dev Psychol* 1990;26:40–50.
23. Fleming JE, Offord DR. Epidemiology of childhood depressive disorders: a critical review. *J Am Acad Child Adolesc Psychiatry* 1990;29:571–580.
24. Fleming JE, Boyle MH, Offord DR. The outcome of adolescent depression in the Ontario child health study follow-up. *J Am Acad Child Adolesc Psychiatry* 1993;32:1:28–33.
25. Geller B, Cooper MA, Graham DL, et al. Double-blind placebo-controlled study of nortriptyline in depressed adolescents using a "fixed plasma level" design. *Psychopharm Bull* 1990;26:85–90.
26. Geller B, Cooper T, Graham DL, Fetner HH, Marsteller FA, Wells JM. Pharmacokinetically designed double-blind placebo-controlled study of nortriptyline in 6- to 12-year-olds with major depressive disorder. *J Am Acad Child Adolesc Psychiatry* 1992;31:34–44.
27. Geller B, Fox LW, Cooper TB, Garrity K. Baseline and 2- to 3-year follow-up characteristics of placebo-washout responders from the nortriptyline study of depressed 6- to 12-year-olds. *J Am Acad Child Adolesc Psychiatry* 1992;31:622–628.
28. Geller B, Fox LW, Fletcher M. Effect of tricyclic antidepressants on switching to mania and on the onset of bipolarity in depressed 6- to 12-year olds. *J Am Acad Child Adolesc Psychiatry* 1993;31:43–50.
29. Giles DE, Roffwarg HP, Kupfer DJ, Rush AJ, Biggs MM, Etzel BA. Secular trend in unipolar depression: a hypothesis. *J Affective Disord* 1989;16:71–75.
30. Goetz RR, Puig-Antich J, Ryan N, et al. Electroencephalographic sleep of adolescents with major depression and normal controls. *Arch Gen Psychiatry* 1987;44:61–68.
31. Gold PW, Loriaux DL, Roy A, et al. Responses to corticotropin-releasing hormone in the hypercortisolism of depression and Cushing's disease. *N Engl J Med* 1986;314:1329–1335.
32. Goldman-Rakic PS, Brown RM. Postnatal development of monoamine content and synthesis in the cerebral cortex of rhesus monkeys. *Dev Brain Res* 1982;4:339–349.
33. Grigoroiu-Serbanescu M, Christodorescu D, Jipescu I, Totoescu A, Marinescu E, Ardelean V. Psychopathology in children aged 10–17 of bipolar parents: psychopathology rate and correlates of the severity of the psychopathology. *J Affective Disord* 1989;16:167–179.
34. Hagnell O, Lanke J, Rorsman B, Ojesjo L. Are we entering an age of melancholy? Depressive illness in a prospective epidemiological study over 25 years: The Lundby Study, Sweden. *Psychol Med* 1982;12:279–289.
35. Hammen C, Burge D, Burney E, Adrian C. Longitudinal study of diagnoses in children of women with unipolar and bipolar affective disorder. *Arch Gen Psychiatry* 1990;47:1112–1117.
36. Harrington R, Fudge H, Rutter M, Pickles A, Hill J. Adult outcomes of childhood and adolescent depression. I. Psychiatric status. *Arch Gen Psychiatry* 1990;47:465–473.
37. Harrington R, Fudge H, Rutter M, Pickles A, Hill J. Adult outcomes of childhood and adolescent depression. II. Links with antisocial disorders. *J Am Acad Child Adolesc Psychiatry* 1991;30:434–439.

38. Hughes CW, Preskorn SH, Weller E, Weller R, Hassanein R, Tucker S. The effect of concomitant disorders in childhood depression on predicting treatment response. *Psychopharmacol Bull* 1990;26:235–238.

39. Jarrett DB, Miewald JM, Kupfer DJ. Recurrent depression is associated with a persistent reduction in sleep-related growth hormone secretion. *Arch Gen Psychiatry* 1990;47:113–118.

40. Jensen JB, Garfinkel BD. Growth hormone dysregulation in children with major depressive order. *J Am Acad Child Adolesc Psychiatry* 1990;29:2:295–301.

41. Kandel DB, Davies M. Adult sequelae of adolescent depressive symptoms. *Arch Gen Psychiatry* 1986;43:255–262.

42. Kashani JH, Shekim WO, Burk JP, Beck NC. Abuse as a predictor of psychopathology in children and adolescents. *J Clin Child Psychology* 1987;16:43–50.

43. Kaufman J. Depressive disorders in maltreated children. *J Am Acad Child Adolesc Psychiatry* 1991;30:257–265.

44. Keller MB, Beardslee WR, Dorer DJ, Lavori PW, Samuelson H, Klerman GR. Impact of severity and chronicity of parental affective illness on adaptive functioning and psychopathology in children. *Arch Gen Psychiatry* 1986;43:930–937.

45. Klein DN, Depue RA, Slater JF. Cyclothymia in the adolescent offspring of parents with bipolar affective disorder. *J Abnorm Psychol* 1985;94:115–127.

46. Klerman GL, Lavori PW, Rice J, et al. Birth-cohort trends in rates of major depressive disorder among relatives of patients with affective disorder. *Arch Gen Psychiatry* 1985;42:689–693.

47. Knowles JB, MacLean AW. Age-related changes in sleep in depressed and healthy subjects: a meta-analysis. *Neuropsychopharmacology* 1990;3:251–259.

48. Kovacs M, Feinberg TL, Crouse-Novak M, Paulsuskas SL, Finkelstein R. Depressive disorders in childhood. I. A longitudinal prospective study of characteristics and recovery. *Arch Gen Psychiatry* 1984;41:229–237.

49. Kovacs M, Feinberg T, Crouse-Novak M, Paulsuskas S, Pollock M, Finkelstein R. Depressive disorders in childhood. II. A longitudinal study of the risk for a subsequent major depression. *Arch Gen Psychiatry* 1984;41:643–649.

50. Kovacs M, Paulsuskas S, Gatsonis C, Richards C. Depressive disorders in childhood. III. A longitudinal study of comorbidity with and risk for conduct disorders. *J Affective Disord* 1988;15:205–217.

51. Kovacs M, Gatsonis C, Paulauskas SL, Richards C. Depressive disorders in childhood. IV. A longitudinal study of comorbidity with and risk for anxiety disorders. *Arch Gen Psychiatry* 1989;46:776–782.

52. Kovacs M, Goldston D, Gatsonis C. Suicidal behaviors and childhood-onset depressive disorders: a longitudinal investigation. *J Am Acad Child Adolesc Psychiatry* 1993;32:1:8–20.

53. Kramer AD, Feiguine RJ. Clinical effects of amitriptyline in adolescent depression. A pilot study. *J Am Acad Child Adolesc Psychiatry* 1981;20:636–644.

54. Kutcher SP, Williamson P, Silverberg J, Marton P, Malkins D, Malkin A. Nocturnal growth hormone secretion in depressed older adolescents. *J Am Acad Child Adolesc Psychiatry* 1988;27:6:751–754.

55. Kutcher S, Malkin D, Silverberg J, et al. Nocturnal cortisol, thyroid stimulating hormone, and growth hormone secretory profiles in depressed adolescents. *J Am Acad Child Adolesc Psychiatry* 1991;30(3):407–414.

56. Kutcher S, Williamson P, Szalai J, Marton P. REM latency in endogenously depressed adolescents. *Br J Psychiatry* 1992;161:399–402.

57. Lahmeyer HW, Poznanski EO, Bellur SN. EEG sleep in depressed adolescents. *Am J Psychiatry* 1983;140:1150–1153.

58. Lesch KP, Laux G, Erb A, Pfuller H, Beckmann H. Growth hormone (GH) responses to GH-releasing hormone in depression: correlation with GH release following clonidine. *Psychiatry Res* 1988;25:301–310.

59. Maes M, Vandewoude M, Schotte C, Maes L, Martin M, Blockx P. Sex-linked differences in cortisol, ACTH and prolactin responses to 5-hydroxy-tryptophan in healthy controls and minor and major depressed patients. *Acta Psychiatr Scand* 1989;80:584–590.

60. Matussek N, Ackenheil M, Hippius F, et al. Effect of clonidine on growth hormone release in psychiatric patients and controls. *Psychiatry Res* 1980;2:25–36.

61. Mendlewicz J, Linkowski P, Kerkhofs, et al. Diurnal hypersecretion of growth hormone in depression. *J Clin Endocrinol Metab* 1985;60:505–512.

62. Merimee TJ, Fineberg SE. Studies of the sex based variation of human growth hormone secretion. *J Clin Endocrinol* 1971;33:896–902.

63. Meyer WJ, Richards GE, Cavallo A, et al. Depression and growth hormone. *J Am Acad Child Adolesc Psychiatry* 1991;30:2:335.

64. Neuhauser H, Laakmann G. Stimulation of growth hormone by GHRH as compared to DMI in depressed patients. *Pharmacopsychiatry* 1988;21:443–444.

65. Orvaschel H. Early onset psychiatric disorder in high risk children and increased familial morbidity. *J Am Acad Child Adolesc Psychiatry* 1990;29:2:184–188.

66. Orvaschel H, Walsh-Allis G, Ye W. Psychopathology in children of parents with recurrent depression. *J Abnorm Child Psychol* 1988;16:17–28.

67. Pfeffer CR. *The Suicidal Child*. New York: Guilford Press, 1986.

68. Pfeffer CR, Stokes P, Shindledecker R. Suicidal behavior and hypothalamic–pituitary–adrenocortical axis indices in child psychiatric patients. *Biol Psychiatry* 1991;29:909–917.

69. Puig-Antich J, Goetz R, Hanlon C, et al. Sleep architecture and REM sleep measures in prepubertal children with major depression: a controlled study. *Arch Gen Psychiatry* 1982;39:932–939.

70. Puig-Antich J, Goetz R, Hanlon C, Tabrizi MA, Davies MA, Weitzman ED. Sleep architecture and REM sleep measures in prepubertal major depressives. Studies during recovery from the depressive episode in a drug-free state. *Arch Gen Psychiatry* 1983;40:187–192.

71. Puig-Antich J, Goetz R, Davies M, et al. Growth hormone secretion in prepubertal children with major depression. II. Sleep-related plasma concentrations during a depressive episode. *Arch Gen Psychiatry* 1984;41:463–466.

72. Puig-Antich J, Goetz D, Davies M, et al. Growth hormone secretion in prepubertal children with major depression. IV. Sleep-related plasma concentrations in a drug-free, fully recovered clinical state. *Arch Gen Psychiatry* 1984;41:479–483.

73. Puig-Antich J, Novacenko MS, Davies M, et al. Growth hormone secretion in prepubertal children with major depression. I. Final report on response to insulin-induced hypoglycemia during a depressive episode. *Arch Gen Psychiatry* 1984;41:455–460.

74. Puig-Antich J, Novacenko MS, Davies M, et al. Growth hormone secretion in prepubertal children with major depression. III. Response to insulin-induced hypoglycemia after recovery from a depressive episode and in a drug-free state. *Arch Gen Psychiatry* 1984;41:471–475.

75. Puig-Antich J, Lukens E, Davies M, Goetz D, Brennan-Quattrock J, Todak G. Psychosocial functioning in prepubertal major depressive disorders. I. Interpersonal relationships during the depressive episode. *Arch Gen Psychiatry* 1985;42:500–507.

76. Puig-Antich J, Lukens E, Davies M, Goetz D, Brennan-Quattrock J, Todak G. Psychosocial functioning in prepubertal major depressive disorders. II. Interpersonal relationships after sustained recovery from affective episode. *Arch Gen Psychiatry* 1985;42:511–517.

77. Puig-Antich J, Perel JM, Lupatkin W, et al. Imipramine in pubertal major depressive disorders. *Arch Gen Psychiatry* 1987;44:81–89.

78. Puig-Antich J, Dahl R, Ryan N. Cortisol secretion in prepubertal children with major depressive disorders. *Arch Gen Psychiatry* 1989;46:801–809.

79. Puig-Antich J, Goetz D, Davies M, et al. A controlled family history study of prepubertal major depressive disorder. *Arch Gen Psychiatry* 1989;46:406–418.

80. Puig-Antich J, Kaufmann J, Ryan ND, et al. The psychosocial functioning and family environment of depressed adolescents. *J Am Acad Child Adolesc Psychiatry* 1993;32(2):244–253.

81. Rao U, Weissman MM, Martin JA, Hammond RW. Childhood depression and risk of suicide: a preliminary report of a longitudinal study. *J Am Acad Child Adolesc Psychiatry* 1993;32:1:21–27.

82. Robbins DR, Alessi NE. Suicide and the dexamethasone suppression test in adolescence. *Biol Psychiatry* 1985;20:107–110.

83. Robbins DR, Alessi NE, Gordon W, Yanchyshyn MD, Colfer MV. The dexamethasone suppression test in psychiatrically hospitalized adolescents. *J Am Acad Child Adolesc Psychiatry* 1983;22:5:467–469.

84. Ryan N, Dahl R. The biology of depression in children and adolescents: In: Mann JJ, Kupfer J, eds. *Biology of depressive disorders, part b: Subtypes of depression and comorbid disorders.* New York: Plenum Press, 1993;37–58.

85. Ryan ND, Puig-Antich J, Cooper T, et al. Imipramine in adolescent major depression: plasma level and clinical response. *Acta Psychiatr Scand* 1986;73:275–288.

86. Ryan ND, Puig-Antich J, Ambrosini P, et al. The clinical picture of major depression in children and adolescents. *Arch Gen Psychiatry* 1987;44:854–861.

87. Ryan ND, Puig-Antich J, Rabinovich H, et al. Growth hormone response to desmethylimipramine in depressed and suicidal adolescents. *J Affective Disord* 1988;15:323–337.

88. Ryan ND, Birmaher B, Perel J, et al. Neuroendocrine response to L-5-hydroxytryptophan challenge in prepubertal major depression. *Arch Gen Psychiatry* 1992;49:843–851.

89. Ryan ND, Williamson DE, Iyengar S, et al. A secular increase in child and adolescent onset affective disorder. *J Am Acad Child Adolesc Psychiatry* 1992;31:4:600–605.

90. Shaffer D, Garland A, Gould M, Fisher P, Trautman P. Preventing teenage suicide: a critical review. *J Am Acad Child Adolesc Psychiatry* 1988;27(6):675–687.

91. Shafii M, Steltz-Lenarsky J, Derrick AM, Beckner C, Whittinghill JR. Comorbidity of mental disorders in the post-mortem diagnosis of completed suicide in children and adolescents. *J Affective Disord* 1988;15:227–233.

92. Siever LJ, Treatman RL, Coccaro EF, et al. The growth hormone response to clonidine in acute and remitted depressed male patients. *Neuropsychopharmacology* 1992;6:165–177.

93. Simeon JG, Dinicola F, Ferguson HB, Copping W. Adolescent depression: a placebo controlled fluoxetine treatment study and follow-up. *Prog Neuropsychopharmacol Biol Psychiatry* 1990;14:791–795.

94. Smals AEM, Pieters GFFM, Smals AGH, Benraad TJ, Van Laarhoven J, Kloppenborg PWC. Sex difference in human growth hormone (GH) response to intravenous human pancreatic GH-releasing hormone administration in young adults. *J Clin Endocrinol Metab* 1986;62:336–341.

95. Strober M, Carlson G. Bipolar illness in adolescents with major depression. Clinical, genetic, and psychopharmacologic predictors in a three- to four-year prospective follow-up investigation. *Arch Gen Psychiatry* 1982;39:549–555.

96. Strober M, Morrell W, Burroughs J, Lampert C, Danforth H, Freeman R. A family study of bipolar I disorder in adolescents. Early onset of symptoms linked to increased familial loading and lithium resistance. *J Affective Disord* 1988;15:255–268.

97. Thase ME, Kupfer DJ. Characteristics of treatment resistant depression. In: Zohar J, Belmaker RH, eds. *Treating resistant depression.* New York: PMA Publishing, 1987;23–45.

98. Warner V, Weissman MM, Fendrich M, Wickramaratne P, Moreau D. The course of major depression in the offspring of depressed parents. Incidence, recurrence, and recovery. *Arch Gen Psychiatry* 1992;49:795–801.

99. Weissman MM, Fendrich M, Warner V, Wickramaratne P. Incidence of psychiatric disorder in offspring at high and low risk for depression. *J Am Acad Child Adolesc Psychiatry* 1992;31:4:640–648.

100. Weller RA, Weller EB, Fristad MA, Bowes JM. Depression in recently bereaved prepubertal children. *Am J Psychiatry* 1991;148:1536–1540.

*Psychopharmacology: The Fourth
Generation of Progress,* edited by
Floyd E. Bloom and David J. Kupfer.
Raven Press, Ltd., New York 1995.

CHAPTER 141

The Interface of Genetics, Neuroimaging, and Neurochemistry in Attention-Deficit Hyperactivity Disorder

Monique Ernst and Alan Zametkin

The application of new technological breakthroughs in basic sciences on problems of children and adolescents presents great challenges to neuroscientists. Despite increasing concerns of using children in research, new advances in family genetics and brain imaging have been applied to children and adolescents diagnosed with attention-deficit hyperactivity disorder (ADHD). The need for enrolling young subjects in neuroscience research is not restricted to the study of childhood disorders. The importance of understanding the developmental origins of such disorders as schizophrenia or bipolar disorder is becoming clearer to researchers studying adult disorders.

This chapter will review progress made in the investigation of ADHD over the past 5 years in three areas: genetics, neuroimaging, and neurochemistry. Our main emphasis is placed in the areas of genetics and neuroimaging because most progress has been done in these fields, in contrast to the lack of new findings in the neurochemistry of ADHD. Advances in genetics and brain imaging may have great impact on research in pharmacology, because they provide means to identify more homogeneous samples for drug trials and enable us to explore more directly drug effects on brain activity and neurotransmitter sys-tems.

Although it is a large topic to be covered in a short chapter, it is our hope that the interface of these three scientific fields would highlight the direction of research not only in child and adolescent psychiatry, but also in adult psychiatry.

The term ADHD will refer to the disorder of attention-deficit hyperactivity disorder as defined by DSM-III (2) or DSM-III-R (3). It is important to keep in mind that these definitions may identify overlapping, and possibly different, syndromes. DSM-III-R is more inclusive because it allows subjects with only two domains of dysfunction to fulfill ADHD criteria in contrast to the impairment in three domains (impulsivity, inattention, and hyperactivity) required in the DSM-III definition (53). For the most part, we will restrict our review to Attention-Deficit Disorder with Hyperactivity, as there is some evidence that Attention-Deficit Disorder without Hyperactivity might be a different disorder (9,36,37). (See Chapters 2, 69, 76, 77, and 119, *this volume,* for related issues.)

GENETICS OF ADHD

There is compelling evidence for the presence of a genetic component to the etiology of ADHD. Familial aggregation of the disorder has been observed for a long time (for review see ref. 11). Recently, family studies attempted to tease out the contribution of familial versus environmental factors to the development of ADHD (for review see ref. 23).

Genetic Models

Several models of genetic transmission have been proposed: single gene, polygenetic, or multifactorial models (13).

M. Ernst and A. Zametkin: Section on Clinical Brain Imaging, Laboratory of Cerebral Metabolism, National Institute of Mental Health, National Institutes of Health, Bethesda, Maryland 20892.

Deutsch et al. (14) performed a genetic latent structure analysis of dysmorphology in attention deficit disorder (ADD), and they found their data to fit an autosomal mode of transmission.

In keeping with this finding, results from a family genetic study of 140 ADHD child probands and their 454 first-degree relatives, compared to 120 normal child probands and their 368 first-degree relatives, were consistent with a model of highly penetrant autosomal dominant gene transmission (23,24). In this study (24), female members of the family (mothers and sisters of male probands) seemed to be linked to an increased familial risk for the disorder. If a parent had ADHD, the risk was 6.6 times greater for sisters and 1.5 times greater for brothers. Also the risk to brothers was 4 times greater than the risk to sisters when no parents were ill. These authors rejected the hypothesis of a more severe genetic disorder in girls, a hypothesis based on the multiple threshold model of familial transmission. This model posits that the expression of the disorder requires more pathogenic genes in girls than in boys. Instead, the authors hypothesized that a proportion of male cases were caused by environmental rather than genetic factors.

In summary, the family studies mentioned above all found positive familial aggregation of ADHD. Although very suggestive of the genetic transmission of the disorder, familial aggregation can also reflect social learning, or other environmental factors transmitted from parent to child.

Adoption Studies

The determination of the relative influence of environmental and genetic factors in the transmission of a disorder is best carried out in adoption studies, where, in a simplistic way, differences are assumed to originate from the environment and similarities from shared genes.

Morrison and Stewart (51) conducted home interviews of the legal parents of 35 adopted hyperactive children who were compared to data previously reported in the groups of biologic parents of 59 hyperactive children and of 41 normal children. The percentage of parents who were retrospectively hyperactive as children were 7.5% in the biologic parents ($N = 97$), 2.1% in the adopting parents ($N = 89$), and 0.8% in the control parents ($N = 41$). The authors cautioned against an overinterpretation of the data because the information was not collected blindly, and the sample of the adopted children was not selected similarly to both other samples.

Deutsch and Swanson (15) compared ADHD symptomatology in first-degree relatives of three groups of probands ($N = 24$ in each group), ADHD non-adoptees, ADHD adoptees, and non-adopted controls. ADHD was found with higher frequency in the biological relatives of non-adopted ADHD probands than in the adoptive relatives of adopted ADHD probands. This finding suggests greater incidence of ADHD in biological than in adoptive parents of ADHD. However, a stronger case could be made if the comparison were between biological and adoptive parents of the same ADHD adoptees.

Twin Studies

Studies of twins represent a third strategy besides family studies and adoptees studies for assessing the role of genetic factors.

Willerman (68) examined activity level in 54 pairs of monozygotic twins (28 males, 26 females) and 39 same-sexed dizygotic pairs (28 males, 11 females) by means of activity and zygosity questionnaires sent to mothers. Zygosity was determined on the basis of the twin zygosity questionnaire, which is less than optimal for assigning twin pairs to either mono- or dizygotic groups. In the pairs with "certain" type of zygosity, correlation between raw scores of activity level were .90 for the monozygotic pairs ($N = 38$) and .52 for the dizygotic pairs ($N = 30$). In pairs where at least one twin was rated "hyperactive" (scores in the upper 20% of the activity scale), the twin–twin intraclass correlation was .71 for the monozygotic pairs ($N = 8$) and 0 for the dizygotic pairs ($N = 16$).

Goodman and Stevenson (28) conducted home interviews in the families of monozygotic and same-sex dizygotic twin pairs. The intraclass correlation for distractibility was .60 for the monozygotic pairs ($N = 186$) and .44 for the dizygotic pairs ($N = 214$). For hyperactivity rated by the teachers, it was 0.62 for the monozygotic pairs ($N = 192$) and 0.26 for the dizygotic pairs ($N = 190$). The scores obtained from mothers were thought to be subjected to significant expectancy effects and were difficult to interpret. On the whole, using a broad definition of hyperactivity, 51% (20/39) of the identical twin and 33% (18/54) of the same-sexed dizygotic twin of the hyperactive probands were also hyperactive.

The higher concordance rate for ADHD in monozygotic than in dizygotic twins is a strong argument for a significant genetic component to ADHD, but does not exclude environmental influences. Unfortunately, data on non-twin siblings in these studies were not collected, and concordance rates for ADHD in monozygotic, dizygotic, and non-twin siblings could not be compared. Increased concordance rates for ADHD in twins compared to non-twin siblings would suggest a role for in utero and perinatal biological environmental factors in the transmission of ADHD. The higher risk for ADHD in the siblings ($N = 117$) of ADHD probands ($N = 73$) than in the siblings ($N = 39$) of normal probands ($N = 26$) (20.8% versus 5.6%) has already been reported (10).

Environmental Factors

In general, environmental factors have not been systematically addressed, although a wide variety of factors have been implicated, such as lead toxicity, early institutional care, psychosocial stress, pregnancy and delivery complications, and prenatal alcohol exposure.

Furthermore, studies of monozygotic twins, with careful assessment of environmental variables, are needed to clarify the nonshared environmental familial factors (59). Any differences between identical twins, who have identical genotype and live in the same household, are assumed to originate from environmental factors (psychosocial and biological), such as parental attitude, classrooms, peer relationships, or medical problems different for each twin.

Biederman's group, in their family studies of ADHD, recorded socioeconomic status and family integrity. They found the families with an ADHD parent to be less cohesive and to have more conflicts (Moos Family Environment Scale) than the families without an ADHD parent (24,26). Parents of ADHD children were more likely to be separated than parents of children with other psychiatric problems or than parents of normal children (10,25). There was no effect of socioeconomic status on pattern of familial transmission.

The recognition of protective factors adds to the complexity of the model of transmission of the disorder. Genetic characteristics can protect from pathogenic environment, and environment can protect individuals from pathogenic genes. Studies tend to focus on identifying adverse factors, and very little is known about protective factors.

Thyroid Receptor-β Gene on Chromosome 3 Linked to ADHD

At present, to our knowledge, there is no information regarding the molecular genetics of ADHD. However, the very interesting finding of an association between ADHD and a specific well-defined autosomal dominant genetic abnormality responsible for a "generalized resistance to thyroid hormone" may provide a model for the study of the biological underpinnings of ADHD (29). "Generalized resistance to thyroid hormone" has been linked to the human thyroid receptor-β gene on chromosome 3 (57) and is characterized by elevated serum thyroxine and triiodothyronine concentrations and decreased responsiveness of the pituitary gland and peripheral tissues to thyroid hormone. This study assessed ADHD in 18 families with a history of "generalized resistance to thyroid hormone," including 49 affected with the thyroid genetic disorder (27 children and 22 adults) and 55 unaffected (23 children and 30 adults). The prevalence rate for ADHD was significantly higher in the affected individuals than in the nonaffected ones (in adults: 50% versus 7%; in children: 70% versus 20%). The gender distribution of ADHD among this population (male/female: 3.2/1 in affected group and 2.7/1 in the unaffected group) was consistent with the distribution of ADHD in the general population reported in the literature (4,12). Comorbidity with other psychiatric disorders also matched the findings in the literature of families of ADHD children. More studies are warranted to separate the possible primary effect of the gene mutation from the secondary effects of the hormonal dysfunction.

In conclusion, we learned from familial studies that both familial and environmental factors contribute to the development of ADHD. We also learned that there is at least one disorder with a well-defined genetic defect, associated with ADHD at an unusually high rate, which can be used to further the understanding of ADHD. Knowledge of the genetic and environmental influences are important not only to clarify etiologies, psychopathogenesis, psychopathology, treatment, and prognosis, but also to validate the syndrome as a separate psychopathological entity. In this regard, brain imaging has a special place. Promising findings have already been reported showing brain metabolism deviance in ADHD subjects (41–43,70).

BRAIN IMAGING

Deficits in attention and abnormal motor activity have been linked to specific brain regions, which constitute the basis for the hypotheses guiding brain imaging studies in ADHD. The symptoms of ADHD have often been compared to those of frontal lesions in humans and animals (7,30,47). Barkley et al. (5) reviewed 22 neuropsychological studies of frontal lobe functions in children with ADD. Tests of response inhibition more reliably distinguished ADHD from normals than did the other tests of frontal lobe function. To date, the regions implicated in attention, motor activation, and arousal include the dorsolateral and medial frontal lobes (including the cingulate gyrus), parietal lobe, striatum, and regions of the reticular formation, including thalamus and mesencephalon (for review, see refs. 30 and 50). It has been noticed that lesions in the right cerebral hemisphere were associated with more attentional problems than were lesions on the left side (30,65). Because brain imaging is a relatively new technology, only relatively few studies of ADHD are available at present.

Brain imaging provides two sets of information, structural and functional, depending on the techniques. Computerized tomography (CT) and magnetic resonance imaging (MRI) are used to assess structures; single photon emission computerized tomography (SPECT) and Positron emission tomography (PET) are used for functional analyses. A new method, functional MRI, may provide simultaneously structural and functional information of cerebral blood flow. Data of brain imaging in ADHD are from structural CT and MRI studies and from functional SPECT and PET studies. Radiation exposure is critical, especially in studies of minors, and explains the absence of PET studies in individuals younger than 12–13 years of age to this date.

Structural Studies

Computerized Tomography

The few CT studies of ADHD (8,52,63) are difficult to compare with each other, because of the use of different diagnostic definitions, different designs (open or blind, with or without a control group), and different methods of analysis (qualitative or quantitative).

Bergström and Bille (8) studied 46 children with minimal brain dysfunction characterized by the presence of "incoordination" and "impairment in sensory–motor integration." Fifteen of these 46 children (32.6%) presented gross CT abnormalities, including cerebral atrophy, ventricular asymmetry, or ventriculomegaly. The detailed description of the clinical presentation of three of these children resembled that of cerebral palsy more than that of ADHD. Also, the analysis was qualitative and the design did not involve controls.

Using quantitative measurement, a control group, and blind analysis, Shaywitz et al. (63) studied 35 children and adolescents ADHD by DSM-III (29 boys and 6 girls; 4–18 years of age, mean 11.0 ± 4.2) and 27 controls (20 boys and 7 girls; 4–19 years of age, mean 11.0 ± 3.5). These control subjects had a normal IQ and had no history of seizures or of ADHD. The authors did not specify the clinical indications for the CT scan in this control group. There was no mention of comorbid psychiatric disorders in the ADHD group. The results showed no significant differences between groups in any of the measurements, which included biventricular width, widths of the left and right anterior horns of the lateral ventricles, width of the brain plus ventricle, widths of the right and left hemispheres, and two derived measures, the cerebroventricular index (Evans index: add: 0.237 ± 0.015, contrasts 0.263 ± 0.016) and the asymmetry index. There was no correlation between brain measurements and IQ, nor was there a correlation between brain measurements and handedness. The authors did not give data on age effect.

Nasrallah et al. (52) studied 24 hyperactive male adults, including 22 with a documented history of childhood ADHD treated with stimulant (mean age 23.2 ± 1.9 years) and 27 control males (mean age 28.7 ± 8.3 years). The hyperactive group was part of a cohort of boys who were diagnosed at the age of 8.7 ± 1.9 years with hyperkinesis/minimal brain dysfunction and who presented primary symptoms of hyperactivity, fidgetiness, inattention, and incoordination. No information was given regarding these symptoms at the time of the CT scan. Seven of the hyperactive group had a history of alcohol abuse. The control group consisted of consecutive victims of vehicle accidents whose neurological exam and CT scan, part of the

medical work-up, were normal. Measurements included lateral ventricular size expressed as the ventricle-to-brain ratio, third ventricular size, sulcal widening visually rated by a neuroradiologist on a 4-point rating scale, and cerebellar atrophy. The hyperactive group showed increased sulcal widening and cerebellar atrophy relative to controls. Although never severe, these abnormalities suggested mild cerebral atrophy. Unfortunately, the inclusion of individuals with a history of alcohol abuse, representing 30% of the sample, confused the interpretation of the results, because the finding mirrored those reported in CT studies of alcoholic adults (19).

In conclusion, one of the three studies was negative. Of the two studies with positive findings of either gross abnormalities or mild cerebral atrophy, one used children with neurological deficits whereas the other used adults with a history of ADHD, comorbid for 30% of the sample with alcohol abuse, and no assessment of the current clinical presentation. There were no abnormalities of left/right ratios, or of the frontal cortex.

Magnetic Resonance Imaging

Most of the MRI studies in ADHD were conducted by Hynd's group in Georgia (31–33,62).

In their first report, Hynd et al. (32) compared three groups, including 10 children with ADHD by DSM-III and DSM-III-R (8 males; age 120.6 ± 40.4 months), 10 children with reading developmental disorder (8 males; age 118.90 ± 24.55 months), and 10 normal controls (8 males; age 141.20 ± 24.07 months). All children had a normal IQ. Comorbidity was present in seven children with ADHD (five conduct disorder/oppositional defiant disorder and two anxiety disorder). The ADHD group had bilaterally smaller anterior cortices, especially on the right, relative to normals. There was a loss of the normal asymmetry of the frontal lobes (L < R) in ADHD children. All other measures were similar to the normal group.

This finding prompted the authors to study the corpus callosum. This structure is composed of connective interhemispheric fibers (34,55), which may reflect the degree of function and lateralization of homologous cerebral hemispheric regions. The anterior region of the corpus callosum contains fibers connecting the premotor, orbitofrontal, and prefrontal cortex (55,56), whereas the posterior part of the corpus callosum is composed of fibers connecting the peri-striate, pro-peri-striate, and juxta-striate regions (1,55). The hypothesis posited that the anterior part of the corpus callosum would be smaller in ADHD individuals than in normal subjects, because this region connects the frontal lobes. In their first study, the authors found that both the anterior (genu) and posterior (splenium) regions of the corpus callosum were significantly smaller in ADHD children ($N = 7$; 5 males; age 109.0 ± 61.07 months) than in normal children ($N = 10$;

8 males; age 141.50 ± 24.36 months) (33). The significant reduction in size of the splenium, but not of the anterior part of the corpus callosum, was replicated in a subsequent study which used a "pure" ADHD group, in contrast to the previous studies whose ADHD sample had comorbid diagnoses (mainly disruptive disorders). There was a trend for the children who did not respond to stimulant medication ($N = 5$) to have smaller corpus callosum than children who responded to medication ($N = 10$).

In a brief report, Hynd et al. (31) showed that the head of the caudate nucleus on the left side was significantly smaller in ADHD subjects ($N = 11$; 8 males) than in normals ($N = 11$; 6 males).

In summary, the right frontal cortex, the corpus callosum (splenium more consistently), and the left head of the caudate nucleus were found reduced in size in ADHD subjects relative to normals. The functional significance and the clinical relevance of these abnormalities remain to be determined.

Functional Imaging

Cerebral Blood Flow

Lou et al. (41–43) presented three studies of cerebral blood flow in ADHD children using xenon-133 inhalation and SPECT in children at rest, with open eyes. This technique gives a quantitative measure of cerebral blood flow in three dimensions, reflecting the metabolic and functional activity of the brain. Resolution of the images in these studies was 17 mm, and the brain slice examined was located 50 mm above the orbitomeatal line.

The first study (41) used a heterogeneous sample of 11 clinically diagnosed ADD children (1 female, 6.5–15 years of age) with various degrees of neonatal/congenital insults (4 of 11), dysphasia (6 of 11), mild mental retardation (2 of 11), and other neuropsychological deficits (7 of 11). Six of these children were also being treated with methylphenidate. The ADD group was compared to 9 normal children (3 females; 7–15 years of age) who were all siblings of the children of the study group.

The results showed hypoperfusion of the frontal lobes in all 11 ADD children, and of the region of the caudate nuclei in 7 of the 11 ADD subjects. In contrast, the occipital lobes were relatively hyperperfused. Six ADD children were scanned before and 30 min after oral administration of their treatment dose of methylphenidate (10–30 mg). They all showed increased perfusion in the frontal and caudate regions after treatment. Absolute or relative values of regional blood flow are not reported by the authors. Also, the findings are difficult to interpret in the face of the heterogeneity of the patient group, the lack of criteria for the diagnosis of ADD, the lack of information regarding comorbid psychiatric disorders, and the fact that the control group was not independent from the study group

because they had genetic and environmental factors in common.

In their second study (43), Lou et al. expanded the patient group from 11 to 19 and divided it into pure ADHD ($N = 6$; 1 female) and ADHD with other neurologic or neuropsychiatric symptoms ($N = 13$; 1 female). The control group was the same as that in the previous study ($N = 9$; 7–15 years old; siblings of patients). Five of the six "pure" ADHD patients had a history of neonatal problems. The findings were consistent with those of the first study: (a) hypoperfusion of the right striatal region (10.6% decrease) and (b) hyperperfusion of the occipital lobe (13.7% increase) and the left sensorimotor and primary auditory region (9.6% increase). Thirty to 60 minutes after methylphenidate administration (10–30 mg) in four "pure" and nine neurologically impaired ADHD children, cerebral blood flow increased significantly: 7% in the left striatal region and in the left and right posterior periventricular regions.

In their third study, Lou et al. (42) used a new control group of 15 normal children (7 females; median age 11 years, range 6–17 years), which included 4 children siblings of patients in the study group. They expanded again the patient group to include children with dysphasia. The extent of overlap of patients between this study and the two preceding ones is unclear. Nine "pure" ADHD children (7 boys and 2 girls) were isolated from the patient group. The findings for this "pure" ADHD group, compared to the control group, were again (a) a decrease in blood flow in the striatal regions without mention of laterality (10.7%) and in the posterior periventricular region (6.8%) and (b) an increase in blood flow in occipital regions.

The consistency of the results within these three studies is not unexpected because there seems to be a significant overlap among samples, which, unfortunately, include patients with history of perinatal brain insults. No standardized instruments were used to make the diagnosis of ADHD. However, the results are in keeping with the theoretical framework of the pathogenesis of ADHD which implicates abnormalities in the frontal cortex and striatum, more so on the right side than on the left side.

Glucose Metabolic Rates

Study in Adults

Zametkin et al. (70) published a study showing, for the first time, definite and quantifiable central neurophysiological differences between ADHD adults and normal adults, using PET and [^{18}F]fluorodeoxyglucose. They studied a very carefully screened sample of 25 adults (18 men, 7 women; 37.4 ± 6.9 years old), who currently met Utah criteria for ADHD, who had a childhood history of ADHD, and who were parents of children diagnosed with

ADHD. This group of 25 patients was compared to 50 normal adults (28 men, 22 females; 36.3 ± 11.7 years old). None of the ADHD adults had ever been treated with stimulants. All studies were done under similar conditions, and the subjects performed an auditory continuous performance task with their eyes patched.

Global glucose metabolism (mean of glucose metabolic rates for all the gray matter-rich areas examined in this study) was 8.1% lower in adults with ADHD than in normals ($p = 0.03$). Half of the brain regions studied (30/60) had significantly reduced glucose metabolic rates in ADHD compared to normal subjects, including four subcortical regions, the right thalamus, right caudate, right hippocampus, and cingulate. The cortical regions were localized bilaterally and predominated in the upper brain. When normalized (divided by global metabolism values), the regional metabolic rates of four regions, in the left premotor and left somatosensory areas, were also significantly decreased. Interestingly, the reduction in brain metabolism was greater in women than in men, but not statistically so.

The decrease in frontal and striatal brain metabolism is consistent with Lou et al.'s finding (42). However, the decreased metabolic rates found in the somatosensory and occipital areas are in contrast to the increased blood flow in these regions reported by Lou et al. (42). It is important to keep in mind, in comparing Lou's and Zametkin's studies, the differences in sample characteristics (children versus adults) and in analysis of the results (single-plane versus five-plane analysis, 17-mm versus 6-mm image resolution, and normalized data versus absolute and normalized values) (see Chapter 58, *this volume*, for background).

Study in Adolescents

Because of the promising results in adults, Zametkin et al. (69) initiated a PET study in adolescents. The authors modified the PET procedure to significantly reduce the amount of radiation exposure to a fifth of the adult exposure. The study of younger subjects, especially in investigations of childhood disorders, is critical. For instance, the interpretation of data collected in adults suffering from a childhood disorder is difficult, because the primary effects of the disorder cannot be sorted out from its secondary effects or long-lasting environmental influences.

Twenty adolescents (14.7 ± 1.7 years old, 5 girls), fulfilling ADHD DSM-III-R criteria, were compared to 19 normal adolescents (14.4 ± 1.4 years old, 6 girls) (29,30). The data originating from the first half of the ADHD and normal samples were analyzed in a preliminary study (69). In the final study (20,21), no significant differences were found in global and absolute glucose metabolic rates between ADHD and normal adolescents. However, similarly to the findings in the adult study,

female adolescents showed greater brain metabolism deviance than did male adolescents. In contrast to boys, ADHD girls ($N = 5$) showed a significant 15% global brain metabolism reduction when compared to normal girls ($N = 6$). Several reasons could have accounted for the overall lack of brain metabolism differences between ADHD and normal teenagers. First, the adolescent control group was not as pure as the control group used in the adult study, because 63% of the normal adolescents had a first-degree relative with ADHD (12/19), in contrast to the absence of ADHD pathology in families of normal adults. Second, 75% adolescents with ADHD had been previously exposed to treatment with stimulants, compared to no history of stimulant treatment in the ADHD adults. Third, an age effect in the development of brain abnormalities in ADHD individuals cannot be ruled out. The results of this study clearly emphasizes the need for studies in females and in children with ADHD.

Effects of Stimulants on Brain Imaging

Besides examining a younger population with ADHD, another question raised by the positive results obtained in ADHD adults (70) was to find out how the reduction in brain metabolism observed in adults with ADHD could be affected by the treatment of choice of this disorder—that is, stimulants (16). The authors expected to observe increased brain glucose metabolism after the administration of a stimulant, especially in the striatal and frontal regions. Matochik et al. (44–46) conducted two studies of acute and chronic stimulant treatment in ADHD adults using PET and [^{18}F]flurorodeoxyglucose.

In the acute study (45), 27 adult outpatients with ADHD were scanned twice: (i) off medication and (ii) after receiving orally a single dose of either dextroamphetamine (0.25 mg/kg) ($N = 13$) or methylphenidate hydrochloride (0.35 mg/kg) ($N = 14$). On-drug and off-drug studies were 1–4 months apart, in counterbalanced order. The PET procedure was identical to the one used in the previous adult study (70), where subjects were studied during an auditory continuous performance task with their eyes patched. The acute administration of an oral dose of stimulant (dextroamphetamine or methylphenidate) had no effect on global glucose metabolic rates. With the data normalized (regional/global), the regional metabolic rates of 7 of 60 regions significantly changed after dextroamphetamine administration. These regions predominated on the right side (5 right, 2 left), and included 4 regions with increased metabolism and 3 with decreased metabolism. Of interest is the increased metabolism in the right caudate nucleus. After methylphenidate, the normalized regional metabolism of 5 regions, all on the left side, were significantly changed: 2 increased and 3 decreased.

The results of the study of the effects of chronic administration of stimulants on brain metabolism (44,46) also showed minimal changes. In this study, a total of 37 adults with ADHD were studied twice, off drug and then on drug, at the end of 6–15 weeks of dextroamphetamine ($N = 18$; mean dose 19 ± 7 mg/day) or methylphenidate ($N = 19$; 28 ± 10 mg/day) treatment. Subjects were randomized to either stimulants, and dosage was individually titrated to optimal therapeutic efficacy. Global and absolute regional brain metabolic rates were unchanged after the administration of stimulants. Normalized metabolic rates were modified in only 2 of the 60 regions studied, and only after methylphenidate treatment (decreased metabolism in the right anterior putamen and increased metabolism in the right posterior orbital frontal region). The lack of effect of the stimulants on brain metabolism was in contrast to the 68% clinical response rate for both drugs combined (positive clinical response defined as an 8-point decrease on the modified self-rated Conners Scale).

Another reason to expect stimulants to increase brain metabolism stemmed from findings in animal studies (6,17,58,67), all reporting an increase in brain activity after stimulant injection.

Zametkin's group undertook a third study to more closely approximate the animal experiments (22). Glucose brain metabolism was measured before and after dextroamphetamine intravenous injection at a dose of 0.15 mg/kg in ADHD adults. Preliminary results in 8 subjects failed to detect any significant changes in global or absolute regional glucose metabolic rates. Only 3 of 60 regional normalized metabolic rates differed between conditions. These 3 regions were on the right side of the brain. Glucose metabolism was decreased in 2 regions (right temporal cortex and right hippocampus), and increased in 1 (right parietal cortex). Here again, the minimal effects on brain metabolism were in contrast to the striking changes in affective (more energetic, increased concentration) and in physiological states (significant increases in diastolic and systolic blood pressure) induced by the intravenous injection of dextroamphetamine. The discrepant results between animal and human studies are not too surprising. For instance, similar findings were reported regarding the effect of cocaine on brain metabolism, where the animal study showed increased brain metabolism (40) and the human study showed a decrease in brain metabolism (39). Many variables may account for the different results in humans and animals, including most importantly the effects of species and of experimental conditions.

The results of the last 4 PET studies described above—assessing brain metabolism in adolescents with ADHD, and after stimulant treatment in ADHD adults—have been somewhat disappointing. However, they clearly illustrate the difficulty of using and interpreting data from functional brain imaging studies. To increase the yield of such studies, it is important to consider (a) the use of behavioral activation tasks tapping the specific areas of deficits of the disorder under study and (b) the use of neurotransmitter-dependent tracers to focus on a specific neurotransmitter system. In ADHD, the activation tasks should target attention and impulsivity. Hyperactivity is now thought to be part of the domain of impulsivity, conceptualized as a motor disinhibition paradigm (DSM-IV). The neurotransmitter system most relevant to ADHD pathology at this time is the dopaminergic system.

Finally, results from the brain imaging studies, along with those of the genetic studies, emphasize the importance of studying females with ADHD, as there is some evidence for greater deviance in brain metabolism and stronger familial risk in females compared to males with ADHD.

NEUROCHEMISTRY UPDATE

In 1987 Zametkin and Rapoport (71) published a review of the neurochemistry of ADHD entitled "Neurobiology of Attention Deficit Disorder with Hyperactivity: Where Have We Come in 50 Years?" The exact cause of ADHD remains elusive, as does the mechanism of action of its treatment of choice (stimulants). Since that review, no new findings have emerged. However, much interesting theoretical writing has appeared.

Our intent in this section is to refer the reader to six most recent reviews of the neurobiochemical basis of ADHD (48,49,54,60,64,66). Each of these reviews offers a model for the understanding and means of studying ADHD. Pharmacological treatments, including stimulants (d-amphetamine, methylphenidate, and magnesium pemoline), antidepressants (tricyclic antidepressants and monoamine oxidase inhibitors), neuroleptics, and the alpha-2 adrenoceptor agonist clonidine, are also presented, and their mechanisms of action are discussed in light of the specific models proposed by the authors. We chose not to repeat the presentation of the various drugs used for the treatment of ADHD, but to highlight one or two points in each of the six reviews:

1. Rogeness et al. (60), in a review of the three neurotransmitter systems—dopaminergic, serotoninergic, and noradrenergic—make the point that no single neurotransmitter hypotheses could fully account for the findings of the large array of data and studies in ADHD. The authors underline the interaction of the norepinephrine with the dopamine systems, whereby dopamine-dependent behaviors are regulated by norepinephrine activity. They suggest that the balance between these systems may be more critical than the individual activity level for the regulation of behavior. For example, decreased activity in both systems, as opposed to the reduction in one system only, would not alter the balance and have no deleterious effect on behavior. The authors also underline the influence of neural maturation on the relative activity of these systems, reflecting the differential maturational rate among neuro-

transmitter systems. Accordingly, dopamine receptor density increases from birth to 2 years of age, and then decreases to reach adult levels by adolescence (61), whereas the index of norpinephrine activity (CSF 3-methoxy-4-hydroxyphenylglycol) remains unchanged after 8 or 9 months of age (38). Both issues of interdependence and differential maturational rates of neurotransmitter systems stress the need to assess neurotransmitter systems simultaneously and to use a sample of narrow age range to be able to interpret studies of the neurochemistry of behavior.

2. In a comprehensive review of the contribution of catecholaminergic activity to ADHD (54), Oades shows how the dysfunction in catecholaminergic systems can lead to various types of symptoms, including inattention, hyperactivity, tics, dyskinesia, and self-mutilation. This is suggested by catecholaminergic abnormalities found in various disorders, including phenylketonuria, Tourette's syndrome, and Lesch Nyhan disease. The type of dysfunction in the neurotransmitter systems, including changes in ''balance'' and time of impairment relative to the developmental stage, account for the variety of symptoms produced by the same neural systems. In addition to the role of neurotransmitters, Oades mentions the putative involvement of estrogen in the development of hyperactivity, because estrogen can act as a dopamine receptor antagonist (35). This finding is in keeping with gender-related differences in incidence of ADHD (4,12) and in brain metabolism of ADHD versus normal subjects (20).

3. Mefford and Potter (49) speculated a dominant role of adrenaline and its inhibitory effect on the locus coeruleus activity in ADHD. This hypothesis stems from the ethological model of behavior stating that ''the orienting response'' (novel stimuli supplant present activity) and ''the orienting reaction'' (motor responses to the novel stimuli) have survival value. The orienting reaction and orienting response, identified as hypervigilance and hyperactivity respectively, have been shown to be regulated through the locus coeruleus activity (27).

4. Voeller (66) reviewed the anatomical substrates of attention and motor control as they apply to ADHD. She proposes the theory of lateralized dysfunction, whereby the right hemisphere of the brain plays a dominant role in the attentional/intentional and arousal/activation systems implicated in ADHD. As more data become available through functional imaging, these hypotheses will be more carefully tested.

5. McCracken (48) submits a neurobiochemical model of ADHD which posits that for the action of a drug to be effective in the treatment of ADHD, there must be simultaneous increases in both (a) dopamine release and (b) inhibited adrenergic tone on the locus coeruleus. The contention by Elia et al. (18) that up to 98% of ADHD children respond to stimulants, when at least two types of stimulants are tried, is not consistent with the requirement for both dopaminergic and noradrenergic effects to occur to achieve therapeutic efficacy, since stimulant

actions are primarily mediated through dopamine release. This is further supported by the lack of specific effect of clonidine on ADHD symptoms as mentioned earlier.

6. Shenker (64), focusing on catecholamine receptor pharmacology, alludes to the function of autoreceptors likely to be implicated in the mechanism of action of stimulants in the treatment of ADHD. This review highlights the dramatic increase in complexity of our understanding about neuropharmacology, which renders earlier speculation about the biochemical basis of ADHD symptomatology woefully constrained.

It is likely that part of the slow progress made in the neurochemistry of ADHD stems from the difficulty in isolating homogeneous samples to study. Advances in genetics and brain imaging may help to refine the selection of uniform groups. It is clear that any significant gain in knowledge about one of the most prevalent disorder in childhood will come from the integrated findings in the three scientific fields of genetics, brain imaging, and neurochemistry (see Chapter 155, *this volume*).

REFERENCES

1. Alexander MP, Warren RL. Localization of callosal auditory pathways: a CT case study. *Neurology* 1988;38:802–804.
2. American Psychiatric Association. *Diagnostic and statistical manual of mental disorders,* 3rd ed. (DSM III). Washington, DC; American Psychiatric Association, 1980.
3. American Psychiatric Association. *Diagnostic and statistical manual of mental disorders,* 3rd ed., revised (DSM-III-R). Washington, DC: American Psychiatric Association, 1987.
4. Anderson JC, Williams S, McGee R, Silva PA. DSM-III disorders in preadolescent children: prevalence in a large sample from the general population. *Arch Gen Psychiatry* 1987;44:69–76.
5. Barkley RA, Grodzinsky G, DuPaul GJ. Frontal lobe functions in attention deficit disorder with and without hyperactivity: a review and research report. *J Abnorm Child Psychol* 1992;20:163–188.
6. Bell RD, Alexander GM, Schwartzman RJ. Methylphenidate decreases local glucose metabolism in the motor cortex. *Pharmacol Biochem Behav* 1983;18:1–5.
7. Benson DF. The role of frontal dysfunction in attention deficit hyperactivity disorder. *J Child Neurol* 1991;6:9–12.
8. Bergström K, Bille B. Computer tomography of the brain in children with minimal brain damage: a preliminary study of 46 children. *Neuropädiatrie* 1978;9:378–384.
9. Berry CA, Shaywitz SE, Shaywitz BA. Girls with attention deficit disorder: a silent minority? A report on behavioral and cognitive characteristics. *Pediatrics* 1985;76:801–809.
10. Biederman J, Faraone SV, Keenan K, Knee D, Tsuang MT. Family-genetic and psychosocial risk factors in DSM-III attention deficit disorder. *J Am Acad Child Adolesc Psychiatry* 1990;29:526–533.
11. Biederman J, Munir K, Knee D, Habelow W, Armentano M, Autor S, Hoge SK, Waternaux C. A family study of patients with attention deficit disorder and normal controls. *J Psychiatr Res* 1986;20:263–274.
12. Bird HR, Canino G, Rubio-Stipec M, Gould MS, Ribera J, Sesman M, Woodbury M, Huertas-Goldman S, Pagan A, Sanchez-Lacay A, Moscoso M. Estimates of the prevalence of childhood maladjustment in a community survey in Puerto Rico. *Arch Gen Psychiatry* 1988;45:1120–1126.
13. Cantwell DP. Genetics of hyperactivity. *J Child Psychol Psychiatry* 1975;16:261–264.
14. Deutsch CK, Matthysse S, Swanson JM, Farkas LG. Genetic latent structure analysis of dysmorphology in attention deficit disorder. *J Am Acad Child Psychiatry* 1990;29:189–194.

15. Deutsch CK, Swanson JM. An adoptive parents and siblings study of attention deficit disorder [Abstract]. *Behav Genet* 1985;15:590–591.
16. DuPaul GJ, Barkley RA. Medication therapy. In: Barkley RA, ed. *Attention-deficit hyperactivity disorder: a handbook for diagnosis and treatment.* New York: Guilford Press, 1990;573–612.
17. Eison MS, Eison AS, Ellison G. The regional distribution of *d*-amphetamine and local glucose utilization in rat brain during continuous amphetamine administration. *Exp Brain Res* 1981;43:281–288.
18. Elia J, Borcherding BG, Rapoport JL, Keysor CS. Methylphenidate and dextroamphetamine treatments of hyperactivity: Are there true nonresponders? *Psychiatry Res* 1991;36:141–155.
19. Epstein P, Pisani V, Fawcett J. Alcoholism and cerebral atrophy. *Alcohol Clin Exp Res* 1977;1:61–65.
20. Ernst M, Liebenauer LL, King AC, Fitzgerald GA, Cohen RM, Zametkin AJ. Reduced brain metabolism in hyperactive teenage girls. *J Am Acad Child Adolesc Psychiatry* [in press].
21. Ernst M, Liebenauer LL, Matochik JA, Fitzgerald GA, Zametkin AJ. Brain metabolism in adolescents with ADHD: effect of gender. Review abstract for a research paper, 40th annual meeting of the American Academy of Child and Adolescent Psychiatry, 1994.
22. Ernst M, Zametkin AJ, Matochik JA, Liebenauer LL, Fitzgerald GL. Intravenous dextroamphetamine on brain metabolism in adults with attention deficit hyperactivity disorder (ADHD). *NCDEU 33rd Annual Meeting* 1993;No. 47.
23. Faraone S, Biederman J, Chen WJ, Krifcher B, Keenan K, Moore C, Sprich S, Tsuang MT. Segregation analysis of attention deficit hyperactivity disorder. *Psychiatr Genet* 1992;2:257–275.
24. Faraone SV, Biederman J, Chen WJ, Tsuang MT. Genetic heterogeneity in attention deficit hyperactivity disorder: gender, psychiatric comorbidity and parental illness. Submitted for publication.
25. Faraone SV, Biederman J, Keenan K, Tsuang MT. A family-genetic study of girls with DSM-III attention deficit disorder. *Am J Psychiatry* 1991;148:112–117.
26. Faraone SV, Biederman J, Lehman BK, Keenan K, Norman D, Seidman LJ, Kolodny R, Kraus I, Perrin J, Chen WJ. Evidence for independent familial transmission of attention deficit hyperactivity disorder and learning disabilities: results from a family genetic study. *Am J Psychiatry* 1993;150:891–895.
27. Foote SL, Bloom FE, Aston-Jones G. Nucleus locus coeruleus: new evidence of anatomical and physiological specificity. *Physiol Rev* 1983;63:844–914.
28. Goodman R, Stevenson J. A twin study of hyperactivity. II. The aetiological role of genes, family relationships and perinatal adversity. *J Child Psychol Psychiatry* 1989;30:691–709.
29. Hauser P, Zametkin AJ, Martinez P, Vitiello B, Matochik JA, Mixson AJ, Weintraub BD. Attention-deficit hyperactivity disorder in people with generalized resistance to thyroid hormone. *N Engl J Med* 1993;328:997–1001.
30. Heilman KM, Voeller KKS, Nadeau SE. A possible pathophysiologic substrate of attention deficit hyperactivity disorder. *J Child Neurol* 1991;6:S76–S81.
31. Hynd GW, Marshall R, Gonzalez JJ. Asymmetry of the caudate nucleus in ADHD: an exploratory study of gender and handedness effects. Presented at the Annual Meeting of the Society for Research in Child and Adolescent Psychopathology, 1993.
32. Hynd GW, Semrud-Clikeman M, Lorys AR, Novey ES, Eliopulos D. Brain morphology in developmental dyslexia and attention deficit disorder/hyperactivity. *Arch Neurol* 1990;47:919–926.
33. Hynd GW, Semrud-Clikeman M, Lorys AR, Novey ES, Eliopulos D, Lyytinen H. Corpus callosum morphology in attention deficit hyperactivity disorder: morphometric analysis of MRI. *J Learning Disabilities* 1991;24:141–146.
34. Innocenti GM. The Development of interhemispheric connections. *Trends Neurol Sci* 1981;142–144.
35. Joyce JN, Montero E, Van Hartesveldt C. Dopamine-mediated behaviors: characteristics of modulation by estrogen. *Pharmacol Biochem Behav* 1984;21:791–800.
36. King C, Young R. Attentional deficits with and without hyperactivity: teacher and peer perceptions. *J Abnorm Child Psychol* 1982;10:483–496.
37. Lahey BB, Schaughency EA, Strauss CC, Frame CL. Are attention deficit disorders with and without hyperactivity similar or disimilar disorders? *J Am Acad Child Psychiatry* 1984;23:302–309.
38. Langlais PJ, Walsh FX, Bird ED, Levy HL. Cerebrospinal fluid neurotransmitter metabolites in neurologically normal infants and children. *Pediatrics* 1985;75:580–586.
39. London ED, Cascella NG, Wong DF, Phillips RL, Dannals RF, Links JM, Herning R, Grayson R, Jaffe JH, Wagner HN. Cocaine-induced reduction of glucose utilization in human brain. *Arch Gen Psychiatry* 1990;47:567–574.
40. London ED, Wilkerson G, Goldberg SR, Risner ME. Effects of 1-cocaine on local cerebral glucose utilization in the rat. *Neurosci Lett* 1986;68:73–78.
41. Lou HC, Henriksen L, Bruhn P. Focal cerebral hypoperfusion in children with dysphasia and/or attention deficit disorder. *Arch Neurol* 1984;41:825–829.
42. Lou HC, Henriksen L, Bruhn P. Focal cerebral dysfunction in developmental learning disabilities. *Lancet* 1990;335:8–11.
43. Lou HC, Henriksen L, Bruhn P, Borner H, Nielsen JB. Striatal dysfunction in attention deficit and hyperkinetic disorder. *Arch Neurol* 1989;46:48–52.
44. Matochik JA, Liebenauer LL, King AC, Szymanski HV, Cohen RM, Zametkin AJ. Cerebral glucose metabolism in adults with attention-deficit hyperactivity disorder after chronic stimulant treatment. *Am J Psychiatry* 1994;151:658–664.
45. Matochik JA, Nordahl TE, Gross M, Semple WE, King AC, Cohen RM, Zametkin AJ. Effects of acute stimulant medication on cerebral metabolism in adults with hyperactivity. *Neuropsychopharmacology* 1993;8:377–386.
46. Matochik JA, Zametkin AJ, Liebenauer LL, Cohen RM. Effects of chronic stimulant treatment on cerebral metabolism in adults with hyperactivity. *Soc Neurosci Abstr* 1992;18:726.
47. Mattes JA. The role of frontal lobe dysfunction in childhood hyperkinesis. *Compr Psychiatry* 1980;21:358–369.
48. McCracken JT. A two part model of stimulant action on attention-deficit hyperactivity disorder in children. *J Neuropsychiatry* 1991;3:201–209.
49. Mefford IN, Potter WZ. A neuroanatomical and biochemical basis for attention deficit disorder with hyperactivity in children: a defect in tonic adrenaline mediated inhibition of locus coeruleus stimulation. *Med Hypotheses* 1989;29:33–42.
50. Mesulam MM. Frontal cortex and behavior. *Ann Neurol* 1986;19:320–325.
51. Morrison JR, Stewart MA. The psychiatric status of the legal families of adopted hyperactive children. *Arch Gen Psychiatry* 1973;28:888–891.
52. Nasrallah HA, Loney J, Olsen SC, McCalley-Whitters M, Kramer J, Jacoby CG. Cortical atrophy in young adults with a history of hyperactivity in childhood. *Psychiatry Res* 1986;17:241–246.
53. Newcorn JH, Halperin JM, Healey JM, O'Brien JD, Pascualvaca DM, Wolf LE, Morganstein A, Sharma V, Young JG. Are ADDH and ADHD the same or different? *J Am Acad Child Adolesc Psychiatry* 1989;28:734–738.
54. Oades RD. Attention deficit disorder with hyperactivity (ADDH): the contribution of catecholaminergic activity. *Prog Neurobiol* 1987;29:365–391.
55. Pandya DN, Karol EA, Heilbronn D. The topographical distribution of interhemispheric projections in the corpus callosum of the rhesus monkey. *Brain Res* 1971;32:31–43.
56. Pandya DN, Seltzer B. The topography of commissural fibers. In: Lepore F, Ptito M, Jasper HH, eds. *Two hemispheres—one brain.* New York: Alan R Liss, 1986;47–73.
57. Pierre Gareau JL, Houle B, Leduc F, Bradley WEC, Dobrovic A. A frequent HindIII RFLP on chromosome 3p21-25 detected by a genomic *erbAβ* sequence. *Nucleic Acids Res* 1988;16:1223.
58. Porrino LJ, Lucignani G, Dow-Edwards D, Sokoloff L. Correlation of dose-dependent effects of acute amphetamine administration on behavior and local cerebral metabolism in rats. *Brain Res* 1984;307:311–320.
59. Reiss D, Plomin R, Hetherington EM. Genetics and psychiatry: an unheralded window on the environment. *Am J Psychiatry* 1991;148:283–291.
60. Rogeness GA, Javors MA, Pliska SR. Neurochemistry and child and adolescent psychiatry. *J Am Acad Child Adolescent Psychiatry* 1992;31,5:765–781.

61. Seeman P, Bzowej NH, Guan HC, Bergeron C, Becker LE, Reynolds GP, Bird ED, Riederer P, Jellinger K, Watanabe S, Tourtelotte W. Human brain dopamine receptors in children and aging adults. *Synapse* 1987;1:399–404.

62. Semrud-Clikeman M, Filipek PA, Biederman J, Steingard R, Kennedy D, Renshaw P, Bekken K. Attention deficit disorder: differences in the corpus callosum by MRI morphometric analysis. Presented at the Annual Meeting of the Society for Research in Child and Adolescent Psychopathology 1993.

63. Shaywitz BA, Shaywitz SE, Byrne T, Cohen DJ, Rothman S. Attention deficit disorder: quantitative analysis of CT. *Neurology* 1983;33:1500–1503.

64. Shenker A. The mechanism of action of drugs used to treat attention deficit hyperactivity disorder: focus on catecholamine receptor pharmacology. *Adv Pediatr* 1992;39:337–382.

65. Voeller KKS. Right hemisphere deficit syndrome in children. *Am J Psychiatry* 1986;143:1004–1009.

66. Voeller KKS. What can neurological models of attention, intention, and arousal tell us about attention-deficit hyperactivity disorder? *J Neuropsychiatry Clin Neurosci* 1991;3:209–216.

67. Wechsler LR, Savaki H, Sokoloff L. Effects of *d*- and *l*-amphetamine on local cerebral glucose utilization in the conscious rat. *J Neurochem* 1979;32:15–22.

68. Willerman L. Activity level and hyperactivity in twins. *Child Dev* 1973;44:288–293.

69. Zametkin AJ, Liebenauer LL, Fitzgerald GA, King AC, Minkunas DV, Herscovitch P, Yamada EM, Cohen RM. Brain metabolism in teenagers with attention deficit hyperactivity disorder. *Arch Gen Psychiatry* 1993;50:333–340.

70. Zametkin AJ, Nordahl TE, Gross M, King AC, Semple WE, Rumsey J, Hamburger S, Cohen RM. Cerebral glucose metabolism in adults with hyperactivity of childhood onset. *N Engl J Med* 1990;323:1361–1366.

71. Zametkin AJ, Rapoport JL. Neurobiology of attention deficit disorder with hyperactivity: where have we come in 50 years? *Am Acad Child Adolesc Psychiatry* 1987;26,5:676–686.

*Psychopharmacology: The Fourth
Generation of Progress,* edited by
Floyd E. Bloom and David J. Kupfer.
Raven Press, Ltd., New York © 1995.

CHAPTER 142

Autism and Pervasive Developmental Disorders

Linda J. Lotspeich

The pervasive developmental disorders (PDD), which include autism, are a heterogeneous group of neurobiological disorders characterized by severe disturbances in the following three areas: (i) social relatedness, (ii) communication, and (iii) routines and interests. PDD has intrigued professionals since the first description of autism by Leon Kanner in 1943 (35). According to the DSM III-R (3), PDD is a category including only two disorders: autistic disorder and pervasive developmental disorder—not otherwise specified (PDD-NOS). PDD may present with either many or few symptoms, and symptom intensity may range from mild to severe. Thus, individuals with PDD exhibit a spectrum of symptoms; generally speaking more severely affected individuals are given the diagnosis of autistic disorder, and the less severely affected are given the diagnosis of PDD-NOS. For example, in a severe case, a child could be mute, mentally retarded, and preoccupied with spinning objects and could actively avoid all social interactions. In a milder case, a child might have normal intelligence and speak in full sentences, but he or she might be unable to carry on a socially appropriate conversation and might be preoccupied with memorizing schedules or sports statistics.

The prevalence of autistic disorder in the general population is approximately 4–5 per 10,000, with a 4:1 predominance of males to females (63). The neurological causes of PDD remain largely unknown, but both clinical experience and research strongly suggest that PDD is a heterogeneous group of neurobiological disorders. Although the pathobiological picture is incomplete, it is clear that PDD is a comprehensive category of medical syndromes arising from diverse neurological causes.

This chapter will summarize what is known today about the neurobiology of PDD. Four major topics will be reviewed: diagnostic issues, associated neurological disorders, neurobiological research, and psychopharmacological treatment. Diagnostic issues are considered first: Which disorders should be included in the spectrum of PDD disorders, and what should be the specific diagnostic criteria? Second, the defined neurological disorders known to be associated with PDD are surveyed. Third, genetic and neurological studies of PDD are reviewed, and, finally, the increasing number of medications useful in the treatment of specific PDD symptoms is discussed. The reader should be aware that, since the diagnostic criteria for PDD-NOS are still imprecise, most of the studies discussed in this chapter have been of autistic subjects (see also Chapters 55, 59, and 60, *this volume*).

DIAGNOSIS

Historical and Current PDD Diagnostic Categories

To better understand how PDD is currently diagnosed, it is helpful to first review the history of the diagnosis of autistic disorder. Autism has long been diagnosed by its clinical presentation, and even today there are no reliable biological markers. Autism cannot be diagnosed at birth but is usually noted or suspected between the first and third years of life. Although diagnosis is based on clinical behaviors, for many years there were no agreed-upon formal criteria. During the 1970s two diagnostic paradigms were developed for diagnosing autism (52,57). However, there still remained a large group of individuals with certain autistic characteristics who did not meet the full criteria for autism. Thus, when autism was included in the International Classification of Diseases, 9th edition (68) and the Diagnostic and Statistical Manual of Mental Disorders III (2), an effort was made to include both the specific and extended definition of autism.

The ICD-9 established a category of disorders—psy-

L. J. Lotspeich: Division of Child Psychiatry and Child Development, Department of Psychiatry and Behavioral Sciences, Stanford University School of Medicine, Stanford, California 94305.

choses with origin specific to childhood—which included the following four disorders: (i) infantile autism, (ii) disintegrative psychosis, (iii) other (atypical childhood psychosis), and (iv) unspecified. In the DSM III, the term *pervasive developmental disorders* (PDD) was introduced to reflect the developmental nature and pervasive deficits of these disorders. The DSM III subdivided the PDD category into five disorders: (i) infantile autism; (ii) residual infantile autism, (iii) child-onset PDD, (iv) residual child-onset PDD, and (v) atypical autism. These groupings subdivided children according to both the age of symptom presentation and symptom severity.

Both the ICD-9 and the DSM III defined infantile autism by narrow criteria, reflecting the more severe and classical Kanner-type of autism. With the revision of the DSM III, the DSM III-R (3), the criteria for autistic disorder became less restrictive, and consequently many more children and adults were given the diagnosis of autism. In the DSM III-R, PDD has been simplified to only two disorders: (i) autistic disorder and (ii) pervasive developmental disorder—not otherwise specified (PDD-NOS). The consensus view of autistic disorder and PDD-NOS was expanded to include individuals with increasingly mild PDD symptoms. Autistic disorder, in turn, was defined by a set of 16 criteria, grouped into the three areas of impaired socialization, impaired communication, and unusual repertoire of interests. To meet the diagnosis of autistic disorder, an individual must exhibit at least 8 of these 16 criteria. Onset of symptoms before 30 months of age is no longer a diagnostic factor in the DSM III-R, as it had been in the DSM IV and ICD-9; however, the DSM III-R does stipulate that onset must occur during childhood. The broader term PDD-NOS implies qualitative impairment in reciprocal social interactions and of verbal or nonverbal communication skills. This diagnosis is applied to a person with only a few symptoms of autism, who had previously been referred to as "autistic-like" or "having autistic features."

The recognition of milder forms of PDD and the increasing realization that PDD symptoms are common features of known neurologic disorders (such as Rett's syndrome) are reflected in the recently published ICD-10 (69) (see Table 1). The ICD-10 moved closer to the DSM III-R by also establishing criteria for autistic disorder similar to those in the DSM III-R. The DSM IV, to be published in the coming year, can be expected to approximate the ICD-10 definition of autistic disorder.

Asperger's Syndrome

Many individuals have symptoms qualitatively similar to those of autistic persons, but to a milder degree; recognizing this, autism researchers have focused on a relatively new diagnosis of Asperger's syndrome (4), which is now considered by many to be part of the PDD spectrum of disorders, as reviewed by Frith (25). Persons with Asperger's syndrome typically have a normal IQ, but are socially awkward, pedantic, and preoccupied with narrow interests, such as memorizing maps or schedules. The syndrome was first described in 1944, only 1 year after Kanner's initial description of autism (35). Thirty-five years later, Wing (65) revived the concept of Asperger's syndrome and recommended that this category be included within childhood autism, because the two disorders shared the symptoms of impaired development of social interaction, communication, and imagination. Asperger's syndrome is not included in either the DSM III-R or the ICD-9, but is included in the ICD-10 and is being considered for inclusion in the DSM IV.

It appears that the PDD diagnoses, though better differentiated than in the past, still lack unambiguous definitions; diagnosis must still be made according to behavioral criteria rather than by specific biological markers. Explicit diagnostic criteria for autistic disorder now exist, but diagnostic criteria for the other forms of PDD, such as PDD-NOS and Asperger's syndrome, remain vague. Thus, by necessity, most neurobiological research studies of PDD are restricted to subjects who meet the full criteria of autistic disorder; to date, there are few neurobiological studies of subjects diagnosed as having PDD-NOS or Asperger's syndrome.

ASSOCIATED NEUROLOGICAL DISORDERS

Autism is associated with a variety of well-described neurological disorders, and these have been reviewed by Young et al. in the previous edition of this ACNP publication (70) and by Lotspeich and Ciaranello (40). Autism has been associated with genetic disorders such as phenylkentonuria, tuberous sclerosis, and Rett's syndrome. The most common chromosomal abnormality associated with autism is fragile X syndrome. Other chromosomal abnormalities have been associated with autism, including other fragile sites, a long Y chromosome, trisomy 21, XYY, and partial trisomy 15. Nongenetic conditions associated with autism include infectious illnesses such as congenital rubella, acute encephalopathy, cytomegalovirus, and possibly perinatal injury. This chapter will review the two neurological disorders most systematically studied: fragile X syndrome and Rett's syndrome.

TABLE 1. *ICD-10 pervasive developmental disorders (69)*

Childhood autism
Atypical autism
Rett's syndrome
Other childhood disintegrative disorder
Overactive disorder associated with mental retardation
 and stereotyped movements
Asperger's syndrome
Other pervasive developmental disorders

Fragile X Syndrome

Fragile X syndrome (fra X) is the most common autism-associated disorder known to be due to defects in a single gene. The estimated prevalence of fra X is 1 per 1000 in males and 1 per 2000 in females (64). It is recognized as a uniquely useful X-linked genetic model for the investigation of both mental retardation and autism. Affected individuals have a characteristic cytological defect of the X chromosome (Xq27.3), accompanied by a clinical picture of mental retardation and dysmorphism. A DNA sequence spanning the fra X site has recently been cloned, and the FMR-1 gene (familial mental retardation-1) was found to be located at the fragile site (44). This FMR-1 gene is known to be expressed in the developing brain, as well as in other organs. Because of our increasing understanding of the genetic basis for fra X, it is perhaps the most relevant genetic prototype for autism and will therefore be reviewed in some detail here.

Fra X genetics is complex. This disorder does not follow the usual pattern of X-linked inheritance. Instead, some females are also affected, and the degree of expression of the disorder increases with successive generations, in both males and females. This phenomenon has been referred to as the *Sherman paradox* (59), or "genetic anticipation." Sherman noted that when an abnormal X chromosome is passed from a carrier male (negative cytogenetically, normal phenotype) through his daughter to her children, the children are likely to develop the symptoms of fra X; boys are at greater risk than girls. Genetic anticipation is explained in terms of the behavior of the fra X candidate gene (FMR-1). Within this gene is a nucleotide triplet, CGG, which is normally repeated 5–50 times; the vast majority of fra X subjects have a mutant gene in which the number of repeats is abnormally large. Carriers of the mutant fra X gene have 50–200 repeats. Males in whom the (CGG)n repeat is amplified more than 200 times almost invariably show clinical and cytogenetic signs of the disease.

The phenomenon of "genetic anticipation" is now reasonably well understood at a molecular level. In families with fra X-positive children, their grandfathers can be demonstrated to have FMR-1 (CGG)n repeats at a level of 50–200. These grandfathers are asymptomatic, and their moderately long (CGG)n repeats are known as *premutations*. The proband's mother inherits the 50–200 (CGG)n repeats, and in most cases she is asymptomatic. During oogenesis in the mother-to-be the premutation of 50–200 (CGG)n repeats is amplified to more than 200 repeats. This amplified (CGG)n repeat is then passed on to her children. Male children born to such a mother have a 50:50 chance of inheriting the defective X chromosome; those who do inherit the fra X copy are almost always symptomatic. Female children also have a 50:50 chance of inheriting the defective gene. Those who inherit the defective gene have both a mutant X chromosome and a normal X chromosome. Only one X chromosome is active in a given cell; thus the greater the fraction of cells expressing the mutant X chromosome, the more likely the individual is to suffer the stigmata of fra X.

The association between fra X and autism remains controversial. The percentage of children/adults with both autism and fra X has been determined in a number of studies. The incidence of fra X syndrome in autistic populations ranges from 0% to 20%. This wide range is probably due to the variety of selection sites (residential versus outpatient), to variable diagnostic criteria for autism, and to differences in the percentage of fra X-positive cells used as a diagnostic criterion. To correct for these biases, Bolton and Rutter (9) pooled results from studies that met the following criteria: at least 30 subjects and at least 4 fra X-positive cells per 100. In this meta-analysis they found the incidence of fra X in the autistic population to be 7% in autistic males and 4% in autistic females. In a review of several studies, Fisch (22) found the prevalence of fra X in an autistic male population to be 5.4%, which is similar to the prevalence of fra X in a mentally retarded male population, 5.5%. For a more extensive review of this work the reader may refer to Bolton and Rutter (9) and Fisch (22). It is, however, clear that fra X puts individuals at increased risk of autism, and it would be of great interest to know exactly how the FMR-1 gene defect leads to autism in this fraction of fra X individuals. However, until the mechanisms by which the gene affects brain development are thoroughly understood, this will remain a moot point.

Rett's Syndrome

The neurodegenerative disorder known as *Rett's syndrome* (RS), first described by Rett in 1966 (51), is also associated with autism. To date, RS has been seen almost exclusively among females; incidence is estimated to be about 1 in 10,000 to 22,000 (29). Infants with RS develop normally until approximately 6 months of age, when developmental delays and regression occur, and acquired microcephaly begin to appear. A striking characteristic of RS is the loss of purposeful hand movement, concurrent with the develop of stereotypic hand movements such as hand wringing. Between the ages of 1 and 4 years, children develop gait ataxia; as they get older, some develop spasticity and lose ambulation. RS is also characterized by a variety of additional symptoms including mental retardation, autistic behaviors, seizures, and hyperventilation.

Comorbidity of autism and RS was noted as early as 1983 (29). During the early stages of the disorder (ages 2–5 years), many children meet the diagnostic criteria for autism. Witt-Engerstrom and Gillberg (66) found that a majority of 47 children with RS had been diagnosed with autistic disorder, or with autistic features, prior to the diagnosis of RS. Because many girls with RS also meet the diagnosis of autism, it is essential that RS be considered in the differential diagnosis of girls with autistic symptoms.

Despite a number of genetic and neurobiological studies, the etiology of this syndrome is not understood, and the genetic basis is uncertain. In a comprehensive review of RS (46), the recent developments and proposed etiologies are discussed and will be briefly summarized in this chapter. Based on patterns of inheritance, RS is considered to be a sex-linked dominant condition, lethal in males, with sporadic new mutations. Many chromosomal abnormalities have been detected in individuals with RS, such as mosaicism for X chromosome terminal deletion. Twin studies reveal 100% concordance in monozygotic (MZ) twins and 0% concordance in dyzygotic (DZ) twins. A handful of families appear to be multiplex for RS; the syndrome may occur in first- and second-degree relatives of unaffected mothers of RS girls. In these familial cases an explanation based on sporadic mutation would seem unlikely. To account for situations like this, other patterns of inheritance have been proposed—for example, nonrandom X chromosome inactivation.

Autistic disorder is associated with many known genetic disorders as well as with a variety of nongenetic disorders. An understanding of these disorders, particularly those with a genetic base, should aid our understanding of the etiology of autism. This chapter has reviewed two such genetic disorders, each representing a different genetic mechanism. Although the gene responsible for fra X syndrome is located on the X chromosome, the disease phenotype does not observe the classical pattern of X-linked inheritance. Fra X thus provides a new model for behavioral genetic disorders based on triplet amplification and genetic anticipation. RS provides a very different model, at present a rather unsettled one; it occurs only in girls and does not follow a traditional mode of inheritance; its untraditional mode of inheritance may be due to the differential X-inactivation process occurring in female cells. Although these two genetic disorders account for only a small fraction of the total cases of autism, they should prove fruitful starting points in unraveling the major genetic mechanisms of the disease.

NEUROBIOLOGICAL INVESTIGATIONS

Genetic Studies

As examples of multiple cases of autism within a single family have accumulated, investigators have increasingly focused their efforts on genetic approaches for the purpose of identifying the gene or genes that cause autism; these approaches now include twin studies, family studies, segregation analysis, and linkage. As with many other psychiatric disorders, studies of the genetics of autism is

problematic. First, the known causes of autism are both genetic and nongenetic (i.e., phenocopies); fragile X syndrome (fra X) is an example of a genetic etiology, and congenital rubella syndrome is an example of a nongenetic etiology. Second, autism may not be a single disorder caused by a single gene, but instead may be a group of similar disorders caused by a variety of aberrant genes (genetic heterogeneity). If so, then subject groups for genetic research must be carefully ascertained, to focus on those in which a single genetic etiology is most likely. It will be necessary to rigorously exclude those families with known genetic or nongenetic disorders. Definition of the phenotype must be consistent, and study design must therefore attend to careful selection of diagnostic instruments, diagnostic reliability, and issues of observer blindness. This section will review twin and family studies, in addition to discussion of segregation and linkage analysis (see also Chapters 2, 59, and 60, *this volume*).

Twin Studies

Twin studies have been reported, and all strongly suggest that autism is a heritable disorder. In the first, Folstein and Rutter (23) examined same-sex twins ascertained from the school-age population of Great Britain. Thirty-six percent (4/11) of the monozygotic (MZ) twins were concordant for autism, whereas none (0/11) of the dyzygotic (DZ) twins were concordant. When cognitive disabilities were included in the definition of the phenotype (such as severe language delay, marked reading disability, and persistent articulation disorder), concordance increased to 82% for MZ and to 10% for DZ twins. Subsequent twin studies confirm the results that concordance rates for MZ are higher than those for DZ (reviewed in ref. 70).

Family Studies

Familial aggregation of autism has been reported for over 20 years. In the last decade, investigators have studied family members of autistic probands to learn whether there is a milder form of autism—or, in other words, an extended phenotype. Because not all autism is genetic (e.g., because of evidence of infectious and traumatic etiologies), studies of singleton families may be misleading. To explore possible genetic etiologies it is much better to study those families with two or more members with autism, because these most likely represent genetic autism. This section will review family studies that help to define such parameters as percent of autism families with more than two affected children, existence of cognitive and psychiatric disorders in siblings of autistic probands, preliminary clinical data of autism multiplex families, and the possible existence of a mild phenotype in parents.

Rutter (56) reported that 2% of children with autism had a sibling with autism; this is 50 times the general population prevalence rate of 4/10,000. Subsequent studies using subjects obtained through clinics, hospitals, and epidemiological studies have found a similar sibling incidence of autism (5,43).

Investigators are also focusing on milder autistic symptoms that may be present in siblings and parents of autism probands. In this connection, August et al. (5) studied the 71 siblings of 41 children with autism and compared them to 38 siblings of 15 children with Down's syndrome. Nine of the 71 siblings (13%) of autistic probands demonstrated cognitive disabilities (e.g., delays in language development, abnormalities of language, low verbal and nonverbal IQ, and special education placement); only one of the 38 controls (3%) was similarly impaired. Later studies have tended to confirm these results. Minton et al. (43) found that siblings of autistic probands had mean full-scale IQ scores 10 points lower than national standards. One study failed to observe cognitive deficits in siblings and parents of autistic probands on full-scale IQ (24).

Family studies have also evaluated the frequency of occurrence of other psychiatric disorders in autism families. DeLong and Dwyer (20) studied 929 first- and second-degree relatives of 44 autistic subjects, using a family history method. Seventeen relatives had Asperger's syndrome, and the majority of these came from families with high functioning autistic probands (IQ > 70). An unexpected result was that 4.2% of the families had a positive history of bipolar disease, a rate 5 times that seen in the general population. Also, 8% of families had a history of depression. Piven et al. (48) also used the family history method to study 67 siblings of 37 autistic probands. They found autism in 3% of siblings, severe social dysfunction and isolation (SSDI, equivalent to Asperger's syndrome) in 4.4%, cognitive disorders in 15%, and treated affective disorder in 15%.

There are obvious advantages in studying multiplex families when the goal is to identify a putative gene for autism. In our own work, Spiker et al. (62) studied autistic probands and their siblings in 44 presumed multiplex autism families, using the Autism Diagnostic Interview (ADI) (39). Thirty-seven of the 44 families were confirmed to be multiplex for autism by ADI criteria. Most of the subjects in these 37 families were unambiguously either autistic or not autistic. Eight of 117 subjects were placed in an ''uncertain'' category because they met some, but not all, ADI criteria for autism. Thus, there were very few siblings with an ''uncertain'' (mild phenotype) for autism. The second part of the study attempted to determine whether there was concordance for specific autistic symptoms within the multiplex families. For most of the individual symptoms there was no evidence of concordance; however, a significant degree of concordance was noted for several individual scores on items reflecting poor emotional expression, lack of expressive gestures, stereotyped utterances, and ritualistic/repetitive activities. Further study of concordant autistic symptoms may point the way to possible behavioral markers for a genetic form of autism.

In genetic studies, the phenotypic status of parents is of course very important. If parents are affected, a dominant model is suggested; if not, then a recessive or more complex model is likely. The possibility that some parents have a mild autism phenotype has been discussed in the literature (9), and several studies now support this notion. Wolff et al. (67) used a structured interview originally devised to diagnose schizoid personality disorder to compare 35 parents of autistic children to 39 parents of nonautistic developmentally delayed children. Forty-six percent of parents of autistic children demonstrated definite schizoid personality traits, whereas none of the 39 control parents demonstrated such traits. Additional evidence for a ''parental phenotype'' comes from studies of Landa et al. (38). Their data indicated that the parents of autistic children exhibited an increase in abnormal social-discourse behaviors and told narratives characterized as ''skeletal or rambling.'' This approach to characterizing the milder phenotype in autism tends to focus on describing and quantifying specific clinical signs rather than assigning diagnostic classifications.

Segregation and Linkage Analysis

There is clear evidence for familial autism, and, though not proven, this is very probably due to genetic factors. In addition, there appears to be a mild subclinical phenotype of autism in parents, and possibly in siblings, of autistic probands. However, this putative phenotype is not explicitly defined. Using the technique of linkage analysis to examine autism multiplex families, it should be possible to map and eventually identify the specific gene or genes responsible for familial autism.

Two studies of segregation analysis in autism have been published; in the first, Ritvo et al. (53) recruited 46 families with multiple incidence of autism. Families were drawn from several sources, including UCLA research files, personal referrals, and advertisement solicitation. The pattern of inheritance revealed in this analysis supported the hypothesis of an autosomal recessive pattern of inheritance for autism and rejected a polygenic model. A second segregation analysis, by Jorde et al. (34), surveyed 185 autism families ascertained in the Utah–UCLA epidemiology study of autism. This survey suggested a multifactorial threshold model, but a major gene effect could not be excluded, particularly if genetic heterogeneity is assumed. These studies appear to be contradictory, but they are only preliminary. In both studies, parents were considered to be unaffected. As discussed in the previous section, some parents may in fact have a mild autism phenotype, as yet not precisely defined.

These preliminary surveys have encouraged a search for a major autism gene, and an attempt has been made at linkage analysis which failed to show linkage between autism and 30 markers (61). More recently, in a statistical study of allelic frequencies, Herault et al. (30) examined four genes on chromosome 11. They determined allelic frequencies of the genes for tyrosine hydroxylase, dopamine-β-hydroxylase, tryptophan hydroxylase, and c-Harvey-Ras-1 (HRAS-1) in both autistic and control children. The frequencies of certain HRAS-1 alleles were greater in the autistic children than in the controls. This is a preliminary finding and will require follow-up by traditional linkage analysis.

The association between autism and fra X has prompted researchers to look for linkage between autism and the FMR-1 gene and to examine the FMR-1 gene of autistic subjects for subtle or occult changes. With this intent, Malmgren et al. (41) studied 22 autistic members of 18 families. Only seven of the autistic subjects were known to be cytologically positive for fra X, and DNA testing revealed a typical pattern of fra X-related (CGG)n amplification among these 7 subjects. The remaining 15 autistic subjects were fra X-negative by DNA testing. In these 15 individuals, autism was clearly occurring in the absence of any changes in the (CGG)n repeats in the FMR-1 gene. In our own laboratory, Hallmayer et al. (*unpublished observations*) used DNA probes to examine the degree of amplification of (CGG)n repeats in a group of 79 autistic subjects from 35 autism multiplex families. No obvious abnormalities were detected in the size of the (CGG)n repeat region. In addition, two microsatellite markers close to the fra X gene were used in linkage analysis on all first-degree relatives from the 35 autism multiplex families; again, no linkage with autism was noted. Thus, autism occurring in the absence of cytological evidence of fra X is not associated with amplification of (CGG)n repeats in the FMR-1 gene, nor is the autism phenotype positionally linked to this gene.

In summary, twin and family studies have strongly indicated a genetic basis for autism, but most cases of autism are not related to fra X. However, if the hypothetical gene for autism behaves like the fra X gene, we can predict that the clinical presentation of individuals harboring the gene will be highly variable. Although some autism multiplex family studies suggest an increased frequency of cognitive, social, and psychiatric disorders in siblings of autistic subjects, the evidence for an extended phenotype in siblings remains tentative. Several studies, however, suggest a mild autism phenotype in some parents; if this is confirmed, then characterizing that phenotype will be critical for genetic linkage studies.

Neuropathological Studies

There have been only a few autopsy studies of autism; to date, the brains of a few subjects have been examined and compared to controls. Kemper and Bauman (36) have completed detailed autopsy studies on the brains of six autistic cases (five males and one female) varying in age from 9 to 29 and have compared them to identically processed age- and sex-matched controls. They identified consistent neuropathologic abnormalities in the cerebellum, the brainstem, and the forebrain of the autistic cases. A marked reduction in Purkinje cell number was seen in the cerebellum of all subjects. This reduction was particularly noted in the posterolateral neocerebellum and adjacent archicerebellar cortex, while the anterolateral cerebellum and vermis were relatively spared (6). A decrease in density of cerebellar granule cells was also noted.

There were age-dependent abnormalities of neuronal cell size both in deep cerebellar nuclei and in the inferior olivary nuclei of the brainstem. In the brains from younger individuals, neurons were abnormally large in both cerebellar and inferior olivary nuclei. The brains of older autistic subjects showed a decrease in cell size in these same nuclei. A possible explanation lies in the developmental history of the cerebellum. The authors point out that the cells of the inferior olivary nuclei of the brainstem project to the cerebellum; they speculate that a developmental failure in the critical interaction between inferior olivary nuclei and Purkinje cells might lead to cell loss or abnormal neuronal development in the olivary and cerebellar nuclei. Kemper and Bauman (36) speculate that as a consequence of the marked early loss of Purkinje cells, the large neuronal cells characteristic of fetal circuitry are retained for an abnormally long time in the deep nuclei of the younger subjects. This immature circuitry may function initially in autistic subjects, but it is not retained into adult life, nor is it replaced by the adult neuronal pattern. The result is a reduction in number and size of neurons in the olivary and cerebellar nuclei of the older subjects.

In the forebrains of four cases, Kemper and Bauman (36) found unusually small and densely packed cells in limbic structures, including the hippocampus and amygdala nuclei. Abnormal cells were also noted in the vertical limb of the diagonal band of Broca, a nucleus with cholinergic projections to the hippocampus and amygdala. As in the cerebellum, age-dependent cellular abnormalities were also noted in the diagonal band of Broca. The cell bodies of this nucleus were abnormally large in the brains of the younger cases but small in the brains of the older cases. This pattern is formally similar to that seen in the inferior olivary and cerebellar nuclei, with the larger cells characteristic of fetal circuitry being abnormally retained into childhood and early youth.

Neuroanatomical Studies

Radiological imaging studies have been performed on autistic subjects using the full spectrum of imaging methodologies. Although it is now clear that brain abnormalities are common in autism, no single abnormality is present in all subjects; indeed, many autistic subjects appear to have grossly normal brains. Earlier studies, using computerized tomography (CT), were reviewed in the previous ANCP edition (70). The more recent studies, including magnetic resonance imaging (MRI), positron emission tomography (PET), and nuclear magnetic resonance spectroscopy (MRS), are briefly reviewed here.

MRI

The pioneering MRI investigations of autism (for review see ref. 40) revealed nonspecific findings of enlarged fourth ventricle, larger fourth ventricle/posterior fossa ratio, small cerebellum/posterior fossa ratio, and small cerebellum/total brain ratio. More recent MRI scans have focused on the cerebellum and structures of the cerebrum.

The histoanatomical studies of Bauman and Kemper (36), describing Purkinje cell loss in autism, called attention to the cerebellum as a probable site of anatomic abnormality in autism. Since then, there have been a number of MRI studies of the cerebellum, particularly those of the cerebellar vermi. Courchesne et al. (17) determined the size of the vermal lobules in 18 autistic subjects as compared to 12 radiographic medical controls. In 14 of the 18 autistic subjects, vermal lobes VI and VII averaged 25% smaller than those of the normal controls. In more recent studies, Holttum et al. (32) and Piven et al. (50) attempted to replicate the studies of Courchesne et al. (17), using volunteer controls matched for age, gender, IQ, and socioeconomic status (SES). When the AD group was compared to the control group (matched for SES and age), vermal lobules VI–VII were found to be smaller in the autistic group, as originally reported by Courchesne et al. (17). However, when a control group matched by IQ and age was used for comparison, no significant differences were seen. Thus the observed abnormalities in size of cerebellar features appear to be correlated with subnormal IQ, rather than with autism itself.

Increasingly, as MRI resolution has improved, investigators have turned their attention to the structures of the cerebrum. Gaffney et al. (26), for instance, reviewed axial scans for evidence of abnormal sizes of cerebral hemispheres, ventricles, thalamus, and structures of the basal ganglia; all were unremarkable, except for the right lenticular nucleus, which was, on average, significantly larger in the autistic group. On axial view, the areas of the frontal horns and the body of the lateral ventricles were significantly greater in the autistic subjects.

There have also been reports of specific malformations of cortical architecture. Piven et al. (47) found evidence of four types of gyria malformations in the cerebral cortex of autistic subjects (polymicrogyria, pachygyria, heterotopia and schizencephaly), whereas no gyria malformations were found in the control group. Gyria malformations are considered to be a result of defects in migration of neurons during the first 6 months of fetal development. Courchesne et al. (18) reported that a significant fraction of autistic subjects (9 of 21, or 43%) had parietal lobe abnormalities absent in normal controls. These included loss of cortical volume, loss of white matter, and thinning of the corpus callosum.

PET and MRS

Positron emission tomography (PET) allows accurate measurement of glucose metabolic rate (GMR) in specific regions of the brain. The short-lived radioactive analogues of glucose used in PET studies are concentrated in the most actively metabolizing cells of the brain; their decay allows investigators to map sites of active glucose metabolism. Results to date have been suggestive, but inconclusive. Rumsey and co-workers (55) studied 10 high-functioning autistic men and 15 age-matched controls. The autistic group showed a significant increase in cortical GMR during rest, but with a considerable overlap between the subject and control groups. De Volder et al. (19) found no significant differences between autistic and control subjects. Siegel et al. (60) found that non-mentally retarded autistic subjects did not differ from controls on average measures of GMR; they did, however, show "outlier" regions—that is, brain regions of significantly increased or decreased metabolic activity that varied from one subject to another.

Using PET methodology, Horwitz et al. (33) had noted paired regions of elevated glucose uptake in the frontal and parietal lobes of the brain in normal subjects. They suggested that these paired regions of elevated glucose metabolism are a reflection of correlated functional activity between lobes of the normal brain. They then determined the level of such functional associations between brain regions in a group of 14 autistic men and age-matched controls; the autistic men had significantly fewer functional associations than did the controls, particularly between homologous regions of the frontal and parietal lobes. These frontal and parietal regions are the location of neural systems associated with directed attention.

Recently, Minshew et al. (42) have reported preliminary evidence for abnormal phosphorous metabolism and increased degradation of brain membranes in autism. By using MRS, which does not require radioisotopes, they were able to measure levels of phosphorous-containing metabolites, including phosphocreatine and phospho mono- and diesters, in the prefrontal cortex of autistic and normal subjects. Briefly, they found that as test performance declined across the spectrum of their autistic subjects, there was a parallel decrease in levels of high-energy phosphates and membrane building blocks, along with an increase in the breakdown products of membranes (phosphodiesters). In the normal control group, no comparable correlation was seen between performance and levels of phosphorous-containing compounds. The authors note that these results are consistent with the existence in autism of a hypermetabolic state, coupled with an undersynthesis of brain membranes. The findings of Minshew et al. (42) are consistent with both (a) the suggestion of Ciaranello et al. (14) that arborization of the neuronal dendritic tree might be abnormal in autism and (b) the observations of Bauman and Kemper (6) of truncation in the development of the neuronal dendritic tree of autistic subjects. Confirmation and elaboration of these results will be anticipated with interest.

To summarize, the failure to observe a uniform anatomical change in the brains of all autistic subjects should not be surprising, because autism is clearly a heterogeneous disorder with a variety of etiologies. Future neurobiological research will benefit from a greater focus on subgroups, perhaps selected by common MRI, PET, or MRS phenotype. The converse is also true; subgroups that share common genetic or nongenetic causal factors are more likely to yield consistent MRI, PET, or MRS findings. One might expect, for instance, that a subgroup assembled from autism multiplex families might demonstrate related abnormalities when examined by these methodologies.

Neurochemical Studies

Neurochemical studies of autism were begun in the 1960s. Although there are clear abnormalities in levels of a number of neurotransmitters, as yet no one has yet put forward a unifying hypothesis of autism based on a specific defect in a single neurotransmitter system. The large body of work on the neurochemistry and immunochemistry of autism is reviewed in the previous edition of this ACNP publication (70); thus, only studies published since then will be reviewed here. These more recent studies have focused on serotonin and the opioids.

Serotonin

Serotonin [5-hydroxytryptamine (5-HT)] has received the most attention in autism. It has been noted during the last 30 years that approximately 30% of autistic subjects have abnormally high levels of whole-blood serotonin (70). More recent studies have focused on families, and several have found evidence that high blood levels of 5-HT are familial. Kuperman et al. (37) measured platelet-rich plasma 5-HT in families with an autistic proband, and they found significant correlation of 5-HT levels between parents and children. Investigators have reported elevated whole-blood 5-HT in a majority of the first-degree relatives of autistic probands who themselves have elevated 5-HT; relatives of autistic probands with normal levels of 5-HT have, for the most part, normal 5-HT levels

(1,15). Autism multiplex families appear to have the highest levels of blood serotonin; Piven et al. (49), for instance, compared 5-HT blood levels in five autistic multiplex children with levels in two control groups (23 singleton autistic children and 10 normal controls). Mean 5-HT levels were highest in the multiplex group and lowest in the normal group. The data thus indicate that high 5-HT blood levels are familial and may be associated with genetic liability to autism (see also Chapters 39 and 41, *this volume*).

Opioids

Many autistic children have a very high pain threshold and exhibit self-abusive behaviors. A parallel has been noted between these behaviors and the behavior of animals addicted to opiates, where there is also a decreased response to pain and an increase in self-injurious behavior (45). Thus there has been considerable interest in determining the levels of endogenous opioids in autism. There have in fact been two reports of elevated endogenous opioids in autism: Gillberg et al. (27) noted higher CSF endorphin fraction II levels in 20 autistic children compared to controls, and Ross et al. (54) also noted high CSF β-endorphin levels in autistic children (6 subjects, 8 controls). Opioid blockers such as naloxone and naltrexone have been examined for their potential effectiveness in modifying self-injurious behavior in autism and will be reviewed in the treatment section of this chapter.

In summary, although there is considerable abnormality in measured levels of neurotransmitters and their metabolites in autism, a unifying theory remains elusive. The elevation of serotonin in blood is the most consistent finding, and it may be significant that drugs able to influence CNS levels of serotonin (16,28) also appear to have therapeutic value in autism. It is also possible that hyperserotonemia can be used as a biological marker for familial autism, and, if so, this could be of great value for genetic research (see also Chapter 46, *this volume*).

TREATMENT

The treatment of autism has focused on extinguishing specific aberrant behaviors (e.g., hyperactivity, temper tantrums, stereotypies, and self-injurious behaviors) and improving social relatedness, use of language, and overall cognitive abilities. There are no cures for autism/PDD, but treatment modalities have been developed to modify specific behaviors. Effective treatment requires an interdisciplinary approach which includes education, speech and language therapy, occupational therapy, behavior modification, and medications. The reader is referred to Berkell (8) for a review of behavioral forms of treatment. This chapter will focus on the psychopharmacology of autism and PDD.

During the last 20 years there have been a number of clinical studies of drugs in autism, principally of children rather than adults. The most studied and most useful agent historically has been haloperidol, which is known to improve many of the aberrant behaviors of autism. Recent studies have also focused on the effects of opioid blockers and serotonin uptake blockers. This review will summarize the systematic studies on effects of these psychopharmacologic agents in autism that have appeared since the publication of Campbell's review in the previous edition of this ACNP publication (10).

Neuroleptics

Campbell (11) has conducted several well-designed double-blind, placebo-controlled studies of haloperidol. The behavioral improvements observed included significant decreases in social withdrawal, stereotypies, hyperactivity, abnormal object relationships, fidgetiness, negativism, angry affect, and liability. Up to 29% of the 82 children treated with haloperidol developed neuroleptic-induced dyskinesias during 2–60 months of treatment (12). The dyskinesias were reversible, and there was no pattern of sex, age, baseline stereotypies, or IQ to separate those children who developed dyskinesias from those who did not. Because haloperidol is sedating, pimozide has been evaluated as a promising substitute in treating autistic children who are hypoactive (21).

Opioid Blockers

Panksepp and Sahley (45) suggested that excessive opioid activity might underlie the symptomatology of autism. As a result there have been several studies investigating the effectiveness of naltrexone and naloxone in treating autism, particularly the self-injurious behavior frequently seen in autistic children (for review see ref. 58). Some children respond well, whereas others do not. Campbell et al. (13) conducted a double-blind, placebo-controlled study of naltrexone in 41 autistic children 3–7 years of age. Naltrexone was superior to placebo in reducing hyperactivity. Herman (31) reported significant improvement in patients with severe self-injurious behaviors of head and face hitting. However, Campbell (13) found no significant improvement over placebo in reduction of self-injurious behaviors.

Serotonergic Agents

Motivated in part by biochemical evidence of hyperserotonemia in autism, researchers have evaluated a variety of serotonergic agents for their effectiveness in treatment of autism. These studies first focused on fenfluramine, an agent which lowers both peripheral and central serotonin levels; the results of these studies are contradictory, but, generally speaking, there appears to be only weak evidence that fenfluramine is an effective treatment for autistic behaviors (10).

More recent studies have examined the role of serotonin reuptake blockers, including fluoxetine and clomipramine. It seems reasonable that serotonin medications effective in the treatment of obsessive–compulsive disorder might also be effective in moderating the perseverative and ritualistic behaviors seen in autism. In the only study published to date, an open trial, a majority of 23 autistic subjects (aged 8–27 years) demonstrated global improvement when treated with fluoxetine (16). Several subjects developed agitation requiring discontinuation of fluoxetine. Clomipramine appears even more promising. Gordon et al. (28) have conducted a double-blind crossover study using clomipramine, desipramine, and placebo. In their study of 24 subjects, they found clomipramine to be superior to both desipramine and placebo in reducing repetitive behaviors, compulsive behaviors, and anger. Clomipramine may produce these behavioral changes through enhancement of central serotonergic transmission; however, clomipramine has additional pharmacologic actions, including significant dopamine blocking activity, and its mechanism of action is at present far from clear.

SUMMARY

Over the past 10 years, methodologic advances in neuroscience have helped us to better define autism/PDD. Though no universal disease mechanism has been identified, certain generalities are emerging. Autism and PDD are brought about by aberrations in brain development, produced by both genetic and nongenetic mechanisms. Although no gene specific for autism has yet been identified, autism subjects demonstrate a variety of anatomical and neurochemical abnormalities that should help us define specific subgroups. These should help, eventually, in the identification of specific genetic factors. Abnormalities in gross brain architecture and in neuronal activity may now be investigated by powerful imaging techniques, sensitive to both brain metabolism and molecular structure. Recent results with MRS seem especially promising in this regard. No useful neurochemical model of autism/PDD has yet emerged; in fact, the explosion of new neurotransmitters and neuroregulators seems to make this an increasingly distant goal. Nonetheless, there are an increasing number of useful pharmacologic agents for treatment of specific symptoms, particularly among the serotonergic agents. None of these, however, can be said to have touched the core behaviors of autism/PDD.

ACKNOWLEDGMENTS

Work from the author's laboratory was supported by grants from the National Alliance for Research on Schizophrenia and Depression (NARSAD) and from the Scottish Rite Benevolent Foundation's Schizophrenia Research Program, N.M.J., U.S.A.

REFERENCES

1. Abramson RK, Wright HH, Carpenter R, et al. Elevated blood serotonin in autistic probands and their first-degree relatives. *J Autism Dev Disord* 1989;19:397–407.
2. American Psychiatric Association. *Diagnostic and statistical manual of mental disorders, DSM III.* Washington, DC: American Psychiatric Association, 1980.
3. American Psychiatric Association. *Diagnostic and statistical manual of mental disorders, DSM III-R.* Washington, DC: American Psychiatric Association, 1987.
4. Asperger H. Die 'autistischen psychopathen' im kindesalter. *Arch Psychiatrie Nervenkrankheiten* 1944;117:76–136.
5. August GJ, Stewart MA, Tsai L. The incidence of cognitive disabilities in the siblings of autistic children. *Br J Psychiatry* 1981;138:416–422.
6. Bauman M, Kemper TL. Histoanatomic observations of the brain in early infantile autism. *Neurology* 1985;35:866–874.
7. Bauman ML. Microscopic neuroanatomic abnormalities in autism. *Pediatrics* 1991;87(Suppl):791–795.
8. Berkell D, ed. *Autism: identification, education and treatment.* Hillsdale, NJ: Lawrence Erlbaum Associates, 1992.
9. Bolton P, Rutter M. Genetic influences in autism. *Int Rev Psychiatry* 1990;2:67–80.
10. Campbell M. Drug treatment of infantile autism: The past decade. In: Meltzer HY, ed. *Psychopharmacology: the third generation of progress.* New York: Raven Press, 1987;1225–1231.
11. Anderson LT, Campbell M, Adams P, Small AM, Perry R, Shell J. The effects of haloperidol on discrimination learning and behavioral symptoms in autistic children. *J Autism Dev Disord* 1989;19:227–239.
12. Campbell M, Adams P, Perry R, Spencer EK, Overall JE. Tardive and withdrawal dyskinesia in autistic children: a prospective study. *Psychopharmacol Bull* 1988;24:251–255.
13. Campbell M, Anderson LT, Small AM, Adams P, Gonzalez NM, Ernst M. Naltrexone in autistic children: behavioral symptoms and attentional learning. *J Am Acad Child Adolesc Psychiatry* 1993:32:1283–1291.
14. Ciaranello RD, Vandenberg SR, Anders TF. Intrinsic and extrinsic determinants of neuronal development: Relation to infantile autism. *J Autism Dev Disord* 1982;12:115–145.
15. Cook EH, Leventhal BL, Hellar W, Metz J, Wainwright M, Freedman DX. Autistic children and their first-degree relatives: relationships between serotonin and norepinephrine levels and intelligence. *J Neuropsychiatry Clin Neurosci* 1990;2:268–274.
16. Cook EH, Rowlet R, Jaselskis C, Leventhal BL. Fluoxetine treatment of children and adults with autistic disorder and mental retardation. *J Am Acad Child Adolesc Psychiatry* 1992;4:739–745.
17. Courchesne E, Yeung-Courchesne R, Press GA, Hesselink JR, Jernigan TL. Hypoplasia of cerebellar vermal lobules VI and VII in autism. *N Engl J Med* 1988;318:1349–1354.
18. Courchesne E, Press GA, Yeung-Courchesne R. Parietal lobe abnormalities detected with MR in patients with infantile autism. *Am J Roentgenol* 1993;160:387–393.
19. De Volder A, Bol A, Michel C, Congneau M, Goffinet AM. Brain glucose metabolism in children with the autistic syndrome: positron tomography analysis. *Brain Dev* 1987;9:581–587.
20. DeLong GR, Dwyer JT. Correlation of family history with specific autistic subgroups: Asperger's syndrome and bipolar affective disease. *J Autism Dev Disord* 1988;18:593–600.
21. Ernst M, Magee HJ, Gonzalez NM, Locascio JJ, Rosenberg CR, Campbell M. Pimozide in autistic children. *Psychopharmacol Bull* 1992;28:187–191.
22. Fisch GS. Is autism associated with the fragile X syndrome? *Am J Med Genet* 1992;43:47–55.
23. Folstein S, Rutter M. Infantile autism: a genetic study of 21 twin pairs. *J Child Psychol Psychiatry* 1977;18:297–321.
24. Freeman BJ, Ritvo ER, Mason-Brothers A, et al. Psychometric assessment of first-degree relatives of 62 autistic probands in Utah. *Am J Psychiatry* 1989;146:361–364.
25. Frith U, ed. *Autism and Asperger syndrome.* Cambridge: Cambridge University Press, 1991.
26. Gaffney GR, Kuperman S, Tsai LY, Minchin S. Forebrain structure in infantile autism. *J Am Acad Child Adolesc Psychiatry* 1989;28:534–537.
27. Gillberg C, Terenius L, Lonnerholm G. Endorphine activity in childhood psychosis. *Arch Gen Psychiatry* 1985;42:780–783.
28. Gordon CT, State RC, Nelson JE, Hamburger SD, Rapoport JL. A double-blind comparison of clomipramine, desipramine, and placebo in the treatment of autistic disorder. *Arch Gen Psychiatry* 1993;50:441–447.
29. Hagberg G, Aicardi F, Dias K, Ramos O. A progressive syndrome of autism, dementia, ataxia, and loss of purposeful hand use in girls: Rett's syndrome—report of 35 cases. *Ann Neurol* 1983;14:471–479.
30. Herault J, Perrot A, Barthelemy C, et al. Possible association of C-Harvey-Ras-1 (HRAS-1) marker with autism. *Psychiatry Res* 1993;46:261–267.
31. Herman BH, Hammock MK, Egan J, Arthur-Smith A, Chatoor R, Werner A. Role for opioid peptides in self-injurious behavior: dissociation from autonomic nervous system functioning. *Dev Pharmacol Ther* 1989;12:81–89.
32. Holttum JR, Minshew NJ, Sanders RS, Phillips NE. Magnetic resonance imaging of the posteriour fossa in autism. *Biol Psychiatry* 1992;32:1091–1101.
33. Horwitz B, Rumsey J, Grady C, et al. Interregional correlations of glucose utilization among brain regions in autistic adults. *Ann Neurol* 1987;22:118.
34. Jorde LB, Mason-Brothers A, Waldmann R, et al. The UCLA–University of Utah epidemiologic survey of autism: genealogical analysis of familial aggregation. *Am J Med Genet* 1990;36:85–88.
35. Kanner L. Autistic disturbances of affective contact. *Nerv Child* 1943;2:217–250.
36. Kemper TL, Bauman ML. The contribution of neuropathologic studies to the understanding of autism. *Behav Neurol* 1993;11:175–187.
37. Kuperman S, Beeghly JH, Burns TL, Tsai LY. Serotonin relationships of autistic probands and their first-degree relatives. *J Am Acad Child Adolesc Psychiatry* 1985;24:186–190.
38. Landa R, Folstein SE, Isaacs C. Spontaneous narrative-discourse performance of parents of autistic individuals. *J Speech Hear Res* 1991;34:1339–1345.
39. LeCouteur A, Rutter M, Lord C, et al. Autism diagnostic interview: a standardized investigator-based instrument. *J Autism Dev Disord* 1989;19:363–387.
40. Lotspeich LJ, Ciaranello RD. The neurobiology and genetics of infantile autism. In: Bradley R, Harris R, eds. *International review of neurobiology.* San Diego: Academic Press, 1993;87–129.
41. Malmgren H, Gustavson K, Wahlstrom J, et al. Infantile autism—fragile X: molecular findings support genetic heterogeneity. *Am J Med Genet* 1992;44:830–833.
42. Minshew NJ, Goldstein G, Dombrowski SM, Panchalingam K, Pettegrew JW. A preliminary ^{31}P MRS study of autism: evidence for undersynthesis and increased degradation of brain membranes. *Biol Psychiatry* 1993;33:762–773.
43. Minton J, Campbell M, Green WH, Jennings S, Samit C. Cognitive assessment of siblings of autistic children. *J Am Acad Child Psychiatry* 1982;21:256–261.
44. Oberlé I, Rousseau F, Heitz D, et al. Instability of a 550-base pair DNA segment and abnormal methylation in fragile X syndrome. *Science* 1991;252:1097–1102.
45. Panksepp J, Sahley TL. Possible brain opioid involvement in disrupted social intent and language development in autism. In: Schopler E, Mesibov GB, eds. *Neurobiological issues in Autism.* New York: Plenum Press, 1987;357–372.
46. Perry A. Rett syndrome: a comprehensive review of the literature. *Am J Ment Retard* 1991;96:275–290.
47. Piven J, Berthier ML, Starkstein SE, Nehme E, Pearlson G, Folstein S. Magnetic resonance imaging evidence for a defect of cerebral cortical development in autism. *Am J Psychiatry* 1990;147:734–739.

48. Piven J, Gayle J, Chase GA, et al. A family history study of neuropsychiatric disorders in the adult siblings of autistic individuals. *J Am Acad Child Adolesc Psychiatry* 1990;29:177–183.

49. Piven J, Tsai G, Nehme E, Coyle JT. Platelet serotonin, a possible marker for familial autism. *J Autism Dev Disord* 1991;21:51–59.

50. Piven J, Nehme E, Simon J, Barta P, Pearlson G, Folstein SE. Magnetic resonance imaging in autism: measurement of the cerebellum, pons, and fourth ventricle. *Biol Psychiatry* 1992;31:491–504.

51. Rett A. Uber ein eigenartiges hirmatrophisches syndrom bei hyperammoniamie in kindesalter. *Wien Med Wochenschr* 1966;116:723–738.

52. Ritvo ER, Freeman BJ. National society for autistic children definition of the syndrome of autism. *J Autism Child Schizophr* 1978;8:162–167.

53. Ritvo ER, Spence MA, Freeman BJ, Mason-Brothers A, Mo A, Marazita ML. Evidence for autosomal recessive inheritance in 46 families with multiple incidences of autism. *Am J Psychiatry* 1985;142:187–192.

54. Ross DL, Klykylo WM, Hitzemann R. Reduction of elevated CSF beta-endorphine by fenfluramine in infantile autism. *Pediatr Neurol* 1987;3:83–86.

55. Rumsey JM, Duara R, Grady C, et al. Brain metabolism in autism. *Arch Gen Psychiatry* 1985;42:448–455.

56. Rutter M. Psychotic disorders in early childhood. In: Coppen AJ, Walk A, eds. *Recent developments in schizophrenia. British Journal of Psychiatry special publication.* 1967;133–158.

57. Rutter M, Hersov R, eds. *Child psychiatry: modern approaches.* Oxford: Blackwell Scientific, 1977.

58. Sandman CA. The opiate hypothesis in autism and self-injury. *J Child Adolesc Psychopharmacol* 1990/1991;1:237–248.

59. Sherman SL, Jacobs PA, Morton NE, et al. Further segregation analysis of the fragile X syndrome with special reference to transmitting males. *Hum Genet* 1985;68:289–299.

60. Siegel BV, Asarnow R, Tanguay P, et al. Regional cerebral glucose metabolism and attention in adults with a history of childhood autism. *J Neuropsychiatry* 1992;4:406–414.

61. Spence MA, Ritvo ER, Marazita ML, Funderburk SJ, Sparkes RS, Freeman BJ. Gene mapping studies with the syndrome of autism. *Behav Genet* 1985;15:1–13.

62. Spiker DK, Lotspeich L, Kraemer HC, et al. The genetics of autism: characteristics of affected and unaffected children from 37 multiplex families. *Neuropsychiatric Genet* 1994;54:27–35.

63. Steffenberg S, Gillberg C. Autism and autistic-like conditions in Swedish rural and urban areas: a population study. *Br J Psychiatry* 1986;149:81–87.

64. Webb TP, Bundey SE, Thake AI, Todd J. Population incidence and segregation ratios in the Martin–Bell syndrome. *Am J Med Genet* 1986;23:573–580.

65. Wing L. Asperger's syndrome: a clinical account. *Psychol Med* 1981;11:115–129.

66. Witt-Engerstrom I, Gillberg C. Rett syndrome in Sweden. *J Autism Dev Disord* 1987;17:149–150.

67. Wolff S, Narayan S, Moyes B. Personality characteristics of parents of autistic children: a controlled study. *J Child Psychol Psychiatry* 1988;29:143–153.

68. World Health Organization. *ICD-9. International classification of diseases,* 9th ed. Geneva: WHO, 1977.

69. World Health Organization. *ICD-10. Classification of mental and behavioural disorders. Clinical description and diagnostic guidelines.* Geneva: WHO, 1992.

70. Young JG, Leven LI, Newcorn JH, Knott PJ. Genetic and neurobiological approaches to the pathophysiology of autism and the pervasive developmental disorders. In: Meltzer HY, eds. *Psychopharmacology: the third generation of progress.* New York: Raven Press, 1987;825–836.

Psychopharmacology: The Fourth
Generation of Progress, edited by
Floyd E. Bloom and David J. Kupfer.
Raven Press, Ltd., New York © 1995.

CHAPTER 143

Tic Disorders

James F. Leckman, David L. Pauls, and Donald J. Cohen

During the course of the past decade, Tourette's syndrome (TS) and related conditions have emerged as model disorders for researchers interested in the interaction of genetic, epigenetic (environmental), and neurobiological factors which shape clinical outcomes from health to chronic disability over the lifespan (35). Figure 1 depicts these interactions and provides a framework for much of the research described in this chapter (see Chapter 155, *this volume*).

PHENOMENOLOGY AND NATURAL HISTORY

TS is a chronic neuropsychiatric disorder of childhood onset that is characterized by (a) tics that wax and wane in severity and (b) an array of behavioral problems including attention-deficit hyperactivity disorder (ADHD) and some forms of obsessive–compulsive disorder (OCD) (28,38). Many of the features of the syndrome—including the age of onset, course, anatomic distribution of tics, the sensory phenomena, the sex ratio, the comorbidity with OCD and ADHD, and the marked diminution of tics during sleep— provide promising clues concerning the underlying neurobiology of this syndrome (see also Chapters 71 and 141, *this volume*).

Tic Symptoms

The range of symptoms is enormous and includes motor and phonic tics (sudden repetitive movements, gestures, or utterances that typically occur in bouts and mimic some aspect of a normal behavioral repertoire). Usually of brief duration, simple motor tics rarely last more than a second. Motor tics vary from abrupt movements such as rapid, forceful eye-blinking, sudden head jerks, and shoulder

shrugs, to more complex and purposive or dystonic behaviors such as gestures of the hands or face or a slow sustained head tilt. Phonic or vocal tics range from simple sniffing or throat-clearing to fragments of words and phrases.

Clinical rating instruments presently in use focus on the number, frequency, intensity, and complexity of tics as well as the degree of interference that they can cause (30). Other useful instruments focus on how noticeable the tics are to others, whether they elicit comments or curiosity, and the extent to which they make the patient's appearance odd or bizarre (58). Videotaped tic counts can also provide valuable information for medication trials (33,59) and acute challenge studies (5,6,39).

Premonitory Urges

Less well appreciated are the sensorimotor phenomena that frequently accompany tics and obsessive–compulsive behavior. These experiences include (a) premonitory feelings or urges that are relieved with the performance of the tic (8,37) and (b) a need to perform tics or compulsions until they are felt to be "just right" (38).

Natural History

As described by Georges Gilles de la Tourette and as is reported in virtually every series, the modal age of onset of motor tics is 6–7 years of age, with a range from 2 to 16 or 17. The symptoms usually begin as transient bouts of motor tics involving the eyes, face, or head. Typically, the phonic symptoms begin somewhat later at 10–11 years of age. This is also the point at which the patient typically begins to have some awareness of the premonitory sensory phenomena. Tics increase during periods of stress and fatigue. Some patients notice an in-

J. F. Leckman, D. L. Pauls, and D. J. Cohen: Yale University, Child Study Center, New Haven, Connecticut 06510.

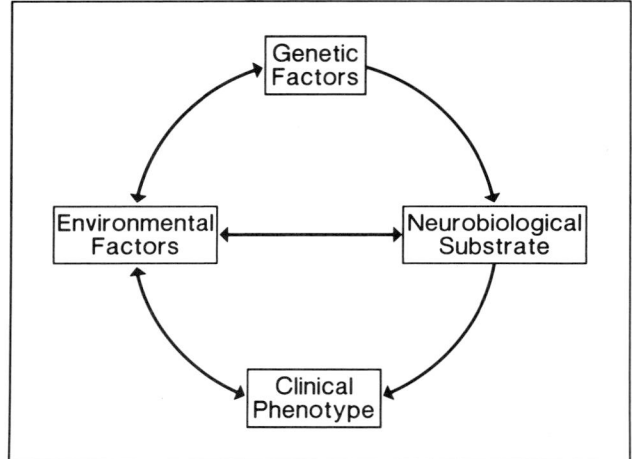

FIG. 1. Pathogenesis of tic disorders. Interactions among genetic factors, neurobiological substrates, and epigenetic or environmental risk and protective factors in the production of clinical phenotypes. (Adapted from ref. 35.)

crease in tics during periods of thermal stress (39). Sleep is associated with a marked reduction in tics (20).

Waxing and waning of the symptoms are characteristic. Although a more or less stable and distinctive repertoire of tics emerges over time for a given individual, the range and variability of these symptoms are remarkable. Tic symptoms are usually at their worst from the time of onset through early puberty, with gradual improvement thereafter. However, in its most extreme form, TS is a lifelong condition that is chronically disabling in adulthood due to nearly constant volleys of motor and phonic tics that interfere with work tasks and verbal communication. Although rare, self-abusive tics such as hitting the face can also occur as can virulent coprolalia and copropraxia.

The factors that influence the natural history of TS have yet to be fully established but are likely to include gender-specific hormonal factors, adverse prenatal conditions, postnatal stress, and drug exposures, as well as comorbid medical and psychiatric conditions (see section entitled "Epigenetic and Environmental Factors," below).

Comorbidity

Tic symptoms are usually not the child's first or only difficulty. Attentional deficits, impulsivity, and motoric hyperactivity are commonplace, affecting 40–50% of all referred TS cases (9). When present, these symptoms are finely interwoven with the tic symptoms and can often have disastrous effects on peer acceptance, school performance, and parental supports (14,66).

For more than 60% of TS patients, persistent obsessive–compulsive symptoms appear a few years after the onset of the tic symptoms (36). Some portion of these

individuals go on to develop full-blown OCD and may experience enduring obsessive–compulsive symptoms even though their TS symptoms have otherwise diminished. As noted below (see section entitled "Genetic Factors"), the OCD associated with TS may be the result of the same underlying genetic vulnerability as the tic symptoms. Tic-related OCD, although quite similar in most respects to other forms of OCD, may be distinctive in terms of (a) its earlier age of onset, (b) the prominence of such symptoms as ritualized touching, tapping, and rubbing, and (c) its relative refractoriness to serotonin reuptake inhibitors and responsiveness to neuroleptic augmentation (22).

In adulthood many TS patients suffer from other comorbid psychiatric disorders, including major depression and various anxiety disorders (9,50).

Epidemiology

Once thought to be a rare condition, the prevalence of TS is now estimated to be between 1 and 6 cases per 1000 boys, and milder variants of the syndrome are likely to occur in 2–10% of the population (3,11,69). Consistent with the course of illness described above, the frequency of TS among adults is reduced by at least an order of magnitude (4).

GENETIC FACTORS

The etiology of TS remains unknown. Twin studies indicate that genetic factors are likely to play an important role in the transmission and expression of TS and related phenotypes (25,54,68). Specifically, monozygotic (MZ) twin pairs have been found to be highly concordant for TS (53%), and if other tic disorders are included, the overall concordance for the MZ pairs is substantially higher (>75%). The concordance of same-sex dizygotic twin pairs is much lower (8% for TS or 23% if other tic disorders are included). These concordance figures are consistent with a genetic etiology with variable phenotypic expression.

In addition to other tic disorders, twin and family studies also provide evidence that some forms of OCD may be etiologically related to TS (48,54,68). The family genetic data have been less helpful in sorting out the relationship between TS and ADHD. In the largest series, ADHD among the first-degree relatives was most strongly associated with the TS proband having ADHD as well, suggesting that the vulnerability to ADHD symptoms is familial in those families (49). In addition, there is a greater than chance association of TS and ADHD among those first-degree relatives who have TS. However, this association is not observed in the case of other first-degree relatives who have tic disorders.

Using mathematical models of genetic transmission and

either a broad or narrow definition of the affected phenotype, the distribution of affected individuals within families follows a pattern consistent with an autosomal dominant form of transmission (15,48). This finding, coupled with recent advances in human genetics, has led directly to the initiation of genetic linkage studies in an effort to identify the chromosomal location of the putative TS gene.

The potential benefits of detecting linkage to a chromosomal region are many and include improved diagnostic capability, the identification of high-risk individuals, and the potential to use molecular genetic techniques to identify the TS vulnerability gene itself and to unravel the pathophysiology of these related disorders from their source. Thus far, more than 80% genome has been excluded (45,47), and the search continues.

Advances in molecular neurobiology make this a propitious time to search for the putative TS vulnerability gene. Numerous candidate genes, such as the family of dopamine receptors, are being characterized (16,17). In addition, it is now possible to use highly efficient polymerase chain reaction (PCR) techniques to generate linkage data.

In addition to their use in linkage studies, the characterization of functional allelic variants of key genes involved in the pathobiology of TS may also prove to be a promising area of investigation. At present, the only polymorphic systems that have been examined in detail are the dopamine D2 receptor locus on chromosome 11 and the dopamine D3 receptor locus on chromosome. Although doubts remain about the functional role of the allelic variants, some investigators have claimed that specific alleles are associated with a more severe course of disease (12). Some of these results, however, have not been confirmed by other investigators (18).

EPIGENETIC AND ENVIRONMENTAL FACTORS

Studies of monozygotic twins indicate that epigenetic or environmental factors play an important role in mediating the extent to which the genetic vulnerability to TS and related disorders is expressed (25,54). Apart from gender (males are 3 to 4 times more likely than females to develop TS) and adverse perinatal conditions (within symptomatically discordant monozygotic twin pairs the more severely affected twin almost always has a lower birth weight than the less severely affected twin), other epigenetic factors that mediate expression have not been unequivocally identified (25,27,31,52). The epigenetic factors may include exposure to high levels of gonadal androgens and stress hormones during early central nervous system (CNS) development, as well as exposure to conditions that affect the delivery of oxygen and nutrients to the developing fetus (25,27,31,52). Other possible candidates include: exposure to chronic intermittent psy-

chosocial stress in the postnatal period (27); exposure to thermal stress (39); exposure to anabolic steroids (32); exposure to cocaine or other CNS stimulants (43); and recurrent streptococcal infections.

The prospects for being able to identify specific or nonspecific risk and/or protective factors will be greatly enhanced when the TS vulnerability gene has been mapped. By selecting biologically homogeneous high-risk carriers, investigators will be able to control for a significant portion of the biological variance so that detecting effects of a risk or protective factor will be more readily accomplished. The successful identification of risk and/or protective factors may lead directly to early interventions that will limit, if not prevent, clinically significant forms of TS and OCD.

NEUROANATOMIC SUBSTRATES

Although there have been relatively few neuropathological studies of TS brains, there is a substantial body of data that implicate the basal ganglia and related cortical and thalamic structures in the pathobiology of Tourette's syndrome and OCD. These data include the ameliorative effects on tic behaviors following neurosurgical lesions to thalamic nuclei and following procedures that isolate regions of the prefrontal cortex (34).

Recent magnetic resonance imaging (MRI) studies have revealed abnormalities in the structural lateralization of basal ganglia structures in both children and adults with TS (52,64). Data have also been presented that indicate that adult TS subjects, on average, have smaller corpus callosi as measured in the midsagittal plane (53). These structural alterations are likely to have functional consequences as well as provide clues concerning the location and timing of events in the developing CNS that directly influence the emergence and course of TS and related symptomatology such as ADHD and the premonitory urges.

Functional brain imaging studies suggest that the abnormalities associated with TS may not be limited to the basal ganglia. Positron emission tomography (PET) studies have demonstrated altered patterns of cerebral metabolism including decreased regional metabolic activity in frontal, cingulate, and insular cortices, as well as in the striatum, in TS subjects (65). Some investigators have also reported increased metabolic rates in the superior cortical convexities including the supplementary motor area (65). Functional neuroimaging studies of cerebral blood flow in TS patients using single photon emission computerize tomography (SPECT) techniques have yielded either similar findings or no differences when compared to normal control subjects (19,55).

It is intriguing to note that many of these same areas have been implicated in other PET studies of OCD and ADHD. OCD appears to involve metabolic changes in orbital frontal cortices and the caudate (2,44), whereas ADHD may involve superior sensorimotor areas centered in the premotor cortices (70).

Functionally, the basal ganglia are composed of fiber tracks that contribute to the multiple parallel cortico-striato-thalamocortical circuits (CSTC) that concurrently subserve a wide variety of sensorimotor, motor, oculomotor, cognitive, and "limbic" processes. Leckman et al. (34) have hypothesized that TS and etiologically related forms of OCD are associated with a failure to inhibit subsets of these CSTC mini-circuits. Based on this hypothesis, it is anticipated that the frequently encountered tics involving the face would be associated with a failure of inhibition of those mini-circuits that include the ventromedian areas of the caudate and putamen that receive topographic projections from the orofacial regions of the primary motor and premotor cortex. Using similar logic, we and others (34) have hypothesized that obsessions with aggressive and sexual themes would be associated with a failure to inhibit portions of the limbic mini-circuits, whereas counting obsessions and obsessive need for symmetry and exactness would be the result of a failure to inhibit some number of prefrontal mini-circuits. The potential role of the corpus callosum in mediating this disinhibition has not been explored.

Other aspects of the circuitry of the basal ganglia may provide important clues concerning the anatomical distribution of motor tics and the "choice" of obsessive themes frequently encountered in forms of OCD related to TS. Specifically, the unidirectional input from the amygdala to widespread areas of the nucleus accumbens and ventral portions of the caudate and putamen appears to overlap those areas most affected in TS-related OCD (26). Studies in primates and humans have also shown that stimulation of the amygdala produces motor and vocal activity reminiscent of the symptoms of TS.

In addition, reciprocal connections between midbrain sites (periaqueductal gray, substantia nigra, and the ventral tegmental area), portions of the hypothalamus, and structures in the basal ganglia and amygdala are likely to play a critical role in the genesis and maintenance of the symptoms of TS. These connections may also contribute to the stress sensitivity (including sensitivity to thermal stress observed in a limited number of subjects) of the disorder and the more frequent expression of TS in males than females (many of these structures contain receptors for gonadal steroids and are responsive to alterations in their hormonal environment) (see subsection entitled "Gender-Specific Endocrine Factors," below).

While the neurophysiological defect that underlies TS and etiologically related conditions remains unknown, a complete understanding of these disorders will likely illuminate mechanisms that regulate the activity of the multiple parallel CSTC circuits that subserve much of our normal cognitive, behavioral, and emotive repertoire. Advances in this area will also lead to the identification of specific neuroanatomical sites that may be crucially involved in the genesis of TS and OCD symptoms which in turn may be of value in isolating candidate genes that are uniquely expressed in these regions.

NEUROCHEMICAL AND NEUROPHARMACOLOGICAL DATA

Among the most remarkable developments in the neurobiology of the basal ganglia and related structures over the past decade are the extensive immunohistochemical studies which have demonstrated the presence of a wide spectrum of differently distributed classic neurotransmitters, neuromodulators, and neuropeptides (23,46). The functional status of a number of these systems has been evaluated in Tourette's syndrome (see ref. 38 for a review). Thus far, the mesencephalic monoaminergic (dopaminergic, noradrenergic, and serotonergic) projections that modulate the activity of the CSTC circuits have received the greatest amount of attention in TS and in related conditions such as OCD and ADHD. Despite their central role in the functioning of the CSTC circuits, the data concerning the roles of various excitatory and inhibitory amino acid neurotransmitter systems are sparse and inconclusive. Other evidence has focused attention on the endogenous opioid projections from the striatum to the pallidum and substantia nigra that form one portion of the CSTC circuits (6,7). Some data implicate cholinergic systems as well. More recently, investigators have focussed their attention on the role of components of intracellular signaling systems and the role of gender-specific hormonal factors.

Dopaminergic Systems

Based largely on parallels between the tics, vocalizations, and obsessive–compulsive behaviors seen in some patients with encephalitis lethargica, Devinsky (13) has suggested that TS is the result of altered dopaminergic function in the midbrain. Other data implicating central dopaminergic mechanisms include clinical trials in which haloperidol and other neuroleptics which preferentially block dopaminergic D2 receptors have been found to be effective in the partial suppression of tics in a majority of TS patients (59). Tic suppression has also been reported following administration of agents that reduce dopamine synthesis (see ref. 28 for a review). Alternatively, increased tics have been reported following withdrawal of neuroleptics and following exposure to agents which increase central dopaminergic activity such as L-DOPA and CNS stimulants including cocaine. The exacerbation of tics with CNS stimulants remains a controversial area (58), with some investigators reporting no change in tic symptoms (67). Transient increases in tics following thermal stress (in a subset of patients) may also be mediated by increased dopaminergic activity (39).

Investigators have also reported that TS patients have lower mean levels of homovanillic acid (HVA), a major metabolite of brain dopamine, in CSF (28) and in certain brain regions (1). Recent preliminary PET studies of brain dopamine D2 receptors, however, do not support the view that there are increased numbers of these receptors in the few TS patients that have been studied (63). Additional imaging studies are needed to address fully the potential abnormalities of receptor number, affinity, and distribution across the growing family of dopamine receptors. Indeed, the recent molecular characterization of a large family of dopaminergic receptors holds considerable promise both in terms of potential treatments and in terms of the development of safe and effective pharmacological probes.

More recently, Singer et al. (62) have reported increased levels of the dopamine transporter sites in the postmortem striatum of a small number of TS subjects. Studies are presently underway to evaluate this finding using radioligands and in vivo neuroimaging techniques.

The role of dopaminergic systems in tic-related OCD has not been as carefully studied as it has in TS, despite both preclinical and clinical evidence implicating dopamine in some obsessive–compulsive behaviors. The preclinical evidence consists of animal models for compulsive behavior that involve the induction of stereotypies by agents that increase dopaminergic activity, such as amphetamine, bromocriptine, the dopamine precursor L-DOPA, and the D2/D3 agonist quinpirole (see ref. 22 for review). Complex repetitive behaviors that resemble naturally occurring obsessive–compulsive symptoms have also been observed in subjects who abuse stimulants. These so-called "punding" behaviors include repetitive cleaning, washing, grooming, and hoarding. In addition, there have been multiple reports of the occurrence of obsessive–compulsive symptoms, alone or in association with tics, in postencephalitic parkinsonian patients (as noted above, the neuropathology of this condition involves the basal ganglia and midbrain dopaminergic systems).

Direct evidence for a role of dopamine in mediating tic-related OCD includes the observations of McDougle and co-workers that many OCD patients with a personal or family history of a tic disorder are less responsive to serotonergic reuptake blocking agents than other OCD patients (41) and that neuroleptic augmentation of the reuptake blocker leads to further improvement in the OCD symptoms (42).

In sum, dopaminergic systems have been repeatedly implicated in the pathophysiology of TS and related disorders. The next decade should bring notable advances in terms of the availability of (a) highly selective pharmacological agents that may have therapeutic value and (b) novel ligands that will permit state-of-the-art neuroimaging studies.

Noradrenergic Systems

Evidence of noradrenergic involvement in the pathophysiology of TS is based, in part, on the reported beneficial effects of clonidine. Although the effectiveness of clonidine remains controversial (21), we have recently completed a large double-blind, placebo-controlled trial in TS subjects that again demonstrated a beneficial effect of this agent on motor tics and some of the symptoms of ADHD (33). Additional support has been based on (a) the rebound exacerbations of tics in patients abruptly withdrawn from clonidine and (b) the finding of blunted growth-hormone response to clonidine challenge in children with TS (28). Most recently, a series of adult TS patients were found to have elevated levels of CSF norepinephrine (NE) and to have excreted high levels of urinary NE in response to the stress of the lumbar puncture (LP) (7). However, studies of central and peripheral levels of 3-methoxy-4-hydroxyphenylethylene glycol (MHPG), a major metabolite of NE, have been inconclusive (28). In addition, no differences in platelet alpha-2 adrenoreceptors or in plasma NE have been found (28).

If noradrenergic mechanisms play an important role in TS, the neurobiological basis for these effects has not been established. A number of reports indicate that the entral tegmental area, a collection of dopamine-containing neurons that innervate mesolimbic areas (nucleus accumbens, olfactory tubercles, amygdala) and mesocortical sites such as the prefrontal cortex, receives noradrenergic afferents from the brainstem and that these inputs may be of functional significance in regulating its activity. As noted above, many of these sites are part of the ventral striatopallidal complex and related neural circuits that are involved in the control of motor behaviors that are responsive to emotional stimuli. Noradrenergic projections to the neocortex may also play some role in modulating the activity of some of the CSTC circuits.

At the level of receptor function, clonidine has been traditionally viewed as a selective alpha-2 adrenoceptor agonist active at either pre- or postsynaptic sites, and previous reports have speculated that the effectiveness of clonidine in treating TS may be due to the ability of alpha-2 adrenoceptor agonists to reduce the firing rate and the release of norepinephrine from central noradrenergic neurons and to modulate indirectly the firing of dopamine neurons in the ventral tegmental area. While this mechanism cannot be discounted at present, mounting evidence of heterogeneity among the alpha-2 class of adrenoceptors and their distinctive distribution within relevant brain regions adds further complexity and suggests that these subtypes may account for the differential responsiveness of particular behavioral features of this syndrome to clonidine treatment.

Serotonergic Systems

Ascending serotonergic projections from the dorsal raphe have been repeatedly invoked as playing a role in the pathophysiology of both TS and OCD. The most compelling evidence relates to OCD and is based largely on the well-established efficacy of potent serotonin reuptake inhibitors (RUIs) such as clomipramine and fluvoxamine in the treatment of OCD (22). However, some investigators have reported that the serotonin RUIs are less effective in treating tic-related OCD compared to other forms of OCD (41). It is also doubtful that treatment with serotonin RUIs diminish tic symptoms given recent data from clinical trials.

Additional evidence has come from pharmacological challenge studies in which serotonergic agonists such as m-chlorophenylpiperazine (m-CPP) were found to exacerbate obsessive–compulsive symptoms in some patients (22) or were associated with a blunted plasma prolactin response. This last observation was interpreted as evidence for down-regulation of postsynaptic 5-HT receptors in some OCD patients, but this variable pattern of response has not been linked to the individual's personal or family history of tics.

Finally, preliminary postmortem brain studies in TS have recently shown that serotonin and the related compounds tryptophan (TRP) and 5-hydroxy-indoleacetic acid (5-HIAA) may be globally decreased in the basal ganglia and other areas receiving projections from the dorsal raphe (1). Although preliminary, these postmortem findings are consistent with previous observations of significantly lower levels of CSF 5-HIAA (28), plasma TRP, whole-blood serotonin, and 24-hr urinary serotonin in TS patients compared to normal controls (10,28) (see Chapters 36–42, this volume, for background).

Excitatory Amino Acid Systems

With few exceptions, the limited data from the examination of postmortem brain material do not indicate that excitatory amino acid systems play a major role in TS. Except for a report of reduced levels of glutamate (GLU) in the globus pallidus, levels of GLU and aspartate in a wide range of telencephalic brain regions appear to be normal as is the level of GLU decarboxylase in the cortex (1). As a result of the reduced levels of GLU in the globus pallidus, Anderson and co-workers have hypothesized that the GLU output from the subthalamic nucleus is abnormal in TS. Further work is needed to clarify the importance of these observations (see Chapter 7, this volume, for background).

Inhibitory Amino Acid Systems

Although inhibitory amino acid neurotransmitters, particularly gamma-aminobutyric acid (GABA), are the principal neurotransmitters of the striatopallidal and pallidothalamic projections that form two major portions of CSTC circuits, neurochemical studies of GABA levels in various brain regions, CSF, and plasma have not shown significant differences between TS and controls (28). Similarly, although the long-acting benzodiazepine clonazepam is frequently used in the treatment of refractory TS, the scientific data supporting its efficacy are limited to small-scale trials. Additional work is needed to document the efficacy of clonazepam or related compounds and to clarify the role of inhibitory amino acids in the pathobiology of TS and related conditions (see Chapter 8, this volume, for background).

Endogenous Opioid Peptides

Endogenous opioid peptides (EOPs) are localized in structures of the extrapyramidal system, are known to interact with central dopaminergic and GABAergic neurons, and are likely to be importantly involved in the gating of motor functions. Two of the three families of EOPs, dynorphin and met-enkephalin, are highly concentrated and similarly distributed in the basal ganglia and substantia nigra. In addition, significant levels of opiate receptor binding have been detected in both primate and human neostriatum and substantia nigra.

EOPs have been directly implicated in the pathophysiology of TS. Haber and co-workers reported decreased levels of dynorphin A(1-17) immunoreactivity in striatal fibers projecting to the globus pallidus in postmortem material from a small number of TS patients (24). This observation, coupled with the neuroanatomic distribution of dynorphin, its broad range of motor and behavioral effects, and its modulatory interactions with striatal dopaminergic systems, suggested that dynorphin may play a role in the pathobiology of TS. Additional evidence comes from a CSF study of dynorphin A(1-8) and from studies of the opiate antagonists and agonists (5,6,29). Data from these studies lend additional support to the hypothesis that opioids exert a modulatory effect on TS symptoms. In particular, the results are most consistent with an effect mediated by mu rather than kappa receptors (see Chapter 46, this volume, for background).

Cholinergic Systems

Throughout the cortex and striatum, local circuit cholinergic neurons are likely to play an important role in modulating the CSTC circuits. The most compelling recent evidence of cholinergic involvement in the pathobiology of TS concerns the augmentation of the tic-reducing effects of D2 dopamine receptor blocking agents by nicotine gum (40). Elevated erythrocyte choline has also been proposed as a trait marker in TS, although the supporting data are equivocal (28). The remaining neurochemical studies (including reports of normal levels of cortical and CSF acetylcholinesterase activity) and psychopharmacological data (involving clinical trials of choline, lecithin, and deanol and challenge studies with physostigmine) have been disappointing (56; see ref. 28 for review of earlier work in this area; see Chapters 9–12, *this volume*, for background).

Second Messenger Systems

Singer et al. (61) have reported reduced levels of cyclic adenosine 3′,5′-monophosphate (cAMP) activity in several areas of the neocortex based on the analysis of four postmortem brain specimens. Additional studies are needed to clarify the potential interactions of cAMP metabolism and TS symptoms.

Gender-Specific Endocrine Factors

The results of genetic studies which have shown that TS is transmitted within families as an autosomal dominant trait suggest that males and females should be at equal risk. However, as previously noted, males are in fact several times more frequently affected than females (58). This observation has led us and others to hypothesize that androgenic steroids acting at key developmental periods (the prenatal period when the brain is being formed, adrenarche when adrenal androgens first appear at age 5 to 7 years, and puberty) may be involved in determining the natural history of TS and related disorders (32,35,51). This may be a direct effect of androgenic steroids, or it may be due in part to the action of estradiol (formed in key brain regions by the aromatization of testosterone).

Normal surges in testosterone and other androgenic steroids during critical periods in male fetal development are known to be involved in the production of long-term functional augmentation of subsequent hormonal challenges (as in adrenarche and during puberty) and in the formation of structural CNS dimorphisms (60). In recent years, several sexually dimorphic brain regions have been described, including portions of the amygdala (and related limbic areas) and the hypothalamus (including the medial preoptic area that mediates the body's response to thermal stress). These regions contain high levels of androgen and estrogen receptors and are known to influence activity in the basal ganglia both directly and indirectly. It is also of note that some of the neurochemical and neuropeptidergic systems implicated in TS and related disorders, such as dopamine, serotonin, and the opioids, are involved with these regions and appear to be regulated by sex-specific factors.

Further support for a role for androgens comes from case reports of tic exacerbation following anabolic steroid abuse (32) and from pilot study data from open trials of antiandrogens in patients with severe OCD and TS (51).

Some evidence also supports a role of estrogens in tic exacerbation. Specifically, Schwabe and Konkol (57) reported that approximately one-quarter of women with TS experience exacerbation of their tics premenstrually during the estrogenic phase of the cycle.

PROMISING AREAS FOR CLINICAL AND BASIC RESEARCH

Building on the advances of the past decade and the synergistic potential among the various areas of active research, substantial progress can be anticipated in the identification of risk and protective factors that mediate the expression of TS. Advances in related fields of developmental neurobiology may also clarify the mechanisms by which these risk and protective factors operate.

Phenomenology and Clinimetrics

Assessment methodologies are critical to clinical research. They are indispensable in family genetic studies and natural history studies as well as in drug trials. Although several valid and reliable clinical rating instruments are now available, further refinements are needed. Special attention needs to be focused on the relationship of clinician severity ratings and various videotaped protocols for tic counting (Chappell et al., *personal communication*). Careful attention to the dynamics of tics and their occurrence in bouts may reveal new avenues for understanding the interface between the activity of specific brain circuits and behavior and may also reveal insights into the waxing and waning of tics over longer time intervals (Peterson et al., *personal communication*).

Further research in the detection of structural and functional CNS abnormalities, undertaken with a fuller appreciation of the range of phenotypic expression and comorbidities associated with TS, will set the stage for a promising set of neuropsychological and neurophysiological studies which focus on specific brain circuits. The determination of structure–function relationships may yield important insights into the pathophysiology of these disorders and may also provide the groundwork for the development of the next generation of assessment procedures. For example, it may be possible to determine whether or not the diminished midsagittal cross-sectional area of the corpus callosum seen in many TS cases (52) has any functional significance in terms of the interhemispheric transfer of information and whether or not such deficits, if they do exist, play a role in the progression of the disorder or the development of certain comorbid symptoms.

With the availability of valid and reliable instruments, the time is ripe for a range of clinical studies using case–control, prospective longitudinal designs to examine in more detail the natural history of these disorders. Some of the most promising critical periods of development include the prenatal period which may well set the stage for later tic severity, middle childhood with the emergence of ADHD, tics, and OC symptoms, and adolescence with the progression of tic and obsessive–compulsive symptoms in some cases and the attenuation of these behaviors in most others.

Genetics

Despite the slow progress of recent years in efforts to identify the gene(s) involved in TS, the opportunities that will accompany breakthroughs in this area are unparalleled. Improved diagnostic procedures will result once a chromosomal locus is established, and, with a full characterization of the abnormal gene and its products, a whole series of possibilities will unfold, including the development of animal models. Identification of genetically at-risk individuals will also enrich prospective longitudinal studies of at-risk children and facilitate the study of epigenetic risk and protective factors by controlling for a crucial and substantial source of biological variation. In the meantime, attention to functionally significant allelic variations that exist at certain loci may yield important information about genes of small effect that impact on the development and course of this syndrome.

Given the recent progress in the development of highly informative genetic markers, a high-resolution map of the human is within view. This will greatly facilitate the search for the TS gene. Other developments in the area of developmental neurobiology may also play an important role in the identification of sets of candidate genes that are uniquely active in specific brain regions of interest such as the basal ganglia.

Neurobiology

The natural history of TS offers many clues concerning the underlying neurobiology of this syndrome. Examples include the role of gender-specific hormonal factors, the reduction of tics during sleep, the exacerbation of tics with stress and fatigue, the existence of premonitory sensory urges, and the frequent co-occurrence of comorbid ADHD and OCD. Clinical studies focusing on these areas, taken together with advances in related fields (e.g., the studies of sexually dimorphic brain regions, advances in our understanding of the neurobiology of stress, fatigue, and sleep), may lead to deeper insights into the pathobiology of TS.

The development of a range of neuroimaging techniques, from ligand-based studies to functional MRI techniques, offers some of the most appealing studies for the next generation of TS research. For example, the recent report of increased levels of the dopamine transporter in postmortem striatal tissue (62) needs to be followed up with functional brain studies with ligands specific for these sites (see Chapters 16 and 28, *this volume*, for background).

Intervention Research

Incremental advances in the treatment and prevention of TS and related disorders can be expected. Hopeful signs on the horizon include the development of pharmacological agents with increased specificity to particular dopamine and serotonin receptors. The most pressing clinical areas include the severely affected individuals, particularly those with comorbid ADHD and OCD that are refractory to currently available agents. Innovative treatments may emerge from the range of studies described above. Examples include the use of antiandrogens such as flutamide (51). The use of combined pharmacological and nonpharmacological treatments also needs to be explored, particularly in children with comorbid ADHD and/or OCD. Efforts to prevent the emergence of severe forms of tic disorder by diminishing the impact of risk factors associated with pregnancy may be worthwhile (25,27,31).

CONCLUSION

TS and related disorders are likely to be associated with detectable alterations in brain function. Systematic and sustained investigation of possible pathobiological mechanisms in TS has led to promising new treatment strategies. Advances in the neurosciences are continuing at a rapid pace. Although the enormous complexity of the neurochemical, neuroendocrine, and neuropharmacological data in TS and OCD does not yield readily to simplistic explanations focused on a single neurotransmitter or neuromodulatory systems, it is likely that significant progress will be made over the next decade with regard to the biological causes and determinants of TS and related disorders and the development of safe and effective treatments.

ACKNOWLEDGMENTS

This work was supported in part, by NIH grants MH44843, MH49351, MH00508, NS16648, HD03008, RR00125, RR06022 (General Clinical Research Centers), and MH30929 (Mental Health Clinical Research Center) and by the Tourette Syndrome Association. The author would also like to acknowledge the many important scientific and practical contributions made to this research program by Drs. Phillip B. Chappell, Wayne K. Goodman, Mark A. Riddle, George M. Anderson, Bradley S. Peterson, James Duncan, John T. Walkup, Dorothy E. Grice, Paul J. Lombroso, Yanki Yazgan, Bruce Wexler, and Robert A. King and by Ms. Sharon I. Ort, Mr. Lawrence D. Scahill, and Ms. Maureen T. McSwiggin-Hardin. A complete set of citations is available from the authors.

REFERENCES

1. Anderson GM, Pollak ES, Chatterjee D, Leckman JF, Riddle MA, Cohen DJ. Postmortem analyses of brain monoamines and amino acids in Tourette's syndrome: a preliminary study of subcortical regions. *Arch Gen Psychiatry* 1992;49:584–586.
2. Baxter LR Jr, Schwartz JA, Bergman KS, et al. Caudate glucose metabolic rate changes with both drug and behavior therapy for obsessive–compulsive disorder. *Arch Gen Psychiatry* 1992;49:681–689.
3. Burd L, Kerbeshian J, Wikenheiser M, et al. A prevalence study of Gilles de la Tourette syndrome in North Dakota school-age children. *J Am Acad Child Adolesc Psychiatry* 1986;25:552–553.
4. Burd L, Kerbeshian J, Wikenheiser M, Fisher W. Prevalence of Gilles de la Tourette's syndrome in North Dakota adults. *Am J Psychiatry* 1986;143:787–788.
5. Chappell PB, Leckman JF, Riddle MA, et al. Neuroendocrine and behavioral effects of naloxone in Tourette syndrome. In: Chase TN, Friedhoff AJ, Cohen DJ, eds. *Advances in neurology,* vol 58. New York: Raven Press, 1992;253–262.
6. Chappell PB, Leckman JF, Scahill L, Hardin MT, Anderson GM, Cohen DJ. Neuroendocrine and behavioral effects of the selective kappa agonist spiradoline mesylate (U-62066E) in Tourette's syndrome. *Psychol Res* 1993;47:267–280.
7. Chappell PB, Riddle MA, Anderson GM, et al. Enhanced stress responsivity of Tourette syndrome patients undergoing lumbar puncture. *Biol Psychol* 1994;[in press].
8. Cohen AJ, Leckman JF. Sensory phenomena associated with Gilles de la Tourette's syndrome. *J Clin Psychiatry* 1992;53:319–323.
9. Comings DE, Comings BG. A controlled study of Tourette syndrome. *Am J Hum Genet* 1987;41:701–741.
10. Comings DE. Blood serotonin and tryptophan in Tourette syndrome. *Am J Med Genet* 1990;36:418–430.
11. Comings DE, Himes JA, Comings BG. An epidemiological study of Tourette's syndrome in a single school district. *J Clin Psychiatry* 1990;51:463–469.
12. Comings DE, Comings BG, Muhleman D, et al. The dopamine D2 receptor locus as a modifying gene in neuropsychiatric disorders. *JAMA* 1991;266:1793–1800.
13. Devinsky O. Neuroanatomy of Gilles de la Tourette's syndrome: possible midbrain involvement. *Arch Neurol* 1983;40:508–514.
14. Dykens E, Leckman JF, Riddle, MA, Hardin MT, Schwartz S, Cohen DJ. Intellectual, academic and adaptive functioning of Tourette syndrome children with and without attention deficit disorder. *J Abnorm Child Psychol* 1990;18:607–615.
15. Eapen V, Pauls DL, Robertson MM. Evidence for autosomal dominant transmission in Gilles de la Tourette syndrome—United Kingdom cohort study. *Br J Psychiatry* 1993;162:593–596.
16. Gelernter J, Pakstis AJ, Pauls DL, et al. Gilles de la Tourette syndrome not linked to D2-dopamine receptor. *Arch Gen Psychiatry* 1990;47:1073–1077.
17. Gelernter J, Kennedy JL, Grandy DK, et al. Exclusion of close linkage of Tourette's syndrome to D1 dopamine receptor. *Am J Psychiatry* 1993;150:449–453.
18. Gelernter J, Pauls DL, Leckman JF, Kidd KK, Kurlan R. D2 dopamine receptor (DRD2) alleles do not influence severity of Tourette syndrome: DRD2 as a gene of no proven effect in neuropsychiatric disorders. *Arch Neurology* 1994;51:397–400.
19. George MS, Trimble MR, Costa DC, Robertson MM, Ring HA, Ell PJ. Elevated frontal cerebral blood flow in Gilles de la Tourette syndrome: a ^{99m}Tc-HMPAO SPECT study. *Psychiatry Res* 1992;45:143–151.
20. Glaze DG, Frost JD, Jankovich J. Sleep in Gilles de la Tourette's syndrome: disorder of arousal. *Neurology* 1983;33:586–592.
21. Goetz CG, Tanner CM, Wilson RS, et al. Clonidine and Gilles de la Tourette syndrome: double-blind study using objective rating method. *Ann Neurol* 1987;21:307–310.
22. Goodman WK, McDougle CJ, Price LH, et al. Beyond the serotonin hypothesis: a role for dopamine in some forms of obsessive–compulsive disorder? *J Clin Psychiatry* 1990;51:36–43.
23. Graybiel AM. Neurotransmitters and neuromodulators in the basal ganglia. *Trends Neurosci* 1990;13:244–251.
24. Haber SN, Wolfer D. Basal ganglia peptidergic staining in Tourette syndrome: a follow-up study. In: Chase TN, Friedhoff AJ, Cohen DJ, eds. *Advances in neurology,* vol 58. New York: Raven Press, 1992;145–150.
25. Hyde TM, Aaronson BA, Randloph C, Rickler KS, Weinberger DR. Relationship of birth weight to the phenotypic expression of Gilles de la Tourette's syndrome in monozygotic twins. *Neurology* 1992;42:652–658.
26. Jadresic D. The role of the amygdaloid complex in Gilles de la Tourette's syndrome. *Br J Psychiatry* 1992;161:532–534.
27. Leckman JF, Price RA, Walkup JT, Ort S, Pauls DL, Cohen DJ. Nongenetic factors in Gilles de la Tourette's syndrome. *Arch Gen Psychiatry* 1987;44:100.
28. Leckman JF, Walkup JT, Riddle MA, et al. Tic disorders. In: Meltzer HY, ed. *Psychopharmacology: the third generation of progress.* New York: Raven Press, 1987;1239–1246.
29. Leckman JF, Riddle MA, Berretini WH, et al. Elevated CSF dynorphin A[1-8] in Tourette's syndrome. *Life Sci* 1988;43:2015–2023.
30. Leckman JF, Riddle MA, Hardin MT, et al. The Yale global tic severity scale: initial testing of a clinician-rated scale of tic severity. *J Am Acad Child Adol Psychiatry* 1989;28:566–573.
31. Leckman JF, Dolnansky ES, Hardin MT, et al. Perinatal factors in the expression of Tourette's syndrome: an exploratory study. *J Am Acad Child Adolesc Psychiatry* 1990;29:220–226.
32. Leckman JF, Scahill L. Possible exacerbation of tics by androgenic steroids. *N Engl J Med* 1990;322:1674.
33. Leckman JF, Hardin MT, Riddle MA, Stevenson J, Ort SI, Cohen DJ. Clonidine treatment of Gilles de la Tourette's syndrome. *Arch Gen Psychiatry* 1991;48:324–328.
34. Leckman JF, Knorr AM, Rasmusson AM, Cohen DJ. Basal ganglia research and Tourette's syndrome. *Trends Neurosci* 1991;14:94.
35. Leckman JF, Pauls DL, Peterson BS, Riddle MA, Anderson GM, Cohen DJ. Pathogenesis of Tourette's syndrome: clues from the clinical phenotype and natural history. In: Chase TN, Friedhoff AJ, DJ Cohen, eds. *Advances in neurology,* vol 58. New York: Raven Press, 1992;15–23.
36. Leckman JF. Tourette's syndrome. In: Hollander E, ed. *Obsessive–compulsive related disorders.* Washington, DC: American Psychiatric Press, 1993;113–138.
37. Leckman JF, Walker DE, Cohen DJ. Premonitory urges in Tourette's syndrome. *Am J Psychiatry* 1993;150:98–102.
38. Leckman JF, Walker DE, Goodman WK, Pauls DL, Cohen DJ. ''Just right'' perceptions associated with compulsive behavior in Tourette's syndrome. *Am J Psychiatry* 1994;151:675–680.
39. Lombroso PJ, Mack G, Scahill L, King R, Leckman JF. Exacerbation of Tourette's syndrome associated with thermal stress: a family study. *Neurology* 1991;41:1984–1987.
40. McConville BJ, Sanberg PR, Fogelson MH, et al. The effects of nicotine plus haloperidol compared to nicotine only and placebo in reducing tic severity and frequency in Tourette's disorder. *Biol Psychiatry* 1992;31:832–840.
41. McDougle CJ, Goodman WK, Leckman JF, Barr LC, Heninger GR, Price LH. The efficacy of fluvoxamine in obsessive–compulsive disorder: effects of comorbid chronic tic disorder. *J Clin Psychopharmacol* 1993;13:354–358.
42. McDougle CJ, Goodman WK, Leckman JF, Lee NC, Heninger GR, Price LH. Haloperidol addition in fluvoxamine-refractory obsessive–compulsive disorder: a double-blind, placebo-controlled study in patients with and without tics. *Arch Gen Psychiatry* 1994;51:302–308.
43. Mesulam MM. Cocaine and Tourette's syndrome. *N Engl J Med* 1986;315:398.
44. Nordahl TE, Benkelfat C, Semple WE, et al. Cerebral glucose metabolic rates in obsessive compulsive disorder. *Neuropsychopharmacology* 1989;2:23–28.
45. Pakstis AJ, Heutinik P, Pauls DL, et al. Progress in the search for genetic linkage with Tourette syndrome: an exclusion map covering more than 50% of the autosomal genome. *Am J Hum Genet* 1991;48:281–294.
46. Parent A. *Comparative neurobiology of the basal ganglia.* New York: John Wiley & Sons, 1986.
47. Pauls DL, Pakstis AJ, Kurlan R, et al. Segregation and linkage analysis of Gilles de la Tourette's syndrome and related disorders. *J Am Acad Child Adolesc Psychiatry* 1990;29:195–203.
48. Pauls DL, Raymond CL, Stevenson J, Leckman JF. A family study

of Gilles de la Tourette syndrome. *Am J Hum Genet* 1991;48:154–163.

49. Pauls DL, Leckman JF, Cohen DJ. The familial relationship between Gilles de la Tourette's syndrome, attention deficit disorder, learning disabilities, speech disorders, and stuttering. *J Am Acad Child Adolesc Psychiatry* 1993;32:1044–1050.

50. Pauls DL, Leckman JF, Cohen DJ. Evidence against a genetic relationship between Gilles de la Tourette's syndrome and anxiety, depression, panic and phobic disorders. *Br J Psychiatry* 1994; 164:215–221.

51. Peterson BS, Leckman JF, Scahill L, et al. Steroid hormones and CNS sexual dimorphisms modulate symptom expression in Tourette's syndrome. *Psychoneuroendocrinology* 1992;6:553–563.

52. Peterson BS, Riddle MA, Cohen DJ, et al. Reduced basal ganglia volumes in Tourette's syndrome using 3-dimensional reconstruction techniques from magnetic resonance images. *Neurology* 1993;43:941–949.

53. Peterson BS, Leckman JF, Wetzels R, et al. Corpus callosum morphology from MR images in Tourette's syndrome. *Psychol Res* 1994;[in press].

54. Price AR, Kidd KK, Cohen DJ, Pauls DL, Leckman JF. A twin study of Tourette syndrome. *Arch Gen Psychiatry* 1985;42:815–882.

55. Riddle MA, Rasmusson AM, Woods SW, Hoffer PB. SPECT imaging of cerebral blood flow in Tourette syndrome. In: Chase TN, Friedhoff AJ, Cohen DJ, eds. *Advances in neurology,* vol 58. New York: Raven Press, 1992;207–211.

56. Sallee FR, Kopp U, Hanin I. Controlled study of erythrocyte choline in Tourette syndrome. *Biol Psychiatry* 1992;31:1204–1212.

57. Schwabe MJ, Konkol RJ. Menstrual cycle-related fluctuations of tics in Tourette syndrome. *Pediatr Neurol* 1992;8:43–46.

58. Shapiro AK, Shapiro ES, Young JG, Feinberg TE, eds. In: *Gilles de la Tourette syndrome,* 2nd ed. New York: Raven Press, 1988;451–480.

59. Shapiro ES, Shapiro AK, Fulop G, et al. Controlled study of halo-

peridol, pimozide and placebo for the treatment of Gilles de la Tourette's syndrome. *Arch Gen Psychiatry* 1989;46:722–730.

60. Sikich L, Todd RD. Are neurodevelopmental effects of gonadal hormones related to sex differences in psychiatric illnesses. *Psychiatr Dev* 1988;6:277–310.

61. Singer HS, Hahn IH, Krowiak E, Nelson E, Moran T. Tourette's syndrome: a neurochemical analysis of postmortem cortical brain tissue. *Ann Neurol* 1990;27:443–446.

62. Singer HS, Hahn IH, Moran TH. Abnormal dopamine uptake sites in postmortem striatum from patients with Tourette's syndrome. *Ann Neurol* 1991;30:558–562.

63. Singer HS, Wong DF, Brown JE, et al. Positron emission tomography evaluation of dopamine D2 receptors in adults with Tourette syndrome In: Chase TN, Friedhoff AJ, Cohen DJ, eds. *Advances in neurology,* vol 58. New York: Raven Press, 1992;233–239.

64. Singer HS, Reiss AL, Brown JB, et al. Volumetric MRI changes in basal ganglia of children with Tourette syndrome. *Neurology* 1993;43:950–956.

65. Stoetter B, Braun AR, Randolph C, et al. Functional neuroanatomy of Tourette syndrome: limbic–motor interactions studied with FDG PET. In: Chase TN, Friedhoff AJ, Cohen DJ, eds. *Advances in neurology,* vol 58. New York: Raven Press, 1992;213–226.

66. Stokes A, Bawden HN, Camfield PR, Backman JE, Dooley MB. Peer problems in Tourette's syndrome. *Pediatrics* 1991;87:936–942.

67. Sverd J, Gadow KD, Nolan EE, Sprafkin J, Ezor SN. Methylphenidate in hyperactive boys with comorbic tic disorder. I. clinic evaluations. *Advances in neurology,* vol 58. New York: Raven Press, 1992;271–281.

68. Walkup JT, Leckman JF, Price AR, et al. The relationship between obsessive compulsive disorder and Tourette's syndrome. *Psychopharmacol Bull* 1988;24:375–379.

69. Zahner GEP, Clubb MM, Leckman JF, Pauls DL. The epidemiology of Tourette's syndrome. In: Cohen DJ, Bruun RD, Leckman JF, eds. *Tourette's syndrome and tic disorders.* New York: John Wiley & Sons, 1988;79–89.

70. Zametkin AJ, Nordahl TE, Gross M, et al. Cerebral glucose metabolism in adults with hyperactivity of childhood onset. *N Engl J Med* 1990;323:1361–1366.

Psychopharmacology: The Fourth
Generation of Progress, edited by
Floyd E. Bloom and David J. Kupfer.
Raven Press, Ltd., New York © 1995.

CHAPTER 144

Eating Disturbances and Eating Disorders in Childhood

Regina C. Casper

Whereas eating problems in children are fairly common (74), the classical eating disorders occur rarely (1,31,49). Nevertheless, cases of prepubertal anorexia nervosa as early as age 7 have been reliably documented for over a century (20,49,65). As yet, no clear evidence exists that bulimia nervosa as a syndrome has been observed in children except for two possible retrospectively determined cases recently reported by Kent et al. (41). Overeating episodes, on the other hand, have been described in male and female children in the course of anorexia nervosa, albeit infrequently (28,37,41,73) (see Chapters 136, 137, 138, *this volume*).

In the forthcoming fourth edition of the Diagnostic and Statistical Manual (4), eating disorders will no longer be classified under disorders usually first evident in infancy, childhood, or adolescence as in DSM-III-R (3); instead they have been moved into a separate category. This reclassification is unfortunate because it ignores the evidence that anorexia nervosa does occur in childhood, typically has its onset during adolescence, and is a disorder of childhood and adolescence intricately related to growth and development. "Feeding" disorders of infancy or early childhood remain in the childhood section and will comprise the following three syndromes: pica, rumination disorder, and feeding disorder of infancy or early childhood.

In point of fact, recent retrospective analyses of hospital records have noted an increase in childhood cases. Whether this finding is due to a true increase in incidence or reflects previous underdiagnosis of childhood anorexia nervosa will require more study. For instance, Bryant-Waugh and Lask (12) have shown that few medical practitioners in England are familiar with anorexia nervosa in

childhood. A mere 31% among pediatricians and only 3% of family practitioners in a geographical area mentioned a possible diagnosis of anorexia nervosa when they were asked to evaluate two case vignettes of childhood anorexia nervosa.

Another factor which could contribute to underdiagnosis is the paucity of current diagnostic criteria. Irwin (37) considered the DSM-III diagnostic criteria (2) as too restrictive and insufficiently specific for diagnosing children. On the assumption that excessive fear of becoming obese in the presence of severe underweight was a universally accepted core symptom, Irwin (37) argued that the amount of body weight loss required for the diagnosis in children was too high, because the smaller percentage of total body fat in the prepubescent girl resulted in greater emaciation with less weight loss than in the postpubertal female. These concerns led to a revision of the weight criteria in DSM-III-R (3), with a reduction of the weight loss requirements to 15% instead of 25%. The criteria requiring amenorrhea in females or impotence for males of course do not apply to children.

This chapter, then, in reviewing eating disturbances in infancy and early childhood—pica, rumination disorder, and the principal eating disorder recorded in childhood, anorexia nervosa—relies on clinical evidence rather than a diagnostic schema. The information regarding children's attitudes towards body shape and food, as well as those developmental and environmental factors in childhood which might increase the risk for eating disturbances or an eating disorder to develop, will be presented. Lastly, the problems inherent in previous work and directions for future work will be commented on.

FOOD REFUSAL, WEIGHT CONCERNS, AND FEAR OF FATNESS IN CHILDREN

Children refuse food for all kinds of reasons—aversion to the sight, taste, or form of food; little appetite; or

R. C. Casper: Department of Psychiatry and Behavioral Sciences, Stanford University, Stanford, California 94305-5546.

distractions with more interesting activities, such as play—but food refusal seldom lasts long.

Research has shown that infants and children from a very early age on can control their own food intake and grow normally, given proper guidance and emotional support. Clara Davis (23) demonstrated that newly weaned infants, 6–8 months old, when offered natural food materials, whole grain, fruit, vegetables, eggs, fish, and meat, could feed themselves and grow normally. Birch et al. (8) more recently reported similar observations for children from 2 to 5 years of age. The children's intake was found to be highly variable at individual meals, but the total daily energy intake was relatively constant for each child, because the children tended to adjust their energy intake at successive meals.

In the Western Hemisphere, young children seem to absorb the prevailing cultural values about food and beauty. Worsley (75) reported that 10-year-old Australian boys and girls noticed first the fattening, then the healthy characteristics of food and only lastly expressed sensory preferences. In a study of British school girls aged 12–20 years, Crisp et al. (21) noted that 26% of premenarchal girls compared to 48% in postmenarchal girls were concerned about fatness. Pugliese et al. (55) described ''fear of fatness'' in children as a reason for stunted growth. Out of 201 children evaluated for short stature or delayed puberty or both at the Department of Pediatrics at Cornell Medical College, 14 children (9 boys, 5 girls) aged 9–17, all coming from middle-class families, showed growth failure due to malnutrition as a result of self-imposed restriction of caloric intake arising out of fear of becoming obese. The youngsters resumed normal growth when they were counseled and given an age-appropriate diet.

EPIDEMIOLOGICAL STUDIES ON DIETING, WEIGHT CONCERNS, AND BODY IMAGE

Studies on dieting in adolescence have consistently shown a high prevalence of dieting in the Western Hemisphere, about 60–80% since the early 1970s (51,60,63). A recent study (47) of upper-middle-class white children found that over 40% wanted to be thinner and about 30% had attempted to lose weight, mostly through increasing their activity level. Newspaper reports have conveyed the impression that children are beginning to pay more attention to their weight and that more might be dieting. For example, the *Wall Street Journal* reported that 75% of fourth-grade girls complained that they weighed too much (76), while *Newsweek* quoted a study that half of fourth-grade girls in a middle-class school in San Francisco described themselves as overweight, although only 15% were actually overweight; among the 9-year-olds, 31% thought themselves too fat and almost half were on a diet (52). Richards et al. (58) surveyed nearly 500 students

from fifth to ninth grade from middle- and working-class families in Chicago schools. Between fifth and seventh grade, a mere 15% among the girls expressed extreme weight concerns or dieting attempts, but this proportion increased to 32% by the eighth and ninth grade. The opposite trend was observed for boys: 8–12% expressed weight and eating concerns between the fifth and the seventh grade, and only 3% by the ninth grade.

Few studies of body image perception and satisfaction before the onset of puberty have been conducted. Most have chosen the onset of menarche as a critical variable for research purposes because of its close association with hormonal variables, self-image, body image, and peer and parental relationships during adolescence (11). Koff et al. (42) found that premenarchal girls indicated less satisfaction with body parts than did postmenarchal girls, while Gargiulo et al. (29) found no relationship between menarchal status and body satisfaction. In a comparison of premenarchal and postmenarchal girls on perceptual and subjective measures of body image, few differences were found; premenarchal girls overestimated their thighs to a greater degree than did postmenarchal girls (26). Interestingly, in both groups, a history of having been teased was positively associated with body dissatisfaction. Studies on the association between the timing of onset of menarche and body image have suggested that girls who experience menarche after the age of 14 have a more positive body image than those who have their first menstrual period before the age of 11 (11). Contributing to the negative effects of menarche for girls may be the observation that early maturers are generally shorter than late maturers, but usually weigh more (30).

Staffieri (66) reported that children early on incorporate certain beliefs and expectations in relation to body configuration. Boys 6–10 years old considered the mesomorph (muscular) image most favorable. The thin (ectomorph) figure was viewed as quiet, weak, and fearful, whereas the endomorph (overweight body type) was seen as combative, lazy, and cheating. A recent survey of 36 public schools grades 4–10, commissioned by the American Association of University Women (22), reported a pronounced loss of self-confidence in white girls from prepuberty to middle adolescence, but no change for boys. Whereas most 9-year-old girls were happy with themselves, only 29% still felt that way by high school. For boys, the proportion dropped from 67% to 46%, leaving more boys with more self-esteem than girls. Interestingly, black girls retained their self-confidence into high school.

THE RELATIONSHIP BETWEEN WEIGHT AND DIETING CONCERNS AND PSYCHOLOGICAL WELL-BEING

Negative emotions have been shown to be correlated with body shape dissatisfaction (51,63). Richards et al.

(58) reported positive correlations between body image dissatisfaction and depressive symptoms in fifth- to sixth-grade girls and boys, and in girls only they reported negative correlations between body image satisfaction and weight and eating concerns. Fifth- and sixth-grade boys, who reported more dysphoric affect and lower daily levels of energy and arousal, expressed greater weight and eating concerns.

EATING DISTURBANCES IN INFANTS AND YOUNG CHILDREN WITH FAILURE TO THRIVE

The term *feeding* instead of *eating* disturbance in DSM-IV seeks to recognize the dyadic nature of the process in which both mother and infant are active participants. Although the distinction between organic and nonorganic eating problems of infancy and early childhood is conveniently accepted, the distinction is not always clear. Any medical problem—for example, gastroesophageal reflux—can disrupt the mother–child interaction during feeding. Furthermore, childhood eating problems can have profound consequences for physical growth and the child's development.

Failure to thrive (FTT) refers to infants who fail to make expected and age-appropriate gains in weight. Failure to thrive has been reported in 1–5% of pediatric hospital admissions, but organic factors seem to account for less than 10% of the cases (64). The evaluation of nonorganic FTT nowadays is no longer based on weight and height alone, but seeks to determine the infant's developmental level and the quality of the infant–mother or caretaker interaction. Malnutrition, socioeconomic factors, and emotional deprivation have been implicated as etiological in nonorganic FTT; nevertheless, many infants grow normally despite these conditions, whereas other infants or children show delayed development in the presence of normal weight gain. FTT is not included as a DSM-III-R diagnostic entity, nor is psychosocial dwarfism, a syndrome of decelerated linear growth which can be associated with bizarre eating habits.

In view of the controversy surrounding the heterogeneity of FTT, a developmental classification of feeding disorders based on observations of the mother–infant interaction outlined by Chatoor et al. (18) will be briefly described here.

Disorders of Homeostasis

Disorders of homeostasis are said to occur during the time from birth to 2 months, when basic functional cycles and rhythms of sleep and wakefulness, nursing, and elimination are established. Temperamental differences, a high level of irritability, and oversensitivity to stimulation can give rise to the colicky infant, and in other instances the

integration of the sucking and breathing response may be delayed. In such cases a mother's inability or inflexibility to respond to the child's particular needs may disrupt the infant's attempt to establish a regular feeding pattern.

Disorders of Attachment

Between 2 and 6 months, the infant's capacity to emotionally engage the mother determines the feeding experience. Regulation of food intake is closely linked to the bodily and visual cues guiding the interaction between mother and infant. Mothers who remain detached or disinterested because of depression or character disorders, or because of deprivation in their own childhood, may have children who are withdrawn and listless during feedings or who show vomiting, diarrhea, and poor weight gain.

Disorders of Autonomy and Separation

Physical and cognitive maturation which occurs during the age of 6 months to 3 years has led Mahler (46) to characterize this period as the first separation–individuation phase. Chatoor et al. (18) have called the disturbed eating during this time a separation disorder. If the mother cannot respond to the expressions of the infant's beginning autonomy, the infant may assert his will by refusing to eat through rejecting food.

Post-traumatic Eating Disturbances

Bernal (7) and Chatoor et al. (19) have described food refusal following an incident of choking. Eating problems due to trauma bear similarities to post-traumatic stress disorder and to phobia, because children demonstrate acute anxiety about food ingestion and consequently refuse to eat.

EATING DISORDERS IN CHILDHOOD

Pica

Pica derives from the Latin term for the "magpie," a bird noted for its habit of carrying away inedible objects. Pica denotes the eating of any foreign substances and includes earth eating (geophagia). Parry-Jones and Parry-Jones (53) recently published an excellent and exhaustive overview of the phenomenon of pica throughout history. During past centuries, pica has been regarded as a symptom (i.e., a sign of a morbid appetite), and the question remains whether turning pica into a diagnosis is of any value. For instance, geophagia (34) is a worldwide practice. Nosologically, pica captured attention when it was recognized that young children, especially black children in inner cities, were ingesting paint chips in older houses painted with lead-base paint, thereby exposing themselves to toxic lead levels. Three criteria will be necessary to diagnose pica in DSM-IV (4): (a) persistent eating of non-nutritive substances for at least 1 month, (b) the eating of non-nutritive substances is inappropriate to the developmental level, and (c) the eating behavior is not part of a culturally sanctioned practice. There is no agreement among researchers about the etiology of pica and its appropriate treatment. When children experience symptoms of abdominal pain and anemia or failure to thrive, pica should be suspected. Undoubtedly, pica frequently has become a habit, and thus treatment efforts need to be directed towards removing non-nutritive substances which can be eaten and are toxic from the house and towards feeding children properly and taking care of their emotional needs.

Rumination Disorder in Childhood

This rare disorder which occurs primarily during the first year of life is defined by repeated regurgitation and chewing of food (in the absence of associated gastrointestinal illness) for a period of at least 1 month following a period of normal functioning.

Because the disorder is rare, no epidemiological studies exist. A study by Mayes et al. (50) suggests a slight male predominance for rumination disorder. The differential diagnosis of rumination disorder includes pyloric stenosis and other congenital gastrointestinal abnormalities, as well as normal vomiting of early infancy. The typical characteristic preparatory movements interpreted as voluntary movements can help to distinguish the disorder from ordinary vomiting. Gastroesophageal reflux is associated with high rates of rumination disorder in infancy. The most common type is psychogenic rumination. If treated successfully, it is associated with normal cognitive development, whereas a second type called self-stimulatory rumination occurs mainly in mental retardation.

ANOREXIA NERVOSA IN CHILDHOOD

Our knowledge about anorexia nervosa in childhood is incomplete in part because of its rarity. Table 1 lists published case series reliably diagnosed from information in hospital records. The confusion over interchangeably used terms creates another problem. Some authors use premenarchal anorexia nervosa, which is not synonymous with prepubertal anorexia nervosa, because pubertal changes in girls precede the onset of menarche by about 3 years; other authors seem to include pubescent cases. Use of the Tanner (71) stages for standardizing sexual development would provide the most reliable distinction between childhood and adolescence, especially because anorexia nervosa rises dramatically with the evolution of puberty.

Incidence and Age at Onset

To our knowledge, no epidemiological studies on anorexia nervosa in childhood exist; therefore, incidence and prevalence rates are unknown. When the few retrospective case surveys which contain information about prepubertal anorexia nervosa are pooled (38), 4–8% of all anorexia nervosa cases seem to have had an onset in childhood. Considering that the incidence of anorexia nervosa is low [0.15 new cases in 100,000 per year (70)], childhood anorexia nervosa is infrequent. Because most epidemiological surveys rely on psychiatric case records, it is possible that the inclusion of milder cases who are seen by pediatricians would increase the estimate. Before age 7, anorexia nervosa in the traditional sense is virtually unheard of. In childhood, the restricting or fasting type of anorexia nervosa (13) prevails, but it appears that the phenomenology may differ somewhat across cultures. A Russian report described seventeen 9- to 11-year-old girls who regularly engaged in vomiting with the purpose of slimming down and improving dysphoric mood after eating. All suffered stunted growth as a result of their caloric restriction, but none became cachectic. Remarkably, with treatment all girls recovered without relapse (43).

Sex Ratio

As Table 2 indicates, the proportion of boys who present with childhood anorexia nervosa, on average about 26–28%, seems considerably higher than the percentage of boys who present with anorexia nervosa after puberty, which has been estimated to be 4–6%. The reasons for this prepubertal/postpubertal difference are unknown.

Precipitating Events

Psychological Precursors

Disruptive life events precede the onset of anorexia nervosa more commonly in childhood than in adolescence (35). Such events might be the birth of a sibling, moving, losing a friend, death in the family, family quarrel, parental divorce, or disappointment in a relationship. All cause anxiety or depressive symptoms and undermine the child's faith in his control and sense of security and can lead to a reduction in appetite. Once the parents and/or the pediatrician become alarmed, the child may discover, not always consciously, the controlling power in the refusal to eat (61) and thus precipitate weight loss and through it, if a predisposition exists, anorexia nervosa.

Physical Precursors and Eating Problems

Food fads and picky eating in early childhood have been associated with anorexia nervosa (40,61), whereas

TABLE 1. Cases of childhood anorexia nervosa in mostly retrospective surveys of hospital records

Reference	Number of cases (Total)	M:F ratio	Age at onset (years)	Age at presentation (years)	Core symptoms	Comorbidity	Treatment	Outcome	Period cases reviewed	Comments
Lesser et al. 1960	3 (15)	Not reported	Before age 13	Not reported	+	Hysterical obsessive-compulsive schizoid	Hospitalization	"Good"	1960	Youngest 10 years
Blitzer et al. 1961	9 (15)	3:15	7–14	10–16	+	Anxiety anger	Hospitalization	1/27 died	1960–68	9 premenarchal
Warren 1968	8 prepubertal 4 premenarchal (20)	No boys	10–15	12–16	Less weight loss +	Depression anxiety tension	Hospitalization	2/8 prepubertal pts. died	1949–64	10% of all patients admitted to Maudsley Hospital
Galdston 1972	? (50) 8–16 years	9:41	Number of prepubertal cases not reported	Not reported	3 suicidal +	Moderate depression euphoria	Hospitalization psychotherapy	All discharged with weight gain	1960–72	Children's Hospital Boston
Hahmi 1974	7 (94)	6:88	8% <10 years	29% 10–15 41% 16–25 25% >25	+	Anxiety obsessive-compulsive depression	Hospitalization	Not reported	1920–72	Hospitals U. of Iowa
Goetz et al. 1977	? (30)	2:28		9.5–16	+	Hysterical obsessive-compulsive schizoid	Hospitalization	Good	1954–70	Children's Hospital Pittsburgh
Irwin 1984	13 (54)	Males excluded	?	9–12	Less weight loss +	Depression	Hospitalization	Not reported	1960–80	7% under age 10
Hawley 1985	10 prepubescent 7 pubescent (21)	4:21	7.2–13.5	Not reported	+	Not reported	Hospitalization	67% good outcome	1964–82	All boys prepubertal Children's Hospital Birmingham
Jacobs & Isaacs 1986	20	6:14	7.2–13.9	Not reported	+	Sexual anxiety disturbed peer relationships	Hospitalization	Poor prognosis low social class, family psychopathology	1963–81	Maudsley Hospital
Fosson et al. 1987	23 prepubertal (48)	13:35	7.7–13.7	8.2–13.9	+	Depression family conflict	Hospitalization	Good	1960–84	Hospital for Sick Children 7:16 prepubescent 6:14 pubescent
Higgs et al. 1989	(27)	8:19	8–16	Not reported	+	Higher obsessionality than comparison group	Hospitalization	50% good or intermediate outcome, boys better outcome	1958–84	Children's Hospital Manchester
Atkins and Silber 1990	9 (21)	0:21	9 Tanner stage I	7–12	+ in 16	71% additional diagnosis	Hospitalization	All prepubertal cases good outcome	1978–89	Children's Hospital
Gowers et al. 1991	30 premenarchal	Males excluded	13.6 ± 2.2	16.3 ± 5.3	+	Not described	Hospitalization	Anxiety about pubertal development	Not indicated	St. George's Hospital

TABLE 2. *Gender distribution in prepubertal (or in cases <16 years old*) versus postpubertal series of patients with anorexia nervosa*

Anorexia nervosa	Male %	Female %	Total number of cases	Reference
Prepubertal	26	74	15	Blitzer et al. 1961 (9)
	18	82	50	Galdston 1974* (28)
	9	91	30	Goetz et al. 1977* (32)
	25	75	4	Anyan & Schowalter 1983 (5)
	40	60	10	Hawley 1985 (33)
	30	70	20	Jacobs & Isaacs 1986 (40)
	18	82	90	Pfeiffer et al. 1986* (54)
	27	73	48	Fosson et al. 1987 (27)
	27	73	33	Gislason 1988 (31)
	30	70	27	Higgs et al. 1989 (35)
	10	90	20	Rastam 1989* (56)
Postpubertal	4–6	94–96	>300	Dally 1969; Jacobs & Isaacs 1986 (29,50)
				Suematsu 1985 (68), Szmuckler et al. 1986 (70)

pica and family conflicts during meals in early childhood seem to be precursors for bulimia nervosa (48). Early physical maturation may enhance bodily awareness and body size (14) and lead to conscious or unconscious fears of uncontrollable overweight, resulting in food refusal and thus enhancing the risk for anorexia nervosa during early puberty.

The Vulnerable Child Syndrome

A minority of children who develop anorexia nervosa tend to be sickly or frail or have experienced early physical threats or perinatal trauma (6).

Symptomatology

The symptoms of childhood and postpubertal anorexia nervosa are remarkably similar: refusal to eat out of fear of fatness, based on a deliberate personal decision, although children sometimes convincingly state that eating is bad. The voluntary food restriction in children often extends to life-threatening fluid restriction. Their smaller body proportions make weight loss more noticeable early on. Typically, children fail to gain weight commensurate with their previous growth rate rather than lose weight. A second diagnostic sign is indifference to or denial that lack of expected weight gain is of any importance, which suggests partial unawareness of the bodily changes. Vague abdominal pain and avoidance of high caloric food or idiosyncratic ideas about food, such as avoiding eggs because of their connotations with fertility, are not uncommon in children. Failure to grow more often alarms children, and the danger of growth arrest will motivate some children, unfortunately not all, to eat more. By and large, children tend to be less fixated on thinness per se. The only appropriate way to study the effects of food deprivation in children is to fit growth curves to the weight

and height data for each individual child usually available from the child's pediatrician. This curve then serves as the individual's own control and basis for predicted growth and for the calculations of deceleration of expected growth in height and size (39). Children are generally hospitalized for persistent refusal to eat and intractable weight loss in the absence of demonstrable organic pathology. Overactive behavior can be observed in pre- and postpubertal anorexia nervosa cases, in contrast to prepubertal neurotic children (27,40).

Personality Dimensions

The clinical description of the personality of children with anorexia nervosa, shyness, lack of pleasure, compliance, rigidity, and perfectionism (13,16,17,28) is consistent with personality traits of adolescents with the restricting type of anorexia nervosa (16). Casper et al. (16) have suggested that these personalities tendencies which would be expected to facilitate food abstention may place youngsters at risk for developing the restricting type of anorexia nervosa.

Comorbidity

Despite the presence of sadness and withdrawal, many children appear euphoric and many do not fit any diagnosis. Jacobs and Isaacs (40) reported disturbed peer relations in two-thirds of prepubertal anorectic as opposed to one-third of neurotic children. Fosson et al. (27) found obsessions and compulsions in roughly a third. In a prospective study, Atkins and Silber (6) applied DSM-III-R criteria to 21 children with anorexia nervosa who were diagnosed at the age of 12 or under. Nine were prepubertal, whereas pubertal development had begun in the remaining ones. Comorbidity was reported for the group without specifying pubertal stages, six patients had no other psychiatric diagnosis, four had signs of a depressive disorder, three were considered to have either a narcissistic personality disorder or an overanxious disorder, two were diagnosed with obsessive–compulsive or oppositional disorder, and one was diagnosed with a borderline personality disorder.

Family Functioning

Roughly half the children are said to have families which manifest conflict, intrafamilial social stress, discordant intrafamiliar relationships, or overinvolvement. Birth, death, illness, and sometimes alcoholism create family crises (59). Jacobs and Isaacs (40) reported more frequent food fads and familial overinvolvement in prepubertal anorectic families compared to neurotic controls, but no differences with respect to postpubertal anorectic families were observed. Fosson et al. (27), whose report includes early adolescents up to age 15 years, reported family dysfunction in the majority of cases.

DEVELOPMENTAL ARREST: THE TOLL OF ANOREXIA NERVOSA IN CHILDHOOD

Effects on Emotional Development

To date, to our knowledge, no prospective outcome study on children alone has been published. The outcome information on ''children,'' referring mainly to youngsters under the age of 16 at the time of hospitalization, is variable. Only 2 of 20 had recovered in one study 1–9 years later, whereas Goetz et al. (32) reported normal weight and good psychological adjustment in 26 of 30 assessed 5–20 years after hospitalization. Similar variability has been reported in recent outcome studies. Hawley (33) and Steinhausen and Glanville (67) observed a good nutritional outcome in 67% and good psychological adjustment for about 50% at 3- to 15-year follow-up. By contrast, only a third of Higgs et al.'s (35) patients evaluated 5 years after hospitalization qualified for a good outcome, and Fosson et al. (27) reported a poorer outcome for children whose age at referral was less than 11 years.

The controversy as to whether prepubertal anorexia nervosa is a milder disorder than anorexia nervosa with pubertal or postpubertal onset (33,44,45,67) will remain undecided as long as outcome studies are based on hospital records or drawn from specialized referral centers (69), and as long as milder cases of children treated in pediatric practices and as outpatients are not included in the follow-up.

Endocrine and Metabolic Changes

To our knowledge, the endocrine changes associated with anorexia nervosa in childhood have not been studied.

On the whole, the starvation-induced endocrine and physical changes in children can be expected to be similar to those observed in adolescents (17). Support for this claim is provided by the fact that with profound weight loss the hypothalamic–pituitary–gonadal axis invariably regresses, even in mature women, to prepubertal functioning. However, it is not known whether the activation of the hypothalamic–pituitary–adrenocortical axis is as pronounced in children as it is in adults (10). The cardiac changes (e.g., severe bradycardia) require closer monitoring in children than in adolescents. Although sleep studies have not been published in childhood anorexia nervosa, sleep abnormalities in children with poor growth as a result of psychosocial deprivation, showing significant decreases in the percentage of stage IV sleep and an increased amount of rapid eye movement sleep, have been well documented (72).

Effects on Physical Maturation and on Linear Growth

In chronically ill anorexia nervosa patients who had premenarchal illness onset, Russell (62) reported delay of puberty, delayed breast development, and interference with growth and height.

Caloric deficiency alone can lead to slowing or arrest of physical growth. Dreizen et al. (25) studied skeletal maturity through serial roentgenograms of the left hand and wrist every 6 months into adulthood in 30 undernourished girls between the ages of 4 and 5 years in comparison to well-nourished girls. Sustained nutritional deprivation slowed the rate of bone growth and maturation, delayed puberty, and prolonged the growth period. Surprisingly, no differences in adult height were recorded. Davis et al. (24) examined 36 children (25 boys and 11 girls) aged 2–15 years, who were below the third percentile for height. Most displayed a poor appetite and had long-standing feeding or eating problems. Retarded growth in these otherwise healthy children was associated with a long-standing, albeit modest, caloric deficiency. A sustained increase in caloric content resulted in renewed, more rapid growth.

Whether ultimate linear growth is impaired seems to depend on long-term nutrition. Casper and Jabine (15) reported that anorexia nervosa patients with good outcome 8–10 years after illness onset were as tall as their sisters, but that those who were still symptomatic were slightly, yet not significantly, lower in height than their sisters. Root and Powers (60) reported growth retardation in three adolescents with anorexia nervosa as did Higgs et al. (35) in 5 of 23 childhood cases. But Pfeiffer et al. (54) reported that the mean percentile for height was higher at follow-up than at the time of diagnosis in those adolescents who had had anorexia nervosa at or before age 16 years, suggesting significant late growth acceleration.

CONCLUSIONS AND RECOMMENDATIONS FOR TREATMENT AND FURTHER RESEARCH

There is no doubt that the continued debate about diagnostic standards for feeding and eating disturbances in infancy and childhood has hampered comparative studies. Other obstacles to data collection have been the difficulties and ethical considerations for conducting research in young children.

The profound effects of disordered feeding and eating on the physical and psychological growth and development of children are indisputable. Treatment of these disorders needs to be swift and to respond to individual needs. Supervised refeeding often takes precedence over the introduction of treatments which would address the psychological issues.

In general, the behavioral and attitudinal diagnostic criteria for anorexia nervosa can be applied to children, if one keeps in mind that the motivation and reasoning of the child may differ and tends to reflect individual stages of development as well as the child's upbringing. Individually plotted growth curves are necessary to accurately determine body weight loss and growth deceleration in children.

Most of the information about anorexia nervosa in childhood has come from single case reports or from retrospective chart reviews of hospitalized patients and only lately from cases seen at children hospitals. This literature has tended to be overinclusive in the sense that premenarchal cases and those between the ages of 13 and 16 years have been considered as childhood cases. For the purpose of this chapter, we have taken the position that childhood comes to an end with the appearance of any sign of puberty (71).

The treatment of anorexia nervosa in children requires special adjustments (5,9,28,57), because apprehension about growing up, fears of bodily changes, and the sexual implications of puberty (14) color the clinical picture. On the other hand, the treatment of children is made easier by the infinitely greater willingness of nursing staff to mother an 11-year-old, even a hostile and obstinate 11-year-old anorectic patient, than to care for a 20-year old anorectic patient.

In childhood, just as much as in adolescence, the severity of the eating disorder seems to be determined by the severity of the psychiatric impairment. No drug that treats the core symptoms of anorexia nervosa is yet available, but food seems to have pharmacological properties, because good nutrition and weight gain do ameliorate the core symptoms. Unfortunately, the children's response to medication which might be indicated for a comorbid condition is not as reliable as in adults, and therefore supportive and family treatment to explore long-standing dysfunctional family interactions and to evaluate parental psychopathology become all the more important.

The need for epidemiological, clinical, endocrine, genetic (36), and outcome data is obvious, but unless milder cases seen as outpatients or in pediatric practice can be included into the database, studies cannot be considered representative of the full syndrome.

The observed differences in the prevalence rates between prepubertal and postpubertal males stand in need of investigation. Likely hypotheses explore the significant rise of androgens during male puberty as well as contemporary gender-related cultural factors.

REFERENCES

1. Alessi NE, Krahn D, Brehm D, Wittekindt J. Prepubertal anorexia nervosa and major depressive disorder. *J Am Acad Child Adolesc Psychiatry* 1989;28:380–384.
2. American Psychiatric Association. *Diagnostic and statistical manual of mental disorders,* 3rd ed. Washington, DC: APA, 1980.
3. American Psychiatric Association. *Diagnostic and statistical manual of mental disorders,* 3rd ed. (revised). Washington, DC: APA, 1987.
4. American Psychiatric Association. *Diagnostic and statistical manual of mental disorders IV draft criteria: task force on DSM-IV.* Washington, DC: APA, 1993.
5. Anyan WR Jr, Schowalter JE. A comprehensive approach to anorexia nervosa. *Child Psychiatry* 1983;22:122–127.
6. Atkins DM, Silber TJ. Anorexia nervosa in preadolescent youngsters. Abstract: Fourth International Conference on Eating Disorders, April 27–29, 1990.
7. Bernal ME. Behavioral treatment of a child's eating problem. *J Behav Ther Exp Psychiatry* 1972;3:43–50.
8. Birch LL, Johnson SL, Anderson G, Peters JC, Schulte MC. The variability of young children's energy intake. *N Engl J Med* 1991;324:232–235.
9. Blitzer JR, Rollins N, Blackwell A. Children who starve themselves: anorexia nervosa. *Psychosom Med* 1961;23:369–383.
10. Boyar RM, Hellman LD, Roffwarg HP, et al. Cortisol secretion and metabolism in anorexia nervosa. *N Engl J Med* 1977;296:190–193.
11. Brooks-Gunn J, Warren MP. Effects of delayed menarche in different contexts: dance and nondance students. *J Youth Adolesc* 1985;14:285–300.
12. Bryant-Waugh RJ, Lask BD. Can paediatricians and family practitioners recognize anorexia nervosa in children? New York: Fourth International Conference on Eating Disorders, April 27–29, 1990.
13. Casper RC, Eckert ED, Halmi KA, Goldberg SC, Davis JM. Bulimia: its incidence and clinical significance in patients with anorexia nervosa. *Arch Gen Psychiatry* 1980;37:1030–1035.
14. Casper RC, Offer D, Ostrov E. The self-image of adolescents with acute anorexia nervosa. *J Pediatr* 1981;98:656–661.
15. Casper RC, Jabine LN. Psychological functioning in anorexia nervosa: a comparison between anorexia nervosa patients on follow-up and their sisters. In: Lacey JH, Sturgeon DA, eds. *Proceedings of the 15th european conference on psychosomatic research.* London: John Libbey & Co, 1986;172–178.
16. Casper RC, Hedeker D, McClough JF. Personality dimensions in eating disorders and their relevance for subtyping. *J Am Acad Child Adolesc Psychiatry* 1992;31:830–840.
17. Casper RC. Neuroendocrine aspects of anorexia nervosa and bulimia nervosa. In: JL Woolston, ed. *Child and adolescent psychiatric clinics of North America: eating and growth disorders.* Philadelphia: WB Saunders, 1993;161–174.
18. Chatoor I, Egan J, Getson P, Menvielle E, O'Donnell R. Mother-infant interactions in infantile anorexia nervosa. *J Am Acad Child Adolesc Psychiatry* 1988;27:535–540.
19. Chatoor I, Conley C, Dickson L. Food refusal after an incident of choking: a posttraumatic eating disorder. *J Am Acad Child Adolesc Psychiatry* 1988;27:105–110.
20. Collins WJ. Anorexia nervosa. *Lancet* 1894;1:202–203.

21. Crisp AH, Palmer RL, Kalucy RS. How common is anorexia nervosa? A prevalence study. *Br J Psychiatry* 1976;128:549–554.
22. Daley S. Girls' self-esteem is lost on way to adolescence—new study finds. *Chicago Tribune,* Wednesday, January 9, 1991;B1.
23. Davis C. Self selection of diet by newly weaned infants: an experimental study. *Am J Dis Child* 1928;36:651–679.
24. Davis DR, Apley J, Fill G. Diet and retarded growth. *Br Med J* 1978;1:539–542.
25. Dreizen S, Spirakis CN, Stone RE. A comparison of skeletal growth and maturation in undernourished and well-nourished girls before and after menarche. *J Pediatr* 1967;70:256–263.
26. Fabian LJ, Thompson JK. Body image and eating disturbance in young females. *Int J Eating Disord* 1989;8:63–74.
27. Fosson A, Knibbs J, Bryant-Waugh R, Lask B. Early onset anorexia nervosa. *Arch Dis Child* 1987;62:114–118.
28. Galdston R. Mind over matter. Observations on 50 patients hospitalized with anorexia nervosa. *J Am Acad Child Psychiatry* 1974;13:246–263.
29. Gargiulo J, Brooks-Gunn J, Attie I, Warren MP. Girls' dating behavior as a function of social context and maturation. *Dev Psychol* 1987;23:730–737.
30. Garn SM, LaVelle M, Rosenberg KR, Hawthorne VM. Maturational timing as a factor in female fatness and obesity. *Am J Clin Nutrition* 1986;43:879–883.
31. Gislason IL. Eating disorders in childhood (ages 4 through 11 years). In: Blinder BJ, Chaitin BF, Goldstein R, eds. *The eating disorders.* PMA Publishing Corporation, 1988;285–293.
32. Goetz PL, Succop RA, Reinhart JB, Miller A. Anorexia nervosa in children. A follow-up study. *Am J Orthopsychiatry* 1977;47:597–603.
33. Hawley RM. The outcome of anorexia nervosa in younger subjects. *Br J Psychiatry* 1985;146:657–660.
34. Halsted JA. Geophagia in man: its nature and nutritional effects. *Am J Clin Nutr* 1968;21:1384–1393.
35. Higgs JF, Goodyer IM, Birch J. Anorexia nervosa and food avoidance emotional disorder. *Arch Dis Child* 1989;64:346–351.
36. Holland AJ, Sicotte N, Treasure JL. Anorexia nervosa: evidence for a genetic basis. *J Psychosom Res* 1988;32:561–571.
37. Irwin M. Diagnosis of anorexia nervosa in children and the validity of DSM-III. *Am J Psychiatry* 1981;138:1382–1383.
38. Irwin M. Early onset of anorexia nervosa. *South Med J* 1984;77:611–614.
39. Jackson RL, Kelby AG. Growth charts for use in pediatric practice. *J Pediatr* 1945;27:215–229.
40. Jacobs BW, Isaacs S. Pre-pubertal anorexia: a retrospective controlled study. *J Child Psychol Psychiatry* 1986;27:237–250.
41. Kent A, Lacey H, McCluskey. Pre-menarchal bulimia nervosa. *J Psychosom Res* 1992;36:205–210.
42. Koff E, Rierdan J, Silverstone E. Changes in representation of body image as a function of menarchal status. *Dev Psychol* 1978;14:635–642.
43. Korkina MV, Marilov VV. Pre-pubertal anorexia. *Zh Nevropatol Psikhiatr* 1981;81:1536–1540.
44. Kreipe RE, Churchill BH, Strauss J. Long-term outcome of adolescents with anorexia nervosa. *Am J Dis Child* 1989;143:1322–1327.
45. Lesser LI, Ashenden B, Debuskey M, Eisenberg L. Anorexia nervosa in children. *Am J Orthopsychiatry* 1960;30:572–580.
46. Mahler MS. Thoughts about development and individuation. *Psychoanal Study Child* 1963;18:307–324.
47. Maloney MJ, McGuire J, Daniels SR, Specker B. Dieting behavior and eating attitudes in children. *Pediatrics* 1989;84:482–489.
48. Marchi M, Cohen P. Early childhood eating behaviors and adolescent eating disorders. *J Am Acad Child Adolesc Psychiatry* 1990;29:112–117.
49. Marshall CF. A fatal case of anorexia nervosa. *Lancet* 1895;1:817.
50. Mayes SD, Humphrey FJ II, Handford HA, Mitchell JF. Rumination disorder: differential diagnosis. *J Am Acad Child Adolesc Psychiatry* 1988;27:300–302.
51. Nylander I. The feelings of being fat and dieting in a school population: epidemiologic interview investigation. *Acta Sociomed Scand* 1971;3:17–26.
52. Ogintz E. Winning by losing. *Chicago Tribune,* Friday, October 12, 1990, Tempo Section, p. 1.
53. Parry-Jones B, Parry-Jones WLL. Pica: symptom or eating disorder? A historical assessment. *Br J Psychiatry* 1992;160:341–354.
54. Pfeiffer RJ, Lucas AR, Ilstrip DM. Effect of anorexia nervosa on linear growth. *Clin Pediatr* 1986;25:7–12.
55. Pugliese MT, Lifshitz F, Grad G, Fort P, Marks-Katz M. Fear of obesity: a cause of short stature and delayed puberty. *N Engl J Med* 1983;309:513–518.
56. Rastam M, Gillberg C, Garton M. Anorexia nervosa in a Swedish urban region: a population-based study. *Br J Psychiatry* 1989;155:642–646.
57. Reinhart JB, Kenna MD, Succop RA. Anorexia nervosa in children: outpatient management. *J Acad Child Psychiatry* 1972;11:114–131.
58. Richards MH, Casper RC, Larson R. Weight and eating concerns among pre- and young adolescent boys and girls. *J Adolesc Health Care* 1990;11:203–209.
59. Rollins N, Blackwell A. The treatment of anorexia nervosa in children and adolescents: stage 1. *J Child Psychol Psychiatry* 1968;9:81–91.
60. Root AW, Powers PS. Anorexia nervosa presenting as growth retardation in adolescents. *J Adolesc Health Care* 1983;4:25–30.
61. Rose JA. Eating inhibitions in children in relation to anorexia nervosa. *Psychosom Med* 1943;5:117–124.
62. Russell GFM. Delayed puberty due to anorexia nervosa of early onset. In: Darby PL, Garfinkel PE, Garner DM, Coscina DV, eds. *Anorexia nervosa: recent developments in research.* New York: Alan R Liss, 1983;331–42.
63. Schleimer K. Dieting in teenage schoolgirls: a longitudinal prospective study. *Acta Paediatr Scand* 1983;312(Suppl):1–54.
64. Skuse D. Epidemiologic and definitional issues in failure to thrive. In: Woolston JL, ed. *Child and adolescent psychiatric clinics of North America: eating and growth disorders.* Philadelphia: WB Saunders, 1993;37–59.
65. Soltman O. Anorexia cerebralis und centrale Nutritionsneurosen. *Jahrb Kinderheilk* 1894;38:1–13.
66. Staffieri JR. A study of social stereotype of body image in children. *J Person Soc Psychol* 1967;7:101–104.
67. Steinhausen HC, Glanville K. Follow-up studies of anorexia nervosa: a review of research findings. *Psychol Med* 1983;13:239–249.
68. Suematsu H, Ishikawa H, Kuboki T, Ito T. Statistical studies on anorexia nervosa in Japan: detailed clinical data on 1,011 patients. *Psychother Psychosom* 1985;43:96–103.
69. Swift WJ. The long-term outcome of early onset anorexia nervosa: a critical review. *J Am Acad Child Psychiatry* 1982;21:38–46.
70. Szmuckler G, McCance C, McCrone L, Hunter D. Anorexia nervosa: a psychiatric case register study from Aberdeen. *Psychol Med* 1986;16:49–58.
71. Tanner JM. *Growth at adolescence.* Oxford: Blackwell, 1962.
72. Taylor BJ, Brook CGD. Sleep EEG in growth disorders. *Arch Dis Child* 1986;61:754–760.
73. Tolstrup K. Psychogenic anorexia and hyperorexia among siblings. *Acta Paediatr* 1952;41:360–372.
74. Woolston JL. Eating and growth disorders in infants and children. *Dev Clin Psychol Psychiatry* 1991;24:1–91.
75. Worsley A. In the eye of the beholder: social and personal characteristics of teenagers and their impressions of themselves and fat and slim people. *Br J Med Psychol* 1981;54:231–242.
76. Zaslow J. Fourth-grade girls these days ponder weighty matters. *The Wall Street Journal,* February 11, 1986;1, 28.

Psychopharmacology: The Fourth
Generation of Progress, edited by
Floyd E. Bloom and David J. Kupfer.
Raven Press, Ltd., New York 1995.

CHAPTER 145

Cocaine

Chris-Ellyn Johanson and Charles R. Schuster

Cocaine remains a major drug of abuse in the view of the public and is blamed for many of the nation's ills, including the deterioration of families and cities and increases in violent crime. Neuropsychopharmacological research has focused on cocaine, and several reviews of its actions have been written in the last decade (34,48,84,96). The present review concentrates on areas of research where significant advances have been made since the *Third Generation of Progress* was written and assumes that the reader is familiar with earlier literature.

EPIDEMIOLOGY AND ETIOLOGY*

At the time of the writing of the *Third Generation of Progress,* cocaine use in the United States was near peak levels. National surveys conducted over the last two decades indicated that past-year and past-30-day prevalence rates reached a peak in 1985 and then steadily declined, reaching the lowest levels in the most recent National Household Survey on Drug Abuse (NHSDA) in 1992. For example, the 1985 NHSDA reported that almost 6 million people had used cocaine (including crack) at least once in the past 30 days. By 1991, this number had decreased by over 70% to less than two million. This decline was found at all age levels, including the 12- to 17-year-old age group. On the other hand, among respondents reporting use in the past year, the numbers of those who had used it at least once a week or more remained the same (between 650,000 to 800,000) over this same time period. Thus, the more frequent, problematic use of cocaine remains at peak levels.

Another United States national survey of drug use, called Monitoring the Future (MTF), which has been conducted since 1975, uses high school seniors as respondents (63).† This survey has also shown that the use of cocaine (including crack) has declined over the same period. It must be recognized, however, that the prevalence rates for the use of cocaine are most likely higher among those who dropped out of school. Unfortunately, systematic data on dropouts are not available, although the NHSDA provides evidence that they are a vulnerable population. Nevertheless, it is encouraging that the overall trend noted by both the MTF and the NHSDA indicates a decline in cocaine use in adolescents.

In addition to decreases in overall prevalence, there has been a change in the demographic characteristics of those who use cocaine today, compared to the late 1970s and early 1980s. Although cocaine was then the ''drug of choice'' among the ''elite,'' its use has become increasingly prevalent in other portions of the population. Data from the 1991 NHSDA showed that the past-year and past-month prevalence rates for cocaine use were significantly higher in those who had not completed high school compared to those who had received a high school diploma, supporting the concern that the MTF may be underestimating actual numbers of users. These differences were particularly striking for crack cocaine use, where there was a fourfold greater past-month prevalence rate among those who did not finish high school in comparison to college graduates. This is in contrast to the situation in 1982 when high school and college graduates were two to three times more likely to have used cocaine in the past 30 days than age-matched respondents who had not finished high school. Furthermore, in 1991, cocaine use in the past month among the unemployed was 4.6 times higher than in the employed. This difference was

---

* References for the major national surveys including DAWN can be obtained from the authors or directly from the National Institute on Drug Abuse, the Substance Abuse Mental Health Services Administration, or the National Institute of Justice.

C.-E. Johanson and C. R. Schuster: National Institute on Drug Abuse, Intramural Research Program, National Institutes of Health, Baltimore, Maryland 21224.

† Eighth- and tenth-grade students were studied in the most recent surveys. However, there are not sufficient data to discuss trends in prevalence rates in these age groups.

even greater with crack cocaine. Recent statistics from the National Institute of Justice show that the rates of cocaine-positive urines among both male and female arrestees in major cities remain near peak levels of 40–80%. It would thus appear that the decreasing trend in prevalence rates of cocaine use observed in the general population is absent or significantly less in the educationally, economically, and socially disadvantaged. These prevalence rates must be put in proper perspective, however, by noting that these disadvantaged groups are relatively small in numbers. Thus, it remains the case that the majority of cocaine users are employed high school graduates who would not be characterized as disadvantaged.

Although the yearly trends in the NHSDA and in the MTF may very well be accurate, it is likely that both surveys underestimate the actual numbers of regular crack cocaine users. Newspaper and magazine accounts estimate the number to be somewhere between 500,000 and one million. Regardless of the exact numbers, however, the impact on the health delivery systems in already overcrowded urban hospitals has been overwhelming. Lindenbaum et al. (54) reported that more than half of the patients at the Albert Einstein Medical trauma center tested positive for cocaine and approximately 50% had been involved in a violent crime. Publicly funded treatment programs have experienced a sixfold increase from 1985 to 1990 in the numbers of people seeking treatment for their cocaine problem (3). The number of reported emergency room (ER) admissions reported to the Drug Abuse Warning Network (DAWN) associated with cocaine use has also increased dramatically over this same time span. The total number of cocaine-related ER mentions in 1992 was 119,800 (28% of ER drug-related admissions) compared to approximately 28,800 (9% of ER drug-related admissions) in 1985. At the present time, cocaine ranks a close second to alcohol-in-combination-with-other-drugs in ER mentions.

Although prevalence rates for the use of cocaine in the past 30 days were significantly lower in women than in men, the use of cocaine by women in their child-bearing years is of vital concern. Estimates of the numbers of women who use cocaine during pregnancy have varied widely. Furthermore, there are many reasons to believe that these estimates are unreliable, not the least of which is that women may deny drug use in states where they face criminal sanctions or the loss of custody of their newborn for cocaine use during pregnancy (84). That there is a significant number of fetuses exposed to cocaine during pregnancy is attested to by a recent large-scale prospective drug screening study (65). Meconium samples from 3010 neonates born to women coming to an urban obstetrics service were analyzed for the presence of cocaine. Although only 11% of the women reported the use of illicit drugs during their pregnancy, 31% of the infants' meconium tested positive for cocaine.

There has been an increasing effort to probe the meaning of differences in prevalence rates in drug use in groups varying in demographic characteristics. One demographic characteristic that has received attention in this regard is race/ethnicity. In both the 1988 and 1990 NHSDA, lifetime prevalence rates for crack cocaine use were over twice as high among black Americans compared to white Americans. However, analyses of these data designed to understand underlying factors of etiologic significance demonstrated that when the survey respondents were grouped into neighborhood clusters, thereby holding shared characteristics such as drug availability and social conditions constant, the odds of crack cocaine use did not differ by race/ethnicity (7,53). Thus, it appears that neighborhood characteristics that promote the use of crack cocaine are equally effective, independently of racial or ethnic status. There is, however, a disproportionately larger percentage of black Americans than white Americans living in neighborhoods with these characteristics, thus leading to the higher prevalence rates. It must be remembered, however, that because of the relatively smaller size of the black American population compared to the white American population in the United States (11% versus 81%), the majority of crack users are white. Differences in reported use of crack have also been noted in Hispanic populations. In 1988, the lifetime prevalence rate for Hispanic Americans was 2.1% compared to a percentage of 1.0 for white Americans. However, there was no difference in odds ratios when neighborhood factors were controlled (53). In addition, in the 1990 NHSDA the lifetime prevalence rate of Hispanic Americans was found to have declined to 1.6%, which was not significantly different from the prevalence rate of white Americans. In fact, when Chilcoat et al. (7) adjusted for neighborhood, Hispanic Americans were found to have a significantly lower odds ratio for being crack users.

In addition to environmental influences, a variety of studies have suggested that individual-level characteristics play a role in the etiology of cocaine abuse. Studies of community samples have shown that the diagnosis of alcoholism or drug abuse/dependence is associated with higher prevalence rates of a wide variety of psychiatric disorders (43). In a recent study that evaluated the psychiatric status of individuals seeking treatment for cocaine abuse or dependence (80), both high current (55.7%) and lifetime (73.5%) prevalence rates for psychiatric disorders other than substance abuse were reported. The principal types of coexisting psychiatric disorders were: major depression, minor bipolar conditions, anxiety disorders, antisocial personality, and a history of attention-deficit hyperactivity disorder (ADHD). Prospective studies have shown that adolescents who show residual symptoms of ADHD have higher rates of substance abuse problems (58). In follow-up studies into adulthood, those diagnosed with antisocial personality showed increased rates of drug abuse (58). However, for those who reached adulthood and no longer showed symptoms of ADHD or antisocial personality, the odds of being a drug abuser were no different than those in controls (58).

One of the complications in determining the role of psychiatric disorders in the development of substance abuse problems is that drug use itself can cause psychiatric sequelae. While there is continuing debate about the etiologic significance of psychiatric disorders in the development of substance abuse, there is general agreement that substance abuse and other psychiatric problems coexist and that substance abuse treatment clients with coexistent psychiatric disorders have poorer treatment outcome. Appropriate pharmacological or psychotherapeutic treatment of the comorbid psychiatric disorder has been shown to improve the outcome of substance abuse treatment (98).

Another risk factor for the initiation of the use of cocaine is the use of other psychoactive substances that are legal, less costly, or more easily obtained. Epidemiological studies have provided evidence that there is a sequence of drug use stages leading up to the use of cocaine and opiates. Kandel and Faust (41) showed that the use of legal drugs, such as beer and cigarettes, preceded the use of marijuana, which preceded the use of cocaine. There had been a concern that young people might initiate crack cocaine smoking earlier in the developmental sequence than previously found for intranasal or intravenous cocaine because of its availability, ease of ingestion, and relatively cheap price. However, a recent study by Kandel and Yamaguchi (42) reported that crack smoking was the last member of the chain of substances to be used, after powdered cocaine itself. Furthermore, Chilcoat and Schutz (7) showed that peak use of crack cocaine occurs in individuals over 20 years of age, with very little crack use being reported by individuals under 20. Although previous drug use per se may not be an etiologic factor, early use of licit substances, such as beer and cigarettes, can be used as a marker for identifying children who are at risk of developing problematic drug use, including the use of cocaine.

PHARMACOKINETICS

The pharmacokinetics of cocaine has been extensively investigated because of the purported differences in the dependence potential and toxicity associated with different routes of administration. Although the intranasal route of administration (insufflation) remains the most common route, the smoked and intravenous routes are associated with a higher frequency of ER mentions (DAWN) and number of people entering treatment for cocaine abuse or dependence.

Pharmacokinetic studies of intravenous and intranasal cocaine have been reviewed previously (34). Following nasal insufflation of 96 mg of cocaine, peak venous plasma levels between 150 and 200 ng/ml were reached in approximately 30 min. Intravenous administration of 32 mg of cocaine produced peak venous plasma levels of approximately 250–300 ng/ml after 4 min. A similar rise to between 200 and 250 ng/ml was found in venous plasma levels following the smoking of 50 mg of cocaine base (18). Regardless of the route of administration, the elimination half-life was approximately 40 min, although longer half-lives of 60 min have been reported.

Recent studies of the pharmacokinetics of smoked and intravenously administered cocaine have compared venous and arterial plasma levels (15). When a dose of cocaine base of 50 mg was smoked or an intravenous injection of 32 mg of cocaine hydrochloride (HCl) was given, arterial plasma levels reached a peak within a few seconds whereas venous plasma levels did not reach their peak until after several minutes. Furthermore, the peak arterial levels reached by either route of administration were substantially higher than the peak venous plasma levels. Thus, the levels of cocaine reaching the heart and brain after either smoking cocaine base or the intravenous administration of cocaine HCl were much greater than would have been predicted from prior data on venous plasma levels.

Cocaine is metabolized by cholinesterases present in the plasma and liver into two principal metabolites, benzoylecognine and ecgonine methyl ester, which are excreted in the urine. The major metabolites of cocaine can be found in the urine for periods up to 36 h after the last administration of the drug. Cocaine can also be measured in saliva and in hair. Furthermore, cocaine and its metabolites have been found in the meconium of infants born to woman who have used cocaine during pregnancy (65). The smoking of cocaine base produces a pyrolysis product, anhydroecgonine methyl ester, which can be detected in the urine and thereby serve as a marker for the use of cocaine by the smoking route. These various means of detecting drug use each have their own advantages and disadvantages for monitoring of patients, for drug testing in the workplace, and for forensic purposes.

Although cocaethylene was identified in 1978 in urine samples that contained both cocaine and alcohol, its spectrum of pharmacological activity and significance for dependence on (and toxicity of) cocaine and alcohol combinations has only recently been investigated (25). It is estimated that between 60% and 90% of cocaine abusers consume alcohol concomitantly with cocaine. It has been assumed that the reinforcing effects of alcohol and cocaine combinations could be understood as the summation of their separate reinforcing properties or due to alcohol's sedative effects counteracting excessive stimulation from cocaine. Cocaethylene, however, has been found to be a psychoactive substance with a pharmacological profile similar to cocaine but with a significantly longer duration of action. In addition, the LD_{50} in mice for cocaethylene is significantly lower than that for cocaine (26). The combination of cocaine and alcohol also has been shown to produce greater changes in heart rate and blood pressure than either drug alone (17). These experimental studies may help explain the fact that many cases of death apparently associated with cocaine use have reported very low blood levels of cocaine. That is, it is likely that these individuals had also consumed alcohol, leading to the formation of cocaethylene which subsequently produced excess toxicity. In fact, recent studies (28) of postmortem blood and tissue levels of cocaine and cocaethylene have reported cases of low levels of cocaine and very high levels of cocaethylene.

The interaction of cocaine and alcohol is further complicated by the fact that alcohol has been shown to increase the blood levels of cocaine administered intransally (67). Whether this is an effect of alcohol on the absorption of cocaine through the nasal mucosa, secondary to alcohol-induced vasodilation, remains to be determined. Interestingly, in that same study, cocaethylene levels in venous plasma rose slowly and were increasing at the time that the subjective and physiological effects of cocaine were returning to baseline. It would thus appear that the formation of cocaethylene after a single insufflation of cocaine (1.25 or 1.9 mg/kg) following the ingestion of alcohol (0.85 g/kg) does not contribute to the physiological or subjective effects observed over the next 2 h. However, one could speculate that with repeated administrations within a relatively short time period, cocaethylene levels could continue to rise and reach toxic levels.

NEUROBIOLOGY OF COCAINE DEPENDENCE

A major consequence of the cocaine epidemic and enhanced public concern about its abuse has been an acceleration in the number of investigations designed to increase the understanding of cocaine's central nervous system (CNS) effects, particularly those related to its ability to produce dependence. Although it has been known for a number of years that dopamine (DA) plays a major role in the behavioral actions of cocaine (e.g., see refs. 34, 48, and 96), research in the 1990s has provided even more definitive evidence of DA's role in mediating the reinforcing effects of cocaine and other psychomotor stimulant drugs, as well as drugs of abuse from other classes (12). This has given rise to the so-called "dopamine hypothesis" of cocaine's reinforcing actions (51). The implications of the DA hypothesis are extremely important because it suggests the target neurochemical system for medications for the treatment of cocaine dependence.

There are several areas of research where advances have occurred in the 1990s that have contributed to an increased confidence that DA mediates cocaine's dependence-related behavioral actions. These include the identification and characterization of its site of action at the dopamine transporter, the cloning of the dopamine transporter, additional findings of cocaine's acute and chronic effects on DA neurotransmission, particularly those that have utilized in vivo techniques, and, finally, further evidence of the role of DA in mediating the behavioral effects of cocaine related to dependence. Because there are reviews of the earlier findings in these areas (34,48), this review will concentrate exclusively on more recent ones.* (See Chapter 66, *this volume*, for related discussion).

Dopamine Transporter

Cocaine blocks the uptake of DA, 5-hydroxytryptamine (5-HT), and norepinephrine (NE) in the CNS. However, the determination of which of these actions is associated with its reinforcing effects has only recently been elucidated. There is a significant positive correlation between the potencies of cocaine and some related compounds as DA uptake blockers and their ability to serve as reinforcers in self-administration studies in the rhesus monkey (76). In contrast, significant correlations between the reinforcing effects and blockade of uptake of NE and 5-HT have not been found. These data strongly suggest that it is the blockade of the uptake of DA that is an essential step in the mediation of the reinforcing effects of cocaine. Further support for this DA hypothesis comes from evidence supporting the conclusion that the cocaine "receptor" and the DA transporter are identical proteins. Particularly strong evidence has come from cloning experiments. Transfection of COS cells, which do not take up DA or bind cocaine, with a single cDNA for the DA transporter confers both DA uptake and cocaine binding activity simultaneously on the cells (86). Other studies have shown that several DA uptake inhibitors, such as high-affinity analogues of cocaine, mazindol, and several analogues of GBR 12909, bind to a single common site and interact competitively, which leads to the parsimonious conclusion that they bind to the dopamine transporter (5,74). Furthermore, Grilli et al. (24) have shown that the expression of cocaine binding sites and dopamine uptake sites occurs at the same time during in vitro cellular development. Another indication that cocaine binding sites and the dopamine transporter are intimately related is the fact that cocaine binding sites are distributed within the CNS in areas of high concentrations of DA nerve terminals. While these data indicate a prominent role for DA, it remains likely that significant interactions between different neurochemical mediator systems will be discovered that modulate the reinforcing actions of cocaine and related compounds.

Progress has also been made in elucidating the charac-

---

* References included in ref. 34 are not repeated in the present chapter.

teristics of the cocaine structure that are significant for its binding activity at the DA transporter. The important structural features include a levorotatory configuration, a beta-oriented substituent at C-2 and C-3, and a benzene ring at the C-3 carbon (75). The effects of changes in these structural features, in terms of reduction in pharmacological activity, are described by Carroll et al. (5).

In addition to the characterization of the structure of cocaine relevant to its binding, several laboratories have been involved in characterizing the DA transporter protein itself. These studies led to the development of techniques that eventually resulted in the cloning and expression of cDNA for the cocaine-sensitive DA transporter (44,86). This finding provides an opportunity to elucidate the molecular sequelae that result in DA uptake and to determine how this process is disrupted by cocaine. Ultimately this knowledge may be useful for the development of medications for treating cocaine dependence. One approach, stemming from this research, that appears promising for the development of a cocaine antagonist is based upon the possibility that the binding sites for DA and cocaine on the DA transporter are overlapping, but not identical. By altering the DA transporter through site-directed mutagenesis, it is possible to determine whether the changes differentially alter the binding of cocaine and DA. The finding that an aspartic acid residue lying within a particular region is crucial for both DA transport and cocaine binding whereas other areas are only important for DA transport supports the possibility of being able to develop a cocaine antagonist that does not interfere with normal DA transport (45) (see also Chapter 16, *this volume*).

Neural Bases of Cocaine Sensitization

With repeated exposure to a fixed dose, the locomotor and stereotypic effects of cocaine have been shown to increase in magnitude, a phenomenon known as *sensitization*. Sensitization was an early observation and has been shown with a variety of psychomotor stimulants besides cocaine (78). Conditioning processes appear to play an important role in the development of sensitization, at least under certain circumstances, because it is not always found if animals are tested for the occurrence of sensitization following repeated cocaine administration in a novel environment—that is, a place where they have never received an injection of cocaine before (71). Because the DA systems mediating the locomotor effects of cocaine appear to be the same as those for its reinforcing effects, and because sensitization is a long-lasting effect (78), an understanding of sensitization and conditioned sensitization has been suggested to have relevance for cocaine abuse and the difficulty of treating abusers (39).

In recent years, there have been a number of studies on the neurobiology of sensitization (for a review see ref. 39). The development of in vivo methods, such as microdialysis and voltammetry, which allow the monitoring of changes in extracellular DA levels and behavior simultaneously has made a major contribution to our understanding of the CNS actions of repeatedly administered cocaine. Studies employing standard approaches, such as synaptosomal preparations, tissue slice preparations, and electrophysiological techniques, have also contributed substantially to this area of research.

Initially, in vivo techniques were used to demonstrate that acute administrations of cocaine increased extracellular DA levels in several brain regions, including the nucleus accumbens. Of more relevance to sensitization, Pettit et al. (70) showed that the elevation of synaptic levels of DA in response to cocaine was augmented to an even greater extent in the nucleus accumbens after repeated administration. Kalivas et al. (39,40) measured both DA efflux and locomotor activity *simultaneously* in the same animals and found a correlation between changes in these two measures, both of which increased over a period of repeated cocaine treatment. In a subsequent study which examined more carefully the time course of the two effects, Kalivas and Duffy (37) found that following a 5-day regimen of 15 mg/kg cocaine, locomotor activity became augmented as evidenced by increased levels 24 hr after the regimen was terminated. In addition, similar levels of augmented activity were observed 4, 10, and 20 days later when cocaine was again tested. However, elevated levels of DA in the nucleus accumbens in response to an injection of cocaine were only observed 10 and 20 days post regimen, not during the earlier tests. A study by Koob and his associates (94) also provided information about changes in drug-induced DA efflux as well as in basal levels of DA following repeated cocaine. This study showed that basal DA levels were increased on day 1 following a 10-day regimen of 10 mg/kg or 30 mg/kg cocaine in rats but returned to saline-treated levels by day 7 post repeated cocaine regimen. These investigators also noted that while absolute levels of cocaine-induced DA were augmented on day 1, the percentage increase *relative to baseline* was less compared to chronically treated saline rats given cocaine because of this difference in baseline levels. The authors postulated that this difference may have been due to increased activation of presynaptic autoreceptors (94).

In addition to changes in DA efflux, Ng et al. (62) also provided evidence that DA uptake rate was increased with repeated cocaine administration. Using the in vitro technique of examining ^{3}H-DA uptake in tissue slices, others have also found evidence of an increase in DA uptake rate following chronic cocaine (e.g., ref. 101), while others have found persistent inhibition, at least in the nucleus accumbens (31).

Kalivas and Duffy (38) placed dialysis probes in the area of DA cell bodies (A10) of the VTA whose projections terminate in the nucleus accumbens. They found that levels of extracellular DA in the VTA and locomotor activity in response to an injection of cocaine both were augmented 24 hr after the drug regimen was terminated. Thirteen days later, however, the locomotor response still showed sensitization to an injection of cocaine, but the levels of extracellular DA in the VTA did not. At this time, however, increased levels of DA in the terminal fields are seen. Based on evidence of this type, Kalivas and his colleagues have postulated that changes in DA processes related to sensitization involve several mechanisms that occur sequentially (39). Initially, changes in the DA-containing cell bodies in the VTA underlie sensitization. The mechanism involves increased somatodendritic release of DA in the VTA. As a consequence of this increased release, there is a decrease in the sensitivity of D2 autoreceptors that regulate impulse generation. Because activation of these autoreceptors normally inhibits neuronal firing, their decreased sensitivity results in increased neuronal firing and subsequent increases in extracellular DA in the nucleus accumbens (40).

Several studies using local administration of substances into the VTA have provided supporting evidence for the importance of the cell bodies in the VTA in the initiation of sensitization. For instance, injections of stimulants directly into the VTA result in augmented responses to *systemically* administered stimulants, whereas injections into the nucleus accumbens do not (39,40). Furthermore, the administration of a DA antagonist into the VTA prevents the development of sensitization to the repeated administration of cocaine (88). Using electrophysiological techniques, White and his colleagues (27) have also shown that inhibitory impulse-regulating somatodendritic D2 autoreceptors in the VTA become subsensitive with repeated cocaine administration. This subsensitivity, which results in increased levels of neuronal firing, lasts less than 8 days (27) and thus supports the conception that these changes may be important in the initiation of sensitization, but not in its long-term maintenance. Electrophysiological studies by White and his colleagues have also shown the involvement of postsynaptic elements in the nucleus accumbens in sensitization. More specifically, DA receptors become supersensitive to the effects of extracellular DA (27). This increased sensitivity appears to be limited to D1 receptors (27).

Changes in the 5-HT system related to cocaine sensitization have also been demonstrated. Cunningham et al. (10) have described changes in serotonergic systems using behavioral, electrophysiological, and autoradiographic techniques that occur after chronic administration and appear to be correlated with behavioral sensitization. One consequence of uptake blockade of 5-HT in the dorsal raphe by acute administration of cocaine is decreased spontaneous 5-HT neuronal firing. This decrease appears to be a result of enhanced inhibition due to increased stimulation of $5-HT_{1A}$ impulse-modulating autoreceptors (10). Furthermore, this decreased firing in response to cocaine is augmented over a 7-day chronic cocaine regimen that concurrently produces behavioral sensitization (10). These authors have speculated that the decreased neuronal firing would result in decreased release of 5-HT in neuronal projections to areas such as the VTA and nucleus accumbens. As a result, the inhibitory influence of 5-HT would be diminished, further increasing DA neurotransmission and thus contributing to behavioral sensitization.

It appears that the mechanism(s) underlying sensitization are complex. A recent highly informative review by Kalivas et al. (39) gives a more complete description of the entire circuitry that may be involved in both the initiation and maintenance of sensitization. In addition, the chapter by Nestler et al. in this volume describes cellular changes, such as decreased G-protein coupling, that are related to sensitization. As Kalivas points out, a clear picture of neurobiological changes which produce sensitization has not yet emerged, in part because researchers have used different treatment regimens, different techniques to measure changes, and different times of assessment. Each of the mechanisms proposed to mediate sensitization is supported by empirical evidence. However, additional studies are needed to differentiate and determine the interactions among these changes in the developmental course and long-term expression of sensitization. Nevertheless, a great deal has already been learned about the cascade of neurobiological events that affect behavioral responses following repeated cocaine treatment. Given the progress over the last 5 years (see ref. 34), it is likely that the next few years will yield a more definitive picture. It is also likely that this research, which is spurred in large part by an interest in cocaine abuse, will reveal facts about the molecular biology of sensitization which have importance for much broader areas of mental health disorders.

Neural Basis of Reinforcement

Cocaine is a robust positive reinforcer, and it is generally agreed that its reinforcing effects are mediated by mesolimbic/mesocortical dopaminergic neuronal systems. Several reviews on the behavioral determinants of cocaine self-administration and the important role of DA in the neurochemical mediation of these actions are available (34,35,48). To briefly summarize,* other DA uptake blockers and D2 DA agonists support self-administration behavior. Second, both D1 and D2 DA antagonists have been shown to modify cocaine self-administration, whereas noradrenergic antagonists do not. Third, depletions of DA produced by injections of the neurotoxin 6-OHDA into the mesolimbic/mesocortical dopaminergic neuronal pathway, including the VTA, nucleus accumbens, and ventral pallidum, attenuate cocaine self-

---

* See ref. 34 for references to earlier studies.

administration, whereas depletions of norepinephrine do not. Furthermore, Dworkin and Smith (13) showed that DA depletions in the nucleus accumbens, while attenuating cocaine self-administration, did not have any effects on food- and water-maintained responding. Finally, direct injections of cocaine into the medial prefrontal cortex, a rostral projection of the mesolimbic/mesocortical pathway, support self-administration, although direct injections into the nucleus accumbens and VTA do not (23). In addition, the reinforcing effects of direct injections of cocaine into the prefrontal cortex are blocked by DA antagonists. However, depletions of DA in the medial prefrontal cortex produced by the neurotoxin 6-OHDA have produced a variety of effects that are difficult to reconcile.

In summary, although the data are not completely consistent (see ref. 34), the confluence of evidence from this earlier research supports the view that mesolimbic/mesocortical DA pathways mediate the initial steps in the cascade of neural events underlying cocaine's reinforcing effects. More recent evidence supporting this view has come from microdialysis studies. Pettit and Justice (68), using a microdialysis probe located in the nucleus accumbens, showed that extracellular DA levels were increased when cocaine was self-administered. For individual animals the levels remained constant across sessions, suggesting the attainment of an optimal level of DA (68). However, the DA levels attained were dose-dependent and correlated with increased levels of cocaine intake that resulted as dose was increased (69).

In contrast to Pettit and Justice (68,69), Hurd et al. (30) have reported that with repeated exposure to cocaine during self-administration sessions (9–10 daily sessions), the increases in extracellular DA following cocaine self-administration were diminished relative to those following initial administrations. The authors speculated that this tolerance-like effect may have been due to changes in uptake, release mechanisms, or postsynaptic receptor sensitivity. Others have suggested that the disparity between these studies was due to methodological differences (69). Thus, as with sensitization, there still remains the need for additional studies to clarify the role of DA in the long-term maintenance of cocaine self-administration.

The role of D1 and D2 receptors in the mediation of the reinforcing effects of cocaine has also been studied. As reviewed by Johanson and Fischman (34), much of the earlier self-administration work using DA agonists and antagonists pointed to a prominent role for postsynaptic D2 receptors, although the specificity of this role had been questioned (100). However, it has been reported that SCH 23390, a relatively specific D1 antagonist, also blocks cocaine's reinforcing effects in rats when delivered systemically, as well as directly into the nucleus accumbens (49,57), although in the rhesus monkey, Woolverton (99) failed to show that SCH 23390 affected cocaine self-administration. Furthermore, studies in rats using progres-

sive ratio schedules have concluded that both D1 and D2 antagonists specifically decrease the reinforcing effects of cocaine, suggesting that both receptor subtypes are important in cocaine reinforcement (29,77). There is also a recent study demonstrating that at least one D1 agonist, SKF 81297, has reinforcing effects in rhesus monkeys (92). Finally, there is recent evidence that D3 receptors also have a role in mediating the reinforcing effects of cocaine (4). Thus, at the present time, the interactions among the various DA receptors mediating cocaine's reinforcing effects have not been completely delineated. Undoubtedly, all three receptors, and perhaps others as well, play some role, but there are differences among studies as a function of species and paradigms.

Although self-administration paradigms are the most direct means for evaluating reinforcing effects, drug discrimination studies can provide complementary information, based upon the conception that they are related to the subjective effects of drugs in humans. Johanson and Fischman (34) reviewed earlier studies that indicated that cocaine's discriminative stimulus (DS) effects, like its reinforcing effects, are mediated by DA. Recent studies have augmented these findings and have begun to elucidate the relative importance of different DA receptor subtypes. Spealman et al. (87) demonstrated that cocaine analogues that were more potent than cocaine in binding to cocaine binding sites and in inhibiting uptake of DA were also more potent substitutes for cocaine as DS in squirrel monkeys. However, neither D1 nor D2 agonists, nor a combination of the two, completely substituted for cocaine, although both D1 and D2 antagonists blocked its DS effects. Spealman et al. (87) suggested that the activation of both receptor subtypes was important in cocaine's actions. Similar results were found in pigeons (33). However, studies in rats and rhesus monkeys (46,97) have not replicated all of these findings, suggesting that there may be species differences in the DA receptor subtypes mediating cocaine's DS effects.

In addition to the evidence of a role for DA in cocaine reinforcement and discrimination studies, there have also been some recent studies suggesting at least a modulatory role for 5-HT. Cunningham and Callahan (9), using a drug discrimination paradigm, showed that fluoxetine, a 5-HT uptake blocker, shifted the cocaine dose–response function to the left, indicative of potentiation. In a drug discrimination study with pigeons, both fluoxetine and 8-OH-DPAT, a 5-HT$_{1A}$ agonist, partially substituted for, and the putative 5-HT$_{1A}$ antagonist NAN-190 partially blocked, the DS effects of cocaine (33). In addition to evidence of 5-HT's modulatory effects from drug discrimination studies, self-administration studies have also indicated a role for 5-HT. Loh and Roberts (55) showed that depletions of 5-HT in the medial forebrain bundle or amygdala, induced by injections of the neurotoxin 5,7-dihydroxytryptamine, increased the reinforcing effects of cocaine as indicated by an increase in break-point under a progressive ratio schedule. Similarly, Carroll et al. (6) reported that rate of cocaine self-administration was reduced by fluoxetine. However, these investigators wisely concluded that this change may have been due to either a decrease (blockade) or an increase in the reinforcing effects of cocaine. Given the finding by Ritz et al. (76) that there is an inverse correlation between binding of compounds to 5-HT binding sites and their ability to maintain self-administration, it is possible that 5-HT influences cocaine self-administration. It is also clear that further research is needed to clarify the nature of its modulatory effect.

Other neurotransmitters may also affect cocaine self-administration as a consequence of their interaction with dopaminergic systems. Injections of APV (2-amino-5-phosphonovaleric acid), a selective N-methyl-D-aspartate (NMDA) receptor antagonist, into the nucleus accumbens decreases the effective reinforcing dose of cocaine, and MK-801, a noncompetitive NMDA antagonist, also has been shown to interfere with both the acquisition and maintenance of cocaine self-administration (72,83). Because there is evidence of glutamatergic projections to the nucleus accumbens which interact with dopamine systems, these results suggest a modulatory role for glutamate on the reinforcing effects of cocaine.

It is also well known that endogenous opioid and DA systems interact in the CNS (48). An interesting series of studies on the effects of opiate agonists/antagonists on cocaine self-administration has been instrumental in shaping a new approach to the treatment of cocaine dependence, at least in clients that are also dependent on opiates. Mello et al. (60) showed that buprenorphine, a mixed opioid agonist/antagonist, specifically reduced the self-administration of cocaine in rhesus monkeys, and this reduction was maintained over time. The specificity, durability, and interpretation of this effect as indicating an antagonism of cocaine's reinforcing effects by buprenorphine has been questioned (95). In an open clinical trial, buprenorphine was reported to significantly reduce both opiate and cocaine abuse by patients who had been abusing these drugs for over 10 years (19). However, in a controlled clinical trial that demonstrated that buprenorphine was effective in reducing heroin abuse, no decreases in coexistent cocaine abuse were noted (36). Further research is necessary to determine whether buprenorphine has any clinical effectiveness in the treatment of cocaine abuse and dependence.

Pharmacotherapy

In 1985, Dackis and Gold (11) postulated that the prolonged use of cocaine resulted in a depletion of brain DA. This depletion resulted in symptoms of anergia, anhedonia, depression, and cocaine-craving during cocaine abstinence. Further detailed descriptions of a cocaine withdrawal syndrome were provided by Gawin and Kleber (21). These clinicians interviewed outpatients who retrospectively described the phasic nature and sequence of withdrawal symptoms following abrupt discontinuation of cocaine. Gawin and Kleber (21), like Dackis and Gold (11), attributed these withdrawal symptoms to disturbances in DA function. Furthermore, they hypothesized that these withdrawal symptoms would lead to craving for cocaine and relapse to cocaine use. Therefore, pharmacotherapies which would increase DA brain levels or activate DA receptors should alleviate the mood changes during withdrawal, thereby decreasing craving for cocaine and the probability of relapse (11). Later studies, conducted under controlled conditions (i.e., in an inpatient unit), however, have failed to find evidence of a phasic cocaine withdrawal pattern and, in fact, have only reported mild changes in mood and cocaine-craving during withdrawal (e.g., see ref. 82). It should be noted that these studies were done with inpatients where environmental influences on withdrawal (i.e., conditioned cues) were not present.

Although the idea that brain levels of DA are depleted as a result of chronic cocaine administration and that the functional consequences of this depletion becomes manifest upon the termination of cocaine use continues to be accepted by many clinical investigators, the support for this conception is weak. There are data in humans demonstrating that prolactin release, which is under central inhibitory DA control, is increased during the first weeks of cocaine abstinence (11,61). However, the controlled study of cocaine withdrawal by Satel et al. (82) showed only modest neuroendocrine changes indicative of DA depletion, and these were not correlated with craving for cocaine. On the other hand, position emission tomography (PET) studies of human cocaine abusers have provided support for the role of dopaminergic dysfunction during cocaine withdrawal. Volkow et al. (90) showed decreased cerebral blood flow in the prefrontal cortex in humans with a history of cocaine use. Although this deficit might be a consequence of a cerebral accident, the authors suggested that this effect was due to changes in neuronal functioning indicative of neurotoxic changes in DA neurons. A subsequent study using PET with [^{18}F]-fluorodeoxyglucose showed that glucose metabolism was increased in the orbitofrontal cortex and basal ganglia shortly following cessation of cocaine use in humans, which is also consistent with decreased DA activity (89). Activity levels were normal in subjects that were tested 2–4 weeks after cessation when symptoms of withdrawal had decreased.

Although the neuroendocrine and PET studies in humans are cited to support the idea that DA is depleted as a consequence of repeated cocaine exposure, these measures of DA levels are indirect. More definitive evidence can be obtained from animal experiments where DA levels can be measured directly. In fact, long-term depletion of brain DA and 5-HT has been found following the repeated administration of methamphetamine (MA) in a variety of animal species (85). Because MA and cocaine are pharmacologically similar, evidence of depletions following MA gives credence to the idea that brain DA may also be depleted by cocaine. However, while other MA-like drugs have also been shown to have similar long-lasting neurotoxic effects, cocaine does not decrease brain levels of DA or its metabolites in animal experiments (e.g., see ref. 47).

Although there does not appear to be evidence from animal studies of DA depletion, there have been recent data from animal studies indicating a *functional* DA depletion. That is, there is evidence, obtained using microdialysis techniques, of a decrease in basal levels of extracellular DA following chronic cocaine, at least at certain times periods. For instance, although Parsons et al. (66) showed no change in basal extracellular DA levels immediately after a 10-day regimen of 20 mg/kg/day cocaine, after 10 days of abstinence these levels were significantly reduced, which the investigators attributed to reduced release, not increases in uptake. Rossetti et al. (79), using a high-dose regimen of 15 mg/kg twice daily for 16 days, found a similar time course of effects and also reported decreases in basal extracellular DA following other drugs of abuse. Rossetti et al. (79) related these decreases in basal DA levels to the findings of Markou and Koob (59), who demonstrated that immediately following a period of prolonged cocaine self-administration, there was an increase in the threshold for electrical intracranial self-stimulation which was prolonged. Furthermore, the magnitude and duration of the increase were dose- and time-dependent. On the other hand, other investigators have shown *increased* levels of basal extracellular DA immediately following a chronic regimen, which, however, were not maintained over time (94). However, when expressed as a percent of basal DA levels, the chronic cocaine regimen resulted in a *diminished* increase in DA levels extracellularly in response to cocaine (94). Most provocative is the finding that within hours following a short regimen of intravenous cocaine self-administration, there were decreases in basal extracellular DA levels (93); these decreases were directly related to the duration of self-administration. These authors also related these findings to the changes reported in threshold for intracranial electrical stimulation reinforcement.

Although the exact nature and importance of DA dysfunction in the maintenance of cocaine dependence and withdrawal is not clear, the possibility of DA dysfunction has had a major impact on the strategy for the development of medications for the treatment of cocaine abuse. Furthermore, the evidence that cocaine's reinforcing effects are mediated by DA provides a rationale for pursuing the use of dopaminergic agonists or antagonists in the treatment of cocaine dependence, in a manner analogous to the use of methadone or naltrexone for the treatment

of heroin addiction (see Chapter 148, *this volume*). Hence, both bromocriptine, a dopamine agonist, and amantadine, which presumably releases DA and blocks its uptake, have been assessed in clinical trials for their ability to decrease withdrawal symptoms. Although there are reports that these medications decrease craving for cocaine, more recent double-blind placebo-controlled trials have failed to confirm a positive effect (e.g., see ref. 91). In addition, a variety of other types of dopaminergic agonists (e.g., pergolide, mazindol, methylphenidate) have been suggested for the treatment of cocaine dependence. Unfortunately controlled clinical trials have failed to establish their usefulness in promoting cocaine abstinence. Despite evidence that D1 and D2 receptor antagonists decrease the reinforcing effects of cocaine (see previous section), there have been no controlled trials using antagonists. There has been a report of success in an open trial with the blocker flupenthixol decanoate, but as yet this drug has not been evaluated in a more rigorous trial (20). Furthermore, because this antagonist differentially blocks inhibitory autoreceptors at low doses, the authors attribute its success to increasing DA activity, which has been decreased due to autoreceptor supersensitivity (14). On the other hand, Gawin et al. (22) have demonstrated the efficacy of desipramine, a tricyclic antidepressant, for treating cocaine dependence in a carefully conducted clinical trial. Gawin et al. (22) have speculated that desipramine's effectiveness in promoting abstinence is based on its ability to reverse the neurochemical changes produced by chronic exposure to cocaine, perhaps as a result of its ability to block DA uptake. In fact, a meta-analysis of nine placebo-controlled studies of the effectiveness of desipramine has claimed that, although this drug did not improve retention in treatment, it did promote greater rates of abstinence than placebo (52). The meta-analysis, however, included only two reports which showed that desipramine was more effective than placebo in promoting abstinence, one of which was an interim report of an ongoing study (64). When the study was completed, the investigators concluded that desipramine was not more effective than placebo (1). Thus, the conclusions of the meta-analysis by Levin and Lehman (52) may no longer be tenable. Furthermore, a later 12-week study comparing amantadine, desipramine, and placebo in different groups of methadone-maintained patients showed no differences across groups in numbers of cocaine-free urines (50). It would thus appear that the effectiveness of desipramine for the treatment of cocaine dependence is not established, although it may be useful in cocaine-dependent people with coexisting depression. It is also interesting to note that in a human self-administration study, desipramine appeared to have no effect on cocaine self-administration, although there were indications that it increased cocaine's aversive effects (16).

In summary, despite optimism based in part upon the success in the treatment of opiate addiction with agonists or antagonists and early indications of success in open clinical trials and a few controlled trials, to date, there is no pharmacological agent that appears to be effective for the treatment of cocaine dependence. The failure to find an effective medication for the treatment of cocaine dependence may be due to our limited knowledge of the neurobiological basis of cocaine reinforcement and dependence. It may also be the case, however, that the neural substrates of cocaine reinforcement and dependence are more difficult to selectively manipulate pharmacologically than those underlying opiate reinforcement and dependence. Thus, limiting treatment research to pharmacotherapy of any type may not be the most useful strategy (see Chapter 154, *this volume*).

ORGAN TOXICITY

Clinical studies conducted since the *Third Generation of Progress* have confirmed earlier observations that cocaine abuse produces a wide variety of toxic effects, including: toxic psychosis; increased incidence of panic disorder and suicide; convulsions; brain damage; cardiovascular problems; liver toxicity; hyperthermia; muscle damage leading to rhabdomyolysis; deviated nasal septum from snorting cocaine, as a result of its vasoconstrictive properties; and burns of the larynx from crack cocaine smoking. Cocaine has also been implicated as a cause of traumatic accidents in urban areas (54). Several recent reviews on organ toxicity are available (2), and therefore the coverage in this section will be selective.

By far the most common toxic effects of cocaine involve the cardiovascular system. There have been numerous case reports of neurovascular complications associated with the use of cocaine by all routes of administration (32). These include cerebral parenchymal hemorrhages, subarachnoid hemorrhages, and ischemic cerebral manifestations. In a large percentage of cases, there was evidence of underlying vascular abnormalities which, in association with the systemic hypertension produced by cocaine, may have led to hemorrhagic stroke. The pathological changes in the vasculature that place individuals at increased risk for neurovascular accidents with cocaine include arteriolar thickening, increased perivascular deposits of collagen and glycoprotein, and inflammatory cellular infiltrates (8).

The cardiovascular toxicity of cocaine and the mechanisms underlying the pathological changes have been extensively reviewed elsewhere (8). This review concluded that more than one mechanism accounts for the deleterious effects of cocaine on the myocardium and that a subgroup of the population may be more vulnerable to the cardiotoxic effects of cocaine. It is difficult to determine at present, for example, whether the atherosclerotic changes seen in young cocaine users are a function of their cocaine use or a preexisting condition. This preexisting condition

is then exacerbated by cocaine use, resulting in a cardiac emergency that brings the individual to the attention of researchers.

There have been a number of recent reports showing an association between nontraumatic rhabdomyolysis and cocaine abuse. Although the exact mechanism responsible for this association is not known, it is important clinically for several reasons. First, chest pain associated with rhabdomyolysis may be misdiagnosed as cocaine-induced myocardial infarction; second, rhabdomyolysis may lead to fatal kidney failure (81).

The use of cocaine by women during pregnancy is a major public health concern, although the evidence for teratogenic and mutagenic effects is controversial. Furthermore, estimates of the incidence of neonatal exposure to cocaine in utero vary widely and are increasingly difficult to obtain (84). In addition, much of the early clinical research giving rise to the concern about "crack babies" was seriously flawed and failed to consider that pregnant cocaine users are often polydrug abusers, nutritionally deprived, and infected with sexually transmitted diseases, and that they rarely obtain adequate prenatal care. A meta-analysis of studies on the effects of cocaine on fetal development found few perinatal effects, other than low birth weight, that could be specifically attributed to the mother's use of cocaine (56). Importantly, the low birth weight seen in many neonates that are born to cocaine-using mothers can be significantly attenuated if the mother receives adequate prenatal care (73). It is thus of the utmost importance that in our attempts to protect the developing fetus from cocaine exposure, we do not have policies which will lead drug-using women to avoid contact with medical services. In addition, it is now time to focus research efforts on developmental outcomes because even if there are no discernible perinatal effects, the long-term outcome of exposure to cocaine in utero as well as subsequent exposure to a drug-using lifestyle is unknown.

Because it is extremely difficult to determine the specific effects of cocaine on pregnancy outcome and later postnatal development, animal research would seem to be the obvious answer for controlling many of the confounding variables. The use of animal models for studying the effects of drugs of abuse on fetal development, however, raises its own set of difficulties. For a discussion of these problems, see Schuster and Gust (84).

SUMMARY

Although the use of cocaine in the general population has declined markedly in the last few years, the abuse of cocaine by regular users has not. Furthermore, since the introduction of crack cocaine in the mid-1980s, there has been a tremendous increase in (a) the number of ER mentions in association with cocaine (DAWN) and (b) the numbers of people presenting for treatment with cocaine dependence as their primary problem. During this same period of time, rapid advances in our understanding of the molecular, cellular, physiological, and behavioral bases of cocaine-dependence-producing effects have been made. This research has clearly shown the importance of DA systems in mediating these effects. It is also clear, however, that a full understanding of the dependence-producing properties will not emerge until the complex interactions among the multiple neuronal systems that cocaine affects are understood. Furthermore, these neuronal mechanisms must be studied in conjunction with environmental manipulations which modify cocaine's reinforcing efficacy. This research will also provide insights into the interactions of neurochemical systems and their interaction with environmental determinants of behavior that will have implications far beyond the phenomenon of cocaine dependence. These insights may also aid us in our search for a medication to decrease the reinforcing efficacy of cocaine, decrease withdrawal signs and symptoms that are related to relapse, and help maintain longer-term abstinence. Such medications would help to make the cocaine-dependent individual more "available" for behavioral and psychosocial interventions which are essential if the individual is to achieve a cocaine-free lifestyle.

ACKNOWLEDGMENTS

This chapter was prepared during the same period of time that another chapter on the same topic was being prepared by CEJ. That chapter will appear in *Handbook of Experimental Pharmacology, Volume 116: Pharmacological Aspects of Drug Dependence: Toward an Integrated Neurobehavioral Approach*, edited by C. R. Schuster and M. Kuhar, publisher Springer-Verlag. The authors are M. W. Fischman and C.-E. Johanson. Portions of the two chapters overlap and all authors have agreed to this arrangement. In addition, the editors of both books have been informed.

REFERENCES

1. Arndt IO, Dorozynsky L, Woody GE, McLellan AT, O'Brien CP. Desipramine treatment of cocaine dependence in methadone-maintained patients. *Arch Gen Psychiatry* 1992;49:888–893.
2. Benowitz NL. How toxic is cocaine? In: *Cocaine: scientific and social dimensions*. Chichester: John Wiley & Sons, Ciba Foundation Symposium 166, 1992;125–148.
3. Butynski W, Reda JL, Canova D, et al. *State resources and services related to alcohol and drug abuse profile data*. Washington, DC: National Association of State Alcohol and Drug Abuse Directors, 1991.
4. Caine SG, Koob GF. Modulation of cocaine self-administration in the rat through D-3 dopamine receptors. *Science* 1993;260:1814–1816.
5. Carroll FI, Lewin AH, Boja JW, Kuhar MJ. Cocaine receptor: biochemical characterization and structure-activity relationships of cocaine analogues at the dopamine transporter. *J Med Chem* 1992;35:969–981.
6. Carroll ME, Lac ST, Acensio M, Kragh R. Fluoxetine reduces intravenous cocaine self-administration in rats. *Pharmacol Biochem Behav* 1990;35:237–244.
7. Chilcoat HD, Schutz CG. Racial/ethnic differences in crack use within neighborhoods. *Addiction Res* 1994; in press.
8. Chow JM, Menchen SL, Paul BD, Stein RJ. Vascular changes in the nasal submucosa of chronic cocaine addicts. *Am J Forensic Med Pathol* 1990;11:136–143.
9. Cunningham KA, Callahan PM. Monoamine reuptake inhibitors enhance the discriminative state induced by cocaine in the rat. *Psychopharmacology* 1991;104:177–180.
10. Cunningham KA, Paris JM, Goeders NE. Serotonin neurotransmission in cocaine sensitization. In: Kalivas PW, Samson HH, eds. *The neurobiology of drug and alcohol addiction*. New York: The New York Academy of Sciences, 1992;117–127.
11. Dackis CA, Gold MS. Pharmacological approaches to cocaine addiction. *J Subst Abuse Treat* 1985;2:139–145.
12. Di Chiara G, Imperato A. Drugs abused by humans preferentially increase synaptic dopamine concentrations in the mesolimbic system of freely moving rats. *Proc Natl Acad Sci USA* 1988;85:5274–5278.
13. Dworkin SI, Smith JE. Neurobehavioral pharmacology of cocaine. In: Clouet D, Asghar K, Brown R, eds. *Mechanisms of cocaine abuse and toxicity*. Washington, DC: U.S. Government Printing Office, 1988;185–198.
14. Dwoskin LP, Peris J, Yasuda RP, Philpott K, Zahniser NR. Repeated cocaine administration results in supersensitivity of striatal D-2 autoreceptors to pergolide. *Life Sci* 1988;42:255–262.
15. Evans SM, Cone EJ, Marco AP, Henningfield JE. A comparison of the arterial kinetics of smoked and intravenous cocaine. In: Harris L, eds. *Problems of drug dependence, 1992*. Rockville, MD: U.S. Department of Health and Human Services, 1993;343.
16. Fischman MW, Foltin RW. The effects of desipramine maintenance on cocaine self-administration in humans. *Psychopharmacology* 1988;96:S20.
17. Foltin RW, Fischman MW. Ethanol and cocaine interactions in humans: cardiovascular consequences. *Pharmacol Biochem Behav* 1989;31:877–883.
18. Foltin RW, Fischman MW. Smoked and intravenous cocaine in humans: acute tolerance, cardiovascular and subjective effects. *J Pharmacol Exp Ther* 1991;257:247–261.
19. Gastfriend D, Mendelson J, Mello N, Teoh S, Reif S. Buprenorphine pharmacotherapy for concurrent heroin and cocaine dependence. *Am J Addict* 1993;2:269–278.
20. Gawin F, Allen D, Hurnblestone B. Outpatient treatment of "crack" cocaine smoking with flupenthixol decanoate. *Arch Gen Psychiatry* 1989;46:322–325.
21. Gawin FH, Kleber HD. Abstinence symptomatology and psychiatric diagnosis in cocaine abusers. Clinical observations. *Arch Gen Psychiatry* 1986;43:107–113.
22. Gawin FH, Kleber HD, Byck R, et al. Desipramine facilitation of initial cocaine abstinence. *Arch Gen Psychiatry* 1989;46:117–121.
23. Goeders NE, Smith JE. Intracranial cocaine self-administration into the medial prefrontal cortex increases dopamine turnover in the nucleus accumbens. *J Pharmacol Exp Ther* 1993;265:592–600.
24. Grilli M, Wright AG, Hanbauer I. Characterization of [³H]-dopamine uptake sites and [³H]cocaine recognition sites in primary cultures of mesencephalic neurons during in vitro development. *J Neurochem* 1991;56:2108–2115.
25. Hearn WL, Flynn DD, Hime GW, et al. Cocaethylene: a unique cocaine metabolite displays high affinity for the dopamine transporter. *J Neurochem* 1991;56:698–701.
26. Hearn WL, Rose S, Wagner J, Ciarleglios A, Mash DC. Cocaethylene is more potent that cocaine in mediating lethality. *Pharmacol Biochem Behav* 1991;3:531–533.
27. Henry DJ, White FJ. Electrophysiological correlates of psychomotor stimulant-induced sensitization. In: Kalivas PW, Samson HH, eds. *The neurobiology of drug and alcohol addiction*. New York: The New York Academy of Sciences, 1992;654:88–100.
28. Hime GW, Hearn WL, Rose S, Cofino J. Analysis of cocaine and cocaethylene in blood and tissues by GD-NPD and GC-ion trap mass spectrometry. *J Anal Toxicol* 1991;15:241–245.
29. Hubner CB, Moreton JE. Effects of selective D1 and D2 dopamine

antagonists on cocaine self-administration in the rat. *Psychopharmacology* 1991;105:151–156.

30. Hurd YL, Weiss F, Anden N-E, Koob GF, Ungerstedt U. Cocaine reinforcement and extracellular dopamine overflow in rat nucleus accumbens: an in vivo microdialysis study. *Brain Res* 1989;498:199–203.
31. Izenwasser S, Cox BM. Daily cocaine treatment produces a persistent reduction of [³H]dopamine uptake in vitro in rat nucleus accumbens but not in striatum. *Brain Res* 1990;531:338–341.
32. Jacobs IG, Roszler MH, Kelly JK, Klein MA, Kling GA. Cocaine abuse: neurovascular complications. *Radiology* 1989;170:223–227.
33. Johanson CE, Barrett JE. The discriminative stimulus effects of cocaine in pigeons. *J Pharmacol Exp Ther* 1993;267:1–8.
34. Johanson CE, Fischman MF. The pharmacology of cocaine related to its abuse. *Pharmacol Rev* 1989;41:3–52.
35. Johanson CE, Schuster CR. Animal models of drug self-administration. In: Mello NK, ed. *Advances in substance abuse: behavioral and biological research.* Greenwich, CT, JAI Press, 1981; 219–297.
36. Johnson RE, Jaffe JH, Fudala PJ. A controlled trial of buprenorphine treatment for opioid dependence. *JAMA* 1992;267:2750–2755.
37. Kalivas PW, Duffy P. Time course of extracellular dopamine and behavioral sensitization to cocaine. I. Dopamine axon terminals. *J Neurosci* 1993;13:266–275.
38. Kalivas PW, Duffy P. Time course of extracellular dopamine and behavioral sensitization to cocaine. II. Dopamine perikarya. *J Neurosci* 1993;13:276–284.
39. Kalivas PW, Sorg BA, Hooks MS. The pharmacology and neural circuitry of sensitization to psychostimulants. *Behav Pharmacol* 1993;4:315–334.
40. Kalivas PW, Striplin CD, Steketee JD, Klitenick MA, Duffy P. Cellular mechanisms of behavioral sensitization to drugs of abuse. In: Kalivas PW, Samson HH, eds. *The neurobiology of drug and alcohol addiction.* New York: The New York Academy of Sciences, 1992;654:128–135.
41. Kandel DB, Faust R. Sequences and stages in patterns of adolescent drug use. *Arch Gen Psychiatry* 1975;32:923–932.
42. Kandel DB, Yamaguchi K. From beer to crack: developmental patterns of involvement in drugs. *Am J Public Health* 1993;83:851–855.
43. Kilbey MM, Breslau N, Andreski P. Cocaine use and dependence in young adults: associated psychiatric disorders and personality traits. *Drug Alcohol Depend* 1992;29:283–290.
44. Kilty JE, Lorang D, Amara SG. Cloning and expression of a cocaine-sensitive rat dopamine transporter. *Science* 1991;254:578–579.
45. Kitayama S, Shimada S, Xu H, Markham L, Donovan DM, Uhl GR. Dopamine transporter site-directed mutations differentially alter substrate transport and cocaine binding. *Proc Natl Acad Sci USA* 1992;89:7782–7785.
46. Kleven MS, Anthony EW, Woolverton WL. Pharmacological characterization of the discriminative stimulus effects of cocaine in rhesus monkeys. *J Pharmacol Exp Ther* 1990;254:312–317.
47. Kleven MS, Woolverton WL, Seiden LS. Lack of long-term monoamine depletions following continuous or repeated exposure to cocaine. *Brain Res Bull* 1988;21:233–237.
48. Koob GF, Bloom FE. Cellular and molecular mechanisms of drug dependence. *Science* 1988;242:715–723.
49. Koob GF, Le HT, Creese I. The D1 dopamine receptor antagonist SCH 23390 increases cocaine self-administration in the rat. *Neurosci Lett* 1987;79:315–320.
50. Kosten RT, Morgan CM, Falcione J, Schottenfeld RS. Pharmacotherapy for cocaine-abusing methadone-maintained patients using amantadine or desipramine. *Arch Gen Psychiatry* 1992;49:894–898.
51. Kuhar MJ, Ritz MC, Boja JW. The dopamine hypothesis of the reinforcing properties of cocaine. *Trends Neurosci* 1991;14:299–302.
52. Levin FR, Lehman AF. Meta-analysis of desipramine as an adjunct in the treatment of cocaine addiction. *J Clin Psychopharmacol* 1991;11:374–378.
53. Lillie-Blanton M, Anthony JC, Schuster CR. Probing the meaning of racial/ethnic group comparisons in crack-cocaine smoking. *JAMA* 1993;269:993–997.
54. Lindenbaum GA, Carroll SF, Daskal I, Kapusnick R. Patterns of alcohol and drug abuse in an urban trauma center: the increasing role of cocaine abuse. *J Trauma* 1989;29:1654–1658.
55. Loh EA, Roberts DCS. Break-points on a progressive ratio schedule reinforced by intravenous cocaine increase following depletion of forebrain serotonin. *Psychopharmacology* 1990;101:262–266.
56. Lutiger B, Graham K, Einarson TR, Koren G. Relationship between gestational cocaine use and pregnancy outcome: a meta-analysis. *Teratology* 1991;44:405–414.
57. Maldonado R, Robledo P, Chover AJ, Caine SB, Koob GF. D1 dopamine receptors in the nucleus accumbens modulate cocaine self-administration in the rat. *Pharmacol Biochem Behav* 1993;45:239–242.
58. Mannuzza S, Klein RG, Bessler A, Malloy P, LaPadula M. Adult outcome of hyperactive boys. *Arch Gen Psychiatry* 1993;50:565–576.
59. Markou A, Koob GF. Postcocaine anhedonia: an animal model of cocaine withdrawal. *Neuropsychopharmacology* 1991;4:17–26.
60. Mello NK, Mendelson JH, Bree MP, Lukas SE. Buprenorphine suppresses cocaine self-administration by rhesus monkeys. *Science* 1989;245:859–862.
61. Mendelson JH, Mello NK, Teoh SK, Elingboe J, Cochin J. Cocaine effects on pulsatile secretion of anterior pituitary, gonadal, and adrenal hormones. *J Clin Endocrinol Metab* 1989;69:1256–1260.
62. Ng JP, Hubert GW, Justice JB. Increased stimulated release and uptake of dopamine in nucleus accumbens after repeated cocaine administration as measured by in vivo voltammetry. *J Neurochem* 1991;56:1485–1492.
63. National Institute on Drug Abuse. National survey results on drug use from The Monitoring the Future Study, 1975–1992. Government Publication Number 93-3597, 1993.
64. O'Brien CP, Childress AR, Arndt IO, McLellan AT, Woody GE, Maany I. Pharmacological and behavioral treatments of cocaine dependence: controlled studies. *J Clin Psychiatry* 1988;49(Suppl):17–22.
65. Ostrea EM, Brady M, Gause S, Raymundo AL, Stevens M. Drug screening of newborns by meconium analysis: a large-scale, prospective, epidemiologic study. *Pediatrics* 1992;89:107–113.
66. Parsons LH, Smith AD, Justice JB. Basal extracellular dopamine is decreased in the rat nucleus accumbens during abstinence from chronic cocaine. *Synapse* 1991;9:60–65.
67. Perez-Reyes M, Jeffcoat AR. Ethanol/cocaine interaction: cocaine and cocaethylene plasma concentrations and their relationship to subjective and cardiovascular effects. *Life Sci* 1992;51:553–563.
68. Pettit H, Justice J Jr. Dopamine in the nucleus accumbens during cocaine self-administration as studied by in vivo microdialysis. *Pharmacol Biochem Behav* 1989;34:899–904.
69. Pettit HO, Justice JB. Effect of dose on cocaine self-administration behavior and dopamine levels in the nucleus accumbens. *Brain Res* 1991;539:94–102.
70. Pettit HO, Pan H-T, Parsons LH, Justice JB. Extracellular concentrations of cocaine and dopamine are enhanced during chronic cocaine administration. *J Neurochem* 1990;55:798–804.
71. Post RM, Lickfeld A, Squillace KM, Contel NR. Drug–environment interaction: context dependency of cocaine induced behavioral sensitization. *Life Sci* 1981;28:755–760.
72. Pulverenti L, Maldonado-Lopez R, Koob GF. MNDA receptors in the nucleus accumbens modulate intravenous cocaine but not heroin self-administration in the rat. *Brain Res* 1992;594:327–330.
73. Racine A, Joyce T, Anderson R. The association between prenatal care and birth weight among women exposed to cocaine in New York City. *JAMA* 1993;270:13.
74. Reith MEA, de Costa B, Rice KC, Jacobson AE. Evidence for mutually exclusive binding of cocaine, BTCP, GBR 12935, and dopamine to the dopamine transporter. *Eur J Pharmacol* 1992;227:417–425.
75. Ritz MC, Cone EJ, Kuhar MJ. Cocaine inhibition of ligand binding at dopamine, norepinephrine and serotonin transporters: a structure–activity study. *Life Sci* 1990;46:635–645.
76. Ritz MC, Lamb RJ, Goldberg SR, Kuhar MJ. Cocaine receptors on dopamine transporters are related to self-administration of cocaine. *Science* 1987;237:1219–1223.

77. Roberts DCS, Loh EA, Vickers G. Self-administration of cocaine on a progressive ratio schedule in rats: dose–response relationship and effect of haloperidol pretreatment. *Psychopharmacology* 1989;97:535–538.

78. Robinson TE. Stimulant drugs and stress: factors influencing individual differences in the susceptibility to sensitization. In: Kalivas PW, Barnes CD, eds. *Sensitization in the nervous systems.* Caldwell, NJ: Telford Press, 1988;145–173.

79. Rossetti ZL, Hmaidan Y, Gessa GL. Marked inhibition of mesolimbic dopamine release: a common feature of ethanol, morphine, cocaine and amphetamine abstinence in rats. *Eur J Pharmacol* 1992;221:227–234.

80. Rounsaville BJ, Foley-Anton S, Carroll K, Budde D, Pursoff BA, Gawin F. Psychiatric diagnosis of treatment-seeking cocaine abusers. *Arch Gen Psychiatry* 1991;48:43–51.

81. Rubin RB, Neugarten J. Cocaine rhabdomyolysis masquerading as myocardial ischemis. *Am J Med* 1989;86:551–553.

82. Satel SL, Price LH, Palumbo JM, et al. Clinical phenomenology and neurobiology of cocaine abstinence: a prospective inpatient study. *Am J Psychiatry* 1991;148:1712–1716.

83. Schenk S, Valadez A, McNamara C, et al. Development and expression of sensitization to cocaine's reinforcing properties: role of NMDA receptors. *Psychopharmacology* 1993;111:332–338.

84. Schuster CR, Gust S. Cocaine: challenges to research. In: Edwards G, Strang J, Jaffe JH, eds. *Drugs, alcohol, and tobacco.* Oxford: Oxford University Press, 1993;146–155.

85. Seiden LS, Ricaurte GA. Neurotoxicity of methamphetamine and related drugs. In: Meltzer HY, ed. *Psychopharmacology: the third generation of progress.* New York: Raven Press, 1987;359–366.

86. Shimada S, Kitayama S, Lin C-L, et al. Cloning and expression of a cocaine-sensitive dopamine transporter complementary DNA. *Science* 1991;254:576–577.

87. Spealman RD, Bergman J, Madras BK, Melia KF. Discriminative stimulus effects of cocaine in squirrel monkeys: involvement of dopamine receptor subtypes. *J Pharmacol Exp Ther* 1991;258:945–953.

88. Stewart J, Vezina P. Microinjections of SCH-23390 into the ventral tegmental area and substantia nigra pars reticulata attenuate the development of sensitization to the locomotor activating effects of systemic amphetamine. *Brain Res* 1989;495:401–406.

89. Volkow ND, Fowler JS, Wolf AP, et al. Changes in brain glucose metabolism in cocaine dependence and withdrawal. *Am J Psychiatry* 1991;148:621–626.

90. Volkow ND, Mullani N, Gould KL, Adler S, Krajewski K. Cerebral blood flow in chronic cocaine users: a study with positron emission tomography. *Br J Psychiatry* 1988;152:641–648.

91. Weddington WW, Brown BS, Haertzen CA, et al. Comparison of amantadine and desipramine combined with psychotherapy for treatment of cocaine dependence. *Am J Drug Alcohol Abuse* 1991;17:137–152.

92. Weed MR, Vanover KE, Woolverton WL. Reinforcing effect of the D1 dopamine agonist SKF 81297 in rhesus monkeys. *Psychopharmacology* 1993;113:51–52.

93. Weiss F, Markou A, Lorang MT, Koob GF. Basal extracellular dopamine levels in the nucleus accumbens are decreased during cocaine withdrawal after unlimited-access self-administration. *Brain Res* 1992;593:314–318.

94. Weiss F, Paulus MP, Lorang MR, Koob GF. Increases in extracellular dopamine in the nucleus accumbens by cocaine are inversely related to basal levels: effects of acute and repeated administration. *J Neurosci* 1992;12:4372–4380.

95. Winger G, Skjoldager P, Woods JH. Effects of buprenorphine and other opioid agonists and antagonists on alfentanil- and cocaine-reinforced responding in rhesus monkeys. *J Pharmacol Exp Ther* 1992;261:311–317.

96. Wise RA, Bozarth MA. A psychomotor stimulant theory of addiction. *Psychol Rev* 1987;94:469–492.

97. Witkin JM, Nichols DE, Terry P, Katz JL. Behavioral effects of selective dopaminergic compounds in rats discriminating cocaine injection. *J Pharmacol Exp Ther* 1991;257:706–713.

98. Woody GE, McLellan AT, Luborsky L, O'Brien CP. Sociopathy and psychotherapy outcome. *Arch Gen Psychiatr* 1985;42:1081–1086.

99. Woolverton WL. Effects of a D1 and a D2 dopamine antagonist on the self-administration of cocaine and piribedil by rhesus monkeys. *Pharmacol Biochem Behav* 1986;24:531–535.

100. Woolverton WL, Virus RM. The effects of a D1 and a D2 dopamine antagonist on behavior maintained by cocaine or food. *Pharmacol Biochem Behav* 1989;32:691–697.

101. Yi S-J, Johnson KM. Effects of acute and chronic administration of cocaine on striatal uptake, compartmentalization and release of [^{3}H]dopamine. *Neuropharmacology* 1990;29:475–486.

Psychopharmacology: The Fourth Generation of Progress, edited by Floyd E. Bloom and David J. Kupfer. Raven Press, Ltd., New York © 1995.

CHAPTER 146

Caffeine—A Drug of Abuse?

Roland R. Griffiths and Geoffrey K. Mumford

The widespread use of culturally sanctioned caffeine-containing foods presents an intriguing paradox. On one hand, it is the experience of most regular caffeine users that caffeine produces only rather subtle effects that are generally so well-woven into the fabric of daily experience that they are not clearly differentiated from the changes in mood and behavior associated with normal experience.

On the other hand, however, caffeine is arguably the most robust form of drug self-administration known to man. Consider the facts: (a) Historically, use of caffeine-containing foods has been long-term (possibly dating back 4700 years), with use of these foods spreading worldwide despite recurring efforts, motivated on moral, economic, medical, or political grounds, to restrict or eliminate their use (4,45). (b) Currently, regular daily consumption of behaviorally active doses [e.g., >80% of adults in the United States (44,69)] is widespread throughout the world (38); the extent of caffeine usage far exceeds that estimated for alcohol and nicotine, which rank second and third, respectively, as the most widely consumed psychotropic drugs worldwide (39). (c) Habitual consumption of behaviorally active doses of caffeine occurs in widely different vehicles (e.g., drinking of coffee, tea, soft drinks, maté; chewing kola nuts) and under widely different social and cultural conditions; therefore, caffeine ingestion is a remarkably generalized form of drug self-administration occurring across a broad range of dietary and contextual conditions.

It is this paradox of seemingly subtle pharmacological effects juxtaposed against its robustness as a self-adminis-

tered drug that makes caffeine among the most intriguing psychotropic substances for research into the behavioral–pharmacological mechanisms underlying the habitual use of drugs generally, and possibly drugs of abuse in particular. The purpose of this chapter is to provide an updated review of the rapidly emerging research literature concerning the behavioral pharmacology of caffeine as it relates to our understanding of self-administered and abused substances. Specifically, the chapter will review infrahuman and human research on the reinforcing effects of caffeine and human research on caffeine subjective effects, tolerance, and physical dependence. The review will conclude with a discussion about whether it is meaningful to consider caffeine to be a drug of abuse. Neurochemical mechanisms underlying some of caffeine's pharmacological effects are discussed in Chapter 57 on purinoceptors in this volume.

REINFORCING EFFECTS OF CAFFEINE IN LABORATORY ANIMALS

Reinforcing efficacy of a drug refers to the relative effectiveness in establishing or maintaining behavior on which the delivery of the drug is dependent (52). Over the last 25 years, reliable experimental models of drug-taking behavior in laboratory animals have been developed that provide valid information about the relative reinforcing effects of psychoactive drugs (10,48) (see Chapter 66, *this volume*).

Intravenous self-injection has a high degree of face validity and is often regarded by specialists as providing the most direct and unequivocal assessment of a drug's reinforcing effect (11). Intravenous self-injection involves implanting a venous catheter in animals and allowing them to self-administer a drug. A behavioral response (often a lever press) is followed by intravenous drug injection. The ability of the injection to reinforce behavior is assessed by examining the establishment or maintenance of responding, usually relative to vehicle control.

R. R. Griffiths: Department of Psychiatry and Behavioral Sciences and Department of Neurosciences, Behavioral Biology Research Center, Johns Hopkins University School of Medicine, Baltimore, Maryland 21224.

G. K. Mumford: Department of Psychiatry and Behavioral Sciences, Behavioral Biology Research Center, Johns Hopkins University School of Medicine, Baltimore, Maryland 21224.

TABLE 1. *Reinforcing effects of caffeine in laboratory animals—intravenous self-injection*[a]

Reference	Species	Method	Results
Nonhuman primates			
Deneau, Yanagita, and Seevers, 1969 (25)	Rhesus monkeys	Intravenous injections (1–5 mg/kg, as an unspecified caffeine salt) were dependent on a lever-press response under FR 1 schedule; 24-hr access for as long as 18 weeks; if self-injection was not spontaneously initiated, then animals received programmed injections.	Self-injection was maintained in all 5 monkeys at one or more dose(s), although programmed injections were required to initiate self-injection on some occasions; the pattern of self-injection was sporadic, with irregular intervals of self-injection alternating with periods of abstinence.
Schuster, Woods, and Seevers, 1969 (96)	Rhesus monkeys	Intravenous injections (1–5 mg/kg caffeine) were dependent on lever-press response; 24-hr access; some animals tested after 1-month of programmed administration.	Self-injection was maintained in 1 of 4 monkeys.
Yanagita, 1970 (110)	Rhesus monkeys	Intravenous injections (0.25–4 mg/kg caffeine) were dependent on lever-press response; 4-hr access for 3 days after substitution for SPA.	Self-injection was not maintained in 4 monkeys when caffeine was substituted for SPA, a CNS stimulant which maintains high rates of self-injection.
Hoffmeister and Wuttke, 1973 (61)	Rhesus monkeys	Intravenous injections (0.2 mg/kg caffeine) were dependent on lever-press response under FR 10 schedule; 3-hr access for 6 days after substitution for codeine.	Self-injection was not maintained at the single dose level tested in 3 monkeys when caffeine was substituted for codeine.
Griffiths, Brady, and Bradford, 1979 (52)	Baboons	Intravenous injections (0.1–10.0 mg/kg caffeine citrate) were dependent on lever-press response under FR 160 schedule 3-hr time-out; 24-hr access for 15 days after substitution for cocaine.	Self-injection was maintained in all 3 baboons at 3.2 mg/kg/inj; self-injection performance was sporadic across days in 2 of 3 baboons.
Griffiths, Sannerud, and Kaminski, (Figure 1, previously unpublished data)	Baboons	Intravenous injections (0.1 mg/kg caffeine citrate) were dependent on lever-press response under FR 2 schedule; 50 injections or 2 hr, whichever came first, for 9–13 weeks.	Self-injection was maintained in all 3 baboons; self-injection was sporadic across days in all 3 baboons.
Rats			
Atkinson and Enslen, 1976 (3)	Rats	Intravenous injections (0.3–5 mg/kg caffeine) were dependent on lever-press response under FR 1 schedule of 24-hr access for 3–7 days; some rats received forced pretreatment with caffeine for up to 98 hr before self-injection.	Self-injection of caffeine was maintained in 5 of an estimated total of 18 rats tested at doses of 1–5 mg/kg; self-injection was maintained up to 4 days and decreased thereafter, self-injection occurred in animals with and without caffeine pretreatment.
Collins, Weeks, Cooper, Good, and Russell, 1984 (20)	Rats	Intravenous injections (1 mg/kg caffeine) were dependent on lever-press response under FR 1 schedule; 24-hr access for 9 days, with the dose reduced to 0.1 mg/kg on day 6.	Self-injection was maintained in 2 of 6 rats.
Dworkin, Vrana, Broadbent, and Robinson, 1993 (28)	Rats	Intravenous injections (0.25 mg/injection caffeine) were dependent on lever-press response under FR 1 schedule; 1- to 3-hr access for 30 days after training food-maintained responding.	Self-injection of caffeine was maintained in the 3 rats tested at about 15 and 8 responses/hr over first 5 and 30 days, respectively; maintenance of self-injection was concluded, although no vehicle control data were presented.

[a] Doses are expressed as the free drug, except as noted. Except where otherwise noted, self-injection was concluded if rate of responding under the drug condition was higher than that under control (usually vehicle) conditions in the same or different animals.

As shown in Table 1, intravenous drug self-injection studies indicate that caffeine can function as a reinforcer under some conditions. Of the nine self-injection studies (all of which were conducted in nonhuman primates and rats), all but two demonstrated caffeine self-injection in at least a portion of the animals studied. The two negative studies either tested only one dose level of caffeine (61) or tested caffeine self-injection for a relatively short period (1 or 3 days) after substitution for a psychomotor stimulant drug (SPA) that maintained high rates of self-injection (110).

Of the seven positive studies, four demonstrated self-

Intravenous Caffeine Self-Injection in Baboons

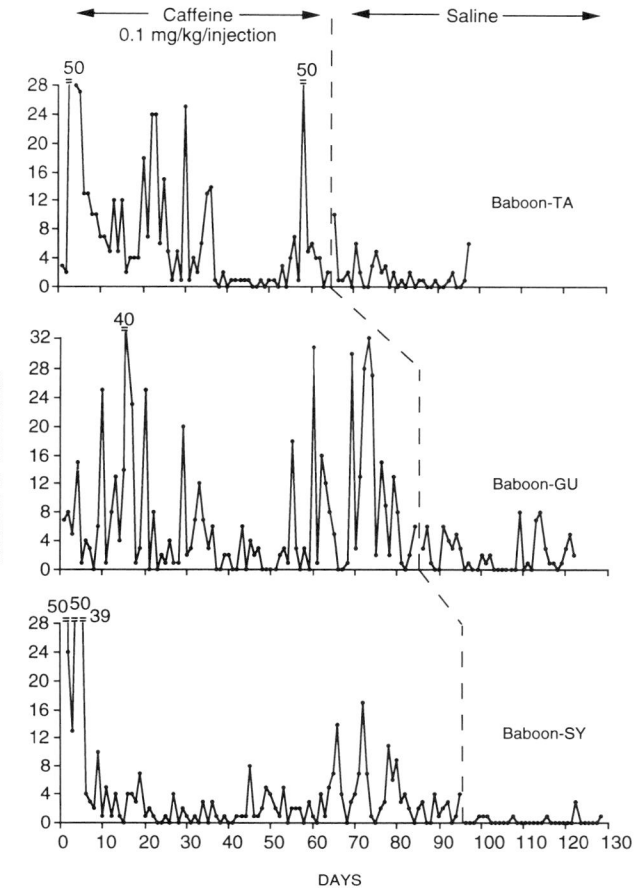

FIG. 1. Intravenous self-injection of caffeine in each of three male baboons with histories of self-injection of various stimulant and sedative drugs. Using methods similar to those described previously (52), injections were dependent on a lever-press response under fixed-ratio 2 (FR 2) schedule of reinforcement; daily sessions were terminated after 50 injections or after 2 hr, whichever came first. *Data points* show number of injections self-administered each day; numerals above points indicate number of injections when that number exceeded 32. *Dashed line* indicates the point at which saline (caffeine vehicle) was substituted for caffeine (Griffiths, Sannerud, and Kaminski, *unpublished data;* see Table 2).

injection in all animals (25,28,52; Griffiths, Sannerud, and Kaminski, *unpublished data;* Table 1), whereas three (3,20,96) showed that only a subset of animals (25–33%) self-injected caffeine. A characteristic sporadic pattern of caffeine self-injection has emerged in three studies with nonhuman primates that examined self-injection over an extended period of consecutive days (25,52; Griffiths, Sannerud, and Kaminski, *unpublished data;* Table 1). This pattern is characterized by periods of relatively high rates of intake alternating irregularly with periods of low intake. Figure 1 illustrates this pattern in three baboons.

These intravenous self-injection studies clearly show that caffeine can function as a reinforcer under some con-

ditions. However, the inconsistent results across animals and studies contrast with the results reported with the classic abused stimulants (e.g., amphetamine and cocaine) that have more consistently been shown to maintain intravenous self-injection across a wide range of species and conditions (52). The variation in results with caffeine is analogous to that reported in self-injection studies with nicotine: Nicotine has not reliably maintained self-injection across animals and studies. It has been concluded that although nicotine can serve as a reinforcer (40,59), it does so under a more limited range of conditions than do drugs such as cocaine (28,40). A similar conclusion seems warranted for caffeine (28).

REINFORCING EFFECTS OF CAFFEINE IN HUMANS

As in the animal drug self-administration laboratory, over the last 25 years, reliable procedures have been developed in the human laboratory for examining the reinforcing effects of drugs (7,23,48,60). These procedures have permitted the demonstration of drug reinforcement and the examination of correlates and determinants of reinforcement.

Demonstration of Caffeine Reinforcement

Although the circumstantial evidence suggesting the reinforcing effects of caffeine is compelling (see introductory paragraphs at beginning of this chapter), clear experimental evidence has only recently been reported. Table 2 summarizes 10 studies that examined whether caffeine could function as a reinforcer in humans. These studies provide unequivocal evidence of the reinforcing effects of caffeine. These studies demonstrated caffeine reinforcement under double-blind conditions using various subject populations (moderate and heavy caffeine users with and without histories of alcohol or drug abuse), using a variety of different methodological approaches (variations on both choice and ad libitum self-administration procedures), when caffeine was available in coffee, soda, or capsules, when subjects did and did not have immediate past histories of chronic caffeine exposure, and in the context of different behavioral requirements after drug ingestion (vigilance versus relaxation activities). Figure 2 illustrates caffeine reinforcement in three subjects who chose between capsules containing caffeine and placebo.

Incidence of Caffeine Reinforcement

Table 2 shows that caffeine reinforcement has been demonstrated in 100% of subjects with histories of heavy caffeine use and abuse of alcohol or drugs (49–51) and in a somewhat lower proportion (about 45%) of subjects

TABLE 2. *Reinforcing effects of caffeine in humans[a,b]*

Reference	Subjects	Method	Results
Griffiths, Bigelow, Liebson, O'Keeffe, O'Leary, and Russ, 1986 (51)	Three male subjects with histories of heavy coffee drinking (mean prestudy caffeine intake, 1530 mg/day) and alcohol abuse.	Subjects lived on a residential research ward where access to coffee was experimentally controlled; the caffeine dose per cup of coffee was varied in a mixed sequence across days (decaff, 25, 50, 100, 200, and 400 mg/cup).	Low caffeine doses (25 or 50 mg/cup) were correlated with a slightly higher number of cups consumed than the decaffeinated condition in all three subjects; for all 3 subjects, higher doses of caffeine (50–400 mg) produced orderly dose-related decreases in cups consumed.
Griffiths, Bigelow, and Liebson, 1986 (49)	Six male subjects with histories of heavy coffee drinking (mean prestudy caffeine intake, 1020 mg/day), most of whom had histories of alcohol or drug abuse.	Subjects lived on a residential research ward where access to coffee was experimentally controlled; an across-day choice procedure was used to compare the reinforcing effects of caffeinated (100 mg/cup) versus decaffeinated coffee; on forced-exposure days the available coffee was identified to subjects by letter code; on choice days, subjects made a mutually exclusive choice between two letter-coded coffees.	Caffeinated coffee was chosen over decaffeinated coffee in all 6 subjects (11 out of a total of 12 tests) when testing was done under conditions in which subjects had been receiving caffeinated coffee daily for a week or more before forced-exposure and choice days.
Griffiths and Woodson, 1988 (57)	Twelve normal subjects with a mean prestudy caffeine intake of 361 mg/day.	An across-day choice procedure was used to compare the reinforcing effects of capsules containing caffeine (100, 200, 400, or 600 mg) versus placebo; on forced-exposure days the available capsules were identified to subjects by a color code; on choice days, subjects made a mutually exclusive choice between two types of color-coded capsules; subjects made 10 experimentally independent choices at each of several dose levels; testing occurred when subjects were overnight abstinent from their normal caffeine intake.	Significant caffeine choice was demonstrated in 5 of 12 subjects at one or more dose(s); percentage selection of caffeine was inversely related to dose, with 4 subjects showing significant caffeine avoidance at 400 and/or 600 mg.
Griffiths, Bigelow, and Liebson, 1989 (50)	Ten male subjects with histories of heavy coffee drinking (mean prestudy caffeine intake, 1081 mg/day), most of whom had histories of alcohol or drug abuse.	Subjects lived on a residential research ward where access to coffee was experimentally controlled; in one experiment, 6 subjects had 13 opportunities daily to ingest either a caffeine (100 mg) or a placebo capsule; in a second experiment, 6 subjects had 10 opportunities daily to ingest a cup of coffee or (on different days) a capsule, dependent upon completing a work requirement that progressively increased and then decreased over days; in the second experiment, one of four conditions was studied each day: caffeinated coffee (100 mg/cup), decaffeinated coffee, caffeine capsules (100 mg/capsule), or placebo capsules.	In the first experiment, all 6 subjects developed a clear preference for caffeine capsules; in the second experiment, caffeinated coffee maintained the most self-administration, significantly higher than decaffeinated coffee and placebo capsules but not different from caffeine capsules; both caffeine capsules and decaffeinated coffee were significantly higher than placebo capsules but not different from each other.
Hughes, Higgins, Bickel, Hunt, Fenwick, Gulliver, and Mireault, 1991 (65)	Twenty-two normal, predominately female subjects with mean prestudy coffee intake of 5.3 cups/day (~451 mg/day caffeine).	A choice procedure was used to compare the reinforcing effects of caffeinated (100 mg/cup) versus decaffeinated coffee; on forced-exposure days the available coffee was identified to subjects by letter code; on 2-day choice tests, subjects could self-administer both coffees; subjects were exposed to six experimentally independent choice tests; subjects abstained from their normal coffee intake on forced-exposure and choice days; subjects were required to consume at least 4 cups/day on forced-exposure and choice test days.	Significant choice of caffeinated coffee over decaffeinated coffee was demonstrated in 10 of 22 subjects; occurrence of headache on forced-exposure day tended to predict subsequent caffeine preference.

TABLE 2. *Continued*

Reference	Subjects	Method	Results
Hughes, Hunt, Higgins, Bickel, Fenwick, and Pepper, 1992 (66)	Eight normal, predominately female subjects who had already participated in Hughes et al., 1991 (65).	A choice procedure identical to that of Hughes et al., 1991 (65) was used, except that subjects were exposed to up to 6 experimentally independent choice tests at each of several caffeine doses (25, 50, 150, and 200 mg/cup).	Significant choice of caffeinated coffee over decaffeinated coffee was demonstrated at 25, 50, 150, and 200 mg/cup in 2 of 6, 4 of 8, 3 of 6, and 0 of 3 subjects, respectively; occurrence of headache on forced-exposure day predicted subsequent caffeine preference.
Oliveto, Hughes, Pepper, Bickel, and Higgins, 1991 (89)	Eleven normal subjects who consumed 1.5 to 7 cups coffee/day (~128–595 mg/ day caffeine).	A choice procedure similar to that of Hughes et al., 1991 (65) was used, except that subjects were not required to drink a minimum number of cups of coffee; subjects were exposed to 6 experimentally independent choice tests at each of several caffeine doses (12.5, 25, 50, and 100 mg/cup).	Significant choice of caffeinated coffee over decaffeinated coffee was demonstrated at 12.5, 25, 50, and 100 mg/cup in 0 of 2, 2 of 11, 5 of 11, and 5 of 10 subjects, respectively.
Oliveto, Hughes, Higgins, Bickel, Pepper, Shea, and Fenwick, 1992 (88)	Ten normal subjects with mean prestudy coffee intake of 3.9 cups/day (~332 mg/day caffeine).	A choice procedure similar to that of Hughes et al., 1991 (65) was used to compare the reinforcing effects of caffeinated (100 mg/ cup) versus decaffeinated coffee, except that in one condition the subjects were not required to drink a minimum number of cups of coffee.	Significant choice of caffeinated coffee over decaffeinated coffee was demonstrated in only 1 of 10 subjects, and this occurred only in the condition in which subjects were not required to drink a minimum number of cups of coffee.
Hughes, Oliveto, Bickel, Higgins, and Valliere, 1992 (68)	Nine normal subjects with mean prestudy caffeinated soda intake of 5.4 sodas/day (~194 mg/day caffeine).	A choice procedure similar to that of Hughes et al., 1991 (65) was used to compare the reinforcing effects of caffeinated soda (25, 50, or 100 mg/soda) versus decaffeinated soda.	Significant choice of caffeinated soda over decaffeinated soda was demonstrated in 4 of 9 subjects at one or more dose(s).
Silverman, Mumford, and Griffiths, 1994 (100)	Eight normal subjects with mean prestudy intake of 214 mg/ day.	Subjects were initially trained in a 100-mg caffeine versus placebo drug discrimination using letter-coded capsules; using the same letter codes, across-day drug versus drug and drug versus money choice procedures were used to assess caffeine reinforcing effects when subjects were required to engage in a computer vigilance activity or a relaxation activity following capsule ingestion; subjects made 10 choices in each condition; choices were not experimentally independent.	In a condition in which subjects could choose to take either caffeine or placebo with either vigilance or relaxation activities, significant caffeine choice was demonstrated in 6 of 6 subjects with vigilance but with only 1 of 6 with relaxation; in a condition in which subjects could choose between capsules and money, in 6 of 7 subjects, the maximum monetary value at which capsules were chosen over money was significantly higher for caffeine in vigilance than for placebo in either activity; in contrast, for 2 of 7 subjects, this value was higher for caffeine in relaxation than for placebo in either activity.

[a] Unless otherwise noted, studies were conducted on a nonresidential (i.e. outpatient) basis in which subjects periodically came to the research laboratory.

[b] Five reports of caffeine choice or self-administration have been excluded from the table because their methods or results did not allow for an unambiguous interpretation of whether or not caffeine reinforcement had been demonstrated (6,32,74,90,102).

with histories of moderate and heavy caffeine use alone (57,65,66,68,88,89,100). However, one recent study (100) demonstrated caffeine reinforcement in 100% of moderate users when they were given caffeine discrimination training and required to perform a vigilance task after capsule administration.

Caffeine Reinforcement Is an Inverted U-Shaped Function of Dose

Caffeine reinforcement appears to be an inverted U-shaped function of dose. A dose as low as 25 mg per cup of coffee has been shown to function as a reinforcer un-

Reinforcing Effects of Caffeine in Humans

● Caffeine
○ Placebo

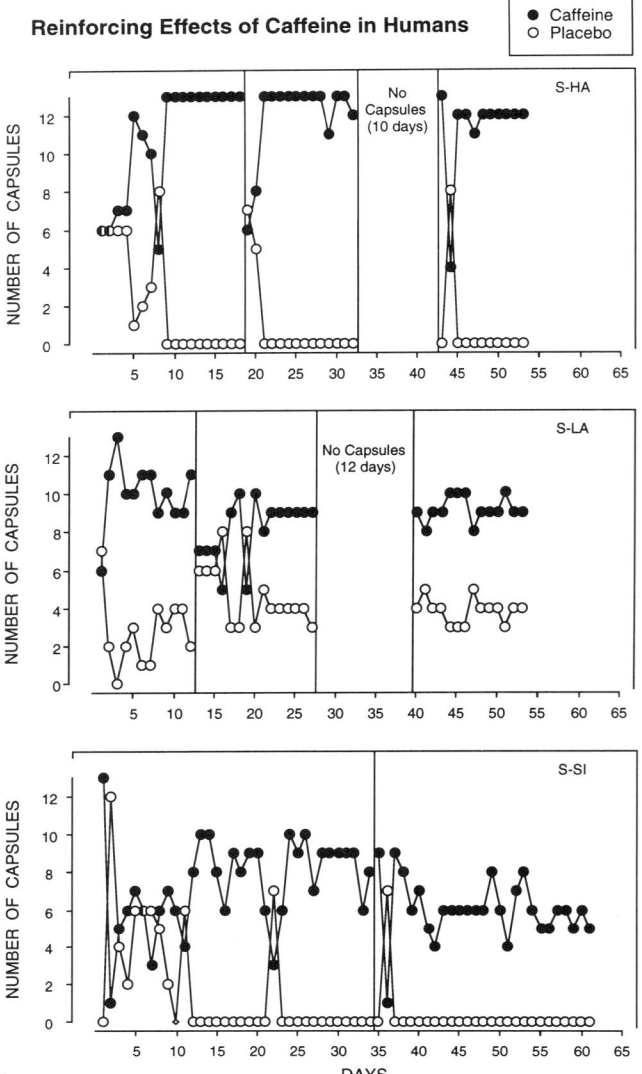

FIG. 2. Oral self-administration of caffeine capsules in each of three male volunteers with histories of heavy coffee drinking who resided in a residential laboratory. Subjects had 13 opportunities each day to self-administer either a caffeine (100 mg) or a placebo capsule. *Vertical lines* indicate a change in condition: Either novel double-blind color codes associated with caffeine and placebo capsules were introduced or a period of capsule unavailability was initiated. (Redrawn from ref. 50.)

der conditions in which subjects could repeatedly self-administer that dose within the day (66,89). A robust finding has been that increasing doses beyond 50 or 100 mg tends to decrease choice of caffeine or rates of caffeine self-administration (51,57,66,74,102). Relatively high doses of caffeine (e.g., 400 or 600 mg as a single dose) have been shown to produce significant caffeine avoidance (57).

Subjective Effects of Caffeine and Placebo Co-vary with Reinforcement or Choice

A robust finding from studies of caffeine reinforcement has been that qualitative ratings of subjective effects have generally co-varied with measures of reinforcement or choice. A good example is provided from a choice study by Evans and Griffiths (32) that examined the subjective effects of placebo and caffeine on forced-exposure days. When these data were retrospectively categorized into caffeine choosers and nonchoosers, a face-valid profile of changes in subjective effects emerged. It was found that (a) choosers showed "positive" subjective effects of caffeine relative to placebo (e.g., increased alert, content, energetic, liking), (b) nonchoosers showed "negative" effects of caffeine relative to placebo (e.g., increased anxiety, mood disturbance, jittery), and (c) choosers showed "negative" effects of placebo (e.g., increased headache, fatigue).

The results of most caffeine reinforcement and choice studies reported to date are consistent with these generalities drawn from Evans and Griffiths (32). For example, in studies involving subjects with histories of heavy coffee drinking and drug abuse, experimental conditions that have maintained higher levels of self-administration or greater choice have generally been associated with higher ratings of liking or "positive" subjective effects (49–51). Analysis of subjective effect data from a choice study by Stern et al. (102) also showed that caffeine produced positive subjective effects in choosers and negative effects in nonchoosers. That study provided little evidence that placebo was associated with negative effects in choosers, probably because subjects were not abstinent from their normal dietary caffeine. Also consistent, Griffiths and Woodson (57) reported that caffeine choice was positively related to ratings of content/satisfied and negatively related to ratings of mood disturbance and dislike effects following caffeine. Finally, Hughes et al. (67) analyzed data from a series of four previous choice studies and showed that caffeine choice was positively related to ratings of headache and drowsiness following placebo.

Despite these reasonably consistent findings across a range of different studies, it is important to recognize that the relationship between reinforcement or choice and subjective effects has not been invariant. For example, although Hughes et al. (67) demonstrated an inverse relationship between caffeine choice and the occurrence of drowsiness, they also provided examples in which this relationship was absent.

Future research should determine whether subjective effect changes in response to caffeine and placebo challenges can prospectively predict subsequent, experimentally independent caffeine reinforcement. The measures of subjective effects in all of the studies cited above have been obtained at the same time that reinforcement or choice has been assessed. In the choice studies, for example, subjective effects have been obtained during the same forced-exposure days which provided the basis for the subsequent choice.

Finally, as a historical note, the profile of subjective effects that have emerged from reinforcement studies to date are entirely consistent with the results of a survey study (41) and a companion caffeine administration study (43) that did not investigate reinforcement per se. These studies showed that after overnight caffeine abstinence, heavy coffee users reported positive subjective effects of coffee drinking or caffeine administration in contrast to coffee abstainers or light users, who reported unpleasant and undesirable subjective effects. In addition, compared to abstainers or light users, heavy users reported undesirable dysphoric effects of coffee abstinence or placebo.

Behavioral Context Modulates Caffeine Reinforcement

One recent study demonstrated that caffeine reinforcement can be enhanced by explicitly manipulating the behavioral requirements following drug ingestion (100). In that study, all subjects demonstrated caffeine reinforcement in one condition or more when a computer vigilance activity was required following drug ingestion. In contrast, only two of seven subjects showed caffeine reinforcement when a relaxation activity was required following drug ingestion.

Physical Dependence May Potentiate Caffeine Reinforcement

An important implication of the findings described above showing a relationship between abstinence-associated headache, fatigue and drowsiness, and either choice/reinforcement or heavy caffeine use is that physical dependence may potentiate the reinforcing effects of caffeine. In this regard, a retrospective analysis by Hughes et al. (67) of data from four previous studies involving choice between caffeinated coffee (100 mg/cup) and decaffeinated coffee showed that subjects who reliably reported more headache with decaffeinated than with caffeinated coffee were 2.6 times more likely to show reliable choice of caffeinated coffee.

A direct experimental test of the hypothesis linking physical dependence to reinforcement was provided in a choice study by Griffiths et al. (49) in heavy caffeine users who first received forced exposure to caffeinated and decaffeinated coffee on different days and then, on a subsequent choice day, made a mutually exclusive choice between the two coffees. When subjects had received only caffeinated coffee for a week or more before the choice tests (and presumably were physically dependent), subjects reliably chose, and reported more liking for, caffeinated over decaffeinated coffee. In contrast, when subjects had received only decaffeinated coffee for a week or more before the choice tests (and presumably were not physically dependent), subjects did not reliably choose caffeinated coffee, nor were there pronounced differences in ratings of liking.

Evans and Griffiths (32) failed to replicate the effect of caffeine physical dependence on caffeine choice in a study in which two groups of normal subjects had a choice test between capsules containing 600 mg caffeine or placebo after being exposed to either 900 mg/day caffeine or placebo for 18 days. Although the chronic caffeine group was shown to be both tolerant and physically dependent (i.e., showed withdrawal), the groups did not differ in the percentage choice of caffeine (44% versus 31% in the chronic caffeine and placebo groups, respectively). The authors speculated that the duration of placebo exposure was too short to result in maximal withdrawal after the high chronic dose of caffeine (900 mg/day). Also, the dose of caffeine used in the choice tests (600 mg) was higher than that shown to be a reinforcer in previous dose–effect studies (57,66).

Thus, although individuals who report caffeine withdrawal are more likely to show caffeine reinforcement, the two studies (32,49) that attempted to demonstrate a potentiation of caffeine reinforcement by providing a history of chronic caffeine administration have provided equivocal results. Finally, it is also clear that a history of chronic caffeine administration is not a necessary condition for caffeine to function as a reinforcer. One study demonstrated caffeine reinforcement in a subject who normally abstained from all caffeine (57), and two other studies demonstrated caffeine reinforcement in subjects after they were caffeine-free for several weeks (50,100).

Effects of Prestudy Caffeine Intake on Caffeine Reinforcement

Although a reasonable a priori prediction would be that amount of prestudy caffeine use should predict the incidence of reinforcement in experimental studies, such a relationship has not been demonstrated (57,67,102), and there has been one instance in which caffeine reinforcement was demonstrated in an individual who normally abstained from caffeine use (57). Given that subjective effects have been shown to co-vary with caffeine reinforcement, these results would appear to be at variance with studies by Goldstein and colleagues (41,43), who showed that after overnight caffeine abstinence, heavy coffee users (5 or more cups/day) reported pleasant and desirable effects of coffee drinking and caffeine in contrast to coffee abstainers or light users, who reported more unpleasant and undesirable subjective effects. It seems likely that the subject samples investigated to date in caffeine reinforcement studies have been too small and homogeneous to demonstrate what appears to be a relatively weak relationship between prestudy caffeine use and caffeine reinforcement.

Effects of Prestudy Anxiety Levels on Caffeine Reinforcement

In two studies, caffeine choice has been significantly negatively correlated with prestudy anxiety levels (32,57). In one of these studies, the two subjects with the highest prestudy anxiety had the lowest incidence of caffeine choice and demonstrated significant caffeine avoidance at a lower dose than any other subject (57). These results are consistent with questionnaire studies that have shown that anxiety and panic disorder patients report less consumption of caffeine than controls (9,76,77,104), presumably because such patients are particularly sensitive to anxiogenic and related dysphoric subjective effects of caffeine (13,17,104).

SUBJECTIVE EFFECTS OF CAFFEINE IN HUMANS

Subjective effects of a drug usually refer to drug-induced changes in an individual's experiences or feelings that are not accessible to independent verification by an observer. Reasonably sophisticated methods for assessing human subjective effects of drugs were first developed about 40 years ago (5,72) and have been extensively used to evaluate caffeine. Typically, these methods involve having subjects self-rate their moods, feelings, or behaviors on questionnaires after double-blind administration of drug.

Qualitative Subjective Effects of Caffeine

Laboratory examination of subjective effects (i.e., self-reported ratings of mood) of caffeine has often led to equivocal and sometimes confusing results. Many studies have failed to find significant subjective effects of caffeine either at usual dietary doses (40–100 mg) (e.g., see refs. 14,18, and 79) or at doses as high as 200–500 mg (e.g., see refs. 18,79,81,82, and 86). Other studies have shown that high doses of caffeine (200–800 mg) produce a predominantly "dysphoric" profile of subjective effects characterized by increases in anxiety, nervousness, or jittery (e.g., see refs. 15,16,30,80,83,87, and 91).

The total lack of subjective effects and the dysphoric subjective effects of caffeine are at variance with the common experience of regular caffeine users who generally report positive or desirable subjective effects after consuming caffeine (41). In contrast to the studies cited above, an increasing number of studies have reported a profile of predominately positive subjective effects after caffeine administration (53,75,78,85,99,100; also see studies cited in section on subjective effects and caffeine reinforcement). The types of positive subjective effects that have been significantly affected by caffeine include (a) increases in ratings of well-being, energy/active, alert,

concentration, self-confidence, motivation for work, and desire to talk to people and (b) decreases in ratings of sleepiness and muzziness/not clearheaded (53,85,99).

There seem to be at least three factors that may increase the likelihood of demonstrating such positive subjective effects of caffeine: (i) testing in caffeine deprivation or total abstinence; (ii) testing low caffeine doses; and (iii) testing under conditions (or in populations) in which caffeine functions as a reinforcer.

First, most studies that demonstrated positive subjective effects of caffeine have tested caffeine after a significant period of caffeine deprivation or abstinence [e.g., overnight or 24 hr (53,75,78,85,99,100)]. That studies have also shown such effects in subjects who were maintained on an otherwise caffeine-free diet (85,99) indicates that physical dependence is not a necessary condition for demonstrating positive subjective effects of caffeine. Second, the positive subjective effects of caffeine have been most often demonstrated at relatively low caffeine doses [e.g., 20–200 mg (53,75,78,85,99,100)]. Although there appear to be wide individual differences in relative sensitivity, it is clear that dysphoric/anxiogenic subjective effects of caffeine emerge in a dose-related fashion (15,30,87). Third, the positive subjective effects of caffeine are more likely to be demonstrated in individuals in whom caffeine is presumably functioning as a reinforcer (32,43,57); see section on subjective effects and caffeine reinforcement).

When caffeine produces positive changes in subjective effects, the profile of these changes (e.g., increases in well-being, energy/active, alert, concentration, self-confidence, motivation for work, desire to talk to people) is remarkably similar to that produced by d-amphetamine and cocaine (34). A major difference in the subjective effect profile appears to be that caffeine is more likely to produce dysphoria/anxiety with increases in dose than d-amphetamine and cocaine.

There is some evidence suggesting a dissociation between the positive/energy effect and the dysphoric/anxiogenic effect of caffeine. Two studies that administered 300 mg of caffeine to a group of subjects showed virtually no correlation between caffeine-induced stimulation and anxiety (14,42). Examination of individual subject data from these and other studies (30,53,99) indicates that these two types of subjective effects can occur alone or together in the same individual.

Finally, results of questionnaire and experimental studies suggest that panic disorder patients may be particularly vulnerable to the anxiety- and panic-producing effects of caffeine. Questionnaire studies indicate that such patients self-report consuming less caffeine and experiencing more anxiety than control subjects (9,76,77,104). An experimental study by Charney et al. (17) showed that, compared to normal controls, panic disorder patients had more anxiety and a greater rate of panic attacks after blind oral administration of caffeine [10 mg/kg caffeine citrate:

equivalent to 5 mg/kg (about 350 mg) caffeine base] after being instructed to follow a caffeine-free diet for 2 weeks. Similar results have been described by Uhde (104), who compared the effects of 480 mg of caffeine in panic disorder patients and normal controls.

TOLERANCE TO CAFFEINE IN HUMANS

Tolerance refers to an acquired change in responsiveness of an individual as a result of exposure to drug such that an increased dose of drug is necessary to produce the same degree of response, or that less effect is produced by the same dose of drug. The development of tolerance is most unambiguously concluded from studies that compare full dose–response curves in the presence and absence of the tolerance-inducing manipulation (73). As reviewed elsewhere (62), preclinical research has clearly demonstrated tolerance to response-rate-decreasing, behavioral stimulant, and discriminative stimulus effects of caffeine, with the extent and rate of tolerance development differing across the different measures.

Information about the development of caffeine tolerance in humans is relatively easily obtained by measuring any pharmacological response before and after caffeine exposure. As described below, "complete" tolerance development (i.e., caffeine effects no longer different from placebo) has been demonstrated after repeated administration of relatively high caffeine doses spread across the day for a number of consecutive days. Beyond these demonstrations, however, detailed quantitative knowledge of caffeine tolerance in humans is quite fragmentary.

Tolerance to Caffeine Subjective Effects

Tolerance to the subjective effects of caffeine has been demonstrated only in one recent study (32), in which two groups of subjects received either caffeine (300 mg t.i.d.) or placebo (t.i.d.) for 18 consecutive days. During the last 14 days of chronic dosing, the caffeine and placebo groups did not differ meaningfully on ratings of mood and subjective effects. Furthermore, after chronic dosing, compared to placebo, caffeine (300 mg b.i.d.) produced significant subjective effects (including increases in tension-anxiety, jittery/nervous shaky, active/stimulated/energetic and strength of drug effect) in the chronic placebo group but not in the chronic caffeine group, suggesting the development of complete tolerance at these doses. Figure 3 shows these effects for ratings of tension-anxiety and strength of drug effect.

Tolerance to Caffeine Sleep Disruption

Unambiguous evidence for the development of tolerance to caffeine sleep-disrupting effects is also quite re-

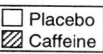
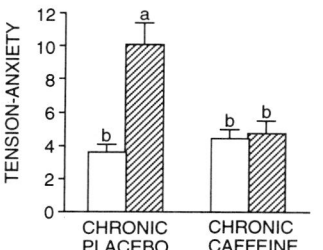
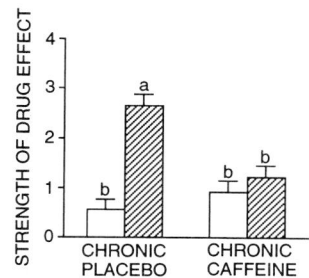

FIG. 3. Complete tolerance development to the subjective effects of caffeine. Subjective ratings of Tension-Anxiety (POMS) and Strength of Drug Effect after receiving placebo (*open bars*) or 300 mg b.i.d. caffeine (*striped bars*). Data are shown for the Chronic Placebo group (*N* = 15) and the Chronic Caffeine group (*N* = 17) (300 mg t.i.d. for 18 days). *Bars* represent means, and *brackets* show +SEM. Letters a and b indicate the results of statistical comparisons; within a panel, any two bars designated with the same letter are not significantly ($p \leq 0.05$) different. Caffeine and placebo were administered double-blind in capsules. (Redrawn from ref. 32.)

cent. Although Colton et al. (21) showed that heavy coffee drinkers were less sensitive to the sleep-disturbing effects of caffeine than light coffee drinkers, the study design did not allow differentiation of tolerance from other pre-existing differences between these self-selected subject populations. Two recent studies provided direct experimental evidence for caffeine tolerance to sleep disruption by demonstrating decreases in caffeine-induced disruption of objective measures of sleep after caffeine dosing of 250 mg b.i.d. for 2 days (111) or 400 mg t.i.d. for 7 days (8). By day 7 in the latter study, a number of sleep measures (e.g., total sleep time, sleep efficiency, number of awakenings) were no longer different from baseline, suggesting the development of complete tolerance at these doses.

Tolerance to Caffeine Physiological Effects

There is good evidence for decreased responsiveness to physiological effects of caffeine with repeated daily caffeine administration. Such tolerance development has been demonstrated to various physiological effects of caffeine, including diuresis (29), parotid gland salivation (108), increased metabolic rate (oxygen consumption) (8), increased blood pressure (2,93), increased plasma norepinephrine and epinephrine, and increased plasma renin activity (93). Compared to a group that received placebo, complete tolerance to caffeine (250 mg t.i.d.) was demonstrated in 1–4 days on blood pressure, plasma norepinephrine and epinephrine, and plasma renin activity (93). Results consistent with these have been reported on other cardiovascular and physiological responses (2,24), although whether complete tolerance development occurs has been questioned (24). The only human study to quantitatively assess the extent of caffeine tolerance by constructing dose–effect curves (as has been done frequently in infrahuman research) was a study that showed a two- to threefold decrease in the minimally effective dose required to produce diuresis after a period of abstinence from caffeine (estimated 170–340 mg/day) (29).

Parametric Determinants of Tolerance

Beyond the several demonstrations of complete tolerance development at high caffeine doses described above, there is little quantitative knowledge about the parameters that determine caffeine tolerance. As with the development of tolerance to most drugs, the degree of tolerance development to caffeine can be expected to depend on the caffeine dose, the dose frequency, the number of doses, and the individual's elimination rate (97). There is some indication that the rate and/or extent of tolerance development differ across different measures (8,24). The rate of tolerance development has been estimated to be quite rapid for blood pressure [$t_{1/2} = 1$ hr (97)], with complete tolerance to various cardiovascular effects occurring in 2–5 days (2,24,93). Little is known about the rate of loss of tolerance except that it was shown to be rapid for blood pressure ($t_{1/2} = 1$ hr) in one study (97), but in another study (29) was suggested to be quite slow for caffeine-induced diuresis.

Relationship Between Caffeine Tolerance and Withdrawal

Tolerance and physical dependence are sometimes thought to be functionally interrelated, reflecting common neuroadaptive changes in response to repeated drug administration. The only relevant study to address this issue is the one described above that demonstrated tolerance to caffeine subjective effects in a group of subjects that received caffeine (300 mg t.i.d.) compared to a group that received only placebo (32). In that study, the group of tolerant subjects showed withdrawal (a time-limited elevation in headache) when switched to placebo compared to the nontolerant placebo group. Overall, this study provides only limited information suggesting the covariation of tolerance and withdrawal.

CAFFEINE PHYSICAL DEPENDENCE IN HUMANS

Physical dependence is manifested by time-limited biochemical, physiological, and behavioral disruptions (i.e., a withdrawal syndrome) upon termination of chronic or repeated drug administration. As has been reviewed elsewhere (56), preclinical research has clearly demonstrated time-limited behavioral disruptions following cessation of chronic caffeine administration. As for human research, 37 case reports and human experimental studies of caffeine withdrawal spanning the period 1833 to 1987 have been reviewed by Griffiths and Woodson (56). The following section updates that review based on 16 additional recent studies that have significantly advanced our understanding of caffeine withdrawal (22,31–33,35,54,63, 65,67–69,84,92,98,103,105).

Signs and Symptoms of Caffeine Withdrawal

The most frequently reported withdrawal symptom is headache (also cerebral fullness), which is characterized as being gradual in development, diffuse, throbbing, and sometimes severe (56). Other symptoms, in roughly decreasing order of prominence, are: (a) drowsiness (increased sleepiness and yawning; decreased energy and alertness), (b) increased work difficulty (decreased motivation for tasks/work, impaired concentration), (c) decreased feelings of well-being/contentment (decreased self-confidence; increased irritability), (d) decreased sociability/friendliness/talkativeness, (e) flu-like feelings (muscle aches/stiffness; hot or cold spells; heavy feelings in arms or legs; nausea), and (f) blurred vision (54,56,98). In addition to these symptoms, composite scales of depression and anxiety may be elevated (98) and psychomotor performance may be impaired (56,92,98). The occurrence of headache as a withdrawal symptom does not necessarily correlate with the occurrence of other symptoms (e.g., tiredness), suggesting that other signs and symptoms are not merely epiphenomena of headache (54,56).

Severity of Caffeine Withdrawal

The severity of caffeine withdrawal is an increasing function of caffeine maintenance dose (31,56). When symptoms of caffeine withdrawal occur, the severity can vary from mild to extreme. At its worst, caffeine withdrawal is incompatible with normal functioning and is sometimes totally incapacitating (56).

Incidence of Caffeine Withdrawal

The incidence of caffeine withdrawal is an increasing function of caffeine maintenance dose (33,35,56). The best estimates of the incidence of caffeine withdrawal in the general population come from a recent survey study and an experimental study. A recent random digit-dial telephone survey in Vermont showed that among current users of caffeine who reported that they had abstained from caffeine for ≥24 hr, 27% reported withdrawal headaches when they abstained (63,69). The experimental study (98) involved 62 individuals from the general community with a distribution of caffeine intake similar to that of the general population in the United States (mean caffeine intake of 235 mg/day). The study involved an approximately 48-hr, double-blind caffeine abstinence trial under conditions which obscured that the purpose of the study was to investigate caffeine. During caffeine withdrawal, 52% reported moderate or severe headache, and 8–11% showed abnormally high scores on standardized depression, anxiety, and fatigue scales. The incidence of headache observed from the survey and experimental study in the general population (27–52%) is in the range of that observed in several other recent studies conducted in special subject populations [19–57%, (54,67,105)].

Minimum Dosing Parameters for Caffeine Withdrawal

Although the incidence and severity of caffeine withdrawal are an increasing function of caffeine dose, two recent studies have shown that caffeine withdrawal can occur after relatively long-term administration of caffeine doses as low as 100 mg/day (31,54). Studies also indicate that caffeine withdrawal headache may occur after termination of high doses of caffeine (terminal doses of ≥600 mg/day) administered for as few as 6–15 days (27,49).

Time Course of Caffeine Withdrawal

The caffeine withdrawal syndrome follows an orderly time course (56). Onset has been usually reported to occur 12–24 hr after terminating caffeine intake, although onset as late as 36 hr has been documented (54). Peak withdrawal intensity has generally been described as occurring 20–48 hr after abstinence. The duration of caffeine withdrawal has most often been described as ranging between 2 days and 1 week, although longer durations have been occasionally noted (32,54,56,105). Figure 4 illustrates the time course of increased headache and decreased energy/active ratings after substitution of placebo capsules for caffeine capsules (100 mg/day).

Clinical Significance of Caffeine Withdrawal

The importance of caffeine withdrawal is derived in part from the large population at risk: 82% of adults in the United States consume caffeine regularly, with mean intake estimated at 227 mg/day (44). Even if a conservative 10% incidence of clinically significant withdrawal were assumed, the size of the vulnerable population is enormous. Caffeine use and abstinence should be consid-

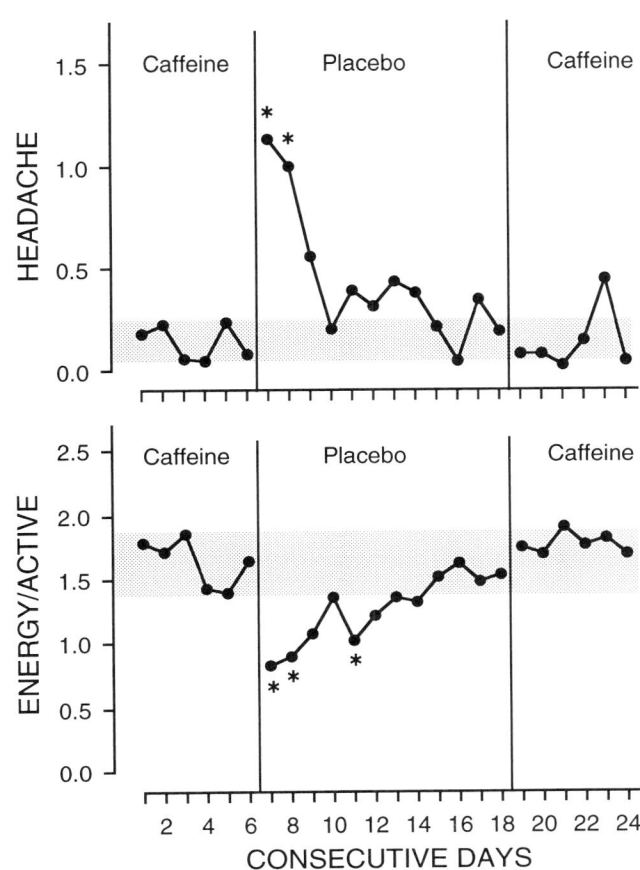

FIG. 4. Effects of double-blind substitution of placebo capsules for caffeine capsules (100 mg/day) on mean ratings of headache and energy/active in four withdrawal-sensitive subjects. *Shaded areas* show the range of means from the initial 6-day caffeine period. *Asterisks* indicate which placebo days are significantly different from the initial caffeine period ($p \leq 0.05$). (Redrawn from ref. 54.)

ered in the differential diagnosis of commonly reported symptoms of headache, fatigue, and mood disturbances. Research is needed to determine the necessity of the common medical practice of requiring short-term caffeine abstinence before various laboratory tests (e.g., serum lipid profiles, fasting blood sugar) as well as in preparation for operations and a variety of procedures such as endoscopies or colonoscopies. Finally, more research is needed to explore possible situations involving caffeine withdrawal morbidity. For example, a neonatal withdrawal syndrome following chronic maternal caffeine ingestion has been proposed (84) and caffeine withdrawal headache has been implicated in postoperative morbidity (33,35), in a weekend migraine syndrome (22), and as a possible mechanism underlying inappropriate chronic daily use of caffeine-containing analgesics (12,19,46).

CAFFEINE AS A DRUG OF ABUSE

Throughout history, caffeine has intermittently been labeled as a drug of abuse (see refs. 4,37, and 58), and analogies have been made to classic abused substances. This suggestion is usually controversial and is rebutted with the following observations: The majority of caffeine use is consistent with socially accepted limits and patterns; gross overconsumption of any article of diet can be harmful; and the adverse effects of excessive intake seem to be largely transient (26). Certainly there is an important distinction to be made between legal, socially domesticated drugs (such as caffeine, nicotine, and alcohol) and illegal drugs (such as cocaine, heroin, and phencyclidine). Instances of appropriate use usually can be identified and agreed upon with the former but not the latter. Beyond the legal distinction, however, definitions of what constitutes a drug of abuse or dependence are often complex and open to alternative interpretations, as has been clearly illustrated in a recent debate about whether or not nicotine is meaningfully considered to be a drug of abuse (94,95,107). Ultimately, whether or not caffeine is labeled as a drug of abuse is a somewhat arbitrary social–political decision subject to revision over time. This section will consider the question of caffeine as a drug of abuse from two current perspectives: a clinical psychiatric perspective and a perspective based on a broader reinforcement/adverse effects analysis.

Clinical Psychiatric Perspective

Generic criteria for making a diagnosis of Psychoactive Substance Dependence Disorder have been developed by the American Psychiatric Association (DSM-III-R and DSM-IV) (1) to facilitate treatment and research on abuse of behaviorally active drugs. In considering caffeine, the most relevant criteria are: (a) persistent desire or unsuccessful efforts to cut down or control use (b) use despite knowledge of physical or psychological problem caused or exacerbated by use, (c) marked tolerance, and (d) characteristic withdrawal syndrome or taking substance to relieve or avoid withdrawal symptoms. These criteria largely overlap with those promulgated by the World Health Organization (ICD-10) (109) for also making a diagnosis of psychoactive substance dependence. Recently, Hughes et al. (70) reviewed studies relevant to making a diagnosis of caffeine dependence and concluded that although there was a substantial research database suggesting the validity of caffeine dependence, an appropriate clinical patient database was almost completely absent. Even more recently, these same investigators (69) reported the results of a random-digit telephone survey in Burlington, Vermont, in which they applied the generic DSM-III-R criteria for drug dependence to current caffeine users. Surprisingly, 44% of current users (about

36% of the general population) were diagnosed as drug-dependent on caffeine by fulfilling three or more of the generic criteria. The most common criterion endorsed was persistent desire or unsuccessful efforts to cut down or control use. Although the sample size from this study was small and the validity of applying to caffeine the generic criteria for psychoactive substance dependence needs to be addressed, the estimate that about one-third of the general population may be dependent on caffeine is startling and worthy of further investigation.

Reinforcement/Adverse Effects Analysis

A broader approach to considering whether it is meaningful to label caffeine as a drug of abuse is to examine the extent to which caffeine has the defining characteristics of a drug of abuse. As discussed elsewhere (55), drugs of abuse have two major characteristics: (i) they have reinforcing effects and (ii) they produce adverse effects (i.e., they have the capacity to harm the individual and/or society). According to this model, the relative abuse liability of a drug can be considered to be a multiplicative function of the degree of reinforcing effect and the degree of adverse effect.

With regard to the first characteristic of abused drugs (i.e., reinforcing effects), as has been reviewed in previous sections, it is now clear from research with laboratory animals and with humans that caffeine can function as a reinforcer under some conditions. The results of intravenous caffeine self-injection studies in nonhuman primates and rats indicate that caffeine functions as a reinforcer under a more limited range of conditions than do classic psychomotor stimulant drugs of abuse such as d-amphetamine or cocaine. This conclusion about caffeine is similar to that previously reached for nicotine (28,40). The results of self-administration and choice studies in humans clearly demonstrate the reinforcing effects of low and moderate doses of caffeine. Studies of subjective effects have demonstrated that amphetamine generally produces greater elevations than caffeine in ratings indicating "euphoria" and "well-being" (14,15,106). The only human study to directly compare the self-administration of caffeine with that of another drug was a study that examined the effects of response requirement on consumption of coffee and cigarettes, and it concluded that the reinforcing effects of coffee and cigarettes were comparable (6). Overall, the available animal and human research suggests that caffeine is a reinforcer, but a less robust reinforcer than cocaine or d-amphetamine, and perhaps most similar to nicotine.

With regard to the second characteristic of abused drugs (i.e., adverse effects), a balanced discussion of adverse effects of caffeine is beyond the scope of this chapter and has been the focus of a number of recent books (36,71,101). Briefly, the adverse effects of caffeine use include caffeine intoxication, caffeine withdrawal signs and symptoms, and exacerbation of medical conditions. Acute or chronic caffeine intoxication, also known as *caffeinism,* is a DSM-IV diagnostic category which may be indistinguishable from manic episodes, panic disorder, and generalized anxiety disorder (1), and which may occur in about 10% of the population (47,69). In chronic or recurrent forms of caffeinism, patients often will not recognize the ingestion of caffeine-containing foods as problematic and may seek medical treatment for anxiety, insomnia, or cardiovascular, gastrointestinal, and other somatic complaints (47). Caffeine withdrawal signs and symptoms, which have been discussed in a previous section, may occur at clinically significant levels in about 10% of caffeine consumers who abruptly abstain. In terms of exacerbating medical conditions, the majority of medical specialists recommend reducing or eliminating caffeine for a variety of conditions including, anxiety, insomnia, palpitations, tachycardia, arrhythmia, fibrocystic disease, esophagitis/hiatal hernia, ulcers, and pregnancy (64), although the scientific basis for at least some of these recommendations appears ambiguous (36,71,101). Importantly, significant health risk from nonreversible pathological consequences of chronic caffeine use (e.g., heart disease, cancer, human reproduction) has not been conclusively demonstrated, although here too the status of the present data remains somewhat ambiguous (36,71,101).

This analysis indicates that caffeine has the two defining characteristics of prototypic drugs of abuse. Inasmuch as the relative abuse liability of a drug can be considered to be a multiplicative function of the degree of reinforcing effect and the degree of adverse effects, the modest reinforcing effect and modest adverse effects documented to date would suggest a low abuse potential relative to more widely recognized drugs of abuse. This analysis also predicts that if future research reveals significant additional caffeine-associated health risk, the perception of the relative abuse liability of caffeine would increase appreciably, as has occurred with nicotine over the last 20 years.

ACKNOWLEDGMENTS

Preparation of this review was supported, in part, by National Institute on Drug Abuse grants RO1 DA01147 and RO1 DA03889.

REFERENCES

1. American Psychiatric Association. *Diagnostic and statistical manual of mental disorders,* 4th ed. Washington, DC: American Psychiatric Association, 1994.
2. Ammon HPT, Bieck PR, Mandalaz D, Verspohl EJ. Adaptation of blood pressure to continuous heavy coffee drinking in young volunteers. A double-blind crossover study. *Br J Clin Pharmacol* 1983;15:701–706.
3. Atkinson J, Enslen M. Self-administration of caffeine by the rat. *Arzneimittelforschung* 1976;26:2059–2061.
4. Austin GA. Perspectives on the history of psychoactive substance use. In: *NIDA research issues,* vol 24. DHEW publication (ADM) 79-810. Washington, DC: US Government Printing Office, 1979;50–66.
5. Beecher HK. *Measurement of subjective responses: quantitative effects of drugs.* New York: Oxford University Press, 1959.
6. Bickel WK, Hughes JR, DeGrandpre RJ, Higgins ST, Rizzuto P. Behavioral economics of drug self-administration. IV. The effects of response requirement on the consumption of and interaction between concurrently available coffee and cigarettes. *Psychopharmacology (Berlin)* 1992;107:211–216.
7. Bigelow GE, Griffiths RR, Liebson I. Experimental human drug self-administration: methodology and application to the study of sedative abuse. *Pharmacol Rev* 1976;27:523–531.
8. Bonnet MH, Arand DL. Caffeine use as a model of acute and chronic insomnia. *Sleep* 1992;15:526–536.
9. Boulenger JP, Uhde TW, Wolff EAI, Post RM. Increased sensitivity to caffeine in patients with panic disorders: preliminary evidence. *Arch Gen Psychiatry* 1984;41:1067–1071.
10. Bozarth MA, ed. *Methods of assessing the reinforcing properties of abused drugs.* New York: Springer-Verlag, 1987.
11. Bozarth MA. An overview of assessing drug reinforcement. In: Bozarth MA, ed. *Methods of assessing the reinforcing properties of abused drugs.* New York: Springer-Verlag, 1987;635–658.
12. Bridges-Webb C, Grounds M. Analgesic use and abuse: the role of caffeine. *Med J Aust* 1976;20:805.
13. Bruce MS, Lader M. Caffeine abstention in the management of anxiety disorders. *Psychol Med* 1989;19:211–214.
14. Chait LD. Factors influencing the subjective response to caffeine. *Behav Pharmacol* 1992;3:219–228.
15. Chait LD, Griffiths RR. Effects of caffeine on human cigarette smoking behavior and subjective response. *Clin Pharmacol Ther* 1983;34:612–622.
16. Charney DS, Galloway MP, Heninger GR. The effects of caffeine on plasma MHPG, subjective anxiety, autonomic symptoms and blood pressure in healthy humans. *Life Sci* 1984;35:135–144.
17. Charney DS, Heninger GR, Jatlow PI. Increased anxiogenic effects of caffeine in panic disorders. *Arch Gen Psychiatry* 1985;42:233–243.
18. Christensen L, Miller J, Johnson D. Efficacy of caffeine versus expectancy in altering caffeine-related symptoms. *J Gen Psychol* 1991;118:5–12.
19. Collins E, Turner G. A suggestion for reducing the incidence of habitual analgesic consumption. *Med J Aust* 1973;1:863.
20. Collins RJ, Weeks JR, Cooper MM, Good PI, Russell RR. Prediction of abuse liability of drugs using IV self-administration by rats. *Psychopharmacology (Berlin)* 1984;82:6–13.
21. Colton T, Gosselin RE, Smith RP. The tolerance of coffee drinkers to caffeine. *Clin Pharmacol Ther* 1968;9:31–39.
22. Couturier EGM, Hering R, Steiner TJ. Weekend attacks in migraine patients: caused by caffeine withdrawal? *Cephalalgia* 1992;12:99–100.
23. de Wit H. Preference procedures for testing the abuse liability of drugs in humans. *Br J Addict* 1991;86:1579–1586.
24. Denaro CP, Brown CR, Jacob P III, Benowitz NL. Effects of caffeine with repeated dosing. *Eur J Clin Pharmacol* 1991;40:273–278.
25. Deneau G, Yanagita T, Seevers MH. Self-administration of psychoactive substances by the monkey: a measure of psychological dependence. *Psychopharmacologia* 1969;16:30–48.
26. Dews PB. Caffeine. *Annu Rev Nutr* 1982;2:323–341.
27. Dreisbach RH, Pfeiffer C. Caffeine-withdrawal headache. *J Lab Clin Med* 1943;28:1212–1219.
28. Dworkin SI, Vrana SL, Broadbent J, Robinson JH. Comparing the reinforcing effects of nicotine, caffeine, methylpheindate and cocaine. *Med Chem Res* 1993;2:593–602.
29. Eddy NB, Downs AW. Tolerance and cross-tolerance in the human subject to the diuretic effect of caffeine, theobromine and theophylline. *J Pharmacol Exp Ther* 1928;33:167–174.
30. Evans SM, Griffiths RR. Dose-related caffeine discrimination in normal volunteers: individual differences in subjective effects and self-reported cues. *Behav Pharmacol* 1991;2:345–356.

31. Evans SM, Griffiths RR. Low-dose caffeine physical dependence in normal subjects: dose-related effects. In: Harris LS, ed. *Problems of drug dependence 1990.* NIDA Research Monograph No. 105, DHHS Publication No. (ADM) 91-1753. Washington, DC: US Government Printing Office, 1991;446.

32. Evans SM, Griffiths RR. Caffeine tolerance and choice in humans. *Psychopharmacology (Berlin)* 1992;108:51–59.

33. Fennelly M, Galletly DC, Puride GI. Is caffeine withdrawal the mechanism of postoperative headache? *Anesth Analg* 1991;72:449–453.

34. Foltin RW, Fischman MW. Assessment of abuse liability of stimulant drugs in humans: a methodological survey. *Drug Alcohol Depend* 1991;28:3–48.

35. Galletly DC, Fennelly M, Whitwam JG. Does caffeine withdrawal contribute to postanaesthetic morbidity? *Lancet* 1989;June 10:1335.

36. Garattini S. *Caffeine, coffee, and health.* New York: Raven Press, 1993.

37. Gilbert RM. Caffeine as a drug of abuse. In: Gibbins RJ, Israel Y, Kalant H, Popham RE, Schmidt W, Smart RG, eds. *Research advances in alcohol and drug problems,* vol 3. New York: John Wiley & Sons, 1976;49–176.

38. Gilbert RM. Caffeine consumption. In: Spiller GA, ed. *The methylxanthine beverages and foods: chemistry, consumption, and health effects.* New York: Alan R Liss, 1984;185–213.

39. Gilbert RM. Betel-nut chewing in Toronto. In: *The Journal.* Toronto: Addiction Research Foundation of Ontario, April 1, 1986;5.

40. Goldberg SR, Henningfield JE. Reinforcing effects of nicotine in humans and experimental animals responding under intermittent schedules of IV drug injection. *Pharmacol Biochem Behav* 1988;30:227–234.

41. Goldstein A, Kaizer S. Psychotropic effects of caffeine in man. III. A questionnaire survey of coffee drinking and its effects in a group of housewives. *Clin Pharmacol Ther* 1969;10:477–488.

42. Goldstein A, Kaizer S, Warren R. Psychotropic effects of caffeine in man. II. Alertness, psychomotor coordination, and mood. *J Pharmacol Exp Ther* 1965;150:146–151.

43. Goldstein A, Kaizer S, Whitby O. Psychotropic effects of caffeine in man. IV. Quantitative and qualitative differences associated with habituation to coffee. *Clin Pharmacol Ther* 1969;10:489–497.

44. Graham DM. Caffeine—its identity, dietary sources, intake and biological effects. *Nutr Rev* 1978;36:97–102.

45. Graham HN. Tea: the plant and its manufacture; chemistry and consumption of the beverage. In: Spiller GA, ed. *The methylxanthine beverages and foods: chemistry, consumption and health effects.* New York: Alan R Liss, 1984;29–74.

46. Greden JF. Anxiety or caffeinism: a diagnostic dilemma. *Am J Psychiatry* 1974;131:1089–1092.

47. Greden JF, Walters A. Caffeine. In: Lowinson JH, Ruiz P, Millman RB, Langrod JG, eds. *Substance abuse—a comprehensive textbook.* Baltimore: Williams & Wilkins, 1992;357–370.

48. Griffiths RR, Bigelow GE, Henningfield JE. Similarities in animal and human drug-taking behavior. In: Mello NK, ed. *Advances in substance abuse,* vol 1. Greenwich, CT: JAI Press, 1980;1–90.

49. Griffiths RR, Bigelow GE, Liebson IA. Human coffee drinking: reinforcing and physical dependence producing effects of caffeine. *J Pharmacol Exp Ther* 1986;239:416–425.

50. Griffiths RR, Bigelow GE, Liebson IA. Reinforcing effects of caffeine in coffee and capsules. *J Exp Anal Behav* 1989;52:127–140.

51. Griffiths RR, Bigelow GE, Liebson IA, O'Keeffe M, O'Leary D, Russ N. Human coffee drinking: manipulation of concentration and caffeine dose. *J Exp Anal Behav* 1986;45:133–148.

52. Griffiths RR, Brady JV, Bradford LD. Predicting the abuse liability of drugs with animal drug self-administration procedures: psychomotor stimulants and hallucinogens. In: Thompson T, Dews PB, eds. *Advances in behavioral pharmacology* vol 2. New York: Academic Press, 1979;163–208.

53. Griffiths RR, Evans SM, Heishman SJ, Preston KL, Sannerud CA, Wolf B, Woodson PP. Low-dose caffeine discrimination in humans. *J Pharmacol Exp Ther* 1990;252:970–978.

54. Griffiths RR, Evans SM, Heishman SJ, Preston KL, Sannerud CA, Wolf B, Woodson PP. Low-dose caffeine physical dependence in humans. *J Pharmacol Exp Ther* 1990;255:1123–1132.

55. Griffiths RR, Lamb RJ, Ator NA, Roache JD, Brady JV. Relative abuse liability of triazolam: experimental assessment in animals and humans. *Neurosci Biobehav Rev* 1985;9:133–151.

56. Griffiths RR, Woodson PP. Caffeine physical dependence: A review of human and laboratory animal studies. *Psychopharmacology (Berlin)* 1988;94:437–451.

57. Griffiths RR, Woodson PP. Reinforcing effects of caffeine in humans. *J Pharmacol Exp Ther* 1988;246:21–29.

58. Guelliot O. Du cafeisme chronique. *Union Med Sci Nordest* 1885;9:221–240.

59. Henningfield JE, Goldberg SR. Nicotine as a reinforcer in human subjects and laboratory animals. *Pharmacol Biochem Behav* 1983;19:989–992.

60. Henningfield JE, Lukas SE, Bigelow GE. Human studies of drugs as reinforcers. In: Goldberg SR, Stolerman IP, eds. *Behavioral analysis of drug dependence.* Orlando, FL: Academic Press, 1986;69–122.

61. Hoffmeister F, Wuttke W. Self-administration of acetylsalicylic acid and combinations with codeine and caffeine in rhesus monkeys. *J Pharmacol Exp Ther* 1973;186:266–275.

62. Holtzman SG, Finn IB. Tolerance to behavioral effects of caffeine in rats. *Pharmacol Biochem Behav* 1988;29:411–418.

63. Hughes JR. Clinical importance of caffeine withdrawal. *N Engl J Med* 1992;327:1160–1161.

64. Hughes JR, Amori G, Hatsukami DK. A survey of physician advice about caffeine. *J Subst Abuse* 1988;1:67–70.

65. Hughes JR, Higgins ST, Bickel WK, Hunt WK, Fenwick JW, Gulliver SB, Mireault GC. Caffeine self-administration, withdrawal, and adverse effects among coffee drinkers. *Arch Gen Psychiatry* 1991;48:611–617.

66. Hughes JR, Hunt WK, Higgins ST, Bickel WK, Fenwick JW, Pepper SL. Effect of dose on the ability of caffeine to serve as a reinforcer in humans. *Behav Pharmacol* 1992;3:211–218.

67. Hughes JR, Oliveto AH, Bickel WK, Higgins ST, Badger GJ. Caffeine self-administration and withdrawal: Incidence, individual differences and interrelationships. *Drug Alcohol Depend* 1993;32:239–246.

68. Hughes JR, Oliveto AH, Bickel WK, Higgins ST, Valliere W. Caffeine self-administration and withdrawal in soda drinkers. *J Addict Dis* 1992;4:178.

69. Hughes JR, Oliveto AH, Helzer JE, Bickel WK, Higgins ST. Indications of caffeine dependence in a population-based sample. In: Harris LS, ed. *Problems of drug dependence, 1992.* NIDA Research Monograph No. 132, NIH Publication No. 93-3505. Washington, DC: US Government Printing Office, 1993;194.

70. Hughes JR, Oliveto AH, Helzer JE, Higgins ST, Bickel WK. Should caffeine abuse, dependence, or withdrawal be added to DSM-IV and ICD-10? *Am J Psychiatry* 1992;149:33–40.

71. James JE. *Caffeine and health.* New York: Academic Press, 1991.

72. Jaffe JH, Jaffe FK. Historical perspectives on the use of subjective effects measures in assessing the abuse potential of drugs. In: Fischman MW, Mello NK, eds. *Testing for abuse liability of drugs.* NIDA Research Monograph No. 105, DHHS Publication No. (ADM) 89-1613. Washington, DC: US Government Printing Office, 1989;43–72.

73. Kalant H, LeBlanc AE, Gibbins RJ. Tolerance to, and dependence on, some nonopiate psychotropic drugs. *Pharmacol Rev* 1971;3:135–191.

74. Kozlowski LT. Effect of caffeine on coffee drinking. *Nature* 1976;264:354–355.

75. Leathwood PD, Pollet P. Diet-induced mood changes in normal populations. *J Psychiatr Res* 1983;17:147–154.

76. Lee MA, Cameron OG, Greden JF. Anxiety and caffeine consumption in people with anxiety disorders. *Psychiatry Res* 1985;15:211–217.

77. Lee MA, Flegel P, Greden JF, Cameron OG. Anxiogenic effects of caffeine on panic and depressed patients. *Am J Psychiatry* 1988;145:632–635.

78. Lieberman HR, Wurtman RJ, Emde GG, Coviella ILG. The effects of caffeine and aspirin on mood and performance. *J Clin Psychopharmacol* 1987;7:315–320.

79. Lieberman HR, Wurtman RJ, Emde GG, Roberts C, Coviella ILG.

The effects of low doses of caffeine on human performance and mood. *Psychopharmacology (Berlin)* 1987;92:308–312.

80. Loke WH. Effects of caffeine on mood and memory. *Physiol Behav* 1988;44:367–372.

81. Loke WH, Hinrichs JV, Ghoneim MM. Caffeine and diazepam: separate and combined effects on mood, memory, and psychomotor performance. *Psychopharmacology (Berlin)* 1985;87:344–350.

82. Loke WH, Meliska CJ. Effects of caffeine use and ingestion on a protracted visual vigilance task. *Psychopharmacology (Berlin)* 1984;84:54–57.

83. Mattila J, Seppala T, Mattila MJ. Anxiogenic effect of yohimbine in healthy subjects: comparison with caffeine and antagonism by clonidine and diazepam. *Int Clin Psychopharmacol* 1988;3:215–229.

84. McGowan JD, Altman RE, Kanto WP. Neonatal withdrawal symptoms after chronic maternal ingestion of caffeine. *South Med J* 1988;81:1092.

85. Mumford GK, Evans SM, Kaminski BJ, Preston KL, Sannerud CA, Silverman K, Griffiths RR. Discriminative stimulus and subjective effects of theobromine and caffeine in humans. *Psychopharmacology (Berlin)* 1994;in press.

86. Nuotto E, Mattila MJ, Seppala T, Konno K. Coffee and caffeine and alcohol effects on psychomotor function. *Clin Pharmacol Ther* 1982;31:68–76.

87. Oliveto AH, Bickel WK, Hughes JR, Terry SY, Higgins ST, Badger GJ. Pharmacological specificity of the caffeine discriminative stimulus in humans: effects of theophylline, methylphenidate and buspirone. *Behav Pharmacol* 1993;4:237–246.

88. Oliveto AH, Hughes JR, Higgins ST, Bickel WK, Pepper SL, Shea PJ, Fenwick JW. Forced-choice versus free-choice procedures: caffeine self-administration in humans. *Psychopharmacology (Berlin)* 1992;109:85–91.

89. Oliveto AH, Hughes JR, Pepper SL, Bickel WK, Higgins ST. Low doses of caffeine can serve as reinforcers in humans. In: Harris LS, ed. *Problems of drug dependence, 1990*. NIDA Research Monograph No. 105, DHHS Publication No. (ADM) 91-1753. Washington, DC: US Government Printing Office, 1991;442.

90. Podboy J, Malloy W. Caffeine reduction and behavior changes in the severely retarded. *Ment Retard* 1977;15:40.

91. Rapoport JL, Jensvold M, Elkins R, Buchsbaum MS, Weingartner H, Ludlow C, Zahn TP, Berg CJ, Neims AH. Behavioral and cognitive effects of caffeine in boys and adult males. *J Nerv Ment Dis* 1981;169:726–732.

92. Rizzo AA, Stamps LE, Fehr LA. Effects of caffeine withdrawal on motor performance and heart rate changes. *Int J Psychophysiol* 1988;6:9–14.

93. Robertson D, Wade D, Workman R, Woosley RL, Oates JA. Toler-
ance to the humoral and hemodynamic effects of caffeine in man. *J Clin Invest* 1981;67:1111–1117.

94. Robinson JH, Pritchard WS. The meaning of addiction: reply to West. *Psychopharmacology (Berlin)* 1992;108:411–416.

95. Robinson JH, Pritchard WS. The role of nicotine in tobacco use. *Psychopharmacology (Berlin)* 1992;108:397–407.

96. Schuster CR, Woods JH, Seevers MH. Self-administration of control stimulants by the monkey. In: Sjoqvist F, Tottie M, eds. *Abuse of central stimulants*. New York: Raven Press, 1969;339–347.

97. Shi J, Benowitz NL, Denaro CP, Sheiner LB. Pharmacokinetic–pharmacodynamic modeling of caffeine: tolerance to pressor effects. *Clin Pharmacol Ther* 1993;53:6–14.

98. Silverman K, Evans SM, Strain EC, Griffiths RR. Withdrawal syndrome after the double-blind cessation of caffeine consumption. *N Engl J Med* 1992;327:1109–1114.

99. Silverman K, Griffiths RR. Low-dose caffeine discrimination and self-reported mood effects in normal volunteers. *J Exp Anal Behav* 1992;57:91–107.

100. Silverman K, Mumford GK, Griffiths RR. Enhancing caffeine reinforcement by behavioral requirements following drug ingestion. *Psychopharmacology (Berlin)* 1994;114:424–432.

101. Spiller GA. *The methylxanthine beverages and foods: chemistry, consumption, and health effects.* New York: Alan R Liss, 1984.

102. Stern KN, Chait LD, Johanson CE. Reinforcing and subjective effects of caffeine in normal human volunteers. *Psychopharmacology (Berlin)* 1989;98:81–88.

103. Stringer KA, Watson WA. Caffeine withdrawal symptoms. *Am J Emerg* 1987;5:469.

104. Uhde TW. Caffeine-induced anxiety: an ideal chemical model of panic disorder? In: Asnis GM, van Praag HM, eds. *Einstein monograph series in psychiatry.* 1994;in press.

105. van Dusseldorp M, Katan MB. Headache caused by caffeine withdrawal among moderate coffee drinkers switched from ordinary to decaffeinated coffee: a 12 week double blind trial. *Br Med J* 1990;300:1558–1559.

106. Weiss B, Laties VG. Enhancement of human performance by caffeine and the amphetamines. *Pharmacol Rev* 1962;14:1–36.

107. West R. Nicotine addiction: a re-analysis of the arguments. *Psychopharmacology (Berlin)* 1992;108:408–410.

108. Winsor AL, Strongin EI. A study of the development of tolerance for caffeinated beverages. *J Exp Psychol* 1933;16:725–744.

109. World Health Organization. *The ICD-10 classification of mental and behavioural disorders, clinical descriptions and diagnostic guidelines.* Geneva: World Health Organization, 1992.

110. Yanagita T. Self-administration studies on various dependence-producing agents in monkeys. *Univ Michigan Med Center J* 1970;36:216–224.

111. Zwyghuizen-Doorenbos A, Roehrs TA, Lipschutz L, Timms V, Roth T. Effects of caffeine on alertness. *Psychopharmacology (Berlin)* 1990;100:36–39.

Psychopharmacology: The Fourth Generation of Progress, edited by Floyd E. Bloom and David J. Kupfer. Raven Press, Ltd., New York 1995.

CHAPTER 147

Pathophysiology of Tobacco Dependence

Jack E. Henningfield, Leslie M. Schuh, and Murray E. Jarvik

In less than two decades since the first volume in this series, our understanding of the pathophysiology of tobacco dependence has progressed enormously. In the first volume, Jaffe and Jarvik (38) essentially summarized the rational basis for considering cigarette smoking as a form of drug dependence or "addiction." By the time the second volume was developed, sufficient new research had been conducted to enable Jones (42) to describe many of the functional relationships between nicotine dose and the behavioral effects that contribute to the dependence process. The field has continued to progress, enabling us to describe the essential pathophysiology of tobacco dependence. We contend that this understanding will provide a rational guide for developing more effective treatment.

A note on the terminology used in this review is necessary. Consistent with the rest of this volume, we use the term *dependence* in the way that the term "addiction" has been more broadly used to refer to compulsive use of psychoactive drugs in which tolerance and physiological dependence may also be present. The term *physiological dependence* will be used to refer more specifically to the physiological adaptation manifested by the emergence of withdrawal symptoms after cessation of use.

The pathophysiological consequences of tobacco smoke exposure include tissue destruction contributing to lung disease, cellular changes contributing to cancer, and the cellular and molecular reinforcing effects leading to dependence. Once the pathophysiological consequences of tobacco use have occurred, it may be no more a matter of personal choice to abstain from tobacco than to reverse metastasizing lung cells. In fact, most smokers identify smoking as harmful and express a desire to reduce or stop

smoking, and nearly 20 million of them (more than one-third of all smokers) make a serious attempt to quit each year. Unfortunately, less than 7% of these smokers attempting to quit (or less than 3% of all smokers) achieve 1-year abstinence each year (17).

The importance, as well as inadequacies, of educational efforts and motivational contingencies is illustrated by the following statistic: Approximately 50% of the survivors of myocardial infarctions, lung removal, and tracheostomy resume smoking (74). This illustrates two important points. First, powerful motivational incentives can lead to cessation; no widely used formal treatment reliably establishes 50% rates of long-term abstinence. Second, this powerful motivational contingency (i.e., threat of death) is inadequate for 50% of cigarette smokers; they may also require medications, behavior modification procedures, or both.

Thus, educational efforts and motivational factors are clearly limited in their ability to induce remission from tobacco dependence by the pathophysiological effects of chronic tobacco exposure. As will be evident from the present review, it is doubtful that complete reversal of all dependence consequences can be accomplished or that all motivated people can achieve lasting abstinence with presently approved medications and medication use guidelines. However, many people can achieve cessation and reduce their risk of tobacco-caused disease with currently available treatment. The purpose of this review is to summarize the present state of knowledge on the pathophysiological basis of tobacco dependence and advances in treatment (see also Chapters 9–12, and 66, *this volume,* for related topics).

J. E. Henningfield and L. M. Schuh: Clinical Pharmacology Branch, National Institute on Drug Abuse, Intramural Research Program, Baltimore, Maryland 21224.
M. E. Jarvik: Psychopharmacology Unit, Veterans Affairs Medical Center, Los Angeles, California 90024.

NATURAL HISTORY AND CLINICAL COURSE

The cigarette-dependence process, like other pathogenically induced diseases, is influenced by host or individual factors, environmental factors, and the level of exposure to the pathogen. Initiation is often mediated by a variety of social and cultural factors. However, over time the reinforcing effects of the drug strengthen and the individual's control over use weakens. Although other factors continue to operate, cigarette dependence is powerfully and critically driven by the positively and negatively reinforcing effects of nicotine, as will be discussed below.

Like other drug dependencies, nicotine dependence is a "progressive," "chronic," "relapsing" disorder. Mean age of cigarette smoking onset is 13–14 years (21). The level of nicotine dependence in adults is inversely related to the age of smoking initiation when measured by diagnostic criteria of the American Psychiatric Association (8).

Continued smoke intake is accompanied by the development of tolerance and physiological dependence. After smoking a few cigarettes, estimates of people who progress to dependence ranges from roughly 33% to 94%. For example, a survey of adults in Great Britain in the early 1960s indicated that 94% of those who smoked more than three cigarettes became "long-term regular smokers" (62). However, these data might not be relevant regarding current risks. Recently collected data in the United States and Great Britain suggest that between 33% and 50% of people who try cigarettes become regular smokers (29,52). Consistent with these observations, the 1991 U.S. National Health Survey determined that approximately 70% of adolescents tried smoking, whereas only 25% smoked each of the 30 days preceding the survey. Improving the precision of risk estimates is problematic because surveys differ in their criteria for initial smoking and dependent smoking. Nonetheless, it seems reasonable to conclude that in the United States, where there is widespread awareness of smoking hazards, the risk of developing dependence after smoking more than one cigarette is at least one in three. Supporting these observations and the low frequency of quitting, the National Household Survey of the National Institute on Drug Abuse found that 38% of people who ever smoked cigarettes reported that they needed tobacco or felt dependent at the time the survey was conducted.

Tobacco use tends to be chronic, with short-lived remission occurring rarely. In fact, studies have shown that, unlike cocaine, heroin, and alcohol use, the progression of cigarette smoking was slowed but not reversed as individuals aged (59). Chronic use is highly resistant to modification. For example, efforts to reduce intake by smoking fewer cigarettes or cigarettes with lower nicotine delivery ratings are usually partially or completely thwarted by compensatory changes in how the cigarettes are smoked (42,74).

Abstinence is usually short-lived; most individuals resume smoking within 3 days (34). Providing minimal assistance prolongs the remission by at least a few more days, and providing nicotine replacement can extend the mean remission duration by 6 months or more (20). One year later, nearly one-third of those surveyed had relapsed, a testament to the persistence of the dependence (17,74). These patterns of relapse are similar to those observed with other drug dependencies (74), but the relapse process has been studied in even finer detail for cigarette smoking than for other dependence-producing substances.

Epidemiology and Trends

There are approximately 45 million cigarette smokers in the United States, 15–20 million of whom try to quit smoking each year (17). This represents a substantial reduction in prevalence from 42% of adults in 1965 to approximately 25% in 1990. Cigarette smoking continues to account for more than 20% of all deaths in the United States, with more than 400,000 cigarette smokers dying each year because of their tobacco intake and more than 50,000 nonsmokers dying from environmental tobacco smoke exposure.

The spread of nicotine dependence follows the course of an infectious disease, with transmission being largely by person-to-person exposure to cigarettes. More than 33% of those who continue smoking will die prematurely as a result of this smoking (51); however, mortality can be significantly reduced by cessation at any age (76). The causes of death in order of incidence are cardiovascular diseases (43%), all forms of tobacco-caused cancer (36%), respiratory diseases (20%), and all other smoking-caused deaths (1%) (51). The three primary causes of mortality are similar for men and women: heart disease, cancer, and stroke, with cigarette smoking being an important contributor to this similarity.

Adolescent Nicotine Dependence

Chronic tobacco use and dependence commonly develop during adolescence and may be considered pediatric medical disorders (69). A Gallup Survey of cigarette smoking and markers of dependence indicated that 40% of teenage cigarette smokers begin smoking within 1 hr of awakening each day (a sign of dependence); 50% of teenage smokers had tried to quit but relapsed; 70% would not start smoking if they could "do it again"; and 38% of teenage smokers would be interested in smoking cessation programs targeted to their needs (21). These observations are consistent with earlier findings from the 1985 National Institute on Drug Abuse Household Survey which showed that 84% of 12- to 17-year-olds who smoked a pack or more each day felt that they "needed" or were "dependent upon" cigarettes (28). These data also showed that 12- to 17-year-olds develop tolerance, dependence, needs, graduating usage, and inability to abstain from nicotine, indicating that the dependence processes are fundamentally the same as those studied in adults (28,74).

Thus, tobacco dependence, not just initiation of smoking, is common during adolescence. Unfortunately, despite the apparent public health problem of adolescent nicotine dependence and the interest by many millions of teenagers in obtaining cessation assistance, there has been little systematic effort to evaluate the efficacy and risks of powerful adult-targeted treatment strategies such as nicotine replacement therapy. This is a challenge that must be met because of the poor prognosis of untreated nicotine dependence.

Severity of Nicotine Dependence

Several studies have found nicotine to be as capable of producing dependence as heroin, cocaine, or alcohol (28,29). Moreover, a higher percentage of cigarette smokers consider themselves to be dependent when compared to users of other abused substances. For example, in a 1990 Gallup Poll, 61% of current smokers reported that they considered themselves to be ''addicted'' to cigarettes (21). These findings are consistent with those of the 1990 National Household Survey which indicated that, among people who had ever smoked in their lifetimes, 38% were smoking at the time of the survey and reported that they needed tobacco or felt dependent at the time the survey was conducted, and approximately 80% of people who smoked at least a pack per day felt that they were dependent. By contrast, among people who had consumed alcoholic beverages in the past year, 30% had consumed at least once in the past week; and among those who had binged (five or more drinks in a row) in the past 30 days, 17% reported they felt they needed to drink or were dependent. For cocaine, the National Household Survey indicated that among people who had used the drug in the past year, 16% had used in the past week, and among people who used 11 times or more in their lives, 7.7% reported they felt they needed the drug or were dependent (28).

The cigarette is distinguished as an abused drug in that the pattern of occasional or low-level use that characterizes most users of other abused drugs is relatively rare for tobacco. For example, whereas only about 10–15% of current alcohol drinkers are considered problem drinkers, approximately 90% of cigarette smokers smoke at least five cigarettes every day (27,29). Part of the reason that only 2–3% of smokers successfully achieve abstinence for 1 year on an annual basis (17) may be that most people who smoke on a daily basis report that they feel dependent and that they have experienced withdrawal symptoms (28,74).

Non-Drug-Related Factors

Factors unrelated to the drug itself can affect the prevalence of drug dependence in society as well as the severity in individuals. Some of the factors are the same as those that determine the prevalence and severity of other medical disorders resulting from exposure to toxins. For example, social factors are important determinants of both the likelihood of initial self-administration and sustained self-administration until the reinforcing effects of the drug can maintain self-administration in their own right. Many non-drug-related factors associated with both achievement of abstinence and relapse appear similarly operative across dependence-producing drugs and include drug-dependence-related illness, learning to manage cravings, social sanctions, availability of the substance, cost of the substance, and perception of the risks of using the substance (74).

Nicotine Delivery System

It is now clear that the nicotine delivery vehicle is a determinant of toxicity and abuse potential (31,74). The vehicle determines these characteristics in two ways: First, it determines the speed of nicotine delivery to the user and also determines the nicotine concentrations to which body tissues are exposed. For example, smoke inhalation essentially mimics the effects of a rapid intravenous injection and exposes the heart, brain, and fetus to high concentrations that dissipate within a few minutes. Psychoactive and cardioactive effects are directly related to the speed of nicotine delivery (4,31). Second, the delivery system determines the nature and quantity of other toxic substances to which the user is exposed.

These issues are not unique to nicotine. Drug dosage form is a determinant of patient acceptability of a medication and compliance with instructions for its use; similarly, it is a determinant of the abuse potential of psychoactive substances (31,74). The drug delivery system determines ease and convenience of use as well as the speed and amount of drug absorbed. For example, tobacco and coca leaves are rarely swallowed and dependence to swallowed formulations is uncommon, presumably because the bioavailability of the nicotine and cocaine is fairly poor via the gastrointestinal system (e.g., 30% of oral nicotine reaches the systemic circulation); furthermore, the drug that is absorbed via this route does not produce the rapid onset and offset of effects that characterize the most powerful dependence-producing drugs and drug forms (31,42,74). Despite the ability of intravenous nicotine injections to simulate many of the pleasurable effects of smoking, smoking appears to provide a more acceptable means of nicotine intake and one in which the individual's control over dosage is probably superior (74). Nicotine polacrilex gum and transdermal patch systems have low abuse liability, in part because rapid absorption is not possible with either system. Moreover, release of nicotine from polacrilex requires a substantial work effort—that is, chewing (31,74). Thus, the cigarette seems to have done for nicotine dependence what crack did for cocaine dependence; in both cases, a highly addictive form of the drug was made readily available and convenient to repeatedly self-administer, and it led to higher rates of morbidity and mortality than did previously abused forms (29,74).

For smokeless tobacco products, the nature of the product is a major determinant of how much nicotine the user obtains and how rapidly absorption occurs. Those products highly effective in the initiation process, termed "starter products" by the smokeless tobacco industry (31), tend to be low in nicotine concentration and low in pH (thus delaying absorption), and some are in a unit dosage form ("tobacco pouch") that helps first-time users avoid placing too much total product in their mouths. Subsequently, users are encouraged through advertising techniques to switch to maintenance products (higher in nicotine concentration and pH) to achieve greater levels of "satisfaction" and "pleasure" as they become increasingly tolerant (31).

NEUROPHARMACOLOGY

Chemistry

Nicotine is a tertiary amine existing in both isomeric forms, but tobacco contains only the more pharmacologically active levorotatory form, namely, (S)-nicotine (4). It is a water- and lipid-soluble weak base with an 8.0 index of ionization. Thus, the nicotine present in the mildly alkaline smoke of cigars, pipes, chewing tobacco, and snuff is readily absorbed across mucosal membranes of the mouth and nose (72). Cigarette smoke is mildly acidic and must be inhaled for effective absorption (4).

Effective nicotine absorption from polacrilex is facilitated by adding a buffer to slightly alkylinate the normally mildly acidic saliva (16), and consuming acidic beverages such as coffee, soft drinks, or fruit drinks while using the polacrilex prevents nicotine absorption (32). Swallowed nicotine is poorly absorbed, with much of that entering circulation detoxified in its first pass through the liver (74), thus providing little therapeutic benefit. Unfortunately, swallowed nicotine can cause nausea and hiccuping and may lead to patient dissatisfaction with nicotine polacrilex when improper use leads to swallowed nicotine-containing saliva (32).

The tobacco cigarette is the most toxic and addictive widely used vehicle for nicotine delivery. Nicotine is distilled at the tip of a burning cigarette where it is carried by particulate matter ("tar" droplets) deep into the lungs with inspired air. The nearly 2000°F microblast at the cigarette's tip is also the source of carbon monoxide and many other toxicologically significant pyrolysis products. Nicotine is rapidly absorbed in the alveoli of the lung, concentrated in the pulmonary veins as a bolus, and pumped by the left ventricle of the heart throughout the body. Absorption characteristics are similar to those of gases (such as oxygen) that are exchanged in the lung from inspired air to venous blood (33). Thus, smoke inhalation produces arterial boli that may be 10 times more concentrated than the levels measured in venous blood (33). A similar phenomenon of arterial boli occurs when cocaine is smoked, adding to the addictiveness and toxicity of "crack" cocaine (13).

Most cigarettes contain about 8–9 mg of nicotine, of which the smoker generally obtains 1–3 mg (4). The typical pack-per-day smoker obtains 20–40 mg of nicotine each day and may achieve venous plasma levels that are substantially higher than values produced by nicotine transdermal systems (6,14).

Nicotine is primarily eliminated through metabolism in the liver, with less than 5% typically excreted unchanged in the urine (74). The major initial nicotine metabolite is cotinine, which has pharmacological activity at the cellular and behavioral level but appears about one-hundredth to one-twentieth as potent as nicotine (23,40,43). Cotinine provides a useful marker of nicotine intake because it has an approximately 20-hr half-life and is readily measurable in blood, urine, or saliva. Carbon monoxide (CO) is eliminated through the lung as a function of respiration rate. The half-life of CO is 4–7 hr; thus, measurement of expired air CO or COHb provides a useful marker of recent cigarette smoke exposure (74).

Tolerance

Nicotine tolerance appears to be substantially acquired during youth as smokers progress from a few to many cigarettes to obtain the same effects (42,75). Administering nicotine to a tobacco-deprived smoker can substantially increase heart rate and euphoria measures and decrease knee-reflex strength. With repeated doses, heart rate stabilizes at a level intermediate to that produced by the first dose and that occurring when nicotine-deprived, subjective effects are minimal, and the knee reflex may appear normal (11,74). Tolerance to a variety of the behavioral, physiological, and subjective effects of nicotine have been studied (74). There are several physiological mechanisms of nicotine tolerance, including decreased responsiveness to the drug at the site of drug action and increased nicotine receptor number and some degree of increased metabolism (7,74).

Cigarette smokers lose a substantial degree of tolerance while sleeping each day and regain it upon resumption of smoking. A single nicotine exposure induces short-lived tolerance to its psychoactive, cardiovascular, and other effects and is thus referred to as *tachyphylaxis* (71). The rapid pharmacodynamic development of tolerance may contribute to the disappointment with nicotine replacement systems expressed by many patients. Specifically, they lose the ability to obtain desirable nicotine effects as quickly as when smoking, thus preventing the desirable moment-to-moment manipulation of mood possible with cigarettes.

Physical Dependence

After at least "several weeks" of nicotine exposure (1), physical dependence on nicotine develops, and, when deprived for more than a few hours, withdrawal symptoms that are generally opposite to the effects initially produced by nicotine are reported (74). The cellular and neurological adaptations that produce tolerance also lead to physical dependence. In actuality, compared to nonsmokers, the cigarette smoker has an elevated pulse (5–7 beats per minute), elevated circulating catecholamines, lower body weight (5–8 pounds), and increased nicotine receptor binding sites (7). Such increases in brain nicotine receptors may affect the smoker's subsequent risk for neuropsychiatric disorders.

Nicotine administration to animals and humans produces altered spontaneous electroencephalogram (EEG) (producing signs of electroencephalographic activation such as increased beta power, decreased alpha and theta power, and increased alpha frequency), evoked brain electrical potentials, and local cerebral glucose metabolism, increased adrenal hormone release (including adrenocorticotropic hormone, β-endorphin, β-lipotropin, growth hormone, vasopressin, and neurophysin), increased heart rate, and caused changes in skeletal muscle tension (55,74). Most, if not all, of these effects are related to the dose of nicotine, and tolerance develops to differing degrees across effects.

The nicotine withdrawal syndrome has been described in detail (1). Onset begins within a few hours of the last cigarette; symptoms include increased craving, anxiety, irritability, and appetite; decreased cognitive capabilities and heart rate; and increased tendency to smoke (37,55). Altered brain electrical potentials and hormonal output are primarily opposite in direction to those produced by acute nicotine administration, and decrements in evoked electrical potentials of the brain indicate impaired information processing capabilities (57,74).

The severity of the syndrome and specific prominent symptoms vary across individuals, but it is generally unpleasant and frequently intolerable (74), with most patients relapsing before the syndrome begins to subside (31,37). The time course varies across individuals and responses, but withdrawal symptoms usually peak within a few days and then begin to subside over the next several weeks. For example, certain measures of brain function (e.g., P300 evoked electrical potential) recover within a few days, whereas others may take weeks or more (e.g., N100 evoked potential) (37,74), and powerful urges to smoke may recur for many years (37,74). Nicotine re-

placement therapy does not appear to shorten the course of the syndrome but can reduce symptom severity to the generally more tolerable levels that are typically reported after about 4–5 weeks of untreated abstinence.

Withdrawal severity is related to prior nicotine intake, although differences in just a few cigarettes may not have an effect (74). It is precipitated by an approximately 50–60% reduction in smoking (78). Similarly, withdrawal symptoms can be relieved by readministering nicotine. In general, the degree of relief appears to be related to the nicotine dose (74): Significant relief of physical withdrawal signs is provided by 60% replacement of plasma nicotine, and greater relief is provided by higher levels of replacement (55). Laboratory studies of the nicotine withdrawal syndrome (55,74) show the time course of measures of brain and cognitive function parallel each other, and symptoms were completely reversed (in dose-related fashion) by nicotine polacrilex gum. Nonlaboratory studies suggest that nicotine given transdermally is similarly effective in alleviating withdrawal symptoms (14), although studies of electrical brain activity have yet to be conducted.

Pharmacokinetics and Pharmacodynamics

Nicotine absorption curves vary across types of delivery systems. Nicotine absorption is rapid for cigarettes, and levels fall quickly because about half of the nicotine is redistributed throughout body compartments within 15–20 min of the last puff from a cigarette. Further decline is more gradual, with a terminal half-life averaging 2 hr, but highly variable across individuals (6). Arterial blood nicotine levels produced by smoking a single cigarette are 3–5 times greater than the maximal levels produced by nicotine transdermal systems (33). Nicotine absorption from smokeless tobacco and noninhaled pipe or cigar smoke is absorbed less rapidly than from inhaled cigarette smoke, and presumably without an arterial bolus. By contrast, plasma levels increase much more slowly when nicotine transdermal systems are used, generally requiring several hours to achieve the venous levels produced in a few minutes by one cigarette. Nicotine polacrilex is capable of somewhat more rapid delivery than transdermal systems but is also slow compared to tobacco products.

Over the course of a day, transdermal systems produce a much less variable pattern of nicotine plasma levels than that associated with cigarette smoking. In general, the pack-per-day cigarette smoker obtains more nicotine than will be obtained from any of the transdermal systems and from typical levels of 2 mg polacrilex use, although there is considerable individual variability. Nicotine levels fall rapidly overnight during smoking abstinence, but fall more slowly when a transdermal system is removed before sleeping. This is consistent with the 4- to 5-hr half-life of transdermally delivered nicotine, which is approximately double that of cigarette-delivered nicotine (14). It may take several days on transdermal nicotine for daily plasma levels to stabilize as the possibly higher nicotine levels obtained from smoking decline (4) and cumulative effects of transdermal dosing develop (61).

There are no medications known to adversely interact with nicotine replacement medications in patients who had already been exposed to daily doses of nicotine from tobacco. However, achieving tobacco abstinence decreases the need for many other medications. Cigarette smoke is a powerful hepatic enzyme inducer, which frequently means that higher doses of many drugs must be administered to smokers than to nonsmokers to obtain similar plasma levels (74). For example, caffeine concentrations can increase by more than 250% during smoking cessation attempts (5). Nicotine replacement medications may not produce the same level of hepatic induction as cigarette smoke; for example, theophylline metabolism is increased by tobacco smoke but not by nicotine only (47). These findings suggest that patients in treatment for nicotine dependence should be warned not to increase their caffeine intake; follow-up evaluations of patient status should include questions about caffeine and other drug intake. It is also worth noting that acute caffeine abstinence results in its own withdrawal syndrome (68) that might complicate simultaneous tobacco withdrawal.

Neurophysiology

Nicotine produces a cascade of behavioral and physiological effects mediated through receptors (C6) at autonomic ganglia, the adrenal medulla, and sensory nerve endings, through neuromuscular (C10) receptors on muscle endplates, and by brain receptors. The powerful conditioning action of nicotine is mediated, at least in part, by (a) the activation of nicotinic cholinergic receptors in the brain (74) and (b) the modulation of levels of hormones such as epinephrine (''adrenalin'') and cortisol (57,74). The mesolimbic dopaminergic reward system, which mediates the ability of cocaine to produce dependence, has also been implicated in nicotine's ability to produce dependence (57,74). The cells of this system are located in the ventral tegmental area of the midbrain. Axons project to the limbic system—specifically, to the nucleus accumbens, olfactory tubercle, nuclei of the stria terminalis, and parts of the amygdala. Behaviors followed by such neural activation can become extremely persistent. Cortical effects of nicotine administration include changes in local cerebral metabolism (49) and EEG (42). Prominent endocrine effects include release of catecholamines, serotonin, prolactin, growth hormone, arginine vasopressin, β-endorphin, and adrenocorticotropic hormone (57,74). These effects mediate both (a) the positive nicotine reinforcement sought by smokers and even animals

(10,30,56,74) and (b) the negative reinforcement of withdrawal symptoms that also fuel the compulsion to smoke (37,57).

Nicotine's observed effects on any given response can appear either stimulant-like or sedative-like depending upon dose administered, time since the last dose, level of tolerance, and degree of physical dependence (31,58). For example, the initial cigarettes of the day produce autonomic arousal, abrupt activation of EEG, and clearly discriminable (often pleasurable) effects. Subsequent cigarettes may produce little change in physiology or behavior (67). The sedative-like effects, however, may be indirect, for example, dependent upon withdrawal relief or behavioral conditioning processes.

Although some nicotine effects may depend little on rate of delivery, the contribution of rapid delivery to dependence-producing psychoactive and reinforcing effects appears to be as important for nicotine as it is for coca-derived products, barbiturates, minor tranquilizers, and opioids, where dependence is directly related to speed of onset. For example, whereas rapid intravenous injections or cigarette smoke inhalation produce psychoactive effects that may be pleasurable, slow infusions or delivery by the transdermal systems produce little, if any, discriminable psychoactive response (31) and blunted or eliminated physiological responses (14).

Mechanisms of Reinforcement

Tolerance and dependence development are not sufficient to establish compulsive smoking of cigarettes, or any other drug for that matter (73). The drug also must be self-administered frequently enough for its reinforcing effects to condition the behavior. Such conditioning processes are maximally effective when the drug effect is discrete, paired with readily discriminable stimuli, and follows a specific behavior within a few seconds (73). The paradigm is optimal for smoking to become powerfully conditioned because each cigarette provides approximately 10 nicotine reinforcers, each carried by a sensorally sating cloud of smoke and delivered to the brain in seconds. Tolerance and physical dependence potentiate the process by establishing a motivational state in the individual which did not preexist. Thus, smoking is reinforced both by the direct positively reinforcing actions of nicotine on the brain and by the necessity of continued nicotine administration to prevent withdrawal symptoms.

In addition to the direct actions of nicotine to strengthen behavior and alleviate withdrawal symptoms, cigarette smokers commonly report benefits that may be at least partially attributable to nicotine. It may not be possible to completely dissociate transient relief of withdrawal from nicotine effects that people with certain vulnerabilities or deficits find addressed by nicotine, but it is important to be aware that smoking cessation will lead to a variety of potential unfulfilled needs that can contribute to relapse. For example, some people claim that smoking enhances their ability to handle stress, helps to control appetite and weight, increases the pleasure of leisure activities such as reading and listening to music, and facilitates social interactions.

At least three kinds of nicotine effects, then, can contribute to the development of dependence: (i) Nicotine delivery produces reinforcing effects mediated by reward systems in the brain; (ii) tolerance and physical dependence are produced such that nicotine abstinence is accompanied by adverse effects; and (iii) at least those dependent on nicotine may derive useful effects on mood, appetite, and cognition. These effects are not mutually exclusive, and they often interact.

When nicotine replacement therapy is viewed from the foregoing perspective, we see that very little of the cigarette is actually replaced by the nicotine delivery medications. Therefore, patients may be disappointed when they find that the medications are neither as pleasurable nor as quickly satisfying as cigarettes. Nonetheless, our understanding of the pathophysiology of tobacco dependence has progressed to the point that it has been possible to develop nicotine replacement pharmaceuticals with impact on the disease process. These medications may not satisfy all the wants and desires of the cigarette smoker, but they can provide many patients with what they need to achieve tobacco abstinence.

PSYCHOPHARMACOLOGY

The observation is not recent nor unique to nicotine that abused drugs may provide their users with effects that are clinically useful, or at least users perceive the effects to be beneficial. In fact, most abused drugs have been used in the practice of medicine. For example, opioids continue to be important in pain control, sedatives are helpful in treating anxiety, and stimulants are valuable in treating narcolepsy. Nonetheless, the diverse psychopharmacological actions of abused drugs have long been understood to be important in the etiology and maintenance of drug dependence (74). The abuse liability of a drug that can directly activate neurological mechanisms of reinforcement would appear to be enhanced by its potential to also provide some sort of benefit, even if the long-term consequences of the substance abuse tend to be disastrous. Some of the apparent benefits of drug exposure may be most appropriately conceptualized as reflecting the reversal of withdrawal symptoms, whereas other benefits may be direct effects of drug administration.

Effects That May Contribute to Chronic Use

As discussed earlier, nicotine administration and withdrawal have diverse effects on brain and endocrine func-

tion that may be of functional significance in the etiology and treatment of psychiatric and neurological disorders such as affective disorders, Alzheimer's and Parkinson's diseases, Tourette's syndrome, and maintenance of cognitive function (39,53). Regarding Parkinson's disease, an analysis of 17 studies supports the conclusion that cigarette smoking provides a weak protective effect (53). There is little evidence that nicotine is an effective treatment for the disorder, or even that the protective effect is specific to nicotine, but the relationship is intriguing and has generated new research on possible mechanisms.

By contrast, cigarette smoking appears to be positively associated with Alzheimer's disease development, although evidence is far from conclusive (53). Preliminary data suggesting that nicotine administration might be of benefit to Alzheimer's patients (53,65) are also intriguing but at present fall far short of supporting a clinical application of nicotine.

Although sufficient epidemiological data are still lacking to determine the relationship between cigarette smoking and Tourette's syndrome, a trial administering nicotine polacrilex and haloperidol to treatment-resistant Tourette's patients produced a therapeutic effect (66). These results are particularly interesting considering data implicating dopaminergic neurons in the reinforcing effects of nicotine as well as in Tourette's syndrome (10,66).

One of the increasingly studied potential therapeutic applications of nicotine is to treat ulcerative colitis. The gastrointestinal tract is rich in receptors for neurotransmitters and is quite responsive to environmental factors. Several studies have now documented that nicotine, administered in tobacco smoke, polacrilex, or transdermal system, can reduce symptoms of ulcerative colitis (70). Continuous nicotine administration appears to suppress the reemergence of colitis symptoms (70).

One of the most common reasons females give for beginning to smoke and for relapsing upon cessation is their belief that tobacco helps control their appetite and body weight (74); this factor appears somewhat less important for males. In fact, there is now a substantial literature that documents the robust effect of nicotine exposure to reduce body weight and prevent developmental weight gain in animals and humans (46). Furthermore, the results of a twin study support the hypothesis that the relationship is a consequence of cigarette smoking and not simply a correlate (12).

Several mechanisms have been postulated to account for the appetite- and weight-suppressing effect of cigarettes (46,74). Those that appear specific to nicotine include a selective decrease in appetite for sweet carbohydrates, increased metabolic rate, and decreased appetite through serotonergic mechanisms. Interestingly, the slowly releasing form of nicotine provided by the transdermal medications does not provide the weight attenuating effect of either continued smoking or nicotine polacrilex use (14). This is not because the total daily dose is inadequate; no weight-suppressing effect was found with up to 22 mg of transdermal nicotine, whereas the effect of nicotine polacrilex appears reliable at a daily intake of approximately 5–8 mg (the expected dose received from the consumption of 6–9 units of 2-mg-containing polacrilex) (24). The more pronounced catecholamine-releasing effects of faster forms of nicotine delivery (4) might account for cigarettes appearing to be particularly efficacious anorectants, polacrilex less so, and transdermal systems without such an effect.

Cognitive Effects

A prominent component of the nicotine withdrawal syndrome is impaired cognitive performance; readministration of nicotine provides rapid relief, thus providing a potentially powerful source of reinforcement for continued smoking. It has even been suggested that nicotine does not really produce dependence but that instead people self-administer cigarettes primarily to provide cognitive benefit (77); however, the presence or lack of therapeutic efficacy is not a criterion for the determination of addiction liability. Furthermore, the only conditions under which reliable cognitive benefits of nicotine administration have been documented are in persons who are cognitively impaired during nicotine withdrawal or possibly by Alzheimer's disease.

In nonsmokers, nicotine administration can increase finger-tapping rate and slightly (but significantly in some studies) attenuate the deterioration in attention that occurs during protracted testing. These effects are scientifically interesting but do not appear to be of either the type or magnitude to explain why at least one in three people exposed to a few cigarettes becomes dependent (74). Moreover, complex cognitive performance may be impaired by nicotine in cigarette smokers as well as in nonsmokers (26).

Vulnerability and Psychiatric Comorbidities

A corollary of the possibility that nicotine can provide certain benefits that then contribute to its overall abuse is that individuals vary in their vulnerability to nicotine dependence. Several studies suggest that the risk of dependence, following the smoking of a few cigarettes, is present in most people. For example, as discussed earlier, in a study in the United Kingdom, 94% of adolescents who smoked at least four cigarettes graduated to regular use persisting for at least 5 years (62). Furthermore, until the 1960s, most male adults in the United States smoked cigarettes; presently, in Japan and other countries, most men smoke cigarettes. On the other hand, with present antismoking educational efforts and policies in the United States, smoking prevalence among men has declined to

approximately 27%. This decline cannot be explained by a reduction in biologically conferred vulnerability occurring within three decades. Rather, it would seem more plausible that most people are vulnerable but that education and prevention efforts can reduce the likelihood of exposure and the progression to dependence after exposure.

Individuals vary in their vulnerability to dependence on nicotine and other drugs just as they vary in their vulnerability to other medical disorders: Some people show a high degree of resistance to the disorder despite multiple exposures to the carrier, whereas others very quickly become dependent or otherwise sick (74). Prominent social and environmental factors have been identified—for example, smoking by a household member, stressful environment, and cost of cigarettes (74). In addition, personality characteristics determined by age 6 (44), as well as genetic heritage (45), are associated with the risk of dependence.

Certain psychiatric comorbidities have also been identified as significant concomitants of cigarette smoking. Depression, possibly certain anxiety disorders, and other forms of drug abuse or dependence occur in approximately one in three cigarette smokers (9). Particularly interesting is the direct relationship between nicotine dependence severity, as determined using *Diagnostic and Statistical Manual III-R* criteria (DSM-III-R; 1), and depression, anxiety, and other drug abuse (9).

There are several potential explanations for the coincidence of these disorders that are not mutually exclusive. Most plausible are that common factors (inherited or environmental) may elevate the risk of developing nicotine dependence as well as the comorbid disorder, the risk of smoking may have been elevated by early premorbid symptoms of another disorder (which could have been alleviated to some degree by smoking), or chronic alteration of dopaminergic and endocrine function resulting from chronic smoking during adolescence may alter the risk of developing certain comorbid disorders.

TREATMENT

The basic principles of nicotine-dependence treatment are the same as those of other drug abuse treatment, discussed elsewhere in this volume. These include the use of behavioral techniques and medications to reduce or eliminate drug use, alleviate withdrawal symptoms, and prevent relapse. A difference in the population of tobacco users from other drug abusers should be considered because of its implications for understanding the etiology and treatment course; that is, epidemiological information suggests that most tobacco users are employed, well adjusted in society without legal problems, and highly motivated to quit. These factors are prominent correlates of success in the treatment of abusers of other drugs (40,74), and attention to these factors is a major, if not the primary, target of treatment efforts for them but is probably less important for treatment of most tobacco-dependent persons.

The often severe consequences of untreated nicotine dependence have been important stimuli for the search for more effective treatments. Making effective treatments more widely available is vital, particularly because cancer chemotherapy, surgery, and other medical treatments for tobacco-caused diseases are often less efficacious and are invariably far more toxic than nicotine-dependence treatments that may prevent the development of these disorders. Helping people achieve abstinence is also important from the perspective of containing health care costs because cessation at any age reduces the risk of most forms of tobacco-caused morbidity as well as mortality (76). For example, in 1993 the U.S. Office of Technology Assessment reported to the U.S. Congress that tobacco-attributable health care costs were 68 billion dollars in 1990 and that these costs could be reduced by more effective treatment and prevention.

Pharmacological approaches to treating nicotine dependence were surely one of the important medical advances of the 1980s and 1990s. However, pharmacological approaches are generally viewed as medications to supplement some type of behaviorally oriented approach because the goal is to assist in modifying smoking behavior. This is not meant to imply, however, that medications should only be used by persons trained in behavior modification techniques or that extensive behavioral counseling is necessary to incur some level of benefit. Several studies have documented long-term benefits of nicotine polacrilex and transdermal systems in general practice settings that administered only a brief behavioral intervention package (64). The basic elements of such interventions will be summarized below.

Diagnostic Advances

The first step in determining the appropriate treatment course is to diagnose the severity of the nicotine dependence and determine if complicating comorbidities are present. No strong rational basis exists for prescribing nicotine replacement therapy if there is little or no nicotine dependence or withdrawal symptoms. If this is the case or if the patient has never tried to quit, the patient should be strongly advised to attempt to quit without medication. Some patients will succeed; those who do not will at least be able to provide useful diagnostic information about their degree of dependence. This is also one of the ways patients learn to cope with life without cigarettes.

Several potential predictive measures of dependence severity tend to co-vary. These include: cotinine level in biological fluid such as saliva, blood, or urine; number of cigarettes smoked per day (e.g., 16 versus 25 may be significant, whereas 21 versus 25 may not be significant); score on the Fagerstrom Tolerance Questionnaire; and number of symptoms from the American Psychiatric Association's DSM-III-R (1). As discussed in the 1988 Report of the Surgeon General (74), these measures tend to predict the following: difficulty achieving abstinence, severity of withdrawal symptoms, rapidity of relapse, and efficacy of replacement therapy. The probability of spontaneous remission (i.e., quitting without formal treatment intervention) is inversely related to the predicted strength of the dependence.

Each of the aforementioned measures has a particular area of utility. The Fagerstrom Tolerance Questionnaire takes only a minute or two to administer and provides remarkably predictive information about the level of dependence and appropriateness of nicotine replacement therapy. Expired air carbon monoxide (or carboxyhemoglobin) provides a quantitative marker of smoke intake and may be useful in monitoring treatment efficacy and potential reduction in smoke-delivered toxins over the course of treatment. Cotinine (assessed in saliva, urine, or blood) may be the single most useful measure of dependence but is not generally worth the expense of collection except in cases where nicotine replacement will be used, and it is especially important to document that the overall exposure to nicotine is lower during therapy than during pretreatment smoking (e.g., pregnancy, active heart disease, and adolescent treatment).

The two medical disorders pertaining to nicotine dependence are identified by the American Psychiatric Association:

1. *Nicotine dependence,* which is a type of *psychoactive-substance-use disorder.* The essential feature is "a cluster of cognitive, behavioral, and physiologic symptoms that indicate the person has impaired control of psychoactive substance use and continues use of the substance despite adverse consequences" (1, p. 166). The most common form is cigarette smoking, in part due to the rapid onset of nicotine effects via this route which "facilitate the conditioning of an intensive habit" (1, pp. 181–182). However, it is noted that dependence to other forms of nicotine delivery, including smokeless tobacco and nicotine gum, may also occur.

2. *Nicotine withdrawal,* which is a type of *psychoactive-substance-induced organic mental disorder.* The essential feature is "a characteristic withdrawal syndrome due to the abrupt cessation of, or reduction in, the use of nicotine-containing substances (e.g., cigarettes, cigars, pipes, chewing tobacco, or nicotine gum) that has been at least moderate in duration and amount. The syndrome includes craving for nicotine, irritability, frustration, anger, anxiety, difficulty concentrating, restlessness, decreased heartrate, and increased appetite or weight gain." (1, pp. 150–151).

The American Psychiatric Association criteria are useful in estimating the likely severity of withdrawal symptoms (if the patient can accurately remember symptoms from prior cessation attempts) and appear most useful in predicting the likelihood of comorbid depression and anxiety (9).

Behavioral Treatment Strategies

Behavioral intervention is the cornerstone of all forms of effective smoking cessation intervention. Even high-dose administration of nicotine to smokers not attempting to quit does not induce spontaneous cessation and generally produces reductions in smoke intake that, although scientifically important, are probably of little health benefit (e.g., reduction of cigarette intake from 27 to 23 cigarettes per day). Several behavioral forms of intervention varying both in type and intensity have been demonstrated to substantially enhance cessation rates above the 3–7% baseline cessation rate detected in several population studies. These interventions range from briefly administered physician advice and guidance to intensive behavior modification (63). The more widely studied forms are summarized in this section.

Individual behavioral counseling often includes the provision of self-help materials providing strategies for achieving and sustaining remission. Dependence level, possible withdrawal severity, and putative relapse factors that vary across individuals (e.g., weight gain, stress, friends who smoke, and alcohol consumption) are important factors in the development of a behavioral prescription. Setting a target quit date 1–3 weeks from the initial intervention appears critical to give the person time to prepare for the possible trauma, but it is critical not to leave the quit date's occurrence open-ended. Behavioral approaches may also include skills training, relaxation training, recommendations for exercise, and contingency contracting.

Group counseling approaches are used in a variety of health care settings and by many voluntary agencies. Specific protocols vary, but there appear to be at least three important elements: information about smoking risks and the benefits of quitting to provide additional motivation; strategies to cope with relapse situations and sustain abstinence; and social settings which may constitute a contingency program for achieving and sustaining cessation. The latter factor is probably subsumed under what is often referred to as *group dynamics* and appears to be powerful in some groups and weak or counterproductive in others. A major problem with this approach is that it appears that less than 10% of cigarette smokers who want to quit would actually participate in a group program.

Nicotine fading approaches attempt to achieve gradual reduction of smoke intake by decreasing puffs per cigarette, number of cigarettes smoked per day, and smoking brands of cigarettes that deliver lower doses of nicotine. Special cigarette filters and approaches to dilute the smoke may also be incorporated. Although nicotine fading can be helpful when done carefully, the main problem with these approaches is that the goal of reduced tobacco intake may be easily defeated by subtle changes in how each cigarette is smoked because it is possible to extract several milligrams of nicotine from nearly any brand of cigarettes sold in the United States (74).

Aversion treatments are designed to condition a cigarette aversion by pairing smoking with either unpleasant imagery (covert sensitization), electric shock, or unpleasant effects of smoking itself through directed smoking procedures. Directed smoking techniques include satiation, rapid smoking, and focused smoking. The usefulness of aversion procedures is limited because the aversions are rarely permanent, and it is difficult to condition aversion to a substance that has had repeated past use.

Acupuncture and hypnosis are two widely marketed techniques that have never been proven efficacious as specific procedures to induce lasting cessation. However, clinics offering such services range from those that apply the procedure with little additional support to those that apply the procedure ancillary to extensive individual or group counseling. It is plausible that clinics offering a comprehensive approach (some hypnosis programs even incorporate nicotine-delivering medications) may be effective, although there has been little systematic study of this possibility. Controlled clinical trials of acupuncture have not demonstrated significant efficacy (63,74).

Pharmacological Treatment Strategies

The major pharmacological approaches are *nicotine replacement, symptomatic treatment, nicotine blockade,* and *deterrent treatment.* Nicotine replacement and symptomatic treatment have become part of general medical practice. Until further information is collected, blockade and deterrent treatment must still be considered experimental. These will be summarized in what we believe is reverse order of their presently known efficacy.

Nicotine blockade therapy is based on the rationale that if one blocks the rewarding aspects of nicotine by administering an antagonist, the person who smokes for the pleasant effects nicotine produces will be more likely to stop smoking. To be effective, the drug must be centrally active. Thus, mecamylamine, which acts at both central and peripheral nervous system sites, may increase rates of abstinence, whereas hexamethonium and pentolinium, which block peripheral receptors only, should have no effect on abstinence. Preliminary data suggest that mecamylamine might be used to antagonize the nicotine-mediated reinforcing effects of smoking (40). Unfortunately, there are presently no pure nicotine antagonists clinically available. Drugs like mecamylamine produce side effects such as sedation, low blood pressure, and fainting that probably limit their role to experimental tools but not for clinical treatment (40).

The rationale for *deterrent therapy* is that pretreatment with a drug may transform smoking from a rewarding experience to an aversive one if the unpleasant consequences are immediate and strong enough. Disulfiram treatment for alcoholism is an example of this type of treatment. After pretreatment, even a small quantity of alcohol can produce discomfort and acute illness. Silver acetate administration is a potential deterrent treatment for smokers. When silver acetate contacts the sulfides in tobacco smoke, the resulting sulfide salts are very distasteful to most people. Although many over-the-counter deterrent smoking prevention treatments are available, their effectiveness has not been scientifically validated. Additionally, a severe limitation to this treatment is compliance. It has been difficult to ensure that patients continue to take the medication as needed (74).

Nicotine administration and withdrawal produce a number of neurohormonal and other physiological effects. *Symptomatic treatment* methods are nonspecific pharmacotherapies to relieve the discomforts and mood changes associated with withdrawal. If the potential quitter relapses to escape withdrawal, these methods should help to prevent such relapse. There is a long history of pharmacological treatment of smokers. Sedatives, tranquilizers, anticholinergics, sympathomimetics, and anticonvulsants have all been used to reduce withdrawal, but they failed to increase chances of quitting relative to placebo. Clonidine has been used in attempts to treat withdrawal discomfort. Glassman et al. (22) administered clonidine to heavy smokers on days they abstained from smoking and found that clonidine reduced anxiety, irritability, restlessness, tension, and cigarette craving. Moreover, there was a significantly greater rate of smoking cessation among women, but not among men, 6 months after clonidine treatment. The mechanism of the gender difference was not elucidated. For example, it was not clear whether this lack of efficacy in men was due to gender or insufficient dose (the same doses were given to all subjects regardless of body weight). Before recommending clonidine for smokers, potential side effects such as drowsiness, hypotension, and discontinuation-related hypertension must also be considered.

Among nicotine's effects is the regulation of mood. Smokers have been shown to smoke more during stressful situations, and people trying to quit often relapse during stressful situations. These observations suggest that treating the mood changes associated with abstinence with, for example, benzodiazepine tranquilizers, antidepressants, or psychomotor stimulants may improve abstinence rates. The benzodiazepine tranquilizer alprazolam was also examined by Glassman et al. (22) and found to reduce anxiety, irritability, tension, and restlessness, but it had no effect on cravings in heavy cigarette smokers abstain-

ing from smoking for one day. Although clonidine and other medications with potential utility in treating symptoms of nicotine abstinence do not have Food and Drug Administration (FDA) approval, they may still merit attention for some people not helped by other means (40).

The rationale for administering *nicotine replacement medications* is to substitute a safer, more manageable, and, ideally, less addictive form of the drug to alleviate withdrawal symptoms and facilitate abstinence. The ability of health professionals to effectively treat nicotine dependence was greatly enhanced by the appearance of nicotine replacement medications. The first generation of such medications was nicotine polacrilex (''gum''), approved by the FDA for marketing in 1984. The second generation was the transdermal delivery system, four of which were approved from December 1991 to August 1992. Another generation is in development, encouraged by the proven utility as well as limitations of the first two generations. This includes a nicotine vapor inhaler, nasal nicotine spray (gel droplets), and lozenge.

The scientific foundations for administering nicotine as a substitute for cigarette smoke included work by Johnston (41) in the 1940s and Luchessi et al. in the 1960s (50). However, it was not until the 1970s that the first non-tobacco nicotine-delivering formulation intended as a medicinal replacement for tobacco, a chewable nicotine resin complex (nicotine polacrilex), was developed by the Swedish pharmaceutical company A.B. Leo (16). The main limitation of nicotine polacrilex is difficulty maintaining adequate self-administration to provide a viable means of nicotine replacement for smoking (40).

The constraints on the utility of nicotine polacrilex were partially addressed by the transdermal delivery system. The transdermal nicotine delivery approach was initially developed to treat nicotine dependence in research supported by the National Institute on Drug Abuse (60). By August 1992, four pharmaceutical companies in the United States received approval by the FDA to market their transdermal systems.

Lobeline is a putative nicotine agonist present in several aids for smoking cessation such as CigArrest™, Bantron™, and Nicoban™. These and other such aids were removed from the market in December 1992 by the FDA until they are established to be efficacious in scientific studies. Lobeline is a weak nicotinic receptor agonist, but it is of unproven efficacy for smoking cessation treatment; it appears to act at cholinergic receptor sites other than those mediating the discriminative effects of nicotine (40). It is possible that higher doses than those tested might be helpful, but studies have yet to be conducted.

The clinical use of nicotine replacement medication may be advanced by considering research on the correlates of efficacy of methadone treatment of heroin dependence. Particularly valuable is the information provided by the study of Ball and Ross (2), which showed that heroin treatment efficacy was related to factors such as daily methadone dose, duration of treatment, level of support, and characteristics of the counselors themselves. Similar factors appear important in treating nicotine dependence using nicotine-delivering medications.

Nicotine Replacement Therapy: Clinical Issues

Mechanism of Action and Limitations

The goal of nicotine replacement therapy is to help the patient establish remission and sustain it long enough to develop prophylactic strategies to avoid relapse. The physiological mechanisms of action of nicotine replacement must be understood to predict the possible benefits as well as probable limitations of the medication. Nicotine replacement is used to facilitate the cessation of tobacco use, but there is no evidence that nicotine replacement would induce smoking cessation in persons not attempting to quit. In fact, spontaneous smoking in persons not attempting to quit is only slightly reduced (54,74).

There appear to be three pharmacological mechanisms by which nicotine facilitates smoking cessation. Nicotine replacement reduces withdrawal symptoms that can motivate relapse. This mechanism provides a secondary, albeit controversial, indication for nicotine replacement—that is, relief of withdrawal symptoms in those who must undergo intermittent periods of abstinence but who are not attempting to cease smoking (e.g., this application is practiced in many hospitals for short-term inpatients and by some military pilots). Nicotine replacement also partially sates the appetite for cigarettes by sustaining nicotine tolerance and thereby reduces the acute reinforcing effects of smoke-delivered doses (74).

Besides reducing the pharmacological reinforcing effects of cigarettes, nicotine replacement may provide some of the effects the smoker had come to rely upon cigarettes to provide, such as sustaining desirable mood and attentional states and handling stressful or boring situations. Nicotine gum, but not transdermal systems, also reduces the weight gain accompanying smoking cessation (14). These effects are at least partially related to withdrawal reduction, but many other uses of cigarettes do not involve withdrawal relief. There is little reason to believe that nicotine replacement would reduce these pressures to smoke. Most apparent may be the social situations in which smoking had come to serve as a lubricant and common bond. Equally prominent would be the private pleasures of sensorium satisfaction established over hundreds of thousands of smoking episodes. For many, these pleasures may be no more satisfied by nicotine polacrilex or transdermal systems than were the pleasures of eating satisfied by nutritional substitutes for normal food in volunteers kept healthy by these substitutes.

There do not appear to be any residual pharmacological effects of nicotine replacement to protect against relapse;

unfortunately, the pressures to relapse are constant, and the likelihood of cigarette smoke exposure is virtually guaranteed for most people in remission. Therefore, establishing new patterns of behavior (i.e., of learning to handle life without cigarettes) during the replacement-aided period of remission would act as the primary protection from relapse.

Rational Basis for Dosing

Diagnosis of nicotine dependence level and determination whether previous cessation attempts have resulted in withdrawal symptoms are essential to provide individualized guidance to the patient, as well as provide a rational basis for dosing decisions. The need for appropriate dosing is the same as that for other medications—namely, to ensure adequate doses to provide therapeutic benefit while minimizing the risks associated with doses that are too high. The importance of the latter concern is that smokers are a high-risk population for nicotine-attributable mortality, and risks do not immediately cease with the cessation of smoking. Thus, clinicians should perform an appropriate diagnosis to confirm that their prescribed dosing regimen does not expose patients to higher levels of nicotine than they obtained by smoking.

Efficacy of Nicotine Replacement

Nicotine polacrilex and transdermal systems have been approved by the FDA as safe and effective, and the medications have been suggested as important and cost-effective components of an emerging health care system (3). The efficacy of the medications in helping to achieve cessation and manage withdrawal symptoms has been repeatedly demonstrated under a broad range of conditions, although some level of structured behavioral support is critical (14,18,40). In addition, several reviews have concluded that 1-year quit rates following transdermal medications are approximately 20–30%, or double those of placebo treatment and approximately five times greater than spontaneous quitting rates (14,18,19). Similar short- and moderate-term success rates have been reported with nicotine polacrilex, but long-term efficacy with this medication appears to be more dependent on its incorporation into a systematic behavioral treatment approach than are transdermal systems (36).

In treatment trials, the level of behavioral intervention is generally correlated with efficacy rates among both nicotine-medicated and placebo-receiving groups (25). What is unclear, however, is the level of behavioral intervention beyond which no further reliable benefit occurs, or if certain kinds of interventions are generally more effective than others (63).

Two studies have reported increased withdrawal relief by combining a nicotine transdermal system with polacrilex (15,48). Rationale for this combination is that the transdermal system provides stable nicotine levels that can then be supplemented as needed by polacrilex. Although long-term benefits are not yet known, this regime appears reasonable for highly dependent patients and those not helped by either alone.

Dependence Potential

Nicotine polacrilex and transdermal systems can sustain tolerance and some degree of physical dependence but do not produce the highly reinforcing effects of rapid delivery systems (31,74). In fact, transdermal systems deliver nicotine so slowly that they are almost devoid of the psychoactive effects characteristic of drugs with significant abuse potential (31,54). Nicotine polacrilex takes considerable effort to produce such a limited response compared to tobacco products and has proven to be low in abuse liability (31). In addition, there is no evidence that the widespread availability of nicotine replacement systems has led to dependence in people not already dependent on nicotine. Among people prescribed nicotine polacrilex, less than 5% continue their use for a year of more, and approximately 20% of people who have sustained abstinence continue to use the polacrilex. When there appears to be minimal danger of smoking relapse, available data suggest that most of these persons can end their nicotine medication usage without undue difficulty (35).

SUMMARY AND CONCLUSIONS

The pathophysiological consequences of tobacco use produce changes in body tissues that contribute to heart disease, cancer, respiratory diseases, and dependence. These disorders are not inevitable consequences of tobacco exposure, but tobacco exposure is a causal factor in their etiology. Approximately one in three adolescents who smoke a few cigarettes develop nicotine dependence; of these, approximately one in three die of tobacco-related disease. Thus, the relationship between tobacco exposure and death is not unlike that seen with other pathogens such as *Mycobacterium tuberculosis,* in which approximately one in ten carriers of the bacteria develop tuberculosis disease. Among the disorders resulting from tobacco use, dependence is unique because its primary manifestation is behavioral; this has implications for treatment that were discussed.

Understanding of the pathophysiological basis of tobacco dependence has progressed as rapidly as the understanding of cancer and other tobacco-related disorders. The pathophysiology of nicotine dependence includes tolerance development, receptor up-regulation, physiological dependence, and reinforcing effects, as well as the many other effects of nicotine on behavior and physiolog-

ical functioning. The reinforcing effects of nicotine, in turn, are related to the method of nicotine delivery. Genetic constitution appears to contribute to the vulnerability to nicotine dependence as well as to the vulnerability to comorbid disorders.

These recent advances in knowledge have contributed to our understanding of nicotine dependence as a chronic disorder. Insufficient motivation or inadequate knowledge of risks do not adequately explain why most cigarette smokers continue tobacco use. Most tobacco users are aware of the risks, and they frequently attempt abstinence; however, they usually fail, even when motivated by the near-death experience of a heart attack. It seems reasonable to conclude that once nicotine dependence is established, the seemingly irrational behavior of continued tobacco use is no more governed by free choice and rational decision-making than is the behavior of metastasizing cells once cancer onset has occurred. In both cases, systematic treatment can enhance the individual's prognosis. However, treatments for nicotine dependence are generally more effective and less toxic than treatments for heart disease and cancer. Therefore, greater availability of nicotine-dependence treatment will be an important means of lowering the overall health cost burden of a nation.

REFERENCES

1. American Psychiatric Association. *Diagnostic and statistical manual of mental disorders,* 3rd ed. (revised). Washington, DC: American Psychiatric Association, 1987.
2. Ball JC, Ross A. *The effectiveness of methadone maintenance therapy.* New York: Springer-Verlag, 1991.
3. Becker DM, Windsor R, Ockene JK, Berman B, Best JA. *Setting the policy, education, and research agenda to reduce tobacco use. Circulation* 1994;88:1381–1386.
4. Benowitz NL. Pharmacokinetics considerations in understanding nicotine dependence. In: *The biology of nicotine dependence 1990.* Ciba Foundation Symposium 152. Chichester: Wiley, 1990;186–209.
5. Benowitz NL, Hall SM, Modin G. Persistent increase in caffeine concentrations in people who stop smoking. *Br Med J* 1989;298:1075–1076.
6. Benowitz NL, Jacob P, Denaro C, Jenkins R. Stable isotope studies of nicotine kinetics and bioavailability. *Clin Pharmacol Ther* 1991;49:270–277.
7. Benwell MM, Balfour DJ, Anderson JM. Evidence that tobacco smoking increases the density of (−)-[³H] nicotine binding sites in human brain. *J Neurochem* 1988;50:1243–1247.
8. Breslau N, Fenn N, Peterson EL. Early smoking initiation and nicotine dependence in a cohort of young adults. *Drug Alcohol Depend* 1994; in press.
9. Breslau N, Kilbey M, Andreski P. Nicotine dependence, major depression, and anxiety in young adults. *Arch Gen Psychiatry* 1991;48:1069–1074.
10. Corrigall WA. Regulation of intravenous nicotine self-administration—dopamine mechanisms. In: Adlkofer F, Thurau K, eds. *Effects of nicotine on biological systems. Advances in pharmacological sciences.* Boston: Berkhauser Verlag, 1991;423–432.
11. Domino EF, von Baumgarten AM. Tobacco cigarette smoking and patellar reflex depression. *Clin Pharmacol Ther* 1969;10:72–78.
12. Eisen SA, Lyons MJ, Goldberg J, True WR. The impact of cigarette and alcohol consumption on weight and obesity: an analysis of 1911

monozygotic male twin pairs. *Arch Intern Med* 1993;153:2457–2463.

13. Evans S, Cone E, Marco AP, Henningfield JE. A comparison of the arterial kinetics of smoked and intravenous cocaine. In: Harris L, ed. *Problems of drug dependence 1992*. NIDA research monograph. Washington DC: US Government Printing Office, NIH publication no. 93-3505, 1993;343.

14. Fagerström KO, Hurt RD, Säwe U, Tönnesen P. Therapeutic use of nicotine patches: efficacy and safety. *J Smoking-Related Dis* 1992;3:247–261.

15. Fagerström KO, Schneider NG, Lunell E. Effectiveness of nicotine patch and nicotine gum as individual versus combined treatments for tobacco withdrawal symptoms. *Psychopharmacology* 1993;111:271–277.

16. Ferno O. The development of chewing gum containing nicotine and some comments on the role played by nicotine in the smoking habit. In: Steinfeld J, Griffiths W, Ball K, Taylor RM, eds. *Smoking and health. Proceedings of the 3rd world congress on smoking and health*. Washington, DC: US Government Printing Office, DHEW publication no. (NIH) 77-1413, 1977;569–573.

17. Fiore MC. Trends in cigarette smoking in the United States. The epidemiology of tobacco use. *Med Clin North Am* 1992;76:289–303.

18. Fiore MC, Jorenby DE, Baker TB, Kenford SL. Tobacco dependence and the nicotine patch. *JAMA* 1992;268:1–9.

19. Foulds J. Does nicotine replacement therapy work? [editorial] *Addiction* 1993;88:1473–1478.

20. Foulds J, Stapleton J, Hayward M, Russell MAH, Feyerabend C, Fleming T, Costello J. Transdermal nicotine patches with low-intensity support to aid smoking cessation in outpatients in a general hospital. *Arch Fam Med* 1993;2:417–423.

21. George H. Gallup International Institute. *Teen-age attitudes and behavior concerning tobacco. Report of the findings*. Princeton, NJ, September 1992.

22. Glassman AH, Stetner F, Walsh T, Raizman PS, Fleiss JL, Cooper TB, Covey LS. Heavy smokers, smoking cessation, and clonidine. *JAMA* 1988;259:2863–2866.

23. Goldberg SR, Risner ME, Stolerman IP, Reavill C, Garcha HS. Nicotine and some related compounds: effects on schedule-controlled behavior and discriminative properties in rats. *Psychopharmacology* 1989;97:295–302.

24. Gross J, Stitzer ML. Nicotine replacement: ten-week effects on tobacco withdrawal symptoms. *Psychopharmacology* 1989;98:334–341.

25. Hatsukami D, Lando H. Behavioral treatment for smoking cessation. *Health Values* 1993;17:32–40.

26. Heishman SJ, Snyder FR, Henningfield JE. Performance, subjective, and physiological effects of nicotine in nonsmokers. *Drug Alcohol Depend* 1993;34:11–18.

27. Henningfield JE. Occasional drug use: comparing nicotine with other addictive drugs. *Tobacco Control* 1992;1:161–162.

28. Henningfield JE, Clayton R, Pollin W. The involvement of tobacco in alcoholism and illicit drug use. *Br J Addict* 1990;85:279–292.

29. Henningfield JE, Cohen C, Slade JD. Is nicotine more addictive than cocaine? *Br J Addict* 1991;86:565–569.

30. Henningfield JE, Goldberg SR. Nicotine as a reinforcer in human subjects and laboratory animals. *Pharmacol Biochem Behav* 1983;19:989–992.

31. Henningfield JE, Keenan RM. Nicotine delivery kinetics and abuse liability. *J Consult Clin Psychol* 1993;61:1–8.

32. Henningfield JE, Radzius A, Cooper TM, Clayton RR. Drinking coffee and carbonated beverages blocks absorption of nicotine from nicotine polacrilex gum. *JAMA* 1990;264:1560–1564.

33. Henningfield JE, Stapleton JM, Benowitz NL, Grayson RF, London ED. Higher levels of nicotine in arterial than in venous blood after cigarette smoking. *Drug Alcohol Depend* 1993;33:23–29.

34. Hughes JR, Gulliver SB, Fenwick JW, Valliere WA, Cruser K, Pepper S, Shea P, Solomon LJ, Flynn BS. Smoking cessation among self-quitters. *Health Psychol* 1992;11:331–334.

35. Hughes JR, Gust SW, Keenan R, et al. Long-term use of nicotine vs placebo gum. *Arch Intern Med* 1991;151:1993–1998.

36. Hughes JR, Gust SW, Keenan M, Fenwick JW, Healey ML. Nicotine vs placebo gum in general medical practice. *JAMA* 1989;261:1300–1305.

37. Hughes JR, Hatsukami DK. The nicotine withdrawal syndrome: a brief review and update. *Int J Smoking Cessation* 1992;1:21–26.

38. Jaffe JH, Jarvik ME. Tobacco use and tobacco use disorder. In: Lipton MA, DiMascio A, Killam KF, eds. *Psychopharmacology: a generation of progress*. New York: Raven Press, 1978;1665–1676.

39. Jarvik ME. Beneficial effects of nicotine. *Br J Addict* 1991;86:571–575.

40. Jarvik ME, Henningfield JE. Pharmacological adjuncts for the treatment of nicotine dependence. In: Slade JD, Orleans CT, eds. *Nicotine addiction: principles and management*. New York: Oxford University Press, 1993.

41. Johnston LM. Tobacco smoking and nicotine. *Lancet* 1942;2:742.

42. Jones RT. Tobacco dependence. In: Meltzer HY, ed. *Psychopharmacology: the third generation of progress*. New York: Raven Press, 1987.

43. Keenan RM, Hatsukami DK, Pentel PR, Thompson T, Grillo MA. Pharmacodynamic effects of cotinine in abstinent smokers. *Clin Pharmacol Ther* 1994;55:581–590.

44. Kellam SG, Ensminger ME, Simon MB. Mental health in first grade and teenage drug, alcohol, and cigarette use. *Drug Alcohol Depend* 1980;5:273–304.

45. Kendler KS, Neale MC, MacLean CJ, et al. Smoking and major depression. A causal analysis. *Arch Gen Psychiatry* 1993;50:36–43.

46. Klesges RC, Meyers AW, Klesges LM, LaVasque ME. Smoking, body weight, and their effects on smoking behavior: a comprehensive review of the literature. *Psychol Bull* 1989;106:204–230.

47. Lee BL, Benowitz NL, Jacob P. Cigarette abstinence, nicotine gum, and theophylline disposition. *Ann Intern Med* 1987;106:553–555.

48. Leischow SJ, Valente SN, Hill AL, Otte PS, Aickin M, Kligman EW. Nicotine patch and gum: withdrawal symptoms, side effects, and medication preference. In: Harris L, ed. *Problems of drug dependence 1993*. NIDA research monograph. Washington, DC: US Government Printing Office, 1994;(in press).

49. London ED, Morgan MJ. Positron emission tomographic studies on the acute effects of psychoactive drugs on brain metabolism and mood. In: London ED, ed. *Imaging drug action in the brain*. Boca Raton, FL: CRC Press, 1993;265–280.

50. Luchessi BR, Schuster CR, Emley AB. The role of nicotine as a determinant of cigarette smoking frequency in man with observations of certain cardiovascular effects associated with the tobacco alkaloid. *Clin Pharmacol Ther* 1967;789–796.

51. McGinnis JM, Foege WH. Actual causes of death in the United States. *JAMA* 1993;270:2207–2212.

52. McNeill AD. The development of dependence on smoking in children. *Br J Addict* 1991;86:589–592.

53. Newhouse PA, Hughes JR. The role of nicotine and nicotinic mechanisms in neuropsychiatric disease. *Br J Addict* 1991;86:521–526.

54. Pickworth WB, Bunker EB, Henningfield JE. Transdermal nicotine: Reduction of smoking with minimum abuse liability. *Psychopharmacology* 1994;in press.

55. Pickworth WB, Herning RI, Henningfield JE. Spontaneous EEG changes during tobacco abstinence and nicotine substitution. *J Pharmacol Exp Ther* 1989;251:976–982.

56. Pomerleau OF. Nicotine and the central nervous system: Biobehavioral effects of cigarette smoking. *Am J Med* 1992;93(suppl 1A):2A–7S.

57. Pomerleau OF, Pomerleau CS. Neuroregulators and the reinforcement of smoking: towards a biobehavioral explanation. *Neurosci Biobehav Rev* 1984;8:503–513.

58. Pomerleau OF, Rosecrans J. Neuroregulatory effects of nicotine. *Psychoneuroendocrinology* 1989;14:407–423.

59. Raveis VH, Kandel DB. Changes in drug behavior from middle to late 20s: initiation, persistence and cessation of use. *Am J Public Health* 1987;77:607–611.

60. Rose JE, Jarvik ME, Rose KD. Transdermal administration of nicotine. *Drug Alcohol Depend* 1984;13:209–213.

61. Ross HD, Chan KH, Piraino AJ, John VA. Pharmacokinetics of multiple daily transdermal doses of nicotine in healthy smokers. *Pharmacol Res* 1991;8:385–388.

62. Russell MAH. The nicotine addiction trap: a 40-year sentence for four cigarettes. *Br J Addiction* 1990;85:295–300.

63. Sachs DPL. Advances in smoking cessation treatment. *Curr Pulmonol* 1991;12:139–198.

64. Sachs DPL, Leischow SJ. Pharmacologic approaches to smoking cessation. *Clin Chest Med* 1991;12:769–791.

65. Sahakian B, Jones G, Levy R, Gray J, Warburton D. The effects of nicotine on attention, information processing, and short-term memory in patients with dementia of the Alzheimer's type. *Br J Psychiatry* 1989;154:797–800.

66. Sanberg PR, Fogelson HM, Mandersheid PZ, Parker KW, Norman AB, McConville BJ. Nicotine gum and haloperidol in Tourette's syndrome. *Lancet* 1988;1:592.

67. Sheiner LB. Clinical pharmacology and the choice between theory and empiricism. *Clin Pharmacol Ther* 1989;46:605–615.

68. Silverman K, Evans SM, Strain EC, Griffiths RR. Withdrawal syndrome after the double-blind cessation of caffeine consumption. *N Engl J Med* 1992;327:1109–1114.

69. Slade J. Nicotine addiction. Blakeman EM, Engelberg AL, eds. *Tobacco use in America conference.* Washington, DC: American Medical Association, 1991;7–11.

70. Srivastava ED, Russell MAH, Feyerabend C, Williams GT, Masterson JG, Rhodes J. Transdermal nicotine in active ulcerative colitis. *Eur J Gastroenterol Hepatol* 1991;3:815–818.

71. Srivastava ED, Russell MAH, Feyerabend C, Masterson JG, Rhodes J. Sensitivity and tolerance to nicotine in smokers and nonsmokers. *Psychopharmacology* 1991;105:63–68.

72. Svensson CK. Clinical pharmacokinetics of nicotine. *Clin Pharmacokinet* 1987;12:30–40.

73. Thompson TI, Schuster CR. *Behavioral pharmacology.* Englewood Cliffs, NJ: Prentice–Hall, 1968.

74. United States Department of Health and Human Services (US DHHS), Public Health Service. *The health consequences of smoking: nicotine addiction: a report of the Surgeon General.* Washington, DC: US Government Printing Office, DHHS publication no. (CDC) 88-8406, 1988.

75. United States Department of Health and Human Services (US DHHS), Public Health Services. *Drug abuse and drug abuse research.* The Second Triennial Report to Congress from the Secretary, Department of Health and Human Services. Washington, DC: US Government Printing Office, DHHS publication no. (ADM) 87-1486, 1987.

76. United States Department of Health and Human Services (US DHHS), Public Health Service. *The health benefits of smoking cessation: a report of the Surgeon General.* Washington, DC: US Government Printing Office, DHHS publication no. (CDC) 90-8416, 1990.

77. Warburton DM. Nicotine: an addictive substance or a therapeutic agent? *Prog Drug Res* 1989;33:9–41.

78. West RJ, Russell MAH, Jarvis MJ, Feyerabend C. Does switching to an ultra-low nicotine cigarette induce nicotine withdrawal effects? *Psychopharmacology* 1984;84:120–123.

Psychopharmacology: The Fourth Generation of Progress, edited by Floyd E. Bloom and David J. Kupfer. Raven Press, Ltd., New York 1995.

CHAPTER 148

Opioids

George E. Bigelow and Kenzie L. Preston

Drug-abuse-related research with opioids pursues two primary clinical goals: (i) the development of effective analgesics with reduced abuse liability and (ii) the development of medications for treatment of opioid abuse and dependence. The purpose of the present chapter is to review selected recent human research developments in these two areas. These are closely related, often overlapping, areas. A major goal of medications development research is to identify medications that reduce the abuse liability of opioids. Recent research pursuing these two goals has produced an extensive body of knowledge concerning the clinical and behavioral pharmacology of opioids and of opioid abuse and dependence.

PREVALENCE OF ABUSE

Because opioid abuse is both illegal and often over represented in marginalized segments of society, its prevalence is difficult to determine accurately. It is commonly estimated that there are 600,000 opioid addicts in the United States, but estimates of the number of opioid abusers approach 2 million. Though the population prevalence of opioid dependence is relatively low, the prevalence of vulnerability to dependence appears substantially higher. Historical experience prior to the legal restriction of opioid availability is that substantial portions of the population became regular users when opioids were readily available (39). Similarly, 15–20% of American military enlisted men serving in Vietnam, where opioids were widely and cheaply available, reported having become

addicted (54). The lower current population prevalence of opioid dependence is presumably attributable to education, social and legal sanctions, and restrictions on availability, as well as to research that identified drugs with significant abuse potential prior to their introduction into general use.

There is a risk that antidrug education, sanctions, and restrictions, by emphasizing the risk side of opioid use, may deter physicians and patients from using opioids when medically appropriate and may thereby result in inadequate treatment of clinical pain. In fact, the risk that the behavioral disorder of opioid abuse will result from appropriate medical use of opioid analgesics is quite small. A study of 11,882 hospitalized patients who received opioids found only four cases of subsequent new addictions—an incidence of 0.03% (41). Most opioid abuse develops with illicit opioids such as heroin. Of course, medically used opioids have high abuse liability, and they will be sought by abusers, who may feign need; therefore caution in medical use is essential. In addition, opioids pose a significant occupational hazard for abuse among health professionals who may have convenient access and be tempted either to self-medicate or to experiment.

ABUSE LIABILITY ASSESSMENT

The sections below describe and review the methods that have been developed for assessing opioid abuse liability in humans and summarize the data these methods have generated concerning the clinical pharmacology of opioid agonists, antagonists, and mixed agonist–antagonists. Drug-abuse-related research interests have been the dominant force in studying and characterizing the clinical pharmacology of opioids. The utility of these methods has been broad. They have served an important descriptive function in simply analyzing and quantifying

G. E. Bigelow: Behavioral Pharmacology Research Unit, Department of Psychiatry and Behavioral Sciences, Johns Hopkins University School of Medicine, Baltimore, Maryland 21224.

K. L. Preston: Behavioral Pharmacology Research Unit, Department of Psychiatry and Behavioral Sciences, Johns Hopkins University School of Medicine, and National Institute on Drug Abuse, Intramural Research Program, Baltimore, Maryland 21224.

aspects of opioid action and opioid dependence. They have served an important basic science function in developing methods and indices that have permitted examination in humans of the specific behavioral and physiological functions controlled by the increasingly complex neurobiological processes and actions involved in opioid pharmacology, and they have served as a stimulus to advanced basic science conceptualization of how opioids act in brain. They have served an important practical and public health function in assessing the potential abuse liability of new compounds and thereby insuring proper prior professional education about abuse risks and/or proper prior societal restriction or regulation of drug availability. Finally, they have more recently served an important applied research and therapeutic function as they have been adapted and utilized in the task of assessing and developing new pharmacotherapies for opioid abuse and dependence.

Methodology

Much of the developmental work in human opioid psychopharmacology was conducted at the Addiction Research Center (ARC) in Lexington, Kentucky (2). Many of the methods and principles used today to assess abuse liability in humans are derived from this ARC work. While the emphasis of ARC research was on opioids, the methods developed have served as the model from which adaptations have been derived for assessment of other drug classes.

The major modern methods include: assessment of subjective effect profiles; assessment of discriminative drug effects; assessment of behavioral reinforcing properties and self-administration; assessment of degree of antagonist activity; and assessment of physical dependence capacity. Inclusion of placebo as a negative control and the use of double-blind procedures are critical elements of these procedures. To provide positive reference values against which to interpret the effects of the test drug, it is also critical to include appropriate positive control drugs; these would normally be prototypic drugs of known high and/or low abuse liability, such as morphine or naloxone. This section reviews methods used to evaluate drugs on these dimensions and summarizes results for the clinically available mixed agonist–antagonist opioids.

Subjective Effects

The most thoroughly developed and most frequently used psychopharmacological technique for evaluating opioids in humans is assessment of subjective effects through questionnaires. The purpose of subjective effect indices is to provide qualitative and quantitative characterization of changes produced by test drugs in subjects' mood, feelings, perceptions, and symptoms. The five basic types of information most frequently collected in subjective effect questionnaires are: whether and/or how much the subject feels a drug effect; whether and/or how much the subject likes the drug effect; what symptoms are produced by the drug; what pharmacological class is the drug most like; and what mood effects does the drug produce. The questionnaires most commonly used to study opioids include the ARC Single-Dose Questionnaire, the Morphine–Benzedrine Group (MBG), Pentobarbital–Chloropromazine–Alcohol Group (PCAG), LSD scales of the Addiction Research Center Inventory (ARCI) (widely used as indices of "euphoria," "apathetic sedation," and "dysphoria," respectively), global drug effect scales (e.g., magnitudes of drug effect, liking of the drug, good and bad effects, and withdrawal sickness), adjective rating scales, and drug class identification scales (e.g., see refs. 8,21,44, and 48). The adjectives used have depended on the class of drugs being studied and their expected effects. In opioid studies, symptoms associated with opioid agonist effects (such as itching, nodding, and talkativeness), agonist–antagonist effects (such as floating, confused, and numb), and opioid abstinence (such as watery eyes, chills, and gooseflesh) have been used. To evaluate the type of drug they have received, subjects identify the pharmacological class of the test drug from a list of eight to ten choices. In most studies, subjective effect questionnaires are completed before drug administration to determine a baseline and then again at specified intervals after administration to determine the time course of effects.

The major recent change in subjective effects assessment has been their increased incorporation as concurrent measures in behavioral studies such as drug discrimination and self-administration. Use of subjective effects indices to predict abuse potential has been criticized because questionnaire responses are quite indirect predictors of reinforcing efficacy. Better understanding of the relationship between subjective effects and behavioral indices may improve our ability to interpret subjective effect data as they relate to abuse liability assessment.

Drug Discrimination

In drug discrimination studies, subjects are typically trained to emit one response in the presence of a training drug and to emit an alternate response in the absence of the training drug. The method has been used extensively in nonhumans to study the pharmacology of opioids and to assess abuse liability of new drugs. In the last decade, investigators have adapted these paradigms to study opioid pharmacology in humans (for review see ref. 43). These studies have combined the collection of behavioral drug discrimination data with the traditional subjective effect questionnaire data. Drug discrimination itself provides a novel procedure for characterizing human opioid pharmacology, and concomitant collection of subjective effect data permits study of the relationship between subjective and discriminative effects of opioids.

Human opioid drug discrimination studies have used either two or three training drugs, and they have used participants with extensive histories of opioid abuse (43). In the discrimination training phase, each training drug administration is paired with an identifying label (frequently an arbitrary letter code). An extrinsic reinforcer (money) is provided contingent on correct discrimination performance. Acquisition of the discrimination is verified by re-exposing subjects to the training drugs and determining whether their correct drug labels (letter codes) are identified. Generalization testing sessions are then conducted to assess the dose–effect function of one or more test drugs. Drugs are not identifiable by appearance or volume and are given under double-blind conditions. In addition to discrimination responses, subjective, physiological, and psychomotor task performance measures can be collected.

A series of studies has been conducted in opioid abusers trained to discriminate between intramuscularly administered placebo and various opioid agonists and mixed agonist–antagonists (45,50,53; Preston et al., submitted). The training conditions (e.g., number and types of training drugs and dependence level of the subjects) were systematically varied across the studies, and they included two-choice (hydromorphone/placebo) and three-choice (saline/hydromorphone/pentazocine or saline/hydromorphone/butorphanol) discriminations in nonphysiologically dependent opioid abusers and three-choice saline/hydromorphone/naloxone discriminations in opioid-dependent subjects. Hydromorphone, pentazocine, butorphanol, nalbuphine, and buprenorphine dose–response curves were determined in each study to assess cross-generalization. One significant finding was that opioid abusers had no difficulty discriminating between a mu agonist and a mixed agonist–antagonist with both mu and kappa agonist activity (pentazocine or butorphanol). Not unexpectedly, methadone-dependent subjects had no difficulty discriminating an opioid agonist from an opioid antagonist.

A second major finding was that the results of generalization tests of the agonist–antagonists were highly dependent on the specific discriminations that had been trained. For example, under some conditions (nondependent subjects in a two-choice hydromorphone/placebo discrimination), hydromorphone, pentazocine, butorphanol, nalbuphine, and buprenorphine were all discriminated as hydromorphone-like at one or more doses (53); in contrast, under other conditions (a three-choice saline–hydromorphone–pentazocine discrimination), none of the mixed agonist-antagonists were discriminated as hydromorphone-like (45). It was concluded that three-choice discrimination procedures permit a more precise and refined differentiation among test drugs than do two-choice procedures. Selection of specific discrimination training procedures permits one to focus the experimental question and to assess and detect differences among drugs which also possess similarities. Thus, drug discrimination can be a valuable tool for studying the agonist–antagonist opioids, but assessment under multiple procedural/training conditions may be necessary to characterize fully their pharmacological properties.

Generalization across routes of administration and across drug class has been evaluated by testing oral doses in volunteers trained to discriminate among intramuscular saline, hydromorphone, and pentazocine (4). Results are consistent with the view that drug discrimination performance is controlled by the central pharmacological actions of study drugs and not by peripheral effects that might be related to the route of administration.

Studies of opioids have provided extensive data on the covariation of subjective and discriminative responses over a range of test doses (43). These studies suggest a rather strong relationship between subjective and discriminative effects. Opioids discriminated as similar had similar subjective profiles, and opioids with similar subjective profiles were discriminated as similar. Novel drugs had subjective effects that overlapped with those of the drugs to which they were discriminated as similar. Thus, these human data are supportive of the view that drug discrimination effects in animals may be analogous to subjective effects in human. However, the data also make clear that there are circumstances where subjective and discriminative effects may diverge. This phenomenon clearly supports the value of using multiple methods for assessing abuse liability and the value of incorporating subjective effect assessment as a concurrent and complementary procedure along with other methods.

The utility of human drug discrimination procedures in abuse liability assessment has been reviewed by Preston (42). Drug stimulus similarity, like subjective effect profile, is an indirect predictor of relative reinforcing efficacy and is not a direct index of abuse liability. However, if appropriate discriminations are trained and if appropriate reference drugs of known abuse liability are included, drug discrimination methods can yield quite specific information about relative abuse potential. This is a method that should prove quite valuable in assessing new opioids as they are developed.

Drug Self-Administration

There has been extensive development and use of drug self-administration technology as a tool for assessing opioid abuse liability in animals. In contrast, there has been little opioid self-administration research in humans. This now promises to be a fertile new research area.

Studies in the 1970s and 1980s showed that opioid addicts would complete operant work requirements to obtain doses of opioids (38). This self-administration methodology was used in the human laboratory to document the therapeutic efficacy of methadone, naltrexone, and buprenorphine by showing that pretreatment with these agonists, antagonists, and agonist–antagonists decreased the self-administration of opioid agonists (27,37,38).

More recently, Lamb et al. (30) examined the self-administration of different doses of morphine and concurrently evaluated subjective effects following drug administration. Subjects could respond on a fixed-ratio, second-order operant schedule to obtain a single daily intramuscular injection of placebo or morphine (3.75, 7.5, 15, and 30 mg). Placebo was not self-administered, but all active doses were self-administered by the majority of subjects. Interestingly, there was a dissociation between self-administration behavior and subjective report of drug effects; only the highest morphine dose reliably increased scores on subjective effects scales. These data suggest that self-administration procedures may be more sensitive indices of abuse liability than are the traditional subjective effects procedures.

The drug self-administration method provides direct assessment of drug-taking behavior and drug reinforcement, and thus it has substantial face validity as an index of abuse liability. Self-administration methods for opioid abuse liability assessment have not yet received sufficient use to develop the necessary validation of their predictive accuracy. Much work is needed to understand the relationships among self-administration, discriminative stimuli, and subjective effects and to develop practical self-administration methods that reliably predict abuse liability.

Far more opioid self-administration work has been done in recent years in the context of patient-controlled analgesia (19). This procedure permits patients with clinical pain to control (within limits) the frequency and timing of opioid analgesic administration. Safe and effective use of patient-controlled analgesia depends on knowledge of dose effects, onset latency, potency, intrinsic activity, duration of action, elimination rate, and relative receptor activity. These same parameters are critical to the understanding of opioid self-administration in the drug abuse context. Thus, increased interactions between researchers across these two areas may significantly enhance our knowledge of the principles of human opioid self-administration (see Chapter 66, *this volume*, for related discussion.)

Physical Dependence, Tolerance, and Abstinence

Opioids are well known for their capacity to produce tolerance and physical dependence, and these are important dimensions to assess in characterizing the complete abuse liability profile of any opioid. Methods for studying the development of tolerance and physical de-

pendence and their physiological and behavioral consequences in humans have been reviewed by Jasinski (21).

Effects of Repeated Administration of Opioid Agonists

Historically, the method used at the ARC (the direct addiction procedure) involved administration of increasing doses of a test drug to subjects over time until a predetermined maximum stabilization level was reached, then testing with known agonists and/or known antagonists, and then examining the effects of abrupt discontinuation of the maintenance test drug. The dose escalation period provided information about tolerance development, as did the response to supplemental opioid challenges during the maintenance period. Antagonist challenges (the abstinence precipitation procedure) and abrupt substitution of placebo for the maintenance test drug (the spontaneous abstinence procedure) provided information about physical dependence and about the nature of the abstinence syndrome. Both physiological and subjective effect data were assessed throughout these studies. In a modification of the direct addiction procedures, the ability of test drugs to substitute for morphine and suppress abstinence in morphine-dependent humans was tested (the substitution procedure). The series of direct addiction and substitution studies conducted at the ARC from the 1930s through the 1970s was critical to establishing the existence and character of opioid physical dependence and the abstinence syndrome, defining differences between the effects of chronic administration and abstinence syndromes of mu and kappa agonists, and determining effective treatments of abstinence signs and symptoms. These studies were also integral parts of the abuse liability assessment of novel opioids. For a variety of reasons, direct addiction studies are no longer being conducted.

Studies of opioid physical dependence, tolerance, and abstinence in humans have continued in the last decade by combining methods adapted and modified from the ARC direct addiction and substitution procedures with newer research techniques. For example, to evaluate the cross-tolerance to the subjective and physiological effects of supplemental opioids conferred by methadone maintenance treatment, McCaul et al. (36) compared the acute subjective and physiological effects of challenge doses of intravenously administered hydromorphone in methadone-maintained and in non-physiologically dependent opioid abusers. The primary innovation has been to use volunteer methadone maintenance patients or morphine-maintained opioid abusers as the dependent subjects and to conduct substitution studies assessing whether test drugs suppress the opioid abstinence syndrome. Thus, human laboratory studies of physical dependence show good promise for screening of potential treatment agents and for selection of doses for clinical trials of new pharmacological treatments of opioid abuse. (See Chapter 64, *this volume,* for related discussion.)

Effects of Opioid Antagonists

Administration of an opioid antagonist to individuals who are physically dependent on opioids produces the signs and symptoms of abstinence. Methods for quantifying opiate abstinence precipitated by antagonists were developed at the ARC (for review see ref. 21). The methods involve administering placebo and one or more antagonists or agonist/antagonists to subjects physically dependent on an opioid agonist such as morphine or methadone. Although the opiate abstinence scoring system developed by Himmelsbach still serves as a basis for the quantifying physiological abstinence signs, subjective measures of abstinence are now included in most studies (51). Precipitation studies can sometimes be complicated by the fact that precipitation of abstinence, while not life-threatening, does involve some physical discomfort to opioid dependent volunteers. Care must be used in designing these studies to minimize this discomfort.

Opioid antagonists have proven to be useful tools in human opioid pharmacology research. Antagonist-precipitated abstinence is similar in profile, but more rapid in onset and shorter in duration than that produced by abrupt discontinuation of the maintenance agonist. Naloxone is the most frequently used antagonist in abstinence precipitation studies. At doses of 0.1–0.2 mg i.m., naloxone produces dose-related abstinence-like effects that last 30–60 min (48,49). Naloxone-precipitated abstinence has been shown to serve as a discriminative stimulus in opioid-dependent humans (50). In studies comparing the antagonist activity of the agonist-antagonist opioids, butorphanol, nalbuphine, and pentazocine were shown to precipitate abstinence syndromes that differed somewhat from that produced by naloxone (48,49,62). Information about the antagonist potency of these drugs may be used in conjunction with analgesic potency to calculate an antagonist/analgesic potency ratio (the dose precipitating abstinence divided by the analgesic dose). This ratio provides a useful index for comparing among the agonist–antagonists and provides a basis for predicting abuse liability.

Acute Physical Dependence

While the phenomenon of physical dependence following chronic administration of opioids is well established, the number of repeated administrations necessary to produce physical dependence is less clear. Evidence now indicates that the physical dependence process begins after even a single opioid agonist administration. Acute physical dependence refers to the abstinence syndrome precipitated by the administration of an opioid antagonist after either a single dose or a short-term administration of an opioid agonist. Acute physical dependence has been demonstrated in humans as well as in mice, rats, dogs, and monkeys (7). The procedure consists of giving a single administration of an opioid to a nondependent subject, followed usually several hours later by administration of an opioid antagonist, and then measuring the response. The measures used to assess the precipitated abstinence are the same as those used in the studies of opioid antagonist administration in subjects receiving chronic administration of opioid agonists.

The doses of agonist used in the paradigm are at those used therapeutically for analgesia and above—for example, 10–30 mg of morphine (7,17). The doses of opioid antagonist necessary to precipitate abstinence after a single morphine dose are larger than those used to precipitate abstinence after chronic agonist treatment—for example, 10 mg versus 0.2 mg of naloxone, respectively. The signs and symptoms of abstinence produced in the acute physical dependence paradigm are generally similar to those of opioid antagonist-precipitated abstinence in chronically treated subjects, though they tend to be milder. The intensity of the response is directly related to the dose of morphine pretreatment (7) and directly related to dose of the antagonist (17). Precipitated abstinence can be produced as early as 45 min and as late as 24 hr after a single intramuscular injection of morphine (18,28). Naloxone-precipitated abstinence may be observed even longer (up to 96 hr) after a single dose of the longer-acting agonist methadone, and at much lower doses (approximately 1 mg) of naloxone (60); this suggests that the physical dependence produced by methadone is more intense and protracted than that produced by comparable doses of morphine. Additional studies are needed to understand fully the relationship between duration of agonist action and the time course of acute physical dependence, but it appears that the acute physical dependence paradigm may be quite useful as an index of physical dependence capacity.

Studies in Opioid Abusers

The discovery of the agonist–antagonist opioids was a major advance in the development of analgesics with low abuse potential and as tools for pharmacological research, leading to the postulated existence of multiple opioid receptors, the description of the functional consequences of activation of the mu and kappa receptors, and descriptions of the mu and kappa abstinence syndromes (35). A number of agonist–antagonists have been marketed as analgesics and have been extensively studied or have recently become available for therapeutic use. Human behavioral pharmacology abuse liability assessment results and the pharmacological activities of these drugs are summarized in Table 1 and described below.

Pentazocine

Pentazocine is an agonist–antagonist with both mu and non-mu agonist activity in humans. It produces both

---

1736 / OPIOIDS

TABLE 1. *Summary of human behavioral pharmacology abuse liability assessment*

	Mu agonists	Mixed agonist–antagonists				Opioid antagonists
	Morphine and hydromorphone	Buprenorphine	Pentazocine	Butorphanol	Nalbuphine	Naloxone and naltrexone
Subjective and discriminative effects						
Nondependent subjects						
Morphine-like	Yes	Yes	Yes	Some	Some	No
Non-morphine-like[a]	No	No	Yes	Yes	Yes	No
Physically dependent subjects						
Morphine-like	Attenuated	Attenuated	No	No	No	No
Withdrawal-like	No	Variable	Yes	Yes	Yes	Yes
Antagonist activity						
Precipitates withdrawal	No	Variable	Yes	Yes	Yes	Yes
Antagonist/analgesic ratio	Infinite	>26.67	2	0.75	0.3	0
Physical dependence capacity						
Suppresses abstinence	Yes	Yes	No	No	No	No
Abstinence syndrome						
Morphine-like	Yes	Mild	Yes	Yes	Yes	None
Non-morphine-like[a]	No	No	Yes	Yes	Yes	None
Putative receptor activity						
Mu	Agonist	Partial Ag	Partial Ag	Partial Ag	Partial Ag	Antagonist
Kappa	None	Antagonist	Ag/partial Ag	Ag/partial Ag	Ag/partial Ag	Antagonist
Evidence of abuse	Yes	Yes	Yes, limited	Infrequent	No	No

[a] Possibly kappa agonist effects.

morphine-like and non-morphine-like subjective effects, with the non-morphine-like effects predominantly occurring at higher doses (25,46). Naltrexone, which is more potent in blocking mu-receptor activity than kappa-receptor activity, antagonized the effects of hydromorphone to a greater extent that those of pentazocine, supporting the suggestion that pentazocine has kappa agonist activity (44). Drug discrimination studies have also shown a mixed mu and non-mu profile of effects. Pentazocine was discriminated as hydromorphone-like in subjects trained in a two-choice discrimination between the effects of intramuscularly administered saline and hydromorphone (53). On the other hand, the stimulus effects of pentazocine were sufficiently different from those of hydromorphone to permit training of a reliable discrimination in subjects trained in a three-choice saline–hydromorphone–pentazocine discrimination (4,45). Butorphanol, but not nalbuphine or buprenorphine, produced pentazocine-appropriate responding. Repeated administration of pentazocine produces physical dependence characterized by both mu and non-mu characteristics during chronic treatment and on abrupt abstinence (25). Pentazocine appears to have significant antagonist effects as well. Pentazocine precipitated abstinence in morphine-dependent and methadone-dependent subjects at doses of 60–120 mg i.m. (25,62), and although tested under a number of morphine dose levels, pentazocine did not suppress abstinence in morphine-dependent subjects (25).

In spite of its significant non-mu-like subjective effects and antagonist activity, an outbreak of pentazocine abuse occurred in the mid 1970s in the form of "T's and Blues," intravenously injected combinations with the antihistamine tripelennamine (55). A laboratory study showed that combinations of pentazocine and tripelenamine were identified as opioids more frequently and produced greater euphoria and liking and less dysphoria than either drug alone (31). After pentazocine was moved from unscheduled status to control under Schedule IV of the Controlled Substances Act, and a pentazocine 50 mg/naloxone 0.5 mg combination product was marketed in place of the original pentazocine 50 mg tablets, the incidence of pentazocine abuse significantly declined.

Butorphanol

Butorphanol, like the other marketed agonist–antagonists, has similarities to mu agonists as well as differences. Both morphine and butorphanol increased subjects' liking scale scores and increased opiate symptom scale scores, but butorphanol produced other, non-morphine-like effects as well (51). The subjective effects of butorphanol were more similar to those of the agonist–antagonists cyclazocine and pentazocine. Drug discrimination studies have also shown a mixed mu and non-mu profile of effects. Butorphanol was discriminated as hydromorphone-like in nondependent subjects trained in a two-choice saline–hydromorphone discrimination (52). In a three-choice saline–hydromorphone–pentazocine discrimination, butorphanol produced pentazocine-appropriate responding (45). In opioid-dependent individuals, butorphanol acts primarily as an antagonist. The results of precipitation studies with butorphanol have yielded inconsistent results. Butorphanol precipitated abstinence in methadone-dependent subjects (48) but failed to precipitate abstinence in morphine-dependent subjects (51). Interestingly, although butorphanol produced effects generally similar to the effects of naloxone, there were some differences in the abstinence syndromes precipitated by naloxone versus butorphanol. The stimulus properties of butorphanol, however, are clearly abstinence-like in opioid-dependent individuals; butorphanol produced naloxone-appropriate responding in methadone-maintained subjects trained in a three-choice (saline–hydromorphone–naloxone) discrimination (50). Butorphanol also failed to substitute for morphine and to suppress abstinence in humans maintained on a relatively low dose of morphine (60 mg/day) (51). Physical dependence on butorphanol was both morphine-like and nalorphine-like during chronic dosing and more similar to cyclazocine than to morphine after abrupt abstinence (51). Subjects requested morphine for relief of their symptoms; however, when offered butorphanol or a sedative, subjects refused the butorphanol and, instead, chose the sedative.

Butorphanol was recently marketed in a novel transnasal formulation. A study comparing the effects of butorphanol given by the transnasal and intramuscular routes showed that, while the overall profile of effects were not substantially different, transnasal butorphanol had a slower onset and a decreased potency relative to i.m. butorphanol (53). Dysphoric sedation was prominent after administration of 4 mg by the i.m., but not the transnasal, route. The results suggest that there is a ceiling on the effects of transnasal butorphanol, perhaps due to limited absorption.

Nalbuphine

Nalbuphine produced (a) a profile of subjective effects different from that of the prototypic agonist morphine and (b) a very shallow dose–response curve on acute administration (24). In drug discrimination studies, nalbuphine was discriminated as hydromorphone-like in subjects trained in a two-choice discrimination between i.m. saline and hydromorphone (52). When tested in non-physically dependent subjects trained in a three-choice saline–hydromorphone–pentazocine discrimination, nalbuphine was consistently discriminated from placebo but produced mixed hydromorphone- and pentazocine-appropriate responding, not consistently discriminated as either (50).

Nalbuphine has strong antagonist activity relative to its agonist activity. It precipitated abstinence in morphine-dependent subjects at doses of 6 and 12 mg/70 kg (24) and in doses of 2 mg/70 kg and higher in methadone-dependent subjects (49,50), doses less than its therapeutic dose for analgesia (10 mg). In opioid-dependent humans trained in a three-choice drug discrimination between i.m. saline, hydromorphone, and naloxone, nalbuphine was discriminated as naloxone-like (50). The ability of nalbuphine to substitute for morphine and suppress abstinence in humans has been tested in subjects maintained on morphine 30 mg/day using the 24-hr substitution technique (Jasinski, personal communication). Nalbuphine failed to suppress the intensity of the abstinence syndrome. In direct addiction studies, nalbuphine administered up to 51 days in increasing doses to 147–240 mg/day produced morphine-like effects at low doses but produced disturbing side effects at higher doses (24). Abrupt abstinence from nalbuphine was followed by a mild abstinence syndrome that was characterized by both morphine-like and nalorphine-like signs and symptoms. Subjects requested opiates for relief from the abstinence.

Buprenorphine

Buprenorphine, administered parenterally in doses to 2 mg, produced morphine-like effects including increases in drug liking, opiate symptoms, and MBG scale scores (26). Administered sublingually to doses of 32 mg, buprenorphine produced long-lasting, morphine-like subjective effects, without serious side effects (65). In drug discrimination studies, buprenorphine was discriminated as hydromorphone-like in nondependent subjects trained to discriminate saline and hydromorphone. In nondependent subjects trained to discriminate among saline, hydromorphone, and pentazocine, there was not complete generalization to either hydromorphone or pentazocine at any dose tested, though buprenorphine was clearly discriminated from saline (45). Buprenorphine does not have strong antagonist effects. In subjects maintained on relatively low doses of methadone, sublingual buprenorphine to 4 mg (22) and intramuscular buprenorphine to 8 mg (61) failed to produce naloxone-like subjective effects, though reports from circumstances of higher methadone maintenance doses indicate that under some conditions buprenorphine does precipitate abstinence-like effects in dependent patients. The physical dependence capacity of buprenorphine was tested in a direct addiction study in doses increasing to 8 mg over 45–52 days (26). Buprenorphine produced morphine-like effects including liking of the drug effect and was identified as "dope." On abrupt withdrawal the intensity of abstinence from buprenorphine was greater than that produced by placebo but milder than that produced by morphine, cyclazocine, nalorphine, nalbuphine, pentazocine, butorphanol, profadol, and propiram. Overall, buprenorphine appears to have the most morphine-like effects of the marketed agonist–antagonists. Buprenorphine–naloxone combinations have been studied as part of an effort to develop a buprenorphine formulation with low abuse potential. Buprenorphine administered to methadone-maintained subjects in combination with naloxone slightly attenuated the antagonist effects of naloxone (47). Concurrent naloxone administration attenuated the opioid effects of buprenorphine in nondependent subjects (67).

Studies in Nonabusers

The majority of human behavioral pharmacology research on opioids has been conducted in subjects with histories of opioid abuse. Reports of experienced opioid abusers have been argued to be the best predictors of abuse liability because abusers have histories of self-administration of opioids and presumably are sensitive to their positive mood effects. Until recently, there has been only limited information on the subjective effects of opioids in individuals without substance abuse. Zacny et al. (68–71) have recently begun to publish a series of studies in which opioids have been tested in healthy, nonabuser volunteers using the methods developed for assessing abuse potential. Intravenously administered morphine, fentanyl, meperidine, and dezocine have been fairly consistent in producing constellations of effects in nonabuser volunteers that are similar to those produced in experienced opioid abusers.

DRUG ABUSE TREATMENT MEDICATIONS

A great deal of research attention in recent years has been directed toward the goal of developing new and/or improved pharmacological treatments for drug abuse. Consequently, there have been significant advances in pharmacotherapies for opioid abuse and dependence.

Short-Term Pharmacotherapies

The purposes of short-term pharmacotherapies for opioid abuse or dependence are as follows: (a) live-saving reversal of acute opioid intoxication and respiratory depression and (b) palliative care to ease the process of opioid withdrawal and detoxification and to suppress the opioid abstinence syndrome. Naloxone remains the treatment of choice for the first of these. Described below are recent developments in opioid detoxification.

Clonidine-Assisted Detoxification

Clonidine is an alpha-2-adrenergic agonist, marketed for treatment of hypertension, which has been shown to suppress many of the signs and symptoms of opioid withdrawal. Research with clonidine has been quite informative concerning the neurobiological mechanisms involved in opioid physical dependence and withdrawal. Clonidine acts via autoreceptors in the locus coeruleus to suppress adrenergic hyperactivity there that is involved in the expression of the opioid withdrawal syndrome. Its efficacy is limited primarily to suppression of autonomic signs and symptoms such as sweating, diarrhea, intestinal cramping, and nausea; it is relatively ineffective in suppressing insomnia, muscle aches, and drug craving (23). Clonidine-assisted opioid detoxification involves abrupt cessation of opioids and initiation of clonidine; there is greater symptomatic discomfort than with gradual opioid dose reduction, but much less than with abrupt opioid withdrawal alone. Clonidine's major advantage is that it is a non-narcotic and has low abuse liability; thus, it is especially attractive in settings where diversion and abuse might be of concern or where the legal restrictions on narcotic use present a problem.

Antagonist-Assisted Rapid Detoxification

Opioid detoxification may be hastened and the duration of the opioid abstinence syndrome shortened by administration of opioid antagonists (such as naloxone or naltrexone), which displace the opioid agonist from the receptor. The precise mechanisms involved in the shortening of the abstinence syndrome are not yet known and require further research. Antagonist administration and clonidine administration have been combined to provide a rapid inpatient detoxification procedure that results in patients' being converted, in approximately 4 days, from opioid physical dependence to maintenance on full blocking doses of narcotic antagonist (11). It has been suggested that this procedure might be further improved by first switching patients to maintenance on the partial agonist buprenorphine, because the abstinence syndrome following buprenorphine discontinuation is less intense than that following discontinuation of pure agonists such as heroin, morphine, or methadone (58).

Longer-Term Pharmacotherapies

The purpose of longer-term pharmacotherapy of opioid abuse and dependence is to reduce or eliminate illicit opioid self-administration. Medications achieve this goal by reducing or eliminating the reinforcing effects of illicit opioids. This is done via mechanisms of either opioid tolerance and substitution or opioid receptor blockade. Since the mid-1960s the primary medication for long-term treatment of opioid abuse has been methadone. The available pharmacotherapeutic options are now increasing. New medications have been made available for clinical use or are under development and expected to be available in the near future. At the same time, systematic research has provided new guidance about how to use these and the previously available treatment medications most effectively. Relevant characteristics of the major treatment medications are summarized in Table 2.

LAAM

In July 1993, levo-alpha-acetyl-methadol (LAAM) was approved by the U.S. Food and Drug Administration for marketing as a maintenance treatment for opioid dependence. Though the research supporting this approval was spread over the preceding four decades, it is worthwhile to review LAAM's characteristics here because its clinical introduction may significantly alter the practice of opioid maintenance treatment of addicts.

LAAM, also sometimes called *levomethadyl acetate,* is a synthetic mu-opioid agonist structurally related to methadone. Its synthesis derived from efforts to develop opioid analgesics of reduced abuse liability (13). It produces typical opioid mu-agonist effects, including analgesia, respiratory depression, miosis, decreased gastrointestinal motility, euphoria, and, in opioid-dependent subjects, suppression of the opioid abstinence syndrome. It produces or sustains opioid physical dependence, and its discontinuation is followed by the characteristic opioid abstinence syndrome, consisting of rhinnorhea, lacrimation, gooseflesh, mydriasis, restlessness, muscle aches, and drug-seeking behavior. After equivalent maintenance doses the abstinence syndromes following LAAM and methadone are of similar intensity and duration, though that following LAAM has a somewhat slower onset (14,57). Its therapeutic efficacy is through the mechanism of opioid tolerance and substitution.

The important features of LAAM that led to its consideration and development as a maintenance treatment for opioid dependence are its good oral bioavailability, its slow onset and long duration of action, and its relatively low parenteral abuse liability (20). From a treatment perspective, LAAM is a pharmacokinetically complex drug. This pharmacokinetic complexity likely accounts for many of its desirable features, but also introduces a need for special cautions. LAAM is metabolized to two active metabolites, nor-LAAM and di-nor-LAAM, both of which are more potent than LAAM itself and both of which have long half-lives (9). Following oral administration, LAAM's opioid effects appear at about 90 min, with peak effect approximately 4 hr post dosing; in contrast, following parenteral administration the onset of LAAM's opioid effects is delayed 4–6 hr and the effects gradually increase over 12–16 hr (10). This difference in onset as a function of route of administration is likely due to first-pass inactivation of LAAM and gradual accumulation of active metabolites following parenteral administration. With chronic dosing there is gradual metabolite accumu-

lation such that 2–3 weeks are required for plasma level stabilization (10). One desirable consequence of this slow onset and gradual accumulation is that LAAM has relatively low abuse liability, especially by the parenteral route. A second, and less desirable, consequence is that the onset of therapeutic effects is similarly delayed. This less-than-optimal pharmacological substitution early in treatment may increase patient dropout and illicit heroin use during this time (56). Therefore, patients must be informed of LAAM's time course, urged to remain in treatment, and cautioned not to use illicit drugs during the initiation of LAAM therapy in a way that might additively interact with LAAM's delayed onset and produce overdose or other toxicity.

LAAM suppresses the opioid abstinence syndrome and prevents the effects of injected opioids for 72 hr, versus 24 hr for methadone (32). LAAM's long duration of action is its greatest benefit in comparison to methadone. LAAM is typically administered thrice weekly—for example, Monday, Wednesday, Friday, with the Friday dose being increased by 30–40% to compensate for the longer duration to be covered. Daily dosing with LAAM must be avoided because there is a risk of toxic—even fatal—accumulation of active metabolites. LAAM's longer duration of action, less frequent dosing, and less frequent clinic visits are a convenience to patients and to clinicians, may make treatment more comfortable and acceptable to patients, may decrease per-patient treatment costs (or increase treatment availability) and, because U.S. regulations prohibit LAAM take-home medication, may eliminate the problem of diversion and abuse of take-home medications which has sometimes been a problem in methadone treatment.

Numerous clinical trials have supported the conclusion that thrice-weekly LAAM treatment is equi-efficacious to daily methadone treatment (15,20,33,34,56,57,72). Outcome indices have included opioid-positive urines, withdrawal symptoms, and treatment retention. It appears that 1.2–1.3 mg LAAM thrice weekly is equivalent to 1 mg methadone daily. Thus, typical thrice-weekly LAAM maintenance doses might be 70/70/100 mg or 100/100/140 mg; these maintenance levels should be attained via 2–4 weeks of gradual dose escalation.

Because the majority of the clinical research supporting LAAM's safety and efficacy was one to two decades old at the time, prior to granting approval for general clinical use the Food and Drug Administration required the gathering and assessment of some modern experience. This so-called "labeling assessment study" was an open-label, multisite assessment of the ability of typical treatment clinics (i.e., not specialized research centers) to provide LAAM treatment guided simply by the instructions in the proposed LAAM package insert. No special problems were encountered in the treatment of females (who had been largely absent from older trials) or in the treatment of patients with substantial concurrent cocaine abuse (as

TABLE 2. Summary of characteristics of major treatment medications for opioid abuse and dependence

Drug	Action	Suppress w/d?[a]	Physical dependence?	Precipitate w/d?	Abuse liability?	Treatment retention	Risk of overdose	Dosing frequency	Route of administration	Take-homes?	Analgesic dose	Drug abuse treatment dose
Methadone	Agonist	Yes	Yes	No	Yes	Good	Yes	Every 24 hr	Oral	Yes	10–20 mg	60–80 mg/day
LAAM	Agonist	Yes	Yes	No	Modest	Good	Yes	Every 48–72 hr	Oral	No	NA[b]	70–120 mg × 3/week
Buprenorphine	Partial agonist	Yes	Mild	Variable	Yes	Good	No	Every 24–48 hr	Sublingual	No	0.3 mg	4–16 mg/day
Naltrexone	Antagonist	No	No	Yes	No	Poor	No	Every 24–72 hr	Oral	Yes	NA	50 mg/day

[a] w/d, opioid withdrawal or abstinence syndrome.
[b] NA, not applicable.

is common now). However, presumably because of symptomatic withdrawal complaints, a substantial proportion of patients received take-home methadone doses as a supplement to help them through the long 72-hr interdose interval. This raises some questions about how successful LAAM treatment will be in eliminating the need for take-home medications.

Buprenorphine

Buprenorphine is an opioid partial agonist exerting its primary pharmacological effects at the mu receptor and producing a morphine-like profile of effects (26). It is being very actively studied and developed as a treatment for opioid dependence. Over the range of 2–16 mg/day, s.l. buprenorphine produces dose-related attenuation of response to parenteral opioid challenge (6). Several double-blind outpatient clinical trials have reported buprenorphine to be equi-efficacious to methadone treatment (5,64). The primary features of buprenorphine that make it attractive as a potential treatment medication are its combination of agonist and antagonist actions, and consequent reduced abuse liability, its mild abstinence syndrome following discontinuation, and its improved safety profile relative to full opioid agonists.

As a partial agonist, buprenorphine has the potential to display either agonist-like or antagonist-like effects, depending upon the circumstances. In nondependent subjects buprenorphine acts as an opioid agonist (26); in moderately dependent subjects it may show neither agonist nor antagonist effects (61); and in more highly-dependent subjects it may display antagonist-like abstinence-precipitation effects (June et al., submitted). This potential for antagonist activity is seen as reducing the abuse potential of buprenorphine below that of full agonists; however, further study of this relationship is needed in order to clarify the conditions and parameters under which opioid-dependent patients may be treated with buprenorphine without precipitating the opioid abstinence syndrome. It is not clear at this time whether buprenorphine's clinical efficacy occurs via a mechanism of opioid tolerance and substitution or via opioid receptor blockade. It may be that different aspects of its efficacy derive from each of these mechanisms.

Several studies have reported that discontinuation of chronic buprenorphine treatment results in a minimal-to-mild opioid abstinence syndrome with onset 5–13 days after the last dose of buprenorphine (16,26). This suggests that buprenorphine may be of significant benefit in opioid detoxification treatment. It also suggests that patients may feel no need to attend treatment regularly. One study has reported buprenorphine attendance/retention rates to be equivalent to those with methadone (64). Another has reported inferior attendance/retention with buprenorphine, but this may have been due to an inadequate dose of buprenorphine (29).

Buprenorphine appears to have quite a favorable safety profile as a consequence of its being a partial agonist. Its limited ability to activate opioid mechanisms results in a ceiling on the magnitude of its effects, and it appears that this ceiling is below that of opioid toxicity. Buprenorphine challenges up to 32 mg s.l.—that is, up to 100 times the analgesic dose—were tolerated by nondependent opioid abusers without adverse effect other than prolonged sedation (65).

Buprenorphine has several potential disadvantages as a treatment medication. Chief among these are its low oral bioavailability and the fact that it has significant morphine-like abuse liability. Buprenorphine's oral bioavailability is about 15%. Because it is expensive to produce, this low oral availability has the consequence that buprenorphine is given sublingually—clinically a somewhat inconvenient procedure, but one with bioavailability of about 50%. This route requires that buprenorphine be provided in a water-soluble dosage form that has the potential for diversion to parenteral administration. Buprenorphine analgesic preparations have been diverted to parenteral abuse by heroin abusers where they have been marketed. This potential for parenteral diversion, combined with the large doses of buprenorphine used in addiction treatment, has resulted in buprenorphine treatment's being designed as a clinic-only procedure—that is, without the opportunity for take-home dosages.

The feasibility and efficacy of less-than-daily dosing with buprenorphine are under active investigation. The slow onset and mild characteristics of the opioid abstinence syndrome in buprenorphine-treated subjects suggest that less-than-daily dosing should be acceptable. However, one study of alternate-day dosing found corresponding fluctuations in symptom reports (16). Another study has reported that doubling the buprenorphine dose prior to omitting a daily dose results in stable symptom profiles across both days (1). These latter data suggest that for a partial agonist, with a ceiling on the magnitude of agonist effects, dosage level may function as a surrogate variable for controlling duration of action. It remains necessary, however, to replicate these data and to determine whether response to opioid challenge is similarly attenuated throughout the 2-day period.

Methadone

Approximately 90,000 patients are enrolled in methadone maintenance treatment in the United States. The primary pharmacological mechanism of methadone's clinical efficacy is opioid tolerance and substitution. In human laboratory studies methadone produces dose-related attenuation of opioid self-administration (27). Extensive clinical research documents both the efficacy of methadone treatment and the fact that nonpharmacological factors have a substantial influence on that efficacy

(3). Controlled double-blind studies have documented the dose-related efficacy of outpatient methadone treatment (63). At the same time, surveys of clinical practice have documented that a large proportion of clinics use dosages that are below optimal (12). Optimal dosage appears to be in the range of 60–100 mg/day orally.

Despite its demonstrated efficacy, methadone treatment is not without its limitations. Opioid abusers and society at large both have some ambivalence toward treatment with a medication that sustains substantial physical dependence. Some opioid abusers decline methadone treatment, and some communities restrict or prohibit methadone treatment availability. The abstinence syndrome following methadone discontinuation is somewhat less intense but of a longer duration than that following discontinuation of pharmacologically comparable doses of morphine or heroin. However, the relatively high doses of methadone required for optimal efficacy may result in a greater degree of physical dependence during methadone treatment than abusers are able to sustain with illicit drug supplies. These differences in time course and degree of dependence result in patients' reporting that methadone withdrawal is more difficult than heroin withdrawal.

Because methadone's duration of withdrawal suppression is approximately 24 hr, it must be administered daily. To reduce the frequency of required clinic visits, to make treatment more convenient for patients, and to support their employment and social rehabilitation, methadone take-home doses may be provided. Because methadone is an opioid agonist, these take-home doses have abuse potential and may be used inappropriately or diverted to the illicit market. This, of course, produces adverse community consequences for this treatment modality.

Despite its imperfections, methadone treatment remains unsurpassed in efficacy. It has good patient acceptability and treatment retention; it dramatically reduces both illicit opioid use and the criminal activity often associated with acquiring illicit opioids; it substantially improves employment rates, and it substantially improves morbidity and mortality (including HIV infection rates). Pharmacotherapeutic alternatives to methadone are being developed not because methadone is ineffective but because it is not universally delivered, not universally effective, and not universally appropriate. The goal of developing pharmacotherapeutic alternatives is to permit individualized treatment selection in response to the heterogeneous characteristics and goals of patients and of communities.

Naltrexone

Naltrexone is an instructive example of what can at times be a great disparity between pharmacological efficacy and clinical efficacy. As a long-acting, orally effective, opioid antagonist that blocks opioid receptors and prevents acute opioid effects as well as the development

of physical dependence, naltrexone would appear to be a pharmacological wonder drug ideally suited to addiction treatment; however, it has had relatively little clinical impact. This is due to poor patient compliance with use of the medication (40). A depot dosage form that would be effective for 1 month is under development and may partially overcome this compliance problem. At present, effective clinical use of naltrexone appears to be limited to highly motivated patients, or to circumstances where medication use can be supervised (66). Recent clinical trials indicating efficacy of naltrexone in alcoholism treatment suggest involvement of opioid mechanisms in alcohol abuse.

Compatibility with Concurrent Behavioral Therapies

Drug abuse pharmacotherapies are not in themselves sufficient to treat the wide range of personal and psychosocial problems that so frequently accompany opioid dependence. While pharmacotherapy alone may be beneficial, concurrent behavioral or psychosocial treatment is generally indicated. Different pharmacotherapies may have differing compatibilities with such concurrent psychosocial treatment. Thus, selection of pharmacotherapies should not be guided solely by the pharmacological aspects of treatment. For example, the frequency of required clinic attendance, which may co-vary implicitly with the selection of treatment medication, may itself be therapeutically important. Also, the potential benefit of using medication take-home privileges as contingent behavioral incentives to motivate therapeutic behavior change (59) will be absent with medications, such as LAAM, for which medication take-homes are prohibited. It is not yet known whether these differing compatibilities with concurrent behavioral therapies will have important clinical consequences. Behavioral treatments for drug abuse are discussed in the chapter by Stitzer and Higgins, in this volume.

CONCLUSIONS AND FUTURE DIRECTIONS

One of the implications to be drawn from this review is that drug abuse and drug abuse treatment involve the complex interplay of both pharmacological and environmental/behavioral factors. Pharmacology, though critical, is not sufficient to determine whether a drug will be abused, or whether a pharmacotherapy will be clinically useful. We are struck by the overwhelming importance of practical, logistical, and behavioral factors as determinants of the abuse and/or the clinical efficacy of opioids. Such factors as dosage form and route of administration play major roles, as do such factors as fads, patient compliance, and community standards. Basic and systematic clinical pharmacological information is an essential element in predicting abuse liability, in preventing drug abuse, and in developing effective therapies.

Areas in which we expect to see important advances in the next decade include the following:

1. *More refined data concerning the specific functions controlled by various opioid receptors.* In particular, we would expect advances in the recognition of subtypes of the mu, kappa, and delta opioid receptors, and possibly identification of other opioid receptor classes, and characterization of their behavioral and physiological functions. We would expect to see data characterizing the clinical effects of delta receptor ligands. And we would expect to see advances in our understanding of the interrelationships and interactions among different classes of opioid receptors. We would expect to see greater bridging of the gap between preclinical and clinical research, so that knowledge about the neurobiology of opioid receptors and about the pharmacology of endogenous ligands can be more fully tested and utilized in humans. In particular, we would expect to see advances in our understanding of how various opioidergic systems interact to control and to modulate the development and expression of physical dependence and the opioid abstinence syndrome, as well as the basic behavioral reinforcement process that is at the heart of drug abuse. Such data may lead to identification of new therapeutic uses for opioids—especially for mixed agonist–antagonists and drug combinations.

2. *More refined data concerning comparative efficacy of various pharmacotherapies.* Now that opioid dependence pharmacotherapy has moved beyond the "one therapy fits all" stage, it is essential that we develop comparative efficacy data and examine efficacy in relation to the heterogeneous characteristics of patients. This should include comparative assessment of the acceptability to patients of various treatments. We will likely see increasing recognition of the role of practical, logistical, and behavioral factors in determining the clinical efficacy of pharmacotherapies. This may involve the development of new dosage forms and the development of pharmacotherapies specifically for their compatibility with concurrent behavioral and psychosocial treatments.

ACKNOWLEDGMENTS

This work was supported, in part, by NIH grants K05-DA00050, R01-DA04089, R18-DA06120, R18-DA06165, and P50-DA05273 from the National Institute on Drug Abuse.

REFERENCES

1. Amass L, Bickel WK, Higgins ST, Badger GJ. Alternate-day dosing during buprenorphine. *Life Sci* 1994;54:1215–1228.
2. *Annotated Bibliography of Papers From the Addiction Research Center 1935–1975.* National Institute on Drug Abuse, Rockville, Maryland. Washington, DC: U.S. Department of Health, Education, and Welfare, 1978, ADM 77-435.
3. Ball JC, Ross A. *The effectiveness of methadone treatment.* New York: Springer-Verlag, 1991.
4. Bickel WK, Bigelow GE, Preston KL, Liebson IA. Opioid drug discrimination in humans: stability, specificity, and relation to self-reported drug effect. *J Pharmacol Exp Ther* 1989;251:1053–1063.
5. Bickel WK, Stitzer ML, Bigelow GE, Liebson IA, Jasinski DR, Johnson RE. A clinical trial of buprenorphine: comparison with methadone in the detoxification of heroin addicts. *J Clin Pharmacol Ther* 1988;43:72–78.
6. Bickel WK, Stitzer ML, Bigelow GE, Liebson IA, Jasinski DR, Johnson RE. Buprenorphine: dose-related blockade of opioid challenge effects in opioid dependent humans. *J Pharmacol Exp Ther* 1988;247:47–53.
7. Bickel WK, Stitzer ML, Liebson IA, Bigelow GE. Acute physical dependence in man: effects of naloxone after brief morphine exposure. *J Pharmacol Exp Ther* 1988;244:126–132.
8. Bigelow GE. Human drug abuse liability assessment: opioids and analgesics. *Br J Addict* 1991;86:1615–1628.
9. Billings RE, McMahon RE, Blake DA. l-Acetylmethadol (LAM) treatment of opiate dependence: plasma and urine levels of two pharmacologically active metabolites. *Life Sci* 1974;14:1437–1446.
10. Blaine JD, Thomas DB, Barnett G, Whysner JA, Renault PF. Levo-alpha acetylmethadol (LAAM): clinical utility and pharmaceutical development. In: Lowinson J, Ruiz P, eds. *Substance abuse—clinical problems and perspectives.* Baltimore: Williams & Wilkins, 1981:360–388.
11. Charney DS, Heninger GR, Kleber HD. The combined use of clonidine and naltrexone as a rapid, safe, and effective treatment of abrupt withdrawal from methadone. *Am J Psychiatry* 1986;143:831–837.
12. Cooper JR. Ineffective use of psychoactive drugs: methadone treatment is no exception. *JAMA* 1992;267:281–282.
13. Eddy NB, May EL, Mosetig E. Chemistry and pharmacology of the methadols and acetylmethadols. *J Organ Chem* 1952;17:321–326.
14. Fraser HF, Isbell H. Actions and addiction liabilities of alpha-acetylmethadols in man. *J Pharmacol Exp Ther* 1952;105:458–465.
15. Freedman RR, Czertko G. A comparison of thrice weekly LAAM and daily methadone in employed heroin addicts. *Drug Alcohol Depend* 1981;8:215–222.
16. Fudala PJ, Jaffe JE, Dax EM, Johnson RE. Use of buprenorphine in the treatment of opioid addiction II: physiologic and behavioral effects of daily and alternate-day administration and abrupt withdrawal. *J Clin Pharmacol Ther* 1990;47:525–534.
17. Heishman SJ, Stitzer ML, Bigelow GE, Liebson IA. Acute opioid physical dependence in postaddict humans: naloxone dose effects after brief morphine exposure. *J Pharmacol Exp Ther* 1989;248:127–134.
18. Heishman SJ, Stitzer ML, Bigelow GE, Liebson IA. Acute opioid physical dependence in humans: effect of varying the morphine-naloxone interval. *J Pharmacol Exp Ther* 1989;250:485–491.
19. Hill HF, Mather LW. Patient-controlled analgesia: pharmacokinetic and therapeutic considerations. *Clin Pharmacokinet* 1993;24:124–140.
20. Jaffe JH, Schuster CR, Smith BB, Blachley PH. Comparison of acetylmethadol and methadone in the treatment of long-term heroin users—a pilot study. *JAMA* 1970;211:1834–1836.
21. Jasinski DR. Assessment of the abuse potential of morphine-like drugs (methods used in man). In: Martin WR, ed. *Drug addiction I,* vol 45/1. Heidelberg: Springer-Verlag, 1977;197–258.
22. Jasinski DR, Henningfield JE, Hickey JE, Johnson RE. Progress report of the NIDA Addiction Research Center, Baltimore, Maryland, 1982. In: Harris LS, ed. *Problems of drug dependence, 1982.* National Institute on Drug Abuse Research Monograph 43. Washington, DC: DHHS, 1983;92–98 (ADM) 83-1264.
23. Jasinski DR, Johnson RE, Kocher TR. Clonidine in morphine withdrawal: differential effects on signs and symptoms. *Arch Gen Psychiatry* 1985;42:1063–1065.
24. Jasinski DR, Mansky PA. Evaluation of nalbuphine for abuse potential. *Clin Pharmacol Ther* 1972;13:78–90.
25. Jasinski DR, Martin WR, Hoeldtke RD. Effects of short- and long-

term administration of pentazocine in man. *Clin Pharmacol Ther* 1970;11:385–403.

26. Jasinski DR, Pevnick JS, Griffith JD. Human pharmacology and abuse potential of the analgesic buprenorphine. *Arch Gen Psychiatry* 1978;35:501–516.

27. Jones BE, Prada JA. Drug-seeking behavior during methadone maintenance. *Psychopharmacologia* 1975;41:7–10.

28. Kirby KC, Stitzer ML, Heishman SJ. Acute opioid physical dependence in humans: effect of varying the morphine–naloxone interval. *J Pharmacol Exp Ther* 1990;255:730–737.

29. Kosten TR, Schottenfeld R, Ziedonis D, Falcioni J. Buprenorphine versus methadone for opioid dependence. *J Nerv Ment Dis* 1993;181:358–364.

30. Lamb RJ, Preston KL, Henningfield JE, Schindler CW, Meisch RL, Davis F, Katz JL, Goldberg SR. The reinforcing and subjective effects of morphine in post-addicts: a dose–response study. *J Pharmacol Exp Ther* 1991;259:1165–1173.

31. Lange WR, Jasinski DR. The clinical pharmacology of pentazocine and tripelennamine (T's and Blues). *Adv Alcohol Subst Abuse* 1986;5:71–83.

32. Levine R, Zaks A, Fink M, Freedman AM. Levomethadyl acetate: prolonged duration of opioid effects, including cross tolerance to heroin, in man. *JAMA* 1973;226:316–318.

33. Ling W, Charuvastra VC, Kaim SC, Klett CJ. Methadyl acetate and methadone as maintenance treatments for heroin addicts: a Veterans Administration cooperative study. *Arch Gen Psychiatry* 1976; 33:709–720.

34. Ling W, Klett J, Gillis RD. A cooperative clinical study of methadyl acetate I. Three-times-a-week regimen. *Arch Gen Psychiatry* 1978;35:345–353.

35. Martin WR. Pharmacology of opioids. *Pharmacol Rev* 1983; 35:283–323.

36. McCaul ME, Stitzer ML, Bigelow GE, Liebson IA. Intravenous hydromorphone: effects in opiate-free and methadone maintenance subjects. In: Harris LS, ed. *Problems of drug dependence, 1982. Proceedings of the 44th annual scientific meeting.* The Committee on Problems of Drug Dependence, Inc. NIDA Research Monograph 43, ADM 83-1264. Washington, DC: Department of Health and Human Services, 1983;238–244.

37. Mello NK, Mendelson JH, Kuehnle JC, Sellers MS. Operant analysis of human heroin self-administration and the effects of naltrexone. *J Pharmacol Exp Ther* 1981;216:45–54.

38. Mello NK, Mendelson JH, Kuehnle JC. Buprenorphine effects on human heroin self-administration: an operant analysis. *J Pharmacol Exp Ther* 1982;223:30–39.

39. Musto DF. *The American disease: origins of narcotic control.* New Haven, CT: Yale University Press, 1973.

40. NRC Committee on Clinical Evaluation of Narcotic Antagonists. Clinical evaluation of naltrexone treatment of opiate-dependent individuals. *Arch Gen Psychiatry* 1978;35:335–340.

41. Porter J, Jick H. Addiction rare in patients treated with narcotics. *N Engl J Med* 1980;302:123.

42. Preston KL. Drug discrimination methods in abuse liability evaluation. *Br J Addiction* 1991;86:1587–1594.

43. Preston KL, Bigelow GE. Subjective and discriminative effects of drugs. *Behav Pharmacol* 1991;2:293–313.

44. Preston KL, Bigelow GE. Differential naltrexone antagonism of hydromorphone and pentazocine in human volunteers. *J Pharmacol Exp Ther* 1993;264:813–823.

45. Preston KL, Bigelow GE, Bickel WK, Liebson IA. Drug discrimination in human post-addicts: agonist-antagonist opioids. *J Pharmacol Exp Ther* 1989;250:184–196.

46. Preston KL, Bigelow GE, Liebson IA. Comparative evaluation of morphine, pentazocine and ciramadol in postaddicts. *J Pharmacol Exp Ther* 1987;240:900–910.

47. Preston KL, Bigelow GE, Liebson IA. Buprenorphine and naloxone alone and in combination in opioid-dependent humans. *Psychopharmacol* 1988;94:484–490.

48. Preston KL, Bigelow GE, Liebson IA. Butorphanol-precipitated withdrawal in opioid-dependent humans. *J Pharmacol Exp Ther* 1988;246:441–448.

49. Preston KL, Bigelow GE, Liebson IA. Antagonist effects of nalbuphine in opioid-dependent humans. *J Pharmacol Exp Ther* 1989;248:929–937.

50. Preston KL, Bigelow GE, Liebson IA. Discriminative stimulus properties of naloxone, butorphanol, nalbuphine, and hydromorphone in opioid-dependent humans. *Pharmacol Biochem Behav* 1990;37:511–522.

51. Preston KL, Jasinski DR. Abuse liability studies of opioid agonist–antagonists in humans. *Drug Alcohol Depend* 1991;28:49–82.

52. Preston KL, Liebson IA, Bigelow GE. Discrimination of agonist-antagonist opioids in humans trained on a two-choice saline-hydromorphone discrimination. *J Pharmacol Exp Ther* 1992;261: 62–71.

53. Preston KL, Sullivan JT, Testa MP, Jasinski DR. Psychopharmacology and abuse potential of transnasal butorphanol. *Drug Alcohol Depend* 1994;35:159–167.

54. Robins LN, Davis DH, Goodwin DW. Drug use by U.S. Army enlisted men in Vietnam: a follow-up on their return home. *Am J Epidemiol* 1974;99:235–249.

55. Senay EC. Clinical experience with T's and B's. *Drug Alcohol Depend* 1985;14:305–311.

56. Senay EC, Dorus W, Renault PF. Methadyl acetate and methadone. *JAMA* 1977;237:138–142.

57. Sorensen JL, Hargreaves WA, Weinberg JA. Withdrawal from heroin in three or six weeks—comparison of methadyl acetate and methadone. *Arch Gen Psychiatry* 1982;39:167–171.

58. Stine SM, Kosten TR. Use of drug combinations in treatment of opioid withdrawal. *J Clin Psychopharmacol* 1992;12:203–209.

59. Stitzer ML, Iguchi MY, Felch LJ. Contingent take-home incentive: effects on drug use of methadone maintenance patients. *J Consult Clin Psychol* 1992;60:927–934.

60. Stitzer ML, Wright C, Bigelow GE, June HL, Felch LJ. Time course of naloxone-precipitated withdrawal after acute methadone exposure in humans. *Drug Alcohol Depend* 1991;29:39–46.

61. Strain EC, Preston KL, Liebson IA, Bigelow GE. Effects of buprenorphine, hydromorphone, and naloxone in methadone-maintained volunteers. *J Pharmacol Exp Ther* 1992;261:985–993.

62. Strain EC, Preston KL, Liebson IA, Bigelow GE. Precipitated withdrawal by pentazocine in methadone-maintained volunteers. *J Pharmacol Exp Ther* 1993;267:624–634.

63. Strain EC, Stitzer ML, Liebson IA, Bigelow GE. Dose–response effects of methadone in the treatment of opioid dependence. *Ann Intern Med* 1993;119:23–27.

64. Strain EC, Stitzer ML, Liebson IA, Bigelow GE. A comparison of buprenorphine to methadone in the treatment of opioid dependence. *Am J Psychiatry* 1994;151:1025–1030.

65. Walsh SL, Preston KL, Stitzer ML, Cone E, Bigelow GE. Clinical pharmacology of buprenorphine: ceiling effects at high doses. *Clin Pharmacol Ther* 1994; (*in press*).

66. Washton AM, Pottash AC, Gold MS. Naltrexone in addicted business executives and physicians. *J Clin Psychiatry* 1984;45:39–41.

67. Weinhold LL, Preston KL, Farre M, Liebson IA, Bigelow GE. Buprenorphine alone and in combination with naloxone in nón-dependent humans. *Drug Alcohol Depend* 1992;30:263–274.

68. Zacny JP, Lichtor JL, Binstock W, Coalson DW, Cutter T, Flemming DC, Glosten B. Subjective, behavioral, and physiologic responses to intravenous meperidine in healthy volunteers. *Psychopharmacology* 1993;111:306–314.

69. Zacny JP, Lichtor JL, de Wit H. Subjective, behavioral, and physiologic responses to intravenous dezocine in healthy volunteers. *Anesth Analg* 1992;74:523–530.

70. Zacny JP, Lichtor JL, Flemming D, Coalson DW, Thompson WK. A dose–response analysis of the subjective, psychomotor, and physiologic effects of intravenous morphine in healthy volunteers. *J Pharmacol Exp Ther* 1994;268:1–9.

71. Zacny JP, Lichtor JL, Zaragoza JG, de Wit H. Effects of fasting on responses to intravenous fentanyl in healthy volunteers. *J Subst Abuse* 1992;4:197–207.

72. Zaks A, Fink M, Freedman AM. Levomethadyl in maintenance treatment of opiate dependence. *JAMA* 1972;220:811–813.

Psychopharmacology: The Fourth Generation of Progress, edited by Floyd E. Bloom and David J. Kupfer. Raven Press, Ltd., New York 1995.

CHAPTER 149

Pharmacotherapy of Alcoholism

Charles P. O'Brien, Michael J. Eckardt, and V. Markku I. Linnoila

Alcohol abuse and dependence (alcoholism) are serious health problems throughout the world. In the United States alone, excessive alcohol ingestion costs society more than about 150 billion dollars annually and results in over 40,000 deaths (75). Household surveys show the lifetime prevalence of alcohol abuse/dependence to be between 11% and 16%, amounting to over 30 million Americans afflicted with this disorder at some time in their lives (79). Until recently, medical approaches to the treatment of alcoholism focused on detoxification, while long-term rehabilitation was the province of drug-free, nonmedical programs based on the 12 Steps/Alcoholics Anonymous philosophy. Some patients have been treated successfully with this approach, but the overall rate of relapse is substantial even in the best drug-free programs. During the past decade, even therapists who have strongly opposed all medications as a "crutch" have begun to see the potential for an approach that combines psychotherapy and a medication that decreases the tendency to resume alcohol drinking. Psychopharmacologists have approached alcoholism by developing animal models of excessive alcohol drinking, analyzing the neurochemical factors involved in the reinforcement produced by alcohol and then testing medications that block or diminish this reinforcement. The implicit hypothesis has been that if a medication acceptable to patients could be found that reduces the urges to resume alcohol drinking or diminishes the rewarding effects of alcohol, the results of treatment could be improved. In this chapter we will describe some of the progress that has been made in classifying subcategories of alcoholics, in understanding the pharmacology of alcohol, and in testing new and possibly more effective treatments. (See Chapters 64, 66, 68, and 69, *this volume*, for related topics.)

CLASSIFICATION OF ALCOHOLICS

Various subpopulations of alcoholics have been defined by clinical researchers in recent years, the characteristics of which suggest specific pharmacotherapies. Tarter et al. (90) described primary alcoholics as experiencing more severe alcohol-related problems, and at an earlier age, than secondary alcoholics. Primary alcoholics were also described as more energized and disinhibited with a history of more childhood signs and symptoms suggestive of hyperactivity/minimal brain dysfunction. Cloninger (10) also described two subgroups of alcoholics. Type II was characterized as male-limited, with an onset of alcohol-related problems before the age of 25, and was often accompanied by aggressive behavior. Type I was characterized as milieu-limited, with an onset of alcohol-related problems after age 25. von Knorring et al. (99) classified alcoholics into either Type 1 or Type 2 using more clinically based criteria, with Type 2 differentially including impaired social or occupational functioning due to alcohol use before 25 years of age. Cloninger (10) has suggested that certain personality characteristics such as novelty seeking, harm avoidance, and reward dependence differentiate the subtypes in their interactions with the environment.

It is well documented that alcoholism is more prevalent in relatives of alcoholics than relatives of nonalcoholics (14). A significant heritability for an increased vulnerability to alcoholism is suggested by twin studies wherein the concordance of alcoholism in monozygotic twins is much higher than in dizygotic twins (48,78). Adoption studies also suggest a significant genetic component related to excessive consumption of alcoholic beverages (9,12,34). Although some genetic marker studies have

C. P. O'Brien: Department of Psychiatry, University of Pennsylvania, VAMC, Philadelphia, Pennsylvania 19104-6178.

M. J. Eckardt and V. M. I. Linnoila: National Institute on Alcohol Abuse and Alcoholism, National Institutes of Health, Bethesda, Maryland 20892.

proposed that certain biological characteristics may be associated with risk of excessive alcohol consumption, to date, none has been widely accepted (33). The complexity of gene–environment interactions is apparent in the observations that many people at risk for alcoholism do not develop the disorder and that several traits associated with alcoholism (length of sobriety, frequency of consumption, and quantity consumed) may be inherited separately (40,41).

It seems reasonable to postulate that the aggressive behavioral traits of Type 2 alcoholics described above could be produced by dysfunction in a neurotransmitter system such as serotonin and that this dysfunction might respond to appropriate pharmacotherapy. Similar alcoholics have been described as type B (4) and have been shown to respond better to coping skills treatment than to interactional therapy (52). In contrast, the behavioral presentations of Type 1 alcoholics suggest the potential for a different type of pharmacotherapy directed toward relieving chronic, low-grade anxiety and dysphoria. The Type I alcoholics are similar to those described as type A (4) who respond better to interactional therapy than to coping skills treatment (52).

BASIC PHARMACOLOGY OF ALCOHOL

Ethyl alcohol, called alcohol in this chapter, is pharmacologically nonspecific and of low potency. Pharmacokinetically, it is characterized by its relatively low first-pass metabolism and quick distribution throughout body water. Alcohol's elimination approximates zero-order kinetics, with most of the metabolism occurring in the liver. The pharmacological effects of alcohol that are of particular interest for understanding the mechanisms of its excessive ingestion are the reinforcing effects produced by this drug. *Reinforcement* refers to the effects produced by a drug that increase the likelihood that once having experienced these effects, the user will continue to take the drug. In general, these effects are interpreted by the user as pleasant or rewarding. It is likely that development of medications for the treatment of alcoholism would be aided by a better understanding of how alcohol affects behavior.

In intoxicating doses to humans, alcohol has major effects on ion channels and ion channel–receptor complexes. This is particularly true for the N-methyl-D-aspartate (NMDA) and GABA$_A$ receptors. Alcohol decreases the NMDA receptor agonist-induced cation currents (54) and enhances the GABA$_A$ receptor agonist-induced chloride flux (89). Alcohol's effects on these ion fluxes are thought to be particularly relevant to its intoxicating, amnesic and ataxic effects (64,88,89). These effects are reversed during alcohol withdrawal (38,65). The full meaning of the effects on ion fluxes is, however, not clear at this time. For instance, pigeons performing a drug dis-

crimination task are unable to distinguish between the effects of low doses of alcohol and the effects of the hallucinogenic drug phencyclidine (37). Phencyclidine is an irreversible inhibitor of the NMDA receptor, and it is a known substance of abuse in humans. Furthermore, the benzodiazepine receptor partial inverse agonist Ro 15-4513, which antagonizes alcohol-induced ataxia in rats (88), in low doses reduces alcohol consumption by alcohol-preferring rats (59). Lastly, no relationship has been established between alcohol's effects on these ion channels and its reinforcing effects in humans. Thus, most investigators at this time consider the effects on ion fluxes to be of doubtful importance to alcohol reinforcement.

Alcohol's reinforcing effects are currently thought to be primarily related to the release of dopamine and serotonin. In this context, particular attention has been focused on the effects of alcohol on extracellular dopamine concentrations in the nucleus accumbens. Alcohol administered either locally into the nucleus accumbens in anesthetized animals (104) or systemically in freely moving rats (16,45) increases extracellular dopamine concentrations in the nucleus accumbens. Alcohol also increases the firing rate of ventral tegmental dopamine neurons which project to the limbic forebrain including the nucleus accumbens (30,63). Although these effects are observed at alcohol concentrations which are relevant to human social alcohol consumption, the direct demonstration of alcohol increasing extracellular dopamine concentrations in the nucleus accumbens in humans is still lacking. During acute alcohol withdrawal, extracellular dopamine concentrations are reduced in the nucleus accumbens of rats. This finding has been suggested to explain alcohol-withdrawal-associated aversive effects in rodents and, by inference, dysphoric mood during alcohol withdrawal in humans (80). Certain behavioral experiments, however, appear to yield evidence that conflicts with the notion that extracellular dopamine concentrations in the nucleus accumbens are important for alcohol reinforcement. For example, destruction of the dopamine neurons projecting to the nucleus accumbens has been reported to be without effect on alcohol preference in rats (49). Moreover, low-dose dopamine-2 receptor blockers do not alter alcohol-induced place preference (15). Additional behavioral studies are clearly needed to settle this issue (see Chapters 66 and 68, *this volume*).

ENDOGENOUS OPIOIDS IN ALCOHOL REINFORCEMENT

Extensive behavioral evidence links the endogenous opioid system to alcohol reinforcement. Alcohol-preferring strains of mice and rats have increased basal β-endorphin levels in the pituitary gland and increased metenkephalin and β-endorphin in some brain areas relative to alcohol-nonpreferring rodents (31). The μ/δ opiate receptor antagonist naltrexone has been found to reduce alcohol drinking in monkeys (3,67) and in strains of rodents selected for alcohol preference (24,44,58,81) and to block the post-stress drinking of alcohol observed in rats (96,98). Low doses of morphine have been reported to stimulate alcohol drinking in rats (43), whereas higher doses suppress the drinking of alcohol (85).

Studies in human subjects support the concept that alcohol affects the endogenous opioid system. Gianoulakis et al. (31) (Fig. 1) studied nonalcoholic volunteers with a strong family history of alcoholism (high risk) and compared them to volunteers with no family history of alcoholism (low risk). Baseline levels of plasma β-endorphin were lower in the high-risk subjects, but a 0.5 g/kg test dose of alcohol produced a significantly greater rise in plasma β-endorphin in the high-risk group. In another study of plasma β-endorphin, alcoholics were found to

have depressed levels shortly after cessation of drinking, but these returned to normal range after 6 weeks of abstinence (95). Of course, plasma β-endorphin levels reflect pituitary rather than brain activity, but the results support an effect of alcohol on the endogenous opioid system.

These data taken together are consistent with the hypothesis that alcohol ingestion stimulates the release of endogenous opioids, which increases some of the rewarding effects of alcohol through opioid mechanisms. A small amount of morphine may produce alcohol drinking in rodents by priming this effect, but larger doses of an opioid drug would replace alcohol and thus reduce alcohol preference. Naltrexone, by blocking opiate receptors, would block this mechanism of reinforcement and thus reduce or eliminate alcohol preference. This hypothesis is supported by data from clinical trials of naltrexone in alcoholics reviewed below. Because opioid reinforcement has also been linked to limbic dopamine activation (101), the opioid effects on alcohol drinking behavior are consistent with the data implicating dopamine in the alcohol reinforcement mechanism.

CONDITIONED DOPAMINE INCREASE

There is a long history of experiments showing that the effects of alcohol and other abused drugs can be classically conditioned (76). Environmental cues may serve as conditioned stimuli, which may be important determinants of expected reinforcing effects of substances of abuse including alcohol (56). Recently, environmentally conditioned expectancy of alcohol in rats has been reported to decrease dopamine-2 receptor binding in the nucleus accumbens, suggesting a conditioned increase of endogenous dopamine that competes with the radioligand (93). In another study, rats who had received alcohol in a specific environment began to show increased dopamine levels in the nucleus accumbens measured by microdialysis when placed in the environment before receiving any alcohol (100). This finding, if replicated, may have implications for relapse in abstinent alcoholics. If environmental cues such as the sights and smells of people drinking can produce an alcohol-like effect in the brain, this could act to prime the dopamine system, similar to the effects of a small dose of morphine in rats, and produce urges to drink.

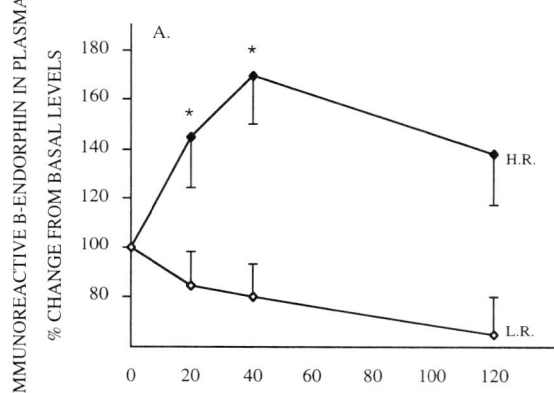

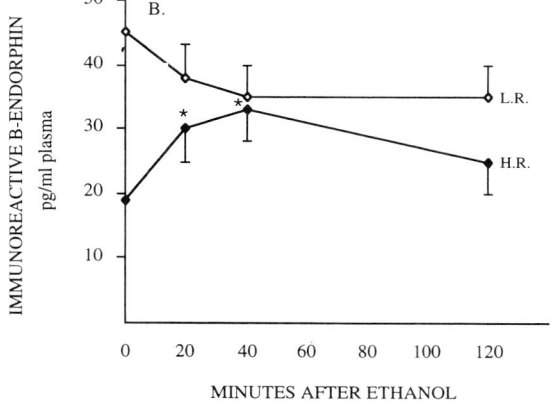

MINUTES AFTER ETHANOL

FIG. 1. A: Following a test dose of alcohol (0.5 g/kg) plasma immunoreactive β-endorphin is plotted for 120 min. High-risk (*H.R.*) subjects (positive family history for alcoholism) subjects show a significantly greater response than low-risk (*L.R.*) subjects (negative family history). Levels are expressed as percent change from baseline, and bars indicate the standard error of the mean. **B:** Graph showing actual plasma levels. High-risk subjects are lower than low-risk subjects at baseline, but the test dose of alcohol brings them to within the range of the low-risk group. (From ref. 31.)

SEROTONIN

Serotonin is yet another neurotransmitter that has been intensively investigated as a possible mediator of alcohol's reinforcing effects. Relatively low concentrations of alcohol increase the firing rate of the primarily serotonergic raphé neurons (94) and increase extracellular serotonin concentrations in the nucleus accumbens (106). Alcohol also directly increases cation flux at the serotonin-3 receptor-associated ion channel (53). On the behavioral level, serotonin reuptake inhibitors (which may desensitize serotonin-3 receptors during chronic administration) and serotonin-3 receptor antagonists reduce alcohol consumption by alcohol preferring and accepting rats (21,59). Serotonin-3 receptor antagonists also disrupt ethanol discrimination in pigeons (36).

RECEPTOR INTERACTIONS

There are also important interactions between and among different neurotransmitter systems. The importance of alcohol's serotonergic effects on the alcohol-induced increase in extracellular dopamine concentrations in the nucleus accumbens has not been fully elucidated, but serotonin-3 receptor blockers attenuate alcohol-induced dopamine release in the nucleus accumbens (13,104). Extracellular dopamine concentrations in the nucleus accumbens are known to be physiologically regulated by opiates, serotonin, amino acids, and neuropeptides. Pharmacological antagonism (1,25,101) at opiate receptors decreases extracellular dopamine concentrations. Agonism at serotonin-3 receptors increases stimulated dopamine release (103).

As briefly reviewed above, the dopamine-alcohol reinforcement hypothesis itself has not been established beyond some doubt. Nevertheless, an extensive literature on effects of alcohol in experimental animals has been based on this hypothesis. Findings of these studies suggest that dopaminergic, serotonergic, and opiate receptor manipulations may yield effective pharmacotherapies for alcoholism. In humans, blocking catecholamine synthesis has been reported to block the ''high'' or euphoria associated with alcohol-induced intoxication (2). The relative importance of dopamine and norepinephrine for this finding has not, however, been elucidated. Even though acute alcohol-induced intoxication increases cerebrospinal fluid concentrations of 3-methoxy-4-hydroxyphenylglycol concentrations in humans (6), noradrenergic mechanisms are currently thought to play only a minor role, if any, in alcohol reinforcement (92).

ALCOHOL CONSUMPTION STUDIES

There have been numerous experiments involving the effects of manipulation of the serotonergic and dopaminergic systems on alcohol preference. These studies have been the subject of numerous recent reviews (19,28,32,35, 42,60,61,68,82,107). A reader wishing to gain a comprehensive picture of the field is encouraged to examine all the cited reviews in addition to the key original data publications.

Animal Self-Administration Studies

The alcohol research field has been characterized by an extensive and successful investment in the development of animal models for alcohol abuse and dependence. The most extensively investigated products of these efforts are the AA (Alko alcohol) and ANA (Alko nonalcohol) (20) and the P (preferring) and NP (nonpreferring) (60) rat lines. The P animals orally self-administer alcohol to reach intoxicating blood alcohol concentrations. The P rats develop dependence and tolerance to alcohol when it is freely available, and they show withdrawal symptoms upon removal of alcohol. Therefore, the P rats are thought to represent a reasonable animal model for alcoholism.

The P rats have about 20% lower serotonin concentrations in the nucleus accumbens, frontal cortex, and anterior striatum than do the NP rats (108). Furthermore, a strong negative correlation has been reported across several inbred mouse strains between brain serotonin content and alcohol consumption and preference (105). The P rats also have a higher $5HT_1$ receptor density in cortical and hippocampal cell membrane preparations than do the NP rats (102). Serotonin uptake inhibitors (61) and mixed serotonin 1B and 1C receptor agonists (61) have been reported to reduce voluntary alcohol self-administration in the P rats. Moreover, fluoxetine reduced intragastric self-infusion rate of alcohol in the P rats (66). This last experiment is mechanistically important, because the results indicate that fluoxetine is not reducing alcohol self-administration by means of a taste aversion, which is a common effect of many functional serotonin agonists.

Studies describing the effects of opiate receptor antagonists on animal models of alcohol self-administration are cited above.

Human Experiments Involving Alcohol Consumption

Following the lead provided by the animal data, Naranjo and Sellers at the Addiction Research Foundation of Ontario in Toronto (70,72,83) have conducted a series of innovative studies administering various serotonin uptake inhibitors to male heavy ''social drinkers,'' most of whom fulfilled DSM III-R criteria for alcohol dependence. The investigators recruited their subjects by newspaper advertisements, screened them medically and psychiatrically, and asked them to continue their usual alcohol consumption and to document the level of consumption carefully. Subjects were then administered zimelidine, citalopram 20 or 40 mg, fluoxetine, and viqualone, each in controlled, double-blind, crossover studies with placebo. The general findings can be summarized as follows:

1. All serotonin uptake inhibitors except citalopram 20 mg reduced significantly the amount of alcohol consumed.

2. The quantitative effect was modest, but clinically meaningful, in the 50–70% of subjects who were classified as responders.
3. The effect was immediate.
4. There was a reduction of body weight which coincided with the administration of serotonin uptake inhibitors, but was independent of their effect on alcohol consumption.
5. Cigarette smoking was not reduced by the serotonin uptake inhibitors.
6. The 40-mg dose of citalopram seemed to reduce reinforcing effects of alcohol.

Even though theoretically interesting, clinically these studies present the reader with several problems. The first question involves whether a study of this nature is in accord with guidelines for studies of human subjects. Is it reasonable for an investigator studying alcohol-dependent subjects consuming in excess of six drinks per day to implicitly condone their continued drinking for experimental reasons on an outpatient basis for 2 months or more? Clearly the study was conducted with appropriate committee review and oversight, but the issues presented by the protocol are difficult and debatable. Second, the clinical applicability of these data is limited, because the current treatment of alcoholism involves initial cessation of consumption and treatment of withdrawal followed by treatments conducive to abstinence. An important insight gained from the Naranjo and Sellers studies is that the mechanism for reducing alcohol consumption and the antidepressant mechanisms of action of serotonin uptake inhibitors are probably different. The alcohol-consumption-reducing effect is immediate, whereas the antidepressant effect is delayed and the alcohol-consumption-reducing effect may require higher doses than the antidepressant effect. As such, the Naranjo and Sellers results parallel somewhat the results of studies on the efficacy of fluoxetine in bulimia (23).

In several abstracts, serotonin-3 receptor antagonists have been reported to reduce voluntary alcohol consumption in rats. Therefore, Sellers studied ondansetron, a drug from this category that has already been approved for the treatment of vomiting. Using the paradigm described above, Sellers found that in a very low but not in a medium dose, ondansetron reduced alcohol consumption in heavy social drinkers.

Gorelick (35) performed an inpatient study in very heavily drinking alcohol-dependent men in a Veterans' Administration Medical Center. He administered placebo and up to 80 mg fluoxetine/24 hr for 4 weeks on a research ward where alcohol was available according to a fixed interval procedure. Fluoxetine reduced alcohol consumption by 14%, but only during the first week. The author attributes the lack of efficacy during the last 3 weeks of the study to the development of tolerance to fluoxetine. An equally plausible explanation is an alcohol–fluoxetine

interaction. The initial effects of fluoxetine alone could have been overcome by the adaptation produced by the combination of alcohol and fluoxetine. In animal studies, co-administration of alcohol reverses receptor changes produced by noradrenergic antidepressants and neuroleptics.

TREATMENT OF ALCOHOLISM

The preclinical studies described above have stimulated clinical research that integrates medication into the existing treatment approaches for alcoholism. There are two distinct phases in the current treatment of alcohol dependence: detoxification and rehabilitation. Detoxification consists of stopping the ingestion of alcohol so that alcohol in the body is metabolized and the various organ systems affected by alcohol can readjust to the absence of alcohol. During this readjustment after abrupt stopping of alcohol, withdrawal symptoms consisting of rebound effects may occur. In most cases these symptoms are mild and do not require hospitalization. Depending on the dose of alcohol and the general health of the patient, the withdrawal syndrome can be severe and life-threatening and medical evaluation is important. Benzodiazepines are so effective in the management of the alcohol syndrome that the majority of alcoholics with uncomplicated withdrawal can be managed on an outpatient basis (41). For a full description of the management of withdrawal, see Jaffe et al. (46). While the withdrawal phase of treatment can be treated very successfully with modern medications, most patients will quickly relapse unless they are engaged in the rehabilitation phase.

Rehabilitation of alcoholics and other drug-dependent patients should consist of a long-term (years) structured program aimed at helping the patient cope with the life problems likely to provoke relapse. Currently there are many 28-day treatment programs that promote abstinence via group and individual therapy sessions in a hospital or residential sheltered living arrangement. Follow-up care frequently consists only of referral to a local Alcoholics Anonymous (AA) group. The AA program is extremely helpful to many patients, but without an individualized program directed by a therapist experienced in the management of substance abuse, relapse to uncontrolled drinking is common. Even in good outpatient programs that combine AA and individualized treatment, relapse rate at 3 months is in the neighborhood of 50% (18,22,26,27,74,77). Clearly there is a need for medications that could be used in conjunction with psychosocial rehabilitation programs.

CLINICAL TRIALS

Methodological Issues

The course of alcoholism is quite variable, so in any test of a medication or treatment approach, a randomly assigned control group is essential. Evaluation prior to beginning treatment should be comprehensive. Simply recording the daily intake of alcohol is not adequate. Important variables that may influence outcome include: presence of another psychiatric disorder; age; history of prior treatment; use of other drugs; and the degree of problems in the family, social, occupational, legal, or medical areas. The sample size should be large enough so that there is general equality across all of these important areas between treatment and control groups. Evaluations before, during, and after treatment should be conducted by investigators who are not aware of the patients' group assignment.

Compliance with medication is an important variable in any clinical trial. Studies conducted in populations of alcoholics or drug abusers should be carefully evaluated for compliance because those who are sufficiently motivated to comply with the medication regimen may be more likely to remain abstinent irrespective of medication. It is particularly misleading to measure compliance in the medication group without also measuring it in the placebo group. Thus any compliance measure must apply equally to drug and placebo groups. With most medications, one can measure compliance directly by monitoring plasma levels of the compound, but measures of placebo compliance are problematic. In some studies, riboflavin has been added to both drug and placebo, and urine fluorescence is tested on each clinic visit. This procedure presents several practical problems because of an inability to monitor riboflavin-containing dietary supplements and because the urine may be falsely negative if it is obtained within 1 hr or more than 12 hr of ingesting the study medication. Also, the addition of riboflavin to a drug in the investigational phase is regarded as a new formulation, and thus data from a study where riboflavin has been added could not be used for potential FDA approval of a new medication. Residual pill counts are another method to assess compliance that does not interfere with the drug development process. Of course, this method can be misleading if a patient is determined to deceive the investigator while not dropping out of the study. Comparisons of the riboflavin method and pill counts indicate comparable accuracy (87). Pill counts can be enhanced by giving research patients a container that has a different number of pills each week and determining how many were ingested by counting the remainder. Yet another method involves special pill bottles containing a microchip in the lid that records the dates and times that the lid is removed. Clearly, compliance should be addressed in some fashion during all clinical trials of new medications.

Another variable that should be quantitated in clinical trials is the level of psychosocial intervention. Because some detoxified alcoholics do very well while receiving no medication or when assigned to placebo, the nonmedical aspects of a rehabilitation program should be assessed. Of course, in a clinical trial the amount of psychosocial treatment should be specified and equal for all research patients. In order to ensure this equality and to assess the psychosocial component in all patients, a treatment assessment instrument (62) has been developed that is patterned on the addiction severity index (ASI). Data are obtained directly from the patient as the number of minutes spent each week with a helping person or a self-help group working on problems in each of the seven areas of the ASI.

Any discussion of clinical trials methodology should include a consideration of the population that volunteers for a treatment requiring random assignment. Studies (86) of the alcoholics who refuse to volunteer after the study is explained to them indicate that, in general, the volunteer study subjects are more severely ill than the refusers. Thus double-blind trials may underestimate medication efficacy because of the nature of the patients being treated.

The clinical trials to be discussed in the remainder of this chapter have strengths and weaknesses, and none has solved all of the methodological issues mentioned above. Unless trials are replicated in several different research centers, one cannot give them high credibility.

Serotonin 1A Receptor Partial Agonists

Buspirone, a serotonin 1A receptor partial agonist, which has weak dopamine-2 receptor antagonist potency and is quickly metabolized to 1-pyrimidinylpiperazine (1-PP), which is an α_2 receptor antagonist, has been investigated in three studies on abstinence maintenance. Bruno in Italy investigated buspirone 20 mg/24 hr for 8 weeks in a double-blind, placebo-controlled study (8). There were significantly fewer dropouts, and the patients reported greater anxiety reduction in the buspirone than in the placebo group. The patients reported a significant reduction in their alcohol intake during the buspirone treatment. Tollefson et al. (91) conducted a double-blind, placebo-controlled investigation of buspirone 40 mg/24 hr of 24 weeks' duration. All patients had an anxiety disorder in addition to alcohol dependence, and they had maintained abstinence for 30 days prior to the start of the medication. More patients on buspirone than on placebo attained clinically meaningful anxiety reduction and were retained in the study, but no data were given on maintenance of abstinence. Malcolm et al. (57) treated 67 anxious, alcohol-dependent patients in a Veterans Affairs Medical Center in a double-blind, placebo-controlled, parallel groups study for 6 months with 45–60 mg/24 hr buspirone. In this carefully conducted study, which used several outcome measures, no benefit over placebo could be documented for buspirone on either alcohol consumption or anxiety-related variables.

The main criticisms of the buspirone studies are twofold: (i) Buspirone administered chronically is a relatively nonspecific compound to test the importance of the serotonergic system in the relapse process in alcohol-dependent patients. (ii) Anxious alcoholics are more likely to represent late-onset or Type I alcoholics, who, in biochemical and neuroendocrinological studies, have been found to demonstrate only subtle, if any, serotonergic abnormalities. Thus, the very alcoholics who have shown the clearest signs of serotonergic dysfunction, who have early-onset antisocial traits, who are called Type II by Cloninger et al. (11) and von Knorring et al. (99), and who rarely have clinically significant levels of anxiety have been excluded from these studies. Partial serotonin 1A receptor agonists with a greater specificity than buspirone need to be tested for their efficacy as adjunctive pharmacotherapy in sobriety maintenance in early-onset alcoholics with antisocial traits.

In summary, there are several interesting leads in the animal and clinical literature that are suggestive of potential efficacy of serotonergic agents in reducing alcohol intake and perhaps preventing relapse in alcohol-dependent patients. Experiments in animals and in humans given serotonergic medications described above suggest that serotonergic systems play a role in alcohol reinforcement. There is a tremendous need for controlled clinical trials of serotonergic medications such as fluoxetine and citalopram to determine whether the reductions of alcohol drinking reported in the Naranjo and Sellers (68,69,71,73) and Gorelick (35) experiments can be clinically significant.

GABA$_A$ Receptor Agonists

Calcium bisacetyl homotaurine, acamprosate, which has been claimed to function as a direct GABA receptor agonist, has in two controlled studies shown efficacy in the treatment of alcoholism. The first study involved 85 alcoholics who were considered "hopeless" due to the severity of their illness and who were therefore not considered to be good candidates for psychotherapy. The dose of acamprosate was 25 mg/kg of body weight/24 hr, and duration of treatment was 90 days. Twenty of 33 patients on acamprosate and 12 of 37 on placebo ($p <$ 0.02 by χ^2 test) did not relapse during the study (50).

The second multicenter study on sobriety maintenance with acamprosate enrolled 356 patients, 181 on acamprosate and 175 on placebo (51). The dose of acamprosate was significantly higher than in the prior study at 1.3 g/ 24 hr, and the duration of treatment was similar, namely, 90 days. The main dependent variable was the liver enzyme, γ-glutamyltransferase (γGT). At the end of the study the γGT concentration was significantly higher in the placebo than in the γGT group, suggesting that there was more alcohol use in the placebo group, but the number of subjects maintaining abstinence is not given in the article. The results of these two studies appear promising. Further controlled clinical trials of acamprosate in alcoholics are warranted.

Dopamine Precursors

L-DOPA + carbidopa combination in doses up to 100 mg of carbidopa and 800 mg of L-DOPA titrated according to patient's tolerance to side effects was compared to placebo in a 1-year follow-up study on sobriety maintenance (29). A total of 30 patients started the trial after an intensive 6-week inpatient treatment program. All were encouraged to take advantage of AA meetings during the outpatient follow-up period, and they visited the outpatient clinic regularly. The study was discontinued after an interim analysis that showed no efficacy of L-DOPA and carbidopa over placebo.

Serotonin Precursors

The above-mentioned L-DOPA and carbidopa study included also a 5-hydroxytryptophan and carbidopa cell which consisted of 15 alcoholics. The dose was titrated up to 100 mg of carbidopa and 400 mg of 5-hydroxytryptophan according to the patients' tolerance. The combination was no more effective than placebo.

Dopamine Receptor Agonists

In the past, apomorphine has been used as an emetic to produce aversion to alcohol in alcoholics. No controlled studies of apomorphine's efficacy used in aversion treatment are available. Apomorphine in relatively low doses, which do not provoke nausea or vomiting, has in uncontrolled studies been reported to enhance sobriety maintenance. In a 2-week controlled clinical study of 40 patients, started immediately after treatment for alcohol withdrawal, apomorphine 36 or 108 mg/24 hr was, however, no better than placebo in maintaining sobriety (47). Thus, there appears to be no evidence based on controlled studies that shows apomorphine to be efficacious in sobriety maintenance.

Bromocriptine, a relatively nonspecific dopamine-2 receptor agonist which undergoes extensive first-pass metabolism in humans, has been used in two controlled, double-blind studies to enhance sobriety maintenance. The two studies have yielded conflicting results. Borg (7) treated 50 alcoholics using a parallel group design for 6 months with 2.5 mg bromocriptine three times a day. During months 4 through 6, the dose was increased to 5 mg three times a day. Borg reported significant efficacy for bromocriptine. The bromocriptine group reported reduced craving and fewer depressive reactions, and only one of 19 patients reported drinking at the end of the trial. The study had a remarkably low dropout rate in both the placebo and bromocriptine groups.

Dongier et al. (17) administered 2.5 mg bromocriptine three times a day for 8 weeks to 84 alcoholics of whom 38 were available for analysis at the end of the treatment phase. Twenty patients could be investigated after a further 8-week medication-free follow-up. In this study, which had a more typical dropout rate than did the Borg study, bromocriptine did not improve relapse rate compared to placebo. However, various measures of psychiatric symptoms showed significant advantage for bromocriptine over placebo.

Dopamine Receptor Antagonists

Shaw et al. (84) reported a 6-month double-blind comparison of 100 mg tiapride three times a day and placebo in 32 alcoholic-dependent patients. Tiapride is a substituted benzamide which acts primarily as a dopamine-2 receptor antagonist. All patients had high anxiety and depression ratings at the end of their detoxification. Twenty patients completed the study. Tiapride halved the amount of ethanol consumed by the patients and roughly doubled the number of abstinent days compared to placebo. Both findings were statistically significant. Depression and anxiety ratings were also significantly reduced in the tiapride group. These promising results have not been replicated, but the size of the claimed therapeutic effect definitely warrants further studies.

γ-Hydroxybutyrate

This endogenous substance is a sedative whose exact mechanism of action is not known. Low doses have been demonstrated to increase dopamine turnover in the central nervous system, whereas high doses have been shown to reduce it. Thus, it has been postulated to mimic alcohol's reinforcing effects. In a double-blind, placebo-controlled, parallel group study with a 90-day treatment period, 36 patients received 50 mg/kg of body weight/24 hr of γ-hydroxybutyrate and 35 patients received placebo (5). During the third month, but not earlier, the number of patients abstaining or practicing "controlled drinking" was significantly ($p < 0.001$) higher in the group receiving γ-hydroxybutyrate. If γ-hydroxybutyrate is not self-administered by animals, these exciting results clearly deserve to be confirmed or refuted in a large-scale follow-up study.

Opioid Antagonists

As reviewed above, there are several animal models of alcohol drinking that suggest a role for endogenous opioids in the reinforcement produced by alcohol. It was these reports from animal studies that caused Volpicelli et al. (97) to conduct a double-blind trial of naltrexone versus placebo in chronic alcoholics. The patients in the study were applying for treatment at the Philadelphia Veterans Affairs Medical Center. The 70 male subjects were,

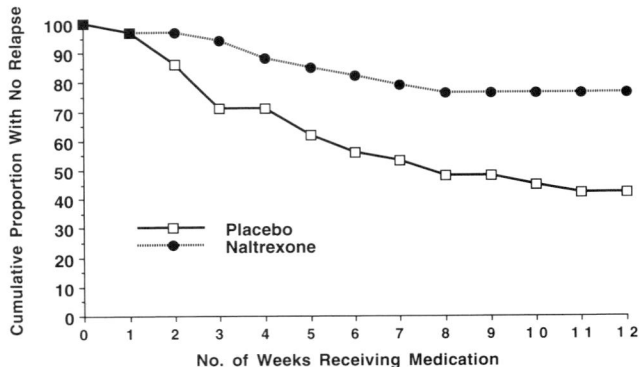

FIG. 2. "Survival" as defined by nonrelapse for the two treatment groups. All patients were receiving intensive psychosocial intervention. Relapse to alcoholic drinking in the patients randomized to placebo was 54% at 12 weeks, whereas for those randomized to naltrexone, the proportion relapsing was 23%. (From ref. 96.)

on average, 43 years old with a 20-year history of heavy drinking, and all met at least five of the nine DSM-III-R criteria for alcohol dependence, including physical signs of withdrawal sufficient to require medication. After completion of detoxification, the patients began an outpatient rehabilitation program that consisted of 1 month of daily day hospital participation tapering to weekly counseling sessions during months 2 and 3. At the time of entering the rehabilitation program, the patients were randomly assigned to 50 mg naltrexone daily or to placebo. During the 3 months of the study, the naltrexone-treated patients reported significantly less craving for alcohol and they reported significantly fewer days of alcohol use. The overall survival curve during the 3-month study is shown in Fig. 2. As is typical of chronic alcoholics in a rehabilitation program, 54% of the placebo patients met criteria for relapse whereas only 23% of those in the naltrexone group met these criteria. Among the patients randomized to placebo, having a "slip" and drinking any alcohol almost invariably (95%) led to a relapse. In contrast, those receiving naltrexone who used any alcohol had only a 23% relapse rate. Two naltrexone patients who dropped out due to nausea were included in the outcome analysis. There was no evidence that naltrexone impaired liver function. To the contrary, there were more improvements in liver enzyme data in the naltrexone group, probably reflecting their greater abstinence, but the differences did not reach statistical significance.

Positive results in a single study of a new treatment for alcoholism would not be remarkable because of the variability in the course of this disorder. O'Malley et al. (77), however, heard a preliminary report of the Philadelphia group and conducted a similar study among 97 alcohol-dependent subjects in New Haven. Instead of a day hospital, the rehabilitation program consisted of coping skills/relapse prevention or supportive psychotherapy.

The results of this independent study involving a predominantly white male population were quite similar to those of the Philadelphia group. Naltrexone was found to be clearly superior to placebo irrespective of the type of psychosocial intervention to which the patients were assigned. Those randomly assigned to naltrexone drank on half as many days and consumed one-third the number of standard drinks during the trial as did subjects who received placebo. Craving for alcohol was significantly decreased only in those subjects who completed the study. Relapse rates were significantly lower in the naltrexone-treated patients. As in the Volpicelli et al. (97) study, relapse rate differences were particularly high among patients who drank some alcohol. Among the patients who had at least one drink, those randomized to naltrexone and coping skills therapy had one-fourth the risk of relapse compared with subjects taking placebo who received coping skills treatment. Medication compliance was measured by the addition of riboflavin to the study medication and the testing of urines weekly with ultraviolet light. This method indicated high compliance for both groups, but significantly higher for the naltrexone treated patients. As in the previous study, there was no evidence of naltrexone-induced hepatotoxicity. Aspartate aminotransferase levels were significantly lower in the naltrexone-treated patients at endpoint, and a similar trend was noted for alanine aminotransferase.

The patients in the Volpicelli et al. (97) study who had a ''lapse'' and drank some alcohol were asked about the effects of the alcohol. Those receiving placebo reported that the effects were no different from those experienced prior to the study. Those receiving naltrexone reported significantly less euphoria from their drinking than they expected based on prior experience. This finding, which suggests an effect of naltrexone on the immediate subjective effects of alcohol, may give a clue as to the mechanism of action by which naltrexone might decrease relapse rates in alcoholics. Double-blind studies in human subjects of the acute effects of alcohol and alcohol placebo in the presence of naltrexone or naltrexone placebo are needed. These studies should be conducted in normal volunteers, in alcoholics, and in nonalcoholics with a family history of alcoholism.

These two studies of naltrexone in middle-aged alcoholics involved in good outpatient rehabilitation programs, and receiving adjunctive medication consisting of either naltrexone or placebo had strikingly similar results. More studies are required, but the available clinical evidence is completely consistent with evidence from rodent and nonhuman primate models. It suggests that by blocking μ and δ opiate receptors, naltrexone is able to reduce the reinforcement produced by alcohol drinking. Both studies had total abstinence as the stated goal of treatment, and there was no intention of using naltrexone to teach controlled drinking. Naltrexone clearly does not prevent alcoholics from relapsing. Patients can stop the medication at any time with no withdrawal symptoms and resume drinking. Naltrexone may, however, interact with the effects of the rehabilitation program and, by reducing the reward produced by alcohol, enable the patient to remain in treatment longer and receive the benefits of long-term behavior change.

REFERENCES

1. Acquas E, Meloni M, DiChiara G. Blockage of δ-opioid receptors in the nucleus accumbens prevents ethanol-induced stimulation of dopamine release. *Eur J Pharmacol* 1993;230:239–241.
2. Ahlenius S, Carlsson A, Engel J, Svensson T, Sodersten P. Antagonism by alphamethyltyrosine of the ethanol-induced stimulation and euphoria in man. *Clin Pharmacol Ther* 1973;14:586–591.
3. Altshuler HL, Phillips PE, Feinhandler DA. Alteration of ethanol self-administration by naltrexone. *Life Sci* 1980;26:679–688.
4. Babor TF, Hoffman M, DelBoca FK, Hesselbrock V, Meyer RE, Dolinsky ZS, Rounsaville B. Types of alcoholics, I: evidence for an empirically derived typology based on indicators of vulnerability and severity. *Arch Gen Psychiatry* 1992;49:599–608.
5. Biggio G, Cibin M, Diana M, et al. Suppression of voluntary alcohol intake in rats and alcoholics by gamma-hydroxybutyric acid: a non-GABAergic mechanism. In: Biggio G, Concas C, Costa E, eds. *GABAergic synaptic transmission.* New York: Raven Press, 1992;281–288.
6. Borg S, Kvande H, Sedvall G. Central norepinephrine metabolism during alcohol intoxication in addicts and healthy volunteers. *Science* 1981;213:1135–1137.
7. Borg V. Bromocriptine in the prevention of alcohol abuse. *Acta Psychiatr Scand* 1983;68:110–110.
8. Bruno F. Buspirone and the treatment of alcoholic patients. *Psychopathology* 1989;22(1):49–59.
9. Cadoret RJ, Cain CA, Grove WM. Development of alcoholism in adoptees raised apart from alcoholic biologic relatives. *Arch Gen Psychiatry* 1980;37:561–563.
10. Cloninger CR. Neurogenetic adaptive mechanisms in alcoholism. *Science* 1987;236:410–416.
11. Cloninger CR, Bohman M, Sigvardsson S. Inheritance of alcohol abuse: cross-fostering analysis of adopted men. *Arch Gen Psychiatry* 1981;38:861–868.
12. Cloninger CR, Bohman M, Sigvardsson S, von Knorring AL. Psychopathology in adopted-out children of alcoholics: the Stockholm adoption study. In: Galanter M, ed. *Recent developments in alcoholism.* New York: Plenum Press, 1985;3.
13. Corbin E, Acquas E, Frau R, DiChiara G. Differential inhibitory effects of 5HT$_3$ antagonist on drug-induced stimulation of dopamine. *Eur J Pharmacol* 1989;164:515–519.
14. Cotton NS. The familial incidence of alcoholism: a review. *J Stud Alcohol* 1979;40:89–116.
15. Cunningham CL, Malott DH, Dickinson SD, Risinger FO. Haloperidol does not alter expression of ethanol-induced conditioned place preference. *Behav Brain Res* 1992;50:1–5.
16. DiChiara G, Imperato A. Ethanol preferentially stimulates dopamine release in the nucleus accumbens of freely moving rats. *Eur J Pharmacol* 1985;115:131–132.
17. Dongier M, Vachon L, Schwartz G. Bromocriptine in the treatment of alcohol dependence. *Alcohol Clin Exp Res* 1991;15:970–977.
18. Dorus W, Ostrow DG, Anton R, Cushman P, Collins JF, Schaefer M, Charles HL, Desai P, Hayashida M, Malkerneker U, Willenbrug O, Fiscella R, Sather MR. Lithium treatment of depressed and nondepressed alcoholics. *JAMA* 1989;262:1646–1652.
19. Engel JA, Enerback C, Fahlke C, Hulthe P, Hard E, Johannessen K, Swensson L, Soderpalm B. Serotonergic and dopaminergic involvement in ethanol intake. In: Naranjo CA, Sellers EM, eds. *Model pharmacological interventions for alcoholism.* New York: Springer-Verlag, 1992;68–82.
20. Eriksson K. Genetic selection for voluntary alcohol consumption in the albino rat. *Science* 1968;159:105–120.
21. Fadda F, Garau B, Marchei F, et al. MDL 7222, a selective 5-HT$_3$

receptor antagonist, suppresses voluntary ethanol consumption in alcohol-preferring rats. *Alcohol* 1991;26:107–1110.

22. Fawcett J, Clark DC, Gibbons RD, Aagesen CA, Pisani VD, Tilkin JM, Sellers D, Stulzman D. Evaluation of lithium therapy for alcoholism. *J Clin Psychiatry* 1984;45:494–499.

23. Fluoxetine Bulimia Nervosa Collaboration Study Group. Fluoxetine in the treatment of bulimia nervosa: a multicenter, placebo-controlled, double-blind trial. *Arch Gen Psychiatry* 1992;49:139–147.

24. Froehlich JC, Harts J, Lumeng L, Li TK. Naloxone attenuates voluntary ethanol intake in rats selectively bred for high ethanol preference. *Pharmacol Biochem Behav* 1990;35:385–390.

25. Fuchs V, Coper H, Rommelspacher H. The effect of ethanol and haloperidol on dopamine receptor (D2) density. *Neuropharmacology* 1987;26:1231–1233.

26. Fuller RK, Branchey L, Brightwell DR, Derman RM, Emrick CD, Iber FL, James KE, Lacoursiere RB, Lee KK, Lowenstam I, Manny I, Neiderhiser D, Nocks S, Shaw JJ. Disulfiram treatment of alcoholism: a Veterans Administration cooperative study. *JAMA* 1986;256:1449–1455.

27. Fuller RK, Roth HP. Disulfiram for the treatment of alcoholism: an evaluation in 128 men. *Ann Intern Med* 1979;90:901–904.

28. George DR, Wozniak K, Linnoila M. Basic and clinical studies on serotonin, alcohol and alcoholism. In: Naranjo CA, Sellers EM, eds. *Novel pharmacological interventions for alcoholism.* New York: Springer-Verlag, 1992;92–104.

29. George DT, Lindguist T, Rawlings RR, et al. Pharmacologic maintenance of abstinence in patients with alcoholism: no efficacy of 5-hydroxytryptophan or levodopa. *Clin Pharmacol Ther* 1992;52:553–560.

30. Gessa GL, Muntoni F, Collu M, et al. Low doses of ethanol activate dopaminergic neurons in the ventral tegmental area. *Brain Res* 1985;348:201–203.

31. Gianoulakis C, Angelogianni P, Meaney M, Thavundayil J, Tawar V. Endorphins in individuals with high and low risk for development of alcoholism. In: Reid LD, ed. *Opioids, bulimia and alcohol abuse and alcoholism.* New York: Springer-Verlag, 1990;229–246.

32. Gill K, Amit Z. Serotonin uptake blockers and voluntary alcohol consumption a review of recent studies. In: Galanter M, ed. *Recent developments in alcoholism,* vol 7. New York: Plenum Press, 1989;225–248.

33. Goldman D. Molecular markers for linkage of genetic loci contributing to alcoholism. In: Galanter M, ed. *Recent developments in alcoholism.* New York: Plenum Press, 1988;6.

34. Goodwin DW, Schulsinger F, Hermansen L, Guze S, Winokur G. Alcohol problems in adoptees raised apart from alcoholic biological parents. *Arch Gen Psychiatry* 1973;28:238–243.

35. Gorelick DA. Serotonin uptake blockers and the treatment of alcoholism. In: Galanter M, ed. *Recent developments in alcoholism.* New York: Plenum Press, 1989;267–278.

36. Grant KA, Barrett JE. Blockade of the discriminative stimulus effects of ethanol with 5-HT₃ receptor antagonists. *Psychopharmacology* 1991;104:451–456.

37. Grant KA, Colombo G. Discriminative stimulus effects of ethanol: effect of training dose on the substitution of N-methyl-D-aspartate antagonists. *J Pharmacol Exp Ther* 1992;264:1241–1247.

38. Gubya K, Grant KA, Valverius P, Hoffman PL, Tabakoff B. Brain regional specificity and time course of changes in the NMDA receptor–ionophore complex during ethanol withdrawal. *Brain Res* 1991;547:129–134.

39. Hayashida M, Alterman A, McLellan AT, O'Brien CP, Purtil J, Volpicelli J. Comparative effectiveness of inpatient and outpatient detoxification of patients with mild to moderate alcohol withdrawal syndrome. *N Engl J Med* 1989;320:358–365.

40. Heath AC, Meyer J, Jardine R, Martin NG. The inheritance of alcohol consumption patterns in a general population twin sample. I. Multidimensional scaling of quantity/frequency data. *J Stud Alcohol* 1991;52:345–352.

41. Heath AC, Meyer J, Jardine R, Martin NG. The inheritance of alcohol consumption patterns in a general population twin sample. II. Determinants of consumption frequency and quantity consumed. *J Stud Alcohol* 1991;52:425–433.

42. Higgin GA, Lawrin MO, Sellers EM. Serotonin and alcohol con-

sumption. In: Naranjo CA, Sellers EM, eds. *Novel pharmacological interventions for alcoholism.* New York: Springer-Verlag, 1992:83–91.

43. Hubbell CL, Abelson ML, Burkhardt CA, Herlands SE, Reid LD. Constant infusions of morphine and intakes of sweetened ethanol solution among rats. *Alcohol* 1988;5:409–415.

44. Hyytia P, Sinclair JD. Responding for oral ethanol after naloxone treatment by alcohol-preferring AA rats. *Alcohol Clin Exp Res* 1993;17:631–636.

45. Imperato A, DiChiara G. Preferential stimulation of dopamine release in the nucleus accumbens of freely moving rats by ethanol. *J Pharmacol Exp Ther* 1986;239:219–228.

46. Jaffe JH, Kranzler HR, Ciraulo DA. Drugs used in the treatment of alcoholism. In: Mendelson JH, Mello MK, eds. *Medical diagnosis and treatment of alcoholism.* New York: McGraw–Hill, 1992;12:421–461.

47. Jensen SB, Christoffersen CB, Noerregaard A. Apomorphine in outpatient treatment of alcohol intoxication and abstinence: a double-blind study. *Br J Addiction* 1977;72:325–330.

48. Kendler KS, Heath AC, Neale MC, Kessler RC, Eaves LJ. A population-based twin study of alcoholism in women. *JAMA* 1992;268:1877–1882.

49. Kiianmaa K, Andersson K, Fuxe K. On the role of ascending dopamine systems in the control of voluntary enthanol intake and ethanol intoxication. *Pharmacol Biochem Behav* 1979;10:603–608.

50. Lhuintre JP, Moore N, Saligaut C, et al. Ability of calcium bis acetyl homotauraine, a GABA agonist, to prevent relapse in weaned alcoholics. *Lancet* 1985:1014–1016.

51. Lhuintre JP, Moore N, Tran G, et al. Acamprosate appears to decrease alcohol intake in weaned alcoholics. *Alcohol* 1990;25:613–622.

52. Litt MD, Babor TF, DelBoca FK, Kadden RM, Cooney NL. Types of alcoholics, II: application of an empiricallay derived typology to treatment matching. *Arch Gen Psychiatry* 1992;49:609–614.

53. Lovinger DM. Ethanol potentiation of 5-HT₃ receptor-mediated ion current in NCB-20 neuroblastoma cells. *Neurosci Lett* 1991;122:57–60.

54. Macfarlane SJ, White JM. Acquisition and extinction of an alcohol-opposite conditioned response in humans. *Psychopharmacology.* 1989;97:355–357.

55. Lovinger DM, White G. Ethanol potentiation of 5-hydroxytryptamine₃ receptor-mediated ion current in neuroblastoma cells and isolated adult mammalian neurons. *Mol Pharmacol* 1991;40:263–270.

56. Malcolm R, Anton RF, Randall CL, Johnston A, Brady K, Thevos A. A placebo-controlled trial of buspirone in anxious inpatient alcoholics. *Alcohol Clin Exp Res* 1992;16:1007–1013.

57. Malcolm R, Anton RF, Randall CL, Johnston A, Brady K, Thevos A. A placebo-controlled trial of buspirone in anxious inpatient alcoholics. *Alcohol Clin Exp Res* 1992;16:1007–1013.

58. Marfaing-Jallet P, Miceli D, Le Magnen J. Decrease in ethanol consumption by naloxone in naive and dependent rats. *Pharmacol Biochem Behav* 1983;18:537–539.

59. McBride WJ, Murphy JM, Lumeng L, Li TK. Effects of Ro 15-45B, fluoxetine and desipramine on the intake of ethanol, water and food by the alcohol preferring (P) and non-preferring (NP) lines of rats. *Pharmacol Biochem Behav* 1988;30:1045–1050.

60. McBride WJ, Murphy JM, Lumeng L, Li TK. Serotonin and ethanol preference. In: Galanter M, ed. *Recent developments in alcoholism,* vol 7. New York: Plenum Press, 1989;187–205.

61. McBride WJ, Murphy WJ, Lumeng L, Li TK. Serotonin and alcohol consumption. In: Naranjo CA, Sellers EM, eds. *Novel pharmacological interventions for alcoholism.* New York: Springer-Verelag, 1992;59–67.

62. McLellan AT, Alterman AI, Cacciola J, Metzger D, O'Brien CP. A new measure of substance abuse treatment: initial studies of the treatment services review. *J Nerv Ment Dis* 1992;180:101–110.

63. Mereu G, Fadda F, Gessa GL. Ethanol stimulates the firing rate of nigral dopaminergic neurons in unanesthetized rats. *Brain Res* 1984;292:63–69.

64. Morriset RA, Swartzwelder HS. Attenuation of hippocampal long-term potentiation by ethanol: a patch-clamp of glutamatergic and GABAergic mechanisms. *J Neurosci* 1993;13:2264–2272.

65. Morrow AL, Suzdak PD, Karanian JW, Paul SM. Chronic ethanol administration alters gamma-aminobutyric acid, pentobarbital and ethanol-mediated ^{36}CL uptake in cerebral cortical synaptoneurosomes. *J Pharmacol Exp Ther* 1988;246:158–164.

66. Murphy JM, Waller MB, Gatto GJ, McBride WJ, Lumeng L, Li TK. Effects of fluoxetine on the intragastric self-administration of ethanol in the alcohol preferring P line of rats. *Alcohol* 1988;5:283–286.

67. Myers RD, Borg S, Mossberg R. Antagonism by naltrexone of voluntary alcohol selection in the chronically drinking macaque monkey. *Alcohol* 1986;3:383–388.

68. Naranjo CA, Bremner KE. Evaluation of the effects of serotonin uptake inhibitors in alcoholics: a review. In: Naranjo CA, Sellers EM, eds. *Novel pharmacological interventions for alcoholism.* New York: Springer-Verlag, 1992;105–120.

69. Naranjo CA, Kadlec KE, Sanheuza P, Woodley-Remus D, Sellers EM. Fluoxetine differentially alters alcohol intake and other consummatory behaviors in problem drinkers. *Clin Pharmacol Ther* 1990;47:490–498.

70. Naranjo CA, Sellers EM, Sullivan JT, Woodley DV, Kadlec K, Sykora K. The serotonin uptake inhibitor citalopram attenuates ethanol intake. *Clin Pharmacol Ther* 1987;41:266–274.

71. Naranjo CA, Sellers EM. Serotonin uptake inhibitors attenuate ethanol intake in problem drinkers. In: Galanter M, ed. *Alcoholism.* New York: Plenum Press, 1989;7:255–266.

72. Naranjo CA, Sellers EM, Roach CA, Woodley DV, Sanchez-Craig M, Sykora K. Zimelidine-induced variations in alcohol intake by nondepressed heavy drinkers. *Clin Pharmacol Ther* 1984;35:374–381.

73. Naranjo CA, Sullivan JT, Kadlec KE, Woodley-Remus DC, Kennedy G, Sellers EM. Differential effects of viqualine on alcohol intake and other consummatory behaviors. *Clin Pharmacol Ther* 1989;46:301–309.

74. Nathan PE. Outcomes of treatment for alcoholism: current data. *Ann Behav Med* 1986;8:40–46.

75. National Institute on Alcohol Abuse and Alcoholism. Economic costs of alcohol abuse. *Seventh Special Report to the Congress on Alcohol and Health* 1990;Jan:174.

76. O'Brien CP, Childress AR, McLellan AT, Ehrman R. Classical conditioning in drug dependent humans. The neurology of drug and alcohol addiction. In: Galanter M, ed. *Ann NY Acad Sci* 1992;654:400–415.

77. O'Malley SS, Jaffe AJ, Chang G, Schottenfeld RS, Meyer RE, Rounsaville B. Naltrexone and coping skills therapy for alcohol dependence. *Arch Gen Psychiatry* 1992;49:881–887.

78. Pickens RW, Svikis DS, McGue M, Lykken DT, Heston LL, Clayton PJ. Heterogeneity in the inheritance of alcoholism. *Arch Gen Psychiatry* 1991;48:19–28.

79. Robbins LN, Helzer JE, Weissman MM, Orvaschel H, Gruenberg E, Burke JD, Regier DA. Lifetime prevalence of specific psychiatric disorders in three sites. *Arch Gen Psychiatry* 1984;41:949–958.

80. Rossetti ZL, Hmaidan Y, Gessa GL. Marked inhibition of mesolimbic release: a common feature of ethanol, morphine, cocaine and amphetamine abstinence in rats. *Eur J Pharmacol* 1992;221:227–234.

81. Samson HH, Doyle TF. Oral ethanol self-administration in the rat: effect of naloxone. *Pharmacol Biochem Behav* 1985;22:91–99.

82. Sellers EM, Higgins GA, Sobell, MG. 5-HT and alcohol abuse. *Trends Pharmacol Sci* 1992;13:69–75.

83. Sellers EM, Naranjo CA, Kadlec K. Do serotonin uptake inhibitors decrease smoking? Observations in a group of heavy drinkers. *J Clin Psychopharmacol* 1987;7:417–420.

84. Shaw GK, Majumdar SK, Waller S, MacGarvie J, Dunn G. Tiapride in the long-term management of alcoholics of anxious or depressive temperament. *Br J Psychiatry* 1987;150:164–168.

85. Sinclair JD, Adkins J, Walker S. Morphine-induced suppression of voluntary alcohol drinking in rats. *Nature* 1973;246:425–427.

86. Strohmetz DB, Alterman AI, Walter D. Selection factors in alcoholics volunteering for a treatment study. *Alcoholism Clin Exp Res* 1990;14:736–738.

87. Sullivan JT, Naranjo CA, Sellers EM. Compliance among heavy alcohol users in clinical drug trials. *J Subst Abuse* 1989;1:184–194.

88. Suzdak PD, Glowa JR, Crawley JN, Schwartz RD, Skolnick P, Paul SM. A selective imidazobenzodiazepine antagonist of ethanol in the rat. *Science* 1986;234:1243–1247.

89. Suzdak PD, Schwartz RD, Skolnick P, Paul SM. Ethanol stimulates gamma-aminobutyric acid receptor-mediated chloride transport in rat brain synaptoneurosomes. *Proc Natl Acad Sci USA* 1986;83:4071–4075.

90. Tarter R, McBride H, Buonpane N, Schneider D. Differentiation of alcoholics according to childhood history of minimal brain dysfunction, family history and drinking pattern. *Arch Gen Psychiatry* 1977;34:761–768.

91. Tollefson GD, Montagu-Clouse J, Lancaster SP. Busiprone in comorbid alcohol dependency and generalized anxiety disorders. *Ther Bull* 1990;Suppl Aug:35–50.

92. Turkka J, Gurguis G, Karanian J, Potter WZ, Linnoila M. Effects of chronic exposure to ethanol alone and in combination with desipramine on β-adrenoceptors of rat brain. *Eur J Pharmacol* 1990;177:171–179.

93. Vavrousek-Jakuba E, Cohen CA, Shoemaker WJ. Ethanol effects of CNS dopamine receptors: in vivo binding following voluntary ethanol (ETOH) intake in rats. In: Naranjo CA, Sellers EM, eds. *Novel pharmacological interventions for alcoholism.* New York: Springer-Verlag, 1992;372–374.

94. Verbanck P, Sentin V, Dresse A, Scuvee J, Massotte L, Giesbers I, Kornreich C. Electrophysiological effects of ethanol on monoaminergic neurons: an in vivo and in vitro study. *Alcohol Clin Exp Res* 1990;14:728–735.

95. Vescovi PP, Coiro V, Volpi R, Giannini A, Passeri M. Plasma beta-endorphin but not met-enkephalin levels are abnormal in chronic alcoholics. *Alcohol Alcoholism* 1992;27(5):471–175.

96. Volpicelli JR. Uncontrollable events and alcohol drinking. *Br J Addict* 1987;82:385–396.

97. Volpicelli JR, Alterman AI, Hayashida M, O'Brien CP. Naltrexone in the treatment of alcohol dependence. *Arch Gen Psychiatry* 1992;49:876–880.

98. Volpicelli JR. Davis MA, Olin JE. Naltrexone blocks the post-shock increase of ethanol consumption. *Life Sci* 1986;38:841–847.

99. von Knorring L, von Knorring AL, Smigan L, Lindberg U, Edholm M. Personality traits in subtypes of alcoholics. *J Stud Alcohol* 1987;48:523–527.

100. Weiss F, Hurd YL, Ungerstedt U, Markou A, Plotsky PM, Koob GF. Neurochemical correlates of cocaine and ethanol self-administration. *Ann NY Acad Sci* 1992;654:220–241.

101. Widdowson PS, Holman RB. Ethanol-induced increase in endogenous dopamine release may involve endogenous opiates. *J Neurochem* 1992;59:157–162.

102. Wong DT, Threlkeld PG, Lumeng L, Li TK. Higher density of serotonin-1A receptors in the hippocampus and cerebral cortex of alcohol-preferring P rats. *Life Sci* 1990;146:231–235.

103. Wozniak KM, Pert A, Linnoila M. Antagonism of 5HT$_3$ receptors attenuates the effects of ethanol on extracellular dopamine. *Eur J Pharmacol* 1990;187:287–289.

104. Wozniak KM, Pert A, Mele A, Linnoila M. Focal application of alcohol elevates extracellular dopamine in rat brain: a microdialysis study. *Brain Res* 1991;540:31–40.

105. Yoshimoto K, Komura S. Reexamination of the relationship between alcohol preference and brain monoamines in inbred strains of mice including senescence-accelerated mice. *Pharmacol Biochem Behav* 1987;27:317–322.

106. Yoshimoto K, McBride WJ, Lumeng L, Li TK. Ethanol enhances the release of dopamine and serotonin in the nucleus accumbens of HAD and LAA lines of rats. *Alcohol Clin Exp Res* 1992;16:781–785.

107. Zabik JE. Use of serotonin-active drugs in alcohol preference studies. In: Galanter M, ed. *Recent developments in alcoholism*, vol 7. New York: Plenum Press, 1989;211–220.

108. Zhou FC, Bledsoe S, Luming L, Li TK. Immunostained serotonergic fibers are decreased in selected brain regions of alcohol-preferring rats. *Alcohol* 1991;8:425–431.

*Psychopharmacology: The Fourth
Generation of Progress,* edited by
Floyd E. Bloom and David J. Kupfer.
Raven Press, Ltd., New York © 1995.

CHAPTER 150

Marijuana

Billy R. Martin

Marijuana continues to be the most frequently abused illicit drug in America. Despite modest declines from the pinnacle of its use in the mid-1970s, marijuana smoking is prevalent regardless of age, ethnicity, and sex. Marijuana usage by juveniles and young adults still poses a major problem. Nearly 15 years have passed since the peak period of marijuana use in the United States. Approximately 70% of adults between the ages of 27 and 32 have used marijuana during their lifetime. One of the most important statistics is the current daily use, which is estimated to be at the 2–3% level. The health consequences of marijuana still defy simple characterization and remain controversial. One objective of this review is to discuss current reports dealing with the adverse actions of marijuana, with particular emphasis on the reasons for the continuing ambiguity. The clinical utility of cannabinoids, albeit limited, will also be discussed. The biochemical and pharmacological actions of cannabinoids attracted considerable interest in the 1970s, only to be followed by a quiescent period in the early 1980s. During the past few years, numerous breakthroughs have occurred that have greatly increased our understanding of the cannabinoids. It is now evident that an endogenous cannabinoid system exists. A receptor has been characterized and cloned, second messenger systems have been identified, and a putative endogenous ligand has been isolated and synthesized. Our concept now extends beyond the notion that cannabinoids are producing their behavioral effects by directly interfering with neurotransmitter systems. This review will also summarize these findings and discuss their implications for future research (see Chapter 53, *this volume,* for related topic).

HUMAN PHARMACOLOGY

Effects on Performance

It is well recognized that cannabinoids affect sensory, psychomotor, and cognitive function, and therefore it is

B. R. Martin: Department of Pharmacology and Toxicology, Medical College of Virginia, Commonwealth University, Richmond, Virginia 23298-0613.

not surprising that the ability to perform certain tasks would be compromised in some individuals following marijuana smoking. There is little dispute that high doses of marijuana can disrupt performance when the task is difficult. Cannabinoid-induced impairment of flying and driving has been documented. As might be expected, the effects of marijuana on performance become more variable as the complexity of the task is simplified and the dose of marijuana is reduced. In a recent review, Chait and Pierri (4) concluded that marijuana, at doses that produce moderate levels of intoxication, can affect a wide range of learned and unlearned behaviors, including simple motor tasks and more complex psychomotor and cognitive tasks. Their evaluation of the literature indicated that although marijuana adversely affects gross and simple motor function (body sway and hand tremor) and psychomotor behaviors (rotary pursuit, Digit Symbol Substitution Test, reaction time, accuracy in divided attention tasks, and sustained attention), it does not adversely affect simple reaction time and hand–eye coordination. Therefore, it is not surprising that motor impairment and diminution of cognition could easily lead to accidents and traffic fatalities and that accidents have been linked to abuse of marijuana.

There are factors that confound the interpretation of marijuana-induced impairment, such as co-abuse with other agents, individual variability, development of tolerance, and the normal difficulties associated with a systematic evaluation conducted in the general population. For the above reasons, it has been difficult to assess the consequences of millions of individuals smoking marijuana in terms of personal injury, lost productivity, and so on. Although it is indisputable that tolerance develops during chronic exposure to high quantities of Δ^9-tetrahydrocannabinol (Δ^9-THC), it is certainly less definitive following intermittent exposure to marijuana (20). As for motor performance, cannabis intoxication of experienced abusers may be difficult to detect except in difficult performance tasks or for those tasks in which they have had little previous training (4). On the other hand, cannabis intoxication in an inexperienced individual can be readily detectable on some performance measures. The other complicating factor in assessing marijuana effects on function is that marijuana is frequently co-abused with other drugs, such as alcohol, that are likely to augment its effects (20). Perez-Reyes et al. (46) reported that ethanol dose-dependent decrements in performance skill necessary for automobile driving were further exacerbated by marijuana. Needless to say, establishing a direct correlation between the degree of impairment and blood concentrations of cannabinoids would be of tremendous benefit in establishing causality in accidents. Given the individual sensitivity to marijuana and the confounding factors discussed above, it not likely that measures of Δ^9-THC or its major metabolites in either blood or urine will become standards for intoxication.

Memory and Learning

There is lack of consensus regarding the effects of Δ^9-THC on memory and learning in that results are often inconsistent and test specific (4,51). THC appears to produce its greatest decrement in free recall or short-term memory, and it has been proposed that chronic marijuana use in adolescents may result in long-term memory impairment (51). There are also indications that individuals with learning disabilities may be more susceptible to memory deficits (51). Almost all studies have shown that marijuana has no effect on retrieval of already-learned material. THC reliably alters the perception of time, with subjects overestimating elapsed time or experiencing an increase in the subjective rate of time (4).

Psychiatric Disorders

The relationship between marijuana use and mental illness has always received attention because of the frequency of drug use in individuals with psychological disorders. Despite suggestions that marijuana induces several psychopathological states (42), a ''cannabis psychosis'' has not been successfully characterized. It is certainly not surprising that marijuana exacerbates preexisting mental disorders. The detrimental effects of marijuana in schizophrenics are widely recognized, and a significant proportion of these individuals continue to ''self-medicate'' with marijuana even after recognizing its negative effects (43). Schizophrenics abusing marijuana have been reported to be more difficult to treat effectively, or their symptoms worsen even when appropriate neuroleptic levels were maintained. The question of the causal relationship between abuse of marijuana and the development of schizophrenia has not been established, although some investigators believe that marijuana use is a causative factor

(1,43). It has been pointed out that individuals abusing marijuana who also develop psychiatric problems suffer from rapid-onset schizophrenia (1). A systematic study will be required in order to establish the relative risk of developing psychiatric problems in marijuana abusers. Until proven otherwise, the risk appears to be relatively small given the widespread abuse of marijuana in the general population.

Central Nervous System Physiology

One of the most notable findings in recent years has been the effects of cannabinoids on cerebral blood flow and electroencephalographic measures. Mathew and Wilson (34) summarized the recent literature and concluded that marijuana smoking increased cerebral blood flow, with the greatest increases in the frontal region and right hemisphere. Marijuana also increases cerebral artery velocity, which is thought to be due to increased capillary perfusion. There is continued interest in the effects of marijuana on EEG. Struve et al. (53) reported that THC produced an increase in absolute power of all frequencies over all cortical areas.

Reproduction

The effects of marijuana and cannabinoids on hormonal functions in laboratory animals and humans during pregnancy were reviewed in the last edition and has been updated recently by Wenger et al. (60). Reproduction studies in both animals and humans have produced conflicting results and widely varying conclusions, which may be due in great part to a combination of differences in experimental design and interspecies differences in drug tolerance (60). However, Δ^9-THC has been described as a reproductive toxicant in both humans and animals in various studies. In animal studies, THC produces adverse effects on gametogenesis, embryogenesis, and postnatal development (55). Earlier conclusions that marijuana may be linked to infertility were based on (a) reductions in sperm concentrations following administration of 4–16 marijuana joints per week for a 4-week period and (b) oligospermia with Leydig and Sertoli cell dysfunction. Wenger (60) concluded that marijuana can produce reversible and irreversible effects on the reproductive system of both sexes. Marijuana attenuation of luteinizing hormone has been well documented in females (38) and males (57). It is still unclear whether marijuana has direct toxic effects on the embryo and fetus.

Adverse Consequences

Our understanding of the potential adverse consequences of marijuana has remained largely unchanged from that presented in the last edition. There are always reasons to be concerned about drug abuse during pregnancy and in adolescents. The dangers of inhalation of foreign substances have been well documented. Concern regarding the pathophysiology of marijuana on these and other organ systems has been expressed by several investigators (42). However, little new information regarding specific detrimental effects of marijuana has appeared in the past few years.

CHEMISTRY

Although the chemistry of marijuana has been well-characterized for many years, interest in the levels of Δ^9-THC continues to increase. Evaluation of confiscated material indicates that the average Δ^9-THC content in marijuana has remained relatively stable during the past 10–15 years. However, occasional samples containing as much as 15% Δ^9-THC have been seized. What impact this variation in THC content has had on marijuana abuse pattern is uncertain.

The development of highly potent cannabinoid agonists has lagged behind the progress made for many other centrally acting agents. Fortunately, potent cannabinoid agonists have begun to emerge and indeed have played key roles in recent advances regarding cannabinoid pharmacology. The research group at Pfizer embarked on a synthetic strategy that resulted in novel bicyclic structures that proved to be 4–25 times more potent than Δ^9-THC, depending upon the pharmacological measure (5). The success of Johnson and Melvin (24) not only helped redefine many of the structural determinants of cannabinoid action, it also resulted in novel bi- and tricyclic analogues that are as much as 700 times more potent than Δ^9-THC (28). A second group of compounds with potent agonists properties has also been developed. Mechoulam et al. (36) prepared 11-OH-Δ^8-THC-DMH (Fig. 1) that, as they had predicted, proved to be several hundred times more potent than Δ^8-THC in several behavioral tests (29). The corresponding 11-OH-Δ^9-THC-DMH also exhibited similar high potency (33). Equally important was the preparation of highly pure enantiomers of 11-OH-Δ^8-THC-DMH. These enantiomers were used to finally establish that cannabinoids indeed exhibit high enantioselectivity (36). Findings of high potency and high enantioselectivity reinforced the notion that cannabinoids are acting through receptor mechanisms.

A future challenge is to develop a competitive cannabinoid antagonist. If the indications that cannabinoids are interacting with a specific receptor are correct, then it should be possible to synthesize an antagonist that interferes with cannabinoid–receptor interactions. Despite years of effort, such an antagonist has not yet emerged. The availability of antagonists would greatly aid in exploring the biochemical processes responsible for canna-

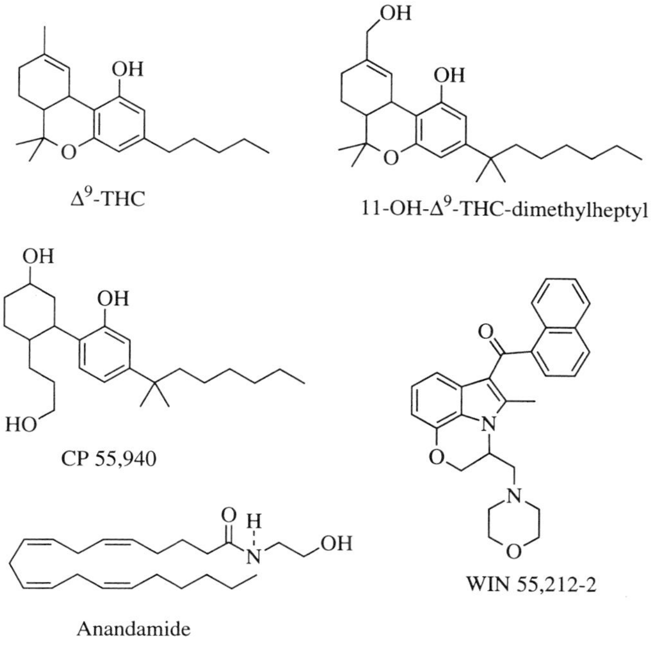

FIG. 1. Structures of Δ^9-THC, potent analogues, and the putative endogenous ligand.

binoid pharmacological effects. The other major goal of the chemist and pharmacologist is to develop therapeutically useful cannabinoids that are devoid of unwarranted side effects.

CANNABINOID RECEPTORS

The development of potent cannabinoids, such as CP-55,940, provided new opportunities to explore cannabinoid receptors (37). Indeed, it was not until the potent analgesic CP-55,940 was radiolabeled and used as the ligand that a specific saturable cannabinoid binding site was shown to exist (7). Behaviorally active cannabinoids, including Δ^9-THC, exhibit high affinity for this site, lending credence to its being the cannabinoid receptor. Subsequently, this receptor has been characterized using other radiolabeled ligands such as ^{3}H-11-OH-Δ^9-THC-DMH, ^{3}H-WIN 55212-2, and ^{3}H-11-OH-hexahydro-THC-DMH. Δ^9-THC has been reported to compete with these ligands, with K_I values in the range of 1–40 nM. Although there are subtle differences in the binding characteristics of these various ligands, they all appear to be binding to the same site in a similar fashion. It has now been well established that there is an excellent correlation between the pharmacological potency of cannabinoids and their affinity for this binding site. The most extensive study has been conducted by Compton et al. (6), who demonstrated that the binding affinities of 60 cannabinoids were consistent with the pharmacological potencies of these agents in numerous pharmacological assays in mice and rats. Their findings suggested that this single receptor type could account for all of the behavioral and pharmacological effects of the cannabinoids. Similarly, computer modeling studies indicate that a single pharmacophore could accommodate all of the agents that interact at this cannabinoid site (54). Although it is reasonable to speculate that multiple cannabinoid receptors might exist, evidence has not yet been forthcoming.

A key issue for any receptor is that it exhibits selectivity for a given class of compounds. This point is particularly important for the cannabinoids in that they have been shown to share numerous pharmacological properties with neurotransmitters and other centrally acting agents (9,31). Howlett et al. (22) have examined an impressive array of centrally acting compounds and have found that the following agents do not compete for cannabinoid binding: adrenergic, dopaminergic, opioid, sigma, cholinergic, neuroleptics, GABAergic, serotonergic, hormones, steroids, amino acids, peptides, nonsteroidal antiinflammatory agents, arachidonic acid and metabolites, prostaglandins, and leukotrienes, as well as numerous other agents.

The anatomical distribution of the receptor throughout the brain, as well as the localization within the neuron, has been determined by autoradiography (19). The binding sites are densest in the basal ganglia (substantia nigra pars reticulata, globus pallidus, entopeduncular nucleus, and regions of the caudate-putamen) and cerebellum (molecular layer). Low levels of binding were observed in discrete brain regions, including the brainstem (medulla and pons), thalamic nuclei, hypothalamus, corpus callosum, and the deep nuclear layer of the cerebellum. Intermediate levels of binding were seen in layers I and VI of the cortex, as well as in the dentate gyrus and CA pyramidal cell regions of the hippocampus.

The discrete distribution of receptors throughout the brain can provide some insight into their functional significance. High receptor densities in the extrapyramidal motor system and the cerebellum are consistent with the actions of cannabinoids on many forms of movement. The hippocampal formation is also a brain region demonstrating relatively dense binding of cannabinoids. The hippocampus has been shown to be a brain region involved in coding sensory information and storing memory. Importantly, Δ^9-THC has been shown to disrupt short-term memory in humans, as discussed earlier. Therefore, the effects of cannabinoids on cognition and memory may be due to the relatively dense receptors in the hippocampus and cortex. The presence of cannabinoid receptors in the ventromedial striatum and nucleus accumbens suggests an association with dopamine neurons, which have been hypothesized to mediate brain reward (15). Δ^9-THC has been shown to augment self-administered electrical stimulation in the rat medial forebrain bundle and to enhance both potassium-stimulated presynaptic dopamine efflux in rat neostriatum and presynaptic basal dopamine efflux

in the nucleus accumbens of freely moving rats. Despite the rather low density of receptors in the hypothalamus, cannabinoids produce hypothermia in mice when given intravenously (28), after intracerebroventricular administration, or when administered directly into the preoptic area (13). Lastly, the low density of cannabinoid receptors in medullary nuclei would be expected given that there are almost no reports of marijuana producing fatal overdoses in humans.

Convincing evidence for a cannabinoid receptor was provided by cloning experiments of Matsuda et al. (35). These investigators isolated a clone from a rat brain library that had a high degree of homology with other G-protein-coupled receptors. This receptor gained "orphan" status when all of the traditional agonists of G-protein-coupled receptors failed to interact with it. However, discovery that the distribution of mRNA of the clone paralleled that of the cannabinoid receptor, as reported by Herkenham et al. (19), led them to speculate that they had cloned the cannabinoid receptor. When cells were transfected with this clone, CP-55,940, Δ^9-THC, and other psychoactive cannabinoids were able to inhibit adenylyl cyclase, whereas untransfected cells were nonresponsive. The human cannabinoid receptor was subsequently cloned (17). The cannabinoid receptor appears to be part of a G-protein-coupled receptor subfamily that also includes the adrenocorticotropin and melanotropin receptors (39). Knowledge of the structure of the cannabinoid receptor provides the opportunity to study its interactions with both ligands and second messenger systems. More importantly, it demonstrates that the cannabinoid receptor is a constituent of the brain that undoubtedly plays an important functional role.

All evidence points to the brain cannabinoid receptor as being coupled to G proteins. Ligand binding at the cannabinoid receptor was found to be reduced by the nonhydrolyzable guanine nucleotide analogue Gpp(NH)p (7). The most likely candidate for a second messenger system is adenylyl cyclase (21). Numerous laboratories have demonstrated that cannabinoids inhibit adenylyl cyclase both in vivo and in vitro, most likely by interaction with G_i. However, it does not appear that the effects of cannabinoids are confined to adenylyl cyclase. Electrophysiological studies in neuroblastoma cells indicate that cannabinoids inhibit an omega-conotoxin-sensitive, high-voltage-activated calcium channel, an effect that is blocked by the administration of pertussis toxin and is independent of the formation of cAMP (30). It was hypothesized that N-type calcium channels were affected because the L-type calcium channel blocker, nitrendipine, failed to alter the effect of the cannabinoids. It has also been reported recently that calcium influx stimulates the release of an endogenous factor that displaces cannabinoid binding (11) (see Chapters 11, 27, and 38, *this volume*, for related topics).

Although multiple cannabinoid receptors have not been

identified in the brain, a peripheral receptor has been identified that is structurally different from the brain receptor (40). This cloned receptor is expressed in macrophages in the marginal zone of the spleen. It is too early to determine what functional role it may play in the spleen. The limited pharmacological analysis conducted to date suggests that it is indeed different from the brain receptor. The discovery of this cannabinoid receptor in the spleen raises the possibility that other receptor subtypes with entirely unique functional roles may exist.

PUTATIVE ENDOGENOUS LIGANDS

Devane et al. (8) postulated that an endogenous cannabinoid ligand is likely to be a highly lipophilic agent, and therefore they undertook to isolate THC-like substances from lipid extracts of porcine brain. An ethanolamine derivative of arachidonic acid was isolated and found to bind to the cannabinoid receptor and to inhibit electrically stimulated contractions of smooth muscle much in the same fashion as Δ^9-THC. This compound has been named *anandamide* (Fig. 1). Studies with mice also indicate that anandamide shares some of the pharmacological effects of Δ^9-THC (14) and similarly inhibits adenylyl cyclase and N-type calcium channels (12). Because fatty acids are so plentiful, it is not unreasonable to predict that an entire family of anandamide-like compounds may exist. Indeed, Hanus et al. (18) have identified homo-γ-linolenylethanolamide and docosatetraenylethanolamide as constituents in porcine brain that also compete for cannabinoid receptor binding.

The future challenge is establishing the physiological role for the endogenous cannabinoids. Is anandamide a neurotransmitter or a neuromodulator? Does an entire cannabinoid family of amide derivatives of fatty acids exist, each of which has a distinct neurochemical role? If cannabinoids serve a normal physiological role, then what are the consequences of an imbalance in this system? Answers to these and related questions will likely provide an entirely new perspective on the way we view cannabinoids (see also Chapter 53, *this volume*).

NEUROCHEMICAL INTERACTIONS

The interactions of cannabinoids with central neurotransmitters and neuromodulators has been reviewed recently by Pertwee (47), who pointed out that although there is a well-established cannabinoid interaction with these systems, the nature of the interactions is less well defined. The cholinergic nervous system appears to be involved in the production of cannabinoid-induced catalepsy in that cholinergic agonists will potentiate this effect, whereas antagonists will attenuate it. The cholinergic system is not involved in all of the actions of the cannabinoids in that cholinergic antagonists fail to alter the

discriminative stimulus of Δ^9-THC. The cholinergic system also does not appear to be involved in the antinociceptive effects of Δ^9-THC. Efforts to characterize a role for the cholinergic system in the production of cannabinoid-induced hypothermia have been somewhat equivocal.

Considerable interest has been directed toward the interactions between cannabinoids and dopamine and norepinephrine. One measure of motor function that has received considerable attention has been cannabinoid-induced catalepsy. Numerous laboratories have demonstrated that agents that stimulate the dopaminergic system attenuate cannabinoid-induced catalepsy, whereas dopamine antagonists enhance catalepsy. The adrenergic system has been implicated in the antinociceptive effects of cannabinoids. For example, the α_2 antagonist yohimbine administered intrathecally will block cannabinoid antinociception (26). As mentioned earlier, Gardner (15) summarized the findings of cannabinoids on brain reward. He and his colleagues have previously shown that cannabinoids do enhance brain-stimulating reward in the Lewis rat. A strong argument was made that Δ^9-THC enhances both basal and potassium-stimulated extracellular dopamine efflux in brain loci involved in reward mechanisms.

There are relatively few studies implicating the serotonergic system in the actions of the cannabinoids. As Pertwee notes (47), consistent results have not emerged from studies characterizing the influence of serotonergic agonists and antagonists on cannabinoid-induced hypothermia. On the other hand, there are numerous results suggesting that activation of the serotonergic system enhances, whereas serotonergic antagonists attenuate, the cataleptic effects of the cannabinoids. Spinally administered methysergide has no effect on Δ^9-THC-induced antinociception (26).

Several lines of research suggest a link between GABAergic compounds and cannabinoids. First, Δ^9-THC acts synergistically with both $GABA_A$ (muscimol) and $GABA_B$ [(−)-baclofen] agonists in producing catalepsy (48). Additionally, benzodiazepines, which facilitate GABA interaction with $GABA_A$ receptors, act synergistically with Δ^9-THC in producing catalepsy, which can be blocked by flumazenil. Studies from our own laboratory have shown that cannabinoids that exhibit anxiogenic properties (increased aversion to open arms of the elevated plus maze) can be blocked by either diazepam or flumazenil (44). Furthermore, there are reports of partial generalization by diazepam to the THC discriminative cue and a report of cannabinoids influencing benzodiazepine receptor binding. Childer and coworkers (32) have found that $GABA_B$ receptor agonists and cannabinoids decrease cAMP levels in cerebellar granule cells in a nonadditive fashion, whereas they act in an additive fashion in stimulating GTPase in cerebellar membranes. They interpreted these findings as a case of receptor convergence in which both classes of drugs share common adenylyl cyclase catalytic units without sharing common G proteins.

The observations that cannabinoids and opioids exhibit several similar pharmacological properties has prompted speculation that they share a common mechanism of action. There are indications that opioids and cannabinoids may produce some cross-tolerance in selected tests; however, the data are far from conclusive. The cannabinoids, like the opioids, produce antinociception and analgesia. Human subjects receiving oral doses of 10 and 20 mg/kg Δ^9-THC exhibited analgesia comparable to that of codeine, and they suffered a significant degree of undesirable side effects. Intravenous administration of Δ^9-THC to human dental patients produced analgesia that was accompanied by dysphoria and anxiety. Animal studies have also revealed spinal and supraspinal antinociception. Several potent cannabinoid analogues have been shown to produce antinociceptive effects upon intrathecal (i.t.) administration to rats and dogs. Studies conducted in mice and rats also indicate that the cannabinoid-induced antinociceptive effects are mediated at both spinal and supraspinal sites (27,59).

The localization of cannabinoid receptors allow for an interaction with the opioid system. The binding of CP-55,940 has been shown to be dense in the striatum (19), an area associated with dense binding of the opioids. Although cannabinoid receptors are relatively sparse in the medulla, there are moderate concentrations in the periaqueductal gray, a structure that contains high concentrations of opioid receptors and plays an important role in analgesia. Binding of CP-55,940 in the substantia gelatinosa of the spinal cord has been shown, although it is rather low (19). Nonetheless, it is much higher than the binding in the dorsal horn of the spinal cord of substance P, a major transmitter involved with pain processing in the spinal cord. The substantia gelatinosa is also the principal binding site of the opioids in the dorsal horn and is the major site of the processing of pain signals for transmission to the spinothalamic tract.

Although there have been a few suggestions that opioid antagonists such as naloxone can block the antinociceptive effects of cannabinoids, most of the studies have failed to support such a contention. Indeed, no studies have demonstrated that cannabinoids and opioids have high affinity for each other's receptor (56). It has been shown that the antinociceptive effect of Δ^9-THC and morphine are additive following intravenous (i.v.) administration, thus implying distinct mechanisms of action (16). Recently, Welch (58) published the intriguing observation that cannabinoid antinociception was blocked by the κ opioid antagonist, nor-binaltorphimine (nor-BNI). The δ antagonist, ICI 174,864 (10 μg/mouse, administered i.t.), failed to block the effects of any of the cannabinoids administered i.v. Moreover, the nor-BNI blockade of the Δ^9-THC (i.t.) antinociception was specific for antinociception and did not block catalepsy, hypothermia, or hypoactivity (52). The lack of naloxone blockade of the cannabinoid-induced antinociception leads to the question

of opioid involvement in the effects of nor-BNI. To date, all κ-opioid antinociceptive effects are blocked by naloxone, albeit at high doses of naloxone. In addition, κ-opioid binding has been shown to remain unaltered by cannabinoids (56), and cannabinoid binding in the brain is not displaced by nor-BNI or the κ agonist, U50,488H (58). Thus, the exact nature of the nor-BNI blockade is not known.

Enkephalinergic neurons are shown to synapse on dopaminergic neurons in the nucleus accumbens, the site proposed to modulate the reward system for all addicting drugs (15). The cannabinoids appear to interact with opioids allosterically, either presynaptically on the enkephalinergic neuron or with the opioid receptor on the dopaminergic neuron to enhance reinforcing effects. Although there are numerous distinct differences in their mechanisms of action, opioid–cannabinoid interactions cannot be ruled out.

A great deal of information has been generated regarding the actions of cannabinoids on prostaglandin synthesis, a topic that has been recently reviewed by Burstein (3). As pointed out by Burstein, interest initially arose because these two classes of compounds share some similar pharmacological properties, namely, analgesia and hypothermia. Additionally, discovery of abundant quantities of arachidonic acid and prostaglandins in the central nervous system led to speculation that they may play a role in normal brain function. Several investigators have shown that blockers of prostaglandin formation, such as aspirin and indomethacin, attenuate the antinociceptive, cataleptic, and hypotensive effects of Δ^9-THC (3). More recently, similar findings have been reported to occur in humans (45), where selected behavioral effects of the cannabinoids were blocked by indomethacin. Immunization of mice against PGE_2 led to reduced responsiveness to cannabinoids (23), and administration of Δ^9-THC produced a rise in levels of PGE_2 and $PGF_{2\alpha}$ (2). Despite these indications that eicosanoids are involved in the actions of the cannabinoids, defining a precise role for them has not been possible. Needless to say, the discovery of an arachidonic acid metabolite as a putative endogenous cannabinoid intensifies interest in this area.

The influence of cannabinoids on the adrenal–pituitary has been reviewed by Eldridge and Landfield (10), who point out that the Δ^9-THC-induced release of glucocorticoids is most likely regulated by central mechanisms. Although marijuana is typically perceived as reducing anxiety, it has been reported to have anxiogenic properties that are probably dependent upon the environmental situation and individual reaction to marijuana. Interest has been revived in the possible interaction between glucocorticoids and cannabinoids because of the observations that chronic administration of Δ^9-THC to rats resulted in aging-like degenerative changes in the hippocampus that strongly resembled that produced by either stress or elevated glucocorticoid secretion. These authors suggest that cannabinoids either produce glucocorticoid agonist effects or inhibit the negative feedback control that produces enhanced output of adrenocorticol steroids.

POTENTIAL THERAPEUTIC USES

Although the above-mentioned analogues have proven to be extremely valuable as receptor probes in laboratory studies, none has emerged as clinically useful agents. The lack of pharmacological specificity remains as a major impediment to the therapeutic use of cannabinoids, as discussed later. The primary cannabinoid that is used clinically is Δ^9-THC itself, which has been given the generic name *dronabinol.*

There has been considerable interest in the therapeutic potential of cannabinoids for several reasons. First, there have always been folklore and anecdotal reports of cannabis treatment for a wide range of disorders. Some of the more likely therapeutic uses include treatment of pain, convulsions, glaucoma, muscle spasticity, bronchial asthma, loss of appetite, nausea, and vomiting (20). Second, cannabinoids most likely represent a distinctively different means of therapy because they differ from the agents traditionally used to treat these disorders. This latter point is important from the standpoint that new strategies are crucial for treating patients who are unresponsive to current therapy or who suffer severe side effects.

There have been impassioned pleas on both sides of the argument as to the merits of using Δ^9-THC and marijuana as therapeutic agents. There are those who argue that marijuana is a highly efficacious agent without serious side effects, whereas others contend that marijuana and Δ^9-THC lack sufficient efficacy to warrant therapeutic use and that they are highly dangerous substances. There may be a bit of truth in both sides of this argument. It is a well-known fact that development of abused substances for medical uses has far more hurdles to overcome than other medications. Until the mid-1980s, Δ^9-THC was a Schedule I drug—in other words, an abused substance without any medical use—but was reclassified as a Schedule II drug. Δ^9-THC was formulated in sesame oil, given the name *dronabinol* and marketed as Marinol (Roxane Laboratories, Columbus, OH).

Nausea and Vomiting

The indication studied most extensively has been nausea and vomiting. It is generally thought that marijuana, Δ^9-THC, and some analogues (nabilone and levonantradol) are effective in managing chemotherapy-induced vomiting (25). In 1987, Δ^9-THC (dronabinol) was introduced in the United States for use as an antiemetic in patients suffering from nausea and vomiting induced by cancer chemotherapy and who were refractory to the usual antiemetic drugs. Although it is less certain that Δ^9-THC is effective in patients refractory to other treatments, it has proven to be a useful antiemetic. More recently, marijuana has been used by AIDS victims to block the nausea of chemotherapy and to stimulate their appetite. The FDA has granted orphan status to Δ^9-THC for stimulating appetite and preventing weight loss in AIDS patients. Clinical trials with dronabinol in AIDS patients have suggested improved appetite at a dose that was tolerated during chronic administration (49). However, it would appear that sanctioning the use of marijuana and Δ^9-THC for appetite stimulation was based more on political expediency than on sound scientific principles. Even though there is a lack of conclusive evidence that Δ^9-THC adversely effects the immune system in healthy adults, there is a wealth of information demonstrating cannabinoid-induced alterations in the immune system in laboratory animals (41). It should be obvious that AIDS patients are at a higher risk than the normal population to potentially immunosuppressive drugs. With the development of any therapeutic agent, the next required step is evaluation of the drug in the targeted population for both efficacy and adverse effects.

Analgesia

Cannabinoids are potent antinociceptive agents in laboratory animal models, as indicated in the above description of cannabinoid-opioid interactions. However, cannabinoid analgesia can only be elicited at doses producing other behavioral side effects, and these agents are no more potent than the more commonly used opioid analgesics; a goal has been to develop therapeutically useful cannabinoids with significantly fewer undesirable side effects (50). There is ample evidence thus far that cannabinoids can be highly potent antinociceptive agents. Most studies also demonstrate that the production of antinociception is usually accompanied by catalepsy and hypothermia as well as sedation. The pharmacological profile of these drugs and their diversity of effects may indicate that multiple mechanisms of action are involved. In addition, the pharmacological profile and the known mechanisms of action of the cannabinoids appear to be distinguishable from other antinociceptive agents. Thus, these drugs may work via a unique mechanism for controlling pain. The results with *nor*-BNI blockade of cannabinoid-induced antinociception are important because the other behaviors of cannabinoids were not affected. The use of *nor*-BNI may prove to be a useful tool in the delineation of the mechanism of the antinociceptive effects of the cannabinoids.

SUMMARY

The recreational use of marijuana and our understanding of its health consequences have largely remained unchanged from that described in the last edition. Although there is a downward trend in use, a large segment of the population is still abusing this drug. Consistent use of high quantities of marijuana has a detrimental effect on social and interpersonal skills and likely impedes the normal development of young individuals. The adverse consequences of infrequent use of marijuana are less clearly defined. Concerns remain regarding marijuana-induced pulmonary damage and possible lung cancer. Despite the absence of definitive studies demonstrating a direct role of marijuana in producing detrimental effects on reproduction and development, there is sufficient evidence to discourage marijuana use during pregnancy. As for long-term effects induced by marijuana, reports of other pathophysiological disorders have been described in selected groups of individuals but have not been confirmed in the general population.

The therapeutic potential of cannabinoids continues to attract interest. Unfortunately, synthetic analogues have not emerged that are devoid of cannabinoid behavioral effects. Drug development strategy is to avoid agents that produce a wide spectrum of effects, even if they are not severely toxic to the patient. With the advent of potent new cannabinoid derivatives, it may be possible in the near future to develop cannabinoids that lack undesirable side effects.

Tremendous progress has been made in the past 5 years regarding our understanding of the mechanism of action of cannabinoids. A cannabinoid receptor has been characterized using traditional in vitro binding methodology, and its distribution has been mapped throughout the central nervous system. This receptor has also been cloned and appears to be a member of G-protein-associated receptors. Moreover, a putative endogenous ligand, anandamide, has been identified from porcine brain that appears to share most of the pharmacological properties of Δ^9-THC. We hope that our understanding of the cannabinoid system in the brain will continue to grow in an exponential fashion.

ACKNOWLEDGMENT

Preparation of his chapter was supported in part by National Institute on Drug Abuse grant DA-03672.

REFERENCES

1. Allebeck P. Schizophrenia and cannabis: cause–effect relationship? In: Nahas GG, Latour C, eds. *Cannabis: physiopathology, epidemiology, detection.* Boca Raton, FL: CRC Press, 1993;113–117.
2. Bhattacharya SK. Δ^9-Tetrahydrocannabinol increases brain prostaglandins in the rat. *Psychopharmacology* 1986;90:499.
3. Burstein S. Eicosanoids as mediators of cannabinoid action. In: Murphy L, and Bartke A, eds. *Marijuana/cannabinoids: neurobiology and neurophysiology.* Boca Raton, FL: CRC Press, 1992;73–91.
4. Chait LD, Pierri J. Effects of smoked marijuana on human performance: a critical review. In: Murphy L, Bartke A, eds. *Marijuana/*
cannabinoids: neurobiology and neurophysiology.* Boca Raton, FL. CRC Press, 1992;387–423.
5. Compton DR, Johnson MR, Melvin LS, Martin BR. Pharmacological profile of a series of bicyclic cannabinoid analogs: classification as cannabimimetic agents. *J Pharmacol Exp Ther* 1992; 260:201–209.
6. Compton DR, Rice KC, De Costa BR, et al. Cannabinoid structure–activity relationships: correlation of receptor binding and in vivo activities. *J Pharmacol Exp Ther* 1993;265:218–226.
7. Devane WA, Dysarz II, FA, Johnson MR, Melvin LS, Howlett AC. Determination and characterization of a cannabinoid receptor in rat brain. *Mol Pharmacol* 1988;34:605–613.
8. Devane WA, Hanus L, Breuer A, et al. Isolation and structure of a brain constituent that binds to the cannabinoid receptor. *Science* 1992;258:1946–1949.
9. Dewey WL. Cannabinoid pharmacology. *Pharmacol Rev* 1986;38: 151–178.
10. Eldridge JC, Landfield PW. Cannabinoid–glucocorticoid interactions in the hippocampal region of the brain. In: Murphy L, Bartke A, ed. *Marijuana/cannabinoids: neurobiology and neurophysiology.* Boca Raton, FL: CRC Press, 1992;93–117.
11. Evans DM, Johnson MR, Howlett AC. Ca^{2+}-dependent release from rat brain of a cannabinoid receptor binding activity. *J Neurochem* 1992;58:780–782.
12. Felder CC, Briley EM, Axelrod J, Simpson JT, Mackie K, Devane WA. Anandamide, an endogenous cannabimimetic eicosanoid, binds to the cloned human cannabinoid receptor and stimulates receptor-mediated signal transduction. *Proc Natl Acad Sci USA* 1993;90:7656–7660.
13. Fitton AG, Pertwee RG. Changes in body temperature and oxygen consumption rate of conscious mice produced by intrahypothalamic and intracerebroventricular injections of Δ^9-tetrahydrocannabinol. *Br J Pharmacol* 75:409–414.
14. Fride E, Mechoulam R. Pharmacological activity of the cannabinoid receptor agonist, anandamide, a brain constituent. *Eur J Pharmacol* 1993;231:313–314.
15. Gardner EL. Cannabinoid interaction with brain reward systems—the neurobiological basis of cannabinoid abuse. In: Murphy L, Bartke A, eds. *Marijuana/cannabinoids: neurobiology and neurophysiology.* Boca Raton, FL: CRC Press, 1992;275–335.
16. Gennings C, Carter J, WH, Martin BR. Response-surface analysis of morphine sulfate and Δ^9-tetrahydrocannabinol interaction in mice. In: Lange N, Ryan L, eds. *Case studies in biometry.* New York: John Wiley & Sons, [in press].
17. Gérard CM, Mollereau C, Vassart G, Parmentier M. Molecular cloning of a human cannabinoid receptor which is also expressed in testis. *Biochem J* 1991;279:129–134.
18. Hanus L, Gopher A, Almog S, Mechoulam R. Two new unsaturated fatty acid ethanolamides in brain that bind to the cannabinoid receptor. *J Med Chem* 1993;36:3032–3034.
19. Herkenham M, Lynn AB, Little MD, et al. Cannabinoid receptor localization in the brain. *Proc Natl Acad Sci USA* 1990;87:1932–1936.
20. Hollister LE. Health aspects of cannabis. *Pharmacol Rev* 1986;38:1–20.
21. Howlett AC, Bidaut-Russell M, Devane WA, Melvin LS, Johnson MR, Herkenham M. The cannabinoid receptor: biochemical, anatomical and behavioral characterization. *Trends Neurosci* 1990;13: 420–423.
22. Howlett AC, Evans DM, Houston DB. The cannabinoid receptor. In: Murphy L, Bartke A, eds. *Marijuana/cannabinoids: neurobiology and neurophysiology.* Boca Raton, FL: CRC Press, 1992; 35–72.
23. Hunter SA, Audette CA, Burstein S. Elevation of brain prostaglandin E_2 levels in rodents by Δ^1-THC. *Prostaglandins Leukot Essent Fatty Acids* 1991;43:185.
24. Johnson MR, Melvin LS. The discovery of nonclassical cannabinoid analgetics. In: Mechoulam R, ed. *Cannabinoids as therapeutic agents.* Boca Raton, FL: CRC Press, 1986;121–144.
25. Levitt M. Cannabinoids as antiemetics in cancer chemotherapy. In: Mechoulam R, ed. *Cannabinoids as therapeutic agents.* Boca Raton, FL: CRC Press, 1986;71–103.
26. Lichtman AH, Martin BR. Cannabinoid induced antinociception

is mediated by a spinal α_2 noradrenergic mechanism. *Brain Res* 1991;559:309–314.

27. Lichtman AH, Martin BR. Spinal and supraspinal mechanisms of cannabinoid-induced antinociception. *J Pharmacol Exp Ther* 1991; 258:517–523.
28. Little PJ, Compton DR, Johnson MR, Melvin LS, Martin BR. Pharmacology and stereoselectivity of structurally novel cannabinoids in mice. *J Pharmacol Exp Ther* 1988;247:1046–1051.
29. Little PJ, Compton DR, Mechoulam R, Martin BR. Stereochemical effects of 11-OH-dimethylheptyl-Δ^8-tetrahydrocannabinol. *Pharmacol Biochem Behav* 32:661–666.
30. Mackie K, Hille B. Cannabinoids inhibit N-type calcium channels in neuroblastoma-glioma cells. *Proc Natl Acad Sci USA* 1992;89:3825–3829.
31. Martin BR. Cellular effects of cannabinoids. *Pharmacol Rev* 1986;38:45–74.
32. Martin BR, Cabral G, Childers SR, Deadwyler S, Mechoulam R, Reggio P. International Cannabis Research Society meeting summary, Keystone, CO (June 19–20, 1992). *Drug Alcohol Depend* 1993;31:219–227.
33. Martin BR, Compton DR, Thomas BF, et al. Behavioral, biochemical, and molecular modeling evaluations of cannabinoid analogs. *Pharmacol Biochem Behav* 1991;40:471–478.
34. Mathew RJ, Wilson WH. The effects of marijuana on cerebral blood flow and metabolism. In: Murphy L, Bartke A, eds. *Marijuana/cannabinoids: neurobiology and neurophysiology.* Boca Raton, FL: CRC Press, 1992;337–386.
35. Matsuda LA, Lolait SJ, Brownstein MJ, Young AC, Bonner TI. Structure of a cannabinoid receptor and functional expression of the cloned cDNA. *Nature* 1990;346:561–564.
36. Mechoulam R, Feigenbaum JJ, Lander N, et al. Enantiomeric cannabinoids: stereospecificity of psychotropic activity. *Experientia* 1988;44:762–764.
37. Melvin LS, Johnson MR. Structure–activity relationships of tricyclic and nonclassical bicyclic cannabinoids. In: Rapaka RS, Makriyannis A, eds. *Structure–activity relationships of the cannabinoids.* Washington, DC: U.S. Government Printing Office, 1987;31–47.
38. Mendelson JH, Mello NK, Ellingboe J, Skupny AS, Lex BW, Griffin M. Marijuana smoking suppresses luteinizing hormone in women. *J Pharmacol Exp Ther* 1986;237:862–866.
39. Mountjoy KG, Robbins LS, Mortrud MT, and Cone RD. The cloning of a family of genes that encode the melanocortin receptors. *Science* 1992;257:1248–1251.
40. Munro S, Thomas KL, Abu-Shaar M. Molecular characterization of a peripheral receptor for cannabinoids. *Nature* 1993;365:61–64.
41. Munson AE, Fehr KO. Immunological effects of cannabis. In: Fehr KO, Kalant H, eds. *Cannabis and health hazards. Proceedings of an ARF/WHO scientific meeting on adverse health and behavioral consequences of cannabis use.* Toronto: Addiction Research Foundation, 1983;257–354.
42. Nahas G. Historical outlook of the psychopathology of cannabis. In: Nahas GG, Latour C, eds. *Cannabis: physiopathology, epidemiology, detection.* Boca Raton, FL: CRC Press, 1993;95–99.
43. Negrete JC. Effects of cannabis on schizophrenia. In: Nahas GG, Latour C, eds. *Cannabis: physiopathology, epidemiology, detection.* Boca Raton, FL: CRC Press, 1993;105–112.
44. Onaivi ES, Green MR, Martin BR. Pharmacological characterization of cannabinoids in the elevated plus maze. *J Pharmacol Exp Ther* 1990;253:1002–1009.
45. Perez-Reyes M, Burstein SH, White WR, McDonald SA, Hicks RE. Antagonism of marihuana effects by indomethacin in humans. *Life Sci* 1991;48:507–515.
46. Perez-Reyes M, Hicks RE, Bumberry J, Jeffcoat AR, Cook CE. Interaction between marihuana and ethanol: effects on psychomotor performance. *Alcohol Clin Exp Res* 1988;12:268–276.
47. Pertwee R. In vivo interactions between psychotropic cannabinoids and other drugs involving central and peripheral neurochemical mediators. In: Murphy L, Bartke A, eds. *Marijuana/cannabinoids: neurobiology and neurophysiology.* Boca Raton, FL: CRC Press, 1992;165–218.
48. Pertwee RG, Greentree SG, Swift PA. Drugs which stimulate or facilitate central GABAergic transmission interact synergistically with Δ^9-tetrahydrocannabinol to produce marked catalepsy in mice. *Neuropharmacology* 1988;27:1265–1270.
49. Plasse TF, Gorter RW, Krasnow SH, Lane M, Shepard KV, Wadleigh RG. Recent clinical experience with Dronabinol. *Pharmacol Biochem Behav* 1991;40:695–700.
50. Razdan RK. Structure–activity relationships in cannabinoids. *Pharmacol Rev* 1986;38:75–149.
51. Schwartz RH. Chronic marihuana smoking and short-term memory impairment. In: Nahas GG, Latour C, eds. *Cannabis: physiopathology, epidemiology, detection.* Boca Raton, FL: CRC Press, 1993;61–71.
52. Smith PB, Welch SP, Martin BR. Interactions between Δ^9-tetrahydrocannabinol and kappa opioids in mice. *J Pharmacol Exp Ther* 1994;268:1381–1387.
53. Struve FA, Straumanis JJ, Patrick G, Price L. Topographic mapping of quantitative EEG variables in chronic heavy marihuana users: empirical findings with psychiatric patients. *Clin Electroencephalogr* 1989;20:6–23.
54. Thomas BF, Compton DR, Martin BR, Semus SF. Modeling the cannabinoid receptor: a three-dimensional quantitative structure–activity analysis. *Mol Pharmacol* 1991;40:656–665.
55. Tuchmann-Duplessis H. Effects of cannabis on reproduction. In: Nahas GG, Latour C, eds. *Cannabis: physiopathology, epidemiology, detection.* Boca Raton, FL: CRC Press, 1993;187–192.
56. Vaysse PJ, Gardner EL, Zukin RS. Modulation of rat brain opioid receptors by cannabinoids. *J Pharmacol Exp Ther* 1987;241:534–539.
57. Vescovi PP, Pedrazzoni M, Michelini M, Maninetti L, Bernardelli F, Passeri M. Chronic effects of marihuana smoking on luteinizing hormone, follicle-stimulating hormone and prolactin levels in human males. *Drug Alcohol Depend* 1992;30:59–62.
58. Welch SP. Blockade of cannabinoid-induced antinociception by nor-binaltorphimine, but not N,N-diallyl-tyrosine-Aib-phenylalanine-leucine, ICI 174,864 or naloxone in mice. *J Pharmacol Exp Ther* 1993;256:633–640.
59. Welch SP, Stevens DL. Antinociceptive activity of intrathecally administered cannabinoids alone, and in combination with morphine, in mice. *J Pharmacol Exp Ther* 1992;262:10–18.
60. Wenger T, Croix D, Tramu G, Leonardelli J. Effects of Δ^9-tetrahydrocannabinol on pregnancy, puberty, and the neuroendocrine system. In: Murphy L, Bartke A, eds. *Marijuana/cannabinoids: neurobiology and neurophysiology.* Boca Raton, FL: CRC Press, 1992;539–560.

Psychopharmacology: The Fourth Generation of Progress, edited by Floyd E. Bloom and David J. Kupfer. Raven Press, Ltd., New York 1995.

CHAPTER 151

Phencyclidine (PCP)

David A. Gorelick and Robert L. Balster

Phencyclidine (commonly known as PCP or "angel dust") is a synthetic arylcyclohexylamine with a complex and unusual pharmacology that has captured the interest of researchers, clinicians, recreational drug users, and illegal drug dealers alike. Although human therapeutic use in the United States has ended and illicit use has waned over the past decade, scientific interest remains high, focused on the use of PCP as a probe for certain neurotransmitter systems (see Chapter 7, *this volume*) and as a model for certain psychiatric disorders (see Chapter 101, *this volume*). This chapter selectively reviews the basic neuropharmacology of PCP and its animal and human psychopharmacology.

PCP was developed in the 1950s as an injectable anesthetic. Animal testing revealed its unusual "cataleptoid anesthetic" properties; that is, in addition to producing anesthesia and analgesia, it made animals tranquil and serene—hence its trade names Sernyl and Sernylan (2). Clinical testing as an anesthetic revealed disturbing behavioral side effects during postoperative emergence, including dysphoria, confusion, delirium, and psychosis (8,51,66). These side effects attracted the interest of psychiatric researchers, who viewed PCP as producing a model psychosis useful in understanding schizophrenia (29). Subanesthetic doses administered to normal volunteers produced many schizophrenia-like symptoms, whereas schizophrenic patients suffered exacerbation of their symptoms. This research stopped when clinical trials were terminated in 1965, although PCP was later marketed for a time as a veterinary anesthetic (86).

Illicit recreational use of PCP first appeared during the mid-1960s on the West Coast in the form of oral capsules (2,8,51,66). Its propensity for causing unpredictable dysphoric reactions gave PCP a bad street reputation, and

use waned. It was classified as a Schedule III controlled substance in 1970. By the mid-1970s, illicit use had increased again, both because it could be easily and cheaply synthesized from legally available precursor chemicals and because users began smoking the drug, allowing individual titration of dosage to better control effects. In response, PCP and several analogues were reclassified into Schedule II, and controls were placed on the distribution of precursor chemicals. To prevent diversion of legal supplies, PCP was withdrawn from veterinary use in the United States in 1978. The close analogue ketamine, which has similar pharmacological properties, remains a legally marketed dissociative anesthetic not regulated under the Controlled Substances Act.

Illicit PCP use peaked in the United States in 1979, when prevalence of lifetime use was around 14% among high school seniors and young adults 18–25 years old, and recent (past 30 days) use prevalence was 2.4% for high school seniors (31). By 1992, lifetime and recent use prevalence had declined to 2.4% and 0.6%, respectively, among high school seniors and to 2.0% and 0.2% among young adults 19–28 years old. However, daily use has remained relatively stable among high school seniors over the past decade (0.1–0.3% prevalence), and PCP remains an important drug of abuse in some metropolitan areas and among certain sociodemographic groups, either taken alone or together with other illicit drugs such as marijuana ("primos," "wac," "zoom") or cocaine ("space base," "space cadet," "tragic magic"). Most PCP users also use or abuse other illicit drugs and alcohol, complicating efforts to identify effects of PCP from studies of clinical populations (13,22,23). Pharmacokinetic and pharmacodynamic interactions between smoked PCP and other concurrently smoked drugs (e.g., marijuana) may also complicate interpretation of PCP effects in drug users (41).

CHEMISTRY

PCP and ketamine are arylcycloalkylamines, as are at least 20 identified PCP analogues and metabolites, some

D. A. Gorelick: Treatment Branch, National Institutes of Health, NIDA/Intramural Program Research Center, Baltimore, Maryland 21224.

R. L. Balster: Department of Pharmacology, Medical College of Virginia, Richmond, Virginia 23298.

of which are themselves psychoactive and sold as "designer drugs" (1,2). The structure–activity relationships among arylcycloalkylamines are well understood (38). As a lipophilic weak base, PCP readily crosses cell membranes and the blood–brain barrier, and its renal clearance is strongly dependent on urine pH (1,7).

Compounds that structurally differ from the arylcycloalkylamines, but share significant aspects of PCP's neuropharmacological and behavioral effects, have proven to be useful tools for exploring the neuropsychopharmacology of PCP. For example, the 1,3-substituted dioxolanes, etoxadrol and dexoxadrol, which produce a profile of effects nearly identical to that of PCP (2,3), have been very useful for studying stereoselectivity and for modeling the PCP pharmacophore (71). Dizocilpine (MK-801), a potent ligand for PCP sites of action in the brain, is used extensively as a selective probe for the PCP receptor (2,30).

The similarities in the cellular and pharmacological actions of PCP and sigma-agonist benzomorphans led to great confusion in the literature when it was discovered, using radioligand binding, that N-allylnormetazocine (NANM) bound with high affinity to a site in nervous tissue that was clearly not the same as the historical PCP/sigma receptor thought responsible for their shared pharmacology (30). Nonetheless, this site quickly came to be called a sigma receptor (56). There are now hundreds of drugs identified with high affinity for this site (77), including (+)-3-PPP, di-tolyl guanidine, and certain potential novel antipsychotics. There is also evidence for heterogeneity of sigma sites (77). It is increasingly clear that these high-affinity sigma sites are not responsible for the behavioral/psychological effects of PCP, and may not mediate the psychotomimetic effects of any drug class (30,47).

CELLULAR PHARMACOLOGY

PCP administration in animals has effects on a number of neurotransmitter systems, including dopaminergic agonist effects, complex actions on both nicotinic and muscarinic cholinergic systems, N-methyl-D-aspartate (NMDA) antagonist effects, and poorly understood interactions with noradrenergic and serotonergic neurotransmission (30). Determining which of these neuropharmacological effects are responsible for which of the pharmacological, behavioral, and psychological effects of PCP has been the subject of extensive investigation.

PCP acts as an indirect-acting dopaminergic agonist in many model systems (15,30). It remains unclear whether this is primarily an effect of PCP acting directly on sites within dopaminergic synapses or an indirect consequence of PCP activating presynaptic dopaminergic neurons, presumably through its primary actions at the NMDA receptor complex.

The best-characterized cellular action of PCP results from its interaction with a specific and unique binding site in neural tissues which satisfies many of the biochemical and pharmacological criteria for a physiologically relevant receptor (30,87). Because of the affinity of benzomorphan sigma-agonist opioids for this site, this "PCP receptor" was known for a time as the PCP/sigma receptor. Actions at this site are an important neural basis for the behavioral effects of PCP-like drugs (2,30). This conclusion is primarily based on the excellent concordance between binding site affinity and the potency and efficacy of arylcyclohexylamines and PCP-like drugs from other chemical classes for the production of PCP-like behavioral effects in animal studies.

The structure and physiological function of this PCP binding site have been clarified over the past decade. PCP has been identified as a noncompetitive NMDA antagonist probably acting as a channel blocker in the NMDA receptor complex. The previously identified PCP receptor is this site in the channel of the glutamate ionophore; there is an excellent correlation between the potencies of arylcyclohexylamines and other PCP-like drugs as NMDA antagonists and their activities at the PCP receptor site (35). In addition, there is a substantial overlap in the anatomical distribution of PCP and NMDA binding sites. The best evidence of a PCP-associated site on the NMDA receptor complex comes from expression cloning studies of NMDA receptor subunits that contain PCP-sensitive channels (46). By implication, this also suggests that NMDA antagonism probably plays an important role in producing the behavioral and psychological effects of PCP (82).

The explosion of knowledge in recent years regarding the neuropharmacology of glutamatergic receptors (see Chapters 7 and 101, this volume) and the structure, distribution, and function of the NMDA-receptor complex (35,45) has helped clarify many of the pharmacological actions of PCP-like drugs. The key features of the NMDA receptor complex that explain PCP pharmacology include the following: Glutamate activates the NMDA site, leading to the opening of cationic channels resulting in Ca^{2+} and Na^+ influx. Currents resulting from NMDA site activation are voltage-sensitive due to a block by Mg^{2+}, which is overcome when the neuron is sufficiently depolarized. Thus, the use dependency of NMDA receptors provides a means by which they may participate in neuroplasticity and in the destabilization of membranes during convulsions. Excessive Ca^{2+} flux resulting from NMDA receptor activation during neural injury also appears to play an important role in excitotoxicity.

Another important feature of the NMDA receptor is the large number of allosteric modulatory sites on the receptor complex. In addition to the PCP site in the channel that blocks ion flux, there is a well-characterized glycine co-agonist site. The presence of glycine facilitates channel opening by agonists at the NMDA site, and competitive antagonists at the glycine site can function as noncompetitive NMDA antagonists. There also appears to be a polyamine regulatory site. The development of drugs with selective agonist or antagonist actions at each of these sites has provided a means of studying the pharmacology of the NMDA receptor.

Endogenous PCP-like Compounds

During the 1980s, endogenous PCP-like activity was isolated from a variety of animal and human tissues, including cerebrospinal fluid (CSF), brain, and gastrointestinal (GI) tract (11). This activity was characterized as PCP-like because of its specific binding to PCP receptors and its ability to block NMDA-induced dopamine release in vitro. Initial attempts to isolate, purify, and identify the endogenous PCP-like ligand resulted in a small polypeptide. These results have never been convincingly replicated, so that the existence of an endogenous PCP-like compound remains uncertain.

BEHAVIORAL PHARMACOLOGY

PCP and other arylcyclohexylamines (such as ketamine) produce a unique profile of psychopharmacological effects (2) that may be conceptualized as having dopaminergic stimulant, depressant-like, and other unique components. (See also Chapters 64, 66, and 68, *this volume*, for related discussions.)

Stimulant Effects

PCP produces many amphetamine-like stimulant effects, particularly in rodent species, including sympathetic nervous system stimulation, increased locomotor activity, stereotyped behavior, ipsilateral rotation in substantia nigra-lesioned rats, suppression of plasma prolactin levels, increases in low rates of scheduled-controlled operant behavior, and enhancement of effects of amphetamine-like drugs (2). The locomotor effects, at least, are mediated by dopamine release in the nucleus accumbens (6,68), but this may be less a result of any direct PCP action at the dopamine synapse than of PCP's NMDA antagonist effects, which block NMDA receptors on dopaminergic VTA neurons (78). PCP itself has little affinity for postsynaptic dopamine receptors, but does have some affinity for the dopamine transporter through a low-affinity, PCP2 binding site (30,60). The discovery of a potent dopamine uptake inhibitor, BTCP, which is a structural analogue of PCP, lends support to the idea that PCP may exert some of its dopaminergic actions this way (44). On the other hand, PCP typically has a much higher in vitro affinity for the NMDA channel site ($K_i = 50-100$ nM) than it does for the dopamine transporter ($K_i \approx 0.1$ μM) (30). It is even less potent as a dopamine-releasing agent. Furthermore, some drugs, such as dizocilpine, which produce PCP-like dopaminergic behavioral effects, have little, if any, in vitro affinity for the dopamine transporter (58),

yet have high affinity for the PCP site on the NMDA receptor (30). This suggests that the dopaminergic effects of PCP-like drugs seen in vivo, and in many functional in vitro assays, may be secondary to NMDA antagonism (30). There are many studies showing functional interrelationships between glutamatergic and dopaminergic systems in brain (see Chapter 101, *this volume*). The cellular basis for the dopaminergic actions of PCP may be relevant to the possible relationship between PCP and schizophrenia, a question of considerable current research interest (6,15,18,78).

Depressant and Anxiolytic Effects

PCP produces many effects similar to those produced by classical depressant drugs, such as the barbiturates, benzodiazepines, and ethanol (2). These include motor incoordination and muscle relaxation, anticonvulsant effects, and enhancement of the toxic, anesthetic, and behavioral effects of depressant drugs. Although PCP's anesthetic effects might be included here, it is clear that the dissociative anesthesia produced by PCP-like drugs differs qualitatively from anesthesia produced by depressant drugs and volatile anesthetics.

Another depressant-like effect of PCP that has attracted recent interest is its activity in various animal models predictive of anxiolytic activity. PCP and related drugs such as ketamine and dizocilpine generally increase punished behaviors in rats and pigeons, although the magnitude and range of effective doses is typically less than is seen with benzodiazepines under comparable conditions (81), and antipunishment effects are not seen in squirrel monkeys (39). Dizocilpine is also active in a variety of nonpunishment procedures, as are other types of NMDA antagonists (81), suggesting (a) the possibility that NMDA antagonists may be developed as anxiolytics and (b) a possible role for the NMDA receptor in anxiety disorders.

Analgesic Effects

PCP and ketamine produce antinociceptive effects in a variety of animal tests through a nonopioid mechanism (17). The potency relationships among PCP-like drugs suggest that NMDA antagonism is the basis for their antinociceptive effects. This is consistent with the increasing evidence for a role for NMDA receptors in nociception. The poor separation of antinociceptive from other behavioral effects of PCP-like drugs suggests why they may not be clinically useful analgesics.

Effects on Sensorimotor Gating

PCP and other PCP-like NMDA antagonists produce deficits in sensorimotor gating in several animal models, deficits similar to those produced by dopaminergic agonists that are considered models for the analogous deficits found in schizophrenic patients (2). Evidence from brain lesion, drug interaction, and structure–activity studies suggests that PCP's effects in the pre-pulse inhibition of the startle model are mediated through its NMDA-antagonist actions (33).

Discriminative Stimulus Effects

In animal studies, PCP produces a unique profile of discriminative stimulus effects different from its stimulant and depressant effects (2,3). In animals trained to discriminate PCP or another PCP-like drug such as ketamine, drugs from other classes, including stimulants, depressants, and hallucinogens, fail to fully substitute (3). Despite numerous attempts, no drug has been found that consistently antagonizes PCP discrimination. This failure to obtain substitution or antagonism with selective agonists and antagonists for a large number of known receptor systems is an important basis for ruling out these systems as mediating PCP discrimination.

PCP- or ketamine-like discriminative stimulus effects are consistently produced by compounds with PCP-site-selective NMDA antagonist effects (2,3,82,83). The fact that all potent and selective NMDA channel blockers produce PCP or ketamine-like discriminative stimulus effects with a potency consistent with their affinity for the PCP site in the channel is strong support of the hypothesis that this blockade is an important neural mechanism for PCP discrimination (3). PCP-site NMDA channel blockers that have been tested in humans (NANM, dexoxadrol, dextrorphan, dizocilpine) tend to produce dysphoric psychological effects (3,47,73), and a number of arylcyclohexylamine analogues of PCP (TCP and PCE) have appeared as "designer drugs" of abuse. Taken together, these data support the hypothesis that the ability of drugs to produce PCP-like discriminative stimulus effects in animals is predictive of their potential to produce PCP-like subjective effects and abuse liability in humans and that this effect is the result of NMDA channel blockade.

Reinforcing Effects

PCP has reinforcing effects in all animal species in which it has been studied (2), a characteristic that distinguishes its behavioral pharmacology from that of classical hallucinogens. It appears that all NMDA channel blockers studied, including other arylcyclohexylamines, (+)-NANM, dizocilpine, dexoxadrol, and etoxadrol, have reinforcing effects (2,82,83). As with a number of other classes of drug reinforcers, the self-administration of PCP-like drugs by animals can be modified by changing food deprivation conditions, response requirements per injection, and the availability of alternative reinforcers

(2). The sensitivity of PCP self-administration to these and other variables suggests that animal studies can be used to explore the complex interactions between pharmacology and context that underlie individual differences in vulnerability to PCP abuse (9).

Tolerance and Dependence

Tolerance to the behavioral effects of PCP in animals has been shown in a number of studies (2). Generally, only two- to fourfold shifts in dose–effect curves are seen when moderate, behaviorally active doses are given repeatedly. This magnitude of tolerance is less than is generally seen with other classes of drugs of abuse, such as the opioids and sympathomimetic stimulants. Most tolerance is pharmacodynamic, rather than biodispositional, and learning plays an important role in the development and persistence of tolerance (2,80) and its situational specificity (67).

PCP can produce physical dependence in animal studies (2)—for example, in rhesus monkeys who self-administered very large daily doses. The excitatory discontinuation syndrome included tremors, oculomotor hyperactivity, bruxism, fearfulness, vocalizations, diarrhea, and, in some animals, emesis and convulsions. The time course of the syndrome corresponded to clearance of drug from the body. At lower, less behaviorally toxic doses, an easily observable withdrawal syndrome is not typically produced, but subtler changes in learned behavior following cessation of repeated PCP administration can be reliably demonstrated (2,10,80). There is some evidence for cross-dependence between PCP and other PCP-like NMDA antagonists, such as ketamine and (+)-NANM. The neural basis of dependence on PCP is not known. Studies of possible changes in PCP/NMDA receptor regulation with repeated dosing have yielded conflicting results (42,79).

Physical dependence on PCP may occur in some human chronic daily users, but is not common in psychologically dependent users presenting for drug abuse treatment, and has never been systematically studied in humans (2,22,23). Burn patients do show tolerance to the analgesic effects of ketamine, and up to fourfold tolerance to PCP's behavioral/psychological effects has been reported anecdotally in some abusers (1,8). No obvious PCP withdrawal syndrome has been reported in human users, although one group has described a possible discontinuation syndrome occurring within 1 day of drug cessation among outpatients who were daily users for at least 3 months (8). The syndrome included depression, anxiety, irritability, anergia, hypersomnia, increased appetite, poor memory, confused thoughts, and increased craving for PCP. Given the nonspecific nature of these symptoms, it remains unclear to what extent they represent a true drug-withdrawal syndrome.

Modification of Drug Tolerance and Dependence

PCP, or other PCP-like NMDA antagonists such as dizocilpine, given repeatedly in combination with other drugs of abuse, can block or reduce development of tolerance and dependence [e.g., to opioids (74)] and sensitization [e.g., to effects of amphetamines, cocaine, and nicotine (32,63)]. Competitive as well as noncompetitive NMDA antagonists are able to block tolerance development (72). Although the neural basis by which NMDA antagonists modify tolerance and dependence development is not known, it is possible that their interference with NMDA-receptor-mediated neuroadaptive processes is involved.

Learning and Memory

The functionality of NMDA receptor activation is activity-dependent, as evidenced by voltage-dependent Mg^{2+} blockade of the associated ion channel. This suggests their possible important role in integration of cell firing and neuronal plasticity. Consistent with this role is evidence that NMDA receptors are involved in long-term potentiation (LTP) in the hippocampus, a form of activity-dependent synaptic plasticity (40). Inhibition of LTP by PCP and other NMDA antagonists could account for their consistent disruption of learning and memory in a wide variety of animal models (82,83).

CLINICAL PHARMACOLOGY

Pharmacokinetics

PCP is well-absorbed and readily penetrates the central nervous system after intravenous, inhalational (smoked), intranasal, oral, and percutaneous administration (7,53), and it can be passively absorbed from the environment (61). The rapidity of onset of action varies with the route of administration: Within 1 min with intravenous and inhalation, several minutes with intranasal, and 20–40 min after oral (7). The time to peak effect also varies: 10 min with intravenous, 5–30 min with inhalation, and 90 min with oral administration (7).

PCP intoxication may last 4–8 hr after recreational doses, with some users reporting subjective effects for 24–48 hr (51,66). This prolonged duration of action contrasts with PCP's rapid clearance from blood (distribution [alpha] half-life: 1–4 hr) by uptake into brain and other fatty tissues, and may be related to tissue stores and a gastroenteric circulation facilitated by pH-dependent GI absorption (7). The plasma [beta] elimination half-life is 7–50 hr (mean: 17.6 hr) in normal volunteers and somewhat longer (11–89 hr) in overdose patients (7). Chronic users often show an asymptotic [gamma] elimination phase lasting several weeks, which probably represents prolonged, slow release of PCP from saturated fatty tissue stores. (PCP and metabolites have been shown to persist for weeks in rat brain and other fatty tissue.) This may account for positive urine toxicology results occurring several weeks after the last PCP use (22,64).

PCP is metabolized mainly by cytochrome P-450-dependent mixed function oxidases in liver (and placenta), resulting in about 75% of an administered dose becoming polar (chiefly ring hydroxylated) metabolites that are eliminated in the urine (7,41). None of these polar metabolites are known to contribute to the behavioral effects of PCP administration, but more than a third of minor metabolites are still not chemically identified.

PCP's pharmacokinetic parameters and metabolite patterns appear to be similar over a wide range of doses regardless of route of administration or chronicity of use (7). Inhalation introduces a new set of compounds by pyrolysis of PCP to 1-phenyl-1-cyclohexene (PC) and piperidine, which then undergo their own oxidative metabolism (41). In mice, PC and its metabolites are 100 times less behaviorally active than PCP, but their human pharmacology is unknown. PCP metabolism shows substantial individual variation. One factor may be cigarette smoking, which is associated with increased in vitro PCP hydroxylation by human liver (54). Pregnant and postpartum women and neonates tend to have different metabolite patterns from other subjects studied, suggesting that there may be hormonal influences on PCP metabolism (7). Genetics may also be a factor, because rate of PCP metabolism in mouse liver is controlled by a single gene on the X chromosome or chromosome 17 (26).

Pharmacodynamics

As described above for animals, PCP produces a variety of behavioral and psychological effects in human recreational users, effects which may be influenced by dose, rate, route of administration, and prior experience with the drug (51,66) (see section entitled "Tolerance and Dependence," above). These include hypesthesia and analgesia, sedative or depressant-like effects (feelings of calmness, depression, psychic numbing, anergia, impaired concentration, ataxia, and analgesia), stimulant-like effects (feelings of euphoria, power, invulnerability, anxiety, insomnia, and anorexia), and hallucinogenic or psychotomimetic effects (distortions of time perception and body image, synesthesias, illusions and hallucinations, depersonalization, derealization, thought disorganization, paranoid ideation, and bizarre behavior).

There is little direct human data indicating which neuropharmacological mechanisms mediate these psychopharmacological effects of PCP. In experimental studies with normal volunteers, these effects occur at doses up to 5 mg orally and 1–2 mg i.v. or by inhalation, producing serum concentrations up to 100 ng/ml (0.4 μM) (29). At these concentrations, PCP has significant interactions only with its NMDA receptor and dopamine transporter binding sites. Such pharmacokinetic correlations, as well as limited human structure–activity correlation studies with PCP analogues, suggest that analgesic and psychotomimetic effects are mediated by the PCP binding site in the NMDA receptor complex. PCP NMDA receptor sites are widely distributed in human brain, with highest densities in cerebellum, hippocampus, and temporal cortex (79). The contribution of PCP's dopaminergic actions to its human stimulant-like and reinforcing effects remains unknown.

Consistent dose–effect or concentration–effect correlations have never been established in clinical studies (29,51,66). Serum concentrations in several case series of intoxicated patients have ranged from 0 to 800 ng/ml, whereas subjects arrested for public intoxication or driving under the influence have had concentrations from 7 to 240 ng/ml. The reasons for this wide variation in tolerated plasma concentrations are not well understood, but probably include (a) poor correspondence between PCP concentrations in body fluids and binding at the sites of action in the brain and (b) individual variation in sensitivity to phencyclidine. No relevant data on human brain or CSF PCP concentrations are available in the literature.

ADVERSE CONSEQUENCES

Consequences of Acute Use

Behavioral/Psychological

Acute PCP intoxication can produce three stages of behavioral/psychological toxicity: (i) behavioral toxicity with only mild neurologic and physiologic abnormalities, (ii) stupor or light coma with responsiveness to pain, and (iii) deep coma with unresponsiveness to pain (1,51,66,86). Manifestations of behavioral toxicity can be loosely grouped into several clinical patterns that resemble psychiatric syndromes, and thus should be considered in the differential diagnosis of many newly presenting psychiatric patients. The commonest pattern seen in health care settings is that of delirium (i.e., disorientation, confusion, impaired recent memory, labile and inappropriate affect, and impaired judgment), without other evidence of psychosis. Delirium lasting up to several days is quite common in patients recovering from PCP-induced coma, and may occur transiently as the final phase of any episode of PCP intoxication. Other common patterns include (a) psychosis, with hallucinations and (usually paranoid) delusions occurring in an alert and oriented patient, and (b) catatonia, with negativism, mutism, blank staring, and catalepsy. The rarest patterns in health care settings (but much commoner in users not seeking or needing acute treatment) are (a) euphoria occurring in oriented patients without psychosis and (b) lethargy or sedation, also occurring without psychosis.

PCP intoxication may be accompanied by agitated or bizarre behavior regardless of the primary symptom pattern (1,51,66). PCP has gained a reputation as causing violent behavior (5,13). Coupled with the drug's alleged analgesic and strength-enhancing effects, this has given PCP users a reputation for being especially dangerous to interact with. The bases for this reputation have never been confirmed by direct scientific evidence (5). All published case series lack one or more methodologic factors needed to support firm conclusions, including objective confirmation of PCP use around the time of the violent behavior, exclusion of concurrent use of other drugs, distinction between intended violence and agitation or psychosis, and knowledge of any prior history of violent behavior. Large-sample, population-based studies do not suggest a special propensity for violence or criminal behavior among PCP users. For example, lifetime and prior-month PCP users are overrepresented four- to eightfold compared to the general population among state prison inmates, but this is no greater than the four- to twelvefold overrepresentation of users of other illicit drugs such as cocaine and heroin (37). Also among state prison inmates, 5.6% of lifetime PCP users reported being under the influence of the drug while committing their crime, compared with 29% of lifetime cocaine users and 23% of lifetime opiate users (37). Data such as these are consistent with the association between illicit drug use and antisocial, including violent, behavior, but do not suggest any special risk for such behaviors in PCP users. Animal studies using experimental models of aggression also do not support any special propensity for PCP to produce aggression (2).

PCP users may be more at risk for trauma (including accidents) in general. Substantially more PCP users who present to hospital emergency departments do so because of trauma (7.7% in 1991) than do users of opiates (3.4%) or cocaine (5.3%) (48), and more PCP users whose deaths are investigated by medical examiners die because of a contributing external physical event (36.4% in 1991) than do users of opiates (8.1%) or cocaine (25.2%) (49). These findings may reflect the ability of PCP to impair both psychomotor function and judgment.

Physical

PCP intoxication produces a variety of neurological and cardiovascular effects mostly related to its sympathomimetic actions and disruption of cerebellar function (1,51,66). Common neurological effects include increased muscle tone, tremor, brisk deep tendon reflexes, nystagmus (especially vertical), and ataxia. Pupil size is variable: It is often normal or enlarged, and it is usually reduced only during actual coma. Common cardiovascular effects, probably due to both sympathomimetic action and decreased baroreceptor activity, include moderate elevations in heart rate (typically 20–30 beats/min) and blood pressure (typically 10–20 mm Hg, with systolic greater than diastolic), resulting in increased cardiac output. Noncardiovascular sympathomimetic effects include diaphoresis, lacrimation, and increased bronchial and salivary secretions.

At doses intentionally taken by PCP users, the drug does not significantly influence respiration, metabolic rate, or GI motility (1,51,66). At higher doses, PCP causes a variety of serious medical complications, including coma, seizures, hyperthermia, intracranial hemorrhage, apnea, and acute rhabdomyolysis (often resulting in myoglobinuria and acute renal failure). Direct depression of myocardial contractility and decreased peripheral vascular resistance may cause hypotension and circulatory collapse. Other medical complications, such as diarrhea, abdominal cramps, and hematemesis, may be due to byproducts of synthesis or pyrolysis and other contaminants in street samples, rather than PCP itself (62).

In the absence of clinically usable antagonists, treatment of acute PCP intoxication—that is, reduction of environmental stimulation and control of remaining behavioral toxicity with sedatives (for anxiety, agitation) or high-potency neuroleptics (for psychosis), as appropriate (1,51,66)—remains symptomatic. A variety of other medications, such as calcium channel blockers, have seen scattered use (55). There are no comparative controlled clinical trials to favor the use of any particular medication over others. In severe intoxication with serious physiologic abnormalities, enhancement of PCP renal clearance by aggressive acidification of the urine can be useful (16,36), although care must be taken to avoid producing metabolic acidosis (with consequent risk of renal compromise) and to exclude the presence of other drugs whose renal clearance might be retarded by urine acidification.

Consequences of Chronic Use

Behavioral/Psychological

PCP use clearly can produce psychological dependence, as manifested in users who enter drug abuse treatment reporting that use is rewarding for them and who have great difficulty in stopping use despite knowledge of adverse consequences (2,22,23). The specific subjective effect of PCP that reinforces drug-taking may vary with the individual. Three patterns of acute intoxication responses have been described as desirable by PCP abusers in treatment: euphoria/stimulation, depression/sedation, and hallucinogenic effects (including religious experiences) (13,22,23). Two psychological effects commonly reported by PCP abusers as motivating their continued drug use are: (i) feelings of power, strength, and invulnerability; and (ii) psychic numbing used as self-medication for dysphoria (22,23). In the absence of relevant epidemiologic data, it is unknown what proportion of PCP users become dependent, or what frequency or duration of PCP use is associated with dependence. Among high school

seniors in 1992, 25% of lifetime PCP users used the drug within a 30-day period, compared with 22%, 21%, and 25% of lifetime LSD, cocaine, and heroin users, respectively, using their drug within a 30-day period (31). By contrast, 17% of current (within past 30 days) PCP users were daily users, compared with 5%, 8%, and 17%, respectively, of current LSD, cocaine, and heroin users. Almost all PCP abusers in drug abuse treatment have been using the drug for several years, although only about one-third have been using it daily (22,23).

There is little available data on the treatment of PCP abuse/dependence and few controlled clinical trials (13). Most published studies describe psychosocial treatment methods such as outpatient group therapy and long-term residential treatment, chiefly in adolescents and young adults. Clinical experience and the available outcome data suggest that currently used treatment methods tend to have low long-term success rates (13,22,23). Even less data are available on pharmacological treatment of PCP abuse/dependence. Desipramine (150 mg daily) and buspirone (10 mg t.i.d.) have been used in conjunction with counseling in small, double-blind, placebo-controlled outpatient trials, with significant improvement in psychological symptoms (especially depression) but no effect on PCP use (all groups had high retention and abstinence rates) (19,20).

A variety of persisting behavioral/psychological changes have been associated with PCP use, including psychosis, depression, anxiety, personality change, and neuropsychological impairment (1,2,12,13,24). Persistent depressed mood, sometimes severe enough to require psychiatric treatment, can follow any episode of PCP intoxication. Persisting psychosis may follow acute PCP-induced psychosis, especially in patients with preexisting schizophrenia (24). One recent test–retest study found some neuropsychological impairment persisting over several weeks of drug abstinence (12). Most studies have used retrospective data collection, lacked appropriate comparison groups, or had other methodological flaws making it impossible to distinguish actual PCP effects from preexisting conditions or from the consequences of other factors frequently associated with PCP use, such as other substance use, head injury, and a drug-abusing lifestyle. When an appropriate comparison group is used, there is often no significant difference between the PCP users and non-PCP-using drug users.

Physical

PCP causes a variety of degenerative changes in rat and human neurons and astrocytes in vitro, including vacuolization, inhibition of microtubule function, suppression of axon outgrowth, and cell death (43,50). These effects are time- and concentration-dependent, tending to occur only after several days of exposure to PCP concentrations (100–500 μM) substantially higher than the plasma concentrations found in human PCP users, but probably closer to concentrations achieved in the fetuses of PCP-abusing mothers. These neuropathic effects may be mediated by blockade of inactivating potassium channels rather than by other actions of PCP because they occur only at concentrations far above those required for action at PCP's NMDA and dopaminergic receptor sites and are produced by other potassium channel blockers but not by other NMDA or sigma receptor ligands.

There is currently no information directly linking the PCP-induced neuropathologic effects observed in animal and in vitro studies with the behavioral/psychological effects observed in human PCP users. Children born to PCP-using mothers exhibit hypertonicity, coarse tremor, irritability, poor visual tracking, and impaired attention as neonates and may continue to have abnormal EEG patterns, nystagmus, and impaired interactive behavior and organizational responses to environmental stimuli through several years of age (21,57,70,75,76). Prospective longitudinal studies are needed to determine the persistence and consequences of these abnormalities, along with appropriate comparison groups to distinguish specific effects of PCP exposure in utero from general effects of maternal drug use and a drug-using lifestyle.

Brain imaging studies in small numbers of adult chronic PCP users suggest that they may have decreased right cerebral cortical blood flow and frontal glucose metabolism, abnormalities similar to those found in schizophrenic patients (25,84). The affinity and density of brain PCP and sigma receptor sites has been reported to be normal in adult chronic PCP users who died traumatically (79).

Maternal PCP use during pregnancy is associated with intrauterine growth retardation, precipitate labor, and fetal distress (reflected in meconium staining), but not with prematurity or any specific congenital malformation or teratogenic risk (21). Because these pregnancy-related problems also occur frequently with maternal use of other illicit drugs, it is unclear to what extent they represent a specific pharmacologic action of PCP.

Adult chronic PCP users do not generally show evidence of clinically significant cardiovascular, hematologic, renal, or hepatic toxicity (1). Although PCP in vitro has been shown to block epinephrine-induced activation and aggregation of platelets and to depress stimulated antibody and interleukin production (possibly mediated by sigma receptors on leukocytes) (28,52), it has not been associated clinically with coagulation or immune dysfunction.

THERAPEUTIC POTENTIAL

Although PCP itself will not see therapeutic use because of its adverse psychoactive effects, its use as an experimental tool for increasing understanding of the neuropsychopharmacology of NMDA receptors is likely to

bear therapeutic fruit in the future. The development of potent and specific ligands for the PCP receptor and other sites associated with the NMDA–receptor complex is likely to result in improved anticonvulsants, neuroprotective agents for the treatment of stroke and other ischemic and anoxic brain injuries, and novel antipsychotic medications free of the side effects associated with the currently available antidopaminergic neuroleptics (14,29,30,69).

FUTURE CHALLENGES

1. *Separating PCP-like effects from therapeutic effects of NMDA antagonists.* To maximize therapeutic utility, an NMDA antagonist should not produce significant PCP-like behavioral/psychological side effects or have PCP-like abuse liability. All NMDA antagonists tested to date that act at the PCP site in the channel are very likely to produce PCP-like side effects in humans. However, two lines of evidence suggest that separation of therapeutic from adverse PCP-like effects may be possible. First, different classes of site-selective NMDA antagonists produce different profiles of neurochemical and behavioral effects in animals (18,82,83); for example, competitive NMDA antagonists may have a better "therapeutic index" than noncompetitive antagonists. Second, early results with systemically active drugs that act as glycine-site and polyamine-site NMDA antagonists show that they may produce behavioral effects that are even more dissimilar from those of PCP than are obtained with competitive antagonists (4,65).

2. *Subtypes of NMDA/PCP receptors.* The NMDA receptor is composed of a number of different subunits. Different heteromeric NMDA channels, created by oocyte expression, show differential sensitivities to PCP, ketamine, dizocilpine, and NANM (85). Biochemical and neuroimaging studies have shown differences among PCP and NMDA receptors in different brain regions (27,58) and between agonist- and antagonist-preferring forms (45). These early findings suggest that identification of subtypes of PCP receptor sites may allow development of PCP-site antagonists with more selective pharmacological properties.

3. *Pharmacodynamics of PCP intoxication.* The most recent human experimental studies of PCP intoxication occurred over a decade ago, without use of brain imaging, electroencephalographic brain mapping, or computerized neuropsychological testing. Future studies using these modern techniques, correlated with pharmacokinetic measurements, should help clarify the neuropsychopharmacological mechanisms of acute PCP intoxication, as well as provide experimental models for studying the neuropsychopharmacology of psychosis and for developing potential treatments for acute PCP intoxication. Such studies are already underway using the PCP analogue ketamine, thereby avoiding some of the potential problems posed by using PCP itself (34). Comparative controlled clinical

trials are needed to evaluate treatments for PCP intoxication. Prospective, longitudinal studies with appropriate comparison groups, such as non-PCP-abusing drug users, are needed to identify the incidence, nature, and course of long-term consequences of PCP use.

4. *Treatment of PCP abuse/dependence.* Both pilot studies and controlled clinical trials are needed to develop and evaluate (a) improved treatments for PCP abuse/dependence, including both psychosocial methods such as cognitive therapy and behavior modification, and (b) new pharmacotherapies based on knowledge of the neuropharmacology of PCP.

REFERENCES

1. Baldridge EB, Bessen HA. Phencyclidine. *Emergency Med Clin North Am* 1990;8:541–550.
2. Balster RL. The behavioral pharmacology of phencyclidine. In: Meltzer HY, ed. *Psychopharmacology: the third generation of progress.* New York: Raven Press, 1987;1573–1579.
3. Balster RL. Discriminative stimulus properties of phencyclidine and other NMDA antagonists. In: Glennon RA, Järbe TUC, Frankenheim J, eds. *Drug discrimination: applications to drug abuse research.* National Institute on Drug Abuse Research Monograph Series 116. DHHS publication no. (ADM) 92-1878. Washington, DC: U.S. Government Printing Office, 1991;163–180.
4. Balster RL, Nicholson KL, Sanger DJ. Evaluation of the reinforcing effects of eliprodil in rhesus monkeys and its discriminative stimulus effects in rats. *Drug Alcohol Depend,* 1994;[in press].
5. Brecher M, Wang BW, et al. Phencyclidine and violence: clinical and legal issues. *J Clin Psychopharmacol* 1988;8:397–401.
6. Bristow LJ, Hutson PH, Thorn HL, Trickelbank MD. The glycine/NMDA receptor antagonist, R-(+)-HA-966, blocks activation of the mesolimbic dopaminergic system induced by phencyclidine and dizocilpine (MK-801) in rodents. *Br J Pharmacol* 1993;108:1156–1163.
7. Busto U, Bendayan R, and Sellers EM. Clinical pharmacokinetics of non-opiate abused drugs. *Clinical Pharmacokinetics* 1989;16:1–26.
8. Carroll ME. PCP and hallucinogens. *Adv Alcohol Subst Abuse* 1990;9:167–190.
9. Carroll ME. The economic context of drug and non-drug reinforcers affects acquisition and maintenance of drug-reinforced behavior and withdrawal effects. *Drug Alcohol Depend* 1993;33:201–210.
10. Carroll ME, Carmona G. Effects of food FR and food deprivation on disruptions in food-maintained performance of monkeys during phencyclidine withdrawal. *Psychopharmacology* 1991;104:143–149.
11. Contreras PC, Gray NM, DiMaggio DA, et al. Isolation and characterization of an endogenous ligand for the PCP and receptors from porcine, rat, and human tissue. *Sigma, PCP, and NMDA receptors.* National Institute on Drug Abuse Research Monograph Series 133. NIH publication no. 93-3587. Washington, DC: U.S. Government Printing Office, 1993;207–223.
12. Cosgrove J, Newell TG. Recovery of neuropsychological functions during reduction in use of phencyclidine. *J Clin Psychol* 1991;47:159–169.
13. Daghestani AN, Schnoll SH. Phencyclidine abuse and dependence. *Treatments of psychiatric disorders, vol 2. A task force report of the American Psychiatric Association.* Washington, DC: American Psychiatric Association 1989;1209–1218.
14. De Sarro GB, De Sarro A. Anticonvulsant properties of non-competitive antagonists of the N-methyl-D-aspartate receptor in genetically epilepsy-prone rats: comparison with CPPene. *Neuropharmacology* 1993;32:51–68.
15. Dimpfel W, Spuler M. Dizocilpine (MK-801), ketamine and phencyclidine: low doses affect brain field potentials in the freely moving rat in the same way as activation of dopaminergic transmission. *Psychopharmacology* 1990;101:317–323.
16. Done AK, Aronow R, Miceli JN. Pharmacokinetic bases for the

diagnosis and treatment of acute PCP intoxication. *J Psychedelic Drugs* 1980;12:253–258.
17. France CP, Snyder AM, Woods JH. Analgesic effects of phencyclidine-like drugs in rhesus monkeys. *J Pharmacol Exp Ther* 1989;250:197–201.
18. French ED, Mura A, Wang T. MK-801, phencyclidine (PCP), and PCP-like drugs increase burst firing in rat A10 dopamine neurons: Comparison to competitive NMDA antagonists. *Synapse* 1993;13:108–116.
19. Giannini AJ, Loiselle RH, Graham BH, et al. Behavioral response to buspirone in cocaine and phencyclidine withdrawal. *J Subst Abuse Treat* 1993;10:523–527.
20. Giannini AJ, Malone DA, Giannini MC, et al. Treatment of depression in chronic cocaine and phencyclidine abuse with desipramine. *J Clin Pharmacol* 1986;26:211–214.
21. Glantz JC, Woods JR. Cocaine, heroin, and phencyclidine: obstetric perspectives. *Clin Obstet Gynecol* 1993;36:279–301.
22. Gorelick DA, Wilkins JN. Inpatient treatment of PCP abusers and users. *Am J Drug Alcohol Abuse* 1989;15:1–12.
23. Gorelick DA, Wilkins JN, Wong C. Outpatient treatment of PCP abusers. *Am J Drug Alcohol Abuse* 1989;15:367–374.
24. Gwirtsman HE, Wittkop W, Gorelick DA, et al. Phencyclidine intoxication incidence, clinical patterns, and course of treatments. *Res Commun Psychol Psychiatry Behav* 1984;9:405–410.
25. Hertzman M, Reba RC, Kotlyarove EV. Single photon emission computed tomography in phencyclidine and related drug abuse. *Am J Psychiatry* 1990;147:255–256.
26. Holsztynska EJ, Weber WW, Domino EF. Genetic polymorphism of cytochrome P-450-dependent phencyclidine hydroxylation in mice. *Drug Metab Disposition,* 1991;19:48–53.
27. Itzhak Y. Different modulation of the binding to two phencyclidine (PCP) receptor subtypes: effects of N-methyl-D-aspartate agonists and antagonists. *Neurosci Lett* 1989;104:314–319.
28. Jamieson GA, Agrawal AK, Greco NJ, et al. Phencyclidine binds to blood platelets with high affinity and specifically inhibits their activation by adrenaline. *Biochem J* 1992;285:35–39.
29. Javitt DC, Zukin SR. Recent advances in the phencyclidine model of schizophrenia. *Am J Psychiatry* 1991;148:1301–1308.
30. Johnson KM, Jones SM. Neuropharmacology of phencyclidine: basic mechanisms and therapeutic potential. *Annu Rev Pharmacol Toxicol* 1990;30:707–750.
31. Johnston LD, O'Malley PM, Bachman JG. *National survey results on drug use from the Monitoring the Future Study, 1975–1992.* National Institutes of Health, Publication no. 93-3598, 1993.
32. Karler R, Calder LD, Chaudhry IA, Turkanis SA. Blockade of reverse tolerance to cocaine and amphetamine by MK-801. *Life Sci* 1989;45:599–606.
33. Keith VA, Mansbach RS, Geyer MA. Failure of haloperidol to block the effects of phencyclidine and dizocilpine on prepulse inhibition of startle. *Biol Psychiatry* 1991;30:557–566.
34. Krystal JH, Karper L, Seibyl JP, et al. Subanesthetic effects of the noncompetitive NMDA antagonist, ketamine in humans. *Arch Gen Psychiatry* 1994;51:199–214.
35. Lodge D, Johnson KM. Noncompetitive excitatory amino acid receptor antagonists. *Trends Pharmacol Sci* 1990;11:81–86.
36. Lyddane JE, Thomas BF, Compton DR, et al. Modification of phencyclidine intoxification and biodisposition by charcoal and other treatments. *Pharmacol Biochem Behav* 1988;30:371–377.
37. Maguire K, Pastore AL, Flanagan TJ, eds. *Sourcebook of criminal justice statistics, 1994.* Washington, DC: U.S. US Dept of Justice, Bureau of Justice Statistics, 1993.
38. Manallack DT, Davies JW, Beart PM, Saunders MR, Livingstone DJ. Analysis of the biological and molecular properties of phencyclidine-like compounds by chemometrics. *Arzneimittelforschung* 1993;43:1029–1032.
39. Mansbach RS, Willetts J, Jortani SA, Balster RL. NMDA antagonists: lack of an antipunishment effect in squirrel monkeys. *Pharmacol Biochem Behav* 1991;39:977–981.
40. Maren S, Baudry M, Thompson RF. Differential effects of ketamine and MK-801 on the induction of long-term potentiation. *Neuroreport* 1991;2:239–242.
41. Martin BR, Boni J. Pyrolysis and inhalation studies with phencyclidine and cocaine. *Research findings on smoking of abused substances.* NIDA Research Monograph 99. Washington, DC: NIDA, 1990;141–158.
42. Massey BM, Wessinger WD. Alterations in rat brain [³H]-TCP

binding following chronic phencyclidine administration. *Life Sci* 1990;47:139–143.

43. Mattson MP, Rychlik B, Cheng B. Degenerative and axon outgrowth-altering effects of phencyclidine in human fetal cerebral cortical cells. *Neuropharmacology* 1992;31:279–291.

44. Maurice T, Vignon J, Kamenka JM, Chicheportiche R. Differential interaction of phencyclidine-like drugs with the dopamine uptake complex *in vivo. J Neurochem* 1991;56:533–559.

45. Monaghan DT, Bridges RJ, Cotman CW. The excitatory amino acid receptors: their classes, pharmacology, and distinct properties in the function of the central nervous system. *Annu Rev Pharmacol Toxicol* 1989;29:365–402.

46. Moriyoshi K, Masu M, Ishii T, Shigemoto R, Mizuno N, Nakanishi S. Molecular cloning and characterization of the rat NMDA receptor. *Nature* 1991;354:31–37.

47. Musacchio JM. The psychotomimetic effects of opiates and the σ receptor. *Neuropsychopharmacology* 1990;3:191–200.

48. NIDA Statistical Series, Series I, Number 11-A. *Annual emergency room data, 1991.* DHHS publication no. (ADM) 92-1955, 1992.

49. NIDA Statistical Series, Series I, Number 11-B. *Annual medical examiner data, 1991.* DHHS publication no. (ADM) 92-1956, 1992.

50. Olney JW, Labruyere J, Price MT. Pathological changes induced in cerebrocortical neurons by phencyclidine and related drugs. *Science* 1989;244:1360–1362.

51. Pearlson GD. Psychiatric and medical syndromes associated with phencyclidine (PCP) abuse. *Johns Hopkins Med J* 1981;148: 25–33.

52. Pillai R, Nair BS, Watson RR, et al. AIDS, drugs of abuse and the immune system: a complex immunotoxicological network. *Arch Toxicol* 1991;65:609–617.

53. Pitts FN, Allen RE, Aniline O, et al. Occupational intoxication and long-term persistence of phencyclidine (PCP) in law enforcement personnel. *Clin Toxicol* 1981;18:1015–1020.

54. Pohorecki R, Rayburn W, Coon WW, et al. Some factors affecting phencyclidine biotransformation by human liver and placenta. *Drug Metab Dispos* 1989;17:271–274.

55. Price WA, Giannini AJ, Krishen A. Management of acute PCP intoxication with verapamil. *Clin Toxicol* 1986;24:85–87.

56. Quirion R, Chicheportiche R, Contreras PC, Johnson KM, Lodge D, Tam SW, Woods JH, Zukin SR. Classification and nomenclature of phencyclidine and sigma receptor sites. *Trends Neurosci* 1987;10:444–446.

57. Rahbar F, Fomufod A, White D, et al. Impact of intrauterine exposure to phencyclidine (PCP) and cocaine on neonates. *J Natl Med Assoc* 1985;85:349–352.

58. Rao TS, Kim HC, Lehmann J, Martin LL, Wood PL. Selective activation of dopaminergic pathways in the mesocortex by compounds that act at the phencyclidine (PCP) binding site: tentative evidence for PCP recognition sites not coupled to *N*-methyl-D-aspartate (NMDA) receptors. *Neuropharmacology* 1990;29: 225–230.

59. Renfroe CL, Messinger TA. Street drug analysis: an eleven year perspective on illicit drug alteration. *Semin Adolesc Med* 1985;1:247–257.

60. Rothman RB, Reid AA, Monna JA, Jacobson AE, Rice KC. The psychotomimetic drug phencyclidine labels 2 high affinity binding sites in guinea pig brain: evidence for *N*-methyl-D-aspartate coupled and dopamine reuptake carrier-associated phencyclidine binding sites. *Mol Pharmacol* 1989;36:887–896.

61. Schwartz RH. Passive inhalation of marijuana, phencyclidine, and freebase. *Am J Dis Child* 1989;143:644.

62. Shesser R, Jotte R, Olshaker J. The contribution of impurities to the acute morbidity of illegal drug use. *Am J Emerg Med* 1991;9:336–342.

63. Shoaib M, Stolerman IP. MK-801 attenuates behavioural adaptation to chronic nicotine administration in rats. *Br J Pharmacol* 1991;105:514–515.

64. Simpson GM, Khajawall AM, Alatorre E, et al. Urinary phencyclidine excretion in chronic abusers. *J Toxicol Clin Toxicol* 1982–1983;19:1051–1059.

65. Singh L, Menzies R, Tricklebank MD. The discriminative stimulus properties of (+)-HA-966, an antagonist at the glycine/*N*-methyl-D-aspartate receptor. *Eur J Pharmacol* 1990;186:129–132.

66. Sioris L, Krenzelok E. Phencyclidine intoxication: literature review. *Am J Hosp Pharm* 1978;35:1362–1367.

67. Smith JB. Situational specificity of tolerance to effects of phencyclidine on responding of rats under fixed-ratio and spaced-responding schedules. *Psychopharmacology* 1991;103:121–128.

68. Steinpreis RE, Salamone JD. The role of nucleus accumbens dopamine in the neurochemical and behavioral effects of phencyclidine: a microdialysis and behavioral study. *Brain Res* 1993;612:263–270.

69. Sveinbjornsdottir S, Sander JWAS, Upton D, Thompson PJ, Patsalos PN, Hirt D, Emre M, Lowe D, Duncan JS. The excitatory amino acid antagonist D-CPPene (SDZ EAA-494) in patients with epilepsy. *Epilepsy Res* 1993;16:165–174.

70. Tabor BL, Smith-Wallace T, Yonekura ML. Perinatal outcome associated with PCP versus cocaine use. *Am J Drug Alcohol Abuse* 1990;16:337–348.

71. Thurkauf A, Zenk PC, Balster RL, May EL, George C, Caroll FI, Mascarella SW, Rice KC, Jacobson AE, Mattson MV. Synthesis, absolute configuration, and molecular modeling study of etoxadrol, a potent phencyclidine-like agonist. *J Med Chem* 1988;31: 2257–2263.

72. Tiseo PJ, Inturrisi CE. Attenuation and reversal of morphine tolerance by competitive *N*-methyl-D-aspartate receptor antagonist, LY274614. *J Pharmacol Exp Ther* 1992;264:1090–1096.

73. Troupin AS, Mendius JR, Cheng F, Risinger MW. MK-801. In: Meldrum B, Porter R, eds. *New Anticonvulsant drugs.* London: John Libby, 1986;191–201.

74. Trujillo KA, Akil H. Inhibition of morphine tolerance and dependence by the NMDA receptor antagonist MK-801. *Science* 1991;251:85–87.

75. Van Dyke DC, Fox AA. Fetal drug exposure and its possible implications for learning in the preschool and school-age population. *J Learn Disabil* 1990;23:160–163.

76. Wachsman L, Schuetz S, Chan LS, et al. What happens to babies exposed to phencyclidine (PCP) in utero? *Am J Drug Alcohol Abuse* 1989;15:31–39.

77. Walker JM, Bowen WD, Walker FO, Matsumoto RR, de Costa R, Rice KC. Sigma receptors: biology and function. *Pharmacol Rev* 1990;42:355–402.

78. Wang T, French ED. Effects of phencyclidine on spontaneous and excitatory amino acid-induced activity of ventral tegmental dopamine neurons: an extracellular in vitro study. *Life Sci* 1993;53: 49–56.

79. Weissman AD, Casanova MF, Kleinman JE, DeSouza EB. PCP and sigma receptors in brain are not altered after repeated exposure to PCP in humans. *Neuropsychopharmacology* 1991;4:95–102.

80. Wessinger SD, Owens SM. Phencyclidine dependence: The relationship of dose and serum concentrations to operant behavior effects. *J Pharmacol Exp Ther* 1991;258:207–215.

81. Wiley JL, Balster RL. Preclinical evaluation of *N*-methyl-D-aspartate antagonists for antianxiety effects: a review. In: Kamenka J-M, Domino EF, eds. *Multiple sigma and PCP receptor ligands: mechanisms for neuromodulation and neuroprotection?* Ann Arbor, MI: NPP Books, 1992;801–815.

82. Willetts J, Balster RL, Leander JD. The behavioral pharmacology of NMDA receptor antagonists. *Trends Pharmacol Sci* 1990;11:423–428.

83. Woods JH, Koek W, France CP, Moerschbaecher JM. Behavioural effects of NMDA antagonists. In: Meldrum BS, ed. *Excitatory amino acid antagonists.* Oxford: Blackwell Scientific Publications, 1991;237–264.

84. Wu JC, Buchsbaum MS, Bunney WE. Positron emission tomography study of phencyclidine users as a possible drug model of schizophrenia. *Jpn J Psychopharmacol* 1991;11:47–48.

85. Yamakura T, Mori H, Masaki H, Shimoji K, Mishina M. Different sensitivities of NMDA receptor channel subtypes to noncompetitive antagonists. *Neuroreport* 1993;4:687–90.

86. Young T, Lawson GW, et al. Clinical aspects of phencyclidine (PCP). *Int J Addict* 1987;22:1–15.

87. Zukin RS, Zukin SR. Phencyclidine, σ and NMDA receptors: Emerging concepts. In: Domino EF, Kamenka J-M, eds. *Sigma and phencyclidine-like compounds as molecular probes in biology.* Ann Arbor, MI: NPP Books, 1988;407–424.

Psychopharmacology: The Fourth Generation of Progress, edited by Floyd E. Bloom and David J. Kupfer. Raven Press, Ltd., New York 1995.

CHAPTER 152

Abuse and Therapeutic Use of Benzodiazepines and Benzodiazepine-Like Drugs

James H. Woods, Jonathan L. Katz, and Gail Winger

Since their introduction over 30 years ago, benzodiazepines have largely replaced older sedative–hypnotic agents in most countries. Because these drugs are used primarily for their therapeutic effects, abuse and misuse of benzodiazepines are best conceptualized in the context of their appropriate use. This chapter will therefore review pharmacological, clinical, and epidemiological studies of both appropriate use of benzodiazepines and their liability for abuse.

Research has of course continued in the effort to develop new anxiolytics with lesser sedative effects or liability for abuse. The most fruitful of these efforts have continued to focus on the benzodiazepine receptor system. In the context of what is known about established benzodiazepines, this chapter will consider some newer sedative/anxiolytic drugs (i.e., zopiclone, zolpidem, abecarnil, and bretazenil) that act on the benzodiazepine receptor.

There have been several recent reviews of the pharmacology of benzodiazepines. For a broader discussion of the basic pharmacological mechanisms of action of these drugs, the interested reader is referred to reviews by Haefely (e.g., see refs. 29–31). Hollister et al. (35) have recently published a comprehensive review of therapeutic uses of benzodiazepines, to which this chapter refers. With respect to the abuse liability of benzodiazepines,

this chapter draws extensively from our previous reviews (76,77).

Because of editorial limitations on the number of references that can be cited in this chapter, we refer to literature considered in our earlier reviews (76,77) or in that of Hollister et al. (35) as follows: Rather than citing individual studies, we generally cite review articles, including numbers of the pages on which the relevant studies were discussed. We regret that we cannot cite all individual studies.

CHEMISTRY

Established Agents

The first marketed benzodiazepines, chlordiazepoxide and diazepam, have a 1,4-diazepine ring that contains a 5-aryl substitutent ring and is fused to a benzene ring (Fig. 1). This has become known as the classic 1,4-benzodiazepine structure. A number of modifications of this structure have produced compounds with similar binding characteristics and, typically, similar spectra of action. Midazolam, the shortest-acting of the benzodiazepines, has an imidazo ring fused to the diazepine ring. The benzodiazepine antagonist flumazenil also possesses an imidazo ring in this position. The triazolobenzodiazepines, including alprazolam and triazolam, are more recently developed anxiolytic and sedative compounds, which have a triazolo ring fused to the diazepine ring.

Newer Compounds

A number of newer anxiolytic or sedative compounds act at the benzodiazepine site or at a subset of this site,

This chapter is dedicated to Mitchell Balter, a truly outstanding and pioneering epidemiologist. His contributions to psychopharmacology will be missed greatly.

J. H. Woods: Department of Pharmacology, University of Michigan Medical School, Ann Arbor, Michigan 48109.
J. L. Katz: Psychobiology Laboratory, NIDA Addiction Research Center, Baltimore, Maryland 21224.
G. Winger: Department of Pharmacology, University of Michigan Medical School, Ann Arbor, Michigan 48109.

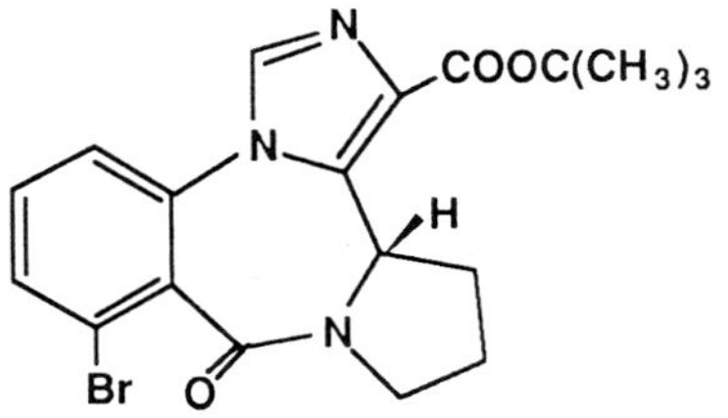

Bretazenil

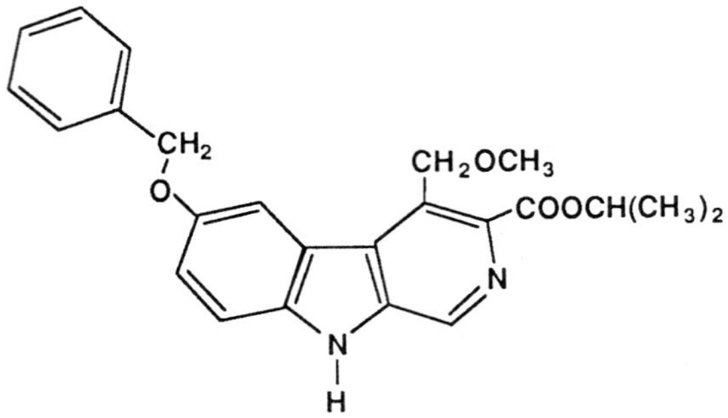

Abecarnil

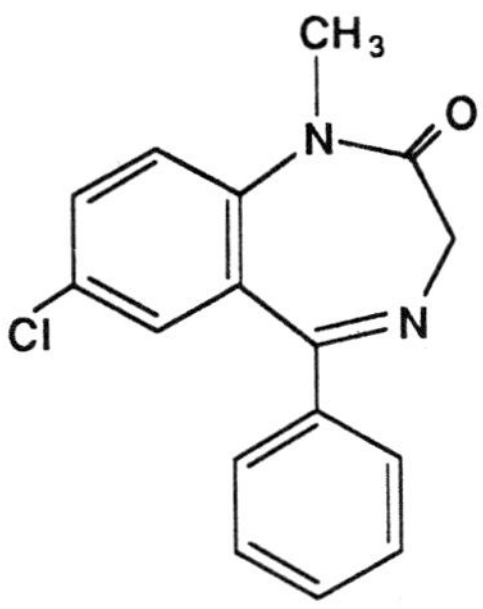

Diazepam

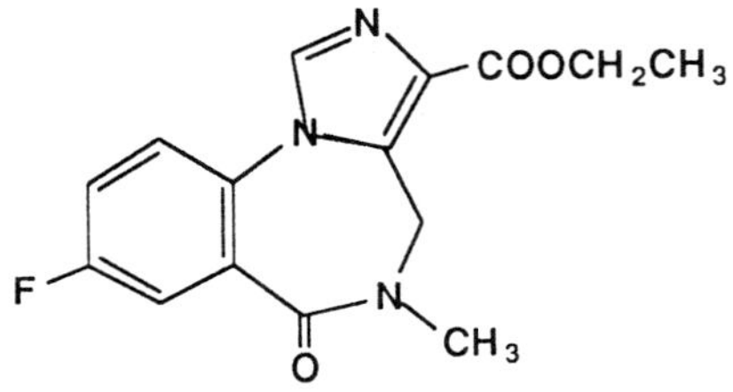

Flumazenil

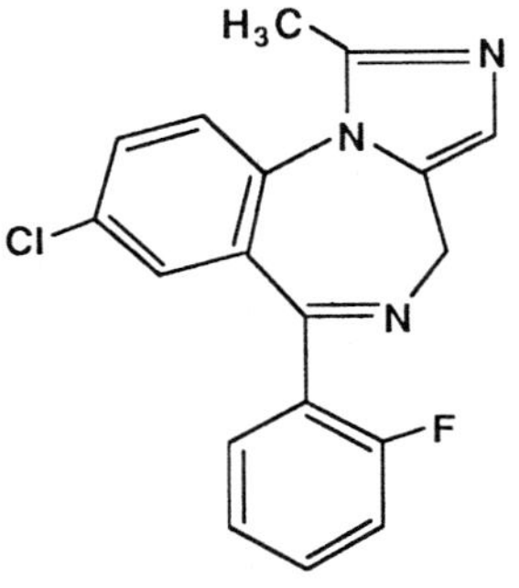

Midazolam

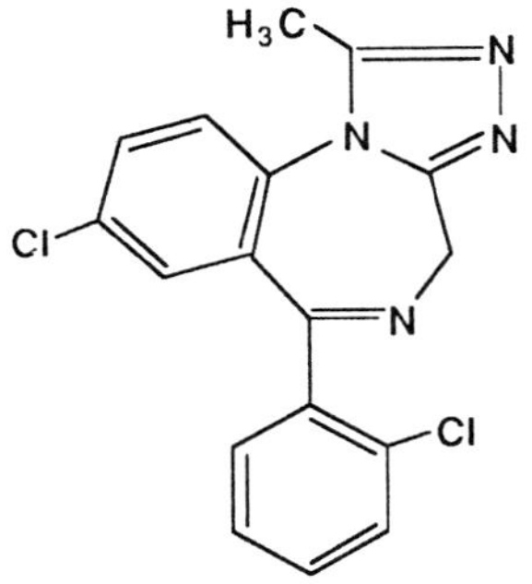

Triazolam

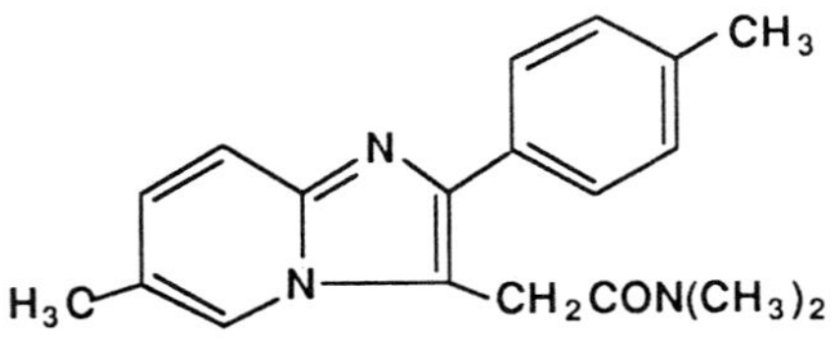

Zolpidem

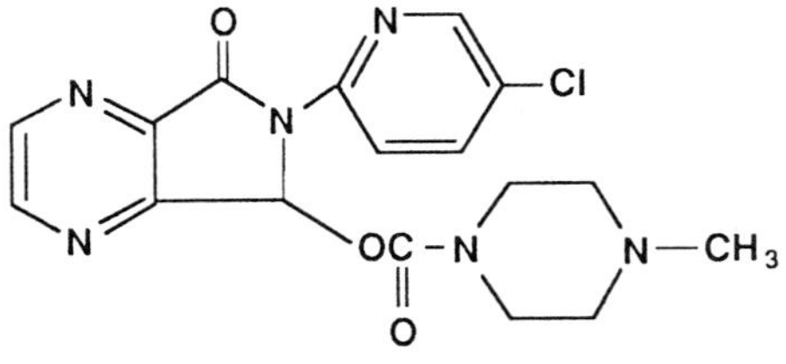

Zopiclone

FIG. 1. Structures of benzodiazepines and benzodiazepine-like substances.

but they do not share the classic benzodiazepine chemical structure. One of the first such compounds to be developed was zopiclone, a cyclopyrrolone. The imidazopryidine class has also yielded sedative compounds, of which zolpidem is an example. Also among the newer sedatives is abecarnil, which has a beta-carboline structure. Another example of the newer sedative compounds to be considered here is bretazenil, which is a tetracyclic 1,4-benzodiazepine.

RECEPTOR CHARACTERISTICS

Benzodiazepine agonists and other agonist ligands at the benzodiazepine site achieve their therapeutic effects by enhancing the actions of the inhibitory neurotransmitter gamma-aminobutyric acid (GABA) at its receptor. The benzodiazepines have a binding site on the GABA receptor, which forms a channel through the membrane and opens and closes to control chloride flow into the cell. When benzodiazepine agonists are on their receptor site, GABA produces a more rapid pulsatile opening of the channel, and the flow of chloride is increased. The central GABA receptor, known as the $GABA_A$ receptor, consists of at least four subunits; three of these—alpha, beta, and gamma—each contains three to six variants. The multiplicity of variants suggests that there are a number of different GABA receptors, but the subunit makeup of the native receptor has not yet been determined.

Two GABA receptors have been identified anatomically and pharmacologically. These receptors—variably called type I and type II, benzodiazepine I and benzodiazepine II, or omega I and omega II—are located throughout much of the central nervous system (CNS). The omega I site has been associated with the alpha-1 subunit, whereas the omega II site appears to be heterogeneous, located on receptors with alpha-2, alpha-3, and alpha-5 subunits (75). The ratio of omega I to omega II binding sites is greater in the cerebellar and cerebral cortices, whereas omega II sites predominate in the spinal cord. Pharmacological studies indicate that the 1,4-benzodiazepines bind with relative nonselectivity to both omega I and omega II sites. The triazolobenzodiazepines tend to have a greater affinity for omega I and II receptors than do the other benzodiazepines, and they are more potent. Zopiclone, despite its unusual chemical structure, has a binding profile much like that of the classic benzodiazepines. Zolpidem, however, binds with much greater affinity to the omega I site (e.g., see ref. 49), and there is evidence that abecarnil may have some specificity for the omega I site as well (69).

Most of the benzodiazepines currently available for therapeutic use are considered to be full agonists at the benzodiazepine site; a full benzodiazepine agonist is a drug that produces the maximum effect in all biological assays, although it occupies less than the maximum number of benzodiazepine receptors. Recently, partial agonists at the benzodiazepine site have been identified; a partial benzodiazepine agonist is a drug that produces less effect than a full agonist when it occupies the same number of benzodiazepine receptors. Benzodiazepine antagonists are drugs with affinity for the benzodiazepine modulatory site but no efficacy. A unique aspect of the benzodiazepine-related modulatory site on the $GABA_A$ receptor is that it is bidirectional; there are agents that bind here that decrease the effects of GABA at its site on this receptor, and thus have effects opposite to those of classical benzodiazepines.

There is of course great interest in the possibility of developing compounds that offer the therapeutic effects of the classic benzodiazepines, but with less risk of the adverse effects associated with these drugs. Identification of site-selective compounds, such as zolpidem, is one strategy that has been tried in this pursuit. Another is to develop compounds with a partial agonist profile, either at both omega I and omega II receptors (e.g., bretazenil) or selectively at the omega I receptor (e.g., abecarnil). As discussed in this chapter, agents with either site-selective or partial agonist activity appear to have behavioral profiles that differ in interesting ways from those of the classic benzodiazepines (see also Chapters 8 and 69, *this volume*).

THERAPEUTICS

Therapeutic Effects

Established Agents

Benzodiazepines have been found useful in a remarkably wide and varied array of clinical applications. Most traditional clinical use has been based on their anxiolytic, hypnotic, anticonvulsant, and antispastic effects. Other, possibly related effects demonstrated in clinical trials and practice include antipanic, antidepressant, amnestic, and anesthetic effects.

In view of the diversity of these effects, it is remarkable that, as demonstrated by numerous clinical comparisons, benzodiazepines are distinguished much more by their similarities than by their differences. This supports the hypothesis that the activity of agonists at the benzodiazepine receptor is in fact the dominant mechanism underlying the clinical effects of these drugs.

The most important differences with respect to clinical use pertain to relative potency and to onset and duration of action. When equipotent doses of the various agents can be used, however, they tend to exhibit similar effects. For example, early studies had found that the older benzodiazepines were generally ineffective in treatment of panic disorder. Thus when the newer agent, alprazolam, showed antipanic efficacy, this was speculatively attributed to the compound's novel triazolo ring. However, alprazolam is also relatively more potent than the older agents; more recent studies have found that, when used at higher dosages, older benzodiazepines are effective against panic disorder as well (35, pp. 16S–17S).

With respect to clinical utility, differences pertaining to onset and offset of action are probably most important. In some uses, including various medical and psychiatric emergencies, rapid onset of action is of course a necessity. Short duration of action may be useful (e.g., for outpatient surgical and diagnostic procedures), although longer duration of action may be desired (e.g., in treatment of sleep-maintenance disturbances or for seizure control). Differences of onset and offset of action also have important implications with respect to adverse effects as discussed below.

The following brief description of therapeutic effects of benzodiazepines summarizes the conclusions of the recent review by Hollister et al. (35), which is certainly the most comprehensive review of the clinical uses of these drugs. A large number of placebo-controlled studies have demonstrated the efficacy of benzodiazepines in treatment of anxiety disorders, including generalized anxiety disorder (GAD) and panic disorder; benzodiazepines are also useful in facilitating the behavioral treatment of phobias (35, pp. 2S–23S). They are also effective in management of anxiety and other symptoms of psychological distress associated with various medical disorders (35, pp. 64S–72S). As shown in sleep laboratory and controlled clinical trials, benzodiazepines are effective in treatment of disturbances of falling asleep and of maintaining sleep (35, pp. 23S–51S). Alprazolam has been shown effective in treatment of major depressive disorder of mild or moderate severity. Although they do not appear to have specific antimanic activity, clonazepam and lorazepam provide rapid control of manic episodes (35, pp. 23S–51S). Used alone or in combination with neuroleptics, benzodiazepines have proved valuable for management of various psychiatric emergencies involving agitation or hostility. They also provide acute relief of catatonic symptoms, and they are sometimes useful "neuroleptic-sparing" adjuncts in treatment of schizophrenia (35, pp. 72S–81S).

Objective measures demonstrate the rapid and dramatic resolution of symptoms of many convulsive and spastic disorders with administration of benzodiazepines. Intravenous diazepam is frequently life-saving in various convulsive emergencies, such as status epilepticus or tetanus spasms. Benzodiazepines afford prompt control of neonatal seizures resulting from perinatal hypoxia, and they provide effective prophylaxis in children susceptible to prolonged seizure activity. Chronic administration of benzodiazepines as adjuncts to other anticonvulsants can significantly improve control of many cases of epilepsy (35, pp. 81S–94S). Benzodiazepines frequently bring substantial relief of spasticity associated with chronic conditions, such as multiple sclerosis and paraplegia resulting from

spinal trauma. They are also of benefit in some patients with cerebral palsy, particularly younger patients with athetoid movements (35, pp. 100S–107S). The drugs are often effective in treatment of involuntary movement disorders, including restless legs syndrome, choreas, intention myoclonus, and some dyskinesias and dystonias associated with use of neuroleptic medications (35, pp. 94S–100S). It has long been recognized that benzodiazepines are effective in managing acute withdrawal from alcohol; they reduce the incidence of potentially fatal complications, such as alcoholic delirium, seizures, and hyperpyrexia (35, pp. 107S–113S).

Benzodiazepines are important adjuncts in medical and dental procedures. When administered prior to surgical anesthesia, they reduce anxiety, provide sedation, facilitate anesthetic induction, and produce amnesia for the events surrounding induction; they also often reduce the required doses of anesthetic agents. They provide safe and effective sedation for mechanical ventilation following cardiac surgery. Lorazepam and other benzodiazepines can help to control nausea and vomiting associated with cancer chemotherapy. Benzodiazepines are commonly used for their anxiolytic, sedative, and amnestic effects in a wide range of stressful diagnostic procedures (35, pp. 118S–135S).

In many of their uses, benzodiazepines are required for only short periods of treatment; as discussed below, the vast majority of actual use of these drugs lasts for only a few weeks. However, some disorders for which benzodiazepines are indicated are recurrent or chronic. Although the effects of long-term benzodiazepine treatment have not been systematically studied, the results of a number of studies provide some interesting suggestions about long-term effects. Therapeutic effects of benzodiazepines are usually or often sustained over months or years, without the need for increased dosage, in treatment of GAD and panic disorder (35, pp. 19S–21S). Relief of insomnia has been documented during periods of regular nightly use for up to 6 months (35, p. 138S). Although benzodiazepines are not indicated as sole therapy for chronic convulsive disorders, such as epilepsies, because they are known to lose effect fairly rapidly in a large proportion of cases, it is of interest that tolerance is not seen to develop in all cases; in some patients, the drugs have continued to control seizures for years (35, pp. 85S–88S). Similar evidence of interindividual variation in tolerance development has been described in benzodiazepine treatment of spastic and dyskinetic disorders (35, pp. 95S–99S). This evidence that tolerance does not develop to these effects in some individuals is compelling in that the sustained benefit can be verified objectively. However, there has been no attempt to study this interindividual variation in tolerance development directly.

Newer Compounds

Zopiclone is the oldest of the "new" compounds considered here, having been introduced in the late 1970s.

Accordingly, there have been many more studies of the clinical effects of this drug than of the others. Most controlled studies of zopiclone have compared the hypnotic effects of a 7.5-mg dose with those of benzodiazepine hypnotics (13). Sleep laboratory studies, in which zopiclone was compared with flurazepam 30 mg (35, p. 25S), triazolam 0.25 mg (35, p. 32S), or nitrazepam 5 mg (35, p. 29S), showed each compound to be effective, with no significant differences between them on any parameters of effect. In studies using subjective ratings, zopiclone was equivalent to flurazepam 30 mg (35, p. 25S), triazolam 0.25 mg (35, p. 32S), temazepam 20 mg (35, p. 38S), and nitrazepam 5 mg (35, p. 29S) on most or all measures. Among other comparative studies using patient questionnaires, some found zopiclone to be superior to benzodiazepines on some parameters (35, pp. 29S, 32S–33S), whereas others found the benzodiazepines to be superior (35, pp. 32S–33S, 36S).

Sleep laboratory studies have also provided objective evidence of the hypnotic efficacy of the newer agent, zolpidem (15,39); the latter study found that zolpidem produced fewer alterations of sleep "architecture" than did flunitrazepam. Other controlled studies have also shown the efficacy of zolpidem as compared with triazolam (60), flunitrazepam (23), or placebo (67). Zolpidem also appears to be useful as a preanesthetic medication, producing good sedation as well as anterograde amnesia (14,56).

In the single placebo-controlled study of the anxiolytic efficacy of abecarnil reported to date (3), patients with GAD who received 3–9 mg daily for 3 weeks were significantly more improved than controls, according to global evaluations as well as scores on the Hamilton Anxiety Rating Scale. Higher doses of abecarnil were not more effective and were associated with a higher incidence of sedative side effects.

Adverse Effects

The most common side effects of benzodiazepines in routine clinical use are manifestations of excessive depression of the CNS; adverse effects on other physiological systems are rare. Sedative side effects most frequently include drowsiness, muscle weakness, lightheadedness, vertigo, ataxia, dysarthria, diplopia, blurring of vision, confusion, apathy, and vertigo (e.g., see refs. 57 and 66). The relative risk of such effects varies with individual patient susceptibility; because of pharmacokinetic changes associated with aging, for example, the elderly may be at increased risk (27).

Adverse Behavioral Effects

A large number of experimental and clinical studies have attempted to assess the liability of benzodiazepines to impair psychomotor performance. Various tests of performance in normal, anxious, and insomniac subjects have shown effects of single doses of benzodiazepines within the therapeutic range. When administration is repeated over several days, these effects diminish. Effects over much longer periods of time have not been adequately studied. There is remarkably little agreement among studies with respect to the types of performance most susceptible to the effects of benzodiazepines (76, pp. 290–300; 77, pp. 207–214).

With respect to the newer compounds considered here, a significant number of studies have assessed the effects on psychomotor performance of zopiclone, and somewhat fewer studies have assessed such effects of zolpidem. As with most of the benzodiazepines that have been studied, zopiclone at therapeutic doses produced a decrement in performance on various psychomotor tests when these tests were administered shortly after treatment (25,40). When the drug was given at night, performances on the following morning were usually not disrupted (32,54,58; but also see refs. 10 and 12). A similar profile has been demonstrated for zolpidem (7,19,23,50). These findings are consistent with the relatively short durations of actions of these drugs. Only one study (17) has assessed effects of abecarnil on performance. Performance was disrupted by 20 and 40 mg of abecarnil, with recovery at 24 hr after treatment; when the drug was administered over 9 days, patients developed some tolerance to these effects. Bretazenil has been reported to produce dose-related disruptions in psychomotor performance; however, the slope of the dose–response curve was not as steep as that for diazepam or alprazolam (64).

Among the experimental behaviors affected by benzodiazepines are performances in simulated or real automobile driving. However, whether such drug effects actually contribute to driving accidents can be established only by case–control epidemiological studies of drivers involved in accidents. The few studies of this kind that have attempted to address the question have not found evidence that benzodiazepines contribute to automobile accidents (76, pp. 308–315; 77, pp. 229–233). This conclusion has been substantiated in a recent study comparing accident victims that were and were not responsible for the accidents; there was no difference between these groups with respect to presence of benzodiazepines in blood (8).

A number of recent epidemiological studies have examined the association between use of benzodiazepines and the risk of falls and/or hip fractures in elderly populations. Some, but not all, of these studies have found a significant positive association (77, pp. 233–237). In sum, the research suggests that benzodiazepines can contribute to the risk of falls among elderly patients, although the extent of this contribution alone is apparently not great.

The greatest recent advance in our understanding of the psychomotor effects of benzodiazepines comes from increasingly sophisticated research on human recall. It can now be shown reliably that acute doses of these drugs can markedly impair recall, especially delayed recall (77, pp. 215–216). Further study is needed to establish whether and to what extent tolerance to any or all of the drugs' amnestic effects may develop. Benzodiazepines produce decrements in recall in elderly subjects, but these decrements are not greater than those produced in younger subjects; however, because of baseline deficits in recall in the elderly, the additional impairment produced by benzodiazepines may represent a more severe compromise (77, p. 219). Further research is needed to pursue important recent suggestions that benzodiazepines may vary substantially in their effects on recall (77, pp. 216–217).

A number of early case reports of hostile behavior in patients taking benzodiazepines prompted several experimental investigations of the older, longer-acting agents, with conflicting results. Some of the case reports described increased hostility and aggression following ingestion of these drugs (76, pp. 316–317). It is possible that these reports reflected phenomena similar to those described in the numerous and notorious case reports of untoward behavioral reactions to the short-acting, relatively more potent agent, triazolam. On the basis of these reports, triazolam has been subject to various official restrictions in several countries. Regardless of their numbers, however, case reports cannot substitute for controlled studies.

Very few controlled studies have inquired into the incidence or nature of daytime distress during and after periods of nightly administration of triazolam. Some studies found certain adverse effects during and/or after treatment, including increased anxiety (38,52) and apparent idiosyncratic reactions such as panic attacks, personality changes, and delusional episodes (1); others have found no increased anxiety (11,45,61) or hostility (61) during triazolam treatment or upon discontinuation. Further controlled research is certainly needed to establish whether triazolam and/or other short-acting benzodiazepines can produce such adverse effects, and, if so, what their nature and incidence might be.

Overdose

The relative safety of the benzodiazepines is most clearly evident in cases of overdose. Even massive overdoses, if taken without other CNS depressants, are almost never fatal. Morbidity and mortality associated with drug overdoses declined dramatically as benzodiazepines replaced older sedative–hypnotics; this has been one of the most important and least controversial advantages of this drug class (26,57; 76, pp. 377–385; 77, pp. 302–314).

There is as yet no reliable evidence regarding the incidence or characteristics of overdoses of the newer compounds considered here. It will be especially interesting to learn whether overdoses of zolpidem are associated with less risk than are overdoses of other hypnotics.

EPIDEMIOLOGY OF USE AND ABUSE

In view of the extensive worldwide experience with benzodiazepines during the past 30 years, epidemiology should be our most important guide in assessing their risks, including their liability for abuse. This is particularly appropriate in view of the remarkable agreement among a great many diverse sources of information about how these drugs are used, which permits a high degree of confidence in the reliability of the patterns described.

Use

History and Appropriateness of Use

In most countries for which data are available, sales of benzodiazepines increased steadily from the time of their introduction until the mid- to late 1970s; during this period they largely displaced the barbiturates (76, pp. 324–334). Sales then declined substantially until the early 1980s, after which there was some increase throughout the decade. In the 1980s, sales of benzodiazepine hypnotics increased far more rapidly than sales of benzodiazepine anxiolytics (77, pp. 239–250). Cross-national surveys conducted in 1981 indicated that an average of 12% of the adult populations of a number of Western European countries and the United States reported using anxiolytics (of which more than 80% were benzodiazepines) during the previous year (4). National data indicating trends in use are available for the United States, where the overall prevalence of annual use of anxiolytics declined from 11.1% of the adult population in 1979 to 8.3% in 1990; use of hypnotics meanwhile remained stable, at about 2.5% of adults (5).

As benzodiazepines originally came to be widely used, and indeed long thereafter, it was commonly perceived that this widespread use of psychoactive drugs was a uniquely contemporary phenomenon. This perception led many observers to assume that the benzodiazepines were overprescribed and overused, without consideration of the prevalence of the disorders for which the drugs were indicated. However, a historical review of United States prescription surveys indicates that benzodiazepines have not accounted for a greater proportion of prescriptions than have other sedative–hypnotics over the course of at least a century. Similarly, prescription data for the United Kingdom show that sedative–hypnotics accounted for about 15% of all prescriptions dispensed in 1949–1951 (chiefly bromides and barbiturates) as well as in 1975 (chiefly benzodiazepines). It seems reasonable to assume that the relative stability of sedative–hypnotic consumption is a function of the relatively stable morbidity that motivates use of these drugs (76, pp. 321–324).

Surveys comparing drug use and psychiatric morbidity in the general population have found that actual use of anxiolytics is generally appropriate, in that users report high levels of emotional distress. On the other hand, the vast majority of people afflicted by psychiatric problems do not seek or receive treatment (76, pp. 346–348). Thus, the problem is not contemporary overmedication, but rather the continued history of undertreatment of psychiatric illness.

Demographics and Patterns of Use

Although rates of use of benzodiazepines vary widely across geographic areas, the demographics and patterns of use within populations are strikingly similar. In virtually every population studied, women receive about twice as many prescriptions for these drugs as do men. Also, use of anxiolytics increases to a peak prevalence in people aged about 50–65 years and declines somewhat in older people, whereas use of hypnotics is most frequent in the oldest age range (77, pp. 254–260).

Most people who receive benzodiazepine prescriptions use the drugs for relatively short periods of time—for example, 4 weeks or less. Patients tend to use lower doses than those prescribed, and to reduce use over time. However, a substantial minority of those who receive benzodiazepine prescriptions continue to use the drugs on a regular basis for longer than a year (76, pp. 355–361).

As suggested above, elderly patients receive a disproportionately large fraction of benzodiazepine prescriptions. They are also more likely than younger patients to use benzodiazepines on a daily basis and to continue use for long periods of time, often for years. Surveys show that long-term users are likely to be elderly patients with multiple chronic physical disorders; they receive prescriptions for benzodiazepines concurrently with multiple other medications (76, pp. 356–357, 367–369; 77, pp. 273–275).

Recent Trends; Focuses for Further Study

In the United States and some Western European nations, which have historically led trends in drug use, rates of use of anxiolytics have declined in recent years, whereas use of hypnotics has remained stable or increased (77, p. 262). Because hypnotic use is particularly prevalent among older patients, the stability of use of these drugs may largely reflect a contingent of elderly patients who use hypnotics regularly for long periods. Although the last few years have brought a considerable increase in epidemiological information about older patients' use of benzodiazepines in general, there has been little attention specifically to use of hypnotics among these patients;

because hypnotic use may be basically distinct from anxiolytic use in many respects, this represents an important focus for future study.

Recent years have also seen a dramatic increase in many countries in use of the benzodiazepines introduced in the late 1970s and later, particularly those with short elimination half-lives; this increase has come at the expense of a proportional decline in use of the older compounds, particularly those with long half-lives (77, pp. 240–250). An important result of this shift is that many patients are now taking single daily doses of benzodiazepine hypnotics with short half-lives, and may thus be exposed to the risk of interdose withdrawal or rebound (discussed further below); the liability for such risks should be assessed in animals as well as in humans. Interview surveys with patients using the short-acting hypnotics could also be designed to provide useful insights into the correlates and effects of this regimen.

Abuse

History of Abuse

Despite the wide availability and extensive medical use of benzodiazepines, there has been very little misuse or recreational use of the drugs among adults or youths in the general population (76, pp. 371–373; 77, pp. 286–297). There has been some nonmedical use of the drugs among populations of drug abusers, though benzodiazepines have usually not been the primary drugs of abuse (76, pp. 373–375; 77, pp. 297–302). These findings from epidemiological research parallel the results of experimental studies (described below) that have demonstrated no preference for benzodiazepines in normal subjects. In subjects with histories of sedative abuse, although there are virtually no reinforcing effects of doses within the therapeutic range, modest reinforcing effects are seen at higher doses.

Benzodiazepines are found with some frequency in overdose surveys, usually in combination with other drugs (76, pp. 377–385; 77, pp. 302–314). When the frequency of overdose cases is examined in relation to the volume and patterns of prescriptions, the frequency of cases involving benzodiazepines is substantially lower than that of other prescribed drugs (e.g., analgesics), and the relative frequency of cases involving individual benzodiazepines is generally proportional to their respective medical availability (76, p. 384; 77, p. 311). These drugs are rarely implicated in fatal overdoses (76, pp. 383–384; 77, p. 311). Overdoses involving benzodiazepines are most likely to result from suicide attempts rather than from accidental consequences of recreational use; in this respect, these overdoses are like those typical of other psychotherapeutic agents and distinct from those typical of benchmark drugs of abuse (76, pp. 384–385; 77, pp. 308–311).

Recent Trends

Survey data from the United States have documented continuing declines in nonmedical use of benzodiazepines in the general population. Periodic household surveys by the National Institute on Drug Abuse have shown that, between 1985 and 1992, annual rates of nonmedical use of tranquilizers decreased by more than half among adolescents (12–17 years old), young adults (18–25 years old), and adults (26 years of age and older) (72,73); in 1992, between 1% and 3% of a national sample reported nonmedical use within the previous year, and 0.6% or less within the previous month (73). Periodic surveys in the United States and Canada have shown that nonmedical use of tranquilizers among youth has declined fairly steadily since the late 1970s (36,37; 77, pp. 288–289); in 1992, the monthly prevalence of such use among United States high school seniors and college students, respectively, was 1.0% and 0.6% (36,37). Data from the Drug Abuse Warning Network (DAWN) show that the frequency of mentions of benzodiazepines in overdose cases in the United States has been decreasing since the mid-1970s (77, pp. 308–309).

Newer Compounds

To date, there is no appreciable epidemiological evidence regarding abuse of the newer compounds considered here. It will surely be some considerable time before we know, for example, how abuse of these drugs may differ from abuse of the established benzodiazepines.

ABUSE LIABILITY

We define the abuse liability of a compound as its capacity to produce psychological dependence (which we prefer to address in terms of objective measures of drug taking), or physiological dependence, in conjunction with the capacity to alter behavior in a manner that is detrimental to the individual or to his or her social environment. The following section reviews experimental and clinical studies of the reinforcing effects of benzodiazepines and of their potential to produce physiological dependence.

Reinforcing Effects

When a subject takes (or "self-administers") a drug, the pharmacological effects are a consequence of the behavior. If this behavior subsequently increases in frequency, or if frequent self-administration is maintained, the behavior is considered to have been reinforced by the drug. This psychological process is an essential determinant of the abuse liability of a drug. Studies of reinforcing effects of drugs have largely supplanted studies of "psychological dependence" and have proven to have predictive value in identifying drugs of abuse.

Studies in Animals

Established Agents

In self-administration studies imposing a wide variety of experimental conditions, benzodiazepines appear only marginally effective as reinforcers. There is little or no preference for benzodiazepines in oral forms, even in physiologically dependent subjects (77, pp. 158–159, 162). Studies in which multiple responses are required for each intravenous injection, which represent relatively stringent measures of reinforcing effects, have demonstrated that benzodiazepines maintain response rates above those maintained by vehicle alone; however, these rates are typically lower than those maintained by reference drugs such as cocaine, codeine, or several barbiturates (76, pp. 258–260; 77, pp. 161–162).

Some studies have suggested that relative onset of action may be a critical factor in determining whether benzodiazepines will function as reinforcers (76, pp. 259–260; 77, p. 162). This suggestion, from studies comparing several compounds, has not been supported by systematic evaluation of all benzodiazepines; nevertheless, the possibility is important and should be pursued directly in experimental studies. There is also some evidence that self-administration of diazepam might be maintained more readily in subjects trained to self-administer barbiturates than in those trained to self-administer stimulants (76, p. 259; 77, pp. 161–162). The influence of drug use history on the reinforcing effects of benzodiazepines is an important question that has also been raised in human studies (see below) and that deserves systematic study in animals. Similarly, as described below, clinical observations suggest that reinforcing effects of benzodiazepines are increased in patients undergoing withdrawal. Relevant studies in animals do not support this conclusion (77, pp. 159 and 162). However, these studies were not designed explicitly to assess reinforcing effects of benzodiazepines during withdrawal; such studies are clearly needed.

Newer Compounds

Only a few studies have examined the reinforcing effects of the newer compounds in animals. Zopiclone self-administration was maintained in rhesus monkeys at rates higher than those maintained by vehicle (79). Bretazenil did not maintain responding in cynomolgus monkeys trained to self-administer pentobarbital (47). In baboons trained to self-administer cocaine, abecarnil failed to maintain responding (62), whereas zolpidem maintained self-administration at rates similar to those obtained with cocaine or methohexital and considerably greater than those shown previously with most other benzodiazepines (28,78). Thus, drugs (such as zolpidem) that act as full agonists on a subset of benzodiazepine receptors appear to have marked reinforcing effects, whereas drugs that act as partial agonists may have reduced reinforcing effects.

Studies in Humans

Evidence in humans pertaining to the liability of benzodiazepines for abuse is largely limited to experimental and epidemiological studies. Few of these studies have examined indices of inappropriate use in clinical populations, or in conditions of therapeutic use. This section considers experimental evidence of abuse liability of benzodiazepines in normal and anxious subjects and in subjects with histories of sedative abuse.

Established Agents

A number of studies have consistently shown that, when given a choice between diazepam and placebo, normal volunteers prefer to take placebo. Even anxious subjects tend to choose placebo over diazepam, at least if they are not actively seeking treatment for their anxiety. Anxious subjects seeking treatment were more likely to choose diazepam over placebo, although only a minority always selected the active drug (76, pp. 261–262; 77, pp. 164–165). These findings suggest that it is unlikely that most use of these drugs in patient populations is associated with a significant risk of abuse.

On the other hand, patients undergoing withdrawal following abrupt discontinuation of diazepam show an increased tendency to self-administer the drug (77, p. 165). This suggests that physiological dependence to benzodiazepines, and the withdrawal signs resulting from their discontinuation, may maintain ingestion of these drugs. However, studies of dependent patients (see below) have found no tendency to escalate doses. Self-administration of benzodiazepines during withdrawal appears to reflect an effort to relieve distressing symptoms; after the withdrawal syndrome abates, patients do not exhibit continued "craving" to resume benzodiazepine use (43).

Perhaps the most interesting recent finding is that subjects who were moderate users of alcohol (consuming an average of 11 drinks weekly), in contrast to lighter drinkers, consistently chose to take diazepam rather than placebo (16). Previous studies had shown consistent preference for benzodiazepines only in populations of sedative abusers (76, pp. 261–267; 77, pp. 164–167). It will be of great interest to determine the specific conditions associated with diazepam selection in these experiments with moderate drinkers and to explore whether moderate use of

other classes of drugs (e.g., other sedatives or stimulants) might also be associated with increased preference for benzodiazepines.

Subjects with histories of sedative abuse show a preference for benzodiazepines over saline or vehicle; this preference is less than that induced by short- or intermediate-acting barbiturates. Sedative abusers also express greater "liking" for benzodiazepines than for placebo (76, pp. 263–265). Studies of sedative abusers often examine effects of only a single dose of each drug tested, which may be a limitation of this research. In addition, studies of sedative abusers have increasingly tended to focus on subjective effects to the exclusion of behavioral effects; although there appears to be a reasonably good correlation between drug-liking and drug-taking in these subjects, it remains important to observe actual drug selection and ingestion in order to assess reinforcing effects. Also, because studies of this population have indicated that reinforcing effects of benzodiazepines tend to decrease over time (76, p. 263), experimental observations of subjective and reinforcing effects of these drugs should be assessed for a period sufficient to obtain stable evaluations of effects.

Newer Compounds

There have been few studies of the abuse liability of the newer benzodiazepine receptor ligands in humans. Forty inpatients recently detoxified from alcohol were trained to distinguish 0.25 mg triazolam from 3.75 mg zopiclone. When given a choice of which to take, 25 chose triazolam and 15 chose zopiclone. The preference for triazolam appeared to be due to the perception that this drug had greater antianxiety effects. The drugs produced nearly equal reports of hypnotic effects and euphoric effects (6).

Effects of several doses of triazolam and zolpidem were studied in subjects with histories of sedative abuse. At the two highest doses tested (0.5 and 0.75 mg triazolam, and 30 and 45 mg zolpidem), subjects reported "drug-liking" greater than that with placebo, with no significant difference between the drugs. Interestingly, drug-liking as rated the next day was not different from placebo for either drug; this finding supports the need for assessment of such effects over time. Neither zolpidem nor triazolam produced increases in the MBG scale of the ARCI questionnaire, a scale that traditionally measures drug-induced "euphoria" (19).

Sellers et al. (64) compared the effects of several doses of diazepam, alprazolam, and bretazenil on subjective measures in sedative abusers. Although each drug produced effects greater than those of placebo on most scales, the effects of diazepam and alprazolam were dose-related, whereas those of bretazenil were not clearly related to dose. On the basis of the subjective effects measured, bretazenil appeared to have less liability for abuse than did diazepam or alprazolam.

Physiological Dependence

Physiological dependence is a condition of the organism, induced by drug treatment, that results in a time-limited withdrawal reaction when treatment is discontinued or when an antagonist (e.g., flumazenil) is administered.

Studies in Animals

Established Agents

Several studies in animals have shown that large doses of benzodiazepines can produce physiological dependence. These studies have also provided some information about the extent to which this physiological dependence conforms to the general rules derived from studies of this phenomenon with opioids, barbiturates, and ethanol. The general rules suggest that withdrawal signs are more frequent or of greater magnitude (a) following administration of doses with greater effects, (b) following treatment for longer periods of time, and (c) following continuous rather than periodic drug administration.

Most studies of benzodiazepines have found results consistent with the first general rule (68; 76, pp. 271 and 276; 77, pp. 173–174). However, some findings suggest that the magnitude of the withdrawal may reach some asymptote beyond which increases in dose have no effect, or have different effects on a composite withdrawal score (76, pp. 271 and 276) or on individual withdrawal signs (68).

The rule that the frequency or intensity of withdrawal should vary as a function of the duration of treatment has been borne out consistently in studies of benzodiazepines (76, pp. 271 and 276–277; 77, p. 174).

Whether benzodiazepine dependence is more frequent or of greater magnitude following continuous rather than periodic administration has not been systematically investigated. It seems particularly important to conduct such studies since the advent of short-acting compounds, which are often used clinically as hypnotics (i.e., in single daily doses). This has introduced the phenomenon of repeated intermittent, rather than continuous, exposure to the agonist. Some animal studies have indicated that dependence can develop to single daily exposures to midazolam (20), although this compound is eliminated within a few hours. However, studies have not addressed the possibility, suggested by some clinical observations, that once-daily administration of short-acting benzodiazepines might produce repeated episodes of acute dependence and withdrawal. The behavioral and biochemical correlates and

consequences of this pattern of benzodiazepine use should be pursued systematically.

Results of several studies have suggested that benzodiazepines might differ in their potential to produce physiological dependence. Of particular interest is a series of studies of precipitated withdrawal by Martin et al. (48), which suggest that the withdrawal syndromes following exposure to different benzodiazepine agonists may consist of overlapping but distinct constellations of signs. Following chronic treatment with several agonists in dogs, flumazenil was administered and the nature and intensity of withdrawal was assessed by scoring individual signs. Withdrawal was most intense in subjects treated with diazepam, less intense with flunitrazepam or halazepam, lesser still with nordiazepam or alprazolam, and least for those treated with oxazepam. Seizures were most frequent in dogs treated with alprazolam, diazepam, or flunitrazepam, less frequent with nordiazepam, and least frequent with halazepam or lorazepam. The investigators identified three different syndromes associated with different agonists, characterized by relative frequency of seizures and relative magnitude of withdrawal scores. They suggested that differences among these syndromes may be due to differences in the mechanisms and sites of action of the benzodiazepines or their metabolites.

Newer Compounds

The capacity of some of the newer sedative/anxiolytic agents to produce physiological dependence has been evaluated to a limited extent in animals. Following chronic treatment with abecarnil subcutaneously at doses that elevated seizure threshold, flumazenil produced few signs of withdrawal in dogs, and only one of seven subjects showed a lowered threshold for pentylenetetrazol-induced seizures after treatment was discontinued (41). In a subsequent study in dogs, abecarnil and diazepam were chronically administered subcutaneously at doses with approximately equal anticonvulsant effects; antagonists produced signs of withdrawal in all subjects treated with diazepam, but signs of precipitated withdrawal were much less frequent in subjects treated with abecarnil (42; see also ref. 65). In baboons given abecarnil by continuous intragastric infusion, two of four subjects exhibited "mild" signs of withdrawal upon administration of flumazenil and after discontinuation of 6–8 weeks of treatment (62). Steppuhn et al. (71) examined mice treated with subcutaneous depot injections of abecarnil or diazepam at doses producing equivalent time courses and receptor occupancy. Only the mice treated with diazepam showed signs of withdrawal after discontinuation. This study reveals the importance of relating response to receptor occupancy; by including this comparison, the authors could strongly suggest an intrinsic difference in the potential of these drugs to produce physiological dependence.

Flumazenil produced clear withdrawal signs in squirrel monkeys treated with diazepam, but not in those treated with bretazenil (46). In another study (47), squirrel monkeys treated with a range of doses of bretazenil or alprazolam were challenged with the benzodiazepine partial agonist, sarmazenil (Ro 15-3505); sarmazenil produced convulsions in a smaller proportion of the subjects treated with the various doses of bretazenil compared with alprazolam. Because bretazenil is more potent than alprazolam in producing a range of pharmacological effects, these findings led the authors to conclude that it has a greater potential to produce physiological dependence.

Moreau et al. (51) compared bretazenil with triazolam, alprazolam, and diazepam in convulsion-prone DBA/2J mice. After 1 week of continuous treatment using osmotic minipumps, sarmazenil produced signs of withdrawal that varied in frequency with dose of triazolam, alprazolam, or diazepam; withdrawal signs were not observed in animals treated with bretazenil or vehicle alone. These investigators also conducted in vivo studies of receptor occupancy, which established that both bretazenil and alprazolam were bioavailable in the CNS; this represents important evidence that the difference between the drugs in producing dependence is a function of differences in their intrinsic efficacy, rather than their relative CNS bioavailability. Additional evidence of an intrinsic difference in the dependence potential of these drugs was provided by a further study in which mice were treated with doses of bretazenil and alprazolam that were roughly equivalent multiples of their anticonvulsant ED_{50} values; sarmazenil precipitated withdrawal in mice treated with alprazolam, but not in mice treated with bretazenil.

In a procedure for rapid evaluation of dependence-producing effects of benzodiazepines, after 3 days of treatment mice were injected with flumazenil and the threshold for electric-shock-induced seizure was determined. Flumazenil substantially reduced seizure threshold following treatment with several benzodiazepine agonists and related compounds, including chlordiazepoxide, diazepam, flurazepam, alprazolam, triazolam, midazolam, and zopiclone, as well as the partial agonists bretazenil and Ro 17-1812. In contrast, seizure threshold was not altered after treatment with zolpidem, tracazolate, or CL 218, 872. In addition, although bretazenil and alprazolam had similar ED_{50} values for inhibition of in vivo binding, the dose of bretazenil required to produce any sign of dependence was 10 times greater than that of alprazolam. Similarly, the ED_{50} values of the full agonist triazolam and the partial agonist Ro 17-1812 were similar, though 10-fold-higher doses of Ro 17-1812 were required to produce signs of dependence (74). These data are consistent with the conclusion that drugs with limited efficacy are also limited in their liability for producing physiological dependence.

In another study in mice, zolpidem or midazolam was administered for 10 days at pharmacologically equivalent

doses, based on time course and effectiveness in suppression of locomotor activity. Latency to isoniazid-induced convulsions was used as an index of withdrawal. Both precipitated and spontaneous withdrawal was observed in mice treated with midazolam; neither was observed in those treated with zolpidem (55).

In contrast to the above studies, Griffiths et al. (28) obtained a result that might indicate a physiological dependence on zolpidem. Baboons were trained to earn food pellets during and after periods of zolpidem self-administration. When zolpidem was replaced with vehicle, five of seven baboons substantially decreased their responses for food. The suppression of this behavior proved to be time-limited and may therefore have represented withdrawal; to confirm this interpretation, it would have been useful to determine whether the effect could have been reversed by resumption of treatment. In earlier studies, Yanagita (80) rated the magnitude of withdrawal from zopiclone, diazepam, and nitrazepam in rhesus monkeys. Discontinuation of chronic administration of zopiclone and nitrazepam produced withdrawal of intermediate intensity, whereas withdrawal from diazepam was rated as severe. The author noted that the lower intensity of withdrawal ratings of zopiclone may have been due to its relatively short time course (76, pp. 272–273).

Discussion

A number of studies have suggested that benzodiazepines may differ in their potential to produce dependence or in the characteristics of the dependence they produce. For example, results of studies by W. R. Martin and co-workers suggest that the withdrawal syndromes following administration of different benzodiazepine agonists may consist of overlapping but distinct constellations of signs. Studies with the beta-carboline abecarnil and the imidazopyridine zolpidem, as well as studies with benzodiazepine partial agonists, suggest that these compounds may have less potential to produce dependence than do classical benzodiazepine agonists. In addition, as noted above, there have been suggestions that the partial agonists are not effective as reinforcers.

It has also been suggested that the onset of withdrawal might be more rapid and the intensity of withdrawal might be greater following discontinuation of short-acting benzodiazepines than after discontinuation of long-acting compounds. However, when the short-acting benzodiazepine midazolam was administered for a period equivalent to the duration of the effects of a single dose of the long-acting chlordiazepoxide, spontaneous withdrawal from the two regimens was comparable in intensity (12). Further studies that equate the benzodiazepines according to all dosing parameters, except their speed of elimination, will be of importance in verifying these results. Meanwhile, the available evidence from animal studies is not consistent with clinical data (see below) indicating that withdrawal is more intense following termination of short-acting as compared with long-acting benzodiazepines. However, animal and human studies appear to concur that the onset of withdrawal is more rapid following discontinuation of the short-acting agents (77, pp. 178–180 and 187–195).

Finally, it may be noted that an increasing number of behavioral procedures purport to assess rebound anxiety using animal models (77, pp. 183–184). In the majority of these procedures, the models used have not been validated according to standard pharmacological criteria for establishing behaviors as withdrawal phenomena. Moreover, the behaviors measured have not been shown to be functionally equivalent to human anxiety; nor have they been shown to have any utility for prediction of clinical outcomes. Few of these studies to date have made a substantial contribution to the understanding of benzodiazepine withdrawal.

Studies in Humans

Established Agents

A withdrawal syndrome following abrupt discontinuation of high doses of chlordiazepoxide was first described in 1961 (33). The possibility that dependence could develop at therapeutic doses of benzodiazepines was recognized only around 1980 (66; 76, pp. 279–285). Although high-dose benzodiazepine dependence surprised no one familiar with the pharmacology of sedative drugs, the phenomenon of dependence at therapeutic doses had not been anticipated (34); systematic study of barbiturates and other older sedatives had shown that dependence developed only at doses far above the therapeutic range (18,22). Although dependence on therapeutic doses of benzodiazepines has now been documented in numerous studies and remains a focus of widespread concern, our understanding of this phenomenon has not advanced appreciably.

The studies that established the potential of benzodiazepines to produce physiological dependence at therapeutic doses also found that not all patients using these drugs became dependent; that is, some did not show signs of withdrawal when the drugs were discontinued (76, p. 280). More recent studies have supported this finding, although they have not clarified what proportion of users do become dependent nor have they confirmed the determinants of dependence (77, pp. 195–198). Most studies of therapeutic-dose dependence examined the effects of discontinuation in patients who had used the drugs for relatively long periods, and it was often assumed that the risk increased with duration of use; studies in animals supported that view (76, pp. 279–285). However, more recent human studies have demonstrated withdrawal after relatively brief periods of use (e.g., 2 weeks), and some studies comparing discontinuation after different periods of treatment have found no difference in the incidence of withdrawal (53; 77, pp. 197–198). Other factors that have been considered as possible determinants of the development of physiological dependence have included duration of drug action, magnitude of dose, patients' prior drug use, age, and personality traits; although some of these factors have influenced the development of dependence in animals, none has yet been shown to be clearly related to the risk of dependence in patients (77, pp. 204–205). As described previously, the development of tolerance to therapeutic effects of benzodiazepines evidently varies widely among individuals. This suggests the importance of examining individual variables as they may interact with the pharmacological determinants of benzodiazepine dependence.

Upon abrupt discontinuation of benzodiazepine treatment, dependent patients are likely to experience increased anxiety and/or insomnia. Other characteristics of the benzodiazepine withdrawal syndrome include alterations in taste and smell sensations, tremor, restlessness, gastrointestinal distress, sweating, tachycardia, and mild systolic hypertension. The syndrome and associated discomfort are usually mild, reaching peak severity in 2–10 days and abating within 4 weeks after discontinuation (59,66; 76, pp. 289–290). Some recent studies have suggested that symptoms and signs of benzodiazepine withdrawal can persist for many months or for years, but the available evidence is not convincing (66; 77, p. 205).

Although it has not been established whether dependence is more or less likely to develop with short- versus long-half-life benzodiazepines, recent studies have shown that withdrawal from the short-acting drugs develops more rapidly and may be more intense than withdrawal from benzodiazepines with longer durations of action. It has also been found that effective discontinuation of short-acting benzodiazepines, to minimize the risk of rebound symptoms and other effects of withdrawal, requires a particularly gradual and prolonged tapering regimen and that, at least in the short term, patients discontinued from these drugs are more likely to resume use than are patients discontinued from long-acting agents (77, pp. 187 and 192–195).

Despite concerns about the risk of physiological dependence on benzodiazepines, there has been little consideration of ways in which dependence might be prevented from the onset of treatment. Clinical authorities have long recommended that use should be interrupted by occasional "drug holidays," which would permit reassessment of the need to continue treatment and might also reduce the risk of dependence development; however, the effect of drug-free intervals on the development of dependence has not been studied under controlled conditions. Another possible approach to prevention has been suggested by studies of chronic benzodiazepine treatment in animals; periodic injections of a benzodiazepine antagonist significantly reduced the intensity of the subsequent withdrawal syndrome (24). The suggestion that it might be possible in this way to "reset the clock" for the initiation of dependence needs to be pursued through studies of a variety of benzodiazepines in both animals and humans.

Newer Compounds

The potential of zopiclone to produce physiological dependence in humans has not been extensively studied. A review by Bianchi and Musch (9) found that in 25 studies of zopiclone including assessments of possible withdrawal phenomena, only a small minority found such effects. Nervousness, anxiety, or vertigo appeared as possible withdrawal signs in seven (1.6%) of 441 patients treated with zopiclone, whereas possible withdrawal signs were observed in 6%, 7%, and 10% of patients treated with flunitrazepam, triazolam, and flurazepam, respectively. In comparative trials of hypnotic use, rebound insomnia was observed following discontinuation of nitrazepam, flurazepam, and triazolam, but not after discontinuation of zopiclone. Among patients with insomnia associated with GAD, nightly treatment with zopiclone was associated with less daytime anxiety than was treatment with nitrazepam (2) or triazolam (21).

The dependence potential of zolpidem has likewise received little study in humans. However, the available data are consistent in reflecting no rebound insomnia or withdrawal signs in insomniac patients receiving zolpidem daily for periods from 7 to 180 days (44,63,67).

Abecarnil was administered in three different dosage ranges to patients with GAD. Following 3 weeks of treatment, insomnia, anxiety, and other possible signs of withdrawal were observed among patients who received active medication, but not among a placebo control group. The incidence of withdrawal signs was positively related to the dose administered (3).

FUTURE CHALLENGES

Benzodiazepines have been on the market for over 30 years and have achieved remarkable clinical success. The introduction of these drugs in clinical practice represented a very significant advance over previous generations of sedative–hypnotics. Some problems of course remain, associated with both abuse and therapeutic use of benzodiazepines. From our current perspective, it appears that it may be difficult to overcome these problems.

Therapeutic use has largely shifted from the older, longer-acting benzodiazepines to the shorter-acting agents that became available more recently. However, it is not clear that this represents an advance in the appropriate use of these drugs. This massive shift in prescribing should be regarded as a compelling stimulus to well-controlled assessments of the relative advantages and disadvantages of the longer- versus the shorter-acting agents in a variety of clinical applications.

Similarly, it is not clear that efforts to develop newer sedative–hypnotics, such as those considered in this chapter, will readily resolve the kinds of problems associated with established benzodiazepines. There are multiple genetic forms of the benzodiazepine receptor. It will be no easy matter to find ligands selective for them. Moreover, if such ligands can be identified, there is a long and arduous path, from in vitro pharmacology through pharmacodynamics, to establish whether they bear pharmacological characteristics that are relevant to therapeutic or adverse effects. Although the prospect of this work is daunting, it is certainly one of the most exciting challenges for the future of benzodiazepine research.

The partial agonist compounds bretazenil and abecarnil may well represent the most interesting leads to date. The available information on both of these compounds suggests that they may represent significant progress toward reducing the risks associated with reinforcing effects, subjective effects associated with abuse liability, and potential to produce physiological dependence. Human trials of abecarnil are likely to provide new challenges to animal pharmacology and the concept of partial agonism, as well as information about therapeutic effects of this compound (e.g., see ref. 70).

The amalgamation of new molecular developments in receptorology and research toward development of new ligands for the benzodiazepine receptor should prove to be one of the most productive avenues for the growth of knowledge in this area of therapeutics.

ACKNOWLEDGMENT

The authors thank Kaim Associates, Inc., for support in collection, organization, and management of the literature reviewed and for administrative and editorial assistance.

REFERENCES

1. Adam K, Oswald I. Can a rapidly-eliminated hypnotic cause daytime anxiety? *Pharmacopsychiatry* 1989;22:115–119.
2. Agnoli A, Manna V, Martucci N. Double-blind study on the hypnotic and antianxiety effects of zopiclone compared with nitrazepam in the treatment of insomnia. *Int J Clin Pharmacol Res* 1989;9: 277–281.
3. Ballenger JC, McDonald S, Noyes R Jr, et al. The first double-blind, placebo-controlled trial of a partial benzodiazepine agonist, abecarnil (ZK 112-119), in generalized anxiety disorder. *Adv Biochem Psychopharmacol* 1992;47:431–447.
4. Balter MB, Levine J, Manheimer DI. Cross-national study of the extent of anti-anxiety/sedative drug use. *N Engl J Med* 1974; 290:769–774.
5. Balter MB. Benzodiazepine use/abuse: an epidemiologic appraisal. Presented at symposium, Triplicate Prescription: Issues and Answers, New York, February 28, 1991.
6. Bechelli LPDC, Navas F, Pierangelo SA. Comparison of the rein-

forcing properties of zopiclone and triazolam in former alcoholics. *Pharmacology* 1983;27(Suppl 2):235–241.

7. Bensimon G, Foret J, Warot D, Lacomblez L, Thiercelin JF, Simon P. Daytime wakefulness following a bedtime oral dose of zolpidem 20 mg, flunitrazepam 2 mg and placebo. *Br J Clin Pharmacol* 1990;30(3):463–469.

8. Benzodiazepine/Driving Collaborative Group. Are benzodiazepines a risk factor for road accidents? *Drug Alcohol Depend* 1993;33:19–22.

9. Bianchi M, Musch B. Zopiclone discontinuation: review of 25 studies assessing withdrawal and rebound phenomena. *Int Clin Psychopharmacol* 1990;5(Suppl 2):139–145.

10. Billiard M, Besset A, de Lustrac C, Brissaud L, Cadilhac J. Effects of zopiclone on sleep, daytime somnolence and nocturnal and daytime performance in healthy volunteers. *Neurophysiol Clin* 1989;19(2):131–143.

11. Bliwise DL, Seidel WF, Cohen SA, Bliwise NG, Dement WC. Profile of mood states changes during and after 5 weeks of nightly triazolam administration. *J Clin Psychiatry* 1988;49:349–355.

12. Boisse NR, Quaglietta N, Samoriski GM, Guarini JJ. Tolerance and physical dependence to a short-acting benzodiazepine, midazolam. *J Pharmacol Exp Ther* 1990;252:1125–1133.

13. Broadhurst A, Cushnaghan RC. Residual effects of zopiclone (Imovane). *Sleep* 1987;10(Suppl 1):48–53.

14. Cashman JN, Power SJ, Jones RM. Assessment of a new hypnotic imidazo-pyridine (zolpidem) as oral premedication. *Br J Clin Pharmacol* 1987;24:85–92.

15. Declerck AC, Ruwe F, O'Hanlon JF, Wauquier A. Effects of zolpidem and flunitrazepam on nocturnal sleep of women subjectively complaining of insomnia. *Psychopharmacology (Berl)* 1992;106:497–501.

16. De Wit H, Pierri J, Johanson C-E. Reinforcing and subjective effects of diazepam in nondrug-abusing volunteers. *Pharmacol Biochem Behav* 1989;33:205–213.

17. Duka T, Schütt B, Krause W, Dorow R, McDonald S, Fichte K. Human studies on abecarnil a new β-carboline anxiolytic: safety, tolerability and preliminary pharmacological profile. *Br J Clin Pharmacol* 1993;35:386–394.

18. Eddy N, Isbell H. *Public Health Rep* 1959;74:755–763.

19. Evans SM, Funderburk FR, Griffiths RR. Zolpidem and triazolam in humans: behavioral and subjective effects and abuse liability. *J Pharmacol Exp Ther* 1990;255(3):1246–1255.

20. Falk JL, Tang M. Development of physical dependence on midazolam by oral self-administration. *Pharmacol Biochem Behav* 1987;26:797–800.

21. Fontaine R, Beaudry P, Le Morvan P, Beauclair L, Chouinard G. Zopiclone and triazolam in insomnia associated with generalized anxiety disorder: a placebo-controlled evaluation of efficacy and daytime anxiety. *Int Clin Psychopharmacol* 1990;5:173–183.

22. Fraser HF, Wikler A, Essig CF, Isbell H. Degree of physical dependence induced by secobarbital or pentobarbital. *JAMA* 1958;166:126–129.

23. Frattola L, Maggioni M, Cesana B, Priore P. Double blind comparison of zolpidem 20 mg versus flunitrazepam 2 mg in insomniac inpatients. *Drugs Exp Clin Res* 1990;16:371–376.

24. Gallager DW, Heninger K, Heninger G. Periodic benzodiazepine antagonist administration prevents benzodiazepine withdrawal symptoms in primates. *Eur J Pharmacol* 1986;132:31–38.

25. Gorenstein C, Tavares SM, Gentil V, Peres C, Moreno RA, Dreyfus JF. Psychophysiological effects and dose equivalence of zopiclone and triazolam administered to healthy volunteers: methodological considerations. *Braz J Med Biol Res* 1990;23(10):941–951.

26. Greenblatt DJ, Shader RI, Abernethy DR. Drug therapy: current status of benzodiazepines. *N Engl J Med* 1983;309:354–358.

27. Greenblatt DJ, Shader RI, Harmatz JS. Implications of altered drug disposition in the elderly: studies of benzodiazepines. *J Clin Pharmacol* 1989;29:866–872.

28. Griffiths RR, Sannerud CA, Ator NA, Brady JV. Zolpidem behavioral pharmacology in baboons: self-injection, discrimination, tolerance and withdrawal. *J Pharmacol Exp Ther* 1992;260:1199–1208.

29. Haefely WE. Pharmacology of the benzodiazepine receptor. *Eur Arch Psychiatry Neurol Sci* 1989;238:294–301.

30. Haefely WE. Pharmacology of the allosteric modulation of GABAa receptors by benzodiazepine receptor ligands. In: Barnard EA, Costa

E, eds. *Allosteric modulation of amino acid receptors: therapeutic implications.* New York: Raven Press, 1989;47–69.

31. Haefely WE. The GABA–benzodiazepine interaction fifteen years later. *Neurochem Res* 1990;15:169–174.

32. Hindmarch I. Immediate and overnight effects of zopiclone 7.5 mg and nitrazepam 5 mg with ethanol, on psychomotor performance and memory in healthy volunteers. *Int Clin Psychopharmacol* 1990;5(Suppl 2):105–113.

33. Hollister LE, Motzenbecker FP, Degan RO. Withdrawal reactions from chlordiazepoxide ("Librium"). *Psychopharmacologia* 1961;2:63–68.

34. Hollister LE. Dependence on benzodiazepines. In: Szara I, Ludford JP, eds. *Benzodiazepines: a review of research results, 1980.* NIDA research monograph series 33. Washington, DC: U.S. Government Printing Office, 1981;70–82.

35. Hollister LE, Müller-Oerlinghausen B, Rickels K, Shader RI. Clinical uses of benzodiazepines. *J Clin Psychopharmacol* 1993;13(Suppl 1):1S–169S.

36. Johnston LD, O'Malley PM, Bachman JG. *National survey results on drug use from the "monitoring the future" study, 1975–1992, vol I: Secondary school students.* NIH publication no. 93-3597. Washington, DC: U.S. Government Printing Office, 1993.

37. Johnston LD, O'Malley PM, Bachman JG. *National survey results on drug use from the "monitoring the future" study, 1975–1992, volume II: College students and young adults.* NIH publication no. 93-3598. Washington, DC: U.S. Government Printing Office, 1993.

38. Kales A, Soldatos CR, Bixler EO, Kales JD. Early morning insomnia with rapidly eliminated benzodiazepines. *Science* 1983;220:95–97.

39. Kryger MH, Steljes D, Pouliot Z, Neufeld H, Odynski T. Subjective versus objective evaluation of hypnotic efficacy: experience with zolpidem. *Sleep* 1991;14:399–407.

40. Kuitunen T, Mattila MJ, Seppala T. Actions and interactions of hypnotics on human performance: single doses of zopiclone, triazolam and alcohol. *Int Clin Psychopharmacol* 1990;5(Suppl 2):115–130.

41. Loscher W, Honack D, Scherkl R, Hashem A, Frey H-H. Pharmacokinetics, anticonvulsant efficacy and adverse effects of the β-carboline abecarnil, a novel ligand for benzodiazepine receptors, after acute and chronic administration in dogs. *J Pharmacol Exp Ther* 1990;255:541–548.

42. Löscher W, Hönack D. Withdrawal precipitation by benzodiazepine receptor antagonists in dogs chronically treated with diazepam or the novel anxiolytic and anticonvulsant β-carboline abecarnil. *Naunyn Schmiedebergs Arch Pharmacol* 1992;345:452–460.

43. Lucki I, Volpicelli JR, Schwiezer E. Differential craving between abstinent alcohol-dependent subjects and therapeutic users of benzodiazepines. Proceedings of the Annual Meeting of the Committee on Problems of Drug Dependence, June 1990. *Natl Inst Drug Abuse Res Monogr Ser* 1991;105:322–323.

44. Maarek L, Cramer P, Attali P, Coquelin JP, Morselli PL. The safety and efficacy of zolpidem in insomniac patients: a long-term open study in general practice. *J Int Med Res* 1992;20:162–170.

45. Mamelak M, Csima A, Price V. A comparative 25-night sleep laboratory study on the effects of quazepam and triazolam on chronic insomniacs. *J Clin Pharmacol* 1984;24:65–75.

46. Martin JR, Cumin R, Haefely WE. Precipitated withdrawal in monkeys after repeated daily administration of different benzodiazepines. *Soc Neurosci Abstr* 1988;14:1109.

47. Martin JR, Kuwahara A, Horii I, Moreau JL, Jenck F, Sepenwall J, Haefley W. Evidence that the benzodiazepine receptor partial agonist RO 16-6028 has minimal abuse and physical dependence liability. *Soc Neurosci Abstr* 1990;16:1104.

48. Martin WR, Sloan JW, Wala E. Precipitated abstinence in orally dosed benzodiazepine-dependent dogs. *J Pharmacol Exp Ther* 1990;255:744–755.

49. Massotti M, Schlichting JL, Antonacci MD, Giusti P, Memo M, Costa E, Guidotti A. Gamma-aminobutyric acid$_A$ receptor heterogeneity in rat central nervous system: studies with clonazepam and other benzodiazepine ligands. *J Pharmacol Exp Ther* 1991;256:1154–1160.

50. Monti JM. Effect of zolpidem on sleep in insomniac patients. *Eur J Clin Pharmacol* 1989;36(5):461–466.

51. Moreau JL, Jenck F, Pieri L, Schoch P, Martin JR, Haefely WE.

Physical dependence induced in DBA/2J mice by benzodiazepine receptor full agonists, but not by partial agonist Ro 16-6028. *Eur J Pharmacol* 1990;190:269–273.

52. Morgan K, Oswald I. Anxiety caused by a short-life hypnotic. *Br Med J* 1982;284:942.

53. Murphy SM, Owen R, Tyrer P. Comparative assessment of efficacy and withdrawal symptoms after 6 and 12 weeks' treatment with diazepam or buspirone. *Br J Psychiatry* 1989;154:529–534.

54. Nicholson AN, Stone BM. Efficacy of zopiclone in middle age. *Sleep* 1987;10(Suppl 1):35–39.

55. Perrault G, Morel E, Sanger DJ, Zivkovic B. Lack of tolerance and physical dependence upon repeated treatment with the novel hypnotic zolpidem. *J Pharmacol Exp Ther* 1992;263:298–303.

56. Praplan-Pahud J, Forster A, Gamulin Z, Tassonyi E, Sauvanet JP. Preoperative sedation before regional anaesthesia: comparison between zolpidem, midazolam and placebo. *Br J Anaesth* 1990;64:670–674.

57. Rall TW, Hypnotics and sedatives; ethanol. In: Gilman AG, Rall TW, Nies AS, Taylor P, eds. *Goodman and Gilman's: The pharmacological basis of therapeutics,* 8th ed. New York: Pergamon Press, 1990;345–382.

58. Rettig HC, de Haan P, Zuurmond WW, von Leeuwen L. Effects of hypnotics on sleep and psychomotor performance. A double-blind randomised study of lormetazepam, midazolam and zopiclone. *Anaesthesia* 1990;45(12):1079–1082.

59. Rickels K, Schweizer E, Case WG. Benzodiazepines: tolerance and withdrawal: the clinician's point of view. *Clin Neuropharmacol* 1992;15(Suppl 1, Part A):102A–103A.

60. Roger M, Attali P, Coquelin JP. Multicenter, double-blind, controlled comparison of zolpidem and triazolam in elderly patients with insomnia. *Clin Ther* 1993;15:127–136.

61. Roth T, Kramer M, Lutz T. Intermediate use of triazolam: a sleep laboratory study. *J Int Med Res* 1976;4:59–63.

62. Sannerud CA, Ator NA, Griffiths RR. Behavioral pharmacology of abecarnil in baboons: self-injection, drug discrimination and physical dependence. *Behavioural Pharmacology* 1992;3:507–516.

63. Schlich D, L'Heritier C, Coquelin JP, Attali P. Long-term treatment of insomnia with zolpidem: a multicentre general practitioner study of 107 patients. *J Int Med Res* 1991;19:271–279.

64. Sellers EM, Kaplan HL, Busto UE. Abuse liability of bretazenil and other partial agonists. *Clin Neuropharmacol* 1992;15(Suppl):409A.

65. Serra M, Ghiani CA, Foddi MC, Galici R, Motzo C, Biggio G. Failure of flumazenil to precipitate a withdrawal syndrome in cats chronically treated with the new anxioselective β-carboline derivative abecarnil. *Behav Pharmacol* 1993;4:529–533.

66. Shader RI, Greenblatt DJ. Use of benzodiazepines in anxiety disorders. *N Engl J Med* 1993;328:1398–1405.

67. Shaw SH, Curson H, Coquelin JP. A double-blind, comparative study of zolpidem and placebo in the treatment of insomnia in elderly psychiatric in-patients. *J Int Med Res* 1992;20:150–161.

68. Sloan JW, Martin WR, Wala E. Effect of the chronic dose of diazepam on the intensity and characteristics of the precipitated abstinence syndrome in the dog. *J Pharmacol Exp Ther* 1993;265:1152–1162.

69. Stephens DN, Turski L, Hillman M, Turner JD, Schneider HH, Yamaguchi M. What are the differences between abecarnil and conventional benzodiazepine anxiolytics? *Adv Biochem Psychopharmacol* 1992;47:395–405.

70. Stephens DN, Turski L, Jones GH, Steppuhn KG, Schneider HH. Abecarnil: a novel anxiolytic with mixed full agonist/partial agonist properties in animal models of anxiety and sedation. In: *Anxiolytic β-carbolines: from molecular biology to the clinic.* Berlin: Springer-Verlag, 1993;79–95.

71. Steppuhn KG, Schneider HH, Turski L, Stephens DN. Long-term treatment with abecarnil does not induce diazepam-like dependence in mice. *J Pharmacol Exp Ther* 1993;264:1395–1400.

72. Substance Abuse and Mental Health Services Administration. *National household survey on drug abuse: main findings 1991. Revised November 20, 1992.* DHHS publication no. (SMA) 93-1980. Washington, DC: U.S. Government Printing Office, 1993.

73. Substance Abuse and Mental Health Services Administration. *National household survey on drug abuse: population estimates 1992.* DHHS publication no. (SMA) 93-2053. Washington, DC: U.S. Government Printing Office, 1993.

74. Von Voigtlander PF, Lewis RA. A rapid screening method for the assessment of benzodiazepine related-agonist and partial agonist. *J Pharmacol Methods* 1991;26:1–5.

75. Wieland HA, Luddens H, Seeburg PH. Molecular determinants in GABAA/BZ receptor subtypes. *Adv Biochem Psychopharmacol* 1992;47:29–40.

76. Woods JH, Katz JL, Winger GD. Abuse liability of benzodiazepines. *Pharmacol Rev* 1987;39:251–419.

77. Woods JH, Katz JL, Winger GD. Benzodiazepines: use, abuse and consequences. *Pharmacol Rev* 1992;44:151–347.

78. Woolverton WL, Nader MA, Winger G, Woods JH, Patrick GA, Harris LS. *Progress report from the Testing Program for Stimulant and Depressant Drugs 1992.* NIDA research monograph, 1994;132:579–594.

79. Yanagita T, Kato S, Oinuma N. Dependence potential of triazolam tested in rhesus monkeys. *CIEA (Cent Inst Exp Anim) Preclin Rep* 1983;9:175–186.

80. Yanagita T. Dependence potential of zopiclone tested in monkeys. *Pharmacology* 1983;27(Suppl 2):216–227.

Psychopharmacology: The Fourth Generation of Progress, edited by Floyd E. Bloom and David J. Kupfer. Raven Press, Ltd., New York 1995.

CHAPTER 153

Genetic Influences in Drug Abuse

George R. Uhl, Gregory I. Elmer, Michele C. LaBuda, and Roy W. Pickens

HUMAN SUBSTANCE ABUSE VULNERABILITY AND GENETIC INFLUENCES

Individuals are differentially vulnerable to substance abuse. Everyone has access to addictive substances. Not everyone who has an opportunity to use an addictive substance does so, and not everyone who uses an addictive substance becomes addicted. Sixty-three percent of individuals 12 years of age or older report never using illicit drugs or psychotherapeutics, 29% never use cigarettes, and 17% never use alcohol (1992 National Household Survey; Substance Abuse and Mental Health Services Administration, 1993). Sixty-five percent of individuals reporting access to marijuana use the substance, while only 16% of those having access to heroin report use (National Institute on Drug Abuse, 1991).

The likelihood of continuing drug use also varies from individual to individual. Illicit drug use often begins in early teen years, peaks in the late teens and early twenties, and can decline substantially thereafter (e.g., see ref. 39). However, some individuals continue to use drugs into later adulthood. Ninety-three percent of individuals who used alcohol, 60% of cigarette smokers, 19% of heroin users, and 8% of hallucinogen users continued to use drugs at the end of their third decades of life (57).

The frequency and consequences of illicit drug use, factors that underlie most definitions of drug addiction, also vary from user to user. Forty-five percent of individuals using marijuana report using it 12 times or more; half of these report using it once a week or more (National Institute on Drug Abuse, 1992). Variability can also be seen in reports of symptoms of dependence, even among

G. R. Uhl, G. I. Elmer, and R. W. Pickens: Intramural Research Program, Addiction Research Center, National Institute of Drug Abuse, National Institutes of Health, Baltimore, Maryland 21224.
M. C. LaBuda: Department of Psychiatry and Behavioral Sciences, Johns Hopkins University School of Medicine, Baltimore, Maryland 21287.

regular users. Forty-two percent of regular cocaine users did not report any symptom of cocaine dependence (National Institute on Drug Abuse, 1991).

Observations such as these suggest that genetic and environmental conditions that differentially predispose individuals to drug-taking behavior and to the transition from drug-taking behavior to established and maintained drug abuse might be found.

Processes involved in substance abuse are likely to be behaviorally complex; genetic mechanisms contributing to interindividual differences in substance abuse vulnerability are thus likely to be equally complex. Genetic influences on drug use and dependence might operate at a variety of levels. Genetic influences that contribute to the initiation of drug use may differ from those that contribute to heavier drug use or drug dependence (30). Drug use vulnerability might also be modified by protective factors that could contribute to drug abstinence or protect from development of regular use patterns or drug dependence (30). Allelic variants of specific genes could mediate differential drug reinforcing properties, alter drug pharmacodynamics or pharmacokinetics, influence "sensation-seeking" personality traits that may facilitate exposure to drugs, exacerbate drug toxicities, or minimize "protective" factors such as hangovers. Individuals also differ in their specific drugs of choice. Ideal investigations of the genetic components of addictions might therefore separately investigate the neurobiological substrates of vulnerability to drug use acquisition, maintenance, or resistance to extinction for each abused substance. In practice, however, individuals meeting substance abuse criteria which largely center on the extent and duration of consumption of addictive substances are the focus of most attention in studies attempting to identify components of the genetic bases of substance abuse vulnerability.

Familial and population genetic studies are beginning to reveal possible genetic bases for some of the interindividual differences in vulnerability to substance abuse.

Studies of related individuals can provide evidence of the proportionate contributions of genes and environment to a behavioral disorder such as substance abuse. Data from these approaches can also be used to suggest whether a hypothesized simple genetic pattern of familial transmission fits with observed data to suggest mendelizing inheritance. Several differing methodologies are employed. Each is based upon a set of assumptions, and the results of each must therefore be interpreted in light of specific methodological limitations (51; see Table 1). Twin and adoption studies have determined that both genetic and environmental influences are involved in drug use or dependence and have indicated the extent of their involvement (see below). Perhaps the most convincing evidence for the nature and degree of genetic bases for substance abuse comes from the convergence of results obtained through methodologically-distinct approaches.

Application of molecular genetic approaches to studies of substance abuse is relatively recent. Nevertheless, recent studies with polymorphic genetic markers at several candidate gene loci have initiated the search for specific genes whose alleles could contribute to genetic differences in substance abuse vulnerability (see below). Indeed, substantial collective work on markers at the dopamine D2 receptor gene locus (DRD2) has continued to suggest differences between substance abusers and controls in work from several, but not all, groups (66,67; but see ref. 23). Because molecular genetic studies in this area are likely to assume increasing prominence, the second portion of this chapter describes possible approaches to identifying candidate or anonymous genes that could contribute to substance abuse vulnerability. It also details evidence at the DRD2 locus, the single site most explored as a candidate for contributions to substance abuse vulnerability.

Animal studies have shown that a variety of species can be bred for drug-accepting preferences, and they have attempted to identify likely candidate gene loci for symptoms of drug dependence. Such studies cannot provide direct evidence concerning human genetic polymorphisms relevant to substance abuse. However, these studies can reveal some of the behavioral parameters susceptible to genetic variability. Some of the genetic possibilities for human substance abuse vulnerability, derived from animal studies, are thus detailed in the concluding section of this chapter.

Several reviews of the large body of classical genetic studies of alcoholism have recently appeared (e.g., see refs. 15,44, and 61; also see Chapter 69, *this volume*), but little has been done to summarize data that focus on drug abusers. This chapter will therefore review the genetics of drug abuse. Because few drug abusers abstain from alcohol, and because alcoholism is present in almost half

TABLE 1. *Classical and molecular genetic approaches for studying human vulnerability to substance abuse*

Method	Purpose	Problems and limitations[a]
Classical Genetic Studies		
Family studies	• Determine if family members of substance abusers are at increased risk for substance abuse. • Provide evidence consistent with a genetic basis for the disorder (not conclusive).	• Generational and secular trends in drug use. • Nonpaternity. • Inability to separate genetic from family environmental effects.
Segregation analyses	• Use the diagnostic status of family members to determine the relative likelihood of alternative modes of transmission for a familial disorder (e.g., polygenic, single major locus, mixed).	• Affected by statistical non-normality. • No direct test of single locus versus polygenic model of transmission.
Twin studies	• Determine if within-pair similarity for substance abuse is greater in genetically identical twins than in 50% genetically identical fraternal twins.	• Requires accurate zygosity determination. • Assumes equal relevant environments in identical and fraternal twins. • Rare subjects.
Adoption studies	• Separate the effects of genes and environment by studying the similarity between biological parents, their adopted-away children, and their adoptive parents.	• Assumes no selective placement. • Places prenatal environmental effects in the "genetic" component. • Rarity of subjects.
Molecular genetic studies		
Linkage analyses	• To use family data to statistically link a trait to a genetic marker on a particular chromosome.	• Multiple statistical comparisons. • Assumes particular mode of transmission. • Rare multigenerational drug abuse pedigrees. • Generational and secular trends.
Association studies	• To compare genetic variation at a specific site in affected and unaffected individuals.	• Appropriate control group.

[a] Problems common to all methods include: diagnostic imprecision, variable age of onset, etiological heterogeneity, assortative mating, and ascertainment bias.

of drug abusers in population-based surveys (58), these approaches in fact often focus on polysubstance abusers.

This review's focus on genetic influences should not obscure the significant environmental nature of many risk factors for drug abuse. Drugs must be available for drug abuse to develop. The type of drug available can also be important, because drugs can differ considerably in their reinforcing effects and abuse liabilities. Risk factors reported to contribute to drug use include laws, social norms, drug availability, economic deprivation, neighborhood disorganization, family drug-related behavior, family management practices, family conflict, low family bonding, early and persistent problem behaviors, academic failure, low commitment to school, peer rejection in elementary grades, association with drug-using peers, alienation and rebelliousness, attitudes favorable to drug use, and early onset of drug use (32). One major fruit of the labors of elucidating genetic influences of drug abuse behaviors will be that the environmental components of vulnerability will be more readily identified so that their independent and interactive components can be more easily assessed (40). Appropriate recognition of genetic and environmental vulnerabilities can lead to improvements and better targeting of treatment and prevention strategies.

CLASSICAL GENETIC STUDIES

Approaches

Family studies analyze transmission of substance abuse disorders from generation to generation through families (Table 1). The basic approach determines if family members of substance abusers are at increased risk for substance abuse. A variant, segregation analysis, uses the diagnostic status of family members to determine the relative likelihoods of different modes of genetic transmission. These studies display limitations noted in Table 1. Noting these limitations is especially important in substance abuse disorders in which marked generational and secular trends in drug of choice, nonpaternity, and assortative mating can all provide confounding factors. Family studies do not conclusively separate genetic from family environmental bases for these disorders. Adoption and twin study data are thus of additional importance.

Adoption studies aim to separate the effects of genes and environment by studying the similarity between adopted-away children, their biological parents, and their adoptive parents. Although prenatal environment is confounded with genetic influences, this approach also displays substantial power in differentiating between environmental and genetic contributions to substance abuse disorders (Table 1).

Twin studies determine if within-pair similarity for substance abuse is greater in genetically identical monozygotic (MZ) twins than in less genetically similar fraternal

dizygotic (DZ) twins (Table 1). Careful studies of these relatively rare subjects have allowed the first tentative estimates of the magnitude of the genetic components of drug abuse vulnerability (e.g., see ref. 56).

Classical Genetic Studies of Drug Abuse

There are now family, twin, and adoption studies of drug abuse. However, it is important to keep in mind the extensive alcoholism comorbidity found in drug abusers (58). Alcoholism and drug abuse display substantial comorbidity both in clinical samples and in the general population. Abuse of cocaine, sedatives, opiates, hallucinogens, and amphetamines, for example, was found to be 10 times higher in alcoholics than in nonalcoholics in the epidemiological catchment area (ECA) survey (35). Almost half of drug abusers attained DSM III-R criteria for alcohol abuse or dependence in this ECA sample (58).

Family Studies

Extensive family study work now supports enhanced frequencies of drug abuse in families of drug abuser probands when compared to general population base rates. Most of these workers have utilized family history and family structure data obtained from the proband, and varying diagnostic criteria have been employed.

Several studies of the families of drug abusers now strongly suggest familial influences on drug abuse, although different diagnostic criteria and ascertainment methodologies have been used in different time periods (see references in refs. 13,41–43,45, and 59) (Table 2). These data are supported by results of family studies that cannot be summarized in the same fashion (e.g., see refs. 20 and 28). The more recent work of Mirin et al. (45), who developed DSM III diagnoses in relatives of 350 substance abusers, provides features typical of many of these studies. These workers found that male relatives were almost twice as likely as female relatives to display substance abuse. Furthermore, this increased risk for male relatives was observed whether the proband preferred opiates or cocaine, although female relatives of sedative–hypnotic abusers were more likely than male relatives to abuse drugs. Unfortunately, this work also resembles most of the other reports in that appropriate control populations interviewed in the same fashion as the relatives of drug abusers were not included. ECA data suggest prevalences of 7% and 4% for drug abuse or dependence in males and females, respectively (58). Therefore data from studies with control populations assessed using similar instruments are of special value in helping to interpret these frequency estimates.

Rounsaville and co-workers (41,42,59) studied relatives of 201 opiate addicts and 82 controls obtained in a similar population area. Between 18% and 23% of first-

TABLE 2. *Family studies of drug abuse*

Investigators	Year	N	Proband's primary drug dependence	Father	Mother	Father or mother	Brother	Sister	Brother or sister	First degree
Drug abusers										
Polisch[a]	1933	66	Opiate	2	5	3[b]	4	5	4[b]	
Smith et al.[a]	1966	100	Opiate			4			14	
Vaillant[a]	1966	100	Opiate			1			24[c]	
Ellinwood et al.[a]	1966	111	Opiate	3	0	2[c]	14	4	9[c]	
O'Donnell[a]	1969	266	Opiate	3	2	3[c]			5[c]	
Hawks et al.	1969	74	Amphetamines	3	4	4[c]			16	
Willis[a]	1969	50	Opiate			6[c]			8[c]	
Willis[a]	1971	100	Opiate	0	0	0			8	
Hill et al.	1977	114	Opiate	1	0	1[c]	18	5	12	
Maddux et al.[a]	1989	235	Opiate	0	0[b]	0[b]	20[b]	3[b]	12[b]	8[b]
Mirin et al.	1991	350	Mixed							9
Rounsaville	1991	201	Opiate			12			37	20
Luthar et al.	1992									
Luthar et al.	1993	298	Cocaine	6	4	5[c]	40	22	33[c]	

Controls		N		Male	Female	Either				
ECA Sample		9339		7	4	6				
Rounsaville		360[d]				3				

[a] See references in ref. 15.
[b] Opiate dependence of relatives assessed; data omitted from summary.
[c] Estimated from presented data.
[d] 80 probands.

degree relatives of addicts, as well as 3% of first-degree relatives of normal controls, manifested drug abuse. These data suggested an odds ratio of almost 14-fold for drug abuse in first-degree relatives of drug abusers, compared to the normal controls examined (59). Rates of drug abuse in siblings were almost three times higher than those in parents, and gender differences were significant (59). Luthar and Rounsaville (43) used similar approaches to study first-degree relatives of 298 cocaine abuser probands. They found that 40% of male and 22% of female sibs of cocaine users, as well as 5% of parents, displayed drug abuse or dependence. These values were thus significantly different from ECA data and from previously studied control populations.

Several conclusions concerning the familial nature of drug abuse now seem reasonably well supported by this accumulated family study data:

1. A substantial degree of familiality of substance abuse vulnerability fits best with the accumulated data. Family studies, standing alone, cannot separate family environment from genetic contributions to familial resemblance, however.

2. The marked secular trends in abused substances of choice and male/female differences in substance abuse muddy these data. Family studies of "vertical," transgenerational transmission of substance abuse can thus be significantly limited due to differences in the pattern of availability of drugs across generations, and due to gender differences in substance use. Anecdotal data obtained

from studying pedigrees of families of drug abusers reveals frequent multigenerational patterns of abuse of alcohol and drugs, suggesting that certain underlying genetic and/or environmental determinants might predispose to abuse of both categories of substances (but see below). Control for these generational and gender factors in studies of the familial aggregation of drug abuse may be exerted by restricting analyses to individuals within the same temporal and gender cohort, such as siblings or twins of the same sex.

Adoption Studies

Cadoret et al. (8) studied almost 450 adopted individuals, finding 40 with drug abuse, 75 with alcohol abuse, and 46 with antisocial personality problems. There was a significant correlation between drug abuse in the adoptee and alcohol problems in the biological parent (odds ratio = 4.3), but there was no increased risk if only the adoptive parent drank (8). This evidence for a genetic basis for substance abuse heritability was accompanied by an enhanced risk for alcoholism if the biological parent was alcoholic (odds ratio = 5.9). Interestingly, while antisocial personality in the biological parent enhanced the relative risk of antisocial personality, it did not significantly increase the risk of drug abuse. This work, as well as a recent replication of the results in a different group of subjects (R. Cadoret, *personal communication*, 1993), suggests a significant genetic component to heritability of substance abuse.

Twin Studies

Pickens et al. (56) examined twin concordance for drug abuse in a sample of 50 monozygotic and 64 dizygotic twins in which the proband was identified in drug and alcoholism rehabilitation programs. These workers found a significantly greater concordance for substance abuse in monozygotic males than in dizygotic males. These workers then used ECA data concerning population prevalences to estimate components of liability variance. These analyses provide, for the first time, an estimate of the proportion of genetic contribution to substance abuse in these individuals. When substance abuse and/or dependence in men was considered, 31% of the variance could be attributed to genetic components. The corresponding figures for alcohol dependence were 60%. Trends in the same direction in a smaller female population did not reach statistical significance (56).

A study of over 2600 Vietnam Era twin-pair registrants also indicated genetic components to drug abuse (31). Significant heritability (h^2 values ranging from 0.4 to 0.6) for abuse of hallucinogens, stimulants, opiates, sedatives, and marijuana was found. Only cannabis users displayed shared environmental components. This large twin study thus provides the first evidence that vulnerability to each of these classes of addictive substances may display a genetic component. Equally striking is the conclusion that vulnerability to no substance could be attributed to shared environmental features alone. There is thus little evidence from either twin study to suggest that environmental factors shared within a twin pair, such as neighborhood characteristics, religious affiliation or common friends are significant causes of twin pair resemblance for drug usage.

Similar data is found in studies of nicotine abuse, although relative risk estimates from genetic twin studies are substantially more modest. Studies in the United States and Scandinavia suggest modest genetic contributions to relative risks of smoking (e.g., see ref. 9). Interestingly, stronger genetic components were identified in individuals who had never smoked and in those who successfully stopped (9). These data concerning a substance with wide environmental availability provide some of the only information concerning the possibility that genetic influences on resistance to substance use and on substance abuse cessation might be as robust as those impacting on more typical measures of quantity and frequency of substance use.

In summary, twin data now provide significant support for the idea that drug abuse vulnerability displays significant genetic components. Genetic components appear to be more prominent in the more severe abusers. However, environmental influences on drug abuse susceptibility are underscored by the failure of concordance for drug abuse in more than one-third of identical male twins and more than two-thirds of identical female twins (e.g., see ref. 56).

Levels at Which Further Classical Genetic Studies of Substance Abuse Vulnerability Can Be Focused

Relationship Between Alcohol and Drug Abuse

Alcoholism and drug abuse display substantial comorbidity both in clinical samples and in the general population. Abuse of cocaine, sedatives, opiates, hallucinogens, and amphetamines, for example, was found to be 10 times higher in alcoholics than in nonalcoholics in the ECA survey (35). Many family pedigrees contain both alcohol and drug abusers (see above). However, tentative evidence from two studies suggests caution in assuming that possible genetic bases for predisposition to alcoholism are identical to genetic bases for predisposition to substance abuse.

Hill et al. (36) found that alcoholism clustered in families to a greater extent than did opiate addiction, although secular trends with more striking opiate use in sibs than in parents may have obscured the analyses. Rounsaville et al. (59) also identified higher rates of alcoholism in relatives of opiate addict probands who had comorbid alcoholism than in relatives of opiate addicts lacking this comorbidity. Such data would mitigate against a single, identical genetic determinant underlying both alcoholism and substance abuse. Anecdotal pedigree studies do suggest that both of these disorders occur in many of the same families and thus probably share some genetic components. Identification of the specific genetic determinants shared by drug abuse and alcoholism and those that might be specific to each group of agents remains an area of current interest.

Segregation Analyses: Investigating Possible Modes of Genetic Transmission for Substance Abuse

Familial patterns of polysubstance abuse are documented by the family studies undertaken to date, as noted above. Unfortunately, the striking secular trends in the substances used have rendered attempts to identify the familial patterns of transmission difficult. Indeed, even with alcoholism, two attempts to characterize the transmission of the underlying genetic vulnerability to alcoholism have reached dissimilar conclusions (3,29). Gilligan et al. (29) found evidence to support a recessive major locus in families of male alcoholics. However, Aston and Hill (3) concluded that the major effect transmitted within the families of male alcoholics was either nonmendelian or a major environmental effect with a polygenic background. No evidence for a major effect of either genes or environment was found in families of female alcoholics (29). Multifactorial transmission, combining effects at several gene loci with environmental influences, may be the most likely mode of transmission in these families. Although such a pattern appears most likely to also explain drug abuse, direct segregation study data documenting this conclusion is currently lacking. The lack of solid information concerning inheritance pattern provides difficulties for genetic linkage analyses, which require assumptions concerning mode of inheritance.

Specific Features of Drug Abuse Susceptible to Possible Genetic Influences

There are many points, beginning with initial exposure to drugs and leading up to substance abuse or dependence, upon which genetic research could focus. As genetic underpinnings of substance abuse in toto become better established, genetic contributions to specific features of substance abuse will be increasingly studied. Features of interest include the following:

1. *Subjective and objective effects of substances.* Studies in this area investigate whether genetic vulnerability is related to either subjective or objective effects of substances. These aspects have been approached in alcoholism, where results are contradictory. Individuals with positive family histories for alcoholism can report less intense feelings of intoxication at moderate doses of alcohol as well as other behavioral and biochemical effects (46).

2. *Factors affecting exposure.* Factors which lead to initial experimentation with drugs provide another area of research. The impact of genetic and environmental effects on teenage alcohol use have been estimated in a study of Australian twins (33), which found that both genetic and environmental factors shared within twin pairs are important in determining teenage abstinence. Additionally, genetic factors were found to be a major contributor to the observed variance in age of onset of alcohol use in females, whereas shared environmental factors were much more influential in males. Contrastingly, genetic factors were significant contributors to average weekly consumption in both sexes. Just as environmental factors important in exposure to alcohol and drugs may differ from environmental factors important in first use or in escalating use to abuse, the genetic factors important in the degree of alcohol consumption are important only once alcohol use has started but have little to do with the determinants of age of onset. Because this study involved nonalcoholic individuals, there is no evidence to determine whether the genetic factors affecting alcohol use are the same or different from those genetic factors which are involved in alcohol dependence. Studies in drug abusers can also help to tease out such components.

3. *Factors influencing drug metabolism and distribu-*

tion. The pathways by which most drugs are metabolized are known. Genetic variants at some loci, such as the cholinesterase that is responsible for much of cocaine's metabolism, are also known. Studies relating these variants to substance abuse phenotypes are just beginning. However, work on the alcohol metabolism genetics of alcohol dehydrogenase and aldehyde dehydrogenase gene variants has revealed (a) variants occurring more frequently in alcoholics than in controls and (b) variants associated with the characteristic "flushing" response noted in Asians (see ref. 63). Adult, nonalcoholic monozygotic twins are also more similar than dizygotic twins in measures of alcohol absorption, degradation, and elimination (34). Conceivably, similar genetic contributions to drug metabolism could help to explain components of the genetic contribution to substance abuse vulnerability.

4. *Comorbid behavioral factors.* Families with drug abuse and alcoholism are frequently enriched in individuals with other psychiatric diagnoses, especially antisocial personality. Indeed, Cadoret et al. (8) have suggested that drug abuse may occur on three distinct backgrounds in his adoptees: those of biological familial antisocial personality, those of biological familial background of substance abuse, and those with adoptive families providing an environment of disruption and psychiatric disturbance. Twin data also suggest that cross-concordances for alcoholism and antisocial personality in male twins are likely to display significant genetic components (Pickens et al., *personal communication*).

APPROACHES TO FINDING SPECIFIC GENES CONTRIBUTING TO HUMAN SUBSTANCE ABUSE VULNERABILITY

Candidate Genes

Knowledge about the cellular and molecular bases of acute drug action has exploded over the last several years. Information about the genes expressed by brain systems on which drugs act has allowed testing of the possibility that interindividual differences in genes encoding proteins expressed in these systems could contribute to interindividual differences in drug abuse vulnerability (reviewed in ref. 65).

Significant data now support the idea that virtually every abused drug can induce behavioral reinforcing properties by altering function in brain dopamine circuits arising from the ventral midbrain (16). Genes important in the mesolimbic/mesocortical dopaminergic pathways are thus strong candidate genes for possible contributions to interindividual differences in substance abuse vulnerability. The dopamine D2 receptor gene (see below) represents one such candidate gene.

Recent molecular cloning studies have also identified the genes encoding many drug receptors, including the dopamine transporter that is the pharmacologically defined cocaine receptor, G-protein-linked opiate receptors that are the heroin/morphine receptors, the G-protein-linked canabanoid receptor that mediates marijuana action, the *N*-methyl-D-aspartate (NMDA)-glutamate receptor ligand-gated ion channels that mediate phencyclidine actions, the nicotinic acetylcholine receptor ligand-gated ion channel that is the site of action of nicotine, and the gamma-aminobutyric acid (GABA) receptor ligand-gated ion channels that mediate actions of barbiturates and benzodiazepines (see ref. 33 for review). GABA and NMDA receptors are also strong candidate loci for acute ethanol effects.

Polymorphic Anonymous Genetic Markers

We know how addictive processes start: Drug occupies a brain receptor. Processes directly modulating receptor function, however, have not been able to account for significant fractions of the biochemical bases of addiction. Other candidate molecular mechanisms of information storage can be tentatively postulated as possibly involved in addiction (65). However, direct genetic approaches not dependent on biochemical hypotheses may be more likely to identify genes that could contribute to interindividual differences in substance abuse vulnerability than candidate gene approaches that assume greater knowledge of addiction process biochemistry than we may actually possess.

A large number of richly polymorphic genetic markers are now available for use. These markers include variable number polymorphisms such as simple sequence repeats and restriction fragment length polymorphisms (RFLPs). The increasing number of such markers, distributed on each segment of each human chromosome, provides increasing potential power for genetic studies scanning the genome for loci that are associated with substance abuse vulnerability. As noted below, this power may be essential for any approach that aims to detect functional genes with characteristics likely to contribute to substance abuse vulnerabilities.

Familial Linkage and Allelic Association Approaches

Linkage and Association

Linkage analyses use family data to statistically link a trait to a genetic marker on a particular chromosome. Genetic markers at a single gene locus can be identified as *linked* with a disease if, in different generations of families displaying a genetic familial disorder, one form of a genetic polymorphic marker at a gene locus is coinherited with the disease. One gene marker form is thus present in family members with the disease, but not in those displaying normal phenotypes, in the simplest case.

Genetic linkage studies thus involve analysis of the ways in which the disease phenotype and each of a number of genotypic markers cosegregate or appear together in different family members.

Association studies compare genetic variation at a specific site to behavioral variation within affected and unaffected individuals. Genetic markers at a gene locus can also be *associated* with a disease if they are present more often in unrelated individuals displaying the disease than in unaffected individuals.

Power Losses in Linkage and Association Studies with Complex Genetic Bases and Significant Secular Trends

The probable polygenic mode of inheritance of substance abuse vulnerabilities and the large environmental impact on substance abuse outcomes are both likely to dramatically weaken the power of the classical familial molecular genetic linkage approaches, in which tests are made to determine how genotypes at each of many genetic loci cosegregate with substance abuse phenotypes. If substance abuse in any individual could be caused by several different genes, or by strictly environmental influences, then numerous "phenocopy" substance abusers will share the same clinical characteristics but differ in genotype. Mathematical modeling studies indicate dramatic loss of power of genetic linkage studies as more different genes and more diverse environmental influences yield more frequent phenocopies. Thus, true presence of a genetic marker in only substance abusers in one family due to the marker's true linkage with a nearby gene allele causing this substance abuse will be masked by studies in a second phenocopy family in which other genes lead to substance abuse or in a third phenocopy family in which environmental factors lead to nongenetic but still familial patterns of substance abuse.

Each of these genetic and environmental phenocopies also weakens association studies, in which genetic marker presence in populations of substance abusers is compared to marker presence in nonabusers. However, modeling work suggests that the loss of power due to phenocopies may be less severe in association studies than in classical linkage studies. Thus, if a set of genetic markers adequately tags each of the genes potentially implicated in drug abuse vulnerability, association studies should be better able to elucidate the genes that contribute to the disorder. The abilities of genetic markers to provide such informative data about functional gene alleles, however, rests on specific considerations based on recombination between the polymorphic markers and the functional alleles of interest.

The secular trends in abused substances also provide substantial difficulties for linkage studies, which often rely on phenotype characterizations of individuals in different generations maturing in substantially different drug environments (see above). Linkage studies, which study affected and unaffected individuals in the same cohort (e.g., sib-pairs), are less susceptible to these problems.

Recombination, Linkage, Linkage Disequilibrium, and Allelic Association

The abilities of either candidate gene or anonymous polymorphic genetic markers to adequately indicate either genetic linkage or allelic association is based on considerations of chromosomal recombination. The meiotic events forming the chromosomes for each human generation result in "crossing over" recombinant events splicing sequences from one chromosomal copy with those of the other chromosomal copy. The average rate of this process allows 1% of chromosomal loci separated by 1 million base pairs of DNA to recombine in each generation. However, this average rate of recombination can vary substantially across different chromosomal loci (see ref. 66).

For a polymorphic marker to indicate genetic linkage, chromosomal recombination between that marker and a postulated gene leading to familial substance abuse must occur infrequently within the several generations assessed in the family. Markers located within several million base pairs of the functional gene defect causing substance abuse would thus be likely to detect genetic linkage if substance abuse were a mendelizing disorder. However, for allelic association to be detected, chromosomal recombination between a polymorphic marker and a postulated gene contributing to substance abuse in the population must occur infrequently within the many generations separating the inheritance of the population sampled. A polymorphic marker such as a specific RFLP successfully used in association studies could thus lie very close to the functional gene defect contributing to substance abuse vulnerability. Alternatively, such a marker could be in linkage disequilibrium with the functional gene defect. Linkage disequilibrium is a term used to define a process with poorly understood mechanisms that results in the much-lower-than-average rates of recombination observed between some chromosomal loci (see ref. 66). Linkage disequilibrium can thus allow a genetic marker used in an allelic association study to provide information not only about whether closely adjacent DNA contains a functional gene defect, but also about the possibility that DNA many thousands of bases removed from the polymorphic genetic marker but in linkage disequilibrium with it could also contain a functional gene defect. As we shall see below, the linkage disequilibrium that has now been well documented at the dopamine D2 receptor gene locus provides a plausible rationale for allelic association between RFLP markers at this locus and substance abuse vulnerability.

Example: The DRD2 Locus and Substance Abuse Vulnerability

The DRD2 gene encodes a G-protein-linked, seven-transmembrane region receptor protein expressed abundantly in dopaminergic circuits important for behavioral reward (66). Genetic polymorphic markers have been identified at several DRD2 loci. A *Taq*I A RFLP is located in the 3' flanking region of the DRD2 gene, a *Taq*I B RFLP lies more 5', and a *Taq*I C RFLP provides a polymorphic marker for a site lying between *Taq*I A and *Taq*I B (see ref. 66).

Blum et al. (6) provided the first evidence that the DRD2 gene might display population variants influencing susceptibility to alcoholism. These workers found a striking allelic association between the *Taq*I A1 RFLP form and alcoholism. However, these results were viewed with caution for several reasons (25,67). Thousands of different genes are expressed in the human brain; the a priori probability of identifying a vulnerability-enhancing allele of one of these genes was low. Genetic linkage of this marker in several families in which alcohol abuse appeared to pass from generation to generation in nearly mendelizing fashion was not supported (7,52). The *Taq*I A RFLPs used in this study were demonstrated to be inhomogeneously distributed in different human populations (50), with high A1 allele frequencies in black, Asian, and American Indian populations (23,50,67). Spurious associations not indicative of true causal links between DRD2 allelic status and substance abuse could thus result from sample stratification—that is, disproportionate sampling of abusers or controls from population subgroups displaying atypical RFLP frequencies.

Despite these cautions, we and other investigators have examined DRD2 gene markers in drug abusers (Table 3). These data are now joined by results obtained by three other laboratories that have now provided data that allow assessments of DRD2 gene marker frequencies in drug abusers and nonabuser control populations. Several conclusions seem to be supported by the current status of these data:

1. The *Taq*I A1 and B1 DRD2 RFLPs are interesting reporters for events in significant portions of the DRD2 gene locus in Caucasians. Although the *Taq*I A and B RFLP sites are separated by chromosomal distances at which recombination events occurring randomly in the genome would have been expected to render them randomly associated with each other, or with the structural or regulatory regions of the dopamine receptor gene, substantial linkage disequilibrium does preserve the chromosomal connection between *Taq*I A and B RFLPs and, presumably, certain surrounding sites that could include DRD2 coding or regulatory sequences. Quantitative studies indicate that more than 95% of the possible linkage disequilibrium (D'/D_{max}) is maintained between these loci (50). Another poly-

TABLE 3. *DRD2 TaqI A and B RFLP frequencies in drug abusers and controls*

Investigators		%A1		%B1	
		Drug abusers	Controls	Drug abusers	Controls
Smith et al. and O'Hara et al.	1992 1993	41% (96/237)	28% (45/160)	32% (76/237)	22% (35/160)
Noble et al.	1993	51% (27/53)	16% (16/100)	38% (20/52)	13% (7/53)
Comings et al.	1993	42% (45/106)	29% (221/763)		
Gelertner et al.[a]	1993	45% (49/108)	35% (24/68)		
Totals:		**43% (217/504)**	**28% (306/1091)**	**33% (96/289)**	**20% (42/213)**

[a] Estimated from presented data, assuming Hardy–Weinberg equilibrium.

morphic *Taq*I C RFLP locus, intermediate on the physical map of this region, nevertheless displays less linkage disequilibrium with the *Taq*I A and B sites that flank it. *Taq*I A and B genotypes could thus reliably mark a structural or functional gene variant at the DRD2 locus that could be directly involved in altering behavior.

2. A1 and B1 markers appear more frequently in drug abusers than in control populations in each of four currently available studies (10,24,48,50,64). Meta-analyses of these data suggest that differences between drug abuser and control populations are highly significant for both the four studies examining A1 and the two studies examining B1 frequencies.

3. The most severe abusers of addictive substances may manifest higher A1 and B1 DRD2 gene marker frequencies, while "control" comparison groups that are studied carefully to eliminate individuals with significant use of any addictive substance appear to display lower A1 and B1 frequencies than unscreened control populations (see ref. 66).

4. No data available to date derive from true population based sampling techniques. Although the theoretical possibility of false-positive error based on sample stratification thus remains, combining available data from nonpopulation based studies of Caucasians sampled in several centers appears to render unplanned stratification less likely.

Current meta-analyses based on the three studies reported in full suggest that drug abusers may display (a) a 2.4:1 odds ratio of drug abuse likelihood for individuals possessing an A1 allele and (b) a 3.3:1 odds ratio for those having a B1 allele [$p < 0.001$ in both cases; calculated per Smith et al. (66)].

Other Genes

Other genetic and environmental influences remain likely to determine the majority of variance in individual vulnerability to substance abuse.

Association studies for polymorphic markers at loci for other dopaminergic genes have also been carried out. Markers at the dopamine transporter, synaptic vesicular

transporter, and tyrosine hydroxylase loci have not yielded positive allelic association results (6,49,53; C. Surratt, A. Persico, and G. R. Uhl, *in preparation*). However, none of these loci have been documented to display the striking linkage disequilibrium that could conceivably render the *Taq*I A and B DRD2 gene markers accurately reporters for hypothesized DRD2 gene variants at regulatory or coding sequences.

STUDIES IN EXPERIMENTAL ANIMAL MODELS HELP TO DEFINE THE LIMITS OF POSSIBLE GENETIC AND ENVIRONMENTAL FACTORS IN VULNERABILITY RESEARCH

Rationale for Animal Studies

Workers investigating neurobiological factors in human addiction have limited ability to intervene in the genetics, personal environment, or neurobiology of drug abusers. In a complex disorder such as addiction, experimental approaches that can either manipulate or hold constant environmental and biological variables important for drug-taking behavior provide an opportunity to systematically examine the addiction process. Animal models can mimic human drug-taking behavior, perhaps the most basic aspect of addiction, to a remarkable degree. Virtually all drugs abused by humans will serve as positive reinforcers in animals under operant self-administration paradigms. Drug-related phenotypes such as dependence, tolerance, sensitization, and conditioned drug effects can also be experimentally analyzed separately in animal models with precision unavailable in clinical settings. Animal research can help to elucidate possible roles of genetic and environmental constituents in the addiction process that might otherwise be difficult to untangle.

Animal models of addiction are clearly limited in their ability to precisely mimic all aspects of the human condition. However, such studies provide experimental control of genetic and neurobiological manipulations essential to thoroughly explore mechanisms that contribute to vulnerability. Furthermore, they can allow environmental manipulations that would be ethically proscribed in human experimentation. Animal studies can thus help to define the limits of possible genetic contributions to human substance-abusing behaviors. Data from such studies can suggest areas that are likely to prove fruitful for future explorations in humans (see also Chapters 2 and 69, *this volume*).

Genetic Approaches in Experimental Animals

Several behavioral and genetic approaches have been used to determine genetic contributions to drug-related effects in experimental animals (Table 4). Most studies have been performed in rodents, due to the rich repertoire of genetically defined strains currently available and the facility with which transgenic mice can be created.

1. *Correlations across inbred strains and outbred individuals* assess the expression of each of several drug-related phenotypes in several genetically distinct strains and examine how the phenotypic traits covary across genotype. Alternatively, the same phenotypes can be exam-

ined in different individuals within genetically heterogeneous animal stocks, and the extent to which two or more phenotypes covary can be assessed (19).

2. *Classic genetic analysis.* Systematic cross-breeding experiments utilizing inbred strains and first filial "F1" generation individuals can be used to (a) determine the mode of inheritance of specific traits that may vary from parental strain to parental strain and (b) study gene–environment interaction. Congenic strain methodologies place gene(s) of interest from a donor strain into an acceptor strain while successively eliminating background donor genes by repeated backcrossing.

3. *Selective breeding* for a drug-related trait selects individuals of extreme phenotype for breeding over a number of generations to selectively isolate the genes responsible for the trait while randomizing irrelevant genes (19). Selective breeding can provide estimates of heritability (h^2) and even biochemical and behavioral covariates of the selected trait.

4. *Quantitative trait loci (QTL)* analyses compare the strain distribution patterns of a drug-related response to the strain distribution patterns of molecular genetic mark-

TABLE 4. *Representative animal studies of drug abuse genetics[a]*

Drug	Behavior	Genetic approach	Comments
Opioids	Preference	Inbred strain	Significant genetic influence.
		Classical analysis	High heritability and dominance for morphine preference.
		Selection	Bidirectional shift in morphine and ethanol preference.
		Quantative trait locus	Three significant loci: Chromosomes 8, 10, 12; chromosome 8, *ES-1* confirmed within inbreds.
	Conditioned place preference	Inbred strain	Predominantly qualitative differences; not always similar to preference.
	Operant self-administration	Inbred strain	Acquisition dependent upon history, route, and access; differences found in extinction.
Cocaine	Preference	Inbred strain	Significant genetic influence.
	Conditioned place preference	Inbred strain	Significant genetic influence.
		Selection	Bidirectional shift unrelated to high-dose cocaine discrimination.
	Operant self-administration	Inbred strain	Significant genetic influence in similar direction as ethanol, opioids, and diazepam.
Amphetamine	Intracranial self-stimulation		Potency and efficacy significantly influenced by genotype.
	Operant self-administration	Within subjects/randomly inbred rodents	Rate of acquisition correlated with innate locomotor behavior.
Benzodiazapine	Operant self-administration	Inbred strains	Significant genetic influence in similar direction as ethanol, opioids, and cocaine.
THC	Intracranial self-stimulation	Inbred strains	Significant genotype-dependent change; complements operant studies with other drugs.

[a] See text for references.

ers. Multivariate analyses can determine the fraction of strain-to-strain differences in a trait that can be assigned to a particular locus. They also provide information about the location of the affected chromosomal locus. Substantial syntony is now documented between many mouse and human chromosomal regions (11). Although the presence of a behaviorally significant allelic variant in a mouse gene does not automatically predict a comparable behaviorally significant allelic variant in the corresponding human gene, data from such animal studies can provide testable hypotheses about possible roles for allelic variants at these loci that can be tested in human allelic association or other genetic studies.

5. *Transgenic animals* provide strains that overexpress or underexpress one or more introduced genes, so that behavioral consequences of over- or underexpression can be explored (38). As more and more candidate genes for involvement in substance abuse are identified, effects of altered gene structures or altered gene expression levels can thus be tested in vivo. In most transgenic animals, the chromosomal location of the introduced genetic material is random, so that examination of a single line of offspring of a single transgenic animal could provide confounded effects due to disruptions at the site of insertion (38). Homologous recombinant/embryonic stem cell technologies aid in targeting introduced genomic material to known sites whose disruption can thus be planned.

Genetic Variability Is Demonstrable in Drug Self-Administration and Other Aspects of Drug-Reinforced Behavior

Studies investigating vulnerability to drugs in animals have now identified genetic components in several behavioral paradigms for most abused substances.

1. *Opioids.* Inbred mouse strains and selected lines have revealed genotype-dependent differences in virtually every opiate response including analgesia, locomotor stimulation, physical dependence, tolerance, respiratory depression, hypothermia, diuresis, and gastrointestinal motility (see ref. 5). Measures of the motivational effects of opioids such as conditioned place preference can also vary among different rodent strains; Cunningham et al. (14) demonstrated significant morphine-induced place preference that was greater in DBA/2J than in C57BL/6J mice. Quantitative trait locus analyses of inbred and recombinant inbred strains demonstrate association between morphine preference and polymorphic markers at the *Es-1* region of murine chromosome 8 (4). Each of these studies clearly demonstrate genotype-dependent opioid preferences. Although each measure of drug-taking or drug-reinforced behavior differs in its interpretation, the overall results clearly indicate that many aspects of both opioid addiction and opioid side effects are influenced by genetic factors. The degree of genetic covariance

among these opiate phenotypes can vary significantly, however, suggesting independent inheritance of at least several opiate phenotypes.

The combined data from each of these experimental approaches now overwhelmingly supports genotype-dependence of a variety of opioid effects in experimental animals, suggests probable involvement of several genes including those on murine chromosome 8, supports significant environmental influences even in individuals reared in similar fashions, and hint that the genetic bases of vulnerability to opioid reinforcement displays features that are not identical to the genetic bases for reinforcement due to other addictive substances.

2. *Cocaine and amphetamine.* Many aspects of cocaine and amphetamine responses, including locomotor stimulant, sensitizing, hyperthermic, hepatotoxic, and cardiovascular alterations can be influenced by genotype (for review see ref. 62). Inbred strain analyses have demonstrated significant effects of genotype on cocaine preference (1,14,26). Quantitative trait locus studies of amphetamine hyperthermia have localized genes responsible for strain-to-strain differences in this acute drug effect to the chromosome 1 region adjacent to the lamb2 locus (4). Psychostimulant abuse thus displays many signs of genetic predisposition in animal studies, with animal data supporting the same sorts of patterns of polygenic inheritance noted for opiates.

3. *Other drugs.* Inbred mouse strains and animal lines derived from selection studies have revealed genotype-dependent differences in drug abuse phenotypes. Genotype-dependent differences in locomotion induced by phencyclidine in recombinant inbred strains (21) demonstrate varying responses to NMDA or sigma receptor blockade. The cannabanoid Δ^9-THC altered thresholds for intracranial self-stimulation in Lewis but not in F344, Sprague–Dawley, or Wistar rats (22). Lewis rats were also reinforced by diazepam, whereas F344 rats were not reinforced by the drug (37).

Although the reinforcing properties of abused drugs can vary as a function of genotype, evidence for common genetic bases for drug-taking behavior across drug classes and especially across behavioral paradigms is more mixed. C57BL/6J mice and Lewis rats self-administer ethanol, cocaine, and opioids, whereas rodents of several other genotypes will derive conditioned reinforcement from only a single drug class (reviewed by ref. 62).

Animal Studies Can Point to Specific Features of Drug Abuse Vulnerability Susceptible to Genetic Variability and Genetic Covariation

Many differing risk or protective factors may be involved in the acquisition of drug-taking behavior, and these factors may display different mechanisms than those implicated in the maintenance, extinction, or relapse of drug-taking behavior. Genetic approaches in animals can help to suggest possible specific inherited behavioral, neurochemical, neuroendocrinological, or other features that could provide mechanisms for each of these drug related behaviors.

1. *Behavioral correlates.* Several inherited behaviors and stress responses manifest in animals prior to drug administration have now been correlated with the same strains' drug responses. If animals of different genotypes are segregated into two groups based upon a non-drug phenotypic response and if each group is then tested for drug-seeking behavior, the ability of the primary phenotype to predict subsequent drug-seeking behavior can be assessed (54). Animals segregated from populations of randomly inbred rats based on their high locomotor responses to novel environments acquire amphetamine self-administration behavior more rapidly than those with low locomotor responses to novel situations (54). Rats selectively bred for high rates of intracranial self-stimulation or for high "emotional reactivity" in open-field situations displayed stronger opiate-induced conditioned place preferences and two-bottle preference than did rats bred for the opposing characteristics (e.g., see ref. 60). Significant differences in operant self-administration of opioids that can be positively correlated with baseline locomotor activities have now been identified in several mouse and rat strains (2,18).

2. *Neurochemical correlates.* Belknap and Crabbe (4) have used recombinant inbred strains to examine relationships between opioid-induced behaviors and brain opiate receptor densities or activities. In addition, lines of mice selectively bred for opiate-induced analgesia demonstrate significant differences in mu-opioid receptor binding and distribution (see ref. 5). Recombinant inbred mouse strains displaying fewer μ_1-opiate receptors also manifest less potent opiate responses than do other mouse strains including self-administration, while mice with supernormal opiate receptor binding densities are also more sensitive to several opiate drug effects (18; see references in ref. 5).

3. *Neuroendocrinological correlates.* Rats with high locomotor responses in novel environments display both prolonged corticosterone release and enhanced self-administration of amphetamine (55). Exogenous corticosterone administration can also induce more rapid acquisition of amphetamine self-administration (55). Because genotype can significantly affect individual stress responses in animals and humans, these data may thus have significant implications for human drug abuse vulnerabilities. However, inbred rat strains with exaggerated and blunted hormonal responses to stress do not demonstrate the predicted pattern of opioid, ethanol, cocaine, or diazepam self-administration behavior (e.g., see refs. 2, 27, and 37).

4. *Chronic drug effects.* Tolerance to, and repeated withdrawal from, drugs of abuse are important aspects of many human addictions. The chronic effects of a drug involve behaviors present in the maintenance and extinction phase of drug use that may be highly relevant for drug use in humans. However, mechanisms underlying chronic drug effects are likely to differ substantially from those underlying the acute effects of even the same drugs, although some common mechanisms might be identified as well.

Studies using selectively bred murine lines suggest that the genes which determine ethanol withdrawal severity can be involved in the ability of ethanol to sustain conditioned place preferences (12). Behavioral sensitization, one possible animal model of certain components of drug addiction, can also be studied in relationship to genotype and to the acquisition of drug-reinforced behaviors. Repeated administration of cocaine results in various degrees of sensitization that depend on the genotype (e.g., see ref. 17). Interestingly, the strain that most readily displays a sensitization response to cocaine also shows significant drug-reinforced behaviors mediated by cocaine, ethanol, and opioids (e.g., see ref. 18). The degree of sensitization following repeated administration of amphetamine can predict the rate of acquisition of amphetamine self-administration behavior (54). Repeated amphetamine administration sensitizes subsequent amphetamine responses in low-activity rats that do not readily acquire self-administration behavior but not in high-activity rats that readily acquire this behavior (54). Interestingly, the sensitization process enhances the rate of acquisition of amphetamine self-administration behavior in low-reactivity rats to the level demonstrated in high-reactivity rats (54,55).

5. *Environmental factors* which can contribute to variance in drug-related behaviors can also be appropriately isolated and studied in animals. Such features as drug availability, schedule of drug reinforcement, and drug history can be conveniently manipulated in animals in a fashion not possible in humans (see ref. 47).

CONCLUSIONS

Animal studies suggest that interindividual differences at several gene loci, together with substantial environmental contributions, can mediate quantitative and qualitative differences in the behavioral effects of almost all drugs of abuse. Shared genetic components, and some differentiable genetic components, could underlie the acquisition, maintenance, and resistance-to-extinction characteristic of addictions to a number of abused substances in humans.

Studies in humans support a substantial role for genetic differences in vulnerability to human substance abuse. No data obtained to date are inconsistent with the picture emerging from animal studies: Actions of alleles at several gene loci are likely to interact with environmental factors to yield substance abuse vulnerabilities. Some genes' alleles may predispose to abuse of multiple substances, whereas others may yield preferential vulnerability to more specific classes of drugs. While molecular genetic studies of family pedigrees may be able to identify genes producing shared vulnerabilities to both alcoholism and drug abuse, secular trends in abuse substance fashion and availability will be more likely to make allelic association studies increasingly prominent in identifying any gene alleles that manifest greater impact on drug abuse than on alcoholism. Data from both animal and human studies will probably be necessary to unravel the complex interactions between multiple genes and environment likely to contribute to the pathogenesis of common and disabling human addictive disorders.

ACKNOWLEDGMENTS

We are indebted to collaborators in this work, including Bruce O'Hara, Antonio Persico, Brian Suarez, and Stevens Smith; to Antonio Persico, Lucinda Miner, Charles Schuster, and Rodney Marley for helpful comments; and to Stevens Smith for help with meta-analyses. Support for the work from the authors' laboratories derives from the intramural program of the National Institute on Drug Abuse.

REFERENCES

1. Alexander RC, Duda J, Garth D, Vogel W, Berrettini WH. Morphine and cocaine preference in inbred mice. *Psychiatr Genet* 1993;3:33–37.
2. Ambrosio EA, Goldberg SR, Elmer GI. Behavior genetic investigation of the relationship between innate locomotor activity and the acquisition of morphine self-administration behavior. *Behav Pharmacol* 1994;[in press].
3. Aston CE, Hill SY. Segregation analysis of alcoholism in families ascertained through a pair of male alcoholics. *Am J Hum Genet* 1990;46:879–887.
4. Belknap JK, Crabbe JC. Chromosome mapping of gene loci affecting morphine and amphetamine responses in the BXD recombinant inbred mice. In: Kalivas PW, Samson HH, eds. *The neurobiology of drug and alcohol addiction.* New York: The New York Academy of Sciences, 1992;311–323.
5. Belknap JK, O'Toole LA. Studies of genetic differences in response to opioid drugs. In: Harris RA, Crabbe JC, eds. *The genetic basis of alcohol and drug actions.* New York: Plenum Press, 1991;225–252.
6. Blum K, Noble EP, Sheridan PJ, et al. Allelic association of human dopamine D2 receptor gene in alcoholism. *JAMA* 1990;263:2055–2060.
7. Bolos AM, Dean M, Lucas-Derse S, Ramsburg M, Brown GL, Goldman D. Population and pedigree studies reveal a lack of association between the dopamine D2 receptor gene and alcoholism. *JAMA* 1990;264:3156–3160.
8. Cadoret RJ, O'Gorman T, Troughton E, Heywood E. An adoption study of genetic and environmental factors in drug abuse. *Arch Gen Psychiatry* 1986;43:1131–1136.
9. Carmelli D, Swan G, Robinette D, Fabsitz R. Genetic influence on smoking: a study of male twins. *N Engl J Med* 1992;327:89–833.
10. Comings DE, MacMurray J, Johnson JP, et al. The dopamine D₂ receptor gene: a genetic risk factor in polysubstance abuse. *Alcohol Drug Depend* 1993;[in press].
11. Copeland NG, Jenkins NA, Gilbert DJ, et al. A genetic linkage map of the mouse: current applications and future prospects. *Science* 1993;262:57–66.
12. Crabbe JC, Phillips TJ, Cunningham CL, Belknap JK. Determinants of ethanol reinforcement. In: Kalivas PW, Samson HH, eds. *The neurobiology of drug and alcohol addiction,* vol 654. New York: New York Academy of Sciences, 1992;302–310.
13. Croughan JL. The contribution of family studies to understanding drug abuse. In: Robbins L, ed. *Studying drug abuse,* vol. 6. New Brunswick: Rutgers University Press, 1985;93–116.
14. Cunningham CL, Niehus DR, Malott DH, Prather LK. Genetic differences in the rewarding and activating effects of morphine and ethanol. *Psychopharmacology* 1992;107:385–393.
15. Di Chiara G, Imperato A. Drugs abused by humans preferentially increase synaptic dopamine concentrations in the mesolimbic system of freely moving rats. *Proc Natl Acad Sci USA* 1988;85:5274–5278.
16. Devor EJ, Cloninger CR. Genetics of alcoholism. *Annu Rev Genet* 1989;23:19–36.
17. Elmer GI, Brockington A, Gorelick D, Goldberg SR, Rothman RB. Acute cocaine-induced locomotor activity and context-dependent sensitization in inbred mice. *NIDA Research Monographs* 1994;141:16.
18. Elmer GI, Pieper JO, Goldberg SR, George FR. Opioid operant self-administration, analgesia, stimulation and respiratory depression in μ-deficient mice. *Psychopharmacology* 1994;[in press].
19. Falconer DS. *Introduction to quantitative genetics.* New York: Longman Scientific and Technical Publishers and John Wiley & Sons, 1989.
20. Fawzy FI, Coombs RH, Gerber B. Generational continuity in the use of substances: the impact of parental substance use on adolescent substance use. *Addict Behav* 1983;8:109–114.
21. Freed WJ, Crump S, Jeste DV. Genetic effects on PCP-induced stimulation in recombinant inbred strains of mice. *Pharmacol Biochem Behav* 1984;21:159–162.
22. Gardner EL, Lowinson JH. Marijuana's interaction with brain reward systems: update 1991. *Pharmacol Biochem Behav* 1991;40:571–580.
23. Gelernter J, Goldman D, Risch N. The A1 allele at the D2 dopamine receptor gene and alcoholism: a reappraisal. *JAMA* 1993;269:1673–1677.
24. Gelernter J, Kranzler H, Satel S. No association between DRD2 alleles and cocaine abuse. Fifty-Fifth Annual Scientific Meeting, College on Problems of Drug Dependence, Inc., poster, June 16, 1993.
25. Gelernter J, O'Malley S, Risch N, et al. No association between an allele at the D2 dopamine receptor gene (DRD2) and alcoholism. *JAMA* 1991;266:1801–1807.
26. George FR, Goldberg SR. Genetic differences in response to cocaine. *NIDA Res Monogr* 1988;239–249.
27. George FR, Goldberg SR. Genetic approaches to the analysis of addiction. *Trends Pharmacol Sci* 1989;10:73–83.
28. Gfroerer J. Correlation between drug use by teenagers and drug use by older family members. *Am J Drug Alcohol Abstr* 1987;95–108.
29. Gilligan SB, Reich R, Cloninger CR. Etiologic heterogeneity in alcoholism. *Genet Epidemiol* 1987;4:395–414.
30. Glantz M, Pickens R. *Vulnerability to drug abuse.* Washington, DC: American Psychological Association, 1992.
31. Goldberg J, Lyons MJ, Eisen SA, True WR, Tsuang M. Genetic influence on drug use: a preliminary analysis of 2674 Vietnam era veteran twins [Abstract]. *Behav Genet Society* 1993.
32. Hawkins JD, Catalano RF, Miller JY. Risk and protective factors for alcohol and other drug problems in adolescence and early adulthood: implications for substance abuse prevention. *Psychol Bull* 1992;112:64–105.
33. Heath AC, Martin NG. Teenage alcohol use in the Australian twin register: genetic and determinants of starting to drink. *Compr Psychiatry* 1988;12:735–741.
34. Heath AC, Phil D, Martin NG. Genetic differences in psychomotor performance decrement after alcohol: a multivariate analysis. *J Stud Alcohol* 1992;53:262–271.
35. Helzer JE, Przybeck TR. Concurrence of alcoholism with other

psychiatric disorders in the general population and its impact on treatment. *J Stud Alcohol* 1988;49:219–224.

36. Hill SY, Cloninger CR, Ayre FR. Independent familial transmission of alcoholism and opiate abuse. *Alcohol Clin Exp Res* 1977;1:335–342.

37. Inayama M, Suzuki T, Misawa M, Meisch RA. Diazepam oral self-administration in Lewis and Fischer 344 inbred rat strains. *Eur J Pharmacol* 1991;183:1983.

38. Jaenisch R. Transgenic animals. *Science* 1988;240:1468–1474.

39. Kandel DB, Raveis VH. Cessation of illicit drug use in young adulthood. *Arch Gen Psychiatry* 1989;46:109–116.

40. Khoury MJ, James LM. Population and familial relative risks of disease associated with environmental factors in the presence of gene–environment interaction. *Am J Epidemiol* 1993;137:1241–1250.

41. Luthar SS, Anton SF, Merikangas KR, Rounsaville BJ. Vulnerability to drug abuse among opioid addict's siblings: individual, familial, and peer influences. *Compr Psychiatry* 1992;33:190–196.

42. Luthar SS, Anton SF, Merikangas KR, Rounsaville BJ. Vulnerability to substance abuse and psychopathology among siblings of opioid abusers. *J Nerv Ment Dis* 1992;180:153–161.

43. Luthar SS, Rounsaville BJ. Substance misuse and comorbid psychopathology in a high-risk group: A study of siblings of cocaine misusers. *Int J Addict* 1993;28:415–434.

44. Merikangas KR. The genetic epidemiology of alcoholism. *Psychol Med* 1990;20:11–22.

45. Mirin SM, Weiss RD, Griffin ML, Michael JL. Psychopathology in drug abusers and their families. *Compr Psychiatry* 1991;32:36–51.

46. Moss HB, Yao JK, Maddock JM. Responses by sons of alcoholic fathers to alcoholic and placebo drinks: perceived mood, intoxication, and plasma prolactin. *Alcohol Clin Exp Res* 1989;13:252–257.

47. Nader MA, Tatham TA, Barrett JE. Behavioral and pharmacological determinants of drug abuse. In: Kalivas PW, Samson HH, eds. *The neurobiology of drug and alcohol addiction,* vol 654. New York: New York Academy of Sciences, 1992;368–385.

48. Noble EP, Blum K, Khalsa ME, et al. D_2 dopamine receptor gene alleles in treatment-seeking cocaine dependent caucasian subjects. *Drug Alcohol Depend* 1993;[in press].

49. Noble EP, Blum K, Ritchie T, Montgomery A, Sheridan PF. Allelic association of the D2 dopamine receptor gene with receptor-binding characteristics in alcoholism. *Arch Gen Psychiatry* 1991;48:648–654.

50. O'Hara BF, Smith SS, Bird G, et al. Dopamine D2 receptor RFLPs, Haplotypes and their association with substance use in black and caucasian research volunteers. *Hum Hered* 1993;43:209–218.

51. Ott J. *Analysis of human genetic linkage.* Baltimore: Johns Hopkins University Press, 1991.

52. Parsian A, Todd RD, Devor EJ, et al. Alcoholism and alleles of the human D2 dopamine receptor locus. *Arch Gen Psychiatry* 1991;48:655–663.

53. Persico AM, O'Hara BF, Farmer S, Gysin R, Flanagan S, Uhl GR. Dopamine D2 receptor gene TaqI "A" locus map including A4 variant: relevance for alcoholism and drug abuse. *Drug Alcohol Depend* 1993;31:229–234.

54. Piazza PV, Deminiere JM, Le Moal M, Simon H. Factors that predict individual vulnerability to amphetamine self-administration. *Science* 1989;245:1511–1513.

55. Piazza PV, Deminiere JM, Le Moal M, Simon H. Stress- and pharmacologically-induced behavioral sensitization increases vulnerability to acquisition of amphetamine self-administration. *Brain Res* 1990;514:22–26.

56. Pickens RW, Svikis DS, McGue M, Lykken DT, Heston LL, Clayton PJ. Heterogeneity in the inheritance of alcoholism: a study of male and female twins. *Arch Gen Psychiatry* 1991;48:19–28.

57. Raveis VH, Kandel DB. Changes in drug behavior from the middle to the late twenties: initiation, persistence, and cessation of use. *J Public Health* 1987;77:607–611.

58. Regier DA, Farmer ME, Rae DS, et al. Comorbidity of mental disorders with alcohol and other drug abuse. *JAMA* 1990;264:2511–2518.

59. Rounsaville BJ, Kosten TR, Weissman MM, et al. Psychiatric disorders in relatives of probands with opiate addiction. *Arch Gen Psychiatry* 1991;48:33–42.

60. Satinder KP. Oral intake of morphine in selectively bred rats. *Pharmacol Biochem Behav* 1977;7:43–49.

61. Schuckit MA. Biology of risk for alcoholism. In: Meltzer H, ed. *Psychopharmacology: a third generation of progress,* New York: Raven Press, 1987;1527–1533.

62. Seale TW. Genetic differences in response to cocaine and stimulant drugs. In: Crabbe JC, Harris RA, eds. *The genetic basis of alcohol and drug actions.* New York: Plenum Press, 1991;279–321.

63. Smith M. Genetics of human alcohol and aldehyde dehydrogenases. *Adv Hum Genet* 1986;15:249–290.

64. Smith SS, O'Hara BF, Persico AM, et al. Genetic vulnerability to drug abuse: the dopamine D2 receptor TaqI B1 RFLP is more frequent in polysubstance abusers. *Arch Gen Psychiatry* 1992;49:723–727.

65. Uhl GR. Molecular and genetic studies of the targets of acute drug action, substrates for interindividual differences in vulnerability to substance abuse, and candidate mechanisms for addiction. *NIDA Monogr* 1993;[in press].

66. Uhl GR, Blum K, Smith SS. Substance abuse vulnerability and D2 receptor genes. *Trends Neurosci* 1993;16:83–88.

67. Uhl GR, Persico AM, Smith SS. Current excitement with D2 dopamine receptor gene alleles in substance abuse. *Arch Gen Psychiatry* 1992;49:157–160.

Psychopharmacology: The Fourth Generation of Progress, edited by Floyd E. Bloom and David J. Kupfer. Raven Press, Ltd., New York © 1995.

CHAPTER 154

Behavioral Treatment of Drug and Alcohol Abuse

Maxine L. Stitzer and Stephen T. Higgins

Drug abuse treatments generally derive from a conceptual and theoretical definition of the problems to be treated and of their underlying causes. Two primary schools of thought have been advanced to explain the clinical characteristics of substance dependence and have led to different treatment approaches. These contrasting views have been reviewed and discussed more fully by Marlatt and Gordon (43). The "disease model" postulates that substance-dependent individuals have a biological abnormality (possibly genetic) that predisposes them to seek and use chemical substances to excess. In this view, drug-seeking behavior is outside the control of the afflicted individual. The treatment approach that has derived from the disease model emphasizes admitting powerlessness over drugs or alcohol, accepting total abstinence as the goal of change, and adopting the norms and values of a new social group, the Alcoholics Anonymous (AA) self-help group, in order to achieve and sustain abstinence (20). The disease model is highly regarded by clinicians, but it has not been extensively researched and therefore currently lacks strong empirical support.

The "learning model," which flows mainly from an academic research tradition, rests on recent scientific evidence that drugs act as primary reinforcers directly on brain reward systems and that orderly learning processes, both classical and operant, underlie the acquisition and maintenance of drug self-administration behavior. Treatments developed under a learning model acknowledge the chronic relapsing nature of dependence, as well as the important role of the physical and social environment in promoting relapse versus abstinence. Furthermore,

these treatments call for development of new behavioral strategies on the part of the substance abuser, as well as reorganization of the physical and social environment, to counteract relapse tendencies engendered by learned drug associations. Consistent with its roots in academia, the behavioral approach has received considerable evaluation, much of which supports the effectiveness of this general approach to treatment. The purpose of the present chapter is to review recent developments in learning-based approaches to treatment of heroin, cocaine, and alcohol dependence (see Chapters 64 and 66, *this volume*).

LEARNING-BASED TREATMENTS IN METHADONE MAINTENANCE

Methadone is an important modality for opioid abusers, with close to 100,000 people presently in treatment within the United States (56). Methadone treatment has demonstrated efficacy in suppressing heroin use and associated criminal activity (5,31), but does not directly address the full range of problems that drug abusers bring to treatment. Polysubstance abuse is common among methadone patients, with illicit use of cocaine (12,24,38) replacing benzodiazepines (33,71) as the most serious and prevalent secondary substance of abuse. Nevertheless, methadone brings polydrug-abusing patients into a therapeutic setting and provides the context for contingency management procedures that are well-suited to addressing the clinical problem of illicit drug supplementation, and that have been shown effective for improving treatment outcome. Methadone treatment also provides an excellent model for the integration of behavioral and pharmacological treatments. The use of contingency management procedures in methadone programs demonstrates how behavioral and pharmacological treatments, which address dif-

M. L. Stitzer: Behavioral Biology Research Center, Johns Hopkins Bayview Medical Center, Baltimore, Maryland 21224.
S. T. Higgins: Department of Psychiatry, University of Vermont, Burlington, Vermont 05401.

ferent aspects of the clinical problems of drug abusers, can be successfully integrated to produce outcomes that are better than those obtained with either therapy alone.

Methadone Take-Home Incentive Procedures

A number of potential rewards and punishments can be identified within the context of a daily methadone dispensing clinic for use in contingency management procedures. The methadone take-home privilege, in which an extra daily dose of methadone is dispensed to the patient for ingestion on the following day, offers a convenient and valued (by clients) incentive for use in abstinence reinforcement protocols (68) and is one of the most potent positive reinforcers available within the context of routine clinic operation. An early study by Stitzer et al. (70), as well as a more recent study by Iguchi et al. (34), examined take-home incentives in methadone patients who chronically supplemented with benzodiazpines. When take-home privileges could be earned for providing drug-free urines, temporary abstinence was observed in about 50% of study patients during the contingent take-home intervention lasting 12–20 weeks. Magura et al. (40) found that 1-month contracting for contingent take-home privileges resulted in 34% of their polydrug-abusing subjects achieving abstinence, whereas Milby et al. (51) found a similar percentage of clients responding to a take-home incentive program with increased numbers of consecutive drug-free urines, as required by the contingent intervention. Most of these studies focused on selected groups of identified polydrug abusers and used within-subject designs to evaluate effectiveness of contingent take-home programs for improving treatment outcomes.

A more recent controlled clinical trial was conducted by Stitzer et al. (72) to examine take-home incentive effects in 54 newly admitted methadone maintenance patients randomly assigned to receive take-home privileges under contingent or noncontingent conditions. In the contingent condition, the first take-home privilege was available after a relatively short (2-week) period of demonstrated abstinence from supplemental drugs, in an attempt to provide an immediate reward for positive behavior change. The conditional probability that a patient would improve on drug use was 2.5 times greater for the contingent than for the noncontingent study condition, whereas the probability of worsening on the drug use measure was two times greater for the noncontingent than for the contingent group. Overall, 32% of contingent patients achieved sustained periods of abstinence during the intervention (mean 9.4 weeks; range 5–15 weeks). The beneficial effect of contingent take-home delivery was replicated within the group of noncontingent patients who switched to the contingent intervention after their 6-month evaluation in the main study (partial crossover design). In this case, 28% improved substantially and

achieved, on average, 15.5 drug-free weeks. In both the main study and the partial crossover, as well as in a recent analysis of the characteristics of take-home earners in clinical practice (37), lower rates of drug-positive urines early in treatment predicted improvement under the contingent take-home program, but patients using cocaine and benzodiazepines were equally likely to respond.

Incentive Procedures with Other Reinforcers

A study by McCaul et al. (47) examined effects of an incentive package on relapse to opiate drug use during a 90-day ambulatory methadone detoxification. Patients selected for the study had submitted ≤50% opiate-positive urines during a baseline period and were randomly assigned to a control or contingent intervention condition. In the latter, opiate-free urines resulted in $10 cash and a take-home day, whereas opiate-positive urines resulted in increased counseling contact, urine sample collection, and data questionnaire requirements for patients. The contingent procedure was shown to be effective for promoting sustained periods of opiate abstinence and delaying relapse. Reductions in drug use during ambulatory detoxification were also reported in a controlled trial by Hall et al. (21) using small amounts of money ($4 to $10 per sample) as the reward for drug-free urines.

Methadone dose changes have also been used in contingent arrangements and have been shown to be effective for suppressing supplemental drug use. Impressive suppression of opiate use during ambulatory methadone detoxification was achieved in a study by Higgins et al. (30) under conditions where the contingent incentive for opiate-free urines was the opportunity to increase the methadone dose by up to 20 mg, an opportunity that remained active only so long as urines were opiate-free. Suppression of opiate use was shown to be specifically related to the contingency between increased methadone dose and drug use, because the benefits were not apparent in a group that could receive noncontingent increases in their methadone dose. Another study by Stitzer et al. (69) extended evaluation of dose change incentives by showing that decreases in polydrug abuse could be demonstrated during methadone maintenance both when methadone dose was increased above original maintenance levels as a result of drug-free urines and when dose was decreased below original maintenance levels as a consequence of drug-positive urines.

Structured contingency programs appear to hold considerable promise as a means to begin making inroads into the chronic supplemental drug use of methadone patients. The studies reviewed demonstrate that incentives, including methadone take-home privilege, money, and methadone dose changes, when used in a contingent fashion, can delay relapse during detoxification and promote improvements in supplemental drug use during treatment.

However, the effectiveness of these contingent incentive programs generally appears limited to patients with less severe polydrug abuse. Future research needs to focus on ways to optimize the utility and cost-effectiveness of incentives that are readily available in the context of methadone clinic operation, to further characterize patients who do and do not respond to treatment, and to develop and evaluate more potent reinforcers for their ability to influence the drug use of more severely dependent polydrug abusers.

Treatment Termination Contracting

Another commonly used intervention that has received research evaluation is the contingent availability of further methadone treatment. Treatment termination contracting provides a means of formulating specific behavioral improvement objectives for poorly performing methadone patients, with the consequence of noncompliance being dose reduction and termination from treatment. Liebson et al. (39), in an elegant early study, showed that treatment outcome could be dramatically improved for severely alcoholic methadone patients by using the threat of treatment termination to motivate participation in a monitored disulfiram program at the clinic. McCarthy and Borders (46) showed that structured treatment involving the threat of termination for failure to meet specified standards of drug-free urine submissions could improve outcomes on measures of opiate drug use during treatment. Two other studies using pre- versus post-intervention evaluation designs have demonstrated the effectiveness of contingent treatment termination approaches. Dolan et al. (14) showed that 50% of study patients ($N = 21$), all with histories of demonstrated failure at controlling illicit drug supplementation, improved and submitted drug-free urines during a 30-day treatment contracting period. Similarly, Saxon et al. (66) have recently shown that 40% of a VA methadone maintenance population with ongoing supplemental drug use during treatment responded to termination contracts by slowing or stopping illicit drug use. In both the Dolan and Saxon studies (15,66), patients most likely to succeed had been in treatment a longer time, submitted relatively fewer drug-positive samples prior to contract initiation, and were less likely to be abusing cocaine or an opiate–cocaine combination than other classes of illicit drugs. Thus, although treatment termination contracting is clearly effective with some proportion of methadone patients, these interventions pose an ethical dilemma, because they inevitably result in voluntary or involuntary treatment termination for those patients who will not or cannot conform to the demands of the contingent treatment contract (34,69).

Overall, the studies reviewed indicate that both positive and negative incentives can be used in contingent arrangements to promote at least temporary periods of abstinence

from supplemental drug use among methadone patients. Both approaches are effective with a subgroup of patients (generally 30–50% of the total treatment sample), who are typically the less severely dependent polydrug abusers. However, positive incentives have the advantage of keeping patients in treatment, whereas negative incentives, particularly those involving methadone dose decrease or threat of treatment termination, result in treatment dropout. One interesting issue that deserves additional research is whether there are any patient characteristics associated with response to positive versus negative incentive procedures. A second issue is whether multiple incentives can be utilized together to increase the potency of contingency management procedures for improving outcomes during methadone treatment.

Drug Abuse Counseling with Contingent Incentives

Ever since its inception in the late 1960s, drug abuse counseling has been a part of methadone treatment. Only recently, however, has research begun to define the elements of drug abuse counseling and to assess the effectiveness of these counseling services. In a recent landmark study, McLellan et al. (50) have specifically investigated treatment outcomes for methadone patients as a function of the amount and type of counseling treatment offered. Male intravenous-opiate-abusing veterans ($N = 92$) were randomly assigned to receive methadone with minimal, standard, or enhanced counseling services. The minimal counseling group received perfunctory contact with therapists focused on satisfying routine requests for information transfer to outside agencies, requests for methadone dose change, and enforcement of program rules. These patients could receive take-home privileges based on employment and independent of urine test results. Standard and enhanced care patients met routinely with counselors to discuss their drug use and life adjustment issues. Treatment for these groups included contingencies targeted on drug use; take-home medication privileges could be earned by employed clients who were also drug-free. Furthermore, the number of counseling sessions per week was increased for those submitting drug-positive urines.

A primary outcome examined during the 24-week study was the percent of patients meeting predetermined criteria for treatment failure. The criteria included unremitting illicit drug use and/or multiple emergency situations requiring immediate health care. Sixty-nine percent of patients receiving methadone with minimal counseling met these criteria and were transferred to standard care within the first 12 weeks of the study. In contrast, only 41% of the standard counseling patients and 19% of the enhanced counseling patients met treatment failure criteria during the course of the study. Furthermore, 90–100% of standard and enhanced care patients were able to sustain 8 weeks of abstinence from opiates and cocaine during the study as compared with only 30% of clients in the minimal services condition. These findings clearly support the utility of structured drug abuse counseling services that include contingencies targeted on objective evidence of drug use versus abstinence.

Drug Abuse Counseling with Professional Services

The McLellan et al. (50) study discussed above also provided a contrast between standard counseling and counseling enhanced by psychiatric, family, and employment counseling resources. Although not all services were provided in the amounts intended, the groups did differ significantly in the planned direction on amounts of family therapy and psychiatric (but not employment) services received. Enhanced care patients submitted significantly fewer opiate- (but not cocaine)-positive urines during the treatment episode. Furthermore, outcome measures of drug use, psychiatric status, and social functioning generally favored the enhanced care over the standard care group in data gathered at the end of treatment.

Similar outcomes were shown in an earlier related study by this same group (75,78), in which methadone-maintained volunteers ($N = 110$) were randomly assigned to receive 6 months of drug abuse counseling alone or counseling supplemented with psychotherapy (supportive–expressive or cognitive behavioral). Outcome assessments, both during therapy and after therapy ended, showed generally better performance for the psychotherapy-plus-counseling than for counseling-alone subjects, with psychotherapy subjects requesting fewer methadone dose increases and fewer psychiatric medications during treatment. It should be noted that in this study, psychotherapy patients attended twice the number of sessions as did counseling-only patients, so that extra attention rather than any specific content of the psychotherapy cannot be ruled out as a mechanism for the effects. In further analysis of the data from this study, the investigators found that differential benefits of the added psychotherapy were most apparent in patients with highest prestudy levels of psychiatric symptoms, as measured by the Addiction Severity Index (76). In contrast, patients diagnosed with antisocial personality disorder did not benefit from added psychotherapy treatment (77).

Taken together, these findings support the conclusion that treatment outcomes for a subgroup of methadone patients may be improved by providing extra therapy (independent of contingency management interventions) and suggest that it may be possible to target ancillary treatments to patients who can best benefit from these treatments. Future research needs to determine how added services and psychotherapy can best be integrated with contingency management techniques to enhance the broadest array of treatment outcomes.

Skills Training

A specialized form of behavior therapy that could be especially beneficial to drug abusers involves training in the social skills necessary to function effectively as a nonabuser. Programs have been developed to train drug abusers in relapse prevention skills (26,44) and in skills necessary to seek and obtain employment (22,23,61). Relapse prevention skills programs are designed to bolster drug-free support systems and to teach drug abusers the skills needed to handle problematic situations that might lead to relapse. Hawkins et al. (25,26) delivered relapse prevention skills training to therapeutic community patients before they left residential treatment. The program effectively enhanced interpersonal and problem-solving skills, as assessed in post-treatment role-play tests (26). However, there was little evidence of skills training effects on post-treatment drug use or relapse rates (25). McAuliffe and colleagues (44,45) evaluated an aftercare treatment package called *Recovery Training and Self-Help*, which combined skills training with participation in self-help groups after formal treatment ended. The package was administered to opiate abusers drawn from a variety of program types (methadone, drug-free, detoxification, and residential treatment) both in the United States and China. Outcome evaluation during a 1-year follow-up found significantly more good outcomes (abstinent or using opiates less than once a month) among subjects in the experimental group than among control group subjects, with a 15–17% improvement in abstinence rates. In each group, however, there was no assessment of treatment impact on nonopiate illicit drug use, including cocaine. The diversity of study populations makes it difficult to draw conclusions about impact on any particular subgroup.

Hall et al. (22,23) developed and evaluated a Job Seekers Workshop for drug abusers. The program was shown to effectively teach the desired skills (including preparing applications and interviewing) and to result in higher employment rates for experimental than for control subjects. However, there was no evaluation of impact on drug use.

Overall, research on skills training for heroin abusers is at an early stage. However, this approach appears promising for teaching skills needed to adopt a drug-free lifestyle (e.g., job-seeking), as well as for relapse prevention. Future research needs to consider integration and timing of effective treatment elements—including contingency management, psychotherapy, and skills training—to best achieve positive long-term outcomes.

LEARNING-BASED TREATMENTS FOR COCAINE ABUSE: OUTPATIENT NONMETHADONE

Important recent advances have been made in learning-based interventions for outpatient treatment of cocaine abuse. Across several controlled trials, learning-based interventions have resulted in clinically significant reductions in cocaine use in dependent patients. These reports have focused almost exclusively on during-treatment abstinence and relatively short follow-up periods. These projects were initiated in the midst of the U.S. cocaine epidemic, and the pressing clinical challenge was to identify interventions that could effectively retain patients in treatment and establish even an initial period of cocaine abstinence. Longer-term outcome (1 year after treatment entry) has been assessed in recent trials (7,27); now that an empirical base has been established and investigators are more familiar with cocaine abuse, other trials are planned.

Community-Reinforcement Approach (CRA)

In a series of controlled trials conducted in the same clinic by Higgins et al. (27–29), an outpatient treatment combining CRA and contingency-management procedures was demonstrated to be effective in retaining patients in treatment and establishing clinically significant periods of cocaine abstinence. CRA attempts to eliminate drug use by systematically altering naturalistic contingencies so that reinforcement density is relatively high when the subject is abstinent and low during and immediately following use. Systematic interventions are used to improve marital/family relations, vocation, social, and recreational activities. The common goal across these different treatment components is to enrich the quality of the cocaine user's life when sober and to have him or her experience a time-out from those enriched circumstances when drug use occurs. The primary contingency-management procedure used in this treatment is one in which patients earn vouchers exchangeable for retail items contingent on documentation via urinalysis testing that they have recently abstained from cocaine. The voucher system is in effect for weeks 1–12 of treatment, whereas a $1.00 state lottery ticket is awarded for each cocaine-negative urinalysis test during treatment weeks 13–24. The value of the vouchers increases with each consecutive cocaine-negative specimen delivered, and cocaine-positive specimens reset the value of vouchers back to their initial level. Those who are continuously abstinent (all cocaine-negative urine tests) could earn the equivalent of $997.50 during weeks 1–12 and $24 during weeks 13–24. This translates to an average maximum earning of $6.08 per day for those who are continuously abstinent from cocaine; in practice, the average earning has been approximately $3.50 per day.

Two of the trials examining the efficacy of this treatment compared it against standard outpatient drug counseling based on the disease model of drug dependence and the 12 steps of recovery (28,29). The first trial was limited to 12 weeks, whereas the second trial was 24

weeks. Both treatments were delivered by experts in the respective approaches during twice-weekly sessions during weeks 1–12 of treatment and, in the randomized trial, once-weekly sessions during weeks 13–24. Patients were assigned to the two treatments as consecutive admissions in the first trial and randomly in the second trial. In both trials, the behavioral treatment retained patients significantly longer and documented significantly longer periods of continuous cocaine abstinence than did standard counseling. For example, in the randomized trial, 58% of patients assigned to the behavioral treatment completed 24 weeks versus 11% of those assigned to standard counseling. Furthermore, 68% and 42% of patients in the behavioral group achieved 8 and 16 weeks of documented, continuous cocaine abstinence versus 11% and 5% of those in the counseling group.

In a third trial conducted with this treatment, patients were randomly assigned to receive the behavioral treatment with or without the voucher program (27). Treatment was 24 weeks in duration and the voucher versus no-voucher difference was in effect during weeks 1–12 only. Both treatment groups were treated the same after week 12. Both treatment groups were followed for an additional 6 months after treatment termination so as to cover a 1-year period from the point of treatment entry. This study was the first in a series of studies planned to dismantle this multicomponent treatment to determine which components actively contribute to outcome. Vouchers significantly improved treatment retention and cocaine abstinence. Seventy-five percent of patients in the group with vouchers completed 24 weeks of treatment versus 40% in the group without vouchers, and average duration of continuous cocaine abstinence were 11.7 ± 2.0 weeks in the former versus 6.0 ± 1.5 in the latter. At the end of the 24-week treatment period, significant decreases from pretreatment scores were observed in both treatment groups on the Addiction Severity Index (ASI) family/social and alcohol scales, with no differences between the groups. Both groups also decreased on the ASI drug scale, but the magnitude of change was significantly greater in the voucher group than in the no-voucher group. Only the voucher group showed a significant improvement on the ASI psychiatric scale. Those significant pretreatment to post-treatment changes and between-group differences on the ASI remained stable through follow-ups conducted at 9 and 12 months after treatment entry.

Because these studies were conducted in a clinic located in Burlington, Vermont with almost exclusively Caucasian patients, questions could be raised about the generality of these findings to inner-city, minority cocaine abusers. A recent, well-controlled study conducted with cocaine-abusing methadone maintenance patients in a clinic located in Baltimore, Maryland extended the generality of the voucher program to inner-city, primarily minority abusers (67). During a 12-week study, patients in the experimental group ($N = 19$) received vouchers exchangeable for retail items contingent on cocaine-negative urinalysis tests. A matched control group ($N = 18$) received the vouchers according to a schedule that was yoked to the experimental group and not contingent on urinalysis results. Both groups received a standard form of outpatient drug and alcohol abuse counseling. Cocaine use was substantially reduced in the experimental group, but remained relatively unchanged in the control group. For example, 47% and 42% of patients in the experimental group achieved 4 and 8 weeks of continuous cocaine abstinence, whereas only a single control subject was abstinent for 4 weeks and none were abstinent for 8 weeks.

Overall, there are four controlled trials supporting the efficacy of the community reinforcement approach to outpatient treatment of cocaine abuse. Future studies will focus on (a) which components of this multicomponent treatment other than the voucher program actively contribute to positive outcomes, (b) longer-term outcomes, and (c) the generality of this treatment to other settings and populations. The voucher program thus far appears to have generality to a fairly broad array of patients and settings. Whether that is true for other components is unknown. Application of this approach to pregnant abusers, in whom even short-term abstinence is very important, appears to be an especially promising avenue for future research.

Relapse Prevention

Another treatment demonstrated in controlled clinical trials to be efficacious as an outpatient intervention for cocaine dependence is relapse prevention. This is a cognitive-behavioral treatment that teaches patients to recognize high-risk situations for drug use, to implement alternative coping strategies when confronted with high-risk events, and to apply strategies to prevent a full-blown relapse should an episode of drug use occur (43). In a randomized trial conducted by Carroll et al. (8), 42 cocaine-dependent patients were assigned to relapse prevention treatment or interpersonal psychotherapy, which teaches strategies for improving social and interpersonal problems. Both treatments were delivered by professional therapists during weekly sessions. Outcomes achieved with relapse prevention during the 12-week trial were significantly better than those obtained with interpersonal psychotherapy: 67% of those assigned to relapse prevention versus 38% assigned to interpersonal psychotherapy completed treatment, and 57% of those in relapse prevention versus 33% in interpersonal psychotherapy achieved 3 or more weeks of continuous cocaine abstinence.

In a subsequent randomized trial conducted by the same group, relapse prevention and case management were compared in a two-by-two design in which patients also received either desipramine or placebo (9). One hundred

thirty-nine patients were randomized to one of four treatment groups (relapse prevention plus desipramine, relapse prevention plus placebo, case management plus desipramine, case management plus placebo); data analyses were based on 110 patients who received at least two sessions of their respective treatments. Case management was designed to provide a nonspecific therapeutic relationship and an opportunity to monitor patients' clinical status. Both treatments were delivered in weekly therapy sessions during the 12 weeks of treatment. All treatment groups improved from pretreatment to post-treatment on measures of cocaine use and the ASI drug, alcohol, family/social, and psychiatric scales; however, there were no significant main effects for psychosocial (relapse prevention versus case management) or drug treatment (desipramine versus placebo). An interesting retrospective analysis suggested outcome differences as a function of whether patients reported using high (>4.5 g) or low ($1-2.5$ g) amounts of cocaine per week at pretreatment. With relapse prevention, high-use patients were retained for a significantly greater mean number of sessions than were low-use patients (8.6 versus 6.0). For clinical management, there was a nonsignificant trend in the opposite direction; that is, mean number of sessions with high-severity patients was less than with low-severity patients (6.1 versus 8.0). Comparable, nonsignificant trends in the same directions were noted when continuous cocaine abstinence in the two treatments was analyzed as a function of severity of cocaine use. In a follow-up of patients during the year after treatment, patients who received relapse prevention achieved significantly higher levels of cocaine abstinence at 12-month follow-up than did patients who received case management (7).

Overall, evidence exists supporting the efficacy of relapse prevention as an outpatient treatment for cocaine dependence, but further studies will be needed to determine its reliability in producing positive during-treatment and longer-term outcomes. That is, the initial trial by Carroll et al. (8) supports its efficacy during treatment, but follow-up data were not reported. The subsequent trial (7,9) supports its efficacy at 1-year follow-up but not during the treatment period. Obviously, both areas are necessary to recover from cocaine dependence; and if relapse prevention is demonstrated to reliably facilitate one or both, it would be an important contribution to cocaine abuse treatment research.

Other Learning-Based Treatments

In addition to CRA and relapse prevention, four other learning-based treatment approaches appear promising based on preliminary results, including active cue exposure (11), coping skills training (63), chemical aversion therapy (16), and neurobehavioral treatment (62). The first three in this list are designed to serve as adjuncts to more comprehensive treatments, whereas the fourth is a comprehensive treatment.

Active cue-exposure teaches patients to engage in coping behaviors (e.g., relaxation) when confronted with environmental stimuli that elicit a conditioned drug response (e.g., craving) or that otherwise have previously set the occasion for drug use. Coping skills training is similar to active-cue exposure, but is designed to teach specific drug refusal and social skills deemed important for accessing alternatives to drug use and for coping with events that place the patient at high risk for drug use. Chemical aversion therapy is designed to establish an aversion to cocaine use by repeatedly pairing use in the clinic with a strong chemically induced nausea. To approximate cocaine use during therapy sessions, patients use an inactive placebo substance that closely resembles cocaine in appearance. Neurobehavioral treatment emphasizes many of the elements described above in relapse prevention and coping skills training in an attempt to provide the user with the skills necessary to abstain from cocaine use and avoid relapse. The prefix *neuro* is included to note special attention in the treatment process to difficulties likely to arise due to putative neurobiological changes that accompany initial and sustained abstinence from cocaine following chronic use. Each of these treatments address important areas of concern or interest in the quest to develop empirically based and effective treatments for cocaine abuse. Additionally, each is currently being evaluated in one or more controlled clinical trials, and thus their efficacy should be known in the near future.

Obviously, much remains to be learned about treatment of cocaine abuse, but, considered together, the aforementioned treatments represent a promising start. That optimism is bolstered by the fact that most of the treatments that appear promising with cocaine abuse have been previously demonstrated to be efficacious in the treatment of other forms of substance abuse.

LEARNING-BASED TREATMENTS FOR ALCOHOLISM

The literature on learning-based treatments for alcoholism and problem drinking has been developing over the past two to three decades. The phrase *problem drinking* is used here to refer to a continuum of drinking-induced problems ranging from mild disruptions in functions to severe alcohol dependence. Learning-based treatments for problem drinking include an array of empirically based and effective treatments. Some are comprehensive treatments, whereas others are designed as treatment adjuncts. No one of these treatments can be touted as the superior intervention. It is true of alcoholism treatment in general that not all patients uniformly respond positively to any particular treatment. Problem drinking is a complex condition with multiple determinants, and no one intervention

should be expected to be effective with everyone. Importantly, this perspective has spurred a large-scale research initiative aimed at systematically matching patients to optimal treatments (53). Matching is a plausible concept with some empirical support, but its practical utility awaits thorough experimental evaluation. A multisite trial (Project Match) sponsored by the National Institute on Alcohol Abuse and Alcoholism is currently underway to examine the merits of this intriguing concept.

The specific treatments described below are interventions demonstrated to be efficacious in controlled clinical trials conducted with problem drinkers enrolled in treatment. Other promising primary and secondary prevention strategies aimed at reducing alcohol-related harm in those exhibiting early signs or risk factors for developing serious alcohol-related problems are not covered below because they fall outside the treatment focus of this chapter (e.g., see refs. 3 and 4).

Behavioral Self-Control Training

In behavioral self-control training, patients are taught to monitor their drinking, set ingestion limits, use strategies to control their alcohol intake, reward successes in achieving goals, analyze and learn from failed efforts, and develop alternative coping skills for achieving some of the benefits previously derived from drinking. Treatment is usually conducted in small groups during approximately eight weekly 1 to 1.5-hr sessions, with periodic follow-ups. The treatment can be used to achieve outcomes of controlled drinking or total abstinence.

Behavioral self-control training is based on a position that drinking patterns, be they light, moderate, or excessive, are determined, at least in part, by one's learning history and current environmental circumstances. Hence, those with excessive or otherwise problematic drinking patterns should be able to acquire a moderate, problem-free drinking style given the requisite skills and alterations in pertinent aspects of their drinking environment. A relatively extensive research literature provides empirical support for that position, with the important qualification that a goal of controlled, asymptomatic drinking is contraindicated in severely dependent alcoholics (19,55).

A series of experimental studies reported over a 10-year period indicated that approximately 20–70% of clinical samples could learn to drink moderately and that those effects could be sustained for up to 2 years (52,65,73,74). A recent longer-term study conducted by Miller et al. (55) with 140 patients meeting criteria for alcohol abuse and/or dependence revealed more modest, but nevertheless clinically important, outcomes. Follow-up conducted 3.5–8 years post treatment with 99 of the originally treated patients revealed that 14% were asymptomatic drinkers, 23% were totally abstinent, 22% were clinically improved but still impaired drinkers, 35% were unremitted problem drinkers, and 5% were deceased. Aysmptomatic drinking was most likely to be achieved by those without severe alcohol dependence or without a family history of alcoholism.

An important clinical trial in this area by Sanchez et al. (65) demonstrated that among less-dependent problem drinkers, outcome was not influenced by treatment goals of asymptomatic drinking versus abstinence. Subjects were randomly assigned to receive behavioral self-control training with treatment goals of moderate drinking or total abstinence. Approximately 75% of subjects in both treatment groups were asymptomatic drinkers or abstinent at 2-year follow-up with no significant differences in outcome resulting from the different treatment goals.

Studies comparing outcomes when behavioral self-control training was delivered in individual versus group formats or by therapist- versus client-guided use of a treatment manual consistently have demonstrated substantial clinical improvements with no significant differences related to the mode of treatment delivery (52,54).

An important caveat is that none of the aforementioned results quantify the direct contributions of behavioral self-control training to the observed outcomes. Such an assessment can only be gleaned from clinical trials comparing behavioral self-control training versus a no-treatment or standard-treatment control group, but relatively few such studies have been reported. One published trial conducted with a sample of 60 drunk drivers demonstrated a superior outcome with behavioral self-control training compared to drunk driver education or no treatment control (6). The controlled drinking group showed a 52% reduction from pretreatment baseline in amount of drinking reported at 12-month follow-up, compared to a 28% reduction and 14% increase in drinking in the standard education and untreated control groups, respectively.

Behavioral self-control training appears to be a promising approach for curtailing heavy drinking and its related problems. More thorough quantification of the contribution of the therapy to long-term outcomes would be an issue to address in future studies.

Community Reinforcement Approach (CRA)

As was noted above, CRA is a multicomponent treatment developed within an operant conceptual framework, with a basic goal of decreasing substance use by systematically altering naturalistic contingencies so that reinforcement density is relatively high when the subject is abstinent and low during and immediately following use. In CRA studies with alcoholics, an alcohol-free social club that resembled a bar in atmosphere was sometimes made available to patients for socializing, parties, and so on. Patients had to be sober to attend. CRA was initially developed and tested in alcoholics residing in a state hospital, which often includes a treatment-recalcitrant population. The treatment for alcoholics is typically 6–8 weeks in duration with periodic follow-up sessions and a treatment goal of total abstinence.

Four controlled studies have all supported the efficacy of this intervention. In the seminal study by Hunt and Azrin (32), 16 males admitted to a state hospital for alcoholism were divided into matched pairs and randomly assigned to receive CRA plus standard hospital care or the standard care alone. Following discharge from the hospital, CRA patients received a tapered schedule of counseling sessions beginning on a once-weekly basis during the first month and then a once-monthly basis over the next several months. During the 6-month follow-up period, patients who received CRA reported approximately 6- to 14-fold less time drinking, unemployed, away from their families, or institutionalized than did control patients.

CRA was subsequently refined to include monitored disulfiram therapy, some additional crisis counseling after hospital discharge, and a "buddy" system wherein individuals in the alcoholic's neighborhood were available to give assistance with practical issues such as repairing cars, and so on. In a second study by Azrin (1), CRA was compared to a standard inpatient hospital program. Twenty matched pairs of alcoholic males were randomly assigned to receive CRA or the standard hospital program. During the 6 months after discharge, the CRA group spent 3- to 28-fold less time drinking, unemployed, or away from home compared to controls. The CRA group spent no time in an institutional setting (hospital, jail), whereas controls spent 45% of their time in such settings during the 6-month follow-up. During the 2 years following discharge, the CRA group spent 90% or more time abstinent; comparable data were not reported for controls. Compared to the prior CRA treatment package, this refined treatment involved less counseling time and resulted in greater abstinence levels.

A subsequent study by Mallams et al. (41) examined the effects of adding the social club to a standard regimen of outpatient counseling for alcoholism. Forty alcoholics were randomly assigned to receive systematic encouragement to attend the social club described above or to a control group that was informed about the existence of the club but received no encouragement to attend. A great deal of effort also was made to socially integrate the experimental subjects with other club members when they did attend. Similar efforts apparently were not made with controls. Subjects were assessed at intake and 3 months later. There were no differences between the two groups in subject characteristics at intake. Mean attendance at the social club during the 3 months was 2.47 ± 2.43 for the experimental group and 0.13 ± 0.5 for the control group. The experimental group showed significant improvements from intake to 3-month follow-up on measures of quantity–frequency of drinking, behavioral impairment, and time spent in heavy-drinking situations, whereas the control group did not improve significantly on any of those measures.

The fourth study by this group (2) was designed to assess the contribution of disulfiram and other aspects of CRA to outcome. Forty-three alcoholic outpatients were randomly assigned to receive (a) traditional treatment and traditional disulfiram therapy, (b) traditional therapy plus monitored disulfiram therapy, or (c) monitored disulfiram therapy plus the other components of CRA. Outcome was best with the full treatment of CRA plus monitored disulfiram, intermediate with monitored disulfiram alone, and poorest with the traditional treatment and disulfiram. Outcomes with the full CRA treatment were comparable to those reported in earlier studies, providing a third replication. When the results were analyzed according to patients' marital status, a potentially important interaction was noted. Married patients did equally well with the full CRA treatment or monitored disulfiram; it was only the single subjects who needed the complete CRA treatment to achieve abstinence.

The outcomes achieved with CRA equal or exceed the results of any controlled treatment-outcome study in the alcoholism literature. Its efficacy with severely dependent alcoholics makes it an important addition to learning-based treatments for problem drinking. Notable limitations are that all of the published studies supporting the efficacy of this approach were conducted by a single group of investigators in a rural area of Illinois. Whether these results can be replicated by other investigators in other settings remains an important question. A replication effort is currently underway in Albuquerque, New Mexico. As was described above, CRA has been adapted as an effective outpatient treatment for cocaine dependence (28,29).

Behavioral Marital Counseling

Involving spouses and family in alcoholism treatment is supported by at least three lines of reasoning: (a) family members may engage in behaviors that initiate or reinforce drinking; (b) family members may be able to acquire skills that promote decreased drinking; and (c) family members are an important potential source of alternative reinforcement once drinking stops.

Three recent well-controlled studies by O'Farrell et al. have assessed the effects of behavioral marital therapy on treatment outcomes. One study (60), that included a 2-year follow-up (59) involved 36 couples, in which the husbands had recently begun individual alcoholism treatment and received a prescription for disulfiram. Couples were randomly assigned to a no-marital therapy control group, a behavioral couples group, or an interactional couples group. Couples in the behavioral group signed a contract regarding disulfiram compliance, and they received counseling to increase positive family activities

and improve communication. Couples in the interactional group primarily shared feelings about their relationship during therapy sessions. Behavioral couples therapy produced better outcomes on marital adjustment ratings than did other therapies, but there were no significant differences in abstinence among the three groups. For example, percent of days abstinent during the 10-week treatment, as reported by subjects, was 99.4%, 82.7%, and 90.6% for the behavioral, interactional, and control therapies, respectively.

In a similar study by another research group, McCrady et al. (48,49) randomly assigned 45 patients to one of three groups: (a) minimal spouse involvement, which consisted of individual counseling with the spouse present for support; (b) alcohol-focused spouse involvement, in which spouses learned specific therapeutic skills such as how to reinforce abstinence and decrease behaviors that might occasion drinking; or (c) alcohol behavioral marital therapy, which involved all of the above elements plus skills training on how to improve other aspects of the marriage. There were no significant differences between the three groups in overall abstinence levels either during or after treatment. However, time trend analysis revealed that while the percentage of days abstinent decreased steadily over 18 months in the minimal and alcohol-focused spouse involvement groups, this trend was reversed in the behavioral marital therapy group during the second half of the follow-up period. Those between-group differences were statistically significant, and based on graphic display they appeared to represent approximately 10–15% more abstinent days in the behavioral marital group during the second half of the follow-up period. Several measures of marital and personal adjustment also indicated better outcomes during follow-up with behavioral marital therapy.

A more recent study by the O'Farrell group (58) has added insight regarding the potential importance of post-treatment relapse prevention maintenance sessions. Fifty-nine couples, defined by the inclusion of an alcoholic husband, were randomly assigned to receive or not receive 15 maintenance sessions following completion of 5 months of weekly behavioral marital therapy that included a contract for disulfiram compliance. Abstinence improved significantly from pretreatment levels in both groups during the follow-up period, but couples who received the maintenance sessions reported significantly greater abstinence and greater use of the disulfiram contract than did those who did not receive the extra sessions. Improvements in marital adjustment outcomes during follow-up as compared with pretreatment also tended to favor the group that received extra sessions.

Two studies have specifically examined the use of behavioral procedures involving spouses to increase disulfiram compliance, with one reporting positive (2) and the other negative (36) outcomes. The studies differed along numerous dimensions, making it difficult to speculate on what might account for the different outcomes.

Considered together, the results obtained using behavioral marital therapy in alcoholism treatment give grounds for cautious optimism. Although the magnitude of improvement in abstinence outcomes has not been particularly impressive, the relatively small number of studies and some between-study discrepancies underscore the importance of further research. Studies are needed that address the apparent discrepancies concerning the efficacy of using spouses to improve disulfiram compliance. Recent findings about the importance of longer-term therapy should be pursued. Finally, it is possible that the issue of overriding importance is whether or not a spouse is involved in treatment, rather than the particular brand of treatment delivered. Studies that compare couples and individual therapy would be useful in this regard.

Skills Training

Problem drinkers often report that they use alcohol to cope with unpleasant or stressful events, and such events have been reported to influence relapse (42). For these and other reasons, behavior therapists have examined whether social and problem-solving skills training would improve outcomes of problem drinkers. A series of clinical trials have clearly demonstrated that skills training can be an efficacious adjunct treatment for problem drinkers. The majority of trials have examined coping skills as an adjunct to inpatient treatment, and they have focused on assertiveness and related social skills as well as on general problem-solving skills. Positive outcomes have been reported both when patients were specifically selected because they exhibited certain skill deficits (18) and when training was done with general alcoholic samples (17).

In an important, well-controlled study on this topic, Chaney et al. (10) randomly assigned 40 inpatient, male alcoholics to either (a) an eight-session skills-training group focused on drinking-related problem-solving or (b) a discussion control condition in which similar topics were discussed but no specific training was provided. During a 1-year follow-up period, the skills group as compared to the combined control groups (which did not differ from each other) reported, on average, fourfold fewer drinks taken, sixfold fewer days drunk (11 versus 64 days during the 12-month follow-up), and a ninefold reduction in duration of drinking episodes (averaging 5 versus 44 days).

Similarly positive outcomes have been reported in clinical trials in which assertiveness rather than problem-solving skills was the focus of the intervention. In one study by Oei and Jackson (57), 32 alcoholics residing in an inpatient program were selected for participation based on low scores on an assertiveness scale. Patients were matched on several relevant characteristics and assigned to one of four treatment groups: (a) social skills training; (b) cognitive restructuring; (c) a combination of social skills training and cognitive restructuring; or (d) a control group consisting of traditional supportive therapy. All of the experimental groups had better outcomes than the control group on measures of assertiveness and drinking during a 1-year follow-up, but the combined group fared best and the social skills group had poorest outcomes. During the week preceding the 12-month follow-up, for example, mean ethanol ingestion levels in the control, social skills, cognitive restructuring, and combined groups were 34, 17, 11, and 5 ounces, respectively.

In one of the few negative trials on skills training, training in problem-solving strategies was compared to covert sensitization and a discussion control in chronic alcoholics residing in a half-way house (64). There were no outcome differences across the three treatment groups at 6-, 12-, or 18-month follow-up. During treatment, subjects assigned to the skills-training group could recite the strategies they were taught, but they showed marked decrements in their ability to do so at follow-up. Whether those decrements account for the failure to discern positive effects at follow-up is unclear, but seems plausible.

One recent study in the coping-skills literature by Kadden et al. (35) has illustrated the potential importance of patient-treatment matching for achieving positive outcomes. Ninety-six male and female problem drinkers who recently completed an inpatient treatment were randomly assigned to receive coping skills or interactional therapy during aftercare. Subjects in both treatment groups improved on measures of drinking and social stability, and there were no significant differences between the treatments. The investigators then looked post hoc for interactions between treatment group and patient characteristics. Coping-skills therapy was more effective for patients higher in psychiatric severity (measured by Addiction Severity Index psychological scale) and sociopathy (measured by California Psychological Inventory Socialization Scale), whereas interactional therapy was more effective for patients with lower psychopathology. Patients who scored higher on neuropsychological impairment (derived from several scales) did better with interactional therapy. The same treatment–outcome interactions were still evident at 2-year follow-up (13). Of course, retrospective analyses of this type must be treated cautiously pending replication in prospective trials, but they underscore the importance of anticipating that particular subgroups of problem drinkers may respond differently to skills training as well as any other treatment for problem drinking.

Overall, this literature is quite positive in demonstrating that skills training can produce significant and enduring improvements in outcome. More needs to be learned regarding the efficacy of different types of skills training, whether outcomes could be further improved through greater systematic matching of the interventions to particular skill deficits, and specification of any boundary conditions on the type of patient who benefits from skills training.

SUMMARY/FUTURE DIRECTIONS

Significant advances have recently been made with regard to the behavioral treatment of heroin, cocaine, and alcohol abusers. The beneficial effects of including contingency-based drug abuse counseling in methadone treatment have been demonstrated. In both methadone and outpatient cocaine treatment, contingent reinforcement interventions have been shown effective for promoting sustained periods of abstinence during treatment. Some of the most impressive findings have come from an outpatient treatment for cocaine abusers that involves abstinence reinforcement (vouchers that can be traded for retail items in the community) offered in the context of an aggressive behavioral treatment program that attempts to enhance sources of nondrug reinforcement in the environment (CRA). In general, however, influencing environmental factors that may hold the key to abstinence versus relapse continues to be a challenge to behavior therapists. Learning-based relapse-prevention and skills-training therapies have shown some efficacy for teaching drug abusers skills that can help to insulate them from the insidious influence of social and other environmental stimulus factors that promote drug use. Also, involvement of significant others during treatment (BMT for alcoholism, CRA for cocaine) appears to be a promising way to exert a positive influence on the immediate environment of the abuser. More research is needed in all these promising areas to systematically assess the dose and elements of behavioral treatment that are effective, to compare potency (effect sizes) of different types of treatment when delivered to similar populations, and to examine hypotheses related to patient–treatment matching.

REFERENCES

1. Azrin NH. Improvements in the community-reinforcement approach to alcoholism. *Behav Res Ther* 1976;14(5):339–348.
2. Azrin NH, Sisson RW, Meyers R, Godley M. Alcoholism treatment by disulfiram and community reinforcement therapy. *J. Behav Ther Exp Psychiatry* 1982;13(2):105–112.
3. Babor TF, Grant M. *Project on identification and management of alcohol-related problems. Report on Phase II: a randomized clinical trial or brief interventions in primary health care.* Geneva: World Health Organization, 1991.
4. Baer JS, Marlatt GA, Kivlahan DR, Fromme K, Larimer ME, Williams E. An experimental test of three methods of alcohol risk reduction with young adults. *J Consult Clin Psychol* 1992; 60(6):974–979.
5. Ball JC, Ross A. *The effectiveness of methadone maintenance treatment.* New York: Springer-Verlag, 1991.
6. Brown RA. Conventional education and controlled drinking education courses with convicted drunken drivers. *Behav Ther* 1980;11:632–642.
7. Carroll KM. Psychotherapy and pharmacotherapy for ambulatory cocaine abusers. Paper presented at the NIDA Technical Review Meeting on "Outcomes for Treatment of Cocaine Dependence," Bethesda, MD, September 1993.
8. Carroll KM, Rounsaville BJ, Gawin FH. A comparative trial of psychotherapies for ambulatory cocaine abusers: relapse prevention and interpersonal psychotherapy. *Am J Drug Alcohol Abuse* 1991;17(3):229–247.
9. Carroll KM, Rounsaville BJ, Gordon LT, Nich C, Jatlow P, Bisighinni RM, Gawin FH. Psychotherapy and pharmacotherapy for ambulatory cocaine abusers. *Arch Gen Psychiatry* 1994;51:177–187.
10. Chaney EF, O'Leary MR, Marlatt GA. Skill training with alcoholics. *J Consult Clin Psychol* 1978;46(5):1092–1104.
11. Childress AR. Using active strategies to cope with cocaine cue reactivity: preliminary treatment outcomes. Paper presented at the NIDA Technical Review Meeting on "Outcomes for Treatment of Cocaine Dependence," Bethesda, MD, September 1993.
12. Condelli WS, Fairbank JA, Dennis ML, Rachal JV. Cocaine use by clients in methadone programs: significance, scope, and behavioral interventions [Review]. *J Subst Abuse Treat* 1991;8(4):203–212.
13. Cooney NL, Kadden RM, Litt MD, Getter H. Matching alcoholics to coping skills or interactional therapies: two-year follow-up results. *J Consult Clin Psychol* 1991;59(4):598–601.
14. Dolan MP, Black JL, Penk WE, Rabinowitz R, DeFord HA. Contracting for treatment termination to reduce illicit drug use among methadone maintenance treatment failures. *J Consult Clin Psychol* 1985;53(4):549–551.
15. Dolan MP, Black JL, Penk WE, Rabinowitz R, DeFord HA. Predicting the outcome of contingency contracting for drug abuse. *Behav Ther* 1986;17:470–474.
16. Elkins RL. Aversion therapy treatment of cocaine dependent individuals. Paper presented at the NIDA Technical Review Meeting on "Outcomes for Treatment of Cocaine Dependence," Bethesda, MD, September 1993.
17. Eriksen L, Bjornstad S, Gotestam KG. Social skills training in groups for alcoholics: one-year treatment outcome for groups and individuals. *Addict Behav* 1986;11(3):309–329.
18. Ferrell WL, Galassi JP. Assertion training and human relations training in the treatment of chronic alcoholics. *Int J Addict* 1981;16(5):959–968.
19. Foy DW, Nunn LB, Rychtarik RG. Broad-spectrum behavioral treatment for chronic alcoholics: effects of training controlled drinking skills. *J Consult Clin Psychol* 1984;52(2):218–230.
20. Greil AL, Rudy DR. Conversion to the world view of Alcoholics Anonymous: a refinement of conversion theory. *Qual Sociol* 1983;6:5–28.
21. Hall SM, Bass A, Hargreaves WA, Loeb P. Contingency management and information feedback in outpatient heroin detoxification. *Behav Ther* 1979;10:443–451.
22. Hall SM, Loeb P, Coyne K, Cooper J. Increasing employment in ex-heroin addicts. I. Criminal justice sample. *Behav Ther* 1981;12:443–452.
23. Hall SM, Loeb P, LeVois M, Cooper J. Increasing employment in ex-heroin addicts. II. Methadone maintenance sample. *Behav Ther* 1981;12:453–460.
24. Hanbury R, Sturiano V, Cohen M, Stimmel B, Aguillaume C. Cocaine use in persons on methadone maintenance. *Adv Alcohol Subst Abuse* 1986;6(2):97–106.
25. Hawkins JD, Catalano RF, Gillmore MR, Wells EA. Skills training for drug abusers: generalization, maintenance and effects on drug use. *J Consult Clin Psychol* 1981;57:559–563.
26. Hawkins JD, Catalano RF, Wells EA. Measuring effects of a skills training intervention for drug abusers. *J Consult Clin Psychol* 1986;54(5):661–664.
27. Higgins ST, Budney AJ, Bickel WK, Foerg FE, Donham R, Badger GJ. Incentives improve treatment retention and cocaine abstinence in ambulatory cocaine-dependent patients. *Arch Gen Psychiatry* 1994;51:568–576.
28. Higgins ST, Budney AJ, Bickel WK, Hughes JR, Foerg F, Badger G. Achieving cocaine abstinence with a behavioral approach. *Am J Psychiatry* 1993;150(5):763–769.
29. Higgins ST, Delaney DD, Budney AJ, et al. A behavioral approach to achieving initial cocaine abstinence. *Am J Psychiatry* 1991;148(9):1218–1224.
30. Higgins ST, Stitzer ML, Bigelow GE, Liebson IA. Contingent meth-

adone delivery: effects on illicit-opiate use. *Drug Alcohol Depend* 1986;17(4):311–322.

31. Hubbard RL, Marsden ME, Rachal JV, Harwood HJ, Cavanaugh ER, Genzberg HM. *Drug abuse treatment: a national study of effectiveness.* Chapel Hill, NC: University of North Carolina Press, 1989.

32. Hunt GM, Azrin NH. A community-reinforcement approach to alcoholism. *Behav Res Ther* 1973;11(1):91–104.

33. Iguchi MY, Handelsman L, Bickel WK, Griffiths RR. Benzodiazepine and sedative use/abuse by methadone maintenance clients. *Drug Alcohol Depend* 1993;32(3):257–266.

34. Iguchi MY, Stitzer ML, Bigelow GE, Liebson IA. Contingency management in methadone maintenance: effects of reinforcing and aversive consequences on illicit polydrug use. *Drug Alcohol Depend* 1988;22:1–7.

35. Kadden RM, Cooney NL, Getter H, Litt MD. Matching alcoholics to coping skills or interactional therapies: posttreatment results. *J Consult Clin Psychol* 1989;57(6):698–704.

36. Keane TM, Foy DW, Nunn B, Rychtarik RG. Spouse contracting to increase antabuse compliance in alcoholic veterans. *J Clin Psychol* 1984;40(1):340–344.

37. Kidorf M, Stitzer ML. Characteristics of methadone patients responding to take-home incentives. *Behav Ther* 1994;25:109–121.

38. Kosten TR, Gawin FH, Rounsaville BJ, Kleber HD. Cocaine abuse among opioid addicts: demographic and diagnostic factors in treatment. *Am J Drug Alcohol Abuse* 1986;12(1–2):1–16.

39. Liebson IA, Tommasello A, Bigelow GE. A behavioral treatment of alcoholic methadone patients. *Ann Intern Med* 1978;89(3):342–344.

40. Magura S, Casriel C, Goldsmith DS, Strug DL, Lipton DS. Contingency contracting with polydrug-abusing methadone patients. *Addict Behav* 1988;13(1):113–118.

41. Mallams JH, Godley MD, Hall GM, Meyers RJ. A social-systems approach to resocializing alcoholics in the community. *J Stud Alcohol* 1982;43(11):1115–1123.

42. Marlatt GA. Stress as a determinant of excessive drinking and relapse. In: Pohorecky L, Brick J, eds. *Stress and alcohol use.* New York: Elsevier, 1983;279–294.

43. Marlatt GA, Gordon JR, eds. *Relapse prevention: maintenance strategies in the treatment of addictive behaviors.* New York: Guilford Press, 1985.

44. McAuliffe WE, Ch'ien JM. Recovery training and self help: a relapse-prevention program for treated opiate addicts. *J Subst Abuse Treat* 1986;3(1):9–20.

45. McAuliffe WE, Ch'ien, JMN, Launer E, Friedman R, Feldman B. The Harvard group aftercare program: preliminary evaluation results and implementation issues. In: Ashery RS, ed. *Progress in the development of cost-effective treatment for drug abusers.* National Institute on Drug Abuse Research Monograph 58. DHHS publication no. (ADM)88-1401. Washington, DC: U.S. Government Printing Office, 1985;147–155.

46. McCarthy JJ, Borders OT. Limit setting on drug abuse in methadone maintenance patients. *Am J Psychiatry* 1985;142(12):1419–1423.

47. McCaul ME, Stitzer ML, Bigelow GE, Liebson IA. Contingency management interventions: effects on treatment outcome during methadone detoxification. *J Appl Behav Anal* 1984;17(1):35–43.

48. McCrady BS, Noel NE, Abrams DB, Stout RL, Nelson HF, Hay WM. Comparative effectiveness of three types of spouse involvement in outpatient behavioral alcoholism treatment. *J Stud Alcohol* 1986;47(6):459–467.

49. McCrady BS, Stout R, Noel N, Abrams D, Nelson HF. Effectiveness of three types of spouse-involved behavioral alcoholism treatment. *Br J Addict* 1991;86(11):1415–1424.

50. McLellan AT, Arndt IO, Metzger DS, Woody GE, O'Brien CP. The effects of psychosocial services in substance abuse treatment. *JAMA* 1993;269(15):1953–1959.

51. Milby JB, Garrett C, English C, Fritschi O, Clarke C. Take-home methadone: contingency effects on drug-seeking and productivity of narcotic addicts. *Addict Behav* 1978;3(3–4):215–220.

52. Miller WR, Baca LM. Two year follow-up of bibliotherapy and therapist-directed controlled drinking training for problem drinkers. *Behav Ther* 1983;14:441–448.

53. Miller WR, Hester RK. Matching problem drinkers with optimal treatments. In: Miller WR, Heather N, eds. *Treating addictive behaviors: processes of change.* New York: Plenum, 1986;175–203.

54. Miller WR, Taylor CA. Relative effectiveness of bibliotherapy, individual and group self-control training in the treatment of problem drinkers. *Addict Behav* 1980;5(1):13–24.

55. Miller WR, Leckman AL, Delaney HD, Tinkcom M. Long-term follow-up of behavioral self-control training. *J Stud Alcohol* 1992;53(3):249–261.

56. National Institute on Drug Abuse. *National Drug and Alcoholism Treatment Unit Survey (NDATUS).* Publication no. 91-1729. Rockville, MD: DHHS, 1990.

57. Oei TP, Jackson PR. Social skills and cognitive behavioral approaches to the treatment of problem drinking. *J Stud Alcohol* 1982;43(5):532–547.

58. O'Farrell TJ, Choquette KA, Cutter HSG, Brown ED, McCourt WF. Behavioral marital therapy with and without additional couples relapse prevention sessions for alcoholics and their wives. *J Stud Alcohol* 1994;3;54:652–666.

59. O'Farrell TJ, Cutter HSG, Choquette KA, Floyd FJ, Bayog RD. Behavioral marital therapy for male alcoholics: marital and drinking adjustment during the two years after treatment. *Behav Ther* 1992;23:529–549.

60. O'Farrell TJ, Cutter HSG, Floyd FJ. Evaluating behavioral marital therapy for male alcoholics: effects on marital adjustment and communication from before to after therapy. *Behav Ther* 1985;16:147–167.

61. Platt JJ, Megzger D. The role of employment in the rehabilitation of heroin addicts. In: Ashery RS, ed. *Progress in the development of cost-effective treatment for drug abusers. NIDA Res Monogr* 1985;58:111–145.

62. Rawson RA. The Matrix neurobehavioral model: evidence of efficacy. Paper presented at the NIDA Technical Review Meeting on *Outcomes for Treatment of Cocaine Dependence,* September 1993, Bethesda, MD.

63. Rohsenow D. Social skills training for cocaine dependent individuals. Paper presented at the NIDA Technical Review Meeting on *Outcomes for Treatment of Cocaine Dependence,* September 1993, Bethesda, MD.

64. Sanchez CM, Walker K. Teaching coping skills to chronic alcoholics in a coeducational halfway house. I. Assessment of programme effects. *Br J Addict* 1982;77(1):35–50.

65. Sanchez CM, Annis HM, Bornet AR, MacDonald KR. Random assignment to abstinence and controlled drinking: evaluation of a cognitive-behavioral program for problem drinkers. *J Consult Clin Psychol* 1984;52(3):390–403.

66. Saxon AJ, Calsyn DA, Kivlahan DR, Roszell DK. Outcome of contingency contracting for illicit drug use in a methadone maintenance program. *Drug Alcohol Depend* 1993;31(3):205–214.

67. Silverman K, Schuster CR, Brooner RK, Montoya ID, Preston KL. Contingency management of cocaine use in a methadone maintenance program. Paper presented at the annual meeting of the Association for the Advancement of Behavior Therapy, November 1993, Atlanta, GA.

68. Stitzer ML, Bigelow GE. Contingency management in a methadone maintenance program: availability of reinforcers. *Int J Addict* 1978;13:737–746.

69. Stitzer ML, Bickel WK, Bigelow GE, Liebson IA. Effect of methadone dose contingencies on urinalysis test results of polydrug-abusing methadone-maintenance patients. *Drug Alcohol Depend* 1986;18(4):341–348.

70. Stitzer ML, Bigelow GE, Liebson IA, Hawthorne JW. Contingent reinforcement for benzodiazepine-free urines: evaluation of a drug abuse treatment intervention. *J Appl Behav Anal* 1982;15(4):493–503.

71. Stitzer ML, Griffiths RR, McLellan AT, Grabowski J, Hawthorne JW. Diazepam use among methadone maintenance patients: patterns and dosages. *Drug Alcohol Depend* 1981;8(3):189–199.

72. Stitzer ML, Iguchi MY, Felch LJ. Contingent take-home incentive: effects on drug use of methadone maintenance patients. *J Consult Clin Psychol* 1992;60(6):927–934.

73. Vogler RE, Compton JV, Weissbach TA. Integrated behavior change techniques for alcoholics. *J Consult Clin Psychol* 1975;43(2):233–243.

74. Vogler RE, Weissbach TA, Compton JV, Martin GT. Integrated behavior change techniques for problem drinkers in the community. *J Consult Clin Psychol* 1977;45(2):267–279.

75. Woody GE, Luborsky L, McLellan T, et al. Psychotherapy for opiate addicts. *Arch Gen Psychiatry* 1983;40:639–645.

76. Woody GE, McLellan AT, Luborsky L, et al. Severity of psychiatry symptoms as a predictor of benefits from psychotherapy: the Veterans Administration–Penn study. *Am J Psychiatry* 1984; 141(10):1172–1177. [Published erratum appears in *Am J Psychiatry* 1989;146(12):1651.]

77. Woody GE, McLellan AT, Luborsky L, O'Brien CP. Sociopathy and psychotherapy outcome. *Arch Gen Psychiatry* 1985; 42(11):1081–1086.

78. Woody GE, McLellan AT, Luborsky L, O'Brien CP. Twelve-month follow-up of psychotherapy for opiate dependence. *Am J Psychiatry* 1987;144(5):590–596. [Published erratum appears in *Am J Psychiatry* 1989;146(12):1651.]

Psychopharmacology: The Fourth Generation of Progress, edited by Floyd E. Bloom and David J. Kupfer. Raven Press, Ltd., New York © 1995.

CHAPTER 155

Genetics

Raymond R. Crowe

Recombinant DNA technology has enabled us to explore the human genome in ways that would not have been thought possible 20 years ago. Widespread DNA polymorphism has been exploited through the use of restriction enzymes and, more recently, the polymerase chain reaction to create genetic markers and detect linkage to a growing list of human disease genes. These genetic markers are defining a human linkage map of increasingly greater resolution. Genes expressed in the brain are being cloned in large numbers and will ultimately be placed on the linkage map. This progress with the human genome is being paralleled by similar developments in rodents and other potential animal models. The end result of all of these efforts will be the creation of a set of tools that will enable us to identify disease-producing mutations in increasingly complex genetic diseases.

These developments have obvious implications for psychiatry. Collaborative efforts are underway to collect pedigrees and bank cell lines and to search for genes contributing to schizophrenia, bipolar illness, alcoholism, and Alzheimer's disease. Unlike the diseases that have been successfully mapped, behavioral disorders present unique challenges for molecular genetic strategies. These are illustrated by the number of linkage findings in psychiatry that cannot be replicated. The special problems of applying molecular strategies to complex traits can be appreciated with an understanding of the genetic epidemiology of mental disorders and the theoretical underpinnings of the molecular genetic strategies. Understanding the interrelationship of these two disciplines is crucial to designing strategies that will avoid the pitfalls of the past and maximize the chances of success in the future (see also Chapters 2, 69, and 153, *this volume*).

R. R. Crowe: Department of Psychiatry, University of Iowa College of Medicine, Iowa City, Iowa 52242.

PSYCHIATRIC GENETICS

Family, twin and adoption studies have supplied the raw material for a substantial foundation of genetic epidemiology. Family and twin studies can provide information on the penetrance of the genotype, as well as on its full range of expression. Twin and adoption studies separate genetic from environmental transmission. Segregation analyses define the range of genetic hypotheses that can account for the observed transmission patterns. A growing number of molecular genetic studies aimed at identifying disease genes is now being added to this foundation of classical genetics.

Manic–Depressive Illness

McGuffin and Katz (39) reviewed 12 family studies of bipolar illness and found the average morbidity risk among first-degree relatives to be 7.8% for bipolar and 11.4% for unipolar illness. This is a substantial increase over the respective population rates of approximately 1% and 3%, cited by the same authors. Probandwise monozygotic twin concordance rates for bipolar illness range from 62% to 72%, and an additional 18–25% have unipolar illness (8,67). Comparative dizygotic concordance rates range from 0% to 8% for bipolar illness, with an additional unipolar range from 0% to 11%. The role of genes in bipolar illness is further supported by observations on adoptees. Increased rates of both bipolar and unipolar illness are seen in biological parents but not in adoptive parents of bipolar adoptees, indicating that the family and twin data indeed reflect the action of genes (41). Collectively, the evidence points to a genetic predisposition with a relatively high penetrance and a range of expression including bipolar and unipolar affective disorder.

The most extensive observations on the bipolar phenotype and its transmission come from a comprehensive family study of bipolar I, bipolar II, schizoaffective, unipolar, and control probands (22). The first four disorders, with the possible addition of cyclothymic personality disorder, aggregate in the families of schizoaffective and bipolar probands. Genetic analyses of these pedigrees indicate that a multifactorial-threshold model provides a plausible explanation of the transmission and that a single-locus model can be excluded (22,23). According to the model, schizoaffective disorder is the most severe form of the illness, followed by bipolar I, bipolar II, and unipolar depressive disorder.

The discovery of large bipolar pedigrees among the Old Order Amish provides a rare opportunity to study manic–depressive illness in a population isolate with an apparently autosomal dominant form of the disease. Such genetically isolated populations are ideal for linkage studies because their gene pools are typically more homogeneous than those of the general population. Indeed, a gene appeared to have been found when linkage was reported between bipolar illness and two DNA markers (HRAS and INS) on the short arm of chromosome 11 (18).

In retrospect, failures to replicate the finding should have sounded a note of caution, but at that time the discrepancy between the studies was felt to be evidence of genetic heterogeneity. This explanation seemed plausible because of the isolated nature of the Amish population; the linkage could represent a rare gene that would be difficult to replicate outside of that group. Therefore, the pedigree was extended to include two new branches and, at the same time, the diagnoses were updated (30). Linkage analyses based on these revisions resulted in a decisive erosion of the original logarithm of the odds (lod) score to the point that a disease locus for bipolar illness could now be excluded from the region in question. The lod scores at the two marker loci that had previously supported linkage, HRAS and INS, fell from 4.08 to −9.31 and from 2.63 to −7.75, respectively. The reversal of support for linkage was accounted for predominantly by two changes: Two relatives who were unaffected in the original analyses subsequently became ill, and the two pedigree extensions introduced a number of new affected relatives. The net effect of both changes was to introduce a number of obligate recombinants—that is, crossovers between affectation status and marker typings.

How can the steep fall in the lod scores be reconciled with the strong original evidence of linkage? One possible explanation is the inclusion of unipolar depression in the affected phenotype. Though unipolar depression is an expression of the bipolar genotype, the high population prevalence of depression could introduce cases into the pedigree that are unrelated to the bipolar gene. Indeed, it was unipolar depressives in the new pedigree extensions that were most responsible for the lod score changes.

Alternatively, a second gene for bipolar illness could have entered the pedigree through marriage. The existence of positive assortative mating for mood disorder makes this a plausible possibility. Finally, the lod scores supporting linkage may have represented a false-positive finding. The failure of other linkage reports in psychiatry to be replicated supports this explanation.

The X-linkage hypothesis of manic–depressive illness has been an intriguing and elusive one since evidence for it first appeared over 25 years ago. Since that time, attempts to replicate X linkage have produced a confusing melange of supportive and contradictory results. A report of five Israeli pedigrees provided remarkably strong evidence for linkage to the G6PD and color blindness loci (located at Xq27-q28), supported by lod scores of 7.52 and greater (5). However, when three of the original pedigrees were reinterviewed and retyped with DNA markers, the overall evidence for linkage declined dramatically. Lod scores in two of the pedigrees became negative, and in the third pedigree the score remained in the range of 2.00 (6).

Several reasons for the change in lod scores were identified (6). Females could not be typed at the G6PD and color blindness loci in the first study because DNA markers were not used. When these pedigree members were typed in the reanalysis, a number of new recombinants were found. Diagnostic changes resulting from new interviews created additional recombinants. In addition, several key family members that had supported linkage were lost to reanalysis. Finally, a mother of two affected male offspring was found to be homozygous at the G6PD locus, and thus her sons, who had supported linkage in the first analysis, became uninformative. These changes, plus several minor ones, resulted in the virtual disappearance of a lod score favoring linkage with an odds ratio of over 33 million to one.

Schizophrenia

Recent family studies using current interview methods and diagnostic criteria have arrived at reasonably similar estimates of the recurrence risk for schizophrenia. The Roscommon Family Study was based on a complete ascertainment of all cases of schizophrenia in county Roscommon, Ireland, and it found a morbidity risk for schizophrenia of 6.5% (S.E. 1.6%) among interviewed relatives (34). This rate is 13 times the rate of 0.5% found among the relatives of control probands, and it is 7.6 times the usually quoted population rate of schizophrenia of 0.85%.

Twin studies provide further evidence of genetic vulnerability. Despite the wide diagnostic variation across studies, when monozygotic (MZ) and dizygotic (DZ) concordances are compared within studies the MZ/DZ ratios are remarkably consistant and indicate that genes account for a median of 65% of the variance in the transmission of schizophrenia (31). Adoption studies further support the role of genes by demonstrating a correlation in liability between biological relatives separated at birth (32).

The full expression of the genetic liability to schizophrenia is seen in MZ cotwins of schizophrenics. Therefore, the spectrum of illnesses that maximizes the MZ:DZ concordance ratio provides a genetic definition of the schizophrenia spectrum. In the Maudsley twin series, the range of DSM-III diagnoses that maximizes this ratio includes schizophrenia, schizotypal personality disorder, affective disorder with mood incongruent psychosis, atypical psychosis, and schizophreniform disorder (20). Although schizoaffective disorder was not placed in the spectrum in this series, a consensus exists that *chronic* schizoaffective disorder is related to schizophrenia. In the Roscommon Family Study, increased rates of schizophrenia were found in the relatives of probands with schizoaffective disorder, schizotypal personality disorder, psychotic affective disorder, and other nonaffective psychoses (34).

When schizophrenia is considered as a unitary syndrome, the preponderance of the evidence supports polygenic, rather than mendelian, inheritance (56). Mendelian diseases tend to be rare because of genetic selection against the gene, whereas the prevalence of schizophrenia is nearly 1%. MZ concordance rates of mendelian diseases are approximately twice the DZ rates, so the observed ratios of over 4:1 for schizophrenia are more consistent with polygenes. Familial morbidity risks of mendelian diseases decrease by one-half with each increasing degree of genetic distance from the proband (i.e., from first- to second- to third-degree relatives). The more rapid regression seen in families of schizophrenics suggests polygenic inheritance. Finally, segregation analyses have not supported a mendelian model (4). If schizophrenia is genetically homogeneous, the evidence argues convincingly against mendelian inheritance, but it is unlikely to be homogeneous. If, as is likely, the causes are multiple, it is possible that rare mendelian genes for schizophrenia exist and could be found in multiply affected pedigrees. This possibility has fueled interest in searching for vulnerability genes with linkage.

The search for a major gene effect received an impetus from the report of a pedigree segregating a chromosome 5 translocation with schizophrenia (7). As a result of the translocation, both the proband and a maternal uncle were trisomic for $5q_{11}-q_{13}$, raising the possibility that excess activity of a gene in this region might have contributed to the schizophrenia. A linkage study with DNA markers in this region in seven Icelandic and English pedigrees resulted in what appeared to be convincing evidence of linkage: a lod score of 3.22 (60). Moreover, when the affected phenotype was broadened to include schizophrenia spectrum disorders, the lod score increased to 4.33,

and when all psychiatric disorders were considered as affected, it reached 6.49. The last finding is puzzling because the inclusion of genetically unrelated disorders should result in a reduction in the lod score.

At first, when the chromosome 5 finding could not be replicated, the nonreplications were attributed to genetic heterogeneity, but as failures to replicate continued to appear, heterogeneity became an increasingly unlikely explanation. Another argument against heterogeneity as an explanation is that it should be detectable *within* studies, but a meta-analysis found that the published studies were internally homogeneous but demonstrated heterogeneity *between* studies. The heterogeneity was accounted for by differences between the study reporting linkage and those attempting to replicate it (40). Because the genetic structure of the Icelandic population is not unique, there should be no reason for finding heterogeneity between these studies, and the most likely explanation is that the original lod scores were spuriously elevated.

Tourette's Syndrome

Tourette's syndrome (TS) is often familial, and extensive pedigrees of the disease have been reported (35) (see also Chapter 143, *this volume*). Family members have an increased risk of TS, chronic motor tics, and obsessive–compulsive disorder. In one study of first-degree relatives of TS probands, the morbidity risk for TS was 8.7%, for chronic tics 17.3%, and for obsessive–compulsive disorder 11.5%. Thus, the aggregate morbidity risk was 37.5%, which was over seven times the population rate of 5.2% found in the same study (53). The ratio of affected males to females was 4:1 for TS and 1:2 for obsessive–compulsive disorder.

The genetic vulnerability is underscored by an MZ twin concordance rate of 53% for TS among cotwins of TS probands and 77% for TS or chronic motor tics. The respective DZ concordances are 8% and 23% (55). Segregation analysis supports an autosomal dominant gene as the most likely mode of transmission (52).

The close fit to autosomal dominant transmission, the high penetrance, and the existance of large multiplex pedigrees make TS an ideal choice for linkage studies, and the interim results of a collaborative genome search have been published (50). Ten large pedigrees typed with 228 markers have covered at least half, and perhaps as much as two-thirds, of the genome, but no convincing evidence of linkage has been found. Now that more informative and detailed human genome maps are available, a complete genome search of TS should be forthcoming.

Panic Disorder

The familial nature of panic disorder is supported by family history, with patients reporting secondary cases in

12–15% of their first-degree relatives (14). Interviews with family members found an age-corrected morbidity risk of 17% for panic disorder or agoraphobia with panic attacks, and the rate was 24% when subsyndromal panic attacks were included (14). The mean age of onset is 25 years, and the sex ratio (F/M) is approximately 2:1. The range of disorders found in family members was limited to panic disorder, agoraphobia, and subsyndromal panic attacks (46).

Limited twin data, based on 13 MZ and 16 DZ pairs, are consistent with the familial findings, both with respect to a genetic predisposition and with respect to its range of expression. Panic disorder, subsyndromal panic attacks, and agoraphobia appeared among MZ cotwins of panic disorder twins, and the aggregate concordance rate was 31%, compared with 0% for dizygotic cotwins (66). Segregation analyses of pedigrees and threshold models applied to aggregate recurrence rates are consistent with either a single-locus or a multifactorial mode of transmission (14,51). Linkage studies of panic disorder are currently underway at a number of centers. In one study, approximately 30% of the genome has been screened with RFLP markers in 10–14 pedigrees, but no evidence of linkage was found (15).

Alcoholism

Controlled family studies of alcoholism based on current interview methods and diagnostic criteria support (a) a sevenfold increase in risk of alcoholism in first-degree relatives of alcoholics over controls and (b) a fivefold risk increase in male relatives over females (43). A representative study found the following rates of alcoholism among first-degree relatives of alcoholic probands: fathers 16.1%, brothers 12.4%, mothers 1.6%, and sisters 1.0% (54). The aggregate control rate was 1.2%.

Kendler's sample of female twins provides the best available estimate of the heritability of alcoholism because it was drawn from a population sample and all participating twins were interviewed (33). Probandwise MZ concordance rates ranged from 26% to 47%, depending on strictness of diagnosis, and the corresponding DZ rates ranged from 12% to 32%. These findings indicate that genes account for 50–60% of the variance in the transmission of alcoholism (33).

The role of genes in the etiology of alcoholism is further supported by adoption studies. Biological relatives separated by adoption show strong correlations in the diagnosis of alcoholism (25) and in temperance board registrations for alcohol abuse (13). The last study identified two patterns of inheritance: Type 1 alcoholism was correlated with postnatal environment but not with criminality in biological fathers, whereas type 2 alcoholism followed the opposite pattern. In contrast to type 2 alco-

holism, type 1 was more common, had a later onset, was less severe, and was more likely to include women.

A segregation analysis of 35 pedigrees found that neither a mendelian nor a polygenic model could account for the transmission (1). Because the disease is demonstrably genetic, it is puzzling that neither single nor multiple locus models could explain the transmission. The authors speculated that this result could reflect oligogenic inheritance (i.e., a small number of loci), phenocopies, sex effects, or genetic heterogeneity.

Ethanol is eliminated from the body by first being converted to acetaldehyde by the enzyme alcohol dehydrogenase (ADH), and acetaldehyde is then broken down to acetate and water by aldehyde dehydrogenase (ALDH). Genetic polymorphisms in both enzymes correlate with their activity. Three ADH alleles (ADH1-3) are responsible for marked variation in the elimination rate of ethanol. The breakdown of acetaldehyde is catalyzed primarily by the mitochondrial enzyme ALDH2. A dominant allele (ALDH2*2) confers an absence of detectable enzyme activity. The ALDH2*2 allele is prevalent in Asians and causes a flushing response to ethanol ingestion, similar to that caused by the drug disulfuram, which inhibits ALDH activity. This mechanism appears to contribute to the low rate of alcoholism among Asians (61). Interestingly, compared to nonalcoholics, Chinese alcoholics may have a lower allele frequency of two ADH genes (ADH2*2 and ADH3*1) in addition to a lower frequency of ALDH2*2 (65). These three alleles have the net effect of decreasing blood acetaldehyde levels after ethanol ingestion by retarding production while accelerating elimination. These important findings demonstrate a mechanism by which genetic variation appears to influence drinking behavior in Asians. Since the ALDH2*2 allele is absent in Caucasians it cannot account for their drinking behavior.

The role of polymorphism at the dopamine D2 receptor locus (DRD2) in the pathogenesis of alcoholism has been a source of continuing controversy (68). Mesolimbic and mesocortical dopaminergic systems appear to be involved in the mediation of reward, suggesting that dopamine could play a role in addictive behaviors. This hypothesis was supported by the report of an association between a restriction fragment length polymorphism (RFLP) allele (A2) at the DRD2 locus and alcoholism (10). A consensus of the literature supports a number of conclusions about the association. First, it has been replicated more often than would be expected by chance. Second, the association is stronger with more severe cases of alcoholism. Third, it is not limited to alcoholism but includes other substance abuse disorders and possibly an even broader spectrum of psychopathology. Finally, the DRD2 locus is not linked to alcoholism.

What do these results tell us about the genetics of substance abuse? If the association is real, the most likely explanation is that variation in receptor kinetics contributes to the liability to substance abuse and the variation is correlated with DRD2 alleles the way ADH and ALDH enzyme activity correlate with alleles at their respective loci. Even if D2 receptor kinetics contribute to alcoholism, a simple cause-and-effect relationship between DRD2 alleles and the disease is excluded by the lack of linkage. This implies that the allele would have to act epistatically—that is, by modifying the effects of other genes that have a more direct causal role. This explanation is consistent with the association appearing stronger with more severe cases of alcoholism. It could also account for the D2 receptor influencing the pathogenesis of a broader range of diseases than alcoholism. This theoretical explanation for the DRD2 association is supported by observations that the A2 allele alters receptor kinetics (45).

GENETIC RESEARCH IN OTHER NEUROPSYCHIATRIC DISEASES

Examining how molecular genetic strategies have made inroads into several neuropsychiatric diseases that share many of the complexities of typical psychiatric disorders may provide clues to what can be anticipated in psychiatry. Alzheimer's disease is reviewed in detail elsewhere in this volume (Chapter 115). The appearance of an Alzheimer-like dementia in persons with Down's syndrome, the location of the amyloid precursor protein gene (APP) on the long arm of chromosome 21, and the existence of apparently autosomal dominant forms of Alzheimer's disease led to an intense search for disease vulnerability genes on chromosome 21q. The search resulted in the discovery of mutations in APP which account for a rare, early-onset, chromosome-21-linked form of the disease. A systematic genome scan identified (a) a second locus on chromosome 14 responsible for early-onset, familial cases and (b) a third locus on chromosome 19 causing a late-onset, familial form of the disease. Although the genetics of Alzheimer's disease are proving to be complex, they still follow known genetic mechanisms by which point mutations cause mendelian inheritance of a disorder. In the case of the fragile X syndrome and Huntington's disease, an entirely new genetic mechanism was uncovered.

The Fragile-X Syndrome

Families with male-limited mental retardation with dysmorphic features and X-linked recessive inheritance have been noted since the 1940s. Subsequently, the fragile-X syndrome, X-linked mental retardation associated with a fragile site on the long arm of X, was recognized as the most common cause of hereditary mental retardation, accounting for 1 in 1250 retarded males and

an additional 1 in 2000 females with mild retardation (17). The fragile site created a biological marker for the fragile-X syndrome, and when family studies included an assessment of the fragile site a curious phenomenon was discovered (59). Twenty percent of males with the fragile site are unaffected, and, conversely, 30% of female heterozygotes are mildly affected, so the gene is neither completely dominant nor fully recessive. When the gene passes from unaffected males through their daughters to their grandsons, the penetrance in grandsons is 40%. Yet, brothers of nonpenetrant males have a 9% penetrance. The low penetrance in brothers compared with the high penetrance in grandsons cannot be explained by mendelian inheritance and became known as the *Sherman paradox*.

The Sherman paradox was finally explained when the mutation responsible for the fragile-X syndrome was discovered (21). It is a (CGG)n trinucleotide repeat located in the coding sequence of a gene of unknown function. The repeat is capable of expanding as it passes to successive generations. The number of repeats in normals ranges from 6 to 50. When the number expands into the range of 50–200 repeats, it is termed a *premutation* because it is prone to further expansion into a range of from 200 to over 1000 repeats. This last expansion causes the fragile-X syndrome. The Sherman paradox was explained by the observation that premutations must pass through females to expand and cause the syndrome. The probability of expansion increases with the existing size of the repeat, and this explains another genetic paradox—anticipation: the tendency for some diseases to exhibit earlier onset, increased severity, or greater penetrance in successive generations. It should be reassuring to behavior geneticists that a complex pattern of inheritance at the phenotypic level was accounted for by a simple mechanism once the genetics were understood.

Huntington's Disease

Huntington's disease is an autosomal dominant trait with complete penetrance, provided that persons at risk live long enough to develop it. Although the genetics are mendelian, it manifests some of the complexities of psychiatric diseases. Penetrance is age-dependent, with an average age of onset of approximately 45 years. Although juvenile-onset cases exist, their symptoms differ from those in the adult, with rigidity being more prominent than choreiform movements.

The gene has been localized to the short arm of chromosome 4 by linkage (27). The first step in moving from a linkage to the disease gene is to flank the locus with a second marker and narrow the flanked region by walking new markers toward the center. Once the region was flanked and narrowed to about 2 million base pairs, the search for candidate genes began. Eventually, a candidate was found that contained a mutation in all patients tested but not in normals. The type of mutation proved to be as exciting as the discovery itself because it belongs to the recently identified class of triplet repeats (64). The (CAG)n repeat is present in all copies of the gene, but the repeat number varies from person to person. The number is capable of expanding during meiosis, and when it becomes large enough it inactivates the gene, causing the disease. Furthermore, the more severe, early-onset cases have larger numbers of repeats than do the more typical cases. These findings illustrate how the phenotypic complexities of Huntington's disease can be explained by a simple genetic mechanism. The next step will be to clarify the normal function of the gene and how it causes Huntington's disease. Meanwhile, the DNA diagnosis of Huntington's disease has become a reality.

Conclusion

The problem of why genetic strategies have delivered so many false starts in psychiatry has been the subject of intense analysis. As a result, the field has achieved a more critical understanding of the difficulties of applying linkage to diseases of ambiguous etiology, genetics, and phenotype (i.e., "complex" genetic traits). A number of factors may have contributed to the difficulties. Lod scores based on small numbers of pedigrees can be particularly labile in the face of new information, such as diagnostic changes and pedigree extensions. Because the lod score is a parametric test, ambiguity over the genetic parameters of the disease invalidates the conventional significance level of 3.00. When multiple analyses are done to cover a range of inheritance models and disease phenotypes, they can inflate the lod score. Basing a linkage decision on the genetic and diagnostic model that maximizes the lod score increases the risk of false-positives further by confusing exploratory with confirmatory analyses. Failure to appreciate the profound effect of the prior odds of linkage on the posterior odds, represented by the lod score, can prompt premature conclusions that linkage has been found.

The importance of the prior odds for *any* molecular genetic strategy is illustrated by the three examples of successful gene searches in neuropsychiatry. In each case a successful search began with a sound biological clue: in Huntington's disease, mendelian inheritance; in Alzheimer's disease, mendelian inheritance and amyloid plaques; and in fragile-X syndrome, the fragile site. These clues focused the research so that the prior probability of success was favorable. Biological findings of this nature do not exist currently for any psychiatric disorder. The absence of such clues to help dissect the genetic complexity of behavior disorders has been the Achilles' heel of psychiatric genetics.

MOLECULAR GENETIC STRATEGIES

Linkage

The usual test for linkage is the lod score. This statistic is derived by calculating the binomial probability of the observed distribution of pedigree members who show recombination between the trait and the marker locus and those who do not. (Formally, the lod score at any recombination fraction is the logarithm to the base 10 of the ratio of the probability of the pedigree assuming linkage at the given recombination fraction divided by the probability assuming no linkage.) The lod score is dependent on the correct specification of the mode of inheritance, disease allele frequency, penetrance, and the frequency of new mutations and nongenetic cases. Furthermore, the critical value of the lod score for linkage detection (3.00) is based on the assumption that a disease locus exists and will be detected if enough markers are tested; thus, the probability of false-positive lod scores due to testing multiple markers is offset by the increasing probability of a true-positive as the genome is systematically searched. When linkage analysis is limited to simple mendelian diseases, these requirements are satisfied, and the analysis and interpretation of the results are straightforward. However, when it is applied to nonmendelian diseases the lod score and its interpretation can be seriously compromised by the need to specify information that is not known about the genetic transmission and phenotypic expression of the disease.

The Genotype

The mode of inheritance is not known for any of the major psychiatric disorders. Although it is hoped that major loci account for a large enough proportion of pedigrees to be detected by linkage, this may not be the case, and inheritance may be due to two or more additive loci. In polygenic inheritance, a large number of loci contribute small, equal, and additive effects to disease liability. No single locus produces an effect great enough to be detected by linkage. In practice, most polygenic traits have proven to be oligogenic when the loci were accounted for. In oligogenic inheritance a small number of loci contribute additively to the phenotype. Theoretically, oligogenic loci are detectable by linkage; however, the smaller the effect of a locus, the larger the number of pedigrees needed to detect it.

The allele frequency of the disease gene must also be known to calculate the lod score accurately. When penetrance is incomplete, unaffected carriers marrying into the pedigree can produce affected descendents who could appear as recombinants and adversely affect the lod score. Etiologic heterogeneity may pose the most serious obstacle to finding genes through linkage. Mendelian diseases tend to be rare because selection against the gene keeps the allele frequency low. Therefore, common diseases are likely to be nonmendelian, and if mendelian forms exist, they are likely to account for a minority of the pedigrees. These arguments predict considerable etiological heterogeneity of psychiatric disorders.

Heterogeneity can be either genetic or environmental. Environmental heterogeneity causes phenocopies, which are considered under the discussion of the phenotype. Genetic heterogeneity can occur within loci when multiple alleles cause the disease, or it can occur between loci as illustrated by Alzheimer's disease. Of the two, only interlocus heterogeneity complicates linkage. Multiple disease loci can confound linkage analysis by occurring either within or between pedigrees. Heterogeneity between pedigrees weakens positive lod scores by contributing negative scores to the total. Heterogeneity within pedigrees weakens lod scores by creating false recombinants. In both cases the net effect is loss of power to detect linkage.

The Phenotype

Pedigree members must be dichotomized into affected and unaffected cases for linkage analysis. Misclassification due to either false-positive or false-negative diagnoses weakens the lod score, and this can happen in a number of ways.

Incomplete penetrance causes genetically affected persons to appear unaffected. Penetrance can vary with age, sex, and birth cohort. Incomplete penetrance is typical of psychiatric disorders, as demonstrated by MZ twin concordances for psychiatric syndromes being consistently less than 100%.

One effect of incomplete penetrance on linkage analysis is illustrated by the Amish study of bipolar illness already discussed (30). Two pedigree members who had not developed symptoms at the time of the first analysis decreased the lod score by almost two lod units when they were counted as affected in the reanalysis. The usual effect of incomplete penetrance is to weaken the power to detect and exclude linkage. The lod score can be corrected for incomplete penetrance; but the lower the penetrance, the less the unaffected relatives contribute to the lod score.

Variable expressivity also causes diagnostic misclassification. *Expressivity* refers to the range of clinical features the genotype can assume. The diagnostic boundaries of many psychiatric disorders are obscured by a spectrum of conditions that are genetically related to the core illness. For example, bipolar I illness may be genetically related to bipolar II, major depressive disorder, schizoaffective disorder, and cyclothymic disorder (22). The prob-

lem with including borderline and subclinical disorders in the affected phenotype definition is that some have high population prevalences (e.g., major depressive disorder) and are likely to introduce heterogeneity into the study. Expressivity also includes such phenotypes as biological markers, but, at present, none of the biological markers in psychiatry can replace or extend clinical diagnosis in linkage studies.

Phenocopies are environmental copies of genetic traits. Diseases as common as depression and alcoholism are likely to include a large proportion of these. Obviously, phenocopies will also be created by inappropriately broad definitions of the disease. They create another source of false recombinants. The phenocopy rate can be modeled in linkage analyses; but the greater it is, the less the affected relatives contribute to the lod score. Whether the phenocopy rate is modeled in the analysis or not, the net effect is to weaken the power to detect linkage.

Practical Issues of Linkage

How can linkage studies be designed to minimize these limitations and maximize the chances of finding disease genes? Now that the availability of dense, highly informative genetic maps has ceased to be a limiting factor, linkage studies will succeed or fail on the grounds of pedigree ascertainment, clinical assessment, and statistical analysis.

The pedigree ascertainment strategy is the first line of defense against genetic heterogeneity. Not surprisingly, it has received considerable attention, and a number of solutions have been proposed (26,70). One suggestion for minimizing heterogeneity is to study a single pedigree. This requires an extensive pedigree, such as the Venezuelan kindred used to map Huntington's disease (27). In psychiatry, this strategy might be suitable for TS and perhaps for bipolar illness, but pedigrees of this size have not been reported for other psychiatric illnesses. This strategy has the added advantage that the genetic model can be estimated by a segregation analysis of the pedigree.

Extended pedigrees also have a number of disadvantages (26). By their multigenerational nature, they select against recessive genes. Furthermore, they are not immune to the effects of heterogeneity because of multiple persons marrying into the pedigree. In addition, lod scores in these pedigrees can be highly dependent on diagnostic changes in key pedigree members. This last phenomenon is illustrated by the reanalysis of the chromosome 11 linkage findings in bipolar illness already discussed (30). Finally, linkage in such pedigrees may be difficult to replicate because the pedigrees, by virtue of their unusual nature, may represent a rare form of the disease.

Genetic isolates provide another means of minimizing heterogeneity. Isolated populations that are descended from a small group of founders tend to be genetically more homogeneous than the general population. The genetic model can be estimated by segregation analysis with the assurance that it will be appropriate for linkage pedigrees selected from the same population. However, a major disadvantage of this approach is that findings might prove difficult to replicate in other populations.

Another strategy for overcoming the effects of heterogeneity is to exploit the sheer statistical power of large samples. The lod scores of individual pedigrees can be analyzed for heterogeneity and linkage can be detected, provided that the proportion of the pedigrees that are transmitting the same gene is large enough. Linkage to Alzheimer's disease was detected in this way, despite appreciable genetic heterogeneity. If less than 50% of the pedigrees are transmitting the linked form of the illness, the pedigree set would need to be quite large to detect linkage, and this consideration has prompted a number of collaborative linkage studies in psychiatry.

Ambiguous disease phenotypes present a different set of problems. These can be subsumed under the categories of incomplete penetrance and variable expressivity. Incomplete penetrance due to age, sex, and cohort effects can be modeled in the linkage analysis. Alternatively, the analysis can be restricted to affected persons, and analytical methods have been developed for this strategy (24,69).

With regard to expressivity, multiple phenotypes can be analyzed or the analyses can be restricted to definite cases of the disease. An alternative approach is to include all phenotypic categories in a single analysis by weighting each one with the probability of its being an expression of the genotype (48). One strategy for coping with both types of phenotypic ambiguity is the affected sib-pair strategy (24). Pedigrees of two or more affected siblings are collected, and the linkage analysis is based on those individuals only. Another advantage of affected pedigree member methods is that the results do not depend on an assumed genetic model because they are nonparametric. The tradeoff is that they are less powerful than the lod score method.

Clinical assessment is another critical issue in designing linkage studies, and broad agreement exists on a number of optimal methods to be used (42,70). Standardized interview instruments, operationalized diagnostic criteria, and explicit diagnostic hierarchies facilitate replication of results and comparison of studies. Instruments that assess a broad range of psychopathology and accommodate multiple diagnostic systems are more likely to capture the full expression of the genotype. Periodically updating the diagnoses keeps the database current when penetrance is incomplete. Assessing the families of persons marrying into the pedigree helps to identify bilineal transmission. Keeping assessments blind to the marker typing protects against diagnostic contamination. The value of aug-

menting the clinical assessments with biological markers is demonstrated by juvenile myoclonic epilepsy, where electroencephalograms (EEGs) greatly increased the power to detect linkage (26). However, none of the current biological markers in psychiatry have achieved the same level of validity that the EEG has achieved in diagnosing epilepsy.

The data analysis strategy needs to be chosen as carefully as the strategies for ascertainment and assessment. If a parametric analysis is used, genetic parameters must be estimated or else several models must be tested to cover the range of possibilities. On the other hand, the lod score method has several distinct advantages because it is parametric: It is a more powerful statistic, it can be used to map loci, and it can exclude a disease locus. In principle, a map of closely linked markers can be used to systematically exclude a disease locus from all of the genome except where linkage exists.

Unfortunately, the ambiguities of psychiatric data affect all three strengths of the method (49). Although misspecification of the genetic model does not inflate the lod score, it does weaken it and inflates the estimate of genetic distance. At the same time, the critical lod score levels for both linkage detection and exclusion are unknown. Therefore, in psychiatry the differences between parametric and nonparametric methods may not be as critical as they are in mendelian genetics. Even with the more powerful lod score method, a large pedigree set may be needed to find linkage.

The genetic model can be estimated by segregation analysis, but only if the pedigrees are systematically ascertained and extended, and even then many of the same ambiguities that frustrate linkage analysis will complicate segregation analysis as well. If the genetic model cannot be estimated, a number of models may need to be analyzed, in addition to several diagnostic definitions. This creates the danger of lod score inflation. One solution is to adjust the score by subtracting the $\log_{10}$ of the number of models analyzed. Alternatively, the correct adjustment can be derived from simulations with the pedigrees used in the analysis.

The effect of analyzing multiple markers on the lod score needs to be considered as well. This is not a problem with mendelian diseases because as the probability of a false-positive increases with each new marker tested, the probability of finding the gene increases correspondingly, and a lod score of 3.00 is adjusted for the prior probability to give a 5% posterior probability of a false-positive result (49). However, in psychiatry the prior probability is unknown, and therefore the lod score may not be self-correcting. For this reason, the lod score may need to be adjusted by as much as two lod units for a complete genome search. The net effect of all the lod score corrections may be that the lod score method has little advantage over nonparametric methods in psychiatry.

Given the limitations of the lod score method under these circumstances, nonparametric methods may provide a reasonable screening tool. They are based on the principle that if the disease and marker loci are linked, affected family members will share alleles at the marker locus more frequently than expected by chance. For example, the probability of a pair of siblings sharing 0, 1, or 2 alleles identical by descent is 0.25, 0.50, and 0.25, respectively. A significant departure from this expected distribution in the direction of increased allele sharing is evidence of linkage. With a sufficiently large sample, this method is more robust to intralocus heterogeneity and oligogenic inheritance than is the lod score method. This consideration and its short computation time make sib-pair analyses an attractive screening tool for linkage.

These linkage strategies have been presented as competing alternatives when, in practice, studies typically incorporate features of several methods. Thus, ascertainment may be based on an affected sib-pair strategy, but the pedigrees may be extended to include more relatives. Similarly, the primary analytical tool may be the lod score with a nonparametric analysis added to check its validity.

STRATEGIES NOT BASED ON LINKAGE

Candidate Genes

Candidate genes offer an alternative to an exhaustive genome search. A gene may be considered a candidate by virtue of its location near a linkage, its involvement in the disease pathogenesis, or both. The amyloid precursor protein exemplifies both types of candidate by its location on chromosome 21 and its role in the pathogenesis of amyloid plaques. Until recently, candidate gene approaches were felt to be too unlikely to succeed for serious consideration. A third to a half of the estimated 100,000 human genes are expressed in brain (63), whereas the genome can be screened with 300 markers at a 10-centimorgan level of resolution; thus, if 300 markers can exclude 100,000 genes, it makes little sense to examine candidates individually. However, experience with Alzheimer's disease, where the amyloid precursor protein gene, which was thought to have been excluded by linkage, proved to be responsible for the disease in several families, demonstrates how easily exclusion maps can miss rare disease genes.

One appeal of candidate genes is their ability to circumvent the tedious task of positional cloning—the process of proceeding from a linkage to finding a disease gene. It consists of flanking the disease locus with additional markers and then progressively narrowing the intermarker region until it is small enough to clone and begin the gene search. For the process to work, genetic distance must be measured by linkage and association, but the

accuracy of these measurements depends on the accuracy of the genetic model and disease phenotype. Therefore, psychiatric disorders will complicate positional cloning for the same reasons that they complicate linkage analysis.

Candidate gene strategies fall into three categories: association (linkage disequilibrium), mutation screening (e.g., single-strand conformational polymorphisms and denaturing gradient gel electrophoresis) (47,58), and direct sequencing. Mutation screening procedures are based on electrophoresis methods that can detect single base-pair changes through altered mobility of DNA fragments. Sequencing detects mutations by reading the genetic code. Association studies depend on the detection of linkage disequilibrium.

Linkage disequilibrium results from a marker polymorphism occurring so close to a disease mutation that meiotic recombination has not had time to establish equilibrium among the allele frequencies at the two loci. Consequently, allele frequencies at the marker locus differ between affected and unaffected populations. This disequilibrium can be detected by a simple test of association between the disease and the marker allele. Because the test is nonparametric, it is more robust than the lod score to the confounding effects of complex diseases. The effects of interlocus heterogeneity, oligogenic inheritance, incomplete penetrance, variable expressivity, and phenocopies can, in principle, be overcome with large, narrowly diagnosed samples.

For linkage disequilibrium to occur, the loci must be less than 2.0 centimorgans apart (i.e., less than 2% recombination), and therefore the approach is best suited to candidate genes. Linkage disequilibrium is one cause of disease-marker associations; others include sampling cases from either ethnic subgroups or inbred populations, interaction between the two loci, and evolutionary selection for alleles at both loci. Ethnic stratification is a potential source of false-positive results. Allele frequencies can vary widely across ethnic groups, and if cases and controls differ on this critical variable, a spurious association will result. This bias can be avoided by sampling parents of cases and estimating population allele frequencies from the parental alleles that were not transmitted to the cases (the haplotype relative risk method) (19).

Mutation screening is more sensitive than association and linkage because it can detect mutation in a single patient, but its time-intensiveness limits its general applicability. Still, it can play an important role in the overall search for disease genes (62). When a provisional linkage is found, candidate genes in the region can be screened for mutation in linked pedigrees; and if the disease gene is found, the task of positional cloning will be circumvented.

If a proven linkage or some other biological mechanism existed for any psychiatric disorder, a compelling case could be made for studying candidate genes. However, without a biological basis with which to prioritize candidates, any of the 30,000 to 50,000 genes expressed in brain is a potential candidate. When the prior odds of a gene being pathogenic are so low, the posterior odds of a nominally significant result being correct can be discouragingly low (16). For example, if the 20,000 genes nonconstitutively expressed in brain are all considered potential candidates, 98.5% of associations at the 0.05 significance level will be spurious. The same reasoning holds for sequence variants identified through mutation screening. Demonstrating that a sequence variant occurs in an evolutionarily conserved region of the gene or that it affects the protein structure of the gene product provides only circumstantial evidence connecting the variant with the disease. Sequence variation can be tied to a behavioral phenotype only by demonstrating association in the population or linkage in pedigrees. Ironically, the lack of biological clues to help focus molecular genetic strategies in psychiatry, the same problem that complicates linkage research and makes candidate gene approaches attractive, also complicates candidate gene approaches.

Triplet Repeats

Trinucleotide repeats have now been identified as the cause of five neuropsychiatric diseases (Huntington's disease, fragile-X syndrome, myotonic dystrophy, spinobulbar muscular atrophy, and spinocerebellar ataxia type 1) (38). Finding a mechanism that can explain genetic and phenotypic complexities in such diseases as the fragile-X syndrome has generated enthusiasm for searching for triplet repeats in psychiatric disorders. Such repeats appear to be common in genes expressed in brain, being found in 35% of 40 cDNA clones tested in one study (36). Moreover, methods have been developed to detect triplet expansions in genomic DNA, opening the way to screening populations of psychiatric disorders (57). Indeed, this mechanism could be the biological clue needed to increase the prior odds of a candidate gene being etiologic.

Genomic Mismatch Scanning

The essence of linkage is to identify regions of the genome shared by affected family members through inheritance from a common ancestor. Genomic mismatch scanning is a promising strategy that could revolutionize the search for genes underlying complex diseases by delivering a complete set of DNA clones from these regions (44). Genomic DNA from an affected pair of relatives is digested with a restriction enzyme to yield restriction fragments, and these are mixed under conditions that permit the formation of heteroduplex molecules (consisting of one strand from each individual). Enzymatic treatment is then used to degrade homoduplex molecules (those composed of both strands from the same individual). The

remaining heteroduplexes are treated with an *Escherichia coli* exonuclease that recognizes single basepair mismatches and nicks one strand of the DNA near the mismatch. Further enzymatic digestion strips off runs of bases from the nicked strand, and intact strands are separated from partially stripped ones by column separation. The final product is a collection of DNA molecules representing all regions of the genome where the two relatives match. These molecules can be labeled and used to probe a genomic library to identify matching genomic clones to search for candidate genes. Thus far, the method has only been applied to yeast; but if it can be adapted to affected relative pairs in humans, it could become a powerful tool for finding candidate genes.

Animal Models

The Human Genome Project has created maps of the rat and mouse genomes in addition to the human map, and these maps can be used to find genes controlling behavioral traits in these organisms. Linkage analysis is far more controllable in laboratory animals than it is in humans. Animals are easily bred to provide the sample sizes needed. Inbred strains are isogenic: Each strain is homozygous at all loci, and therefore all members of any strain are genetically identical, eliminating the problem of genetic heterogeneity. Phenotypes can be carefully measured, and laboratory conditions can be held uniform to reduce phenotypic variation. The same strengths of the method will make it far easier to positionally clone genes once linkages are found. Alternatively, linkage in rodents may facilitate a search for linkage or candidate genes in homologous regions of the human genome.

Animal strains can be exploited in two ways (2). Strains bred to maximize and minimize a trait can be crossed and the offspring, which are heterozygous at all loci, backcrossed with a parental strain or intercrossed with each other. The trait then can be measured in the progeny and analyzed for linkage. Alternatively, the trait of interest can be measured in a number of inbred strains that are already typed with a genome map. Linkage can be detected by correlations between the trait and the genetic marker typings.

Detection of a locus for hypertension in the spontaneously hypertensive rat has sparked interest in using similar approaches in behavior disorders (29). Two examples of relevant animal models are (i) the Maudsley reactive and nonreactive strains as a model of anxiety and (ii) alcohol-preferring and -nonpreferring strains as a model of alcoholism (9,37). Although animal models have many features of an attractive experimental system for linkage, their greatest weakness is uncertainty over whether the animal behavior accurately models the disease in question. If not, genes contributing to the animal behavior may be unrelated to the disease in humans. However, a counterbalancing strength is the immense importance of cloning any gene that determines a behavioral trait.

CONCLUSION

Genetics is a rapidly evolving field, and considerable flexibility is required to adapt to the new technologies and insights. Our understanding of the complexities of applying linkage and other molecular methods in psychiatry has matured greatly. This maturation is the product of a productive interaction of theoretical, population, and laboratory genetics. Deploying new technologies effectively requires careful analysis to identify optimal research designs and analytical methods to complement the technologies, as well as to avoid hidden pitfalls inherent in them. Likewise, new disease mechanisms, such as triplet repeats, necessitate a reanalysis of epidemiological data to identify candidate diseases for the mechanism. Thus, psychiatric genetics rests on a foundation of molecular, clinical, and statistical science.

Finding disease genes in psychiatry is likely to require not only collaboration of these three sciences, but also a productive interaction of existing methods and strategies. If linkage searches do not deliver a confirmed linkage, they will certainly identify provisional linkages, both in the entire pedigree set and in subsets of it. These regions will then become target regions for candidate gene strategies. Association studies with candidate loci in large populations may have the power to replicate provisional linkages that are based on a small subsample of the pedigree set. Furthermore, the ability to study candidate genes in pedigrees where the candidate and disease are cosegregating will greatly enhance the chances of finding etiological mutations.

Several thousand cDNA clones have now been partially sequenced and mapped as expressed sequence tags (ESTs), and the pace will certainly accelerate in the future. This effort will create a map of anonymous genes as candidates for diseases whenever a region is spotlighted by human or animal linkage studies. This change in candidate gene technology has prompted the speculation that the positional cloning strategy may become a positional candidate approach in the future (3). What is envisioned is that as more is known about these anonymous genes, their characteristics can be matched to those of the disease being studied. Genes expressed preferentially in limbic structures will be of considerable interest. Those containing triplet repeats will be candidates for diseases demonstrating anticipation. Membrane-spanning domains suggest a receptor function. Developmentally expressed genes will be a priority for mental diseases thought to have a developmental etiology. The positional candidate strategy is certainly an attractive scenario in

psychiatry, where the complexities of the disorders make it unlikely that linkage and association could narrow a region of interest to the point where a search for candidate sequences could be contemplated.

Two recent developments in psychiatric genetics will close the chapter on a note of optimism. The first is an association between familial thyroid hormone resistance and attention-deficit hyperactivity disorder (ADHD) (28). Symptoms of ADHD are often seen in persons with familial thyroid hormone resistance, an autosomal dominant disease caused by a variety of mutations in exons 9 and 10 of the receptor gene (hTR_{beta}). When ADHD was assessed in a number of these families, strong cosegregation of DSM-III-R ADHD with hTR_{beta} mutations was found. Although the finding accounts for a small minority of ADHD cases, understanding the mechanism may put investigators on the trail of other causes of ADHD.

The second development is new insight into the genetics of an unusual X-linked form of mental retardation (11). The disease is a nondysmorphic mental retardation characterized by aggressive and impulsive behavior that follows an X-linked recessive pattern of inheritance in a large Dutch pedigree. A gene for the disease was localized by linkage to Xp21-p11. Because monoamine oxidase A (MAOA) is located in this region, urinary monoamine metabolites were analyzed in several affected cases and found to be markedly abnormal. A point mutation in the eighth exon of the MAOA gene was identified in five of the affected males (12). The next step is to determine how frequently MAOA mutations account for mental retardation and aggressive behavior in the population.

Both of these developments are examples of the kind of biological insights that could reveal the etiology of two rare forms of behavior disorder. Insights like these have made molecular genetic strategies powerful tools for finding disease etiologies in other areas of medicine. More work will need to be done with both diseases before the genetic etiology of the disorder is considered to be found. If it is found, identifying the genetic code responsible for a behavior disorder will be a major advance in psychiatric genetics.

REFERENCES

1. Aston CE, Hill SY. Segregation analysis of alcoholism in families ascertained through a pair of male alcoholics. *Am J Hum Genet* 1990;46:879–887.
2. Bailey DW. Strategic uses of recombinant inbred and congenic strains in behavior genetics research. In: Gershon ES, Matthysse S, Breakefield XO, Ciaranello RD, eds. *Genetic research strategies in psychobiology and psychiatry.* Boxwood Press, Pacific Grove, CA, 1981;189–198.
3. Ballabio A. The rise and fall of positional cloning. *Nature Genet* 1993;3:277–279.
4. Baron M. Genetics of schizophrenia. I. Familial patterns and mode of inheritance. *Biol Psychiatry* 1986;21:1051–1066.
5. Baron M, Risch N, Hamburger R, Mandel B, Kushner S, New-

man M, Drumer D, Belmaker RH. Genetic linkage between X-chromosome markers and bipolar affective illness. *Nature* 1987; 326:289–292.

6. Baron M, Freimer NF, Risch N, Lerer B, Alexander JR, Straub RE, Asokan S, et al. Diminished support for linkage between manic depressive illness and X-chromosome markers in three Israeli pedigrees. *Nature Genet* 1993;3:49–55.

7. Bassett AS, McGillivray BC, Jones BD, Pantzar JT. Partial trisomy chromosome 5 cosegregating with schizophrenia. *Lancet* 1988; 1:799–800.

8. Bertelsen A, Harvald B, Hauge M. A Danish twin study of manic-depressive disorders. *Br J Psychiatry* 1977;130:330–354.

9. Blizard DA. The Maudsley reactive and nonreactive strains: a North American perspective. *Behavior Genet* 1981;5:469–489.

10. Blum K, Noble EP, Sheridan PJ, Montgomery A, Ritchie T, Jagadeeswaran P, Nogami H, et al. Allelic association of human dopamine D₂ receptor gene in alcoholism. *JAMA* 1990;263:2055–2060.

11. Brunner HG, Nelen MR, Van Zandvoort P, Abeling NGGM, van Gennip AH, Wolters EC, Kuiper MA, et al. X-linked borderline mental retardation with prominent behavioral disturbance: phenotype, genetic localization, and evidence for disturbed monoamine metabolism. *Am J Hum Genet* 1993;52:1032–1039.

12. Brunner HG, Nelen M, Breakefield XO, Ropers HH, Van Oost BA. Abnormal behavior associated with a point mutation in the structural gene for monoamine oxidase A. *Science* 1993;262:578–580.

13. Cloninger CR, Bohman M, Sigvardsson S. Inheritance of alcohol abuse: cross-fostering analysis of adopted men. *Arch Gen Psychiatry* 1981;38:861–868.

14. Crowe RR, Noyes R, Pauls DL, Slymen D. A family study of panic disorder. *Arch Gen Psychiatry* 1983;40:1065–1069.

15. Crowe RR. Linkage studies of panic disorder. In: Gershon E, Cloninger CR, eds. *Genetic approaches to mental disorders*. Washington, DC: American Psychiatric Press, 1994.

16. Crowe RR. Candidate genes in psychiatry: an epidemiological perspective. *Neuropsychiatr Genet* 1993;48:74–77.

17. Davies K. Breaking the fragile X. *Nature* 1991;351:439–440.

18. Egeland JA, Gerhard DS, Pauls DL, Sussex JN, Kidd KK, Allen CR, Hostetter AM, Housman DE. Bipolar affective disorders linked to DNA markers on chromosome 11. *Nature* 1987;325:783–787.

19. Falk CT, Rubenstein P. Haplotype relative risks: easy reliable way to construct a proper control sample for risk calculations. *Ann Hum Genet* 1987;51:227–233.

20. Farmer AD, McGuffin P, Gottesman II. Twin concordance for DSM-III schizophrenia: scrutinising the validity of the definition. *Arch Gen Psychiatry* 1987;44:634–641.

21. Fu Y-H, Kuhl DP, Pizzuti A, Pieretti M, Sutcliffe JS, Richards S, Verkerk AJMH, et al. Variation of the CGG repeat at the fragile X site results in genetic instability: resolution of the Sherman paradox. *Cell* 1991;67:1047–1058.

22. Gershon ES, Hamovit J, Guroff JJ, Dibble E, Leckman JF, Sceery W, Targum SD, Nurnberger JI, Goldin LR, Bunney WE. A family study of schizoaffective, bipolar I, bipolar II, unipolar, and normal control probands. *Arch Gen Psychiatry* 1982;39:1157–1167.

23. Goldin LR, Gershon ES, Targum SD, Sparkes RS, McGinniss M. Segregation and linkage analyses in families of patients with bipolar, unipolar, and schizoaffective mood disorders. *Am J Hum Genet* 1983;35:274–287.

24. Goldin LR, Gershon ES. Power of the affected-sib-pair method for heterogeneous disorders. *Genet Epidemiol* 1988;5:35–42.

25. Goodwin DW, et al. Alcohol problems in adoptees raised apart from alcoholic biological parents. *Arch Gen Psychiatry* 1973; 28:238–255.

26. Greenberg DA. There is more than one way to collect data for linkage analysis. *Arch Gen Psychiatry* 1992;49:745–750.

27. Guesella JF, Wexler NS, Conneally PM, Naylor SL, Anderson MA, Tanzi RE, Watkins PC, et al. A polymorphic DNA marker genetically linked to Huntington's disease. *Nature* 1983;306:234–238.

28. Hauser P, Zametkin AJ, Martinez P, Vitiello B, Matochik JA, Mixson AJ, Weintraub BD. Attention deficit-hyperactivity disorder in people with generalized resistance to thyroid hormone. *N Engl J Med* 1993;328:997–1001.

29. Hilbert P, Lindpaintner K, Beckmann JS, Serikawa T, Soubrier F,

30. Dulbay C, Cartwright P, et al. Chromosomal mapping of two genetic loci associated with blood-pressure regulation in hereditary hypertensive rats. *Nature* 1991;353:521–529.

30. Kelsoe JR, Ginns EI, Egeland JA, Gerhard DS, Goldstein AM, Bale SJ, Pauls DL, et al. Re-evaluation of the linkage relationship between chromosome 11p loci and the gene for bipolar affective disorder in the Old Order Amish. *Nature* 1989;342:238–243.

31. Kendler KS. Overview: a current perspective on twin studies of schizophrenia. *Am J Psychiatry* 1983;140:1413–1425.

32. Kendler KS, Gruenberg AM. An independent analysis of the Danish adoption study of schizophrenia. *Arch Gen Psychiatry* 1984; 41:555–564.

33. Kendler KS, Heath AC, Neale MC, Kessler RC, Eaves LJ. A population-based twin study of alcoholism in women. *JAMA* 1992; 268:1877–1882.

34. Kendler KS, McGuire M, Gruenberg AM, O'Hare A, Spellman M, Walsh D. The Roscommon Family Study. I. Methods, diagnosis of probands, and risk of schizophrenia in relatives. *Arch Gen Psychiatry* 1993;50:527–540.

35. Kurlan R, Behr J, Medved L, Shoulson I, Pauls DL, Kidd JR, Kidd KK. Familial Tourette's syndrome: report of a large pedigree and potential for linkage analysis. *Neurology* 1986;36:772–776.

36. Li S-H, McInnis MG, Margolis RL, Antonarakis SE, Ross CA. Novel triplet repeat containing genes in human brain: cloning, expression, and length polymorphisms. *Genomics* 1993;16:572–579.

37. Li TK. Genetic animals models for the study of alcoholism. In: Cloninger CR, Begleiter H, eds. *Genetics and biology of alcoholism*. Cold Spring Harbor, NY: Cold Spring Harbor Laboratory Press, 1990;217–226.

38. Martin JB. Molecular genetics of neurological diseases. *Science* 1993;262:674–676.

39. McGuffin P, Katz R. The genetics of depression and manic-depressive illness. *Br J Psychiatry* 1989;155:294–304.

40. McGuffin P, Sargeant M, Hetti G, Tidmarsh S, Whatley S, Marchbanks RM. Exclusion of a schizophrenia susceptibility gene from the chromosome 5q₁₁-q₁₃ region: new data and a reanalysis of previous reports. *Am J Hum Genet* 1990;47:524–535.

41. Mendlewicz J, Rainer J. Adoption study supporting genetic transmission in manic-depressive illness. *Nature* 1977;268:326–329.

42. Merikangas KR, Spense MA, Kupfer DJ. Linkage studies of bipolar disorder: methodologic and analytic issues. *Arch Gen Psychiatry* 1989;46:1137–1141.

43. Merikangas KR. The genetic epidemiology of alcoholism. *Psychol Med* 1990;20:11–22.

44. Nelson SF, McCusker JH, Sander MA, Kee Y, Modrich P, Brown PO. Genomic mismatch scanning: a new approach to genetic linkage mapping. *Nature Genetics* 1993;4:11–18.

45. Noble E, Blum K, Ritchie T, Montgomery A, Sheridan PJ. Allelic association of the D₂ dopamine receptor gene with receptor-binding characteristics in alcoholism. *Arch Gen Psychiatry* 1991;48:648–654.

46. Noyes R, Crowe RR, Harris EL, Hamra BJ, McChesney CM, Chaudhry DR. Relationship between panic disorder and agoraphobia: a family study. *Arch Gen Psychiatry* 1986;43:227–232.

47. Orita M, Iwahana H, Kanazawa H, Hayashi K, Sekiya T. Detection of polymorphisms of human DNA by gel electrophoresis as single-strand conformation polymorphisms. *Proc Natl Acad Sci USA* 1989;86:2766–2770.

48. Ott J. Genetic linkage and complex diseases: a comment. *Genet Epidemiol* 1990;7:35–36.

49. Ott J. *Analysis of human genetic linkage*. Baltimore, MD: The Johns Hopkins University Press, 1991;74–76.

50. Pakstis AJ, Heutink P, Pauls DL, Kurlan R, Van de Wetering BJM, Leckman, Sandkuyl LA, et al. Progress in the search for genetic linkage with Tourette syndrome: an exclusion map covering more than 50% of the autosomal genome. *Am J Hum Genet* 1991;48:281–294.

51. Pauls DL, Bucher KD, Crowe RR, Noyes R. A genetic study of panic disorder pedigrees. *Am J Hum Genet* 1980;32:639–644.

52. Pauls DL, Leckman JF. The inheritance of Gilles de la Tourette's syndrome and associated behaviors. *N Engl J Med* 1986;315:993–997.

53. Pauls DL, Raymond CL, Stevenson JM, Leckman JF. A family

study of Gilles de la Tourette syndrome. *Am J Hum Genet* 1991; 48:154–163.

54. Pitts FN, Winokur G. Affective disorder—VII: alcoholism and affective disorder. *J Psychiatry Res* 1966;4:37–50.

55. Price RA, Kidd KK, Cohen DJ, Pauls DL, Leckman JF. A twin study of Tourette syndrome. *Arch Gen Psychiatry* 1985;42:815–820.

56. Risch N. Genetic linkage and complex diseases, with special reference to psychiatric disorders. *Genet Epidemiol* 1990;7:3–16.

57. Schalling M, Hudson TJ, Buetow KH, Housman DE. Direct detection of novel expanded trinucleotide repeats in the human genome. *Nature Genet* 1993;4:135–139.

58. Sheffield VC, Cox DR, Lerman LS, Myers RM. Attachment of a 40-base-pair G + C rich sequence (GC-clamp) to genomic DNA fragments by the polymerase chain reaction results in improved detection of single-base changes. *Proc Natl Acad Sci USA* 1989; 6:232–236.

59. Sherman SL, Jacobs PA, Morton NE, Froster-Iskenius U, Howard-Peebles PH, Nielsen KB, Partington GR, et al. Further segregation analysis of the fragile X syndrome with special reference to transmitting males. *Hum Genet* 1985;69:289–299.

60. Sherrington R, Brynjolfsson J, Petursson H, Potter M, Dudleston K, Barraclough B, Wasmuth J, et al. Localization of a susceptibility locus for schizophrenia on chromosome 5. *Nature* 1988;336:164–167.

61. Shibuya A, Yoshida A: Genotypes of alcohol-metabolizing enzymes in Japanese with alcohol liver diseases: a strong association of the usual Caucasian-type aldehyde dehydrogenase gene (ALDH21) with the disease. *Am J Hum Genet* 1988;43:744–748.

62. Sobell JL, Heston LL, Sommer SS. Delineation of genetic predisposition to multifactorial disease: a general approach on the threshold of feasibility. *Genomics* 1992;12:1–6.

63. Sutcliffe JG. mRNA in the mammalian central nervous system. *Annu Rev Neurosci* 1988;11:157–198.

64. The Huntington's Disease Collaborative Research Group: a novel gene containing a trinucleotide repeat that is expanded and unstable on Huntington's disease chromosomes. *Cell* 1993;72:971–983.

65. Thomasson HR, Edenberg HJ, Crabb DW, Mai X-L, Jerome RE, Li T-K, Wang S-P, et al. Alcohol and aldehyde dehydrogenase genotypes and alcoholism in Chinese men. *Am J Hum Genet* 1991;48:677–681.

66. Torgersen S. Genetic factors in anxiety disorder. *Arch Gen Psychiatry* 1983;40:1085–1089.

67. Torgersen S. Genetic factors in moderately severe and mild affective disorders. *Arch Gen Psychiatry* 1986;43:222–226.

68. Uhl GR, Persico AM, Smith SS. Current excitement with D_2 dopamine receptor gene alleles in substance abuse. *Arch Gen Psychiatry* 1992;49:157–160.

69. Weeks DE, Lange K. The affected-pedigree-member method of linkage analysis. *Am J Hum Genet* 1988;42:315–326.

70. Weeks DE, Brzustowicz L, Squires-Wheeler E, Cornblatt B, Lehner T, Stefanovich M, Bassett A, et al. Report of a workshop on genetic linkage studies in schizophrenia. *Schizophr Bull* 1990;4:673–686.

Psychopharmacology: The Fourth Generation of Progress, edited by Floyd E. Bloom and David J. Kupfer. Raven Press, Ltd., New York © 1995.

CHAPTER **156**

Strategies for Multimodality Research

Ellen Frank, David J. Kupfer, and Jordan Karp

This chapter addresses treatment outcome research involving both pharmacotherapeutic and psychotherapeutic treatment modalities. We will begin by describing the rationale for such studies and the patient populations to which they might be applicable. We will then address a number of questions relating to the design and implementation of such investigations, including patient selection and the preparation of patients for study participation. We will discuss a number of issues relating to outcome assessment in multimodality research, including the choice of outcome measures, the timing of assessments, and the importance of assessing variables which might be important mediators or moderators of outcome. We discuss magnitude of effects in terms of both statistical and clinical significance. We note the importance of consistency of terminology in describing outcomes and the methodological problems associated with assessing outcome in uncontrolled follow-up. A number of specific design issues are discussed, including types of trials, appropriate ''doses'' and durations of treatments, strategies for achieving comparability across treatments, and the possible utility of assessing psychosocial variables in pharmacotherapy-only trials. We raise methodologic concerns specific to the study of nonsomatic therapies, including the choice of appropriate controls for psychosocial treatments, assessment of the adequacy of the psychosocial treatment, and standardization of the nonpharmacotherapeutic treatments. Finally, we discuss several ethical considerations relevant to multimodality research.

RATIONALE: WHY PERFORM COMBINATION TREATMENT STUDIES?

Surveys of actual clinical practice suggest that the majority of psychiatric practitioners, regardless of their theo-

retical persuasion, practice some form of combination treatment with the majority of their patients. Today, even the most psychoanalytically oriented physician prescribes medication for a portion of her or his patients, whereas the biologically oriented physician typically dispenses both psychoeducation and supportive psychotherapy along with medication.

There have been a number of reasons for the trend toward combination treatment strategies throughout the last two decades. Following the early enthusiasm for psychopharmacologic agents, pharmacotherapeutically oriented clinicians recognized that medications were less than completely effective for a large percentage of their patients. Furthermore, they discovered that by educating the patient about the disorder under treatment and by providing substantial amounts of psychological support, they could improve the patient's adherence to the prescribed drug regimen while awaiting evidence of a therapeutic response. Psychotherapeutically oriented clinicians, on the other hand, came to recognize that pharmacotherapy did not necessarily lead to negative interactions when used along with psychotherapeutic techniques. Rather than diminishing the patients' capacity to participate in the psychotherapeutic process, particularly in the case of the mood disorders, pharmacotherapy actually facilitated patients' participation in the therapeutic work. Thus, clinicians of both orientations came to suspect that they were most likely to achieve optimal results through a combination of medication and psychosocial intervention.

Rush and Hollon (51) have argued that there are two ways in which the combination of pharmacotherapy and psychotherapy might result in an outcome superior to that achieved by either treatment alone: the ''magnitude'' model and the ''frequency'' model. According to the magnitude model, the combination provides a *greater degree of symptom relief* for most or all patients being treated when compared to either modality offered alone.

E. Frank, D. J. Kupfer, and J. Karp: Department of Psychiatry, University of Pittsburgh, Western Psychiatric Institute and Clinic, Pittsburgh, Pennsylvania 15213-2593.

The frequency model posits that combined treatment leads to an *increased likelihood that any given patient will receive the treatment modality to which he or she would have been responsive* had that treatment been offered alone. In truth, any benefit observed for the combination of medication and psychotherapy in a randomized control trial undoubtedly results from a combination of "magnitude" and "frequency" effects.

The Rush and Hollon arguments apply well to acute treatment strategies. When long-term maintenance strategies are under consideration, the typical argument advanced for the superiority of combination treatment is that pharmacotherapy prevents relapse/recurrence *directly* through symptomatic prophylaxis whereas psychotherapy prevents return of symptomatology *indirectly* through improvement in social functioning and capacity for coping with stressful life events. Interestingly, in controlled trials where both pharmacotherapy and psychotherapy have been maximized, it has often been difficult to demonstrate a statistically significant and sustained advantage for combination treatment with respect to relapse recurrence outcomes (7,14,24).

TO WHICH POPULATIONS ARE SUCH STUDIES APPLICABLE?

As implied above, combination treatment strategies are appropriate for both short-term treatment aimed at the resolution of acute symptomatology and prophylactic maintenance aimed at the prevention of new episodes of illness. Combination treatment strategies have been applied successfully in patients suffering from schizophrenia (22–24) and unipolar major depression (7,14,15,58). Studies examining the benefits of combination strategies in bipolar illness and anxiety disorders are ongoing. The eating disorders represent another area where combination treatment might be applicable.

PATIENT SELECTION

Treatment Responsiveness and Representativeness of Patients

Two sometimes conflicting requirements face the investigator selecting patients for a combination treatment trial. Patients selected should, at minimum, represent a population with some likelihood of responsivity to either treatment alone and, perhaps, particularly to the combination. Thus, they must represent a relatively homogeneous, well-defined diagnostic group. On the other hand, for the study results to be of practical value, the patient population selected must be sufficiently representative of populations seen in actual practice to allow for generalization. As Elkin et al. (8) have pointed out, such requirements have implications for both the inclusion and exclusion

criteria for combination treatment trials. Structured diagnostic interviews such as the Schedule for Affective Disorders and Schizophrenia (53) and the accompanying Research Diagnostic Criteria (54), the Diagnostic Interview Schedule (49), and the Structured Clinical Interview for DSM (55) have markedly enhanced the reliability of psychiatric diagnoses and the interpretability of outcomes from controlled treatment trials. Nonetheless, even diagnostic categories as apparently distinct as bipolar 1 disorder are plagued with considerable heterogeneity. In their 1988 paper, Elkin et al. (8) argued for the importance of the inclusion of subtypes of patients presumed to be responsive to each type of treatment in any combination treatment trial in depression. They pointed, for example, to the need to include endogenous patients (presumed to be responsive to drug therapy) but not to the exclusion of other subtypes. More recent studies, however, such as those of Thase et al. (56), suggest that the *same* subtypes are likely to be overrepresented among the responders to *both* psychotherapy and drugs. Some of our own studies (11,13,47) suggest that it is the inclusion of patients with Axis II comorbidity which may be most helpful in demonstrating the efficacy of combination treatments.

In terms of exclusion criteria, many investigators have used the strategy of excluding patients with a previous history of nonresponse to the experimental treatment. In selecting patients for combination treatment studies, however, it might be advantageous to include at least a subset of patients with a history of nonresponse to one or the other treatment alone, stratifying on this variable in order to be certain that equivalent numbers of such patients are included in each treatment condition. Indeed, a failure to find large effects for the combination in comparison to either treatment alone may be a result of the failure in previous trials to include a sufficient number of patients who had previously been nonresponsive to either treatment alone.

Determination of Who Will Benefit from Combination Therapy

Determination of benefit in any treatment protocol will always be dependent on the choice of the outcome measures. Choosing the outcome measures for combination treatment trials can be especially difficult because those measures must reflect the expected mode of action of each of the treatments individually. For example, in a trial combining cognitive therapy for depression (1) and some form of antidepressant pharmacotherapy, one would probably want to use both (a) the Beck Depression Inventory to assess the more cognitive aspects of depression and (b) a measure such as the Hamilton Depression Rating Scale (21) to assess the more somatic aspects of the depressive syndrome. In addition, one might choose to assess dysfunctional attitudes, the presumed etiologic mechanism according to Beck's theory, more directly through a measure such as the Dysfunctional Attitudes Scale (A. N. Weissman, *unpublished dissertation*). The problem is how to combine or weight these measures as outcomes and, as the number of measures expands, how to avoid multiplicity. Needless to say, in such a protocol, the weighting or means of combining outcome measures should be determined a priori.

The treatment paradigm will also, in some respects, determine who benefits from combination therapy. In their earliest trial, Weissman et al. (58) assigned depressed women who had responded to 4 weeks of amitriptyline alone to the combination of amitriptyline and psychotherapy in comparison to medication alone, psychotherapy alone, psychotherapy with a placebo tablet, placebo alone, or low-contact without a tablet. In this design it is likely that those who benefited from the combination would differ from those who would benefit from the combination in a protocol in which patients were assigned to the various treatments from the outset.

A large number of potential biological and psychosocial predictor variables could also enter into the determination of who will benefit from combination treatment strategies. For example, in the area of schizophrenia research, some studies suggest that the level of expressed emotion in the patient's family may predict benefit from family therapy and/or family psychoeducational intervention in combination with pharmacotherapy (18,31). Data from the laboratories of Michael Goldstein and David Miklowitz suggest that the same variables may be important in the prediction of relapse in young manic patients (42). Personality variables (21,42) and recent experience of a stressful life event (29) appear to be related to a slower response to combination treatment in recurrent unipolar patients. It remains an empirical question whether patients with personality pathology or a recent severe life event would have failed to respond altogether had those same investigations included only pharmacotherapy.

In the area of mood disorders, for example, a host of biological predictors has been identified for prediction of response for pharmacotherapy. Electroencephalographic (EEG) sleep parameters (33), failure to suppress cortisol following dexamethasone administration (19), and thyroid function (34) have all been related to outcome in pharmacotherapy trials. Biological predictors have rarely been examined in relation to response to psychosocial interventions for mood disorder patients. Exceptions to this rule are the examination of EEG sleep variables and response to acute cognitive therapy (52) and interpersonal psychotherapy (2,3), maintenance interpersonal psychotherapy in depression (32), and psychophysiologic testing in treatment of anxiety disorders (4,39–41). The investigator who has a strong belief in the predictive capacity of any or several of these variables may wish to carry out pretreatment assessments in order to stratify on these variables.

PREPARATION OF PATIENTS FOR CLINICAL TRIALS

There are three important aspects to preparing patients for a combination treatment study. The first is explaining the rationale for each of the individual treatment modalities, as well as the rationale for combining them. The second aspect of patient preparation has to do with those maneuvers that the investigator goes through to ensure patient adherence to each of the treatment modalities. Finally, and not unrelated to ensuring adherence, is the investigator's responsibility to address possible patient biases regarding each of the individual treatments.

Explaining the Rationale for Each Modality and the Combination

One of the important advances of modern psychiatric treatment is the general demystification of the treatment process for the patient. Whether modern clinicians choose a pharmacotherapeutic approach, a disorder-specific psychotherapeutic approach, or a combination of the two, they typically spend some part of the early phase of treatment in explaining the rationale for the treatment strategy they have chosen. This can be even more important in the conduct of treatment research where a good understanding on the part of the patient of the theoretical basis of the treatment appears to have positive effects on adherence to the treatment regimen and on remaining in the study. Needless to say, explanations of the rationale and/or mechanism of action of each of the treatments should be provided in a manner consistent with the intelligence and education level of the individual patient. It is also necessary to take into account the patient's clinical state at the time such an explanation is offered. For symptomatic patients whose ability to concentrate and remember may be seriously impaired, it is often helpful to provide both an oral and a written description of the rationale for the treatment, giving the patient the opportunity to read and reread the written description as cognitive functioning improves. It may also be important to repeat the oral description of the treatment rationale at several points in time as the patient's clinical state is improving. The clinician should ask for feedback as to what the patient understands the rationale to be so that any misconceptions can be corrected.

Once the clinician feels reasonably confident that the patient understands the rationale for each treatment individually, she or he can then develop the rationale for combining the two treatments. In many instances this rationale will simply take the form of increasing the chance that the patient will respond (the "frequency" model of Rush and Hollon) (51); however, there may actually be a rationale for the "magnitude" model—that is, that the pharmacotherapeutic intervention is likely to act on one aspect of the disorder while the psychotherapeutic intervention is likely to act on a second.

Maneuvers to Ensure Adherence to Each Type of Treatment

A second important maneuver for ensuring patient compliance is the setting of reasonable expectations for the time course of recovery. As Elkin et al. (8) have pointed out, expectations about the time course of recovery can influence both therapist and patient morale and may have subtle and not-so-subtle effects on the behavior of both. In the treatment of depression, for example, it has been helpful not only to set reasonable expectations for how long either drug therapy or psychotherapy is likely to take, but also to explain that the course of recovery is rarely a linear trajectory and more often saw-toothed in nature. Such an explanation prevents patients from becoming demoralized when a modest improvement is followed by a temporary setback. Another important aspect of expectation-setting is informing the patient that different symptoms will remit on different time courses and that this is also modality-specific. For example, in the treatment of mood and anxiety disorders, the symptoms which remit earliest with pharmacotherapy may be different from the symptoms which remit early in the course of treatment with psychotherapy.

In addition to the maneuvers described above, we have found it helpful to involve family members as "ex officio" members of the treatment team. This can be done by meeting with one family member at a time or through workshops conducted for groups of family members and significant others. In our own work we have found that such educational workshops offered early in the treatment course have led to some of the lowest reported attrition rates of modern treatment research (12,27). By providing family members and friends with a rationale for each of the treatments, a rationale for the conduct of the investigation (i.e., what the investigator hopes to learn), and reasonable expectations about the course of recovery, it appears possible to make family members important allies of the treatment team. In this role they can support the patient when she or he becomes discouraged, remind the patient to take medication, and watch for changes in the patient's clinical state of which the patient may be unaware but which may be important to continued protocol adherence.

Addressing Patient Biases Regarding Each Treatment Modality

Patients' willingness to consent to a treatment trial in which they might receive either pharmacotherapy, psy-

chotherapy, or the combination does not mean that they have no treatment preferences or biases regarding which treatment is likely to be most effective. Such attitudes and expectations can affect patient behavior (and ultimately treatment outcome) in a variety of important ways. If a treatment facility is known for one form of treatment or another, patients coming to that facility are likely to be seeking that form of treatment and, although they agree to random assignment, are hoping for the form of treatment they originally sought. Patient expectations and biases can affect patient behavior in the treatment itself, response to any self-report evaluations of treatment efficacy, and attrition rates. The most sensible approach to these potential attitudinal confounds is to conduct an explicit assessment of patient expectations and attitudes and analyze outcome results as a function of such attitudes. An investigator might even consider stratification of subjects on the basis of their beliefs and biases regarding the biological versus psychosocial nature of the etiology of their illness and/or their desire for one form of treatment or the other.

An important counterbalance to biases on the part of patients is the neutral or, more properly, equally enthusiastic stance of the treating clinicians with respect to the treatments being provided. In the area of psychotherapy research, there have been endless debates as to whether clinicians should be crossed with treatments or whether clinicians should provide only the treatment at which they are most expert and about which they are most enthusiastic. This debate applies equally to the combination treatment trials in which medication, psychotherapy, and the combination are being provided. Whichever choice an investigator makes, it is essential to ensure that clinicians convey enthusiasm and optimism about each form of treatment they are being asked to provide.

OUTCOME CRITERIA ISSUES

Treatment Combinations Suggest a Spectrum of Outcomes

Outcome Measurement Choices

Kasdin (30) has argued that in the ideal case outcome should be multifaceted, involving the perspectives of (a) the patients under study, (b) their significant others, and (c) the clinician. In addition, assessments should address different facets of the individual and consequences of the individual's psychopathology. Thus, assessments should be made of subjective distress, overt symptomatology, and impairment in functioning. Finally, in the ideal case, assessment will involve self-report instruments, clinician ratings, and observational measures. Finally, as Waskow and Parloff (57) pointed out, a core assessment battery—particularly in a combination or multimodality treatment study—should be applicable to outcomes viewed from a variety of theoretical orientations.

Having argued for such a battery, one must acknowledge that the analysis of such a large and diversified assessment battery presents both practical and philosophical problems. It is incumbent on the investigator using such a battery to specify at the outset how such data will be examined. Does the investigator, for example, have a specific hypothesis that different treatments will affect different domains (i.e., distress versus symptoms versus functioning)? Does the investigator hypothesize that only one of the modalities, perhaps the combination, will lead to effects observable by significant others? While combination treatment studies, in particular, appear to require such multifaceted assessment, unless a clearly defined set of hypotheses is stated a priori, the investigator using such a battery runs the risk of having different analyses lead to different conclusions about the relative efficacy of the treatments under study.

A final issue in the area of measurement choices has to do with the tendency in the field of treatment research to continue to use old, established measures despite clear evidence that they are not particularly sensitive to the outcomes of interest. A prominent example of this is the continued use of the Hamilton Rating Scale for Depression (HRSD) (21). The HRSD was originally designed for the assessment of change in inpatient populations with melancholic unipolar depression. Wanting to be in a position to compare their results to those of previous studies, investigators have continued to use this measure despite considerable evidence that it is relatively insensitive to change in milder, outpatient nonmelancholic depressions and particularly inadequate in the substantial proportion of unipolar outpatients with reverse vegetative signs.

Timing of Assessments

Another critical decision in the development of an assessment protocol for all treatment outcome research is that of the timing of assessments. Particularly in combination or multimodality research where the presumed effects of the different treatments are also presumed to operate on differing time courses, the more frequently the core assessment battery can be performed, the more likely it is that such differential effects can be observed. The additional value of multiple assessment points is that a much better understanding of the effects of treatment on those patients who ultimately drop out or are terminated from the study can be obtained. This is especially true when survival analytic or random effects models can be applied to the data. Under ideal circumstances, short-term treatment studies should include weekly or biweekly assessments. Longer-term studies, as well as long-term follow-up of acute treatment effects, should obtain at least some portion of the assessment battery on a monthly or bimonthly basis.

End-of-treatment and follow-up evaluations provide a particular dilemma in studies in which one of the modalities under investigation is short-term pharmacotherapy. While Elkin et al. (8) argued in 1988 that one might consider end-of-treatment evaluation of such subjects both prior to and following drug taper, today we would probably consider any evaluation following the tapering of pharmacotherapy to be a follow-up rather than end-of-treatment evaluation. Follow-up evaluations are discussed more fully below.

Other Measures to Be Considered

As implied above in the discussion of patient preparation for a treatment protocol, a number of variables which may mediate or moderate treatment outcome should be assessed as well as outcome per se. As noted above, patient expectations and biases regarding the likely efficacy of biological versus psychosocial versus combination treatments fall into this category. In our own work, measures of treatment specificity have proven to be particularly useful in the interpretation of psychotherapy and combination treatment outcome (15). Particularly important in interpreting "placebo" effects in studies crossing psychotherapy versus no psychotherapy with drug versus placebo would be measures of treatment "process" in the non-psychotherapeutic condition. For example, had data from the Treatment of Depression Collaborative Research Program (9) been analyzed in this way, it might be possible to make a more sensible interpretation of the equivalence of the clinical management with placebo condition in the less severely depressed subjects.

One aspect of measurement which is almost universally lacking in treatment outcome studies is an assessment of the costs versus benefits of the interventions as seen from the perspective of health economists. Kasdin (30) pointed out that a better understanding of such variables as the cost of providing the treatment, the cost of training clinicians to carry out the treatment, and the requirements for ongoing supervision of clinicians would complement more traditional measures of efficacy and facilitate a more complete assessment of the actual costs and benefits of each of the treatments under study. Health economists tend to be interested in other "costs" of treatment, such as the time required for patient participation, the side-effect and nuisance profile of each of the treatments under consideration, and the evaluation of extreme outcomes such as suicide. Under such an analysis, treatments that were less effective from the symptom reduction or probability of remission standpoint but were more effective from the suicide prevention standpoint might be judged more effective overall.

Magnitude of Effect/Response

Assessment of Statistical Significance

The conventional approach to the assessment of treatment outcome has been to examine the statistical significance of pre- to post-treatment change and/or of differences between the treatment groups. Typically, in studies of this nature, the outcome of primary interest has been the end-of-treatment score on a single measure or a variety of measures. This outcome evaluation is then compared to baseline in a paired *t* test within a group of subjects or between groups using a *t* test or analysis of variance, sometimes adjusting for baseline scores. There are numerous problems with this method of examining treatment effects (none of which are specific to multimodality research). The most prominent of these problems have to do with (a) how dropouts and early terminators should be handled in such an analysis and (b) how much confidence one should have in any value or combination of values taken from a single assessment.

With respect to the problem of handling dropouts and early terminators, one approach has been to analyze data by the principle of intention-to-treat, carrying forward the last observation available on any subject who drops out or is terminated prematurely. All too often the observation being carried forward is the baseline, pretreatment evaluation of the subject and, thus, really tells us nothing about the efficacy of the treatment for that particular subject. A second common approach has been to analyze only those subjects who complete the full course or a specified minimum proportion of the course of treatment. Finally, some investigators (26) have chosen to present analyses based on all three of these approaches. Such a presentation may leave the reader confused as to what lesson is, in fact, to be drawn from the investigation, particularly if the three sets of analyses lead to somewhat different conclusions.

A relatively new, but much more satisfying, approach to the analysis of such data involves the use of random effects models such as those proposed by Gibbons et al. (17). By analyzing treatment response trajectories averaged across subjects within a treatment for as long as any given subject is under treatment, these models allow the investigator to incorporate all of the data obtained from a given subject for as long as the subject is continued in the protocol. Random effects models thus provide for a more rational way of handling the problems associated with dropouts and early terminators. This can be particularly important in multimodality research where subjects in different treatment groups are likely to drop out or be terminated at different rates and for different reasons. The use of a random effects or random regression analysis approach allows the investigator to model those differences.

Assessment of Clinical Significance

While generally thought of as another approach to the assessment of *statistical* significance, methods involving life-table or survival analytic techniques might be conceptualized as falling somewhere *between* the analysis of clinical and statistical significance. When such models are used, the investigator is required to make a single, categorical determination with respect to the outcome of interest. In the case of a short-term treatment study, this outcome would likely be response or clinical remission. In prophylactic maintenance studies the outcome of interest is likely to be relapse, recurrence, or rehospitalization. In any case, a clinically based determination as to whether a subject meets criteria for this categorical outcome represents the outcome of interest. To the extent that this determination is made on the basis of clinical judgment, the *statistical* analysis of such outcomes through survival analytic methods can be thought of as having substantial *clinical* significance as well.

The more common meaning of the term *clinical significance* grows out of the work of several investigators (26,28,60). These investigators have sought to define ways of (a) measuring and analyzing the extent to which a treatment results in a return to functioning comparable to that of some normative sample, (b) examining the *magnitude* of change, and/or (c) determining the degree to which change is apparent to nonclinical observers, such as family members or friends. While some of these methods have been well worked out from a statistical standpoint, they have not gained wide acceptance. Few papers, other than those written by the developers of these methods themselves, have presented analyses of clinical significance.

There is also a more informal way in which clinical significance is discussed among researchers and clinicians familiar with a given outcome measure. For example, such individuals might conclude that despite the fact that an investigator achieved a statistically significant difference between two large groups of subjects on the Brief Psychiatric Rating Scale (BPRS) (45), the difference is not clinically meaningful in terms of the size of the change achieved. They would therefore conclude that the result is statistically but not clinically significant.

Distinguishing Response/Remission/Recovery and Relapse/Recurrence

Prien et al. (48) have demonstrated the extent to which the mood disorders outcome literature is riddled with inconsistent use of terms describing outcome. One investigator's "response" is another's "remission." We suspect that a similar situation exists in the outcome literature for other major psychiatric disorders.

As an attempt at an antidote to this problem, a task

force of the MacArthur Foundation Network I on the Psychobiology of Affective Disorders offered conceptual definitions differentiating among these terms in order to reduce the amount of confusion in the mood disorders literature (16). Similar efforts have been made or are underway with respect to several other diagnostic categories including substance abuse and anxiety disorders. At the very least, within a single report or series of reports from a single study, investigators should attempt to make clear how such terms are being used and to use them in a consistent fashion.

Problems Associated with Follow-Up in Acute Treatment Studies

It has recently become apparent how problematic the interpretation is of follow-up evaluations of treatment responders in a randomized trial. Several years ago, Elkin et al. (8) argued that such evaluations may reveal delayed effects of one treatment or the other. More recently, however, a number of methodologists including Lavori (*unpublished paper,* presented 1992) have argued that any follow-up evaluation is of limited interpretability. Because only responders to the various modalities are included in the follow-up assessments, the various groups can no longer be considered to have been randomly sampled from the same population and thus cannot be compared statistically. An important area of future work for multimodality research will be to define acceptable methods for the examination of uncontrolled, naturalistic follow-up data. If such methods cannot be developed, one must question whether the time and expense involved in such evaluations is warranted.

STUDY DESIGN ISSUES

This section on issues relating to study design will address the types of trials the multimodality researcher may consider conducting, what the optimal design for such trials might be, the appropriate dose and duration of the various types of interventions, the problems associated with equating the various interventions, and, finally, the value of examining psychosocial outcomes in studies involving only pharmacotherapy.

Types of Trials

At the most basic level, treatment trials sort themselves into two varieties: (i) those that assess the extent to which a treatment or treatments improve patients' clinical condition and/or bring about a full remission of symptoms and (ii) those that assess the extent to which treatments prevent a return of symptoms. Studies of the first variety, often referred to as *short-term* or *acute* treatment studies

in the psychopharmacology literature, have generally taken the form of a randomized controlled comparison of one or more active treatments with a placebo tablet in acutely ill patients. Typically carried primarily for the purpose of obtaining FDA approval for the use of a compound for a particular indication, these trials have often been very brief (a few weeks in duration) and have simply explored the question of whether there is a difference between the active treatment(s) and the control condition on some rating scale. Moving this paradigm to multimodality research has changed the nature of the research enterprise, because psychotherapy generally operates on a much more extended time course. While the pharmacotherapy-only trials tended to look simply for *response* to the treatment (i.e., a difference between the active and control condition), multimodality trials involving a psychotherapy comparison have typically defined the minimum or ideal length of the psychotherapeutic intervention and then compared the drug, the psychotherapy, and, in some cases, the combination over the time course needed to complete the short-term psychotherapeutic intervention (37,50,59).

Particularly in the areas of mood and substance abuse disorders, there has been increasing recognition of the importance of relapse following initial treatment success. This has led to the emergence of the concept of continuation treatment—that is, interventions aimed at the prevention of relapse once a remission of symptoms has been achieved. While various parameters of continuation treatment, including its appropriate duration for unipolar depression (20), have been described, to our knowledge we are yet to see a trial in which patients brought to remission by various controlled or uncontrolled routes are randomly assigned to a set of continuation treatment strategies. Although the term "relapse" has often been applied to severe symptomatic exacerbations in patients suffering from schizophrenia, the duration of most (i.e., several years) makes them more like maintenance treatment studies.

The concept of maintenance treatment probably first emerged in the mood disorder area with the early study of Weissman et al. (58), which they characterized as a "maintenance" trial. Because this followed on only 4 weeks of amitriptyline treatment, however, in current parlance it would be considered a continuation treatment study. As implied above, the true maintenance studies have focused on years rather than months of prophylaxis and, as will be described below, have led to some very substantial controversies with respect to appropriate design.

Optimal Design

The issue of primary concern in multimodality research is which and how many treatment conditions ought to be considered. Issues of secondary concern relate to blocking or stratifying variables. In the area of continuation and maintenance treatment studies, the investigator not only must make a determination as to which treatment conditions are to be evaluated, but also must determine at which point in the course of treatment the experiment is to begin.

The naive (or, at least, simple) answer to the question of the ideal design for multimodality research is the two-by-two factorial in which active pharmacotherapy and placebo are crossed with active psychotherapy and some form of psychotherapy control condition. From a pure design standpoint, this is clearly the ideal paradigm. Unfortunately, however, the treatment conditions created in such a design (especially the no-active drug/no-active psychotherapy condition and the psychotherapy with placebo tablet condition) may not actually be applicable to several clinical conditions or generalize to real clinical practice. For example, the placebo tablet/placebo psychotherapy condition would probably rarely be applied to patients with psychotic disorders, including schizophrenia and bipolar 1 disorder. With respect to the representativeness of design conditions vis-à-vis clinical practice, Hollon and Beck (25) and many other psychotherapy researchers have argued that psychotherapy with a placebo tablet is not representative of psychotherapy in actual clinical practice, where a placebo tablet would never be given.

Is the Six-Cell Design the Solution?

This has led Hollon and Beck (25) to propose a six-cell design in which psychotherapy and a psychotherapy-control condition are crossed with active medication, placebo tablet, and no pill. While from a purely objective standpoint this could be considered an "ideal" design, it raises at least as many practical problems as the two-by-two factorial. For example, is the no-pill/no-active psychosocial treatment condition a viable option? For some conditions (e.g., depression following bereavement) it might be possible to convince subjects that a regularly scheduled visit intended simply to check on the progress of their recovery is a reasonable treatment option. However, it is difficult to imagine how one would present the rationale for such a condition to, for example, an individual with severe, incapacitating panic disorder.

Recognition of the difficulties associated with the perfectly balanced factorial designs leads to the recommendation of a variety of unbalanced designs for the conduct of multimodality research. For example, in our own work we have carried out a five-cell comparison of psychotherapy and medication in which the conditions were (a) maintenance interpersonal psychotherapy (IPT-M) and active medication, (b) IPT-M and placebo tablet, (c) IPT-M alone, (d) medication clinic visits and active imipramine, and (e) medication clinic visits and placebo tablet. Post-hoc analyses revealed absolutely no differences be-

tween the IPT-M alone and the IPT-M-plus-placebo condition for any of the outcome or outcome-mediating variables (10). In light of the amount of time required to recruit the additional 20% of subjects needed for this fifth condition and in light of our difficulty in analyzing a variety of interaction effects because of the reduced power resulting from the smaller cell sizes, we concluded in retrospect that it would have been preferable to limit the study to four treatment conditions.

In the end the investigator must balance scientific purity, interpretability, and generalizability. Certain designs may be less than ideal from a scientific standpoint. The information yield may, nonetheless, be high relative to the cost of mounting the trial. In contrast, other designs with perfect scientific credibility may be so costly as to render them useless in an environment of shrinking resources for clinical research.

A discussion of design decisions would not be complete without addressing the problem of statistical power in multimodality treatment research. Studies examining multiple treatment modalities are almost always underpowered when one considers anything beyond the primary outcome measures. The presumed moderators and mediators of treatment outcome invariably differ for the pharmacotherapy and psychotherapy conditions, leading to a profusion of assessment measures. While the investigator typically had an appropriate rationale for each measure, there is rarely sufficient power to examine the relationship of these measures to outcome.

The most common solution to the problem of inadequate power has been the multicenter trial. However, multicenter trials raise serious problems of their own. Achieving consistency among treatment providers and raters is difficult enough in a single-site investigation, but it represents a major challenge in multicenter trials. How investigators and funding agencies should make a determination as to whether the likely additional yield from a multicenter trial outweighs the additional complexity and expense is not clear. The development of criteria for decision-making in this arena could be a useful addition to the field.

Appropriate Doses and Durations of Interventions in Trials Involving Both Pharmacotherapy and Psychotherapy

One of the many decisions facing the investigator, once the specific treatments to be investigated have been decided upon, is what the duration of those treatments should be. As Elkin et al. (8) pointed out, the appropriate length of most of the disorder-specific, manualized psychotherapies is reasonably well defined. In contrast, there is still considerable controversy over what the ideal length of any given pharmacotherapeutic intervention should be. Equally, there are disputes as to the appropriate "dose" of each intervention. For most of the disorder-specific psychotherapies the modal frequency of contact appears to be once a week. However, there are circumstances under which treatment might be more or less frequent. In the pharmacotherapy domain, the investigator must consider whether to employ a titrated dose or a fixed dose or whether to key the intervention to a targeted blood level of the compound.

For studies of long-term prophylaxis, the duration of treatment may be more easily defined by the expected time to relapse/recurrence in the study population. However, the question of dose remains problematic for both the pharmacotherapeutic and the psychotherapeutic intervention. Should the medication be maintained at a constant dose comparable to that used in acute therapy or is a reduced, "maintenance" dose (or blood level) more appropriate to the study population in question? How frequently should the psychosocial intervention be offered: as often as practical for subject retention or as often as seems likely to be required for prophylaxis?

Equally perplexing in the design of combination trials is the issue of the *equivalence* of the interventions, both in terms of the duration of individual sessions and in terms of the amount and source of attention given to individuals in each treatment condition. A recurrent theme in the critiques of multimodality treatment research is the time differential between the active psychosocial intervention and the psychosocial control condition. For example, when a psychotherapy is being contrasted with a clinical management/medication clinic condition, the investigator must decide whether the control condition sessions will be of a duration equal to that of the active psychotherapy. Choosing to make them equivalent removes the confound of time differential but may introduce the very practical problem of how the clinician providing the control condition can fill the time of the session without providing something that (a) is not representative of a real-world pharmacotherapeutic clinical management and (b) is not contaminated with the aspects of either the active psychosocial treatment under study or some other active psychosocial intervention. In the end, in most circumstances we would come down on the side of recommending the more ecologically valid choice; that is, each modality should be representative of how it is likely to be provided in actual clinical practice. Because the ultimate goal of all clinical research is to provide information that is generalizable to the real world of treatment provision, the more representative the modality, the better.

Achieving Comparability Among Psychosocial, Medication, and Combination Treatments

A good argument can be made that the goal in multimodality research should be achieving *comparably good operationalization* of each of the modalities rather than achieving *comparability* across modalities. When the operationalization of each of the individual treatments is maximized—that is, when pharmacotherapy, psychotherapy, and the combination are each being provided by well-trained, well-monitored enthusiastic clinicians—the fairest test of the treatments in comparison to one another can occur. In order to do this, the investigator must specify each of the interventions with equal clarity. The interpersonal interaction through which pharmacotherapy is to be provided must be defined as clearly as the manner in which the psychotherapy is to be provided. Clinicians carrying out these treatments (and the combination) must be trained to equivalent levels of competence, and ongoing monitoring (preferably in the form of objective rating of audio or video tapes of treatment sessions) should be employed to verify the continued adherence of the clinicians in each modality.

Multimodality treatment studies invariably raise the issue of what the specific duties of physician and nonphysician clinicians will be during the trial. Will both physicians and nonphysicians provide the psychosocial treatment? If so, does the investigator need to have sufficient power to examine clinician discipline as a variable in the analysis? The more common approach is probably to have physicians provide pharmacotherapy, while nonphysicians provide the psychotherapy. Does this then mean that those individuals assigned to a combined treatment condition will have two clinicians rather than one? And how, then, should any superior efficacy of the combination be interpreted? As a function of the intervention or the additional clinicians presence?

One solution which undoubtedly adds to the expense and complexity of the trial but provides for a certain amount of equivalence across conditions is to assign each subject a physician and a nonphysician clinician. The nonphysician might then be given the role of primary clinician, and the physician might be given the role of consulting psychiatrist. The nonphysician has responsibility for the provision of the psychosocial treatment or its contrast condition, and the physician has the responsibility for prescribing in those treatment conditions where medication or pill placebo is being provided and for monitoring the symptoms and side effects being experienced by the subject even in those treatment conditions where no pill is offered. Depending upon the disorder under investigation, such a design may have considerable ecological validity. For example, in the long-term management of schizophrenia or bipolar disorder, it is quite likely that most of the treatment will be provided by a nonphysician, with the physician seeing the patient less frequently and primarily for the purpose of adjusting medication. In the treatment of panic disorder, however, a purely behavioral intervention might be offered in the absence of any pharmacotherapy. In the "real world" there would be no role for the physician in the provision of this treatment, making the physician's participation in the subject's care questionable in terms of generalizability. In designing a study where psychosocial treatment of panic disorder is compared with pharmacotherapy, the investigator must decide whether to opt for balance across conditions versus ecological validity in giving the physician a consulting role in the psychosocial intervention.

A related issue is whether, setting aside discipline as a variable, all clinicians should be crossed with treatments or whether clinicians should provide only those interventions in which they have the greatest expertise and for which they have the highest level of enthusiasm. For example, in a study where family psychoeducation is compared with an individual medication management approach, one might choose to have very different types of clinicians carrying out the two treatments because this is more consistent with the relative expertise and enthusiasms of, for example, psychiatric social workers and psychiatrists.

Assessment of Psychosocial Outcomes in Pharmacotherapy-Only Studies

It is altogether possible that one might wish to examine a variety of psychosocial parameters in a study in which only pharmacotherapy is being provided. These parameters might occur in two domains: (i) in the patient–clinician interaction itself and (ii) in the patient's life outside of the treatment setting. Even with very severe illnesses such as schizophrenia and psychotic mania, it would appear that the nature of the patient–clinician interaction can have an impact on outcome. Thus, we would argue that even in pharmacotherapy-only studies it is critical that the investigator specify the nature of the clinician–patient interaction and monitor this interaction throughout the trial in order to investigate adherence to the specifications of the interaction and the extent to which adherence or other "process" parameters affect outcome. "Clinician" is almost never inspected as a variable in a single-site drug–placebo study. If it were, interesting differences might emerge. In many multicenter medication trials (D. Stangl, *unpublished dissertation*) the center differences are actually more striking than the differences between treatment conditions. This is almost certainly attributable to uncontrolled differences in the nature of the clinician–patient interactions at various sites. Had the nature of that interaction been more carefully specified and monitored throughout the trial, we would at least be able to determine whether the center differences are attributable to unmeasured differences in the patient populations recruited at the various sites or, more probably, to unmeasured differences in clinician behavior.

A related problem is how one makes the determination as to whether a supportive medication management intervention has somehow crossed into the realm of psychotherapy. A frequent observation in recent years has been

the steady decline in the drug–placebo difference observed in pharmacotherapy trials (C. M. Beasley, Jr., *unpublished paper*, 1991). This has been particularly true in outpatient treatment of mood and anxiety disorders. One hypothesis is that this decline is attributable to the increasing sophistication with which pharmacotherapeutically oriented clinicians are providing psychological support along with medication management. This raises the question of when such support, in fact, becomes supportive psychotherapy. In their search for adequate and ethical control conditions, psychotherapy researchers have noted the vagueness of this boundary; however, little attention has been paid to this issue the pharmacotherapy-alone research enterprise.

The measurement of change in the psychosocial realm has rarely been a feature of pharmacotherapy-only trials. The possible exceptions are those studies which have included a "quality of life" measure. Occasionally, assessment is made of more specific aspects of social functioning or social adjustment. There are particular areas of pharmacotherapy research where such assessment seems especially relevant. For example, it would appear that clozapine not only provides a level of symptomatic relief not seen with other antipsychotic medication but also leads to improvements in social adjustment that are unlike those observed with other treatments for schizophrenia (6,35,38). Prior to clozapine there was probably little reason to think that one agent would lead to psychosocial outcomes that are markedly different from those observed with another. With the advent of the new antipsychotics and the selective serotonin reuptake inhibitor antidepressants, much more sophisticated assessment of various aspects of social and interpersonal functioning would seem warranted.

METHODOLOGICAL CONSIDERATIONS SPECIFIC TO THE STUDY OF NONSOMATIC THERAPIES

Establishment of Appropriate Controls for the Psychotherapy/Psychosocial Treatment

As implied above, in recent years the psychotherapy research community has been particularly concerned about the development of appropriate controls for active psychotherapeutic conditions. Up to now most contrast or control conditions for active psychosocial interventions have been inadequate in one way or another. This concern applies equally to multimodality research. As Parloff (46) pointed out in his classic paper on psychotherapy "placebos," the term *placebo* historically has referred to inactive medications prescribed primarily for the purpose of placating or soothing the patient rather than directly treating any real disorder. In trying to conceptualize a psychotherapy placebo we run directly into the traditional medical distinction between core somatic pathology and psychological symptoms which might be associated with the experience of that pathology. In psychiatry, whether we are treating with medication, with psychotherapy, or with the combination, we are interested in *both* the somatic pathology and the psychological symptoms. Therefore, what constitutes a "placebo effect" in physical medicine may be synonomous with a treatment goal in psychiatry. The reduction of anxiety is a clear example of this. Up to the present time there have been approximately a half-dozen types of controls used in psychotherapy research, only some of which apply to the multimodality treatment research enterprise. These have included: (a) dropout waiting-list controls, (b) attention controls (the nonspecific support, medication clinic, clinical management paradigm would fit in here), (c) alternative treatment controls, (d) crossover controls, (e) the mirror image or "patient as own control" paradigm, and (f) dismantling the treatment package. With respect to multimodality research, the most applicable of these paradigms are the attention controls, alternative treatment controls, and, in the case of highly chronic disorders, the mirror image design. While a dismantling paradigm has many attractive features in a psychotherapy-alone study, the level of complexity involved in a study involving both medication and psychotherapy which at the same time attempts to dismantle the psychotherapeutic treatment package seems to preclude the actual conduct of such a trial.

Multimodality investigators do generally have the advantage of being able to contrast the psychotherapeutic condition or the combined treatment condition with an attention control (clinical or medication management). While this has many of the features of an adequate control condition, as noted above, there are design problems which must ,be addressed in terms of "equating" this condition with the psychotherapy condition both with respect to the amount of time spent in the treatment session and with respect to the discipline of the clinician providing the control intervention.

Measuring the "Blood Level" or "Take" of the Psychosocial Treatment

It has been typical of well-designed pharmacotherapy trials to examine the blood level of the compound under investigation both as a measure of patient compliance and as a measure of the potential for therapeutic effect. Recently, psychotherapy researchers have begun to address similar issues.

Luborsky et al. (36) investigated the relationship of treatment quality to efficacy of drug counseling, cognitive-behavioral psychotherapy, and supportive–expressive psychotherapy with methadone-maintained, opioid-dependent patients. These investigators found that there was a positive relationship between the presence of supportive–expressive elements and 7-month outcome even among patients who were assigned to the other two conditions. However, the strongest relationship to outcome was for their measure of "purity" (the ratio of the intended therapy rating to the total of all ratings). This was especially true for the two psychotherapy conditions. They noted that this finding can be interpreted as follows: The more therapists did what they were "supposed to do," the better the outcome, *or* the better the outcome, the more therapists did what they were supposed to do.

O'Malley et al. (44) examined the relationship of therapist competence to efficacy of IPT in patients with unipolar depression. These investigators used multiple regression analyses to predict outcome and found that supervisors' ratings of the fourth treatment session, which took into account quality of problem-oriented strategies, quality of techniques, general IPT skills, and overall session quality, made a significant contribution to explained variance in patient-rated change at termination beyond the contribution of pretreatment patient characteristics. While competence ratings did not add to the explained variance (after pretreatment characteristics) in total Hamilton Depression Rating Scale (HDRS) (21) scores at termination, they did contribute significantly to the termination apathy factor of the HDRS. Thus, they found that higher treatment specificity was related to greater improvement on at least some measures. In this study, treatment purity was not examined directly.

More recently, Crits-Cristoph et al. (5) examined the extent to which accuracy of interpretations, errors in technique, and "positive-helping alliance" scores were related to treatment outcomes of residual gain and rated benefits among patients in individual psychodynamic psychotherapy. Accuracy of interpretation and positive-helping alliance were both significantly related to outcome, with one measure of accuracy ("wish plus response from other") being the best predictor of outcome. Although the results did not lend themselves quite as well as the findings from the earlier study of Luborsky et al. (36) to a conceptualization in terms of specificity versus purity, it would appear that, in this instance, it was specificity of the therapy that was more strongly related to outcome. For individual studies, then, it remains an empiric question whether, if outcome is found to be related to treatment quality, it is specificity or purity that is the better predictor of outcome.

Finally, our own research group has reported that in a long-term trial examining the prophylactic capacity of IPT-M, patients whose monthly therapy sessions were rated above the median on specificity of IPT had a median survival time of almost 2 years, while those below the median on IPT specificity had a median survival time of less than 5 months (45). Clearly, some measure of the extent to which the specific ingredients of a therapy are being provided by the clinician and/or absorbed by the patient should be included in any multimodality research design.

Standardizing Nonpharmacotherapeutic Treatments

As noted above and as Elkin et al. (8) have pointed out, it is critical to multimodality research that the pharmacotherapy provision condition be "defined with sufficient clarity to ensure the adequate delivery of the active ingredients of this treatment." Treatment manuals and specific treatment training, along with ongoing monitoring of therapist's behavior, represent important methodologic advances in the direction of ensuring the adequate delivery of such treatment. Furthermore, actual ratings of the content of the pharmacotherapy/clinical management sessions have the potential to greatly enhance the interpretability of the results.

ETHICAL CONSIDERATIONS

Justification for the Double-Placebo Condition

In relatively short-term trials with relatively milder conditions it is not difficult to justify a treatment condition in which the patient can expect to receive neither active pharmacotherapy nor active psychotherapy, provided that the subject is fully informed as to the nature of all the treatment conditions included in the trial. When it comes to more severe conditions and to longer-term trials even in less severe conditions, the investigator must consider carefully whether there is ethical justification for the double-placebo condition. In discussing this issue, O'Leary and Borkovec (43) argued that one approach to this ethical dilemma (admittedly, a rationalization) is to argue that if there is no scientific evidence of the efficacy of the active treatment, then it is not unethical to withhold it. The problem comes in the severe disorders where we do have treatments known to be effective. In these circumstances, asking a subject to consent to random assignment in a trial testing one or several new treatments and forego known effective treatments represents an ethical dilemma with no easy rationalization. It is around this very issue that the demands of science and the values of an ethical clinician investigator most often come into conflict, often with no fully satisfying solution.

If the investigator concludes that the scientific gains of a no-active-treatment condition outweigh the ethical concerns associated with it, it is then incumbent on the investigator to (a) do everything possible to maximize the extent to which the patient and family members are fully informed about the nature of the investigation and the probability of receiving the inactive drug/inactive therapy condition and (b) be prepared to provide active intervention as soon as treatment failure has been established. In our own work we have employed an *ongoing* consent process involving an initial informed consent while the patient is acutely ill, whenever possible including both the patient and a well family member in the consent process. This initial consent is followed by a second full disclosure of the nature of the investigation which takes place at a patient/family educational workshop timed to coincide with the early phase of clinical remission. At this time, subjects and their family members are reminded of the existence of the double-placebo condition and of the patient's freedom to withdraw from the investigation at any time. Finally, just prior to random assignment, the various treatment conditions are once again reviewed with the subject. While not all investigators may wish to mount a family educational workshop, at a minimum a process of ongoing consent which reminds patients and, when possible, family members of what it is they have consented to seems a reasonable way to proceed, particularly when one is concerned about the inclusion of a fully inactive condition.

Weighing the Costs and Benefits of Combination Strategies in Describing Results

A second ethical problem arises for the multimodality researcher in describing the results of an investigation in which the combination strategy has proven more effective than either of the single modalities alone. Here we must once again concern ourselves with the distinction between statistical and clinical significance. First, the investigator must decide whether the standard of clinical as well as statistical significance of superiority of the combination has been achieved. If this is the case, then it is incumbent on the investigator to describe the added therapeutic benefit measured against the additional cost incurred in the provision of the combined treatment. Only when the results are described in this way is the investigator fully meeting her or his responsibility to assess the results of the investigation.

ACKNOWLEDGMENTS

This work is supported in part by NIMH grants MH29618, MH49115 (Dr. Frank), and MH30915 (Dr. Kupfer). Portions of this chapter were adapted from the following sources:

Frank E, Kupfer DJ, Levenson J. Continuation therapy of unipolar depression: the case for combined treatment. In: Manning D, Frances A, eds. *Combination drug and psychotherapy in depression.* Washington, DC: American Psychiatric Press, 1990;133–149.
Frank E, Kupfer DJ, Wagner EF, McEachran A, Cornes C. Efficacy of interpersonal psychotherapy as a maintenance treatment for recurrent depression: contributing factors. *Arch Gen Psychiatry* 1991;48:1053–1059.

Frank E, Kupfer DJ, Thase ME. Combining psychotherapy and psychopharmacology. In: Elliott GR, Ciaranello RD, Barchas JD, eds. *Psychopharmacology: from theory to practice*. New York: Oxford University Press (*in press*).

REFERENCES

1. Beck AT, Mahoney M. Schools of 'thought.' *Am Psychol* 1979;34:93–98.
2. Buysse DJ, Kupfer DJ, Frank E, Monk TH, Ritenour A, Ehlers CL. Electroenephalographic sleep studies in depressed outpatients treated with interpersonal psychotherapy. I. Baseline studies in responders and non-responders. *Psychiatr Res* 1992;40:13–26.
3. Buysse DJ, Kupfer DJ, Frank E, Monk TH, Ritenour A. Electroencephalographic sleep studies in depressed outpatients treated with interpersonal psychotherapy. II. Longitudinal studies at baseline and recovery. *Psychiatr Res* 1992;40:27–40.
4. Clark DB, Agras WS. The assessment and treatment of performance anxiety in musicians. *Am J Psychiatry* 1991;148:598–605.
5. Crits-Cristoph P, Cooper A, Luborsky L. The accuracy of therapists' interpretations and the outcome of dynamic psychotherapy. *J Consult Clin Psychol* 1988;56:490–495.
6. Davies MA, Conley RR, Schulz SC, Bell-Delaney J. One-year follow-up of 24 patients in a clinical trial of clozapine. *Hosp Community Psychiatry* 1991;42(6):628–629.
7. Dimascio A, Weissman MM, Prusoff BA, Neu C, Zwilling M, Klerman GL. Differential symptom reduction by drugs and psychotherapy in acute depression. *Arch Gen Psychiatry* 1979;36:1450–1456.
8. Elkin I, Pilkonis P, Docherty J, Sotsky S. Conceptual and methodological issues in comparative studies of psychotherapy and pharmacotherapy. II. Nature and timing of treatment effects. *Am J Psychiatry* 1988;145:1070–1076.
9. Elkin I, Shea T, Watkins J, et al. NIMH treatment of depression collaborative research program: comparative outcome findings. *Arch Gen Psychiatry* 1989;49:971–982.
10. Frank E, Kupfer DJ. Does a placebo tablet affect psychotherapeutic treatment outcome? Results from the Pittsburgh study of maintenance therapies in recurrent depression. *Psychotherapy Res* 1992;2:102–111.
11. Frank E, Jarrett DB, Kupfer DJ, Grochocinski VJ. Biological and clinical predictors of response in recurrent depression (a preliminary report). *Psychiatry Res* 1984;13:315–324.
12. Frank E, Prien R, Kupfer DJ. Implications of non-compliance on research in affective disorders. *Psychopharmacol Bull* 1985;21:37–42.
13. Frank E, Kupfer DJ, Jacob M, Jarrett D. Personality features and response to acute treatment in recurrent depression. *J Pers Dis* 1987;1:14–26.
14. Frank E, Kupfer DJ, Perel JM, et al. Three year outcomes for maintenance therapies in recurrent depression. *Arch Gen Psychiatry* 1990;47:1093–1099.
15. Frank E, Kupfer DJ, Wagner EF, McEachran A, Cornes C. Efficacy of interpersonal psychotherapy as a maintenance treatment for recurrent depression: contributing factors. *Arch Gen Psychiatry* 1991;48:1053–1059.
16. Frank E, Prien R, Jarrett RB, et al. Conceptualization and rationale for consensus definitions of terms in major depressive disorder: response, remission, recovery, relapse and recurrence. *Arch Gen Psychiatry* 1991;48:851–855.
17. Gibbons RD, Hedokor D, Elkin I, et al. Some conceptual and statistical issues in analysis of longitudinal psychiatric data. *Arch Gen Psychiatry* 1993;50:739–750.
18. Glick ID, Clarkin JF, Haas GL, Spencer JH Jr, Chen CL. A randomized clinical trial of inpatient family intervention. VI. Mediating variables and outcome. *Fam Process* 1991;30:85–99.
19. Greden JF, Gardner R, King D, et al. Dexamethasone suppression test in antidepressant treatment of melancholia. *Arch Gen Psychiatry* 1983;40:493–500.
20. Greenhouse JB, Stangl D, Kupfer DJ, Prien RF. Methodological issues in maintenance therapy clinical trials. *Arch Gen Psychiatry* 1991;48:313–318.
21. Hamilton M. A rating scale for depression. *J Neurol Neurosurg Psychiatry* 1960;23:56–62.
22. Hogarty GE, Schooler NR, Ulrich RF, Mussare F, Herron E, Ferro P. Fluphenazine and social therapy in the aftercare of schizophrenic patients. *Arch Gen Psychiatry* 1979;36:1283–1294.
23. Hogarty GE, Anderson CM, Reiss DJ, et al. Family psychoeducation, social skills training and maintenance chemotherapy in the aftercare treatment of schizophrenia. I. One year effects of a controlled study on relapse and expressed emotion. *Arch Gen Psychiatry* 1986;43:633–642.
24. Hogarty GE, Anderson CM, Reiss DJ, et al. Family psychoeducation, social skills training and maintenance chemotherapy in the aftercare treatment of schizophrenia. *Arch Gen Psychiatry* 1991;48:340–347.
25. Hollon S, Beck AT. Psychotherapy and drug therapy: comparisons and combinations. In: Garfield SL, Bergin AE, eds. *Handbook of psychotherapy and behavior change: an empirical analysis*, 2nd ed. New York: Wiley, 1978;437–490.
26. Hugdahl K, Ost L. On the difference between statistical and clinical significance. *Behav Assess* 1981;3:289–295.
27. Jacob M, Frank E, Kupfer DJ, Cornes C, Carpenter LL. A psychoeducational workshop for depressed patients, family and friends: description and evaluation. *Hosp Community Psychiatry* 1987;38:968–972.
28. Jacobson NS, Follette WC, Revenstorf D. Psychotherapy outcome research: methods for reporting variability and evaluating clinical significance. *Behav Ther* 1984;15:336–352.
29. Karp JF, Frank E, Anderson B, et al. Time to remission in late-life depression: analysis of effects of demographic, treatment, and life-events measures. *Depression* 1993;1:250–256.
30. Kasdin AE. Comparative outcomes studies of psychotherapy: methodological issues and strategies. *J Consult Clin Psychol* 1986;54:95–105.
31. Kavanagh DJ. Recent developments in expressed emotion and schizophrenia. *Br J Psychiatry* 1992;160:601–620.
32. Kupfer DJ, Frank E, Grochocinski VJ, Messiano M, McEachran AB. EEG sleep profiles in recurrent depression: a longitudinal investigation. *Arch Gen Psychiatry* 1988;45:678–681.
33. Kupfer DJ, Frank E, Grochocinski VJ, McEachran AB. Delta sleep ratio: a biological correlate of early recurrence in unipolar affective disorder. *Arch Gen Psychiatry* 1990;47:1100–1105.
34. Langer G, Konig G, Hatzinger R, et al. Response of thyrotropin to thyrotropin-releasing hormone as a predictor of treatment outcome: prediction of recovery and relapse in treatment with antidepressants and neuroleptics. *Arch Gen Psychiatry* 1986;43:861–868.
35. Levin H, Chengappa KN, Kambhampati RK, Mahdavi N, Ganguli R. Should chronic treatment refractory akathisia be an indication for the use of clozapine in schizophrenic patients? *J Clin Psychiatry* 1992;53(7):248–251.
36. Luborsky L, McLellan AT, Woody GE, O'Brien CP, Auerbach A. Therapist success and its determinants. *Arch Gen Psychiatry* 1985;42:602–611.
37. Mavissakalian M, Michelson L. Agoraphobia: relative and combined effectiveness of therapist-assisted in vivo exposure and imipramine. *J Clin Psychiatry* 1986;47:117–122.
38. Meltzer HY, Burnett S, Bastani B, Ramirez LF. Effects of six months of clozapine treatment on the quality of life of chronic schizophrenic patients. *Hosp Community Psychiatry* 1990;41(8):892–897.
39. Michelson L, Mavissakalian M. Psychophysiological outcome of behavioral and pharmacologic treatments of agoraphobia. *J Consult Clin Psychol* 1985;53:229–236.
40. Michelson L, Mavissakalian M, Marchione K. Cognitive-behavioral treatment of agoraphobia: clinical, behavioral, and psychophysiological outcome. *J Consult Clin Psychol* 1985;53:913–925.
41. Michelson L. Treatment consonance and response profiles in agoraphobia: the role of individual differences in Cancelede, behavioral and physiological treatments. *Behav Res Ther* 1986;24:263–275.
42. Miklowitz DJ, Goldstein MJ. Behavioral family treatment for patients with bipolar affective disorder. Special Issue: Recent develop-

ments in the behavioral treatment of chronic psychiatric illness. *Behav Mod* 1990;14:457–589.

43. O'Leary KD, Borkovec TD. Conceptual, methodological and ethical problems of placebo groups in psychotherapy research. *Am Psychol* 1978;Sept:821–830.

44. O'Malley SS, Foley SH, Rounsaville BJ, et al. Therapist competence and patient outcome in interpersonal psychotherapy of depression. *J Consult Clin Psychol* 1988;56:496–501.

45. Overall JE, Gorham DR. The brief psychiatric rating scale. *Psychol Rep* 1962;10:799–812.

46. Parloff MB. Placebo controls in psychotherapy research: a sine qua non or a placebo for research problems? *J Consult Clin Psychol* 1986;54(1):79–87.

47. Pilkonis PA, Frank E. Personality pathology in recurrent depression: nature, prevalence, and relationship to treatment response. *Am J Psychiatry* 1988;145(4):435–441.

48. Prien R, Carpenter LL, Kupfer DJ. The definition and operational criteria for treatment outcome of major depressive disorder: a review of the current research literature. *Arch Gen Psychiatry* 1991; 48:796–800.

49. Robins LN, Helzer JE, Croughan JL. *The NIMH diagnostic interview schedule (DIS).* St Louis: Washington University, 1979.

50. Rush AJ, Beck AT, Kovacs M, Hollon S. Comparative efficacy of cognitive therapy and imipramine in the treatment of depressed outpatients. *Cognitive Ther Res* 1977;1:17–37.

51. Rush AJ, Hollon SD. Clinical implications of research into specific disorders: depression. In: Beitman BD, Klerman GL, eds. *Integrating pharmacotherapy and psychotherapy.* Washington, DC: American Psychiatric Press, 1991;121–142.

52. Simons AD, Thase ME. Biological markers: treatment outcome and one-year follow-up of endogenous depression. Electroencephalographic sleep studies in response to cognitive therapy. *J Consult Clin Psychiatry* 1992;60:392–401.

53. Spitzer RL, Endicott J. *Schedule for affective disorders and schizophrenia.* New York: New York State Psychiatric Institute, 1975.

54. Spitzer RL, Endicott J, Robbins E. Research diagnostic criteria: rationale and reliability. *Arch Gen Psychiatry* 1978;35:733–782.

55. Spitzer RL, Williams JBW, Gibbon M, First MB. The structured clinical interview for DSM-III-R, I: history, rationale and description. *Arch Gen Psychiatry* 1992;49:624–629.

56. Thase ME, Simons AD, Cahalane J, McGeary J. Cognitive behavior therapy of endogenous depression, part 1: an outpatient clinical replication series. *Behav Ther* 1991;22:457–467.

57. Waskow IE, Parloff MB. *Psychotherapy change measures.* Washington, DC: Department of Health, Education, and Welfare, 1975.

58. Weissman MM, Klerman GL, Paykel ES, Prusoff BA, Hanson B. Treatment effects on the social adjustments of depressed patients. *Arch Gen Psychiatry* 1974;30:771–778.

59. Weissman MM, Prusoff BA, DiMascio A, Neu C, Goklaney M, Klerman GL. The efficacy of drugs and psychotherapy in the treatment of acute depressive episodes. *Am J Psychiatry* 1979;136:555–558.

60. Yeaton WH, Sechrest L. Critical dimensions in the choice and maintenance of successful treatments: strength, integrity and effectiveness. *J Consult Clin Psychol* 1981;49:156–167.

Psychopharmacology: The Fourth Generation of Progress, edited by Floyd E. Bloom and David J. Kupfer. Raven Press, Ltd., New York © 1995.

CHAPTER 157

Methodological and Statistical Progress in Psychiatric Clinical Research

A Statistician's Perspective

Helena Chmura Kraemer

A generation or two ago, there was still active debate as to whether clinical questions in psychiatry could be addressed with scientific research. Such questions arose from a premise that the interaction between a clinician and a patient in a psychiatric framework was so specific to that particular clinician and that particular patient that it was inappropriate to generalize from any sample of patients or any sample of clinicians. One hears little such debate now, and recent years have seen the scientific research standards of excellence in psychiatric clinical research become as stringent as those in any other area of clinical research.

One result of this evolution is that all the considerable armamentarium of methodological and statistical tools developed in other areas of medical research have become available to psychiatric research. This includes tools relevant to issues of (a) research question conceptualization and specification, (b) representativeness of samples and of generalization from particular samples to populations, (c) measurement and classification, (d) powerful and cost-effective research designs, and (e) statistical analysis and presentation and documentation of results. At the same time, research methods developed within the context of psychiatry to cope with the special problems of studying human behavior are being "exported" to other areas of medical research, particularly because behavioral issues (e.g., diet, exercise, smoking, coping with stress, affect, quality of life) have become more and more relevant to

the prevention and to the successful treatment of physical disorders such as heart disease, cancer, and acquired immune deficiency syndrome (AIDS). This blurring of the lines between clinical research in psychiatry and in other fields of medicine promises to continue and to increase, with benefits to all fields concerned.

In psychiatric research journals of recent years, we have seen many randomized clinical trials assessing the efficacy or the effectiveness of pharmacological and psychotherapeutic treatments for mental disorders, including several multisite studies. We have seen epidemiological studies with a national and international perspective. We have seen application of new and powerful genetic models, such as those underlying linkage analysis, to psychiatric disorders. We have seen the DSM-IV move toward a more empirical basis than was true of earlier DSM versions as a result of serious and thoughtful reconsideration of the problems of accurate diagnosis and prognosis of psychiatric disorders. We have seen a refocusing of thinking about psychiatric disorders with a more developmental perspective, and we have witnessed a growing emphasis on prevention, on detection of disorders, and on cost-effectiveness of both detection and treatments. We have seen cross-disciplinary interactions bring new insights and strengths to the study of mental disorders.

That's the good news. Now here's the bad news: The availability of such methodological riches, however, has not translated into their wide and consistent usage. While there are many methodological "gems," the statistical methods used in most research papers in the psychiatric research literature are generally those that were current in medical research 50 or more years ago: one- and two-

H. C. Kraemer: Department of Psychiatry and Behavioral Sciences, Stanford University School of Medicine, Stanford, California 94305.

sample t tests, Pearson product moment correlation coefficients, simple chi-square tests of independence in contingency tables, simple analysis of variance, or linear regression models (3). To make matters worse, frequently even these classic statistical procedures are misapplied, yielding potentially invalid results (24). Even more frequently, these procedures are applied when much more powerful and informative methods are available (17).

At a meeting not too long ago, one psychiatric researcher stated: "Who cares whether the statistical analysis is done right or not? The proof is in the pudding." Because a primary goal of statistical methodology is to identify strategies to ensure the reproducibility, validity, and generalizability of research results, the natural result of misuse and abuse of statistical methods is nonreplicability.

How tasty is the resulting "psychiatric pudding"? The introductory sections of psychiatric research papers or proposals often extensively tally the inconsistencies within the body of previous work on a particular research issue: Five papers say "yea," and five say "nay," and the remaining 20 were inconclusive. Practice guidelines in psychiatry (e.g., see Chapter 73, *this volume*) sound a recurrent theme: ". . . it is unclear . . ."; ". . . currently no clear consensus . . ."; ". . . more definitive strategies cannot be suggested. . . ." In fact, the basis of much of psychiatric practice guidelines continues not to be clinical research results but, instead, what is "intuitively appealing," "expert opinion," and "conventional wisdom." Over and over again, the plea is made for more definitive data and for more specific and convincing studies.

Even more disturbing is the recent spate of research results published by prestigious research groups, particularly in psychiatric genetics, later retracted or contradicted. Such results carry serious messages about the inadequacy of sampling, design, measurement, or analytic procedures used in those studies. Who cares whether the statistical and methodological issues are well dealt with? We all should: patients, policy makers, psychiatric clinicians, researchers, and statisticians.

Those who consider ourselves statisticians with special interest in psychiatric research must share in the responsibility for this situation. It may well be that (17):

1. There are too few of us, and those few make ourselves inaccessible to psychiatric researchers.
2. We communicate or teach badly or reluctantly. There is a certain arrogance and contemptuousness in our interactions that is off-putting.
3. We are impatient with dealing with the real problems of psychiatric researchers, and we ask for the impossible: sample size in the thousands where only tens are available, absolutely reliable measures where the best fall short of that, and so on.
4. We are more concerned with elegant and complex

mathematical methods than with whether those methods serve the needs of psychiatric research.

Another major source of these problems lies in the quantity and quality of training of psychiatric researchers. Many psychiatrists receive no training at all in statistical methodology, nor do they seek any. One psychiatry resident (hopefully a rare case) complained that he was required to take a quarter course in elementary research methodology, because he claimed that sampling, measurement, design, estimation, testing, "and all that crap" were simply tokens in a game played by academic psychiatrists to achieve tenure and other signs of academic prestige. "Real" psychiatrists never read the journals, nor did they need to know "that stuff" to be good psychiatrists. Most trainees are not so extreme or so outspoken. However, psychiatrists who lack sensitivity to the ways poor statistical approaches can produce misleading results remain poorly equipped to read the psychiatric research literature or to produce important and reproducible research findings. For example, too many have no clear understanding of what "statistically significant" does and does not mean; they often mistakenly interpret the term to mean true, big, or important (see Chapter 156, *this volume*).

When psychiatrists are given statistical training, the emphasis of that training is frequently on "number crunching": how to compute a t-test statistic or a product moment correlation coefficient and, most of all, how to generate those all-important "asterisks" indicating statistical significance. There is little coverage of the more fundamental concepts—namely, vital sampling, measurement, and analytic issues. Instead, particularly with today's ready access to computer statistical packages and today's psychiatrists' greater comfort with the use of computers, the emphasis is on which computer buttons to push. Very complex statistical methods are frequently implemented by computer programs that are widely distributed to researchers who know little or nothing of their underlying assumptions, the robustness of the results to deviations from those assumptions, and hence any of the caveats to using the methods. (The disquietude statisticians feel about this situation is analogous to what physicians might feel if all drugs currently available only with physician's prescription were made available over-the-counter.) Under these circumstances, nonreproducibility and nonvalidity of results are inevitable.

In the journal review process, not infrequently a paper submitted with "state-of-the-art" statistical approaches, clearly explained and documented, is rejected by reviewers and editors on the claim that the readers of the journal would not understand or would not be interested. Reviewers and editors sometimes even demand as a condition of publication that t tests or Pearson r tests be used instead of the state-of-the-art methods, even when these simple methods are neither appropriate nor optimal. Frequently, but not always, the same results can be validly achieved with less complex statistical approaches, in which case they should be (application of Occam's razor). However, to routinely reject papers for necessary complexity or to routinely sacrifice results by demanding less-than-optimal approaches, merely because they are more simple, in essence insulates the psychiatric community from ever upgrading methodological skills. Thus the "horse and buggy" methods remain the mainstay of the field, even with the ready availability not only of "horseless buggies" but also of modern high-speed cars, trains, jets, and perhaps even spaceships.

The focus of this discussion will not be on the general range of statistical methods commonly seen in the psychiatric research literature in the last generation, nor will it be on the range of statistical methods available, because that information is currently readily available to those interested. Instead the focus will be on those issues that within this last generation have become most salient in addressing psychiatric clinical research questions. It is not the *practice* but the *pitfalls and potential* of statistical methods in psychiatric clinical research that will be considered—namely, those factors that are likely to have the greatest impact on future progress in this field.

DIAGNOSIS AND DISORDER

Most fundamental to all psychiatric research is the reliability (precision) and validity (accuracy) of a psychiatric diagnosis. Psychiatric diagnoses are used for selection of patients for a study, defining both inclusion and exclusion criteria. They are used as outcome measures in epidemiological assessment of risk factors, in genetic studies, and in clinical trials. Diagnoses are used in monitoring subjects over time to either (a) assess the development of a disorder, (b) assess the natural history of a disorder or its resolution with treatment, or (c) remove subjects from a study because of emergence of side effects. In short, the quality of diagnosis affects every aspect of every type of psychiatric clinical research. If a diagnosis is not valid (accurate), subjects may be inappropriately included in (or excluded from) a study, and the outcome measures may simply be wrong, possibly biasing all the conclusions based on that study. On the other hand, if the diagnosis is valid but not very reliable (precise), signals are muddled. Sample sizes necessary to detect what is going on must be very large, because the result of low reliability is low power. Therefore, research becomes less efficient. That barrier can sometimes be overcome by enormous expenditure of time or money to generate sample sizes in the hundreds or thousands. But then what is seen in the results of such studies may seem very weak and unimpressive, because effect sizes as well as power are attenuated by unreliability (12). Inadequate reliability and validity of diagnoses used in different studies may be one of the

major sources of inconsistent and nonreproducible results. For all these reasons, the potential of statistical methodology in psychiatric research is fundamentally related to how well the issue of quality of diagnosis can be addressed (see Chapter 71, *this volume*).

Reliability and Validity

A Diagnosis Is Not the Same Thing as a Disorder

A disorder represents something wrong (a disease, an abnormality, an injury, etc.) in the patient. A diagnosis, on the other hand, represents the opinion of a clinician as to whether or not that disorder is present. One can think of a diagnosis as having three independent components:

Diagnosis = Disorder in the patients (A)

+ Characteristics of the patients irrelevant

to the disorder(contaminants) (B)

+ Random error (noninformative

about the patients) (C)

The proportion of variability among patients of a population in the diagnosis directly due to variability among the patient in the disorder is the classical definition of "validity" or accuracy of the diagnosis (schematically $A/(A + B + C)$). The proportion of variability among patients of a population in the diagnosis due to variability either among the patients in disorder or among contaminants is the classical definition of "reliability" or precision of the diagnosis (schematically $(A + B)/(A + B + C)$). It is important to note that under these definitions (from classical measurement theory; e.g., see ref. 18) one cannot speak of the reliability or validity of an individual patient's diagnosis, but only of the reliability or validity of a diagnosis in a population of subjects. Moreover, it should also be clear that, by definition, reliability is always greater than validity. A totally unreliable diagnosis cannot be valid, but a totally reliable diagnosis can be totally invalid. You cannot be completely inconsistent yet always right, but you can be consistently wrong.

Moreover, both the reliability and validity of a diagnosis can and does vary from one population to another. In a population in which the disorder is either very rare or very common, there will be little variability among the subjects in the diagnosis (A), and this variability is easily overcome even by moderate contamination (B) or minor error (C), leading to the so-called base-rate problem.

The base-rate problem is a "red-herring," but it serves as an illustration of how and why misuse of statistical methods arises in psychiatric research.

The Base-Rate Problem

In a 1979 (12) paper on the theoretical underpinnings of the kappa coefficient as a measure of diagnostic reliability, three special cases were used to illustrate a general principle. The first of these asked the reader to fantasize (technical term: assume) a population of subjects made up of two absolutely homogeneous subgroups. In one subgroup, the probability of a positive diagnosis for every single subject on repeated blinded diagnosis was a constant, namely, the sensitivity. In the other subgroup the probability of a positive diagnosis for every single subject was another constant, namely, the complement of specificity or the "false alarm rate." This was a fantasy, because earlier papers in the psychiatric literature had already presented strong evidence that these assumptions seldom approached reality. In the years since, the evidence of the fantastic nature of these assumptions has only become stronger.

In any case, what was shown was that in that fantasized situation, if one selected any subpopulation, no matter how, the kappa coefficient was mathematically related by a specific formula to the prevalence in that subgroup and approached zero in a predictable way whenever the prevalence became very small or very large.

That case was followed by two other illustrations, in which the reader was asked to fantasize (assume) other different situations. The results of the last two cases were quite different from those of the first. In fact, the latter two cases, although based on different fantasies (i.e., assumptions), seem much closer to reality. However, the first case has been repeatedly cited and developed in the psychiatric research literature, and other cases and the fact that all special cases here and elsewhere are limited were ignored. Eventually the results based on that fantasy became some sort of "truth," namely, the base-rate problem.

Reaction to the base-rate problem takes on two forms. One is the claim that the kappa coefficient is a poor choice of measure of reliability because it makes the diagnostician look bad when the base rate (prevalence) is low. That's not the diagnostician's fault. Under this argument, it is suggested that measures other than kappa be used to describe reliability that are kinder and fairer to the diagnosticians, even some that do not well characterize the reproducibility of the diagnosis or the effect of diagnostic error on power or effect size. The other type of reaction is that one should simply learn to live with low kappas for low-base-rate populations. Under this argument, one should be sanguine about a high false-positive and -negative rate in clinical applications when the disorder is a rare (and frequently very serious) one.

The truth of the matter is that every diagnostic procedure has a reliability that may vary from one clinical population to another. In general, the reliability cannot be predicted simply from the prevalence. Actually, reliability depends more on the homogeneity of the population. Low- and high-prevalence populations tend to be homogeneous, and thus tend to have low reliability, but very homogeneous moderate-prevalence populations will also demonstrate low reliability. Generally it is more difficult to detect faint signals. Thus empirically it is more difficult to develop highly reliable procedures for very-low-prevalence or very-high-prevalence populations. However, that merely sounds a warning that it will be very difficult to find true effects of any clinical or policy significance in populations in which the disorder of interest is very rare without investing major effort to find diagnostic procedures for that population that are very reliable.

What types of major effort are necessary are well known. The diagnostic protocol (definitions and rules) must be made clear, the conditions under which the diagnostic protocol can validly be applied should be stipulated and adhered to; and diagnosticians should be well-trained to be consistent in their application of the diagnostic protocol. And if all this does not produce acceptable reliability in a low-prevalence population, it has been known since 1910 (2,22), and most clinicians intuitively understand, that consensus of repeated independent assessments has greater reliability than any one such assessment. Then one can use consensus diagnoses based on the same diagnostic procedure to build up the reliability. This principle has been shown to apply to diagnosis (12), and methods have been proposed as to how to form the appropriate consensus to accomplish this purpose (13). The procedure of having a second or third opinion on each subject in a study may well be costly and time-consuming but may spell the difference between clear, unambiguous findings and non-statistically significant results difficult to publish, statistically significant results that appear to have little clinical significance, or simply inconsistent and confusing results. This becomes all the more important in studying low-prevalence disorders.

To summarize: First, there was an incomplete reading of the statistical literature and the psychiatric research literature, then a poor coordination between the two. What was a special case (defined by certain mathematical assumptions) in the statistical literature, which should have been known from the psychiatric literature seldom to represent clinical reality, was taken as the general case. Then inferences and methodological recommendations were made and applied based on this misreading. When statistical methods are misapplied in psychiatric research, this seems often the process by which such misapplication evolves.

The Problem of Validity of Psychiatric Diagnoses

The same general principles apply to validity. Contaminants of a diagnosis (*B* above) may include factors such as education level, facility with the language, level of cooperation of the patients or their families, and so on. Random error (*C* above) may include patient inconsistencies in the manifestation of symptoms or in the report of patients and their families used in the diagnosis. (When the patient is examined in the morning she says or does one thing, whereas in the afternoon she says or does another, but the disorder remains present or absent.) It may include observer (diagnostician) error or instrumental error (i.e., some problem intrinsic to the diagnostic method). How one designs a study to assess reliability and validity of a diagnostic procedure in a population depends on which B and C sources one is concerned about, and in what population.

Consequently, how strong the influence of irrelevant information (B) is may also vary from population to population, and thus the validity of a diagnosis may vary as well. If a major source of such irrelevant information is related to sociodemographic differences, the reliability or validity in a population of middle-class white subjects may be considerably higher than in a population more heterogeneous in terms of education, race, and income level. It is an inconvenient fact of life that the reliability and validity of a diagnosis must be reestablished for each different population to which it is applied, and by each different research unit who seeks to apply it.

To Establish the Reliability of a Diagnosis

There is considerable disagreement on this related to which sources of error (C) are admitted and omitted, but let me propose minimal standards for the assessment of diagnostic reliability.

1. *Take a sample of subjects from the population to which the results are to apply.* Thus for use in an epidemiological study, one would be typically sampling a low-prevalence population perhaps with major heterogeneity in contaminating factors. For use in a clinical study such as a randomized clinical trial (RCT) evaluating efficacy or effectiveness of a treatment, one would be sampling a clinical population with much higher prevalence and sometimes greater homogeneity. The results from the two reliability studies, even using exactly the very same diagnostic procedure, should be expected to be different, with the same diagnostic procedure likely to prove more reliable in the clinical population than in the epidemiological population. Moreover, how one defines the clinical or the epidemiological population (inclusion and exclusion criteria and site sampled) may also often change the reliability and/or the validity.

2. *For each subject sampled, obtain two or more "blinded" diagnoses from different diagnosticians on separate occasions within a period short enough so that the disorder status of the patient is unlikely to change, but long enough to ensure independence of errors.* Inconsistency within subjects either in the manifestations of signs and symptoms or in their reports seems frequently to be the major source of error, not observer or instrumental error. Thus to judge the reliability of a diagnosis by having two observers review the same mate-

rials (e.g., transcript, videotape) precludes adequate assessment of what may be the major source of error. The resulting inflation of reliability would tend to mislead researchers both in designing their studies and in interpreting their results.

If the period of time between repeated assessments is long enough so that patient's disorder may come or go, what is assessed is a combination of reliability and stability that cannot be separated. If the period of time between repeated assessments is short enough so that the errors of the first assessment are likely simply to be repeated in the second, what is assessed is a combination of reliability and patient consistency in behavior or report that cannot be separated. In either case, the results may be interesting, but not an assessment of diagnostic reliability that would reflect the adequacy of the diagnosis for purposes of clinical decision-making or research.

3. *Use an intraclass kappa as the measure of diagnostic reliability.* The documentation of why kappa (and not some other measure of association between test and retest) is the best advice is extensive and clear (12,15,16) and need not be repeated here.

Questions of the quality of diagnosis have attracted far more research attention in psychiatry than in other medical fields, suggesting that there may be more problems with psychiatric diagnosis than with medical diagnosis in general. Psychiatric clinicians and researchers are typically very surprised to find out that what evidence there is on reliability of diagnosis in other medical fields suggests strongly that the reliability of psychiatric diagnosis in general is neither much better nor much worse than that in other fields of medicine (11). This is an important observation, because one recurrent argument used to delay looking into the validity of psychiatric diagnoses has been that the reliability remains too low to start such studies. It may well be that reluctance to aggressively pursue the issue of validity will, in the long run, make the difference.

4. *If the reliability is not high enough (say greater than 0.4), one could use signal detection methods to assess how many opinions should be used and how they should be combined to obtain acceptable reliability, and then proceed to follow that recommendation in research studies on this population and in clinical applications (13).*

To Establish the Validity of a Diagnosis

It is relatively easy, at least in principle, to establish the reliability of a diagnosis, to increase that reliability if it is not adequate, and to cope with its effects on power and effect size in research. The real challenge is the assessment of validity (21). There has been very little systematic attention to the validity of psychiatric diagnosis. Because the validity of a diagnosis depends on how closely the diagnosis corresponds to the disorder (A

above), there must be some criterion of the presence/absence of the disorder—that is, a "gold standard"—against which to assess the diagnosis. It is repeatedly and correctly stated that such "gold standards" for psychiatric diagnoses do not exist. *Nor do they for other medical diagnoses!*

What differentiates the situation for psychiatric versus other medical disorder seems to be some sort of nonsystematic process of "triangulation." Generally one starts with a "face valid" diagnosis, a diagnostic definition that incorporates the clinical view of the range and importance of symptoms involved in the disorder (as in the DSM approach), often suggested by clinical observation of subjects and their responses to treatment. Then, as one uses that diagnosis in research studies, one slowly gains greater understanding of the etiology, the risk factors, the biological concomitants, the symptomatology, the natural course, or response to treatment that characterizes that disorder and differentiates it from other disorders. This knowledge can then be cycled back to be included in an upgraded diagnostic procedure, thus cycling closer and closer to the goal. As the diagnosis improves, the quality of the research information improves, and thus the diagnosis improves further and faster than before, until some upper limit (usually considerably short of perfection) is reached.

What seems to be missing for psychiatric diagnosis is that process of "cycling back" the results of research studies to upgrade diagnostic procedures. Thus while diagnosis of, for example, coronary artery disease today is far different from what it was a generation ago, having progressed far beyond simple observation and classification of clinical signs and symptoms (and it continues to be updated), the process of diagnosis of schizophrenia and depression over the same period of time has changed very little. It is still focused on simple observation and classification of signs and symptoms.

Fundamentally there is no *one* "gold standard" for the validity of any diagnosis, but instead there are many; none of them are pure "gold," and all of them are changing over time. It is reasonable to use the DSM IIIR as a "gold standard" for the DSM IV if the clinical evidence supports that the DSM IIIR "works," and then to propose to supplant the DSM IIIR by the DSM IV diagnosis if it can also be shown using other "gold standards" that the DSM IV is better than the DSM IIIR (more reliable; more consistent over sites; more closely related to functional impairment; less subject to certain types of contamination; more homogeneous etiology, course, response to treatment, etc.). If that can be done, then the DSM IV becomes the "gold standard" for the next generation of studies. Then if the next generation of studies discloses biological concomitants of a disorder, then perhaps blood and urine tests, imaging, genetic screens, and the like could ultimately become part of the DSM V or VI.

The implementation of such validation studies is greatly facilitated by application of signal detection methods (14,23). These are a body of exploratory procedures in which a "gold standard" (however faulty) is used to assess a set of signs, symptoms, contaminants, biological responses (collectively called "tests"), and any other readily obtained information thought to be relevant to the disorder. The goal is to determine the best choice of "tests," the optimal way of combining these "tests" (symptoms A and B, for example, or symptoms A or B?), and the optimal cutpoints (5 out of 7 symptoms, for example, or 3 out of 7?) to generate optimally sensitive tests, as well as to determine specific or efficient tests for the "gold standard," depending on the relative clinical importance of false-negatives and false-positives. Moreover, one can include considerations of test cost as well as accuracy. Signal detection methods provide tools to do all such tasks that in the formulation of the DSM and other psychiatric diagnostic systems have been done subjectively and without adequate scientific documentation.

Clearly, if such a process were ever to take place in the development of psychiatric diagnoses, what we "know" about the disorders will also change. If the sensitivity of the diagnosis of the disorder increases (and specificity holds steady), one would expect prevalences to increase, onset times to occur earlier, durations of illness to increase, and relapse times to become shorter. If the specificity of the diagnosis of the disorder increases (and sensitivity holds steady), the opposite effects will occur. If both sensitivity and specificity increase, smaller sample sizes will be needed to detect effects of all kinds in research studies, and the effects detected will seem of greater clinical significance, but, most of all, it will be easier to replicate true findings and to achieve consistent results across studies.

Currently a great deal of emphasis is placed on setting criteria so that the prevalence does not change, or setting criteria so that the ICD and the DSM systems are more comparable, or setting criteria to reflect social norms. What would happen if the decision not to use mammography were based on the argument that with its increased sensitivity to early cancers, the prevalence of breast cancer would increase? Or what would happen if we proposed not to use mammography because it is generally not used in Europe (or some other locale) and we want to ensure comparability between diagnosis of cancer in the United States and Europe, or if we proposed not to use mammography because some powerful political pressure group opposed it? Guidelines for use of routine mammography are currently quite controversial, but the basis of the controversy is the question about the accuracy and value of the test to protect the interests of the patients, not considerations such as those above.

THE VALUE AND IMPORTANCE OF LONGITUDINAL RESEARCH

It is much cheaper and easier to do cross-sectional than longitudinal clinical research studies. By far, most psychiatric clinical research studies are, if not strictly cross-sectional (observation of a subject at only one point of time), then, at most, very short term. Even in longitudinal studies, many have analyzed their data in cross-sectional manner. Such studies then have, at best, the same value as serial cross-sectional studies which would have been cheaper, less time-consuming, and less subject to sampling bias (due to dropout over the follow-up time in longitudinal studies). Many of the studies that attempt to present longitudinal perspectives do so with cross-sectional designs using retrospective recall data, or data from records to recreate the history of a subject.

Clinical and research evidence indicates that there are major individual differences among those who at some time during their lifetimes suffer from a psychiatric disorder. Some have quite early onset, others quite late. Some may have a single episode, whereas others may have a succession of episodes. Some, but not all, patients may seek and receive treatment and do so during some episodes and not others. What treatment is received may differ from one episode to another for a subject, and from one subject to another. Whether the effect of the treatment is evanescent, or has influence on all that is to follow for that patient, may vary. Duration of episodes and/or remissions may differ both within and between subjects. Some subjects may completely recover, whereas others may not.

Thus for each subject who ever experiences a psychiatric disorder at any time during the lifetime, the disorder is a process taking place over the lifetime of that individual that can only be fully understood by following that patient over time and observing the time course or trajectory (see Chapter 156, *this volume*). Differences in age of onset, number and duration of episodes, duration of remissions, and occurrence of recovery may be manifestations of fundamentally different disorders (i.e., disorders with different etiology, course, and/or response to treatment) which we may be inadvertently lumping under one diagnostic title. It may also be that certain disorders to which we now assign different diagnostic titles may in fact be manifestations of essentially the same disorder. Without access to a lifetime perspective on the disorder that could only be gained in longitudinal studies, it is difficult to see how such problems can be resolved. Certainly, progress to date does not encourage blind trust that current common research methodologies will rapidly resolve such problems.

Attempts to study certain aspects of lifetime course using retrospective recall in cross-sectional studies generate all the usual problems both with retrospective sampling (Is the availability of the subject sampled into the study itself affected by the disorder?) and with retrospective data and recall. What one recalls may be affected by events that occur between the event and the report. Thus, for example, a brief bout of depression during one's teen years followed by many disorder-free years may be more

likely forgotten by the age of 50 than is one followed by unpleasant subsequent related events (e.g., a suicide attempt) or many later episodes of depression or depression-related outcomes. Analysis of retrospective recall data might then suggest that early-onset depression has a high association with unpleasant subsequent related events and many recurrences when compared to later-onset depression. But that may be purely a statistical artifact.

Use of clinical records to recreate history creates other problems. Experience, particularly in multisite clinical research studies, demonstrates the difficulty in training diagnosticians to acceptable standards of consistency and reliability. That experience makes it less credible that psychiatric diagnoses recorded by psychiatrists and psychologists (and others), who are not trained to uniform standards and who operate over many sites and many years, could be expected to produce consistent, reliable, and valid diagnoses as a basis of clinical research studies done 5, 10, or 20 years later.

Yet, it is unrealistic to propose prospective lifetime follow-up of nationally representative samples for a variety of reasons. Not the least of these is the prohibitive cost of, and delay in, achieving even partial answers to crucial clinical questions. However, it is quite feasible to follow each subject in a study for 3–5 years or so (much longer than current follow-up time), and then (depending on the nature of the research question) to "piece together" information from different cohorts of subjects to begin to understand longer time-course patterns. Such designs have come to be called "accelerated lifetime studies" or "cohort-sequential designs" (1) or "overlapping cohort designs" (20). It is also quite possible in RCTs not merely to follow the subject to the end of treatment, as is typically done, but to follow the subject for a period of 1–3 years later, to check for delayed effects of treatment or maintenance or relapse effects.

Within recent years, excellent and exciting statistical analytic methods have become readily available to deal with such follow-up studies. Two general approaches deserve mention.

Survival methods (8,10,25) deal with research questions concerning time to an event: age of onset, duration of episode or duration of remission, latency to treatment response, and so on. These methods require a well-defined zero point (birth for age of onset, beginning of episode or remission for duration; beginning of treatment for latency to response) and a well-defined event (onset, remission, relapse, response). These methods deal well with irregular follow-up frequency or duration and with censored follow-ups (e.g., patient loss to follow-up or death from a competing cause), some of the most common problems in longitudinal research designs. Such methods concern complete description of survival (Kaplan–Meier curves) under minimal restrictive assumptions, as well as comparisons of survival curves and with identification of factors that predict survival (e.g., Cox proportional hazards model).

Random regression models (growth models, hierarchical linear models, etc.) deal with repeated measures of subjects over time (5,7) (see also Chapter 156, *this volume*). These methods require a well-defined outcome measure that can be validly, reliably, and repeatedly obtained from each subject over the follow-up time. The basic principle of all such methods is that the first step in the analysis examines the trajectory of each individual subject and characterizes that trajectory in one or more clinically meaningful ways (e.g., rate of change over time, peak response over time), and the second step compares subjects on those characterizations (Are subjects in the treatment group likely to improve more rapidly than subjects in the control group?) or assesses the predictors of those characterizations (Is the initial severity of the disorder predictive of the rate of response to treatment?). These methods may be quite simple or, depending on what mathematical assumptions can be reasonably made in a particular context, quite mathematically complex. However, well-applied, they cope well with the problems typical of longitudinal research (irregular follow-up, dropouts, unreliability of measurements, etc.), and offer great power and sensitivity to detect the type of effects most important to psychiatric advances.

Perhaps the most crucial issue to be dealt with in longitudinal studies is that of onset of disorders, both (a) the issue of time of onset and (b) factors predicting onset. This is urgent for three reasons: (i) Understanding the etiology of psychiatric disorders may fundamentally require observations before, at, or immediately after the onset of the disorder; (ii) efforts to prevent mental disorders absolutely require knowing the time and risk factors for onset; and (iii) it may be, as it is in cancer, heart disease, and other disorders, that responsivity to treatment is closely related to how early in the course of the disorder the treatment is initiated. It may be that the lack of effectiveness of many psychiatric treatments may be related simply to the fact that they are initiated too late in the disease process.

FITTING MATHEMATICAL MODELS TO THE "REAL WORLD" VERSUS FITTING THE "REAL WORLD" TO MATHEMATICAL MODELS

A Problem in Analysis

Long ago, Feinstein (6) most eloquently summarized an issue now most crucial to the future of psychiatric clinical research: ". . . mathematics has only the secondary role of providing lines and colors for the map; the main goal is the identification of different clinical terrains. Mathematics has no value in helping us understand nature

unless we begin by understanding nature. To start with mathematical formulations and to alter nature so that it fits the assumptions is a procrustean 'non sequitur' unfortunately all too prevalent in 'contemporary science.' What emerges is tenable and sometimes even elegant as mathematics, but is too distorted by its initial assumptions to be a valid representation of what goes on in nature."

Without exception, every statistical inference procedure (i.e., any procedure by which we try to understand what goes on in a population of subjects by studying a sample from that population) is based on a certain number of mathematical assumptions. These assumptions are of four types:

1. *Those guaranteed by the design.* The assumption that subjects were randomly assigned to treatment and control groups is guaranteed by implementing a random process to do so. The assumption that errors or measurement are independent is guaranteed by blinding all assessors to data coming from other sources.

2. *Those empirically shown to correspond reasonably well to reality in the context.* Thus the assumption of equal variance in two groups of subjects can be checked by comparing the observed variances in the two groups. The assumption that two variables are linearly related can be checked by examining a scatter diagram of those variables.

3. *Those assumptions from which it can be mathematically demonstrated deviations do not seriously compromise the inference (robustness).* Thus, for example, if the sample sizes are equal, the two-sample *t* test is remarkably robust to deviations from equal variance assumptions. There are many studies showing that a Pearson product moment correlation coefficient is quite robust to deviations from the assumption that both variables being correlated have normal distribution (but nonrobust to deviations from the assumption that they are linearly related and equal variance assumptions).

4. *Those assumptions that are fantasies; that is, they do not correspond to reality, and there is no robustness to protect the inferences.* As suggested above, fantastic assumptions are dangerous. In a purely mathematical or logical exercise, one can make any assumptions one wishes, because what follows is understood to be true only conditional on the assumptions (i.e., the conclusions are just as fantastic as the assumptions, no more and no less). Thus in a mathematical or logical exercise, if one wished to assume that the sun rose in the west, or that objects fall up instead of down, there is no impediment to doing so. It is clearly understood that what follows has no validity in the real world because the assumptions are clearly untrue in the real world. It is only a mathematical or logical exercise, no more.

However, when one is dealing with issues related to the health and well-being of patients, as one does in clinical practice or research, one cannot be casual about what assumptions are made. It is the responsibility of the ethical medical researcher to check those assumptions, lest fantastic ones do harm, and it is the responsibility of the ethical biostatistician to bring those assumptions to the attention of the medical researchers to make sure they are checked.

The consequences of not avoiding fantasies in psychiatric clinical research has been given a resounding empirical demonstration in recent years: Either every reported finding of a linkage for a psychiatric disorder to date has been refuted upon attempt to replicate or confirm, or, worse yet, the results have had to be retracted by those researchers reporting the finding. This situation is exactly what sound biostatistics in medical clinical research is meant to prevent.

The mathematical models used in these studies are sound, having proven their value in other fields of medicine in finding linkages for breast cancer, for Huntington's chorea, and so on. It is their application to psychiatric disorders that seems to foment the problem. What's so different about their application to psychiatric disorders?

First of all, genetic linkage analysis is based on the assumption that those labeled "affected" have the disorder and those "nonaffected" do not—that is, diagnoses are (at least reasonably) valid and reliable. In psychiatric linkage studies, whatever the disorder, there are multiple diagnoses that can be used to create these labels and that often conflict with each other. Indeed many research proposals suggest trying several different ways of labeling those with and without one disorder in the same study. Just that fact calls into question the validity of the labeling of "affected" versus "nonaffected."

For any one of these diagnostic procedures, the evidence is clear that there is substantial unreliability of diagnosis; that is, if someone labeled "affected" were independently evaluated by several other expert diagnosticians using the same diagnostic system, there would frequently be disagreement. When the label of "affected" is applied based on either self-report, family report, or abstracted clinical records from the distant past, one encounters even more serious questions about validity and reliability. The fact that multiple readers of the same, possibly flawed, clinical report or record would draw the same conclusion, often reported as the "reliability" of the diagnosis, is not assurance of either the precision or accuracy of what appears in the record or the report.

The effect of unreliability (taking validity for granted for the moment) is to attenuate the power of statistical tests. Therefore, in the case of genetic linkage analysis, unreliability will attenuate the logarithm of the odds (LOD) score, making it harder to find positive results (false or true). Consequently, if unreliability were the only problem, and the only purpose of a genetics linkage analysis was to decide whether there is evidence sufficient to support a claim of linkage, the assumption of reliability

would tend to fall under the third category of assumptions above, because the reports of positive results would be robust to deviations from this assumption.

However, such robustness provides little real protection here, because that protection applies only if *one* genetic linkage analysis were applied using only *one* diagnostic rule, and examining only *one* locus. Then the current methods would have *less than* a 5% chance of a false-positive finding. However, when *multiple* different diagnostic rules are used and *multiple* loci are tested, and frequently *multiple* assessments of each locus, the probability of a false-positive finding increases directly with the number of multiple tests. Given enough families, enough different diagnostic rules, enough different loci, and enough different analytic approaches, it is almost certain that a false-positive finding will result. (This has been called the "Gambler's Ruin" problem in classical statistics.)

The statistical methods underlying genetic linkage analyses (and many of the other most common statistical tests) are based on likelihood ratio theory. The fundamental step in such methods is multiplying together the probabilities of *independent* outcomes (e.g, see ref. 19, p. 27ff). In practice, this means that the diagnosis of each member of a family must be made "blind" to all other diagnoses and to genetic typing, and that genetic typing must be made "blind" to diagnoses, so that the errors of classification are independent.

One cannot label one subject with an ambiguous clinical picture "affected" because the diagnostician knows that the subject's mother and both sisters have already been labeled "affected," when another subject, whose clinical picture is similar, is labeled "unaffected" because there are no other known "affected" members in the same family. Obtaining diagnoses from recall and clinical records becomes even more troublesome than usual, because one can never guarantee the independence necessary. How can one be sure that Dr. X, 20 years ago, did not decide to label this subject "depressed" partially because he knew that depression "ran in the family"?

Without independence of errors, guaranteed by "blinded" diagnoses, the likelihood functions are invalid and all the estimation and testing procedures based on them are also invalid. Thus if "blindness" is not guaranteed in the design of a genetic study, since existing methods require blindness and the results are not robust to deviations from this assumption, there are no known valid methods for analyzing for genetic linkage.

Finally, many genetic linkage analyses are based on an assumption of known mode of inheritance. As is true in many other areas of science, there is a progression of studies necessary to resolve a question (like Phase 1, 2, 3 drug trials, for example). There is a natural progression of genetic studies as well: (i) family studies (or the like) to show that there is some sort of familial transmission; (ii) twin or adoption studies (or the like) to show that the familial transmission detected above is indeed to some extent genetic transmission; (iii) segregation studies (or the like) to delineate the nature of the genetic transmission found above; (iv) linkage studies (or the like) to locate the general locus of the particular genetic transmission delineated above; and (v) molecular biology studies to locate the gene and its products.

In the absence of segregation studies (in the same population with the same diagnosis), the mode of transmission necessary for linkage studies can be assumed, but the assumption may be a fantasy. Frequently the analysis of each diagnosis, each locus, and each method is repeated under several different fantastic assumptions of mode of inheritance, which even further increases the probability of a false-positive.

In short, that false-positive reports of psychiatric genetic linkages abound is no surprise. In any research context in which mathematical assumptions so crucial to the validity of results have been so casually dealt with, false-positive and false-negative results can be anticipated, but, of course, it is the false-positive results that are published.

Moreover, this problem is probably not restricted to psychiatric genetic linkage studies. Complex mathematical models, such as those in structural equation models, in Lisrel models, in path analyses models, and so on, are based on many mathematical assumptions that either must be guaranteed in the design of the research or must be checked against empirical evidence, or the inferences must be mathematically demonstrated to be robust against deviations from those assumptions (9). However, there are so many such assumptions that generally few are guaranteed and few are checked. It may be that the only reason this problem has become recently so salient in psychiatric genetics and not much earlier in other such complex mathematical modeling is simply that it is more customary in genetic research to seek immediate replication than it has been in other research areas.

The easiest solution to such problems is simply to restrict use of such complex analytic models only to *exploratory* studies to generate one very specific hypotheses (one diagnosis, one mode of inheritance, one locus, one analytic approach). When that specific hypothesis appears clear to the researchers from the exploratory study, they would be required to test that one hypothesis in a carefully designed independent focused study before publication of the "finding." In the genetic linkage framework, for example, this would mean that the initial studies reporting linkage would have been considered pilot studies, and publication would have been delayed until after independent confirmation. If this had earlier been the case, none of the earlier findings would ever have appeared in the literature. However, such a strategy would require that there would have to be a new willingness to invest major funding resources in pilot studies, and perhaps new design strategies that would provide for independent replication

concomitant with the pilot study proposal would have to be evolved.

A Problem in Design

Another aspect of problems with the relationship between what clinical research does and the "real world" has to do with efficacy, effectiveness, and efficiency of treatments (e.g., see ref. 4). Because these terms are not precisely and consistently defined in clinical research publications and often seem to be used interchangeably, but carry important implications for clinical research, let us begin with some proposed definitions.

To demonstrate *efficacy,* a study must show that in ideally selected subjects under ideal conditions the treatment "works." To demonstrate *effectiveness,* a study must show that in typical subjects with the disorder under conditions that can apply in the real world, the treatment "works" in some clinically meaningful sense. To demonstrate *efficiency,* a study must show that the effectiveness is achieved at reasonable cost.

For a variety of reasons, most clinical research studies of treatment have focused on efficacy. Exclusion criteria used in sampling are frequently so strict that the sample may actually represent a small and unrepresentative minority of the clinical population with the disorder. The conditions of delivering treatment are often those that would be impossible to enact in "real world" application. Such restrictions (a) maximize the probability that the treatment will "work" in the study and (b) minimize the probability that it will work in the real world. In an efficacy study, the sample sizes needed to detect effects will be smaller, both because the size of effects is maximized and the heterogeneity is minimized. Consequently the time and effort needed to do such studies are more limited. Because demonstration of efficacy is generally all that the FDA requires of drug companies to licence new drugs, this approach is very attractive for drug-company-sponsored pharmacologic RCTs, and such studies are emulated in other contexts.

With no requirement that the outcome measures (which define that the treatment "work") have clear clinical interpretation (which would be needed to demonstrate effectiveness) and no requirement for cost/risk measures (needed to demonstrate efficiency), treatments found to "work" in efficacy studies run a high risk that, when applied in the "real world," they will not live up to their billing. Thus the result of a "successful" efficacy study may be a recommendation for an ineffective and inefficient treatment. In the absence of emphasis on checking such results for effectiveness and efficiency, there is no protection against noneffective treatments going into widespread use, and there is little protection against unnecessary costs and risks to the patients.

This problem is probably not more common in evaluations of psychiatric than of other medical treatments. However, in this era of health care reform, this problem may have greater impact on psychiatry than on other medical areas, because the somewhat negative perceptions of the cost–benefit balance of psychiatry treatments in "real world" applications may have a major impact in the years to come on coverage and availability of psychiatry treatments and funding for psychiatric research. The research materials (efficacy studies) that psychiatric clinical research has forged to fight these perceptions and to document the value of psychiatric treatments may well be found ineffectual to counteract current perceptions.

This is not to argue against studies of efficacy. It is extraordinarily difficult to design cost-effective research studies of effectiveness or efficiency of treatments without preliminary studies of efficacy. Efficacy studies are needed to (a) establish the feasibility of effectiveness and efficiency studies, (b) estimate clinical effect sizes needed for power calculations, and (c) field-test the methodologies (e.g., measurements, designs). For this reason, efficacy studies must continue to be supported. However, they should be short-term and low-cost studies, done as a preliminary to effectiveness and efficiency studies, not as an end in themselves. Then effectiveness and efficiency studies should (a) deal with samples representative of the clinical population with the disorder, (b) deliver treatments under the conditions that can be duplicated in ordinary clinical settings, (c) evaluate the effects of the treatments using measures that have clinical meaning, and (d) strive to evaluate the costs and risks to the patients. Then their results are more likely to generalize to the "real world." The risk, of course, is that many treatments now favored may prove to be ineffective or inefficient, and studies documenting this will be used to decrease patients' access to such treatments. Perhaps it is this fear that makes studies of effectiveness or efficiency so unattractive to psychiatric researchers.

A MORE FLEXIBLE STRUCTURE IN PSYCHIATRIC RESEARCH?

The above discussions clarify that a major unresolved problem in the future of psychiatric clinical research is that of the value placed on exploratory research and the support afforded for such studies. Exploratory studies are often labeled with derogatory terms such as "fishing expeditions," "data dredging," and so on, and are not generally favorably viewed for funding, nor are their results favorably viewed for publication. Consequently, there is little incentive to propose or to do such studies.

Yet there is little chance of designing cost-effective *confirmatory* research projects without the data and experience that can only be gained from *exploratory* studies of various kinds. The discouragement of well-designed and well-executed exploratory studies may have contrib-

uted to the tendency to make premature jumps to confirmatory analyses (e.g., jumping to linkage studies without segregation studies) or to make premature generalization from limited confirmatory analyses (e.g., recommending for or against treatments on the basis of efficacy studies in absence of effectiveness or efficiency studies). Well-done exploratory studies submitted for review are often inappropriately reported by reviewers and editors to be confirmatory studies; this is done by presenting hypotheses as if they were a priori when they are in fact post hoc, or by presenting invalid p values.

Clearly there are exploratory studies that merit derogatory labels, studies whose sampling, design, measurement, and analytic approaches are so poorly formulated or executed that one should not accept any results, even as preliminary indications or hypotheses generated for later testing. But there are poorly done confirmatory studies as well. Perhaps the time has come, and perhaps the need is urgent, that the distinction be made between good and bad studies; furthermore, it must be acknowledged that a good study may be either exploratory or confirmatory, but admitted that a bad study may be either exploratory or confirmatory as well. Both approaches, exploratory and confirmatory, have their important place in clinical research, and neither approach can be excellently done without the other.

CONCLUSIONS

To resolve the methodological/statistical problems that have been identified or have arisen in the last generation of psychiatric research, there seem to be three urgent needs:

1. Better training of psychiatrists in statistical principles and better training of statisticians in psychiatric principles.
2. Changes in funding and publication policy to foster a greater tolerance for well-done exploratory research and a greater intolerance for badly done research whether exploratory or confirmatory. This would, of course, require a clear understanding of the differences between exploratory and confirmatory research approaches, and the place and value of both.
3. Better communication between psychiatric researchers and statisticians working in psychiatric research areas. Proposals of mathematical models based on assumptions that misrepresent psychiatric situations should not be tolerated by either the psychiatrists or the statisticians involved. Because one would not expect the usual statistician to be expert in psychiatry, nor would one expect the usual psychiatrist to be expert in statistics, this means a very close interactive collaboration, so that each expertise is well-represented.

George Santayana said: "Progress, far from consisting

in change, depends on retentiveness. . . . When experience is not retained, as among savages, infancy is perpetual. Those who cannot remember the past are condemned to repeat it.'' It would be most interesting to see what the next generation of progress in psychiatric clinical research might be if we remembered and learned from our methodological errors of the past.

REFERENCES

1. Anderson ER. Analyzing change in short-term longitudinal research using cohort-sequential designs. *J Consult Clin Psychol* 1993; 61:929–940.
2. Brown W. Some experimental results in the correlation of mental abilities. *Br J Psychol* 1910;3:296–322.
3. De Groot MH, Mezzich JE. Psychiatric Statistics. In: Atkinson AC, Feinberg SE, eds. *A celebration of statistics.* New York: Springer-Verlag, 1985;146–165.
4. Donabedian A. The seven pillars of quality. *Arch Pathol Lab Med* 1990;114:1115–1118.
5. Ekstrom D, Quade D, Golden R. Statistical analysis of repeated measures in psychiatric research. *Arch Gen Psychiatry* 1990; 47:770–774.
6. Feinstein AR. *Clinical judgment.* New York: Robert E Krieger Publishing Company, 1967;16.
7. Gibbons RD, Hedeker D, Watermaux C, Kraemer HC, Greenhouse JB. Some conceptual and statistical issues in the analysis of longitudinal psychiatric data. *Arch Gen Psychiatry* 1993;50:739–750.
8. Greenhouse J, Stangl D, Bromberg J. An introduction to survival analysis: statistical methods for the analysis of clinical trial data. *J Consult Clin Psychol* 1989;57:536–544.
9. Junker B, Pilkonis P. Personality and depression: modeling and measurement issues. In: Klein MH, Kupfer DJ, Shea MT, eds. *Personality and depression.* New York: Guilford Press, 1993;171–177.
10. Kalbfleisch JD, Prentice RL. *The statistical analysis of failure time data.* New York: John Wiley & Sons, 1980.
11. Koran LM. The reliability of clinical methods, data, and judgments. *N Engl J Med* 1975;293:642–646, 695–701.
12. Kraemer HC. Ramifications of a population model for k as a coefficient of reliability. *Psychometrika* 1979;44:461–472.
13. Kraemer HC. How many raters? Toward the most reliable diagnostic consensus. *Stat Med* 1992;11:317–331.
14. Kraemer HC. *Evaluating medical tests: objective and quantitative guidelines.* Newbury Park: Sage Publications, 1992.
15. Kraemer HC. Measurement of reliability for categorical data in medical research. *Stat Methods Med Res* 1992;1:183–199.
16. Kraemer HC, Bloch DA. Kappa coefficients in epidemiology: an appraisal of a reappraisal. *J Clin Epidemiol* 1988;41:959–968.
17. Kraemer HC, Pruyn JP, Gibbons RD, Greenhouse JB, Grochocinski VJ, Waternaux C, Kupfer D. Methodology in psychiatric research: report on the 1986 MacArthur Foundation Network I Methodology Institute. *Arch Gen Psychiatry* 1987;44:1100–1106.
18. Lord FM, Novick MR. *Statistical theories of mental test scores.* Reading, MA: Addison–Wesley, 1968.
19. Ott J. *Analysis of human genetic linkage.* Baltimore: Johns Hopkins University Press, 1985.
20. Raudenbush SW, Chan W-S. Application of a hierarchical linear model to the study of adolescent deviance in an overlapping cohort design. *J Consult Clin Psychol* 1993;61:941–951.
21. Robins LN, Barrett JE. *The validity of psychiatric diagnosis.* New York: Raven Press, 1989.
22. Spearman C. Correlation calculated from faulty data. *Br J Psychol* 1910;3:271–295.
23. Swets JA, Pickett RM. *Evaluation of diagnostic systems: methods from signal detection theory.* New York: Academic Press, 1982.
24. White SF. Statistical errors in papers in the *British Journal of Psychiatry. Br J Psychiatry* 1979;135:336–342.
25. Willet JB, Singer JD. Investigation onset, cessation, relapse, and recovery: why you should, and how you can, use discrete-time survival analysis to examine even occurrence. *J Consult Clin Psychol* 1993;61:952–965.

Psychopharmacology: The Fourth Generation of Progress, edited by Floyd E. Bloom and David J. Kupfer. Raven Press, Ltd., New York © 1995.

CHAPTER 158

New Drug Design in Psychopharmacology

The Impact of Molecular Biology

John F. Tallman and Svein G. Dahl

The design of therapeutics for the treatment of neurological and psychiatric disorders has undergone a number of epochs or phases in the modern era. One of the earliest examples in the first generation was the discovery (36) that antihistamines (promethazine) could lead to drowsiness which might be useful in the treatment of psychiatric disorders, including schizophrenia. This serendipitous discovery led to the development of chlorpromazine. By demonstrating that a drug could influence the course of a chronic disorder, chlorpromazine not only revolutionized treatment in psychiatry but also brought legitimacy to the concept of biological psychiatry.

A second phase of progress involved the use of in vivo animal models in the setting of pharmaceutical discovery research that led to the discovery (again serendipitous) of the sedating, muscle-relaxant, and taming effects of chlordiazepoxide, and ultimately to many other benzodiazepines (51). The increasing use of biochemical models (e.g., monoamine reuptake and metabolism) and the incorporation of biochemistry into pharmacological receptor theory (e.g., the discovery of adenylate cyclase) led to a third phase of progress in which in vitro methodology was used to discover drug candidate leads. This list (L-dopa, tricyclic antidepressants, etc.) is quite long and contains many of the therapeutics discussed throughout this volume.

A landmark study for drug identification and design was the discovery of specific radioligand binding to the opiate receptor (47); this study ultimately led to the biochemical identification of the multiple receptor subtypes within a number of neurotransmitter families. Such a multiplicity of subtypes had previously been predicted indirectly through pharmacological measurements of both in vivo and in vitro activities of agonists and antagonists. Over the last 20 years, the precision of drug design has been assisted by the study of receptor binding affinities and receptor localization.

The cloning of receptor molecules and other advances in molecular biology, together with the development of high-powered computers and software for calculation of three-dimensional molecular structures, holds promise for the fourth and perhaps the most precise period where new drug candidates are developed by rational design from the three-dimensional structures of target molecules. The isolation of individual receptor proteins by virtue of their pharmacological and high-affinity binding properties has allowed the determination of portions of their primary amino acid sequence. In turn, this has resulted in the isolation of the primary nucleic acid sequence coding for these receptors and the discovery of hitherto undetected similarities between receptors for distantly related neurotransmitter receptors and differences within what were thought to be single receptor subtypes. It is these studies in this fourth phase of progress that are the focus of this review with the particular perspective of indicating how they will impact molecular design and discovery within the pharmaceutical industry (see Chapters 2, 3, 9, 10, 11, 27, 38, and 61, *this volume,* for related issues).

THE TOOLS OF MODERN DRUG DISCOVERY

Isolation of Cloned Receptors

Four techniques have been of value in identifying the novel lead clones in individual receptor and channel fami-

J. F. Tallman: Neurogen Corporation, Branford, Connecticut 06405.

S. G. Dahl: Department of Pharmacology, Institute of Medical Biology, University of Tromsö, N-9037 Tromsö, Norway.

lies. Each has its advantages and disadvantages and its proponents. All are characterized by the need for a great degree of cleverness, persistence, and luck for their success. A flow chart for proceeding from pharmacological activity to clone is shown in Fig. 1.

The first technique is to identify a partial amino acid sequence of the receptor protein to be cloned; the immediate limitation is that enough protein must be available for microsequencing. Using degenerate oligonucleotides covering all the possibilities of cDNA coding for this protein sequence, a cDNA library prepared from mRNA of a tissue enriched for the receptor of interest is screened and a number of partial- or full-length clones are identified, isolated, and sequenced. The open reading frames are identified and the full length of the receptor is determined.

The advantage of this approach is that the sequence of the cDNA codes exactly for the protein that is expressed in the tissue of interest. If the screening is done at high stringency, unique clones are identified and the full amino acid structure of the receptor is elucidated. One of the first receptor clones on record, that of the α subunit of the *Torpedo californica* acetylcholine receptor, was obtained this way over 10 years ago (45).

The disadvantages of this method of screening for clones is that if the known sequence of amino acids is not unique or if the amino acids are coded for by highly degenerate triplets, multiple inconsistent clones are identified. A second problem is that partial sequences from non-full-length clones are identified but full-length sequences cannot be obtained. This problem arises because of the nature of the construction of the library from mRNA by reverse transcriptase and its lack of specific proofreading mechanisms or large amounts of nontranslated RNA that may be in the native mRNA. This is a persistent problem

with any type of screen that does not rely on functional activity and particularly hampered the original identification of dopamine D4 receptors (64). The solution chosen by these investigators was to splice a portion of sequence derived from the genomic form of the receptor to the cloned cDNA; while this was a clever approach at the time, recent studies of the AMPA-type glutamate receptor subunits indicate that post-transcriptional modifications may alter critical amino acids due to base modification as the mRNA is processed in the cell (56). This modification is enzymatic and appears to be under specific control separate from that of the gene being expressed; the prevalence and distribution of this enzyme and its function are obscure at the present time. A more vexing problem for the resulting D4 receptor clone was the presence of an intron in the genomic sequence that limited high-level expression of this clone in some cell lines. An intron-deleted form of the dopamine D4 receptor or synthetic gene has led to much higher levels of receptor expression (*unpublished results*).

The use of functional expression of a receptor to be cloned without significant structural information would appear to circumvent many of the problems described above. Here a constructed library in an expression vector or mRNA itself is used to create a receptor protein in a recipient cell. The cells are then screened for a particular pharmacological activity and the library is subdivided; successive iterations lead to a pure clone. The difficulties of this approach beyond library construction are the need to have very specific assay systems that can determine receptor presence through binding or functional activity. For the biochemical approach, a very-high-affinity ligand of high specific activity, usually iodine-labeled, is needed to allow the detection of a vanishingly small number of positive cells among many possible false leads. For the functional approach, an expression system (such as the *Xenopus* oocytes) and a specific functional assay are needed. Ionotropic receptor family members for which a single subunit can create a channel are the best candidates for this approach. In this case the response element is built into the protein itself and exogenous transducers, like G proteins, are not required. A real limitation of this approach is that proteins which require other subunits to function (multimeric proteins) or interact with other proteins that are not expressed in the cell to carry out their function are not amenable to cloning in this way. As examples, this approach has led to the cloning of (a) the only serotonin receptor (5-HT$_3$) in the ionotropic or ligand-gated superfamily (41) and (b) the 5HT$_{2c}$ (formerly called 5HT$_{1c}$) receptor, a G-protein-linked receptor. The 5HT$_{1c}$ receptor was identified by using its specific pharmacology along with multistep activation (G-protein-mediated) of an endogenous Ca^{2+}-gated Cl$^-$ channel in *Xenopus* oocytes (37).

The third approach derives intellectually from the old studies of inborn errors of metabolism and the isolation

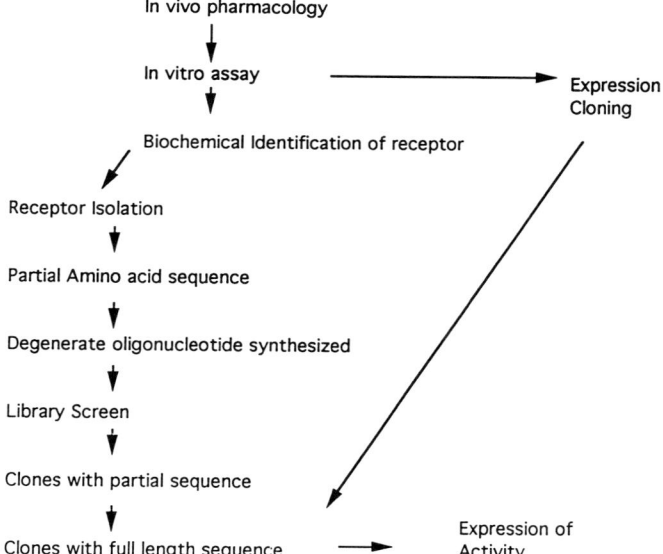

FIG. 1. Steps in the process from pharmacological activity to clone.

of mutant proteins from patients with such disorders. The major success thus far in the channel area has been the isolation of voltage-dependent potassium channels from a *Drosophila* mutant *Shaker,* identified phenotypically because the flies convulsively twitch their legs upon exposure to ether. The identification of the A current and the isolation of genomic clones in the vicinity of the *Shaker* mutation led (by chromosomal walking) to the *Shaker* gene. Here the nucleic acid sequence and gene were cloned before the protein was isolated and identified as the potassium channel (29). No novel receptor genes have yet been identified in this precise way.

The fourth major method for discovering novel clones is through screening of libraries with previously discovered clones at reduced stringency, by using sequences common to members of the superfamily as probes, or by using these sequences as primers for polymerase chain reaction (PCR)-based techniques (16). These are by far the most widely used techniques and account for the discovery and identification of most monoamine and peptide receptor genes described to date. Here investigators have been assisted by the unexpectedly large similarities across a great variety of receptors in the G-protein-linked superfamily. Such techniques also account for the discovery of most of the GABA, glutamate, and other ionotropic receptor subunits. Most of the later references of this chapter report receptors identified by these methods. Clearly, the methods are efficient at proliferating subtypes, but are dependent upon a starting point within a family and some knowledge of a potential relationship between receptors (see Chapters 7, 8, 11, 27, and 38, *this volume*).

PCR-based techniques can identify novel orphan clones of unknown sequence (43). However, almost everyone who has worked with these techniques also can report the amplification of unknown sequences from contaminating materials in their libraries or reagents. This can be most vexing because subcloning and sequencing are needed to separate new and interesting sequences from the false leads. Most frequently these PCR-generated sequences are not long enough to contain the entire coding sequence of a receptor, and these sequences are used for further library screens. The list of full-length putative receptor proteins in search of a function, or orphan clones, is increasing and provide unique challenges to those who discover them. Among the receptors that were identified as orphan clones is the cannabinoid receptor, derived first from a tachykinin receptor (27). Some of the mas oncogenes related to the seven-transmembrane spanning region proteins have been found as orphan clones (67).

Expression Systems and Their Applications

A number of methods to express the protein coded for by the cDNA after it has been cloned have been used.

While yeast and bacterial systems can yield the largest amounts of protein for study, their use in expression of mammalian receptors has been limited. In an interesting series of experiments, two forms of human β-adrenergic receptor cDNA have been expressed in *Escherichia coli* and show insertion into bacterial membranes and interactions with G proteins (14). However, bacteria do not generally carry out post-translational modification such as leader sequence removal, intron deletion, glycosylation, and so on, and animal cells are generally much more useful.

Xenopus oocytes are the traditional cells for expression of ion channels and ionotropic receptors. Each oocyte is individually injected with mRNA prepared in vitro from the cDNA; this allows functional studies to be easily carried out, but oocytes are not very useful for biochemical studies. One of us (JFT) has adapted this system to routine drug screening as part of a drug discovery program. Affinity and efficacy at several GABA$_a$ receptor subtypes can be determined for a single drug in one day's work; structure–activity relationships can be developed. Large-scale screening of libraries of compounds is not possible with this technique, and it is most useful for lead optimization and modeling.

Mammalian expression systems have been useful for the G-protein-linked family of receptors, and many cell lines permanently expressing single receptors have been developed. Large amounts of cell membrane and passage of cells through a number of generations yield enough material for large-scale screens. Frequently, the specific G protein that the native receptor interacts with is not present in the recipient cell, and this is a limitation of the mammalian cell expression. While adenylate cyclase is used in many cases as a surrogate measure, it is known that a much wider diversity of intracellular messages are controlled by receptors in vivo. Almost any fibroblastoid cell can serve as a recipient, and cookbooks of molecular biology describe the many methods for transfection. The expression of multisubunit proteins is more difficult because of the statistical possibilities for expression of one, two,or more subunits in a single cell. A recent advance in virology and molecular biology of insect viruses has allowed the development of a method based upon the baculovirus infection of insect cells to be applied to receptor expression. The advantages of this system are that very high levels of multimeric proteins can be produced and that control of the absolute levels of infection and ratios of subunits used can be obtained (38). The disadvantage is that the cells that express the receptors are insect cells and may not be identical to mammalian cells in their processing of proteins. This system can easily produce enough receptor protein for library screening of either a pharmaceutical library (archives of compounds synthesized by a company), natural product libraries, or various combinatorial libraries (peptides, nucleic acids, heterocyclic compounds). From these libraries, leads can be obtained for the identification of novel receptor-specific drugs.

Computational Chemistry and Molecular Modeling

When the three-dimensional structure of a receptor molecule is known, new potential drug molecules may be custom-tailored, by molecular modeling techniques, to precisely fit into a binding pocket on the receptor. This approach has been called "structure-based" or "rational" drug design, as opposed to more random synthesis and screening of a series of substances. Over the last 20 years, three-dimensional structures of many proteins have been determined by x-ray crystallographic methods, which has shed new light on their mode of action. Methods of modern molecular biology have made it possible to produce larger quantities of pure receptor material than did previous conventional methods. However, neurotransmitter receptors have several hydrophobic segments in the peptide chain, which probably represent domains of the protein that are embedded into the cell membrane. This makes it difficult to purify and crystallize receptor proteins, and a detailed x-ray crystallographic structure determination of any such receptor has not yet been reported. We and others have therefore used molecular modeling techniques to build three-dimensional receptor models from the amino acid sequences, and have used these models to study the molecular mechanisms of drug–receptor interactions.

Modern molecular modeling techniques contain four key elements: computer graphics, quantum mechanical calculations, molecular mechanical calculations, and molecular dynamics simulations. Computer graphic visualization of the spatial arrangement of atoms and the distribution of electrostatic potentials in molecules has proven to be a powerful tool for explaining structure–activity relationships of biologically active compounds. High-resolution graphics computers offering stereo viewing, real-time translation, and rotation of molecular models are now available for prices not much higher than those for common workstations. Such computers enable assembly of various parts of a receptor model (such as a seven- or five-helical bundle), as well as inspection of how the various receptor segments fit to each other, to be done by interactive computer graphics techniques.

Energy Minimization of Molecular Models

Quantum mechanical methods allow relatively accurate calculation of molecular structures and electrostatic potentials of small molecules, but require far too much computing time to be applicable for calculations of protein structures. Molecular mechanics calculations are less accurate but a lot faster, and they enable refinement of a protein structure with several hundred amino acid residues

to be done on a workstation. The method requires a set of atomic coordinates to start the calculation from. This may be a crystal structure, a molecular model built by interactive computer graphics, or a structure obtained during a molecular dynamics simulation.

Structure refinement by molecular mechanics calculations separates overlapping atoms and usually corrects unrealistic bond lengths and angles. The method does not, however, change a molecular structure across conformational energy barriers, but merely searches for the nearest minimum in the potential energy of the molecule. Once a receptor model has been built by interactive computer graphics or by other methods, it therefore more or less retains its overall structure after molecular mechanical energy minimization.

Molecular Dynamics Simulations

Most of the receptor models that have been proposed up to now were built and examined as static structures. However, proteins in their native state in cells have constantly changing geometries, with movements occurring on a femtosecond (10^{-15} sec) time scale. Molecular dynamics simulations have been used to (a) study the naturally occurring internal movements in proteins and other biologically active molecules and (b) refine three-dimensional molecular structures. Such simulations, which always are started from an energy-minimized molecular structure, involve a large number of computational steps. Simulations of macromolecules, even over a period of a few picoseconds (10^{-12} sec), are therefore facilitated by using a supercomputer. In molecular dynamics simulations, kinetic energy is added to the molecular system. A structure may therefore move across conformational barriers and undergo substantial changes during such simulations. For example, a seven-helical protein model may change from an initial circular arrangement of the helices into a more oval and bacteriorhodopsin-like shape during 20–25 psec of molecular dynamics simulation (10,28)

Receptor Modeling

The classical experiments of Anfinsen (1) suggested that all information required to direct the folding of a protein into its tertiary structure lies in the amino acid sequence. Prediction of secondary and tertiary structures from the amino acid sequence has, however, proven to be extremely difficult, and no generally applicable method for accurate prediction of tertiary protein structures has yet been found. Receptor models therefore have to be based on structural data in addition to the primary structure of the protein. Results from cloning, expression, and ligand binding studies of site-specific mutants and chimeric receptors have been particularly useful for construction and refinement of neurotransmitter receptor models.

Such receptor models are often built from α-helical models of each membrane-spanning segment. These are constructed from the amino acid sequence, and they are assembled by interactive computer graphics or by automated superposition upon an other receptor model. Particular residues postulated to be directly involved in ligand binding are often used to determine the relative positions of individual helices. Several models of G-protein-linked receptors that have been published contain only the seven transmembrane α-helices; these models were constructed by superposition on a model of the membrane-spanning α-helices in bacteriorhodopsin, based on electron diffraction data (22). Other receptor models have also included the loops between helices and the terminal parts (3,10,39,60). The receptor models are usually refined by molecular mechanical energy minimization. Some have also been refined by molecular dynamics simulations, which may lead to a tighter packing of transmembrane (TM) helices and a certain tilt in some of the helices.

However, regardless of the computational procedure used for structure refinement, the features of the starting model are crucial for the final, energy-minimized receptor model. At present, the lack of any detailed ionotropic or metabotropic receptor structure from x-ray crystallographic studies limits the accuracy of all available receptor models. It has now become a trivial task to calculate minimum-energy conformations of a protein and examine how various ligands fit into a known binding site, once the three-dimensional protein structure is known at atomic resolution. Similar calculations may easily be performed on any receptor model, but the validity of the results depends on the accuracy of the model and has to be verified by experimental methods.

STRUCTURE OF NEUROTRANSMITTER RECEPTORS IN TWO MAJOR SUPERFAMILIES

While the discovery technologies simplify the identification of new receptors, and molecular modeling has reached a new level of sophistication, knowledge of the structure of members of the receptor superfamilies is needed to apply these techniques. Some of the common and unique properties of two major receptor superfamilies are discussed next. Chemical communication involves the release of a pulse of neurotransmitter that results in the brief attainment of a very high concentration of transmitter at its receptor in the synaptic cleft. This results in the direct opening of an ion channel in the case of fast transmission mediated by the ionotropic receptors. In the case of slower transmission, this receptor activation of second messenger systems via a G-protein mediator results in metabolic events within the cell or mediation of indirect channel opening.

Ionotropic Receptors and Their Modulators

The transmitters that currently are known as fast transmitters are acetylcholine, glycine, glutamate, GABA, and serotonin. Almost all of these transmitters can also mediate slow transmission through a separate set of G-protein-linked receptors. Structural and functional data that have been derived from molecular biological studies of the sequence and activity of expressed receptors have pointed out the unexpected nature of the phylogenetic relationship of these receptors and allow the information derived from the study of one receptor to be applied to the others. Thus, much of our interpretation of data gathered about glycine, GABA, glutamate, and 5-HT$_3$ receptors is based on the hard-won knowledge about acetylcholine receptors. Some modification of these interpretations will be needed as each receptor and the component proteins are studied in turn, but we can classify the ionotropic receptors together as a superfamily.

Figure 2 shows a generic representation of how we think the transmembrane organization of a ligand-gated channel subunit occurs. A pentameric structure of the nicotinic cholinergic receptor composed of five of these subunits is thought to be the standard form. Evidence for this is based upon electron microscopic and cross-linking studies (63). By analogy, this structure is thought to be the form of other members of the superfamily.

Each member of the superfamily shows significant amino acid sequence homology in TM1–TM4 (transmembrane segment). The amino acids of TM2 are of particular interest because they are thought to form the pore or ion channel for all members of this receptor superfamily; it is these amino acids that have been highly conserved between and within each family. The secondary structure of the protein segment forming the channel is thought to be helical. These amino acids include a high proportion of hydrophobic amino acids; and at spaced

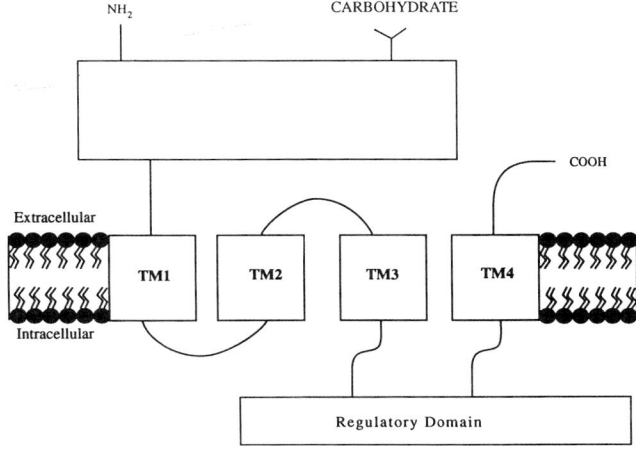

FIG. 2. Transmembrane organization of a ligand-gated channel subunit.

intervals they include neutral amino acids, such as serine and threonine. These may contribute to the inner components of the walls of the ionic channel. Charged amino acids at the ends of these sequences and other amino acids within the channel appear to control ion selectivity both through direct ionic interactions and through control of the geometry of the channel. Specific mutations of these charged amino acids have been carried out in the α_7 nAChR (nicotinic acetylcholine receptor), which can form a homomeric channel and thus has been a useful model for mutagenesis because of its simple $(\alpha_7)5$ structure. Some of these mutations alter which cations are allowed to enter (permeability Ca^{2+} versus permeability Na^+), which might be expected. Other mutations of α_7 nAChR with homologous amino acids of the glycine receptor actually convert α_7 ion channel selectivity from cationic to anionic (19).

Within this superfamily, the amino acids lining the channel form the binding pockets for drugs such as chlorpromazine (nAChR), phencyclidine (NMDA), MK801 (NMDA), some anesthetic barbiturates (GABA and glycine), ondansetron ($5HT_3$), and some insecticides (nAChR and GABA). Because of the great structural similarity of the channel amino acids within a single family, pharmacological subtyping has not been tried and the development of subtype specific drugs would be a difficult effort. However, some interesting naturally occurring point mutations have been identified, including one within the TM2 that may account for pesticide resistance in *Drosophila* (15). Such molecular studies as these also answer some of the questions of cross-relationships for drugs acting in the channel, but still remaining are the more philosophical questions: When did the nAChR and the other receptors diverge, and why did the ion selectivities change? (See Chapter 9, *this volume*).

GABAₐ Receptors

Some of the most divergent parts of the ionotropic receptor superfamily are the extracellular domain and the loop between TM3 and TM4. The extracellular domains contain the neurotransmitter binding sites and some of the modulatory sites. The intracellular loop contains consensus sequences for various protein kinases which control assembly and function of each receptor. Space does not permit us to focus on all the functions of these receptor domains and all the members of this superfamily, so we have chosen to focus on the GABA and part of the glutamate family. These have provided, and continue to provide, some of the most interesting drugs in psychopharmacology.

The GABAₐ receptor subunits have been classified into five separate groups. For example, the α subunits have been classified together solely based upon homology to one another versus lower homology to the β, γ, and δ

subunits (4). Much similarity is found in the putative transmembrane regions. Comparison of all the N-terminal amino acids of the subunits of the GABAₐ receptor complex at an amino acid level show little overall homology; however, some of the most interesting binding and modulatory sites are found here. The assembly of homomeric subunits is poorly accomplished, and for GABA it appears that more than one subunit is needed to express the interesting pharmacology of this receptor system. Using the baculovirus expression system, the addition of β subunits to α subunits yields a muscimol binding site and a fully functional channel. The further addition of a γ subunit (γ_2) to the baculovirus infection yields a receptor that also contains a benzodiazepine receptor (20).

The conclusion that we draw is that at least part of the benzodiazepine binding site or structure required for the formation of the benzodiazepine binding site is conferred by the coexpression of the γ subunits with α and β. Expression of α with γ or β with γ in this system does not result in a functional benzodiazepine receptor. Thus we can account for three of the five subunits of the GABAₐ receptor complex. Is there more than one of each subunit? The baculovirus system allows an approach to this problem by using varying multiplicities of infection. If the ratio of γ is increased beyond one, the number of Ro15-1788 sites does not increase, it decreases; one tentative thought is that a single γ is part of the complex (20). More than one α or β subunit per receptor still remain the more likely possibilities, while a fourth potential subunit, a δ, does not significantly change the pharmacology of the complex. The inclusion of the $\alpha\beta$ with a γ lowered the number of sites for muscimol, indicating the likely interaction of α and β to form a GABA binding site. The whole issue of receptor assembly is still under investigation. In an interesting series of experiments with nAChR subunits (18), the normal routes of receptor assembly were shown to involve the formation of intermediate forms of the receptor complex with fewer number of subunits; these forms of the receptor are not mature; the subunit insertion and conformational changes that allow this to occur may take hours to days. The study of assembly of subunits is a topic of great interest to cell biologists and will be an important future research area.

The GABA binding site appears to be coded for in the N-terminal portion of the GABAₐ receptor; and photoaffinity labeling with muscimol, a rigid analogue of GABA, has identified phenylalanine 61 in the α subunit as intimately involved in the binding site (57). Because the determinants of GABA that are required for binding are relatively simple, subtyping of this site, by combining different α subunits with β and γ, has not yet appeared in the literature. Examination of large libraries of more rigid GABA analogues with receptor subtypes reconstructed from clones should be useful in identifying any subtle differences in the binding site for GABA. If they exist and are substantial, these differences could be exploited by developing a pharmacophore model for each subtype that can be used pharmacologically in the development of directly acting agonists with subtype specificity.

One subtyping of the benzodiazepine response at GABA$_a$ receptors preceded the era of molecular biology; that was the type I/II difference originally seen with a Lederle compound (CL218,872) and more recently seen with the hypnotic zolpidem (Ambien) and its weaker analogue, the anxiolytic alpidem (50). For zolpidem, the pharmacology is clear from a binding perspective. Zolpidem is much more potent in displacing from an α_1-containing construct (e.g., $\alpha_1\beta_1\gamma_2$) than from other constructs. A molecular basis of glutamate (α_2, etc.) substituting for glycine (α_1) at amino acid position 201 accounts for this difference (50). From a functional point of view, some of these differences are less clear. Zolpidem at high doses produces an agonist activity at more than the one subtype, and at higher doses the specificity of the response disappears. Expression of subtypes and screening with individual GABA$_a$ receptor subtypes can discover drugs with different receptor subtype specificities. Within the next year, drugs that have been discovered in the current period of discovery that possess substantially greater specificity for one or another GABA$_a$ receptor subtype will enter the clinic. Then, we will be able to find out if subtype-specific, rather than subtype-selective, modulatory sites on the GABA$_a$ receptor complex analogous to the benzodiazepine site can have similar modes of action or represent improvements over existing medications.

A second question for the drug developer in the GABA$_a$ receptor field is whether a single drug can have a multiplicity of actions at different receptor subtypes? Here we return to the concept of agonist, antagonist, and inverse agonist developed originally to encompass the benzodiazepine blocking activities of flumazenil and the anxiogenic and proconvulsant activities of the β-carbolines (61). The answer to this question is yes. For the full agonists, the subtype differences are not interesting because at pharmacological doses in animals all of the subtypes effects are blurred or overwhelmed by the most active form. A more interesting situation is in the case of drugs with agonist activities at one subtype and inverse agonist activities at another. Is there an anxiolytic cognitive enhancer in the group? The answer is perhaps; again we will know when these agents enter the clinic.

What do the clinician and behavioral pharmacologist need to do to adjust to the era where drugs are discovered by their molecular properties rather than by their in vivo activities? Perhaps the focus should be on new ways of assessing pharmacological activities. Because sedation may not be a component of these anxiolytics, tasks where sedation is a measure of component activity are not appropriate. In a similar way, anxiety and proconvulsant activity are not a component of cognitive enhancement; there-fore, proconvulsant or anxiogenic activities should not be used to measure preclinical efficacy of inverse agonists as cognitive enhancers. Rating scales related to the disorder and new ways of specifically determining clinical efficacy will be needed. The magic bullets of the near future will possess these activities and will allow the clinician to return with confidence to GABA$_a$ mechanisms that have proven relatively safe over the last 30 years, and with these refinements they are likely to be even safer (see also Chapter 8, *this volume*).

Glutamate Receptors

The opposite of inhibition is excitation. A large number of neurons in the central nervous system use glutamate as a transmitter to produce neuronal excitation; in parallel, glutamate may also influence neuronal plasticity and cause neurotoxicity. The glutamate receptors also consist of two groups: (i) the ionotropic receptors including *N*-methyl-D-aspartate (NMDA) receptors and the α-amino-3-hydroxy-5-methyl-4 isoxazole propionate (AMPA)-kainate receptor and (ii) the metabotropic glutamate receptors that are coupled to G proteins and modulate the production of intracellular messengers. Over 15 different members of the glutamate family of receptors are known to exist (56).

Within the ionotropic glutamate receptors there are a number of classes. One class consists of four subunits (GluR1-4) and shows high affinity for AMPA, whereas another very similar set consists of two kinds of kainate-selective subunits (Glu 5-7 and KA 1-2). A further related set of clones δ_1 and δ_2 has also been found. All of these subunits are substantially larger than the other members of the family (glycine, GABA, nAChR): >100 kD as opposed to 50 kD (56).

Expression of the AMPA subunits show differences in current–voltage relations and permeability to Ca^{2+}. Thus, they are true subtypes controlling different ions in addition to different kinetics in vivo. In particular, GluR2 subunits have particularly weak Ca^{2+} permeability and dominate the electrical properties of a complex in which they are found. GluR2 has an arginine within TM2 at position, whereas the other subunits contain a glutamate residue. In certain regions of the brain, absence of this form translates to an AMPA-kainate receptor on cells with a permeability to Ca^{2+}, rather than just monovalent cations. More surprising is the finding that the genomic forms of all the AMPA subunits contain glutamate codon (CAG) at the Glu-Arg position even though an arginine codon (CGG) is found in cDNAs for GluR2, GluR5, and GluR6. Apparently, the adenosine-to-guanosine alteration and amino acid change is caused by an RNA editing mechanism, which is enzyme-driven and post-transcriptional. This mechanism occurs with varying efficiency and has an impact on the Ca^{2+} permeability of the resulting receptor. For the drug discoverer, this type of post-transcriptional editing points out a potential pitfall of clones obtained when molecular biologists use genomic sequences instead of cDNAs for cloning (56).

A further complexity of the AMPA-kainate receptors is increased by alternate splicing between TM3 and TM4. The two alternate splice molecules, flip and flop, import distinct kinetic and amplitudes of response to the AMPA-kainate family. Clearly this family of receptors is diverse and widely distributed in brain and does much of the day-to-day work of glutamate transmission. No drugs in the clinic are yet available to modulate this system, and it takes a back seat to the more glamorous cousins, the NMDA receptors. However, specific modulation of the subtypes of this receptor system could possess many of the advantages (and disadvantages) of the modulators of the GABA$_a$ receptors.

NMDA receptors can be reconstituted as heteromeric structures of two subunit types, namely, NR1 along with one of four separate NR2 subunits. In molecular terms, the NR1 are only slightly related to the NR2 subunits (18% sequence identity). The NR2 subunits are also different from the rest of this class because their carboxy-terminal regions have about 550 extra amino acids. Structural models, based upon the nAChR and GABA$_a$ receptors, thus may not be applicable here. NR1 is the most common form of NMDA receptor and exists in different splice forms. It can form homomeric receptors but also more efficiently forms heteromeric receptor sites. The important conceptual framework for NMDA receptors is that the NMDA receptor may be viewed as primarily an NR1 receptor widely distributed throughout brain, uniquely modulated in different areas by the formation of heteromeric NR1–NR2 combinations. Here again, we don't know the specific subunits composition of the complex or even the number of subunits per complex. Drug discovery depends upon the mix and match of these subunits (probably in twos) for screening purposes.

Drugs with specificity for the ion channel, like MK-801 and phencyclidine, have been shown routinely to cause psychotomimetic effects at low doses and strong sedation in the therapeutic range (53). The competitive NMDA binding site blockers also seem to share similar properties. Both classes of drug cause a strange transient phenomena called *vacuolization* in rodent cingulate cortex (46). This finding has slowed regulatory review of most drugs in this class.

The modulatory sites of the NMDA receptors (analogous but not identical to benzodiazepine sites on GABA$_a$ receptors) appear to be places to start in drug discovery for the NMDA receptor (33). One such site has been termed the *nonstrychnine glycine binding site*. This modulatory site normally responds to tonic levels of glycine, and its occupancy by glycine is absolutely required for NMDA agonist activity. Antagonists and agonists for this site already exist (inverse agonist?). All modulatory drugs

at the nonstrychnine glycine site studied to date have been free of the vacuolization phenomena and thus are improvements on the competitive and noncompetitive inhibitors.

The methodology that went into their discovery is traditional medicinal chemistry in which the requirements for an antagonist and agonist pharmacophore are defined and then subtlely modified to enhance the fit in the glycine site of the NMDA receptor (33). The first agonists were simple derivatives of glycine, lacking enantioselectivity. The antagonists (such as kynurenic acid) and weak partial agonists (including R-(+)-HA-966 and L 687414) also contain the structural elements of glycine, but with additional groups that confer stereospecificity on the resulting derivatives. Some of the partial agonists have been shown to have potent anticonvulsant effects, and some of the antagonists have been shown to be of interest as neuroprotective agents. Probably for these uses, relatively nonsubtype-selective drugs are needed. However, anxiolytic activity could require subtype-specific agents, and a general cognitive enhancing function of agonists would certainly need some greater degree of specificity. Before we see the subtype-specific generation of compounds, we will see the relatively nonspecific drugs in the clinic. Those that are useful will continue in development. Some modulation of mesolimbic dopamine by drugs at the nonstrychnine glycine site may indicate a use for nonstrychnine glycine site modulators in schizophrenia. Active subtyping would follow in the next generation of drugs much faster than in the case of the GABA$_a$ modulators (see also Chapters 7 and 8, *this volume*).

G-Protein-Linked Receptors

More than 200 different G-protein-linked receptors have now been cloned, and the number of cloned receptors belonging to this superfamily continues to increase at a seemingly exponential rate. As for the ionotropic receptors, the metabotropic receptors show highest sequence similarity in the putative membrane-spanning regions.

Structure of Membrane-Spanning Regions

The generally accepted concept of G-protein-linked receptors as proteins with seven transmembrane α-helices was originally based on the pioneering work of Henderson and Unwin (21). They demonstrated that the membrane protein bacteriorhodopsin in *Halobacterium halobium*, which has been characterized as a ''photon-driven proton pump'' because it translocates protons in response to light, contains seven membrane-spanning α-helices, closely packed in an oval arrangement with the chromophore, retinal, located in a central pore between the helices. This structure was later confirmed by more accurate

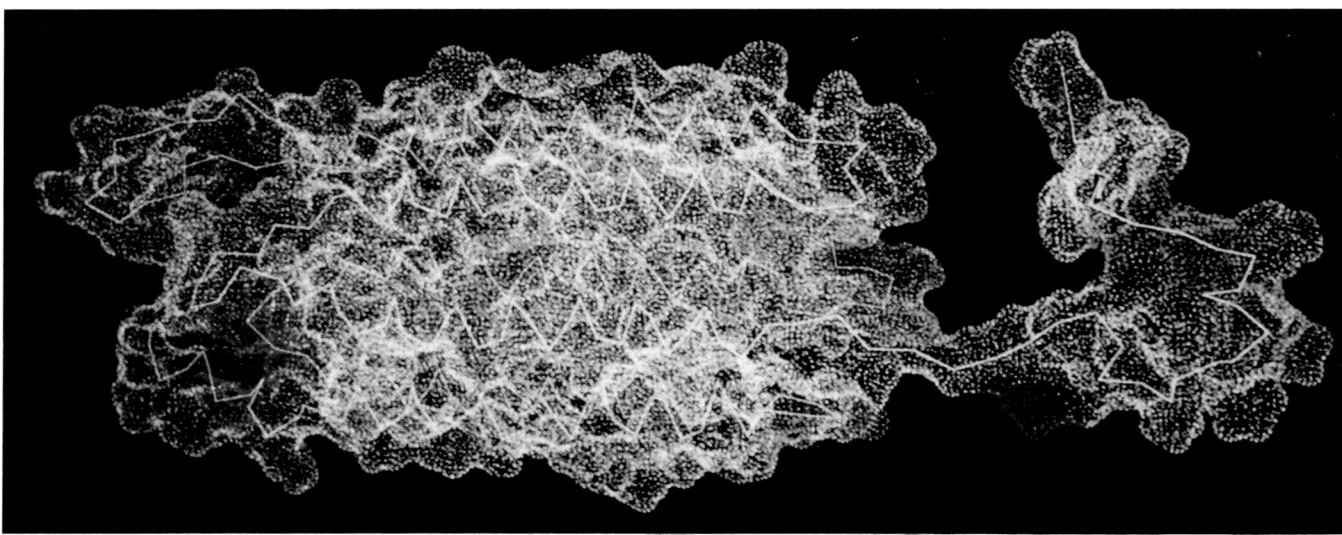

FIG. 3. Possible molecular model of the rat dopamine D_2 receptor. The dots show the water-accessible surface of the receptor molecule, color coded according to the electrostatic field around the protein: Blue, $e < -15$ kcal/mol; white, -15 kcal/mol $< e < 15$ kcal/mol; red, $e > 15$ kcal/mol. (*e:* electrostatic potential 1.4 Å outside the molecular surface.) (From ref. 2.)

electron microscopic and electron diffraction studies by the same group (22).

Bacteriorhodopsin is not linked to any G protein, and it has been questioned whether G-protein-linked receptors may have the same overall architecture as bacteriorhodopsin, because their amino acid sequences have only 10–15% identity with that of bacteriorhodopsin. However, the available information from a number of structural, biochemical, and biological studies has suggested a seven-membrane-spanning α-helical topography as a general structure also of G-protein-linked receptors. This has recently been confirmed by Henderson and collaborators (55) for visual rhodopsin, the photoreceptor in retinal rod cells, which activates transducin (G_t) in the visual signal transduction process (34). Two-dimensional projection maps of crystalline rhodopsin at 9-Å resolution were interpreted to show seven transmembrane helices, four being nearly perpendicular to the membrane plane.

The approximate locations of the putative membrane-spanning domains in a receptor sequence are usually determined from hydropathy indices, which may be calculated by different methods (26,35). We have calculated such indices for the photosynthetic reaction center of *Rhodopseudomonas viridis,* a membrane protein for which the three-dimensional structure is known from x-ray crystallographic experiments (6). The hydropathy indices predicted the correct number of putative membrane-spanning α-helices in the protein, but not their exact length or localization in the sequence. It seems that the exact start and end points of each TM helix in a membrane protein may only be determined by x-ray crystallographic, nuclear magnetic resonance (NMR)-spectroscopic, or other physical chemistry methods. However, molecular biological alteration of amino acid sequences and expression in cells has provided valuable information about the organization of synaptic, membrane-spanning, and cytoplasmic domains of various G-protein-linked receptors (49,54). In a review of his structure–function studies of bacteriorhodopsin and rhodopsin, Khorana (34) suggested that the membrane-spanning α-helices in bacteriorhodopsin have 20–27 residues (average 23) and that the seven α-helices in rhodopsin have 24–30 residues with an average length of 27 residues.

Structure of Synaptic and Cytoplasmic Domains

While there is at least indirect information about the three-dimensional structure of the membrane-spanning domains, there is virtually no available information about the tertiary structure of the synaptic and cytoplasmic domains of G-protein-linked receptors. Molecular biology studies with rhodopsin have suggested that the extracellular domains may have a crucial role in the folding and stabilization of the protein structure (34). A disulfide bond between cysteine residues in the extracellular domain

has a functional role in rhodopsin (31) and in the α_2-adrenergic receptor (8). These two cysteine residues are conserved and may have a similar function in most G-protein-linked receptors (49).

Molecular dynamics simulations have been used to model the loops between the TM helices and the N- and C-terminal parts in G-protein-linked receptors (3,10,39). In principle, such simulations may lead to more energetically favorable conformations than do models built only by secondary structure predictions from the amino acid sequence. It is difficult to judge how well the folding of loops and terminal parts after such simulations mimic the real structures, due to the lack of tertiary structural data for these receptor domains.

Addition of synaptic and cytoplasmic loops and terminals to receptor models has, however, demonstrated that dopamine and 5-HT receptors have a bipolar overall structure, with mainly negative electrostatic potentials at the synaptic side and positive electrostatic potentials in the cytoplasmic domains (3,10,60). This is illustrated in Fig. 3 for the rat dopamine D2 receptor. From this it seems likely that negative electrostatic fields around certain domains at the synaptic side may guide the positively charged neurotransmitter molecules and the protonated receptor antagonists to their receptor binding sites. Similar mechanisms have been demonstrated for substrate–enzyme interactions (66). Rational drug design from three-dimensional receptor models must therefore take into consideration that both the molecular electrostatic potentials and the three-dimensional structure of ligand molecules must fulfill certain requirements for receptor recognition and binding.

Ligand Binding Sites

Individual G-protein-linked receptors are similar in overall structure and function, but differ in key amino acid residues. Shortly after the cloning of a β_2-adrenergic receptor (7), site-specific mutagenesis experiments demonstrated that residues within the postulated membrane-spanning domains were involved in ligand binding and signal transduction (58). From this, and from the proposed seven-membrane-spanning topograpny of the receptor, it was suggested that the β_2-adrenergic receptor has a bacteriorhodopsin-like arrangement of seven α-helices, each with (a) a length of 20–28 amino acids and (b) a ligand binding pocket in the central pore between the helices (9,59). The suggestion from site-directed mutagenesis studies that the antagonist binding site lies within the membrane-spanning domain of the β_2-adrenergic receptor (9) has since been confirmed by fluorescence emission spectroscopic experiments (62), which have shown that the antagonist binding site lies within the membrane-spanning segment, about 12 Å from the synaptic membrane surface.

Site-directed mutagenesis studies have shown that two conserved serine residues in TM helix 5 are involved in agonist binding and activation of β_2-adrenergic (59), dopamine D1 (48), and dopamine D2 (40) receptors. It has been postulated that these serine residues are involved in ligand binding and may form hydrogen bonds with the hydroxyl groups in catecholamines (59).

Site-directed mutagenesis studies have also demonstrated that aspartic acid residues in TM helices 2 and 3 have functional roles in metabotropic receptors. An aspartic acid residue in TM3, which is conserved in G-protein-linked neurotransmitter receptors, is required for antagonist and agonist binding, and it has been postulated that this residue acts as a counterion in the binding of protonated ligands (54). A conserved aspartic acid residue in TM2 plays an important role in agonist-induced signal transduction in G-protein-linked neurotransmitter receptors. It is not clear, however, whether this residue is directly involved in agonist binding. It has been suggested that the corresponding residue acts as a counterion for agonist binding to β_2-adrenergic (65) and 5-HT$_{1A}$ receptors (24) and for binding of Na$^+$ to α_2-adrenergic and dopamine D$_2$ receptors (54).

It is possible that agonists and antagonists may have different but overlapping binding sites in G-protein-linked neurotransmitter receptors. Many receptor models place the conserved Asp residue in TM2 further down in the central core of the receptor than the conserved Asp residue in TM3. This arrangement offers a steric explanation of how the Asp in TM2 may be involved in signal transduction, and possibly also in agonist binding, without affecting antagonist binding. In this mode, the neurotransmitter moves down the central core of the receptor, as its own positive electrostatic potentials are attracted to negative potentials created by aspartate residues in TM3 and TM2, to "dock" the transmitter in the receptor. This attraction between the transmitter and the receptor changes the conformation of the receptor protein, leading to G-protein stimulation and subsequent intracellular biochemical changes.

Acetylcholine, dopamine, 5-HT, norepinephrine, and other receptor ligands have flexible structures, which move rapidly between various conformations as the ligand approaches the receptor. Our molecular dynamics simulation of ligand–receptor complexes suggests that transmitters as well as antagonists bind to metabotropic receptors by a "zipper" mechanism, in which the ligand adjusts its conformation as it approaches and binds to the receptor. These simulations also suggest that the amine groups of dopamine and serotonin may interact with more than one site in the receptor.

Because of their flexibility and ability to change conformation as a result of binding, the interaction of neuropeptides with their receptors, most of which are in the G-protein-linked family, are likely to be quite complex to model using the above techniques. However, a few unify-

ing principles are beginning to emerge from studies of the molecular biology of their receptors. The first is the continuation of the discovery of unexpected relationships between seemingly unrelated peptide receptors. This is exemplified by the high degree (37%) of identity of delta opiate receptors to somatostatin, angiotensin (31% identity), and the chemotactic receptors (about 20%). This may indicate that they control similar processes in the cell, and more importantly for the drug discoverer, they partly explain observations like the interactions of somatostatin analogues with the opiate receptor (12). That common motifs exist within the peptide family is supported by studies that implicate an amino–aromatic interaction between his-197 of the NK-1 receptor and a low-molecular-weight antagonist, CP 96,345. This amino acid is located at the extracellular surface of the fifth transmembrane helical domain and may indicate a more superficial area of binding for peptides to their receptors than the biogenic amines (13). It also indicated that there may exist common areas on peptide receptors similar to those on the biogenic amine receptors that are hot spots for drug design (see also Chapters 11, 27, 38, 45–52, and 61, *this volume,* for related issues).

G-Protein Interactions

The three-dimensional structures of two guanine nucleotide binding proteins, EF-Tu and p21^{ras}, have been determined by x-ray crystallography (5,30). These structures, together with data from various biochemical experiments, have been used to model α subunits of G proteins (25,42), which are coupled to membrane receptors (32). A model of transducin (G$_{t\alpha}$), constructed from the crystal structure of Cu–Zn superoxide dismutase (52), was used to propose a possible mechanism for interaction between transducin and rhodopsin (23).

Biological experiments have produced substantial information about which receptor domains are interacting with G proteins. As the receptor models become more refined, and more information about the structure of various G proteins becomes available, a next step may be to build models of receptor–G-protein complexes, use these models to suggest new site-directed mutagenesis experiments, and use the results of such experiments to refine the models of G-protein–receptor complexes.

RECEPTOR MODELING AND DRUG DESIGN

One of the aims of receptor modeling is to explain the specificity of various ligands and to make correct predictions about receptor binding affinities of ligands which have not yet been examined in receptor binding assays. Despite the theoretical effort to fold G-protein-linked receptors based upon a knowledge of their amino acid sequences, the determination of protein structure requires the application of additional techniques to confirm such folding. X-ray crystallographic techniques and protein NMR are two of the most advanced analytical techniques currently being implemented in drug design; however, the hurdles blocking their application to the study of receptors for psychotherapeutics are formidable.

Except for the models described earlier, x-ray crystallographic study of receptors is at a primitive level. While the steps needed in a structure determination are clear, the first step of obtaining receptor protein crystals is the major limitation for these studies to be successful. Because of the extensive transmembrane structure required for their function, even the solubilization of many receptors has not been possible; this includes several receptors whose amino acid sequences are known. There is little question that x-ray crystallography can be powerful in producing atomic resolution of proteins and their complexes with ligands or transmitter substances. This information can be used either (a) a posteriori to rationalize structure–activity relationships as has been done in the design of human rhinovirus inhibitors or (b) a priori as has been done in the production of inhibitors of human immunodeficiency viral proteases (HIV PR) that are required for viral replication (11). Here crystallographic information led to the realization that HIV PR was structurally related to aspartic proteases such as renin and that a reduced or simplified renin inhibitor could serve as a starting point for discovery efforts. A second starting point was the search of a database for structures that show complementarity to the active site; from this study (11), the surprising finding that haloperidol could inhibit HIV PR was made. A third approach attempted to mimic the pharmacophoric aspects of the inhibitor enzyme interactions (11); from these studies a central OH (hydroxy), two hydrogen bonds, and an aromatic group along with their spacing were identified.

Besides x-ray crystallography, NMR is the only other technique with the ability to produce details at the atomic level. An advantage is that crystals are not required. However, at present, NMR is limited to proteins with molecular weight less that about 40 kD due to the broad signals obtained for proteins of this size. An additional limitation is the need for high concentrations and solubility (about 1 mM) of proteins being studied. The results with solution NMR when it has been applied to suitable problems are spectacular. The interactions of the immunosuppressant cyclosporin with its target cyclophilin have been visualized, and conformation of cyclosporin bound to cyclophilin has been determined. This is quite different from the conformation previously determined in solution both by x-ray crystallography and by NMR spectroscopy (11). This also can provide a starting point for additional structure–activity determination and development of additional drug candidates.

While advances like these are still in the future for the discoverer of psychotherapeutics, the ability to obtain

human receptor subtypes and to express these subtypes in cell lines at high levels provides a powerful screening tool for existing and novel drug libraries. In addition to conventional libraries of drugs that most pharmaceutical companies have prepared in the course of drug discovery, new libraries based upon small building blocks have been prepared (44). These blocks can be nucleic acids, amino acids, or heterocyclic precursors. What is unique about all these approaches is the random nature of the compounds formed; these libraries can be classified as diversity libraries, and the approach is a combinatorial approach. Because no a priori assumptions are made about the compounds, their structures can theoretically fill all or any space. With a high-throughput screen using a cloned receptor expressed in a cell line, it is literally possible to screen millions of possible drug candidates for a lead structure. While not as intellectually satisfying as a purely rational approach, it has resulted in the discovery of important drug candidates and the identification of a number of useful templates for solving diverse problems in drug design. One such template is the 1,4-benzodiazepine template (Fig. 4); closely related compounds have solved problems that cross a diverse group of receptor families, including GABA, cholecystokinin, opiate, PAF receptor, and HIV PR (2). Perhaps common motifs of binding crossing families of receptors exist; and there are common sites for these templates to interact with, along with unique elements that are specific to each receptor.

CONCLUSIONS

The use of cloned receptors as targets for drug discovery is both an evolution and a revolution. It is an evolution because their use is a logical outgrowth of the historical progress in the pursuit of rational drug design by pharmaceutical firms. While we have not yet reached a point where a purely rational approach is possible, the use of cloned expressed receptors allows a previously unattainable level of chemical precision in drug design. It allows not only the attainment of high affinity for the target receptor, but also specificity through lowering affinity for other receptor subtypes through the use of reverse screening techniques. This may result in the diminution of unwanted side effects in the next generation of drugs. The importance of side effects can be underscored by the focus that continues to be placed on them and their interference with dosing both acutely and during chronic treatment. These are major themes of several chapters in this volume.

Another evolution in drug design is in the use of human receptor homologues for design of new therapeutic entities. The recent experience of the Pfizer group in the discovery and development of nonpeptidic substance P antagonists underscores the importance of having activity at human receptors for potential human therapeutics. The high affinity of CP 96,345 as a potential human therapeu-

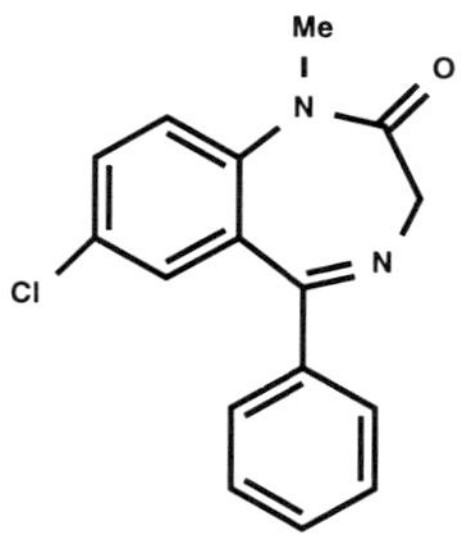

Diazepam- Anxiolytic

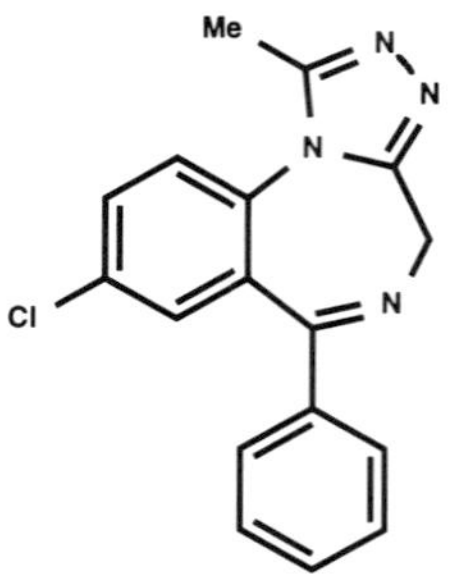

Alprazolam - Sedative

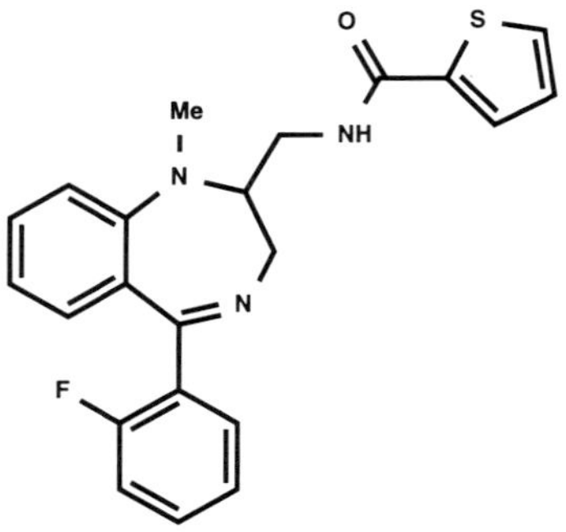

Tifluadom - Opiate receptor antagonist

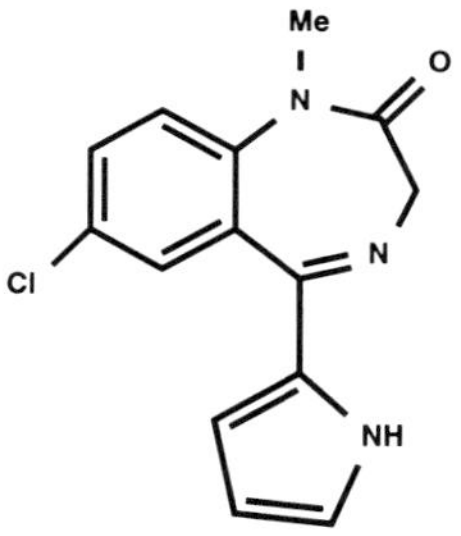

HIV Tat Antagonist

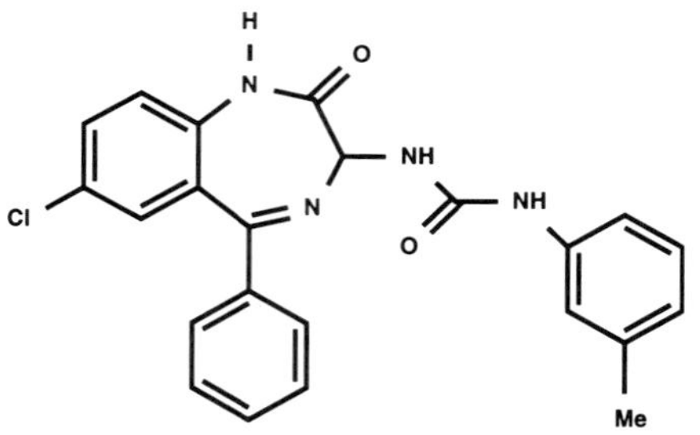

L365,260 - CCK B Antagonist

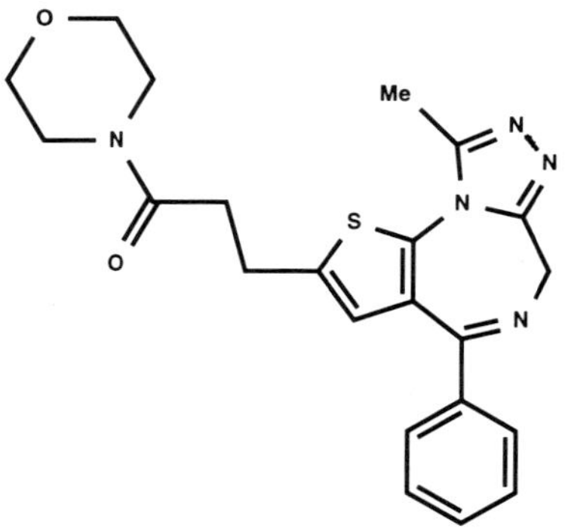

Apafant - PAF Antagonist

FIG. 4. The benzodiazepine nucleus: a universal template for many receptors

tic would not have been discovered through the use of substance P receptor assays with rat brain membranes, where its affinity is 100-fold lower (or rat clones for that matter), nor could it have even been easily identified though traditional pharmacological models in rodents. These differences have been explored through the use of chimeric receptors and have a clear molecular basis (17). Enough similar experiences are emerging to indicate that human receptor testing should be the norm in choosing a clinical candidate in the future.

The use of receptor clones has been revolutionary also. It has led to the discovery of unexpected relationships between the receptors for distinct transmitter families (e.g., the ionotropic receptors) and a realignment of traditional pharmacological classifications of subtypes within the monoamine families of receptors (e.g., the reclassified 5-HT_{2c} receptors are more related to 5-HT_{2a} than type 1 forms). An emerging theme (exemplified by the relation of δ-opiate receptors to somatostatin receptors) is that commonality of biochemical function (whether channel opening or activation of second messenger system) may indicate closer phylogenetic relationships than the transmitter that interacts to activate the receptor; this has implications for the starting point of drug design and choice of targets. The complexity of the second messenger systems also remains for further exploration.

The use of receptor clones most significantly expands our horizons for drug discovery. It identifies new members within a family where the older drugs may have exerted parts of their therapeutic actions (e.g., clozapine's action at dopamine D4 receptors) and thus new and specific targets for therapeutics. It allows totally novel receptors to be identified within a family where no therapeutics yet exist [e.g., the many new serotonin ($5\text{HT}_{4-?}$) receptors] and should spur interest in novel mechanisms. Finally, the technology allows sufficient amounts of rare receptors to be produced to allow them to be explored for their biological and future therapeutic importance.

Receptor modeling techniques have provided new insight into receptor mechanisms, and they have been used to design biological experiments. Modeling of receptor molecules, along with molecular dynamics simulations of ligand–receptor interactions, has provided some clues both to the nature of ligand–receptor associations and to the structural transitions that occur upon agonist binding. Until a detailed crystal structure and related biological activity of an ionotropic or metabotropic receptor molecule is available, molecular modeling techniques may not be expected to provide information about the fine structure of such proteins and detailed receptor mechanisms. Molecular modeling of receptor molecules, based on the amino acid sequences of the protein and other available structural data, may still provide information which may be used in a rational design of potential drug molecules. The rapid development of molecular modeling applications indicate that such techniques will play an increasingly important role in future drug design.

The presence of advanced technologies for drug discovery and design can lead to the discovery of magic bullets. How these magic bullets can be used in the clinic and what disorders can be treated with these receptor-specific drugs still remains the domain of the astute and observant clinician. Perhaps we have come full circle with a new generation of precise agents whose ultimate utility in the clinic will be determined not only rationally, but also serendipitously.

REFERENCES

1. Anfinsen CB. Principles that govern the folding of protein chains. *Science* 1973;181:223–230.
2. Bunin BA, Ellman JA. A general and expedient method for the solid-phase synthesis of 1,4-benzodiazepine derivatives. *J Am Chem Soc* 1992;114:10997–10998.
3. Dahl SG, Edvardsen Ø, Sylte I. Molecular dynamics of dopamine at the D2 receptor. *Proc Natl Acad Sci USA* 1991;88:8111–8115.
4. DeLorey TM, Olsen RW. γ-Aminobutyric acid receptor structure and function. *J Biol Chem* 1992;267:16747–16751.
5. DeVos AM, Tong L, Milburn MV, Matias PM, Jancarik J, Noguchi S, Nishimura S, Miura K, Ohtsuka K, Kim S-H. Three dimensional structure of an oncogene protein. Catalytic domain of human C-H-ras p21. *Science* 1988;239:888–893.
6. Deisenhofer J, Epp O, Miki K, Huber R, Michel H. Structure of the protein subunits in the photosynthetic reaction centre of *Rhodopseudomonas viridis* at 3 Å resolution. *Nature* 1985;318:618–624.
7. Dixon RA, Kobilka BK, Strader DJ, Benovic JL, Dohlman HG, Frielle T, Bolanowski MA, Bennett CD, Rands E, Diehl RE, Mumford RA, Slater EE, Sigal IS, Caron MG, Lefkowitz RJ, Strader CD. Cloning of the gene and cDNA for mammalian β-adrenergic receptor and homology with rhodopsin. *Nature* 1986;321:75–79.
8. Dixon RA, Sigal IS, Rands E, Register RB, Candelore MR, Blake AD, Strader CD. Ligand binding to the β-adrenergic receptor involves its rhodopsin-like core. *Nature* 1987;326:73–77.
9. Dixon RA, Sigal IS, Candelore MR, Register RB, Scattergood W, Rands E, Strader CD. Structural features required for ligand binding to the β-adrenergic receptor. *EMBO J* 1987;6:3269–3275.
10. Edvardsen Ø, Style I, Dahl SG. Molecular dynamics of serotonin and ritanserin interacting with the 5-HT$_2$ receptor. *Mol Brain Res* 1992;14:166–178.
11. Erickson JW, Fesik SW. Macromolecular x-ray crystallography and NMR as tools for structure-based drug design. *Annu Rep Med Chem* 1992;27:271–287.
12. Evans CJ, Keith, DE, Morrison H, Magendzo K, Edwards RH. Cloning of a delta opioid receptor by functional expression. *Science* 1992;258:1952–1955.
13. Fong YM, Cascieri MA, Yu H, Bansai A, Swain C, Strader C. Amino-aromatic interaction between histidine 197 of the neurokinin-1 receptor and CP 96345. *Nature* 1993;362:350–353.
14. Freissmuth M, Selzer E, Marullo S, Shutz W, Strosberg D. Expression of two human β-adrenergic receptors in *E. coli* a: functional interaction with two forms of the stimulatory G protein. *Proc Natl Acad Sci USA* 1991;88:8548–8552.
15. Ffrench-Constant R, Rocheleau T, Steichen J, Chalmers A. Molecular basis of resistance to picrotoxinin and cyclodiene insecticides in a *Drosophila* GABA receptor. *Soc Neurosci Abstr* 1993;19:852.
16. Frohman M, Dush M, Martin G. Rapid production of full-length cDNAs from rare transcripts: amplification using a single gene-specific oligonucleotide primer. *Proc Natl Acad Sci USA* 1988;85:8998–9002.
17. Gether U, Yokota Y, Edmonds-Alt X, Brelaiere J, Lowe J, Snider R, Nakanishi S, Schwartz T. Two non peptide tachykinin antagonists act through epitopes on corresponding segments of the NK1 and NK2 receptors. *Proc Natl Acad Sci USA* 1993;90:6194–6198.
18. Green W, Claudio T. Acetylcholine receptor assembly, subunit folding and oligomerization occur sequentially. *Cell* 1993;74:57–69.
19. Galzi J, Devillers-Thiery A, Hussy N, Bertrand S, Changoux J, Bertrand D. Mutations in the channel domain of a neuronal nicotinic receptor convert ion selectivity from cationic to anionic. *Nature* 1992;359:500–504.
20. Hartnett C, Yu J, Brown M, Gerber K, Primus R, Ramabhadran R, Gallager D. Effect of subunit composition on GABA/benzodiazepine receptor binding characteristics in a baculovirus expression system. *Soc Neurosci Abstr* 1993;19(1):477.
21. Henderson R, Unwin PNT. Three-dimensional model of purple membrane obtained by electron microscopy. *Nature* 1975;257:28–32.
22. Henderson R, Baldwin JM, Ceska TA, Zemlin F, Beckmann E, Downing KH. Model for the structure of bacteriorhodopsin based on high-resolution electron cryomicroscopy. *J Mol Biol* 1990;213:899–929.
23. Hingorani VN, Ho Y-K. A structural model for the α-subunit of transducin. Implications of its role as a molecular switch in the visual signal transduction mechanism. *FEBS Lett* 1987;220:15–22.
24. Ho BY, Karschin A, Branchek T, Davidson N, Lester HA. The role of conserved aspartate and serine residues in ligand binding and in function of the 5-HT$_{1A}$ receptor: a site-directed mutation study. *FEBS Lett* 1992;312:259–262.
25. Holbrook SR, Kim S-H. Molecular model of the G protein or a subunit based on the crystal structure of the HRAS protein. *Proc Natl Acad Sci USA* 1989;86:1751–1755.
26. Hopp TP, Woods KR. Prediction of protein antigenic determinants from amino acid sequences. *Proc Natl Acad Sci USA* 1981;78:3824–3828.
27. Howlett A, Bidaut-Russel M, Devane W, Melvin L, Johnson M, Herkenham M. The cannabinoid receptor: biochemical, anatomical and behavioral characterization *Trends Neurosci* 1990;13:420–423.
28. Jähnig F, Edholm O. Modeling of the structure of bacteriorhodopsin. A molecular dynamics study. *J Mol Biol* 1992;226:837–850.
29. Jan L, Jan Y. Voltage sensitive ion channels. *Cell* 1989;56:13–25.
30. Jurnak F. Structure of the GDP domain of EF-Tu and location of the amino acids homologous to ras oncogene proteins. *Science* 1985;230:32–36.
31. Karnik SS, Khorana HG. Assembly of functional rhodopsin requires a disulfide bond between cysteine residues 110 and 187. *J Biol Chem* 1990;265:17520–17524.
32. Kaziro Y, Itoh H, Kozasa T, Nakafuku M, Satoh T. Structure and function of signal-transducing GTP-binding proteins. *Annu Rev Biochem* 1991;60:349–400.
33. Kemp JA, Lesson PD. The glycine site of the NMDA receptor-five years on. *Trends Pharmacol Sci* 1993;14:20–25.
34. Khorana HG. Two light-transducing membrane proteins: Bacteriorhodopsin and the mammalian rhodopsin. *Proc Natl Acad Sci USA* 1993;90:1166–1171.
35. Kyte J, Doolittle RF. A simple method for displaying the hydropathic character of a protein. *J Mol Biol* 1982;157:105–132.
36. Laborit H. Sur l'utilization de certain agents pharmacodynamiques à action neuro-vegetative en periode per-et postoperatoire. *Acta Chir Belg* 1949;48:485–492.
37. Lubbert H, Hoffman B, Snutch T, vanDyke T, Levine A, Hartig, P, Lester H, Davidson N. cDNA cloning of a serotonin 1c receptor by electrophysiological assays of mRNA-injected *Xenopus* oocytes. *Proc Nat Acad Sci USA* 1987;87:928–932.
38. Luckow V. Protein production and processing from baculovirus expression vectors. In: Granados RR, Hammer DA, Wood HA, Shuler M, eds. *Insect cell cultures: biopesticide and protein production.* New York: Wiley, 1993.
39. Maloney Huss K, Lybrand TP. Three-dimensional structure for the β$_2$ adrenergic receptor protein based on computer modeling studies. *J Mol Biol* 1992;225:859–871.
40. Mansour A, Meng F, Meador-Woodruff JH, Taylor LP, Civelli O, Akil H. Site directed mutagenesis of the human dopamine D$_2$ receptor. *Eur J Pharmacol Mol Pharmacol* 1992;227:205–214.
41. Maricq A, Peterson A, Brake A, Myers R, Julius D. Primary struc-

ture and functional expression of the 5HT₃ receptor, a serotonin-gated ion channel. *Science* 1991;254:432–437.

42. Masters SB, Stroud RM, Bourne HR. Family of G protein α chains: amphipathic analysis and predicted structure of functional domains. *Protein Eng* 1986;1:47–54.

43. Mills A, Duggan M. Orphan seven transmembrane domain receptors: reversing pharmacology. *Trends Pharmacol Sci* 1993;14:394–396.

44. Moos WH, Green G, Pavia MR. Recent advances in the generation of molecular diversity. *Annu Rep Med Chem* 1993;28:315–324.

45. Noda M, Takahashi H, Tanabe T, Toyosato M, Furutani Y, Hirose T, Asai M, Inayama S, Miyata T, Numa S. Primary structure of α-subunit precursor of *Torpedo californica* acetylcholine receptor deduced from cDNA sequence. *Nature* 1982;299:793–797.

46. Olney J, Labruyere J, Price M. Phencyclidine, dizocilpine, and cerebrocortical neurons. *Science* 1990;247:221.

47. Pert C, Snyder S. Opiate receptor: demonstration in nervous system. *Science* 1973;179:1011–1014.

48. Pollock NJ, Manelli AM, Hutchins CW, Steffey ME, MacKenzie RG, Frail DE. Serine mutations in transmembrane V of the dopamine D1 receptor affect ligand interactions and receptor activation. *J Biol Chem* 1992;267:17780–17786.

49. Probst WC, Snyder LA, Schuster DI, Brosius J, Sealfon SC. Sequence alignment of the G-protein coupled receptor superfamily. *DNA Cell Biol* 1992;11:1–20.

50. Prittchett D, Luddens B, Seeburg P. Type I and II GABAa benzodiazepine receptors produced by transfected cells. *Science* 1989;245:1389–1392.

51. Randall LO. Discovery of benzodiazepines. In: Usdin E, Skolnick P, Tallman J, Greenblatt D, Paul S, eds. *Pharmacology of benzodiazepines*. London: Macmillan, 1982;15–21.

52. Richardson JS, Thomas KA, Rubin BH, Richardson DC. Crystal structure of bovine Cu, Zn superoxide dismutase at 3 Angstroms resolution, chain tracing and metal ligands. *Proc Natl Acad Sci USA* 1975;72:1349–1353.

53. Rogawski M, Porter R. Antiepileptic drugs: pharmacological mechanisms and clinical efficacy with consideration of promising developmental stage compounds. *Pharm Rev* 1990;42:223–286.

54. Savarese TM, Fraser CM. *In vitro* mutagenesis and the search for structure–function relationships among G protein-coupled receptors. *Biochem J* 1992;283:1–19.

55. Schertler GFX, Villa C, Henderson R. Projection structure of rhodopsin. *Nature* 1993;362:770–772.

56. Seeburg, P. The molecular biology of the mammalian glutamate receptor channels. *Trends Neurosci* 1993;16:359–365.

57. Smith G, Olsen R. Identification of a 3H muscimol photoaffinity substrate in GABAa receptor alpha subunit. *Soc Neurosci Abstr* 1993;19:476.

58. Strader CD, Sigal IS, Register RB, Candelore MR, Rands E, Dixon RA. Identification of residues required for ligand binding to the β-adrenergic receptor. *Proc Natl Acad Sci USA* 1987;84:4384–4388.

59. Strader CD, Candelore MR, Hill WS, Sigal IS, Dixon RAF. Identification of two serine residues involved in agonist activation of the β-adrenergic receptor. *J Biol Chem* 1989;264:13572–13578.

60. Sylte I, Edvardsen Ø, Dahl SG. Molecular dynamics of the 5-HT₁ₐ receptor and ligands. *Protein Eng* 1993;6:691–700.

61. Tallman, J, Gallager, D. The GABA-ergic system: a locus of benzodiazepine action. *Annu Rev Neurosci* 1985;8:21–44.

62. Tota MR, Strader CD. Characterization of the binding domain of the β-adrenergic receptor with the fluorescent antagonist carazolol. *J Biol Chem* 1990;265:16891–16897.

63. Unwin N. The nicotinic acetylcholine receptor at 9 Å resolution. *J Membr Biol* 1993;229:1101–1124.

64. Van Tol H, Bunzow J, Guan H, Sunahara R, Seeman P, Niznik H, Civelli O. Cloning of the gene for a human dopamine D4 receptor with high affinity for the antipsychotic clozapine. *Nature* 1991;350:610–614.

65. Venter JC, Fraser CM, Kerlavage AR, Buck MA. Molecular biology of adrenergic and muscarinic cholinergic receptors. A perspective. *Biochem Pharmacol* 1989;38:1197–1208.

66. Wade RC, Luty BA, Demchuk E, Madura JD, Davis ME, Briggs JM, McCammon JA. Simulation of enzyme–substrate encounter with gated active sites. *Struct Biol* 1994;1:65–69.

67. Young D, Waitches G, Birchmeier C. Isolation and characterization of a new cellular oncogene encoding a protein with multiple potential transmembrane domains. *Cell* 1986;45:711–716.

Psychopharmacology: The Fourth Generation of Progress, edited by Floyd E. Bloom and David J. Kupfer. Raven Press, Ltd., New York © 1995.

CHAPTER 159

Ethical Issues in Genetic Screening and Testing, Gene Therapy, and Scientific Conduct

Lisa S. Parker and Elizabeth Gettig

Bioethics, as an interdisciplinary field involving clinicians, lawyers, philosophers, theologians, and other humanists, was born in the early 1970s amid technological advances in medicine and growing respect for persons in society. The era was marked by the end of the Tuskegee syphilis study, the first widespread use of hemodialysis and mechanical ventilation, abortion reform, and the first human heart transplant. Technological capabilities clashed with individuals' values. In short, bioethics was born of conflict (26).

Respect for individuals' rights of self-determination came into conflict with some social values and with the medical profession's previously largely unchallenged paternalistic concern for patient welfare, as the medical profession and individual professionals—not patients—defined that well-being. In 1970, for example, Paul Ramsey published his patient-centered medical ethics treatise, *The Patient as Person* (31). The field of bioethics emerged in the wake of landmark legal cases, such as Karen Quinlan's parents' bid to remove her from her respirator (30) or the paralyzed Mr. Canterbury's suit claiming that he had not been fully informed of the risks of his surgery (7). Bioethics evolved to provide a legal and ethical framework within which to resolve conflicts between physician and patient and between social consensus and individual values. The individual patient's values came to trump the traditional values of medicine, and the privacy both of individuals and of the physician–patient relationship erected a boundary against the intrusion of society's interests.

Historically, the physician–patient relationship has been the primary focus of bioethics, but it is clear that the crisis of funding health care is emerging as the funda-

mental challenge of the 1990s (9,22,35). Social policies and institutional contexts are now considered in association with, or occasionally instead of, the physician or health-care provider and patient relationship (21).

Developments in theoretical ethics, specifically feminist ethics, support bioethics' new focus. Feminist philosophers suggest that in order to provide just answers to ethical questions, ethics must pay increased attention to their social context and political dynamics, the balance of power, and the history of oppression (14,15,33).

So it was in this intellectual and social climate that the Human Genome Project (HGP) was initiated in 1990 to support and coordinate efforts of the National Institutes of Health (NIH) and the Department of Energy (DOE) to produce a complete genetic map of all human genes. The Ethical, Legal, and Social Implications (ELSI) Program of the HGP was charged with anticipating the social consequences of the acquisition of this knowledge and developing policies to guide its use. With 5% of the genome budget supporting ELSI activities, the ELSI Program is both the first federally supported extramural research initiative in ethical issues and the largest source of public funds for bioethics (44).

However, the bioethical issues of the HGP are not unique. The topics of informed consent, justice, gender justice, privacy, confidentiality, discrimination, genetic discrimination, health-care needs, or private health insurance versus a national health service are familiar ones. Even those challenges to the premises of a private health insurance system presented by genetic screening are, for example, also presented by other predictive medical tests—for example, cholesterol screening for hypertension.

Advances in genetics may, however, place ethical concerns on a grander scale because everyone is at an increased risk for developing some disease. New genetic

L. S. Parker and E. Gettig: Department of Human Genetics, University of Pittsburgh, Pittsburgh, Pennsylvania 15261.

1876 / ETHICAL ISSUES IN GENETIC STUDIES

technologies may cause ethical concerns to arise at a different stage of life or of decision-making (e.g., prior to conception or at a presymptomatic stage of a disease).

If the conflict between paternalism and autonomy is seen to have been played out in the context of the doctor–patient relationship since the 1970s, the genetic counselor–consultand relationship of the 1980s and 1990s seems to reflect the resolution of that conflict. Prior to the 1970s, a priestly model accurately described the typical, paternalistic doctor–patient relationship. According to this model, decision-making is taken from the patient and placed in the hands of the expert professional who is charged with benefiting the patient; in the extreme, the physician's "moral authority so dominates the patient that the patient's freedom and dignity are extinguished" (39). In contrast, the physician–patient relationship model which is currently advocated is a contractual model: "The basic norms of freedom, dignity, truth-telling, promise-keeping, and justice are essential to a contractual relationship. The promise is trust and confidence even though it is recognized that there is not a full mutuality of interests. . . . With the contractual relationship there is a sharing in which the physician recognizes that the patient must maintain freedom of control over his own life and destiny when significant choices are to be made" (39).

The relationship between professional genetic counselors and their consultands reflects this shared decision-making process which guarantees to consultands the authority to make choices reflecting their own values. The Code of Ethics of the National Society of Genetic Counselors (NSGC) states that genetic counselors strive to: "respect their clients' beliefs, cultural traditions, inclinations, circumstances, and feelings . . . and refer clients to other competent professionals when they are unable to support the clients" (25). Thus, the consultand-centered, autonomy-oriented conception of the genetic counseling relationship reflects the outcome of at least two decades of bioethical discussions of patients' rights, of the therapeutic advantage of involving patients in their own care, and of value pluralism.

The nonpaternalistic, nondirective process of genetic counseling also embodies aspects of the doctrine of informed consent, the most prominent bioethical and legal doctrine to emerge in the early years of bioethics. Informed consent is the process whereby competent patients or research subjects are informed of the risks and benefits of proposed therapeutic or research protocols ("disclosure"), are asked to weigh these risks and benefits in light of their own values and desires, and are asked to give their informed, voluntary consent to undertake the therapy or participate in the research (2). Health-care professionals and researchers are obligated to (a) disclose the information in a manner so that a reasonable layperson can understand it and (b) answer the specific questions which the individual client or research subject may raise. Insofar as the professional or researcher becomes aware of a par-

ticular client's or subject's desire to have additional information disclosed, the professional or researcher incurs an obligation to make reasonable attempts to satisfy that desire ("dialogue"). The doctrine of informed consent has two justifications: first and most fundamentally, respect for persons and their autonomy; and second, protection of individuals' welfare by requiring their consent as a prerequisite to incur the risks of research or treatment (5).

The fundamental role of genetic counselors is to provide information to enable consultands to make free and informed reproductive and health care decisions. The NSGC Code of Ethics states that counselors "strive to enable their clients to make informed independent decisions, free of coercion, by providing or illuminating the necessary facts and clarifying alternatives and anticipated consequences" (25). Supplying information in an understandable manner, answering consultands' questions, helping consultands develop the understanding necessary to make their own decisions, and supporting those choices are the primary tasks of genetic counselors. Whereas these tasks, which comprise the disclosure and dialogue stages of the process of informed consent, are just one facet of other health care providers' jobs, they constitute, in broad outline, the primary tasks of genetic counselors.

Thus, in an important sense, the first two decades of bioethics not only provided background for current ethical consideration of issues arising from genetic research and the management of genetic disease, but actually laid the foundation for the process of modern genetic counseling. As the HGP progresses and genetic services become a more integral part of health care, ethical analysis of issues concerning these rapid advances in genetic technology and knowledge will continue to reflect this individual-oriented bioethical tradition.

Growing attention to more socially oriented bioethical concerns, such as allocation of health-care resources, however, also coincides with, and will be influenced by, advances in genetics. Allocation issues, for example, are no longer primarily questions of micro-allocation or triage, but instead focus on macro-allocation concerns, such as how to provide a decent minimum of health care to all of society's members, what constitutes a decent minimum, and whether certain types of health care should be available at all ("should organ transplantation research or gene therapy trials receive funding?").

PREVENTIVE ETHICS

Although the field of bioethics was born in an atmosphere of conflict and was initially concerned with the resolution of ethical conflicts, it is gradually beginning to address the social and institutional factors which may create or exacerbate ethical problems. Thus bioethics may be said to parallel preventive medicine (10,27). The practice of "preventive ethics," including its anticipatory stance and its attention to social and institutional factors, mirrors the practice of preventive medicine (12).

Waiting until a conflict arises makes resolving ethical quandaries more difficult, because by then medical and institutional factors may limit options or opposing parties may have become deeply entrenched and personally identified with their (conflicting) positions. The inadvertent disclosure of confidential information to family members about their risk for having or transmitting a genetic condition can result in long-term dysfunction in family dynamics which might be avoided by establishing and observing preventive ethics policies for information management. Therefore, even successfully resolved crises incur high human costs in terms of time and emotion expended in their resolution.

Furthermore, the crisis-resolution approach measures success in terms of whether a settlement to the particular crisis can be found and thus too readily accepts patterns of recurring ethical problems. In its early years, bioethics neglected the underlying causes of ethical conflicts, such as routine aspects of health care or social and institutional structures which have exacerbated or even directly caused ethical conflicts in the provision of health care (4). The traditional approach defines the scope of bioethics in terms of discrete problems; thus, it necessarily fails to attend adequately to the ethical aspects of health care in which no specific "problem" has been identified. Outside of genetic counseling, for example, even though the process of informed consent is important in defining the ethical character of every provider–patient interaction, the disclosure and dialogue inherent in informed consent are often ignored until the physician and patient disagree about the proper treatment.

In contrast, a preventive approach to bioethical issues can help overcome these limitations of early crisis-oriented bioethics by placing a greater emphasis on preventing the development of ethical conflicts (28). A preventive approach seeks to detect potential ethical conflicts at stages where "symptoms" of the conflicts are not yet present or are relatively mild. By identifying the predictable patterns of "pathophysiology" (3) and "ethical risk factors" shared by common ethical problems (e.g., institutional structures or differences in cultural or religious views), preventive ethics facilitates the development of mechanisms to avert serious conflicts or to reach ethically defensible plans more readily, thereby minimizing unnecessary personal anguish and social conflict.

Because preventive ethics correctly recognizes that the absence of ethical conflict is an inadequate measure of the ethical provision of health care or conduct of research, preventive ethics not only seeks to avoid conflicts, but also strives to create and preserve relationships of trust and understanding between health-care providers and recipients and between researchers and the public (12). It seeks to maximize opportunities for the exercise of auton-

omy and the provision of quality patient or consultand-centered care.

According to a preventive bioethics approach, alternative social policies should be judged not merely according to whether they will prevent open ethical conflicts, but also according to their capacity to promote ethical health care and the opportunity for society's members to pursue life plans reflecting their own values. In expanding the focus of bioethics from decisions in problematic cases to a general concern with both the routine aspects of health care and the social and institutional factors which affect health care, preventive ethics more fully integrates ethical considerations into health care and research.

By identifying recurrent problems, a preventive ethics approach enables researchers and health-care providers to develop ethics "protocols" for addressing them, particularly in advance of individual occurrences. Thus, the preventive approach (i) may avoid some individual hardship (or at least permit individuals to anticipate and prepare for future hardships), (ii) may, by identifying the problems, invite their innovative solution, and (iii) may prompt changes in existing structures and policies, if they are themselves contributing to the problems.

PREVENTIVE ETHICS IN GENETIC RESEARCH

In genetic research, practicing preventive ethics in the presymptomatic testing of individuals at risk for Huntington's disease (HD) has led to a tentative code of conduct for genetic researchers (17). The code evolved from research on samples from families with genetic disease and from the development of new molecular tests. The proposed code of conduct intends to protect both the subject and researchers. Harper (17) admits that most problems encountered in genetic testing are a result of not paying adequate attention to the ethics of gene testing and therapy. HD protocols have been examined by review committees, often (unfortunately) with more attention given to the risks of the sampling procedure (dangers and discomfort of venipuncture) than to the social, psychological, and economic consequences of the test results (e.g., the detection of a genetic defect).

The proposed code also addresses the conflicts of interest between the patient's needs and the physician's or researcher's interests. Financial ties with industry, through research, personal investment in commercial ventures, or consulting fees, appear to be greater in genetics than in other fields of medicine due to the technology-driven nature of genetic research. Norman Fost (13) has written that "sometimes it is difficult to distinguish a conflict of interest from a congruence of interest. The scientist's desire of fame and fortune may drive him or her to the extra effort that results in a discovery that benefits others. The physician's desire for income may stimulate him or her to work long hours and provide beneficial services to others. But there is also evidence that self-interest can adversely affect clinical judgement, whether it be for suggesting elective surgery or for ordering expensive diagnostic tests.''

Disclosure statements have become commonplace to minimize the possible effects of conflicts of interest; and some groups, notably a multicenter clinical trial of treatment after coronary-artery bypass-graft surgery, have moved toward prohibiting ties with industry when such ties are not necessary for the practice of medicine or the advancement of science (20).

The code of conduct proposed by Harper (18) also points to some of the difficulties that will be faced as genetic technologies developed in the research context are applied in the clinical diagnostic or therapeutic context. The code states the following:

1. Family members ''at risk'' for a genetic disorder should not be sampled unless strictly necessary for the research, especially in late-onset or variable disorders. This statement applies particularly to children. Proposals should clearly justify the testing of unaffected subjects and should include a clear plan stating what will be done in the event that a genotypic abnormality is detected.

2. When consent is given for sampling by an unaffected person to assist a family member in determining his/her risk status, it should be made clear that the risk status of the unaffected person will not be disclosed and that the result of the test should not be expected nor will it be sent to his/her doctor nor placed in his/her medical record unless specifically requested.

3. If the sample is to be stored and used for future tests, new consent should be obtained if the implications for the person at risk resulting from the new research are likely to be considerably different; for example, if direct mutations analysis, rather than a general linkage analysis, is possible.

4. If the possibility of identifying defects in people at risk is foreseeable or inevitable, then such samples should be coded or made anonymous for the purpose of these tests unless the person concerned has specifically requested that relevant information should be disclosed and has received information that allows him/her to fully understand the implications of such disclosure.

5. If a person at risk who gave a research sample later requests presymptomatic testing or other genetic services, a new sample should be taken and the request handled in the same way as it would be for any other person electing presymptomatic testing.

6. When a test may show a specific genetic defect in people affected by a disorder not previously known to be genetic, the possible genetic implications (as well as psychosocial implications) should be made clear and new consent obtained if samples previously obtained are being restudied.

7. Ethics committees should pay at least as much attention to the consequences of a sample being taken as to the risks attached to the sampling procedure.

The presymptomatic HD testing programs have attempted to create and preserve trust and understanding between researchers and test providers. Presymptomatic testing is a multistep process involving numerous visits to testing centers. The HD protocols prescribe review of the subject's family history, neurologic examination, psychiatric examination, review of medical charts of extended family members for confirmation of diagnostic information, psychological testing, pre-test counseling, and disclosure of results. Follow-up both clinically and for research purposes is a standard feature of presymptomatic testing protocols (11).

The HD model sometimes limited the subject's right to privacy because of the need for extensive review of family medical data and the need for samples for linkage analysis (prior to the recent discovery of the HD gene). The protocol was born from the traditional pre-1970s model of the physician–patient relationship. It is therefore criticized on paternalistic grounds. The protocols were neither publicly reviewed nor discussed. As individuals have ''graduated'' from the testing program, the protocols are being revisited. Suggestions and recommendations from participants are being sought in order to evaluate and possibly to modify the protocols. Moreover, the recent discovery of the gene responsible for HD has pushed the scientific community to reevaluate the protocols because extended family review is no longer necessary.

The HD model represents the first testing program which enables a person to choose to know with a high degree of certainty that he or she will die of a fatal, inherited, and presently untreatable disease. The psychiatric and social consequences of having such knowledge were anticipated and prompted the rigid protocol structure to preserve the most basic of ethical tenets—that is, to do no harm. Experience with the HD protocols has shown that explaining genetic risks is a complex subject and that understanding comes slowly (24).

The counseling steps of the HD protocols may be included in future genetic testing models. Testing without giving information, counseling, and support must be agreed to be unacceptable. Concern about stigmatization and discrimination in employment, insurance, and personal relationships should provoke society to monitor and regulate the availability and use of genetic testing to ensure that abuse or coercion does not occur (18). A preventive ethics approach allows for better planning and more open discussion of these ethical concerns.

GENE THERAPY

The creation of the NIH's Recombinant DNA Advisory Committee (RAC) represents an attempt to anticipate and address ethical concerns pertaining to gene therapy. The RAC was responsible for what some consider one of the most important milestones in the history of medicine— namely, the approval of a human gene transfer study and human gene therapy protocols (40). The gene therapy protocols currently involve only somatic cell gene therapy. Somatic cell gene therapy refers to the insertion of new DNA into a particular tissue (such as bone marrow) of an affected individual. The reproductive system is not targeted, so the new DNA material serves the individual only and is not transmitted to progeny.

A preventive ethics approach is evident in the RAC's public review process. By serving to inform the public of perhaps the most controversial advances in genetics and permitting public comment on the use of gene therapy technology, the RAC provides a mechanism to minimize public concern and social conflict. The guidelines of the RAC evolved over a decade.

The RAC is not, however, without its critics. The RAC is a committee of the NIH, which, in turn, is the primary funding agent for biomedical research. The initial protocols were submitted by NIH scientists. The RAC has acknowledged the conflict in simultaneously promoting and regulating a single field of research.

In addition, because RAC review provides a safeguard against employment of potentially high risk gene therapy in the absence of safety and efficacy data, the 1992 decision to exempt one therapeutic protocol on a compassionate plea basis raises concern (20,36,37). By responding to the crisis of the moment and not fully addressing the precedent-setting ramifications of its departure from its peer review protocol, the NIH's departure from its preventive ethics stance invited criticism concerning the susceptibility of the NIH's peer review process to political pressure and constituted a potentially serious breach of public trust (8,19).

Still, the RAC again embraced the notion of preventive ethics by introducing for public debate the concept of germ-line gene therapy. Germ-line gene therapy means that the new DNA introduced into an individual may be passed to future generations. In 1990 Francis Collins, now director of the Human Genome Project, stated that "germ-line gene therapy ... is an approach that carries such risks of unknown damage to future generations that virtually all geneticists and lay organizations have concluded that it would not be appropriate to attempt it in humans" (16).

The very next year LeRoy Walters stated that "the time has now come to begin a formal public process for the ethical assessment of germ line genetic intervention" (40). Organizations such as the Council for Responsible Genetics oppose the use of germ-line gene modification in humans (29). RAC chairman Nelson Wivel (writing as a citizen and not in his official capacity) and Walters state that, "it would, in our view, be a useful investment of time and energy to continue and in fact intensify the

public discussion of germ line gene modification for disease prevention, even though the application of this new technology to humans is not likely to be proposed in the near future" (43). The debate continues regarding gene therapy and its application to human subjects.

SCREENING FOR GENETIC DISEASES

A national policy has yet to be developed governing population-based screening of genetic disease. The debate over population-based screening for the gene for cystic fibrosis (CF) has begun. Earlier screening programs, particularly screening for the gene for sickle cell anemia in the African-American population, failed to clearly establish program goals, failed to distinguish promotion of patient autonomy from the motivation of the public health community (i.e., distinguish reproductive choices from the public health concern to decrease the incidence of the disease or the gene in the population), and led to discrimination by employers, including the military, as well as the loss of insurance. The development of the screening program for gene for Tay–Sachs disease in the Jewish community benefited from the sickle cell experience and has resulted in successful population-based screening with high community acceptance and minimal adverse effects (23).

Before population-based screening for genetic conditions occurs, programs should consider five points (41). First, screening programs should clearly state their purpose and goal. Second, peer-reviewed pilot studies are necessary to demonstrate that the stated goals of the program can be achieved at a reasonable cost and with few adverse effects. This proposed safeguard may come under pressure, because the potential of screening for literally hundreds of genetic traits or susceptibilities creates pressure to begin screening prior to either adequate review of pilot studies or public debate. Third, the target population must be educated about the disease or condition in question and receive counseling about the risks and benefits of screening. Fourth, the traditional standards of informed consent must be observed. Screening should remain voluntary. Individuals must be able to exercise their "right not to know." Fifth, confidentiality of the individual must be maintained. In addition, although Fost does not specifically address this concern, universal access to testing must be ensured by public health agencies if genetic technologies are not to exacerbate existing social inequalities.

A national policy for genetic screening should have procedural mechanisms in place at both the state and federal levels to prevent harm to the individual being screened (42). Discrimination as a consequence of genetic testing has been documented (6). The health and life insurance industries use genetic test results to deny coverage, and the presence of preexisting condition clauses in many policies have led to "job lock" for families or the loss of coverage for either the individual with a genetic disease or the carrier of a gene for a disease. Stigmatization in the form of loss of services or entitlement has also been reported.

TRANSPLANTS

The use of fetal tissue transplants for Parkinson's disease has prompted considerable debate by the public and within scientific communities. In 1987 the NIH submitted a request to the Assistant Secretary of Health seeking approval for fetal tissue transplantation. In May 1988, however, a moratorium on federal funding was declared on fetal tissue transplant research. Although at least one center voluntarily discontinued its research in response to the moratorium, two centers, at Yale and at the University of Colorado, elected to use private funds to continue research efforts with fetal tissue transplants (1). The central objection to the use of fetal tissue is political rather than scientific. Because the tissue is obtained from aborted fetuses, it is the source of the tissue rather than its use that creates conflict.

Political responses and both public and scientific debate about fetal tissue transplants for Parkinson's disease patients clearly illustrates the shift from the physician and patient-based bioethic to one influenced by social and political interests. Indeed, the 1993 lifting of the ban on fetal tissue research by the Clinton administration both was responsive to public debate and guarantees that the debate will continue, while permitting research protocols to be judged on scientific merit rather than political precepts.

PSYCHIATRIC DISORDERS

The genes responsible for schizophrenia, bipolar disorders, and Alzheimer's disease have yet to be clearly elucidated, though familial predispositions have been identified. The etiology of schizophrenia and affective disorders is unknown. These conditions are probably heterogeneous, resulting from both biologic and environmental components. The cause of Alzheimer's disease is also unknown but may have several genetic etiologies.

Family studies involving the affective disorders have confirmed clear genetic factors, including: increased risks for early-onset probands versus late-onset probands; an increased risk for unipolar depression in women and a slightly increased risk for bipolar depression in women; an increased risk for women who have first-degree relatives with a bipolar disorder for developing bipolar disease while no such association has been noted for unipolar conditions; relatives of bipolar probands have a higher risk of affective disorders (primarily unipolar) than do relatives of unipolar probands; affected relatives of unipolar probands usually have unipolar depression; and an increased risk (50–75%) is present when both parents have bipolar disorders (32).

Hereditary risks are also present in schizophrenia. Empiric risks are dependent upon the relationship to the affected individual. Second-degree relatives have the lowest risk (about 2–3%), whereas an individual with an affected identical twin has a 40–60% chance of developing the condition. The individual with one affected parent has about a 10–15% risk for schizophrenia.

In the late 1980s, the genetic material responsible for schizophrenia was mapped to chromosome 5 and bipolar disorders were mapped to chromosome 11. This work could not be replicated, and the initial findings were discovered to have been reversed in the original samples. The data further polarized the debate of the role of genetics in psychiatric conditions. The arguments of nurture versus nature resurfaced in the mental health community.

Alzheimer's disease fared better with pathophysiological characterization of β-amyloid-containing plaques and eventual mutation identification of early-onset Alzheimer's disease on chromosome 21 and another early-onset gene on chromosome 14. A late-onset gene has been mapped to chromosome 19.

Alzheimer's disease demonstrates that genetic studies can be applied to psychiatric conditions despite the confounding factors of genetic heterogeneity, ascertainment of late-onset conditions, and variable ages of onset.

Psychiatric disorders are complex and will probably result in the identification of complicated rather than straightforward modes of inheritance and uncertainty in defining inherited psychiatric conditions (38).

The preventive ethics model is again well-suited to these complex conditions. Psychiatric genetic research poses two specific issues that other genetic conditions do not—namely, the subject's competence to participate in research and determining the legal and ethical acceptability of substituted judgment for subjects not competent to consent (34).

Legal requirements of competence must be met; and if a research participant is not competent to consent, provisions could be obtained from a legally authorized representative approved by the local internal review board (IRB) in accordance with prevailing state regulations. Harper's guidelines previously reviewed do not address the competency issue. Psychiatric conditions also may involve the circumstance where clinical information is communicated to a third party for the subject's safety. Consent documents might include a section allowing the subject to designate a physician or allowing another individual to receive such information.

The protection of the rights of the individual are not unique to psychiatric disorders or genetic conditions but pose significant issues in the context of genetic research and discovery of the genes responsible for psychiatric disorders.

CONCLUSION

The preventive ethics paradigm provides a model for considering clinical and scientific conduct which accommodates more than the factors immediately apparent in a particular circumstance. By anticipating ethical concerns, seeking comment from the relevant parties, and examining background social factors and institutional structures, preventive ethics anticipates the effects of policies and practices on people of different social, economic, and educational backgrounds. By adopting an anticipatory (rather than a reactive) stance, the preventive ethics model encourages the development of policies governing genetic research and the provision of genetic services which build upon the experience of health-care providers and researchers in nongenetic contexts. Finally, in seeking to anticipate and minimize ethical conflict and to explore possible ethical solutions to problems before actual conflicts develop, preventive ethics seeks to provide individuals with the opportunity to make use of genetic and other medical technologies in the pursuit of their life plans in accordance with their sets of values.

REFERENCES

1. Annas GJ. *Standard of care.* New York: Oxford University Press, 1993;154–159, 164–166, 181–186.
2. Appelbaum PS, Lidz CW, Meisel A. *Informed consent: legal theory and clinical practice.* New York: Oxford University Press, 1987.
3. Appelbaum PS, Roth LH. Patients who refuse treatment in medical hospitals. *JAMA* 1983;250:1296–1301.
4. Barnard D. Unsung questions of medical ethics. *Soc Sci Med* 1985;21:243–249.
5. Beauchamp TL, Childress JF. *Principles of biomedical ethics.* 3rd ed. New York: Oxford University Press, 1989.
6. Billings P, et al. Discrimination as a consequence of genetic testing. *Am J Hum Genet* 1992;51(4):899–901.
7. *Canterbury v. Spence.* 464 F.2d 772, 1972.
8. Emmitt RJ. Tardy compassion [Letter]. *Lancet* 1993;341:1157–1158.
9. Epstein AN. Changes in the delivery of care under comprehensive health care reform. *N Engl J Med* 1993;329:1672–1676.
10. Fisher M, ed. *U.S. Preventive Services Task Force. Guide to clinical preventive services; an assessment of the effectiveness of 169 interventions.* Baltimore: Williams & Wilkins, 1989.
11. Folstein S. *Huntington disease.* Baltimore: Johns Hopkins University Press, 1989;177–187.
12. Forrow L, Arnold RM, Parker LS. Preventive ethics: expanding the horizons of clinical ethics. *J Clin Ethics* 1993;4:287–294.
13. Fost N. Genetic diagnosis and treatment. *AJDC* 1993;146:1190–1195.
14. Friedman M. Care and context in moral reasoning. In: Kittay EF, Meyers DT, eds. *Women and moral theory.* Totowa, NJ: Rowman & Littlefield, 1987.
15. Frye M. *The politics of reality: essays in feminist theory.* Trumansburg, NY: Crossing Press, 1983.
16. Gelehrter T, Collins F. *Principles of medical genetics.* Baltimore: Williams & Wilkins, 1990;289–297.
17. Harper P. Research samples from families with genetic diseases: a proposed code of conduct. *Br Med J* 1993;306:1391–1394.
18. Harper P. Clinical consequences of isolating the gene for Huntington's disease. *Br Med J* 1993;307:397–398.
19. Hasty compassion [Editorial]. *Lancet* 1993;341:663.
20. Healy B. Remarks for the RAC committee meeting of January 14, 1993, regarding compassionate use exemption. *Hum Gene Ther* 1993;4:196–197.
21. Jennings B. Bioethics and democracy. *Centennial Rev* 1990; 35(2):207–225.
22. *Journal of the American Medical Association.* Special Issue: Caring for the Uninsured and Underinsured *JAMA* 1993;265:2437–2624.
23. Kaback MM, Zeiger RS. The John Kennedy Institute Tay Sachs Program: practical and ethical issues in an adult genetic screening program. In: Condliffe P, Callanhan D, Hilton B, eds. *Ethical issues in genetic counseling and the use of genetic knowledge.* New York: Plenum Press, 1972.
24. Murray T. Ethical issues in human genome research. *FASEB* 1991;5:55–60.
25. National Society of Genetic Counselors. *Code of ethics.* Wallingford, PA, 1992.
26. Parker L. Bioethics for human geneticists: models for reasoning and methods for teaching. *Am J Hum Genet* 1994;54:137–147. [Portions of this chapter have appeared previously in this article.]
27. Payer L. *Medicine and culture.* New York: Henry Holt and Company, 1988.
28. Pincoffs E. Quandary ethics. *Mind* 1971;80:552–571.
29. Position paper on human germ line manipulation presented by Council for Responsible Genetics, Human Genetic Committee, Fall 1992. *Hum Gene Ther* 1993;4:35–37.
30. *In the matter of Karen Quinlan.* 70 NJ 10, 1976.
31. Ramsey P. *The patient as person.* New Haven: Yale University Press, 1970.
32. Robinson A, Linden M. *Clinical genetic handbook.* 2nd ed. Boston: Blackwell Scientific Publications, 1993;465–469.
33. Sherwin SS. *No longer patient: feminist ethics and health care.* Philadelphia: Temple University Press, 1992.
34. Shore D, Berg K, Wynne O, Folstein MF. Legal and ethical issues in psychiatric genetic research. *Am J Med Gen* 1993;48(1):17–21.
35. Starr P. The framework of health care reform. *N Engl J Med* 1993;329:1666–1672.
36. Thompson L. Harkin seeks compassionate use of unproven treatments. *Science* 1992;258:1728.
37. Thompson L. Healy approves an unproven treatment. *Science* 1993;259:172.
38. Tsuang MT, Faraone SV. Neuropsychiatric genetics: a new specialty section of the American Journal of Medical Genetics [Editorial]. *Am J Med Genet* 1993;48(1):1–3.
39. Veatch RM. Models for ethical medicine in a revolutionary age. *Hastings Center Rep* 1972;2(3):5–7.
40. Walters L. Human gene therapy: ethics and public policy. *Hum Gene Ther* 1991;2:115–122.
41. Wilfond BS, Fost N. The introduction of cystic fibrosis carrier screening into clinical practice: policy considerations. *Milbank Q* 1992;70(4):629–59.
42. Wilfond BS, Nolan K. National policy development for the clinical application of genetic diagnostic technologies. Lessons from cystic fibrosis. *JAMA* 1993;270(24):2948–2954.
43. Wivel N, Walters, L. Germ line gene modification and disease prevention: some medical and ethical perspectives. *Science* 1993;262:533–538.
44. Yesley MS. *Bibliography: ethical legal and social implications of the human genome project.* U.S. Department of Energy, Washington, DC, 1992.

Psychopharmacology: The Fourth Generation of Progress, edited by Floyd E. Bloom and David J. Kupfer. Raven Press, Ltd., New York © 1995.

CHAPTER 160

The Economics of Psychotropic Drug Development

Joseph A. DiMasi and Louis Lasagna

The benefits that drugs, often in conjunction with psychotherapy or other adjunctive therapy, have brought since the 1950s to the treatment of many psychiatric disorders are substantial. It has been estimated that two to four million people in the United States are severely mentally ill (1), with nearly two-thirds of them suffering from schizophrenia (30). In the late 1950s, two-thirds of schizophrenics spent most of their lives in mental hospitals; in the late 1980s, however, 95% of schizophrenic patients were treated on an outpatient basis (2). In the United States the inpatient schizophrenic population fell by more than 400,000 from the mid-1950s, when chlorpromazine was introduced, to the late 1980s (2). While not the only factor, the development of chlorpromazine and other antipsychotics surely played a major role in the deinstitutionalization.

Similarly, lithium has transformed the treatment of bipolar disorder, so that now the majority of manic–depressive patients can effectively cope with their condition. The introduction of tricyclic antidepressants, monoamine oxidase (MAO) inhibitors, and, more recently, the selective serotonin reuptake inhibitors has provided effective means for relieving the symptoms of many patients suffering from major depression or dysthymia.

While substantial progress has been made over the last four decades in developing new psychotropic drugs with improved side effect profiles and, to some extent, in finding expanded uses for already available drugs, relatively few breakthroughs have been achieved. Notable exceptions are clomipramine for obsessive–compulsive disorder and clozapine for refractory schizophrenia. This has led some to argue for increased government/industry collaboration in this area, the creation of an expert panel that would assess the potential contribution to public health

of therapeutic agents that are used in other countries, or additional economic incentives to develop novel, but seemingly unprofitable, psychotropic drugs (11,21,33).

Clearly, some of the obstacles to the development of new drugs that would be useful to patients who are refractory to current treatments are economic. In general, new drug development is a costly, lengthy, and risky endeavor. Psychotropic drug development is no exception to the rule. The evidence on changing development costs is striking. DiMasi et al. (4) examined the research and development (R&D) costs of 12 U.S. pharmaceutical firms for their new chemical entities (NCEs) that began clinical testing during 1970–1982. They found the fully allocated cost per drug approved in the United States to be $279 million (in 1992 dollars). A comparable study by Hansen (15) covering an earlier time period (NCEs entering clinical testing during 1963–1975) found the average R&D cost for NCEs to be $121 million (in 1992 dollars).

The average U.S. approval date for NCEs in the Hansen (15) sample was in 1975, while the average U.S. approval for the DiMasi et al. (4) sample occurred in 1984. Thus, R&D costs have more than doubled in inflation-adjusted dollars in approximately one decade. This remarkable rate of increase in the resources devoted to new drug development cannot continue indefinitely. There is, however, no indication as yet that these costs will decline. Costs of this magnitude present imposing barriers that developers of new drugs must surmount. High R&D costs and uncertainties in the drug development process can be particularly problematic for biotechnology firms because they often depend on frequent infusions of large amounts of venture capital.

The length of the entire drug development process, from discovery of a compound to its approval for marketing, can also serve as a disincentive to innovation. Lengthier development times are generally associated with higher development costs (both out-of-pocket and in

---

J. A. DiMasi and L. Lasagna: Center for the Study of Drug Development, Tufts University, Boston, Massachusetts 02111.

terms of lost investment income from alternative uses of the funds). In addition, the longer it takes to test a drug and get it approved, the shorter will be the period of patent exclusivity and, therefore, the less time a firm will have to recoup the large fixed costs associated with modern new drug development. DiMasi et al. (5,6) have shown how protracted the process has become for drugs approved in the United States. The mean time from synthesis to U.S. marketing approval rose from approximately 8 years for drugs approved in the mid- to late 1960s to approximately 14 years for drugs approved in the 1980s.

The high risks faced by developers of new drugs can also inhibit innovation. The number of compounds synthesized for every one that proves to be marketable has been estimated to be in the thousands (8,14,17,36,37). Although the adoption of "rational drug design" techniques may reduce the number of compounds that are investigated, the risks are likely to remain high. Even for drugs that are judged promising enough to warrant testing in humans, substantial uncertainty remains. Only about one in five new drugs that reach the clinical testing stage in the United States will eventually be approved for marketing (4–6,32) (see also Chapter 158, *this volume*).

Whether psychotropic drug development is, in some economic sense, more or less problematic than drug development in general is a question that we can answer adequately only by appeal to the facts. In this chapter we investigate some of the factors that affect the economics of psychotropic drug development and review what is known about the benefits and costs of treating mental illness. Specifically, in the section entitled "Discovery to Marketing: A Lengthy Process" we compare results on development and regulatory review times for marketed drugs in the major psychotropic drug subclasses to one another and to results for all new drugs. Data on U.S. investigational drugs are used in the section entitled "Trends in Psychotropic Drug Innovation" to measure trends in psychotropic drug innovation and success rates for psychotropic drugs. The section entitled "The Cost of New Drug Development" presents some results on the cost of developing new psychotropic drugs. In the section entitled "The Availability of Psychotropic Drugs in the United States" we review the literature on the availability of psychotropic drugs in the United States in comparison to other countries. We discuss some of the practical problems and ethical concerns in conducting clinical research on psychotropic drugs in the section entitled "Operational and Ethical Impediments to Psychotropic Drug Development." Studies on the cost of mental illness are critically assessed in the section entitled "The Cost of Mental Illness." Finally, we offer some conclusions in the section entitled "Conclusions."

DISCOVERY TO MARKETING: A LENGTHY PROCESS

The length of the development process for drugs as a whole has been well documented (4–6). The literature, though, lacks specifics about psychotropic drugs. The Center for the Study of Drug Development (CSDD) maintains a database of NCEs that have received U.S. marketing approval since 1963. The database contains both publicly available and proprietary information obtained from surveys of pharmaceutical firms. We use information in this database to determine average development and regulatory review times for psychotropic drugs and compare them to similar data for all new drugs.

For the purposes of this chapter, an NCE is defined as a new molecular compound not previously tested in humans. Excluded are new salts and esters of existing compounds, diagnostics, and biologics. We confined our analysis of psychotropic drugs to the NCEs in the antianxiety, antipsychotic, sedative/hypnotic, and miscellaneous psychotherapeutic categories in *Drug Facts and Comparisons* (7). Information on milestones in the development process were obtained from the CSDD database for 45 psychotropic NCEs approved in the United States from 1963 through 1992. Table 1 lists those drugs by subclass. For each drug it also shows the date on which a new drug application (NDA) was submitted to the Food and Drug Administration (FDA) for marketing approval, the date of NDA approval, and the review time for the drug, defined as the time from NDA submission to NDA approval.

The period of analysis (1963–1992) is long, and studies have found increases in the length of the new drug development process over this time frame (5,6). Proportionately more of the psychotropics have been approved in the first half of the study period than is the case for all NCEs (51% versus 41%). As a class, psychotropics have had development time trends that are qualitatively similar to those of NCEs in general. Under the assumption then that the trends reflect meaningful changes over time in the development process, comparison of psychotropic drug development times to those of all NCEs over the study period may understate the extent to which psychotropic development times exceed the overall averages for recent development.

The psychotropic subclasses differ, however, in terms of how their approvals are distributed over time. The antianxiety and antipsychotic approvals are concentrated in the first half of the study period, while the antidepressants and sedative/hypnotics have been approved predominantly in the second half of the period. The number of approvals for the subclasses in the two periods, though, tend to be small, thus limiting the ability to do meaningful analysis by subperiod. We do, however, report results in the text for more recent approvals when the results differ substantially from those for the whole period. In addition, a regression analysis was conducted that allows comparisons of development and review times for psychotropics and NCEs in other therapeutic classes, while controlling for the year of approval.

Clinical Development and Regulatory Review

Mean clinical phase times for psychotropic subclasses and for all NCEs in the CSDD database are shown in

TABLE 1. *Psychotropic new chemical entities approved in the United States, 1963–1992*

Generic name	Trade name	Company	NDA submitted	NDA approved	NDA review time (months)
Antianxiety					
Diazepam	Valium	Roche	12/15/61	11/15/63	23.0
Tybamate	Solacen	Wallace	6/11/63	3/10/65	21.0
Oxazepam	Serax	Wyeth	1/13/64	6/04/65	16.7
Clorazepate dipotassium	Tranxene	Abbott	11/09/71	6/23/72	7.5
Prazepam	Verstran	Warner-Lambert	12/29/72	12/14/76	47.5
Lorazepam	Ativan	Wyeth	10/08/75	9/30/77	23.8
Halazepam	Paxipam	Schering-Plough	5/13/75	9/24/81	76.4
Alprazolam	Xanax	Upjohn	3/02/79	10/16/81	31.5
Buspirone HCl	Buspar	Bristol-Myers	12/15/82	9/29/86	45.5
Antidepressant					
Pargyline HCl	Eutonyl	Abbott	3/07/62	2/14/63	11.3
Nortriptyline HCl	Aventyl HCl	Lilly	6/03/63	11/06/64	17.1
Desipramine HCl	Norpramin	Merrell	4/09/63	11/20/64	19.4
Protriptyline HCl	Vivactil HCl	Merck	2/25/64	9/27/67	43.0
Doxepin HCl	Sinequan	Pfizer	7/05/68	9/23/69	14.6
Trimipramine maleate	Surmontil	Ives	6/20/68	6/12/79	131.7
Amoxapine	Asendin	Lederle	4/14/77	9/22/80	41.3
Maprotiline HCl	Ludiomil	Ciba-Geigy	11/01/73	12/01/80	85.0
Trazodone	Desyrel	Mead Johnson	10/11/78	12/21/81	38.3
Nomifensine maleate	Merital	Hoechst	12/28/78	12/31/84	72.1
Bupropion HCl	Wellbutrin	Burroughs Wellcome	12/23/81	12/30/85	48.2
Fluoxetine HCl	Prozac	Lilly	9/06/83	12/29/87	51.7
Clomipramine	Anafranil	Ciba-Geigy	6/16/89	12/29/89	6.4
Sertralline HCl	Zoloft	Pfizer	4/13/88	12/30/91	44.6
Paroxetine HCl	Paxil	SmithKline Beecham	11/20/89	12/29/92	37.3
Antipsychotic					
Carphenazine maleate	Proketazine	Wyeth	1/30/61	1/29/63	24.0
Haloperidol	Haldol	McNeil	12/17/63	4/12/67	39.8
Thiothixene	Navane	Pfizer	11/17/66	7/24/67	8.2
Butaperazine maleate	Repoise	Robins	5/05/64	9/26/67	40.7
Piperacetazine	Quide	Dow	5/29/62	2/03/69	80.2
Mesoridazine	Serentil	Sandoz	4/30/68	2/27/70	21.9
Lithium carbonate	Eskalith	SmithKline & French	5/09/69	4/06/70	10.9
Molindone HCl	Moban	Du Pont	11/11/71	1/18/74	26.3
Loxapine succinate	Loxitane	Lederle	9/25/73	2/25/75	17.0
Pimozide	Orap	McNeil	4/06/73	7/31/84	135.8
Clozapine	Clozaril	Sandoz	9/01/87	9/26/89	24.8
Sedative/Hypnotic					
Flurazepam HCl	Dalmene	Roche	11/20/67	4/07/70	28.6
Triclofos sodium	Triclos	Merrell	8/05/68	3/22/72	43.5
Temazepam	Restoril	Sandoz	6/21/78	2/27/81	32.3
Etomidate	Amidate	Abbott	11/21/78	9/07/82	45.5
Triazolam	Halcion	Upjohn	5/11/76	11/15/82	78.2
Midazolam HCl	Versed	Roche	12/15/82	12/20/85	36.2
Quazepam	Dormalin	Schering-Plough	4/09/82	12/27/85	44.6
Estazolam	Proscom	Abbott	12/19/83	12/26/90	84.2
Nedecromil sodium	Tilade	Fisons	1/30/89	12/16/92	46.5
Miscellaneous					
Pemoline	Cylert	Abbott	11/25/68	1/27/75	74.1

Fig. 1. We report results only for those NCEs for which we have complete phase data. Phase length is defined as the time from the start of testing in the phase to the start of the next phase. These phase lengths may overestimate or underestimate actual phase testing times. Testing in a phase may end before the next phase begins, or it may overlap with the next phase. DiMasi et al. (4) found small differences, on average, between phase lengths defined in this way and actual phase lengths for Phases I and II. However, Phase III extended, on average, 6 months into the NDA review period. Thus, the Phase III times in Fig. 1 may underestimate the actual amount of time spent in Phase III clinical testing.

Mean Phase I time for psychotropics for the whole period (12.7 months) is close to the average for all NCEs. Average Phase I time for the last 15 years of the study period, however, is 4.4 months longer for psychotropics. Among the subclasses, only the antidepressant category has longer-than-average Phase I times for both halves of the study period. The psychotropics tended to spend much

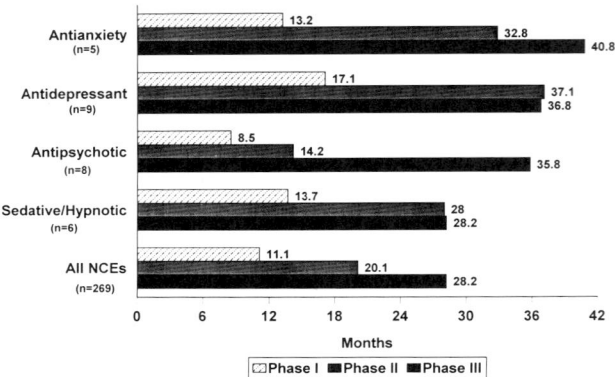

FIG. 1. Mean clinical phase development times for psychotropic and all new chemical entities (NCEs) approved in the United States during 1963–1992. The length of a phase is determined as the time from when the phase begins to when the next phase begins. Phase length for Phase III is the time from the start of Phase III to new drug application (NDA) submission. Only those NCEs with complete phase time data are included.

more time in testing than NCEs as a whole in Phases II and III (27.1 and 35.1 months, respectively), where efficacy is explored and established. For the most part, however, this is a recent phenomenon. Phase II and Phase III mean times are 2.2 and 3.6 months longer than those for all NCEs for the first 15 years, respectively. For the last 15 years, however, mean Phase II time is 11.7 months longer than that for all NCEs, and mean Phase III time is 10.2 months longer.

We have more data on investigational new drug application (IND) and NDA filing dates than we do on phase starting dates. Clinical development time can be measured as the time from IND filing to NDA submission. We define this period to be the IND phase. Similarly, we measure the regulatory review period as the NDA phase—that is the time from NDA submission to NDA approval. Mean IND and NDA phases for the psychotropic subclasses and for all NCEs are shown in Fig. 2. Medians, ranges, and sample sizes are shown in Table 2.

Clinical development periods for psychotropics (a mean of 68.1 months for 1963–1992) tend to be longer than average. This is especially true for the more recent approvals. The mean IND phase for psychotropics approved during 1978–1992 is 94.1 months, compared to 66.8 months for all NCEs. Over the whole study period, with the exception of antipsychotics, clinical development times for the psychotropic subclasses tend to be much longer than those for NCEs in general. For the last half of the study period, all subclasses have mean clinical development times that are much longer than those for all NCEs.

Each of the psychotropic subclasses have average regulatory review times that are longer than those for all NCEs. However, during the first half of the study period, the antidepressant and antianxiety categories had below

average review times. Average review time for all psychotropics during this period, though, is 2.2 months longer than the average for all NCEs (28.7 versus 26.5 months). The difference in review times between psychotropics and other NCEs is striking for the more recent subperiod. Mean review time is substantially greater for each psychotropic subclass than for all NCEs during this period. The 22 psychotropic NCEs approved during 1978–1992 have a mean review time of 56.3 months, compared to 32.1 months for all NCEs.

Preclinical and Total Development Time

While psychotropics appear to have, on average, longer clinical testing and regulatory reviews than do other NCEs, the evidence does not suggest the same for preclinical testing. Our measure of the length of preclinical testing is the time from the first tests for pharmacologic activity to the first human tests. Figure 3 shows average preclinical time, measured in this way, for psychotropic subclasses and for all NCEs (medians and ranges are given in Table 3). Although mean preclinical time is longer for the antipsychotics than for all NCEs, the other subclasses (and psychotropics as a whole) tend to move from first pharmacologic testing to human testing quicker than do NCEs in general. Mean preclinical time for psychotropics (29.5 months) is 7.4 months shorter than it is for all NCEs. The differences in average preclinical time between psychotropics and all NCEs are nearly identical for both halves of the study period.

Development costs, and thus the economic viability of new drug development, depend on the entire period from discovery of a compound to marketing approval. In Fig. 4 we show the mean time from synthesis of a new drug to its approval for marketing in the United States

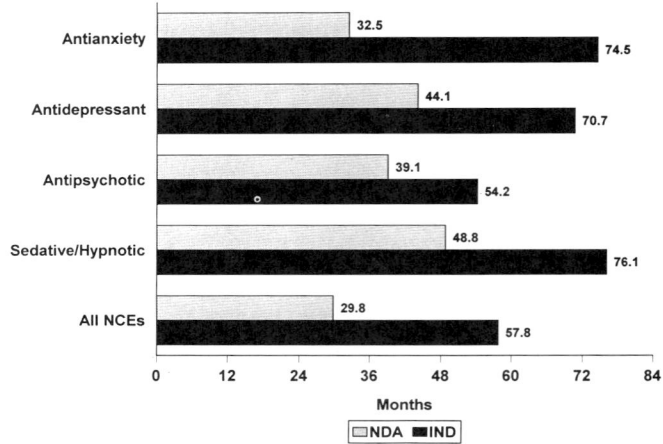

FIG. 2. Mean clinical and regulatory review phase times for psychotropic and all NCEs approved in the United States during 1963–1992. The investigational new drug application (IND) phase is the time from IND filing to NDA submission. The NDA phase is the time from NDA submission to NDA approval.

TABLE 2. *Median clinical development and regulatory review times (months) for psychotropic and all new chemical entities approved in the United States, 1963–1992*

Drug	IND phase[a] Median (range)	N	NDA phase[a] Median (range)	N	Total phase[a] Median (range)	N
Antianxiety	65.9 (19.0–128.0)	9	23.8 (7.5–76.4)	9	134.8 (35.6–173.4)	9
Antidepressant	54.6 (13.7–234.0)	15	41.3 (6.4–131.7)	15	129.1 (25.0–240.5)	15
Antipsychotic	47.7 (6.3–189.4)	10	24.8 (8.2–135.8)	11	81.5 (28.7–214.2)	10
Sedative/hypnotic	71.9 (36.9–142.9)	9	44.6 (28.6–84.2)	9	121.7 (79.6–175.1)	9
All NCEs	48.2 (3.5–300.2)	455	23.7 (2.9–135.8)	496	77.9 (11.8–331.5)	455

[a] The IND phase is the time from IND filing to NDA submission. The NDA phase is the time from NDA submission to NDA approval. The total phase is the time from IND filing to NDA approval.

for psychotropic subclasses and for all NCEs (medians and ranges are given in Table 3). For the whole study period, mean synthesis-to-approval time is moderately longer for psychotropics than for all NCEs (155.2 months versus 146.6 months). However, for the last half of the study period, psychotropic time from synthesis to approval averages 212.4 months, while the mean for all NCEs approved during that period is 171.5 months. For the first half of the study period, the psychotropic subclasses had average to below-average synthesis-to-approval times. Thus, psychotropic total development time has increased markedly in relation to other NCEs in more recent years.

Regression Analysis

As noted above, the new drug development process has tended to lengthen over time. For a thorough analysis of development and regulatory review times for a class of drugs, we should therefore allow for trends in the data. There may also be other characteristics of new drugs that

should be accounted for in isolating the length of the process for a group of drugs. Regression analysis allows us to control for multiple factors that may affect the length of the development or regulatory review periods. We use regression analysis to evaluate the major components of the process: the NDA phase, the IND phase, and the time from synthesis to marketing approval.

One characteristic that may partially explain development and review times is the therapeutic rating that the drug receives from the Food and Drug Administration (FDA). From 1976 to 1991 the FDA gave NCEs that were thought to represent a significant gain over existing therapy (a 1A rating), a modest gain over existing therapy (a 1B rating), and little or no gain over existing therapy (a 1C rating). Drugs to treat acquired immunodeficiency syndrome (AIDS) and AIDS-related conditions were given a 1AA rating. The FDA retroactively rated NCEs approved during 1963–1975 in accordance with this rating scheme. Since 1992 the FDA has simplified its rating scheme; New drugs receive either a priority (1P) or a standard (1S) rating.* For the regression analysis, we created a dummy variable (RATING) that takes on the value one if the NCE has a 1AA, 1A, 1B, or 1P rating and zero otherwise.

The regression format allows us to compare psychotropic development and review times to those for other therapeutic classes. We formed dummy variables for major therapeutic categories. Specifically, we use the variables ANINF for antiinfectives, ANALG/ANEST for analgesic-anesthetics, ANTINEO for antineoplastic NCEs, CARDIO for cardiovascular NCEs, ENDO for endocrine NCEs, GI for gastrointestinal NCEs, OCNS for central nervous system NCEs that are not psychotropics, RESP

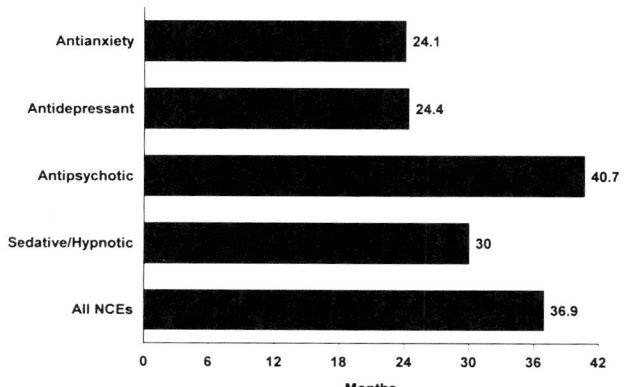

FIG. 3. Mean preclinical phase time for psychotropic and all NCEs approved in the United States during 1963–1992. The preclinical phase is the time from first pharmacologic testing of a compound to its first testing in humans.

*The distribution of psychotropic drugs by therapeutic rating is substantially different than it is for all NCEs. For example, while 47% of the NCEs approved between 1963 and 1992 have a 1C or 1S rating, 80% of the psychotropics have such ratings. Only three of 45 psychotropics have a 1A rating [lithium (given retrospectively), clomipramine, and clozapine]; 20% of all NCEs approved between 1963 and 1991 have 1A ratings (15% for those NCEs that have received prospective ratings).

TABLE 3. *Median preclinical and synthesis-to-approval times (months) for psychotropic and all new chemical entities approved in the United States, 1963–1992*

Drug	Preclinical phase[a]		Synthesis-to-approval phase[a]	
	Median (range)	N	Median (range)	N
Antianxiety	18.5 (6.0–50.0)	8	124.9 (48.0–223.0)	8
Antidepressant	24.5 (0.0–49.0)	14	192.5 (43.0–294.5)	14
Antipsychotic	38.0 (3.9–120.0)	10	128.0 (57.0–351.4)	9
Sedative/hypnotic	24.0 (13.0–59.0)	4	154.0 (99.0–186.0)	4
All NCEs	25.1 (0.0–240.0)	326	133.0 (31.9–359.7)	341

[a] The preclinical phase is the time from first pharmacologic testing to first administration in humans anywhere. The synthesis-to-approval phase is the time from synthesis of the compound to U.S. marketing approval.

for respiratory NCEs, and MISC for a miscellaneous category of NCEs. The regressions also include the explanatory variable YEAR—the year in which the NCE was approved.

Table 4 shows ordinary least-squares regression estimates for the NDA phase, the IND phase, and synthesis-to-approval time for the period 1963–1992. The regressions support the hypothesis of increasing trends in development and review times, independent of shifts over time in therapeutic classes or therapeutic significance. The year of approval is positively and significantly related to the length of each of the phases. The coefficients of the YEAR variable imply that, other things being equal, the NDA phase increased at the rate of 1 month every 3.3 years, the IND phase increased 1.7 months per year, and the synthesis-to-approval phase increased 3.7 months per year.

The coefficients of the therapeutic rating variable are statistically significant. As has been suggested elsewhere (6,20), the results indicate that NDA review times are shorter and that development times are longer for priority-rated NCEs. The shorter review times support the notion that the FDA has been successful in evaluating more ex-

peditiously drugs that it believes represent significant gains over existing therapy. The longer development times could be explained, in part, if priority-rated NCEs are more often singular in their therapeutic effects or pharmacologic mechanisms of action than are standard-rated NCEs.

The psychotropic class is the omitted therapeutic category in the regressions in Table 4. Thus, the coefficients of the therapeutic class variables can be interpreted as the differences in review or development times between the class in question and the psychotropic class. With a small number of exceptions, the therapeutic class coefficients are negative and the majority are statistically significant. None of the positive coefficients are statistically significant. Thus the results indicate that psychotropic drug development and regulatory review are lengthier than for many other classes, with no evidence that they are shorter than those of any of the other classes. The data are too thin to use the regression format to analyze differences with and among psychotropic subclasses.

Separate regressions using only data from the last half of the study period support the observations made above about review and development times for psychotropic drugs in relation to other NCEs for this subperiod. The therapeutic class coefficients for these regressions are much larger in absolute value than they are in Table 4. For example, the results in Table 4 imply that for the whole study period, psychotropics took (other things being equal) 19 months longer than antiinfectives to be reviewed, 34 months longer than antiinfectives in clinical testing up to NDA submission, and 45 months longer than antiinfectives from synthesis to marketing approval. The regressions for the last half of the study period, however, indicate that the differences between psychotropics and antiinfectives for 1978–1992 approvals are 31 months for review, 51 months for the IND phase, and 73 months from synthesis to approval.*

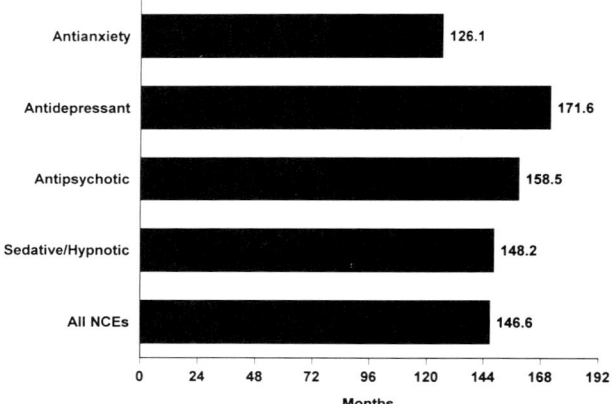

FIG. 4. Mean time from synthesis of a compound to NDA approval for psychotropic and all NCEs approved in the United States during 1963–1992.

*We also ran regressions with interaction variables, where the therapeutic class and RATING variables were multiplied by YEAR. The overall fits of the regressions and the statistical significance levels of the variables were almost identical to those reported here.

TABLE 4. *Regression analysis of development and regulatory review times for psychotropic drugs approved in the United States, 1963–1992*

Dependent variable	NDA phase[a]		IND phase[a]		Synthesis-to-approval phase[a]	
	Coefficient (t statistic)	p value	Coefficient (t statistic)	p value	Coefficient (t statistic)	p value
CONSTANT	20.225 (2.353)	0.0190	−67.120 (−3.880)	<0.0001	−131.544 (−5.955)	<0.0001
YEAR	0.305 (2.912)	0.0038	1.732 (8.191)	<0.0001	3.706 (10.285)	<0.0001
RATING	−7.005 (−3.667)	0.0003	8.872 (2.404)	0.0166	13.948 (2.075)	0.0387
ANINF	−18.766 (−5.209)	<0.0001	−34.237 (−5.076)	<0.0001	−44.538 (3.720)	0.0002
ANALG/ANEST	−9.389 (−2.362)	0.0185	−21.086 (−2.860)	0.0044	−23.144 (−1.827)	0.0686
ANTINEO	−14.170 (−3.159)	0.0017	0.884 (0.106)	0.9159	5.761 (0.370)	0.7114
CARDIO	−7.392 (−1.961)	0.0504	−12.008 (−1.701)	0.0897	−16.221 (−1.295)	0.1961
ENDO	−8.584 (−1.896)	0.0585	−13.478 (−1.538)	0.1247	−10.992 (−0.728)	0.4672
GI	−14.499 (−2.467)	0.0140	−32.113 (−2.769)	0.0059	−61.799 (−2.708)	0.0071
MISC	−8.090 (−1.597)	0.1109	−24.258 (−2.344)	0.0195	28.085 (1.497)	0.1354
OCNS	−10.337 (−1.989)	0.0473	−15.939 (−1.62)	0.1058	−20.391 (−1.207)	0.2283
RESP	−4.366 (−0.764)	0.4454	−15.971 (−1.486)	0.1380	−7.868 (−0.427)	0.6699
R^2	0.1267		0.2052		0.3000	
F	6.382		10.397		12.818	
N	496		455		341	

[a] The IND phase is the time from IND filing to NDA submission. The NDA phase is the time from NDA submission to NDA approval. The synthesis-to-approval phase is the time from synthesis of the compound to U.S. marketing approval.

TRENDS IN PSYCHOTROPIC DRUG INNOVATION

The final output of pharmaceutical firm new drug development can be measured by the number of NCE approvals. If, however, we examine investigational NCEs, then we can also glimpse where firms had invested their hopes and form expectations about how much innovation we will see in the near future. The CSDD maintains a database of investigational NCEs. We examined this database for trends in the number and kinds of psychotropic NCEs entering clinical testing in the United States.

The CSDD database contains information on commercial IND filings for NCEs by 36 U.S. pharmaceutical firms during the period 1963–1989. We divided this period into three decade-long subperiods. In the first decade these firms filed INDs on 847 NCEs. The number of IND filings declined 35% to 550 in the second decade, and then increased 17% to 645 for the last decade. As can be seen in Fig. 5, the pattern was different for psychotropics. While there was a decline of roughly the same proportions for psychotropics from the first decade to the second as

was observed for all NCEs, the number of psychotropic NCEs tested did not increase for the last decade. One factor that may have affected the incentive to pursue psychotropic drug development is the lengthening of the process over time in relative as well as absolute terms, as noted above.

The IND filing trends differ for psychotropic drug subclasses. The largest group of psychotropics investigated is the antidepressant category. The pattern for antidepressant development is similar to that for psychotropics as a whole. However, activity on anxiolytics and antipsychotics increased in the last decade analyzed, whereas activity on sedative/hypnotics dropped dramatically.

The disparate patterns for the subclasses may reflect, in part, differing scientific and economic opportunities. In particular, the developmental and commercial success of clozapine and a potentially large market for drugs to treat schizophrenia may have spurred development of antipsychotics. For example, the world market for drugs to treat schizophrenia is forecast to be valued at $2 billion (1992 dollars) in 2002 (28). The use of neuroleptics for psychoses is expected to increase 2.8% per year from

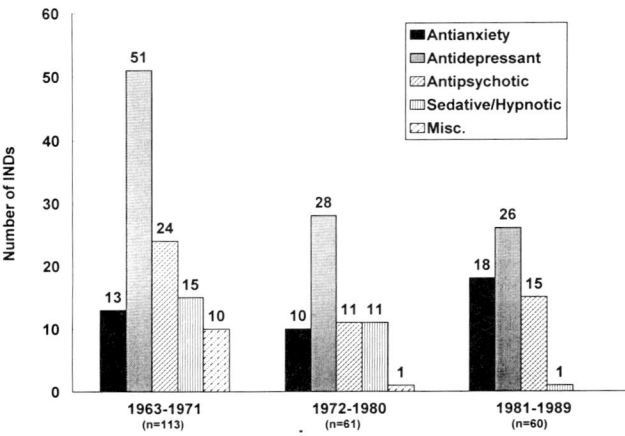

FIG. 5. Number of IND filings by 36 U.S. pharmaceutical firms in four specific and one miscellaneous psychotropic drug categories by period of IND filing.

1992 to 2002, with most of the growth fueled by the introduction of clozapine in markets where it has not been launched and the approval of new drugs (dopamine antagonists, serotonin antagonists, and dual-action serotonin–dopamine antagonists).

Success Rates for Psychotropic Clinical Development

Output from the new drug development process depends not only on the number of drugs investigated, but also on the probability that an investigational drug will be approved. We used the CSDD database on investigational NCEs to examine clinical success rates for psychotropics and for all NCEs. A clinical success rate is defined as the percentage of NCEs with INDs filed that are given U.S. marketing approval.

Figure 6 shows clinical success rates (as of December 31, 1992) for psychotropics and for all NCEs for three IND filing periods.* Success rates for psychotropics relative to other NCEs declined over time. Psychotropic success rates are clearly higher for the 1960s filings. None of the psychotropics from this period are still in active testing. A number of the other NCEs from this period are still active; but even if all of them eventually get approved, the success rate for all NCEs would increase only to 14.3%. Success rates for the two groups for the early 1970s are nearly identical. None of the psychotropics with INDs filed during 1970 to 1974 are still active, so 19.4% is a final success rate. The final success rate for all NCEs with early 1970s IND filings will be between 18.1% and 19.7%.

The clinical success rate for late 1970s psychotropic filings is well below average. Only one of the 28 psy-

chotropics from this group is still active. Thus, the final psychotropic success rate will be either 10.7% or 14.3%. If all of the active NCEs for this period are approved, then the final success rate for all NCEs will be 25.6%. Long development times, particularly for psychotropics, make analysis for the 1980s filings problematic. Even considering that development times for recent psychotropic approvals are much longer than average, the available evidence on psychotropic filings in the 1980s is not favorable. Only one of the 50 psychotropics with an IND filed in the 1980s has been approved.

It is not clear why psychotropic clinical success rates have declined. However, what is certain is that, other things being equal, a lower clinical success rate does imply a higher development cost per approved drug. The reason is that a lower success rate means that the costs of research failures are greater for every drug that does get approved.

THE COST OF NEW DRUG DEVELOPMENT

As noted above, DiMasi et al. (4) estimated average R&D costs for sample NCEs that were first tested in humans during 1970–1982. The costs of research failures and income foregone from investing in development for a period before any returns are earned (time costs) were included. Unpublished data from this sample on clinical phase costs for neuropharmacologic and all NCEs are shown in Fig. 7. The neuropharmacologic class includes more than psychotropics. However, small sample sizes precluded further decomposition of costs by therapeutic category.

Phase III costs for neuropharmacologics are about average. However, costs for the earlier phases and animal testing done during the clinical period are lower for neuropharmacologics. Each phase cost includes the costs of every drug that entered the phase, whether the drug was eventually abandoned or approved. The fully allocated cost per approved drug, however, depends critically on success rates, phase attrition rates, and the time spent in the various testing phases.

The clinical period out-of-pocket, time, and total costs per approved NCE for neuropharmacologics and for all NCEs in the sample are shown in Fig. 8. Lower-than-average success rates and longer development and regulatory review times for neuropharmacologics account for the fact that total cost per approved neuropharmacologic is 11% above average. The regressions presented above suggest that clinical testing and regulatory review have been longer for psychotropics than for other central nervous system drugs. Thus, the average cost of developing psychotropic drugs may be even higher than the average cost for all neuropharmacologics.

---

*We begin the analysis at 1964 instead of 1963 because many of the 1963 IND filings were for NCEs that had begun clinical testing in the United States prior to 1963. The 1962 Amendments to the Food, Drug, and Cosmetic Act of 1938 established the IND process.

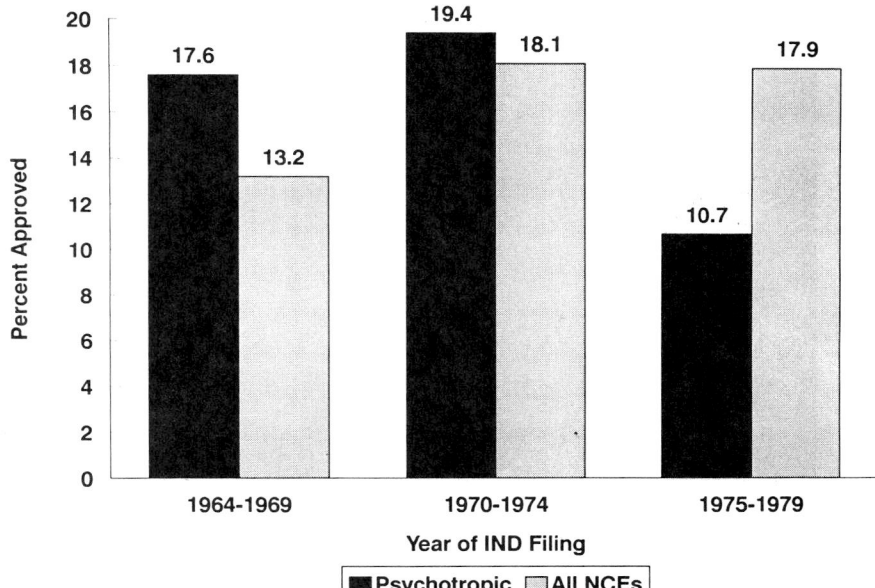

FIG. 6. Clinical success rates for self-originated (i.e., discovered and developed by the same firm) NCEs by period of IND filing. A clinical success rate is the percentage of NCEs with INDs filed in a period that obtained U.S. marketing approval as of the end of 1992.

THE AVAILABILITY OF PSYCHOTROPIC DRUGS IN THE UNITED STATES

Psychopharmacological innovations are not disseminated to all countries at even roughly the same time. In some instances, the lag between the availability of a psychotropic drug in two countries is substantial. A number of studies have specifically examined the availability of new drugs in the United States in relation to other industrialized countries. Wardell (34) documented a U.S. lag with respect to the United Kingdom in the availability of new drugs introduced in either market during 1962–1971. He found that, of 28 psychotropic NCEs approved in either country, 13 were exclusively available in the United Kingdom, while only four were exclusively available in the United States.

Later studies updated the Wardell analysis for more recent periods. Wardell (35) examined NCEs approved in the United States and the United Kingdom during

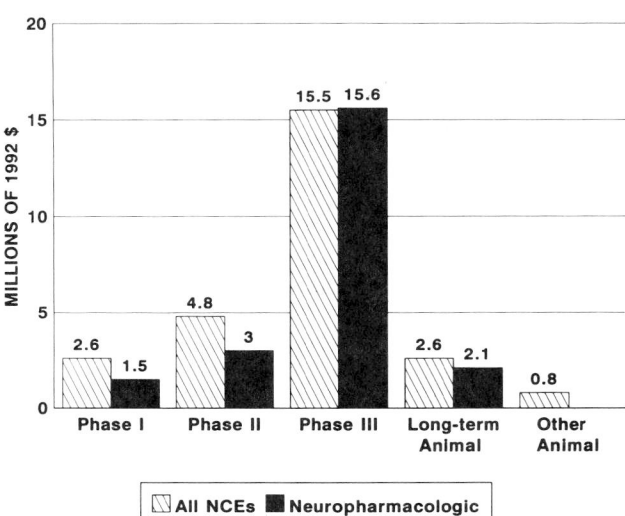

FIG. 7. Mean phase costs for investigational self-originated NCEs. Data are for a sample of NCEs that first entered clinical testing anywhere in the world during 1970–1982. The all-category results are for the full sample of 93 NCEs. Animal costs were incurred during the clinical period. Other animal costs are for animal testing that firms did not classify as long-term carcinogenicity or teratogenicity testing.

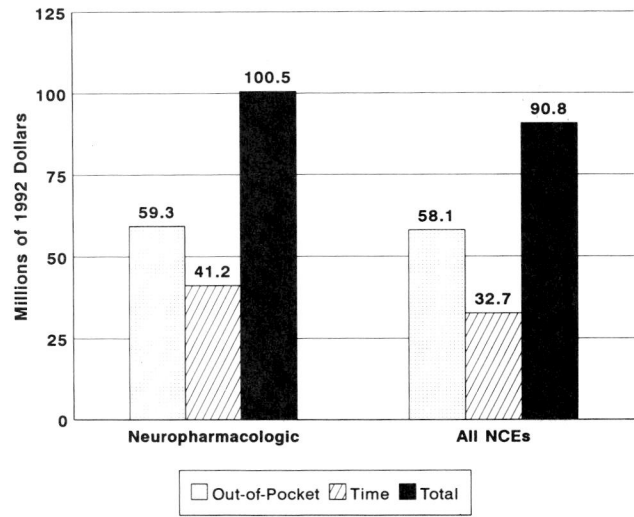

FIG. 8. Capitalized clinical period cost per approved NCE. The all-category results cover the full sample of 93 NCEs. Data are for a sample of NCEs that first entered clinical testing anywhere in the world during 1970–1982. A 9% real discount rate was used to capitalize out-of-pocket cost per approved NCE. Time cost is a measure of the income forgone from investing in development for a period before returns are earned. Total is the sum of out-of-pocket and time cost.

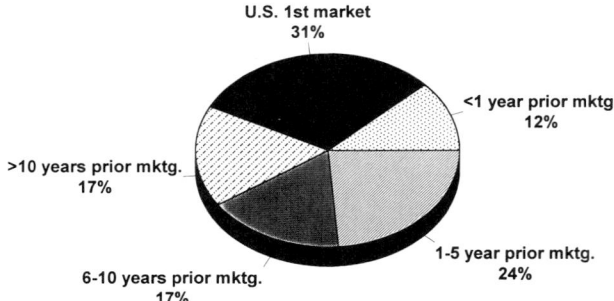

FIG. 9. Percentages of psychotropic NCEs approved for marketing in the United States during 1963–1992 that were first marketed in the United States and those that were first marketed in other countries for varying amounts of time prior to U.S. approval.

1972–1976. Of the 14 psychotropic NCEs made available during this period, eight were exclusively available in the United Kingdom and three were exclusively available in the United States. The most recent update in this series (19) found that, of 29 psychotropic NCEs made available during 1977–1987, 12 were exclusively available in the United Kingdom and five were exclusively available in the United States. Of the 12 psychotropic NCEs that were mutually available during this period, nine had been introduced in the United Kingdom first.

More recently, Vinar et al. (33) surveyed clinical pharmacologists about the usefulness of 50 psychotropic drugs that were either marketed or in late-stage clinical trials in Europe, but not available in the United States, for therapy or as a research tool. Twenty of these drugs were judged to be of particular interest after experts rated the drugs on the basis of novelty of mechanism of action and probable safety in comparison with drugs available in the United States. Some of the drugs have been available in Europe for decades. As of the end of 1993, none of these drugs had been approved in the United States. A search of the *NDA Pipeline* (26) indicated that only one of these drugs was in active testing at the end of 1992: fluvoxamine was in Phase III trials for depression and had an NDA submitted for obsessive–compulsive disorder.

Many of the drugs in the Vinar et al. (33) list have lost, or are close to losing, patent protection. They therefore likely have limited economic potential. Vinar et al. (33) argue for the creation of a board of pharmacological experts that would make recommendations to the FDA about foreign drugs that should be considered for accelerated regulatory review and, like compounds now given orphan drug designation, be granted a period of marketing exclusivity.

Many of the psychotropic drugs that do make it to the U.S. market had lengthy periods of prior foreign marketing. The CSDD database on NCEs approved in the United States contains information on the country in which the NCE was first marketed and the date of first marketing. Figure 9 shows how psychotropic NCEs approved in the

United States are distributed according to the number of years of prior foreign marketing. The United States was the first market for only 31% of the drugs. The proportions of drugs approved first in the United States or within 1 year of approval in the United States are virtually the same for all NCEs as for psychotropic drugs (30% approved in the United States first and 13% approved within 1 year of first foreign marketing for all NCEs). Proportionately many more of the psychotropic drugs that have been approved in the United states, however, have been available in a foreign market for a very long time. Only 12% of all NCEs have 6–10 years of prior marketing, and 9% of all NCEs have been marketed in another country for more than 10 years prior to U.S. approval. The lengthiest periods of prior foreign marketing for the psychotropics were for some of the most innovative drugs in this class. Clozapine was available in a foreign market (Switzerland) 17 years prior to U.S. approval, and clomipramine was first available 20 years before U.S. approval (Finland).

OPERATIONAL AND ETHICAL IMPEDIMENTS TO PSYCHOTROPIC DRUG DEVELOPMENT

As shown above, clinical development of psychotropic drugs is a lengthy and costly process. Significant improvements in the process can therefore pay off handsomely for society as well as for developers. There are a number of impediments to efficient and effective clinical development of psychotropic drugs that are worth noting. The problems include the allocation and adequacy of resources, special patient population characteristics, proper trial design, legal considerations, and ethical concerns.

For example, schizophrenic patients are often treated in a number of settings depending on the severity and the stage of the illness. Thus, the development of antipsychotics often requires extensive coordination and capabilities across varied facilities. A Phase II multicenter trial for an antipsychotic compound could, for example, easily require 20 sites (18).

The impaired cognitive capabilities of schizophrenic patients also present some difficulties for clinical research. The accuracy of symptoms reported by psychotic patients is questionable. Investigators, however, must often rely on these subjective reports. The accuracy of the reports may improve after treatment, but this makes it difficult to establish a baseline. In some cases, it may be important to recruit subjects who have not been previously treated. Results from animal studies, for example, have suggested that the effects of dopamine D_1 antagonists might differ according to whether the subject had been pretreated with a D_2 dopamine antagonist (18). Finally, the inclination of some psychotic patients to cooperate with clinical investigators or their capacity to give truly informed consent can be affected by their condition.

Klein (22) has identified a number of problems associated with Phase II trials for many psychotropic drugs that are potentially correctable. These include (a) selecting incorrect target populations, (b) study periods that are too short to detect beneficial effects, (c) recruitment difficulties, and (d) ignoring drug-withdrawal problems. Klein offers a number of suggestions to ameliorate these and other problems that would, hopefully, lead to more useful Phase III trials.

Finally, for almost two decades, certain kinds of research were greatly hampered by an FDA pronouncement that women of child-bearing potential should not be exposed to a drug candidate until some evidence of safety and efficacy was in hand from the study of other populations. The basis for this regulation was the residual anxieties that followed the thalidomide teratogenicity tragedies of the 1960s.

This restriction was a serious one in the case (for example) of antidepressants, where women of child-bearing potential represented the largest experimental population. The 1993 revised status of this population has seemingly eliminated this problem. The worry now is that advocates for clinical trials in diverse populations (women, blacks, the elderly, etc.) will force sponsors to pursue clinical benefit and safety assessments in such varied populations as to still further delay drug development and approval.

THE COST OF MENTAL ILLNESS

The potential for psychotropic drugs to relieve pain and suffering, and even to reduce the economic burden of mental illness on society, is substantial. While pain and suffering are difficult to assess quantitatively, we can more easily measure the economic costs to society of mental illness in general or of specific psychiatric disorders in particular. We review here the primary methodological approaches that have been used to measure the cost of illness and discuss the results of some of the more recent studies of the cost of mental illness.

Cost of illness studies have typically attempted to measure both direct costs of treatment (payments made) and indirect costs (resources lost). Two basic methodological approaches to valuing human life have been used: (i) the human capital approach, which measures an individual's lost productivity due to morbidity or mortality, and (ii) the willingness-to-pay approach, which measures what an individual would be willing to pay to avoid an increased risk of death or morbidity. Each of these approaches has conceptual problems. There have also been attempts, however, to combine the two approaches (24).

The human capital approach only counts economic loss in the marketplace. It excludes the value to individuals of reduced pain and suffering, changes in leisure time, and changes in risk per se. Typically, indirect costs of disease are measured partly on the basis of expected future lifetime earnings. This biases downward cost estimates for children, the elderly, and unpaid household workers. The approach is also problematic if there are

imperfections in labor markets. The value of the output of some individuals will be underestimated if, for example, wage discrimination on the basis of race or gender exists. For these and other reasons, many analysts have rejected the human capital approach. It still may be useful, however, as long as one realizes what it does and does not measure.

The willingness-to-pay approach has a conceptual basis in economic theory. Life is valued according to what individuals would be willing to pay to reduce the probability of illness. However, the results of willingness-to-pay analyses depend on the income distribution of the individuals who would be affected by the illness. The approach also has substantive measurement problems. Typically, individuals are asked hypothetical questions about valuing very small reductions in the probability of death. In addition, the approach is usually operationally very difficult to undertake. The relative ease with which human capital studies can be conducted has helped make it the most commonly used methodology in cost-of-illness studies.

Seminal work on the economic cost of mental illness was done by Fain (9), who estimated the direct and indirect cost of mental illness to be at least $2.4 billion in the mid-1950s. Since then, the trend in estimates of the cost of mental illness has been decidedly upward. The estimates actually fluctuate quite a bit, but this is undoubtedly due to differences in how and what costs were included (27).

Table 5 shows some of the more recent estimates of the cost of various illnesses. The costs of mental illness are roughly on a par with those of such major diseases as cancer and cardiovascular disease. Costs for depression

TABLE 5. *The economic cost of mental illness and other selected major illnesses in the United States*

Illness	Cost[a]	Study period
Mental illness		
Rice et al. (27)	104	1985
NMHAC (16)[b]	148	1990
Depression		
Stoudemire et al. (31)	16	1980
Greenberg et al. (12)	44	1990
Schizophrenia		
NMHAC (16)	33	1990
Arthritis		
Boston Consulting Group (2)	38	1987
Coronary heart disease		
National Institutes of Health (3)	43	1987
AIDS		
Scitovsky and Rice (29)	66	1991
Cancer		
Boston Consulting Group (2)	104	1987
Cardiovascular disease		
NMHAC (16)	160	1990

[a] Billions of dollars.
[b] NMHAC, National Mental Health Advisory Council.

and schizophrenia are similar to those for arthritis and coronary heart disease. A major portion of the costs of mental illness are attributable to indirect costs. For example, the indirect costs of depression in Greenberg et al. (12,13) account for 72% of the total cost of $44 billion. In fact, one of the indirect costs reported in Greenberg et al. (12) accounts for a significant portion of the difference in total cost between that study and the Stoudemire et al. (31) study. Greenberg et al. (12) included an estimate of the reductions in productive capacity (20%) of depressed individuals while at work during episodes of depression. While quality-of-life changes are not measured in these studies, these are undoubtedly important costs of depression and of other mental illnesses (see Chapter 161, *this volume*).

CONCLUSIONS

New drug development is a complex and uncertain process that depends on a mix of economic factors, regulation, the progress of science, and serendipity. The economic considerations include not only the R&D costs that are paid out-of-pocket, but also the length of the development process and the returns that can be expected from successful development. The data presented here show that psychotropic drug development in the United States has been lengthier than average, particularly for clinical development and regulatory review. We also found clinical development to be riskier than average, in the sense that proportionately fewer psychotropic drugs investigated clinically make it to marketing approval than is the case for investigational drugs as a whole. Both of these factors contribute to above-average clinical development costs for psychotropics. Longer-than-average development times also tend to reduce the period of patent protection.

While the costs and risks of psychotropic drug development are substantial, the markets for new psychotropic drugs that are demonstrably more effective are potentially lucrative. Even drugs that offer markedly improved side-effect profiles can pay off well. Markets for psychotropic drugs have been growing strongly in recent years. The world market for psychotropics has expanded at a 17% compound annual rate of growth from $2 billion in 1986 to $4.4 billion in 1991 (23). This growth was led by antidepressants, with sales that grew at a 42% compound annual rate during this period. The introduction of fluoxetine and other selective serotonin reuptake inhibitors accounted for much of this growth.

The considerable potential value to society of effective psychotropic drugs is clearly illustrated by the economic costs to society of depression, schizophrenia, and other mental illnesses that some studies have demonstrated. In an era when cost containment is a widespread objective, developers will have to make convincing cases for the kinds of reimbursement levels that are needed to make

further development economically worthwhile. At least in the published literature, studies examining the cost-effectiveness of psychotropic drugs have been few and far between. One exception is clozapine, where recent published studies have shown it to be cost-effective for treatment-resistant schizophrenia when used for long-term maintenance therapy, despite prices that some argue are unjustifiably high (10,25). In the current economic environment, developers will also find it increasingly necessary to find ways to make the psychotropic development process more efficient and fruitful.

If the unmet needs of psychiatric patients are to be met with new drugs or new uses for old drugs, industry, academic, and government researchers must vigilantly explore new avenues. The search for new psychotropic drugs has invited a number of strategies. The most successful, in fact, has been the serendipitous discovery of useful therapeutic activity by astute clinical observers administering NCEs to psychiatrically ill patients. A second approach has been to follow up on serendipitous discoveries by molecular modification of first-generation discoveries. A third approach is to devise animal models, usually constructed so that they *would* have identified standard drugs. The latter two techniques have the theoretical limitation that they may propose as candidates those drugs that are only marginally different from already available medications. The more recent attempt to identify drug receptors as a basis for selecting new candidates is conceptually exciting but awaits empiric testing to confirm or reject biotechnological guesses and the current optimism about this approach.

Because there is general agreement that predicting psychotropic activity with precision remains a difficult challenge, the drug developer is left with an unattractive scenario: a potentially valuable drug will be expensive to test in numerous different clinical settings, but picking ''*the*'' correct type of patient in advance is difficult if not impossible. Some have proposed that we go back to the practices of earlier days, and let experienced clinicians expose small numbers of patients with different psychiatric problems to a drug candidate in ''*open*'' clinical trials rather than conduct formal controlled clinical trials. Opponents of this view argue that false-positives will be frequently encountered with the ''open'' proposition and lead to wasted resources. The solution to this dilemma is not apparent.

REFERENCES

1. *Caring for people with severe mental disorders: a national plan of research to improve services.* National Institute of Mental Health, DHHS publication no. (ADM) 91-1762. Washington, DC: U.S. Government Printing Office, 1991.
2. *The contribution of pharmaceutical companies: what's at stake for America.* Boston, MA: Boston Consulting Group, September 1993.
3. *Data fact sheet: morbidity from coronary heart disease in the United States.* Washington, DC: National Institutes of Health, May 1992.
4. DiMasi JA, Hansen RW, Grabowski HG, Lasagna L. Cost of inno-

vation in the pharmaceutical industry. *J Health Econ* 1991;10:107–142.

5. DiMasi JA, Bryant NR, Lasagna L. New drug development in the United States from 1963 to 1990. *Clin Pharmacol Ther* 1991; 50:471–486.

6. DiMasi JA, Seibring MA, Lasagna L. New drug development in the United States, 1963 to 1992. *Clin Pharmacol Ther* 1994; 55:609–622 .

7. *Drug facts and comparisons.* St. Louis: Facts and Comparisons, 1993.

8. Faust RE, Harris MR, Lee KI. Factors which can harm the patient: economic restraints on research and development in the pharmaceutical industry. In: L'Etang H, ed. *Regulation and restraint in contemporary medicine in the UK and USA.* London: Published jointly by the Royal Society of Medicine and MacMillan Press, 1983.

9. Fein R. *Economics of mental illness: a report to the staff director. Jack R. Ewalt.* New York: Basic Books, 1958.

10. Fitton A, Benfield P. Clozapine: an appraisal of its pharmacoeconomic benefits in the treatment of schizophrenia. *Pharmacoeconomics* 1993;4:131–156.

11. Freedman DX, Stahl SM. Pharmacology: policy implications of new psychiatric drugs. *Health Aff (Millwood)* 1992;11:157–163.

12. Greenberg PE, Stiglin LE, Finkelstein SN, Berndt ER. The economic burden of depression in 1990. *J Clin Psychiatry* 1993;54:405–418.

13. Greenberg PE, Stiglin LE, Finkelstein SN, Berndt ER. Depression: a neglected major illness. *J Clin Psychiatry* 1993;54:419–424.

14. Halliday RG, Walker SR, Lumley CE. R&D philosophy and management in the world's leading pharmaceutical companies. *J Pharm Med* 1992;2:139–154.

15. Hansen RW. The pharmaceutical development process: estimates of current development costs and times and the effects of regulatory changes. In: Chien RI, ed. *Issues in pharmaceutical economics.* Lexington, MA: Heath, 1979;151–187.

16. *Health care reform for Americans with severe mental illnesses.* Washington, DC: National Mental Health Advisory Council, March 3, 1993.

17. James B. *The future of the multinational pharmaceutical industry to 1990.* New York: John Wiley & Sons, 1977.

18. Kane JM. Obstacles to clinical research and new drug development in schizophrenia. *Schizophr Bull* 1991;7:353–356.

19. Kaitin KI, Mattison N, Northington FK, Lasagna L. The drug lag: an update of new drug introductions in the United States and in the United Kingdom, 1977 through 1987. *Clin Pharmacol Ther* 1989;46:121–138.

20. Kaitin KI, Walsh HL. Are initiatives to speed the new drug approval process working? *Drug Inf J* 1992;26:341–349.

21. Klein DF. Psychotropic drug development: challenge and promise. *Biol Psychiatry* 1990;27:1061–1064.

22. Klein DF. Improvement of phase III drug trials by intensive phase II work. *Neuropsychopharmacology* 1991;4:251–258.

23. The market for psychotropic drugs. *Scrip* May 22, 1992;1720:26.

24. Landefeld JS, Seskin EP. The economic value of life: linking theory to practice. *Am J Public Health* 1982;72:555–566.

25. Meltzer HY, Cola P, Way L, Thompson PA, Bastani B, Davies MA, Snitz B. Cost-effectiveness of clozapine in neuroleptic-resistant schizophrenia. *Am J Psychiatry* 1993;150:1630–1638.

26. *The NDA pipeline—1992.* Chevy Chase, MD: F-D-C Development Corp., 1993.

27. Rice DP, Kalman S, Miller LS, Dunnmeyer S. *The economic costs of alcohol and drug abuse and mental illness, 1985.* Rockville, MD: U.S. Department of Health and Human Services, Public Health Service, Alcohol, Drug Abuse, and Mental Health Administration, 1990.

28. Schizophrenia market worth $2 billion by 2002. *Marketletter* May 17, 1993;20:15.

29. Scitovsky AA, Rice DP. Estimates of the direct and indirect costs of acquired immunodeficiency syndrome in the United States, 1985, 1986, and 1991. *Public Health Rep* 1987;102:5–17.

30. Steinwachs DM, Kasper JD, Skinner EA. Patterns of use and costs among severely mentally ill people. *Health Aff (Millwood)* 1992;11:178–185.

31. Stoudemire A, Frank R, Hedemark N, Kamlet M, Blazer D. The economic burden of depression. *Gen Hosp Psychiatry* 1986;8:387–394.

32. Tucker SA, Blozan C, Coppinger P. *The outcome of research on new molecular entities commencing clinical research in the years 1976–1978.* Rockville, MD: Food and Drug Administration, Office of Planning and Evaluation, Economics Staff, OPE Study 77, May 1988.

33. Vinar O, Klein DF, Potter WZ, Gause EM. A survey of psychotropic medications not available in the United States *Neuropsychopharmacology* 1991;5:201–217.

34. Wardell WM. Introduction of new therapeutic drugs in the United States and Great Britain: an international comparison. *Clin Pharmacol Ther* 1973;14:773–790.

35. Wardell WM. The drug lag revisited: comparison by therapeutic area of patterns of drugs marketed in the United States and Great Britain from 1972 through 1976. *Clin Pharmacol Ther* 1978;24:499–524.

36. Wardell WM. The history of drug discovery, development, and regulation. In: Chien RI, ed. *Issues in pharmaceutical economics.* Lexington, MA: Heath, 1979;3–11.

37. Wardell WM, DiRaddo J, Trimble, AG. Development of new drugs originated and acquired by United States-owned pharmaceutical firms, 1963–1976. *Clin Pharmacol Ther* 1980;28:270–277.

Psychopharmacology: The Fourth Generation of Progress, edited by Floyd E. Bloom and David J. Kupfer. Raven Press, Ltd., New York © 1995.

CHAPTER 161

Economic Evaluation of Drug Treatment for Psychiatric Disorders:

The New Clinical Trial Protocol

Gary A. Zarkin, Henry G. Grabowski, Josephine Mauskopf, Heather A. Bannerman, and Richard H. Weisler

During the 1980s and continuing into the 1990s, health-care cost containment has received increasing attention as health care costs have risen more rapidly than inflation. At the same time, many new drugs have been introduced at such high prices that they have become a target for third-party payer and government efforts for cost containment.

In response to the public outcry over drug prices, many researchers have designed and performed studies to evaluate the costs and outcomes of new drug therapies (e.g., see refs. 15,23,32,38–40) These cost and outcome studies, which we refer to as drug valuation or economic evaluation studies, are important to drug companies, clinicians, patients, and public policymakers. Valuation studies can provide marketing information and enhance pharmaceutical companies' competitive advantage (17). For patients and their physicians, valuation studies can identify whether new therapies justify their potentially greater financial expense. In addition, valuation studies can help patients assess whether future health benefits justify a reduction in the quality of life caused by a current therapy. For policymakers who must make resource allocation decisions, a valuation study that reflects a more complete picture of societal benefits can help differentiate between therapies with marginal differences in clinical efficacy.

The Food and Drug Administration (FDA) currently requires clinical trials to demonstrate the safety and clinical efficacy of new drugs. Although safety and clinical efficacy data clearly are of primary importance, they provide policymakers with insufficient information about the economic implications of approving a new drug. Pharmaceutical companies have not had the incentive to collect the data required for economic valuation studies, at least for drug approval in the U.S. market. However, in several countries (e.g., Australia), pricing and reimbursement decisions for new drugs are based on economic valuation studies (2,6,12). In the United States, insurance providers are indicating the desire for economic valuation studies of drugs (12), and health-care reform in the United States may bring an increased demand for economic evaluations of clinical trial data. These trends have induced U.S. pharmaceutical companies to include economic measures as an integral component of clinical trial protocols.

Thus far, these new protocols have been primarily introduced for treatment of nonpsychiatric conditions. Published economic studies of psychotherapeutic medications are just beginning to emerge. To understand the role economics plays in the evaluation of new drug treat-

G. A. Zarkin: Center for Economics Research, Research Triangle Institute, Research Triangle Park, North Carolina 27709.
H. G. Grabowski: Department of Economics, Duke University, Durham, North Carolina 27708.
J. Mauskopf: Burroughs Wellcome, Research Triangle Park, North Carolina 27709.
H. A. Bannerman: Department of Health Behavior and Health Education, School of Public Health, University of North Carolina, Chapel Hill, North Carolina 27599.
R. H. Weisler: Department of Psychology, Duke University Medical Center, Durham, North Carolina 27710.

ments for psychiatric disorders, we reviewed economic evaluations of drug treatment for schizophrenia, major depression, and anxiety disorders. Although psychiatric disorders are prevalent and impose substantial individual and societal costs, we found relatively few published economic evaluations of psychotherapeutic drugs (18,22,26,27,29,31).

This chapter describes the type of economic data that are being collected in trials of drug treatment for psychiatric disorders and discusses the use of these data in economic valuation studies. Possible economic outcomes in clinical trials include changes in patient well-being (defined as the patient's quality of life), work days gained for patients and caregivers, and changes in medical resource use and associated medical care costs. We also describe how these enhanced clinical trials data can be used to develop decision-tree models. These models are useful because they capture the dynamics of disease/treatment patterns over the entire course of the disease, providing a basis for evaluating the effects of alternative therapeutic interventions over a patient's lifetime. Many of the initial parameters required for these models can be estimated using clinical trial outcome data. After the drug has been introduced to the market, however, the initial model parameters may be validated and improved with data from actual clinical practice and post-marketing studies.

This chapter is organized as follows. The section entitled "Cost–Outcome Valuation Methods" briefly reviews economic valuation methods, including cost-effectiveness, benefit–cost, and cost–utility analyses as well as the recently introduced idea of healthy-years equivalent. The section entitled "Outcome Data Collected in Traditional Clinical Trial Protocols" discusses the outcomes collected in traditional clinical trial protocols for depression, schizophrenia, and anxiety disorders and discusses their limitations in economic valuation studies. In the section entitled "Recent Enhancements to Clinical Trial Protocols for Psychiatric Disorders," we highlight recent additions to clinical trial protocols and their use in valuation studies. The section entitled "Using the Results of Clinical Trials" describes how clinical trials data can be used to develop decision-tree models. Finally, the section entitled "Conclusion" summarizes our discussion and reviews our suggestions for using clinical trial data in economic analyses of drug therapy for psychiatric disorders (see Chapters 72, 73, and 160, *this volume*).

COST–OUTCOME VALUATION METHODS

Cost–outcome analysis aids policymakers in deciding whether the costs of a new drug treatment are justified by the benefits it generates. One method of analyzing the benefits of a new drug therapy is to list the relevant clinical endpoints and compare the differences in clinical endpoints between an old drug therapy and a new drug therapy. For example, analysts might compare the differences in symptoms and side effects between two alternative drug therapies. If the new drug therapy results in more symptomatic improvement and fewer side effects compared to an older drug, the new drug would be more valuable from a purely clinical viewpoint. However, the clinical viewpoint neglects changes in the patient's overall quality of life and differences in resource use, including differences in the cost of the treatment regimens. An expanded value analysis might compare the differences between an old drug therapy and a new drug therapy in terms of the relevant clinical, quality-of-life, and resource-use endpoints.

For many purposes, comparing all the relevant outcomes may be sufficient to demonstrate that one drug is more valuable than another. For example, if a new drug has better clinical outcomes, uses fewer resources (including expenditures for the drug itself), and is associated with a better quality of life than an older drug, the new drug is more valuable and should be used in place of the older drug. More often, a new drug may improve clinical outcomes and the qualify of life, but cost more than a competing drug. In these cases, researchers must perform "cost–outcome" studies to account for changes in both costs and outcomes attributable to drug therapy, and to provide a rational basis for assessing whether a drug's extra expense justifies the improvements in clinical and quality-of-life outcomes. Three cost–outcome valuation methods can be applied to drug valuation studies: cost-effectiveness analysis, benefit–cost analysis, and cost–utility analysis.

Economists often employ an alternative method of valuing drugs: individuals' willingness to pay for a drug rather than go without it. Although this willingness-to-pay definition is considerably more encompassing than cost–outcome analyses, and it captures economists' fundamental definition of value, willingness to pay must be measured by a preference elicitation method such as questionnaire-based models or revealed preference method (14). Because these elicitation methods are still relatively new, they are not yet widely accepted by the medical community (14). Consequently, in this chapter we will focus on cost–outcome methods for measuring the value of drugs.

Cost-effectiveness analysis compares the differences in cost and outcome across alternative therapies. The outcome generally refers to a clinical outcome and is measured in its natural units. The results are usually expressed as the incremental cost (relative to an alternative treatment) per unit of incremental outcome change, yielding ratios such as cost per averted sick day or cost per life-year(s) gained.

To perform a cost-effectiveness analysis, a researcher

should have one unambiguous objective of the intervention yielding a single outcome measure of effectiveness (4). If there are many outcomes of interest, cost-effectiveness measures are often computed for each of the alternative outcomes (4); but if the therapy under study is not clearly superior for all possible outcomes, decisionmakers are left in a quandary as to the desirability of the therapy. Under these circumstances, a *benefit–cost analysis* may be performed. By translating all the costs and benefits (including the health-outcome and quality-of-life improvements, days of work loss averted, days of caregiver time saved, hospital and physician days avoided) into dollars, benefit–cost analysis allows researchers to assess directly whether the benefits of treatment justify the treatment costs.

Benefit–cost analysis potentially provides the broadest estimate of the total value to society attributable to a drug therapy. In practice, however, measuring and quantifying all the costs and benefits of a drug therapy—especially the dollar value of quality-of-life changes—is extremely difficult and often controversial. For example, some analysts have raised concerns about assigning dollar values to improvements in labor market productivity (5). Furthermore, analysts are often uncomfortable assigning dollar values to changes in people's well-being (10).

Because of these concerns, many analysts turn to *cost–utility analysis.* Cost–utility analysis is similar to cost-effectiveness analysis in that it compares the incremental cost and outcome attributable to a particular therapy, but cost–utility analysis also accounts for changes in the quality of health caused by drug treatment (4). Thus, cost–utility analysis incorporates changes in the *quality of life* resulting from the clinical effect in addition to changes in the *length* of life. In cost–utility analysis, the entire array of health improvements is converted to a single common unit, most commonly qualify-adjusted life-years (QALYs) gained, which makes comparing alternative treatments easier. Recently, researchers have developed an alternative to QALYs—health-years-equivalent (HYE)—that reflects the number of years in good health that is equivalent to a longer lifetime in poor health (3,13). Gafni et al. (13) claim that HYEs are more consistent with economists' utility maximization paradigm, but others are not persuaded that HYEs are better than QALYs (3).

Recently, researchers have designed models to simulate the effect of therapeutic interventions on outcomes such as incidence, mortality, and resource use. The transition patterns between severity levels are estimated using state-transition or decision-tree models that capture the dynamics of treatment patterns over the entire course of the disorder. For example, Weinstein et al. (41) used a state-transition model to simulate future trends in incidence, prevalence, mortality, and resource cost under alternative assumptions about preventive and therapeutic interventions for coronary heart disease (CHD). Their model allows for simulation of the initial outcomes attributable to the CHD event, as well as subsequent events (such as recurrence) in persons suffering from CHD.

Given that psychiatric disorders tend to be chronic and recurring, we recommend using state-transition or decision-tree models in economic analyses of psychotherapeutic drugs. These models allow researchers to consider economic outcomes in a dynamic context over the lifetime of the individual. These models incorporate (a) the potential resource savings from reducing the intensity and length of acute episodes and (b) the gains from preventing future acute episodes.

In the section entitled "Using the Results of Clinical Trials" we present an example of a decision-tree model applied to the acute and maintenance phases of major depression.

OUTCOME DATA COLLECTED IN TRADITIONAL CLINICAL TRIAL PROTOCOLS

Although hundreds of clinical trials have been conducted to determine the efficacy of medications for major depression, schizophrenia, and anxiety disorders, there are very few published economic valuation studies of these drugs. A review of the literature on health-care cost–benefit and cost-effective analyses between 1979 and 1990 found only nine published studies on psychiatric medications, compared to close to 200 studies on medications for nonpsychiatric diseases (9).

The small number of economic evaluations of psychotherapeutic drugs may be attributable to the difficulty in measuring psychological states with reliability and validity. Disease states and concomitant economic outcomes may be easier to measure for nonpsychiatric illness than for psychiatric disorders. Another problem is that, until recently, clinical trials have not collected the data needed by economists to conduct valuation studies. Traditionally, clinical trials for pharmacotherapy of depression, schizophrenia, and anxiety disorders focused on safety and clinical efficacy. For acute treatment, efficacy was determined by general or disease-specified psychometric measures indicating the presence, frequency, and intensity of symptoms, behaviors, or feelings (30). Common clinical outcome measures of general psychopathology include the Brief Psychiatric Rating Scale, Hopkins Symptom Checklist, Global Assessment Scale, and Clinical Global Impressions scale. Disease-specific scales, such as the Hamilton Rating Scales for Depression and Anxiety and the Schedule for Affective Disorders and Schizophrenia, are more popular among clinical researchers (7).

Similarly, trials of maintenance drugs have not collected the specific economic outcomes required for valuation studies. Maintenance therapies generally have measured outcomes such as relapse rates, time between episodes (survival time), number and severity of subsequent episodes after treatment, and duration and severity of symptoms.

Social functioning (e.g., Social Adjustment Scale) and quality-of-life scales have been more widely used in recent years. Quality-of-life instruments are available to measure emotional and social functioning, well-being, disability, and overall health status attributable to diseases and their treatments (16,19). These instruments usually include questions about (a) physical, social, and role functioning, (b) bodily pain, and (c) overall well-being. Although these measures provide more meaningful information about the drug's effect on functioning and well-being, they still do not provide the direct quantifiable utility-based, quality-of-life measure that economists prefer (described in the following section), nor are they substitutes for direct, quantifiable measures of productivity and resource use that are necessary for economic valuation studies. Apart from using an expert elicitation process to link scores on these scales to utility-based, quality-of-life measures, resources used, or productivity levels, there is no direct way to determine a drug's economic value based on these scales.

Thus, until recently, clinical trials for pharmacotherapy of psychiatric disorders have not provided the data economists need to conduct drug valuation studies. Because of these data limitations, most published economic studies of the costs of psychiatric disorders have relied on secondary data for their estimates (e.g., see refs. 1 and 33). Very few have been able to determine the economic value of alleviating a psychotic episode or preventing recurrence.

RECENT ENHANCEMENTS TO CLINICAL TRIAL PROTOCOLS FOR PSYCHIATRIC DISORDERS

Recently, researchers have started to collect economic outcomes as part of their clinical trial protocols, especially for expensive drugs with improved efficacy relative to alternative treatments. For example, clozapine, a new treatment for neuroleptic-resistant schizophrenia, has instigated several cost-effectiveness studies in the past several years (18,24,26,31).

Many clinical trial protocols are now collecting the following economic outcomes for psychotherapeutic drugs:

1. Mortality
2. Resource-use measures
   a. Hospital admissions and days
   b. Housing costs (nursing home or group home)
   c. Visits to health professionals
   d. Other outpatient costs (e.g., case management, day care)
   e. Lab procedures
   f. Drugs prescribed
   g. Other costs related to illness (e.g., transportation, legal fees)
   h. Unit costs of resource use measures
3. Labor market and household productivity measures
   a. Working time
   b. Paid and nonpaid caregiver time
   c. Patient's time (including transportation time) associated with treatment
4. Quality-of-life measures

Conducting a resource-use analysis for treating psychiatric disorders entails collecting data during the clinical trial on inpatient and outpatient resource use. Health-care resource costs can be estimated separately from the clinical trial using standard charge schedules and cost-to-charge ratios. Examples of economic outcome studies that have collected data on hospitalization costs and physician charges for psychiatric disorders include Meltzer et al. (26), Revicki et al. (31), and Kamlet et al. (20).

Other important endpoints that should be collected in clinical trials are labor market and household productivity effects. These measures include the days of work the patient gained, the level of function of those days gained, and the paid and nonpaid caregiver time avoided as a result of treatment. Examples of questions that might be added to assess these effects include: "Since we saw you last, how many days of work did you miss because of panic attacks?"; and "Since we saw you last, how many days did a nonpaid caregiver miss work to take care of you while you felt depressed?"

A dollar value of lost work time can be calculated by multiplying the foregone days of work attributable to the disorder by a wage measure. However, this method has some limitations. First, if the patient is not employed, no wage measure exists. Thus, an estimated wage would have to be developed for those patients who are too ill to work, are unemployed, are retired, or who work as homemakers. Second, patients may be reluctant to provide income information during the clinical trial. Finally, this method of valuing productivity changes, known as the *human capital approach,* is controversial. Grabowski and Hansen (14) suggest that such a procedure "measures health and quality of life as though they are a unit of production, not something of intrinsic value." As a result, the human capital approach to valuing the productivity gains of a new depression drug treatment gives more weight to high-wage earners than to low-wage earners.

Many clinical trial protocols for new medications (including those mandated in Australia) do not currently collect productivity measures. However, in spite of the limitations, we believe that valuing productivity gains or losses is important and we recommend routinely including productivity questions in clinical trial protocols.

Because psychiatric disorders can have pervasive effects on individuals' lives, changes in patients' quality of life are also important endpoints being measured during many clinical trials (25,42). Most economists prefer to measure quality-of-life changes as the difference in the patient's utility between perfect health and alternative impaired health states (4,36,37). Several techniques exist to elicit individuals' utility of alternative health states. One technique, category scaling, asks a person to place several alternative health states in the appropriate place on a line bounded by zero (death) and one (perfect health). Other quality-of-life valuation techniques include the standard gamble and time trade-off methods (4). Using the standard gamble method, people are asked to choose between a certain less-than-perfect health outcome and an outcome of either perfect health with probability $1 - p$ or death with probability p. The probability of death at which the person is indifferent between the choices is equal to the utility of the certain less-than-perfect outcome (4). A typical standard gamble question might be: "Imagine that there is a new, free medication available which will either completely cure your mental illness or kill you. Suppose that 50% of the people who take the new medication are cured of the disease, and 50% die. Would you risk taking the new medication?" If the individual answered "yes," the probability of dying would be successively increased until the individual answered "no." Similarly, if the individual initially answered "no," the probability of death would be successively reduced until their answer changed to "yes." In either case, the probability at which the answer to the question changes represents the utility of being mentally ill (34). In the time trade-off method a person is asked to give the length of time in perfect health that is equivalent to a full lifetime in selected, less-than-perfect health states (37). These methods may be limited, however, because people do not give necessarily give consistent or sensible answers to these elicitation methods (34).

Another method of determining value is the willingness-to-pay method, which quantifies the utility of alternative health states in dollar values. This method determines the amounts of money people are willing to pay for various possible health states (34). For example, an investigator might ask the patient (35): "Consider all the effects of your anxiety on your life. How much would you currently be willing to pay each week, realistically, to get rid of your anxiety and all the problems it brings?" As above, this method is potentially limited because respondents may not be able to give consistent or rational personal judgments on their willingness to pay (34). Furthermore, willingness-to-pay estimates are controversial because the magnitude of the estimates is likely affected by the income level of the respondents, such that higher-income respondents may have a greater willingness to pay for good health (and hence a greater value of good health) than would lower-income respondents.

We recognize that methods of valuing economic outcomes, particularly productivity and utility-based quality-of-life changes, have limitations and are currently controversial. Although none of these techniques or scales has been widely used or accepted as standard, conceptual work to advance their use in clinical trials for mentally ill persons is underway. The development of common definitions and standards of measurement will allow researchers to accumulate comparable data across studies and across populations (21). In turn, these data will help economists improve their economic valuation studies of drug treatment.

USING THE RESULTS OF CLINICAL TRIALS

Clinical trials data can be used in conjunction with other data sources to develop decision-tree models that highlight clinical decision points, alternative treatment choices, and the resulting possible outcomes. Using these models, researchers can illustrate the temporal and logical sequence of the disease/treatment dynamics, combine the results of acute and maintenance clinical trials, and control for natural recovery that may occur apart from drug treatment.

We suggest that clinicians develop decision trees concurrently with clinical trial protocols to help guide choices of outcome measures and to ensure that the trials collect data on the appropriate economic endpoints. Well-designed clinical trial protocols can estimate the transition probabilities between alternative disease states that are needed for decision-tree models.

Figures 1 and 2 illustrate treatment choices, disease/treatment dynamics, and outcomes using a simplified example of a decision-tree model. Our focus in these figures is on modeling the treatment of major depression, but this is meant to be illustrative of modeling psychiatric disorders more generally. The basic structure of this decision-tree model would be essentially the same for anxiety disorders or schizophrenia.

Figure 1 represents the disorder/treatment dynamics for an acute depressive episode, while Figure 2 represents a phase in which the patient is stable and under maintenance therapy. We make several simplifying assumptions in this model: (a) Depression occurs at four basic severity levels (i.e., mild, moderate, severe without psychotic symptoms, and severe with psychotic symptoms); (b) the patient is only affected by unipolar depression; (c) four treatment choices (i.e., drugs only, psychotherapy only, drugs and psychotherapy combined, and electroconvulsive therapy) are available; and (d) treatment-switching decisions are made only at 8 weeks and 6 months after initial treatment.

As illustrated in Fig. 1, the patient enters treatment in

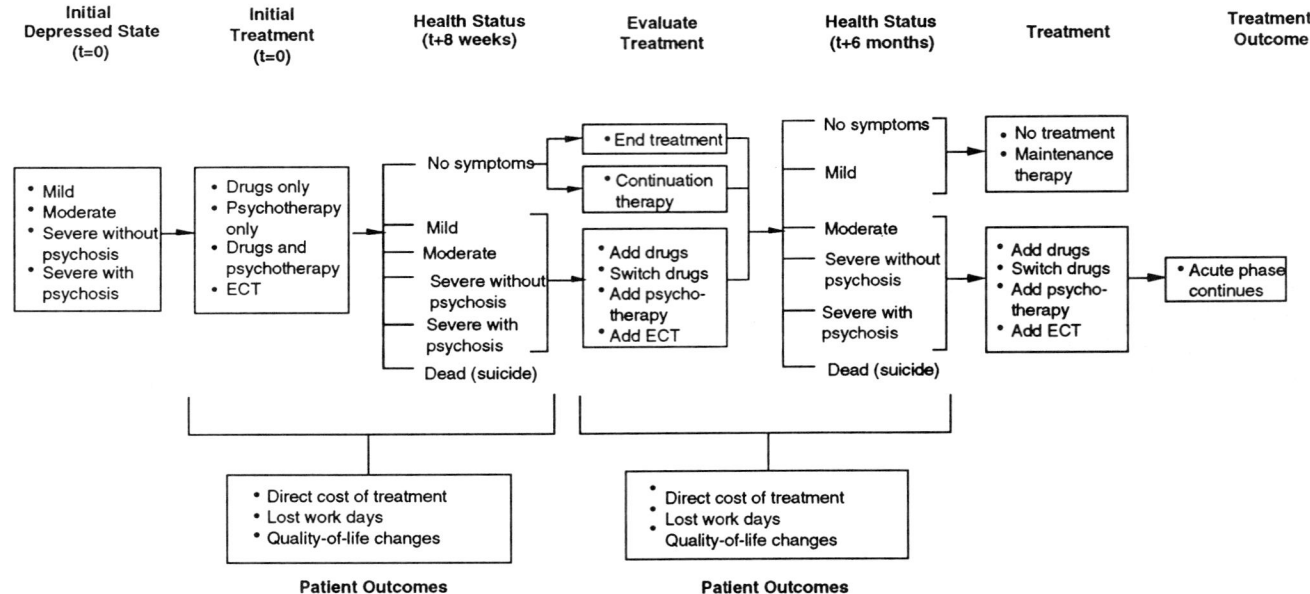

| Initial Depressed State (t=0) | Initial Treatment (t=0) | Health Status (t+8 weeks) | Evaluate Treatment | Health Status (t+6 months) | Treatment | Treatment Outcome |

FIG. 1. A decision-tree model for evaluating the acute phase of treatment for depression.

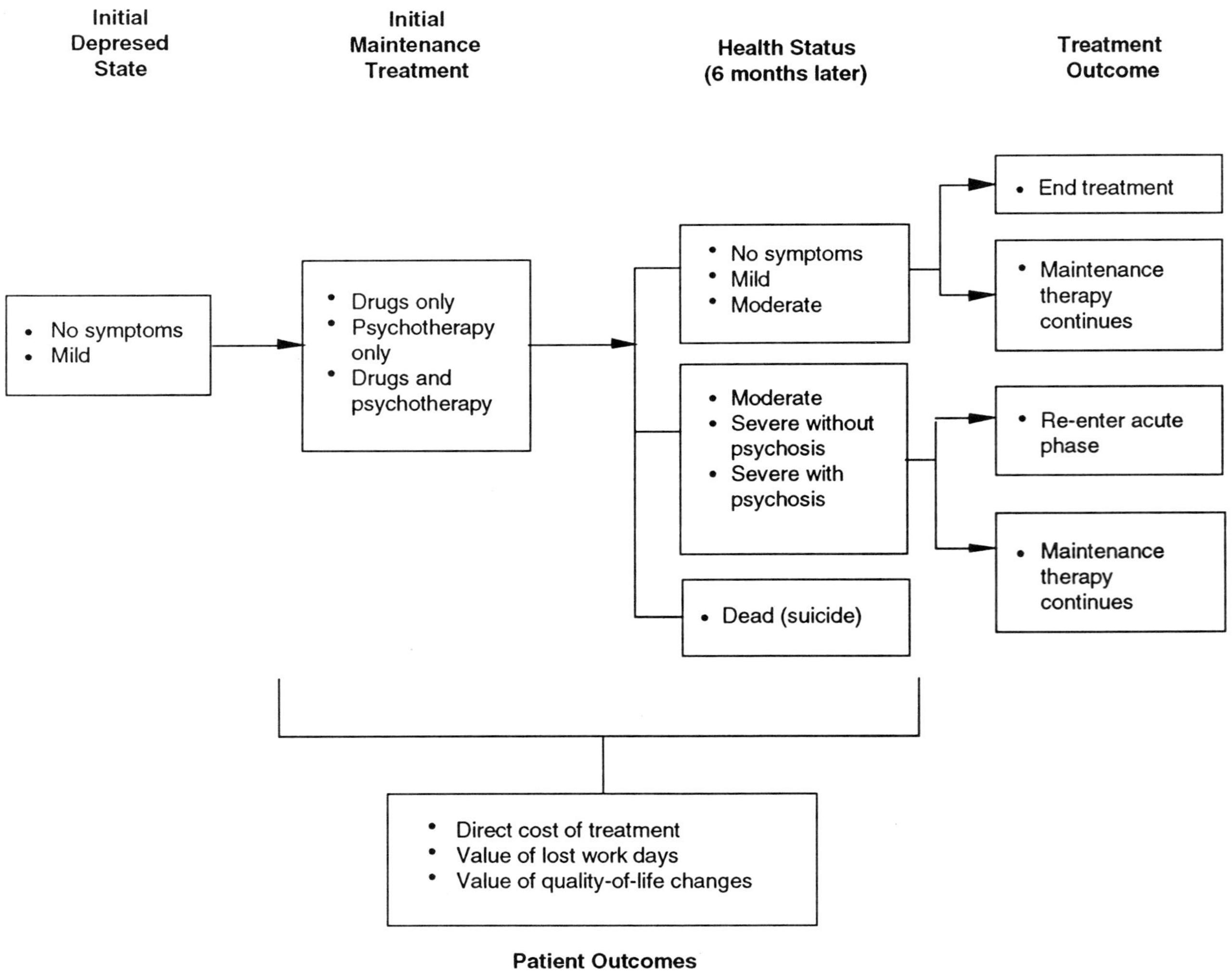

FIG. 2. A decision-tree model for evaluating the maintenance phase of treatment of depression.

one of the four possible severity levels. Based on the patient's initial severity level, the physician selects a treatment. After the initial treatment visit, the patient is reexamined periodically; in subsequent visits, the patient's health status will have improved, worsened, or remained the same. Alternative treatments may affect the length of time spent in each severity level and, hence, the functional loss of the patient. Each severity level is associated with health-care resource use, days of lost work or reduced productivity, and quality-of-life-changes that can be measured at various time intervals.

Depending on the success of the acute treatment and the patient's history of depression, several treatment paths may be taken at the 8-week and 6-month time points. Those patients who are asymptomatic after 8 weeks or 6 months and have no previous history of depression may end treatment at either point. Those patients who still have mild depression or worse at the 8-week or 6-month time points are still in the acute phase; their treatment will be evaluated and possibly changed. Asymptomatic or mildly depressed patients with a history of three or more prior depressive episodes may be treated with continuation therapy to avoid relapse at the 8-week point, or these patients may enter maintenance therapy to avoid recurrence at the 6-month point. Most patients with a history of recurrent depressive episodes will likely proceed to maintenance therapy.

Figure 2 summarizes the disorder/treatment dynamics for the maintenance phase of depression treatment. Patients enter maintenance therapy with either mild residual symptoms or no symptoms. After the initial maintenance treatment visit, the patient periodically visits the physician, who assesses the efficacy of the treatment. At the 6-month assessment point, the patient's mental status will have either improved, worsened, or stayed the same.

This example of depression/treatment dynamics illustrates the connection between changes in disease stages, resource use, and quality-of-life endpoints. Measuring the movements between severity levels provides estimates of transition probabilities for decision-tree models. These estimates can then be used in conjunction with estimates of resource use to simulate the costs and benefits of new drugs in the context of the complete drug/treatment dynamics.

Kamlet et al. (20) recently operationalized this type of decision model in their cost–utility analysis of maintenance therapy for recurrent depression. They drew on results from the Pittsburgh Recurrent Depression Project (11), in which the clinical effectiveness of alternative treatments in delaying recurrence of depression was evaluated. Although the trial lasted only 3 years, Kamlet et al. developed a lifetime model of acute episodes followed by stable periods under maintenance treatment. To implement their cost–utility model, they required estimates of the following variables: time until recurrence, time spent in a depressive episode, probability of suicide, quality of life during a depressed episode and during maintenance treatment, and direct costs per episode of acute and maintenance treatment. Because their clinical trial data were limited to the maintenance phase, the analysis had to base the other parameter values on secondary data supplemented with assumptions or consensus of expert opinion.

Although decision-tree models are useful tool for economic evaluation of new drugs, analysts must use caution when attempting to generalize the results of clinical trials beyond the trial setting. First, the results of individual clinical trials—which often evaluate short-term effects and are directed at the acute phase of a disorder—may provide a misleading picture of the entire disorder/treatment dynamics of that drug. This is especially likely to be a problem for drugs used for treating either (a) diseases with a prolonged duration or (b) chronic diseases that recur over a person's lifetime (as with many psychiatric disorders). Another limitation of clinical trials data is that patients in a clinical trial may not be representative of the diseased population. Because trials are typically conducted in tertiary care settings, patients participating in the trial are a highly selected subset of all those who have the disorder being studied. Furthermore, the clinical trial takes place in an idealized setting, where patient compliance with dosage is monitored more closely than with typical patients in an actual clinical setting. Thus, the drug's efficacy is likely to be overestimated when applied to patients outside the clinical trial setting. Finally, clinical trials usually compare the new drug to placebo rather than to an existing drug or the suggested medical therapy, leaving policymakers with little information about comparative outcomes (12,28).

Because of these limitations, we suggest performing a sensitivity analysis of model parameters and validating parameter estimates from clinical trials against other data. Sensitivity analysis involves substituting a range of estimates for the probabilities and resource-use estimates to see whether they alter the model's conclusions. Eisenberg et al. (8) suggest comparing clinical trial data with data from other trials, expert opinion, and information from large databases such as Medicare claims files. Finally, researchers can validate decision-tree models with data from actual clinical practice or from post-marketing economics studies. For example, randomized trials may be developed with the primary purpose of estimating differential resource use across alternative drugs. As more information becomes available, researchers will be able to build better models of the mental disease/treatment dynamics.

CONCLUSION

Improved economic valuation studies will help patients, physicians, pharmaceutical companies, and policymakers decide whether new therapies justify their additional expense. Given the advent of expensive new drugs and limited health-care resources, comprehensive economic evaluation studies based on clinical trials data are critical to sound decisionmaking.

In the past, clinical trials have not provided adequate data for economic analysis of psychotherapeutic drugs. However, researchers are increasingly recognizing the importance of incorporating economic outcomes into clinical trial protocols. Trials are now collecting data on the resource use, lost labor market productivity, and quality of life that are needed for sound economic analysis.

These enhanced data can be used to develop decision-tree models to guide a comparison of the costs and outcomes of alternative drug therapies. Decision-tree models can be developed that incorporate the results of separate acute and maintenance trials into a single model. These models can be validated and improved with data from other trials, expert opinion, post-marketing studies, and large databases such as Medicare claims files. As clinical trial protocols continue evolving to collect more economic information, researchers will be able to build more sophisticated economic models that evaluate the merits of new psychotherapeutic drugs in the context of the mental disorder/treatment dynamics.

ACKNOWLEDGMENTS

This study was supported, in part, with funds from Glaxo, Inc. Dr. Mauskopf was employed by Research Triangle Institute when this work began. The views expressed do not necessarily represent those of Research Triangle Institute, Burroughs Wellcome or Glaxo, Inc.

REFERENCES

1. Andrews G, Hall W, Goldstein G, Lapsley H, Bartels R, Silove D. The economic costs of schizophrenia: implications for public policy. *Arch Gen Psychiatry* 1985;42:537–543.
2. Bloom B. Issues in mandatory economic assessment of pharmaceuticals. *Health Aff (Milewood)* 1992;11(4):197–201.
3. Buckingham K. A note on HYE (health years equivalent). *Health Econ* 1993;11:301–309.
4. Drummond GW, Stoddart GL, Torrance GW. *Methods for the economic evaluation of health care programs*. Oxford, England: Oxford University Press, 1987.
5. Drummond M. Cost-of-illness studies: a major headache? *Pharmacoeconomics* 1992;2(1):1–4.
6. Drummond MF. Basing prescription drug payment on economic analysis: the case of Australia. *Health Aff (Millwood)* 1992;11(4):191–196.
7. Drummond MF, Davies L. 1991. Economics analysis alongside clinical trials: revisiting the methodological issues. *Int J Technol Assess Health Care* 1991;7(4):561–573.
8. Eisenberg JM, Glcik H, Koffer H. Pharmacoeconomics: economic evaluation of pharmaceuticals. In: Strom B, ed. *Pharmacoepidemiology*. New York: Churchill Livingstone, 1989.
9. Elixhauser A. Health care cost-benefit and cost-effectiveness analysis from 1979 to 1990: a bibliography. *Med Care (Suppl)* 1993;31(7).
10. Feeny D, Labelle R, Torrance G. Integrating economic evaluations and quality of life assessments. In: Spilker B, ed. *Quality of life assessments in clinical trials*. New York: Raven Press, 1990:71–83.
11. Frank E, Kupfer D, Perel J, Cornes C, Jarrett D, Mallinger A, Thase M, McEachran A, Grochocinski V. Three-year outcomes for maintenance therapies in recurrent depression. *Arch Gen Psychiatry* 1990;47:1093–1099.
12. Freund DA, Evans D, Henry D, Dittus R. Implications of the Australian guidelines for the United States. *Health Aff (Milewood)* 1992;11(4):202–206.
13. Gafni A, Birch S, Mehrez A. Economics, health and health economics: HYEs versus OALYs. *J Health Econ* 1993;11:325–339.
14. Grabowski H, Hansen R. Economic scales and tests. In: Spilker B, ed. *Quality of life assessments in clinical trials*. New York: Raven Press, 1990;61–69.
15. Guiati SC, Bennett CL. Granulocyte-macrophage colony-stimulating factor (GM-CSF) as adjunct therapy in relapsed Hodgkin disease. *Ann Intern Med* 1992;116:177.
16. Guyatt G, Jaeschke R. Measurements in clinical trials: choosing the appropriate approach. In: Spilker B, ed. *Quality of life assessments in clinical trials*. New York: Raven Press, 1990;37–46.
17. Henderson-James D, Pilker B. An industry perspective. In: Spilker B, ed. *Quality of life assessments in clinical trials*. New York: Raven Press. 1990;183–192.
18. Honigfeld G, Patin J. A 2-year clinical and economic follow-up of patients on clozapine. *Hosp Community Psychiatry* 1990;41(8):882–885.
19. Hunt S. McKenna S. The QLDS: a scale for the measurement of quality of life in depression. *Health Policy* 1992;22:307–319.
20. Kamlet M, Paul N, Greenhouse J, Kupfer D, Frank E, Wade M. *Cost utility analysis of maintenance treatment for recurrent depression*. Technical Report, Mental Health Clinic Research Center, March 26, 1992.
21. Lehman AF, Burns BJ. Severe mental illness in the community. In: Spilker B, ed. *Quality of life assessments in clinical trials*. New York: Raven Press, 1990.
22. Lyons JS, Larson DB, Hromco J. Clinical and economic evaluation of benzodiazepines. *Pharmacoeconomics* 1992;2(5):397–407.
23. Maniscaico WM, Kendig JW, Shapiro DL. Surfactant replacement therapy: impact on hospital charges for premature infants with respiratory distress syndrome. *Pediatrics* 1989;83:1.
24. Marder SR, Van Putten T, Mintz J, McKenzie J, Lebell M, Faltico G, May PRA. Costs and benefits of two doses of fluphenazine. *Arch Gen Psychiatry* 1984;41:1025–1029.
25. Meltzer HY, Burnett S, Bastani B, Ramire LF. Effects of 6 months of clozapino treatment on the quality of life of chronic schizophrenic patients. *Hosp Community Psychiatry* 1990;41(8):892–897.
26. Meltzer HY, Cola P, Way L, Thompson PA, Bastani B, Davies MA, Snitz B. Cost effectiveness of clozapine in neuroleptic-resistant schizophrenia. *Am J Psychiatry* 1993;150(11):1630–1638.
27. Mintz J, Mintz LI, Arruda MJ, Hwang SS. Treatments of depression and the function capacity to work. *Arch Gen Psychiatry* 1992;49:761–768.
28. Ray WA, Griffin MR, Avorn J. Evaluating drugs after their approval for clinical use. *N Engl J Med* 1993;329(27):2029–2032.
29. Reifman A, Wyatt RJ. Lithium: a brake in the rising cost of mental illness. *Arch Gen Psychiatry* 1980;37:385–388.
30. Revicki D. Relationship between health utility and psychometric health status measures. *Med Care* 1992;30(5):274–282.
31. Revicki DA, Luce BR, Weschler JM, Brown RE, Adler MA. Cost-effectiveness of clozapine for treatment-resistant schizophrenic patients. *Hosp Community Psychiatry* 1990;41(8):850–854.
32. Showstock J, Katz P, Amend W, Salvatierra O. The association of cyclosporine with the 1-year costs of cadaver-donor kidney transplants. *JAMA* 1990;264:1818–1823.
33. Stoudemire A. Frank R, Hedemark N, Kamlet M, Blazer D. The economic burden of depression. *Gen Hosp Psychiatry* 1986;8:387–394.
34. Thompson M. Willingness to pay and accept risks to cure chronic disease. *Am J Public Health* 1986;76(4):392–396.

35. Thompson M, Read JL, Liang M. Feasibility of willingness-to-pay measurement for chronic arthritis. *Med Decis Making* 1984;4:195–215.

36. Torrance GW. Measurement of health state utilities for economic appraisal. *J Health Econ* 1986;5:1–30.

37. Torrance GW, Boyle MH, Horwood SP. Application of multi-attribute utility theory to measure social preferences for health states. *Oper Res* 1982;30(6):1043–1069.

38. Tsevat J, Snydman DR, Pauker SG, Durand-Zaleski I, Werner BG, Levey AS. Which renal transplant patients should receive cytomegalovirus immune globulin? *Transplantation* 1991;52:259–265.

39. Tubman TRJ, Halliday HL, Norman C. Cost of surfactant replacement treatment for severe neonatal respiratory distress syndrome; a randomized controlled trial. *BMJ* 1990;301:842.

40. Vermeer F, Simoons ML, deZwaan C, van Es GA, Verheugt FWA, van der Laarse A, van Hoogenhuyze DCA, Azar AJ, van Dalen FJ, Jubsen J, Hugenholtz PG. Cost benefit analysis of early thrombolytic treatment with intracoronary streptokinase. *Br Heart J* 1987;59:527–534.

41. Weinstein MC, Coxson PG, Williams LW, Pass TM, Statson WB, Goldman L. Forecasting coronary heart disease incidence, mortality, and cost: the coronary heart disease policy model. *Am J Public Health* 1987;77(11):1417–1426.

42. Wells KB, Stewart A, Hays RD, Burnam MA, Rogers W, Daniels M, Berry S, Greenfield S, Ware J. The functioning and well-being of depressed patients—results from the medical outcomes study. *JAMA* 1989;262(7):914–919.

Psychopharmacology: The Fourth Generation of Progress, edited by Floyd E. Bloom and David J. Kupfer. Raven Press, Ltd., New York © 1995.

CHAPTER 162

Ethnicity, Culture, and Psychopharmacology

Keh-Ming Lin and Russell E. Poland

One of the most important issues in clinical pharmacology that perhaps has not received sufficient attention in research, as well as in the day-to-day clinical care setting, is the remarkably large interindividual variability in drug responses and side effect profiles. Such variability, which can be 40-fold or more, has been demonstrated with practically all classes of psychotropics, making it difficult to formulate rational guidelines for the dosing and the interpretation of biological parameters (such as the plasma or serum drug concentrations) that might be associated with therapeutic response (28,37,49,62). Although much remains unknown, a number of factors have been demonstrated to be important determinants of such variability. These include not only genetics, disease state, nutritional status, concurrent use of drugs, and other pharmacoactive substances, but also demographic factors such as age, gender, and ethnicity (49,72,79).

The primary focus of this chapter will be to briefly review the influence of ethnicity—and, to a lesser extent, culture—on psychotropic responses. It will start with an overview of the various mechanisms that could be responsible for ethnic and cultural differences in psychotropic response. This will be followed by a review of the literature which already provides substantial evidence of ethnic variations in response to major classes of psychotropics. Finally, the clinical and theoretical implications of these findings, as well as future research directions, will be discussed (see also Chapter 74, *this volume*).

MECHANISMS AFFECTING DRUG RESPONSES

As has been described in greater detail in Chapter 74, (*this volume*), the effects of pharmacoactive agents are determined by pharmacokinetic and pharmacodynamic factors (see Fig. 1). While pharmacodynamics deals with the interactions of pharmacoactive substances with the target organ (various receptor systems in the central nervous system in the case of psychopharmacology), pharmacokinetic principles describe the disposition and fate of pharmacoactive substances inside the body. The pharmacokinetics of most drugs are determined by four basic processes: absorption, distribution, biotransformation, and excretion (28,65). Of these, the biotransformation process (metabolism) shows considerable interindividual as well as cross-ethnic variations (36,49) and has been an exceptionally active and productive area of research. The rate of biotransformation is determined by both genetic and environmental factors. Evidence suggests that ethnicity and culture exert substantial influences on drug response through both mechanisms.

Ethnicity and Pharmacogenetics

The development of the field of pharmacogenetics as an academic discipline has been closely intertwined with findings of dramatic ethnic differences in drug responses that were found to be genetically determined (34,36). Through these efforts, the genetic control of a large number of drug-metabolizing enzymes has been established (Table 1). The activities of many of these enzymes also show substantial cross-ethnic differences. Classic examples include:

1. *Differential rates of "isoniazid toxicity" between Asians and Caucasians.* This led to the finding of slow versus rapid acetylation across ethnic groups, which accounted for the toxic effects of this drug in certain individuals and which, more recently, accounted for the identification of ethnospecific loci of point mutations responsible for slow acetylation (80). Acetylation represents an important metabolic pathway for a large number of medici-

K.-M. Lin and R. E. Poland: Research Center on the Psychobiology of Ethnicity and the Department of Psychiatry, Harbor–UCLA Medical Center, Torrance, California 90509.

Pharmacokinetics and Pharmacodynamics of a Drug

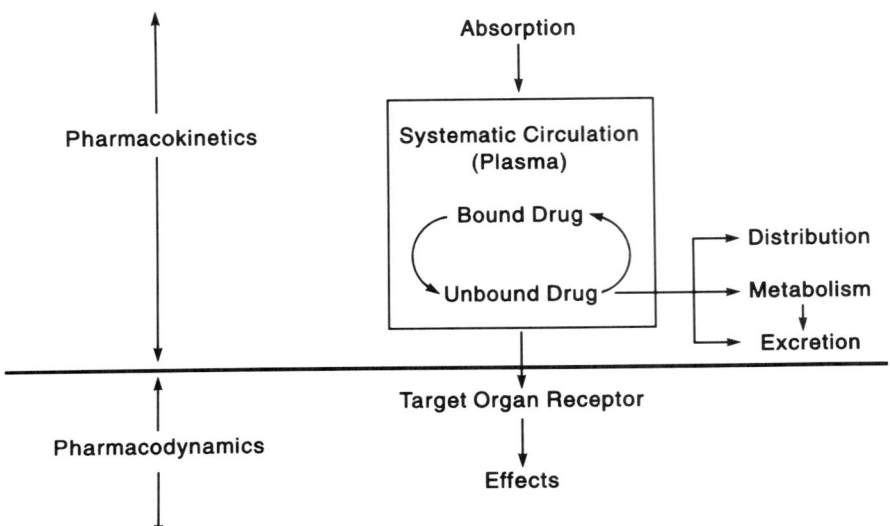

FIG 1. Schematic presentation of the pharmacokinetics and pharmacodynamics of a drug.

nal agents, including some frequently encountered psychoactive agents such as caffeine, phenelzine and nitrazepam.

2. *"Primaquine hemolysis" found among African-American soldiers fighting in Southeast Asia during World War II* (34,37). This led to the discovery of an inborn deficiency of glucose-6-phosphate dehydrogenase, a condition that could result in severe hemolytic anemia when the afflicted is exposed to a variety of substances, including primaquine, an antimalarial agent.

3. *The "flushing response" in Asians exposed to alcohol.* Subsequent studies demonstrated that this was mainly due to a genetically determined deficiency of aldehyde dehydrogenase, which is accentuated further in some indi-

TABLE 1. *Genetically variable enzymes of drug metabolism[a]*

Butyryl cholinersterase
Serum paroxanase/arylesterase[b]
Debrisoquin-sparteine oxidase (CYP2D6)[b]
Mephenytoin hydroxylase (CYP$_{mp}$)[b]
Dopamine-β-hydroxylase
Catalase
Superoxide dismutase
Monoamine oxidase
Alcohol dehydrogenase[b]
Aldehyde dehydrogenase[b]
Dihydropyrimidine dehydrogenase (DPD)
N-Acetyltransferase (NAT2)[b]
Glucuronyl transferase (UDPGT)[b]
Thiol methyltranferase[b]
Thiopurine methyltransferase
Phenol sulfotransferase (thermal stability)[b]
Glutathione-*S*-transferase (class mu)[b]

[a] Adapted from ref. 36.
[b] Indicates polymorphic variation.

viduals by an overactivity of alcohol dehydrogenase. The molecular basis of these mechanisms has been elucidated by a series of studies in recent years (3,85).

The cytochrome P-450 enzyme system represents a major focus of contemporary research in pharmacogenetics (25–27,35,37). Together, isozymes belonging to this system are responsible for the metabolism and detoxification (usually) of the majority of modern chemotherapeutic agents, including practically all psychotropics that require oxidation prior to conjugation and excretion. At least two of these isozymes, the CYP2D6 (debrisoquine hydroxylase) and the CYP$_{mp}$ (mephenytoin hydroxylase), have been found to be bimodally distributed. It has further been demonstrated that the bimodal distribution of the activities of these important enzymes is genetically controlled and can be traced to mutations in the nucleic acid sequence in the DNA, leading consequently to alterations in the amino acid structure and activity of the enzymes. Because of these mutations, a certain proportion of any given population can be classified as poor metabolizers (PMs)—in contrast to extensive metabolizers (EMs), who do not have such deficiencies.

Interestingly, substantial cross-ethnic differences in the frequency of the PM phenotype exist with these enzymes (37,49). Table 2 summarizes the frequency of PMs of CYP2D6 in studies involving different populations. The rate ranges from less than 1% in some of the Asians studies to as high as 19% among Sans Bushmen, with the majority of the studies demonstrating a consistent and substantial contrast between Asians (0.5–2.4%) and Caucasians (2.9–10%). Recent genotyping studies have further demonstrated that the majority of the Caucasian PMs have a 44-kb gene insertion associated with several

TABLE 2. *Worldwide distribution of the percentage of poor metabolizers (PMs) of debrisoquine hydroxylase (CYP2D6) and mephenytoin hydroxylase (CYP$_{mp}$)*

Population	Debrisoquine hydroxylase	Mephenytoin hydroxylase
Caucasians	3–9.2%	2.5–6.7%
Arabians/Egyptians	1–1.4%	?
Asian Indians	?	20.8%
East Asians	0–2.4%	17.4–22%
Amerindians	0–5.2%	0%
Hispanics	4.5%	4.8%
Subsaharan Africans	0–8.1%	?
Sans Bushman	19%	?
African-Americans	1.9%	18.5%

types of point mutations that render the enzyme completely inactive. In contrast, the same 44-kb gene insertion is highly prevalent (34%) among Asians, albeit without the associated point mutations. Phenotypically the Asians with 44-kb gene insertion were classified as EMs. However, their CYP2D6 metabolic capacity was significantly lower than that of either Caucasian EMs or Asian EMs without gene insertion. This led to an overall lower CYP2D6 activity in Asians as compared to Caucasians, although not low enough to be considered PMs. In a recent study with African-Americans, similar results were found, with a high prevalence (33%) of gene-insertion-related slower metabolism. Thus, EM and PM are relative terms and are not necessarily quantitatively or qualitatively comparable across ethnic groups (52).

As also shown in Table 2, the frequency of PM of CYP$_{mp}$ also varies substantially across ethnic groups (37,49). While PMs of CYP$_{mp}$ are relatively rare among Caucasians, they have been found to be quite prevalent in Asian populations, with approximately 20% of Japanese and Chinese being classified as PMs. A recent study on African-Americans also reported a rate significantly higher than that in Caucasians (52).

The remarkable diversity of the genotypes of drug-metabolizing enzymes poses a challenging question for evolutionary biologists (26,27,36). The historical survival value of the inborn deficiency of glucose-6-phosphate dehydrogenase is easier to explain, because those possessing such a trait are more resistant to malarial infection. More puzzling is the case for the cytochrome P-450 isozymes. However, these isozymes together represent one of the most important defense systems that evolved in our ancestors through the millennia to protect against potentially harmful xenobiotics to which they were routinely exposed in their habitat (27). It has been argued (36) that, just as genetic variability in susceptibility to infectious diseases has been shown to be conducive to the survival of populations, so does pharmacogenetic variability help to ensure the survival of a population facing an onslaught of toxic chemicals in the environment.

In contrast to the uncertainties surrounding the phylogenetic basis of ethnic diversity of these drug-metabolizing enzymes, their clinical implications have been more clearly delineated. To greater and lesser extents, both enzymes are involved in the metabolism of a large number of psychotropics (Table 3). Recent studies have demonstrated that these pharmacogenetic traits significantly af-

TABLE 3. *Substrates of debrisoquin hydroxylase (CYP2D6) and mephenytoin hydroxylase (CYP$_{mp}$)*

Substrates of CYP2D6			
Psychoactive agents	Cardiovascular agents	Other agents	Substrates of CYP$_{mp}$
Neuroleptics	*Antiarrhythmics*	Codeine	Desipramine
Clozapine	Encainide	Dextromethorphan[a]	Diazepam
Fluphenazine	Flecainide	Methoxyamphetamine	Demethyldiazepam
Haloperidol	Mexiletine	Perhexilene	Hexobarbital
Perphenazine	*N*-Propylajmaline	Phenformin	Imipramine
Risperidone	Sparteine		Mephebarbital
Thioridazine	*Beta-blockers*		Mephenytoin
Trifluperidol	Bufuralol		Omeprazole
Heterocyclic antidepressants	Metoprolol		Propranolol
Amitriptyline	Propranolol		
Clomipramine	Timolol		
Desipramine	*Antihypertensives*		
Imipramine	Indoramin		
Nortriptyline	Debrisoquine		
Selective serotonin-receptor inhibitors	Guanoxan		
Fluoxetine			
Paroxetine			
Tomoxetine			
Monoamine inhibitors			
Amiflamine			
Methoxyphenamine			

[a] Frequently used instead of debrisoquine to characterize the polymorphic status of CYP2D6.

fect the pharmacokinetics of a number of psychotrophics, and are likely clinically important. For example, as compared to EMs, PMs of CYP2D6 exhibit significantly higher serum concentrations of tricyclics when given comparable doses of the medication, and PMs of CYP_{mp} show significant differences in the metabolism of diazepam (37). Ethnic variations in regard to these, as well as other cytochrome P-450 isozymes, might explain, at least in part, some of the ethnic differences in psychotropic response that will be reviewed below.

Ethnicity, Environmental Factors, and Drug Metabolism

The activities of many, but probably not all, of the cytochrome P-450 isozymes can be inhibited, as well as induced, by a wide variety of substances (57,58). These include not only some of the highly specific and often extremely potent drugs that have been utilized for research in this area, but also commonly used pharmaceutical agents (cimetidine and carbamazepine are prime examples), herbal medicines, environmental toxins, steroid and sex hormones, alcohol, caffeine, constituents of tobacco, substances in charcoal-broiled beef, brussels sprouts and cabbage, and dietary compositions (i.e., high-protein versus high-carbohydrate diets). The mechanisms responsible for inhibition include competitive interaction (reversible inhibition), autocatalytic inactivation (irreversible inhibition), and possibly repression of gene transcription. Induction is most likely the result of increased gene transcription, leading to an increased synthesis of P-450 proteins. However, it is possible that stabilization of these proteins, and/or their corresponding mRNAs, also plays a role.

A major advance in recent years in this regard is the discovery of the ''Ah (aromatic hydrocarbon) receptor,'' a cytosolic receptor responsible for recognizing the inducing agent and triggering the induction response by functioning as an enhancer at the 5'-flanking region of the P-450 genes (58). This results in an increase in gene transcription, in the production of mRNAs, and consequently in the enhancement of the production of the enzymes. As the name ''Ah receptor'' indicates, most of the substrates of this receptor are aromatic hydrocarbons, many of them carcinogens. Two P-450 isozymes, CYP1A1 and CYP1A2, which are mainly responsible for the metabolism of these substances, are readily induced through this mechanism. Although the Ah receptor is structurally very similar to the receptors for steroid hormones, cDNA and protein sequencing studies suggest that the former might be more ancient than the latter. In fact, Ah receptor has been found in virtually all organisms, presumably has existed ever since life first emerged on earth, and thus likely serves an extremely vital function in protecting the organisms from harmful environmental chemicals. In addition to inductions mediated by the Ah receptor, there are several other major types of inductions that are also physiologically important, including the induction by phenobarbital-like compounds (P-450b and P-450e, equivalent to human CYP2B), by glucocortocoids (P-450p or CYP3A1), and by ethanol (CPY2E1). Although receptors have been speculated for these inductions, their existence has not been proven.

Remarkable cross-strain differences in the Ah-receptor-mediated inducibility have been demonstrated in inbred mice. This has led to speculation that similar heritable differences could be present in human populations, resulting from postulated polymorphisms in the Ah receptor gene(s). However, this hypothesis remains to be tested.

At the clinical level, a number of studies have demonstrated substantial cross-ethnic differences in drug metabolism that appear to be environmentally determined. Branch et al. (6) compared the rate of the biotransformation of antipyrine and found a significantly longer antipyrine half-life among Sudanese living in their home villages as compared to Sudanese residing in Great Britain and to Caucasian British subjects. The latter two groups metabolized antipyrine at similar rates, suggesting that environmental rather than genetic factors were responsible for the pharmacokinetic profiles observed among Sudanese residing in their native land. Similar findings were reported in subsequent studies involving Asian Indians living in India, Asian Indian immigrants residing in Great Britain, and Caucasian British subjects (19). When Asian Indian immigrants were divided into those who continued to follow their traditional vegetarian diet and those who had switched to a British diet, it became evident that diet was the determining factor underlying the change of the pharmacokinetic profiles in the Indians. Similar results have been found in studies utilizing clomipramine as the test drug (1).

Steroids, including sex hormones, also are predominantly metabolized by cytochrome P-450 isozymes (25,37), which are inducible by some of the same agents listed above with proven efficacy in inducing drug-metabolizing enzymes. Interestingly, dramatic cross-ethnic differences also have been reported in the metabolism and physiological effects of these compounds, both endogenous and exogenous. For example, Asian women were demonstrated to have 30–75% lower plasma estrone and estradiol concentrations as compared to their Caucasian counterparts. Similar findings with plasma testosterone levels in males with different ethnic backgrounds have been reported (16). In a WHO sponsored multinational study of the efficacy of male contraceptive hormones, it was found that the efficacy of these preparations was much greater in subjects living in nonindustrialized countries than in those residing in western industrialized sites (R. Swerdloff, *personal communication*). Although much remains to be elucidated, it appears that at least part of these differences might be explained by ethnic differences in dietary practice.

Ethnicity and Other Pharmacokinetic Factors

Conjugation

The majority of drugs that utilize P-450 enzymes as the first step in their metabolism also subsequently undergo another metabolic step involving conjugation with endogenous substances (glucuronidation and sulfation) which biotransforms these compounds to more polar ones, so as to further increase their water solubility and excretion (12,75). Contrary to earlier beliefs, emerging recent data indicate that conjugated compounds might play a significant role in determining the clinical or adverse effects of medications such as haloperidol (76). Mechanisms involved in the control of conjugation remain largely unexplored. Little is known regarding ethnic differences in conjugation. However, a recent study did report significantly slower glucuronidation of codeine in Asians, leading to heightened sensitivity to this analgesic in many of the Asians (37,84).

Volume of Distribution

As one of the major components of the pharmacokinetic processes, the distribution of drugs also has been found to manifest significant cross-ethnic variability. Because most psychotropics are highly lipophilic, they generally have a large volume of distribution, the size of which is a reflection of the body composition, especially the proportion of fat to water. Diversity in body build across ethnic groups is expected to lead to differences in the volume of distribution and thus the pharmacokinetics of drugs that are lipophilic. This in fact has been identified as one of the reasons for the greater effect of diazepam in Asians than in Caucasians (42).

Protein Binding

Protein binding represents another important factor that could significantly influence the distribution of many drugs. Among the proteins in plasma that provide binding sites, and thus function as carriers for these pharmacoactive agents, α_1-acid glycoproteins (5,41,69) and albumins (67) are most important. Variations in the concentration of these drug-binding proteins in plasma can significantly influence the effect of the drug by changing the free fraction and thus the amount of the unbound (free) drug concentrations in the plasma (44). Because (usually) only the free (unbound) fraction of drug is pharmacologically active and capable of crossing the blood–brain barrier,

changes in the concentrations of drug-binding proteins might have profound clinical significance (13).

The structures of these plasma proteins are genetically determined. They are polymorphic, and they have been shown to vary across ethnic group in several studies (32). Cross-ethnic studies (13) of plasma protein-binding have thus far focused only on Asian–Caucasian comparisons and have revealed conflicting results. Zhou et al. (88) reported that, as compared to Caucasians, Asians had significantly lower plasma α_1-acid glycoprotein but similar albumin concentrations. Kumana et al. (42), however, reported that their Hong Kong Chinese subjects had significantly lower albumin levels than did their Caucasian counterparts. Similarly, some, but not all, of the cross-ethnic protein binding studies reported lower degree of protein binding, leading to higher free drug fraction in Asians than in Caucasians (49).

Red Blood Cell (RBC)/Serum Lithium Ratio

The distribution of lithium across cellular membranes is controlled by several membrane transport and countertransport mechanisms (7). Among these, the sodium–lithium countertransport system appears to play a particularly pivotal role. The status of this membrane transport system is clearly under genetic control and is strongly associated with the risk for hypertension (81). This system also is significantly less active in African-Americans and African Blacks than in Caucasians, which might contribute to the higher prevalence of hypertension among Blacks (7). More recent studies have shown that, in addition to its hemodynamic implications, ethnic variability in the activity of this system also leads to significant differences in the RBC/serum lithium ratio (59,60,77). This ratio is likely correlated with the intracellular concentration of lithium, which might have important meaning not only in terms of the genetic control of cell membrane permeability to lithium, but also in terms of the clinical and side effects of lithium. Thus, the difference between Blacks and other ethnic groups in the RBC/serum lithium ratio might have important clinical significance. Such a possibility has been recently demonstrated by a study conducted by our group; this study revealed that significant differences in the lithium ratio exist between African-American and Caucasian bipolar patients, and it further demonstrated a higher rate of central nervous system (CNS)-related side effects in African-American patients, suggesting that the higher lithium ratio in this group might indeed lead to higher central toxicity (77).

Other Pharmacokinetics Factors

Although, at least in theory, ethnic variations could also exist in terms of absorption, excretion, and the movement of drugs across the blood–brain barrier, little information currently exists to confirm such possibilities.

Similarly, recent studies (37) have indicated that cytochrome P-450 isozymes also exist in the CNS. Although the amount and activity of these enzymes are much smaller than those found in liver, they directly influence the concentration of their substrates at the receptor sites. Thus, they might be responsible for variations in drug response not readily explainable by peripheral pharmacokinetics. Although it is conceivable and likely that some of the ethnic variations in P-450 isozymes (e.g., CYP2D6) would also exist at the CNS level, this hypothesis has not been directly examined thus far.

Ethnicity and Pharmacodynamics

Contrasting the remarkably rich literature on ethnic variations in the structure and function of various drug-metabolizing enzymes with the relative paucity of information on receptors, Kalow (34,36) recently suggested that while diversity in the former is evolutionarily adaptive because the substrates of the enzymes are predominantly xenobiotics, organisms can ill afford substantive variability in receptors, because their substrates are endogenous. This persuasive argument not withstanding, some of the recently emerging information does suggest that ethnic variations in receptors (4) and receptor-coupled responses also exist, although their functional implications have not been fully clarified.

At a more global level, ethnic differences in the pharmacodynamics of various medications have long been reported. As far back as the 1920s, researchers have observed dramatic ethnic differences in the mydriatic responses to various classes of drugs including cocaine, ephedrine, atropine, and scopolamine (2,20). When the same amount of medication was applied locally, Blacks were consistently least responsive, Asians in the middle, and Caucasians on the other extreme. This reduction in the mydriatic effect appeared to be correlated with the degree of pigmentation of the iris, and it was not seen among albino Africans. The fact that these were all applied locally, and that so many compounds with divergent chemical structures were involved, suggested that this phenomenon was not pharmacokinetically mediated. Recent studies involving the intramuscular administration of atropine and scopolamine (20) confirmed this suspicion. Thus, although the mechanism responsible for this phenomenon has not been fully determined, it appears that it is pharmacodynamic in nature.

Another prominent example of how ethnicity and pharmacodynamics interact is found for beta-blockers such as propranolol, which have been found to be relatively ineffective in treating hypertension in African-American patients (55). In contrast, the doses of propranolol required for the effective treatment of hypertension in

Asians were substantially smaller than those required for Caucasians (87). Subsequent studies objectively demonstrated that the effects of propranolol on blood pressure and heart rate were most pronounced in Asians, and least prominent in African-Americans, with Caucasians falling in between (14). These differences could not be explained by pharmacokinetic factors (87). Studies which have demonstrated that Blacks have significantly higher concentrations of cyclic AMP, both at baseline and after the administration of propranolol, suggest that Blacks might have a higher degree of β_2-adrenoceptor activity (73). This in turn has led to the hypothesis that differences in the sensitivity of adrenoceptors might be the major cause for the differential effects of propranolol and other beta blockers in various ethnic groups (33).

Clozapine-induced agranulocytosis serves as a different type of example of ethnic differences in drug responses (in this case, adverse responses) that are mediated through nonpharmacokinetic mechanisms. In earlier drug trials, it was observed that this potentially life-threatening condition was significantly more prevalent among Azkenazi Jews. This phenomenon led to the finding that a special cluster of human lymphocyte antigen (HLA) typings (45), which is present among Azkenazi Jews with a significantly higher frequency, is associated with substantially increased risk of clozapine-induced agranulocytosis. In a recent report, such an association also has been observed in an American Indian patient (61).

Observations of the ethnic differences in therapeutic concentrations of various psychotropics (29,78,82) and their neurohormonal effects have led to speculation about the existence of ethnic differences in pharmacodynamics of these drugs. These will be discussed below in relation to specific classes of psychotropics.

Culture and "Nonbiological" Issues

Compared to the relatively rich data-set reviewed above on ethnic diversity in drug responses that are mediated by biological mechanisms, there is practically no information regarding how, and to what extent, cultural and symbolic processes affect drug responses in general, and psychotropic responses in particular (49). This is most unfortunate because culture and symbolic forces exert powerful influences on treatment outcome (40). It is to be expected that the clinical effect of psychotropics, as well as most other drugs, is determined to a large extent by factors such as physicians' biases, patients' beliefs, expectations, placebo effects, and compliance, rather than by their "real" pharmacological properties (49).

Prescription biases are most clearly demonstrated in a series of studies (15,51,66,90) consistently demonstrating that African-American patients are not only far more likely to be assigned a more severe diagnosis such as schizophrenia, but also far more likely to be treated with neuroleptics irrespective of diagnosis. Given the same diagnosis, they are significantly more likely to be placed on depot rather than oral medications, presumably reflecting the clinicians' heightened concern with problems of compliance.

As demonstrated by earlier large-scale drug trials involving multiple ethnic groups or cross-national comparisons, there is some evidence suggesting that non-Caucasians may be more responsive to placebo treatment than Caucasians (17,24). Several studies also have elegantly demonstrated that the perception and report of side effects are intimately influenced by the patients' culturally determined beliefs and expectations (49). Sporadic reports (15,16,23,38,51,66) also have shown that medication compliance might be a particularly serious problem in cross-cultural clinical settings. In addition, level of stress, quality and quantity of social support, and personality styles all have been reported to significantly influence psychotropic response (49). Cultural forces impinge upon all of these factors, although systematic research has not been performed in these interesting and important areas (49).

ETHNICITY AND PSYCHOTROPIC RESPONSE

Reports of ethnic differences in psychotropic response can be traced back to the 1950s, when these potent therapeutic agents were developed and quickly introduced worldwide (56). Throughout the last four decades, reports of such nature, mostly based on clinical impressions and surveys, have been numerous (49). However, it is only in the last decade that researchers started to tackle these issues with vigorous study designs and sophisticated methodologies. Although many controversies remain unresolved, the results of these studies, taken together, clearly demonstrate that ethnicity is an important issue that should be considered in clinical settings for most, if not all, classes of psychotropics. Because of space limitations, only selected studies will be highlighted and/or discussed.

Neuroleptics

Several carefully designed studies have demonstrated that Asians and Caucasians differ significantly in terms of haloperidol pharmacokinetics and pharmacodynamics. Asian normal volunteers (46) and schizophrenic patients (64) had approximately 50% higher plasma haloperidol concentrations than their Caucasian counterparts when given comparable doses of medication. As depicted in Fig. 2, this ethnic contrast is superimposed upon an already quite remarkable interindividual variability in both ethnic groups. Thus, although trends for each group were clearly different, there was at the same time considerable overlap in the middle ranges.

The mechanisms responsible for such ethnic differences have not been elucidated. A series of recent studies (10,30,31) have indicated that Asians had lower reduced haloperidol/haloperidol ratios, suggesting that a lower rate of reduction (a major metabolic pathway for haloperidol) in Asians might be responsible for the slower rate of metabolism, and consequently for the more prominent effects observed when given equivalent doses. Alternatively, ethnic differences in the activities of CYP2D6 might also play a role, although such a possible association has yet to be tested.

Pharmacodynamic differences between Asians and Caucasians were suggested by the larger prolactin responses to haloperidol challenge in Asians in the above-mentioned study with normal volunteers (46), which remained statistically significant after controlling for differences in haloperidol concentrations, suggesting the existence of ethnic differences in receptor-coupled responses. In a subsequent clinical treatment study (48), Asian schizophrenic patients responded optimally to significantly lower plasma haloperidol concentrations as compared to their Caucasian counterparts, again suggesting that pharmacodynamic factors contribute to ethnic differences in response to haloperidol.

In a comparison study including four patient groups treated with therapeutic doses of haloperidol, Jann et al. (31) reported significantly different pharmacokinetic profiles for Chinese and African-Americans as compared to Caucasians and Hispanics. In contrast, however, Midha et al. (53,54) found no differences between Canadian Blacks and Caucasians in the pharmacokinetics of two phenothiazines (trifluoroperazine and fluphenazine).

Tricyclic Antidepressants (TCAs)

In contrast to neuroleptics, studies of ethnic differences in the pharmacokinetics of the TCAs have led to inconclusive results. Among the six previous studies comparing Asians with Caucasians, three (39,71,74) revealed that Asians metabolize TCAs significantly slower than their Caucasian counterparts. Although the other three studies (62,63; Silver and Potkin, *unpublished data*) showed differences in the same direction, these differences did not reach statistical significance, particularly after controlling for body weight. In a recently completed study, Lin and colleagues (*unpublished data*) compared the pharmacokinetics of imipramine among Asians, African-Americans, Hispanics, and Caucasians. With the exception of higher desipramine concentrations in the African-American group, they did not find any significant differences among the four comparison groups. These results were in agreement with earlier study demonstrating lack of difference in the pharmacokinetics of nortriptyline between Mexican-Americans and Caucasians (21). The elevation of secondary amine concentrations also has been previously reported among African-American patients (89).

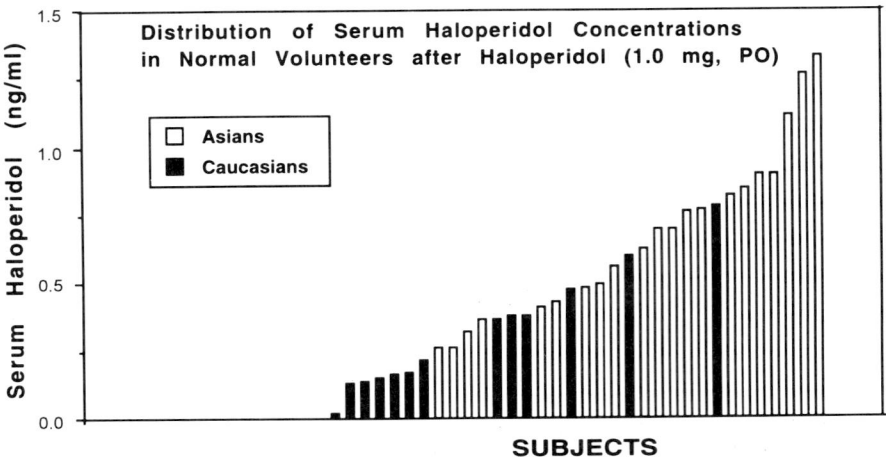

FIG 2. Distribution of serum haloperidol concentrations in normal volunteers after the administration of a single oral dose of haloperidol (1.0 mg) in 26 Asian and 14 Caucasian normal volunteers.

Pharmacodynamic factors have not been formally examined in studies comparing the use of antidepressants across ethnic groups. However, results from two clinical studies in Asia (29, 82) indicated that severely depressed hospitalized Asian patients responded clinically to lower combined concentrations of imipramine and desipramine (130 ng/ml) than had been previously reported in North American and European studies (180–200 ng/ml), thereby suggesting that differential brain receptor responsivity might also play a role in determining ethnic differences in tricyclic dosage requirement. Although clinical reports have suggested that African-Americans were more susceptible to CNS side effects of TCAs (50,70), the mechanisms that might be responsible for such a phenomenon have not been carefully evaluated.

Lithium

Several recent cross-national comparison studies have replicated earlier reports from Japanese researchers regarding the need for lower doses of lithium as well as lower therapeutic lithium levels among Asians (49,77). Yang (83) studied 101 Taiwanese bipolar patients treated over a 2-year period with clinically determined doses of lithium. He found that the plasma lithium level of the majority of good responders ranged between 0.5 and 0.79 mEq/L. More recently, Lee (43) reported that bipolar patients in Hong Kong were stabilized on an average lithium concentration of 0.63 mmol/L. In two studies conducted separately in Shanghai and in Taipei, Chang et al. (8,9) reported remarkably similar pharmacokinetic profiles and therapeutic lithium concentrations for these two Chinese groups residing in drastically divergent socioeconomic environments. These Chinese patients did not differ from Caucasians in terms of pharmacokinetics. However, these patients responded optimally to mean lithium concentrations of 0.71 and 0.73 mEq/L, respectively. These were significantly lower than the mean level of 0.98 mEq/L for the matched Caucasian-American patients, as well as

significantly lower than the 0.8–1.2 Meq/L therapeutic levels generally reported in Europe and North America. Thus, it appears that, compared to their Caucasian counterparts, Asian bipolar patients may require lower doses of lithium because of pharmacodynamic reasons ("increased CNS responsivity").

As mentioned above, higher RBC/plasma lithium ratio in African-Americans and African Blacks may lead to higher central toxicity (77). This suggests that their therapeutic serum or plasma lithium concentrations might have to be lowered as compared to patients from other ethnic backgrounds. However, this remains a hypothesis that needs to be further examined.

Benzodiazepines

Confirming earlier clinical and survey reports (49,68), four recent studies (22,42,47,86) involving Asians and Caucasians demonstrated significant pharmacokinetic differences between the two ethnic groups. Three of the studies used diazepam as the test drug, and one utilized alprazolam. These studies involved the administration of the test drugs by either oral or intravenous routes, or both. Furthermore, they were conducted in Asians residing in diverse areas of the world, including Los Angeles, St. Louis, Hong Kong, and Beijing. Given the diversity of sites and research methodology, the consistency in these reports of a slower metabolism of benzodiazepines is quite remarkable, suggesting that genetic factors are more important than environmental factors in the control of benzodiazepine metabolism.

In a recent study of the pharmacokinetics and pharmacodynamics of adinazolam, a triazolobenzodiazepine currently being investigated as an anxiolytic and antidepressant, African-Americans were found to have increased clearance of adinazolam, resulting in significantly higher concentrations of N-desmethyladinazolam, a metabolite of adinazolam, and greater drug effects on psychomotor performance (18,49). Adinazolam is almost exclusively eliminated by hepatic oxidation to *N*-desmethyladinazolam, so these findings suggested that African-Americans may have a higher metabolic capacity for adinazolam. Because *N*-desmethyladinazolam is cleared directly by renal excretion in addition to hepatic metabolism, increases in oxidative capacity are expected to have a lesser effect on *N*-desmethyladinazolam AUC values. *N*-Desmethyladinazolam has been shown primarily to mediate the benzodiazepine-like side effects, including effects on psychomotor performance, after adinazolam administration (18). This might explain the greater drug effects on African-Americans despite their higher metabolic capacity for adinazolam.

SUMMARY AND CONCLUSIONS

As reviewed above, multiple mechanisms—not only those belonging to the realm of pharmacokinetics and pharmacodynamics, but also various psychosocial factors—could be responsible for differences in psychotropic response. Although remarkable progress has been made in clarifying the mechanisms by which ethnicity and culture influence drug response, much remains unexplored and/or unresolved. This notwithstanding, the available information clearly indicates that ethnicity and culture are important variables that should not be neglected in the practice of psychopharmacology for several important reasons.

Clinically, the importance of culture and ethnicity has been significantly intensified because of the rapid and accelerating population shifts occurring in all metropolitan areas of the world. Furthermore, because of the rapid pace of intercontinental transportation and large-scale migration, most psychiatrists no longer have the luxury of practicing their trades in culturally or ethnically homogeneous settings. Patients seeking help enter the clinic with divergent beliefs, expectations, dietary practices, and genetic constitution. These all have the potential of significantly affecting the outcome of psychopharmacotherapy and should not be ignored. This is part of the reason that the National Institutes of Health and the Food and Drug Administration have started to pay attention to ethnicity as a factor in the research activities that fall under their aegis.

Along with the escalating cost of drug development and marketing, international collaboration becomes increasingly important in such endeavors. However, in order for pharmacokinetic and clinical trial results to be shared cross-nationally, potential ethnic and cultural influences need to be identified. Failure to do so might lead to the inappropriate application of findings derived from one population to another, sometimes leading to unforeseen and potentially disastrous results. Similar arguments could be made with regard to using safety and efficacy data derived from one particular group (in this country,

most often "young male Whites") for approval of pharmaceutical agents, which then are used widely in other populations. Not only are these issues beginning to be addressed early on in clinical trials, but some of these issues are currently being addressed even earlier at the molecular level. For example, in order to tailor-make a new pharmaceutical agent, the availability of cDNA-expressed P-450s will allow for in vitro studies to be performed on newly designed drugs before Phase I studies are even undertaken (11).

Finally, in terms of research, it should be again emphasized that throughout the history of the development of the field of pharmacogenetics, as well as many other fields of medicine, ethnic diversity serves as a major source of stimulus for new discoveries. It is to be expected that this will continue, with cross-ethnic research designs serving as a powerful tool for psychopharmacological research in the future.

ACKNOWLEDGMENTS

This work was supported, in part, by the Research Center on the Psychobiology of Ethnicity (grant MH47193) and by NIMH Research Scientist Development Award MH00534 (Dr. Poland). The authors thank Dora Anderson, R.N. for her helpful comments and editorial assistance.

REFERENCES

1. Allen JJ, Rack PH, Vaddadi KS. Differences in the effects of clomipramine on English and Asian volunteers: preliminary report on a pilot study. *Postgrad Med J* 1977;53(Suppl 4):79–86.
2. Angenent WJ, Koelle GB. A possible enzymatic basis for the differential action of mydriatics on light and dark irises. *J Physiol* 1953;119:102–117.
3. Argawal DP, Goedde HW. *Alcohol metabolism, alcohol intolerance and alcoholism.* Berlin: Springer-Verlag, 1990.
4. Bar CL, Kidd KK. Population frequencies of the Tag I A-system alleles at the dopamine D2 receptor locus [Abstract]. *Am J Hum Genetic* 1992;51(Suppl):145.
5. Baumann P, Eap CB. *Alpha₁-acid glycoprotein genetics, biochemistry, physiological functions, and pharmacology.* New York: Alan R Liss, 1988.
6. Branch RA, Salih SY, Homeida M. Racial differences in drug metabolizing ability: a study with antipyrine in the Sudan. *Clin Pharmacol Ther* 1978;24:283–286.
7. Bunker CH, Mallinger AG, Adams LL, Kuller LH. Red blood cell sodium–lithium countertransport and cardiovascular risk factors in black and white college students. *J Hypertens* 1987;5:7–15.
8. Chang SS, Pandey GN, Zhang MY, Ku NF, Davis JM. Racial differences in plasma and RBC lithium levels (paper no 27 presented at the annual meeting of the American Psychiatric Association). *Continuing Medical Education Syllabus and Scientific Proceedings* 1984;239–240.
9. Chang SS, Pandey GN, Yang YY, Yeh EK, Davis JM. Lithium pharmacokinetics: interracial comparison. Presented at the 138th Annual Meeting of the American Psychiatric Association, Dallas, Texas, May 19–24, 1985.
10. Chang W-H, Chen T-Y, Lee C-F, Hu WH, Yeh EK. Low plasma reduced haloperidol/haloperidol ratios in Chinese patients. *Biol Psychiatry* 1987;22:1406–1408.
11. Cholerton S, Daly AK, Idle JR. The role of individual human cyto-

chormes P450 in drug metabolism and clinical response. *Trends Pharmacol Sci Rev* 1992;13:434–439.

12. Clark WG, Brater DG, Johnson AR, eds. *Goth's medical pharmacology*, 12th ed. St. Louis: CV Mosby, 1988.

13. Crabtree BL, Jann MW, Pitts WM. Alpha, acid glycoprotein levels in patients with schizophrenia: effect of treatment with haloperidol. *Biol Psychiatry* 1991;29:43A–185A.

14. Dimsdale J, Ziegler M, Graham R. The effect of hypertension, sodium, and race on isoproterenol sensitivity. *Clin Exp Hypertens Theory Pract* 1988;A10:747–756.

15. D'Mello DA, McNeil JA, Harris W. Multiethnic variance in psychiatric diagnosis and neuroleptic dosage. APA 142nd Annual Meeting, San Francisco, California, May 6–11, 1989.

16. Ellis L, Nyborg H. Racial/ethnic variations in male testosterone levels: a probable contributor to group differences in health. *Steroids* 1992;57:72–75.

17. Escobar JI, Tuason VB. Antidepressant agents: a cross cultural study. *Psychopharmacol Bull* 1980;16:49–52.

18. Fleishaker JC, Smith TC, Friedman HL, Hulst. LK. Separation of the pharmacokinetic/pharmacodynamic properties of oral and IV adinazolam mesylate and N-desmethyladinazolam mesylate in healthy volunteers. *Drug Invest* 1992;4:155–165.

19. Fraser HS, Mucklow JC, Bulpitt CJ, Kahn C, Mould G, Dollery CT. Environmental factors affecting antipyrine metabolism in London factory and office workers. *Br J Clin Pharmacol* 1979;7:237–243.

20. Garde JF, Aston R, Endler GC, Sison OS. Racial mydriatic response to belladonna premedication. *Anesth Analg* 1978;57:572–576.

21. Gaviria M, Gil AA, Javaid JI. Nortriptyline kinetics in Hispanic and Anglo subjects. *J Clin Psychopharmacol* 1986;6:227–231.

22. Ghoneim MM, Korttila K, Chiang CK, Jacobs L, Schoenwald RD, Newaldt SP, Lauaba KO. Diazepam effects and kinetics in Caucasians and Orientals. *Clin Pharmacol Ther* 1981;29:749–756.

23. Gillis LS, Trollip D, Jakoet A, et al. Non-compliance with psychotropic medication. *S Afr Med J* 1987;72:602–606.

24. Goldberg SC, Schooler NR, Davidson EM, et al. Sex and race differences in response to drug treatment among schizophrenics. *Psychopharmacologia (Berl)* 1966;9:31–47.

25. Gonzalez FJ. The molecular biology of cytochrome P450s. *Pharmacol Rev* 1989;40:243–288.

26. Gonzalez FJ. Human cytochormes P450: problem and prospects. *Trends Pharmacol Sci Rev* 1992;13:346–352.

27. Gonzalez FJ, Nebert DW. Evolution of the P450 gene superfamily: animal–plant "warfare," molecular drive and human genetic differences in drug oxidation. *Trends Genet* 1990;6:182–186.

28. Greenblatt, DJ. Basic pharmacokinetic principles and their application to psychotropic drugs. *J Clin Psychiatry* 1993;54(Suppl):8–13.

29. Hu WH, Lee CF, Yang YY, Tseng YT. Imipramine plasma levels and clinical response. *Bull Chinese Soc Neurol Psychiatry* 1983;9:40–49.

30. Jann MW, Chang WH, Davis CM, Chen TY, Deng HC, Lung FW, Ereshefsky L, Saklad SR, Richards AL. Haloperidol and reduced haloperidol plasma levels in Chinese vs. non-Chinese psychiatric patients. *Psychiatry Res* 1989;30:45–52.

31. Jann MW, Lam YW, Chang WH. Haloperidol and reduced haloperidol plasma concentrations in different ethnic populations and inter-individual variabilities in haloperidol metabolism. In: Lin KM, Poland RE, Nakasaki G, eds. *Psychopharmacology and psychobiology of ethnicity*. Washington, DC: American Psychiatric Press, 1993;133–152.

32. Juneja RK, Weitkamp LR, Stratil A, et al. Further studies of the plasma α_1 B-glycoprotein polymorphism: two new alleles and allele frequencies in Caucasians and in American blacks. *Hum Hered* 1988;38:267–272.

33. Kalow W. Race and therapeutic drug response. *N Eng J Med* 1989;320:588–589.

34. Kalow W. Pharmacogenetics: past and future. *Life Sci* 1990;47:1385–1397.

35. Kalow W. Interethnic variation of drug metabolism. *Trends Pharmacol Sci Rev* 1991;12:102–107.

36. Kalow W. Pharmacogenetics: its biologic roots and the medical challenge. *Clin Pharmacol Ther* 1993;54:235–241.

37. Kalow W, ed. *Pharmacogenetics of drug metabolism*. New York: Pergamon Press, 1992.

38. Kinzie JD, Leung P, Boehnlein J, Fleck J. Tricyclic antidepressant plasma levels in Indochinese refugees: clinical implication. *J Nerv Ment Dis* 1987;175:480–485.

39. Kishimoto A, Hollister LE. Nortriptyline kinetics in Japanese and Americans [Letter to the editor]. *J Clin Psychopharmacol* 1984;4:171–172.

40. Kleinman A. *Rethinking psychiatry*. New York: The Free Press, 1988.

41. Kremer JMH, Wilting J, Janssen LHM. Drug binding to human alpha-1-acid glycoprotein in health and disease. *Pharmacol Rev* 1988;40:1–45.

42. Kumana CR, Lauder IJ, Chan M, Ko W, Lin HJ. Differences in diazepam pharmacokinetics in Chinese and white Caucasians—relation to body lipid stores. *Eur J Clin Pharmacol* 1987;32:211–215.

43. Lee S. Side effects of lithium therapy in Hong Kong Chinese: an ethnopsychiatric perspective. *Cult Psychiatry Med* 1993;17:301–320.

44. Levy RH, Moreland TA. Rationale for monitoring free drug levels. *Clin Pharmacokinet* 1984;9(Suppl 1):1–9.

45. Lieberman JA, Yunis J, Egea E, et al. HLA-B38, DR4, DQw3 and clozapine-induced agranulocytosis in Jewish patients with schizophrenia. *Arch Gen Psychiatry* 1990;47:945–948.

46. Lin KM, Poland RE, Lau JK, Rubin RT. Haloperidol and prolactin concentrations in Asians and Caucasians. *J Clin Psychopharmacol* 1988;8:195–201.

47. Lin KM, Lau JK, Smith R, Poland RE. Comparison of alprazolam plasma levels and behavioral effects in normal Asian and Caucasian male volunteers. *Psychopharmacology* 1988;96:365–369.

48. Lin KM, Poland RE, Nuccio I, Matsuda K, Hathuc N, Su TP, Fu P. Longitudinal assessment of haloperidol dosage and serum concentration in Asian and Caucasian schizophrenic patients. *Am J Psychiatry* 1989;146:1307–1311.

49. Lin KM, Poland RE, Nakasaki, G. *Psychopharmacology and psychobiology of ethnicity*. Washington, DC: American Psychiatric Press, 1993.

50. Livingston RL, Zucker DK, Isenberg K, Wetzel RD. Tricyclic antidepressants and delirium. *J Clin Psychiatry* 1983;44:173–176.

51. Marcolin MA, Stiers W, Chung YS. Racial differences in schizophrenia when controlling for economic status. *Continuing Medical Education Syllabus and Scientific Proceedings*, 80-81. American Psychiatric Association, 144th Annual Meeting, New Orleans, Louisiana, May 11–16, 1991.

52. Meyer UA. Molecular genetics and the future of pharmacogenetics. In: Kalow W, ed. *Pharmacogenetics of drug metabolism*. New York: Pergamon Press, 1992.

53. Midha KK, Hawes EM, Hubbard JW, Korchinski ED, McKay G. A pharmacokinetic study of trifluoperazine in two ethnic populations. *Psychopharmacology* 1988;95:333–338.

54. Midha KK, Hawes EM, Hubbard JW, Korchinski ED, McKay G. Variation in the single dose pharmacokinetics of fluphenazine in psychiatric patients. *Psychopharmacology* 1988;96:206–211.

55. Moser M, Lunn J. Comparative effects of pindolol and hydrochlorothiazide in black hypertensive patients. *Angiology* 1981;32:561–566.

56. Murphy HBM. Ethnic variations in drug responses. *Transcul Psychiatric Res Rev* 1969;6:6–23.

57. Murray M, Reidy GF. Selectivity in the inhibition of mammalian cytochromes P-450 by chemical agents. *Pharmacol Rev* 1990;42:2–101.

58. Okey, AB. Enzyme induction in the cytochrome P-450 system. In: Kalow W, ed. *Pharmacogenetics of drug metabolism*. New York: Pergamon Press, 1992.

59. Okpaku S, Frazer A, Mendels J. A pilot study of racial differences in erythrocyte lithium transport. *Am J Psychiatry* 1980;137:120–121.

60. Ostrow DG, Dorus W, Okonek A, Desai P, Bauer J, Bresolin LB, Davis JM. The effect of alcoholism on membrane lithium transport. *J Clin Psychiatry* 1986;47:350–353.

61. Pfister GM, Hanson DR, Roerig JL, Landbloom R, Popkin MK. Clozapine-induced agranulocytosis in a Native American: HLA typing and further support for an immune-mediated mechanism. *J Clin Psychiatry* 1992;53:242–244.

62. Pi EH, Simpson GH, Cooper MA. Pharmacokinetics of desipramine

in Caucasian and Asian volunteers. *Am J Psychiatry* 1986;143:1174–1176.

63. Pi EH, Tran-Johnson TK, Walker NR, Cooper RB, Suckow RF, Gray GE. Pharmacokinetics of desipramine in Asian and Caucasian volunteers. *Psychopharmacol Bull* 1989;25:483–487.

64. Potkin SG, Shen Y, Pardes H, Phelps BH, Zhou D, Shu L, Korpi E, Wyatt RJ. Haloperidol concentrations elevated in Chinese patients. *Psychiatry Res* 1984;12:167–172.

65. Preskorn, SH. Pharmacokinetics of antidepressants: why and how they are relevant to treatment. *J Clin Psychiatry* 1993;54(Suppl): 14–34.

66. Price ND, Glazer WM, Morgenstern H. Race and the use of flu-phenazine decanoate. *Am J Psychiatry* 1985;142:1491–1492.

67. Reidenberg MM, Erill S, eds. *Drug-protein binding*. New York: Oxford University Press, 1986.

68. Rosenblat R, Tang SW. Do Oriental psychiatric patients receive different dosages of psychotropic medication when compared with Occidentals? *Can J Psychiatry* 1987;32:270–274.

69. Routledge PA. The plasma protein binding of basic drugs. *Br J Clin Pharmacol* 1986;22:499–506.

70. Rudorfer MV, Robins E. Amitriptyline overdose: clinical effects on tricyclic antidepressant plasma levels. *J Clin Psychiatry* 1982;43:457–460.

71. Rudorfer MV, Lane EA, Chang WH, Zhang MD, Potter WZ. Desi-pramine pharmacokinetics in Chinese and Caucasian volunteers. *Br J Clin Pharmacol* 1984;17:433–440.

72. Rudorfer, MV. Pharmacokinetics of psychotropic drugs in special populations. *J Clin Psychiatry* 1993;54(Suppl):50–54.

73. Rutledge DR, Steinberg MB, Cardozo L. Racial differences in drug response: isoproterenol effects on heart rate following intravenous metoprolol. *Clin Pharmacol Ther* 1989;45:380–386.

74. Schneider L, Pawluczyk S, Dopheide J, Lyness SA, Suckow RF, Copper TB. *Ethnic differences in portriptyline metabolism*. New Research Program and Abstracts, American Psychiatric Association, 144th Annual Meeting, New Orleans, Louisiana, May 1991.

75. Shen WW, Lin KM. Cytochrome P-450 monooxygenases and inter-actions of psychotropic drugs. *Int J Psychiatry Med* 1990;21:21–30.

76. Someya T, Sibasaki M, Noguchi T, et al. Haloperidol metabolism in psychiatric patients: importance of glucuronidation and carbonyl reduction. *J Clin Psychopharmacol* 1992;12:169–174.

77. Strickland T, Lin KM, Fu P, Anderson D, Zheng YP, RBC lithium ratio variation among African American and Caucasian bipolar pa-tients [*in press*]

78. Takahashi R. Lithium treatment in affective disorders: therapeutic plasma level. *Psychopharmacol Bull* 1979;15:32–35.

79. Vesell ES. The model drug approach in clinical pharmacology. *Clin Pharmacol Ther* 1991;50:239–248.

80. Weber WW. *The acetylator genes and drug responses*. New York: Oxford University Press, 1987.

81. Weinberger MH, Smith JB, Fineberg NS, Luft FC. Red cell so-dium–lithium countertransport and fractional excretion of lithium in normal and hypertensive humans. *Hypertension* 1989;13(3):206–212.

82. Yamashita I, Asano Y. Tricyclic antidepressants: therapeutic plasma level. *Psychopharmacol Bull* 1979;15:40–41.

83. Yang YY. Prophylactic efficacy of lithium and its effective plasma levels in Chinese bipolar patients. *Acta Psyhiatr Scand* 1985;71:171–175.

84. Yue QY, Svensson JO, Sjoqvist F, Sawe J. A comparison of the pharmacokinetics of codeine and its metabolites in healthy Chinese and Caucasian extensive hydroxylators of debrisoquin. *Brit J Clin Pharmacol* 1991;31:643–647.

85. Yoshida A. Genetic polymorphisms of alcohol-metabolizing en-zymes related to alcohol sensitivity and alcoholic diseases. In: Lin KM, Poland RE, Nakasaki G, eds. *Psychopharmacology and psy-chobiology of ethnicity*. Washington, DC: American Psychiatric Press, 1993;169–186.

86. Zhang Y, Reviriego J, Lou Y, Sjoqvist F, Bertilsson L. Diazepam metabolism in native Chinese poor and extensive hydroxylators of *S*-mephenytoin: interethnic differences in comparison with white subjects. *Clin Pharmacol Ther* 1990;48:496–502.

87. Zhou HH, Koshakji RP, Siolberstein DJ, Wilkinson GR, Wood AJJ. Altered sensitivity to and clearance of propranolol in men of Chi-nese descent as compared with American whites. *N Engl J Med* 1989;320:565–570.

88. Zhou HH, Adedoyin A, Wilkinson GR. Differences in plasma bind-ing of drugs between Caucasians and Chinese subjects. *Clin Phar-macol Ther* 1990;48:10–17.

89. Ziegler VE, Biggs JT. Tricyclic plasma levels—effect of age, race, sex, and smoking. *JAMA* 1977;438:2167–2169.

90. Zito JM, Craig TJ, Wanderling J, Seigel C. Pharmaco-epidemiology in 136 hospitalized schizophrenic patients. *Am J Psychiatry* 1987;144:778–782.

Psychopharmacology: The Fourth Generation of Progress, edited by Floyd E. Bloom and David J. Kupfer. Raven Press, Ltd., New York © 1995.

CHAPTER 163

Violence And Aggression

J. John Mann

This chapter will address the question of violence and aggression by a consideration of physical acts that are directed by an individual toward other persons with the goal of causing them physical harm, or towards the self with the goal of suicide. Externally directed aggressive acts will be confined to those occurring in the context of an affect such as anger or fear and will exclude acts towards others that are planned in the context of deliberate criminal behavior. The emphasis will be on a review of (a) neurobiological mechanisms involved in such self-directed or outwardly directed aggression and (b) the implications of these mechanisms for possible pharmacological treatment approaches. The reason for this emphasis is to be consistent with the overall theme of the volume — that is, neuropsychopharmacology. Social, cognitive, behavioral, and other psychological mechanisms are also of fundamental importance in understanding violence and aggression (48), but careful treatment of these important areas is beyond the scope of this chapter.

With regard to externally directed aggression there is a considerable animal literature, and this will be reviewed and integrated with clinical findings. With regard to suicidal behavior there is no significant animal literature, and the review will therefore concentrate on human studies. There is, however, a relationship between internal and externally directed aggression based partly on the observation of a statistically significant association of both types of aggression within the same individual. Therefore, externally directed violence will not be discussed independently of internally directed violence or suicidal behavior, and common and different features will

be noted where relevant (see also Chapters 41 and 42, *this volume*).

MAGNITUDE OF THE PROBLEM

Based on data for 1991 reported by the National Center for Health Statistics, suicide is the eighth leading cause of death and homicide is the tenth highest cause of death. According to data from the Federal Bureau of Investigation there were 23,760 homicides in the United States in 1992. Poverty and drug abuse are associated with a higher rate of violence and may contribute to the elevated homicide rate in minorities such as young African-American males. Over 90% of murderers are males. Violent crime by females appears to be increasing (19), but the gender difference demands explanation.

In contrast, suicides occur most frequently amongst the young white males. The Centers for Disease Control report that in 1990 there were 30,906 suicides in the United States: 24,724 of these occurred in males, 22,448 of whom were white. The reason for these racial and sex differences in the proportions of suicide and homicide is unclear, but may provide clues as to how to favorably alter the rates of both problems. For example, males make up a majority of both suicide victims and murderers. The Epidemiological Catchment Area (ECA) Study found that violent behavior in the year prior to interview was two times more prevalent in males than in females (71). Studies in noncriminal populations find that males are more aggressive than females. Understanding these behavioral differences in males and females may also help to identify ways of reducing serious aggression.

In many cases the violence appears to be clearly directed inwardly or outwardly; however, a closer examination of the data indicates that this separation is not a strong as it may first appear. First, there are cases involv-

J. J. Mann: Laboratories of Neuropharmacology and MHCRC for the Study of Suicidal Behavior, Department of Psychiatry, University of Pittsburgh School of Medicine, Pittsburgh, Pennsylvania; Department of Neuroscience, New York State Psychiatric Institute, New York, New York 10032.

ing homicide followed by suicide (16). In these cases there are a disproportionate number of multiple homicides before the perpetrator kills themself. At a less extreme level, examination of murderers indicates a significant rate of previous suicide attempts or at least self-destructive acts that have threatened the life of the individual and that may be interpreted as suicidal acts. About 30% of violent individuals have a history of self-destructive acts. Conversely, 10–20% of suicidal individuals have a past history of violent behavior towards others.

The problem of violence extends beyond the extremes of homicide. Whereas in 1984 the rate of murder was 7.9 per 100,000 people per year, the rate of aggravated assault was estimated at 290 per 100,000 per year, and the rate of forcible rape was 35.7 per 100,000 per year. Thus, the extent of the problem of aggression and violence is enormous and has led to considerable controversy in terms of seeking methods for controlling violence, including legislating gun control, increasing prison capacity, mandatory sentences for violent offenses, attempts to control drug-related sales and purchases, lobbying to reduce violence on television and films, and public education. There is no evidence that these measures are being pursued to the full extent that is possible, nor is there evidence that the attempts to pursue these avenues have been particularly successful.

The type of externally directed violence addressed in this chapter may well account for only a small fraction of the type of violence that has placed the nation in crisis. Psychiatric illness is associated with a minority of violent acts (48), whereas psychiatric illness is associated with suicide in over 90% of cases. Thus, this chapter addresses mechanisms that are involved in a minority of cases of violence against other persons but is applicable to the vast majority of cases of suicide.

The chapter is organized into two major parts. The first part addresses externally directed aggression and begins with animal studies of aggression, followed by clinical studies of serenics or antiaggression pharmacotherapy, and concludes with the neurobiology of human aggression. The second part covers suicidal behavior beginning with the neurobiology of completed suicide and then deals with attempted suicide. The reader is referred to the chapter by B. Eichelman (22) in the 1987 ACNP volume, *Psychopharmacology: A Third Generation of Progress.* Because of the reference limit in this volume, all relevant aggression references in that earlier chapter are referenced via that chapter in the text.

Part I: Externally Directed Aggression

ANIMAL STUDIES OF AGGRESSION

Animal models of aggression are generated in two major ways. The first involves development of models of aggression through manipulation of the brain pharmacologically or by lesioning in order to induce aggressive states. A second approach utilizes behavioral manipulation to produce a model of aggressive behavior. These animal models of aggression have been used to test a variety of pharmacological agents that may have potential in the treatment of human aggression (for reviews see refs. 22, 32, and 52).

There are two major types of animal models of aggression, namely, offensive and defensive aggressive behavior. A third domain of behavior that has been associated with aggression or aggressivity is dominance. It is assumed that more dominant animals are more aggressive. This is an oversimplification because dominant animals may merely frighten other animals in their group without actual physical contact. Models of offensive aggression include isolation-induced aggression, the resident–intruder paradigm (i.e., territorial aggression), and maternal aggression. In isolation-induced aggression, male mice are isolated for 2–6 weeks and then placed together for fighting. The latency, duration, and intensity of the fighting are measured, and then effects of pharmacological intervention can be assessed. In territorial aggression models, a male rat or mice is housed with a female. When another male is introduced into the territory, heavy fighting may be triggered. Lesions of the hypothalamus of male or female rats can produce similar behavior. Another model involving maternal aggression is created when a mouse is killed by a rat, referred to as *muricide*. A related model involves philicidal behavior, which involves pup killing. In most of these models including shock-induced aggression, decreasing serotonergic activity results in an increase in aggression, whereas increasing serotonergic activity results in a decrease in the aggressive behavior. These data have been reviewed extensively by other investigators (14,18,22,23,32,69,76).

Defensive aggression models include the characteristic of the lack of an active approach, and usually no wounds are made on the attacker (22,52). Examples of this model are (a) footshock- or pain-induced aggression and (b) the rat resident–intruder paradigm or maternal aggression in response to an intruder. Therefore, this kind of defensive behavior model reflects a different form of aggression to the offensive aggression models. However, this behavior may also be manipulated by serotonergic activity. Defensive aggression models have not been as extensively used in pharmacological drug development, perhaps because they are viewed as less "pathological."

In recent years, two sets of developments have reawakened the interest in the study of aggression in animal models. The first is a series of studies carried out in nonhuman primates, and the second involves the cloning of multiple serotonin-receptor subtypes whose specific role in mediating aggression can be studied.

With regards to the serotonin-receptor subtypes of interest, it has been known for a number of years that 5-HT$_2$-receptor antagonists, which include most antipsychotic drugs, may have antiaggressive properties. Of considerable interest is the recent report by Hen et al. (28) that deleting the 5-HT$_{1B}$ gene in mice produced a decrease in latency to attack and an increase in attack behavior using the intruder–resident mouse model. This raises the possibility that the 5-HT$_{1B}$ receptor mediates the antiaggressive effects of the transmitter serotonin.

The nonhuman primate studies have demonstrated a relationship between low levels of serotonin and aggressive behavior and potentially either a state or trait-dependent relationship with dominance hierarchy. Cerebrospinal-fluid 5-hydroxyindoleacetic acid (CSF 5-HIAA) has been reported to be lower in dominant monkeys, and platelet serotonin content has been reported to be higher in dominant monkeys in a state-dependent fashion (60). A high-cholesterol diet has been shown to raise CSF 5-HIAA levels and increase the prolactin response to serotonin in monkeys. These biochemical effects are accompanied by differences in levels of overt aggression and socialization. Thus, cholesterol appears to be one mechanism whereby the serotonergic system can be manipulated independently of the nonadrenergic and dopaminergic systems, and these manipulations appear to have behavioral consequences which involve overt aggression and degree of social contact with peers. The serotonergic system has been found to be under significant genetic control both in monkeys (59) and in humans (47,54) and may represent a biochemical trait with behavioral trait consequences.

SERENICS OR ANTIAGGRESSION DRUGS

Assessment of the efficacy of pharmacological agents for the treatment of aggressive and violent behavior requires that a distinction be made between specific antiaggressive effects and nonspecific effects such as the induction of sedation, hypotension, extrapyramidal symptoms such as hypokinesia, and other nonspecific effects. Drugs that have been widely used as serenics include benzodiazepines, anticonvulsants, antipsychotics, and beta-adrenergic receptor (BAR) antagonists, and all have such nonspecific effects. Several published reviews discuss the efficacy of drugs in animal models of aggression (22,52). This chapter will focus on human studies.

Antipsychotic medications have been used for many years as antiaggressive drugs (22); however, studies in animals suggest that their action may be more nonspecific than commonly appreciated. While we and others have found a relationship between dopaminergic activity and dominance, it is more difficult to find direct relationships of dopaminergic activity with aggressivity. Many antipsychotic drugs are not only dopamine-receptor antagonists, but they also have sedating effects and antiserotonin effects and reduce blood pressure through α_1-adrenergic blockade. Newer antipsychotic drugs that have more selective effects for dopamine-receptor subtypes—such as the action of clozapine on D$_2$ and D$_4$ receptors, as well as the action of clozapine and other antipsychotics on 5-HT$_2$ receptors—raise the possibility of more specific antiaggression agents; therefore, controlled clinical trials are warranted. Lithium carbonate has been found to be of use in the treatment of certain types of aggressive disorders (22), an effect attributed to its serotonin-enhancing action. Anticonvulsants have been used to treat aggressive behavior (22), initially based on the observation that certain types of seizure disorders were associated with aggressive behavior. This raised the possibility that subictal discharges could be associated with behavioral discontrol or aggressivity. However, the data supporting the usefulness of anticonvulsants is relatively weak outside the context of a clear-cut seizure disorder. Benzodiazepines have also been used for treating aggressive behavior (22) and have both sedative and anticonvulsant properties as well as an effect on the GABAergic system. BAR antagonists have been used for treating acute aggressive outbursts. Antiandrogen drugs have been used to treat aggression (22). Most of the studies have been carried out in Europe, and there is a lack of double-blind, placebo-controlled studies to determine whether these approaches are efficacious.

Conversely, naturalistic and some controlled studies have demonstrated that alcohol, cocaine, and amphetamines can potentially increase aggressive behavior (22,25,58). Drugs such as amphetamines release norepinephrine, dopamine, and serotonin. Drugs such as cocaine are monoamine reuptake inhibitors of particularly dopamine and norepinephrine. It is hypothesized that enhancement of transmission in dopaminergic and noradrenergic systems is related to aggressivity. Paradoxically, acute alcohol administration also causes release of serotonin. All of these agents share the common feature of a depletion state following an initial excess of transmitter. This depletion state appears to be associated with depression. One formulation of these results is that the pronounced release of dopamine and perhaps norepinephrine leads to the increase in aggression. That release overwhelms any restraining or modulating effect of serotonin release. Another, related formulation is that significant aggression results from the use of these agents in individuals who are already vulnerable due to brain damage or other neurobiological predispositions. In such individuals, drugs are only one of an array of potential triggers of aggression (25).

THE NEUROBIOLOGY OF AGGRESSION IN HUMAN SUBJECTS

This review will focus on the potential role of the noradrenergic, serotonergic, and dopaminergic systems in aggression. In addition, the role of brain injury and genetics in aggression is discussed.

Human studies of the noradrenergic system have involved two major methodologies. The first is the neuroendocrine strategy such as the use of growth hormone response to the α_2-adrenergic agonist clonidine. Siever and Trestman (68) have shown that clonidine-stimulated growth hormone responses are increased in patients with personality disorders and that this increase correlates with sensation-seeking and risk-taking behaviors. They did not find a correlation of clonidine-stimulated growth hormone response with overt aggression or impulsivity. This finding of an enhanced growth hormone response to clonidine contrasts with reports by the same group and others of a blunted growth hormone response in depressed patients which persists into the well state. Thus, opposite findings were made in depression and aggression. A second strategy has involved the measurement of CSF levels of 3-hydroxy-4-methoxyphenylglycol (MHPG). Brown et al. (11) have reported a positive correlation between a history of aggressive behavior in military personnel with a personality disorder and levels of CSF MHPG. Consistent with these findings there have been reports that the β-adrenergic antagonist, propranolol, may be effective in the treatment of episodic aggressive behavior. This kind of behavior is frequently associated with head injuries.

As indicated previously, there is some evidence that the noradrenergic system is involved in aggression from animal studies. Stimulation of the amygdala produces sham rage (61), and this behavior has been associated with a fall in brainstem and brain levels of norepinephrine. Presumably the drop in levels of norepinephrine is a reflection of norepinephrine release. Other animal models have supported a role for increased norepinephrine in aggression. What is paradoxical is that certain animal models of aggression such as shock-induced fighting are induced more readily with lowered brain norepinephrine levels.

The most consistent data address the role of the serotonergic system in human aggression. In a study of subjects with personality disorders, Brown et al. (11) found that CSF 5-HIAA was inversely correlated with clinician or self-reports of lifetime aggression. Other investigators have reported negative correlations of CSF 5-HIAA with irritability (14), hostility (14), impulsive homicide (38),

fire setting (75), and maternal aggression, as well as with self-rated behavioral difficulties during childhood. Recidivism of murderers has also been showed to be correlated with low levels of CSF 5-HIAA (75). Neuroendocrine studies using the agent fenfluramine have found an inverse correlation between the prolactin response to fenfluramine and irritable, impulsive aggression in patients with personality disorder (14), but the same investigators were not able to demonstrate the presence of such a relationship in depressed patients. There is also evidence for a similar negative correlation between the prolactin response to the direct $5\text{-HT}_2/5\text{-HT}_{1C}$-receptor agonist, m-chlorophenylpiperazine, and impulsive aggression. There is also a significant positive correlation between the prolactin response to mCPP and to fenfluramine, suggesting that a significant part of the variance in the prolactin response to fenfluramine is accounted for by $5\text{-HT}_2/5\text{-HT}_{1C}$-receptor responsivity (15). More recently, a correlation has been found between the genotype for a polymorphism of an intron (noncoding section) in the gene for tryptophan hydroxylase and levels of CSF 5-HIAA in impulsive aggressive individuals (49). This suggests a link between a gene involved in the serotonergic system and impulsive aggression. Because the serotononergic system is under significant control (47,54) and there is a genetic contribution to aggressivity (46,66), part of the basis for a genetic vulnerability to aggression may be explained by low CSF 5-HIAA as an inherited trait.

Head injuries involving the prefrontal cortex are associated with aggressive behavior. Seizure disorders of various types, particularly involving the temporal lobe, are also associated with episodic and impulsive aggression. These studies suggest that organic injuries to the brain, particularly prefrontal cortex and perhaps certain limbic areas, somehow interfere with mechanisms involving inhibition of aggressive behavior, and the failure of such inhibitory mechanisms results in an increased likelihood of aggression and violence.

There is a genetic component involved in aggression (46,66). The mechanism of this genetic component remains uncertain. We have already suggested that a reduced level of serotonin function may be one way in which genetic effects could predispose an individual to aggressive behavior. Because there is evidence that the dopaminergic system is also under genetic control (59) and greater dopaminergic activity has been associated with dominance and aggressivity, it is conceivable that genetic factors could also result in increased dopaminergic activity leading to greater aggressivity. There have been few direct studies of the dopaminergic system in aggressive individuals. Pharmacological data from the effects of amphetamine (22) and the antiaggressive effects of dopamine antagonists (22) support the hypothesis that increased dopaminergic activity may underlie some forms of aggression. Two other observations are relevant. Individuals with additional Y chromosomes are more common in violent, criminal populations. Because males are more aggressive than females, there may be a role for the Y chromosome in aggression. Testosterone may play a role in mediating aggression. A recent study (12) reported that a point mutation in the eighth exon of the gene on the X chromosome for monoamine oxidase (MAO) A causes a failure in transcription and results in an absence of MAO A in affected males. In this single family the absence of MAO A is associated with lower intelligence and impulsive, aggressive behavior.

The lack of MAO A activity would result in reduced levels of 5-HIAA, homovanillic acid, and vanillyl-mandelic acid and increased levels of norepinephrine, dopamine, and serotonin (12).

It is highly probable that multiple transmitters are involved in modulation of aggressive behavior. The serotonergic system does have some inhibitory effects on the dopaminergic system, and reduced serotonergic function may thereby result in increased dopaminergic function. Such a formulation may explain the potential coexistence of these two transmitter system abnormalities.

Part 2: The Neurobiology of Suicidal Behavior or Self-Directed Aggression

There are approximately 31,000 suicides per year in the United States. The majority of these suicides occur in the context of a major depressive episode. Schizophrenia, personality disorders, alcoholism, and substance abuse are other frequently associated psychiatric disorders. Over 90% of suicide victims suffer from a psychiatric disorder, and it is uncommon for suicide to occur in a individual who is not psychiatrically ill. Conversely, many patients with psychiatric disorders may experience suicidal ideation but do not commit suicide. It raises the following important question: What is it that distinguishes psychiatrically ill individuals who commit suicide from those who do not? A second related question is whether there is a common predisposing factor or set of factors across psychiatric diagnoses that predispose individuals to commit suicide, or whether there are other factors related to suicide risk in psychiatric disorders that are specific for each disorder. We will discuss in some detail the results of studies in postmortem brain tissue from suicide victims and data from studies comparing suicide attempters with psychiatric controls.

SELF-INJURIOUS BEHAVIOR IN MONKEYS

There are no models of suicidal behavior in animals. One approximation is self-injurious behavior in monkeys. This model has been reviewed in detail by Kraemer and Clarke (34). Essentially isolation has been found to increase the probability of self-injurious behavior during adolescence and adulthood. There is evidence of abnormalities in both the serotonergic and noradrenergic systems in self-injuring monkeys. This behavior tends to get worse as the monkey matures and is principally modified by pharmacological agents acting on the serotonergic system. Kraemer and Clarke (34) report that improvement with serotonergic agents seems to be somewhat individual. The relationship of self-injurious behavior to human

models as a model of suicide attempts is questionable, and it may be a better model of Lesch–Nyhan disorder (51) and other such unusual biochemical abnormalities in humans. It also may be a model of self-injurious behavior displayed by certain patients with personality disorders or cognitive deficits.

NEUROBIOLOGY OF COMPLETED SUICIDE

In the ever-increasing literature describing postmortem studies of suicide victims, the majority of the work has concentrated on the serotonergic system and to a much lesser extent on the noradrenergic system. Other neurotransmitters, including the GABAergic system, the cholinergic system, the dopaminergic system, and peptide modulators and transmitters, have been studied to a far lesser degree, thus preventing definite conclusions. This review will be confined to the serotonergic and the noradrenergic system where there is greatest information available. Transmitter turnover and receptor studies and their relationship to the type of suicidal behavior (i.e., violent versus nonviolent), or to the underlying psychiatric disorder, will be themes that guide this review.

There have been approximately 14 studies of concentration of serotonin (5-HT) and its major metabolite 5-hydroxyindoleacetic acid (5-HIAA) in brain tissue from suicide victims (see ref. 43 for a review). Five out of the seven studies of the brainstem of suicide victims found reductions in either 5-HT or 5-HIAA in the brainstem. In contrast, studies of the prefrontal cortex found a reduction in 5-HIAA levels in only three out of eight studies, and no study found a reduction in serotonin. Studies of other brain regions reported reductions in 5-HT or 5-HIAA in four out of seven studies. The degree of reduction in 5-HT or 5-HIAA appears to be similar in depressed patients, schizophrenics, personality disorder patients, and alcoholics (35). Similarly, violent suicides are not associated with a greater degree of decrease in serotonin or 5-HIAA than are nonviolent suicides (41). Therefore, the method of suicide appears to be unrelated to the biochemical findings.

In summary, there appears to be evidence for a modest reduction in levels of 5-HT and 5-HIAA in the brainstem of suicide victims, independent of psychiatric diagnosis. It is an open question as to whether 5-HT and 5-HIAA are altered in the prefrontal cortex or other brain regions.

The serotonin receptor that has received the greatest attention is the serotonin transporter. There have been at least 15 studies published of serotonin transporter binding or of [³H]-imipramine binding in suicide victims (see ref. 43 for a review). Four of these studies reported a decrease in imipramine binding. None of the studies that used more specific ligands than [³H]imipramine, or used a more selective displacer than desipramine, have found a reduction in binding, with the notable exception of a study by Laruelle et al. (36), who used [³H]paroxetine combined with clomipramine as a displacing agent. These findings suggest that the reductions reported in earlier studies may in fact have involved a binding site other than the physiologically relevant transporter site. The functional role of this other binding site is unclear. The nontransporter site is found in greater numbers than the transporter site itself, and further research is required to determine whether or not it has a physiological role. Another factor to consider is the brain region that is being studied. For example, an autoradiographic study of suicide victims by Gross-Isseroff et al. (27) found regions of unchanged, increased, and decreased [³H]imipramine binding. Our own studies using autoradiography find that the reduction in cyanoimipramine binding to the transporter site is confined to orbital and lateral prefrontal cortex. This suggests that in addition to ligand specificity, there may indeed be a reduction in transporter binding, but that the reduction appears to be located in areas of prefrontal cortex different from those commonly previously studied.

The 5-HT$_2$ serotonin receptor is one of the earliest identified postsynaptic serotonin receptors in cortical tissue. In 1983 we first reported a 44% increase in [³H] spiroperidol binding to the 5-HT$_2$ receptor as defined by mianserine in prefrontal cortex (43). We replicated the same result in two other series of brains in 1986 and 1990 (1,42). The later study (1) was carried out using both membrane binding with ^{125}I-LSD and autoradiography studies. That study not only confirmed an increase in binding in the prefrontal cortex, but also involved a greater number of binding sites with no difference in the K_D. Moreover, the degree of difference between the suicides and the controls appears to be greater in prefrontal cortex than in temporal cortex, suggesting regional specificity of the suicide effect. Of the five studies that did not replicate the result (13,27,53), four came from a single research group and one was an independent autoradiographic study by Gross-

Isseroff et al. (27). However, three other studies investigators have replicated this finding, including Laruelle (36), and Yates et al. (78). The latter study involves a series of depressed patients dying of natural causes. Thus, there is evidence both for and against this finding. Further work is needed to map the distribution of change in 5-HT$_2$ receptors in suicide victims throughout the prefrontal cortex as well as in other cortical brain regions.

There have been at least five published studies of 5-HT$_{1A}$ receptors in suicide victims (see ref. 43 for a review). In prefrontal cortex, the 5-HT$_{1A}$ receptor is predominantly postsynaptic. Of the five published studies, two reported an increase in suicide victims and three did not. One factor that may be relevant for explaining these discrepant results is that the two studies that found an increase in 5-HT$_{1A}$ receptor binding, namely those of Arango et al. (3) and Joyce et al. (31), both found this increase to be confined to very discrete brain regions. Thus, techniques such as autoradiography, which can map the regions likely to show receptor binding changes, are essential for detecting highly localized alterations.

Other serotonin receptor subtypes have barely begun to be investigated, and studies are ongoing of 5-HT$_{1C}$, 5-HT$_{1B}$ and 5-HT$_{1D}$ receptors in suicide victims. Overall, the preponderance of data suggests that there are alterations in the serotonin system in suicide victims, and the use of techniques such as autoradiography coupled with gene expression studies will help to clarify the range and extent of the receptor and transmitter changes, as well as identifying where in the brain these changes are most pronounced.

Too few postmortem studies of cortical or brainstem norepinephrine concentrations have been carried out in suicide victims to draw firm conclusions. No change in norepinephrine concentrations have been found in the brainstem, and increased norepinephrine in the cerebral cortex provides little guide as to norepinephrine levels available for release or as to what the level of noradrenergic activity might be. Other investigators examined the CSF of suicide attempters as a way of avoiding the postmortem degradation of neurotransmitter and obtaining an index of neuronal activity. Except for a couple of studies (4,5), the majority (11,57,64,65,67) did not find reduced concentrations of the principal norepinephrine metabolite MHPG in the CSF of suicide attempters. Excretion of MHPG may be reduced in the urine of suicide attempters (4,5).

Increased binding to β-adrenergic receptors in the cerebral cortex in suicide victims compared to controls has been reported by some investigators (1,10,42), but not by others (20,39,70). Although few studies have examined the α-adrenergic receptor subtypes, α_1-adrenergic and/or α_2-adrenergic receptor binding in suicide victims in cerebral cortex has been reported to be increased (2,45) or decreased (26). Additional studies are warranted, particularly because different ligands were used by different studies to define the α_2-adrenergic receptor subtype.

These findings are a snapshot of brain function at the moment of suicide and therefore include effects of genetics, development and early life processes, the associated psychiatric disease and any treatment, environmental stresses, and the artifacts of the postmortem delay. However, several other questions which will be critical to the interpretation of our existing knowledge can be asked and should serve to direct future studies. Are the serotonergic changes genetic in origin, and are the noradrenergic changes state-dependent? Is there a highly specific and sensitive serotonergic trait marker which will identify the person at risk for suicide? Identification of the brain systems most affected by, or predictive of, suicide may then provide the opportunity for effective pharmacological intervention. Much remains to be learned through further systematic postmortem neurochemical studies of tissue from individuals where clinical information is available.

NEUROBIOLOGY OF ATTEMPTED SUICIDE

Reduced levels of CSF 5-HIAA appear to be associated with higher rates of a history of planned, nonimpulsive suicide attempts as well as higher rates of suicide attempts resulting in more medical damage. It was originally reported that CSF levels of 5-HIAA are distributed bimodally in depressed patients (6) and that the group with lower levels of CSF 5-HIAA are distinguished by a higher rate of serious suicide attempts and a higher rate of future suicide. However, suicide intent and medical damage were not quantified in that study. Since that report, many other studies have been published examining the relationship of CSF 5-HIAA to suicidal behavior in depressed and other psychiatric populations. Ten previous studies (4,6,21,30,40,55,73) found lower levels of CSF 5-HIAA in patients with a major depressive disorder who had also carried out a suicide attempt compared to depressed patients who had not attempted suicide. Five studies did not find lower CSF 5-HIAA in suicide attempters (63,67,77). Four out of seven studies found lower CSF 5-HIAA levels in schizophrenics who attempted suicide (17,37,50,57,64,74,77). However, all six studies (7,11,24,72) of personality disorders and violent criminals [if the study of a mixed group of psychiatric patients by Banki and Arató (7) is included] found lower CSF 5-HIAA in suicide attempters. Three studies that did not find reduced CSF 5-HIAA levels in depressed patients who attempted suicide had included a significant number with bipolar disorder. One study found lower CSF 5-HIAA levels in association with suicidal behavior in unipolar but not in bipolar depressed patients (4). However, a second study where the depressed population comprised about 50% bipolar cases did find reduced CSF 5-HIAA

in the attempters (7). Thus, there is significant disagreement in the literature as to whether CSF 5-HIAA is lower in depressed or schizophrenic patients who have made a suicide attempt. This disagreement does not appear to be explained by diagnostic group because it applies to both schizophrenia and depression. It now appears that suicidal behavior involving planning and resulting in greater medical damage is significantly associated with lower CSF 5-HIAA levels, and therefore the type of suicidal behavior exhibited by the study population may potentially explain some of the differences in results in published studies.

With regard to suicidal behavior and CSF levels of HVA or MHPG, no consistent pattern has emerged in the literature. Some, but not all, studies report lower levels of CSF HVA in attempters (4,63,72), and in addition there is disagreement as to whether this relationship holds true only for major depressive disorder, or whether it is also present in other diagnostic groups (63). CSF MHPG appears to have a unimodal distribution in affective disorders, with levels tending to be elevated relative to controls (33). One study found a complex relationship between CSF MHPG and suicidal behavior (4) but our study found no correlation. We found that, unlike CSF 5-HIAA, CSF MHPG and HVA did not have statistically significant relationships with planning or medical damage, indicating a biochemical selectivity for this biobehavioral correlation.

It has also been hypothesized that the dimension of the suicidal behavior related to low CSF 5-HIAA is the degree of violence of the attempt as opposed to some other aspect of suicidal behavior such as suicidal intent. Only three out of eight studies with available data reported that violent suicide attempts are associated with lower levels of CSF 5-HIAA. Therefore, the weight of the evidence is against this hypothesis. It is therefore relevant to note that we have reported (44) that availability of method is a major factor determining choice of suicide method. Thus, selection of a violent method for suicide may not be biologically determined. If so, then another dimension of suicidal behavior may be biologically determined.

Although impulsive violence correlates with reduced serotonin activity (38,75), previous studies have not directly examined the relationship between the degree of impulsivity involved in the suicidal act and CSF 5-HIAA. It has been reported (8) that Beck Suicide Intent Scale scores are higher in patients who complete suicide than in patients who have attempted suicide, and this scale assigns higher scores to planning in contrast to impulsivity. Moreover, Suicide Intent Scale scores are higher in patients who reattempt suicide in the future (8) and in those who ultimately complete suicide (9). Because degree of planning, and not impulsivity, is associated more frequently with greater medical damage, from a behavioral standpoint suicide attempters who plan resemble completed suicides more so than do impulsive suicide attempters. Thus, nonimpulsive suicide attempters resemble suicide completers both biologically and behaviorally.

The observation that greater planning is associated with more severe medical damage, means that failed suicides appears to be related to completed suicide not only in terms of behavioral aspects but also in terms of biological measures of serotonin function. Further evidence in favor of such a category of suicide attempters is provided by our findings that the degree of planning correlated with the degree of medical damage, such that more highly planned suicide attempts result in greater medical damage. Others have also reported that degree of medical damage correlates with the score on the Suicide Intent Scale (56).

Levels of CSF 5-HIAA do not correlate with the recency of the suicide attempt, but only with the characteristics of the suicide attempt. When taken together with data indicating that CSF 5-HIAA levels are stable in individuals tested on multiple occasions (29,47), it suggests that CSF 5-HIAA reflects a biochemical trait that may be determined genetically or as a result of developmental effects (54). Some studies suggest that suicide risk is at least partly genetically determined or familial (62). Thus, CSF 5-HIAA may be a biochemical trait related to the threshold for suicidal behavior, and can be measured even if the suicide attempt was carried out some time earlier. Pharmacological elevation of serotonergic activity during periods of higher risk may protect patients from suicide or serious suicide attempts and perhaps mitigate the degree of medical damage in the event of a suicide attempt.

CONCLUSIONS

Aggression can be self-directed (suicidal acts) or externally directed. Aggression of both types tend to coexist in the same individual. The neurotransmitter correlates of aggression include decreased serotonergic activity and increased noradrenergic and dopaminergic activity. Whereas it is impulsive violence that has the strongest correlation with reduced serotonergic activity, it is more highly planned and medically damaging suicidal behavior that correlates with reduced serotonergic activity. Genetic factors and acquired brain injuries also contribute to violent behavior and suicide risk. Studies of the neurobiology of aggression must seek to distinguish state and trait factors and develop methods for detecting high-risk patients who are candidates for pharmacotherapy. The neurobiological component that determines the predominant direction of aggression, namely inward (suicide) or outward, remains to be identified. Development of drug treatment for aggression requires a greater emphasis on controlled clinical trials in high-risk populations. Identification of new serotonin and dopamine receptor subtypes offers the possibility of more specific serenic drugs.

ACKNOWLEDGMENT

This work was supported by the MHCRC for the Study of Suicidal Behavior (grant MH46745).

REFERENCES

1. Arango V, Ernsberger P, Marzuk PM, Chen J-S, Tiemney H, Stanley M, Reis DJ, et al. Autoradiographic demonstration of increased serotonin 5-HT$_2$ and β-adrenergic receptor binding sites in the brain of suicide victims. *Arch Gen Psychiatry* 1990;47:1038–1047.
2. Arango V, Ernsberger P, Sved AF, Mann JJ. Quantitative autoradiography of α_1- and α_2-adrenergic receptors in the cerebral cortex of controls and suicide victims. *Brain Res* 1993;630:271–282.
3. Arango V, Miller WE, Miller ML, Underwood MD, Smith RW, Mann JJ. Quantitative autoradiography of 5-HT$_{1A}$ binding in suicide. [Abstract]. *Soc Neurosci Abstr* 1991;17:1472.
4. Ågren H. Symptom patterns in unipolar and bipolar depression correlating with monoamine metabolites in the cerebrospinal fluid. II. Suicide. *Psychiatry Res* 1980;3:225–236.
5. Ågren H. Depressive symptom patterns and urinary MHPG excretion. *Psychiatry Res* 1982;6:185–196.
6. Åsberg M, Thorén P, Träskman L, Bertilsson L, Ringberger V. "Serotonin depression"—a biochemical subgroup within the affective disorders? *Science* 1976;191:478–480.
7. Banki CM, Arató M. Amine metabolites and neuroendocrine responses related to depression and suicide. *J Affect Disord* 1983;5:223–232.
8. Beck A, Schuyler D, Herman J. Development of suicidal intent scales. In: Beck A, Resnick K, Letierri D, eds. *The prediction of suicide.* Bowie, MD: Charles Press, 1974.
9. Beck AT, Steer RA. Clinical predictors of eventual suicide: a 5- to 10-year prospective study of suicide attempters. *J Affect Disord* 1989;17:203–209.
10. Biegon A, Israeli M. Regionally selective increases in β-adrenergic receptor density in the brains of suicide victims. *Brain Res* 1988;442:199–203.
11. Brown GL, Ebert MH, Goyer PF, Jimerson DC, Klein WJ, Bunney WEJ, Goodwin FK. Aggression, suicide and serotonin: relationships to CSF amine metabolites. *Am J Psychiatry* 1982;139:741–746.
12. Brunner HG, Nelen M, Breakefield XO, Ropers HH, van Oost BA. Abnormal behavior associated with a point mutation in the structural gene for monoamine oxidase. A. *Science* 1993;262:578–580.
13. Cheetham SC, Cromptom MR, Katona CLE, Horton RW. Brain 5-HT$_2$ receptor binding sites in depressed suicide victims. *Brain Res* 1988;443:272–280.
14. Coccaro EF. Central serotonin and impulsive aggression. *Br J Psychiatry* 1989;155:52–62.
15. Coccaro EF, Kavoussi RJ, Hauger R. PRL responses to D-fenfluramine and D,L-fenfluramine in man [Abstract]. *American College of Neuropsychopharmacology 32nd Annual Meeting, Honolulu, Hawaii* 1993;160.
16. Coid J. The epidemiology of abnormal homicide and murder followed by suicide. *Psychol Med* 1983;13:855–860.
17. Cooper SJ, Kelly CB, King DJ. 5-Hydroxyindoleacetic acid in cerebrospinal fluid and prediction of suicidal behavior in schizophrenia. *Lancet* 1992;340: 940–941.
18. Copenhaver JH, Schalock RL, Carver MJ. Parachloro-D,L-phenylalanine induced filicidal behavior in the female rat. *Pharmacol Biochem Behav* 1978;8:263–270.
19. Daniel AE, Kashani JH. Women who commit crimes of violence. *Psychiatr Ann* 1983;13(9):697–708.
20. De Paermentier F, Cheetham SC, Crompton MR, Katona CLE, Horton RW. Brain β-adrenoceptor binding sites in antidepressant-free depressed suicide victims. *Brain Res* 1990;525:71–77.
21. Edman G, Asberg M, Levander S, Schalling D. Skin conductance habituation and cerebrospinal fluid 5-hydroxyindoleacetic acid in suicidal patients. *Arch Gen Psychiatry* 1986;43:586–592.
22. Eichelman B. Neurochemical and psychopharmacologic aspects of aggressive behavior. In: Meltzer HY, ed. *Psychopharmacology: the*

third generation of progress. New York: Raven Press, 1987;697–704.

23. Garattini S, Giacolone E, Valzelli L. Biochemical changes during isolation-induced aggressiveness in mice. In: Garattini S, Sigg EG, eds. *Aggressive behavior*. New York: John Wiley & Sons, 1969;179–187.

24. Gardner DL, Lucas PB, Cowdry RW. CSF metabolites in borderline personality disorder compared with normal controls. *Biol Psychiatry* 1990;28:247–254.

25. Gomey B. Domestic violence and chemical dependency: dual problems, dual interventions. *J Psychoactive Drugs* 1989;21:229–238.

26. Gross-Isseroff R, Dillon KA, Fieldust SJ, Biegon A. Autoradiographic analysis of α_1-noadrenergic receptors in the human brain postmortem. *Arch Gen Psychiatry* 1990;47:1049–1053.

27. Gross-Isseroff R, Salama D, Israeli M, Biegon A. Autoradiographic analysis of [^{3}H]ketanserin binding in the human brain postmortem: effect of suicide. *Brain Res* 1990;507:208–215.

28. Hen R, Boschert U, Lemeur M, Dierich A, Ait Amara D, Buhot MC, Segu L, et al. 5-HT1B receptor "KNOCK OUT": pharmacological and behavioral consequences [Abstract]. *Society for Neuroscience 23rd Annual Meeting, Washington, DC* 1993;19:632.

29. Hildebrand J, Bourgeois F, Buyse M, Przedborski S, Goldman S. Reproducibility of monoamine metabolite measurements in human cerebrospinal fluid. *Acta Neurol Scand* 1990;81:427–430.

30. Jones JS, Stanley B, Mann JJ, Frances AJ, Guido JR, Träskman-Bendz L, Winchel R, et al. CSF 5-HIAA and HVA concentrations in elderly depressed patients who attempted suicide. *Am J Psychiatry* 1990;147:1225–1227.

31. Joyce JN, Shane A, Lexow N, Winokur A, Casanova MF, Kleinman JE. Serotonin uptake sites and serotonin receptors are altered in the limbic system of schizophrenics. *Neuropsychopharmacology* 1993;8:315–336.

32. Katz RJ. Role of serotonergic mechanisms in animal models of predation. *Prog Neuropsychopharmacol* 1980;4:219–231.

33. Koslow SH, Maas JW, Bowden CL, David JM, Hanin I, Javaid J. CSF and urinary biogenic amines and metabolism in depression and mania. A controlled univariate analysis. *Arch Gen Psychiatry* 1983;40:999–1010.

34. Kraemer GW, Clarke AS. The behavioral neurobiology of self-injurious behavior in rhesus monkeys. *Prog Neuropsychopharmacol Biol Psychiatry* (Suppl) 1990;14:S141–S168.

35. Lagattuta TF, Henteleff RA, Arango V, Mann JJ. Reduction in cortical serotonin transporter site number in suicide victims in the absence of altered levels of serotonin, its precursors or metabolite [Abstract]. *Soc Neurosci Abstr* 1992;18:1598.

36. Laruelle M, Abi-Dargham A, Casanova MF, Toti R, Weinberger DR, Kleinman JE. Selective abnormalities of prefrontal serotonergic receptors in schizophrenia: a postmortem study. *Arch Gen Psychiatry* 1993;50:810–818.

37. Lemus CZ, Lieberman JA, Johns CA, Pollack S, Bookstein P, Cooper TB. CSF 5-hydroxyindoleacetic acid levels and suicide attempts in schizophrenia. *Biol Psychiatry* 1990;27:926–929.

38. Linnoila M, Virkkunen M, Scheinin M, Nuutila A, Rimond R, Goodwin FK. Low cerebrospinal fluid 5-hydroxyindoleacetic acid concentration differentiates impulsive from non-impulsive violent behaviour. *Life Sci* 1983;33:2609–2614.

39. Little KY, Clark TB, Ranc J, Duncan GE. β-Adrenergic receptor binding in frontal cortex from suicide victims. *Biol Psychiatry* 1993;34:596–605.

40. Lopez-Ibor JJ, Saiz-Ruiz R, Perez de los Cobos JC. Biological correlations of suicide and aggressivity in major depressions (with melancholia): 5-hydroxyindoleacetic acid and cortisol in cerebral spinal fluid, dexamethasone suppression test and therapeutic response to 5-hydroxytryptophan. *Neuropsychobiology* 1985;14:67–74.

41. Mann JJ, Marzuk PM, Arango V, McBride PA, Leon AC, Tierney H. Neurochemical studies of violent and nonviolent suicide. *Psychopharmacol Bull* 1989;25:407–413.

42. Mann JJ, Stanley M, McBride PA, McEwen BS. Increased serotonin$_2$ and β-adrenergic receptor binding in the frontal cortices of suicide victims. *Arch Gen Psychiatry* 1986;43:954–959.

43. Mann JJ, Underwood MD, Arango V. Postmortem studies of suicide

44. Marzuk PM, Leon AC, Tardiff K, Morgan EB, Stajic M, Mann JJ. The effect of access to lethal methods of injury on suicide rates. *Arch Gen Psychiatry* 1992;49:451–458.

45. Meana JJ, Garcia-Sevilla JA. Increased α_2-adrenoceptor density in the frontal cortex of depressed suicide victims. *J Neural Transm* 1987;70:377–381.

46. Mednick SA, Gabrielli WF, Hutchings B. Genetic influences in criminal convictions: evidence from an adoption cohort. *Science* 1984;224:891–894.

47. Menachem BE, Persson L, Schechter PJ, Haegele KD, Huebert N, Hardenberg J. Cerebrospinal fluid parameters in healthy volunteers during serial lumbar punctures. *J Neurochem* 1989;52:632–635.

48. Monahan J. Mental disorder and violent behavior: perceptions and evidence. *Am Psychol* 1992;47:511–521.

49. Nielsen DA, Goldman D, Virkkunen M, Tokola R, Rawlings R, Linnoila M. Suicidality and 5-hydroxyindoleacetic acid concentration associated with a tryptophan hydroxylase polymorphism. *Arch Gen Psychiatry* 1994;51:34–38.

50. Ninan PT, van Kammen DP, Scheinin M, Linnoila M, Bunney WEJ, Goodwin FK. CSF 5-hydroxyindoleacetic acid levels in suicidal schizophrenic patients. *Am J Psychiatry* 1984;141:566–569.

51. Nylan WL, Johnson HG, Kaufman IA, Jones KL. Serotonergic approaches to the modification of behavior in the Lesch–Nyhan syndrome. *Appl Res Ment Retard* 1980;1:25–40.

52. Olivier B, Mos J, Tulp M, Schipper J, den Daas S, van Oortmerssen G. Serotonergic involvement in aggressive behavior in animals. In: van Praag HM, Plutchik R, Apter A, eds. *Violence and suicidality*. New York: Brunner/Mazel Publishers, 1990;79–137.

53. Owen F, Chambers DR, Cooper SJ, Crow TJ, Johnson JA, Lofthouse R, Poulter M. Serotonergic mechanisms in brains of suicide victims. *Brain Res* 1986;362:185–188.

54. Oxenstierna G, Edman G, Iselius L, Oreland L, Ross SB, Sedvall G. Concentrations of monoamine metabolites in the cerebrospinal fluid of twins and unrelated individuals. A genetic study. *J Psychiatr Res* 1986;20:19–29.

55. Palaniappan V, Ramachandran V, Somasundaram O. Suicidal ideation and biogenic amines in depression. *Indian J Psychiatry* 1983;25(4):286–292.

56. Pallis DJ, Sainsbury P. The value of assessing intent in attempted suicide. *Psychol Med* 1976;6:487–492.

57. Pickar D, Roy A, Breier A, Doran A, Wolkowitz O, Colison J, Argen H. Suicide and aggression in schizophrenia. Neurobiologic correlates. *Ann NY Acad Sci* 1986;487:189–196.

58. Pihl RO, Peterson JB, Lau MA. A biosocial model of the alcohol–aggression relationship. *J Stud Alcohol* 1993;11:128–139.

59. Raleigh MJ, Brammer GL, McGuire MT, Pollack DB, Yuwiler A. Individual differences in basal cisternal cerebrospinal fluid 5-HIAA and HVA in monkeys: the effects of gender, age, physical characteristics, and matrilineal influences. *Neuropsychopharmacology* 1992;7:295–304.

60. Raleigh MJ, McGuire MT, Brammer GL, Yuwiler A. Social and environmental influences on blood serotonin concentrations in monkeys. *Arch Gen Psychiatry* 1984;41:405–410.

61. Reis DJ. The relationship between brain norepinephrine and aggressive behavior. *Res Publ Assoc Res Nerv Ment Dis* 1972;50:266–297.

62. Roy A. Family history of suicide. *Arch Gen Psychiatry* 1983;40:971–974.

63. Roy A, Ågren H, Pickar D, Linnoila M, Doran A, Cutler N, Paul SM. Reduced CSF concentrations of homovanillic acid and homovanillic acid to 5-hydroxyindoleacetic acid ratios in depressed patients: relationship to suicidal behavior and dexamethasone nonsuppression. *Am J Psychiatry* 1986;143:1539–1545.

64. Roy A, Ninan PT, Mazonson A, Pickar D, van Kammen DP, Linnoila M, Paul SM. CSF monoamine metabolites in chronic schizophrenic patients who attempt suicide. *Psychol Med* 1985;15:335–340.

65. Roy A, Pickar D, De Jong J, Karoum F, Linnoila M. Suicidal behavior in depression: relationship to noradrenergic function. *Biol Psychiatry* 1989;25:341–350.

66. Schiavi RC, Theilgaard A, Owen DR, White D. Sex chromosome

victims. In: Watson SJ, ed. *Biology of schizophrenia and affective disease*. New York: Raven Press, 1994;[*in press*].

anomalies, hormones, and aggressivity. *Arch Gen Psychiatry* 1984;41:93–99.

67. Secunda SK, Cross CK, Koslow S, Katz MM, Kocsis J, Maas JW, Landis H. Biochemistry and suicidal behavior in depressed patients. *Biol Psychiatry* 1986;21:756–767.

68. Siever L, Trestman RL. The serotonin system and aggressive personality disorder. *Int Clin Psychopharmacol* 1993;8:33–39.

69. Soubrie P, Martin P, el-Mestikawy S, Thiebot MH, Simon P, Hamon M. The lesion of sertonergic neurons does not prevent antidepressant-induced reversal of escape failure produced by inescapable shocks in rats. *Pharmacol Biochem Behav* 1986;25:1–6.

70. Stockmeier CA, Metlzer HY. β-Adrenergic receptor binding in frontal cortex of suicide victims. *Biol Psychiatry* 1991;29:183–191.

71. Swanson J, Holzer C, Ganju V, Jono R. Violence and psychiatric disorder in the community: evidence from the Epidemiologic Catchment Area surveys. *Hosp Community Psychiatry* 1990;41:761–770.

72. Träskman-Bendz L, Åsberg M, Schalling D. Serotonergic function and suicidal behavior in personality disorders. *Ann NY Acad Sci* 1986;487:168–174.

73. van Praag HM. Depression, suicide and the metabolism of serotonin in the brain. *J Affect Disord* 1982;4:275–290.

74. van Praag HM. CSF 5-HIAA and suicide in non-depressed schizophrenics. *Lancet* 1983;ii:977–978.

75. Virkkunen M, De Jong J, Bartko J, Goodwin FK, Linnoila M. Relationship of psychobiological variables to recidivism in violent offenders and impulsive fire setters. A follow-up study. *Arch Gen Psychiatry* 1989;46:600–603.

76. Waldbillig RJ. The role of the dorsale and median raphe in the inhibition of muricide. *Brain Res* 1979;160:341–346.

77. Westenberg HG, Verhoeven WM. CSF monoamine metabolites in patients and controls: support for a bimodal distribution in major affective disorders. *Acta Psychiatr Scand* 1988;78:541–549.

78. Yates M, Leake A, Candy JM, Fairbairn AF, McKeith IG, Ferrier IN. 5-HT$_2$ receptor changes in major depression. *Biol Psychiatry* 1990;27:489–496.

Subject Index

A

A1/A2 noradrenergic cells, neuropeptides, 349
A_1 adenosine receptor
  allosteric modulation, 647
  carbamazepine action, 649
  chronic stress effects, 703
  clonidine response, development, 692
  cloning, 644
  distribution, CNS, 648
  electroconvulsive shock effects, 1138
  NMDA receptors colocalization, hippocampus, 649
  pharmacology, 644
A_2 adenosine receptor
  clonidine developmentally-determined response, 692
  cloning, 645–646
  distribution, CNS, 648
  dopaminergic interactions, 650–651
  Huntington's disease, 650
  pharmacology, 644–645
  and premenstrual syndrome, 1038
  subtypes, 644–646
A_{2a} adenosine receptor, 644–646
  cloning, 646
  distribution, CNS, 648
  dopaminergic interactions, 650–651
A_{2b} adenosine receptor, 644–646
  cloning, 646
  distribution, CNS, 648
A_3 adenosine receptor, 646
A_4 adenosine receptor, 646
A10 dopamine cells, 235
Abdominal fat. See Waist-to-hip circumference
Abecarnil
  anxiolytic potential, 1316, 1781
  binding profile, 1779
  GABA-A partial agonist, 1344
  psychomotor effects, 1781
  self-administration, 1784–1785
  structure, 1778
  withdrawal, 1786–1787, 1789
Absolute treatment resistance, 1082
Abstract reasoning
  mild and moderate dementia, 1402
  schizophrenia deficits, 1252, 1254
  specificity, 1254
ABT-418
  in Alzheimer's disease animal model, 106
  antianxiety effects, 107
  behavioral effects, 106
  nicotinic receptor agonist, 104–105

  safety, 106
  in smoking cessation, 107
  structure, 96
Academic examination stress, 987
Acamprosate, alcoholism treatment, 1751
"Accelerated lifetime studies," 1855
Acetoacetate
  brain utilization, 658
  food intake block, 1600
Acetophenazine
  in Alzheimer's psychosis, 1431
  in late-onset schizophrenia, 1443
N-Acetylaspartate, 1537–1538
N-Acetylaspartylglutamate, 1537–1538
N-Acetyl-β-endorphin, 723
Acetylcholine, 945–956. See also Cholinergic system
  attention role, 150–151
  developmental neurochemistry, 684, 687
  dopamine interactions, midbrain, 235
  electroconvulsive therapy effects, 1137
  magnetic resonance spectroscopy, 947–948
  mood disorders role, 945–946
  nicotinic receptor ligand, 98
  noradrenergic system relationship, depression, 917, 945–946
  stress link, 952–953
Acetylcholinesterase
  Alzheimer's disease, 1389–1390, 1419
    CSF measures, 1389–1390
  cholinergic pathways, primate brain, 136–140
  dopamine neuron colocalization, 202
  schizophrenia versus Alzheimer's pathology, 1454
Acetylcholinesterase inhibitors. See Cholinesterase inhibitors
3-Acetylpyridine, 1535
Acidic fibroblast growth factor, 620
  dopamine neuron colocalization, 202
  long-term potentiation effects, 625
  motor neuron effects, 620
  tyrosine hydroxylase modulation, 193
Acoustic startle response
  anxiety paradigm, animals, 1329–1330
  glutamate antagonist drugs, 1211
  neural circuitry, 1239–1240
  prepulse inhibition, 1238–1240
Acquired immunodeficiency syndrome. See AIDS
Acromegaly, growth hormone secretion, 967
Acromelic acid, 80
ACTH

  anorexia and bulimia nervosa, 1613
  baseline measures, 958
  cholecystokinin regulation, 592
  corticotropin-releasing factor regulation, 511, 723, 773–774
  baseline measures, 958
  5-HT2 receptor upregulation, 939
  immune system effects, 723–725, 993
  oxytocin and vasopressin effects, 536–537
Action potentials, dopamine neurons, 169–170
Activating transcription factors, 635
Activator protein-1. See AP-1
Active avoidance behavior, 284
Active cue-exposure treatment, 1812–1813
Activin A, gene expression, 621
Activities of daily living. See also Functional level
  Alzheimer's disease, 1378, 1424
  measures of, 1385–1386
Activity cycle. See Rest-activity cycle
Activity dependence, neural development, 676, 690
Activity levels. See Physical activity
Acupuncture, in smoking cessation, 1724
Acute-phase proteins, Alzheimer's disease, 1421–1422
Acute physical dependence paradigm, 1735
Acute schizophrenia
  adjunctive treatments, 1262–1265
  atypical neuroleptics, 1264–1265
  neuroleptic dosage, 1260–1262
Acute treatment, 839–848. See also under specific disorders
  anxiety disorders, 845
  depression, 1068
  mood disorders, 842–844
  strategies, 839–848
  study design, 1841
Acutely isolated neuron model, 47–48
Addictive Research Center Inventory, 1732
Addiction severity index, 1750
Adenosine, 643–655. See also $A_1 \ldots A_4$ adenosine receptors
  agonist tolerance issue, 653
  antiinflammatory effects, 650
  anxiety role, 649
  CNS activity, 648
  depression potentiation, 652
  dopaminergic interactions, 650–651
  electroconvulsive therapy effects, 1138
  homeostatic role, 647
  and neurodegeneration, 649–650

Alzheimer's disease (contd.)
and corticotropin-releasing hormone,
514–515, 974
cholinergic interactions, 515
depression, 1396–1397
biological substrates, 1396
drug treatment, 1427–1429
prognosis, 1396–1397
drug treatment approaches, 1417–1425
cholinergic system, 1417–1420
methodological problems, 1423–1424
experimental therapeutics, 1417–1425
function, 1405–1414
asymmetries, 1408–1411
parietal/frontal gradients, 1408–1411
galanin antagonist potential, 569
galanin levels, 351
genetics, 1361–1369
glutamate transport, 83
imaging, 1401–1416
immune system involvement,
1421–1422
muscarinic signal transduction, 131
neuropeptides, 1361
neuroprotective strategies, 1420–1423
neuropsychological assessment,
1377–1388
neurotensin amygdala concentrations,
580
noradrenergic system, 1420
nicotine effect, 100, 105–106, 1418
pharmacologic probes, 1393–1396
psychotic symptoms, 1429–1432
biological substrates, 1396
drug treatment, 1430–1432
prevalence, 1429
REM sleep, 1620
second messenger systems, 1395–1396
selective cholinergic channel activators
in, 106
serotonergic system, 1390–1391, 1394,
1433
sleep disorders, mortality, 1619–1620
somatostatin levels, 557–558, 976
structural imaging, 1403–1405
tardive dyskinesia prevalence, 1444
thyrotropin-releasing hormone treatment,
500
vascular dementia distinction,
1403–1404, 1516
PET imaging, 1406, 1516
SPECT imaging, 1413, 1516
structural imaging, 1403–1404
vasopressin and oxytocin effects, 537
Alzheimer's Disease Assessment Scale-
Cognitive Portion
annual rate of change scores,
1383–1384
antidementia drug assessment,
1381–1382, 1424
longitudinal data, 1383
strengths and weaknesses, 1381, 1424
Alzheimer's disease caregivers, immune
function, 987
Amantadine
akathisia treatment, 1271
cocaine withdrawal treatment, 1693
AMBP, 645
American Indians, and clozapine, 1912
Amfebutamone, 181

Amineptine
animal screening, 1148
antidepressant effects, 924, 1148
structure, 1145
tianeptine similarity, 1147
Amino acid load, 473–476
Amino acid sequencing, 1862
1-Aminocyclobutane, 1421
Amino glutethamide, 1151
Aminoketones. See also Bupropion
selective efficacy, 1058
N^6-2(4-Aminophenyl)ethyladenosine, 646
structure, 644
2-Amino-7-phosphoheptanoic acid. See
AP-7
Aminotetralins
serotonin receptor binding, 417
structure, 418
Amish pedigree, 1822
Amitriptyline
adolescent depression, 1637
aggressive behavior exacerbation, 1573
anorexia nervosa acute treatment, 1582
binding affinities, 1059
bulimia nervosa, 1583
comparator trials difficulties,
1056–1057
elderly depressed efficacy, 1475
elderly metabolism, 1471–1473
gender factors, 1114
maintenance use efficacy, 1072
mineralocorticoid receptor changes, 963
muscarinic receptor binding, 129, 132
neurotransmitter uptake inhibition
potency, 1059
orthostatic hypotension in elderly, 1474
Parkinson's disease depression, 1483
serotonin transporter binding, 323
therapeutic drug monitoring guidelines,
1060–1061
Ammonia homeostases, 1531
Amnesic effects
benzodiazepines, 1355, 1782
electroconvulsive therapy, 1132–1133,
1139–1140
mechanisms, 1139
pharmacologic treatment, 1139–1140
AMPA-induced lesions, 150
AMPA receptor. See also Kainate
receptors
agonists, 79–80, 1533
antagonists, 80, 1533
distribution, 79
molecular characterization, 78–79
in new drug development, 1867–1868
tuboinfundibular dopaminergic role, 250
Amperozide, 1283–1284
^{123}I-amphetamine, major depression, 1023
Amphetamine challenge
borderline personality disorder, 1575
mood response, 924, 1575
Amphetamine hyperthermia, genetics, 807
Amphetamine-induced psychosis, 1490
Amphetamine-induced stereotypy,
794–795
Amphetamines. See also
Dextroamphetamine;
Levoamphetamine;
Methamphetamine

caffeine comparison as reinforcer, 1706,
1710
cognitive enhancement, schizophrenia,
1255
dopamine autoreceptor effects, 290–291
dopamine transporter interactions, 182
5-HT and NE transporter binding,
323–324
inbred mouse strain analysis, 1803
locus coeruleus effects, 380
mesocorticolimbic dopamine system
effect, 287–292
behavior sensitization, plasticity,
290–292
mood effects, 923–924
schizophrenia model, 794–795
face validity, 794–795
schizotypal personality disorder
worsening, 1569
self-administration, vulnerability,
291–292
Amygdala
autism pathology, 1658
cholinergic innervation, 138
dopamine neuron ultrastructure, 265
dopamine receptor expression, 211–212
locus coeruleus interactions, behavior,
367
Tourette's syndrome, 1668
Amygdala central nucleus
corticotropin-releasing factor, 507
neuropeptide Y anxiolytic action, 549
pericoerulear projections, 378
Amygdala kindling
contingent tolerance, carbamazepine,
1162–1166
cortical spread, 1158
differential pharmacology, 1162
Amyloid angiopathy, imaging, 1404
Amyloid beta protein. See Beta-amyloid
protein
Amyloid precursor protein
Alzheimer's disease pathology, 1361,
1371–1374
amyloidogenesis, 1372
biology, 1371–1372
carboxyl terminal degradation products,
1393
CSF levels, 1390–1391
experimental therapeutics, 1422
genetics, 1361–1364, 1372
interleukin influences, 1421
in olfactory neuroblasts, 1393
proteolytic processing, 1365, 1371
transgenic mice, 1373–1374
Amyloidogenesis
aged nonhuman primates, 1372–1373
Alzheimer's disease, 1371–1375
experimental therapeutics, 1422
mechanisms, 1372
transgenic mice, 1373–1374
Amyotrophic lateral sclerosis, 1531–1543
glutamate role, 83, 1531–1541
CSF levels, 1536–1541
pathophysiology, 1538–1539
plasma levels, 1536–1539
transport, 83
glycine hypothesis, 1540–1541
incidence, 1531

in acute bipolar depression, 1100
in acute mania, 1099–1100
  carbamazepine comparison, 1102–1103
    dosage, 1100
adverse effects, 1101–1102
AIDS mania treatment, 1553
Alzheimer's mania behaviors, 1433
anorexia nervosa acute treatment, 1582
augmentation of, 1075
augmentation with, 1088–1090
  elderly, 1473
  neuroleptics, 1263
bipolar disorder maintenance treatment, 1074–1075, 1099–1110
  alternatives, 1074–1075, 1099, 1103
  carbamazepine comparison, 1103
  dosage, 1076
  and kindling, 1162
  predictors of response, 1074, 1100–1101, 1161
  tolerance development, 1162
  valproate comparison, 1106
bulimia nervosa, 1586
carbamazepine augmentation, acute mania, 1103
carbamazepine comparison, acute mania, 1102–1103
catecholamine effects, 916
circadian period changes, 1014
clozapine interactions, 1280
discontinuation-induced refractoriness, 1076, 1100
  kindling model, 1161–1162, 1165–1166
  predictors, 1166
dosage therapeutic range, 1108
drug interactions, 1101
ECT comparison, mania, 1126–1127
elderly depressed, 1473–1474
ethnic variations in response to, 1914
kindling model of refractory response, 1161–1162
long-term use, 844, 1072–1075, 1100–1101
membrane phospholipid effects, 129
and muscarinic signal transduction, 131–132
pharmacokinetics, 1101, 1108
postpartum mood disorder, prophylaxis, 1034–1035
prediction of response, 1074, 1100–1101
in pregnancy, 1101–1102
premenstrual syndrome treatment, 1038
psychosocial response predictors, 1114, 1116
in rapid cycling, 1101
renal clearance, 1462
response rats, 1099
retinal sensitivity, 1014
sex differences in response, 1114
short-term use, mania, 843
subjective side effects, 1102
substance abuser response, 1156
tardive dyskinesia, 1492, 1507
tolerance development, 1162
valproate comparison, acute mania, 1104–1105
Lithium augmentation, 1088–1090, 1473

elderly, 1473–1474
Lithium-induced hypothyroidism, 1030
Litoxetine, 1147
Lobeline
  nicotinic receptor activity, 102, 104
  smoking cessation use, 107, 1725
  structure, 96
Local drug application
  behavioral electrophysiology role, 61
  and in vivo single-cell electrophysiology, 54–55
Locomotor activity
  circadian cycle physiology, 1003
  corticotropin-releasing hormone effect, 512
  gene inactivation studies, 72
  inbred rat strains, 1804
  mesocorticolimbic dopaminergic system, 284, 288–292
  serotonin role, 463
  somatostatin effects, 556
  and thyrotropin-releasing hormone, 498
Locus coeruleus
  afferents, 373–375, 387–388
    physiology, 377–378
    and stress, 381–383
  anatomy, 373–377, 387–388
  anxiety role, 369, 387–393, 1326
  behavioral functions, 338–339, 343, 363–370
  chronic stress sensitization, noradrenergic neurons, 356–357
  coexisting transmitters, noradrenergic neurons, 347–352
  and cognitive function, 369–370
  cortical projection, and behavior, 363–370
  corticotropin-releasing factor effects, EEG, 512
  depression role, 369, 383
  drug dependence/withdrawal role, 380–381
  efferents, 375–377, 387–388
    divergence property, 376
    physiology, 378–379
    and stress, 383
    typography, 376–377
    ultrastructure, 377
  and forebrain EEG, 340–341, 363–364, 383
  lesion studies, behavior, 389
  neocortical target neuron input, 339–340
  neurotransmitter candidates, 374–375
  nicotine effects, 380
  norepinephrine release, 378–379
  oddball paradigm studies, 338–339, 364
  opiate addiction model system, 697–700
  pain role, 379–380
  primary dementia and depression, 1396
  and psychopathology, 369–370, 383–384
  serotonin receptor, electrophysiology, 452, 454
  stimulation of, 339–343
Locus coeruleus slices
  alpha2 adrenoceptor mechanisms, 335–337
  applications, 53
Locus of rise, 762

Lod score, 1826–1828
  bipolar disorder linkage studies, 1822
  diagnostic reliability problem, 1857
  linkage test, 1826–1829
    limitations, 1828
  as parametric method, 1828
  and prior odds, 1826
  schizophrenia linkage studies, 1823
Long half-life benzodiazepines
  animal studies, 1787–1788
  withdrawal, 1356, 1787–1788
Long/short sleep mice
  characteristics, 800, 803
  $GABA_A$ receptor, ethanol, 804–805
  genetic map, 808
Long-term potentiation
  arachidonic acid role, 603–604
  behavioral pharmacology, knockout studies, 72
  cholinergic role, 143
  cytokines role, 625
  glucocorticoid enhancement, 710
  metabotropic glutamate receptors, 82
  nitric oxide retrograde regulation, 616
  opioid peptide role, 524–525
Long-term treatment. See also
    Continuation treatment;
    Maintenance treatment
  anxiety disorders, 845–846, 1349–1359
    risks, 1354–1357
  attrition problem, 831–832
  design of studies, 831–832
  kindling model predictions, 1166
  mood disorders, 844–845, 1067–1079
  obstacles to studies of, 1077
  rationale, 839
  schizophrenia indications, 840–842
  strategies, 839–848
Longitudinal studies
  clinical trials, 831–832
  general principles, 1854–1856
  value of, 1854–1856
Lophotoxins, 103
Loprazolam, clearance in elderly, 1467
Lorazepam
  clinical development and review time, 1885
  HIV infection anxiety, 1554
  withdrawal, animals, 1786
Lorazepam probe, Alzheimer's disease, 1394
Lordosis behavior
  antisense studies, 754–755
  dopaminergic influence, 746
  hormonal regulation, 709
  opiate/opioid effects, 750–751
  oxytocin facilitation, 751
  norepinephrine effects, 747
  serotonergic effects, 747
Low birth weight, and cocaine, 1694
Low-density lipoprotein cholesterol, 1605
Low-density-lipoprotein receptor, 1366–1367
Low-dose neuroleptics
  acute treatment, 1260–1261
  Alzheimer's disease, 1431–1432
  HIV-1 related psychosis, 1554
  intermittent treatment, 1268
  maintenance treatment, 841, 1267–1268
  schizotypal personality disorder, 1569